LEXI-COMP'S

Drug Information Handbook FOR Advanced Practice Nursing

Ideal for:

Nurse Practitioners
Nurse Midwives
Clinical Nurse Specialists

6ᵗʰ Edition

LEXI-COMP

Drug Information Handbook FOR Advanced Practice Nursing

Ideal for:

Nurse Practitioners
Nurse Midwives
Clinical Nurse Specialists

6th Edition

Beatrice B. Turkoski, RN, PhD
Associate Professor, Graduate Faculty,
Advanced Pharmacology
College of Nursing
Kent State University
Kent, Ohio

Brenda R. Lance, RN, MSN
Program Development Director
Northcoast HealthCare Management Company
Northcoast Infusion Therapies
Oakwood Village, Ohio

Mark F. Bonfiglio, BS, PharmD, RPh
Director of Pharmacotherapy Resources
Lexi-Comp, Inc
Hudson, Ohio

Foreword by:
Margaret A. Fitzgerald, MS, APRN, BC, NP-C, FAANP

LEXI-COMP

NOTICE

Drug information is constantly evolving because of ongoing research and clinical experience and is often subject to interpretation. While great care has been taken to ensure the accuracy of the information presented, the reader is advised that the authors, editors, reviewers, contributors, and publishers cannot be responsible for the continued currency of the information or for any errors, omissions, or the application of this information, or for any consequences arising therefrom. Therefore, the author(s) and/or the publisher shall have no liability to any person or entity with regard to claims, loss, or damage caused, or alleged to be caused, directly or indirectly, by the use of information contained herein. Because of the dynamic nature of drug information, readers are advised that decisions regarding drug therapy must be based on the independent judgment of the clinician, changing information about a drug (eg, as reflected in the literature and manufacturer's most current product information), and changing medical practices. The authors are not responsible for any inaccuracy of quotation or for any false or misleading implication that may arise due to the text or formulas as used or due to the quotation of revisions no longer official.

Further, the *Drug Information Handbook for Advanced Practice Nursing* is not offered as a guide to dosing. The reader, herewith, is advised that information shown under the heading **Dosing** is provided only as an indication of the amount of the drug typically given or taken during therapy. Actual dosing amount for any specific drug should be based on an in-depth evaluation of the individual patient's therapy requirement and strong consideration given to such issues as contraindications, warnings, precautions, adverse reactions, along with the interaction of other drugs. The manufacturers most current product information or other standard recognized references should always be consulted for such detailed information prior to drug use.

The authors and contributors have written this book in their private capacities. No official support or endorsement by any federal agency or pharmaceutical company is intended or inferred.

If you have any suggestions or questions regarding any information presented in this handbook, please contact our drug information pharmacist at **1-877-837-LEXI (5394)**.

This manual was produced using the FormuLex™ Program —
a complete publishing service of Lexi-Comp Inc.

ISBN 1-59195-112-7

LEXI-COMP
1100 Terex Road
Hudson, Ohio 44236
(330) 650-6506

TABLE OF CONTENTS

FOREWORD

Nationwide, there are now more than 175,000 advanced practice nurses (APNs). As our ranks grow, so do our practice responsibilities. We write thousands of prescriptions daily as we provide care, often to the most vulnerable members of society. As with all busy clinicians, an APN needs references to help guide care, especially in the fast-changing field of pharmacotherapeutics.

During the course of APN practice, prescribing questions need to be answered quickly and precisely. When the question is about drug therapy, often the answer is hard to find:

- *Where can you find information on both FDA-approved and unlabeled uses of a drug?*

- *When prescribing a certain agent, are there food, herbal, ethanol, or drug interactions?*

- *How should the drug be started?*

- *How should the dose be adjusted?*

- *How long until a therapeutic dose is reached and therapeutic effect realized?*

- *What is the critical information the prescriber needs to convey to the patient and family in order to ensure safety and facilitate an optimum outcome?*

The *Drug Information Handbook for Advanced Practice Nursing* provides this valuable information and much more, in a clear, concise format. Seldom has so much rich information been found in a single source. A section on pharmacokinetics, pharmacodynamics, and therapeutics sets the stage in this helpful handbook. Each drug monograph features a clear guide to safe prescribing, highlighting important issues, such as information on prescribing for children, adults, geriatrics, and during pregnancy/lactation. All generic drug names and cross-references are highlighted in red, a helpful feature in an information-intensive text. There are 54 fields of pertinent data that can appear in each monograph, including effects on laboratory values, as well as, information on monitoring for adverse reactions and required ongoing monitoring. Features of this 6th edition include improved patient education and physical assessment fields; the addition of 33 new drug monographs; numerous updates for previously-approved medications; and completely revised cytochrome P450 enzyme interactions with the most up-to-date information available.

The appendix is one of the most valuable portions of this book, providing critical information to informed APN practice. Found here are concise summaries of important documents, such as the OBRA Guidelines for use of psychotropic medications in long-term care, as well as, nationally-recognized standards of care for common diseases including asthma, diabetes, obesity, community-acquired pneumonia, sexually-transmitted diseases, and hyperlipidemia. This edition includes the newest JNC VII Hypertension Guidelines and updated immunization recommendations with a revised immunization table. Given the current focus on evidenced-based healthcare, a ready-reference for this type of information is critically-important.

The publication of the *Drug Information Handbook for Advanced Practice Nursing* comes at an exciting and challenging time. The increasing complexity of clinical care and development of new therapies contribute to the challenges of prescriptive practice. The need for quality references to enhance APN practice continues. In this regard, the *Drug Information Handbook for Advanced Practice Nursing* is a valuable asset.

Margaret A. Fitzgerald, MS, APRN, BC, NP-C, FAANP

Ms Fitzgerald is the President and Principal Lecturer with Fitzgerald Health Education Associates, a national provider of NP Certification and Practice Preparation and ongoing continuing education for NPs and other healthcare providers. In addition, she is a family nurse practitioner at the Greater Lawrence Family Health Center in Lawrence, Massachusetts, where her clinical practice focuses on the primary care of multigenerational Latino families and adults with chronic physical and mental health problems and adjunct faculty to the Health Center's Family Practice Residency Program.

PREFACE

The ever-expanding roles of Advanced Practice Nurses require them to be informed and knowledgeable about safe and therapeutic pharmacotherapy. Yet, at the same time, there is an expanding number and complexity of pharmacotherapeutic agents used in both outpatient and institutional settings. In addition, there is an increased availability of over-the-counter (OTC) agents and nonregulated biological and herbal products used by the public, whose information about use and safety may or may not be accurate. The information about current drug therapy is voluminous and the quality of that information varies greatly. Compiling reliable information into a logical guide for therapy when facing the complexities of diverse disease states and the demands of today's changing healthcare environment is difficult. The authors of this book have extensively reviewed the available literature and have developed the *Drug Information Handbook for Advanced Practice Nursing* with the intent to provide pertinent information related to pharmacotherapeutic agents.

In addition to the helpful descriptions of the organization and use of the *Drug Information Handbook for Advanced Practice Nursing*, the introductory section reviews basic pharmacokinetic and pharmacodynamic principles necessary for understanding drug therapy and provides guidelines and approved abbreviations/symbols for safe prescription writing.

The individual drug monographs present information in a concise and consistent manner with cross-referencing to an extensive appendix of helpful information. Each monograph contains pertinent pharmacokinetics, therapeutic purpose, dosing guidelines, and possible adverse effects. Fields highlighted in red contain special issues which may be of particular concern. The FDA-proposed "tall-man letters" in generic names help distinguish those drugs with look-alike names.

The extensive appendix includes information on diagnostics and surgical aids; calculations and conversions; overdose and toxicology; immunization recommendations and vaccines; common herbal products; food and fluid concerns; maternal and fetal guidelines; OBRA guidelines for long-term care; and selected treatment guidelines for various conditions. Standard laboratory values are provided, along with updated lists of adverse reactions, and comparison charts of drugs in specific classes. In addition to the newest cytochrome P450 lists found in the appendix, the information in the drug interaction field of the monographs has been extensively revised and reformatted to more clearly indicate relevant isoenzyme interactions.

The introductory information, format of drug monographs, valuable appendices, and index information in the *Drug Information Handbook for Advanced Practice Nursing* have all been designed to provide the Advanced Practice Nurse with information to facilitate safe clinical decision-making.

ABOUT THE AUTHORS

Beatrice B. Turkoski, RN, PhD

Dr Turkoski received her BSN from Alverno College in Wisconsin, an MS in Community Health Nursing from the University of Wisconsin-Milwaukee School of Nursing, and a PhD from the University of Wisconsin. Her extensive professional nursing experience includes several years as a clinician in critical care in Wisconsin and Israel, Director of Nursing, clinician, and researcher in gerontology and chronic adult illness in Wisconsin and Ohio, and clinical nurse specialist in family/community practice in Israel.

In her graduate faculty role at Kent State University College of Nursing, Dr Turkoski developed and teaches the Advanced Pharmacology course for graduate students in the Nurse Practitioner and Clinical Nurse Specialist programs. Her expertise in this area is highly regarded by both students and faculty. She also conducts continuing education programs and workshops in pharmacology and nursing practice, both in person and on the internet.

Dr Turkoski is an active member and past officer in several national and international professional organizations. She has made presentations at scientific conferences in the United States, Europe, China, Korea, Canada, and Israel. Dr. Turkoski is also a frequent contributor to professional journals.

Brenda R. Lance, RN, MSN

Ms Lance received a diploma in nursing from Methodist Hospital School of Nursing in Lubbock, Texas. She also has earned bachelor's and master's degrees in nursing from Kent State University, Kent, Ohio.

Ms Lance's nursing experiences and expertise are numerous and varied. Her nursing career spans over 30 years, having worked in intensive care, emergency room, ambulatory care clinics, home health, and home infusion. She is currently the Program Development Director for Northcoast HealthCare Management Company and Northcoast Infusion Therapies located in Oakwood Village, Ohio.

In addition to many years of direct patient care experience, she is also certified in risk management, has extensive experience in Joint Commission on Accreditation of Healthcare Organizations standards and Medicare regulations for home health, and has been a military nurse for the past 30 years. She retired with the rank of Captain (0-6) from the U.S. Naval Reserve Nurse Corps.

Ms Lance is a member of the Sigma Theta Tau (National Honor Society of Nursing) and National Home Infusion Association.

Mark F. Bonfiglio, BS, PharmD, RPh

Dr Bonfiglio received his bachelor's degrees and undergraduate training from the University of Toledo (BA in Biology/BS in Pharmacy) and his PharmD from the Ohio State University. He completed a residency in Critical Care Pharmacy at University Hospitals in Columbus, Ohio. On completion of his training, he worked for several years as a Clinical Specialist in Critical Care in the SUMMA Health System, followed by a position as Pharmacotherapy Specialist in Internal Medicine at Akron General Medical Center. In both of these positions he was concurrently employed by the College of Pharmacy at Ohio Northern University where he attained the rank of Associate Clinical Professor. In addition to his current responsibilities at Lexi-Comp, he has continued to remain active in science and healthcare education. He currently coordinates the Advanced Pharmacology course for the College of Nursing at Malone College, and serves as a Part-Time Faculty in the Department of Biological Sciences at Kent State University, serving as the primary lecturer for the Department's course in Immunology.

Dr Bonfiglio is currently the Director of the Medical Science Division of Lexi-Comp, Inc. He coordinates the development and maintenance of the core pharmacology database and serves as an author for several printed titles, including the *Drug Information Handbook for Advanced Practice Nursing* and *Drug Interactions Handbook*. He is also a contributing author to the *Pharmacogenomics Handbook*. Dr Bonfiglio maintains memberships in the Society for Critical Care Medicine (SCCM), the American Pharmacists Association (APhA), the American Society of Health-System Pharmacists (ASHP), the Ohio College of Clinical Pharmacy (OCCP), the American Society for Automation in Pharmacy (ASAP), and the American Association for the Advancement of Science (AAAS).

EDITORIAL ADVISORY PANEL

Tracey Hagemann, PharmD
Associate Professor
College of Pharmacy
The University of Oklahoma
Oklahoma City, Oklahoma

Charles E. Hawley, DDS, PhD
Professor Emeritus
Department of Periodontics
University of Maryland
Consultant on Periodontics
Commission on Dental Accreditation of the American Dental Association

Martin D. Higbee, PharmD, CGP
Associate Professor
Department of Pharmacy Practice and Science
The University of Arizona
Tucson, Arizona

Jane Hurlburt Hodding, PharmD
Director, Pharmacy
Miller Children's Hospital
Long Beach, California

Rebecca T. Horvat, PhD
Assistant Professor of Pathology and Laboratory Medicine
University of Kansas Medical Center
Kansas City, Kansas

Collin A. Hovinga, PharmD
Neuropharmacologist
Miami Children's Hospital
Miami, Florida

Darrell T. Hulisz, PharmD
Department of Family Medicine
Case Western Reserve University
Cleveland, Ohio

Sana Isa-Pratt, MD
Attending Physician
Department of Medicine
Overlake Hospital
Bellevue, Washington

David S. Jacobs, MD
President, Pathologists Chartered
Consultant in Pathology and Laboratory Medicine
Overland Park, Kansas

Bernard L. Kasten, Jr, MD, FCAP
Vice-President/Chief Medical Officer
Quest Diagnostics Inc
Teteroboro, New Jersey

Polly E. Kintzel, PharmD, BCPS, BCOP
Clinical Pharmacy Specialist-Oncology
Spectrum Health
Grand Rapids, Michigan

Jill Kolesar, PharmD, FCCP, BCPS
Associate Professor of Pharmacy
University of Wisconsin
Madison, Wisconsin

Donna M. Kraus, PharmD, FAPhA
Associate Professor of Pharmacy Practice
Departments of Pharmacy Practice and Pediatrics
Pediatric Clinical Pharmacist
University of Illinois
Chicago, Illinois

Daniel L. Krinsky, RPh, MS
Director, Pharmacotherapy Sales and Marketing
Lexi-Comp, Inc
Hudson, Ohio

EDITORIAL ADVISORY PANEL *(Continued)*

Franklin A. Michota, Jr, MD
Head, Section of Hospital and Preoperative Medicine
Department of General Internal Medicine
The Cleveland Clinic Foundation
Cleveland, Ohio

Michael A. Militello, PharmD, BCPS
Clinical Cardiology Specialist
Department of Pharmacy
The Cleveland Clinic Foundation
Cleveland, Ohio

J. Robert Newland, DDS, MS
Professor
Department of Diagnostic Sciences
University of Texas Health Science Center
Houston, Texas

Cecelia O'Keefe, PharmD
Pharmacotherapy Specialist
Lexi-Comp, Inc.
Hudson, Ohio

Eugene S. Olsowka, MD, PhD
Pathologist
Institute of Pathology PC
Saginaw, Michigan

Dwight K. Oxley, MD
Consultant in Pathology and Laboratory Medicine
Wichita, Kansas

Frank P. Paloucek, PharmD, DABAT
Clinical Associate Professor in Pharmacy Practice
Director, Residency Programs
University of Illinois
Chicago, Illinois

Christopher J. Papasian, PhD
Director of Diagnostic Microbiology and Immunology Laboratories
Truman Medical Center
Kansas City, Missouri

Alpa Patel, PharmD
Clinical Specialist, Infectious Diseases
Johns Hopkins Hospital
Baltimore, Maryland

Luis F. Ramirez, MD
Adjunct Associate Professor of Psychiatry
Case Western Reserve University
Cleveland, Ohio

A.J. (Fred) Remillard, PharmD
Assistant Dean, Research and Graduate Affairs
College of Pharmacy and Nutrition
University of Saskatchewan
Saskatoon, Saskatchewan

Martha Sajatovic, MD
Associate Professor of Psychiatry
Case Western Reserve University
Cleveland, Ohio

Todd P. Semla, PharmD, BCPS, FCCP
Clinical Pharmacy Specialist
Department of Veterans Affairs
Pharmacy Benefits Management
Associate Professor of Clinical Psychiatry
Feinberg School of Medicine
Northwestern University
Chicago, Illinois

Francis G. Serio, DMD, MS
Professor & Chairman
Department of Periodontics
University of Mississippi
Jackson, Mississippi

EDITORIAL ADVISORY PANEL *(Continued)*

ACKNOWLEDGMENTS

This handbook exists in its present form as the result of the concerted efforts of the following individuals: Robert D. Kerscher, publisher and president of Lexi-Comp, Inc; Mark Bonfiglio, PharmD, director of pharmacotherapy resources; Stacy S. Robinson, editorial manager; Barbara F. Kerscher, production manager; Robin L. Farabee, project manager; David C. Marcus, director of information systems; Tracey J. Henterly, graphic designer; Alexandra Hart, composition specialist; Leslie Jo Hoppes, pharmacology database manager; Matthew C. Kerscher, product manager.

Much of the material contained in this book was a result of pharmacy contributors throughout the United States and Canada. Lexi-Comp has assisted many medical institutions to develop hospital-specific formulary manuals that contain clinical drug information as well as dosing. Working with clinical pharmacists, hospital pharmacy and therapeutics committees, and hospital drug information centers, Lexi-Comp has developed an evolutionary drug database that reflects the practice of pharmacy in these major institutions.

The authors wish to thank Penelope L. Cukr, RN, DNSc, cANP, Director of the Adult Nurse Practitioner Program at Kent State University and Scott Fleming, RN, MSN, cFNP, Instructor in the Nurse Practitioner Program at Kent State University, for their suggestions and review of this handbook. (Dr Cukr passed away before this edition was published. Her constant support and valuable contributions from the 1st edition to this edition will always be appreciated.)

The authors also thank their families, friends, and colleagues, who supported them in their efforts to complete this handbook.

DESCRIPTION OF SECTIONS AND FIELDS

Introduction

This and other documents in this section provide guidelines for the use of the handbook including descriptions of Safe Prescription Writing; Basic Pharmacotherapeutic Concepts (Pharmacokinetics, Pharmacodynamics, Patient Factors That Influence Drug Therapy, and Pharmacotherapeutics); Therapeutic Nursing Management of Side Effects.

Individual Drug Monographs

Medications are arranged alphabetically by generic name. Abbreviated monographs contain unique information, commonly for combination formulations. U.S. brand names and synonyms are cross-referenced between monographs.

Monograph Fields

Generic Name	U.S. adopted name
Pronunciation	Phonetic pronunciation of generic name
U.S. Brand Names	Trade names (manufacturer-specific) found in the United States. The symbol [DSC] appears after trade names that have been recently discontinued.
Synonyms	Other name(s) or accepted abbreviation(s) of the generic drug
Controlled Substance	The controlled substance classification from the Drug Enforcement Agency (DEA); U.S. schedules are I-V; schedules vary by country and sometimes state (ie, Massachusetts uses I-VI)
Restrictions	Information pertaining to dispensing and availability restrictions
Generic Available	Indicated by "Yes" or "No"; may include specific forms or exceptions
Pharmacologic Category	Indicates one or more systematic classifications of the drug
Medication Safety Issues	In an effort to promote the safe use of medications, this field is intended to highlight possible sources of medication errors such as look-alike/sound-alike drugs or highly concentrated formulations which require vigilance on the part of healthcare professionals. In addition, medications which have been associated with severe consequences in the event of a medication error are also identified in this field.
Use	Description of FDA-approved indications of the drug
Unlabeled/Investigational Use	Information pertaining to non-FDA approved and investigational indications of the drug
Mechanism of Action/Effect	A brief description of how the drug works
Contraindications	Inappropriate use(s) of the drug or disease states and patient populations in which the drug should not be used, according to the FDA
Warnings/Precautions	Warnings include hazardous conditions related to use of the drug. Precautions include disease states or patient populations in which the drug should be used with caution.
Drug Interactions	Agents that, when combined with the drug, may affect therapy; may include the following:
Cytochrome P450 Effect	Drugs which are involved in possible interactions due to their activity with the hepatic cytochrome P450 system are identified, and their role for a specific isoenzyme is listed according to the degree of effect. Substrates are described as major or minor. Inhibitors are classified as weak, moderate, or strong. Inducers are defined as weak or strong.
Decreased Effect	Drug combinations that result in a decreased therapeutic effect between the drug listed in the monograph and other drugs or drug classes
Increased Effect/Toxicity	Drug combinations that result in a increased or toxic therapeutic effect between the drug listed in the monograph and other drugs or drug classes

Nutritional/Ethanol Interactions	Information regarding potential interactions with food, nutritional supplements (including herbal products and vitamins), ethanol, or cigarette smoking
Lab Interactions	Effect drug may have on assays during therapy
Adverse Reactions	Only side effects >1% are included and are grouped by percentage of incidence (if known) and/or body system
Overdose/Toxicology	Comment or considerations with signs/symptoms of excess drug ingestion
Pharmacodynamics/Kinetics	
Onset of Action	The time after drug administration when therapeutic effect is observed; may also include time for peak therapeutic effect
Duration of Action	Length of therapeutic effect
Absorption	The amount of absorbed drug, including rate and route for the drug listed
Bioavailability	Fraction of administered drug dose that enters systemic circulation
Time to Peak	Describes the relative time after ingestion when concentration achieves the highest serum concentration
Protein Binding	The percent of drug listed in the monograph bound to circulating proteins (ie, albumin, etc)
Half-Life Elimination	The reported half-life of elimination for the parent or metabolites of the drug
Metabolism	Describes the site of metabolism and may include the percentage of active metabolites.
Excretion	Route of drug elimination
Pharmacokinetic Note	Provides additional pharmacokinetic information when needed.
Dosing	The amount of drug to be typically given or taken during therapy; may include the following:
Adults	The recommended amount of drug to be given to adult patients
Adults and Elderly	This combined field is only used to indicate that no specific adjustments for elderly patients were identified. However, other issues should be considered (ie, renal or hepatic impairment). Also refer to Geriatric Considerations for additional information related to the elderly.
Elderly	A suggested amount of drug to be given to elderly patients which may include adjustments from adult dosing; lack of information in the monograph may imply that the drug is not used in the elderly patient or no specific adjustments could be identified
Pediatrics	Suggested amount of drug to be given to neonates, infants, and children
Renal Impairment	Suggested dosage adjustments or comments based on compromised renal function; may include dosing instructions for patients on dialysis
Hepatic Impairment	Suggested dosage adjustments or comments based on compromised liver function
Available Dosage Forms	A description of the product form(s), including strength and formulation (ie, tablet, capsule, injection, syrup, etc)
Monitoring and Teaching Issues	
Physical Assessment	Monitoring guidelines
Monitoring Laboratory Tests	Suggested laboratory tests to monitor for safety and efficacy of the drug
Patient Education	Suggested items to discuss with the patient or caregiver when taking the medication; may include issues regarding contraception, self-monitoring, precautions, and administration
Dietary Considerations	Includes information on how the medication should be taken relative to meals or food

DESCRIPTION OF SECTIONS AND FIELDS *(Continued)*

Geriatric Considerations	Comments or suggestions of drug use in elderly patients; may include monitoring, dose adjustments, precautions, or comments on appropriateness of use
Pregnancy Risk Factor	Indicates one or more of the five categories established by the FDA to indicate the potential of a systemically absorbed drug for causing birth defects
Pregnancy Issues	Comments related to safe drug administration during pregnancy, if appropriate
Lactation	Information regarding use of the drug while breast-feeding (where recommendation of American Academy of Pediatrics differs, notation is made); the following distinctions are made:
	Does not enter breast milk
	Enters breast milk (may include: /compatible, use caution, not recommended, contraindicated, or consult prescriber)
	Excretion in breast milk unknown (may include: /compatible, use caution, not recommended, contraindicated, or consult prescriber)
	Not indicated for use in women
	No data available (may include: /use caution)
Breast-feeding Issues	Provides further information relating to taking the drug while nursing
Other Issues	Additional pertinent information regarding nursing issues
Administration	
Oral I.M. I.V. Inhalation Topical Other	The administration field contains subfields by route regarding issues relative to appropriately giving a medication; includes suggestions on final drug concentrations and/or rates of infusion for parenteral medications and comments regarding the timing of drug administration relative to meals. Also see Compatibility.
Reconstitution	Includes comments on solution choice with time or conditions for the mixture to maintain full potency before administration
Compatibility	Provides information regarding stability of the drug in different solutions; known incompatibilities when admixed or coadministered with other drugs; and when it is administered through Y-site administration sets
Storage	Information relating to appropriate storage of the medication prior to opening the manufacturers original packaging; information is only given if recommendations are for storage at other than room temperature; includes storage requirements for reconstituted products
Additional Information	Information about sodium content and/or pertinent information about specific brands
Related Information	Cross-reference to other pertinent drug information in this handbook

Controlled Substance Index

A list of drug names and their corresponding controlled substance classification

Pharmacologic Category Index

Lists all drugs by their unique pharmacologic category and includes cross-references to the monographs

Appendix

The last section is an extensive appendix of useful information that includes conversion laboratory information, adverse reactions, comparison charts for selected classes of drugs, maternal and fetal guidelines, OBRA recommendations for long-term care, toxicology information, and treatment guidelines for selected therapy.

FDA NAME DIFFERENTIATION PROJECT: THE USE OF TALL-MAN LETTERS

Confusion between similar drug names is an important cause of medication errors. For years, The Institute For Safe Medication Practices (ISMP), has urged generic manufacturers use a combination of large and small letters as well as bolding (ie, chlorpro**MAZINE** and chlorpro**PAMIDE**) to help distinguish drugs with look-alike names, especially when they share similar strengths. Recently the FDA's Division of Generic Drugs began to issue recommendation letters to manufacturers suggesting this novel way to label their products to help reduce this drug name confusion. Although this project has had marginal success, the method has successfully eliminated problems with products such as diphenhydr**AMINE** and dimenhy**DRINATE**. Hospitals should also follow suit by making similar changes in their own labels, preprinted order forms, computer screens and printouts, and drug storage location labels.

Lexi-Comp Medical Publishing has adopted the use of these "Tall-Man" letters for the drugs suggested by the FDA.

The following is a list of product names and recommended FDA revisions.

DRUG PRODUCT	RECOMMENDED REVISION
acetazolamide	aceta**ZOLAMIDE**
acetohexamide	aceto**HEXAMIDE**
bupropion	bu**PROP**ion
buspirone	bus**PIR**one
chlorpromazine	chlorpro**MAZINE**
chlorpropamide	chlorpro**PAMIDE**
clomiphene	clomi**PHENE**
clomipramine	clomi**PRAMINE**
cycloserine	cyclo**SERINE**
cyclosporine	cyclo**SPORINE**
daunorubicin	**DAUNO**rubicin
dimenhydrinate	dimenhy**DRINATE**
diphenhydramine	diphenhydr**AMINE**
dobutamine	**DOBUT**amine
dopamine	**DOP**amine
doxorubicin	**DOXO**rubicin
glipizide	glipi**ZIDE**
glyburide	gly**BURIDE**
hydralazine	hydr**ALAZINE**
hydroxyzine	hydr**OXY**zine
medroxyprogesterone	medroxy**PROGESTER**one
methylprednisolone	methyl**PREDNIS**olone
methyltestosterone	methyl**TESTOSTER**one
nicardipine	ni**CAR**dipine
nifedipine	**NIFE**dipine
prednisolone	predniso**LONE**
prednisone	predni**SONE**
sulfadiazine	sulfa**DIAZINE**
sulfisoxazole	sulfi**SOXAZOLE**
tolazamide	**TOLAZ**amide
tolbutamide	**TOLBUT**amide
vinblastine	vin**BLAS**tine
vincristine	vin**CRIS**tine

Institute for Safe Medication Practices. "New Tall-Man Lettering Will Reduce Mix-Ups Due to Generic Drug Name Confusion," *ISMP Medication Safety Alert*, September 19, 2001. Available at: http://www.ismp.org.

Institute for Safe Medication Practices. "Prescription Mapping, Can Improve Efficiency While Minimizing Errors With Look-Alike Products," *ISMP Medication Safety Alert*, October 6, 1999. Available at: http://www.ismp.org.

U.S. Pharmacopeia, "USP Quality Review: Use Caution-Avoid Confusion," March 2001, No. 76. Available at: http://www.usp.org.

FDA PREGNANCY CATEGORIES

Throughout this book there is a field labeled Pregnancy Risk Factor and the letter A, B, C, D, or X, immediately following, which signifies a category. The FDA has established these five categories to indicate the potential of a systemically-absorbed drug for causing birth defects. The key differentiation among the categories rests upon the reliability of documentation and the risk:benefit ratio. Category **X** is particularly notable, in that if any data exists that may implicate a drug as a teratogen, and the risk:benefit ratio is clearly negative, the drug is **contraindicated** during pregnancy.

These categories are summarized as follows:

A   Controlled studies in pregnant women fail to demonstrate a risk to the fetus in the first trimester with no evidence of risk in later trimesters. The possibility of fetal harm appears remote.

B   Either animal-reproduction studies have not demonstrated a fetal risk but there are no controlled studies in pregnant women, or animal-reproduction studies have shown an adverse effect (other than a decrease in fertility) that was not confirmed in controlled studies in women in the first trimester and there is no evidence of a risk in later trimesters.

C   Either studies in animals have revealed adverse effects on the fetus (teratogenic or embryocidal effects or other) and there are no controlled studies in women, or studies in women and animals are not available. Drugs should be given only if the potential benefits justify the potential risk to the fetus.

D   There is positive evidence of human fetal risk, but the benefits from use in pregnant women may be acceptable despite the risk (eg, if the drug is needed in a life-threatening situation or for a serious disease for which safer drugs cannot be used or are ineffective).

X   Studies in animals or human beings have demonstrated fetal abnormalities or there is evidence of fetal risk based on human experience, or both, and the risk of the use of the drug in pregnant women clearly outweighs any possible benefit. The drug is contraindicated in women who are or may become pregnant.

SAFE WRITING

Health professionals and their support personnel frequently produce handwritten copies of information they see in print; therefore, such information is subjected to even greater possibilities for error or misinterpretation on the part of others. Thus, particular care must be given to how drug names and strengths are expressed when creating written healthcare documents.

The following are a few examples of safe writing rules suggested by the Institute for Safe Medication Practices, Inc.*

1. There should be a space between a number and its units as it is easier to read. There should be no periods after the abbreviations mg or mL.

Correct	Incorrect
10 mg	10mg
100 mg	100mg

2. Never place a decimal and a zero after a whole number (2 mg is correct and 2.0 mg is **incorrect**). If the decimal point is not seen because it falls on a line or because individuals are working from copies where the decimal point is not seen, this causes a tenfold overdose.

3. Just the opposite is true for numbers less than one. Always place a zero before a naked decimal (0.5 mL is correct, .5 mL is **incorrect**).

4. Never abbreviate the word unit. The handwritten U or u, looks like a 0 (zero), and may cause a tenfold overdose error to be made.

5. IU is not a safe abbreviation for international units. The handwritten IU looks like IV. Write out international units or use int. units.

6. Q.D. is not a safe abbreviation for once daily, as when the Q is followed by a sloppy dot, it looks like QID which means four times daily.

7. O.D. is not a safe abbreviation for once daily, as it is properly interpreted as meaning "right eye" and has caused liquid medications such as saturated solution of potassium iodide and Lugol's solution to be administered incorrectly. There is no safe abbreviation for once daily. It must be written out in full.

8. Do not use chemical names such as 6-mercaptopurine or 6-thioguanine, as sixfold overdoses have been given when these were not recognized as chemical names. The proper names of these drugs are mercaptopurine or thioguanine.

9. Do not abbreviate drug names (5FC, 6MP, 5-ASA, MTX, HCTZ, CPZ, PBZ, etc) as they are misinterpreted and cause error.

10. Do not use the apothecary system or symbols.

11. Do not abbreviate microgram as µg; instead use mcg as there is less likelihood of misinterpretation.

12. When writing an outpatient prescription, write a complete prescription. A complete prescription can prevent the prescriber, the pharmacist, and/or the patient from making a mistake and can eliminate the need for further clarification. The legible prescriptions should contain:

    a. patient's full name

    b. for pediatric or geriatric patients: their age (or weight where applicable)

    c. drug name, dosage form and strength; if a drug is new or rarely prescribed, print this information

    d. number or amount to be dispensed

    e. complete instructions for the patient, including the purpose of the medication

    f. when there are recognized contraindications for a prescribed drug, indicate to the pharmacist that you are aware of this fact (ie, when prescribing a potassium salt for a patient receiving an ACE inhibitor, write "K serum level being monitored")

*From "Safe Writing" by Davis NM, PharmD and Cohen MR, MS, Lecturers and Consultants for Safe Medication Practices, 1143 Wright Drive, Huntington Valley, PA 19006. Phone: (215) 947-7566.

COMMON SYMBOLS AND ABBREVIATIONS

Abbreviation	Meaning
°C	degrees Celsius (Centigrade)
<	less than
>	greater than
≤	less than or equal to
≥	greater than or equal to
μg	microgram
μmol	micromole
$\overline{aa}$, aa	of each
AAPC	antibiotic associated pseudomembranous colitis
ABG	arterial blood gas
ABMT	autologous bone marrow transplant
ac	before meals or food
ACE	angiotensin-converting enzyme
ACLS	advanced cardiac life support
ad	to, up to
a.d.	right ear
ADH	antidiuretic hormone
ad lib	at pleasure
AED	antiepileptic drug
AIDS	acquired immunodeficiency syndrome
a.l.	left ear
ALL	acute lymphoblastic leukemia
ALT	alanine aminotransferase (formerly called SGPT)
AM	morning
AML	acute myeloblastic leukemia
amp	ampul
amt	amount
ANA	antinuclear antibodies
ANC	absolute neutrophil count
ANLL	acute nonlymphoblastic leukemia
APTT	activated partial thromboplastin time
aq	water
aq. dest.	distilled water
a.s.	left ear
ASA (class I-IV)	American Society of Anesthesiology physical status classification of surgical patients according to their baseline health
	ASA I: Normal healthy patients
	ASA II: Patients having controlled disease states (eg, controlled hypertension)
	ASA III: Patients having a disease which compromises their organ function (eg, decompensated CHF, end stage renal failure)
	ASA IV: Patients who are extremely critically ill
ASAP	as soon as possible
AST	aspartate aminotransferase (formerly called SGOT)
a.u.	each ear
AUC	area under the curve (area under the serum concentration-time curve)
A-V	atrial-ventricular
bid	twice daily
bm	bowel movement
BMT	bone marrow transplant
bp	blood pressure
BPH	benign prostatic hyperplasia
BSA	body surface area
BUN	blood urea nitrogen
c	a gallon
$\overline{c}$	with
cal	calorie
cAMP	cyclic adenosine monophosphate
cap	capsule
CBC	complete blood count
cc	cubic centimeter

(continued)

Abbreviation	Meaning
CHF	congestive heart failure
CI	cardiac index
CI_{cr}	creatinine clearance
cm	centimeter
CMV	cytomegalovirus
CNS	central nervous system
comp	compound
cont	continue
COPD	chronic obstructive pulmonary disease
CSF	cerebrospinal fluid
CT	computed tomography
CVA	cerebral vascular accident
CVP	central venous pressure
d	day
D_5W	dextrose 5% in water
$D_5/1/2NS$	dextrose 5% in sodium chloride 0.45%
$D_{10}W$	dextrose 10% in water
d/c	discontinue
DIC	disseminated intravascular coagulation
dil	dilute
disp	dispense
div	divide
DL_{co}	pulmonary diffusion capacity for carbon monoxide
DNA	deoxyribonucleic acid
dtd	give of such a dose
DVT	deep vein thrombosis
ECHO	echocardiogram
ECMO	extracorporeal membrane oxygenation
EEG	electroencephalogram
EKG	electrocardiogram
elix, el	elixir
emp	as directed
ESR	erythrocyte sedimentation rate
et	and
E.T.	endotracheal
ex aq	in water
f, ft	make, let be made
FDA	Food and Drug Administration
FEV_1	forced expiratory volume exhaled after 1 second
FSH	follicle-stimulating hormone
FVC	forced vital capacity
g	gram
G6PD	glucose-6-phosphate dehydrogenase
GA	gestational age
GABA	gamma-aminobutyric acid
GE	gastroesophageal
GI	gastrointestinal
gr	grain
gtt	a drop
GU	genitourinary
h	hour
HIV	human immunodeficiency virus
HPLC	high performance liquid chromatography
hs	at bedtime
IBW	ideal body weight
ICP	intracranial pressure
IgG	immune globulin G
I.M.	intramuscular
INR	international normalized ratio
int. unit	international units
I.O.	intraosseous
I & O	input and output
IOP	intraocular pressure

COMMON SYMBOLS AND ABBREVIATIONS *(Continued)*

(continued)

Abbreviation	Meaning
I.T.	intrathecal
I.V.	intravenous
IVH	intraventricular hemorrhage
IVP	intravenous push
JRA	juvenile rheumatoid arthritis
kcal	kilocalorie
kg	kilogram
L	liter
LDH	lactate dehydrogenase
LE	lupus erythematosus
LH	luteinizing hormone
liq	a liquor, solution
LP	lumbar puncture
LR	lactated Ringer's
M.	mix
MAC	*Mycobacterium avium* complex
MAO	monoamine oxidase
MAP	mean arterial pressure
mcg	microgram
m. dict	as directed
mEq	milliequivalent
mg	milligram
MI	myocardial infarction
min	minute
mixt	a mixture
mL	milliliter
mm	millimeter
mo	month
mOsm	milliosmoles
MRI	magnetic resonance image
MRSA	methicillin-resistant *Staphylococcus aureus*
NCI	National Cancer Institute
ND	nasoduodenal
NF	National Formulary
ng	nanogram
NG	nasogastric
NMDA	n-methyl-d-aspartate
nmol	nanomole
no.	number
noc	in the night
non rep	do not repeat, no refills
NPO	nothing by mouth
NSAID	nonsteroidal anti-inflammatory drug
O, Oct	a pint
o.d.	right eye
o.l.	left eye
O.R.	operating room
o.s.	left eye
OTC	over-the-counter (nonprescription)
o.u.	each eye
PABA	para-aminobenzoic acid
PALS	pediatric advanced life support
pc, post cib	after meals
PCA	postconceptional age
PCP	*Pneumocystis carinii* pneumonia
PCWP	pulmonary capillary wedge pressure
PDA	patent ductus arteriosus
per	through or by
PIP	peak inspiratory pressure
PM	afternoon or evening
PNA	postnatal age
P.O.	by mouth

(continued)

Abbreviation	Meaning
P.R.	rectally
prn	as needed
PSVT	paroxysmal supraventricular tachycardia
PT	prothrombin time
PTT	partial thromboplastin time
PUD	peptic ulcer disease
pulv	a powder
PVC	premature ventricular contraction
PVR	peripheral vascular resistance
q	every
qad	every other day
qd	every day
qh	every hour
qid	four times a day
qod	every other day
qs	a sufficient quantity
qs ad, qsad	a sufficient quantity to make, add amount to equal
qty	quantity
qv	as much as you wish
RAP	right arterial pressure
RIA	radioimmunoassay
RNA	ribonucleic acid
Rx	take, a recipe
rep	let it be repeated
$\bar{s}$	without
S-A	sino-atrial
sa	according to art
sat	saturated
S_{cr}	serum creatinine
SIADH	syndrome of inappropriate antidiuretic hormone
sig	label, or let it be printed
SL	sublingual
SLE	systemic lupus erythematosus
sol	solution
solv	dissolve
$\overline{ss}$	one-half
sos	if there is need
stat	at once, immediately
supp	suppository
SubQ	subcutaneous
SVR	systemic vascular resistance
SVT	supraventricular tachycardia
SWI	sterile water for injection
syr	syrup
T_3	triiodothyronine
T_4	thyroxine
tab	tablet
tal	such
TIBC	total iron binding capacity
tid	three times a day
TPN	total parenteral nutrition
tr, tinct	tincture
trit	triturate
TSH	thyroid stimulating hormone
tsp	teaspoonful
TT	thrombin time
u.d., ut dict	as directed
ung	ointment
USAN	United States Adopted Names
USP	United States Pharmacopeia
UTI	urinary tract infection
V_d	volume of distribution
V_{dss}	volume of distribution at steady-state

COMMON SYMBOLS AND ABBREVIATIONS *(Continued)*

(continued)

Abbreviation	Meaning
VMA	vanillylmandelic acid
v.o.	verbal order
w.a.	while awake
w/w	weight for weight
x3	3 times
x4	4 times
y, yr	year

BASIC PHARMACOTHERAPEUTIC CONCEPTS

Safe and effective drug therapy requires an understanding of the basic principles of pharmacokinetics and pharmacodynamics and an awareness of how individual patient traits and lifestyles influence the actions and effects of drugs. A brief overview of basic concepts is discussed on the following pages.

1. Pharmacokinetics and Pharmacodynamics
2. Patient Factors That Influence Drug Therapy (pregnancy, age, weight, lifestyle)
3. Pharmacotherapeutics

PHARMACOKINETICS

The pharmacokinetics principles of absorption, distribution, and elimination govern how quickly a drug becomes available to the target organ and how long the drug will remain available.

Absorption

Absorption refers to how a drug progresses from the dosage form given into one bodily compartment into the blood stream to be distributed to the target site of action. The rate and degree of absorption depends on the formulation of the drug, the route of drug administration, and physiological variables. Drugs administered by the I.V. route require no absorption since they enter the circulatory system directly. Intramuscularly or subcutaneously administered drugs involve differing degrees of absorption. For instance, formulations in oil or microfine crystals (long-acting) have longer absorption times than other formulations and drugs administered into the deltoid muscle are absorbed faster than those administered into the gluteus muscle because of the increased blood flow in the deltoid muscle.

The oral route of drug administration is the preferred route for most drug therapy because it is more comfortable for the patient and usually safer and easier to use. The enteral route however, has a longer absorption time than other routes of absorption. This is, in part, related to the particular drug formulation (compressed tablet, extended release, repeat action). Anything that reduces systemic blood flow can reduce absorption rates, strenuous exercise decreases splanchnic blood flow as more blood is diverted to the muscles; pain and stress can also reduce blood flow in this area. Prolonged intestinal transit time (experienced with high-fat meals, solid food, anticholinergic drugs) may delay absorption rate, but increase the amount of total drug absorption. In addition, drug-drug interactions or drug-food interactions can reduce absorption; substances that significantly alter the gastric pH (eg, H_2-blockers, such as famotidine or proton pump inhibitors such as omeprazole, etc) can, in turn effect the absorption rates of some drugs. Absorption from the gastrointestinal tract may involve active transport across membranes. Some enzymes actually "pump" drug back into the GI lumen, opposing their absorption. One such enzyme is p-glycoprotein. Drugs which inhibit p-glycoprotein abolish this "pumping" action, and may lead to dramatic increases in the absorption of some drugs.

Orally administered drugs must pass through the portal system before they enter the systemic circulation. Many drugs undergo metabolic changes as they pass through the liver prior to reaching the systemic circulation. This means a substantial portion of the dose will never reach its target tissue (first-pass effect). The orally administered dose required to achieve a specific therapeutic response may, therefore be much larger than the dose for a route that bypasses portal circulation (parenteral or transdermal). Enterohepatic recycling (reabsorption) may occur with some drugs and may be a particular concern in some cases of toxicity. A few drugs (eg, digoxin, leflunomide, levothyroxine) re-enter the gastrointestinal tract (via excretion in the bile) from the bloodstream. They are then reabsorbed from the intestine and re-enter the circulatory system. Administration of substances, such as charcoal or cholestyramine resin (Questran®) or sodium polystyrene sulfonate (Kayexalate®), that bind the recycled drug in the GI tract, may be necessary to rapidly reduce the toxic serum levels of the recycled drug.]

Other routes of drug administration (eg, vaginal, rectal, topical, buccal, inhalation) all have positive and negative aspects of absorption. Advantages of drug absorption via these alternative sites include the ability to establish relatively high local concentrations of drugs at target tissues as well as the ability to bypass the "first-pass" metabolism of orally administered drugs. Drugs administered by inhalation must be formulated in microsized particles and are typically administered by nebulization or aerosolization in order to reach the terminial airways. Rectal absorption for systemic drugs is generally slow and administration of these drugs is often uncomfortable or painful. However, for some drugs and for some patients (for example, in severe nausea where oral medications cannot be administered), this is either the only route available or may be the route of choice. Topical absorption has the advantage of continuous absorption, although onset of action is generally slower than other forms of administration and degree of absorption may differ considerably depending on patient characteristics. Transdermal formulations have been designed to work together with the absorptive properties of the skin and may allow the delivery of a consistent rate of drug absorption for several days. Drugs for ophthalmic and otic administration are highly

BASIC PHARMACOTHERAPEUTIC CONCEPTS *(Continued)*

specific and are designed to produce high local concentrations, however healthcare professionals should also take the absorption properties and systemic effects of drugs administered by these routes into consideration.

Distribution

Distribution of an absorbed drug is dependent on several physical and/or chemical characteristics of the drug, including affinity for lipid or aqueous tissue and ability to permeate various tissue barriers (sometimes through the assistance of specific transport proteins), pH differences, blood flow, and degree of protein binding. The size and charge of the drug molecules will also help determine to which bodily compartment they are distributed. Drugs localize to specific tissues according to the combined properties of both drug and tissue. Drug concentrations can vary considerably between organs.

Drugs enter the system by one or another means of absorption, circulate (distribute) through the body via the circulatory system, interact with target receptors, and are excreted from the body in due course. When blood flow is impeded, the distribution of any substance in the blood is also impeded. Anything that alters the concentration of blood (eg, dehydration or edema) may also impact the distribution of drug molecules to the target site.

Albumin levels may also influence the distribution of some drugs that have a potential for binding to large proteins. Usually, the degree to which any drug binds to albumin remains predictable (eg, gentamicin <30% bound and warfarin >97% bound). Dosing recommendations are predicated on the idea that a certain level of unbound molecules remain "free" in the circulation when albumin levels are "normal." When disease states, nutritional status, or other drugs significantly change the amount of albumin available for binding or the ability to bind to this "carrier" protein, toxic serum levels of free (unbound) drug may occur.

Physiological barriers also influence distribution. One example is the blood-brain barrier that is a continuous network of cells with tight junctions that make the brain impermeable to some drugs according to their degree of water or lipid solubility. This makes the brain less accessible to drugs that are able to accumulate in other tissues (eg, many chemotherapeutic drugs and many antibiotics). In addition to this physical barrier, a substantial part of the ability of the brain to exclude certain chemicals is related to the presence of specialized transport proteins which actively "pump" these chemicals out of the CSF. Drugs which inhibit transport enzymes may influence the ability of drug to accumulate in tissues such as the brain.

Elimination via Metabolism

Elimination via metabolism is the process of biotransformation that occurs when a drug changes from its parent form to a more water-soluble form.

Some drugs are not metabolized and are excreted from the body unchanged (aminoglycosides, gabapentin). However, most drugs are metabolized in the liver, in tissues, in the gastric system, or in the lungs. The metabolites are most often inactive forms of the parent that are more water soluble than the parent drug and can therefore be excreted in the urine. In some instances, metabolism is required to convert a biologically inactive drug (prodrug) to an active form. Dopamine does not cross the blood-brain barrier; however, levodopa, an inactive precursor of dopamine, does cross the blood-brain barrier where it is metabolized to dopamine. In other cases, metabolism results in active metabolites (imipramine metabolizes to desipramine).

Hepatic metabolism is a result of specific enzymes and can be influenced by other drugs. In particular, enzymes belonging to the cytochrome P450 family are frequently involved in drug metabolism. Some drugs stimulate an increase in specific enzyme activity which increases the metabolism breakdown of other drugs; thereby decreasing the availability of the second drug (eg, phenobarbital induces the enzyme that metabolizes theophylline). Conversely, when a drug inhibits the enzyme activity necessary for metabolism of a second drug, toxic levels of the second drug can result (eg, cimetidine inhibits the enzyme that metabolizes theophylline; theophylline metabolism is inhibited thereby causing an elevated theophylline level). Much has been learned about the specific pathways by which certain drugs are metabolized, allowing more accurate prediction of potential interactions. Knowing that a drug is either an enzyme inhibitor or an enzyme inducer should cause a nurse monitoring drug effects to be alert for the effects of any other drugs that may be potentially affected.

Elimination via Excretion

Elimination via excretion is the process by which a drug or its metabolites is removed from the body.

Drugs can be eliminated through the lungs, kidneys, liver, skin, intestinal tract, or via excretory glands – in sweat, tears, saliva, or breast milk. Peritoneal dialysis or hemodialysis may also be used to remove drugs from the body.

Half-life is the time required for the blood levels of a drug to be diminished by one-half. This can be expressed as the percentage of the original concentration over time (eg, after one half-life 50% remains, after the second half-life 25%, third half-life 12.5%, etc). With normal functioning excretion, the half-life of a drug will help to determine spacing of dosing schedules. While a true half-life of a drug is specific to its persistence in an individual patient, it is a common practice to express this value as a population average measured in clinical trials.

Because of this, it is important to recognize that the half-life in an individual patient can vary considerably, and may be substantially different in patients with organ dysfunction or deficiencies in metabolizing enzymes. For example, in the presence of decreased kidney function, elimination is slowed or delayed and more of the drug remains in the body than half-life figures from an otherwise healthy population would indicate. The actual half-life in these persons may be several times longer than the population average. Extended half-lives may result in higher drug accumulation. Elderly persons frequently have decreased kidney function as a part of the aging process – drugs excreted primarily via the kidneys thereby hold the potential for toxic levels for elderly persons when given in "normal" doses.

PHARMACODYNAMICS

Pharmacodynamics refers to the time course and relationships which determine how a drug brings about biophysical or biochemical changes.

Drug molecules must interact with specific receptors on target cell membranes in order to effect some biochemical or biophysical action. The drug-receptor interaction may alter or modify cellular function, at times activating new responses and/or previously unexpressed potential of the cell; however, drugs do not cause a new function in a cell or tissue. Action at the cellular level then impacts the tissue function in measurable or observable ways. For instance, insulin interacts with receptors to facilitate glucose transport across cellular membranes, this in turn causes a measurable increase in serum glucose levels; atropine blocks acetylcholine receptors, which results in a decrease in the effects of acetylcholine (anticholinergic response; see Pharmacologic Category Index). The effects of drug and receptor interactions may be desired (beneficial) or nonbeneficial (adverse or side effects).

Most drug molecules can only interact with specific receptors. These may be located within the cell or on cellular membranes for which they have an affinity in a "lock-and-key" type bond. Following interaction with a receptor, a sequence of events may occur within the cell. Pathways in the cell may be activated to alter the production or activity of the cellular enzymes. In some cases, this involves the activation of specific genes. Drugs that stimulate receptor actions are called agonists. Drugs that fit to receptors and prevent or inhibit cellular responses to other drugs or endogenous compounds are called antagonists. In some instances, antagonist action is desirable (eg, naloxone competes with opioids for opioid receptors and may be used to reverse an opioid overdose).

Some drugs are extremely specific for one kind of receptor and some drugs are less specific so that they nonselectively stimulate all of a particular class of receptors. For instance, epinephrine will stimulate all beta-adrenergic receptors resulting in stimulation of both cardiac tissue and pulmonary smooth muscle tissue whereas terbutaline is more selective for $beta_2$ adrenergic receptors and resulting action is primarily on the smooth muscle of the lungs.

Several factors may also influence the number of specific receptors (up-regulation or down-regulation) and their ability to couple with other drugs or endogenous substances. The changes in number of receptors (increase or decrease) or sensitivity may result in drug tolerance (eg, biogenic amines [antidepressants]). The rebound phenomena that follows abrupt withdrawal of some drugs is related to an increase in the availability of receptor sites as the drug is released from the receptor (ie, clonidine). Disease states can influence number and responsiveness of receptors (eg, thyroid hormones can increase the number of beta receptors and their sensitivity to catecholamines in cardiac muscle, which may account for the tachycardia of thyrotoxicosis). Age can decrease responsiveness to insulin. Pharmacodynamics are normally associated with changes in drug concentrations (pharmacokinetics). In other words, the concentration of available drug in systemic circulation as determined by pharmacokinetic properties (bioavailability, metabolism, and excretion) have direct influence on the degree of biophysical or biochemical changes effected by drugs or pharmacodynamics.

Ideally, the dose of a drug should achieve the desired response without the occurrence of adverse effects. Unfortunately, with some drugs, the onset of adverse effects occurs before therapeutic dosage levels can be reached. This precludes the use of this drug. Fortunately, many drugs have a fairly wide window of safety (eg, the relationship between effective dosing levels and adverse effects is wide enough so that adverse or toxic responses can be minimized). Some drugs, however, have a very narrow therapeutic index (TI); the range between therapeutic effect and toxic response is very small. Drugs with a narrow TI should be monitored (physical assessment and/or serum drug levels) on a regular basis (eg, lithium, digoxin, phenytoin, theophylline, etc).

PATIENT FACTORS THAT INFLUENCE DRUG THERAPY

Many factors related to an individual patient, or a group of similar patients, can impact the pharmacokinetics of drugs and relate to adverse reactions.

Pregnancy / Lactation

The changes that occur during pregnancy may necessitate dosage changes for some drugs. Decreased gastric tract motility, increased blood volume, decreased protein binding sites, and increased glomerular filtration rates may alter the degree of anticipated pharmacotherapeutic response.

BASIC PHARMACOTHERAPEUTIC CONCEPTS *(Continued)*

Primarily, the concern about drugs during pregnancy is the effect of drugs on the fetus, either teratogenic (causing birth defects) or systemic (causing addiction). Although many drugs cross the placenta, the type of drug, the concentration of that drug, and the gestational age at time of exposure of the fetus are primary determinants of fetal reaction. When prescribing or administering drugs to any childbearing age female, it is vital to ask when her last menstrual period was and, if necessary, to wait for the results of a pregnancy test before starting any drug therapy. Of course, it is best to avoid all drugs during pregnancy, however, in some cases, the physiological context (ie, cardiac output, renal blood flow, etc) may be altered enough to require the use of drugs that are not needed by the same woman when not pregnant.

Most systematically absorbed drugs have been assigned a pregnancy risk factor based on the drugs potential to cause birth defects. This permits an evaluation of the risk:benefit ratio when prescribing or administering drugs becomes necessary. Drugs in the risk factor class "A" are generally considered to be safe for use during pregnancy, class "X" drugs are never safe and are known to be positively teratogenic. See FDA Pregnancy Categories *on page 16*.

Contraception note: Many drugs will interact with and decrease the effect of oral contraceptives (eg, barbiturates, protease inhibitors, rifampin, and carbamazepine). When a second drug will decrease the effect of oral contraceptives, the patient needs to be educated about the necessity for using a "barrier" (nonhormonal) form of contraception. Barrier contraception (alone or in combination with some form of oral contraception) is often recommended for the patient who must take selected drugs with pregnancy risk factors "D" (idarubicin) or class "X" (isotretinoin).

Because many drugs and substances used by a mother appear in breast milk, care must be taken to evaluate the drug effects on the lactating woman and the infant. Some drugs are identified as being clearly contraindicated during lactation, others may cross into breast milk but adverse side effects on the fetus have not been identified, and for some drugs the administration times should be distanced from nursing time. Nurses should advise lactating women about the effects that drugs may have on the infant.

Age

All pharmacokinetics (absorption, distribution, metabolism, and excretion) are different in infants, young adults, and elderly patients. Elderly patients may have mildly decreased or severely decreased blood flow to all organs, gastric motility may be slowed, kidney function may be reduced, decreased nutrition may result in decreased albumin, and sedentary lifestyles may have an impact on drug response. Slower gastric motility means that absorption is slowed, resulting in longer time periods to clinical response. Decreased blood flow means that distribution is altered, resulting in decreased response or longer response time. Excretion may be altered with decreased glomerular filtration rates or slower gastric emptying which can result in increased levels of drug remaining in the system.

The ratio between total body water and total body fat also changes with age; older persons have decreased amounts of total body water and higher body fat. This aspect of aging also influences the blood concentration of some drugs. In a person with increased body fat, fat-soluble drugs are distributed to tissues more than to plasma; resulting in a longer response time as the drug must then be redistributed from tissue to plasma. The idiosyncratic response incidence also increases with an aging population. Responses to drugs may be both more exaggerated or diminished with the "usual" doses of some drugs.

In addition, and of major concern with elderly patients, is the incidence of poly-pharmacy; the increased numbers of drugs the patient may be taking. Older patients may have 2, 3, 4, or 5 (or more) chronic conditions for which they are taking medication. In addition, they may be seeing a different prescriber for each of these conditions. Often, it is a nurse who identifies and coordinates the care of these elderly patients, and the nurse must be aware of the possibility for increased incidence of adverse effects.

Body Weight / Build

Most "recommended" dosages of drugs are based on the average size, young or middle aged adult (usually males). Extremely obese or extremely thin patients may be prone to adverse effects as a result of "nonindividualized" prescribing. Serum creatinine is a breakdown product of skeletal muscle and its levels in the serum are frequently used to estimate renal function. Decreased muscle mass can result in reduced creatinine from muscle breakdown, leading to a serum creatinine, which is artificially low or appears normal. When dosing is based on estimated creatinine clearance (which is calculated based on the serum creatinine) rather than on "actual" creatinine clearance, normal doses may be administered to patients with a diminished capacity for excretion, potentially leading to accumulation and toxicity. This is a particular problem in elderly and/or debilitated patients.

Smoking, Alcohol, Nutrition, and Hydration

Smoking has a direct impact on liver enzyme activity, blood flow, and the central nervous system. Excessive alcohol intake impacts liver enzymes, renal function, and has an additive effect with most antipsychotic, sedative, or anxiolytic medications, as well as altering responses to many other medications. Nutrition and hydration also play an important part in drug responses and possible adverse reactions. Poor hydration may result in reduced blood flow and excretion. Decreased or prolonged gastric motility can result in slowed excretion and/or prolonged absorption. Poor or inadequate nutrition may result in decreased protein available for binding.

It is vital that a patient's current habits are considered when prescribing, administering, or monitoring drug therapy, but in addition, patients must be aware of the need to inform their professional care provider that they have changed their smoking, alcohol, or dietary patterns. When dosage of theophylline is based on the fact that the patient is a smoker, the theophylline dosage must be adjusted to prevent overdose, if the patient quits smoking. When a patient is on warfarin, drastic increases in the amount of vitamin K intake through increased green leafy vegetables can dramatically alter the dose of warfarin.

Other Patient Factors That Influence Drug Response

– Genetic variations

– Differences in circadian patterns

– Disease states

– Psychological temperament

Genetic differences in enzymes may influence the effectiveness of therapy or the incidence of adverse effects (fast acetylators or slow acetylators). The emerging science of pharmacogenomics is devoted to the investigation of these genetic differences in drug response, and offers the hope of truly individualized therapy. Circadian rhythms differ among individuals and have an impact on absorption patterns, hormone secretion, or urinary excretion patterns. Disease states can and do change all aspects of pharmacokinetics. Cirrhosis can impair liver enzyme metabolism rate. Kidney disease will reduce excretion rates for many drugs. Abnormal thyroid function can influence drug metabolism. Diseases which affect blood circulation (eg, hypertension, CHF, Raynaud's phenomena, malignancies, etc) can have an impact on absorption, distribution, and excretion. Diabetes impacts the response to many drugs. Malnutrition, commonly associated with disease, can drastically reduce albumin levels.

See Therapeutic Nursing Management of Side Effects *on page 29.*

PHARMACOTHERAPEUTICS

Drug therapy is used for treatment of disease or symptoms of diseases (empiric, supportive, maintenance, or palliative), for prevention (immunization), and for diagnosis (iodine, barium). In some cases, drugs may be used to correct imbalances or improve regulation of excessive physiological responses.

Optimal drug therapy should be both effective and safe. It needs to be tailored to the patient and the problem (see Patient Factors That Influence Drug Therapy). Assessing the problem is the first step, this involves identifying the problem (eg, etiology, laboratory confirmation, subjective and objective symptoms, urgency, severity, and prognosis) and determining what is the goal of therapy. Identifying and assessing the various options require knowledge of what drug therapy is appropriate. These steps lead to clinical decision-making (eg, selecting the drug regimen that is appropriate to meet the goal for this patient).

While professionals responsible for prescribing medications usually select therapy, the implementing of therapy is often a responsibility of nurses, in collaboration with pharmacists. Implementing therapy includes not only the preparation and dispensing of the drug, but also the education of those individual(s) who will administer the drug: nurses, patients, and family members. A major aspect of the education of patients includes how to administer the drug, when to administer the drug, and any dietary or drug-related precautions.

Monitoring the results of that therapy is a major responsibility that involves the prescriber, pharmacist, nurse, patient, and other healthcare providers. A major aspect of monitoring is communicating the subjective and objective responses to the responsible prescriber. Patients, nurses, and other caregivers must know the anticipated results of drug therapy and how to assess and report possible adverse effects.

The design, implementation, and monitoring of drug therapy in an individual patient is a complex and time-consuming task, requiring participation of many members of the healthcare team. Several common types of problems may be encountered in drug therapy. These include omissions of potentially beneficial drugs from the regimen, duplications in therapy, selection/titration to the appropriate dosage, the identification and management of drug interactions, and the identification and management of adverse reactions. An awareness of these potential problems is essential to enhance the safety of drug therapy.

Drug Interactions

Drug interactions are a major concern in drug therapy. Interactions may occur between food and drugs or between different drugs (ie, over-the-counter drugs, herbals, home remedies, and prescription drugs). Careful assessment of **ALL** substances patients are using to treat themselves is imperative for safe drug therapy. Patients may not consider some of the substances they use to treat themselves as drugs and nurses may need to be highly sensitive and very aware when they discuss this subject with the patient.

The potential for drug interactions increases exponentially with the number of drugs a person is taking. Thus, the more illnesses a patient has, the more likely it is he/she will be taking multiple drugs, and the more likely he/she will be to experience drug interactions.

BASIC PHARMACOTHERAPEUTIC CONCEPTS *(Continued)*

Drugs can interact with other drugs to produce additive effects (when combined they produce similar cumulative effects with a lesser dose of either drug than they would alone), synergistic effects (the combination produces a greater response than either alone), or antagonistic effect (one drug negates or reverses the effect of the other drug). Such interactions can be a result of altering the pharmacokinetics of the drugs involved; increasing or decreasing either the rate or the quantity in absorption, altering the distribution through competitive receptor binding, changing the metabolism by inducing or reducing actions of liver enzymes, altering blood flow, or excretion by altering renal clearance.

Food, alcohol, and cigarette smoking can interact with drugs. Absorption of some drugs is enhanced with high fat meals (griseofulvin) or by low protein or high carbohydrate meals (theophylline). Whereas, absorption of some drugs is slowed, rather than blocked, when the stomach is full and gastric transport is slowed. Other drugs can bind with food to impair or prevent absorption of food byproducts such as carbohydrates or vitamins (eg, cholestyramine, mineral oil). Some drugs, such as isotretinoin, are isomers of vitamins and dietary intake of vitamin A can cause overdose reactions.

Other foods can produce pharmacologic activity on their own and when the patient is also taking a medication that is designed to result in that same pharmacologic activity the result may be life-threatening. For instance, patients using a monoamine oxidase (MAO) inhibitor should avoid foods containing tyramines or tryptophan (see Tyramine Content of Foods list *on page 1758*) to prevent excess release of catecholamines resulting in severe potentially life-threatening effects.

Drugs can also impact the results of laboratory tests. This is the basis for instructions from the laboratory to "hold" certain medications prior to some laboratory tests.

Adverse Drug Reactions

Adverse reactions to drug therapy can range from mild to debilitating and life-threatening. Mild reactions may either be not severe enough to discontinue the drug or will disappear when the drug is discontinued. Severe or life-threatening reactions may require immediate discontinuance, treatment with other drugs, or dialysis. Adverse reactions may be related to the dosing, they may be inherent in the drug's primary actions, they may be iatrogenic to the drug, or they may be related to individual patient sensitivity or genetics.

Dose-related side effects can be addressed through careful dosage adjustment. Adverse effects associated with inherent properties of the drugs (constipation with opiates or some pain medications) can be addressed through appropriate interventions (ie, increasing fluids, fiber in diets, increased exercise, or stool softeners). Iatrogenic effects (ie, GI irritation and bleeding from aspirin or indomethacin, orthostatic hypotension from antihypertensives) can be reduced by taking a complete patient history, by patient administration and precaution education (eg, safe dose, time, diet, activity, etc), by prescribing another drug to address the anticipated iatrogenic response, or by choosing another drug for treatment. Thorough knowledge of the possible adverse effects, coupled with anticipatory action, will reduce the incidence of adverse side effects.

True allergic responses usually result from previous exposure to one drug or drugs with related chemical composition that sensitizes the patient's immune system. Careful drug histories and assessment of a patient's reported previous adverse responses will help in averting allergic reactions. Idiosyncratic responses are those that are specific to that patient and are generally unpredictable, although many times these are genetically determined.

THERAPEUTIC NURSING MANAGEMENT OF SIDE EFFECTS

MANAGEMENT OF DRUG-RELATED PROBLEMS

Patients may experience some type of side effect or adverse drug reaction as a result of their drug therapy. The type of effect, the severity, and the frequency of occurrence is dependent on the medication and dose being used, as well as the individual's response to therapy. The following information is presented as helpful tips to assist the patient through these drug-related problems. Pharmacological support may also be required for their management.

Alopecia

- Your hair loss is temporary. Hair usually will begin to grow within 3-6 months of completing drug therapy.
- Your hair may come back with a different texture, color, or thickness.
- Avoid excessive shampooing and hair combing, or harsh hair care products.
- Avoid excessive drying of hair.
- Avoid use of permanents, dyes, or hair sprays.
- Always cover head in cold weather or sunshine.

Anemia

- Observe all bleeding precautions (see Thrombocytopenia).
- Get adequate sleep and rest.
- Be alert for potential for dizziness, fainting, or extreme fatigue.
- Maintain adequate nutrition and hydration.
- Have laboratory tests done as recommended.
- If unusual bleeding occurs, notify prescriber.

Anorexia

- Small frequent meals containing favorite foods may tempt appetite.
- Eat simple foods such as toast, rice, bananas, mashed potatoes, scrambled eggs.
- Eat in a pleasant environment conducive to eating.
- When possible, eat with others.
- Avoid noxious odors when eating.
- Use nutritional supplements high in protein and calories.
- Freezing nutritional supplements sometimes makes them more palatable.
- A small glass of wine (if not contraindicated) may stimulate appetite.
- Mild exercise or short walks may stimulate appetite.
- Request antiemetic medication to reduce nausea or vomiting.

Diarrhea

- Include fiber, high protein foods, and fruits in dietary intake.
- Drink plenty of liquids.
- Buttermilk, yogurt, or boiled milk may be helpful.
- Antidiarrheal agents may be needed. Consult your prescriber.
- Include regular rest periods in your activities.
- Institute skin care regimen to prevent breakdown and promote comfort.

Fluid Retention/Edema

- Elevate legs when sitting.
- Wear support hose.
- Increase physical exercise.
- Maintain adequate hydration; avoiding fluids will not reduce edema.
- Weigh yourself regularly.
- If your prescriber has advised you to limit your salt intake, avoid foods such as ham, bacon, processed meats, and canned foods. Many foods are high in salt content. Read labels carefully.
- Report to prescriber if any of the following occur: sudden weight gain, decrease in urination, swelling of hands or feed, increase in waist size, wet cough, or difficulty breathing.

Headache

- Lie down.
- Use cool cloth on forehead.
- Avoid caffeine.
- Use mild analgesics. Consult prescriber.

THERAPEUTIC NURSING MANAGEMENT OF SIDE EFFECTS
(Continued)

Leukopenia/Neutropenia

- Monitor for signs of infections: persistent sore throat, fever, chills, fatigue, headache, flu-like symptoms, vaginal discharge, foul-smelling stools.
- Prevent infection. Maintain strict handwashing at all times. Avoid crowds when possible. Avoid exposure to infected persons.
- Avoid exposure to temperature changes.
- Maintain adequate nutrition and hydration.
- Maintain good personal hygiene.
- Avoid injury or skin breaks.
- Avoid vaccinations (unless recommended by healthcare provider).
- Avoid sunburn.

Nausea and Vomiting

- Eat food served cold or at room temperature. Ice chips are sometimes helpful.
- Drink clear liquids in severe cases of nausea. Avoid carbonated beverages.
- Sip liquids slowly.
- Avoid spicy food. Bland foods are easier to digest.
- Rinse mouth with lemon water. Practice good oral hygiene.
- Avoid sweet, fatty, salty foods and foods with strong odors.
- Eat small frequent meals rather than heavy meals.
- Use relaxation techniques and guided imagery.
- Use distractions such as meals, television, reading, games, etc.
- Sleep during intense periods of nausea.
- Chew gum or suck on hard candy or lozenges.
- Eat in an upright (sitting position), rather than semirecumbant.
- Avoid tight constrictive clothing at meal time.
- Use some mild exercise following light meals rather than lying down.
- Request antiemetic medication to reduce nausea or vomiting.

Postural Hypotension

- Use care and rise slowly from sitting or lying position to standing.
- Use care when climbing stairs.
- Initiate ambulation slowly. Get your bearings before you start walking.
- Do not bend over; always squat slowly if you must pick up something from floor.
- Use caution when showering or bathing (use secure handrails).

Stomatitis

- Perform good oral hygiene frequently, especially before and after meals.
- Avoid use of strong or alcoholic commercial mouthwashes.
- Keep lips well lubricated.
- Avoid tobacco or other products that are irritating to the oral mucosa.
- Avoid hot, spicy, excessively salty foods.
- Eat soft foods and drink adequate fluids.
- Request topical or systemic analgesics for painful ulcerations.
- Be alert for and report signs of oral fungal infections.

Thrombocytopenia

- Avoid aspirin and aspirin-containing products.
- Use electric or safety razor and blunt scissors.
- Use soft toothbrush or cotton swabs for oral care. Avoid use of dental floss.
- Avoid use of enemas, cathartics, and suppositories unless approved by prescriber.
- Avoid valsalva maneuvers such as straining at stool.
- Use stool softeners if necessary to prevent constipation. Consult prescriber.
- Avoid blowing nose forcefully.
- Never go barefoot, wear protective foot covering.
- Use care when trimming nails (if necessary).
- Maintain safe environment; arrange furniture to provide safe passageway.
- Maintain adequate lighting in darkened areas to avoid bumping into objects.
- Avoid handling sharp tools or instruments.
- Avoid contact sports or activities that might result in injury.
- Promptly report signs of bleeding; abdominal pain; blood in stool, urine, or vomitus; unusual fatigue; easy bruising; bleeding around gums; or nosebleeds.
- If injection or bloodsticks are necessary, inform healthcare provider that you may have excess bleeding.

Vertigo

- Observe postural hypotension precautions.
- Use caution when driving or using any machinery.
- Avoid sudden position shifts; do not "rush".
- Utilize appropriate supports (eg, cane, walker) to prevent injury.

ALPHABETICAL LISTING OF DRUGS

ABACAVIR

♦ **A200® Lice [OTC]** *see* Permethrin *on page 1190*

Abacavir (a BAK a veer)
U.S. Brand Names Ziagen®
Synonyms Abacavir Sulfate; ABC
Restrictions An FDA-approved medication guide is available at www.fda.gov/cder/Offices/ODS/labeling.htm; distribute to each patient to whom this medication is dispensed.
Generic Available No
Pharmacologic Category Antiretroviral Agent, Reverse Transcriptase Inhibitor (Nucleoside)
Use Treatment of HIV infections in combination with other antiretroviral agents
Mechanism of Action/Effect Nucleoside reverse transcriptase inhibitor which interferes with HIV viral RNA dependent DNA polymerase resulting in inhibition of viral replication
Contraindications Hypersensitivity to abacavir (or carbovir) or any component of the formulation (do not rechallenge patients who have experienced hypersensitivity to abacavir); moderate-to-severe hepatic impairment
Warnings/Precautions Should always be used as a component of a multidrug regimen. Serious and sometimes fatal hypersensitivity reactions have occurred. **Patients exhibiting symptoms from two or more of the following: Fever, skin rash, constitutional symptoms (malaise, fatigue, aches), respiratory symptoms (eg, pharyngitis, dyspnea, cough) and GI symptoms (eg, abdominal pain, diarrhea, nausea, vomiting) should discontinue therapy immediately and call for medical attention. Abacavir should be permanently discontinued if hypersensitivity cannot be ruled out, even when other diagnoses are possible. Abacavir SHOULD NOT be restarted because more severe symptoms may occur within hours, including LIFE-THREATENING HYPOTENSION AND DEATH. Fatal hypersensitivity reactions have occurred following the reintroduction of abacavir in patients whose therapy was interrupted (interruption in drug supply, temporary discontinuation while treating other conditions). Reactions occurred within hours. In some cases, signs of hypersensitivity may have been previously present, but attributed to other medical conditions (acute onset respiratory diseases, gastroenteritis, reactions to other medications). If abacavir is restarted following an interruption in therapy, evaluate the patient for previously unsuspected symptoms of hypersensitivity. Do not restart if hypersensitivity is suspected or if hypersensitivity cannot be ruled out. To report these events on abacavir hypersensitivity, a registry has been established (1-800-270-0425).** Use with caution in patients with mild hepatic dysfunction (contraindicated in moderate-to-severe dysfunction) Lactic acidosis and severe hepatomegaly with steatosis (sometimes fatal) have occurred with antiretroviral nucleoside analogues; female gender, obesity, and prolonged treatment may increase the risk of hepatotoxicity.

Drug Interactions
  Increased Effect/Toxicity: Abacavir increases the blood levels of amprenavir. Abacavir may decrease the serum concentration of methadone in some patients. Concomitant use of ribavirin and nucleoside analogues may increase the risk of developing lactic acidosis (includes adefovir, didanosine, lamivudine, stavudine, zalcitabine, zidovudine).
Nutritional/Ethanol Interactions Ethanol: Ethanol may increase the risk of toxicity.
Adverse Reactions Hypersensitivity reactions (which may be fatal) occur in ~5% of patients (see Warnings/Precautions). Symptoms may include anaphylaxis, fever, rash (including erythema multiforme), fatigue, diarrhea, abdominal pain; respiratory symptoms (eg, pharyngitis, dyspnea, cough, adult respiratory distress syndrome, or respiratory failure); headache, malaise, lethargy, myalgia, myolysis, arthralgia, edema, paresthesia, nausea and vomiting, mouth ulcerations, conjunctivitis, lymphadenopathy, hepatic failure, and renal failure.

Note: Rates of adverse reactions were defined during combination therapy with other antiretrovirals (lamivudine and efavirenz **or** lamivudine and zidovudine). Only reactions which occurred at a higher frequency than in the comparator group are noted. Adverse reaction rates attributable to abacavir alone are not available.

>10%:
  Central nervous system: Headache (7% to 13%), fatigue and malaise (7% to 12%)
  Gastrointestinal: Nausea (7% to 19%, children 9%)
1% to 10%:
  Central nervous system: Depression (6%), dizziness (6%), fever (6%, children 9%), anxiety (5%), abnormal dreams (10%)
  Dermatologic: Rash (5% to 6%, children 7%)
  Gastrointestinal: Diarrhea (7%), vomiting (2% to 10%, children 9%), abdominal pain (6%)
  Hematologic: Thrombocytopenia (1%)
  Hepatic: AST increased (6%)
  Neuromuscular and skeletal: Musculoskeletal pain (5% to 6%)
  Respiratory: Bronchitis (4%), respiratory viral infection (5%)
  Miscellaneous: Hypersensitivity reactions (9%; may include reactions to other components of antiretroviral regimen), infection (EENT 5%)
Pharmacodynamics/Kinetics
  Absorption: Rapid and extensive absorption
  Bioavailability: 83%
  Time to Peak: 0.7-1.7 hours
  Protein Binding: 50%
  Half-Life Elimination: 1.5 hours
  Metabolism: Hepatic via alcohol dehydrogenase and glucuronyl transferase to inactive carboxylate and glucuronide metabolites
  Excretion: Primarily urine (as metabolites, 1.2% as unchanged drug); feces (16% total dose)
Dosing
  Adults & Elderly: HIV treatment: Oral: 300 mg twice daily or 600 mg once daily in combination with other antiretroviral agents

Pediatrics: HIV treatment: Oral: 3 months to 16 years: 8 mg/kg body weight twice daily (maximum 300 mg twice daily) in combination with other antiretroviral agents

Hepatic Impairment:
Mild dysfunction (Child-Pugh score 5-6): 200 mg twice daily (oral solution is recommended)
Moderate-to-severe dysfunction: Use is contraindicated by the manufacturer

Available Dosage Forms
Solution, oral: 20 mg/mL (240 mL) [strawberry-banana flavor]
Tablet: 300 mg

Monitoring and Teaching Issues

Physical Assessment: Assess closely for any previous exposure/allergy to abacavir prior to beginning treatment. Assess other prescriptions, OTC medications, or herbal products patient may be taking for potential interactions (see Drug Interactions) Patient must be closely monitored for any sign of hypersensitivity reaction (anaphylaxis, fever, rash, fatigue, diarrhea, abdominal pain; pharyngitis, dyspnea, cough, adult respiratory distress syndrome, or respiratory failure; headache, malaise, lethargy, myalgia, myolysis, arthralgia, edema, paresthesia, nausea and vomiting, mouth ulcerations, conjunctivitis, lymphadenopathy, hepatic failure, and renal failure). Hypersensitivity can occur within hours and may be fatal (see Warnings/Precautions). If hypersensitivity occurs, infusion should be stopped and prescriber notified. Assess effectiveness of therapy (decrease in infections and progress of disease [viral load and CD4 count]), adverse reactions (see Adverse Reactions). Teach patient proper use as part of combination drug regimen, possible side effects/interventions, and adverse symptoms to report (eg, signs and symptoms of hypersensitivity).

Patient Education: Do not take any new medications during treatment without consulting prescriber. This drug will not cure HIV; use appropriate precautions to prevent spread to other persons. This drug is prescribed as one part of a multidrug combination; take exactly as directed, for full course of therapy. Maintain adequate hydration (2-3 L/day of fluids) unless advised by prescriber to restrict fluids. Avoid alcohol to decrease risk of hypersensitivity reaction. You may be susceptible to infection (avoid crowds and exposure to known infections and do not have any vaccinations without consulting prescriber). May cause dizziness or weakness (use caution when driving or engaging in tasks requiring alertness until response to drug is known); or nausea or vomiting (small frequent meals, frequent mouth care, chewing gum, or sucking lozenges may help). Report immediately symptoms of hypersensitivity (eg, fever; rash; fatigue or lethargy; persistent nausea, vomiting, diarrhea, or abdominal pain; mouth sores; sore throat, cough, difficulty breathing, headache, malaise, swelling of face, mouth or throat; numbness or loss of sensation; headache; loss of sensation, pain, tingling, or numbness in toes, feet, muscles or joints; swollen glands, alterations in urinary pattern; swelling of extremities or weight gain). If you are instructed to stop the medication, do not take this medication in the future. Do not restart without specific instruction by your prescriber. **Pregnancy/breast-feeding precautions:** Inform prescriber if you are or intend to become pregnant. Do not breast-feed.

Dietary Considerations: May be taken with or without food.

Pregnancy Risk Factor: C

Pregnancy Issues: It is not known if abacavir crosses the human placenta. Cases of lactic acidosis/hepatic steatosis syndrome have been reported in pregnant women receiving nucleoside analogues. It is not known if pregnancy itself potentiates this known side effect; however, pregnant women may be at increased risk of lactic acidosis and liver damage. Hepatic enzymes and electrolytes should be monitored frequently during the 3rd trimester of pregnancy in women receiving nucleoside analogues. The pharmacokinetics of abacavir during pregnancy are currently under study. The Perinatal HIV Guidelines Working Group considers abacavir to be an alternative NRTI in dual nucleoside combination regimens. Health professionals are encouraged to contact the antiretroviral pregnancy registry to monitor outcomes of pregnant women exposed to antiretroviral medications (1-800-258-4263 or www.APRegistry.com).

Lactation: Excretion in breast milk unknown/contraindicated

Breast-Feeding Issues: HIV-infected mothers are discouraged from breast-feeding to decrease potential transmission of HIV.

Administration

Oral: May be administered with or without food.

Storage: Store oral solution and tablets at controlled room temperature of 20°C to 25°C (68°F to 77°F). Oral solution may be refrigerated; do not freeze.

Additional Information A medication guide is available and should be dispensed with each prescription or refill for abacavir. A warning card is also available and patients should be instructed to carry this card with them.

A high rate of early virologic nonresponse was observed when abacavir, lamivudine, and tenofovir were used as the initial regimen in treatment-naive patients. Use of this combination is not recommended; patients currently on this regimen should be closely monitored for modification of therapy.

Abacavir and Lamivudine (a BAK a veer & la MI vyoo deen)

U.S. Brand Names Epzicom™

Synonyms Abacavir Sulfate and Lamivudine; Lamivudine and Abacavir

Restrictions An FDA-approved medication guide is available at www.fda.gov/cder/Offices/ODS/labeling.htm; distribute to each patient to whom this medication is dispensed.

Generic Available No

Pharmacologic Category Antiretroviral Agent, Reverse Transcriptase Inhibitor (Nucleoside)

Use Treatment of HIV infections in combination with other antiretroviral agents

Dosing

Adults: Oral: HIV: One tablet (abacavir 600 mg and lamivudine 300 mg) once daily

Renal Impairment: Cl_{cr} <50 mL/minute: Use not recommended

Hepatic Impairment: Use not recommended

Available Dosage Forms Tablet, film-coated: Abacavir 600 mg and lamivudine 300 mg (Continued)

Abacavir and Lamivudine *(Continued)*

Monitoring and Teaching Issues
Physical Assessment: See individual agents.
Pregnancy Risk Factor: C
Lactation: Enters breast milk/contraindicated

Abacavir, Lamivudine, and Zidovudine
(a BAK a veer, la MI vyoo deen, & zye DOE vyoo deen)

U.S. Brand Names Trizivir®

Synonyms Azidothymidine, Abacavir, and Lamivudine; AZT, Abacavir, and Lamivudine; Compound S, Abacavir, and Lamivudine; Lamivudine, Abacavir, and Zidovudine; 3TC, Abacavir, and Zidovudine; ZDV, Abacavir, and Lamivudine; Zidovudine, Abacavir, and Lamivudine

Restrictions An FDA-approved medication guide is available at www.fda.gov/cder/Offices/ODS/labeling.htm; distribute to each patient to whom this medication is dispensed.

Generic Available No

Pharmacologic Category Antiretroviral Agent, Reverse Transcriptase Inhibitor (Nucleoside)

Use Treatment of HIV infection (either alone or in combination with other antiretroviral agents) in patients whose regimen would otherwise contain the components of Trizivir®

Dosing
Adults: HIV treatment: Oral: 1 tablet twice daily. **Note:** Not recommended for patients <40 kg.
Elderly: Use with caution.
Pediatrics: HIV treatment: Adolescents: Refer to adult dosing (not recommended for patients <40 kg).
Renal Impairment: Cl_{cr} ≤50 mL/minute: Avoid use.

Available Dosage Forms Tablet [film coated]: Abacavir 300 mg, lamivudine 150 mg, and zidovudine 300 mg

Monitoring and Teaching Issues
Physical Assessment: See individual agents.
Patient Education: This is not a cure for HIV infection, nor will it reduce the risk of transmission of HIV to others. Take exactly as prescribed without regard to food or water. Do not discontinue even if feeling better. You will need to have frequent blood tests to identify possible blood cell problems. You may experience headache, muscle pain, weakness, insomnia, unusual bleeding (eg, tarry stools, easy bruising, blood in stool, urine, or mouth), dizziness, or numbness; report these to your prescriber. **Note:** Trizivir® contains abacavir (also called Ziagen®). About 1 in 20 patients who take abacavir will have a serious allergic reaction that can result in death if the drug is not stopped right away. You may be having this reaction if you get a skin rash or if you get one or more symptoms from at least two of the following groups: fever; nausea, vomiting, diarrhea, stomach pain; extreme tiredness, achiness, general ill feeling; or sore throat, shortness of breath, cough. If you think you are having this reaction contact your prescriber immediately. If you stop Trizivir® because of this reaction, **never** take Trizivir® or Ziagen® (abacavir) again or you could die within hours. If you stop Trizivir® therapy for any other reason, consult your prescriber before restarting therapy. **Pregnancy/breast-feeding precautions:** Inform your prescriber if you are or intend to become pregnant. Breast-feeding is not recommended. HIV-infected mothers are discouraged from breast-feeding to decrease potential transmission of HIV.

Pregnancy Risk Factor: C
Lactation: See individual agents.
Related Information
    Abacavir *on page 32*
    Lamivudine *on page 861*
    Zidovudine *on page 1585*

♦ **Abacavir Sulfate** *see* Abacavir *on page 32*
♦ **Abacavir Sulfate and Lamivudine** *see* Abacavir and Lamivudine *on page 33*

Abarelix (a ba REL iks)

U.S. Brand Names Plenaxis™
Synonyms PPI-149; R-3827

Restrictions Abarelix is not distributed through retail pharmacies. Prescribing and distribution of abarelix is limited to physicians and hospital pharmacies participating in the Plenaxis™ PLUS program. See Additional Information, or contact Praecis Pharmaceuticals at www.plenaxisplus.com or by calling 1-877-772-3247.

Generic Available No

Pharmacologic Category Gonadotropin Releasing Hormone Antagonist

Use Palliative treatment of advanced symptomatic prostate cancer; treatment is limited to men who are not candidates for LHRH therapy, refuse surgical castration, and have one or more of the following complications due to metastases or local encroachment: 1) risk of neurological compromise, 2) ureteral or bladder outlet obstruction, or 3) severe bone pain (persisting despite narcotic analgesia)

Mechanism of Action/Effect Competes with naturally occurring GnRH for binding on receptors of the pituitary. Suppresses LH and FSH, resulting in decreased testosterone. Unlike LHRH agonists, does not induce an initial rise in serum testosterone.

Contraindications Hypersensitivity to abarelix or any component of the formulation

Warnings/Precautions The U.S. Food and Drug Administration (FDA) currently recommends that procedures for proper handling and disposal of antineoplastic agents be considered. Has been associated with immediate-onset allergic reactions; may occur with initial dose and risk increases with duration of treatment. Observe for signs/symptoms of allergic reactions (which may include hypotension and/or syncope) for at least 30 minutes following each injection. Abarelix may cause prolongation of the QT interval; consider risk:benefit in patients with baseline QT_c values >450 msec or patients receiving concurrent medications which prolong the QT_c interval (class Ia and class III antiarrhythmics). Efficacy may diminish during prolonged treatment, particularly in patients weighing >225 pounds; monitor serum testosterone levels to identify treatment failures. Monitor transaminase levels and hepatic function during therapy. Extended treatment may result in a decrease in bone mineral density. Not indicated for use in women or children.

Drug Interactions

Increased Effect/Toxicity: When used with other QT_c-prolonging agents, additive effects QT_c prolongation may occur with concurrent therapy. Life-threatening ventricular arrhythmias may result; example drugs include class Ia and class III antiarrhythmics, cisapride, selected quinolones, erythromycin, pimozide, mesoridazine, and thioridazine.

Adverse Reactions

>10%:

Cardiovascular: Hot flushes (79%), peripheral edema (15%)

Central nervous system: Sleep disturbance (44%), pain (31%), dizziness (12%), headache (12%)

Endocrine & metabolic: Breast enlargement (30%), nipple discharge/tenderness (20%)

Gastrointestinal: Constipation (15%), diarrhea (11%)

Neuromuscular & skeletal: Back pain (17%)

Respiratory: Upper respiratory infection (12%)

1% to 10%:

Central nervous system: Fatigue (10%)

Endocrine & metabolic: Serum triglycerides increased (10%)

Gastrointestinal: Nausea (10%)

Genitourinary: Dysuria (10%), micturition frequency (10%), urinary retention (10%), urinary tract infection (10%)

Hepatic: Transaminases increased (2% to 8%)

Miscellaneous: Allergic reactions (urticaria, pruritus, syncope, hypotension): risk increases with prolonged treatment (in clinical trials, cumulative risk increased from 0.5% at 56 days to 2.9% at 676 days of therapy)

Overdosage/Toxicology No experience in overdose. Treatment is symptomatic and supportive.

Pharmacodynamics/Kinetics

Time to Peak: 3 days (following I.M. administration)

Half-Life Elimination: 13 days

Metabolism: Hepatic, via peptide hydrolysis

Excretion: Urine (13% unchanged drug)

Dosing

Adults & Elderly: Male prostate cancer: I.M.: 100 mg administered on days 1, 15, 29 (week 4), then every 4 weeks

Available Dosage Forms Injection, powder for reconstitution [preservative free]: 113 mg [provides 100 mg/2 mL depot suspension when reconstituted; packaged with diluent and syringe]

Monitoring and Teaching Issues

Physical Assessment: Refer to Additional Information for **required Plenaxis™ PLUS program** prior to prescribing. Assess potential for interactions with other prescriptions, OTC medications, or herbal products patient may be using. Assess results of laboratory tests, therapeutic effectiveness, and adverse reactions with each injection and frequently throughout therapy. **Note:** Patient must be monitored for adverse reactions for a minimum of 30 minutes following each injection. Teach patient possible side effects/appropriate interventions and adverse symptoms to report. **Pregnancy risk factor X:** Not indicated for use in women. May cause fetal harm if administered to a pregnant woman.

Monitoring Laboratory Tests: Obtain transaminase levels at baseline and periodically during treatment. Serum testosterone (to identify treatment failure) just prior to abarelix administration, beginning on day 29 and every 8 weeks thereafter. PSA and bone mineral density may be monitored as needed.

Patient Education: Do not take any new medications during therapy without consulting prescriber. This drug must be administered via injections. You will be monitored closely following the injections. Report immediately any feelings of flushing, dizziness, difficulty swallowing difficulty breathing, or chest tightness. You will be scheduled for injections and frequent laboratory tests. It is important to maintain adequate nutrition (frequent small meals) and hydration (2 L/day) unless advised to restrict fluids by prescriber. You may experience hot flashes (cool clothes and temperatures may help); swelling of extremities; sleep disturbances, dizziness, headache (use caution when driving or engaging in hazardous tasks until response to drug is known); breast enlargement, nipple tenderness/ discharge; gastrointestinal disturbances (frequent small meals and frequent mouth care may help); constipation (increased dietary fiber and fluid and increased exercise may help); diarrhea (boiled milk or yogurt may help); back pain (consult prescriber for analgesic). Report any palpitations or chest pain, respiratory difficulty, rash, or any other persistent adverse reaction.

Pregnancy Risk Factor: X

Lactation: Excretion in breast milk unknown/not indicated in women

Breast-Feeding Issues: Not indicated for use in women

Administration

I.M.: Administer intramuscularly (to the buttock).

Reconstitution: Reconstitute vial with 2.2 mL of NS; reconstituted solutions contain abarelix 50 mg/mL.

Storage: Store at room temperature: 25°C (77°F), excursions permitted to 15°C to 30°C (58°F to 86°F). Reconstituted solution is stable for at least 8 hours at 30°C. Because it contains no preservative, manufacturer recommends administration within 1 hour of reconstitution.

Additional Information Prior to distribution, Praecis Pharmaceuticals must enroll prescribing physicians and/or hospital pharmacies in the Plenaxis™ user safety program (Plenaxis™ PLUS). A Physician Attestation form must be used to document the physician's qualifications and acceptance of responsibilities concerning patient education and adverse effect reporting.

(Continued)

Abarelix *(Continued)*

Physicians must obtain the patient's signature and personally cosign the two-part Plenaxis™ Patient Information leaflet. The original signed copy should be retained in the patient's medical record while the other copy should be given to the patient. Hospital pharmacies must submit a hospital pharmacy agreement form to allow dispensing, which will be limited to physicians enrolled in the prescriber's registry. Confirmation of physician enrollment may be obtained by calling 1-866-753-6294. All doses must be dispensed with a Patient Information leaflet. Distributors must restrict shipment to physicians or hospital pharmacies enrolled in the Plenaxis™ prescribing program. Additional details and/or forms may be obtained through Praecis Pharmaceuticals at www.plenaxisplus.com or by calling 1-877-772-3247.

- ◆ **Abbokinase**® **[DSC]** *see* Urokinase *on page 1536*
- ◆ **Abbott-43818** *see* Leuprolide *on page 876*
- ◆ **ABC** *see* Abacavir *on page 32*
- ◆ **ABCD** *see* Amphotericin B Cholesteryl Sulfate Complex *on page 107*
- ◆ **Abelcet**® *see* Amphotericin B (Lipid Complex) *on page 111*
- ◆ **Abilify**® *see* Aripiprazole *on page 137*
- ◆ **ABLC** *see* Amphotericin B (Lipid Complex) *on page 111*
- ◆ **Abraxane**™ *see* Paclitaxel (Protein Bound) *on page 1146*

Acamprosate *(a kam PROE sate)*

U.S. Brand Names Campral®
Synonyms Acamprosate Calcium; Calcium Acetylhomotaurinate
Generic Available No
Pharmacologic Category GABA Agonist/Glutamate Antagonist
Use Maintenance of alcohol abstinence
Mechanism of Action/Effect Mechanism not fully defined. Structurally similar to GABA, acamprosate appears to restore balance to GABA and glutamate activities which are disrupted in alcohol dependence. During therapeutic use, alcohol intake is reduced, but does not cause a disulfiram-like reaction following alcohol ingestion.
Contraindications Hypersensitivity to acamprosate or any component of the formulation; severe renal impairment (Cl$_{cr}$ <30 mL/minute)
Warnings/Precautions Should be used as part of a comprehensive program to treat alcohol dependence. Treatment should be initiated as soon as possible following the period of alcohol withdrawal, when the patient has achieved abstinence. Acamprosate does not eliminate or diminish the symptoms of alcohol withdrawal. Use caution in moderate renal impairment (Cl$_{cr}$ 30-50 mL/minute). Suicidal ideation, attempts and completed suicides have occurred in acamprosate-treated patients; monitor for depression and/or suicidal thinking. Traces of sulfites may be present in the formulation. Safety and efficacy have not been established in pediatric patients.
Drug Interactions
  Decreased Effect: No clinically significant drug-drug interactions have been identified.
Nutritional/Ethanol Interactions
  Ethanol: Abstinence is required during treatment. Ethanol does not affect the pharmacokinetics of acamprosate; however, the continued use of ethanol will decrease desired efficacy of acamprosate.
  Food: Food decreases absorption of acamprosate (not clinically significant).
Adverse Reactions
  Note: Many adverse effects associated with treatment may be related to alcohol abstinence; reported frequency range may overlap with placebo.
  >10%: Gastrointestinal: Diarrhea (10% to 17%)
  1% to 10%:
    Cardiovascular: Syncope, palpitation, edema (peripheral)
    Central nervous system: Insomnia (6% to 9%), anxiety (5% to 8%), depression (4% to 8%), dizziness (3% to 4%), pain (2% to 4%), paresthesia (2% to 3%), headache, somnolence, amnesia, tremor, chills
    Dermatologic: Pruritus (3% to 4%), rash
    Endocrine and metabolic: Weight gain, libido decreased
    Gastrointestinal: Anorexia (2% to 5%), flatulence (1% to 3%), nausea (3% to 4%), abdominal pain, dry mouth (1% to 3%), vomiting, dyspepsia, constipation, appetite increased, taste perversion
    Genitourinary: Impotence
    Neuromuscular & skeletal: Weakness (5% to 7%), back pain, myalgia, arthralgia
    Ocular: Abnormal vision
    Respiratory: Rhinitis, dyspnea, pharyngitis, bronchitis
    Miscellaneous: Diaphoresis (2% to 3%), suicide attempt
Overdosage/Toxicology Symptoms may include diarrhea and (in chronic overdose) hypocalcemia. Treatment is symptom-directed and supportive.
Pharmacodynamics/Kinetics
  Bioavailability: 11%
  Protein Binding: Negligible
  Half-Life Elimination: 20-33 hours
  Metabolism: Not metabolized
  Excretion: Urine (as unchanged drug)
Dosing
  Adults & Elderly: Alcohol abstinence: Oral: 666 mg 3 times/day (a lower dose may be effective in some patients).
    Adjustment in patients with low body weight (unlabeled): A lower dose (4 tablets/day) may be considered in patients with low body weight (eg, <60 kg).
    Note: Treatment should be initiated as soon as possible following the period of alcohol withdrawal, when the patient has achieved abstinence.

Renal Impairment: Initial dose should be reduced to 333 mg 3 times/day in patients with moderate renal impairment (Cl_{cr} 30-50 mL/minute). Contraindicated in severe renal impairment (Cl_{cr} <30 mL/minute).

Available Dosage Forms Tablet, enteric coated, delayed release, as calcium: 333 mg [contains calcium 33 mg and sulfites]

Monitoring and Teaching Issues

Physical Assessment: Assess other medications patient may be taking for effectiveness and potential interactions. May cause depression. Monitor for suicide ideation.

Patient Education: Taking this medication helps maintain abstinence only when used as part of a treatment program that includes counseling and support. Swallow tablet whole. Do not chew or crush. Maintain adequate hydration (2-3 L/day of fluids) unless instructed to restrict fluid intake by prescriber. Can cause drowsiness (use caution when driving or engaging in activities requiring alertness until response to drug is known). You may experience diarrhea (buttermilk, boiled milk, or yogurt may help), peripheral edema, insomnia, anxiety, depression, and generalized weakness. Report persistent diarrhea, excessive or sudden weight gain, swelling of extremities, respiratory difficulties, fainting, or thoughts of suicide. **Pregnancy/breast-feeding precautions:** Inform prescriber if you are or intend to become pregnant. Consult prescriber before breast-feeding.

Dietary Considerations: May be taken without regard to meals. Each 333 mg tablet contains 33 mg of elemental calcium.

Geriatric Considerations: Initial studies did not include sufficient geriatric patients to be able to derive sufficient data to compare elderly to younger adults. Only 41 out of 4234 patients in clinical trials were ≥65 years of age with none ≥75 years. However, since this medication is cleared renally exclusively, caution should be used since many elderly have Cl_{cr} 30-50 mL/minute where dosage reduction is required (see Dosing).

Pregnancy Risk Factor: C

Lactation: Excretion in breast milk unknown/use caution

Administration

Oral: May be administered without regard to meals. Tablet should be swallowed whole; do not crush or chew.

Storage: Store at 25°C (77°F); excursions permitted to 15°C to 30°C (59°F to 86°F)

♦ **Acamprosate Calcium** *see Acamprosate on page 36*

Acarbose (AY car bose)

U.S. Brand Names Precose®

Generic Available No

Pharmacologic Category Antidiabetic Agent, Alpha-Glucosidase Inhibitor

Medication Safety Issues

Sound-alike/look-alike issues:
Precose® may be confused with PreCare®

Use

Monotherapy, as indicated as an adjunct to diet to lower blood glucose in patients with type 2 diabetes mellitus (noninsulin dependent, NIDDM) whose hyperglycemia cannot be managed on diet alone

Combination with a sulfonylurea, metformin, or insulin in patients with type 2 diabetes mellitus (noninsulin dependent, NIDDM) when diet plus acarbose do not result in adequate glycemic control. The effect of acarbose to enhance glycemic control is additive to that of other hypoglycemic agents when used in combination.

Mechanism of Action/Effect Delays glucose absorption and lowers postprandial hyperglycemia.

Contraindications Hypersensitivity to acarbose or any component of the formulation; patients with diabetic ketoacidosis or cirrhosis; patients with inflammatory bowel disease, colonic ulceration, partial intestinal obstruction, or in patients predisposed to intestinal obstruction; patients who have chronic intestinal diseases associated with marked disorders of digestion or absorption, and in patients who have conditions that may deteriorate as a result of increased gas formation in the intestine

Warnings/Precautions Acarbose given in combination with a sulfonylurea will cause a further lowering of blood glucose and may increase the hypoglycemic potential of the sulfonylurea. If hypoglycemia occurs, appropriate adjustments in the dosage of these agents should be made. Oral glucose (dextrose) should be used in the treatment of mild to moderate hypoglycemia.

Treatment-emergent elevations of serum transaminases (AST and/or ALT) occurred in 15% of acarbose-treated patients in long-term studies. These serum transaminase elevations appear to be dose related and were asymptomatic, reversible, more common in females, and, in general, were not associated with other evidence of liver dysfunction.

Drug Interactions

Decreased Effect: The effect of acarbose is antagonized/decreased by thiazide and related diuretics, corticosteroids, phenothiazines, thyroid products, estrogens, oral contraceptives, phenytoin, nicotinic acid, sympathomimetics, calcium channel-blocking drugs, isoniazid, intestinal adsorbents (eg, charcoal), and digestive enzyme preparations (eg, amylase, pancreatin). Acarbose decreases the absorption/serum concentration of digoxin.

Increased Effect/Toxicity: Acarbose may increase the risk of hypoglycemia when used with oral hypoglycemics. See Warnings/Precautions.

Nutritional/Ethanol Interactions Ethanol: Limit ethanol.

Adverse Reactions >10%:

Gastrointestinal: Abdominal pain (21%) and diarrhea (33%) tend to return to pretreatment levels over time, and the frequency and intensity of flatulence (77%) tend to abate with time

Hepatic: Transaminases increased

Overdosage/Toxicology An overdose of acarbose will not result in hypoglycemia. An overdose may result in transient increases in flatulence, diarrhea, and abdominal discomfort which shortly subside. However, acarbose may complicate the treatment of hypoglycemia from other causes, since it will inhibit the absorption of oral disaccharides (sucrose). Oral (Continued)

37

Acarbose *(Continued)*

glucose (dextrose) should be used in mild to moderate hypoglycemia; severe hypoglycemia should be treated with I.V. glucose.

Pharmacodynamics/Kinetics
Absorption: <2% as active drug
Bioavailability: Low systemic bioavailability of parent compound; acts locally in GI tract
Metabolism: Exclusively via GI tract, principally by intestinal bacteria and digestive enzymes; 13 metabolites identified
Excretion: Urine (~34%)

Dosing
Adults & Elderly: Type 2 diabetes: Oral:
Initial: 25 mg 3 times/day
Maintenance dose: Should be adjusted at 4- to 8-week intervals based on 1-hour postprandial glucose levels and tolerance until maintenance dose is reached; maintenance dose: 50-100 mg 3 times/day. Dosage must be individualized on the basis of effectiveness and tolerance while not exceeding the maximum recommended dose.
Maximum:
≤60 kg: 50 mg 3 times/day
>60 kg: 100 mg 3 times/day
Patients receiving sulfonylureas: Acarbose given in combination with a sulfonylurea will cause a further lowering of blood glucose and may increase the hypoglycemic potential of the sulfonylurea. If hypoglycemia occurs, appropriate adjustments in the dosage of these agents should be made.
Renal Impairment: Cl$_{cr}$ <25 mL/minute: Peak plasma concentrations were 5 times higher and AUCs were 6 times larger than in volunteers with normal renal function; however, long-term clinical trials in diabetic patients with significant renal dysfunction have not been conducted and treatment of these patients with acarbose is not recommended

Available Dosage Forms Tablet: 25 mg, 50 mg, 100 mg

Monitoring and Teaching Issues
Physical Assessment: Assess potential for interactions with other prescriptions, OTC medications, or herbal products patient may be taking. Assess results of laboratory tests, therapeutic effectiveness, and adverse response on a regular basis throughout therapy. Teach patient proper use (or refer patient to diabetic educator), possible side effects/appropriate interventions (eg, importance of adequate hydration), and adverse symptoms to report.
Monitoring Laboratory Tests: Postprandial glucose, glycosylated hemoglobin levels, and serum transaminase levels should be checked every 3 months during the first year of treatment and periodically thereafter.
Patient Education: Do not take any new medication during therapy unless approved by prescriber. Take this medication exactly as directed, with the first bite of each main meal. Do not change dosage or discontinue without first consulting prescriber. Do not take other medications with or within 2 hours of this medication unless advised by prescriber. Avoid alcohol. It is important to follow dietary and lifestyle recommendations of prescriber. You will be instructed in signs of hypo- or hyperglycemia by prescriber or diabetic educator. If combining acarbose with other diabetic medication (eg, sulfonylureas, insulin), keep source of glucose (sugar) on hand in case hypoglycemia occurs. May cause mild side effects during first weeks of acarbose therapy (eg, bloating, flatulence, diarrhea, abdominal discomfort); these should diminish over time. Report severe or persistent side effects, fever, extended vomiting or flu, or change in color of urine or stool. **Breast-feeding precaution:** Consult prescriber if breast-feeding.
Geriatric Considerations: Monitor change in preprandial blood glucose concentrations to account for potential age-related changes in postprandial glucose.
Pregnancy Risk Factor: B
Pregnancy Issues: Abnormal blood glucose levels are associated with a higher incidence of congenital abnormalities. Insulin is the drug of choice for the control of diabetes mellitus during pregnancy.
Lactation: Excretion in breast milk unknown

Administration
Oral: Should be **administered with the first bite of each main meal.**
Storage: Store at <25°C (77°F) and protect from moisture.

Related Information
Diabetes Mellitus Management *on page 1819*

♦ **Accolate**® *see* Zafirlukast *on page 1577*
♦ **AccuNeb**™ *see* Albuterol *on page 59*
♦ **Accupril**® *see* Quinapril *on page 1294*
♦ **Accuretic**® *see* Quinapril and Hydrochlorothiazide *on page 1296*
♦ **Accutane**® *see* Isotretinoin *on page 842*
♦ **ACE** *see* Captopril *on page 246*
♦ **Aceon**® *see* Perindopril Erbumine *on page 1188*
♦ **Acephen**® **[OTC]** *see* Acetaminophen *on page 38*
♦ **Acetadote**® *see* Acetylcysteine *on page 45*

Acetaminophen *(a seet a MIN oh fen)*

U.S. Brand Names Acephen® [OTC]; Aspirin Free Anacin® Maximum Strength [OTC]; Cetafen® [OTC]; Cetafen Extra® [OTC]; Comtrex® Sore Throat Maximum Strength [OTC]; ElixSure™ Fever/Pain [OTC]; FeverALL® [OTC]; Genapap® [OTC]; Genapap® Children [OTC]; Genapap® Extra Strength [OTC]; Genapap® Infant [OTC]; Genebs® [OTC]; Genebs® Extra Strength [OTC]; Mapap® [OTC]; Mapap® Arthritis [OTC]; Mapap® Children's [OTC]; Mapap® Extra Strength [OTC]; Mapap® Infants [OTC]; Redutemp® [OTC]; Silapap® Children's [OTC]; Silapap® Infants [OTC]; Tylenol® [OTC]; Tylenol® 8 Hour [OTC]; Tylenol® Arthritis Pain [OTC]; Tylenol® Children's [OTC]; Tylenol® Extra Strength [OTC]; Tylenol®

Infants [OTC]; Tylenol® Junior Strength [OTC]; Tylenol® Sore Throat [OTC]; Valorin [OTC]; Valorin Extra [OTC]

Synonyms APAP; N-Acetyl-P-Aminophenol; Paracetamol

Generic Available Yes

Pharmacologic Category Analgesic, Miscellaneous

Medication Safety Issues

Sound-alike/look-alike issues:

Acephen® may be confused with AcipHex®

FeverALL® may be confused with Fiberall®

Tylenol® may be confused with atenolol, timolol, Tuinal®, Tylox®

Use Treatment of mild to moderate pain and fever (antipyretic/analgesic); does not have antirheumatic or anti-inflammatory effects

Mechanism of Action/Effect Reduces fever by acting on the hypothalamus to cause vasodilatation and sweating

Contraindications Hypersensitivity to acetaminophen or any component of the formulation

Warnings/Precautions Limit dose to <4 g/day. May cause severe hepatic toxicity on acute overdose; in addition, chronic daily dosing in adults has resulted in liver damage in some patients. Use with caution in patients with alcoholic liver disease; consuming ≥3 alcoholic drinks/day may increase the risk of liver damage. Use caution in patients with known G6PD deficiency.

OTC labeling: When used for self-medication, patients should be instructed to contact healthcare provider if used for fever lasting >3 days or for pain lasting >10 days in adults or >5 days in children.

Drug Interactions

Cytochrome P450 Effect: Substrate (minor) of CYP1A2, 2A6, 2C8/9, 2D6, 2E1, 3A4; **Inhibits** CYP3A4 (weak)

Decreased Effect: Barbiturates, carbamazepine, hydantoins, rifampin, sulfinpyrazone may decrease the analgesic effect of acetaminophen; cholestyramine may decrease acetaminophen absorption (separate dosing by at least 1 hour)

Increased Effect/Toxicity: Barbiturates, carbamazepine, hydantoins, isoniazid, rifampin, sulfinpyrazone may increase the hepatotoxic potential of acetaminophen; chronic ethanol abuse increases risk for acetaminophen toxicity; effect of warfarin may be enhanced

Nutritional/Ethanol Interactions

Ethanol: Excessive intake of ethanol may increase the risk of acetaminophen-induced hepatotoxicity. Avoid ethanol or limit to <3 drinks/day.

Food: Rate of absorption may be decreased when given with food.

Herb/Nutraceutical: St John's wort may decrease acetaminophen levels.

Lab Interactions Increased chloride, bilirubin, uric acid, glucose, ammonia (B), chloride (S), uric acid (S); alkaline phosphatase (S), chloride (S); decreased sodium, bicarbonate, calcium (S)

Adverse Reactions Frequency not defined.

Dermatologic: Rash

Endocrine & metabolic: May increase chloride, uric acid, glucose; may decrease sodium, bicarbonate, calcium

Hematologic: Anemia; blood dyscrasias (neutropenia, pancytopenia, leukopenia)

Hepatic: May increase bilirubin, alkaline phosphatase

Renal: May increase ammonia, nephrotoxicity with chronic overdose, analgesic nephropathy

Miscellaneous: Hypersensitivity reactions (rare)

Overdosage/Toxicology Symptoms of overdose include hepatic necrosis, transient azotemia, renal tubular necrosis with acute toxicity, anemia, and GI disturbances with chronic toxicity. Treatment consists of acetylcysteine 140 mg/kg orally (loading) followed by 70 mg/kg every 4 hours for 17 doses; therapy should be initiated based upon laboratory analysis suggesting a high probability of hepatotoxic potential. Activated charcoal is very effective at binding acetaminophen. Intravenous acetylcysteine should be reserved for patients unable to take oral forms.

Pharmacodynamics/Kinetics

Onset of Action: <1 hour

Duration of Action: 4-6 hours

Absorption: Incomplete; varies by dosage form

Time to Peak: Serum: Oral: 10-60 minutes; may be delayed in acute overdoses

Protein Binding: 8% to 43% at toxic doses

Half-Life Elimination: Prolonged following toxic doses

Neonates: 2-5 hours; Adults: 1-3 hours (may be increased in elderly; however, this should not affect dosing)

Metabolism: At normal therapeutic dosages, hepatic to sulfate and glucuronide metabolites, while a small amount is metabolized by CYP to a highly reactive intermediate (acetylimidoquinone) which is conjugated with glutathione and inactivated; at toxic doses (as little as 4 g daily) glutathione conjugation becomes insufficient to meet the metabolic demand causing an increase in acetylimidoquinone concentration, thought to cause hepatic cell necrosis

Excretion: Urine (2% to 5% unchanged; 55% as glucuronide metabolites; 30% as sulphate metabolites)

Dosing

Adults & Elderly: Pain or fever: Oral, rectal: 325-650 mg every 4-6 hours or 1000 mg 3-4 times/day; do **not** exceed 4 g/day.

Pediatrics: Pain or fever: Oral, rectal Children <12 years: 10-15 mg/kg/dose every 4-6 hours as needed; do **not** exceed 5 doses (2.6 g) in 24 hours; alternatively, the following doses may be used; see table on next page.

Note: Higher rectal doses have been studied for use in preoperative pain control in children. However, specific guidelines are not available and dosing may be product dependent. The safety and efficacy of alternating acetaminophen and ibuprofen dosing has not been established.

(Continued)

Acetaminophen *(Continued)*

Acetaminophen Dosing

Age	Dosage (mg)	Age	Dosage (mg)
0-3 mo	40	4-5 y	240
4-11 mo	80	6-8 y	320
1-2 y	120	9-10 y	400
2-3 y	160	11 y	480

Renal Impairment:
Cl_{cr} 10-50 mL/minute: Administer every 6 hours.
Cl_{cr} <10 mL/minute: Administer every 8 hours (metabolites accumulate).
Moderately dialyzable (20% to 50%)

Hepatic Impairment: Use with caution. Limited, low-dose therapy usually well tolerated in hepatic disease/cirrhosis. However, cases of hepatotoxicity at daily acetaminophen dosages <4 g/day have been reported. Avoid chronic use in hepatic impairment.

Available Dosage Forms

Caplet (Cetafen Extra® Strength, Genapap® Extra Strength, Genebs® Extra Strength, Mapap® Extra Strength, Tylenol® Extra Strength): 500 mg

Caplet, extended release (Mapap® Arthritis, Tylenol® Arthritis Pain): 650 mg

Capsule (Mapap® Extra Strength): 500 mg

Elixir: 160 mg/5 mL (120 mL, 480 mL, 3780 mL)
  Mapap® Children's: 160 mg/5 mL (120 mL) [alcohol free; contains benzoic acid and sodium benzoate; cherry flavor]

Gelcap (Mapap® Extra Strength, Tylenol® Extra Strength): 500 mg

Geltab (Mapap® Extra Strength, Tylenol® Extra Strength): 500 mg

Geltab, extended release (Tylenol® 8 Hour): 650 mg

Liquid, oral: 500 mg/15 mL (240 mL)
  Comtrex® Sore Throat Maximum Strength: 500 mg/15 mL (240 mL) [contains sodium benzoate; honey lemon flavor]
  Genapap® Children: 160 mg/5 mL (120 mL) [contains sodium benzoate; cherry and grape flavors]
  Silapap®: 160 mg/5 mL (120 mL, 240 mL, 480 mL) [sugar free; contains sodium benzoate; cherry flavor]
  Tylenol® Extra Strength: 500 mg/15 mL (240 mL) [contains sodium benzoate; cherry flavor]
  Tylenol® Sore Throat: 500 mg/15 mL (240 mL) [contains sodium benzoate; cherry and honey-lemon flavors]

Solution, oral drops: 80 mg/0.8 mL (15 mL) [droppers are marked at 0.4 mL (40 mg) and at 0.8 mL (80 mg)]
  Genapap® Infant: 80 mg/0.8 mL (15 mL) [fruit flavor]
  Silapap® Infant's: 80 mg/0.8 mL (15 mL, 30 mL) [contains sodium benzoate; cherry flavor]

Solution, oral: 160 mg/5 mL (120 mL, 480 mL)

Suppository, rectal: 120 mg, 325 mg, 650 mg
  Acephen®: 120 mg, 325 mg, 650 mg
  FeverALL®: 80 mg, 120 mg, 325 mg, 650 mg
  Mapap®: 125 mg, 650 mg

Suspension, oral:
  Mapap® Children's: 160 mg/5 mL (120 mL) [contains sodium benzoate; cherry flavor]
  Tylenol® Children's: 160 mg/5 mL (120 mL, 240 mL) [contains sodium benzoate; bubble gum, cherry, and grape flavors]

Suspension, oral drops:
  Mapap® Infants 80 mg/0.8 mL (15 mL, 30 mL) [contains sodium benzoate; cherry flavor]
  Tylenol® Infants: 80 mg/0.8 mL (15 mL, 30 mL) [contains sodium benzoate; cherry and grape flavors]

Syrup, oral (ElixSure™ Fever/Pain): 160 mg/5 mL (120 mL) [bubble gum, cherry, and grape flavors]

Tablet: 325 mg, 500 mg
  Aspirin Free Anacin® Extra Strength, Genapap® Extra Strength, Genebs® Extra Strength, Mapap® Extra Strength, Redutemp®, Tylenol® Extra Strength, Valorin Extra: 500 mg
  Cetafen®, Genapap®, Genebs®, Mapap®, Tylenol®, Valorin: 325 mg

Tablet, chewable: 80 mg
  Genapap® Children: 80 mg [contains phenylalanine 6 mg/tablet; fruit and grape flavors]
  Mapap® Children's: 80 mg [contains phenylalanine 3 mg/tablet; bubble gum, fruit, and grape flavors]
  Mapap® Junior Strength: 160 mg [contains phenylalanine 12 mg/tablet; grape flavor]
  Tylenol® Children's: 80 mg [fruit and grape flavors contain phenylalanine 3 mg/tablet; bubble gum flavor contains phenylalanine 6 mg/tablet]
  Tylenol® Junior Strength: 160 mg [contains phenylalanine 6 mg/tablet; fruit and grape flavors]

Monitoring and Teaching Issues

Physical Assessment: Assess patient for history of liver disease or ethanol abuse (acetaminophen and excessive ethanol may have adverse liver effects). Assess other medications patient may be taking for additive or adverse interactions. Assess knowledge/teach patient appropriate use. Teach patient to monitor for adverse reactions and appropriate interventions to reduce side effects.

Monitoring Laboratory Tests: Serum APAP levels with long-term use in patients with hepatic disease

Patient Education: Take exactly as directed; do not increase dose or frequency. Most adverse effects are related to excessive use. Take with food or milk. While using this medication, avoid or limit alcohol to <3 drinks/day and avoid other prescription or OTC medications that contain acetaminophen. Maintain adequate hydration (2-3 L/day of fluids) unless instructed to restrict fluid intake. This medication will not reduce inflammation; consult prescriber for anti-inflammatory, if needed. Report unusual bleeding (stool, mouth, urine) or bruising; unusual fatigue and weakness; change in elimination patterns; or change in color of urine or stool.

Dietary Considerations: Chewable tablets may contain phenylalanine (amount varies, ranges between 3-12 mg/tablet); consult individual product labeling.

Pregnancy Risk Factor: B

Lactation: Enters breast milk/compatible

Administration

Oral: Shake suspension well before pouring dose.

Storage: Do not freeze suppositories.

Related Information

Overdose and Toxicology *on page 1775*

Acetaminophen and Codeine (a seet a MIN oh fen & KOE deen)

U.S. Brand Names Capital® and Codeine; Tylenol® With Codeine

Synonyms Codeine and Acetaminophen

Controlled Substance C-III; C-V

Note: In countries outside of the U.S., some formulations of Tylenol® with Codeine (eg, Tylenol® No. 3) include caffeine.

Generic Available Yes

Pharmacologic Category Analgesic, Narcotic

Medication Safety Issues

Sound-alike/look-alike issues:

Capital® may be confused with Capitrol®

Tylenol® may be confused with atenolol, timolol, Tuinal®, Tylox®

"T3" abbreviation should not be used when writing orders for this medication; has been misread as liothyronine

Use Relief of mild to moderate pain

Dosing

Adults: Doses should be adjusted according to severity of pain and response of the patient. Adult doses ≥60 mg codeine fail to give commensurate relief of pain but merely prolong analgesia and are associated with an appreciably increased incidence of side effects.

Cough (Antitussive): Oral: Based on codeine (15-30 mg/dose) every 4-6 hours

Pain (Analgesic): Oral: Based on codeine (30-60 mg/dose) every 4-6 hours

1-2 tablets every 4 hours to a maximum of 12 tablets/24 hours

Elderly: Doses should be titrated to appropriate analgesic effect.

1 Tylenol® [#3] or 2 Tylenol® [#2] tablets every 4 hours; do **not** exceed 4 g/day acetaminophen.

Pediatrics:

Analgesic: Oral:

Codeine: 0.5-1 mg codeine/kg/dose every 4-6 hours

Acetaminophen: 10-15 mg/kg/dose every 4 hours up to a maximum of 2.6 g/24 hours for children <12 years

3-6 years: 5 mL 3-4 times/day as needed of elixir

7-12 years: 10 mL 3-4 times/day as needed of elixir

Children >12 years: 15 mL every 4 hours as needed of elixir

Renal Impairment: See individual monographs for Acetaminophen and Codeine.

Hepatic Impairment: Use with caution. Limited, low-dose therapy is usually well tolerated in hepatic disease/cirrhosis; however, cases of hepatotoxicity at daily acetaminophen dosages <4 g/day have been reported. Avoid chronic use in hepatic impairment.

Available Dosage Forms [DSC] = Discontinued product; [CAN] = Canadian brand name

Caplet:

ratio-Lenoltec No. 1 [CAN], Tylenol No. 1 [CAN]: Acetaminophen 300 mg, codeine phosphate, 8 mg and caffeine 15 mg [not available in the U.S.]

Tylenol No. 1 Forte [CAN]: Acetaminophen 500 mg, codeine phosphate 8 mg, and caffeine 15 mg [not available in the U.S.]

Elixir, oral [C-V]: Acetaminophen 120 mg and codeine phosphate 12 mg per 5 mL (5 mL, 10 mL, 12.5 mL, 15 mL, 120 mL, 480 mL) [contains alcohol 7%]

Tylenol® with Codeine [DSC]: Acetaminophen 120 mg and codeine phosphate 12 mg per 5 mL (480 mL) [contains alcohol 7%; cherry flavor]

Tylenol Elixir with Codeine [CAN]: Acetaminophen 160 mg and codeine phosphate 8 mg per 5 mL (500 mL) [contains alcohol 7%, sucrose 31%; cherry flavor; not available in the U.S.]

Suspension, oral [C-V] (Capital® and Codeine): Acetaminophen 120 mg and codeine phosphate 12 mg per 5 mL (480 mL) [alcohol free; fruit punch flavor]

Tablet [C-III]: Acetaminophen 300 mg and codeine phosphate 15 mg; acetaminophen 300 mg and codeine phosphate 30 mg; acetaminophen 300 mg and codeine phosphate 60 mg

ratio-Emtec [CAN], Triatec-30 [CAN]: Acetaminophen 300 mg and codeine phosphate 30 mg [not available in the U.S.]

ratio-Lenoltec No. 1 [CAN]: Acetaminophen 300 mg, codeine phosphate 8 mg, and caffeine 15 mg [not available in the U. S.]

ratio-Lenoltec No. 2 [CAN], Tylenol No. 2 with Codeine [CAN]: Acetaminophen 300 mg, codeine phosphate 15 mg, and caffeine 15 mg [not available in the U.S.]

ratio-Lenoltec No. 3 [CAN], Tylenol No. 3 with Codeine [CAN]: Acetaminophen 300 mg, codeine phosphate 30 mg, and caffeine 15 mg [not available in the U.S.]

ratio-Lenoltec No. 4 [CAN], Tylenol No. 4 with Codeine [CAN]: Acetaminophen 300 mg and codeine phosphate 60 mg [not available in the U.S.]

Triatec-8 [CAN]: Acetaminophen 325 mg, codeine phosphate 8 mg, and caffeine 30 mg [not available in the U.S.]

Triatec-8 Strong [CAN]: Acetaminophen 500 mg, codeine phosphate 8 mg, and caffeine 30 mg [not available in the U.S.]

(Continued)

Acetaminophen and Codeine *(Continued)*

Tylenol® with Codeine No. 3: Acetaminophen 300 mg and codeine phosphate 30 mg [contains sodium metabisulfite]
Tylenol® with Codeine No. 4: Acetaminophen 300 mg and codeine phosphate 60 mg [contains sodium metabisulfite]

Monitoring and Teaching Issues
Physical Assessment: See individual agents.
Patient Education: See individual agents. **Pregnancy/breast-feeding precautions:** Inform prescriber if you are or intend to become pregnant. Consult prescriber if breast-feeding.
Pregnancy Risk Factor: C
Lactation: Enters breast milk/use caution

Related Information
Acetaminophen *on page 38*
Codeine *on page 366*

♦ **Acetaminophen and Hydrocodone** *see* Hydrocodone and Acetaminophen *on page 754*

♦ **Acetaminophen and Oxycodone** *see* Oxycodone and Acetaminophen *on page 1138*

♦ **Acetaminophen and Pentazocine** *see* Pentazocine and Acetaminophen *on page 1181*

♦ **Acetaminophen, Butalbital, and Caffeine** *see* Butalbital, Acetaminophen, and Caffeine *on page 225*

♦ **Acetaminophen, Caffeine, Codeine, and Butalbital** *see* Butalbital, Acetaminophen, Caffeine, and Codeine *on page 226*

♦ **Acetaminophen, Dichloralphenazone, and Isometheptene** *see* Acetaminophen, Isometheptene, and Dichloralphenazone *on page 42*

Acetaminophen, Isometheptene, and Dichloralphenazone

(a seet a MIN oh fen, eye soe me THEP teen, & dye KLOR al FEN a zone)
U.S. Brand Names Amidrine; Duradrin®; Midrin®; Migrin-A
Synonyms Acetaminophen, Dichloralphenazone, and Isometheptene; Dichloralphenazone, Acetaminophen, and Isometheptene; Dichloralphenazone, Isometheptene, and Acetaminophen; Isometheptene, Acetaminophen, and Dichloralphenazone; Isometheptene, Dichloralphenazone, and Acetaminophen
Controlled Substance C-IV
Generic Available Yes
Pharmacologic Category Analgesic, Miscellaneous
Medication Safety Issues
Sound-alike/look-alike issues:
Midrin® may be confused with Mydfrin®
Use Relief of migraine and tension headache
Contraindications Hypersensitivity to acetaminophen, isometheptene, dichloralphenazone, or any component of the formulation; glaucoma; severe renal disease; hypertension; organic heart disease; hepatic disease; MAO inhibitor therapy
Drug Interactions
Cytochrome P450 Effect: Acetaminophen: **Substrate** (minor) of CYP1A2, 2A6, 2C8/9, 2D6, 2E1, 3A4; **Inhibits** CYP3A4 (weak)
Nutritional/Ethanol Interactions Ethanol: Excessive intake of ethanol may increase the risk of acetaminophen-induced hepatotoxicity. Avoid ethanol or limit to <3 drinks/day.
Adverse Reactions Frequency not defined.
Central nervous system: Transient dizziness
Dermatological: Rash
Dosing
Adults & Elderly:
Migraine headache: Oral: 2 capsules to start, followed by 1 capsule every hour until relief is obtained (maximum: 5 capsules/12 hours)
Tension headache: Oral: 1-2 capsules every 4 hours (maximum: 8 capsules/24 hours)
Hepatic Impairment: Use with caution. Limited, low-dose therapy usually well tolerated in hepatic disease/cirrhosis; however, cases of hepatotoxicity at daily acetaminophen dosages <4 g/day have been reported. Avoid chronic use in hepatic impairment.
Available Dosage Forms Capsule: Acetaminophen 325 mg, isometheptene mucate 65 mg, dichloralphenazone 100 mg
Monitoring and Teaching Issues
Physical Assessment: Monitor therapeutic effectiveness. Instruct patient in appropriate use.
Patient Education: Can cause dizziness. Use caution when driving or engaging in hazardous tasks until response to drug is known. **Breast-feeding precaution:** Consult prescriber if breast-feeding.
Lactation: Excretion in breast milk unknown/use caution
Breast-Feeding Issues: Acetaminophen and dichloralphenazone are excreted in breast milk; excretion of isometheptene is not known.
Related Information
Acetaminophen *on page 38*

♦ **Acetasol® HC** *see* Acetic Acid, Propylene Glycol Diacetate, and Hydrocortisone *on page 44*

AcetaZOLAMIDE (a set a ZOLE a mide)
U.S. Brand Names Diamox® Sequels®
Generic Available Yes: Injection, tablet
Pharmacologic Category Anticonvulsant, Miscellaneous; Carbonic Anhydrase Inhibitor; Diuretic, Carbonic Anhydrase Inhibitor; Ophthalmic Agent, Antiglaucoma

Medication Safety Issues

Sound-alike/look-alike issues:

AcetaZOLAMIDE may be confused with acetoHEXAMIDE

Diamox® Sequels® may be confused with Dobutrex®, Trimox®

Use Treatment of glaucoma (chronic simple open-angle, secondary glaucoma, preoperatively in acute angle-closure); drug-induced edema or edema due to congestive heart failure (adjunctive therapy); centrencephalic epilepsies (immediate release dosage form); prevention or amelioration of symptoms associated with acute mountain sickness

Unlabeled/Investigational Use Urine alkalinization; respiratory stimulant in COPD

Mechanism of Action/Effect Reversible inhibition of the enzyme carbonic anhydrase resulting in reduction of hydrogen ion secretion at renal tubule and an increased renal excretion of sodium, potassium, bicarbonate, and water. Decreases production of aqueous humor; also inhibits carbonic anhydrase in central nervous system to retard abnormal and excessive discharge from CNS neurons.

Contraindications Hypersensitivity to acetazolamide, sulfonamides, or any component of the formulation; hepatic disease or insufficiency; decreased sodium or potassium levels; adrenocortical insufficiency, cirrhosis; hyperchloremic acidosis, severe renal disease or dysfunction; severe pulmonary obstruction; long-term use in noncongestive angle-closure glaucoma

Warnings/Precautions Use in impaired hepatic function may result in coma. Use with caution in patients with respiratory acidosis and diabetes mellitus. Impairment of mental alertness and/or physical coordination may occur. I.M. administration is painful (use by this route is not recommended). Drug may cause substantial increase in blood glucose in some diabetic patients. Malaise and complaints of tiredness and myalgia are signs of excessive dosing and acidosis in the elderly. Cross-sensitivity between sulfonamide antibiotics and sulfonamide diuretics including various thiazide diuretics. **Sustained release is not recommended for anticonvulsant use.**

Drug Interactions

Cytochrome P450 Effect: Inhibits CYP3A4 (weak)

Decreased Effect: Use of acetazolamide may increase lithium excretion and alter excretion of other drugs by alkalinization of urine (eg, amphetamines, quinidine, methenamine, salicylates). Primidone serum concentrations may be decreased.

Increased Effect/Toxicity: Concurrent use with diflunisal may increase the effect of acetazolamide causing a significant decrease in intraocular pressure. Cyclosporine concentrations may be increased by acetazolamide. Salicylate use may result in carbonic anhydrase inhibitor accumulation and toxicity. Acetazolamide-induced hypokalemia may increase the risk of toxicity with digoxin.

Lab Interactions May cause false-positive results for urinary protein with Albustix®, Labstix®, Albutest®, Bumintest®. Interferes with HPLC theophylline assay.

Adverse Reactions Frequency not defined.

Cardiovascular: Flushing

Central nervous system: Ataxia, confusion, convulsions, depression, dizziness, drowsiness, excitement, fatigue, headache, malaise

Dermatologic: Allergic skin reactions, photosensitivity, Stevens-Johnson syndrome, toxic epidermal necrolysis, urticaria

Endocrine & metabolic: Electrolyte imbalance, growth retardation (children), hyperglycemia, hypoglycemia, hypokalemia, hyponatremia, metabolic acidosis

Gastrointestinal: Appetite decreased, diarrhea, melena, nausea, taste alternation, vomiting

Genitourinary: Crystalluria, glycosuria, hematuria, polyuria, renal failure

Hematologic: Agranulocytosis, aplastic anemia, leukopenia, thrombocytopenia, thrombocytopenic purpura

Hepatic: Cholestatic jaundice, fulminant hepatic necrosis, hepatic insufficiency, liver function tests abnormal

Neuromuscular & skeletal: Flaccid paralysis, paresthesia

Ocular: Myopia

Otic: Hearing disturbance, tinnitus

Miscellaneous: Anaphylaxis

Overdosage/Toxicology Symptoms of overdose include low blood sugar, tingling of lips and tongue, nausea, yawning, confusion, agitation, tachycardia, sweating, convulsions, stupor, and coma. Hypoglycemia should be managed with 50 mL I.V. dextrose 50% followed immediately with a continuous infusion of 10% dextrose in water (administer at a rate sufficient enough to approach a serum glucose level of 100 mg/dL). The use of corticosteroids to treat hypoglycemia is controversial, however, adding 100 mg of hydrocortisone to the dextrose infusion may prove helpful.

Pharmacodynamics/Kinetics

Onset of Action: Capsule, extended release: 2 hours; I.V.: 2 minutes

Peak effect: Capsule, extended release: 8-12 hours; I.V.: 15 minutes; Tablet: 2-4 hours

Duration of Action: Inhibition of aqueous humor secretion: Capsule, extended release: 18-24 hours; I.V.: 4-5 hours; Tablet: 8-12 hours

Excretion: Urine (70% to 100% as unchanged drug)

Dosing

Adults: Note: I.M. administration is not recommended.

Glaucoma:

Chronic simple (open-angle): Oral: 250 mg 1-4 times/day or 500 mg sustained release capsule twice daily

Secondary, acute (closed-angle): I.V.: 250-500 mg, may repeat in 2-4 hours to a maximum of 1 g/day

Edema: Oral, I.V.: 250-375 mg once daily

Epilepsy: Oral: 8-30 mg/kg/day in 1-4 divided doses, not to exceed 1 g/day. *Sustained release capsule is not recommended for treatment of epilepsy.*

Mountain sickness: Oral: 250 mg every 8-12 hours (or 500 mg extended release capsules every 12-24 hours). Therapy should begin 24-48 hours before and continue during ascent and for at least 48 hours after arrival at the high altitude.

(Continued)

AcetaZOLAMIDE *(Continued)*

Urine alkalinization (unlabeled use): Oral: 5 mg/kg/dose repeated 2-3 times over 24 hours

Respiratory stimulant in COPD (unlabeled use): Oral, I.V.: 250 mg twice daily

Elderly: Oral: Initial: 250 mg once or twice daily; use lowest effective dose possible.

Pediatrics: Note: I.M. administration is not recommended.

Glaucoma:
Oral: 8-30 mg/kg/day or 300-900 mg/m^2/day divided every 8 hours
I.V.: 20-40 mg/kg/24 hours divided every 6 hours, not to exceed 1 g/day

Edema: Oral, I.V.: 5 mg/kg or 150 mg/m^2 once every day

Epilepsy: Oral: Refer to adult dosing.

Renal Impairment:
Cl_{cr} 10-50 mL/minute: Administer every 12 hours.
Cl_{cr} <10 mL/minute: Avoid use (ineffective).
Moderately dialyzable (20% to 50%)

Available Dosage Forms

Capsule, sustained release (Diamox® Sequels®): 500 mg
Injection, powder for reconstitution: 500 mg
Tablet: 125 mg, 250 mg

Monitoring and Teaching Issues

Physical Assessment: Assess allergy history prior to beginning therapy. Assess effectiveness and interactions of other medications patient may be taking. Monitor for signs of excessive dosing and acidosis (especially in elderly). Measure intraocular pressure at the beginning of therapy and periodically while on this medication. Assess results of laboratory tests, therapeutic effectiveness, and adverse response. Monitor blood glucose levels closely if diabetic. Assess knowledge/teach patient appropriate use, possible side effects/appropriate interventions, and adverse symptoms to report.

Monitoring Laboratory Tests: Serum electrolytes, periodic CBC with differential

Patient Education: Take as directed; do not chew or crush long-acting capsule (contents may be sprinkled on soft food). May be administered with food to decrease GI upset. You will need periodic ophthalmic examinations while taking this medication. You may experience drowsiness, dizziness, or weakness (use caution when driving or engaging in tasks that require alertness until response to drug is known); nausea, loss of appetite, or altered taste (small frequent meals, frequent mouth care, sucking lozenges, or chewing gum may help). Monitor serum glucose closely (may cause altered blood glucose in some patients with diabetes, or unusual response to some forms of glucose testing). You may experience increased sensitivity to sunlight (use sunblock, protective clothing, and avoid exposure to direct sunlight). Report unusual and persistent tiredness; numbness, burning, or tingling of extremities or around mouth, lips, or anus; muscle weakness; black stool; or excessive depression. **Pregnancy/breast-feeding precautions:** Inform prescriber if you are or intend to become pregnant. Consult prescriber if breast-feeding.

Dietary Considerations: May be taken with food to decrease GI upset. Sodium content of 500 mg injection: 47.2 mg (2.05 mEq).

Geriatric Considerations: Malaise and complaints of tiredness and myalgia are signs of excessive dosing and acidosis in the elderly. Assess blood pressure (orthostatic hypotension can occur).

Pregnancy Risk Factor: C

Lactation: Enters breast milk/not recommended (AAP rates "compatible")

Administration

Reconstitution: Injection: Reconstitute with at least 5 mL sterile water to provide a solution containing not more than 100 mg/mL. Further dilute in D_5W or NS for I.V. infusion.

Compatibility: Stable in dextran 6% in D_5W, dextran 6% in NS, D_5LR, D_5NS, $D_5^1/_2NS$, $D_5^1/_4NS$, D_5W, $D_{10}W$, LR, NS, $^1/_2NS$

Compatibility when admixed: Incompatible with multivitamins

Storage:
Capsules, tablets: Store at controlled room temperature.
Injection: Store vial for injection (prior to reconstitution) at controlled room temperature. Stability of IVPB solution is 5 days at room temperature (25°C) and 44 days at refrigeration (5°C).

Related Information

Anticonvulsants By Seizure Type *on page 1712*
FDA Name Differentiation Project: The Use of Tall-Man Letters *on page 15*
Glaucoma Drug Therapy *on page 1827*

♦ **Acetic Acid, Hydrocortisone, and Propylene Glycol Diacetate** *see* Acetic Acid, Propylene Glycol Diacetate, and Hydrocortisone *on page 44*

Acetic Acid, Propylene Glycol Diacetate, and Hydrocortisone

(a SEE tik AS id, PRO pa leen GLY kole dye AS e tate, & hye droe KOR ti sone)

U.S. Brand Names Acetasol® HC; VoSol® HC

Synonyms Acetic Acid, Hydrocortisone, and Propylene Glycol Diacetate; Hydrocortisone, Acetic Acid, and Propylene Glycol Diacetate; Hydrocortisone, Propylene Glycol Diacetate, and Acetic Acid; Propylene Glycol Diacetate, Acetic Acid, and Hydrocortisone; Propylene Glycol Diacetate, Hydrocortisone, and Acetic Acid

Generic Available Yes

Pharmacologic Category Otic Agent, Anti-infective

Use Treatment of superficial infections of the external auditory canal caused by organisms susceptible to the action of the antimicrobial, complicated by swelling

Dosing

Adults & Elderly: Otitis externa (superficial): Instill 4 drops in ear(s) 3-4 times/day

Pediatrics: Refer to adult dosing.

Available Dosage Forms Solution, otic drops: Acetic acid 2%, propylene glycol diacetate 3%, and hydrocortisone 1% (10 mL)

Monitoring and Teaching Issues
Physical Assessment: Refer to Hydrocortisone monograph.
Related Information
Hydrocortisone *on page 760*

♦ **Acetoxymethylprogesterone** *see* MedroxyPROGESTERone *on page 938*

Acetylcysteine (a se teel SIS teen)
U.S. Brand Names Acetadote®; Mucomyst®
Synonyms Acetylcysteine Sodium; Mercapturic Acid; NAC; *N*-Acetylcysteine; *N*-Acetyl-L-Cysteine
Generic Available Yes: Solution for inhalation
Pharmacologic Category Antidote; Mucolytic Agent
Medication Safety Issues
Sound-alike/look-alike issues:
Acetylcysteine may be confused with acetylcholine
Mucomyst® may be confused with Mucinex®
Use Adjunctive mucolytic therapy in patients with abnormal or viscid mucous secretions in acute and chronic bronchopulmonary diseases; pulmonary complications of surgery and cystic fibrosis; diagnostic bronchial studies; antidote for acute acetaminophen toxicity
Unlabeled/Investigational Use Prevention of radiocontrast-induced renal dysfunction (oral); distal intestinal obstruction syndrome (DIOS, previously referred to as meconium ileus equivalent)
Mechanism of Action/Effect Exerts mucolytic action through its free sulfhydryl group which opens up the disulfide bonds in the mucoproteins thus lowering mucous viscosity. The exact mechanism of action in acetaminophen toxicity is unknown. It is thought to act by providing substrate for conjugation with the toxic metabolite.
Contraindications Hypersensitivity to acetylcysteine or any component of the formulation
Warnings/Precautions
Inhalation: Since increased bronchial secretions may develop after inhalation, percussion, postural drainage and suctioning should follow; if bronchospasm occurs, administer a bronchodilator; discontinue acetylcysteine if bronchospasm progresses
Intravenous: Acute flushing and erythema have been reported; usually occurs within 30-60 minutes and may resolve spontaneously. Serious anaphylactoid reactions have also been reported. Acetylcysteine infusion may be interrupted until treatment of allergic symptoms is initiated; the infusion can then be carefully restarted. Treatment for anaphylactic reactions should be immediately available. Use caution with asthma or history of bronchospasm.
Drug Interactions
Decreased Effect: Adsorbed by activated charcoal; clinical significance is minimal, though, once a pure acetaminophen ingestion requiring N-acetylcysteine is established; further charcoal dosing is unnecessary once the appropriate initial charcoal dose is achieved (5-10 g:g acetaminophen)
Adverse Reactions
Inhalation: Frequency not defined.
Central nervous system: Drowsiness, chills, fever
Gastrointestinal: Vomiting, nausea, stomatitis
Local: Irritation, stickiness on face following nebulization
Respiratory: Bronchospasm, rhinorrhea, hemoptysis
Miscellaneous: Acquired sensitization (rare), clamminess, unpleasant odor during administration

Intravenous:
>10%: Miscellaneous: Anaphylactoid reaction (~17%; reported as severe in 1% or moderate in 10% of patients within 15 minutes of first infusion; severe in 1% or mild-to-moderate in 6% to 7% of patients after 60-minute infusion)
1% to 10%:
Cardiovascular: Angioedema (2% to 8%), vasodilation (1% to 6%), hypotension (1% to 4%), tachycardia (1% to 4%), syncope (1% to 3%), chest tightness (1%), flushing (1%)
Central nervous system: Dysphoria (<1% to 2%)
Dermatologic: Urticaria (2% to 7%), rash (1% to 5%), facial erythema (≤1%), palmar erythema (≤1%), pruritus (≤1% to 3%), pruritus with rash and vasodilation (2% to 9%)
Gastrointestinal: Vomiting (<1% to 10%), nausea (1% to 10%), dyspepsia (≤1%)
Neuromuscular & skeletal: Gait disturbance (<1% to 2%)
Ocular: Eye pain (<1% to 3%)
Otic: Ear pain (1%)
Respiratory: Bronchospasm (1% to 6%), cough (1% to 4%), dyspnea (<1% to 3%), pharyngitis (1%), rhinorrhea (1%), rhonchi (1%), throat tightness (1%)
Miscellaneous: Diaphoresis (≤1%)
Overdosage/Toxicology Treatment of acetylcysteine toxicity is usually aimed at reversing anaphylactoid symptoms or controlling nausea and vomiting. The use of epinephrine, antihistamines, and steroids may be beneficial.
Pharmacodynamics/Kinetics
Onset of Action: Inhalation: 5-10 minutes
Duration of Action: Inhalation: >1 hour
Time to Peak: Plasma: Oral: 1-2 hours
Protein Binding: 83%
Half-Life Elimination: Reduced acetylcysteine: 2 hours; Total acetylcysteine: Adults: 5.5 hours; Newborns: 11 hours
Excretion: Urine
Dosing
Adults & Elderly:
Acetaminophen poisoning:
Oral: 140 mg/kg; followed by 17 doses of 70 mg/kg every 4 hours; repeat dose if emesis occurs within 1 hour of administration; therapy should continue until all doses are
(Continued)

Acetylcysteine *(Continued)*

administered even though the acetaminophen plasma level has dropped below the toxic range

I.V. (Acetadote®): Loading dose: 150 mg/kg over 15 minutes. Maintenance dose: 50 mg/kg infused over 4 hours followed by 100 mg /kg infused over 16 hours. **Note:** To avoid fluid overload in patients <40 kg and those requiring fluid restriction, decrease volume of D_5W proportionally.

Alternatively, the following dose has been reported using solution for oral inhalation (unlabeled route): Loading dose: 140 mg/kg, followed by 70 mg/kg every 4 hours, for a total of 13 doses (loading dose and 48 hours of treatment); infuse each dose over 1 hour

Adjuvant therapy in respiratory conditions:

Note: Patients should receive bronchodilator 15 minutes prior to dose.

Inhalation, nebulization (face mask, mouth piece, tracheostomy): Acetylcysteine 10% and 20% solution (Mucomyst®) (dilute 20% solution with sodium chloride or sterile water for inhalation); 10% solution may be used undiluted: 3-5 mL of 20% solution or 6-10 mL of 10% solution until nebulized given 3-4 times/day; dosing range: 1-10 mL of 20% solution or 2-20 mL of 10% solution every 2-6 hours

Inhalation, nebulization (tent, croupette): Dose must be individualized; may require up to 300 mL solution/treatment

Direct instillation:

Into tracheostomy: 1-2 mL of 10% to 20% solution every 1-4 hours

Through percutaneous intrathecal catheter: 1-2 mL of 20% or 2-4 mL of 10% solution every 1-4 hours via syringe attached to catheter

Diagnostic bronchogram: Nebulization or intrathecal: 1-2 mL of 20% solution or 2-4 mL of 10% solution administered 2-3 times prior to procedure

Prevention of radiocontrast-induced renal dysfunction (unlabeled use): Oral: 600 mg twice daily for 2 days (beginning the day before the procedure); may be given as powder in capsules, some centers use solution (diluted in cola beverage or juice). Hydrate patient with saline concurrently.

Pediatrics:

Acetaminophen poisoning: Refer to adult dosing.

Adjuvant therapy in respiratory conditions:

Note: Patients should receive an aerosolized bronchodilator 10-15 minutes prior to acetylcysteine

Inhalation, nebulization (face mask, mouth piece, tracheostomy): Acetylcysteine 10% and 20% solution (Mucomyst®) (dilute 20% solution with sodium chloride or sterile water for inhalation); 10% solution may be used undiluted:

Infants: 1-2 mL of 20% solution or 2-4 mL 10% solution until nebulized given 3-4 times/day

Children: Refer to adult dosing.

Inhalation, nebulization (tent, croupette): Children: Refer to adult dosing.

Available Dosage Forms

Injection, solution (Acetadote®): 20% [200 mg/mL] (30 mL) [contains disodium edetate]

Solution, as sodium (Mucomyst®): 10% [100 mg/mL] (4 mL, 10 mL, 30 mL); 20% [200 mg/mL] (4 mL, 10 mL, 30 mL)

Monitoring and Teaching Issues

Physical Assessment: Instruct patient on appropriate use, adverse effects to report, and interventions to reduce side effects. Monitor pulmonary function and response to therapy. If giving I.V., monitor for possible anaphylactoid reactions and be prepared to treat appropriately if needed.

Monitoring Laboratory Tests: Acetaminophen overdose: AST, ALT, bilirubin, PT, serum creatinine, BUN, serum glucose and electrolytes. Acetaminophen levels at ~4 hours postingestion (~8 hours if extended release acetaminophen), and 4-6 hours later to assess for possible hepatotoxicity.

Patient Education: Pulmonary treatment: Prepare solution (may dilute with sterile water to reduce concentrate from impeding nebulizer) and use as directed. Clear airway by coughing deeply before using aerosol. Wash face and face mask after treatment to remove any residual. You may experience drowsiness (use caution when driving), nausea, or vomiting (small frequent meals may help). Report persistent chills or fever, adverse change in respiratory status, palpitations, or extreme anxiety or nervousness.

Pregnancy Risk Factor: B

Pregnancy Issues: Based on limited reports using acetylcysteine to treat acetaminophen overdose in pregnant women, acetylcysteine has been shown to cross the placenta and may provide protective levels in the fetus.

Lactation: Excretion in breast milk unknown/use caution

Administration

Oral: For treatment of acetaminophen overdosage, administer orally as a 5% solution. Dilute the 20% solution 1:3 with a cola, orange juice, or other soft drink. Use within 1 hour of preparation. Unpleasant odor becomes less noticeable as treatment progresses. If patient vomits within 1 hour of dose, readminister.

I.V.: Recommended procedure for I.V. administration of **ORAL** N-acetylcysteine:

Obtain informed consent.

Using D_5W, dilute acetylcysteine 20% oral solution to a 3% solution.

Administer loading dose of NAC: 140 mg/kg infused through a peripheral intravenous catheter over 1 hour using an in-line 0.2-μ millipore filter

Administer maintenance doses of NAC (first maintenance dose 4 hours after initiating the loading dose): 70 mg/kg/dose: Doses administered every 4 hours, each infused over 1 hour through an in-line 0.2-μ millipore filter for a total of 13 doses (loading dose and 48 hours of treatment)

Inhalation: Acetylcysteine is incompatible with tetracyclines, erythromycin, amphotericin B, iodized oil, chymotrypsin, trypsin, and hydrogen peroxide. Administer separately. Intermittent aerosol treatments are commonly given when patient arises, before meals, and just before retiring at bedtime.

Reconstitution:
Solution for injection (Acetadote®): To avoid fluid overload in patients <40 kg and those requiring fluid restriction, decrease volume of D_5W proportionally. Discard unused portion.
Loading dose: Dilute 150 mg/kg in D_5W 200 mL
Initial maintenance dose: Dilute 50 mg/kg in D_5W 500 mL
Second maintenance dose: Dilute 100 mg/kg in D_5W 1000 mL
Solution for inhalation (Mucomyst®): The 20% solution may be diluted with sodium chloride or sterile water; the 10% solution may be used undiluted.
Intravenous administration of solution for inhalation (unlabeled route): Using D_5W, dilute acetylcysteine 20% oral solution to a 3% solution.

Compatibility:
Inhalation: **Incompatible** with rubber and metals (particularly iron, copper, and nickel); do not mix with ampicillin, tetracycline, oxytetracycline, erythromycin
Intravenous: **Incompatible** with rubber and metals (particularly iron, copper, and nickel)

Storage:
Solution for injection (Acetadote®): Store vials at room temperature, 20°C to 25°C (68°F to 77°F); following reconstitution with D_5W, solution is stable for 24 hours at room temperature
Solution for inhalation (Mucomyst®): Store unopened vials at room temperature; once opened, store under refrigeration and use within 96 hours. A color change may occur in opened vials (light purple) and does not affect the safety or efficacy.

Acrivastine and Pseudoephedrine (AK ri vas teen & soo doe e FED rin)

U.S. Brand Names Semprex®-D
Synonyms Pseudoephedrine and Acrivastine
Generic Available No
Pharmacologic Category Antihistamine
Use Temporary relief of nasal congestion, decongest sinus openings, running nose, itching of nose or throat, and itchy, watery eyes due to hay fever or other upper respiratory allergies

Dosing
Adults & Elderly: Rhinitis, nasal congestion, allergic symptoms: Oral: 1 capsule 3-4 times/day
Pediatrics: Refer to adult dosing.
Renal Impairment: Do not use.

Available Dosage Forms Capsule: Acrivastine 8 mg and pseudoephedrine hydrochloride 60 mg

Monitoring and Teaching Issues
Physical Assessment: Assess effectiveness and interactions of other medications patient may be taking. Monitor effectiveness of therapy and adverse reactions at beginning of therapy and periodically with long-term use. Assess knowledge/teach patient appropriate use, interventions to reduce side effects, and adverse symptoms to report.
Patient Education: Take as directed; do not exceed recommended dose. Avoid use of other depressants, alcohol, or sleep-inducing medications unless approved by prescriber. You may experience drowsiness or dizziness (use caution when driving or engaging in hazardous activity until response to drug is known); or dry mouth, nausea, or vomiting (small frequent meals, frequent mouth care, chewing gum, or sucking lozenges may help). Report persistent dizziness, sedation, or agitation; chest pain, rapid heartbeat, or palpitations; respiratory difficulty or increased cough; changes in urinary pattern; muscle weakness; or lack of improvement or worsening or condition. **Breast-feeding precaution:** Do not breast-feed.

Pregnancy Risk Factor: B
Lactation: Enters breast milk/contraindicated

Related Information
Pseudoephedrine on page 1282

- ◆ **Activated Ergosterol** *see Ergocalciferol on page 538*
- ◆ **Activated Protein C, Human, Recombinant** *see Drotrecogin Alfa on page 501*
- ◆ **Activella®** *see Estradiol and Norethindrone on page 557*
- ◆ **Actonel®** *see Risedronate on page 1331*
- ◆ **Actos®** *see Pioglitazone on page 1217*
- ◆ **Acular®** *see Ketorolac on page 853*
- ◆ **Acular LS™** *see Ketorolac on page 853*
- ◆ **Acular® PF** *see Ketorolac on page 853*
- ◆ **ACV** *see Acyclovir on page 48*
- ◆ **Acycloguanosine** *see Acyclovir on page 48*

Acyclovir (ay SYE kloe veer)

U.S. Brand Names Zovirax®
Synonyms Aciclovir; ACV; Acycloguanosine
Generic Available Yes: Excludes cream, ointment
Pharmacologic Category Antiviral Agent
Medication Safety Issues
  Sound-alike/look-alike issues:
    Zovirax® may be confused with Zostrix®, Zyvox™
Use Treatment of genital herpes simplex virus (HSV), herpes labialis (cold sores), herpes zoster (shingles), HSV encephalitis, neonatal HSV, mucocutaneous HSV, varicella-zoster (chickenpox)
Unlabeled/Investigational Use Prevention of HSV reactivation in HIV positive patients; prevention of HSV reactivation in hematopoietic stem cell transplant (HSCT); prevention of CMV infection after bone marrow transplants in HSV and CMV seropositive individuals
Mechanism of Action/Effect Inhibits DNA synthesis and viral replication
Contraindications Hypersensitivity to acyclovir, valacyclovir, or any component of the formulation
Warnings/Precautions Use with caution in immunocompromised patients; thrombocytopenic purpura/hemolytic uremic syndrome (TTP/HUS) has been reported. Use caution in the elderly, pre-existing renal disease or in those receiving other nephrotoxic drugs. Maintain adequate hydration during I.V. therapy. Use I.V. preparation with caution in patients with underlying neurologic abnormalities, serious hepatic or electrolyte abnormalities, or substantial hypoxia.

Chickenpox: Treatment should begin within 24 hours of appearance of rash; oral route not recommended for routine use in otherwise healthy children with varicella, but may be effective in patients at increased risk of moderate to severe infection (>12 years of age, chronic cutaneous or pulmonary disorders, long-term salicylate therapy, corticosteroid therapy).

Genital herpes: Physical contact should be avoided when lesions are present; transmission may also occur in the absence of symptoms. Treatment should begin with the first signs or symptoms.

Herpes labialis: For external use only to the lips and face; do not apply to eye or inside the mouth or nose. Treatment should begin with the first signs or symptoms.

Herpes zoster: Acyclovir should be started within 72 hours of appearance of rash to be effective.
Drug Interactions
  Increased Effect/Toxicity: Increased CNS side effects when taken with zidovudine or probenecid.
Nutritional/Ethanol Interactions Food: Does not appear to affect absorption of acyclovir.
Adverse Reactions
  Systemic: Oral:
    1% to 10%:
      Central nervous system: Lightheadedness, headache
      Gastrointestinal: Diarrhea, nausea, vomiting, abdominal pain
  Systemic: Parenteral:
    >10%:
      Central nervous system: Lightheadedness
      Gastrointestinal: Anorexia
    1% to 10%:
      Dermatologic: Hives, itching, rash
      Gastrointestinal: Nausea, vomiting
      Hepatic: Liver function tests increased
      Local: Inflammation at injection site or phlebitis
      Renal: Acute renal failure, BUN increased, creatinine increased
  Topical:
    >10%: Mild pain, burning, or stinging
    1% to 10%: Itching
Overdosage/Toxicology Symptoms of overdose include seizures, somnolence, confusion, elevated serum creatinine, and renal failure. In the event of overdose, sufficient urine flow must be maintained to avoid drug precipitation within renal tubules. Hemodialysis has resulted in up to 60% reduction in serum acyclovir levels.
Pharmacodynamics/Kinetics
  Absorption: Oral: 15% to 30%
  Bioavailability: Oral: 10% to 20% with normal renal function (bioavailability decreases with increased dose)
  Time to Peak: Serum: Oral: Within 1.5-2 hours
  Protein Binding: 9% to 33%
  Half-Life Elimination: Terminal: Neonates: 4 hours; Children 1-12 years: 2-3 hours; Adults: 3 hours

Metabolism: Converted by viral enzymes to acyclovir monophosphate, and further converted to diphosphate then triphosphate (active form) by cellular enzymes

Excretion: Urine (62% to 90% as unchanged drug and metabolite)

Dosing

Adults & Elderly: Note: Obese patients should be dosed using ideal body weight

Genital HSV:

I.V.: Immunocompetent: Initial episode, severe: 5 mg/kg every 8 hours for 5-7 days

Oral:

Initial episode: 200 mg every 4 hours while awake (5 times/day) for 10 days (per manufacturer's labeling); 400 mg 3 times/day for 5-10 days has also been reported

Recurrence: 200 mg every 4 hours while awake (5 times/day) for 5 days (per manufacturer's labeling; begin at earliest signs of disease); 400 mg 3 times/day for 5 days has also been reported

Chronic suppression: 400 mg twice daily or 200 mg 3-5 times/day, for up to 12 months followed by re-evaluation (per manufacturer's labeling); 400-1200 mg/day in 2-3 divided doses has also been reported

Topical: Immunocompromised: Ointment: Initial episode: $^1/_2$" ribbon of ointment for a 4" square surface area every 3 hours (6 times/day) for 7 days

Herpes labialis (cold sores): Topical: Apply 5 times/day for 4 days

Herpes zoster (shingles):

Oral: Immunocompetent: 800 mg every 4 hours (5 times/day) for 7-10 days

I.V.: Immunocompromised: 10 mg/kg/dose or 500 mg/m^2/dose every 8 hours for 7 days

HSV encephalitis: I.V.: 10 mg/kg/dose every 8 hours for 10 days (per manufacturer's labeling); 10-15 mg/kg/dose every 8 hours for 14-21 days also reported

Mucocutaneous HSV:

I.V.: Immunocompromised: 5 mg/kg/dose every 8 hours for 7 days (per manufacturer's labeling); dosing for up to 14 days also reported

Oral: Immunocompromised (unlabeled use): 400 mg 5 times a day for 7-14 days

Topical: Ointment: Nonlife-threatening, immunocompromised: $^1/_2$" ribbon of ointment for a 4" square surface area every 3 hours (6 times/day) for 7 days

Varicella-zoster (chickenpox): Begin treatment within the first 24 hours of rash onset:

Oral: >40 kg (immunocompetent): 800 mg/dose 4 times a day for 5 days

I.V.: Immunocompromised (unlabeled use): 1500 mg/m^2/day divided every 8 hours or 10 mg/kg/dose every 8 hours for 7-10 days

Prevention of HSV reactivation in HIV-positive patients, for use only when recurrences are frequent or severe (unlabeled use): Oral: 200 mg 3 times/day or 400 mg 2 times/day

Prevention of HSV reactivation in HSCT (unlabeled use): Note: Start at the beginning of conditioning therapy and continue until engraftment or until mucositis resolves (~30 days)

Oral: 200 mg 3 times/day

I.V.: 250 mg/m^2/dose every 12 hours

Bone marrow transplant recipients (unlabeled use): I.V.: Allogeneic patients who are HSV and CMV seropositive: 500 mg/m^2/dose (10 mg/kg) every 8 hours; for clinically-symptomatic CMV infection, consider replacing acyclovir with ganciclovir

Pediatrics: Note: Obese patients should be dosed using ideal body weight

Genital HSV:

I.V.: Children ≥12 years: Refer to adult dosing.

Oral:

Initial episode (unlabeled use): 40-80 mg/kg/day divided into 3-4 doses for 5-10 days (maximum: 1 g/day)

Chronic suppression (unlabeled use; limited data): 80 mg/kg/day in 3 divided doses (maximum: 1 g/day), re-evaluate after 12 months of treatment

Herpes labialis (cold sores): Topical: Children ≥12 years: Refer to adult dosing.

Herpes zoster (shingles): I.V.:

Children <12 years (immunocompromised): 20 mg/kg/dose every 8 hours for 7 days

Children ≥12 years: Refer to adult dosing.

HSV encephalitis: I.V.:

Children 3 months to 12 years: 20 mg/kg/dose every 8 hours for 10 days (per manufacturer's labeling); dosing for 14-21 days also reported

Children ≥12 years: Refer to adult dosing.

Mucocutaneous HSV: I.V.:

Children <12 years (immunocompromised): 10 mg/kg/dose every 8 hours for 7 days

Children ≥12 years: Refer to adult dosing.

Neonatal HSV: I.V.: Neonate: Birth to 3 months: 10 mg/kg/dose every 8 hours for 10 days (manufacturer's labeling); 15 mg/kg/dose or 20 mg/kg/dose every 8 hours for 14-21 days has also been reported

Varicella-zoster (chickenpox): Begin treatment within the first 24 hours of rash onset:

Oral:

Children ≥2 years and ≤40 kg (immunocompetent): 20 mg/kg/dose (up to 800 mg/dose) 4 times/day for 5 days

Children >40 kg: Refer to adult dosing.

I.V.:

Children <1 year (immunocompromised, unlabeled use): 10 mg/kg/dose every 8 hours for 7-10 days

Children ≥1 year: Refer to adult dosing.

Prevention of HSV reactivation in HIV-positive patients, for use only when recurrences are frequent or severe (unlabeled use): Oral: 80 mg/kg/day in 3-4 divided doses

Prevention of HSV reactivation in HSCT (unlabeled use): Note: Start at the beginning of conditioning therapy and continue until engraftment or until mucositis resolves (~30 days): I.V.: 250 mg/m^2/dose every 8 hours or 125 mg/m^2/dose every 6 hours

Bone marrow transplant recipients (unlabeled use): I.V.: Refer to adult dosing.

(Continued)

Acyclovir *(Continued)*

Renal Impairment:

Oral:

Cl_{cr} 10-25 mL/minute: Normal dosing regimen 800 mg every 4 hours: Administer 800 mg every 8 hours

Cl_{cr} <10 mL/minute:

Normal dosing regimen 200 mg every 4 hours, 200 mg every 8 hours, or 400 mg every 12 hours: Administer 200 mg every 12 hours

Normal dosing regimen 800 mg every 4 hours: Administer 800 mg every 12 hours

I.V.:

Cl_{cr} 25-50 mL/minute: Administer recommended dose every 12 hours

Cl_{cr} 10-25 mL/minute: Administer recommended dose every 24 hours

Cl_{cr} <10 mL/minute: Administer 50% of recommended dose every 24 hours

Hemodialysis: Administer dose after dialysis

Peritoneal dialysis: No supplemental dose needed

CAVH: 3.5 mg/kg/day

CVVHD/CVVH: Adjust dose based upon Cl_{cr} 30 mL/minute

Available Dosage Forms

Capsule: 200 mg

Cream, topical: 5% (2 g)

Injection, powder for reconstitution, as sodium: 500 mg, 1000 mg

Zovirax®: 500 mg

Injection, solution, as sodium [preservative free]: 25 mg/mL (20 mL, 40 mL); 50 mg/mL (10 mL, 20 mL)

Ointment, topical: 5% (15 g)

Suspension, oral: 200 mg/5 mL (480 mL) [banana flavor]

Tablet: 400 mg, 800 mg

Monitoring and Teaching Issues

Physical Assessment: Assess for use cautions (eg, immunocompromised patients and those with underlying neurologic abnormalities, serious hepatic or electrolyte abnormalities, or substantial hypoxia; see Warnings/Precautions). Assess results of laboratory tests, therapeutic response according to purpose for use, and adverse responses (eg, headache, dizziness, rash, gastrointestinal upset or pain, renal failure [BUN/Cr increased]; see Adverse Reactions). Teach patient appropriate use (if self-administered), possible side effects/appropriate interventions, and adverse symptoms to report.

Monitoring Laboratory Tests: Urinalysis, BUN, serum creatinine, liver enzymes, CBC

Patient Education: Do not take any new prescriptions, OTC medications, or herbal products during therapy (including creams, lotions, or ointments) unless approved by prescriber. This is not a cure for herpes (recurrences tend to continually reappear every 3-6 months after original infection), nor will this medication reduce the risk of transmission to others when lesions are present; avoid sexual intercourse when visible lesions are present. Use as directed for full course of therapy; do not discontinue even if feeling better. Oral doses may be taken with or without food. Maintain adequate hydration (2-3 L/day of fluids) unless instructed to restrict fluid intake. May cause nausea or vomiting (small frequent meals, frequent mouth care, sucking lozenges, or chewing gum may help); lightheadedness or dizziness (use caution when driving or engaging in tasks that require alertness until response to drug is known); or headache, fever, muscle pain (consult prescriber for approved analgesic). Report any change in urination (difficulty urinating, dark colored or concentrated urine); persistent lethargy; acute headache; severe nausea or vomiting; confusion or hallucinations; rash; or respiratory difficulty.

Topical: Apply as directed. Use gloves or finger cot when applying.

Dietary Considerations: May be taken with or without food. Acyclovir 500 mg injection contains sodium ~50 mg (~2 mEq).

Geriatric Considerations: Calculate creatinine clearance. Dose adjustment may be necessary depending on renal function.

Pregnancy Risk Factor: B

Pregnancy Issues: Teratogenic effects were not observed in animal studies. Acyclovir has been shown to cross the human placenta. Results from a pregnancy registry, established in 1984 and closed in 1999, did not find an increase in the number of birth defects with exposure to acyclovir when compared to those expected in the general population. However, due to the small size of the registry and lack of long-term data, the manufacturer recommends using during pregnancy with caution and only when clearly needed. Data from the pregnancy registry may be obtained from GlaxoSmithKline.

Lactation: Enters breast milk/use with caution (AAP rates "compatible")

Breast-Feeding Issues: Nursing mothers with herpetic lesions near or on the breast should avoid breast-feeding.

Administration

Oral: May be administered with or without food.

I.V.: For I.V. infusion only. Avoid rapid infusion. Infuse over 1 hour to prevent renal damage. Maintain adequate hydration of patient. Check for phlebitis and rotate infusion sites.

Topical: Not for use in the eye. Apply using a finger cot or rubber glove to avoid transmission to other parts of the body or to other persons.

Reconstitution: Powder for injection: Reconstitute acyclovir 500 mg with SWFI 10 mL; do not use bacteriostatic water containing benzyl alcohol or parabens. For intravenous infusion, dilute to a final concentration of ≤7 mg/mL. Concentrations >10 mg/mL increase the risk of phlebitis.

Compatibility: Stable in D_5W, D_5NS, $D_5\frac{1}{4}NS$, $D_5\frac{1}{2}NS$, LR, NS

Incompatible with blood products and protein-containing solutions

Y-site administration: Incompatible with amifostine, amsacrine, aztreonam, cefepime, dobutamine, dopamine, fludarabine, foscarnet, gemcitabine, idarubicin, levofloxacin, ondansetron, piperacillin/tazobactam, sargramostim, vinorelbine

Compatibility when admixed: Incompatible with dobutamine, dopamine

Storage:
Capsule, tablet: Store at controlled room temperature of 15°C to 25°C (59°F to 77°F); protect from moisture.
Cream, suspension: Store at controlled room temperature of 15°C to 25°C (59°F to 77°F).
Ointment: Store at controlled room temperature of 15°C to 25°C (59°F to 77°F) in a dry place.
Injection: Store powder at controlled room temperature of 15°C to 25°C (59°F to 77°F). Reconstituted solutions remain stable for 12 hours at room temperature. Do not refrigerate reconstituted solutions as they may precipitate. Once diluted for infusion, use within 24 hours.

♦ **AD3L** *see* Valrubicin *on page 1546*
♦ **Adalat® CC** *see* NIFEdipine *on page 1081*

Adalimumab (a da LIM yoo mab)

U.S. Brand Names Humira®
Synonyms Antitumor Necrosis Factor Apha (Human); D2E7; Human Antitumor Necrosis Factor-Alpha
Generic Available No
Pharmacologic Category Antirheumatic, Disease Modifying; Monoclonal Antibody; Tumor Necrosis Factor (TNF) Blocking Agent
Medication Safety Issues
Sound-alike/look-alike issues:
Humira® may be confused with Humulin®
Use Treatment of active rheumatoid arthritis (moderate to severe) in patients with inadequate response to one or more disease-modifying antirheumatic drugs (DMARDs)
Mechanism of Action/Effect Adalimumab decreases signs and symptoms of rheumatoid arthritis and inhibits progression of structural damage.
Contraindications Hypersensitivity to adalimumab or any component of the formulation
Warnings/Precautions Tuberculosis (disseminated or extrapulmonary) has been reactivated while on adalimumab. Most cases have been reported within the first 8 months of treatment. Patients should be evaluated for latent tuberculosis infection with a tuberculin skin test prior to therapy. Treatment of latent tuberculosis should be initiated before adalimumab is used. Use caution with chronic infection, history of recurrent infection, or predisposition to infection. Do not give to patients with a clinically-important, active infection. Adalimumab may affect defenses against infections and malignancies; serious infections (including sepsis and fatal infections) have been reported in patients receiving TNF-blocking agents, including adalimumab. Many of the serious infections have occurred in patients on concomitant immunosuppressive therapy. Other opportunistic infections (*Histoplasma*, *Aspergillus*, and *Nocardia*) have occurred during therapy. Use caution in patients who have resided in regions where histoplasmosis is endemic. Patients who develop a new infection while undergoing treatment with adalimumab should be monitored closely. If a patient develops a serious infection or sepsis, adalimumab should be discontinued. Impact on the development and course of malignancies is not fully defined. Rare cases of lymphoma have also been reported in association with adalimumab.

May exacerbate pre-existing or recent-onset demyelinating CNS disorders. Use caution in patients with CHF. Patients should be brought up to date with all immunizations before initiating therapy. Live vaccines should not be given concurrently. Rare cases of pancytopenia (including aplastic anemia) have been reported with TNF-blocking agents; with significant hematologic abnormalities, consider discontinuing therapy. Safety and efficacy have not been established in pediatric patients.

Drug Interactions
Decreased Effect: Concomitant use with vaccines (live) has not be studied; currently recommended not to administer live vaccines during adalimumab therapy.
Increased Effect/Toxicity: Concomitant use with anakinra may increase risk of infections; not recommended.
Adverse Reactions
>10%:
Central nervous system: Headache (12%)
Dermatologic: Rash (12%)
Local: Injection site reaction (20%; includes erythema, itching, hemorrhage, pain, swelling)
Respiratory: Upper respiratory tract infection (17%), sinusitis (11%)
5% to 10%:
Cardiovascular: Hypertension (5%)
Endocrine & metabolic: Hyperlipidemia (7%), hypercholesterolemia (6%)
Gastrointestinal: Nausea (9%), abdominal pain (7%)
Genitourinary: Urinary tract infection (8%)
Hepatic: Alkaline phosphatase increased (5%)
Local: Injection site reaction (8%)
Neuromuscular & skeletal: Back pain (6%)
Renal: Hematuria (5%)
Miscellaneous: Accidental injury (10%), flu-like syndrome (7%)
<5%:
Cardiovascular: Arrhythmia, atrial fibrillation, chest pain, CHF, coronary artery disorder, heart arrest, hypertensive encephalopathy, myocardial infarct, palpitation, pericardial effusion, pericarditis, peripheral edema, syncope, tachycardia, thrombosis (leg), vascular disorder
Central nervous system: Confusion, fever, multiple sclerosis, pain in extremity, paresthesia, subdural hematoma, tremor
Dermatologic: Cellulitis
Endocrine & metabolic: Dehydration, menstrual disorder, parathyroid disorder
Gastrointestinal: Esophagitis, gastroenteritis, gastrointestinal hemorrhage, vomiting
Genitourinary: Cystitis, pelvic pain
Hematologic: Agranulocytosis, granulocytopenia, leukopenia, pancytopenia, polycythemia
(Continued)

Adalimumab (Continued)

Hepatic: Cholecystitis, cholelithiasis, hepatic necrosis

Neuromuscular & skeletal: Arthritis, bone fracture, bone necrosis, joint disorder, muscle cramps, myasthenia, pyogenic arthritis, synovitis, tendon disorder

Ocular: Cataract

Renal: Kidney calculus, paraproteinemia, pyelonephritis

Respiratory: Asthma, bronchospasm, dyspnea, lung function decreased, pleural effusion, pneumonia

Miscellaneous: Adenoma, allergic reactions; carcinoma (including breast, gastrointestinal, skin, urogenital); cytopenia, erysipelas, healing abnormality, herpes zoster, ketosis, lupus erythematosus syndrome, lymphoma, melanoma, sepsis, tuberculosis (reactivation of latent infection)

Overdosage/Toxicology Doses of up to 10 mg/kg have been tolerated in clinical trials. In case of overdose, treatment should be symptomatic and supportive.

Pharmacodynamics/Kinetics

Bioavailability: Absolute: 64%

Time to Peak: SubQ: 131 ± 56 hours

Half-Life Elimination: Terminal: ~2 weeks (range 10-20 days)

Excretion: Clearance increased in the presence of antiadalimumab antibodies; decreased in patients 40 to >75 years

Dosing

Adults: Rheumatoid arthritis: SubQ: 40 mg every other week; may be administered with other DMARDs; patients not taking methotrexate may increase dose to 40 mg/weekly

Available Dosage Forms Injection, solution [preservative free]: 40 mg/0.8 mL (1 mL) [prefilled glass syringe; packaged with alcohol preps]

Monitoring and Teaching Issues

Physical Assessment: Perform tuberculin skin test prior to initiating therapy. Monitor for signs and symptoms of infection. Assess for liver dysfunction. Assess potential for interactions with other prescriptions, OTC medications, and herbal products patient may be taking. Assess results of laboratory tests (PDD), therapeutic effectiveness (eg, pain, range of movement, mobility), and adverse response at regular intervals during treatment. Teach patient proper use if self-injected (appropriate injection technique and syringe/needle disposal), possible side effects/appropriate interventions, and adverse symptoms to report.

Patient Education: Inform prescriber of all prescriptions, OTC medications, or herbal products you are taking, allergies, history of tuberculosis, or any kind of infection you have. Do not take any new medication during therapy without consulting prescriber. If self-administered, follow directions for injection and needle/syringe disposal exactly. Do not have any vaccinations while using this medication without consulting prescriber first. May cause headache or dizziness (use caution when driving or engaged in potentially hazardous tasks); if persistent, consult prescriber for approved analgesic. Report persistent fever, respiratory tract infection, unhealed or infected wounds, urinary tract infection, or flu-like symptoms. Stop drug and report immediately persistent nausea, abdominal pain; numbness or tingling; problems with vision; weakness in legs; chest pains, respiratory difficulty; joint pain; skin rash; redness, swelling, or pain at injection site.

Pregnancy Risk Factor: B

Pregnancy Issues: Teratogenic effects were not observed in animal studies, however, there are no adequate and well-controlled studies in pregnant women. Use during pregnancy only if clearly needed. A pregnancy registry has been established to monitor outcomes of women exposed to adalimumab during pregnancy (877-311-8972).

Lactation: Excretion in breast milk unknown/not recommended

Administration

Other: For SubQ injection; rotate injection sites. Do not use if solution is discolored. Do not administer to skin which is red, tender, bruised, or hard.

Storage: Store under refrigeration at 2°C to 8°C (36°F to 46°F). Do not freeze. Protect from light.

♦ **Adamantanamine Hydrochloride** *see* Amantadine *on page 83*

Adapalene (a DAP a leen)

U.S. Brand Names Differin®

Generic Available No

Pharmacologic Category Acne Products

Use Treatment of acne vulgaris

Mechanism of Action/Effect Retinoid-like compound which is a modulator of cellular differentiation, keratinization and inflammatory processes, all of which represent important features in the pathology of acne vulgaris

Contraindications Hypersensitivity to adapalene or any component in the vehicle gel

Warnings/Precautions Use with caution in patients with eczema. Avoid excessive exposure to sunlight and sunlamps. Avoid contact with abraded skin, mucous membranes, eyes, mouth, and angles of the nose.

Adverse Reactions >10%: Dermatologic: Erythema, scaling, dryness, pruritus, burning, pruritus or burning immediately after application

Overdosage/Toxicology Toxic signs of overdose commonly respond to drug discontinuation, with spontaneous resolution in a few days to weeks. When confronted with signs of increased intracranial pressure, treatment with mannitol (0.25 g/kg I.V. up to 1 g/kg/dose repeated every 5 minutes as needed), dexamethasone (1.5 mg/kg I.V. load followed with 0.375 mg/kg every 6 hours for 5 days), and/or hyperventilation should be employed.

Pharmacodynamics/Kinetics
Absorption: Topical: Minimal

Excretion: Bile

Dosing
Adults & Elderly: Acne: Topical: Apply once daily before bedtime; results appear after 8-12 weeks of therapy.

Pediatrics: Children >12 years: Refer to adult dosing.

Available Dosage Forms
Cream, topical: 0.1% (15 g, 45 g)

Gel, topical: 0.1% (15 g, 45 g) [alcohol free]

Pledget, topical: 0.1% (60s)

Solution, topical: 0.1% (30 mL)

Monitoring and Teaching Issues
Physical Assessment: Assess knowledge/teach patient appropriate use and adverse symptoms to report.

Patient Education: For external use only. Apply with gloves in thin film at night to thoroughly clean/dry skin; avoid area around eyes or mouth. Do not apply occlusive dressing. Results may take 8-12 weeks to appear. You may experience transient burning or stinging immediately after applying. Report worsening of condition or skin redness, dryness, peeling, or burning that persists between applications. Avoid excessive exposure to sunlight or sunlamps.

Pregnancy Risk Factor: C

Lactation: Excretion in breast milk unknown/use caution

- Adderall® *see* Dextroamphetamine and Amphetamine *on page 436*
- Adderall XR™ *see* Dextroamphetamine and Amphetamine *on page 436*

Adefovir (a DEF o veer)

U.S. Brand Names Hepsera™

Synonyms Adefovir Dipivoxil

Generic Available No

Pharmacologic Category Antiretroviral Agent, Reverse Transcriptase Inhibitor (Nucleoside)

Use Treatment of chronic hepatitis B with evidence of active viral replication (based on persistent elevation of ALT/AST or histologic evidence), including patients with lamivudine-resistant hepatitis B

Mechanism of Action/Effect Acyclic nucleotide reverse transcriptase inhibitor (adenosine analog) which interferes with HBV viral DNA polymerase resulting in inhibition of viral replication

Contraindications Hypersensitivity to adefovir or any component of the formulation

Warnings/Precautions Use with caution in patients with renal dysfunction or in patients at risk of renal toxicity (including concurrent nephrotoxic agents or NSAIDs). Chronic administration may result in nephrotoxicity. Dosage adjustment is required in patients with renal dysfunction or in patients who develop renal dysfunction during therapy. May cause the development of resistance in patients with unrecognized or untreated HIV infection. Lactic acidosis and severe hepatomegaly with steatosis (sometimes fatal) have occurred with antiretroviral nucleoside analogues; female gender, obesity, and prolonged treatment may increase the risk of hepatotoxicity. Treatment should be discontinued in patients with lactic acidosis or signs/symptoms of hepatotoxicity (which may occur without marked transaminase elevations). Acute exacerbations of hepatitis may occur (in up to 25% of patients) when antihepatitis therapy is discontinued. Exacerbations typically occur within 12 weeks; monitor patients following discontinuation of therapy. Safety and efficacy in pediatric patients have not been established.

Drug Interactions
Increased Effect/Toxicity: Ibuprofen increases the bioavailability of adefovir. Concurrent use of nephrotoxic agents (including aminoglycosides, cyclosporine, NSAIDs, tacrolimus, vancomycin) may increase the risk of nephrotoxicity.

Nutritional/Ethanol Interactions
Ethanol: Should be avoided in hepatitis B infection due to potential hepatic toxicity.

Food: Does not have a significant effect on adefovir absorption.

Adverse Reactions
>10%: Renal: Hematuria (11% vs. 10% in placebo-treated)

1% to 10%:

Central nervous system: Fever, headache,

Dermatologic: Rash, pruritus

Gastrointestinal: Dyspepsia (3%), nausea, vomiting, flatulence, diarrhea, abdominal pain

Hepatic: AST/ALT increased, abnormal liver function, hepatic failure

Neuromuscular & skeletal: Weakness

Renal: Serum creatinine increased (4%), renal failure, renal insufficiency

> Note: In patients with baseline renal dysfunction, frequency of increased serum creatinine has been observed to be as high as 26% to 37%; the role of adefovir in these changes could not be established.

Respiratory: Cough increased, sinusitis, pharyngitis

Overdosage/Toxicology Limited experience in acute overdose. Chronic overdose may be associated with renal toxicity and gastrointestinal adverse effects. Hemodialysis may be effective in the removal of adefovir (35% of a 10 mg dose removed in 4 hours). *(Continued)*

Adefovir *(Continued)*

Pharmacodynamics/Kinetics
Bioavailability: 59%
Protein Binding: ≤4%
Half-Life Elimination: 7.5 hours; prolonged in renal impairment
Metabolism: Prodrug; rapidly converted to adefovir (active metabolite) in intestine
Excretion: Urine (45% as active metabolite within 24 hours)

Dosing
Adults & Elderly: Hepatitis B (chronic): Oral: 10 mg once daily
Renal Impairment:
Cl$_{cr}$ 20-49 mL/minute: 10 mg every 48 hours
Cl$_{cr}$ 10-19 mL/minute: 10 mg every 72 hours
Hemodialysis: 10 mg every 7 days (following dialysis)
Hepatic Impairment: Refer to adult dosing. No adjustment required.

Available Dosage Forms Tablet, as dipivoxil: 10 mg

Monitoring and Teaching Issues
Physical Assessment: Assess for use cautions (eg, renal dysfunction, risk of renal toxicity, unrecognized or untreated HIV, history of hepatitis; see Warnings/Precautions). Monitor other prescriptions, OTC medications, or herbal products patient may be taking for potential nephrotoxicity (see Drug Interactions). Assess results of laboratory tests, therapeutic response, and adverse responses (eg, hepatic or renal failure; see Adverse Reactions). Teach patient proper use, possible side effects/interventions, and adverse symptoms to report immediately.
Monitoring Laboratory Tests: HIV status (prior to initiation of therapy); serum creatinine (prior to initiation and during therapy)
Patient Education: Do not take any new medication during therapy without consulting prescriber. Use appropriate precautions to prevent spread to other persons. Take as directed. Do not discontinue without consulting prescriber. You will require frequent blood tests; follow recommended schedule. Maintain adequate hydration (2-3 L/day of fluids) unless instructed to restrict fluid intake. You may be more susceptible to infection (avoid crowds and exposure to infection; do not have any vaccinations without consulting prescriber). May cause headache or abdominal pain (consult prescriber for approved analgesia); or nausea or vomiting (small frequent meals, frequent mouth care, sucking lozenges, or chewing gum may help). Report unusual bleeding (blood in urine, tarry stools, or easy bruising); dark colored urine or light colored stools, yellowing of eyes; unresolved nausea or vomiting; signs of infection (eg, fever, chills, sore throat, burning urination, flu-like symptoms); persistent fatigue; muscle weakness; changes in urinary pattern; rash or skin irritation; unusual cough; or other persistent adverse effects. **Pregnancy/breast-feeding precautions:** Inform prescriber if you are or intend to become pregnant. Breast-feeding is not recommended.
Dietary Considerations: May be taken without regard to food.
Pregnancy Risk Factor: C
Lactation: Excretion in breast milk unknown/not recommended

Administration
Oral: May be administered without regard to food.
Storage: Store at 25°C (77 °F); excursions permitted to 15°C to 30°C (59°F to 86°F).

Additional Information Adefovir dipivoxil is a prodrug, rapidly converted to the active component (adefovir). It was previously investigated as a treatment for HIV infections (at dosages substantially higher than the approved dose for hepatitis B). The NDA was withdrawn, and no further studies in the treatment of HIV are anticipated (per manufacturer).

♦ **Adefovir Dipivoxil** *see* Adefovir *on page 53*
♦ **Adenocard®** *see* Adenosine *on page 54*
♦ **Adenoscan®** *see* Adenosine *on page 54*

Adenosine *(a DEN oh seen)*

U.S. Brand Names Adenocard®; Adenoscan®
Synonyms 9-Beta-D-Ribofuranosyladenine
Generic Available Yes
Pharmacologic Category Antiarrhythmic Agent, Class IV; Diagnostic Agent
Use
Adenocard®: Treatment of paroxysmal supraventricular tachycardia (PSVT) including that associated with accessory bypass tracts (Wolff-Parkinson-White syndrome); when clinically advisable, appropriate vagal maneuvers should be attempted prior to adenosine administration; **not effective in atrial flutter, atrial fibrillation, or ventricular tachycardia**
Adenoscan®: Pharmacologic stress agent used in myocardial perfusion thallium-201 scintigraphy
Mechanism of Action/Effect Slows conduction time through the AV node and restores normal sinus rhythm
Contraindications Hypersensitivity to adenosine or any component of the formulation; second- or third-degree AV block or sick sinus syndrome (except in patients with a functioning artificial pacemaker), atrial flutter, atrial fibrillation, and ventricular tachycardia (this drug is not effective in converting these arrhythmias to sinus rhythm). The manufacturer states that Adenoscan® should be avoided in patients with known or suspected bronchoconstrictive or bronchospastic lung disease.
Warnings/Precautions Patients with pre-existing SA nodal dysfunction may experience prolonged sinus pauses after adenosine. There have been reports of atrial fibrillation/flutter in patients with PSVT associated with accessory conduction pathways after adenosine. Adenosine decreases conduction through the AV node and may produce a short-lasting first-, second-, or third-degree heart block. Because of the very short half-life, the effects are generally self-limiting. Rare, prolonged episodes of asystole have been reported, with fatal

outcomes in some cases. At the time of conversion to normal sinus rhythm, a variety of new rhythms may appear on the ECG. A limited number of patients with asthma have received adenosine and have not experienced exacerbation of their asthma. Adenosine may cause bronchoconstriction in patients with asthma, and should be used cautiously in patients with obstructive lung disease not associated with bronchoconstriction (eg, emphysema, bronchitis).

Drug Interactions

Decreased Effect: Methylxanthines (eg, caffeine, theophylline) antagonize the effect of adenosine.

Increased Effect/Toxicity: Dipyridamole potentiates effects of adenosine. Use with carbamazepine may increase heart block.

Nutritional/Ethanol Interactions Food: Avoid food or drugs with caffeine. Adenosine's therapeutic effect may be decreased if used concurrently with caffeine.

Adverse Reactions

>10%:

Cardiovascular: Facial flushing (18%), palpitation, chest pain, hypotension
Central nervous system: Headache
Respiratory: Dyspnea (12%)
Miscellaneous: Diaphoresis

1% to 10%:

Central nervous system: Dizziness
Gastrointestinal: Nausea (3%)
Neuromuscular & skeletal: Paresthesia, numbness
Respiratory: Chest pressure (7%)

Overdosage/Toxicology Since adenosine half-life is <10 seconds, adverse effects are rapidly self-limiting. Treatment of prolonged effects requires individualization. Theophylline and other methylxanthines are competitive inhibitors of adenosine and may have a role in reversing its toxic effects.

Pharmacodynamics/Kinetics

Onset of Action: Rapid

Duration of Action: Very brief

Half-Life Elimination: <10 seconds

Metabolism: Blood and tissue to inosine then to adenosine monophosphate (AMP) and hypoxanthine

Dosing

Adults:

Paroxysmal supraventricular tachycardia (Adenocard®): I.V. (rapid - over 1-2 seconds, via peripheral line): 6 mg; if not effective within 1-2 minutes, 12 mg may be given; may repeat 12 mg bolus if needed; maximum single dose: 12 mg.

Follow each I.V. bolus of adenosine with normal saline flush.

Note: Preliminary results in adults suggest adenosine may be administered via a central line at lower doses (ie, initial adult dose: 3 mg).

Pharmacologic stress agent (Adenoscan®): I.V.: Continuous I.V. infusion via peripheral line: 140 mcg/kg/minute for 6 minutes using syringe or columetric infusion pump; total dose: 0.84 mg/kg. Thallium-201 is injected at midpoint (3 minutes) of infusion.

Elderly: Refer to adult dosing. Elderly may be more sensitive to effects of adenosine.

Pediatrics:

Paroxysmal supraventricular tachycardia (Adenocard®): Rapid I.V. push (over 1-2 seconds) via peripheral line: Infants and Children (Manufacturer's recommendation):

Children <50 kg: 0.05 to 0.1 mg/kg. If conversion of PSVT does not occur within 1-2 minutes, may increase dose by 0.05 to 0.1 mg/kg. May repeat until sinus rhythm is established or to a maximum single dose of 0.3 mg/kg or 12 mg. Follow each dose with normal saline flush.

Children ≥50 kg: Refer to adult dosing.

Pediatric advanced life support (PALS): Treatment of SVT: I.V., I.O.: 0.1 mg/kg; if not effective, administer 0.2 mg/kg; maximum single dose: 12 mg. Follow each dose with normal saline flush.

Available Dosage Forms Injection, solution [preservative free]: 3 mg/mL (2 mL)

Adenocard®: 3 mg/mL (2 mL, 4 mL)
Adenoscan®: 3 mg/mL (20 mL, 30 mL)

Monitoring and Teaching Issues

Physical Assessment: Assess other medications patient may be taking for effectiveness and interactions. Requires use of infusion pump and continuous cardiac and hemodynamic monitoring during infusion. Monitor for adverse reactions. Note that adenosine could produce bronchoconstriction in patients with asthma.

Patient Education: Adenosine is administered in emergencies, patient education should be appropriate to the situation.

Geriatric Considerations: Geriatric patients may be more sensitive to the effects of this medication.

Pregnancy Risk Factor: C

Lactation: Excretion in breast milk unknown

Other Issues: Confirm labeling before administration. **Do not use adenosine phosphate (given I.M. for symptomatic relief of varicose veins complications). Have emergency resuscitation and equipment available when using this drug.**

Administration

I.V.: For rapid bolus I.V. use only. Administer I.V. push over 1-2 seconds at a peripheral I.V. site as proximal as possible to trunk (ie, not in lower arm, hand, lower leg, or foot).

Compatibility: Stable in D$_5$LR, D$_5$W, LR, NS

Storage: Store at controlled room temperature of 15°C to 30°C (59°F to 86°F). Do **not** refrigerate, precipitation may occur (may dissolve by warming to room temperature).

Related Information

Antiarrhythmic Drugs *on page 1708*

- **ADH** *see* Vasopressin *on page 1554*
- **Adoxa**™ *see* Doxycycline *on page 496*
- **ADR** *see* DOXOrubicin *on page 491*
- **Adrenalin**® *see* Epinephrine *on page 525*
- **Adrenaline** *see* Epinephrine *on page 525*
- **Adria** *see* DOXOrubicin *on page 491*
- **Adriamycin PFS**® *see* DOXOrubicin *on page 491*
- **Adriamycin RDF**® *see* DOXOrubicin *on page 491*
- **Adrucil**® *see* Fluorouracil *on page 647*
- **Adsorbent Charcoal** *see* Charcoal *on page 302*
- **Advair Diskus**® *see* Fluticasone and Salmeterol *on page 664*
- **Advate** *see* Antihemophilic Factor (Recombinant) *on page 127*
- **Advil**® **[OTC]** *see* Ibuprofen *on page 777*
- **Advil**® **Children's [OTC]** *see* Ibuprofen *on page 777*
- **Advil**® **Infants' [OTC]** *see* Ibuprofen *on page 777*
- **Advil**® **Junior [OTC]** *see* Ibuprofen *on page 777*
- **Advil**® **Migraine [OTC]** *see* Ibuprofen *on page 777*
- **AeroBid**® *see* Flunisolide *on page 642*
- **AeroBid**®**-M** *see* Flunisolide *on page 642*
- **Afeditab**™ *see* NIFEdipine *on page 1081*
- **AG** *see* Aminoglutethimide *on page 91*
- **Agenerase**® *see* Amprenavir *on page 119*
- **Aggrastat**® *see* Tirofiban *on page 1486*
- **Aggrenox**® *see* Aspirin and Dipyridamole *on page 147*
- **Agoral**® **Maximum Strength Laxative [OTC]** *see* Senna *on page 1365*
- **AGT** *see* Aminoglutethimide *on page 91*
- **AHF (Human)** *see* Antihemophilic Factor (Human) *on page 124*
- **AHF (Porcine)** *see* Antihemophilic Factor (Porcine) *on page 126*
- **AHF (Recombinant)** *see* Antihemophilic Factor (Recombinant) *on page 127*
- **A-hydroCort** *see* Hydrocortisone *on page 760*
- **AK-Dilate**® *see* Phenylephrine *on page 1200*
- **AK-Fluor**® **Injection** *see page 1625*
- **AK-Nefrin**® *see* Phenylephrine *on page 1200*
- **Akne-Mycin**® *see* Erythromycin *on page 543*
- **AK-Pentolate**® *see page 1625*
- **AK-Poly-Bac**® *see* Bacitracin and Polymyxin B *on page 171*
- **AK-Pred**® *see* PrednisoLONE *on page 1245*
- **AK-Spore**® **H.C. [DSC]** *see* Bacitracin, Neomycin, Polymyxin B, and Hydrocortisone *on page 172*
- **AK-Sulf**® *see* Sulfacetamide *on page 1403*
- **AK-Taine**® *see page 1625*
- **AKTob**® *see* Tobramycin *on page 1489*
- **AK-Tracin**® **[DSC]** *see* Bacitracin *on page 169*
- **Alavert**™ **[OTC]** *see* Loratadine *on page 918*
- **Alavert**™ **Allergy and Sinus [OTC]** *see* Loratadine and Pseudoephedrine *on page 919*

Albendazole (al BEN da zole)

U.S. Brand Names Albenza®
Generic Available No
Pharmacologic Category Anthelmintic
Use Treatment of parenchymal neurocysticercosis caused by *Taenia solium* and cystic hydatid disease of the liver, lung, and peritoneum caused by *Echinococcus granulosus*
Unlabeled/Investigational Use Albendazole has activity against *Ascaris lumbricoides* (roundworm); *Ancylostoma caninum*; *Ancylostoma duodenale* and *Necator americanus* (hookworms); cutaneous larva migrans; *Enterobius vermicularis* (pinworm); *Gnathostoma spinigerum*; *Gongylonema* sp; *Hymenolepis nana* sp (tapeworms); *Mansonella perstans* (filariasis); *Opisthorchis sinensis* and *Opisthorchis viverrini* (liver flukes); *Strongyloides stercoralis* and *Trichuris trichiura* (whipworm); visceral larva migrans (toxocariasis); activity has also been shown against the liver fluke *Clonorchis sinensis*, *Giardia lamblia*, *Cysticercus cellulosae*, and *Echinococcus multilocularis*. Albendazole has also been used for the treatment of intestinal microsporidiosis (*Encephalitozoon intestinalis*), disseminated microsporidiosis (*E. hellem, E. cuniculi, E. intestinalis, Pleistophora* sp, *Trachipleistophora* sp, *Brachiola vesicularum*), and ocular microsporidiosis (*E. hellem, E. cuniculi, Vittaforma corneae*).
Mechanism of Action/Effect Active metabolite, albendazole, causes selective degeneration of cytoplasmic microtubules in intestinal and tegmental cells of intestinal helminths and larvae; glycogen is depleted, glucose uptake and cholinesterase secretion are impaired, and desecratory substances accumulate intracellulary. ATP production decreases causing energy depletion, immobilization, and worm death.
Contraindications Hypersensitivity to albendazole or any component of the formulation
Warnings/Precautions Discontinue therapy if LFT elevations are significant; may restart treatment when decreased to pretreatment values. Becoming pregnant within 1 month following therapy is not advised.

Neurocysticercosis: Corticosteroids should be administered 1-2 days before albendazole therapy to minimize inflammatory reactions. Steroid and anticonvulsant therapy should be used concurrently during the first week of therapy to prevent cerebral hypertension. If retinal lesions exist, weigh risk of further retinal damage due to albendazole-induced changes to the retinal lesion vs benefit of disease treatment.

Drug Interactions

Cytochrome P450 Effect: Substrate (minor) of CYP1A2, 3A4; **Inhibits** CYP1A2 (weak)

Nutritional/Ethanol Interactions Food: Albendazole serum levels may be increased if taken with a fatty meal (increases the oral bioavailability by 4-5 times).

Adverse Reactions

N = Neurocysticercosis; H = Hydatid disease

>10%:
  Central nervous system: Headache (11% - N; 1% - H)
  Hepatic: LFTs Increased (~15% - H; <1% - N)
1% to 10%:
  Central nervous system: Dizziness, vertigo, fever (≤1%); intracranial pressure increased (1% - N); meningeal signs (1% - N)
  Dermatologic: Alopecia (2% - H; <1% - N)
  Gastrointestinal: Abdominal pain (6% - H; 0% - N); nausea/vomiting (3% to 6%)
  Hematologic: Leukopenia (reversible) (<1%)
  Miscellaneous: Allergic reactions (<1%)

Pharmacodynamics/Kinetics

Absorption: <5%; may increase up to 4-5 times when administered with a fatty meal

Time to Peak: Serum: 2-2.4 hours

Protein Binding: 70%

Half-Life Elimination: 8-12 hours

Metabolism: Hepatic; extensive first-pass effect; pathways include rapid sulfoxidation (major), hydrolysis, and oxidation

Excretion: Urine (<1% as active metabolite); feces

Dosing

Adults & Elderly:

Neurocysticercosis:
  <60 kg: 15 mg/kg/day in 2 divided doses (maximum: 800 mg/day) for 8-30 days
  ≥60 kg: 400 mg twice daily for 8-30 days
  Note: Give concurrent anticonvulsant and steroid therapy during first week.

Hydatid:
  <60 kg: 15 mg/kg/day in 2 divided doses (maximum: 800 mg/day)
  ≥60 kg: 400 mg twice daily
  Note: Administer dose for three 28-day cycles with a 14-day drug-free interval in between

Ancylostoma caninum, Ascaris lumbricoides **(roundworm),** *Ancylostoma duodenale,* **and** *Necator americanus* **(hookworms) (unlabeled use):** 400 mg as a single dose

Clonorchis sinensis **(Chinese liver fluke) (unlabeled use):** 400 mg twice daily for 7 days

Cutaneous larva migrans (unlabeled use): 400 mg once daily for 3 days

Enterobius vermicularis **(pinworm) (unlabeled use):** 400 mg as a single dose; may repeat in 2 weeks

Gnathostoma spinigerum **(unlabeled use):** 400 mg twice daily for 21 days

Gongylonemiasis (unlabeled use): 10 mg/kg/day for 3 days

Mansonella perstans **(unlabeled use):** 400 mg twice daily for 10 days

Visceral larva migrans (toxocariasis) (unlabeled use): 400 mg twice daily for 5 days

Cysticercus cellulosae **(unlabeled use):** 400 mg twice daily for 8-30 days; may be repeated as necessary

Disseminated microsporidiosis (unlabeled use): 400 mg twice daily

Echinococcus granulosus **(tapeworm) (unlabeled use):** 400 mg twice daily for 1-6 months

Intestinal microsporidiosis (unlabeled use): 400 mg twice daily for 21 days

Ocular microsporidiosis (unlabeled use): 400 mg twice daily, in combination with fumagillin

Pediatrics:

Neurocysticercosis: Oral: Refer to adult dosing.

Hydatid: Oral: Refer to adult dosing.

Cysticercus cellulosae **(unlabeled use):** Oral: 15 mg/kg/day (maximum: 800 mg/day) in 2 divided doses for 8-30 days; may be repeated as necessary

Echinococcus granulosus **(tapeworm) (unlabeled use):** Oral: 15 mg/kg/day (maximum: 800 mg) divided twice daily for 1-6 months

For the following unlabeled uses, refer to adult dosing:
  Ancylostoma caninum, Ascaris lumbricoides (roundworm), *Ancylostoma duodenale, Clonorchis sinensis* (Chinese liver fluke), cutaneous larva migrans, *Enterobius vermicularis* (pinworm), *Gnathostoma spinigerum*, gongylonemiasis, *Mansonella perstans, Necator americanus* (hookworms), visceral larva migrans (toxocariasis)

Available Dosage Forms Tablet: 200 mg

Monitoring and Teaching Issues

Physical Assessment: Dosing based on identification of parasite. See Warnings/Precautions for pretreatment suggestions. Monitor laboratory results for therapeutic effectiveness (reduction or elimination of ova and parasites) and adverse reactions (eg, elevated LFTs, leukopenia; see Adverse Reactions). Teach patient appropriate use, possible side effects/appropriate interventions, and adverse symptoms to report.

Monitoring Laboratory Tests: Monitor fecal specimens for ova and parasites prior to and 3 weeks after treatment; LFTs and CBC at start of each 28 day cycle and every 2 weeks during therapy

Patient Education: You may be prescribed other medications to take during first week of therapy. Do not take any other new medication during therapy unless approved by prescriber. Laboratory tests may be required; maintain recommended schedule. Take as directed, with a high-fat meal. Follow prescriber's suggestions to prevent reinfection. May cause loss of hair (reversible); nausea or vomiting (small frequent meals, frequent mouth care, sucking lozenges, or chewing gum may help); or dizziness or headaches (use caution when driving or engaging in tasks that require alertness until response to drug is known). Report unusual fever, persistent or unresolved abdominal pain, vomiting, yellowing of skin (Continued)

Albendazole *(Continued)*

or eyes, darkening of urine, or light colored stools. **Pregnancy/breast-feeding precautions:** Inform prescriber if you are or intend to become pregnant. Breast-feeding is not recommended. Becoming pregnant within 1 month following therapy is not advised.

Dietary Considerations: Should be taken with a high-fat meal.

Pregnancy Risk Factor: C

Pregnancy Issues: Albendazole has been shown to be teratogenic in laboratory animals and should not be used during pregnancy, if at all possible. Women should be advised to avoid pregnancy for at least 1 month following therapy. Discontinue if pregnancy occurs during treatment.

Lactation: Excretion in breast milk unknown/not recommended

Administration

Oral: Administer with meals; administer anticonvulsant and steroid therapy during first week of neurocysticercosis therapy

♦ **Albenza®** *see* Albendazole *on page 56*

♦ **Albumarc®** *see* Albumin *on page 58*

Albumin (al BYOO min)

U.S. Brand Names Albumarc®; Albuminar®; Albutein®; Buminate®; Plasbumin®

Synonyms Albumin (Human); Normal Human Serum Albumin; Normal Serum Albumin (Human); Salt Poor Albumin; SPA

Generic Available Yes

Pharmacologic Category Blood Product Derivative; Plasma Volume Expander, Colloid

Medication Safety Issues

Sound-alike/look-alike issues:

Albutein® may be confused with albuterol

Buminate® may be confused with bumetanide

Use Plasma volume expansion and maintenance of cardiac output in the treatment of certain types of shock or impending shock; may be useful for burn patients, ARDS, and cardiopulmonary bypass; other uses considered by some investigators (but not proven) are retroperitoneal surgery, peritonitis, and ascites; unless the condition responsible for hypoproteinemia can be corrected, albumin can provide only symptomatic relief or supportive treatment

Unlabeled/Investigational Use In cirrhotics, administered with diuretics to help facilitate diuresis; large volume paracentesis; volume expansion in dehydrated, mildly-hypotensive cirrhotics

Mechanism of Action/Effect Restores plasma volume

Contraindications Hypersensitivity to albumin or any component of the formulation; patients with severe anemia or cardiac failure

Warnings/Precautions Use with caution in patients with hepatic or renal failure because of added protein load; rapid infusion of albumin solutions may cause vascular overload. All patients should be observed for signs of hypervolemia such as pulmonary edema. Use with caution in those patients for whom sodium restriction is necessary. Avoid 25% concentration in preterm infants due to risk of intraventricular hemorrhage. Nutritional supplementation is not an appropriate indication for albumin.

Drug Interactions

Increased Effect/Toxicity: ACE inhibitors: May have increased risk of atypical reactions; withhold ACEIs for at least 24 hours prior to plasma exchanges using large volumes of albumin

Adverse Reactions Frequency not defined.

Cardiovascular: CHF precipitation, edema, hyper-/hypotension, hypervolemia, tachycardia

Central nervous system: Chills, fever, headache

Dermatologic: Pruritus, rash, urticaria

Gastrointestinal: Nausea, vomiting

Respiratory: Bronchospasm, pulmonary edema

Miscellaneous: Anaphylaxis

Overdosage/Toxicology Symptoms of overdose include hypervolemia, congestive heart failure, and pulmonary edema.

Dosing

Adults & Elderly:

Note: Use **5%** solution in hypovolemic patients or intravascularly-depleted patients. Use **25%** solution in patients in whom fluid and sodium intake is restricted.

Usual dose: 25 g; initial dose may be repeated in 15-30 minutes if response is inadequate; no more than 250 g should be administered within 48 hours.

Hypoproteinemia: I.V.: 0.5-1 g/kg/dose; repeat every 1-2 days as calculated to replace ongoing losses.

Hypovolemia: I.V.: 0.5-1 g/kg/dose; repeat as needed; maximum: 6 g/kg/day.

Pediatrics:

Note: **5%** should be used in hypovolemic patients or intravascularly-depleted patients. **25%** should be used in patients in whom fluid and sodium intake must be minimized.

Dose depends on condition of patient: Hypovolemia: I.V.: 0.5-1 g/kg/dose (10-20 mL/kg/ dose of albumin 5%); maximum dose: 6 g/kg/day

Available Dosage Forms Injection, solution, human: 5% [50 mg/mL] (50 mL, 250 mL, 500 mL); 25% [250 mg/mL] (50 mL, 100 mL)

Albumarc®: 5% [50 mg/mL] (250 mL, 500 mL); 25% [250 mg/mL] (50 mL, 100 mL)

Albuminar®: 5% [50 mg/mL] (50 mL, 250 mL, 500 mL, 1000 mL); 25% [250 mg/mL] (20 mL, 50 mL, 100 mL)

Albutein®, Buminate®: 5% [50 mg/mL]: (250 mL, 500 mL); 25% [250 mg/mL] (20 mL, 50 mL, 100 mL)

Plasbumin®: 5% [50 mg/mL] (50 mL, 250 mL, 500 mL); 25% [250 mg/mL] (20 mL, 50 mL, 100 mL)

Monitoring and Teaching Issues

Physical Assessment: Assess patient for hepatic or renal failure (see Warnings/Precautions). Patient should be monitored closely for pulmonary edema and cardiac failure (vital signs, central venous pressure) during administration, with frequent assessment for hypovolemia or fluid overload (see Adverse Reactions). If adverse reactions (eg, fever, tachycardia, hypotension, dyspnea) occur, infusion should be stopped and prescriber notified. Teach patient adverse symptoms to report.

Monitoring Laboratory Tests: Hematocrit

Patient Education: Education is provided as appropriate for patient condition. This medication can only be administered intravenously. You will be monitored closely during the infusion. Report immediately any pain or reaction at infusion site; acute headache, difficulty breathing, chills, chest pain or tightness, palpitations, or sudden pain. **Pregnancy precaution:** Inform prescriber if you are pregnant.

Pregnancy Risk Factor: C

Lactation: Excretion in breast milk unknown/compatible

Administration

I.V.: For I.V. administration only. Use within 4 hours after opening vial; discard unused portion. In emergencies, may administer as rapidly as necessary to improve clinical condition. After initial volume replacement:

5%: Do not exceed 2-4 mL/minute in patients with normal plasma volume; 5-10 mL/minute in patients with hypoproteinemia

25%: Do not exceed 1 mL/minute in patients with normal plasma volume; 2-3 mL/minute in patients with hypoproteinemia

Do not dilute 5% solution. Rapid infusion may cause vascular overload. Albumin 25% may be given undiluted or diluted in normal saline. May give in combination or through the same administration set as saline or carbohydrates. Do not use with ethanol or protein hydrolysates, precipitation may form.

Reconstitution: If 5% human albumin is unavailable, it may be prepared by diluting 25% human albumin with 0.9% sodium chloride or 5% dextrose in water. Do not use sterile water to dilute albumin solutions, as this has been associated with hypotonic-associated hemolysis.

Compatibility: Stable in dextran 6% in D_5W, dextran 6% in NS, D_5LR, D_5NS, $D_5^{1}/_2NS$, $D_5^{1}/_4NS$, D_5W, $D_{10}W$, LR, NS, $^{1}/_2NS$; **incompatible** with sterile water
Y-site administration: Incompatible with midazolam, vancomycin, verapamil
Compatibility when admixed: Incompatible with verapamil

Storage: Store at a temperature ≤30°C (86°F); do not freeze. Do not use solution if it is turbid or contains a deposit; use within 4 hours after opening vial; discard unused portion.

Additional Information Albumin 5% and 25% solutions contain 130-160 mEq/L sodium and are considered isotonic with plasma. Dilution of albumin 25% solution with sterile water produces a hypotonic solution; administration of such can cause hemolysis and/or renal failure. An albumin 5% solution is osmotically equivalent to an equal volume of plasma, whereas a 25% solution is osmotically equivalent to 5 times its volume of plasma. Albumin solutions are heated to 60°C for 10 hours, decreasing any possible risk of viral hepatitis transmission. To date, there have been no reports of viral transmission using these products.

♦ **Albuminar®** see Albumin on page 58
♦ **Albumin (Human)** see Albumin on page 58
♦ **Albutein®** see Albumin on page 58

Albuterol (al BYOO ter ole)

U.S. Brand Names AccuNeb™; Proventil®; Proventil® HFA; Proventil® Repetabs®; Ventolin® HFA; Volmax® [DSC]; VoSpire ER™

Synonyms Albuterol Sulfate; Salbutamol

Generic Available Yes: Excludes extended release

Pharmacologic Category Beta₂-Adrenergic Agonist

Medication Safety Issues
Sound-alike/look-alike issues:
Albuterol may be confused with Albutein®, atenolol
Proventil® may be confused with Bentyl®, Prilosec® Prinivil®
Salbutamol may be confused with salmeterol
Ventolin® may be confused with phentolamine, Benylin®, Vantin®
Volmax® may be confused with Flomax®

Use Bronchodilator in reversible airway obstruction due to asthma or COPD; prevention of exercise-induced bronchospasm

Mechanism of Action/Effect Relaxes bronchial smooth muscle by action on beta₂-receptors with little effect on heart rate

Contraindications Hypersensitivity to albuterol, adrenergic amines, or any component of the formulation

Warnings/Precautions Optimize anti-inflammatory treatment before initiating maintenance treatment with albuterol. Do not use as a component of chronic therapy without an anti-inflammatory agent. Only the mildest forms of asthma (Step 1 and/or exercise-induced) would not require concurrent use based upon asthma guidelines. Patient must be instructed to seek medical attention in cases where acute symptoms are not relieved or a previous level of response is diminished. The need to increase frequency of use may indicate deterioration of asthma, and treatment must not be delayed.

Use caution in patients with cardiovascular disease (arrhythmia or hypertension or CHF), convulsive disorders, diabetes, glaucoma, hyperthyroidism, or hypokalemia. Beta agonists may cause elevation in blood pressure, heart rate, and result in CNS stimulation/excitation. Beta₂ agonists may increase risk of arrhythmia, increase serum glucose, or decrease serum potassium.

Do not exceed recommended dose; serious adverse events including fatalities, have been associated with excessive use of inhaled sympathomimetics. Rarely, paradoxical bronchospasm may occur with use of inhaled bronchodilating agents; this should be distinguished (Continued)

Albuterol *(Continued)*

from inadequate response. All patients should utilize a spacer device when using a metered-dose inhaler; in addition, face masks should be used in children <4 years of age.

Because of its minimal effect on beta$_1$-receptors and its relatively long duration of action, albuterol is a rational choice in the elderly when an inhaled beta agonist is indicated. Oral use should be avoided in the elderly due to adverse effects. Patient response may vary between inhalers that contain chlorofluorocarbons and those which are chlorofluorocarbon-free.

Drug Interactions
Cytochrome P450 Effect: Substrate of CYP3A4 (major)

Decreased Effect: When used with nonselective beta-adrenergic blockers (eg, propranolol) the effect of albuterol is decreased. Levels/effects of albuterol may be decreased by aminoglutethimide, carbamazepine, nafcillin, nevirapine, phenobarbital, phenytoin, rifamycins, and other CYP3A4 inducers.

Increased Effect/Toxicity: When used with inhaled ipratropium, an increased duration of bronchodilation may occur. Cardiovascular effects are potentiated in patients also receiving MAO inhibitors, tricyclic antidepressants, and sympathomimetic agents (eg, amphetamine, dopamine, dobutamine). Albuterol may increase the risk of malignant arrhythmias with inhaled anesthetics (eg, enflurane, halothane).

Nutritional/Ethanol Interactions
Food: Avoid or limit caffeine (may cause CNS stimulation).
Herb/Nutraceutical: Avoid ephedra, yohimbe (may cause CNS stimulation).

Lab Interactions
Increased renin (S), aldosterone (S)

Adverse Reactions
Incidence of adverse effects is dependent upon age of patient, dose, and route of administration.

Cardiovascular: Angina, atrial fibrillation, chest discomfort, extrasystoles, flushing, hypertension, palpitation, tachycardia

Central nervous system: CNS stimulation, dizziness, drowsiness, headache, insomnia, irritability, lightheadedness, migraine, nervousness, nightmares, restlessness, sleeplessness, tremor

Dermatologic: Angioedema, erythema multiforme, rash, Stevens-Johnson syndrome, urticaria

Endocrine & metabolic: Hypokalemia, serum glucose increased, serum potassium decreased

Gastrointestinal: Diarrhea, dry mouth, gastroenteritis, nausea, unusual taste, vomiting, tooth discoloration

Genitourinary: Micturition difficulty

Neuromuscular & skeletal: Muscle cramps, weakness

Otic: Otitis media, vertigo

Respiratory: Asthma exacerbation, bronchospasm, cough, epistaxis, laryngitis, oropharyngeal drying/irritation, oropharyngeal edema

Miscellaneous: Allergic reaction, lymphadenopathy

Overdosage/Toxicology
Symptoms of overdose include tachycardia, tremor, hypertension, angina, and seizures. Hypokalemia also may occur. Cardiac arrest and death may be associated with abuse of beta-agonist bronchodilators. Treatment includes immediate discontinuation and symptomatic and supportive therapies. Cautious use of beta-adrenergic blocking agents may be considered in severe cases.

Pharmacodynamics/Kinetics
Onset of Action: Peak effect: Nebulization/oral inhalation: 0.5-2 hours; Oral: 2-3 hours

Duration of Action: Nebulization/oral inhalation: 3-4 hours; Oral: 4-6 hours

Half-Life Elimination: Inhalation: 3.8 hours; Oral: 3.7-5 hours

Metabolism: Hepatic to an inactive sulfate

Excretion: Urine (30% as unchanged drug)

Dosing
Adults:

Acute treatment of bronchospasm:
Inhalation: MDI 90 mcg/puff: 4-8 puffs every 20 minutes for up to 4 hours, then every 1-4 hours as needed
Nebulization: 2.5 mg, diluted to a total of 3 mL, 3-4 times/day over 5-15 minutes
NIH guidelines: 1.25-5 mg every 4-8 hours

Bronchospasm in ICU patients (acute):
Nebulization: 2.5-5 mg every 20 minutes for 3 doses, then 2.5-10 mg every 1-4 hours as needed, **or** 10-15 mg/hour continuously

Chronic treatment of bronchospasm:
Inhalation: MDI 90 mcg/puff: 1-2 inhalations every 4-6 hours; maximum: 12 inhalations/day
NIH guidelines: 2 puffs 3-4 times a day as needed; may double dose for mild exacerbations
Oral:
Regular release: 2-4 mg/dose 3-4 times/day; maximum dose not to exceed 32 mg/day (divided doses)
Extended release: 8 mg every 12 hours; maximum dose not to exceed 32 mg/day (divided doses). A 4 mg dose every 12 hours may be sufficient in some patients, such as adults of low body weight.

Prophylaxis of exercise-induced bronchospasm: Inhalation: MDI 90 mcg/puff: 2 puffs 5-30 minutes prior to exercise

Elderly:
Inhalation: Refer to adult dosing.
Bronchospasm (treatment): Oral: 2 mg 3-4 times/day; maximum: 8 mg 4 times/day

Pediatrics:

Bronchospasm (acute):
Inhalation: MDI 90 mcg/puff:
Children ≤12 years: 4-8 puffs every 20 minutes for 3 doses, then every 1-4 hours; spacer/holding-chamber device should be used

Children >12 years: Refer to adult dosing.

Nebulization:

Children ≤12 years: Solution 0.5%: 0.15 mg/kg (minimum dose: 2.5 mg) every 20 minutes for 3 doses, then 0.15-0.3 mg/kg (up to 10 mg) every 1-4 hours as needed; may also use 0.5 mg/kg/hour by continuous infusion. Continuous nebulized albuterol at 0.3 mg/kg/hour has been used safely in the treatment of severe status asthmaticus in children; continuous nebulized doses of 3 mg/kg/hour ± 2.2 mg/kg/hour in children whose mean age was 20.7 months resulted in no cardiac toxicity; the optimal dosage for continuous nebulization remains to be determined.

Children >12 years: Refer to adult dosing.

Prophylaxis of exercise-induced bronchospasm:

Inhalation: MDI 90 mcg/puff:

Children ≤12 years: 1-2 puffs 5 minutes prior to exercise

Children >12 years: Refer to adult dosing.

Chronic treatment of bronchospasm:

Inhalation: MDI 90 mcg/puff: Children ≥4 years: Refer to adult dosing.

Oral:

Children: 2-6 years: 0.1-0.2 mg/kg/dose 3 times/day; maximum dose not to exceed 12 mg/day (divided doses)

Children: 6-12 years: 2 mg/dose 3-4 times/day; maximum dose not to exceed 24 mg/day (divided doses)

Extended release: 4 mg every 12 hours; maximum dose not to exceed 24 mg/day (divided doses)

Children >12 years: Refer to adult dosing.

Nebulization:

Children ≤12 years: 0.05 mg/kg every 4-6 hours; minimum dose: 1.25 mg, maximum dose: 2.5 mg

2-12 years: AccuNeb™: 0.63 mg or 1.25 mg 3-4 times/day, as needed, delivered over 5-15 minutes

Note: Use of the 0.5% solution should be used for bronchospasm (acute or treatment) in children <15 kg.

Children >40 kg, patients with more severe asthma, or children 11-12 years: May respond better with a 1.25 mg dose

Children >12 years: Refer to adult dosing.

Renal Impairment: Not removed by hemodialysis

Available Dosage Forms [DSC] = Discontinued product

Aerosol, oral: 90 mcg/dose (17 g) [200 doses]

Proventil®: 90 mcg/dose (17 g) [200 doses]

Aerosol, oral, as sulfate [chlorofluorocarbon free]:

Proventil® HFA: 90 mcg/dose (6.7 g) [200 doses]

Ventolin® HFA: 90 mcg/dose (18 g) [200 doses]

Solution for oral inhalation, as sulfate: 0.083% (3 mL); 0.5% (20 mL)

AccuNeb™: 0.63 mg/3 mL (3 mL); 1.25 mg/3 mL (3 mL)

Proventil®: 0.083% (3 mL); 0.5% (20 mL)

Syrup, as sulfate: 2 mg/5 mL (480 mL)

Tablet, as sulfate: 2 mg, 4 mg

Tablet, extended release, as sulfate:

Proventil® Repetabs®: 4 mg

Volmax® [DSC], VoSpire ER™: 4 mg, 8 mg

Monitoring and Teaching Issues

Physical Assessment: Assess effectiveness and interactions of other medications patient may be taking. Monitor vital signs, effectiveness of therapy, and adverse reactions at beginning of therapy and periodically with long-term use. Assess knowledge/teach patient appropriate use, interventions to reduce side effects, and adverse symptoms to report.

Monitoring Laboratory Tests: Arterial or capillary blood gases (if patients condition warrants); FEV$_1$, peak flow, and/or other pulmonary function tests; serum potassium, serum glucose (in selected patients)

Patient Education: Use exactly as directed; do not use more often than recommended. Take oral medicine with water 1 hour before or 2 hours after meals. Maintain adequate hydration (2-3 L/day of fluids) unless instructed to restrict fluid intake. You may experience nervousness, dizziness, or fatigue (use caution when driving or engaging in hazardous activities until response to drug is known); dry mouth, unpleasant taste, stomach upset (frequent, small meals, frequent mouth care, chewing gum, or sucking lozenges may help); or difficulty urinating (always void before treatment). Report unresolved GI upset, dizziness or fatigue, vision changes, chest pain or palpitations, persistent inability to void, nervousness or insomnia, muscle cramping or tremor, or unusual cough.

Self-administered inhalation: Do not freeze. Shake canister before using. Sit when using medication. Close eyes when administering albuterol to avoid spray getting into eyes. Exhale slowly and completely through nose; inhale deeply through mouth while administering aerosol. Hold breath for 5-10 seconds after inhalation. Wait at least 1 full minute between inhalations. Wash mouthpiece between use. If more than one inhalation medication is used, use albuterol first and wait 5 minutes between medications. Prime inhaler prior to first use, and whenever the inhaler has not been used for more than 2 weeks, by releasing 4 test sprays into the air (away from face). Discard inhaler after labeled number of doses are used, even if the canister does not feel empty. **Ventolin® HFA:** Discard canister after 200 actuations or 3 months after removal from foil pouch, whichever comes first. Store with mouthpiece down. Do not allow metal canister to become wet.

Self-administered nebulizer: Wash hands before and after treatment. Wash and dry nebulizer after each treatment. Twist open the top of one unit dose vial and squeeze contents into nebulizer reservoir. Connect nebulizer reservoir to the mouthpiece or face mask. Connect nebulizer to compressor. Sit in comfortable, upright position. Place mouthpiece in your mouth or put on face mask and turn on compressor. If face mask is used, avoid leakage around the mask to avoid mist getting into eyes which may cause vision problems.

(Continued)

Albuterol *(Continued)*

Breathe calmly and deeply until no more mist is formed in nebulizer (about 5 minutes). At this point treatment is finished.

Volmax®: Tablets should be swallowed whole; do not crush or chew. Outer coating of tablet is not absorbed and may be found eliminated in stool.

Dietary Considerations: Oral forms should be administered with water 1 hour before or 2 hours after meals.

Geriatric Considerations: Because of its minimal effect on beta₁-receptors and its relatively long duration of action, albuterol is a rational choice in the elderly when a beta agonist is indicated. Elderly patients may find it beneficial to utilize a spacer device when using a metered dose inhaler. The Ventolin Rotahaler® is an alternative for patients who have difficulty using the metered dose inhaler. Oral use should be avoided due to adverse effects.

Pregnancy Risk Factor: C

Pregnancy Issues: Albuterol crosses the placenta; tocolytic effects, fetal tachycardia, fetal hypoglycemia secondary to maternal hyperglycemia with oral or intravenous routes reported. Available evidence suggests safe use during pregnancy.

Lactation: Excretion in breast milk unknown/use caution

Administration

Oral: Do not crush or chew extended release tablets.

Inhalation: MDI: Shake well before use; prime prior to first use, and whenever inhaler has not been used for >2 weeks, by releasing 4 test sprays into the air (away from face)

Reconstitution: Nebulization 0.5% solution: To prepare a 2.5 mg dose, dilute 0.5 mL of solution to a total of 3 mL with normal saline; also compatible with cromolyn or ipratropium nebulizer solutions.

Storage:

Syrup, nebulization 0.5% solution: Store at 2°C to 30°C (36°F to 86°F)

HFA aerosols: Store at 15°C to 25°C (59°F to 77°F)

Ventolin® HFA: Discard after using 200 actuations or 3 months after removal from protective pouch, whichever comes first. Store with mouthpiece down.

Inhalation solution: AccuNeb™: Store at 2°C to 25°C (36°F to 77°F). Do not use if solution changes color or becomes cloudy. Use within 1 week of opening foil pouch.

Related Information

Inhalant Agents *on page 1734*

♦ **Albuterol and Ipratropium** *see* Ipratropium and Albuterol *on page 827*

♦ **Albuterol Sulfate** *see* Albuterol *on page 59*

♦ **Alcaine®** *see page 1625*

♦ **Alcalak [OTC]** *see* Calcium Carbonate *on page 235*

♦ **Aldactazide®** *see* Hydrochlorothiazide and Spironolactone *on page 753*

♦ **Aldactone®** *see* Spironolactone *on page 1391*

♦ **Aldara™** *see* Imiquimod *on page 792*

Aldesleukin *(al des LOO kin)*

U.S. Brand Names Proleukin®

Synonyms Epidermal Thymocyte Activating Factor; ETAF; IL-2; Interleukin-2; Lymphocyte Mitogenic Factor; NSC-373364; T-Cell Growth Factor; TCGF; Thymocyte-Stimulating Factor

Generic Available No

Pharmacologic Category Biological Response Modulator

Medication Safety Issues

Sound-alike/look-alike issues:

Aldesleukin may be confused with oprelvekin

Proleukin® may be confused with oprelvekin

Use Treatment of metastatic renal cell cancer, melanoma

Unlabeled/Investigational Use Investigational: Multiple myeloma, HIV infection, and AIDS; may be used in conjunction with lymphokine-activated killer (LAK) cells, tumor-infiltrating lymphocyte (TIL) cells, interleukin-1, and interferons; colorectal cancer; non-Hodgkin's lymphoma

Mechanism of Action/Effect Aldesleukin promotes proliferation, differentiation, and recruitment of T and B cells, natural killer (NK) cells, and thymocytes; also causes cytolytic activity in a subset of lymphocytes and subsequent interactions between the immune system and malignant cells; can stimulate lymphokine-activated killer (LAK) cells and tumor-infiltrating lymphocytes (TIL) cells. LAK cells (which are derived from lymphocytes from a patient and incubated in aldesleukin) have the ability to lyse cells which are resistant to NK cells; TIL cells (which are derived from cancerous tissue from a patient and incubated in aldesleukin) have been shown to be 50% more effective than LAK cells.

Contraindications Hypersensitivity to aldesleukin or any component of the formulation; patients with abnormal thallium stress or pulmonary function tests; patients who have had an organ allograft; retreatment in patients who have experienced sustained ventricular tachycardia (≥5 beats), refractory cardiac rhythm disturbances, recurrent chest pain with ECG changes consistent with angina or myocardial infarction, intubation ≥72 hours, pericardial tamponade, renal dialysis for ≥72 hours, coma or toxic psychosis lasting ≥48 hours, repetitive or refractory seizures, bowel ischemia/perforation, GI bleeding requiring surgery

Warnings/Precautions Has been associated with capillary leak syndrome (CLS). CLS results in hypotension and reduced organ perfusion which may be severe and can result in death. Therapy should be restricted to patients with normal cardiac and pulmonary functions as defined by thallium stress and formal pulmonary function testing. Extreme caution should be used in patients with normal thallium stress tests and pulmonary functions tests who have a history of prior cardiac or pulmonary disease.

Intensive aldesleukin treatment is associated with impaired neutrophil function (reduced chemotaxis) and with an increased risk of disseminated infection, including sepsis and bacterial endocarditis, in treated patients. Consequently, pre-existing bacterial infections should be adequately treated prior to initiation of therapy. Additionally, all patients with indwelling central lines should receive antibiotic prophylaxis effective against *S. aureus*.

May exacerbate pre-existing or initial presentation of autoimmune diseases and inflammatory disorders. Patients should be evaluated and treated for CNS metastases and have a negative scan prior to treatment. Mental status changes (irritability, confusion, depression) can occur and may indicate bacteremia, hypoperfusion, CNS malignancy, or CNS toxicity.

Disseminated infections acquired in the course of treatment are a major contributor to treatment morbidity and use of antibiotic prophylaxis, and aggressive treatment of suspected and documented infections may reduce the morbidity of aldesleukin treatment.

Drug Interactions
Decreased Effect: Corticosteroids have been shown to decrease toxicity of aldesleukin, but have not been used since there is concern that they may reduce the efficacy of the lymphokine.

Increased Effect/Toxicity: Aldesleukin may affect central nervous function; therefore, interactions could occur following concomitant administration of psychotropic drugs (eg, narcotics, analgesics, antiemetics, sedatives, tranquilizers).

Concomitant administration of drugs possessing nephrotoxic (eg, aminoglycosides, indomethacin), myelotoxic (eg, cytotoxic chemotherapy), cardiotoxic (eg, doxorubicin), or hepatotoxic (eg, methotrexate, asparaginase) effects with aldesleukin may increase toxicity in these organ systems. The safety and efficacy of aldesleukin in combination with chemotherapies has not been established.

Beta-blockers and other antihypertensives may potentiate the hypotension seen with aldesleukin.

Nutritional/Ethanol Interactions
Ethanol: Avoid ethanol (due to CNS adverse effects)

Adverse Reactions
>10%:
Cardiovascular: Hypotension (85%), dose-limiting, possibly fatal; sinus tachycardia (70%); arrhythmia (22%); edema (47%); angina

Central nervous system: Mental status changes (transient memory loss, confusion, drowsiness) (73%); dizziness (17%); cognitive changes, fatigue, malaise, somnolence and disorientation (25%); headaches, insomnia, paranoid delusion

Dermatologic: Macular erythematous rash (100% of patients on high-dose therapy); pruritus (48%); erythema (41%); rash (26%); exfoliative dermatitis (14%); dry skin (15%)

Endocrine & metabolic: Fever and chills (89%); low electrolyte levels (magnesium, calcium, phosphate, potassium, sodium) (1% to 15%)

Gastrointestinal: Nausea and vomiting (87%); diarrhea (76%); stomatitis (32%); GI bleeding (13%); weight gain (23%), anorexia (27%)

Hematologic: Anemia (77%); thrombocytopenia (64%); leukopenia (34%) - may be dose-limiting; coagulation disorders (10%)

Hepatic: Transient elevations of bilirubin (64%) and enzymes (56%); jaundice (11%)

Neuromuscular & skeletal: Weakness; rigors - respond to acetaminophen, diphenhydramine, an NSAID, or meperidine

Renal: Oliguria/anuria (63%, severe in 5% to 6%), proteinuria (12%); renal failure (dose-limiting toxicity) manifested as oliguria noted within 24-48 hours of initiation of therapy; marked fluid retention, azotemia, and increased serum creatinine seen, which may return to baseline within 7 days of discontinuation of therapy; hypophosphatemia

Respiratory: Congestion (54%); dyspnea (27% to 52%)

Miscellaneous: Pain (54%), infection (including sepsis and endocarditis) due to neutrophil impairment (23%)

1% to 10%:
Cardiovascular: Capillary leak syndrome, including peripheral edema, ascites, pulmonary infiltration, and pleural effusion (2% to 4%), may be dose-limiting and potentially fatal; MI (2%)

Central nervous system: Seizures (1%)

Endocrine & metabolic: Hypo- and hyperglycemia (2%); increased electrolyte levels (magnesium, calcium, phosphate, potassium, sodium) (1%), hypothyroidism

Hepatic: Ascites (4%)

Neuromuscular & skeletal: Arthralgia (6%), myalgia (6%)

Renal: Hematuria (9%), increased creatinine (5%)

Respiratory: Pleural effusions, edema (10%)

Overdosage/Toxicology
Side effects following the use of aldesleukin are dose related. Administration of more than the recommended dose has been associated with a more rapid onset of expected dose-limiting toxicities. Adverse reactions generally will reverse when the drug is stopped particularly because of its short serum half-life. Provide supportive treatment of any continuing symptoms. Life-threatening toxicities have been ameliorated by the I.V. administration of dexamethasone, but may result in a less than therapeutic effect of aldesleukin.

Pharmacodynamics/Kinetics
Bioavailability: I.M.: 37%

Half-Life Elimination: Initial: 6-13 minutes; Terminal: 80-120 minutes

Dosing
Adults & Elderly: Refer to individual protocols.

Renal cell carcinoma: I.V.: 600,000 int. units/kg every 8 hours for a maximum of 14 doses; repeat after 9 days of rest for a total of 28 doses per course. Re-evaluate at 4 weeks. Retreat if needed 7 weeks after hospital discharge from previous course.

Melanoma:
I.V.:
Single-agent use: 600,000 int. units/kg every 8 hours for a maximum of 14 doses; repeat after 9 days of rest for a total of 28 doses per course. Re-evaluate at 4 weeks. Retreat if needed 7 weeks after hospital discharge from previous course.

In combination with cytotoxic agents: 24 million int. units/m^2 days 12-16 and 19-23

(Continued)

Aldesleukin *(Continued)*

SubQ:

Single-agent doses: 3-18 million int. units/day for 5 days weekly and repeated weekly up to 6 weeks

In combination with interferon:

5 million int. units/m² 3 times/week

1.8 million int. units/m² twice daily 5 days/week for 6 weeks

Investigational regimen: SubQ: 11 million int. units (flat dose) daily x 4 days per week for 4 consecutive weeks; repeat every 6 weeks

Available Dosage Forms Injection, powder for reconstitution: 22 x 10⁶ int. units [18 million int. units/mL = 1.1 mg/mL when reconstituted]

Monitoring and Teaching Issues

Physical Assessment: Assess potential for interactions with other prescriptions, OTC medications, or herbal products patient may be taking. See I.V. Administration specifics. Infusion site should be monitored for extravasation. Vital signs; cardiac, respiratory, and CNS status; fluid balance; signs of systemic sepsis, changes in mental status, and laboratory reports should be assessed daily prior to beginning infusion and for 2 hours following infusion. Teach patient possible side effects/appropriate interventions and adverse symptoms to report.

Monitoring Laboratory Tests: CBC, differential, and platelet counts; blood chemistries including electrolytes, renal and hepatic function; chest x-rays

Patient Education: Do not take any new medication during therapy unless approved by prescriber. Avoid alcohol. Maintain adequate hydration (2-3 L/day of fluids) unless instructed to restrict fluid intake. You will be susceptible to infection (avoid crowds and exposure to infection and do not have any vaccinations without consulting prescriber). May cause increased sensitivity to sunlight (use sunblock 15 SPF or greater, wear protective clothing, avoid direct sun exposure); or nausea, vomiting, stomatitis, anorexia (frequent mouth care, small frequent meals, chewing gum, or sucking lozenges may help). This drug may result in many side effects; you will be monitored and assessed closely during therapy, however, it is important that you report any changes or problems for evaluation. Report any changes in urination, unusual bruising or bleeding, chest pain or palpitations, acute dizziness, respiratory difficulty, fever or chills, changes in cognition, rash, feelings of pain or numbness in extremities, severe or persistent GI upset or diarrhea, vaginal discharge or mouth sores, yellowing of eyes or skin, or changes in color of urine or stool.

Pregnancy/breast-feeding precautions: Inform prescriber if you are pregnant. Do not breast-feed.

Pregnancy Risk Factor: C

Pregnancy Issues: Use during pregnancy only if benefits to the mother outweigh potential risk to the fetus. Contraception is recommended for fertile males or females using this medication.

Lactation: Enters breast milk/contraindicated

Administration

I.V.: Infuse over 15 minutes.

Other: May be administered by SubQ injection.

Reconstitution: Reconstituted or diluted solution should be refrigerated. Gently swirl, do not shake.

Concentrations <30 mcg/mL **OR** concentrations between ≥30-70 mcg/mL for infusion via ambulatory infusion pump require addition of albumin (final albumin concentration: 0.1%), see table.

Final Dilution Concentration (mcg/mL)	Final Dilution Concentration (10⁶int. units/mL)	Stability
<30	<0.49	Albumin must be added to bag **prior to addition** of aldesleukin at a final concentration of 0.1% (1 mg/mL) albumin; stable at room temperature or at ≥32°C (89°F) for 6 days[1,2]
≥30 to ≤70	≥0.49 to ≤1.1	Stable at room temperature at 6 days without albumin added or at ≥32°C (89°F) for 6 days only if albumin is added (0.1%)[1,2]
70-100	1.2-1.6	Unstable; avoid use
>100-500	1.7-8.2	Stable at room temperature and at ≥32°C (89°F) for 6 days[1,2]

[1]These solutions do not contain a preservative; use for more than 24 hours may not be advisable.

[2]Continuous infusion via ambulatory infusion device raises aldesleukin to this temperature.

Note: As with most biological proteins, solutions containing aldesleukin should not be filtered; filtration will result in significant loss of bioactivity.

Compatibility: Stable in D₅W

Y-site administration: Incompatible with ganciclovir, lorazepam, pentamidine, prochlorperazine edisylate, promethazine

Compatibility when admixed: Incompatible with NS

Storage: Store vials of lyophilized injection in a refrigerator at 2°C to 8°C (36°F to 46°F).

Additional Information

1 Cetus unit = 6 int. units

1.1 mg = 18 x 10⁶ int. units (or 3 x 10⁶ Cetus units)

1 Roche unit (Teceleukin) = 3 int. units

♦ Aldomet *see* Methyldopa *on page 980*

♦ Aldoril® *see* Methyldopa and Hydrochlorothiazide *on page 981*

Alefacept *(a LE fa sept)*

U.S. Brand Names Amevive®

Synonyms B 9273; BG 9273; Human LFA-3/IgG(1) Fusion Protein; LFA-3/IgG(1) Fusion Protein, Human

Restructions Alefacept will be distributed directly to physician offices or to a specialty pharmacy; injections are intended to be administered in the physician's office

Generic Available No

Pharmacologic Category Monoclonal Antibody

Use Treatment of moderate to severe plaque psoriasis in adults who are candidates for systemic therapy or phototherapy

Mechanism of Action/Effect Alefacept is a monoclonal antibody against a specific receptor on T-lymphocytes, and reduces the number of both CD4+ and CD8+ T-lymphocytes. It improves symptoms of psoriasis by decreasing the number of activated T-lymphocytes, and their production of inflammatory mediators such as interferon gamma.

Contraindications Hypersensitivity to alefacept or any component of the formulation; patients with a pretreatment depression in CD4 T-lymphocytes; history of severe malignancy; clinically-important infection

Warnings/Precautions Alefacept induces a decline in circulating T-lymphocytes (CD4+ and CD8+); CD4+ lymphocyte counts should be monitored weekly throughout therapy. Do not initiate in pre-existing depression of CD4+ lymphocytes and withhold treatment in any patient who develops a depressed CD4+ lymphocyte count (<250 cells/μL) during treatment; permanently discontinue if CD4+ lymphocyte counts remain <250 cells/μL for 1 month.

Alefacept may increase the risk of malignancies; use caution in patients at high risk for malignancy. Discontinue if malignancy develops during therapy. Alefacept may increase the risk of infection and may reactivate latent infection; monitor for new infections. Avoid use in patients receiving other immunosuppressant drugs or phototherapy. Safety and efficacy of live or attenuated vaccines have not been evaluated. Not indicated for use in pediatric patients.

Drug Interactions

Decreased Effect: No formal drug interaction studies have been completed.

Increased Effect/Toxicity: No formal drug interaction studies have been completed.

Adverse Reactions

≥10%:

Hematologic: Lymphopenia (up to 10% of patients required temporary discontinuation, up to 17% during a second course of therapy)

Local: Injection site reactions (up to 16% of patients; includes pain, inflammation, bleeding, edema, or other reaction)

1% to 10%:

Central nervous system: Chills (6%; primarily during intravenous administration), dizziness

Dermatologic: Pruritus

Gastrointestinal: Nausea

Neuromuscular & skeletal: Myalgia

Respiratory: Pharyngitis, cough increased

Miscellaneous: Malignancies (1% vs 0.2% in placebo), antibodies to alefacept (3%; significance unknown), infection (1% to 2% requiring hospitalization)

Overdosage/Toxicology No specific experience in overdose. Symptoms may include chills, headache, arthralgia, and sinusitis. Reductions in lymphocyte populations should be closely monitored. Treatment is supportive.

Pharmacodynamics/Kinetics

Bioavailability: 63% (following I.M. administration)

Half-Life Elimination: 270 hours (following I.V. administration)

Excretion: Clearance: 0.25 mL/hour/kg

Dosing

Adults & Elderly: Psoriasis (moderate to severe plaque psoriasis):

I.V.: 7.5 mg once weekly; usual duration of treatment: 12 weeks

I.M.: 15 mg once weekly; usual duration of treatment: 12 weeks

Second course: A second course of treatment may be initiated at least 12 weeks after completion of the initial course of treatment, provided CD4+ T-lymphocyte counts are within the normal range.

Note: CD4+ T-lymphocyte counts should be monitored before initiation of treatment and weekly during therapy. Dosing should be withheld if CD4+ counts are <250 cells/μL, and dosing should be permanently discontinued if CD4+ lymphocyte counts remain at <250 cell/μL for longer than 1 month.

Renal Impairment: No dosage adjustment required.

Available Dosage Forms [DSC] = Discontinued product

Injection, powder for reconstitution: 7.5 mg [for I.V. administration; supplied with SWFI] [DSC]

Injection, powder for reconstitution: 15 mg [for I.M. administration; supplied with SWFI]

Monitoring and Teaching Issues

Physical Assessment: Monitor closely for the development of malignancies or infections. Assess results of laboratory tests. Assess effectiveness and adverse response. Teach patient possible side effects/appropriate interventions and adverse symptoms to report.

Monitoring Laboratory Tests: Baseline lymphocyte counts prior to initiation and weekly during treatment course

Patient Education: This medication can only be administered by infusion or injection; report immediately any pain, redness, swelling at injection or infusion site, chills, rash, difficulty swallowing or breathing, or feelings of tightness in chest. You will need weekly blood tests while taking this medication. May cause nausea or muscle pain. Report unusual feelings of fatigue or weakness; signs of infection (eg, cough, runny nose, sore throat, unusual cough, swollen glands, mouth sores, vaginal itching or discharge, burning on urination, fever, chills, or unhealed sores). Notify prescriber if pregnancy occurs during therapy or within 8 weeks of treatment. **Breast-feeding precaution:** Breast-feeding is not recommended.

Pregnancy Risk Factor: B

Pregnancy Issues: Patients who become pregnant during therapy or within 8 weeks of treatment are advised to enroll in pregnancy registry (866-263-8483).

(Continued)

Alefacept (Continued)

Lactation: Excretion in breast milk unknown/not recommended

Breast-Feeding Issues: It is not known whether alefacept is excreted in breast milk. Since alefacept is an immunosuppressant, and transfer of proteins into breast milk may occur, breast-feeding women are cautioned to discontinue breast-feeding or to discontinue use of the drug while breast-feeding (recommendations per manufacturer).

Administration

I.M.: I.M. injections should be administered at least 1 inch from previous administration sites.

I.V.: Do not filter alefacept solutions. I.V. administration set should be primed with 3 mL NS and the line should be flushed with 3 mL NS following the dose. Administer over ≤5 seconds.

Reconstitution: Reconstitute 15 mg vial for I.M. solution with 0.6 mL of SWFI (supplied); 0.5 mL of reconstituted solution contains 15 mg of alefacept. Reconstitute 7.5 mg vial for I.V. administration with 0.6 mL of SWFI (supplied); 0.5 mL of reconstituted solution contains 7.5 mg alefacept.

Gently swirl to avoid foaming. Do not filter reconstituted solutions. Do not mix with other medications or solutions.

Compatibility: Do not mix with other medications or solutions.

Storage: Store at 15°C to 30°C (59°F to 86°F). Protect from light. Following reconstitution, may be stored for up to 4 hours at 2°C to 8°C (36°F to 46°F). Discard any unused solution after 4 hours.

Alendronate (a LEN droe nate)

U.S. Brand Names Fosamax®

Synonyms Alendronate Sodium

Generic Available No

Pharmacologic Category Bisphosphonate Derivative

Medication Safety Issues

Sound-alike/look-alike issues:

Fosamax® may be confused with Flomax®

Use Treatment and prevention of osteoporosis in postmenopausal females; treatment of osteoporosis in males; Paget's disease of the bone in patients who are symptomatic, at risk for future complications, or with alkaline phosphatase ≥2 times the upper limit of normal; treatment of glucocorticoid-induced osteoporosis in males and females with low bone mineral density who are receiving a daily dosage ≥7.5 mg of prednisone (or equivalent)

Mechanism of Action/Effect A bisphosphonate which inhibits bone resorption via actions on osteoclasts or on osteoclast precursors; decreases the rate of bone resorption, leading to an indirect increase in bone mineral density. In Paget's disease, characterized by disordered resorption and formation of bone, inhibition of resorption leads to an indirect decrease in bone formation; but the newly-formed bone has a more normal architecture.

Contraindications Hypersensitivity to alendronate, other bisphosphonates, or any component of the formulation; hypocalcemia; abnormalities of the esophagus which delay esophageal emptying such as stricture or achalasia; inability to stand or sit upright for at least 30 minutes; oral solution should not be used in patients at risk of aspiration

Warnings/Precautions Use caution in patients with renal impairment; hypocalcemia must be corrected before therapy initiation; ensure adequate calcium and vitamin D intake. May cause irritation to upper gastrointestinal mucosa. Esophagitis, esophageal ulcers, esophageal erosions, and esophageal stricture (rare) have been reported; risk increases in patients unable to comply with dosing instructions. Use with caution in patients with dysphagia, esophageal disease, gastritis, duodenitis, or ulcers (may worsen underlying condition).

Drug Interactions

Decreased Effect: Oral medications (especially those containing multivalent cations, including calcium and antacids): May interfere with alendronate absorption; wait at least 30 minutes after taking alendronate before taking any oral medications

Increased Effect/Toxicity: I.V. ranitidine has been shown to double the bioavailability of alendronate. Estrogen replacement therapy, in combination with alendronate, may enhance the therapeutic effects of both agents on the maintenance of bone mineralization. An increased incidence of adverse GI effects has been noted when >10 mg alendronate is used in patients taking aspirin-containing products.

Nutritional/Ethanol Interactions Food: All food and beverages interfere with absorption. Coadministration with caffeine may reduce alendronate efficacy. Coadministration with dairy products may decrease alendronate absorption. Beverages (especially orange juice and coffee), food, and medications (eg, antacids, calcium, iron, and multivalent cations) may reduce the absorption of alendronate as much as 60%.

Adverse Reactions Note: Incidence of adverse effects increases significantly in patients treated for Paget's disease at 40 mg/day, mostly GI adverse effects.

>10%: Endocrine & metabolic: Hypocalcemia (transient, mild, 18%); hypophosphatemia (transient, mild, 10%)

1% to 10%:

Central nervous system: Headache (0.2% to 3%)

Gastrointestinal: Abdominal pain (1% to 7%), acid reflux (1% to 5%), dyspepsia (1% to 4%), nausea (1% to 4%), flatulence (0.2% to 4%), diarrhea (0.6% to 3%), constipation (0.3% to 3%), esophageal ulcer (0.1% to 2%), abdominal distension (0.2% to 1%), gastritis (0.2% to 1%), vomiting (0.2% to 1%), dysphagia (0.1% to 1%), gastric ulcer (1%), melena (1%)

Neuromuscular & skeletal: Musculoskeletal pain (0.4% to 4%), muscle cramps (0.2% to 1%)

Overdosage/Toxicology Symptoms of overdose include hypocalcemia, hypophosphatemia, and upper GI adverse affects (eg, upset stomach, heartburn, esophagitis, gastritis, or ulcer). Treat with milk or antacids to bind alendronate. Dialysis would not be beneficial.

Pharmacodynamics/Kinetics
  Bioavailability: Fasting: Female: 0.7%; Male: 0.6%; reduced 60% with food or drink
  Protein Binding: ~78%
  Half-Life Elimination: Exceeds 10 years
  Metabolism: None
  Excretion: Urine; feces (as unabsorbed drug)

Dosing
  Adults & Elderly: Note: Patients treated with glucocorticoids and those with Paget's disease should receive adequate amounts of calcium and vitamin D.
    Osteoporosis in postmenopausal females: Oral:
      Prophylaxis: 5 mg once daily **or** 35 mg once weekly
      Treatment: 10 mg once daily **or** 70 mg once weekly
    Osteoporosis in males: Oral: 10 mg once daily **or** 70 mg once weekly
    Osteoporosis secondary to glucocorticoids in males and females: Oral: Treatment: 5 mg once daily; a dose of 10 mg once daily should be used in postmenopausal females who are not receiving estrogen.
    Paget's disease of bone in males and females: Oral: 40 mg once daily for 6 months
      Retreatment: Relapses during the 12 months following therapy occurred in 9% of patients who responded to treatment. Specific retreatment data are not available. Retreatment with alendronate may be considered, following a 6-month post-treatment evaluation period, in patients who have relapsed based on increases in serum alkaline phosphatase, which should be measured periodically. Retreatment may also be considered in those who failed to normalize their serum alkaline phosphatase.
  Renal Impairment:
    Cl$_{cr}$ 35-60 mL/minute: None necessary.
    Cl$_{cr}$ <35 mL/minute: Alendronate is not recommended due to lack of experience.
  Hepatic Impairment: No adjustment necessary.

Available Dosage Forms
  Solution, oral, as monosodium trihydrate: 70 mg/75 mL [contains parabens; raspberry flavor]
  Tablet, as sodium: 5 mg, 10 mg, 35 mg, 40 mg, 70 mg

Monitoring and Teaching Issues
  Physical Assessment: See Contraindications, Warnings/Precautions, and Dosing for use cautions. Assess results of laboratory tests, therapeutic effectiveness, and adverse reactions (eg, hypocalcemia). Teach patient appropriate use and administration of medications (see Administration), lifestyle and dietary changes that will have a beneficial impact on Paget's disease or osteoporosis, possible side effects, interventions to reduce side effects, and adverse reactions to report.
  Monitoring Laboratory Tests: Alkaline phosphatase should be periodically measured; serum calcium and phosphorus; hormonal status (male and female) prior to therapy; bone mineral density (should be done prior to initiation of therapy and after 6-12 months of combined glucocorticoid and alendronate treatment)
  Patient Education: Inform prescriber of all prescriptions, OTC medications, or herbal products you are taking, and any allergies you have. Do not take any new medication during therapy unless approved by prescriber. Take as directed, with a full glass of water first thing in the morning and at least 30 minutes before the first food or beverage of the day. Wait at least 30 minutes after taking alendronate before taking anything else. Stay in sitting or standing position for 30 minutes following administration and until after the first food of the day to reduce potential for esophageal irritation. Consult prescriber to determine necessity of lifestyle changes (eg, decreased smoking, decreased alcohol intake, dietary supplements of calcium or vitamin D). May cause flatulence, bloating, nausea, or acid regurgitation; small frequent meals may help. Report acute headache or gastric pain, unresolved GI upset, or acid stomach. **Pregnancy/breast-feeding precautions:** Inform prescriber if you are or intend to become pregnant. Consult prescriber if breast-feeding.
  Dietary Considerations: Ensure adequate calcium and vitamin D intake; however, wait at least 30 minutes after taking alendronate before taking any supplement. Must be taken with plain water first thing in the morning and at least 30 minutes before the first food or beverage of the day.
  Geriatric Considerations: Since many elderly patients receive diuretics, evaluation of electrolyte status (calcium, phosphate, magnesium, potassium) may need to be done periodically due to the drug class (bisphosphonate). Should assure immobile patients are at least sitting up for 30 minutes after swallowing tablets. Drink a full glass of water with each dose.
  Pregnancy Risk Factor: C
  Pregnancy Issues: Safety and efficacy have not been established in pregnant women. Animal studies have shown delays in delivery and fetal/neonatal death (secondary to hypocalcemia). Bisphosphonates are incorporated into the bone matrix and gradually released over time. Theoretically, there may be a risk of fetal harm when pregnancy follows the completion of therapy. Based on limited case reports with pamidronate, serum calcium levels in the newborn may be altered if administered during pregnancy.
  Lactation: Excretion in breast milk unknown/use caution

Administration
  Oral: Alendronate must be taken with plain water (tablets 6-8 oz; oral solution 2 oz) first thing in the morning and ≥30 minutes before the first food, beverage, or other medication of the day. Patients should be instructed to stay upright (not to lie down) for at least 30 minutes **and** until after first food of the day (to reduce esophageal irritation). Patients should receive supplemental calcium and vitamin D if dietary intake is inadequate.
  Storage: Store tablets and oral solution at room temperature of 15°C to 30°C (59°F to 86°F). Keep in well-closed container.

♦ **Alendronate Sodium** *see* Alendronate *on page 66*

♦ **Aler-Cap [OTC]** *see* DiphenhydrAMINE *on page 463*

♦ **Aler-Dryl [OTC]** *see* DiphenhydrAMINE *on page 463*

♦ **Aler-Tab [OTC]** *see* DiphenhydrAMINE *on page 463*

♦ **Alesse**® *see* Ethinyl Estradiol and Levonorgestrel *on page 585*

♦ **Aleve**® [OTC] *see* Naproxen *on page 1056*

Alfuzosin (al FYOO zoe sin)

U.S. Brand Names Uroxatral™

Synonyms Alfuzosin Hydrochloride

Generic Available No

Pharmacologic Category Alpha$_1$ Blocker

Use Treatment of the functional symptoms of benign prostatic hyperplasia (BPH)

Mechanism of Action/Effect An antagonist of alpha$_1$ adrenoreceptors in the lower urinary tract. Blockade of these adrenoreceptors can cause smooth muscles in the bladder neck and prostate to relax, resulting in an improvement in urine flow rate and a reduction in symptoms of BPH.

Contraindications Hypersensitivity to alfuzosin or any component of the formulation; moderate or severe hepatic insufficiency (Child-Pugh class B and C); potent CYP3A4 inhibitors (eg, itraconazole, ketoconazole, ritonavir)

Warnings/Precautions Not intended for use as an antihypertensive drug. May cause orthostasis, syncope, or dizziness. Patients should avoid situations where injury may occur as a result of syncope. Discontinue if symptoms of angina occur or worsen. Use caution with history of QT prolongation or use with medications which may prolong the QT interval. Rule out prostatic carcinoma before beginning therapy. Use caution with renal or mild hepatic impairment.

Drug Interactions

Cytochrome P450 Effect: Substrate of CYP3A4 (major)

Decreased Effect: Levels/effects of alfuzosin may be decreased by aminoglutethimide, carbamazepine, nafcillin, nevirapine, phenobarbital, phenytoin, rifamycins, and other CYP3A4 inducers.

Increased Effect/Toxicity: Alfuzosin levels/effects may be increased by azole antifungals, ciprofloxacin, clarithromycin, diclofenac, doxycycline, erythromycin, imatinib, isoniazid, nefazodone, nicardipine, propofol, protease inhibitors, quinidine, verapamil, and other CYP3A4 inhibitors. Concurrent use of itraconazole, ketoconazole, or ritonavir is contraindicated.

Nutritional/Ethanol Interactions

Food: Food increases the extent of absorption.

Adverse Reactions

1% to 10%:

Central nervous system: Dizziness (6%), fatigue (3%), headache (3%), pain (1% to 2%)

Gastrointestinal: Abdominal pain (1% to 2%), constipation (1% to 2%), dyspepsia (1% to 2%), nausea (1% to 2%)

Genitourinary: Impotence (1% to 2%)

Respiratory: Upper respiratory tract infection (3%), bronchitis (1% to 2%), pharyngitis (1% to 2%), sinusitis (1% to 2%)

Overdosage/Toxicology Hypotension would be expected in case of overdose. Treatment is supportive.

Pharmacodynamics/Kinetics

Absorption: Decreased 50% under fasting conditions

Bioavailability: 49% following a meal

Time to Peak: Plasma: 8 hours following a meal

Protein Binding: 82% to 90%

Half-Life Elimination: 10 hours

Metabolism: Hepatic, primarily via CYP3A4; metabolism includes oxidation, O-demethylation and N-dealkylation; forms metabolites (inactive)

Excretion: Feces (69%); urine (24%)

Dosing

Adults & Elderly: Benign prostatic hyperplasia (BPH): Oral: 10 mg once daily

Renal Impairment: Bioavailability and maximum serum concentrations are increased by ~50% with mild, moderate, or severe renal impairment.

Note: Safety has not been evaluated in patients with creatinine clearances <30 mL/minute.

Hepatic Impairment:

Mild hepatic impairment: Use has not been studied.

Moderate or severe hepatic impairment (Child-Pugh class B and C): Clearance is decreased 1/3 to 1/4 and serum concentration is increased three- to fourfold; use is contraindicated.

Available Dosage Forms Tablet, extended release, as hydrochloride: 10 mg

Monitoring and Teaching Issues

Physical Assessment: Prostatic carcinoma should be ruled out before beginning therapy. Assess for use cautions (eg, history of QT prolongation, renal or hepatic impairment; see Warnings/Precautions). Assess potential for interactions with other medications (see Drug Interactions). Monitor for patient response (eg, improved urine flow) and adverse reactions at beginning of therapy and on a regular basis with long-term therapy. Teach patient proper use, possible side effects/appropriate interventions, and adverse symptoms to report.

Patient Education: Do not take any new medication during therapy without consulting prescriber. Take exactly as directed, with a meal at the same time each day. Swallow tablet whole; do not crush or chew. May cause drowsiness, dizziness, impaired judgment (use caution when driving or engaging in tasks that require alertness until response to drug is known); or postural hypotension (use caution when rising from sitting or lying position or when climbing stairs). Report unusual chest pain, respiratory difficulty, or any persistent adverse reactions.

Dietary Considerations: Take following a meal at the same time each day.

Pregnancy Risk Factor: B

Lactation: Not indicated for use in women

Administration

Oral: Tablet should be swallowed whole; do not crush or chew. Administer once daily (with a meal); should be taken at the same time each day.

Storage: Store at controlled room temperature of 15°C to 30°C (59°F to 86°F). Protect from light and moisture.

♦ **Alfuzosin Hydrochloride** see Alfuzosin on page 68

Alglucerase (al GLOO ser ase)

U.S. Brand Names Ceredase®

Synonyms Glucocerebrosidase

Generic Available No

Pharmacologic Category Enzyme

Medication Safety Issues

Sound-alike/look-alike issues:

Ceredase® may be confused with Cerezyme®

Use Replacement therapy for Gaucher's disease (type 1)

Mechanism of Action/Effect Replaces the missing enzyme, glucocerebrosidase associated with Gaucher's disease

Contraindications Hypersensitivity to any component of the formulation

Warnings/Precautions Prepared from pooled human placental tissue that may contain the causative agents of some viral diseases. Patients who develop IgG antibodies may be at a higher risk for developing hypersensitivity. Use caution with androgen sensitive malignancies or prior allergies to hCG. May cause early virilization in males <10 years of age.

Lab Interactions False positive pregnancy tests

Adverse Reactions Frequency not defined.

Cardiovascular: Peripheral edema

Central nervous system: Chills, fatigue, fever, headache, lightheadedness

Endocrine & metabolic: Hot flashes, menstrual abnormalities

Gastrointestinal: Abdominal discomfort, diarrhea, nausea, oral ulcerations, vomiting

Local: Injection site: Abscess, burning, discomfort, pruritus, swelling

Neuromuscular & skeletal: Backache, weakness

Miscellaneous: Dysosmia; hypersensitivity reactions (abdominal cramping, angioedema, chest discomfort, flushing, hypotension, nausea, pruritus, respiratory symptoms, urticaria); IgG antibody formation (~13%)

Overdosage/Toxicology No obvious toxicity has been detected after single doses up to 234 units/kg.

Pharmacodynamics/Kinetics

Half-Life Elimination: ~3-11 minutes

Dosing

Adults & Elderly: Gaucher's disease: I.V.: Initial: 30-60 units/kg every 2 weeks; dosing is individualized based on disease severity; average dose: 60 units/kg every 2 weeks. Range: 2.5 units/kg 3 times/week to 60 units/kg 1-4 times/week. Once patient response is well established, dose may be reduced every 3-6 months to determine maintenance therapy.

Pediatrics: Refer to adult dosing.

Available Dosage Forms Injection, solution [preservative free]: 10 units/mL (5 mL); 80 units/mL (5 mL) [contains human albumin 1%]

Monitoring and Teaching Issues

Physical Assessment: Use caution with androgen sensitive malignancies or prior allergies to hCG (see Warnings/Precautions). Assess results of laboratory tests and therapeutic effectiveness (eg, energy level, change in bleeding tendency, reduced joint swelling, or bone pain). Teach patient possible side effects/appropriate interventions and adverse symptoms to report.

Monitoring Laboratory Tests: CBC, platelets, acid phosphatase (AP), plasma glucocerebroside, IgG antibody formation

Patient Education: Do not take any new medication during therapy unless approved by prescriber. This medication will not cure Gaucher's disease, but rather, may help control the disease. Treatment is required for life. May cause abdominal discomfort, nausea, or vomiting (small frequent meals, good mouth care, chewing gum, or sucking lozenges may help); these symptoms should go away with continued use. Inform prescriber if pain, swelling, or redness occurs at injection site or if GI symptoms persist. **Pregnancy/breast-feeding precautions:** Inform prescriber if you are or intend to become pregnant. Consult prescriber if breast-feeding.

Pregnancy Risk Factor: C

Lactation: Excretion in breast milk unknown/use caution

Administration

I.V.: Infuse I.V. over 1-2 hours; use of an in-line filter is recommended.

Reconstitution: Dilute with NS to a final volume ≤200 mL. Do not shake.

Storage: Refrigerate (4°C), do not freeze. Contains no preservatives. Do not store opened vials for future use. Once diluted, 100 mL and 200 mL solutions for infusion are stable for 18 hours when stored at 2°C to 8°C.

♦ **Alimta®** see Pemetrexed on page 1169

♦ **Alinia®** see Nitazoxanide on page 1087

Alitretinoin (a li TRET i noyn)

U.S. Brand Names Panretin®

Generic Available No

Pharmacologic Category Antineoplastic Agent, Miscellaneous

(Continued)

Alitretinoin (Continued)

Medication Safety Issues
Sound-alike/look-alike issues:
Panretin® may be confused with pancreatin

Use Orphan drug: Topical treatment of cutaneous lesions in AIDS-related Kaposi's sarcoma

Unlabeled/Investigational Use Cutaneous T-cell lymphomas

Mechanism of Action/Effect Binds to retinoid receptors to inhibit growth of Kaposi's sarcoma

Contraindications Hypersensitivity to alitretinoin, other retinoids, or any component of the formulation; pregnancy

Warnings/Precautions Do not use concurrently with topical products containing DEET (a common component of insect repellent products); increased toxicity may result. A common component of insect repellent products. Safety in pediatric patients or geriatric patients has not been established.

Drug Interactions
Increased Effect/Toxicity: Increased toxicity of DEET may occur if products containing this compound are used concurrently with alitretinoin. Due to limited absorption after topical application, interaction with systemic medications is unlikely.

Adverse Reactions
>10%:
Central nervous system: Pain (0% to 34%)
Dermatologic: Rash (25% to 77%), pruritus (8% to 11%)
Neuromuscular & skeletal: Paresthesia (3% to 22%)
5% to 10%:
Cardiovascular: Edema (3% to 8%)
Dermatologic: Exfoliative dermatitis (3% to 9%), skin disorder (0% to 8%)

Overdosage/Toxicology There has been no experience with human overdosage of alitretinoin, and overdose is unlikely following topical application. Treatment is symptomatic and supportive.

Pharmacodynamics/Kinetics
Absorption: Not extensive

Dosing
Adults & Elderly:
Kaposi's sarcoma: Topical: Apply gel twice daily to cutaneous lesions.
T-cell lymphomas (unlabeled use): Topical: Apply gel twice daily to cutaneous lesions.

Available Dosage Forms Gel: 0.1% (60 g tube)

Monitoring and Teaching Issues
Physical Assessment: Assess effectiveness of therapy and adverse reactions at beginning and periodically during therapy. Teach patient appropriate use/application, need to avoid DEET-containing insect repellents, and adverse symptoms to report.

Patient Education: For external use only. Use exactly as directed; do not overuse. Avoid use of any product, such as insect repellents, containing DEET (check with your pharmacist). Wear protective clothing and/or avoid exposure to direct sun or sunlamps. Wash hands thoroughly before applying. Avoid applying skin products that contain alcohol or harsh chemicals during treatment. Do not apply occlusive dressings. Stop treatment and inform prescriber if rash, skin irritation, redness, scaling, or excessive dryness appears.
Pregnancy/breast-feeding precautions: Do not get pregnant while taking this medication. Consult prescriber for appropriate contraceptive measures. Breast-feeding is not recommended.

Pregnancy Risk Factor: D

Pregnancy Issues: Potentially teratogenic and/or embryotoxic; limb, craniofacial, or skeletal defects have been observed in animal models. If used during pregnancy or if the patient becomes pregnant while using alitretinoin, the woman should be advised of potential harm to the fetus. Women of childbearing potential should avoid becoming pregnant.

Lactation: Excretion in breast milk unknown/not recommended

Breast-Feeding Issues: Excretion in human breast milk is unknown; women are advised to discontinue breast-feeding prior to using this medication.

Administration
Topical: Do not use occlusive dressings.
Storage: Store at room temperature.

Allopurinol (al oh PURE i nole)

U.S. Brand Names Aloprim™; Zyloprim®

Synonyms Allopurinol Sodium

Generic Available Yes

Pharmacologic Category Xanthine Oxidase Inhibitor

Medication Safety Issues
Sound-alike/look-alike issues:
Allopurinol may be confused with Apresoline
Zyloprim® may be confused with Xylo-Pfan®, ZORprin®

Use
Oral: Prevention of attack of gouty arthritis and nephropathy; treatment of secondary hyperuricemia which may occur during treatment of tumors or leukemia; prevention of recurrent calcium oxalate calculi

I.V.: Treatment of elevated serum and urinary uric acid levels when oral therapy is not tolerated in patients with leukemia, lymphoma, and solid tumor malignancies who are receiving cancer chemotherapy

Mechanism of Action/Effect Allopurinol inhibits xanthine oxidase, the enzyme responsible for the conversion of hypoxanthine to xanthine to uric acid. Allopurinol is metabolized to oxypurinol which is also an inhibitor of xanthine oxidase; allopurinol acts on purine catabolism, reducing the production of uric acid without disrupting the biosynthesis of vital purines.

Contraindications Hypersensitivity to allopurinol or any component of the formulation

Warnings/Precautions Do not use to treat asymptomatic hyperuricemia. Discontinue at first signs of rash. Reduce dosage in renal insufficiency. Reinstate with caution in patients who have had a previous mild allergic reaction. Monitor liver function and complete blood counts before initiating therapy and periodically during therapy. Use with caution in patients taking diuretics concurrently. Risk of skin rash may be increased in patients receiving amoxicillin or ampicillin. The risk of hypersensitivity may be increased in patients receiving thiazides, and possibly ACE inhibitors. Use caution with mercaptopurine or azathioprine; dosage adjustment required.

Drug Interactions
Decreased Effect: Ethanol decreases effectiveness.

Increased Effect/Toxicity: Allopurinol may increase the effects of azathioprine, chlorpropamide, mercaptopurine, theophylline, and oral anticoagulants. An increased risk of bone marrow suppression may occur when given with myelosuppressive agents (cyclophosphamide, possibly other alkylating agents). Amoxicillin/ampicillin, ACE inhibitors, and thiazide diuretics have been associated with hypersensitivity reactions when combined with allopurinol (rare), and the incidence of rash may be increased with penicillins (ampicillin, amoxicillin). Urinary acidification with large amounts of vitamin C may increase kidney stone formation.

Nutritional/Ethanol Interactions
Ethanol: Avoid ethanol (may decrease effectiveness).
Iron supplements: Hepatic iron uptake may be increased.
Vitamin C: Large amounts of vitamin C may acidify urine and increase kidney stone formation.

Adverse Reactions The most common adverse reaction to allopurinol is a skin rash (usually maculopapular; however, more severe reactions, including Stevens-Johnson syndrome, have also been reported). While some studies cite an incidence of these reactions as high as >10% of cases (often in association with ampicillin or amoxicillin), the product labeling cites a much lower incidence, reflected below. Allopurinol should be discontinued at the first appearance of a rash or other sign of hypersensitivity.
>1%:
Dermatologic: Rash (1.5%)
Gastrointestinal: Nausea (1.3%), vomiting (1.2%)
Renal: Renal failure/impairment (1.2%)

Overdosage/Toxicology If significant amounts of allopurinol have been absorbed, it is theoretically possible that oxypurinol stones could form, but no record of such occurrence exists. Alkalinization of urine and forced diuresis can help prevent potential xanthine stone formation.

Pharmacodynamics/Kinetics
Onset of Action: Peak effect: 1-2 weeks
Absorption: Oral: ~80%; Rectal: Poor and erratic
Bioavailability: 49% to 53%
Time to Peak: Plasma: Oral: 30-120 minutes
Protein Binding: <1%
Half-Life Elimination:
Normal renal function: Parent drug: 1-3 hours; Oxypurinol: 18-30 hours
End-stage renal disease: Prolonged
Metabolism: ~75% to active metabolites, chiefly oxypurinol
Excretion: Urine (76% as oxypurinol, 12% as unchanged drug)
Allopurinol and oxypurinol are dialyzable

Dosing
Adults: Doses >300 mg should be given in divided doses.
Gout: Oral: Mild: 200-300 mg/day; Severe: 400-600 mg/day; to reduce the possibility of acute gouty attacks, initiate dose at 100 mg/day and increase weekly to recommended dosage. Maximum daily dose: 800 mg/day.
Secondary hyperuricemia associated with chemotherapy:
Oral: 600-800 mg/day in 2-3 divided doses for prevention of acute uric acid nephropathy for 2-3 days starting 1-2 days before chemotherapy
I.V.: 200-400 mg/m^2/day (maximum: 600 mg/day)
Note: Intravenous daily dose can be given as a single infusion or in equally divided doses at 6-, 8-, or 12-hour intervals. A fluid intake sufficient to yield a daily urinary output of at least 2 L in adults and the maintenance of a neutral or, preferably, slightly alkaline urine are desirable.
Recurrent calcium oxalate stones: 200-300 mg/day in single or divided doses
Elderly: Oral: Initial: 100 mg/day; increase until desired uric acid level is obtained. Refer to adult dosing.
Pediatrics:
Gout: Children >10 years: Refer to adult dosing.
Recurrent calcium oxalate stones: Children >10 years: Refer to adult dosing.
Secondary hyperuricemia associated with chemotherapy:
Oral: Children ≤10 years: 10 mg/kg/day in 2-3 divided doses **or** 200-300 mg/m^2/day in 2-4 divided doses, maximum: 800 mg/24 hours, for prevention of acute uric acid nephropathy (begin 1-2 days before chemotherapy)
Alternative (manufacturer labeling):
<6 years: 150 mg/day in 3 divided doses
6-10 years: 300 mg/day in 2-3 divided doses
>10 years: Refer to adult dosing.

(Continued)

Allopurinol *(Continued)*

I.V.:

Children ≤10 years: Starting dose: 200 mg/m²/day

Note: Intravenous daily dose can be given as a single infusion or in equally divided doses at 6-, 8-, or 12-hour intervals. Adequate fluid intake and the maintenance of a neutral or, preferably, slightly alkaline urine are desirable.

Children >10 years: Refer to adult dosing.

Renal Impairment:

Oral:

Must be adjusted due to accumulation of allopurinol and metabolites; see table.

Adult Maintenance Doses of Allopurinol[1]

Creatinine Clearance (mL/min)	Maintenance Dose of Allopurinol (mg)
140	400 daily
120	350 daily
100	300 daily
80	250 daily
60	200 daily
40	150 daily
20	100 daily
10	100 every 2 days
0	100 every 3 days

[1]This table is based on a standard maintenance dose of 300 mg of allopurinol per day for a patient with a creatinine clearance of 100 mL/min.

Hemodialysis: Administer dose after hemodialysis or administer 50% supplemental dose.

I.V.:

Cl_{cr} 10-20 mL/minute: Administer 200 mg/day.

Cl_{cr} 3-10 mL/minute: Administer 100 mg/day.

Cl_{cr} <3 mL/minute: Administer 100 mg/day at extended intervals.

Available Dosage Forms

Injection, powder for reconstitution, as sodium (Aloprim™): 500 mg

Tablet (Zyloprim®): 100 mg, 300 mg

Monitoring and Teaching Issues

Physical Assessment: Assess effectiveness and interactions of other medications patient may be taking. Monitor laboratory values, effectiveness of therapy, and adverse reactions at beginning of therapy and periodically with long-term use. Assess knowledge/teach patient appropriate use, interventions to reduce side effects, and adverse symptoms to report.

Monitoring Laboratory Tests: CBC, serum uric acid levels, hepatic and renal function, especially at start of therapy

Patient Education: Take as directed. Maintain adequate hydration (2-3 L/day of fluids) unless instructed to restrict fluid intake. While using this medication, do not use alcohol, other prescriptions, OTC medications, or vitamins without consulting prescriber. You may experience drowsiness (use caution when driving or engaging in tasks requiring alertness until response to drug is known); nausea, vomiting, or heartburn (small frequent meals, frequent mouth care, chewing gum, or sucking lozenges may help); or hair loss (reversible). Report skin rash or lesions; painful urination or blood in urine or stool; unresolved nausea or vomiting; numbness of extremities; pain or irritation of the eyes; swelling of lips, mouth, or tongue; unusual fatigue; easy bruising or bleeding; yellowing of skin or eyes; or any change in color of urine or stool. **Pregnancy precaution:** Inform prescriber if you are or intend to become pregnant. Consult prescriber if breast-feeding.

Dietary Considerations: Should administer oral forms after meals with plenty of fluid. Fluid intake should be administered to yield neutral or slightly alkaline urine and an output of ~2 L (in adults).

Geriatric Considerations: Adjust dose based on renal function.

Pregnancy Risk Factor: C

Lactation: Enters breast milk/use caution (AAP rates "compatible")

Administration

Oral: Should be administered after meals.

I.V.: The rate of infusion depends on the volume of the infusion. Whenever possible, therapy should be initiated at 24-48 hours before the start of chemotherapy known to cause tumor lysis (including adrenocorticosteroids). I.V. daily dose can be administered as a single infusion or in equally divided doses at 6-, 8-, or 12-hour intervals.

Reconstitution: Allopurinol injection must be reconstituted and diluted. Each 30 mL vial should be reconstituted with 25 mL sterile water for injection, USP. It may then be added to NS or D_5W. A final concentration of no greater than 6 mg/mL is recommended.

Compatibility: Stable in D_5W, NS, SWFI

Y-site administration: Incompatible with amikacin, amphotericin B, carmustine, cefotaxime, chlorpromazine, cimetidine, clindamycin, cytarabine, dacarbazine, daunorubicin, diphenhydramine, doxorubicin, doxycycline, droperidol, floxuridine, gentamicin, haloperidol, hydroxyzine, idarubicin, imipenem/cilastatin, mechlorethamine, meperidine, methylprednisolone sodium succinate, metoclopramide, minocycline, nalbuphine, netilmicin, ondansetron, prochlorperazine edisylate, promethazine, sodium bicarbonate, streptozocin, tobramycin, vinorelbine

Storage:
Powder for injection: Store at controlled room temperature of 15°C to 30°C (59°F to 86°F). Following reconstitution, intravenous solutions should be stored at 20°C to 25°C. Do not refrigerate reconstituted and/or diluted product. Must be administered within 10 hours of solution preparation.
Tablet: Store at controlled room temperature of 15°C to 25°C (59°F to 77°F).

♦ **Allopurinol Sodium** *see* Allopurinol *on page 70*

♦ **All-*trans*-Retinoic Acid** *see* Tretinoin (Oral) *on page 1514*

♦ **Almora® [OTC]** *see* Magnesium Gluconate *on page 930*

Almotriptan (al moh TRIP tan)

U.S. Brand Names Axert™
Synonyms Almotriptan Malate
Generic Available No
Pharmacologic Category Serotonin 5-HT$_{1D}$ Receptor Agonist
Medication Safety Issues
Sound-alike/look-alike issues:
Axert™ may be confused with Antivert®
Use Acute treatment of migraine with or without aura
Mechanism of Action/Effect The therapeutic effect for migraine is due to serotonin agonist activity.
Contraindications Hypersensitivity to almotriptan or any component of the formulation; use as prophylactic therapy for migraine; hemiplegic or basilar migraine; cluster headache; known or suspected ischemic heart disease (angina pectoris, MI, documented silent ischemia, coronary artery vasospasm, Prinzmetal's variant angina); peripheral vascular syndromes (including ischemic bowel disease); uncontrolled hypertension; use within 24 hours of another 5-HT$_1$ agonist; use within 24 hours of ergotamine derivative; concurrent administration or within 2 weeks of discontinuing an MAO inhibitor (specifically MAO type A inhibitors)
Warnings/Precautions Indicated for migraine headaches only. Not for patients with risk factors for coronary artery disease; need cardiac evaluation first. If patient's cardiovascular evaluation is good, healthcare provider should administer the first dose and cardiovascular status should be periodically evaluated. Vasospastic events may occur in the heart, peripheral vascular, or gastrointestinal system. Cerebral/subarachnoid hemorrhage, stroke, and hypertensive crisis have occurred. Use with caution in liver or renal dysfunction. Safety and efficacy in pediatric patients have not been established.
Drug Interactions
Cytochrome P450 Effect: Substrate (minor) of CYP2D6, 3A4
Increased Effect/Toxicity: Ergot-containing drugs prolong vasospastic reactions; ketoconazole increases almotriptan serum concentration; select serotonin reuptake inhibitors may increase symptoms of hyper-reflexia, weakness, and incoordination; MAO inhibitors may increase toxicity
Adverse Reactions 1% to 10%:
Central nervous system: Headache (>1%), dizziness (>1%), somnolence (>1%)
Gastrointestinal: Nausea (1% to 2%), xerostomia (1%)
Neuromuscular & skeletal: Paresthesia (1%)
Overdosage/Toxicology Hypertension or more serious cardiovascular symptoms may occur. Clinical and electrocardiographic monitoring needed for at least 20 hours even if patient asymptomatic. Treatment is symptom-directed and supportive.
Pharmacodynamics/Kinetics
Absorption: Well absorbed
Bioavailability: 70%
Time to Peak: 1-3 hours
Protein Binding: ~35%
Half-Life Elimination: 3-4 hours
Metabolism: MAO type A oxidative deamination (~27% of dose); via CYP3A4 and 2D6 (~12% of dose) to inactive metabolites
Excretion: Urine: 40% (as unchanged drug); feces (13% unchanged and metabolized)
Dosing
Adults & Elderly: Migraine: Oral: Initial: 6.25-12.5 mg in a single dose; if the headache returns, repeat the dose after 2 hours; no more than 2 doses in 24-hour period
Note: If the first dose is ineffective, diagnosis needs to be re-evaluated. Safety of treating more than 4 migraines/month has not been established.
Renal Impairment: Initial: 6.25 mg in a single dose; maximum daily dose: ≤12.5 mg
Hepatic Impairment: Initial: 6.25 mg in a single dose; maximum daily dose: ≤12.5 mg
Available Dosage Forms Tablet, as malate: 6.25 mg, 12.5 mg
Monitoring and Teaching Issues
Physical Assessment: Clear diagnosis of migraines and cardiac status should be determined before beginning treatment. Assess for use cautions (eg, risk factors for coronary artery disease; liver or renal dysfunction; see Warnings/Precautions). Monitor for use of ergot-containing drugs, SSRIs, or MAO inhibitors (see Drug Interactions). Assess effectiveness of therapy (relief of migraines) and adverse response (eg, hypertension or more serious cardiovascular symptoms; see Adverse Reactions). Teach patient proper use, possible side effects/appropriate interventions, and adverse symptoms to report.
Patient Education: This drug is to be used to reduce your migraine, not to prevent or reduce the number of attacks. Follow exact instructions for use. Do not use more than 2 doses in 24 hours and do not take within 24 hours of any other migraine medication without consulting prescriber. May cause dizziness, fatigue, or drowsiness (use caution when driving or engaging in tasks requiring alertness until response to drug is known). Report immediately any chest pain, palpitations, or throbbing; feelings of tightness or pressure in jaw or throat; acute headache or dizziness; muscle cramping, pain, or tremors; skin rash; hallucinations, anxiety, panic; or other adverse reactions. **Pregnancy/breast-feeding** (Continued)

Almotriptan *(Continued)*

precautions: Inform prescriber if you are or intend to become pregnant. Consult prescriber if breast-feeding.

Dietary Considerations: May be taken without regard to meals

Pregnancy Risk Factor: C

Lactation: Excretion in breast milk unknown/use caution

Administration
Storage: Store at 15°C to 30°C (59°F to 86°F).

Related Information
Antimigraine Drugs: 5-HT$_1$ Receptor Agonists *on page 1716*

- ◆ **Almotriptan Malate** *see Almotriptan on page 73*
- ◆ **Alocril®** *see Nedocromil on page 1062*
- ◆ **Aloe Vesta® 2-n-1 Antifungal [OTC]** *see Miconazole on page 999*
- ◆ **Alomide®** *see Lodoxamide on page 911*
- ◆ **Aloprim™** *see Allopurinol on page 70*
- ◆ **Alora®** *see Estradiol on page 552*
- ◆ **Aloxi™** *see Palonosetron on page 1148*
- ◆ **Alphagan® P** *see Brimonidine on page 206*
- ◆ **Alphanate®** *see Antihemophilic Factor (Human) on page 124*
- ◆ **Alphaquin HP** *see Hydroquinone on page 768*

Alprazolam *(al PRAY zoe lam)*

U.S. Brand Names Alprazolam Intensol®; Xanax®; Xanax XR®

Controlled Substance C-IV

Generic Available Yes: Immediate release tablet

Pharmacologic Category Benzodiazepine

Medication Safety Issues
Sound-alike/look-alike issues:
Alprazolam may be confused with alprostadil, lorazepam, triazolam
Xanax® may be confused with Lanoxin®, Tenex®, Tylox®, Xopenex®, Zantac®, Zyrtec®

Use Treatment of anxiety disorder (GAD); panic disorder, with or without agoraphobia; anxiety associated with depression

Unlabeled/Investigational Use Anxiety in children

Mechanism of Action/Effect Binds to stereospecific benzodiazepine receptors on the post-synaptic GABA neuron at several sites within the central nervous system, including the limbic system, reticular formation. Enhancement of the inhibitory effect of GABA on neuronal excitability results by increased neuronal membrane permeability to chloride ions. This shift in chloride ions results in hyperpolarization (a less excitable state) and stabilization.

Contraindications Hypersensitivity to alprazolam or any component of the formulation (cross-sensitivity with other benzodiazepines may exist); narrow-angle glaucoma; concurrent use with ketoconazole or itraconazole; pregnancy

Warnings/Precautions Rebound or withdrawal symptoms, including seizures may occur 18 hours to 3 days following abrupt discontinuation or large decreases in dose (more common in patients receiving >4 mg/day or prolonged treatment). Breakthrough anxiety may occur at the end of dosing interval. Use with caution in patients receiving concurrent CYP3A4 inhibitors. Use with caution in renal impairment or predisposition to urate nephropathy. Use with caution in elderly or debilitated patients, patients with hepatic disease (including alcoholics), renal impairment, or obese patients.

Causes CNS depression (dose-related) which may impair physical and mental capabilities. Patients must be cautioned about performing tasks that require mental alertness (eg, operating machinery or driving). Effects with other sedative drugs or ethanol may be potentiated. Benzodiazepines have been associated with falls and traumatic injury and should be used with extreme caution in patients who are at risk of these events (especially the elderly). Use with caution in patients with respiratory disease or impaired gag reflex.

Use caution in patients with depression, particularly if suicidal risk may be present. Episodes of mania or hypomania have occurred in depressed patients treated with alprazolam. May cause physical or psychological dependence. Acute withdrawal may be precipitated in patients after administration of flumazenil.

Benzodiazepines have been associated with anterograde amnesia. Paradoxical reactions have been reported with benzodiazepines, particularly in adolescent/pediatric or psychiatric patients. Does not have analgesic, antidepressant, or antipsychotic properties.

Drug Interactions

Cytochrome P450 Effect: Substrate of CYP3A4 (major)

Decreased Effect: Aminoglutethimide, carbamazepine, nafcillin, nevirapine, phenobarbital, phenytoin, rifamycins and other CYP3A4 inducers may decrease the levels/effects of alprazolam.

Increased Effect/Toxicity: Alprazolam serum levels/effects may be increased by azole antifungals, ciprofloxacin, clarithromycin, diclofenac, doxycycline, erythromycin, imatinib, isoniazid, nefazodone, nicardipine, propofol, protease inhibitors, quinidine, telithromycin, verapamil, and other inhibitors of CYP3A4. Contraindicated with itraconazole or ketoconazole. Alprazolam potentiates the CNS depressant effects of narcotic analgesics, barbiturates, phenothiazines, ethanol, antihistamines, MAO inhibitors, sedative-hypnotics, and cyclic antidepressants. Alprazolam increases plasma concentrations of imipramine and desipramine.

Nutritional/Ethanol Interactions
Cigarette smoking: May decrease alprazolam concentrations up to 50%.
Ethanol: Avoid ethanol (may increase CNS depression).
Food: Alprazolam serum concentration is unlikely to be increased by grapefruit juice because of alprazolam's high oral bioavailability. The C_{max} of the extended release formulation is increased by 25% when a high-fat meal is given 2 hours before dosing. T_{max} is decreased

30% when food given immediately prior to dose. T_{max} is increased by 30% when food is given ≥1 hour after dose.

Herb/Nutraceutical: St John's wort may decrease alprazolam levels. Avoid valerian, St John's wort, kava kava, gotu kola (may increase CNS depression).

Lab Interactions Increased with alkaline phosphatase

Adverse Reactions

>10%:

Central nervous system: Depression, drowsiness, dysarthria, fatigue, headache, irritability, lightheadedness, memory impairment, sedation

Endocrine & metabolic: Libido decreased, menstrual disorders

Gastrointestinal: Appetite increased/decreased, salivation decreased, weight gain/loss, xerostomia

1% to 10%:

Cardiovascular: Hypotension

Central nervous system: Abnormal coordination, akathisia, attention disturbance, confusion, derealization, disorientation, disinhibition, dizziness, hypersomnia, nightmares, vertigo

Dermatologic: Dermatitis, pruritus, rash

Endocrine & metabolic: Libido increased

Gastrointestinal: Diarrhea, dyspepsia, salivation increased, vomiting

Genitourinary: Incontinence, micturition difficulty, sexual dysfunction

Neuromuscular & skeletal: Arthralgia, ataxia, muscle cramps, muscle twitching, myalgia, paresthesia, rigidity, tremor

Ophthalmic: Blurred vision

Otic: Tinnitus

Respiratory: Allergic rhinitis, dyspnea, nasal congestion

Miscellaneous: Diaphoresis

Overdosage/Toxicology Symptoms of overdose include somnolence, confusion, coma, and diminished reflexes. Treatment for benzodiazepine overdose is supportive. Flumazenil has been shown to selectively block the binding of benzodiazepines to CNS receptors, resulting in a reversal of benzodiazepine-induced sedation; however, its use may not reverse respiratory depression.

Pharmacodynamics/Kinetics

Bioavailability: 90%

Time to Peak: Serum: 1-2 hours

Protein Binding: 80%

Half-Life Elimination: Healthy adults: 11.2 hours (range: 6.3-26.9); Elderly: 16.3 hours (range: 9-26.9 hours); Alcoholic liver disease: 19.7 hours (range: 5.8-65.3 hours); Obesity: 21.8 hours (range: 9.9-40.4 hours)

Metabolism: Hepatic via CYP3A4; forms 2 active metabolites (4-hydroxyalprazolam and α-hydroxyalprazolam)

Excretion: Urine (as unchanged drug and metabolites)

Dosing

Adults: Note: Treatment >4 months should be re-evaluated to determine the patient's continued need for the drug

Anxiety: Oral: *Immediate release:* Effective doses are 0.5-4 mg/day in divided doses; the manufacturer recommends starting at 0.25-0.5 mg 3 times/day; titrate dose upward; maximum: 4 mg/day

Anxiety associated with depression: Oral: *Immediate release:* Average dose required: 2.5-3 mg/day in divided doses

Ethanol withdrawal (unlabeled use): Oral: *Immediate release:* Usual dose: 2-2.5 mg/day in divided doses

Panic disorder: Oral:

Immediate release: Initial: 0.5 mg 3 times/day; dose may be increased every 3-4 days in increments ≤1 mg/day; many patients obtain relief at 2 mg/day, as much as 10 mg/day may be required

Extended release: 0.5-1 mg once daily; may increase dose every 3-4 days in increments ≤1 mg/day (range: 3-6 mg/day)

Switching from immediate release to extended release: Patients may be switched to extended release tablets by taking the total daily dose of the immediate release tablets and giving it once daily using the extended release preparation.

Dose reduction: Abrupt discontinuation should be avoided. Daily dose may be decreased by 0.5 mg every 3 days, however, some patients may require a slower reduction. If withdrawal symptoms occur, resume previous dose and discontinue on a less rapid schedule.

Elderly: Initial: 0.125-0.25 mg twice daily; increase by 0.125 mg/day as needed. The smallest effective dose should be used.

Immediate release: Initial 0.25 mg 2-3 times/day

Extended release: Initial: 0.5 mg once daily

Pediatrics:

Anxiety (unlabeled use): Oral: Immediate release: Initial: 0.005 mg/kg/dose or 0.125 mg/dose 3 times/day; increase in increments of 0.125-0.25 mg, up to a maximum of 0.02 mg/kg/dose or 0.06 mg/kg/day (0.375-3 mg/day)

Note: Treatment >4 months should be re-evaluated to determine the patient's continued need for the drug

Hepatic Impairment: Oral: Reduce dose by 50% to 60% or avoid in cirrhosis.

Available Dosage Forms

Solution, oral (Alprazolam Intensol®): 1 mg/mL (30 mL)

Tablet (Xanax®): 0.25 mg, 0.5 mg, 1 mg, 2 mg

Tablet, extended release (Xanax XR®): 0.5 mg, 1 mg, 2 mg, 3 mg

Monitoring and Teaching Issues

Physical Assessment: Assess other medications patient may be taking for effectiveness and interactions. Assess for signs of CNS depression. Assess for history of addiction; long-term use can result in dependence, abuse, or tolerance; periodically evaluate need for (Continued)

Alprazolam *(Continued)*

continued use. For inpatient use, institute safety measures and monitor effectiveness and adverse reactions. For outpatients, monitor therapeutic effectiveness and adverse reactions at beginning of therapy and periodically with long-term use. Taper dosage slowly when discontinuing. Assess knowledge/teach patient appropriate use, interventions to reduce side effects, and adverse symptoms to report.

Patient Education: Take exactly as directed; do not increase dose or frequency. Drug may cause physical and/or psychological dependence. Avoid alcohol and do not take other prescription or OTC medications (especially pain medications, sedatives, antihistamines, or hypnotics) without consulting prescriber. Maintain adequate hydration (2-3 L/day of fluids) unless instructed to restrict fluid intake. You may experience drowsiness, lightheadedness, impaired coordination, dizziness, or blurred vision (use caution when driving or engaging in hazardous tasks until response to drug is known); nausea, vomiting, or dry mouth (small frequent meals, frequent mouth care, chewing gum, or sucking lozenges may help); constipation (increased exercise, fluids, fruit, and fiber may help); altered sexual drive or ability (reversible); or photosensitivity (use sunscreen, wear protective clothing and eyewear, and avoid direct sunlight). Report persistent CNS effects (eg, confusion, depression, increased sedation, excitation, headache, agitation, insomnia or nightmares, dizziness, fatigue, impaired coordination, changes in personality, or changes in cognition); changes in urinary pattern; muscle cramping, weakness, tremors, or rigidity; ringing in ears or visual disturbances; chest pain, palpitations, or rapid heartbeat; excessive perspiration; excessive GI symptoms (eg, cramping, constipation, vomiting, anorexia); or worsening of condition. **Pregnancy/breast-feeding precautions:** Do not get pregnant while taking this medication; use appropriate contraceptive measures as recommended by your prescriber. Breast-feeding is not recommended.

Geriatric Considerations: Due to short duration of action, it is considered to be a benzodiazepine of choice in the elderly.

Pregnancy Risk Factor: D

Pregnancy Issues: Benzodiazepines cross the placenta. The association between benzodiazepine exposure and malformations remains controversial. A number of types of malformation have been reported (oral cleft, inguinal hernia, cardiac defects, spina bifida, dysmorphic facial features, skeletal defects); however, confounding factors make a clear association difficult. Overall, the risk to the fetus may be low. Nonteratogenic effects (including neonatal flaccidity, respiratory and feeding problems, and withdrawal symptoms) during the postnatal period have also been reported with benzodiazepine use.

Lactation: Enters breast milk/not recommended (AAP rates "of concern")

Breast-Feeding Issues: Symptoms of withdrawal, lethargy, and loss of body weight have been reported in infants exposed to alprazolam and/or benzodiazepines while nursing. Breast-feeding is not recommended.

Administration

Oral:

Immediate release preparations: Can be administered sublingually with comparable onset and completeness of absorption.

Extended release tablet: Should be taken once daily in the morning; do not crush, break or chew.

Additional Information Not intended for management of anxieties and minor distresses associated with everyday life. Treatment longer than 4 months should be re-evaluated to determine the patient's need for the drug. Patients who become physically dependent on alprazolam tend to have a difficult time discontinuing it; withdrawal symptoms may be severe. To minimize withdrawal symptoms, taper dosage slowly; do not discontinue abruptly. Abrupt discontinuation after sustained use (generally >10 days) may cause withdrawal symptoms.

Related Information

Anxiolytic / Hypnotic Use in Long-Term Care Facilities *on page 1769*
Benzodiazepines *on page 1719*
Federal OBRA Regulations: Recommended Maximum Doses *on page 1773*

♦ **Alprazolam Intensol®** *see Alprazolam* *on page 74*

Alprostadil *(al PROS ta dill)*

U.S. Brand Names Caverject®; Caverject® Impulse™; Edex®; Muse®; Prostin VR Pediatric®

Synonyms PGE₁; Prostaglandin E₁

Generic Available Yes

Pharmacologic Category Prostaglandin

Medication Safety Issues

Sound-alike/look-alike issues:

Alprostadil may be confused with alprazolam

Use

Prostin VR Pediatric®: Temporary maintenance of patency of ductus arteriosus in neonates with ductal-dependent congenital heart disease until surgery can be performed. These defects include cyanotic (eg, pulmonary atresia, pulmonary stenosis, tricuspid atresia, Fallot's tetralogy, transposition of the great vessels) and acyanotic (eg, interruption of aortic arch, coarctation of aorta, hypoplastic left ventricle) heart disease

Caverject®: Treatment of erectile dysfunction of vasculogenic, psychogenic, or neurogenic etiology; adjunct in the diagnosis of erectile dysfunction

Edex®, Muse®: Treatment of erectile dysfunction of vasculogenic, psychogenic, or neurogenic etiology

Unlabeled/Investigational Use Investigational: Treatment of pulmonary hypertension in infants and children with congenital heart defects with left-to-right shunts

Mechanism of Action/Effect

Erectile dysfunction: Causes vasodilation by dilation of cavernosal arteries when injected along the penile shaft, allowing blood flow to, and entrapment in, the lacunar spaces of the penis (ie, corporeal veno-occlusive mechanism)

Neonate: Has direct effects on smooth muscle of ductus arteriosus.

Contraindications Hypersensitivity to alprostadil or any component of the formulation; hyaline membrane disease or persistent fetal circulation and when a dominant left-to-right shunt is present; respiratory distress syndrome; conditions predisposing patients to priapism (sickle cell anemia, multiple myeloma, leukemia); patients with anatomical deformation of the penis, penile implants; use in men for whom sexual activity is inadvisable or contraindicated; pregnancy

Warnings/Precautions Use cautiously in neonates with bleeding tendencies. Apnea may occur in 10% to 12% of neonates with congenital heart defects, especially in those weighing <2 kg at birth. Apnea usually appears during the first hour of drug infusion.

When used in erectile dysfunction: priapism may occur. Patient must be instructed to report to physician or seek immediate medical assistance if an erection persists for longer than 4 hours. Treat immediately to avoid penile tissue damage and permanent loss of potency; discontinue therapy if signs of penile fibrosis develop (penile angulation, cavernosal fibrosis, or Peyronie's disease). Syncope occurring within 1 hour of administration, has been reported; the potential for drug-drug interactions may occur when prescribed concomitantly with antihypertensives; some lowering of blood pressure may occur without symptoms, and swelling of leg veins, leg pain, perineal pain, and rapid pulse have been reported in <2% of patients during in-clinic titration and home treatment.

Drug Interactions
Increased Effect/Toxicity: Risk of hypotension and syncope may be increased with antihypertensives.

Nutritional/Ethanol Interactions Ethanol: Avoid concurrent use (vasodilating effect).

Adverse Reactions
Intraurethral:
>10%: Genitourinary: Penile pain, urethral burning
2% to 10%:
Central nervous system: Headache, dizziness, pain
Genitourinary: Vaginal itching (female partner), testicular pain, urethral bleeding (minor)

Intracavernosal injection:
>10%: Genitourinary: Penile pain
1% to 10%:
Cardiovascular: Hypertension
Central nervous system: Headache, dizziness
Genitourinary: Prolonged erection (>4 hours, 4%), penile fibrosis, penis disorder, penile rash, penile edema
Local: Injection site hematoma and/or bruising

Intravenous:
>10%:
Cardiovascular: Flushing
Central nervous system: Fever
Respiratory: Apnea
1% to 10%:
Cardiovascular: Bradycardia, hyper-/hypotension, tachycardia, cardiac arrest, edema
Central nervous system: Seizures, headache, dizziness
Endocrine & metabolic: Hypokalemia
Gastrointestinal: Diarrhea
Hematologic: Disseminated intravascular coagulation
Neuromuscular & skeletal: Back pain
Respiratory: Upper respiratory infection, flu syndrome, sinusitis, nasal congestion, cough
Miscellaneous: Sepsis, localized pain in structures other than the injection site

Overdosage/Toxicology Symptoms of overdose when treating patent ductus arteriosus include apnea, bradycardia, hypotension, and flushing. If hypotension or pyrexia occurs, the infusion rate should be reduced until symptoms subside. Apnea or bradycardia requires drug discontinuation. If intracavernous overdose occurs, supervise until systemic effects have resolved or until penile detumescence has occurred.

Pharmacodynamics/Kinetics
Onset of Action: Rapid
Duration of Action: <1 hour
Protein Binding: Plasma: 81% to albumin
Half-Life Elimination: 5-10 minutes
Metabolism: ~75% by oxidation in one pass via lungs
Excretion: Urine (90% as metabolites) within 24 hours

Dosing
Adults & Elderly:
Erectile dysfunction:
Intracavernous (Caverject®, Edex®): Individualize dose by careful titration; doses >40 mcg (Edex®) or >60 mcg (Caverject®) are not recommended: Initial dose must be titrated in physicians office. Patient must stay in the physician's office until complete detumescence occurs; if there is no response, then the next higher dose may be given within 1 hour; if there is still no response, a 1-day interval before giving the next dose is recommended; increasing the dose or concentration in the treatment of impotence results in increasing pain and discomfort
Vasculogenic, psychogenic, or mixed etiology: Initiate dosage titration at 2.5 mcg, increasing by 2.5 mcg to a dose of 5 mcg and then in increments of 5-10 mcg depending on the erectile response until the dose produces an erection suitable for intercourse, not lasting >1 hour; if there is absolutely no response to initial 2.5 mcg dose, the second dose may be increased to 7.5 mcg, followed by increments of 5-10 mcg
Neurogenic etiology (eg, spinal cord injury): Initiate dosage titration at 1.25 mcg, increasing to a dose of 2.5 mcg and then 5 mcg; increase further in increments 5 mcg until the dose is reached that produces an erection suitable for intercourse, not lasting >1 hour

(Continued)

Alprostadil *(Continued)*

Maintenance: Once appropriate dose has been determined, patient may self-administer injections at a frequency of no more than 3 times/week with at least 24 hours between doses

Intraurethral (Muse® Pellet):

Initial: 125-250 mcg

Maintenance: Administer as needed to achieve an erection; duration of action is about 30-60 minutes; use only two systems per 24-hour period

Pediatrics:

Patent ductus arteriosus I.V.:

Prostin VR Pediatric®: I.V. continuous infusion into a large vein, or alternatively through an umbilical artery catheter placed at the ductal opening: 0.05-0.1 mcg/kg/minute with therapeutic response, rate is reduced to lowest effective dosage. With unsatisfactory response, rate is increased gradually; maintenance: 0.01-0.4 mcg/kg/minute.

Note: PGE$_1$ is usually given at an infusion rate of 0.1 mcg/kg/minute, but it is often possible to reduce the dosage to $1/2$ or even $1/10$ without losing the therapeutic effect. The mixing schedule is shown in the table.

Alprostadil

Add 1 Ampul (500 mcg) to:	Concentration (mcg/mL)	Infusion Rate	
		mL/min/kg Needed to Infuse 0.1 mcg/kg/min	mL/kg/24 h
250 mL	2	0.05	72
100 mL	5	0.02	28.8
50 mL	10	0.01	14.4
25 mL	20	0.005	7.2

Note: Therapeutic response is indicated by increased pH in those with acidosis or by an increase in oxygenation (PO$_2$) usually evident within 30 minutes.

Available Dosage Forms [DSC] = Discontinued product

Injection, powder for reconstitution:

Caverject®: 10 mcg, 20 mcg, 40 mcg [contains lactose; diluent contains benzyl alcohol]

Caverject® Impulse™: 10 mcg, 20 mcg [prefilled injection system; contains lactose; diluent contains benzyl alcohol]

Edex®: 10 mcg, 20 mcg, 40 mcg [contains lactose; diluent contains benzyl alcohol; also packaged in kits containing diluent, syringe, and alcohol swab]

Injection, solution: 500 mcg/mL (1 mL)

Caverject® [DSC]: 20 mcg/mL (2 mL)

Prostin VR Pediatric®: 500 mcg/mL (1 mL) [contains dehydrated alcohol]

Pellet, urethral (Muse®): 125 mcg, 250 mcg, 500 mcg, 1000 mcg

Monitoring and Teaching Issues

Physical Assessment: Neonate: Monitor closely; apnea has occurred during first hour after administration. **Erectile dysfunction:** After individual dose titration is determined by physician, the Caverject® injection (or Muse®) is generally self-administered. Teach patient proper use if self-administered (appropriate injection technique and syringe/needle disposal), possible side effects/appropriate interventions, and adverse symptoms to report. **Pregnancy risk factor X:** See Pregnancy Issues.

Patient Education: Use only as directed, no more than 3 times/week, allowing 24 hours between injections. Avoid alcohol. Store in refrigerator and dilute with supplied diluent immediately before use. Use alternate sides of penis with each injection. Dispose of syringes and needle and single dose vials in a safe manner (do not share medication, syringes, or needles). Note that the risk of transmitting blood-borne disease is increased with use of alprostadil injections since a small amount of bleeding at injection site is possible. Stop using and contact prescriber immediately if signs of priapism occur, erections last more than 4 hours, or you experience moderate to severe penile pain. Report penile problems (eg, nodules, new penile pain, rash, bruising, numbness, swelling, signs of infection, abnormal ejaculations); cardiac symptoms (hypo- or hypertension, chest pain, palpitations, irregular heartbeat); flushing, fever, flu-like symptoms; respiratory difficulty or wheezing; or other adverse reactions. Refer to prescriber every 3 months to ensure proper technique and for dosage evaluation. **Pregnancy precautions:** Consult prescriber about use of contraceptives. Do not give blood while taking this medication and for 1 month following discontinuance.

Geriatric Considerations: Elderly may have concomitant diseases which would contraindicate the use of alprostadil. Other forms of attaining penile tumescence are recommended.

Pregnancy Risk Factor: X/C (Muse®)

Pregnancy Issues: Alprostadil is embryotoxic in animal studies. It is not indicated for use in women. The manufacturer of Muse® recommends a condom barrier when being used during sexual intercourse with a pregnant women.

Lactation: Not indicated for use in women

Administration

Other: Erectile dysfunction: Use a $1/2$ inch, 27- to 30-gauge needle. Inject into the dorsolateral aspect of the proximal third of the penis, avoiding visible veins; alternate side of the penis for injections.

Reconstitution:

Caverject® powder: Use only the supplied diluent for reconstitution (ie, bacteriostatic/sterile water with benzyl alcohol 0.945%).

Caverject® Impulse™: Provided as a dual-chamber syringe with diluent in one chamber. To mix, hold syringe with needle pointing upward and turn plunger clockwise; turn upside down several times to mix. Device can be set to deliver specified dose, each device can be set at various increments.

Edex®: Reconstitute with NS.

Storage:

Caverject® Impulse™: Store at controlled room temperature of 15°C to 30°C (59°F to 86°F). Following reconstitution, use within 24 hours and discard any unused solution.

Caverject® powder: The 5 mcg, 10 mcg, and 20 mcg vials should be stored at or below 25°C (77°F); The 40 mcg vial should be stored at 2°C to 8°C until dispensed. After dispensing, stable for up to 3 months at or below 25°C. Following reconstitution, all strengths should be stored at or below 25°C (77°F); do not refrigerate or freeze; use within 24 hours.

Caverject® solution: Prior to dispensing, store frozen at -20°C to -10°C (-4°F to -14°F). Once dispensed, may be stored frozen for up to 3 months, or under refrigeration at 2°C to 8°C (36°F to 46°F) for up to 7 days. Do not refreeze. Once removed from foil wrap, solution may be allowed to warm to room temperature prior to use. If not used immediately, solution should be discarded. Shake well prior to use.

Edex®: Store at controlled room temperature of 15°C to 30°C (59°F to 86°F); following reconstitution, use immediately and discard any unused solution.

Muse®: Refrigerate at 2°C to 8°C (36°F to 46°F); may be stored at room temperature for up to 14 days

Prostin VR Pediatric®: Refrigerate at 2°C to 8°C (36°F to 46°F). Prior to infusion, dilute with D_5W or NS; use within 24 hours.

+ **Alrex®** *see* Loteprednol *on page 924*

+ **Altace®** *see* Ramipril *on page 1304*

+ **Altarussin DM [OTC]** *see* Guaifenesin and Dextromethorphan *on page 731*

Alteplase (AL te plase)

U.S. Brand Names Activase®; Cathflo™ Activase®

Synonyms Alteplase, Recombinant; Alteplase, Tissue Plasminogen Activator, Recombinant; tPA

Generic Available No

Pharmacologic Category Thrombolytic Agent

Medication Safety Issues

Sound-alike/look-alike issues:

Alteplase may be confused with Altace®

"tPA" abbreviation should not be used when writing orders for this medication; has been misread as TNKase (tenecteplase)

Use Management of acute myocardial infarction for the lysis of thrombi in coronary arteries; management of acute massive pulmonary embolism (PE) in adults

Acute myocardial infarction (AMI): Chest pain ≥20 minutes, ≤12-24 hours; S-T elevation ≥0.1 mV in at least two ECG leads

Acute pulmonary embolism (APE): Age ≤75 years: Documented massive pulmonary embolism by pulmonary angiography or echocardiography or high probability lung scan with clinical shock

Cathflo™ Activase®: Restoration of central venous catheter function

Unlabeled/Investigational Use Acute peripheral arterial occlusive disease

Mechanism of Action/Effect Dissolves thrombus (clot)

Contraindications Hypersensitivity to alteplase or any component of the formulation

Treatment of acute MI or PE: Active internal bleeding; history of CVA; recent intracranial or intraspinal surgery or trauma; intracranial neoplasm; arteriovenous malformation or aneurysm; known bleeding diathesis; severe uncontrolled hypertension

Treatment of acute ischemic stroke: Evidence of intracranial hemorrhage or suspicion of subarachnoid hemorrhage on pretreatment evaluation; recent (within 3 months) intracranial or intraspinal surgery; prolonged external cardiac massage; suspected aortic dissection; serious head trauma or previous stroke; history of intracranial hemorrhage; uncontrolled hypertension at time of treatment (eg, >185 mm Hg systolic or >110 mm Hg diastolic); seizure at the onset of stroke; active internal bleeding; intracranial neoplasm; arteriovenous malformation or aneurysm; known bleeding diathesis including but not limited to: current use of anticoagulants or an INR >1.7, administration of heparin within 48 hours preceding the onset of stroke and an elevated aPTT at presentation, platelet count <100,000/mm³.

Other exclusion criteria (NINDS recombinant tPA study): Stroke or serious head injury within 3 months, major surgery or serious trauma within 2 weeks, GI or urinary tract hemorrhage within 3 weeks, aggressive treatment required to lower blood pressure, glucose level <50 mg/dL or >400 mg/dL, arterial puncture at a noncompressible site or lumbar puncture within 1 week, clinical presentation suggesting post-MI pericarditis, pregnancy; breast-feeding.

Warnings/Precautions Concurrent heparin anticoagulation may contribute to bleeding. Monitor all potential bleeding sites. Doses >150 mg are associated with increased risk of intracranial hemorrhage. Intramuscular injections and nonessential handling of the patient should be avoided. Venipunctures should be performed carefully and only when necessary. If arterial puncture is necessary, use an upper extremity vessel that can be manually compressed. If serious bleeding occurs then the infusion of alteplase and heparin should be stopped.

For the following conditions the risk of bleeding is higher with use of alteplase and should be weighed against the benefits of therapy: recent major surgery (eg, CABG, obstetrical delivery, organ biopsy, previous puncture of noncompressible vessels), cerebrovascular disease, recent gastrointestinal or genitourinary bleeding, recent trauma, hypertension (systolic BP >175 mm Hg and/or diastolic BP >110 mm Hg), high likelihood of left heart thrombus (eg, mitral stenosis with atrial fibrillation), acute pericarditis, subacute bacterial endocarditis, hemostatic defects including ones caused by severe renal or hepatic dysfunction, significant hepatic dysfunction, pregnancy, diabetic hemorrhagic retinopathy or other

(Continued)

Alteplase *(Continued)*

hemorrhagic ophthalmic conditions, septic thrombophlebitis or occluded AV cannula at seriously infected site, advanced age (eg, >75 years), patients receiving oral anticoagulants, any other condition in which bleeding constitutes a significant hazard or would be particularly difficult to manage because of location.

Coronary thrombolysis may result in reperfusion arrhythmias. In treatment of patients with acute ischemic stroke more than 3 hours after symptom onset is not recommended; treatment of patients with minor neurological deficit or with rapidly improving symptoms is not recommended.

Cathflo™ Activase®: When used to restore catheter function, use Cathflo™ cautiously in those patients with known or suspected catheter infections. Evaluate catheter for other causes of dysfunction before use. Avoid excessive pressure when instilling into catheter. Use of Cathflo™ in children <2 years of age (or weighing <10 kg) has not been studied.

Drug Interactions

Decreased Effect: Aminocaproic acid (an antifibrinolytic agent) may decrease the effectiveness of thrombolytic therapy. Nitroglycerin may increase the hepatic clearance of alteplase, potentially reducing lytic activity (limited clinical information).

Increased Effect/Toxicity: The potential for hemorrhage with alteplase is increased by oral anticoagulants (warfarin), heparin, low molecular weight heparins, and drugs which affect platelet function (eg, NSAIDs, dipyridamole, ticlopidine, clopidogrel, IIb/IIIa antagonists). Concurrent use with aspirin and heparin may increase the risk of bleeding. However, aspirin and heparin were used concomitantly with alteplase in the majority of patients in clinical studies.

Nutritional/Ethanol Interactions Herb/Nutraceutical: Avoid cat's claw, dong quai, evening primrose, feverfew, red clover, horse chestnut, garlic, green tea, ginseng, ginkgo (all have additional antiplatelet activity).

Lab Interactions Altered results of coagulation and fibrinolytic agents

Adverse Reactions As with all drugs which may affect hemostasis, bleeding is the major adverse effect associated with alteplase. Hemorrhage may occur at virtually any site. Risk is dependent on multiple variables, including the dosage administered, concurrent use of multiple agents which alter hemostasis, and patient predisposition. Rapid lysis of coronary artery thrombi by thrombolytic agents may be associated with reperfusion-related atrial and/or ventricular arrhythmia. **Note:** Lowest rate of bleeding complications expected with dose used to restore catheter function.

1% to 10%:

Cardiovascular: Hypotension

Central nervous system: Fever

Dermatologic: Bruising (1%)

Gastrointestinal: GI hemorrhage (5%), nausea, vomiting

Genitourinary: GU hemorrhage (4%)

Local: Bleeding at catheter puncture site (15.3%, accelerated administration)

Hematologic: Bleeding (0.5% major, 7% minor: GUSTO trial)

Additional cardiovascular events associated **with use in MI:** AV block, cardiogenic shock, heart failure, cardiac arrest, recurrent ischemia/infarction, myocardial rupture, electromechanical dissociation, pericardial effusion, pericarditis, mitral regurgitation, cardiac tamponade, thromboembolism, pulmonary edema, asystole, ventricular tachycardia, bradycardia, ruptured intracranial AV malformation, seizure, hemorrhagic bursitis, cholesterol crystal embolization

Additional events associated **with use in pulmonary embolism:** Pulmonary re-embolization, pulmonary edema, pleural effusion, thromboembolism

Additional events associated **with use in stroke:** Cerebral edema, cerebral herniation, seizure, new ischemic stroke

Overdosage/Toxicology Increased incidence of intracranial bleeding.

Pharmacodynamics/Kinetics

Duration of Action: >50% present in plasma cleared ~5 minutes after infusion terminated, ~80% cleared within 10 minutes

Excretion: Clearance: Rapidly from circulating plasma (550-650 mL/minute), primarily hepatic; >50% present in plasma is cleared within 5 minutes after the infusion is terminated, ~80% cleared within 10 minutes

Dosing

Adults & Elderly:

Coronary artery thrombi: I.V. Front loading dose (weight-based):

Patients >67 kg: Total dose: 100 mg over 1.5 hours; infuse 15 mg over 1-2 minutes. Infuse 50 mg over 30 minutes. See "Note."

Patients ≤67 kg: Total dose: 1.25 mg/kg; infuse 15 mg I.V. bolus over 1-2 minutes, then infuse 0.75 mg/kg (not to exceed 50 mg) over next 30 minutes, followed by 0.5 mg/kg over next 60 minutes (not to exceed 35 mg). See "Note."

Note: Concurrently, begin heparin 60 units/kg bolus (maximum: 4000 units) followed by continuous infusion of 12 units/kg/hour (maximum: 1000 units/hour) and adjust to aPTT target of 1.5-2 times the upper limit of control. Infuse remaining 35 mg of alteplase over the next hour.

Acute pulmonary embolism: I.V.: 100 mg over 2 hours.

Acute ischemic stroke: I.V.: Doses should be given within the first 3 hours of the onset of symptoms; recommended total dose: 0.9 mg/kg (maximum dose should not exceed 90 mg) infused over 60 minutes.

Load with 0.09 mg/kg (10% of the 0.9 mg/kg dose) as an I.V. bolus over 1 minute, followed by 0.81 mg/kg (90% of the 0.9 mg/kg dose) as a continuous infusion over 60 minutes. Heparin should not be started for 24 hours or more after starting alteplase for stroke.

Central venous catheter clearance: Intracatheter (Cathflo™ Activase®):

Patients ≥10 to <30 kg: 110% of the internal lumen volume of the catheter (≤2 mg [1 mg/mL]); retain in catheter for ≤2 hours; may instill a second dose if catheter remains occluded

Patients ≥30 kg: 2 mg (1 mg/mL); retain in catheter for ≤2 hours; may instill a second dose if catheter remains occluded

Acute peripheral arterial occlusive disease (unlabeled use): Intra-arterial: 0.02-0.1 mg/kg/hour for up to 36 hours

Advisory Panel to the Society for Cardiovascular and Interventional Radiology on Thrombolytic Therapy recommendation: ≤2 mg/hour and subtherapeutic heparin (aPTT <1.5 times baseline)

Pediatrics: Central venous catheter clearance: Intracatheter: ≥10 to <30 kg: 110% of the internal lumen volume of the catheter (≤2 mg [1 mg/mL]); retain in catheter for ≤2 hours; may instill a second dose if catheter remains occluded

Available Dosage Forms Injection, powder for reconstitution, recombinant:

Activase®: 50 mg [29 million int. units]; 100 mg [58 million int. units]

Cathflo™ Activase®: 2 mg

Monitoring and Teaching Issues

Physical Assessment: See Contraindications, Warnings/Precautions, and Dosing for use cautions. Assess potential for interactions with other medications that may affect coagulation or platelet function (see Drug Interactions). Assess vital signs, results of laboratory tests, and ECG prior to, during, and after therapy. Arrhythmias may occur; antiarrhythmic drugs should be immediately available. Infusion site should be monitored and patient assessed for hemorrhage every 10 minutes (or according to institutional policy) during therapy and for 1 hour following therapy (see Adverse Reactions). Strict bedrest should be maintained and bleeding precautions should be instituted; avoid invasive procedures and activities that could cause trauma. Patient instructions determined by patient condition.

Monitoring Laboratory Tests: CBC, PTT

Patient Education: Inform prescriber of all prescriptions, OTC medications, or herbal products you are taking, and any allergies you have. This medication can only be administered by infusion; you will be monitored closely during and after treatment. You will have a tendency to bleed easily; use caution to prevent injury (use electric razor, soft toothbrush, and use caution with knives, needles, or anything sharp). Follow instructions for strict bedrest to reduce the risk of injury. If bleeding occurs, report immediately and apply pressure to bleeding spot until bleeding stops completely. Report unusual pain (acute headache, joint pain, chest pain); unusual bruising or bleeding; blood in urine, stool, or vomit; bleeding gums; vision changes; or respiratory difficulty. **Pregnancy/breast-feeding precautions:** Inform prescriber if you are or intend to become pregnant. Consult prescriber if breast-feeding.

Pregnancy Risk Factor: C

Lactation: Excretion in breast milk unknown

Other Issues: Drug is frequently administered with heparin. Discontinue both if serious bleeding occurs. Avoid invasive procedures.

Administration

I.V.: Activase®: Acute MI: Accelerated infusion:

Bolus dose may be prepared by one of three methods:

1) removal of 15 mL reconstituted (1 mg/mL) solution from vial

2) removal of 15 mL from a port on the infusion line after priming

3) programming an infusion pump to deliver a 15 mL bolus at the initiation of infusion

Remaining dose may be administered as follows:

50 mg vial: Either PVC bag or glass vial and infusion set

100 mg vial: Insert spike end of the infusion set through the same puncture site created by transfer device and infuse from vial

If further dilution is desired, may be diluted in equal volume of 0.9% sodium chloride or D₅W to yield a final concentration of 0.5 mg/mL AD

Other: Cathflo™ Activase®: Intracatheter: Instill dose into occluded catheter. Do not force solution into catheter. After a 30-minute dwell time, assess catheter function by attempting to aspirate blood. If catheter is functional, aspirate 4-5 mL of blood to remove Cathflo™ Activase® and residual clots. Gently irrigate the catheter with NS. If catheter remains nonfunctional, let Cathflo™ Activase® dwell for another 90 minutes (total dwell time: 120 minutes) and reassess function. If catheter function is not restored, a second dose may be instilled.

Reconstitution:

Activase®:

50 mg vial: Use accompanying diluent (50 mL sterile water for injection); do not shake; final concentration: 1 mg/mL

100 mg vial: Use transfer set with accompanying diluent (100 mL vial of sterile water for injection); no vacuum is present in 100 mg vial; final concentration: 1 mg/mL

Cathflo™ Activase®: Add 2.2 mL SWFI to vial; do not shake. Final concentration: 1 mg/mL. Once reconstituted, store at 2°C to 30°C (36°F to 86°F).

Compatibility: Stable in NS, SWFI; **incompatible** with bacteriostatic water

Y-site administration: Incompatible with dobutamine, dopamine, heparin, nitroglycerin

Compatibility when admixed: Incompatible with dobutamine, dopamine, heparin

Storage:

Activase®: The lyophilized product may be stored at room temperature (not to exceed 30°C/86°F), or under refrigeration; once reconstituted it must be used within 8 hours

Cathflo™ Activase®: Store lyophilized product in refrigerated; protect from excessive exposure to light when stored for extended periods of time. Once reconstituted, store at 2°C to 30°C (36°F to 86°F).

♦ **Altocor™ [DSC]** *see* Lovastatin *on page 925*

♦ **Altoprev™** *see* Lovastatin *on page 925*

Altretamine (al TRET a meen)

U.S. Brand Names Hexalen®

Synonyms Hexamethylmelamine; HEXM; HMM; HXM; NSC-13875

Generic Available No

Pharmacologic Category Antineoplastic Agent, Miscellaneous

Use Palliative treatment of persistent or recurrent ovarian cancer

Mechanism of Action/Effect Exact mechanism of action that causes cell death is not known. Metabolism in the liver is required for cytotoxicity. Although altretamine clinical antitumor spectrum resembles that of alkylating agents, the drug has demonstrated activity in alkylator-resistant patients. The drug selectively inhibits the incorporation of radioactive thymidine and uridine into DNA and RNA, inhibiting DNA and RNA synthesis. Reactive intermediates covalently bind to microsomal proteins and DNA; can spontaneously degrade to demethylated melamines and formaldehyde which are also cytotoxic.

Contraindications Hypersensitivity to altretamine or any component of the formulation; pre-existing severe bone marrow suppression or severe neurologic toxicity; pregnancy

Warnings/Precautions The U.S. Food and Drug Administration (FDA) currently recommends that procedures for proper handling and disposal of antineoplastic agents be considered. Use with caution in patients previously treated with other myelosuppressive drugs or with pre-existing neurotoxicity. Use with caution in patients with renal or hepatic dysfunction. Altretamine may be slightly mutagenic.

Drug Interactions

Decreased Effect: Phenobarbital may increase metabolism of altretamine which may decrease the effect.

Increased Effect/Toxicity: Altretamine may cause severe orthostatic hypotension when administered with MAO inhibitors. Cimetidine may decrease metabolism of altretamine.

Nutritional/Ethanol Interactions Ethanol: Avoid ethanol (due to GI irritation).

Adverse Reactions

>10%:

Central nervous system: Peripheral sensory neuropathy, neurotoxicity (21%; may be progressive and dose-limiting)

Gastrointestinal: Nausea/vomiting (50% to 70%), anorexia (48%), diarrhea (48%)

Hematologic: Anemia, thrombocytopenia (31%), leukopenia (62%), neutropenia

1% to 10%:

Central nervous system: Seizures

Gastrointestinal: Stomach cramps

Hepatic: Alkaline phosphatase increased

Overdosage/Toxicology Symptoms of overdose include nausea, vomiting, peripheral neuropathy, severe bone marrow suppression. Treatment is supportive.

Pharmacodynamics/Kinetics

Absorption: Well absorbed (75% to 89%)

Time to Peak: Plasma: 0.5-3 hours

Half-Life Elimination: 13 hours

Metabolism: Hepatic; rapid and extensive demethylation; active metabolites

Excretion: Urine (<1% as unchanged drug)

Dosing

Adults & Elderly: Ovarian cancer (palliative): Oral:

4-12 mg/kg/day in 3-4 divided doses for 21-90 days

Alternatively: 240-320 mg/m²/day in 3-4 divided doses per day for 21 days, repeated every 6 weeks

Alternatively: 260 mg/m²/day in 4 divided doses per day for 14-21 days of a 28-day cycle

Available Dosage Forms Gelcap: 50 mg [contains lactose]

Monitoring and Teaching Issues

Physical Assessment: Assess for use cautions (eg, patients previously treated with other myelosuppressive drugs or with pre-existing neurotoxicity; renal or hepatic dysfunction; see Warnings/Precautions). Monitor for potential for drug interactions (see Drug Interactions). Assess results of laboratory tests, therapeutic effectiveness, and adverse response (eg, neuropathy, gastrointestinal upset, anemia; see Adverse Reactions). Teach patient appropriate use, possible side effects/appropriate interventions, and adverse symptoms to report.

Monitoring Laboratory Tests: CBC with platelet count and differential should be done routinely before and after drug therapy.

Patient Education: Do not take anything new (including aspirin or any aspirin-containing products) during treatment unless approved by prescriber. Take exactly as directed, preferably after meals. Avoid alcohol. May cause nausea or vomiting (small frequent meals, good mouth care, chewing gum, or sucking lozenges may help). You will be more susceptible to infection (avoid crowds and exposure to infection). Report any numbness, tingling, or pain in extremities; unrelieved nausea or vomiting; tremors; yellowing of skin or eyes; fever; chills; easy bruising or unusual bleeding; extreme weakness; or increased fatigue. **Pregnancy/breast-feeding precautions:** Do not get pregnant while taking this medication. Consult prescriber for appropriate contraceptive measures. Consult prescriber if breast-feeding.

Dietary Considerations: Should be taken after meals at bedtime.

Pregnancy Risk Factor: D

Lactation: Excretion in breast milk unknown

Administration

Oral: Administer total daily dose as 3-4 divided doses after meals and at bedtime.

♦ **Alu-Cap® [OTC]** *see* Aluminum Hydroxide *on page 83*

Aluminum Hydroxide (a LOO mi num hye DROKS ide)

U.S. Brand Names ALternaGel® [OTC]; Alu-Cap® [OTC]

Generic Available Yes: Suspension

Pharmacologic Category Antacid; Antidote

Use Treatment of hyperacidity; hyperphosphatemia

Mechanism of Action/Effect Neutralizes or reduces gastric acidity, resulting in increased gastric pH and inhibition of pepsin activity

Contraindications Hypersensitivity to aluminum salts or any component of the formulation

Warnings/Precautions Binds with phosphate ions. Hypophosphatemia may occur with prolonged administration or large doses. Use with caution in patients with CHF, renal failure, edema, cirrhosis, and low sodium diets, and patients who have recently suffered GI hemorrhage. Uremic patients not receiving dialysis may develop aluminum intoxication or osteomalacia and osteoporosis due to phosphate depletion.

Drug Interactions

Decreased Effect: Aluminum hydroxide may decrease the absorption of allopurinol, antibiotics (tetracyclines, quinolones, some cephalosporins), bisphosphonate derivatives, corticosteroids, cyclosporine, delavirdine, iron salts, imidazole antifungals, isoniazid, mycophenolate, penicillamine, phosphate supplements, phenytoin, phenothiazines, trientine. Absorption of aluminum hydroxide may be decreased by citric acid derivatives.

Lab Interactions Decreased phosphorus, inorganic (S); may interfere with some gastric imaging techniques or gastric acid secretion tests

Adverse Reactions Frequency not defined.

Gastrointestinal: Constipation, stomach cramps, fecal impaction, nausea, vomiting, discoloration of feces (white speckles)

Endocrine & metabolic: Hypophosphatemia, hypomagnesemia

Overdosage/Toxicology Aluminum antacids may cause constipation, phosphate depletion, and bezoar or fecalith formation. In patients with renal failure, aluminum may accumulate to toxic levels. Deferoxamine, traditionally used as an iron chelator, has been shown to increase urinary aluminum output. Deferoxamine chelation of aluminum has resulted in improvement of clinical symptoms and bone histology; however, this remains an experimental treatment for aluminum poisoning and has significant potential for adverse effects.

Dosing

Adults & Elderly:

Hyperphosphatemia: Oral: Initial: 300-600 mg 3 times/day with meals

Hyperacidity: Oral: 600-1200 mg between meals and at bedtime

Pediatrics: Hyperphosphatemia: Oral: 50-150 mg/kg/24 hours in divided doses every 4-6 hours, titrate dosage to maintain serum phosphorus within normal range

Renal Impairment: Aluminum may accumulate in renal impairment.

Available Dosage Forms

Capsule (Alu-Cap®): 400 mg

Suspension, oral: 320 mg/5 mL (473 mL)

ALternaGel®: 600 mg/5 mL (360 mL)

Monitoring and Teaching Issues

Physical Assessment: Assess results of laboratory tests and therapeutic effectiveness. Assess for constipation and treat accordingly.

Monitoring Laboratory Tests: Calcium and phosphate levels periodically when patient is on chronic therapy

Patient Education: Take as directed, preferably 1-3 hours after meals (when used as an antacid) or with any other medications. When used to decrease phosphorus, take within 20 minutes of a meal. Do not increase sodium intake and maintain adequate hydration (2-3 L/day of fluids) unless instructed to restrict fluid intake. You may experience constipation (increased exercise, fluids, fruit, or fiber may help; if unresolved, contact prescriber). Report unresolved nausea, malaise, muscle weakness, blood in stool or black stool, or abdominal pain. **Pregnancy/breast-feeding precautions:** Inform prescriber if you are or intend to become pregnant. Consult prescriber if breast-feeding.

Dietary Considerations: Should be taken 1-3 hours after meals when used as an antacid. When used to decrease phosphorus, should be taken within 20 minutes of a meal.

Geriatric Considerations: Elderly, due to disease and/or drug therapy, may be predisposed to constipation and fecal impaction. This may be managed with a stool softener or laxatives. Careful evaluation of possible drug interactions must be done. Consider renal insufficiency (<30 mL/minute) as predisposition to aluminum toxicity.

Pregnancy Risk Factor: C

Lactation: Excretion in breast milk unknown

Administration

Oral: Dose should be followed with water.

♦ **Aluminum Sucrose Sulfate, Basic** *see* Sucralfate *on page 1402*

Amantadine (a MAN ta deen)

U.S. Brand Names Symmetrel®

Synonyms Adamantanamine Hydrochloride; Amantadine Hydrochloride

Generic Available Yes

Pharmacologic Category Anti-Parkinson's Agent, Dopamine Agonist; Antiviral Agent

Medication Safety Issues

Sound-alike/look-alike issues:

Amantadine may be confused with ranitidine, rimantadine

Symmetrel® may be confused with Synthroid®

Use Prophylaxis and treatment of influenza A viral infection; treatment of parkinsonism; treatment of drug-induced extrapyramidal symptoms

Unlabeled/Investigational Use Creutzfeldt-Jakob disease

Mechanism of Action/Effect As an antiviral, blocks the uncoating of influenza A virus preventing penetration of virus into host; antiparkinsonian activity may be due to its blocking *(Continued)*

Amantadine *(Continued)*

the reuptake of dopamine into presynaptic neurons or by increasing dopamine release from presynaptic fibers

Contraindications Hypersensitivity to amantadine or any component of the formulation

Warnings/Precautions Use with caution in patients with liver disease, history of recurrent and eczematoid dermatitis, uncontrolled psychosis or severe psychoneurosis, seizures, and in those receiving CNS stimulant drugs. Reduce dose in renal disease. When treating Parkinson's disease, do not discontinue abruptly. In many patients, the therapeutic benefits of amantadine are limited to a few months. Elderly patients may be more susceptible to CNS effects (using 2 divided daily doses may minimize this effect). Has been associated with neuroleptic malignant syndrome (associated with dose reduction or abrupt discontinuation). Has not been shown to prevent bacterial infection or complications when used as prophylaxis or treatment of influenza A. Use with caution in patients with CHF, peripheral edema, or orthostatic hypotension. Avoid in angle closure glaucoma.

Drug Interactions

Increased Effect/Toxicity: Anticholinergics (benztropine and trihexyphenidyl) may potentiate CNS side effects of amantadine. Hydrochlorothiazide, triamterene, and/or trimethoprim may increase toxicity of amantadine; monitor for altered response.

Nutritional/Ethanol Interactions Ethanol: Avoid ethanol (may increase CNS adverse effects).

Adverse Reactions 1% to 10%:

Cardiovascular: Orthostatic hypotension, peripheral edema

Central nervous system: Insomnia, depression, anxiety, irritability, dizziness, hallucinations, ataxia, headache, somnolence, nervousness, dream abnormality, agitation, fatigue, confusion

Dermatologic: Livedo reticularis

Gastrointestinal: Nausea, anorexia, constipation, diarrhea, xerostomia

Respiratory: Dry nose

Overdosage/Toxicology Symptoms of overdose include nausea, vomiting, slurred speech, blurred vision, lethargy, hallucinations, seizures, and myoclonic jerking. Acute toxicity may be primarily due to anticholinergic effects. The minimum lethal dose may be as low as 1 g. Treatment should be directed at reducing CNS stimulation, controlling seizures, and maintaining cardiovascular function.

Pharmacodynamics/Kinetics

Onset of Action: Antidyskinetic: Within 48 hours

Absorption: Well absorbed

Bioavailability: 86% to 90%

Time to Peak: 1-4 hours

Protein Binding: Normal renal function: ~67%; Hemodialysis: ~59%

Half-Life Elimination: Normal renal function: 16 ± 6 hours (9-31 hours); End-stage renal disease: 7-10 days

Metabolism: Not appreciable; small amounts of an acetyl metabolite identified

Excretion: Urine (80% to 90% unchanged) by glomerular filtration and tubular secretion; Total clearance: 2.5-10.5 L/hour

Dosing

Adults:

Influenza A treatment: Oral: 100 mg twice daily; initiate within 24-48 hours after onset of symptoms; discontinue as soon as possible based on clinical response (generally within 3-5 days or within 24-48 hours after symptoms disappear).

Influenza A prophylaxis: Oral: 100 mg twice daily; continue treatment throughout the peak influenza activity in the community or throughout the entire influenza season in patients who cannot be vaccinated. Development of immunity following vaccination takes ~2 weeks; amantadine therapy should be considered for high-risk patients from the time of vaccination until immunity has developed.

Drug-induced extrapyramidal symptoms: Oral: 100 mg twice daily; may increase to 300-400 mg/day, if needed

Parkinson's disease or Creutzfeldt-Jakob disease (unlabeled use): Oral: 100 mg twice daily as sole therapy; may increase to 400 mg/day if needed with close monitoring; initial dose: 100 mg/day if with other serious illness or with high doses of other anti-Parkinson drugs

Elderly: Adjust dose based on renal function; some patients tolerate the drug better when it is given in 2 divided daily doses (to avoid adverse neurologic reactions).

Pediatrics:

Influenza A treatment: Oral: Children: **Note:** Initiate within 24-48 hours after onset of symptoms; discontinue as soon as possible based on clinical response (generally within 3-5 days or within 24-48 hours after symptoms disappear)

1-9 years: 5 mg/kg/day in 2 divided doses (manufacturers range: 4.4-8.8 mg/kg/day); maximum dose: 150 mg/day

≥10 years and <40 kg: 5 mg/kg/day; maximum dose: 150 mg/day

10-12 years and ≥40 kg: 100 mg twice daily.

≥13 years: Refer to adult dosing.

Influenza A prophylaxis: Oral: Refer to "Influenza A treatment" dosing. Continue treatment throughout the peak influenza activity in the community or throughout the entire influenza season in patients who cannot be vaccinated. Development of immunity following vaccination takes ~2 weeks; amantadine therapy should be considered for high-risk patients from the time of vaccination until immunity has developed. For children <9 years receiving influenza vaccine for the first time, amantadine prophylaxis should continue for 6 weeks (4 weeks after the first dose and 2 weeks after the second dose)

Renal Impairment:

Cl_{cr} 30-50 mL/minute: Administer 200 mg on day 1, then 100 mg/day

Cl_{cr} 15-29 mL/minute: Administer 200 mg on day 1, then 100 mg on alternate days

Cl_{cr} <15 mL/minute: Administer 200 mg every 7 days

Hemodialysis: Administer 200 mg every 7 days

Peritoneal dialysis: No supplemental dose is needed
Continuous arteriovenous or venous-venous hemofiltration: No supplemental dose is needed

Available Dosage Forms
Capsule, as hydrochloride: 100 mg
Syrup, as hydrochloride (Symmetrel®): 50 mg/5 mL (480 mL) [raspberry flavor]
Tablet, as hydrochloride (Symmetrel®): 100 mg

Monitoring and Teaching Issues
Physical Assessment: Assess effectiveness and interactions of other medications patient may be taking. Monitor renal function, therapeutic effectiveness, and adverse reactions at beginning of therapy and periodically throughout therapy. Assess blood pressure; monitor for signs of fluid retention. When treating Parkinson's disease, taper slowly when discontinuing. Assess knowledge/teach patient appropriate use, interventions to reduce side effects, and adverse symptoms to report.

Monitoring Laboratory Tests: Renal function

Patient Education: Take as directed; do not increase dosage, take more often than prescribed, or discontinue without consulting prescriber. Maintain adequate hydration (2-3 L/day of fluids) unless instructed to restrict fluid intake and void before taking medication. Take last dose of day in the afternoon to reduce incidence of insomnia. Avoid alcohol, sedatives, or hypnotics unless consulting prescriber. You may experience decreased mental alertness or coordination (use caution when driving, climbing stairs, or engaging in tasks requiring alertness until response to drug is known); or nausea or dry mouth (small frequent meals, frequent mouth care, sucking lozenges, or chewing gum may help). Report unusual swelling of extremities, respiratory difficulty or shortness of breath, change in gait or increased tremors, or changes in mentation (eg, depression, anxiety, irritability, hallucination, slurred speech). **Pregnancy/breast-feeding precautions:** Inform prescriber if you are pregnant. Breast-feeding is not recommended.

Geriatric Considerations: Elderly patients may be more susceptible to the CNS effects of amantadine; using 2 divided daily doses may minimize this effect. The syrup may be used to administer doses <100 mg.

Pregnancy Risk Factor: C

Pregnancy Issues: Impaired fertility has also been reported during animal studies and during human *in vitro* fertilization.

Lactation: Enters breast milk/not recommended

Administration
Storage: Store at 15°C to 30°C (59°F to 86°F). Protect from freezing.

Additional Information Patients with intolerable CNS side effects often do better with rimantadine.

♦ Amantadine Hydrochloride see Amantadine on page 83
♦ Amaryl® see Glimepiride on page 713

Ambenonium (am be NOE nee um)

U.S. Brand Names Mytelase®
Synonyms Ambenonium Chloride
Generic Available No
Pharmacologic Category Cholinergic Agonist
Use Treatment of myasthenia gravis
Mechanism of Action/Effect Action increases acetylcholine concentration at transmission sites in parasympathetic neurons and skeletal muscles by inhibiting acetylcholinesterase
Contraindications Routine administration of atropine or other belladonna alkaloids with ambenonium is contraindicated because they may suppress the muscarinic symptoms of excessive gastrointestinal stimulation, leaving only the more serious symptoms of muscle fasciculations and paralysis as signs of overdosage; should not be administered to patients receiving mecamylamine
Warnings/Precautions Prolonged action after cholinergics, drug should be discontinued until the patient is stabilized. Use with caution in patients with asthma, epilepsy, bradycardia, hyperthyroidism, or peptic ulcer. Differentiation of cholinergic/myasthenia crisis is critical, use edrophonium and clinical judgment. Anticholinergic insensitivity may develop for brief or prolonged periods. Reduce or withhold dosages until the patient becomes sensitive again. May require respiratory support.

Drug Interactions
Decreased Effect: Corticosteroids antagonize effects of anticholinesterases in myasthenia gravis. Procainamide or quinidine may reverse ambenonium cholinergic effects on muscle.
Increased Effect/Toxicity: Succinylcholine neuromuscular blockade may be prolonged.
Lab Interactions Increased aminotransferase [ALT (SGPT)/AST (SGOT)] (S), amylase (S)

Adverse Reactions Frequency not defined.
Cardiovascular: Arrhythmias (especially bradycardia), hypotension, decreased carbon monoxide, tachycardia, AV block, nodal rhythm, nonspecific ECG changes, cardiac arrest, syncope, flushing
Central nervous system: Convulsions, dysarthria, dysphonia, dizziness, loss of consciousness, drowsiness, headache
Dermatologic: Skin rash, thrombophlebitis (I.V.), urticaria
Gastrointestinal: Hyperperistalsis, nausea, vomiting, salivation, diarrhea, stomach cramps, dysphagia, flatulence
Genitourinary: Urinary urgency
Neuromuscular & skeletal: Weakness, fasciculations, muscle cramps, spasms, arthralgia
Ocular: Small pupils, lacrimation
Respiratory: Increased bronchial secretions, laryngospasm, bronchiolar constriction, respiratory muscle paralysis, dyspnea, respiratory depression, respiratory arrest, bronchospasm
Miscellaneous: Diaphoresis (increased), anaphylaxis, allergic reactions

Overdosage/Toxicology Have atropine on hand to reverse cholinergic crisis or hypersensitivity reaction.
(Continued)

Ambenonium (Continued)

Dosing
Adults & Elderly: Myasthenia gravis: Oral: 5-25 mg 3-4 times/day

Available Dosage Forms Caplet, as chloride [scored]: 10 mg [contains lactose and sucrose]

Monitoring and Teaching Issues
Physical Assessment: Assess bladder and sphincter adequacy prior to administering medication. Assess other medications patient may be taking for effectiveness and interactions. Monitor therapeutic effectiveness and adverse reactions (cholinergic crisis). Assess knowledge/teach patient appropriate use, interventions to reduce side effects, and adverse symptoms to report.

Patient Education: This drug will not cure myasthenia gravis, but it may reduce the symptoms. Use as directed; do not increase dose or discontinue without consulting prescriber. Maintain adequate hydration (2-3 L/day of fluids) unless instructed to restrict fluid intake. May cause dizziness, drowsiness, or postural hypotension (rise slowly from sitting or lying position and use caution when driving or climbing stairs); vomiting or loss of appetite (small frequent meals, frequent mouth care, sucking lozenges, or chewing gum may help); or diarrhea (boiled milk, yogurt, or buttermilk may help). Report persistent abdominal discomfort; significantly increased salivation, sweating, tearing, or urination; flushed skin; chest pain or palpitations; acute headache; unresolved diarrhea; excessive fatigue, insomnia, dizziness, or depression; increased muscle, joint, or body pain; vision changes or blurred vision; or shortness of breath or wheezing. **Pregnancy/breast-feeding precautions:** Inform prescriber if you are or intend to become pregnant. Breast-feeding is not recommended.

Pregnancy Risk Factor: C

Lactation: Excretion in breast milk unknown/not recommended

- **Ambenonium Chloride** *see* Ambenonium *on page 85*
- **Ambien®** *see* Zolpidem *on page 1595*
- **Ambifed-G** *see* Guaifenesin and Pseudoephedrine *on page 733*
- **AmBisome®** *see* Amphotericin B (Liposomal) *on page 113*
- **Amerge®** *see* Naratriptan *on page 1058*
- **Americaine® [OTC]** *see* Benzocaine *on page 181*
- **Americaine® Anesthetic Lubricant [DSC]** *see* Benzocaine *on page 181*
- **Americaine® Hemorrhoidal [OTC]** *see* Benzocaine *on page 181*
- **A-Methapred** *see* MethylPREDNISolone *on page 986*
- **Amethopterin** *see* Methotrexate *on page 974*
- **Amevive®** *see* Alefacept *on page 64*
- **Amfepramone** *see* Diethylpropion *on page 449*
- **AMG 073** *see* Cinacalcet *on page 326*
- **Amibid DM** *see* Guaifenesin and Dextromethorphan *on page 731*
- **Amidrine** *see* Acetaminophen, Isometheptene, and Dichloralphenazone *on page 42*

Amifostine (am i FOS teen)
U.S. Brand Names Ethyol®

Synonyms Ethiofos; Gammaphos; WR-2721; YM-08310

Generic Available No

Pharmacologic Category Adjuvant, Chemoprotective Agent (Cytoprotective); Antidote

Medication Safety Issues
Sound-alike/look-alike issues:
Ethyol® may be confused with ethanol

Use Reduce the incidence of moderate to severe xerostomia in patients undergoing postoperative radiation treatment for head and neck cancer, where the radiation port includes a substantial portion of the parotid glands. Reduce the cumulative renal toxicity associated with repeated administration of cisplatin in patients with advanced ovarian cancer or nonsmall cell lung cancer.

Mechanism of Action/Effect Reduces the toxic effects of cisplatin, cyclophosphamide, radiation therapy

Contraindications Hypersensitivity to aminothiol compounds, mannitol, or any component of the formulation

Warnings/Precautions Patients who are hypotensive or in a state of dehydration should not receive amifostine. Interrupt antihypertensive therapy for 24 hours before amifostine. Patients receiving antihypertensive therapy that cannot be stopped for 24 hours preceding amifostine treatment also should not receive amifostine.

It is recommended that antiemetic medication, including dexamethasone 20 mg I.V. and a serotonin 5-HT$_3$ receptor antagonist be administered prior to and in conjunction with amifostine. Rare hypersensitivity reactions, including anaphylaxis and severe cutaneous reaction, have been reported with a higher frequency in patients receiving amifostine as a radioprotectant. Discontinue if allergic reaction occurs; do not rechallenge.

Reports of clinically relevant hypocalcemia are rare, but serum calcium levels should be monitored in patients at risk of hypocalcemia, such as those with nephrotic syndrome.

Drug Interactions
Increased Effect/Toxicity: Special consideration should be given to patients receiving antihypertensive medications or other drugs that could potentiate hypotension.

Adverse Reactions >10%:
Cardiovascular: Flushing; hypotension (62%)
Central nervous system: Chills, dizziness, somnolence
Gastrointestinal: Nausea/vomiting (may be severe)
Respiratory: Sneezing
Miscellaneous: Feeling of warmth/coldness, hiccups

Overdosage/Toxicology Symptoms of overdose include hypotension, nausea, and vomiting. Treatment includes supportive measures as clinically indicated.

Pharmacodynamics/Kinetics

Half-Life Elimination: 9 minutes

Metabolism: Hepatic dephosphorylation to two metabolites (active-free thiol and disulfide)

Excretion: Urine

Clearance, plasma: 2.17 L/minute

Dosing

Adults & Elderly:

Cisplatin-induced renal toxicity, reduction: I.V.: 740-910 mg/m^2 once daily 30 minutes prior to cytotoxic therapy

Note: Doses >740 mg/m^2 are associated with a higher incidence of hypotension and may require interruption of therapy or dose modification for subsequent cycles. For 910 mg/m^2 doses, the manufacturer suggests the following blood pressure-based adjustment schedule:

The infusion of amifostine should be interrupted if the systolic blood pressure decreases significantly from baseline, as defined below:

Decrease of 20 mm Hg if baseline systolic blood pressure <100

Decrease of 25 mm Hg if baseline systolic blood pressure 100-119

Decrease of 30 mm Hg if baseline systolic blood pressure 120-139

Decrease of 40 mm Hg if baseline systolic blood pressure 140-179

Decrease of 50 mm Hg if baseline systolic blood pressure ≥180

If the blood pressure returns to normal within 5 minutes (assisted by fluid administration and postural management) and the patient is asymptomatic, the infusion may be restarted so that the full dose of amifostine may be administered. If the full dose of amifostine cannot be administered, the dose of amifostine for subsequent cycles should be 740 mg/m^2.

Xerostomia from head and neck cancer, reduction:

I.V.: 200mg/m^2/day during radiation therapy **or**

SubQ: 500 mg/day during radiation therapy

Available Dosage Forms Injection, powder for reconstitution: 500 mg

Monitoring and Teaching Issues

Physical Assessment: Monitor blood pressure closely during infusion (continuously or every 5-7 minutes; see Dosing). Can cause hypotension. Monitor nausea and treat with antiemetic as appropriate.

Patient Education: This I.V. medication is given to help reduce side effects of your chemotherapy and/or radiation therapy. Report immediately any nausea; you will be given medication. Report chills, severe dizziness, tremors or shaking, or sudden onset of hiccups. **Breast-feeding precaution:** Do not breast-feed.

Pregnancy Risk Factor: C

Lactation: Excretion in breast milk unknown/contraindicated

Administration

I.V.: Administer over 3-15 minutes; administration as a longer infusion is associated with a higher incidence of side effects.

Reconstitution: Reconstitute with 9.5 mL of sterile 0.9% sodium chloride. For SubQ administration, reconstitute with 2.4 mL NS or SWFI.

Compatibility: Stable in NS

Y-site administration: Incompatible with acyclovir, amphotericin B, cefoperazone, chlorpromazine, cisplatin, ganciclovir, hydroxyzine, minocycline, prochlorperazine edisylate

Storage: Reconstitute with 9.5 mL of sterile 0.9% sodium chloride. The reconstituted solution (500 mg/10 mL) is chemically stable for up to 5 hours at room temperature (25°C) or up to 24 hours under refrigeration 2°C to 8°C. Amifostine should be further diluted in 0.9% sodium chloride to a concentration of 5-40 mg/mL; diluted solutions (5-40 mg/mL) are stable for up to 5 hours at room temperature (25°C) or up to 24 hours when stored under refrigeration 2°C to 8°C.

Additional Information Mean onset of hypotension is 14 minutes into the 15-minute infusion and the mean duration was 6 minutes.

♦ **Amigesic®** *see* Salsalate *on page 1354*

Amikacin (am i KAY sin)

U.S. Brand Names Amikin®

Synonyms Amikacin Sulfate

Generic Available Yes

Pharmacologic Category Antibiotic, Aminoglycoside

Medication Safety Issues

Sound-alike/look-alike issues:

Amikacin may be confused with Amicar®, anakinra

Amikin® may be confused with Amicar®

Use Treatment of serious infections due to organisms resistant to gentamicin and tobramycin including *Pseudomonas*, *Proteus*, *Serratia*, and other gram-positive bacilli (bone infections, respiratory tract infections, endocarditis, and septicemia); documented infection of mycobacterial organisms susceptible to amikacin

Mechanism of Action/Effect Inhibits protein synthesis in susceptible bacteria by binding to ribosomal subunits

Contraindications Hypersensitivity to amikacin sulfate or any component of the formulation; cross-sensitivity may exist with other aminoglycosides

Warnings/Precautions Dose and/or frequency of administration must be monitored and modified in patients with renal impairment. Drug should be discontinued if signs of ototoxicity, nephrotoxicity, or hypersensitivity occur. Ototoxicity is proportional to the amount of drug given and the duration of treatment. Tinnitus or vertigo may be indications of vestibular injury and impending bilateral **irreversible** damage. Renal damage is usually reversible. May contain sulfites, use with caution in patients with asthma.

(Continued)

Amikacin *(Continued)*

Drug Interactions

Increased Effect/Toxicity: Amikacin may increase or prolong the effect of neuromuscular blocking agents. Concurrent use of amphotericin (or other nephrotoxic drugs) may increase the risk of amikacin-induced nephrotoxicity. The risk of ototoxicity from amikacin may be increased with other ototoxic drugs.

Lab Interactions Penicillin may decrease aminoglycoside serum concentrations *in vitro*

Adverse Reactions 1% to 10%:

Central nervous system: Neurotoxicity

Otic: Ototoxicity (auditory), ototoxicity (vestibular)

Renal: Nephrotoxicity

Overdosage/Toxicology Symptoms of overdose include ototoxicity, nephrotoxicity, and neuromuscular toxicity. Treatment of choice following a single acute overdose appears to be maintenance of urine output of at least 3 mL/kg/hour during the acute treatment phase. Dialysis is of questionable value in enhancing aminoglycoside elimination. If required, hemodialysis is preferred over peritoneal dialysis in patients with normal renal function.

Pharmacodynamics/Kinetics

Absorption: I.M.: May be delayed in the bedridden patient

Time to Peak: Serum: I.M.: 45-120 minutes

Half-Life Elimination: Renal function and age dependent:

Infants: Low birth weight (1-3 days): 7-9 hours; Full-term >7 days: 4-5 hours

Children: 1.6-2.5 hours

Adults: Normal renal function: 1.4-2.3 hours; Anuria/end-stage renal disease: 28-86 hours

Excretion: Urine (94% to 98%)

Dosing

Adults & Elderly: Individualization is critical because of the low therapeutic index

Note: Use of ideal body weight (IBW) for determining the mg/kg/dose appears to be more accurate than dosing on the basis of total body weight (TBW)

In morbid obesity, dosage requirement may best be estimated using a dosing weight of IBW + 0.4 (TBW - IBW)

Susceptible infections: I.M., I.V.: 5-7.5 mg/kg/dose every 8 hours

Adjustment: Initial and periodic peak and trough plasma drug levels should be determined, particularly in critically-ill patients with serious infections or in disease states known to significantly alter aminoglycoside pharmacokinetics (eg, cystic fibrosis, burns, or major surgery)

Note: Some clinicians suggest a daily dose of 15-20 mg/kg for all patients with normal renal function. This dose is at least as efficacious with similar, if not less, toxicity than conventional dosing.

Pediatrics: Infants and Children: Refer to adult dosing.

Renal Impairment: Individualization is critical because of the low therapeutic index. Some patients may require larger or more frequent doses if serum levels document the need (ie, cystic fibrosis or febrile granulocytopenic patients).

Cl_{cr} ≥60 mL/minute: Administer every 8 hours.

Cl_{cr} 40-60 mL/minute: Administer every 12 hours.

Cl_{cr} 20-40 mL/minute: Administer every 24 hours.

Cl_{cr} 10-20 mL/minute: Administer every 48 hours.

Cl_{cr} <10 mL/minute: Administer every 72 hours.

Dialyzable (50% to 100%)

Administer dose postdialysis or administer $^2/_3$ normal dose as a supplemental dose postdialysis and follow levels.

Peritoneal dialysis effects: Dose as for Cl_{cr} <10 mL/minute: Follow levels.

Continuous arteriovenous or venovenous hemodiafiltration effects: Dose as for Cl_{cr} 10-40 mL/minute: Follow levels.

Available Dosage Forms Injection, solution, as sulfate: 50 mg/mL (2 mL, 4 mL); 62.5 mg/mL (8 mL); 250 mg/mL (2 mL, 4 mL) [contains metabisulfite]

Monitoring and Teaching Issues

Physical Assessment: Assess allergy history prior to beginning therapy. Assess potential for interactions with other prescriptions, OTC medications, or herbal products patient may be taking. Assess results of laboratory tests, therapeutic effectiveness, and adverse response. Monitor for ototoxicity, nephrotoxicity, neurotoxicity. Hearing and renal status should be assessed before, during, and after therapy. Teach patient possible side effects/appropriate interventions and adverse symptoms to report.

Monitoring Laboratory Tests: Perform culture and sensitivity testing prior to initiating therapy. Urinalysis, BUN, serum creatinine, appropriately timed peak and trough concentrations. Initial and periodic peak and trough plasma drug levels should be determined, particularly in critically-ill patients with serious infections or in disease states known to significantly alter aminoglycoside pharmacokinetics (eg, cystic fibrosis, burns, or major surgery). Aminoglycoside levels measured from blood taken from Silastic® central catheters can sometimes give falsely high readings (draw levels from alternate lumen or peripheral stick, if possible).

Patient Education: Do not take any new medication during therapy unless approved by prescriber. This drug can only be administered by I.V. or I.M. injection. It is important to maintain adequate hydration (2-3 L/day of fluids) unless instructed to restrict fluid intake. Report immediately any change in hearing acuity, ringing or roaring in ears, alteration in balance, vertigo, feeling of fullness in head; pain, tingling, or numbness of any body part; or change in urinary pattern or decrease in urine. Report signs of opportunistic infection (eg, white plaques in mouth, vaginal discharge, unhealed sores, sore throat, unusual fever, chills); pain, redness, or swelling at injection site; or other adverse reactions. **Pregnancy precaution:** Inform prescriber if you are or intend to become pregnant.

Dietary Considerations: Sodium content of 1 g: 29.9 mg (1.3 mEq)

Geriatric Considerations: Adjust dose based on renal function.

Pregnancy Risk Factor: D

Lactation: Enters breast milk/compatible

Breast-Feeding Issues: No specific recommendations. However, aminoglycosides are not systemically available when taken orally. Therefore, the risk to the infant is minimal if ingested with breast milk.

Administration

I.M.: Administer I.M. injection in large muscle mass. Administer around-the-clock to promote less variation in peak and trough serum levels. Do not mix with other drugs, administer separately.

I.V.: Infuse over 30-60 minutes.

Compatibility: Stable in dextran 75 6% in NS, D_5LR, $D_5^{1}/_4NS$, $D_5^{1}/_3NS$, $D_5^{1}/_2NS$, D_5NS, $D_{10}NS$, D_5W, $D_{10}W$, $D_{20}W$, mannitol 20%, $^{1}/_4NS$, $^{1}/_2NS$, NS

    Y-site administration: Incompatible with allopurinol, amphotericin B cholesteryl sulfate complex, hetastarch, propofol

    Compatibility in syringe: Incompatible with heparin

    Compatibility when admixed: Incompatible with amphotericin B, ampicillin, cefazolin, chlorothiazide, heparin, phenytoin, thiopental, vitamin B complex with C

Storage: Stable for 24 hours at room temperature and 2 days at refrigeration when mixed in D_5W, $D_5^{1}/_4NS$, $D_5^{1}/_2NS$, NS, LR.

Additional Information Aminoglycoside levels measured from blood taken from Silastic® central catheters can sometimes give falsely high readings (draw levels from alternate lumen or peripheral stick, if possible)

Related Information

Antimicrobial Drugs of Choice *on page 1792*
Peak and Trough Guidelines *on page 1694*
Tuberculosis *on page 1864*

♦ **Amikacin Sulfate** *see* Amikacin *on page 87*

♦ **Amikin**® *see* Amikacin *on page 87*

Amiloride *(a MIL oh ride)*

U.S. Brand Names Midamor® [DSC]

Synonyms Amiloride Hydrochloride

Generic Available Yes

Pharmacologic Category Diuretic, Potassium-Sparing

Medication Safety Issues

Sound-alike/look-alike issues:

    Amiloride may be confused with amiodarone, amlodipine, amrinone

Use Counteracts potassium loss induced by other diuretics in the treatment of hypertension or edematous conditions including CHF, hepatic cirrhosis, and hypoaldosteronism; usually used in conjunction with more potent diuretics such as thiazides or loop diuretics

Unlabeled/Investigational Use Investigational: Cystic fibrosis; reduction of lithium-induced polyuria

Mechanism of Action/Effect Decreases potassium and calcium excretion in distal tubule, cortical collecting tubule, and collecting direct by inhibiting sodium, potassium, and ATPase; increases sodium, magnesium, and water excretion

Contraindications Hypersensitivity to amiloride or any component of the formulation; presence of elevated serum potassium levels (>5.5 mEq/L); if patient is receiving other potassium-conserving agents (eg, spironolactone, triamterene) or potassium supplementation (medicine, potassium-containing salt substitutes, potassium-rich diet); anuria; acute or chronic renal insufficiency; evidence of diabetic nephropathy. Patients with evidence of renal impairment or diabetes mellitus should not receive this medicine without close, frequent monitoring of serum electrolytes and renal function.

Warnings/Precautions May cause hyperkalemia (patients with renal impairment, diabetes and the elderly are at greatest risk). Should be stopped at least 3 days before glucose tolerance testing. Use caution in severely ill patients in whom respiratory or metabolic acidosis may occur.

Drug Interactions

Decreased Effect: Decreased effect of amiloride with use of NSAIDs. Amoxicillin's absorption may be reduced with concurrent use.

Increased Effect/Toxicity: Increased risk of amiloride-associated hyperkalemia with triamterene, spironolactone, ACE inhibitors or angiotensin receptor antagonists, potassium preparations, cyclosporine, tacrolimus, and indomethacin. Amiloride may increase the toxicity of amantadine and lithium by reduction of renal excretion. Quinidine and amiloride together may increase risk of malignant arrhythmias.

Nutritional/Ethanol Interactions Food: Hyperkalemia may result if amiloride is taken with potassium-containing foods.

Lab Interactions Increased potassium (S)

Adverse Reactions 1% to 10%:

Central nervous system: Headache, fatigue, dizziness

Endocrine & metabolic: Hyperkalemia (up to 10%; risk reduced in patients receiving kaliuretic diuretics), hyperchloremic metabolic acidosis, dehydration, hyponatremia, gynecomastia

Gastrointestinal: Nausea, diarrhea, vomiting, abdominal pain, gas pain, appetite changes, constipation

Genitourinary: Impotence

Neuromuscular & skeletal: Muscle cramps, weakness

Respiratory: Cough, dyspnea

Overdosage/Toxicology Clinical signs of toxicity are consistent with dehydration and electrolyte disturbance. Large amounts may result in life-threatening hyperkalemia (>6.5 mEq/L). This can be treated with I.V. glucose (dextrose 25% in water), rapid-acting insulin, concurrent *(Continued)*

Amiloride *(Continued)*

I.V. sodium bicarbonate, and (if needed) Kayexalate® oral or rectal solution in sorbitol. Persistent hyperkalemia may require dialysis.

Pharmacodynamics/Kinetics

Onset of Action: 2 hours

Duration of Action: 24 hours

Absorption: ~15% to 25%

Time to Peak: Serum: 6-10 hours

Protein Binding: 23%

Half-Life Elimination: Normal renal function: 6-9 hours; End-stage renal disease: 8-144 hours

Metabolism: No active metabolites

Excretion: Urine and feces (equal amounts as unchanged drug)

Dosing

Adults: Hypertension, edema (to limit potassium loss): Oral: Initial: 5-10 mg/day (up to 20 mg)

Hypertension (JNC 7): 5-10 mg/day in 1-2 divided doses

Elderly: Oral: Initial: 5 mg once daily or every other day

Pediatrics: Edema, hypertension: Oral: Although safety and efficacy in children have not been established by the FDA, a dosage of 0.625 mg/kg/day has been used in children weighing 6-20 kg.

Renal Impairment: Oral:

Cl_{cr} 10-50 mL/minute: Administer 50% of normal dose.

Cl_{cr} <10 mL/minute: Avoid use.

Available Dosage Forms Tablet, as hydrochloride: 5 mg

Monitoring and Teaching Issues

Physical Assessment: Assess for use cautions (eg, patients at risk for hyperkalemia; see Contraindications and Warnings/Precautions). Monitor for interactions with other prescriptions, OTC medications, or herbal products patient may be taking. Assess results of laboratory tests (electrolytes), fluid status (I & O, weight blood pressure), therapeutic effectiveness, and adverse response (eg, dehydration, hyperkalemia, hyperchloremic metabolic acidosis, hyponatremia; see Adverse Reactions). Teach patient proper use, possible side effects/appropriate interventions, and adverse symptoms to report.

Monitoring Laboratory Tests: Serum electrolytes

Patient Education: Do not take any new medication during therapy unless approved by prescriber. Take as directed, preferably early in day with food. Do not increase dietary intake of potassium unless instructed by prescriber (too much potassium can be as harmful as too little). May cause dizziness or fatigue (use caution when driving or engaging in tasks that require alertness until response to drug is known); constipation (increased exercise, fluids, fruit, and fiber may help); impotence (reversible); or loss of hair (rare). Report muscle cramping or weakness, unresolved nausea or vomiting, palpitations, or respiratory difficulty. **Breast-feeding precaution:** Do not breast-feed.

Dietary Considerations: Take with food or meals to avoid GI upset. Do not use salt substitutes or low salt milk without checking with your healthcare provider, too much potassium can be as harmful as too little.

Geriatric Considerations: Use lower initial dose, and adjust dose for renal impairment.

Pregnancy Risk Factor: B

Lactation: Excretion in breast milk unknown/contraindicated

Administration

Oral: Administer with food or meals to avoid GI upset.

Additional Information Medication should be discontinued if potassium level exceeds 6.5 mEq/L. Combined with hydrochlorothiazide as Moduretic®. Amiloride is considered an alternative to triamterene or spironolactone.

Related Information

Heart Failure *on page 1828*

Amiloride and Hydrochlorothiazide

(a MIL oh ride & hye droe klor oh THYE a zide)

U.S. Brand Names Moduretic® [DSC]

Synonyms Hydrochlorothiazide and Amiloride

Generic Available Yes

Pharmacologic Category Diuretic, Combination

Use Potassium-sparing diuretic; antihypertensive

Dosing

Adults: Hypertension, edema: Oral: Initial: 1 tablet/day, then may be increased to 2 tablets/day if needed; usually given in a single dose

Elderly: Oral: Initial: $1/2$ to 1 tablet/day

Available Dosage Forms Tablet: Amiloride hydrochloride 5 mg and hydrochlorothiazide 50 mg

Monitoring and Teaching Issues

Physical Assessment: See individual agents.

Patient Education: See individual agents. **Breast-feeding precaution:** Do not breast-feed.

Pregnancy Risk Factor: B

Lactation: Excretion in breast milk unknown/contraindicated

Related Information

Amiloride *on page 89*

Hydrochlorothiazide *on page 751*

♦ **Amiloride Hydrochloride** *see* Amiloride *on page 89*

♦ **2-Amino-6-Mercaptopurine** *see* Thioguanine *on page 1462*

♦ **2-Amino-6-Trifluoromethoxy-Benzothiazole** *see* Riluzole *on page 1328*

♦ **Aminobenzylpenicillin** *see* Ampicillin *on page 115*

Aminoglutethimide (a mee noe gloo TETH i mide)

U.S. Brand Names Cytadren®
Synonyms AG; AGT; BA-16038; Elipten
Generic Available No
Pharmacologic Category Aromatase Inhibitor; Enzyme Inhibitor; Hormone Antagonist, Anti-Adrenal; Nonsteroidal Aromatase Inhibitor
Medication Safety Issues
Sound-alike/look-alike issues:
   Cytadren® may be confused with cytarabine
Use Suppression of adrenal function in selected patients with Cushing's syndrome
Unlabeled/Investigational Use Treatment of prostate cancer (androgen synthesis inhibitor)
Mechanism of Action/Effect Blocks the conversion of cholesterol to delta-5-pregnenolone, thereby reducing the synthesis of adrenal glucocorticoids, mineralocorticoids, estrogens, aldosterone, and androgens. This inhibits growth of tumors that need estrogen to thrive.
Contraindications Hypersensitivity to aminoglutethimide, glutethimide, or any component of the formulation; pregnancy; breast-feeding
Warnings/Precautions Monitor blood pressure in all patients at appropriate intervals. Hypothyroidism may occur. **Mineralocorticoid replacement is necessary in up to 50% of patients.** Glucocorticoid replacement is necessary in most patients.
Drug Interactions
   Cytochrome P450 Effect: Induces CYP1A2 (strong), 2C19 (strong), 3A4 (strong)
   Decreased Effect: Aminoglutethimide may decrease therapeutic effect of dexamethasone, digitoxin (after 3-8 weeks), warfarin, medroxyprogesterone, megestrol, and tamoxifen. Aminoglutethimide may decrease the levels/effects of aminophylline, benzodiazepines, calcium channel blockers, citalopram, clarithromycin, cyclosporine, diazepam, erythromycin, estrogens, fluvoxamine, methsuximide, mirtazapine, nateglinide, nefazodone, nevirapine, phenytoin, proton pump inhibitors, protease inhibitors, ropinirole, sertraline, tacrolimus, theophylline, venlafaxine, voriconazole and other drugs metabolized by CYP1A2, 2C19, or 3A4.
Lab Interactions Increased alkaline phosphatase (S), AST (SGOT), TSH; decreased plasma cortisol, thyroxine (S), and urinary aldosterone
Adverse Reactions Most adverse effects will diminish in incidence and severity after the first 2-6 weeks
   >10%:
      Central nervous system: Headache, dizziness, drowsiness, lethargy, clumsiness
      Dermatologic: Skin rash
      Gastrointestinal: Nausea, anorexia
      Hepatic: Cholestatic jaundice
      Neuromuscular & skeletal: Myalgia
      Renal: Nephrotoxicity
      Respiratory: Pulmonary alveolar damage
   1% to 10%:
      Cardiovascular: Hypotension, tachycardia, orthostasis
      Dermatologic: Hirsutism, pruritus
      Endocrine & metabolic: Adrenocortical insufficiency
      Gastrointestinal: Vomiting
Overdosage/Toxicology Symptoms of overdose include ataxia, somnolence, lethargy, dizziness, distress, fatigue, coma, hyperventilation, respiratory depression, hypovolemia, and shock. Treatment is supportive.
Pharmacodynamics/Kinetics
   Onset of Action: Adrenal suppression: 3-5 days; following withdrawal of therapy, adrenal function returns within 72 hours
   Absorption: 90%
   Protein Binding: Plasma: 20% to 25%
   Half-Life Elimination: 7-15 hours; shorter following multiple doses
   Metabolism: Major metabolite is N-acetylaminoglutethimide; induces its own metabolism
   Excretion: Urine (34% to 50% as unchanged drug, 25% as metabolites)
Dosing
   Adults & Elderly:
      Cushing disease: Oral: 250 mg every 6 hours may be increased at 1- to 2-week intervals to a total of 2 g/day
      Prostate cancer (unlabeled use): Oral: 250 mg 4 times/day
   Renal Impairment: Dose reduction may be necessary.
Available Dosage Forms Tablet [scored]: 250 mg
Monitoring and Teaching Issues
   Physical Assessment: Assess potential for interactions with other medications patient may be taking (see Drug Interactions). Assess results of laboratory tests, therapeutic effectiveness (suppression of adrenal function), and adverse reactions (eg, ataxia, hypotension, mood swings, susceptibility to infection; see Adverse Reactions). Teach patient proper use, possible side effects/appropriate interventions, and adverse symptoms to report.
   Monitoring Laboratory Tests: Thyroid function tests, CBC, liver function, electrolytes. Follow adrenal cortical response by careful monitoring of plasma cortisol until the desired level of suppression is achieved.
   Patient Education: Do not take any new medication during therapy unless approved by prescriber. Take exactly as directed; may be taken with food to reduce incidence of nausea. May cause drowsiness or dizziness (avoid driving or engaging in tasks that require alertness until response to drug is known); nausea or vomiting (small frequent meals, frequent mouth care, chewing gum or sucking lozenges may reduce incidence of nausea or vomiting); hypotension (use caution when rising from sitting or lying position or when
(Continued)

Aminoglutethimide *(Continued)*

climbing stairs); or masculinization (reversible when treatment is discontinued). Report persistent lethargy or fatigue, rash, unresolved nausea or vomiting, yellowing of skin or eyes, easy bruising or bleeding, change in color of urine or stool, increased growth of facial hair, thick tongue, severe mood swings, palpitations, or respiratory difficulty. **Pregnancy/breast-feeding precautions:** Do not get pregnant while taking this medication. Consult prescriber for appropriate contraceptive measures. Do not breast-feed.

Pregnancy Risk Factor: D

Pregnancy Issues: Suspected of causing virilization when given throughout pregnancy

Lactation: Excretion in breast milk unknown/contraindicated

Administration

Oral: Administer every 6 hours to reduce incidence of nausea and vomiting.

Storage: Store at controlled room temperature not >30°C (86°F).

♦ **Aminosalicylate Sodium** *see* Aminosalicylic Acid *on page 92*

Aminosalicylic Acid *(a mee noe sal i SIL ik AS id)*

U.S. Brand Names Paser®

Synonyms Aminosalicylate Sodium; 4-Aminosalicylic Acid; Para-Aminosalicylate Sodium; PAS; Sodium PAS

Generic Available No

Pharmacologic Category Salicylate

Use Adjunctive treatment of tuberculosis used in combination with other antitubercular agents

Unlabeled/Investigational Use Crohn's disease

Mechanism of Action/Effect Aminosalicylic acid (PAS) is a highly specific bacteriostatic agent active against *M. tuberculosis*. Most strains of *M. tuberculosis* are sensitive to a concentration of 1 mcg/mL. Structurally related to para-aminobenzoic acid (PABA) and its mechanism of action is thought to be similar to the sulfonamides, a competitive antagonism with PABA. Disrupts plate biosynthesis in sensitive organisms.

Contraindications Hypersensitivity to aminosalicylic acid or any component of the formulation

Warnings/Precautions Use with caution in patients with hepatic or renal dysfunction and patients with gastric ulcer.

Drug Interactions

Decreased Effect: Aminosalicylic acid may decrease serum levels of digoxin and vitamin B_{12}.

Adverse Reactions Frequency not defined.

Cardiovascular: Pericarditis, vasculitis

Central nervous system: Encephalopathy, fever

Dermatologic: Skin eruptions

Endocrine & metabolic: Goiter (with or without myxedema), hypoglycemia

Gastrointestinal: Abdominal pain, diarrhea, nausea, vomiting

Hematologic: Agranulocytosis, anemia (hemolytic), leukopenia, thrombocytopenia

Hepatic: Hepatitis, jaundice

Ocular: Optic neuritis

Respiratory: Eosinophilic pneumonia

Overdosage/Toxicology Acute overdose results in crystalluria and renal failure, nausea, and vomiting. Alkalinization of urine with sodium bicarbonate and forced diuresis can prevent crystalluria and nephrotoxicity.

Pharmacodynamics/Kinetics

Absorption: Readily, >90%

Time to Peak: Serum: 6 hours

Protein Binding: 50% to 60%

Half-Life Elimination: Reduced with renal impairment

Metabolism: Hepatic (>50%) via acetylation

Excretion: Urine (>80% as unchanged drug and metabolites)

Dosing

Adults & Elderly:

Tuberculosis: Oral: 150 mg/kg/day in 2-3 equally divided doses

Crohn's disease: 1.5 g/day

Pediatrics: Tuberculosis: Oral: Children: 200-300 mg/kg/day in 3-4 equally divided doses

Renal Impairment:

Cl_{cr} 10-50 mL/minute: Administer 50% to 75% of dose.

Cl_{cr} <10 mL/minute: Administer 50% of dose.

Administer after hemodialysis: Administer 50% of dose.

Continuous arteriovenous hemofiltration: Dose for Cl_{cr} <10 mL/minute

Hepatic Impairment: Use with caution.

Available Dosage Forms Granules: 4 g/packet (30s) [contains talc]

Monitoring and Teaching Issues

Physical Assessment: Monitor for effectiveness of treatment and indications of adverse effects.

Patient Education: May be taken with food; may sprinkle on applesauce or yogurt, or suspend in tomato or orange juice. Do not use granules if discolored (brown or purple) or if packet is swollen; see pharmacist for new prescription. Do not stop taking without consulting prescriber. Report persistent sore throat, fever, unusual bleeding or bruising, persistent nausea or vomiting, or abdominal pain. **Pregnancy/breast-feeding precautions:** Inform prescriber if you are or intend to become pregnant. Breast-feeding is not recommended.

Dietary Considerations: May be taken with food.

Geriatric Considerations: See Warnings/Precautions; elderly may require lower recommended dose.

Pregnancy Risk Factor: C

Lactation: Enters breast milk/not recommended

Administration

Oral: Do not use granules if packet is swollen or if granules are discolored (ie, brown or purple). Granules may be sprinkled on applesauce or yogurt (do not chew) or suspended in tomato or orange juice.

Storage: Prior to dispensing, store granules below 15°C (59°F). Once dispensed, packets may be stored at room temperature for short periods of time. Do not use if packet is swollen or if granules are dark brown or purple.

♦ **4-Aminosalicylic Acid** *see* Aminosalicylic Acid *on page 92*

♦ **5-Aminosalicylic Acid** *see* Mesalamine *on page 957*

♦ **Aminoxin® [OTC]** *see* Pyridoxine *on page 1289*

Amiodarone (a MEE oh da rone)

U.S. Brand Names Cordarone®; Pacerone®

Synonyms Amiodarone Hydrochloride

Restrictions An FDA-approved medication guide is available at www.fda.gov/cder/Offices/ODS/labeling.htm; distribute to each patient to whom this medication is dispensed.

Generic Available Yes

Pharmacologic Category Antiarrhythmic Agent, Class III

Medication Safety Issues

Sound-alike/look-alike issues:

Amiodarone may be confused with amiloride, amrinone

Cordarone® may be confused with Cardura®, Cordran®

High alert medication: The Institute for Safe Medication Practices (ISMP) includes this medication among its list of drugs which have a heightened risk of causing significant patient harm when used in error.

Use

Oral: Management of life-threatening recurrent ventricular fibrillation (VF) or hemodynamically unstable ventricular tachycardia (VT)

I.V.: Initiation of treatment and prophylaxis of frequency recurring VF and unstable VT in patients refractory to other therapy. Also, used for patients when oral amiodarone is indicated, but who are unable to take oral medication.

Unlabeled/Investigational Use

Conversion of atrial fibrillation to normal sinus rhythm; maintenance of normal sinus rhythm

Prevention of postoperative atrial fibrillation during cardiothoracic surgery

Paroxysmal supraventricular tachycardia (SVT)

Control of rapid ventricular rate due to accessory pathway conduction in pre-excited atrial arrhythmias [ACLS guidelines]

After defibrillation and epinephrine in cardiac arrest with persistent ventricular tachycardia (VT) or ventricular fibrillation (VF) [ACLS guidelines]

Control of hemodynamically stable VT, polymorphic VT or wide-complex tachycardia of uncertain origin [ACLS guidelines]

Mechanism of Action/Effect Class III antiarrhythmic agent which inhibits adrenergic stimulation, prolongs the action potential and refractory period in myocardial tissue; decreases AV conduction and sinus node function. antiarrhythmic activity may result from both parent compound and active metabolite DEA.

Contraindications Hypersensitivity to amiodarone, iodine, or any component of the formulation; severe sinus-node dysfunction; second- and third-degree heart block (except in patients with a functioning artificial pacemaker); bradycardia causing syncope (except in patients with a functioning artificial pacemaker); pregnancy

Warnings/Precautions Monitor for pulmonary toxicity, liver toxicity, or exacerbation of the arrhythmia. Use very cautiously and with close monitoring in patients with thyroid or liver disease. May cause hyper- or hypothyroidism. Hyperthyroidism may aggravate or cause breakthrough arrhythmias. Significant heart block or sinus bradycardia can occur. Patients should be hospitalized when amiodarone is initiated. Amiodarone is a potent inhibitor of CYP enzymes, and may lead to increased serum concentrations/toxicity of a number of medications. Particular caution must be used when a drug with QT_c-prolonging potential relies on metabolism via these enzymes, since the effect of elevated concentrations may be additive with the effect of amiodarone. Carefully assess risk:benefit of coadministration of other drugs which may prolong QT_c interval. Correct electrolyte disturbances, especially hypokalemia or hypomagnesemia, prior to use and throughout therapy.

Pre-existing pulmonary disease does not increase risk of developing pulmonary toxicity, but if pulmonary toxicity develops then the prognosis is worse. Due to complex pharmacokinetics, it is difficult to predict when an arrhythmia or interaction with a subsequent treatment will occur following discontinuation of amiodarone. May cause optic neuropathy and/or optic neuritis, usually resulting in visual impairment. Corneal microdeposits occur in a majority of patients, and may cause visual disturbances in some patients (blurred vision, halos); these are not generally considered a reason to discontinue treatment.

Caution in surgical patients; may enhance hemodynamic effect of anesthetics; associated with increased risk of adult respiratory distress syndrome (ARDS) postoperatively. Injection contains benzyl alcohol, which has been associated with "gasping syndrome" in neonates. Safety and efficacy of amiodarone in children has not been fully established.

Drug Interactions

Cytochrome P450 Effect: Substrate of CYP1A2 (minor), 2C8/9 (major at low concentration), 2C19 (minor), 2D6 (minor), 3A4 (major); **Inhibits** CYP1A2 (strong), 2A6 (moderate), 2B6 (weak), 2C8/9 (moderate), 2C19 (weak), 2D6 (moderate), 3A4 (moderate)

Decreased Effect: Levels/effects of amiodarone may be decreased by aminoglutethimide, carbamazepine, nafcillin, nevirapine, phenobarbital, phenytoin, rifampin, rifapentine, secobarbital, and other CYP2C8/9 inducers or and CYP3A4 inducers. Amiodarone may decrease the levels/effects of codeine, hydrocodone, oxycodone, tramadol, and other

(Continued)

Amiodarone *(Continued)*

prodrug substrates of CYP2D6. Amiodarone may alter thyroid function and response to thyroid supplements; monitor closely.

Increased Effect/Toxicity: Note: Due to the long half-life of amiodarone, drug interactions may take 1 or more weeks to develop. The effect of drugs which prolong the QT interval, including amitriptyline, azole antifungals, bepridil, cisapride, clarithromycin, disopyramide, erythromycin, gatifloxacin, haloperidol, imipramine, moxifloxacin, quinidine, pimozide, procainamide, sotalol, sparfloxacin, theophylline, and thioridazine may be increased. Cisapride and sparfloxacin are contraindicated. Use of amiodarone with diltiazem, verapamil, digoxin, beta-blockers, and other drugs which delay AV conduction may cause excessive AV block (amiodarone may also decrease the metabolism of some of these agents - see below).

Amiodarone may increase the levels of digoxin (reduce dose by 50% on initiation), flecainide (decrease dose up to 33%), phenothiazines, procainamide (reduce dose), and quinidine. Amiodarone may increase the levels/effects of aminophylline, amphetamines, selected benzodiazepines, selected beta-blockers, calcium channel blockers, cyclosporine, dexmedetomidine, dextromethorphan, fluoxetine, fluvoxamine, glimepiride, glipizide, ifosfamide, lidocaine, mexiletine, mirtazapine, nateglinide, nefazodone, paroxetine, phenytoin, pioglitazone, risperidone, ritonavir, ropinirole, rosiglitazone, sildenafil (and other PDE-5 inhibitors), sertraline, tacrolimus, theophylline, thioridazine, tricyclic antidepressants, trifluoperazine, venlafaxine, warfarin, and other CYP1A2, 2A6, 2C8/9, CYP2D6, and/or CYP3A4 substrates. Selected benzodiazepines (midazolam, triazolam), cisapride, ergot alkaloids, selected HMG-CoA reductase inhibitors (lovastatin and simvastatin), mesoridazine, pimozide, and thioridazine are generally contraindicated with strong CYP3A4 inhibitors. When used with strong CYP3A4 inhibitors, dosage adjustment/limits are recommended for sildenafil and other PDE-5 inhibitors; consult individual monographs.

The levels/effects of amiodarone may be increased by amprenavir, cimetidine, delavirdine, fluconazole, gemfibrozil, indinavir, ketoconazole, nelfinavir, nicardipine, NSAIDs, pioglitazone, ritonavir, sulfonamides, and other CYP2C8/9 inhibitors.

Concurrent use of fentanyl may lead to bradycardia, sinus arrest, and hypotension. Amiodarone may alter thyroid function and response to thyroid supplements. Amiodarone enhances the myocardial depressant and conduction defects of inhalation anesthetics (monitor). During concomitant ropivacaine therapy, cardiac effects may be additive.

Nutritional/Ethanol Interactions

Food: Increases the rate and extent of absorption of amiodarone. Grapefruit juice increases bioavailability of oral amiodarone by 50% and decreases the conversion of amiodarone to N-DEA (active metabolite); altered effects are possible; use should be avoided during therapy.

Herb/Nutraceutical: St John's wort may decrease amiodarone levels or enhance photosensitization. Avoid ephedra (may worsen arrhythmia). Avoid dong quai.

Lab Interactions Thyroid function tests: Amiodarone partially inhibits the peripheral conversion of thyroxine (T_4) to triiodothyronine (T_3); serum T_4 and reverse triiodothyronine (rT_3) concentrations may be increased and serum T_3 may be decreased. Most patients remain clinically euthyroid, however, clinical hypothyroidism or hyperthyroidism may occur.

Adverse Reactions In a recent meta-analysis, patients taking lower doses of amiodarone (152-330 mg daily for at least 12 months) were more likely to develop thyroid, neurologic, skin, ocular, and bradycardic abnormalities than those taking placebo. Pulmonary toxicity was similar in both the low dose amiodarone group and in the placebo group but there was a trend towards increased toxicity in the amiodarone group. Gastrointestinal and hepatic events were seen to a similar extent in both the low dose amiodarone group and placebo group.

>10%:

Cardiovascular: Hypotension (I.V. 16%, refractory in rare cases)

Central nervous system (3% to 40%): Abnormal gait/ataxia, dizziness, fatigue, headache, malaise, impaired memory, involuntary movement, insomnia, poor coordination, peripheral neuropathy, sleep disturbances, tremor

Dermatologic: Photosensitivity (10% to 75%)

Endocrine & Metabolic: Hypothyroidism (1% to 22%)

Gastrointestinal: Nausea, vomiting, anorexia and constipation (10% to 33%), AST or ALT level >2X normal (15% to 50%)

1% to 10%:

Cardiovascular: CHF (3%), bradycardia (3% to 5%), AV block (5%), conduction abnormalities, SA node dysfunction (1% to 3%), cardiac arrhythmia, flushing, edema. Additional effects associated with I.V. administration include asystole, cardiac arrest, electromechanical dissociation, ventricular tachycardia, and cardiogenic shock.

Dermatologic: Slate blue skin discoloration (<10%)

Endocrine & metabolic: Hyperthyroidism (<3%), libido decreased

Gastrointestinal: Abdominal pain, abnormal salivation, abnormal taste (oral)

Hematologic: Coagulation abnormalities

Hepatic: Hepatitis and cirrhosis (<3%)

Local: Phlebitis (I.V., with concentrations >3 mg/mL)

Ocular: Visual disturbances (2% to 9%), corneal microdeposits (occur in a majority of patients and lead to visual disturbance in ~10%), halo vision (<5% occurring especially at night), optic neuritis (1%)

Respiratory: Pulmonary toxicity has been estimated to occur at a frequency between 2% and 7% of patients (some reports indicate a frequency as high as 17%). Toxicity may present as hypersensitivity pneumonitis; pulmonary fibrosis (cough, fever, malaise); pulmonary inflammation; interstitial pneumonitis; or alveolar pneumonitis. ARDS has been reported in up to 2% of patients receiving I.V. amiodarone, and postoperatively in patients receiving oral amiodarone.

Miscellaneous: Abnormal smell (oral)

Overdosage/Toxicology Symptoms include extension of pharmacologic effects, sinus bradycardia and/or heart block, hypotension, and QT prolongation. Patients should be monitored for several days following ingestion. Intoxication with amiodarone necessitates ECG monitoring. Bradycardia may be atropine resistant. Injectable isoproterenol or a temporary pacemaker may be required.

Pharmacodynamics/Kinetics
Onset of Action: Oral: 3 days to 3 weeks; I.V.: May be more rapid; Peak effect: 1 week to 5 months

Duration of Action: After discontinuing therapy: 7-50 days

Note: Mean onset of effect and duration after discontinuation may be shorter in children than adults

Bioavailability: Oral: ~50%

Protein Binding: 96%

Half-Life Elimination: Terminal: 40-55 days (range: 26-107 days); shorter in children than adults

Metabolism: Hepatic via CYP2C8 and 3A4, major metabolite active; possible enterohepatic recirculation

Excretion: Feces; urine (<1% as unchanged drug)

Dosing
Adults & Elderly: Note: Lower loading and maintenance doses are preferable in women and all patients with low body weight.

Ventricular arrhythmias: Oral: 800-1600 mg/day in 1-2 doses for 1-3 weeks, then 600-800 mg/day in 1-2 doses for 1 month; maintenance: 400 mg/day; lower doses are recommended for supraventricular arrhythmias.

Breakthrough VF or VT: I.V.: 150 mg supplemental doses in 100 mL D_5W over 10 minutes

Pulseless VF or VT: I.V. push: Initial: 300 mg in 20-30 mL NS or D_5W; if VF or VT recurs, supplemental dose of 150 mg followed by infusion of 1 mg/minute for 6 hours, then 0.5 mg/minute (maximum daily dose: 2.2 g)

Note: When switching from I.V. to oral therapy, use the following as a guide:
<1 week I.V. infusion: 800-1600 mg/day
1- to 3-week I.V. infusion: 600-800 mg/day
>3 week I.V. infusion: 400 mg

Recommendations for conversion to intravenous amiodarone after oral administration: During long-term amiodarone therapy (ie, ≥4 months), the mean plasma-elimination half-life of the active metabolite of amiodarone is 61 days. Replacement therapy may not be necessary in such patients if oral therapy is discontinued for a period <2 weeks, since any changes in serum amiodarone concentrations during this period may **not** be clinically significant.

Unlabeled uses:

Prophylaxis of atrial fibrillation following open heart surgery (unlabeled use):
Note: A variety of regimens have been used in clinical trials, including oral and intravenous regimens:
Oral: 400 mg twice daily (starting in postop recovery) for up to 7 days. An alternative regimen of amiodarone 600 mg/day for 7 days prior to surgery, followed by 200 mg/day until hospital discharge has also been shown to decrease the risk of postoperative atrial fibrillation.
I.V.: 1000 mg infused over 24 hours (starting at postop recovery) for 2 days has been shown to reduce the risk of postoperative atrial fibrillation

Recurrent atrial fibrillation (unlabeled use): No standard regimen defined; examples of regimens include: Oral: Initial: 10 mg/kg/day for 14 days; followed by 300 mg/day for 4 weeks, followed by maintenance dosage of 100-200 mg/day. Other regimens have been described and are used clinically (ie, 400 mg 3 times/day for 5-7 days, then 400 mg/day for 1 month, then 200 mg/day).

Stable VT or SVT (unlabeled use): First 24 hours: 1000 mg according to following regimen
Step 1: 150 mg (100 mL) over first 10 minutes (mix 3 mL in 100 mL D_5W)
Step 2: 360 mg (200 mL) over next 6 hours (mix 18 mL in 500 mL D_5W): 1 mg/minute
Step 3: 540 mg (300 mL) over next 18 hours: 0.5 mg/minute
Note: After the first 24 hours: 0.5 mg/minute utilizing concentration of 1-6 mg/mL

Pediatrics:

Arrhythmias (unlabeled use):
Loading dose: 10-20 mg/kg/day in 1-2 doses for 4-14 days or until adequate control of arrhythmia or prominent adverse effects occurs; alternative loading dose in children <1 year: 600-800 mg/1.73 m^2/day in 1-2 divided doses/day.
Maintenance dose: Dose may be reduced to 5 mg/kg/day for several weeks (or 200-400 mg/1.73 m^2/day given once daily); if no recurrence of arrhythmia, dose may be further reduced to 2.5 mg/kg/day; maintenance doses may be given 5-7 days/week.

Arrhythmias (unlabeled use, dosing based on limited data): I.V.:
Loading dose: 5 mg/kg over 30 minutes; may repeat up to 3 times if no response.
Maintenance dose: 2-20 mg/kg/day (5-15 mcg/kg/minute) by continuous infusion.
Note: I.V. administration at low flow rates (potentially associated with use in pediatrics) may result in leaching of plasticizers (DEHP) from intravenous tubing. DEHP may adversely affect male reproductive tract development. Alternative means of dosing and administration (1 mg/kg aliquots) may need to be considered.

Pulseless VF or VT (PALS dosing): 5 mg/kg rapid I.V. bolus or I.O.

Perfusing tachycardias (PALS dosing): Loading dose: 5 mg/kg I.V. over 20-60 minutes or I.O.; may repeat up to maximum dose of 15 mg/kg/day

Renal Impairment:
Hemodialysis effects: Not removed by hemodialysis or peritoneal dialysis (0% to 5%); no supplemental doses required.

Hepatic Impairment: Dosage adjustment is probably necessary in substantial hepatic impairment. No specific guidelines available.

Available Dosage Forms
Injection, solution, as hydrochloride: 50 mg/mL (3 mL, 18 mL) [contains benzyl alcohol and polysorbate (Tween®) 80]
(Continued)

Amiodarone *(Continued)*

Cordarone®: 50 mg/mL (30 mL) [contains benzyl alcohol and polysorbate (Tween®) 80]
Tablet, as hydrochloride [scored]: 200 mg
Cordarone®: 200 mg
Pacerone®: 100 mg [not scored], 200 mg, 400 mg

Monitoring and Teaching Issues

Physical Assessment: Assess other medications patient may be taking for effectiveness and interactions. Eye examinations should be performed periodically. Monitor cardiac status closely and assess for CNS changes. **I.V.:** Requires continuous cardiac/hemodynamic monitoring and observation for adverse reactions. **Oral:** Assess results of laboratory tests, therapeutic effectiveness, and symptoms of adverse effects at beginning of therapy and regularly during long-term therapy.

Monitoring Laboratory Tests: Thyroid function, pulmonary function, liver enzymes, serum electrolytes (potassium, magnesium)

Patient Education: Emergency use: Patient condition will determine amount of patient education.

Oral: May be taken with food to reduce GI disturbance, but be consistent. Always take with food or always take without food. Do not change dosage or discontinue drug without consulting prescriber. Regular blood work, ophthalmic exams, and cardiac assessment will be necessary while taking this medication on a long-term basis. You may experience dizziness, weakness, or insomnia (use caution when driving, climbing stairs, or engaging in tasks requiring alertness until response to drug is known); hypotension (use caution when rising from sitting or lying position); nausea, vomiting, loss of appetite, stomach discomfort, or abnormal taste (small frequent meals, frequent mouth care, chewing gum, or sucking lozenges may help); photosensitivity (use sunscreen, wear protective clothing and eyewear, and avoid direct sunlight); or decreased libido (reversible). Report persistent dry cough or shortness of breath; chest pain, palpitations, irregular or slow heartbeat; unusual bruising or bleeding; blood in urine, feces (black stool), vomitus; warmth, swelling, pain, in in calves; muscle tremor, weakness, numbness, or changes in gait; skin rash or irritation; or changes in urinary patterns. **Pregnancy/breast-feeding precautions:** Do not get pregnant while taking this medication; use appropriate contraceptive measures. Do not breast-feed.

Dietary Considerations: Administer consistently with regard to meals. Amiodarone contains iodine 37.3% by weight. Grapefruit juice is not recommended.

Geriatric Considerations: Elderly may be predisposed to toxicity (see Drug Interactions). Half-life may be prolonged due to decreased clearance (see Hepatic/Renal Impairment).

Pregnancy Risk Factor: D

Pregnancy Issues: May cause fetal harm when administered to a pregnant woman, leading to congenital goiter and hypo- or hyperthyroidism.

Lactation: Enters breast milk/not recommended (AAP rates "of concern")

Breast-Feeding Issues: Hypothyroidism may occur in nursing infants. Both amiodarone and its active metabolite are excreted in human milk. Breast-feeding may lead to significant infant exposure and potential toxicity.

Administration

Oral: Administer consistently with regard to meals. Take in divided doses with meals if high daily dose or if GI upset occurs. If GI intolerance occurs with single-dose therapy, use twice daily dosing.

I.V.: Give I.V. therapy using an infusion pump at a concentration of <2 mg/mL. Slow the infusion rate if hypotension develops. Infusions >2 hours must be administered in glass or polyolefin bottles. **Note:** I.V. administration at low flow rates (potentially associated with use in pediatrics) may result in leaching of plasticizers (DEHP) from intravenous tubing. DEHP may adversely affect male reproductive tract development. Alternative means of dosing and administration (1 mg/kg aliquots) may need to be considered.

Compatibility:
Y-site administration: **Incompatible** with aminophylline, cefamandole, heparin, sodium bicarbonate
Compatibility in syringe: **Incompatible** with heparin
Compatibility when admixed: **Incompatible** with floxacillin

Storage: Store at room temperature and protect from light.

Related Information

Antiarrhythmic Drugs *on page 1708*

♦ **Amiodarone Hydrochloride** *see Amiodarone on page 93*
♦ **Ami-Tex PSE** *see Guaifenesin and Pseudoephedrine on page 733*
♦ **Amitone® [OTC]** *see Calcium Carbonate on page 235*

Amitriptyline *(a mee TRIP ti leen)*

U.S. Brand Names Elavil® [DSC]

Synonyms Amitriptyline Hydrochloride

Restrictions A medication guide should be dispensed with each prescription. A template for the required MedGuides can be found on the FDA website at: http://www.fda.gov/cder/drug/antidepressants/labelTemplate.pdf

Generic Available Yes

Pharmacologic Category Antidepressant, Tricyclic (Tertiary Amine)

Medication Safety Issues
Sound-alike/look-alike issues:
Amitriptyline may be confused with aminophylline, imipramine, nortriptyline
Elavil® may be confused with Aldoril®, Eldepryl®, enalapril, Equanil®, Mellaril®, Oruvail®, Plavix®

Use Relief of symptoms of depression

Unlabeled/Investigational Use Analgesic for certain chronic and neuropathic pain; prophylaxis against migraine headaches; treatment of depressive disorders in children

Mechanism of Action/Effect Increases the synaptic concentration of serotonin and/or norepinephrine in the central nervous system by inhibition of their reuptake by the presynaptic neuronal membrane

Contraindications Hypersensitivity to amitriptyline or any component of the formulation (cross-sensitivity with other tricyclics may occur); use of MAO inhibitors within past 14 days; acute recovery phase following myocardial infarction; concurrent use of cisapride

Warnings/Precautions Antidepressants increase the risk of suicidal thinking and behavior in children and adolescents with major depressive disorder (MDD) and other depressive disorders; consider risk prior to prescribing. All patients must be closely monitored for clinical worsening, suicidality, or unusual changes in behavior, especially during the initiation of therapy or following an increase or decrease in dosage. When used in children, the child's family or caregiver should be instructed to closely observe the patient and communicate condition with healthcare provider. A medication guide should be dispensed with each prescription. **Amitriptyline is not FDA approved for use in children <12 years of age.**

The possibility of a suicide attempt is inherent in major depression and may persist until remission occurs. Use caution in high-risk patients. Worsening depression and severe abrupt suicidality that are not part of the presenting symptoms may require discontinuation or modification of drug therapy. The patient's family or caregiver should be alerted to monitor patients for the emergence of suicidality and associated behaviors (such as agitation, irritability, hostility, impulsivity, and hypomania) and notify healthcare provider.

May worsen psychosis in some patients or precipitate a shift to mania or hypomania in patients with bipolar disorder. Patients presenting with depressive symptoms should be screened for bipolar disorder. Monotherapy in patients with bipolar disorder should be avoided. **Amitriptyline is not FDA approved for bipolar depression.**

The degree of sedation, anticholinergic effects, orthostasis, and conduction abnormalities are high relative to other antidepressants. Amitriptyline often causes drowsiness/sedation, resulting in impaired performance of tasks requiring alertness (eg, operating machinery or driving). Sedative effects may be additive with other CNS depressants and/or ethanol. Use with caution in patients with a history of cardiovascular disease (including previous MI, stroke, tachycardia, or conduction abnormalities). Use with caution in patients with urinary retention, benign prostatic hyperplasia, narrow-angle glaucoma, xerostomia, visual problems, constipation, or a history of bowel obstruction.

May alter glucose control - use with caution in patients with diabetes. May cause hyponatremia/SIADH. Consider discontinuing, when possible, prior to elective surgery. Therapy should not be abruptly discontinued in patients receiving high doses for prolonged periods. May lower seizure threshold - use caution in patients with a previous seizure disorder or condition predisposing to seizures such as brain damage, alcoholism, or concurrent therapy with other drugs which lower the seizure threshold. May increase the risks associated with electroconvulsive therapy. Use with caution in hyperthyroid patients or those receiving thyroid supplementation. Use with caution in patients with hepatic or renal dysfunction and in elderly patients.

Drug Interactions

Cytochrome P450 Effect: Substrate of CYP1A2 (minor), 2B6 (minor), 2C8/9 (minor), 2C19 (minor), 2D6 (major), 3A4 (minor); **Inhibits** CYP1A2 (weak), 2C8/9 (weak), 2C19 (weak), 2D6 (weak), 2E1 (weak)

Decreased Effect: Amitriptyline inhibits the antihypertensive response to bethanidine, clonidine, debrisoquin, guanadrel, guanethidine, guanabenz, or guanfacine. Cholestyramine and colestipol may bind TCAs and reduce their absorption.

Increased Effect/Toxicity: Amitriptyline increases the effects of amphetamines, anticholinergics, other CNS depressants (sedatives, hypnotics, or ethanol), carbamazepine, tolazamide, chlorpropamide, and warfarin. When used with MAO inhibitors, hyperpyrexia, hypertension, tachycardia, confusion, seizures, and **deaths have been reported** (serotonin syndrome). Serotonin syndrome has also been reported with ritonavir (rare). Levels/effects of amitriptyline may be increased by chlorpromazine, delavirdine, fluoxetine, miconazole, paroxetine, pergolide, quinidine, quinine, ritonavir, ropinirole, and other CYP2D6 inhibitors. Cimetidine, fenfluramine, grapefruit juice, indinavir, methylphenidate, diltiazem, valproate, and verapamil may increase the serum concentrations of tricyclic antidepressants (TCAs). Use of lithium with a TCA may increase the risk for neurotoxicity. Phenothiazines may increase concentration of some TCAs and TCAs may increase the concentration of phenothiazines. Pressor response to I.V. epinephrine, norepinephrine, and phenylephrine may be enhanced in patients receiving TCAs (**Note:** Effect is unlikely with epinephrine or levonordefrin dosages typically administered as infiltration in combination with local anesthetics). Combined use of beta-agonists or drugs which prolong QT_c (including quinidine, procainamide, disopyramide, cisapride, sparfloxacin, gatifloxacin, moxifloxacin) with TCAs may predispose patients to cardiac arrhythmias.

Nutritional/Ethanol Interactions

Ethanol: Avoid ethanol (may increase CNS depression).

Food: Grapefruit juice may inhibit the metabolism of some TCAs and clinical toxicity may result.

Herb/Nutraceutical: St John's wort may decrease amitriptyline levels. Avoid valerian, St John's wort, kava kava, gotu kola (may increase CNS depression).

Lab Interactions Amitriptyline may increase or decrease serum glucose levels, may elevate liver function tests, and may prolong conduction time.

Adverse Reactions Anticholinergic effects may be pronounced; moderate to marked sedation can occur (tolerance to these effects usually occurs).

Frequency not defined.

Cardiovascular: Orthostatic hypotension, tachycardia, nonspecific ECG changes, changes in AV conduction, cardiomyopathy (rare), MI, stroke, heart block, arrhythmia, syncope, hypertension, palpitation

Central nervous system: Restlessness, dizziness, insomnia, sedation, fatigue, anxiety, impaired cognitive function, seizure, extrapyramidal symptoms, coma, hallucinations, (Continued)

Amitriptyline *(Continued)*

confusion, disorientation, impaired coordination, ataxia, headache, nightmares, hyperpyrexia

Dermatologic: Allergic rash, urticaria, photosensitivity, alopecia

Endocrine & metabolic: Syndrome of inappropriate ADH secretion

Gastrointestinal: Weight gain, xerostomia, constipation, paralytic ileus, nausea, vomiting, anorexia, stomatitis, peculiar taste, diarrhea, black tongue

Genitourinary: Urinary retention

Hematologic: Bone marrow depression, purpura, eosinophilia

Neuromuscular & skeletal: Numbness, paresthesia, peripheral neuropathy, tremor, weakness

Ocular: Blurred vision, mydriasis, ocular pressure increased

Otic: Tinnitus

Miscellaneous: Diaphoresis; withdrawal reactions (nausea, headache, malaise)

Overdosage/Toxicology Symptoms of overdose include agitation, confusion, hallucinations, urinary retention, hypothermia, hypotension, ventricular tachycardia, and seizures. Treatment is symptomatic and supportive. Alkalinization by sodium bicarbonate and/or hyperventilation may limit cardiac toxicity.

Pharmacodynamics/Kinetics

Onset of Action: Migraine prophylaxis: 6 weeks, higher dosage may be required in heavy smokers because of increased metabolism; Depression: 4-6 weeks, reduce dosage to lowest effective level

Time to Peak: Serum: ~4 hours

Half-Life Elimination: Adults: 9-27 hours (average: 15 hours)

Metabolism: Hepatic to nortriptyline (active), hydroxy and conjugated derivatives; may be impaired in the elderly

Excretion: Urine (18% as unchanged drug); feces (small amounts)

Dosing

Adults:

Depression:

Oral: 50-150 mg/day single dose at bedtime or in divided doses; dose may be gradually increased up to 300 mg/day.

I.M.: 20-30 mg 4 times/day

Chronic pain management (unlabeled use): Oral: Initial: 25 mg at bedtime; may increase as tolerated to 100 mg/day.

Migraine prophylaxis (unlabeled use): Oral: Initial: 10-25 mg at bedtime; usual dose: 150 mg; reported dosing ranges: 10-400 mg/day

Elderly: Depression: Oral: Initial: 10-25 mg at bedtime; dose should be increased in 10-25 mg increments every week if tolerated; dose range: 25-150 mg/day. See Renal/Hepatic Impairment.

Pediatrics:

Chronic pain management (unlabeled use): Oral: Initial: 0.1 mg/kg at bedtime, may advance as tolerated over 2-3 weeks to 0.5-2 mg/kg at bedtime

Depressive disorders:

Children (unlabeled use): Oral: Initial doses of 1 mg/kg/day given in 3 divided doses with increases to 1.5 mg/kg/day have been reported in a small number of children (n=9) 9-12 years of age; clinically, doses up to 3 mg/kg/day (5 mg/kg/day if monitored closely) have been proposed

Adolescents: Initial: 25-50 mg/day; may administer in divided doses; increase gradually to 100 mg/day in divided doses.

Migraine prophylaxis (unlabeled use): Oral: Initial: 0.25 mg/kg/day, given at bedtime; increase dose by 0.25 mg/kg/day to maximum 1 mg/kg/day. Reported dosing ranges: 0.1-2 mg/kg/day; maximum suggested dose: 10 mg

Renal Impairment: Nondialyzable

Hepatic Impairment: Use with caution and monitor plasma levels and patient response.

Available Dosage Forms [DSC] = Discontinued product

Injection, as hydrochloride: 10 mg/mL (10 mL) [DSC]

Tablet, as hydrochloride: 10 mg, 25 mg, 50 mg, 75 mg, 100 mg, 150 mg

Monitoring and Teaching Issues

Physical Assessment: Assess other medications patient may be taking for effectiveness and interactions. Assess for suicidal tendencies or unusual changes in behavior before beginning therapy and periodically thereafter. May cause physiological or psychological dependence, tolerance, or abuse; evaluate need for continued use periodically. Caution patients with diabetes; may alter serum glucose levels. Monitor therapeutic response and adverse reactions at beginning of therapy and periodically with long-term use. Taper dosage slowly when discontinuing. Teach patient appropriate use, interventions to reduce side effects, and adverse symptoms to report.

Patient Education: Take exactly as directed; do not increase dose or frequency. It may take several weeks to achieve desired results. Restrict use of alcohol or caffeine; avoid grapefruit juice. Maintain adequate hydration (2-3 L/day of fluids) unless instructed to restrict fluid intake. If you have diabetes, monitor glucose levels closely; this medication may alter glucose levels. May turn urine blue-green (normal). May cause drowsiness, lightheadedness, impaired coordination, dizziness, or blurred vision (use caution when driving or engaging in tasks requiring alertness until response to drug is known); constipation (increased exercise, fluids, fruit, or fiber may help); urinary retention (void before taking medication); postural hypotension (use caution climbing stairs or when changing position from lying or sitting to standing); altered sexual drive or ability (reversible); or photosensitivity (use sunscreen, wear protective clothing and eyewear, and avoid direct sunlight). Report persistent CNS effects (eg, nervousness, restlessness, insomnia, headache, agitation, impaired coordination, changes in cognition); muscle cramping, weakness, tremors, or rigidity; ringing in ears or visual disturbances; chest pain, palpitations, or irregular heartbeat; blurred vision; or worsening of condition. **Pregnancy/breast-feeding precautions:** Do not get pregnant while taking this medication. Consult prescriber for appropriate contraceptive measures. Breast-feeding is not recommended.

Geriatric Considerations: The most anticholinergic and sedating of the antidepressants. Due to pronounced effects on the cardiovascular system (hypotension), many psychiatrists agree it is best to avoid in the elderly.

Pregnancy Risk Factor: C

Pregnancy Issues: Teratogenic effects have been observed in animal studies. Amitriptyline crosses the human placenta; CNS effects, limb deformities and developmental delay have been noted in case reports.

Lactation: Enters breast milk/not recommended (AAP rates "of concern")

Breast-Feeding Issues: Generally, it is not recommended to breast-feed if taking antidepressants because of the long half-life, active metabolites, and the potential for side effects in the infant.

Administration
I.V.: Do **not** administer I.V.

Related Information
Antidepressant Agents *on page 1713*
Antidepressant Medication Guidelines *on page 1765*
Federal OBRA Regulations: Recommended Maximum Doses *on page 1773*
Peak and Trough Guidelines *on page 1694*

♦ **Amitriptyline Hydrochloride** *see* Amitriptyline *on page 96*

Amlexanox (am LEKS an oks)

U.S. Brand Names Aphthasol®
Generic Available No
Pharmacologic Category Anti-inflammatory, Locally Applied
Use Treatment of aphthous ulcers (ie, canker sores)
Unlabeled/Investigational Use Allergic disorders
Mechanism of Action/Effect As a benzopyrano-bipyridine carboxylic acid derivative, amlexanox has anti-inflammatory and antiallergic properties; it inhibits chemical mediatory release of the slow-reacting substance of anaphylaxis (SRSA) and may have antagonistic effects on interleukin-3
Contraindications Hypersensitivity to amlexanox or any component of the formulation
Warnings/Precautions Discontinue therapy if rash or contact mucositis develops.
Adverse Reactions 1% to 2%:
Dermatologic: Allergic contact dermatitis
Gastrointestinal: Oral irritation
Pharmacodynamics/Kinetics
Absorption: Some from swallowed paste
Time to Peak: Serum: 2 hours
Half-Life Elimination: 3.5 hours
Metabolism: Hydroxylated and conjugated metabolites
Excretion: Urine (17% as unchanged drug)
Dosing
Adults & Elderly: Aphthous ulcers: Topical: Administer (0.5 cm - ¼") directly on ulcers 4 times/day following oral hygiene, after meals, and at bedtime.
Available Dosage Forms Paste: 5% (5 g) [contains benzyl alcohol]
Monitoring and Teaching Issues
Physical Assessment: Assess knowledge/teach patient appropriate application and use, adverse effects to report, and interventions for side-effects.
Patient Education: This medication is only for treatment of mouth ulcers; do not apply to ulcers of the eye or any other part of the body. Use as directed. Apply after eating. Wash hands before and after use. Brush teeth and rinse mouth before applying directly to ulcers. Squeeze a small amount of paste on your clean finger tip and dab paste onto each ulcer in the mouth, using gentle pressure. Wash eyes immediately if any paste should come into contact with eyes. Notify prescriber or dentist if rash or irritation occurs, or if condition does not improve after 10 days use. **Breast-feeding precaution:** Consult prescriber if breast-feeding.
Pregnancy Risk Factor: B
Lactation: Excretion in breast milk unknown/use caution

Amlodipine (am LOE di peen)

U.S. Brand Names Norvasc®
Synonyms Amlodipine Besylate
Generic Available No
Pharmacologic Category Calcium Channel Blocker
Medication Safety Issues
Sound-alike/look-alike issues:
Amlodipine may be confused with amiloride
Norvasc® may be confused with Navane®, Norvir®, Vascor®
Use Treatment of hypertension and angina
Mechanism of Action/Effect Inhibits calcium ion from entering the "slow channels" or select voltage-sensitive areas of vascular smooth muscle and myocardium during depolarization
Contraindications Hypersensitivity to amlodipine or any component of the formulation
Warnings/Precautions Increased angina and/or MI has occurred with initiation or dosage titration of calcium channel blockers. Use caution in severe aortic stenosis. Use caution in patients with severe hepatic impairment. Dosage titration should occur after 7-14 days on a given dose.
Drug Interactions
Cytochrome P450 Effect: Substrate of CYP3A4 (major); **Inhibits** CYP1A2 (moderate), 2A6 (weak), 2B6 (weak), 2C8/9 (weak), 2D6 (weak), 3A4 (weak)
(Continued)

Amlodipine *(Continued)*

Decreased Effect: Calcium may reduce the calcium channel blocker's hypotensive effects. Levels/effects of amlodipine may be decreased by aminoglutethimide, carbamazepine, nafcillin, nevirapine, phenobarbital, phenytoin, rifamycins, and other CYP3A4 inducers.

Increased Effect/Toxicity: Amlodipine may increase the levels/effects of aminophylline, fluvoxamine, mexiletine, mirtazapine, ropinirole, theophylline, trifluoperazine and other CYP1A2 substrates. Levels/effects of amlodipine may be increased by azole antifungals, ciprofloxacin, clarithromycin, diclofenac, doxycycline, erythromycin, imatinib, isoniazid, nefazodone, nicardipine, propofol, protease inhibitors, quinidine, telithromycin, verapamil, and other CYP3A4 inhibitors. Cyclosporine levels may be increased by amlodipine. Blood pressure-lowering effects of sildenafil, tadalafil, and vardenafil are additive with amlodipine (use caution).

Nutritional/Ethanol Interactions

Food: Grapefruit juice may modestly increase amlodipine levels.

Herb/Nutraceutical: St John's wort may decrease amlodipine levels. Avoid dong quai if using for hypertension (has estrogenic activity). Avoid ephedra, yohimbe, ginseng (may worsen hypertension). Avoid garlic (may have increased antihypertensive effects).

Adverse Reactions

>10%: Cardiovascular: Peripheral edema (2% to 15% dose related)

1% to 10%:

Cardiovascular: Flushing (1% to 3%), palpitation (1% to 4%)

Central nervous system: Headache (7%; similar to placebo 8%), dizziness (1% to 3%), fatigue (4%), somnolence (1% to 2%)

Dermatologic: Rash (1% to 2%), pruritus (1% to 2%)

Endocrine & metabolic: Male sexual dysfunction (1% to 2%)

Gastrointestinal: Nausea (3%), abdominal pain (1% to 2%), dyspepsia (1% to 2%), gingival hyperplasia

Neuromuscular & skeletal: Muscle cramps (1% to 2%), weakness (1% to 2%)

Respiratory: Dyspnea (1% to 2%), pulmonary edema (15% from PRAISE trial, CHF population)

Overdosage/Toxicology Primary cardiac symptoms of calcium channel blocker overdose include hypotension and bradycardia. Noncardiac symptoms include confusion, stupor, nausea, vomiting, metabolic acidosis, and hyperglycemia. Treat other signs and symptoms symptomatically.

Pharmacodynamics/Kinetics

Onset of Action: 30-50 minutes; Peak effect: 6-12 hours

Duration of Action: 24 hours

Absorption: Oral: Well absorbed

Bioavailability: 64% to 90%

Protein Binding: 93%

Half-Life Elimination: 30-50 hours

Metabolism: Hepatic (>90%) to inactive metabolite

Excretion: Urine

Dosing

Adults:

Hypertension: Initial dose: 5 mg once daily; maximum dose: 10 mg once daily. In general, titrate in 2.5 mg increments over 7-14 days. Usual dosage range (JNC 7): 2.5-10 mg once daily.

Angina: Usual dose: 5-10 mg

Elderly: Dosing should start at the lower end of dosing range due to possible increased incidence of hepatic, renal, or cardiac impairment. Elderly patients also show decreased clearance of amlodipine.

Hypertension: Oral: 2.5 mg once daily

Angina: Oral: 5 mg once daily

Pediatrics: Hypertension: Oral: Children 6-17 years: 2.5-5 mg once daily

Hepatic Impairment:

Hypertension: Administer 2.5 mg once daily

Angina: Administer 5 mg once daily

Available Dosage Forms Tablet, as besylate [equivalent to amlodipine base]: 2.5 mg, 5 mg, 10 mg

Monitoring and Teaching Issues

Physical Assessment: Assess potential for interactions with prescriptions, OTC medications, or herbal products patient may be taking (eg, nitrates or other drugs that effect blood pressure; see Drug Interactions). Assess therapeutic effectiveness (blood pressure, cardiac rhythm, frequency and intensity of angina, I & O ratio, weight, edema) according to purpose for use and signs of adverse reactions at beginning of therapy, when changing dose, and periodically during long-term therapy (see Adverse Reactions). Teach patient proper use, possible side effects/appropriate interventions, and adverse symptoms to report.

Patient Education: Do not take any new medication during therapy unless approved by prescriber. Take exactly as directed; do not alter dose or discontinue without consulting prescriber. May cause headache (if unrelieved, consult prescriber); nausea or vomiting (small frequent meals, frequent mouth care, chewing gum or sucking lozenges may help); constipation (increased dietary bulk and fluids may help); drowsiness (use caution when driving or engaging in tasks that require alertness until response to drug is known); or postural hypotension (use caution when rising from sitting or lying position or when climbing stairs). Report unrelieved headache; vomiting, constipation; palpitations; peripheral or facial swelling; weight gain >5 lb/week; or respiratory changes. **Pregnancy/breast-feeding precautions:** Inform prescriber if you are or intend to become pregnant. Consult prescriber if breast-feeding.

Dietary Considerations: May be taken without regard to meals.

Geriatric Considerations: Elderly or debilitated persons may experience a greater hypotensive response. Theoretically, constipation may be more of a problem with elderly.

Pregnancy Risk Factor: C

Lactation: Excretion in breast milk unknown/not recommended

Administration

Oral: May be administered without regard to meals.

Storage: Store at room temperature of 15°C to 30°C (59°F to 86°F).

Related Information

Calcium Channel Blockers *on page 1722*

Amlodipine and Atorvastatin (am LOW di peen & a TORE va sta tin)

U.S. Brand Names Caduet®

Synonyms Atorvastatin Calcium and Amlodipine Besylate

Generic Available No

Pharmacologic Category Antilipemic Agent, HMG-CoA Reductase Inhibitor; Calcium Channel Blocker

Use For use when treatment with both agents is appropriate:

Amlodipine is used for the treatment of hypertension and angina.

Atorvastatin is used with dietary therapy for the following:

Hyperlipidemias: To reduce elevations in total cholesterol, LDL-C, apolipoprotein B, and triglycerides in patients with primary hypercholesterolemia (elevations of 1 or more components are present in Fredrickson type IIa, IIb, III, and IV hyperlipidemias); treatment of homozygous familial hypercholesterolemia

Heterozygous familial hypercholesterolemia (HeFH): In adolescent patients (10-17 years of age, females >1 year postmenarche) with HeFH having LDL-C ≥190 mg/dL **or** LDL ≥160 mg/dL with positive family history of premature cardiovascular disease (CVD) or with 2 or more CVD risk factors in the adolescent patient

Primary prevention of CVD in high-risk patients

Dosing

Adults: Treatment of hypertension/angina and hyperlipidemias: Oral: Dose is individualized, given once daily and substituted for each individual component. See individual agents. Maximum dose: Amlodipine 10 mg/day, atorvastatin 80 mg/day.

Pediatrics: Treatment of hypertension/angina and hyperlipidemias: Oral: Children 10-17 years (females >1 year postmenarche): Refer to adult dosing.

Renal Impairment: See individual agents.

Hepatic Impairment: Use of atorvastatin is contraindicated.

Available Dosage Forms

Tablet:

2.5/10: Amlodipine 2.5 mg and atorvastatin 10 mg
2.5/20: Amlodipine 2.5 mg and atorvastatin 20 mg
2.5/40: Amlodipine 2.5 mg and atorvastatin 40 mg
5/10: Amlodipine 5 mg and atorvastatin 10 mg
5/20: Amlodipine 5 mg and atorvastatin 20 mg
5/40: Amlodipine 5 mg and atorvastatin 40 mg
5/80: Amlodipine 5 mg and atorvastatin 80 mg
10/10: Amlodipine 10 mg and atorvastatin 10 mg
10/20: Amlodipine 10 mg and atorvastatin 20 mg
10/40: Amlodipine 10 mg and atorvastatin 40 mg
10/80: Amlodipine 10 mg and atorvastatin 80 mg

Monitoring and Teaching Issues

Physical Assessment: See individual agents. **Pregnancy risk factor X: Determine that** patient is not pregnant before starting therapy. Do not give to childbearing-age females unless capable of complying with effective contraceptive measures. Breast-feeding is contraindicated.

Patient Education: See individual agents. **Pregnancy/breast-feeding precautions:** Inform prescriber if you are pregnant. Do not get pregnant during therapy. Consult prescriber for instructions in appropriate contraceptive measures. This drug can cause severe fetal defects. Do not donate blood while taking this medication and for some period of time after discontinuing. Do not breast-feed.

Pregnancy Risk Factor: X

Lactation: Excretion in breast milk unknown/contraindicated

Amlodipine and Benazepril (am LOE di peen & ben AY ze pril)

U.S. Brand Names Lotrel®

Synonyms Benazepril and Amlodipine

Generic Available No

Pharmacologic Category Antihypertensive Agent, Combination

Use Treatment of hypertension

Dosing

Adults: Hypertension: Oral: Dosage is individualized, given once daily.

Elderly: Initial dose: 2.5 mg (based on amlodipine component). Refer to adult dosing.

Renal Impairment: Cl$_{cr}$ ≤30 mL/minute: Use of combination product is not recommended.

Hepatic Impairment: Initial dose: 2.5 mg based on amlodipine component.

Available Dosage Forms

Capsule:

Amlodipine 2.5 mg and benazepril hydrochloride 10 mg
Amlodipine 5 mg and benazepril hydrochloride 10 mg
Amlodipine 5 mg and benazepril hydrochloride 20 mg
Amlodipine 10 mg and benazepril hydrochloride 20 mg

(Continued)

Amlodipine and Benazepril (Continued)

Monitoring and Teaching Issues
Physical Assessment: See individual agents.

Patient Education: See individual agents. **Pregnancy/breast-feeding precautions:** Inform prescriber if you are or intend to become pregnant. Consult prescriber if breast-feeding.

Pregnancy Risk Factor: C/D (2nd and 3rd trimesters)

Lactation:
Amlodipine: Excretion in breast milk unknown
Benazepril: Enters breast milk

Related Information
Amlodipine on page 99
Benazepril on page 178

♦ **Amlodipine Besylate** see Amlodipine on page 99

♦ **Amnesteem™** see Isotretinoin on page 842

♦ **AMO Vitrax®** see page 1625

Amoxicillin (a moks i SIL in)

U.S. Brand Names Amoxil®; DisperMox™; Moxilin®; Trimox®

Synonyms Amoxicillin Trihydrate; Amoxycillin; p-Hydroxyampicillin

Generic Available Yes: Excludes tablet for oral suspension

Pharmacologic Category Antibiotic, Penicillin

Medication Safety Issues
Sound-alike/look-alike issues:
Amoxicillin may be confused with amoxapine, Amoxil®, Atarax®
Amoxil® may be confused with amoxapine, amoxicillin
Trimox® may be confused with Diamox®, Tylox®

Use Treatment of otitis media, sinusitis, and infections caused by susceptible organisms involving the respiratory tract, skin, and urinary tract; prophylaxis of bacterial endocarditis in patients undergoing surgical or dental procedures; as part of a multidrug regimen for *H. pylori* eradication

Unlabeled/Investigational Use Postexposure prophylaxis for anthrax exposure with documented susceptible organisms

Mechanism of Action/Effect Interferes with bacterial cell wall synthesis during active multiplication, causing cell wall death and resultant bactericidal activity against susceptible bacteria

Contraindications Hypersensitivity to amoxicillin, penicillin, or any component of the formulation

Warnings/Precautions In patients with renal impairment, doses and/or frequency of administration should be modified in response to the degree of renal impairment. A high percentage of patients with infectious mononucleosis have developed rash during therapy with amoxicillin.

Drug Interactions
Decreased Effect: Decreased effectiveness with tetracyclines and chloramphenicol. Although anecdotal reports suggest oral contraceptive efficacy could be reduced by penicillins, this has been refuted by more rigorous scientific and clinical data.

Increased Effect/Toxicity: Disulfiram and probenecid may increase amoxicillin levels. Amoxicillin may increase the effects of oral anticoagulants (warfarin). Theoretically, allopurinol taken with amoxicillin has an additive potential for amoxicillin rash. Penicillins may increase the exposure to methotrexate during concurrent therapy; monitor.

Lab Interactions Increased AST, ALT, protein; altered response to Benedict's reagent in Clinitest®

Adverse Reactions Frequency not defined.
Central nervous system: Hyperactivity, agitation, anxiety, insomnia, confusion, convulsions, behavioral changes, dizziness
Dermatologic: Acute exanthematous pustulosis, erythematous maculopapular rash, erythema multiforme, Stevens-Johnson syndrome, exfoliative dermatitis, toxic epidermal necrolysis, hypersensitivity vasculitis, urticaria
Gastrointestinal: Nausea, vomiting, diarrhea, hemorrhagic colitis, pseudomembranous colitis, tooth discoloration (brown, yellow, or gray; rare)
Hematologic: Anemia, hemolytic anemia, thrombocytopenia, thrombocytopenia purpura, eosinophilia, leukopenia, agranulocytosis
Hepatic: Elevated AST (SGOT) and ALT (SGPT), cholestatic jaundice, hepatic cholestasis, acute cytolytic hepatitis
Renal: Crystalluria

Overdosage/Toxicology Symptoms of penicillin overdose include neuromuscular hypersensitivity (eg, agitation, hallucinations, asterixis, encephalopathy, confusion, and seizures). Electrolyte imbalance may occur if the preparation contains potassium or sodium salts, especially in renal failure. Hemodialysis may be helpful to aid in removal of the drug from blood; otherwise, treatment is symptom-directed and supportive.

Pharmacodynamics/Kinetics
Absorption: Oral: Rapid and nearly complete; food does not interfere
Time to Peak: Capsule: 2 hours; Suspension: 1 hour
Protein Binding: 17% to 20%
Half-Life Elimination:
Neonates, full-term: 3.7 hours
Infants and Children: 1-2 hours
Adults: Normal renal function: 0.7-1.4 hours
Cl_{cr} <10 mL/minute: 7-21 hours

Metabolism: Partially hepatic

Excretion: Urine (80% as unchanged drug); lower in neonates

Dosing

Adults & Elderly:

Susceptible infections: Oral: Dosing range: 250-500 mg every 8 hours or 500-875 mg twice daily; maximum dose: 2-3 g/day

Ear, nose, throat, genitourinary tract or skin/skin structure infections:
Mild to moderate: 500 mg every 12 hours **or** 250 mg every 8 hours
Severe: 875 mg every 12 hours **or** 500 mg every 8 hours

Lower respiratory tract infections: 875 mg every 12 hours **or** 500 mg every 8 hours

Endocarditis prophylaxis: 2 g 1 hour before procedure

Peptic ulcer disease: Eradication of *Helicobacter pylori:* Oral: 1000 mg twice daily; requires combination therapy with at least one other antibiotic and an acid-suppressing agent (proton pump inhibitor or H$_2$ blocker)

Anthrax exposure (unlabeled use): Oral: **Note:** Postexposure prophylaxis only with documented susceptible organisms: 500 mg every 8 hours

Pediatrics:

Susceptible infections: Oral:
Children ≤3 months: 20-30 mg/kg/day divided every 12 hours
Children: >3 months and <40 kg: Dosing range: 20-50 mg/kg/day in divided doses every 8-12 hours

Ear, nose, throat, genitourinary tract, or skin/skin structure infections: Oral:
Mild to moderate: 25 mg/kg/day in divided doses every 12 hours **or** 20 mg/kg/day in divided doses every 8 hours
Severe: 45 mg/kg/day in divided doses every 12 hours **or** 40 mg/kg/day in divided doses every 8 hours

Acute otitis media: Due to highly-resistant strains of *S. pneumoniae:* Oral: Doses as high as 80-90 mg/kg/day divided every 12 hours have been used

Lower respiratory tract infections: Oral: 45 mg/kg/day in divided doses every 12 hours **or** 40 mg/kg/day in divided doses every 8 hours

Subacute bacterial endocarditis prophylaxis: Oral: 50 mg/kg 1 hour before procedure

Anthrax exposure (unlabeled use): Oral: **Note:** Postexposure prophylaxis only with documented susceptible organisms:
<40 kg: 15 mg/kg every 8 hours
≥40 kg: 500 mg every 8 hours

Renal Impairment:
The 875 mg tablet should not be used in patients with Cl$_{cr}$ <30 mL/minute.
Cl$_{cr}$ 10-30 mL/minute: 250-500 mg every 12 hours
Cl$_{cr}$ <10 mL/minute: 250-500 mg every 24 hours
Moderately dialyzable (20% to 50%) by hemodialysis or peritoneal dialysis; approximately 50 mg of amoxicillin per liter of filtrate is removed by continuous arteriovenous or venovenous hemofiltration. Dose as per Cl$_{cr}$ <10 mL/minute guidelines.

Available Dosage Forms [DSC] = Discontinued product

Capsule, as trihydrate: 250 mg, 500 mg
Amoxil®: 250 mg [DSC], 500 mg
Moxilin®, Trimox®: 250 mg, 500 mg

Powder for oral suspension, as trihydrate: 125 mg/5 mL (80 mL, 100 mL, 150 mL); 200 mg/5 mL (50 mL, 75 mL, 100 mL); 250 mg/5 mL (80 mL, 100 mL, 150 mL); 400 mg/5 mL (50 mL, 75 mL, 100 mL)
Amoxil®: 125 mg/5 mL (150 mL) [contains sodium benzoate; strawberry flavor] [DSC]; 200 mg/5 mL (5 mL, 50 mL, 75 mL, 100 mL) [contains sodium benzoate; bubble gum flavor]; 250 mg/5 mL (100 mL, 150 mL) [contains sodium benzoate; bubble gum flavor]; 400 mg/5 mL (5 mL, 50 mL, 75 mL, 100 mL) [contains sodium benzoate; bubble gum flavor]
Moxilin®: 250 mg/5 mL (100 mL, 150 mL)
Trimox®: 125 mg/5 mL (80 mL, 100 mL, 150 mL); 250 mg/5 mL (80 mL, 100 mL, 150 mL) [contains sodium benzoate; raspberry-strawberry flavor]
Powder for oral suspension, as trihydrate [drops] (Amoxil®): 50 mg/mL (15 mL [DSC], 30 mL) [bubble gum flavor]
Tablet, as trihydrate [film coated] (Amoxil®): 500 mg, 875 mg
Tablet, chewable, as trihydrate: 125 mg, 200 mg, 250 mg, 400 mg
Amoxil®: 200 mg [contains phenylalanine 1.82 mg/tablet; cherry banana peppermint flavor]; 400 mg [contains phenylalanine 3.64 mg/tablet; cherry banana peppermint flavor]
Tablet, for oral suspension, as trihydrate (DisperMox™): 200 mg [contains phenylalanine 5.6 mg; strawberry flavor]; 400 mg [contains phenylalanine 5.6 mg; strawberry flavor]; 600 mg [contains phenylalanine 11.23 mg; strawberry flavor]

Monitoring and Teaching Issues

Physical Assessment: Assess culture and sensitivity report and patient allergy history prior to starting therapy. Assess potential for interactions with other medications patient may be taking (see Drug Interactions). Caution patients with diabetes about altered response to Clinitest®. Assess for therapeutic effectiveness and adverse reactions (eg, opportunistic infection; fever, chills, unhealed sores, white plaques in mouth or vagina, purulent vaginal discharge, fatigue; see Adverse Reactions and Overdose/Toxicology). Teach patient proper use, possible side effects/appropriate interventions, and adverse symptoms to report.

Monitoring Laboratory Tests: Perform culture and sensitivity testing prior to initiating therapy.

Patient Education: Do not take any new medication during therapy unless approved by prescriber. Take entire prescription, even if you are feeling better. Take at equal intervals around-the-clock. May be taken with milk, juice, or food. If you have diabetes, drug may cause false test results with Clinitest® urine glucose monitoring; use of another type of glucose monitoring is preferable. May cause nausea or vomiting (small frequent meals, frequent mouth care, sucking lozenges, or chewing gum may help). Report rash; unusual diarrhea; vaginal itching, burning, or pain; unresolved vomiting or constipation; fever or

(Continued)

Amoxicillin (Continued)

chills; abdominal pain; jaundice; unusual bruising or bleeding; or if condition being treated worsens or does not improve by the time prescription is completed.

Dietary Considerations: May be taken with food. Amoxil® chewable contains phenylalanine 1.82 mg per 200 mg tablet, phenylalanine 3.64 mg per 400 mg tablet. DisperMox™ contains phenylalanine 5.6 mg in each 200 mg and 400 mg tablet.

Geriatric Considerations: Resistance to amoxicillin has been a problem in patients on frequent antibiotics or in nursing homes. Alternative antibiotics may be necessary in these populations. Consider renal function.

Pregnancy Risk Factor: B

Lactation: Enters breast milk/compatible

Administration

Oral: Administer around-the-clock to promote less variation in peak and trough serum levels. The appropriate amount of suspension may be mixed with formula, milk, fruit juice, water, ginger ale or cold drinks; administer dose immediately after mixing.

DisperMox™: Dissolve 1 tablet in ~10 mL of water immediately before administration. Rinse container with additional water and drink entire contents to ensure that complete dose is taken. Do not chew or swallow tablet whole.

Reconstitution: DisperMox™: Dissolve 1 tablet in ~10 mL water immediately before use.

Storage: Amoxil®: Oral suspension remains stable for 14 days at room temperature or if refrigerated (refrigeration preferred); unit-dose antibiotic oral syringes are stable for 48 hours.

Related Information

Antimicrobial Drugs of Choice *on page 1792*
Community-Acquired Pneumonia in Adults *on page 1807*
Helicobacter pylori Treatment *on page 1835*

Amoxicillin and Clavulanate Potassium

(a moks i SIL in & klav yoo LAN ate poe TASS ee um)

U.S. Brand Names Augmentin®; Augmentin ES-600®; Augmentin XR™

Synonyms Amoxicillin and Clavulanic Acid

Generic Available Yes: Excludes extended release

Pharmacologic Category Antibiotic, Penicillin

Medication Safety Issues

Sound-alike/look-alike issues:
Augmentin® may be confused with Azulfidine®

Use Treatment of otitis media, sinusitis, and infections caused by susceptible organisms involving the lower respiratory tract, skin and skin structure, and urinary tract; spectrum same as amoxicillin with additional coverage of beta-lactamase producing *B. catarrhalis*, *H. influenzae*, *N. gonorrhoeae*, and *S. aureus* (not MRSA). The expanded coverage of this combination makes it a useful alternative when amoxicillin resistance is present and patients cannot tolerate alternative treatments.

Mechanism of Action/Effect Interferes with bacterial cell wall synthesis during active multiplication, causing cell wall death and resultant bactericidal activity against susceptible bacteria. Clavulanic acid binds and inhibits beta-lactamases that inactivate amoxicillin resulting in amoxicillin having an expanded spectrum of activity.

Contraindications Hypersensitivity to amoxicillin, clavulanic acid, penicillin, or any component of the formulation; history of cholestatic jaundice or hepatic dysfunction with amoxicillin/clavulanate potassium therapy

Warnings/Precautions Prolonged use may result in superinfection; in patients with renal impairment, doses and/or frequency of administration should be modified in response to the degree of renal impairment; high percentage of patients with infectious mononucleosis have developed rash during therapy; a low incidence of cross-allergy with cephalosporins exists; incidence of diarrhea is higher than with amoxicillin alone. Use caution in patients with hepatic dysfunction. Hepatic dysfunction, although rare, is more common in elderly and/or males, and occurs more frequently with prolonged treatment, and may occur after therapy is complete. Due to differing content of clavulanic acid, not all formulations are interchangeable. Some products contain phenylalanine.

Drug Interactions

Decreased Effect: Although anecdotal reports suggest oral contraceptive efficacy could be reduced by penicillins, this has been refuted by more rigorous scientific and clinical data.

Increased Effect/Toxicity: Probenecid may increase amoxicillin levels. Increased effect of anticoagulants with amoxicillin. Allopurinol taken with Augmentin® has an additive potential for rash. Penicillins may increase the exposure to methotrexate during concurrent therapy; monitor.

Lab Interactions Urinary glucose (Benedict's solution, Clinitest®)

Adverse Reactions

>10%: Gastrointestinal: Diarrhea (3% to 34%; incidence varies upon dose and regimen used)

1% to 10%:

Dermatologic: Diaper rash, skin rash, urticaria

Gastrointestinal: Abdominal discomfort, loose stools, nausea, vomiting

Genitourinary: Vaginitis

Miscellaneous: Moniliasis

Additional adverse reactions seen with **ampicillin-class antibiotics:** Agitation, agranulocytosis, ALT elevated, anaphylaxis, anemia, angioedema, anxiety, AST elevated, behavioral changes, black "hairy" tongue, confusion, convulsions, crystalluria, dizziness, enterocolitis, eosinophilia, erythema multiforme, exanthematous pustulosis, exfoliative dermatitis, gastritis, glossitis, hematuria, hemolytic anemia, hemorrhagic colitis, indigestion, insomnia, hyperactivity, interstitial nephritis, leukopenia, mucocutaneous candidiasis, pruritus, pseudomembranous colitis, serum sickness-like reaction, Stevens-Johnson syndrome, stomatitis, thrombocytopenia, thrombocytopenic purpura, tooth discoloration, toxic epidermal necrolysis

Overdosage/Toxicology Symptoms of overdose may include abdominal pain, diarrhea, drowsiness, rash, hyperactivity, stomach pain, and vomiting. Electrolyte imbalance may occur, especially in renal failure. Hemodialysis may be helpful to aid in removal of the drug from blood; otherwise, treatment is supportive or symptom-directed.

Pharmacodynamics/Kinetics
  Metabolism:
    Clavulanic acid: Hepatic
  Excretion:
    Clavulanic acid: Urine (30% to 40% as unchanged drug)
  Pharmacokinetic Note: Amoxicillin pharmacokinetics are not affected by clavulanic acid. See Amoxicillin monograph.

Dosing
  Adults & Elderly: Note: Dose is based on the amoxicillin component; see "Augmentin® Product-Specific Considerations table".
    Susceptible infections: Oral: Children >40 kg and Adults: 250-500 mg every 8 hours or 875 mg every 12 hours

Augmentin® Product-Specific Considerations

Strength	Form	Consideration
125 mg	CT, S	q8h dosing
	S	For adults having difficulty swallowing tablets, 125 mg/5 mL suspension may be substituted for 500 mg tablet.
200 mg	CT, S	q12h dosing
	CT	Contains phenylalanine
	S	For adults having difficulty swallowing tablets, 200 mg/5 mL suspension may be substituted for 875 mg tablet.
250 mg	CT, S, T	q8h dosing
	CT	Contains phenylalanine
	T	Not for use in patients <40 kg
	CT, T	Tablet and chewable tablet are not interchangeable due to differences in clavulanic acid.
	S	For adults having difficulty swallowing tablets, 250 mg/5 mL suspension may be substituted for 500 mg tablet.
400 mg	CT, S	q12h dosing
	CT	Contains phenylalanine
	S	For adults having difficulty swallowing tablets, 400 mg/5 mL suspension may be substituted for 875 mg tablet.
500 mg	T	q8h or q12h dosing
600 mg	S	q12h dosing
		Contains phenylalanine
		Not for use in adults or children ≥40 kg
		600 mg/5 mL suspension is not equivalent to or interchangeable with 200 mg/5 mL or 400 mg/5 mL due to differences in clavulanic acid.
875 mg	T	q12h dosing; not for use in Cl$_{cr}$ <30 mL/minute
1000 mg	XR	q12h dosing
		Not for use in children <16 years of age
		Not interchangeable with two 500 mg tablets
		Not for use in Cl$_{cr}$ <30 mL/minute or hemodialysis

Legend: CT = chewable tablet, S = suspension, T = tablet, XR = extended release.

  Acute bacterial sinusitis: Oral: Extended release tablet: Two 1000 mg tablets every 12 hours for 10 days
  Community-acquired pneumonia: Oral: Extended release tablet: Two 1000 mg tablets every 12 hours for 7-10 days
  Pediatrics: Note: Dose is based on the amoxicillin component; see "Augmentin® Product-Specific Considerations table".
    Susceptible infections: Oral: Infants <3 months: 30 mg/kg/day divided every 12 hours using the 125 mg/5 mL suspension
    Otitis media: Oral: Children ≥3 months and <40 kg: 90 mg/kg/day divided every 12 hours for 10 days
    Lower respiratory tract infections, severe infections, sinusitis: Oral: Children ≥3 months and <40 kg: 45 mg/kg/day divided every 12 hours **or** 40 mg/kg/day divided every 8 hours
    Less severe infections: Oral:
      Children ≥3 months and <40 kg: 25 mg/kg/day divided every 12 hours or 20 mg/kg/day divided every 8 hours
      Children >40 kg: Refer to adult dosing.
  Renal Impairment:
    Cl$_{cr}$ <30 mL/minute: Do not use 875 mg tablet or extended release tablets.
    Cl$_{cr}$ 10-30 mL/minute: 250-500 mg every 12 hours
    Cl$_{cr}$ <10 mL/minute: 250-500 mg every 24 hours
    Hemodialysis: Moderately dialyzable (20% to 50%)
      250-500 mg every 24 hours; administer dose during and after dialysis. Do not use extended release tablets.
    Peritoneal dialysis: Moderately dialyzable (20% to 50%)
      Amoxicillin: Administer 250 mg every 12 hours
      Clavulanic acid: Dose for Cl$_{cr}$ <10 mL/minute
    Continuous arteriovenous or venovenous hemofiltration effects:
      Amoxicillin: ~50 mg of amoxicillin/L of filtrate is removed
      Clavulanic acid: Dose for Cl$_{cr}$ <10 mL/minute
(Continued)

Amoxicillin and Clavulanate Potassium *(Continued)*

Available Dosage Forms

Powder for oral suspension: 200: Amoxicillin 200 mg and clavulanate potassium 28.5 mg per 5 mL (100 mL) [contains phenylalanine]; 400: Amoxicillin 400 mg and clavulanate potassium 57 mg per 5 mL (100 mL) [contains phenylalanine]

Augmentin®:

125: Amoxicillin 125 mg and clavulanate potassium 31.25 mg per 5 mL (75 mL, 100 mL, 150 mL) [banana flavor]

200: Amoxicillin 200 mg and clavulanate potassium 28.5 mg per 5 mL (50 mL, 75 mL, 100 mL) [contains phenylalanine 7 mg/5 mL; orange-raspberry flavor]

250: Amoxicillin 250 mg and clavulanate potassium 62.5 mg per 5 mL (75 mL, 100 mL, 150 mL) [orange flavor]

400: Amoxicillin 400 mg and clavulanate potassium 57 mg per 5 mL (50 mL, 75 mL, 100 mL) [contains phenylalanine 7 mg/5 mL; orange-raspberry flavor]

Augmentin ES-600®: Amoxicillin 600 mg and clavulanic potassium 42.9 mg per 5 mL (75 mL, 125 mL, 200 mL) [contains phenylalanine 7 mg/5 mL; orange flavor]

Tablet: 500: Amoxicillin trihydrate 500 mg and clavulanate potassium 125 mg; 875: Amoxicillin trihydrate 875 mg and clavulanate potassium 125 mg

Augmentin®:

250: Amoxicillin trihydrate 250 mg and clavulanate potassium 125 mg

500: Amoxicillin trihydrate 500 mg and clavulanate potassium 125 mg

875: Amoxicillin trihydrate 875 mg and clavulanate potassium 125 mg

Tablet, chewable: 200: Amoxicillin trihydrate 200 mg and clavulanate potassium 28.5 mg [contains phenylalanine]; 400: Amoxicillin trihydrate 400 mg and clavulanate potassium 57 mg [contains phenylalanine]

Augmentin®:

125: Amoxicillin trihydrate 125 mg and clavulanate potassium 31.25 mg [lemon-lime flavor]

200: Amoxicillin trihydrate 200 mg and clavulanate potassium 28.5 mg [contains phenylalanine 2.1 mg/tablet; cherry-banana flavor]

250: Amoxicillin trihydrate 250 mg and clavulanate potassium 62.5 mg [lemon-lime flavor]

400: Amoxicillin trihydrate 400 mg and clavulanate potassium 57 mg [contains phenylalanine 4.2 mg/tablet; cherry-banana flavor]

Tablet, extended release (Augmentin XR™): Amoxicillin 1000 mg and clavulanic acid 62.5 mg

Monitoring and Teaching Issues

Physical Assessment: Assess for allergy history prior to starting therapy. See Contraindications and Warnings/Precautions for use cautions. Assess potential for interactions with other prescriptions, OTC medications, or herbal products patient may be taking (see Drug Interactions). Caution patients with diabetes about altered response to Clinitest®. Assess results of laboratory tests, therapeutic effectiveness, and adverse reactions (eg, opportunistic infection: fever, chills, unhealed sores, white plaques in mouth or vagina, purulent vaginal discharge, fatigue; see Adverse Reactions and Overdose/Toxicology). Teach patient proper use, possible side effects/appropriate interventions, and adverse symptoms to report (see Patient Education). Note breast-feeding caution.

Monitoring Laboratory Tests: Renal, hepatic, and hematologic function periodically with prolonged therapy. Perform culture and sensitivity testing prior to initiating therapy.

Patient Education: Inform prescriber of all prescriptions, OTC medications, or herbal products you are taking, and any allergies you have. Do not take any new medication during therapy unless approved by prescriber. Take as directed, for as long as directed, even if you are feeling better. (For small children, bottles may contain more suspension than needed, take for number of days prescribed.) Take at equal intervals around-the-clock; may be taken with milk, juice, or food. Extended release tablets should be taken with food. If you have diabetes, drug may cause false test results with Clinitest® urine glucose monitoring; use of another type of glucose monitoring is preferable. May cause nausea or vomiting (small frequent meals, frequent mouth care, sucking lozenges, or chewing gum may help). Report rash; unusual diarrhea; vaginal itching, burning, or pain; unresolved vomiting or constipation; fever or chills; abdominal pain; jaundice; unusual bruising or bleeding; or if condition being treated worsens or does not improve by the time prescription is completed. Some products contain phenylalanine. Avoid use in phenylketonurics. **Breast-feeding precaution:** Consult prescriber if breast-feeding.

Dietary Considerations: May be taken with meals or on an empty stomach; take with meals to increase absorption and decrease GI intolerance; may mix with milk, formula, or juice. Extended release tablets should be taken with food. Some products contain phenylalanine; avoid use in phenylketonurics. All dosage forms contain potassium.

Geriatric Considerations: Resistance to amoxicillin has been a problem in patients on frequent antibiotics or in nursing homes. However, expanded coverage of this combination makes it a useful alternative when amoxicillin resistance is present and patients cannot tolerate alternative treatments. Consider renal function. Considered one of the drugs of choice in the outpatient treatment of community-acquired pneumonia in older adults.

Pregnancy Risk Factor: B

Pregnancy Issues: Both amoxicillin and clavulanate potassium cross the human placenta. Teratogenic effects have not been reported. Use in women with premature rupture of fetal membranes may increase risk of necrotizing enterocolitis in neonates.

Lactation: Enters breast milk/use caution (AAP rates "compatible")

Breast-Feeding Issues: The AAP considers amoxicillin to be "compatible" with breast-feeding.

Administration

Oral: Administer around-the-clock to promote less variation in peak and trough serum levels. Administer with food to decrease stomach upset; shake suspension well before use. Extended release tablets should be administered with food.

Reconstitution: Reconstitute powder for oral suspension with appropriate amount of water as specified on the bottle. Shake vigorously until suspended. Reconstituted oral suspension should be kept in refrigerator. Discard unused suspension after 10 days. Unit-dose antibiotic oral syringes are stable for 48 hours.

Storage:
Powder for oral suspension: Store dry powder at room temperature of 25°C (77°F).
Tablet: Store at room temperature of 25°C (77°F).

Additional Information Two 250 mg tablets are not equivalent to a 500 mg tablet (both tablet sizes contain equivalent clavulanate). Two 500 mg tablets are not equivalent to a single 1000 mg extended release tablet.

Related Information
Amoxicillin *on page 102*
Community-Acquired Pneumonia in Adults *on page 1807*

♦ **Amoxicillin and Clavulanic Acid** *see* Amoxicillin and Clavulanate Potassium *on page 104*

♦ **Amoxicillin, Lansoprazole, and Clarithromycin** *see* Lansoprazole, Amoxicillin, and Clarithromycin *on page 868*

♦ **Amoxicillin Trihydrate** *see* Amoxicillin *on page 102*

♦ **Amoxil®** *see* Amoxicillin *on page 102*

♦ **Amoxycillin** *see* Amoxicillin *on page 102*

♦ **Amphetamine and Dextroamphetamine** *see* Dextroamphetamine and Amphetamine *on page 436*

♦ **Amphocin®** *see* Amphotericin B (Conventional) *on page 109*

♦ **Amphotec®** *see* Amphotericin B Cholesteryl Sulfate Complex *on page 107*

Amphotericin B Cholesteryl Sulfate Complex
(am foe TER i sin bee kole LES te ril SUL fate KOM plecks)

U.S. Brand Names Amphotec®
Synonyms ABCD; Amphotericin B Colloidal Dispersion
Generic Available No
Pharmacologic Category Antifungal Agent, Parenteral
Medication Safety Issues
Safety issues:
Lipid-based amphotericin formulations (Amphotec®) may be confused with conventional formulations (Amphocin®, Fungizone®)
Large overdoses have occurred when conventional formulations were dispensed inadvertently for lipid-based products. Single daily doses of conventional amphotericin formulation never exceed 1.5 mg/kg.

Use Treatment of invasive aspergillosis in patients who have failed amphotericin B deoxycholate treatment, or who have renal impairment or experience unacceptable toxicity which precludes treatment with amphotericin B deoxycholate in effective doses.

Unlabeled/Investigational Use Effective in patients with serious *Candida* species infections

Mechanism of Action/Effect Binds to ergosterol altering cell membrane permeability in susceptible fungi and causing leakage of cell components with subsequent cell death

Contraindications Hypersensitivity to amphotericin B or any component of the formulation

Warnings/Precautions Anaphylaxis has been reported. Facilities for cardiopulmonary resuscitation should be available. Infusion reactions, sometimes severe, usually subside with continued therapy.

Drug Interactions

Decreased Effect: Pharmacologic antagonism may occur with azole antifungals (eg, ketoconazole, miconazole).

Increased Effect/Toxicity: Toxic effect with other nephrotoxic drugs (eg, cyclosporine and aminoglycosides) may be additive. Corticosteroids may increase potassium depletion caused by amphotericin. Amphotericin B may predispose patients receiving digitalis glycosides or neuromuscular blocking agents to toxicity secondary to hypokalemia.

Adverse Reactions
>10%: Central nervous system: Chills, fever
1% to 10%:
Cardiovascular: Hypotension, tachycardia
Central nervous system: Headache
Dermatologic: Rash
Endocrine & metabolic: Hypokalemia, hypomagnesemia
Gastrointestinal: Nausea, diarrhea, abdominal pain
Hematologic: Thrombocytopenia
Hepatic: LFT change
Neuromuscular & skeletal: Rigors
Renal: Elevated creatinine
Respiratory: Dyspnea

Note: Amphotericin B colloidal dispersion has an improved therapeutic index compared to conventional amphotericin B, and has been used safely in patients with amphotericin B-related nephrotoxicity; however, continued decline of renal function has occurred in some patients.

Overdosage/Toxicology Symptoms of overdose include renal dysfunction, anemia, thrombocytopenia, granulocytopenia, fever, nausea, and vomiting. Treatment is supportive.

Pharmacodynamics/Kinetics
Half-Life Elimination: 28-29 hours; prolonged with higher doses

Dosing
Adults & Elderly:
Note: Premedication: For patients who experience chills, fever, hypotension, nausea, or other nonanaphylactic infusion-related immediate reactions, premedicate with the following drugs, 30-60 minutes prior to drug administration: a nonsteroidal (eg, ibuprofen, choline magnesium trisalicylate) with or without diphenhydramine; or acetaminophen

(Continued)

Amphotericin B Cholesteryl Sulfate Complex *(Continued)*

with diphenhydramine; or hydrocortisone 50-100 mg. If the patient experiences rigors during the infusion, meperidine may be administered.

Susceptible infections: I.V.: Usual range: 3-4 mg/kg/day (infusion of 1 mg/kg/hour); maximum: 7.5 mg/kg/day

A regimen of 6 mg/kg/day has been used for treatment of life-threatening invasive mold infections in immunocompromised patients; maximum: 7.5 mg/kg/day.

Initially infuse at 1 mg/kg/hour. Rate of infusion may be increased with subsequent doses to 3 mg/kg/hour as patient tolerance allows. Treatment should continue as patient tolerance allows, until complete resolution of microbiologic and clinical evidence of fungal disease.

Pediatrics: Refer to adult dosing.

Available Dosage Forms Injection, powder for reconstitution: 50 mg, 100 mg

Monitoring and Teaching Issues

Physical Assessment: Assess culture and sensitivity report and patient's previous exposure to amphotericin B prior to starting therapy. Assess potential for interactions with other medications patient may be taking (eg, other nephrotoxic drugs; see Drug Interactions). See I.V. Details for premedication recommendations and specifics of administration and compatibility prior to administering first dose. Patient should be monitored closely for infusion-related reactions (eg, anaphylaxis, chills, fever, nausea, vomiting, rigors, hypotension, acute respiratory distress) and cardiopulmonary resuscitation should be available. If acute respiratory distress occurs, infusion should be stopped and prescriber notified. Assess results of laboratory tests, therapeutic effectiveness, and adverse response (see Adverse Reactions) frequently during therapy. Teach patient possible side effects/appropriate interventions and adverse symptoms to report.

Monitoring Laboratory Tests: Monitor serum electrolytes (especially potassium and magnesium), liver function, and CBC. Perform culture and sensitivity testing prior to initiating therapy.

Patient Education: Do not take any new medication during therapy unless approved by prescriber. This medication can only be administered by infusion and therapy may last several weeks. You will be monitored closely during and after infusion; report immediately any pain or selling at infusion site; chills, nausea, chest pain, swelling of face or mouth, difficulty breathing, muscle cramping, acute anxiety or other infusion reactions. Maintain adequate hydration (2-3 L/day of fluids) unless instructed to restrict fluid intake. May cause postural hypotension (use caution when changing from lying or sitting position to standing or when climbing stairs); or nausea or vomiting (small frequent meals, frequent mouth care, sucking lozenges, or chewing gum may help). Report chest pain or palpitations; CNS disturbances; skin rash; unusual chills or fever; persistent nausea, vomiting, or abdominal pain; sore throat; excessive fatigue; swelling of extremities or unusual weight gain; difficulty breathing; pain at infusion site; muscle cramping or weakness; or other adverse reactions.
Breast-feeding precaution: Do not breast-feed.

Geriatric Considerations: The pharmacokinetics and dosing of amphotericin have not been studied in the elderly. It appears that use is similar to young adults. Caution should be exercised and renal function and desired effect monitored closely.

Pregnancy Risk Factor: B

Lactation: Excretion in breast milk unknown/contraindicated

Breast-Feeding Issues: Due to limited data, consider discontinuing nursing during therapy.

Administration

I.V.: For a patient who experiences chills, fever, hypotension, nausea, or other nonanaphylactic infusion-related reactions, premedication with the following drugs, 30-60 minutes prior to drug administration: A nonsteroidal (eg, ibuprofen, choline magnesium trisalicylate) with or without diphenhydramine; or acetaminophen with diphenhydramine, or hydrocortisone 50-100 mg. If the patient experiences rigors during the infusion, meperidine may be administered. If severe respiratory distress occurs, the infusion should be immediately discontinued.

Compatibility: Stable in D$_5$W; **incompatible** with NS

Y-site administration: Incompatible with alfentanil, amikacin, ampicillin, ampicillin/sulbactam, atenolol, aztreonam, bretylium, buprenorphine, butorphanol, calcium chloride, calcium gluconate, carboplatin, cefazolin, cefepime, cefoperazone, ceftazidime, ceftriaxone, chlorpromazine, cimetidine, cisatracurium, cisplatin, cyclophosphamide, cyclosporine, cytarabine, diazepam, digoxin, diphenhydramine, dobutamine, dopamine, doxorubicin, doxorubicin liposome, droperidol, enalaprilat, esmolol, famotidine, fluconazole, fluorouracil, gatifloxacin, gentamicin, haloperidol, heparin, hydromorphone, hydroxyzine, imipenem/cilastatin, labetalol, leucovorin, lidocaine, magnesium sulfate, meperidine, mesna, metoclopramide, metoprolol, metronidazole, midazolam, mitoxantrone, morphine, nalbuphine, naloxone, ofloxacin, ondansetron, paclitaxel, pentobarbital, phenobarbital, phenytoin, piperacillin, piperacillin/tazobactam, potassium chloride, prochlorperazine, promethazine, propranolol, ranitidine, remifentanil, sodium bicarbonate, ticarcillin, ticarcillin/clavulanate, tobramycin, vancomycin, vecuronium, verapamil, vinorelbine

Additional Information Controlled trials which compare the original formulation of amphotericin B to the newer liposomal formulations (ie, Amphotec®) are lacking. Thus, comparative data discussing differences among the formulations should be interpreted cautiously. Although the risk of nephrotoxicity and infusion-related adverse effects may be less with Amphotec®, the efficacy profiles of Amphotec® and the original amphotericin formulation are comparable. Consequently, Amphotec® should be restricted to those patients who cannot tolerate or fail a standard amphotericin B formulation.

Related Information

Compatibility of Drugs *on page 1723*

♦ **Amphotericin B Colloidal Dispersion** *see* Amphotericin B Cholesteryl Sulfate Complex *on page 107*

Amphotericin B (Conventional) (am foe TER i sin bee con VEN sha nal)

U.S. Brand Names Amphocin®; Fungizone®

Synonyms Amphotericin B Desoxycholate

Generic Available Yes: Powder for reconstitution

Pharmacologic Category Antifungal Agent, Parenteral; Antifungal Agent, Topical

Medication Safety Issues

Safety issues:

Conventional amphotericin formulations (Amphocin®, Fungizone®) may be confused with lipid-based formulations (AmBisome®, Abelcet®, Amphotec®).

Large overdoses have occurred when conventional formulations were dispensed inadvertently for lipid-based products. Single daily doses of conventional amphotericin formulation never exceed 1.5 mg/kg.

Use Treatment of severe systemic and central nervous system infections caused by susceptible fungi such as *Candida* species, *Histoplasma capsulatum*, *Cryptococcus neoformans*, *Aspergillus* species, *Blastomyces dermatitidis*, *Torulopsis glabrata*, and *Coccidioides immitis*; fungal peritonitis; irrigant for bladder fungal infections; and topically for cutaneous and mucocutaneous candidal infections; used in fungal infection in patients with bone marrow transplantation, amebic meningoencephalitis, ocular aspergillosis (intraocular injection), candidal cystitis (bladder irrigation), chemoprophylaxis (low-dose I.V.), immunocompromised patients at risk of aspergillosis (intranasal/nebulized), refractory meningitis (intrathecal), coccidioidal arthritis (intra-articular/I.M.)

Low-dose amphotericin B 0.1-0.25 mg/kg/day has been administered after bone marrow transplantation to reduce the risk of invasive fungal disease. Alternative routes of administration and extemporaneous preparations have been used when standard antifungal therapy is not available (eg, inhalation, intraocular injection, subconjunctival application, intracavitary administration into various joints and the pleural space).

Mechanism of Action/Effect Binds to ergosterol altering cell membrane permeability in susceptible fungi and causing leakage of cell components with subsequent cell death

Contraindications Hypersensitivity to amphotericin or any component of the formulation

Warnings/Precautions Avoid additive toxicity with other nephrotoxic drugs. Monitor BUN and serum creatinine, potassium, and magnesium levels every 2-4 days, and daily in patients at risk for acute renal dysfunction. I.V. amphotericin is used primarily for the treatment of patients with progressive and potentially fatal fungal infections. Topical preparations may stain clothing. The standard dosage of lipid-based amphotericin B formulations, including amphotericin B cholesteryl sulfate (Amphotec®), amphotericin B lipid complex (Abelcet®), and liposomal amphotericin B (AmBisome®) is many fold greater than the dosage of conventional amphotericin B. To prevent inadvertent overdose, the product name and dosage must be verified for any amphotericin B dosage exceeding 1.5 mg/kg. Amphotericin B has been administered to pregnant women without obvious deleterious effects to the fetus, but the number of cases reported is small. Use during pregnancy only if absolutely necessary.

Drug Interactions

Decreased Effect: Pharmacologic antagonism may occur with azole antifungal agents (ketoconazole, miconazole).

Increased Effect/Toxicity: Use of amphotericin with other nephrotoxic drugs (eg, cyclosporine and aminoglycosides) may result in additive toxicity. Amphotericin may increase the toxicity of flucytosine. Antineoplastic agents may increase the risk of amphotericin-induced nephrotoxicity, bronchospasms, and hypotension. Corticosteroids may increase potassium depletion caused by amphotericin. Amphotericin B may predispose patients receiving digitalis glycosides or neuromuscular-blocking agents to toxicity secondary to hypokalemia.

Lab Interactions Increased BUN (S), serum creatinine, alkaline phosphate, bilirubin; decreased magnesium, potassium (S)

Adverse Reactions

>10%:

Central nervous system: Fever, chills, headache, malaise, generalized pain

Endocrine & metabolic: Hypokalemia, hypomagnesemia

Gastrointestinal: Anorexia

Hematologic: Anemia

Renal: Nephrotoxicity

1% to 10%:

Cardiovascular: Hypotension, hypertension, flushing

Central nervous system: Delirium, arachnoiditis, pain along lumbar nerves

Gastrointestinal: Nausea, vomiting

Genitourinary: Urinary retention

Hematologic: Leukocytosis

Local: Thrombophlebitis

Neuromuscular & skeletal: Paresthesia (especially with I.T. therapy)

Renal: Renal tubular acidosis, renal failure

Overdosage/Toxicology Symptoms of overdose include renal dysfunction, cardiac arrest, anemia, thrombocytopenia, granulocytopenia, fever, nausea, and vomiting. Treatment is supportive.

Pharmacodynamics/Kinetics

Time to Peak: Within 1 hour following a 4- to 6-hour dose

Protein Binding: Plasma: 90%

Half-Life Elimination: Biphasic: Initial: 15-48 hours; Terminal: 15 days

Excretion: Urine (2% to 5% as biologically active form); ~40% eliminated over a 7-day period and may be detected in urine for at least 7 weeks after discontinued use

Dosing

Adults & Elderly:

Note: Premedication: For patients who experience chills, fever, hypotension, nausea, or other nonanaphylactic infusion-related immediate reactions, premedicate with the following drugs, 30-60 minutes prior to drug administration: a nonsteroidal (eg, ibuprofen, (Continued)

Amphotericin B (Conventional) *(Continued)*

choline magnesium trisalicylate) with or without diphenhydramine; or acetaminophen with diphenhydramine; or hydrocortisone 50-100 mg. If the patient experiences rigors during the infusion, meperidine may be administered.

Test dose: I.V.: 1 mg infused over 20-30 minutes. Many clinicians believe a test dose is unnecessary.

Systemic fungal infections: I.V.: Maintenance dose: Usual: 0.25-1.5 mg/kg/day; 1-1.5 mg/kg over 4-6 hours every other day may be given once therapy is established. Aspergillosis, mucormycosis, rhinocerebral phycomycosis often require 1-1.5 mg/kg/day; do not exceed 1.5 mg/kg/day.

Duration of therapy varies with nature of infection: Usual duration is 4-12 weeks or cumulative dose of 1-4 g.

Meningitis, coccidioidal or cryptococcal: I.T.:

Initial: 25-300 mcg every 48-72 hours; increase to 500 mcg to 1 mg as tolerated; maximum total dose: 15 mg has been suggested.

Oral candidiasis: Oral (suspension): 1 mL (100 mg) 4 times/day

Dermal infection: Topical: Apply to affected areas 2-4 times/day for 1-4 weeks of therapy depending on nature and severity of infection.

Cystitis (Candidal): Bladder irrigation: Irrigate with 50 mcg/mL solution instilled periodically or continuously for 5-10 days or until cultures are clear.

Bone marrow transplantation (prophylaxis): I.V.: Low-dose amphotericin B 0.1-0.25 mg/kg/day has been administered after bone marrow transplantation to reduce the risk of invasive fungal disease.

Note: Alternative routes of administration and extemporaneous preparations have been used when standard antifungal therapy is not available (eg, inhalation, intraocular injection, subconjunctival application, intracavitary administration into various joints and the pleural space).

Pediatrics:

Note: Premedication: For patients who experience chills, fever, hypotension, nausea, or other nonanaphylactic infusion-related immediate reactions, premedicate with the following drugs, 30-60 minutes prior to drug administration: a nonsteroidal (eg, ibuprofen, choline magnesium trisalicylate) with or without diphenhydramine; or acetaminophen with diphenhydramine; or hydrocortisone 50-100 mg. If the patient experiences rigors during the infusion, meperidine may be administered.

Test dose: I.V.: Infants and Children: 0.1 mg/kg/dose to a maximum of 1 mg; infuse over 30-60 minutes. Many clinicians believe a test dose is unnecessary.

Susceptible fungal infections: I.V.: Infants and Children: Maintenance dose: 0.25-1 mg/kg/day given once daily; infuse over 2-6 hours. Once therapy has been established, amphotericin B can be administered on an every-other-day basis at 1-1.5 mg/kg/dose; cumulative dose: 1.5-2 g over 6-10 week

Note: Duration of therapy varies with nature of infection: Usual duration is 4-12 weeks or cumulative dose of 1-4 g.

Meningitis, coccidioidal or cryptococcal: I.T.: Children: 25-100 mcg every 48-72 hours; increase to 500 mcg as tolerated

Renal Impairment:

If renal dysfunction is due to the drug, the daily total can be decreased by 50% or the dose can be given every other day. I.V. therapy may take several months.

Poorly dialyzed; no supplemental dose is necessary when using hemo- or peritoneal dialysis or CAVH/CAVHD.

Administration in dialysate: 1-2 mg/L of peritoneal dialysis fluid either with or without low-dose I.V. amphotericin B (a total dose of 2-10 mg/kg given over 7-14 days).

Available Dosage Forms

Cream (Fungizone®): 3% (20 g)

Injection, powder for reconstitution, as desoxycholate (Amphocin®; Fungizone®): 50 mg

Lotion (Fungizone®): 3% (30 mL)

Monitoring and Teaching Issues

Physical Assessment: Assess culture and sensitivity report and patient's previous exposure to amphotericin B prior to starting therapy. Assess potential for interactions with other medications patient may be taking (eg, other nephrotoxic drugs; see Drug Interactions). See I.V. Details for premedication recommendations and specifics of administration and compatibility prior to administering first dose. Patient should be monitored closely for infusion-related reactions (eg, anaphylaxis, chills, fever, nausea, vomiting, rigors, hypotension, acute respiratory distress) and cardiopulmonary resuscitation should be available. If acute respiratory distress occurs, infusion should be stopped and prescriber notified. Assess results of laboratory tests, therapeutic effectiveness, and adverse response (see Adverse Reactions) frequently during therapy. Teach patient appropriate use (topical application or oral solution), possible side effects/appropriate interventions, and adverse symptoms to report.

Monitoring Laboratory Tests: BUN and serum creatinine levels should be determined every other day when therapy is increased and at least weekly thereafter. Monitor serum electrolytes (especially potassium and magnesium), liver function, and CBC. Perform culture and sensitivity testing prior to initiating therapy.

Patient Education: Do not take any new medication during therapy unless approved by prescriber. I.V.: You will be monitored closely during and after infusion; report immediately any pain or swelling at infusion site; chills, nausea, chest pain, swelling of face or mouth, difficulty breathing, muscle cramping, acute anxiety or other infusion reactions. Oral: Take entire prescription, even if you are feeling better. Most skin lesions may take 1-3 weeks of therapy; maintain good personal hygiene to reduce spread and recurrence of lesions. Maintain adequate hydration (2-3 L/day of fluids) unless instructed to restrict fluid intake. May cause nausea, vomiting, or anorexia (small frequent meals, frequent mouth care, sucking lozenges, or chewing gum may help); generalized muscle or joint paint (consult prescriber for approved analgesic); or hypotension (use caution when rising from sitting or lying position or when climbing stairs). Report severe muscle cramping or weakness; chest pain or palpitations; CNS disturbances; skin rash; change in urinary patterns or difficulty voiding; black stool; unusual bruising or bleeding; or pain, redness, swelling at infusion site. **Breast-feeding precaution:** Do not breast-feed.

Topical: Amphotericin cream may slightly discolor skin and stain clothing; use gloves when applying. Avoid covering topical application with occlusive bandages. Most skin lesions require 1-3 weeks of therapy. Maintain good personal hygiene to reduce the spread and recurrence of lesions.

Geriatric Considerations: Caution should be exercised and renal function and desired effect monitored closely in older adults.

Pregnancy Risk Factor: B

Lactation: Excretion in breast milk unknown/contraindicated

Administration

I.V.: May be infused over 4-6 hours. For a patient who experiences chills, fever, hypotension, nausea or other nonanaphylactic infusion-related reactions, premedication with the following drugs, 30-60 minutes prior to drug administration: A nonsteroidal (eg, ibuprofen, choline magnesium trisalicylate) with or without diphenhydramine; or acetaminophen with diphenhydramine, or hydrocortisone 50-100 mg. If the patient experiences rigors during the infusion, meperidine may be administered. Bolus infusion of normal saline immediately preceding, or immediately preceding and following amphotericin B may reduce drug-induced nephrotoxicity. Risk of nephrotoxicity increases with amphotericin B doses >1 mg/kg/day. Infusion of admixtures more concentrated than 0.25 mg/mL should be limited to patients absolutely requiring volume contraction.

Topical: Wear gloves to administer. Amphotericin may stain skin and clothing.

Reconstitution: Reconstitute only with sterile water without preservatives, not bacteriostatic water. **Benzyl alcohol, sodium chloride, or other electrolyte solutions may cause precipitation.** Short-term exposure (<24 hours) to light during I.V. infusion does **not** appreciably affect potency. Reconstituted solutions with sterile water for injection and kept in the dark remain stable for 24 hours at room temperature and 1 week when refrigerated. Stability of parenteral admixture at room temperature (25°C) is 24 hours; at refrigeration (4°C) is 2 days.

Standard diluent: Dose per 250-500 mL D_5W

Admixture concentration: Standard admixture concentrations are 0.1 mg/mL (peripheral infusion) and 0.25 mg/mL (central administration). Although 0.8 mg/mL in D_5W is physically compatible and chemically stable, the safety of infusing amphotericin B >0.25 mg/mL has not been formally evaluated.

Compatibility:

Solution is **incompatible** with ampicillin, calcium gluconate, carbenicillin, cimetidine, dopamine, gentamicin, lidocaine, potassium chloride, tetracycline, verapamil.

Compatibility when admixed: Some sterile evacuated glass containers have small amounts of ionic liquid buffer that may cause precipitation.

Storage: Amphotericin B does not have a bacteriostatic constituent, subsequently admixture expiration is determined by sterility more than chemical stability.

Additional Information Premedication with diphenhydramine and acetaminophen may reduce the severity of acute infusion-related reactions. Meperidine reduces the duration of amphotericin B-induced rigors and chilling. Hydrocortisone may be used in patients with severe or refractory infusion-related reactions. Bolus infusion of normal saline immediately preceding, or immediately preceding and following amphotericin B may reduce drug-induced nephrotoxicity. Risk of nephrotoxicity increases with amphotericin B doses >1 mg/kg/day. Infusion of admixtures more concentrated than 0.25 mg/mL should be limited to patients absolutely requiring volume restriction. Amphotericin B does not have a bacteriostatic constituent, subsequently admixture expiration is determined by sterility more than chemical stability.

Related Information

Compatibility of Drugs *on page 1723*

♦ **Amphotericin B Desoxycholate** *see* Amphotericin B (Conventional) *on page 109*

Amphotericin B (Lipid Complex) (am foe TER i sin bee LIP id KOM pleks)

U.S. Brand Names Abelcet®

Synonyms ABLC

Generic Available No

Pharmacologic Category Antifungal Agent, Parenteral

Medication Safety Issues

Safety issues:

Lipid-based amphotericin formulations (Abelcet®) may be confused with conventional formulations (Amphocin®, Fungizone®)

Large overdoses have occurred when conventional formulations were dispensed inadvertently for lipid-based products. Single daily doses of conventional amphotericin formulation never exceed 1.5 mg/kg.

Use Treatment of aspergillosis or any type of progressive fungal infection in patients who are refractory to or intolerant of conventional amphotericin B therapy

Unlabeled/Investigational Use Effective in patients with serious *Candida* species infections

Mechanism of Action/Effect Mechanism is like amphotericin - includes binding to ergosterol altering cell membrane permeability in susceptible fungi and causing leakage of cell components with subsequent cell death.

Contraindications Hypersensitivity to amphotericin or any component of the formulation

Warnings/Precautions Anaphylaxis has been reported with amphotericin B-containing drugs. If severe respiratory distress occurs, the infusion should be immediately discontinued. During the initial dosing, the drug should be administered under close clinical observation. Acute reactions (including fever and chills) may occur 1-2 hours after starting an intravenous infusion. These reactions are usually more common with the first few doses and generally diminish with subsequent doses.

(Continued)

Amphotericin B (Lipid Complex) *(Continued)*

Drug Interactions

Decreased Effect: See Drug Interactions - Decreased Effect in Amphotericin B (Conventional) *on page 109*.

Increased Effect/Toxicity: See Drug Interactions - Increased Effect/Toxicity in Amphotericin B (Conventional) *on page 109*.

Lab Interactions Increased BUN (S), serum creatinine, alkaline phosphate, bilirubin; decreased magnesium, potassium (S)

Adverse Reactions Nephrotoxicity and infusion-related hyperpyrexia, rigor, and chilling are reduced relative to amphotericin deoxycholate.

>10%:
Central nervous system: Chills, fever
Renal: Increased serum creatinine

1% to 10%:
Cardiovascular: Hypotension, cardiac arrest
Central nervous system: Headache, pain
Dermatologic: Rash
Endocrine & metabolic: Bilirubinemia, hypokalemia, acidosis
Gastrointestinal: Nausea, vomiting, diarrhea, gastrointestinal hemorrhage, abdominal pain
Renal: Renal failure
Respiratory: Respiratory failure, dyspnea, pneumonia

Pharmacodynamics/Kinetics

Half-Life Elimination: ~24 hours

Excretion: Clearance: Increases with higher doses (5 mg/kg/day): 400 mL/hour/kg

Dosing

Adults & Elderly:

Note: Premedication: For patients who experience chills, fever, hypotension, nausea, or other nonanaphylactic infusion-related immediate reactions, premedicate with the following drugs, 30-60 minutes prior to drug administration: a nonsteroidal (eg, ibuprofen, choline magnesium trisalicylate) with or without diphenhydramine; or acetaminophen with diphenhydramine; or hydrocortisone 50-100 mg. If the patient experiences rigors during the infusion, meperidine may be administered.

Susceptible infections: I.V.: 2.5-5 mg/kg/day as a single infusion. Test dose is not recommended.

Pediatrics: Refer to adult dosing.

Renal Impairment: The effects of renal impairment on drug pharmacokinetics or pharmacodynamics are currently unknown. The dose of amphotericin B lipid complex may be adjusted or drug administration may have to be interrupted in patients with acute kidney dysfunction to reduce the magnitude of renal impairment.

Hemodialysis: Supplemental dose is not necessary.
Peritoneal dialysis: Supplemental dose is not necessary.
Continuous arteriovenous or venovenous hemofiltration: Supplemental dose is not necessary.

Available Dosage Forms Injection, suspension: 5 mg/mL (20 mL)

Monitoring and Teaching Issues

Physical Assessment: Assess culture and sensitivity report and patient's previous exposure to amphotericin B prior to starting therapy. Assess potential for interactions with other medications patient may be taking (eg, other nephrotoxic drugs; see Drug Interactions). See I.V. Details for premedication recommendations and specifics of administration and compatibility prior to administering first dose. Patient should be monitored closely for infusion-related reactions (eg, anaphylaxis, chills, fever, nausea, vomiting, rigors, hypotension, acute respiratory distress) and cardiopulmonary resuscitation should be available. If acute respiratory distress occurs, infusion should be stopped and prescriber notified. Assess results of laboratory tests, therapeutic effectiveness, and adverse response (see Adverse Reactions) frequently during therapy. Teach patient possible side effects/appropriate interventions and adverse symptoms to report.

Monitoring Laboratory Tests: BUN and serum creatinine levels should be determined every other day while therapy is increased and at least weekly thereafter. Monitor serum electrolytes (especially potassium and magnesium), liver function, and CBC. Perform culture and sensitivity testing prior to initiating therapy.

Patient Education: Do not take any new medication during therapy unless approved by prescriber. This medication can only be administered by infusion and therapy may last several weeks. You will be monitored closely during and after infusion; report immediately and pain or selling at infusion site; chills, nausea, chest pain, swelling of face or mouth, difficulty breathing, muscle cramping, acute anxiety or other infusion reactions. Maintain adequate hydration (2-3 L/day of fluids) unless instructed to restrict fluid intake. May cause postural hypotension (use caution when changing from lying or sitting position to standing or when climbing stairs); or nausea or vomiting (small frequent meals, frequent mouth care, sucking lozenges, or chewing gum may help). Report chest pain or palpitations; CNS disturbances; skin rash; unusual chills or fever; persistent nausea, vomiting, or abdominal pain; sore throat; excessive fatigue; swelling of extremities or unusual weight gain; difficulty breathing; pain at infusion site; muscle cramping or weakness; or other adverse reactions. **Breast-feeding precaution:** Do not breast-feed.

Geriatric Considerations: Caution should be exercised and renal function and desired effect monitored closely in older adults.

Pregnancy Risk Factor: B

Lactation: Enters breast milk/contraindicated

Breast-Feeding Issues: Due to limited data, consider discontinuing nursing during therapy.

Administration

I.V.: For a patient who experiences chills, fever, hypotension, nausea, or other nonanaphylactic infusion-related reactions, premedication with the following drugs, 30-60 minutes prior to drug administration: A nonsteroidal (eg, ibuprofen, choline magnesium trisalicylate) with or without diphenhydramine; or acetaminophen with diphenhydramine, or hydrocortisone 50-100 mg. If the patient experiences rigors during the infusion, meperidine may be administered. If infusion time exceeds 2 hours, mix contents by shaking infusion bag every 2 hours.

Reconstitution: Shake vial gently to disperse yellow sediment at bottom of container. Withdraw correct volume to prepare dose. Inject into appropriate volume of D_5W through 5-micron filter needle provided by manufacturer. Each filter needle may be used to filter the contents of up to four vials. The final infusion concentration should be 1 mg/mL in D_5W, and is stable for 48 hours at 2°C to 8°C, then an additional 6 hours at room temperature; 2 mg/mL in D_5W may be used for pediatric patients or patients with cardiovascular disease. Infuse 2.5 mg/kg/hour. Do not use an in-line filter during administration. Admixture must be inverted several times before infusion, then every 2 hours, to prevent settling or aggregation of lipid particles. Protect from light.

Compatibility: Do not admix or Y-site with any blood products, intravenous drugs, or intravenous fluids other than D_5W.

Storage: 100 mg vials in 20 mL of suspension in single-use vials (no preservative is present). Intact vials should be stored at 2°C to 8°C (35°F to 46°F) and protected from exposure to light; do not freeze intact vials.

Additional Information As a modification of dimyristoyl phosphatidylcholine:dimyristoyl phosphatidylglycerol 7:3 (DMPC:DMPG) liposome, amphotericin B lipid-complex has a higher drug to lipid ratio and the concentration of amphotericin B is 33 M. ABLC is a ribbon-like structure, not a liposome.

Controlled trials which compare the original formulation of amphotericin B to the newer liposomal formulations (ie, Abelcet®) are lacking. Thus, comparative data discussing differences among the formulations should be interpreted cautiously. Although the risk of nephrotoxicity and infusion-related adverse effects may be less with Abelcet®, the efficacy profiles of Abelcet® and the original amphotericin formulation are comparable. Consequently, Abelcet® should be restricted to those patients who cannot tolerate or fail a standard amphotericin B formulation.

Related Information
Compatibility of Drugs *on page 1723*

Amphotericin B (Liposomal) (am foe TER i sin bee lye po SO mal)

U.S. Brand Names AmBisome®

Synonyms L-AmB

Generic Available No

Pharmacologic Category Antifungal Agent, Parenteral

Medication Safety Issues

Safety issues:

Lipid-based amphotericin formulations (AmBisome®) may be confused with conventional formulations (Amphocin®, Fungizone®)

Large overdoses have occurred when conventional formulations were dispensed inadvertently for lipid-based products. Single daily doses of conventional amphotericin formulation never exceed 1.5 mg/kg.

Use Empirical therapy for presumed fungal infection in febrile, neutropenic patients. Treatment of patients with *Aspergillus* species, *Candida* species and/or *Cryptococcus* species infections refractory to amphotericin B desoxycholate, or in patients where renal impairment or unacceptable toxicity precludes the use of amphotericin B desoxycholate. Treatment of cryptococcal meningitis in HIV-infected patients. Treatment of visceral leishmaniasis.

Unlabeled/Investigational Use Effective in patients with serious *Candida* species infections

Mechanism of Action/Effect Amphotericin B, the active ingredient, acts by binding to the sterol component of a cell membrane leading to alterations in cell permeability and cell death. While amphotericin B has a higher affinity for the ergosterol component of the fungal cell membrane, it can also bind to the cholesterol component of the mammalian cell leading to cytotoxicity. AmBisome®, the liposomal preparation of amphotericin B, has been shown to penetrate the cell wall of both extracellular and intracellular forms of susceptible fungi.

Contraindications Hypersensitivity to amphotericin B or any component of the formulation unless, in the opinion of the treating physician, the benefit of therapy outweighs the risk

Warnings/Precautions Although amphotericin B (liposomal) has been shown to be significantly less toxic than amphotericin B desoxycholate, adverse events may still occur. Patients should be under close clinical observation during initial dosing. As with other amphotericin B-containing products, anaphylaxis has been reported. Facilities for cardiopulmonary resuscitation should be available during administration, and the drug should be administered by medically-trained personnel. Acute reactions (including fever and chills) may occur 1-2 hours after starting infusions; reactions are more common with the first few doses and generally diminish with subsequent doses. Immediately discontinue infusion if severe respiratory distress occurs; the patient should not receive further infusions. Safety and efficacy have not been established in patients <1 year of age.

Drug Interactions

Increased Effect/Toxicity: Drug interactions have not been studied in a controlled manner; however, drugs that interact with conventional amphotericin B may also interact with amphotericin B liposome for injection. See Drug Interactions - Increased Effect/Toxicity in Amphotericin B (Conventional) monograph.

Adverse Reactions Percentage of adverse reactions is dependent upon population studied and may vary with respect to premedications and underlying illness. Incidence of decreased renal function and infusion-related events are lower than rates observed with amphotericin B deoxycholate.

>10%:

Cardiovascular: Peripheral edema (15%), edema (12% to 14%), tachycardia (9% to 18%), hypotension (7% to 14%), hypertension (8% to 20%), chest pain (8% to 12%), hypervolemia (8% to 12%)

(Continued)

Amphotericin B (Liposomal) *(Continued)*

Central nervous system: Chills (29% to 48%), insomnia (17% to 22%), headache (9% to 20%), anxiety (7% to 14%), pain (14%), confusion (9% to 13%)

Dermatologic: Rash (5% to 25%), pruritus (11%)

Endocrine & metabolic: Hypokalemia (31% to 51%), hypomagnesemia (15% to 50%), hyperglycemia (8% to 23%), hypocalcemia (5% to 18%), hyponatremia (8% to 12%)

Gastrointestinal: Nausea (16% to 40%), vomiting (10% to 32%), diarrhea (11% to 30%), abdominal pain (7% to 20%), constipation (15%), anorexia (10% to 14%)

Hematologic: Anemia (27% to 48%), blood transfusion reaction (9% to 18%), leukopenia (15% to 17%), thrombocytopenia (6% to 13%)

Hepatic: Increased alkaline phosphatase (7% to 22%), increased BUN (7% to 21%), bilirubinemia (9% to 18%), increased ALT (15%), increased AST (13%), abnormal liver function tests (not specified) (4% to 13%)

Local: Phlebitis (9% to 11%)

Neuromuscular & skeletal: Weakness (6% to 13%), back pain (12%)

Renal: Increased creatinine (18% to 40%), hematuria (14%)

Respiratory: Dyspnea (18% to 23%), lung disorder (14% to 18%), increased cough (2% to 18%), epistaxis (8% to 15%), pleural effusion (12%), rhinitis (11%)

Miscellaneous: Sepsis (7% to 14%), infection (11% to 12%)

2% to 10%:

Cardiovascular: Arrhythmia, atrial fibrillation, bradycardia, cardiac arrest, cardiomegaly, facial swelling, flushing, postural hypotension, valvular heart disease, vascular disorder

Central nervous system: Agitation, abnormal thinking, coma, convulsion, depression, dysesthesia, dizziness (7% to 8%), hallucinations, malaise, nervousness, somnolence

Dermatologic: Alopecia, bruising, cellulitis, dry skin, maculopapular rash, petechia, purpura, skin discoloration, skin disorder, skin ulcer, urticaria, vesiculobullous rash

Endocrine & metabolic: Acidosis, increased amylase, fluid overload, hypernatremia (4%), hyperchloremia, hyperkalemia, hypermagnesemia, hyperphosphatemia, hypophosphatemia, hypoproteinemia, increased lactate dehydrogenase, increased nonprotein nitrogen

Gastrointestinal: Constipation, dry mouth, dyspepsia, enlarged abdomen, eructation, fecal incontinence, flatulence, gastrointestinal hemorrhage (10%), hematemesis, hemorrhoids, gum/oral hemorrhage, ileus, mucositis, rectal disorder, stomatitis, ulcerative stomatitis

Genitourinary: Vaginal hemorrhage

Hematologic: Coagulation disorder, hemorrhage, decreased prothrombin, thrombocytopenia

Hepatic: Hepatocellular damage, hepatomegaly, veno-occlusive liver disease

Local: Injection site inflammation

Neuromuscular & skeletal: Arthralgia, bone pain, dystonia, myalgia, neck pain, paresthesia, rigors, tremor

Ocular: Conjunctivitis, dry eyes, eye hemorrhage

Renal: Abnormal renal function, acute kidney failure, dysuria, kidney failure, toxic nephropathy, urinary incontinence

Respiratory: Asthma, atelectasis, cough, dry nose, hemoptysis, hyperventilation, lung edema, pharyngitis, pneumonia, respiratory alkalosis, respiratory insufficiency, respiratory failure, sinusitis, hypoxia (6% to 8%)

Miscellaneous: Allergic reaction, cell-mediated immunological reaction, flu-like syndrome, graft versus host disease, herpes simplex, hiccup, procedural complication (8% to 10%), diaphoresis (7%)

Overdosage/Toxicology The toxicity due to overdose has not been defined. Repeated daily doses up to 7.5 mg/kg have been administered in clinical trials with no reported dose-related toxicity. If overdose should occur, cease administration immediately. Symptomatic supportive measures should be instituted. Particular attention should be given to monitoring renal function.

Pharmacodynamics/Kinetics

Half-Life Elimination: Terminal: 174 hours

Dosing

Adults & Elderly:

Note: Premedication: For patients who experience chills, fever, hypotension, nausea, or other nonanaphylactic infusion-related immediate reactions, premedicate with the following drugs, 30-60 minutes prior to drug administration: a nonsteroidal (eg, ibuprofen, choline magnesium trisalicylate) with or without diphenhydramine; or acetaminophen with diphenhydramine; or hydrocortisone 50-100 mg. If the patient experiences rigors during the infusion, meperidine may be administered.

Empiric therapy: I.V.: Recommended initial dose: 3 mg/kg/day

Systemic fungal infections (*Aspergillus*, *Candida*, *Cryptococcus*): I.V.: Recommended initial dose of 3-5 mg/kg/day

Cryptococcal meningitis in HIV-infected patients: I.V.: 6 mg/kg/day

Treatment of visceral leishmaniasis: I.V.:

Immunocompetent patients: 3 mg/kg/day on days 1-5, and 3 mg/kg/day on days 14 and 21; a repeat course may be given in patients who do not achieve parasitic clearance

Immunocompromised patients: 4 mg/kg/day on days 1-5, and 4 mg/kg/day on days 10, 17, 24, 31, and 38

Pediatrics: Refer to adult dosing.

Renal Impairment:

Dosing adjustment in renal impairment: None necessary; effects of renal impairment are not currently known.

Hemodialysis: Supplemental dose is not necessary.

Peritoneal dialysis effects: Supplemental dose is not necessary.

Continuous arteriovenous or venovenous hemofiltration: Supplemental dose is not necessary.

Available Dosage Forms Injection, powder for reconstitution: 50 mg

Monitoring and Teaching Issues

Physical Assessment: Assess culture and sensitivity report and patient's previous exposure to amphotericin B prior to starting therapy. Assess potential for interactions with other medications patient may be taking (eg, other nephrotoxic drugs; see Drug Interactions). See I.V. Details for premedication recommendations and specifics of administration and compatibility prior to administering first dose. Patient should be monitored closely for infusion-related reactions (eg, anaphylaxis, chills, fever, nausea, vomiting, rigors, hypotension, acute respiratory distress) and cardiopulmonary resuscitation should be available. If acute respiratory distress occurs, infusion should be stopped and prescriber notified. Assess results of laboratory tests, therapeutic effectiveness, and adverse response (see Adverse Reactions) frequently during therapy. Teach patient possible side effects/appropriate interventions and adverse symptoms to report.

Monitoring Laboratory Tests: BUN and serum creatinine levels should be determined every other day while therapy is increased and at least weekly thereafter. Serum potassium and magnesium should be monitored closely. Monitor electrolytes, liver function, hematocrit, and CBC regularly.

Patient Education: Do not take any new medication during therapy unless approved by prescriber. This medication can only be administered by infusion and therapy may last several weeks. You will be monitored closely during and after infusion; report immediately any pain or swelling at infusion site; chills, nausea, chest pain, swelling of face or mouth, difficulty breathing, muscle cramping, acute anxiety, or other infusion reactions. Maintain adequate hydration (2-3 L/day of fluids) unless instructed to restrict fluid intake. May cause postural hypotension (use caution when changing from lying or sitting position to standing or when climbing stairs); or nausea or vomiting (small frequent meals, frequent mouth care, sucking lozenges, or chewing gum may help). Report chest pain or palpitations; CNS disturbances; skin rash; unusual chills or fever; persistent nausea, vomiting, or abdominal pain; sore throat; excessive fatigue; swelling of extremities or unusual weight gain; difficulty breathing; pain at infusion site; muscle cramping or weakness; or other adverse reactions.
Breast-feeding precaution: Do not breast-feed.

Pregnancy Risk Factor: B

Lactation: Excretion in breast milk unknown/contraindicated

Administration

I.V.: Should be administered by intravenous infusion, using a controlled infusion device, over a period of approximately 2 hours. Infusion time may be reduced to approximately 1 hour in patients in whom the treatment is well-tolerated. If the patient experiences discomfort during infusion, the duration of infusion may be increased. Administer at a rate of 2.5 mg/kg/hour. Discontinue if severe respiratory distress occurs.

For a patient who experiences chills, fever, hypotension, nausea, or other nonanaphylactic infusion-related reactions, premedication with the following drugs, 30-60 minutes prior to drug administration: A nonsteroidal (eg, ibuprofen, choline magnesium trisalicylate) with or without diphenhydramine; or acetaminophen with diphenhydramine, or hydrocortisone 50-100 mg. If the patient experiences rigors during the infusion, meperidine may be administered.

Reconstitution: Must be reconstituted using sterile water for injection, USP (without a bacteriostatic agent). Vials containing 50 mg of amphotericin B are prepared as follows.

1. Aseptically add 12 mL of sterile water for injection, USP to each vial to yield a preparation containing 4 mg amphotericin B/mL. **Caution:** Do not reconstitute with saline or add saline to the reconstituted concentration, or mix with other drugs. The use of any solution other than those recommended, or the presence of a bacteriostatic agent in the solution, may cause precipitation.

2. Immediately after the addition of water, **shake the vial vigorously** for 30 seconds to completely disperse the powder, it then forms a yellow, translucent suspension. Visually inspect the vial for particulate matter and continue shaking until completely dispersed.

Filtration and Dilution:

3. Calculate the amount of reconstituted (4 mg/mL) to be further diluted.

4. Withdraw this amount of reconstituted powder into a sterile syringe.

5. Attach the 5-micron filter, provided, to the syringe. Inject the syringe contents through the filter, into the appropriate amount of 5% Dextrose Injection. (Use only one filter per vial.)

6. Must be diluted with 5% dextrose injection to a final concentration of 1-2 mg/mL prior to administration. Lower concentrations (0.2-0.5 mg/mL) may be appropriate for infants and small children to provide sufficient volume for infusion. **Discard partially used vials.** Injection should commence within 6 hours of dilution with 5% dextrose injection. An in-line membrane filter may be used for the intravenous infusion; provided, **the mean pore diameter of the filter should not be less than 1 micron.**

Storage: Unopened vials should be stored at temperatures ≤25°C (77°F).

Additional Information Amphotericin B (liposomal) is a true single bilayer liposomal drug delivery system. Liposomes are closed, spherical vesicles created by mixing specific proportions of amphophilic substances such as phospholipids and cholesterol so that they arrange themselves into multiple concentric bilayer membranes when hydrated in aqueous solutions. Single bilayer liposomes are then formed by microemulsification of multilamellar vesicles using a homogenizer. Amphotericin B (liposomal) consists of these unilamellar bilayer liposomes with amphotericin B intercalated within the membrane. Due to the nature and quantity of amphophilic substances used, and the lipophilic moiety in the amphotericin B molecule, the drug is an integral part of the overall structure of the amphotericin B liposomal liposomes. Amphotericin B (liposomal) contains true liposomes that are <100 nm in diameter.

Ampicillin (am pi SIL in)

U.S. Brand Names Principen®
Synonyms Aminobenzylpenicillin; Ampicillin Sodium; Ampicillin Trihydrate
Generic Available Yes
(Continued)

Ampicillin (Continued)

Pharmacologic Category Antibiotic, Penicillin

Medication Safety Issues
Sound-alike/look-alike issues:
Ampicillin may be confused with aminophylline

Use Treatment of susceptible bacterial infections (nonbeta-lactamase-producing organisms); susceptible bacterial infections caused by streptococci, pneumococci, nonpenicillinase-producing staphylococci, *Listeria*, meningococci; some strains of *H. influenzae*, *Salmonella*, *Shigella*, *E. coli*, *Enterobacter*, and *Klebsiella*

Mechanism of Action/Effect Interferes with bacterial cell wall synthesis during active multiplication, causing cell wall death and resultant bactericidal activity against susceptible bacteria

Contraindications Hypersensitivity to ampicillin, any component of the formulation, or other penicillins

Warnings/Precautions Dosage adjustment may be necessary in patients with renal impairment. A low incidence of cross-allergy with other beta-lactams exists. High percentage of patients with infectious mononucleosis have developed rash during therapy with ampicillin. Appearance of a rash should be carefully evaluated to differentiate a nonallergic ampicillin rash from a hypersensitivity reaction. Ampicillin rash is a generalized dull red, maculopapular rash, generally appearing 3-14 days after the start of therapy. It normally begins on the trunk and spreads over most of the body. It may be most intense at pressure areas, elbows, and knees.

Drug Interactions

Decreased Effect: Although anecdotal reports suggest oral contraceptive efficacy could be reduced by penicillins, this has been refuted by more rigorous scientific and clinical data.

Increased Effect/Toxicity: Ampicillin increases the effect of disulfiram and anticoagulants. Probenecid may increase penicillin levels. Theoretically, allopurinol taken with ampicillin has an additive potential for rash. Penicillins may increase the exposure to methotrexate during concurrent therapy; monitor.

Nutritional/Ethanol Interactions Food: Food decreases ampicillin absorption rate; may decrease ampicillin serum concentration.

Lab Interactions Increased protein, positive Coombs' [direct]; alters result of urinary glucose (Benedict's solution, Clinitest®)

Adverse Reactions Frequency not defined.
Central nervous system: Fever, penicillin encephalopathy, seizure
Dermatologic: Erythema multiforme, exfoliative dermatitis, rash, urticaria
Note: Appearance of a rash should be carefully evaluated to differentiate (if possible) nonallergic ampicillin rash from hypersensitivity reaction. Incidence is higher in patients with viral infection, *Salmonella* infection, lymphocytic leukemia, or patients that have hyperuricemia.
Gastrointestinal: black hairy tongue, diarrhea, enterocolitis, glossitis, nausea, pseudomembranous colitis, sore mouth or tongue, stomatitis, vomiting
Hematologic: Agranulocytosis, anemia, hemolytic anemia, eosinophilia, leukopenia, thrombocytopenia purpura
Hepatic: AST increased
Renal: Interstitial nephritis (rare)
Respiratory: Laryngeal stridor
Miscellaneous: Anaphylaxis, serum sickness-like reaction

Overdosage/Toxicology Symptoms of penicillin overdose include neuromuscular hypersensitivity (eg, agitation, hallucinations, asterixis, encephalopathy, confusion, and seizures). Electrolyte imbalance may occur if the preparation contains potassium or sodium salts, especially in renal failure. Hemodialysis may be helpful to aid in removal of the drug from blood; otherwise, treatment is supportive or symptom-directed.

Pharmacodynamics/Kinetics

Absorption: Oral: 50%

Time to Peak: Oral: Within 1-2 hours

Protein Binding: 15% to 25%

Half-Life Elimination:
Children and Adults: 1-1.8 hours
Anuria/end-stage renal disease: 7-20 hours

Excretion: Urine (~90% as unchanged drug) within 24 hours

Dosing

Adults:

Susceptible infections:
Oral: 250-500 mg every 6 hours
I.M., I.V.: 250-500 mg every 6 hours

Sepsis/meningitis: I.M., I.V.: 150-250 mg/kg/24 hours divided every 3-4 hours (range: 6-12 g/day)

Endocarditis prophylaxis: I.M., I.V.:
Dental, oral, respiratory tract, or esophageal procedures: 2 g within 30 minutes prior to procedure in patients unable to take oral amoxicillin
Genitourinary and gastrointestinal tract (except esophageal) procedures:
High-risk patients: 2 g within 30 minutes prior to procedure, followed by ampicillin 1 g (or amoxicillin 1 g orally) 6 hours later; must be used in combination with gentamicin.
Moderate-risk patients: 2 g within 30 minutes prior to procedure.

Elderly: Administer usual adult dose unless renal function is markedly reduced.

Pediatrics:

Mild-to-moderate infections: Infants and Children:
I.M., I.V.: 100-150 mg/kg/day in divided doses every 6 hours (maximum: 2-4 g/day)
Oral: 50-100 mg/kg/day in doses divided every 6 hours (maximum: 2-4 g/day)

Severe infections/meningitis: Infants and Children: I.M., I.V.: 200-400 mg/kg/day in divided doses every 6 hours (maximum: 6-12 g/day)

Endocarditis prophylaxis: Infants and Children: I.M., I.V.:
  Dental, oral, respiratory tract, or esophageal procedures: 50 mg/kg within 30 minutes prior to procedure in patients unable to take oral amoxicillin
  Genitourinary and gastrointestinal tract (except esophageal) procedures:
    High-risk patients: 50 mg/kg (maximum: 2 g) within 30 minutes prior to procedure, followed by ampicillin 25 mg/kg (or amoxicillin 25 mg/kg orally) 6 hours later; must be used in combination with gentamicin.
    Moderate-risk patients: 50 mg/kg within 30 minutes prior to procedure.

Renal Impairment:
  Cl_{cr} >50 mL/minute: Administer every 6 hours
  Cl_{cr} 10-50 mL/minute: Administer every 6-12 hours
  Cl_{cr} <10 mL/minute: Administer every 12-24 hours
  Hemodialysis: Moderately dialyzable (20% to 50%); administer dose after dialysis
  Peritoneal dialysis: Moderately dialyzable (20% to 50%)
    Administer 250 mg every 12 hours
  Continuous arteriovenous or venovenous hemofiltration effects: Dose as for Cl_{cr} 10-50 mL/minute; ~50 mg of ampicillin per liter of filtrate is removed

Available Dosage Forms
  Capsule (Principen®): 250 mg, 500 mg
  Injection, powder for reconstitution, as sodium: 125 mg, 250 mg, 500 mg, 1 g, 2 g, 10 g
  Powder for oral suspension (Principen®): 125 mg/5 mL (100 mL, 200 mL); 250 mg/5 mL (100 mL, 200 mL)

Monitoring and Teaching Issues
  Physical Assessment: Assess results of culture and sensitivity tests and patient's allergy history prior to starting therapy. Assess potential for interactions with other medication, patient may be taking (see Drug Interactions). Caution patients with diabetes about altered response to Clinitest®. Assess therapeutic effectiveness and adverse reactions (eg, opportunistic infection; fever, chills, unhealed sores, white plaques in mouth or vagina, purulent vaginal discharge, fatigue; see Adverse Reactions and Overdose/Toxicology). Teach patient proper use, possible side effects/appropriate interventions, and adverse symptoms to report.
  Monitoring Laboratory Tests: Perform culture and sensitivity testing prior to initiating therapy.
  Patient Education: Do not take any new medication during therapy unless approved by prescriber. Take entire prescription, even if you are feeling better. Take at equal intervals around-the-clock; preferably on an empty stomach with a full glass of water (1 hour before or 2 hours after meals). Maintain adequate hydration (2-3 L/day of fluids) unless instructed to restrict fluid intake. If you have diabetes, this drug may cause false test results with Clinitest® urine glucose monitoring; use of another type of glucose monitoring is preferable. May cause nausea or vomiting (small frequent meals, frequent mouth care, sucking lozenges, or chewing gum may help); or diarrhea (buttermilk, boiled milk, or yogurt may help). Report immediately any rash; swelling of face, tongue, mouth, or throat; or chest tightness. Report if condition being treated worsens or does not improve by the time prescription is completed.
  Dietary Considerations: Take on an empty stomach 1 hour before or 2 hours after meals.
    Sodium content of 5 mL suspension (250 mg/5 mL): 10 mg (0.4 mEq)
    Sodium content of 1 g: 66.7 mg (3 mEq)
  Geriatric Considerations: See Drug Interactions and Renal Impairment. Adjust dose for renal impairment.
  Pregnancy Risk Factor: B
  Lactation: Enters breast milk/use caution

Administration
  Oral: Administer around-the-clock to promote less variation in peak and trough serum levels. Administer on an empty stomach (ie, 1 hour prior to, or 2 hours after meals) to increase total absorption.
  I.V.: Administer around-the-clock to promote less variation in peak and trough serum levels. Administer over 3-5 minutes (125-500 mg) or over 10-15 minutes (1-2 g). More rapid infusion may cause seizures. Ampicillin and gentamicin should not be mixed in the same I.V. tubing or administered concurrently.
  Reconstitution:
    Oral: Oral suspension is stable for 7 days at room temperature or for 14 days under refrigeration.
    I.V.:
      Minimum volume: Concentration should not exceed 30 mg/mL due to concentration-dependent stability restrictions.
      Solutions for I.M. or direct I.V. should be used within 1 hour. Solutions for I.V. infusion will be inactivated by dextrose at room temperature. If dextrose-containing solutions are to be used, the resultant solution will only be stable for 2 hours versus 8 hours in the 0.9% sodium chloride injection. D_5W has limited stability.
      Stability of parenteral admixture in NS at room temperature (25°C) is 8 hours.
      Stability of parenteral admixture in NS at refrigeration temperature (4°C) is 2 days.
      Standard diluent: 500 mg/50 mL NS; 1 g/50 mL NS; 2 g/100 mL NS.
  Compatibility: Incompatible with D_5W, D_5NS, $D_{10}W$, fat emulsion 10%, hetastarch 6%, LR
    Y-site administration: Incompatible with amphotericin B cholesteryl sulfate complex, epinephrine, fluconazole, hydralazine, midazolam, ondansetron, sargramostim, verapamil, vinorelbine
    Compatibility in syringe: Incompatible with erythromycin lactobionate, gentamicin, hydromorphone, kanamycin, lincomycin, metoclopramide
    Compatibility when admixed: Incompatible with amikacin, chlorpromazine, dopamine, gentamicin, hydralazine, prochlorperazine

Related Information
  Antimicrobial Drugs of Choice *on page 1792*
  Community-Acquired Pneumonia in Adults *on page 1807*
  Compatibility of Drugs *on page 1723*
  I.V. to Oral Conversion *on page 1688*

Ampicillin and Sulbactam (am pi SIL in & SUL bak tam)

U.S. Brand Names Unasyn®

Synonyms Sulbactam and Ampicillin

Generic Available Yes

Pharmacologic Category Antibiotic, Penicillin

Use Treatment of susceptible bacterial infections involved with skin and skin structure, intra-abdominal infections, gynecological infections; spectrum is that of ampicillin plus organisms producing beta-lactamases such as *S. aureus*, *H. influenzae*, *E. coli*, *Klebsiella*, *Acinetobacter*, *Enterobacter*, and anaerobes

Mechanism of Action/Effect Interferes with bacterial cell wall synthesis during active multiplication, causing cell wall death and resultant bactericidal activity against susceptible bacteria. The addition of sulbactam, a beta-lactamase inhibitor, to ampicillin extends the spectrum of ampicillin to include beta-lactamase producing organisms.

Contraindications Hypersensitivity to ampicillin, sulbactam, penicillins, or any component of the formulations

Warnings/Precautions Dosage adjustment may be necessary in patients with renal impairment. A low incidence of cross-allergy with other beta-lactams exists. A high percentage of patients with infectious mononucleosis have developed rash during therapy with ampicillin. Appearance of a rash should be carefully evaluated to differentiate a nonallergic ampicillin rash from a hypersensitivity reaction.

Drug Interactions

Decreased Effect: Although anecdotal reports suggest oral contraceptive efficacy could be reduced by penicillins, this has been refuted by more rigorous scientific and clinical data.

Increased Effect/Toxicity: Disulfiram or probenecid can increase ampicillin levels. Theoretically, allopurinol taken with ampicillin has an additive potential for rash. Penicillins may increase the exposure to methotrexate during concurrent therapy; monitor.

Lab Interactions False-positive urinary glucose levels (Benedict's solution, Clinitest®); may cause temporary decreases in serum estrogens in pregnant women.

Adverse Reactions Also see Ampicillin monograph

>10%: Local: Pain at injection site (I.M.)

1% to 10%:

Dermatologic: Rash

Gastrointestinal: Diarrhea

Local: Pain at injection site (I.V.), thrombophlebitis

Miscellaneous: Allergic reaction (may include serum sickness, urticaria, bronchospasm, hypotension, etc)

Overdosage/Toxicology Symptoms of penicillin overdose include neuromuscular hypersensitivity (eg, agitation, hallucinations, asterixis, encephalopathy, confusion, and seizures). Electrolyte imbalance may occur if the preparation contains potassium or sodium salts, especially in renal failure. Hemodialysis may be helpful to aid in removal of the drug from blood; otherwise, treatment is supportive or symptom-directed.

Pharmacodynamics/Kinetics

Protein Binding:

Sulbactam: 38%

Half-Life Elimination:

Sulbactam: Normal renal function: 1-1.3 hours

Excretion:

Sulbactam: Urine (~75% to 85% as unchanged drug) within 8 hours

Pharmacokinetic Note: See Ampicillin monograph.

Dosing

Adults & Elderly: Note: Unasyn® (ampicillin/sulbactam) is a combination product. Dosage recommendations for Unasyn® are based on the ampicillin component.

Susceptible infections: I.M., I.V.: 1-2 g ampicillin (1.5-3 g Unasyn®) every 6 hours; maximum: 8 g ampicillin/day (12 g Unasyn®)

Pediatrics: Note: Unasyn® (ampicillin/sulbactam) is a combination product. Dosage recommendations for Unasyn® are based on the ampicillin component.

Mild-to-moderate infections: Children ≥1 year: I.V.: 100-150 mg ampicillin/kg/day (150-300 mg Unasyn®) divided every 6 hours; maximum: 8 g ampicillin/day (12 g Unasyn®)

Severe infections: Children ≥1 year: I.V.: 200-400 mg ampicillin/kg/day divided every 6 hours; maximum: 8 g ampicillin/day (12 g Unasyn®)

Renal Impairment:

Cl_{cr} 15-29 mL/minute: Administer every 12 hours

Cl_{cr} 5-14 mL/minute: Administer every 24 hours

Available Dosage Forms Injection, powder for reconstitution: 3 g [ampicillin sodium 2 g and sulbactam sodium 1 g]; 15 g [ampicillin sodium 10 g and sulbactam sodium 5 g] [bulk package]

Unasyn®: 1.5 g [ampicillin sodium 1 g and sulbactam sodium 0.5 g]; 3 g [ampicillin sodium 2 g and sulbactam sodium 1 g]; 15 g [ampicillin sodium 10 g and sulbactam sodium 5 g] [bulk package]

Monitoring and Teaching Issues

Physical Assessment: Assess for allergy history prior to starting therapy. See Contraindications, Warnings/Precautions, and Dosing for use cautions. Assess potential for interactions with other prescriptions, OTC medications, or herbal products patient may be taking (see Drug Interactions). Caution patients with diabetes about altered response to Clinitest®. Assess results of laboratory tests, therapeutic effectiveness, and adverse reactions (eg, opportunistic infection: fever, chills, unhealed sores, white plaques in mouth or vagina, purulent vaginal discharge, fatigue; see Adverse Reactions and Overdose/Toxicology).

Teach possible side effects/appropriate interventions and adverse symptoms to report (see Patient Education). Note breast-feeding caution.

Monitoring Laboratory Tests: Hematologic, renal, and hepatic function with prolonged therapy. Perform culture and sensitivity testing prior to initiating therapy.

Patient Education: Inform prescriber of all prescriptions, OTC medications, or herbal products you are taking, and any allergies you have. Do not take any new medication during therapy unless approved by prescriber. This medication is administered by infusion/injection. Report immediately pain, redness, swelling, or burning at injection/infusion site or feelings of acute anxiety, chest tightness, or difficulty swallowing. Maintain adequate hydration (2-3 L/day of fluids) unless instructed to restrict fluid intake. If you have diabetes, drug may cause false test results with Clinitest® urine glucose monitoring; use of another type of glucose monitoring is preferable. May cause diarrhea (if persistent, consult prescriber for approved medication). Report rash or persistent, opportunistic infection (eg, fever, chills, unhealed sores, white plaques in mouth or vagina, purulent vaginal discharge, fatigue). **Breast-feeding precaution:** Consult prescriber if breast-feeding caution.

Dietary Considerations: Sodium content of 1.5 g injection: 115 mg (5 mEq)

Geriatric Considerations: Adjust dose for renal function.

Pregnancy Risk Factor: B

Lactation: Enters breast milk/use caution

Administration

I.V.: Administer around-the-clock to promote less variation in peak and trough serum levels. Administer by slow injection over 10-15 minutes or I.V. over 15-30 minutes. Ampicillin and gentamicin should not be mixed in the same I.V. tubing or administered concurrently.

Reconstitution: I.M. and direct I.V. administration: Use within 1 hour after preparation. Reconstitute with sterile water for injection or 0.5% or 2% lidocaine hydrochloride injection (I.M.). Sodium chloride 0.9% (NS) is the diluent of choice for I.V. piggyback use. Solutions made in NS are stable up to 72 hours when refrigerated whereas dextrose solutions (same concentration) are stable for only 4 hours.

Compatibility: Stable in NS

Y-site administration: Incompatible with aminoglycosides (eg, gentamicin, tobramycin), amphotericin B cholesteryl sulfate complex, ciprofloxacin, idarubicin, ondansetron, sargramostim

Compatibility when admixed: Incompatible with aminoglycosides

Storage: Prior to reconstitution, store at ≤30°C (86°F).

Related Information

Ampicillin *on page 115*
Antimicrobial Drugs of Choice *on page 1792*
I.V. to Oral Conversion *on page 1688*

♦ **Ampicillin Sodium** *see* Ampicillin *on page 115*

♦ **Ampicillin Trihydrate** *see* Ampicillin *on page 115*

Amprenavir (am PREN a veer)

U.S. Brand Names Agenerase®

Generic Available No

Pharmacologic Category Antiretroviral Agent, Protease Inhibitor

Use Treatment of HIV infections in combination with at least two other antiretroviral agents; oral solution should only be used when capsules or other protease inhibitors are not therapeutic options

Mechanism of Action/Effect Binds to the protease activity site and inhibits the activity of the enzyme. HIV protease is required for the cleavage of viral polyprotein precursors into individual functional proteins found in infectious HIV. Inhibition prevents cleavage of these polyproteins, resulting in the formation of immature, noninfectious viral particles.

Contraindications Hypersensitivity to amprenavir or any component of the formulation; concurrent therapy with cisapride, ergot derivatives, midazolam, pimozide, and triazolam; severe previous allergic reaction to sulfonamides; oral solution is contraindicated in infants or children <4 years of age, pregnant women, patients with renal or hepatic failure, and patients receiving concurrent metronidazole or disulfiram

Warnings/Precautions Because of hepatic metabolism and effect on cytochrome P450 enzymes, amprenavir should be used with caution in combination with other agents metabolized by this system (see Contraindications and Drug Interactions). Avoid use of lovastatin or simvastatin (risk of rhabdomyolysis increases). Avoid concurrent use of hormonal contraceptives, rifampin, and/or St John's wort. Use with caution in patients with diabetes mellitus, sulfonamide allergy, hepatic impairment, or hemophilia. Redistribution of fat may occur (eg, buffalo hump, peripheral wasting, cushingoid appearance). Additional vitamin E supplements should be avoided. Certain ethnic populations (Asians, Eskimos, Native Americans) may be at increased risk of propylene glycol-associated adverse effects; use of the oral solution of amprenavir should be avoided. Use oral solution only when capsules or other protease inhibitors are not options.

Drug Interactions

Cytochrome P450 Effect: Substrate of CYP2C8/9 (minor), 3A4 (major); **Inhibits** CYP2C19 (weak), 3A4 (strong)

Decreased Effect: Serum concentrations of estrogen (oral contraceptives) may be decreased, use alternative (nonhormonal) forms of contraception. Dexamethasone may decrease the therapeutic effect of amprenavir. Serum concentrations of delavirdine may be decreased; may lead to loss of virologic response and possible resistance to delavirdine; concomitant use is not recommended. Efavirenz and nevirapine may decrease serum concentrations of amprenavir (dosing for combinations not established). Avoid St John's wort (may lead to subtherapeutic concentrations of amprenavir). Effect of amprenavir may be diminished when administered with methadone (consider alternative antiretroviral); in addition, effect of methadone may be reduced (dosage increase may be required). The levels/effects of amprenavir may be decreased by include aminoglutethimide, carbamazepine, nafcillin, nevirapine, phenobarbital, phenytoin, rifamycins, and other CYP3A4 (Continued)

Amprenavir *(Continued)*

inducers. The administration of didanosine (buffered formulation) should be separated from amprenavir by 1 hour to limit interaction between formulations.

Increased Effect/Toxicity: Concurrent use of cisapride, midazolam, pimozide, quinidine, or triazolam is contraindicated. Concurrent use of ergot alkaloids (dihydroergotamine, ergotamine, ergonovine, methylergonovine) with amprenavir is also contraindicated (may cause vasospasm and peripheral ischemia). Concurrent use of oral solution with disulfiram or metronidazole is contraindicated, due to the risk of propylene glycol toxicity.

Serum concentrations of amiodarone, bepridil, lidocaine, quinidine and other antiarrhythmics may be increased, potentially leading to toxicity; when amprenavir is coadministered with ritonavir, flecainide and propafenone are contraindicated. HMG-CoA reductase inhibitors serum concentrations may be increased by amprenavir, increasing the risk of myopathy/rhabdomyolysis; lovastatin and simvastatin are not recommended; fluvastatin and pravastatin may be safer alternatives.

Amprenavir may increase the levels/effects of selected benzodiazepines (midazolam and triazolam are contraindicated), calcium channel blockers, cyclosporine, mirtazapine, nateglinide, nefazodone, quinidine, sildenafil (and other PDE-5 inhibitors), tacrolimus, venlafaxine, and other CYP3A4 substrates. When used with strong CYP3A4 inhibitors, dosage adjustment/limits are recommended for sildenafil and other PDE-5 inhibitors; refer to individual monographs.

Concurrent therapy with ritonavir may result in increased serum concentrations: dosage adjustment is recommended; avoid concurrent use of amprenavir and ritonavir oral solutions due to metabolic competition between formulation components. Clarithromycin, indinavir, nelfinavir may increase serum concentrations of amprenavir.

Nutritional/Ethanol Interactions

Ethanol: Avoid ethanol with amprenavir oral solution.

Food: Levels increased sixfold with high-fat meals.

Herb/Nutraceutical: Amprenavir serum concentration may be decreased by St John's wort; avoid concurrent use. Formulations contain vitamin E; avoid additional supplements.

Adverse Reactions Protease inhibitors cause dyslipidemia which includes elevated cholesterol and triglycerides and a redistribution of body fat centrally to cause increased abdominal girth, buffalo hump, facial atrophy, and breast enlargement. These agents also cause hyperglycemia.

>10%:

Central nervous system: Paresthesia (peripheral 10% to 14%)

Dermatologic: Rash (22%)

Endocrine & metabolic: Hyperglycemia (>160 mg/dL: 37% to 41%), hypertriglyceridemia (>399 mg/dL: 36% to 47%; >750 mg/dL: 8% to 13%)

Gastrointestinal: Nausea (43% to 74%), vomiting (24% to 34%), diarrhea (39% to 60%), abdominal symptoms

Miscellaneous: Perioral tingling/numbness (26% to 31%)

1% to 10%:

Central nervous system: Depression (4% to 15%), headache, fatigue, depression, mood disorder

Dermatologic: Stevens-Johnson syndrome (1% of total, 4% of patients who develop a rash)

Endocrine & metabolic: Hyperglycemia (>251 mg/dL: 2% to 3%)

Gastrointestinal: Taste disorders (2% to 10%)

Hepatic: AST increased (3% to 5%), ALT increased (4%), amylase increased (3% to 4%)

Overdosage/Toxicology Monitor for signs and symptoms of propylene glycol toxicity if the oral solution is administered.

Pharmacodynamics/Kinetics

Absorption: 63%

Bioavailability: Not established; increased sixfold with high-fat meal

Time to Peak: 1-2 hours

Protein Binding: 90%

Half-Life Elimination: 7.1-10.6 hours

Metabolism: Hepatic via CYP (primarily CYP3A4)

Excretion: Feces (75%); urine (14% as metabolites)

Dosing

Adults & Elderly: Note: Capsule and oral solution are **not** interchangeable on a mg-per-mg basis.

HIV infection: Oral:

Capsule:

<50 kg: 20 mg/kg twice daily (maximum: 2400 mg/day)

≥50 kg: 1200 mg twice daily

Dosage adjustments for amprenavir when administered in combination therapy:

Efavirenz: Adjustments necessary for both agents:

Amprenavir 1200 mg 3 times/day (single protease inhibitor) **or**

Amprenavir 1200 mg twice daily plus ritonavir 200 mg twice daily

Ritonavir: Adjustments necessary for both agents:

Amprenavir 1200 mg plus ritonavir 200 mg once daily **or**

Amprenavir 600 mg plus ritonavir 100 mg twice daily

Solution:

<50 kg: 22.5 mg/kg (maximum: 2800 mg/day)

≥50 kg: 1400 mg twice daily

Pediatrics: Note: Capsule and oral solution are **not** interchangeable on a mg-per-mg basis.

HIV infection: Oral:

Capsule:

Children 4-12 years and older (<50 kg): 20 mg/kg twice daily or 15 mg/kg 3 times daily; maximum: 2400 mg/day

Children >13 years (>50 kg): 1200 mg twice daily
Solution:
    Children 4-12 years or older (up to 16 years weighing <50 kg): 22.5 mg/kg twice daily or 17 mg/kg 3 times daily; maximum: 2800 mg/day
    Children 13-16 years (weighing at least 50 kg) or >16 years: 1400 mg twice daily

Renal Impairment: Oral solution is contraindicated in renal failure.

Hepatic Impairment:
Child-Pugh score between 5-8:
    Capsule: 450 mg twice daily
    Solution: 513 mg twice daily; contraindicated in hepatic failure.
Child-Pugh score between 9-12:
    Capsule: 300 mg twice daily
    Solution: 342 mg twice daily; contraindicated in hepatic failure.

Available Dosage Forms [DSC] = Discontinued product
Capsule: 50 mg, 150 mg [DSC]
Solution, oral [use only when there are no other options]: 15 mg/mL (240 mL) [contains propylene glycol 550 mg/mL and vitamin E 46 int. units/mL; grape-bubble gum-peppermint flavor]

Monitoring and Teaching Issues

Physical Assessment: Assess closely for potential interactions with other pharmacological agents or herbal products patient may be taking (eg, ergot alkaloids, antiarrhythmics, HMG-CoA reductase inhibitors). Assess therapeutic response and adverse reactions (eg, peripheral paresthesia, persistent gastrointestinal upset leading to dehydration and weight loss, hyperglycemia; see Adverse Reactions) at regular intervals during therapy. Caution patients to monitor glucose levels closely; protease inhibitors may cause hyperglycemia or new-onset diabetes. Teach patient proper use, possible side effects/appropriate interventions, and adverse symptoms to report.

Monitoring Laboratory Tests: Viral load

Patient Education: Do not take any new medication during therapy unless approved by prescriber. This drug is not a cure for HIV, nor has it been found to reduce transmission. Take as directed, at regular intervals around-the-clock. May take with light meal (eg, dry toast, skim milk, corn flakes) to reduce GI upset. Avoid alcohol. Maintain adequate hydration (2-3 L/day of fluids) unless instructed to restrict fluid intake. Amprenavir may be prescribed with a combination of other medications; time these medications as directed by prescriber. You may be advised to check your glucose levels (this drug can cause exacerbation or new-onset diabetes). You will be more susceptible to infection (avoid crowds and exposure to infection and do not have any vaccinations unless approved by prescriber). May cause body changes due to redistribution of body fat, facial atrophy, or breast enlargement (normal effects of drug); nausea, vomiting, or flatulence (small frequent meals, frequent mouth care, chewing gum, or sucking lozenges may help); muscle weakness or flank pain (consult prescriber for approved analgesic); headache or insomnia (consult prescriber for medication); or diarrhea (boiled milk, buttermilk, or yogurt may help). Inform prescriber if you experience muscle numbness or tingling; unresolved persistent vomiting, diarrhea, or abdominal pain; respiratory difficulty or chest pain; unusual skin rash; or change in color of stool or urine. **Pregnancy/breast-feeding precautions:** Inform prescriber if you are pregnant and do not get pregnant while taking this medicine. This drug decreases the effect of oral contraceptives; consult prescriber for use of appropriate contraceptives. Do not breast-feed.

Dietary Considerations: May be taken with or without food; do not take with high-fat meal.

Pregnancy Risk Factor: C

Pregnancy Issues: It is not known if amprenavir crosses the human placenta and there are no clinical studies currently underway to evaluate its use in pregnant women. Pregnancy and protease inhibitors are both associated with an increased risk of hyperglycemia. Glucose levels should be closely monitored. Health professionals are encouraged to contact the antiretroviral pregnancy registry to monitor outcomes of pregnant women exposed to antiretroviral medications (1-800-258-4263 or www.APRegistry.com).

Lactation: Excretion in breast milk unknown/contraindicated

Breast-Feeding Issues: HIV-infected mothers are discouraged from breast-feeding to decrease potential transmission of HIV.

Additional Information The 150 mg capsules contain 109 int. units of vitamin E per capsule; oral solution contains 46 int. units of vitamin E per mL. Propylene glycol is included in the oral solution; a dose of 22.5 mg/kg twice daily corresponds to an intake of 1650 mg/kg of propylene glycol. Capsule and oral solution are not interchangeable on a mg-per-mg basis.

Related Information
Tuberculosis *on page 1864*

♦ **Amvisc®** *see page 1625*
♦ **Amvisc® Plus** *see page 1625*
♦ **AN100226** *see Natalizumab on page 1059*
♦ **Anafranil®** *see ClomiPRAMINE on page 350*
♦ **Anaprox®** *see Naproxen on page 1056*
♦ **Anaprox® DS** *see Naproxen on page 1056*
♦ **Anaspaz®** *see Hyoscyamine on page 775*

Anastrozole (an AS troe zole)

U.S. Brand Names Arimidex®
Synonyms ICI-D1033; ZD1033
Generic Available No
Pharmacologic Category Aromatase Inhibitor
Use Treatment of locally-advanced or metastatic breast cancer (ER-positive or hormone receptor unknown) in postmenopausal women; treatment of advanced breast cancer in postmenopausal women with disease progression following tamoxifen therapy; adjuvant treatment of early ER-positive breast cancer in postmenopausal women
(Continued)

Anastrozole *(Continued)*

Mechanism of Action/Effect Potent and selective nonsteroidal aromatase inhibitor. By inhibiting aromatase, the conversion of androstenedione to estrone, and testosterone to estradiol, is prevented. Anastrozole causes an 85% decrease in estrone sulfate levels.

Contraindications Hypersensitivity to anastrozole or any component of the formulation; pregnancy

Warnings/Precautions Use with caution in patients with hyperlipidemias; total cholesterol and LDL-cholesterol increase in patients receiving anastrozole. Exclude pregnancy before initiating therapy. Tamoxifen should not be used concurrently. Anastrozole may be associated with a reduction in bone mineral density. Safety and efficacy in premenopausal women or pediatric patients have not been established.

Drug Interactions

Cytochrome P450 Effect: Inhibits CYP1A2 (weak), 2C8/9 (weak), 3A4 (weak)

Decreased Effect:

Estrogens: Concurrent use may decrease efficacy of anastrozole.

Tamoxifen: Decreased plasma concentration of anastrozole; avoid concurrent use.

Nutritional/Ethanol Interactions Herb/Nutraceutical: Avoid black cohosh, hops, licorice, red clover, thyme, and dong quai.

Lab Interactions Lab test abnormalities: GGT, AST, ALT, alkaline phosphatase, total cholesterol and LDL increased; threefold elevations of mean serum GGT levels have been observed among patients with liver metastases. These changes were likely related to the progression of liver metastases in these patients, although other contributing factors could not be ruled out. Mean serum total cholesterol levels increased by 0.5 mmol/L among patients.

Adverse Reactions

>10%:

Cardiovascular: Vasodilatation (25% to 35%)

Central nervous system: Pain (11% to 15%), headache (9% to 13%), depression (5% to 11%)

Endocrine & metabolic: Hot flashes (12% to 35%)

Neuromuscular & skeletal: Weakness (16% to 17%), arthritis (14%), arthralgia (13%), back pain (8% to 12%), bone pain (5% to 11%)

Respiratory: Cough increased (7% to 11%), pharyngitis (6% to 12%)

1% to 10%:

Cardiovascular: Peripheral edema (5% to 10%), hypertension (5% to 9%), chest pain (5% to 7%)

Central nervous system: Insomnia (6% to 9%), dizziness (6%), anxiety (5%), lethargy (1%), fever, malaise, confusion, nervousness, somnolence

Dermatologic: Rash (6% to 10%), alopecia, pruritus

Endocrine & metabolic: Hypercholesteremia (7%)

Gastrointestinal: Vomiting (8% to 9%), constipation (7% to 9%), abdominal pain (7% to 8%), diarrhea (7% to 8%), anorexia (5% to 7%), xerostomia (6%), dyspepsia (5%), weight gain (2% to 8%), weight loss

Genitourinary: Urinary tract infection (6%), vulvovaginitis (6%), vaginal bleeding (5%) leukorrhea (2%), vaginal hemorrhage (2%), vaginal dryness (2%)

Hematologic: Anemia, leukopenia

Hepatic: Liver function tests increased, alkaline phosphatase increased

Local: Deep vein thrombosis, thrombophlebitis

Neuromuscular & skeletal: Osteoporosis (7%), fracture (7%), arthrosis (6%), paresthesia (5% to 6%), hypertonia (3%), myalgia, arthralgia

Ocular: Cataracts (4%)

Respiratory: Dyspnea (6% to 10%), sinusitis, bronchitis, rhinitis

Miscellaneous: Lymph edema (9%), infection (7%), flu-like syndrome (5% to 7%), diaphoresis (2% to 4%)

Overdosage/Toxicology Symptoms of overdose include severe irritation to the stomach (necrosis, gastritis, ulceration, and hemorrhage). There is no specific antidote; treatment must be symptomatic. Dialysis may be helpful because anastrozole is not highly protein bound.

Pharmacodynamics/Kinetics

Onset of Action: Onset of estradiol reduction: 24 hours

Duration of Action: Duration of estradiol reduction: 6 days

Absorption: Well absorbed (80%); not affected by food

Protein Binding: Plasma: 40%

Half-Life Elimination: 50 hours

Metabolism: Extensively hepatic (85%) via N-dealkylation, hydroxylation, and glucuronidation; primary metabolite inactive

Excretion: Urine (10% as unchanged drug; 60% as metabolites)

Dosing

Adults & Elderly: Breast cancer: Oral (refer to individual protocols): 1 mg once daily

Renal Impairment: Dosage adjustment is not necessary.

Hepatic Impairment: Plasma concentrations in subjects with stable hepatic cirrhosis were within the range concentrations in normal subjects across all clinical trials; therefore, no dosage adjustment is needed.

Available Dosage Forms Tablet: 1 mg

Monitoring and Teaching Issues

Physical Assessment: See Contraindications and Warnings/Precautions for use cautions. Assess potential for interactions with other pharmacological agents and herbal products patient may be using. Assess results of laboratory results, therapeutic effectiveness, and adverse reactions (eg, hyperlipidemia, hypotension, CNS changes, thrombophlebitis, bone pain or fracture; see Adverse Reactions) periodically during therapy. Teach patient proper use, possible side effects/appropriate interventions, and adverse symptoms to report.

Monitoring Laboratory Tests: CBC with differential and platelet count

Patient Education: Do not take any new medication during therapy unless approved by prescriber. Take exactly as directed. Maintain adequate hydration (2-3 L/day of fluids) unless instructed to restrict fluid intake. May cause headache (consult prescriber for approved analgesic); drowsiness, dizziness, anxiety (use caution when driving or engaging in tasks that require alertness until response to drug is known); mild nausea or vomiting (small frequent meals, frequent mouth care, chewing gum, or sucking lozenges may help); or increased pelvic, bone or tumor pain (may lessen with continued use; if not, consult prescriber for approved analgesic). Report rash; unresolved nausea or vomiting; pain or burning on urination; severe mood swings, confusion, anxiety; palpitations; flu-like symptoms; persistent bone of joint pain; or respiratory difficulty. **Pregnancy/breast-feeding precautions:** Do not get pregnant while taking this medication. Consult prescriber for appropriate contraceptive measures. Consult prescriber if breast-feeding.

Pregnancy Risk Factor: D

Pregnancy Issues: Anastrozole can cause fetal harm when administered to a pregnant woman.

Lactation: Excretion in breast milk unknown/use caution

Administration
  Storage: Store at 20°C to 25°C (68°F to 77°F).

♦ **Anbesol® [OTC]** see Benzocaine on page 181
♦ **Anbesol® Baby [OTC]** see Benzocaine on page 181
♦ **Anbesol® Cold Sore Therapy [OTC]** see Benzocaine on page 181
♦ **Anbesol® Jr. [OTC]** see Benzocaine on page 181
♦ **Anbesol® Maximum Strength [OTC]** see Benzocaine on page 181
♦ **Ancef®** see Cefazolin on page 268
♦ **Ancobon®** see Flucytosine on page 636
♦ **Andehist NR Drops** see Carbinoxamine and Pseudoephedrine on page 254
♦ **Androderm®** see Testosterone on page 1450
♦ **AndroGel®** see Testosterone on page 1450
♦ **Android®** see MethylTESTOSTERone on page 988
♦ **Anectine® [DSC]** see Succinylcholine on page 1400
♦ **Anectine® Chloride Injection** see page 1625
♦ **Anectine® Flo-Pack®** see page 1625
♦ **Anestacon®** see Lidocaine on page 898
♦ **Aneurine Hydrochloride** see Thiamine on page 1461
♦ **Anexsia®** see Hydrocodone and Acetaminophen on page 754
♦ **Angiotensin Agents** see page 1704
♦ **Anolor 300** see Butalbital, Acetaminophen, and Caffeine on page 225
♦ **Ansaid®** see Flurbiprofen on page 656
♦ **Ansamycin** see Rifabutin on page 1322
♦ **Antabuse®** see Disulfiram on page 469
♦ **Antagon®** see Ganirelix on page 697
♦ **Antara™** see Fenofibrate on page 615

Anthralin (AN thra lin)

U.S. Brand Names Drithocreme®; Dritho-Scalp®; Psoriatec™
Synonyms Dithranol
Generic Available No
Pharmacologic Category Antipsoriatic Agent; Keratolytic Agent
Use Treatment of psoriasis (quiescent or chronic psoriasis)
Mechanism of Action/Effect Inhibits synthesis of nucleic protein from inhibition of DNA synthesis to affected areas
Contraindications Hypersensitivity to anthralin or any component of the formulation; acute psoriasis (acutely or actively inflamed psoriatic eruptions)
Warnings/Precautions If redness is observed, reduce frequency of dosage or discontinue application; avoid eye contact; should generally not be applied to opposing skin surfaces that may rub or touch (eg, skin folds of the groin, axilla, and breasts) and high strengths should not be used on these sites; do not apply to genitalia. Use caution in patients with renal disease and in those having extensive and prolonged applications. May stain skin, hair, fingernails (temporary); or fabrics (may be permanent).
Drug Interactions
  Increased Effect/Toxicity: Long-term use of topical corticosteroids may destabilize psoriasis and withdrawal may also give rise to a "rebound" phenomenon. Allow an interval of at least 1 week between the discontinuance of topical corticosteroids and the commencement of therapy.
Adverse Reactions Frequency not defined: Dermatologic: Transient primary irritation of uninvolved skin; temporary discoloration of skin, hair and fingernails; contact allergic reactions; erythema
Dosing
  Adults & Elderly:
    Psoriasis: Topical: Generally, apply once a day or as directed. The irritant potential of anthralin is directly related to the strength being used and each patient's individual tolerance. Always commence treatment using a short, daily contact time (5-10 minutes) for at least 1 week using the lowest strength possible. Contact time may be gradually increased (to 20-30 minutes) as tolerated.
    Skin application: Apply sparingly only to psoriatic lesions and rub gently and carefully into the skin until absorbed. Avoid applying an excessive quantity which may cause unnecessary soiling and staining of the clothing or bed linen.
(Continued)

Anthralin *(Continued)*

> *Scalp application:* Comb hair to remove scalar debris, wet hair and, after suitably parting, rub cream well into the lesions, taking care to prevent the cream from spreading onto the forehead,

Note: Remove by washing or showering; optimal period of contact will vary according to the strength used and the patient's response to treatment. Continue treatment until the skin is entirely clear (ie, when there is nothing to feel with the fingers and the texture is normal).

Pediatrics: Unlabeled use: Refer to adult dosing.

Available Dosage Forms
Cream:
Drithocream®, Psoriatec™: 1% (50 g)
Dritho-Scalp®: 0.5% (50 g)

Monitoring and Teaching Issues
Physical Assessment: When applied to large areas of skin or for extensive periods of time, monitor for adverse skin or systemic reactions. Assess knowledge/teach patient appropriate application and use and adverse symptoms (see Adverse Reactions) to report.
Patient Education: For external use only. Use exactly as directed; do not overuse. Before using, wash and dry area gently. Wear gloves to apply a thin film to affected area and rub in gently. Remove by washing; may discolor fabric, skin, or hair. Use a porous dressing if necessary. For lesions on scalp, comb hair to remove scalar debris, part hair, and rub cream into lesions. Do not allow cream to spread to forehead or onto neck. Remove by washing hair. Avoid contact with eyes. Avoid exposing treated areas to direct sunlight; sunburn can occur. Optimal period of contact will vary according to strength used and response to treatment. Report increased swelling, redness, rash, itching, signs of infection, worsening of condition, or lack of healing. **Pregnancy/breast-feeding precautions:** Inform prescriber if you are or intend to become pregnant. Breast-feeding is not recommended.

Pregnancy Risk Factor: C
Lactation: Excretion in breast milk unknown/not recommended

Administration
Topical: May apply using latex gloves to prevent staining of fingers. Apply directly to plaques; rub in gently but thoroughly; avoid application to unaffected skin. When applying to scalp, part hair in one-inch segments to reach plaques. Remove by washing after conclusion of prescribed contact period. When rinsing, take care to avoid contact with eyes. Immediately clean tub or shower to prevent staining. Dry off using old towel (stains on fabric may be permanent) Petroleum jelly may be used around the edges of plaques, in body folds, or skin creases to prevent irritation of unaffected skin.
Storage: Store at controlled room temperature of 15°C to 30°C (59°F to 86°F). Avoid excessive heat.

♦ **Anthrax Vaccine (Adsorbed)** *see page 1660*

♦ **Anti-4 Alpha Integrin** *see* Natalizumab *on page 1059*

♦ **Antiarrhythmic Drugs** *see page 1708*

♦ **AntibiOtic® Ear** *see* Neomycin, Polymyxin B, and Hydrocortisone *on page 1069*

♦ **Anti-CD11a** *see* Efalizumab *on page 508*

♦ **Anti-CD20 Monoclonal Antibody** *see* Rituximab *on page 1338*

♦ **Anti-CD20-Murine Monoclonal Antibody I-131** *see* Tositumomab and Iodine I 131 Tositumomab *on page 1501*

♦ **Anticoagulants, Injectable** *see page 1711*

♦ **Anticoagulant Therapy Guidelines** *see page 1784*

♦ **Anticonvulsants By Seizure Type** *see page 1712*

♦ **Antidepressant Agents** *see page 1713*

♦ **Antidepressant Medication Guidelines** *see page 1765*

♦ **Antidigoxin Fab Fragments, Ovine** *see* Digoxin Immune Fab *on page 455*

♦ **Antidiuretic Hormone** *see* Vasopressin *on page 1554*

♦ **Antiemetics for Chemotherapy-Induced Nausea and Vomiting** *see page 1788*

Antihemophilic Factor (Human) *(an tee hee moe FIL ik FAK tor HYU man)*

U.S. Brand Names Alphanate®; Hemofil® M; Humate-P®; Koāte®-DVI; Monarc® M; Monoclate-P®
Synonyms AHF (Human); Factor VIII (Human)
Generic Available Yes
Pharmacologic Category Antihemophilic Agent; Blood Product Derivative
Use Management of hemophilia A for patients in whom a deficiency in factor VIII has been demonstrated; can be of significant therapeutic value in patients with acquired factor VIII inhibitors not exceeding 10 Bethesda units/mL
Humate-P®: In addition, indicated as treatment of spontaneous bleeding in patients with severe von Willebrand disease and in mild and moderate von Willebrand disease where desmopressin is known or suspected to be inadequate
Orphan status: Alphanate®: Management of von Willebrand disease
Mechanism of Action/Effect Protein (factor VIII) in normal plasma which is necessary for clot formation and maintenance of hemostasis; activates factor X in conjunction with activated factor IX; activated factor X converts prothrombin to thrombin, which converts fibrinogen to fibrin, and with factor XIII forms a stable clot
Contraindications Hypersensitivity to any component of the formulation or to mouse protein (Monoclate-P®, Hemofil® M)
Warnings/Precautions Risk of viral transmission is not totally eradicated. Because antihemophilic factor is prepared from pooled plasma, it may contain the causative agent of viral hepatitis and other viral diseases. Hepatitis B vaccination is recommended for all patients. Hepatitis A vaccination is also recommended for seronegative patients. Antihemophilic factor

contains trace amounts of blood groups A and B isohemagglutinins and when large or frequently repeated doses are given to individuals with blood groups A, B, and AB, the patient should be monitored for signs of progressive anemia and the possibility of intravascular hemolysis should be considered. Natural rubber latex is a component of Hemofil® M packaging. Products vary by preparation method; final formulations contain human albumin.

Overdosage/Toxicology Massive doses have been reported to cause acute hemolytic anemia, increased bleeding tendency, or hyperfibrinogenemia. Occurrence is rare.

Pharmacodynamics/Kinetics

Half-Life Elimination: Mean: 12-17 hours with hemophilia A; consult specific product labeling

Dosing

Adults: Hemophilia: I.V.: Individualize dosage based on coagulation studies performed prior to treatment and at regular intervals during treatment. 1 AHF unit is the activity present in 1 mL of normal pooled human plasma. Dosage should be adjusted to actual vial size currently stocked in the pharmacy. (General guidelines presented; consult individual product labeling for specific dosing recommendations.)

Dosage based on desired factor VIII increase (%):
To calculate dosage needed based on desired factor VIII increase (%):
Body weight (kg) x 0.5 int. units/kg x desired factor VIII increase (%) = int. units factor VIII required
For example:
50 kg x 0.5 int. units/kg x 30 (% increase) = 750 int. units factor VIII

Dosage based on expected factor VIII increase (%):
It is also possible to calculate the **expected** % factor VIII increase:
(# int. units administered x 2%/int. units/kg) divided by body weight (kg) = expected % factor VIII increase
For example:
(1400 int. units x 2%/int. units/kg) divided by 70 kg = 40%

General guidelines:
Minor hemorrhage: Required peak postinfusion AHF level: 20% to 40% (10-20 int. units/kg), repeat dose every 12-24 hours for 1-3 days until bleeding is resolved or healing achieved; mild superficial or early hemorrhages may respond to a single dose.

Moderate hemorrhage: Required peak postinfusion AHF level: 30% to 60% (15-30 int. units/kg): Infuse every 12-24 hours for ≥3 days until pain and disability are resolved. Alternatively, a loading dose to achieve 50% (25 int. units/kg) may be given, followed by 10-15 int. units/kg dose given every 8-12 hours; may be needed for >7 days.

Severe/life-threatening hemorrhage: Required peak postinfusion AHF level: 60% to 100% (30-50 int. units/kg): Infuse every 8-24 hours until threat is resolved.
Alternatively, a loading dose to achieve 80% to 100% (40-50 int. units/kg) may be given, followed by 20-25 int. units/kg dose given every 8-12 hours for ≥14 days.

Minor surgery: Required peak postinfusion AHF level: 30% to 80% (15-40 int. units/kg): Highly dependent upon procedure and specific product recommendations; for some procedures, may be administered as a single infusion plus oral antifibrinolytic therapy within 1 hour. In other procedures, may repeat dose every 12-24 hours as needed.

Major surgery: Required peak pre- and postsurgery AHF level: 80% to 100% (40-50 int. units/kg): Administer every 6-24 hours until healing is complete (10-14 days).

Prophylaxis: May also be given on a regular schedule to prevent bleeding.

If bleeding is not controlled with adequate dose, test for presence of inhibitor. It may not be possible or practical to control bleeding if inhibitor titers >10 Bethesda units/mL; antihemophilic factor (porcine) may be considered as an alternative.

von Willebrand disease:
Treatment of hemorrhage in von Willebrand disease (Humate-P®): 1 int. units of factor VIII per kg of body weight would be expected to raise circulating vWF:RC of approximately 3.5-4 int. units/dL.

Type 1, mild (if desmopressin is not appropriate): Major hemorrhage:
Loading dose: 40-60 int. units/kg
Maintenance dose: 40-50 int. units/kg every 8-12 hours for 3 days, keeping vWF:RC of nadir >50%; follow with 40-50 int. units/kg daily for up to 7 days

Type 1, moderate or severe:
Minor hemorrhage: 40-50 int. units/kg for 1-2 doses
Major hemorrhage:
Loading dose: 50-75 int. units/kg
Maintenance dose: 40-60 int. units/kg daily for up to 7 days

Types 2 and 3:
Minor hemorrhage: 40-50 int. units/kg for 1-2 doses
Major hemorrhage:
Loading dose: 60-80 int. units/kg
Maintenance dose: 40-60 int. units/kg every 8-12 hours for 3 days, keeping vWF:RC of nadir >50%; follow with 40-60 int. units/kg daily for up to 7 days

Elderly: Refer to adult dosing. Dosage should be individualized.

Pediatrics: Refer to adult dosing.

Available Dosage Forms Injection, human [single-dose vial]: Labeling on cartons and vials indicates number of int. units

Monitoring and Teaching Issues

Physical Assessment: Assess potential for interactions with other pharmacological agents patient may be taking that may affect coagulation or platelet function. Patient should be monitored closely during and after infusion for any change in vital signs, cardiac and CNS status, or hypersensitivity reactions (chills, fever, chest pain, respiratory difficulty). Assess patient response (eg, results of laboratory tests [hematocrit and coagulation studies], therapeutic effectiveness [bleeding and coagulation status], and adverse reactions [eg, signs of intravascular hemolysis, increased bleeding or anemia]; see Adverse Reactions). Provide patient education according to patient condition.

Monitoring Laboratory Tests: In patients with circulating inhibitors, the inhibitor level should be monitored; hematocrit

(Continued)

Antihemophilic Factor (Human) *(Continued)*

Patient Education: This medication can only be administered by infusion; you will be monitored during and after infusion. Report immediately any sudden onset of headache, rash, chest or back pain, wheezing or respiratory difficulties, hives, itching, low-grade fever, stomach pain, or nausea/vomiting to prescriber. Wear identification indicating that you have a hemophilic condition. **Pregnancy/breast-feeding precautions:** Inform prescriber if you are or intend to become pregnant. Consult prescriber if breast-feeding.

Pregnancy Risk Factor: C

Pregnancy Issues: Safety and efficacy in pregnant women have not been established. Use during pregnancy only if clearly needed. Parvovirus B19, which may be present in the solution, may seriously affect a pregnant woman.

Lactation: Excretion in breast milk unknown/use caution

Administration

I.V.: Total dose may be administered over 5-10 minutes (maximum: 10 mL/minute); infuse Monoclate-P® at 2 mL/minute. Adapt based on patient response.

Storage: Store under refrigeration, 2°C to 8°C (36°F to 46°F); avoid freezing. Use within 3 hours of reconstitution; gently agitate or rotate vial after adding diluent, do not shake vigorously. Do not refrigerate after reconstitution, precipitation may occur.

Alphanate®: May be stored at room temperature for ≤2 months.

Hemofil® M: May be stored at room temperature for ≤12 months.

Humate-P®, Koāte®-DVI; Monoclate-P®: May also be stored at room temperature for ≤6 months.

If refrigerated, the dried concentrate and diluent should be warmed to room temperature before reconstitution.

Antihemophilic Factor (Porcine) (an tee hee moe FIL ik FAK ter POR seen)

U.S. Brand Names Hyate:C®

Synonyms AHF (Porcine); Factor VIII (Porcine)

Generic Available No

Pharmacologic Category Antihemophilic Agent

Use Management of hemophilia A in patients with antibodies to human factor VIII (consider use of human factor VIII in patients with antibody titer of <5 Bethesda units/mL); management of previously nonhemophilic patients with spontaneously-acquired inhibitors to human factor VIII, regardless of initial antihuman inhibitor titer

Mechanism of Action/Effect Factor VIII is the coagulation portion of the factor VIII complex in plasma. Factor VIII acts as a cofactor for factor IX to activate factor X in the intrinsic pathway of blood coagulation.

Contraindications Hypersensitivity to porcine or any component of the formulation

Warnings/Precautions Rarely administration has been associated with anaphylaxis. Epinephrine, hydrocortisone, and facilities for cardiopulmonary resuscitation should be available in case such a reaction occurs. Infusion may be followed by a rise in plasma levels of antibody to both human and porcine factor VIII. Inhibitor levels should be monitored both pre- and post-treatment.

Adverse Reactions Reactions tend to lessen in frequency and severity as further infusions are given; hydrocortisone and/or antihistamines may help to prevent or alleviate side effects and may be prescribed as precautionary measures.

1% to 10%:

Central nervous system: Fever, headache, chills

Dermatologic: Rashes

Gastrointestinal: Nausea, vomiting

Overdosage/Toxicology Massive doses of antihemophilic factor (human) have been reported to cause acute hemolytic anemia, increased bleeding tendency, or hyperfibrinogenemia. Occurrence is rare.

Pharmacodynamics/Kinetics

Half-Life Elimination: 10-11 hours (patients without detectable inhibitors)

Dosing

Adults & Elderly: Clinical response should be used to assess efficacy.

Factor VIII deficiency: I.V.: Initial dose:

Antibody level to human factor VIII <50 Bethesda units/mL: 100-150 porcine units/kg (body weight) is recommended.

Antibody level to human factor VIII >50 Bethesda units/mL: Activity of the antibody to antihemophilic (porcine) should be determined. **An antiporcine antibody level** >20 Bethesda units/mL indicates that the patient is unlikely to benefit from treatment; for lower titers, a dose of 100-150 porcine units/kg is recommended.

The initial dose may also be calculated using the following method:

1. Determine patient's antibody titer against porcine factor VIII.

2. Calculate average plasma volume:

(body weight kg) (average blood volume) (1 - hematocrit) = plasma volume

(body weight kg) (80 mL/kg) (1 - hematocrit) = plasma volume

Note: A hematocrit of 50% = 0.5 for the equation

3. Neutralizing dose:

(plasma volume mL) (antibody titer Bethesda units/mL) = neutralizing dose units

This is the predicted dose required to neutralize the circulating antibodies. An incremental dose must be added to the neutralizing dose in order to increase the plasma factor VIII to the desired level.

4. Incremental dose:

(desired plasma factor VIII level) (body weight) divided by 1.5 = incremental dose units

5. Total dose = neutralizing dose + incremental dose = total dose units

Note: If a patient has previously been treated with Hyate:C®, this may provide a guide to his likely response and, therefore, assist in estimation of the preliminary dose.

Subsequent doses: Following administration of the initial dose, if the recovery of factor VIII in the patient's plasma is not sufficient, another larger dose should be administered. If recovery after the second dose is still insufficient, a third and larger dose may prove effective. Once appropriate factor VIII levels are achieved, dosing can be repeated every 6-8 hours.

Pediatrics: Refer to adult dosing.

Available Dosage Forms Injection, powder for reconstitution: 400-700 porcine units [to be reconstituted with 20 mL SWFI]

Monitoring and Teaching Issues

Physical Assessment: Identify any patient allergies to antihemophilic factor or porcine substances prior to starting therapy. See Warnings/Precautions for use cautions. Assess potential for interactions with other pharmacological agents or herbal products patient may be taking that may affect coagulation or platelet function. Vital signs and cardiac and CNS status should be monitored during and after therapy. Patient should be monitored closely during infusion for adverse reactions. Administration has been associated with rare anaphylactic reactions. Epinephrine, hydrocortisone, and facilities for cardiopulmonary resuscitation should be available in case such a reaction occurs (see Adverse Reactions). Provide patient education according to patient condition (see Patient Education).

Monitoring Laboratory Tests: Factor VIII levels pre- and postinfusion; inhibitor levels to human and/or porcine factor VIII pre- and postinfusion; bleeding

Antibody levels to human factor VIII >50 Bethesda units/mL: Activity of the antibody to antihemophilic factor (porcine) should be determined.

Antiporcine antibody level >20 Bethesda units/mL: Patient may not benefit from treatment.

Patient Education: This medication can only be given intravenously. Report sudden onset headache, rash, chest or back pain, wheezing or respiratory difficulties, hives, itching, low-grade fever, stomach pain, nausea, or vomiting to prescriber. Wear identification indicating that you have a hemophilic condition. **Pregnancy/breast-feeding precautions:** Inform prescriber if you are or intend to become pregnant. Consult prescriber if breast-feeding.

Pregnancy Risk Factor: C

Lactation: Excretion in breast milk unknown/use caution

Administration

I.V.: Administer by I.V. route only; infuse slowly, 2-5 mL/minute.

Storage: Store at -15°C to -20°C (5°F to -4°F); warm to 20°C to 37°C (68°F to 98.6°F) prior to reconstitution; use within 3 hours of mixing.

Additional Information Sodium ion concentration is not more than 200 mmol/L. The assayed amount of activity is stated on the label, but may vary depending on the type of assay and hemophilic substrate plasma used.

Antihemophilic Factor (Recombinant)
(an tee hee moe FIL ik FAK tor ree KOM be nant)

U.S. Brand Names Advate; Helixate® FS; Kogenate® FS; Recombinate™; ReFacto®

Synonyms AHF (Recombinant); Factor VIII (Recombinant); rAHF

Generic Available No

Pharmacologic Category Antihemophilic Agent

Use Management of hemophilia A (classic hemophilia) for patients in whom a deficiency in factor VIII has been demonstrated; prevention and control of bleeding episodes; perioperative management of hemophilia A; can be of significant therapeutic value in patients with acquired factor VIII inhibitors not exceeding 10 Bethesda units/mL

Mechanism of Action/Effect Protein (factor VIII) in normal plasma which is necessary for clot formation and maintenance of hemostasis; activates factor X in conjunction with activated factor IX; activated factor X converts prothrombin to thrombin, which converts fibrinogen to fibrin, and with factor XIII forms a stable clot

Contraindications Hypersensitivity to mouse or hamster protein (Advate, Helixate® FS, Kogenate® FS); hypersensitivity to mouse, hamster, or bovine protein (Recombinate™, ReFacto®); hypersensitivity to any component of the formulation

Warnings/Precautions Monitor for signs of formation of antibodies to factor VIII; may occur at anytime but more common in young children with severe hemophilia. Monitor for allergic hypersensitivity reactions. Products vary by preparation method. Recombinate™ is stabilized using human albumin. Helixate® FS and Kogenate® FS are stabilized with sucrose.

Overdosage/Toxicology Massive doses of antihemophilic factor (human) have been reported to cause acute hemolytic anemia, increased bleeding tendency, or hyperfibrinogenemia. Occurrence is rare.

Pharmacodynamics/Kinetics

Half-Life Elimination: Mean: 14-16 hours

Dosing

Adults: Hemophilia: I.V.: Individualize dosage based on coagulation studies. performed prior to treatment and at regular intervals during treatment; 1 AHF unit is the activity present in 1 mL of normal pooled human plasma; dosage should be adjusted to actual vial size currently stocked in the pharmacy. (General guidelines presented; consult individual product labeling for specific dosing recommendations.)

Dosage based on desired factor VIII increase (%):
To calculate dosage needed based on desired factor VIII increase (%):
Body weight (kg) x 0.5 int. units/kg x desired factor VIII increase (%) = int. units factor VIII required
For example:
50 kg x 0.5 int. units/kg x 30 (% increase) = 750 int. units factor VIII

Dosage based on expected factor VIII increase (%):
It is also possible to calculate the **expected** % factor VIII increase:
(# int. units administered x 2%/int. units/kg) divided by body weight (kg) = expected % factor VIII increase
For example:
(1400 int. units x 2%/int. units/kg) divided by 70 kg = 40%

(Continued)

Antihemophilic Factor (Recombinant) *(Continued)*

General guidelines:

Minor hemorrhage: Required peak postinfusion AHF level: 20% to 40% (10-20 int. units/kg); mild superficial or early hemorrhages may respond to a single dose; may repeat dose every 12-24 hours for 1-3 days until bleeding is resolved or healing achieved

Moderate hemorrhage/minor surgery: Required peak postinfusion AHF level: 30% to 60% (15-30 int. units/kg); repeat dose at 12-24 hours if needed; some products suggest continuing for ≥3 days until pain and disability are resolved

Severe/life-threatening hemorrhage: Required peak postinfusion AHF level: Initial dose: 80% to 100% (40-50 int. units/kg); maintenance dose: 40% to 50% (20-25 int. units/kg) every 8-12 hours until threat is resolved

Major surgery: Required peak pre- and postsurgery AHF level: ~100% (50 int. units/kg) give first dose prior to surgery and repeat every 6-12 hours until healing complete (10-14 days)

Prophylaxis: May also be given on a regular schedule to prevent bleeding

If bleeding is not controlled with adequate dose, test for presence of inhibitor. It may not be possible or practical to control bleeding if inhibitor titers >10 Bethesda units/mL; antihemophilic factor (porcine) may be considered as an alternative

Elderly: Refer to adult dosing. Dosage should be individualized.

Pediatrics: Refer to adult dosing.

Available Dosage Forms

Injection, powder for reconstitution, recombinant [preservative free]:

Advate: 250 int. units, 500 int. units, 1000 int. units, 1500 int. units [plasma/albumin free]

Helixate® FS, Kogenate® FS: 250 int. units, 500 int. units, 1000 int. units [contains sucrose 28 mg/vial]

Recombinate™: 250 int. units, 500 int. units, 1000 int. units [contains human albumin 12.5 mg/mL; packaging contains natural rubber latex]

ReFacto®: 250 int. units, 500 units, 1000 int. units, 2000 int. units [contains sucrose]

Monitoring and Teaching Issues

Physical Assessment: Assess potential for interactions with other pharmacological agents patient may be taking that may affect coagulation or platelet function. Patient should be monitored closely during and after infusion for any change in vital signs, cardiac and CNS status, or hypersensitivity reactions (chills, fever, chest pain, respiratory difficulty). Assess patient response (eg, results of laboratory tests [hematocrit and coagulation studies]), therapeutic effectiveness (bleeding and coagulation status), and adverse reactions (eg, bleeding or anemia; see Adverse Reactions). Provide patient education according to patient condition.

Monitoring Laboratory Tests: Development of circulating inhibitors; bleeding

Patient Education: This medication can only be administered by infusion; you will be monitored during and after infusion. Report immediately any sudden onset of headache, rash, chest or back pain, wheezing or respiratory difficulties, hives, itching, low-grade fever, stomach pain, or nausea/vomiting to prescriber. Wear identification indicating that you have a hemophilic condition. **Pregnancy/breast-feeding precautions:** Inform prescriber if you are or intend to become pregnant. Consult prescriber if breast-feeding.

Pregnancy Risk Factor: C

Lactation: Excretion in breast milk unknown/use caution

Administration

I.V.: Total dose may be administered over 5-10 minutes (maximum: 10 mL/minute); adapt based on patient response

Advate: Infuse over ≤5 minutes (maximum: 10 mL/minute)

Storage: Store under refrigeration, 2°C to 8°C (36°F to 46°F); avoid freezing. Use within 3 hours of reconstitution; gently agitate or rotate vial after adding diluent, do not shake vigorously. Do not refrigerate after reconstitution, a precipitation may occur.

Advate: May also be stored at room temperature for up to 6 months.

Kogenate® FS: Avoid prolonged exposure to light during storage.

Recombinate™, ReFacto®: May also be stored at room temperature for up to 3 months; avoid prolonged exposure to light during storage

If refrigerated, the dried concentrate and diluent should be warmed to room temperature before reconstitution.

Anti-inhibitor Coagulant Complex

(an tee in HI bi tor coe AG yoo lant KOM pleks)

U.S. Brand Names Autoplex® T; Feiba VH®

Synonyms Coagulant Complex Inhibitor

Generic Available No

Pharmacologic Category Antihemophilic Agent; Blood Product Derivative

Use Patients with factor VIII inhibitors who are to undergo surgery or those who are bleeding

Contraindications Disseminated intravascular coagulation; patients with normal coagulation mechanism

Warnings/Precautions Products are prepared from pooled human plasma; such plasma may contain the causative agents of viral diseases. Tests used to control efficacy such as aPTT, WBCT, and TEG do not correlate with clinical efficacy. Dosing to normalize these values may result in DIC. Identification of the clotting deficiency as caused by factor VIII inhibitors is essential prior to starting therapy. Use with extreme caution in patients with impaired hepatic function.

Lab Interactions Increased/decreased PT, PTT; increased fibrin split products; decreased WBCT, fibrin, platelets

Overdosage/Toxicology Rapid infusion may cause hypotension. Excessive administration can cause DIC.

Dosing

Adults & Elderly: Bleeding or surgery in patients with factor VIII inhibitors: I.V.: Dosage range: 25-100 factor VIII correctional units per kg depending on the severity of hemorrhage

Note: Tests used to control efficacy such as aPTT, WBCT, and TEG do not correlate with clinical efficacy. Dosing to normalize these values may result in DIC. Identification of the clotting deficiency as caused by factor VIII inhibitors is essential prior to starting therapy.
Pediatrics: Refer to adult dosing.
Hepatic Impairment: Use with extreme caution.

Available Dosage Forms

Injection, powder for reconstitution:

Autoplex® T: Each bottle is labeled with correctional units of factor VIII [with heparin 2 units/mL; packaging contains natural rubber latex]

Feiba VH®: Each bottle is labeled with correctional units of factor VIII [heparin free; packaging contains natural rubber latex]

Monitoring and Teaching Issues

Physical Assessment: Assess potential for interactions with other pharmacological agents patient may be taking that may affect coagulation or platelet function. Patient should be monitored closely during and after infusion for any change in vital signs, cardiac and CNS status, or hypersensitivity reactions (chills, fever, chest pain, respiratory difficulty). **Caution:** See Monitoring Laboratory Tests. If hypotension develops, the rate of infusion should be slowed and prescriber notified. Provide patient education is according to patient condition.

Monitoring Laboratory Tests: Note: Tests used to control efficacy such as aPTT, WBCT, and TEG do not correlate with clinical efficacy. Dosing to normalize these values may result in DIC.

Patient Education: This medication can only be administered by infusion; you will be monitored during and after infusion. Report immediately any sudden-onset headache, rash, chest or back pain, wheezing or respiratory difficulties, hives, itching, low-grade fever, stomach pain, or nausea/vomiting to prescriber. Wear identification indicating that you have a hemophilic condition. **Pregnancy/breast-feeding precautions:** Inform prescriber if you are or intend to become pregnant. Consult prescriber if breast-feeding.

Pregnancy Risk Factor: C
Lactation: Excretion in breast milk unknown/use caution

Administration

I.V.: I.V. push (maximum rate: 2 units/kg/minute or 2.5-7.5 mL/minutes).
Reconstitution: Do **not** shake or refrigerate after reconstitution. Use within 1-3 hours after reconstitution.
Storage: Store at 2°C to 8°C (36°F to 46°F)

♦ **Antimicrobial Drugs of Choice** *see page 1792*
♦ **Antimigraine Drugs: 5-HT$_1$ Receptor Agonists** *see page 1716*
♦ **Antipsychotic Agents** *see page 1717*
♦ **Antipsychotic Medication Guidelines** *see page 1766*

Antithymocyte Globulin (Equine) (an te THY moe site GLOB yu lin, E kwine)

U.S. Brand Names Atgam®
Synonyms Antithymocyte Immunoglobulin; ATG; Horse Antihuman Thymocyte Gamma Globulin; Lymphocyte Immune Globulin
Generic Available No
Pharmacologic Category Immunosuppressant Agent
Medication Safety Issues
Sound-alike/look-alike issues:
Atgam® may be confused with Ativan®
Use Prevention and treatment of acute renal allograft rejection; treatment of moderate to severe aplastic anemia in patients not considered suitable candidates for bone marrow transplantation
Unlabeled/Investigational Use Prevention and treatment of other solid organ allograft rejection; prevention of graft-versus-host disease following bone marrow transplantation
Mechanism of Action/Effect May involve elimination of antigen-reactive T lymphocytes (killer cells) in peripheral blood or alteration of T-cell function
Contraindications Hypersensitivity to lymphocytic immune globulin, any component of the formulation, or other equine gamma globulins
Warnings/Precautions For I.V. use only. Must be administered via central line due to chemical phlebitis. Should only be used by physicians experienced in immunosuppressive therapy or management of solid organ or bone marrow transplant patients. Adequate laboratory and supportive medical resources must be readily available in the facility for patient management. Rash, dyspnea, hypotension, or anaphylaxis precludes further administration of the drug. Discontinue if severe and unremitting thrombocytopenia and/or leukopenia occur. Dose must be administered over at least 4 hours. Patient may need to be pretreated with an antipyretic, antihistamine, and/or corticosteroid.

Adverse Reactions

>10%:
Central nervous system: Fever, chills
Dermatologic: Pruritus, rash, urticaria
Hematologic: Leukopenia, thrombocytopenia
1% to 10%:
Cardiovascular: Bradycardia, chest pain, CHF, edema, encephalitis, hyper-/hypotension, myocarditis, tachycardia
Central nervous system: Agitation, headache, lethargy, lightheadedness, listlessness, seizure
Gastrointestinal: Diarrhea, nausea, stomatitis, vomiting
Hepatic: Hepatosplenomegaly, liver function tests abnormal
Local: Pain at injection site, phlebitis, thrombophlebitis, burning soles/palms
Neuromuscular & skeletal: Myalgia, back pain, arthralgia
Ocular: Periorbital edema
Renal: Abnormal renal function tests
(Continued)

Antithymocyte Globulin (Equine) *(Continued)*

Respiratory: Dyspnea, respiratory distress

Miscellaneous: Anaphylaxis, serum sickness, viral infection, night sweats, diaphoresis, lymphadenopathy

Pharmacodynamics/Kinetics

Half-Life Elimination: Plasma: 1.5-12 days

Excretion: Urine (~1%)

Dosing

Adults & Elderly: Note: An intradermal skin test is recommended prior to administration of the initial dose of ATG; use 0.1 mL of a 1:1000 dilution of ATG in normal saline. A positive skin reaction consists of a wheal ≥10 mm in diameter. If a positive skin test occurs, the first infusion should be administered in a controlled environment with intensive life support immediately available. A systemic reaction precludes further administration of the drug. The absence of a reaction does **not** preclude the possibility of an immediate sensitivity reaction.

Note: Premedication with diphenhydramine, hydrocortisone, and is recommended prior to first dose.

Aplastic anemia protocol: I.V.: 10-20 mg/kg/day for 8-14 days, then give every other day for 7 more doses for a total of 21 doses in 28 days.

Renal allograft rejection, prevention: I.V.: 15 mg/kg/day for 14 days, then give every other day for 7 more doses for a total of 21 doses in 28 days; initial dose should be administered within 24 hours before or after transplantation.

Renal allograft rejection, treatment: I.V.: 10-15 mg/kg/day for 14 days, then give every other day for 7 more doses.

Pediatrics: Note: See adult dosing for notes on intradermal skin testing and premedication.

Aplastic anemia protocol: I.V.: 10-20 mg/kg/day for 8-14 days; then administer every other day for 7 more doses; addition doses may be given every other day for 21 total doses in 28 days.

Renal allograft: I.V.: 5-25 mg/kg/day

Available Dosage Forms Injection, solution: 50 mg/mL (5 mL)

Monitoring and Teaching Issues

Physical Assessment: Assess for history of previous allergic reactions. Monitor vital signs during infusion and observe for adverse or allergic reactions. Teach patient adverse symptoms to report.

Monitoring Laboratory Tests: Lymphocyte profile, CBC with differential, platelet count

Patient Education: This medication can only be administered by infusion. You will be monitored closely during the infusion. Do not get up alone; ask for assistance if you must get up or change position. Do not have any vaccinations for the next 3 months without consulting prescriber. Immediately report chills; persistent dizziness or nausea; itching or stinging; acute back pain; chest pain, tightness, or rapid heartbeat; or respiratory difficulty. **Pregnancy/breast-feeding precautions:** Inform prescriber if you are pregnant. Consult prescriber if breast-feeding.

Pregnancy Risk Factor: C

Pregnancy Issues: Reproduction studies have not been conducted; use during pregnancy is not recommended. Women exposed to Atgam® during pregnancy may be enrolled in the National Transplantation Pregnancy Registry (877-955-6877).

Lactation: Excretion in breast milk unknown/use caution

Administration

I.V.: Infuse dose over at least 4 hours. Any severe systemic reaction to the skin test such as generalized rash, tachycardia, dyspnea, hypotension, or anaphylaxis should preclude further therapy. Epinephrine and resuscitative equipment should be nearby. Patient may need to be pretreated with an antipyretic, antihistamine, and/or corticosteroid. Mild itching and erythema can be treated with antihistamines. Infuse into a vascular shunt, arterial venous fistula or high-flow central vein through a 0.2-1 micron in-line filter

First dose: Premedicate with diphenhydramine orally 30 minutes prior to and hydrocortisone I.V. 15 minutes prior to infusion and acetaminophen 2 hours after start of infusion

Reconstitution: Dilute into inverted bottle of sterile vehicle to ensure that undiluted lymphocyte immune globulin does not contact air. Gently rotate or swirl to mix. Final concentration should be 4 mg/mL. May be diluted in NS, D$_5$1/4NS, D$_5$1/2NS.

Storage: Ampuls must be refrigerated; do not freeze. Diluted solution is stable for 24 hours (including infusion time) at refrigeration.

Apomorphine (a poe MOR feen)

U.S. Brand Names Apokyn™

Synonyms Apomorphine Hydrochloride; Apomorphine Hydrochloride Hemihydrate

Generic Available No

Pharmacologic Category Anti-Parkinson's Agent, Dopamine Agonist

Use Treatment of hypomobility, "off" episodes with Parkinson's disease

Unlabeled/Investigational Use Treatment of erectile dysfunction

Mechanism of Action/Effect Improves motor function in Parkinson's disease

Contraindications Hypersensitivity to apomorphine or any component of the formulation; concomitant use with 5HT$_3$ antagonists; intravenous administration

Warnings/Precautions May cause orthostatic hypotension especially during dosage escalation; use extreme caution, especially in patients on antihypertensives and/or vasodilators. Orthostasis peaks 20 minutes after dosing and lasts at least 90 minutes. If patient develops clinically-significant orthostatic hypotension with test dose, then apomorphine should not be used. **Pretreatment with antiemetic is necessary;** avoid pretreatment with antidopaminergic and antiserotonin antiemetic agents. (antiemetic experience is greatest with trimethobenzamide). Monitor patients for drowsiness; patients may not be aware of drowsiness and may fall asleep without warning. Use caution in patients with risk factors for torsade de pointes (hypokalemia, hypomagnesemia, bradycardia, concurrent use of drugs that prolong QT$_c$, or genetic predisposition).

Use caution in cardiovascular and cerebrovascular disease; hypotension may cause coronary and/or cerebral ischemia. Use caution in patients with hepatic or renal dysfunction. Neuroleptic malignant syndrome has been reported with other dopamine agonists. Retinal degeneration has been observed in animal studies when using dopamine agonists for prolonged periods. Rare cases of abuse have been reported. Contains metabisulfite which may cause allergic reactions in some individuals. Safety and efficacy in pediatric patients have not been established.

Drug Interactions

Cytochrome P450 Effect: Substrate (minor) of CYP1A2, 3A4, 2C19; **Inhibits** CYP1A2 (weak), 3A (weak), 2C19 (weak)

Decreased Effect: Typical antipsychotics may decrease the efficacy of apomorphine.

Increased Effect/Toxicity: Antihypertensives, vasodilators, and 5HT$_3$ antagonists may increase risk of hypotension. QT$_c$ prolongation may rarely occur with concurrent use of QT$_c$-prolonging agents. Effects of concomitant levodopa may be increased.

Nutritional/Ethanol Interactions

Ethanol: Caution with ethanol consumption; may increase risk of hypotension.

Adverse Reactions

>10%:

Cardiovascular: Chest pain/pressure or angina (15%)

Central nervous system: Drowsiness or somnolence (35%), dizziness or orthostatic hypotension (20%)

Gastrointestinal: Nausea and/or vomiting (30%)

Neuromuscular & skeletal: Falls (30%), dyskinesias (24% to 35%)

Respiratory: Yawning (40%), rhinorrhea (20%)

1% to 10%:

Cardiovascular: Edema (10%), vasodilation (3%), hypotension (2%), syncope (2%), CHF

Central nervous system: Hallucinations or confusion (10%), anxiety, depression, fatigue, headache, insomnia, pain

Dermatologic: Bruising

Endocrine & metabolic: Dehydration

Gastrointestinal: Constipation, diarrhea

Local: Injection site reactions

Neuromuscular & skeletal: Arthralgias, weakness

Miscellaneous: Diaphoresis increased

Overdosage/Toxicology An accidental overdose of 25 mg SubQ was reported resulting in nausea, loss of consciousness, bradycardia, and hypotension. Treatment should be supportive and symptomatic.

Pharmacodynamics/Kinetics

Onset of Action: SubQ: Rapid

Time to Peak: Plasma: Improved motor scores: 20 minutes

Half-Life Elimination: Terminal: 40 minutes

Metabolism: Not established; potential routes of metabolism include sulfation, N-demethylation, glucuronidation, and oxidation; catechol-O methyltransferase and nonenzymatic oxidation. CYP isoenzymes do not appear to play a significant role.

Excretion: Urine 93% (as metabolites); feces 16%

Dosing

Adults & Elderly: Begin antiemetic therapy 3 days prior to initiation and continue for 2 months before reassessing need.

Parkinson's disease, "off" episode: SubQ: Initial test dose 2 mg, **medical supervision required; see "Note".** Subsequent dosing is based on both tolerance and response to initial test dose.

If patient tolerates test dose and responds: Starting dose: 2 mg as needed; may increase dose in 1 mg increments every few days; maximum dose: 6 mg

If patient tolerates but does not respond to 2 mg test dose: Second test dose: 4 mg

If patient tolerates and responds to 4 mg test dose: Starting dose: 3 mg, as needed for "off" episodes; may increase dose in 1 mg increments every few days; maximum dose 6 mg

If patient does not tolerate 4 mg test dose: Third test dose: 3 mg

If patient tolerates 3 mg test dose: Starting dose: 2 mg as needed for "off" episodes; may increase dose in 1 mg increments to a maximum of 3 mg

If therapy is interrupted for >1 week, restart at 2 mg and gradually titrate dose.

(Continued)

Apomorphine *(Continued)*

Note: Medical supervision is required for all test doses with standing and supine blood pressure monitoring predose and 20-, 40-, and 60 minutes postdose. If subsequent test doses are required, wait >2 hours before another test dose is given; next test dose should be timed with another "off" episode. If a single dose is ineffective for a particular "off" episode, then a second dose should not be given. The average dosing frequency was 3 times/day in the development program with limited experience in dosing >5 times/day and with total daily doses >20 mg. Apomorphine is intended to treat the "off" episodes associated with levodopa therapy of Parkinson's disease and has not been studied in levodopa-naive Parkinson's patients.

Renal Impairment:
Mild-to-moderate impairment: Reduce test dose and starting dose: 1 mg
Severe impairment: Has not been studied

Hepatic Impairment:
Mild-to-moderate: Use caution
Severe impairment: Has not been studied

Available Dosage Forms Injection, solution, as hydrochloride: 10 mg/mL (2 mL) [contains sodium metabisulfite]; (3 mL) [multidose cartridge; contains sodium metabisulfite and benzyl alcohol]

Monitoring and Teaching Issues

Physical Assessment: Assess potential for interactions with other prescriptions, OTC medications, or herbal products patient may be taking. See Dosing and Administration for specifics about "test" doses and necessity of premedication with antiemetic prior to each dose. Patient must be monitored closely for minimum of 90 minutes following each test dose (eg, orthostatic hypotension). Assess therapeutic effectiveness and adverse response (eg, orthostatic hypotension, nausea, vomiting, dyskinesias, excessive sedation or somnolence) at beginning of therapy, with each change in dose, and at regular intervals during therapy. Teach patient (or caregiver) proper use (injection pen or syringe, needle disposal), possible side effects/appropriate interventions, and adverse symptoms to report.

Patient Education: Do not take any new medications during therapy without consulting prescriber. Follow specific directions for administration with injection pen or syringe and needle disposal. Avoid alcohol while taking Apokyn™. An antiemetic may be prescribed to reduce nausea or vomiting; take as directed. May cause headache, drowsiness or dizziness (use caution when climbing stairs, driving, or engaged in potentially hazardous tasks until response to drug is known); postural hypotension (use caution climbing stairs or when changing position from lying or sitting to standing); nausea or vomiting (if antiemetic medication does not relieve this, contact prescriber). Report immediately any irregular or rapid heartbeat, chest pain, palpitations, difficulty breathing, shortness of breath; unusual or sudden sleepiness; unusual muscle or skeletal movements or weakness, tremors, or altered gait; CNS changes (hallucinations, confusion, insomnia, anxiety, or depression); redness, swelling, or irritation at injection site, or other persistent side effects. **Pregnancy/breast-feeding precautions:** Inform prescriber if you are or intend to become pregnant. Breast-feeding is contraindicated.

Dietary Considerations: Avoid ethanol consumption.

Pregnancy Risk Factor: C

Lactation: Excretion in breast milk unknown/contraindicated

Administration

I.V.: Not for I.V. administration.

Other: SubQ: Initiate antiemetic 3 days before test dose of apomorphine and continue for 2 months (if patient to be treated) before reassessment. Administer in abdomen, upper arm, or upper leg; change site with each injection. 3 mL cartridges are used with a manual, reusable, multidose injector pen. Injector pen can deliver doses up to 1 mL in 0.02 mL increments. Do not give intravenously; thrombus formation or pulmonary embolism may occur.

Storage: Store at 15°C to 30°C (59°F to 86°F).

- ♦ **Apomorphine Hydrochloride** *see Apomorphine on page 131*
- ♦ **Apomorphine Hydrochloride Hemihydrate** *see Apomorphine on page 131*
- ♦ **Apothecary / Metric Equivalents** *see page 1683*
- ♦ **APPG** *see Penicillin G Procaine on page 1175*
- ♦ **Apraclonidine** *see page 1625*

Apraclonidine *(a pra KLOE ni deen)*

U.S. Brand Names Iopidine®

Synonyms Aplonidine; Apraclonidine Hydrochloride; p-Aminoclonidine

Generic Available No

Pharmacologic Category Alpha$_2$ Agonist, Ophthalmic

Medication Safety Issues
Sound-alike/look-alike issues:
Iopidine® may be confused with indapamide, iodine, Lodine®

Use Prevention and treatment of postsurgical intraocular pressure (IOP) elevation; short-term, adjunctive therapy in patients who require additional reduction of IOP

Contraindications Hypersensitivity to apraclonidine, clonidine, or any component of the formulation; use with or with 14 days of MAO inhibitors

Warnings/Precautions IOP-lowering efficacy decreases over time in some patients; most patients will experience decreased benefit from therapy lasting longer than 1 month. Closely monitor patients who develop exaggerated reductions in intraocular pressure; use with caution in patients with cardiovascular disease, coronary insufficiency, recent myocardial infarction, cerebrovascular disease, history of vasovagal reactions, Raynaud's disease, thromboangiitis obliterans, depression, chronic renal failure, or severe renal or hepatic impairment.

Drug Interactions
Increased Effect/Toxicity: Topical beta-blockers, pilocarpine may have an additive effect on intraocular pressure. Apraclonidine may reduce pulse and blood pressure; use systemic agents with caution. Adverse effects may be additive with CNS-depressant agents. Use with MAO inhibitors is contraindicated.

Adverse Reactions
Ocular:
5% to 15%: Discomfort, hyperemia, pruritus
1% to 5%: Blanching, blurred vision, conjunctivitis, discharge, dry eye, foreign body sensation, lid edema, tearing

Other body systems:
1% to 10%: Gastrointestinal: Dry mouth (10%)
<3%:
Cardiovascular: Arrhythmia, chest pain, facial edema, peripheral edema
Central nervous system: Depression, dizziness, headache, insomnia, malaise, nervousness, somnolence
Dermatologic: Contact dermatitis, dermatitis
Gastrointestinal: Constipation, nausea, taste perversion
Neuromuscular & skeletal: Abnormal coordination, myalgia, paresthesia, weakness
Respiratory: Asthma, dry nose, dyspnea, parosmia, pharyngitis, rhinitis

Overdosage/Toxicology Bradycardia, drowsiness, and hypothermia have been reported following ingestion of the ophthalmic solution.

Pharmacodynamics/Kinetics
Onset of Action: 1 hour; Peak effect: Decreased intraocular pressure: 3-5 hours
Absorption: Ocular: Systemically absorbed
Half-Life Elimination: Systemic: 8 hours

Dosing
Adults & Elderly: Postsurgical intraocular pressure elevation (prevention/treatment): Ophthalmic:
0.5%: Instill 1-2 drops in the affected eye(s) 3 times/day
1%: Instill 1 drop in operative eye 1 hour prior to anterior segment laser surgery, second drop in eye immediately upon completion of procedure

Renal Impairment: Although the topical use of apraclonidine has not been studied in renal failure patients, structurally related clonidine undergoes a significant increase in half-life in patients with severe renal impairment. Close monitoring of cardiovascular parameters in patients with impaired renal function is advised.

Hepatic Impairment: Close monitoring of cardiovascular parameters in patients with impaired liver function is advised because the systemic dosage form of clonidine is partially metabolized in the liver.

Available Dosage Forms Solution, ophthalmic, as hydrochloride: 0.5% (5 mL, 10 mL); 1% (0.1 mL) [contains benzalkonium chloride]

Monitoring and Teaching Issues
Physical Assessment: See Warnings/Precautions for use cautions (eg, patients with cardiovascular disease, cerebrovascular disease, Raynaud's disease, depression, renal failure, or severe renal or hepatic impairment). Assess potential for interactions with other pharmacological agents patient may be taking. Monitor therapeutic response (intraocular pressure) and adverse effects (ocular and other systems; see Adverse Reactions). Teach patient proper use, side effects/appropriate interventions, and adverse symptoms to report.

Patient Education: For use in eyes only; use exactly as directed. May sting on instillation; do not touch dropper to eye. Visual acuity may be decreased after administration; night vision may be decreased and distance vision may be altered (use caution, especially when driving) until response to medication is known. Read package instructions for administration. **Pregnancy/breast-feeding precautions:** Inform prescriber if you are or intend to become pregnant. Consult prescriber if breast-feeding.

Pregnancy Risk Factor: C
Lactation: Excretion in breast milk unknown/use caution

Administration
Other: Wait 5 minutes between instillation of other ophthalmic agents to avoid washout of previous dose. After topical instillation, finger pressure should be applied to lacrimal sac to decrease drainage into the nose and throat and minimize possible systemic absorption.

Storage: Store between 2°C to 27°C (36°F to 80°F). Protect from freezing and light.

Related Information
Glaucoma Drug Therapy *on page 1827*

♦ **Apraclonidine Hydrochloride** *see Apraclonidine on page 132*

Aprepitant *(ap RE pi tant)*
U.S. Brand Names Emend®
Synonyms L 754030; MK 869
Generic Available No
Pharmacologic Category Antiemetic; Substance P/Neurokinin 1 Receptor Antagonist
Use Prevention of acute and delayed nausea and vomiting associated with highly-emetogenic chemotherapy in combination with a corticosteroid and $5-HT_3$ receptor antagonist
Mechanism of Action/Effect Prevents acute and delayed vomiting at the substance P/neurokinin 1 (NK_1) receptor.
Contraindications Hypersensitivity to aprepitant or any component of the formulation; use with cisapride or pimozide
Warnings/Precautions Use caution with agents primarily metabolized via CYP3A4. Use caution with hepatic impairment. Not intended for treatment of nausea and vomiting or for chronic continuous therapy. Safety and efficacy in pediatric patients have not been established.
(Continued)

Aprepitant *(Continued)*

Drug Interactions

Cytochrome P450 Effect: Substrate of CYP1A2 (minor), 2C19 (minor), 3A4 (major); **Inhibits** CYP2C8/9 (weak), 2C19 (weak), 3A4 (moderate); **Induces** CYP2C9 (weak), 3A4 (weak)

Decreased Effect: CYP3A4 inducers may decrease the levels/effects of aprepitant; example inducers include aminoglutethimide, carbamazepine, nafcillin, nevirapine, phenobarbital, phenytoin, and rifamycins. Metabolism of warfarin may be induced; monitor INR following the start of each cycle. Efficacy of oral contraceptives may be decreased (plasma levels of ethinyl estradiol and norethindrone decreased with concomitant use). Plasma levels of both paroxetine and aprepitant are decreased with concomitant use.

Increased Effect/Toxicity: Use with cisapride or pimozide is contraindicated. CYP3A4 inhibitors may increase the levels/effects of aprepitant; example inhibitors include azole antifungals, ciprofloxacin, clarithromycin, diclofenac, diltiazem, doxycycline, erythromycin, imatinib, isoniazid, nefazodone, nicardipine, propofol, protease inhibitors, quinidine, and verapamil. Aprepitant may increase the bioavailability of corticosteroids; dose adjustment of dexamethasone and methylprednisolone is needed. Aprepitant may increase the levels/effects of CYP3A4 substrates; example substrates include benzodiazepines, calcium channel blockers, ergot derivatives, mirtazapine, nateglinide, nefazodone, tacrolimus, and venlafaxine.

Nutritional/Ethanol Interactions

Food: Aprepitant serum concentration may be increased when taken with grapefruit juice; avoid concurrent use.

Herb/Nutraceutical: St John's wort may decrease aprepitant levels.

Adverse Reactions Percentages reported as part of combination therapy.

>10%:
Central nervous system: Fatigue (18%)
Gastrointestinal: Nausea (13%)
Neuromuscular & skeletal: Weakness (18%)
Miscellaneous: Hiccups (11%)

1% to 10%:
Central nervous system: Dizziness (7%)
Endocrine & metabolic: Dehydration (6%)
Gastrointestinal: Diarrhea (10%), abdominal pain (5%), epigastric discomfort (4%), gastritis (4%)
Hepatic: ALT increased (6%), AST increased (3%)
Renal: BUN increased (5%), proteinuria (7%), serum creatinine increased (4%)

Overdosage/Toxicology Limited data available; single doses up to 600 mg were well-tolerated, drowsiness was noted at a dose of 1440 mg. In case of overdose, treatment should be symptom-directed and supportive. Not removed by hemodialysis.

Pharmacodynamics/Kinetics

Bioavailability: 60% to 65%

Time to Peak: Plasma: 4 hours

Protein Binding: >95%

Half-Life Elimination: Terminal: 9-13 hours

Metabolism: Extensively hepatic via CYP3A4 (major); CYP1A2 and CYP2C19 (minor); forms seven metabolites (weakly active)

Dosing

Adults & Elderly: Antiemetic: Oral: 125 mg on day 1, followed by 80 mg on days 2 and 3; should be used in combination with a corticosteroid and 5-HT$_3$ receptor antagonist

In clinical trials, the following regimen was used:
Aprepitant: Oral: 125 mg day 1, followed by 80 mg on days 2 and 3
Dexamethasone: Oral: 12 mg on day 1, followed 8 mg on days 2, 3, and 4
Ondansetron: I.V.: 32 mg on day 1

Renal Impairment: No dose adjustment necessary in patients with renal disease or end-stage renal disease maintained on hemodialysis.

Hepatic Impairment:
Mild to moderate impairment (Child-Pugh score 5-9): No adjustment necessary.
Severe impairment (Child-Pugh score >9): No data available.

Available Dosage Forms

Capsule: 80 mg, 125 mg
Combination package: Capsule 80 mg (2s), capsule 125 mg (1s)

Monitoring and Teaching Issues

Physical Assessment: Should be used in combination with other medications (see Dosing). Assess potential for interactions with other pharmacological agents or herbal products patient may be taking (see Warnings/Precautions and Drug Interactions). Assess for therapeutic effectiveness (decreased nausea/vomiting) and adverse reactions (eg, fatigue, weakness, gastrointestinal disturbance, dehydration; see Adverse Reactions). Teach proper use, possible side effects/appropriate interventions, and adverse symptoms to report.

Patient Education: This medication will be prescribed in combination with other medications; follow directions and timing exactly. May take with or without food; avoid grapefruit juice and St John's Wort while taking this medication. Report unusual fatigue, weakness, dizziness, disorientation, abdominal discomfort, chest pain, respiratory distress or other persistent side effects to prescriber. **Breast-feeding precaution:** Breast-feeding is not recommended.

Dietary Considerations: May be taken with or without food.

Geriatric Considerations: In two studies by the manufacturer, with a total of 544 patients, 31% were >65 years of age, while 5% were >75 years. No differences in safety and efficacy were noted between elderly subjects and younger adults. No dosing adjustment is necessary.

Pregnancy Risk Factor: B

Lactation: Excretion in breast milk unknown/not recommended

Administration

Oral: May be administered with or without food. First dose should be given 1 hour prior to chemotherapy; subsequent doses should be given in the morning.

Storage: Store at controlled room temperature of 20°C to 25°C (68°F to 77°F).

♦ **Apresazide [DSC]** see Hydralazine and Hydrochlorothiazide on page 751
♦ **Apresoline [DSC]** see HydrALAZINE on page 749
♦ **Apri®** see Ethinyl Estradiol and Desogestrel on page 578
♦ **Aquachloral® Supprettes®** see Chloral Hydrate on page 303
♦ **Aqua Gem E®[OTC]** see Vitamin E on page 1569
♦ **Aquanil™ HC [OTC]** see Hydrocortisone on page 760
♦ **Aquasol E® [OTC]** see Vitamin E on page 1569
♦ **Aquatab® D [DSC]** see Guaifenesin and Pseudoephedrine on page 733
♦ **Aquatab® DM [DSC]** see Guaifenesin and Dextromethorphan on page 731
♦ **Aqueous Procaine Penicillin G** see Penicillin G Procaine on page 1175
♦ **Arabinosylcytosine** see Cytarabine on page 389
♦ **Ara-C** see Cytarabine on page 389
♦ **Aralen®** see Chloroquine on page 310
♦ **Aranelle™** see Ethinyl Estradiol and Norethindrone on page 589
♦ **Aranesp®** see Darbepoetin Alfa on page 405
♦ **Arava®** see Leflunomide on page 870
♦ **Aredia®** see Pamidronate on page 1149

Argatroban (ar GA troh ban)

Generic Available No

Pharmacologic Category Anticoagulant, Thrombin Inhibitor

Medication Safety Issues

Sound-alike/look-alike issues:

Argatroban may be confused with Aggrastat®

Use Prophylaxis or treatment of thrombosis in adults with heparin-induced thrombocytopenia; adjunct to percutaneous coronary intervention (PCI) in patients who have or are at risk of thrombosis associated with heparin-induced thrombocytopenia

Mechanism of Action/Effect A direct, highly selective thrombin inhibitor. Reversibly binds to the active thrombin site of free and clot-associated thrombin. Inhibits fibrin formation; activation of coagulation factors V, VIII, and XIII; protein C; and platelet aggregation.

Contraindications Hypersensitivity to argatroban or any component of the formulation; overt major bleeding

Warnings/Precautions Hemorrhage can occur at any site in the body. Extreme caution should be used when there is an increased danger of hemorrhage, such as severe hypertension, immediately following lumbar puncture, spinal anesthesia, major surgery (including brain, spinal cord, or eye surgery), congenital or acquired bleeding disorders, and gastrointestinal ulcers. Use caution in critically-ill patients; reduced clearance may require dosage reduction. Use caution with hepatic dysfunction. Concomitant use with warfarin will cause increased prolongation of the PT and INR greater than that of warfarin alone; alternative guidelines for monitoring therapy should be followed. Safety and efficacy for use with other thrombolytic agents has not been established. Discontinue all parenteral anticoagulants prior to starting therapy. Allow reversal of heparin's effects before initiation. Patients with hepatic dysfunction may require >4 hours to achieve full reversal of argatroban's anticoagulant effect following treatment. Avoid use during PCI in patients with elevations of ALT/AST (>3 times ULN); the use of argatroban in these patients has not been evaluated. Safety and efficacy in children <18 years of age have not been established.

Drug Interactions

Cytochrome P450 Effect: Substrate of CYP3A4 (minor)

Increased Effect/Toxicity: Drugs which affect platelet function (eg, aspirin, NSAIDs, dipyridamole, ticlopidine, clopidogrel), anticoagulants, or thrombolytics may potentiate the risk of hemorrhage. Sufficient time must pass after heparin therapy is discontinued; allow heparin's effect on the aPTT to decrease

Concomitant use of argatroban with warfarin increases PT and INR greater than that of warfarin alone. Argatroban is commonly continued during the initiation of warfarin therapy to assure anticoagulation and to protect against possible transient hypercoagulability.

Lab Interactions Argatroban produces dose-dependent effects on PT, INR, ACT, and TT, however, therapeutic ranges are not established.

Adverse Reactions As with all anticoagulants, bleeding is the major adverse effect of argatroban. Hemorrhage may occur at virtually any site. Risk is dependent on multiple variables, including the intensity of anticoagulation and patient susceptibility.

>10%:

Gastrointestinal: Gastrointestinal bleed (minor, 14%; <1% in PCI)

Genitourinary: Genitourinary bleed and hematuria (minor, 12%)

1% to 10%:

Cardiovascular: Hypotension (7%), cardiac arrest (6%), ventricular tachycardia (5%), atrial fibrillation (3%), cerebrovascular disorder (2%)

Central nervous system: Fever (7%), pain (7%), intracranial bleeding (1%, only observed in patients also receiving streptokinase or tissue plasminogen activator)

Gastrointestinal: Diarrhea (6%), nausea (5%), vomiting (4%), abdominal pain (3%), bleeding (major, 2%)

Genitourinary: Urinary tract infection (5%)

Hematologic: Decreased hemoglobin <2 g/dL and hematocrit (minor, 10%)

Local: Bleeding at the injection site (minor, 2% to 5%)

Renal: Abnormal renal function (3%)

(Continued)

Argatroban *(Continued)*

Respiratory: Dyspnea (8% to 10%), cough (3% to 10%), hemoptysis (minor, 3%), pneumonia (3%)

Miscellaneous: Sepsis (6%), infection (4%)

Overdosage/Toxicology No specific antidote is available. Treatment should be symptomatic and supportive. Discontinue or decrease infusion to control excessive anticoagulation with or without bleeding. Reversal of anticoagulant effects may be longer than 4 hours in patients with hepatic impairment.

Pharmacodynamics/Kinetics

Onset of Action: Immediate

Time to Peak: Steady-state: 1-3 hours

Protein Binding: Albumin: 20%; α_1-acid glycoprotein: 35%

Half-Life Elimination: 39-51 minutes; Hepatic impairment: ≤181 minutes

Metabolism: Hepatic via hydroxylation and aromatization. Metabolism via CYP3A4/5 to four known metabolites plays a minor role. Unchanged argatroban is the major plasma component. Plasma concentration of metabolite M1 is 0% to 20% of the parent drug and is three-to fivefold weaker.

Excretion: Feces (65%); urine (22%); low quantities of metabolites M2-4 in urine

Dosing

Adults & Elderly:

Prophylaxis of thrombosis (heparin-induced thrombocytopenia): I.V.:

Initial dose: 2 mcg/kg/minute

Maintenance dose: Measure aPTT after 2 hours, adjust dose until the steady-state aPTT is 1.5-3.0 times the initial baseline value, not exceeding 100 seconds; dosage should not exceed 10 mcg/kg/minute

Conversion to oral anticoagulant: Because there may be a combined effect on the INR when argatroban is combined with warfarin, loading doses of warfarin should not be used. Warfarin therapy should be started at the expected daily dose.

Patients receiving ≤2 mcg/kg/minute of argatroban: Argatroban therapy can be stopped when the combined INR on warfarin and argatroban is >4; repeat INR measurement in 4-6 hours; if INR is below therapeutic level, argatroban therapy may be restarted. Repeat procedure daily until desired INR on warfarin alone is obtained.

Patients receiving >2 mcg/kg/minute of argatroban: Reduce dose of argatroban to 2 mcg/kg/minute; measure INR for argatroban and warfarin 4-6 hours after dose reduction; argatroban therapy can be stopped when the combined INR on warfarin and argatroban is >4. Repeat INR measurement in 4-6 hours; if INR is below therapeutic level, argatroban therapy may be restarted. Repeat procedure daily until desired INR on warfarin alone is obtained.

Note: Critically-ill patients with normal hepatic function became excessively anticoagulated with FDA-approved or lower starting doses of argatroban. Doses between 0.15-1.3 mcg/kg/minute were required to maintain aPTTs in the target range. Another report of a cardiac patient with anasarca secondary to acute renal failure had a reduction in argatroban clearance similar to patient with hepatic dysfunction. Reduced clearance may have been attributed to reduced perfusion to the liver. Consider reducing starting dose to 0.5-1 mcg/kg/minute in critically-ill patients who may have impaired hepatic perfusion (eg, patients requiring vasopressors, having decreased cardiac output, having fluid overload).

Percutaneous coronary intervention (PCI): I.V.:

Initial: Begin infusion of 25 mcg/kg/minute and administer bolus dose of 350 mcg/kg (over 3-5 minutes). ACT should be checked 5-10 minutes after bolus infusion; proceed with procedure if ACT >300 seconds. Following initial bolus:

ACT <300 seconds: Give an additional 150 mcg/kg bolus, and increase infusion rate to 30 mcg/kg/minute (recheck ACT in 5-10 minutes)

ACT >450 seconds: Decrease infusion rate to 15 mcg/kg/minute (recheck ACT in 5-10 minutes)

Once a therapeutic ACT (300-450 seconds) is achieved, infusion should be continued at this dose for the duration of the procedure.

Impending abrupt closure, thrombus formation during PCI, or inability to achieve ACT >300 sec: An additional bolus of 150 mcg/kg, followed by an increase in infusion rate to 40 mcg/kg/minute may be administered.

Renal Impairment: No adjustment is necessary.

Hepatic Impairment: Decreased clearance and increased elimination half-life are seen with hepatic impairment; dose should be reduced. Initial dose for moderate hepatic impairment is 0.5 mcg/kg/minute. **Note:** During PCI, avoid use in patients with elevations of ALT/AST (>3 times ULN); the use of argatroban in these patients has not been evaluated.

Available Dosage Forms Injection, solution: 100 mg/mL (2.5 mL) [contains dehydrated alcohol 1000 mg/mL]

Monitoring and Teaching Issues

Physical Assessment: Use caution with patients at increased danger of hemorrhage, critically-ill patients; patients with hepatic dysfunction (see Warnings/Precautions). Assess potential for interactions with other pharmacological agents patient may be taking(especially drugs which affect platelet function or coagulation). Assess for therapeutic effectiveness according to purpose for use and adverse reactions (eg, abnormal bleeding, GI pain, hematuria, infusion site; see Adverse Reactions) frequently during therapy. Observe bleeding precautions and teach patient interventions to reduce side effects and adverse reactions to report.

Monitoring Laboratory Tests: Hemoglobin, hematocrit

Patient Education: This medication can only be administered by intravenous infusion; you will observed closely and monitored with blood tests during therapy. You may have a tendency to bleed easily; use electric razor, brush teeth with soft brush, floss with waxed floss, avoid all scissors or sharp instruments (knives, needles, etc), and avoid injury or bruising. Report stomach cramping or pain; dark or bloody stools; blood in urine; acute

headache or confusion; respiratory difficulty; nosebleed; or bleeding from gums.
Breast-feeding precaution: Breast-feeding is not recommended.

Pregnancy Risk Factor: B

Lactation: Excretion in breast milk unknown/not recommended

Breast-Feeding Issues: It is not known if argatroban is excreted in human milk. Because of the serious potential of adverse effects to the nursing infant, a decision to discontinue nursing or discontinue argatroban should be considered.

Administration

I.V.: Solution **must be diluted to 1 mg/mL** prior to administration.

Reconstitution: May be mixed with 0.9% sodium chloride injection, 5% dextrose injection, or lactated Ringer's injection. Do not mix with other medications. To prepare solution for I.V. administration, dilute each 250 mg vial with 250 mL of diluent. Mix by repeated inversion for one minute. Once mixed, final concentration should be 1 mg/mL. A slight but brief haziness may occur prior to mixing.

Compatibility: Stable in 0.9% NS, D_5W, LR; do not expose diluted solution to direct sunlight (light-resistant containers are not necessary with exposure to ambient light)
Y-site administration: Incompatible with other medications
Compatibility when admixed: Incompatible with other medications

Storage: Store at 25°C (77°F). Protect from light. The prepared solution is stable for 24 hours at 25°C (77°F) in ambient indoor light. Do not expose to direct sunlight. Prepared solutions are stable for 48 hours at 2°C to 8°C when stored in the dark.

Additional Information Platelet counts recovered by day 3 in 53% of patients with heparin-induced thrombocytopenia and in 58% of patients with heparin-induced thrombocytopenia with thrombosis syndrome.

♦ **8-Arginine Vasopressin** *see* Vasopressin *on page 1554*

♦ **Aricept**® *see* Donepezil *on page 480*

♦ **Arimidex**® *see* Anastrozole *on page 121*

Aripiprazole (ay ri PIP ray zole)

U.S. Brand Names Abilify®

Synonyms BMS 337039; OPC-14597

Generic Available No

Pharmacologic Category Antipsychotic Agent, Atypical

Medication Safety Issues

Sound-alike/look-alike issues:

Aripiprazole may be confused with rabeprazole

Use Treatment of schizophrenia; stabilization and maintenance therapy of bipolar disorder (with acute manic or mixed episodes)

Unlabeled/Investigational Use Depression with psychotic features

Mechanism of Action/Effect Aripiprazole (quinolinone antipsychotic) is a dopamine-serotonin system stabilizer with activity at dopamine and serotonin receptors. It improves symptoms of schizophrenia.

Contraindications Hypersensitivity to aripiprazole or any component of the formulation

Warnings/Precautions Patients with dementia-related behavioral disorders treated with atypical antipsychotics are at an increased risk of death compared to placebo. Aripiprazole is not approved for this indication.

May cause extrapyramidal symptoms, including pseudoparkinsonism, acute dystonic reactions, akathisia, and tardive dyskinesia (risk of these reactions is very low relative to typical/conventional antipsychotics, frequencies reported are similar to placebo). May be associated with neuroleptic malignant syndrome (NMS). The possibility of suicide attempt is inherent in psychosis and bipolar disorder.

May be sedating, use with caution in disorders where CNS depression is a feature. May cause orthostatic hypotension (although reported rates are similar to placebo); use caution in patients at risk of this effect or those who would not tolerate transient hypotensive episodes (cerebrovascular disease, cardiovascular disease, or other medications which may predispose). Clinical data have demonstrated an increased incidence of serious, including fatal, cardiovascular events in elderly patients.

Use caution in patients with Parkinson's disease; hemodynamic instability; bone marrow suppression; predisposition to seizures; subcortical brain damage; severe cardiac, hepatic, renal, or respiratory disease. Esophageal dysmotility and aspiration have been associated with antipsychotic use; use caution in patients at risk of pneumonia (ie, Alzheimer's disease). May alter temperature regulation or mask toxicity of other drugs due to antiemetic effects. Use caution in patients with a history of drug abuse.

Atypical antipsychotics have been associated with development of hyperglycemia; in some cases may be extreme and associated with ketoacidosis, hyperosmolar coma, or death. Reports of hyperglycemia with aripiprazole therapy have been few and specific risk associated with this agent is not known. Use caution in patients with diabetes or other disorders of glucose regulation; monitor for worsening of glucose control.

The possibility of a suicide attempt is inherent in psychotic illness or bipolar disorder; use caution in high-risk patients during initiation of therapy. Prescriptions should be written for the smallest quantity consistent with good patient care. Safety and efficacy in pediatric patients have not been established.

Drug Interactions

Cytochrome P450 Effect: Substrate (major) of CYP2D6, 3A4

Decreased Effect: CYP3A4 inducers may decrease the levels/effects of aripiprazole; example inducers include aminoglutethimide, carbamazepine, nafcillin, nevirapine, phenobarbital, phenytoin, and rifamycins. Manufacturer recommends a doubling of the aripiprazole dose when carbamazepine is added. Similar increases may be required with other inducers.

(Continued)

Aripiprazole *(Continued)*

Increased Effect/Toxicity: CYP2D6 inhibitors may increase the levels/effects of aripiprazole; example inhibitors include chlorpromazine, delavirdine, fluoxetine, miconazole, paroxetine, pergolide, quinidine, quinine, ritonavir, and ropinirole. CYP3A4 inhibitors may increase the levels/effects of aripiprazole; example inhibitors include azole antifungals, ciprofloxacin, clarithromycin, diclofenac, doxycycline, erythromycin, imatinib, isoniazid, nefazodone, nicardipine, propofol, protease inhibitors, quinidine, and verapamil. Manufacturer recommends a 50% reduction in dose during concurrent ketoconazole therapy. Similar reductions in dose may be required with other potent inhibitors.

Nutritional/Ethanol Interactions
Ethanol: Avoid ethanol (may increase CNS depression).
Food: Ingestion with a high-fat meal delays time to peak plasma level.
Herb/Nutraceutical: St John's wort may decrease aripiprazole levels. Avoid kava kava, gotu kola, valerian, St John's wort (may increase CNS depression).

Adverse Reactions
>10%:
  Central nervous system: Headache (31%), agitation (25%), anxiety (20%), insomnia (20%), somnolence (12%), akathisia (15%), lightheadedness (11%)
  Endocrine & metabolic: Weight gain (8% to 30%; highest frequency in patients with BMI <23)
  Gastrointestinal: Nausea (16%), dyspepsia (15%), constipation (13%), vomiting (11%)
1% to 10%:
  Cardiovascular: Edema (peripheral 2%), hypertension (2%), tachycardia, hypotension, bradycardia, chest pain
  Central nervous system: Extrapyramidal symptoms (6%), fever, depression, nervousness, mania, confusion, hallucination, hostility, paranoid reaction, suicidal thought, delusion, abnormal dream
  Dermatologic: Rash (6%), dry skin, skin ulcer
  Endocrine & metabolic: Dehydration, hypothyroidism
  Gastrointestinal: Salivation increased (3%), anorexia
  Genitourinary: Urinary incontinence, pelvic pain
  Hematologic: Anemia, bruising
  Neuromuscular & skeletal: Weakness (8%), myalgia (4%), tremor (4%), neck pain, neck rigidity, muscle cramp, CPK increased, abnormal gait
  Ocular: Blurred vision (3%), conjunctivitis
  Respiratory: Rhinitis (4%), pharyngitis (4%), asthma, cough (3%), dyspnea, pneumonia, sinusitis
  Miscellaneous: Accidental injury (6%), flu-like syndrome

Overdosage/Toxicology Symptoms of overdose include nausea, weakness, diarrhea, somnolence, and vomiting. Treatment is supportive; an ECG should be obtained and monitored if abnormalities are present. Due to the high degree of protein binding, hemodialysis is unlikely to be effective in removing aripiprazole.

Pharmacodynamics/Kinetics
  Onset of Action: Initial: 1-3 weeks
  Absorption: Well absorbed
  Bioavailability: 87%
  Time to Peak: Plasma: 3-5 hours; delayed 3 hours with high-fat meal
  Protein Binding: 99%, primarily to albumin
  Half-Life Elimination: Aripiprazole: 75 hours; dehydro-aripiprazole: 94 hours
  Metabolism: Hepatic, via CYP2D6, CYP3A4 (dehydro-aripiprazole metabolite has affinity for D2 receptors similar to the parent drug and represents 40% of the parent drug exposure in plasma)
  Excretion: Feces (55%), urine (25%); primarily as metabolites

Dosing
  Adults & Elderly: Note: Oral solution may be substituted for the oral tablet on a mg-per-mg basis, up to 25 mg. Patients receiving 30 mg tablets should be given 25 mg oral solution.

  Schizophrenia: Oral: 10-15 mg once daily; may be increased to a maximum of 30 mg once daily (efficacy at dosages above 10-15 mg has not been shown to be increased). Dosage titration should not be more frequent than every 2 weeks.
  Bipolar disorder (acute manic or mixed episodes):
    Stabilization: Oral: 30 mg once daily; may require a decrease to 15 mg based on tolerability (15% of patients had dose decreased); safety of doses >30 mg/day has not been evaluated
    Maintenance: Continue stabilization dose for up to 6 weeks; efficacy of continued treatment >6 weeks has not been established.
  Dosage adjustment with concurrent CYP3A4 inducer therapy: With the addition of CYP3A4 inducers (eg, carbamazepine), aripiprazole dose should be doubled. If CYP3A4 inducers are withdrawn from therapy with aripiprazole, aripiprazole dose should be decreased by one-half.
  Renal Impairment: No dosage adjustment required.
  Hepatic Impairment: No dosage adjustment required.

Available Dosage Forms
  Solution, oral: 1 mg/mL (50 mL, 150 mL, 480 mL) [contains sucrose 400 mg/mL and fructose 200 mg/mL; orange flavor]
  Tablet: 5 mg, 10 mg, 15 mg, 20 mg, 30 mg [contains lactose]

Monitoring and Teaching Issues
  Physical Assessment: Assess personal/family history of diabetes vital signs, blood pressure; mental status, thoughts of suicide ideation, abnormal involuntary movement scale (AIMS), extrapyramidal symptoms (EPS). Weight and waist circumference should be assessed prior to treatment, at 4 weeks, 8 weeks, 12 weeks, and then at quarterly intervals. Consider titrating to a different antipsychotic agent for a weight gain greater than or equal to 5% of the initial weight. This drug may alter glucose regulation and control. Monitor

closely. Assess potential for interactions with other prescriptions, OTC medications, or herbal products patient may be taking. Assess results of laboratory tests prior to and periodically during therapy (eg, ophthalmic hematological, cardiovascular). Assess therapeutic effectiveness and adverse response (eg, extrapyramidal symptoms, neuroleptic malignant syndrome) at beginning of and at regular intervals during therapy. Teach patient proper use, possible side effects/appropriate interventions, and adverse symptoms to report.

Monitoring Laboratory Tests: Fasting lipid profile and fasting blood glucose/Hgb A$_{1c}$ (prior to treatment, at 3 months, then annually); BMI

Patient Education: Do not take any new medication during therapy without consulting prescriber. Take exactly as directed at the same time of day, without regard to meals. Do not alter dose; it may take some time to achieve desired results. Avoid alcohol. May cause headache, dizziness, lightheadedness, anxiety (use caution when driving or engaged in potentially hazardous tasks until response to drug is known), nausea or vomiting (small frequent meals and frequent mouth care may help), orthostatic hypotension (use caution when changing position from lying or sitting to standing and when climbing stairs). Report chest pain or palpitations; persistent gastrointestinal effects; muscle or skeletal pain, weakness, cramping, or tremors; involuntary movements, altered gait; change in vision; change in mental status (especially suicide ideation); increased weight gain or loss; respiratory changes or flu-like symptoms.

Dietary Considerations: May be taken with or without food. Oral solution contains sucrose 400 mg/mL and fructose 200 mg/mL.

Geriatric Considerations: Not approved for treatment of psychosis associated with Alzheimer's dementia; elderly patients may be at greater risk of serious, and possibly fatal cerebrovascular events

Pregnancy Risk Factor: C

Lactation: Excretion in breast milk unknown/not recommended

Breast-Feeding Issues: Excretion in breast milk is unknown (excreted in animal models). Breast-feeding is not recommended.

Administration

Oral: May be administered with or without food. Tablet and oral solution may be interchanged on a mg-per-mg basis, up to 25 mg. Doses using 30 mg tablets should be exchanged for 25 mg oral solution.

Storage:

Capsule: Store under refrigeration of 2°C to 8°C (36°F to 46°F); use within 6 months after opening

Tablet: Store at 25°C (77°F); excursions permitted to 15°C to 30°C (59°F to 86°F)

Related Information

Antipsychotic Agents *on page 1717*

Arsenic Trioxide (AR se nik tri OKS id)

U.S. Brand Names Trisenox™

Synonyms NSC-706363

Generic Available No

Pharmacologic Category Antineoplastic Agent, Miscellaneous

Use Induction of remission and consolidation in patients with acute promyelocytic leukemia (APL) which is specifically characterized by t(15;17) translocation or PML/RAR-alpha gene expression. Should be used only in those patients who have relapsed or are refractory to retinoid and anthracycline chemotherapy.

Orphan drug: Treatment of myelodysplastic syndrome; multiple myeloma; chronic myeloid leukemia (CML); acute myelocytic leukemia (AML)

Mechanism of Action/Effect Not fully understood; causes *in vitro* morphological changes and DNA fragmentation to NB4 human promyelocytic leukemia cells; also damages or degrades the fusion protein PML-RAR alpha

Contraindications Hypersensitivity to arsenic or any component of the formulation; pregnancy

Warnings/Precautions The U.S. Food and Drug Administration (FDA) currently recommends that procedures for proper handling and disposal of antineoplastic agents be considered. For use only by physicians experienced with the treatment of acute leukemia. A baseline 12-lead ECG, serum electrolytes (potassium, calcium, magnesium), and creatinine should be obtained. Correct electrolyte abnormalities prior to treatment and monitor potassium and magnesium levels during therapy (potassium should stay >4 mEq/dL and magnesium >1.8 mg/dL). Correct QT$_c$ >500 msec prior to treatment. Discontinue therapy and hospitalize patient if QT$_c$ >500 msec, syncope or irregular heartbeats develop during therapy. May prolong the QT interval. May lead to torsade de pointes or complete AV block. Risk factors for torsade de pointes include CHF, a history of torsade de pointes, pre-existing QT interval prolongation, patients taking potassium-wasting diuretics, and conditions which cause hypokalemia or hypomagnesemia. If possible, discontinue all medications known to prolong the QT interval. May cause retinoic-acid-acute promyelocytic leukemia (RA-APL) syndrome or APL differentiation syndrome (high-dose steroids have been used for treatment). May lead to the development of hyperleukocytosis. Use with caution in renal impairment. Safety and efficacy in children <5 years of age have not been established (limited experience with children 5-16 years of age).
(Continued)

Arsenic Trioxide *(Continued)*

Drug Interactions

Increased Effect/Toxicity: Use caution with medications causing hypokalemia or hypomagnesemia (ampho B, aminoglycosides, diuretics, cyclosporin). Use caution with medications that prolong the QT interval, avoid concurrent use if possible; includes type Ia and type III antiarrhythmic agents, selected quinolones (sparfloxacin, gatifloxacin, moxifloxacin, grepafloxacin), cisapride, thioridazine, and other agents.

Nutritional/Ethanol Interactions

Food: Avoid seafood (due to presence of arsenic as arsenobetaine and arsenocholine).

Herb/Nutraceutical: Avoid homeopathic products (arsenic is present in some homeopathic medications).

Adverse Reactions

>10%:

Cardiovascular: Tachycardia (55%), edema (40%), QT interval >500 msec (38%), chest pain (25%), hypotension (25%)

Central nervous system: Fatigue (63%), fever (63%), headache (60%), insomnia (43%), anxiety (30%), dizziness (23%), depression (20%), pain (15%)

Dermatologic: Dermatitis (43%), pruritus (33%), bruising (20%), dry skin (13%)

Endocrine & metabolic: Hypokalemia (50%), hyperglycemia (45%), hypomagnesemia (45%), hyperkalemia (18%)

Gastrointestinal: Nausea (75%), abdominal pain (58%), vomiting (58%), diarrhea (53%), sore throat (40%), constipation (28%), anorexia (23%), decreased appetite (15%), weight gain (13%)

Genitourinary: Vaginal hemorrhage (13%)

Hematologic: Leukocytosis (50%), APL differentiation syndrome (23%), thrombocytopenia (19%), anemia (14%), febrile neutropenia (13%)

Hepatic: Elevated ALT (20%), elevated AST (13%)

Local: Injection site: Pain (20%), erythema (13%)

Neuromuscular & skeletal: Rigors (38%), arthralgia (33%), paresthesia (33%), myalgia (25%), bone pain (23%), back pain (18%), limb pain (13%), neck pain (13%), tremor (13%)

Respiratory: Cough (65%), dyspnea (53%), epistaxis (25%), hypoxia (23%), pleural effusion (20%), sinusitis (20%), postnasal drip (13%), upper respiratory tract infection (13%), wheezing (13%)

Miscellaneous: Herpes simplex (13%)

1% to 10%:

Cardiovascular: Hypotension (10%), flushing (10%), pallor (10%), palpitation (10%), facial edema (8%), abnormal ECG (not QT prolongation) (7%)

Central nervous system: Convulsion (8%), somnolence (8%), agitation (5%), coma (5%), confusion (5%)

Dermatologic: Erythema (10%), hyperpigmentation (8%), petechia (8%), skin lesions (8%), urticaria (8%), local exfoliation (5%)

Endocrine & metabolic: Hypocalcemia (10%), hypoglycemia (8%), acidosis (5%)

Gastrointestinal: Dyspepsia (10%), loose stools (10%), abdominal distension (8%), abdominal tenderness (8%), dry mouth (8%), fecal incontinence (8%), gastrointestinal hemorrhage (8%), hemorrhagic diarrhea (8%), oral blistering (8%), weight loss (8%), oral candidiasis (5%)

Genitourinary: Intermenstrual bleeding (8%), incontinence (5%)

Hematologic: Neutropenia (10%), DIC (8%), hemorrhage (8%), lymphadenopathy (8%)

Neuromuscular & skeletal: Weakness (10%)

Ocular: Blurred vision (10%), eye irritation (10%), dry eye (8%), eyelid edema (5%), painful eye (5%)

Otic: Earache (8%), tinnitus (5%)

Renal: Renal failure (8%), renal impairment (8%), oliguria (5%)

Respiratory: Crepitations (10%), decreased breath sounds (10%), rales (10%), hemoptysis (8%), rhonchi (8%), tachypnea (8%), nasopharyngitis (5%)

Miscellaneous: Diaphoresis increased (10%), injection site edema (10%), bacterial infection (8%), herpes zoster (8%), night sweats (8%), hypersensitivity (5%), sepsis (5%)

Overdosage/Toxicology

Symptoms of arsenic toxicity include convulsions, muscle weakness, and confusion. Discontinue treatment and begin chelation therapy. One suggested adult protocol: Dimercaprol 3 mg/kg I.M. every 4 hours, continue until life-threatening toxicity has subsided; follow with penicillamine 250 mg orally up to 4 times/day (total daily dose ≤1 g).

Pharmacodynamics/Kinetics

Metabolism: Hepatic; pentavalent arsenic is reduced to trivalent arsenic (active) by arsenate reductase; trivalent arsenic is methylated to monomethylarsinic acid, which is then converted to dimethylarsinic acid via methyltransferases

Excretion: Urine (as methylated metabolite); disposition not yet studied

Dosing

Adults:

Antineoplastic:

Induction: I.V.: 0.15 mg/kg/day; administer daily until bone marrow remission; maximum induction: 60 doses

Consolidation: I.V.: 0.15 mg/kg/day starting 3-6 weeks after completion of induction therapy; maximum consolidation: 25 doses over 5 weeks

Elderly: Safety and efficacy have not been established. Clinical trials included patients ≤72 years of age. Use with caution due to the increased risk of renal impairment in the elderly.

Pediatrics: Children >5 years: Refer to adult dosing.

Renal Impairment: Safety and efficacy have not been established; use with caution due to renal elimination.

Hepatic Impairment: Safety and efficacy have not been established.

Available Dosage Forms Injection, solution [preservative free]: 1 mg/mL (10 mL)

Monitoring and Teaching Issues

Physical Assessment: To be used only by physicians experienced with the treatment of acute leukemia. See Warnings/Precautions for use cautions. Assess potential for interactions with other pharmacological agents or herbal products patient may be using; especially anything that may cause hypokalemia or hypomagnesemia, or antiarrhythmic agents. Assess results of laboratory tests at baseline and during therapy (see Monitoring Laboratory Tests). Assess patient response at beginning and periodically during therapy (especially cardiac and electrolyte status; see Adverse Reactions). Teach patient possible side effects/appropriate interventions and adverse symptoms to report.

Monitoring Laboratory Tests: Baseline then weekly 12-lead ECG, baseline then twice weekly serum electrolytes, hematologic and coagulation profiles at least twice weekly; more frequent monitoring may be necessary in unstable patients.

Patient Education: Do not take any new medication during therapy unless approved by prescriber. This medication can only be administered by intravenous infusion. Report immediately any redness, swelling, pain, or burning at infusion site. May cause dizziness, fatigue, blurred vision (use caution when driving or engaging in tasks requiring alertness until response to drug is known); or nausea, vomiting, diarrhea, or decreased appetite (small frequent meals, frequent mouth care, sucking lozenges, or chewing gum may help). Report immediately unexplained fever; respiratory difficulty; chest pain or palpitations; confusion, lightheadedness, or fainting; or other persistent adverse effects. **Pregnancy/breast-feeding precautions:** Inform prescriber if you are pregnant. Do not get pregnant while take this medication. Consult prescriber for appropriate contraceptive methods. Do not breast-feed.

Pregnancy Risk Factor: D

Lactation: Excretion in breast milk unknown/contraindicated

Administration

I.V.: Dilute in 100-250 mL D_5W or 0.9% sodium chloride. Does not contain a preservative; properly discard unused portion. Do not mix with other medications. Infuse over 1-2 hours. If acute vasomotor reactions occur, may infuse over a maximum of 4 hours. Does not require administration via a central venous catheter.

Storage: Store at room temperature, 25°C (77°F); do not freeze. Following dilution, stable for 24 hours at room temperature or 48 hours when refrigerated.

Additional Information Arsenic is stored in liver, kidney, heart, lung, hair, and nails. Arsenic trioxide is a human carcinogen.

* **Artane** *see* Trihexyphenidyl *on page 1526*
* **Arthrotec®** *see* Diclofenac and Misoprostol *on page 444*
* **ASA** *see* Aspirin *on page 143*
* **5-ASA** *see* Mesalamine *on page 957*
* **Asacol®** *see* Mesalamine *on page 957*
* **Ascriptin® [OTC]** *see* Aspirin *on page 143*
* **Ascriptin® Extra Strength [OTC]** *see* Aspirin *on page 143*

Asparaginase (a SPEAR a ji nase)

U.S. Brand Names Elspar®

Synonyms *E. coli* Asparaginase; *Erwinia* Asparaginase; L-asparaginase; NSC-106977 (*Erwinia*); NSC-109229 (*E. coli*)

Generic Available No

Pharmacologic Category Antineoplastic Agent, Miscellaneous

Medication Safety Issues
Sound-alike/look-alike issues:
Asparaginase may be confused with pegaspargase

Use Treatment of acute lymphocytic leukemia, lymphoma

Mechanism of Action/Effect Asparaginase inhibits protein synthesis by hydrolyzing asparagine to aspartic acid and ammonia. Leukemia cells, specially lymphoblasts, require exogenous asparagine; normal cells can synthesize asparagine. Asparaginase is cycle-specific for the G_1 phase.

Contraindications Hypersensitivity to asparaginase or any component of the formulation; history of anaphylaxis to asparaginase; if a reaction occurs to Elspar®, obtain **Erwinia L-asparaginase** and use with caution; pancreatitis (active or any history of)

Warnings/Precautions The U.S. Food and Drug Administration (FDA) currently recommends that procedures for proper handling and disposal of antineoplastic agents be considered. Monitor for severe allergic reactions. May alter hepatic function. Use cautiously in patients with an underlying coagulopathy. Up to 33% of patients who have an allergic reaction to *E. coli* asparaginase will also react to the *Erwinia* form or pegaspargase.

A test dose is often recommended prior to the first dose of asparaginase, or prior to restarting therapy after a hiatus of several days. **False-negative rates of up to 80% to test doses of 2-50 units are reported.** Desensitization may be performed in patients found to be hypersensitive by the intradermal test dose or who have received previous courses of therapy with the drug. See Administration.

Drug Interactions

Decreased Effect: Asparaginase terminates methotrexate action.

Increased Effect/Toxicity: Increased toxicity has been noticed when asparaginase is administered with vincristine (neuropathy) and prednisone (hyperglycemia). Decreased metabolism when used with cyclophosphamide. Increased hepatotoxicity when used with mercaptopurine.

Lab Interactions Decreased thyroxine and thyroxine-binding globulin

Adverse Reactions Note: Immediate effects: Fever, chills, nausea, and vomiting occur in 50% to 60% of patients.

>10%:
Central nervous system: Fatigue, somnolence, depression, hallucinations, agitation, disorientation or convulsions (10% to 60%), stupor, confusion, coma (25%)

(Continued)

Asparaginase *(Continued)*

Endocrine & metabolic: Fever, chills (50% to 60%), hyperglycemia (10%)

Gastrointestinal: Nausea, vomiting (50% to 60%), anorexia, abdominal cramps (70%), acute pancreatitis (15%, may be severe in some patients)

Hematologic: Hypofibrinogenemia and depression of clotting factors V and VIII, variable decreased in factors VII and IX, severe protein C deficiency and decrease in antithrombin III (may be dose-limiting or fatal)

Hepatic: Transaminases, bilirubin, and alkaline phosphatase increased (transient)

Hypersensitivity: Acute allergic reactions (fever, rash, urticaria, arthralgia, hypotension, angioedema, bronchospasm, anaphylaxis (15% to 35%); may be dose-limiting in some patients, may be fatal)

Renal: Azotemia (66%)

1% to 10%:

Endocrine & metabolic: Hyperuricemia

Gastrointestinal: Stomatitis

Overdosage/Toxicology Symptoms of overdose include nausea and diarrhea.

Pharmacodynamics/Kinetics

Absorption: I.M.: Produces peak blood levels 50% lower than those from I.V. administration

Half-Life Elimination: 8-30 hours

Metabolism: Systemically degraded

Excretion: Urine (trace amounts)

Clearance: Unaffected by age, renal or hepatic function

Dosing

Adults & Elderly: Refer to individual protocols.

Single agent induction:

I.V. infusion:

200 units/kg/day for 28 days **or**

5000-10,000 units/m^2/day for 7 days every 3 weeks **or**

10,000-40,000 units every 2-3 weeks

I.M.: 6000-12,000 units/m^2; reconstitute to 10,000 units/mL may be necessary

Notes: Some institutions recommended the following precautions for asparaginase administration: Have parenteral epinephrine, diphenhydramine, and hydrocortisone available at the bedside. Have a freely running I.V. in place. Have a physician readily accessible. Monitor the patient closely for 30-60 minutes. Avoid administering the drug at night.

Test dose: A test dose is often recommended prior to the first dose of asparaginase, or prior to restarting therapy after a hiatus of several days. Most commonly, 0.1-0.2 mL of a 20-250 units/mL (2-50 units) is injected intradermally, and the patient observed for 15-30 minutes. False-negative rates of up to 80% to test doses of 2-50 units are reported.

Some practitioners recommend a desensitization regimen for patients who react to a test dose, or are being retreated following a break in therapy. Doses are doubled and given every 10 minutes until the total daily dose for that day has been administered.

One schedule begins with a total of 1 unit given I.V. and doubles the dose every 10 minutes until the total amount given in the planned dose for that day. For example, if a patient was to receive a total dose of 4000 units, he/she would receive injections 1 through 12 during the desensitization. See table.

Asparaginase Desensitization

Injection No.	Elspar Dose (int. units)	Accumulated Total Dose
1	1	1
2	2	3
3	4	7
4	8	15
5	16	31
6	32	63
7	64	127
8	128	255
9	256	511
10	512	1023
11	1024	2047
12	2048	4095
13	4096	8191
14	8192	16,383
15	16,384	32,767
16	32,768	65,535
17	65,536	131,071
18	131,072	262,143

Pediatrics: Refer to individual protocols.

Infusion for induction:

I.V.: 1000 units/kg/day for 10 days; consolidation: 6000-10,000 units/m^2/day for 14 days

I.M.: 6000 units/m^2 on days 4, 7, 10, 13, 16, 19, 22, 25, 28

Note: Refer to information in adult dosing.

Available Dosage Forms Injection, powder for reconstitution: 10,000 units

Monitoring and Teaching Issues

Physical Assessment: See Warnings/Precautions, Dosing, and Administration for specific use cautions and information related to skin tests and desensitization. Assess potential for interactions with other pharmacological agents patient may be taking (see Drug Interactions). Assess results of skin tests and regular laboratory tests prior to and frequently during therapy. With each dose, patient should be monitored closely for adverse reactions (acute hypersensitivity reactions [may occur in 10% to 40% of patients and can be fatal]; hyperglycemia; CNS changes; nausea or vomiting; see Adverse Reactions). In the event of hypersensitivity or hyperglycemia, infusion should be stopped and prescriber notified immediately. Teach patient possible side effects/appropriate interventions and adverse symptoms to report.

Monitoring Laboratory Tests: CBC, serum amylase, blood glucose, uric acid, liver function prior to and frequently during therapy

Patient Education: Do not take any new medication during therapy unless approved by prescriber. This medication can only be given I.M. or I.V. Report immediately any pain or burning at infusion/injection site, rash, chest pain, respiratory difficulty or chest tightness, difficulty swallowing, or sharp back pain. It is vital to maintain adequate hydration (2-3 L/ day of fluids) unless instructed to restrict fluid intake and good nutritional status (small frequent meals may help). May cause acute nausea or vomiting (small frequent meals, frequent mouth care, chewing gum, or sucking lozenges may help; or consult prescriber for approved antiemetic). Report unusual fever or chills; confusion, agitation, depression; yellowing of skin or eyes; unusual bleeding or bruising; unhealed sores; or vaginal discharge. **Pregnancy/breast-feeding precautions:** Inform prescriber if you are or intend to become pregnant. Consult prescriber if breast-feeding.

Pregnancy Risk Factor: C

Pregnancy Issues: Based on limited reports in humans, the use of asparaginase does not seem to pose a major risk to the fetus when used in the 2nd and 3rd trimesters, or when exposure occurs prior to conception in either females or males. Because of the teratogenicity observed in animals and the lack of human data after the 1st trimester exposure, asparaginase should be used cautiously, if at all, during this period.

Lactation: Excretion in breast milk unknown

Administration

I.M.: Doses should be given as a deep intramuscular injection into a large muscle.

I.V.: The following precautions should be taken when administering. Administer in 50-250 mL of D_5W over at least 60 minutes. Give a small test dose (0.1 mL of a dilute 20 unit/mL solution) first. Note that a negative skin test does not preclude the possibility of an allergic reaction. Desensitization may be performed in patients who have been found to be hypersensitive by the intradermal skin test or who have received previous courses of therapy with the drug. Have epinephrine, diphenhydramine, and hydrocortisone at the bedside. Have a running I.V. in place. A physician should be readily accessible.

Reconstitution: Lyophilized powder should be reconstituted with 1-5 mL sterile water for I.V. administration or NS for I.M. use.

Standard I.M./SubQ dilution: 2000, 5000, or 10,000 units/mL: 2 mL/syringe

Standard I.V. dilution: Dose in 50-250 mL NS or D_5W

Compatibility: Stable in D_5W, NS

Storage: Intact vials of powder should be refrigerated (<8°C); reconstituted solutions are stable 1 week at room temperature; shake well but not too vigorously; use of a 5 micron in-line filter is recommended to remove fiber-like particles in the solution (not 0.2 micron filter - has been associated with some loss of potency). Solutions for I.V. infusion are stable for 8 hours at room temperature or under refrigeration.

Additional Information The *E. coli* and the *Erwinia* strains of asparaginase differ slightly in their gene sequencing, and have slight differences in their enzyme characteristics. Both are highly specific for asparagine and have <10% activity for the D-isomer. The *E. coli* form is more commonly used, with the *Erwinia* variety usually being used only in patients who demonstrate allergic reactions to the other form.

♦ **Aspart, Insulin** *see* Insulin Preparations *on page 805*

♦ **Aspercin [OTC]** *see* Aspirin *on page 143*

♦ **Aspercin Extra [OTC]** *see* Aspirin *on page 143*

♦ **Aspergum® [OTC]** *see* Aspirin *on page 143*

Aspirin (AS pir in)

U.S. Brand Names Ascriptin® [OTC]; Ascriptin® Extra Strength [OTC]; Aspercin [OTC]; Aspercin Extra [OTC]; Aspergum® [OTC]; Bayer® Aspirin [OTC]; Bayer® Aspirin Extra Strength [OTC]; Bayer® Aspirin Regimen Adult Low Strength [OTC]; Bayer® Aspirin Regimen Children's [OTC]; Bayer® Aspirin Regimen Regular Strength [OTC]; Bayer® Extra Strength Arthritis Pain Regimen [OTC]; Bayer® Plus Extra Strength [OTC]; Bayer® Women's Aspirin Plus Calcium [OTC]; Bufferin® [OTC]; Bufferin® Extra Strength [OTC]; Buffinol [OTC]; Buffinol Extra [OTC]; Easprin® [OTC]; Ecotrin® [OTC]; Ecotrin® Low Strength [OTC]; Ecotrin® Maximum Strength [OTC]; Halfprin® [OTC]; St. Joseph® Adult Aspirin [OTC]; Sureprin 81™ [OTC]; ZORprin®

Synonyms Acetylsalicylic Acid; ASA

Generic Available Yes: Excludes gum

Pharmacologic Category Salicylate

Medication Safety Issues

Sound-alike/look-alike issues:

Aspirin may be confused with Afrin®, Asendin®

Ascriptin® may be confused with Aricept®

Ecotrin® may be confused with Akineton®, Edecrin®, Epogen®

Halfprin® may be confused with Halfan®, Haltran®

ZORprin® may be confused with Zyloprim®

Use Treatment of mild-to-moderate pain, inflammation, and fever; may be used as prophylaxis of myocardial infarction; prophylaxis of stroke and/or transient ischemic episodes; management of rheumatoid arthritis, rheumatic fever, osteoarthritis, and gout (high dose); adjunctive

(Continued)

Aspirin *(Continued)*

therapy in revascularization procedures (coronary artery bypass graft [CABG], percutaneous transluminal coronary angioplasty [PTCA], carotid endarterectomy), stent implantation

Unlabeled/Investigational Use Low doses have been used in the prevention of pre-eclampsia, complications associated with autoimmune disorders such as lupus or anti-phospholipid syndrome

Mechanism of Action/Effect Inhibits prostaglandin synthesis, acts on the hypothalamus heat-regulating center to reduce fever, blocks prostaglandin synthetase action which prevents formation of the platelet-aggregating substance thromboxane A_2

Contraindications Hypersensitivity to salicylates, other NSAIDs, or any component of the formulation; asthma; rhinitis; nasal polyps; inherited or acquired bleeding disorders (including factor VII and factor IX deficiency); do not use in children (<16 years of age) for viral infections (chickenpox or flu symptoms), with or without fever, due to a potential association with Reye's syndrome; pregnancy (3rd trimester especially)

Warnings/Precautions Use with caution in patients with platelet and bleeding disorders, renal dysfunction, dehydration, erosive gastritis, or peptic ulcer disease. Heavy ethanol use (>3 drinks/day) can increase bleeding risks. Avoid use in severe renal failure or in severe hepatic failure. Discontinue use if tinnitus or impaired hearing occurs. Caution in mild-moderate renal failure (only at high dosages). Patients with sensitivity to tartrazine dyes, nasal polyps and asthma may have an increased risk of salicylate sensitivity. Surgical patients should avoid ASA if possible, for 1-2 weeks prior to surgery, to reduce the risk of excessive bleeding.

When used for self-medication (OTC labeling): Children and teenagers who have or are recovering from chickenpox or flu-like symptoms should not use this product. Changes in behavior (along with nausea and vomiting) may be an early sign of Reye's syndrome; patients should be instructed to contact their healthcare provider if these occur.

Drug Interactions

Cytochrome P450 Effect: Substrate of CYP2C8/9 (minor)

Decreased Effect: The effects of ACE inhibitors may be blunted by aspirin administration (may be significant only at higher aspirin dosages). Aspirin may decrease the effects of beta-blockers, loop diuretics (furosemide), thiazide diuretics, and probenecid. Aspirin may cause a decrease in NSAIDs serum concentration and decrease the effects of probenecid. Increased serum salicylate levels when taken with with urine acidifiers (ammonium chloride, methionine).

Increased Effect/Toxicity: Aspirin may increase methotrexate serum levels/toxicity and may displace valproic acid from binding sites which can result in toxicity. NSAIDs and aspirin increase GI adverse effects (ulceration). Aspirin with oral anticoagulants (warfarin), thrombolytic agents, heparin, low molecular weight heparins, and antiplatelet agents (ticlopidine, clopidogrel, dipyridamole, NSAIDs, and IIb/IIIa antagonists) may increase risk of bleeding. Bleeding times may be additionally prolonged with verapamil. The effects of older sulfonylurea agents (tolazamide, tolbutamide) may be potentiated due to displacement from plasma proteins. This effect does not appear to be clinically significant for newer sulfonylurea agents (glyburide, glipizide, glimepiride).

Nutritional/Ethanol Interactions

Ethanol: Avoid ethanol (may enhance gastric mucosal damage).

Food: Food may decrease the rate but not the extent of oral absorption.

Folic acid: Hyperexcretion of folate; folic acid deficiency may result, leading to macrocytic anemia.

Iron: With chronic aspirin use and at doses of 3-4 g/day, iron-deficiency anemia may result.

Sodium: Hypernatremia resulting from buffered aspirin solutions or sodium salicylate containing high sodium content. Avoid or use with caution in CHF or any condition where hypernatremia would be detrimental.

Benedictine liqueur, prunes, raisins, tea, and gherkins: Potential salicylate accumulation.

Fresh fruits containing vitamin C: Displace drug from binding sites, resulting in increased urinary excretion of aspirin.

Herb/Nutraceutical: Avoid cat's claw, dong quai, evening primrose, feverfew, garlic, ginger, ginkgo, red clover, horse chestnut, green tea, ginseng (all have additional antiplatelet activity). Limit curry powder, paprika, licorice; may cause salicylate accumulation. These foods contain 6 mg salicylate/100 g. An ordinarily American diet contains 10-200 mg/day of salicylate.

Lab Interactions False-negative results for glucose oxidase urinary glucose tests (Clinistix®). Interferes with Gerhardt test, VMA determination; 5-HIAA, xylose tolerance test and T_3 and T_4.

Adverse Reactions As with all drugs which may affect hemostasis, bleeding is associated with aspirin. Hemorrhage may occur at virtually any site. Risk is dependent on multiple variables including dosage, concurrent use of multiple agents which alter hemostasis, and patient susceptibility. Many adverse effects of aspirin are dose related, and are rare at low dosages. Other serious reactions are idiosyncratic, related to allergy or individual sensitivity. Accurate estimation of frequencies is not possible. The reactions listed below have been reported for aspirin (frequency not defined).

Cardiovascular: Hypotension, tachycardia, dysrhythmias, edema

Central nervous system: Fatigue, insomnia, nervousness, agitation, confusion, dizziness, headache, lethargy, cerebral edema, hyperthermia, coma

Dermatologic: Rash, angioedema, urticaria

Endocrine & metabolic: Acidosis, hyperkalemia, dehydration, hypoglycemia (children), hyperglycemia, hypernatremia (buffered forms)

Gastrointestinal: Nausea, vomiting, dyspepsia, epigastric discomfort, heartburn, stomach pain, gastrointestinal ulceration (6% to 31%), gastric erosions, gastric erythema, duodenal ulcers

Hematologic: Anemia, disseminated intravascular coagulation, prolongation of prothrombin times, coagulopathy, thrombocytopenia, hemolytic anemia, bleeding, iron deficiency anemia

Hepatic: Hepatotoxicity, transaminases increased, hepatitis (reversible)

Neuromuscular & skeletal: Rhabdomyolysis, weakness, acetabular bone destruction (OA)

Otic: Hearing loss, tinnitus

Renal: Interstitial nephritis, papillary necrosis, proteinuria, renal impairment, renal failure (including cases caused by rhabdomyolysis), increased BUN, increased serum creatinine

Respiratory: Asthma, bronchospasm, dyspnea, laryngeal edema, hyperpnea, tachypnea, respiratory alkalosis, noncardiogenic pulmonary edema

Miscellaneous: Anaphylaxis, prolonged pregnancy and labor, stillbirths, low birth weight, peripartum bleeding, Reye's syndrome

Overdosage/Toxicology Symptoms of overdose include tinnitus, headache, dizziness, confusion, metabolic acidosis, hyperpyrexia, hypoglycemia, and coma. Treatment should be based upon symptomatology.

Pharmacodynamics/Kinetics

Duration of Action: 4-6 hours

Absorption: Rapid

Bioavailability: 50% to 75% reaches systemic circulation

Time to Peak: Serum: ~1-2 hours

Half-Life Elimination: Parent drug: 15-20 minutes; Salicylates (dose dependent): 3 hours at lower doses (300-600 mg), 5-6 hours (after 1 g), 10 hours with higher doses

Metabolism: Hydrolyzed to salicylate (active) by esterases in GI mucosa, red blood cells, synovial fluid, and blood; metabolism of salicylate occurs primarily by hepatic conjugation; metabolic pathways are saturable

Excretion: Urine (75% as salicyluric acid, 10% as salicylic acid)

Dosing

Adults & Elderly:

Analgesic and antipyretic: Oral, rectal: 325-650 mg every 4-6 hours up to 4 g/day

Anti-inflammatory: Oral: Initial: 2.4-3.6 g/day in divided doses; usual maintenance: 3.6-5.4 g/day; monitor serum concentrations

Acute myocardial infarction: 160-325 mg/day (have patient chew tablet if not taking aspirin before presentation)

Myocardial infarction prophylaxis: 75-325 mg/day; use of a lower aspirin dosage has been recommended in patients receiving ACE inhibitors

CABG: 75-325 mg/day starting 6 hours following procedure; if bleeding prevents administration at 6 hours after CABG, initiate as soon as possible

PTCA: Initial: 80-325 mg/day starting 2 hours before procedure; longer pretreatment durations (up to 24 hours) should be considered if lower dosages (80-100 mg) are used

Stent implantation: Oral: 325 mg 2 hours prior to implantation and 160-325 mg daily thereafter

Carotid endarterectomy: 81-325 mg/day preoperatively and daily thereafter

Acute stroke: 160-325 mg/day, initiated within 48 hours (in patients who are not candidates for thrombolytics and are not receiving systemic anticoagulation)

Stroke prevention/TIA: 30-325 mg/day (dosages up to 1300 mg/day in 2-4 divided doses have been used in clinical trials)

Pre-eclampsia prevention (unlabeled use): 60-80 mg/day during gestational weeks 13-26 (patient selection criteria not established)

Pediatrics:

Analgesic and antipyretic: Oral, rectal: Children: 10-15 mg/kg/dose every 4-6 hours, up to a total of 4 g/day

Anti-inflammatory: Oral: Children: Initial: 60-90 mg/kg/day in divided doses; usual maintenance: 80-100 mg/kg/day divided every 6-8 hours; monitor serum concentrations

Antiplatelet effects: Oral: Children: Adequate pediatric studies have not been performed; pediatric dosage is derived from adult studies and clinical experience and is not well established; suggested doses have ranged from 3-5 mg/kg/day to 5-10 mg/kg/day given as a single daily dose. Doses are rounded to a convenient amount (eg, $1/2$ of 80 mg tablet).

Mechanical prosthetic heart valves: Oral: Children: 6-20 mg/kg/day given as a single daily dose (used in combination with an oral anticoagulant in children who have systemic embolism despite adequate oral anticoagulation therapy (INR 2.5-3.5) and used in combination with low-dose anticoagulation (INR 2-3) and dipyridamole when full-dose oral anticoagulation is contraindicated)

Blalock-Taussig shunts: Oral: Children: 3-5 mg/kg/day given as a single daily dose

Kawasaki disease: Oral: Children: 80-100 mg/kg/day divided every 6 hours; monitor serum concentrations; after fever resolves: 3-5 mg/kg/day once daily; in patients without coronary artery abnormalities, give lower dose for at least 6-8 weeks or until ESR and platelet count are normal; in patients with coronary artery abnormalities, low-dose aspirin should be continued indefinitely

Antirheumatic: Oral: Children: 60-100 mg/kg/day in divided doses every 4 hours

Renal Impairment:

Cl_{cr} <10 mL/minute: Avoid use.

Dialyzable (50% to 100%)

Hepatic Impairment: Avoid use in severe liver disease.

Available Dosage Forms

Caplet:

Bayer® Aspirin: 325 mg [film coated]

Bayer® Aspirin Extra Strength: 500 mg [film coated]

Bayer® Extra Strength Arthritis Pain Regimen: 500 mg [enteric coated]

Bayer® Women's Aspirin Plus Calcium: 81 mg [contains elemental calcium 300 mg]

Caplet, buffered (Ascriptin® Extra Strength): 500 mg [contains aluminum hydroxide, calcium carbonate, and magnesium hydroxide]

Gelcap (Bayer® Aspirin Extra Strength): 500 mg

Gum (Aspergum®): 227 mg [cherry or orange flavor]

Suppository, rectal: 300 mg, 600 mg

Tablet: 325 mg

Aspercin: 325 mg

Aspercin Extra: 500 mg

(Continued)

Aspirin *(Continued)*

Bayer® Aspirin: 325 mg [film coated]

Tablet, buffered: 325 mg

Ascriptin®: 325 mg [contains aluminum hydroxide, calcium carbonate, and magnesium hydroxide]

Bayer® Plus Extra Strength: 500 mg [contains calcium carbonate]

Bufferin®: 325 mg [contains citric acid]

Bufferin® Extra Strength: 500 mg [contains citric acid]

Buffinol®: 325 mg [contains magnesium oxide]

Buffinol Extra: 500 mg [contains magnesium oxide]

Tablet, chewable: 81 mg

Bayer® Aspirin Regimen Children's Chewable: 81 mg [cherry, mint or orange flavor]

St. Joseph® Adult Aspirin: 81 mg [orange flavor]

Tablet, controlled release (ZORprin®): 800 mg

Tablet, enteric coated: 81 mg, 325 mg, 500 mg, 650 mg

Bayer® Aspirin Regimen Adult Low Strength, Ecotrin® Low Strength, St. Joseph Adult Aspirin: 81 mg

Bayer® Aspirin Regimen Regular Strength, Ecotrin® Regular Strength: 325 mg

Easprin®: 975 mg

Ecotrin® Maximum Strength: 500 mg

Halfprin®: 81 mg, 162 mg

Sureprin 81™: 81 mg

Monitoring and Teaching Issues

Physical Assessment: Do not use for persons with allergic reaction to salicylate or other NSAIDs. Assess other medications patient may be taking for additive or adverse interactions. Monitor therapeutic effectiveness and for signs of adverse reactions or overdose at beginning of therapy and periodically with long-term therapy. Assess knowledge/ teach patient appropriate use. Teach patient to monitor for adverse reactions, adverse reactions to report, and appropriate interventions to reduce side effects.

Patient Education: If self-administered, use exactly as directed; do not increase dose or frequency. Adverse reactions can occur with overuse. Take with food or milk. Do not use aspirin with strong vinegar-like odor. Do not crush or chew extended release products. While using this medication, avoid alcohol, excessive amounts of vitamin C, or salicylate-containing foods (eg, curry powder, prunes, raisins, tea, or licorice), other prescription or OTC medications containing aspirin or salicylate, or other NSAIDs without consulting prescriber. Maintain adequate hydration (2-3 L/day of fluids) unless instructed to restrict fluid intake. You may experience nausea, vomiting, gastric discomfort (frequent mouth care, small frequent meals, sucking lozenges, or chewing gum may help); GI bleeding, ulceration, or perforation (can occur with or without pain); or discoloration of stool (pink/red). Stop taking aspirin and report ringing in ears; persistent stomach pain; unresolved nausea or vomiting; respiratory difficulty or shortness of breath; unusual bruising or bleeding (mouth, urine, stool); or skin rash. **Pregnancy/breast-feeding precautions:** Inform prescriber if you are or intend to become pregnant. Consult prescriber if breast-feeding.

Dietary Considerations: Take with food or large volume of water or milk to minimize GI upset.

Geriatric Considerations: Elderly are at high risk for adverse effects from NSAIDs. Elderly with GI complications can develop peptic ulceration and/or hemorrhage asymptomatically. The concomitant use of H_2 blockers and sucralfate is not effective as prophylaxis with the exception of NSAID-induced duodenal ulcers which may be prevented by the use of ranitidine. Misoprostol and proton pump inhibitors are the only prophylactic agents proven effective. Also, concomitant disease and drug use contribute to the risk for GI adverse effects. Use lowest effective dose for shortest period possible. Consider renal function decline with age. Use of NSAIDs can compromise existing renal function especially when Cl_{cr} is ≤30 mL/minute. Tinnitus may be a difficult and unreliable indication of toxicity due to age-related hearing loss or eighth cranial nerve damage. CNS adverse effects such as confusion, agitation, and hallucination are generally seen in overdose or high-dose situations, but elderly may demonstrate these adverse effects at lower doses than younger adults.

Pregnancy Risk Factor: C/D (full-dose aspirin in 3rd trimester - expert analysis)

Pregnancy Issues: Salicylates have been noted to cross the placenta and enter fetal circulation. Adverse effects reported in the fetus include mortality, intrauterine growth retardation, salicylate intoxication, bleeding abnormalities, and neonatal acidosis. Use of aspirin close to delivery may cause premature closure of the ductus arteriosus. Adverse effects reported in the mother include anemia, hemorrhage, prolonged gestation, and prolonged labor. Aspirin has been used for the prevention of pre-eclampsia; however, the ACOG currently recommends that it not be used in low-risk women. Low-dose aspirin is used to treat complications resulting from antiphospholipid syndrome in pregnancy (either primary or secondary to SLE). In general, low doses during pregnancy needed for the treatment of certain medical conditions have not been shown to cause fetal harm, however, discontinuing therapy prior to delivery is recommended. Use of safer agents for routine management of pain or headache should be considered.

Lactation: Enters breast milk/use caution

Breast-Feeding Issues: Low amounts of aspirin can be found in breast milk. Milk/plasma ratios ranging from 0.03-0.3 have been reported. Peak levels in breast milk are reported to be at ~9 hours after a dose. Metabolic acidosis reported in one infant following an aspirin dose of 3.9 g/day in the mother. The AAP states that aspirin should be used with caution while breast-feeding. The WHO considers occasional doses of aspirin to be compatible with breast-feeding, but to avoid long-term therapy and consider monitoring the infant for adverse effects. Other sources suggest avoiding aspirin while breast-feeding due to the theoretical risk of Reye's syndrome.

Administration
Oral: Do not crush sustained release or enteric coated tablet. Administer with food or a full glass of water to minimize GI distress. For acute myocardial infarction, have patient chew tablet.

Storage: Keep suppositories in refrigerator; do not freeze. Hydrolysis of aspirin occurs upon exposure to water or moist air, resulting in salicylate and acetate, which possess a vinegar-like odor. Do not use if a strong odor is present.

◆ **Aspirin and Carisoprodol** *see Carisoprodol and Aspirin on page 259*

Aspirin and Codeine (AS pir in & KOE deen)
Synonyms Codeine and Aspirin
Controlled Substance C-III
Generic Available Yes
Pharmacologic Category Analgesic, Narcotic
Use Relief of mild to moderate pain
Dosing
Adults: Management of pain: Oral: 1-2 tablets (#3 tablet) every 4-6 hours as needed for pain
Elderly: One ASA with codeine 30 mg (#3 tablet), or two ASA with codeine 15 mg (#2 tablet) every 4-6 hours as needed for pain
Renal Impairment:
Cl_{cr} 10-50 mL/minute: Administer 75% of dose.
Cl_{cr} <10 mL/minute: Avoid use.
Hepatic Impairment: Avoid use in severe liver disease.
Available Dosage Forms Tablet:
#3: Aspirin 325 mg and codeine phosphate 30 mg
#4: Aspirin 325 mg and codeine phosphate 60 mg
Monitoring and Teaching Issues
Physical Assessment: See individual agents.
Patient Education: See individual agents. **Pregnancy/breast-feeding precautions:** Inform prescriber if you are or intend to become pregnant. Consult prescriber if breast-feeding.
Pregnancy Risk Factor: D
Lactation: Enters breast milk/use caution
Related Information
Aspirin *on page 143*
Codeine *on page 366*

Aspirin and Dipyridamole (AS pir in & dye peer ID a mole)
U.S. Brand Names Aggrenox®
Synonyms Aspirin and Extended-Release Dipyridamole; Dipyridamole and Aspirin
Generic Available No
Pharmacologic Category Antiplatelet Agent
Medication Safety Issues
Sound-alike/look-alike issues:
Aggrenox® may be confused with Aggrastat®
Use Reduction in the risk of stroke in patients who have had transient ischemia of the brain or completed ischemic stroke due to thrombosis
Dosing
Adults & Elderly: Stroke prevention: Oral: 1 capsule (200 mg dipyridamole, 25 mg aspirin) twice daily.
Renal Impairment: Avoid use in patients with severe renal dysfunction (Cl_{cr} <10 mL/minute).
Hepatic Impairment: Avoid use in patients with severe hepatic impairment.
Available Dosage Forms Capsule: Dipyridamole (extended release) 200 mg and aspirin 25 mg [contains lactose]
Monitoring and Teaching Issues
Physical Assessment: Assess for previous drug allergies before administering first dose. Assess other medications patient may be taking for effectiveness and interactions (see Drug Interactions). See Contraindications and Warnings/Precautions for use cautions. Monitor for signs of stroke or bleeding, laboratory results, therapeutic effect, adverse reactions, and overdose (see Monitoring Laboratory Tests, Adverse Reactions, and Overdose/Toxicology). Assess knowledge/teach patient appropriate use, interventions to reduce side effects, and adverse reactions to report (see Patient Education).
Patient Education: See individual agents. **Pregnancy/breast-feeding precautions:** Notify prescriber if you are or intend to become pregnant. Do not breast-feed.
Pregnancy Risk Factor: D
Lactation: Enters breast milk/use caution
Related Information
Aspirin *on page 143*
Dipyridamole *on page 468*

◆ **Aspirin and Extended-Release Dipyridamole** *see Aspirin and Dipyridamole on page 147*
◆ **Aspirin and Hydrocodone** *see Hydrocodone and Aspirin on page 757*

Aspirin and Meprobamate (AS pir in & me proe BA mate)
U.S. Brand Names Equagesic®
Synonyms Meprobamate and Aspirin
Controlled Substance C-IV
Generic Available No
Pharmacologic Category Antianxiety Agent, Miscellaneous
Use Adjunct to treatment of skeletal muscular disease in patients exhibiting tension and/or anxiety
(Continued)

Aspirin and Meprobamate *(Continued)*

Dosing

Adults: Muscular disorders, anxiety (adjunct): Oral: 1 tablet 3-4 times/day

Elderly: Refer to dosing in individual monographs; use with caution.

Available Dosage Forms Tablet: Aspirin 325 mg and meprobamate 200 mg

Monitoring and Teaching Issues

Physical Assessment: See individual agents.

Patient Education: See individual agents. **Pregnancy/breast-feeding precautions:** Inform prescriber if you are or intend to become pregnant. Consult prescriber if breast-feeding.

Pregnancy Risk Factor: D

Lactation: Enters breast milk/use caution due to aspirin content

Related Information

Aspirin *on page 143*

Meprobamate *on page 952*

♦ **Aspirin and Oxycodone** *see* Oxycodone and Aspirin *on page 1139*

Aspirin and Pravastatin *(AS pir in & PRA va stat in)*

U.S. Brand Names Pravigard™ PAC

Synonyms Buffered Aspirin and Pravastatin Sodium; Pravastatin and Aspirin

Generic Available No

Pharmacologic Category Antilipemic Agent, HMG-CoA Reductase Inhibitor; Salicylate

Use Combination therapy in patients who need treatment with aspirin and pravastatin to reduce the incidence of cardiovascular events, including myocardial infarction, stroke, and death.

Dosing

Adults:

Initial: Oral: Pravastatin 40 mg with aspirin (either 81 mg or 325 mg); both medications taken once daily. If pravastatin 40 mg does not achieve the desired cholesterol result, dosage may be increased to 80 mg once daily with aspirin (either 81 mg or 325 mg) once daily. Some patients may achieve/maintain goal cholesterol levels at a pravastatin dosage of 20 mg.

See Pravastatin *on page 1241* monograph for dosing in renal or hepatic impairment, as well as, dosing with concurrent immunosuppressant therapy.

Renal Impairment: Initial pravastatin dosage: 10 mg

Hepatic Impairment: Initial pravastatin dosage: 10 mg

Available Dosage Forms Combination package (Pravigard™ PAC) [each administration card contains]:

81/20:

Tablet: Aspirin, buffered 81 mg (5/card) [contains calcium carbonate, and magnesium oxide, and magnesium carbonate]

Tablet (Pravachol®): Pravastatin sodium 20 mg (5/card) [contains lactose]

81/40:

Tablet: Aspirin, buffered 81 mg (5/card) [contains calcium carbonate, and magnesium oxide, and magnesium carbonate]

Tablet (Pravachol®): Pravastatin sodium 40 mg (5/card) [contains lactose]

81/80:

Tablet: Aspirin, buffered 81 mg (5/card) [contains calcium carbonate, and magnesium oxide, and magnesium carbonate]

Tablet (Pravachol®): Pravastatin sodium 80 mg (5/card) [contains lactose]

325/20:

Tablet: Aspirin, buffered 325 mg (5/card) [contains calcium carbonate, and magnesium oxide, and magnesium carbonate]

Tablet (Pravachol®): Pravastatin sodium 20 mg (5/card) [contains lactose]

325/40:

Tablet: Aspirin, buffered 325 mg (5/card) [contains calcium carbonate, and magnesium oxide, and magnesium carbonate]

Tablet (Pravachol®): Pravastatin sodium 40 mg (5/card) [contains lactose]

325/80:

Tablet: Aspirin, buffered 325 mg (5/card) [contains calcium carbonate, and magnesium oxide, and magnesium carbonate]

Tablet (Pravachol®): Pravastatin sodium 80 mg (5/card) [contains lactose]

Monitoring and Teaching Issues

Physical Assessment: See individual agents. **Pregnancy risk factor X: Determine that patient is not pregnant before starting therapy. Do not give to females of childbearing age unless capable of complying with contraceptive use. Breast-feeding is contraindicated.**

Patient Education: See individual agents. **Pregnancy/breast-feeding precautions:** Inform prescriber if you are pregnant. Consult prescriber for appropriate contraceptive measures to use during and for 1 month following therapy. This drug may cause severe fetal defects. Do not donate blood during or for 1 month following therapy. Do not breast-feed during or for 1 month following therapy.

Pregnancy Risk Factor: X

Lactation: Enters breast milk/contraindicated

Related Information

Aspirin *on page 143*

Pravastatin *on page 1241*

♦ **Aspirin, Caffeine, and Butalbital** *see* Butalbital, Aspirin, and Caffeine *on page 226*

♦ **Aspirin, Caffeine, and Propoxyphene** *see* Propoxyphene, Aspirin, and Caffeine *on page 1273*

♦ **Aspirin, Carisoprodol, and Codeine** *see* Carisoprodol, Aspirin, and Codeine *on page 259*

♦ **Aspirin Free Anacin® Maximum Strength [OTC]** *see* Acetaminophen *on page 38*

ATENOLOL

- **Aspirin, Orphenadrine, and Caffeine** *see* Orphenadrine, Aspirin, and Caffeine *on page 1125*
- **Asthma** *see page 1799*
- **Astramorph/PF™** *see* Morphine Sulfate *on page 1031*
- **Atacand®** *see* Candesartan *on page 242*
- **Atacand HCT™** *see* Candesartan and Hydrochlorothiazide *on page 243*
- **Atarax®** *see* HydrOXYzine *on page 773*

Atenolol (a TEN oh lole)

U.S. Brand Names Tenormin®
Generic Available Yes: Tablet
Pharmacologic Category Beta Blocker, Beta₁ Selective
Medication Safety Issues
Sound-alike/look-alike issues:
Atenolol may be confused with albuterol, Altenol®, timolol, Tylenol®
Tenormin® may be confused with Imuran®, Norpramin®, thiamine, Trovan®
Use Treatment of hypertension, alone or in combination with other agents; management of angina pectoris, postmyocardial infarction patients
Unlabeled/Investigational Use Acute ethanol withdrawal, supraventricular and ventricular arrhythmias, and migraine headache prophylaxis
Mechanism of Action/Effect Competitively blocks response to beta-adrenergic stimulation, selectively blocks beta₁-receptors with little or no effect on beta₂-receptors except at high doses
Contraindications Hypersensitivity to atenolol or any component of the formulation; sinus bradycardia; sinus node dysfunction; heart block greater than first-degree (except in patients with a functioning artificial pacemaker); cardiogenic shock; uncompensated cardiac failure; pulmonary edema; pregnancy
Warnings/Precautions Administer cautiously in compensated heart failure and monitor for a worsening of the condition (efficacy of atenolol in heart failure has not been established). Use caution with concurrent use of beta-blockers and either verapamil or diltiazem; bradycardia or heart block can occur. Avoid concurrent I.V. use of both agents. Beta-blockers should be avoided in patients with bronchospastic disease (asthma) and peripheral vascular disease (may aggravate arterial insufficiency). Atenolol, with B1 selectivity, has been used cautiously in bronchospastic disease with close monitoring. Use cautiously in patients with diabetes - may mask hypoglycemic symptoms. May mask signs of thyrotoxicosis. May cause fetal harm when administered in pregnancy. Use cautiously in the renally impaired (dosage adjustment required). Use care with anesthetic agents which decrease myocardial function. Caution in patients with myasthenia gravis. Beta-blocker therapy should not be withdrawn abruptly (particularly in patients with CAD), but gradually tapered to avoid acute tachycardia, hypertension, and/or ischemia.
Drug Interactions
Decreased Effect: Decreased effect of atenolol with aluminum salts, barbiturates, calcium salts, cholestyramine, colestipol, NSAIDs, penicillins (ampicillin), rifampin, salicylates, and sulfinpyrazone due to decreased bioavailability and plasma levels. Beta-blockers may decrease the effect of sulfonylureas.
Increased Effect/Toxicity: Atenolol may increase the effects of other drugs which slow AV conduction (digoxin, verapamil, diltiazem), alpha-blockers (prazosin, terazosin), and alpha-adrenergic stimulants (epinephrine, phenylephrine). Atenolol may mask the tachycardia from hypoglycemia caused by insulin and oral hypoglycemics. In patients receiving concurrent therapy, the risk of hypertensive crisis is increased when either clonidine or the beta-blocker is withdrawn. Reserpine has been shown to enhance the effect of atenolol. Beta-blockers may increase the action or levels of ethanol, disopyramide, nondepolarizing muscle relaxants, and theophylline although the effects are difficult to predict.
Nutritional/Ethanol Interactions
Food: Atenolol serum concentrations may be decreased if taken with food.
Herb/Nutraceutical: Avoid dong quai if using for hypertension (has estrogenic activity). Avoid ephedra, yohimbe, ginseng (may worsen hypertension). Avoid garlic (may have increased antihypertensive effect).
Lab Interactions Increased glucose; decreased HDL
Adverse Reactions 1% to 10%:
Cardiovascular: Persistent bradycardia, hypotension, chest pain, edema, heart failure, second- or third-degree AV block, Raynaud's phenomenon
Central nervous system: Dizziness, fatigue, insomnia, lethargy, confusion, mental impairment, depression, headache, nightmares
Gastrointestinal: Constipation, diarrhea, nausea
Genitourinary: Impotence
Miscellaneous: Cold extremities
Overdosage/Toxicology Symptoms of toxicity include lethargy, respiratory drive disorder, wheezing, sinus pause and bradycardia. Additional effects associated with any beta-blocker are congestive heart failure, hypotension, bronchospasm, and hypoglycemia. Treatment includes removal of unabsorbed drug by induced emesis, gastric lavage, or administration of activated charcoal and symptomatic treatment of toxic responses. Atenolol can be removed by hemodialysis.
Pharmacodynamics/Kinetics
Onset of Action: Peak effect: Oral: 2-4 hours
Duration of Action: Normal renal function: 12-24 hours
Absorption: Incomplete
Protein Binding: 3% to 15%
Half-Life Elimination: Beta:
Neonates: ≤35 hours; Mean: 16 hours
Children: 4.6 hours; children >10 years may have prolonged half-life (>5 hours) compared to children 5-10 years (<5 hours)
(Continued)

149

Atenolol *(Continued)*

Adults: Normal renal function: 6-9 hours, prolonged with renal impairment; End-stage renal disease: 15-35 hours

Metabolism: Limited hepatic

Excretion: Feces (50%); urine (40% as unchanged drug)

Dosing

Adults & Elderly:

Hypertension:

Oral: 25-50 mg once daily, may increase to 100 mg/day. Doses >100 mg are unlikely to produce any further benefit.

I.V.: Dosages of 1.25-5 mg every 6-12 hours have been used in short-term management of patients unable to take oral enteral beta-blockers

Angina pectoris: Oral: 50 mg once daily, may increase to 100 mg/day. Some patients may require 200 mg/day.

Postmyocardial infarction:

I.V.: Early treatment: 5 mg slow I.V. over 5 minutes; may repeat in 10 minutes. If both doses are tolerated, may start oral atenolol 50 mg every 12 hours or 100 mg/day for 6-9 days postmyocardial infarction.

Oral: Follow I.V. dose with 100 mg/day or 50 mg twice daily for 6-9 days postmyocardial infarction.

Pediatrics:

Hypertension: Oral: Children: 0.8-1 mg/kg/dose given daily; range of 0.8-1.5 mg/kg/day; maximum dose: 2 mg/kg/day

Renal Impairment:

Cl_{cr} 15-35 mL/minute: Administer 50 mg/day maximum.

Cl_{cr} <15 mL/minute: Administer 50 mg every other day maximum.

Hemodialysis effects: Moderately dialyzable (20% to 50%) via hemodialysis. Administer dose postdialysis or administer 25-50 mg supplemental dose. Elimination is not enhanced with peritoneal dialysis. Supplemental dose is not necessary.

Available Dosage Forms

Injection, solution: 0.5 mg/mL (10 mL)

Tablet: 25 mg, 50 mg, 100 mg

Monitoring and Teaching Issues

Physical Assessment: Assess potential for interactions with other prescriptions, OTC medications, or herbal products patient may be taking. I.V. administration requires cardiac and hemodynamic monitoring and hypotensive precautions. For oral administration, assess blood pressure and heart rate prior to and following first dose and any change in dosage. Assess therapeutic effectiveness and adverse effects (eg, CHF, edema, new cough, dyspnea, unresolved fatigue). Advise patients with diabetes to monitor glucose levels closely (beta-blockers may alter glucose tolerance). Do not discontinue abruptly; taper dose gradually. Teach patient appropriate use, possible side effects/interventions (hypotension precautions), and adverse symptoms to report.

Patient Education: Do not take any new medication during therapy unless approved by prescriber. Take exactly as directed; with or without regard to meals; do not take with antacids. Do not adjust dosage or discontinue without consulting prescriber. Take pulse daily (prior to medication) and follow prescriber's instruction about holding medication. If you have diabetes, monitor serum sugar closely (drug may alter glucose tolerance or mask signs of hypoglycemia). May cause fatigue, dizziness, or postural hypotension (use caution when changing position from lying or sitting to standing, when driving, or climbing stairs until response to medication is known). Alteration in sexual performance (reversible); or constipation (increased dietary bulk and fluids and exercise may help). Report unresolved swelling of extremities, respiratory difficulty or new cough, unresolved fatigue, unusual weight gain, unresolved constipation, or unusual muscle weakness. **Pregnancy/breast-feeding precautions:** Do not get pregnant or cause a pregnancy (males) while using this medication. Consult prescriber for appropriate contraceptive measures. Consult prescriber if breast-feeding.

Dietary Considerations: May be taken without regard to meals.

Geriatric Considerations: Due to alterations in the beta-adrenergic autonomic nervous system, beta-adrenergic blockade may result in less hemodynamic response than seen in younger adults.

Pregnancy Risk Factor: D

Pregnancy Issues: Atenolol crosses the placenta; beta-blockers have been associated with persistent bradycardia, hypotension, and IUGR; IUGR is probably related to maternal hypertension. Available evidence suggests beta-blockers are generally safe during pregnancy (JNC 7). Cases of neonatal hypoglycemia have been reported following maternal use of beta-blockers at parturition or during breast-feeding. Monitor breast-fed infant for symptoms of beta-blockade.

Lactation: Enters breast milk/use caution

Breast-Feeding Issues: Symptoms of beta-blockade including cyanosis, hypothermia, and bradycardia have been reported in nursing infants.

Administration

I.V.: When administered acutely for cardiac treatment, monitor ECG and blood pressure. The injection can be administered undiluted or diluted with a compatible I.V. solution. May administer by rapid infusion (I.V. push) at a rate of 1 mg/minute or by slow infusion over ~30 minutes. Necessary monitoring for surgical patients who are unable to take oral beta-blockers (prolonged ileus) has not been defined. Some institutions require monitoring of baseline and postinfusion heart rate and blood pressure when a patient's response to beta-blockade has not been characterized (ie, the patient's initial dose or following a change in dose). Consult individual institutional policies and procedures.

Compatibility: Stable in D_5W, NS

Y-site administration: Incompatible with amphotericin B cholesteryl sulfate complex

Related Information

Beta-Blockers *on page 1720*

Atenolol and Chlorthalidone (a TEN oh lole & klor THAL i done)

U.S. Brand Names Tenoretic®
Synonyms Chlorthalidone and Atenolol
Generic Available Yes
Pharmacologic Category Antihypertensive Agent, Combination
Use Treatment of hypertension with a cardioselective beta-blocker and a diuretic
Dosing

Adults & Elderly: Hypertension: Oral: Initial: 1 (50) tablet once daily, then individualize dose until optimal dose is achieved

Renal Impairment:
Cl_{cr} 15-35 mL/minute: Administer 50 mg/day.
Cl_{cr} <15 mL/minute: Administer 50 mg every other day.

Available Dosage Forms Tablet:
50: Atenolol 50 mg and chlorthalidone 25 mg
100: Atenolol 100 mg and chlorthalidone 25 mg

Monitoring and Teaching Issues

Physical Assessment: See individual agents.

Patient Education: See individual agents. **Pregnancy/breast-feeding precautions:** Inform prescriber if you are or intend to become pregnant. Consult prescriber if breast-feeding.

Pregnancy Risk Factor: D

Lactation: Excretion in breast milk unknown

Related Information
Atenolol on page 149
Chlorthalidone on page 314

♦ **ATG** see Antithymocyte Globulin (Equine) on page 129
♦ **Atgam®** see Antithymocyte Globulin (Equine) on page 129
♦ **Ativan®** see Lorazepam on page 919

Atomoxetine (AT oh mox e teen)

U.S. Brand Names Strattera™
Synonyms Atomoxetine Hydrochloride; LY139603; Methylphenoxy-Benzene Propanamine; Tomoxetine
Generic Available No
Pharmacologic Category Norepinephrine Reuptake Inhibitor, Selective
Use Treatment of attention deficit/hyperactivity disorder (ADHD)
Unlabeled/Investigational Use Treatment of depression
Mechanism of Action/Effect Selectively inhibits the reuptake of norepinephrine (Ki 4.5nM) with little to no activity at the other neuronal reuptake pumps or receptor sites.
Contraindications Hypersensitivity to atomoxetine or any component of the formulation; use of MAO inhibitors within 14 days; narrow-angle glaucoma
Warnings/Precautions Use caution with hepatic and renal impairment (dosage adjustments necessary in hepatic impairment). Use may be associated with rare hepatotoxicity; discontinue if signs or symptoms of hepatotoxic reaction (eg, jaundice, pruritus, flu-like symptoms) are noted. May cause increased heart rate or blood pressure, use caution with hypertension or other cardiovascular disease. Use caution in patients who are "poor metabolizers" (CYP2D6), bioavailability increases. May cause urinary retention/hesitancy, use caution in patients with history of urinary retention or bladder outlet obstruction. Allergic reactions (including angioneurotic edema, urticaria, and rash) may occur. Growth should be monitored during treatment. Safety and efficacy have not been evaluated in pediatric patients <6 years of age; safety and efficacy of long-term use have not been established.

Drug Interactions

Cytochrome P450 Effect: Substrate of CYP2C19 (minor), 2D6 (major)

Increased Effect/Toxicity: MAO inhibitors may increase risk of CNS toxicity (combined use is contraindicated). CYP2D6 inhibitors may increase the levels/effects of atomoxetine; example inhibitors include chlorpromazine, delavirdine, fluoxetine, miconazole, paroxetine, pergolide, quinidine, quinine, ritonavir, and ropinirole. Albuterol may increase risk of cardiovascular toxicity.

Adverse Reactions Percentages as reported in children and adults; some adverse reactions may be increased in "poor metabolizers" (CYP2D6).

>10%:
Central nervous system: Headache (17% to 27%), insomnia (16%)
Gastrointestinal: Xerostomia (4% to 21%), abdominal pain (20%), vomiting (15%), appetite decreased (10% to 14%), nausea (12%)
Respiratory: Cough (11%)

1% to 10%:
Cardiovascular: Palpitations (4%), systolic blood pressure increased (2% to 9%), orthostatic hypotension (2%), tachycardia (2%)
Central nervous system: Fatigue/lethargy (7% to 9%), irritability (8%), somnolence (7%), dizziness (6%), mood swings (5%), abnormal dreams (4%), sleep disturbance (4%), pyrexia (3%), rigors (3%), crying (2%)
Dermatologic: Dermatitis (2% to 4%)
Endocrine & metabolic: Dysmenorrhea (7%), libido decreased (6%), menstruation disturbance (3%), orgasm abnormal (2%), weight loss (2%)
Gastrointestinal: Dyspepsia (6% to 8%), diarrhea (4%), flatulence (2%), constipation (3% to 10%)
Genitourinary: Erectile disturbance (7%), ejaculatory disturbance (5%), prostatitis (3%), impotence (3%)
Neuromuscular & skeletal: Paresthesia (4%), myalgia (3%)
Otic: Ear infection (3%)
Renal: Urinary retention/hesitation (8%)
Respiratory: Rhinorrhea (4%), sinus headache (3%), sinusitis (6%)

(Continued)

Atomoxetine *(Continued)*

Miscellaneous: Diaphoresis increased (4%), influenza (3%)

Overdosage/Toxicology Effects of overdose unknown; gastric emptying and use of activated charcoal may prevent drug absorption; monitor patient and provide supportive care

Pharmacodynamics/Kinetics

Absorption: Rapid

Bioavailability: 63% in extensive metabolizers; 94% in poor metabolizers

Time to Peak: Plasma: 1-2 hours

Protein Binding: 98%, primarily albumin

Half-Life Elimination: Atomoxetine: 5 hours (up to 24 hours in poor metabolizers); Active metabolites: 4-hydroxyatomoxetine: 6-8 hours; N-desmethylatomoxetine: 6-8 hours (34-40 hours in poor metabolizers)

Metabolism: Hepatic, via CYP2D6 and CYP2C19; forms metabolites (4-hydroxyatomoxetine, active, equipotent to atomoxetine; N-desmethylatomoxetine in poor metabolizers, limited activity)

Excretion: Urine (80%, as conjugated 4-hydroxy metabolite); feces (17%)

Dosing

Adults:

Treatment of ADHD: Oral: Initial: 40 mg/day, increased after minimum of 3 days to ~80 mg/day; may administer as either a single daily dose or two evenly divided doses in morning and late afternoon/early evening. May increase to 100 mg in 2-4 additional weeks to achieve optimal response. In patients receiving effective CYP2D6 inhibitors (eg, paroxetine, fluoxetine, quinidine), do not exceed 80 mg/day.

Treatment of depression (unlabeled use): Oral: 40-65 mg/day

Elderly: Use has not been evaluated in the elderly.

Pediatrics:

Treatment of ADHD:

Children and Adolescents ≤70 kg: Oral: Initial: 0.5 mg/kg/day, increase after minimum of 3 days to ~1.2 mg/kg/day; may administer as either a single daily dose or two evenly divided doses in morning and late afternoon/early evening. Maximum daily dose: 1.4 mg/kg or 100 mg, whichever is less. In patients receiving effective CYP2D6 inhibitors (eg, paroxetine, fluoxetine, quinidine), do not exceed 1.2 mg/kg.

Children and Adolescents >70 kg: Refer to adult dosing.

Renal Impairment: No adjustment needed.

Hepatic Impairment:

Moderate hepatic insufficiency (Child-Pugh class B): All doses should be reduced to 50% of normal.

Severe hepatic insufficiency (Child-Pugh class C): All doses should be reduced to 25% of normal.

Available Dosage Forms Capsule: 10 mg, 18 mg, 25 mg, 40 mg, 60 mg

Monitoring and Teaching Issues

Physical Assessment: Use with caution in presence of hepatic and renal impairment, hypertension or other cardiovascular disease, or history of urinary retention or bladder outlet obstruction (see Contraindications and Warnings/Precautions). Assess potential for interactions with other pharmacological agents patient may be taking. Assess therapeutic effectiveness and adverse response (see Adverse Reactions) at regular intervals during therapy. Teach patient proper use, possible side effects/appropriate interventions, and adverse symptoms to report.

Patient Education: Do not take any new medication during therapy without consulting prescriber. Take exactly as directed at the same time of day, without regard for meals. Do not discontinue or alter dose without consulting prescriber. Avoid alcohol. May cause CNS changes; fatigue/lethargy, irritability, sleep disturbances (use caution when driving or engaged in potentially hazardous tasks until response to drug is known); diarrhea or constipation; menstrual disturbances, abnormal orgasm, erectile or ejaculatory disturbance, impotence; muscle, bone, or joint pain. Report chest pain, palpitations, rapid heartbeat; persistent CNS changes; gastrointestinal effects; muscle or skeletal pain or weakness; or other persistent adverse effects. **Pregnancy/breast-feeding precautions:** Inform prescriber if you are or intend to become pregnant. Consult prescriber if breast-feeding.

Dietary Considerations: May be taken with or without food.

Pregnancy Risk Factor: C

Lactation: Excretion in breast milk unknown/use caution

Administration

Oral: May be administered with or without food.

Storage: Store at room temperature of 25°C (77°F).

♦ **Atomoxetine Hydrochloride** *see* Atomoxetine *on page 151*

Atorvastatin *(a TORE va sta tin)*

U.S. Brand Names Lipitor®

Generic Available No

Pharmacologic Category Antilipemic Agent, HMG-CoA Reductase Inhibitor

Medication Safety Issues

Sound-alike/look-alike issues:

Lipitor® may be confused with Levatol®

Use

Primary prevention of CVD in high-risk patients

Used with dietary therapy for the following:

Hyperlipidemias: To reduce elevations in total cholesterol, LDL-C, apolipoprotein B, and triglycerides in patients with primary hypercholesterolemia (elevations of 1 or more components are present in Fredrickson type IIa, IIb, III, and IV hyperlipidemias)

Treatment of homozygous familial hypercholesterolemia

Heterozygous familial hypercholesterolemia (HeFH): In adolescent patients (10-17 years of age, females >1 year postmenarche) with HeFH having LDL-C ≥190 mg/dL **or** LDL ≥160 mg/dL with positive family history of premature cardiovascular disease (CVD) or with 2 or more CVD risk factors in the adolescent patient

Mechanism of Action/Effect Inhibitor of 3-hydroxy-3-methylglutaryl coenzyme A (HMG-CoA) reductase, the rate limiting enzyme in cholesterol synthesis (reduces the production of mevalonic acid from HMG-CoA); this then results in a compensatory increase in the expression of LDL receptors on hepatocyte membranes and a stimulation of LDL catabolism

Contraindications Hypersensitivity to atorvastatin or any component of the formulation; active liver disease; unexplained persistent elevations of serum transaminases; pregnancy; breast-feeding

Warnings/Precautions Secondary causes of hyperlipidemia should be ruled out prior to therapy. Liver function must be monitored by periodic laboratory assessment. Rhabdomyolysis with acute renal failure has occurred. Risk is dose-related and is increased with concurrent use of lipid-lowering agents which may cause rhabdomyolysis (gemfibrozil, fibric acid derivatives, or niacin at doses ≥1 g/day) or during concurrent use with potent CYP3A4 inhibitors (including amiodarone, clarithromycin, cyclosporine, erythromycin, itraconazole, ketoconazole, nefazodone, grapefruit juice in large quantities, verapamil, or protease inhibitors such as indinavir, nelfinavir, or ritonavir). Weigh the risk versus benefit when combining any of these drugs with atorvastatin. Discontinue in any patient experiencing an acute or serious condition predisposing to renal failure secondary to rhabdomyolysis. Use with caution in patients who consume large amounts of ethanol or have a history of liver disease. Safety and efficacy have not been established in patients <10 years or in premenarcheal girls.

Drug Interactions

Cytochrome P450 Effect: Substrate of CYP3A4 (major); **Inhibits** CYP3A4 (weak)

Decreased Effect: Colestipol, antacids decreased plasma concentrations but effect on LDL-cholesterol was not altered. Cholestyramine may decrease absorption of atorvastatin when administered concurrently.

Increased Effect/Toxicity: CYP3A4 inhibitors may increase the levels/effects of atorvastatin; example inhibitors include azole antifungals, ciprofloxacin, clarithromycin, diclofenac, doxycycline, erythromycin, imatinib, isoniazid, nefazodone, nicardipine, propofol, protease inhibitors, quinidine, and verapamil. The risk of myopathy and rhabdomyolysis due to concurrent use of a CYP3A4 inhibitor with atorvastatin is probably less than lovastatin or simvastatin. Cyclosporine, clofibrate, fenofibrate, gemfibrozil, and niacin also may increase the risk of myopathy and rhabdomyolysis. The effect/toxicity of levothyroxine may be increased by atorvastatin. Levels of digoxin and ethinyl estradiol may be increased by atorvastatin.

Nutritional/Ethanol Interactions

Ethanol: Avoid excessive ethanol consumption (due to potential hepatic effects).

Food: Atorvastatin serum concentrations may be increased by grapefruit juice; avoid concurrent intake of large quantities (>1 quart/day).

Herb/Nutraceutical: St John's wort may decrease atorvastatin levels.

Adverse Reactions

>10%: Central nervous system: Headache (3% to 17%)

2% to 10%:

Cardiovascular: Chest pain, peripheral edema

Central nervous system: Insomnia, dizziness

Dermatologic: Rash (1% to 4%)

Gastrointestinal: Abdominal pain (up to 4%), constipation (up to 3%), diarrhea (up to 4%), dyspepsia (1% to 3%), flatulence (1% to 3%), nausea

Genitourinary: Urinary tract infection

Hepatic: Transaminases increased (2% to 3% with 80 mg/day dosing)

Neuromuscular & skeletal: Arthralgia (up to 5%), arthritis, back pain (up to 4%), myalgia (up to 6%), weakness (up to 4%)

Respiratory: Sinusitis (up to 6%), pharyngitis (up to 3%), bronchitis, rhinitis

Miscellaneous: Infection (3% to 10%), flu-like syndrome (up to 3%), allergic reaction (up to 3%)

Overdosage/Toxicology Treatment is supportive.

Pharmacodynamics/Kinetics

Onset of Action: Initial changes: 3-5 days; Maximal reduction in plasma cholesterol and triglycerides: 2 weeks

Absorption: Rapid

Time to Peak: Serum: 1-2 hours

Protein Binding: 98%

Half-Life Elimination: Parent drug: 14 hours

Metabolism: Hepatic; forms active ortho- and parahydroxylated derivates and an inactive beta-oxidation product

Excretion: Bile; urine (2% as unchanged drug)

Dosing

Adults & Elderly:

Hyperlipidemias: Oral: Initial: 10-20 mg once daily; patients requiring >45% reduction in LDL-C may be started at 40 mg once daily; range: 10-80 mg once daily

Note: Doses should be individualized according to the baseline LDL-cholesterol levels, the recommended goal of therapy, and patient response; adjustments should be made at intervals of 2-4 weeks

Primary prevention of CVD: Oral: 10 mg once daily

Pediatrics:

HeFH: Children 10-17 years (females >1 year postmenarche): Oral: 10 mg once daily (maximum: 20 mg/day)

Note: Doses should be individualized according to the baseline LDL-cholesterol levels, the recommended goal of therapy, and patient response; adjustments should be made at intervals of 2-4 weeks

(Continued)

Atorvastatin *(Continued)*

Renal Impairment: No adjustment is necessary.

Hepatic Impairment: Decrease dosage with severe disease (eg, chronic alcoholic liver disease).

Available Dosage Forms Tablet: 10 mg, 20 mg, 40 mg, 80 mg

Monitoring and Teaching Issues

Physical Assessment: Note Contraindications and Warnings/Precautions for use cautions (eg, liver disease, large alcohol intake). Assess risk potential for interactions with other prescriptions or herbal products patient may be taking (eg, risk of myopathy and rhabdomyolysis; see Drug Interactions). Laboratory tests should be scheduled and results assessed prior to initiation and at regular intervals (eg, lipid levels, CPK). Assess for therapeutic response and adverse effects (see Adverse Reactions). Teach patient proper use, possible side effects/appropriate interventions, and adverse symptoms to report. **Pregnancy risk factor X:** Determine that patient is not pregnant before beginning treatment. Instruct patients of childbearing age about appropriate contraceptive measures.

Monitoring Laboratory Tests: Monitor lipid levels after 2-4 weeks; LFTs prior to initiation and 12 weeks after initiation or first dose or dose elevation, and periodically (semiannually) thereafter; CPK

Patient Education: Do not take any new medication during therapy unless approved by prescriber. May take without regard to food. Maintain adequate hydration (2-3 L/day of fluids) unless instructed to restrict fluid intake. You will need laboratory evaluation during therapy. May cause headache (consult prescriber for approved analgesic); diarrhea (buttermilk, boiled milk, or yogurt may help); euphoria, giddiness, or confusion (use caution when driving or engaging in tasks that require alertness until response to medication is known). Report immediately any unusual muscle cramping or weakness. Report persistent diarrhea; changes in mood or memory, yellowing of skin or eyes, unusual bruising or bleeding, or unusual fatigue. **Pregnancy/breast-feeding precautions:** Inform prescriber if you are pregnant. Do not get pregnant during therapy. Consult prescriber for instructions on appropriate contraceptive measures. This drug can cause severe fetal defects. Do not donate blood while taking this medication and for some period of time after discontinuing. Do not breast-feed.

Dietary Considerations: May take with food if desired; may take without regard to time of day. Before initiation of therapy, patients should be placed on a standard cholesterol-lowering diet for 3-6 months and the diet should be continued during drug therapy.

Geriatric Considerations: Effective and well tolerated in elderly. The definition of and, therefore, when to treat hyperlipidemia in the elderly is a controversial issue. The National Cholesterol Education Program recommends that all adults maintain a plasma cholesterol <160 mg/dL. In elderly patients with one additional risk factor, goal LDL would decrease to <130 mg/dL. Pharmacologic treatment should be reserved for those who are unable to obtain a desirable plasma cholesterol concentration by diet alone and for whom the benefits of treatment are believed to outweigh the potential adverse effects, drug interactions, and cost of treatment.

Pregnancy Risk Factor: X

Lactation: Enters breast milk/contraindicated

Administration

Oral: May be administered with food if desired; may take without regard to time of day

Related Information

Hyperlipidemia Management *on page 1836*

Lipid-Lowering Agents *on page 1738*

♦**Atorvastatin Calcium and Amlodipine Besylate** *see* Amlodipine and Atorvastatin *on page 101*

Atovaquone *(a TOE va kwone)*

U.S. Brand Names Mepron®

Generic Available No

Pharmacologic Category Antiprotozoal

Use Acute oral treatment of mild to moderate *Pneumocystis carinii* pneumonia (PCP) in patients who are intolerant to co-trimoxazole; prophylaxis of PCP in patients intolerant to co-trimoxazole; treatment/suppression of *Toxoplasma gondii* encephalitis, primary prophylaxis of HIV-infected persons at high risk for developing *Toxoplasma gondii* encephalitis

Mechanism of Action/Effect Has not been fully elucidated; may inhibit electron transport in mitochondria inhibiting metabolic enzymes

Contraindications Life-threatening allergic reaction to the drug or formulation

Warnings/Precautions Has only been used in mild to moderate PCP. Use with caution in elderly patients due to potentially impaired renal, hepatic, and cardiac function.

Drug Interactions

Decreased Effect: Rifamycins (rifampin) used concurrently decrease the steady-state plasma concentrations of atovaquone.

Increased Effect/Toxicity: Possible increased toxicity with other highly protein-bound drugs.

Nutritional/Ethanol Interactions Food: Ingestion with a fatty meal increases absorption.

Adverse Reactions Note: Adverse reaction statistics have been compiled from studies including patients with advanced HIV disease; consequently, it is difficult to distinguish reactions attributed to atovaquone from those caused by the underlying disease or a combination, thereof.

>10%:

Central nervous system: Headache, fever, insomnia, anxiety

Dermatologic: Rash

Gastrointestinal: Nausea, diarrhea, vomiting

Respiratory: Cough

1% to 10%:

Central nervous system: Dizziness

Dermatologic: Pruritus
Endocrine & metabolic: Hypoglycemia, hyponatremia
Gastrointestinal: Abdominal pain, constipation, anorexia, dyspepsia, increased amylase
Hematologic: Anemia, neutropenia, leukopenia
Hepatic: Elevated liver enzymes
Neuromuscular & skeletal: Weakness
Renal: Elevated BUN/creatinine
Miscellaneous: Oral moniliasis

Pharmacodynamics/Kinetics
Absorption: Significantly increased with a high-fat meal
Bioavailability: Tablet: 23%; Suspension: 47%
Protein Binding: >99%
Half-Life Elimination: 2-3 days
Metabolism: Undergoes enterohepatic recirculation
Excretion: Feces (94% as unchanged drug)

Dosing
Adults & Elderly:
Prevention of PCP: Oral: 1500 mg once daily with food
Treatment of mild to moderate PCP: Oral: 750 mg twice daily with food for 21 days
Pediatrics: Adolescents 13-16 years: Refer to adult dosing.
Available Dosage Forms Suspension, oral: 750 mg/5 mL (5 mL, 210 mL) [contains benzyl alcohol; citrus flavor]

Monitoring and Teaching Issues
Physical Assessment: Monitor for CNS and respiratory changes and patient's knowledge of adverse reactions. Assess for interactions with other prescription or OTC medications.
Patient Education: Take as directed. Take with high-fat meals. You may experience dizziness or lightheadedness; use caution when driving or engaging in tasks that require alertness until response to drug is known. Small meals may help reduce nausea. Report unresolved diarrhea, fever, mouth sores (use good mouth care), unresolved headache, or vomiting. **Pregnancy/breast-feeding precautions:** Inform prescriber if you are or intend to become pregnant. Consult prescriber if breast-feeding.
Pregnancy Risk Factor: C
Lactation: Excretion in breast milk unknown/use caution

Administration
Storage: Do not freeze.

Atovaquone and Proguanil (a TOE va kwone & pro GWA nil)
U.S. Brand Names Malarone®
Synonyms Proguanil and Atovaquone
Generic Available No
Pharmacologic Category Antimalarial Agent
Use Prevention or treatment of acute, uncomplicated *P. falciparum* malaria
Mechanism of Action/Effect
Atovaquone: Selectively inhibits parasite mitochondrial electron transport.
Proguanil: The metabolite cycloguanil inhibits dihydrofolate reductase, disrupting deoxythymidylate synthesis. Together, atovaquone/cycloguanil affect the erythrocytic and exoerythrocytic stages of development.
Contraindications Hypersensitivity to atovaquone, proguanil, or any component of the formulation; prophylactic use in severe renal impairment
Warnings/Precautions Not indicated for severe or complicated malaria. Absorption of atovaquone may be decreased in patients who have diarrhea or vomiting; monitor closely and consider use of an antiemetic. If severe, consider use of an alternative antimalarial. Do not use with other medications containing proguanil. Administer with caution to patients with pre-existing renal disease. Not for use in patients <5 kg (treatment) or <11 kg (prophylaxis). Delayed cases of *P. falciparum* malaria may occur after stopping prophylaxis; travelers returning from endemic areas who develop febrile illnesses should be evaluated for malaria. Recrudescent infections or infections following prophylaxis with this agent should be treated with alternative agent(s).
Drug Interactions
Cytochrome P450 Effect: Proguanil: **Substrate** (minor) of 1A2, 2C19, 3A4
Decreased Effect: Metoclopramide decreases bioavailability of atovaquone. Rifabutin decreases atovaquone levels by 34%. Rifampin decreases atovaquone levels by 50%. Tetracycline decreases plasma concentrations of atovaquone by 40%.
Nutritional/Ethanol Interactions Food: Atovaquone taken with dietary fat increases the rate and extent of absorption.
Adverse Reactions The following adverse reactions were reported in patients being treated for malaria. When used for prophylaxis, reactions are similar to those seen with placebo.
>10%: Gastrointestinal: Abdominal pain (17%), nausea (12%), vomiting (children 10% to 13%, adults 12%)
1% to 10%:
Central nervous system: Headache (10%), dizziness (5%)
Dermatologic: Pruritus (children 6%)
Gastrointestinal: Diarrhea (children 6%, adults 8%), anorexia (5%)
Neuromuscular & skeletal: Weakness (8%)
Overdosage/Toxicology
Atovaquone: Overdoses of up to 31,500 mg have been reported. Rash has been reported as well as methemoglobinemia in one patient also taking dapsone. There is no known antidote and it is unknown if it is dialyzable.
Proguanil: Single doses of 1500 mg and 700 mg twice daily for two weeks have been reported without toxicity. Reversible hair loss, scaling of skin, reversible aphthous ulceration, and hematologic side effects have occurred. Epigastric discomfort and vomiting would also be expected.
There have been no reported overdoses with the atovaquone/proguanil combination.
(Continued)

Atovaquone and Proguanil *(Continued)*

Pharmacodynamics/Kinetics
Absorption: Proguanil: Extensive

Protein Binding: Proguanil: 75%

Half-Life Elimination: Proguanil: 12-21 hours

Metabolism: Proguanil: Hepatic to active metabolites, cycloguanil (via CYP2C19) and 4-chlorophenylbiguanide

Excretion: Proguanil: Urine (40% to 60%)

Pharmacokinetic Note: See Atovaquone monograph.

Dosing
Adults: Doses given in mg of atovaquone and proguanil:

Prevention of malaria: Oral: Atovaquone/proguanil 250 mg/100 mg once daily; start 1-2 days prior to entering a malaria-endemic area, continue throughout the stay and for 7 days after returning.

Treatment of acute malaria: Oral: Atovaquone/proguanil 1 g/400 mg as a single dose, once daily for 3 consecutive days

Elderly: Refer to adult dosing. Use with caution due to possible decrease in renal and hepatic function, as well as possible decreases in cardiac function, concomitant diseases, or other drug therapy.

Pediatrics: Doses given in mg of atovaquone and proguanil (dosage based on body weight):

Prevention of malaria: Oral: Children: Start 1-2 days prior to entering a malaria-endemic area, continue throughout the stay and for 7 days after returning. Take as a single dose, once daily.
11-20 kg: Atovaquone/proguanil 62.5 mg/25 mg
21-30 kg: Atovaquone/proguanil 125 mg/50 mg
31-40 kg: Atovaquone/proguanil 187.5 mg/75 mg
>40 kg: Atovaquone/proguanil 250 mg/100 mg

Treatment of acute malaria: Oral: Children: Take as a single dose, once daily for 3 consecutive days.
5-8 kg: Atovaquone/proguanil 125 mg/50 mg
9-10 kg: Atovaquone/proguanil 187.5 mg/75 mg
11-20 kg: Atovaquone/proguanil 250 mg/100 mg
21-30 kg: Atovaquone/proguanil 500 mg/200 mg
31-40 kg: Atovaquone/proguanil 750 mg/300 mg
>40 kg: Atovaquone/proguanil 1 g/400 mg

Renal Impairment: Should not be used as prophylaxis in severe renal impairment (Cl_{cr} <30 mL/minute). Alternative treatment regimens should be used in patients with Cl_{cr} <30 mL/minute. No dosage adjustment required in mild to moderate renal impairment.

Hepatic Impairment: No dosage adjustment required in mild to moderate hepatic impairment. No data available for use in severe hepatic impairment.

Available Dosage Forms
Tablet: Atovaquone 250 mg and proguanil hydrochloride 100 mg
Tablet, pediatric: Atovaquone 62.5 mg and proguanil hydrochloride 25 mg

Monitoring and Teaching Issues
Physical Assessment: See Contraindications, Warnings/Precautions, and Dosing for safe use. Assess potential for interactions with other prescriptions, OTC medications, or herbal products patient may be taking (see Drug Interactions and Nutritional/Ethanol Interactions). Teach patient appropriate administration, possible side effects, interventions to reduce side effects, and adverse symptoms to report (see Patient Education).

Patient Education: Inform prescriber of all prescriptions, OTC medications, or herbal products you are taking, and any allergies you have. Do not take any new medication during therapy without consulting prescriber. Complete full course of therapy; do not discontinue or alter dosage without consulting prescriber. Take at the same time each day with full glass of milk or food. If vomiting occurs within 1 hour of taking dose, you may repeat the dose. You may experience nausea, vomiting, or loss of appetite (small frequent meals may help); or headache (If persistent, contact prescriber). Follow recommended precautions to avoid malaria exposure (use insect repellent, bednets, protective clothing). Notify prescriber if you develop fever after returning from or while visiting a malaria-endemic area. **Pregnancy/breast-feeding precautions:** Inform prescriber if you are or intend to become pregnant. Consult prescriber if breast-feeding.

Dietary Considerations: Must be taken with food or a milky drink.

Pregnancy Risk Factor: C

Pregnancy Issues: Because falciparum malaria can cause maternal death and fetal loss, pregnant women traveling to malaria-endemic areas must use personal protection against mosquito bites.

Lactation:
Atovaquone: Excretion in breast milk unknown
Proguanil: Enters breast milk (small amounts)/use caution

Administration
Oral: Administer with food or milk at the same time each day. If patient vomits within 1 hour of administration, repeat the dose. For children who have difficulty swallowing tablets, tablets may be crushed and mixed with condensed milk just prior to administration.

Storage: Store tablets at 25°C (77°F).

Related Information
Atovaquone *on page 154*

◆ **ATRA** *see* Tretinoin (Oral) *on page 1514*

Atracurium (a tra KYOO ree um)

U.S. Brand Names Tracrium®

Synonyms Atracurium Besylate

Generic Available Yes

Pharmacologic Category Neuromuscular Blocker Agent, Nondepolarizing

Use Adjunct to general anesthesia to facilitate endotracheal intubation and to relax skeletal muscles during surgery; to facilitate mechanical ventilation in ICU patients; does not relieve pain or produce sedation

Mechanism of Action/Effect Blocks neural transmission at the myoneural junction by binding with cholinergic receptor sites

Contraindications Hypersensitivity to atracurium besylate or any component of the formulation

Warnings/Precautions Reduce initial dosage and inject slowly (over 1-2 minutes) in patients in whom substantial histamine release would be potentially hazardous (eg, patients with clinically important cardiovascular disease); maintenance of an adequate airway and respiratory support is critical; certain clinical conditions may result in potentiation or antagonism of neuromuscular blockade:

> Potentiation: Electrolyte abnormalities, severe hyponatremia, severe hypocalcemia, severe hypokalemia, hypermagnesemia, neuromuscular diseases, acidosis, acute intermittent porphyria, renal failure, hepatic failure
>
> Antagonism: Alkalosis, hypercalcemia, demyelinating lesions, peripheral neuropathies, diabetes mellitus

Increased sensitivity in patients with myasthenia gravis, Eaton-Lambert syndrome; resistance in burn patients (>30% of body) for period of 5-70 days postinjury; resistance in patients with muscle trauma, denervation, immobilization, infection, chronic treatment with atracurium. Cross-sensitivity with other neuromuscular-blocking agents may occur; use extreme caution in patients with previous anaphylactic reactions. Bradycardia may be more common with atracurium than with other neuromuscular-blocking agents since it has no clinically significant effects on heart rate to counteract the bradycardia produced by anesthetics.

Drug Interactions

Decreased Effect: Effect of nondepolarizing neuromuscular blockers may be reduced by carbamazepine (chronic use), corticosteroids (also associated with myopathy - see increased effect), phenytoin (chronic use), sympathomimetics, and theophylline.

Increased Effect/Toxicity: Increased effects are possible with aminoglycosides, beta-blockers, clindamycin, calcium channel blockers, halogenated anesthetics, imipenem, ketamine, lidocaine, loop diuretics (furosemide), macrolides (case reports), magnesium sulfate, procainamide, quinidine, quinolones, tetracyclines, and vancomycin. May increase risk of myopathy when used with high- dose corticosteroids for extended periods.

Adverse Reactions Mild, rare, and generally suggestive of histamine release

1% to 10%: Cardiovascular: Flushing

Causes of prolonged neuromuscular blockade: Excessive drug administration; cumulative drug effect, decreased metabolism/excretion (hepatic and/or renal impairment); accumulation of active metabolites; electrolyte imbalance (hypokalemia, hypocalcemia, hypermagnesemia, hypernatremia); hypothermia

Overdosage/Toxicology

Symptoms of overdose include respiratory depression and cardiovascular collapse.

Neostigmine 1-3 mg slow I.V. push in adults (0.5 mg in children) antagonizes the neuromuscular blockade, and should be administered with or immediately after atropine 1-1.5 mg I.V. push (adults). This may be especially useful in the presence of bradycardia.

Pharmacodynamics/Kinetics

Onset of Action: Dose dependent: 2-3 minutes

Duration of Action: Recovery begins in 20-35 minutes following initial dose of 0.4-0.5 mg/kg under balanced anesthesia; recovery to 95% of control takes 60-70 minutes

Half-Life Elimination: Biphasic: Adults: Initial (distribution): 2 minutes; Terminal: 20 minutes

Metabolism: Undergoes ester hydrolysis and Hofmann elimination (nonbiologic process independent of renal, hepatic, or enzymatic function); metabolites have no neuromuscular blocking properties; laudanosine, a product of Hofmann elimination, is a CNS stimulant and can accumulate with prolonged use. Laudanosine is hepatically metabolized.

Excretion: Urine (<5%)

Dosing

Adults & Elderly: For I.V. administration only (not to be used I.M.): Dose to effect; doses must be individualized due to interpatient variability; use ideal body weight for obese patients.

Adjunct to surgical anesthesia (neuromuscular blockade):

> *I.V. (bolus):* 0.4-0.5 mg/kg, then 0.08-0.1 mg/kg 20-45 minutes after initial dose to maintain neuromuscular block, followed by repeat doses of 0.08-0.1 mg/kg at 15- to 25-minute intervals
>
> Initial dose after succinylcholine for intubation (balanced anesthesia): Adults: 0.2-0.4 mg/kg
>
> Pretreatment/priming: I.V.: 10% of intubating dose given 3-5 minutes before initial dose
>
> *I.V. continuous infusion:* Initial: 9-10 mcg/kg/minute at initial signs of recovery from bolus dose; block is usually maintained by a rate of 5-9 mcg/kg/minute under balanced anesthesia.

ICU neuromuscular blockade: I.V.: Initial (bolus) 0.4-0.5 mg/kg, followed by I.V. continuous infusion at an initial rate of 5-10 mcg/kg/min; block is usually maintained by rate of 11-13 mcg/kg/minute (rates for pediatric patients may be higher).

Pediatrics:

Adjunct to surgical anesthesia: I.V. (not to be used I.M.): Dose to effect; doses must be individualized due to interpatient variability; use ideal body weight for obese patients

(Continued)

Atracurium *(Continued)*

Children 1 month to 2 years: Initial: 0.3-0.4 mg/kg followed by maintenance doses as needed to maintain neuromuscular blockade

Children >2 years: Refer to adult dosing.

Renal Impairment: No adjustment is necessary.

Hepatic Impairment: No adjustment is necessary.

Available Dosage Forms

Injection, as besylate: 10 mg/mL (10 mL) [contains benzyl alcohol]

Injection, as besylate [preservative free]: 10 mg/mL (5 mL)

Monitoring and Teaching Issues

Physical Assessment: Only clinicians experienced in the use of neuromuscular blocking drugs should administer and/or manage the use of atracurium. Dosage and rate of administration should be individualized and titrated to the desired effect, according to relevant clinical factors, premedication, concomitant medications, age, and general condition of the patient. Ventilatory support must be instituted and maintained until adequate respiratory muscle function and/or airway protection are assured. Assess other medications for effectiveness and safety. Other drugs that affect neuromuscular activity may increase/decrease neuromuscular block induced by atracurium. This drug does not cause anesthesia or analgesia; pain must be treated with appropriate analgesic agents. Continuous monitoring of vital signs, cardiac status, respiratory status, and degree of neuromuscular block (objective assessment with peripheral external nerve stimulator) is mandatory during infusion and until full muscle tone has returned. Muscle tone returns in a predictable pattern, starting with diaphragm, abdomen, chest, limbs, and finally muscles of the neck, face, and eyes. Safety precautions must be maintained until full muscle tone has returned. **Note:** It may take longer for return of muscle tone in obese or elderly patients or patients with renal or hepatic disease, myasthenia gravis, myopathy, other neuromuscular disease, dehydration, electrolyte imbalance, or severe acid/base imbalance. Provide appropriate patient teaching/support prior to and following administration.

Long-term use: Monitor fluid levels (intake and output) during and following infusion. Reposition patient and provide appropriate skin care, mouth care, and care of patient's eyes every 2-3 hours while sedated. Provide appropriate emotional and sensory support (auditory and environmental).

Monitoring Laboratory Tests: Renal function (serum creatinine, BUN) and liver function when in ICU

Patient Education: Patient will usually be unconscious prior to administration. Patient education should be appropriate to individual situation. Reassurance of constant monitoring and emotional support to reduce fear and anxiety should precede and follow administration. Following return of muscle tone, do not attempt to change position or rise from bed without assistance. Report immediately any skin rash or hives, pounding heartbeat, respiratory difficulty, or muscle tremors. **Pregnancy/breast-feeding precautions:** Inform prescriber if you are pregnant. Consult prescriber if breast-feeding.

Pregnancy Risk Factor: C

Lactation: Excretion in breast milk unknown/use caution

Administration

I.M.: Not for I.M. injection due to tissue irritation.

I.V.: May be given undiluted as a bolus injection. Administration via infusion requires the use of an infusion pump. Use infusion solutions within 24 hours of preparation.

Compatibility: Stable in D_5W, NS, D_5NS; **incompatible** with LR

Y-site administration: **Incompatible** with diazepam, propofol, thiopental

Compatibility when admixed: **Incompatible** with aminophylline, cefazolin, heparin, quinidine gluconate, ranitidine, sodium nitroprusside

Storage: Refrigerate; unstable in alkaline solutions.

Additional Information Atracurium is classified as an intermediate-duration neuromuscular-blocking agent. It does not appear to have a cumulative effect on the duration of blockade. It does not relieve pain or produce sedation.

♦ **Atracurium Besylate** *see Atracurium on page 157*

♦ **AtroPen®** *see Atropine on page 158*

Atropine *(A troe peen)*

U.S. Brand Names AtroPen®; Atropine-Care®; Isopto® Atropine; Sal-Tropine™

Synonyms Atropine Sulfate

Restrictions The AtroPen® formulation is available for use primarily by the Department of Defense.

Generic Available Yes: Excludes tablet

Pharmacologic Category Anticholinergic Agent; Anticholinergic Agent, Ophthalmic; Antidote; Antispasmodic Agent, Gastrointestinal; Ophthalmic Agent, Mydriatic

Use

Injection: Preoperative medication to inhibit salivation and secretions; treatment of symptomatic sinus bradycardia; AV block (nodal level); ventricular asystole; antidote for organophosphate pesticide poisoning

Ophthalmic: Produce mydriasis and cycloplegia for examination of the retina and optic disc and accurate measurement of refractive errors; uveitis

Oral: Inhibit salivation and secretions

Unlabeled/Investigational Use Pulseless electric activity, asystole, neuromuscular blockade reversal; treatment of nerve agent toxicity (chemical warfare) in combination with pralidoxime

Mechanism of Action/Effect Blocks the action of acetylcholine at parasympathetic sites in smooth muscle, secretory glands and the CNS; increases cardiac output, dries secretions, antagonizes histamine and serotonin

Contraindications Hypersensitivity to atropine or any component of the formulation; narrow-angle glaucoma; adhesions between the iris and lens; tachycardia; obstructive GI disease; paralytic ileus; intestinal atony of the elderly or debilitated patient; severe ulcerative colitis; toxic megacolon complicating ulcerative colitis; hepatic disease; obstructive uropathy; renal disease; myasthenia gravis (unless used to treat side effects of acetylcholinesterase inhibitor); asthma; thyrotoxicosis; Mobitz type II block

Warnings/Precautions Heat prostration can occur in the presence of a high environmental temperature. Psychosis can occur in sensitive individuals. The elderly may be sensitive to side effects. Use caution in patients with myocardial ischemia. Use caution in hyperthyroidism, autonomic neuropathy, BPH, CHF, tachyarrhythmias, hypertension, and hiatal hernia associated with reflux esophagitis. Use with caution in children with spastic paralysis.

AtroPen®: There are no absolute contraindications for the use of atropine in organophosphate poisonings, however, use caution in those patients where the use of atropine would be otherwise contraindicated. Formulation for use by trained personnel only.

Drug Interactions

Decreased Effect: Effect of some phenothiazines may be antagonized. Levodopa effects may be decreased (limited clinical validation). Drugs with cholinergic mechanisms (metoclopramide, cisapride, bethanechol) decrease anticholinergic effects of atropine.

Increased Effect/Toxicity: Antihistamines, phenothiazines, TCAs, and other drugs with anticholinergic activity may increase anticholinergic effects of atropine when used concurrently. Sympathomimetic amines may cause tachyarrhythmias; avoid concurrent use.

Adverse Reactions Severity and frequency of adverse reactions are dose related and vary greatly; listed reactions are limited to significant and/or life-threatening.

Cardiovascular: Arrhythmia, flushing, hypotension, palpitation, tachycardia

Central nervous system: Ataxia, coma, delirium, disorientation, dizziness, drowsiness, excitement, fever, hallucinations, headache, insomnia, nervousness

Dermatologic: Anhidrosis, urticaria, rash, scarlatiniform rash

Gastrointestinal: Bloating, constipation, delayed gastric emptying, loss of taste, nausea, paralytic ileus, vomiting, xerostomia

Genitourinary: Urinary hesitancy, urinary retention

Neuromuscular & skeletal: Weakness

Ocular: Angle-closure glaucoma, blurred vision, cycloplegia, dry eyes, mydriasis, ocular tension increased

Respiratory: Dyspnea, laryngospasm, pulmonary edema

Miscellaneous: Anaphylaxis

Overdosage/Toxicology Symptoms of overdose include dilated, unreactive pupils; blurred vision; hot, dry flushed skin; dryness of mucous membranes; difficulty swallowing; foul breath; diminished or absent bowel sounds; urinary retention; tachycardia; hyperthermia; hypertension; and increased respiratory rate. For anticholinergic overdose with severe life-threatening symptoms, physostigmine 1-2 mg SubQ or I.V. slowly, may be given to reverse these effects.

Pharmacodynamics/Kinetics

Onset of Action: I.V.: Rapid

Absorption: Complete

Half-Life Elimination: 2-3 hours

Metabolism: Hepatic

Excretion: Urine (30% to 50% as unchanged drug and metabolites)

Dosing

Adults: Doses <0.5 mg have been associated with paradoxical bradycardia.

Asystole:

I.V.: 1 mg; repeat in 3-5 minutes if asystole persists; total dose of 0.04 mg/kg.

Intratracheal: Administer 2-2.5 times the recommended I.V. dose; dilute in 10 mL NS or distilled water. **Note:** Absorption is greater with distilled water, but causes more adverse effects on PaO_2.

Inhibit salivation and secretions (preanesthesia):

I.M., I.V., SubQ: 0.4-0.6 mg 30-60 minutes preop and repeat every 4-6 hours as needed.

Oral: 0.4 mg, may repeat every 4-6 hours

Bradycardia: I.V.: 0.5-1 mg every 5 minutes, not to exceed a total of 3 mg or 0.04 mg/kg; may give intratracheal in 1 mg/10 mL dilution only, intratracheal dose should be 2-2.5 times the I.V. dose.

Neuromuscular blockade reversal: I.V.: 25-30 mcg/kg 30 seconds before neostigmine or 10 mcg/kg 30 seconds before edrophonium

Organophosphate or carbamate poisoning:

I.V.: 2 mg, followed by 2 mg every 15 minutes until adequate atropinization has occurred; initial doses of up to 6 mg may be used in life-threatening cases

I.M.: AtroPen®: Mild symptoms: Administer 2 mg as soon as exposure is known or suspected. If severe symptoms develop after first dose, 2 additional doses should be repeated in 10 minutes; do not administer more than 3 doses. Severe symptoms: Immediately administer three 2 mg doses.

Nerve agent toxicity management (unlabeled use): I.M.: See **Note.** Prehospital ("in the field") or hospital/emergency department: Mild-to-moderate symptoms: 2-4 mg; severe symptoms: 6 mg

Note: Pralidoxime is a component of the management of nerve agent toxicity; consult pralidoxime monograph for specific route and dose.

Prehospital ("in the field") management: Repeat atropine I.M. (2 mg) at 5-10 minute intervals until secretions have diminished and breathing is comfortable or airway resistance has returned to near normal.

Hospital management: Repeat atropine I.M. (2 mg) at 5-10 minute intervals until secretions have diminished and breathing is comfortable or airway resistance has returned to near normal.

Mydriasis, cycloplegia (preprocedure): Ophthalmic (1% solution): Instill 1-2 drops 1 hour before the procedure.

Uveitis: Ophthalmic:

1% solution: Instill 1-2 drops 4 times/day.

(Continued)

Atropine *(Continued)*

Ointment: Apply a small amount in the conjunctival sac up to 3 times/day. Compress the lacrimal sac by digital pressure for 1-3 minutes after instillation.

Elderly: Refer to adult dosing.

Nerve agent toxicity management (unlabeled use): I.M.: Elderly and frail patients: also see "**Note**" in adult dosing:

Prehospital ("in the field"): Mild-to-moderate symptoms: 1 mg; severe symptoms: 2-4 mg

Hospital/emergency department: Mild-to-moderate symptoms: 1 mg; severe symptoms: 2 mg

Pediatrics: Note: Doses <0.1 mg have been associated with paradoxical bradycardia.

Inhibit salivation and secretions (preanesthesia): Oral, I.M., I.V., SubQ: Neonates, Infants, and Children:

Children <5 kg: 0.02 mg/kg/dose 30-60 minutes preop then every 4-6 hours as needed. Use of a minimum dosage of 0.1 mg in neonates <5 kg will result in dosages >0.02 mg/kg. There is no documented minimum dosage in this age group.

Children >5 kg: 0.01-0.02 mg/kg/dose to a maximum 0.4 mg/dose 30-60 minutes preop; minimum dose: 0.1 mg

Alternate dosing:

3-7 kg (7-16 lb): 0.1 mg

8-11 kg (17-24 lb): 0.15 mg

11-18 kg (24-40 lb): 0.2 mg

18-29 kg (40-65 lb): 0.3 mg

>30 kg (>65 lb): 0.4 mg

Bradycardia: I.V., intratracheal: Neonates, Infants, and Children:

0.02 mg/kg, minimum dose 0.1 mg, maximum single dose: 0.5 mg in children and 1 mg in adolescents; may repeat in 5-minute intervals to a maximum total dose of 1 mg in children or 2 mg in adolescents. (**Note:** For intratracheal administration, the dosage must be diluted with normal saline to a total volume of 1-5 mL). When treating bradycardia in neonates, reserve use for those patients unresponsive to improved oxygenation and epinephrine.

Organophosphate or carbamate poisoning:

I.V.: Children: 0.03-0.05 mg/kg every 10-20 minutes until atropine effect, then every 1-4 hours for at least 24 hours

I.M. (AtroPen®): Children: Mild symptoms: Administer dose listed below as soon as exposure is known or suspected. If severe symptoms develop after first dose, 2 additional doses should be repeated in 10 minutes; do not administer more than 3 doses. Severe symptoms: Immediately administer 3 doses as follows:

<6.8 kg (15 lb): Use of **AtroPen® formulation not recommended**; administer atropine 0.05 mg/kg

6.8-18 kg (15-40 lb): 0.5 mg/dose

18-41 kg (40-90 lb): 1 mg/dose

>41 kg (>90 lb): 2 mg/dose

Nerve agent toxicity management (unlabeled use): I.M.: Infants and Children: See "**Note**" in adult dosing.

Prehospital ("in the field"):

Birth to <2 years: Mild-to-moderate symptoms: 0.05 mg/kg; severe symptoms: 0.1 mg/kg

2-10 years: Mild-to-moderate symptoms: 1 mg; severe symptoms: 2 mg

>10 years: Mild-to-moderate symptoms: 2 mg; severe symptoms: 4 mg

Hospital/emergency department:

Birth to <2 years: Mild-to-moderate symptoms: 0.05 mg/kg I.M. **or** 0.02 mg/kg I.V.; severe symptoms: 0.1 mg/kg I.M. **or** 0.02 mg/kg I.V

2-10 years: Mild-to-moderate symptoms: 1 mg; severe symptoms: 2 mg

>10 years: Mild-to-moderate symptoms: 2 mg; severe symptoms: 4 mg

Available Dosage Forms

Injection, solution, as sulfate: 0.05 mg/mL (5 mL); 0.1 mg/mL (5 mL, 10 mL); 0.4 mg/mL (0.5 mL, 1 mL, 20 mL); 0.5 mg/mL (1 mL); 1 mg/mL (1 mL)

AtroPen® [prefilled autoinjector]: 0.5 mg/0.7 mL (0.7 mL); 1 mg/0.7 mL (0.7 mL); 2 mg/0.7 mL (0.7 mL)

Ointment, ophthalmic, as sulfate: 1% (3.5 g)

Solution, ophthalmic, as sulfate: 1% (5 mL, 15 mL)

Atropine-Care®: 1% (2 mL)

Isopto® Atropine: 1% (5 mL, 15 mL)

Tablet, as sulfate (Sal-Tropine™): 0.4 mg

Monitoring and Teaching Issues

Physical Assessment: Assess other medications patient may be taking for effectiveness and interactions. Monitor for tachycardia, hypotension especially if cardiac problems are present. Be alert to the potential of heat prostration in the presence of high temperatures. Assess knowledge/teach patient appropriate use, interventions to reduce side effects, and adverse symptoms to report.

Patient Education: Take oral forms exactly as directed, 30 minutes before meals. Maintain adequate hydration (2-3 L/day of fluids) unless instructed to restrict fluid intake. Void before taking medication. You may experience dizziness, blurred vision, sensitivity to light (use caution when driving or engaging in tasks requiring alertness until response to drug is known); dry mouth, nausea, or vomiting (small frequent meals, frequent mouth care, sucking lozenges, or chewing gum may help); orthostatic hypotension (use caution when climbing stairs and when rising from lying or sitting position); constipation (increased exercise, fluids, fruit, or fiber may help; if not effective, consult prescriber); increased sensitivity to heat and decreased perspiration (avoid extremes of heat, reduce exercise in hot weather); or decreased milk if breast-feeding. Report hot, dry, flushed skin; blurred vision or vision changes; difficulty swallowing; chest pain, palpitations, or rapid heartbeat; painful or difficult urination; increased confusion, depression, or loss of memory; rapid or difficult respirations; muscle weakness or tremors; or eye pain.

Ophthalmic: Instill as often as recommended. Wash hands before using. Sit or lie down, open eye, look at ceiling, and instill prescribed amount of solution. Do not blink for 30 seconds, close eye and roll eye in all directions, and apply gentle pressure to inner corner of eye for 1-2 minutes. Do not let tip of applicator touch eye; do not contaminate tip of applicator (may cause eye infection, eye damage, or vision loss). Temporary stinging or blurred vision may occur.

Pregnancy/breast-feeding precautions: Inform prescriber if you are or intend to become pregnant. Consult prescriber if breast-feeding.

Geriatric Considerations: Anticholinergic agents are generally not well tolerated in the elderly and their use should be avoided when possible (see Warnings/Precautions, Adverse Reactions). In the elderly, anticholinergic agents should not be used as prophylaxis against extrapyramidal symptoms.

Pregnancy Risk Factor: C

Lactation: Enters breast milk (trace amounts)/use caution (AAP rates "compatible")

Breast-Feeding Issues: Anticholinergic agents may suppress lactation.

Administration

I.M.: AtroPen®: Administer to outer thigh. May be given through clothing as long as pockets at the injection site are empty. Hold autoinjector in place for 10 seconds following injection; massage the injection site.

I.V.: Administer undiluted by rapid I.V. injection; slow injection may result in paradoxical bradycardia

Other: Intratracheal: Dilute in NS or distilled water. Absorption is greater with distilled water, but causes more adverse effects on PaO_2. Pass catheter beyond tip of tracheal tube, stop compressions, spray drug quickly down tube. Follow immediately with several quick insufflations and continue chest compressions.

Compatibility:

Y-site administration: **Incompatible** with thiopental

Compatibility in syringe: **Incompatible** with cimetidine/pentobarbital

Compatibility when admixed: **Incompatible** with floxacillin, metaraminol, methohexital, norepinephrine

Storage: Store injection at controlled room temperature of 15°C to 30°C (59°F to 86°F); avoid freezing. In addition, AtroPen® should be protected from light.

Related Information

Compatibility of Drugs *on page 1723*

Compatibility of Drugs in Syringe *on page 1725*

Azacitidine (ay za SYE ti deen)

U.S. Brand Names Vidaza™

Synonyms AZA-CR; 5-Azacytidine; 5-AZC; Ladakamycin; NSC-102816

Generic Available No

Pharmacologic Category Antineoplastic Agent, Antimetabolite (Pyrimidine)

Use Treatment of myelodysplastic syndrome (MDS)

(Continued)

Azacitidine *(Continued)*

Unlabeled/Investigational Use Investigational: Refractory acute lymphocytic and myelogenous leukemia

Mechanism of Action/Effect Antineoplastic effects may be a result of azacitidine's ability to promote hypomethylation of DNA leading to direct toxicity of abnormal hematopoietic cells in the bone marrow.

Contraindications Hypersensitivity to azacitidine, mannitol, or any component of the formulation; advanced malignant hepatic tumors; pregnancy

Warnings/Precautions The U.S. Food and Drug Administration (FDA) currently recommends that procedures for proper handling and disposal of antineoplastic agents be considered. Azacitidine may be hepatotoxic, use caution with hepatic impairment. Progressive hepatic coma leading to death has been reported (rare) in patients with extensive tumor burden, especially those with a baseline albumin <30 g/L. Use caution with renal impairment; dose adjustment may be required.

Adverse Reactions Note: Percentages reported following SubQ administration unless otherwise noted:

>10%:

Cardiovascular: Hypotension (7%; I.V. 6% to 66% - incidence may be related to dose and rate of infusion), chest pain (16%), pallor (15%), peripheral edema (19%), pitting edema (14%)

Central nervous system: Pyrexia (52%), fatigue (13% to 36%), headache (22%), dizziness (19%), anxiety (13%), depression (12%), insomnia (11%), malaise (11%), pain (11%)

Dermatologic: Alopecia (I.V. 20%), bruising (30%), petechiae (24%), erythema (17%), skin lesion (14%), rash (14%)

Gastrointestinal: Nausea (70%; more common/more severe with I.V. administration), vomiting (54%; more common/more severe with I.V. administration), mucositis (I.V. 23% to 45%), diarrhea (36%), constipation (34%), anorexia (21%), weight loss (16%), abdominal pain (15%), appetite decreased (13%), abdominal tenderness (12%)

Hematologic: Anemia (70%), thrombocytopenia (66%), leukopenia (48%), neutropenia (32%), febrile neutropenia (16%)

Nadir: Day 10-17

Recovery: Day 28-31

Hepatic: Hepatic enzymes increased (I.V. 37%)

Local: Injection site:

I.V.: Redness, irritation, and induration (80%)

SubQ: Erythema (35%), pain (23%), bruising (14%)

Neuromuscular & skeletal: Weakness (30%), rigors (26%), arthralgia (22%), limb pain (20%), back pain (19%), myalgia (16%)

Respiratory: Cough (30%), dyspnea (5% to 30%), pharyngitis (20%), epistaxis (16%), nasopharyngitis (14%), upper respiratory tract infection (13%), productive cough (11%), pneumonia (11%)

Miscellaneous: Contusion (19%)

5% to 10%:

Cardiovascular: Cardiac murmur (10%), tachycardia (9%) peripheral swelling (7%), syncope (6%), chest wall pain (5%), hypoesthesia (5%), postprocedural pain (5%)

Central nervous system: Lethargy (8%)

Dermatologic: Cellulitis (8%), urticaria (6%), dry skin (5%), skin nodule (5%)

Gastrointestinal: Upper abdominal pain (10%), gingival bleeding (9%), oral mucosal petechiae (8%), stomatitis (8%), dyspepsia (7%), hemorrhoids (7%), abdominal distension (6%), loose stools (5%), dysphagia (5%), tongue ulceration (5%)

Genitourinary: Dysuria (8%), urinary tract infection (8%)

Hematologic: Hematoma (9%), postprocedural hemorrhage (6%)

Local: Injection site: Pruritus (7%), granuloma (5%), pigmentation change (5%), swelling (5%)

Neuromuscular & skeletal: Muscle cramps (6%)

Respiratory: Crackles (10%), rhinorrhea (10%), wheezing (9%), breath sounds decreased (8%), pleural effusion (6%), postnasal drip (6%), rhonchi (6%), nasal congestion (5%), atelectasis (5%), sinusitis (5%)

Miscellaneous: Diaphoresis (10%), lymphadenopathy (9%), herpes simplex (9%), night sweats (7%), transfusion reaction (7%), mouth hemorrhage (5%)

Overdosage/Toxicology Diarrhea, nausea, and vomiting were reported following a single I.V. dose of 290 mg/m². Treatment should be supportive.

Pharmacodynamics/Kinetics

Absorption: SubQ: Rapid and complete

Bioavailability: SubQ: 89%

Time to Peak: 30 minutes

Half-Life Elimination: ~4 hours

Metabolism: Hepatic; hydrolysis to several metabolites

Excretion: Urine (50% to 85%); feces (minor)

Dosing

Adults & Elderly: Note: I.V. administration is an unlabeled use; doses reported in combination regimens.

Acute leukemia: I.V.:

50-150 mg/m² days 1 through 5 of induction

200 mg/m² CIVI days 7 through 9 of induction

AML induction: I.V.: 150 mg/m² days 3 through 5 and 8 through 10, **then**
150 mg/m² days 1 through 5 and 8 through 10 (cycle 2 consolidation)

AML consolidation: I.V.: 150 mg/m² CIVI days 1 through 7 for 3 cycles

AML maintenance: I.V.: 150 mg/m² days 1 through 3 every 6 weeks

CML (accelerated phase and blast crisis): I.V.: 50-150 mg/m² days 1 through 5 of induction

MDS: I.V.: 75-150 mg/m² CIVI days 1 through 7 every 4 weeks

MDS: SubQ: 75 mg/m^2/day for 7 days repeated every 4 weeks. Dose may be increased to 100 mg/m^2/day if no benefit is observed after 2 cycles and no toxicity other than nausea and vomiting have occurred. Treatment is recommended for at least 4 cycles.

Dosage adjustment based on hematology: SubQ:

For baseline WBC ≥3.0 x 10^9/L, ANC ≥1.5 x 10^9/L, and platelets ≥75 x 10^9/L:

Nadir count: ANC <0.5 x 10^9/L and platelets <25 x 10^9/L: Administer 50% of dose during next treatment course

Nadir count: ANC 0.5-1.5 x 10^9/L and platelets 25-50 x 10^9/L: Administer 67% of dose during next treatment course

Nadir count: ANC >1.5 x 10^9/L and platelets >50 x 10^9/L: Administer 100% of dose during next treatment course

For baseline WBC <3 x 10^9/L, ANC 1.5 x 10^9/L, or platelets <75 x 10^9/L: Adjust dose as follows based on nadir counts and bone marrow biopsy cellularity at the time of nadir, unless clear improvement in differentiation at the time of the next cycle:

WBC or platelet nadir decreased 50% to 75% from baseline and bone marrow biopsy cellularity at time of nadir 30% to 60%: Administer 100% of dose during next treatment course

WBC or platelet nadir decreased 50% to 75% from baseline and bone marrow biopsy cellularity at time of nadir 15% to 30%: Administer 50% of dose during next treatment course

WBC or platelet nadir decreased 50% to 75% from baseline and bone marrow biopsy cellularity at time of nadir <15%: Administer 33% of dose during next treatment course

WBC or platelet nadir decreased >75% from baseline and bone marrow biopsy cellularity at time of nadir 30% to 60%: Administer 75% of dose during next treatment course

WBC or platelet nadir decreased >75% from baseline and bone marrow biopsy cellularity at time of nadir 15% to 30%: Administer 50% of dose during next treatment course

WBC or platelet nadir decreased >75% from baseline and bone marrow biopsy cellularity at time of nadir <15%: Administer 33% of dose during next treatment course

Note: If a nadir defined above occurs, administer the next treatment course 28 days after the start of the preceding course as long as WBC and platelet counts are >25% above the nadir and rising. If a >25% increase above the nadir is not seen by day 28, reassess counts every 7 days. If a 25% increase is not seen by day 42, administer 50% of the scheduled dose.

Dosage adjustment base on serum electrolytes: If serum bicarbonate falls to <20 mEq/L (unexplained decrease): Reduce dose by 50% for next treatment course

Pediatrics: Note: Unlabeled use, doses reported in combination regimens:

Pediatric AML and ANLL: I.V.: 250 mg/m^2 days 4 and 5 every 4 weeks

Pediatric AML induction: I.V.: 300 mg/m^2 days 5 and 6

Renal Impairment: Adults: If unexplained increases in BUN or serum creatinine occur, delay next cycle until values reach baseline or normal, then reduce dose by 50% for next treatment course.

Available Dosage Forms Injection, powder for suspension: 100 mg [contains mannitol 100 mg]

Monitoring and Teaching Issues

Physical Assessment: Use with caution in presence of hepatic or renal impairment (eg, may be hepatotoxic; see Warnings/Precautions). Pretreatment with antiemetic is recommended to reduce nausea and vomiting. Solutions have limited stability; note specific administration, reconstitution, and storage instructions. Assess results of laboratory tests prior to beginning therapy and prior to each cycle (see Monitoring Laboratory Tests). Patient should be monitored closely for adverse effects (eg, hypotension, CNS changes, GI, hematologic, and hepatic effects; see Adverse Reactions). Teach patient (or caregiver) possible side effects/appropriate intervention and adverse symptoms to report.

Monitoring Laboratory Tests: Liver function tests, electrolytes, CBC, renal function tests (BUN and serum creatinine) should be obtained prior to initiation of therapy. Electrolytes, renal function (BUN and creatinine), CBC should be monitored periodically to monitor response and toxicity. At a minimum, CBC should be repeated prior to each cycle.

Patient Education: Do not take anything new during treatment unless approved by prescriber. This medication can only be administered by injection or infusion; report immediately any pain, burning, swelling at injection/infusion site. Limit oral intake for 4-6 hours before therapy to reduce potential for nausea/vomiting. It is important that you maintain adequate nutrition between treatments (small frequent meals may help) and adequate hydration (2-3 L/day of fluids), unless advised by prescriber to restrict fluids. You may be susceptible to infection (avoid crowds and exposure to infection and do not have any vaccinations without consulting prescriber). May cause nausea, vomiting, or anorexia (small frequent meals, frequent mouth care, chewing gum, or sucking lozenges may help; if nausea/vomiting are severe, request antiemetic); mouth sores (use soft toothbrush or cotton swabs for mouth care); loss of hair (reversible). Report chest pain or palpitations; sore throat, fever, chills, unusual weakness or fatigue; unusual bruising/bleeding; change in color of urine or stool; difficulty breathing; change in visual acuity; or pain, redness, or swelling at injection site, or any other adverse reactions. **Pregnancy/breast-feeding precautions:** Inform prescriber if you are pregnant. Do not get pregnant or cause a pregnancy (males) during therapy. Consult prescriber for instruction on appropriate contraceptive measures. This drug may cause severe fetal defects. Breast-feeding is not recommended.

Geriatric Considerations: Monitor renal function

Pregnancy Risk Factor: D

Pregnancy Issues: Embryotoxicity, fetal death, and fetal abnormalities were observed in animal studies. Women of childbearing potential should be advised to avoid pregnancy during treatment. In addition, males should be advised to avoid fathering a child while on azacitidine therapy.

Lactation: Excretion in breast milk unknown/not recommended

Administration

I.V.: Premedication for nausea and vomiting is recommended. Administer as short (15 minutes to 2 hours) bolus or continuous (24 hour) infusion. Due to azacitidine's limited (Continued)

Azacitidine *(Continued)*

stability, for continuous infusions the daily dose should be divided by 12, and a freshly prepared bag, using a freshly reconstituted vial, started every 2 hours.

Other: SubQ: Premedication for nausea and vomiting is recommended. Doses >50 mg (2 mL) should be divided into 2 syringes and injected into 2 separate sites. Allow refrigerated suspensions to come to room temperature (up to 30 minutes) prior to administration. Resuspend by gently rolling the syringe between the palms for 30 seconds. If azacitidine suspension comes in contact with the skin, immediately wash with soap and water.

Reconstitution:

SubQ: Slowly add 4 mL SWFI to each vial. Invert vial 2-3 times and gently rotate until a suspension is formed.

I.V.: Reconstitute vial with 19.9 mL of lactated Ringer's injection, 0.9% sodium chloride, or 5% dextrose to form a 5 mg/mL solution. Mix in 50-250 mL (final concentration ≥2 mg/mL) lactated Ringer's injection for infusion.

Storage:

SubQ: Prior to reconstitution, store powder at room temperature of 15°C to 30°C (59°F to 86°F). Following reconstitution, suspension may be stored at room temperature for up to 1 hour, or immediately refrigerated at 2°C to 8°C (36°F to 46°F) and stored for up to 8 hours.

I.V.: Solutions for injection have very limited stability and must be prepared fresh immediately prior to each dose. Solutions (≥2 mg/mL) in lactated Ringer's injection are stable for 3 hours; solutions in 5% dextrose in water or 0.9% sodium chloride injection are only stable for ~1 hour.

♦ **AZA-CR**   *see* Azacitidine *on page 161*

♦ **Azactam®**   *see* Aztreonam *on page 168*

♦ **5-Azacytidine**   *see* Azacitidine *on page 161*

♦ **Azasan®**   *see* Azathioprine *on page 164*

Azathioprine *(ay za THYE oh preen)*

U.S. Brand Names Azasan®; Imuran®

Synonyms Azathioprine Sodium

Generic Available Yes

Pharmacologic Category Immunosuppressant Agent

Medication Safety Issues

Sound-alike/look-alike issues:

Azathioprine may be confused with azatadine, azidothymidine, Azulfidine®

Imuran® may be confused with Elmiron®, Enduron®, Imdur®, Inderal®, Tenormin®

Use Adjunct with other agents in prevention of rejection of kidney transplants; also used in severe active rheumatoid arthritis unresponsive to other agents; other autoimmune diseases (ITP, SLE, MS, Crohn's disease)

Unlabeled/Investigational Use Adjunct in prevention of rejection of solid organ (nonrenal) transplants

Mechanism of Action/Effect Antagonizes purine metabolism and may inhibit synthesis of DNA, RNA, and proteins; may also interfere with cellular metabolism and inhibit mitosis

Contraindications Hypersensitivity to azathioprine or any component of the formulation; pregnancy

Warnings/Precautions Chronic immunosuppression increases the risk of neoplasia. Has mutagenic potential to both men and women and with possible hematologic toxicities. Use with caution in patients with liver disease, renal impairment. Monitor hematologic function closely. Patients with genetic deficiency of thiopurine methyltransferase (TPMT) or concurrent therapy with drugs which may inhibit TPMT may be sensitive to myelosuppressive effects.

Drug Interactions

Decreased Effect: Azathioprine may result in decreased action of warfarin.

Increased Effect/Toxicity: Allopurinol may increase serum levels of azathioprine's active metabolite (mercaptopurine). Decrease azathioprine dose to $\frac{1}{3}$ to $\frac{1}{4}$ of normal dose. Azathioprine and ACE inhibitors may induce severe leukopenia. Aminosalicylates (olsalazine, mesalamine, sulfasalazine) may inhibit TPMT, increasing toxicity/myelosuppression of azathioprine.

Nutritional/Ethanol Interactions Herb/Nutraceutical: Avoid cat's claw, echinacea (have immunostimulant properties).

Adverse Reactions Frequency not defined.

Central nervous system: Fever, chills

Dermatologic: Alopecia, erythematous or maculopapular rash

Gastrointestinal: Nausea, vomiting, anorexia, diarrhea, aphthous stomatitis, pancreatitis

Hematologic: Leukopenia, thrombocytopenia, anemia, pancytopenia (bone marrow suppression may be determined, in part, by genetic factors, ie, patients with TPMT deficiency are at higher risk)

Hepatic: Hepatotoxicity, jaundice, hepatic veno-occlusive disease

Neuromuscular & skeletal: Arthralgias

Ocular: Retinopathy

Miscellaneous: Rare hypersensitivity reactions which include myalgia, rigors, dyspnea, hypotension, serum sickness, rash; secondary infection may occur secondary to immunosuppression

Overdosage/Toxicology Symptoms of overdose include nausea, vomiting, diarrhea, and hematologic toxicity. Following initiation of essential overdose management, symptomatic and supportive treatment should be instituted. Dialysis has been reported to remove significant amounts of the drug and its metabolites, and should be considered as a treatment option in those patients who deteriorate despite established forms of therapy.

Pharmacodynamics/Kinetics

Protein Binding: ~30%

Half-Life Elimination: Parent drug: 12 minutes; mercaptopurine: 0.7-3 hours; End-stage renal disease: Slightly prolonged

Metabolism: Extensively hepatic via xanthine oxidase to mercaptopurine (active); mercaptopurine requires detoxification by thiopurine methyltransferase (TPMT)

Excretion: Urine (primarily as metabolites)

Dosing

Adults & Elderly: I.V. dose is equivalent to oral dose.

Renal transplantation: Oral, I.V.: 2-5 mg/kg/day to start, then 1-3 mg/kg/day maintenance

Rheumatoid arthritis: Oral: 1 mg/kg/day for 6-8 weeks; increase by 0.5 mg/kg every 4 weeks until response or up to 2.5 mg/kg/day

Pediatrics: Children: Refer to adult dosing.

Renal Impairment:

Cl$_{cr}$ 10-50 mL/minute: Administer 75% of normal dose.

Cl$_{cr}$ <10 mL/minute: Administer 50% of normal dose.

Hemodialysis: Slightly dialyzable (5% to 20%) Administer dose posthemodialysis.

CAPD effects: Unknown; CAVH effects: Unknown

Available Dosage Forms

Injection, powder for reconstitution, as sodium: 100 mg

Tablet [scored]: 50 mg

Azasan®: 25 mg, 50 mg, 75 mg, 100 mg

Imuran®: 50 mg

Monitoring and Teaching Issues

Physical Assessment: Assess effectiveness and interactions of other medications patient may be taking. Assess results of laboratory tests therapeutic effectiveness (according to purpose for use) and adverse reactions at beginning of therapy and periodically throughout therapy, especially opportunistic infection. Assess knowledge/teach patient appropriate use, interventions to reduce side effects, and adverse symptoms to report.

Monitoring Laboratory Tests: CBC, platelet counts, total bilirubin, alkaline phosphatase

Patient Education: Take as prescribed (may take in divided doses or with food if GI upset occurs). You will be susceptible to infection (avoid crowds and exposure to infection and do not have any vaccinations unless approved by prescriber). You may experience nausea, vomiting, loss of appetite (small frequent meals, frequent mouth care, chewing gum, or sucking lozenges may help). Report abdominal pain and unresolved GI upset (eg, persistent vomiting or diarrhea); unusual fever or chills; bleeding or bruising; sore throat, unhealed sores, or signs of infection; yellowing of skin or eyes; or change in color of urine or stool.

Rheumatoid arthritis: Response may not occur for up to 3 months; do not discontinue without consulting prescriber.

Organ transplant: Azathioprine will usually be prescribed with other antirejection medications.

Pregnancy/breast-feeding precautions: Do not get pregnant while taking this medication; use appropriate contraceptive measures. Breast-feeding is not recommended.

Dietary Considerations: May be taken with food.

Geriatric Considerations: Immunosuppressive toxicity is increased in the elderly. Signs or symptoms of infection may differ in the elderly. Lethargy or confusion may be the first signs of infection.

Pregnancy Risk Factor: D

Lactation: Excretion in breast milk unknown/not recommended

Administration

I.V.: Can be administered IVP over 5 minutes at a concentration not to exceed 10 mg/mL **or** azathioprine can be further diluted with normal saline or D$_5$W and administered by intermittent infusion over 15-60 minutes.

Compatibility: Stable in neutral or acid solutions, but is hydrolyzed to mercaptopurine in alkaline solutions. Stable in D$_5$W, $^1/_2$NS, NS.

Storage: Stability of parenteral admixture at room temperature (25°C) is 24 hours. Stability of parenteral admixture at refrigeration temperature (4°C) is 16 days.

◆ **Azathioprine Sodium** see Azathioprine on page 164

◆ **5-AZC** see Azacitidine on page 161

◆ **Azidothymidine** see Zidovudine on page 1585

◆ **Azidothymidine, Abacavir, and Lamivudine** see Abacavir, Lamivudine, and Zidovudine on page 34

Azithromycin (az ith roe MYE sin)

U.S. Brand Names Zithromax®

Synonyms Azithromycin Dihydrate; Zithromax® TRI-PAK™; Zithromax® Z-PAK®

Generic Available No

Pharmacologic Category Antibiotic, Macrolide

Medication Safety Issues

Sound-alike/look-alike issues:

Azithromycin may be confused with erythromycin

Zithromax® may be confused with Zinacef®

Use Treatment of acute otitis media due to *H. influenzae*, *M. catarrhalis*, or *S. pneumoniae*; pharyngitis/tonsillitis due to *S. pyogenes*; treatment of mild-to-moderate upper and lower respiratory tract infections, infections of the skin and skin structure, community-acquired pneumonia, pelvic inflammatory disease (PID), sexually-transmitted diseases (urethritis/cervicitis), pharyngitis/tonsillitis (alternative to first-line therapy), and genital ulcer disease (chancroid) due to susceptible strains of *C. trachomatis*, *M. catarrhalis*, *H. influenzae*, *S.*

(Continued)

Azithromycin *(Continued)*

aureus, S. pneumoniae, Mycoplasma pneumoniae, and *C. psittaci;* acute bacterial exacerbations of chronic obstructive pulmonary disease (COPD) due to *H. influenzae, M. catarrhalis,* or *S. pneumoniae;* acute bacterial sinusitis

Unlabeled/Investigational Use Prevention of (or to delay onset of) or treatment of MAC in patients with advanced HIV infection; prophylaxis of bacterial endocarditis in patients who are allergic to penicillin and undergoing surgical or dental procedures

Mechanism of Action/Effect Inhibits RNA-dependent protein synthesis at the chain elongation step; binds to the 50S ribosomal subunit resulting in blockage of transpeptidation

Contraindications Hypersensitivity to azithromycin, other macrolide antibiotics, or any component of the formulation

Warnings/Precautions Use with caution in patients with hepatic dysfunction; hepatic impairment with or without jaundice has occurred chiefly in older children and adults; it may be accompanied by malaise, nausea, vomiting, abdominal colic, and fever; discontinue use if these occur. May mask or delay symptoms of incubating gonorrhea or syphilis, so appropriate culture and susceptibility tests should be performed prior to initiating azithromycin. Pseudomembranous colitis has been reported with use of macrolide antibiotics; use caution with renal dysfunction. Prolongation of the QT$_c$ interval has been reported with macrolide antibiotics; use caution in patients at risk of prolonged cardiac repolarization. Safety and efficacy have not been established in children <6 months of age with acute otitis media, acute bacterial sinusitis, or community-acquired pneumonia, or in children <2 years of age with pharyngitis/tonsillitis.

Drug Interactions

Cytochrome P450 Effect: Substrate of CYP3A4 (minor); **Inhibits** CYP3A4 (weak)

Decreased Effect: Decreased azithromycin peak serum concentrations with aluminum- and magnesium-containing antacids (by 24%), however, total absorption is unaffected.

Increased Effect/Toxicity: Concurrent use of pimozide is contraindicated due to potential cardiotoxicity. The manufacturer warns that azithromycin potentially may increase levels of tacrolimus, phenytoin, ergot alkaloids, alfentanil, bromocriptine, carbamazepine, cyclosporine, digoxin, disopyramide, and triazolam. However, azithromycin did not affect the response/levels of carbamazepine, theophylline, or warfarin in specific interaction studies; caution is advised when administered together. Nelfinavir may increase azithromycin serum levels (monitor for adverse effects).

Nutritional/Ethanol Interactions Food: Rate and extent of GI absorption may be altered depending upon the formulation. Azithromycin suspension, not tablet form, has significantly increased absorption (46%) with food.

Adverse Reactions 1% to 10%: Gastrointestinal: Diarrhea, nausea, abdominal pain, cramping, vomiting (especially with high single-dose regimens)

Overdosage/Toxicology Symptoms of overdose include nausea, vomiting, diarrhea, and prostration. Treatment is supportive and symptomatic.

Pharmacodynamics/Kinetics

Absorption: Rapid

Bioavailability: 37%; variable effect with food (increased with oral suspension, unchanged with tablet)

Time to Peak: Serum: 2.3-4 hours

Protein Binding: Concentration dependent: 7% to 50%

Half-Life Elimination: Terminal: 68 hours

Metabolism: Hepatic

Excretion: Feces (50% as unchanged drug); urine (~5% to 12%)

Dosing

Adults & Elderly:

Mild to moderate respiratory tract, skin, and soft tissue infections: Oral: 500 mg in a single loading dose on day 1 followed by 250 mg/day as a single dose on days 2-5
Alternative regimen: Bacterial exacerbation of COPD: 500 mg/day for a total of 3 days

Bacterial sinusitis: Oral: 500 mg/day for a total of 3 days

Community-acquired pneumonia: I.V.: 500 mg as a single dose for at least 2 days, follow I.V. therapy by the oral route with a single daily dose of 500 mg to complete a 7- to 10-day course of therapy.

Urethritis/cervicitis:
Due to *C. trachomatis:* Oral: 1 g as a single dose
Due to *N. gonorrhoeae:* Oral: 2 g as a single dose

Chancroid due to *H. ducreyi:* Oral: 1 g as a single dose

Pelvic inflammatory disease (PID): I.V.: 500 mg as a single dose for 1-2 days, follow I.V. therapy by the oral route with a single daily dose of 250 mg to complete a 7-day course of therapy.

Prophylaxis for bacterial endocarditis (unlabeled use): Oral: 500 mg 1 hour prior to the procedure

Disseminated *M. avium* complex disease in patient with advanced HIV infection (unlabeled use):
Prophylaxis: Oral: 1200 mg once weekly (may be combined with rifabutin)
Treatment: Oral: 600 mg daily in combination with ethambutol 15 mg/kg

Pediatrics:

Note: Adolescents ≥16 years: Refer to adult dosing.

Community-acquired pneumonia: Oral: Children ≥6 months: 10 mg/kg on day 1 (maximum: 500 mg/day) followed by 5 mg/kg/day once daily on days 2-5 (maximum: 250 mg/day)

Bacterial sinusitis: Oral: Children ≥6 months: 10 mg/kg once daily for 3 days (maximum: 500 mg/day)

Otitis media: Oral: Children ≥6 months:
1-day regimen: 30 mg/kg as a single dose (maximum dose: 1500 mg)
3-day regimen: 10 mg/kg once daily for 3 days (maximum: 500 mg/day)

5-day regimen: 10 mg/kg on day 1 (maximum: 500 mg/day) followed by 5 mg/kg/day once daily on days 2-5 (maximum: 250 mg/day)

Pharyngitis, tonsillitis: Oral: Children ≥2 years: 12 mg/kg/day once daily for 5 days (maximum: 500 mg/day)

Disseminated *M. avium*-infected patients with acquired immunodeficiency syndrome (unlabeled use): Oral: 5 mg/kg/day once daily (maximum dose: 250 mg/day) or 20 mg/kg (maximum dose: 1200 mg) once weekly given alone or in combination with rifabutin

Treatment and secondary prevention of disseminated MAC (unlabeled use): Oral: 5 mg/kg/day once daily (maximum dose: 250 mg/day) in combination with ethambutol, with or without rifabutin

Prophylaxis for bacterial endocarditis (unlabeled use): Oral: 15 mg/kg 1 hour before procedure

Uncomplicated chlamydial urethritis or cervicitis (unlabeled use): Children ≥45 kg: 1 g as a single dose

Renal Impairment: Use caution in patients with Cl$_{cr}$ <10 mL/minute

Hepatic Impairment: Use with caution due to potential for hepatotoxicity (rare). Specific guidelines for dosing in hepatic impairment have not been established.

Available Dosage Forms

Injection, powder for reconstitution, as dihydrate: 500 mg

Powder for oral suspension, as dihydrate: 100 mg/5 mL (15 mL); 200 mg/5 mL (15 mL, 22.5 mL, 30 mL) [cherry creme de vanilla and banana flavor]; 1 g [single-dose packet; cherry creme de vanilla and banana flavor]

Tablet, as dihydrate: 250 mg, 500 mg, 600 mg

Zithromax® TRI-PAK™ [unit-dose pack]: 500 mg (3s)

Zithromax® Z-PAK® [unit-dose pack]: 250 mg (6s)

Monitoring and Teaching Issues

Physical Assessment: Assess results of culture and sensitivity tests and patient's allergy history prior to beginning therapy. Note Warnings/Precautions for use cautions. Assess potential for interactions with other pharmacological agents patient may be taking (see Drug Interactions). Assess results of laboratory tests (LFTs, CBC with differential), therapeutic effectiveness, and adverse effects (see Adverse Reactions and Overdose/Toxicology). Instruct patients being treated for STDs about preventing transmission. Teach patient appropriate use, possible side effects/appropriate interventions, and adverse symptoms to report.

Monitoring Laboratory Tests: Liver function, CBC with differential. Perform culture and sensitivity testing prior to initiating therapy.

Patient Education: Do not take any new medication during therapy unless approved by prescriber. Take as directed. Take entire prescription and do not discontinue until prescription is completed. Take capsule form 1 hour before or 2 hours after meals; suspension may be taken with or without food; tablet form may be taken with meals to decrease GI effects. Do not take with antacids that contain aluminum or magnesium. Maintain adequate hydration (2-3 L/day of fluids) unless instructed to restrict fluid intake. If taken to treat a sexually-transmitted disease, follow advice of prescriber related to sexual intercourse and preventing transmission. May cause transient abdominal distress, diarrhea, and headache. Report signs of additional infections (eg, sores in mouth or vagina, vaginal discharge, unresolved fever, severe vomiting, or loose or foul smelling stools). **Breast-feeding precaution:** Consult prescriber if breast-feeding.

Dietary Considerations:

Powder for oral suspension may be administered with or without food.

Tablet may be administered with food to decrease GI effects.

Sodium content:

Injection: 114 mg (4.96 mEq) per vial

Powder: 3.7 mg per 100 mg/5 mL of constituted solution; 7.4 mg per 200 mg/5 mL of constituted solution; 37 mg per 1 g single-dose packet

Tablet: 0.9 mg/250 mg tablet; 1.8 mg/500 mg tablet; 2.1 mg/600 mg tablet

Geriatric Considerations: Dosage adjustment does not appear to be necessary in the elderly. Considered one of the drugs of choice in the treatment of outpatient treatment of community-acquired pneumonia in older adults.

Pregnancy Risk Factor: B

Lactation: Enters breast milk/use caution

Breast-Feeding Issues: Based on one case report, azithromycin has been shown to accumulate in breast milk.

Administration

Oral: Suspension and tablet may be taken without regard to food.

I.V.: Other medications should not be infused simultaneously through the same I.V. line.

Reconstitution: Injection: Prepare initiation solution by adding 4.8 mL of sterile water for injection to the 500 mg vial (resulting concentration: 100 mg/mL). Use of a standard syringe is recommended due to the vacuum in the vial (which may draw additional solution through an automated syringe).

The initial solution should be further diluted to a concentration of 1 mg/mL (500 mL) to 2 mg/mL (250 mL) in 0.9% sodium chloride, 5% dextrose in water, or lactated Ringer's. The diluted solution is stable for 24 hours at or below room temperature (30°C or 86°F) and for 7 days if stored under refrigeration (5°C or 41°F).

Compatibility: Other medications should not be infused simultaneously through the same I.V. line.

Storage:

Injection: Store intact vials of injection at room temperature. Reconstituted solution is stable for 24 hours when stored below 30°C/86°F.

Suspension: Store dry powder below 30°C (86°F); following reconstitution, store suspension at 5°C to 30°C (41°F to 86°F).

Tablets: Store between 15°C to 30°C (59°F to 86°F).

Additional Information Capsules are no longer being produced in the United States.

(Continued)

Azithromycin *(Continued)*

Related Information
Antimicrobial Drugs of Choice *on page 1792*
Community-Acquired Pneumonia in Adults *on page 1807*
I.V. to Oral Conversion *on page 1688*

♦ **Azithromycin Dihydrate** *see Azithromycin on page 165*

♦ **Azmacort®** *see Triamcinolone on page 1518*

♦ **Azo-Gesic® [OTC]** *see Phenazopyridine on page 1193*

♦ **Azopt®** *see Brinzolamide on page 207*

♦ **Azo-Standard® [OTC]** *see Phenazopyridine on page 1193*

♦ **AZT** *see Zidovudine on page 1585*

♦ **AZT + 3TC** *see Zidovudine and Lamivudine on page 1587*

♦ **AZT, Abacavir, and Lamivudine** *see Abacavir, Lamivudine, and Zidovudine on page 34*

♦ **Azthreonam** *see Aztreonam on page 168*

Aztreonam *(AZ tree oh nam)*
U.S. Brand Names Azactam®
Synonyms Azthreonam
Generic Available No
Pharmacologic Category Antibiotic, Miscellaneous
Medication Safety Issues
Sound-alike/look-alike issues:
Aztreonam may be confused with azidothymidine
Use Treatment of patients with urinary tract infections, lower respiratory tract infections, septicemia, skin/skin structure infections, intra-abdominal infections, and gynecological infections caused by susceptible gram-negative bacilli
Mechanism of Action/Effect Monobactam which is active only against gram-negative bacilli; inhibits bacterial cell wall synthesis during active multiplication, causing cell wall destruction
Contraindications Hypersensitivity to aztreonam or any component of the formulation
Warnings/Precautions Rare cross-allergenicity to penicillins and cephalosporins has been reported. Use caution in renal impairment; dosing adjustment required.
Drug Interactions
Decreased Effect: Avoid antibiotics that induce beta-lactamase production (cefoxitin, imipenem).
Lab Interactions Urine glucose (Clinitest®)
Adverse Reactions As reported in adults:
1% to 10%:
Dermatologic: Rash
Gastrointestinal: Diarrhea, nausea, vomiting
Local: Thrombophlebitis, pain at injection site
Overdosage/Toxicology Symptoms of overdose include seizures. Treatment is supportive. If necessary, dialysis can reduce the drug concentration in the blood.
Pharmacodynamics/Kinetics
Absorption: I.M.: Well absorbed; I.M. and I.V. doses produce comparable serum concentrations
Time to Peak: I.M., I.V. push: Within 60 minutes; I.V. infusion: 1.5 hours
Protein Binding: 56%
Half-Life Elimination:
Children 2 months to 12 years: 1.7 hours
Adults: Normal renal function: 1.7-2.9 hours
End-stage renal disease: 6-8 hours
Metabolism: Hepatic (minor %)
Excretion: Urine (60% to 70% as unchanged drug); feces ($\sim$13% to 15%)
Dosing
Adults & Elderly:
Urinary tract infection: I.M., I.V.: 500 mg to 1 g every 8-12 hours
Moderately severe systemic infections:
I.M.: 1 g every 8-12 hours
I.V.: 1-2 g I.V. every 8-12 hours
Severe systemic or life-threatening infections (especially caused by *Pseudomonas aeruginosa*): I.V.: 2 g every 6-8 hours; maximum: 8 g/day
Pediatrics:
Susceptible infections: I.M., I.V.: Children >1 month:
Mild-to-moderate infections: 30 mg/kg every 8 hours
Moderate-to-severe infections: 30 mg/kg every 6-8 hours; maximum: 120 mg/kg/day (8 g/day)
Infection in children with cystic fibrosis: I.V.: Children >1 month: 50 mg/kg/dose every 6-8 hours (ie, up to 200 mg/kg/day); maximum: 8 g/day
Renal Impairment: Adults: Following initial dose, maintenance doses should be given as follows:
Cl_{cr} 10-30 mL/minute: 50% of usual dose at the usual interval
Cl_{cr} <10 mL/minute: 25% of usual dosage at the usual interval
Hemodialysis: Moderately dialyzable (20% to 50%); $^1/_8$ of initial dose after each hemodialysis session (given in addition to the maintenance doses)
Peritoneal dialysis: Administer as for Cl_{cr} <10 mL/minute
Continuous arteriovenous or venovenous hemofiltration: Dose as for Cl_{cr} 10-30 mL/minute
Available Dosage Forms
Infusion [premixed]: 1 g (50 mL); 2 g (50 mL)
Injection, powder for reconstitution: 500 mg, 1 g, 2 g

Monitoring and Teaching Issues

Physical Assessment: Assess results of culture and sensitivity tests and patient's allergy history before initiating therapy (see Warnings/Precautions). I.V. infusion site should be monitored closely. Assess therapeutic effectiveness and adverse response (see Adverse Reactions). Caution patients with diabetes about altered response to Clinitest®. Teach patient possible side effects/appropriate interventions and adverse symptoms to report.

Monitoring Laboratory Tests: Obtain specimens for culture and sensitivity before the first dose.

Patient Education: Do not take any new medication during therapy unless approved by prescriber. This medication can only be administered by injection or infusion. Report immediately any burning, pain, swelling, or redness at infusion/injection site. May cause nausea or GI distress (frequent mouth care, frequent small meals, sucking lozenges, or chewing gum may help relieve these symptoms). If you have diabetes, drug may cause false tests with Clinitest® urine glucose monitoring; use of another type of glucose monitoring is preferable. Report rash, persistent and unrelieved diarrhea or vomiting, pain at injection site, unresolved fever, unhealed or new sores in mouth or vagina, vaginal discharge, or acute onset of respiratory difficulty. **Breast-feeding precaution:** Consult prescriber if breast-feeding.

Geriatric Considerations: Adjust dose relative to renal function.

Pregnancy Risk Factor: B

Lactation: Enters breast milk/not recommended (AAP rates "compatible")

Breast-Feeding Issues: Aztreonam is excreted in breast milk at levels <1% of the maternal serum concentration. The manufacturer recommends temporary discontinuation of nursing during therapy.

Administration

I.M.: Administer by deep injection into large muscle mass, such as upper outer quadrant of gluteus maximus or the lateral part of the thigh. Doses >1 g should be administered I.V.

I.V.: I.V. route is preferred for doses >1 g or in patients with severe life-threatening infections. Administer by IVP over 3-5 minutes or by intermittent infusion over 20-60 minutes at a final concentration not to exceed 20 mg/mL.

Reconstitution: Reconstituted solutions are colorless to light yellow straw and may turn pink upon standing without affecting potency. Use reconstituted solutions and I.V. solutions (in NS and D_5W) within 48 hours if kept at room temperature (25°C) or 7 days if kept in refrigerator (4°C).

    I.M.: Reconstitute with at least 3 mL SWFI, sterile bacteriostatic water for injection, NS, or bacteriostatic sodium chloride.

    I.V.:

        Bolus injection: Reconstitute with 6-10 mL SWFI.

        Infusion: Reconstitute to a final concentration ≤2%. Solution for infusion may be frozen at less than -2°C (less than -4°F) for up to 3 months. Thawed solution should be used within 24 hours if thawed at room temperature or within 72 hours if thawed under refrigeration. **Do not refreeze.**

Compatibility: Solution for infusion: Stable in D_5LR, $D_5^1/_4NS$, $D_5^1/_2NS$, D_5NS, D_5W, $D_{10}W$, mannitol 5%, mannitol 10%, LR, NS

    Y-site administration: Incompatible with acyclovir, alatrofloxacin, amphotericin B, amphotericin B cholesteryl sulfate complex, amsacrine, chlorpromazine, daunorubicin, ganciclovir, lorazepam, metronidazole, mitomycin, mitoxantrone, prochlorperazine edisylate, streptozocin

    Compatibility when admixed: Incompatible with metronidazole, nafcillin

Storage: Prior to reconstitution, store at room temperature. Avoid excessive heat.

Additional Information Although marketed as an agent similar to aminoglycosides, aztreonam is a monobactam antimicrobial with almost pure gram-negative aerobic activity. It cannot be used for gram-positive infections. Aminoglycosides are often used for synergy in gram-positive infections.

Related Information

Antimicrobial Drugs of Choice *on page 1792*
Community-Acquired Pneumonia in Adults *on page 1807*

- ♦ **Azulfidine®** *see Sulfasalazine on page 1409*
- ♦ **Azulfidine® EN-tabs®** *see Sulfasalazine on page 1409*
- ♦ **B1** *see Tositumomab and Iodine I 131 Tositumomab on page 1501*
- ♦ **B1 Antibody** *see Tositumomab and Iodine I 131 Tositumomab on page 1501*
- ♦ **B2036-PEG** *see Pegvisomant on page 1167*
- ♦ **B 9273** *see Alefacept on page 64*
- ♦ **BA-16038** *see Aminoglutethimide on page 91*
- ♦ **Bacid® [OTC]** *see Lactobacillus on page 859*
- ♦ **Baciguent® [OTC]** *see Bacitracin on page 169*
- ♦ **BaciIM®** *see Bacitracin on page 169*

Bacitracin (bas i TRAY sin)

U.S. Brand Names AK-Tracin® [DSC]; Baciguent® [OTC]; BaciIM®

Generic Available Yes

Pharmacologic Category Antibiotic, Ophthalmic; Antibiotic, Topical; Antibiotic, Miscellaneous

Medication Safety Issues

Sound-alike/look-alike issues:

    Bacitracin may be confused with Bactrim®, Bactroban®

Use Treatment of susceptible bacterial infections mainly; has activity against gram-positive bacilli; due to toxicity risks, systemic and irrigant uses of bacitracin should be limited to situations where less toxic alternatives would not be effective

Unlabeled/Investigational Use Oral administration: Successful in antibiotic-associated colitis; has been used for enteric eradication of vancomycin-resistant enterococci (VRE) (Continued)

Bacitracin *(Continued)*

Mechanism of Action/Effect Inhibits bacterial cell wall synthesis by preventing transfer of mucopeptides into the growing cell wall

Contraindications Hypersensitivity to bacitracin or any component of the formulation; I.M. use is contraindicated in patients with renal impairment

Warnings/Precautions Prolonged use may result in overgrowth of nonsusceptible organisms. I.M. use may cause renal failure due to tubular and glomerular necrosis. **Do not administer intravenously** because severe thrombophlebitis occurs.

Drug Interactions

Increased Effect/Toxicity: Nephrotoxic drugs, neuromuscular blocking agents, and anesthetics (increased neuromuscular blockade).

Adverse Reactions 1% to 10%:

Cardiovascular: Hypotension, edema of the face/lips, tightness of chest

Central nervous system: Pain

Dermatologic: Rash, itching

Gastrointestinal: Anorexia, nausea, vomiting, diarrhea, rectal itching

Hematologic: Blood dyscrasias

Miscellaneous: Diaphoresis

Overdosage/Toxicology Symptoms of overdose include nephrotoxicity (parenteral), nausea, and vomiting (oral). Treatment is symptomatic and supportive.

Pharmacodynamics/Kinetics

Duration of Action: 6-8 hours

Absorption: Poor from mucous membranes and intact or denuded skin; rapidly following I.M. administration; not absorbed by bladder irrigation, but absorption can occur from peritoneal or mediastinal lavage

Time to Peak: Serum: I.M.: 1-2 hours

Protein Binding: Plasma: Minimal

Excretion: Urine (10% to 40%) within 24 hours

Dosing

Adults & Elderly: Do not administer I.V.:

Antibiotic-associated colitis: Oral: 25,000 units 4 times/day for 7-10 days

VRE eradication (unlabeled use): Oral: 25,000 units 4 times/day for 7-10 days

Superficial dermal infection: Topical: Apply 1-5 times/day.

Ophthalmic infection: Ophthalmic (ointment): Instill $^1/_4$" to $^1/_2$" ribbon every 3-4 hours into conjunctival sac for acute infections, or 2-3 times/day for mild to moderate infections for 7-10 days.

Local irrigation: Solution: 50-100 units/mL in normal saline, lactated Ringer's, or sterile water for irrigation; soak sponges in solution for topical compresses 1-5 times/day or as needed during surgical procedures.

Pediatrics: Do not administer I.V.

Infants: I.M.:

≤2.5 kg: 900 units/kg/day in 2-3 divided doses

>2.5 kg: 1000 units/kg/day in 2-3 divided doses

Children: I.M.: 800-1200 units/kg/day divided every 8 hours

Available Dosage Forms [DSC] = Discontinued product

Injection, powder for reconstitution (BaciIM®): 50,000 units

Ointment, ophthalmic (AK-Tracin® [DSC]): 500 units/g (3.5 g)

Ointment, topical: 500 units/g (0.9 g, 15 g, 30 g, 120 g, 454 g)

Baciguent®: 500 units/g (15 g, 30 g)

Monitoring and Teaching Issues

Physical Assessment: Do not administer I.V. Assess potential for interactions with other pharmacological agents patient may be taking (eg, nephrotoxic drugs, neuromuscular blocking agents, anesthetics; see Drug Interactions). **Oral, I.M.:** Monitor laboratory results (urinalysis), renal function, effectiveness of therapy, and adverse reactions (see Adverse Reactions). **Ophthalmic/topical:** Instruct patient on appropriate application and use, possible adverse reactions, and symptoms to report.

Monitoring Laboratory Tests: I.M.: Urinalysis

Patient Education:

Oral/I.M.: Maintain adequate hydration (2-3 L/day of fluids) unless instructed to restrict fluid intake. Report rash, redness, or itching; change in urinary pattern; acute dizziness; swelling of face or lips; chest pain or tightness; acute nausea or vomiting; or loss of appetite (small frequent meals or frequent mouth care may help).

Ophthalmic: Instill as many times per day as directed. Wash hands before using. Gently pull lower eyelid forward, instill prescribed amount of ointment into lower eyelid. Close eye and roll eyeball in all directions. May cause blurred vision; use caution when driving or engaging in tasks that require clear vision. Report any adverse reactions such as rash or itching, swelling of face or lips, burning or pain in eye, worsening of condition, or if condition does not improve.

Topical: Apply a thin film as many times per day as prescribed to the affected area. May cover with porous sterile bandage (avoid occlusive dressings). Do not use longer than 1 week unless advised by prescriber.

Pregnancy Risk Factor: C

Lactation: Excretion in breast milk unknown/use caution

Administration

Oral: The injection formulation is extemporaneously prepared and flavored to improve palatability.

I.M.: For I.M. administration only. pH of urine should be kept >6 by using sodium bicarbonate. Bacitracin sterile powder should be dissolved in 0.9% sodium chloride injection containing 2% procaine hydrochloride. Do not use diluents containing parabens.

I.V.: Not for I.V. administration.

Reconstitution: For I.M. use only. Bacitracin sterile powder should be dissolved in 0.9% sodium chloride injection containing 2% procaine hydrochloride. Once reconstituted, bacitracin is stable for 1 week under refrigeration (2°C to 8°C). Sterile powder should be stored in the refrigerator. Do not use diluents containing parabens.

Additional Information 1 unit is equivalent to 0.026 mg

Bacitracin and Polymyxin B (bas i TRAY sin & pol i MIKS in bee)

U.S. Brand Names AK-Poly-Bac®; Betadine® First Aid Antibiotics + Moisturizer [OTC]; Polysporin® Ophthalmic; Polysporin® Topical [OTC]

Synonyms Polymyxin B and Bacitracin

Generic Available Yes

Pharmacologic Category Antibiotic, Ophthalmic; Antibiotic, Topical

Medication Safety Issues

Sound-alike/look-alike issues:

Betadine® may be confused with Betagan®, betaine

Use Treatment of superficial infections caused by susceptible organisms

Dosing

Adults & Elderly:

Ophthalmic infection: Ophthalmic (ointment): Instill ½" ribbon in the affected eye(s) every 3-4 hours for acute infections or 2-3 times/day for mild to moderate infections for 7-10 days.

Superficial dermal infection: Topical ointment/powder: Apply to affected area 1-4 times/day; may cover with sterile bandage if needed.

Pediatrics: Refer to adult dosing.

Available Dosage Forms

Ointment, ophthalmic (AK-Poly-Bac®, Polysporin®): Bacitracin 500 units and polymyxin B sulfate 10,000 units per g (3.5 g)

Ointment, topical [OTC]: Bacitracin 500 units and polymyxin B sulfate 10,000 units per g in white petrolatum (15 g, 30 g)

Betadine® First Aid Antibiotics + Moisturizer: Bacitracin 500 units and polymyxin B sulfate 10,000 units per g (14 g)

Polysporin®: Bacitracin 500 units and polymyxin B sulfate 10,000 units per g (15 g, 30 g)

Powder, topical (Polysporin®): Bacitracin 500 units and polymyxin B sulfate 10,000 units per g (10 g)

Monitoring and Teaching Issues

Physical Assessment: See individual agents.

Patient Education: See individual agents. **Pregnancy/breast-feeding precautions:** Inform prescriber if you are or intend to become pregnant. Consult prescriber if breast-feeding.

Pregnancy Risk Factor: C

Lactation: Excretion in breast milk unknown/use caution

Related Information

Bacitracin *on page 169*

Polymyxin B *on page 1228*

Bacitracin, Neomycin, and Polymyxin B

(bas i TRAY sin, nee oh MYE sin, & pol i MIKS in bee)

U.S. Brand Names Neosporin® Neo To Go® [OTC]; Neosporin® Ophthalmic Ointment; Neosporin® Topical [OTC]

Synonyms Neomycin, Bacitracin, and Polymyxin B; Polymyxin B, Bacitracin, and Neomycin; Triple Antibiotic

Generic Available Yes

Pharmacologic Category Antibiotic, Ophthalmic; Antibiotic, Topical

Use Helps prevent infection in minor cuts, scrapes and burns; short-term treatment of superficial external ocular infections caused by susceptible organisms

Dosing

Adults & Elderly:

Ophthalmic infection: Ophthalmic ointment: Instill ½" into the conjunctival sac every 3-4 hours for 7-10 days for acute infections

Superficial dermal infection: Topical: Apply 1-3 times/day to infected area; may cover with sterile bandage if necessary.

Pediatrics: Refer to adult dosing.

Available Dosage Forms

Ointment, ophthalmic (Neosporin®): Bacitracin 400 units, neomycin 3.5 mg, and polymyxin B 10,000 units per g (3.5 g)

Ointment, topical: Bacitracin 400 units, neomycin 3.5 mg, and polymyxin B 5000 units per g (0.9 g, 15 g, 30 g, 454 g)

Neosporin®: Bacitracin 400 units, neomycin 3.5 mg, and polymyxin B 5000 units per g (15 g, 30 g)

Neosporin® Neo To Go®: Bacitracin 400 units, neomycin 3.5 mg, and polymyxin B 5000 units per g (0.9 g)

Monitoring and Teaching Issues

Physical Assessment: See individual agents.

Patient Education: See individual agents. **Pregnancy/breast-feeding precautions:** Inform prescriber if you are or intend to become pregnant. Consult prescriber if breast-feeding.

Pregnancy Risk Factor: C

Lactation: Excretion in breast milk unknown/use caution

Related Information

Bacitracin *on page 169*

Neomycin *on page 1067*

Polymyxin B *on page 1228*

Bacitracin, Neomycin, Polymyxin B, and Hydrocortisone
(bas i TRAY sin, nee oh MYE sin, pol i MIKS in bee, & hye droe KOR ti sone)

U.S. Brand Names AK-Spore® H.C. [DSC]; Cortisporin® Ointment

Synonyms Hydrocortisone, Bacitracin, Neomycin, and Polymyxin B; Neomycin, Bacitracin, Polymyxin B, and Hydrocortisone; Polymyxin B, Bacitracin, Neomycin, and Hydrocortisone

Generic Available Yes: Ophthalmic ointment

Pharmacologic Category Antibiotic, Ophthalmic; Antibiotic, Otic; Antibiotic, Topical; Corticosteroid, Ophthalmic; Corticosteroid, Otic; Corticosteroid, Topical

Use Prevention and treatment of susceptible inflammatory conditions where bacterial infection (or risk of infection) is present

Dosing
Adults & Elderly:
Ophthalmic infection: Ophthalmic (ointment): Instill ½" ribbon to inside of lower lid every 3-4 hours until improvement occurs.
Superficial dermal infection: Topical: Apply sparingly 2-4 times/day.
Pediatrics: Refer to adult dosing.

Available Dosage Forms [DSC] = Discontinued product
Ointment, ophthalmic (AK-Spore® H.C. [DSC], Cortisporin®): Bacitracin 400 units, neomycin sulfate 3.5 mg, polymyxin B 10,000 units, and hydrocortisone 10 mg per g (3.5 g)
Ointment, topical (Cortisporin®): Bacitracin 400 units, neomycin 3.5 mg, polymyxin B 5000 units, and hydrocortisone 10 mg per g (15 g)

Monitoring and Teaching Issues
Physical Assessment: See individual agents.
Patient Education: See individual agents. **Pregnancy/breast-feeding precautions:** Inform prescriber if you are or intend to become pregnant. Consult prescriber if breast-feeding.

Pregnancy Risk Factor: C

Lactation: Excretion in breast milk unknown/use caution

Related Information
Bacitracin *on page 169*
Hydrocortisone *on page 760*
Neomycin *on page 1067*
Polymyxin B *on page 1228*

Baclofen (BAK loe fen)

U.S. Brand Names Lioresal®

Generic Available Yes: Tablets only

Pharmacologic Category Skeletal Muscle Relaxant

Medication Safety Issues
Sound-alike/look-alike issues:
Baclofen may be confused with Bactroban®
Lioresal® may be confused with lisinopril, Loniten®, Lotensin®

Use Treatment of reversible spasticity associated with multiple sclerosis or spinal cord lesions
Orphan drug: Intrathecal: Treatment of intractable spasticity caused by spinal cord injury, multiple sclerosis, and other spinal disease (spinal ischemia or tumor, transverse myelitis, cervical spondylosis, degenerative myelopathy)

Unlabeled/Investigational Use Intractable hiccups, intractable pain relief, bladder spasticity, trigeminal neuralgia, cerebral palsy, Huntington's chorea

Mechanism of Action/Effect Inhibits the transmission of both monosynaptic and polysynaptic reflexes at the spinal cord level, possibly by hyperpolarization of primary afferent fiber terminals, with resultant relief of muscle spasticity

Contraindications Hypersensitivity to baclofen or any component of the formulation

Warnings/Precautions Use with caution in patients with seizure disorder or impaired renal function. Avoid abrupt withdrawal of the drug; abrupt withdrawal of intrathecal baclofen has resulted in severe sequelae (hyperpyrexia, obtundation, rebound/exaggerated spasticity, muscle rigidity, and rhabdomyolysis), leading to organ failure and some fatalities. Risk may be higher in patients with injuries at T-6 or above, history of baclofen withdrawal, or limited ability to communicate. Elderly are more sensitive to the effects of baclofen and are more likely to experience adverse CNS effects at higher doses.

Drug Interactions
Increased Effect/Toxicity: Effects may be additive with CNS depressants.

Nutritional/Ethanol Interactions
Ethanol: Avoid ethanol (may increase CNS depression).
Herb/Nutraceutical: Avoid valerian, St John's wort, kava kava, gotu kola.

Lab Interactions Increased alkaline phosphatase, AST, glucose, ammonia (B); decreased bilirubin (S)

Adverse Reactions
>10%:
Central nervous system: Drowsiness, vertigo, psychiatric disturbances, insomnia, slurred speech, ataxia, hypotonia
Neuromuscular & skeletal: Weakness
1% to 10%:
Cardiovascular: Hypotension
Central nervous system: Fatigue, confusion, headache
Dermatologic: Rash
Gastrointestinal: Nausea, constipation
Genitourinary: Polyuria

Overdosage/Toxicology Symptoms of overdose include vomiting, muscle hypotonia, salivation, drowsiness, coma, seizures, and respiratory depression. Atropine has been used to improve ventilation, heart rate, blood pressure, and core body temperature. Treatment is symptom-directed and supportive.

BACLOFEN

For toxicity following intrathecal administration: For adults, administer physostigmine 2 mg I.M. or I.V. (not to exceed 1 mg/minute). For pediatric patients, administer physostigmine 0.02 mg/kg I.M. or I.V. (not to exceed 0.5 mg/minute). Consider withdrawal of 30-40 mL of CSF to reduce baclofen concentration. Abrupt withdrawal of intrathecal baclofen has resulted in severe sequelae (hyperpyrexia, obtundation, muscle rigidity, and rhabdomyolysis)

Pharmacodynamics/Kinetics
Onset of Action: 3-4 days; Peak effect: 5-10 days
Absorption: Oral: Rapid; dose dependent
Time to Peak: Serum: Oral: Within 2-3 hours
Protein Binding: 30%
Half-Life Elimination: 3.5 hours
Metabolism: Hepatic (15% of dose)
Excretion: Urine and feces (85% as unchanged drug)

Dosing
Adults:
Spasticity:
Oral: 5 mg 3 times/day, may increase 5 mg/dose every 3 days to a maximum of 80 mg/day
Intrathecal:
Test dose: 50-100 mcg, doses >50 mcg should be given in 25 mcg increments, separated by 24 hours. A screening dose of 25 mcg may be considered in very small patients. Patients not responding to screening dose of 100 mcg should not be considered for chronic infusion/implanted pump.
Maintenance: After positive response to test dose, a maintenance intrathecal infusion can be administered via an implanted intrathecal pump. Initial dose via pump: Infusion at a 24-hourly rate dosed at twice the test dose. Avoid abrupt discontinuation.
Hiccups (unlabeled use): 10-20 mg 2-3 times/day
Elderly: Oral (the lowest effective dose is recommended): Initial: 5 mg 2-3 times/day, increasing gradually as needed; if benefits are not seen withdraw the drug slowly.
Pediatrics:
Spasticity:
Oral (avoid abrupt withdrawal of drug): Children:
2-7 years: Initial: 10-15 mg/24 hours divided every 8 hours; titrate dose every 3 days in increments of 5-15 mg/day to a maximum of 40 mg/day.
≥8 years: Maximum: 60 mg/day in 3 divided doses
Intrathecal: Refer to adult dosing.
Renal Impairment: May be necessary to reduce dosage; no specific guidelines have been established

Available Dosage Forms
Injection, solution, intrathecal [preservative free] (Lioresal®): 50 mcg/mL (1 mL); 500 mcg/mL (20 mL); 2000 mcg/mL (5 mL)
Tablet: 10 mg, 20 mg

Monitoring and Teaching Issues
Physical Assessment: Assess effectiveness and interactions of other medications patient may be taking. Monitor effectiveness of therapy and adverse reactions at beginning of therapy and periodically with long-term use. Assess knowledge/teach patient appropriate use, interventions to reduce side effects, and adverse symptoms to report.
Patient Education: Take this drug as prescribed. Do not discontinue without consulting prescriber (abrupt discontinuation may cause hallucinations). Do not take any prescription or OTC sleep-inducing drugs, sedatives, or antispasmodics without consulting prescriber. Avoid alcohol use. You may experience transient drowsiness, lethargy, or dizziness; use caution when driving or engaging in tasks requiring alertness until response to drug is known. Frequent small meals or lozenges may reduce GI upset.

Intrathecal use: Keep scheduled pump refill visits; abrupt interruption can cause serious withdrawal symptoms. Report increased spasticity, itching, numbness, unresolved insomnia, painful urination, change in urinary patterns, constipation, high fever, or persistent confusion.

Pregnancy precaution: Inform prescriber if you are or intend to become pregnant.
Geriatric Considerations: The elderly are more sensitive to the effects of baclofen and are more likely to experience adverse CNS effects at higher doses. Two cases of encephalopathy were reported after inadvertent high doses (50 mg/day and 90 mg/day) were given to elderly patients.
Pregnancy Risk Factor: C
Lactation: Enters breast milk (small amounts)/compatible

Administration
Other: Intrathecal: For screening dosages, dilute with preservative-free sodium chloride to a final concentration of 50 mcg/mL for bolus injection into the subarachnoid space; for maintenance infusions, concentrations of 500-2000 mcg/mL may be used
Compatibility: Stable in sterile, preservative free NS

- **Bactrim™** *see* Sulfamethoxazole and Trimethoprim *on page 1407*
- **Bactrim™ DS** *see* Sulfamethoxazole and Trimethoprim *on page 1407*
- **Bactroban®** *see* Mupirocin *on page 1038*
- **Bactroban® Nasal** *see* Mupirocin *on page 1038*
- **Baking Soda** *see* Sodium Bicarbonate *on page 1380*
- **BAL in Oil®** *see page 1625*
- **Bancap HC®** *see* Hydrocodone and Acetaminophen *on page 754*
- **Band-Aid® Hurt-Free™ Antiseptic Wash [OTC]** *see* Lidocaine *on page 898*
- **Banophen [OTC]** *see* DiphenhydrAMINE *on page 463*
- **Basic Pharmacotherapeutic Concepts** *see page 23*

Basiliximab (ba si LIK si mab)

U.S. Brand Names Simulect®

Generic Available No

Pharmacologic Category Monoclonal Antibody

Use Prophylaxis of acute organ rejection in renal transplantation

Mechanism of Action/Effect Mouse-derived monoclonal IgG antibody which blocks the alpha-chain of the interleukin-2 (IL-2) receptor complex; this receptor is expressed on activated T lymphocytes and is a critical pathway for activating cell-mediated allograft rejection

Contraindications Hypersensitivity basiliximab, murine proteins, or any component of the formulation

Warnings/Precautions To be used as a component of immunosuppressive regimen which includes cyclosporine and corticosteroids. Only physicians experienced in transplantation and immunosuppression should prescribe, and patients should receive the drug in a facility with adequate equipment and staff capable of providing the laboratory and medical support required for transplantation.

The incidence of lymphoproliferative disorders and/or opportunistic infections may be increased by immunosuppressive therapy. Severe hypersensitivity reactions, occurring within 24 hours, have been reported. Reactions, including anaphylaxis, have occurred both with the initial exposure and/or following re-exposure after several months. Use caution during re-exposure to a subsequent course of therapy in a patient who has previously received basiliximab. Discontinue the drug permanently if a reaction occurs. Medications for the treatment of hypersensitivity reactions should be available for immediate use. Treatment may result in the development of human antimurine antibodies (HAMA); however, limited evidence suggesting the use of muromonab-CD3 or other murine products is not precluded.

Drug Interactions

Decreased Effect: Basiliximab is an immunoglobulin; specific drug interactions have not been evaluated, but are not anticipated. It is not known if the immune response to vaccines will be impaired during or following basiliximab therapy.

Increased Effect/Toxicity: Basiliximab is an immunoglobulin; specific drug interactions have not been evaluated, but are not anticipated.

Adverse Reactions Administration of basiliximab did not appear to increase the incidence or severity of adverse effects in clinical trials. Adverse events were reported in 96% of both the placebo and basiliximab groups.

>10%:

Cardiovascular: Peripheral edema, hypertension, atrial fibrillation

Central nervous system: Fever, headache, insomnia, pain

Dermatologic: Wound complications, acne

Endocrine & metabolic: Hypokalemia, hyperkalemia, hyperglycemia, hyperuricemia, hypophosphatemia, hypercholesterolemia

Gastrointestinal: Constipation, nausea, diarrhea, abdominal pain, vomiting, dyspepsia

Genitourinary: Urinary tract infection

Hematologic: Anemia

Neuromuscular & skeletal: Tremor

Respiratory: Dyspnea, infection (upper respiratory)

Miscellaneous: Viral infection

3% to 10%:

Cardiovascular: Chest pain, cardiac failure, hypotension, arrhythmia, tachycardia, generalized edema, abnormal heart sounds, angina pectoris

Central nervous system: Hypoesthesia, neuropathy, agitation, anxiety, depression, malaise, fatigue, rigors, dizziness

Dermatologic: Cyst, hypertrichosis, pruritus, rash, skin disorder, skin ulceration

Endocrine & metabolic: Dehydration, diabetes mellitus, fluid overload, hypercalcemia, hyperlipidemia, hypoglycemia, hypomagnesemia, acidosis, hypertriglyceridemia, hypocalcemia, hyponatremia

Gastrointestinal: Flatulence, gastroenteritis, GI hemorrhage, gingival hyperplasia, melena, esophagitis, stomatitis, enlarged abdomen, moniliasis, ulcerative stomatitis, weight gain

Genitourinary: Impotence, genital edema, albuminuria, bladder disorder, hematuria, urinary frequency, oliguria, abnormal renal function, renal tubular necrosis, ureteral disorder, urinary retention, dysuria

Hematologic: Hematoma, hemorrhage, purpura, thrombocytopenia, thrombosis, polycythemia, leukopenia

Neuromuscular & skeletal: Arthralgia, arthropathy, cramps, fracture, hernia, myalgia, paresthesia, weakness, back pain, leg pain

Ocular: Cataract, conjunctivitis, abnormal vision

Respiratory: Bronchitis, bronchospasm, pneumonia, pulmonary edema, sinusitis, rhinitis, cough, pharyngitis

Miscellaneous: Accidental trauma, facial edema, sepsis, infection, increased glucocorticoids, herpes infection

Overdosage/Toxicology There have been no reports of overdose.

Pharmacodynamics/Kinetics

Duration of Action: Mean: 36 days (determined by IL-2R alpha saturation)

Half-Life Elimination: Children: 9.4 days; Adults: Mean: 7.2 days

Excretion: Clearance: Children: 20 mL/hour; Adults: Mean: 41 mL/hour

Dosing

Adults & Elderly: Note: Patients previously administered basiliximab should only be re-exposed to a subsequent course of therapy with extreme caution.

Renal transplantation: I.V.: 20 mg within 2 hours prior to transplant surgery, followed by a second 20 mg dose 4 days after transplantation. The second dose should be withheld if complications occur (including severe hypersensitivity reactions or graft loss).

Pediatrics: Note: Patients previously administered basiliximab should only be re-exposed to a subsequent course of therapy with extreme caution.

Renal transplantation: I.V.:

Children <35 kg: 10 mg within 2 hours prior to transplant surgery, followed by a second 10 mg dose 4 days after transplantation; the second dose should be withheld if complications occur (including severe hypersensitivity reactions or graft loss)

Children ≥35 kg: Refer to adult dosing

Renal Impairment: No specific dosing adjustment is recommended.

Hepatic Impairment: No specific dosing adjustment is recommended.

Available Dosage Forms Injection, powder for reconstitution: 10 mg, 20 mg

Monitoring and Teaching Issues

Physical Assessment: Monitor cardiorespiratory function, renal function, and adverse reactions during infusion and periodically following infusion. Be alert to opportunistic infections. Assess knowledge/teach patient possible side effects/interventions and adverse symptoms to report as inpatient or following discharge.

Patient Education: This medication, which may help to reduce transplant rejection, can only be given by infusion. You will be monitored and assessed closely during infusion and thereafter. It is important that you report any changes or problems for evaluation. You will be susceptible to infection (avoid crowds and exposure to infection). Frequent mouth care and small frequent meals may help counteract any GI effects you may experience and will help maintain adequate nutrition and fluid intake. Report any changes in urination; unusual bruising or bleeding; chest pain or palpitations; acute dizziness; respiratory difficulty; fever or chills; changes in cognition; rash; feelings of pain or numbness in extremities; severe GI upset or diarrhea; unusual back or leg pain or muscle tremors; vision changes; or any sign of infection (eg, chills, fever, sore throat, easy bruising or bleeding, mouth sores, unhealed sores, vaginal discharge). **Breast-feeding precaution:** Breast-feeding is not recommended.

Pregnancy Risk Factor: B (manufacturer)

Pregnancy Issues: IL-2 receptors play an important role in the development of the immune system. Use in pregnant women only when benefit exceeds potential risk to the fetus. Women of childbearing potential should use effective contraceptive measures before beginning treatment and for 2 months after completion of therapy with this agent.

Lactation: Excretion in breast milk unknown/not recommended

Breast-Feeding Issues: It is not known whether basiliximab is excreted in human milk. Because many immunoglobulins are secreted in milk and the potential for serious adverse reactions exists, a decision should be made whether to discontinue nursing or discontinue the drug, taking into account the importance of the drug to the mother.

Administration

I.V.: For intravenous administration only. Infuse over 20-30 minutes.

Reconstitution: Reconstitute vials with sterile water for injection. Dilute reconstituted contents in normal saline or 5% dextrose.

Storage: Store vials under refrigeration 2°C to 8°C (36°F to 46°F). Reconstituted vials are stable under refrigeration for 24 hours, but only 4 hours at room temperature.

♦ **Bayer® Aspirin [OTC]** *see Aspirin on page 143*
♦ **Bayer® Aspirin Extra Strength [OTC]** *see Aspirin on page 143*
♦ **Bayer® Aspirin Regimen Adult Low Strength [OTC]** *see Aspirin on page 143*
♦ **Bayer® Aspirin Regimen Children's [OTC]** *see Aspirin on page 143*
♦ **Bayer® Aspirin Regimen Regular Strength [OTC]** *see Aspirin on page 143*
♦ **Bayer® Extra Strength Arthritis Pain Regimen [OTC]** *see Aspirin on page 143*
♦ **Bayer® Plus Extra Strength [OTC]** *see Aspirin on page 143*
♦ **Bayer® Women's Aspirin Plus Calcium [OTC]** *see Aspirin on page 143*
♦ **BayGam®** *see page 1660*
♦ **BayHepB™** *see page 1660*
♦ **BayRab®** *see page 1660*
♦ **BayRho-D® Full-Dose** *see Rh₀(D) Immune Globulin on page 1316*
♦ **BayRho-D® Mini-Dose** *see Rh₀(D) Immune Globulin on page 1316*
♦ **BayTet™** *see page 1660*
♦ **Baza® Antifungal [OTC]** *see Miconazole on page 999*
♦ **BCG Vaccine** *see page 1660*
♦ **BCNU** *see Carmustine on page 260*

Beclomethasone (be kloe METH a sone)

U.S. Brand Names Beconase® [DSC]; Beconase® AQ; QVAR®

Synonyms Beclomethasone Dipropionate

Generic Available No

Pharmacologic Category Corticosteroid, Inhalant (Oral); Corticosteroid, Nasal

Medication Safety Issues

Sound-alike/look-alike issues:

Vanceril® may be confused with Vancenase®

Use

Oral inhalation: Maintenance and prophylactic treatment of asthma; includes those who require corticosteroids and those who may benefit from a dose reduction/elimination of systemically administered corticosteroids. Not for relief of acute bronchospasm

Nasal aerosol: Symptomatic treatment of seasonal or perennial rhinitis and to prevent recurrence of nasal polyps following surgery

Mechanism of Action/Effect Acts at cellular level to prevent or control inflammation

Contraindications Hypersensitivity to beclomethasone or any component of the formulation; status asthmaticus

Warnings/Precautions Not to be used in status asthmaticus or for the relief of acute bronchospasm. May cause suppression of hypothalamic-pituitary-adrenal (HPA) axis, particularly in younger children or in patients receiving high doses for prolonged periods. Fatalities have occurred due to adrenal insufficiency in asthmatic patients during and after transfer from

(Continued)

Beclomethasone *(Continued)*

systemic corticosteroids to aerosol steroids; aerosol steroids do **not** provide the systemic steroid needed to treat patients having trauma, surgery, or infections. Withdrawal and discontinuation of the corticosteroid should be done slowly and carefully.

Controlled clinical studies have shown that orally-inhaled and intranasal corticosteroids may cause a reduction in growth velocity in pediatric patients, which appears to be related to dose and duration of exposure.

May suppress the immune system, patients may be more susceptible to infection. Use with caution in patients with systemic infections or ocular herpes simplex. Avoid exposure to chickenpox and measles. Corticosteroids should be used with caution in patients with diabetes, hypertension, osteoporosis, peptic ulcer, glaucoma, cataracts, or tuberculosis. Use caution in hepatic impairment. Safety and efficacy in children <6 years of age have not been established.

Drug Interactions
Increased Effect/Toxicity: The addition of salmeterol has been demonstrated to improve response to inhaled corticosteroids (as compared to increasing steroid dosage).

Adverse Reactions Frequency not defined.
Central nervous system: Agitation, depression, dizziness, dysphonia, headache, lightheadedness, mental disturbances

Dermatologic: Acneiform lesions, angioedema, atrophy, bruising, pruritus, purpura, striae, rash, urticaria

Endocrine & metabolic: Cushingoid features, growth velocity reduction in children and adolescents, HPA function suppression, weight gain

Gastrointestinal: Dry/irritated nose, throat and mouth, hoarseness, localized *Candida* or *Aspergillus* infection, loss of smell, loss of taste, nausea, unpleasant smell, unpleasant taste, vomiting

Local: Nasal spray: Burning, epistaxis, localized *Candida* infection, nasal septum perforation (rare), nasal stuffiness, nosebleeds, rhinorrhea, sneezing, transient irritation, ulceration of nasal mucosa (rare)

Ocular: Cataracts, glaucoma, increased intraocular pressure

Respiratory: Cough, paradoxical bronchospasm, pharyngitis, sinusitis, wheezing

Miscellaneous: Anaphylactic/anaphylactoid reactions, death (due to adrenal insufficiency, reported during and after transfer from systemic corticosteroids to aerosol in asthmatic patients), immediate and delayed hypersensitivity reactions

Overdosage/Toxicology Symptoms of overdose include irritation and burning of the nasal mucosa, sneezing, intranasal and pharyngeal *Candida* infections, nasal ulceration, epistaxis, rhinorrhea, nasal stuffiness, and headache. When consumed in high doses over prolonged periods, systemic hypercorticism and adrenal suppression may occur. In those cases, discontinuation of the corticosteroid should be done judiciously.

Pharmacodynamics/Kinetics
Onset of Action: Therapeutic effect: 1-4 weeks

Absorption: Readily; quickly hydrolyzed by pulmonary esterases prior to absorption

Bioavailability: Of active metabolite, 44% following nasal inhalation (43% from swallowed portion)

Protein Binding: 87%

Half-Life Elimination: Initial: 3 hours

Metabolism: Hepatic via CYP3A4 to active metabolites

Excretion: Feces (60%); urine (12%)

Dosing
Adults & Elderly: Nasal inhalation and oral inhalation dosage forms are not to be used interchangeably.

Rhinitis:
Intranasal aqueous inhalation (Beconase® AQ): 1-2 inhalations each nostril twice daily; total dose 168-336 mcg/day

Intranasal aerosol (Beconase®): 1 inhalation in each nostril 2-4 times/day or 2 inhalations each nostril twice daily (total dose 168-336 mcg/day); usual maximum maintenance: 1 inhalation in each nostril 3 times/day (252 mcg/day)

Asthma: Oral inhalation (doses should be titrated to the lowest effective dose once asthma is controlled) (QVAR®):
Patients previously on bronchodilators only: Initial dose 40-80 mcg twice daily; maximum dose 320 mcg twice day

Patients previously on inhaled corticosteroids: Initial dose 40-160 mcg twice daily; maximum dose 320 mcg twice daily

Pediatrics: Nasal inhalation and oral inhalation dosage forms are not to be used interchangeably.

Rhinitis:
Intranasal aqueous solution (Beconase® AQ): Children ≥6 years: 1-2 inhalations each nostril twice daily; total dose 168-336 mcg/day

Intranasal aerosol (Beconase®):
Children 6-12 years: 1 inhalation in each nostril 3 times/day; total dose 252 mcg/day
Children ≥12 years: 1 inhalation in each nostril 2-4 times/day or 2 inhalations each nostril twice daily (total dose 168-336 mcg/day); usual maximum maintenance: 1 inhalation in each nostril 3 times/day (252 mcg/day)

Asthma: Oral inhalation (doses should be titrated to the lowest effective dose once asthma is controlled) (QVAR®):
Children 5-11 years: Initial: 40 mcg twice daily; maximum dose: 80 mcg twice daily
Children ≥12 years:
Patients previously on bronchodilators only: Initial dose 40-80 mcg twice daily; maximum dose: 320 mcg twice day
Patients previously on inhaled corticosteroids: Initial dose 40-160 mcg twice daily; maximum dose: 320 mcg twice daily

Available Dosage Forms [DSC] = Discontinued product

Aerosol for oral inhalation, as dipropionate (QVAR®): 40 mcg/inhalation [100 metered doses] (7.3 g); 80 mcg/inhalation [100 metered doses] (7.3 g)

Aerosol, intranasal, as dipropionate (Beconase® [DSC]): 42 mcg/inhalation: [80 metered doses] (6.7 g); [200 metered doses] (16.8 g)

Suspension, intranasal, aqueous, as dipropionate [spray] (Beconase® AQ): 42 mcg/inhalation [180 metered doses] (25 g)

Monitoring and Teaching Issues

Physical Assessment: Not to be used to treat status asthmaticus or fungal infections of nasal passages. Monitor therapeutic effectiveness and adverse reactions. When changing from systemic steroids to inhalational steroids, taper reduction of systemic medication slowly. Growth should be routinely monitored in pediatric patients. Assess knowledge/teach patient appropriate use, interventions to reduce side effects, and adverse symptoms to report.

Patient Education: Use as directed; do not increase dosage or discontinue abruptly without consulting prescriber. It may take 1-4 weeks for you to realize full effects of treatment. Review use of inhaler or spray with prescriber or follow package insert for directions. Keep oral inhaler clean and unobstructed. Always rinse mouth and throat after use of inhaler to prevent infection. If you are also using an inhaled bronchodilator, wait 10 minutes before using this steroid aerosol. Report adverse effects such as skin redness, rash, or irritation; pain or burning of nasal mucosa; white plaques in mouth or fuzzy tongue; unresolved headache; or worsening of condition or lack of improvement. Discard after date calculated by prescriber; the amount of medication in canister cannot be guaranteed after using the labeled number of actuations (sprays) even though it may not feel empty. **Pregnancy/breast-feeding precautions:** Inform prescriber if you are or intend to become pregnant. Consult prescriber if breast-feeding.

Inhalation: Sit when using. Take deep breaths for 3-5 minutes, and clear nasal passages before administration (use decongestant as needed). Hold breath for 5-10 seconds after use, and wait 1-3 minutes between inhalations. Follow package insert instructions for use. Do not exceed maximum dosage. If also using inhaled bronchodilator, use before beclomethasone. Rinse mouth and throat after use to reduce aftertaste and prevent candidiasis.

Geriatric Considerations: Older patients may have difficulty with oral metered dose inhalers and may benefit from the use of a spacer or chamber device.

Pregnancy Risk Factor: C

Lactation: Enters breast milk (oral)/use caution

Administration

Inhalation: Shake well before use. Keep oral inhaler clean and unobstructed, wash in warm water and dry thoroughly. Rinse mouth and throat after use to prevent *Candida* infection.

Storage: Do not store near heat or open flame. Do not puncture canisters. Store at room temperature. Rest QVAR® on concave end of canister with actuator on top.

Additional Information Effects of inhaled/intranasal steroids on growth have been observed in the absence of laboratory evidence of HPA axis suppression, suggesting that growth velocity is a more sensitive indicator of systemic corticosteroid exposure in pediatric patients than some commonly used tests of HPA axis function. The long-term effects of this reduction in growth velocity associated with orally-inhaled and intranasal corticosteroids, including the impact on final adult height, are unknown. The potential for "catch up" growth following discontinuation of treatment with inhaled corticosteroids has not been adequately studied.

Related Information

Asthma *on page 1799*
Inhalant Agents *on page 1734*

♦ **Beclomethasone Dipropionate** *see* Beclomethasone *on page 175*
♦ **Beconase® [DSC]** *see* Beclomethasone *on page 175*
♦ **Beconase® AQ** *see* Beclomethasone *on page 175*
♦ **Belladonna Alkaloids With Phenobarbital** *see* Hyoscyamine, Atropine, Scopolamine, and Phenobarbital *on page 777*

Belladonna and Opium (bel a DON a & OH pee um)

U.S. Brand Names B&O Supprettes®
Synonyms Opium and Belladonna
Controlled Substance C-II
Generic Available Yes
Pharmacologic Category Analgesic Combination (Narcotic); Antispasmodic Agent, Urinary
Use Relief of moderate to severe pain associated with rectal or bladder tenesmus that may occur in postoperative states and neoplastic situations; pain associated with ureteral spasms not responsive to non-narcotic analgesics and to space intervals between injections of opiates

Mechanism of Action/Effect Anticholinergic alkaloids act primarily by competitive inhibition of the muscarinic actions of acetylcholine on structures innervated by postganglionic cholinergic neurons and on smooth muscle; resulting effects include antisecretory activity on exocrine glands and intestinal mucosa and smooth muscle relaxation. Contains many narcotic alkaloids including morphine; its mechanism for gastric motility inhibition is primarily due to this morphine content, resulting in a decrease in digestive secretions, an increase in GI muscle tone, and therefore a reduction in GI propulsion.

Contraindications Glaucoma; severe renal or hepatic disease; bronchial asthma; respiratory depression; convulsive disorders; acute alcoholism; premature labor

Warnings/Precautions Usual precautions of opiate agonist therapy should be observed. Use with caution and generally in reduced doses in the very young or geriatric patients.

Drug Interactions

Decreased Effect: May decrease effects of drugs with cholinergic mechanisms. Antipsychotic efficacy of phenothiazines may be decreased.

Increased Effect/Toxicity: Additive effects with CNS depressants. May increase effects of digoxin and atenolol. Coadministration with other anticholinergic agents (phenothiazines, (Continued)

Belladonna and Opium *(Continued)*

tricyclic antidepressants, amantadine, and antihistamines) may increase effects such as dry mouth, constipation, and urinary retention.

Nutritional/Ethanol Interactions Ethanol: Avoid ethanol (may increase sedation).

Lab Interactions Increased aminotransferase [ALT (SGPT)/AST (SGOT)] (S)

Adverse Reactions

>10%:

Dermatologic: Dry skin

Gastrointestinal: Constipation, dry throat, xerostomia

Respiratory: Dry nose

Miscellaneous: Diaphoresis (decreased)

1% to 10%:

Dermatologic: Increased sensitivity to light

Endocrine & metabolic: Decreased flow of breast milk

Gastrointestinal: Dysphagia

Overdosage/Toxicology Primary attention should be directed to ensuring adequate respiratory exchange. Opiate agonist-induced respiratory depression may be reversed with parenteral naloxone hydrochloride. Anticholinergic toxicity may be caused by strong binding of a belladonna alkaloid to cholinergic receptors. Physostigmine 1-2 mg given slowly SubQ or I.V. may be administered to reverse overdose with life-threatening effects.

Pharmacodynamics/Kinetics

Onset of Action:

Opium: Within 30 minutes

Metabolism:

Opium: Hepatic, with formation of glucuronide metabolites

Dosing

Adults & Elderly: Rectal/bladder tenesmus or ureteral spasm: Rectal: 1 suppository 1-2 times/day, up to 4 doses/day

Available Dosage Forms Suppository:

#15 A: Belladonna extract 16.2 mg and opium 30 mg

#16 A: Belladonna extract 16.2 mg and opium 60 mg

Monitoring and Teaching Issues

Physical Assessment: Assess other medications patient may be taking for additive or adverse interactions. Monitor therapeutic effectiveness, signs of overdose, and adverse effects at beginning of therapy and at regular intervals with long-term use. May cause physical and/or psychological dependence. For inpatients, implement safety measures. Assess knowledge/teach patient appropriate use if self-administered. Teach patient to monitor for adverse reactions, adverse reactions to report, and appropriate interventions to reduce side effects.

Patient Education: If self-administered, use exactly as directed; do not increase dose or frequency. Drug may cause physical and/or psychological dependence. While using this medication, do not use alcohol and other prescription or OTC medications (especially sedatives, tranquilizers, antihistamines, or pain medications) without consulting prescriber. Maintain adequate hydration (2-3 L/day of fluids) unless instructed to restrict fluid intake. May cause hypotension, dizziness, or drowsiness; use caution when driving, climbing stairs, or changing position (rising from sitting or lying to standing) or when engaging in tasks requiring alertness (until response to drug is known); dry mouth or throat (frequent mouth care, frequent sips of fluids, chewing gum, or sucking lozenges may help); constipation (increased exercise, fluids, fruit, or fiber may help; if unresolved, consult prescriber about use of stool softeners); photosensitivity (use sunscreen, wear protective clothing and eyewear, and avoid direct sunlight); or decreased perspiration (avoid extremes in temperature or excessive activity in hot environments). Report chest pain or palpitations; persistent dizziness; changes in mentation; changes in gait; blurred vision; shortness of breath or respiratory difficulty. **Pregnancy/breast-feeding precautions:** Inform prescriber if you are or intend to become pregnant. Consult prescriber if breast-feeding.

Pregnancy Risk Factor: C

Lactation: Excretion in breast milk unknown/use caution

Administration

Other: Prior to rectal insertion, the finger and suppository should be moistened. Assist with ambulation.

Storage: Store at 15°C to 30°C; avoid freezing.

Related Information

Opium Tincture *on page 1122*

♦ Benadryl® Allergy [OTC] *see* DiphenhydrAMINE *on page 463*
♦ Benadryl® Children's Allergy [OTC] *see* DiphenhydrAMINE *on page 463*
♦ Benadryl® Children's Allergy Fastmelt® [OTC] *see* DiphenhydrAMINE *on page 463*
♦ Benadryl® Dye-Free Allergy [OTC] *see* DiphenhydrAMINE *on page 463*
♦ Benadryl® Injection *see* DiphenhydrAMINE *on page 463*
♦ Benadryl® Itch Stopping [OTC] *see* DiphenhydrAMINE *on page 463*
♦ Benadryl® Itch Stopping Extra Strength [OTC] *see* DiphenhydrAMINE *on page 463*

Benazepril *(ben AY ze pril)*

U.S. Brand Names Lotensin®

Synonyms Benazepril Hydrochloride

Generic Available Yes

Pharmacologic Category Angiotensin-Converting Enzyme (ACE) Inhibitor

Medication Safety Issues

Sound-alike/look-alike issues:

Benazepril may be confused with Benadryl®

Lotensin® may be confused with Lioresal®, Loniten®, lovastatin

Use Treatment of hypertension, either alone or in combination with other antihypertensive agents

Mechanism of Action/Effect Competitive inhibitor of angiotensin-converting enzyme (ACE); prevents conversion of angiotensin I to angiotensin II, a potent vasoconstrictor; results in lower levels of angiotensin II which causes an increase in plasma renin activity and a reduction in aldosterone secretion

Contraindications Hypersensitivity to benazepril or any component of the formulation; angioedema or serious hypersensitivity related to previous treatment with an ACE inhibitor; bilateral renal artery stenosis; patients with idiopathic or hereditary angioedema; pregnancy (2nd and 3rd trimesters)

Warnings/Precautions Anaphylactic reactions can occur. Angioedema can occur at any time during treatment (especially following first dose). Angioedema may involve head and neck (potentially affecting the airway) or the intestine (presenting with abdominal pain). Careful blood pressure monitoring with first dose (hypotension can occur especially in volume depleted patients). Dosage adjustment needed in renal impairment. Use with caution in hypovolemia; collagen vascular diseases; valvular stenosis (particularly aortic stenosis); hyperkalemia; or before, during, or immediately after anesthesia. Avoid rapid dosage escalation which may lead to renal insufficiency. Rare toxicities associated with ACE inhibitors include cholestatic jaundice (which may progress to hepatic necrosis) and neutropenia/agranulocytosis with myeloid hyperplasia. Hypersensitivity reactions may be seen during hemodialysis with high-flux dialysis membranes (eg, AN69). Deterioration in renal function can occur with initiation. Use with caution in unilateral renal artery stenosis and pre-existing renal insufficiency.

Drug Interactions

Decreased Effect: Aspirin (high dose) may reduce the therapeutic effects of ACE inhibitors; at low dosages this does not appear to be significant. Rifampin may decrease the effect of ACE inhibitors. Antacids may decrease the bioavailability of ACE inhibitors (may be more likely to occur with captopril); separate administration times by 1-2 hours. NSAIDs, specifically indomethacin, may reduce the hypotensive effects of ACE inhibitors.

Increased Effect/Toxicity: Potassium supplements, co-trimoxazole (high dose), angiotensin II receptor antagonists (eg, candesartan, losartan, irbesartan) or potassium-sparing diuretics (amiloride, spironolactone, triamterene) may result in elevated serum potassium levels when combined with benazepril. ACE inhibitor effects may be increased by phenothiazines or probenecid (increases levels of captopril). ACE inhibitors may increase serum concentrations/effects of digoxin, lithium, and sulfonylureas. Diuretics have additive hypotensive effects with ACE inhibitors, and hypovolemia increases the potential for adverse renal effects of ACE inhibitors. In patients with compromised renal function, coadministration with NSAIDs may result in further deterioration of renal function. Allopurinol and ACE inhibitors may cause a higher risk of hypersensitivity reaction when taken concurrently.

Nutritional/Ethanol Interactions Herb/Nutraceutical: Avoid dong quai if using for hypertension (has estrogenic activity). Avoid ephedra, yohimbe, ginseng (may worsen hypertension). Avoid garlic (may have increased antihypertensive effect).

Adverse Reactions 1% to 10%:
Cardiovascular: Postural dizziness (2%)
Central nervous system: Headache (6%), dizziness (4%), fatigue (3%), somnolence (2%)
Endocrine & metabolic: Hyperkalemia (1%), increased uric acid
Gastrointestinal: Nausea (2%)
Renal: Increased serum creatinine (2%), worsening of renal function may occur in patients with bilateral renal artery stenosis or hypovolemia
Respiratory: Cough (1% to 10%)

Overdosage/Toxicology Mild hypotension has been the primary toxic effect seen with acute overdose. Bradycardia may also occur. Hyperkalemia occurs even with therapeutic doses, especially in patients with renal insufficiency and those taking NSAIDs. Treatment is symptom-directed and supportive.

Pharmacodynamics/Kinetics

Onset of Action:
Reduction in plasma angiotensin-converting enzyme (ACE) activity: Peak effect: 1-2 hours after 2-20 mg dose
Reduction in blood pressure: Peak effect: Single dose: 2-4 hours; Continuous therapy: 2 weeks

Duration of Action: Reduction in plasma angiotensin-converting enzyme (ACE) activity: >90% inhibition for 24 hours after 5-20 mg dose

Absorption: Rapid (37%); food does not alter significantly; metabolite (benazeprilat) itself unsuitable for oral administration due to poor absorption

Time to Peak: Parent drug: 0.5-1 hour

Half-Life Elimination: Benazeprilat: Effective: 10-11 hours; Terminal: Children: 5 hours, Adults: 22 hours

Metabolism: Rapidly and extensively hepatic to its active metabolite, benazeprilat, via enzymatic hydrolysis; extensive first-pass effect

Excretion: Clearance: Nonrenal clearance (ie, biliary, metabolic) appears to contribute to the elimination of benazeprilat (11% to 12%), particularly patients with severe renal impairment; hepatic clearance is the main elimination route of unchanged benazepril

Dialysis: ~6% of metabolite removed in 4 hours of dialysis following 10 mg of benazepril administered 2 hours prior to procedure; parent compound not found in dialysate

Dosing

Adults: Hypertension: Oral: Initial: 10 mg/day in patients not receiving a diuretic; 20-40 mg/day as a single dose or 2 divided doses; the need for twice-daily dosing should be assessed by monitoring peak (2-6 hours after dosing) and trough responses.
Note: Patients taking diuretics should have them discontinued 2-3 days prior to starting benazepril. If they cannot be discontinued, then initial dose should be 5 mg; restart after blood pressure is stabilized if needed.

Elderly: Oral: Initial: 5-10 mg/day in single or divided doses; usual range: 20-40 mg/day; adjust for renal function. Also see "Note" in adult dosing.
(Continued)

Benazepril *(Continued)*

Pediatrics: Hypertension: Children ≥6 years: Oral: Initial: 0.2 mg/kg/day as monotherapy; dosing range: 0.1-0.6 mg/kg/day (maximum dose: 40 mg/day)

Renal Impairment:
Cl_{cr} <30 mL/minute:
Children: Use is not recommended.
Adults: Administer 5 mg/day initially; maximum daily dose: 40 mg.
Hemodialysis: Moderately dialyzable (20% to 50%); administer dose postdialysis or administer 25% to 35% supplemental dose.
Peritoneal dialysis: Supplemental dose is not necessary.

Available Dosage Forms Tablet, as hydrochloride: 5 mg, 10 mg, 20 mg, 40 mg

Monitoring and Teaching Issues

Physical Assessment: Refer to Contraindications and Warnings/Precautions for use cautions (eg, renal impairment, hereditary angioedema). Assess potential for interactions with other pharmacological agents or herbal products patient may be taking (see Drug Interactions). Assess results of laboratory tests, therapeutic effectiveness (blood pressure should be monitored after first doses and periodically during therapy), and adverse response (see Adverse Reactions) on a regular basis during therapy. Teach patient proper use, possible side effects/appropriate interventions, and adverse symptoms to report.

Monitoring Laboratory Tests: CBC, renal function tests, electrolytes

Patient Education: Do not take any new medication during therapy without consulting prescriber. Take exactly as directed; do not alter dose or discontinue without consulting prescriber. Take first dose at bedtime. Do not take potassium supplements or salt substitutes containing potassium without consulting prescriber. This drug does not eliminate need for diet or exercise regimen as recommended by prescriber. May cause dizziness, fainting, or lightheadedness (use caution when driving or engaging in tasks that require alertness until response to drug is known); postural hypotension (use caution when rising from lying or sitting position or climbing stairs); nausea, vomiting, abdominal pain, dry mouth, or transient loss of appetite (small frequent meals, frequent mouth care, sucking lozenges, or chewing gum may help); report if these side effects persist. Report mouth sores; fever or chills; swelling of extremities, face, mouth, or tongue; respiratory difficulty or unusual cough; or other persistent adverse reactions. **Pregnancy precaution:** Inform prescriber if you are or intend to become pregnant. This drug should not be used in the 2nd or 3rd trimester of pregnancy. Consult prescriber for appropriate contraceptive measures.

Geriatric Considerations: Due to frequent decreases in glomerular filtration (also creatinine clearance) with aging, elderly patients may have exaggerated responses to ACE inhibitors. Differences in clinical response due to hepatic changes are not observed. ACE inhibitors may be preferred agents in elderly patients with congestive heart failure and diabetes mellitus. Diabetic proteinuria is reduced and insulin sensitivity is enhanced. In general, the side effect profile is favorable in elderly and causes little or no CNS confusion. Use lowest dose recommendations initially.

Pregnancy Risk Factor: C/D (2nd and 3rd trimesters)

Pregnancy Issues: ACE inhibitors can cause fetal injury or death if taken during the 2nd or 3rd trimester. Discontinue ACE inhibitors as soon as pregnancy is detected.

Lactation: Enters breast milk/compatible

Related Information
Angiotensin Agents *on page 1704*

♦ **Benazepril and Amlodipine** *see Amlodipine and Benazepril on page 101*

Benazepril and Hydrochlorothiazide

(ben AY ze pril & hye droe klor oh THYE a zide)

U.S. Brand Names Lotensin® HCT

Synonyms Hydrochlorothiazide and Benazepril

Generic Available Yes

Pharmacologic Category Antihypertensive Agent, Combination

Use Treatment of hypertension

Dosing

Adults: Hypertension: Oral: Dose is individualized (range: benazepril: 5-20 mg; hydrochlorothiazide: 6.25-25 mg/day)

Elderly: Dose is individualized.

Renal Impairment: Cl_{cr} <30 mL/minute: Not recommended; loop diuretics are preferred.

Available Dosage Forms Tablet:
5/6.25: Benazepril 5 mg and hydrochlorothiazide 6.25 mg
10/12.5: Benazepril 10 mg and hydrochlorothiazide 12.5 mg
20/12.5: Benazepril 20 mg and hydrochlorothiazide 12.5 mg
20/25: Benazepril 20 mg and hydrochlorothiazide 25 mg

Monitoring and Teaching Issues

Physical Assessment: See individual agents.

Patient Education: See individual agents. **Pregnancy precaution:** Do not get pregnant while taking this medication; use appropriate contraceptive measures.

Pregnancy Risk Factor: C/D (2nd and 3rd trimesters)

Lactation: Enters breast milk/compatible

Related Information
Benazepril *on page 178*
Hydrochlorothiazide *on page 751*

♦ **Benazepril Hydrochloride** *see Benazepril on page 178*

♦ **Benemid [DSC]** *see Probenecid on page 1253*

♦ **Benicar™** *see Olmesartan on page 1112*

♦ **Benicar HCT™** *see Olmesartan and Hydrochlorothiazide on page 1113*

♦ **Benylin® Expectorant [OTC]** *see Guaifenesin and Dextromethorphan on page 731*

♦ **Benzamycin®** *see Erythromycin and Benzoyl Peroxide on page 546*

- **Benzamycin® Pak**   see Erythromycin and Benzoyl Peroxide *on page 546*
- **Benzathine Benzylpenicillin**   see Penicillin G Benzathine *on page 1172*
- **Benzathine Penicillin G**   see Penicillin G Benzathine *on page 1172*
- **Benzene Hexachloride**   see Lindane *on page 902*
- **Benzhexol Hydrochloride**   see Trihexyphenidyl *on page 1526*
- **Benzmethyzin**   see Procarbazine *on page 1257*

Benzocaine (BEN zoe kane)

U.S. Brand Names Americaine® [OTC]; Americaine® Anesthetic Lubricant [DSC]; Americaine® Hemorrhoidal [OTC]; Anbesol® [OTC]; Anbesol® Baby [OTC]; Anbesol® Cold Sore Therapy [OTC]; Anbesol® Jr. [OTC]; Anbesol® Maximum Strength [OTC]; Benzodent® [OTC]; Cēpacol® Sore Throat [OTC]; Chiggerex® [OTC]; Chiggertox® [OTC]; Cylex® [OTC]; Dentapaine [OTC]; Dent's Extra Strength Toothache [OTC]; Dent's Maxi-Strength Toothache [OTC]; Dermoplast® Antibacterial [OTC]; Dermoplast® Pain Relieving [OTC]; Detane® [OTC]; Foille® [OTC]; HDA® Toothache [OTC]; Hurricaine®; Ivy-Rid® [OTC]; Kanka® Soft Brush™ [OTC]; Lanacane® [OTC]; Lanacane® Maximum Strength [OTC]; Mycinettes® [OTC]; Orabase®-B with Benzocaine [OTC]; Orajel® [OTC]; Orajel® Baby Teething [OTC]; Orajel® Baby Teething Nighttime [OTC]; Orajel® Denture Plus [OTC]; Orajel® Maximum Strength [OTC]; Orajel® Medicated Toothache [OTC]; Orajel® Mouth Sore [OTC]; Orajel® Multi-Action Cold Sore [OTC]; Orajel PM® [OTC]; Orajel® Ultra Mouth Sore [OTC]; Oticaine; Otocaine™; Outgro® [OTC]; Red Cross™ Canker Sore [OTC]; Rid-A-Pain Dental Drops [OTC]; Skeeter Stik [OTC]; Solarcaine® [OTC]; Sting-Kill [OTC]; Thorets [OTC]; Trocaine® [OTC]; Zilactin®-B [OTC]; Zilactin® Baby [OTC]

Synonyms Ethyl Aminobenzoate

Generic Available Yes: Lozenge, oral gel, otic drops

Pharmacologic Category Local Anesthetic

Medication Safety Issues
Sound-alike/look-alike issues:
Orabase®-B may be confused with Orinase®

Use Temporary relief of pain associated with local anesthetic for pruritic dermatosis, pruritus, minor burns, acute congestive and serous otitis media, swimmer's ear, otitis externa, toothache, minor sore throat pain, canker sores, hemorrhoids, rectal fissures, anesthetic lubricant for passage of catheters and endoscopic tubes; nonprescription diet aid

Mechanism of Action/Effect Benzocaine blocks both the initiation and conduction of nerve impulses by decreasing the neuronal membrane's permeability to sodium ions, which results in inhibition of depolarization with resultant blockade of conduction. As a diet aide, the anesthetic effect appears to decrease the ability to detect degrees of sweetness by taste perception.

Contraindications Hypersensitivity to benzocaine, other ester-type local anesthetics, or any component of the formulation; secondary bacterial infection of area; ophthalmic use; see package labeling for specific contraindications

Warnings/Precautions Not intended for use when infections are present.

Drug Interactions
Decreased Effect: May antagonize actions of sulfonamides.

Adverse Reactions Dose-related and may result in high plasma levels
1% to 10%:
Dermatologic: Angioedema, contact dermatitis
Local: Burning, stinging

Overdosage/Toxicology Methemoglobinemia has been reported with benzocaine in oral overdose. Treatment is primarily symptomatic and supportive; termination of anesthesia by pneumatic tourniquet inflation should be attempted when the agent is administered by infiltration or regional injection. Methemoglobinemia may be treated with methylene blue, 1-2 mg/kg I.V. infused over several minutes. Seizures commonly respond to diazepam, while hypotension responds to I.V. fluids and Trendelenburg positioning. Bradyarrhythmias (when the heart rate is <60) can be treated with I.V., I.M., or SubQ atropine 15 mcg/kg. With the development of metabolic acidosis, I.V. sodium bicarbonate 0.5-2 mEq/kg and ventilatory assistance should be instituted.

Pharmacodynamics/Kinetics
Absorption: Topical: Poor to intact skin; well absorbed from mucous membranes and traumatized skin
Metabolism: Hepatic (to a lesser extent) and plasma via hydrolysis by cholinesterase
Excretion: Urine (as metabolites)

Dosing
Adults & Elderly:
Local anesthetic: Mucous membranes: Dosage varies depending on area to be anesthetized and vascularity of tissues.
Oral mouth/throat preparations: Do not administer for >2 days unless directed by a physician; refer to specific package labeling. **Note:** Do not administer for >2 days or use in children <2 years of age, unless directed by physician.
Topical: Apply to affected area as needed.
Pediatrics: Children: Refer to adult dosing.

Available Dosage Forms
Aerosol, oral spray (Hurricaine®): 20% (60 mL) [dye free]; cherry flavor]
Aerosol, topical spray:
Americaine®: 20% (60 mL)
Dermoplast® Antibacterial: 20% (83 mL) [contains aloe vera, benzethonium chloride, menthol]
Dermoplast® Pain Relieving: 20% (83 mL) [contains menthol]
Foille®: 5% (97.5 mL) [contains chloroxylenol 0.63% and corn oil]
Ivy-Rid®: 5% (83 mL)
Lanacane® Maximum Strength: 20% (120 mL) [contains alcohol]
Solarcaine®: 20% (120 mL) [contains triclosan 0.13%, alcohol 35%]
(Continued)

Benzocaine *(Continued)*

Cream, oral:
- Benzodent®: 20% (7.5 g, 30 g)
- Orajel PM®: 20% (5.3 g)

Cream, topical:
- Lanacane®: 6% (30 g, 60 g)
- Lanacane® Maximum Strength: 20% (30 g)

Gel, oral:
- Anbesol®: 10% (7.5 g) [cool mint flavor]
- Anbesol® Baby: 7.5% (7.5 g) [contains benzoic acid; grape flavor]
- Anbesol® Jr.: 10% (7 g) [contains benzyl alcohol; bubble gum flavor]
- Anbesol® Maximum Strength: 20% (7.5 g, 10 g) [contains benzyl alcohol]
- Dentapaine: 20% (11 g) [contains clove oil]
- HDA® Toothache: 6.5% (15 mL) [contains benzyl alcohol]
- Hurricaine®: 20% (5 g) [dye free; wild cherry flavor]; (30 g) dye free; mint, pina colada, watermelon, and wild cherry flavors]
- Kanka® Soft Brush™: 20% (2 mL) [packaged in applicator with brush tip]
- Orabase® with Benzocaine®: 20% (7 g) [contains ethyl alcohol 48%; mild mint flavor]
- Orajel® 10% (7.5 g)
- Orajel® Baby Teething: 7.5% (9.4 g) [cherry flavor]
- Orajel® Baby Teething Nighttime: 10% (5.3 g)
- Orajel® Denture Plus: 15% (9 g) [contains menthol 2%, ethyl alcohol 66.7%]
- Orajel® Maximum Strength: 20% (5.3 g, 9.4 g)
- Orajel® Mouth Sore: 20% (5.3 g, 9.4 g) [contains benzalkonium chloride 0.02%, zinc chloride 0.1%]
- Orajel® Multi-Action Cold Sore: 20% (9.4 g) [contains allantoin 0.5%, camphor 3%, dimethicone 2%]
- Orajel® Ultra Mouth Sore: 15% (9.4 g) [contains ethyl alcohol 66.7%, menthol 2%]
- Zilactin®-B: 10% (7.5 g)
- Zilactin® Baby: 10% (10 g) [alcohol free, dye free; grape flavor]

Gel, topical:
- Americaine® Anesthetic Lubricant: 20% (2.5 g, 28 g) [contains 0.1% benzethonium chloride [DSC]
- Detane®: 7.5% (15 g)
- Gum [oral wax] (Dent's Extra Strength Toothache): 20% (1 g)

Liquid, oral:
- Anbesol®: 10% (9 mL) [cool mint flavor]
- Anbesol® Maximum Strength: 20% (9 mL) [contains benzyl alcohol]
- Hurricaine®: 20% (30 mL) [pina colada and wild cherry flavors]
- Orajel®: 10% (13 mL) [contains ethyl alcohol 44%, tartrazine]
- Orajel® Baby Teething: 7.5% (13 mL) [very berry flavor]
- Orajel® Maximum Strength: 20% (13 mL) [contains ethyl alcohol 44%, tartrazine]

Liquid, oral drop:
- Dent's Maxi-Strength Toothache: 20% (3.7 mL) [contains alcohol 74%]
- Rid-A-Pain Dental Drops: 6.3% (30 mL) [contains alcohol]

Liquid, topical:
- Chiggertox®: 2% (30 mL)
- Outgro®: 20% (9 mL)
- Skeeter Stik: 5% (14 mL) [contains menthol]

Lozenge: 6 mg (18s) [contains menthol]; 15 mg (10s)
- Cepacol® Sore Throat: 10 mg (18s) [contains cetylpyridinium, menthol; cherry, citrus, honey lemon, and menthol flavors]
- Cepal® Sore Throat: 10 mg (16s) [sugar free; contains cetylpyridinium, menthol; cherry and menthol flavors]
- Cylex: 15 mg [sugar free; contains cetylpyridinium chloride 5 mg; cherry flavor]
- Mycinettes®: 15 mg (12s) [sugar free; contains sodium 9 mg; cherry or regular flavor]
- Thorets: 18 mg (500s) [sugar free]
- Trocaine®: 10 mg (40s, 400s)

Ointment, oral:
- Anbesol® Cold Sore Therapy: 20% (7.1 g) [contains benzyl alcohol, aloe, camphor, menthol, vitamin E]
- Red Cross™ Canker Sore: 20% (7.5 g) [contains coconut oil]

Ointment, rectal (Americaine® Hemorrhoidal): 20% (30 g)

Ointment, topical:
- Chiggerex®: 2% (52 g) [contains aloe vera]
- Foille®: 5% (3.5 g, 14 g, 28 g) [contains chloroxylenol 0.1%, benzyl alcohol; corn oil base]

Pads, topical (Sting-Kill): 20% (8s) [contains menthol]

Paste, oral (Orabase® with Benzocaine): 20% (6 g)

Solution, otic drops (Oticaine, Otocaine™): 20% (15 mL)

Swabs, oral:
- Hurricaine®: 20% (6s, 100s) [dye free]
- Orajel® Baby Teething: 7.5% (12s) [berry flavor]
- Orajel® Medicated Mouth Sore, Orajel® Medicated Toothache: 20% (8s) [contains tartrazine]
- Zilactin®: 20% (8s)

Swabs, topical (Sting-Kill): 20% (5s) [contains menthol]

Monitoring and Teaching Issues

Physical Assessment: Monitor for effectiveness of application and adverse reactions.

Oral: Use caution to prevent gagging or choking and avoid food or drink for 1 hour. Teach patient adverse reactions to report; use and teach appropriate interventions to promote safety.

Patient Education: Use as directed; do not overuse. Do not apply when infections are present and do not apply to large areas of broken skin. Do not eat or drink for 1 hour following oral application. Discontinue application and report if swelling of mouth, lips, tongue, or throat occurs; or if skin irritation occurs at application site. **Pregnancy/ breast-feeding precautions:** Inform prescriber if you are pregnant. Consult prescriber if breast-feeding.

Dietary Considerations: When used as a nonprescription diet aid, take just prior to food consumption.

Pregnancy Risk Factor: C

Lactation: Excretion in breast milk unknown

Administration

Topical: Do not eat for 1 hour after application to oral mucosa. Chemical burns should be neutralized before application of benzocaine. Avoid application to large areas of broken skin, especially in children.

♦ Benzodent® [OTC] *see* Benzocaine *on page 181*

♦ Benzodiazepines *see page 1719*

Benzonatate (ben ZOE na tate)

U.S. Brand Names Tessalon®

Generic Available Yes

Pharmacologic Category Antitussive

Use Symptomatic relief of nonproductive cough

Mechanism of Action/Effect Suppresses cough by topical anesthetic action on the respiratory stretch receptors

Contraindications Hypersensitivity to benzonatate, related compounds (such as tetracaine), or any component of the formulation

Adverse Reactions 1% to 10%:
Central nervous system: Sedation, headache, dizziness
Dermatologic: Rash
Gastrointestinal: GI upset
Neuromuscular & skeletal: Numbness in chest
Ocular: Burning sensation in eyes
Respiratory: Nasal congestion

Overdosage/Toxicology Symptoms of overdose include restlessness, tremor, and CNS stimulation. Benzonatate's local anesthetic activity can reduce the patient's gag reflex and, therefore, may contradict the use of ipecac following ingestion. Treatment is supportive and symptomatic.

Pharmacodynamics/Kinetics

Onset of Action: Therapeutic: 15-20 minutes

Duration of Action: 3-8 hours

Dosing

Adults & Elderly: Cough: Oral: 100 mg 3 times/day or every 4 hours up to 600 mg/day

Pediatrics: Children >10 years: Refer to adult dosing.

Available Dosage Forms

Capsule: 100 mg
Tessalon®: 100 mg, 200 mg

Monitoring and Teaching Issues

Physical Assessment: Assess patient response (effectiveness of therapy [relief of cough, lung sounds, and respiratory pattern] and adverse reactions [eg, CNS changes]; see Adverse Reactions) at beginning of therapy and periodically with long-term use. Teach patient proper use, possible side effects/ interventions, and adverse symptoms to report.

Patient Education: Do not take any new medications (especially depressants or sleep-inducing agents) without consulting prescriber. Take only as prescribed; do not exceed prescribed dose or frequency. Do not break or chew capsule. Maintain adequate hydration (2-3 L/day of fluids) unless instructed to restrict fluid intake. You may experience drowsiness, impaired coordination, blurred vision, or increased anxiety (use caution when driving or engaging in tasks requiring alertness until response to drug is known); or upset stomach or nausea (small frequent meals, frequent mouth care, chewing gum, or sucking hard candy may help). Report persistent CNS changes (dizziness, sedation, tremor, or agitation); numbness in chest or feeling of chill; visual changes or burning in eyes; numbness of mouth or difficulty swallowing; or lack of improvement or worsening or condition. **Pregnancy/breast-feeding precautions:** Inform prescriber if you are or intend to become pregnant. Consult prescriber if breast-feeding.

Geriatric Considerations: No specific geriatric information is available about benzonatate. Avoid use in patients with impaired gag reflex or who cannot swallow the capsule whole.

Pregnancy Risk Factor: C

Lactation: Excretion in breast milk unknown

Administration

Oral: Swallow capsule whole (do not break or chew).

♦ Benzoyl Peroxide and Erythromycin *see* Erythromycin and Benzoyl Peroxide *on page 546*

Benzoyl Peroxide and Hydrocortisone

(BEN zoe il peer OKS ide & hye droe KOR ti sone)

U.S. Brand Names Vanoxide-HC®

Synonyms Hydrocortisone and Benzoyl Peroxide

Generic Available No

Pharmacologic Category Topical Skin Product; Topical Skin Product, Acne

Use Treatment of acne vulgaris and oily skin

Dosing

Adults & Elderly: Acne vulgaris: Topical: Apply thin film 1-3 times/day, gently massage into skin.

(Continued)

Benzoyl Peroxide and Hydrocortisone *(Continued)*

Pediatrics: Adolescents: Refer to adult dosing.

Available Dosage Forms Lotion: Benzoyl peroxide 5% and hydrocortisone acetate 0.5% (25 mL)

Monitoring and Teaching Issues

Physical Assessment: See individual agents.

Patient Education: See individual agents. **Pregnancy precaution:** Inform prescriber if you are or intend to become pregnant.

Pregnancy Risk Factor: C

Lactation: For topical use

Related Information

Hydrocortisone *on page 760*

Benztropine *(BENZ troe peen)*

U.S. Brand Names Cogentin®

Synonyms Benztropine Mesylate

Generic Available Yes: Tablet

Pharmacologic Category Anticholinergic Agent; Anti-Parkinson's Agent, Anticholinergic

Medication Safety Issues

Sound-alike/look-alike issues:

Benztropine may be confused with bromocriptine

Use Adjunctive treatment of Parkinson's disease; treatment of drug-induced extrapyramidal symptoms (except tardive dyskinesia)

Mechanism of Action/Effect Possesses both anticholinergic and antihistaminic effects. *In vitro* anticholinergic activity approximates that of atropine; *in vivo* it is only about half as active as atropine. Animal data suggest its antihistaminic activity and duration of action approach that of pyrilamine maleate. May also inhibit the reuptake and storage of dopamine and thereby, prolong the action of dopamine.

Contraindications Hypersensitivity to benztropine or any component of the formulation; pyloric or duodenal obstruction, stenosing peptic ulcers; bladder neck obstructions; achalasia; myasthenia gravis; children <3 years of age

Warnings/Precautions Use with caution in older children (dose has not been established). Use with caution in hot weather or during exercise. May cause anhydrosis and hyperthermia, which may be severe. The risk is increased in hot environments, particularly in the elderly, alcoholics, patients with CNS disease, and those with prolonged outdoor exposure.

Elderly patients frequently develop increased sensitivity and require strict dosage regulation - side effects may be more severe in elderly patients with atherosclerotic changes. Use with caution in patients with tachycardia, cardiac arrhythmias, hypertension, hypotension, prostatic hyperplasia (especially in the elderly), any tendency toward urinary retention, liver or kidney disorders, and obstructive disease of the GI or GU tract. When given in large doses or to susceptible patients, may cause weakness and inability to move particular muscle groups.

May be associated with confusion or hallucinations (generally at higher dosages). Intensification of symptoms or toxic psychosis may occur in patients with mental disorders. Benztropine does not relieve symptoms of tardive dyskinesia.

Drug Interactions

Cytochrome P450 Effect: Substrate of CYP2D6 (minor)

Decreased Effect: May increase gastric degradation of levodopa and decrease the amount of levodopa absorbed by delaying gastric emptying. Therapeutic effects of cholinergic agents (tacrine, donepezil) and neuroleptics may be antagonized.

Increased Effect/Toxicity: Central and/or peripheral anticholinergic syndrome can occur when benztropine is administered with amantadine, rimantadine, narcotic analgesics, phenothiazines and other antipsychotics (especially with high anticholinergic activity), tricyclic antidepressants, quinidine and some other antiarrhythmics, and antihistamines. Benztropine may increase the absorption of digoxin.

Nutritional/Ethanol Interactions Ethanol: Avoid ethanol (may increase CNS depression).

Adverse Reactions Frequency not defined.

Cardiovascular: Tachycardia

Central nervous system: Confusion, disorientation, memory impairment, toxic psychosis, visual hallucinations

Dermatologic: Rash

Endocrine & metabolic: Heat stroke, hyperthermia

Gastrointestinal: Xerostomia, nausea, vomiting, constipation, ileus

Genitourinary: Urinary retention, dysuria

Ocular: Blurred vision, mydriasis

Miscellaneous: Fever

Overdosage/Toxicology Symptoms of overdose include CNS depression, confusion, nervousness, hallucinations, dizziness, blurred vision, nausea, vomiting, and hyperthermia. For anticholinergic overdose with severe life-threatening symptoms, physostigmine 1-2 mg SubQ or I.V. slowly, may be given to reverse these effects.

Pharmacodynamics/Kinetics

Onset of Action: Oral: Within 1 hour; Parenteral: Within 15 minutes

Duration of Action: 6-48 hours

Bioavailability: 29%

Metabolism: Hepatic (N-oxidation, N-dealkylation, and ring hydroxylation)

Dosing

Adults:

Drug-induced extrapyramidal symptom: Oral, I.M., I.V.: 1-4 mg/dose 1-2 times/day

Acute dystonia: I.M., I.V.: 1-2 mg

Parkinsonism: Oral: 0.5-6 mg/day in 1-2 divided doses; if one dose is greater, give at bedtime. Titrate dose in 0.5 mg increments at 5- to 6-day intervals.

Elderly: Oral: Initial: 0.5 mg once or twice daily; titrate dose in 0.5 mg increments at every 5-6 days; maximum: 4 mg/day.

Pediatrics: Note: Use in children <3 years of age should be reserved for life-threatening emergencies.

Drug-induced extrapyramidal symptoms: Oral, I.M., I.V.: Children >3 years: 0.02-0.05 mg/kg/dose 1-2 times/day

Available Dosage Forms

Injection, solution, as mesylate (Cogentin®): 1 mg/mL (2 mL)

Tablet, as mesylate: 0.5 mg, 1 mg, 2 mg

Monitoring and Teaching Issues

Physical Assessment: Assess effectiveness and interactions of other medications patient may be taking. Monitor therapeutic effectiveness and adverse reactions at beginning of therapy and at regular intervals throughout therapy. Assess knowledge/teach patient appropriate use, interventions to reduce side effects, and adverse symptoms to report.

Patient Education: Take exactly as directed; do not increase, decrease, or discontinue without consulting prescriber. Take at the same time each day. Do not use alcohol and any prescription or OTC sedatives or CNS depressants without consulting prescriber. You may experience drowsiness, dizziness, confusion, and blurred vision (use caution when driving, climbing stairs, or engaging in tasks requiring alertness until response to drug is known); increased susceptibility to heat stroke, decreased perspiration (use caution in hot weather, maintain adequate fluids and reduce exercise activity); or constipation (increased exercise, fluids, fruit, or fiber may help). Report unresolved nausea, vomiting, or gastric disturbances; rapid or pounding heartbeat, chest pain, or palpitation; respiratory difficulty; CNS changes (hallucination, loss of memory, nervousness, etc); eye pain; prolonged fever; painful or difficult urination; unresolved constipation; increased muscle spasticity or rigidity; skin rash; or significant worsening of condition. **Pregnancy/breast-feeding precautions:** Inform prescriber if you are or intend to become pregnant. Consult prescriber if breast-feeding.

Geriatric Considerations: Anticholinergic agents are generally not well tolerated in the elderly and their use should be avoided when possible (see Warnings/Precautions and Adverse Reactions). In the elderly, anticholinergic agents should not be used as prophylaxis against extrapyramidal symptoms.

Pregnancy Risk Factor: C

Lactation: Excretion in breast milk unknown

Additional Information No significant difference in onset of I.M. or I.V. injection, therefore, there is usually no need to use the I.V. route. Improvement is sometimes noticeable a few minutes after injection.

- ♦ **Benztropine Mesylate** *see* Benztropine *on page 184*
- ♦ **Benzylpenicillin Benzathine** *see* Penicillin G Benzathine *on page 1172*
- ♦ **Benzylpenicillin Potassium** *see* Penicillin G (Parenteral/Aqueous) *on page 1174*
- ♦ **Benzylpenicillin Sodium** *see* Penicillin G (Parenteral/Aqueous) *on page 1174*
- ♦ **Benzylpenicilloyl-Polylysine** *see page 1625*
- ♦ **Beta-Blockers** *see page 1720*
- ♦ **Betadine® First Aid Antibiotics + Moisturizer [OTC]** *see* Bacitracin and Polymyxin B *on page 171*
- ♦ **9-Beta-D-Ribofuranosyladenine** *see* Adenosine *on page 54*
- ♦ **Beta-HC®** *see* Hydrocortisone *on page 760*

Betamethasone (bay ta METH a sone)

U.S. Brand Names Beta-Val®; Celestone®; Celestone® Soluspan®; Diprolene®; Diprolene® AF; Luxiq®; Maxivate®

Synonyms Betamethasone Dipropionate; Betamethasone Dipropionate, Augmented; Betamethasone Sodium Phosphate; Betamethasone Valerate; Flubenisolone

Generic Available Yes: Excludes foam, injection, syrup

Pharmacologic Category Corticosteroid, Systemic; Corticosteroid, Topical

Medication Safety Issues

Sound-alike/look-alike issues:

Luxiq® may be confused with Lasix®

Use Inflammatory dermatoses such as seborrheic or atopic dermatitis, neurodermatitis, anogenital pruritus, psoriasis, inflammatory phase of xerosis

Mechanism of Action/Effect Binds to corticosteroid receptors in cell and acts to prevent or control inflammation

Contraindications Hypersensitivity to betamethasone or any component of the formulation; systemic fungal infections

Warnings/Precautions Not to be used in status asthmaticus or for the relief of acute bronchospasm; topical use in patients ≤12 years of age is not recommended. May cause suppression of hypothalamic-pituitary-adrenal (HPA) axis, particularly in younger children or in patients receiving high doses for prolonged periods. Particular care is required when patients are transferred from systemic corticosteroids to inhaled products due to possible adrenal insufficiency or withdrawal from steroids, including an increase in allergic symptoms. Patients receiving 20 mg per day of prednisone (or equivalent) may be most susceptible. Fatalities have occurred due to adrenal insufficiency in asthmatic patients during and after transfer from systemic corticosteroids to aerosol steroids; aerosol steroids do **not** provide the systemic steroid needed to treat patients having trauma, surgery, or infections. Withdrawal and discontinuation of the corticosteroid should be done slowly and carefully

Controlled clinical studies have shown that orally-inhaled and intranasal corticosteroids may cause a reduction in growth velocity in pediatric patients. (In studies of orally-inhaled corticosteroids, the mean reduction in growth velocity was approximately 1 centimeter per year [range 0.3-1.8 cm per year] and appears to be related to dose and duration of exposure.) The growth of pediatric patients receiving inhaled corticosteroids, should be monitored routinely (Continued)

Betamethasone *(Continued)*

(eg, via stadiometry). To minimize the systemic effects of orally-inhaled and intranasal corticosteroids, each patient should be titrated to the lowest effective dose.

May suppress the immune system, patients may be more susceptible to infection. Use with caution in patients with systemic infections or ocular herpes simplex. Avoid exposure to chickenpox and measles.

Use with caution in patients with hypothyroidism, cirrhosis, ulcerative colitis; do not use occlusive dressings on weeping or exudative lesions and general caution with occlusive dressings should be observed; discontinue if skin irritation or contact dermatitis should occur; do not use in patients with decreased skin circulation.

Drug Interactions

Cytochrome P450 Effect: Inhibits CYP3A4 (weak)

Decreased Effect: May induce cytochrome P450 enzymes, which may lead to decreased effect of any drug metabolized by P450 (ie, barbiturates, phenytoin, rifampin). Decreased effectiveness of salicylates when taken with betamethasone.

Increased Effect/Toxicity: Inhibitors of CYP3A4 (including erythromycin, diltiazem, itraconazole, ketoconazole, quinidine, and verapamil) may decrease metabolism of betamethasone.

Nutritional/Ethanol Interactions

Ethanol: Avoid ethanol (may enhance gastric mucosal irritation).

Food: Betamethasone interferes with calcium absorption.

Herb/Nutraceutical: Avoid cat's claw, echinacea (have immunostimulant properties).

Adverse Reactions

Systemic:

>10%:

Central nervous system: Insomnia, nervousness

Gastrointestinal: Increased appetite, indigestion

1% to 10%:

Central nervous system: Dizziness or lightheadedness, headache

Dermatologic: Hirsutism, hypopigmentation

Endocrine & metabolic: Diabetes mellitus

Neuromuscular & skeletal: Arthralgia

Ocular: Cataracts, glaucoma

Respiratory: Epistaxis

Miscellaneous: Diaphoresis

Topical:

1% to 10%:

Dermatologic: Itching, allergic contact dermatitis, erythema, dryness papular rash, folliculitis, furunculosis, pustules, pyoderma, vesiculation, hyperesthesia, skin infection (secondary)

Local: Burning, irritation

Overdosage/Toxicology When consumed in high doses for prolonged periods, systemic hypercorticism and adrenal suppression may occur. In those cases, discontinuation of the corticosteroid should be done judiciously.

Pharmacodynamics/Kinetics

Time to Peak: Serum: I.V.: 10-36 minutes

Protein Binding: 64%

Half-Life Elimination: 6.5 hours

Metabolism: Hepatic

Excretion: Urine (<5% as unchanged drug)

Dosing

Adults: Base dosage on severity of disease and patient response

Inflammatory conditions:

Oral: 2.4-4.8 mg/day in 2-4 doses; range: 0.6-7.2 mg/day

I.M.: Betamethasone sodium phosphate and betamethasone acetate: 0.6-9 mg/day (generally, $\frac{1}{3}$ to $\frac{1}{2}$ of oral dose) divided every 12-24 hours

Psoriasis (scalp): Topical (foam): Apply twice daily, once in the morning and once at night to scalp.

Rheumatoid arthritis/osteoarthritis:

Intrabursal, intra-articular, intradermal: 0.25-2 mL

Intralesional:

Very large joints: 1-2 mL

Large joints: 1 mL

Medium joints: 0.5-1 mL

Small joints: 0.25-0.5 mL

Steroid-responsive dermatoses: Topical: Apply thin film 2-4 times/day. Therapy should be discontinued when control is achieved; if no improvement is seen, reassessment of diagnosis may be necessary.

Elderly: Refer to adult dosing. Use the lowest effective dose.

Pediatrics: Base dosage on severity of disease and patient response.

Inflammatory conditions: Note: Use lowest dose listed as initial dose for adrenocortical insufficiency (physiologic replacement).

I.M.: 0.0175-0.125 mg base/kg/day divided every 6-12 hours **or** 0.5-7.5 mg base/m²/day divided every 6-12 hours

Oral: 0.0175-0.25 mg/kg/day divided every 6-8 hours **or** 0.5-7.5 mg/m²/day divided every 6-8 hours

Topical:

≤12 years: Use is not recommended.

>12 years: Apply a thin film twice daily; use minimal amount for shortest period of time to avoid HPA axis suppression

Hepatic Impairment: Adjustments may be necessary in patients with liver failure because betamethasone is extensively metabolized in the liver

Available Dosage Forms [DSC] = Discontinued product

Note: Potency expressed as betamethasone base.

Cream, topical, as dipropionate: 0.05% (15 g, 45 g)

  Maxivate®: 0.05% (45 g)

Cream, topical, as dipropionate augmented (Diprolene® AF): 0.05% (15 g, 50 g)

Cream, topical, as valerate: 0.1% (15 g, 45 g)

  Beta-Val®: 0.1% (15 g, 45 g)

Foam, topical, as valerate (Luxiq®): 0.12% (50 g, 100 g, 150 g) [contains alcohol 60.4%]

Gel, topical, as dipropionate augmented: 0.05% (15 g, 50 g)

  Diprolene® [DSC]: 0.05% (15 g, 50 g)

Injection, suspension (Celestone® Soluspan®): Betamethasone sodium phosphate 3 mg/mL and betamethasone acetate 3 mg/mL [6 mg/mL] (5 mL)

Lotion, topical, as dipropionate: 0.05% (60 mL)

  Maxivate®: 0.05% (60 mL)

Lotion, topical, as dipropionate augmented (Diprolene®): 0.05% (30 mL, 60 mL)

Lotion, topical, as valerate (Beta-Val®): 0.1% (60 mL)

Ointment, topical, as dipropionate: 0.05% (15 g, 45 g)

  Maxivate®: 0.05% (45 g)

Ointment, topical, as dipropionate augmented: 0.05% (15 g, 50 g)

  Diprolene®: 0.05% (15 g, 50 g)

Ointment, topical, as valerate: 0.1% (15 g, 45 g)

Syrup, as base (Celestone®): 0.6 mg/5 mL (118 mL)

Monitoring and Teaching Issues

Physical Assessment: Assess potential for interactions with other prescriptions, OTC medications, or herbal products patient may be taking. Assess therapeutic response and adverse effects according to indications for therapy, dose, route (systemic or topical), and duration of therapy. When used for long-term therapy (>10-14 days), do not discontinue abruptly; decrease dosage incrementally. Growth should be routinely monitored in pediatric patients. With systemic administration, caution patients with diabetes to monitor glucose levels closely (corticosteroids may alter glucose levels). Teach patient proper use (according to formulation), side effects/appropriate interventions, and symptoms to report.

Patient Education: Do not take any new medication during therapy unless approved by prescriber. Take exactly as directed; do not increase dose or discontinue abruptly without consulting prescriber. Take oral medication with or after meals. Avoid alcohol and limit intake of caffeine or stimulants. Prescriber may recommend increased dietary vitamins, minerals, or iron. If you have diabetes, monitor glucose levels closely (antidiabetic medication may need to be adjusted). Inform prescriber if you are experiencing greater-than-normal levels of stress (medication may need adjustment). You may be more susceptible to infection (avoid crowds and exposure to infection and do not have any vaccination without consulting prescriber). Some forms of this medication may cause GI upset (small frequent meals and frequent mouth care may help or oral medication may be taken with meals to reduce GI upset). Report promptly excessive nervousness or sleep disturbances; signs of infection (eg, sore throat, unhealed injuries); excessive growth of body hair or loss of skin color; vision changes; excessive or sudden weight gain (>3 lb/week); swelling of face or extremities; respiratory difficulty; muscle weakness; change in color of stools (tarry) or persistent abdominal pain; or worsening of condition or failure to improve.

Topical: For external use only. Do not use for eyes, mucous membranes, or open wounds. Use exactly as directed. Before using, wash and dry area gently. Apply in a thin layer (may rub in lightly). Apply light dressing (if necessary) to area being treated. Do not use occlusive dressing unless so advised by prescriber. Avoid prolonged or excessive use around sensitive tissues, genital, or rectal areas. Avoid exposing treated area to direct sunlight. Inform prescriber if condition worsens (redness, swelling, irritation, signs of infection, or open sores) or fails to improve.

Pregnancy/breast-feeding precautions: Inform prescriber if you are or intend to become pregnant. Consult prescriber if breast-feeding.

Dietary Considerations: May be taken with food to decrease GI distress.

Geriatric Considerations: Because of the risk of adverse effects, systemic corticosteroids should be used cautiously in the elderly, in the smallest possible dose, and for the shortest possible time.

Pregnancy Risk Factor: C

Pregnancy Issues: There are no reports linking the use of betamethasone with congenital defects in the literature. Betamethasone is often used in patients with premature labor [26-34 weeks gestation] to stimulate fetal lung maturation.

Lactation: Excretion in breast milk unknown/use caution

Breast-Feeding Issues: Systemic corticosteroids are excreted in human milk. The extent of topical absorption is variable. Use with caution while breast-feeding; do not apply to nipples.

Administration

Oral: Not for alternate day therapy; once daily doses should be given in the morning.

I.M.: Do **not** give injectable sodium phosphate/acetate suspension I.V.

Topical: Apply topical sparingly to areas. Not for use on broken skin or in areas of infection. Do not apply to wet skin unless directed. Do not apply to face or inguinal area. Do not cover with occlusive dressing.

Related Information

Corticosteroids *on page 1731*

Betamethasone and Clotrimazole (bay ta METH a sone & kloe TRIM a zole)

U.S. Brand Names Lotrisone®

Synonyms Clotrimazole and Betamethasone

Generic Available Yes

Pharmacologic Category Antifungal Agent, Topical; Corticosteroid, Topical

(Continued)

Betamethasone and Clotrimazole *(Continued)*

Medication Safety Issues
Sound-alike/look-alike issues:
Lotrisone® may be confused with Lotrimin®

Use Topical treatment of various dermal fungal infections (including tinea pedis, cruris, and corpora in patients ≥17 years of age)

Dosing
Adults:
Tinea corporis, tinea cruris: Topical: Massage into affected area twice daily, morning and evening. Do not use for longer than 2 weeks; re-evaluate after 1 week if no clinical improvement. Do not exceed 45 g cream/week or 45 mL lotion/week.
Tinea pedis: Topical: Massage into affected area twice daily, morning and evening. Do not use for longer than 4 weeks; re-evaluate after 2 weeks if no clinical improvement. Do not exceed 45 g cream/week or 45 mL lotion/week.

Elderly: Use with caution. Skin atrophy and skin ulceration (rare) have been reported in patients with thinning skin. Do not use for diaper dermatitis or under occlusive dressings.

Pediatrics:
Children <17 years: Do not use.
Children ≥17 years: Refer to adult dosing.

Available Dosage Forms
Cream: Betamethasone dipropionate 0.05% and clotrimazole 1% (15 g, 45 g) [contains benzyl alcohol]
Lotion: Betamethasone dipropionate 0.05% and clotrimazole 1% (30 mL) [contains benzyl alcohol]

Monitoring and Teaching Issues
Physical Assessment: See individual agents.
Patient Education: This medication is for topical use only. Avoid contact with the eyes or mouth. Do not use intravaginally. Do not use longer than recommended. Do not use under dressings or diapers. Shake lotion well before use. Notify prescriber if the condition does not improve or if side effects occur. **Pregnancy/breast-feeding precautions:** Inform prescriber if you are or intend to become pregnant. Consult prescriber if breast-feeding.

Pregnancy Risk Factor: C
Lactation: Excretion in breast milk unknown/use caution

Related Information
Betamethasone *on page 185*
Clotrimazole *on page 360*

♦ **Betamethasone Dipropionate** *see* Betamethasone *on page 185*

♦ **Betamethasone Dipropionate, Augmented** *see* Betamethasone *on page 185*

♦ **Betamethasone Sodium Phosphate** *see* Betamethasone *on page 185*

♦ **Betamethasone Valerate** *see* Betamethasone *on page 185*

♦ **Betapace®** *see* Sotalol *on page 1386*

♦ **Betapace AF®** *see* Sotalol *on page 1386*

♦ **Betaseron®** *see* Interferon Beta-1b *on page 821*

♦ **Beta-Val®** *see* Betamethasone *on page 185*

Betaxolol *(be TAKS oh lol)*

U.S. Brand Names Betoptic® S; Kerlone®
Synonyms Betaxolol Hydrochloride
Generic Available Yes: Solution, tablet
Pharmacologic Category Beta Blocker, Beta₁ Selective
Medication Safety Issues
Sound-alike/look-alike issues:
Betaxolol may be confused with bethanechol, labetalol

Use Treatment of chronic open-angle glaucoma and ocular hypertension; management of hypertension

Mechanism of Action/Effect Competitively blocks $beta_1$-receptors, with little or no effect on $beta_2$-receptors; ophthalmic reduces intraocular pressure by reducing the production of aqueous humor

Contraindications Hypersensitivity to betaxolol or any component of the formulation; sinus bradycardia; heart block greater than first-degree (except in patients with a functioning artificial pacemaker); cardiogenic shock; uncompensated cardiac failure; pulmonary edema; pregnancy (2nd and 3rd trimester)

Warnings/Precautions Administer cautiously in compensated heart failure and monitor for a worsening of the condition (efficacy has not been demonstrated in heart failure). Use caution with concurrent use of beta-blockers and either verapamil or diltiazem; bradycardia or heart block can occur. Use caution in patients with PVD (can aggravate arterial insufficiency). In general, beta-blockers should be avoided in patients with bronchospastic disease. Betaxolol, with B1 selectivity, has been used cautiously in some patients with bronchospastic disease. Use with caution in patients with diabetes, beta-blockers may mask prominent hypoglycemic symptoms. May mask signs of thyrotoxicosis. Dosage adjustment required in severe renal impairment and those on dialysis. Use care with anesthetic agents which decrease myocardial function. Beta-blocker therapy should not be withdrawn abruptly (particularly in patients with CAD), but gradually tapered to avoid acute tachycardia, hypertension, and/or ischemia.

Drug Interactions
Cytochrome P450 Effect: Substrate (major) of CYP1A2, 2D6; **Inhibits** CYP2D6 (weak)
Decreased Effect: CYP1A2 inducers may decrease the levels/effects of betaxolol; example inducers include aminoglutethimide, carbamazepine, phenobarbital, and rifampin. Decreased effect of betaxolol with aluminum salts, barbiturates, calcium salts, cholestyramine, colestipol, NSAIDs, penicillins (ampicillin), rifampin, salicylates, and sulfinpyrazone due to decreased bioavailability and plasma levels. Beta-blockers may decrease the effect of sulfonylureas.

Increased Effect/Toxicity: CYP1A2 Inhibitors may increase the levels/effects of betaxolol; example inhibitors include amiodarone, ciprofloxacin, fluvoxamine, ketoconazole, norfloxacin, ofloxacin, and rofecoxib. CYP2D6 inhibitors may increase the levels/effects of betaxolol; example inhibitors include chlorpromazine, delavirdine, fluoxetine, miconazole, paroxetine, pergolide, quinidine, quinine, ritonavir, and ropinirole. The heart rate-lowering effects of betaxolol are additive with other drugs which slow AV conduction (digoxin, verapamil, diltiazem). Reserpine increases the effects of betaxolol. Concurrent use of betaxolol may increase the effects of alpha-blockers (prazosin, terazosin), alpha-adrenergic stimulants (epinephrine, phenylephrine), and the vasoconstrictive effects of ergot alkaloids. Betaxolol may mask the tachycardia from hypoglycemia caused by insulin and oral hypoglycemics. In patients receiving concurrent therapy, the risk of hypertensive crisis is increased when either clonidine or the beta-blocker is withdrawn. Beta-blockers may increase the action or levels of ethanol, disopyramide, nondepolarizing muscle relaxants, and theophylline although the effects are difficult to predict.

Nutritional/Ethanol Interactions Herb/Nutraceutical: Avoid dong quai if using for hypertension (has estrogenic activity). Avoid ephedra, yohimbe, ginseng (may worsen hypertension). Avoid garlic (may have increased antihypertensive effect).

Adverse Reactions

Ophthalmic:

>10%: Ocular: Conjunctival hyperemia

1% to 10%:

Ocular: Anisocoria, corneal punctate keratitis, keratitis, corneal staining, decreased corneal sensitivity, eye pain, vision disturbances

Systemic:

>10%:

Central nervous system: Drowsiness, insomnia

Endocrine & metabolic: Decreased sexual ability

1% to 10%:

Cardiovascular: Bradycardia, palpitation, edema, CHF, reduced peripheral circulation

Central nervous system: Mental depression

Gastrointestinal: Diarrhea or constipation, nausea, vomiting, stomach discomfort

Respiratory: Bronchospasm

Miscellaneous: Cold extremities

Overdosage/Toxicology Symptoms of significant overdose include bradycardia, hypotension, AV block, CHF, bronchospasm, hypoglycemia. Treat initially with fluids. Sympathomimetics (eg, epinephrine or dopamine), glucagon, or a pacemaker can be used to treat toxic bradycardia, asystole, and/or hypotension.

Pharmacodynamics/Kinetics

Onset of Action: Ophthalmic: 30 minutes; Oral: 1-1.5 hours

Duration of Action: Ophthalmic: ≥12 hours

Absorption: Ophthalmic: Some systemic; Oral: ~100%

Bioavailability: Oral: 89%

Time to Peak: Ophthalmic: ~2 hours; Oral: 1.5-6 hours

Protein Binding: Oral: 50%

Half-Life Elimination: Oral: 12-22 hours

Metabolism: Hepatic to multiple metabolites

Excretion: Urine

Dosing

Adults:

Glaucoma: Ophthalmic: Instill 1 drop twice daily.

Hypertension, angina: Oral: 5-10 mg/day; may increase dose to 20 mg/day after 7-14 days if desired response is not achieved

Elderly:

Ophthalmic: Refer to adult dosing.

Hypertension: Oral: Initial: 5 mg/day

Renal Impairment: Oral: Administer 5 mg/day; can increase every 2 weeks up to a maximum of 20 mg/day.

Cl$_{cr}$ <10 mL/minute: Administer 50% of usual dose.

Available Dosage Forms

Solution, ophthalmic, as hydrochloride: 0.5% (5 mL, 10 mL, 15 mL) [contains benzalkonium chloride]

Suspension, ophthalmic, as hydrochloride (Betoptic® S): 0.25% (2.5 mL, 5 mL, 10 mL, 15 mL) [contains benzalkonium chloride]

Tablet, as hydrochloride (Kerlone®): 10 mg, 20 mg

Monitoring and Teaching Issues

Physical Assessment: Assess potential for interactions with other prescriptions, OTC medications, or herbal products patient may be taking (especially products that affects cardiac function or blood pressure). Assess therapeutic response and adverse effects. Patients with diabetes should be cautioned that beta-blockers may mask prominent hypoglycemic symptoms. Teach patient proper use (according to formulation), side effects/appropriate interventions, and symptoms to report. Systemic absorption from ophthalmic instillation is minimal. Intraocular pressure should be measured periodically.

Monitoring Laboratory Tests: Ophthalmic: Intraocular pressure

Patient Education: Do not take any new medication during therapy unless approved by prescriber.

Oral: Use as directed and do not discontinue without consulting prescriber. May cause dizziness or blurred vision (use caution when driving or engaging in tasks requiring alertness until response to drug is known); or nausea or vomiting (small frequent meals, frequent mouth care, sucking lozenges, or chewing gum may help). If diabetic, may mask prominent hypoglycemic symptoms. Monitor blood glucose levels closely. Report chest (Continued)

Betaxolol *(Continued)*

pain, palpitations or irregular heartbeat; persistent GI upset (eg, nausea, vomiting, diarrhea, or constipation); unusual cough; respiratory difficulty; swelling or coolness of extremities; or unusual mental depression. **Pregnancy/breast-feeding precautions:** Inform prescriber if you are or intend to become pregnant. Consult prescriber if breast-feeding.

Ophthalmic: Shake suspension well before using. Tilt head back and instill in eye. Keep eye open; do not blink for 30 seconds. Apply gentle pressure to corner of eye for 1 minute. Wipe away excess from skin. Do not let tip of applicator touch eye; do not contaminate tip of applicator (may cause eye infection, eye damage, or vision loss). Report if condition does not improve or if you experience eye pain, vision changes, or other adverse eye response.

Geriatric Considerations: Oral: Due to alterations in the beta-adrenergic autonomic nervous system, beta-adrenergic blockade may result in less hemodynamic response than seen in younger adults.

Pregnancy Risk Factor: C (manufacturer); D (2nd and 3rd trimesters - expert analysis)

Lactation: Oral: Enters breast milk/use caution

Administration

Other: Ophthalmic: Shake well before using. Tilt head back and instill in eye. Keep eye open and do not blink for 30 seconds. Apply gentle pressure to lacrimal sac for 1 minute. Wipe away excess from skin. Do not touch applicator to eye and do not contaminate tip of applicator.

Storage: Avoid freezing.

Related Information

Beta-Blockers *on page 1720*
Glaucoma Drug Therapy *on page 1827*

- **Betaxolol Hydrochloride** *see* Betaxolol *on page 188*

Bethanechol *(be THAN e kole)*

U.S. Brand Names Urecholine®

Synonyms Bethanechol Chloride

Generic Available Yes

Pharmacologic Category Cholinergic Agonist

Medication Safety Issues

Sound-alike/look-alike issues:

Bethanechol may be confused with betaxolol

Use Nonobstructive urinary retention and retention due to neurogenic bladder

Unlabeled/Investigational Use Treatment and prevention of bladder dysfunction caused by phenothiazines; diagnosis of flaccid or atonic neurogenic bladder; gastroesophageal reflux

Mechanism of Action/Effect Stimulates cholinergic receptors in the smooth muscle of the urinary bladder and GI tract resulting in increased peristalsis, increased GI and pancreatic secretions, bladder muscle contraction, and increased ureteral peristaltic waves

Contraindications Hypersensitivity to bethanechol or any component of the formulation; mechanical obstruction of the GI or GU tract or when the strength or integrity of the GI or bladder wall is in question; hyperthyroidism, peptic ulcer disease, epilepsy, obstructive pulmonary disease, bradycardia, vasomotor instability, atrioventricular conduction defects, hypotension, or parkinsonism

Warnings/Precautions Potential for reflux infection if the sphincter fails to relax as bethanechol contracts the bladder; safety and efficacy in children have not been established.

Drug Interactions

Decreased Effect: Procainamide, quinidine may decrease the effects of bethanechol. Anticholinergic agents (atropine, antihistamines, TCAs, phenothiazines) may decrease effects.

Increased Effect/Toxicity: Bethanechol and ganglionic blockers may cause a critical fall in blood pressure. Cholinergic drugs or anticholinesterase agents may have additive effects with bethanechol.

Lab Interactions Increased lipase, AST, amylase (S), bilirubin, aminotransferase [ALT (SGPT)/AST (SGOT)] (S)

Adverse Reactions Frequency not defined.

Cardiovascular: Hypotension, tachycardia, flushed skin

Central nervous system: Headache, malaise

Gastrointestinal: Abdominal cramps, diarrhea, nausea, vomiting, salivation, eructation

Genitourinary: Urinary urgency

Ocular: Lacrimation, miosis

Respiratory: Asthmatic attacks, bronchial constriction

Miscellaneous: Diaphoresis

Overdosage/Toxicology Symptoms of overdose include nausea, vomiting, abdominal cramps, diarrhea, involuntary defecation, flushed skin, hypotension, and bronchospasm. Treat symptomatically; atropine for severe muscarinic symptoms, epinephrine to reverse severe cardiovascular or pulmonary sequelae.

Pharmacodynamics/Kinetics

Onset of Action: 30-90 minutes

Duration of Action: Up to 6 hours

Absorption: Variable

Dosing

Adults:

Urinary retention, neurogenic bladder, and/or bladder atony:

Oral: Initial: 10-50 mg 2-4 times/day (some patients may require dosages of 50-100 mg 4 times/day). To determine effective dose, may initiate at a dose of 5-10 mg, with additional doses of 5-10 mg hourly until an effective cumulative dose is reached. Cholinergic effects at higher oral dosages may be cumulative.

SubQ: Initial: 2.575 mg, may repeat in 15-30 minutes (maximum cumulative initial dose: 10.3 mg); subsequent doses may be given 3-4 times daily as needed (some patients may require more frequent dosing at 2.5- to 3-hour intervals). Chronic neurogenic atony may require doses of 7.5-10 every 4 hours.

Gastroesophageal reflux (unlabeled): Oral: 25 mg 4 times/day

Elderly: Use the lowest effective dose.

Pediatrics:

Urinary retention (unlabeled use): Oral: 0.6 mg/kg/day divided 3-4 times/day

Gastroesophageal reflux (unlabeled use): Oral: 0.1-0.2 mg/kg/dose given 30 minutes to 1 hour before each meal to a maximum of 4 times/day

Available Dosage Forms Tablet, as chloride: 5 mg, 10 mg, 25 mg, 50 mg

Monitoring and Teaching Issues

Physical Assessment: Assess bladder and sphincter adequacy prior to administering medication. Assess other medications patient may be taking for effectiveness and interactions. Assess therapeutic effectiveness and adverse reactions. Assess knowledge/teach patient appropriate use, interventions to reduce side effects, and adverse symptoms to report.

Patient Education: Take as directed, on an empty stomach to avoid nausea or vomiting. Do not discontinue without consulting prescriber. Maintain adequate hydration (2-3 L/day of fluids) unless instructed to restrict fluid intake. May cause dizziness or hypotension (rise slowly from sitting or lying position and use caution when driving or climbing stairs); or vomiting or loss of appetite (small frequent meals, frequent mouth care, sucking lozenges, or chewing gum may help). Report persistent abdominal discomfort; significantly increased salivation, sweating, tearing, or urination; flushed skin; chest pain or palpitations; acute headache; unresolved diarrhea; excessive fatigue, insomnia, dizziness, or depression; increased muscle, joint, or body pain; vision changes or blurred vision; or respiratory difficulty or wheezing. **Pregnancy/breast-feeding precautions:** Inform prescriber if you are or intend to become pregnant. Do not breast-feed.

Dietary Considerations: Should be taken 1 hour before meals or 2 hours after meals.

Geriatric Considerations: Urinary incontinence in an elderly patient should be investigated. Bethanechol may be used for overflow incontinence (dribbling) caused by an atonic or hypotonic bladder, but clinical efficacy is variable (see Contraindications, Warnings/Precautions, and Adverse Reactions).

Pregnancy Risk Factor: C

Lactation: Excretion in breast milk unknown/contraindicated

Administration

Storage: Store at room temperature of 15°C to 30°C (59°F to 86°F).

♦ **Bethanechol Chloride** *see* Bethanechol *on page 190*

♦ **Betimol®** *see* Timolol *on page 1478*

♦ **Betoptic® S** *see* Betaxolol *on page 188*

Bevacizumab (be vuh SIZ uh mab)

U.S. Brand Names Avastin™

Synonyms Anti-VEGF Monoclonal Antibody; rhuMAb-VEGF

Generic Available No

Pharmacologic Category Antineoplastic Agent, Monoclonal Antibody; Vascular Endothelial Growth Factor (VEGF) Inhibitor

Use Treatment of metastatic colorectal cancer as a component of multidrug therapy

Unlabeled/Investigational Use Breast cancer, malignant mesothelioma, prostate cancer

Mechanism of Action/Effect Bevacizumab is a monoclonal antibody which binds to (and neutralizes) vascular endothelial growth factor (VEGF), preventing its association with endothelial receptors. It blocks the formation of new blood vessels which in turn may slow the growth of all tissues (including metastatic tissue).

Contraindications Hypersensitivity to bevacizumab, murine products, or any component of the formulation

Warnings/Precautions Gastrointestinal perforation, intra-abdominal abscess, and wound dehiscence have been reported in patients receiving bevacizumab; monitor patients for signs/symptoms of abdominal pain, constipation or vomiting. Permanent discontinuation is recommended in patients who develop these complications. The appropriate intervals between administration of bevacizumab and surgical procedures to avoid impairment in wound healing has not been established. Do not initiate therapy within 28 days of major surgery and only following complete healing of the incision. Bevacizumab should be discontinued prior to elective surgery and the estimated half-life (20 days) should be considered.

Avoid use in patients with recent hemoptysis; significant pulmonary bleeding has been reported in patients receiving bevacizumab (primarily in patients with nonsmall cell lung cancer). Avoid use in patients with CNS metastases; patients with CNS metastases were excluded from clinical trials due to concerns for bleeding. Other serious bleeding events may occur, but with a lower frequency; discontinuation of treatment is recommended in all patients with serious hemorrhage.

An increased risk for arterial thromboembolic events (eg, stroke, MI, TIA, angina) is associated with bevacizumab use with combination chemotherapy. History of arterial thromboembolism or ≥65 years of age may present an even greater risk; permanently discontinue if serious arterial thromboembolic events occur.

May cause CHF and/or potentiate cardiotoxic effects of anthracyclines. Use with caution in patients with cardiovascular disease; patients with significant cardiovascular disease were excluded from clinical trials. Bevacizumab may cause and/or worsen hypertension; use caution in patients with pre-existing hypertension and monitor BP closely in all patients. Permanent discontinuation is recommended in patients who experience a hypertensive crisis. Temporarily discontinue in patients who develop uncontrolled hypertension. Interrupt therapy in patients experiencing severe infusion reactions; there are no data to address reinstitution of therapy in patients who experience CHF and/or severe infusion reactions. Proteinuria and/ (Continued)

Bevacizumab *(Continued)*

or nephrotic syndrome has been associated with bevacizumab; discontinuation of therapy is recommended in patients with nephrotic syndrome. Safety and efficacy in pediatric patients have not been established.

Drug Interactions

Increased Effect/Toxicity: Bevacizumab may potentiate the cardiotoxic effects of anthracyclines. Serum concentrations of irinotecan's active metabolite may be increased by bevacizumab; an approximate 33% increase has been observed.

Adverse Reactions No data are available concerning the frequency of adverse reactions to bevacizumab alone. The frequencies noted below are from two controlled clinical trials of bevacizumab in combination with irinotecan, fluorouracil, and leucovorin (IFL). These frequencies, where noted, are compared to the incidence in the placebo-controlled arms of the trials.

>10%:

Cardiovascular: Hypertension (23% to 34% vs 14%, severe/life-threatening 12% vs 2%); hypotension (7% to 15% vs 7%); thromboembolism (18% vs 15%)

Central nervous system: Pain (61% to 62% vs 55%, severe 8% vs 5%); abdominal pain (50% to 61% vs 55%, severe/life-threatening 8% vs 5%); headache (26% vs 19%); dizziness (19% to 26% vs 20%)

Dermatologic: Alopecia (6% to 32% vs 26%), dry skin (7% to 20% vs 7%), exfoliative dermatitis (3% to 19% vs 3%), skin discoloration (2% to 16% vs 3%)

Endocrine & metabolic: Weight loss (15% to 16% vs 10%), hypokalemia (12% to 16% vs 11%)

Gastrointestinal: Diarrhea (severe/life-threatening 34% vs 25%); vomiting (47% to 52% vs 47%); anorexia (35% to 43% vs 30%); constipation (29% to 40% vs 29%, severe/life-threatening 4% vs 2%); stomatitis (30% to 32% vs 18%); dyspepsia (17% to 24% vs 15%); flatulence (11% to 19% vs 10%); taste disorder (14% to 21% vs 9%)

Hematologic: Leukopenia (severe/life-threatening 37% vs 31%), epistaxis (32% to 35% vs 10%), gastrointestinal hemorrhage (19% to 24% vs 6%), neutropenia (severe/life-threatening 21% vs 14%)

Neuromuscular & skeletal: Weakness (73% to 74% vs 70%, severe/life-threatening 10% vs 7%); myalgia (8% to 15% vs 7%)

Ocular: Tearing increased (6% to 18% vs 2%)

Renal: Proteinuria includes nephrotic syndrome in some patients (36% vs 24%)

Respiratory: Upper respiratory infection (40% to 47% vs 39%), dyspnea (25% to 26% vs 15%)

1% to 10%:

Cardiovascular: DVT (6% to 9% vs 3%, severe/life-threatening 9% vs 5%); intra-arterial thrombosis (severe/life-threatening 3% vs 1%)

Central nervous system: Confusion (1% to 6% vs 1%), syncope (severe/life-threatening 3% vs 1%), abnormal gait (1% to 5% vs 0%)

Dermatologic: Skin ulcer (6% vs 1%), nail disorders (2% to 8% vs 3%)

Endocrine & metabolic: Infusion reactions (<3%)

Gastrointestinal: Dry mouth (4% to 7% vs 2%), colitis (1% to 6% vs 1%)

Hematologic: Thrombocytopenia (5% vs 0%)

Hepatic: Bilirubinemia (1% to 6% vs 0%)

Renal: Urinary frequency/urgency (3% to 6% vs 1%)

Respiratory: Voice alteration (6% to 9% vs 2%)

Pharmacodynamics/Kinetics

Half-Life Elimination: Half-life elimination: 20 days (range: 11-50 days)

Excretion: Clearance: 2.75-5 mL/kg/day

Dosing

Adults & Elderly:

Colorectal cancer: I.V.: 5-10 mg/kg every 2 weeks

Breast cancer (unlabeled use): I.V.: 3 mg/kg or 10 mg/kg or 20 mg/kg every 2 weeks

Head and neck cancer (unlabeled use): 5 mg/kg or 10 mg/kg, or 15 mg/kg every 3 weeks

Prostate cancer (unlabeled use): I.V.: 10 mg/kg every 2 weeks

Renal cell cancer (unlabeled use): 3 mg/kg or 10 mg/kg every 2 weeks

Dosage adjustment for toxicity: Temporary suspension is recommended in moderate-to-severe proteinuria or in patients with severe hypertension which is not controlled with medical management. Permanent discontinuation is recommended (by the manufacturer) in patients who develop wound dehiscence requiring intervention, gastrointestinal perforation, hypertensive crisis, serious bleeding, or nephrotic syndrome.

Available Dosage Forms Injection, solution [preservative free]: 25 mg/mL (4 mL, 16 mL)

Monitoring and Teaching Issues

Physical Assessment: See Warnings/Precautions for specific use cautions. Assess potential for interactions with other pharmacological agents patient may be taking (see Drug Interactions). Patient must be monitored closely during and following infusion for infusion reaction, abdominal pain, constipation, vomiting, bleeding events, hypertension, nephrotic syndrome (see Adverse Reactions). Teach patient proper use, possible side effects/appropriate interventions, and adverse symptoms to report.

Monitoring Laboratory Tests: CBC with differential; urinalysis

Patient Education: Do not take any new medication during therapy unless approved by prescriber. This medication can only be administered by infusion; you will be closely monitored during infusion; report immediately unusual back or abdominal pain, acute headache, difficulty breathing or chest tightness, difficulty swallowing, itching or rash, redness, swelling, or pain at infusion site. Maintain adequate hydration (2-3 L/day of fluids) unless instructed to restrict fluid intake and nutrition (small frequent meals). You may experience dry mouth or taste changes (frequent oral care, sucking lozenges, or chewing gum may help); loss of hair (will grow back when therapy is completed). Report any chest pain, palpitations or change in heart rate; acute headache, dizziness; abdominal pain, vomiting or constipation; changes in urinary pattern; pain, redness or swelling or loss of sensation in extremities; any unusual bleeding; skin rash, or any other adverse reactions. **Pregnancy precautions:** Inform prescriber if you are or intend to become pregnant or breast-feed.

Geriatric Considerations: Elderly patients ≥65 years of age had an increased incidence of arterial thromboembolic events; other serious adverse events occurring often include weakness, sepsis, hyper-/hypotension, CHF, constipation, anorexia, anemia, hyper-/hypokalemia, and diarrhea.

Pregnancy Risk Factor: C

Pregnancy Issues: There are no adequate or well-controlled studies in pregnant women. Angiogenesis is of critical importance to fetal development, and bevacizumab is likely to have adverse consequences in terms of fetal development. Adequate contraception during therapy is recommended. The risk and benefit of treatment should be evaluated in pregnant women. Patients should also be counseled regarding prolonged exposure following discontinuation of therapy due to the long half-life of bevacizumab.

Lactation: Excretion in breast milk unknown/not recommended

Breast-Feeding Issues: Immunoglobulins are excreted in breast milk, and it is assumed that bevacizumab may appear in breast milk. Due to concerns for effects on the infant, breast-feeding is not recommended. The half-life of bevacizumab is up to 50 days (average 20 days), and this should be considered when decisions are made concerning breast-feeding resumption.

Administration
I.V.: Do not administer as I.V. push or rapid I.V. bolus. Infuse the initial dose over 90 minutes (administer following chemotherapy). Infusion may be shortened to 60 minutes if the initial infusion is well tolerated. The third and subsequent infusions may be shortened to 30 minutes if the 60 minute infusion is well tolerated.

Reconstitution: Prior to infusion, dilute prescribed dose of bevacizumab in 100 mL NS. Do not mix with dextrose-containing solutions.

Storage: Store vials at 2°C to 8°C (36°F to 46°F). Protect from light; do not freeze or shake. Diluted solutions are stable for up to 8 hours under refrigeration.

Bexarotene (beks AIR oh teen)
U.S. Brand Names Targretin®

Generic Available No

Pharmacologic Category Antineoplastic Agent, Miscellaneous

Use

Oral: Treatment of cutaneous manifestations of cutaneous T-cell lymphoma in patients who are refractory to at least one prior systemic therapy

Topical: Treatment of cutaneous lesions in patients with refractory cutaneous T-cell lymphoma (stage 1A and 1B) or who have not tolerated other therapies

Mechanism of Action/Effect Exact mechanism in is unknown. Acts to inhibit the growth of some tumor cell lines of hematopoietic and squamous cell origin.

Contraindications Hypersensitivity to bexarotene or any component of the formulation; pregnancy

Warnings/Precautions Pregnancy test needed 1 week before initiation and every month thereafter. Effective contraception must be in place one month before initiation, during therapy, and for at least 1 month after discontinuation. Male patients with sexual partners who are pregnant, possibly pregnant, or who could become pregnant, must use condoms during sexual intercourse during treatment and for 1 month after last dose. Induces significant lipid abnormalities in a majority of patients (triglyceride, total cholesterol, and HDL); reversible on discontinuation. Use extreme caution in patients with underlying hypertriglyceridemia. Pancreatitis secondary to hypertriglyceridemia has been reported. Monitor for liver function test abnormalities and discontinue drug if tests are three times the upper limit of normal values for AST (SGOT), ALT (SGPT) or bilirubin. Hypothyroidism occurs in about a third of patients. Monitor for signs and symptoms of infection about 4-8 weeks after initiation (leukopenia may occur). Any new visual abnormalities experienced by the patient should be evaluated by an ophthalmologist (cataracts can form, or worsen, especially in the geriatric population). May cause photosensitization. Safety and efficacy are not established in the pediatric population. Avoid use in hepatically impaired patients. Limit additional vitamin A intake to <15,000 int. units/day. Use caution with diabetic patients; monitor for hypoglycemia.

Drug Interactions

Cytochrome P450 Effect: Substrate of CYP3A4 (minor); **Induces** CYP3A4 (weak)

Decreased Effect: Bexarotene may decrease the plasma levels of hormonal contraceptives and tamoxifen.

Increased Effect/Toxicity: Bexarotene plasma concentrations may be increased by gemfibrozil. Bexarotene may increase the toxicity of DEET.

Nutritional/Ethanol Interactions

Food: Take with a fat-containing meal. Bexarotene serum levels may be increased by grapefruit juice; avoid concurrent use.

Herb/Nutraceutical: Avoid dong quai, St John's wort (may also cause photosensitization). St John's wort may decrease bexarotene levels. Additional vitamin A supplements may lead to vitamin A toxicity (dry skin, irritation, arthralgias, myalgias, abdominal pain, hepatic changes).

Adverse Reactions First percentage is at a dose of 300 mg/m²/day; the second percentage is at a dose >300 mg/m²/day.

>10%:

Cardiovascular: Peripheral edema (13% to 11%)

Central nervous system: Headache (30% to 42%), chills (10% to 13%)

Dermatologic: Rash (17% to 23%), exfoliative dermatitis (10% to 28%)

Endocrine & metabolic: Hyperlipidemia (about 79% in both dosing ranges), hypercholesteremia (32% to 62%), hypothyroidism (29% to 53%)

Hematologic: Leukopenia (17% to 47%)

(Continued)

Bexarotene *(Continued)*

Neuromuscular & skeletal: Weakness (20% to 45%)

Miscellaneous: Infection (13% to 23%)

<10%:

Cardiovascular: Hemorrhage, hypertension, angina pectoris, right heart failure, tachycardia, cerebrovascular accident

Central nervous system: Fever (5% to 17%), insomnia (5% to 11%), subdural hematoma, syncope, depression, agitation, ataxia, confusion, dizziness, hyperesthesia

Dermatologic: Dry skin (about 10% for both dosing ranges), alopecia (4% to 11%), skin ulceration, acne, skin nodule, maculopapular rash, serous drainage, vesicular bullous rash, cheilitis

Endocrine & metabolic: Hypoproteinemia, hyperglycemia, weight loss/gain, serum amylase (elevated), breast pain

Gastrointestinal: Abdominal pain (11% to 4%), nausea (16% to 8%), diarrhea (7% to 42%), vomiting (4% to 13%), anorexia (2% to 23%), constipation, xerostomia, flatulence, colitis, dyspepsia, gastroenteritis, gingivitis, melena, pancreatitis,

Genitourinary: Albuminuria, hematuria, urinary incontinence, urinary tract infection, urinary urgency, dysuria, kidney function abnormality

Hematologic: Hypochromic anemia (4% to 13%), anemia (6% to 25%), eosinophilia, thrombocythemia, coagulation time increased, lymphocytosis, thrombocytopenia

Hepatic: LDH increase (7% to 13%), hepatic failure

Neuromuscular & skeletal: Back pain (2% to 11%), arthralgia, myalgia, bone pain, myasthenia, arthrosis, neuropathy

Ocular: Dry eyes, conjunctivitis, blepharitis, corneal lesion, visual field defects, keratitis

Otic: Ear pain, otitis externa

Renal: Creatinine (elevated)

Respiratory: Pharyngitis, rhinitis, dyspnea, pleural effusion, bronchitis, increased cough, lung edema, hemoptysis, hypoxia

Miscellaneous: Flu-like syndrome (4% to 13%), bacterial infection (1% to 13%)

Topical:

Cardiovascular: Edema (10%)

Central nervous system: Headache (14%), weakness (6%), pain (30%)

Dermatologic: Rash (14% to 72%), pruritus (6% to 40%), contact dermatitis (14%), exfoliative dermatitis (6%)

Hematologic: Leukopenia (6%), lymphadenopathy (6%)

Neuromuscular & skeletal: Paresthesia (6%)

Respiratory: Cough (6%), pharyngitis (6%)

Miscellaneous: Diaphoresis (6%), infection (18%)

Overdosage/Toxicology Doses up to 1000 mg/m^2/day have been used in humans without acute toxic effects. Any overdose should be treated with supportive care focused on the symptoms exhibited.

Pharmacodynamics/Kinetics

Absorption: Significantly improved by a fat-containing meal

Time to Peak: 2 hours

Protein Binding: >99%

Half-Life Elimination: 7 hours

Metabolism: Hepatic via CYP3A4 isoenzyme; four metabolites identified; further metabolized by glucuronidation

Excretion: Primarily feces; urine (<1% as unchanged drug and metabolites)

Dosing

Adults & Elderly:

Cutaneous T-cell lymphoma:

Oral: 300 mg/m^2/day taken as a single daily dose. If there is no tumor response after 8 weeks and the initial dose was well tolerated, then an increase to 400 mg/m^2/day can be made with careful monitoring. Maintain as long as the patient is deriving benefit. If the initial dose is not tolerated, then it may be adjusted to 200 mg/m^2/day, then to 100 mg/m^2/day or temporarily suspended if necessary to manage toxicity.

Cutaneous lesions of T-cell lymphoma: Topical: Apply to lesions once every other day for first week, then increase on a weekly basis to once daily, 2 times/day, 3 times/day, and finally 4 times/day, according to tolerance.

Renal Impairment: No studies have been conducted; however, renal insufficiency may result in significant protein binding changes and alter pharmacokinetics of bexarotene.

Hepatic Impairment: No studies have been conducted; however, hepatic impairment would be expected to result in decreased clearance of bexarotene due to the extensive hepatic contribution to elimination.

Available Dosage Forms

Capsule: 75 mg

Gel: 1% (60 g)

Monitoring and Teaching Issues

Physical Assessment: See Warnings/Precautions prior to starting therapy. Assess potential for interactions with other pharmacological agents or herbal products patient may be taking (see Drug Interactions). Assess results of laboratory tests (pregnancy, lipid panel, LFTs, thyroid function, CBC) prior to and during therapy (see Monitoring Laboratory Tests). Assess therapeutic response (reduction of cutaneous lesions) and adverse reactions (eg, CNS or cardiovascular effects, opportunistic infection, visual abnormalities, hypoglycemia; see Warnings/Precautions and Adverse Reactions). Teach patient proper use according to formulation, side effects/appropriate interventions, and symptoms to report. **Pregnancy risk factor X:** Determine that patient is not pregnant before beginning treatment. Instruct female patients of childbearing age and males who may have intercourse with females of childbearing age about appropriate use of contraceptives 1 month prior to, during, and 1 month following treatment.

Monitoring Laboratory Tests: If female, pregnancy test 1 week before initiation then monthly while on bexarotene; lipid panel before initiation, then weekly until lipid response established and then at 8-week intervals thereafter; baseline LFTs, repeat at 1, 2, and 4 weeks after initiation then at 8-week intervals thereafter if stable; baseline and periodic thyroid function tests; baseline CBC with periodic monitoring

Patient Education: Do not take any new medication during therapy unless approved by prescriber. Use exactly as directed; it is preferable to take capsules after a fat-containing meal. Maintain adequate hydration (2-3 L/day of fluids) unless instructed to restrict fluid intake. Avoid grapefruit juice, St John's wort, or additional vitamin A supplements while using this medication. You may be more susceptible to infection (avoid crowds and exposure to infection and do not have any vaccinations without consulting prescriber). May cause nausea, vomiting, anorexia, flatulence (frequent, small meals, good mouth care, chewing gum, or sucking lozenges may help); constipation (increased exercise, fluid, fruit, or fiber may help); diarrhea (buttermilk, boiled milk, or yogurt may help); headache, back or muscle pain (consult prescriber for mild analgesic); or photosensitivity (avoid direct sunlight, wear protective clothing and hat, use sunblock, and protective eyewear). Report chest pain, rapid heartbeat; unresolved GI effects; headache, back or muscle pain; skin dryness, skin rash or peeling; mucous membrane lesions; altered urinary patterns; flu syndrome or opportunistic infection (eg, weakness, fatigue, white plaques or sores in mouth, vaginal discharge, chills, fever); CNS disturbances (insomnia, dizziness, agitation, confusion, depression); vision or hearing changes; or any other adverse effects. **Pregnancy/breast-feeding precautions:** Pregnancy test is needed 1 week before initiation of therapy and every month during therapy. Consult prescriber for appropriate contraceptives. Effective contraception must be in place 1 month before initiation, during therapy, and for at least 1 month after discontinuation. Male patients with sexual partners who are pregnant, possibly pregnant, or who could become pregnant, must use condoms when having sexual intercourse while using this medication and for 1 month after last dose. Do not breast-feed.

Oral: Take exactly as directed, at the same time each day with a fat-containing meal. If you miss a dose, take as soon as possible. If it is almost time for next dose, skip the missed dose and continue on regular schedule. Do not double doses.

Topical: Apply as directed. Allow gel to dry before covering. Avoid applying to normal skin or mucous membranes. Do not use occlusive dressings.

Dietary Considerations: It is preferable to take the oral capsule following a fat-containing meal.

Pregnancy Risk Factor: X

Pregnancy Issues: Bexarotene caused birth defects when administered orally to pregnant rats. It must not be given to a pregnant woman or a woman who intends to become pregnant. If a woman becomes pregnant while taking the drug, it must be stopped immediately and appropriate counseling be given.

Lactation: Excretion in breast milk unknown/contraindicated

Administration

Oral: Administer capsule following a fat-containing meal.

Topical: Allow gel to dry before covering with clothing. Avoid application to normal skin. Use of occlusive dressings is not recommended.

Storage: Store at 2°C to 25°C (36°F to 77°F). Protect from light.

- ◆ **Bextra®** see Valdecoxib on page 1540
- ◆ **Bexxar®** see Tositumomab and Iodine I 131 Tositumomab on page 1501
- ◆ **BG 9273** see Alefacept on page 64
- ◆ **BI-007** see Paclitaxel (Protein Bound) on page 1146
- ◆ **Biaxin®** see Clarithromycin on page 342
- ◆ **Biaxin® XL** see Clarithromycin on page 342

Bicalutamide (bye ka LOO ta mide)

U.S. Brand Names Casodex®

Synonyms CDX; ICI-176334

Generic Available No

Pharmacologic Category Antineoplastic Agent, Antiandrogen

Use In combination therapy with LHRH agonist analogues in treatment of advanced prostatic carcinoma

Mechanism of Action/Effect Nonsteroidal antiandrogen that inhibits androgen uptake or inhibits binding of androgen in target tissues

Contraindications Hypersensitivity to bicalutamide or any component of the formulation; pregnancy

Warnings/Precautions Rare cases of death or hospitalization due to hepatitis have been reported postmarketing. Use with caution in moderate to severe hepatic dysfunction. Hepatotoxicity generally occurs within the first 3-4 months of use. Baseline liver function tests should be obtained and repeated regularly during the first 4 months of treatment, and periodically thereafter. Additionally, patients should be monitored for signs and symptoms of liver dysfunction. Bicalutamide should be discontinued if patients have jaundice or ALT is two times the upper limit of normal. May cause gynecomastia in a high percentage of patients.

Drug Interactions

Increased Effect/Toxicity: Bicalutamide may displace warfarin from protein binding sites which may result in an increased anticoagulant effect, especially when bicalutamide therapy is started after the patient is already on warfarin.

Adverse Reactions

10%: Endocrine & metabolic: Hot flashes (8% to 24% in combination with LHRH agonists), gynecomastia (23% to 62%), breast tenderness (25% to 60%)

≥2% to <5%:

Cardiovascular: Angina pectoris, CHF, edema

Central nervous system: Anxiety, depression, confusion, somnolence, nervousness, fever, chills

Dermatologic: Dry skin, pruritus, alopecia

Endocrine & metabolic: Breast pain, diabetes mellitus, decreased libido, dehydration, gout

(Continued)

Bicalutamide *(Continued)*

Gastrointestinal: Anorexia, dyspepsia, rectal hemorrhage, xerostomia, melena, weight gain
Genitourinary: Polyuria, urinary impairment, dysuria, urinary retention, urinary urgency
Hepatic: Alkaline phosphatase increased
Neuromuscular & skeletal: Myasthenia, arthritis, myalgia, leg cramps, pathological fracture, neck pain, hypertonia, neuropathy
Renal: Creatinine increased
Respiratory: Cough increased, pharyngitis, bronchitis, pneumonia, rhinitis, lung disorder
Miscellaneous: Sepsis, neoplasma

Overdosage/Toxicology Symptoms of overdose include hypoactivity, ataxia, anorexia, vomiting, slow respiration, and lacrimation. Management is supportive. Dialysis is of no benefit.

Pharmacodynamics/Kinetics
Absorption: Rapid and complete
Protein Binding: 96%
Half-Life Elimination: Up to 10 days; active enantiomer 5.8 days
Metabolism: Extensively hepatic; stereospecific metabolism
Excretion: Urine and feces (as unchanged drug and metabolites)

Dosing
Adults & Elderly: Advanced prostatic carcinoma: Oral: 50-150 mg/day
Hepatic Impairment: Limited data in subjects with severe hepatic impairment suggest that excretion of bicalutamide may be delayed and could lead to further accumulation. Use with caution in patients with moderate to severe hepatic impairment.

Available Dosage Forms Tablet: 50 mg

Monitoring and Teaching Issues
Physical Assessment: See Warnings/Precautions and Drug Interactions for use cautions (hepatic or renal impairment, use of warfarin). Assess results of laboratory tests at baseline and periodically during therapy (see Monitoring Laboratory Tests). Assess patient response (therapeutic effectiveness and adverse effects; see Adverse Reactions). Advise patients with diabetes to monitor glucose levels closely (may induce hyperglycemia). Teach patient appropriate use, possible side effects/appropriate interventions, and adverse symptoms to report. **Pregnancy risk factor X:** Instruct patient on absolute need for contraceptives. Note breast-feeding caution.

Monitoring Laboratory Tests: Liver function tests should be obtained at baseline and repeated regularly during the first 4 months of treatment, and periodically thereafter (in addition to monitoring signs/symptoms of liver dysfunction). Discontinue if jaundice is noted or ALT is two or more times the upper limit of normal. CBC, ECG, echocardiograms, and serum testosterone and luteinizing hormone (periodically).

Patient Education: Do not take any new medication during therapy unless approved by prescriber. Take as directed, at the same time each day, with or without food. Do not alter dose or discontinue without consulting prescriber. Void before taking medication. If you have diabetes, monitor serum glucose closely and notify prescriber of changes (this medication may alter glucose levels). May cause dizziness, confusion, or drowsiness (use caution when driving or engaging in tasks that require alertness until response to drug is known); nausea or vomiting (small frequent meals, frequent mouth care, sucking lozenges, or chewing gum may help); constipation (increased exercise, fluids, fruit, or fiber may help); hair loss; or impotence. Report easy bruising or bleeding; yellowing of skin or eyes; change in color of urine or stool; unresolved CNS changes (eg, nervousness, chills, insomnia, somnolence); skin rash, redness, or irritation; chest pain or palpitations; respiratory difficulty; urinary retention or inability to void; muscle weakness, tremors, or pain; persistent nausea, vomiting, diarrhea, constipation; or other unusual signs or adverse reactions. **Pregnancy/breast-feeding precautions:** This drug will cause fetal abnormalities; consult prescriber for effective contraceptives.

Dietary Considerations: May be taken with or without food.

Geriatric Considerations: Renal impairment has no clinically significant changes in elimination of the parent compound or active metabolite; therefore, no dosage adjustment is needed in the elderly. In dosage studies, no difference was found between young adults and elderly with regard to steady-state serum concentrations for bicalutamide and its active R-enantiomer metabolite.

Pregnancy Risk Factor: X
Lactation: Excretion in breast milk unknown

Administration
Oral: Dose should be taken at the same time each day with or without food.
Storage: Store at room temperature.

♦ **Bicillin® L-A** *see* Penicillin G Benzathine *on page 1172*
♦ **Bicitra®** *see* Sodium Citrate and Citric Acid *on page 1382*
♦ **BiCNu®** *see* Carmustine *on page 260*

Bimatoprost *(bi MAT oh prost)*
U.S. Brand Names Lumigan®
Generic Available No
Pharmacologic Category Ophthalmic Agent, Miscellaneous
Use Reduction of intraocular pressure (IOP) in patients with open-angle glaucoma or ocular hypertension; should be used in patients who are intolerant of other IOP-lowering medications or failed treatment with another IOP-lowering medication
Mechanism of Action/Effect Decreases intraocular pressure by increasing outflow of aqueous humor
Contraindications Hypersensitivity to bimatoprost or any component of the formulation
Warnings/Precautions May cause permanent changes in eye color (increases the amount of brown pigment in the iris), the eyelid skin, and eyelashes. In addition, may increase the length and/or number of eyelashes (may vary between eyes). Use caution in patients with

intraocular inflammation, aphakic patients, pseudophakic patients with a torn posterior lens capsule, or patients with risk factors for macular edema. Contains benzalkonium chloride (may be adsorbed by contact lenses). Safety and efficacy have not been determined for use in patients with renal impairment, angle-closure-, inflammatory-, or neovascular glaucoma. Safety and efficacy in pediatric patients have not been established.

Adverse Reactions
>10%: Ocular (15% to 45%): Conjunctival hyperemia, growth of eyelashes, ocular pruritus
1% to 10%:
Central nervous system: Headache (1% to 5%)
Dermatologic: Hirsutism (1% to 5%)
Hepatic: Abnormal liver function tests (1% to 5%)
Neuromuscular & skeletal: Weakness (1% to 5%)
Ocular:
3% to 10%: Blepharitis, burning, cataract, dryness, eyelid redness, eyelash darkening, foreign body sensation, irritation, pain, pigmentation of periocular skin, superficial punctate keratitis, visual disturbance
1% to 3%: Allergic conjunctivitis, asthenopia, conjunctival edema, discharge, increased iris pigmentation, photophobia, tearing
Respiratory: Upper respiratory tract infection (10%)

Overdosage/Toxicology No information available; treatment is symptom-directed and supportive

Pharmacodynamics/Kinetics
Onset of Action: Reduction of IOP: ~4 hours; Peak effect: Maximum reduction of IOP: ~8-12 hours
Time to Peak: 10 minutes
Protein Binding: ~88%
Half-Life Elimination: I.V.: 45 minutes
Metabolism: Undergoes oxidation, N-demethylation, and glucuronidation after reaching systemic circulation; forms metabolites
Excretion: Urine (67%); feces (25%)

Dosing
Adults & Elderly: Open-angle glaucoma or ocular hypertension: Ophthalmic: Instill 1 drop into affected eye(s) once daily in the evening; do not exceed once-daily dosing (may decrease IOP-lowering effect). If used with other topical ophthalmic agents, separate administration by at least 5 minutes.

Available Dosage Forms Solution, ophthalmic: 0.03% (2.5 mL, 5 mL, 7.5 mL) [contains benzalkonium chloride]

Monitoring and Teaching Issues
Physical Assessment: Assess potential for interactions with other prescriptions, OTC medications, or herbal products patient may be taking. Assess therapeutic response and adverse effects. Teach patient proper use, side effects/appropriate interventions, and symptoms to report.
Patient Education: For use in eyes only. Wash hands before instilling. Sit or lie down to instill. Open eye, look at ceiling, and instill prescribed amount of solution. Apply gentle pressure to inner corner of eye. Do not let tip of applicator touch eye; do not contaminate tip of applicator (may cause eye infection, eye damage, or vision loss). Contact prescriber concerning continued use of drops if eye infection develops, trauma occurs to the eye, and prior to eye surgery. This product contains benzalkonium chloride which may be adsorbed by contact lenses; remove contacts prior to administration and wait 15 minutes before reinserting. May cause permanent changes in eye color (increases the amount of brown pigment in the iris), eyelid, and eyelashes. May also increase the length and/or number of eyelashes. Changes may occur slowly (months to years). May be used with other eye drops to lower intraocular pressure. If using more than one eye drop medicine, wait at least 5 minutes in between application of each medication. Notify prescriber if conjunctivitis or eyelid reactions occur with use of this product. **Pregnancy/breast-feeding precautions:** Inform prescriber if you are pregnant or breast-feeding.
Pregnancy Risk Factor: C
Lactation: Excretion in breast milk unknown/use caution

Administration
Other: May be used with other eye drops to lower intraocular pressure. If using more than one ophthalmic product, wait at least 5 minutes in between application of each medication. Remove contact lenses prior to administration and wait 15 minutes before reinserting.
Storage: Store between 2°C to 25°C (36°F to 77°F).
Additional Information The IOP-lowering effect was shown to be 7-8 mm Hg in clinical studies.

Related Information
Glaucoma Drug Therapy on page 1827

♦ **Biocef®** see Cephalexin on page 294
♦ **Biofed [OTC]** see Pseudoephedrine on page 1282
♦ **Bio-Statin®** see Nystatin on page 1103
♦ **BioThrax™** see page 1660
♦ **bis-chloronitrosourea** see Carmustine on page 260
♦ **Bismatrol** see Bismuth on page 197

Bismuth (BIZ muth)

U.S. Brand Names Children's Kaopectate® *(reformulation)* [OTC] [DSC]; Diotame® [OTC]; Kaopectate® [OTC]; Kaopectate® Extra Strength [OTC]; Kaopectolin *(new formulation)* [OTC]; Pepto-Bismol® [OTC]; Pepto-Bismol® Maximum Strength [OTC]
Synonyms Bismatrol; Bismuth Subgallate; Bismuth Subsalicylate; Pink Bismuth
Generic Available Yes
Pharmacologic Category Antidiarrheal
(Continued)

Bismuth *(Continued)*

Medication Safety Issues
Sound-alike/look-alike issues:
Kaopectate® may be confused with Kayexalate®

Use
Subsalicylate formulation: Symptomatic treatment of mild, nonspecific diarrhea; control of traveler's diarrhea (enterotoxigenic *Escherichia coli*); as part of a multidrug regimen for *H. pylori* eradication to reduce the risk of duodenal ulcer recurrence

Subgallate formulation: An aid to reduce fecal odors from a colostomy or ileostomy

Mechanism of Action/Effect Bismuth subsalicylate exhibits both antisecretory and antimicrobial action. This agent may provide some anti-inflammatory action as well. The salicylate moiety provides antisecretory effect and the bismuth exhibits antimicrobial directly against bacterial and viral gastrointestinal pathogens.

Contraindications Hypersensitivity to bismuth or any component of the formulation

Subsalicylate formulation: Do not use subsalicylate in patients with influenza or chickenpox because of risk of Reye's syndrome; hypersensitivity to salicylates or any component of the formulation; history of severe GI bleeding; history of coagulopathy; pregnancy (3rd trimester)

Warnings/Precautions Subsalicylate should be used with caution if patient is taking aspirin. Use with caution in children, especially those <3 years of age and those with viral illness. May be neurotoxic with very large doses.

When used for self-medication (OTC labeling): Children and teenagers who have or are recovering from chickenpox or flu-like symptoms should not use subsalicylate. Changes in behavior (along with nausea and vomiting) may be an early sign of Reye's syndrome; patients should be instructed to contact their healthcare provider if these occur. Patients should be instructed to contact healthcare provider for diarrhea lasting >2 days, hearing loss, or ringing in the ears. Not labeled for OTC use in children <12 years of age.

Drug Interactions
Decreased Effect: The effects of tetracyclines and uricosurics may be decreased.

Increased Effect/Toxicity: Toxicity of aspirin, warfarin, and/or hypoglycemics may be increased.

Lab Interactions Increased uric acid, AST; may interfere with radiologic tests since bismuth is radiopaque.

Adverse Reactions Frequency not defined; subsalicylate formulation:
Central nervous system: Anxiety, confusion, headache, mental depression, slurred speech
Gastrointestinal: Discoloration of the tongue (darkening), grayish black stools, impaction may occur in infants and debilitated patients
Neuromuscular & skeletal: Muscle spasms, weakness
Ocular: Hearing loss, tinnitus

Overdosage/Toxicology
Symptoms of toxicity:
Subsalicylate: Hyperpnea, nausea, vomiting, tinnitus, hyperpyrexia, metabolic acidoses/respiratory alkalosis, tachycardia, and confusion; seizures in severe overdose, pulmonary or cerebral edema, respiratory failure, cardiovascular collapse, coma, and death. **Note:** Each 262.4 mg tablet of bismuth subsalicylate contains an equivalent of 130 mg aspirin (150 mg/kg of aspirin is considered to be toxic; serious life-threatening toxicity occurs with >300mg/kg)

Bismuth: Rare with short-term administrations of bismuth salts; encephalopathy, methemoglobinemia, seizures

Treatment: Gastrointestinal decontamination (activated charcoal for immediate release formulations (10 x dose of ASA in g), whole bowel irrigation for enteric coated tablets or when serially increasing ASA plasma levels indicate the presence of an intestinal bezoar), supportive and symptomatic treatment with emphasis on correcting fluid, electrolyte, blood glucose and acid-base disturbances; elimination is enhanced with urinary alkalinization (sodium bicarbonate infusion with potassium), multiple dose activated charcoal, and hemodialysis. Chelation with dimercaprol in doses of 3 mg/kg or penicillamine 100 mg/kg/day for 5 days can hasten recovery from bismuth-induced encephalopathy; methylene blue 1-2 mg/kg in a 1% sterile aqueous solution I.V. push over 4-6 minutes for methemoglobinemia. This may be repeated within 60 minutes if necessary, up to a total dose of 7 mg/kg. Seizures usually respond to I.V. diazepam.

Pharmacodynamics/Kinetics
Absorption: Bismuth: <1%; Subsalicylate: >90%

Half-Life Elimination: Terminal: Bismuth: Highly variable

Metabolism: Bismuth subsalicylate is converted to salicylic acid and insoluble bismuth salts in the GI tract.

Excretion: Bismuth: Urine and feces; Salicylate: Urine

Dosing
Adults & Elderly:
Treatment of nonspecific diarrhea, control/relieve traveler's diarrhea: Oral: Subsalicylate (doses based on 262 mg/15 mL liquid or 262 mg tablets): 2 tablets or 30 mL every 30 minutes to 1 hour as needed up to 8 doses/24 hours

Helicobacter pylori **eradication:** Oral: 524 mg 4 times/day with meals and at bedtime; requires combination therapy

Control of fecal odor in ileostomy or colostomy: Oral: Subgallate: 200-400 mg up to 4 times/day

Pediatrics:
Nonspecific diarrhea: Subsalicylate (doses based on 262 mg/5 mL liquid or 262 mg tablet): Oral:
Children: Up to 8 doses/24 hours:
3-6 years: 1/3 tablet or 5 mL every 30 minutes to 1 hour as needed
6-9 years: 2/3 tablet or 10 mL every 30 minutes to 1 hour as needed
9-12 years: 1 tablet or 15 mL every 30 minutes to 1 hour as needed

Renal Impairment: Should probably be avoided in patients with renal impairment.

Available Dosage Forms [DSC] = Discontinued product

Caplet, as subsalicylate (Pepto-Bismol®): 262 mg [sugar free; contains sodium 2 mg]

Liquid, as subsalicylate: 262 mg/15 mL (240 mL, 360 mL, 480 mL); 525 mg/15 mL (240 mL, 360 mL)

Children's Kaopectate®: 87 mg/5 mL (180 mL) [contains sodium 3.3 mg/5 mL; cherry flavor] [DSC]

Diotame®: 262 mg/15 mL (30 mL)

Kaopectate®: 262 mg/15 mL (180 mL, 240 mL, 360 mL) [contains sodium 10 mg/15 mL; regular and peppermint flavor]

Kaopectate® Extra Strength: 525 mg/15 mL (240 mL) [contains sodium 11 mg/15 mL; peppermint flavor]

Pepto-Bismol®: 262 mg/15 mL (120 mL, 240 mL, 360 mL, 480 mL) [sugar free; contains sodium 6 mg/15 mL and benzoic acid; wintergreen flavor]

Pepto-Bismol® Maximum Strength: 525 mg/15 mL (120 mL, 240 mL, 360 mL) [sugar free; contains sodium 6 mg/15 mL and benzoic acid; wintergreen flavor]

Suspension (Kaopectolin): 262 mg/15 mL (480 mL)

Tablet, as subgallate: 200 mg

Tablet, chewable, as subsalicylate: 262 mg

Diotame®: 262 mg

Pepto-Bismol®: 262 mg [sugar free; contains sodium <1 mg; cherry flavor]

Monitoring and Teaching Issues

Physical Assessment: See Contraindications and Warnings/Precautions for use cautions (eg, history of GI bleed or coagulopathy, risk of Reye's syndrome). Assess potential for interactions with other pharmacological agents patient may be taking (eg, aspirin products; see Drug Interactions). Assess therapeutic effectiveness (reduction in diarrhea) and adverse response (eg, CNS changes, impactions, tinnitus; see Adverse Reactions). Teach patient appropriate use, possible side effects/appropriate interventions, and adverse symptoms to report.

Patient Education: Do not take any new medication during therapy unless approved by prescriber. Chew tablet well or shake suspension well before using. Maintain adequate fluid intake to prevent dehydration (2-3 L/day of fluids, unless instructed to restrict fluid intake). May darken stools and turn tongue black. If diarrhea persists for more than 2 days, consult healthcare provider. If tinnitus (ringing in the ears) occurs this may indicate toxicity; discontinue use and notify healthcare provider. **Pregnancy/breast-feeding precautions:** Inform prescriber if you are or intend to become pregnant or breast-feed.

Dietary Considerations: Drink plenty of fluids to help prevent dehydration caused by diarrhea. Different dosage forms contain variable amounts of sodium; consult individual product labeling.

Pregnancy Risk Factor: C/D (3rd trimester)

Lactation: Excretion in breast milk unknown (salicylates enter breast milk)/use caution

Administration

Oral: Subsalicylate tablets should be taken at least 3 hours apart from other medications.

Related Information

Helicobacter pylori Treatment *on page 1835*

♦ **Bismuth Subgallate** *see* Bismuth *on page 197*

♦ **Bismuth Subsalicylate** *see* Bismuth *on page 197*

Bismuth Subsalicylate, Metronidazole, and Tetracycline

(BIZ muth sub sa LIS i late, me troe NI da zole, & tet ra SYE kleen)

U.S. Brand Names Helidac®

Synonyms Bismuth Subsalicylate, Tetracycline, and Metronidazole; Metronidazole, Bismuth Subsalicylate, and Tetracycline; Metronidazole, Tetracycline, and Bismuth Subsalicylate; Tetracycline, Bismuth Subsalicylate, and Metronidazole; Tetracycline, Metronidazole, and Bismuth Subsalicylate

Generic Available No

Pharmacologic Category Antibiotic, Tetracycline Derivative; Antidiarrheal

Use In combination with an H_2 antagonist, as part of a multidrug regimen for *H. pylori* eradication to reduce the risk of duodenal ulcer recurrence

Dosing

Adults & Elderly: Duodenal ulcer associated with *H. pylori* infection: Oral: Chew 2 bismuth subsalicylate 262.4 mg tablets, swallow 1 metronidazole 250 mg tablet, and swallow 1 tetracycline 500 mg capsule plus an H_2 antagonist 4 times/day at meals and bedtime for 14 days; follow with 8 oz of water.

Available Dosage Forms Combination package [each package contains 14 blister cards (2-week supply); each card contains the following]:

Capsule: Tetracycline hydrochloride: 500 mg (4)

Tablet: Bismuth subsalicylate [chewable]: 262.4 mg (8)

Tablet: Metronidazole: 250 mg (4)

Monitoring and Teaching Issues

Physical Assessment: See individual agents.

Patient Education: See individual agents. **Pregnancy/breast-feeding precautions:** Inform prescriber if you are or intend to become pregnant. Do not breast-feed.

Pregnancy Risk Factor: D (tetracycline); B (metronidazole)

Lactation: Enters breast milk/contraindicated

Related Information

Bismuth *on page 197*

Metronidazole *on page 995*

Tetracycline *on page 1452*

♦ **Bismuth Subsalicylate, Tetracycline, and Metronidazole** *see* Bismuth Subsalicylate, Metronidazole, and Tetracycline *on page 199*

Bisoprolol (bis OH proe lol)

U.S. Brand Names Zebeta®

Synonyms Bisoprolol Fumarate

Generic Available Yes

Pharmacologic Category Beta Blocker, Beta₁ Selective

Medication Safety Issues
  Sound-alike/look-alike issues:
    Zebeta® may be confused with DiaBeta®

Use Treatment of hypertension, alone or in combination with other agents

Unlabeled/Investigational Use Angina pectoris, supraventricular arrhythmias, PVCs

Mechanism of Action/Effect Selective inhibitor of beta₁-adrenergic receptors; little or no effect on beta₂-receptors at doses <10 mg

Contraindications Hypersensitivity to bisoprolol or any component of the formulation; sinus bradycardia; heart block greater than first-degree (except in patients with a functioning artificial pacemaker); cardiogenic shock; uncompensated cardiac failure; pulmonary edema; pregnancy (2nd and 3rd trimesters)

Warnings/Precautions Administer cautiously in compensated heart failure and monitor for a worsening of the condition. Beta-blocker therapy should not be withdrawn abruptly (particularly in patients with CAD), but gradually tapered to avoid acute tachycardia, hypertension, and/or ischemia. Use caution in patients with PVD (can aggravate arterial insufficiency). Use caution with concurrent use of beta-blockers and either verapamil or diltiazem; bradycardia or heart block can occur. In general, beta-blockers should be avoided in patients with bronchospastic disease. Bisoprolol, with B1 selectivity, has been used cautiously in bronchospastic disease with close monitoring. Use cautiously in patients with diabetes because it can mask prominent hypoglycemic symptoms. Can mask signs of thyrotoxicosis. Can cause fetal harm when administered in pregnancy. Dosage adjustment is required in patients with significant hepatic or renal dysfunction. Use care with anesthetic agents which decrease myocardial function.

Drug Interactions

  Cytochrome P450 Effect: Substrate of CYP2D6 (minor), 3A4 (major)

  Decreased Effect: Decreased effect of bisoprolol with aluminum salts, calcium salts, cholestyramine, colestipol, NSAIDs, penicillins (ampicillin), and salicylates due to decreased bioavailability and plasma levels. The effect of sulfonylureas may be decreased by beta-blockers. CYP3A4 inducers may decrease the levels/effects of bisoprolol; example inducers include aminoglutethimide, carbamazepine, nafcillin, nevirapine, phenobarbital, phenytoin, and rifamycins.

  Increased Effect/Toxicity: Bisoprolol may increase the effects of other drugs which slow AV conduction (digoxin, verapamil, diltiazem), alpha-blockers (prazosin, terazosin), and alpha-adrenergic stimulants (epinephrine, phenylephrine). Bisoprolol may mask the tachycardia from hypoglycemia caused by insulin and oral hypoglycemics. In patients receiving concurrent therapy, the risk of hypertensive crisis is increased when either clonidine or the beta-blocker is withdrawn. Reserpine has been shown to enhance the effect of beta-blockers. Beta-blockers may increase the action or levels of ethanol, disopyramide, nondepolarizing muscle relaxants, and theophylline although the effects are difficult to predict. CYP3A4 inhibitors may increase the levels/effects of bisoprolol; example inhibitors include azole antifungals, ciprofloxacin, clarithromycin, diclofenac, doxycycline, erythromycin, imatinib, isoniazid, nefazodone, nicardipine, propofol, protease inhibitors, quinidine, and verapamil.

Nutritional/Ethanol Interactions Herb/Nutraceutical: Avoid dong quai if using for hypertension (has estrogenic activity). Avoid ephedra, yohimbe, ginseng (may worsen hypertension). Avoid garlic (may have increased antihypertensive effect).

Lab Interactions Increased thyroxine (S), cholesterol (S), glucose, triglycerides, uric acid; decreased HDL; possible false glucose tolerance tests

Adverse Reactions

  >10%:
    Central nervous system: Drowsiness, insomnia
    Endocrine & metabolic: Decreased sexual ability

  1% to 10%:
    Cardiovascular: Bradycardia, palpitation, edema, CHF, reduced peripheral circulation
    Central nervous system: Mental depression
    Gastrointestinal: Diarrhea or constipation, nausea, vomiting, stomach discomfort
    Ocular: Mild ocular stinging and discomfort, tearing, photophobia, decreased corneal sensitivity, keratitis
    Respiratory: Bronchospasm
    Miscellaneous: Cold extremities

Overdosage/Toxicology Symptoms of overdose include severe hypotension, bradycardia, heart failure, bronchospasm, and hypoglycemia. Treat initially with I.V. fluids. Sympathomimetics (eg, epinephrine or dopamine), glucagon, or a pacemaker can be used to treat the toxic bradycardia, asystole, and/or hypotension. Bisoprolol may be removed by hemodialysis. Other treatment is symptomatic and supportive.

Pharmacodynamics/Kinetics

  Onset of Action: 1-2 hours

  Absorption: Rapid and almost complete

  Time to Peak: 1.7-3 hours

  Protein Binding: 26% to 33%

  Half-Life Elimination: 9-12 hours

  Metabolism: Extensively hepatic; significant first-pass effect

  Excretion: Urine (3% to 10% as unchanged drug); feces (<2%)

Dosing

  Adults: Hypertension: Oral: 2.5-5 mg once daily, may be increased to 10 mg, and then up to 20 mg once daily, if necessary; usual dose range (JNC 7): 2.5-10 mg once daily

Elderly: Oral: Initial: 2.5 mg/day; may be increased by 2.5-5 mg/day; maximum recommended dose: 20 mg/day

Renal Impairment: Oral: Initial: 2.5 mg/day; increase cautiously.
Not dialyzable

Available Dosage Forms Tablet, as fumarate: 5 mg, 10 mg

Monitoring and Teaching Issues

Physical Assessment: Assess potential for interactions with other prescriptions, OTC medications, or herbal products patient may be taking. Blood pressure and heart rate should be assessed prior to and following first dose and with any change in dosage. Assess for therapeutic effectiveness and adverse effects. Instruct patients with diabetes to monitor glucose levels closely (beta-blockers may alter glucose tolerance). Teach patient proper use, possible side effects/appropriate interventions (hypotension precautions), and adverse symptoms to report.

Monitoring Laboratory Tests: Serum glucose regularly (if diabetic)

Patient Education: Do not take any new medication during therapy unless approved by prescriber. Take exactly as directed, with or without regard to meals. Do not take with antacids. Do not adjust dosage or discontinue without consulting prescriber. Take pulse daily (prior to medication) and follow prescriber's instruction about holding medication. If you have diabetes, monitor serum sugar closely (drug may alter glucose tolerance or mask signs of hypoglycemia). May cause fatigue, dizziness, or postural hypotension (use caution when changing position from lying or sitting to standing, when driving, or climbing stairs until response to medication is known); alteration in sexual performance (reversible); or constipation (increased dietary bulk and fluids and exercise may help). Report unresolved swelling of extremities, respiratory difficulty or new cough, unresolved fatigue, unusual weight gain, unresolved constipation, or unusual muscle weakness. **Pregnancy/breast-feeding precautions:** Inform prescriber if you are or intend to become pregnant. Consult prescriber if breast-feeding.

Dietary Considerations: May be taken without regard to meals.

Geriatric Considerations: Due to alterations in the beta-adrenergic autonomic nervous system, beta-adrenergic blockade may result in less hemodynamic response than seen in younger adults.

Pregnancy Risk Factor: C (manufacturer); D (2nd and 3rd trimesters - expert analysis)

Pregnancy Issues: No data available on whether bisoprolol crosses the placenta. Beta-blockers have been associated with persistent bradycardia, hypotension, and IUGR; IUGR is probably related to maternal hypertension. Available evidence suggests beta-blockers are generally safe during pregnancy (JNC 7). Cases of neonatal hypoglycemia have been reported following maternal use of beta-blockers at parturition or during breast-feeding. Monitor breast-fed infant for symptoms of beta-blockade.

Lactation: Enters breast milk/use caution

Related Information
Beta-Blockers *on page 1720*
Heart Failure *on page 1828*

Bisoprolol and Hydrochlorothiazide
(bis OH proe lol & hye droe klor oh THYE a zide)

U.S. Brand Names Ziac®

Synonyms Hydrochlorothiazide and Bisoprolol

Generic Available Yes

Pharmacologic Category Antihypertensive Agent, Combination

Medication Safety Issues
Sound-alike/look-alike issues:
Ziac® may be confused with Tiazac®, Zerit®

Use Treatment of hypertension

Dosing

Adults & Elderly: Hypertension: Oral: Dose is individualized, given once daily.

Hepatic Impairment: Caution should be used in dosing/titrating patients.

Available Dosage Forms
Tablet:
2.5/6.25: Bisoprolol fumarate 2.5 mg and hydrochlorothiazide 6.25 mg
5/6.25: Bisoprolol fumarate 5 mg and hydrochlorothiazide 6.25 mg
10/6.25: Bisoprolol fumarate 10 mg and hydrochlorothiazide 6.25 mg

Monitoring and Teaching Issues

Physical Assessment: See individual agents.

Patient Education: See individual agents. **Pregnancy/breast-feeding precautions:** Inform prescriber if you are or intend to become pregnant. Consult prescriber if breast-feeding.

Pregnancy Risk Factor: C/D (2nd and 3rd trimesters)

Lactation: Enters breast milk/use caution

Related Information
Bisoprolol *on page 200*
Hydrochlorothiazide *on page 751*

♦ **Bisoprolol Fumarate** *see Bisoprolol on page 200*

♦ **Blenoxane®** *see Bleomycin on page 201*

♦ **Bleo** *see Bleomycin on page 201*

Bleomycin (blee oh MYE sin)

U.S. Brand Names Blenoxane®

Synonyms Bleo; Bleomycin Sulfate; BLM; NSC-125066

Generic Available Yes

Pharmacologic Category Antineoplastic Agent, Antibiotic
(Continued)

Bleomycin *(Continued)*

Medication Safety Issues

Sound-alike/look-alike issues:

Bleomycin may be confused with Cleocin®

Use Treatment of squamous cell carcinomas, melanomas, sarcomas, testicular carcinoma, Hodgkin's lymphoma, and non-Hodgkin's lymphoma

Orphan drug: Sclerosing agent for malignant pleural effusion

Mechanism of Action/Effect Inhibits synthesis of DNA

Contraindications Hypersensitivity to bleomycin sulfate or any component of the formulation; severe pulmonary disease; pregnancy

Warnings/Precautions The U.S. Food and Drug Administration (FDA) currently recommends that procedures for proper handling and disposal of antineoplastic agents be considered. Occurrence of pulmonary fibrosis is higher in elderly patients and in those receiving >400 units total and in smokers and patients with prior radiation therapy. A severe idiosyncratic reaction consisting of hypotension, mental confusion, fever, chills, and wheezing is possible. Check lungs prior to each treatment for fine rales (crackles), which may be the first symptom of pulmonary toxicity.

Drug Interactions

Decreased Effect: Bleomycin may decrease plasma levels of digoxin. Concomitant therapy with phenytoin results in decreased phenytoin levels.

Increased Effect/Toxicity: Lomustine increases severity of leukopenia. Cisplatin may decrease bleomycin elimination.

Adverse Reactions

>10%:

Cardiovascular: Raynaud's phenomenon

Dermatologic: Pain at the tumor site, phlebitis. About 50% of patients develop erythema, induration, hyperkeratosis, and peeling of the skin, particularly on the palmar and plantar surfaces of the hands and feet. Hyperpigmentation (50%), alopecia, nailbed changes may also occur. These effects appear dose related and reversible with discontinuation of the drug.

Gastrointestinal: Stomatitis and mucositis (30%), anorexia, weight loss

Respiratory: Tachypnea, rales, acute or chronic interstitial pneumonitis and pulmonary fibrosis (5% to 10%), hypoxia and death (1%). Symptoms include cough, dyspnea, and bilateral pulmonary infiltrates. The pathogenesis is not certain, but may be due to damage of pulmonary, vascular, or connective tissue. Response to steroid therapy is variable and somewhat controversial.

Miscellaneous: Acute febrile reactions (25% to 50%); anaphylactoid reactions characterized by hypotension, confusion, fever, chills, and wheezing. Onset may be immediate or delayed for several hours.

1% to 10%:

Dermatologic: Rash (8%), skin thickening, diffuse scleroderma, onycholysis

Miscellaneous: Acute anaphylactoid reactions

Overdosage/Toxicology Symptoms of overdose include chills, fever, pulmonary fibrosis, and hyperpigmentation. Treatment is supportive.

Pharmacodynamics/Kinetics

Absorption: I.M. and intrapleural administration: 30% to 50% of I.V. serum concentrations; intraperitoneal and SubQ routes produce serum concentrations equal to those of I.V.

Time to Peak: Serum: I.M.: Within 30 minutes

Protein Binding: 1%

Half-Life Elimination: Biphasic: Renal function dependent:

Normal renal function: Initial: 1.3 hours; Terminal: 9 hours

End-stage renal disease: Initial: 2 hours; Terminal: 30 hours

Metabolism: Via several tissues including hepatic, GI tract, skin, pulmonary, renal, and serum

Excretion: Urine (50% to 70% as active drug)

Dosing

Adults & Elderly: Refer to individual protocols; 1 unit = 1 mg; may be administered I.M., I.V., SubQ, or intracavitary.

Test dose for lymphoma patient: I.M., I.V., SubQ: 1-5 units of bleomycin before the first dose; monitor vital signs every 15 minutes; wait a minimum of 1 hour before administering remainder of dose.

Single agent therapy:

I.M./I.V./SubQ: Squamous cell carcinoma, lymphosarcoma, reticulum cell sarcoma, testicular carcinoma: 0.25-0.5 units/kg (10-20 units/m^2) 1-2 times/week

Continuous intravenous infusion: 15 units/m^2 over 24 hours/day for 4 days

Combination agent therapy:

I.M./I.V.: 3-4 units/m^2

I.V.: ABVD: 10 units/m^2 on days 1 and 15

Maximum cumulative lifetime dose: 400 units

Pleural sclerosing: Intracavitary: 60-240 units as a single infusion. Dose may be repeated at intervals of several days if fluid continues to accumulate (mix in 50-100 mL of D$_5$W, NS, or SWFI); may add lidocaine 100-200 mg to reduce local discomfort.

Pediatrics: Refer to adult dosing.

Renal Impairment:

Cl$_{cr}$ 10-50 mL/minute: Administer 75% of normal dose.

Cl$_{cr}$ <10 mL/minute: Administer 50% of normal dose.

Available Dosage Forms Injection, powder for reconstitution, as sulfate: 15 units, 30 units

Monitoring and Teaching Issues

Physical Assessment: Assess pulmonary and pregnancy status prior to beginning therapy (see Contraindications and Warnings/Precautions). Assess potential for interactions with other pharmacological agents patient may be taking (see Drug Interactions). Lungs should be checked prior to each treatment for fine rales (may be the first symptom of pulmonary toxicity) and prescriber notified of any changes. Lymphoma patients should be closely monitored for one hour following test dose before remainder of dose is administered. Infusion or injection site must be monitored closely to avoid extravasation. Assess results of laboratory tests (pulmonary, renal, and hepatic function; see Monitoring Laboratory Tests). Monitor patient response (therapeutic effectiveness and adverse effects; see Adverse Reactions). Teach patient possible side effects/appropriate interventions and adverse symptoms to report.

Monitoring Laboratory Tests: Pulmonary function (total lung volume, forced vital capacity, carbon monoxide diffusion), renal function, chest x-ray, liver function

Patient Education: Do not take any new medications during treatment unless approved by prescriber. This medication can only be administered by injection or infusion; report immediately any redness, burning, pain, or swelling at injection/infusion site. May cause loss of appetite, nausea, or vomiting (small frequent meals, sucking lozenges, or chewing gum may help); mouth sores (frequent mouth care with soft swabs and mouth rinses may help); fever or chills (will usually resolve); redness, peeling, or increased color of skin; or loss of hair (reversible after cessation of therapy). Report any change in respiratory status; respiratory difficulty; wheezing; air hunger; increased secretions; difficulty expectorating secretions; confusion; unresolved fever or chills; sores in mouth; vaginal itching, burning, or discharge; sudden onset of dizziness; acute headache; or burning, stinging, redness, or swelling at injection site. **Pregnancy/breast-feeding precautions:** Inform prescriber if you are pregnant. Do not get pregnant during or for 1 month following therapy. Consult prescriber for instruction on appropriate contraceptives. This drug may cause severe fetal defects. Breast-feeding is not recommended.

Geriatric Considerations: Pulmonary toxicity has been reported more frequently in geriatric patients (>70 years of age).

Pregnancy Risk Factor: D

Lactation: Excretion in breast milk unknown/not recommended

Administration

I.M.: May cause pain at injection site.

I.V.: May be an irritant. I.V. doses should be administered slowly (manufacturer recommends giving over a period of 10 minutes).

Other: SubQ: May cause pain at injection site.

Reconstitution: Reconstitute powder with 1-5 mL BWFI or BNS which is stable at room temperature or under refrigeration for 28 days.

Standard I.V. dilution: Dose/50-1000 mL NS or D_5W
Stable for 96 hours at room temperature and 14 days under refrigeration.

Compatibility: Stable in NS

Compatibility when admixed: Incompatible with aminophylline, ascorbic acid injection, cefazolin, diazepam, hydrocortisone sodium succinate, methotrexate, mitomycin, nafcillin, penicillin G sodium, terbutaline

Storage: Refrigerate intact vials of powder; intact vials are stable for up to one month at 45°C

♦ **Bleomycin Sulfate** see Bleomycin on page 201

♦ **Bleph®-10** see Sulfacetamide on page 1403

♦ **Blephamide®** see Sulfacetamide and Prednisolone on page 1404

♦ **BLM** see Bleomycin on page 201

♦ **Blocadren®** see Timolol on page 1478

♦ **BMS 337039** see Aripiprazole on page 137

♦ **Body Surface Area of Adults and Children** see page 1685

♦ **Bonine® [OTC]** see Meclizine on page 937

Bortezomib (bore TEZ oh mib)

U.S. Brand Names Velcade™

Synonyms LDP-341; MLN341; PS-341

Generic Available No

Pharmacologic Category Proteasome Inhibitor

Use Treatment of multiple myeloma in patients who have had at least one prior therapy

Mechanism of Action/Effect Reversibly inhibits enzyme complexes (proteosomes) which control intracellular protein homeostasis. Inhibition leads to cell death (apoptosis).

Contraindications Hypersensitivity to bortezomib, boron, mannitol, or any component of the formulation; pregnancy

Warnings/Precautions The U.S. Food and Drug Administration (FDA) currently recommends that procedures for proper handling and disposal of antineoplastic agents be considered. May cause peripheral neuropathy (usually sensory but may be mixed sensorimotor); risk may be increased with previous use of neurotoxic agents or pre-existing peripheral neuropathy; adjustment of dose and schedule may be required. May cause orthostatic/postural hypotension; use caution with dehydration, history of syncope or medications associated with hypotension. Has been associated with the development or exacerbation of congestive heart failure; use caution in patients with risk factors or existing heart disease. May cause tumor lysis syndrome; risk is increased in patients with large tumor burden prior to treatment. Hematologic toxicity with severe thrombocytopenia may occur; risk is increased in patients with pretreatment platelet counts <75,000 μL; frequent monitoring is required throughout treatment. Use caution with hepatic or renal impairment. Safety and efficacy have not been established in pediatric patients.

Drug Interactions

Cytochrome P450 Effect: Substrate of CYP1A2 (minor), 2C8/9 (minor), 2C19 (minor), 2D6 (minor), 3A4 (major); **Inhibits** CYP1A2 (weak), 2C8/9 (weak), 2C19 (moderate), 2D6 (weak), 3A4 (weak)

Decreased Effect: Levels/effects of bortezomib may be decreased by aminoglutethimide, carbamazepine, nafcillin, nevirapine, phenobarbital, phenytoin, rifamycins, and other CYP3A4 inducers.

(Continued)

Bortezomib *(Continued)*

Increased Effect/Toxicity: Bortezomib may increase the levels/effects citalopram, diazepam, methsuximide, phenytoin, propranolol, sertraline, and other CYP2C19 substrates. Levels/effects of bortezomib may be increased by azole antifungals, ciprofloxacin, clarithromycin, diclofenac, doxycycline, erythromycin, imatinib, isoniazid, nefazodone, nicardipine, propofol, protease inhibitors, quinidine, telithromycin, verapamil, and other CYP3A4 inhibitors.

Adverse Reactions

>10%:

Cardiovascular: Edema (25%), hypotension (12%)

Central nervous system: Pyrexia (36%), psychiatric disturbance (35%), headache (28%), insomnia (27%), dizziness (21%, excludes vertigo), anxiety (14%)

Dermatologic: Rash (21%), pruritus (11%)

Endocrine & metabolic: Dehydration (18%)

Gastrointestinal: Nausea (64%), diarrhea (51%), appetite decreased (43%), constipation (43%), vomiting (36%), abdominal pain (13%), abnormal taste (13%), dyspepsia (13%)

Hematologic: Thrombocytopenia (43%, Grade 3: 27%, Grade 4: 3%; Nadir: Day 11); anemia (32%, Grade 3: 9%); neutropenia (24%, Grade 3: 13%, Grade 4: 3%)

Neuromuscular & skeletal: Asthenic conditions (65%, Grade 3: 18% - includes fatigue, malaise, weakness); peripheral neuropathy (37%, Grade 3: 14%), arthralgia (26%); limb pain (26%); paresthesia and dysesthesia (23%); bone pain (16%); back pain (14%); muscle cramps (14%); myalgia (14%); rigors (12%)

Ocular: Blurred vision (11%)

Respiratory: Dyspnea (22%), upper respiratory tract infection (18%), cough (17%), lower respiratory infection (15%), nasopharyngitis (14%)

Miscellaneous: Herpes zoster (11%)

1% to 10%: Respiratory: Pneumonia (10%)

Overdosage/Toxicology In case of overdose, treatment should be symptom directed and supportive.

Pharmacodynamics/Kinetics

Protein Binding: ~83%

Half-Life Elimination: 9-15 hours

Metabolism: Hepatic via CYP 1A2, 2C9, 2C19, 2D6, 3A4; forms metabolites (inactive)

Dosing

Adults: Multiple myeloma: I.V.: 1.3 mg/m^2 twice weekly for 2 weeks on days 1, 4, 8, 11, followed by a 10-day rest period on days 12-21. Consecutive doses should be separated by at least 72 hours. One treatment cycle is equal to 21 days.

Dosage adjustment for toxicity:

Grade 3 nonhematological (excluding neuropathy) or Grade 4 hematological toxicity: Withhold until toxicity resolved; may reinitiate at a 25% reduced dose

Neuropathic pain and/or peripheral sensory neuropathy:

Grade 1 without pain or loss of function: No action needed

Grade 1 with pain or Grade 2 interfering with function but not activities of daily living: Reduce dose to 1 mg/m^2

Grade 2 with pain or Grade 3 interfering with activities of daily living: Withhold until toxicity resolved, may reinitiate at 0.7 mg/m^2 once weekly

Grade 4: Discontinue therapy

Renal Impairment: Specific guidelines are not available; studies did not include patients with Cl$_{cr}$ <13 mL/minute and patients on hemodialysis. Monitor closely for toxicity.

Hepatic Impairment: Specific guidelines are not available; clearance may be decreased; monitor closely for toxicity.

Available Dosage Forms Injection, powder for reconstitution [preservative free]: 3.5 mg [contains mannitol 35 mg]

Monitoring and Teaching Issues

Physical Assessment: Assess potential for interactions with other prescriptions, OTC medications, or herbal products patient may be taking. See Administration specifics. Assess results of laboratory tests, effectiveness of therapy, and adverse reactions on regular basis during therapy (eg, peripheral neuropathy, postural hypotension, dehydration, congestive heart failure). Teach patient possible side effects/appropriate interventions and adverse symptoms to report.

Monitoring Laboratory Tests: CBC

Patient Education: Do not take any new medication during therapy without consulting prescriber. This medication can only be administered intravenously; you will be monitored during and following infusion. Report immediately any chest pain, respiratory difficulty, itching, rash, acute headache, throat tightness, pain, redness, or swelling at infusion site. Maintain adequate hydration (2-3 L/day of fluids) unless instructed to restrict fluid intake. May cause headache, dizziness, anxiety, or fatigue (use caution when driving or engaging in hazardous tasks until response to drug is known); nausea, vomiting or abnormal taste (small frequent meals, frequent mouth care, chewing gum, or sucking lozenges may help). Report chest pain or shortness of breath, swelling in extremities, recent weight gain, persistent headache; muscle, bone, or back pain; cramping or loss of sensation; changes in vision; or other persistent adverse reactions. **Pregnancy/breast-feeding precautions:** Inform prescriber if you are pregnant. Do not get pregnant or cause a pregnancy (males) during therapy or for 1 month following therapy. Consult prescriber for instructions on appropriate nonhormonal contraceptive measures. This drug may cause fetal defects. Breast-feeding is not recommended.

Pregnancy Risk Factor: D

Pregnancy Issues: Adverse effects were observed in animal studies. Effective contraception is recommended for women of childbearing potential.

Lactation: Excretion in breast milk unknown/not recommended

Breast-Feeding Issues: Breast-feeding should be avoided.

Administration

I.V.: Administer via rapid I.V. push (3-5 seconds).

Reconstitution: Dilute each 3.5 mg vial with 3.5 mL NS.

Storage: Prior to reconstitution, store at controlled room temperature, 15°C to 30°C (59°F to 86°F). Protect from light. Once reconstituted, may be stored at room temperature for up to 8 hours in vial or 3 hours in syringe; solution should be administered within 8 hours

Additional Information Bortezomib was FDA approved under an accelerated approval program. Clinical trials have shown safety and efficacy as well as a decrease in tumor size. Studies addressing clinical benefit (including impact on survival) are ongoing.

♦ **B&O Supprettes®** *see Belladonna and Opium on page 177*

♦ **Bravelle™** *see Follitropins on page 670*

♦ **Brethaire [DSC]** *see Terbutaline on page 1445*

♦ **Brethine®** *see Terbutaline on page 1445*

Bretylium (bre TIL ee um)

Synonyms Bretylium Tosylate

Generic Available No

Pharmacologic Category Antiarrhythmic Agent, Class III

Medication Safety Issues

Sound-alike/look-alike issues:

Bretylium may be confused with Brevibloc®

Use Treatment of ventricular tachycardia and fibrillation; treatment of other serious ventricular arrhythmias resistant to lidocaine

Mechanism of Action/Effect Class III antiarrhythmic; after an initial release of norepinephrine at the peripheral adrenergic nerve terminals, bretylium inhibits further release by post-ganglionic nerve endings in response to sympathetic nerve stimulation

Contraindications Hypersensitivity to bretylium or any component of the formulation; severe aortic stenosis; severe pulmonary hypertension

Warnings/Precautions Use only in areas where there is equipment and staff familiar with management of life-threatening arrhythmias. Use continuous cardiac and blood pressure monitoring. Keep patients supine (postural hypotension common). Initially, may see transient hypertension and increased frequency of arrhythmias. Adjust dose in patients with impaired renal function. Give to a pregnant woman only if clearly needed. Rapid I.V. administration may cause nausea and vomiting, and a higher risk of orthostatic hypotension (particularly in elderly patients).

Drug Interactions

Increased Effect/Toxicity: Other antiarrhythmic agents may potentiate or antagonize cardiac effects of bretylium. Toxic effects may be additive. The vasopressor effects of catecholamines may be enhanced by bretylium. Toxicity of agents which may prolong QT interval (including cisapride, tricyclic antidepressants, antipsychotics, erythromycin, Class Ia and Class III antiarrhythmics) and specific quinolones (sparfloxacin, gatifloxacin, moxifloxacin) may be increased. Digoxin toxicity may be aggravated by bretylium.

Adverse Reactions

>10%: Cardiovascular: Hypotension (both postural and supine)

1% to 10%: Gastrointestinal: Nausea, vomiting

Overdosage/Toxicology Symptoms of overdose include significant hypertension followed by severe hypotension. Administration of a short-acting hypotensive agent should be used for the hypertensive response. Treatment is symptomatic and supportive. Dialysis is not useful.

Pharmacodynamics/Kinetics

Onset of Action: I.M.: May require 2 hours; I.V.: 6-20 minutes; Peak effect: 6-9 hours

Duration of Action: 6-24 hours

Protein Binding: 1% to 6%

Half-Life Elimination: 7-11 hours; Mean: 4-17 hours; End-stage renal disease: 16-32 hours

Metabolism: None

Excretion: Urine (70% to 80% as unchanged drug) within 24 hours

Dosing

Adults & Elderly: (Note: Patients should undergo defibrillation/cardioversion before and after bretylium doses as necessary.)

Immediate life-threatening ventricular arrhythmias, ventricular fibrillation, unstable ventricular tachycardia: I.V.: Initial: 5 mg/kg (undiluted) over 1 minute; if arrhythmia persists, give 10 mg/kg (undiluted) over 1 minute and repeat as necessary (usually at 15- to 30-minute intervals) up to a total dose of 30-35 mg/kg

Other life-threatening ventricular arrhythmias: I.M., I.V.:

Initial: 5-10 mg/kg, may repeat every 1-2 hours if arrhythmia persist; give I.V. dose (diluted) over 8-10 minutes

Maintenance dose: I.M.: 5-10 mg/kg every 6-8 hours; I.V. (diluted): 5-10 mg/kg every 6 hours; I.V. infusion (diluted): 1-2 mg/minute (little experience with doses >40 mg/kg/day)

Pediatrics: Note: Patients should undergo defibrillation/cardioversion before and after bretylium doses as necessary.

Arrhythmias:

Note: Not well established, although the following dosing has been suggested:

I.M.: Children: 2-5 mg/kg as a single dose

I.V.: Children: Acute ventricular fibrillation: Initial: 5 mg/kg, then attempt electrical defibrillation; repeat with 10 mg/kg if ventricular fibrillation persists at 15- to 30-minute intervals to maximum total of 30 mg/kg

Maintenance dose: I.M., I.V.: 5 mg/kg every 6 hours

(Continued)

Bretylium *(Continued)*

Renal Impairment:
Cl$_{cr}$ 10-50 mL/minute: Administer 25% to 50% of dose.
Cl$_{cr}$ <10 mL/minute: Administer 25% of dose.
Not dialyzable

Available Dosage Forms [DSC] = Discontinued product
Injection, solution, as tosylate: 50 mg/mL (10 mL) [DSC]
Injection, solution, as tosylate [premixed in D$_5$W]: 2 mg/mL (250 mL); 4 mg/mL (250 mL) [DSC]

Monitoring and Teaching Issues

Physical Assessment: Assess other medications patient may be taking for effectiveness and interactions. **I.V.:** Requires use of infusion pump and continuous cardiac and hemodynamic monitoring. Be alert for adverse cardiovascular reactions. Patient education/instruction is according to patient condition.

Patient Education: Emergency use: Patient education is determined by patient condition. You may experience nausea or vomiting (call for assistance if this occurs, do not try to get out of bed or change position on your own). Report chest pain, acute dizziness, or respiratory difficulty immediately. **Breast-feeding precaution:** Consult prescriber if breast-feeding.

Geriatric Considerations: Elderly are particularly at risk of orthostatic hypotension. See Warnings/Precautions and Adverse Reactions.

Pregnancy Risk Factor: C

Lactation: Excretion in breast milk unknown

Administration

I.M.: I.M. injection in adults should not exceed 5 mL volume in any one site.

I.V.: 2 g/250 mL D$_5$W (infusion pump should be used for I.V. infusion)
Bolus, emergency: Infuse rapidly (1 minute).
Bolus, nonemergency: May be given over 8-10 minutes.
Suggested rate of I.V. infusion: 1-4 mg/minute.
1 mg/minute = 7 mL/hour
2 mg/minute = 15 mL/hour
3 mg/minute = 22 mL/hour
4 mg/minute = 30 mL/hour

Reconstitution: Standard diluent: 2 g/250 mL D$_5$W

Compatibility: Stable in D$_5$LR, D$_5$½NS, D$_5$NS, D$_5$W, mannitol 20%, LR, sodium bicarbonate 5%, NS
Y-site administration: Incompatible with amphotericin B cholesteryl sulfate complex, propofol, warfarin
Compatibility when admixed: Incompatible with phenytoin

Storage: The premix infusion should be stored at room temperature and protected from freezing.

Related Information
Antiarrhythmic Drugs *on page 1708*

♦ **Bretylium Tosylate** *see Bretylium on page 205*
♦ **Brevibloc®** *see Esmolol on page 549*
♦ **Brevicon®** *see Ethinyl Estradiol and Norethindrone on page 589*
♦ **Bricanyl [DSC]** *see Terbutaline on page 1445*

Brimonidine *(bri MOE ni deen)*

U.S. Brand Names Alphagan® P

Synonyms Brimonidine Tartrate

Generic Available Yes

Pharmacologic Category Alpha$_2$ Agonist, Ophthalmic; Ophthalmic Agent, Antiglaucoma

Medication Safety Issues
Sound-alike/look-alike issues:
Brimonidine may be confused with bromocriptine

Use Lowering of intraocular pressure (IOP) in patients with open-angle glaucoma or ocular hypertension

Mechanism of Action/Effect Decreases IOP by reducing aqueous humor formation and increasing uveoscleral outflow

Contraindications Hypersensitivity to brimonidine tartrate or any component of the formulation; patients receiving MAO-inhibitor therapy

Warnings/Precautions Exercise caution in treating patients with severe cardiovascular disease. Use with caution in patients with depression, cerebral or coronary insufficiency, Raynaud's phenomenon, orthostatic hypotension or thromboangiitis obliterans. Use with caution in patients with hepatic or renal impairment. Safety and efficacy in children <2 years of age have not been established.

Alphagan® contains benzalkonium chloride which may be absorbed by contact lenses; remove contacts prior to administration and wait 15 minutes before reinserting. The IOP-lowering efficacy observed with brimonidine tartrate during the first of month of therapy may not always reflect the long term level of IOP reduction. Routinely monitor IOP.

Drug Interactions

Decreased Effect: Tricyclic antidepressants can affect the metabolism and uptake of circulating amines

Increased Effect/Toxicity: CNS depressants (eg, ethanol, barbiturates, opiates, sedatives, anesthetics) may have additive or potentiating effect; topical beta-blockers, pilocarpine may have additive decreased intraocular pressure; antihypertensives, cardiac glycosides may increase effects

Adverse Reactions
>10%:
Central nervous system: Headache, fatigue/drowsiness

Gastrointestinal: Xerostomia

Ocular: Ocular hyperemia, burning and stinging, blurring, foreign body sensation, conjunctival follicles, ocular allergic reactions and ocular pruritus

1% to 10%:

Central nervous system: Dizziness

Ocular: Corneal staining/erosion, photophobia, eyelid erythema, ocular ache/pain, ocular dryness, tearing, eyelid edema, conjunctival edema, blepharitis, ocular irritation, conjunctival blanching, abnormal vision, lid crusting, conjunctival hemorrhage, abnormal taste, conjunctival discharge

Respiratory: Upper respiratory symptoms

Pediatric use: Somnolence and lethargy were reported in up to 83% of patients 2-6 years of age. Children ≥7 years of age experienced somnolence less frequently (25%).

Alphagan® P:

>10%: Ocular: Allergic conjunctivitis, conjunctival hyperemia, eye pruritus

1% to 10%: (unless otherwise noted 1% to 4%)

Cardiovascular: Hypertension (5% to 9%)

Central nervous system: Dizziness, headache

Dermatologic: Rash

Gastrointestinal: Xerostomia (5% to 9%), dyspepsia

Ocular: Burning sensation (5% to 9%), conjunctival folliculosis (5% to 9%), visual disturbance (5% to 9%), blepharitis, conjunctival edema, conjunctival hemorrhage, conjunctivitis, eye discharge, irritation, eyelid edema, eyelid erythema, follicular conjunctivitis, foreign body sensation, pain, photophobia, stinging, superficial punctate keratopathy, visual field defect, vitreous floaters, watery eyes, worsened visual acuity

Respiratory: Bronchitis, cough, dyspnea, pharyngitis, rhinitis, sinus infection

Miscellaneous: Allergic reaction, flu-like syndrome

Overdosage/Toxicology No information is available on overdosage in humans. Treatment is supportive and symptomatic.

Pharmacodynamics/Kinetics

Onset of Action: Peak effect: 2 hours

Time to Peak: Plasma: Alphagan®: 1-4 hours; Alphagan® P: 0.5-2.5 hours

Half-Life Elimination: 2-3 hours

Metabolism: Hepatic

Excretion: Urine (74%)

Dosing

Adults & Elderly: Glaucoma: Ophthalmic (Alphagan®, Alphagan® P):Instill 1 drop in affected eye(s) 3 times/day (approximately every 8 hours)

Pediatrics: Children ≥2 years of age: Refer to adult dosing.

Available Dosage Forms

Solution, ophthalmic, as tartrate:

Alphagan® P: 0.15% (5 mL, 10 mL, 15 mL) [contains Purite® 0.005% as preservative]

Monitoring and Teaching Issues

Physical Assessment: Assess potential for interactions with other prescriptions, OTC medications, or herbal products patient may be taking. Monitor intraocular pressure periodically. Assess therapeutic response and adverse effects. Teach patient proper use, side effects/appropriate interventions, and symptoms to report.

Patient Education: For use in eyes only. Wash hands before instilling. Sit or lie down to instill. Open eye, look at ceiling, and instill prescribed amount of solution. Apply gentle pressure to inner corner of eye. Do not let tip of applicator touch eyes; do not contaminate tip of applicator (may cause eye infection, eye damage, or vision loss). Brimonidine tartrate may cause fatigue or drowsiness in some patients. Avoid engaging in hazardous activities due to potential for decreased mental alertness. Wait at least 15 minutes after instilling brimonidine tartrate before reinserting soft contact lenses. **Breast-feeding precaution:** Do not breast-feed.

Pregnancy Risk Factor: B

Lactation: Excretion in breast milk unknown/contraindicated

Administration

Other: Alphagan®: Remove contact lenses prior to administration; wait 15 minutes before reinserting

Storage: Store between 15°C to 25°C (59°F to 77°F)

Additional Information The use of Purite® as a preservative in Alphagan® P has lead to a reduced incidence of certain adverse effects associated with Alphagan®, which uses benzalkonium chloride as a preservative.

Related Information

Glaucoma Drug Therapy *on page 1827*

♦ **Brimonidine Tartrate** *see* Brimonidine *on page 206*

Brinzolamide (brin ZOH la mide)

U.S. Brand Names Azopt®

Generic Available No

Pharmacologic Category Carbonic Anhydrase Inhibitor; Ophthalmic Agent, Antiglaucoma

Use Lowers intraocular pressure in patients with ocular hypertension or open-angle glaucoma

Mechanism of Action/Effect Brinzolamide inhibits carbonic anhydrase, leading to decreased aqueous humor secretion. This results in a reduction of intraocular pressure.

Contraindications Hypersensitivity to brinzolamide, sulfonamides, or any component of the formulation

Warnings/Precautions Effects of prolonged use on corneal epithelial cells have not been evaluated; has not been studied in acute angle-closure glaucoma. Use caution with renal impairment (parent and metabolite may accumulate). Systemic absorption may cause serious hypersensitivity reactions to recur. Chemical similarities are present among sulfonamides, sulfonylureas, carbonic anhydrase inhibitors, thiazides, and loop diuretics (except ethacrynic acid). In patients with allergy to one of these compounds, a risk of cross-reaction (Continued)

Brinzolamide *(Continued)*

exists; avoid use when previous reaction has been severe. Safety and efficacy have not been established with hepatic impairment or in pediatric patients.

Drug Interactions
Cytochrome P450 Effect: Substrate of CYP3A4 (minor)
Increased Effect/Toxicity: Concurrent use of oral carbonic anhydrase inhibitors (CAIs) may lead to additive effects and toxicity (use is not recommended). High-dose salicylates may result in toxicity from CAIs.

Adverse Reactions
1% to 10%:
Dermatologic: Dermatitis (1% to 5%)
Gastrointestinal: Taste disturbances (5% to 10%)
Ocular: Blurred vision (5% to 10%), blepharitis (1% to 5%), dry eye (1% to 5%), foreign body sensation (1% to 5%), eye discharge (1% to 5%), eye pain (1% to 5%), itching of eye (1% to 5%)
Respiratory: Rhinitis (1% to 5%)

Overdosage/Toxicology Theoretically, overdose could lead to electrolyte imbalance, acidosis and CNS effects; monitor serum electrolytes and blood pH. Treatment is supportive.

Pharmacodynamics/Kinetics
Onset of Action: Peak effect: 2 hours
Duration of Action: 8-12 hours
Absorption: Topical: Into systemic circulation
Metabolism: To N-desmethyl brinzolamide
Excretion: Urine (as unchanged drug and metabolites)

Dosing
Adults & Elderly: Glaucoma: Ophthalmic: Instill 1 drop in affected eye(s) 3 times/day
Available Dosage Forms Suspension, ophthalmic: 1% (5 mL, 10 mL, 15 mL) [contains benzalkonium chloride]

Monitoring and Teaching Issues
Physical Assessment: Assess potential for interactions with other prescriptions, OTC medications, or herbal products patient may be taking. Assess therapeutic response and adverse effects. Measure intraocular pressure periodically. Teach patient proper use, side effects/appropriate interventions, and symptoms to report
Patient Education: For use in eyes only. Tilt head back, place medication in conjunctival sac, and close eyes. Apply finger pressure at corner of eye for 1 minute following application. Do not let tip of applicator touch eye; do not contaminate tip of applicator (may cause eye infection, eye damage, or vision loss). If using other ophthalmic preparations, administer 10 minutes apart. Avoid excessive use of aspirin or aspirin-containing medications (may cause toxicity). May cause taste changes; runny nose; or vision changes (blurred vision, dry eye, foreign body sensation, eye discharge, temporary sensitivity to bright light, blurring or stinging, altered distance perception, reduced night vision acuity). Report persistent dizziness or headache, skin rash, loss of hair, unresolved GI disturbance, difficulty breathing, or persistent sore throat. **Pregnancy/breast-feeding precautions:** Inform prescriber if you are or intend to become pregnant. Breast-feeding is not recommended.
Pregnancy Risk Factor: C
Lactation: Excretion in breast milk unknown/not recommended

Administration
Other: May be used concomitantly with other topical ophthalmic drug products to lower intraocular pressure. If more than one topical ophthalmic drug is being used, administer drugs at least 10 minutes apart.
Storage: Store at 4°C to 30°C (39°F to 86°F). Shake well before use.

Related Information
Glaucoma Drug Therapy *on page 1827*

♦ **Brioschi® [OTC]** *see* Sodium Bicarbonate *on page 1380*
♦ **BRL 43694** *see* Granisetron *on page 726*

Bromocriptine *(broe moe KRIP teen)*
U.S. Brand Names Parlodel®
Synonyms Bromocriptine Mesylate
Generic Available Yes: Tablet
Pharmacologic Category Anti-Parkinson's Agent, Dopamine Agonist; Ergot Derivative
Medication Safety Issues
Sound-alike/look-alike issues:
Bromocriptine may be confused with benztropine, brimonidine
Parlodel® may be confused with pindolol, Provera®
Use
Amenorrhea with or without galactorrhea; infertility or hypogonadism; prolactin-secreting adenomas; acromegaly; Parkinson's disease
A previous indication for prevention of postpartum lactation was withdrawn voluntarily by Sandoz Pharmaceuticals Corporation.
Unlabeled/Investigational Use Neuroleptic malignant syndrome
Mechanism of Action/Effect Semisynthetic ergot alkaloid derivative and a dopamine receptor agonist which activates postsynaptic dopamine receptors in the tuberoinfundibular and nigrostriatal pathways
Contraindications Hypersensitivity to bromocriptine, ergot alkaloids, or any component of the formulation; ergot alkaloids are contraindicated with potent inhibitors of CYP3A4 (includes protease inhibitors, azole antifungals, and some macrolide antibiotics); uncontrolled hypertension; severe ischemic heart disease or peripheral vascular disorders; pregnancy (risk to benefit evaluation must be performed in women who become pregnant during treatment for acromegaly, prolactinoma, or Parkinson's disease - hypertension during treatment should generally result in efforts to withdraw)

Warnings/Precautions Use with caution in patients with impaired renal or hepatic function, a history of psychosis, or cardiovascular disease (myocardial infarction, arrhythmia). Patients who receive bromocriptine during and immediately following pregnancy as a continuation of previous therapy (ie, acromegaly) should be closely monitored for cardiovascular effects. Discontinuation of bromocriptine in patients with macroadenomas has been associated with rapid regrowth of tumor and increased prolactin serum levels. Use with caution in patients with a history of peptic ulcer disease, dementia, or concurrent antihypertensive therapy. Pleural and peritoneal fibrosis have been reported with prolonged daily use. Cardiac valvular fibrosis has also been associated with ergot alkaloids. Safety and effectiveness in patients <15 years of age have not been established.

Drug Interactions

Cytochrome P450 Effect: Substrate of CYP3A4 (major); **Inhibits** CYP1A2 (weak), 3A4 (weak)

Decreased Effect: Effects of bromocriptine may be diminished by antipsychotics, metoclopramide.

Increased Effect/Toxicity: Effects of bromocriptine may be increased by antifungals (azole derivatives); macrolide antibiotics; protease inhibitors; MAO inhibitors. Bromocriptine may increase the effects of sibutramine and other serotonin agonists (serotonin syndrome). CYP3A4 inhibitors may increase the levels/effects of bromocriptine; example inhibitors include azole antifungals, ciprofloxacin, clarithromycin, diclofenac, doxycycline, erythromycin, imatinib, isoniazid, nefazodone, nicardipine, propofol, protease inhibitors, quinidine, and verapamil.

Nutritional/Ethanol Interactions

Ethanol: Avoid ethanol (may increase GI side effects or ethanol intolerance).

Herb/Nutraceutical: St John's wort may decrease bromocriptine levels.

Adverse Reactions

>10%:

Central nervous system: Headache, dizziness

Gastrointestinal: Nausea

1% to 10%:

Cardiovascular: Orthostatic hypotension

Central nervous system: Fatigue, lightheadedness, drowsiness

Gastrointestinal: Anorexia, vomiting, abdominal cramps, constipation

Respiratory: Nasal congestion

Overdosage/Toxicology Symptoms of overdose include nausea, vomiting, and hypotension. Treatment is symptomatic and supportive.

Pharmacodynamics/Kinetics

Time to Peak: Serum: 1-2 hours

Protein Binding: 90% to 96%

Half-Life Elimination: Biphasic: Initial: 6-8 hours; Terminal: 50 hours

Metabolism: Primarily hepatic

Excretion: Feces; urine (2% to 6% as unchanged drug)

Dosing

Adults & Elderly:

Parkinsonism: Oral: 1.25 mg 2 times/day, increased by 2.5 mg/day in 2- to 4-week intervals (usual dose range is 30-90 mg/day in 3 divided doses), though elderly patients can usually be managed on lower doses.

Neuroleptic malignant syndrome: Oral: 2.5-5 mg 3 times/day

Hyperprolactinemia: Oral: 2.5 mg 2-3 times/day

Acromegaly: Initial: Oral: 1.25-2.5 mg increasing as necessary every 3-7 days; usual dose: 20-30 mg/day

Prolactin-secreting adenomas: Oral: Initial: 1.25-2.5 mg/day; may be increased as tolerated every 2-7 days until optimal response (range: 2.5-15 mg/day)

Pediatrics:

Prolactin-secreting adenoma: Oral:

Children 11-15 years (based on limited information): Initial: 1.25-2.5 mg daily. Dosage may be increased as tolerated to achieve a therapeutic response (range 2.5-10 mg daily).

Children ≥16 years: Refer to adult dosing.

Hepatic Impairment: No guidelines are available, however, adjustment may be necessary.

Available Dosage Forms

Capsule, as mesylate: 5 mg

Tablet, as mesylate: 2.5 mg

Monitoring and Teaching Issues

Physical Assessment: Assess effectiveness and interactions of other medications patient may be taking. Assess therapeutic effectiveness (eg, mental status, involuntary movements) and adverse reactions at beginning of therapy and periodically throughout therapy. Assess knowledge/teach patient appropriate use, interventions to reduce side effects, and adverse symptoms to report.

Patient Education: Take exactly as directed (may be prescribed in conjunction with levodopa/carbidopa); do not change dosage or discontinue without consulting prescriber. Therapeutic effects may take several weeks or months to achieve and you may need frequent monitoring during first weeks of therapy. Take with meals if GI upset occurs, before meals if dry mouth occurs, or after eating if drooling or if nausea occurs. Take at the same time each day. Maintain adequate hydration (2-3 L/day of fluids) unless instructed to restrict fluid intake; void before taking medication. Do not use alcohol, prescription or OTC sedatives or CNS depressants without consulting prescriber. Urine or perspiration may appear darker. You may experience drowsiness, dizziness, confusion, or vision changes (use caution when driving, climbing stairs, or engaging in tasks requiring alertness until response to drug is known); orthostatic hypotension (use caution when rising from sitting or lying position); constipation (increased exercise, fluids, fruit, or fiber may help); nasal congestion (consult prescriber for appropriate relief); or nausea, vomiting, loss of appetite, or stomach discomfort (small frequent meals, frequent mouth care, chewing gum, or sucking lozenges may help). Report unresolved constipation or vomiting; chest pain or irregular heartbeat; (Continued)

Bromocriptine *(Continued)*

acute headache or dizziness; CNS changes (eg, hallucination, loss of memory, seizures, acute headache, nervousness); painful or difficult urination; increased muscle spasticity, rigidity, or involuntary movements; skin rash; or significant worsening of condition.

Breast-feeding precaution: Do not breast-feed.

Dietary Considerations: May be taken with food to decrease GI distress.

Geriatric Considerations: See Adverse Reactions; elderly patients are usually managed on lower doses.

Pregnancy Risk Factor: B

Lactation: Enters breast milk/contraindicated

Additional Information Usually used with levodopa or levodopa/carbidopa to treat Parkinson's disease. When adding bromocriptine, the dose of levodopa/carbidopa can usually be decreased.

- ◆ **Bromocriptine Mesylate** *see* Bromocriptine *on page 208*
- ◆ **Brontex®** *see* Guaifenesin and Codeine *on page 731*
- ◆ **B-Type Natriuretic Peptide (Human)** *see* Nesiritide *on page 1071*
- ◆ **Bubbli-Pred™** *see* PrednisoLONE *on page 1245*

Budesonide *(byoo DES oh nide)*

U.S. Brand Names Entocort™ EC; Pulmicort Respules®; Pulmicort Turbuhaler®; Rhinocort® Aqua®

Generic Available No

Pharmacologic Category Corticosteroid, Inhalant (Oral); Corticosteroid, Nasal; Corticosteroid, Systemic

Use

Intranasal: Children ≥6 years of age and Adults: Management of symptoms of seasonal or perennial rhinitis

Nebulization: Children 12 months to 8 years: Maintenance and prophylactic treatment of asthma

Oral capsule: Treatment of active Crohn's disease (mild to moderate) involving the ileum and/or ascending colon

Oral inhalation: Maintenance and prophylactic treatment of asthma; includes patients who require corticosteroids and those who may benefit from systemic dose reduction/elimination

Mechanism of Action/Effect Anti-inflammatory effect on nasal tissues

Contraindications Hypersensitivity to budesonide or any component of the formulation

Inhalation: Contraindicated in primary treatment of status asthmaticus, acute episodes of asthma; not for relief of acute bronchospasm

Warnings/Precautions May cause hypercorticism and/or suppression of hypothalamic-pituitary-adrenal (HPA) axis, particularly in younger children or in patients receiving high doses for prolonged periods. Particular care is required when patients are transferred from systemic corticosteroids to products with lower systemic bioavailability (ie, inhalation). May lead to possible adrenal insufficiency or withdrawal from steroids, including an increase in allergic symptoms. Patients receiving prolonged therapy of ≥20 mg per day of prednisone (or equivalent) may be most susceptible. Aerosol steroids do **not** provide the systemic steroid needed to treat patients having trauma, surgery, or infections.

Controlled clinical studies have shown that orally-inhaled and intranasal corticosteroids may cause a reduction in growth velocity in pediatric patients. (In studies of orally-inhaled corticosteroids, the mean reduction in growth velocity was approximately 1 centimeter per year [range 0.3-1.8 cm per year] and appears to be related to dose and duration of exposure.) To minimize the systemic effects of orally-inhaled and intranasal corticosteroids, each patient should be titrated to the lowest effective dose. Growth should be routinely monitored in pediatric patients.

May suppress the immune system, patients may be more susceptible to infection. Use with caution in patients with systemic infections or ocular herpes simplex. Avoid exposure to chickenpox and measles. Corticosteroids should be used with caution in patients with diabetes, hypertension, osteoporosis, peptic ulcer, glaucoma, cataracts, or tuberculosis. Use caution in hepatic impairment. Enteric-coated capsules should not be crushed or chewed.

Drug Interactions

Cytochrome P450 Effect: Substrate of CYP3A4 (major)

Decreased Effect: Theoretically, proton pump inhibitors (omeprazole, pantoprazole) alter gastric pH may affect the rate of dissolution of enteric-coated capsules. Administration with omeprazole did not alter kinetics of budesonide capsules.

Increased Effect/Toxicity: Cimetidine may decrease the clearance and increase the bioavailability of budesonide, increasing its serum concentrations. In addition, CYP3A4 inhibitors may increase the serum level and/or toxicity of budesonide this effect was shown with ketoconazole, but not erythromycin. Other potential inhibitors include amiodarone, cimetidine, clarithromycin, delavirdine, diltiazem, dirithromycin, disulfiram, fluoxetine, fluvoxamine, grapefruit juice, indinavir, itraconazole, ketoconazole, nefazodone, nevirapine, propoxyphene, quinupristin-dalfopristin, ritonavir, saquinavir, verapamil, zafirlukast, zileuton. The addition of salmeterol has been demonstrated to improve response to inhaled corticosteroids (as compared to increasing steroid dosage).

Nutritional/Ethanol Interactions

Food: Grapefruit juice may double systemic exposure of orally-administered budesonide. Administration of capsules with a high-fat meal delays peak concentration, but does not alter the extent of absorption.

Herb/Nutraceutical: St John's wort may decrease budesonide levels.

Adverse Reactions Reaction severity varies by dose and duration; not all adverse reactions have been reported with each dosage form.

>10%:

Central nervous system: Oral capsule: Headache (up to 21%)

Gastrointestinal: Oral capsule: Nausea (up to 11%)

Respiratory: Respiratory infection, rhinitis

Miscellaneous: Symptoms of HPA axis suppression and/or hypercorticism (acne, easy bruising, fat redistribution, striae, edema) may occur in >10% of patients following administration of dosage forms which result in higher systemic exposure (ie, oral capsule), but may be less frequent than rates observed with comparator drugs (prednisolone). These symptoms may be rare (<1%) following administration via methods which result in lower exposures (topical).

1% to 10%:

Cardiovascular: Syncope, edema, hypertension

Central nervous system: Chest pain, dysphonia, emotional lability, fatigue, fever, insomnia, migraine, nervousness, pain, dizziness, vertigo

Dermatologic: Bruising, contact dermatitis, eczema, pruritus, pustular rash, rash

Endocrine & metabolic: Hypokalemia, adrenal insufficiency

Gastrointestinal: Abdominal pain, anorexia, diarrhea, dry mouth, dyspepsia, gastroenteritis, oral candidiasis, taste perversion, vomiting, weight gain, flatulence

Hematologic: Cervical lymphadenopathy, purpura, leukocytosis

Neuromuscular & skeletal: Arthralgia, fracture, hyperkinesis, hypertonia, myalgia, neck pain, weakness, paresthesia, back pain

Ocular: Conjunctivitis, eye infection

Otic: Earache, ear infection, external ear infection

Respiratory: Bronchitis, bronchospasm, cough, epistaxis, nasal irritation, pharyngitis, sinusitis, stridor

Miscellaneous: Allergic reaction, flu-like syndrome, herpes simplex, infection, moniliasis, viral infection, voice alteration

Overdosage/Toxicology

Inhaled formulations: Symptoms of overdose include irritation and burning of the nasal mucosa, sneezing, intranasal and pharyngeal *Candida* infections, nasal ulceration, epistaxis, rhinorrhea, nasal stuffiness, headache.

When consumed in excessive quantities, systemic hypercorticism and adrenal suppression may occur, in those cases discontinuation and withdrawal of the corticosteroid should be done judiciously. Treatment should be symptomatic and supportive.

Pharmacodynamics/Kinetics

Onset of Action: Respules®: 2-8 days; Rhinocort Aqua®: ~10 hours; Turbuhaler®: 24 hours

Peak effect: Respules®: 4-6 weeks; Rhinocort Aqua®: ~2 weeks; Turbuhaler®: 1-2 weeks

Absorption: Capsule: Rapid and complete

Bioavailability: Limited by high first-pass effect; Capsule: 9% to 21%; Respules®: 6%; Turbuhaler®: 6% to 13%; Nasal: 34%

Time to Peak: Capsule: 30-600 minutes (variable in Crohn's disease); Respules®: 10-30 minutes; Turbuhaler®: 1-2 hours; Nasal: 1 hour

Protein Binding: 85% to 90%

Half-Life Elimination: 2-3.6 hours

Metabolism: Hepatic via CYP3A4 to two metabolites: 16 alpha-hydroxyprednisolone and 6 beta-hydroxybudesonide; minor activity

Excretion: Urine (60%) and feces as metabolites

Dosing

Adults & Elderly:

Asthma: Inhalation: 1- to 4-inhalations twice daily using Pulmicort Turbuhaler® device; maintenance therapy may be gradually reduced to a single daily inhalation. See table.

Budesonide

Previous Therapy	Recommended Starting Dose	Highest Recommended Dose
Bronchodilators alone	200-400 mcg twice daily	400 mcg twice daily
Inhaled corticosteroids[1]	200-400 mcg twice daily	800 mcg twice daily
Oral corticosteroids	400-800 mcg twice daily	800 mcg twice daily

[1]In patients with mild to moderate asthma who are well controlled on inhaled corticosteroids, dosing with Pulmicort® Turbuhaler® 200 mcg or 400 mcg once daily may be considered. Pulmicort® Turbuhaler® can be administered once daily either in the morning or in the evening.

Crohn's disease: Oral: 9 mg once daily in the morning; safety and efficacy have not been established for therapy duration >8 weeks; recurring episodes may be treated with a repeat 8-week course of treatment

Note: Treatment may be tapered to 6 mg once daily for 2 weeks prior to complete cessation. Patients receiving CYP3A4 inhibitors should be monitored closely for signs and symptoms of hypercorticism; dosage reduction may be required.

Rhinitis: Nasal inhalation (Rhinocort Aqua®): 64 mcg/day as a single 32 mcg spray in each nostril. Some patients who do not achieve adequate control may benefit from increased dosage. A reduced dosage may be effective after initial control is achieved. Maximum dose: Children <12 years: 129 mcg/day; Adults: 256 mcg/day

Pediatrics:

Asthma:

Nasal inhalation: ≥6 years: Refer to adult dosing.

Oral inhalation: ≥6 years:

Previous therapy of bronchodilators alone: 200 mcg twice initially which may be increased up to 400 mcg twice daily

Previous therapy of inhaled corticosteroids: 200 mcg twice initially which may be increased up to 400 mcg twice daily

Previous therapy of oral corticosteroids: The highest recommended dose in children is 400 mcg twice daily

NIH Guidelines (give in divided doses twice daily):

"Low" dose: 100-200 mcg/day

(Continued)

Budesonide *(Continued)*

"Medium" dose: 200-400 mcg/day (1-2 inhalations/day)

"High" dose: >400 mcg/day (>2 inhalation/day)

Nebulization: Children 12 months to 8 years: Pulmicort Respules®: Titrate to lowest effective dose once patient is stable; start at 0.25 mg/day or use as follows:

Previous therapy of bronchodilators alone: 0.5 mg/day administered as a single dose or divided twice daily (maximum daily dose: 0.5 mg)

Previous therapy of inhaled corticosteroids: 0.5 mg/day administered as a single dose or divided twice daily (maximum daily dose: 1 mg)

Previous therapy of oral corticosteroids: 1 mg/day administered as a single dose or divided twice daily (maximum daily dose: 1 mg)

Hepatic Impairment: Monitor closely for signs and symptoms of hypercorticism; dosage reduction may be required.

Available Dosage Forms

Capsule, enteric coated (Entocort™ EC): 3 mg

Powder for oral inhalation (Pulmicort Turbuhaler®): 200 mcg/inhalation (104 g) [delivers ~160 mcg/inhalation; 200 metered doses]

Additional dosage strengths available in Canada: 100 mcg/inhalation, 400 mcg/inhalation

Suspension, nasal spray (Rhinocort® Aqua®): 32 mcg/inhalation (8.6 g) [120 metered doses]

Suspension for oral inhalation (Pulmicort Respules®): 0.25 mg/2 mL (30s), 0.5 mg/2 mL (30s)

Monitoring and Teaching Issues

Physical Assessment: Monitor therapeutic effectiveness and adverse reactions. When changing from systemic steroids to inhalational steroids, taper reduction of systemic medication slowly (may take several months). Growth should be routinely monitored in pediatric patients. Assess knowledge/teach patient appropriate use, interventions to reduce side effects, and adverse symptoms to report.

Patient Education: Use as directed; do not increase dosage or discontinue abruptly without consulting prescriber. May be more susceptible to infection; avoid exposure to chickenpox and measles unless immunity has been established. If exposure to measles or chickenpox occurs, notify your prescriber immediately. Report acute nervousness or inability to sleep; severe sneezing or nosebleed; respiratory difficulty, sore throat, hoarseness, or bronchitis; respiratory difficulty or bronchospasms; disturbed menstrual pattern; vision changes; loss of taste or smell perception; or worsening of condition or lack of improvement. **Pregnancy/breast-feeding precautions:** Inform prescriber if you are or intend to become pregnant. Consult prescriber if breast-feeding.

Oral capsule: Swallow whole; do not crush or chew capsule.

Inhalation/nebulization: This is not a bronchodilator and will not relieve acute asthma attacks. It may take several days for you to realize full effects of treatment. If you are also using an inhaled bronchodilator, wait 10 minutes before using this steroid aerosol. Take 5-10 deep breaths. Use inhaler on inspiration. Hold breath for 5-10 seconds after inhalation. Allow 1 full minute between inhalations. You may experience dizziness, anxiety, or blurred vision (rise slowly from sitting or lying position and use caution when driving or engaging in tasks requiring alertness until response to drug is known); or taste disturbance or aftertaste (frequent mouth care and mouth rinses may help). Rinse mouth with water following oral treatments to decrease risk of oral candidiasis (wash face if using a face mask).

Dietary Considerations: Avoid grapefruit juice when using oral capsules.

Geriatric Considerations: Ensure that patients can correctly use nasal inhaler.

Pregnancy Risk Factor: C/B (Pulmicort Respules® and Turbuhaler®, Rhinocort® Aqua®)

Pregnancy Issues: There are no adequate and well-controlled studies in pregnant women; use only if potential benefit to the mother outweighs the possible risk to the fetus. Hypoadrenalism has been reported in infants.

Lactation: Enters breast milk/use caution

Administration

Oral: Oral capsule: Capsule should be swallowed whole; do not crush or chew.

Inhalation:

Inhalation: Inhaler should be shaken well immediately prior to use; while activating inhaler, deep breathe for 3-5 seconds, hold breath for ~10 seconds and allow ≥1 minute between inhalations. Rinse mouth with water after use to reduce aftertaste and incidence of candidiasis.

Nebulization: Shake well before using. Use Pulmicort Respules® with jet nebulizer connected to an air compressor; administer with mouthpiece or facemask. Do not use ultrasonic nebulizer. Do not mix with other medications in nebulizer. Rinse mouth following treatments to decrease risk of oral candidiasis (wash face if using face mask).

Storage:

Nebulizer: Store upright at 20°C to 25°C (68°F to 77°F) and protect from light. Do not refrigerate or freeze. Once aluminum package is opened, solution should be used within 2 weeks. Continue to protect from light.

Nasal inhaler: Store with valve up at 15°C to 30°C (59°F to 86°F). Use within 6 months after opening aluminum pouch. Protect from high humidity.

Nasal spray: Store with valve up at 20°C to 25°C (68°F to 77°F) and protect from light. Do not freeze.

Additional Information Effects of inhaled/intranasal steroids on growth have been observed in the absence of laboratory evidence of HPA axis suppression, suggesting that growth velocity is a more sensitive indicator of systemic corticosteroid exposure in pediatric patients than some commonly used tests of HPA axis function. The long-term effects of this reduction in growth velocity associated with orally-inhaled and intranasal corticosteroids, including the impact on final adult height, are unknown. The potential for "catch up" growth following discontinuation of treatment with inhaled corticosteroids has not been adequately studied.

Related Information

Asthma *on page 1799*

Inhalant Agents *on page 1734*

- ♦ **Buffered Aspirin and Pravastatin Sodium** *see* Aspirin and Pravastatin *on page 148*
- ♦ **Bufferin®** [OTC] *see* Aspirin *on page 143*
- ♦ **Bufferin® Extra Strength** [OTC] *see* Aspirin *on page 143*
- ♦ **Buffinol** [OTC] *see* Aspirin *on page 143*
- ♦ **Buffinol Extra** [OTC] *see* Aspirin *on page 143*

Bumetanide (byoo MET a nide)
U.S. Brand Names Bumex®
Generic Available Yes
Pharmacologic Category Diuretic, Loop
Medication Safety Issues
Sound-alike/look-alike issues:
Bumetanide may be confused with Buminate®
Bumex® may be confused with Brevibloc®, Buprenex®, Permax®

Use Management of edema secondary to congestive heart failure or hepatic or renal disease including nephrotic syndrome; may be used alone or in combination with antihypertensives in the treatment of hypertension; can be used in furosemide-allergic patients

Mechanism of Action/Effect Inhibits reabsorption of sodium and chloride in the ascending loop of Henle and proximal renal tubule, causing increased excretion of water, sodium, chloride, magnesium, phosphate and calcium

Contraindications Hypersensitivity to bumetanide, any component of the formulation, or sulfonylureas; anuria; patients with hepatic coma or in states of severe electrolyte depletion until the condition improves or is corrected; pregnancy (based on expert analysis)

Warnings/Precautions In cirrhosis, avoid electrolyte and acid/base imbalances that might lead to hepatic encephalopathy. Ototoxicity is associated with I.V. rapid administration, renal impairment, excessive doses, and concurrent use of other ototoxins. Hypersensitivity reactions can rarely occur. Monitor fluid status and renal function in an attempt to prevent oliguria, azotemia, and reversible increases in BUN and creatinine. May cause significant electrolyte disturbances or volume depletion. Coadministration of antihypertensives may increase the risk of hypotension.

Chemical similarities are present among sulfonamides, sulfonylureas, carbonic anhydrase inhibitors, thiazides, and loop diuretics (except ethacrynic acid). Use in patients with sulfonylurea allergy is specifically contraindicated in product labeling, however, a risk of cross-reaction exists in patients with allergy to any of these compounds; avoid use when previous reaction has been severe.

Drug Interactions
Decreased Effect: Glucose tolerance may be decreased by loop diuretics, requiring adjustment of hypoglycemic agents. Cholestyramine or colestipol may reduce bioavailability of bumetanide. Indomethacin (and other NSAIDs) may reduce natriuretic and hypotensive effects of diuretics. Hypokalemia may reduce the efficacy of some antiarrhythmics.

Increased Effect/Toxicity: Bumetanide-induced hypokalemia may predispose to digoxin toxicity and may increase the risk of arrhythmia with drugs which may prolong QT interval, including type Ia and type III antiarrhythmic agents, cisapride, and some quinolones (sparfloxacin, gatifloxacin, and moxifloxacin). The risk of toxicity from lithium and salicylates (high dose) may be increased by loop diuretics. Hypotensive effects and/or adverse renal effects of ACE inhibitors and NSAIDs are potentiated by bumetanide-induced hypovolemia. The effects of peripheral adrenergic-blocking drugs or ganglionic blockers may be increased by bumetanide.

Bumetanide may increase the risk of ototoxicity with other ototoxic agents (aminoglycosides, cis-platinum), especially in patients with renal dysfunction. Synergistic diuretic effects occur with thiazide-type diuretics. Diuretics tend to be synergistic with other antihypertensive agents, and hypotension may occur.

Nutritional/Ethanol Interactions Herb/Nutraceutical: Avoid ephedra, yohimbe, ginseng (may worsen hypertension). Avoid dong quai if using for hypertension (has estrogenic activity). Avoid garlic (may have increased antihypertensive effect).

Adverse Reactions
>10%:
Endocrine & metabolic: Hyperuricemia (18%), hypochloremia (15%), hypokalemia (15%)
Renal: Azotemia (11%)
1% to 10%:
Central nervous system: Dizziness (1%)
Endocrine & metabolic: Hyponatremia (9%), hyperglycemia (7%), variations in phosphorus (5%), CO_2 content (4%), bicarbonate (3%), and calcium (2%)
Neuromuscular & skeletal: Muscle cramps (1%)
Otic: Ototoxicity (1%)
Renal: Increased serum creatinine (7%)

Overdosage/Toxicology Symptoms of overdose include electrolyte depletion and volume depletion. Treatment is symptomatic and supportive.

Pharmacodynamics/Kinetics
Onset of Action: Oral, I.M.: 0.5-1 hour; I.V.: 2-3 minutes
Duration of Action: 6 hours
Protein Binding: 95%
Half-Life Elimination: Neonates: ~6 hours; Infants (1 month): ~2.4 hours; Adults: 1-1.5 hours
Metabolism: Partially hepatic
Excretion: Primarily urine (as unchanged drug and metabolites)

Dosing
Adults:
Edema:
Oral: 0.5-2 mg/dose (maximum dose: 10 mg/day) 1-2 times/day
I.M., I.V.: 0.5-1 mg/dose; may repeat in 2-3 hours for up to 2 doses if needed (maximum dose: 10 mg/day)
Continuous I.V. infusion: 0.9-1 mg/hour
(Continued)

Bumetanide *(Continued)*

Hypertension: Oral: 0.5 mg daily (maximum dose: 5 mg/day)
Usual dosage range (JNC 7): 0.5-2 mg/day in 2 divided doses
Elderly: Initial: Oral: 0.5 mg once daily, increase as necessary.
Pediatrics: Edema (diuresis); Not FDA-approved for use in children <18 years of age:
<6 months: Dose not established
>6 months:
Oral: Initial: 0.015 mg/kg/dose once daily or every other day; maximum dose: 0.1 mg/kg/
day
I.M., I.V.: Dose not established

Available Dosage Forms
Injection, solution: 0.25 mg/mL (2 mL, 4 mL, 10 mL) [contains benzyl alcohol]
Tablet (Bumex®): 0.5 mg, 1 mg, 2 mg

Monitoring and Teaching Issues
Physical Assessment: Assess history of allergies, renal, electrolyte, hepatic, and pregnancy status prior to use (see Contraindications and Warnings/Precautions). Assess
potential for interactions with other pharmacological agents and herbal products patient
may be taking (eg, increased risk hyperglycemia, hypotension, arrhythmias, ototoxicity;
see Drug Interactions). Blood pressure, weight, and fluid status should be monitored at
beginning of therapy and periodically during therapy. Glucose levels for patients with
diabetes should be monitored closely (glucose tolerance may be decreased by loop
diuretics, requiring adjustment of hypoglycemic agents). Assess results of laboratory tests
(electrolytes and renal function), therapeutic effectiveness (reduced edema and cardiopulmonary symptoms), and adverse effects (hypotension, electrolyte imbalance, ototoxicity;
see Adverse Reactions). Teach patient proper use, possible side effects/appropriate interventions, and adverse symptoms to report.

Monitoring Laboratory Tests: Serum electrolytes, renal function

Patient Education: Do not take any new medication during therapy unless approved by
prescriber. May be taken with food to reduce GI effects. If taking one dose daily, take single
dose early in day; if taking twice daily, take last dose early in afternoon to prevent sleep
interruptions. Include orange juice or bananas (or other sources of potassium-rich foods) in
your daily diet but do not take supplemental potassium without consulting prescriber. If you
have diabetes, monitor glucose levels closely (glucose tolerance may be decreased by
loop diuretics) and notify prescriber of noted changes (hypoglycemic agent may need to be
adjusted). May cause dizziness, hypotension, lightheadedness, or weakness (use caution
when changing position from sitting or lying position, when driving, exercising, climbing
stairs, or performing hazardous tasks until response to drug is known). Report palpitations
or chest pain; swelling of ankles or feet, weight increase or decrease (>3 lb in any one
day), increased fatigue, muscle cramps or trembling, changes in hearing, or other persistent adverse effects. **Pregnancy/breast-feeding precautions:** Inform prescriber if you are
or intend to become pregnant (contraceptives may be recommended) or breast-feed.

Dietary Considerations: May require increased intake of potassium-rich foods.

Geriatric Considerations: See Warnings/Precautions. Severe loss of sodium and/or
increases in BUN can cause confusion. For any change in mental status in patients on
bumetanide, monitor electrolytes and renal function.

Pregnancy Risk Factor: C (manufacturer); D (expert analysis)

Lactation: Excretion in breast milk unknown/use caution

Administration
I.V.: Administer I.V. slowly, over 1-2 minutes; an alternate-day schedule or a 3-4 daily dosing
regimen with rest periods of 1-2 days in between may be the most tolerable and effective
regimen for the continued control of edema; reserve I.V. administration for those unable to
take oral medications

Compatibility: Stable in D_5W, NS, LR
Y-site administration: Incompatible with midazolam
Compatibility when admixed: Incompatible with dobutamine, milrinone

Storage:
I.V.: Store vials at 15°C to 30°C (59°F to 86°F). Infusion solutions should be used within 24
hours after preparation; light sensitive, discoloration may occur when exposed to light.
Tablet: Store at 15°C to 30°C (59°F to 86°F).

Related Information
Heart Failure *on page 1828*

♦ **Bumex®** *see Bumetanide on page 213*
♦ **Buminate®** *see Albumin on page 58*

Bupivacaine *(byoo PIV a kane)*

U.S. Brand Names Marcaine®; Marcaine® Spinal; Sensorcaine®; Sensorcaine®-MPF
Synonyms Bupivacaine Hydrochloride
Generic Available Yes
Pharmacologic Category Local Anesthetic
Medication Safety Issues
Sound-alike/look-alike issues:
Bupivacaine may be confused with mepivacaine, ropivacaine
Marcaine® may be confused with Narcan®
Use Local anesthetic (injectable) for peripheral nerve block, infiltration, sympathetic block,
caudal or epidural block, retrobulbar block
Mechanism of Action/Effect Blocks both the initiation and conduction of nerve impulses by
decreasing the neuronal membrane's permeability to sodium ions, which results in inhibition
of depolarization with resultant blockade of conduction
Contraindications Hypersensitivity to bupivacaine hydrochloride, amide-type local anesthetics (etidocaine, lidocaine, mepivacaine, prilocaine, ropivacaine) or any component of the

formulation (para-aminobenzoic acid or parabens in specific formulations); not to be used for obstetrical paracervical block anesthesia

Warnings/Precautions Use with caution in patients with hepatic impairment. Some commercially available formulations contain sodium metabisulfite, which may cause allergic-type reactions. Pending further data, should not be used in children <12 years of age and the solution for spinal anesthesia should not be used in children <18 years of age. **Do not use solutions containing preservatives for caudal or epidural block**. Convulsions due to systemic toxicity leading to cardiac arrest have been reported, presumably following unintentional intravascular injection. The 0.75% is **not** recommended for obstetrical anesthesia. A test dose is recommended prior to epidural administration (prior to initial dose) and all reinforcing doses with continuous catheter technique.

Drug Interactions

Cytochrome P450 Effect: Substrate (minor) of CYP1A2, 2C19, 2D6, 3A4

Increased Effect/Toxicity: Increased effect if used with hyaluronidase. Bupivacaine used in conjunction with epinephrine in patients on beta-blockers, ergot-type oxytocics, MAO inhibitors, tricyclic antidepressants, phenothiazines, vasopressors, or isoproterenol may result in prolonged hypotension or hypertension.

Adverse Reactions Note: Incidence of adverse reactions is difficult to define. Most effects are dose related, and are often due to accelerated absorption from the injection site, unintentional intravascular injection, or slow metabolic degradation. The development of any central nervous system symptoms may be an early indication of more significant toxicity (seizure).

Cardiovascular: Hypotension, bradycardia, palpitation, heart block, ventricular arrhythmia, cardiac arrest

Central nervous system: Restlessness, anxiety, dizziness, seizure (0.1%); rare symptoms (usually associated with unintentional subarachnoid injection during high spinal anesthesia) include persistent anesthesia, paresthesia, paralysis, headache, septic meningitis, and cranial nerve palsies

Gastrointestinal: Nausea, vomiting; rare symptoms (usually associated with unintentional subarachnoid injection during high spinal anesthesia) include fecal incontinence and loss of sphincter control

Genitourinary: Rare symptoms (usually associated with unintentional subarachnoid injection during high spinal anesthesia) include urinary incontinence, loss of perineal sensation, and loss of sexual function

Neuromuscular & skeletal: Weakness

Ocular: Blurred vision, pupillary constriction

Otic: Tinnitus

Respiratory: Apnea, hypoventilation (usually associated with unintentional subarachnoid injection during high spinal anesthesia)

Miscellaneous; Allergic reactions (urticaria, pruritus, angioedema), anaphylactoid reactions

Overdosage/Toxicology Treatment is symptomatic and supportive. Termination of anesthesia by pneumatic tourniquet inflation should be attempted when bupivacaine is administered by infiltration or regional injection. Treatment is symptomatic and supportive. Methemoglobinemia should be treated with methylene blue 1-2 mg/kg in a 1% sterile aqueous solution by I.V. push over 4-6 minutes, repeated up to a total dose of 7 mg/kg.

Pharmacodynamics/Kinetics

Onset of Action: Anesthesia (route dependent): 4-10 minutes

Duration of Action: 1.5-8.5 hours

Half-Life Elimination: Age dependent: Neonates: 8.1 hours; Adults: 1.5-5.5 hours

Metabolism: Hepatic

Excretion: Urine (~6%)

Dosing

Adults & Elderly: Note: Dose varies with procedure, depth of anesthesia, vascularity of tissues, duration of anesthesia and condition of patient. Do not use solutions containing preservatives for caudal or epidural block.

Caudal block (with or without epinephrine): 15-30 mL of 0.25% or 0.5%
Epidural block (other than caudal block): 10-20 mL of 0.25% or 0.5%
Peripheral nerve block: 5 mL dose of 0.25% or 0.5% (12.5-25 mg); maximum: 2.5 mg/kg (plain); 3 mg/kg (with epinephrine); up to a maximum of 400 mg/day
Sympathetic nerve block: 20-50 mL of 0.25% (no epinephrine) solution

Pediatrics: Dose varies with procedure, depth of anesthesia, vascularity of tissues, duration of anesthesia, and patient condition. Metabisulfites (in epinephrine-containing injection); do not use solutions containing preservatives for caudal or epidural block.

Caudal block (with or without epinephrine): Children: 1-3.7 mg/kg
Epidural block (other than caudal block): Children: 1.25 mg/kg/dose

Available Dosage Forms

Injection, solution, as hydrochloride [preservative free]: 0.25% [2.5 mg/mL] (10 mL, 20 mL, 30 mL, 50 mL); 0.5% [5 mg/mL] (10 mL, 20 mL, 30 mL); 0.75% [7.5 mg/mL] (10 mL, 20 mL, 30 mL)
Marcaine®: 0.25% [2.5 mg/mL] (10 mL, 30 mL, 50 mL); 0.5% [5 mg/mL] (10 mL, 30 mL); 0.75% [7.5 mg/mL] (10 mL, 30 mL)
Marcaine® Spinal: 0.75% [7.5 mg/mL] (2 mL) [in dextrose 8.25%]
Sensorcaine®-MPF: 0.25% [2.5 mg/mL] (10 mL, 30 mL); 0.5% [5 mg/mL] (10 mL, 30 mL); 0.75% [7.5 mg/mL] (10 mL, 30 mL)
Injection, solution, as hydrochloride (Marcaine®, Sensorcaine®): 0.25% [2.5 mg/mL] (50 mL); 0.5% [5 mg/mL] (50 mL) [contains methylparaben]
Injection, solution, with epinephrine 1:200,000, as hydrochloride [preservative free]: 0.25% [2.5 mg/mL] (10 mL, 30 mL); 0.5 % [5 mg/mL] (30 mL)
Marcaine®: 0.25% [2.5 mg/mL] (10 mL, 30 mL); 0.5% [5 mg/mL] (3 mL, 10 mL, 30 mL); 0.75% [7.5 mg/mL] (30 mL) [contains sodium metabisulfite]
Sensorcaine®-MPF: 0.25% [2.5 mg/mL] (10 mL, 30 mL); 0.5% [5 mg/mL] (10 mL, 30 mL); 0.75% [7.5 mg/mL] (30 mL) [contains sodium metabisulfite]

(Continued)

Bupivacaine *(Continued)*

Injection, solution, with epinephrine 1:200,000, as hydrochloride [with preservative] (Marcaine®, Sensorcaine®): 0.25% [2.5 mg/mL] (50 mL); 0.5% [5 mg/mL] (50 mL) [contains methylparaben and sodium metabisulfite]

Monitoring and Teaching Issues

Physical Assessment: Assess other medications patient may be taking for additive or adverse interactions. Monitor for effectiveness of anesthesia and adverse reactions. Monitor for return of sensation. Teach patient adverse reactions to report; use and teach appropriate interventions to promote safety.

Patient Education: This medication is given to reduce sensation in the injected area. You will experience decreased sensation to pain, heat, or cold in the area and/or decreased muscle strength (depending on area of application) until the effects wear off; use necessary caution to reduce incidence of possible injury until full sensation returns. If used in mouth, do not eat or drink until full sensation returns. Immediately report chest pain or palpitations; increased restlessness, anxiety, or dizziness; skeletal or muscle weakness; respiratory difficulty; ringing in ears; or vision changes. **Pregnancy/breast-feeding precautions:** Inform prescriber if you are pregnant. Do not breast-feed.

Pregnancy Risk Factor: C

Lactation: Enters breast milk/contraindicated

Administration

Compatibility: Stable in NS

Storage: Solutions with epinephrine should be protected from light.

♦ **Bupivacaine Hydrochloride** *see Bupivacaine on page 214*
♦ **Buprenex®** *see Buprenorphine on page 216*

Buprenorphine *(byoo pre NOR feen)*

U.S. Brand Names Buprenex®; Subutex®

Synonyms Buprenorphine Hydrochloride

Controlled Substance Injection: C-V; Tablet: C-III

Prescribing of tablets for opioid dependence is limited to physicians who have met the qualification criteria and have received a DEA number specific to prescribing this product. Tablets will be available through pharmacies and wholesalers which normally provide controlled substances.

Generic Available Yes: Injection

Pharmacologic Category Analgesic, Narcotic

Medication Safety Issues

Sound-alike/look-alike issues:
Buprenex® may be confused with Brevibloc®, Bumex®

Use

Injection: Management of moderate to severe pain
Tablet: Treatment of opioid dependence

Unlabeled/Investigational Use Injection: Heroin and opioid withdrawal

Mechanism of Action/Effect Buprenorphine exerts its analgesic effect via high affinity binding to μ opiate receptors in the CNS; displays both agonist and antagonist activity

Contraindications Hypersensitivity to buprenorphine or any component of the formulation

Warnings/Precautions An opioid-containing analgesic regimen should be tailored to each patient's needs and based upon the type of pain being treated (acute versus chronic), the route of administration, degree of tolerance for opioids (naive versus chronic user), age, weight, and medical condition. The optimal analgesic dose varies widely among patients. Doses should be titrated to pain relief/prevention.

May cause CNS depression, which may impair physical or mental abilities. Effects with other sedative drugs or ethanol may be potentiated. Elderly may be more sensitive to CNS depressant and constipating effects. May cause respiratory depression - use caution in patients with respiratory disease or pre-existing respiratory depression. Potential for drug dependency exists; abrupt cessation may precipitate withdrawal. Use caution in elderly, debilitated, pediatric patients, depression or suicidal tendencies, or in patients with a history of drug abuse. Tolerance, psychological and physical dependence may occur with prolonged use. Partial antagonist activity may precipitate acute narcotic withdrawal in opioid-dependent individuals.

Use with caution in patients with hepatic, pulmonary, or renal function impairment. Also use caution in patients with head injury or increased ICP, biliary tract dysfunction, pancreatitis, patients with history of ileus or bowel obstruction, glaucoma, hyperthyroidism, adrenal insufficiency, prostatic hyperplasia, urinary stricture, CNS depression, toxic psychosis, alcoholism, delirium tremens, or kyphoscoliosis.

Tablets, which are used for induction treatment of opioid dependence, should not be started until effects of withdrawal are evident.

Drug Interactions

Cytochrome P450 Effect: Substrate of CYP3A4 (major); **Inhibits** CYP1A2 (weak), 2A6 (weak), 2C19 (weak), 2D6 (weak)

Decreased Effect: CYP3A4 inducers may decrease the levels/effects of buprenorphine; example inducers include aminoglutethimide, carbamazepine, nafcillin, nevirapine, phenobarbital, phenytoin, and rifamycins. Naltrexone may antagonize the effect of narcotic analgesics; concurrent use or use within 7-10 days of injection for pain relief is contraindicated.

Increased Effect/Toxicity: Barbiturate anesthetics and other CNS depressants may produce additive respiratory and CNS depression. Respiratory and CV collapse was reported in a patient who received diazepam and buprenorphine. Effects may be additive with other CNS depressants. CYP3A4 inhibitors may increase the levels/effects of buprenorphine; example inhibitors include azole antifungals, ciprofloxacin, clarithromycin, diclofenac, doxycycline, erythromycin, imatinib, isoniazid, nefazodone, nicardipine, propofol, protease inhibitors, quinidine, and verapamil.

Nutritional/Ethanol Interactions

Ethanol: Avoid ethanol (may increase CNS depression).

Herb/Nutraceutical: Avoid valerian, St John's wort, kava kava, gotu kola (may increase CNS depression).

Adverse Reactions

Injection:
>10%: Central nervous system: Sedation

1% to 10%:
Cardiovascular: Hypotension
Central nervous system: Respiratory depression, dizziness, headache
Gastrointestinal: Vomiting, nausea
Ocular: Miosis
Otic: Vertigo
Miscellaneous: Diaphoresis

Tablet:
>10%:
Central nervous system: Headache (30%), pain (24%), insomnia (21% to 25%), Orality (12%), depression (11%)
Gastrointestinal: Nausea (10% to 14%), abdominal pain (12%), constipation (8% to 11%)
Neuromuscular & skeletal: Back pain (14%), weakness (14%)
Respiratory: Rhinitis (11%)
Miscellaneous: Withdrawal syndrome (19%; placebo 37%), infection (12% to 20%), diaphoresis (12% to 13%)

1% to 10%:
Central nervous system: Chills (6%), nervousness (6%), somnolence (5%), dizziness (4%), fever (3%)
Gastrointestinal: Vomiting (5% to 8%), diarrhea (5%), dyspepsia (3%)
Ocular: Lacrimation (5%)
Respiratory: Cough (4%), pharyngitis (4%)
Miscellaneous: Flu-like syndrome (6%)

Overdosage/Toxicology Symptoms of overdose include CNS depression, pinpoint pupils, hypotension, and bradycardia. Treatment is supportive. Naloxone may have limited effects in reversing respiratory depression; doxapram has also been used to stimulate respirations.

Pharmacodynamics/Kinetics
Onset of Action: Analgesic: 10-30 minutes
Duration of Action: 6-8 hours
Absorption: I.M., SubQ: 30% to 40%
Protein Binding: High
Half-Life Elimination: 2.2-3 hours
Metabolism: Primarily hepatic; extensive first-pass effect
Excretion: Feces (70%); urine (20% as unchanged drug)

Dosing
Adults: Long-term use is not recommended
Note: These are guidelines and do not represent the maximum doses that may be required in all patients. Doses should be titrated to pain relief/prevention. In high-risk patients (eg, elderly, debilitated, presence of respiratory disease) and/or concurrent CNS depressant use, reduce dose by one-half. Buprenorphine has an analgesic ceiling.
Acute pain (moderate to severe):
I.M.: Initial: Opiate-naive: 0.3 mg every 6-8 hours as needed; initial dose (up to 0.3 mg) may be repeated once in 30-60 minutes after the initial dose if needed; usual dosage range: 0.15-0.6 mg every 4-8 hours as needed
Slow I.V.: Initial: Opiate-naive: 0.3 mg every 6-8 hours as needed; initial dose (up to 0.3 mg) may be repeated once in 30-60 minutes after the initial dose if needed
Heroin or opiate withdrawal (unlabeled use): I.M., slow I.V.: Variable; 0.1-0.4 mg every 6 hours
Opioid dependence: Sublingual:
Induction: Range: 12-16 mg/day (doses during an induction study used 8 mg on day 1, followed by 16 mg on day 2; induction continued over 3-4 days). Treatment should begin at least 4 hours after last use of heroin or short-acting opioid, preferably when first signs of withdrawal appear. Titrating dose to clinical effectiveness should be done as rapidly as possible to prevent undue withdrawal symptoms and patient drop-out during the induction period.
Maintenance: Target dose: 16 mg/day; range: 4-24 mg/day; patients should be switched to the buprenorphine/naloxone combination product for maintenance and unsupervised therapy
Elderly: Moderate to severe pain: I.M., slow I.V.: 0.15 mg every 6 hours; elderly patients are more likely to suffer from confusion and drowsiness compared to younger patients. **Long-term use is not recommended.**
Pediatrics:
Children 2-12 years: Moderate to severe pain: I.M., slow I.V.: 2-6 mcg/kg every 4-6 hours
Children ≥13 years: Management of moderate to severe pain or opioid dependence: Refer to adult dosing.

Available Dosage Forms
Injection, solution (Buprenex®): 0.3 mg/mL (1 mL)
Tablet, sublingual (Subutex®): 2 mg, 8 mg

Monitoring and Teaching Issues
Physical Assessment: Assess other medications patient may be taking for possible additive or adverse interactions. Monitor for effectiveness of pain relief and adverse reactions or overdose (can cause respiratory depression) at beginning of therapy and at regular intervals with long-term use. For inpatients, implement safety measures. Assess knowledge/teach patient appropriate use (if self-administered). Teach patient to monitor and report adverse reactions and appropriate interventions to reduce side effects.
Monitoring Laboratory Tests: LFTs
Patient Education: If self-administered, use exactly as directed; do not increase dose or frequency. While using this medication, do not use alcohol and other prescription or OTC
(Continued)

Buprenorphine *(Continued)*

medications (especially sedatives, tranquilizers, antihistamines, or pain medications) without consulting prescriber. May cause dizziness, drowsiness, confusion, or blurred vision (use caution when driving, climbing stairs, rising from sitting or lying position, or engaging in tasks requiring alertness until response to drug is known). You may experience nausea or vomiting (frequent mouth care, small frequent meals, sucking lozenges, or chewing gum may help); or constipation (increased exercise, fluids, or dietary fruit and fiber may help). If constipation is unresolved, consult prescriber about use of stool softeners and/or laxatives. Report unresolved nausea or vomiting; respiratory difficulty or shortness of breath; excessive sedation or unusual weakness; or rapid heartbeat or palpitations. **Pregnancy/breast-feeding precautions:** Inform prescriber if you are or intend to become pregnant. Breast-feeding is not recommended.

Pregnancy Risk Factor: C

Pregnancy Issues: Withdrawal has been reported in infants of women receiving buprenorphine during pregnancy. Onset of symptoms ranged from day 1 to day 8 of life, most occurring on day 1.

Lactation: Enters breast milk/not recommended

Administration

Oral: Sublingual: Tablet should be placed under the tongue until dissolved; should not be swallowed. If 2 or more tablets are needed per dose, all may be placed under the tongue at once, or 2 at a time; to ensure consistent bioavailability, subsequent doses should always be taken the same way.

I.V.: Administer slowly, over at least 2 minutes.

Compatibility: Injection:

Y-site administration: Incompatible with amphotericin B cholesteryl sulfate complex, doxorubicin liposome

Compatibility when admixed: Incompatible with diazepam, floxacillin, furosemide, lorazepam

Storage:

Injection: Protect from excessive heat of >40°C (>104°F) and light.

Tablet: Store at room temperature of 25°C (77°F).

Additional Information

Buprenorphine injection: 0.3 mg = 10 mg morphine or 75 mg meperidine, has longer duration of action than either agent

Subutex® (buprenorphine) should be limited to supervised use whenever possible; patients should be switched to Suboxone® (buprenorphine/naloxone) for maintenance and unsupervised therapy

Related Information

Narcotic / Opioid Analgesic Comparison *on page 1739*

Buprenorphine and Naloxone *(byoo pre NOR feen & nal OKS one)*

U.S. Brand Names Suboxone®

Synonyms Buprenorphine Hydrochloride and Naloxone Hydrochloride Dihydrate; Naloxone and Buprenorphine; Naloxone Hydrochloride Dihydrate and Buprenorphine Hydrochloride

Controlled Substance C-III; Prescribing of tablets for opioid dependence is limited to physicians who have met the qualification criteria and have received a DEA number specific to prescribing this product. Tablets will be available through pharmacies and wholesalers which normally provide controlled substances.

Generic Available No

Pharmacologic Category Analgesic, Narcotic

Use Treatment of opioid dependence

Dosing

Adults: Opioid dependence: Sublingual: **Note:** This combination product is not recommended for use during the induction period; initial treatment should begin using buprenorphine oral tablets. Patients should be switched to the combination product for maintenance and unsupervised therapy.

Maintenance: Target dose (based on buprenorphine content): 16 mg/day; range: 4-24 mg/day

Pediatrics: Children ≥16 years: Opioid dependence: Refer to adult dosing.

Available Dosage Forms Tablet, sublingual: Buprenorphine 2 mg and naloxone 0.5 mg; buprenorphine 8 mg and naloxone 2 mg [lemon-lime flavor]

Monitoring and Teaching Issues

Physical Assessment: See individual agents.

Patient Education: If self-administered, use exactly as directed; do not increase dose or frequency. While using this medication, do not use alcohol, other prescriptions, or OTC medications (especially sedatives, tranquilizers, antihistamines, or pain medications) without consulting prescriber. May cause dizziness, drowsiness, confusion, or blurred vision (use caution when driving, climbing stairs, or changing position - rising from sitting or lying to standing, or when engaging in tasks requiring alertness until response to drug is known). You may experience nausea or vomiting (frequent mouth care, small frequent meals, sucking lozenges, or chewing gum may help); or constipation (increased exercise, fluids, or dietary fruit and fiber may help). If constipation is unresolved, consult prescriber about use of stool softeners and/or laxatives. Report unresolved nausea or vomiting; respiratory difficulty or shortness of breath; excessive sedation or unusual weakness; rapid heartbeat or palpitations. In case of an emergency, notify prescriber and emergency room staff you are taking this medication. **Pregnancy/breast-feeding precautions:** Inform prescriber if you are or intend to become pregnant. Breast-feeding is not recommended.

Pregnancy Risk Factor: C

Lactation: Buprenorphine: Enters breast milk/not recommended

Related Information

Buprenorphine *on page 216*
Naloxone *on page 1052*

♦ **Buprenorphine Hydrochloride** *see* Buprenorphine *on page 216*
♦ **Buprenorphine Hydrochloride and Naloxone Hydrochloride Dihydrate** *see* Buprenorphine and Naloxone *on page 218*

BuPROPion (byoo PROE pee on)

U.S. Brand Names Wellbutrin®; Wellbutrin SR®; Wellbutrin XL™; Zyban®

Restrictions A medication guide should be dispensed with each prescription. A template for the required MedGuides can be found on the FDA website at: http://www.fda.gov/cder/drug/antidepressants/labelTemplate.pdf

Generic Available Yes: Excludes Wellbutrin XL™

Pharmacologic Category Antidepressant, Dopamine-Reuptake Inhibitor; Smoking Cessation Aid

Medication Safety Issues
Sound-alike/look-alike issues:
BuPROPion may be confused with busPIRone
Wellbutrin SR® may be confused with Wellbutrin XL™
Wellbutrin XL™ may be confused with Wellbutrin SR®
Zyban® may be confused with Zagam®

Use Treatment of depression; adjunct in smoking cessation

Unlabeled/Investigational Use Attention-deficit/hyperactivity disorder (ADHD)

Mechanism of Action/Effect Antidepressant structurally different from all other marketed antidepressants; like other antidepressants the mechanism of bupropion's activity is not fully understood; relatively weak inhibitor of the neuronal uptake of serotonin, norepinephrine, and dopamine

Contraindications Hypersensitivity to bupropion or any component of the formulation; seizure disorder; anorexia/bulimia; use of MAO inhibitors within 14 days; patients undergoing abrupt discontinuation of ethanol or sedatives (including benzodiazepines); patients receiving other dosage forms of bupropion

Warnings/Precautions Antidepressants increase the risk of suicidal thinking and behavior in children and adolescents with major depressive disorder (MDD) and other depressive disorders; consider risk prior to prescribing. All patients must be closely monitored for clinical worsening, suicidality, or unusual changes in behavior, especially during the initiation of therapy or following an increase or decrease in dosage. When used in children, the child's family or caregiver should be instructed to closely observe the patient and communicate condition with healthcare provider. A medication guide should be dispensed with each prescription. **Bupropion is not FDA approved for use in children.**

The possibility of a suicide attempt is inherent in major depression and may persist until remission occurs. Use caution in high-risk patients. Worsening depression and severe abrupt suicidality that are not part of the presenting symptoms may require discontinuation or modification of drug therapy. The patient's family or caregiver should be alerted to monitor patients for the emergence of suicidality and associated behaviors (such as agitation, irritability, hostility, impulsivity, and hypomania) and notify the healthcare provider.

May worsen psychosis in some patients or precipitate a shift to mania or hypomania in patients with bipolar disorder. Patients presenting with depressive symptoms should be screened for bipolar disorder. Monotherapy in patients with bipolar disorder should be avoided. **Bupropion is not FDA approved for bipolar depression.**

When using immediate release tablets, seizure risk is increased at total daily dosage >450 mg, individual dosages >150 mg, or by sudden, large increments in dose. Data for the immediate-release formulation of bupropion revealed a seizure incidence of 0.4% in patients treated at doses in the 300-450 mg/day range. The estimated seizure incidence increases almost 10-fold between 450 mg and 600 mg per day. Data for the sustained release dosage form revealed a seizure incidence of 0.1% in patients treated at a dosage range of 100-300 mg/day, and increases to ~0.4% at the maximum recommended dose of 400 mg/day. The risk of seizures is increased in patients with a history of seizures, anorexia/bulimia, head trauma, CNS tumor, severe hepatic cirrhosis, abrupt discontinuation of sedative-hypnotics or ethanol, medications which lower seizure threshold (antipsychotics, antidepressants, theophyllines, systemic steroids), stimulants, or hypoglycemic agents. Discontinue and do not restart in patients experiencing a seizure. May cause CNS stimulation (restlessness, anxiety, insomnia) or anorexia. May increase the risks associated with electroconvulsive therapy. Consider discontinuing, when possible, prior to elective surgery. May cause weight loss; use caution in patients where weight loss is not desirable. The incidence of sexual dysfunction with bupropion is generally lower than with SSRIs.

Use caution in patients with cardiovascular disease, history of hypertension, or coronary artery disease; treatment-emergent hypertension (including some severe cases) has been reported, both with bupropion alone and in combination with nicotine transdermal systems. Use with caution in patients with hepatic or renal dysfunction and in elderly patients. Elderly patients may be at greater risk of accumulation during chronic dosing. May cause motor or cognitive impairment in some patients, use with caution if tasks requiring alertness such as operating machinery or driving are undertaken. Arthralgia, myalgia, and fever with rash and other symptoms suggestive of delayed hypersensitivity resembling serum sickness reported.

Drug Interactions
Cytochrome P450 Effect: Substrate of CYP1A2 (minor), 2A6 (minor), 2B6 (major), 2C8/9 (minor), 2D6 (minor), 2E1 (minor), 3A4 (minor); **Inhibits** CYP2D6 (weak)
Decreased Effect: CYP2B6 inducers may decrease the levels/effects of bupropion; example inducers include carbamazepine, nevirapine, phenobarbital, phenytoin, and rifampin. Effect of warfarin may be altered by bupropion.
Increased Effect/Toxicity: Treatment-emergent hypertension may occur in patients treated with bupropion and nicotine patch. Cimetidine may inhibit the metabolism (increase clinical/adverse effects) of bupropion. Toxicity of bupropion is enhanced by levodopa and phenelzine (MAO inhibitors). Risk of seizures may be increased with agents that may lower seizure threshold (antipsychotics, antidepressants, theophylline, abrupt discontinuation of benzodiazepines, systemic steroids). Effect of warfarin may be altered by bupropion.
(Continued)

BuPROPion (Continued)

Concurrent use with amantadine appears to result in a higher incidence of adverse effects; use caution. CYP2B6 inhibitors may increase the levels/effects of bupropion; example inhibitors include desipramine, paroxetine, and sertraline. Combined use of CYP2B6 inhibitors (orphenadrine, thiotepa, cyclophosphamide) with bupropion may increase serum concentrations and may result in seizures.

Nutritional/Ethanol Interactions

Ethanol: Ethanol (may increase CNS depression).

Herb/Nutraceutical: Avoid valerian, St John's wort, SAMe, gotu kola, kava kava (may increase CNS depression).

Lab Interactions Decreased prolactin levels

Adverse Reactions Frequencies, when reported, reflect highest incidence reported with sustained release product.

>10%:

Central nervous system: Dizziness (11%), headache (25%), insomnia (16%)

Gastrointestinal: Nausea (18%), xerostomia (24%)

Respiratory: Pharyngitis (11%)

1% to 10%:

Cardiovascular: Arrhythmias, chest pain (4%), flushing, hypertension (may be severe), hypotension, palpitation (5%), syncope, tachycardia

Central nervous system: Agitation (9%), anxiety (6%), confusion, depression, euphoria, hostility, irritability (2%), memory decreased (3%), migraine, nervousness (3%), sleep disturbance, somnolence (3%)

Dermatologic: Pruritus (4%), rash (4%), sweating increased (5%), urticaria (1%)

Endocrine & metabolic: Hot flashes, libido decreased, menstrual complaints

Gastrointestinal: Abdominal pain, anorexia (3%), appetite increased, constipation (5%), diarrhea (7%), dyspepsia, dysphagia (2%), taste perversion (4%), vomiting (2%)

Genitourinary: Urinary frequency (5%)

Neuromuscular & skeletal: Arthralgia (4%), arthritis (2%), myalgia (6%), neck pain, paresthesia (2%), tremor (3%), twitching (2%)

Ocular: Amblyopia (2%), blurred vision

Otic: Auditory disturbance, tinnitus (6%)

Respiratory: Cough increased (2%), sinusitis (1%)

Miscellaneous: Allergic reaction (including anaphylaxis, pruritus, urticaria), infection

Overdosage/Toxicology Symptoms of overdose include labored breathing, salivation, ataxia, and convulsions. Dialysis may be of limited value after drug absorption because of slow tissue-to-plasma diffusion. Treatment is symptomatic and supportive.

Pharmacodynamics/Kinetics

Absorption: Rapid

Bioavailability: 5% to 20% in animals

Time to Peak: Bupropion: ~3 hours; Bupropion extended release: ~5 hours

Metabolites (hydroxybupropion, erythrohydrobupropion, threohydrobupropion): 6 hours

Protein Binding: 82% to 88%

Half-Life Elimination: Half-life:

Distribution: 3-4 hours

Elimination: 21 ± 9 hours; Metabolites: Hydroxybupropion: 20 ± 5 hours; Erythrohydrobupropion: 33 ± 10 hours; Threohydrobupropion: 37 ± 13 hours

Metabolism: Extensively hepatic to 3 active metabolites: Hydroxybupropion, erythrohydrobupropion, threohydrobupropion (metabolite activity ranges from $^1/_5$ to $^1/_2$ potency of bupropion)

Excretion: Urine (87%); feces (10%)

Dosing

Adults:

Depression: Oral:

Immediate release: 100 mg 3 times/day; begin at 100 mg twice daily; may increase to a maximum dose of 450 mg/day.

Sustained release: Initial: 150 mg/day in the morning; may increase to 150 mg twice daily by day 4 if tolerated; target dose: 300 mg/day given as 150 mg twice daily; maximum dose: 400 mg/day given as 200 mg twice daily.

Extended release: Initial: 150 mg/day in the morning; may increase as early as day 4 of dosing to 300 mg/day; maximum dose: 450 mg/day

Smoking cessation (Zyban®): Oral: Initiate with 150 mg once daily for 3 days; increase to 150 mg twice daily; treatment should continue for 7-12 weeks.

Elderly:

Depression: Oral: Initial: 37.5 mg of immediate release tablets twice daily or 100 mg/day of sustained release tablets; increase by 37.5-100 mg every 3-4 days as tolerated. **Note:** There is evidence that the elderly respond at 150 mg/day in divided doses, but some may require a higher dose.

Smoking cessation: Refer to adult dosing.

Pediatrics: ADHD (unlabeled use): Oral: Children and Adolescents: 1.4-6 mg/kg/day

Renal Impairment: Effect of renal disease on bupropion's pharmacokinetics has not been studied; elimination of the major metabolites of bupropion may be affected by reduced renal function. Patients with renal failure should receive a reduced dosage initially and be closely monitored.

Hepatic Impairment:

Mild to moderate hepatic impairment: Use with caution and/or reduced dose/frequency

Severe hepatic cirrhosis: Use with extreme caution; maximum dose:

Wellbutrin®: 75 mg/day;

Wellbutrin SR®: 100 mg/day or 150 mg every other day;

Wellbutrin XL™: 150 mg every other day

Zyban®: 150 mg every other day

Note: The mean AUC increased by ~1.5-fold for hydroxybupropion and ~2.5-fold for erythro/threohydrobupropion; median T_{max} was observed 19 hours later for hydroxybupropion, 31 hours later for erythro/threohydrobupropion; mean half-life for hydroxybupropion increased fivefold, and increased twofold for erythro/threohydrobupropion in patients with severe hepatic cirrhosis compared to healthy volunteers.

Available Dosage Forms
Tablet, as hydrochloride (Wellbutrin®): 75 mg, 100 mg
Tablet, extended release, as hydrochloride (Wellbutrin XL™): 150 mg, 300 mg
Tablet, sustained release, as hydrochloride: 100 mg, 150 mg [equivalent to Wellbutrin® SR], 150 mg [equivalent to Zyban®]
Wellbutrin® SR: 100 mg, 150 mg, 200 mg
Zyban®: 150 mg

Monitoring and Teaching Issues
Physical Assessment: Assess other medications patient may be taking for effectiveness and interactions. Monitor therapeutic effectiveness and adverse reactions at beginning of therapy and periodically with long-term use. Monitor for clinical worsening and suicidality, especially at the beginning of therapy or when dose changes occur. Taper dosage slowly when discontinuing. Assess knowledge/teach patient appropriate use, interventions to reduce side effects, and adverse symptoms to report.

Patient Education: Be aware that bupropion is marketed under different names and should not be taken together; Zyban® is for smoking cessation and Wellbutrin® is for treatment of depression. **Note:** Excessive use or abrupt discontinuation of alcohol or sedatives may alter seizure threshold.

Depression: Take as directed, in equally divided doses; do not take in larger dose or more often than recommended. Do not discontinue without consulting prescriber. Do not use alcohol or OTC medications not approved by prescriber. May cause drowsiness, clouded sensorium, headache, restlessness, or agitation (use caution when driving or engaging in tasks requiring alertness until response to drug is known); nausea, vomiting, or dry mouth (small frequent meals, frequent mouth care, chewing gum, or sucking lozenges may help); constipation (increased exercise, fluids, fruit, or fiber may help); or impotence (reversible). Report persistent CNS effects (eg, agitation, confusion, anxiety, restlessness, insomnia, psychosis, hallucinations, seizures); suicidal ideation; muscle weakness or tremor; skin rash or irritation; chest pain or palpitations, abdominal pain or blood in stools; yellowing of skin or eyes; or respiratory difficulty, bronchitis, or unusual cough.

Smoking cessation: Use as directed; do not take extra doses. Do not combine nicotine patches with use of Zyban® unless approved by prescriber. May cause dry mouth and insomnia (these may resolve with continued use). Report any respiratory difficulty, unusual cough, dizziness, or muscle tremors.

Breast-feeding precaution: Breast-feeding is not recommended.
Geriatric Considerations: Limited data is available about the use of bupropion in the elderly. Two studies have found it equally effective when compared to imipramine. Its side effect profile (minimal anticholinergic and blood pressure effects) may make it useful in persons who do not tolerate traditional cyclic antidepressants.
Pregnancy Risk Factor: B
Lactation: Enters breast milk/not recommended (AAP rates "of concern")
Breast-Feeding Issues: Generally, it is not recommended to breast-feed if taking antidepressants because of the long half-life, active metabolites, and the potential for side effects in the infant.

Administration
Oral: May be taken without regard to meals. Zyban® and extended release tablets should be swallowed whole; do not crush, chew, or divide. The insoluble shell of the extended-release tablet may remain intact during GI transit and is eliminated in the feces. Wellbutrin® SR may be divided, but not crushed or chewed.
Storage: Store at controlled of 20°C to 25°C (68°F to 77°F).

Related Information
Antidepressant Agents on page 1713
Antidepressant Medication Guidelines on page 1765
FDA Name Differentiation Project: The Use of Tall-Man Letters on page 15

♦ **Burnamycin [OTC]** see Lidocaine on page 898
♦ **Burn Jel [OTC]** see Lidocaine on page 898
♦ **Burn-O-Jel [OTC]** see Lidocaine on page 898
♦ **BuSpar®** see BusPIRone on page 221

BusPIRone (byoo SPYE rone)
U.S. Brand Names BuSpar®
Synonyms Buspirone Hydrochloride
Generic Available Yes
Pharmacologic Category Antianxiety Agent, Miscellaneous
Medication Safety Issues
Sound-alike/look-alike issues:
BusPIRone may be confused with buPROPion
Use Management of generalized anxiety disorder (GAD)
Unlabeled/Investigational Use Management of aggression in mental retardation and secondary mental disorders; major depression; potential augmenting agent for antidepressants; premenstrual syndrome
Mechanism of Action/Effect The mechanism of action of buspirone is unknown. Buspirone has a high affinity for serotonin 5-HT$_{1A}$ and 5-HT$_2$ receptors, without affecting benzodiazepine-GABA receptors. Buspirone has moderate affinity for dopamine D$_2$ receptors.
Contraindications Hypersensitivity to buspirone or any component of the formulation
Warnings/Precautions Safety and efficacy not established in children <18 years of age; use in hepatic or renal impairment is not recommended; does not prevent or treat withdrawal from (Continued)

BusPIRone (Continued)

benzodiazepines; low potential for cognitive or motor impairment. Use with MAO inhibitors may result in hypertensive reactions.

Drug Interactions

Cytochrome P450 Effect: Substrate of CYP2D6 (minor), 3A4 (major)

Decreased Effect: CYP3A4 inducers may decrease the levels/effects of buspirone; example inducers include aminoglutethimide, carbamazepine, nafcillin, nevirapine, phenobarbital, phenytoin, and rifamycins.

Increased Effect/Toxicity: Concurrent use of buspirone with SSRIs or trazodone may cause serotonin syndrome. Buspirone should not be used concurrently with an MAO inhibitor due to reports of increased blood pressure; theoretically, a selective MAO type B inhibitors (selegiline) has a lower risk of this reaction. Concurrent use of buspirone with nefazodone may increase risk of CNS adverse events; limit buspirone initial dose (eg, 2.5 mg/day). CYP3A4 inhibitors may increase the levels/effects of buspirone; example inhibitors include azole antifungals, ciprofloxacin, clarithromycin, diclofenac, doxycycline, erythromycin, imatinib, isoniazid, nefazodone, nicardipine, propofol, protease inhibitors, quinidine, and verapamil.

Nutritional/Ethanol Interactions

Ethanol: Ethanol (may increase CNS depression).

Food: Food may decrease the absorption of buspirone, but it may also decrease the first-pass metabolism, thereby increasing the bioavailability of buspirone. Grapefruit juice may cause increased buspirone concentrations; avoid concurrent use.

Herb/Nutraceutical: St John's wort may decrease buspirone levels or increase CNS depression. Avoid valerian, gotu kola, kava kava (may increase CNS depression).

Lab Interactions Increased AST, ALT, growth hormone(s), prolactin (S)

Adverse Reactions

>10%: Central nervous system: Dizziness

1% to 10%:

Central nervous system: Drowsiness, EPS, serotonin syndrome, confusion, nervousness, lightheadedness, excitement, anger, hostility, headache

Dermatologic: Rash

Gastrointestinal: Diarrhea, nausea

Neuromuscular & skeletal: Muscle weakness, numbness, paresthesia, incoordination, tremor

Ocular: Blurred vision, tunnel vision

Miscellaneous: Diaphoresis, allergic reactions

Overdosage/Toxicology Symptoms of overdose include dizziness, drowsiness, pinpoint pupils, nausea, and vomiting. There is no known antidote for buspirone. Treatment is supportive.

Pharmacodynamics/Kinetics

Absorption: Oral: ~100%

Bioavailability: ~4%

Time to Peak: Serum: Within 0.7-1.5 hours

Protein Binding: 95%

Half-Life Elimination: Mean: 2.4 hours (range: 2-11 hours)

Metabolism: Hepatic via oxidation; extensive first-pass effect

Excretion: Urine: 65%; feces: 35%; ~1% dose excreted unchanged

Dosing

Adults: Anxiety disorders (GAD): Oral: 15 mg/day (7.5 mg twice daily); may increase in increments of 5 mg/day every 2-4 days to a maximum of 60 mg/day. Target dose for most people is 30 mg/day (15 mg twice daily).

Elderly: Oral: Initial: 5 mg twice daily, increase by 5 mg/day every 2-3 days as needed up to 20-30 mg/day; maximum daily dose: 60 mg/day (see Geriatric Considerations).

Pediatrics:

Generalized anxiety disorder (GAD): Oral: Children and Adolescents: Initial: 5 mg daily; increase in increments of 5 mg/day at weekly intervals as needed, to a maximum dose of 60 mg/day divided into 2-3 doses

Renal Impairment: Use in patients with severe renal impairment cannot be recommended.

Hepatic Impairment: Buspirone is metabolized by the liver and excreted by the kidneys. Patients with impaired hepatic or renal function demonstrated increased plasma levels and a prolonged half-life of buspirone. Therefore, use in patients with severe hepatic or renal impairment cannot be recommended.

Available Dosage Forms Tablet, as hydrochloride: 5 mg, 7.5 mg, 10 mg, 15 mg, 30 mg

BuSpar®: 5 mg, 10 mg, 15 mg, 30 mg

Monitoring and Teaching Issues

Physical Assessment: Assess other medications patient may be taking for effectiveness and interactions. Monitor therapeutic effectiveness and adverse reactions at beginning of therapy and periodically with long-term use. Assess knowledge/teach patient appropriate use, interventions to reduce side effects, and adverse symptoms to report.

Patient Education: Take only as directed; do not increase dose or take more often than prescribed. May take 2-3 weeks to see full effect; do not discontinue without consulting prescriber. Do not use alcohol or other prescription or OTC medications (especially pain medications, sedatives, antihistamines, or hypnotics) without consulting prescriber. Maintain adequate hydration (2-3 L/day of fluids) unless instructed to restrict fluid intake. You may experience drowsiness, lightheadedness, impaired coordination, dizziness, or blurred vision (use caution when driving or engaging in tasks requiring alertness until response to drug is known); or upset stomach, nausea (small frequent meals, frequent mouth care, chewing gum, or sucking lozenges may help). Report persistent vomiting; chest pain or rapid heartbeat; persistent CNS effects (eg, confusion, restlessness, anxiety, insomnia, excitation, headache, dizziness, fatigue, impaired coordination); or worsening of condition.

Breast-feeding precaution: Breast-feeding is not recommended.

Geriatric Considerations: Because buspirone is less sedating than other anxiolytics, it may be a useful agent in geriatric patients when an anxiolytic is indicated.

Pregnancy Risk Factor: B

Lactation: Excretion in breast milk unknown/not recommended

Additional Information Has shown little potential for abuse; needs continuous use. Because of slow onset, not appropriate for "as needed" (prn) use or for brief, situational anxiety. Ineffective for treatment of benzodiazepine or ethanol withdrawal.

Related Information
FDA Name Differentiation Project: The Use of Tall-Man Letters *on page 15*

♦ Buspirone Hydrochloride *see BusPIRone on page 221*

Busulfan (byoo SUL fan)

U.S. Brand Names Busulfex®; Myleran®

Generic Available No

Pharmacologic Category Antineoplastic Agent, Alkylating Agent

Medication Safety Issues
Sound-alike/look-alike issues:
Busulfan may be confused with Butalan®
Myleran® may be confused with melphalan, Mylicon®

Use
Oral: Chronic myelogenous leukemia; conditioning regimens for bone marrow transplantation
I.V.: Combination therapy with cyclophosphamide as a conditioning regimen prior to allogeneic hematopoietic progenitor cell transplantation for chronic myelogenous leukemia

Unlabeled/Investigational Use Oral: Bone marrow disorders, such as polycythemia vera and myeloid metaplasia; thrombocytosis

Mechanism of Action/Effect Interferes with DNA function; cytotoxic

Contraindications Hypersensitivity to busulfan or any component of the formulation; failure to respond to previous courses; pregnancy

Warnings/Precautions The U.S. Food and Drug Administration (FDA) currently recommends that procedures for proper handling and disposal of antineoplastic agents be considered. May induce severe bone marrow hypoplasia; reduce or discontinue dosage at first sign, as reflected by an abnormal decrease in any of the formed elements of the blood; use with caution in patients recently given other myelosuppressive drugs or radiation treatment. If white blood count is high, hydration and allopurinol should be employed to prevent hyperuricemia. Use caution in patients predisposed to seizures. Discontinue if lung toxicity develops. Busulfan has been causally related to the development of secondary malignancies (tumors and acute leukemias). Busulfan has been associated with ovarian failure (including failure to achieve puberty) in females. Avoid I.M. injections if platelet count falls to <100,000/mm³. High busulfan area under the concentration versus time curve (AUC) values (>1500 µM/minute) are associated with increased risk of hepatic veno-occlusive disease during conditioning for allogenic BMT.

Drug Interactions
Cytochrome P450 Effect: Substrate of CYP3A4 (major)
Decreased Effect: CYP3A4 inducers may decrease the levels/effects of busulfan; example inducers include aminoglutethimide, carbamazepine, nafcillin, nevirapine, phenobarbital, phenytoin, and rifamycins.
Increased Effect/Toxicity: CYP3A4 inhibitors may increase the levels/effects of busulfan; example inhibitors include azole antifungals, ciprofloxacin, clarithromycin, diclofenac, doxycycline, erythromycin, imatinib, isoniazid, nefazodone, nicardipine, propofol, protease inhibitors, quinidine, and verapamil. Metronidazole may increase busulfan plasma levels.

Nutritional/Ethanol Interactions
Ethanol: Avoid ethanol due to GI irritation.
Food: No clear or firm data on the effect of food on busulfan bioavailability.
Herb/Nutraceutical: St John's wort may decrease busulfan levels.

Adverse Reactions
Fertility/carcinogenesis: Sterility, ovarian suppression, amenorrhea, azoospermia, and testicular atrophy; malignant tumors have been reported in patients on busulfan therapy.

>10%: Hematologic: Severe pancytopenia, leukopenia, thrombocytopenia, anemia, and bone marrow suppression are common and patients should be monitored closely while on therapy. Since this is a delayed effect (busulfan affects the stem cells), the drug should be discontinued temporarily at the first sign of a large or rapid fall in any blood element. Some patients may develop bone marrow fibrosis or chronic aplasia which is probably due to the busulfan toxicity. In large doses, busulfan is myeloablative and is used for this reason in BMT. Myelosuppressive:
WBC: Moderate
Platelets: Moderate
Onset: 7-10 days
Nadir: 14-21 days
Recovery: 28 days
1% to 10%:
Dermatologic: Hyperpigmentation skin (busulfan tan), urticaria, erythema, alopecia
Endocrine & metabolic: Amenorrhea
Gastrointestinal: Nausea, vomiting, diarrhea; drug has little effect on the GI mucosal lining
Neuromuscular & skeletal: Weakness

Overdosage/Toxicity Symptoms of overdose include leukopenia and thrombocytopenia. Induction of vomiting or gastric lavage with charcoal is indicated for recent ingestion; the effects of dialysis are unknown.
(Continued)

Busulfan *(Continued)*

Pharmacodynamics/Kinetics
Duration of Action: 28 days

Absorption: Rapid and complete

Time to Peak: Serum: Oral: Within 4 hours; I.V.: Within 5 minutes

Protein Binding: ~14%

Half-Life Elimination: After first dose: 3.4 hours; After last dose: 2.3 hours

Metabolism: Extensively hepatic (may increase with multiple dosing)

Excretion: Urine (10% to 50% as metabolites) within 24 hours (<2% as unchanged drug)

Dosing
Adults: Refer to individual protocols.

  Note: Busulfan should be based on adjusted ideal body weight because actual body weight, ideal body weight, or other factors can produce significant differences in busulfan clearance among lean, normal, and obese patients.

  CML remission induction: Oral: 4-8 mg/day (may be as high as 12 mg/day); Maintenance doses: Controversial, range from 1-4 mg/day to 2 mg/week; treatment is continued until WBC reaches 10,000-20,000 cells/mm³ at which time drug is discontinued; when WBC reaches 50,000/mm³, maintenance dose is resumed

  BMT marrow-ablative conditioning regimen:
    Oral: 1 mg/kg/dose (ideal body weight) every 6 hours for 16 doses
    I.V.: 0.8 mg/kg (ideal body weight or actual body weight, whichever is lower) every 6 hours for 4 days (a total of 16 doses)
    I.V. dosing in morbidly obese patients: Dosing should be based on adjusted ideal body weight (AIBW) which should be calculated as ideal body weight (IBW) + 0.25 times (actual weight minus ideal body weight)
    AIBW = IBW + 0.25 x (AW - IBW)

  Polycythemia vera (unlabeled use): Oral: 2-6 mg/day

  Thrombocytosis (unlabeled use): Oral: 4-6 mg/day

Elderly: Oral (refer to individual protocols): Start with lowest recommended doses for adults.

Pediatrics: Refer to individual protocols.

  Note: Busulfan should be based on adjusted ideal body weight because actual body weight, ideal body weight, or other factors can produce significant differences in busulfan clearance among lean, normal, and obese patients. Refer to individual protocols.

  CML remission: Oral: Children: Induction: 0.06-0.12 mg/kg/day **or** 1.8-4.6 mg/m²/day; titrate dosage to maintain leukocyte count above 40,000/mm³; reduce dosage by 50% if the leukocyte count reaches 30,000-40,000/mm³; discontinue drug if counts fall to ≤20,000/mm³.

  BMT marrow-ablative conditioning regimen:
    Oral: 1 mg/kg/dose (ideal body weight) every 6 hours for 16 doses
    I.V.:
      ≤12 kg: 1.1 mg/kg/dose (ideal body weight) every 6 hours for 16 doses
      >12 kg: 0.8 mg/kg/dose (ideal body weight) every 6 hours for 16 doses
      Adjust dose to desired AUC [1125 μmol(min)] using the following formula:
      Adjusted dose (mg) = Actual dose (mg) x [target AUC μmol(min) / actual AUC μmol(min)]

Available Dosage Forms
Injection, solution (Busulfex®): 6 mg/mL (10 mL)

Tablet (Myleran®): 2 mg

Monitoring and Teaching Issues
Physical Assessment: Identify any history of seizures, recent myelosuppressive therapy or radiation treatment, and pregnancy status prior to therapy (see Contraindications and Warnings/Precautions). Assess potential for interactions with other pharmacological agents or herbal products patient may be taking that may increase or decrease levels/effects of busulfan (see Drug Interactions). Dosing should be based on adjusted ideal body weight (refer to individual protocols). Use phenytoin or clonazepam to reduce risk of seizures (see Administration). Assess results of laboratory tests (CBC with differential, platelet count, LFT) and adverse pulmonary (pulmonary fibrosis) or hematologic effects (pancytopenia, leukopenia, thrombocytopenia, anemia, and bone marrow suppression; see Adverse Reactions) during therapy and for several months following therapy. Teach patient proper use (oral), possible side effects/appropriate interventions, and adverse symptoms to report.

Monitoring Laboratory Tests: CBC with differential and platelet count, liver function

Patient Education: Inform prescriber of all prescriptions, OTC medications, or herbal products you are taking, and any allergies you have. Do not take any new medication during therapy unless approved by prescriber. Take oral medication as directed with chilled liquids. Maintain adequate hydration (2-3 L/day of fluids) unless instructed to restrict fluid intake. Avoid alcohol and acidic or spicy foods. You will be more susceptible to infection (avoid crowds and exposure to infection and do not have any vaccinations unless approved by prescriber). May cause mouth sores (brush teeth with soft toothbrush or cotton swab); loss of hair or darkening of skin color (reversible when medication is discontinued); nausea, vomiting, or anorexia (small frequent meals, chewing gum, or sucking hard candy may help); constipation (increased exercise, fruit, fluids, or fiber may help); amenorrhea; sterility; or skin rash. Report palpitations or chest pain, excessive dizziness, confusion, respiratory difficulty, numbness or tingling of extremities, unusual bruising or bleeding, pain or changes in urination, or other adverse effects. **Pregnancy/breast-feeding precautions:** Inform prescriber if you are pregnant. Do not get pregnant during or for 1 month following therapy. Consult prescriber for instruction on appropriate barrier contraceptive measures. This drug may cause severe fetal defects. Do not breast-feed.

Geriatric Considerations: Toxicity to immunosuppressives is increased in the elderly. Start with lowest recommended adult doses. Signs of infection, such as fever and rise in WBCs, may not occur. Lethargy and confusion may be more prominent signs of infection.

Pregnancy Risk Factor: D
Lactation: Contraindicated

Administration

Oral: BMT only: Phenytoin or clonazepam should be administered prophylactically during and for at least 48 hours following completion of busulfan. Risk of seizures is increased in patients with sickle cell disease. Increased risk of VOD when busulfan AUC >3000 μmol(min)/L (mean AUC, 2012 μmol(min)/L). To facilitate ingestion of high doses, insert multiple tablets into clear gel capsules.

I.V.: Intravenous busulfan should be administered via a **central** venous catheter as a 2-hour infusion, every 6 hours for 4 consecutive days for a total of 16 doses. Do not use polycarbonate syringes.

BMT only: Phenytoin or clonazepam should be administered prophylactically during and for at least 48 hours following completion of busulfan. Risk of seizures is increased in patients with sickle cell disease. Increased risk of VOD when busulfan AUC >3000 μmol(min)/L (mean AUC, 2012 μmol(min)/L). To facilitate ingestion of high doses, insert multiple tablets into clear gel capsules.

Reconstitution: Filter busulfan using the 5 micron syringe filter provided, using one filter per ampul. If using the enclosed syringe filter in the forward flow direction, allow for ~0.16 mL of residual busulfan to remain in the filter. Dilute busulfan injection in 0.9% sodium chloride injection or dextrose 5% in water. The dilution volume should be ten times the volume of busulfan injection, ensuring that the final concentration of busulfan is 0.5 mg/mL.

Storage: Store unopened ampuls (injection) under refrigeration (2°C to 8°C). Final solution is stable for up to 8 hours at room temperature (25°C) but the infusion must also be completed within that 8-hour time frame. Dilution of busulfan injection in 0.9% sodium chloride is stable for up to 12 hours at refrigeration (2°C to 8°C) but the infusion must also be completed within that 12-hour time frame. Do not use polycarbonate syringes.

Related Information
Maternal / Fetal Toxicology *on page 1762*

♦ **Busulfex**® *see* Busulfan *on page 223*

Butalbital, Acetaminophen, and Caffeine
(byoo TAL bi tal, a seet a MIN oh fen, & KAF een)

U.S. Brand Names Anolor 300; Dolgic® LQ; Dolgic® Plus; Esgic®; Esgic-Plus™; Fioricet®; Medigesic®; Repan®; Zebutal™

Synonyms Acetaminophen, Butalbital, and Caffeine

Generic Available Yes: Excludes elixir

Pharmacologic Category Barbiturate

Medication Safety Issues
Sound-alike/look-alike issues:
Fioricet® may be confused with Fiorinal®, Lorcet®
Repan® may be confused with Riopan®

Use Relief of the symptomatic complex of tension or muscle contraction headache

Dosing

Adults: Tension or muscle contraction headache: Oral: 1-2 tablets or capsules (or 15-30 mL elixir) every 4 hours; not to exceed 6 tablets or capsules (or 180 mL elixir) daily

Elderly: Not recommended for use in the elderly.

Renal Impairment: Dosage should be reduced.

Hepatic Impairment: Dosage should be reduced.

Available Dosage Forms
Capsule:
Anolor 300, Esgic®, Medigesic®: Butalbital 50 mg, caffeine 40 mg, and acetaminophen 325 mg
Dolgic® Plus: Butalbital 50 mg, caffeine 40 mg, and acetaminophen 750 mg
Esgic-Plus™, Zebutal™: Butalbital 50 mg, caffeine 40 mg, and acetaminophen 500 mg
Elixir (Dolgic® LQ): Butalbital 50 mg, caffeine 40 mg, and acetaminophen 325 mg per 15 mL (480 mL) [contains alcohol 7%; fruit flavor]
Tablet: Butalbital 50 mg, caffeine 40 mg, and acetaminophen 325 mg; butalbital 50 mg, caffeine 40 mg, and acetaminophen 500 mg
Esgic®, Fioricet®, Repan®: Butalbital 50 mg, caffeine 40 mg, and acetaminophen 325 mg

Monitoring and Teaching Issues

Physical Assessment: Assess patient for history of liver disease or ethanol abuse. Assess other medications patient may be taking for additive or adverse interactions. Monitor therapeutic effectiveness. Assess knowledge/teach patient appropriate use, adverse reactions to report, and appropriate interventions to reduce side effects.

Patient Education: If self-administered, use exactly as directed; do not increase dose or frequency. Drug may cause physical and/or psychological dependence. Take with food or milk. While using this medication, do not use alcohol and other prescription or OTC medications (especially sedatives, tranquilizers, antihistamines, or pain medications) without consulting prescriber. Maintain adequate hydration (2-3 L/day of fluids) unless instructed to restrict fluid intake. May cause dizziness, lightheadedness, confusion, or drowsiness (use caution when driving, climbing stairs, or changing position - rising from sitting or lying to standing, or when engaging in tasks requiring alertness until response to drug is known); heartburn or epigastric discomfort (frequent mouth care, frequent sips of fluids, chewing gum, or sucking lozenges may help); or constipation (increased exercise, fluids, fruit, or fiber may help). Report chest pain or palpitations; persistent dizziness; confusion; nightmares, excitation, or changes in mentation; shortness of breath or respiratory difficulty; skin rash; unusual bleeding or bruising; or unusual fatigue and weakness.

Pregnancy Risk Factor: C

Lactation: Enters breast milk/not recommended

Related Information
Acetaminophen *on page 38*

Butalbital, Acetaminophen, Caffeine, and Codeine
(byoo TAL bi tal, a seet a MIN oh fen, KAF een, & KOE deen)

U.S. Brand Names Fioricet® with Codeine

Synonyms Acetaminophen, Caffeine, Codeine, and Butalbital; Caffeine, Acetaminophen, Butalbital, and Codeine; Codeine, Acetaminophen, Butalbital, and Caffeine

Controlled Substance C-III

Generic Available Yes

Pharmacologic Category Analgesic Combination (Narcotic); Barbiturate

Medication Safety Issues
Sound-alike/look-alike issues:
Fioricet® may be confused with Fiorinal®, Lorcet®

Use Relief of symptoms of complex tension (muscle contraction) headache

Dosing
Adults & Elderly: Oral: Adults: 1-2 capsules every 4 hours. Total daily dosage should not exceed 6 capsules.

Hepatic Impairment: Use with caution. Limited, low-dose therapy usually well tolerated in hepatic disease/cirrhosis. However, cases of hepatotoxicity at daily acetaminophen dosages <4 g/day have been reported. Avoid chronic use in hepatic impairment.

Available Dosage Forms Capsule: Butalbital 50 mg, caffeine 40 mg, acetaminophen 325 mg, and codeine phosphate 30 mg

Monitoring and Teaching Issues
Physical Assessment: See Contraindications, Warnings/Precautions, and Dosing for use cautions. Assess effectiveness and interactions of other prescription, OTC, or herbal medication patient may be taking (see Drug Interactions). Assess history for allergies (see Contraindications). Monitor for effectiveness of pain relief, signs of overdose, and adverse reactions (see Adverse Reactions and Overdose/Toxicology). Discontinue slowly after long-term use. For inpatient use, safety precautions should be implemented. Teach patient proper use, appropriate interventions to reduce side effects, and adverse symptoms to report (see Adverse Reactions and Patient Education).

Patient Education: Inform prescriber of all prescriptions, OTC medications, or herbal products you are taking, and any allergies you have. Do not take any new medication during therapy unless approved by prescriber. Take oral medication as directed with chilled liquids. Use exactly as directed; do not increase dose or frequency. Drug may cause physical and/or psychological dependence. Take with food or milk. Do not use alcohol, other prescriptions, OTC medications, or herbal products (especially sedatives, tranquilizers, antihistamines, or pain medications) without consulting prescriber. Maintain adequate hydration (2-3 L/day of fluids) unless instructed to restrict fluid intake. May cause dizziness, lightheadedness, confusion, or drowsiness (use caution when driving, climbing stairs, or changing position sitting or lying to standing, or when engaging in tasks requiring alertness until response to drug is known); heartburn, nausea (small frequent meals, frequent mouth care, chewing gum, or sucking lozenges may help); or constipation (increased exercise, fluids, fruit, or fiber may help; if unresolved, contact prescriber). Report chest pain or palpitation; persistent dizziness; confusion; nightmares; excitation or changes in mentation; shortness of breath or respiratory difficulty; skin rash or irritation; unusual muscle weakness or leg pain; or ringing in ears. **Pregnancy/breast-feeding precautions:** Inform prescriber if you are or intend to become pregnant. Breast-feeding is not recommended.

Pregnancy Risk Factor: C (per manufacturer); D (prolonged use or high doses at term)
Lactation: Enters breast milk/not recommended

Related Information
Acetaminophen on page 38
Codeine on page 366

Butalbital, Aspirin, and Caffeine (byoo TAL bi tal, AS pir in, & KAF een)
U.S. Brand Names Fiorinal®

Synonyms Aspirin, Caffeine, and Butalbital; Butalbital Compound

Controlled Substance C-III

Generic Available Yes

Pharmacologic Category Barbiturate

Medication Safety Issues
Sound-alike/look-alike issues:
Fiorinal® may be confused with Fioricet®, Florical®, Florinef®

Use Relief of the symptomatic complex of tension or muscle contraction headache

Dosing
Adults: Tension or muscle contraction headache: Oral: 1-2 tablets or capsules every 4 hours; not to exceed 6 tablets or capsules/day

Elderly: Not recommended for use in the elderly.

Renal Impairment: Dosage should be reduced.

Hepatic Impairment: Dosage should be reduced.

Available Dosage Forms Capsule (Fiorinal®): Butalbital 50 mg, caffeine 40 mg, and aspirin 325 mg

Monitoring and Teaching Issues
Physical Assessment: Monitor for effectiveness of pain relief. Monitor CNS status, heart rate, blood pressure, fluid balance, and elimination regularly. Combination drug contains aspirin; assess for aspirin sensitivity.

Patient Education: Take as directed; do not exceed prescribed amount. Avoid alcohol, aspirin or aspirin-containing medications, or any OTC medications unless approved by prescriber. Maintain adequate hydration to prevent constipation (2-3 L/day) unless instructed to restrict fluid intake. You may experience drowsiness, impaired judgment or coordination; use caution when driving or engaging in tasks that require alertness until response to drug is known. Small frequent meals may help reduce GI upset. Report any ringing in ears; abdominal pain; easy bruising or bleeding; blood in urine; severe weakness; acute unresolved dizziness or confusion, nervousness, nightmares, insomnia; or skin rash. **Pregnancy/breast-feeding precautions:** Inform prescriber if you are or intend to become pregnant. Consult prescriber if breast-feeding.

Pregnancy Risk Factor: C/D (prolonged use or high doses at term)

Lactation: Enters breast milk/use caution due to aspirin content

Related Information

Aspirin *on page 143*

Butalbital, Aspirin, Caffeine, and Codeine
(byoo TAL bi tal, AS pir in, KAF een, & KOE deen)

U.S. Brand Names Fiorinal® With Codeine; Phrenilin® With Caffeine and Codeine

Synonyms Butalbital Compound and Codeine; Codeine and Butalbital Compound; Codeine, Butalbital, Aspirin, and Caffeine

Controlled Substance C-III

Generic Available Yes

Pharmacologic Category Analgesic Combination (Narcotic); Barbiturate

Medication Safety Issues

Sound-alike/look-alike issues:

Fiorinal® may be confused with Fioricet®, Florical®, Florinef®

Phrenilin® may be confused with Phenergan®, Trinalin®

Use Mild to moderate pain when sedation is needed

Dosing

Adults: Mild to moderate pain (sedation desired): Oral: 1-2 capsules every 4 hours as needed; up to 6 capsules/day

Elderly: Not recommended for use in the elderly.

Available Dosage Forms Capsule: Butalbital 50 mg, caffeine 40 mg, aspirin 325 mg, and codeine phosphate 30 mg

Fioricet® with Codeine: Butalbital 50 mg, caffeine 40 mg, acetaminophen 325 mg, and codeine phosphate 30 mg [may contain benzyl alcohol]

Phrenilin® with Caffeine and Codeine: Butalbital 50 mg, caffeine 40 mg, acetaminophen 325 mg, and codeine phosphate 30 mg [contains benzyl alcohol and lactose]

Monitoring and Teaching Issues

Physical Assessment: Do not use for persons with allergic reaction to aspirin, opium, or codeine. Assess other medications patient may be taking for additive or adverse interactions Monitor for effectiveness of pain relief, signs of overdose, and adverse reactions at beginning of therapy and at regular intervals with long-term use. May cause physical and/or psychological dependence. Discontinue slowly after long-term use. For inpatients, implement safety. Assess knowledge/teach patient appropriate use if self-administered. Teach patient to monitor for adverse reactions, adverse reactions to report, and appropriate interventions to reduce side effects.

Patient Education: If self-administered, use exactly as directed; do not increase dose or frequency. Drug may cause physical and/or psychological dependence. Take with food or milk. While using this medication, do not use alcohol and other prescription or OTC medications (especially sedatives, tranquilizers, antihistamines, or pain medications) without consulting prescriber. Maintain adequate hydration (2-3 L/day of fluids) unless instructed to restrict fluid intake. May cause dizziness, lightheadedness, confusion, or drowsiness (use caution when driving, climbing stairs, or changing position - rising from sitting or lying to standing, or when engaging in tasks requiring alertness until response to drug is known); heartburn or epigastric discomfort (frequent mouth care, frequent sips of fluids, chewing gum, or sucking lozenges may help); or constipation (increased exercise, fluids, fruit, or fiber may help; if unresolved, consult prescriber about use of stool softeners). Report chest pain or palpitations; persistent dizziness; confusion; nightmares, excitation, or changes in mentation; shortness of breath or respiratory difficulty; skin rash, unusual bleeding or bruising; or unusual fatigue and weakness. **Pregnancy/ breast-feeding precautions:** Inform prescriber if you are or intend to become pregnant. Consult prescriber if breast-feeding.

Pregnancy Risk Factor: C/D (prolonged use or high doses at term)

Lactation: Excretion in breast milk unknown/use caution

Related Information

Aspirin *on page 143*

Codeine *on page 366*

◆ **Butalbital Compound** *see* Butalbital, Aspirin, and Caffeine *on page 226*

◆ **Butalbital Compound and Codeine** *see* Butalbital, Aspirin, Caffeine, and Codeine *on page 227*

Butorphanol (byoo TOR fa nole)

U.S. Brand Names Stadol®; Stadol® NS [DSC]

Synonyms Butorphanol Tartrate

Controlled Substance C-IV

Generic Available Yes

Pharmacologic Category Analgesic, Narcotic

Medication Safety Issues

Sound-alike/look-alike issues:

Stadol® may be confused with Haldol®, sotalol

Use

Parenteral: Management of moderate to severe pain; preoperative medication; supplement to balanced anesthesia; management of pain during labor

Nasal spray: Management of moderate to severe pain, including migraine headache pain

Mechanism of Action/Effect Mixed narcotic agonist-antagonist with central analgesic actions; binds to opiate receptors in the CNS, causing inhibition of ascending pain pathways, altering the perception of and response to pain; produces generalized CNS depression

(Continued)

Butorphanol *(Continued)*

Contraindications Hypersensitivity to butorphanol or any component of the formulation; avoid use in opiate-dependent patients who have not been detoxified, may precipitate opiate withdrawal; pregnancy (prolonged use or high doses at term)

Warnings/Precautions An opioid-containing analgesic regimen should be tailored to each patient's needs and based upon the type of pain being treated (acute versus chronic), the route of administration, degree of tolerance for opioids (naive versus chronic user), age, weight, and medical condition. The optimal analgesic dose varies widely among patients. Doses should be titrated to pain relief/prevention. May cause CNS depression, which may impair physical or mental abilities. Effects with other sedative drugs or ethanol may be potentiated. Use with caution in patients with hepatic/renal dysfunction. Tolerance or drug dependence may result from extended use. Concurrent use of sumatriptan nasal spray and butorphanol nasal spray may increase risk of transient high blood pressure.

Drug Interactions
Increased Effect/Toxicity: Increased toxicity with CNS depressants, phenothiazines, barbiturates, skeletal muscle relaxants, alfentanil, guanabenz, and MAO inhibitors.

Nutritional/Ethanol Interactions
Ethanol: Avoid or limit ethanol (may increase CNS depression). Watch for sedation.
Herb/Nutraceutical: Avoid valerian, St John's wort, kava kava, gotu kola (may increase CNS depression).

Adverse Reactions
>10%:
Central nervous system: Drowsiness (43%), dizziness (19%), insomnia (Stadol® NS)
Gastrointestinal: Nausea/vomiting (13%)
Respiratory: Nasal congestion (Stadol® NS)
1% to 10%:
Cardiovascular: Vasodilation, palpitation
Central nervous system: Lightheadedness, headache, lethargy, anxiety, confusion, euphoria, somnolence
Dermatologic: Pruritus
Gastrointestinal: Anorexia, constipation, xerostomia, stomach pain, unpleasant aftertaste
Neuromuscular & skeletal: Tremor, paresthesia, weakness
Ocular: Blurred vision
Otic: Ear pain, tinnitus
Respiratory: Bronchitis, cough, dyspnea, epistaxis, nasal irritation, pharyngitis, rhinitis, sinus congestion, sinusitis, upper respiratory infection
Miscellaneous: Diaphoresis (increased)

Overdosage/Toxicology Symptoms of overdose include respiratory depression, cardiac and CNS depression. Treatment is supportive. Naloxone, 2 mg I.V. with repeat administration as necessary up to a total of 10 mg, can also be used to reverse toxic effects of the opiate.

Pharmacodynamics/Kinetics
Onset of Action: I.M.: 5-10 minutes; I.V.: <10 minutes; Nasal: Within 15 minutes
Peak effect: I.M.: 0.5-1 hour; I.V.: 4-5 minutes
Duration of Action: I.M., I.V.: 3-4 hours; Nasal: 4-5 hours
Absorption: Rapid and well absorbed
Bioavailability: Nasal: 60% to 70%
Protein Binding: 80%
Half-Life Elimination: 2.5-4 hours
Metabolism: Hepatic
Excretion: Primarily urine

Dosing
Adults: Note: These are guidelines and do not represent the maximum doses that may be required in all patients. Doses should be titrated to pain relief/prevention. Butorphanol has an analgesic ceiling.
Acute pain (moderate to severe):
I.M.: Initial: 2 mg, may repeat every 3-4 hours as needed; usual range: 1-4 mg every 3-4 hours as needed
I.V.: Initial: 1 mg, may repeat every 3-4 hours as needed; usual range: 0.5-2 mg every 3-4 hours as needed
Intranasal (spray) (includes use for migraine headache pain): Initial: 1 spray (~1 mg per spray) in 1 nostril; if adequate pain relief is not achieved within 60-90 minutes, an additional 1 spray in 1 nostril may be given; may repeat initial dose sequence in 3-4 hours after the last dose as needed
Note: In some clinical trials, an initial dose of 2 mg (as 2 doses 1 hour apart or 2 mg initially - 1 spray in each nostril) has been used, followed by 1 mg in 1 hour; side effects were greater at these dosages
Migraine: Nasal spray: Refer to "moderate to severe pain" indication
Preoperative medication: I.M.: 2 mg 60-90 minutes before surgery
Supplement to balanced anesthesia: I.V.: 2 mg shortly before induction and/or an incremental dose of 0.5-1 mg (up to 0.06 mg/kg), depending on previously administered sedative, analgesic, and hypnotic medications
Pain during labor (fetus >37 weeks gestation and no signs of fetal distress):
I.M., I.V.: 1-2 mg; may repeat in 4 hours
Note: Alternative analgesia should be used for pain associated with delivery or if delivery is anticipated within 4 hours
Elderly:
I.M., I.V.: 0.5-2 mg every 6-8 hours, increase as necessary
Nasal spray: Initial dose should not exceed 1 mg; after 90-120 minutes, assess whether a second dose is needed; may repeat in 3-4 hours.

Available Dosage Forms
Injection, solution, as tartrate [preservative free] (Stadol®): 1 mg/mL (1 mL); 2 mg/mL (1 mL, 2 mL)
Injection, solution, as tartrate [with preservative] (Stadol®): 2 mg/mL (10 mL)

Solution, intranasal spray, as tartrate: 10 mg/mL (2.5 mL) [14-15 doses]
Stadol® NS [DSC]: 10 mg/mL (2.5 mL)

Monitoring and Teaching Issues

Physical Assessment: Assess other medications patient may be taking for possible additive or adverse interactions. Monitor for effectiveness of pain relief, signs of overdose, vital signs, and adverse effects at beginning of therapy and at regular intervals with long-term use. For inpatients, implement safety measures. May cause physical and/or psychological dependence. Assess knowledge/teach patient appropriate use (if self-administered), adverse reactions to report, and appropriate interventions to reduce side effects.

Patient Education: If self-administered, use exactly as directed; do not increase dose or frequency. Drug may cause physical and/or psychological dependence. While using this medication, do not use alcohol and other prescription or OTC medications (especially sedatives, tranquilizers, antihistamines, or pain medications) without consulting prescriber. May cause dizziness, drowsiness, confusion, or blurred vision (use caution when driving, climbing stairs, or changing position - rising from sitting or lying to standing, or when engaging in tasks requiring alertness until response to drug is known); nausea or vomiting, or loss of appetite (frequent mouth care, small frequent meals, sucking lozenges, or chewing gum may help). Report unresolved nausea or vomiting; respiratory difficulty or shortness of breath; restlessness, insomnia, euphoria, or nightmares; excessive sedation or unusual weakness; facial flushing, rapid heartbeat, or palpitations; urinary difficulty; or vision changes.

Nasal administration: Do not use more frequently than prescribed. Blow nose prior to administering. Follow directions on package insert. Insert nozzle of applicator gently into one nostril and exhale. With next breath, squeeze applicator once firmly and quickly once as you breath in. If adequate relief from headache is not achieved within 60-90 minutes, an additional 1 spray may be given. May be repeated in 3-4 hours following last dose, as needed. **Alternately:** Two sprays may be given - one spray in each nostril, if you are able to remain lying down (in the event of drowsiness or dizziness). Additional doses should not be taken for 3-4 hours. Avoid using simultaneously with intranasal migraine sprays. Separate by at least 30 minutes.

Pregnancy/breast-feeding precautions: Inform prescriber if you are or intend to become pregnant. If you are breast-feeding, take dose immediately after breast-feeding or 3-4 hours prior to next feeding.

Geriatric Considerations: Adjust dose for renal function in the elderly.

Pregnancy Risk Factor: C/D (prolonged use or high doses at term)

Lactation: Enters breast milk/use caution (AAP rates "compatible")

Administration

Inhalation: See Dosing.

Topical: Intranasal: Consider avoiding simultaneous intranasal migraine sprays; may want to separate by at least 30 minutes

Compatibility:

Y-site administration: Incompatible with amphotericin B cholesteryl sulfate complex, midazolam

Compatibility in syringe: Incompatible with dimenhydrinate, pentobarbital

Storage: Store at room temperature; protect from freezing.

Related Information

Compatibility of Drugs in Syringe *on page 1725*
Narcotic / Opioid Analgesic Comparison *on page 1739*

◆ **Butorphanol Tartrate** *see Butorphanol on page 227*
◆ **BW-430C** *see Lamotrigine on page 863*
◆ **BW524W91** *see Emtricitabine on page 514*
◆ **C2B8** *see Rituximab on page 1338*
◆ **C2B8 Monoclonal Antibody** *see Rituximab on page 1338*
◆ **311C90** *see Zolmitriptan on page 1593*
◆ **C225** *see Cetuximab on page 299*
◆ **Caduet®** *see Amlodipine and Atorvastatin on page 101*
◆ **Cafcit®** *see Caffeine on page 229*
◆ **Caffedrine® [OTC]** *see Caffeine on page 229*

Caffeine (KAF een)

U.S. Brand Names Cafcit®; Caffedrine® [OTC]; Enerjets [OTC]; Lucidex [OTC]; No Doz® Maximum Strength [OTC]; Vivarin® [OTC]

Synonyms Caffeine and Sodium Benzoate; Caffeine Citrate; Sodium Benzoate and Caffeine

Generic Available Yes: Caffeine and sodium benzoate injection

Pharmacologic Category Stimulant

Use

Caffeine citrate: Treatment of idiopathic apnea of prematurity

Caffeine and sodium benzoate: Treatment of acute respiratory depression (not a preferred agent)

Caffeine [OTC labeling]: Restore mental alertness or wakefulness when experiencing fatigue

Unlabeled/Investigational Use Caffeine and sodium benzoate: Treatment of spinal puncture headache; CNS stimulant; diuretic

Mechanism of Action/Effect CNS stimulant which increases respiratory center sensitivity to carbon dioxide, stimulates central inspiratory drive, and improves skeletal muscle contraction (diaphragmatic contractility); prevention of apnea may occur by competitive inhibition of adenosine

Contraindications Hypersensitivity to caffeine or any component of the formulation; sodium benzoate is not for use in neonates

Warnings/Precautions Use with caution in patients with a history of peptic ulcer, gastroesophageal reflux, impaired renal or hepatic function, seizure disorders, or cardiovascular (Continued)

Caffeine *(Continued)*

disease. Avoid use in patients with symptomatic cardiac arrhythmias, agitation, anxiety or tremor. Over-the-counter [OTC] products contain an amount of caffeine similar to one cup of coffee; limit the use of other caffeine-containing beverages or foods.

Caffeine citrate should not be interchanged with caffeine and sodium benzoate. Avoid use of products containing sodium benzoate in neonates; has been associated with a potentially fatal toxicity ("gasping syndrome"). Neonates receiving caffeine citrate should be closely monitored for the development of necrotizing enterocolitis. Caffeine serum levels should be closely monitored to optimize therapy and prevent serious toxicity.

Drug Interactions

Cytochrome P450 Effect: Substrate of CYP1A2 (major), 2C8/9 (minor), 2D6 (minor), 2E1 (minor), 3A4 (minor); **Inhibits** CYP1A2 (weak), 3A4 (moderate)

Decreased Effect: Caffeine may diminish the sedative or anxiolytic effects of benzodiazepines. CYP1A2 inducers may decrease the levels/effects of caffeine; example inducers include aminoglutethimide, carbamazepine, phenobarbital, and rifampin.

Increased Effect/Toxicity: Quinolones (specifically ciprofloxacin, norfloxacin, ofloxacin) and CYP1A2 inhibitors may increase the levels/effects of caffeine; example inhibitors include amiodarone, fluvoxamine, ketoconazole, and rofecoxib

Adverse Reactions Frequency not specified; primarily serum-concentration related.

Cardiovascular: Angina, arrhythmia (ventricular), chest pain, flushing, palpitation, sinus tachycardia, tachycardia (supraventricular), vasodilation

Central nervous system: Agitation, delirium, dizziness, hallucinations, headache, insomnia, irritability, psychosis, restlessness

Dermatologic: Urticaria

Gastrointestinal: Esophageal sphincter tone decreased, gastritis

Neuromuscular & skeletal: Fasciculations

Ocular: Intraocular pressure increased (>180 mg caffeine), miosis

Renal: Diuresis

Overdosage/Toxicology Symptoms may include CNS stimulation, tachyarrhythmias, and tremor. Treatment is symptomatic and supportive.

Pharmacodynamics/Kinetics

Time to Peak: Oral: Within 30 minutes to 2 hours

Protein Binding: 17% (children) to 36% (adults)

Half-Life Elimination:

Neonates: 72-96 hours (range: 40-230 hours)

Children >9 months and Adults: 5 hours

Metabolism: Hepatic, via demethylation by CYP1A2. **Note:** In neonates, interconversion between caffeine and theophylline has been reported (caffeine levels are ~25% of measured theophylline after theophylline administration and ~3% to 8% of caffeine would be expected to be converted to theophylline)

Excretion:

Neonates ≤ month: 86% excreted unchanged in urine

Infants >1 month and Adults: In urine, as metabolites

Dosing

Adults & Elderly:

Note: Caffeine citrate should not be interchanged with the caffeine sodium benzoate formulation.

Caffeine and sodium benzoate:

Respiratory depression: I.M., I.V.: 250 mg as a single dose; may repeat as needed. Maximum single dose should be limited to 500 mg; maximum amount in any 24-hour period should generally be limited to 2500 mg

Spinal puncture headache (unlabeled use):

I.V.: 500 mg in 1000 mL NS infused over 1 hour, followed by 1000 mL NS infused over 1 hour; a second course of caffeine can be given for unrelieved headache pain in 4 hours.

Oral: 300 mg as a single dose

Stimulant/diuretic (unlabeled use): I.M., I.V.: 500 mg, maximum single dose: 1 g

OTC labeling (stimulant): Oral: 100-200 mg every 3-4 hours as needed

Pediatrics:

Note: Caffeine citrate should not be interchanged with the caffeine sodium benzoate formulation.

Caffeine citrate: Apnea of prematurity: Neonates: Oral, I.V.:

Loading dose: 10-20 mg/kg as caffeine citrate (5-10 mg/kg as caffeine base). If theophylline has been administered to the patient within the previous 3 days, a full or modified loading dose (50% to 75% of a loading dose) may be given.

Maintenance dose: 5 mg/kg/day as caffeine citrate (2.5 mg/kg/day as caffeine base) once daily starting 24 hours after the loading dose. Maintenance dose is adjusted based on patient's response and serum caffeine concentrations.

Caffeine and sodium benzoate: Stimulant:

I.M., I.V., SubQ: 8 mg/kg every 4 hours as needed

Oral: OTC labeling: Children ≥12 years: Refer to adult dosing.

Renal Impairment: No dosage adjustment required.

Available Dosage Forms

Caplet (Caffedrine®, Vivarin®): 200 mg [OTC]

Injection, solution, as citrate [preservative free] (Cafcit®): 20 mg/mL (3 mL) [equivalent to 10 mg/mL caffeine base]

Injection, solution [with sodium benzoate]: Caffeine 125 mg/mL and sodium benzoate 125 mg/mL (2 mL); caffeine 121 mg/mL and sodium benzoate 129 mg/mL (2 mL)

Lozenge: 75 mg [OTC; Hazelnut coffee or mochamint flavor]

Solution, oral, as citrate (Cafcit®): 20 mg/mL (3 mL) [equivalent to 10 mg/mL caffeine base]

Tablet:

Lucidex: 100 mg [OTC]

NoDoz® Maximum Strength, Vivarin®: 200 mg [OTC]

Monitoring and Teaching Issues

Physical Assessment: Assess other prescription and OTC medications the patient may be taking to avoid duplications and interactions. Assess knowledge/teach patient appropriate use, side effects, and symptoms to report.

Patient Education: Take as directed. Do not exceed recommended dosage. Maintain adequate hydration (2-3 L/day of fluids) unless instructed to restrict fluid intake by prescriber. You may experience CNS stimulation, excitability, sensorium changes, flushing, dizziness, insomnia, or agitation. Report excessive excitability or nervousness, rapid heartbeat or palpitations, chest pain, or respiratory difficulty. **Pregnancy/breast-feeding precaution:** Inform prescriber if you are or intend to become pregnant. Consult prescriber if breast-feeding.

Pregnancy Risk Factor: C

Lactation: Enters breast milk/use caution (AAP rates "compatible")

Breast-Feeding Issues: Irritability and poor sleeping patterns have been reported following maternal consumption of large amounts of caffeine. Moderate intake (2-3 cups/day) is considered to be compatible with breast-feeding.

Administration

Oral: May be administered without regard to feedings or meals; may administer injectable formulation (caffeine citrate) orally

I.M.: Parenteral: **Caffeine and sodium benzoate:** May administer I.M. undiluted

I.V.: Parenteral:

Caffeine citrate: Infuse loading dose over at least 30 minutes; maintenance dose may be infused over at least 10 minutes; may administer without dilution or diluted with D_5W to 10 mg caffeine citrate/mL

Caffeine and sodium benzoate: I.V. as slow direct injection; for spinal headaches, dilute in 1000 mL NS and infuse over 1 hour; follow with 1000 mL NS, infuse over 1 hour; may administer I.M. undiluted

Storage: Store at 20°C to 25°C (68°F to 77°F).

Calcipotriene (kal si POE try een)

U.S. Brand Names Dovonex®

Generic Available No

Pharmacologic Category Topical Skin Product; Vitamin D Analog

Use Treatment of moderate plaque psoriasis

Mechanism of Action/Effect Synthetic vitamin D_3 analog which regulates skin cell production and proliferation

Contraindications Hypersensitivity to calcipotriene or any component of the formulation; patients with demonstrated hypercalcemia or evidence of vitamin D toxicity; use on the face

Warnings/Precautions Use may cause irritations of lesions and surrounding uninvolved skin. If irritation develops, discontinue use. Transient, rapidly reversible elevation of serum calcium has occurred during use. If elevation in serum calcium occurs above the normal range, discontinue treatment until calcium levels are normal. For external use only; not for ophthalmic, oral, or intravaginal use.

Adverse Reactions

>10%: Dermatologic: Burning, itching, skin irritation, erythema, dry skin, peeling, rash, worsening of psoriasis

1% to 10%: Dermatologic: Dermatitis

Dosing

Adults & Elderly: Psoriasis: Topical: Apply in a thin film to the affected skin twice daily and rub in gently and completely.

Available Dosage Forms

Cream: 0.005% (60 g, 120 g)

Ointment: 0.005% (60 g, 120 g)

Solution, topical: 0.005% (60 mL)

Monitoring and Teaching Issues

Physical Assessment: When applied to large areas of skin or for extensive periods of time, monitor for adverse skin or systemic reactions. Assess knowledge/teach patient appropriate application and use and adverse symptoms to report.

Monitoring Laboratory Tests: Serum calcium

Patient Education: For external use only. Use exactly as directed; do not overuse. Before using, wash and dry area gently. Wear gloves to apply a thin film to affected area and rub in gently. If dressing is necessary, use a porous dressing. Avoid contact with eyes. Avoid exposing treated area to direct sunlight; sunburn can occur. Report increased swelling, redness, rash, itching, signs of infection, worsening of condition, or lack of healing. **Pregnancy/breast-feeding precautions:** Inform prescriber if you are or intend to become pregnant. Consult prescriber if breast-feeding.

(Continued)

Calcipotriene *(Continued)*

Pregnancy Risk Factor: C
Lactation: Excretion in breast milk unknown
Administration
  Topical: For external use only; apply with gloves.

Calcitonin *(kal si TOE nin)*

U.S. Brand Names Miacalcin®
Synonyms Calcitonin (Salmon)
Generic Available No
Pharmacologic Category Antidote
Medication Safety Issues
  Sound-alike/look-alike issues:
    Calcitonin may be confused with calcitriol
    Miacalcin® may be confused with Micatin®
Use Calcitonin (salmon): Treatment of Paget's disease of bone (osteitis deformans); adjunctive therapy for hypercalcemia; used in postmenopausal osteoporosis and osteogenesis imperfecta
Mechanism of Action/Effect Structurally similar to human calcitonin; it directly inhibits osteoclastic bone resorption; promotes the renal excretion of calcium, phosphate, sodium, magnesium and potassium by decreasing tubular reabsorption; increases the jejunal secretion of water, sodium, potassium, and chloride
Contraindications Hypersensitivity to salmon protein or gelatin diluent
Warnings/Precautions A skin test should be performed prior to initiating therapy of calcitonin salmon. Have epinephrine immediately available for a possible hypersensitivity reaction. Use caution with renal insufficiency, pernicious anemia.
Drug Interactions
  Decreased Effect: Calcitonin may be antagonized by calcium and vitamin D in treating hypercalcemia.
  Nutritional/Ethanol Interactions Ethanol: Avoid ethanol (may increase risk of osteoporosis).
Adverse Reactions
  >10%:
    Cardiovascular: Facial flushing
    Gastrointestinal: Nausea, diarrhea, anorexia
    Local: Edema at injection site
  1% to 10%:
    Genitourinary: Polyuria
    Neuromuscular & skeletal: Back/joint pain
    Respiratory: Nasal bleeding/crusting (following intranasal administration)
Overdosage/Toxicology Symptoms of overdose include nausea, vomiting, hypocalcemia, and hypocalcemic tetany. Treat symptomatically.
Pharmacodynamics/Kinetics
  Onset of Action: Hypercalcemia: ~2 hours
  Duration of Action: Hypercalcemia: 6-8 hours
  Half-Life Elimination: SubQ: 1.2 hours
  Excretion: Urine (as inactive metabolites)
Dosing
  Adults & Elderly:
    Paget's disease:
      I.M., SubQ: 100 units/day to start, 50 units/day or 50-100 units every 1-3 days maintenance dose
    Hypercalcemia:
      I.M., SubQ: Initial: 4 units/kg every 12 hours; may increase up to 8 units/kg every 12 hours to a maximum of every 6 hours
    Osteoporosis prevention (in postmenopausal women):
      I.M., SubQ: 100 units/day
      Intranasal: 200 units (1 spray)/day
  Pediatrics: Osteogenesis imperfecta: I.M., SubQ: 2 units/kg 3 times/week
Available Dosage Forms
  Injection, solution, calcitonin-salmon: 200 int. units/mL (2 mL)
  Solution, nasal spray, calcitonin-salmon: 200 int. units/0.09 mL (3.7 mL) [contains benzalkonium chloride]
Monitoring and Teaching Issues
  Physical Assessment: Skin test should be administered before initiating therapy (increased erythema or skin wheal indicates positive reaction and allergy). Assess potential for interactions with other prescriptions, OTC medications, or herbal products patient may be taking. Assess results of laboratory tests and patient response (eg, hypocalcemic tetany, hypercalcemia) at regular intervals during therapy. Teach appropriate administration (eg, subcutaneous or I.M. injections or nasal spray), dietary requirements (low calcium diet if used for hypercalcemia), possible side effects/appropriate interventions, and adverse symptoms to report.
  Monitoring Laboratory Tests: Serum electrolytes and calcium, alkaline phosphatase and 24-hour urine collection for hydroxyproline excretion (Paget's disease)
  Patient Education: Do not take any new medication during therapy unless approved by prescriber. If administered by injection, you or a significant other will be instructed on how to give the injections and dispose of syringes/needles (follow directions exactly). Keep drug vials in refrigerator; do not freeze. May cause increased warmth and flushing (this should only last about 1 hour after administration; taking drug in evening may minimize these discomforts). Report significant nasal irritation if using nasal spray. Immediately report twitching, muscle spasm, dark-colored urine, hives, significant skin rash, palpitations, or

respiratory difficulty. **Pregnancy/breast-feeding precautions:** Inform prescriber if you are or intend to become pregnant. Consult prescriber if breast-feeding.

Dietary Considerations: Adequate vitamin D and calcium intake is essential for osteoporosis. Patients with Paget's disease and hypercalcemia should follow a low calcium diet as prescribed.

Geriatric Considerations: Calcitonin may be the drug of choice for postmenopausal women unable to take estrogens to increase bone density and reduce fractures. Calcium and vitamin D supplements should also be given. Calcitonin may also be effective in steroid-induced osteoporosis and other states associated with high bone turnover.

Pregnancy Risk Factor: C

Lactation: Excretion in breast milk unknown

Breast-Feeding Issues: Has been shown to decrease milk production in animals.

Administration

I.M.: I.M. route is preferred if volume exceeds 2 mL.

Reconstitution: Salmon calcitonin: Injection: NS has been recommended for the dilution to prepare a skin test.

Storage: Salmon calcitonin:

Injection: Store under refrigeration at 2°C to 6°C (36°F to 43°F); stable for up to 2 weeks at room temperature.

Nasal: Store unopened bottle under refrigeration at 2°C to 8°C. Once the pump has been activated, store at room temperature.

- ◆ Calcitonin (Salmon) *see* Calcitonin *on page 232*
- ◆ Cal-Citrate® 250 [OTC] *see* Calcium Citrate *on page 238*

Calcitriol (kal si TRYE ole)

U.S. Brand Names Calcijex®; Rocaltrol®

Synonyms 1,25 Dihydroxycholecalciferol

Generic Available Yes

Pharmacologic Category Vitamin D Analog

Medication Safety Issues

Sound-alike/look-alike issues:

Calcitriol may be confused with calcifediol, Calciferol®, calcitonin

Dosage is expressed in mcg (micrograms), **not** mg (milligrams); rare cases of acute overdose have been reported

Use Management of hypocalcemia in patients on chronic renal dialysis; management of secondary hyperparathyroidism in moderate-to-severe chronic renal failure; management of hypocalcemia in hypoparathyroidism and pseudohypoparathyroidism

Unlabeled/Investigational Use Decrease severity of psoriatic lesions in psoriasis vulgaris; vitamin D resistant rickets

Mechanism of Action/Effect Promotes absorption of calcium in the intestines and retention at the kidneys thereby increasing calcium levels in the serum; decreases excessive serum phosphatase levels, parathyroid hormone levels, and decreases bone resorption; increases renal tubule phosphate resorption

Contraindications Hypercalcemia; vitamin D toxicity; abnormal sensitivity to the effects of vitamin D; pregnancy (dose exceeding RDA)

Warnings/Precautions Adequate dietary (supplemental) calcium is necessary for clinical response to vitamin D. Monitor serum calcium and phosphate concentrations; avoid hypercalcemia; calcium-phosphate product (serum calcium times phosphorus) must not exceed 70. Immobilization or excessive dosage may increase risk of hypercalcemia and/or hypercalciuria. Maintain adequate hydration. Use caution in patients with malabsorption syndromes (efficacy may be limited and/or response may be unpredictable).

Drug Interactions

Cytochrome P450 Effect: Induces CYP3A4 (weak)

Decreased Effect: Cholestyramine and colestipol decrease absorption/effect of calcitriol. Thiazide diuretics and corticosteroids may reduce the effect of calcitriol.

Increased Effect/Toxicity: Risk of hypercalcemia with thiazide diuretics. Risk of hypermagnesemia with magnesium-containing antacids. Risk of digoxin toxicity may be increased (if hypercalcemia occurs).

Lab Interactions Increased calcium, cholesterol, magnesium, BUN, AST, ALT, calcium (S), cholesterol (S); decreased alkaline phosphatase

Adverse Reactions

>10%: Endocrine & metabolic: Hypercalcemia (33%)

Frequency not defined:

Cardiovascular: Cardiac arrhythmia, hyper-/hypotension

Central nervous system: Headache, irritability, seizure (rare), somnolence, psychosis

Dermatologic: Pruritus, erythema multiforme

Endocrine & metabolic: Hypermagnesemia, hyperphosphatemia, polydipsia

Gastrointestinal: Anorexia, constipation, metallic taste, nausea, pancreatitis, vomiting, xerostomia

Hepatic: LFTs increased

Neuromuscular & skeletal: Bone pain, myalgia, dystrophy, soft tissue calcification

Ocular: Conjunctivitis, photophobia

Renal: Polyuria

Overdosage/Toxicology Toxicity rarely occurs from acute overdose. Symptoms of chronic overdose include hypercalcemia, hypercalciuria with weakness, altered mental status, GI upset, renal tubular injury, and occasionally cardiac arrhythmias. Following withdrawal of the drug, treatment consists of bed rest, liberal fluid intake, reduced calcium intake, and cathartic administration. Severe hypercalcemia requires I.V. hydration and forced diuresis. I.V. saline may increase excretion of calcium. Calcitonin, cholestyramine, prednisone, sodium EDTA, bisphosphonates, and mithramycin have all been used successfully to treat the more resistant cases of vitamin D-induced hypercalcemia. Use of peritoneal dialysis against a calcium-free dialysate has been reported.

(Continued)

Calcitriol (Continued)

Pharmacodynamics/Kinetics

Onset of Action: ~2-6 hours

Duration of Action: 3-5 days

Absorption: Oral: Rapid

Protein Binding: 99.9%

Half-Life Elimination: 3-8 hours

Metabolism: Primarily to 1,24,25-trihydroxycholecalciferol and 1,24,25-trihydroxy ergocalciferol

Excretion: Primarily feces; urine (4% to 6%)

Dosing

Adults & Elderly: Individualize dosage to maintain calcium levels of 9-10 mg/dL.

Renal failure:

Oral: 0.25 mcg/day or every other day (may require 0.5-1 mcg/day)

I.V.: 0.5 mcg (0.01 mcg/kg) 3 times/week; most doses in the range of 0.5-3 mcg (0.01-0.05 mcg/kg) 3 times/week

Hypoparathyroidism/pseudohypoparathyroidism: Oral: 0.5-2 mcg/day

Vitamin D-dependent rickets: Oral: 1 mcg once daily

Vitamin D-resistant rickets (familial hypophosphatemia): Oral: Initial: 0.015-0.02 mcg/kg once daily; maintenance: 0.03-0.06 mcg/kg once daily; maximum dose: 2 mcg once daily

Dosage adjustment for toxicity: Hypercalcemia:

Dialysis or hypoparathyroidism: Discontinue calcitriol and calcium supplements; initiate low-calcium diet. In dialysis patients with persistent hypercalcemia, may dialyze against calcium-free dialysate.

Predialysis:

Discontinue or reduce calcium supplements.

If taking calcitriol 0.5 mcg once daily, reduce to 0.25 mcg once daily.

If taking calcitriol 0.25 mcg once daily, discontinue until serum calcium normalizes. Restart at 0.25 mcg every other day.

Pediatrics: Individualize dosage to maintain calcium levels of 9-10 mg/dL.

Renal failure:

Children:

Oral: 0.25-2 mcg/day have been used (with hemodialysis); 0.014-0.041 mcg/kg/day (not receiving hemodialysis); increases should be made at 4- to 8-week intervals.

I.V.: 0.01-0.05 mcg/kg 3 times/week if undergoing hemodialysis

Hypoparathyroidism/pseudohypoparathyroidism: Oral (evaluate dosage at 2- to 4-week intervals):

Children:

<1 year: 0.04-0.08 mcg/kg once daily

1-5 years: 0.25-0.75 mcg once daily

Children >6 years: 0.5-2 mcg once daily

Vitamin D-dependent rickets: Refer to adult dosing.

Vitamin D-resistant rickets (familial hypophosphatemia): Refer to adult dosing.

Available Dosage Forms

Capsule (Rocaltrol®): 0.25 mcg, 0.5 mcg [each strength contains coconut oil]

Injection, solution: 1 mcg/mL (1 mL); 2 mcg/mL (2 mL)

Calcijex®: 1 mcg/mL (1 mL)

Solution, oral (Rocaltrol®): 1 mcg/mL (15 mL) [contains palm seed oil]

Monitoring and Teaching Issues

Physical Assessment: Assess effectiveness and interactions of other medications patient may be taking. Assess results of laboratory tests, therapeutic effectiveness, and adverse effects at beginning of therapy and regularly with long-term use. Assess knowledge/teach patient appropriate use, appropriate nutritional counseling, possible side effects/interventions, and adverse symptoms to report.

Monitoring Laboratory Tests: Serum calcium and phosphorus, and renal function. The serum calcium times phosphate product should not be allowed to exceed 70.

Patient Education: Take exact dose as prescribed; do not increase dose. Maintain recommended diet and calcium supplementation. Avoid taking magnesium-containing antacids. You may experience nausea, vomiting, loss of appetite, or metallic taste (small frequent meals, frequent mouth care, chewing gum, or sucking lozenges may help); or hypotension (use caution when rising from sitting or lying position or when climbing stairs or bending over). Report chest pain or palpitations; acute headache; skin rash; change in vision or eye irritation; CNS changes; unusual weakness or fatigue; persistent nausea, vomiting, cramps, or diarrhea; or muscle or bone pain. **Pregnancy/breast-feeding precautions:** Inform prescriber if you are or intend to become pregnant. Breast-feeding is not recommended.

Dietary Considerations: May be taken without regard to food. Give with meals to reduce GI problems.

Geriatric Considerations: Appetite and caloric requirements may decrease with advanced age. Assess diet for adequate nutrient intake with regard to vitamins and minerals. (Daily vitamin supplements are sometimes recommended). Persons >65 years of age have decreased absorption and may have decreased intake of vitamin D. This may require supplement with daily vitamin D intake, especially for those with high risk for osteoporosis.

Pregnancy Risk Factor: C (manufacturer); A/D (dose exceeding RDA recommendation) (expert analysis)

Lactation: Enters breast milk/not recommended

Administration

Oral: May be administered without regard to food. Give with meals to reduce GI problems.

I.V.: May be administered as a bolus dose I.V. through the catheter at the end of hemodialysis.

Compatibility: Stable in D₅W, NS, SWFI

Storage: Store in tight, light-resistant container. Calcitriol degrades upon prolonged exposure to light.

Calcium Acetate (KAL see um AS e tate)
U.S. Brand Names PhosLo®
Generic Available Yes: Solution for injection
Pharmacologic Category Antidote; Calcium Salt; Electrolyte Supplement, Parenteral
Medication Safety Issues
Sound-alike/look-alike issues:
PhosLo® may be confused with Phos-Flur®, ProSom™
Use
Oral: Control of hyperphosphatemia in end-stage renal failure; does not promote aluminum absorption
I.V.: Calcium supplementation in parenteral nutrition therapy
Dosing
Adults & Elderly:
Dietary Reference Intake:
Adults, Male/Female:
19-50 years: 1000 mg/day
≥51 years: 1200 mg/day
Female: Pregnancy: Same as for Adults, Male/Female
Female: Lactating: Same as for Adults, Male/Female

Control of hyperphosphatemia (ESRD, on dialysis): Oral: Initial: 1334 mg with each meal, can be increased gradually to bring the serum phosphate value <6 mg/dL as long as hypercalcemia does not develop (usual dose: 2001-2868 mg calcium acetate with each meal); do not give additional calcium supplements
Calcium supplementation (parenteral): I.V.: Dose is dependent on the requirements of the individual patient; in central venous total parental nutrition (TPN), calcium is administered at a concentration of 5 mEq (10 mL)/L of TPN solution
Pediatrics:
Dietary Reference Intake:
0-6 months: 210 mg/day
7-12 months: 270 mg/day
1-3 years: 500 mg/day
4-8 years: 800 mg/day
9-18 years: 1300 mg/day

Calcium supplementation (parenteral): I.V.: Dose is dependent on the requirements of the individual patient; in central venous total parental nutrition (TPN), calcium is administered at a concentration of 5 mEq (10 mL)/L of TPN solution; the additive maintenance dose in neonatal TPN is 0.5 mEq calcium/kg/day (1.0 mL/kg/day)
Neonates: 70-200 mg/kg/day
Infants and Children: 70-150 mg/kg/day
Adolescents: 18-35 mg/kg/day
Renal Impairment: Refer to adult dosing.
Available Dosage Forms Note: Elemental calcium listed in brackets:
Gelcap (PhosLo®): 667 mg [169 mg]
Injection, solution: 0.5 mEq/mL (10 mL, 50 mL, 100 mL)
Tablet (PhosLo®): 667 mg [169 mg]
Monitoring and Teaching Issues
Patient Education: Inform prescriber of any other medications or dietary supplements you are taking. Do not take any new medication during therapy without consulting prescriber. Follow exact instructions for dosing. Take with a full glass of water or juice, 1-3 hours after meals and other medications, and 1-2 hours before any approved iron supplements. Avoid alcohol, other antacids, caffeine, or other calcium supplements unless approved by prescriber. May cause constipation (increased exercise, fluids, fiber, or fruits may help) or dry mouth (frequent mouth care, chewing gum, or sucking lozenges may help). Report severe, unresolved GI disturbances and unusual emotional lability (mood swings). **Pregnancy precaution:** Inform prescriber if you are or intend to become pregnant.
Pregnancy Risk Factor: C

♦ **Calcium Acetylhomotaurinate** see Acamprosate on page 36

Calcium Carbonate (KAL see um KAR bun ate)
U.S. Brand Names Alcalak [OTC]; Alka-Mints® [OTC]; Amitone® [OTC]; Calcarb 600 [OTC]; Calci-Chew® [OTC]; Calci-Mix® [OTC]; Cal-Gest [OTC]; Cal-Mint [OTC]; Caltrate® 600 [OTC]; Chooz® [OTC]; Florical® [OTC]; Mylanta® Children's [OTC]; Nephro-Calci® [OTC]; Os-Cal® 500 [OTC]; Oysco 500 [OTC]; Oyst-Cal 500 [OTC]; Titralac™ [OTC]; Titralac™ Extra Strength [OTC]; Tums® [OTC]; Tums® 500 [OTC]; Tums® E-X [OTC]; Tums® Extra Strength Sugar Free [OTC]; Tums® Smooth Dissolve [OTC]; Tums® Ultra [OTC]
Generic Available Yes: Excludes capsule
Pharmacologic Category Antacid; Antidote; Calcium Salt; Electrolyte Supplement, Oral
Medication Safety Issues
Sound-alike/look-alike issues:
Florical® may be confused with Fiorinal®
Mylanta® may be confused with Mynatal®
Nephro-Calci® may be confused with Nephrocaps®
Os-Cal® may be confused with Asacol®
Use As an antacid, and treatment and prevention of calcium deficiency or hyperphosphatemia (eg, osteoporosis, osteomalacia, mild/moderate renal insufficiency, hypoparathyroidism, postmenopausal osteoporosis, rickets); has been used to bind phosphate
Contraindications Hypercalcemia, renal calculi, hypophosphatemia
(Continued)

Calcium Carbonate *(Continued)*

Warnings/Precautions Calcium carbonate absorption is impaired in achlorhydria (common in elderly - use alternate salt, administer with food); administration is followed by increased gastric acid secretion within 2 hours of administration; while hypercalcemia and hypercalciuria may result when therapeutic replacement amounts are given for prolonged periods, they are most likely to occur in hypoparathyroid patients receiving high doses of vitamin D.

Drug Interactions

Decreased Effect: Absorption of tetracycline, atenolol (and potentially other beta-blockers), iron, quinolone antibiotics, alendronate, sodium fluoride, and zinc absorption may be significantly decreased; space administration times. Effects of calcium channel blockers (eg, verapamil) effects may be diminished. Polystyrene sulfonate's potassium-binding ability may be reduced; avoid concurrent administration.

Increased Effect/Toxicity: High doses of calcium with thiazide diuretics may result in milk-alkali syndrome and hypercalcemia; monitor response. Calcium salts may decrease T_4 absorption; separate dose from levothyroxine by at least 4 hours. Calcium acetate may potentiate digoxin toxicity.

Nutritional/Ethanol Interactions

Ethanol: Avoid ethanol (may increase risk of osteoporosis).

Food: Food may increase calcium absorption. Calcium may decrease iron absorption. Bran, foods high in oxalates, or whole grain cereals may decrease calcium absorption.

Lab Interactions Increased calcium (S); decreased magnesium

Adverse Reactions Well tolerated

1% to 10%:

Central nervous system: Headache

Endocrine & metabolic: Hypophosphatemia, hypercalcemia

Gastrointestinal: Constipation, laxative effect, acid rebound, nausea, vomiting, anorexia, abdominal pain, xerostomia, flatulence

Miscellaneous: Milk-alkali syndrome with very high, chronic dosing and/or renal failure (headache, nausea, irritability, and weakness or alkalosis, hypercalcemia, renal impairment)

Overdosage/Toxicology

Acute single ingestions of calcium salts may produce mild gastrointestinal distress, but hypercalcemia or other toxic manifestations are extremely unlikely

Treatment is supportive

Pharmacodynamics/Kinetics

Absorption: Requires vitamin D; minimal unless chronic, high doses are given; calcium is absorbed in soluble, ionized form; solubility of calcium is increased in an acid environment

Excretion: Primarily feces (as unabsorbed calcium); urine (20%)

Dosing

Adults & Elderly: Dosage is in terms of elemental calcium:

Dietary Reference Intake:

Adults, Male/Female:

19-50 years: 1000 mg/day

≥51 years: 1200 mg/day

Female: Pregnancy: Same as for Adults, Male/Female

Female: Lactating: Same as for Adults, Male/Female

Hypocalcemia (dose depends on clinical condition and serum calcium level): Dose expressed in mg of **elemental calcium:** 1-2 g or more/day in 3-4 divided doses

Dietary supplementation: 500 mg to 2 g divided 2-4 times/day

Antacid: Dosage based on acid-neutralizing capacity of specific product; generally, 1-2 tablets or 5-10 mL every 2 hours; maximum: 7000 mg calcium carbonate per 24 hours; specific product labeling should be consulted

Osteoporosis: Adults >51 years: 1200 mg/day

Pediatrics: Dosage is in terms of elemental calcium:

Dietary Reference Intake:

0-6 months: 210 mg/day

7-12 months: 270 mg/day

1-3 years: 500 mg/day

4-8 years: 800 mg/day

9-19 years: 1300 mg/day

Hypocalcemia (dose depends on clinical condition and serum calcium level): Dose expressed in mg of **elemental calcium**

Neonates: 50-150 mg/kg/day in 4-6 divided doses; not to exceed 1 g/day

Children: 45-65 mg/kg/day in 4 divided doses

Renal Impairment: Cl_{cr} <25 mL/minute: Dosage adjustments may be necessary depending on the serum calcium levels.

Available Dosage Forms

Capsule:

Calci-Mix®: 1250 mg [equivalent to elemental calcium 500 mg]

Florical®: 364 mg [equivalent to elemental calcium 145.6 mg; contains sodium fluoride 8.3 mg]

Powder: 1600 mg/teaspoonful (960 g)

Suspension, oral: 1250 mg/5 mL (5 mL, 500 mL) [equivalent to elemental calcium 500 mg/5 mL; mint flavor]

Tablet: 1250 mg [equivalent to elemental calcium 500 mg]; 1500 mg [equivalent to elemental calcium 600 mg]

Calcarb 600, Caltrate® 600, Nephro-Calci®: 1500 mg [equivalent to elemental calcium 600 mg]

Florical®: 364 mg [equivalent to elemental calcium 145.6 mg; contains sodium fluoride 8.3 mg]

Os-Cal® 500, Oysco 500, Oyst-Cal 500: 1250 mg [equivalent to elemental calcium 500 mg]

Tablet, chewable: 500 mg [equivalent to elemental calcium 200 mg]; 650 mg [equivalent to elemental calcium 260 mg]; 750 mg [equivalent to elemental calcium 300 mg]

Alcalak: 420 mg [equivalent to elemental calcium 168 mg]

Alka-Mints®: 850 mg [equivalent to elemental calcium 340 mg; assorted and spearmint flavors]

Amitone®: 420 mg [equivalent to elemental calcium 168 mg; spearmint flavor]

Cal-Gest: 500 mg [equivalent to elemental calcium 200 mg]

Calci-Chew®: 1250 mg [equivalent to elemental calcium 500 mg; cherry, lemon, and orange flavors]

Cal-Mint: 650 mg [equivalent to elemental calcium 260 mg; mint flavor]

Chooz®: 500 mg [equivalent to elemental calcium 200 mg; contains phenylalanine]

Mylanta® Children's: 400 mg [equivalent to elemental calcium 160 mg; bubble gum flavor]

Os-Cal® 500: 1250 mg [equivalent to elemental calcium 500 mg; Bavarian cream flavor]

Titralac™: 420 mg [equivalent to elemental calcium 168 mg; sugar free; mint flavor]

Titralac™ Extra Strength: 750 mg [equivalent to elemental calcium 300 mg; sugar free; mint flavor]

Tums®: 500 mg [equivalent to elemental calcium 200 mg; assorted fruit (contains tartrazine) and peppermint flavors]

Tums® E-X: 750 mg [equivalent to elemental calcium 300 mg; assorted fruit (contains tartrazine), fresh blend, tropical assorted fruit, wintergreen (contains tartrazine), and assorted berry flavors]

Tums® Extra Strength Sugar Free: 750 mg [equivalent to elemental calcium 300 mg; sugar free; contains phenylalanine <1 mg/tablet; orange cream flavor]

Tums® Smooth Dissolve: 750 mg [equivalent to elemental calcium 300 mg; assorted fruit (contains tartrazine) and peppermint flavors]

Tums® Ultra®: 1000 mg [equivalent to elemental calcium 400 mg; assorted mint, assorted berry, and tropical assorted berry (contains tartrazine) flavors]

Monitoring and Teaching Issues

Physical Assessment: Assess other medications patient may be taking for effectiveness and interactions. Assess results of laboratory tests, therapeutic effect, and adverse/toxic effects. Assess knowledge/teach patient proper use, appropriate interventions to reduce side effects, and adverse symptoms to report. If administered I.V., monitor ECG, vital signs, and CNS.

Patient Education: Oral: Follow instructions for dosing. Take with a full glass of water or juice 1-2 hours before any iron supplements and 1-3 hours after meals or other medications. Avoid alcohol, other antacids, caffeine, or other calcium supplements, unless approved by prescriber. You may experience constipation (increased exercise, fluids, fiber, or fruit may help) or dry mouth (sucking lozenges or hard candy may help). Report severe, unresolved GI disturbances and unusual emotional liability (mood swings). **Pregnancy precaution:** Inform prescriber if you are or intend to become pregnant.

Dietary Considerations: As a dietary supplement, should be given with meals to increase absorption. May decrease iron absorption, so should be administered 1-2 hours before or after iron supplementation; limit intake of with bran, foods high in oxalates or whole grain cereals which may decrease calcium absorption.

Additional Information 20 mEq calcium/g; 400 mg elemental calcium/g calcium carbonate (40% elemental calcium)

♦ Calcium Channel Blockers *see page 1722*

Calcium Chloride (KAL see um KLOR ide)

Generic Available Yes

Pharmacologic Category Calcium Salt; Electrolyte Supplement, Parenteral

Use Cardiac resuscitation when epinephrine fails to improve myocardial contractions, cardiac disturbances of hyperkalemia, hypocalcemia, or calcium channel blocking agent toxicity; emergent treatment of hypocalcemic tetany, treatment of hypermagnesemia

Dosing

Adults & Elderly: Note: Calcium chloride is 3 times as potent as calcium gluconate

Cardiac arrest in the presence of hyperkalemia or hypocalcemia, magnesium toxicity, or calcium antagonist toxicity: I.V.: 2-4 mg/kg (10% solution), repeated every 10 minutes if necessary

Hypocalcemia: I.V.: 500 mg to 1 g (7-14 mEq)/dose repeated every 4-6 hours if needed

Hypocalcemic tetany: I.V.: 1 g over 10-30 minutes; may repeat after 6 hours

Hypocalcemia secondary to citrated blood transfusion: I.V.: 2.7-6.8 mEq (2-5 mL of a 10% solution) per 500 mL of blood (infused into another vein).

Note: Routine administration of calcium, in the absence of signs/symptoms of hypocalcemia, is generally not recommended. A number of recommendations have been published seeking to address potential hypocalcemia during massive transfusion of citrated blood; however, many practitioners recommend replacement only as guided by clinical evidence of hypocalcemia and/or serial monitoring of ionized calcium.

Pediatrics: Note: Calcium chloride is 3 times as potent as calcium gluconate

Cardiac arrest in the presence of hyperkalemia or hypocalcemia, magnesium toxicity, or calcium antagonist toxicity: I.V.:

Infants and Children: 20 mg/kg; may repeat in 10 minutes if necessary

Hypocalcemia: I.V.:

Children (manufacturer's recommendation): 2.7-5 mg/kg/dose every 4-6 hours

Alternative pediatric dosing: Infants and Children: 10-20 mg/kg/dose (infants <1 mEq; children 1-7 mEq), repeat every 4-6 hours if needed

Hypocalcemic tetany: I.V.:

Infants and Children: 10 mg/kg (0.5-0.7 mEq/kg) over 5-10 minutes; may repeat after 6-8 hours or follow with an infusion with a maximum dose of 200 mg/kg/day

Hypocalcemia secondary to citrated blood transfusion: I.V.: Neonates, Infants, and Children: Give 0.45 mEq **elemental** calcium for each 100 mL citrated blood infused. See "**Note**" in adult dosing.

Renal Impairment: Cl$_{cr}$ <25 mL/minute: Dosage adjustments may be necessary depending on the serum calcium levels.

(Continued)

Calcium Chloride *(Continued)*

Available Dosage Forms Injection, solution [preservative free]: 10% [100 mg/mL] (10 mL) [equivalent to elemental calcium 27.2 mg/mL, calcium 1.36 mEq/mL]

Monitoring and Teaching Issues

Patient Education: This medication can only be given intravenously. Do not make rapid postural changes while calcium is infusing. Report any feelings of excitation, chest pain, irregular or pounding heartbeat, vomiting, acute headache, or dizziness.

Pregnancy Risk Factor: C

Calcium Citrate *(KAL see um SIT rate)*

U.S. Brand Names Cal-Citrate® 250 [OTC]; Citracal® [OTC]

Generic Available Yes

Pharmacologic Category Calcium Salt

Medication Safety Issues

Sound-alike/look-alike issues:

Citracal® may be confused with Citrucel®

Use Antacid; treatment and prevention of calcium deficiency or hyperphosphatemia (eg, osteoporosis, osteomalacia, mild/moderate renal insufficiency, hypoparathyroidism, postmenopausal osteoporosis, rickets)

Contraindications Hypersensitivity to any component of the formulation; hypercalcemia, renal calculi, ventricular fibrillation

Warnings/Precautions Calcium absorption is impaired in achlorhydria (citrate may be preferred due to limited impact on absorption). Hypercalcemia and hypercalciuria may result when therapeutic replacement amounts are given for prolonged periods, they are most likely to occur in hypoparathyroid patients receiving high doses of vitamin D. Use with caution in digitalized patients, respiratory failure, or acidosis. Hypercalcemia may occur in patients with renal failure, and frequent determination of serum calcium is necessary.

Drug Interactions

Decreased Effect: Absorption of tetracycline, atenolol (and potentially other beta-blockers), iron, quinolone antibiotics, alendronate, sodium fluoride, and zinc absorption may be significantly decreased; space administration times. Effects of calcium channel blockers (eg, verapamil) effects may be diminished. Polystyrene sulfonate's potassium-binding ability may be reduced; avoid concurrent administration.

Increased Effect/Toxicity: High doses of calcium with thiazide diuretics may result in milk-alkali syndrome and hypercalcemia; monitor response. Calcium salts may decrease T_4 absorption; separate dose from levothyroxine by at least 4 hours. Calcium acetate may potentiate digoxin toxicity.

Nutritional/Ethanol Interactions Ethanol: Avoid ethanol (may increase risk of osteoporosis).

Adverse Reactions Frequency not defined:

Mild hypercalcemia (calcium: >10.5 mg/dL) may be asymptomatic or manifest itself as constipation, anorexia, nausea, and vomiting

More severe hypercalcemia (calcium: >12 mg/dL) is associated with confusion, delirium, stupor, and coma

Frequency not defined:

Central nervous system: Headache

Endocrine & metabolic: Hypophosphatemia, hypercalcemia

Gastrointestinal: Nausea, anorexia, vomiting, abdominal pain, constipation

Miscellaneous: Thirst

Pharmacodynamics/Kinetics

Absorption: Requires vitamin D

Dosing

Adults & Elderly: Oral: Dosage is in terms of elemental calcium

Dietary Reference Intake:

Adults, Male/Female:

19-50 years: 1000 mg/day

≥51 years: 1200 mg/day

Female: Pregnancy: Same as for Adults, Male/Female

Female: Lactating: Same as for Adults, Male/Female

Dietary supplement: Oral: Usual dose: 500 mg to 2 g 2-4 times/day

Pediatrics: Oral: Dosage is in terms of elemental calcium

Dietary Reference Intake:

0-6 months: 210 mg/day

7-12 months: 270 mg/day

1-3 years: 500 mg/day

4-8 years: 800 mg/day

9-18 years: 1300 mg/day

Available Dosage Forms

Granules: 760 mg/teaspoonful (480 g)

Tablet: Elemental calcium 200 mg, 250 mg

Cal-Citrate®: Elemental calcium 250 mg

Citracal®: 950 mg [equivalent to elemental calcium 200 mg]

Monitoring and Teaching Issues

Physical Assessment: Assess other medications patient may be taking for effectiveness and interactions. Assess therapeutic effect and adverse/toxic effects. Assess knowledge/teach patient proper use, appropriate interventions to reduce side effects, and adverse symptoms to report.

Patient Education: Inform prescriber of any other medications or dietary supplements you are taking. Do not take any new medication during therapy without consulting prescriber. Follow exact instructions for dosing. Take with a full glass of water or juice, 1-3 hours after other medications, and 1-2 hours before any approved iron supplements. Avoid alcohol, other antacids, caffeine, or other calcium supplements unless approved by prescriber. May cause constipation (increased exercise, fluids, fiber, or fruits may help) or dry mouth (frequent mouth care, chewing gum, or sucking lozenges may help). Report severe, unresolved GI disturbances and unusual emotional lability (mood swings). **Pregnancy precaution:** Inform prescriber if you are or intend to become pregnant.

Pregnancy Risk Factor: C

Calcium Glubionate (KAL see um gloo BYE oh nate)

Generic Available Yes

Pharmacologic Category Calcium Salt

Medication Safety Issues
Sound-alike/look-alike issues:
Calcium glubionate may be confused with calcium gluconate

Use Adjunct in treatment and prevention of postmenopausal osteoporosis; treatment and prevention of calcium depletion or hyperphosphatemia (eg, osteoporosis, osteomalacia, mild/moderate renal insufficiency, hypoparathyroidism, rickets)

Dosing
Adults & Elderly: Dosage is in terms of **elemental** calcium
Dietary Reference Intake:
Adults, Male/Female:
19-50 years: 1000 mg/day
≥51 years: 1200 mg/day
Female: Pregnancy: Same as for Adults, Male/Female
Female: Lactating: Same as for Adults, Male/Female

Syrup is a hyperosmolar solution; dosage is in terms of calcium glubionate, elemental calcium is in parentheses: 6-18 g (~0.5-1 g Ca^{++})/day in divided doses

Pediatrics: Dosage is in terms of **elemental** calcium
Dietary Reference Intake:
0-6 months: 210 mg/day
7-12 months: 270 mg/day
1-3 years: 500 mg/day
4-8 years: 800 mg/day
9-18 years: 1300 mg/day

Note: Syrup is a hyperosmolar solution; dosage is in terms of calcium glubionate, elemental calcium is in parentheses

Neonatal hypocalcemia: 1200 mg (77 mg Ca^{++})/kg/day in 4-6 divided doses
Maintenance: Infants and Children: 600-2000 mg (38-128 mg Ca^{++})/kg/day in 4 divided doses up to a maximum of 9 g (575 mg Ca^{++})/day

Renal Impairment: Cl$_{cr}$ <25 mL/minute: Dosage adjustments may be necessary depending on the serum calcium levels.

Available Dosage Forms Syrup: 1.8 g/5 mL (480 mL) [equivalent to elemental calcium 115 mg/5 mL]

Monitoring and Teaching Issues
Patient Education: Do not take any new medication during therapy without consulting prescriber. Follow exact instructions for dosing. Take with a full glass of water or juice, 1-3 hours after meals and other medications, and 1-2 hours before any approved iron supplements. Avoid alcohol, other antacids, caffeine, or other calcium supplements unless approved by prescriber. May cause constipation (increased exercise, fluids, fiber, or fruits may help) or dry mouth (frequent mouth care, chewing gum, or sucking lozenges may help). Report severe, unresolved GI disturbances and unusual emotional lability (mood swings). **Pregnancy precaution:** Inform prescriber if you are or intend to become pregnant.

Pregnancy Risk Factor: C

Calcium Gluconate (KAL see um GLOO koe nate)

Generic Available Yes

Pharmacologic Category Calcium Salt; Electrolyte Supplement, Oral; Electrolyte Supplement, Parenteral

Medication Safety Issues
Sound-alike/look-alike issues:
Calcium gluconate may be confused with calcium glubionate

Use Treatment and prevention of hypocalcemia; treatment of tetany, cardiac disturbances of hyperkalemia, cardiac resuscitation when epinephrine fails to improve myocardial contractions, hypocalcemia, or calcium channel blocker toxicity; calcium supplementation

Contraindications In ventricular fibrillation during cardiac resuscitation; patients with risk of digitalis toxicity, renal or cardiac disease, hypercalcemia, renal calculi, hypophosphatemia

Warnings/Precautions Avoid too rapid I.V. administration and avoid extravasation. Use with caution in digitalized patients, severe hyperphosphatemia, respiratory failure or acidosis. May produce cardiac arrest. Hypercalcemia may occur in patients with renal failure, frequent determination of serum calcium is necessary.

Drug Interactions
Decreased Effect: Absorption of tetracycline, atenolol (and potentially other beta-blockers), iron, quinolone antibiotics, alendronate, sodium fluoride, and zinc absorption may be significantly decreased by oral calcium administration; space administration times. Effects of calcium channel blockers (eg, verapamil) effects may be diminished. Polystyrene sulfonate's potassium-binding ability may be reduced; avoid concurrent oral administration.

Increased Effect/Toxicity: High doses of calcium with thiazide diuretics may result in milk-alkali syndrome and hypercalcemia; monitor response. Oral administration of calcium salts may decrease T$_4$ absorption; separate dose from levothyroxine by at least 4 hours. Calcium acetate may potentiate digoxin toxicity.

Lab Interactions Increased calcium (S); decreased magnesium

(Continued)

Calcium Gluconate *(Continued)*

Overdosage/Toxicology

Acute single oral ingestions of calcium salts may produce mild gastrointestinal distress, but hypercalcemia or other toxic manifestations are extremely unlikely. Symptoms of hypercalcemia include lethargy, nausea, vomiting, and coma.

Treatment is supportive. Severe hypercalcemia following parenteral overdose requires I.V. hydration. Urine output should be monitored and maintained at >3 mL/kg/hour. I.V. saline and natriuretic agents (eg, furosemide) can quickly and significantly increase excretion of calcium into urine.

Pharmacodynamics/Kinetics

Absorption: Requires vitamin D; minimal unless chronic, high doses are given; calcium is absorbed in soluble, ionized form; solubility of calcium is increased in an acid environment

Excretion: Primarily feces (as unabsorbed calcium); urine (20%)

Dosing

Adults & Elderly: Dosage is in terms of **elemental** calcium

Dietary Reference Intake:

Adults, Male/Female:

19-50 years: 1000 mg/day

≥51 years: 1200 mg/day

Female: Pregnancy: Same as for Adults, Male/Female

Female: Lactating: Same as for Adults, Male/Female

Hypocalcemia: I.V.: 2-15 g/24 hours as a continuous infusion or in divided doses

Hypocalcemia: Oral: 500 mg to 2 g 2-4 times/day

Osteoporosis/bone loss: Oral: 1000-1500 mg in divided doses/day

Hypocalcemia secondary to citrated blood infusion: I.V.: 2.3-4.5 mEq (5-10 mL of a 10% solution) per 500 mL of blood (infused into another vein). Single doses up to 9 mEq (20 mL of a 10% solution) have also been recommended.

Note: Routine administration of calcium, in the absence of signs/symptoms of hypocalcemia, is generally not recommended. A number of recommendations have been published seeking to address potential hypocalcemia during massive transfusion of citrated blood; however, many practitioners recommend replacement only as guided by clinical evidence of hypocalcemia and/or serial monitoring of ionized calcium.

Hypocalcemic tetany: I.V.: 1-3 g (4.5-16 mEq) may be administered until therapeutic response occurs

Calcium antagonist toxicity, magnesium intoxication, or cardiac arrest in the presence of hyperkalemia or hypocalcemia: Calcium chloride is recommended calcium salt: I.V.: 500-800 mg; maximum: 3 g/dose

Maintenance electrolyte requirements for TPN: I.V.: Daily requirements: 8-16 mEq/1000 kcal/24 hours

Pediatrics: Dosage is in terms of **elemental** calcium

Dietary Reference Intake:

0-6 months: 210 mg/day

7-12 months: 270 mg/day

1-3 years: 500 mg/day

4-8 years: 800 mg/day

9-18 years: 1300 mg/day

Hypocalcemia:

I.V.:

Neonates: 200-800 mg/kg/day as a continuous infusion or in 4 divided doses

Infants and Children: 200-500 mg/kg/day as a continuous infusion or in 4 divided doses

Oral: Children: 200-500 mg/kg/day divided every 6 hours

Hypocalcemia secondary to citrated blood infusion: I.V.: Neonates, Infants, and Children: Give 0.45 mEq **elemental** calcium for each 100 mL citrated blood infused. See **"Note"** in adult dosing.

Hypocalcemic tetany: I.V.:

Infants and Children: 100-200 mg/kg/dose (0.5-0.7 mEq/kg/dose) over 5-10 minutes; may repeat every 6-8 hours **or** follow with an infusion of 500 mg/kg/day

Calcium antagonist toxicity, magnesium intoxication or cardiac arrest in the presence of hyperkalemia or hypocalcemia: Calcium chloride is recommended calcium salt: I.V.: Infants and Children: 60-100 mg/kg/dose (maximum: 3 g/dose)

Renal Impairment: Cl_{cr} <25 mL/minute: Dosage adjustments may be necessary depending on the serum calcium levels.

Available Dosage Forms

Injection, solution [preservative free]: 10% [100 mg/mL] (10 mL, 50 mL, 100 mL, 200 mL) [equivalent to elemental calcium 9 mg/mL; calcium 0.46 mEq/mL]

Powder: 347 mg/tablespoonful (480 g)

Tablet: 500 mg [equivalent to elemental calcium 45 mg]; 650 mg [equivalent to elemental calcium 58.5 mg]; 975 mg [equivalent to elemental calcium 87.75 mg]

Monitoring and Teaching Issues

Physical Assessment: Assess other medications patient may be taking for effectiveness and interactions. Assess results of laboratory tests, therapeutic effect, and adverse/toxic effects. Assess knowledge/teach patient proper use, appropriate interventions to reduce side effects, and adverse symptoms to report. If administered I.V., monitor ECG, vital signs, and CNS. Observe infusion site closely. Avoid extravasation.

Patient Education: Do not take any new medication during therapy without consulting prescriber. Follow exact instructions for dosing. Take with a full glass of water or juice, 1-3 hours after other medications, and 1-2 hours before any approved iron supplements. Avoid alcohol, other antacids, caffeine, or other calcium supplements unless approved by prescriber. May cause constipation (increased exercise, fluids, fiber, or fruits may help) or dry mouth (frequent mouth care, chewing gum, or sucking lozenges may help). Report severe, unresolved GI disturbances and unusual emotional lability (mood swings). **Pregnancy precaution:** Inform prescriber if you are or intend to become pregnant.

Pregnancy Risk Factor: C
Administration
Compatibility: Stable in D₅LR, D₅NS, D₅W, D₁₀W, D₂₀W, LR, NS; **incompatible** in fat emulsion 10%
Y-site administration: Incompatible with amphotericin B cholesteryl sulfate complex, fluconazole, indomethacin
Compatibility in syringe: Incompatible with metoclopramide
Compatibility when admixed: Incompatible with amphotericin B, cefamandole, cefazolin, clindamycin, dobutamine, floxacillin, methylprednisolone sodium succinate
Related Information
Compatibility of Drugs *on page 1723*

Calcium Lactate (KAL see um LAK tate)
Generic Available Yes
Pharmacologic Category Calcium Salt
Use Adjunct in prevention of postmenopausal osteoporosis; treatment and prevention of calcium depletion
Dosing
Adults & Elderly: Dosage in terms of calcium lactate
Dietary Reference Intake (in terms of elemental calcium):
Adults, Male/Female:
19-50 years: 1000 mg/day
≥51 years: 1200 mg/day
Female: Pregnancy: Same as Adults, Male/Female
Female: Lactating: Same as Adults, Male/Female

Calcium supplement, osteoporosis prevention: Oral: 1.5-3 g divided every 8 hours
Pediatrics: Oral (in terms of calcium lactate)
Dietary Reference Intake (in terms of elemental calcium):
0-6 months: 210 mg/day
7-12 months: 270 mg/day
1-3 years: 500 mg/day
4-8 years: 800 mg/day
9-18 years: 1300 mg/day

Children: 500 mg/kg/day divided every 6-8 hours; maximum daily dose: 9 g
Renal Impairment: Cl_cr <25 mL/minute: Dosage adjustments may be necessary depending on the serum calcium levels.
Available Dosage Forms Tablet: 650 mg [equivalent to elemental calcium 84.5 mg]
Monitoring and Teaching Issues
Patient Education: Do not take any new medication during therapy without consulting prescriber. Follow exact instructions for dosing. Take with a full glass of water or juice, 1-3 hours after other medications, and 1-2 hours before any approved iron supplements. Avoid alcohol, other antacids, caffeine, or other calcium supplements unless approved by prescriber. May cause constipation (increased exercise, fluids, fiber, or fruits may help) or dry mouth (frequent mouth care, chewing gum, or sucking lozenges may help). Report severe, unresolved GI disturbances and unusual emotional lability (mood swings). **Pregnancy precaution:** Inform prescriber if you are or intend to become pregnant.
Pregnancy Risk Factor: C

♦ **Calcium Leucovorin** *see Leucovorin on page 875*

Calcium Phosphate (Tribasic) (KAL see um FOS fate tri BAY sik)
U.S. Brand Names Posture® [OTC]
Synonyms Tricalcium Phosphate
Generic Available No
Pharmacologic Category Calcium Salt
Use Adjunct in prevention of postmenopausal osteoporosis; treatment and prevention of calcium depletion
Dosing
Adults & Elderly: Oral (dosage is in terms of elemental calcium):
Dietary Reference Intake:
Adults, Male/Female:
19-50 years: 1000 mg/day
≥51 years: 1200 mg/day
Female: Pregnancy: Same as for Adults, Male/Female
Female: Lactating: Same as for Adults, Male/Female

Calcium supplement, prevention of osteoporosis: 1-2 g/day
Pediatrics: Oral (dosage is in terms of elemental calcium):
Dietary Reference Intake:
0-6 months: 210 mg/day
7-12 months: 270 mg/day
1-3 years: 500 mg/day
4-8 years: 800 mg/day
9-18 years: 1300 mg/day

Prevention of osteoporosis: 45-65 mg/kg/day
Renal Impairment: Cl_cr <25 mL/minute: Dosage adjustments may be necessary depending on the serum calcium levels.
Available Dosage Forms Tablet: 1565.2 mg [equivalent to elemental calcium 600 mg; sugar free]
Monitoring and Teaching Issues
Patient Education: Do not take any new medication during therapy without consulting prescriber. Follow exact instructions for dosing. Take with a full glass of water or juice, 1-3
(Continued)

Calcium Phosphate (Tribasic) *(Continued)*

hours after meals and other medications, and 1-2 hours before any approved iron supplements. Avoid alcohol, other antacids, caffeine, or other calcium supplements unless approved by prescriber. May cause constipation (increased exercise, fluids, fiber, or fruits may help) or dry mouth (frequent mouth care, chewing gum, or sucking lozenges may help). Report severe, unresolved GI disturbances and unusual emotional lability (mood swings). **Pregnancy precaution:** Inform prescriber if you are or intend to become pregnant.

Pregnancy Risk Factor: C

♦ **Caldecort®** [OTC] *see* Hydrocortisone *on page 760*

♦ **Cal-Gest** [OTC] *see* Calcium Carbonate *on page 235*

♦ **Cal-Mint** [OTC] *see* Calcium Carbonate *on page 235*

♦ **Caltrate®** 600 [OTC] *see* Calcium Carbonate *on page 235*

♦ **Camila™** *see* Norethindrone *on page 1096*

♦ **Camphorated Tincture of Opium** *see* Paregoric *on page 1158*

♦ **Campral®** *see* Acamprosate *on page 36*

♦ **Camptosar®** *see* Irinotecan *on page 829*

♦ **Camptothecin-11** *see* Irinotecan *on page 829*

♦ **Canasa™** *see* Mesalamine *on page 957*

♦ **Cancidas®** *see* Caspofungin *on page 264*

Candesartan *(kan de SAR tan)*

U.S. Brand Names Atacand®

Synonyms Candesartan Cilexetil

Generic Available No

Pharmacologic Category Angiotensin II Receptor Blocker

Use Alone or in combination with other antihypertensive agents in treating essential hypertension; treatment of heart failure (NYHA class II-IV)

Unlabeled/Investigational Use Congestive heart failure

Mechanism of Action/Effect Blocks the vasoconstrictor and aldosterone-secreting effects of angiotensin II by binding of angiotensin II at the AT1 receptor in many tissues, such as vascular smooth muscle and the adrenal gland. Independent of pathways for angiotensin II synthesis. Does not affect the response to bradykinin; does not bind to block other hormone receptors or ion channels known to be important in cardiovascular regulation.

Contraindications Hypersensitivity to candesartan or any component of the formulation; hypersensitivity to other A-II receptor antagonists; bilateral renal artery stenosis; pregnancy (2nd and 3rd trimesters)

Warnings/Precautions Avoid use or use a smaller dose in patients who are volume depleted. Drugs which alter renin-angiotensin system have been associated with deterioration in renal function, including oliguria, acute renal failure and progressive azotemia. Deterioration in renal function can occur with initiation. Use with caution in unilateral renal artery stenosis and pre-existing renal insufficiency; significant aortic/mitral stenosis. Use caution when initiating in heart failure; may need to adjust dose because of candesartan-induced hypotension.

Drug Interactions

Cytochrome P450 Effect: Substrate of CYP2C8/9 (minor); **Inhibits** CYP2C8/9 (weak)

Increased Effect/Toxicity: The risk of lithium toxicity may be increased by candesartan; monitor lithium levels. Concurrent use with potassium-sparing diuretics (amiloride, spironolactone, triamterene), potassium supplements, or trimethoprim (high-dose) may increase the risk of hyperkalemia.

Nutritional/Ethanol Interactions

Food: Food reduces the time to maximal concentration and increases the C_{max}.

Herb/Nutraceutical: Avoid dong quai if using for hypertension (has estrogenic activity). Avoid ephedra, yohimbe, ginseng (may worsen hypertension). Avoid garlic (may have increased antihypertensive effect).

Adverse Reactions

Cardiovascular: Angina, hypotension (CHF 19%), MI, palpitation, tachycardia

Central nervous system: Dizziness, lightheadedness, drowsiness, headache, vertigo, anxiety, depression, somnolence, fever

Dermatologic: Angioedema, rash

Endocrine & metabolic: Hyperglycemia, hyperkalemia (CHF <1% to 6%), hypertriglyceridemia, hyperuricemia

Gastrointestinal: Dyspepsia, gastroenteritis

Genitourinary: Hematuria

Neuromuscular & skeletal: Back pain, CPK increased, myalgia, paresthesia, weakness

Renal: Serum creatinine increased

Respiratory: Dyspnea, epistaxis, pharyngitis, rhinitis, upper respiratory tract infection

Miscellaneous: Diaphoresis (increased)

Overdosage/Toxicology Symptoms of overdose include hypotension and tachycardia. Treatment is supportive.

Pharmacodynamics/Kinetics

Onset of Action: 2-3 hours; Peak effect: 6-8 hours

Duration of Action: >24 hours

Bioavailability: 15%

Time to Peak: 3-4 hours

Protein Binding: 99%

Half-Life Elimination: Dose dependent: 5-9 hours

Metabolism: To candesartan by the intestinal wall cells

Excretion: Urine (26%)

Clearance: Total body: 0.37 mL/kg/minute; Renal: 0.19 mL/kg/minute

Dosing

Adults & Elderly:

Hypertension: Oral: 4-32 mg once daily. Dosage must be individualized. Blood pressure response is dose-related over the range of 2-32 mg. The usual recommended starting dose is 16 mg once daily when it is used as monotherapy in patients who are not volume depleted. It can be administered once or twice daily with total daily doses ranging from 8-32 mg; larger doses do not appear to have a greater effect and there is relatively little experience with such doses.

Congestive heart failure: Oral: Initial: 4 mg once daily; double the dose at 2-week intervals, as tolerated; target dose: 32 mg

Hepatic Impairment: No initial dosage adjustment required in mild hepatic impairment. Consider initiation at lower dosages in moderate hepatic impairment (AUC increased by 145%). No data available concerning dosing in severe hepatic impairment.

Available Dosage Forms Tablet, as cilexetil: 4 mg, 8 mg, 16 mg, 32 mg

Monitoring and Teaching Issues

Physical Assessment: Use caution in patients who have volume depleted, unilateral renal artery insufficiency, or significant aortic/mitral stenosis (see Warnings/Precautions). Assess potential for interactions with other pharmacological agents or herbal products patient may be taking (eg, increased risk for hypotension, hyperkalemia; see Drug Interactions). Assess results of laboratory tests (electrolytes, serum creatinine, BUN, urinalysis), effectiveness of therapy (reduced hypertension), and adverse response (eg, tachycardia, CNS changes, hyperglycemia, hypotension; see Adverse Reactions) at beginning of therapy, when changing dose, and on a regular basis during long-term therapy. Teach patient proper use, possible side effects/appropriate interventions, and adverse symptoms to report.

Monitoring Laboratory Tests: Electrolytes, serum creatinine, BUN, urinalysis

Patient Education: Do not take any new medication during therapy unless approved by prescriber. Take exactly as directed and do not discontinue without consulting prescriber. Preferable to take on an empty stomach (1 hour before or 2 hours after meals). This drug does not eliminate need for diet or exercise regimen as recommended by prescriber. May cause dizziness, fainting, or lightheadedness (use caution when driving or engaging in tasks that require alertness until response to drug is known); postural hypotension (use caution when rising from lying or sitting position or climbing stairs); nausea or vomiting (small frequent meals, frequent mouth care, chewing gum, or sucking lozenges may help); or diarrhea (boiled milk, buttermilk, or yogurt may help). Report chest pain or palpitations; unusual weight gain or swelling of ankles and hands; persistent fatigue; unusual flu or cold symptoms or dry cough; respiratory difficulty; swelling of eyes, face, or lips; skin rash; muscle pain or weakness; unusual bleeding (blood in urine or stool, or from gums); or excessive sweating. **Pregnancy/breast-feeding precautions:** Inform prescriber if you are or intend to become pregnant. This drug should not be used in the 2nd or 3rd trimester of pregnancy. Consult prescriber for appropriate contraceptive measures if necessary. Do not breast-feed.

Geriatric Considerations: High concentrations occur in the elderly compared to younger subjects. AUC may be doubled in patients with renal impairment.

Pregnancy Risk Factor: C/D (2nd and 3rd trimesters)

Pregnancy Issues: The drug should be discontinued as soon as possible when pregnancy is detected. Drugs which act directly on renin-angiotensin can cause fetal and neonatal morbidity and death.

Lactation: Enters breast milk/contraindicated

Additional Information May have an advantage over losartan due to minimal metabolism requirements and consequent use in mild to moderate hepatic impairment

Related Information

Angiotensin Agents *on page 1704*

Candesartan and Hydrochlorothiazide

(kan de SAR tan & hye droe klor oh THYE a zide)

U.S. Brand Names Atacand HCT™

Synonyms Candesartan Cilexetil and Hydrochlorothiazide

Generic Available No

Pharmacologic Category Angiotensin II Receptor Blocker Combination

Use Treatment of hypertension; combination product should not be used for initial therapy

Dosing

Adults & Elderly: Hypertension, replacement therapy: Oral: Combination product can be substituted for individual agents; maximum therapeutic effect would be expected within 4 weeks

Usual dosage range:

Candesartan: 8-32 mg/day, given once daily or twice daily in divided doses

Hydrochlorothiazide: 12.5-50 mg once daily

Renal Impairment: Serum levels of candesartan are increased and the half-life of hydrochlorothiazide is prolonged in patients with renal impairment. Do not use if Cl_{cr} is <30 mL/minute.

Hepatic Impairment: Use with caution.

Available Dosage Forms Tablet:

16-12.5: Candesartan 16 mg and hydrochlorothiazide 12.5 mg

32-12.5: Candesartan 32 mg and hydrochlorothiazide 12.5 mg

Monitoring and Teaching Issues

Physical Assessment: See individual agents.

Patient Education: See individual agents. **Pregnancy/breast-feeding precautions:** Inform prescriber if you are or intend to become pregnant; contraceptives may be recommended. Do not breast-feed.

(Continued)

Candesartan and Hydrochlorothiazide *(Continued)*

Pregnancy Risk Factor: C/D (2nd and 3rd trimesters)
Lactation: Enters breast milk/contraindicated
Related Information
  Candesartan *on page 242*
  Hydrochlorothiazide *on page 751*

♦ **Candesartan Cilexetil** *see* Candesartan *on page 242*

♦ **Candesartan Cilexetil and Hydrochlorothiazide** *see* Candesartan and Hydrochlorothiazide *on page 243*

♦ *Candida albicans* **(Monilia)** *see page 1625*

Capecitabine *(ka pe SITE a been)*

U.S. Brand Names Xeloda®
Generic Available No
Pharmacologic Category Antineoplastic Agent, Antimetabolite
Use Treatment of metastatic colorectal cancer, metastatic breast cancer
Mechanism of Action/Effect Capecitabine is a prodrug of fluorouracil. It undergoes hydrolysis in the liver and tissues to form fluorouracil. It interferes with DNA (and to a lesser degree RNA) synthesis. Appears to be specific for G_1 and S phases of the cell cycle.
Contraindications Hypersensitivity to capecitabine, fluorouracil, or any component of the formulation; known deficiency of dihydropyrimidine dehydrogenase (DPD); severe renal impairment (Cl_{cr} <30 mL/minute); pregnancy
Warnings/Precautions The U.S. Food and Drug Administration (FDA) currently recommends that procedures for proper handling and disposal of antineoplastic agents be considered. Use with caution in patients with bone marrow suppression, poor nutritional status, on warfarin therapy, ≥80 years of age, or renal or hepatic dysfunction. Use with caution in patients who have received extensive pelvic radiation or alkylating therapy. Use cautiously with warfarin; altered coagulation parameters and bleeding have been reported.

Capecitabine can cause severe diarrhea; median time to first occurrence is 31 days; subsequent doses should be reduced after grade 3 or 4 diarrhea

If grade 2 or 3 hand-and-foot syndrome occurs, interrupt administration of capecitabine until the event resolves or decreases in intensity to grade 1. Following grade 3 hand-and-foot syndrome, decrease subsequent doses of capecitabine.

Use caution in patients with coronary artery disease. Cardiotoxicity has been associated with fluorinated pyrimidine therapy, including myocardial infarction, angina, dysrhythmias, cardiogenic shock, sudden death, and ECG changes (increased risk in CAD).
Drug Interactions
  Increased Effect/Toxicity: Response to warfarin may be increased by capecitabine.
Nutritional/Ethanol Interactions Food: Food reduced the rate and extent of absorption of capecitabine.
Adverse Reactions Frequency listed derived from monotherapy trials.
  >10%:
    Cardiovascular: Edema (9% to 15%)
    Central nervous system: Fatigue (~40%), fever (12% to 18%), pain (colorectal cancer: 12%)
    Dermatologic: Palmar-plantar erythrodysesthesia (hand-and-foot syndrome) (~55%, may be dose limiting), dermatitis (27% to 37%)
    Gastrointestinal: Diarrhea (~55%, may be dose limiting), mild to moderate nausea (43% to 53%), vomiting (27% to 37%), stomatitis (~25%), decreased appetite (colorectal cancer: 26%), anorexia (23%), abdominal pain (20% to 35%), constipation (~15%)
    Hematologic: Lymphopenia (94%), anemia (72% to 80%; Grade 3/4: <1% to 3%), neutropenia (13% to 26%; Grade 3/4: 1% to 2%), thrombocytopenia (24%; Grade 3/4: 1% to 3%)
    Hepatic: Increased bilirubin (22% to 48%)
    Neuromuscular & skeletal: Paresthesia (21%)
    Ocular: Eye irritation (~15%)
    Respiratory: Dyspnea (colorectal cancer: 14%)
  5% to 10%:
    Cardiovascular: Venous thrombosis (colorectal cancer: 8%), chest pain (colorectal cancer: 6%)
    Central nervous system: Headache (~10%), dizziness (~8%), insomnia (8%), mood alteration (colorectal cancer: 5%), depression (colorectal cancer: 5%)
    Dermatologic: Nail disorders (7%), skin discoloration (colorectal cancer: 7%), alopecia (colorectal cancer: 6%)
    Endocrine & metabolic: Dehydration (7%)
    Gastrointestinal: Motility disorder (colorectal cancer: 10%), oral discomfort (colorectal cancer: 10%), dyspepsia (8%), upper GI inflammatory disorders (colorectal cancer: 8%), hemorrhage (colorectal cancer: 6%), ileus (colorectal cancer: 6%), taste disturbance (colorectal cancer: 6%)
    Neuromuscular & skeletal: Back pain (colorectal cancer: 10%), myalgia (9%), neuropathy (colorectal cancer: 10%), arthralgia (colorectal cancer: 8%), limb pain (colorectal cancer: 6%)
    Respiratory: Cough (7%), sore throat (2%), epistaxis (3%)
    Ocular: Abnormal vision (colorectal cancer: 5%)
    Miscellaneous: Viral infection (colorectal cancer: 5%)
Overdosage/Toxicology Symptoms of overdose include myelosuppression, nausea, vomiting, diarrhea, and alopecia. No specific antidote exists. Monitor hematologically for at least 4 weeks. Treatment is supportive.

Pharmacodynamics/Kinetics
Absorption: Rapid and extensive
Time to Peak: 1.5 hours; Fluorouracil: 2 hours
Protein Binding: <60%; 35% to albumin
Half-Life Elimination: 0.5-1 hour
Metabolism: Hepatic: Inactive metabolites: 5′-deoxy-5-fluorocytidine, 5′-deoxy-5-fluorouridine; Tissue: Active metabolite: Fluorouracil
Excretion: Urine (96%, 50% as α-fluoro-β-alanine)

Dosing
Adults: Metastatic breast carcinoma, metastatic colorectal cancer: Oral: 2500 mg/m^2/day in 2 divided doses (~12 hours apart) at the end of a meal for 2 weeks followed by a 1- or 2-week rest period
Dosage modification guidelines: See table.

Recommended Dose Modifications

Toxicity NCI Grades	During a Course of Therapy	Dose Adjustment for Next Cycle (% of starting dose)
Grade 1	Maintain dose level	Maintain dose level
Grade 2		
1st appearance	Interrupt until resolved to grade 0-1	100%
2nd appearance	Interrupt until resolved to grade 0-1	75%
3rd appearance	Interrupt until resolved to grade 0-1	50%
4th appearance	Discontinue treatment permanently	
Grade 3		
1st appearance	Interrupt until resolved to grade 0-1	75%
2nd appearance	Interrupt until resolved to grade 0-1	50%
3rd appearance	Discontinue treatment permanently	
Grade 4		
1st appearance	Discontinue permanently **or** If physician deems it to be in the patient's best interest to continue, interrupt until resolved to grade 0-1	50%

Elderly: The elderly may be pharmacodynamically more sensitive to the toxic effects of fluorouracil. Insufficient data are available to provide dosage modifications.

Renal Impairment:
Cl$_{cr}$ 50-80 mL/minute: No adjustment of initial dose.
Cl$_{cr}$ 30-50 mL/minute: Reduce dose by 25%.
Cl$_{cr}$ <30 mL/minute: Do not use.

Hepatic Impairment:
Mild to moderate impairment: No starting dose adjustment is necessary; however, carefully monitor patients.
Severe hepatic impairment: Patients have not been studied.

Available Dosage Forms Tablet: 150 mg, 500 mg

Monitoring and Teaching Issues
Physical Assessment: See Contraindications, Warnings/Precautions for specific use cautions. Assess results of laboratory tests (renal and hepatic function, CBC with differential; see Monitoring Laboratory Tests). Monitor therapeutic response and adverse reactions (eg, gastrointestinal [diarrhea, nausea, vomiting, pain, dehydration], hematologic [lymphopenia, anemia, thrombocytopenia], cardiovascular [edema, chest pain], paresthesia) at beginning and periodically during therapy. Teach patient proper use, possible side effects/appropriate interventions, and adverse symptoms to report.

Monitoring Laboratory Tests: Renal function should be estimated at baseline to determine initial dose. During therapy, CBC with differential, hepatic function, and renal function should be monitored.

Patient Education: Do not take any new medication during therapy unless approved by prescriber. Take with food or within 30 minutes after meal. Avoid use of antacids within 2 hours of taking this medication. Do not crush, chew, or dissolve tablets. Maintain adequate hydration (2-3 L/day of fluids) unless instructed to restrict fluid intake. You will be more susceptible to infection (avoid crowds and exposure to infection and do not have any vaccinations without consulting prescriber). May cause lethargy, dizziness, visual changes, confusion, anxiety (avoid driving or engaging in tasks requiring alertness until response to drug is known); nausea, vomiting, loss of appetite, or dry mouth (small frequent meals, frequent mouth care, chewing gum, or sucking lozenges may help); loss of hair (will grow back when treatment is discontinued); photosensitivity (use sunscreen, wear protective clothing and eyewear, and avoid direct sunlight); or dry, itchy, skin, and dry or irritated eyes (avoid contact lenses). Report persistent diarrhea or abdominal pain; skin rash, pain, tenderness, or peeling (especially hands and feet); chills or fever, confusion, persistent or violent vomiting; respiratory difficulty; chest pain or palpitations; unusual bleeding or bruising; bone pain; muscle spasms/tremors; or vision changes immediately. **Pregnancy/breast-feeding precautions:** Inform prescriber if you are pregnant. Do not get pregnant while taking this medication. Consult prescriber for appropriate contraceptive measures. Breast-feeding is not recommended.

Dietary Considerations: Because current safety and efficacy data are based upon administration with food, it is recommended that capecitabine be administered with food. In all clinical trials, patients were instructed to administer capecitabine within 30 minutes after a meal.

(Continued)

Capecitabine *(Continued)*

Geriatric Considerations: Patients ≥80 years of age may experience a greater incidence of grade 3 or 4 adverse events (diarrhea, hand-and-foot syndrome, nausea/vomiting).

Pregnancy Risk Factor: D

Lactation: Excretion in breast milk unknown/not recommended

Breast-Feeding Issues: It is not known if the drug is excreted in breast milk. Because of the potential for serious adverse reactions in nursing infants, it is recommended that nursing be discontinued when receiving capecitabine therapy.

Administration

Oral: Capecitabine is administered orally, usually in two divided doses taken 12 hours apart. Doses should be taken after meals with water.

Storage: Store tablets at room temperature of 25°C (77°F).

♦ **Capex™** *see Fluocinolone on page 643*

♦ **Capital® and Codeine** *see Acetaminophen and Codeine on page 41*

♦ **Capoten®** *see Captopril on page 246*

♦ **Capozide®** *see Captopril and Hydrochlorothiazide on page 248*

Captopril *(KAP toe pril)*

U.S. Brand Names Capoten®

Synonyms ACE

Generic Available Yes

Pharmacologic Category Angiotensin-Converting Enzyme (ACE) Inhibitor

Medication Safety Issues

Sound-alike/look-alike issues:

Captopril may be confused with Capitrol®, carvedilol

Use Management of hypertension; treatment of congestive heart failure, left ventricular dysfunction after myocardial infarction, diabetic nephropathy

Unlabeled/Investigational Use Treatment of hypertensive crisis, rheumatoid arthritis; diagnosis of anatomic renal artery stenosis, hypertension secondary to scleroderma renal crisis; diagnosis of aldosteronism, idiopathic edema, Bartter's syndrome, postmyocardial infarction for prevention of ventricular failure; increase circulation in Raynaud's phenomenon, hypertension secondary to Takayasu's disease

Mechanism of Action/Effect Competitive inhibitor of angiotensin-converting enzyme (ACE); prevents conversion of angiotensin I to angiotensin II, a potent vasoconstrictor; results in lower levels of angiotensin II which causes an increase in plasma renin activity and a reduction in aldosterone secretion

Contraindications Hypersensitivity to captopril or any component of the formulation; angioedema related to previous treatment with an ACE inhibitor; idiopathic or hereditary angioedema; bilateral renal artery stenosis; pregnancy (2nd or 3rd trimester)

Warnings/Precautions Angioedema can occur at any time during treatment (especially following first dose). Angioedema may involve head and neck (potentially affecting the airway) or the intestine (presenting with abdominal pain). Careful blood pressure monitoring with first dose (hypotension can occur especially in volume depleted patients). Dosage adjustment needed in renal impairment. Use with caution in hypovolemia; collagen vascular diseases; valvular stenosis (particularly aortic stenosis); hyperkalemia; or before, during, or immediately after anesthesia. Avoid rapid dosage escalation which may lead to renal insufficiency. Rare toxicities associated with ACE inhibitors include cholestatic jaundice (which may progress to hepatic necrosis) and neutropenia/agranulocytosis with myeloid hyperplasia. Additional hematologic monitoring required in patients with baseline renal impairment. Deterioration in renal function can occur with initiation. Use with caution in unilateral renal artery stenosis and pre-existing renal insufficiency.

Drug Interactions

Cytochrome P450 Effect: Substrate of CYP2D6 (major)

Decreased Effect: Aspirin (high dose) may reduce the therapeutic effects of ACE inhibitors; at low dosages this does not appear to be significant. Rifampin may decrease the effect of ACE inhibitors. Antacids may decrease the bioavailability of ACE inhibitors (may be more likely to occur with captopril); separate administration times by 1-2 hours. NSAIDs, specifically indomethacin, may reduce the hypotensive effects of ACE inhibitors. More likely to occur in low renin or volume dependent hypertensive patients.

Increased Effect/Toxicity: Potassium supplements, co-trimoxazole (high dose), angiotensin II receptor antagonists (candesartan, losartan, irbesartan, etc), or potassium-sparing diuretics (amiloride, spironolactone, triamterene) may result in elevated serum potassium levels when combined with captopril. CYP2D6 inhibitors may increase the levels/effects of captopril; example inhibitors include chlorpromazine, delavirdine, fluoxetine, miconazole, paroxetine, pergolide, quinidine, quinine, ritonavir, and ropinirole. ACE inhibitor effects may be increased by phenothiazines or probenecid (increases levels of captopril). ACE inhibitors may increase serum concentrations/effects of digoxin, lithium, and sulfonlyureas.

Diuretics have additive hypotensive effects with ACE inhibitors, and hypovolemia increases the potential for adverse renal effects of ACE inhibitors. In patients with compromised renal function, coadministration with NSAIDs may result in further deterioration of renal function. Allopurinol and ACE inhibitors may cause a higher risk of hypersensitivity reaction when taken concurrently.

Nutritional/Ethanol Interactions

Food: Captopril serum concentrations may be decreased if taken with food. Long-term use of captopril may result in a zinc deficiency which can result in a decrease in taste perception.

Herb/Nutraceutical: Avoid dong quai if using for hypertension (has estrogenic activity). Avoid ephedra, yohimbe, ginseng (may worsen hypertension). Avoid garlic (may have increased antihypertensive effect).

Lab Interactions Increased BUN, creatinine, potassium, positive Coombs' [direct]; decreased cholesterol (S); may cause false-positive results in urine acetone determinations using sodium nitroprusside reagent

Adverse Reactions

1% to 10%:

Cardiovascular: Hypotension (1% to 3%), tachycardia (1%), chest pain (1%), palpitation (1%)

Dermatologic: Rash (maculopapular or urticarial) (4% to 7%), pruritus (2%); in patients with rash, a positive ANA and/or eosinophilia has been noted in 7% to 10%.

Endocrine & metabolic: Hyperkalemia (1% to 11%)

Hematologic: Neutropenia may occur in up to 4% of patients with renal insufficiency or or collagen-vascular disease.

Renal: Proteinuria (1%), increased serum creatinine, worsening of renal function (may occur in patients with bilateral renal artery stenosis or hypovolemia)

Respiratory: Cough (<1% to 2%)

Miscellaneous: Hypersensitivity reactions (rash, pruritus, fever, arthralgia, and eosinophilia) have occurred in 4% to 7% of patients (depending on dose and renal function); dysgeusia - loss of taste or diminished perception (2% to 4%)

Frequency not defined:

Cardiovascular: Angioedema, cardiac arrest, cerebrovascular insufficiency, rhythm disturbances, orthostatic hypotension, syncope, flushing, pallor, angina, MI, Raynaud's syndrome, CHF

Central nervous system: Ataxia, confusion, depression, nervousness, somnolence

Dermatologic: Bullous pemphigus, erythema multiforme, Stevens-Johnson syndrome, exfoliative dermatitis

Endocrine & metabolic: Alkaline phosphatase increased, bilirubin increased, gynecomastia

Gastrointestinal: Pancreatitis, glossitis, dyspepsia

Genitourinary: Urinary frequency, impotence

Hematologic: Anemia, thrombocytopenia, pancytopenia, agranulocytosis, anemia

Hepatic: Jaundice, hepatitis, hepatic necrosis (rare), cholestasis, hyponatremia (symptomatic), transaminases increased

Neuromuscular & skeletal: Asthenia, myalgia, myasthenia

Ocular: Blurred vision

Renal: Renal insufficiency, renal failure, nephrotic syndrome, polyuria, oliguria

Respiratory: Bronchospasm, eosinophilic pneumonitis, rhinitis

Miscellaneous: Anaphylactoid reactions

Overdosage/Toxicology
Mild hypotension has been the primary toxic effect seen with acute overdose. Bradycardia may also occur. Hyperkalemia occurs even with therapeutic doses, especially in patients with renal insufficiency and those taking NSAIDs. Treatment is symptom-directed and supportive.

Pharmacodynamics/Kinetics

Onset of Action: Peak effect: Blood pressure reduction: 1-1.5 hours after dose

Duration of Action: Dose related, may require several weeks of therapy before full hypotensive effect

Absorption: 60% to 75%; reduced 30% to 40% by food

Protein Binding: 25% to 30%

Half-Life Elimination: Renal and cardiac function dependent: Adults: Healthy volunteers: 1.9 hours; Congestive heart failure: 2.06 hours; Anuria: 20-40 hours

Metabolism: 50%

Excretion: Urine (95%) within 24 hours

Dosing

Adults & Elderly: Note: Dosage must be titrated according to patient's response

Acute hypertension (urgency/emergency): Oral: 12.5-25 mg, may repeat as needed (may be given sublingually but no therapeutic advantage demonstrated)

Hypertension: Oral: Initial: 12.5-25 mg 2-3 times/day; may increase by 12.5-25 mg/dose at 1- to 2-week intervals up to 50 mg 3 times/day. Maximum: 150 mg 3 times/day. Add diuretic before further dosage increases.

Usual dose range (JNC 7): 25-100 mg/day in 2 divided doses

Congestive heart failure: Oral:

Initial: 6.25-12.5 mg 3 times/day in conjunction with cardiac glycoside and diuretic therapy. Initial dose depends upon patient's fluid/electrolyte status.

Target: 50 mg 3 times/day

Maximum: 100 mg 3 times/day

Prevention of LV dysfunction following MI: Oral: Initial: 6.25 mg; followed by 12.5 mg 3 times/day; increase to 25 mg 3 times/day over the next few days; following by gradual increase to a goal of 50 mg 3 times/day (Some dosage schedules increase the dosage more aggressively to achieve goal dosage within the first few days of initiation).

Diabetic nephropathy: Oral:

25 mg 3 times/day. May be taken with other antihypertensive therapy if required to further lower blood pressure.

Pediatrics: Note: Dosage must be titrated according to patient's response.

Hypertension: Oral:

Infants: Initial: 0.15-0.3 mg/kg/dose; titrate dose upward to maximum of 6 mg/kg/day in 1-4 divided doses; usual required dose: 2.5-6 mg/kg/day

Children: Initial: 0.5 mg/kg/dose; titrate upward to maximum of 6 mg/kg/day in 2-4 divided doses.

Older Children: Initial: 6.25-12.5 mg/dose every 12-24 hours; titrate upward to maximum of 6 mg/kg/day.

Adolescents: Initial: 12.5-25 mg/dose given every 8-12 hours; increase by 25 mg/dose to maximum of 450 mg/day.

Renal Impairment:

Cl_{cr} 10-50 mL/minute: Administer 75% of normal dose.

Cl_{cr} <10 mL/minute: Administer 50% of normal dose.

Note: Smaller dosages given every 8-12 hours are indicated in patients with renal dysfunction. Renal function and leukocyte count should be carefully monitored during therapy.

Hemodialysis effects: Moderately dialyzable (20% to 50%); administer dose postdialysis or administer 25% to 35% supplemental dose.

Peritoneal dialysis: Supplemental dose is not necessary.

(Continued)

Captopril *(Continued)*

Available Dosage Forms Tablet: 12.5 mg, 25 mg, 50 mg, 100 mg

Monitoring and Teaching Issues

Physical Assessment: See Contraindications and Warnings/Precautions for use cautions (eg, renal impairment, hypovolemia, valvular stenosis, hyperkalemia; anesthesia). Assess potential for interactions with other pharmacological agents or herbal products patient may be taking (especially those that may impact renal function; see Drug Interactions). Assess results of laboratory tests, therapeutic effectiveness (blood pressure should be monitored after first doses and periodically during therapy), and adverse response (eg, hypovolemia, angioedema, postural hypotension; see Adverse Reactions) on a regular basis during therapy. Teach patient proper use, possible side effects/appropriate interventions, and adverse symptoms to report.

Monitoring Laboratory Tests: BUN, serum creatinine, urine dipstick for protein, CBC, electrolytes. If patient has renal impairment, a baseline WBC with differential and serum creatinine should be evaluated and monitored closely during the first 3 months of therapy.

Patient Education: Do not take any new medication during therapy unless approved by prescriber. Do not use potassium supplement or salt substitutes without consulting prescriber. Take exactly as directed; do not discontinue without consulting prescriber. Take first dose at bedtime. Take all doses on an empty stomach, 1 hour before or 2 hours after meals. This drug does not eliminate need for diet or exercise regimen as recommended by prescriber. May cause dizziness, fainting, or lightheadedness (use caution when driving or engaging in tasks that require alertness until response to drug is known); postural hypotension (use caution when rising from lying or sitting position or climbing stairs); or nausea, vomiting, abdominal pain, dry mouth, or transient loss of appetite (small frequent meals, frequent mouth care, sucking lozenges, or chewing gum may help). Report chest pain or palpitations; mouth sores; fever or chills; swelling of extremities, face, mouth, or tongue; skin rash; numbness, tingling, or pain in muscles; respiratory difficulty or unusual cough; and other persistent adverse reactions. **Pregnancy precautions:** Inform prescriber if you are or intend to become pregnant. This drug should not be used in the 2nd or 3rd trimester of pregnancy. Consult prescriber for appropriate contraceptive measures if necessary.

Dietary Considerations: Should be taken at least 1 hour before or 2 hours after eating.

Geriatric Considerations: Due to frequent decreases in glomerular filtration (also creatinine clearance) with aging, elderly patients may have exaggerated responses to ACE inhibitors. Differences in clinical response due to hepatic changes are not observed.

Pregnancy Risk Factor: C/D (2nd and 3rd trimesters)

Pregnancy Issues: ACE inhibitors can cause fetal injury or death if taken during the 2nd or 3rd trimester. Discontinue ACE inhibitors as soon as pregnancy is detected.

Lactation: Enters breast milk/compatible

Breast-Feeding Issues: Crosses into breast milk. AAP considers **compatible** with breast-feeding.

Administration

Oral: Unstable in aqueous solutions; to prepare solution for oral administration, mix prior to administration and use within 10 minutes.

Related Information

Angiotensin Agents *on page 1704*
Heart Failure *on page 1828*

Captopril and Hydrochlorothiazide

(KAP toe pril & hye droe klor oh THYE a zide)

U.S. Brand Names Capozide®

Synonyms Hydrochlorothiazide and Captopril

Generic Available Yes

Pharmacologic Category Antihypertensive Agent, Combination

Use Management of hypertension and treatment of congestive heart failure

Dosing

Adults: Hypertension, CHF: May be substituted for previously titrated dosages of the individual components; alternatively, may initiate as follows: Oral:

Initial: Single tablet (captopril 25 mg/hydrochlorothiazide 15 mg) taken once daily; daily dose of captopril should not exceed 150 mg; daily dose of hydrochlorothiazide should not exceed 50 mg

Elderly: Refer to dosing in individual monographs.

Renal Impairment: May respond to smaller or less frequent doses.

Available Dosage Forms Tablet:

25/15: Captopril 25 mg and hydrochlorothiazide 15 mg

25/25: Captopril 25 mg and hydrochlorothiazide 25 mg

50/15: Captopril 50 mg and hydrochlorothiazide 15 mg

50/25: Captopril 50 mg and hydrochlorothiazide 25 mg

Monitoring and Teaching Issues

Physical Assessment: See individual agents.

Patient Education: See individual agents. **Pregnancy precaution:** Inform prescriber if you are or intend to become pregnant.

Pregnancy Risk Factor: C/D (2nd and 3rd trimesters)

Lactation: Enters breast milk/compatible

Related Information

Captopril *on page 246*
Hydrochlorothiazide *on page 751*

♦ Carac™ *see* Fluorouracil *on page 647*
♦ Carafate® *see* Sucralfate *on page 1402*

Carbamazepine (kar ba MAZ e peen)

U.S. Brand Names Carbatrol®; Epitol®; Equetro™; Tegretol®; Tegretol®-XR

Synonyms CBZ; SPD417

Generic Available Yes: Excludes capsule (extended release), tablet (extended release)

Pharmacologic Category Anticonvulsant, Miscellaneous

Medication Safety Issues
Sound-alike/look-alike issues:
Carbatrol® may be confused with Cartrol®
Epitol® may be confused with Epinal®
Tegretol® may be confused with Mebaral®, Tegrin®, Toradol®, Trental®

Use
Carbatrol®, Tegretol®, Tegretol®-XR: Partial seizures with complex symptomatology (psychomotor, temporal lobe), generalized tonic-clonic seizures (grand mal), mixed seizure patterns, trigeminal neuralgia
Equetro™: Acute manic and mixed episodes associated with bipolar 1 disorder

Unlabeled/Investigational Use Treatment of resistant schizophrenia, ethanol withdrawal, restless leg syndrome, psychotic behavior associated with dementia, post-traumatic stress disorders

Mechanism of Action/Effect In addition to anticonvulsant effects, carbamazepine has anticholinergic, antineuralgic, antidiuretic, muscle relaxant, antimanic, antidepressive, and and antiarrhythmic properties; may depress activity in the nucleus ventralis of the thalamus or decrease synaptic transmission or decrease summation of temporal stimulation leading to neural discharge by limiting influx of sodium ions across cell membrane or other unknown mechanisms; stimulates the release of ADH and potentiates its action in promoting reabsorption of water; chemically related to tricyclic antidepressants

Contraindications Hypersensitivity to carbamazepine, tricyclic antidepressants, or any component of the formulation; bone marrow depression; with or within 14 days of MAO inhibitor use; pregnancy

Warnings/Precautions Administer carbamazepine with caution to patients with history of cardiac damage, hepatic or renal disease; potentially fatal blood cell abnormalities have been reported; patients with a previous history of adverse hematologic reaction to any drug may be at increased risk. Prescriptions should be written for the smallest quantity consistent with good patient care. The smallest effective dose is suggested for use in bipolar disorder to reduce the risk for overdose; high-risk patients should be monitored. Actuation of latent psychosis is possible.

Carbamazepine is not effective in absence, myoclonic or akinetic seizures; exacerbation of certain seizure types have been seen after initiation of carbamazepine therapy in children with mixed seizure disorders. Abrupt discontinuation is not recommended in patients being treated for seizures. Dizziness or drowsiness may occur; caution should be used when performing tasks which require alertness until the effects are known. Coadministration of carbamazepine and delavirdine may lead to loss of virologic response and possible resistance. Elderly may have increased risk of SIADH-like syndrome. Carbamazepine has mild anticholinergic activity; use with caution in patients with increased intraocular pressure, or sensitivity to anticholinergic effects. Severe dermatologic reactions, including Lyell and Stevens-Johnson syndromes, although rarely reported, have resulted in fatalities. Discontinue if there are any signs of hypersensitivity.

Drug Interactions
Cytochrome P450 Effect: Substrate of CYP2C8/9 (minor), 3A4 (major); **Induces** CYP1A2 (strong), 2B6 (strong), 2C8/9 (strong), 2C19 (strong), 3A4 (strong)

Decreased Effect: The levels/effects of carbamazepine may be decreased by aminoglutethimide, nafcillin, nevirapine, phenobarbital, phenytoin, and rifamycins, and other CYP3A4 inducers. Carbamazepine may induce its own metabolism. Carbamazepine suspension is incompatible with chlorpromazine solution and thioridazine liquid. Schedule carbamazepine suspension at least 1-2 hours apart from other liquid medicinals. Concomitant use of antimalarial drugs (chloroquine, mefloquine) with carbamazepine may reduce seizure control by lowering plasma levels.

Carbamazepine may decrease the effect of clozapine, corticosteroids, cyclosporine, doxycycline, ethosuximide, felbamate, felodipine, haloperidol, mebendazole, methadone, oral contraceptives, thyroid hormones, tricyclic antidepressants, and valproic acid. Carbamazepine may decrease the levels/effects of aminophylline, amiodarone, benzodiazepines, bupropion, calcium channel blockers, citalopram, clarithromycin, cyclosporine, diazepam, efavirenz, erythromycin, estrogens, fluoxetine, fluvoxamine, glimepiride, glipizide, losartan, methsuximide, mirtazapine, nateglinide, nefazodone, nevirapine, pioglitazone, promethazine, propranolol, protease inhibitors, proton pump inhibitors, ropinirole, rosiglitazone, selegiline, sertraline, sulfonamides, tacrolimus, theophylline, venlafaxine. voriconazole, warfarin, zafirlukast, and other CYP1A2, 2B6, 2C8/9, 2C19 or 3A4 substrates.

Increased Effect/Toxicity: Carbamazepine may enhance the hepatotoxic potential of acetaminophen. Neurotoxicity may result in patients receiving lithium and carbamazepine concurrently. CYP3A4 inhibitors may increase the levels/effects of carbamazepine; example inhibitors include azole antifungals, ciprofloxacin, clarithromycin, diclofenac, doxycycline, erythromycin, imatinib, isoniazid, nefazodone, nicardipine, propofol, protease inhibitors, quinidine, and verapamil. Carbamazepine may increase the levels/effects of phenytoin.

Nutritional/Ethanol Interactions
Ethanol: Avoid ethanol (may increase CNS depression).
Food: Carbamazepine serum levels may be increased if taken with food. Carbamazepine serum concentration may be increased if taken with grapefruit juice; avoid concurrent use.
Herb/Nutraceutical: Avoid evening primrose (seizure threshold decreased). Avoid valerian, St John's wort, kava kava, gotu kola (may increase CNS depression).

Lab Interactions May interact with some pregnancy tests; increased BUN, AST, ALT, bilirubin, alkaline phosphatase (S); decreased calcium, T_3, T_4, sodium (S)
(Continued)

Carbamazepine *(Continued)*

Adverse Reactions Frequency not defined, unless otherwise specified.

Cardiovascular: Arrhythmias, AV block, bradycardia, chest pain (bipolar use), CHF, edema, hyper-/hypotension, lymphadenopathy, syncope, thromboembolism, thrombophlebitis

Central nervous system: Amnesia (bipolar use), anxiety (bipolar use), aseptic meningitis (case report), ataxia (bipolar use 15%), confusion, depression (bipolar use), dizziness (bipolar use 44%), fatigue, headache (bipolar use 22%), sedation, slurred speech, somnolence (bipolar use 32%)

Dermatologic: Alopecia, alterations in skin pigmentation, erythema multiforme, exfoliative dermatitis, photosensitivity reaction, pruritus (bipolar use 8%), purpura, rash, Stevens-Johnson syndrome, toxic epidermal necrolysis, urticaria

Endocrine & metabolic: Chills, fever, hyponatremia, syndrome of inappropriate ADH secretion (SIADH)

Gastrointestinal: Abdominal pain, anorexia, constipation, diarrhea, dyspepsia (bipolar use), gastric distress, nausea (bipolar use 29%), pancreatitis, vomiting (bipolar use 18%), xerostomia (bipolar use)

Genitourinary: Azotemia, impotence, renal failure, urinary frequency, urinary retention

Hematologic: Acute intermittent porphyria, agranulocytosis, aplastic anemia, bone marrow suppression, eosinophilia, leukocytosis, leukopenia, pancytopenia, thrombocytopenia

Hepatic: Abnormal liver function tests, hepatic failure, hepatitis, jaundice

Neuromuscular & skeletal: Back pain, pain (bipolar use 12%), peripheral neuritis, weakness

Ocular: Blurred vision, conjunctivitis, lens opacities, nystagmus

Otic: Hyperacusis, tinnitus

Miscellaneous: Diaphoresis, hypersensitivity (including multi-organ reactions, may include disorders mimicking lymphoma, eosinophilia, hepatosplenomegaly, vasculitis); infection (bipolar use 12%)

Overdosage/Toxicology Symptoms of overdose include dizziness ataxia, drowsiness, nausea, vomiting, tremor, agitation, nystagmus, urinary retention, dysrhythmias, coma, seizures, twitches, respiratory depression, and neuromuscular disturbances. Severe cardiac complications occur with very high doses. Activated charcoal is effective at binding certain chemicals and this is especially true for carbamazepine. Other treatment is supportive and symptomatic.

Pharmacodynamics/Kinetics

Absorption: Slow

Bioavailability: 85%

Time to Peak: Unpredictable:

Immediate release: Suspension: 1.5 hour; tablet: 4-5 hours

Extended release: Carbatrol®, Equetro™: 12-26 hours (single dose), 4-8 hours (multiple doses); Tegretol®-XR: 3-12 hours

Protein Binding: Carbamazepine: 75% to 90%, may be decreased in newborns; Epoxide metabolite: 50%

Half-Life Elimination:

Carbamazepine: Initial: 18-55 hours; Multiple doses: Children: 8-14 hours; Adults: 12-17 hours

Epoxide metabolite: Initial: 25-43 hours

Metabolism: Hepatic via CYP3A4 to active epoxide metabolite; induces hepatic enzymes to increase metabolism

Excretion: Urine 72% (1% to 3% as unchanged drug); feces (28%)

Dosing

Adults: Dosage must be adjusted according to patient's response and serum concentrations. Administer tablets (chewable or conventional) in 2-3 divided doses daily and suspension in 4 divided doses daily. (See Additional Information for investigational oral loading dose and rectal maintenance dose information.) Oral:

Epilepsy: Initial: 200 mg twice daily (tablets, extended release tablets, or extended release capsules) or 100 mg of suspension 4 times/day (400 mg daily); increase by up to 200 mg/day at weekly intervals using a twice daily regimen of extended release tablets or capsules, or a 3-4 times/day regimen of other formulations until optimal response and therapeutic levels are achieved; usual dose: 800-1200 mg/day

Maximum recommended dose: 1600 mg/day; however, some patients have required up to 1.6-2.4 g/day

Trigeminal or glossopharyngeal neuralgia: Oral: Initial: 100 mg twice daily with food, gradually increasing in increments of 100 mg twice daily as needed

Maintenance: Usual: 400-800 mg daily in 2 divided doses; maximum dose: 1200 mg/day

Bipolar disorder (Equetro™): Oral: Initial: 400 mg/day in divided doses, twice daily; may adjust by 200 mg daily increments; maximum dose: 1600 mg/day

Elderly: 100 mg 1-2 times daily, increase in increments of 100 mg/day at weekly intervals until therapeutic level is achieved; usual dose: 400-1000 mg/day

Pediatrics: Dosage must be adjusted according to patient's response and serum concentrations. Administer tablets (chewable or conventional) in 2-3 divided doses daily and suspension in 4 divided doses daily. (See Additional Information for investigational oral loading dose and rectal maintenance dose information.)

Epilepsy: Oral:

Children <6 years: Initial: 10-20 mg/kg/day divided twice or 3 times daily as tablets or 4 times/day as suspension; increase dose every week until optimal response and therapeutic levels are achieved

Maintenance dose: Divide into 3-4 doses daily (tablets or suspension); maximum recommended dose: 35 mg/kg/day

Children 6-12 years: Initial: 100 mg twice daily (tablets or extended release tablets) or 50 mg of suspension 4 times/day (200 mg/day); increase by up to 100 mg/day at weekly intervals using a twice daily regimen of extended release tablets or 3-4 times daily regimen of other formulations until optimal response and therapeutic levels are achieved

Maintenance: Usual: 400-800 mg/day; maximum recommended dose: 1000 mg/day

Note: Children <12 years who receive ≥400 mg/day of carbamazepine may be converted to extended release capsules (Carbatrol®) using the same total daily dosage divided twice daily

Children >12 years: Refer to adult dosing.

Maximum recommended doses:
Children 12-15 years: 1000 mg/day
Children >15 years: 1200 mg/day

Available Dosage Forms

Capsule, extended release (Carbatrol®, Equetro™): 100 mg, 200 mg, 300 mg
Suspension, oral: 100 mg/5 mL (10 mL, 450 mL)
Tegretol®: 100 mg/5 mL (450 mL) [citrus vanilla flavor]
Tablet (Epitol®, Tegretol®): 200 mg
Tablet, chewable (Tegretol®): 100 mg
Tablet, extended release (Tegretol®-XR): 100 mg, 200 mg, 400 mg

Monitoring and Teaching Issues

Physical Assessment: Assess effectiveness and interactions of other medications patient may be taking. Monitor therapeutic effectiveness, laboratory values, and adverse reactions at beginning of therapy and periodically with long-term use. Taper dosage slowly when discontinuing. Observe and teach seizure/safety precautions. Monitor for mental and CNS changes, excessive sedation (especially when initiating or increasing therapy), suicide ideation. Baseline and periodic eye exams (slit lamp, funduscopy, and tonometry) are recommended. Assess knowledge/teach patient appropriate use, interventions to reduce side effects, and adverse symptoms to report.

Monitoring Laboratory Tests: CBC with platelet count, reticulocytes, serum iron, liver function tests, urinalysis, BUN, serum carbamazepine levels, thyroid function tests, serum sodium

Patient Education: Take exactly as directed; do not increase dose or frequency or discontinue without consulting prescriber. Do not use extended release tablets which have been damaged or crushed. While using this medication, do not use alcohol and other prescription or OTC medications (especially pain medications, sedatives, antihistamines, or hypnotics) without consulting prescriber. Maintain adequate hydration (2-3 L/day of fluids) unless instructed to restrict fluid intake. You may experience drowsiness, dizziness, or blurred vision (use caution when driving or engaging in tasks requiring alertness until response to drug is known); or nausea, vomiting, loss of appetite, or dry mouth (small frequent meals, frequent mouth care, chewing gum, or sucking lozenges may help). Wear identification of epileptic status and medications. Report CNS changes, mentation changes, or changes in cognition; muscle cramping, weakness, tremors, sore throat, mouth ulcers, swollen glands, jaundice, changes in gait; persistent GI symptoms (cramping, constipation, vomiting, anorexia); rash or skin irritations; unusual bruising or bleeding (mouth, urine, stool); or worsening of seizure activity, or loss of seizure control.

Pregnancy/breast-feeding precautions: Inform prescriber if you are or intend to become pregnant. Breast-feeding is not recommended.

Dietary Considerations: Drug may cause GI upset, take with large amount of water or food to decrease GI upset. May need to split doses to avoid GI upset.

Geriatric Considerations: Elderly may have increased risk of SIADH-like syndrome.

Pregnancy Risk Factor: D

Pregnancy Issues: Crosses the placenta. Dysmorphic facial features, cranial defects, cardiac defects, spina bifida, IUGR, and multiple other malformations have been reported. Epilepsy itself, number of medications, genetic factors, or a combination of these probably influence the teratogenicity of anticonvulsant therapy. Benefit:risk ratio usually favors continued use during pregnancy.

Lactation: Enters breast milk/not recommended (AAP rates "compatible")

Breast-Feeding Issues: Carbamazepine and its metabolites are found in breast milk. The manufacturer does not recommend use while breast-feeding.

Other Issues:

Timing of serum samples: Absorption is slow, peak levels occur 6-8 hours after ingestion of the first dose. The half-life ranges from 8-60 hours; therefore, steady-state is achieved in 2-5 days.

Therapeutic levels: 6-12 mcg/mL (SI: 25-51 µmol/L)

Toxic concentration: >15 mcg/mL. Patients who require higher levels of 8-12 mcg/mL (SI: 34-51 µmol/L) should be watched closely. Side effects including CNS effects occur commonly at higher dosage levels. If other anticonvulsants are given therapeutic range is 4-8 mcg/mL.

Administration

Oral:

Suspension: Must be given on a 3-4 times/day schedule versus tablets which can be given 2-4 times/day. When carbamazepine suspension has been combined with chlorpromazine or thioridazine solutions a precipitate forms which may result in loss of effect. Therefore, it is recommended that the carbamazepine suspension dosage form not be administered at the same time with other liquid medicinal agents or diluents. Since a given dose of suspension will produce higher peak levels than the same dose given as the tablet form, patients given the suspension should be started on lower doses and increased slowly to avoid unwanted side effects. Should be administered with meals.

Extended release capsule (Carbatrol®, Equetro™): Consists of three different types of beads: Immediate release, extended-release, and enteric release. The bead types are combined in a ratio to allow twice daily dosing. May be opened and contents sprinkled over food such as a teaspoon of applesauce; may be administered with or without food; do not crush or chew.

Extended release tablet: Should be inspected for damage. Damaged extended release tablets (without release portal) should not be administered. Should be administered with meals; swallow whole, do not crush or chew.

Additional Information Investigationally, loading doses of the suspension (10 mg/kg for children <12 years of age and 8 mg/kg for children >12 years of age) were given (via NG or ND tubes followed by 5-10 mL of water to flush through tube) to PICU patients with frequent

(Continued)

Carbamazepine *(Continued)*

seizures/status. Five of 6 patients attained mean Cp of 4.3 mcg/mL and 7.3 mcg/mL at 1 and 2 hours postload. Concurrent enteral feeding or ileus may delay absorption.

Related Information

Anticonvulsants By Seizure Type *on page 1712*
Maternal / Fetal Toxicology *on page 1762*
Overdose and Toxicology *on page 1775*
Peak and Trough Guidelines *on page 1694*

♦ **Carbaphen 12®** *see* Carbatapentane, Phenylephrine, and Chlorpheniramine *on page 253*

♦ **Carbaphen 12 Ped®** *see* Carbatapentane, Phenylephrine, and Chlorpheniramine *on page 253*

♦ **Carbatrol®** *see* Carbamazepine *on page 249*

♦ **Carbaxefed RF** *see* Carbinoxamine and Pseudoephedrine *on page 254*

Carbenicillin *(kar ben i SIL in)*

U.S. Brand Names Geocillin®
Synonyms Carbenicillin Indanyl Sodium; Carindacillin
Generic Available No
Pharmacologic Category Antibiotic, Penicillin
Use Treatment of serious urinary tract infections and prostatitis caused by susceptible gram-negative aerobic bacilli
Mechanism of Action/Effect Interferes with bacterial cell wall synthesis during active multiplication
Contraindications Hypersensitivity to carbenicillin, penicillins, or any component of the formulation
Warnings/Precautions Do not use in patients with severe renal impairment (Cl$_{cr}$ <10 mL/minute); dosage modification required in patients with impaired renal and/or hepatic function; oral carbenicillin should be limited to treatment of urinary tract infections. Use with caution in patients with history of hypersensitivity to cephalosporins.

Drug Interactions

Decreased Effect: Decreased effectiveness with tetracyclines. Although anecdotal reports suggest oral contraceptive efficacy could be reduced by penicillins, this has been refuted by more rigorous scientific and clinical data.

Increased Effect/Toxicity: Increased bleeding effects if taken with high doses of heparin or oral anticoagulants. Aminoglycosides may be synergistic against selected organisms. Penicillins may increase the exposure to methotrexate during concurrent therapy; monitor. Probenecid and disulfiram may increase levels of penicillins (carbenicillin).

Lab Interactions Increased AST (SGOT), ALT (SGPT)

Adverse Reactions

>10%: Gastrointestinal: Diarrhea

1% to 10%: Gastrointestinal: Nausea, bad taste, vomiting, flatulence, glossitis

Overdosage/Toxicology Symptoms of overdose include neuromuscular hypersensitivity and convulsions. Hemodialysis may be helpful to aid in removal of the drug from blood; otherwise, treatment is supportive or symptom-directed.

Pharmacodynamics/Kinetics

Absorption: 30% to 40%
Time to Peak: Serum: Normal renal function: 0.5-2 hours; concentrations are inadequate for treatment of systemic infections
Protein Binding: ~50%
Half-Life Elimination: Children: 0.8-1.8 hours; Adults: 1-1.5 hours, prolonged to 10-20 hours with renal insufficiency
Excretion: Urine (~80% to 99% as unchanged drug)

Dosing

Adults & Elderly:

Urinary tract infection: Oral: 1-2 tablets every 6 hours
Prostatitis: Oral: 2 tablets every 6 hours for prostatitis

Pediatrics: Susceptible infections: Oral: Children: 30-50 mg/kg/day divided every 6 hours; maximum dose: 2-3 g/day

Renal Impairment:

Cl$_{cr}$ 10-50 mL/minute: Administer every 12-24 hours.
Cl$_{cr}$ <10 mL/minute: Administer every 24-48 hours.
Moderately dialyzable (20% to 50%)

Available Dosage Forms Tablet [film coated]: 382 mg [contains sodium 23 mg/tablet]

Monitoring and Teaching Issues

Physical Assessment: Assess results of culture/sensitivity tests and patient's allergy history prior to beginning treatment. Use caution in presence of renal or hepatic impairment (see Warnings/Precautions). Assess potential for interactions with other pharmacological agents patient may be taking (see Drug Interactions). Assess therapeutic effectiveness and adverse response (see Adverse Reactions). Advise patients with diabetes about use of Clinitest®. Teach patient proper use, possible side effects/appropriate interventions, and adverse symptoms to report.

Monitoring Laboratory Tests: Renal and hepatic function, CBC, serum potassium, bleeding times. Perform culture and sensitivity testing prior to initiating therapy.

Patient Education: Do not take any new medication during therapy unless approved by prescriber. Take as prescribed, at equal intervals around-the-clock, with a full glass of water, and preferably on an empty stomach, 1 hour before or 2 hours after meals. Do not skip doses and take full course of treatment even if feeling better. If you have diabetes, drug may cause false test results with Clinitest® urine glucose monitoring; use of another form of glucose monitoring is preferable. May cause diarrhea (boiled milk, buttermilk, or yogurt may help); if diarrhea persists for more than 2 days, contact prescriber for approved antidiarrhea medication); or dry mouth and bitter aftertaste (frequent mouth care may help).

Report respiratory difficulty; easy bruising or bleeding; rash, itching, hives; or signs of opportunistic infection (eg, sore throat, fever, chills, fatigue, thrush, vaginal discharge). **Breast-feeding precaution:** Consult prescriber if breast-feeding.

Dietary Considerations: Should be taken with water on empty stomach. Sodium content of 382 mg tablet: 23 mg (1 mEq).

Geriatric Considerations: Has not been studied in the elderly.

Pregnancy Risk Factor: B

Lactation: Enters breast milk/use caution

Administration

Oral: Administer around-the-clock to promote less variation in peak and trough serum levels. Give at least 1 hour before aminoglycosides.

Compatibility: Solution is **incompatible** with aminophylline, amphotericin B, epinephrine, erythromycin, gentamicin, levarterenol, tetracycline, vitamin B and C complex.

Related Information

Compatibility of Drugs *on page 1723*

♦ **Carbenicillin Indanyl Sodium** *see* Carbenicillin *on page 252*

Carbetapentane and Chlorpheniramine
(kar bay ta PEN tane & klor fen IR a meen)

U.S. Brand Names Tannate 12 S; Tannic-12; Tannic-12 S; Tannihist-12 RF; Tussi-12®; Tussi-12 S™; Tussizone-12 RF™

Synonyms Carbetapentane Tannate and Chlorpheniramine Tannate; Chlorpheniramine and Carbetapentane

Generic Available Yes

Pharmacologic Category Antihistamine/Antitussive

Use Symptomatic relief of cough associated with upper respiratory tract conditions, such as the common cold, bronchitis, bronchial asthma

Dosing

Adults: Cough and upper respiratory symptoms: Oral (based on carbetapentane 60 mg and chlorpheniramine 5 mg per tablet): 1-2 tablets every 12 hours

Pediatrics: Cough and upper respiratory symptoms: Oral (based on carbetapentane 30 mg and chlorpheniramine 4 mg per 5 mL suspension): Children:
2-6 years: 2.5-5 mL every 12 hours
>6 years: 5-10 mL every 12 hours

Available Dosage Forms

Suspension:

Tannate 12 S: Carbetapentane tannate 30 mg and chlorpheniramine tannate 4 mg per 5 mL (120 mL, 480 mL)

Tannic-12 S: Carbetapentane tannate 30 mg and chlorpheniramine tannate 4 mg per 5 mL (120 mL) [contains benzoic acid; strawberry flavor]

Tannihist-12 RF: Carbetapentane tannate 30 mg and chlorpheniramine tannate 4 mg per 5 mL (120 mL, 480 mL) [strawberry-black currant flavor]

Tussi-12 S™: Carbetapentane tannate 30 mg and chlorpheniramine tannate 4 mg per 5 mL (120 mL) [contains benzoic acid and tartrazine; strawberry-currant flavor]

Tussizone-12 RF™: Carbetapentane tannate 30 mg and chlorpheniramine tannate 4 mg per 5 mL (120 mL, 480 mL) [contains benzoic acid and tartrazine; strawberry-black currant flavor]

Tablet (Tannic-12, Tussi-12®, Tussizone-12 RF™): Carbetapentane tannate 60 mg and chlorpheniramine tannate 5 mg

Monitoring and Teaching Issues

Pregnancy Risk Factor: C

Lactation: Excretion in breast milk unknown/contraindicated

Carbetapentane, Phenylephrine, and Chlorpheniramine
(kar bay ta PEN tane, fen il EF rin, & klor fen IR a meen)

U.S. Brand Names Carbaphen 12®; Carbaphen 12 Ped®; XiraTuss

Synonyms Chlorpheniramine, Carbetapentane, and Phenylephrine; Phenylephrine, Chlorpheniramine, and Carbetapentane

Generic Available Yes

Pharmacologic Category Antihistamine/Decongestant/Antitussive; Antitussive; Histamine H₁ Antagonist; Sympathomimetic

Use Symptomatic relief of cough, nasal congestion, and discharge associated with the common cold, bronchial asthma, acute and chronic bronchitis, and other respiratory tract conditions

Dosing

Adults: Relief of cough, congestion: Oral:
Carbaphen 12®: 5-10 mL every 12 hours
XiraTuss tablet: 1-2 tablets every 12 hours

Pediatrics: Relief of cough, congestion: Oral:
Children 2-6 years:
Carbaphen 12 Ped®: 1-2 mL every 12 hours
XiraTuss suspension: 2.5-5 mL every 12 hours
Children 6-12 years:
Carbaphen 12 Ped®: 2-4 mL every 12 hours
XiraTuss suspension: 5-10 mL every 12 hours
Children >12 years: Refer to adult dosing.

Available Dosage Forms

Suspension:

Carbaphen 12®: Carbetapentane tannate 60 mg, phenylephrine tannate 20 mg, and chlorpheniramine tannate 8 mg per 5 mL (480 mL) [contains benzoic acid, phenylalanine 1 mg/5 mL; alcohol free, sugar free; blueberry-banana flavor]

(Continued)

Carbetapentane, Phenylephrine, and Chlorpheniramine
(Continued)

    Carbaphen 12 Ped®: Carbetapentane tannate 15 mg, phenylephrine tannate 2.5 mg, and chlorpheniramine tannate 2 mg per mL (60 mL) [contains benzoic acid, phenylalanine 1.6 mg/mL; alcohol free, sugar free; blueberry-banana flavor]

    XiraTuss: Carbetapentane tannate 30 mg, phenylephrine tannate 12.5 mg, and chlorpheniramine tannate 4 mg per 5 mL (120 mL) [strawberry flavor]

  Tablet (XiraTuss): Carbetapentane tannate 60 mg, phenylephrine tannate 10 mg, and chlorpheniramine tannate 5 mg

Monitoring and Teaching Issues
Pregnancy Risk Factor: C
Lactation: Excretion in breast milk unknown/contraindicated
Related Information
  Phenylephrine *on page 1200*

- ♦ **Carbetapentane Tannate and Chlorpheniramine Tannate** *see* Carbetapentane and Chlorpheniramine *on page 253*
- ♦ **Carbidopa and Levodopa** *see* Levodopa and Carbidopa *on page 886*
- ♦ **Carbidopa, Levodopa, and Entacapone** *see* Levodopa, Carbidopa, and Entacapone *on page 888*

Carbinoxamine and Pseudoephedrine
  (kar bi NOKS a meen & soo doe e FED rin)
U.S. Brand Names Andehist NR Drops; Carbaxefed RF; Carboxine-PSE; Hydro-Tussin™-CBX; Palgic®-D; Palgic®-DS; Pediatex™-D; Rondec® Drops; Rondec® Tablets; Rondec-TR®; Sildec
Synonyms Pseudoephedrine and Carbinoxamine
Generic Available Yes
Pharmacologic Category Adrenergic Agonist Agent; Antihistamine, H_1 Blocker; Decongestant
Use Seasonal and perennial allergic rhinitis; vasomotor rhinitis
Mechanism of Action/Effect Carbinoxamine is an antihistamine; pseudoephedrine is a decongestant
Contraindications Hypersensitivity to carbinoxamine, pseudoephedrine, or any component of the formulation; severe hypertension or coronary artery disease; MAO inhibitor therapy; GI or GU obstruction; peptic ulcer disease; narrow-angle glaucoma; avoid use in premature or term infants due to a possible association with SIDS; acute asthma attack
Warnings/Precautions Use caution with hypertension, ischemic heart disease, hyperthyroidism, increased intraocular pressure, diabetes mellitus, BPH, and patients >60 years of age. May cause decreased mental alertness; excitation in younger children; paradoxical reactions (manifested by hyperexcitability) in older children. The elderly may be more sensitive to anticholinergic and antihistamine effects and experience increased adverse effects. Use caution in atopic children. Safety and efficacy in children <1 month of age have not been established.
Drug Interactions
  Decreased Effect: May decrease effects of antihypertensive agents.
  Increased Effect/Toxicity: Increased sedation/CNS depression with barbiturates and other CNS depressants; anticholinergic effects may be increased by MAO inhibitors, tricyclic antidepressants
Nutritional/Ethanol Interactions Ethanol: Avoid ethanol (may increase CNS depression).
Adverse Reactions Frequency not defined.
  Cardiovascular: Arrhythmias, cardiovascular collapse, hypertension, pallor, tachycardia
  Central nervous system: Anxiety, convulsions, CNS stimulation, dizziness, excitability (children; rare), fear, hallucinations, headache, insomnia, nervousness, restlessness, sedation
  Gastrointestinal: Anorexia, diarrhea, dyspepsia, nausea, vomiting, xerostomia
  Neuromuscular skeletal: Tremors, weakness
  Ocular: Diplopia
  Renal: Dysuria, polyuria, urinary retention (with BPH)
  Respiratory: Respiratory difficulty
Overdosage/Toxicology Symptoms of overdose include dry mouth, flushed skin, dilated pupils, and CNS depression. There is no specific treatment for antihistamine overdose. Clinical toxicity is due to blockade of cholinergic receptors. For anticholinergic overdose with severe life-threatening symptoms, physostigmine 1-2 mg I.V. slowly, may be given to reverse these effects.
Dosing
  Adults & Elderly: Nasal congestion, allergic symptoms: Oral:
    Liquid (Pediatex™-D): 10 mL 4 times/day
    Syrup (Hydro-Tussin™-CBX, Palgic®-DS): 10 mL 4 times/day
    Tablet (Rondec®): 1 tablet 4 times a day
    Tablet, timed release (Palgic®-D, Rondec-TR®): 1 tablet every 12 hours
  Pediatrics: Nasal congestion, allergic symptoms: Oral:
    Children:
      Drops (Andehist NR, Carbaxefed RF, Rondec®, Sildec):
        1-3 months: 0.25 mL 4 times/day
        3-6 months: 0.5 mL 4 times/day
        6-12 months: 0.75 mL 4 times/day
        12-24 months: 1 mL 4 times/day
      Liquid (Pediatex™-D):
        1-3 months: 1.25 mL up to 4 times/day
        3-6 months: 2.5 mL up to 4 times/day
        6-9 months: 3.75 mL up to 4 times/day
        9-18 months: 3.75-5 mL up to 4 times/day
        18 months to 6 years: 5 mL 3-4 times/day
        >6 years: Refer to adult dosing.

    Syrup (Hydro-Tussin™-CBX, Palgic®-DS):
      1-3 months: 1.25 mL up to 4 times/day
      3-6 months: 2.5 mL up to 4 times/day
      6-9 months: 3.75 mL up to 4 times/day
      9-18 months: 3.75-5 mL up to 4 times/day
      18 months to 6 years: 5 mL 3-4 times/day
      >6 years: Refer to adult dosing.
    Tablet (Rondec®): ≥6 years: Refer to adult dosing.
    Tablet, timed release:
      6-12 years (Palgic®-D): One-half tablet every 12 hours
      ≥12 years (Palgic®-D, Rondec-TR®): Refer to adult dosing.

Available Dosage Forms

Liquid (Pediatex™-D): Carbinoxamine maleate 2 mg and pseudoephedrine hydrochloride 20 mg per 5 mL (480 mL) [alcohol free, dye free, sugar free; cotton candy flavor]

Solution, oral drops:

  Andehist NR: Carbinoxamine maleate 1 mg and pseudoephedrine hydrochloride 15 mg per mL (30 mL) [alcohol and sugar free; raspberry flavor]

  Carbaxefed RF, Rondec®: Carbinoxamine maleate 1 mg and pseudoephedrine hydrochloride 15 mg per mL (30 mL) [alcohol free; contains sodium benzoate; cherry flavor]

  Sildec: Carbinoxamine maleate 1 mg and pseudoephedrine hydrochloride 15 mg per mL (30 mL) [raspberry flavor]

Solution: Carbinoxamine maleate 2 mg and pseudoephedrine hydrochloride 25 mg per 5 mL (480 mL)

  Carboxine-PSE: Carbinoxamine maleate 2 mg and pseudoephedrine hydrochloride 20 mg per 5 mL (480 mL) [peach flavor]

Syrup: Carbinoxamine maleate 2 mg and pseudoephedrine hydrochloride 25 mg per 5 mL (480 mL)

  Hydro-Tussin™-CBX, Palgic®-DS: Carbinoxamine maleate 2 mg and pseudoephedrine hydrochloride 25 mg per 5 mL (480 mL) [alcohol, dye, and sugar free; strawberry/pineapple flavor]

Tablet (Rondec®): Carbinoxamine maleate 4 mg and pseudoephedrine hydrochloride 60 mg

Tablet, timed release:

  Palgic®-D: Carbinoxamine maleate 8 mg and pseudoephedrine hydrochloride 80 mg [dye free]

  Rondec-TR®: Carbinoxamine maleate 8 mg and pseudoephedrine hydrochloride 120 mg

Monitoring and Teaching Issues

Physical Assessment: Assess potential for interactions of other pharmacological agents patient may be taking (see Drug Interactions). See Warnings/Precautions for use cautions (eg, bladder problems, ulcers, narrow-angle glaucoma, or asthma). Monitor effectiveness of therapy and adverse reactions (see Adverse Reactions) at beginning of therapy and periodically with long-term use. Teach patient proper use, possible side effects/appropriate interventions, and adverse symptoms to report.

Patient Education: Take as directed; do not exceed recommended dose. Maintain adequate hydration (2-3 L/day of fluids) unless instructed to restrict fluid intake. Avoid use of other depressants, alcohol, or sleep-inducing medications unless approved by prescriber. You may experience drowsiness, impaired coordination, blurred vision, or increased anxiety (use caution when driving or engaging in tasks requiring alertness until response to drug is known); or dry mouth or nausea (small frequent meals, frequent mouth care, chewing gum, or sucking hard candy may help). Report persistent dizziness, sedation, or agitation; respiratory difficulty or increased cough; changes in urinary pattern; muscle weakness; or lack of improvement or worsening or condition. **Pregnancy/breast-feeding precautions:** Inform prescriber if you are or intend to become pregnant or breast-feed.

Geriatric Considerations: Elderly are more predisposed to adverse effects of sympathomimetics since they frequently have cardiovascular diseases and diabetes mellitus as well as multiple drug therapies. It may be advisable to treat with a short-acting/immediate-release formulation before initiating sustained-release/long-acting formulations.

Pregnancy Risk Factor: C

Lactation: Enters breast milk/contraindicated

Breast-Feeding Issues: Small amounts of antihistamines and pseudoephedrine are excreted in breast milk. Premature infants and newborns have a higher risk of intolerance to antihistamines. Antihistamines may inhibit lactation.

Administration

Oral:

  Palgic®-D: Tablets may be broken in half; do not crush or chew

  Rondec-TR®: Do not crush or chew

Storage: Store at room temperature of 15°C to 30°C (59°F to 86°F).

Related Information

Pseudoephedrine *on page 1282*

♦ **Carbinoxamine, Pseudoephedrine, and Hydrocodone** *see* Hydrocodone, Carbinoxamine, and Pseudoephedrine *on page 759*

Carboplatin (KAR boe pla tin)

U.S. Brand Names Paraplatin®

Synonyms CBDCA

Generic Available Yes

Pharmacologic Category Antineoplastic Agent, Alkylating Agent

Medication Safety Issues

  Sound-alike/look-alike issues:

    Carboplatin may be confused with cisplatin

    Paraplatin® may be confused with Platinol®

Use Treatment of ovarian cancer

(Continued)

Carboplatin *(Continued)*

Unlabeled/Investigational Use Lung cancer, head and neck cancer, endometrial cancer, esophageal cancer, bladder cancer, breast cancer, cervical cancer, CNS tumors, germ cell tumors, osteogenic sarcoma, and high-dose therapy with stem cell/bone marrow support

Mechanism of Action/Effect Carboplatin is an alkylating agent which covalently binds to DNA; possible cross-linking and interference with the function of DNA

Contraindications History of severe allergic reaction to cisplatin, carboplatin, other platinum-containing formulations, mannitol, or any component of the formulation; pregnancy

Warnings/Precautions The U.S. Food and Drug Administration (FDA) currently recommends that procedures for proper handling and disposal of antineoplastic agents be considered. High doses have resulted in severe abnormalities of liver function tests. Bone marrow suppression, which may be severe, and vomiting are dose related; reduce dosage in patients with bone marrow suppression and impaired renal function. Increased risk of allergic reactions in patients previously exposed to platinum therapy. When administered as sequential infusions, taxane derivatives (docetaxel, paclitaxel) should be administered before platinum derivatives (carboplatin, cisplatin) to limit myelosuppression and to enhance efficacy.

Drug Interactions

Increased Effect/Toxicity: Nephrotoxic drugs; aminoglycosides increase risk of ototoxicity. When administered as sequential infusions, observational studies indicate a potential for increased toxicity when platinum derivatives (carboplatin, cisplatin) are administered before taxane derivatives (docetaxel, paclitaxel).

Nutritional/Ethanol Interactions Herb/Nutraceutical: Avoid black cohosh, dong quai in estrogen-dependent tumors.

Adverse Reactions

>10%:

Dermatologic: Alopecia (includes other agents in combination with carboplatin)

Endocrine & metabolic: Hypomagnesemia, hypokalemia, hyponatremia, hypocalcemia; less severe than those seen after cisplatin (usually asymptomatic)

Gastrointestinal: Nausea, vomiting, stomatitis

Hematologic: Myelosuppression is dose related and is the dose-limiting toxicity; thrombocytopenia is the predominant manifestation, with a reported incidence of 37% in patients receiving 400 mg/m^2 as a single agent and 80% in patients receiving 520 mg/m^2; leukopenia has been reported in 27% to 38% of patients receiving carboplatin as a single agent

Nadir: ~21 days following a single dose

Hepatic: Alkaline phosphatase increased, AST increased (usually mild and reversible)

Otic: Hearing loss at high tones (above speech ranges, up to 19%); clinically-important ototoxicity is not usually seen

Renal: Increases in creatinine and BUN have been reported; most of them are mild and they are commonly reversible; considerably less nephrotoxic than cisplatin

1% to 10%:

Gastrointestinal: Diarrhea, anorexia

Hematologic: Hemorrhagic complications

Local: Pain at injection site

Neuromuscular & skeletal: Peripheral neuropathy (4% to 6%; up to 10% in older and/or previously-treated patients)

Otic: Ototoxicity

Overdosage/Toxicology Symptoms of overdose include bone marrow suppression and hepatic toxicity. Treatment is symptomatic and supportive.

Pharmacodynamics/Kinetics

Protein Binding: 0%; platinum is 30% irreversibly bound

Half-Life Elimination: Terminal: 22-40 hours; Cl$_{cr}$ >60 mL/minute: 2.5-5.9 hours

Metabolism: Minimally hepatic to aquated and hydroxylated compounds

Excretion: Urine (~60% to 90%) within 24 hours

Dosing

Adults & Elderly: Protocols have utilized IVPB, I.V. infusion, and intraperitoneal administration (refer to individual protocols).

Autologous BMT: I.V.: 1600 mg/m^2 (total dose) divided over 4 days **requires BMT (ie, FATAL without BMT)**

Ovarian cancer: 300-360 mg/m^2 I.V. every 3-4 weeks

Pediatrics: Refer to individual protocols

Solid tumor: I.V.: Children: 300-600 mg/m^2 once every 4 weeks

Brain tumor: I.V.: Children: 175 mg/m^2 weekly for 4 weeks every 6 weeks, with a 2-week recovery period between courses

Renal Impairment:

Cl$_{cr}$ 41-59 mL/minute: Recommended dose on day 1 is 250 mg/m^2

Cl$_{cr}$ 16-40 mL/minute: Recommended dose on day 1 is 200 mg/m^2

Cl$_{cr}$ <15 mL/minute: The data available for patients with severely-impaired kidney function are too limited to permit a recommendation for treatment

Hepatic Impairment: There are no published studies available on the dosing of carboplatin in patients with impaired liver function.

Available Dosage Forms

Injection, powder for reconstitution: 50 mg, 150 mg, 450 mg

Injection, solution: 10 mg/mL (5 mL, 15 mL, 45 mL, 60 mL)

Monitoring and Teaching Issues

Physical Assessment: Assess patient allergy history prior to therapy and note specific use cautions (eg, bone marrow suppression and renal function; see Warnings/Precautions). Assess potential for interactions with other pharmacological agents and herbal products patient may be taking (especially products that may be ototoxic or nephrotoxic and need for sequencing with taxane derivatives; see Drug Interactions). Assess results of laboratory tests (hematology, electrolytes, renal and hepatic function) prior to treatment and on a regular basis during therapy. Monitor patient response (eg, nausea and vomiting [pretreatment with antiemetic may be required], ototoxicity [audiometry may be advisable], bone marrow depression, anemia, bleeding, peripheral neuropathy; see Adverse Reactions) frequently throughout therapy. Teach patient (or caregiver) possible side effects/ appropriate interventions and adverse symptoms to report.

Monitoring Laboratory Tests: CBC with differential and platelet count, serum electrolytes, creatinine clearance, liver function

Patient Education: Do not take any new medication during therapy unless approved by prescriber. This medicine can only be administered by I.V. Report immediately any redness, burning, pain, or swelling at infusion site or any sudden onset of chest pain, chills, or respiratory difficulty. It is important that you maintain adequate nutrition (small frequent meals may help) and adequate hydration (2-3 L/day of fluids, unless instructed to restrict fluid intake). You will be susceptible to infection (avoid crowds and exposure to infection and do not have any vaccinations without consulting prescriber). May cause nausea and vomiting (small frequent meals, frequent mouth care, chewing gum, or sucking lozenges may help; if unresolved, consult prescriber for antiemetic); mouth sores (use soft toothbrush or cotton swabs for mouth care); or loss of hair (reversible). Report chest pain or palpitations; sore throat, fever, chills, unusual fatigue; unusual bruising/bleeding; respiratory difficulty; numbness, pain, or tingling in extremities; muscle cramps or twitching; change in hearing acuity; or other persistent adverse effects. **Pregnancy/breast-feeding precautions:** Inform prescriber if you are pregnant. Do not get pregnant during or for 1 month following therapy. Male: Do not cause a female to become pregnant. Male/female: Consult prescriber for instruction on appropriate barrier contraceptive measures. This drug may cause severe fetal defects. Do not breast-feed.

Geriatric Considerations: Peripheral neuropathy is more frequent in patients >65 years of age.

Pregnancy Risk Factor: D

Lactation: Excretion in breast milk unknown/contraindicated

Other Issues: Carboplatin is sometimes confused with cisplatin. Institute measures to prevent mix-ups.

Administration

I.V.: Administer as IVPB over 15 minutes up to a continuous intravenous infusion over 24 hours. May also be administered intraperitoneally. When administered as sequential infusions, taxane derivatives (docetaxel, paclitaxel) should be administered before platinum derivatives to limit myelosuppression and to enhance efficacy.

Reconstitution: Reconstitute powder to yield a final concentration of 10 mg/mL; reconstituted carboplatin 10 mg/mL should be further diluted to a final concentration of 0.5-2 mg/mL with D_5W or NS for administration

Compatibility: Stable in $D_5^1/_4NS$, $D_5^1/_2NS$, D_5NS, D_5W, NS

Y-site administration: Incompatible with amphotericin B cholesteryl sulfate complex
Compatibility when admixed: Incompatible with fluorouracil, mesna

Storage: Store intact vials at room temperature of 15°C to 30°C (59°F to 86°F); protect from light. Aluminum needles should not be used for administration due to binding with the platinum ion. Further dilution to a concentration as low as 0.5 mg/mL is stable at room temperature (25°C) or under refrigeration for 8 days in D_5W.

Powder for reconstitution: Reconstituted to a final concentration of 10 mg/mL is stable for 5 days at room temperature (25°C).

Solution for injection: Multidose vials are stable for up to 14 days after opening when stored at room temperature.

♦ Carboprost see Carboprost Tromethamine on page 257

Carboprost Tromethamine (KAR boe prost tro METH a meen)

U.S. Brand Names Hemabate®

Synonyms Carboprost

Generic Available No

Pharmacologic Category Abortifacient; Prostaglandin

Use Termination of pregnancy and refractory postpartum uterine bleeding

Unlabeled/Investigational Use Investigational: Hemorrhagic cystitis

Mechanism of Action/Effect Carboprost tromethamine is a prostaglandin similar to prostaglandin F_2. Carboprost tromethamine stimulates the gravid uterus to contract, which usually results in expulsion of the products of conception. Used to induce abortion between 13-20 weeks of pregnancy.

Contraindications Hypersensitivity to carboprost tromethamine or any component of the formulation; acute pelvic inflammatory disease; pregnancy

Warnings/Precautions Use with caution in patients with history of asthma, hypotension or hypertension, cardiovascular, adrenal, renal or hepatic disease, anemia, jaundice, diabetes, epilepsy, or compromised uterus.

Drug Interactions

Increased Effect/Toxicity: Toxicity may be increased by oxytocic agents.

Adverse Reactions

>10%: Gastrointestinal: Nausea (33%)

1% to 10%: Cardiovascular: Flushing (7%)

Pharmacodynamics/Kinetics

Excretion: Urine

Dosing

Adults & Elderly:

Abortion: I.M.: 250 mcg to start, 250 mcg at $1^1/_2$-hour to $3^1/_2$-hour intervals depending on uterine response; a 500 mcg dose may be given if uterine response is not adequate after several 250 mcg doses; do not exceed 12 mg total dose.

Refractory postpartum uterine bleeding: I.M.: Initial: 250 mcg; may repeat at 15- to 90-minute intervals up to a total dose of 2 mg

Hemorrhagic cystitis: Bladder irrigation (refer to individual protocols): [0.4-1.0 mg/dL as solution] 50 mL instilled into bladder 4 times/day for 1 hour

(Continued)

Carboprost Tromethamine *(Continued)*

Available Dosage Forms Injection, solution: Carboprost 250 mcg and tromethamine 83 mcg per mL (1 mL) [contains benzyl alcohol]

Monitoring and Teaching Issues

Physical Assessment: Premedication with an antiemetic should be considered. Monitor effectiveness and adverse reactions. Assess for complete expulsion of uterine contents (fetal tissue). Assess knowledge/instruct patient on adverse symptoms to report. **Pregnancy risk factor X.**

Patient Education: This medication is used to stimulate expulsion of uterine contents (fetal tissue) or stimulate uterine contractions to reduce uterine bleeding. Report increased blood loss, acute abdominal cramping, foul-smelling vaginal discharge, or persistent elevation of temperature. Increased temperature (elevated temperature) may occur 1-16 hours after therapy and last for several hours. **Pregnancy precaution:** If being treated for hemorrhagic cystitis, inform prescriber if you are pregnant.

Pregnancy Risk Factor: X

Lactation: Excretion in breast milk unknown/opportunity for use is minimal

Administration

I.M.: Give deep I.M.; rotate site if repeat injections are required.

I.V.: Do not inject I.V.; may result in bronchospasm, hypertension, vomiting, and anaphylaxis.

Reconstitution: Bladder irrigation: Dilute immediately prior to administration in NS; stability unknown.

Storage: Refrigerate ampuls.

- ♦ **Carboxine-PSE** *see* Carbinoxamine and Pseudoephedrine *on page 254*
- ♦ **Cardene®** *see* NiCARdipine *on page 1077*
- ♦ **Cardene® I.V.** *see* NiCARdipine *on page 1077*
- ♦ **Cardene® SR** *see* NiCARdipine *on page 1077*
- ♦ **Cardio-Green®** *see page 1625*
- ♦ **Cardizem®** *see* Diltiazem *on page 459*
- ♦ **Cardizem® CD** *see* Diltiazem *on page 459*
- ♦ **Cardizem® LA** *see* Diltiazem *on page 459*
- ♦ **Cardizem® SR [DSC]** *see* Diltiazem *on page 459*
- ♦ **Cardura®** *see* Doxazosin *on page 485*
- ♦ **Carimune™ [DSC]** *see* Immune Globulin (Intravenous) *on page 793*
- ♦ **Carimune™ NF** *see* Immune Globulin (Intravenous) *on page 793*
- ♦ **Carindacillin** *see* Carbenicillin *on page 252*
- ♦ **Carisoprodate** *see* Carisoprodol *on page 258*

Carisoprodol *(kar eye soe PROE dole)*

U.S. Brand Names Soma®

Synonyms Carisoprodate; Isobamate

Generic Available Yes

Pharmacologic Category Skeletal Muscle Relaxant

Use Skeletal muscle relaxant

Mechanism of Action/Effect Precise mechanism is not yet clear, but many effects have been ascribed to its central depressant actions.

Contraindications Hypersensitivity to carisoprodol, meprobamate or any component of the formulation; acute intermittent porphyria

Warnings/Precautions May cause CNS depression, which may impair physical or mental abilities. Effects with other sedative drugs or ethanol may be potentiated. Use with caution in patients with hepatic/renal dysfunction. Tolerance or drug dependence may result from extended use.

Drug Interactions

Cytochrome P450 Effect: Substrate of CYP2C19 (major)

Increased Effect/Toxicity: CYP2C19 inhibitors may increase the levels/effects of carisoprodol; example inhibitors include delavirdine, fluconazole, fluvoxamine, gemfibrozil, isoniazid, omeprazole, and ticlopidine. Ethanol, CNS depressants, psychotropic drugs, and phenothiazines may increase toxicity.

Nutritional/Ethanol Interactions Ethanol: Avoid ethanol (may increase CNS depression).

Adverse Reactions

>10%: Central nervous system: Drowsiness

1% to 10%:

Cardiovascular: Tachycardia, tightness in chest, flushing of face, syncope

Central nervous system: Mental depression, allergic fever, dizziness, lightheadedness, headache, paradoxical CNS stimulation

Dermatologic: Angioedema

Gastrointestinal: Nausea, vomiting, stomach cramps

Neuromuscular & skeletal: Trembling

Ocular: Burning eyes

Respiratory: Dyspnea

Miscellaneous: Hiccups

Overdosage/Toxicology Symptoms of overdose include CNS depression, stupor, coma, shock, and respiratory depression. Treatment is supportive.

Pharmacodynamics/Kinetics
Onset of Action: ~30 minutes
Duration of Action: 4-6 hours
Half-Life Elimination: 8 hours
Metabolism: Hepatic
Excretion: Urine

Dosing
Adults: Muscle spasm (including spasm associated with acute temporomandibular joint pain): Oral: 350 mg 3-4 times/day; take last dose at bedtime; compound: 1-2 tablets 4 times/day
Elderly: Not recommended for use in the elderly (see Geriatric Considerations).

Available Dosage Forms Tablet: 350 mg

Monitoring and Teaching Issues
Physical Assessment: Assess effectiveness and interactions of other medications patient may be taking. Monitor effectiveness of therapy (according to rational for therapy) and adverse reactions. Monitor for excessive drowsiness at beginning of therapy and periodically with long-term use. Do not discontinue abruptly; taper dosage slowly (withdrawal symptoms may occur). Assess knowledge/teach patient appropriate use, interventions to reduce side effects, and adverse symptoms to report.
Patient Education: Take exactly as directed with food. Do not increase dose or discontinue without consulting prescriber. Do not use alcohol, prescriptive or OTC antidepressants, sedatives, and pain medications without consulting prescriber. You may experience drowsiness, dizziness, lightheadedness (avoid driving or engaging in tasks requiring alertness until response to drug is known); nausea, vomiting, or cramping (small frequent meals, frequent mouth care, or sucking hard candy may help); or postural hypotension (change position slowly when rising from sitting or lying or when climbing stairs). Report excessive drowsiness or mental agitation; palpitations, rapid heartbeat, chest pain; skin rash; muscle cramping or tremors; or respiratory difficulty. **Pregnancy/breast-feeding precautions:** Inform prescriber if you are or intend to become pregnant. Breast-feeding is not recommended.
Geriatric Considerations: Because of the risk of orthostatic hypotension and CNS depression, avoid or use with caution in the elderly. Not considered a drug of choice in the elderly.
Pregnancy Risk Factor: C
Lactation: Enters breast milk (high concentrations)/not recommended

Administration
Oral: Give with food to decrease GI upset.

Carisoprodol and Aspirin (kar eye soe PROE dole & AS pir in)
U.S. Brand Names Soma® Compound
Synonyms Aspirin and Carisoprodol
Generic Available Yes
Pharmacologic Category Skeletal Muscle Relaxant
Use Skeletal muscle relaxant

Dosing
Adults: Skeletal muscle relaxant (including TMJ pain/spasm): Oral: 1 or 2 tablets 4 times/day
Elderly: Avoid use in the elderly due to risk of orthostatic hypotension and CNS depression.

Available Dosage Forms Tablet: Carisoprodol 200 mg and aspirin 325 mg

Monitoring and Teaching Issues
Physical Assessment: See individual agents.
Patient Education: See individual agents. **Pregnancy/breast-feeding precautions:** Inform prescriber if you are or intend to become pregnant. Do not breast-feed.
Pregnancy Risk Factor: C/D (full-dose aspirin in 3rd trimester)
Lactation: Enters breast milk/contraindicated

Related Information
Aspirin *on page 143*
Carisoprodol *on page 258*

Carisoprodol, Aspirin, and Codeine
(kar eye soe PROE dole, AS pir in, and KOE deen)
U.S. Brand Names Soma® Compound w/Codeine
Synonyms Aspirin, Carisoprodol, and Codeine; Codeine, Aspirin, and Carisoprodol
Controlled Substance C-III
Generic Available Yes
Pharmacologic Category Skeletal Muscle Relaxant
Use Skeletal muscle relaxant

Dosing
Adults: Skeletal muscle relaxant, analgesic: Oral: 1 or 2 tablets 4 times/day
Elderly: Avoid use in the elderly due to the risk of orthostatic hypotension and CNS depression.

Available Dosage Forms Tablet: Carisoprodol 200 mg, aspirin 325 mg, and codeine phosphate 16 mg

Monitoring and Teaching Issues
Physical Assessment: See individual agents.
Patient Education: See individual agents. **Pregnancy/breast-feeding precautions:** Inform prescriber if you are or intend to become pregnant. Do not breast-feed.
Pregnancy Risk Factor: C/D (full-dose aspirin in 3rd trimester)
Lactation: Enters breast milk/contraindicated

Related Information
Aspirin *on page 143*
Carisoprodol *on page 258*
Codeine *on page 366*

♦ **Carmol® Scalp** *see* Sulfacetamide *on page 1403*

Carmustine (kar MUS teen)

U.S. Brand Names BiCNu®; Gliadel®

Synonyms BCNU; bis-chloronitrosourea; Carmustinum; NSC-409962; WR-139021

Generic Available No

Pharmacologic Category Antineoplastic Agent; Antineoplastic Agent, Alkylating Agent (Nitrosourea); Antineoplastic Agent, DNA Adduct-Forming Agent; Antineoplastic Agent, DNA Binding Agent

Use
Injection: Treatment of brain tumors (glioblastoma, brainstem glioma, medulloblastoma, astrocytoma, ependymoma, and metastatic brain tumors), multiple myeloma, Hodgkin's disease, non-Hodgkin's lymphomas, melanoma, lung cancer, colon cancer
Wafer (implant): Adjunct to surgery in patients with recurrent glioblastoma multiforme; adjunct to surgery and radiation in patients with high-grade malignant glioma

Mechanism of Action/Effect Interferes with the normal function of DNA by alkylation and cross-linking the strands of DNA, and by possible protein modification

Contraindications Hypersensitivity to carmustine or any component of the formulation; myelosuppression; pregnancy

Warnings/Precautions The U.S. Food and Drug Administration (FDA) currently recommends that procedures for proper handling and disposal of antineoplastic agents be considered. Administer with caution to patients with depressed platelet, leukocyte or erythrocyte counts, renal or hepatic impairment. Diluent contains significant amounts of ethanol; use caution with aldehyde dehydrogenase-2 deficiency or history of "alcohol flushing syndrome." Do not give courses more frequently than every 6 week.

Drug Interactions
Increased Effect/Toxicity: Carmustine given in combination with cimetidine is reported to cause bone marrow depression. Carmustine given in combination with etoposide is reported to cause severe hepatic dysfunction with hyperbilirubinemia, ascites, and thrombocytopenia. Diluent for infusion contains alcohol; avoid concurrent use of medications that inhibit aldehyde dehydrogenase-2 or cause disulfiram-like reactions.

Nutritional/Ethanol Interactions Ethanol: Avoid ethanol.

Adverse Reactions
>10%:
Cardiovascular: Hypotension with high dose therapy, due to the alcohol content of the diluent
Central nervous system: Dizziness, ataxia; Wafers: Seizures (54%) postoperatively
Dermatologic: Pain and burning at the injection site (may be relieved by diluting the drug and infusing it through a fast-running dextrose or saline infusion); phlebitis
Gastrointestinal: Severe nausea and vomiting, usually begins within 2-4 hours of drug administration and lasts for 4-6 hours. Patients should receive a prophylactic antiemetic regimen including a serotonin (5-HT$_3$) antagonist and dexamethasone
Hematologic: Myelosuppression - cumulative, dose related, delayed, thrombocytopenia is usually more common and more severe than leukopenia
Onset: 7-14 days
Nadir: 21-35 days
Recovery: 42-56 days
Hepatic: Reversible increases in bilirubin, alkaline phosphatase, and SGOT occur in 20% to 25% of patients
Ocular: Ocular toxicities (transient conjunctival flushing and blurred vision), retinal hemorrhages
Respiratory: Interstitial fibrosis occurs in up to 50% of patients receiving a cumulative dose >1400 mg/m^2, or bone marrow transplantation doses; may be delayed up to 3 years; rare in patients receiving lower doses. A history of lung disease or concomitant bleomycin therapy may increase the risk of this reaction. Patients should have baseline and periodic pulmonary function tests, patients with forced vital capacity (FVC) or carbon monoxide diffusing capacity of the lungs (DLCO) <70% of predicted are at higher risk.

1% to 10%:
Central nervous system: Wafers: Amnesia, aphasia, ataxia, cerebral edema, confusion, convulsion, depression, diplopia, dizziness, headache, hemiplegia, hydrocephalus, insomnia, meningitis, somnolence, stupor
Dermatologic: Facial flushing, probably due to the alcohol diluent; alopecia
Gastrointestinal: Anorexia, constipation, diarrhea, stomatitis
Hematologic: Anemia

Overdosage/Toxicology Symptoms of overdose include nausea, vomiting, thrombocytopenia, and leukopenia. Treatment is symptomatic and supportive.

Pharmacodynamics/Kinetics
Half-Life Elimination: Biphasic: Initial: 1.4 minutes; Secondary: 20 minutes (active metabolites: plasma half-life of 67 hours)
Metabolism: Rapidly hepatic
Excretion: Urine (~60% to 70%) within 96 hours; lungs (6% to 10% as CO$_2$)

Dosing
Adults & Elderly: Refer to individual protocols.
Usual dosage (per manufacturer labeling): I.V.: 150-200 mg/m^2 every 6 weeks as a single dose or divided into daily injections on 2 successive days
Alternative regimens:
75-120 mg/m^2 days 1 and 2 every 6-8 weeks **or**
50-80 mg/m^2 days 1,2,3 every 6-8 weeks

Primary brain cancer:
150-200 mg/m^2 every 6-8 weeks as a single dose **or**
75-120 mg/m^2 days 1 and 2 every 6-8 weeks **or**
20-65 mg/m^2 every 4-6 weeks **or**
0.5-1 mg/kg every 4-6 weeks **or**
40-80 mg/m^2/day for 3 days every 6-8 weeks

Autologous BMT: I.V.: ALL OF THE FOLLOWING DOSES ARE FATAL WITHOUT BMT
Combination therapy: Up to 300-900 mg/m^2
Single-agent therapy: Up to 1200 mg/m^2 (fatal necrosis is associated with doses >2 g/m^2)

Glioblastoma multiforme (recurrent), malignant glioma: Implantation (wafer): Up to 8 wafers may be placed in the resection cavity (total dose 62.6 mg); should the size and shape not accommodate 8 wafers, the maximum number of wafers allowed should be placed

Pediatrics: Refer to individual protocols: Children: I.V.: 200-250 mg/m^2 every 4-6 weeks as a single dose

Hepatic Impairment: Dosage adjustment may be necessary; however, no specific guidelines are available.

Available Dosage Forms

Injection, powder for reconstitution (BiCNu®): 100 mg [packaged with 3 mL of absolute alcohol as diluent]
Wafer (Gliadel®): 7.7 mg (8s)

Monitoring and Teaching Issues

Physical Assessment: See Warnings/Precautions for use cautions (eg, depressed platelet, leukocyte or erythrocyte counts, renal or hepatic impairment, aldehyde dehydrogenase-2 deficiency). Assess potential for interactions with other pharmacological agents patient may be taking (see Drug Interactions). Administer antiemetic (including a serotonin [5-HT$_3$] antagonist and dexamethasone) prior to therapy. Infusion site should be monitored closely to prevent extravasation (see I.V. Detail). Patients should be supine and vital signs closely monitored during high dose infusion (may require the Trendelenburg position, fluid support, and vasopressor support). Assess results of laboratory tests (eg, hematology, pulmonary, hepatic and renal function) baseline and periodically during therapy. Monitor patient response (see Adverse Reactions) regularly during and for some time following therapy. Pulmonary function should be assessed for extended periods following high dose or BMT doses; acute lung injury can occur 1-3 months after treatment and pulmonary fibrosis may be delayed up to 3 years. Teach patient or caregiver possible side effects/appropriate interventions, and adverse symptoms to report.

Monitoring Laboratory Tests: CBC with differential, platelet count, pulmonary function, liver and renal function

Patient Education: Do not take any new medication during therapy unless approved by prescriber. This medication can only be administered by I.V. Report immediately any pain, burning, swelling at infusion site; sudden onset chest pain, respiratory difficult, difficulty swallowing. Limit oral intake for 4-6 hours before therapy to reduce potential for nausea/vomiting. It is important that you maintain adequate nutrition between treatments (small frequent meals may help) and adequate hydration (2-3 L/day of fluids, unless instructed to restrict fluid intake). You will be susceptible to infection (avoid crowds and exposure to infection and do not have any vaccinations without consulting prescriber). May cause nausea, vomiting, or anorexia (small frequent meals, frequent mouth care, chewing gum, or sucking lozenges may help; if nausea/vomiting are severe, request antiemetic); mouth sores (use soft toothbrush or cotton swabs for mouth care); hyperpigmentation of skin and loss of hair (reversible); or sensitivity to sunlight (use sunblock, wear protective clothing and dark glasses, and avoid direct exposure to sunlight). Report immediately any dyspnea, cough, or fever; chest pain or palpitations; sore throat, chills, persistent unusual fatigue; unusual bruising/bleeding; change in color of urine or stool, change in urinary pattern; or change in visual acuity. **Pregnancy/breast-feeding precautions:** Inform prescriber if you are pregnant. Do not get pregnant or cause a pregnancy (males) during therapy or for 1 month following therapy. Consult prescriber for instruction on appropriate barrier contraceptive measures. This drug may cause severe fetal defects. Do not breast-feed.

Pregnancy Risk Factor: D

Pregnancy Issues: Carmustine can cause fetal harm if administered to a pregnant woman.

Lactation: Excretion in breast milk unknown/contraindicated

Breast-Feeding Issues: It is not known if carmustine is excreted in human breast milk. Due to potential harm to infant, breast-feeding is not recommended.

Administration

I.V.: Irritant (alcohol-based diluent). Injection: Significant absorption to PVC containers - should be administered in either glass or Excel® container. I.V. infusion over 1-2 hours is recommended; infusion through a free-flowing saline or dextrose infusion, or administration through a central catheter can alleviate venous pain/irritation

High-dose carmustine: Maximum rate of infusion of ≤3 mg/m^2/minute to avoid excessive flushing, agitation, and hypotension; infusions should run over at least 2 hours; some investigational protocols dictate shorter infusions.

Fatal doses if not followed by bone marrow or peripheral stem cell infusions.

Reconstitution: Injection: Initially, dilute with 3 mL of absolute alcohol. Further dilute with SWFI to a concentration of 3.3 mg/mL.

Compatibility: Stable in NS

Y-site administration: Incompatible with allopurinol

Compatibility when admixed: Incompatible with sodium bicarbonate

Storage:

Injection: Store intact vials under refrigeration; vials are stable for 36 days at room temperature. Reconstituted solutions are stable for 8 hours at room temperature (25°C) and 24 hours under refrigeration (2°C to 8°C) and protected from light. Further dilution in D$_5$W or NS is stable for 8 hours at room temperature (25°C) and 48 hours under refrigeration (4°C) in glass or Excel® protected from light.

(Continued)

Carmustine *(Continued)*

Wafer: Store at or below -20°C (-4°F). May be kept at room temperature for up to 6 hours.

Additional Information Accidental skin contact may cause transient burning and brown discoloration of the skin. Delayed onset pulmonary fibrosis occurring up to 17 years after treatment has been reported in patients who received cumulative >1400 mg/m^2.

- ◆ **Carmustinum** *see Carmustine on page 260*
- ◆ **Carnitor®** *see Levocarnitine on page 884*
- ◆ **Carrington Antifungal [OTC]** *see Miconazole on page 999*
- ◆ **Cartia XT™** *see Diltiazem on page 459*

Carvedilol *(KAR ve dil ole)*

U.S. Brand Names Coreg®

Generic Available No

Pharmacologic Category Beta Blocker With Alpha-Blocking Activity

Medication Safety Issues

Sound-alike/look-alike issues:

Carvedilol may be confused with captopril, carteolol

Use Mild to severe heart failure of ischemic or cardiomyopathic origin (usually in addition to standardized therapy); left ventricular dysfunction following myocardial infarction (MI); management of hypertension

Unlabeled/Investigational Use Angina pectoris

Mechanism of Action/Effect Nonselective beta-adrenoreceptor and alpha-adrenergic blocking agent, lowers heart rate and blood pressure. Has been shown to lower risk of hospitalization and increase survival in patients with mild to severe heart failure.

Contraindications Hypersensitivity to carvedilol or any component of the formulation; patients with decompensated cardiac failure requiring intravenous inotropic therapy; bronchial asthma or related bronchospastic conditions; second- or third-degree AV block, sick sinus syndrome, and severe bradycardia (except in patients with a functioning artificial pacemaker); cardiogenic shock; severe hepatic impairment; pregnancy (2nd and 3rd trimesters)

Warnings/Precautions Initiate cautiously and monitor for possible deterioration in patient status (including symptoms of CHF). Adjustment of other medications (ACE inhibitors and/or diuretics) may be required. In severe chronic heart failure, trial patients were excluded if they had cardiac-related rales, ascites, or a serum creatinine >2.8 mg/dL. Patients should be advised to avoid driving or other hazardous tasks during initiation of therapy due to the risk of syncope. Avoid abrupt discontinuation (may be associated with angina, arrhythmia, or myocardial infarction), particularly in patients with coronary artery disease; dose should be tapered over 1-2 weeks with close monitoring. Manufacturer recommends discontinuation of therapy if liver injury occurs (confirmed by laboratory testing). Use caution in patients with PVD (can aggravate arterial insufficiency). Use caution with concurrent use of verapamil or diltiazem; bradycardia or heart block can occur. Patients with bronchospastic disease should not receive beta-blockers. Use cautiously in patients with diabetes because it can mask prominent hypoglycemic symptoms. May mask signs of thyrotoxicosis. Use care with anesthetic agents that decrease myocardial function. Safety and efficacy in children <18 years of age have not been established.

Drug Interactions

Cytochrome P450 Effect: Substrate of CYP1A2 (minor), 2C8/9 (major), 2D6 (major), 2E1 (minor), 3A4 (minor)

Decreased Effect: CYP2C8/9 inducers may decrease the levels/effects of carvedilol; example inducers include carbamazepine, phenobarbital, phenytoin, rifampin, rifapentine, and secobarbital. Decreased effect of beta-blockers has also occurred with antacids, barbiturates, calcium channel blockers, cholestyramine, colestipol, NSAIDs, penicillins (ampicillin), and salicylates due to decreased bioavailability and plasma levels. Beta-blockers may decrease the effect of sulfonylureas. Nonselective beta-blockers blunt the effect of beta-2 adrenergic agonists (albuterol).

Increased Effect/Toxicity: CYP2C8/9 inhibitors may increase the levels/effects of carvedilol; example inhibitors include delavirdine, fluconazole, gemfibrozil, ketoconazole, nicardipine, NSAIDs, pioglitazone, and sulfonamides. CYP2D6 inhibitors may increase the levels/effects of carvedilol; example inhibitors include chlorpromazine, delavirdine, fluoxetine, miconazole, paroxetine, pergolide, quinidine, quinine, ritonavir, and ropinirole. Clonidine and cimetidine increase the serum levels and effects of carvedilol. Carvedilol may increase the levels of cyclosporine. Carvedilol may increase the effects of other drugs which slow AV conduction (digoxin, verapamil, diltiazem), alpha-blockers (prazosin, terazosin), and alpha-adrenergic stimulants (epinephrine, phenylephrine). Carvedilol may mask the tachycardia from hypoglycemia caused by insulin and oral hypoglycemics. In patients receiving concurrent therapy, the risk of hypertensive crisis is increased when either clonidine or the beta-blocker is withdrawn. Reserpine has been shown to enhance the effect of beta-blockers. Beta-blockers may increase the action or levels of disopyramide, and theophylline although the effects are difficult to predict.

Nutritional/Ethanol Interactions Herb/Nutraceutical: Avoid dong quai if using for hypertension (has estrogenic activity). Avoid ephedra, yohimbe, ginseng (may worsen hypertension). Avoid garlic (may have increased antihypertensive effect).

Lab Interactions Increased hepatic enzymes, BUN, NPN, alkaline phosphatase; decreased HDL

Adverse Reactions Note: Frequency ranges include data from hypertension and heart failure trials. Higher rates of adverse reactions have generally been noted in patients with CHF. However, the frequency of adverse effects associated with placebo is also increased in this population. Events occurring at a frequency > placebo in clinical trials.

>10%:

Cardiovascular: Hypotension (9% to 14%)

Central nervous system: Dizziness (6% to 32%), fatigue (4% to 24%)

Endocrine & metabolic: Hyperglycemia (5% to 12%), weight gain (10% to 12%)

Gastrointestinal: Diarrhea (2% to 12%)
Neuromuscular & skeletal: Weakness (11%)
1% to 10%:
Cardiovascular: Bradycardia (2% to 10%), hypertension (3%), AV block (3%), angina (2% to 6%), postural hypotension (2%), syncope (3% to 8%), dependent edema (4%), palpitation, peripheral edema (1% to 7%), generalized edema (5% to 6%)
Central nervous system: Headache (5% to 8%), fever (3%), paresthesia (2%), somnolence (2%), insomnia (2%), malaise, hypoesthesia, vertigo
Endocrine & metabolic: Alkaline phosphatase increased, gout (6%), hypercholesterolemia (4%), dehydration (2%), hyperkalemia (3%), hypervolemia (2%), hypertriglyceridemia (1%), hyperuricemia, hypoglycemia, hyponatremia
Gastrointestinal: Nausea (4% to 9%), vomiting (6%), melena, periodontitis
Genitourinary: Hematuria (3%), impotence
Hematologic: Thrombocytopenia (1% to 2%), decreased prothrombin, purpura
Hepatic: Transaminases increased
Neuromuscular & skeletal: Back pain (2% to 7%), arthralgia (6%), myalgia (3%), muscle cramps
Ocular: Blurred vision (3% to 5%)
Renal: BUN increased (6%), abnormal renal function, albuminuria, glycosuria, creatinine increased (3%), kidney failure
Respiratory: Rhinitis (2%), increased cough (5%)
Miscellaneous: Injury (3% to 6%), allergy, sudden death
Overdosage/Toxicology Symptoms of intoxication include cardiac disturbances, CNS toxicity, bronchospasm, hypoglycemia, and hyperkalemia. The most common cardiac symptoms include hypotension and bradycardia. Atrioventricular block, intraventricular conduction disturbances, cardiogenic shock, and asystole may occur with severe overdose, especially with membrane-depressant drugs (eg, propranolol). CNS effects include convulsions, coma, and respiratory arrest (commonly seen with propranolol and other membrane-depressant and lipid-soluble drugs). Treatment is symptom-directed and supportive. Carvedilol does not appear to be significantly cleared by hemodialysis.
Pharmacodynamics/Kinetics
Onset of Action: 1-2 hours; Peak antihypertensive effect: ~1-2 hours
Absorption: Rapid; food decreases rate but not extent of absorption; administration with food minimizes risks of orthostatic hypotension
Bioavailability: 25% to 35%
Protein Binding: >98%, primarily to albumin
Half-Life Elimination: 7-10 hours
Metabolism: Extensively hepatic, via **CYP2D6, 2C9,** 3A4, and 2C19 (2% excreted unchanged); three active metabolites (4-hydroxyphenyl metabolite is 13 times more potent than parent drug for beta-blockade); first-pass effect; plasma concentrations in the elderly and those with cirrhotic liver disease are 50% and 4-7 times higher, respectively
Excretion: Primarily feces
Dosing
Adults & Elderly: Reduce dosage if heart rate drops to <55 beats/minute.
Hypertension: Oral: 6.25 mg twice daily; if tolerated, dose should be maintained for 1-2 weeks, then increased to 12.5 mg twice daily. Dosage may be increased to a maximum of 25 mg twice daily after 1-2 weeks. Maximum dose: 50 mg/day
Congestive heart failure: Oral: 3.125 mg twice daily for 2 weeks; if this dose is tolerated, may increase to 6.25 mg twice daily. Double the dose every 2 weeks to the highest dose tolerated by patient. (Prior to initiating therapy, other heart failure medications should be stabilized and fluid retention minimized.)
Maximum recommended dose: Oral:
Mild to moderate heart failure:
<85 kg: 25 mg twice daily
>85 kg: 50 mg twice daily
Severe heart failure: Oral: 25 mg twice daily
Left ventricular dysfunction following MI: Initial 3.125-6.25 mg twice daily; increase dosage incrementally (ie, from 6.25 to 12.5 mg twice daily) at intervals of 3-10 days, based on tolerance, to a target dose of 25 mg twice daily. **Note:** Should be initiated only after patient is hemodynamically stable and fluid retention has been minimized.
Angina pectoris (unlabeled use): Oral: 25-50 mg twice daily
Renal Impairment: None necessary
Hepatic Impairment: Use is contraindicated in severe liver dysfunction.
Available Dosage Forms Tablet: 3.125 mg, 6.25 mg, 12.5 mg, 25 mg
Monitoring and Teaching Issues
Physical Assessment: Assess potential for interactions with other prescriptions, OTC medications, or herbal products patient may be taking (especially anything that will effect blood pressure). Blood pressure and heart rate should be assessed prior to and following first doses and any change in dose. Caution patients with diabetes to monitor glucose levels closely (beta-blockers may alter glucose tolerance). Assess results of laboratory tests, therapeutic effectiveness (eg, reduction of hypertension or angina), and adverse response (eg, CHF). Teach patient proper use, possible side effects/appropriate interventions, and adverse symptoms to report.
Monitoring Laboratory Tests: Renal studies, BUN, liver function
Patient Education: Do not take any new medication during therapy unless approved by prescriber. Take exactly as directed. Do not alter dose or discontinue without consulting prescriber. Take pulse daily, prior to taking medication; follow prescriber's instruction about holding medication. If you have diabetes, monitor serum glucose closely (drug may alter glucose tolerance or mask signs of hypoglycemia). You may experience fatigue, dizziness, or postural hypotension (use caution when changing position from lying or sitting to standing, driving, or climbing stairs until response to medication is known); alteration in sexual performance (reversible); or diarrhea (buttermilk, boiled milk, or yogurt may help). Report unresolved swelling of extremities; respiratory difficulty or new cough; unresolved fatigue; unusual weight gain (>5 lb/week); unresolved constipation or diarrhea; or unusual
(Continued)

Carvedilol *(Continued)*

muscle weakness. **Pregnancy/breast-feeding precautions:** Inform prescriber if you are pregnant. Do not get pregnant while taking this medications. Consult prescriber for appropriate contraceptive use. Do not breast-feed.

Dietary Considerations: Should be taken with food to minimize the risk of orthostatic hypotension.

Geriatric Considerations: Due to alterations in the beta-adrenergic autonomic nervous system, beta-adrenergic blockade may result in less hemodynamic response than seen in younger adults.

Pregnancy Risk Factor: C (manufacturer); D (2nd and 3rd trimesters - expert analysis)

Pregnancy Issues: No data available on whether carvedilol crosses the placenta; beta-blockers have been associated with persistent bradycardia, hypotension, and IUGR; IUGR probably related to maternal hypertension. Cases of neonatal hypoglycemia have been reported following maternal use of beta-blockers at parturition or during breast-feeding. Use during pregnancy only if the potential benefit justifies the risk.

Lactation: Excretion in breast milk unknown/contraindicated

Administration
Oral: Administer with food.
Storage: Store at 30°C (86°F).

Additional Information Fluid retention during therapy should be treated with an increase in diuretic dosage.

Related Information
Beta-Blockers *on page 1720*
Heart Failure *on page 1828*

♦ **Casodex®** *see Bicalutamide on page 195*

Caspofungin *(kas poe FUN jin)*

U.S. Brand Names Cancidas®
Synonyms Caspofungin Acetate
Generic Available No
Pharmacologic Category Antifungal Agent, Parenteral

Use Treatment of invasive *Aspergillus* infections in patients who are refractory or intolerant of other therapy; treatment of candidemia and other *Candida* infections (intra-abdominal abscesses, esophageal, peritonitis, pleural space); empirical treatment for presumed fungal infections in febrile neutropenic patient

Mechanism of Action/Effect Blocks synthesis of a vital component of fungal cell wall, limiting its growth. The cell wall component is unique to specific fungi, limiting any potential for toxicity in mammals.

Contraindications Hypersensitivity to caspofungin or any component of the formulation

Warnings/Precautions Has not been studied as initial therapy for invasive *Aspergillus*. Concurrent use of cyclosporine should be limited to patients for whom benefit outweighs risk, due to a high frequency of hepatic transaminase elevations observed during concurrent use. Limited data are available concerning treatment durations longer than 4 weeks; however, treatment appears to be well tolerated. Use caution in hepatic impairment; dosage reduction required in moderate impairment. Safety and efficacy in pediatric patients have not been established.

Drug Interactions
Decreased Effect: Caspofungin may decrease blood concentrations of tacrolimus. Dosage adjustment of caspofungin to 70 mg is required for patients on rifampin.
Increased Effect/Toxicity: Concurrent administration of cyclosporine may increase caspofungin concentrations; hepatic serum transaminases may be observed.

Adverse Reactions
>10%:
Central nervous system: Headache (up to 11%), fever (3% to 26%), chills (up to 14%)
Endocrine & metabolic: Hypokalemia (4% to 11%)
Hematologic: Hemoglobin decreased (1% to 12%)
Hepatic: Serum alkaline phosphatase (3% to 11%) increased, transaminases increased (up to 13%)
Local: Infusion site reactions (2% to 12%), phlebitis/thrombophlebitis (up to 16%)
1% to 10%:
Cardiovascular: Flushing (2% to 3%), facial edema (up to 3%), hypertension (1% to 2%), tachycardia (1% to 2%), hypotension (1%)
Central nervous system: Dizziness (2%), pain (1% to 5%), insomnia (1%)
Dermatologic: Rash (<1% to 6%), pruritus (1% to 3%), erythema (1% to 2%)
Gastrointestinal: Nausea (2% to 6%), vomiting (1% to 4%), abdominal pain (1% to 4%), diarrhea (1% to 4%), anorexia (1%)
Hematologic: Eosinophils increased (3%), neutrophils decreased (2% to 3%), WBC decreased (5% to 6%), anemia (up to 4%), platelet count decreased (2% to 3%)
Hepatic: Bilirubin increased (3%)
Local: Induration (up to 3%)
Neuromuscular & skeletal: Myalgia (up to 3%), paresthesia (1% to 3%), tremor (≤2%)
Renal: Nephrotoxicity (8%)*, proteinuria (5%), hematuria (2%), serum creatinine increased (<1% to 4%), urinary WBCs increased (up to 8%), urinary RBCs increased (1% to 4%), blood urea nitrogen increased (1%)
*Nephrotoxicity defined as serum creatinine ≥2X baseline value or ≥1 mg/dL in patients with serum creatinine above ULN range (patients with Cl_{cr} <30 mL/minute were excluded)
Miscellaneous: Flu-like syndrome (3%), diaphoresis (up to 3%)

Overdosage/Toxicology No experience with overdosage has been reported. Caspofungin is not dialyzable. Treatment is symptomatic and supportive.

Pharmacodynamics/Kinetics

Protein Binding: 97% to albumin

Half-Life Elimination: Beta (distribution): 9-11 hours; Terminal: 40-50 hours

Metabolism: Slowly, via hydrolysis and *N*-acetylation as well as by spontaneous degradation, with subsequent metabolism to component amino acids. Overall metabolism is extensive.

Excretion: Urine (41% as metabolites, 1% to 9% unchanged) and feces (35% as metabolites)

Dosing

Adults & Elderly: Note: Duration of caspofungin treatment should be determined by patient status and clinical response. Empiric therapy should be given until neutropenia resolves. In patients with positive cultures, treatment should continue until 14 days after last positive culture. In neutropenic patients, treatment should be given at least 7 days after both signs and symptoms of infection **and** neutropenia resolve.

Empiric therapy: Initial dose: 70 mg on day 1; subsequent dosing: 50 mg/day; may increase up to 70 mg/day if tolerated, but clinical response is inadequate.

Invasive *Aspergillus*, candidiasis: I.V.: Initial dose: 70 mg on day 1; subsequent dosing: 50 mg/day

Esophageal candidiasis: I.V.: 50 mg/day; **Note:** The majority of patients studied for this indication also had oropharyngeal involvement.

Dosage adjustment with concomitant use of an enzyme inducer:

Patients receiving rifampin: 70 mg caspofungin daily

Patients receiving carbamazepine, dexamethasone, efavirenz, nevirapine, or phenytoin (and possibly other enzyme inducers) may require an increased daily dose of caspofungin (70 mg/day).

Pediatrics: Safety and efficacy in pediatric patients have not been established.

Renal Impairment: No specific dosage adjustment is required; supplemental dose is not required following dialysis.

Hepatic Impairment:

Mild hepatic insufficiency (Child-Pugh score 5-6): No adjustment necessary.

Moderate hepatic insufficiency (Child-Pugh score 7-9): 35 mg/day; initial 70 mg loading dose should still be administered in treatment of invasive infections.

Severe hepatic insufficiency (Child-Pugh score >9): No clinical experience.

Available Dosage Forms Injection, powder for reconstitution, as acetate: 50 mg [contains sucrose 39 mg], 70 mg [contains sucrose 54 mg]

Monitoring and Teaching Issues

Physical Assessment: Use caution in presence of hepatic impairment (see Warnings/Precautions). Assess therapeutic effectiveness and adverse reactions (see Adverse Reactions). See Administration for I.V. specifics. Teach patient possible side effects/appropriate interventions and adverse symptoms to report.

Patient Education: This medication can only be administered by infusion. Report immediately any pain, burning, or swelling at infusion site, or any signs of allergic reaction (eg, respiratory or swallowing difficulty, back pain, chest tightness, rash, hives, or swelling of lips or mouth). Report nausea, vomiting, abdominal pain, or diarrhea. **Pregnancy/breast-feeding precautions:** Inform prescriber if you are or intend to become pregnant. Consult prescriber if breast-feeding.

Pregnancy Risk Factor: C

Lactation: Excretion in breast milk unknown/use caution

Administration

I.V.: Infuse slowly, over 1 hour. Do not coadminister with other medications.

Reconstitution: Bring refrigerated vial to room temperature. Reconstitute vials using 0.9% sodium chloride for injection, SWFI, or bacteriostatic water for injection. Mix gently until clear solution is formed; do not use if cloudy or contains particles. Solution should be further diluted with 0.9%, 0.45%, or 0.225% sodium chloride or LR. Do not mix with dextrose-containing solutions. Do not coadminister with other medications.

Compatibility: Do not mix with dextrose-containing solutions or coadminister with other medications.

Storage: Store vials at 2°C to 8°C (36°F to 46°F). Reconstituted solution may be stored at less than 25°C (77°F) for 1 hour prior to preparation of infusion solution. Infusion solutions may be stored at less than 25°C (77°F) and should be used within 24 hours; up to 48 hours if stored at 2°C to 8°C (36°F to 46°F).

Cefaclor (SEF a klor)

U.S. Brand Names Ceclor®; Ceclor® CD; Raniclor™

Generic Available Yes

Pharmacologic Category Antibiotic, Cephalosporin (Second Generation)

Medication Safety Issues
Sound-alike/look-alike issues:
Cefaclor may be confused with cephalexin

Use Treatment of susceptible bacterial infections including otitis media, lower respiratory tract infections, acute exacerbations of chronic bronchitis, pharyngitis and tonsillitis, urinary tract infections, skin and skin structure infections

Mechanism of Action/Effect Inhibits bacterial cell wall synthesis by binding to one or more of the penicillin-binding proteins (PBPs)

Contraindications Hypersensitivity to cefaclor, any component of the formulation, or other cephalosporins

Warnings/Precautions Modify dosage in patients with severe renal impairment. Prolonged use may result in superinfection. Use with caution in patients with a history of penicillin allergy especially IgE-mediated reactions (eg, anaphylaxis, urticaria). Beta-lactamase-negative, ampicillin-resistant (BLNAR) strains of *H. influenzae* should be considered resistant to cefaclor. Extended release tablets are not approved for use in children <16 years of age.

Drug Interactions
Increased Effect/Toxicity: Probenecid may decrease cephalosporin elimination. Furosemide, aminoglycosides when taken with cefaclor may result in additive nephrotoxicity.

Nutritional/Ethanol Interactions
Food: Cefaclor serum levels may be decreased slightly if taken with food. The bioavailability of cefaclor extended release tablets is decreased 23% and the maximum concentration is decreased 67% when taken on an empty stomach.

Lab Interactions Positive direct Coombs', false-positive urinary glucose test using cupric sulfate (Benedict's solution, Clinitest®, Fehling's solution), false-positive serum or urine creatinine with Jaffé reaction

Adverse Reactions
1% to 10%:
Dermatologic: Rash (maculopapular, erythematous, or morbilliform) (1% to 2%)
Gastrointestinal: Diarrhea (3%)
Genitourinary: Vaginitis (2%)
Hematologic: Eosinophilia (2%)
Hepatic: Transaminases increased (3%)
Miscellaneous: Moniliasis (2%)
Reactions reported with other cephalosporins include fever, abdominal pain, superinfection, renal dysfunction, toxic nephropathy, hemorrhage, cholestasis

Overdosage/Toxicology Symptoms of overdose include diarrhea, epigastric distress, nausea, and vomiting. Many beta-lactam containing antibiotics have the potential to cause neuromuscular hyperirritability or seizures. Hemodialysis may be helpful to aid in removal of the drug from blood; otherwise, treatment is supportive and symptom-directed.

Pharmacodynamics/Kinetics
Absorption: Well absorbed, acid stable
Time to Peak: Capsule: 60 minutes; Suspension: 45 minutes
Protein Binding: 25%
Half-Life Elimination: 0.5-1 hour; prolonged with renal impairment
Metabolism: Partially hepatic
Excretion: Urine (80% as unchanged drug)

Dosing
Adults & Elderly: Susceptible infection: Oral: Dosing range: 250-500 mg every 8 hours
Extended release tablets:
Acute bacterial exacerbations of or secondary infections with chronic bronchitis: 500 mg every 12 hours for 7 days
Pharyngitis, tonsillitis, uncomplicated skin and skin structure infections: 375 mg every 12 hours for 10 days
Pediatrics: Susceptible infections: Oral: Children >1 month: Dosing range: 20-40 mg/kg/day divided every 8-12 hours; maximum dose: 1 g/day
Otitis media: 40 mg/kg/day divided every 12 hours
Pharyngitis: 20 mg/kg/day divided every 12 hours
Renal Impairment:
Cl_{cr} 10-50 mL/minute: Administer 50% to 100% of dose
Cl_{cr} <10 mL/minute: Administer 50% of dose
Hemodialysis: Moderately dialyzable (20% to 50%)

Available Dosage Forms
Capsule (Ceclor®): 250 mg, 500 mg
Powder for oral suspension: 125 mg/5 mL (75 mL, 150 mL); 187 mg/5 mL (50 mL, 100 mL); 250 mg/5 mL (75 mL, 150 mL); 375 mg/5 mL (50 mL, 100 mL)
Ceclor®: 125 mg/5 mL (150 mL); 187 mg/5 mL (100 mL); 250 mg/5 mL (75 mL, 150 mL); 375 mg/5 mL (100 mL)
Tablet, chewable (Raniclor™): 125 mg [contains phenylalanine 2.8 mg; fruity flavor], 187 mg [contains phenylalanine 4.2 mg; fruity flavor], 250 mg [contains phenylalanine 5.6 mg; fruity flavor], 375 mg [contains phenylalanine 8.4 mg; fruity flavor]
Tablet, extended release (Ceclor® CD): 375 mg, 500 mg

Monitoring and Teaching Issues
Physical Assessment: Assess results of culture/sensitivity tests and patient's allergy history prior to therapy. See Warnings/Precautions for use cautions (eg, renal impairment). Assess potential for interactions with other pharmacological agents patient may be taking (eg, nephrotoxicity; see Drug Interactions). Assess results of laboratory tests (see Monitoring Laboratory Tests), therapeutic response, and adverse effects (hypersensitivity can occur days after therapy is started; see Adverse Reactions). Advise patients with diabetes

about use of Clinitest®. Teach patient proper use, possible side effects/appropriate interventions, and adverse symptoms to report (eg, hypersensitivity, opportunistic infection).

Monitoring Laboratory Tests: Perform culture and sensitivity studies prior to initiating drug therapy; renal function

Patient Education: Do not take any new medication during therapy unless approved by prescriber. Take as directed, at regular intervals around-the-clock (with or without food). Chilling oral suspension improves flavor (do not freeze). Do not chew or crush extended release tablets. Maintain adequate hydration (2-3 L/day of fluids) unless instructed to restrict fluid intake. Complete full course of medication, even if you feel better. May cause false test results with Clinitest®; use of another type of testing is preferable. May cause diarrhea (yogurt, boiled milk, or buttermilk may help). Report rash; breathing or swallowing difficulty; persistent diarrhea, nausea, vomiting, or abdominal pain; changes in urinary pattern or pain on urination; opportunistic infection (eg, vaginal itching or drainage; sores in mouth; blood in stool or urine, unusual fever or chills); CNS changes (eg, irritability, agitation, nervousness, insomnia, hallucinations); or other adverse reactions. **Breast-feeding precaution:** Consult prescriber if breast-feeding.

Dietary Considerations: Capsule, chewable tablet, and suspension may be taken with or without food. Extended release tablet should be taken with food. Raniclor™ contains phenylalanine 2.8 mg/cefaclor 125 mg.

Pregnancy Risk Factor: B

Lactation: Enters breast milk/use caution

Breast-Feeding Issues: Theoretically, drug absorbed by nursing infant may change bowel flora or affect fever work-up result. Small amounts can be detected in breast milk (trace amounts after 1 hour, increasing to 0.16 mcg/mL at 5 hours). **Note:** As a class, cephalosporins are used to treat bacterial infections in infants.

Administration

Oral: Administer around-the-clock to promote less variation in peak and trough serum levels. Chewable tablet: Should be chewed before swallowing; should not be swallowed whole. Extended release tablet: Should not be cut, crushed, or chewed; should be administered with food.

Oral suspension: Shake well before using.

Storage: Store at controlled room temperature. Refrigerate suspension after reconstitution. Discard after 14 days. Do not freeze.

Cefadroxil (sef a DROKS il)

U.S. Brand Names Duricef®

Synonyms Cefadroxil Monohydrate

Generic Available Yes: Capsule, tablet

Pharmacologic Category Antibiotic, Cephalosporin (First Generation)

Use Treatment of susceptible bacterial infections, including those caused by group A beta-hemolytic *Streptococcus*; prophylaxis against bacterial endocarditis in patients who are allergic to penicillin and undergoing surgical or dental procedures

Mechanism of Action/Effect Inhibits bacterial cell wall synthesis by binding to one or more of the penicillin-binding proteins (PBPs)

Contraindications Hypersensitivity to cefadroxil, other cephalosporins, or any component of the formulation

Warnings/Precautions Modify dosage in patients with severe renal impairment; prolonged use may result in superinfection; use with caution in patients with a history of penicillin allergy especially IgE-mediated reactions (eg, anaphylaxis, angioedema, urticaria). May cause antibiotic-associated colitis or colitis secondary to *C. difficile*.

Drug Interactions

Increased Effect/Toxicity: Bleeding may occur when administered with anticoagulants. Probenecid may decrease cephalosporin elimination.

Nutritional/Ethanol Interactions Food: Concomitant administration with food, infant formula, or cow's milk does **not** significantly affect absorption.

Lab Interactions Positive direct Coombs', false-positive urinary glucose test using cupric sulfate (Benedict's solution, Clinitest®, Fehling's solution), false-positive serum or urine creatinine with Jaffé reaction

Adverse Reactions

1% to 10%: Gastrointestinal: Diarrhea

Reactions reported with other cephalosporins include toxic epidermal necrolysis, abdominal pain, superinfection. renal dysfunction, toxic nephropathy, aplastic anemia, hemolytic anemia, hemorrhage, prolonged prothrombin time, increased BUN, increased creatinine, eosinophilia, pancytopenia, seizure

Overdosage/Toxicology Symptoms of overdose include neuromuscular hypersensitivity and convulsions. Many beta-lactam containing antibiotics have the potential to cause neuromuscular hyperirritability or convulsive seizures. Hemodialysis may be helpful to aid in removal of the drug from blood; otherwise, treatment is supportive or symptom-directed.

Pharmacodynamics/Kinetics

Absorption: Rapid and well absorbed

Time to Peak: Serum: 70-90 minutes

Protein Binding: 20%

Half-Life Elimination: 1-2 hours; Renal failure: 20-24 hours

Excretion: Urine (>90% as unchanged drug)

Dosing

Adults & Elderly:

Susceptible infections: Oral: 1-2 g/day in 2 divided doses

Prophylaxis against bacterial endocarditis: Oral: 2 g 1 hour prior to the procedure

Pediatrics:

Susceptible infections: Oral: Children: 30 mg/kg/day divided twice daily up to a maximum of 2 g/day

Prophylaxis against bacterial endocarditis: Oral: Children: 50 mg/kg 1 hour prior to the procedure

(Continued)

Cefadroxil *(Continued)*

Renal Impairment:
Cl$_{cr}$ 10-25 mL/minute: Administer every 24 hours.
Cl$_{cr}$ <10 mL/minute: Administer every 36 hours.

Available Dosage Forms
Capsule, as monohydrate: 500 mg
Powder for oral suspension, as monohydrate: 250 mg/5 mL (50 mL, 100 mL); 500 mg/5 mL (75 mL, 100 mL) [contains sodium benzoate; orange-pineapple flavor]
Tablet, as monohydrate: 1 g

Monitoring and Teaching Issues
Physical Assessment: Assess results of culture/sensitivity tests and patient's allergy history prior to therapy. See Warnings/Precautions for use cautions (eg, renal impairment). Assess potential for interactions with other pharmacological agents patient may be taking (eg, anticoagulants; see Drug Interactions). Assess results of laboratory tests, therapeutic response, and adverse effects (eg, hypersensitivity can occur several days after therapy is started; see Adverse Reactions). Advise patients with diabetes about use of Clinitest®. Teach patient proper use, possible side effects/appropriate interventions, and adverse symptoms to report (eg, hypersensitivity, opportunistic infection, renal dysfunction, anemia).

Monitoring Laboratory Tests: Perform culture and sensitivity studies prior to initiating drug therapy; renal function

Patient Education: Do not take any new medication during therapy unless approved by prescriber. Take as directed, at regular intervals around-the-clock (with or without food). Chilling oral suspension improves flavor (do not freeze). Maintain adequate hydration (2-3 L/day of fluids) unless instructed to restrict fluid intake. Complete full course of medication, even if you feel better. May cause false test results with Clinitest®; use of another type of glucose testing is preferable. May cause diarrhea (yogurt, boiled milk, or buttermilk may help). Report rash; breathing or swallowing difficulty; persistent diarrhea, nausea, vomiting, or abdominal pain; changes in urinary pattern or pain on urination; opportunistic infection (eg, vaginal itching or drainage; sores in mouth; blood in stool or urine, unusual fever or chills); CNS changes (eg, irritability, agitation, nervousness, insomnia, hallucinations); or other adverse reactions. **Breast-feeding precaution:** Consult prescriber if breast-feeding.

Geriatric Considerations: Adjust dose for renal function in the elderly.

Pregnancy Risk Factor: B

Lactation: Enters breast milk (small amounts)/use caution (AAP rates "compatible")

Breast-Feeding Issues: Theoretically, drug absorbed by nursing infant may change bowel flora or affect fever work-up result. **Note:** As a class, cephalosporins are used to treat infections in infants.

Administration
Oral: Administer around-the-clock to promote less variation in peak and trough serum levels.
Reconstitution: Refrigerate suspension after reconstitution. Discard after 14 days.

♦ Cefadroxil Monohydrate *see Cefadroxil on page 267*

Cefazolin *(sef A zoe lin)*
U.S. Brand Names Ancef®
Synonyms Cefazolin Sodium
Generic Available Yes
Pharmacologic Category Antibiotic, Cephalosporin (First Generation)
Medication Safety Issues
Sound-alike/look-alike issues:
Cefazolin may be confused with cefprozil, cephalexin, cephalothin
Kefzol® may be confused with Cefzil®

Use Treatment of respiratory tract, skin and skin structure, genital, urinary tract, biliary tract, bone and joint infections, and septicemia due to susceptible gram-positive cocci (except enterococcus); some gram-negative bacilli including *E. coli*, *Proteus*, and *Klebsiella* may be susceptible; perioperative prophylaxis

Unlabeled/Investigational Use Prophylaxis against bacterial endocarditis

Mechanism of Action/Effect Inhibits bacterial cell wall synthesis by binding to one or more of the penicillin-binding proteins (PBPs)

Contraindications Hypersensitivity to cefazolin sodium, any component of the formulation, or other cephalosporins

Warnings/Precautions Modify dosage in patients with severe renal impairment; prolonged use may result in superinfection; use with caution in patients with a history of penicillin allergy especially IgE-mediated reactions (eg, anaphylaxis, angioedema, urticaria). May cause antibiotic-associated colitis or colitis secondary to *C. difficile*.

Drug Interactions
Increased Effect/Toxicity: High-dose probenecid decreases clearance and increases effect of cefazolin. Aminoglycosides increase nephrotoxic potential when taken with cefazolin. Cefazolin may increase the hypothrombinemic response to warfarin (due to alteration of GI microbial flora).

Lab Interactions Positive direct Coombs', false-positive urinary glucose test using cupric sulfate (Benedict's solution, Clinitest®, Fehling's solution), false-positive serum or urine creatinine with Jaffé reaction

Adverse Reactions Frequency not defined.
Central nervous system: Fever, seizure
Dermatologic: Rash, pruritus, Stevens-Johnson syndrome
Gastrointestinal: Diarrhea. nausea, vomiting, abdominal cramps, anorexia, pseudomembranous colitis, oral candidiasis
Genitourinary: Vaginitis
Hepatic: Transaminases increased, hepatitis
Hematologic: Eosinophilia, neutropenia, leukopenia, thrombocytopenia, thrombocytosis
Local: Pain at injection site, phlebitis

Renal: BUN increased, serum creatinine increased, renal failure
Miscellaneous: Anaphylaxis

Reactions reported with other cephalosporins include toxic epidermal necrolysis, abdominal pain, cholestasis, superinfection, toxic nephropathy, aplastic anemia, hemolytic anemia, hemorrhage, prolonged prothrombin time, pancytopenia

Overdosage/Toxicology Symptoms of overdose include neuromuscular hypersensitivity and convulsions. Many beta-lactam containing antibiotics have the potential to cause neuromuscular hyperirritability or convulsive seizures. Hemodialysis may be helpful to aid in the removal of drug from blood; otherwise, treatment is supportive or symptom-directed.

Pharmacodynamics/Kinetics
Time to Peak: Serum: I.M.: 0.5-2 hours
Protein Binding: 74% to 86%
Half-Life Elimination: 90-150 minutes; prolonged with renal impairment
Metabolism: Minimally hepatic
Excretion: Urine (80% to 100% as unchanged drug)

Dosing
Adults & Elderly:
Susceptible infections: I.M., I.V.: 1-2 g every 8 hours, depending on severity of infection; maximum: 12 g/day
Mild-to-moderate infections: 500 mg to 1 g every 6-8 hours
Mild infection with gram-positive cocci: 250-500 mg every 8 hours
Perioperative prophylaxis: 1 g every 30 minutes prior to surgery (repeat with 500 mg to 1 g during prolonged surgery); followed by 500 mg to 1 g every 6-9 hours for 24 hours postop
Pneumococcal pneumonia: 500 mg every 12 hours
Severe infection: 1-2 g every 6 hours
Prophylaxis against bacterial endocarditis (unlabeled use): 1 g 30 minutes before procedure
UTI (uncomplicated): 1 g every 12 hours
Pediatrics: Susceptible infections: I.M., I.V.: Children >1 month: 25-100 mg/kg/day divided every 6-8 hours; maximum: 6 g/day
Renal Impairment:
Cl_{cr} 10-30 mL/minute: Administer every 12 hours.
Cl_{cr} <10 mL/minute: Administer every 24 hours.
Moderately dialyzable (20% to 50%); administer dose postdialysis or administer supplemental dose of 0.5-1 g after dialysis.
Peritoneal dialysis: Administer 0.5 g every 12 hours.
Continuous arteriovenous or venovenous hemofiltration: Dose as for Cl_{cr} 10-30 mL/minute. Removes 30 mg of cefazolin per liter of filtrate per day.

Available Dosage Forms
Infusion [premixed in D_5W]: 500 mg (50 mL); 1 g (50 mL)
Injection, powder for reconstitution: 500 mg, 1 g, 10 g, 20 g
Ancef®: 1 g, 10 g

Monitoring and Teaching Issues
Physical Assessment: Assess results of culture/sensitivity tests and patient's allergy history prior to therapy. See Warnings/Precautions for use cautions (eg, renal impairment). Assess potential for interactions with other pharmacological agents patient may be taking (eg, anticoagulants; see Drug Interactions). Assess results of laboratory tests, therapeutic effects, and adverse response (eg, hypersensitivity can occur several days after therapy is started; see Adverse Reactions). Advise patients with diabetes about use of Clinitest®. Teach patient proper use, possible side effects/appropriate interventions, and adverse symptoms to report (eg, hypersensitivity, opportunistic infection, renal dysfunction, anemia).
Monitoring Laboratory Tests: Perform culture and sensitivity studies prior to initiating drug therapy; renal function
Patient Education: Do not take any new medication during therapy unless approved by prescriber. This medication is administered by injection or infusion. Report immediately any redness, swelling, burning, or pain at injection/infusion site; rash or hives; or respiratory difficulty, chest pain, or difficulty swallowing. Maintain adequate hydration (2-3 L/day of fluids) unless instructed to restrict fluid intake. If you have diabetes, drug may cause false test results with Clinitest® urine glucose monitoring; use of another type of glucose monitoring is preferable. May cause diarrhea (yogurt, boiled milk, or buttermilk may help). Report rash; breathing or swallowing difficulty; persistent diarrhea, nausea, vomiting, or abdominal pain; changes in urinary pattern or pain on urination; opportunistic infection (eg, vaginal itching or drainage; sores in mouth; blood in stool or urine, unusual fever or chills); CNS changes (eg, irritability, agitation, nervousness, insomnia, hallucinations); or other adverse reactions. **Breast-feeding precautions:** Consult prescriber if breast-feeding.
Dietary Considerations: Sodium content of 1 g: 48 mg (2 mEq)
Geriatric Considerations: Adjust dose for renal function.
Pregnancy Risk Factor: B
Lactation: Enters breast milk (small amounts)/use caution (AAP rates "compatible")
Breast-Feeding Issues: Theoretically, drug absorbed by nursing infant may change bowel flora or affect fever work-up result. **Note:** As a class, cephalosporins are used to treat infections in infants.

Administration
I.M.: Inject deep I.M. into large muscle mass.
I.V.: Inject direct I.V. over 5 minutes. Infuse intermittent infusion over 30-60 minutes.
Reconstitution: Dilute large vial with 2.5 mL SWFI; 10 g vial may be diluted with 45 mL to yield 1 g/5 mL or 96 mL to yield 1 g/10 mL. May be injected or further dilution for I.V. administration in 50-100 mL compatible solution. Standard diluent is 1 g/50 mL D_5W or 2 g/50 mL D_5W.
(Continued)

Cefazolin *(Continued)*

Compatibility: Stable in D_5W, D_5LR, $D_5^1/_4NS$, $D_5^1/_2NS$, D_5NS, $D_{10}W$, LR, NS
  Y-site administration: Incompatible with amphotericin B cholesteryl sulfate complex, idarubicin, pentamidine, vinorelbine
  Compatibility in syringe: Incompatible with ascorbic acid injection, cimetidine, lidocaine
  Compatibility when admixed: Incompatible with amikacin, amobarbital, atracurium, bleomycin, calcium gluconate, clindamycin with gentamicin, colistimethate, kanamycin, pentobarbital, polymyxin B sulfate, ranitidine

Storage: Store intact vials at room temperature and protect from temperatures exceeding 40°C. Reconstituted solutions of cefazolin are light yellow to yellow. Protection from light is recommended for the powder and for the reconstituted solutions. Reconstituted solutions are stable for 24 hours at room temperature and for 10 days under refrigeration. Stability of parenteral admixture at room temperature (25°C) is 48 hours. Stability of parenteral admixture at refrigeration temperature (4°C) is 14 days.
  DUPLEX™: Store at 20°C to 25°C (68°F to 77°F); excursions permitted to 15°C to 30°C (59°F to 86°F) prior to activation. Following activation, stable for 24 hours at room temperature and for 7 days under refrigeration.

Related Information
  Compatibility of Drugs *on page 1723*
  I.V. to Oral Conversion *on page 1688*

♦ **Cefazolin Sodium** *see* Cefazolin *on page 268*

Cefdinir *(SEF di ner)*

U.S. Brand Names Omnicef®
Synonyms CFDN
Generic Available No
Pharmacologic Category Antibiotic, Cephalosporin (Third Generation)
Use Treatment of community-acquired pneumonia, acute exacerbations of chronic bronchitis, acute bacterial otitis media, acute maxillary sinusitis, pharyngitis/tonsillitis, and uncomplicated skin and skin structure infections.
Mechanism of Action/Effect Inhibits bacterial cell wall synthesis by binding to one or more of the penicillin-binding proteins (PBPs) which in turn inhibits the final transpeptidation step of peptidoglycan synthesis in bacterial cell walls, thus inhibiting cell wall biosynthesis. Bacteria eventually lyse due to ongoing activity of cell wall autolytic enzymes (autolysins and murein hydrolases) while cell wall assembly is arrested.
Contraindications Hypersensitivity to cefdinir, other cephalosporins, any component of the formulation, or related antibiotics
Warnings/Precautions Administer cautiously to penicillin-sensitive patients, especially IgE-mediated reactions (eg, anaphylaxis, urticaria). There is evidence of partial cross-allergenicity and cephalosporins cannot be assumed to be an absolutely safe alternative to penicillin in the penicillin-allergic patient. Serum sickness-like reactions have been reported. Signs and symptoms occur after a few days of therapy and resolve a few days after drug discontinuation with no serious sequelae. Pseudomembranous colitis occurs; consider its diagnosis in patients who develop diarrhea with antibiotic use.

Drug Interactions
  Decreased Effect: Coadministration with iron or antacids reduces the rate and extent of cefdinir absorption.
  Increased Effect/Toxicity: Probenecid increases the effects of cephalosporins by decreasing the renal elimination in those which are secreted by tubular secretion. Anticoagulant effects may be increased when administered with cephalosporins.

Adverse Reactions
  1% to 10%:
    Dermatologic: Cutaneous moniliasis (1%)
    Gastrointestinal: Diarrhea (8%), rash (3%), vomiting (1%), increased GGT (1%)
  Reactions reported with other cephalosporins include dizziness, fever, headache, encephalopathy, asterixis, neuromuscular excitability, seizure, aplastic anemia, interstitial nephritis, toxic nephropathy, angioedema, hemorrhage, prolonged PT, serum-sickness reactions, and superinfection
Overdosage/Toxicology After acute overdose, most agents cause only nausea, vomiting, and diarrhea, although neuromuscular hypersensitivity and seizures are possible, especially in patients with renal insufficiency. Hemodialysis may be helpful to aid in the removal of the drug from the blood but not usually indicated, otherwise most treatment is supportive or symptom-directed following GI decontamination.

Pharmacodynamics/Kinetics
  Bioavailability: Capsule: 16% to 21%; Suspension 25%
  Protein Binding: 60% to 70%
  Half-Life Elimination: 100 minutes
  Metabolism: Minimally hepatic
  Excretion: Primarily urine

Dosing
  Adults & Elderly:
    Acute maxillary sinusitis: Oral: 300 mg twice daily **or** 600 mg once daily for 10 days
    Pharyngitis or chronic bronchitis (exacerbation): Oral: 300 mg twice daily for 5-10 days **or** 600 mg once daily for 10 days
    Pneumonia (community-acquired) or skin/skin structure infection (uncomplicated): Oral: 300 mg twice daily for 10 days
  Pediatrics:
    Children 6 months to 12 years:
      Acute maxillary sinusitis: Oral: 7 mg/kg twice daily **or** 14 mg/kg once daily for 10 days
      Otitis media or pharyngitis/tonsillitis: Oral: 7 mg/kg twice daily for 5-10 days **or** 14 mg/kg once daily for 10 days
      Skin/skin structure infection (uncomplicated): Oral: 7 mg/kg twice daily for 10 days
    Children >12 years: Refer to adult dosing.

Renal Impairment: Cl$_{cr}$ <30 mL/minute: 300 mg once daily. Hemodialysis removes cefdinir; recommended initial dose: 300 mg (or 7 mg/kg/dose) every other day. At the conclusion of each hemodialysis session, 300 mg (or 7 mg/kg/dose) should be given. Subsequent doses (300 mg or 7 mg/kg/dose) should be administered every other day.

Available Dosage Forms
Capsule: 300 mg

Powder for oral suspension: 125 mg/5 mL (60 mL, 100 mL) [contains sodium benzoate; strawberry flavor]; 250 mg/5 mL (60 mL, 100 mL) [contains sodium benzoate; strawberry flavor]

Monitoring and Teaching Issues
Physical Assessment: Assess results of culture/sensitivity tests and patient's allergy history prior to therapy (see Warnings/Precautions). Assess potential for interactions with other pharmacological agents patient may be taking (eg, anticoagulants; see Drug Interactions). Assess therapeutic response and adverse effects (see Adverse Reactions). Teach patient proper use, possible side effects/appropriate interventions, and adverse symptoms to report (eg, opportunistic infection, hypersensitivity).

Monitoring Laboratory Tests: Perform culture and sensitivity studies prior to initiating drug therapy; renal function

Patient Education: Take as directed, at regular intervals around-the-clock (with or without food). Chilling oral suspension improves flavor (do not freeze). Complete full course of medication, even if you feel better. Maintain adequate hydration (2-3 L/day of fluids) unless instructed to restrict fluid intake. May cause diarrhea (yogurt, boiled milk, or buttermilk may help); or nausea, vomiting, flatulence (small frequent meals, frequent mouth care, chewing gum, or sucking lozenges may help). Report rash; breathing or swallowing difficulty; persistent diarrhea, nausea, vomiting, or abdominal pain; changes in urinary pattern or pain on urination; opportunistic infection (eg, vaginal itching or drainage; sores in mouth; blood in stool or urine, unusual fever or chills); CNS changes (eg, irritability, agitation, nervousness, insomnia, hallucinations); or other adverse reactions. **Breast-feeding precaution:** Consult prescriber if breast-feeding.

Pregnancy Risk Factor: B

Lactation: Enters breast milk (small amounts)/use caution

Administration
Storage: Oral suspension should be mixed with 38 mL water for the 60 mL bottle and 63 mL of water for the 120 mL bottle. After mixing, the suspension can be stored at room temperature (25°C/77°F). The suspension may be used for 10 days. The suspension should be shaken well before each administration.

Cefditoren (sef de TOR en)
U.S. Brand Names Spectracef™

Synonyms Cefditoren Pivoxil

Generic Available No

Pharmacologic Category Antibiotic, Cephalosporin

Use Treatment of acute bacterial exacerbation of chronic bronchitis or community-acquired pneumonia (due to susceptible organisms including *Haemophilus influenzae*, *Haemophilus parainfluenzae*, *Streptococcus pneumoniae*-penicillin susceptible only, *Moraxella catarrhalis*); pharyngitis or tonsillitis (*Streptococcus pyogenes*); and uncomplicated skin and skin-structure infections (*Staphylococcus aureus* - not MRSA, *Streptococcus pyogenes*)

Mechanism of Action/Effect Has bactericidal activity against susceptible gram-positive and gram-negative pathogens. Inhibits bacterial cell wall synthesis by binding to one or more of the penicillin-binding proteins (PBPs)

Contraindications Hypersensitivity to cefditoren, other cephalosporins, milk protein, or any component of the formulation; carnitine deficiency

Warnings/Precautions Use with caution in patients with a history of penicillin allergy, especially IgE-mediated reactions (eg, anaphylaxis, urticaria). May cause antibiotic-associated colitis or colitis secondary to *C. difficile*. Modify dosage in patients with severe renal impairment. Caution in individuals with seizure disorders. Prolonged use may result in superinfection. Use caution in patients with renal or hepatic impairment. Cefditoren causes renal excretion of carnitine, do not use in patients with carnitine deficiency; not for long-term therapy due to the possible development of carnitine deficiency over time. Cefditoren tablets contain sodium caseinate, which may cause hypersensitivity reactions in patients with milk protein hypersensitivity; this does not affect patients with lactose intolerance. Safety and efficacy have not been established in children <12 years of age.

Drug Interactions
Decreased Effect: Antacids and H$_2$ receptor antagonists decrease cefditoren levels.

Increased Effect/Toxicity: Increased levels of cefditoren with probenecid.

Nutritional/Ethanol Interactions Food: Moderate- to high-fat meals increase bioavailability and maximum plasma concentration.

Lab Interactions May cause a false-negative ferricyanide test; false-positive urine glucose test when using Clinitest®

Adverse Reactions
>10%: Gastrointestinal: Diarrhea (11% to 15%)

1% to 10%:
  Central nervous system: Headache (2% to 3%)
  Endocrine & metabolic: Glucose increased (1%)
  Gastrointestinal: Nausea (4% to 6%), abdominal pain (2%), dyspepsia (1% to 2%), vomiting (1%)
  Genitourinary: Vaginal moniliasis (3% to 6%)
  Hematologic: Hematocrit decreased (2%)
  Renal: Hematuria (3%), urinary white blood cells increased (2%)

Additional adverse effects seen with cephalosporin antibiotics: Anaphylaxis, aplastic anemia, cholestasis, erythema multiforme, hemorrhage, hemolytic anemia, renal dysfunction, (Continued)

Cefditoren (Continued)

reversible hyperactivity, serum sickness-like reaction, Stevens-Johnson syndrome, toxic epidermal necrolysis, toxic nephropathy

Overdosage/Toxicology Specific information not available. Treatment should be symptom-directed and supportive. Hemodialysis may be helpful (removes ~30% from circulation).

Pharmacodynamics/Kinetics

Bioavailability: ~14% to 16%; increased with moderate to high-fat meal
Time to Peak: 1.5-3 hours
Protein Binding: 88% (*in vitro*), primarily to albumin
Half-Life Elimination: 1.6 ± 0.4 hours
Metabolism: Cefditoren pivoxil is hydrolyzed to cefditoren (active) and pivalate
Excretion: Urine (as cefditoren and pivaloylcarnitine)

Dosing

Adults & Elderly:
Acute bacterial exacerbation of chronic bronchitis: Oral: 400 mg twice daily for 10 days
Community-acquired pneumonia: Oral: 400 mg twice daily for 14 days
Pharyngitis, tonsillitis, uncomplicated skin and skin structure infections: Oral: 200 mg twice daily for 10 days
Pediatrics: Children ≥12 years: Refer to adult dosing.
Renal Impairment:
Cl_{cr} 30-49 mL/minute: Maximum dose: 200 mg twice daily
Cl_{cr} <30 mL/minute: Maximum dose: 200 mg once daily
End-stage renal disease: Appropriate dosing not established
Hepatic Impairment:
Mild or moderate impairment: Adjustment not required
Severe impairment (Child-Pugh class C): Specific guidelines not available

Available Dosage Forms Tablet, as pivoxil: 200 mg [equivalent to cefditoren; contains sodium caseinate]

Monitoring and Teaching Issues

Physical Assessment: Assess results of culture/sensitivity tests and patient's allergy history prior to therapy. See Warnings/Precautions for use cautions (eg, renal, hepatic impairment, history of seizures). Assess potential for interactions with other pharmacological agents patient may be taking (see Drug Interactions). Assess therapeutic response and adverse effects (see Adverse Reactions). Advise patients with diabetes about use of Clinitest®. Teach patient proper use, possible side effects/appropriate interventions, and adverse symptoms to report (eg, hypersensitivity, opportunistic infection, gastrointestinal upset, diarrhea).

Monitoring Laboratory Tests: Perform culture and sensitivity studies prior to initiating drug therapy; renal function

Patient Education: Do not take any new medication during therapy without consulting prescriber. Take as directed, at regular intervals around-the-clock, with food. Maintain adequate hydration (2-3 L/day of fluids) unless instructed to restrict fluid intake. Complete full course of medication, even if you feel better. If you have diabetes, monitor glucose levels closely; may cause false test results with Clinitest® urine glucose monitoring; use of another type of glucose monitoring is preferable. May cause diarrhea (yogurt, buttermilk, or boiled milk may help); or nausea or vomiting (small frequent meals, frequent mouth care, sucking lozenges, or chewing gum may help). Report rash; breathing or swallowing difficulty; persistent diarrhea, nausea, vomiting, or abdominal pain; changes in urinary pattern or pain on urination; opportunistic infection (eg, vaginal itching or drainage; sores in mouth; blood in stool or urine, unusual fever or chills); CNS changes (eg, irritability, agitation, nervousness, insomnia, hallucinations); or other adverse reactions. **Breast-feeding precaution:** Consult prescriber if breast-feeding.

Dietary Considerations: Cefditoren should be taken with meals. Plasma carnitine levels are decreased during therapy (39% with 200 mg dosing, 63% with 400 mg dosing); normal concentrations return within 7-10 days after treatment is discontinued.

Pregnancy Risk Factor: B
Lactation: Excretion in breast milk unknown/use caution

Administration

Oral: Should be taken with meals.
Storage: Store at controlled room temperature of 25°C (77°F). Protect from light and moisture.

♦ **Cefditoren Pivoxil** *see* Cefditoren *on page 271*

Cefepime (SEF e pim)

U.S. Brand Names Maxipime®
Synonyms Cefepime Hydrochloride
Generic Available No
Pharmacologic Category Antibiotic, Cephalosporin (Fourth Generation)
Use Treatment of uncomplicated and complicated urinary tract infections, including pyelonephritis caused by typical urinary tract pathogens; monotherapy for febrile neutropenia; uncomplicated skin and skin structure infections caused by *Streptococcus pyogenes*; moderate to severe pneumonia caused by pneumococcus, *Pseudomonas aeruginosa*, and other gram-negative organisms; complicated intra-abdominal infections (in combination with metronidazole). Also active against methicillin-susceptible staphylococci, *Enterobacter* sp, and many other gram-negative bacilli.

Children 2 months to 16 years: Empiric therapy of febrile neutropenia patients, uncomplicated skin/soft tissue infections, pneumonia, and uncomplicated/complicated urinary tract infections.

Mechanism of Action/Effect Inhibits bacterial cell wall synthesis by binding to one or more of the penicillin-binding proteins (PBPs)

Contraindications Hypersensitivity to cefepime, any component of the formulation, or other cephalosporins

Warnings/Precautions Modify dosage in patients with severe renal impairment; prolonged use may result in superinfection; use with caution in patients with a history of penicillin or cephalosporin allergy, especially IgE-mediated reactions (eg, anaphylaxis, urticaria). May cause antibiotic-associated colitis or colitis secondary to *C. difficile*. Use in patients <2 months of age has not been established.

Drug Interactions

Increased Effect/Toxicity: High-dose probenecid decreases clearance and increases effect of cefepime. Aminoglycosides increase nephrotoxic potential when taken with cefepime.

Lab Interactions Positive direct Coombs', false-positive urinary glucose test using cupric sulfate (Benedict's solution, Clinitest®, Fehling's solution), false-positive serum or urine creatinine with Jaffé reaction

Adverse Reactions

>10%: Hematologic: Positive Coombs' test without hemolysis

1% to 10%:

Central nervous system: Fever (1%), headache (1%)

Dermatologic: Rash, pruritus

Gastrointestinal: Diarrhea, nausea, vomiting

Local: Pain, erythema at injection site

Reactions reported with other cephalosporins include aplastic anemia, erythema multiforme, hemolytic anemia, hemorrhage, pancytopenia, prolonged PT, renal dysfunction, Stevens-Johnson syndrome, superinfection, toxic epidermal necrolysis, toxic nephropathy, vaginitis

Overdosage/Toxicology Symptoms of overdose include neuromuscular hypersensitivity and CNS toxicity (including hallucinations, confusion, seizures, and coma). Many beta-lactam containing antibiotics have the potential to cause neuromuscular hyperirritability or convulsive seizures. Hemodialysis may be helpful to aid in removal of the drug from blood; otherwise, treatment is supportive and symptom-directed.

Pharmacodynamics/Kinetics

Absorption: I.M.: Rapid and complete

Time to Peak: 0.5-1.5 hours

Protein Binding: Plasma: 16% to 19%

Half-Life Elimination: 2 hours

Metabolism: Minimally hepatic

Excretion: Urine (85% as unchanged drug)

Dosing

Adults & Elderly:

Susceptible infections: I.V.: 1-2 g every 12 hours for 7-10 days; higher doses or more frequent administration may be required in pseudomonal infections

Urinary tract infections, mild to moderate: I.V., I.M.: 500-1000 mg every 12 hours

Febrile neutropenia: I.V.: 2 g every 8 hours for 7 days or until neutropenia resolves

Pediatrics:

Febrile neutropenia: I.V.: Children >2 months of age: 50 mg/kg every 8 hours for 7-10 days

Uncomplicated skin/soft tissue infections, pneumonia, and complicated/uncomplicated UTI: I.V.: Children >2 months of age: 50 mg/kg twice daily

Renal Impairment:

Adjustment of recommended maintenance schedule is required:

Normal dosing schedule: 500 mg every 12 hours

Cl$_{cr}$ 30-60 mL/minute: 500 mg every 24 hours

Cl$_{cr}$ 11-29 mL/minute: 500 mg every 24 hours

Cl$_{cr}$ <11 mL/minute: 250 mg every 24 hours

Normal dosing schedule: 1 g every 12 hours

Cl$_{cr}$ 30-60 mL/minute: 1 g every 24 hours

Cl$_{cr}$ 11-29 mL/minute: 500 mg every 24 hours

Cl$_{cr}$ <11 mL/minute: 250 mg every 24 hours

Normal dosing schedule: 2 g every 12 hours

Cl$_{cr}$ 30-60 mL/minute: 2 g every 24 hours

Cl$_{cr}$ 11-29 mL/minute: 1 g every 24 hours

Cl$_{cr}$ <11 mL/minute: 500 mg every 24 hours

Normal dosing schedule: 2 g every 8 hours

Cl$_{cr}$ 30-60 mL/minute: 2 g every 12 hours

Cl$_{cr}$ 11-29 mL/minute: 2 g every 24 hours

Cl$_{cr}$ <11 mL/minute: 1 g every 24 hours

Hemodialysis effects: Initial: 1 g (single dose) on day 1. Maintenance: 500 mg once daily (1 g once daily in febrile neutropenic patients). Dosage should be administered after dialysis on dialysis days.

Peritoneal dialysis effects: Removed to a lesser extent than hemodialysis; administer 250 mg every 48 hours.

Continuous arteriovenous hemofiltration: Dose as for Cl$_{cr}$ >30 mL/minute.

Available Dosage Forms Injection, powder for reconstitution, as hydrochloride: 500 mg, 1 g, 2 g

Monitoring and Teaching Issues

Physical Assessment: Assess results of culture/sensitivity tests and patient's allergy history prior to therapy. See Warnings/Precautions for use cautions. Assess potential for interactions with other pharmacological agents patient may be taking (see Drug Interactions). Assess results of laboratory tests, therapeutic response, and adverse effects (see Adverse Reactions). Advise patients with diabetes about use of Clinitest®. Teach patient proper use, possible side effects/appropriate interventions, and adverse symptoms to report (eg, hypersensitivity, nephrotoxicity, opportunistic infection).

(Continued)

Cefepime *(Continued)*

Monitoring Laboratory Tests: Perform culture and sensitivity studies prior to initiating drug therapy; renal function

Patient Education: Do not take any new medication during therapy unless approved by prescriber. This medication is administered by infusion or injection. Report immediately any redness, swelling, burning, or pain at injection/infusion site; itching or hives; chest pain, difficulty swallowing or breathing. Maintain adequate hydration (2-3 L/day of fluids) unless instructed to restrict fluid intake. May cause false test results with Clinitest®; use of another type of glucose testing is preferable. May cause diarrhea (yogurt, boiled milk, or buttermilk may help); nausea, and vomiting (small frequent meals, frequent mouth care, chewing gum, or sucking lozenges may help). Report rash; breathing or swallowing difficulty; persistent diarrhea, nausea, vomiting, or abdominal pain; changes in urinary pattern or pain on urination; opportunistic infection (eg, vaginal itching or drainage; sores in mouth; blood in stool or urine, unusual fever or chills); CNS changes (eg, irritability, agitation, nervousness, insomnia, hallucinations); or other adverse reactions. **Breast-feeding precaution:** Consult prescriber if breast-feeding.

Geriatric Considerations: Adjust dose for changes in renal function.

Pregnancy Risk Factor: B

Lactation: Enters breast milk/use caution

Breast-Feeding Issues: Theoretically, drug absorbed by nursing infant may change bowel flora or affect fever work-up result. **Note:** As a class, cephalosporins are used to treat infections in infants.

Administration

I.M.: Inject deep I.M. into large muscle mass.

I.V.: Inject direct I.V. over 5 minutes. Infuse intermittent infusion over 30-60 minutes.

Compatibility: Stable in D_5LR, D_5NS, D_5W, $D_{10}W$, NS, bacteriostatic water, SWFI

Y-site administration: Incompatible with acyclovir, amphotericin B, amphotericin B cholesteryl sulfate complex, chlordiazepoxide, chlorpromazine, cimetidine, ciprofloxacin, cisplatin, dacarbazine, daunorubicin, diazepam, diphenhydramine, dobutamine, dopamine, doxorubicin, droperidol, enalaprilat, etoposide, etoposide phosphate, famotidine, filgrastim, floxuridine, ganciclovir, haloperidol, hydroxyzine, idarubicin, ifosfamide, magnesium sulfate, mannitol, mechlorethamine, meperidine, metoclopramide, mitomycin, mitoxantrone, morphine, nalbuphine, ofloxacin, ondansetron, plicamycin, prochlorperazine edisylate, promethazine, streptozocin, vancomycin, vinblastine, vincristine

Compatibility when admixed: Incompatible with aminophylline, gentamicin, netilmicin, tobramycin, vancomycin

Related Information

Antimicrobial Drugs of Choice *on page 1792*
Community-Acquired Pneumonia in Adults *on page 1807*

♦ **Cefepime Hydrochloride** *see* Cefepime *on page 272*

Cefixime *(sef IKS eem)*

U.S. Brand Names Suprax®

Generic Available No

Pharmacologic Category Antibiotic, Cephalosporin (Third Generation)

Medication Safety Issues

Sound-alike/look-alike issues:

Suprax® may be confused with Sporanox®, Surbex®

Use Treatment of urinary tract infections, otitis media, respiratory infections due to susceptible organisms including *S. pneumoniae* and *S. pyogenes*, *H. influenzae* and many Enterobacteriaceae; uncomplicated cervical/urethral gonorrhea due to *N. gonorrhoeae*

Mechanism of Action/Effect Inhibits bacterial cell wall synthesis by binding to one or more of the penicillin-binding proteins (PBPs)

Contraindications Hypersensitivity to cefixime, any component of the formulation, or other cephalosporins

Warnings/Precautions Prolonged use may result in superinfection; modify dosage in patients with renal impairment; use with caution in patients with a history of penicillin allergy especially IgE-mediated reactions (eg, anaphylaxis, urticaria). May cause antibiotic-associated colitis or colitis secondary to *C. difficile*.

Drug Interactions

Increased Effect/Toxicity: Aminoglycosides and furosemide may be possible additives to nephrotoxicity. Probenecid increases cefixime concentration. Cefixime may increase carbamazepine. Cefixime may increase prothrombin time when administered with warfarin.

Nutritional/Ethanol Interactions Food: Delays cefixime absorption.

Lab Interactions Positive direct Coombs', false-positive urinary glucose test using cupric sulfate (Benedict's solution, Clinitest®, Fehling's solution), false-positive serum or urine creatinine with Jaffé reaction

Adverse Reactions

>10%: Gastrointestinal: Diarrhea (16%)

2% to 10%: Gastrointestinal: Abdominal pain, nausea, dyspepsia, flatulence, loose stools

Reactions reported with other cephalosporins include interstitial nephritis, aplastic anemia, hemolytic anemia, hemorrhage, pancytopenia, agranulocytosis, colitis, superinfection

Overdosage/Toxicology Symptoms of overdose include neuromuscular hypersensitivity and convulsions. Many beta-lactam containing antibiotics have the potential to cause neuromuscular hyperirritability or convulsive seizures. Hemodialysis may be helpful to aid in the removal of drug from blood; otherwise, treatment is supportive or symptom-directed.

Pharmacodynamics/Kinetics
Absorption: 40% to 50%

Bioavailability: Bioavailability of suspension is higher than that of the tablet.

Time to Peak: Serum: 2-6 hours; delayed with food

Protein Binding: 65%

Half-Life Elimination: Normal renal function: 3-4 hours; Renal failure: Up to 11.5 hours

Excretion: Urine (50% of absorbed dose as active drug); feces (10%)

Dosing
Adults & Elderly:

Susceptible infections: Oral: 400 mg/day divided every 12-24 hours

Uncomplicated cervical/urethral gonorrhea due to *N. gonorrhoeae*: Oral: 400 mg as a single dose

Note: For *S. pyogenes* infections, treat for 10 days; use suspension for otitis media due to increased peak serum levels as compared to tablet form.

Pediatrics:

Susceptible infections: Oral:

Children ≥6 months: 8 mg/kg/day divided every 12-24 hours

Children >50 kg or >12 years: Refer to adult dosing.

Note: For *S. pyogenes* infections, treat for 10 days; use suspension for otitis media due to increased peak serum levels as compared to tablet form.

Renal Impairment:

Cl_{cr} 21-60 mL/minute: Administer 75% of the standard dose.

Cl_{cr} <20 mL/minute: Administer 50% of the standard dose.

10% removed by hemodialysis

Available Dosage Forms
Powder for oral suspension: 100 mg/5 mL (50 mL, 75 mL, 100 mL) [contains sodium benzoate; strawberry flavor]

Tablet [film coated]: 400 mg

Monitoring and Teaching Issues
Physical Assessment: Assess results of culture/sensitivity tests and patient's allergy history prior to therapy. See Warnings/Precautions for use cautions. Assess potential for interactions with other pharmacological agents patient may be taking (see Drug Interactions). Assess results of laboratory tests, therapeutic response, and adverse effects (anemia, hemorrhage, pancytopenia, agranulocytosis, colitis; see Adverse Reactions). Advise patients with diabetes about use of Clinitest®. Teach patient proper use, possible side effects/appropriate interventions, and adverse symptoms to report (eg, hypersensitivity, opportunistic infection).

Monitoring Laboratory Tests: Perform culture and sensitivity studies prior to initiating drug therapy; renal function

Patient Education: Do not take any new medication during therapy unless approved by prescriber. Take as directed, at regular intervals around-the-clock (with or without food). Chilling oral suspension improves flavor (do not freeze); shake suspension thoroughly before using. Maintain adequate hydration (2-3 L/day of fluids) unless instructed to restrict fluid intake. Complete full course of medication, even if you feel better. May cause false test results with Clinitest®; use of another type of glucose testing is preferable. May cause nausea or vomiting (small frequent meals, frequent mouth care, sucking lozenges, or chewing gum may help); or diarrhea (yogurt, boiled milk, or buttermilk may help). Report rash; breathing or swallowing difficulty; persistent diarrhea, nausea, vomiting, or abdominal pain; changes in urinary pattern or pain on urination; opportunistic infection (eg, vaginal itching or drainage; sores in mouth; blood in stool or urine, unusual fever or chills); CNS changes (eg, irritability, agitation, nervousness, insomnia, hallucinations); or other adverse reactions. **Breast-feeding precaution:** Consult prescriber if breast-feeding.

Dietary Considerations: May be taken with food.

Geriatric Considerations: Adjust dose for renal function.

Pregnancy Risk Factor: B

Lactation: Excretion in breast milk unknown/use caution

Breast-Feeding Issues: Theoretically, drug absorbed by nursing infant may change bowel flora or affect fever work-up result. **Note:** As a class, cephalosporins are used to treat infections in infants.

Other Issues: Otitis media should be treated with the suspension since it results in higher peak blood levels than the tablet.

Administration
Oral: Shake oral suspension well before use. May be administered with or without food. Administer with food to decrease GI distress.

Storage: After reconstitution, suspension may be stored for 14 days at room temperature or under refrigeration.

Additional Information Otitis media should be treated with the suspension since it results in higher peak blood levels than the tablet.

♦ **Cefizox**® *see* Ceftizoxime *on page 286*

♦ **Cefotan**® *see* Cefotetan *on page 277*

Cefotaxime (sef oh TAKS eem)
U.S. Brand Names Claforan®

Synonyms Cefotaxime Sodium

Generic Available Yes: Powder

Pharmacologic Category Antibiotic, Cephalosporin (Third Generation)

Medication Safety Issues

Sound-alike/look-alike issues:

Cefotaxime may be confused with cefoxitin, ceftizoxime, cefuroxime

(Continued)

Cefotaxime *(Continued)*

Use Treatment of susceptible infection in respiratory tract, skin and skin structure, bone and joint, urinary tract, gynecologic as well as septicemia, and documented or suspected meningitis. Active against most gram-negative bacilli (not *Pseudomonas*) and gram-positive cocci (not enterococcus). Active against many penicillin-resistant pneumococci.

Mechanism of Action/Effect Inhibits bacterial cell wall synthesis by binding to one or more of the penicillin-binding proteins (PBPs)

Contraindications Hypersensitivity to cefotaxime, any component of the formulation, or other cephalosporins

Warnings/Precautions Modify dosage in patients with severe renal impairment; prolonged use may result in superinfection; a potentially life-threatening arrhythmia has been reported in patients who received a rapid bolus injection via central line. Use caution in patients with colitis; minimize tissue inflammation by changing infusion sites when needed. Use with caution in patients with a history of penicillin allergy especially IgE-mediated reactions (eg, anaphylaxis, urticaria). May cause antibiotic-associated colitis or colitis secondary to *C. difficile*.

Drug Interactions

Increased Effect/Toxicity: Probenecid may decrease cephalosporin elimination resulting in increased levels. Furosemide, aminoglycosides in combination with cefotaxime may result in additive nephrotoxicity.

Lab Interactions Positive direct Coombs', false-positive urinary glucose test using cupric sulfate (Benedict's solution, Clinitest®, Fehling's solution), false-positive serum or urine creatinine with Jaffé reaction

Adverse Reactions

1% to 10%:

Dermatologic: Rash, pruritus

Gastrointestinal: Diarrhea, nausea, vomiting, colitis

Local: Pain at injection site

Reactions reported with other cephalosporins include agranulocytosis, aplastic anemia, cholestasis, hemolytic anemia, hemorrhage, nephropathy, pancytopenia, renal dysfunction, seizure, superinfection.

Overdosage/Toxicology Symptoms of overdose include neuromuscular hypersensitivity and convulsions. Many beta-lactam containing antibiotics have the potential to cause neuromuscular hyperirritability or convulsive seizures. Hemodialysis may be helpful to aid in removal of the drug from blood; otherwise, treatment is supportive or symptom-directed.

Pharmacodynamics/Kinetics

Time to Peak: Serum: I.M.: Within 30 minutes

Half-Life Elimination:

Cefotaxime: Premature neonates <1 week: 5-6 hours; Full-term neonates <1 week: 2-3.4 hours; Adults: 1-1.5 hours, prolonged with renal and/or hepatic impairment

Desacetylcefotaxime: 1.5-1.9 hours; prolonged with renal impairment

Metabolism: Partially hepatic to active metabolite, desacetylcefotaxime

Excretion: Urine (as unchanged drug and metabolites)

Dosing

Adults & Elderly:

Gonorrhea: I.M.: 1 g as a single dose

Uncomplicated infections: I.M., I.V.: 1 g every 12 hours

Moderate/severe infections: I.M., I.V.: 1-2 g every 8 hours

Infections commonly needing higher doses (eg, septicemia): I.V.: 2 g every 6-8 hours

Life-threatening infections: I.V.: 2 g every 4 hours

Preop: I.M., I.V.: 1 g 30-90 minutes before surgery

C-section: 1 g as soon as the umbilical cord is clamped, then 1 g I.M., I.V. at 6- and 12-hours intervals.

Pediatrics:

Susceptible infections: I.M., I.V.: Infants and Children 1 month to 12 years: <50 kg: 50-180 mg/kg/day in divided doses every 4-6 hours

Meningitis: 200 mg/kg/day in divided doses every 6 hours

Children >12 years: Refer to adult dosing.

Renal Impairment:

Cl_{cr} 10-50 mL/minute: Administer every 8-12 hours.

Cl_{cr} <10 mL/minute: Administer every 24 hours.

Moderately dialyzable (20% to 50%)

Continuous arteriovenous hemofiltration: 1 g every 12 hours.

Hepatic Impairment: Moderate dosage reduction is recommended in severe liver disease.

Available Dosage Forms

Infusion, as sodium [premixed in D_5W] (Claforan®): 1 g (50 mL); 2 g (50 mL)

Injection, powder for reconstitution, as sodium: 500 mg, 1 g, 2 g, 10 g, 20 g

Claforan®: 500 mg, 1 g, 2 g, 10 g [contains sodium 50.5 mg (2.2 mEq) per cefotaxime 1 g]

Monitoring and Teaching Issues

Physical Assessment: Assess results of culture/sensitivity tests and patient's allergy history prior to therapy. See Warnings/Precautions for use cautions (eg, renal impairment, arrhythmia, colitis). Assess potential for interactions with other pharmacological agents patient may be taking (eg, nephrotoxicity; see Drug Interactions). Evaluate results of laboratory tests (CBC with differential), therapeutic response, and adverse effects (diarrhea, nausea/vomiting, nephrotoxicity; see Adverse Reactions). Advise patients with diabetes about use of Clinitest®. Teach patient proper use, possible side effects/appropriate interventions, and adverse symptoms to report (eg, hypersensitivity, opportunistic infection).

Monitoring Laboratory Tests: Perform culture and sensitivity studies prior to initiating drug therapy; CBC with differential (especially with long courses); renal function

Patient Education: Do not take any new medication during therapy unless approved by prescriber. This medication is administered by injection or infusion. Report immediately any redness, swelling, burning, or pain at injection/infusion site; chest pain, palpitations, respiratory or swallowing difficulty; or itching or hives. Maintain adequate hydration (2-3 L/day of fluids) unless instructed to restrict fluid intake. May cause false test results with Clinitest®; use of another type of glucose testing is preferable. May cause diarrhea (yogurt, boiled milk, or buttermilk may help); GI distress or nausea (small frequent meals, frequent oral care, chewing gum, or sucking lozenges may help). Report rash; breathing or swallowing difficulty; persistent diarrhea, nausea, vomiting, or abdominal pain; changes in urinary pattern or pain on urination; opportunistic infection (eg, vaginal itching or drainage; sores in mouth; blood in stool or urine, unusual fever or chills); CNS changes (eg, irritability, agitation, nervousness, insomnia, hallucinations); or other adverse reactions. **Breast-feeding precaution:** Consult prescriber if breast-feeding.

Dietary Considerations: Sodium content of 1 g: 50.5 mg (2.2 mEq)

Geriatric Considerations: Adjust dose for renal function.

Pregnancy Risk Factor: B

Lactation: Enters breast milk/use caution (AAP rates "compatible")

Breast-Feeding Issues: Theoretically, drug absorbed by nursing infant may change bowel flora or affect fever work-up result. **Note:** As a class, cephalosporins are used to treat infections in infants.

Administration

I.M.: Inject deep I.M. into large muscle mass.

I.V.: Inject direct I.V. over 3-5 minutes. Infuse intermittent infusion over 30 minutes.

Reconstitution: Reconstituted solution is stable for 12-24 hours at room temperature and 7-10 days when refrigerated and for 13 weeks when frozen; for I.V. infusion in NS or D₅W, solution is stable for 24 hours at room temperature, 5 days when refrigerated, or 13 weeks when frozen in Viaflex® plastic containers; thawed solutions previously of frozen premixed bags are stable for 24 hours at room temperature or 10 days when refrigerated.

Compatibility: Stable in D₅¹/₄NS, D₅¹/₂NS, D₅NS, D₅W, D₁₀W, LR, NS

Y-site administration: Incompatible with allopurinol, filgrastim, fluconazole, gemcitabine, hetastarch, pentamidine

Compatibility in syringe: Incompatible with doxapram

Compatibility when admixed: Incompatible with aminoglycosides, aminophylline, sodium bicarbonate

Related Information

Antimicrobial Drugs of Choice *on page 1792*

Community-Acquired Pneumonia in Adults *on page 1807*

♦ **Cefotaxime Sodium** *see* Cefotaxime *on page 275*

Cefotetan (SEF oh tee tan)

U.S. Brand Names Cefotan®

Synonyms Cefotetan Disodium

Generic Available No

Pharmacologic Category Antibiotic, Cephalosporin (Second Generation)

Medication Safety Issues

Sound-alike/look-alike issues:

Cefotetan may be confused with cefoxitin, Ceftin®

Cefotan® may be confused with Ceftin®

Use Surgical prophylaxis; intra-abdominal infections and other mixed infections; respiratory tract, skin and skin structure, bone and joint, urinary tract and gynecologic as well as septicemia; active against gram-negative enteric bacilli including *E. coli*, *Klebsiella*, and *Proteus*; less active against staphylococci and streptococci than first generation cephalosporins, but active against anaerobes including *Bacteroides fragilis*

Mechanism of Action/Effect Inhibits bacterial cell wall synthesis by binding to one or more of the penicillin-binding proteins (PBPs)

Contraindications Hypersensitivity to cefotetan, any component of the formulation, or other cephalosporins; previous cephalosporin-associated hemolytic anemia

Warnings/Precautions Modify dosage in patients with severe renal impairment; prolonged use may result in superinfection; although cefotetan contains the methyltetrazolethiol side chain, bleeding has not been a significant problem; use with caution in patients with a history of penicillin allergy especially IgE-mediated reactions (eg, anaphylaxis, urticaria). Cefotetan has been associated with a higher risk of hemolytic anemia relative to other cephalosporins (approximately threefold); monitor carefully during use and consider cephalosporin-associated immune anemia in patients who have received cefotetan within 2-3 weeks (either as treatment or prophylaxis). May cause antibiotic-associated colitis or colitis secondary to *C. difficile*.

Drug Interactions

Increased Effect/Toxicity: Disulfiram-like reaction may occur if ethanol is consumed by a patient taking cefotetan. Probenecid may increase cefotetan plasma levels. Cefotetan may increase risk of bleeding in patients receiving warfarin.

Nutritional/Ethanol Interactions Ethanol: Avoid ethanol (may cause a disulfiram-like reaction).

Lab Interactions Positive direct Coombs', false-positive urinary glucose test using cupric sulfate (Benedict's solution, Clinitest®, Fehling's solution), false-positive serum or urine creatinine with Jaffé reaction

Adverse Reactions

1% to 10%:

Gastrointestinal: Diarrhea (1%)

Hepatic: Transaminases increased (1%)

Miscellaneous: Hypersensitivity reactions (1%)

Reactions reported with other cephalosporins include seizure, Stevens-Johnson syndrome, toxic epidermal necrolysis, renal dysfunction, toxic nephropathy, cholestasis, aplastic anemia, hemolytic anemia, hemorrhage, pancytopenia, agranulocytosis, colitis, superinfection

(Continued)

Cefotetan *(Continued)*

Overdosage/Toxicology Symptoms of overdose include neuromuscular hypersensitivity and convulsions. Many beta-lactam containing antibiotics have the potential to cause neuro-muscular hyperirritability or convulsive seizures. Hemodialysis may be helpful to aid in removal of the drug from blood; otherwise, treatment is supportive or symptom-directed.

Pharmacodynamics/Kinetics
Time to Peak: Serum: I.M.: 1.5-3 hours
Protein Binding: 76% to 90%
Half-Life Elimination: 3-5 hours
Excretion: Primarily urine (as unchanged drug); feces (20%)

Dosing
Adults & Elderly:
Susceptible infections: I.M., I.V.: 1-6 g/day in divided doses every 12 hours; usual dose: 1-2 g every 12 hours for 5-10 days; 1-2 g may be given every 24 hours for urinary tract infection
Pelvic inflammatory disease: I.V.: 2 g every 12 hours; used in combination with doxycycline
Preoperative prophylaxis: I.M., I.V.: 1-2 g 30-60 minutes prior to surgery; when used for cesarean section, dose should be given as soon as umbilical cord is clamped

Pediatrics:
Severe infections (unlabeled use): I.M., I.V.: 20-40 mg/kg/dose every 12 hours; maximum: 6 g/day
Preoperative prophylaxis (unlabeled use): I.M., I.V.: 40 mg/kg 30-60 minutes prior to surgery
Pelvic inflammatory disease: Adolescents: I.V.: Refer to adult dosing.

Renal Impairment: I.M., I.V.:
Cl_{cr} 10-30 mL/minute: Administer every 24 hours
Cl_{cr} <10 mL/minute: Administer every 48 hours
Hemodialysis: Dialyzable (5% to 20%); administer $^1/_4$ the usual dose every 24 hours on days between dialysis; administer $^1/_2$ the usual dose on the day of dialysis.
Continuous arteriovenous or venovenous hemodiafiltration effects: Administer 750 mg every 12 hours

Available Dosage Forms [DSC] = Discontinued product
Infusion [premixed iso-osmotic solution]: 1 g (50 mL); 2 g (50 mL) [contains sodium 80 mg/g (3.5 mEq/g)]
Injection, powder for reconstitution: 1 g, 2 g, 10 g [DSC] [contains sodium 80 mg/g (3.5 mEq/g)]

Monitoring and Teaching Issues
Physical Assessment: Assess results of culture/sensitivity tests and patient's allergy history prior to therapy. See Warnings/Precautions for use cautions (eg, renal impairment, hemolytic anemia). Assess potential for interactions with other pharmacological agents patient may be taking (see Drug Interactions). Assess results of laboratory tests (prothrombin time). Monitor for therapeutic response and adverse effects (eg, hemolytic anemia, hypoprothrombinemia, and bleeding; see Adverse Reactions). Advise patients with diabetes about use of Clinitest® (may cause false-positive test). Teach patient possible side effects/appropriate interventions and adverse symptoms to report (eg, nephrotoxicity, opportunistic infection, hypersensitivity reaction).

Monitoring Laboratory Tests: Prothrombin time; perform culture and sensitivity studies prior to initiating drug therapy; renal function

Patient Education: Do not take any new medication during therapy unless approved by prescriber. This medication is administered by injection or infusion. Report immediately any redness, swelling, burning, or pain at injection/infusion site, or immediately report any itching, hives, difficulty swallowing, or respiratory difficulty. Maintain adequate hydration (2-3 L/day of fluids) unless instructed to restrict fluid intake. Avoid alcohol during therapy and for 72 hours after last dose (may cause severe disulfiram-like reactions). May cause false test results with Clinitest®; use of another type of glucose testing is preferable. May cause diarrhea (yogurt, boiled milk, or buttermilk may help). Report rash; breathing or swallowing difficulty; persistent diarrhea, nausea, vomiting, or abdominal pain; changes in urinary pattern or pain on urination; opportunistic infection (eg, vaginal itching or drainage; sores in mouth; blood in stool or urine, unusual fever or chills); CNS changes (eg, irrita-bility, agitation, nervousness, insomnia, hallucinations); or other adverse reactions.
Breast-feeding precaution: Consult prescriber if breast-feeding.

Dietary Considerations: Contains sodium of 80 mg (3.5 mEq) per cefotetan 1 g

Geriatric Considerations: Cefotetan has not been studied in the elderly. Adjust dose for renal function in the elderly.

Pregnancy Risk Factor: B

Lactation: Enters breast milk (small amounts)/use caution

Breast-Feeding Issues: Theoretically, drug absorbed by nursing infant may change bowel flora or affect fever work-up result. **Note:** As a class, cephalosporins are used to treat infections in infants.

Administration
I.M.: Inject deep I.M. into large muscle mass.
I.V.: Inject direct I.V. over 3-5 minutes. Infuse intermittent infusion over 30 minutes.
Reconstitution: Reconstituted solution is stable for 24 hours at room temperature and 96 hours when refrigerated. For I.V. infusion in NS or D_5W solution and after freezing, thawed solution is stable for 24 hours at room temperature or 96 hours when refrigerated. Frozen solution is stable for 12 weeks.
Compatibility: Stable in D_5W, NS
Y-site administration: Incompatible with promethazine, vinorelbine
Compatibility in syringe: Incompatible with doxapram, promethazine
Compatibility when admixed: Incompatible with gentamicin, heparin, tetracyclines

♦ **Cefotetan Disodium** *see* Cefotetan *on page 277*

Cefoxitin (se FOKS i tin)

U.S. Brand Names Mefoxin®

Synonyms Cefoxitin Sodium

Generic Available Yes: Powder for injection

Pharmacologic Category Antibiotic, Cephalosporin (Second Generation)

Medication Safety Issues

Sound-alike/look-alike issues:

Cefoxitin may be confused with cefotaxime, cefotetan, Cytoxan®

Mefoxin® may be confused with Lanoxin®

Use Less active against staphylococci and streptococci than first generation cephalosporins, but active against anaerobes including *Bacteroides fragilis*; active against gram-negative enteric bacilli including *E. coli*, *Klebsiella*, and *Proteus*; used predominantly for respiratory tract, skin and skin structure, bone and joint, urinary tract and gynecologic as well as septicemia; surgical prophylaxis; intra-abdominal infections and other mixed infections; indicated for bacterial *Eikenella corrodens* infections

Mechanism of Action/Effect Inhibits bacterial cell wall synthesis by binding to one or more of the penicillin-binding proteins (PBPs)

Contraindications Hypersensitivity to cefoxitin, any component of the formulation, or other cephalosporins

Warnings/Precautions Use with caution in patients with history of colitis; cefoxitin may increase resistance of organisms by inducing beta-lactamase; modify dosage in patients with severe renal impairment; prolonged use may result in superinfection; use with caution in patients with a history of penicillin allergy especially IgE-mediated reactions (eg, anaphylaxis, urticaria). May cause antibiotic-associated colitis or colitis secondary to *C. difficile*.

Drug Interactions

Increased Effect/Toxicity: Probenecid may decrease cephalosporin elimination. Furosemide, aminoglycosides in combination with cefoxitin may result in additive nephrotoxicity.

Lab Interactions Positive direct Coombs', false-positive urinary glucose test using cupric sulfate (Benedict's solution, Clinitest®, Fehling's solution), false-positive serum or urine creatinine with Jaffé reaction

Adverse Reactions

1% to 10%: Gastrointestinal: Diarrhea

Reactions reported with other cephalosporins include Agranulocytosis, aplastic anemia, cholestasis, colitis, erythema multiforme, hemolytic anemia, hemorrhage, pancytopenia, renal dysfunction, serum-sickness reactions, seizure, Stevens-Johnson syndrome, superinfection, toxic nephropathy, vaginitis

Overdosage/Toxicology Symptoms of overdose include neuromuscular hypersensitivity and convulsions. Many beta-lactam containing antibiotics have the potential to cause neuromuscular hyperirritability or convulsive seizures. Hemodialysis may be helpful to aid in removal of the drug from blood; otherwise, treatment is supportive or symptom-directed.

Pharmacodynamics/Kinetics

Time to Peak: Serum: I.M.: 20-30 minutes

Protein Binding: 65% to 79%

Half-Life Elimination: 45-60 minutes; significantly prolonged with renal impairment

Excretion: Urine (85% as unchanged drug)

Dosing

Adults & Elderly: Susceptible infections: I.M., I.V.: 1-2 g every 6-8 hours (I.M. injection is painful); up to 12 g/day

Pediatrics: Infants >3 months and Children:

Mild to moderate infection: I.M., I.V.: 80-100 mg/kg/day in divided doses every 4-6 hours

Severe infection: I.M., I.V.: 100-160 mg/kg/day in divided doses every 4-6 hours

Maximum dose: 12 g/day

Renal Impairment: I.M., I.V.:

Cl_{cr} 30-50 mL/minute: Administer 1-2 g every 8-12 hours

Cl_{cr} 10-29 mL/minute: Administer 1-2 g every 12-24 hours

Cl_{cr} 5-9 mL/minute: Administer 0.5-1 g every 12-24 hours

Cl_{cr} <5 mL/minute: Administer 0.5-1 g every 24-48 hours

Hemodialysis: Moderately dialyzable (20% to 50%); administer a loading dose of 1-2 g after each hemodialysis; maintenance dose as noted above based on Cl_{cr}

Continuous arteriovenous or venovenous hemodiafiltration effects: Dose as for Cl_{cr} 10-50 mL/minute

Available Dosage Forms

Infusion, as sodium [premixed iso-osmotic solution]: 1 g (50 mL); 2 g (50 mL) [contains sodium 53.8 mg/g (2.3 mEq/g)]

Injection, powder for reconstitution, as sodium: 1 g, 2 g, 10 g [contains sodium 53.8 mg/g (2.3 mEq/g)]

Monitoring and Teaching Issues

Physical Assessment: Assess results of culture/sensitivity tests and patient's allergy history prior to therapy. See Warnings/Precautions for use cautions (eg, colitis, renal impairment). Assess potential for interactions with other pharmacological agents patient may be taking (see Drug Interactions). Assess results of laboratory tests (prothrombin time). Monitor for therapeutic response and adverse effects (eg, hemolytic anemia, hypoprothrombinemia, and bleeding; see Adverse Reactions). Advise patients with diabetes about use of Clinitest® (may cause false-positive test). Teach patient possible side effects/appropriate interventions and adverse symptoms to report (eg, opportunistic infection, hypersensitivity reaction).

Monitoring Laboratory Tests: Prothrombin times; perform culture and sensitivity studies prior to initiating drug therapy; renal function

Patient Education: Do not take any new medication during therapy unless approved by prescriber. This medication is administered by injection or infusion. Report immediately any redness, swelling, burning, or pain at injection/infusion site; chest pain, palpitations, respiratory or swallowing difficulty; itching or hives. Maintain adequate hydration (2-3 L/day of (Continued)

Cefoxitin *(Continued)*

fluids) unless instructed to restrict fluid intake. May cause false test results with Clinitest®; use of another type of glucose testing is preferable. May cause diarrhea (yogurt, boiled milk, or buttermilk may help). Report rash; breathing or swallowing difficulty; persistent diarrhea, nausea, vomiting, or abdominal pain; changes in urinary pattern or pain on urination; opportunistic infection (eg, vaginal itching or drainage; sores in mouth; blood in stool or urine, unusual fever or chills); CNS changes (eg, irritability, agitation, nervousness, insomnia, hallucinations); or other adverse reactions. **Breast-feeding precaution:** Consult prescriber if breast-feeding.

Dietary Considerations: Sodium content of 1 g: 53 mg (2.3 mEq)

Geriatric Considerations: Adjust dose for renal function in the elderly.

Pregnancy Risk Factor: B

Lactation: Enters breast milk (small amounts)/use caution (AAP rates "compatible")

Breast-Feeding Issues: Theoretically, drug absorbed by nursing infant may change bowel flora or affect fever work-up result. **Note:** As a class, cephalosporins are used to treat infections in infants.

Administration

I.M.: Inject deep I.M. into large muscle mass.

I.V.: Can be administered IVP over 3-5 minutes at a maximum concentration of 100 mg/mL or I.V. intermittent infusion over 10-60 minutes at a final concentration for I.V. administration not to exceed 40 mg/mL

Reconstitution: Reconstitute vials with SWFI, bacteriostatic water for injection, NS, or D_5W. For I.V. infusion, solutions may be further diluted in NS, $D_5\frac{1}{4}NS$, $D_5\frac{1}{2}NS$, D_5NS, D_5W, $D_{10}W$, LR, D_5LR, mannitol 10%, or sodium bicarbonate 5%.

Compatibility: Stable in D_5LR, $D_5\frac{1}{4}NS$, $D_5\frac{1}{2}NS$, D_5NS, D_5W, $D_{10}W$, LR, NS, mannitol 10%, sodium bicarbonate 5%

Y-site administration: Incompatible with filgrastim, gatifloxacin, hetastarch, pentamidine

Compatibility when admixed: Incompatible with ranitidine

Storage: Reconstituted solution is stable for 6 hours at room temperature or 7 days when refrigerated; I.V. infusion in NS or D_5W solution is stable for 18 hours at room temperature or 48 hours when refrigerated. Premixed frozen solution, when thawed, is stable for 24 hours at room temperature or 21 days when refrigerated.

♦ **Cefoxitin Sodium** *see Cefoxitin on page 279*

Cefpodoxime *(sef pode OKS eem)*

U.S. Brand Names Vantin®

Synonyms Cefpodoxime Proxetil

Generic Available Yes: Tablet

Pharmacologic Category Antibiotic, Cephalosporin (Third Generation)

Medication Safety Issues

Sound-alike/look-alike issues:

Vantin® may be confused with Ventolin®

Use Treatment of susceptible acute, community-acquired pneumonia caused by *S. pneumoniae* or nonbeta-lactamase producing *H. influenzae*; acute uncomplicated gonorrhea caused by *N. gonorrhoeae*; uncomplicated skin and skin structure infections caused by *S. aureus* or *S. pyogenes*; acute otitis media caused by *S. pneumoniae*, *H. influenzae*, or *M. catarrhalis*; pharyngitis or tonsillitis; and uncomplicated urinary tract infections caused by *E. coli*, *Klebsiella*, and *Proteus*

Mechanism of Action/Effect Inhibits bacterial cell wall synthesis by binding to one or more of the penicillin-binding proteins (PBPs)

Contraindications Hypersensitivity to cefpodoxime, any component of the formulation, or other cephalosporins

Warnings/Precautions Modify dosage in patients with severe renal impairment; prolonged use may result in superinfection. Use with caution in patients with a history of penicillin allergy especially IgE-mediated reactions (eg, anaphylaxis, urticaria).

Drug Interactions

Decreased Effect: Antacids and H_2-receptor antagonists reduce absorption and serum concentration of cefpodoxime.

Increased Effect/Toxicity: Probenecid may decrease cephalosporin elimination. Furosemide, aminoglycosides in combination with cefpodoxime may result in additive nephrotoxicity.

Nutritional/Ethanol Interactions Food: Food delays absorption; cefpodoxime serum levels may be increased if taken with food.

Lab Interactions Positive direct Coombs', false-positive urinary glucose test using cupric sulfate (Benedict's solution, Clinitest®, Fehling's solution), false-positive serum or urine creatinine with Jaffé reaction

Adverse Reactions

>10%:

Dermatologic: Diaper rash (12%)

Gastrointestinal: Diarrhea in infants and toddlers (15%)

1% to 10%:

Central nervous system: Headache (1%)

Dermatologic: Rash (1%)

Gastrointestinal: Diarrhea (7%), nausea (4%), abdominal pain (2%), vomiting (1% to 2%)

Genitourinary: Vaginal infection (3%)

Reactions reported with other cephalosporins include seizure, Stevens-Johnson syndrome, toxic epidermal necrolysis, erythema multiforme, urticaria, serum-sickness reactions, renal dysfunction, interstitial nephritis toxic nephropathy, cholestasis, aplastic anemia, hemolytic anemia, hemorrhage, pancytopenia, agranulocytosis, colitis, vaginitis, superinfection

Overdosage/Toxicology Symptoms of overdose include neuromuscular hypersensitivity and convulsions. Many beta-lactam containing antibiotics have the potential to cause neuro-muscular hyperirritability or convulsive seizures. Hemodialysis may be helpful to aid in removal of the drug from blood; otherwise, treatment is supportive or symptom-directed.

Pharmacodynamics/Kinetics

Absorption: Rapid and well absorbed (50%), acid stable; enhanced in the presence of food or low gastric pH

Time to Peak: Within 1 hour

Protein Binding: 18% to 23%

Half-Life Elimination: 2.2 hours; prolonged with renal impairment

Metabolism: De-esterified in GI tract to active metabolite, cefpodoxime

Excretion: Urine (80% as unchanged drug) in 24 hours

Dosing

Adults & Elderly:

Acute community-acquired pneumonia and bacterial exacerbations of chronic bron-chitis: Oral: 200 mg every 12 hours for 14 days and 10 days, respectively

Acute maxillary sinusitis: Oral: 200 mg every 12 hours for 10 days

Skin and skin structure: Oral: 400 mg every 12 hours for 7-14 days

Uncomplicated gonorrhea (male and female) and rectal gonococcal infections (female): Oral: 200 mg as a single dose

Pharyngitis/tonsillitis: Oral: 100 mg every 12 hours for 5-10 days

Uncomplicated urinary tract infection: Oral: 100 mg every 12 hours for 7 days

Pediatrics:

Acute otitis media: Oral: Children 2 months to 12 years: 10 mg/kg/day divided every 12 hours (400 mg/day) for 5 days (maximum: 200 mg/dose)

Acute maxillary sinusitis: Oral: Children:

2 months to 12 years: 10 mg/kg/day divided every 12 hours for 10 days (maximum: 200 mg/dose)

≥12 years: Refer to adult dosing.

Pharyngitis/tonsillitis: Oral: Children:

2 months to 12 years: 10 mg/kg/day in 2 divided doses for 5-10 days (maximum: 100 mg/dose)

≥12 years: Refer to adult dosing.

Renal Impairment:

Cl$_{cr}$ <30 mL/minute: Administer every 24 hours.

Hemodialysis: Dose 3 times/week following dialysis.

Hepatic Impairment: Dose adjustment is not necessary in patients with cirrhosis.

Available Dosage Forms

Granules for oral suspension: 50 mg/5 mL (50 mL, 75 mL, 100 mL); 100 mg/5 mL (50 mL, 75 mL, 100 mL) [contains sodium benzoate; lemon creme flavor]

Tablet [film coated]: 100 mg, 200 mg

Monitoring and Teaching Issues

Physical Assessment: Assess results of culture/sensitivity tests and patient's allergy history prior to therapy. See Warnings/Precautions for use cautions (eg, renal impairment). Assess potential for interactions with other pharmacological agents patient may be taking (see Drug Interactions). Assess results of laboratory tests. Monitor for therapeutic response and adverse effects (eg, hemolytic anemia, hypoprothrombinemia, and bleeding; see Adverse Reactions). Advise patients with diabetes about use of Clinitest® (may cause false-positive test). Teach patient possible side effects/appropriate interventions and adverse symptoms to report (eg, nephrotoxicity, opportunistic infection, hypersensitivity reaction).

Monitoring Laboratory Tests: Perform culture and sensitivity studies prior to initiating drug therapy; renal function

Patient Education: Do not take any new medication during therapy unless approved by prescriber. Take as directed, at regular intervals around-the-clock (with or without food). Chilling oral suspension improves flavor (do not freeze); shake well before using. Maintain adequate hydration (2-3 L/day of fluids) unless instructed to restrict fluid intake. Complete full course of medication, even if you feel better. May cause false test results with Clin-itest®; use of another type of glucose testing is preferable. May cause nausea or vomiting (small frequent meals, frequent mouth care, sucking lozenges, or chewing gum may help); or diarrhea (yogurt, boiled milk, or buttermilk may help). Report rash; breathing or swal-lowing difficulty; persistent diarrhea, nausea, vomiting, or abdominal pain; changes in urinary pattern or pain on urination; opportunistic infection (eg, vaginal itching or drainage; sores in mouth; blood in stool or urine, unusual fever or chills); CNS changes (eg, irrita-bility, agitation, nervousness, insomnia, hallucinations); or other adverse reactions. **Breast-feeding precaution:** Consult prescriber if breast-feeding.

Dietary Considerations: May be taken with food.

Geriatric Considerations: Considered one of the drugs of choice for outpatient treatment of community-acquired pneumonia in older adults. Adjust dosage with renal impairment.

Pregnancy Risk Factor: B

Lactation: Enters breast milk (small amounts)/use caution

Breast-Feeding Issues: Theoretically, drug absorbed by nursing infant may change bowel flora or affect fever work-up result. **Note:** As a class, cephalosporins are used to treat infections in infants.

Administration

Oral: Administer around-the-clock to promote less variation in peak and trough serum levels.

Reconstitution: After mixing, keep suspension in refrigerator, shake well before using. Discard unused portion after 14 days.

Related Information

Antimicrobial Drugs of Choice *on page 1792*

Community-Acquired Pneumonia in Adults *on page 1807*

♦ **Cefpodoxime Proxetil** *see* Cefpodoxime *on page 280*

Cefprozil (sef PROE zil)

U.S. Brand Names Cefzil®

Generic Available No

Pharmacologic Category Antibiotic, Cephalosporin (Second Generation)

Medication Safety Issues

Sound-alike/look-alike issues:
 Cefprozil may be confused with cefazolin, cefuroxime
 Cefzil® may be confused with Cefol®, Ceftin®, Kefzol®

Use Treatment of otitis media and infections involving the respiratory tract and skin and skin structure; active against methicillin-sensitive staphylococci, many streptococci, and various gram-negative bacilli including *E. coli*, some *Klebsiella*, *P. mirabilis*, *H. influenzae*, and *Moraxella*.

Mechanism of Action/Effect Inhibits bacterial cell wall synthesis by binding to one or more of the penicillin-binding proteins (PBPs)

Contraindications Hypersensitivity to cefprozil, any component of the formulation, or other cephalosporins

Warnings/Precautions Modify dosage in patients with severe renal impairment; prolonged use may result in superinfection; use with caution in patients with a history of penicillin allergy especially IgE-mediated reactions (eg, anaphylaxis, urticaria). May cause antibiotic-associated colitis or colitis secondary to *C. difficile.*

Drug Interactions

Increased Effect/Toxicity: Probenecid may decrease cephalosporin elimination. Furosemide, aminoglycosides in combination with cefprozil may result in additive nephrotoxicity.

Nutritional/Ethanol Interactions Food: Food delays cefprozil absorption.

Lab Interactions Positive direct Coombs', false-positive urinary glucose test using cupric sulfate (Benedict's solution, Clinitest®, Fehling's solution), false-positive serum or urine creatinine with Jaffé reaction

Adverse Reactions

1% to 10%:
 Central nervous system: Dizziness (1%)
 Dermatologic: Diaper rash (2%)
 Gastrointestinal: Diarrhea (3%), nausea (4%), vomiting (1%), abdominal pain (1%)
 Genitourinary: Vaginitis, genital pruritus (2%)
 Hepatic: Transaminases increased (2%)
 Miscellaneous: Superinfection

Reactions reported with other cephalosporins include seizure, toxic epidermal necrolysis, renal dysfunction, interstitial nephritis, toxic nephropathy, aplastic anemia, hemolytic anemia, hemorrhage, pancytopenia, agranulocytosis, colitis, vaginitis, superinfection

Overdosage/Toxicology Symptoms of overdose include neuromuscular hypersensitivity and convulsions. Many beta-lactam containing antibiotics have the potential to cause neuromuscular hyperirritability or convulsive seizures. Hemodialysis may be helpful to aid in removal of the drug from blood; otherwise, treatment is supportive or symptom-directed.

Pharmacodynamics/Kinetics

Absorption: Well absorbed (94%)

Time to Peak: Serum: Fasting: 1.5 hours

Protein Binding: 35% to 45%

Half-Life Elimination: Normal renal function: 1.3 hours

Excretion: Urine (61% as unchanged drug)

Dosing

Adults & Elderly:

Pharyngitis/tonsillitis: Oral: 500 mg every 24 hours for 10 days

Uncomplicated skin and skin structure infections: Oral: 250 mg every 12 hours, or 500 mg every 12-24 hours for 10 days

Secondary bacterial infection of acute bronchitis or acute bacterial exacerbation of chronic bronchitis: Oral: 500 mg every 12 hours for 10 days

Pediatrics:

Otitis media: Oral: Children >6 months to 12 years: 15 mg/kg every 12 hours for 10 days

Pharyngitis/tonsillitis: Oral: Children:
 2-12 years: 7.5 -15 mg/kg/day divided every 12 hours for 10 days (administer for >10 days if due to *S. pyogenes*); maximum: 1 g/day
 >13 years: Refer to adult dosing.

Uncomplicated skin and skin structure infections: Oral:
 2-12 years: 20 mg/kg every 24 hours for 10 days; maximum: 1 g/day
 >13 years: Refer to adult dosing.

Renal Impairment:

Cl$_{cr}$ <30 mL/minute: Reduce dose by 50%.

Hemodialysis effects: 55% is removed by hemodialysis.

Available Dosage Forms

Powder for oral suspension, as anhydrous: 125 mg/5 mL (50 mL, 75 mL, 100 mL); 250 mg/5 mL (50 mL, 75 mL, 100 mL) [contains phenylalanine 28 mg/5 mL and sodium benzoate; bubble gum flavor]

Tablet, as anhydrous: 250 mg, 500 mg

Monitoring and Teaching Issues

Physical Assessment: Assess results of culture/sensitivity tests and patient's allergy history prior to therapy. See Warnings/Precautions for use cautions (eg, renal impairment). Assess potential for interactions with other pharmacological agents patient may be taking (see Drug Interactions). Assess results of laboratory tests, therapeutic response, and adverse effects (eg, interstitial nephritis, hemolytic anemia, hemorrhage; see Adverse Reactions). Advise patients with diabetes about use of Clinitest® (may cause false-positive test). Teach patient possible side effects/appropriate interventions and adverse symptoms to report (eg, opportunistic infection, hypersensitivity reaction).

Monitoring Laboratory Tests: Perform culture and sensitivity studies prior to initiating drug therapy; renal function

Patient Education: Do not take any new medication during therapy unless approved by prescriber. Take as directed, at regular intervals around-the-clock (with or without food). Chilling oral suspension improves flavor (do not freeze). Maintain adequate hydration (2-3 L/day of fluids) unless instructed to restrict fluid intake. Complete full course of medication, even if you feel better. May cause false test results with Clinitest®; use of another type of glucose testing is preferable. May cause dizziness (use caution when driving or engaging in potentially hazardous tasks until response to drug is known); nausea or vomiting (small frequent meals, frequent mouth care, sucking lozenges, or chewing gum may help); or diarrhea (yogurt, boiled milk, or buttermilk may help). Report rash; breathing or swallowing difficulty; persistent diarrhea, nausea, vomiting, or abdominal pain; changes in urinary pattern or pain on urination; opportunistic infection (eg, vaginal itching or drainage; sores in mouth; blood in stool or urine, unusual fever or chills); CNS changes (eg, irritability, agitation, nervousness, insomnia, hallucinations); or other adverse reactions. **Breast-feeding precaution:** Consult prescriber if breast-feeding.

Dietary Considerations: May be taken with food. Oral suspension contains phenylalanine 28 mg/5 mL.

Geriatric Considerations: Has not been studied exclusively in the elderly. Adjust dose for estimated renal function.

Pregnancy Risk Factor: B

Lactation: Enters breast milk/use caution (AAP rates "compatible")

Breast-Feeding Issues: Theoretically, drug absorbed by nursing infant may change bowel flora or affect fever work-up result. **Note:** As a class, cephalosporins are used to treat infections in infants.

Administration

Oral: Administer around-the-clock to promote less variation in peak and trough serum levels. Chilling the reconstituted oral suspension improves flavor (do not freeze).

Related Information

Community-Acquired Pneumonia in Adults *on page 1807*

Ceftazidime (SEF tay zi deem)

U.S. Brand Names Ceptaz® [DSC]; Fortaz®; Tazicef®

Generic Available No

Pharmacologic Category Antibiotic, Cephalosporin (Third Generation)

Medication Safety Issues

Sound-alike/look-alike issues:

Ceftazidime may be confused with ceftizoxime

Ceptaz® may be confused with Septra®

Tazicef® may be confused with Tazidime®

Tazidime® may be confused with Tazicef®

Use Treatment of documented susceptible *Pseudomonas aeruginosa* infection and infections due to other susceptible aerobic gram-negative organisms; empiric therapy of a febrile, granulocytopenic patient

Mechanism of Action/Effect Inhibits bacterial cell wall synthesis by binding to one or more of the penicillin-binding proteins (PBPs)

Contraindications Hypersensitivity to ceftazidime, any component of the formulation, or other cephalosporins

Warnings/Precautions Modify dosage in patients with severe renal impairment; prolonged use may result in superinfection; use with caution in patients with a history of penicillin allergy especially IgE-mediated reactions (eg, anaphylaxis, urticaria). May cause antibiotic-associated colitis or colitis secondary to *C. difficile*.

Drug Interactions

Increased Effect/Toxicity: Probenecid may decrease cephalosporin elimination. Aminoglycosides: *in vitro* studies indicate additive or synergistic effect against some strains of Enterobacteriaceae and *Pseudomonas aeruginosa*. Furosemide, aminoglycosides in combination with ceftazidime may result in additive nephrotoxicity.

Lab Interactions Positive direct Coombs', false-positive urinary glucose test using cupric sulfate (Benedict's solution, Clinitest®, Fehling's solution), false-positive serum or urine creatinine with Jaffé reaction

Adverse Reactions

1% to 10%:

Gastrointestinal: Diarrhea (1%)

Local: Pain at injection site (1%)

Miscellaneous: Hypersensitivity reactions (2%)

Reactions reported with other cephalosporins include seizure, urticaria, serum-sickness reactions, renal dysfunction, interstitial nephritis, toxic nephropathy, elevated BUN, elevated creatinine, cholestasis, aplastic anemia, hemolytic anemia, pancytopenia, agranulocytosis, colitis, prolonged PT, hemorrhage, superinfection

Overdosage/Toxicology Symptoms of overdose include neuromuscular hypersensitivity and convulsions. Many beta-lactam containing antibiotics have the potential to cause neuromuscular hyperirritability or convulsive seizures. Hemodialysis may be helpful to aid in removal of the drug from blood; otherwise, treatment is supportive or symptom-directed.

Pharmacodynamics/Kinetics

Time to Peak: Serum: I.M.: ~1 hour

Protein Binding: 17%

Half-Life Elimination: 1-2 hours, prolonged with renal impairment; Neonates <23 days: 2.2-4.7 hours

Excretion: Urine (80% to 90% as unchanged drug)

Dosing

Adults:

Bone and joint infections: I.V.: 2 g every 12 hours

(Continued)

Ceftazidime *(Continued)*

Cystic fibrosis, lung infection caused by *Pseudomonas* spp: I.V.: 30-50 mg/kg every 8 hours (maximum 6 g/day)

Intra-abdominal or gynecologic infection: I.V.: 2 g every 8 hours

Meningitis: I.V.: 2 g every 8 hours

Pneumonia: I.V.:
Uncomplicated: 500 mg to 1 g every 8 hours
Complicated or severe: 2 g every 8 hours

Skin and soft tissue infections: I.V., I.M.: 500 mg to 1 g every 8 hours

Severe, life-threatening infection (especially in immunocompromised host): I.V.: 2 g every 8 hours

Urinary tract infections: I.V., I.M.:
Uncomplicated: 250 mg every 12 hours
Complicated: 500 mg every 8-12 hours

Elderly: I.M., I.V.: Dosage should be based on renal function with a dosing interval not more frequent then every 12 hours.

Pediatrics: Susceptible infections: I.V.:
Children 1 month to 12 years: 30-50 mg/kg/dose every 8 hours; maximum dose: 6 g/day (higher doses reserved for immunocompromised patients, cystic fibrosis, or meningitis)
Children ≥12 years: Refer to adult dosing.

Renal Impairment:
Cl_{cr} 30-50 mL/minute: Administer every 12 hours
Cl_{cr} 10-30 mL/minute: Administer every 24 hours
Cl_{cr} <10 mL/minute: Administer every 48-72 hours
Hemodialysis: Dialyzable (50% to 100%)
Continuous arteriovenous or venovenous hemodiafiltration effects: Dose as for Cl_{cr} 30-50 mL/minute

Available Dosage Forms [DSC] = Discontinued product
Infusion, as sodium [premixed iso-osmotic solution] (Fortaz®): 1 g (50 mL); 2 g (50 mL)
Injection, powder for reconstitution:
Ceptaz® [DSC]: 10 g [L-arginine formulation]
Fortaz®: 500 mg, 1 g, 2 g, 6 g [contains sodium carbonate]
Tazicef®: 1 g, 2 g, 6 g [contains sodium carbonate]

Monitoring and Teaching Issues

Physical Assessment: Assess results of culture/sensitivity tests and patient's allergy history prior to therapy. See Warnings/Precautions for use cautions (eg, colitis, renal impairment). Assess potential for interactions with other pharmacological agents patient may be taking (eg nephrotoxicity; see Drug Interactions). Assess results of laboratory tests (prothrombin time), therapeutic response, and adverse effects (eg, hemolytic anemia, hypoprothrombinemia, and bleeding; see Adverse Reactions). Advise patients with diabetes about use of Clinitest® (may cause false-positive test). Teach patient possible side effects/appropriate interventions and adverse symptoms to report (eg, opportunistic infection, hypersensitivity reaction).

Monitoring Laboratory Tests: Perform culture and sensitivity studies prior to initiating drug therapy; renal function

Patient Education: Do not take any new medication during therapy unless approved by prescriber. This medication is administered by infusion or injection. Report immediately any redness, swelling, burning, or pain at injection/infusion site. Maintain adequate hydration (2-3 L/day of fluids) unless instructed to restrict fluid intake. May cause false test results with Clinitest®; use of another type of glucose testing is preferable. May cause diarrhea (yogurt, boiled milk, or buttermilk may help). Report rash; breathing or swallowing difficulty; persistent diarrhea, nausea, vomiting, or abdominal pain; changes in urinary pattern or pain on urination; opportunistic infection (eg, vaginal itching or drainage; sores in mouth; blood in stool or urine, unusual fever or chills); CNS changes (eg, irritability, agitation, nervousness, insomnia, hallucinations); or other adverse reactions. **Breast-feeding precautions:** Consult prescriber if breast-feeding.

Dietary Considerations: Sodium content of 1 g: 2.3 mEq

Geriatric Considerations: Changes in renal function associated with aging and corresponding alterations in pharmacokinetics result in every 12-hour dosing being an adequate dosing interval. Adjust dose based on renal function.

Pregnancy Risk Factor: B

Lactation: Enters breast milk (small amounts)/use caution (AAP rates "compatible")

Breast-Feeding Issues: Theoretically, drug absorbed by nursing infant may change bowel flora or affect fever work-up result. **Note:** As a class, cephalosporins are used to treat infections in infants.

Administration

I.M.: Inject deep I.M. into large mass muscle.

I.V.: Ceftazidime can be administered IVP over 3-5 minutes or I.V. intermittent infusion over 15-30 minutes.

Reconstitution: Reconstituted solution and I.V. infusion in NS or D_5W solution are stable for 24 hours at room temperature, 10 days when refrigerated, or 12 weeks when frozen. After freezing, thawed solution is stable for 24 hours at room temperature or 4 days when refrigerated. After mixing for 96 hours refrigerated.

Compatibility: Stable in D_5NS, D_5W, NS, SWFI
Y-site administration: Incompatible with alatrofloxacin, amphotericin B cholesteryl sulfate complex, amsacrine, doxorubicin liposome, fluconazole, idarubicin, midazolam, pentamidine, warfarin
Compatibility when admixed: Incompatible with aminoglycosides in same bottle/bag, aminophylline, ranitidine

Additional Information With some organisms, resistance may develop during treatment (including *Enterobacter* spp and *Serratia* spp); consider combination therapy or periodic susceptibility testing for organisms with inducible resistance

Related Information Antimicrobial Drugs of Choice *on page 1792*

Ceftibuten (sef TYE byoo ten)

U.S. Brand Names Cedax®

Generic Available No

Pharmacologic Category Antibiotic, Cephalosporin (Third Generation)

Use Oral cephalosporin for treatment of bronchitis, otitis media, and pharyngitis/tonsillitis due to *H. influenzae* and *M. catarrhalis*, both beta-lactamase-producing and nonproducing strains, as well as *S. pneumoniae* (weak) and *S. pyogenes*

Mechanism of Action/Effect Inhibits bacterial cell wall synthesis by binding to one or more of the penicillin-binding proteins (PBPs)

Contraindications Hypersensitivity to ceftibuten, any component of the formulation, or other cephalosporins

Warnings/Precautions Modify dosage in patients with severe renal impairment, prolonged use may result in superinfection; use with caution in patients with a history of penicillin allergy, especially IgE-mediated reactions (eg, anaphylaxis, urticaria). May cause antibiotic-associated colitis or colitis secondary to *C. difficile*.

Drug Interactions

Increased Effect/Toxicity: High-dose probenecid decreases clearance. Aminoglycosides in combination with ceftibuten may increase nephrotoxic potential.

Lab Interactions Positive direct Coombs', false-positive urinary glucose test using cupric sulfate (Benedict's solution, Clinitest®, Fehling's solution), false-positive serum or urine creatinine with Jaffé reaction

Adverse Reactions

1% to 10%:

Central nervous system: Headache (3%), dizziness (1%)

Gastrointestinal: Nausea (4%), diarrhea (3%), dyspepsia (2%), vomiting (1%), abdominal pain (1%)

Hematologic: Increased eosinophils (3%), decreased hemoglobin (2%), thrombocytosis

Hepatic: Increased ALT (1%), increased bilirubin (1%)

Renal: Increased BUN (4%)

Reactions reported with other cephalosporins include anaphylaxis, fever, paresthesia, pruritus, Stevens-Johnson syndrome, toxic epidermal necrolysis, erythema multiforme, angioedema, pseudomembranous colitis, hemolytic anemia, candidiasis, vaginitis, encephalopathy, asterixis, neuromuscular excitability, seizure, serum-sickness reactions, renal dysfunction, interstitial nephritis, toxic nephropathy, cholestasis, aplastic anemia, hemolytic anemia, pancytopenia, agranulocytosis, colitis, prolonged PT, hemorrhage, superinfection

Overdosage/Toxicology Symptoms of overdose include neuromuscular hypersensitivity and convulsions. Many beta-lactam containing antibiotics have the potential to cause neuromuscular hyperirritability or convulsive seizures. Hemodialysis may be helpful to aid in the removal of drug from blood; otherwise, treatment is supportive or symptom-directed.

Pharmacodynamics/Kinetics

Absorption: Rapid; food decreases peak concentrations, delays T_{max}, and lowers AUC

Time to Peak: 2-3 hours

Half-Life Elimination: 2 hours

Excretion: Urine

Dosing

Adults & Elderly: Susceptible infections: Oral: 400 mg once daily for 10 days; maximum: 400 mg

Pediatrics: Susceptible infections: Oral:

<12 years: 9 mg/kg/day for 10 days; maximum daily dose: 400 mg

≥12 years: Refer to adult dosing.

Renal Impairment:

Cl_{cr} 30-49 mL/minute: Administer 4.5 mg/kg or 200 mg every 24 hours.

Cl_{cr} 5-29 mL/minute: Administer 2.25 mg/kg or 100 mg every 24 hours.

Available Dosage Forms

Capsule: 400 mg

Powder for oral suspension: 90 mg/5 mL (30 mL, 60 mL, 120 mL) [contains sodium benzoate; cherry flavor]

Monitoring and Teaching Issues

Physical Assessment: Assess results of culture/sensitivity tests and patient's allergy history prior to therapy. See Warnings/Precautions for use cautions (eg, colitis, renal impairment). Assess potential for interactions with other pharmacological agents patient may be taking (eg nephrotoxicity; see Drug Interactions). Assess results of laboratory tests (see Monitoring Laboratory Tests), therapeutic response and adverse effects (eg, hemolytic anemia, hypoprothrombinemia, and bleeding; see Adverse Reactions). Advise patients with diabetes about use of Clinitest® (may cause false-positive test). Teach patient possible side effects/appropriate interventions and adverse symptoms to report (eg, opportunistic infection, hypersensitivity reaction).

Monitoring Laboratory Tests: Renal, hepatic, and hematologic function periodically with prolonged therapy; perform culture and sensitivity studies prior to initiating drug therapy

Patient Education: Do not take any new medication during therapy unless approved by prescriber. Take as directed, at regular intervals around-the-clock (take capsules with or without food, take suspension 2 hours before or 1 hour after meals). Chilling oral suspension improves flavor (do not freeze). Maintain adequate hydration (2-3 L/day of fluids) unless instructed to restrict fluid intake. Complete full course of medication, even if you feel better. May cause false test results with Clinitest®; use of another type of testing is preferable. May cause headache or dizziness (use caution when driving or engaging in potentially hazardous tasks until response to drug is known); nausea or vomiting (small frequent meals, frequent mouth care, sucking lozenges, or chewing gum may help); or diarrhea (yogurt, boiled milk, or buttermilk may help). Report rash; breathing or swallowing difficulty; persistent diarrhea, nausea, vomiting, or abdominal pain; changes in urinary
(Continued)

Ceftibuten *(Continued)*

pattern or pain on urination; opportunistic infection (eg, vaginal itching or drainage; sores in mouth; blood in stool or urine, unusual fever or chills); CNS changes (eg, irritability, agitation, nervousness, insomnia, hallucinations); or other adverse reactions.
Breast-feeding precautions: Consult prescriber if breast-feeding.

Dietary Considerations:
Capsule: Take without regard to food.
Suspension: Take 2 hours before or 1 hour after meals; contains 1 g of sucrose per 5 mL

Geriatric Considerations: Has not been studied specifically in the elderly. Adjust dose for renal function.

Pregnancy Risk Factor: B

Lactation: Excretion in breast milk unknown/use caution

Breast-Feeding Issues: Theoretically, drug absorbed by nursing infant may change bowel flora or affect fever work-up result. **Note:** As a class, cephalosporins are used to treat infections in infants.

Administration
Oral: Administer at the same time each day to maintain adequate blood levels. Shake suspension well before use.

Storage: Reconstituted suspension is stable for 14 days in the refrigerator.

♦ Ceftin® *see* Cefuroxime *on page 290*

Ceftizoxime *(sef ti ZOKS eem)*

U.S. Brand Names Cefizox®

Synonyms Ceftizoxime Sodium

Generic Available No

Pharmacologic Category Antibiotic, Cephalosporin (Third Generation)

Medication Safety Issues
Sound-alike/look-alike issues:
Ceftizoxime may be confused with cefotaxime, ceftazidime, cefuroxime

Use Treatment of susceptible bacterial infection, mainly respiratory tract, skin and skin structure, bone and joint, urinary tract and gynecologic, as well as septicemia; active against many gram-negative bacilli (not *Pseudomonas*), some gram-positive cocci (not *Enterococcus*), and some anaerobes

Mechanism of Action/Effect Inhibits bacterial cell wall synthesis by binding to one or more of the penicillin-binding proteins (PBPs)

Contraindications Hypersensitivity to ceftizoxime, any component of the formulation, or other cephalosporins

Warnings/Precautions Modify dosage in patients with severe renal impairment, prolonged use may result in superinfection; use with caution in patients with a history of penicillin allergy, especially IgE-mediated reactions (eg, anaphylaxis, urticaria). May cause antibiotic-associated colitis or colitis secondary to *C. difficile*.

Drug Interactions
Increased Effect/Toxicity: Probenecid may decrease cephalosporin elimination. Furosemide, aminoglycosides in combination with ceftizoxime may result in additive nephrotoxicity.

Lab Interactions Positive direct Coombs', false-positive urinary glucose test using cupric sulfate (Benedict's solution, Clinitest®, Fehling's solution), false-positive serum or urine creatinine with Jaffé reaction

Adverse Reactions
1% to 10%:
Central nervous system: Fever
Dermatologic: Rash, pruritus
Hematologic: Eosinophilia, thrombocytosis
Hepatic: Alkaline phosphatase increased, transaminases increased
Local: Pain, burning at injection site
Other reactions reported with cephalosporins include Stevens-Johnson syndrome, toxic epidermal necrolysis, erythema multiforme, pseudomembranous colitis, angioedema, hemolytic anemia, candidiasis, encephalopathy, asterixis, neuromuscular excitability, seizure, serum-sickness reactions, renal dysfunction, interstitial nephritis, toxic nephropathy, cholestasis, aplastic anemia, hemolytic anemia, pancytopenia, agranulocytosis, colitis, prolonged PT, hemorrhage, superinfection

Overdosage/Toxicology Symptoms of overdose include neuromuscular hypersensitivity and convulsions. Many beta-lactam containing antibiotics have the potential to cause neuromuscular hyperirritability or convulsive seizures. Hemodialysis may be helpful to aid in removal of the drug from blood; otherwise, treatment is supportive or symptom-directed.

Pharmacodynamics/Kinetics
Time to Peak: Serum: I.M.: 0.5-1 hour
Protein Binding: 30%
Half-Life Elimination: 1.6 hours; Cl_{cr} <10 mL/minute: 25 hours
Excretion: Urine (as unchanged drug)

Dosing
Adults & Elderly: Susceptible infections: I.M., I.V.: 1-2 g every 8-12 hours, up to 2 g every 4 hours or 4 g every 8 hours for life-threatening infections
Pediatrics: Susceptible infections: I.M., I.V.: Children ≥6 months: 150-200 mg/kg/day divided every 6-8 hours (maximum of 12 g/24 hours)
Renal Impairment:
Cl_{cr} 50-79 mL/minute: Administer 500-1500 mg every 8 hours.
Cl_{cr} 5-49 mL/minute: Administer 250-1000 mg every 12 hours.
Cl_{cr} 0-4 mL/minute: Administer 500-1000 mg every 48 hours or 250-500 mg every 24 hours.
Moderately dialyzable (20% to 50%)
Continuous arteriovenous hemofiltration: Dose as for Cl_{cr} 10-50 mL/minute.

Available Dosage Forms

Infusion [premixed iso-osmotic solution]: 1 g (50 mL); 2 g (50 mL)

Injection, powder for reconstitution: 1 g, 2 g, 10 g

Monitoring and Teaching Issues

Physical Assessment: Assess results of culture/sensitivity tests and patient's allergy history prior to therapy. See Warnings/Precautions for use cautions (eg, renal impairment). Assess potential for interactions with other pharmacological agents patient may be taking (see Drug Interactions). Assess results of laboratory tests, therapeutic response, and adverse effects (eg, hemolytic anemia, hypoprothrombinemia, and bleeding; see Adverse Reactions). Advise patients with diabetes about use of Clinitest® (may cause false-positive test). Teach patient possible side effects/appropriate interventions and adverse symptoms to report (eg, opportunistic infection, hypersensitivity reaction).

Monitoring Laboratory Tests: Perform culture and sensitivity studies prior to initiating drug therapy; renal function

Patient Education: Do not take any new medication during therapy unless approved by prescriber. This medication is administered by infusion or injection. Report immediately any redness, swelling, burning, or pain at injection/infusion site; itching or hives; or difficulty swallowing or breathing. Maintain adequate hydration (2-3 L/day of fluids) unless instructed to restrict fluid intake. May cause false test results with Clinitest®; use of another type of glucose testing is preferable. Report rash; breathing or swallowing difficulty; persistent diarrhea, nausea, vomiting, or abdominal pain; changes in urinary pattern or pain on urination; opportunistic infection (eg, vaginal itching or drainage; sores in mouth; blood in stool or urine, unusual fever or chills); CNS changes (eg, irritability, agitation, nervousness, insomnia, hallucinations); or other adverse reactions. **Breast-feeding precaution:** Consult prescriber if breast-feeding.

Dietary Considerations: Sodium content of 1 g: 60 mg (2.6 mEq)

Geriatric Considerations: Adjust dose for renal function in the elderly.

Pregnancy Risk Factor: B

Lactation: Enters breast milk (small amounts)/use caution

Breast-Feeding Issues: Theoretically, drug absorbed by nursing infant may change bowel flora or affect fever work-up result. **Note:** As a class, cephalosporins are used to treat infections in infants.

Administration

I.M.: Inject deep I.M. into large muscle mass.

I.V.: Inject direct I.V. over 3-5 minutes. Infuse intermittent infusion over 30 minutes.

Reconstitution: Reconstituted solution is stable for 24 hours at room temperature and 96 hours when refrigerated. For I.V. infusion in NS or D_5W, solution is stable for 24 hours at room temperature, 96 hours when refrigerated or 12 weeks when frozen. After freezing, thawed solution is stable for 24 hours at room temperature or 10 days when refrigerated.

Compatibility: Stable in $D_5\frac{1}{4}NS$, $D_5\frac{1}{2}NS$, D_5NS, D_5W, $D_{10}W$, LR, NS, sodium bicarbonate 5%

Y-site administration: Incompatible with filgrastim

♦ **Ceftizoxime Sodium** see Ceftizoxime on page 286

Ceftriaxone (sef trye AKS one)

U.S. Brand Names Rocephin®

Synonyms Ceftriaxone Sodium

Generic Available No

Pharmacologic Category Antibiotic, Cephalosporin (Third Generation)

Medication Safety Issues

Sound-alike/look-alike issues:

Rocephin® may be confused with Roferon®

Use Treatment of lower respiratory tract infections, acute bacterial otitis media, skin and skin structure infections, bone and joint infections, intra-abdominal and urinary tract infections, pelvic inflammatory disease (PID), uncomplicated gonorrhea, bacterial septicemia, and meningitis; used in surgical prophylaxis

Unlabeled/Investigational Use Treatment of chancroid, epididymitis, complicated gonococcal infections; sexually-transmitted diseases (STD); periorbital or buccal cellulitis; salmonellosis or shigellosis; atypical community-acquired pneumonia; Lyme disease; used in chemoprophylaxis for high-risk contacts and persons with invasive meningococcal disease; sexual assault

Mechanism of Action/Effect Inhibits bacterial cell wall synthesis by binding to one or more of the penicillin-binding proteins (PBPs)

Contraindications Hypersensitivity to ceftriaxone sodium, any component of the formulation, or other cephalosporins; **do not use in hyperbilirubinemic neonates,** particularly those who are premature since ceftriaxone is reported to displace bilirubin from albumin binding sites

Warnings/Precautions Modify dosage in patients with severe renal impairment, prolonged use may result in superinfection. Use with caution in patients with a history of penicillin allergy, especially IgE-mediated reactions (eg, anaphylaxis, urticaria). May cause antibiotic-associated colitis or colitis secondary to *C. difficile.* Discontinue in patients with signs and symptoms of gallbladder disease.

Drug Interactions

Decreased Effect: Uricosuric agents (eg, probenecid, sulfinpyrazone) may decrease the excretion of cephalosporin; monitor for toxic effects.

Increased Effect/Toxicity: Cephalosporins may increase the anticoagulant effect of coumarin derivatives (eg, dicumarol, warfarin).

Lab Interactions Positive direct Coombs', false-positive urinary glucose test using cupric sulfate (Benedict's solution, Clinitest®, Fehling's solution), false-positive serum or urine creatinine with Jaffé reaction

(Continued)

Ceftriaxone *(Continued)*

Adverse Reactions
1% to 10%:
Dermatologic: Rash (2%)
Gastrointestinal: Diarrhea (3%)
Hematologic: Eosinophilia (6%), thrombocytosis (5%), leukopenia (2%)
Hepatic: Transaminases increased (3.1% to 3.3%)
Local: Pain, induration at injection site (I.V. 1%); warmth, tightness, induration (5% to 17%) following I.M. injection
Renal: Increased BUN (1%)

Overdosage/Toxicology Symptoms of overdose include neuromuscular hypersensitivity and convulsions. Many beta-lactam containing antibiotics have the potential to cause neuromuscular hyperirritability or convulsive seizures. Hemodialysis may be helpful to aid in removal of the drug from blood; otherwise, treatment is supportive or symptom-directed.

Pharmacodynamics/Kinetics
Absorption: I.M.: Well absorbed
Time to Peak: Serum: I.M.: 1-2 hours
Protein Binding: 85% to 95%
Half-Life Elimination: Normal renal and hepatic function: 5-9 hours
Excretion: Urine (33% to 65% as unchanged drug); feces

Dosing
Adults & Elderly:
Susceptible infections: Usual dose: 1-2 g every 12-24 hours, depending on the type and severity of infection
Chemoprophylaxis for high-risk contacts and persons with invasive meningococcal disease (unlabeled use): I.M.: 250 mg in a single dose
Epididymitis, acute (unlabeled use): I.M.: 250 mg in a single dose
Gonococcal conjunctivitis, complicated (unlabeled use): I.M.: 1 g in a single dose
Gonococcal endocarditis (unlabeled use): I.M., I.V.: 1-2 g every 12 hours for at least 28 days
Gonococcal infection, disseminated (unlabeled use): I.M., I.V.: 1 g once daily for 7 days
Gonococcal infection, uncomplicated: I.M.: 125-250 mg in a single dose
PID: I.M.: 250 mg in a single dose
Surgical prophylaxis: I.V.: 1 g 30 minutes to 2 hours before surgery

Pediatrics:
Susceptible infections: Infants and Children: Usual dose: I.M., I.V.:
Mild-to-moderate infections: 50-75 mg/kg/day in 1-2 divided doses every 12-24 hours (maximum: 2 g/day); continue until at least 2 days after signs and symptoms of infection have resolved
Serious infections: 80-100 mg/kg/day in 1-2 divided doses (maximum: 4 g/day)
Gonococcal infection, uncomplicated: I.M.: 125 mg in a single dose
Gonococcal conjunctivitis, complicated (unlabeled use): I.M.:
<45 kg: 50 mg/kg in a single dose (maximum: 1 g)
>45 kg: 1 g in a single dose
Gonococcal endocarditis (unlabeled use):
<45 kg: I.M., I.V.: 50 mg/kg/day every 12 hours (maximum: 2 g/day) for at least 28 days
>45 kg: I.V.: 1-2 g every 12 hours, for at least 28 days
Gonococcal infection, disseminated (unlabeled use): I.M., I.V.:
<45 kg: 25-50 mg/kg once daily (maximum: 1 g)
>45 kg: 1 g once daily for 7 days
Meningitis: I.M., I.V.:
Uncomplicated: Loading dose of 100 mg/kg (maximum: 4 g), followed by 100 mg/kg/day divided every 12-24 hours (maximum: 4 g/day); usual duration of treatment is 7-14 days
Gonococcal, complicated:
<45 kg: 50 mg/kg/day given every 12 hours (maximum: 2 g/day); usual duration of treatment is 10-14 days
>45 kg: I.V.: 1-2 g every 12 hours; usual duration of treatment is 10-14 days
Otitis media: I.M., I.V.:
Acute: 50 mg/kg in a single dose (maximum: 1 g)
Persistent or relapsing (unlabeled use): 50 mg/kg once daily for 3 days
STD, sexual assault (unlabeled uses): 125 mg in a single dose
Chemoprophylaxis for high-risk contacts and persons with invasive meningococcal disease (unlabeled use):
Children ≤15 years: I.M.: 125 mg in a single dose
Children >15 years: Refer to adult dosing.
Epididymitis, acute: Children >8 years (≥45 kg) and Adolescents (unlabeled use): I.M.: 125 mg in a single dose

Renal Impairment:
No adjustment is necessary.
Not dialyzable (0% to 5%)
Administer dose postdialysis.
Peritoneal dialysis effects: Administer 750 mg every 12 hours.
Continuous arteriovenous or venovenous hemofiltration: Removes 10 mg of ceftriaxone of liter of filtrate per day.

Hepatic Impairment: No adjustment necessary.
Available Dosage Forms Note: Contains sodium 83 mg (3.6 mEq) per ceftriaxone 1 g
Infusion [premixed in dextrose]: 1 g (50 mL); 2 g (50 mL)
Injection, powder for reconstitution: 250 mg, 500 mg, 1 g, 2 g, 10 g

Monitoring and Teaching Issues
Physical Assessment: Assess results of culture/sensitivity tests and patient's allergy history prior to therapy. See Warnings/Precautions for use cautions (eg, renal impairment).

Assess potential for interactions with other pharmacological agents patient may be taking (see Drug Interactions). Assess results of laboratory tests (prothrombin times), therapeutic response, and adverse effects (eg, hemolytic anemia, hypoprothrombinemia, and bleeding; see Adverse Reactions). Advise patients with diabetes about use of Clinitest® (may cause false-positive test). Teach patient possible side effects/appropriate interventions and adverse symptoms to report (eg, opportunistic infection, hypersensitivity reaction).

Monitoring Laboratory Tests: Prothrombin times; perform culture and sensitivity studies prior to initiating drug therapy.

Patient Education: Do not take any new medication during therapy unless approved by prescriber. This medication is administered by infusion or injection. Report immediately any redness, swelling, burning, or pain at injection/infusion site; rash, itching, or hives. Maintain adequate hydration (2-3 L/day of fluids) unless instructed to restrict fluid intake. May cause false test results with Clinitest®; use of another type of glucose testing is preferable. May cause diarrhea (yogurt, boiled milk, or buttermilk may help). Report rash; breathing or swallowing difficulty; persistent diarrhea, nausea, vomiting, or abdominal pain; changes in urinary pattern or pain on urination; opportunistic infection (eg, vaginal itching or drainage; sores in mouth; blood in stool or urine, unusual fever or chills); CNS changes (eg, irritability, agitation, nervousness, insomnia, hallucinations); or other adverse reactions. **Breast-feeding precaution:** Consult prescriber if breast-feeding.

Dietary Considerations: Sodium contents: 83 mg (3.6 mEq) per ceftriaxone 1 g

Geriatric Considerations: No adjustment for changes in renal function necessary.

Pregnancy Risk Factor: B

Lactation: Enters breast milk/use caution (AAP rates "compatible")

Breast-Feeding Issues: Theoretically, drug absorbed by nursing infant may change bowel flora or affect fever work-up result. **Note:** As a class, cephalosporins are used to treat infections in infants.

Administration

I.M.: Inject deep I.M. into large muscle mass; a concentration of 250 mg/mL or 350 mg/mL is recommended for all vial sizes except the 250 mg size (250 mg/mL is suggested); can be diluted 1:1 water and 1% lidocaine for I.M. administration

I.V.: Do not admix with aminoglycosides in same bottle/bag. Infuse intermittent infusion over 30 minutes.

Reconstitution:

I.M. injection: Vials should be reconstituted with appropriate volume of diluent (including D_5W, NS, or 1% lidocaine) to make a final concentration of 250 mg/mL or 350 mg/mL. Volume to add to create a **250 mg/mL** solution:
- 250 mg vial: 0.9 mL
- 500 mg vial: 1.8 mL
- 1 g vial: 3.6 mL
- 2 g vial: 7.2 mL

Volume to add to create a **350 mg/mL** solution:
- 500 mg vial: 1.0 mL
- 1 g vial: 2.1 mL
- 2 g vial: 4.2 mL

I.V. infusion: Infusion is prepared in two stages: Initial reconstitution of powder, followed by dilution to final infusion solution.

Vials: Reconstitute powder with appropriate I.V. diluent (including SWFI, D_5W, NS) to create an initial solution of ~100 mg/mL. Recommended volume to add:
- 250 mg vial: 2.4 mL
- 500 mg vial: 4.8 mL
- 1 g vial: 9.6 mL
- 2 g vial: 19.2 mL

Note: After reconstitution of powder, further dilution into a volume of compatible solution (eg, 50-100 mL of D_5W or NS) is recommended.

Piggyback bottle: Reconstitute powder with appropriate I.V. diluent (D_5W or NS) to create a resulting solution of ~100 mg/mL. Recommended initial volume to add:
- 1 g bottle: 10 mL
- 2 g bottle: 20 mL

Note: After reconstitution, to prepare the final infusion solution, further dilution to 50 mL or 100 mL volumes with the appropriate I.V. diluent (including D_5W or NS) is recommended.

Compatibility: Stable in D_5W with KCl 10 mEq, $D_5\frac{1}{4}NS$ with KCl 20 mEq, $D_5\frac{1}{2}$ NS, D_5W, $D_{10}W$, NS, mannitol 5%, mannitol 10%, sodium bicarbonate 5%, bacteriostatic water, SWFI

Y-site administration: Incompatible with alatrofloxacin, amphotericin B cholesteryl sulfate complex, amsacrine, filgrastim, fluconazole, labetalol, pentamidine, vinorelbine

Compatibility when admixed: Incompatible with aminophylline, clindamycin, linezolid, theophylline

Storage:

Powder for injection: Prior to reconstitution, store at room temperature of 25°C (77°F); protect from light.

Premixed solution (manufacturer premixed): Store at -20°C; once thawed, solutions are stable for 3 days at room temperature of 25°C (77°F) or for 21 days refrigerated at 5°C (41°F). Do not refreeze.

Stability of reconstituted solutions:

10-40 mg/mL: Reconstituted in D_5W or NS: Stable for 2 days at room temperature of 25°C (77°F) or for 10 days when refrigerated at 5°C (41°F).

100 mg/mL:

Reconstituted in D_5W or NS: Stable for 2 days at room temperature of 25°C (77°F) or for 10 days when refrigerated at 5°C (41°F). Stable for 26 weeks when frozen at -20°C. Once thawed, solutions are stable for 2 days at room temperature of 25°C (77°F) or for 10 days when refrigerated at 5°C (41°F); does not apply to manufacturer's premixed bags. Do not refreeze.

Reconstituted in lidocaine 1% solution: Stable for 24 hours at room temperature of 25°C (77°F) or for 10 days when refrigerated at 5°C (41°F).

(Continued)

Ceftriaxone *(Continued)*

250-350 mg/mL: Reconstituted in D₅W, NS, lidocaine 1% solution, or SWFI: Stable for 24 hours at room temperature of 25°C (77°F) or for 3 days when refrigerated at 5°C (41°F).

Related Information
Antimicrobial Drugs of Choice *on page 1792*
Community-Acquired Pneumonia in Adults *on page 1807*

◆ **Ceftriaxone Sodium** *see Ceftriaxone on page 287*

Cefuroxime *(se fyoor OKS eem)*
U.S. Brand Names Ceftin®; Zinacef®
Synonyms Cefuroxime Axetil; Cefuroxime Sodium
Generic Available Yes
Pharmacologic Category Antibiotic, Cephalosporin (Second Generation)
Medication Safety Issues
Sound-alike/look-alike issues:
Cefuroxime may be confused with cefotaxime, cefprozil, ceftizoxime, deferoxamine
Ceftin® may be confused with Cefotan®, cefotetan, Cefzil®, Cipro®
Zinacef® may be confused with Zithromax®
Use Treatment of infections caused by staphylococci, group B streptococci, *H. influenzae* (type A and B), *E. coli, Enterobacter, Salmonella,* and *Klebsiella*; treatment of susceptible infections of the lower respiratory tract, otitis media, urinary tract, skin and soft tissue, bone and joint, sepsis and gonorrhea
Mechanism of Action/Effect Inhibits bacterial cell wall synthesis by binding to one or more of the penicillin-binding proteins (PBPs)
Contraindications Hypersensitivity to cefuroxime, any component of the formulation, or other cephalosporins
Warnings/Precautions Modify dosage in patients with severe renal impairment, prolonged use may result in superinfection; use with caution in patients with a history of penicillin allergy, especially IgE-mediated reactions (eg, anaphylaxis, urticaria). May cause antibiotic-associated colitis or colitis secondary to *C. difficile*. May be associated with increased INR, especially in nutritionally-deficient patients, prolonged treatment, hepatic or renal disease. Tablets and oral suspension are not bioequivalent (do not substitute on a mg-per-mg basis).
Drug Interactions
Increased Effect/Toxicity: High-dose probenecid decreases clearance. Aminoglycosides in combination with cefuroxime may result in additive nephrotoxicity.
Nutritional/Ethanol Interactions Food: Bioavailability is increased with food; cefuroxime serum levels may be increased if taken with food or dairy products.
Lab Interactions Positive direct Coombs', false-positive urinary glucose test using cupric sulfate (Benedict's solution, Clinitest®, Fehling's solution), false-positive serum or urine creatinine with Jaffé reaction
Adverse Reactions
1% to 10%:
Endocrine & metabolic: Alkaline phosphatase increased (2%)
Hematologic: Eosinophilia (7%), decreased hemoglobin and hematocrit (10%)
Hepatic: Transaminases increased (4%)
Local: Thrombophlebitis (2%)
Reactions reported with other cephalosporins include agranulocytosis, aplastic anemia, asterixis, encephalopathy, hemorrhage, neuromuscular excitability, serum-sickness reactions, superinfection, toxic nephropathy
Overdosage/Toxicology Symptoms of overdose include neuromuscular hypersensitivity and convulsions. Many beta-lactam containing antibiotics have the potential to cause neuromuscular hyperirritability or convulsive seizures. Hemodialysis may be helpful to aid in removal of the drug from blood; otherwise, treatment is supportive or symptom-directed.
Pharmacodynamics/Kinetics
Absorption: Oral (cefuroxime axetil): Increases with food
Bioavailability: Tablet: Fasting: 37%; Following food: 52%
Time to Peak: Serum: I.M.: ~15-60 minutes; I.V.: 2-3 minutes
Protein Binding: 33% to 50%
Half-Life Elimination: Adults: 1-2 hours; prolonged with renal impairment
Excretion: Urine (66% to 100% as unchanged drug)
Dosing
Adults & Elderly: Note: Cefuroxime axetil film-coated tablets and oral suspension are not bioequivalent and are not substitutable on a mg/mg basis.

Acute bacterial maxillary sinusitis: Oral: 250 mg twice daily for 10 days
Bronchitis, acute (and exacerbations of chronic bronchitis):
Oral: 250-500 mg every 12 hours for 10 days
I.V.: 500-750 mg every 8 hours (complete therapy with oral dosing)
Gonococcal infection, uncomplicated:
Oral: 1 g as a single dose
I.M.: 1.5 g as a single dose (administered at two different sites along with 1 g oral probenecid)
Gonococcal infection, disseminated: I.M., I.V.: 750 mg every 8 hours
Lyme disease (early): Oral: 500 mg twice daily for 20 days
Pharyngitis, tonsillitis: Oral: 250 mg twice daily for 10 days
Skin/skin structure infection, uncomplicated:
Oral: 250-500 mg every 12 hours for 10 days
I.M., I.V.: 750 mg every 8 hours
Urinary tract infection, uncomplicated:
Oral: 125-250 mg twice daily for 7-10 days
I.V., I.M.: 750 mg every 8 hours

Pneumonia, uncomplicated: I.M., I.V.: 750 mg every 8 hours
Severe or complicated infections: I.M., I.V.: 1.5 g every 8 hours (up to 1.5 g every 6 hours in life-threatening infections)
Surgical prophylaxis: I.V.: 1.5 g 30 minutes to 1 hour before procedure; 750 mg every 8 hours I.M. when procedure is prolonged
Open heart surgery: I.V.: 1.5 g at the induction of anesthesia and every 12 hours thereafter to a total of 6 g is recommended
Pediatrics: Note: Cefuroxime axetil film-coated tablets and oral suspension are not bioequivalent and are not substitutable on a mg/mg basis.

Children ≥3 months to 12 years:
Pharyngitis, tonsillitis:
Oral:
Suspension: 20 mg/kg/day (maximum: 500 mg/day) in 2 divided doses for 10 days
Tablet: 125 mg every 12 hours for 10 days
I.M., I.V.: 75-150 mg/kg/day divided every 8 hours; maximum dose: 6 g/day
Acute otitis media, impetigo:
Oral:
Suspension: 30 mg/kg/day (maximum: 1 g/day) in 2 divided doses
Tablet: 250 mg every 12 hours
I.M., I.V.: 75-150 mg/kg/day divided every 8 hours; maximum dose: 6 g/day
Meningitis: NOT recommended (doses of 200-240 mg/kg/day divided every 6-8 hours have been used); maximum dose: 9 g/day
Acute bacterial maxillary sinusitis: Oral:
Suspension: 30 mg/kg/day in 2 divided doses for 10 days; maximum dose: 1 g/day
Tablet: 250 mg twice daily for 10 days
Children ≥13 years: Refer to adult dosing.

Renal Impairment:
Cl_{cr} 10-20 mL/minute: Administer every 12 hours.
Cl_{cr} <10 mL/minute: Administer every 24 hours.
Hemodialysis: Dialyzable (25%)
Note: Cefuroxime axetil film-coated tablets and oral suspension are not bioequivalent and are not substitutable on a mg/mg basis.
Continuous arteriovenous or venovenous hemodiafiltration effects: Dose as for Cl_{cr} 10-20 mL/minute.

Available Dosage Forms [DSC] = Discontinued product
Infusion, as sodium [premixed] (Zinacef®): 750 mg (50 mL); 1.5 g (50 mL) [contains sodium 4.8 mEq (111 mg) per 750 mg]
Injection, powder for reconstitution, as sodium (Zinacef®): 750 mg, 1.5 g, 7.5 g [contains sodium 4.8 mEq (111 mg) per 750 mg]
Powder for oral suspension, as axetil (Ceftin®): 125 mg/5 mL (100 mL) [contains phenylalanine 11.8 mg/5 mL; tutti-frutti flavor]; 250 mg/5 mL (50 mL, 100 mL) [contains phenylalanine 25.2 mg/5 mL; tutti-frutti flavor]
Tablet, as axetil: 250 mg, 500 mg
Ceftin®: 250 mg, 500 mg

Monitoring and Teaching Issues

Physical Assessment: Assess results of culture/sensitivity tests and patient's allergy history prior to therapy. See Warnings/Precautions for use cautions (eg, renal impairment). Assess potential for interactions with other pharmacological agents patient may be taking (nephrotoxicity; see Drug Interactions). Assess results of laboratory tests, therapeutic response, and adverse effects (eg, hemolytic anemia, hypoprothrombinemia, and bleeding; see Adverse Reactions). Advise patients with diabetes about use of Clinitest® (may cause false-positive test). Teach patient possible side effects/appropriate interventions and adverse symptoms to report (eg, opportunistic infection, hypersensitivity reaction).

Monitoring Laboratory Tests: Perform culture and sensitivity studies prior to initiating therapy; renal function

Patient Education: Do not take any new medication during therapy unless approved by prescriber. If administered by injection or infusion, report immediately any swelling, redness, or pain at injection/infusion site; respiratory or swallowing difficulty; chest pain; or rash. Oral tablets or suspension should be taken as directed, at regular intervals around-the-clock (with or without food). Chilling oral suspension improves flavor (do not freeze); shake before use. Complete full course of medication, even if you feel better. Maintain adequate hydration (2-3 L/day of fluids) unless instructed to restrict fluid intake. May cause false test results with Clinitest®; use of another type of glucose testing is preferable. Report rash; breathing or swallowing difficulty; persistent diarrhea, nausea, vomiting, or abdominal pain; changes in urinary pattern or pain on urination; opportunistic infection (eg, vaginal itching or drainage; sores in mouth; blood in stool or urine, unusual fever or chills); CNS changes (eg, irritability, agitation, nervousness, insomnia, hallucinations); or other adverse reactions. **Breast-feeding precaution:** Consult prescriber if breast-feeding.

Dietary Considerations: May be taken with food.
Zinacef®: Sodium content: 4.8 mEq (111 mg) per 750 mg
Ceftin®: Powder for oral suspension 125 mg/5 mL contains phenylalanine 11.8 mg/5 mL; 250 mg/5 mL contains phenylalanine 25.2 mg/5 mL.

Geriatric Considerations: Adjust dose for renal function in the elderly. Considered one of the drugs of choice for outpatient treatment of community-acquired pneumonia in the older adult.

Pregnancy Risk Factor: B
Lactation: Enters breast milk/use caution
Breast-Feeding Issues: Theoretically, drug absorbed by nursing infant may change bowel flora or affect fever work-up result. **Note:** As a class, cephalosporins are used to treat infections in infants.

Administration

Oral: Administer around-the-clock to promote less variation in peak and trough serum levels.
Oral suspension: Administer with food. Shake well before use.
(Continued)

Cefuroxime (Continued)

I.M.: Inject deep I.M. into large muscle mass.

I.V.: Inject direct I.V. over 3-5 minutes. Infuse intermittent infusion over 15-30 minutes.

Reconstitution:

Injectable: Reconstituted solution is stable for 24 hours at room temperature and 48 hours when refrigerated. I.V. infusion in NS or D_5W solution is stable for 24 hours at room temperature, 7 days when refrigerated, or 26 weeks when frozen. After freezing, thawed solution is stable for 24 hours at room temperature or 21 days when refrigerated.

Oral suspension: Store in refrigerator or at room temperature. Discard after 10 days.

Compatibility: Stable in $D_5^{1}/_4NS$, $D_5^{1}/_2NS$, D_5NS, D_5W, $D_{10}W$, LR, NS

Y-site administration: Incompatible with clarithromycin, filgrastim, fluconazole, midazolam, vinorelbine

Compatibility in syringe: Incompatible with doxapram

Compatibility when admixed: Incompatible with aminoglycosides, sodium bicarbonate

Related Information

Antimicrobial Drugs of Choice *on page 1792*
Community-Acquired Pneumonia in Adults *on page 1807*
I.V. to Oral Conversion *on page 1688*

♦ **Cefuroxime Axetil** *see Cefuroxime on page 290*
♦ **Cefuroxime Sodium** *see Cefuroxime on page 290*
♦ **Cefzil®** *see Cefprozil on page 282*
♦ **Celebrex®** *see Celecoxib on page 292*

Celecoxib (se le KOKS ib)

U.S. Brand Names Celebrex®

Generic Available No

Pharmacologic Category Nonsteroidal Anti-inflammatory Drug (NSAID), COX-2 Selective

Medication Safety Issues

Sound-alike/look-alike issues:

Celebrex® may be confused with Celexa™, cerebra, Cerebyx®

Use Relief of the signs and symptoms of osteoarthritis; relief of the signs and symptoms of rheumatoid arthritis in adults; management of acute pain; treatment of primary dysmenorrhea; decreasing intestinal polyps in familial adenomatous polyposis (FAP). **Note:** The Notice of Compliance for the use of celecoxib in FAP has been suspended by Health Canada.

Mechanism of Action/Effect Inhibits prostaglandin synthesis by decreasing the activity of the enzyme, cyclooxygenase-2 (COX-2), which results in decreased formation of prostaglandin precursors. Celecoxib does not inhibit cyclooxygenase-1 (COX-1) at therapeutic concentrations.

Contraindications Hypersensitivity to celecoxib, any component of the formulation, sulfonamides, aspirin, or other NSAIDs; pregnancy (3rd trimester)

Warnings/Precautions Gastrointestinal irritation, ulceration, bleeding, and perforation may occur with NSAIDs (it is unclear whether celecoxib is associated with rates of these events which are similar to nonselective NSAIDs). Use with caution in patients with a history of GI disease (bleeding or ulcers), use lowest dose for shortest time possible. Use with caution in patients with decreased renal function, hepatic disease, CHF, hypertension, or asthma. Carefully evaluate individual cardiovascular risk profiles prior to prescribing COX-2 inhibitors. COX-2 inhibitors may not be appropriate in patients with cardiovascular disease or in patients with significant risk factors for cardiovascular disease.

Anaphylactoid reactions may occur, even with no prior exposure to celecoxib. Use caution in patients with known or suspected deficiency of cytochrome P450 isoenzyme 2C9. Safety and efficacy have not been established in patients <18 years of age.

Drug Interactions

Cytochrome P450 Effect: Substrate (minor) of CYP2C8/9, 3A4; **Inhibits** CYP2D6 (weak)

Decreased Effect: Efficacy of thiazide diuretics, loop diuretics (furosemide), or ACE inhibitors may be diminished by celecoxib.

Increased Effect/Toxicity: Fluconazole increases celecoxib concentrations twofold. Lithium and methotrexate concentrations may be increased by celecoxib. Celecoxib may be used with low-dose aspirin, however, rates of gastrointestinal bleeding may be increased with coadministration. Bleeding events (including rare intracranial hemorrhage in association with increased prothrombin time) have been reported with concomitant warfarin use; monitor closely (especially in the elderly).

Nutritional/Ethanol Interactions

Ethanol: Avoid ethanol (increased GI irritation).

Food: Peak concentrations are delayed and AUC is increased by 10% to 20% when taken with a high-fat meal.

Adverse Reactions

>10%: Central nervous system: Headache (16%)

2% to 10%:

Cardiovascular: Peripheral edema (2%)

Central nervous system: Insomnia (2%), dizziness (2%)

Dermatologic: Skin rash (2%)

Gastrointestinal: Dyspepsia (9%), diarrhea (6%), abdominal pain (4%), nausea (4%), flatulence (2%)

Neuromuscular & skeletal: Back pain (3%)

Respiratory: Upper respiratory tract infection (8%), sinusitis (5%), pharyngitis (2%), rhinitis (2%)

Miscellaneous: Accidental injury (3%)

0.1% to 2%:

Cardiovascular: Hypertension (aggravated), chest pain, MI, palpitation, tachycardia, facial edema

Central nervous system: Migraine, vertigo, hypoesthesia, fatigue, fever, pain, hypotonia, anxiety, depression, nervousness, somnolence

Dermatologic: Alopecia, dermatitis, photosensitivity, pruritus, rash (maculopapular), rash (erythematous), dry skin, urticaria

Endocrine & metabolic: Hot flashes, diabetes mellitus, hyperglycemia, hypercholesterolemia, breast pain, dysmenorrhea, menstrual disturbances, hypokalemia

Gastrointestinal: Constipation, tenesmus, diverticulitis, eructation, esophagitis, gastroenteritis, vomiting, gastroesophageal reflux, hemorrhoids, hiatal hernia, melena, stomatitis, anorexia, increased appetite, taste disturbance, dry mouth, tooth disorder, weight gain

Genitourinary: Prostate disorder, vaginal bleeding, vaginitis, monilial vaginitis, dysuria, cystitis, urinary frequency, incontinence, urinary tract infection,

Hematologic: Anemia, thrombocytopenia, ecchymosis

Hepatic: Alkaline phosphatase increased, transaminases increased

Neuromuscular & skeletal: Leg cramps, increased CPK, neck stiffness, arthralgia, myalgia, bone disorder, fracture, synovitis, tendonitis, neuralgia, paresthesia, neuropathy, weakness

Ocular: Glaucoma, blurred vision, cataract, conjunctivitis, eye pain

Otic: Deafness, tinnitus, earache, otitis media

Renal: Increased BUN, increased creatinine, albuminuria, hematuria, renal calculi

Respiratory: Bronchitis, bronchospasm, cough, dyspnea, laryngitis, pneumonia, epistaxis

Miscellaneous: Allergic reactions, diaphoresis increased, flu-like syndrome, breast cancer, herpes infection, bacterial infection, moniliasis, viral infection

Overdosage/Toxicology Symptoms of overdose may include epigastric pain, drowsiness, lethargy, nausea, and vomiting; gastrointestinal bleeding may occur. Rare manifestations include hypertension, respiratory depression, coma, and acute renal failure. Treatment is symptomatic and supportive. Forced diuresis, hemodialysis and/or urinary alkalinization may not be useful.

Pharmacodynamics/Kinetics
Bioavailability: Absolute bioavailability unknown
Time to Peak: 3 hours
Protein Binding: 97% to albumin
Half-Life Elimination: 11 hours
Metabolism: Hepatic via CYP2C9; forms inactive metabolites
Excretion: Urine (as metabolites, <3% as unchanged drug)

Dosing
Adults & Elderly:
Osteoarthritis: Oral: 200 mg/day as a single dose or in divided dose twice daily
Rheumatoid arthritis: Oral: 100-200 mg twice daily
Familial adenomatous polyposis (FAP): Oral: 400 mg twice daily
Acute pain or primary dysmenorrhea: Oral: Initial dose: 400 mg, followed by an additional 200 mg if needed on day 1; maintenance dose: 200 mg twice daily as needed
Renal Impairment: No specific dosage adjustment is recommended. Not recommended in patients with advanced renal disease.
Hepatic Impairment: Reduced dosage is recommended (AUC may be increased by 40% to 180%). Decrease dose by 50% in patients with moderate hepatic impairment (Child-Pugh class II).

Available Dosage Forms Capsule: 100 mg, 200 mg, 400 mg

Monitoring and Teaching Issues
Physical Assessment: Assess effectiveness and interactions of other medications patient may be taking (ie, monitor patients taking lithium closely). Assess allergy history (aspirin, NSAIDs, salicylates). Monitor effectiveness of therapy. Assess knowledge/teach patient appropriate use, possible side effects/interventions, and adverse symptoms to report.

Patient Education: Do not take more than recommended dose. May be taken with food to reduce GI upset. Do not take with antacids. Avoid alcohol, aspirin, and OTC medication unless approved by prescriber. You may experience dizziness, confusion, or blurred vision (avoid driving or engaging in tasks requiring alertness until response to drug is known); anorexia, nausea, vomiting, taste disturbance, gastric distress (small frequent meals, frequent mouth care, sucking lozenges, or chewing gum may help). GI bleeding, ulceration, or perforation can occur with or without pain. It is unclear whether celecoxib has rates of these events which are similar to nonselective NSAIDs. Stop taking medication and report immediately stomach pain or cramping; unusual bleeding or bruising (blood in vomitus, stool, or urine). Report persistent insomnia; skin rash; unusual fatigue, muscle pain, tremors, or weakness; sudden weight gain or edema; changes in hearing (ringing in ears) or vision; changes in urination pattern; or respiratory difficulty. **Pregnancy/breast-feeding precautions:** Inform your prescriber if you are or intend to become pregnant. This drug should not be used in the 3rd trimester of pregnancy. Breast-feeding is not recommended.

Dietary Considerations: Lower doses (200 mg twice daily) may be taken without regard to meals. Larger doses should be taken with food to improve absorption.

Pregnancy Risk Factor: C/D (3rd trimester)

Pregnancy Issues: In late pregnancy, this drug may cause premature closure of the ductus arteriosus.

Lactation: Enters breast milk/not recommended

Breast-Feeding Issues: Based on limited data, celecoxib has been found to be excreted in milk; a decision should be made whether to discontinue nursing or discontinue the drug, taking into account the importance of the drug to the mother.

Administration
Storage: Store at controlled room temperature of 25°C (77°F).

Related Information
Nonsalicylate / Nonsteroidal Anti-inflammatory Agents *on page 1743*

♦ Centany™ *see* Mupirocin *on page 1038*
♦ Cēpacol® Maximum Strength [OTC] *see* Dyclonine *on page 505*
♦ Cepacol® Sore Throat [OTC] *see* Benzocaine *on page 181*

Cephalexin (sef a LEKS in)

U.S. Brand Names Biocef®; Keflex®; Panixine DisperDose™
Synonyms Cephalexin Monohydrate
Generic Available Yes: Excludes tablet for oral suspension
Pharmacologic Category Antibiotic, Cephalosporin (First Generation)
Medication Safety Issues
Sound-alike/look-alike issues:
Cephalexin may be confused with cefaclor, cefazolin, cephalothin, ciprofloxacin
Use Treatment of susceptible bacterial infections including respiratory tract infections, otitis media, skin and skin structure infections, bone infections and genitourinary tract infections, including acute prostatitis; alternative therapy for acute bacterial endocarditis prophylaxis
Mechanism of Action/Effect Inhibits bacterial cell wall synthesis by binding to one or more of the penicillin-binding proteins (PBPs)
Contraindications Hypersensitivity to cephalexin, any component of the formulation, or other cephalosporins
Warnings/Precautions Modify dosage in patients with severe renal impairment, prolonged use may result in superinfection; use with caution in patients with a history of penicillin allergy, especially IgE-mediated reactions (eg, anaphylaxis, urticaria). May cause antibiotic-associated colitis or colitis secondary to *C. difficile*.
Drug Interactions
Increased Effect/Toxicity: High-dose probenecid may decrease clearance of cephalexin. Aminoglycosides in combination with cephalexin may result in additive nephrotoxicity.
Nutritional/Ethanol Interactions Food: Peak antibiotic serum concentration is lowered and delayed, but total drug absorbed is not affected. Cephalexin serum levels may be decreased if taken with food.
Lab Interactions Positive direct Coombs', false-positive urinary glucose test using cupric sulfate (Benedict's solution, Clinitest®, Fehling's solution), false-positive serum or urine creatinine with Jaffé reaction
Adverse Reactions Frequency not defined.
Central nervous system: Agitation, confusion, dizziness, fatigue, hallucinations, headache
Dermatologic: Angioedema, erythema multiforme (rare), rash, Stevens-Johnson syndrome (rare), toxic epidermal necrolysis (rare), urticaria
Gastrointestinal: Abdominal pain, diarrhea, dyspepsia, gastritis, nausea (rare), pseudomembranous colitis, vomiting (rare)
Genitourinary: Genital pruritus, genital moniliasis, vaginitis, vaginal discharge
Hematologic: Eosinophilia, neutropenia, thrombocytopenia
Hepatic: AST/ALT increased, cholestatic jaundice (rare), transient hepatitis (rare)
Neuromuscular & skeletal: Arthralgia, arthritis, joint disorder
Renal: Interstitial nephritis (rare)
Miscellaneous: Allergic reactions
Overdosage/Toxicology Symptoms of overdose include epigastric distress, diarrhea, hematuria, nausea, and vomiting. Many beta-lactam containing antibiotics have the potential to cause neuromuscular hyperirritability or seizures. Hemodialysis may be helpful to aid in removal of the drug from blood; otherwise, treatment is supportive and symptom-directed.
Pharmacodynamics/Kinetics
Absorption: Delayed in young children
Time to Peak: Serum: ~1 hour
Protein Binding: 6% to 15%
Half-Life Elimination: Adults: 0.5-1.2 hours; prolonged with renal impairment
Excretion: Urine (80% to 100% as unchanged drug) within 8 hours
Dosing
Adults & Elderly:
Dosing range: Oral: 250-1000 mg every 6 hours; maximum: 4 g/day
Streptococcal pharyngitis, skin and skin structure infections: Oral: 500 mg every 12 hours
Uncomplicated cystitis: Oral: 500 mg every 12 hours for 7-14 days
Prophylaxis of bacterial endocarditis (dental, oral, respiratory tract, or esophageal procedures): Oral: 2 g 1 hour prior to procedure
Pediatrics:
Usual dose: Oral: Children >1 year: Dosing range: 25-50 mg/kg/day every 6-8 hours; more severe infections: 50-100 mg/kg/day in divided doses every 6-8 hours; maximum: 4 g/24 hours
Otitis media: 75-100 mg/kg/day in 4 divided doses
Streptococcal pharyngitis, skin and skin structure infections: 25-50 mg/kg/day divided every 12 hours
Uncomplicated cystitis: Children >15 years: Refer to adult dosing.
Prophylaxis of bacterial endocarditis (dental, oral, respiratory tract, or esophageal procedures): 50 mg/kg 1 hour prior to procedure (maximum: 2 g)
Renal Impairment:
Cl_{cr} <10 mL/minute: Adults: 250-500 mg every 12 hours
Hemodialysis: Moderately dialyzable (20% to 50%)
Available Dosage Forms
Capsule: 250 mg, 500 mg
Biocef®: 500 mg
Keflex®: 250 mg, 500 mg
Powder for oral suspension: 125 mg/5 mL (100 mL, 200 mL); 250 mg/5 mL (100 mL, 200 mL)
Biocef®: 125 mg/5 mL (100 mL); 250 mg/5 mL (100 mL)
Tablet, for oral suspension (Panixine DisperDose™): 125 mg [contains phenylalanine 2.8 mg; peppermint flavor], 250 mg [contains phenylalanine 5.6 mg; peppermint flavor]

Monitoring and Teaching Issues

Physical Assessment: Assess results of culture/sensitivity tests and patient's allergy history prior to therapy. See Warnings/Precautions for use cautions (eg, renal impairment). Assess potential for interactions with other pharmacological agents patient may be taking (nephrotoxicity; see Drug Interactions). Assess results of laboratory tests, therapeutic response, and adverse effects (see Adverse Reactions). Advise patients with diabetes about use of Clinitest® (may cause false-positive test). Teach patient possible side effects/appropriate interventions and adverse symptoms to report (eg, opportunistic infection, hypersensitivity reaction; see Patient Education).

Monitoring Laboratory Tests: Renal, hepatic, and hematologic function periodically with prolonged therapy; perform culture and sensitivity studies prior to initiating drug therapy.

Patient Education: Do not take any new medication during therapy unless approved by prescriber. Take as directed, at regular intervals around-the-clock (with or without food); take complete prescription even if feeling better. Maintain adequate hydration (2-3 L/day of fluids) unless instructed to restrict fluid intake. May cause false test results with Clinitest®; use of another type of glucose testing is preferable. May cause diarrhea (yogurt, boiled milk, or buttermilk may help). Report rash; breathing or swallowing difficulty; persistent diarrhea, nausea, vomiting, or abdominal pain; changes in urinary pattern or pain on urination; opportunistic infection (eg, vaginal itching or drainage; sores in mouth; blood in stool or urine, unusual fever or chills); CNS changes (eg, irritability, agitation, nervousness, insomnia, hallucinations); or other adverse reactions. **Breast-feeding precaution:** Consult prescriber if breast-feeding.

Dietary Considerations: Take without regard to food. If GI distress, take with food. Panixine DisperDose™ contains phenylalanine 2.8 mg/cephalexin 125 mg.

Geriatric Considerations: Adjust dose for renal function.

Pregnancy Risk Factor: B

Lactation: Enters breast milk (small amounts)/use caution

Breast-Feeding Issues: Theoretically, drug absorbed by nursing infant may change bowel flora or affect fever work-up result. Cephalexin levels can be detected in breast milk, reaching a maximum concentration 4 hours after a single oral dose and gradually decreasing by 8 hours after administration. **Note:** As a class, cephalosporins are used to treat bacterial infections in infants.

Administration

Oral: Take without regard to food. If GI distress, take with food. Give around-the-clock to promote less variation in peak and trough serum levels.

Panixine DisperDose™: Tablets should be mixed in ~10 mL of water immediately prior to administration. Drink entire solution, then rinse glass with additional water and drink contents to ensure entire dose has been taken. Tablets should not be chewed or swallowed whole.

Reconstitution: Tablets for oral suspension (Panixine DisperDose™): Tablets must be dissolved in ~10 mL water prior to administration.

Storage: Refrigerate suspension after reconstitution; discard after 14 days. Tablets for suspension should be used immediately after dissolving.

♦ **Cephalexin Monohydrate** *see* Cephalexin *on page 294*

Cephradine (SEF ra deen)

U.S. Brand Names Velosef®

Generic Available No

Pharmacologic Category Antibiotic, Cephalosporin (First Generation)

Medication Safety Issues

Sound-alike/look-alike issues:

Cephradine may be confused with cephapirin

Velosef® may be confused with Vasosulf®

Use Treatment of infections when caused by susceptible strains in respiratory, genitourinary, gastrointestinal, skin and soft tissue, bone and joint infections; treatment of susceptible gram-positive bacilli and cocci (never enterococcus); some gram-negative bacilli including *E. coli*, *Proteus*, and *Klebsiella* may be susceptible

Mechanism of Action/Effect Inhibits bacterial cell wall synthesis by binding to one or more of the penicillin-binding proteins (PBPs)

Contraindications Hypersensitivity to cephradine, any component of the formulation, or cephalosporins

Warnings/Precautions Use caution with renal impairment; dose adjustment required. Prolonged use may result in superinfection; use with caution in patients with a history of penicillin allergy, especially IgE-mediated reactions (eg, anaphylaxis, urticaria). May cause antibiotic-associated colitis or colitis secondary to *C. difficile*.

Drug Interactions

Increased Effect/Toxicity: High-dose probenecid decreases clearance of cephradine. Aminoglycosides in combination with cephradine may result in additive nephrotoxicity.

Nutritional/Ethanol Interactions Food: Food delays cephradine absorption but does not decrease extent.

Lab Interactions Positive direct Coombs', false-positive urinary glucose test using cupric sulfate (Benedict's solution, Clinitest®, Fehling's solution), false-positive serum or urine creatinine with Jaffé reaction

Adverse Reactions Frequency not defined.

Central nervous system: Dizziness

Dermatologic: Rash, pruritus

Gastrointestinal: Diarrhea, nausea, vomiting, pseudomembranous colitis

Hematologic: Leukopenia, neutropenia, eosinophilia

Neuromuscular & skeletal: Joint pain

Renal: BUN increased, creatinine increased

Reactions reported with other cephalosporins include anaphylaxis, erythema multiforme, toxic epidermal necrolysis, Stevens-Johnson syndrome, fever, headache, encephalopathy, (Continued)

Cephradine *(Continued)*

asterixis, neuromuscular excitability, seizure, agranulocytosis, pancytopenia, aplastic anemia, hemolytic anemia, interstitial nephritis, toxic nephropathy, vaginitis, angioedema, cholestasis, hemorrhage, prolonged PT, serum-sickness reactions, superinfection

Overdosage/Toxicology Symptoms of overdose include neuromuscular hypersensitivity and convulsions. Many beta-lactam containing antibiotics have the potential to cause neuromuscular hyperirritability or convulsive seizures. Hemodialysis may be helpful to aid in removal of the drug from blood; otherwise, treatment is supportive or symptom-directed.

Pharmacodynamics/Kinetics
Absorption: Well absorbed
Time to Peak: Serum: 1-2 hours
Protein Binding: 18% to 20%
Half-Life Elimination: 1-2 hours; prolonged with renal impairment
Excretion: Urine (~80% to 90% as unchanged drug) within 6 hours

Dosing
Adults & Elderly:
Susceptible infections, usual dose: Oral: 250-500 mg every 6-12 hours
Pediatrics:
Usual dose: Oral: Children ≥9 months: 25-50 mg/kg/day in divided doses every 6 hours
Otitis media: Oral: Children ≥9 months: 75-100 mg/kg/day in divided doses every 6 or 12 hours (maximum: 4 g/day)
Renal Impairment:
Cl_{cr} 10-50 mL/minute: Administer 50% of dose.
Cl_{cr} <10 mL/minute: Administer 25% of dose.

Available Dosage Forms [DSC] = Discontinued product
Capsule: 250 mg, 500 mg [DSC]
Powder for oral suspension: 250 mg/5 mL (100 mL) [fruit flavor]

Monitoring and Teaching Issues
Physical Assessment: Assess results of culture/sensitivity tests and patient's allergy history prior to therapy. See Warnings/Precautions for use cautions (eg, renal impairment). Assess potential for interactions with other pharmacological agents patient may be taking (nephrotoxicity; see Drug Interactions). Assess results of laboratory tests, therapeutic response, and adverse effects (see Adverse Reactions). Advise patients with diabetes about use of Clinitest® (may cause false-positive test). Teach patient possible side effects/ appropriate interventions and adverse symptoms to report (eg, opportunistic infection, hypersensitivity reaction; see Patient Education).

Monitoring Laboratory Tests: Perform culture and sensitivity studies prior to initiating drug therapy; renal function

Patient Education: Do not take any new medication during therapy unless approved by prescriber. Take as directed, at regular intervals around-the-clock (with or without food); take complete prescription even if feeling better. Maintain adequate hydration (2-3 L/day of fluids) unless instructed to restrict fluid intake. May cause false test results with Clinitest®; use of another type of glucose testing is preferable. May cause diarrhea (yogurt, boiled milk, or buttermilk may help). Report rash; breathing or swallowing difficulty; persistent diarrhea, nausea, vomiting, or abdominal pain; changes in urinary pattern or pain on urination; opportunistic infection (eg, vaginal itching or drainage; sores in mouth; blood in stool or urine, unusual fever or chills); CNS changes (eg, irritability, agitation, nervousness, insomnia, hallucinations); or other adverse reactions. Breast-feeding precaution: Consult prescriber if breast-feeding.

Dietary Considerations: May administer with food to decrease GI distress.

Geriatric Considerations: Cephradine has not been studied in the elderly. Adjust dose for renal function in the elderly.

Pregnancy Risk Factor: B

Lactation: Enters breast milk/use caution

Breast-Feeding Issues: Theoretically, drug absorbed by nursing infant may change bowel flora or affect fever work-up result. **Note:** As a class, cephalosporins are used to treat infections in infants.

Administration
Oral: Administer around-the-clock to promote less variation in peak and trough serum levels. Shake oral suspension well.
Storage:
Capsule: Store at controlled room temperature.
Powder for oral suspension: Store at controlled room temperature. Following reconstitution, refrigerated storage of oral suspension maintains potency for 14 days. Room temperature storage maintains potency for 7 days.

♦ **Ceptaz®** [DSC] *see* Ceftazidime *on page 283*
♦ **Cerebyx®** *see* Fosphenytoin *on page 683*
♦ **Ceredase®** *see* Alglucerase *on page 69*
♦ **Cerubidine®** *see* DAUNOrubicin Hydrochloride *on page 410*
♦ **Cervidil®** *see* Dinoprostone *on page 462*
♦ **C.E.S.** *see* Estrogens (Conjugated/Equine) *on page 563*
♦ **Cetacort®** *see* Hydrocortisone *on page 760*
♦ **Cetafen®** [OTC] *see* Acetaminophen *on page 38*
♦ **Cetafen Extra®** [OTC] *see* Acetaminophen *on page 38*
♦ **Ceta-Plus®** *see* Hydrocodone and Acetaminophen *on page 754*

Cetirizine *(se TI ra zeen)*
U.S. Brand Names Zyrtec®
Synonyms Cetirizine Hydrochloride; P-071; UCB-P071
Generic Available No

Pharmacologic Category Antihistamine

Medication Safety Issues

Sound-alike/look-alike issues:

Zyrtec® may be confused with Serax®, Xanax®, Zantac®, Zyprexa®

Use Perennial and seasonal allergic rhinitis and other allergic symptoms including urticaria; chronic idiopathic urticaria

Mechanism of Action/Effect Competes with histamine for H_1-receptor sites on effector cells in the GI tract, blood vessels, and respiratory tract

Contraindications Hypersensitivity to cetirizine, hydroxyzine, or any component of the formulation

Warnings/Precautions Cetirizine should be used cautiously in patients with hepatic or renal dysfunction, or the elderly. May cause drowsiness, use caution performing tasks which require alertness (eg, operating machinery or driving). Safety and efficacy in pediatric patients <6 months of age have not been established.

Drug Interactions

Cytochrome P450 Effect: Substrate of CYP3A4 (minor)

Increased Effect/Toxicity: Increased toxicity with CNS depressants and anticholinergics.

Nutritional/Ethanol Interactions Ethanol: Avoid ethanol (may increase CNS depression).

Adverse Reactions

>10%: Central nervous system: Headache (children 11% to 14%, placebo 12%), somnolence (adults 14%, children 2% to 4%)

2% to 10%:

Central nervous system: Insomnia (children 9%, adults <2%), fatigue (adults 6%), malaise (4%), dizziness (adults 2%)

Gastrointestinal: Abdominal pain (children 4% to 6%), dry mouth (adults 5%), diarrhea (children 2% to 3%), nausea (children 2% to 3%, placebo 2%), vomiting (children 2% to 3%)

Respiratory: Epistaxis (children 2% to 4%, placebo 3%), pharyngitis (children 3% to 6%, placebo 3%), bronchospasm (children 2% to 3%, placebo 2%)

Overdosage/Toxicology Symptoms of overdose may include somnolence, restlessness, or irritability. Treatment is symptomatic and supportive. Cetirizine is not removed by dialysis.

Pharmacodynamics/Kinetics

Onset of Action: 15-30 minutes

Absorption: Rapid

Time to Peak: Serum: 1 hour

Half-Life Elimination: 8 hours

Metabolism: Limited hepatic

Excretion: Urine (70%); feces (10%)

Dosing

Adults: Perennial or seasonal allergic rhinitis, chronic urticaria: Oral: 5-10 mg once daily, depending upon symptom severity

Elderly: Oral: Initial: 5 mg once daily; may increase to 10 mg/day

Note: Manufacturer recommends 5 mg/day in patients ≥77 years of age.

Pediatrics:

Perennial allergic rhinitis, chronic urticaria: Oral: Children:

6-12 months: 2.5 mg once daily

12 months to <2 years: 2.5 mg once daily; may increase to 2.5 mg every 12 hours if needed

Perennial or seasonal allergic rhinitis, chronic urticaria: Oral: Children:

2-5 years: Initial: 2.5 mg once daily; may be increased to 2.5 mg every 12 hours **or** 5 mg once daily

≥6 years Refer to adult dosing.

Renal Impairment:

Children <6 years: Cetirizine use not recommended.

Children 6-11 years: <2.5 mg once daily

Children ≥12 and Adults:

Cl_{cr} 11-31 mL/minute or hemodialysis: Administer 5 mg once daily

Cl_{cr} <11 mL/minute, not on dialysis: Cetirizine use not recommended.

Hepatic Impairment:

Children <6 years: Cetirizine use not recommended.

Children 6-11 years: <2.5 mg once daily

Children ≥12 and Adults: Administer 5 mg once daily

Available Dosage Forms

Syrup, as hydrochloride: 5 mg/5 mL (120 mL, 480 mL) [banana-grape flavor]

Tablet, as hydrochloride: 5 mg, 10 mg

Tablet, chewable, as hydrochloride: 5 mg, 10 mg [grape flavor]

Monitoring and Teaching Issues

Physical Assessment: Assess effectiveness and interactions of other medications patient may be taking. Monitor effectiveness of therapy and adverse reactions at beginning of therapy and periodically with long-term use. Assess knowledge/teach patient appropriate use, interventions to reduce side effects, and adverse symptoms to report. Breast-feeding is not recommended.

Patient Education: Take as directed; do not exceed recommended dose. Avoid use of other depressants, alcohol, or sleep-inducing medications unless approved by prescriber. You may experience drowsiness or dizziness (use caution when driving or engaging in tasks requiring alertness until response to drug is known); or dry mouth (frequent small meals, frequent mouth care, chewing gum, or sucking hard candy may help). Report persistent sedation, confusion, or agitation; persistent nausea or vomiting; changes in urinary pattern; blurred vision; chest pain or palpitations; persistent headaches; or lack of improvement or worsening of condition. **Breast-feeding precaution:** Breast-feeding is not recommended.

(Continued)

Cetirizine (Continued)

Dietary Considerations: May be taken with or without food.
Geriatric Considerations: Adjust dose for renal function.
Pregnancy Risk Factor: B
Lactation: Enters breast milk/not recommended

Administration

Oral: May be administered with or without food.

Storage:

Syrup: Store at room temperature of 15°C to 30°C (59°F to 86°F), or under refrigeration at 2°C to 8°C (36°F to 46°F).

Tablet: Store at room temperature of 15°C to 30°C (59°F to 86°F).

♦ **Cetirizine Hydrochloride** *see* Cetirizine *on page 296*

Cetrorelix (set roe REL iks)

U.S. Brand Names Cetrotide®
Synonyms Cetrorelix Acetate
Generic Available No
Pharmacologic Category Gonadotropin Releasing Hormone Antagonist
Use Inhibits premature luteinizing hormone (LH) surges in women undergoing controlled ovarian stimulation
Mechanism of Action/Effect Competes with naturally occurring GnRH for binding on receptors of the pituitary. This delays luteinizing hormone surge, preventing ovulation until the follicles are of adequate size.
Contraindications Hypersensitivity to cetrorelix or any component of the formulation; extrinsic peptide hormones, mannitol, gonadotropin releasing hormone (GnRH) or GnRH analogs; severe renal impairment; pregnancy
Warnings/Precautions Should only be prescribed by fertility specialists. Monitor carefully after first injection for possible hypersensitivity reactions. Use caution in women with active allergic conditions or a history of allergies; use in women with severe allergic conditions is not recommended. Pregnancy should be excluded before treatment is begun.

Drug Interactions

Decreased Effect: No formal studies have been performed.
Increased Effect/Toxicity: No formal studies have been performed.

Adverse Reactions

1% to 10%:
Central nervous system: Headache (1%)
Endocrine & metabolic: Ovarian hyperstimulation syndrome, WHO grade II or III (4%)
Gastrointestinal: Nausea (1%)
Hepatic: Increased ALT, AST, GGT, and alkaline phosphatase (1% to 2%)

Overdosage/Toxicology No cases of overdose have been reported. In nonfertility studies, single doses of up to 120 mg have been well tolerated.

Pharmacodynamics/Kinetics

Onset of Action: 0.25 mg dose: 2 hours; 3 mg dose: 1 hour
Duration of Action: 3 mg dose (single dose): 4 days
Absorption: Rapid
Bioavailability: 85%
Time to Peak: 0.25 mg dose: 1 hour; 3 mg dose: 1.5 hours
Protein Binding: 86%
Half-Life Elimination: 0.25 mg dose: 5 hours; 0.25 mg multiple doses: 20.6 hours; 3 mg dose: 62.8 hours
Metabolism: Transformed by peptidases; cetrorelix and peptides (1-9), (1-7), (1-6), and (1-4) are found in the bile; peptide (1-4) is the predominant metabolite
Excretion: Feces (5% to 10% as unchanged drug and metabolites); urine (2% to 4% as unchanged drug); within 24 hours

Dosing

Adults:

Controlled ovarian stimulation in conjunction with gonadotropins (FSH, HMG):
Female: SubQ:
Single-dose regimen: 3 mg given when serum estradiol levels show appropriate stimulation response, usually stimulation day 7 (range days 5-9). If hCG is not administered within 4 days, continue cetrorelix at 0.25 mg/day until hCG is administered
Multiple-dose regimen: 0.25 mg morning or evening of stimulation day 5, or morning of stimulation day 6; continue until hCG is administered.

Elderly: Not intended for use in women ≥65 years of age (Phase 2 and Phase 3 studies included women 19-40 years of age).

Renal Impairment:

Severe impairment: Use is contraindicated.
Mild-to-moderate impairment: No specific guidelines are available.

Available Dosage Forms Injection, powder for reconstitution: 0.25 mg, 3 mg [supplied with SWFI in prefilled syringe]

Monitoring and Teaching Issues

Physical Assessment: This medication should only be prescribed by a fertility specialist. Teach patient proper use if self-administered (appropriate injection technique and syringe/needle disposal), possible side effects/appropriate interventions, and adverse symptoms to report. **Pregnancy risk factor X:** Pregnancy must be excluded before starting medication. Breast-feeding is not recommended.

Patient Education: This drug can only be given by injection as demonstrated. An instructional leaflet will be provided if you will be administering this medication to yourself. Instructions will be given on how to administer SubQ injections and proper disposal of syringes and needles. Give at a similar time each day as instructed by prescriber. Do not skip any doses. If you miss an injection, do not double next dose; contact your prescriber.

You must keep all scheduled ultrasound appointments. Store in refrigerator in outer carton. Solution should be used immediately after mixing. You may experience headache (use of mild analgesic may help); or nausea (small frequent meals, good mouth care, chewing gum, or sucking hard candy may help). Report immediately any sudden or acute abdominal pain; shortness of breath; vaginal bleeding; or pain, itching, or signs of infection at injection site. **Pregnancy/breast-feeding precautions:** Do not get pregnant while taking this drug. Breast-feeding is not recommended.

Pregnancy Risk Factor: X

Pregnancy Issues: Animal studies have shown fetal resorption and implantation losses following administration. Resorption resulting in fetal loss would be expected if used in a pregnant woman.

Lactation: Excretion in breast milk unknown/not recommended

Administration

Other: Cetrorelix is administered by SubQ injection following proper aseptic technique procedures. Injections should be to the lower abdomen, preferably around the navel (but staying at least 1 inch from the navel). The injection site should be rotated daily. The needle should be inserted completely into the skin at a 45-degree angle.

Storage: Store in outer carton. Once mixed, solution should be used immediately.
0.25 mg vials: Store under refrigeration at 2°C to 8°C (36°F to 46°F).
3 mg vials: Store at controlled room temperature at 25°C (77°F).

♦ **Cetrorelix Acetate** *see* Cetrorelix *on page 298*

♦ **Cetrotide®** *see* Cetrorelix *on page 298*

Cetuximab (se TUK see mab)

U.S. Brand Names Erbitux™

Synonyms C225; IMC-C225

Generic Available No

Pharmacologic Category Antineoplastic Agent, Monoclonal Antibody; Epidermal Growth Factor Receptor (EGFR) Inhibitor

Use Treatment of epidermal growth factor receptor (EGFR) expressing, metastatic colorectal carcinoma; may be used in combination with irinotecan in patients who are refractory to irinotecan-based chemotherapy or as a single agent in patients who are intolerant to irinotecan-based chemotherapy.

Unlabeled/Investigational Use Breast cancer, head and neck cancer, tumors overexpressing EGFR

Mechanism of Action/Effect Inhibits cell growth, induces apoptosis and decreases matrix metalloproteinase and vascular endothelial growth factor production.

Contraindications Hypersensitivity to cetuximab, murine proteins, or any component of the formulation

Warnings/Precautions Severe infusion reactions have been reported in ~3% of patients; ~90% with the first infusion despite the use of prophylactic antihistamines. **Note:** Although a 20 mg test dose was used in some studies, it did not reliably predict the risk of an infusion reaction, and is not recommended. In case of severe reaction, treatment should be stopped and permanently discontinued. Immediate treatment for anaphylactic/anaphylactoid reactions should be available during administration. Interstitial lung disease (ILD) has been reported; use caution with pre-existing lung disease. Dermatologic toxicities have been reported, including a 90% incidence of acneform rash; sunlight may exacerbate skin reactions. Non-neutralizing anticetuximab antibodies were detected in 5% of evaluable patients. Relationship between the appearance of antibodies and the safety or antitumor activity of the molecule is unknown. Safety and efficacy have not been established in pediatric patients.

Drug Interactions

Increased Effect/Toxicity: Interactions have not been evaluated in clinical trials.

Adverse Reactions

>10%:

Central nervous system: Malaise (49%), fever (33%), headache (25%), pain (19%)

Dermatologic: Acneform rash (90%; ~10% severe), nail disorder (16%)

Gastrointestinal: Nausea (mild-to-moderate 29%), constipation (28%), diarrhea (28%), abdominal pain (25%), vomiting (25%), anorexia (25%), stomatitis (11%)

Neuromuscular & skeletal: Back pain (11%), weakness (49%)

Respiratory: Dyspnea (20%)

Miscellaneous: Infusion reaction (25%; ~3% severe; ~90% with first infusion), infection (11%)

1% to 10%:

Cardiovascular: Peripheral edema (10%)

Central nervous system: Insomnia (10%), depression (9%)

Dermatologic: Pruritus (10%), alopecia (5%), skin disorder (5%)

Endocrine & metabolic: Dehydration (9%)

Gastrointestinal: Weight loss (9%), dyspepsia (7%)

Hematologic: Anemia (10%), leukopenia (1%)

Hepatic: Alkaline phosphatase increased (5% to 10%), transaminases increased (5% to 10%)

Ocular: Conjunctivitis (7%)

Renal: Kidney failure (2%)

Respiratory: Cough increased (10%), pulmonary embolus (1%)

Miscellaneous: Sepsis (3%)

Overdosage/Toxicology There is no experience with overdosage in human clinical trials. Treatment is symptom-directed and supportive.

Pharmacodynamics/Kinetics

Half-Life Elimination: 114 hours (range: 75-188 hours)

Dosing

Adults & Elderly:

Colorectal cancer: I.V.:

Initial loading dose: 400 mg/m^2 infused over 120 minutes

(Continued)

Cetuximab *(Continued)*

    Maintenance dose: 250 mg/m^2 infused over 60 minutes

   Breast cancer (unlabeled use): I.V.: 50-200 mg/m^2 weekly for 6 weeks

   Head and neck cancer (unlabeled use): I.V.:

    Loading dose: 100-500 mg/m^2

    Maintenance dose: 100-250 mg/m^2 weekly for 7 weeks

    or

    200-400 mg/m^2 weekly (no loading dose)

   Tumors overexpressing EGFR (unlabeled use): I.V.:

    5-100 mg/m^2 weekly

    or

    Loading dose: 100-500 mg/m^2

    Maintenance dose: 5-400 mg/m^2 weekly

Dosage adjustment for toxicity:

Mild-to-moderate (grade 1 or 2) infusion reactions: Permanently reduce the infusion rate by 50% and continue to use prophylactic antihistamines

Severe (grade 3 or 4) infusion reactions: Immediately and permanently discontinue treatment

Mild-to-moderate skin toxicity: No dosage modification required

Severe acneform rash:

   First occurrence: Delay cetuximab infusion 1-2 weeks

    If improvement, continue at 250 mg/m^2

    If no improvement, discontinue therapy

   Second occurrence: Delay cetuximab infusion 1-2 weeks

    If improvement, continue at 200 mg/m^2

    If no improvement, discontinue therapy

   Third occurrence: Delay cetuximab infusion 1-2 weeks

    If improvement, continue at 150 mg/m^2

    If no improvement, discontinue therapy

   Fourth occurrence: Delay cetuximab infusion 1-2 weeks

    Discontinue therapy

Renal Impairment: No adjustment required.

Hepatic Impairment: No adjustment required.

Available Dosage Forms Injection, solution [preservative free]: 2 mg/mL (50 mL)

Monitoring and Teaching Issues

Physical Assessment: See Warnings/Precautions for specific use cautions. Patient must be monitored closely for infusion reaction (eg, airway obstruction, hives, hypotension) during infusion and for one hour following infusion; treatment for anaphylactic reactions should be available. In case of severe infusion reaction, treatment should be stopped and prescriber notified. See Dosing recommendations for dose adjustments in event of infusion reaction. Premedication with antihistamines is recommended. See Administration for infusion specifics. Assess therapeutic response and adverse reactions (see Adverse Reactions). Teach patient possible side effects/interventions and adverse symptoms to report (eg, cough, dyspnea, gastrointestinal upset, opportunistic infection; see Patient Education).

Patient Education: Do not take any new medication during therapy unless approved by prescriber. This medication can only be administered by infusion and you will be closely monitored during each infusion; report immediately unusual chest tightness; difficulty breathing or swallowing; itching or skin rash; back pain or acute headache; or redness, swelling, or pain at infusion site. Maintain adequate hydration (2-3 L/day of fluids) unless instructed to restrict fluid intake and nutrition (small frequent meals). You may experience feelings of weakness or fatigue (adequate rest is important); nausea, vomiting, loss of appetite (small frequent meals, sucking lozenges, chewing gum may help); diarrhea (boiled milk or yogurt may help); headache or back pain (consult prescriber for appropriate analgesic); skin rash or dryness (use only mild soap, apply nonmedicated lotion, and wear protective clothing); loss of hair or nail disorder (may grow back after therapy). Report persistent gastrointestinal disturbances (pain, constipation, diarrhea, vomiting); CNS changes (depression or insomnia); skin rash, dryness, or cracking; any signs of infection; or other persistent adverse reactions. **Pregnancy/breast-feeding precautions:** Inform prescriber if you are or intend to become pregnant. Do not breast-feed during therapy or for 60 days following completion.

Pregnancy Risk Factor: C

Lactation: Excretion in breast milk is unknown/not recommended

Breast-Feeding Issues: Breast-feeding should be discontinued during treatment and for 60 days following the last dose.

Administration

I.V.: Administer via I.V. infusion over 1-2 hours. Do not administer as I.V. push or bolus. Do not shake or dilute. May be administered via infusion pump or syringe pump. "Piggyback" into the patient's infusion line. Following the infusion, a 1-hour observation period is recommended. Premedication with antihistamines is recommended. The maximum infusion rate is 5 mL/minute. Administer through a low protein-binding 0.22 micrometer in-line filter and low-sorbing (non-PVC) tubing. Use 0.9% NaCl to flush line at the end of infusion.

Reconstitution: Reconstitution is not required. Appropriate dose should be added to sterile evacuated container or bag.

Storage: Store unopened vials under refrigeration at 2°C to 8°C (36°F to 46°F). Do not freeze. Preparations in infusion containers are stable for up to 12 hours under refrigeration at 2°C to 8°C (36°F to 46°F) and up to 8 hours at controlled room temperature of 20°C to 25°C (68°F to 77°F).

Additional Information Premedication with an H$_1$ antagonist (eg, diphenhydramine 50 mg I.V.) is recommended.

Cevimeline *(se vi ME leen)*

U.S. Brand Names Evoxac®

Synonyms Cevimeline Hydrochloride

Generic Available No
Pharmacologic Category Cholinergic Agonist
Medication Safety Issues
Sound-alike/look-alike issues:
Evoxac® may be confused with Eurax®

Use Treatment of symptoms of dry mouth in patients with Sjögren's syndrome
Mechanism of Action/Effect Binds to muscarinic (cholinergic) receptors, causing an increase in secretion of exocrine glands (including salivary glands)
Contraindications Hypersensitivity to cevimeline or any component of the formulation; uncontrolled asthma; narrow-angle glaucoma; acute iritis; other conditions where miosis is undesirable
Warnings/Precautions May alter cardiac conduction and/or heart rate; use caution in patients with significant cardiovascular disease, including angina, myocardial infarction, or conduction disturbances. Use with caution in patients with controlled asthma, COPD, or chronic bronchitis. May cause decreased visual acuity (particularly at night and in patients with central lens changes) and impaired depth perception. May cause a variety of parasympathomimetic effects, which may be particularly dangerous in elderly patients; excessive sweating may lead to dehydration in some patients.

Use with caution in patients with a history of biliary stones or nephrolithiasis; cevimeline may precipitate cholangitis, cholecystitis, biliary obstruction, renal colic, or ureteral reflux in susceptible patients. Patients with a known or suspected deficiency of CYP2D6 may be at higher risk of adverse effects. Safety and efficacy have not been established in pediatric patients.
Drug Interactions
Cytochrome P450 Effect: Substrate (minor) of CYP2D6, CYP3A4
Decreased Effect: Anticholinergic agents (atropine, TCAs, phenothiazines) may antagonize the effects of cevimeline.
Increased Effect/Toxicity: The effects of other cholinergic agents may be increased during concurrent administration with cevimeline. Concurrent use of cevimeline and beta-blockers may increase the potential for conduction disturbances.
Adverse Reactions
>10%:
Central nervous system: Headache (14%; placebo 20%)
Gastrointestinal: Nausea (14%), diarrhea (10%)
Respiratory: Rhinitis (11%), sinusitis (12%), upper respiratory infection (11%)
Miscellaneous: Diaphoresis increased (19%)
1% to 10%:
Cardiovascular: Peripheral edema, chest pain, edema, palpitation
Central nervous system: Dizziness (4%), fatigue (3%), pain (3%), insomnia (2%), anxiety (1%), fever, depression, migraine, hypoesthesia, vertigo
Dermatologic: Rash (4%; placebo 6%), pruritus, skin disorder, erythematous rash
Endocrine & metabolic: Hot flashes (2%)
Gastrointestinal: Dyspepsia (8%; placebo 9%), abdominal pain (8%), vomiting (5%), excessive salivation (2%), constipation, salivary gland pain, dry mouth, sialoadenitis, gastroesophageal reflux, flatulence, ulcerative stomatitis, eructation, increased amylase, anorexia, tooth disorder
Genitourinary: Urinary tract infection (6%), vaginitis, cystitis
Hematologic: Anemia
Local: Abscess
Neuromuscular & skeletal: Back pain (5%), arthralgia (4%), skeletal pain (3%), rigors (1%), hypertonia, tremor, myalgia, hyporeflexia, leg cramps
Ocular: Conjunctivitis (4%), abnormal vision, eye pain, eye abnormality, xerophthalmia
Otic: Ear ache, otitis media
Respiratory: Coughing (6%), bronchitis (4%), pneumonia, epistaxis
Miscellaneous: Flu-like syndrome, infection, fungal infection, allergy, hiccups
Overdosage/Toxicology Symptoms of toxicity may include headache, visual disturbances, lacrimation, sweating, gastrointestinal spasm, nausea, vomiting, diarrhea, AV block, mental confusion, tremor, cardiac depression, bradycardia, tachycardia, or bronchospasm. Atropine may be of value as an antidote, and epinephrine may be required for bronchoconstriction. Additional treatment is supportive. The effect of hemodialysis is unknown.
Pharmacodynamics/Kinetics
Time to Peak: 1.5-2 hours
Protein Binding: <20%
Half-Life Elimination: 5 hours
Metabolism: Hepatic via CYP2D6 and CYP3A4
Excretion: Urine (as metabolites and unchanged drug)
Dosing
Adults & Elderly: Xerostomia (in Sjögren's syndrome): Oral: 30 mg 3 times/day
Available Dosage Forms Capsule, as hydrochloride: 30 mg
Monitoring and Teaching Issues
Physical Assessment: Assess other medications patient may be taking for effectiveness and interactions. Monitor for therapeutic effect and adverse reactions (especially with elderly persons). Assess knowledge/teach patient appropriate use, interventions to reduce side effects, and adverse reactions to report.
Patient Education: Take exactly as directed; do not alter dosage without consulting prescriber. Take with or without food. You may experience decreased visual acuity (especially at night) (use caution when driving at night or when engaging in other activities in poorly lighted areas until response to medication is known); GI distress or nausea (small frequent meals, frequent mouth care, sucking lozenges, or chewing gum may help); headache (mild analgesic may help); or diarrhea (boiled milk, yogurt, or buttermilk may help). Report unresolved diarrhea or constipation, abdominal pain, flatulence, anorexia, or excessive salivation; excessive sweating; unresolved respiratory distress, runny nose, cold or flu symptoms; joint, bone, or muscle weakness, pain, tremor, or cramping; chest pain or
(Continued)

301

Cevimeline *(Continued)*

palpitations, swelling of extremities, weight gain; or other persistent adverse symptoms.
Pregnancy/breast-feeding precautions: Inform prescriber if you are or intend to become pregnant. Breast-feeding is not recommended.

Dietary Considerations: Take with or without food.

Pregnancy Risk Factor: C

Lactation: Excretion in breast milk unknown/not recommended

Administration

Storage: Store at 25°C (77°F).

♦ **Cevimeline Hydrochloride** *see* Cevimeline *on page 300*

♦ **CFDN** *see* Cefdinir *on page 270*

♦ **CG** *see* Chorionic Gonadotropin (Human) *on page 319*

♦ **CGP-42446** *see* Zoledronic Acid *on page 1591*

♦ **CGP 57148B** *see* Imatinib *on page 785*

♦ **Char-Caps [OTC]** *see* Charcoal *on page 302*

♦ **CharcoAid G® [OTC] [DSC]** *see* Charcoal *on page 302*

Charcoal *(CHAR kole)*

U.S. Brand Names Actidose-Aqua® [OTC]; Actidose® with Sorbitol [OTC]; Char-Caps [OTC]; CharcoAid G® [OTC] [DSC]; Charcoal Plus® DS [OTC]; Charcocaps® [OTC]; EZ-Char™ [OTC]; Kerr Insta-Char® [OTC]

Synonyms Activated Carbon; Activated Charcoal; Adsorbent Charcoal; Liquid Antidote; Medicinal Carbon; Medicinal Charcoal

Generic Available Yes

Pharmacologic Category Antidote

Medication Safety Issues
Sound-alike/look-alike issues:
Actidose® may be confused with Actos®

Use Emergency treatment in poisoning by drugs and chemicals; aids the elimination of certain drugs and improves decontamination of excessive ingestions of sustained -release products or in the presence of bezoars; repetitive doses have proven useful to enhance the elimination of certain drugs (eg, theophylline, phenobarbital, and aspirin); repetitive doses for gastric dialysis in uremia to adsorb various waste products; dietary supplement (digestive aid)

Mechanism of Action/Effect Adsorbs toxic substances or irritants, thus inhibiting GI absorption; adsorbs intestinal gas; the addition of sorbitol results in hyperosmotic laxative action causing catharsis

Contraindications Intestinal obstruction; GI tract not anatomically intact; patients at risk of hemorrhage or GI perforation; if use would increase risk and severity of aspiration; not effective for cyanide, mineral acids, caustic alkalis, organic solvents, iron, ethanol, methanol poisoning, lithium; do not use charcoal with sorbitol in patients with fructose intolerance; charcoal with sorbitol not recommended in children <1 year of age

Warnings/Precautions When using ipecac with charcoal, induce vomiting with ipecac before administering activated charcoal since charcoal adsorbs ipecac syrup; charcoal may cause vomiting which is hazardous in petroleum distillate and caustic ingestions; if charcoal in sorbitol is administered, doses should be limited to prevent excessive fluid and electrolyte losses. Use caution with decreased peristalsis. Most effective when administered within 1 hour of ingestion for most ingestions.

Drug Interactions
Decreased Effect: Charcoal decreases the effect of ipecac syrup.

Nutritional/Ethanol Interactions Food: Do not mix with milk, ice cream, sherbet, or marmalade (may reduce charcoal's effectiveness).

Adverse Reactions Frequency not defined.
Endocrine & metabolic: Hypernatremia, hypokalemia, and hypermagnesemia may occur with coadministration of cathartics
Gastrointestinal: Vomiting (incidence may increase with sorbitol), diarrhea (with sorbitol), constipation, swelling of abdomen, bowel obstruction
Miscellaneous: Fecal discoloration (black)

Pharmacodynamics/Kinetics
Excretion: Feces (as charcoal)

Dosing

Adults & Elderly:
Acute poisoning:
Oral: 25-100 g as a single dose; if multiple doses are needed, additional doses may be given as 12.5 g/hour or equivalent (ie, 25 g every 2 hours)
Note: ~10 g of activated charcoal for each 1 g of toxin is considered adequate; this may require multiple doses. If sorbitol is also used, sorbitol dose should not exceed 1.5 g/kg. When using multiple doses of charcoal, sorbitol should be given with every other dose (not to exceed 2 doses/day)
Dietary supplement: Oral: 500-520 mg after meals; may repeat in 2 hours if needed (maximum 10 g/day)

Pediatrics:
Acute poisoning: Oral:
Children: 1 g/kg as a single dose; if multiple doses are needed, additional doses can be given as 0.25 g/kg every hour or equivalent (ie, 0.5 g/kg every 2 hours) **or**
>1 year to 12 years: 25-50 g as a single dose; smaller doses (10-25 g) may be used in children 1-5 years due to smaller gut lumen capacity
>12 years: Refer to adult dosing.
Note: ~10 g of activated charcoal for each 1 g of toxin is considered adequate; this may require multiple doses. If sorbitol is also used, sorbitol dose should not exceed 1.5 g/kg. When using multiple doses of charcoal, sorbitol should be given with every other dose (not to exceed 2 doses/day).

Available Dosage Forms [DSC] = Discontinued product
Capsule, activated (Char-Caps, Charcocaps®): 260 mg
Granules, activated (CharcoAid G®): 15 g (120 mL) [DSC]
Liquid, activated:
    Actidose-Aqua®: 15 g (72 mL); 25 g (120 mL); 50 g (240 mL)
    Kerr Insta-Char®: 25 g (120 mL) [cherry flavor]; 50 g (240 mL) [unflavored or cherry flavor]
Liquid, activated [with sorbitol]:
    Actidose® with Sorbitol: 25 g (120 mL); 50 g (240 mL)
    Kerr Insta-Char®: 25 g (120 mL); 50 g (240 mL) [cherry flavor]
Pellets, activated (EZ-Char™): 25 g
Powder for suspension, activated: 30 g, 240 g
Tablets, activated (Charcoal Plus® DS): 250 mg

Monitoring and Teaching Issues
    Physical Assessment: Monitor for active bowel sounds prior to administration. If antidote treatment includes ipecac syrup, induce vomiting before administering charcoal. May be administered with sorbitol or chocolate to improve palatability; do not administer with milk products.
    Patient Education: Charcoal will cause your stools to turn black. Do not self-administer as an antidote before calling the poison control center, hospital emergency room, or physician for instructions (charcoal is not the antidote for all poisons). **Pregnancy precaution:** Inform prescriber if you are pregnant.
    Pregnancy Risk Factor: C
    Lactation: Does not enter breast milk/compatible

Administration
    Oral: Flavoring agents (eg, chocolate) and sorbitol can enhance charcoal's palatability. If treatment includes ipecac syrup, induce vomiting prior to administration of charcoal. Often given with a laxative or cathartic; check for presence of bowel sounds before administration.
    Reconstitution: Powder: Dilute with at least 8 mL of water per 1 g of charcoal, or mix in a charcoal to water ratio of 1:4 to 1:8. Mix to form a slurry.
    Storage: Adsorbs gases from air, store in closed container.

Chloral Hydrate (KLOR al HYE drate)

U.S. Brand Names Aquachloral® Supprettes®; Somnote™
Synonyms Chloral; Hydrated Chloral; Trichloroacetaldehyde Monohydrate
Controlled Substance C-IV
Generic Available Yes: Syrup
Pharmacologic Category Hypnotic, Miscellaneous
Use Short-term sedative and hypnotic (<2 weeks), sedative/hypnotic for diagnostic procedures; sedative prior to EEG evaluations
Mechanism of Action/Effect Central nervous system depressant effects are due to its active metabolite trichloroethanol, mechanism unknown
Contraindications Hypersensitivity to chloral hydrate or any component of the formulation; hepatic or renal impairment; gastritis or ulcers; severe cardiac disease
Warnings/Precautions Use with caution in patients with porphyria. Use with caution in neonates, drug may accumulate with repeated use, prolonged use in neonates associated with hyperbilirubinemia. Tolerance to hypnotic effect develops, therefore, not recommended for use longer than 2 weeks. Taper dosage to avoid withdrawal with prolonged use. Trichloroethanol (TCE), a metabolite of chloral hydrate, is a carcinogen in mice; there is no data in humans. Chloral hydrate is considered a second line hypnotic agent in the elderly. Recent interpretive guidelines from the Centers for Medicare and Medicaid Services (CMS) discourage the use of chloral hydrate in residents of long-term care facilities.

Drug Interactions
    Increased Effect/Toxicity: Chloral hydrate and ethanol (and other CNS depressants) have additive CNS depressant effects; monitor for CNS depression. Chloral hydrate's metabolite may displace warfarin from its protein binding sites resulting in an increase in the hypoprothrombinemic response to warfarin; warfarin dosages may need to be adjusted. Diaphoresis, flushing, and hypertension have occurred in patients who received I.V. furosemide within 24 hours after administration of chloral hydrate; consider using a benzodiazepine.

Nutritional/Ethanol Interactions
    Ethanol: Avoid ethanol (may increase CNS depression).
    Herb/Nutraceutical: Avoid valerian, St John's wort, kava kava, gotu kola (may increase CNS depression).

Lab Interactions False-positive urine glucose using Clinitest® method; may interfere with fluorometric urine catecholamine and urinary 17-hydroxycorticosteroid tests
(Continued)

Chloral Hydrate *(Continued)*

Adverse Reactions Frequency not defined.

Central nervous system: Ataxia, disorientation, sedation, excitement (paradoxical), dizziness, fever, headache, confusion, lightheadedness, nightmares, hallucinations, drowsiness, "hangover" effect

Dermatologic: Rash, urticaria

Gastrointestinal: Gastric irritation, nausea, vomiting, diarrhea, flatulence

Hematologic: Leukopenia, eosinophilia, acute intermittent porphyria

Miscellaneous: Physical and psychological dependence may occur with prolonged use of large doses

Overdosage/Toxicology Symptoms of overdose include hypotension, respiratory depression, coma, hypothermia, and cardiac arrhythmias. Treatment is supportive and symptomatic.

Pharmacodynamics/Kinetics

Onset of Action: Peak effect: 0.5-1 hour

Duration of Action: 4-8 hours

Absorption: Oral, rectal: Well absorbed

Half-Life Elimination: Active metabolite: 8-11 hours

Metabolism: Rapidly hepatic to trichloroethanol (active metabolite); variable amounts hepatically and renally to trichloroacetic acid (inactive)

Excretion: Urine (as metabolites); feces (small amounts)

Dosing

Adults:

Sedation, anxiety: Oral, rectal: 250 mg 3 times/day

Hypnotic: Oral, rectal: 500-1000 mg at bedtime or 30 minutes prior to procedure, not to exceed 2 g/24 hours

Discontinuation: Withdraw gradually over 2 weeks if patient has been maintained on high doses for prolonged period of time. Do not stop drug abruptly.

Elderly: Hypnotic: Initial: Oral: 250 mg at bedtime; adjust for renal impairment. See Geriatric Considerations.

Pediatrics:

Sedation, anxiety: Oral, rectal: 5-15 mg/kg/dose every 8 hours, maximum: 500 mg/dose

Prior to EEG: Oral, rectal: 20-25 mg/kg/dose, 30-60 minutes prior to EEG; may repeat in 30 minutes to maximum of 100 mg/kg or 2 g total

Hypnotic: Oral, rectal: 20-40 mg/kg/dose up to a maximum of 50 mg/kg/24 hours or 1 g/dose or 2 g/24 hours

Conscious sedation: Oral: 50-75 mg/kg/dose 30-60 minutes prior to procedure; may repeat 30 minutes after initial dose if needed, to a total maximum dose of 120 mg/kg or 1 g total

Discontinuation: Withdraw gradually over 2 weeks if patient has been maintained on high doses for prolonged period of time. Do not stop drug abruptly.

Renal Impairment:

Cl$_{cr}$ <50 mL/minute: Avoid use.

Hemodialysis effects: Supplemental dose is not necessary; dialyzable (50% to 100%).

Hepatic Impairment: Avoid use in patients with severe hepatic impairment.

Available Dosage Forms

Capsule (Somnote™): 500 mg

Suppository, rectal (Aquachloral® Supprettes®): 325 mg [contains tartrazine], 650 mg

Syrup: 500 mg/5 mL (480 mL) [contains sodium benzoate]

Monitoring and Teaching Issues

Physical Assessment: For short-term use. Assess effectiveness and interactions of other medications patient may be taking. Assess for history of addiction; long-term use can result in dependence, abuse, or tolerance. Monitor for excessive sedation. Evaluate periodically for need for continued use (symptoms of dependence may resemble alcoholism, but usually there is more gastritis). After long-term use, taper dosage slowly when discontinuing. For inpatient use, institute safety measures and monitor effectiveness and adverse reactions. For outpatients, monitor for effectiveness of therapy and adverse reactions at beginning of therapy and periodically with long-term use. Assess knowledge/teach patient appropriate use, interventions to reduce side effects, and adverse symptoms to report.

Patient Education: Use exactly as directed; do not increase dose or frequency or discontinue without consulting prescriber. Drug may cause physical and/or psychological dependence. While using this medication, do not use alcohol and other prescription or OTC medications (especially, pain medications, sedatives, antihistamines, or hypnotics) without consulting prescriber. Maintain adequate hydration (2-3 L/day of fluids) unless instructed to restrict fluid intake. You may experience drowsiness, dizziness, or blurred vision (use caution when driving or engaging in tasks requiring alertness until response to drug is known); nausea, vomiting, unpleasant taste (small frequent meals, frequent mouth care, chewing gum, or sucking lozenges may help); or diarrhea (buttermilk, boiled milk, yogurt may help). Report skin rash or irritation, CNS changes (confusion, depression, increased sedation, excitation, headache, insomnia, or nightmares), unresolved GI distress, chest pain or palpitations, or ineffectiveness of medication. **Pregnancy precaution:** Inform prescriber if you are or intend to become pregnant.

Geriatric Considerations: Chloral hydrate is considered a second- or third-line hypnotic agent in the elderly. Interpretive guidelines from the Centers for Medicare and Medicaid Services (CMS) discourage the use of chloral hydrate in residents of long-term care facilities.

Pregnancy Risk Factor: C

Lactation: Enters breast milk/compatible

Administration

Oral: Chilling the syrup may help to mask unpleasant taste. Do not crush capsule (contains drug in liquid form). Gastric irritation may be minimized by diluting dose in water or other oral liquid.

Storage: Sensitive to light. Exposure to air causes volatilization. Store in light-resistant, airtight container.

Additional Information Not an analgesic
Related Information
Anxiolytic / Hypnotic Use in Long-Term Care Facilities *on page 1769*
Federal OBRA Regulations: Recommended Maximum Doses *on page 1773*

Chlorambucil (klor AM byoo sil)
U.S. Brand Names Leukeran®
Synonyms CB-1348; Chlorambucilum; Chloraminophene; Chlorbutinum; NSC-3088; WR-139013
Generic Available No
Pharmacologic Category Antineoplastic Agent, Alkylating Agent
Medication Safety Issues
Sound-alike/look-alike issues:
Chlorambucil may be confused with Chloromycetin®
Leukeran® may be confused with Alkeran®, leucovorin, Leukine®
Use Management of chronic lymphocytic leukemia, Hodgkin's and non-Hodgkin's lymphoma; breast and ovarian carcinoma; Waldenström's macroglobulinemia, testicular carcinoma, thrombocythemia, choriocarcinoma
Mechanism of Action/Effect Interferes with DNA replication and RNA transcription by alkylation and cross-linking the strands of DNA
Contraindications Hypersensitivity to chlorambucil or any component of the formulation; pregnancy
Warnings/Precautions The U.S. Food and Drug Administration (FDA) currently recommends that procedures for proper handling and disposal of antineoplastic agents be considered. Use with caution in patients with seizure disorder and bone marrow suppression. Reduce initial dosage if patient has received radiation therapy, myelosuppressive drugs, or has a depressed baseline leukocyte or platelet count within the previous 4 weeks. Can severely suppress bone marrow function; effects human fertility; is carcinogenic in humans and probably mutagenic and teratogenic as well. Chromosomal damage has been documented. Secondary AML may be associated with chronic therapy.
Drug Interactions
Decreased Effect: Patients may experience impaired immune response to vaccines; possible infection after administration of live vaccines in patients receiving immunosuppressants.
Nutritional/Ethanol Interactions Food: Avoid acidic foods and hot foods. Avoid spices.
Adverse Reactions
>10%:
Dermatologic: Skin rash
Hematologic: Myelosuppression (common, dose-limiting)
Onset (days): 7
Nadir (days): 14
Recovery (days): 28; may be prolonged to 6-8 weeks in some patients
Hepatic: Transient elevations in liver enzymes
1% to 10%:
Endocrine & metabolic: Hyperuricemia, menstrual cramps
Gastrointestinal: Mild nausea or vomiting, diarrhea, stomatitis
Overdosage/Toxicology Symptoms of overdose include vomiting, ataxia, coma, seizures, and pancytopenia. There are no known antidotes for chlorambucil intoxication. Treatment is mainly supportive and symptomatic.
Pharmacodynamics/Kinetics
Absorption: 70% to 80% with meals
Bioavailability: Reduced 10% to 20% with food
Protein Binding: ~99%
Half-Life Elimination: 1.5 hours; Phenylacetic acid mustard: 2.5 hours
Metabolism: Hepatic; active metabolite, phenylacetic acid mustard
Excretion: Urine (60% primarily as metabolites, <1% as unchanged drug)
Dosing
Adults: Refer to individual protocols.
Usual dose range: Oral: 0.1-0.2 mg/kg/day **or**
3-6 mg/m^2/day for 3-6 weeks, then adjust dose on basis of blood counts **or**
0.4 mg/kg and increased by 0.1 mg/kg biweekly or monthly **or**
14 mg/m^2/day for 5 days, repeated every 21-28 days
Elderly: Oral (refer to individual protocols): Use lowest recommended doses for adults; usual dose for elderly is 2-4 mg/day, particularly for use in treatment of rheumatoid arthritis.
Pediatrics: Refer to individual protocols.
General short courses: Oral: 0.1-0.2 mg/kg/day **or** 4.5 mg/m^2/day for 3-6 weeks for remission induction (usual: 4-10 mg/day); maintenance therapy: 0.03-0.1 mg/kg/day (usual: 2-4 mg/day)
Nephrotic syndrome: Oral: 0.1-0.2 mg/kg/day every day for 5-15 weeks with low-dose prednisone
Chronic lymphocytic leukemia (CLL): Oral:
Biweekly regimen: Initial: 0.4 mg/kg/dose every 2 weeks; increase dose by 0.1 mg/kg every 2 weeks until a response occurs and/or myelosuppression occurs
Monthly regimen: Initial: 0.4 mg/kg, increase dose by 0.2 mg/kg every 4 weeks until a response occurs and/or myelosuppression occurs
Malignant lymphomas: Oral:
Non-Hodgkin's lymphoma: 0.1 mg/kg/day
Hodgkin's lymphoma: 0.2 mg/kg/day
Renal Impairment:
Hemodialysis: Supplemental dose is not necessary.
Peritoneal dialysis: Supplemental dose is not necessary.
Available Dosage Forms Tablet [film coated]: 2 mg
(Continued)

Chlorambucil *(Continued)*

Monitoring and Teaching Issues

Physical Assessment: See Warnings/Precautions for use cautions (eg, seizure disorder, bone marrow suppression). Assess results of laboratory tests, therapeutic effectiveness, and adverse response (eg, hematologic myelosuppression; see Adverse Reactions) on a regular basis throughout therapy. Teach patient (or caregiver) proper use, possible side effects/appropriate interventions, and adverse symptoms to report (refer to Patient Education).

Monitoring Laboratory Tests: Liver function, CBC, platelet count, serum uric acid

Patient Education: Do not take any new medication during therapy unless approved by prescriber. Take exactly as directed. Maintain adequate hydration (2-3 L/day of fluids) unless instructed to restrict fluid intake. Avoid alcohol, acidic, spicy, or hot foods. May cause menstrual irregularities and/or sterility. You will be more susceptible to infection (avoid crowds and exposure to infection and do not have any vaccinations without consulting prescriber). May cause nausea or vomiting (small frequent meals, good mouth care, chewing gum or sucking lozenges may help); or mouth sores (use soft toothbrush or cotton swab for oral care). Report easy bruising or bleeding; unusual rash; persistent nausea, vomiting, or mouth sores; menstrual irregularities; or respiratory difficulty. **Pregnancy/breast-feeding precautions:** Inform prescriber if you are pregnant. Do not get pregnant during therapy. Consult prescriber for instruction on appropriate barrier contraceptive measures. This drug may cause severe fetal defects. Consult prescriber if breast-feeding.

Geriatric Considerations: Toxicity to immunosuppressives is increased in the elderly. Start with lowest recommended adult doses (Dosage). Signs of infection, such as fever and rise in WBCs, may not occur. Lethargy and confusion may be more prominent signs of infection.

Pregnancy Risk Factor: D

Pregnancy Issues: Carcinogenic and mutagenic in humans.

Lactation: Excretion in breast milk unknown

Administration

Oral: Usually administered as a single dose; preferably on an empty stomach

Storage: Store in refrigerator at 2°C to 8°C (36°F to 46°F). Protect from light.

Related Information

Maternal / Fetal Toxicology *on page 1762*

♦ **Chlorambucilum** *see Chlorambucil on page 305*
♦ **Chloraminophene** *see Chlorambucil on page 305*

Chloramphenicol *(klor am FEN i kole)*

U.S. Brand Names Chloromycetin® Sodium Succinate

Generic Available Yes

Pharmacologic Category Antibiotic, Miscellaneous

Medication Safety Issues

Sound-alike/look-alike issues:
Chloromycetin® may be confused with chlorambucil, Chlor-Trimeton®

Use Treatment of serious infections due to organisms resistant to other less toxic antibiotics or when its penetrability into the site of infection is clinically superior to other antibiotics to which the organism is sensitive; useful in infections caused by *Bacteroides*, *H. influenzae*, *Neisseria meningitidis*, *Salmonella*, and *Rickettsia*; active against many vancomycin-resistant enterococci

Mechanism of Action/Effect Reversibly binds to 50S ribosomal subunits of susceptible organisms preventing amino acids from being transferred to growing peptide chains thus inhibiting protein synthesis

Contraindications Hypersensitivity to chloramphenicol or any component of the formulation

Warnings/Precautions Use with caution in patients with impaired renal or hepatic function and in neonates. Reduce dose with impaired liver function. Use with care in patients with glucose 6-phosphate dehydrogenase deficiency. Serious and fatal blood dyscrasias have occurred after both short-term and prolonged therapy. Should not be used when less potentially toxic agents are effective. Prolonged use may result in superinfection.

Drug Interactions

Cytochrome P450 Effect: Inhibits CYP2C8/9 (weak), 3A4 (weak)

Decreased Effect: Phenobarbital and rifampin may decrease serum concentrations of chloramphenicol.

Increased Effect/Toxicity: Chloramphenicol increases serum concentrations of chlorpropamide, phenytoin, and oral anticoagulants.

Nutritional/Ethanol Interactions Food: May decrease intestinal absorption of vitamin B_{12} may have increased dietary need for riboflavin, pyridoxine, and vitamin B_{12}.

Lab Interactions May cause false-positive results in urine glucose tests when using cupric sulfate (Benedict's solution, Clinitest®).

Adverse Reactions

Three (3) major toxicities associated with chloramphenicol include:
Aplastic anemia, an idiosyncratic reaction which can occur with any route of administration; usually occurs 3 weeks to 12 months after initial exposure to chloramphenicol
Bone marrow suppression is thought to be dose related with serum concentrations >25 mcg/mL and reversible once chloramphenicol is discontinued; anemia and neutropenia may occur during the first week of therapy
Gray syndrome is characterized by circulatory collapse, cyanosis, acidosis, abdominal distention, myocardial depression, coma, and death; reaction appears to be associated with serum levels ≥50 mcg/mL; may result from drug accumulation in patients with impaired hepatic or renal function

Additional adverse reactions, frequency not defined:
Central nervous system: Confusion, delirium, depression, fever, headache

Dermatologic: Angioedema, rash, urticaria
Gastrointestinal: Diarrhea, enterocolitis, glossitis, nausea, stomatitis, vomiting
Hematologic: Granulocytopenia, hypoplastic anemia, pancytopenia, thrombocytopenia
Ocular: Optic neuritis
Miscellaneous: Anaphylaxis, hypersensitivity reactions

Overdosage/Toxicology Symptoms of overdose include anemia, metabolic acidosis, hypotension, and hypothermia. Treatment is supportive.

Pharmacodynamics/Kinetics
Protein Binding: 60%
Half-Life Elimination:
Normal renal function: 1.6-3.3 hours
End-stage renal disease: 3-7 hours
Cirrhosis: 10-12 hours
Metabolism: Extensively hepatic (90%) to inactive metabolites, principally by glucuronidation; chloramphenicol sodium succinate is hydrolyzed by esterases to active base
Excretion: Urine (5% to 15%)

Dosing
Adults & Elderly: Systemic infections: I.V.: 50-100 mg/kg/day in divided doses every 6 hours; maximum daily dose: 4 g/day.
Pediatrics:
Meningitis: I.V.: Infants >30 days and Children: 50-100 mg/kg/day divided every 6 hours
Other infections: I.V.: Infants >30 days and Children: 50-75 mg/kg/day divided every 6 hours; maximum daily dose: 4 g/day
Renal Impairment: Slightly dialyzable (5% to 20%) via hemo- and peritoneal dialysis; no supplemental doses are needed in dialysis or continuous arteriovenous or venovenous hemofiltration.
Hepatic Impairment: Avoid use in severe liver impairment as increased toxicity may occur.

Available Dosage Forms Injection, powder for reconstitution (Chloromycetin® Sodium Succinate): 1 g [contains sodium ~52 mg/g (2.25 mEq/g)]

Monitoring and Teaching Issues
Physical Assessment: Assess results of culture and sensitivity tests and patient allergy history prior to beginning treatment. Use caution in presence of hepatic or renal impairment or glucose-6-phosphate dehydrogenase deficiency (see Warnings/Precautions). Assess potential for interactions with other pharmacological agents patient may be taking (see Drug Interactions). Assess results of laboratory tests periodically during therapy. Observe closely for adverse reactions during and following therapy (eg, CNS disturbances, opportunistic infection, bone marrow depression or aplastic anemia [petechiae, sore throat, fatigue, unusual bleeding or bruising, abdominal or bone pain]; see Adverse Reactions). Teach patient appropriate use, possible side effects/appropriate interventions, and adverse symptoms to report (eg, hypersensitivity, opportunistic infection, aplastic anemia (may occur 3 weeks to 12 months after initial exposure to chloramphenicol); see Patient Education).
Monitoring Laboratory Tests: CBC with reticulocyte and platelet counts, periodic liver and renal function, serum drug concentration; culture and sensitivity prior to initiating therapy
Patient Education: I.V.: Do not take any new medication during therapy unless approved by prescriber. This medication can only be administered by infusion and you will be monitored during each infusion; report immediately unusual chest tightness, difficulty breathing or swallowing; itching or skin rash; back pain or acute headache, redness, swelling, or pain at infusion site. You may experience a bitter taste during infusion; this will pass. If you have diabetes, drug may cause false test results with Clinitest® glucose monitoring; use alternative glucose monitoring. May cause nausea, vomiting (small frequent meals, frequent mouth care, sucking lozenges, or chewing gum may help). Report persistent rash, diarrhea; pain, burning, or numbness of extremities; petechiae; sore throat; fatigue; unusual bleeding or bruising; vaginal itching or discharge; mouth sores; yellowing of skin or eyes; dark urine or stool discoloration (blue); CNS disturbances (nightmares, acute headache); lack of improvement or worsening of condition. **Pregnancy/breast-feeding precautions:** Inform prescriber if you are or intend to become pregnant. **Note:** This drug may interfere with effectiveness of oral contraceptives. Breast-feeding is not recommended.
Dietary Considerations: May have increased dietary need for riboflavin, pyridoxine, and vitamin B_{12}. Sodium content of 1 g injection: ~52 mg (2.25 mEq).
Geriatric Considerations: Chloramphenicol has not been studied in the elderly. It is not necessary to adjust the dose based upon the decrease in renal function associated with age. Chloramphenicol should be reserved for serious infections and the oral form avoided.
Pregnancy Risk Factor: C
Pregnancy Issues: Embryotoxic and teratogenic in animals, but there are no adequate and well-controlled trials in pregnant women. Has been shown to cross placental barrier.
Lactation: Enters breast milk/not recommended (AAP rates "of concern")
Breast-Feeding Issues: Excreted in breast milk. Not recommended due to potential bone marrow suppression to the infant.

Administration
I.V.: Do not administer I.M.; can be administered IVP over at least 1 minute at a concentration of 100 mg/mL, or I.V. intermittent infusion over 15-30 minutes at a final concentration for administration of ≤20 mg/mL.
Compatibility: Stable in dextran 6% in dextrose, dextran 6% in NS, D₅LR, D₅¼NS, D₅½NS, D₅NS, D₅W, D₁₀W, fat emulsion 10%, LR, ½NS, NS
Y-site administration: Incompatible with fluconazole
Compatibility in syringe: Incompatible with glycopyrrolate, metoclopramide
Compatibility when admixed: Incompatible with chlorpromazine, hydroxyzine, phenytoin, polymyxin B sulfate, prochlorperazine edisylate, prochlorperazine mesylate, promethazine, vancomycin

(Continued)

Chloramphenicol *(Continued)*

Storage: Store at room temperature prior to reconstitution; reconstituted solutions remain stable for 30 days; use only clear solutions; frozen solutions remain stable for 6 months
Related Information
Antimicrobial Drugs of Choice *on page 1792*

♦ **Chlorbutinum** *see* Chlorambucil *on page 305*

Chlordiazepoxide *(klor dye az e POKS ide)*
U.S. Brand Names Librium®
Synonyms Methaminodiazepoxide Hydrochloride
Controlled Substance C-IV
Generic Available Yes: Capsule
Pharmacologic Category Benzodiazepine
Medication Safety Issues
Sound-alike/look-alike issues:
Librium® may be confused with Librax®

Use Management of anxiety disorder or for the short-term relief of symptoms of anxiety; withdrawal symptoms of acute alcoholism; preoperative apprehension and anxiety

Mechanism of Action/Effect Binds to stereospecific benzodiazepine receptors on the postsynaptic GABA neuron at several sites within the central nervous system, including the limbic system, reticular formation. Enhancement of the inhibitory effect of GABA on neuronal excitability results by increased neuronal membrane permeability to chloride ions. This shift in chloride ions results in hyperpolarization (a less excitable state) and stabilization.

Contraindications Hypersensitivity to chlordiazepoxide or any component of the formulation (cross-sensitivity with other benzodiazepines may also exist); narrow-angle glaucoma; pregnancy

Warnings/Precautions Use with caution in renal impairment or predisposition to urate nephropathy, elderly or debilitated patients, patients with hepatic disease (including alcoholics), renal impairment, respiratory disease, impaired gag reflex, or obese patients. Use with caution in patients receiving concurrent CYP3A4 inhibitors, particularly when these agents are added to therapy. Use with caution in renal impairment or predisposition to urate nephropathy, elderly or debilitated patients, patients with hepatic disease (including alcoholics), renal impairment, respiratory disease, impaired gag reflex, or obese patients.

Parenteral administration should be avoided in comatose patients or shock. Adequate resuscitative equipment/personnel should be available, and appropriate monitoring should be conducted at the time of injection and for several hours following administration. The parenteral formulation should be diluted for I.M. administration with the supplied diluent only. This diluent should not be used when preparing the drug for intravenous administration.

Causes CNS depression (dose-related) which may impair physical and mental capabilities. Use with caution in patients receiving other CNS depressants or psychoactive agents. Benzodiazepines have been associated with falls and traumatic injury and should be used with extreme caution in patients who are at risk of these events (especially the elderly). Active metabolites with extended half-lives may lead to delayed accumulation and adverse effects.

Use caution in patients with depression, particularly if suicidal risk may be present. May cause physical or psychological dependence - use with caution in patients with a history of drug dependence.

Benzodiazepines have been associated with anterograde amnesia. Paradoxical reactions, including hyperactive or aggressive behavior, have been reported with benzodiazepines, particularly in adolescent/pediatric or psychiatric patients. Does not have analgesic, antidepressant, or antipsychotic properties.

Drug Interactions
Cytochrome P450 Effect: Substrate of CYP3A4 (major)
Decreased Effect: CYP3A4 inducers may decrease the levels/effects of chlordiazepoxide; example inducers include aminoglutethimide, carbamazepine, nafcillin, nevirapine, phenobarbital, phenytoin, and rifamycins.
Increased Effect/Toxicity: Chlordiazepoxide potentiates the CNS depressant effects of narcotic analgesics, barbiturates, phenothiazines, ethanol, antihistamines, MAO inhibitors, sedative-hypnotics, and cyclic antidepressants. CYP3A4 inhibitors may increase the levels/effects of chlordiazepoxide; example inhibitors include azole antifungals, ciprofloxacin, clarithromycin, diclofenac, doxycycline, erythromycin, imatinib, isoniazid, nefazodone, nicardipine, propofol, protease inhibitors, quinidine, and verapamil.
Nutritional/Ethanol Interactions
Ethanol: Avoid ethanol (may increase CNS depression).
Food: Serum concentrations/effects may be increased with grapefruit juice, but unlikely because of high oral bioavailability of chlordiazepoxide.
Herb/Nutraceutical: Avoid valerian, St John's wort, kava kava, gotu kola (may increase CNS depression).
Lab Interactions Increased triglycerides (S); decreased HDL
Adverse Reactions
>10%:
Central nervous system: Drowsiness, fatigue, ataxia, lightheadedness, memory impairment, dysarthria, irritability
Dermatologic: Rash
Endocrine & metabolic: Decreased libido, menstrual disorders
Gastrointestinal: Xerostomia, decreased salivation, increased or decreased appetite, weight gain/loss
Genitourinary: Micturition difficulties
1% to 10%:
Cardiovascular: Hypotension
Central nervous system: Confusion, dizziness, disinhibition, akathisia, increased libido
Dermatologic: Dermatitis

Gastrointestinal: Increased salivation

Genitourinary: Sexual dysfunction, incontinence

Neuromuscular & skeletal: Rigidity, tremor, muscle cramps

Otic: Tinnitus

Respiratory: Nasal congestion

Overdosage/Toxicology Symptoms of overdose include hypotension, respiratory depression, coma, hypothermia, and cardiac arrhythmias. Treatment for benzodiazepine overdose is supportive. Flumazenil has been shown to selectively block the binding of benzodiazepines to CNS receptors, resulting in a reversal of benzodiazepine-induced CNS depression. Respiratory depression may not be reversed.

Pharmacodynamics/Kinetics

Time to Peak: Serum: Oral: Within 2 hours; I.M.: Results in lower peak plasma levels than oral

Protein Binding: 90% to 98%

Half-Life Elimination: 6.6-25 hours; End-stage renal disease: 5-30 hours; Cirrhosis: 30-63 hours

Metabolism: Extensively hepatic to desmethyldiazepam (active and long-acting)

Excretion: Urine (minimal as unchanged drug)

Dosing

Adults:

Anxiety:

Oral: 15-100 mg divided 3-4 times/day

I.M., I.V.: Initial: 50-100 mg followed by 25-50 mg 3-4 times/day as needed

Preoperative anxiety: I.M.: 50-100 mg prior to surgery

Ethanol withdrawal symptoms: Oral, I.V.: 50-100 mg to start, dose may be repeated in 2-4 hours as necessary to a maximum of 300 mg/24 hours

Note: Up to 300 mg may be given I.M. or I.V. during a 6-hour period, but not more than this in any 24-hour period.

Elderly: Anxiety: Oral: 5 mg 2-4 times/day; adjust for renal impairment. Avoid use if possible. See Geriatric Considerations.

Pediatrics: Anxiety: Oral, I.M.:

<6 years: Not recommended

>6 years: 0.5 mg/kg/24 hours divided every 6-8 hours

Renal Impairment:

Cl_{cr} <10 mL/minute: Administer 50% of dose.

Not dialyzable (0% to 5%)

Hepatic Impairment: Avoid use.

Available Dosage Forms

Capsule, as hydrochloride: 5 mg, 10 mg, 25 mg

Injection, powder for reconstitution, as hydrochloride: 100 mg [diluent contains benzyl alcohol, polysorbate 80, and propylene glycol]

Monitoring and Teaching Issues

Physical Assessment: Assess other medications patient may be taking for effectiveness and interactions. Assess for CNS depression. Assess for history of addiction; long-term use can result in dependence, abuse, or tolerance; periodically evaluate need for continued use. For inpatient use, institute safety measures and monitor effectiveness and adverse reactions. For outpatients, monitor therapeutic effectiveness and adverse reactions at beginning of therapy and periodically with long-term use. Taper dosage slowly when discontinuing. Assess knowledge/teach patient appropriate use, interventions to reduce side effects, and adverse symptoms to report. **I.V.:** Monitor vital signs frequently during infusion, observe safety precautions, and maintain bedrest for 2-3 hours following infusion.

Patient Education: Oral: Take exactly as directed; do not increase dose or frequency. Drug may cause physical and/or psychological dependence. Do not use alcohol or other prescription or OTC medications (especially pain medications, sedatives, antihistamines, or hypnotics) without consulting prescriber. Maintain adequate hydration (2-3 L/day of fluids) unless instructed to restrict fluid intake. You may experience drowsiness, lightheadedness, impaired coordination, dizziness, or blurred vision (use caution when driving or engaging in tasks requiring alertness until response to drug is known); dry mouth (small frequent meals, frequent mouth care, chewing gum, or sucking lozenges may help); constipation (increased exercise, fluids, fruit, or fiber may help); or altered sexual drive or ability (reversible). Report persistent CNS effects (eg, euphoria, confusion, increased sedation, depression); chest pain, palpitations, or rapid heartbeat; muscle cramping, weakness, tremors, rigidity, or altered gait; or worsening of condition. **Pregnancy/breast-feeding precautions:** Do not get pregnant while taking this medication; use appropriate contraceptive measures. Breast-feeding is not recommended.

Geriatric Considerations: Due to its long-acting metabolite, chlordiazepoxide is not considered a drug of choice in the elderly.

Pregnancy Risk Factor: D

Pregnancy Issues: Benzodiazepines cross the placenta. The association between benzodiazepine exposure and malformations remains controversial. A number of types of malformation have been reported (oral cleft, inguinal hernia, cardiac defects, spina bifida, dysmorphic facial features, skeletal defects); however, confounding factors make a clear association difficult. Overall, the risk to the fetus may be low. Nonteratogenic effects (including neonatal flaccidity, respiratory and feeding problems, and withdrawal symptoms) during the postnatal period have also been reported with benzodiazepine use.

Lactation: Enters breast milk/not recommended

Breast-Feeding Issues: There is no significant data for chlordiazepoxide, but a related compound diazepam has been shown to accumulate in nursing infants. It is recommended to discontinue nursing or the drug.

(Continued)

Chlordiazepoxide *(Continued)*

Administration
I.M.: Administer by deep I.M. injection slowly into the upper outer quadrant of the gluteus muscle; use only the diluent provided for I.M. use; solutions made with SWFI or NS cause pain with I.M. administration

I.V.: Administer slowly over at least 1 minute; do not use the diluent provided for I.M. use; air bubbles form during reconstitution

Reconstitution:
I.M. use: Reconstitute by adding 2 mL of provided diluent; agitate gently until dissolved. Provided diluent is **not** for I.V. use.

I.V. use: Reconstitute by adding 5 mL NS or SWFI; agitate gently until dissolved; **do not administer this dilution I.M.**

Compatibility: Stable in D_5W; **incompatible** (consult detailed reference) in LR, NS
Y-site administration: Incompatible with cefepime

Storage: Injection: Prior to reconstitution, store under refrigeration and protect from light. Solution should be used immediately following reconstitution.

Additional Information Abrupt discontinuation after sustained use (generally >10 days) may cause withdrawal symptoms.

Related Information
Anxiolytic / Hypnotic Use in Long-Term Care Facilities *on page 1769*
Benzodiazepines *on page 1719*
Federal OBRA Regulations: Recommended Maximum Doses *on page 1773*

♦ **Chlorethazine** *see* Mechlorethamine *on page 935*
♦ **Chlorethazine Mustard** *see* Mechlorethamine *on page 935*
♦ **Chlormeprazine** *see* Prochlorperazine *on page 1259*
♦ **2-Chlorodeoxyadenosine** *see* Cladribine *on page 340*
♦ **Chloromag®** *see* Magnesium Chloride *on page 929*
♦ **Chloromycetin® Sodium Succinate** *see* Chloramphenicol *on page 306*

Chloroquine *(KLOR oh kwin)*

U.S. Brand Names Aralen®
Synonyms Chloroquine Phosphate
Generic Available Yes
Pharmacologic Category Aminoquinoline (Antimalarial)
Use Suppression or chemoprophylaxis of malaria; treatment of uncomplicated or mild to moderate malaria; extraintestinal amebiasis
Unlabeled/Investigational Use Rheumatoid arthritis; discoid lupus erythematosus
Mechanism of Action/Effect Chloroquine concentrates within parasite acid vesicles and raises internal pH resulting in inhibition of parasite growth
Contraindications Hypersensitivity to chloroquine or any component of the formulation; retinal or visual field changes
Warnings/Precautions Use with caution in patients with liver disease, G6PD deficiency, alcoholism or in conjunction with hepatotoxic drugs. May exacerbate psoriasis or porphyria. Retinopathy (irreversible) has occurred with long or high-dose therapy; discontinue drug if any abnormality in the visual field or if muscular weakness develops during treatment. Use caution in patients with pre-existing auditory damage; discontinue immediately if hearing defects are noted. Use caution in patients with seizure disorders.
Drug Interactions
Cytochrome P450 Effect: Substrate (major) of CYP2D6, 3A4; **Inhibits** CYP2D6 (moderate)
Decreased Effect: Chloroquine levels may be decreased by antacids or kaolin. Chloroquine may decrease ampicillin and/or praziquantel levels. Chloroquine may decrease the levels/effects of CYP2D6 prodrug substrates; example prodrug substrates include codeine, hydrocodone, oxycodone, and tramadol. The levels/effects of chloroquine may be decreased by aminoglutethimide, carbamazepine, nafcillin, nevirapine, phenobarbital, phenytoin, rifamycins, and other CYP3A4 inducers.
Increased Effect/Toxicity: Chloroquine may increase the levels/effects of dextromethorphan, fluoxetine, lidocaine, mirtazapine, nefazodone, paroxetine, risperidone, ritonavir, thioridazine, tricyclic antidepressants, venlafaxine, and other CYP2D6 substrates. Chloroquine may increase the levels/effects of cyclosporine. The levels/effects of chloroquine may be increased by azole antifungals, chlorpromazine, cimetidine, ciprofloxacin, clarithromycin, delavirdine, diclofenac, doxycycline, erythromycin, fluoxetine, imatinib, isoniazid, miconazole, nefazodone, nicardipine, paroxetine, pergolide, propofol, protease inhibitors, quinidine, quinine, ritonavir, ropinirole, telithromycin, verapamil, and other CYP2D6 or 3A4 inhibitors.
Nutritional/Ethanol Interactions Ethanol: Avoid ethanol (may increase GI irritation).
Adverse Reactions Frequency not defined.
Cardiovascular: Hypotension (rare), ECG changes (rare; including T-wave inversion), cardiomyopathy
Central nervous system: Fatigue, personality changes, headache, psychosis, seizure, delirium, depression
Dermatologic: Pruritus, hair bleaching, pleomorphic skin eruptions, alopecia, lichen planus eruptions, alopecia, mucosal pigmentary changes (blue-black), photosensitivity
Gastrointestinal: Nausea, diarrhea, vomiting, anorexia, stomatitis, abdominal cramps
Hematologic: Aplastic anemia, agranulocytosis (reversible), neutropenia, thrombocytopenia
Neuromuscular & skeletal: Rare cases of myopathy, neuromyopathy, proximal muscle atrophy, and depression of deep tendon reflexes have been reported
Ocular: Retinopathy (including irreversible changes in some patients long-term or high-dose therapy), blurred vision
Otic: Nerve deafness, tinnitus, reduced hearing (risk increased in patients with pre-existing auditory damage)

Overdosage/Toxicology Symptoms of overdose include headache, visual changes, cardio-vascular collapse, shock, seizures, abdominal cramps, vomiting, cyanosis, methemoglobi-nemia, leukopenia, and respiratory and cardiac arrest. Following initial measures (immediate GI decontamination), treatment is supportive and symptomatic.

Pharmacodynamics/Kinetics

Duration of Action: Small amounts may be present in urine months following discontinua-tion of therapy

Absorption: Oral: Rapid (~89%)

Time to Peak: Serum: 1-2 hours

Half-Life Elimination: 3-5 days

Metabolism: Partially hepatic

Excretion: Urine (~70% as unchanged drug); acidification of urine increases elimination

Dosing

Adults & Elderly:

Malaria, suppression or prophylaxis: Oral: 500 mg/week (300 mg base) on the same day each week; begin 1-2 weeks prior to exposure; continue for 4-6 weeks after leaving endemic area; if suppressive therapy is not begun prior to exposure, double the initial loading dose to 1 g (600 mg base) and administer in 2 divided doses 6 hours apart, followed by the usual dosage regimen.

Malaria, acute attack: Oral: 1 g (600 mg base) on day 1, followed by 500 mg (300 mg base) 6 hours later, followed by 500 mg (300 mg base) on days 2 and 3.

Extraintestinal amebiasis: Oral: 1 g/day (600 mg base) for 2 days followed by 500 mg/day (300 mg base) for at least 2-3 weeks.

Rheumatoid arthritis, lupus erythematosus (unlabeled uses): Oral: 250 mg (150 mg base) once daily; reduce dosage following maximal response (taper to discontinue after response in lupus); generally requires 3-6 weeks. **Note:** Not considered first-line agent.

Pediatrics:

Malaria, suppression or prophylaxis: Oral: Administer 5 mg base/kg/week on the same day each week (not to exceed 300 mg base/dose); begin 1-2 weeks prior to exposure; continue for 4-6 weeks after leaving endemic area; if suppressive therapy is not begun prior to exposure, double the initial loading dose to 10 mg base/kg and administer in 2 divided doses 6 hours apart, followed by the usual dosage regimen

Malaria, acute attack: Oral: 10 mg/kg (base) on day 1, followed by 5 mg/kg (base) 6 hours later and 5 mg/kg (base) on days 2 and 3

Extraintestinal amebiasis: Oral: 10 mg/kg (base) once daily for 2-3 weeks (up to 300 mg base/day)

Renal Impairment:

Cl$_{cr}$ <10 mL/minute: Administer 50% of dose.

Hemodialysis effects: Minimally removed by hemodialysis

Available Dosage Forms

Tablet, as phosphate: 250 mg [equivalent to 150 mg base]; 500 mg [equivalent to 300 mg base]

Aralen®: 500 mg [equivalent to 300 mg base]

Monitoring and Teaching Issues

Physical Assessment: Use cautions in presence of liver disease or impairment, G6PD deficiency, seizure disorders (see Warnings/Precautions). Assess potential for interactions with other pharmacological agents patient may be taking (see Drug Interactions). Assess results of laboratory tests (CBC), therapeutic effectiveness (according to purpose for use), and adverse response (eg, retinopathy, hearing loss, myopathy; see Adverse Reactions) regularly during long-term therapy. Teach patient appropriate use, possible side effects/appropriate interventions, and adverse symptoms to report (eg, anemia, muscle weakness, visual or auditory changes; see Patient Education).

Patient Education: Do not take any new medication during therapy unless approved by prescriber. It is important to complete full course of therapy, which may take up to 6 months for full effect. May be taken with meals to decrease GI upset and bitter aftertaste. Avoid alcohol. You should have regular ophthalmic exams (every 4-6 months) if using this medication over extended periods. May cause skin discoloration (blue/black), hair bleaching, or skin rash. If you have psoriasis, may cause exacerbation. May turn urine black/brown (normal). May cause headache (if persistent, consult prescriber for analgesic); nausea, vomiting, or loss of appetite (small frequent meals, frequent mouth care, sucking lozenges, or chewing gum may help); or increased sensitivity to sunlight (wear dark glasses and protective clothing, use sunblock, and avoid direct exposure to sunlight). Report vision or hearing changes; rash or itching; persistent diarrhea or GI disturbances; chest pain or palpitation; CNS changes; unusual fatigue, easy bruising or bleeding; unusual muscle weakness of numbness; or any other persistent adverse reactions. **Pregnancy/breast-feeding precautions:** Inform prescriber if you are or intend to become pregnant or breast-feed.

Dietary Considerations: May be taken with meals to decrease GI upset.

Pregnancy Risk Factor: C

Pregnancy Issues: There are no adequate and well-controlled studies using chloroquine during pregnancy. However, based on clinical experience and because malaria infection in pregnant women may be more severe than in nonpregnant women, chloroquine prophy-laxis may be considered in areas of chloroquine-sensitive *P. falciparum* malaria. Pregnant women should be advised not to travel to areas of *P. falciparum* resistance to chloroquine.

Lactation: Enters breast milk/not recommended (AAP considers "compatible")

Administration

Oral: Chloroquine phosphate tablets have also been mixed with chocolate syrup or enclosed in gelatin capsules to mask the bitter taste.

Storage: Store tablets at 25°C (77°F). Excursions permitted at 15°C to 30°C (59°F to 86°F).

♦ **Chloroquine Phosphate** *see* Chloroquine *on page 310*

♦ **Chlorpheniramine and Carbetapentane** *see* Carbetapentane and Chlorpheniramine *on page 253*

- **Chlorpheniramine, Carbetapentane, and Phenylephrine** *see* Carbetapentane, Phenylephrine, and Chlorpheniramine *on page 253*

- **Chlorpheniramine, Phenylephrine, and Hydrocodone** *see* Phenylephrine, Hydrocodone, and Chlorpheniramine *on page 1202*

- **Chlorpheniramine, Pseudoephedrine, and Hydrocodone** *see* Pseudoephedrine, Hydrocodone, and Chlorpheniramine *on page 1283*

ChlorproMAZINE (klor PROE ma zeen)

U.S. Brand Names Thorazine® [DSC]
Synonyms Chlorpromazine Hydrochloride; CPZ
Generic Available Yes: Tablet
Pharmacologic Category Antipsychotic Agent, Typical, Phenothiazine
Medication Safety Issues
Sound-alike/look-alike issues:
ChlorproMAZINE may be confused with chlorproPAMIDE, clomiPRAMINE, prochlorperazine, promethazine
Thorazine® may be confused with thiamine, thioridazine

Use Control of mania; treatment of schizophrenia; control of nausea and vomiting; relief of restlessness and apprehension before surgery; acute intermittent porphyria; adjunct in the treatment of tetanus; intractable hiccups; combativeness and/or explosive hyperexcitable behavior in children 1-12 years of age and in short-term treatment of hyperactive children

Unlabeled/Investigational Use Management of psychotic disorders

Mechanism of Action/Effect Chlorpromazine is an aliphatic phenothiazine antipsychotic which blocks postsynaptic mesolimbic dopaminergic receptors in the brain; exhibits a strong alpha-adrenergic blocking effect and depresses the release of hypothalamic and hypophyseal hormones; believed to depress the reticular activating system, thus affecting basal metabolism, body temperature, wakefulness, vasomotor tone, and emesis

Contraindications Hypersensitivity to chlorpromazine or any component of the formulation (cross-reactivity between phenothiazines may occur); severe CNS depression; coma

Warnings/Precautions Highly sedating, use with caution in disorders where CNS depression is a feature and in patients with Parkinson's disease. Use with caution in patients with hemodynamic instability, bone marrow suppression, predisposition to seizures, subcortical brain damage, severe cardiac, hepatic, renal, or respiratory disease. Esophageal dysmotility and aspiration have been associated with antipsychotic use - use with caution in patients at risk of aspiration pneumonia (ie, Alzheimer's disease). Caution in breast cancer or other prolactin-dependent tumors (may elevate prolactin levels). May alter temperature regulation or mask toxicity of other drugs due to antiemetic effects. May alter cardiac conduction - life-threatening arrhythmias have occurred with therapeutic doses of neuroleptics.

Use with caution in patients at risk of hypotension (orthostasis is common) or those who would tolerate transient hypotensive episodes (cerebrovascular disease, cardiovascular disease, or other medications which may predispose). Significant hypotension may occur, particularly with parenteral administration. Injection contains sulfites and benzyl alcohol.

Use with caution in patients with decreased gastrointestinal motility, urinary retention, BPH, xerostomia, or visual problems (ie, narrow-angle glaucoma - screening is recommended) and myasthenia gravis. Relative to other neuroleptics, chlorpromazine has a moderate potency of cholinergic blockade.

May cause extrapyramidal symptoms, neuroleptic malignant syndrome (NMS) or pigmentary retinopathy.

Drug Interactions
Cytochrome P450 Effect: Substrate of CYP1A2 (minor), 2D6 (major), 3A4 (minor); **Inhibits** CYP2D6 (strong), 2E1 (weak)
Decreased Effect: Chlorpromazine may decrease the levels/effects of CYP2D6 prodrug substrates; example prodrug substrates include codeine, hydrocodone, oxycodone, and tramadol. Phenothiazines inhibit the ability of bromocriptine to lower serum prolactin concentrations. Benztropine (and other anticholinergics) may inhibit the therapeutic response to chlorpromazine and excess anticholinergic effects may occur. Antihypertensive effects of guanethidine and guanadrel may be inhibited by chlorpromazine. Chlorpromazine may inhibit the antiparkinsonian effect of levodopa. Chlorpromazine and possibly other low potency antipsychotics may reverse the pressor effects of epinephrine.
Increased Effect/Toxicity: The levels/effects of chlorpromazine may be increased by delavirdine, fluoxetine, miconazole, paroxetine, pergolide, quinidine, quinine, ritonavir, ropinirole, and other CYP2D6 inhibitors. Effects on CNS depression may be additive when chlorpromazine is combined with CNS depressants (narcotic analgesics, ethanol, barbiturates, cyclic antidepressants, antihistamines, or sedative-hypnotics). Chlorpromazine may increase the levels/effects of amphetamines, selected beta-blockers, dextromethorphan, fluoxetine, lidocaine, mirtazapine, nefazodone, paroxetine, risperidone, ritonavir, thioridazine, tricyclic antidepressants, and venlafaxine and other CYP2D6 substrates. Chlorpromazine may increase the effects/toxicity of anticholinergics, antihypertensives, lithium (rare neurotoxicity), trazodone, or valproic acid. Concurrent use with TCA may produce increased toxicity or altered therapeutic response. Chloroquine and propranolol may increase chlorpromazine concentrations. Hypotension may occur when chlorpromazine is combined with epinephrine. May increase the risk of arrhythmia when combined with antiarrhythmics, cisapride, pimozide, sparfloxacin, or other drugs which prolong QT interval. Metoclopramide may increase risk of extrapyramidal symptoms (EPS).

Nutritional/Ethanol Interactions
Ethanol: Avoid ethanol (may increase CNS depression).
Herb/Nutraceutical: Avoid St John's wort (may decrease chlorpromazine levels, increase photosensitization, or enhance sedative effect). Avoid dong quai (may enhance photosensitization). Avoid kava kava, gotu kola, valerian (may increase CNS depression).

Lab Interactions False-positives for phenylketonuria, amylase, uroporphyrins, urobilinogen. May cause false-positive pregnancy test.
Adverse Reactions Frequency not defined.

Cardiovascular: Postural hypotension, tachycardia, dizziness, nonspecific QT changes

Central nervous system: Drowsiness, dystonias, akathisia, pseudoparkinsonism, tardive dyskinesia, neuroleptic malignant syndrome, seizure

Dermatologic: Photosensitivity, dermatitis, skin pigmentation (slate gray)

Endocrine & metabolic: Lactation, breast engorgement, false-positive pregnancy test, amenorrhea, gynecomastia, hyper- or hypoglycemia

Gastrointestinal: Xerostomia, constipation, nausea

Genitourinary: Urinary retention, ejaculatory disorder, impotence

Hematologic: Agranulocytosis, eosinophilia, leukopenia, hemolytic anemia, aplastic anemia, thrombocytopenic purpura

Hepatic: Jaundice

Ocular: Blurred vision, corneal and lenticular changes, epithelial keratopathy, pigmentary retinopathy

Overdosage/Toxicology Symptoms of overdose include deep sleep, coma, extrapyramidal symptoms, abnormal involuntary muscle movements, and hypotension. Following initiation of essential overdose management, toxic symptom treatment and supportive treatment should be initiated. Neuroleptics often cause extrapyramidal symptoms (eg, dystonic reactions) requiring management with anticholinergic agents such as benztropine mesylate 1-2 mg for adult patients (oral, I.M., I.V.) or diphenhydramine 25-50 mg (oral, I.M., I.V.) may be effective.

Pharmacodynamics/Kinetics

Onset of Action: I.M.: 15 minutes; Oral: 30-60 minutes

Absorption: Rapid

Bioavailability: 20%

Protein Binding: 92% to 97%

Half-Life Elimination: Biphasic: Initial: 2 hours; Terminal: 30 hours

Metabolism: Extensively hepatic to active and inactive metabolites

Excretion: Urine (<1% as unchanged drug) within 24 hours

Dosing

Adults:

Schizophrenia/psychoses:

Oral: Range: 30-800 mg/day in 1-4 divided doses, initiate at lower doses and titrate as needed; usual dose: 200 mg/day; some patients may require 1-2 g/day

I.M., I.V.: Initial: 25 mg, may repeat (25-50 mg) in 1-4 hours, gradually increase to a maximum of 400 mg/dose every 4-6 hours until patient is controlled; usual dose: 300-800 mg/day

Intractable hiccups: Oral, I.M.: 25-50 mg 3-4 times/day

Nausea and vomiting:

Oral: 10-25 mg every 4-6 hours

I.M., I.V.: 25-50 mg every 4-6 hours

Elderly:

Behavioral symptoms associated with dementia: Initial: 10-25 mg 1-2 times/day; increase at 4- to 7-day intervals by 10-25 mg/day. Increase dose intervals (eg, twice daily, 3 times/day) as necessary to control behavior response or side effects; maximum daily dose: 800 mg; gradual increases (titration) may prevent some side effects or decrease their severity.

Other indications: Refer to adult dosing.

Pediatrics:

Schizophrenia/psychoses: Children ≥6 months:

Oral: 0.5-1 mg/kg/dose every 4-6 hours; older children may require 200 mg/day or higher.

I.M., I.V.: 0.5-1 mg/kg/dose every 6-8 hours; maximum dose for <5 years (22.7 kg): 40 mg/day; maximum for 5-12 years (22.7-45.5 kg): 75 mg/day

Nausea and vomiting: Children ≥6 months:

Oral: 0.5-1 mg/kg/dose every 4-6 hours as needed

I.M., I.V.: 0.5-1 mg/kg/dose every 6-8 hours; maximum dose for <5 years (22.7 kg): 40 mg/day; maximum for 5-12 years (22.7-45.5 kg): 75 mg/day

Renal Impairment: Not dialyzable (0% to 5%)

Hepatic Impairment: Avoid use in severe hepatic dysfunction.

Available Dosage Forms [DSC] = Discontinued product

Injection, solution, as hydrochloride (Thorazine® [DSC]): 25 mg/mL (10 mL) [contains benzyl alcohol, sodium bisulfite, and sodium sulfite]

Tablet, as hydrochloride: 10 mg, 25 mg, 50 mg, 100 mg, 200 mg

Monitoring and Teaching Issues

Physical Assessment: Assess other medications patient is taking for effectiveness and interactions. Review ophthalmic exam and monitor laboratory results, therapeutic effectiveness, and adverse reactions at beginning of therapy and periodically with long-term use.

I.V./I.M.: Significant hypotension may occur. Initiate at lower doses (see Dosing) and taper dosage slowly when discontinuing. Assess knowledge/teach patient appropriate use, interventions to reduce side effects, and adverse symptoms to report. **Note:** Chlorpromazine may cause false-positive pregnancy test.

Monitoring Laboratory Tests: Lipid profile, fasting blood glucose/Hgb A_{1c}; BMI

Patient Education: Use exactly as directed; do not increase dose or frequency. Do not discontinue without consulting prescriber. Tablets may be taken with food. Do not take within 2 hours of any antacid. Store away from light. Avoid alcohol or caffeine and other prescription or OTC medications not approved by prescriber. Maintain adequate hydration (2-3 L/day of fluids) unless instructed to restrict fluid intake. May turn urine red-brown (normal). You may experience excess drowsiness, lightheadedness, dizziness, or blurred vision (use caution driving or when engaging in tasks requiring alertness until response to drug is known); dry mouth, upset stomach, nausea, vomiting, anorexia (small frequent meals, frequent mouth care, sucking lozenges, or chewing gum may help); constipation (increased exercise, fluids, fruit, or fiber may help); postural hypotension (use caution climbing stairs or when changing position from lying or sitting to standing); urinary retention (void before taking medication); ejaculatory dysfunction (reversible); decreased perspiration (avoid strenuous exercise in hot environments); or photosensitivity (use sunscreen, (Continued)

ChlorproMAZINE *(Continued)*

wear protective clothing and eyewear, and avoid direct sunlight). Report persistent CNS effects (trembling fingers, altered gait or balance, excessive sedation, seizures, unusual movements, anxiety, abnormal thoughts, confusion, personality changes); chest pain, palpitations, rapid heartbeat, or severe dizziness; unresolved urinary retention or changes in urinary pattern; altered menstrual pattern, change in libido, swelling or pain in breasts (male or female); vision changes, skin rash, irritation, or changes in color of skin (gray-blue); or worsening of condition. **Pregnancy/breast-feeding precautions:** Inform prescriber if you are or intend to become pregnant. Breast-feeding is not recommended.

Geriatric Considerations: See Warnings/Precautions, Adverse Reactions, and Overdose/Toxicology. Elderly patients have an increased risk of adverse response to side effects or adverse reactions to antipsychotics.

Pregnancy Risk Factor: C

Lactation: Enters breast milk/not recommended (AAP rates "of concern")

Breast-Feeding Issues: Drowsiness and lethargy have been reported in nursing infants; galactorrhea has been reported in mother.

Administration

I.V.: Direct of intermittent infusion: Infuse 1 mg or portion thereof over 1 minute. **Note:** Avoid skin contact with solution; may cause dermatitis.

Reconstitution: Dilute injection (1 mg/mL) with NS for I.V. administration.

Compatibility: Stable in dextran 6% in dextrose, dextran 6% in NS, D_5LR, $D_5^1/_4NS$, $D_5^1/_2NS$, D_5NS, D_5W, $D_{10}W$, LR, $^1/_2NS$, NS

Y-site administration: Incompatible with allopurinol, amifostine, amphotericin B cholesteryl sulfate complex, aztreonam, cefepime, etoposide phosphate, fludarabine, furosemide, linezolid, melphalan, methotrexate, paclitaxel, piperacillin/tazobactam, sargramostim

Compatibility in syringe: Incompatible with cimetidine, dimenhydrinate, heparin, pentobarbital, thiopental

Compatibility when admixed: Incompatible with aminophylline, amphotericin B, ampicillin, chloramphenicol, chlorothiazide, floxacillin, furosemide, methohexital, penicillin G potassium, penicillin G sodium, phenobarbital

Storage: Injection: Protect from light. A slightly yellowed solution does not indicate potency loss, but a markedly discolored solution should be discarded. Diluted injection (1 mg/mL) with NS and stored in 5 mL vials remains stable for 30 days.

Related Information

Antipsychotic Agents *on page 1717*
Antipsychotic Medication Guidelines *on page 1766*
Compatibility of Drugs in Syringe *on page 1725*
FDA Name Differentiation Project: The Use of Tall-Man Letters *on page 15*
Federal OBRA Regulations: Recommended Maximum Doses *on page 1773*

♦ **Chlorpromazine Hydrochloride** *see* ChlorproMAZINE *on page 312*

Chlorthalidone *(klor THAL i done)*

U.S. Brand Names Thalitone®

Synonyms Hygroton

Generic Available Yes

Pharmacologic Category Diuretic, Thiazide

Use Management of mild to moderate hypertension when used alone or in combination with other agents; treatment of edema associated with congestive heart failure or nephrotic syndrome. Recent studies have found chlorthalidone effective in the treatment of isolated systolic hypertension in the elderly.

Mechanism of Action/Effect Sulfonamide-derived diuretic that inhibits sodium and chloride reabsorption in the cortical-diluting segment of the ascending loop of Henle

Contraindications Hypersensitivity to chlorthalidone or any component of the formulation; cross-sensitivity with other thiazides or sulfonamides; anuria; renal decompensation; pregnancy

Warnings/Precautions Use with caution in patients with hypokalemia, renal disease, hepatic disease, gout, lupus erythematosus, or diabetes mellitus. Use with caution in severe renal diseases. Correct hypokalemia before initiating therapy. Chemical similarities are present among sulfonamides, sulfonylureas, carbonic anhydrase inhibitors, thiazides, and loop diuretics (except ethacrynic acid). Use in patients with thiazide or sulfonamide allergy is specifically contraindicated in product labeling, however, a risk of cross-reaction exists in patients with allergy to any of these compounds; avoid use when previous reaction has been severe.

Drug Interactions

Decreased Effect: Effects of oral hypoglycemics may be decreased. Decreased absorption of chlorthalidone with cholestyramine and colestipol. NSAIDs can decrease the efficacy of chlorthalidone, reducing the diuretic and antihypertensive effects.

Increased Effect/Toxicity: Increased effect of chlorthalidone with furosemide and other loop diuretics. Increased hypotension and/or renal adverse effects of ACE inhibitors may result in aggressively diuresed patients. Beta-blockers increase hyperglycemic effects of thiazides in Type 2 diabetes mellitus. Cyclosporine and thiazides can increase the risk of gout or renal toxicity. Digoxin toxicity can be exacerbated if a thiazide induces hypokalemia or hypomagnesemia. Lithium toxicity can occur with thiazides due to reduced renal excretion of lithium. Thiazides may prolong the duration of action with neuromuscular blocking agents.

Nutritional/Ethanol Interactions Herb/Nutraceutical: Avoid dong quai if using for hypertension (has estrogenic activity). Avoid dong quai, St John's Wort (may also cause photosensitization). Avoid ephedra, yohimbe, ginseng (may worsen hypertension).

Lab Interactions Increased creatine phosphokinase [CPK] (S), ammonia (B), amylase (S), calcium (S), chloride (S), cholesterol (S), glucose, acid (S); decreased chloride (S), magnesium, potassium, sodium (S)

Adverse Reactions 1% to 10%:
Dermatologic: Photosensitivity
Endocrine & metabolic: Hypokalemia
Gastrointestinal: Anorexia, epigastric distress

Overdosage/Toxicology Symptoms of overdose include hypermotility, diuresis, lethargy, confusion, muscle weakness, and coma. Treatment is supportive.

Pharmacodynamics/Kinetics
Onset of Action: Peak effect: 2-6 hours
Absorption: 65%
Half-Life Elimination: 35-55 hours; may be prolonged with renal impairment; Anuria: 81 hours
Metabolism: Hepatic
Excretion: Urine ($\sim$50% to 65% as unchanged drug)

Dosing
Adults: Hypertension, edema: Oral: 25-100 mg/day or 100 mg 3 times/week; usual dosage range (JNC 7): 12.5-25 mg/day
Elderly: Oral: Initial: 12.5-25 mg/day or every other day; there is little advantage to using doses >25 mg/day.
Pediatrics: Oral: Children (nonapproved): 2 mg/kg/dose 3 times/week or 1-2 mg/kg/day
Renal Impairment: Cl_{cr} <10 mL/minute: Administer every 48 hours.

Available Dosage Forms
Tablet: 25 mg, 50 mg, 100 mg
Thalitone®: 15 mg

Monitoring and Teaching Issues
Physical Assessment: Assess allergy history prior to beginning therapy. See Contraindications and Warnings/Precautions for use cautions (eg, hypokalemia, renal or hepatic disease, gout, lupus erythematosus, or diabetes mellitus). Assess potential for interactions with other pharmacological agents or herbal products patient may be taking (see Drug Interactions). Monitor electrolyte balance and renal function on a regular basis throughout therapy. Monitor therapeutic effectiveness and adverse response (eg, blood pressure and fluid status; see Adverse Reactions) regularly during long-term therapy. Caution patients with diabetes to monitor glucose levels (may reduce effect of oral hypoglycemics). Teach patient proper use, possible side effects/appropriate interventions, and adverse symptoms to report (see Patient Education).
Monitoring Laboratory Tests: Serum electrolytes, renal function
Patient Education: Do not take any new medication during therapy unless approved by prescriber. Take once-daily dose in morning or last of daily doses early in the day to avoid night-time disturbances. You may need to make dietary changes; your prescriber may recommend a potassium supplement or foods high in potassium; do not increase your potassium intake unless recommended to do so. If using oral hypoglycemics, monitor glucose levels closely (this medication may reduce effect of oral hypoglycemics); contact prescriber with any major changes. May cause sensitivity to sunlight (use sunblock, wear protective clothing, and avoid direct sunlight); or anorexia or GI distress (small frequent meals, frequent mouth care, chewing gum, or sucking lozenges may help). Report muscle twitching or cramps; nausea or vomiting; confusion; numbness of extremities; loss of appetite or GI distress; severe rash, redness, or itching of skin; chest pain or palpitations; respiratory difficulty, unusual weight loss; or other persistent adverse effects. **Pregnancy/breast-feeding precautions:** Do not get pregnant while taking this medication. Consult prescriber for appropriate contraceptive measures. Consult prescriber if breast-feeding.
Dietary Considerations: This product may cause a potassium loss; your healthcare provider may prescribe a potassium supplement, another medication to help prevent the potassium loss, or recommend that you eat foods high in potassium, especially citrus fruits; do not change your diet on your own while taking this medication, especially if you are taking potassium supplements or medications to reduce potassium loss; too much potassium can be as harmful as too little.
Geriatric Considerations: Studies have found chlorthalidone effective in the treatment of isolated systolic hypertension in the elderly.
Pregnancy Risk Factor: B (manufacturer); D (expert analysis)
Lactation: Enters breast milk/use caution (AAP rates "compatible")

Related Information
Heart Failure *on page 1828*

♦ **Chlorthalidone and Atenolol** *see* Atenolol and Chlorthalidone *on page 151*
♦ **Chlorthalidone and Clonidine** *see* Clonidine and Chlorthalidone *on page 357*

Chlorzoxazone (klor ZOKS a zone)

U.S. Brand Names Parafon Forte® DSC
Generic Available Yes
Pharmacologic Category Skeletal Muscle Relaxant
Medication Safety Issues
Sound-alike/look-alike issues:
Parafon Forte® may be confused with Fam-Pren Forte
Use Symptomatic treatment of muscle spasm and pain associated with acute musculoskeletal conditions
Mechanism of Action/Effect Acts on the spinal cord and subcortical levels by depressing polysynaptic reflexes
Contraindications Hypersensitivity to chlorzoxazone or any component of the formulation; impaired liver function
Drug Interactions
Cytochrome P450 Effect: Substrate of CYP1A2 (minor), 2A6 (minor), 2D6 (minor), 2E1 (major), 3A4 (minor); **Inhibits** CYP2E1 (weak), 3A4 (weak)
(Continued)

Chlorzoxazone *(Continued)*

Increased Effect/Toxicity: Effects of CNS depressants may be increased by chlorzoxazone. CYP2E1 inhibitors may increase the levels/effects of chlorzoxazone; example inhibitors include disulfiram, isoniazid, and miconazole. Disulfiram and isoniazid may increase chlorzoxazone concentration; monitor.

Nutritional/Ethanol Interactions Ethanol: Avoid ethanol (may increase CNS depression).

Adverse Reactions Frequency not defined.

Central nervous system: Dizziness, drowsiness lightheadedness, paradoxical stimulation, malaise

Dermatologic: Rash, petechiae, ecchymoses (rare), angioneurotic edema

Gastrointestinal: Nausea, vomiting, stomach cramps

Genitourinary: Urine discoloration

Hepatic: Liver dysfunction

Miscellaneous: Anaphylaxis (very rare)

Overdosage/Toxicology Symptoms of overdose include nausea, vomiting, diarrhea, drowsiness, dizziness, headache, absent tendon reflexes, and hypotension. Treatment is supportive including attempts to enhance drug elimination. Dialysis, hemoperfusion, and osmotic diuresis have all been useful in reducing serum drug concentrations. The patient should be observed for possible relapses due to incomplete gastric emptying.

Pharmacodynamics/Kinetics
Onset of Action: ~1 hour
Duration of Action: 6-12 hours
Absorption: Readily absorbed
Metabolism: Extensively hepatic via glucuronidation
Excretion: Urine (as conjugates)

Dosing
Adults: Muscle spasm: Oral: 250-500 mg 3-4 times/day up to 750 mg 3-4 times/day
Elderly: Oral: Initial: 250 mg 2-4 times/day; increase as necessary to 750 mg 3-4 times/day.
Pediatrics: Muscle spasm: Oral: 20 mg/kg/day or 600 mg/m^2/day in 3-4 divided doses

Available Dosage Forms
Caplet (Parafon Forte® DSC): 500 mg
Tablet: 250 mg, 500 mg

Monitoring and Teaching Issues
Physical Assessment: Assess results of laboratory tests, therapeutic effectiveness (according to rational for therapy), and adverse reactions at beginning of therapy and periodically with long-term use. Do not discontinue abruptly; taper dosage slowly. Assess knowledge/teach patient appropriate use, interventions to reduce side effects, and adverse symptoms to report.

Monitoring Laboratory Tests: Periodic liver functions

Patient Education: Take exactly as directed with food. Do not increase dose or discontinue without consulting prescriber. Do not use alcohol, prescriptive or OTC antidepressants, sedatives, or pain medications without consulting prescriber. May turn urine orange or red (normal). You may experience drowsiness, dizziness, lightheadedness (avoid driving or engaging in tasks that require alertness until response to drug is known); nausea, vomiting, or cramping (small frequent meals, frequent mouth care, or sucking hard candy may help); postural hypotension (change position slowly when rising from sitting or lying or when climbing stairs); or constipation (increased exercise, fluids, fruit, or fiber may help). Report excessive drowsiness or mental agitation; palpitations, rapid heartbeat, or chest pain; skin rash or swelling of mouth or face; persistent diarrhea or constipation; or unusual weakness or bleeding. **Pregnancy/breast-feeding precautions:** Inform prescriber if you are or intend to become pregnant. Breast-feeding is not recommended.

Geriatric Considerations: Start dosing low and increase as necessary. The FDA recently approved a stronger warning about hepatotoxicity in the labeling of chlorzoxazone. Because it can cause unpredictable, fatal hepatic toxicity, the use of chlorzoxazone should be avoided.

Pregnancy Risk Factor: C
Lactation: Excretion in breast milk unknown/not recommended

Cholestyramine Resin *(koe LES teer a meen REZ in)*

U.S. Brand Names Prevalite®; Questran®; Questran® Light
Generic Available Yes
Pharmacologic Category Antilipemic Agent, Bile Acid Sequestrant
Use Adjunct in the management of primary hypercholesterolemia; pruritus associated with elevated levels of bile acids; diarrhea associated with excess fecal bile acids; binding toxicologic agents; pseudomembranous colitis

Mechanism of Action/Effect Forms a nonabsorbable complex with bile acids in the intestine, releasing chloride ions in the process; inhibits enterohepatic reuptake of intestinal bile salts and thereby increases the fecal loss of bile salt-bound low density lipoprotein cholesterol

Contraindications Hypersensitivity to bile acid sequestering resins or any component of the formulation; complete biliary obstruction; bowel obstruction

Warnings/Precautions Not to be taken simultaneously with many other medicines (decreased absorption). Treat any diseases contributing to hypercholesterolemia first. May interfere with fat-soluble vitamins (A, D, E, K) and folic acid. Chronic use may be associated with bleeding problems (especially in high doses). May produce or exacerbate constipation problems. Fecal impaction may occur. Hemorrhoids may be worsened.

Drug Interactions
Decreased Effect:
Cholestyramine can reduce the absorption of numerous medications when used concurrently. Give other medications 1 hour before or 4-6 hours after giving cholestyramine. Medications which may be affected include HMG-CoA reductase inhibitors, thiazide diuretics, propranolol (and potentially other beta-blockers), corticosteroids, thyroid

hormones, digoxin, valproic acid, NSAIDs, loop diuretics, sulfonylureas, troglitazone (and potentially other agents in this class).

Warfarin and other oral anticoagulants: Hypoprothrombinemic effects may be reduced by cholestyramine. Separate administration times (as detailed above) and monitor INR closely when initiating or discontinuing.

Nutritional/Ethanol Interactions
Food: Cholestyramine (especially high doses or long-term therapy) may decrease the absorption of folic acid, calcium, and iron.
Herb/Nutraceutical: Cholestyramine (especially high doses or long-term therapy) may decrease the absorption of fat-soluble vitamins (vitamins A, D, E, and K).

Lab Interactions Increased prothrombin time (S); decreased cholesterol (S), iron (B)

Adverse Reactions
>10%: Gastrointestinal: Constipation, heartburn, nausea, vomiting, stomach pain
1% to 10%:
Central nervous system: Headache
Gastrointestinal: Belching, bloating, diarrhea

Overdosage/Toxicology Symptoms of overdose include GI obstruction. Treatment is supportive.

Pharmacodynamics/Kinetics
Onset of Action: Peak effect: 21 days
Absorption: None
Excretion: Feces (as insoluble complex with bile acids)

Dosing
Adults & Elderly: Dyslipidemia: Oral (dosages are expressed in terms of anhydrous resin): 4 g 1-2 times/day to a maximum of 16-24 g/day (and a maximum of 6 times/day)
Pediatrics: Dyslipidemia: Oral (dosages are expressed in terms of anhydrous resin): Children: 240 mg/kg/day in 3 divided doses; need to titrate dose depending on indication
Renal Impairment: Not removed by hemo- or peritoneal dialysis. Supplemental doses not necessary with dialysis or continuous arteriovenous or venovenous hemofiltration effects.

Available Dosage Forms
Powder for oral suspension: 4 g of resin/5.7 g of powder (5.7 g packets, 240 g can) [light formulation]; 4 g of resin/9 g of powder (9 g packets, 378 g can)
Prevalite®: 4 g of resin/5.5 g of powder (5.5 g packets, 231 g can) [contains phenylalanine 14.1 mg/5.5 g; orange flavor]
Questran®: 4 g of resin/9 g of powder (9 g packets, 378 g can)
Questran® Light: 4 g of resin/5 g of powder (5 g packets, 210 g can) [contains phenylalanine 16.8 g/5 g]

Monitoring and Teaching Issues
Physical Assessment: Assess other medications patient may be taking for effectiveness and interactions. Monitor laboratory results, therapeutic effectiveness, and adverse reactions periodically throughout therapy. Assess knowledge/teach patient appropriate use, interventions to reduce side effects, and adverse symptoms to report.
Monitoring Laboratory Tests: Serum cholesterol and triglyceride levels before initiating treatment and periodically throughout treatment.
Patient Education: Take once or twice a day as directed. Do not take the powder in its dry form; mix with fluid, applesauce, pudding, or jello. Take other medications 1 hour before or 4-6 hours after cholestyramine. Ongoing medical follow-up and laboratory tests may be required. You may experience GI effects (these should resolve after continued use); nausea and vomiting (small frequent meals, frequent mouth care, sucking lozenges, or chewing gum may help); or constipation (increased exercise, fluids, fruit, or fiber may help; consult prescriber about use of stool softener or laxative). Report unusual stomach cramping, pain or blood in stool; unresolved nausea, vomiting, or constipation. **Pregnancy/breast-feeding precautions:** Inform prescriber if you are or intend to become pregnant. Consult prescriber if breast-feeding.
Dietary Considerations: Supplementation of vitamins A, D, E, and K, folic acid, and iron may be required with high-dose, long-term therapy.
Questran® Light contains phenylalanine 16.8 g/5 g powder.
Prevalite® contains phenylalanine 14.1 g/5.5 g powder.
Geriatric Considerations: The definition of and, therefore, when to treat hyperlipidemia in the elderly is a controversial issue. Treatment is best reserved for those who are unable to obtain a desirable plasma cholesterol level by diet alone and for whom the benefits of treatment are believed to outweigh the potential adverse effects, drug interactions, and cost of treatment.
Pregnancy Risk Factor: C
Lactation: Does not enter breast milk/use caution

Administration
Oral: Mix powder with water or other fluid prior to administration; not to be taken in dry form. Suspension should not be sipped or held in mouth for prolonged periods (may cause tooth discoloration or enamel decay).
Storage: Store powder at controlled room temperature of 15°C to 30°C (59°F to 86°F). Mix contents of 1 packet or 1 level scoop of powder with 4-6 oz of beverage. Allow to stand 1-2 minutes prior to mixing. May also be mixed with highly-fluid soups, cereals, applesauce, etc. Suspension may be used for up to 48 hours after refrigeration.

Related Information
Hyperlipidemia Management *on page 1836*
Lipid-Lowering Agents *on page 1738*

Choline Magnesium Trisalicylate
(KOE leen mag NEE zhum trye sa LIS i late)
U.S. Brand Names Trilisate® [DSC]
Synonyms Tricosal
Generic Available Yes
Pharmacologic Category Salicylate
(Continued)

Choline Magnesium Trisalicylate *(Continued)*

Use Management of osteoarthritis, rheumatoid arthritis, and other arthritis; acute painful shoulder

Mechanism of Action/Effect Inhibits prostaglandin synthesis; acts on the hypothalamus heat-regulating center to reduce fever; blocks the generation of pain impulses

Contraindications Hypersensitivity to salicylates, other nonacetylated salicylates, other NSAIDs, or any component of the formulation; bleeding disorders; pregnancy (3rd trimester)

Warnings/Precautions Salicylate salts may not inhibit platelet aggregation and, therefore, should not be substituted for aspirin in the prophylaxis of thrombosis. Use with caution in patients with impaired renal function, dehydration, erosive gastritis, asthma, or peptic ulcer. Discontinue use 1 week prior to surgical procedures. Children and teenagers who have or are recovering from chickenpox or flu-like symptoms should not use this product. Changes in behavior (along with nausea and vomiting) may be an early sign of Reye's syndrome; patients should be instructed to contact their healthcare provider if these occur.

Elderly are a high-risk population for adverse effects from NSAIDs. As many as 60% of elderly can develop peptic ulceration and/or hemorrhage asymptomatically. Use lowest effective dose for shortest period possible. CNS adverse effects may be observed in the elderly at lower doses than younger adults.

Drug Interactions
Decreased Effect: Antacids may decrease choline magnesium trisalicylate absorption/ salicylate concentrations.
Increased Effect/Toxicity: Choline magnesium trisalicylate may increase the hypoprothrombinemic effect of warfarin.

Nutritional/Ethanol Interactions
Ethanol: Avoid ethanol (may enhance gastric mucosal irritation).
Food: May decrease the rate but not the extent of oral absorption.
Herb/Nutraceutical: Avoid cat's claw, dong quai, evening primrose, feverfew, garlic, ginger, ginkgo, red clover, horse chestnut, green tea, ginseng (all have additional antiplatelet activity). Limit curry powder, paprika, licorice, Benedictine liqueur, prunes, raisins, tea, and gherkins; may cause salicylate accumulation. These foods contain 6 mg salicylate/100 g.

Lab Interactions False-negative results for glucose oxidase urinary glucose tests (Clinistix®); false-positives using the cupric sulfate method (Clinitest®); also, interferes with Gerhardt test (urinary ketone analysis), VMA determination; 5-HIAA, xylose tolerance test, and T_3 and T_4; increased PBI; increased uric acid

Adverse Reactions
<20%:
Gastrointestinal: Nausea, vomiting, diarrhea, heartburn, dyspepsia, epigastric pain, constipation
Otic: Tinnitus
<2%:
Central nervous system: Headache, lightheadedness, dizziness, drowsiness, lethargy
Otic: Hearing impairment

Overdosage/Toxicology Symptoms of overdose include tinnitus, vomiting, acute renal failure, hyperthermia, irritability, seizures, coma, and metabolic acidosis. For acute ingestion, determine serum salicylate levels 6 hours after ingestion. Nomograms, such as the "Done" nomogram, may be helpful for estimating the severity of aspirin poisoning and directing treatment using serum salicylate levels. Treatment is based upon symptomatology.

Pharmacodynamics/Kinetics
Onset of Action: Peak effect: ~2 hours
Absorption: Stomach and small intestines
Time to Peak: Serum: ~2 hours
Half-Life Elimination: Dose dependent: Low dose: 2-3 hours; High dose: 30 hours

Dosing
Adults & Elderly: Arthritis, pain: Oral (based on total salicylate content): 500 mg to 1.5 g 2-3 times/day **or** 3 g at bedtime; usual maintenance dose: 1-4.5 g/day
Pediatrics: Children: Oral (based on total salicylate content): <37 kg: 50 mg/kg/day given in 2 divided doses; 2250 mg/day for heavier children
Renal Impairment: Avoid use in severe renal impairment.

Available Dosage Forms
Liquid: 500 mg/5 mL (240 mL) [choline salicylate 293 mg and magnesium salicylate 362 mg per 5 mL; cherry cordial flavor]
Tablet: 500 mg [choline salicylate 293 mg and magnesium salicylate 362 mg]; 750 mg [choline salicylate 440 mg and magnesium salicylate 544 mg]; 1000 mg [choline salicylate 587 mg and magnesium salicylate 725 mg]

Monitoring and Teaching Issues
Physical Assessment: Do not use for persons with allergic reaction to salicylates or other NSAIDs. Assess other medications patient may be taking for additive or adverse interactions. Monitor for effectiveness of pain relief. Monitor for signs of adverse reactions or overdose at beginning of therapy and periodically during long-term therapy. Assess knowledge/teach patient appropriate use. Teach patient to monitor for adverse reactions, adverse reactions to report, and appropriate interventions to reduce side effects.

Monitoring Laboratory Tests: Serum magnesium with high-dose therapy or in patients with impaired renal function, serum salicylate levels, renal function

Patient Education: Use exactly as directed; do not increase dose or frequency. Adverse reactions can occur with overuse. Take with food or milk. While using this medication, do not use alcohol, excessive amounts of vitamin C, or salicylate-containing foods (curry powder, prunes, raisins, tea, or licorice), other prescription or OTC medications containing aspirin or salicylate, or other NSAIDs without consulting prescriber. Maintain adequate hydration (2-3 L/day of fluids) unless instructed to restrict fluid intake. You may experience nausea, vomiting, gastric discomfort (frequent mouth care, small frequent meals, sucking lozenges, or chewing gum may help). GI bleeding, ulceration, or perforation can occur with or without pain. Stop taking medication and report ringing in ears; persistent stomach pain;

unresolved nausea or vomiting; respiratory difficulty or shortness of breath; or unusual bruising or bleeding (mouth, urine, stool); or skin rash. **Pregnancy/breast-feeding precautions:** Inform prescriber if you are or intend to become pregnant. Consult prescriber if breast-feeding.

Dietary Considerations: Take with food or large volume of water or milk to minimize GI upset. Liquid may be mixed with fruit juice just before drinking. Hypermagnesemia resulting from magnesium salicylate; avoid or use with caution in renal insufficiency.

Geriatric Considerations: Elderly are at high risk for adverse effects from nonsteroidal anti-inflammatory agents. As much as 60% of elderly can develop peptic ulceration and/or hemorrhage asymptomatically.

Pregnancy Risk Factor: C/D (3rd trimester)

Pregnancy Issues: Animal reproduction studies have not been conducted. Due to the known effects of other salicylates (closure of ductus arteriosus), use during late pregnancy should be avoided.

Lactation: Enters breast milk/use caution

Breast-Feeding Issues: Excreted in breast milk; peak levels occur 9-12 hours after dose. Use caution if used during breast-feeding.

Administration
 Oral: Liquid may be mixed with fruit juice just before drinking. Do not administer with antacids. Take with a full glass of water and remain in an upright position for 15-30 minutes after administration.
 Storage: Store at controlled room temperature of 15°C to 30°C (59°F to 86°F).

Related Information
 Nonsalicylate / Nonsteroidal Anti-inflammatory Agents *on page 1743*

♦ **Chondroitin Sulfate - Sodium Hyaluronate** *see page 1625*
♦ **Chooz® [OTC]** *see Calcium Carbonate on page 235*
♦ **Choriogonadotropin Alfa** *see Chorionic Gonadotropin (Recombinant) on page 320*

Chorionic Gonadotropin (Human)
(kor ee ON ik goe NAD oh troe pin, HYU man)

U.S. Brand Names Novarel™; Pregnyl®
Synonyms CG; hCG
Generic Available Yes
Pharmacologic Category Ovulation Stimulator
Use Induces ovulation and pregnancy in anovulatory, infertile females; treatment of hypogonadotropic hypogonadism, prepubertal cryptorchidism; spermatogenesis induction with follitropin alfa or follitropin beta
Mechanism of Action/Effect Stimulates production of gonadal steroid hormones by causing production of androgen by the testis; as a substitute for luteinizing hormone (LH) to stimulate ovulation
Contraindications Hypersensitivity to chorionic gonadotropin or any component of the formulation; precocious puberty; prostatic carcinoma or similar neoplasms
Warnings/Precautions Use with caution in asthma, seizure disorders, migraine, cardiac or renal disease. **Not** effective in the treatment of obesity.
Adverse Reactions
 1% to 10%:
  Central nervous system: Mental depression, fatigue
  Endocrine & metabolic: Pelvic pain, ovarian cysts, enlargement of breasts, precocious puberty
  Local: Pain at the injection site
  Neuromuscular & skeletal: Premature closure of epiphyses
Pharmacodynamics/Kinetics
 Half-Life Elimination: Biphasic: Initial: 11 hours; Terminal: 23 hours
 Excretion: Urine (as unchanged drug) within 3-4 days
Dosing
 Adults & Elderly:
  Use with menotropins to stimulate spermatogenesis: I.M.: 5000 units 3 times/week for 4-6 months. With the beginning of menotropins therapy, hCG dose is continued at 2000 units 2 times/week.
  Induction of ovulation and pregnancy: I.M.: 5000-10,000 units 1 day following last dose of menotropins
  Spermatogenesis induction: Male: I.M.: Initial: 1500 int. units twice weekly to normalize serum testosterone levels. If no response in 8 weeks, increase dose to 3000 int. units twice weekly. After normalization of testosterone levels, combine with follitropin beta (Follistim®). Continue hCG at same dose used to normalize testosterone levels. Treatment response was noted at up to 12 months.
 Pediatrics:
  Prepubertal cryptorchidism: I.M.: Children: 1000-2000 units/m²/dose 3 times/week for 3 weeks **or** 4000 units 3 times/week for 3 weeks **or** 5000 units every second day for 4 injections **or** 500 units 3 times/week for 4-6 weeks
  Hypogonadotropic hypogonadism: I.M.: Children: 500-1000 units 3 times/week for 3 weeks, followed by the same dose twice weekly for 3 weeks **or** 1000-2000 units 3 times/week **or** 4000 units 3 times/week for 6-9 months; reduce dosage to 2000 units 3 times/week for additional 3 months.
Available Dosage Forms Injection, powder for reconstitution: 10,000 units [packaged with diluent; diluent contains benzyl alcohol and mannitol]
  Novarel™: 10,000 units [packaged with diluent; diluent contains benzyl alcohol and mannitol]
  Pregnyl®: 10,000 units [packaged with diluent; diluent contains benzyl alcohol]
Monitoring and Teaching Issues
 Physical Assessment: Assess therapeutic effectiveness (according to purpose for use) and adverse response regularly during long-term therapy. Teach patient proper use if (Continued)

Chorionic Gonadotropin (Human) *(Continued)*

self-administered (appropriate injection technique and syringe/needle disposal), possible side effects/appropriate interventions, and adverse symptoms to report.

Patient Education: This medication can only be administered by injection. If self-administered, follow instruction for reconstitution, injection, and needle disposal. Use exactly as directed; do not alter dosage or miss a dose. May cause headache, depression, irritability, or restlessness (use caution when driving or engaging in potentially hazardous tasks until response to drug is known). Contact prescriber if symptoms are severe or do not resolve with use. Contact prescriber if breasts swell; if you experience swelling of legs or feet; or if there is pain, redness, or swelling at injection site. **Pregnancy/breast-feeding precautions:** Inform prescriber if you are or intend to become pregnant. Consult prescriber if breast-feeding.

Pregnancy Risk Factor: C

Lactation: Excretion in breast milk unknown/unlikely to be used

Administration

I.M.: I.M. administration only

Reconstitution: Following reconstitution with the provided diluent, solutions are stable for 30-90 days, depending on the specific preparation, when stored at 2°C to 15°C.

Chorionic Gonadotropin (Recombinant)

(kor ee ON ik goe NAD oh troe pin ree KOM be nant)

U.S. Brand Names Ovidrel®

Synonyms Choriogonadotropin Alfa; r-hCG

Generic Available No

Pharmacologic Category Gonadotropin; Ovulation Stimulator

Use As part of an assisted reproductive technology (ART) program, induces ovulation in infertile females who have been pretreated with follicle stimulating hormones (FSH); induces ovulation and pregnancy in infertile females when the cause of infertility is functional

Contraindications Hypersensitivity to hCG preparations or any component of the formulation; primary ovarian failure; uncontrolled thyroid or adrenal dysfunction; uncontrolled organic intracranial lesion (ie, pituitary tumor); abnormal uterine bleeding, ovarian cyst or enlargement of undetermined origin; sex hormone dependent tumors; pregnancy

Warnings/Precautions For use by infertility specialists; may cause ovarian hyperstimulation syndrome (OHSS); if severe, treatment should be discontinued and patient should be hospitalized. OHSS results in a rapid (<24 hours to 7 days) accumulation of fluid in the peritoneal cavity, thorax, and possibly the pericardium, which may become more severe if pregnancy occurs; monitor for ovarian enlargement; use may lead to multiple births; risk of arterial thromboembolism with hCG products; safety and efficacy in pediatric and geriatric patients have not been established.

Drug Interactions

Increased Effect/Toxicity: Specific drug interaction studies have not been conducted.

Lab Interactions May interfere with interpretation of pregnancy tests; may cross-react with radioimmunoassay of luteinizing hormone and other gonadotropins

Adverse Reactions

2% to 10%:

Endocrine & metabolic: Ovarian cyst (3%), ovarian hyperstimulation (<2% to 3%)

Gastrointestinal: Abdominal pain (3% to 4%), nausea (3%), vomiting (3%)

Local: Injection site: Pain (8%), bruising (3% to 5%), reaction (<2% to 3%), inflammation (<2% to 2%)

Miscellaneous: Postoperative pain (5%)

<2%:

Cardiovascular: Cardiac arrhythmia, heart murmur

Central nervous system: Dizziness, emotional lability, fever, headache, insomnia, malaise

Dermatologic: Pruritus, rash

Endocrine & metabolic: Breast pain, hot flashes, hyperglycemia, intermenstrual bleeding, vaginal hemorrhage

Gastrointestinal: Abdominal enlargement, diarrhea, flatulence

Genitourinary: Cervical carcinoma, cervical lesion, dysuria, genital herpes, genital moniliasis, leukorrhea, urinary incontinence, urinary tract infection, vaginitis

Hematologic: Leukocytosis

Neuromuscular & skeletal: Back pain, paresthesia

Renal: Albuminuria

Respiratory: Cough, pharyngitis, upper respiratory tract infection

Miscellaneous: Ectopic pregnancy, hiccups

In addition, the following have been reported with menotropin therapy: Adnexal torsion, hemoperitoneum, mild to moderate ovarian enlargement, pulmonary and vascular complications. Ovarian neoplasms have also been reported (rare) with multiple drug regimens used for ovarian induction (relationship not established).

Pharmacodynamics/Kinetics

Bioavailability: 40%

Time to Peak: 12-24 hours

Half-Life Elimination: Initial: 4 hours; Terminal: 29 hours

Excretion: Urine (10% of dose)

Dosing

Adults: Assisted reproductive technologies (ART) and ovulation induction in females: SubQ: 250 mcg given 1 day following the last dose of follicle stimulating agent. Use only after adequate follicular development has been determined. Hold treatment when there is an excessive ovarian response.

Elderly: Safety and efficacy have not been established.

Renal Impairment: Safety and efficacy have not been established.

Hepatic Impairment: Safety and efficacy have not been established.

Available Dosage Forms

Injection, powder for reconstitution: 285 mcg [packaged with 1 mL SWFI; delivers 250 mcg r-hCG following reconstitution] [DSC]

Injection, solution: 257.5 mcg/0.515 mL (0.515 mL) [prefilled syringe; delivers 250 mcg r-hCG/0.5 mL]

Monitoring and Teaching Issues

Physical Assessment: For use only under the supervision/direction of an infertility physician. Monitor for adverse reactions. Teach patient proper use if self-administered (storage, reconstitution, injection technique, needle/syringe disposal; recommend return demonstration), monitoring requirements, interventions to reduce side effects, and adverse reactions to report. **Pregnancy risk factor X:** Determine that patient is not pregnant before beginning treatment and monitor ovulation closely during treatment.

Patient Education: Note that there is a risk of multiple births associated with treatment. This drug must be administered exactly as scheduled (1 day following last dose of follicle stimulating agent); maintain a calendar of treatment days. Follow administration directions exactly. Keep all ultrasound and laboratory appointments as instructed by prescriber. Avoid strenuous exercise, especially those with pelvic involvement. You may experience nausea, vomiting, or GI upset (small frequent meals, frequent mouth care, sucking lozenges, or chewing gum may help), hot flashes (cool clothes, cool room, adequate rest may help) if persistent consult prescriber. Report immediately any persistent abdominal pain, vomiting, or acute pelvic pain; chest pain or palpitations; shortness of breath; or urinary tract or vaginal infection or urinary incontinence. **Pregnancy/breast-feeding precautions:** Do not take this medicine if you are pregnant and report to prescriber immediately if you suspect you are pregnant. Consult prescriber if breast-feeding.

Pregnancy Risk Factor: X

Pregnancy Issues: Ectopic pregnancy, premature labor, postpartum fever, and spontaneous abortion have been reported in clinical trials. Congenital abnormalities have also been observed, however, the incidence is similar during natural conception.

Lactation: Excretion in breast milk unknown/use caution

Administration

Reconstitution: Powder for reconstitution: Mix vial with 1 mL sterile water for injection. Gently mix by rotating vial to dissolve powder; do not shake. Use immediately following reconstitution.

Storage:

Powder for reconstitution: Store in original package under refrigeration or at room temperature of 2°C to 25°C (36°F to 77°F). Protect from light.

Prefilled syringe: Prior to dispensing, store at 2°C to 8°C (36°F to 46°F). Patient may store at 25°C (77°F) for up to 30 days. Protect from light.

Additional Information Clinical studies have shown r-hCG to be clinically and statistically equivalent to urinary-derived hCG products.

♦ **Cialis®** see Tadalafil on page 1422

♦ **Cidecin** see Daptomycin on page 404

Cidofovir (si DOF o veer)

U.S. Brand Names Vistide®

Generic Available No

Pharmacologic Category Antiviral Agent

Use Treatment of cytomegalovirus (CMV) retinitis in patients with acquired immunodeficiency syndrome (AIDS). **Note:** Should be administered with probenecid.

Mechanism of Action/Effect Nucleotide analog that selectively inhibits viral DNA polymerase, suppressing viral DNA synthesis

Contraindications Hypersensitivity to cidofovir; history of clinically-severe hypersensitivity to probenecid or other sulfa-containing medications; serum creatinine >1.5 mg/dL; Cl_{cr} <55 mL/minute; urine protein ≥100 mg/dL (≥2+ proteinuria); use with or within 7 days of nephrotoxic agents; direct intraocular injection

Warnings/Precautions Dose-dependent nephrotoxicity requires dose adjustment or discontinuation if changes in renal function occur during therapy (eg, proteinuria, glycosuria, decreased serum phosphate, uric acid or bicarbonate, and elevated creatinine); neutropenia and ocular hypotony have also occurred; safety and efficacy have not been established in children or the elderly; administration must be accompanied by oral probenecid and intravenous saline prehydration; prepare admixtures in a class two laminar flow hood, wearing protective gear; dispose of cidofovir as directed.

Drug Interactions

Increased Effect/Toxicity: Drugs with nephrotoxic potential (eg, amphotericin B, aminoglycosides, foscarnet, and I.V. pentamidine) should not be used with or within 7 days of cidofovir therapy. Due to concomitant probenecid administration, temporarily discontinue or decrease zidovudine dose by 50% on the day of cidofovir administration only.

Adverse Reactions

>10%:

Central nervous system: Chills, fever, headache, pain

Dermatologic: Alopecia, rash

Gastrointestinal: Nausea, vomiting, diarrhea, anorexia

Hematologic: Anemia, neutropenia

Neuromuscular & skeletal: Weakness

Ocular: Intraocular pressure decreased, iritis, ocular hypotony, uveitis

Renal: Creatinine increased, proteinuria, renal toxicity

Respiratory: Cough, dyspnea

Miscellaneous: Infection, oral moniliasis, serum bicarbonate decreased

1% to 10%:

Renal: Fanconi syndrome

(Continued)

Cidofovir *(Continued)*

Respiratory: Pneumonia

Frequency not defined (limited to important or life-threatening reactions):

Cardiovascular: Cardiomyopathy, cardiovascular disorder, CHF, edema, postural hypotension, shock, syncope, tachycardia

Central nervous system: Agitation, amnesia, anxiety, confusion, convulsion, dizziness, hallucinations, insomnia, malaise, vertigo

Dermatologic: Photosensitivity reaction, skin discoloration, urticaria

Endocrine & metabolic: Adrenal cortex insufficiency

Gastrointestinal: Abdominal pain, aphthous stomatitis, colitis, constipation, dysphagia, fecal incontinence, gastritis, GI hemorrhage, gingivitis, melena, proctitis, splenomegaly, stomatitis, tongue discoloration

Genitourinary: Urinary incontinence

Hematologic: Hypochromic anemia, leukocytosis, leukopenia, lymphadenopathy, lymphoma-like reaction, pancytopenia, thrombocytopenia, thrombocytopenic purpura

Hepatic: Hepatomegaly, hepatosplenomegaly, jaundice, liver function tests abnormal, liver damage, liver necrosis

Local: Injection site reaction

Neuromuscular & skeletal: Tremor

Ocular: Amblyopia, blindness, cataract, conjunctivitis, corneal lesion, diplopia, vision abnormal

Otic: Hearing loss

Miscellaneous: Allergic reaction, sepsis

Overdosage/Toxicology Hemodialysis and hydration may reduce drug plasma concentrations. Probenecid may assist in decreasing active tubular secretion.

Pharmacodynamics/Kinetics

Protein Binding: <6%

Half-Life Elimination: Plasma: ~2.6 hours

Metabolism: Minimal; phosphorylation occurs intracellularly

Excretion: Urine

Pharmacokinetic Note: Data is based on a combination of cidofovir administered with probenecid.

Dosing

Adults & Elderly: Treatment of cytomegalovirus (CMV) retinitis: I.V.:

Induction treatment: 5 mg/kg once weekly for 2 consecutive weeks

Maintenance treatment: 5 mg/kg administered once every 2 weeks

Note: Probenecid must be administered orally with each dose of cidofovir.

Probenecid dose: 2 g 3 hours prior to cidofovir dose, 1 g 2 hours and 8 hours after completion of the infusion; patients should also receive 1 L of normal saline intravenously prior to each infusion of cidofovir; saline should be infused over 1-2 hours.

Renal Impairment:

Changes in renal function during therapy: If the creatinine increases by 0.3-0.4 mg/dL, reduce the cidofovir dose to 3 mg/kg; discontinue therapy for increases ≥0.5 mg/dL or development of ≥3+ proteinuria

Pre-existing renal impairment: Use is contraindicated with serum creatinine >1.5 mg/dL, Cl$_{cr}$ <55 mL/minute, or urine protein ≥100 mg/dL (≥2+ proteinuria)

Available Dosage Forms Injection, solution [preservative free]: 75 mg/mL (5 mL)

Monitoring and Teaching Issues

Physical Assessment: Assess patient allergy history (sulfa) prior to beginning therapy. See Warnings/Precautions for use cautions (eg, administration must be accompanied by oral probenecid and intravenous saline prehydration). Assess potential for interactions with other pharmacological agents patient may be taking (especially anything that may be nephrotoxic; see Drug Interactions). Infusion site should be monitored closely to avoid extravasation. Assess results of laboratory tests with each dose, therapeutic effectiveness (ocular symptoms, visual acuity), and adverse response (eg, CNS changes, anemia, renal damage [elevated creatine]; see Adverse Reactions) regularly during therapy. For patients with diabetes, serum glucose should be monitored closely (may cause hyperglycemia). Teach patient possible side effects/appropriate interventions and adverse symptoms to report (eg, infection, persistent gastrointestinal disturbance, change in vision, eye pain, unusual cough or dyspnea; see Patient Education).

Monitoring Laboratory Tests: Serum creatinine, serum bicarbonate, acid-base status, urine protein, WBC should be monitored with each dose; monitor intraocular pressure frequently

Patient Education: Inform prescriber of all prescriptions, OTC medications, or herbal products you are taking, and any allergies you have. Do not take any new medication during therapy unless approved by prescriber. This drug can only be administered I.V. Report immediately any pain, stinging, swelling at infusion site. You may be more susceptible to infection (avoid crowds and exposure to infection and do not have any vaccinations without consulting prescriber). May cause hair loss (reversible); headache, anxiety, confusion (use caution when driving or engaging in tasks that require alertness until response to drug is known); diarrhea (buttermilk or yogurt may help); nausea, heartburn, or vomiting (small frequent meals, frequent mouth care, sucking lozenges, or chewing gum may help); constipation (increased exercise, fluids, fruit, or fiber may help); or postural hypotension (use caution changing from lying to sitting or standing position and when climbing stairs). Report severe unresolved vomiting, constipation, or diarrhea; chills, fever, signs of infection; respiratory difficulty or unusual coughing; palpitations, chest pain, or syncope; CNS changes (eg, hallucinations, depression, excessive sedation, amnesia, seizures, insomnia); vision changes; or other severe side effects. **Pregnancy/breast-feeding precautions:** Inform prescriber if you are pregnant and do not get pregnant while taking this medicine. Consult prescriber for appropriate contraceptives. Do not breast-feed.

Geriatric Considerations: Since elderly individuals frequently have reduced kidney function, particular attention should be paid to assessing renal function before and frequently during administration.

Pregnancy Risk Factor: C

Pregnancy Issues: Cidofovir was shown to be teratogenic and embryotoxic in animal studies, some at doses which also produced maternal toxicity. Reduced testes weight and hypospermia were also noted in animal studies. There are no adequate and well-controlled studies in pregnant women; use during pregnancy only if the potential benefit to the mother outweighs the possible risk to the fetus. Women of childbearing potential should use effective contraception during therapy and for 1 month following treatment. Males should use a barrier contraceptive during therapy and for 3 months following treatment.

Lactation: Excretion in breast milk unknown/contraindicated

Breast-Feeding Issues: The CDC recommends **not** to breast-feed if diagnosed with HIV to avoid postnatal transmission of the virus.

Administration

I.V.: For I.V. infusion only. Infuse over 1 hour. Hydrate with 1 L of 0.9% NS I.V. prior to cidofovir infusion; a second liter may be administered over a 1- to 3-hour period immediately following infusion, if tolerated

Reconstitution: Dilute dose in NS 100 mL prior to infusion.

Compatibility: Stable in $D_5^1/_4$NS, D_5W, NS

Storage: Store at controlled room temperature 20°C to 25°C (68°F to 77°F). Store admixtures under refrigeration for ≤24 hours. Cidofovir infusion admixture should be administered within 24 hours of preparation at room temperature or refrigerated. Admixtures should be allowed to equilibrate to room temperature prior to use.

Cilostazol (sil OH sta zol)

U.S. Brand Names Pletal®

Synonyms OPC-13013

Generic Available Yes

Pharmacologic Category Antiplatelet Agent; Phosphodiesterase Enzyme Inhibitor

Medication Safety Issues

Sound-alike/look-alike issues:

Pletal® may be confused with Plendil®

Use Symptomatic management of peripheral vascular disease, primarily intermittent claudication; currently being investigated for the treatment of acute coronary syndromes and for graft patency improvement in percutaneous coronary interventions with or without stenting

Unlabeled/Investigational Use Investigational: Treatment of acute coronary syndromes and for graft patency improvement in percutaneous coronary interventions with or without stenting

Mechanism of Action/Effect Cilostazol and its metabolites are inhibitors of phosphodiesterase III leading to inhibition of platelet aggregation and vasodilation. Other effects of phosphodiesterase III inhibition include increased cardiac contractility, accelerated AV nodal conduction, increased ventricular automaticity, heart rate, and coronary blood flow.

Contraindications Hypersensitivity to cilostazol or any component of the formulation; heart failure (of any severity)

Warnings/Precautions Use with caution in patients receiving platelet aggregation inhibitors (effects are unknown), hepatic impairment (not studied). Use with caution in patients receiving inhibitors hepatic cytochrome P450 enzymes, particularly CYP3A4 (such as ketoconazole or erythromycin) or inhibitors of CYP2C19 (such as omeprazole).

Drug Interactions

Cytochrome P450 Effect: **Substrate** of CYP1A2 (minor), 2C19 (minor), 2D6 (minor), 3A4 (major)

Increased Effect/Toxicity: Cilostazol serum concentrations may be increased by erythromycin, diltiazem, and omeprazole. Increased concentrations of cilostazol may be anticipated during concurrent therapy with other inhibitors of CYP3A4 (ie, clarithromycin, ketoconazole, itraconazole, fluconazole, miconazole, fluvoxamine, fluoxetine, nefazodone, and sertraline) or inhibitors of CYP2C19. Aspirin-induced inhibition of platelet aggregation is potentiated by concurrent cilostazol. The effect on platelet aggregation with other antiplatelet drugs is unknown.

Nutritional/Ethanol Interactions Food: Taking cilostazol with a high-fat meal may increase peak concentration by 90%. Avoid concurrent ingestion of grapefruit juice due to the potential to inhibit CYP3A4.

Adverse Reactions

>10%:

Central nervous system: Headache (27% to 34%)

Gastrointestinal: Abnormal stools (12% to 15%), diarrhea (12% to 19%)

Miscellaneous: Infection (10% to 14%)

2% to 10%:

Cardiovascular: Peripheral edema (7% to 9%), palpitation (5% to 10%), tachycardia (4%)

Central nervous system: Dizziness (9% to 10%)

Gastrointestinal: Dyspepsia (6%), nausea (6% to 7%), abdominal pain (4% to 5%), flatulence (2% to 3%)

Neuromuscular & skeletal: Back pain (6% to 7%), myalgia (2% to 3%)

Respiratory: Rhinitis (7% to 12%), pharyngitis (7% to 10%), cough (3% to 4%)

Overdosage/Toxicology Experience with overdosage in humans is limited. Headache, diarrhea, hypotension, tachycardia, and/or cardiac arrhythmias may occur. Treatment is symptomatic and supportive. Hemodialysis is unlikely to be of value. In some animal models, high-dose or long-term administration was associated with a variety of cardiovascular lesions, including endocardial hemorrhage, hemosiderin deposition and left ventricular fibrosis, coronary arteritis, and periarteritis.

Pharmacodynamics/Kinetics

Onset of Action: 2-4 weeks; may require up to 12 weeks

Protein Binding: 97% to 98%

Half-Life Elimination: 11-13 hours

Metabolism: Hepatic via CYP3A4 (primarily), 1A2, 2C19, and 2D6; at least one metabolite has significant activity

(Continued)

Cilostazol (Continued)

Excretion: Urine (74%) and feces (20%) as metabolites

Dosing

Adults & Elderly: Peripheral vascular disease: Oral: 100 mg twice daily taken at least 30 minutes before or 2 hours after breakfast and dinner; dosage should be reduced to 50 mg twice daily during concurrent therapy with inhibitors of CYP3A4 or CYP2C19 (see Drug Interactions).

Available Dosage Forms Tablet: 50 mg, 100 mg

Monitoring and Teaching Issues

Physical Assessment: Assess effectiveness and interactions of other medications patient may be taking. Monitor effectiveness of therapy and adverse reactions at beginning of therapy and periodically with long-term use. Assess knowledge/teach patient appropriate use, interventions to reduce side effects, and adverse symptoms to report.

Patient Education: Use exactly as directed; do not discontinue without consulting prescriber. Beneficial effect may take between 2-12 weeks. Take on empty stomach (30 minutes before or 2 hours after meals). Do not take with grapefruit juice. You may experience nervousness, dizziness, or fatigue (use caution when driving or engaging in tasks requiring alertness until response to treatment is known); nausea, vomiting, or flatulence (small frequent meals, frequent mouth care, chewing gum or sucking hard candy may help); or postural hypotension (change position slowly when rising from sitting or lying position or climbing stairs). Report chest pain, palpitations, unusual heartbeat, or swelling of extremities; unusual bleeding; unresolved GI upset or pain; dizziness, nervousness, sleeplessness, or fatigue; muscle cramping or tremor; unusual cough; or other adverse effects. **Pregnancy/breast-feeding precautions:** Inform prescriber if you are or intend to become pregnant. Breast-feeding is not recommended.

Dietary Considerations: It is best to take cilostazol 30 minutes before or 2 hours after meals.

Pregnancy Risk Factor: C

Pregnancy Issues: In animal studies, abnormalities of the skeletal, renal and cardiovascular system were increased. In addition, the incidence of stillbirth and decreased birth weights were increased.

Lactation: Excretion in breast milk unknown/not recommended

Breast-Feeding Issues: It is not known whether cilostazol is excreted in human milk. Because of the potential risk to nursing infants, a decision to discontinue the drug or discontinue nursing should be made.

♦ Ciloxan® see Ciprofloxacin on page 327

Cimetidine (sye MET i deen)

U.S. Brand Names Tagamet®; Tagamet® HB 200 [OTC]

Generic Available Yes

Pharmacologic Category Histamine H_2 Antagonist

Medication Safety Issues

Sound-alike/look-alike issues:

Cimetidine may be confused with simethicone

Use Short-term treatment of active duodenal ulcers and benign gastric ulcers; long-term prophylaxis of duodenal ulcer; gastric hypersecretory states; gastroesophageal reflux; prevention of upper GI bleeding in critically-ill patients; labeled for OTC use for prevention or relief of heartburn, acid indigestion, or sour stomach

Unlabeled/Investigational Use Part of a multidrug regimen for *H. pylori* eradication to reduce the risk of duodenal ulcer recurrence

Mechanism of Action/Effect Competitive inhibition of histamine at H_2-receptors of the gastric parietal cells resulting in reduced gastric acid secretion, gastric volume and hydrogen ion concentration reduced

Contraindications Hypersensitivity to cimetidine, any component of the formulation, or other H_2 antagonists

Warnings/Precautions Adjust dosages in renal/hepatic impairment or patients receiving drugs metabolized through the cytochrome P450 system.

Drug Interactions

Cytochrome P450 Effect: Inhibits CYP1A2 (moderate), 2C8/9 (weak), 2C19 (moderate), 2D6 (moderate), 2E1 (weak), 3A4 (moderate)

Decreased Effect: Cimetidine may decrease the levels/effects of CYP2D6 prodrug substrates (eg, codeine, hydrocodone, oxycodone, and tramadol). Ketoconazole, fluconazole, itraconazole (especially capsule) decrease serum concentration; avoid concurrent use with H_2 antagonists. Delavirdine's absorption is decreased; avoid concurrent use with H_2 antagonists.

Increased Effect/Toxicity: Cimetidine may increase the levels/effects of aminophylline, amphetamines, selected beta-blockers, selected benzodiazepines, calcium channel blockers, citalopram, cyclosporine, dextromethorphan, diazepam, ergot derivatives, fluoxetine, fluvoxamine, lidocaine, methsuximide, mexiletine, mirtazapine, nateglinide, nefazodone, paroxetine, phenytoin, propranolol, risperidone, ritonavir, ropinirole, sertraline, sildenafil (and other PDE-5 inhibitors), tacrolimus, theophylline, thioridazine, tricyclic antidepressants, trifluoperazine, venlafaxine, and other CYP1A2, 2C19, or 2D6 substrates.

Cimetidine increases warfarin's effect in a dose-related manner, and may increase levels/effects of meperidine, metronidazole, moricizine, procainamide, propafenone, quinidine, quinolone antibiotics, tacrine, and triamterene. Cimetidine increases carmustine's myelotoxicity; avoid concurrent use.

Nutritional/Ethanol Interactions

Ethanol: Avoid ethanol (may enhance gastric mucosal irritation).

Food: Cimetidine may increase serum caffeine levels if taken with caffeine. Cimetidine peak serum levels may be decreased if taken with food.

Herb/Nutraceutical: St John's wort may decrease cimetidine levels.

Lab Interactions Increased creatinine (S), AST, ALT

Adverse Reactions 1% to 10%:

Central nervous system: Dizziness, agitation, headache, drowsiness

Gastrointestinal: Diarrhea, nausea, vomiting

Overdosage/Toxicology Treatment is symptomatic and supportive. There is no reported experience with intentional overdose. Reported ingestion of 20 g have had transient side effects seen with recommended doses. Animal data has shown respiratory failure, tachycardia, muscle tremor, vomiting, restlessness, hypotension, salivation, emesis, and diarrhea.

Pharmacodynamics/Kinetics

Onset of Action: 1 hour

Duration of Action: 6 hours

Bioavailability: 60% to 70%

Time to Peak: Serum: Oral: 1-2 hours

Protein Binding: 20%

Half-Life Elimination: Neonates: 3.6 hours; Children: 1.4 hours; Adults: Normal renal function: 2 hours

Metabolism: Partially hepatic

Excretion: Primarily urine (as unchanged drug); feces (some)

Dosing

Adults & Elderly:

Short-term treatment of active ulcers:

Oral: 300 mg 4 times/day or 800 mg at bedtime or 400 mg twice daily for up to 8 weeks

I.M., I.V.: 300 mg every 6 hours or 37.5 mg/hour by continuous infusion; I.V. dosage should be adjusted to maintain an intragastric pH ≥5

Note: *Patients with active bleeding:* Give cimetidine as a continuous infusion (see above)

Duodenal ulcer prophylaxis: Oral: 400-800 mg at bedtime

Gastric hypersecretory conditions: Oral, I.M., I.V.: 300-600 mg every 6 hours; dosage not to exceed 2.4 g/day

Peptic ulcer disease eradication of *Helicobacter pylori* (unlabeled use): Oral: 400 mg twice daily; requires combination therapy with antibiotics

Heartburn, acid indigestion, sour stomach (OTC labeling): Oral: 200 mg up to twice daily; may take 30 minutes prior to eating foods or beverages expected to cause heartburn or indigestion

Pediatrics:

Oral, I.M., I.V.: 20-40 mg/kg/day in divided doses every 6 hours

Heartburn, acid indigestion, sour stomach (OTC labeling): Children ≥12 years: Oral: Refer to adult dosing.

Renal Impairment:

Cl_cr 10-50 mL/minute: Administer 50% of normal dose.

Cl_cr <10 mL/minute: Administer 25% of normal dose.

Slightly dialyzable (5% to 20%)

Hepatic Impairment: Usual dose is safe in mild liver disease but use with caution and in reduced dosage in severe liver disease. Increased risk of CNS toxicity in cirrhosis suggested by enhanced penetration of CNS.

Available Dosage Forms

Infusion, as hydrochloride [premixed in NS]: 300 mg (50 mL)

Injection, solution, as hydrochloride: 150 mg/mL (2 mL, 8 mL) [8 mL size contains benzyl alcohol]

Liquid, oral, as hydrochloride: 300 mg/5 mL (240 mL, 480 mL) [contains alcohol 2.8%; mint-peach flavor]

Tablet: 200 mg [OTC], 300 mg, 400 mg, 800 mg

Tagamet®: 300 mg, 400 mg

Tagamet® HB 200: 200 mg

Monitoring and Teaching Issues

Physical Assessment: Use caution in presence of renal or hepatic impairment (see Warnings/Precautions and Dosing). Assess potential for interactions with other pharmacological agents or herbal products patient may be taking (see Drug Interactions). **I.V.:** See Administration specifics. Assess results of laboratory tests, therapeutic effectiveness (according to purpose for use), and adverse effects (eg, changes in CNS [agitation], gastric bleeding; see Adverse Reactions) regularly during therapy. Teach patient proper use possible side effects/appropriate interventions and adverse symptoms to report (see Patient Education).

Monitoring Laboratory Tests: CBC, gastric pH, occult blood with GI bleeding; monitor renal function to correct dose.

Patient Education: Do not take any new medication during therapy unless approved by prescriber. Take with meals. Do not increase dose or frequency without consulting prescriber. To be effective, continue to take for the prescribed time (possibly 4-8 weeks) even though symptoms may have improved. Smoking decreases the effectiveness of cimetidine (stop smoking if possible). Avoid excess alcohol and caffeine. May cause headache, dizziness, agitation (use caution when driving or engaging in any potentially hazardous tasks until response to drug is known); nausea or vomiting (small frequent meals, frequent mouth care, chewing gum, or sucking lozenges may help); or diarrhea (buttermilk, boiled milk, or yogurt may help). Report CNS changes (confusion, agitation); persistent diarrhea; black tarry stools or coffee ground-like emesis; rash; unusual bleeding or bruising; sore throat; or fever, or other adverse reactions.

Geriatric Considerations: Patients diagnosed with PUD should be evaluated for *Helicobacter pylori*. When H₂-blockers are indicated, they are the preferred drugs for treating PUD in the elderly due to cost and ease of administration and reduced side effects.

(Continued)

Cimetidine *(Continued)*

Pregnancy Risk Factor: B

Lactation: Enters breast milk/compatible

Administration

Oral: Give with meals so that the drug's peak effect occurs at the proper time (peak inhibition of gastric acid secretion occurs at 1 and 3 hours after dosing in fasting subjects and approximately 2 hours in nonfasting subjects. This correlates well with the time food is no longer in the stomach offering a buffering effect). Stagger doses of antacids with cimetidine.

I.V.: May be administered as a slow I.V. push or preferably as an I.V. intermittent or I.V. continuous infusion. Administer each 300 mg (or fraction thereof) over a minimum of 5 minutes when giving I.V. push. Give intermittent infusion over 15-30 minutes for each 300 mg dose. Intermittent infusions are administered over 15-30 minutes at a final concentration not to exceed 6 mg/mL; for patients with an active bleed, preferred method of administration is continuous infusion.

Reconstitution: Stability at room temperature for prepared bags is 7 days. Stable in parenteral nutrition solutions for up to 7 days when protected from light.

Compatibility: Stable in D_5LR, $D_5\frac{1}{4}NS$, $D_5\frac{1}{2}NS$, D_5NS, D_5W, $D_{10}W$, $D_{10}NS$, LR, sodium bicarbonate 5%, NS

Y-site administration: Incompatible with allopurinol, amphotericin B cholesteryl sulfate complex, amsacrine, cefepime, indomethacin, warfarin

Compatibility in syringe: Incompatible with atropine/pentobarbital, cefamandole, cefazolin, chlorpromazine, ioxaglate meglumine and ioxaglate sodium, pentobarbital, secobarbital

Compatibility when admixed: Incompatible with amphotericin B, barbiturates

Storage: Intact vials of cimetidine should be stored at room temperature and protected from light. Cimetidine may precipitate from solution upon exposure to cold but can be redissolved by warming without degradation.

Stability at room temperature for premixed bags: Manufacturer expiration dating and out of overwrap stability: 15 days.

Related Information

Compatibility of Drugs *on page 1723*
Compatibility of Drugs in Syringe *on page 1725*

Cinacalcet *(sin a KAL cet)*

U.S. Brand Names Sensipar™

Synonyms AMG 073; Cinacalcet Hydrochloride

Generic Available No

Pharmacologic Category Calcimimetic

Use Treatment of secondary hyperparathyroidism in dialysis patients; treatment of hypercalcemia in patients with parathyroid carcinoma

Unlabeled/Investigational Use Primary hyperparathyroidism

Mechanism of Action/Effect Increases the sensitivity of the calcium-sensing receptor on the parathyroid gland

Contraindications Hypersensitivity to cinacalcet or any component of the formulation

Warnings/Precautions If hypocalcemia develops during treatment, consider initiating treatment or temporarily withholding cinacalcet. Use caution in patients with a seizure disorder; monitor calcium levels closely. Adynamic bone disease may develop if iPTH levels are suppressed (<100 pg/mL). Use caution in patients with hepatic impairment. Safety and efficacy have not been established in pediatric patients.

Drug Interactions

Cytochrome P450 Effect: Substrate of CYP1A2, 2D6, 3A4; **Inhibits** CYP2D6

Increased Effect/Toxicity: Cinacalcet increases levels of amitriptyline and nortriptyline. Ketoconazole may increase cinacalcet levels.

Nutritional/Ethanol Interactions Food: Food increases bioavailability.

Adverse Reactions

>10%:

Endocrine & metabolic: Hypocalcemia

Gastrointestinal: Nausea (31%), vomiting (27%), diarrhea (21%)

Neuromuscular & skeletal: Myalgia (15%)

1% to 10%:

Cardiovascular: Hypertension (7%)

Central nervous system: Dizziness (10%), seizure (1%)

Endocrine & metabolic: Testosterone decreased

Gastrointestinal: Anorexia (6%)

Neuromuscular & skeletal: Weakness (7%), chest pain (6%)

Overdosage/Toxicology Overdose may cause hypocalcemia. Signs and symptoms may include paresthesias, myalgias, cramping, tetany, and seizures. Treatment is symptom-directed and supportive. Cinacalcet is not removed by dialysis.

Pharmacodynamics/Kinetics

Time to Peak: Nadir in iPTH levels: 2-6 hours postdose

Protein Binding: 93% to 97%

Half-Life Elimination: Terminal: 30-40 hours

Metabolism: Hepatic via CYP3A4, 2D6, 1A2; forms inactive metabolites

Excretion: Urine 80% (as metabolites); feces 15%

Dosing

Adults: Note: Do not titrate dose more frequently than every 2-4 weeks.

Secondary hyperparathyroidism: Oral: Initial: 30 mg once daily (maximum daily dose: 180 mg); increase dose incrementally (60 mg, 90 mg, 120 mg, 180 mg once daily) as necessary to maintain iPTH level between 150-300 pg/mL.

Parathyroid carcinoma: Oral: Initial: 30 mg twice daily (maximum daily dose: 360 mg daily as 90 mg 4 times/day); increase dose incrementally (60 mg twice daily, 90 mg twice daily, 90 mg 4 times/day) as necessary to normalize serum calcium levels.

Dosage adjustment for hypocalcemia:

If serum calcium >7.5 mg/dL but <8.4 mg/dL or if hypocalcemia symptoms occur: Use calcium-containing phosphate binders and/or vitamin D to raise calcium levels.

If serum calcium <7.5 mg/dL or if hypocalcemia symptoms occur and the dose of vitamin D cannot be increased: Discontinue cinacalcet until serum calcium ≥8 mg/dL or symptoms of hypocalcemia resolve. Reinitiate cinacalcet at the next lowest dose.

If iPTH <150-300 pg/mL: Reduce dose or discontinue cinacalcet and/or vitamin D.

Elderly: Refer to adult dosing. No adjustment required.

Renal Impairment: No adjustment required.

Hepatic Impairment: Patients with moderate to severe dysfunction have an increased exposure to cinacalcet and increased half-life.

Available Dosage Forms Tablet [film coated]: 30 mg, 60 mg, 90 mg

Monitoring and Teaching Issues

Physical Assessment: Use caution with history of seizure disorder; assess serum calcium levels closely prior to initiating therapy or dose change and regularly during maintenance therapy (see Warnings/Precautions and Dosing). Assess potential for interactions with other pharmacological agents patient may be taking (see Drug Interactions). Assess therapeutic response (calcium levels and iPTH) and adverse reactions (eg, hypocalcemia [paresthesias, myalgia, cramping, tetany, convulsions]; see Adverse Reactions). Teach patient possible aide effects, interventions to reduce side effects, and adverse symptoms to report (eg, hypocalcemia, myalgia, hypertension; see Patient Education).

Monitoring Laboratory Tests:

Hyperparathyroidism: Serum calcium levels prior to initiation and within a week of initiation or dosage adjustment; iPTH should be measured 1-4 weeks after initiation or dosage adjustment. After the maintenance dose is established, monthly calcium and phosphorus levels and iPTH every 1-3 months are required.

Parathyroid carcinoma: Serum calcium levels prior to initiation and within a week of initiation or dosage adjustment; once maintenance dose is established, obtain serum calcium level every 2 months.

Patient Education: Do not take any new medication during therapy unless approved by prescriber. Take exactly as directed with food; do not break, chew, or crush tablet (swallow whole). Do not take more than prescribed. You may experience dizziness (use caution when driving or engaged in potentially hazards tasks until response to drug is known); nausea, vomiting, or loss of appetite (good mouth care, small frequent meals, sucking lozenges, or chewing gum may help); or diarrhea (yogurt or boiled milk may help). Report any muscle cramping, twitches, tremors, or spasms; chest pain or palpitations; unresolved gastrointestinal disturbance; or other persistent adverse effects. **Pregnancy/ breast-feeding precautions:** Inform prescriber if you are or intend to become pregnant.

Dietary Considerations: Take with food. May be taken with vitamin D and/or phosphate binders.

Pregnancy Risk Factor: C

Lactation: Excretion in breast milk unknown/not recommended

Breast-Feeding Issues: The manufacturer recommends discontinuing nursing or discontinuing cinacalcet.

Administration

Oral: Administer with food. Do not break tablet; should be taken whole.

Storage: Store at 25°C (77°F).

♦ **Cinacalcet Hydrochloride** *see* Cinacalcet *on page 326*

♦ **Cipro®** *see* Ciprofloxacin *on page 327*

♦ **Ciprodex®** *see* Ciprofloxacin and Dexamethasone *on page 331*

Ciprofloxacin (sip roe FLOKS a sin)

U.S. Brand Names Ciloxan®; Cipro®; Cipro® XR

Synonyms Ciprofloxacin Hydrochloride

Generic Available Yes: Suspension, tablet

Pharmacologic Category Antibiotic, Ophthalmic; Antibiotic, Quinolone

Medication Safety Issues

Sound-alike/look-alike issues:

Ciprofloxacin may be confused with cephalexin

Ciloxan® may be confused with cinoxacin, Cytoxan®

Cipro® may be confused with Ceftin®

Use

Children: Complicated urinary tract infections and pyelonephritis due to *E. coli*. **Note:** Although effective, ciprofloxacin is not the drug of first choice in children.

Children and adults: To reduce incidence or progression of disease following exposure to aerolized *Bacillus anthracis*. Ophthalmologically, for superficial ocular infections (corneal ulcers, conjunctivitis) due to susceptible strains

Adults: Treatment of the following infections when caused by susceptible bacteria: Urinary tract infections; acute uncomplicated cystitis in females; chronic bacterial prostatitis; lower respiratory tract infections (including acute exacerbations of chronic bronchitis); acute sinusitis; skin and skin structure infections; bone and joint infections; complicated intra-abdominal infections (in combination with metronidazole); infectious diarrhea; typhoid fever due to *Salmonella typhi* (eradication of chronic typhoid carrier state has not been proven); uncomplicated cervical and urethra gonorrhea (due to *N. gonorrhoeae*); nosocomial pneumonia; empirical therapy for febrile neutropenic patients (in combination with piperacillin)

Unlabeled/Investigational Use Acute pulmonary exacerbations in cystic fibrosis (children); cutaneous/gastrointestinal/oropharyngeal anthrax (treatment, children and adults); disseminated gonococcal infection (adults); chancroid (adults); prophylaxis to *Neisseria meningitidis* following close contact with an infected person

(Continued)

Ciprofloxacin *(Continued)*

Mechanism of Action/Effect Inhibits DNA-gyrase in susceptible organisms; inhibits relaxation of supercoiled DNA and promotes breakage of double-stranded DNA

Contraindications Hypersensitivity to ciprofloxacin, any component of the formulation, or other quinolones

Warnings/Precautions CNS stimulation may occur (tremor, restlessness, confusion, and very rarely hallucinations or seizures). Use with caution in patients with known or suspected CNS disorder. Prolonged use may result in superinfection. Tendon inflammation and/or rupture have been reported with ciprofloxacin and other quinolone antibiotics. Risk may be increased with concurrent corticosteroids, particularly in the elderly. Discontinue at first sign of tendon inflammation or pain. Adverse effects, including those related to joints and/or surrounding tissues, are increased in pediatric patients. Rare cases of peripheral neuropathy may occur.

Severe hypersensitivity reactions, including anaphylaxis, have occurred with quinolone therapy. Quinolones may exacerbate myasthenia gravis, use with caution (rare, potentially life-threatening weakness of respiratory muscles may occur). Use caution in renal impairment. Avoid excessive sunlight; may cause moderate-to-severe phototoxicity reactions.

Drug Interactions

Cytochrome P450 Effect: Inhibits CYP1A2 (strong), 3A4 (weak)

Decreased Effect: Concurrent administration of metal cations, including most antacids, oral electrolyte supplements, quinapril, sucralfate, and some didanosine formulations (chewable/buffered tablets and pediatric powder for oral suspension), may decrease quinolone levels; separate doses. Ciprofloxacin may decrease phenytoin levels.

Increased Effect/Toxicity: Ciprofloxacin may increase the effects/toxicity of caffeine, CYP1A2 substrates (eg, aminophylline, fluvoxamine, mexiletine, mirtazapine, ropinirole, and trifluoperazine), glyburide, methotrexate, ropivacaine, theophylline, and warfarin. Concomitant use with corticosteroids may increase the risk of tendon rupture. Concomitant use with foscarnet may increase the risk of seizures. Probenecid may increase ciprofloxacin levels.

Nutritional/Ethanol Interactions

Food: Food decreases rate, but not extent, of absorption. Ciprofloxacin serum levels may be decreased if taken with dairy products or calcium-fortified juices. Ciprofloxacin may increase serum caffeine levels if taken with caffeine.

Enteral feedings may decrease plasma concentrations of ciprofloxacin probably by >30% inhibition of absorption. Ciprofloxacin should not be administered with enteral feedings. The feeding would need to be discontinued for 1-2 hours prior to and after ciprofloxacin administration. Nasogastric administration produces a greater loss of ciprofloxacin bioavailability than does nasoduodenal administration.

Herb/Nutraceutical: Avoid dong quai, St John's wort (may also cause photosensitization).

Adverse Reactions

1% to 10%:

Central nervous system: Neurologic events (children 2%, includes dizziness, insomnia, nervousness, somnolence); fever (children 2%); headache (I.V. administration); restlessness (I.V. administration)

Dermatologic: Rash (children 2%, adults 1%)

Gastrointestinal: Nausea (children/adults 3%); diarrhea (children 5%, adults 2%); vomiting (children 5%, adults 1%); abdominal pain (children 3%, adults <1%); dyspepsia (children 3%)

Hepatic: ALT/AST increased (adults 1%)

Local: Injection site reactions (I.V. administration)

Respiratory: Rhinitis (children 3%)

Overdosage/Toxicology Symptoms of overdose include acute renal failure and seizures. Treatment is supportive. The drug is not removed by peritoneal or hemodialysis.

Pharmacodynamics/Kinetics

Absorption: Oral: Immediate release tablet: Rapid (~50% to 85%)

Time to Peak: Serum: Oral: Immediate release tablet: 0.5-2 hours; Extended release tablet: 1-2.5 hours

Protein Binding: 20% to 40%

Half-Life Elimination: Children: 2.5 hours; Adults: Normal renal function: 3-5 hours

Metabolism: Partially hepatic; forms 4 metabolites (limited activity)

Excretion: Urine (30% to 50% as unchanged drug); feces (15% to 40%)

Dosing

Adults: Note: Extended release tablets and immediate release formulations are not interchangeable. Unless otherwise specified, oral dosing reflects the use of immediate release formulations.

Urinary tract infection:

Acute uncomplicated: Oral: Immediate release formulation: 100 mg or 250 mg every 12 hours for 3 days

Acute uncomplicated pyelonephritis: Oral: Extended release formulation: 1000 mg every 24 hours for 7-14 days

Uncomplicated/acute cystitis: Oral: Extended release formulation: 500 mg every 24 hours for 3 days

Mild/moderate:

Oral: Immediate release formulation: 250 mg every 12 hours for 7-14 days

I.V.: 200 mg every 12 hours for 7-14 days

Severe/complicated:

Oral:

Immediate release formulation: 500 mg every 12 hours for 7-14 days

Extended release formulation: 1000 mg every 24 hours for 7-14 days

I.V.: 400 mg every 12 hours for 7-14 days

Lower respiratory tract, skin/skin structure infections:

Oral: 500-750 mg twice daily for 7-14 days depending on severity and susceptibility

I.V.:
Mild/moderate: 400 mg every 12 hours for 7-14 days
Severe/complicated: 400 mg every 8 hours for 7-14 days
Nosocomial pneumonia (mild to moderate to severe): I.V.: 400 mg every 8 hours for 10-14 days
Bone/joint infections:
Oral: 500-750 mg twice daily for 4-6 weeks, depending on severity and susceptibility
I.V.:
Mild/moderate: 400 mg every 12 hours for 4-6 weeks
Severe/complicated: 400 mg every 8 hours for 4-6 weeks
Infectious diarrhea: Oral: 500 mg every 12 hours for 5-7 days
Intra-abdominal (in combination with metronidazole):
Oral: 500 mg every 12 hours for 7-14 days
I.V.: 400 mg every 12 hours for 7-14 days
Febrile neutropenia (with piperacillin): I.V.: 400 mg every 8 hours for 7-14 days
Typhoid fever: Oral: 500 mg every 12 hours for 10 days
Gonococcal infections:
Urethral/cervical gonococcal infections: Oral: 250-500 mg as a single dose (CDC recommends concomitant doxycycline or azithromycin due to developing resistance; avoid use in Asian or Western Pacific travelers)
Disseminated gonococcal infection (CDC guidelines): Oral: 500 mg twice daily to complete 7 days of therapy (initial treatment with ceftriaxone 1 g I.M./I.V. daily for 24-48 hours after improvement begins)
Chancroid (CDC guidelines): Oral: 500 mg twice daily for 3 days
Sinusitis (acute):
Oral: 500 mg every 12 hours for 10 days
I.V.: 400 mg every 12 hours for 10 days
Prostatitis (chronic, bacterial):
Oral: 500 mg every 12 hours for 28 days
I.V.: 400 mg every 12 hours for 28 days
Anthrax:
Inhalational (postexposure prophylaxis):
Oral: 500 mg every 12 hours for 60 days
I.V.: 400 mg every 12 hours for 60 days
Cutaneous (treatment, CDC guidelines): Oral: Immediate release formulation: 500 mg every 12 hours for 60 days. **Note:** In the presence of systemic involvement, extensive edema, lesions on head/neck, refer to I.V. dosing for treatment of inhalational/gastrointestinal/oropharyngeal anthrax.
Inhalational/gastrointestinal/oropharyngeal (treatment, CDC guidelines): I.V.: 400 mg every 12 hours. **Note:** Initial treatment should include two or more agents predicted to be effective (per CDC recommendations). Agents suggested for use in conjunction with ciprofloxacin or doxycycline include rifampin, vancomycin, imipenem, penicillin, ampicillin, chloramphenicol, clindamycin, and clarithromycin. May switch to oral antimicrobial therapy when clinically appropriate. Continue combined therapy for 60 days.
Bacterial conjunctivitis:
Ophthalmic solution: Instill 1-2 drops in eye(s) every 2 hours while awake for 2 days and 1-2 drops every 4 hours while awake for the next 5 days
Ophthalmic ointment: Apply a ½" ribbon into the conjunctival sac 3 times/day for the first 2 days, followed by a ½" ribbon applied twice daily for the next 5 days
Corneal ulcer: Ophthalmic solution: Instill 2 drops into affected eye every 15 minutes for the first 6 hours, then 2 drops into the affected eye every 30 minutes for the remainder of the first day. On day 2, instill 2 drops into the affected eye hourly. On days 3-14, instill 2 drops into affected eye every 4 hours. Treatment may continue after day 14 if re-epithelialization has not occurred.
Elderly: Refer to adult dosing. Adjust dose carefully based on renal function.
Pediatrics: See Warnings/Precautions. **Note:** Extended release tablets and immediate release formulations are not interchangeable. Unless otherwise specified, oral dosing reflects the use of immediate release formulations.
Complicated urinary tract infection or pyelonephritis: Children 1-17 years:
Oral: 20-30 mg/kg/day in 2 divided doses (every 12 hours) for 10-21 days; maximum: 1.5 g/day
I.V.: 6-10 mg/kg every 8 hours for 10-21 days (maximum: 400 mg/dose)
Cystic fibrosis (unlabeled use): Children 5-17 years:
Oral: 40 mg/kg/day divided every 12 hours administered following 1 week of I.V. therapy has been reported in a clinical trial; total duration of therapy: 10-21 days
I.V.: 30 mg/kg/day divided every 8 hours for 1 week, followed by oral therapy, has been reported in a clinical trial
Anthrax:
Inhalational (postexposure prophylaxis):
Oral: 15 mg/kg/dose every 12 hours for 60 days; maximum: 500 mg/dose
I.V.: 10 mg/kg/dose every 12 hours for 60 days; do **not** exceed 400 mg/dose (800 mg/day)
Cutaneous (treatment, CDC guidelines): Oral: 10-15 mg/kg every 12 hours for 60 days (maximum: 1 g/day); amoxicillin 80 mg/kg/day divided every 8 hours is an option for completion of treatment after clinical improvement. **Note:** In the presence of systemic involvement, extensive edema, lesions on head/neck, refer to I.V. dosing for treatment of inhalational/gastrointestinal/oropharyngeal anthrax.
Inhalational/gastrointestinal/oropharyngeal (treatment, CDC guidelines): I.V.: Initial: 10-15 mg/kg every 12 hours for 60 days (maximum: 500 mg/dose); switch to oral therapy when clinically appropriate; refer to Adults dosing for notes on combined therapy and duration
Bacterial conjunctivitis:
Ophthalmic solution: Children >1 year: Refer to adult dosing.
Ophthalmic ointment: Children >2 years: Refer to adult dosing.
Corneal ulcer: Children >1 year: Refer to adult dosing.
(Continued)

Ciprofloxacin *(Continued)*

Renal Impairment: Adults:

Cl$_{cr}$ 30-50 mL/minute: Oral: Administer 250-500 mg every 12 hours.

Cl$_{cr}$ <30 mL/minute: Acute uncomplicated pyelonephritis or complicated UTI: Oral: Extended release formulation: 500 mg every 24 hours

Cl$_{cr}$ 5-29 mL/minute:

Oral: Administer 250-500 mg every 18 hours.

I.V.: Administer 200-400 mg every 18-24 hours.

Dialysis: Only small amounts of ciprofloxacin are removed by hemo- or peritoneal dialysis (<10%); usual dose: Oral: 250-500 mg every 24 hours following dialysis.

Continuous arteriovenous or venovenous hemodiafiltration effects: Administer 200-400 mg I.V. every 12 hours.

Hepatic Impairment: Adjustment should be considered in severe hepatic dysfunction.

Available Dosage Forms

Infusion, [premixed in D$_5$W] (Cipro®): 200 mg (100 mL); 400 mg (200 mL) [latex free]

Injection, solution (Cipro®): 10 mg/mL (20 mL, 40 mL, 120 mL)

Microcapsules for oral suspension (Cipro®): 250 mg/5 mL (100 mL); 500 mg/5 mL (100 mL) [strawberry flavor]

Ointment, ophthalmic, as hydrochloride (Ciloxan®): 3.33 mg/g [0.3% base] (3.5 g)

Solution, ophthalmic, as hydrochloride (Ciloxan®): 3.5 mg/mL [0.3% base] (2.5 mL, 5 mL, 10 mL) [contains benzalkonium chloride]

Tablet [film coated]: 250 mg, 500 mg, 750 mg

Cipro®: 100 mg, 250 mg, 500 mg, 750 mg

Tablet, extended release [film coated] (Cipro® XR): 500 mg [equivalent to ciprofloxacin hydrochloride 287.5 mg and ciprofloxacin base 212.6 mg]; 1000 mg [equivalent to ciprofloxacin hydrochloride 574.9 mg and ciprofloxacin base 425.2 mg]

Monitoring and Teaching Issues

Physical Assessment: Assess results of culture and sensitivity tests prior to beginning therapy. Use caution in patients with CNS disorder, myasthenia gravis, or renal impairment (see Warnings/Precautions). Assess potential for interactions with other pharmacological agents or herbal products patient may be taking (see Drug Interactions). **I.V.:** See Administration specifics. Assess results of laboratory tests, therapeutic effectiveness (according to purpose for use), and adverse effects (eg, hypersensitivity reactions [severe reactions, including anaphylaxis, have occurred with quinolone therapy]; changes in CNS, especially in elderly patients; see Adverse Reactions) regularly during therapy. Teach patient proper use, possible side effects/appropriate interventions, and adverse symptoms to report (see Patient Educations).

Monitoring Laboratory Tests: CBC, renal and hepatic function during prolonged therapy; patients receiving concurrent ciprofloxacin, theophylline, or cyclosporine should have serum theophylline or cyclosporine levels monitored. Culture and sensitivity specimen should be taken prior to initiating therapy.

Patient Education: Do not take any new medication during therapy unless approved by prescriber. Take exactly as directed (at least 2 hours before or 6 hours after antacids or other drug products containing calcium, iron, or zinc). Extended release tablet may be taken with meals containing dairy products, but not with dairy products alone; do not crush, split, or chew extended release tablet. Swallow oral suspension; do not chew microcapsules. Shake bottle vigorously with each use. Take entire prescription, even if feeling better. Maintain adequate hydration to avoid concentrated urine and crystal formation (2-3 L/day) unless instructed to restrict fluid intake. You may experience nausea, vomiting, or anorexia (small frequent meals, frequent mouth care, sucking lozenges, or chewing gum may help); or increased sensitivity to sunlight (use sunscreen, wear protective clothing and dark glasses, and avoid direct exposure to sunlight). If signs of inflammation or tendon pain occur, discontinue use immediately and report to prescriber. If signs of allergic reaction (eg, itching urticaria, respiratory difficulty, facial edema, difficulty swallowing, loss of consciousness, tingling, chest pain, palpitations) occur, discontinue use immediately and report to prescriber. Report unusual fever or chills, vaginal itching or foul-smelling vaginal discharge, easy bruising or bleeding, or tendon or muscle pain. **Pregnancy/breast-feeding precautions:** Inform prescriber if you are or intend to become pregnant. Do not breast-feed.

Dietary Considerations:

Food: Drug may cause GI upset; take without regard to meals (manufacturer prefers that immediate release tablet is taken 2 hours after meals). Extended release tablet may be taken with meals that contain dairy products (calcium content <800 mg), but not with dairy products alone.

Dairy products, calcium-fortified juices, oral multivitamins, and mineral supplements: Absorption of ciprofloxacin is decreased by divalent and trivalent cations. The manufacturer states that the usual dietary intake of calcium (including meals which include dairy products) has not been shown to interfere with ciprofloxacin absorption. Ciprofloxacin may be taken 2 hours before or 6 hours after any of these products.

Caffeine: Patients consuming regular large quantities of caffeinated beverages may need to restrict caffeine intake if excessive cardiac or CNS stimulation occurs.

Geriatric Considerations: Ciprofloxacin should not be used as first-line therapy unless the culture and sensitivity findings show resistance to usual therapy. The interactions with caffeine and theophylline can result in serious toxicity in the elderly. Adjust dose for renal function.

Pregnancy Risk Factor: C

Pregnancy Issues: Ciprofloxacin crosses the placenta and concentrates in amniotic fluid; maternal serum levels may be decreased during pregnancy. Reports of arthropathy (observed in immature animals and reported rarely in humans) have limited the use of fluoroquinolones in pregnancy. According to the FDA, the Teratogen Information System concluded that therapeutic doses during pregnancy are unlikely to produce substantial teratogenic risk, but data are insufficient to say that there is no risk. Since safer alternatives are usually available, quinolones should generally be avoided in pregnancy. When considering treatment for life-threatening infection and/or prolonged duration of therapy, the potential risk to the fetus must be balanced against the severity of the potential illness.

Lactation: Enters breast milk/not recommended (AAP rates "compatible")

Breast-Feeding Issues: Ciprofloxacin is excreted in breast milk; however, the exposure to the infant is considered small and one source suggests that the decision to breast-feed be independent of the need for the antibiotic in the mother. Another source recommends the mother wait 48 hours after the last dose of ciprofloxacin to continue nursing. The manufacturer recommends to discontinue nursing or to discontinue ciprofloxacin.

Administration

Oral: May administer with food to minimize GI upset; avoid antacid use; maintain proper hydration and urine output. Administer at least 2 hours before or 6 hours after antacids or other products containing calcium, iron, or zinc (including dairy products or calcium-fortified juices). Separate oral administration from drugs which may impair absorption (see Drug Interactions).

Oral suspension: Should not be administered through feeding tubes (suspension is oil-based and adheres to the feeding tube). Patients should avoid chewing on the microcapsules.

Nasogastric/orogastric tube: Crush immediate-release tablet and mix with water. Flush feeding tube before and after administration. Hold tube feedings at least 1 hour before and 2 hours after administration.

Tablet, extended release: Do not crush, split, or chew. May be administered with meals containing dairy products (calcium content <800 mg), but not with dairy products alone.

I.V.: Administer by slow I.V. infusion over 60 minutes into a large vein.

Reconstitution: Injection, vial: May be diluted with NS, D_5W, SWFI, $D_{10}W$, $D_5\frac{1}{4}$NS, $D_5\frac{1}{2}$NS, LR.

Compatibility: Stable in $D_5\frac{1}{4}$NS, $D_5\frac{1}{2}$NS, D_5W, $D_{10}W$, LR, NS

Y-site administration: Incompatible with aminophylline, ampicillin/sulbactam, cefepime, dexamethasone sodium phosphate, furosemide, heparin, hydrocortisone sodium succinate, methylprednisolone sodium succinate, phenytoin, propofol, sodium phosphates, warfarin

Compatibility when admixed: Incompatible with aminophylline, clindamycin, floxacillin, heparin

Storage:

Injection:

Premixed infusion: Store between 5°C to 25°C (41°F to 77°F). Protect from light. Avoid freezing.

Vial: Store between 5°C to 30°C (41°F to 86°F). Protect from light. Avoid freezing. Diluted solutions of 0.5-2 mg/mL are stable for up to 14 days refrigerated or at room temperature.

Ophthalmic solution/ointment: Store at 36°F to 77°F (2°C to 25°C). Protect from light.

Microcapsules for oral suspension: Prior to reconstitution, store below 25°C (77°F). Protect from freezing. Following reconstitution, store below 30°C (86°F) for up to 14 days. Protect from freezing.

Tablet:

Immediate release: Store below 30°C (86°F).

Extended release: Store at room temperature of 15°C to 30°C (59°F to 86°F).

Related Information

Antimicrobial Drugs of Choice *on page 1792*
Community-Acquired Pneumonia in Adults *on page 1807*
I.V. to Oral Conversion *on page 1688*
Prophylaxis for Exposure to Communicable Diseases *on page 1859*
Tuberculosis *on page 1864*

Ciprofloxacin and Dexamethasone

(sip roe FLOKS a sin & deks a METH a sone)

U.S. Brand Names Ciprodex®

Synonyms Ciprofloxacin Hydrochloride and Dexamethasone; Dexamethasone and Ciprofloxacin

Generic Available No

Pharmacologic Category Antibiotic/Corticosteroid, Otic

Use Treatment of acute otitis media in pediatric patients with tympanostomy tubes or acute otitis externa in children and adults

Dosing

Adults & Elderly: Acute otitis externa: Otic: Instill 4 drops into affected ear(s) twice daily for 7 days

Pediatrics: Acute otitis media in patients with tympanostomy tubes or acute otitis externa: Otic: Instill 4 drops into affected ear(s) twice daily for 7 days

Available Dosage Forms Suspension, otic: Ciprofloxacin 0.3% and dexamethasone 0.1% (7.5 mL) [contains benzalkonium chloride]

Monitoring and Teaching Issues

Physical Assessment: See individual agents.

Patient Education: See individual agents. **Pregnancy/breast-feeding precautions:** Inform prescriber if you are or intend to become pregnant. Breast-feeding is not recommended.

Pregnancy Risk Factor: C

Lactation: Excretion in breast milk unknown/not recommended

Related Information

Ciprofloxacin *on page 327*
Dexamethasone *on page 424*

Ciprofloxacin and Hydrocortisone

(sip roe FLOKS a sin & hye droe KOR ti sone)

U.S. Brand Names Cipro® HC

Synonyms Hydrocortisone and Ciprofloxacin

Generic Available No

(Continued)

Ciprofloxacin and Hydrocortisone *(Continued)*

Pharmacologic Category Antibiotic/Corticosteroid, Otic

Use Treatment of acute otitis externa, sometimes known as "swimmer's ear"

Dosing

Adults & Elderly: Otitis externa: Otic: The recommended dosage for all patients is three drops of the suspension in the affected ear twice daily for seven day; twice-daily dosing schedule is more convenient for patients than that of existing treatments with hydrocortisone, which are typically administered three or four times a day; a twice-daily dosage schedule may be especially helpful for parents and caregivers of young children

Pediatrics: Children ≥1 year: Refer to adult dosing.

Available Dosage Forms Suspension, otic: Ciprofloxacin hydrochloride 0.2% and hydrocortisone 1% (10 mL) [contains benzyl alcohol]

Monitoring and Teaching Issues

Physical Assessment: See individual components listed under Related Information.

Patient Education: Pregnancy/breast-feeding precautions: Inform prescriber if you are or intend to become pregnant. Consult prescriber if breast-feeding.

Related Information

Ciprofloxacin *on page 327*

Hydrocortisone *on page 760*

♦ **Ciprofloxacin Hydrochloride** *see Ciprofloxacin on page 327*

♦ **Ciprofloxacin Hydrochloride and Dexamethasone** *see Ciprofloxacin and Dexamethasone on page 331*

♦ **Cipro® HC** *see Ciprofloxacin and Hydrocortisone on page 331*

♦ **Cipro® XR** *see Ciprofloxacin on page 327*

Cisapride (SIS a pride)

U.S. Brand Names Propulsid®

Restrictions In U.S., available via limited-access protocol only (1-800-JANSSEN).

Generic Available No

Pharmacologic Category Gastrointestinal Agent, Prokinetic

Medication Safety Issues

Sound-alike/look-alike issues:

Propulsid® may be confused with propranolol

Use Treatment of nocturnal symptoms of gastroesophageal reflux disease (GERD); has demonstrated effectiveness for gastroparesis, refractory constipation, and nonulcer dyspepsia

Mechanism of Action/Effect Enhances the release of acetylcholine at the myenteric plexus. *In vitro* studies have shown cisapride to have serotonin-4 receptor agonistic properties which may increase GI motility and cardiac rate; increases lower esophageal sphincter pressure and lower esophageal peristalsis; accelerates gastric emptying of both liquids and solids.

Contraindications

Hypersensitivity to cisapride or any component of the formulations; GI hemorrhage, mechanical obstruction, GI perforation, or other situations when GI motility stimulation is dangerous

Serious cardiac arrhythmias including ventricular tachycardia, ventricular fibrillation, torsade de pointes, and QT prolongation have been reported in patients taking cisapride with other drugs that inhibit CYP3A4. Some of these events have been fatal. Concomitant oral or intravenous administration of the following drugs with cisapride may lead to elevated cisapride blood levels and is contraindicated:

Antibiotics: Oral or I.V. erythromycin, clarithromycin, troleandomycin

Antidepressants: Nefazodone

Antifungals: Oral or I.V. fluconazole, itraconazole, miconazole, oral ketoconazole

Protease inhibitors: Indinavir, ritonavir, amprenavir, atazanavir

Cisapride is also contraindicated for patients with a prolonged electrocardiographic QT intervals (QT_c >450 msec), a history of QT_c prolongation, or known family history of congenital long QT syndrome; clinically significant bradycardia, renal failure, history of ventricular arrhythmias, ischemic heart disease, and congestive heart failure; uncorrected electrolyte disorders (hypokalemia, hypomagnesemia); respiratory failure; and concomitant medications known to prolong the QT interval and increase the risk of arrhythmia, such as certain antiarrhythmics, certain antipsychotics, certain antidepressants, bepridil, sparfloxacin, and terodiline. The preceding lists of drugs are not comprehensive. Cisapride should not be used in patients with uncorrected hypokalemia or hypomagnesemia or who might experience rapid reduction of plasma potassium such as those administered potassium-wasting diuretics and/or insulin in acute settings.

Warnings/Precautions Safety and effectiveness in children have not been established. Serious cardiac ventricular arrhythmias, including ventricular tachycardia, torsade de pointes, and QT prolongation have been reported in patients taking cisapride with other drugs that inhibit P450 3A4 (eg, clarithromycin, erythromycin, fluconazole, itraconazole, ketoconazole, miconazole injection, troleandomycin). Avoid other medications which may prolong QT. Avoid use when stimulation of GI motility may be dangerous (eg, obstruction, perforation, hemorrhage). Extreme caution with use in the elderly.

A 12-lead ECG should be performed prior to administration of cisapride. Treatment with cisapride should not be initiated if the QT_c value exceeds 450 milliseconds. Serum electrolytes (potassium, calcium, and magnesium) and creatinine should be assessed prior to administration of cisapride and whenever conditions develop that may affect electrolyte balance or renal function.

Drug Interactions

Cytochrome P450 Effect: Substrate of CYP1A2 (minor), 2A6 (minor), 2B6 (minor), 2C8/9 (minor), 2C19 (minor), 3A4 (major); **Inhibits** CYP2D6 (weak), 3A4 (weak)

Decreased Effect: Cisapride may decrease the effect of atropine and digoxin.

Increased Effect/Toxicity: Cisapride may increase blood levels of warfarin, diazepam, cimetidine, ranitidine, and CNS depressants. The risk of cisapride-induced malignant arrhythmias may be increased by azole antifungals (fluconazole, itraconazole, ketoconazole, miconazole), antiarrhythmics (Class Ia; quinidine, procainamide, and Class III; amiodarone, sotalol), bepridil, cimetidine, maprotiline, macrolide antibiotics (erythromycin, clarithromycin, troleandomycin), molindone, nefazodone, protease inhibitors (amprenavir, atazanavir, indinavir, nelfinavir, ritonavir), phenothiazines (eg, prochlorperazine, promethazine), sertindole, tricyclic antidepressants (eg amitriptyline), and some quinolone antibiotics (sparfloxacin, gatifloxacin, moxifloxacin). Other strong inhibitors of CYP3A4 (including diclofenac, doxycycline, imatinib, isoniazid, nefazodone, nicardipine, propofol, and verapamil) should be avoided. Cardiovascular disease or electrolyte imbalances (potentially due to diuretic therapy) increase the risk of malignant arrhythmias.

Nutritional/Ethanol Interactions
Ethanol: Avoid ethanol (may increase CNS depression).
Food: Coadministration of grapefruit juice with cisapride increases the bioavailability of cisapride and concomitant use should be avoided.
Herb/Nutraceutical: St John's wort may decrease cisapride levels.

Adverse Reactions
>5%:
  Central nervous system: Headache
  Dermatologic: Rash
  Gastrointestinal: Diarrhea, GI cramping, dyspepsia, flatulence, nausea, xerostomia
  Respiratory: Rhinitis
<5%:
  Cardiovascular: Tachycardia
  Central nervous system: Extrapyramidal effects, somnolence, fatigue, seizure, insomnia, anxiety
  Hematologic: Thrombocytopenia, increased LFTs, pancytopenia, leukopenia, granulocytopenia, aplastic anemia
  Respiratory: Sinusitis, cough, upper respiratory tract infection, increased incidence of viral infection

Pharmacodynamics/Kinetics
Onset of Action: 0.5-1 hour
Bioavailability: 35% to 40%
Protein Binding: 97.5% to 98%
Half-Life Elimination: 6-12 hours
Metabolism: Extensively hepatic to norcisapride
Excretion: Urine and feces (<10%)

Dosing
Adults & Elderly: GERD or gastrointestinal dysmotility: Oral: Initial: 5-10 mg 4 times/day at least 15 minutes before meals and at bedtime; in some patients the dosage will need to be increased to 20 mg to obtain a satisfactory result.
Pediatrics: Gastrointestinal dysmotility: Oral: Children: 0.15-0.3 mg/kg/dose 3-4 times/day; maximum: 10 mg/dose
Hepatic Impairment: Initiate at 50% usual dose.

Monitoring and Teaching Issues
Physical Assessment: See Contraindications and Warnings/Precautions for specific use cautions and limitations prior to beginning treatment. Assess potential for interactions with other pharmacological agents or herbal products patient may be taking (eg, increased risk of cardiac arrhythmias; see Drug Interactions). Assess results of laboratory tests (eg, ECG, electrolyte balance and renal function), therapeutic effectiveness (relief of symptoms), and adverse response (eg, tachycardia, CNS changes, anemia, viral infection; see Adverse Reactions) regularly during therapy. Teach patient proper use, possible side effects/appropriate interventions, and adverse symptoms to report (see Patient Education).
Monitoring Laboratory Tests: A 12-lead ECG should be performed prior to administration of cisapride. Treatment with cisapride should not be initiated if the QT_c value exceeds 450 milliseconds. Serum electrolytes (potassium, calcium, and magnesium) and creatinine should be assessed prior to administration of cisapride and whenever conditions develop that may affect electrolyte balance or renal function.
Patient Education: It is vital for the prescriber know about all other pharmacological agents or herbal products you are taking. Do not take any new medication during therapy unless approved by prescriber. Take before meals. Avoid grapefruit juice; concurrent use with cisapride will increase the potential for dangerous adverse reactions. May cause increased sedation, headache, anxiety (use caution when driving or engaging in hazardous tasks until response to drug is known). Immediately report rapid heartbeat, palpitations, chest pain, or tightness. Report severe abdominal pain, prolonged diarrhea, weight loss, extreme fatigue, or other significant adverse effects. **Pregnancy/breast-feeding precautions:** Inform prescriber if you are or intend to become pregnant or breast-feed.
Geriatric Considerations: Steady-state serum concentrations are higher than those in younger adults; however, the therapeutic dose and pharmacologic effects are the same as those in younger adults and no adjustment in dose recommended for elderly.
Pregnancy Risk Factor: C
Lactation: Enters breast milk/use caution (AAP rates "compatible")

Cisatracurium (sis a tra KYOO ree um)
U.S. Brand Names Nimbex®
Synonyms Cisatracurium Besylate
Generic Available No
Pharmacologic Category Neuromuscular Blocker Agent, Nondepolarizing
Medication Safety Issues
Sound-alike/look-alike issues:
  Nimbex® may be confused with Revex®
Use Adjunct to general anesthesia to facilitate endotracheal intubation and to relax skeletal muscles during surgery; to facilitate mechanical ventilation in ICU patients; does not relieve pain or produce sedation
(Continued)

Cisatracurium *(Continued)*

Mechanism of Action/Effect Blocks neural transmission at the myoneural junction by binding with cholinergic receptor sites

Contraindications Hypersensitivity to cisatracurium besylate or any component of the formulation

Warnings/Precautions Maintenance of an adequate airway and respiratory support is critical; certain clinical conditions may result in potentiation or antagonism of neuromuscular blockade:

> Potentiation: Electrolyte abnormalities, severe hyponatremia, severe hypocalcemia, severe hypokalemia, hypermagnesemia, neuromuscular diseases, acidosis, acute intermittent porphyria, renal failure, hepatic failure
>
> Antagonism: Alkalosis, hypercalcemia, demyelinating lesions, peripheral neuropathies, diabetes mellitus

Increased sensitivity in patients with myasthenia gravis, Eaton-Lambert syndrome; resistance in burn patients (>30% of body) for period of 5-70 days postinjury; resistance in patients with muscle trauma, denervation, immobilization, infection. Cross-sensitivity with other neuromuscular-blocking agents may occur; use extreme caution in patients with previous anaphylactic reactions. Bradycardia may be more common with cisatracurium than with other neuromuscular blocking agents since it has no clinically significant effects on heart rate to counteract the bradycardia produced by anesthetics.

Drug Interactions

Decreased Effect: Effect of nondepolarizing neuromuscular blockers may be reduced by carbamazepine (chronic use), corticosteroids (also associated with myopathy - see increased effect), phenytoin (chronic use), sympathomimetics, and theophylline.

Increased Effect/Toxicity: Increased effects are possible with aminoglycosides, beta-blockers, clindamycin, calcium channel blockers, halogenated anesthetics, imipenem, ketamine, lidocaine, loop diuretics (furosemide), macrolides (case reports), magnesium sulfate, procainamide, quinidine, quinolones, tetracyclines, and vancomycin. May increase risk of myopathy when used with high-dose corticosteroids for extended periods.

Overdosage/Toxicology

Symptoms of overdose include respiratory depression and cardiovascular collapse.

Neostigmine 1-3 mg slow I.V. push in adults (0.5 mg in children) antagonizes the neuromuscular blockade, and should be administered with or immediately after atropine 1-1.5 mg I.V. push (adults). This may be especially useful in the presence of bradycardia.

Pharmacodynamics/Kinetics

Onset of Action: I.V.: 2-3 minutes; Peak effect: 3-5 minutes

Duration of Action: Recovery begins in 20-35 minutes when anesthesia is balanced; recovery is attained in 90% of patients in 25-93 minutes

Half-Life Elimination: 22-29 minutes

Metabolism: Undergoes rapid nonenzymatic degradation in the bloodstream (Hofmann elimination), additional metabolism occurs via ester hydrolysis; some active metabolites

Dosing

Adults & Elderly: Neuromuscular blockade: I.V. (not to be used I.M.):

Operating room administration:

Intubating doses: 0.15-0.2 mg/kg as components of propofol/nitrous oxide/oxygen induction-intubation technique. (**Note:** May produce generally good or excellent conditions for tracheal intubation in 1.5-2 minutes with clinically effective duration of action during propofol anesthesia of 55-61 minutes.) Initial dose after succinylcholine for intubation: 0.1 mg/kg; maintenance dose: 0.03 mg/kg 40-60 minutes after initial dose, then at ~20-minute intervals based on clinical criteria.

Continuous infusion: After an initial bolus, a diluted solution can be given by continuous infusion for maintenance of neuromuscular blockade during extended surgery; adjust the rate of administration according to the patient's response as determined by peripheral nerve stimulation. An initial infusion rate of 3 mcg/kg/minute may be required to rapidly counteract the spontaneous recovery of neuromuscular function; thereafter, a rate of 1-2 mcg/kg/minute should be adequate to maintain continuous neuromuscular block in the 89% to 99% range in most pediatric and adult patients. Consider reduction of the infusion rate by 30% to 40% when administering during stable isoflurane, enflurane, sevoflurane, or desflurane anesthesia. Spontaneous recovery from neuromuscular blockade following discontinuation of infusion of cisatracurium may be expected to proceed at a rate comparable to that following single bolus administration.

Intensive care unit administration: Follow the principles for infusion in the operating room. At initial signs of recovery from bolus dose, begin the infusion at a dose of 3 mcg/kg/minute and adjust rates accordingly; dosage ranges of 0.5-10 mcg/kg/minute have been reported. If patient is allowed to recover from neuromuscular blockade, readministration of a bolus dose may be necessary to quickly re-establish neuromuscular block prior to reinstituting the infusion. See table.

Cisatracurium Besylate Infusion Chart

Drug Delivery Rate (mcg/kg/min)	Infusion Rate (mL/kg/min) 0.1 mg/mL (10 mg/100 mL)	Infusion Rate (mL/kg/min) 0.4 mg/mL (40 mg/100 mL)
1	0.01	0.0025
1.5	0.015	0.00375
2	0.02	0.005
3	0.03	0.0075
5	0.05	0.0125

Pediatrics: Neuromuscular blockade:
Operating room administration:
Children 2-12 years: I.V. (Not to be used I.M.)
Intubating doses: 0.1 mg over 5-15 seconds during either halothane or opioid anesthesia. (**Note:** When given during stable opioid nitrous oxide/oxygen anesthesia, 0.1 mg/kg produces maximum neuromuscular block in an average of 2.8 minutes and clinically effective block for 28 minutes.)
Continuous infusion: Refer to adult dosing.
Intensive care unit administration: Refer to adult dosing.
Renal Impairment: Because slower times to onset of complete neuromuscular block were observed in renal dysfunction patients, extending the interval between the administration of cisatracurium and intubation attempt may be required to achieve adequate intubation conditions.

Available Dosage Forms
Injection, solution: 2 mg/mL (5 mL); 10 mg/mL (20 mL)
Injection, solution: 2 mg/mL (10 mL) [contains benzyl alcohol]

Monitoring and Teaching Issues
Physical Assessment: Only clinicians experienced in the use of neuromuscular blocking drugs should administer and/or manage the use of cisatracurium. Dosage and rate of administration should be individualized and titrated to the desired effect, according to relevant clinical factors, premedication, concomitant medications, age, and general condition of the patient. Ventilatory support must be instituted and maintained until adequate respiratory muscle function and/or airway protection are assured. Assess other medications for effectiveness and safety. Other drugs that affect neuromuscular activity may increase/decrease neuromuscular block induced by cisatracurium. This drug does not cause anesthesia or analgesia; pain must be treated with appropriate analgesic agents. Continuous monitoring of vital signs, cardiac status, respiratory status, and degree of neuromuscular block (objective assessment with peripheral external nerve stimulator) is mandatory during infusion and until full muscle tone has returned. Muscle tone returns in a predictable pattern, starting with diaphragm, abdomen, chest, limbs, and finally muscles of the neck, face, and eyes. Safety precautions must be maintained until full muscle tone has returned. **Note:** It may take longer for return of muscle tone in obese or elderly patients or patients with renal or hepatic disease, myasthenia gravis, myopathy, other neuromuscular disease, dehydration, electrolyte imbalance, or severe acid/base imbalance. Provide appropriate patient teaching/support prior to and following administration.

Long-term use: Monitor fluid levels (intake and output) during and following infusion. Reposition patient and provide appropriate skin care, mouth care, and care of patient's eyes every 2-3 hours while sedated. Provide appropriate emotional and sensory support (auditory and environmental).

Note breast-feeding caution.

Patient Education: Patient will usually be unconscious prior to administration. Patient education should be appropriate to individual situation. Reassurance of constant monitoring and emotional support to reduce fear and anxiety should precede and follow administration. Following return of muscle tone, do not attempt to change position or rise from bed without assistance. Report immediately any skin rash or hives, pounding heartbeat, respiratory difficulty, or muscle tremors. **Breast-feeding precaution:** Consult prescriber if breast-feeding.
Pregnancy Risk Factor: B
Lactation: Excretion in breast milk unknown/use caution

Administration
I.M.: Not for I.M. injection, too much tissue irritation.
I.V.: Administer I.V. only. The use of a peripheral nerve stimulator will permit the most advantageous use of cisatracurium, minimize the possibility of overdosage or underdosage and assist in the evaluation of recovery.

Give undiluted as a bolus injection. Continuous administration requires the use of an infusion pump.
Compatibility: Stable in D₅W, NS, D₅NS
Y-site administration: Incompatible with amphotericin B cholesteryl sulfate complex, cefoperazone
Compatibility when admixed: Incompatible with ketorolac, propofol
Storage: Refrigerate intact vials at 2°C to 8°C/36°F to 46°F. Use vials within 21 days upon removal from the refrigerator to room temperature (25°C to 77°F). Dilutions of 0.1-0.2 mg/mL in 0.9% sodium chloride or dextrose 5% in water are stable for up to 24 hours at room temperature.
Additional Information Cisatracurium is classified as an intermediate-duration neuromuscular-blocking agent. It does not appear to have a cumulative effect on the duration of blockade. Neuromuscular-blocking potency is 3 times that of atracurium; maximum block is up to 2 minutes longer than for equipotent doses of atracurium.

♦ **Cisatracurium Besylate** *see* Cisatracurium *on page 333*

Cisplatin (SIS pla tin)
U.S. Brand Names Platinol®-AQ
Synonyms CDDP
Generic Available Yes
Pharmacologic Category Antineoplastic Agent, Alkylating Agent
Medication Safety Issues
Sound-alike/look-alike issues:
Cisplatin may be confused with carboplatin
Platinol®-AQ may be confused with Paraplatin®, Patanol®, Plaquenil®
Use Treatment of head and neck, breast, testicular, and ovarian cancer; Hodgkin's and non-Hodgkin's lymphoma; neuroblastoma; sarcomas, bladder, gastric, lung, esophageal, (Continued)

Cisplatin *(Continued)*

cervical, and prostate cancer; myeloma, melanoma, mesothelioma, small cell lung cancer, and osteosarcoma

Mechanism of Action/Effect Inhibits DNA synthesis

Contraindications Hypersensitivity to cisplatin, other platinum-containing compounds, or any component of the formulation (anaphylactic-like reactions have been reported); pre-existing renal insufficiency; myelosuppression; hearing impairment; pregnancy

Warnings/Precautions The U.S. Food and Drug Administration (FDA) currently recommends that procedures for proper handling and disposal of antineoplastic agents be considered. All patients should receive adequate hydration prior to and for 24 hours after cisplatin administration, with or without mannitol and/or furosemide, to ensure good urine output and decrease the chance of nephrotoxicity. Reduce dosage in renal impairment. Cumulative renal toxicity may be severe. Dose-related toxicities include myelosuppression, nausea, and vomiting. Ototoxicity, especially pronounced in children, is manifested by tinnitus or loss of high frequency hearing and occasionally, deafness. **Serum magnesium, as well as other electrolytes, should be monitored both before and within 48 hours after cisplatin therapy.** Patients who are magnesium depleted should receive replacement therapy before the cisplatin is administered. If cisplatin contacts the skin, wash and flush thoroughly with water. When administered as sequential infusions, taxane derivatives (docetaxel, paclitaxel) should be administered before platinum derivatives (carboplatin, cisplatin) to limit myelosuppression and to enhance efficacy.

Drug Interactions

Decreased Effect: Sodium thiosulfate theoretically inactivates drug systemically; has been used clinically to reduce systemic toxicity with intraperitoneal administration of cisplatin.

Increased Effect/Toxicity: Cisplatin and ethacrynic acid have resulted in severe ototoxicity in animals. Delayed bleomycin elimination with decreased glomerular filtration rate. When administered as sequential infusions, observational studies indicate a potential for increased toxicity when platinum derivatives (carboplatin, cisplatin) are administered before taxane derivatives (docetaxel, paclitaxel).

Nutritional/Ethanol Interactions Herb/Nutraceutical: Avoid black cohosh, dong quai in estrogen-dependent tumors.

Adverse Reactions

>10%:

Central nervous system: Neurotoxicity: Peripheral neuropathy is dose- and duration-dependent. The mechanism is through axonal degeneration with subsequent damage to the long sensory nerves. Toxicity can first be noted at cumulative doses of 200 mg/m^2, with measurable toxicity at cumulative doses >350 mg/m^2. This process is irreversible and progressive with continued therapy.

Dermatologic: Mild alopecia

Gastrointestinal: Cisplatin is one of the most emetogenic agents used in cancer chemotherapy; nausea and vomiting occur in 76% to 100% of patients and is dose related. Prophylactic antiemetics should always be prescribed; nausea and vomiting may last up to 1 week after therapy.

Hematologic: Myelosuppressive: Mild with moderate doses, mild to moderate with high-dose therapy

WBC: Mild

Platelets: Mild

Onset: 10 days

Nadir: 14-23 days

Recovery: 21-39 days

Hepatic: Elevation of liver enzymes

Renal: Nephrotoxicity: Related to elimination, protein binding, and uptake of cisplatin. Two types of nephrotoxicity: Acute renal failure and chronic renal insufficiency.

Acute renal failure and azotemia is a dose-dependent process and can be minimized with proper administration and prophylaxis. Damage to the proximal tubules by unbound cisplatin is suspected to cause the toxicity. It is manifested as increased BUN/creatinine, oliguria, protein wasting, and potassium, calcium, and magnesium wasting.

Chronic renal dysfunction can develop in patients receiving multiple courses of cisplatin. Slow release of tissue-bound cisplatin may contribute to chronic nephrotoxicity. Manifestations of this toxicity are varied, and can include sodium and water wasting, nephropathy, hyperuricemia, decreased Cl$_{cr}$, and magnesium wasting.

Recommendations for minimizing nephrotoxicity include:

Prepare cisplatin in saline-containing vehicles

Infuse dose over 24 hours

Vigorous hydration (125-150 mL/hour) before, during, and after cisplatin administration

Simultaneous administration of either mannitol or furosemide

Pretreatment with amifostine

Avoid other nephrotoxic agents (aminoglycosides, amphotericin, etc)

Otic: Ototoxicity: Ototoxicity occurs in 10% to 30%, and is manifested as high frequency hearing loss. Baseline audiography should be performed. Ototoxicity is especially pronounced in children.

1% to 10%: Local: Extravasation: May cause thrombophlebitis and tissue damage if infiltrated; may use sodium thiosulfate as antidote, but consult hospital policy for guidelines.

Irritant chemotherapy

Overdosage/Toxicology Symptoms of overdose include severe myelosuppression, intractable nausea and vomiting, kidney and liver failure, deafness, ocular toxicity, and neuritis. There is no known antidote. Hemodialysis appears to have little effect. Treatment is supportive.

Pharmacodynamics/Kinetics

Protein Binding: >90%

Half-Life Elimination: Initial: 20-30 minutes; Beta: 60 minutes; Terminal: ~24 hours; Secondary half-life: 44-73 hours

Metabolism: Nonenzymatic; inactivated (in both cell and bloodstream) by sulfhydryl groups; covalently binds to glutathione and thiosulfate

Excretion: Urine (>90%); feces (10%)

Dosing

Adults & Elderly: Refer to individual protocols.

Note: An estimated Cl_{cr} should be on all cisplatin chemotherapy orders along with other patient parameters (eg, patient's height, weight, and body surface area). Pharmacy and nursing staff should check the Cl_{cr} on the order and determine the appropriateness of cisplatin dosing.

It is recommended that a 24-hour urine creatinine clearance be checked prior to a patient's first dose of cisplatin and periodically thereafter (ie, after every 2-3 cycles of cisplatin).

Pretreatment hydration with 1-2 L of fluid is recommended prior to cisplatin administration. Adequate hydration and urinary output (>100 mL/hour) should be maintained for 24 hours after administration.

Note: If the dose prescribed is a reduced dose, then this should be indicated on the chemotherapy order.

Advanced bladder cancer: 50-70 mg/m^2 every 3-4 weeks

Head and neck cancer: 100-120 mg/m^2 every 3-4 weeks

Malignant pleural mesothelioma (in combination with pemetrexed): 75 mg/m^2 on day 1 of each 21-day cycle; see Pemetrexed monograph for additional details

Metastatic ovarian cancer: 75-100 mg/m^2 every 3 weeks

Intraperitoneal: Cisplatin has been administered intraperitoneal with systemic sodium thiosulfate for ovarian cancer; doses up to 90-270 mg/m^2 have been administered and retained for 4 hours before draining

Testicular cancer: 10-20 mg/m^2/day for 5 days repeated every 3-4 weeks

High dose BMT: Continuous I.V.: 55 mg/m^2/24 hours for 72 hours; total dose: 165 mg/m^2

Pediatrics: Refer to individual protocols.

Note: Various dosing schedules have been used. Examples include:

Intermittent dosing schedule: I.V.: 37-75 mg/m^2 once every 2-3 weeks or 50-100 mg/m^2 over 4-6 hours, once every 21-28 days

Daily dosing schedule: I.V.: 15-20 mg/m^2/day for 5 days every 3-4 weeks

Osteogenic sarcoma or neuroblastoma: I.V.: 60-100 mg/m^2 on day 1 every 3-4 weeks

Recurrent brain tumors: I.V.: 60 mg/m^2 once daily for 2 consecutive days every 3-4 weeks

Bone marrow/blood cell transplantation: Refer to adult dosing.

Renal Impairment:

Cl_{cr} 10-50 mL/minute: Administer 75% of normal dose.

Cl_{cr} <10 mL/minute: Administer 50% of normal dose.

Hemodialysis: Partially cleared by hemodialysis.

Administer dose posthemodialysis.

CAPD effects: Unknown

CAVH effects: Unknown

Available Dosage Forms

Injection, solution: 1 mg/mL (50 mL, 100 mL, 200 mL)

Platinol®-AQ: 1 mg/mL (50 mL, 100 mL)

Monitoring and Teaching Issues

Physical Assessment: Use caution in presence of renal impairment or electrolyte imbalance (see Warnings/Precautions). Assess potential for interactions with other pharmacological agents or herbal products patient may be taking (especially anything that is ototoxic or nephrotoxic; see Drug Interactions). Patient should be vigorously hydrated prior to and for 24 hours following infusion. Cisplatin is highly emetogenic; antiemetic should be administered prior to each treatment and as needed during infusions. Infusion site must be monitored closely to reduce potential for extravasation. See Administration for infusion specifics. Assess results of laboratory tests (see Monitoring Laboratory Tests) and auditory evaluation prior to each treatment and regularly during therapy. Patient response should be closely monitored during and following therapy (eg, renal failure [acute or chronic]; peripheral neuropathy and ototoxicity [may be irreversible]; see Adverse Reactions). Teach patient (or caregiver) possible side effects/appropriate interventions (eg, importance of adequate hydration) and adverse symptoms to report (see Patient Education).

Monitoring Laboratory Tests: Renal function (serum creatinine, BUN, Cl_{cr}); electrolytes (particularly magnesium, calcium, potassium) before and within 48 hours after cisplatin therapy; liver function periodically, CBC with differential and platelet count, urinalysis

Patient Education: Do not take any new medication during therapy unless approved by prescriber. This medication can only be administered by I.V. and numerous side effects can occur. Report immediately any burning, pain, itching, or redness at infusion site. It is important that you maintain adequate hydration (2-3 L/day of fluids) unless instructed to restrict fluid intake and adequate nutrition (small frequent meals may help). May cause severe nausea or vomiting that can be delayed for up to 48 hours after infusion and last for 1 week (consult prescriber for appropriate antiemetic medication); mouth sores (use soft toothbrush or cotton swabs for mouth care); or loss of hair (reversible). You will be susceptible to infection (avoid crowds and exposure to infection and do not have any vaccinations without consulting prescriber). Report promptly any pain, tingling, or loss of sensation in extremities; change in hearing; rash or hives; difficulty breathing or swallowing; fever or chills; chest pain or palpitations; unusual fatigue; unusual bruising/bleeding; muscle cramps or twitching; or any other unusual symptoms. **Pregnancy/breast-feeding precautions:** Inform prescriber if you are pregnant. Do not get pregnant during therapy. Consult prescriber for instruction on appropriate barrier contraceptive measures. This drug may cause severe fetal defects.

Dietary Considerations: Sodium content: 9 mg/mL (equivalent to 0.9% sodium chloride solution)

(Continued)

Cisplatin (Continued)

Pregnancy Risk Factor: D
Lactation: Enters breast milk/contraindicated (AAP rates "compatible")
Administration
    I.V.: Irritant. Perform pretreatment hydration (see Dosing). Aluminum-containing I.V. infusion sets and needles should **not** be used due to binding with the platinum.

    I.V.: Rate of administration has varied from a 15- to 120-minute infusion, 1 mg/minute infusion, 6- to 8-hour infusion, 24-hour infusion, or per protocol. Maximum rate of infusion: 1 mg/minute in patients with CHF.
    When administered as sequential infusions, taxane derivatives (docetaxel, paclitaxel) should be administered before platinum derivatives to limit myelosuppression and to enhance efficacy.

    Reconstitution: Further dilution stability is dependent on the chloride ion concentration and should be mixed in solutions of NS (at least 0.3% NaCl). Further dilution in NS, D_5/0.45% NaCl or D_5/NS to a concentration of 0.05-2 mg/mL are stable for 72 hours at 4°C to 25°C in combination with mannitol; may administer 12.5-50 g mannitol/L.

    Standard I.V. dilution: Dose/250-1000 mL NS, D_5/NS or D_5/0.45% NaCl; stable for 72 hours at 4°C to 25°C (in combination with mannitol).

    Compatibility: Stable in $D_5^1/_4$NS, $D_5^1/_2$NS, D_5NS, $^1/_4$NS, $^1/_3$NS, $^1/_2$NS, NS; **incompatible** with sodium bicarbonate 5%
    Y-site administration: Incompatible with amifostine, amphotericin B cholesteryl sulfate complex, cefepime, piperacillin/tazobactam, thiotepa
    Compatibility when admixed: Incompatible with fluorouracil, mesna, thiotepa

    Storage: Store intact vials at room temperature 15°C to 25°C (59°F to 77°F) and protect from light. Do not refrigerate solution as a precipitate may form. If inadvertently refrigerated, the precipitate will slowly dissolve within hours to days, when placed at room temperature. The precipitate may be dissolved without loss of potency by warming solution to 37°C (98.6°F). After initial entry into the vial, solution is stable for 28 days protected from light or for at least 7 days under fluorescent room light at room temperature.

Additional Information
    Sodium content: 9 mg/mL (equivalent to 0.9% sodium chloride solution)
    Osmolality of Platinol®-AQ = 285-286 mOsm

♦ **13-*cis*-Retinoic Acid** see Isotretinoin *on page 842*

Citalopram (sye TAL oh pram)

    U.S. Brand Names Celexa™
    Synonyms Citalopram Hydrobromide; Nitalapram
    Restrictions A medication guide should be dispensed with each prescription. A template for the required MedGuides can be found on the FDA website at: http://www.fda.gov/cder/drug/antidepressants/labelTemplate.pdf
    Generic Available Yes
    Pharmacologic Category Antidepressant, Selective Serotonin Reuptake Inhibitor
    Medication Safety Issues
    Sound-alike/look-alike issues:
        Celexa™ may be confused with Celebrex®, Cerebra®, Cerebyx®, Zyprexa®
    Use Treatment of depression
    Unlabeled/Investigational Use Treatment of dementia, smoking cessation, ethanol abuse, obsessive-compulsive disorder (OCD) in children, diabetic neuropathy
    Mechanism of Action/Effect A bicyclic phthalein derivative, citalopram selectively inhibits serotonin reuptake in the presynaptic neurons
    Contraindications Hypersensitivity to citalopram or any component of the formulation; hypersensitivity or other adverse sequelae during therapy with other SSRIs; concomitant use with MAO inhibitors or within 2 weeks of discontinuing MAO inhibitors.
    Warnings/Precautions Antidepressants increase the risk of suicidal thinking and behavior in children and adolescents with major depressive disorder (MDD) and other depressive disorders; consider risk prior to prescribing. All patients must be closely monitored for clinical worsening, suicidality, or unusual changes in behavior, especially during the initiation of therapy or following an increase or decrease in dosage. When used in children, the child's family or caregiver should be instructed to closely observe the patient and communicate condition with healthcare provider. A medication guide should be dispensed with each prescription. **Citalopram is not FDA approved for use in children.**

    The possibility of a suicide attempt is inherent in major depression and may persist until remission occurs. Use caution in high-risk patients. Worsening depression and severe abrupt suicidality that are not part of the presenting symptoms may require discontinuation or modification of drug therapy. The patient's family or caregiver should be alerted to monitor patients for the emergence of suicidality and associated behaviors (such as agitation, irritability, hostility, impulsivity, and hypomania) and call healthcare provider.

    May worsen psychosis in some patients or precipitate a shift to mania or hypomania in patients with bipolar disorder. Patients presenting with depressive symptoms should be screened for bipolar disorder. Monotherapy in patients with bipolar disorder should be avoided. **Citalopram is not FDA approved for the treatment of bipolar depression.**

    The potential for severe reaction exists when used with MAO inhibitors; serotonin syndrome (hyperthermia, muscular rigidity, mental status changes/agitation, autonomic instability) may occur. May increase the risks associated with electroconvulsive therapy. Has a low potential to impair cognitive or motor performance; caution operating hazardous machinery or driving.

    Use with caution in patients with hepatic or renal dysfunction, in elderly patients, concomitant CNS depressants, and pregnancy (high doses of citalopram have been associated with teratogenicity in animals). Use caution with concomitant use of NSAIDs, ASA, or other drugs that affect coagulation; the risk of bleeding is potentiated. May cause hyponatremia/SIADH. May cause or exacerbate sexual dysfunction. Upon discontinuation of citalopram therapy, gradually taper dose. If intolerable symptoms occur following a decrease in dosage or upon discontinuation of therapy, then resuming the previous dose with a more gradual taper should be considered.

Drug Interactions

Cytochrome P450 Effect: Substrate of CYP2C19 (major), 2D6 (minor), 3A4 (major); **Inhibits** CYP1A2 (weak), 2B6 (weak), 2C19 (weak), 2D6 (weak)

Decreased Effect: CYP2C19 inducers may decrease the levels/effects of citalopram; example inducers include aminoglutethimide, carbamazepine, phenytoin, and rifampin. Cyproheptadine may inhibit the effects of serotonin reuptake inhibitors. CYP3A4 inducers may decrease the levels/effects of citalopram; example inducers include aminoglutethimide, carbamazepine, nafcillin, nevirapine, phenobarbital, phenytoin, and rifamycins.

Increased Effect/Toxicity: Citalopram should not be used with nonselective MAO inhibitors (phenelzine, isocarboxazid) or other drugs with MAO inhibition (linezolid); fatal reactions have been reported. Wait 5 weeks after stopping citalopram before starting a nonselective MAO inhibitor and 2 weeks after stopping an MAO inhibitor before starting citalopram. Concurrent selegiline has been associated with mania, hypertension, or serotonin syndrome (risk may be reduced relative to nonselective MAO inhibitors).

CYP2C19 inhibitors may increase the levels/effects of citalopram; example inhibitors include delavirdine, fluconazole, fluvoxamine, gemfibrozil, isoniazid, omeprazole, and ticlopidine. CYP3A4 inhibitors may increase the levels/effects of citalopram; example inhibitors include azole antifungals, ciprofloxacin, clarithromycin, diclofenac, doxycycline, erythromycin, imatinib, isoniazid, nefazodone, nicardipine, propofol, protease inhibitors, quinidine, and verapamil.

Combined use of SSRIs and amphetamines, buspirone, meperidine, nefazodone, serotonin agonists (such as sumatriptan), sibutramine, other SSRIs, sympathomimetics, ritonavir, tramadol, and venlafaxine may increase the risk of serotonin syndrome. Risk of hyponatremia may increase with concurrent use of loop diuretics (bumetanide, furosemide, torsemide). Citalopram may increase the hypoprothrombinemic response to warfarin. Concomitant use of citalopram and NSAIDs, aspirin, or other drugs affecting coagulation has been associated with an increased risk of bleeding; monitor.

Combined use of sumatriptan (and other serotonin agonists) may result in toxicity; weakness, hyper-reflexia, and incoordination have been observed with sumatriptan and SSRIs. In addition, concurrent use may theoretically increase the risk of serotonin syndrome; includes sumatriptan, naratriptan, rizatriptan, and zolmitriptan.

Nutritional/Ethanol Interactions

Ethanol: Avoid ethanol (may increase CNS depression).

Herb/Nutraceutical: Avoid valerian, St John's wort, SAMe, kava kava, and gotu kola (may increase CNS depression).

Adverse Reactions

>10%:

Central nervous system: Somnolence, insomnia

Gastrointestinal: Nausea, xerostomia

Miscellaneous: Diaphoresis

<10%:

Central nervous system: Anxiety, anorexia, agitation, yawning

Dermatologic: Rash, pruritus

Endocrine & metabolic: Sexual dysfunction

Gastrointestinal: Diarrhea, dyspepsia, vomiting, abdominal pain, weight gain

Neuromuscular & skeletal: Tremor, arthralgia, myalgia

Respiratory: Cough, rhinitis, sinusitis

Overdosage/Toxicology Symptoms of overdose include dizziness, nausea, vomiting, sweating, tremor, somnolence, and sinus tachycardia. Rare symptoms have included amnesia, confusion, coma, seizures, hyperventilation, and ECG changes (including QT_c prolongation, ventricular arrhythmia, and torsade de pointes). Management is supportive and symptomatic.

Pharmacodynamics/Kinetics

Bioavailability: 80%

Time to Peak: Serum: 1-6 hours, average within 4 hours

Protein Binding: Plasma: ~80%

Half-Life Elimination: 24-48 hours (average: 35 hours); doubled with hepatic impairment

Metabolism: Extensively hepatic, including CYP, to N-demethylated, N-oxide, and deaminated metabolites

Excretion: Urine (10% as unchanged drug)

Note: Clearance was decreased, while AUC and half-life were significantly increased in elderly patients and in patients with hepatic impairment. Mild to moderate renal impairment may reduce clearance (17%) and prolong half-life of citalopram. No pharmacokinetic information is available concerning patients with severe renal impairment.

Dosing

Adults: Depression: Oral: Initial: 20 mg/day, generally with an increase to 40 mg/day; doses of more than 40 mg are not usually necessary. Should a dose increase be necessary, it should occur in 20 mg increments at intervals of no less than 1 week. Maximum dose: 60 mg/day.

Elderly: Oral: Initial dose: 10-20 mg once daily. Increase dose to 40 mg/day only in nonresponders.

Pediatrics: Children and Adolescents: OCD (unlabeled use): Oral: 10-40 mg/day

Renal Impairment: None necessary in mild-moderate renal impairment; best avoided in severely impaired renal function (Cl_{cr} <20 mL/minute).

Hepatic Impairment: Reduce dosage in those with hepatic impairment.

Available Dosage Forms

Solution, oral: 10 mg/5 mL (240 mL) [alcohol free, sugar free; peppermint flavor]

Tablet: 10 mg, 20 mg, 40 mg

(Continued)

Citalopram *(Continued)*

Monitoring and Teaching Issues

Physical Assessment: Assess other medications patient may be taking for possible interaction (especially MAO inhibitors, P450 inhibitors, and other CNS active agents). Monitor for effectiveness of therapy and adverse reactions. Assess mental status for depression, suicidal ideation, anxiety, social functioning, mania, or panic attack. Assess knowledge/teach patient appropriate use, interventions to reduce side effects (eg, hypotensive precautions), and adverse symptoms to report.

Monitoring Laboratory Tests: Liver function tests and CBC with continued therapy

Patient Education: It may take up to 3 weeks to see therapeutic effects from this medication. Take as directed; do not alter dose or frequency without consulting prescriber. May be taken with or without food. Avoid alcohol, caffeine, and CNS stimulants. Avoid use of aspirin or other NSAIDs unless approved by prescriber (may increase risk of bleeding). You may experience sexual dysfunction (reversible). May cause dizziness, anxiety, or blurred vision (rise slowly from sitting or lying position and use caution when driving or engaging in tasks requiring alertness until response to drug is known); or nausea or dry mouth (small frequent meals, frequent mouth care, chewing gum, or sucking lozenges may help). Report confusion or impaired concentration, thoughts of suicide, severe headache, palpitations, rash, insomnia or nightmares, changes in personality, muscle weakness or tremors, altered gait pattern, signs and symptoms of respiratory infection, or excessive perspiration. **Pregnancy/breast-feeding precautions:** Inform prescriber if you are or intend to become pregnant. Do not breast-feed.

Dietary Considerations: May be taken without regard to food.

Geriatric Considerations: Clearance was decreased, while AUC and half-life were significantly increased in elderly patients and in patients with hepatic impairment. Mild to moderate renal impairment may reduce clearance of citalopram (17% reduction noted in trials). No pharmacokinetic information is available concerning patients with severe renal impairment.

Pregnancy Risk Factor: C

Pregnancy Issues: Teratogenic effects have been observed in animal studies. Nonteratogenic effects including respiratory distress, cyanosis, apnea, seizures, temperature instability, feeding difficulty, vomiting, hypoglycemia, hypo- or hypertonia, hyper-reflexia, jitteriness, irritability, constant crying, and tremor have been reported in the neonate immediately following delivery after exposure late in the third trimester. Adverse effects may be due to toxic effects of SSRI or drug discontinuation. In some cases, may present clinically as serotonin syndrome. There are no adequate and well-controlled studies in pregnant women. Use during pregnancy only if the potential benefit to the mother outweighs the possible risk to the fetus. If treatment during pregnancy is required, consider tapering therapy during the third trimester.

Lactation: Enters breast milk/contraindicated

Breast-Feeding Issues: Citalopram is excreted in human milk. Excessive somnolence, decreased feeding, and weight loss have been reported in breast-fed infants. A decision should be made whether to continue or discontinue nursing or discontinue the drug.

Administration

Storage: Store below 25°C.

Related Information

Antidepressant Agents *on page 1713*
Antidepressant Medication Guidelines *on page 1765*

♦ **Citalopram Hydrobromide** *see* Citalopram *on page 338*
♦ **Citracal® [OTC]** *see* Calcium Citrate *on page 238*
♦ **Citrate of Magnesia** *see* Magnesium Citrate *on page 929*
♦ **Citric Acid and Potassium Citrate** *see* Potassium Citrate and Citric Acid *on page 1236*
♦ **Citrovorum Factor** *see* Leucovorin *on page 875*
♦ **CL-118,532** *see* Triptorelin *on page 1533*
♦ **CI-719** *see* Gemfibrozil *on page 704*
♦ **CL-825** *see* Pentostatin *on page 1184*
♦ **CL-184116** *see* Porfimer *on page 1230*
♦ **Cla** *see* Clarithromycin *on page 342*

Cladribine *(KLA dri been)*

U.S. Brand Names Leustatin®

Synonyms 2-CdA; 2-Chlorodeoxyadenosine

Generic Available Yes

Pharmacologic Category Adjuvant, Radiosensitizing Agent; Antineoplastic Agent, Antimetabolite (Purine Antagonist); Antineoplastic Agent, Antimetabolite

Medication Safety Issues
Sound-alike/look-alike issues:
Leustatin® may be confused with lovastatin

Use Treatment of hairy cell leukemia, chronic lymphocytic leukemia (CLL), chronic myelogenous leukemia (CML)

Unlabeled/Investigational Use Non-Hodgkin's lymphomas, progressive multiple sclerosis

Mechanism of Action/Effect A prodrug which incorporates DNA causing breakage of DNA strands and shutdown of DNA synthesis. Cladribine is cell-cycle nonspecific.

Contraindications Hypersensitivity to cladribine or any component of the formulation; pregnancy

Warnings/Precautions The U.S. Food and Drug Administration (FDA) currently recommends that procedures for proper handling and disposal of antineoplastic agents be considered. Because of its myelosuppressive properties, cladribine should be used with caution in patients with pre-existing hematologic or immunologic abnormalities.

Nutritional/Ethanol Interactions Ethanol: Avoid ethanol (due to GI irritation).

Adverse Reactions
>10%:
Allergic: Fever (70%), chills (18%); skin reactions (erythema, itching) at the catheter site (18%)

Central nervous system: Fatigue (17%), headache (13%)

Dermatologic: Rash

Hematologic: Myelosuppression, common, dose-limiting; leukopenia (70%); anemia (37%); thrombocytopenia (12%)
Nadir: 5-10 days
Recovery: 4-8 weeks

1% to 10%:
Cardiovascular: Edema, tachycardia

Central nervous system: Dizziness; pains; chills; malaise; severe infection, possibly related to thrombocytopenia

Dermatologic: Pruritus, erythema

Gastrointestinal: Nausea, mild to moderate, usually not seen at doses <0.3 mg/kg/day; constipation; abdominal pain

Neuromuscular & skeletal: Myalgia, arthralgia, weakness

Renal: Renal failure at high (>0.3 mg/kg/day) doses

Miscellaneous: Diaphoresis, delayed herpes zoster infection, tumor lysis syndrome

Pharmacodynamics/Kinetics
Absorption: Oral: 55%; SubQ: 100%; Rectal: 20%

Protein Binding: Plasma: 20%

Half-Life Elimination: Biphasic: Alpha: 25 minutes; Beta: 6.7 hours; Terminal, mean: Normal renal function: 5.4 hours

Metabolism: Hepatic; 5'-triphosphate moiety-active

Excretion: Urine (21% to 44%); Clearance: Estimated systemic: 640 mL/hour/kg

Dosing
Adults & Elderly: Refer to individual protocols.

Hairy cell leukemia: I.V. Continuous infusion:
0.09-0.1 mg/kg/day days 1-7; may be repeated every 28-35 days **or**
3.4 mg/m²/day SubQ days 1-7

Chronic lymphocytic leukemia: I.V. Continuous infusion:
0.1 mg/kg/day days 1-7 **or**
0.028-0.14 mg/kg/day as a 2-hour infusion days 1-5

Chronic myelogenous leukemia: I.V. 15 mg/m²/day as a 1-hour infusion days 1-5; if no response increase dose to 20 mg/m²/day in the second course.

Pediatrics: Refer to individual protocols.

Acute leukemias: 6.2-7.5 mg/m²/day continuous infusion for days 1-5; maximum tolerated dose was 8.9 mg/m²/day.

Available Dosage Forms Injection, solution [preservative free]: 1 mg/mL (10 mL)

Monitoring and Teaching Issues
Physical Assessment: Use caution in presence of pre-existing hematologic or immunologic abnormalities (see Warnings/Precautions). Assess results of laboratory tests, therapeutic effectiveness, and adverse response (eg, myelosuppression, cardiac changes, renal failure; see Adverse Reactions) prior to therapy, regularly during therapy, and following therapy (patients should be considered immunosuppressed for up to 1 year after cladribine therapy). Teach patient (or caregiver) possible side effects/appropriate interventions and adverse symptoms to report (see Patient Education).

Monitoring Laboratory Tests: Liver and renal function tests, CBC with differential, platelets, uric acid

Patient Education: Do not take any new medication during therapy unless approved by prescriber. This drug is administered by infusion; report any pain, redness, irritation at infusion site; chest pain, rapid heart beat, difficulty breathing or swallowing during infusion. It is important to maintain adequate hydration (2-3 L/day of fluids) unless instructed to restrict fluid intake and nutrition during therapy (small frequent meals may help). You will be more susceptible to infection during therapy and for up to 1 year following therapy (avoid crowds and exposure to infection and do not have any vaccinations without consulting prescriber). May cause nausea or vomiting (small frequent meals, frequent mouth care, sucking lozenges, or chewing gum may help); muscle weakness or pain (consult prescriber for mild analgesics); or mouth sores (use frequent mouth care with soft toothbrush or cotton swabs and frequent mouth rinses). Report immediately rash, unusual excessive fatigue, and/or signs of infection. Report rapid heartbeat or palpitations; unusual bruising or bleeding; persistent GI disturbances; diarrhea or constipation; yellowing of eyes or skin; change in color of urine or stool; swelling, warmth, or pain in extremities; or difficult respirations. **Pregnancy/breast-feeding precautions:** Do not get pregnant while taking this medication. Consult prescriber for appropriate contraceptive measures. Do not breast-feed until prescriber advises it is safe.

Pregnancy Risk Factor: D

Lactation: Enters breast milk/contraindicated

Administration
I.V.: Administer as a 1- to 2-hour infusion or by continuous infusion

Reconstitution: Solutions for 7-day infusion should be prepared in bacteriostatic NS.

Compatibility: Stable in NS; **incompatible** with D₅W

Storage: Store intact vials under refrigeration 2°C to 8°C (36°F to 46°F). Dilutions in 500 mL NS are stable for 72 hours. Stable in PVC containers for 24 hours at room temperature of 15°C to 30°C (59°F to 86°F) and 7 days in Pharmacia Deltec® cassettes.

Clarithromycin (kla RITH roe mye sin)

U.S. Brand Names Biaxin®; Biaxin® XL

Synonyms Cla

Generic Available No

Pharmacologic Category Antibiotic, Macrolide

Medication Safety Issues

Sound-alike/look-alike issues:

Clarithromycin may be confused with erythromycin

Use

Children:

Pharyngitis/tonsillitis, acute maxillary sinusitis, uncomplicated skin/skin structure infections, and mycobacterial infections due to the above organisms

Acute otitis media (*H. influenzae*, *M. catarrhalis*, or *S. pneumoniae*)

Prevention of disseminated mycobacterial infections due to MAC disease in patients with advanced HIV infection

Adults:

Pharyngitis/tonsillitis due to susceptible *S. pyogenes*

Acute maxillary sinusitis and acute exacerbation of chronic bronchitis due to susceptible *H. influenzae*, *M. catarrhalis*, or *S. pneumoniae*

Pneumonia due to susceptible *H. influenzae*, *Mycoplasma pneumoniae*, *S. pneumoniae*, or *Chlamydia pneumoniae* (TWAR)

Uncomplicated skin/skin structure infections due to susceptible *S. aureus*, *S. pyogenes*

Disseminated mycobacterial infections due to *M. avium* or *M. intracellulare*

Prevention of disseminated mycobacterial infections due to *M. avium* complex (MAC) disease (eg, patients with advanced HIV infection)

Duodenal ulcer disease due to *H. pylori* in regimens with other drugs including amoxicillin and lansoprazole or omeprazole, ranitidine bismuth citrate, bismuth subsalicylate, tetracycline, and/or an H₂ antagonist

Alternate antibiotic for prophylaxis of bacterial endocarditis in patients who are allergic to penicillin and undergoing surgical or dental procedures

Mechanism of Action/Effect Exerts its antibacterial action by binding to 50S ribosomal subunit resulting in inhibition of protein synthesis. The 14-OH metabolite of clarithromycin is twice as active as the parent compound against some organisms.

Contraindications Hypersensitivity to clarithromycin, erythromycin, or any macrolide antibiotic; use with ergot derivatives, pimozide, cisapride; combination with ranitidine bismuth citrate should not be used in patients with history of acute porphyria or Cl$_{cr}$ <25 mL/minute

Warnings/Precautions Dosage adjustment required with severe renal impairment, decreased dosage or prolonged dosing interval may be appropriate; antibiotic-associated colitis has been reported with use of clarithromycin. Macrolides (including clarithromycin) have been associated with rare QT prolongation and ventricular arrhythmias, including torsade de pointes. Avoid use of extended release tablets (Biaxin® XL) in patients with known stricture/narrowing of the GI tract. Safety and efficacy in children <6 months of age have not been established.

Drug Interactions

Cytochrome P450 Effect: Substrate of CYP3A4 (major); **Inhibits** CYP1A2 (weak), 3A4 (strong)

Decreased Effect: Clarithromycin may decrease the serum concentrations of zafirlukast. Clarithromycin may antagonize the therapeutic effects of clindamycin and lincomycin. Peak levels (but not AUC) of zidovudine may be increased; other studies suggest levels may be decreased. The levels/effects of clarithromycin may be decreased by aminoglutethimide, carbamazepine, nafcillin, nevirapine, phenobarbital, phenytoin, rifamycins, and other CYP3A4 inducers.

Increased Effect/Toxicity: Avoid concomitant use of the following with clarithromycin due to increased risk of malignant arrhythmias: Cisapride, gatifloxacin, moxifloxacin, pimozide, sparfloxacin, thioridazine. Other agents that prolong the QT$_c$ interval, including type Ia (eg, quinidine) and type III antiarrhythmic agents, and selected antipsychotic agents (eg, mesoridazine, thioridazine) should be used with extreme caution.

Clarithromycin is a strong CYP3A4 inhibitor, and may increase the levels/effects of selected benzodiazepines, calcium channel blockers, cyclosporine, mirtazapine, nateglinide, nefazodone, quinidine, sildenafil (and other PDE-5 inhibitors), tacrolimus, venlafaxine, and other CYP3A4 substrates. Selected benzodiazepines (midazolam, triazolam), cisapride, ergot alkaloids, selected HMG-CoA reductase inhibitors (lovastatin and simvastatin), and pimozide are generally contraindicated with strong CYP3A4 inhibitors. When used with strong CYP3A4 inhibitors, dosage adjustment/limits are recommended for sildenafil and other PDE-5 inhibitors; refer to individual monographs.

The effects of neuromuscular-blocking agents and warfarin have been potentiated by clarithromycin. Clarithromycin serum concentrations may be increased by amprenavir (and possibly other protease inhibitors). Digoxin serum levels may be increased by clarithromycin; digoxin toxicity and potentially fatal arrhythmias have been reported; monitor digoxin levels. Fluconazole increases clarithromycin levels and AUC by ~25%. Peak levels (but not AUC) of zidovudine may be increased; other studies suggest levels may be decreased.

The levels/effects of clarithromycin may be increased by azole antifungals, ciprofloxacin, diclofenac, doxycycline, erythromycin, imatinib, isoniazid, nefazodone, nicardipine, propofol, protease inhibitors, quinidine, telithromycin, verapamil, and other CYP3A4 inhibitors.

Nutritional/Ethanol Interactions

Food: Delays absorption; total absorption remains unchanged.

Herb/Nutraceutical: St John's wort may decrease clarithromycin levels.

Adverse Reactions

1% to 10%:

Central nervous system: Headache (adults and children 2%)

Dermatologic: Rash (children 3%)

Gastrointestinal: Diarrhea (adults 6%, children 6%); vomiting (children 6%); nausea (adults 3%); abnormal taste (adults 7%); heartburn (adults 2%); abdominal pain (adults 2%, children 3%)

Hepatic: Prothrombin time increased (1%)

Renal: BUN increased (4%)

Overdosage/Toxicology Symptoms of overdose include nausea, vomiting, diarrhea, prostration, reversible pancreatitis, hearing loss with or without tinnitus, or vertigo. Treatment includes symptomatic and supportive care.

Pharmacodynamics/Kinetics

Absorption: Highly stable in presence of gastric acid (unlike erythromycin); food delays but does not affect extent of absorption

Bioavailability: 50%

Time to Peak: 2-4 hours

Half-Life Elimination: 5-7 hours

Metabolism: Partially hepatic; converted to 14-OH clarithromycin (active metabolite)

Excretion: Primarily urine

Clearance: Approximates normal GFR

Dosing

Adults & Elderly:

Usual dose: Oral: 250-500 mg every 12 hours **or** 1000 mg (two 500 mg extended release tablets) once daily for 7-14 days

Upper respiratory tract: Oral: 250-500 mg every 12 hours for 10-14 days

Pharyngitis/tonsillitis: 250 mg every 12 hours for 10 days

Acute maxillary sinusitis: 500 mg every 12 hours **or** 1000 mg (two 500 mg extended release tablets) once daily for 14 days

Lower respiratory tract: Oral: 250-500 mg every 12 hours for 7-14 days

Acute exacerbation of chronic bronchitis due to:

M. catarrhalis and *S. pneumoniae:* 250 mg every 12 hours **or** 1000 mg (two 500 mg extended release tablets) once daily for 7-14 days

H. influenzae: 500 mg every 12 hours for 7-14 days

Pneumonia due to:

C. pneumoniae, M. pneumoniae, and *S. pneumoniae:* 250 mg every 12 hours for 7-14 days **or** 1000 mg (two 500 mg extended release tablets) once daily for 7 days

H. influenzae: 250 mg every 12 hours for 7 days **or** 1000 mg (two 500 mg extended release tablets) once daily for 7 days

Mycobacterial infection (prevention and treatment): Oral: 500 mg twice daily (use with other antimycobacterial drugs, eg, ethambutol, clofazimine, or rifampin)

Prophylaxis of bacterial endocarditis: Oral: 500 mg 1 hour prior to procedure

Uncomplicated skin and skin structure: Oral: 250 mg every 12 hours for 7-14 days

Peptic ulcer disease: Eradication of *Helicobacter pylori:* Oral (Combination regimen with bismuth subsalicylate, tetracycline, clarithromycin, and an H$_2$-receptor antagonist; or combination of omeprazole and clarithromycin): 250 mg twice daily to 500 mg 3 times/day

Pediatrics: Oral:

Children ≥6 months: 15 mg/kg/day divided every 12 hours for 10 days

Mycobacterial infection (prevention and treatment): 7.5 mg/kg twice daily, up to 500 mg twice daily

Prophylaxis of bacterial endocarditis: 15 mg/kg 1 hour before procedure (maximum dose: 500 mg)

Renal Impairment:

Cl$_{cr}$ <30 mL/minute: Half the normal dose or double the dosing interval.

In combination with ritonavir:

Cl$_{cr}$ 30-60 mL/minute: Reduce dose by 50%.

Cl$_{cr}$ <30 mL/minute: Reduce dose by 75%.

Hepatic Impairment: No dosing adjustment is needed as long as renal function is normal.

Available Dosage Forms

Granules for oral suspension (Biaxin®): 125 mg/5 mL (50 mL, 100 mL); 250 mg/5 mL (50 mL, 100 mL) [fruit punch flavor]

Tablet [film coated] (Biaxin®): 250 mg, 500 mg

Tablet, extended release [film coated] (Biaxin® XL): 500 mg

Monitoring and Teaching Issues

Physical Assessment: Assess results of culture and sensitivity tests and patient's allergy history prior to therapy. See Contraindications and Warnings/Precautions for use cautions (eg, renal, cardiac, and GI concerns). Assess potential for interactions with other pharmacological agents or herbal products patient may be taking (eg, drugs that affect or affected by CYP3A4 enzyme activity; see Drug Interactions). Assess therapeutic effectiveness (according to purpose for use) and adverse reactions (see Adverse Reactions). Teach patient proper use, possible side effects/appropriate interventions, and adverse symptoms to report (see Patient Education).

Monitoring Laboratory Tests: Perform culture and sensitivity studies prior to initiating drug therapy.

Patient Education: Do not take any new medication during therapy unless approved by prescriber. Take full course of therapy even if feeling better; do not discontinue without consulting prescriber. Tablets or suspension may be taken with or without food or milk. Extended release tablets should be taken with food. Do not crush or chew extended release tablets. Do not refrigerate oral suspension (more palatable at room temperature). Maintain adequate hydration (2-3 L/day of fluids) unless instructed to restrict fluid intake. May cause nausea, heartburn, or abnormal taste (small frequent meals, frequent mouth care, chewing gum or sucking lozenges may help); diarrhea (buttermilk, boiled milk, or yogurt may help); or headache or abdominal cramps (consult prescriber for analgesic). Report rapid heartbeat or palpitations, persistent fever or chills, easy bruising or bleeding, joint pain, severe persistent diarrhea, skin rash, sores in mouth, foul-smelling urine, or

(Continued)

Clarithromycin *(Continued)*

respiratory difficulty. **Pregnancy/breast-feeding precautions:** Inform prescriber if you are or intend to become pregnant. Consult prescriber if breast-feeding.

Dietary Considerations: May be taken with or without meals; may be taken with milk. Biaxin® XL should be taken with food.

Geriatric Considerations: Considered one of the drugs of choice in the outpatient treatment of community-acquired pneumonia in older adults. After doses of 500 mg every 12 hours for 5 days, 12 healthy elderly had significantly increased C_{max} and C_{min}, elimination half-lives of clarithromycin and 14-OH clarithromycin compared to 12 healthy young subjects. These changes were attributed to a significant decrease in renal clearance. At a dose of 1000 mg twice daily, 100% of 13 older adults experienced an adverse event compared to only 10% taking 500 mg twice daily.

Pregnancy Risk Factor: C

Pregnancy Issues: There are no adequate and well-controlled studies in pregnant women. Due to adverse fetal effects reported in animal studies, the manufacturer recommends that clarithromycin not be used in a pregnant woman unless there are no alternatives to therapy.

Lactation: Excretion in breast milk unknown/use caution

Breast-Feeding Issues: Erythromycins may be taken while breast-feeding. Use caution.

Administration

Oral: Clarithromycin may be given with or without meals. Give every 12 hours rather than twice daily to avoid peak and trough variation.

Biaxin® XL: Should be given with food. Do not crush or chew extended release tablet.

Reconstitution: Reconstituted oral suspension should not be refrigerated because it might gel. Microencapsulated particles of clarithromycin in suspension is stable for 14 days when stored at room temperature.

Storage: Store tablets and granules for oral suspension at controlled room temperature.

Related Information

Antimicrobial Drugs of Choice *on page 1792*
Community-Acquired Pneumonia in Adults *on page 1807*
Helicobacter pylori Treatment *on page 1835*

- ◆ **Clarithromycin, Lansoprazole, and Amoxicillin** *see* Lansoprazole, Amoxicillin, and Clarithromycin *on page 868*
- ◆ **Claritin® [OTC]** *see* Loratadine *on page 918*
- ◆ **Claritin-D® 12-Hour [OTC]** *see* Loratadine and Pseudoephedrine *on page 919*
- ◆ **Claritin-D® 24-Hour [OTC]** *see* Loratadine and Pseudoephedrine *on page 919*
- ◆ **Claritin® Hives Relief [OTC]** *see* Loratadine *on page 918*
- ◆ **Cleocin®** *see* Clindamycin *on page 344*
- ◆ **Cleocin HCl®** *see* Clindamycin *on page 344*
- ◆ **Cleocin Pediatric®** *see* Clindamycin *on page 344*
- ◆ **Cleocin Phosphate®** *see* Clindamycin *on page 344*
- ◆ **Cleocin T®** *see* Clindamycin *on page 344*
- ◆ **Climara®** *see* Estradiol *on page 552*
- ◆ **Clindagel®** *see* Clindamycin *on page 344*
- ◆ **ClindaMax™** *see* Clindamycin *on page 344*

Clindamycin *(klin da MYE sin)*

U.S. Brand Names Cleocin®; Cleocin HCl®; Cleocin Pediatric®; Cleocin Phosphate®; Cleocin T®; Clindagel®; ClindaMax™; Clindesse™; Clindets®; Evoclin™

Synonyms Clindamycin Hydrochloride; Clindamycin Palmitate; Clindamycin Phosphate

Generic Available Yes: Excludes foam, vaginal suppositories, vaginal cream

Pharmacologic Category Antibiotic, Miscellaneous

Medication Safety Issues

Sound-alike/look-alike issues:
Cleocin® may be confused with bleomycin, Clinoril®, Lincocin®

Use Treatment against aerobic and anaerobic streptococci (except enterococci), most staphylococci, *Bacteroides* sp and *Actinomyces*; bacterial vaginosis (vaginal cream, vaginal suppository); pelvic inflammatory disease (I.V.); topically in treatment of severe acne; vaginally for *Gardnerella vaginalis*

Unlabeled/Investigational Use May be useful in PCP; alternate treatment for toxoplasmosis

Mechanism of Action/Effect Reversibly binds to 50S ribosomal subunits preventing peptide bond formation thus inhibiting bacterial protein synthesis; bacteriostatic or bactericidal depending on drug concentration, infection site, and organism

Contraindications Hypersensitivity to clindamycin or any component of the formulation; previous pseudomembranous colitis; regional enteritis, ulcerative colitis

Warnings/Precautions Dosage adjustment may be necessary in patients with severe hepatic dysfunction; can cause severe and possibly fatal colitis; discontinue drug if significant diarrhea, abdominal cramps, or passage of blood and mucus occurs. Vaginal products may weaken latex or rubber condoms, or contraceptive diaphragms. Barrier contraceptives are not recommended concurrently or for 3-5 days (depending on the product) following treatment. Some dosage forms contain benzyl alcohol or tartrazine. Use caution in atopic patients.

Drug Interactions

Increased Effect/Toxicity: Increased duration of neuromuscular blockade when given in conjunction with tubocurarine and pancuronium.

Nutritional/Ethanol Interactions

Food: Peak concentrations may be delayed with food.
Herb/Nutraceutical: St John's wort may decrease clindamycin levels.

Adverse Reactions

Systemic:

>10%: Gastrointestinal: Diarrhea, abdominal pain

1% to 10%:
  Cardiovascular: Hypotension
  Dermatologic: Urticaria, rash, Stevens-Johnson syndrome
  Gastrointestinal: Pseudomembranous colitis, nausea, vomiting
  Local: Thrombophlebitis, sterile abscess at I.M. injection site
  Miscellaneous: Fungal overgrowth, hypersensitivity

Topical:
  >10%: Dermatologic: Dryness, burning, itching, scaliness, erythema, or peeling of skin (lotion, solution); oiliness (gel, lotion)
  1% to 10%: Central nervous system: Headache

Vaginal:
  >10%: Genitourinary: Fungal vaginosis, vaginitis or vulvovaginal pruritus (from *Candida albicans*)
  1% to 10%:
    Central nervous system: Back pain, headache
    Gastrointestinal: Constipation, diarrhea
    Genitourinary: Urinary tract infection
    Respiratory: Nasopharyngitis
    Miscellaneous: Fungal infection

Overdosage/Toxicology Symptoms of overdose include diarrhea, nausea, and vomiting. Treatment is supportive.

Pharmacodynamics/Kinetics
  Absorption: Topical: ~10%; Oral: Rapid (90%)
  Bioavailability: Topical: <1%
  Time to Peak: Serum: Oral: Within 60 minutes; I.M.: 1-3 hours
  Half-Life Elimination: Neonates: Premature: 8.7 hours; Full-term: 3.6 hours; Adults: 1.6-5.3 hours (average: 2-3 hours)
  Metabolism: Hepatic
  Excretion: Urine (10%) and feces (~4%) as active drug and metabolites

Dosing
  Adults & Elderly:
    Usual dose:
      Oral: 150-450 mg/dose every 6-8 hours; maximum dose: 1.8 g/day
      I.M., I.V.: 1.2-1.8 g/day in 2-4 divided doses; maximum dose: 4.8 g/day
    Pelvic inflammatory disease: I.V.: 900 mg every 8 hours with gentamicin 2 mg/kg, then 1.5 mg/kg every 8 hours; continue after discharge with doxycycline 100 mg twice daily to complete 14 days of total therapy
    Pneumonia due to *Pneumocystis carinii* (unlabeled use):
      Oral: 300-450 mg 4 times/day with primaquine
      I.M., I.V.: 1200-2400 mg/day with pyrimethamine
      I.V.: 600 mg 4 times/day with primaquine
    Acne: Topical:
      Gel, pledget, lotion, solution: Apply a thin film twice daily
      Foam (Evoclin™): Apply once daily
    Bacterial vaginosis: Intravaginal:
      Suppositories: Insert one ovule (100 mg clindamycin) daily into vagina at bedtime for 3 days
      Cream:
        Cleocin®: One full applicator inserted intravaginally once daily before bedtime for 3 or 7 consecutive days in nonpregnant patients or for 7 consecutive days in pregnant patients
        Clindesse™: One full applicator inserted intravaginally as a single dose at anytime during the day in nonpregnant patients
    Prevention of bacterial endocarditis in patients unable to take amoxicillin (unlabeled use): Oral: 600 mg 1 hour before procedure with no follow-up dose needed; for patients allergic to penicillin and unable to take oral medications: 600 mg I.V. within 30 minutes before procedure
    Orofacial infections: 150-450 mg every 6 hours for at least 7 days; maximum dose: 1.8 g/day
    Patients with prosthesis allergic to penicillin: Oral: 600 mg 1 hour before procedure; for patients with prosthesis allergic to penicillin and unable to take oral medication: I.V.: 600 mg 1 hour before procedure
  Pediatrics:
    Usual dose:
      Oral: Infants and Children: 8-20 mg/kg/day as hydrochloride; 8-25 mg/kg/day as palmitate in 3-4 divided doses; minimum dose of palmitate: 37.5 mg 3 times/day
      I.M., I.V.:
        <1 month: 15-20 mg/kg/day
        >1 month: 20-40 mg/kg/day in 3-4 divided doses
    Prevention of bacterial endocarditis (unlabeled use): Oral: Children: 20 mg/kg 1 hour before procedure with no follow-up dose needed; for patients allergic to penicillin and unable to take oral medications: 20 mg/kg I.V. within 30 minutes before procedure
    Orofacial infections: 8-25 mg/kg in 3-4 equally divided doses
    Acne: Topical: Children ≥12 years: Refer to adult dosing.
    Babesiosis: Oral: 20-40 mg/kg divided every 8 hours for 7 days plus quinine
  Hepatic Impairment: Systemic use: Adjustment is recommended in patients with severe hepatic disease.

Available Dosage Forms Note: Strength is expressed as base
  Capsule, as hydrochloride: 150 mg, 300 mg
  Cleocin HCl®: 75 mg [contains tartrazine], 150 mg [contains tartrazine], 300 mg
  Cream, vaginal, as phosphate:
    Cleocin®: 2% (40 g) [contains benzyl alcohol and mineral oil; packaged with 7 disposable applicators]
    Clindesse™: 2% (5 g) [contains mineral oil; prefilled single disposable applicator]
(Continued)

Clindamycin (Continued)

Foam, topical, as phosphate (Evoclin™): 1% (50 g, 100 g) [contains ethanol 58%]

Gel, topical, as phosphate: 1% [10 mg/g] (30 g, 60 g)

  Cleocin T®: 1% [10 mg/g] (30 g, 60 g)

  Clindagel®: 1% [10 mg/g] (40 mL, 75 mL)

  ClindaMax™: 1% (30 g, 60 g)

Granules for oral solution, as palmitate (Cleocin Pediatric®): 75 mg/5 mL (100 mL) [cherry flavor]

Infusion, as phosphate [premixed in D_5W] (Cleocin Phosphate®): 300 mg (50 mL); 600 mg (50 mL); 900 mg (50 mL)

Injection, solution, as phosphate (Cleocin Phosphate®): 150 mg/mL (2 mL, 4 mL, 6 mL, 60 mL) [contains benzyl alcohol and disodium edetate 0.5 mg]

Lotion, as phosphate (Cleocin T®, ClindaMax™): 1% [10 mg/mL] (60 mL)

Pledgets, topical: 1% (60s) [contains alcohol]

  Clindets®: 1% (69s) [contains isopropyl alcohol 52%]

  Cleocin T®: 1% (60s) [contains isopropyl alcohol 50%]

Solution, topical, as phosphate (Cleocin T®): 1% [10 mg/mL] (30 mL, 60 mL) [contains isopropyl alcohol 50%]

Suppository (ovule), vaginal, as phosphate (Cleocin®): 100 mg (3s) [contains oleaginous base; single reusable applicator]

Monitoring and Teaching Issues

Physical Assessment: Assess previous allergy history prior to beginning therapy. Use caution in presence of severe renal impairment or history of colitis (see Warnings/Precautions). **I.V.:** Cardiac status and blood pressure should be monitored and patient kept recumbent after infusion until blood pressure is stabilized. Assess results of laboratory tests and patient response according to dose, route of administration, and purpose of therapy (see Adverse Reactions). Teach patient proper use, possible side effects/appropriate interventions, and adverse symptoms to report (eg, severe diarrhea, opportunistic infection; see Patient Education).

Monitoring Laboratory Tests: CBC, liver and renal function periodically with prolonged therapy

Patient Education:

Oral: Take each dose with a full glass of water. Complete full prescription, even if feeling better. You may experience nausea or vomiting (small frequent meals, frequent mouth care, chewing gum, or sucking lozenges may help). Report dizziness; persistent GI effects (pain, diarrhea, vomiting); skin redness, rash, or burning; fever; chills; unusual bruising or bleeding; signs of infection; excessive fatigue; yellowing of eyes or skin; change in color of urine or blackened stool; swelling, warmth, or pain in extremities; difficult respirations; bloody or fatty stool (do not take antidiarrheal without consulting prescriber); or lack or improvement or worsening of condition.

Topical: Wash hands before applying or wear gloves. Apply thin film of gel, lotion, or solution to affected area. May apply porous dressing. Report persistent burning, swelling, itching, or worsening of condition.

Vaginal: Wash hands before using. At bedtime, lying down, gently insert full applicator into vagina and expel cream. Wash applicator with soap and water following use. Remain lying down for 30 minutes following administration. Avoid intercourse during therapy. Report adverse reactions (dizziness, nausea, vomiting, stomach cramps, or headache) or lack of improvement or worsening of condition.

Dietary Considerations: May be taken with food.

Geriatric Considerations: Elderly patients are often at a higher risk for developing serious colitis and require close monitoring.

Pregnancy Risk Factor: B

Lactation: Enters breast milk/compatible

Administration

Oral: Administer oral dosage form with a full glass of water to minimize esophageal ulceration. Give around-the-clock to promote less variation in peak and trough serum levels.

I.M.: Deep I.M. sites, rotate sites. Do not exceed 600 mg in a single injection.

I.V.: Never administer as bolus; administer by I.V. intermittent infusion over at least 10-60 minutes, at a rate **not** to exceed 30 mg/minute (not exceed 1200 mg/hour); final concentration for administration should not exceed 18 mg/mL

Topical: Foam: Dispense directly into cap or onto a cool surface. Do not dispense directly into hands.

Other:

Intravaginal:

  Cream: Insertion should be as far as possible into the vagina without causing discomfort

  Ovule: The foil should be removed; if the applicator is used for insertion, it should be washed for additional use

Compatibility: Stable in D_5LR, $D_5^1/_2NS$, D_5NS, D_5W, $D_{10}W$, LR, NS

  Y-site administration: Incompatible with allopurinol, filgrastim, fluconazole, idarubicin

  Compatibility in syringe: Incompatible with tobramycin

  Compatibility when admixed: Incompatible with aminophylline, barbiturates, calcium gluconate, ceftriaxone, ciprofloxacin, gentamicin with cefazolin, magnesium sulfate, phenytoin

Storage:

Capsule: Store at room temperature of 20°C to 25°C (68°F to 77°F).

Cream: Store at room temperature.

Foam: Store at room temperature of 20°C to 25°C (68°F to 77°F). Avoid fire, flame, or smoking during or following application.

Gel: Store at room temperature.

  Clindagel®: Do not store in direct sunlight.

I.V.: Infusion solution in NS or D_5W solution is stable for 16 days at room temperature.

Lotion: Store at room temperature of 20°C to 25°C (68°F to 77°F).

Oral solution: Do not refrigerate reconstituted oral solution (it will thicken). Following reconstitution, oral solution is stable for 2 weeks at room temperature of 20°C to 25°C (68°F to 77°F).

Ovule: Store at room temperature of 15°C to 30°C (68°F to 77°F).

Pledget: Store at room temperature.

Topical solution: Store at room temperature of 20°C to 25°C (68°F to 77°F).

Related Information
Antimicrobial Drugs of Choice *on page 1792*
Community-Acquired Pneumonia in Adults *on page 1807*
Compatibility of Drugs *on page 1723*
I.V. to Oral Conversion *on page 1688*

- ◆ **Clindamycin Hydrochloride** *see* Clindamycin *on page 344*
- ◆ **Clindamycin Palmitate** *see* Clindamycin *on page 344*
- ◆ **Clindamycin Phosphate** *see* Clindamycin *on page 344*
- ◆ **Clindesse™** *see* Clindamycin *on page 344*
- ◆ **Clindets®** *see* Clindamycin *on page 344*
- ◆ **Clinoril®** *see* Sulindac *on page 1414*

Clofazimine (kloe FA zi meen)

U.S. Brand Names Lamprene® [DSC]

Synonyms Clofazimine Palmitate

Restrictions Clofazimine is no longer available through most US pharmacies. Requests for clofazimine to treat leprosy should be directed to the National Hansen's Disease Program (a division of the U.S. Department of Health and Human Services), which holds the IND for this indication. The Administrative Officer may be contacted at 225-578-9861 (phone) or 225-578-9856 (fax). Requests for clofazimine to treat MDRTB must be directed to the Division of Special Pathogen and Immunologic Drug Products (HFD-590) at 301-827-2127 (phone). These requests will be distributed by single-patient INDs administered by the FDA. Physicians must register as an investigator for this indication.

Generic Available No

Pharmacologic Category Leprostatic Agent

Medication Safety Issues
Sound-alike/look-alike issues:
Clofazimine may be confused with clonazepam, clozapine

Use Treatment of lepromatous leprosy including dapsone-resistant leprosy and lepromatous leprosy with erythema nodosum leprosum; multibacillary leprosy

Unlabeled/Investigational Use Investigational: Multidrug-resistant tuberculosis

Dosing
Adults & Elderly:
Dapsone-resistant leprosy: Oral: 100 mg/day in combination with one or more antileprosy drugs for 3 years; then alone 100 mg/day
Dapsone-sensitive multibacillary leprosy: Oral: 100 mg/day in combination with two or more antileprosy drugs for at least 2 years and continue until negative skin smears are obtained, then institute single drug therapy with appropriate agent.
Erythema nodosum leprosum: Oral: 100-200 mg/day for up to 3 months or longer then taper dose to 100 mg/day when possible
Pediatrics: Leprosy: Oral: Children: 1 mg/kg/day every 24 hours in combination with dapsone and rifampin
Hepatic Impairment: Should be considered in severe hepatic dysfunction.

Available Dosage Forms [DSC] = Discontinued product
Capsule: 50 mg [DSC]

Monitoring and Teaching Issues
Physical Assessment: See Contraindications and Warnings/Precautions for use cautions. Assess therapeutic effectiveness and adverse reactions (eg, type 2 reaction state; onset of tender skin nodules with joint and lymph gland swelling or visual disturbances; see Adverse Reactions). Teach patient proper use, possible side effects/appropriate interventions, and adverse symptoms to report (refer to Patient Education).
Patient Education: Take as directed. Take with meals. Drug may cause a pink to brownish-black discoloration of the skin, conjunctiva, tears, sweat, urine, feces, and nasal secretions. Although reversible, it may take months to years for skin discoloration to disappear after therapy is complete. Report promptly bone or joint pain, GI disturbance, or vision changes. **Pregnancy/breast-feeding precautions:** Inform prescriber if you are or intend to become pregnant. Do not breast-feed.
Pregnancy Risk Factor: C
Lactation: Enters breast milk/contraindicated (AAP rates "of concern")

Related Information
Tuberculosis *on page 1864*

- ◆ **Clofazimine Palmitate** *see* Clofazimine *on page 347*

Clofibrate (kloe FYE brate)

Restrictions Not available in U.S.

Generic Available Yes

Pharmacologic Category Antilipemic Agent, Fibric Acid

Medication Safety Issues
Sound-alike/look-alike issues:
Clofibrate may be confused with clorazepate

Use Adjunct to dietary therapy in the management of hyperlipidemias associated with high triglyceride levels (types III, IV, V); primarily lowers triglycerides and very low density lipoprotein
(Continued)

Clofibrate *(Continued)*

Mechanism of Action/Effect Increases breakdown of VLDL to LDL. Decreases liver synthesis of VLDL. Inhibits cholesterol formation, lowering serum lipid levels. Has antiplatelet effect.

Contraindications Hypersensitivity to clofibrate or any component of the formulation; significant hepatic or renal dysfunction; primary biliary cirrhosis

Warnings/Precautions Possible increased risk of malignancy and cholelithiasis. No evidence of cardiovascular mortality benefit. Anemia and leukopenia have been reported. Elevations in serum transaminases can be seen. Discontinue if lipid response is not seen. Use with caution in peptic ulcer disease. Flu-like symptoms may occur. Be careful in patient selection; this is not a first- or second-line choice. Other agents may be more suitable.

Drug Interactions

Cytochrome P450 Effect: Substrate of CYP3A4 (minor); **Inhibits** CYP2A6 (weak); **Induces** CYP2B6 (weak), 2E1 (weak), 3A4 (weak)

Decreased Effect: Rifampin (and potentially other inducers of CYP3A4) may reduce blood levels of clofibrate.

Increased Effect/Toxicity: Clofibrate may increase effects of warfarin, insulin, and sulfonylureas. Clofibrate's levels may be increased with probenecid. HMG-CoA reductase inhibitors (atorvastatin, cerivastatin, fluvastatin, lovastatin, pravastatin, simvastatin) may increase the risk of myopathy and rhabdomyolysis. The manufacturer warns against the concomitant use. However, combination therapy with statins has been used in some patients with resistant hyperlipidemias (with great caution).

Lab Interactions Increased creatine phosphokinase [CPK] (S); decreased alkaline phosphatase (S), cholesterol (S), glucose, uric acid (S)

Adverse Reactions Frequency not defined.

Common: Gastrointestinal: Nausea, diarrhea

Less common:

Central nervous system: Headache, dizziness, fatigue

Gastrointestinal: Vomiting, loose stools, heartburn, flatulence, abdominal distress, epigastric pain

Neuromuscular & skeletal: Muscle cramping, aching, weakness, myalgia

Frequency unknown:

Central nervous system: Fever

Cardiovascular: Chest pain, cardiac arrhythmia

Dermatologic: Rash, urticaria, pruritus, alopecia, toxic epidermal necrolysis, erythema multiforme, Stevens-Johnson syndrome; dry, brittle hair

Endocrine & metabolic: Polyphagia, gynecomastia, hyperkalemia

Gastrointestinal: Stomatitis, gallstones, pancreatitis, gastritis, peptic ulcer, weight gain

Genitourinary: Impotence, decreased libido

Hematologic: Leukopenia, anemia, eosinophilia, agranulocytosis, thrombocytopenic purpura

Hepatic: Hepatomegaly, increased liver function tests, jaundice

Local: Thrombophlebitis

Neuromuscular & skeletal: Myalgia, myopathy, myositis, arthralgia, rhabdomyolysis, increased creatinine phosphokinase (CPK), rheumatoid arthritis, tremor

Ocular: Photophobic

Renal: Dysuria, hematuria, proteinuria, renal toxicity (allergic), rhabdomyolysis-induced renal failure

Miscellaneous: Diaphoresis increased, flu-like syndrome, systemic lupus erythematosus

Overdosage/Toxicology Symptoms of overdose include nausea, vomiting, diarrhea, and GI distress. Treatment is supportive.

Pharmacodynamics/Kinetics

Absorption: Complete

Time to Peak: Serum: 3-6 hours

Protein Binding: 95%

Half-Life Elimination: 6-24 hours; significantly prolonged with renal impairment; Anuria: 110 hours

Metabolism: Hepatic to an inactive glucuronide ester; intestinal transformation required to activate drug

Excretion: Urine (40% to 70%)

Dosing

Adults & Elderly: Dyslipidemia: Oral: 500 mg 4 times/day; some patients may respond to lower doses.

Renal Impairment:

Cl_{cr} >50 mL/minute: Administer every 6-12 hours.

Cl_{cr} 10-50 mL/minute: Administer every 12-18 hours.

Cl_{cr} <10 mL/minute: Avoid use.

Available Dosage Forms Capsule: 500 mg

Monitoring and Teaching Issues

Physical Assessment: Care should be used in patient selection; this is not a first- or second-line choice (see Warnings/Precautions). Assess potential for interactions with other pharmacological agents patient may be taking (see Drug Interactions). Assess results of laboratory tests (lipid panels) and adverse reactions (CNS changes, hepatomegaly, anemia, myopathy, and rhabdomyolysis; see Adverse Reactions). Teach patient proper use, possible side effects/appropriate interventions, and adverse symptoms to report (see Patient Education).

Monitoring Laboratory Tests: Periodic lipid panels

Patient Education: Do not take any new medication during therapy unless approved by prescriber. Take exactly as directed. May take with food or milk to reduce stomach upset. This drug may have to be taken long-term; ongoing follow-up is essential. May cause nausea, vomiting, or stomach upset (small frequent meals, frequent mouth care, chewing gum, or sucking lozenges may help); headache, dizziness, fatigue (use care when driving or engaging in potentially hazardous tasks until response to drug is known); or muscle cramping or pain (if persistent, consult prescriber for analgesic). Report chest pain, shortness of breath, irregular heartbeat, palpitations, severe stomach pain with persistent nausea and vomiting, persistent fever, sore throat, or unusual bleeding or bruising. **Pregnancy/breast-feeding precautions:** Inform prescriber if you are or intend to become pregnant. Do not breast-feed.

Geriatric Considerations: The definition of, and therefore, when to treat hyperlipidemia in the elderly is a controversial issue. Therefore, treatment may be better reserved for those who are unable to obtain a desirable plasma cholesterol level by diet alone and for whom the benefits of treatment are believed to outweigh the potential adverse effects, drug interactions, and cost of treatment. Adjust dose for renal function.

Pregnancy Risk Factor: C

Lactation: Excretion in breast milk unknown/contraindicated

Administration

Oral: Administer with meals or milk if GI upset occurs.

Related Information

Hyperlipidemia Management *on page 1836*
Lipid-Lowering Agents *on page 1738*

♦ **Clomid**® *see* ClomiPHENE *on page 349*

ClomiPHENE (KLOE mi feen)

U.S. Brand Names Clomid®; Serophene®

Synonyms Clomiphene Citrate

Generic Available Yes

Pharmacologic Category Ovulation Stimulator

Medication Safety Issues

Sound-alike/look-alike issues:

ClomiPHENE may be confused with clomiPRAMINE, clonidine

Clomid® may be confused with clonidine

Serophene® may be confused with Sarafem™

Use Treatment of ovulatory failure in patients desiring pregnancy

Unlabeled/Investigational Use Male infertility

Mechanism of Action/Effect Induces ovulation by stimulating the release of pituitary gonadotropins

Contraindications Hypersensitivity to clomiphene citrate or any of its components; liver disease; abnormal uterine bleeding; enlargement or development of ovarian cyst; uncontrolled thyroid or adrenal dysfunction in the presence of an organic intracranial lesion such as pituitary tumor; pregnancy

Warnings/Precautions Use with caution in patients sensitive to pituitary gonadotropins (eg, polycystic ovary disease). Clomiphene may induce multiple pregnancies, ovarian enlargement, ovarian hyperstimulation syndrome, or abdominal pain, blurring or other visual symptoms.

Drug Interactions

Decreased Effect: Decreased response when used with danazol. Decreased estradiol response when used with clomiphene.

Lab Interactions Clomiphene may increase levels of serum thyroxine and thyroxine-binding globulin (TBG)

Adverse Reactions

>10%: Endocrine & metabolic: Hot flashes, ovarian enlargement

1% to 10%:

Cardiovascular: Thromboembolism

Central nervous system: Mental depression, headache

Endocrine & metabolic: Breast enlargement (males), breast discomfort (females), abnormal menstrual flow

Gastrointestinal: Distention, bloating, nausea, vomiting, hepatotoxicity

Ocular: Blurring of vision, diplopia, floaters, after-images, phosphenes, photophobia

Pharmacodynamics/Kinetics

Half-Life Elimination: 5-7 days

Metabolism: Undergoes enterohepatic recirculation

Excretion: Primarily feces; urine (small amounts)

Dosing

Adults & Elderly:

Infertility (in males): Oral: 25 mg/day for 25 days with 5 days rest, or 100 mg every Monday, Wednesday, Friday

Ovulatory failure (females): Oral: 50 mg/day for 5 days (first course); start the regimen on or about the fifth day of cycle. The dose should be increased only in those patients who do not ovulate in response to cyclic 50 mg Clomid®. A low dosage or duration of treatment course is particularly recommended if unusual sensitivity to pituitary gonadotropin is suspected, such as in patients with polycystic ovary syndrome.

Repeat dosing; If ovulation does not appear to occur after the first course of therapy, a second course of 100 mg/day (two 50 mg tablets given as a single daily dose) for 5 days should be given. This course may be started as early as 30 days after the previous one after precautions are taken to exclude the presence of pregnancy. Increasing the dosage or duration of therapy beyond 100 mg/day for 5 days is not recommended. The majority of patients who are going to ovulate will do so after the first course of therapy. If ovulation does not occur after 3 courses of therapy, further treatment is not recommended and the patient should be re-evaluated. If 3 ovulatory responses occur, but pregnancy has not been achieved, further treatment is not recommended. If menses does not occur after an ovulatory response, the patient should be re-evaluated. Long-term cyclic therapy is not recommended beyond a total of about 6 cycles.

Available Dosage Forms Tablet, as citrate: 50 mg

(Continued)

ClomiPHENE *(Continued)*

Monitoring and Teaching Issues

Physical Assessment: Assess results of laboratory tests, therapeutic effectiveness (according to purpose for use), and adverse response regularly during therapy. Teach patient proper use (eg, measuring basal body temperature and timing intercourse), possible side effects/appropriate interventions, and adverse symptoms to report. **Pregnancy risk factor X:** Determine that patient is not pregnant before beginning treatment. Breast-feeding is contraindicated.

Monitoring Laboratory Tests: Urine estrogens and estriol levels; normal levels indicate appropriateness for clomiphene therapy.

Patient Education: Inform prescriber of all prescriptions, OTC medications, or herbal products you are taking, and any allergies you have. Do not take any new medication during therapy unless approved by prescriber. Follow recommended schedule of dosing exactly. May cause hot flashes (cool clothes and cool environment may help). Report acute sudden headache; respiratory difficulty; warmth, swelling, pain, or redness in calves; breast enlargement (male) or breast discomfort (female); abnormal menstrual bleeding; vision changes (blurring, diplopia, photophobia, floaters); acute abdominal discomfort; or fever. **Breast-feeding precaution:** Do not breast-feed.

Pregnancy Risk Factor: X

Lactation: Excretion in breast milk unknown/contraindicated

Administration

Storage: Protect from light.

Related Information

FDA Name Differentiation Project: The Use of Tall-Man Letters *on page 15*

♦ Clomiphene Citrate *see* ClomiPHENE *on page 349*

ClomiPRAMINE *(kloe MI pra meen)*

U.S. Brand Names Anafranil®

Synonyms Clomipramine Hydrochloride

Restrictions A medication guide should be dispensed with each prescription. A template for the required MedGuides can be found on the FDA website at: http://www.fda.gov.cder/drug/antidepressants/labelTemplate.pdf

Generic Available Yes

Pharmacologic Category Antidepressant, Tricyclic (Tertiary Amine)

Medication Safety Issues

Sound-alike/look-alike issues:

ClomiPRAMINE may be confused with chlorproMAZINE, clomiPHENE, desipramine, Norpramin®

Anafranil® may be confused with alfentanil, enalapril, nafarelin

Use Treatment of obsessive-compulsive disorder (OCD)

Unlabeled/Investigational Use Depression, panic attacks, chronic pain

Mechanism of Action/Effect Clomipramine appears to affect serotonin uptake while its active metabolite, desmethylclomipramine, affects norepinephrine uptake

Contraindications Hypersensitivity to clomipramine, other tricyclic agents, or any component of the formulation; use of MAO inhibitors within 14 days; use in a patient during the acute recovery phase of MI

Warnings/Precautions Antidepressants increase the risk of suicidal thinking and behavior in children and adolescents with major depressive disorder (MDD) and other depressive disorders; consider risk prior to prescribing. All patients must be closely monitored for clinical worsening, suicidality, or unusual changes in behavior, especially during the initiation of therapy or following an increase or decrease in dosage. When used in children, the child's family or caregiver should be instructed to closely observe the patient and communicate condition with healthcare provider. A medication guide should be dispensed with each prescription. **Clomipramine is FDA approved for the treatment of OCD in children ≥10 years of age.**

The possibility of a suicide attempt is inherent in major depression and may persist until remission occurs. Use caution in high-risk patients. Worsening depression and severe abrupt suicidality that are not part of the presenting symptoms may require discontinuation or modification of drug therapy. The patient's family or caregiver should be alerted to monitor patients for the emergence of suicidality and associated behaviors (such as agitation, irritability, hostility, impulsivity, and hypomania) and notify the healthcare provider.

May worsen psychosis in some patients or precipitate a shift to mania or hypomania in patients with bipolar disorder. Patients presenting with depressive symptoms should be screened for bipolar disorder. Monotherapy in patients with bipolar disorder should be avoided. **Clomipramine is not FDA approved for bipolar depression.**

May cause seizures (relationship to dose and/or duration of therapy) - do not exceed maximum doses. Use caution in patients with a previous seizure disorder or condition predisposing to seizures such as brain damage, alcoholism, or concurrent therapy with other drugs which lower the seizure threshold. May increase the risks associated with electroconvulsive therapy. Has been associated with a high incidence of sexual dysfunction. Weight gain may occur.

The degree of sedation, anticholinergic effects, and conduction abnormalities are high relative to other antidepressants. Clomipramine often causes drowsiness/sedation, resulting in impaired performance of tasks requiring alertness (eg, operating machinery or driving). Sedative effects may be additive with other CNS depressants and/or ethanol. The risk of orthostasis is moderate-high relative to other antidepressants. Use with caution in patients with a history of cardiovascular disease (including previous MI, stroke, tachycardia, or conduction abnormalities). Use with caution in patients with urinary retention, benign prostatic hyperplasia, narrow-angle glaucoma, xerostomia, visual problems, constipation, or a history of bowel obstruction.

Consider discontinuing, when possible, prior to elective surgery. Therapy should not be abruptly discontinued in patients receiving high doses for prolonged periods. Use with caution in hyperthyroid patients or those receiving thyroid supplementation. Use with caution in patients with hepatic or renal dysfunction and in elderly patients.

Drug Interactions

Cytochrome P450 Effect: Substrate of CYP1A2 (major), 2C19 (major), 2D6 (major), 3A4 (minor); **Inhibits** CYP2D6 (moderate)

Decreased Effect: The levels/effects of clomipramine may be decreased by aminoglutethimide, carbamazepine, phenobarbital, phenytoin, rifampin, and other CYP1A2 or 2C19 inducers. Clomipramine may decrease the levels/effects of CYP2D6 prodrug substrates (eg, codeine, hydrocodone, oxycodone, tramadol). Clomipramine inhibits the antihypertensive response to bethanidine, clonidine, debrisoquin, guanadrel, guanethidine, guanabenz, and guanfacine. Cholestyramine and colestipol may decrease the absorption of clomipramine.

Increased Effect/Toxicity: The levels/effects of clomipramine may be increased by amiodarone, chlorpromazine, ciprofloxacin, delavirdine, fluconazole, fluoxetine, fluvoxamine, gemfibrozil, isoniazid, ketoconazole, miconazole, norfloxacin, ofloxacin, omeprazole, paroxetine, pergolide, quinidine, quinine, ritonavir, rofecoxib, ropinirole, ticlopidine, and other CYP1A2, 2C19, or 2D6 inhibitors. Clomipramine may increase the levels/effects of amphetamines, selected beta-blockers, dextromethorphan, fluoxetine, lidocaine, mirtazapine, nefazodone, paroxetine, risperidone, ritonavir, thioridazine, tricyclic antidepressants, venlafaxine, and other CYP2D6 substrates.

Clomipramine increases the effects of amphetamines, anticholinergics, lithium, other CNS depressants (sedatives, hypnotics, ethanol), chlorpropamide, tolazamide, phenothiazines, and warfarin. When used with MAO inhibitors or other serotonergic drugs, serotonin syndrome may occur. Serotonin syndrome has also been reported with ritonavir (rare). Pressor response to I.V. epinephrine, norepinephrine, and phenylephrine may be enhanced in patients receiving TCAs (**Note:** Effect is unlikely with epinephrine or levonordefrin dosages typically administered as infiltration in combination with local anesthetics). Combined use of beta-agonists or drugs which prolong QT_c (including quinidine, procainamide, disopyramide, cisapride, sparfloxacin, gatifloxacin, moxifloxacin) with TCAs may predispose patients to cardiac arrhythmias.

Nutritional/Ethanol Interactions

Ethanol: Avoid ethanol (may increase CNS depression).

Food: Serum concentrations/toxicity may be increased by grapefruit juice.

Herb/Nutraceutical: Avoid valerian, St John's wort, SAMe, kava kava.

Lab Interactions Increased glucose

Adverse Reactions

>10%:

Central nervous system: Dizziness, drowsiness, headache, insomnia, nervousness

Endocrine & metabolic: Libido changes

Gastrointestinal: Xerostomia, constipation, increased appetite, nausea, weight gain, dyspepsia, anorexia, abdominal pain

Neuromuscular & skeletal: Fatigue, tremor, myoclonus

Miscellaneous: Diaphoresis increased

1% to 10%:

Cardiovascular: Hypotension, palpitation, tachycardia

Central nervous system: Confusion, hypertonia, sleep disorder, yawning, speech disorder, abnormal dreaming, paresthesia, memory impairment, anxiety, twitching, impaired coordination, agitation, migraine, depersonalization, emotional lability, flushing, fever

Dermatologic: Rash, pruritus, dermatitis

Gastrointestinal: Diarrhea, vomiting

Genitourinary: Difficult urination

Ocular: Blurred vision, eye pain

Overdosage/Toxicology Symptoms of overdose include agitation, confusion, hallucinations, urinary retention, hypothermia, hypotension, tachycardia, ventricular tachycardia, seizures, and coma. Following initiation of essential overdose management, toxic symptoms should be treated.

Pharmacodynamics/Kinetics

Absorption: Rapid

Half-Life Elimination: 20-30 hours

Metabolism: Hepatic to desmethylclomipramine (active); extensive first-pass effect

Dosing

Adults & Elderly: Treatment of OCD: Oral: Initial: 25 mg/day and gradually increase, as tolerated, to 100 mg/day the first 2 weeks, may then be increased to a total of 250 mg/day maximum

Pediatrics:

Treatment of OCD: Oral: Children >10 years: Initial: 25 mg/day and gradually increase, as tolerated, to a maximum of 3 mg/kg/day or 200 mg/day, whichever is smaller. **Note:** The safety and efficacy of clomipramine in pediatric patients <10 years of age have not been established and, therefore, dosing recommendations cannot be made.

Available Dosage Forms Capsule, as hydrochloride: 25 mg, 50 mg, 75 mg

Monitoring and Teaching Issues

Physical Assessment: Assess other medications patient may be taking for effectiveness and interactions. Monitor therapeutic effectiveness and adverse reactions at beginning of therapy and periodically with long-term use. Assess mental status, affect, and suicidal tendencies. If history of cardiac problems, monitor cardiac status closely. Be alert to the potential of new or increased seizure activity. Taper dosage slowly when discontinuing. Assess knowledge/teach patient appropriate use, interventions to reduce side effects, and adverse symptoms to report.

Monitoring Laboratory Tests: Monitor ECG/cardiac status in older adults and patients with cardiac disease

(Continued)

ClomiPRAMINE *(Continued)*

Patient Education: Take multiple dose medication with meals to reduce side effects. Take single daily dose at bedtime to reduce daytime sedation. The effect of this drug may take several weeks to appear. Do not use alcohol, caffeine, and other prescriptive or OTC medications without consulting prescriber. May cause dizziness, drowsiness, headache, or seizures (use caution when driving or engaging in tasks that require alertness until response to drug is known); dry mouth or unpleasant aftertaste (sucking lozenges and frequent mouth care may help); constipation (increased exercise, fluids, fruit, or fiber may help); or orthostatic hypotension (use caution when rising from lying or sitting to standing position or when climbing stairs). Report unresolved constipation or GI upset, unusual muscle weakness, palpitations, or persistent CNS disturbances (hallucinations, seizures, delirium, insomnia, or impaired gait). **Pregnancy/breast-feeding precautions:** Inform prescriber if you are or intend to become pregnant. Do not breast-feed.

Geriatric Considerations: Not approved as an antidepressant, clomipramine's anticholinergic and hypotensive effects limit its use versus other preferred antidepressants. Elderly patients were found to have higher dose-normalized plasma concentrations as a result of decreased demethylation (decreased 50%) and hydroxylation (25%).

Pregnancy Risk Factor: C

Pregnancy Issues: There are no adequate and well-controlled studies in pregnant women. Withdrawal symptoms (including dizziness, nausea, vomiting, headache, malaise, sleep disturbance, hyperthermia, and/or irritability) have been observed in neonates whose mothers took clomipramine up to delivery. Use in pregnancy only if the benefits to the mother outweigh the potential risks to the fetus.

Lactation: Enters breast milk/contraindicated (AAP rates "of concern")

Breast-Feeding Issues: Generally, it is not recommended to breast-feed if taking antidepressants because of the long half-life, active metabolites, and the potential for side effects in the infant.

Related Information

Antidepressant Agents *on page 1713*
Antidepressant Medication Guidelines *on page 1765*
FDA Name Differentiation Project: The Use of Tall-Man Letters *on page 15*

♦ **Clomipramine Hydrochloride** *see* ClomiPRAMINE *on page 350*

Clonazepam *(kloe NA ze pam)*

U.S. Brand Names Klonopin®

Controlled Substance C-IV

Generic Available Yes: Tablet

Pharmacologic Category Benzodiazepine

Medication Safety Issues

Sound-alike/look-alike issues:

Clonazepam may be confused with clofazimine, clonidine, clorazepate, Klonopin®, lorazepam

Klonopin® may be confused with clonazepam, clonidine

Use Alone or as an adjunct in the treatment of petit mal variant (Lennox-Gastaut), akinetic, and myoclonic seizures; petit mal (absence) seizures unresponsive to succimides; panic disorder with or without agoraphobia

Unlabeled/Investigational Use Restless legs syndrome; neuralgia; multifocal tic disorder; parkinsonian dysarthria; bipolar disorder; adjunct therapy for schizophrenia

Mechanism of Action/Effect The exact mechanism is unknown, but believed to be related to its ability to enhance the activity of GABA; suppresses the spike-and-wave discharge in absence seizures by depressing nerve transmission in the motor cortex

Contraindications Hypersensitivity to clonazepam or any component of the formulation (cross-sensitivity with other benzodiazepines may exist); significant liver disease; narrow-angle glaucoma; pregnancy

Warnings/Precautions Use with caution in elderly or debilitated patients, patients with hepatic disease (including alcoholics), or renal impairment. Use with caution in patients with respiratory disease or impaired gag reflex or ability to protect the airway from secretions (salivation may be increased). Worsening of seizures may occur when added to patients with multiple seizure types. Concurrent use with valproic acid may result in absence status. Monitoring of CBC and liver function tests has been recommended during prolonged therapy.

Causes CNS depression (dose-related) resulting in sedation, dizziness, confusion, or ataxia which may impair physical and mental capabilities. Use with caution in patients receiving other CNS depressants or ethanol. Benzodiazepines have been associated with falls and traumatic injury and should be used with extreme caution in patients who are at risk of these events (especially the elderly).

Use caution in patients with depression, particularly if suicidal risk may be present. Use with caution in patients with a history of drug dependence. Benzodiazepines have been associated with dependence and acute withdrawal symptoms, including seizures, on discontinuation or reduction in dose.

Benzodiazepines have been associated with anterograde amnesia. Paradoxical reactions, including hyperactive or aggressive behavior, have been reported with benzodiazepines, particularly in adolescent/pediatric or psychiatric patients. Does not have analgesic, antidepressant, or antipsychotic properties.

Drug Interactions

Cytochrome P450 Effect: Substrate of CYP3A4 (major)

Decreased Effect: The combined use of clonazepam and valproic acid has been associated with absence seizures. CYP3A4 inducers may decrease the levels/effects of clonazepam; example inducers include aminoglutethimide, carbamazepine, nafcillin, nevirapine, phenobarbital, phenytoin, and rifamycins.

Increased Effect/Toxicity: Combined use of clonazepam and valproic acid has been associated with absence seizures. Clonazepam potentiates the CNS depressant effects of narcotic analgesics, barbiturates, phenothiazines, ethanol, antihistamines, MAO inhibitors, sedative-hypnotics, and cyclic antidepressants. CYP3A4 inhibitors may increase the levels/ effects of clonazepam; example inhibitors include azole antifungals, ciprofloxacin, clarithromycin, diclofenac, doxycycline, erythromycin, imatinib, isoniazid, nefazodone, nicardipine, propofol, protease inhibitors, quinidine, and verapamil.

Nutritional/Ethanol Interactions

Ethanol: Avoid ethanol (may increase CNS depression).

Food: Clonazepam serum concentration is unlikely to be increased by grapefruit juice because of clonazepam's high oral bioavailability.

Herb/Nutraceutical: St John's wort may decrease clonazepam levels. Avoid valerian, St John's wort, kava kava, gotu kola (may increase CNS depression).

Adverse Reactions Reactions reported in patients with seizure and/or panic disorder. Frequency not defined.

Cardiovascular: Edema (ankle or facial), palpitation

Central nervous system: Amnesia, ataxia (seizure disorder ~30%; panic disorder 5%), behavior problems (seizure disorder ~25%), coma, confusion, depression, dizziness, drowsiness (seizure disorder ~50%), emotional lability, fatigue, fever, hallucinations, headache, hypotonia, hysteria, insomnia, intellectual ability reduced, memory disturbance, nervousness; paradoxical reactions (including aggressive behavior, agitation, anxiety, excitability, hostility, irritability, nervousness, nightmares, sleep disturbance, vivid dreams); psychosis, slurred speech, somnolence (panic disorder 37%), suicidal attempt, vertigo

Dermatologic: Hair loss, hirsutism, skin rash

Endocrine & metabolic: Dysmenorrhea, libido increased/decreased

Gastrointestinal: Abdominal pain, anorexia, appetite increased/decreased, coated tongue, constipation, dehydration, diarrhea, gastritis, gum soreness, nausea, weight changes (loss/ gain), xerostomia

Genitourinary: Colpitis, dysuria, ejaculation delayed, enuresis, impotence, micturition frequency, nocturia, urinary retention, urinary tract infection

Hematologic: Anemia, eosinophilia, leukopenia, thrombocytopenia

Hepatic: Alkaline phosphatase increased (transient), hepatomegaly, serum transaminases increased (transient)

Neuromuscular & skeletal: Choreiform movements, coordination abnormal, dysarthria, muscle pain, muscle weakness, myalgia, tremor

Ocular: Blurred vision, eye movements abnormal, diplopia, nystagmus

Respiratory: Chest congestion, cough, bronchitis, hypersecretions, pharyngitis, respiratory depression, respiratory tract infection, rhinitis, rhinorrhea, shortness of breath, sinusitis

Miscellaneous: Allergic reaction, aphonia, dysdiadochokinesis, encopresis, "glassy-eyed" appearance, hemiparesis, lymphadenopathy

Overdosage/Toxicology May produce somnolence, confusion, ataxia, diminished reflexes, or coma. Treatment for benzodiazepine overdose is supportive. Flumazenil has been shown to selectively block the binding of benzodiazepines to CNS receptors, resulting in a reversal of benzodiazepine-induced CNS depression, but not respiratory depression.

Pharmacodynamics/Kinetics

Onset of Action: 20-60 minutes

Duration of Action: Infants and young children: 6-8 hours; Adults: ≤12 hours

Absorption: Well absorbed

Time to Peak: Serum: 1-3 hours; Steady-state: 5-7 days

Protein Binding: 85%

Half-Life Elimination: Children: 22-33 hours; Adults: 19-50 hours

Metabolism: Extensively hepatic via glucuronide and sulfate conjugation

Excretion: Urine (<2% as unchanged drug); metabolites excreted as glucuronide or sulfate conjugates

Dosing

Adults:

Seizure disorders: Oral:

Initial daily dose not to exceed 1.5 mg given in 3 divided doses; may increase by 0.5-1 mg every third day until seizures are controlled or adverse effects seen (maximum: 20 mg/day)

Usual maintenance dose: 0.05-0.2 mg/kg; do not exceed 20 mg/day

Panic disorder: Oral: 0.25 mg twice daily; increase in increments of 0.125-0.25 mg twice daily every 3 days; target dose: 1 mg/day (maximum: 4 mg/day)

Discontinuation of treatment: To discontinue, treatment should be withdrawn gradually. Decrease dose by 0.125 mg twice daily every 3 days until medication is completely withdrawn.

Elderly: Refer to adult dosing. Initiate with low doses and observe closely.

Pediatrics:

Seizure disorders (see Use): Oral:

Children <10 years or 30 kg:

Initial daily dose: 0.01-0.03 mg/kg/day (maximum: 0.05 mg/kg/day) given in 2-3 divided doses; increase by no more than 0.5 mg every third day until seizures are controlled or adverse effects seen.

Usual maintenance dose: 0.1-0.2 mg/kg/day divided 3 times/day; not to exceed 0.2 mg/ kg/day.

Children >10 years or 30 kg: Refer to adult dosing.

Renal Impairment: Hemodialysis: Supplemental dose is not necessary.

Available Dosage Forms

Tablet: 0.5 mg, 1 mg, 2 mg

Tablet, orally-disintegrating [wafer]: 0.125 mg, 0.25 mg, 0.5 mg, 1 mg, 2 mg

Monitoring and Teaching Issues

Physical Assessment: Assess effectiveness and interactions of other medications patient may be taking. Assess for signs of CNS depression. Assess for history of addiction; long-term use can result in dependence, abuse, or tolerance; periodically evaluate need for continued use. For inpatient use, institute safety measures and monitor effectiveness and (Continued)

Clonazepam *(Continued)*

adverse reactions. For outpatients, monitor therapeutic effectiveness and adverse reactions at beginning of therapy and periodically with long-term use. Taper dosage slowly when discontinuing. Assess knowledge/teach patient seizure precautions (if administered for seizures), appropriate use, interventions to reduce side effects, and adverse symptoms to report.

Monitoring Laboratory Tests: Renal function

Patient Education: Take exactly as directed; do not increase dose or frequency. Drug may cause physical and/or psychological dependence. While using this medication, do not use alcohol and other prescription or OTC medications (especially pain medications, sedatives, antihistamines, or hypnotics) without consulting prescriber. Maintain adequate hydration (2-3 L/day of fluids) unless instructed to restrict fluid intake. You may experience drowsiness, dizziness, or blurred vision (use caution when driving or engaging in tasks requiring alertness until response to drug is known); nausea, vomiting, loss of appetite, or dry mouth (small frequent meals, frequent mouth care, chewing gum, or sucking lozenges may help); or constipation (increased exercise, fluids, fruit, or fiber may help). If medication is used to control seizures, wear identification that you are taking an antiepileptic medication. Report excessive drowsiness, dizziness, fatigue, or impaired coordination; CNS changes (confusion, depression, increased sedation, excitation, headache, agitation, insomnia, or nightmares) or changes in cognition; respiratory difficulty or shortness of breath; changes in urinary pattern, changes in sexual activity; muscle cramping, weakness, tremors, or rigidity; ringing in ears or visual disturbances, excessive perspiration, or excessive GI symptoms (cramping, constipation, vomiting, anorexia); worsening of seizure activity, or loss of seizure control. **Pregnancy/breast-feeding precautions:** Inform prescriber if you are or intend to become pregnant. Breast-feeding is not recommended.

Geriatric Considerations: Hepatic clearance may be decreased allowing accumulation of active drug. Also, metabolites of clonazepam are renally excreted and may accumulate in the elderly as renal function declines with age. Observe for signs of CNS and pulmonary toxicity.

Pregnancy Risk Factor: D

Pregnancy Issues: Benzodiazepines cross the placenta. The association between benzodiazepine exposure and malformations remains controversial. A number of types of malformation have been reported (oral cleft, inguinal hernia, cardiac defects, spina bifida, dysmorphic facial features, skeletal defects); however, confounding factors make a clear association difficult. Overall, the risk to the fetus may be low. Nonteratogenic effects (including neonatal flaccidity, respiratory and feeding problems, and withdrawal symptoms) during the postnatal period have also been reported with benzodiazepine use.

Lactation: Enters breast milk/not recommended

Breast-Feeding Issues: Clonazepam enters breast milk; clinical effects on the infant include CNS depression, respiratory depression reported (no recommendation from the AAP).

Administration

Oral: Orally-disintegrating tablet: Open pouch and peel back foil on the blister; do not push tablet through foil. Use dry hands to remove tablet and place in mouth. May be swallowed with or without water. Use immediately after removing from package.

Additional Information Ethosuximide or valproic acid may be preferred for treatment of absence (petit mal) seizures. Clonazepam-induced behavioral disturbances may be more frequent in mentally handicapped patients. Abrupt discontinuation after sustained use (generally >10 days) may cause withdrawal symptoms. Flumazenil, a competitive benzodiazepine antagonist at the CNS receptor site, reverses benzodiazepine-induced CNS depression.

Related Information

Anticonvulsants By Seizure Type *on page 1712*
Anxiolytic / Hypnotic Use in Long-Term Care Facilities *on page 1769*
Benzodiazepines *on page 1719*

Clonidine *(KLON i deen)*

U.S. Brand Names Catapres®; Catapres-TTS®; Duraclon™

Synonyms Clonidine Hydrochloride

Generic Available Yes: Tablet

Pharmacologic Category Alpha₂-Adrenergic Agonist

Medication Safety Issues

Sound-alike/look-alike issues:

Clonidine may be confused with Clomid®, clomiPHENE, clonazepam, clozapine, Klonopin™, Loniten®, quinidine

Catapres® may be confused with Cataflam®, Cetapred®, Combipres®

Transdermal patch may contain conducting metal (eg, aluminum); remove patch prior to MRI.

Use Management of mild to moderate hypertension; either used alone or in combination with other antihypertensives

Orphan drug: Duraclon™: For continuous epidural administration as adjunctive therapy with intraspinal opiates for treatment of cancer pain in patients tolerant to or unresponsive to intraspinal opiates

Unlabeled/Investigational Use Heroin or nicotine withdrawal; severe pain; dysmenorrhea; vasomotor symptoms associated with menopause; ethanol dependence; prophylaxis of migraines; glaucoma; diabetes-associated diarrhea; impulse control disorder, attention-deficit/hyperactivity disorder (ADHD), clozapine-induced sialorrhea

Mechanism of Action/Effect Stimulates alpha₂-adrenoceptors in the brain stem, thus activating an inhibitory neuron, resulting in reduced sympathetic outflow from the CNS, producing a decrease in peripheral resistance, renal vascular resistance, heart rate, and blood pressure; epidural clonidine may produce pain relief at spinal presynaptic and postjunctional alpha₂-adrenoceptors by preventing pain signal transmission; pain relief occurs only for the body regions innervated by the spinal segments where analgesic concentrations of clonidine exist

Contraindications Hypersensitivity to clonidine hydrochloride or any component of the formulation

Warnings/Precautions Gradual withdrawal is needed (over 1 week for oral, 2-4 days with epidural) if drug needs to be stopped. Patients should be instructed about abrupt discontinuation (causes rapid increase in BP and symptoms of sympathetic overactivity). In patients on both a beta-blocker and clonidine where withdrawal of clonidine is necessary, withdraw the beta-blocker first and several days before clonidine. Then slowly decrease clonidine.

Use with caution in patients with severe coronary insufficiency; conduction disturbances; recent MI, CVA, or chronic renal insufficiency. Caution in sinus node dysfunction. Discontinue within 4 hours of surgery then restart as soon as possible after. Clonidine injection should be administered via a continuous epidural infusion device. Epidural clonidine is not recommended for perioperative, obstetrical, or postpartum pain. It is not recommended for use in patients with severe cardiovascular disease or hemodynamic instability. In all cases, the epidural may lead to cardiovascular instability (hypotension, bradycardia). Transdermal patch may contain conducting metal (eg, aluminum); remove patch prior to MRI. Clonidine cause significant CNS depression and xerostomia. Caution in patients with pre-existing CNS disease or depression. Elderly may be at greater risk for CNS depressive effects, favoring other agents in this population.

Drug Interactions
Decreased Effect: Tricyclic antidepressants (TCAs) antagonize the hypotensive effects of clonidine.

Increased Effect/Toxicity: Concurrent use with antipsychotics (especially low potency), narcotic analgesics, or nitroprusside may produce additive hypotensive effects. Clonidine may decrease the symptoms of hypoglycemia with oral hypoglycemic agents or insulin. Alcohol, barbiturates, and other CNS depressants may have additive CNS effects when combined with clonidine. Epidural clonidine may prolong the sensory and motor blockade of local anesthetics. Clonidine may increase cyclosporine (and perhaps tacrolimus) serum concentrations. Beta-blockers may potentiate bradycardia in patients receiving clonidine and may increase the rebound hypertension of withdrawal. Tricyclic antidepressants may also enhance the hypertensive response associated with abrupt clonidine withdrawal.

Nutritional/Ethanol Interactions
Ethanol: Avoid ethanol (may increase CNS depression).
Herb/Nutraceutical: Avoid dong quai if using for hypertension (has estrogenic activity). Avoid ephedra, yohimbe, ginseng (may worsen hypertension). Avoid valerian, St John's wort, kava kava, gotu kola (may increase CNS depression).

Lab Interactions Increased sodium (S), transient serum glucose; decreased catecholamines (U); positive Coombs'

Adverse Reactions Incidence of adverse events is not always reported.
>10%:
Central nervous system: Drowsiness (35% oral, 12% transdermal), dizziness (16% oral, 2% transdermal)
Dermatologic: Transient localized skin reactions characterized by pruritus, and erythema (15% to 50% transdermal)
Gastrointestinal: Dry mouth (40% oral, 25% transdermal)
1% to 10%:
Cardiovascular: Orthostatic hypotension (3% oral)
Central nervous system: Headache (1% oral, 5% transdermal), sedation (3% transdermal), fatigue (6% transdermal), lethargy (3% transdermal), insomnia (2% transdermal), nervousness (3% oral, 1% transdermal), mental depression (1% oral)
Dermatologic: Rash (1% oral), allergic contact sensitivity (5% transdermal), localized vesiculation (7%), hyperpigmentation (5% at application site), edema (3%), excoriation (3%), burning (3%), throbbing, blanching (1%), papules (1%), and generalized macular rash (1%) has occurred in patients receiving transdermal clonidine.
Endocrine & metabolic: Sodium and water retention, sexual dysfunction (3% oral, 2% transdermal), impotence (3% oral, 2% transdermal), weakness (10% transdermal)
Gastrointestinal: Nausea (5% oral, 1% transdermal), vomiting (5% oral), anorexia and malaise (1% oral), constipation (10% oral, 1% transdermal), dry throat (2% transdermal), taste disturbance (1% transdermal), weight gain (1% oral)
Genitourinary: Nocturia (1% oral)
Hepatic: Liver function test (mild abnormalities, 1% oral)
Miscellaneous: Withdrawal syndrome (1% oral)

Overdosage/Toxicology Symptoms of overdose include bradycardia, CNS depression, hypothermia, diarrhea, respiratory depression, and apnea. Treatment is supportive and symptomatic. Naloxone may be utilized in treating CNS depression and/or apnea and should be given I.V., 0.4-2 mg, with repeated doses as needed up to a total of 10 mg, or as an infusion.

Pharmacodynamics/Kinetics
Onset of Action: Oral: 0.5-1 hour
Duration of Action: 6-10 hours
Bioavailability: 75% to 95%
Time to Peak: 2-4 hours
Protein Binding: 20% to 40%
Half-Life Elimination: Adults: Normal renal function: 6-20 hours; Renal impairment: 18-41 hours
Metabolism: Extensively hepatic to inactive metabolites; undergoes enterohepatic recirculation
Excretion: Urine (65%, 32% as unchanged drug); feces (22%)

Dosing
Adults:
Acute hypertension (urgency): Oral: Initial 0.1-0.2 mg; may be followed by additional doses of 0.1 mg every hour, if necessary, to a maximum total dose of 0.6 mg
Unlabeled route of administration: Sublingual clonidine 0.1-0.2 mg twice daily may be effective in patients unable to take oral medication
(Continued)

Clonidine (Continued)

Hypertension:

Oral: Initial dose: 0.1 mg twice daily (maximum recommended dose: 2.4 mg/day); usual dose range (JNC 7): 0.1-0.8 mg/day in 2 divided doses

Transdermal: Apply once every 7 days; for initial therapy start with 0.1 mg and increase by 0.1 mg at 1- to 2-week intervals (dosages >0.6 mg do not improve efficacy); usual dose range (JNC 7): 0.1-0.3 mg once weekly

Conversion from oral to transdermal:

Day 1: Place Catapres-TTS® 1; administer 100% of oral dose.

Day 2: Administer 50% of oral dose.

Day 3: Administer 25% of oral dose.

Day 4: Patch remains, no further oral supplement necessary.

Nicotine withdrawal symptoms: 0.1 mg twice daily to maximum of 0.4 mg/day for 3-4 weeks

Pain management: Epidural infusion: Starting dose: 30 mcg/hour; titrate as required for relief of pain or presence of side effects; minimal experience with doses >40 mcg/hour; should be considered an adjunct to intraspinal opiate therapy

Elderly: Oral: Initial: 0.1 mg once daily at bedtime, increase gradually as needed.

Pediatrics:

Hypertension: Oral: Initial: 5-10 mcg/kg/day in divided doses every 8-12 hours; increase gradually at 5- to 7-day intervals to 25 mcg/kg/day in divided doses every 6 hours; maximum: 0.9 mg/day.

Clonidine tolerance test (growth hormone release from pituitary): Oral: 0.15 mg/m^2 or 4 mcg/kg as single dose

ADHD (unlabeled use): Oral: Initial: 0.05 mg/day, increase every 3-7 days by 0.05 mg/day to 3-5 mcg/kg/day given in divided doses 3-4 times/day; maximum dose: 0.3-0.4 mg/day

Pain management: Epidural infusion: Reserved for patients with severe intractable pain, unresponsive to other analgesics or epidural or spinal opiates: Initial: 0.5 mcg/kg/hour; adjust with caution, based on clinical effect

Renal Impairment:

Cl$_{cr}$ <10 mL/minute: Administer 50% to 75% of normal dose initially.

Not dialyzable (0% to 5%) via hemo- or peritoneal dialysis; supplemental dose is not necessary.

Available Dosage Forms

Injection, epidural solution, as hydrochloride [preservative free] (Duraclon™): 100 mcg/mL (10 mL); 500 mcg/mL (10 mL)

Patch, transdermal [once-weekly patch]:

Catapres-TTS®-1: 0.1 mg/24 hours (4s)

Catapres-TTS®-2: 0.2 mg/24 hours (4s)

Catapres-TTS®-3: 0.3 mg/24 hours (4s)

Tablet, as hydrochloride (Catapres®): 0.1 mg, 0.2 mg, 0.3 mg

Monitoring and Teaching Issues

Physical Assessment: Use caution with pre-existing cardiovascular disease, hemodynamic instability, and CNS disease or depression (see Warnings/Precautions). Assess potential for interactions with other pharmacological agents or herbal products patient may be taking (eg, potential for additive hypotension, bradycardia, CNS depression; see Drug Interactions). Monitor results of laboratory tests, therapeutic effectiveness (according to purpose for use), and adverse response (see Adverse Reactions) regularly during therapy. Advise patients using oral hypoglycemic agents or insulin to check glucose levels closely; clonidine may decrease the symptoms of hypoglycemia. When discontinuing, monitor blood pressure and taper dose slowly over 1 week or more. Teach patient proper use, possible side effects/appropriate interventions, and adverse symptoms to report (see Patient Education).

Monitoring Laboratory Tests: Liver function tests

Patient Education: Do not take anything new (especially cough or cold remedies and sleep or stay-awake medications that might affect blood pressure) during treatment unless approved by prescriber. Take as directed, at bedtime. If using patch, check daily for correct placement. Do not skip doses or discontinue without consulting prescriber (this drug must be discontinued on a specific schedule to prevent serious adverse effects). Follow dietary restrictions as recommended by prescriber. This medication may cause drowsiness, dizziness, or impaired judgment (use caution when driving or engaging in tasks that require alertness until response is known); decreased libido or sexual function (will resolve when drug is discontinued); postural hypotension (use caution when rising from sitting or lying position or when climbing stairs); constipation (increase roughage, bulk in diet); or dry mouth or nausea (frequent mouth care or sucking lozenges may help). Report difficulty, pain, or burning on urination; increased nervousness or depression; sudden weight gain (weigh yourself in the same clothes at the same time of day once a week); unusual or persistent swelling of ankles, feet, or extremities; wet cough or respiratory difficulty; chest pain or palpitations; muscle weakness, fatigue, or pain; or other persistent side effects. **Pregnancy/breast-feeding precautions:** Inform prescriber if you are or intend to become pregnant. Breast-feeding is not recommended.

Dietary Considerations: Hypertensive patients may need to decrease sodium and calories in diet.

Geriatric Considerations: Because of its potential CNS adverse effects, clonidine may not be considered a drug of choice in the elderly. If the decision is to use clonidine, adjust dose based on response and adverse reactions.

Pregnancy Risk Factor: C

Pregnancy Issues: Clonidine crosses the placenta. Caution should be used with this drug due to the potential of rebound hypertension with abrupt discontinuation.

Lactation: Enters breast milk/not recommended

Breast-Feeding Issues: Enters breast milk; AAP has NO RECOMMENDATION.

Administration

Oral: Do not discontinue clonidine abruptly. if needed, gradually reduce dose over 2-4 days to avoid rebound hypertension.

Topical: Transdermal patches should be applied weekly at bedtime to a clean, hairless area of the upper outer arm or chest. Rotate patch sites weekly. Redness under patch may be reduced if a topical corticosteroid spray is applied to the area before placement of the patch.

Additional Information Transdermal clonidine should only be used in patients unable to take oral medication. The transdermal product is much more expensive than oral clonidine and produces no better therapeutic effects.

Clonidine and Chlorthalidone (KLON i deen & klor THAL i done)

U.S. Brand Names Clorpres®; Combipres® [DSC]

Synonyms Chlorthalidone and Clonidine

Generic Available No

Pharmacologic Category Antihypertensive Agent, Combination

Medication Safety Issues

Sound-alike/look-alike issues:

Combipres® may be confused with Catapres®

Use Management of mild to moderate hypertension

Dosing

Adults: Hypertension: Oral: 1 tablet 1-2 times/day

Elderly: May benefit from lower initial dose; see individual agents.

Available Dosage Forms

Tablet:

0.1: Clonidine hydrochloride 0.1 mg and chlorthalidone 15 mg

0.2: Clonidine hydrochloride 0.2 mg and chlorthalidone 15 mg

0.3: Clonidine hydrochloride 0.3 mg and chlorthalidone 15 mg

Monitoring and Teaching Issues

Physical Assessment: See individual agents.

Patient Education: See individual agents. **Pregnancy/breast-feeding precautions:** Inform prescriber if you are or intend to become pregnant. Breast-feeding is not recommended.

Pregnancy Risk Factor: C

Lactation:

Clonidine: Enters breast milk/not recommended

Chlorthalidone: Enters breast milk/compatible

Related Information

Chlorthalidone *on page 314*

Clonidine *on page 354*

♦ **Clonidine Hydrochloride** *see* Clonidine *on page 354*

Clopidogrel (kloh PID oh grel)

U.S. Brand Names Plavix®

Synonyms Clopidogrel Bisulfate

Generic Available No

Pharmacologic Category Antiplatelet Agent

Medication Safety Issues

Sound-alike/look-alike issues:

Plavix® may be confused with Elavil®, Paxil®

Use Reduce atherosclerotic events (myocardial infarction, stroke, vascular deaths) in patients with atherosclerosis documented by recent myocardial infarction (MI), recent stroke, or established peripheral arterial disease; prevention of thrombotic complications after coronary stenting; acute coronary syndrome (unstable angina or non-Q-wave MI)

Unlabeled/Investigational Use In aspirin-allergic patients, prevention of coronary artery bypass graft closure (saphenous vein)

Mechanism of Action/Effect Blocks the ADP receptors, which prevent fibrinogen binding at that site and thereby reduce the possibility of platelet adhesion and aggregation.

Contraindications Hypersensitivity to clopidogrel or any component of the formulation; active pathological bleeding such as PUD or intracranial hemorrhage; coagulation disorders

Warnings/Precautions Use with caution in patients who may be at risk of increased bleeding, including patients with peptic ulcer disease, trauma, or surgery. Consider discontinuing 5 days before elective surgery. Use caution in mixing with other antiplatelet drugs. Use with caution in patients with severe liver disease (experience is limited). Cases of thrombotic thrombocytopenic purpura (usually occurring within the first 2 weeks of therapy) have been reported.

Drug Interactions

Cytochrome P450 Effect: Substrate (minor) of CYP1A2, 3A4; **Inhibits** CYP2C8/9 (weak)

Decreased Effect: Atorvastatin may attenuate the effects of clopidogrel; monitor. CYP3A4-inhibiting macrolide antibiotics may attenuate the effects of clopidogrel (including clarithromycin, erythromycin, and troleandomycin); monitor.

Increased Effect/Toxicity: At high concentrations, clopidogrel may interfere with the metabolism of amiodarone, cisapride, cyclosporine, diltiazem, fluvastatin, irbesartan, losartan, oral hypoglycemics, paclitaxel, phenytoin, quinidine, sildenafil, tamoxifen, torsemide, verapamil, and some NSAIDs which may result in toxicity. Clopidogrel and naproxen resulted in an increase of GI occult blood loss. Anticoagulants (warfarin, thrombolytics, drotrecogin alfa) or other antiplatelet agents may increase the risk of bleeding. Rifampin may increase the effects of clopidogrel (monitor).

(Continued)

Clopidogrel *(Continued)*

Nutritional/Ethanol Interactions Herb/Nutraceutical: Avoid cat's claw, dong quai, evening primrose, feverfew, garlic, ginger, ginkgo, red clover, horse chestnut, green tea, ginseng (all have additional antiplatelet activity).

Adverse Reactions As with all drugs which may affect hemostasis, bleeding is associated with clopidogrel. Hemorrhage may occur at virtually any site. Risk is dependent on multiple variables, including the concurrent use of multiple agents which alter hemostasis and patient susceptibility.

>10%: Gastrointestinal: The overall incidence of gastrointestinal events (including abdominal pain, vomiting, dyspepsia, gastritis and constipation) has been documented to be 27% compared to 30% in patients receiving aspirin.

3% to 10%:
  Cardiovascular: Chest pain (8%), edema (4%), hypertension (4%)
  Central nervous system: Headache (3% to 8%), dizziness (2% to 6%), depression (4%), fatigue (3%), general pain (6%)
  Dermatologic: Rash (4%), pruritus (3%)
  Endocrine & metabolic: Hypercholesterolemia (4%)
  Gastrointestinal: Abdominal pain (2% to 6%), dyspepsia (2% to 5%), diarrhea (2% to 5%), nausea (3%)
  Genitourinary: Urinary tract infection (3%)
  Hematologic: Purpura (5%), epistaxis (3%)
  Hepatic: Liver function test abnormalities (<3%; discontinued in 0.11%)
  Neuromuscular & skeletal: Arthralgia (6%), back pain (6%)
  Respiratory: Dyspnea (5%), rhinitis (4%), bronchitis (4%), cough (3%), upper respiratory infection (9%)
  Miscellaneous: Flu-like syndrome (8%)

1% to 3%:
  Cardiovascular: Atrial fibrillation, cardiac failure, palpitation, syncope
  Central nervous system: Fever, insomnia, vertigo, anxiety
  Dermatologic: Eczema
  Endocrine & metabolic: Gout, hyperuricemia
  Gastrointestinal: Constipation, GI hemorrhage, vomiting
  Genitourinary: Cystitis
  Hematologic: Hematoma, anemia
  Neuromuscular & skeletal: Arthritis, leg cramps, neuralgia, paresthesia, weakness
  Ocular: Cataract, conjunctivitis

Overdosage/Toxicology

Symptoms of acute toxicity include vomiting, prostration, difficulty breathing, and gastrointestinal hemorrhage. Only one case of overdose with clopidogrel has been reported to date, no symptoms were reported with this case and no specific treatments were required.

Based on its pharmacology, platelet transfusions may be an appropriate treatment when attempting to reverse the effects of clopidogrel. After decontamination, treatment is symptomatic and supportive.

Pharmacodynamics/Kinetics

Onset of Action: Inhibition of platelet aggregation detected: 2 hours after 300 mg administered; after second day of treatment with 50-100 mg/day

  Peak effect: 50-100 mg/day: Bleeding time: 5-6 days; Platelet function: 3-7 days

Absorption: Well absorbed

Time to Peak: Serum: ~1 hour

Half-Life Elimination: ~8 hours

Metabolism: Extensively hepatic via hydrolysis; biotransformation primarily to carboxyl acid derivative (inactive). The active metabolite that inhibits platelet aggregation has not been isolated.

Excretion: Urine

Dosing

Adults & Elderly:

Recent MI, recent stroke, or established arterial disease: Oral: 75 mg once daily

Acute coronary syndrome: Oral: Initial: 300 mg loading dose, followed by 75 mg once daily (in combination with aspirin 75-325 mg once daily). **Note:** A loading dose of 600 mg has been used in some investigations; limited research exists comparing the two doses.

Prevention of coronary artery bypass graft closure (saphenous vein): Aspirin-allergic patients (unlabeled use): Oral: Loading dose: 300 mg 6 hours following procedure; maintenance: 50-100 mg/day

Renal Impairment: No adjustment is necessary.

Hepatic Impairment: Dose adjustment may be necessary for patients with moderate to severe hepatic disease.

Available Dosage Forms Tablet [film coated]: 75 mg

Monitoring and Teaching Issues

Physical Assessment: Assess effectiveness or interactions of other medications patient may be taking. Clopidogrel is a P450 enzyme inhibitor. Monitor for unusual bleeding. Monitor therapeutic effectiveness and instruct patient what symptoms to report.

Monitoring Laboratory Tests: Hemoglobin and hematocrit periodically

Patient Education: Take as directed. May cause headache or dizziness; use caution when driving or engaging in tasks that require alertness until response to drug is known. It may take longer than usual to stop bleeding. Small frequent meals, frequent mouth care, sucking lozenges, or chewing gum may reduce nausea or vomiting. Mild analgesics may reduce arthralgia or back pain. Inform physicians and dentists that you are taking this medication prior to scheduling any surgery or dental procedure. Report immediately unusual or acute chest pain or respiratory difficulties; skin rash; unresolved bleeding, diarrhea, or GI distress; nosebleed; or acute headache. **Breast-feeding precaution:** Breast-feeding is not recommended.

Dietary Considerations: May be taken without regard to meals.

Geriatric Considerations: Plasma levels of the primary clopidogrel metabolite were significantly higher in the elderly (≥75 years). This was not associated with changes in bleeding time or platelet aggregation. No dosage adjustment is recommended.

Pregnancy Risk Factor: B

Lactation: Excretion in breast milk unknown/not recommended

Administration
Storage: Store at 25°C (77°F); excursions permitted to 15°C to 3°C (59°F to 86°F).

♦ Clopidogrel Bisulfate *see* Clopidogrel *on page 357*

Clorazepate (klor AZ e pate)

U.S. Brand Names Tranxene®; Tranxene® SD™; Tranxene® SD™-Half Strength; T-Tab®

Synonyms Clorazepate Dipotassium; Tranxene T-Tab®

Controlled Substance C-IV

Generic Available Yes

Pharmacologic Category Benzodiazepine

Medication Safety Issues
Sound-alike/look-alike issues:
Clorazepate may be confused with clofibrate, clonazepam

Use Treatment of generalized anxiety disorder; management of ethanol withdrawal; adjunct anticonvulsant in management of partial seizures

Mechanism of Action/Effect Binds to stereospecific benzodiazepine receptors on the post-synaptic GABA neuron at several sites within the central nervous system, including the limbic system, reticular formation. Enhancement of the inhibitory effect of GABA on neuronal excitability results in increased neuronal membrane permeability to chloride ions. This shift in chloride ions results in hyperpolarization (a less excitable state) and stabilization.

Contraindications Hypersensitivity to clorazepate or any component of the formulation (cross-sensitivity with other benzodiazepines may exist); narrow-angle glaucoma; pregnancy

Warnings/Precautions
Causes CNS depression (dose-related) which may impair physical and mental capabilities. Use with caution in patients receiving other CNS depressants or psychoactive agents. Benzodiazepines have been associated with falls and traumatic injury and should be used with extreme caution in patients who are at risk of these events (especially the elderly). May cause physical or psychological dependence - use with caution in patients with a history of drug dependence.

Active metabolites with extended half-lives may lead to delayed accumulation and adverse effects. Avoid use in patients with sleep apnea. Use with caution in patients receiving concurrent CYP3A4 inhibitors, particularly when these agents are added to therapy. Use with caution in elderly or debilitated patients, patients with hepatic disease (including alcoholics), renal impairment, respiratory disease, impaired gag reflex, or obese patients.

Benzodiazepines have been associated with anterograde amnesia. Paradoxical reactions, including hyperactive or aggressive behavior, have been reported with benzodiazepines, particularly in adolescent/pediatric or psychiatric patients. Does not have analgesic, antidepressant, or antipsychotic properties. Not recommended for use in patients <9 years of age.

Drug Interactions
Cytochrome P450 Effect: Substrate of CYP3A4 (major)
Decreased Effect: CYP3A4 inducers may decrease the levels/effects of clorazepate; example inducers include aminoglutethimide, carbamazepine, nafcillin, nevirapine, phenobarbital, phenytoin, and rifamycins.
Increased Effect/Toxicity: Clorazepate potentiates the CNS depressant effects of narcotic analgesics, barbiturates, phenothiazines, ethanol, antihistamines, MAO inhibitors, sedative-hypnotics, and cyclic antidepressants. CYP3A4 inhibitors may increase the levels/effects of clorazepate; example inhibitors include azole antifungals, ciprofloxacin, clarithromycin, diclofenac, doxycycline, erythromycin, imatinib, isoniazid, nefazodone, nicardipine, propofol, protease inhibitors, quinidine, and verapamil.

Nutritional/Ethanol Interactions
Ethanol: Avoid ethanol (may increase CNS depression).
Food: Serum concentrations/toxicity may be increased by grapefruit juice.
Herb/Nutraceutical: Avoid valerian, St John's wort, kava kava, gotu kola (may increase CNS depression).

Lab Interactions Decreased hematocrit; abnormal liver and renal function tests

Adverse Reactions Frequency not defined.
Cardiovascular: Hypotension
Central nervous system: Drowsiness, fatigue, ataxia, lightheadedness, memory impairment, insomnia, anxiety, headache, depression, slurred speech, confusion, nervousness, dizziness, irritability
Dermatologic: Rash
Endocrine & metabolic: Decreased libido
Gastrointestinal: Xerostomia, constipation, diarrhea, decreased salivation, nausea, vomiting, increased or decreased appetite
Neuromuscular & skeletal: Dysarthria, tremor
Ocular: Blurred vision, diplopia

Overdosage/Toxicology May produce somnolence, confusion, ataxia, diminished reflexes, and coma. Treatment for benzodiazepine overdose is supportive. Rarely is mechanical ventilation required. Flumazenil has been shown to selectively block the binding of benzodiazepines to CNS receptors, resulting in a reversal of benzodiazepine-induced CNS depression, but not respiratory depression.
(Continued)

Clorazepate *(Continued)*

Pharmacodynamics/Kinetics
Onset of Action: 1-2 hours

Duration of Action: Variable, 8-24 hours

Time to Peak: Serum: ~1 hour

Half-Life Elimination: Adults: Desmethyldiazepam: 48-96 hours; Oxazepam: 6-8 hours

Metabolism: Rapidly decarboxylated to desmethyldiazepam (active) in acidic stomach prior to absorption; hepatically to oxazepam (active)

Excretion: Primarily urine

Dosing
Adults:
Anxiety:
Regular release tablets (Tranxene® T-Tab®): 7.5-15 mg 2-4 times/day
Sustained release (Tranxene® SD): 11.25 or 22.5 mg once daily at bedtime
Ethanol withdrawal: Oral: Initial: 30 mg, then 15 mg 2-4 times/day on first day; maximum daily dose: 90 mg; gradually decrease dose over subsequent days.
Seizures (anticonvulsant): Oral: Initial: Up to 7.5 mg/dose 2-3 times/day; increase dose by 7.5 mg at weekly intervals; not to exceed 90 mg/day
Elderly: Oral: Anxiety: 7.5 mg 1-2 times/day; use is not recommended in the elderly.
Pediatrics:
Seizures (anticonvulsant): Oral:
Children 9-12 years: Initial: 3.75-7.5 mg/dose twice daily; increase dose by 3.75 mg at weekly intervals, not to exceed 60 mg/day in 2-3 divided doses.
Children >12 years: Refer to adult dosing.

Available Dosage Forms Tablet, as dipotassium: 3.75 mg, 7.5 mg, 15 mg
Tranxene® SD™: 22.5 mg [once daily]
Tranxene® SD™-Half Strength: 11.25 mg [once daily]
Tranxene® T-Tab®: 3.75 mg, 7.5 mg, 15 mg

Monitoring and Teaching Issues
Physical Assessment: Assess other medications patient may be taking for effectiveness and interactions. Assess for CNS depression. Assess for history of addiction; long-term use can result in dependence, abuse, or tolerance; periodically evaluate need for continued use. For inpatient use, institute safety measures and monitor effectiveness and adverse reactions. For outpatients, monitor therapeutic effectiveness and adverse reactions at beginning of therapy and periodically with long-term use. Taper dosage slowly when discontinuing. Assess knowledge/teach patient appropriate use, interventions to reduce side effects, and adverse symptoms to report.

Patient Education: Take exactly as directed; do not increase dose or frequency. Drug may cause physical and/or psychological dependence. Do not use alcohol and other prescription or OTC medications (especially pain medications, sedatives, antihistamines, or hypnotics) without consulting prescriber. Maintain adequate hydration (2-3 L/day of fluids) unless instructed to restrict fluid intake. You may experience drowsiness, lightheadedness, impaired coordination, dizziness, or blurred vision (use caution when driving or engaging in tasks requiring alertness until response to drug is known); nausea, vomiting, or dry mouth (small frequent meals, frequent mouth care, chewing gum, or sucking lozenges may help); constipation (increased exercise, fluids, fruit, or fiber may help); altered sexual drive or ability (reversible); or photosensitivity (use sunscreen, wear protective clothing and eyewear, and avoid direct sunlight). Report persistent CNS effects (eg, confusion, depression, increased sedation, excitation, headache, agitation, insomnia or nightmares, dizziness, fatigue, impaired coordination, changes in personality, or changes in cognition); changes in urinary pattern; muscle cramping, weakness, tremors, or rigidity; ringing in ears or visual disturbances; chest pain, palpitations, or rapid heartbeat; excessive perspiration; excessive GI symptoms (cramping, constipation, vomiting, anorexia); or worsening of condition. **Pregnancy/breast-feeding precautions:** Do not get pregnant while using this medication; use appropriate contraceptive measures. Breast-feeding is not recommended.

Geriatric Considerations: Clorazepate is not considered a drug of choice in the elderly. Long-acting benzodiazepines have been associated with falls in the elderly.

Pregnancy Risk Factor: D

Pregnancy Issues: Benzodiazepines cross the placenta. The association between benzodiazepine exposure and malformations remains controversial. A number of types of malformation have been reported (oral cleft, inguinal hernia, cardiac defects, spina bifida, dysmorphic facial features, skeletal defects); however, confounding factors make a clear association difficult. Overall, the risk to the fetus may be low. Nonteratogenic effects (including neonatal flaccidity, respiratory and feeding problems, and withdrawal symptoms) during the postnatal period have also been reported with benzodiazepine use.

Lactation: Excretion in breast milk unknown/not recommended

Breast-Feeding Issues: No specific data for clorazepate; however, other benzodiazepines have been shown to be excreted in breast milk. Therefore, it is recommended not to nurse while taking clorazepate.

Additional Information Abrupt discontinuation after sustained use (generally >10 days) may cause withdrawal symptoms.

Related Information
Anxiolytic / Hypnotic Use in Long-Term Care Facilities *on page 1769*
Benzodiazepines *on page 1719*
Federal OBRA Regulations: Recommended Maximum Doses *on page 1773*

♦ **Clorazepate Dipotassium** *see* Clorazepate *on page 359*
♦ **Clorpres®** *see* Clonidine and Chlorthalidone *on page 357*

Clotrimazole *(kloe TRIM a zole)*
U.S. Brand Names Cruex® Cream [OTC]; Gyne-Lotrimin® 3 [OTC]; Lotrimin® AF Athlete's Foot Cream [OTC]; Lotrimin® AF Athlete's Foot Solution [OTC]; Lotrimin® AF Jock Itch Cream [OTC]; Mycelex®; Mycelex®-7 [OTC]; Mycelex® Twin Pack [OTC]

Generic Available Yes: Cream, solution, troche

Pharmacologic Category Antifungal Agent, Oral Nonabsorbed; Antifungal Agent, Topical; Antifungal Agent, Vaginal

Medication Safety Issues

Sound-alike/look-alike issues:

Clotrimazole may be confused with co-trimoxazole

Lotrimin® may be confused with Lotrisone®, Otrivin®

Mycelex® may be confused with Myoflex®

Use Treatment of susceptible fungal infections, including oropharyngeal candidiasis, dermatophytoses, superficial mycoses, and cutaneous candidiasis, as well as vulvovaginal candidiasis; limited data suggest that clotrimazole troches may be effective for prophylaxis against oropharyngeal candidiasis in neutropenic patients

Mechanism of Action/Effect Binds to phospholipids in the fungal cell membrane altering cell wall permeability resulting in loss of essential intracellular elements

Contraindications Hypersensitivity to clotrimazole or any component of the formulation

Warnings/Precautions Clotrimazole should not be used for treatment of ocular or systemic fungal infection. Use with caution with hepatic impairment. Safety and effectiveness of clotrimazole lozenges (troches) in children <3 years of age have not been established. When using topical formulation, avoid contact with eyes.

Drug Interactions

Cytochrome P450 Effect: Inhibits CYP1A2 (weak), 2A6 (weak), 2B6 (weak), 2C8/9 (weak), 2C19 (weak), 2D6 (weak), 2E1 (weak), 3A4 (moderate)

Increased Effect/Toxicity: Clotrimazole may increase the levels/effects of selected benzodiazepines, calcium channel blockers, cisapride, cyclosporine, ergot derivatives, selected HMG-CoA reductase inhibitors, mesoridazine, mirtazapine, nateglinide, nefazodone, pimozide, quinidine, sildenafil (and other PDE-5 inhibitors), tacrolimus, thioridazine, venlafaxine, and other CYP3A4 substrates.

Adverse Reactions

Oral:

>10%: Hepatic: Abnormal liver function tests

1% to 10%:

Gastrointestinal: Nausea and vomiting may occur in patients on clotrimazole troches

Local: Mild burning, irritation, stinging to skin or vaginal area

Vaginal:

1% to 10%: Genitourinary: Vulvar/vaginal burning

Pharmacodynamics/Kinetics

Absorption: Topical: Negligible through intact skin

Time to Peak: Serum:

Oral topical (troche): Salivary levels occur within 3 hours following 30 minutes of dissolution time

Vaginal cream: High vaginal levels: 8-24 hours

Vaginal tablet: High vaginal levels: 1-2 days

Excretion: Feces (as metabolites)

Dosing

Adults & Elderly:

Oropharyngeal candidiasis: Oral:

Prophylaxis: 10 mg troche dissolved 3 times/day for the duration of chemotherapy or until steroids are reduced to maintenance levels

Treatment: 10 mg troche dissolved slowly 5 times/day for 14 consecutive days

Dermatophytosis, cutaneous candidiasis: Topical (cream, solution): Apply twice daily; if no improvement occurs after 4 weeks of therapy, re-evaluate diagnosis.

Vulvovaginal candidiasis: Intravaginal:

Cream (1%): Insert 1 applicatorful of 1% vaginal cream daily (preferably at bedtime) for 7 consecutive days.

Cream (2%): Insert 1 applicatorful of 2% vaginal cream daily (preferably at bedtime) for 3 consecutive days.

Tablet: Insert 100 mg/day for 7 days or 500 mg single dose.

Dermatologic infection (superficial): Topical (cream, solution): Apply to affected area twice daily (morning and evening) for 7 consecutive days.

Pediatrics:

Oropharyngeal candidiasis: Children >3 years: Refer to adult dosing.

Vaginal, Topical infections: Children >12 years: Refer to adult dosing.

Available Dosage Forms

Combination pack (Mycelex®-7): Vaginal tablet 100 mg (7s) and vaginal cream 1% (7 g)

Cream, topical: 1% (15 g, 30 g, 45 g)

Cruex®: 1% (15 g)

Lotrimin® AF Athlete's Foot: 1% (12 g, 24 g)

Lotrimin® AF Jock Itch: 1% (12 g)

Cream, vaginal: 2% (21 g)

Mycelex®-7: 1% (45 g)

Solution, topical: 1% (10 mL, 30 mL)

Lotrimin® AF Athlete's Foot: 1% (10 mL)

Tablet, vaginal (Gyne-Lotrimin® 3): 200 mg (3s)

Troche (Mycelex®): 10 mg

Monitoring and Teaching Issues

Physical Assessment: Monitor laboratory values, effectiveness of treatment, and adverse reactions. Assess knowledge/teach patient appropriate use, interventions to reduce side effects, and adverse symptoms to report. Assess for opportunistic infection.

Monitoring Laboratory Tests: Periodic liver function during oral therapy with clotrimazole troche

Patient Education: Oral (troche): Do not swallow oral medication whole; allow to dissolve slowly in mouth. You may experience nausea or vomiting (small frequent meals, frequent mouth care, chewing gum, or sucking lozenges may help). Report signs of opportunistic

(Continued)

Clotrimazole *(Continued)*

infection (eg, white plaques in mouth, fever, chills, perianal itching, vaginal itching or discharge, fatigue, unhealed wounds or sores).

Topical: Avoid contact with eyes. Wash hands before applying or wear gloves. Apply thin film to affected area. May apply porous dressing. Report persistent burning, swelling, itching, worsening of condition, or lack of response to therapy.

Vaginal: Wash hands before using. Insert full applicator into vagina gently and expel cream, or insert tablet into vagina, at bedtime. Wash applicator with soap and water following use. Remain lying down for 30 minutes following administration. Avoid intercourse during therapy (sexual partner may experience penile burning or itching). Report adverse reactions (eg, vulvar itching, frequent urination), worsening of condition, or lack of response to therapy. Contact prescriber if symptoms do not improve within 3 days or you do not feel well within 7 days. Do not use tampons until therapy is complete. Contact prescriber immediately if you experience abdominal pain, fever, or foul-smelling discharge.

Pregnancy/breast-feeding precautions: Inform prescriber if you are pregnant. Consult prescriber if breast-feeding.

Geriatric Considerations: Localized fungal infections frequently follow broad spectrum antimicrobial therapy. Specifically, oral and vaginal infections due to *Candida*.

Pregnancy Risk Factor: B (topical); C (troches)

Lactation: Excretion in breast milk unknown

Administration

Oral: Troche: Allow to dissolve slowly over 15-30 minutes.

Topical: For external use only. Apply sparingly. Protect hands with latex gloves. Do not use occlusive dressings.

Other: Avoid contact with eyes.

♦ **Clotrimazole and Betamethasone** *see Betamethasone and Clotrimazole on page 187*

Clozapine *(KLOE za peen)*

U.S. Brand Names Clozaril®; Fazaclo™

Restrictions Patient-specific registration is required to dispense clozapine. Monitoring systems for individual clozapine manufacturers are independent. If a patient is switched from one brand/manufacturer of clozapine to another, the patient must be entered into a new registry (must be completed by the prescriber and delivered to the dispensing pharmacy). Healthcare providers, including pharmacists dispensing clozapine, are encouraged to verify the patient's hematological status and qualification to receive clozapine with all existing registries.

Generic Available Yes

Pharmacologic Category Antipsychotic Agent, Atypical

Medication Safety Issues

Sound-alike/look-alike issues:

Clozapine may be confused with clofazimine, clonidine

Clozaril® may be confused with Clinoril®, Colazal®

Use Treatment-refractory schizophrenia; to reduce risk of recurrent suicidal behavior in schizophrenia or schizoaffective disorder

Unlabeled/Investigational Use Schizoaffective disorder, bipolar disorder, childhood psychosis, severe obsessive-compulsive disorder

Mechanism of Action/Effect Clozapine (dibenzodiazepine antipsychotic) is a weak dopamine$_1$ and dopamine$_2$ receptor blocker; in addition, it blocks D_1-D_5 receptors; in addition, it blocks the serotonin$_2$, alpha-adrenergic, histamine H_1, and cholinergic receptors

Contraindications Hypersensitivity to clozapine or any component of the formulation; history of agranulocytosis or granulocytopenia with clozapine; uncontrolled epilepsy; severe central nervous system depression or comatose state; myeloproliferative disorders or use with other agents which have a well-known risk of agranulocytosis or bone marrow suppression

In patients with WBC ≤3500 cells/mm^3 before therapy; if WBC falls to <3000 cells/mm^3 during therapy the drug should be withheld until signs and symptoms of infection disappear and WBC rises to >3000 cells/mm^3

Warnings/Precautions Patients with dementia-related behavioral disorders treated with atypical antipsychotics are at an increased risk of death compared to placebo. Clozapine is not approved for this indication.

Medication should not be stopped abruptly; taper off over 1-2 weeks. If conditions warrant abrupt discontinuation (leukopenia, myocarditis, cardiomyopathy), monitor patient for psychosis and cholinergic rebound (headache, nausea, vomiting, diarrhea). Elderly patients are more susceptible to adverse effects (including agranulocytosis, cardiovascular, anticholinergic, and tardive dyskinesia).

Significant risk of agranulocytosis, potentially life-threatening. WBC testing should occur weekly for the first 6 months of therapy; thereafter, if acceptable WBC counts are maintained (WBC ≥3000/mm^3, ANC ≥1500/mm^3) then WBC counts can be monitored every other week. WBCs must be monitored weekly for the first 4 weeks after therapy discontinuation. Use with caution in patients receiving other marrow suppressive agents. Eosinophilia has been reported to occur with clozapine and may require temporary or permanent interruption of therapy.

Cognitive and/or motor impairment (sedation) is common with clozapine, resulting in impaired performance of tasks requiring alertness (eg, operating machinery or driving). Use with caution in patients at risk of seizures, including those with a history of seizures, head trauma, brain damage, alcoholism, or concurrent therapy with medications which may lower seizure threshold. Has been associated with benign, self-limiting fever (<100.4°F, usually within first 3 weeks). However, clozapine may also be associated with severe febrile reactions, including neuroleptic malignant syndrome (NMS). Clozapine's potential for extrapyramidal symptoms appears to be extremely low.

May cause anticholinergic effects; use with caution in patients with urinary retention, benign prostatic hyperplasia, narrow-angle glaucoma, xerostomia, visual problems, constipation, or history of bowel obstruction. May cause hyperglycemia; in some cases may be extreme and associated with ketoacidosis, hyperosmolar coma, or death. Use with caution in patients with diabetes or other disorders of glucose regulation; monitor for worsening of glucose control. Use with caution in patients with hepatic disease or impairment; hepatitis has been reported as a consequence of therapy.

May cause orthostatic hypotension and tachycardia; use with caution in patients at risk of hypotension or in patients where transient hypotensive episodes would be poorly tolerated (cardiovascular disease or cerebrovascular disease). Concurrent use of psychotropics and benzodiazepines may increase the risk of severe cardiopulmonary reactions.

Myocarditis, pericarditis, pericardial effusion, cardiomyopathy, and CHF have also been associated with clozapine. Fatalities due to myocarditis have been reported; highest risk in the first month of therapy, however, later cases also reported. Myocarditis or cardiomyopathy should be considered in patients who present with signs/symptoms of heart failure (dyspnea, fatigue, orthopnea, paroxysmal nocturnal dyspnea, peripheral edema), chest pain, palpitations, new electrocardiographic abnormalities (arrhythmias, ST-T wave abnormalities), or unexplained fever. Patients with tachycardia during the first month of therapy should be closely monitored for other signs of myocarditis. Discontinue clozapine if myocarditis is suspected; do not rechallenge in patients with clozapine-related myocarditis. The reported rate of cardiomyopathy in clozapine-treated patients is similar to that in the general population. The majority of patients were over 50 years of age and were taking clozapine for >6 months. Clozapine should be discontinued in patients with confirmed cardiomyopathy unless benefit clearly outweighs risk. Rare cases of thromboembolism, including pulmonary embolism and stroke resulting in fatalities, have been associated with clozapine.

The possibility of a suicide attempt is inherent in psychotic illness or bipolar disorder; use caution in high-risk patients during initiation of therapy. Prescriptions should be written for the smallest quantity consistent with good patient care.

Drug Interactions

Cytochrome P450 Effect: Substrate of CYP1A2 (major), 2A6 (minor), 2C8/9 (minor), 2C19 (minor), 2D6 (minor), 3A4 (minor); **Inhibits** CYP1A2 (weak), 2C8/9 (weak), 2C19 (weak), 2D6 (moderate), 2E1 (weak), 3A4 (weak)

Decreased Effect: Clozapine may decrease the levels/effects of CYP2D6 prodrug substrates; example prodrug substrates include codeine, hydrocodone, oxycodone, and tramadol. The levels/effects of clozapine may be decreased by carbamazepine, phenobarbital, primidone, rifampin, and other CYP1A2 inducers. Cigarette smoking (nicotine) may enhance the metabolism of clozapine. Clozapine may reverse the pressor effect of epinephrine (avoid in treatment of drug-induced hypotension).

Increased Effect/Toxicity: May potentiate anticholinergic and hypotensive effects of other drugs. Benzodiazepines in combination with clozapine may produce respiratory depression and hypotension, especially during the first few weeks of therapy. May potentiate effect/toxicity of risperidone. Clozapine serum concentrations may be increased by inhibitors of CYP1A2; example inhibitors include amiodarone, ciprofloxacin, fluvoxamine, ketoconazole, norfloxacin, ofloxacin, and rofecoxib. Clozapine may increase the levels/effects of amphetamines, selected beta-blockers, substrates; example substrates include dextromethorphan, fluoxetine, lidocaine, mirtazapine, nefazodone, paroxetine, risperidone, ritonavir, thioridazine, tricyclic antidepressants, venlafaxine, and other CYP2D6 substrates. Metoclopramide may increase risk of extrapyramidal symptoms (EPS).

Nutritional/Ethanol Interactions

Ethanol: Avoid ethanol (may increase CNS depression).

Herb/Nutraceutical: St John's wort may decrease clozapine levels. Avoid kava kava, gotu kola, valerian, St John's wort (may increase CNS depression).

Adverse Reactions

>10%:

Cardiovascular: Tachycardia

Central nervous system: Drowsiness, dizziness

Gastrointestinal: Constipation, weight gain, sialorrhea

Genitourinary: Urinary incontinence

1% to 10%:

Cardiovascular: Angina, ECG changes, hyper-/hypotension, syncope

Central nervous system: Akathisia, seizure, headache, nightmares, akinesia, confusion, insomnia, fatigue, myoclonic jerks, restlessness, agitation, lethargy, ataxia, slurred speech, depression, anxiety

Dermatologic: Rash

Gastrointestinal: Abdominal discomfort, anorexia, diarrhea, heartburn, xerostomia, nausea, vomiting

Hematologic: Eosinophilia, leukopenia, leukocytosis

Hepatic: Liver function tests abnormal

Neuromuscular & skeletal: Tremor, rigidity, hyperkinesia, weakness

Ocular: Visual disturbances

Respiratory: Rhinorrhea

Miscellaneous: Diaphoresis (increased), fever

Overdosage/Toxicology Symptoms of overdose include altered states of consciousness, tachycardia, hypotension, hypersalivation, and respiratory depression. Following initiation of essential overdose management, toxic symptom treatment and supportive treatment should be initiated.

(Continued)

Clozapine *(Continued)*

Pharmacodynamics/Kinetics

Bioavailability: 12% to 81%

Time to Peak: 2.5 hours

Protein Binding: 97% to serum proteins

Half-Life Elimination: 12 hours (range: 4-66 hours)

Metabolism: Extensively hepatic

Excretion: Urine (~50%) and feces (30%) with trace amounts of unchanged drug

Dosing

Adults: Schizophrenia or to reduce risk of suicidal behavior: Initial: 12.5 mg once or twice daily; increased, as tolerated in increments of 25-50 mg/day to a target dose of 300-450 mg/day after 2-4 weeks, may require doses as high as 600-900 mg/day for the treatment of schizophrenia; median dose to reduce risk of suicidal behavior is ~300 mg/day (range 12.5-900 mg)

Note: In the event of planned termination of clozapine, gradual reduction in dose over a 1- to 2-week period is recommended. If conditions warrant abrupt discontinuation (leukopenia), monitor patient for psychosis and cholinergic rebound (headache, nausea, vomiting, diarrhea).

Elderly: Oral: Experience in the elderly is limited; initial dose should be 25 mg/day; increase as tolerated by 25 mg/day to desired response. Maximum daily dose in the elderly should probably be 450 mg. Dose titration to 300-450 mg/day may be attained in 2 weeks if tolerated; however, elderly may require slower titration and daily increases may not be tolerated.

Pediatrics: Children and Adolescents: Childhood psychosis (unlabeled use): Oral: Initial: 25 mg/day; increase to a target dose of 25-400 mg/day

Available Dosage Forms

Tablet: 12.5 mg, 25 mg, 100 mg

Clozaril®: 25 mg, 100 mg

Tablet, orally-disintegrating (Fazaclo™): 25 mg [contains phenylalanine 1.75 mg; mint flavor], 100 mg [contains phenylalanine 6.96 mg; mint flavor]

Monitoring and Teaching Issues

Physical Assessment: Assess potential for interactions with other prescriptions, OTC medications, or herbal products patient may be taking. Initiate at lower doses and taper dosage slowly when discontinuing. Instruct patients with diabetes to monitor blood glucose levels closely (may cause hyperglycemia). Be alert to the potential of cardiac abnormalities. Monitor weight prior to initiating therapy and at least monthly. Consider titrating to a different antipsychotic agent for a weight gain ≥5% of initial weight. Review ophthalmic exam periodically and assess results of weekly laboratory tests. Monitor therapeutic effectiveness, and adverse reactions at beginning of therapy and periodically with long-term use. Teach patient appropriate administration, interventions to reduce side effects, and adverse symptoms to report.

Monitoring Laboratory Tests: ECG, fasting lipid profile and fasting blood glucose/Hgb A$_{1c}$ (prior to treatment, at 3 months, then annually). WBC should be obtained at baseline and at least weekly for the first 6 months of continuous treatment. If WBC counts remain acceptable (WBC ≥3000/mm³, ANC ≥1500/mm³) during this time period, then WBC counts may be monitored every other week thereafter. If clozapine is discontinued, a weekly WBC should be completed for an additional 4 weeks. If clozapine therapy is interrupted, the 6-month time period for initiation of biweekly WBCs may need to be reset. This determination depends upon the treatment duration, the length of the break in therapy, and whether or not an abnormal blood event occurred. Consult full prescribing information for determination of appropriate WBC-monitoring interval.

Patient Education: Use exactly as directed; do not increase dose or frequency. Do not discontinue without consulting prescriber. Avoid alcohol or caffeine and other prescription or OTC medications not approved by prescriber. Maintain adequate hydration (2-3 L/day of fluids) unless instructed to restrict fluid intake. If you have diabetes, monitor blood glucose levels frequently. You may experience headache, excess drowsiness, dizziness, or blurred vision (use caution driving or when engaging in tasks requiring alertness until response to drug is known); dry mouth, constipation, diarrhea; nausea, vomiting (small frequent meals, frequent mouth care, sucking lozenges, or chewing gum may help); or postural hypotension (use caution climbing stairs or when changing position from lying or sitting to standing). Report persistent CNS effects (insomnia, depression, altered consciousness); palpitations, rapid heartbeat, severe dizziness; vision changes; hypersalivation, tearing, sweating; respiratory difficulty; or worsening of condition. Report seizures, flu-like symptoms, chest pain, shortness of breath, or excessive fatigue. **Breast-feeding precaution:** Breast-feeding is not recommended.

Dietary Considerations: May be taken without regard to food. Fazaclo™ contains phenylalanine 1.75 mg per 25 mg tablet and phenylalanine 6.96 mg per 100 mg tablet.

Geriatric Considerations: Not recommended for use in nonpsychotic patients. Studies in subjects >65 years of age have not been done. Orthostatic hypotension and sustained tachycardia have been noted in up to 25% of patients taking clozapine; therefore, elderly with cardiovascular disease may be at risk. The anticholinergic effects of clozapine may be prominent in elderly (eg, constipation, confusion, urinary retention).

Pregnancy Risk Factor: B

Pregnancy Issues: Teratogenic effects were not seen in animal studies; however, there are no adequate and well-controlled studies in pregnant women. Use during pregnancy only if clearly needed.

Lactation: Enters breast milk/not recommended (AAP rates "of concern")

Administration

Oral: Orally-disintegrating tablet: Should be removed from foil blister by peeling apart (do not push tablet through the foil). Remove immediately prior to use. Place tablet in mouth and allow to dissolve; swallow with saliva. If dosing requires splitting tablet, throw unused portion away.

Storage: Dispensed in "clozapine patient system" packaging.
Related Information
Antipsychotic Agents *on page 1717*
Antipsychotic Medication Guidelines *on page 1766*
Federal OBRA Regulations: Recommended Maximum Doses *on page 1773*

♦ **Clozaril**® *see* Clozapine *on page 362*
♦ **CMS Guidelines for Unnecessary Drugs in Long-Term Care Facilities** *see page 1772*
♦ **CMV-IGIV** *see* Cytomegalovirus Immune Globulin (Intravenous-Human) *on page 393*
♦ **Coagulant Complex Inhibitor** *see* Anti-inhibitor Coagulant Complex *on page 128*
♦ **Coagulation Factor VIIa** *see* Factor VIIa (Recombinant) *on page 606*

Cocaine (koe KANE)

Synonyms Cocaine Hydrochloride
Controlled Substance C-II
Generic Available Yes
Pharmacologic Category Local Anesthetic
Use Topical anesthesia for mucous membranes
Mechanism of Action/Effect Blocks both the initiation and conduction of nerve impulses
Contraindications Hypersensitivity to cocaine or any component of the topical solution; ophthalmologic anesthesia (causing sloughing of the corneal epithelium); pregnancy (nonmedicinal use)
Warnings/Precautions For topical use only. Limit to office and surgical procedures only. Resuscitative equipment and drugs should be immediately available when any local anesthetic is used. Debilitated, elderly patients, acutely ill patients, and children should be given reduced doses consistent with their age and physical status. Use caution in patients with severely traumatized mucosa and sepsis in the region of the proposed application. Use with caution in patients with cardiovascular disease or a history of cocaine abuse. In patients being treated for cardiovascular complication of cocaine abuse, avoid beta-blockers for treatment.
Drug Interactions
Cytochrome P450 Effect: Substrate of CYP3A4 (major); **Inhibits** CYP2D6 (strong), 3A4 (weak)
Increased Effect/Toxicity: Cocaine may increase the levels/effects of CYP2D6 substrates (eg, amphetamines, selected beta-blockers, dextromethorphan, fluoxetine, lidocaine, mirtazapine, nefazodone, paroxetine, risperidone, ritonavir, thioridazine, tricyclic antidepressants, venlafaxine). Increased toxicity with MAO inhibitors. Use with epinephrine may cause extreme hypertension and/or cardiac arrhythmias. CYP3A4 inhibitors may increase the levels/effects of cocaine (eg, azole antifungals, ciprofloxacin, clarithromycin, diclofenac, doxycycline, erythromycin, imatinib, isoniazid, nefazodone, nicardipine, propofol, protease inhibitors, quinidine, verapamil).
Adverse Reactions
>10%:
Central nervous system: CNS stimulation
Gastrointestinal: Loss of taste perception
Respiratory: Rhinitis, nasal congestion
Miscellaneous: Loss of smell
1% to 10%:
Cardiovascular: Heart rate (decreased) with low doses, tachycardia with moderate doses, hypertension, cardiomyopathy, cardiac arrhythmia, myocarditis, QRS prolongation, Raynaud's phenomenon, cerebral vasculitis, thrombosis, fibrillation (atrial), flutter (atrial), sinus bradycardia, CHF, pulmonary hypertension, sinus tachycardia, tachycardia (supraventricular), arrhythmia (ventricular), vasoconstriction
Central nervous system: Fever, nervousness, restlessness, euphoria, excitation, headache, psychosis, hallucinations, agitation, seizure, slurred speech, hyperthermia, dystonic reactions, cerebral vascular accident, vasculitis, clonic-tonic reactions, paranoia, sympathetic storm
Dermatologic: Skin infarction, pruritus, madarosis
Gastrointestinal: Nausea, anorexia, colonic ischemia, spontaneous bowel perforation
Genitourinary: Priapism, uterine rupture
Hematologic: Thrombocytopenia
Neuromuscular & skeletal: Chorea (extrapyramidal), paresthesia, tremor, fasciculations
Ocular: Mydriasis (peak effect at 45 minutes; may last up to 12 hours), sloughing of the corneal epithelium, ulceration of the cornea, iritis, mydriasis, chemosis
Renal: Myoglobinuria, necrotizing vasculitis
Respiratory: Tachypnea, nasal mucosa damage (when snorting), hyposmia, bronchiolitis obliterans organizing pneumonia
Miscellaneous: "Washed-out" syndrome
Overdosage/Toxicology Symptoms of overdose include anxiety, excitement, confusion, nausea, vomiting, headache, rapid pulse, irregular respiration, delirium, fever, seizures, respiratory arrest, hallucinations, dilated pupils, muscle spasms, sensory aberrations, and cardiac arrhythmias.
Fatal dose: Oral: 500 mg to 1.2 g; severe toxic effects have occurred with doses as low as 20 mg.
Since no specific antidote for cocaine exists, serious toxic effects are treated symptomatically.
Pharmacodynamics/Kinetics
Onset of Action: ~1 minute; Peak effect: ~5 minutes
Duration of Action: Dose dependent: ≥30 minutes; cocaine metabolites may appear in urine of neonates up to 5 days after birth due to maternal cocaine use shortly before birth
Absorption: Well absorbed through mucous membranes; limited by drug-induced vasoconstriction; enhanced by inflammation
(Continued)

Cocaine *(Continued)*

Half-Life Elimination: 75 minutes

Metabolism: Hepatic; major metabolites are ecgonine methyl ester and benzoyl ecgonine

Excretion: Primarily urine (<10% as unchanged drug and metabolites)

Pharmacokinetic Note: Data is based on topical administration to mucosa.

Dosing

Adults: Topical application (ear, nose, throat, bronchoscopy): Dosage depends on the area to be anesthetized, tissue vascularity, technique of anesthesia, and individual patient tolerance; the lowest dose necessary to produce adequate anesthesia should be used; concentrations of 1% to 10% are used (not to exceed 1 mg/kg). Use reduced dosages for children, elderly, or debilitated patients.

Elderly: Refer to adult dosing; use with caution.

Available Dosage Forms

Powder, as hydrochloride: 1 g, 5 g, 25 g

Solution, topical, as hydrochloride: 4% [40 mg/mL] (4 mL, 10 mL); 10% [100 mg/mL] (4 mL, 10 mL)

Monitoring and Teaching Issues

Physical Assessment: Assess other medications patient may be taking for interactions. Monitor adverse effects and teach patient adverse symptoms to report. **Pregnancy risk factor C/X (if nonmedicinal use).** Breast-feeding is contraindicated.

Patient Education: When used orally, do not take anything by mouth until full sensation returns. **Ocular:** Use caution when driving or engaging in tasks that require alert vision (mydriasis may last for several hours). At time of use or immediately thereafter, report any unusual cardiovascular, CNS, or respiratory symptoms. Following use, report skin irritation or eruption; alterations in vision, eye pain, or irritation; persistent GI effects; muscle or skeletal tremors, numbness, or rigidity; urinary or genital problems; or persistent fatigue. **Pregnancy/breast-feeding precautions:** Inform prescriber if you are pregnant. Do not breast-feed.

Pregnancy Risk Factor: C/X (nonmedicinal use)

Lactation: Enters breast milk/contraindicated

Breast-Feeding Issues: Irritability, vomiting, diarrhea, tremors, and seizures have been reported in nursing infants.

Administration

Topical: Use only on mucous membranes of the oral, laryngeal, and nasal cavities. Do not use on extensive areas of broken skin.

Storage: Store in well-closed, light-resistant containers.

Additional Information Cocaine intoxication of infants who are receiving breast milk from their mothers abusing cocaine has been reported.

- ◆ **Cocaine Hydrochloride** *see Cocaine on page 365*
- ◆ **Codafed® Expectorant** *see Guaifenesin, Pseudoephedrine, and Codeine on page 735*
- ◆ **Codafed® Pediatric Expectorant** *see Guaifenesin, Pseudoephedrine, and Codeine on page 735*
- ◆ **Codal-DM [OTC]** *see Phenylephrine, Pyrilamine, and Dextromethorphan on page 1204*

Codeine *(KOE deen)*

Synonyms Codeine Phosphate; Codeine Sulfate; Methylmorphine

Controlled Substance C-II

Generic Available Yes

Pharmacologic Category Analgesic, Narcotic; Antitussive

Medication Safety Issues

Sound-alike/look-alike issues:

Codeine may be confused with Cardene®, Cophene®, Cordran®, iodine, Lodine®

Use Treatment of mild to moderate pain; antitussive in lower doses; dextromethorphan has equivalent antitussive activity but has much lower toxicity in accidental overdose

Mechanism of Action/Effect Inhibits perception of and response to pain; causes cough supression; produces generalized CNS depression

Contraindications Hypersensitivity to codeine or any component of the formulation; pregnancy (prolonged use or high doses at term)

Warnings/Precautions An opioid-containing analgesic regimen should be tailored to each patient's needs and based upon the type of pain being treated (acute versus chronic), the route of administration, degree of tolerance for opioids (naive versus chronic user), age, weight, and medical condition. The optimal analgesic dose varies widely among patients. Doses should be titrated to pain relief/prevention.

Use with caution in patients with hypersensitivity reactions to other phenanthrene derivative opioid agonists (morphine, hydrocodone, hydromorphone, levorphanol, oxycodone, oxymorphone); respiratory diseases including asthma, emphysema, COPD, or severe liver or renal insufficiency; some preparations contain sulfites which may cause allergic reactions; tolerance or drug dependence may result from extended use

Not recommended for use for cough control in patients with a productive cough; not recommended as an antitussive for children <2 years of age; the elderly may be particularly susceptible to the CNS depressant and confusion as well as constipating effects of narcotics

Not approved for I.V. administration (although this route has been used clinically). If given intravenously, must be given slowly and the patient should be lying down. Rapid intravenous administration of narcotics may increase the incidence of serious adverse effects, in part due to limited opportunity to assess response prior to administration of the full dose. Access to respiratory support should be immediately available

Drug Interactions

Cytochrome P450 Effect: Substrate of CYP2D6 (major), 3A4 (minor); **Inhibits** CYP2D6 (weak)

Decreased Effect: CYP2D6 inhibitors may decrease the effects of codeine. Example inhibitors include chlorpromazine, delavirdine, fluoxetine, miconazole, paroxetine, pergolide, quinidine, quinine, ritonavir, and ropinirole. Decreased effect with cigarette smoking.

Increased Effect/Toxicity: May cause severely increased toxicity of codeine when taken with CNS depressants, phenothiazines, tricyclic antidepressants, other narcotic analgesics, guanabenz, MAO inhibitors, and neuromuscular blockers.

Nutritional/Ethanol Interactions

Ethanol: Avoid or limit ethanol (may increase CNS depression). Watch for sedation.

Herb/Nutraceutical: St John's wort may decrease codeine levels. Avoid valerian, St John's wort, kava kava, gotu kola (may increase CNS depression).

Lab Interactions Increased aminotransferase [ALT (SGPT)/AST (SGOT)] (S)

Adverse Reactions

Frequency not defined: Increased AST, ALT

>10%:

Central nervous system: Drowsiness

Gastrointestinal: Constipation

1% to 10%:

Cardiovascular: Tachycardia or bradycardia, hypotension

Central nervous system: Dizziness, lightheadedness, false feeling of well being, malaise, headache, restlessness, paradoxical CNS stimulation, confusion

Dermatologic: Rash, urticaria

Gastrointestinal: Xerostomia, anorexia, nausea, vomiting

Genitourinary: Decreased urination, ureteral spasm

Hepatic: Increased LFTs

Local: Burning at injection site

Neuromuscular & skeletal: Weakness

Ocular: Blurred vision

Respiratory: Dyspnea

Miscellaneous: Histamine release

Overdosage/Toxicology Symptoms of overdose include CNS and respiratory depression, GI cramping, and constipation. Naloxone, 2 mg I.V. with repeat administration as necessary up to a total of 10 mg, can also be used to reverse toxic effects of the opiate.

Pharmacodynamics/Kinetics

Onset of Action: Oral: 0.5-1 hour; I.M.: 10-30 minutes; Peak effect: Oral: 1-1.5 hours; I.M.: 0.5-1 hour

Duration of Action: 4-6 hours

Absorption: Oral: Adequate

Protein Binding: 7%

Half-Life Elimination: 2.5-3.5 hours

Metabolism: Hepatic to morphine (active)

Excretion: Urine (3% to 16% as unchanged drug, norcodeine, and free and conjugated morphine)

Dosing

Adults & Elderly: Note: These are guidelines and do not represent the maximum doses that may be required in all patients. Doses should be titrated to pain relief/prevention. Doses >1.5 mg/kg body weight are not recommended.

Pain management (analgesic):

Oral, regular release: 30 mg every 4-6 hours as needed; patients with prior opiate exposure may require higher initial doses. Usual range: 15-120 mg every 4-6 hours as needed

Oral, controlled release formulation (Codeine Contin®, not available in U.S.): 50-300 mg every 12 hours. **Note:** A patient's codeine requirement should be established using prompt release formulations; conversion to long acting products may be considered when chronic, continuous treatment is required. Higher dosages should be reserved for use only in opioid-tolerant patients.

I.M., SubQ: 30 mg every 4-6 hours as needed; patients with prior opiate exposure may require higher initial doses. Usual range: 15-120 mg every 4-6 hours as needed; more frequent dosing may be needed

Cough (antitussive): Oral (for nonproductive cough): 10-20 mg/dose every 4-6 hours as needed; maximum: 120 mg/day

Pediatrics: Note: These are guidelines and do not represent the maximum doses that may be required in all patients. Doses should be titrated to pain relief/prevention. Doses >1.5 mg/kg body weight are not recommended.

Analgesic: Oral, I.M., SubQ: Children: 0.5-1 mg/kg/dose every 4-6 hours as needed; maximum: 60 mg/dose

Antitussive: Oral (for nonproductive cough): Children: 1-1.5 mg/kg/day in divided doses every 4-6 hours as needed: Alternative dose according to age:

2-6 years: 2.5-5 mg every 4-6 hours as needed; maximum: 30 mg/day

6-12 years: 5-10 mg every 4-6 hours as needed; maximum: 60 mg/day

Renal Impairment:

Cl$_{cr}$ 10-50 mL/minute: Administer 75% of dose.

Cl$_{cr}$ <10 mL/minute: Administer 50% of dose.

Hepatic Impairment: Dosing adjustment is probably necessary in hepatic insufficiency.

Available Dosage Forms

Injection, as phosphate: 15 mg/mL (2 mL); 30 mg/mL (2 mL) [contains sodium metabisulfite]

Solution, oral, as phosphate: 15 mg/5 mL (5 mL, 500 mL) [strawberry flavor]

Tablet, controlled release (Codeine Contin®) [not available in U.S.]: 50 mg, 100 mg, 150 mg, 200 mg

Tablet, as phosphate: 30 mg, 60 mg

Tablet, as sulfate: 15 mg, 30 mg, 60 mg

(Continued)

Codeine *(Continued)*

Monitoring and Teaching Issues

Physical Assessment: Assess other medications patient may be taking for possible additive or adverse interactions. Monitor for effectiveness of pain relief, for signs of overdose, vital signs and CNS status, and adverse reactions at beginning of therapy and at regular intervals with long-term use. May cause physical and/or psychological dependence. For inpatients, implement safety measures. Assess knowledge/teach patient appropriate use (if self-administered). Teach patient to monitor for adverse reactions, adverse reactions to report, and appropriate interventions to reduce side effects.

Patient Education: If self-administered, use exactly as directed; do not increase dose or frequency. Drug may cause physical and/or psychological dependence. While using this medication, do not use alcohol and other prescription or OTC medications (especially sedatives, tranquilizers, antihistamines, or pain medications) without consulting prescriber. Maintain adequate hydration (2-3 L/day of fluids) unless instructed to restrict fluid intake. May cause dizziness, drowsiness, confusion, agitation, impaired coordination, or blurred vision (use caution when driving, climbing stairs, or changing position - rising from sitting or lying to standing, or when engaging in tasks requiring alertness until response to drug is known); nausea or vomiting, or loss of appetite (frequent mouth care, small frequent meals, sucking lozenges, or chewing gum may help); or constipation (increased exercise, fluids, fruit, or fiber may help; if unresolved, consult prescriber about use of stool softeners). Report confusion, insomnia, excessive nervousness, excessive sedation or drowsiness, or shakiness; acute GI upset; respiratory difficulty or shortness of breath; facial flushing, rapid heartbeat, or palpitations; urinary difficulty; unusual muscle weakness; or vision changes.

Pregnancy/breast-feeding precautions: Inform prescriber if you are or intend to become pregnant. If you are breast-feeding, take medication immediately after breast-feeding or 3-4 hours prior to next feeding.

Geriatric Considerations: The elderly may be particularly susceptible to CNS depression and confusion as well as the constipating effects of narcotics.

Pregnancy Risk Factor: C/D (prolonged use or high doses at term)

Lactation: Enters breast milk/use caution (AAP rates "compatible")

Administration

Storage: Store injection between 15°C to 30°C, avoid freezing. Do not use if injection is discolored or contains a precipitate. Protect injection from light.

Related Information

Narcotic / Opioid Analgesic Comparison *on page 1739*

- ◆ **Codeine, Acetaminophen, Butalbital, and Caffeine** *see* Butalbital, Acetaminophen, Caffeine, and Codeine *on page 226*
- ◆ **Codeine and Acetaminophen** *see* Acetaminophen and Codeine *on page 41*
- ◆ **Codeine and Aspirin** *see* Aspirin and Codeine *on page 147*
- ◆ **Codeine and Butalbital Compound** *see* Butalbital, Aspirin, Caffeine, and Codeine *on page 227*
- ◆ **Codeine and Guaifenesin** *see* Guaifenesin and Codeine *on page 731*
- ◆ **Codeine and Promethazine** *see* Promethazine and Codeine *on page 1267*
- ◆ **Codeine, Aspirin, and Carisoprodol** *see* Carisoprodol, Aspirin, and Codeine *on page 259*
- ◆ **Codeine, Butalbital, Aspirin, and Caffeine** *see* Butalbital, Aspirin, Caffeine, and Codeine *on page 227*
- ◆ **Codeine, Guaifenesin, and Pseudoephedrine** *see* Guaifenesin, Pseudoephedrine, and Codeine *on page 735*
- ◆ **Codeine Phosphate** *see* Codeine *on page 366*
- ◆ **Codeine, Promethazine, and Phenylephrine** *see* Promethazine, Phenylephrine, and Codeine *on page 1268*
- ◆ **Codeine Sulfate** *see* Codeine *on page 366*
- ◆ **Codimal® DM [OTC]** *see* Phenylephrine, Pyrilamine, and Dextromethorphan *on page 1204*
- ◆ **Codituss DM [OTC]** *see* Phenylephrine, Pyrilamine, and Dextromethorphan *on page 1204*
- ◆ **Cogentin®** *see* Benztropine *on page 184*
- ◆ **Co-Gesic®** *see* Hydrocodone and Acetaminophen *on page 754*
- ◆ **Cognex®** *see* Tacrine *on page 1418*
- ◆ **Colace® [OTC]** *see* Docusate *on page 474*
- ◆ **ColBenemid** *see* Colchicine and Probenecid *on page 370*

Colchicine *(KOL chi seen)*

Generic Available Yes

Pharmacologic Category Colchicine

Medication Safety Issues

High alert medication: The Institute for Safe Medication Practices (ISMP) includes this medication among its list of drugs which have a heightened risk of causing significant patient harm when used in error.

Use Treatment of acute gouty arthritis attacks and prevention of recurrences of such attacks

Unlabeled/Investigational Use Primary biliary cirrhosis; management of familial Mediterranean fever; pericarditis

Mechanism of Action/Effect Reduces the deposition of urate crystals that perpetuates the inflammatory response

Contraindications Hypersensitivity to colchicine or any component of the formulation; severe renal, gastrointestinal, hepatic, or cardiac disorders; blood dyscrasias; pregnancy (parenteral)

Warnings/Precautions Use with caution in debilitated patients or elderly patients; use caution in patients with mild-to-moderate cardiac, GI, renal, or liver disease. Severe local irritation can occur following SubQ or I.M. administration. Dosage reduction is recommended in patients who develop weakness or gastrointestinal symptoms (anorexia, diarrhea, nausea, vomiting) related to drug therapy.

Intravenous: Use only with extreme caution; potential for serious, life-threatening complications. Should not be administered to patients with renal insufficiency, hepatobiliary obstruction, patients >70 years of age, or recent oral colchicine use. Should be reserved for hospitalized patients who are under the care of a physician experienced in the use of intravenous colchicine.

Drug Interactions

Cytochrome P450 Effect: Substrate of CYP3A4 (major); **Induces** CYP2C8/9 (weak), 2E1 (weak), 3A4 (weak)

Increased Effect/Toxicity: Alkalizing agents potentiate effects of colchicine. CYP3A4 inhibitors may increase the levels/effects of colchicine; example inhibitors include azole antifungals, ciprofloxacin, clarithromycin, diclofenac, doxycycline, erythromycin, imatinib, isoniazid, nefazodone, nicardipine, propofol, protease inhibitors, quinidine, and verapamil. Concurrent use of cyclosporine with colchicine may increase toxicity of colchicine.

CYP3A4 inhibitors: May increase the levels/effects of colchicine. Example inhibitors include azole antifungals, ciprofloxacin, clarithromycin, diclofenac, doxycycline, erythromycin, imatinib, isoniazid, nefazodone, nicardipine, propofol, protease inhibitors, quinidine, and verapamil.

Nutritional/Ethanol Interactions

Ethanol: Avoid ethanol.

Food: Cyanocobalamin (vitamin B_{12}): Malabsorption of the substrate. May result in macrocytic anemia or neurologic dysfunction.

Herb/Nutraceutical: Vitamin B_{12} absorption may be decreased by colchicine.

Lab Interactions May cause false-positive results in urine tests for erythrocytes or hemoglobin

Adverse Reactions

>10%: Gastrointestinal: Nausea, vomiting, diarrhea, abdominal pain

1% to 10%:

Dermatologic: Alopecia

Gastrointestinal: Anorexia

Overdosage/Toxicology Symptoms of overdose include acute nausea, vomiting, abdominal pain, shock, kidney damage, muscle weakness, burning in throat, watery to bloody diarrhea, hypotension, anuria, cardiovascular collapse, delirium, convulsions, and respiratory paralysis. Treatment includes gastric lavage and measures to prevent shock, hemodialysis or peritoneal dialysis. Atropine and morphine may relieve abdominal pain.

Pharmacodynamics/Kinetics

Onset of Action: Oral: Pain relief: ~12 hours if adequately dosed

Time to Peak: Serum: 0.5-2 hours, declining for the next 2 hours before increasing again due to enterohepatic recycling

Protein Binding: 10% to 31%

Half-Life Elimination: 12-30 minutes; End-stage renal disease: 45 minutes

Metabolism: Partially hepatic via deacetylation

Excretion: Primarily feces; urine (10% to 20%)

Dosing

Adults:

Familial Mediterranean fever (unlabeled use): Prophylaxis: Oral: 1-2 mg daily in divided doses (occasionally reduced to 0.6 mg/day in patients with GI intolerance)

Gouty arthritis:

Prophylaxis of acute attacks: Oral: 0.6 mg twice daily; initial and/or subsequent dosage may be decreased (ie, 0.6 mg once daily) in patients at risk of toxicity or in those who are intolerant (including weakness, loose stools, or diarrhea); range: 0.6 mg every other day to 0.6 mg 3 times/day

Acute attacks:

Oral: Initial: 0.6-1.2 mg, followed by 0.6 every 1-2 hours; some clinicians recommend a maximum of 3 doses; more aggressive approaches have recommended a maximum dose of up to 6 mg. Wait at least 3 days before initiating another course of therapy

I.V.: Initial: 1-2 mg, then 0.5 mg every 6 hours until response, not to exceed total dose of 4 mg. If pain recurs, it may be necessary to administer additional daily doses. The amount of colchicine administered intravenously in an acute treatment period (generally ~1 week) should not exceed a total dose of 4 mg. Do not administer more colchicine by any route for at least 7 days after a full course of I.V. therapy.

Note: Many experts would avoid use because of potential for serious, life-threatening complications. Should not be administered to patients with renal insufficiency, hepatobiliary obstruction, patients >70 years of age, or recent oral colchicine use. Should be reserved for hospitalized patients who are under the care of a physician experienced in the use of intravenous colchicine.

Surgery: Gouty arthritis, prophylaxis of recurrent attacks: Oral: 0.6 mg/day or every other day; patients who are to undergo surgical procedures may receive 0.6 mg 3 times/day for 3 days before and 3 days after surgery

Primary biliary cirrhosis (unlabeled use): Oral: 0.6 mg twice daily

Pericarditis (unlabeled use): Oral: 0.6 mg twice daily

Elderly: Refer to adult dosing. Reduce maintenance/prophylactic dose by 50% in individuals >70 years.

Pediatrics: Prophylaxis of familial Mediterranean fever (unlabeled use): Oral:

Children ≤5 years: 0.5 mg/day

Children >5 years: 1-1.5 mg/day in 2-3 divided doses

Renal Impairment:

Gouty arthritis, acute attacks: Oral: Specific dosing recommendations not available from the manufacturer:

Prophylaxis:

Cl_{cr} 35-49 mL/minute: 0.6 mg once daily

Cl_{cr} 10-34 mL/minute: 0.6 mg every 2-3 days

Cl_{cr} <10 mL/minute: Avoid chronic use of colchicine. Use in serious renal impairment is contraindicated by the manufacturer.

(Continued)

Colchicine *(Continued)*

Treatment: Cl_{cr} <10 mL/minute: Use in serious renal impairment is contraindicated by the manufacturer. If a decision is made to use colchicine, decrease dose by 75%.

Peritoneal dialysis: Supplemental dose is not necessary

Hepatic Impairment: Avoid in hepatobiliary dysfunction and in patients with hepatic disease.

Available Dosage Forms
Injection, solution: 0.5 mg/mL (2 mL)
Tablet: 0.6 mg

Monitoring and Teaching Issues
Physical Assessment: Assess effectiveness and interactions of other medications patient may be taking. **I.V.:** Monitor therapeutic effectiveness, laboratory values, and adverse reactions at beginning of therapy and periodically with long-term use. Assess knowledge/ teach patient appropriate use, interventions to reduce side effects, and adverse symptoms to report.

Monitoring Laboratory Tests: CBC and renal function on a regular basis

Patient Education: Take as directed; do not exceed recommended dosage. Consult prescriber about a low-purine diet. Maintain adequate hydration (2-3 L/day of fluids) unless instructed to restrict fluid intake. Do not use alcohol or aspirin-containing medication without consulting prescriber. You may experience nausea, vomiting, or anorexia (small frequent meals, frequent mouth care, chewing gum, or sucking lozenges may help); hair loss (reversible). Stop medication and report to prescriber if severe vomiting, watery or bloody diarrhea, or abdominal pain occurs. Report muscle tremors or weakness; fatigue; easy bruising or bleeding; yellowing of eyes or skin; or pale stool or dark urine. **Pregnancy/ breast-feeding precautions:** Inform prescriber if you are or intend to become pregnant. Consult prescriber if breast-feeding.

Dietary Considerations: May need to supplement with vitamin B_{12}.

Geriatric Considerations: Colchicine appears to be more toxic in the elderly, particularly in the presence of renal, gastrointestinal, or cardiac disease. The most predictable oral side effects are (gastrointestinal) vomiting, abdominal pain, and nausea. If colchicine is stopped at this point, other more severe adverse effects may be avoided, such as bone marrow suppression, peripheral neuritis, etc.

Pregnancy Risk Factor: C (oral); D (parenteral)

Lactation: Enters breast milk/use caution (AAP rates "compatible")

Administration
Oral: Administer tablet orally with water and maintain adequate fluid intake.

I.V.: Injection should be made over 2-5 minutes into tubing of free-flowing I.V. with compatible fluid. Do not administer I.M. or SubQ; severe local irritation can occur following SubQ or I.M. administration. Extravasation can cause tissue irritation.

Compatibility: I.V. colchicine is **incompatible** with dextrose or I.V. solutions with preservatives.

Storage: Protect tablets from light.

Colchicine and Probenecid *(KOL chi seen & proe BEN e sid)*
Synonyms ColBenemid; Probenecid and Colchicine

Generic Available Yes

Pharmacologic Category Antigout Agent; Anti-inflammatory Agent; Uricosuric Agent

Use Treatment of chronic gouty arthritis when complicated by frequent, recurrent acute attacks of gout

Dosing
Adults & Elderly: Gout: Oral: 1 tablet/day for 1 week, then 1 tablet twice daily thereafter

Renal Impairment: Probenecid may not be effective in patients with chronic renal insufficiency particularly when Cl_{cr} is ≤30 mL/minute.

Available Dosage Forms Tablet: Colchicine 0.5 mg and probenecid 0.5 g

Monitoring and Teaching Issues
Physical Assessment: See individual agents.

Patient Education: See individual agents. **Pregnancy/breast-feeding precautions:** Inform prescriber if you are or intend to become pregnant. Consult prescriber if breast-feeding.

Pregnancy Risk Factor: C

Lactation:
Colchicine: Compatible
Probenecid: Excretion in breast milk unknown

Related Information
Colchicine *on page 368*
Probenecid *on page 1253*

♦ **Coldcough HC** *see* Pseudoephedrine, Hydrocodone, and Chlorpheniramine *on page 1283*

Colesevelam *(koh le SEV a lam)*
U.S. Brand Names WelChol®

Generic Available No

Pharmacologic Category Antilipemic Agent, Bile Acid Sequestrant

Use Adjunctive therapy to diet and exercise in the management of elevated LDL in primary hypercholesterolemia (Fredrickson type IIa) when used alone or in combination with an HMG-CoA reductase inhibitor

Mechanism of Action/Effect Colesevelam binds bile acids including glycocholic acid in the intestine, impeding their reabsorption. Increases the fecal loss of bile salt-bound LDL-C.

Contraindications Hypersensitivity to colesevelam or any component of the formulation; bowel obstruction

Warnings/Precautions Use caution in treating patients with triglyceride levels >300 mg/dL (excluded from trials). Safety and efficacy not established in pediatric patients. Use caution in dysphagia, swallowing disorders, severe GI motility disorders, major GI tract surgery, or in patients susceptible to fat soluble vitamin deficiencies. Minimal effects are seen on HDL-C and triglyceride levels. Secondary causes of hypercholesterolemia should be excluded before initiation.

Drug Interactions

Decreased Effect: Sustained-release verapamil AUC and C_{max} were reduced. Clinical significance unknown.

Digoxin, lovastatin, metoprolol, quinidine, valproic acid, or warfarin absorption was not significantly affected with concurrent administration.

Clinical effects of atorvastatin, lovastatin, and simvastatin were not changed by concurrent administration.

Increased Effect/Toxicity: Refer to Decreased Effect.

Adverse Reactions

>10%: Gastrointestinal: Constipation (11%)

2% to 10%:

Gastrointestinal: Dyspepsia (8%)

Neuromuscular & skeletal: Weakness (4%), myalgia (2%)

Respiratory: Pharyngitis (3%)

Incidence less than or equal to placebo: Infection, headache, pain, back pain, abdominal pain, flu syndrome, flatulence, diarrhea, nausea, sinusitis, rhinitis, cough

Overdosage/Toxicology Systemic toxicity low since it is not absorbed.

Pharmacodynamics/Kinetics

Onset of Action: Peak effect: Therapeutic: ~2 weeks

Absorption: Insignificant

Half-Life Elimination: 0.05% was excreted in the urine after 1 month of chronic dosing

Excretion: Urine (0.05%) after 1 month of chronic dosing

Dosing

Adults & Elderly:

Dyslipidemia: Oral:

Monotherapy: 3 tablets twice daily with meals or 6 tablets once daily with a meal; maximum dose: 7 tablets/day

Combination therapy with an HMG-CoA reductase inhibitor: 4-6 tablets daily; maximum dose: 6 tablets/day

Available Dosage Forms Tablet, as hydrochloride [film coated]: 625 mg

Monitoring and Teaching Issues

Physical Assessment: Assess other medications patient may be taking for effectiveness and interactions. Assess results of laboratory tests prior to and on a regular basis during therapy. Assess knowledge/teach patient appropriate use, possible adverse reactions and interventions, and symptoms to report.

Monitoring Laboratory Tests: Serum cholesterol, LDL, and triglyceride levels should be obtained before initiating treatment and periodically thereafter (in accordance with NCEP guidelines).

Patient Education: Take medication exactly as directed; do not alter dosage without consulting prescriber. Other medications should be taken 1 hour before or 2 hours after colesevelam. You may experience constipation (increased exercise, increased exercise, fluids, fruit, fiber, or stool softener may help). Report persistent GI upset, skeletal or muscle pain or weakness, or respiratory difficulties. **Breast-feeding precaution:** Inform prescriber if breast-feeding.

Dietary Considerations: Should be taken with meal(s). Follow dietary guidelines.

Pregnancy Risk Factor: B

Lactation: Excretion in breast milk unknown

Administration

Oral: Administer with meal(s). Make sure patient understands dietary guidelines.

Storage: Store at room temperature. Protect from moisture.

Related Information

Hyperlipidemia Management *on page 1836*

Lipid-Lowering Agents *on page 1738*

♦ **Colestid**® *see* Colestipol *on page 371*

Colestipol (koe LES ti pole)

U.S. Brand Names Colestid®

Synonyms Colestipol Hydrochloride

Generic Available No

Pharmacologic Category Antilipemic Agent, Bile Acid Sequestrant

Use Adjunct in management of primary hypercholesterolemia; regression of arteriolosclerosis; relief of pruritus associated with elevated levels of bile acids; possibly used to decrease plasma half-life of digoxin in toxicity

Mechanism of Action/Effect Increases fecal loss of low density lipoprotein cholesterol

Contraindications Hypersensitivity to bile acid sequestering resins or any component of the formulation; bowel obstruction

Warnings/Precautions Not to be taken simultaneously with many other medicines (decreased absorption). May interfere with fat soluble vitamins (A, D, E, K) and folic acid. Chronic use may be associated with bleeding problems. May produce or exacerbate constipation problems; fecal impaction may occur, hemorrhoids may be worsened.

Drug Interactions

Decreased Effect: Colestipol can reduce the absorption of numerous medications when used concurrently. Give other medications 1 hour before or 4 hours after giving colestipol. Medications which may be affected include HMG-CoA reductase inhibitors, thiazide diuretics, propranolol (and potentially other beta-blockers), corticosteroids, thyroid hormones, digoxin, valproic acid, NSAIDs, loop diuretics, sulfonylureas, troglitazone (and potentially other agents in this class - pioglitazone and rosiglitazone).

(Continued)

Colestipol (Continued)

Warfarin and other oral anticoagulants: Absorption is reduced by cholestyramine and may also be reduced by colestipol. Separate administration times (as detailed above).

Lab Interactions Increased prothrombin time (S); decreased cholesterol (S)

Adverse Reactions

>10%: Gastrointestinal: Constipation

1% to 10%:

Central nervous system: Headache, dizziness, anxiety, vertigo, drowsiness, fatigue

Gastrointestinal: Abdominal pain and distention, belching, flatulence, nausea, vomiting, diarrhea

Overdosage/Toxicology Symptoms of overdose include GI obstruction, nausea, and GI distress. Treatment is supportive.

Pharmacodynamics/Kinetics

Absorption: None

Excretion: Feces

Dosing

Adults & Elderly: Dyslipidemia: Oral: 5-30 g/day in divided doses 2-4 times/day

Available Dosage Forms

Granules, as hydrochloride:

5 g/7.5 g packet (30s, 90s) [unflavored]

5 g/7.5 g (300 g, 500 g) [unflavored]

5 g/7.5 g packet (60s) [contains phenylalanine 18.2 mg/7.5 g; orange flavor]

5 g/7.5 g (450 g) [contains phenylalanine 18.2 mg/7.5 g; orange flavor]

Tablet, as hydrochloride: 1 g

Monitoring and Teaching Issues

Physical Assessment: Assess other medications the patient may be taking for effectiveness and interactions. Monitor knowledge/teach patient appropriate preparation and use, possible adverse reactions, and symptoms to report. Monitor bowel function. Be alert to potential of constipation or hemorrhoid problems.

Patient Education: Take with 3-4 oz of water or fruit juice. Rinse glass with small amount of water to ensure full dose is taken. Take tablets one at a time. Other medications should be taken 1 hour before or 4 hours after colestipol. You may experience constipation (increased exercise, fluids, fruit, fiber, or stool softener may help); or drowsiness or dizziness (use caution when driving or engaging in tasks that require alertness until response to drug is known). Report acute gastric pain, tarry stools, or respiratory difficulty. **Pregnancy/breast-feeding precautions:** Inform prescriber if you are or intend to become pregnant. Breast-feeding is not recommended.

Dietary Considerations: Granules, orange flavor, contain phenylalanine 18.2 mg/7.5 g.

Geriatric Considerations: Pharmacologic treatment should be reserved for those who are unable to obtain a desirable plasma cholesterol level by diet alone and for whom the benefits of treatment are believed to outweigh the potential adverse effects, drug interactions, and cost of treatment.

Pregnancy Risk Factor: C

Lactation: Not recommended

Administration

Oral: Dry powder should be added to at least 90 mL of liquid and stirred until completely mixed. Other drugs should be administered at least 1 hour before or 4 hours after colestipol.

Related Information

Hyperlipidemia Management on page 1836

Lipid-Lowering Agents on page 1738

♦ **Colestipol Hydrochloride** see Colestipol on page 371

♦ **Colistin, Neomycin, Hydrocortisone, and Thonzonium** see Neomycin, Colistin, Hydrocortisone, and Thonzonium on page 1069

Collagenase (KOL la je nase)

U.S. Brand Names Santyl®

Generic Available No

Pharmacologic Category Enzyme, Topical Debridement

Use Promotes debridement of necrotic tissue in dermal ulcers and severe burns

Orphan drug: Injection: Treatment of Peyronie's disease; treatment of Dupytren's disease

Mechanism of Action/Effect Digests collagen in injured tissue. Collagenase will not attack collagen in healthy tissue or newly formed granulation tissue. In addition, it does not act on fat, fibrin, keratin, or muscle.

Contraindications Hypersensitivity to collagenase or any component of the formulation

Warnings/Precautions For external use only. Avoid contact with eyes. Monitor debilitated patients for systemic bacterial infections because debriding enzymes may increase the risk of bacteremia.

Drug Interactions

Decreased Effect: Enzymatic activity is inhibited by detergents, benzalkonium chloride, hexachlorophene, nitrofurazone, tincture of iodine, and heavy metal ions (silver and mercury).

Adverse Reactions Frequency not defined.

Local: Irritation, Pain and burning may occur at site of application

Overdosage/Toxicology Action of enzyme may be stopped by applying Burow's solution.

Dosing

Adults & Elderly: Dermal ulcers, burns: Topical: Apply once daily.

Pediatrics: Refer to adult dosing.

Available Dosage Forms Ointment (Santyl®): 250 units/g (15 g, 30 g)

Monitoring and Teaching Issues

Physical Assessment: For external use only. Clean target area of all interfering agents (eg, detergents, benzalkonium chloride, hexachlorophene, nitrofurazone, tincture of iodine, and heavy metal ions [silver and mercury]). If infection is persistent, apply powdered antibiotic first. Do not introduce into major body cavities. Monitor debilitated patients for systemic bacterial infections. When applied to large areas or for extensive periods of time, monitor for adverse reactions. Teach patient if self-administered (or caregiver) appropriate application and adverse symptoms to report (see Patient Education).

Patient Education: Use exactly as directed; do not overuse. Clean target area of all interfering agents (eg, detergents, benzalkonium chloride, hexachlorophene, nitrofurazone, tincture of iodine, and heavy metal ions [silver and mercury]). Wear gloves to apply a thin film to affected area. If dressing is necessary, use a porous dressing. Avoid contact with eyes. Report increased swelling, redness, rash, itching, signs of infection, worsening of condition, or lack of healing. **Pregnancy/breast-feeding precautions:** Inform prescriber if you are or intend to become pregnant. Consult prescriber if breast-feeding.

Geriatric Considerations: Preventive skin care should be instituted in all older patients at high risk for pressure ulcers. Collagenase is indicated in stage 3 and 4 pressure ulcers.

Pregnancy Risk Factor: C

Lactation: Excretion in breast milk unknown

Administration

Topical: For external use only. Clean target area of all interfering agents listed above. If infection is persistent, apply powdered antibiotic first. Do not introduce into major body cavities. Monitor debilitated patients for systemic bacterial infections.

- **Colocort®** *see* Hydrocortisone *on page 760*
- **Coly-Mycin® S** *see* Neomycin, Colistin, Hydrocortisone, and Thonzonium *on page 1069*
- **Colyte®** *see* Polyethylene Glycol-Electrolyte Solution *on page 1226*
- **CombiPatch®** *see* Estradiol and Norethindrone *on page 557*
- **Combipres® [DSC]** *see* Clonidine and Chlorthalidone *on page 357*
- **Combivent®** *see* Ipratropium and Albuterol *on page 827*
- **Combivir®** *see* Zidovudine and Lamivudine *on page 1587*
- **Combunox™** *see* Oxycodone and Ibuprofen *on page 1140*
- **Commit™ [OTC]** *see* Nicotine *on page 1079*
- **Community-Acquired Pneumonia in Adults** *see page 1807*
- **Compatibility of Drugs** *see page 1723*
- **Compatibility of Drugs in Syringe** *see page 1725*
- **Compazine® [DSC]** *see* Prochlorperazine *on page 1259*
- **Compound F** *see* Hydrocortisone *on page 760*
- **Compound S** *see* Zidovudine *on page 1585*
- **Compound S, Abacavir, and Lamivudine** *see* Abacavir, Lamivudine, and Zidovudine *on page 34*
- **Compoz® Nighttime Sleep Aid [OTC]** *see* DiphenhydrAMINE *on page 463*
- **Compro™** *see* Prochlorperazine *on page 1259*
- **Comtan®** *see* Entacapone *on page 523*
- **Comtrex® Sore Throat Maximum Strength [OTC]** *see* Acetaminophen *on page 38*
- **Concerta®** *see* Methylphenidate *on page 983*
- **Congestac® [OTC]** *see* Guaifenesin and Pseudoephedrine *on page 733*
- **Constulose®** *see* Lactulose *on page 860*
- **Contac® Cold [OTC]** *see* Pseudoephedrine *on page 1282*
- **Controlled Substances** *see page 1727*
- **Copaxone®** *see* Glatiramer Acetate *on page 712*
- **Copegus®** *see* Ribavirin *on page 1318*
- **Copolymer-1** *see* Glatiramer Acetate *on page 712*
- **Cordarone®** *see* Amiodarone *on page 93*
- **Cordron-HC** *see* Pseudoephedrine, Hydrocodone, and Chlorpheniramine *on page 1283*
- **Coreg®** *see* Carvedilol *on page 262*
- **Corgard®** *see* Nadolol *on page 1045*
- **CortaGel® Maximum Strength [OTC] [DSC]** *see* Hydrocortisone *on page 760*
- **Cortaid® Intensive Therapy [OTC]** *see* Hydrocortisone *on page 760*
- **Cortaid® Maximum Strength [OTC]** *see* Hydrocortisone *on page 760*
- **Cortaid® Sensitive Skin [OTC]** *see* Hydrocortisone *on page 760*
- **Cortef®** *see* Hydrocortisone *on page 760*
- **Corticool® [OTC]** *see* Hydrocortisone *on page 760*
- **Corticosteroids** *see page 1731*
- **Corticotropin** *see page 1625*
- **Cortifoam®** *see* Hydrocortisone *on page 760*
- **Cortisol** *see* Hydrocortisone *on page 760*
- **Cortisporin® Cream** *see* Neomycin, Polymyxin B, and Hydrocortisone *on page 1069*
- **Cortisporin® Ointment** *see* Bacitracin, Neomycin, Polymyxin B, and Hydrocortisone *on page 172*
- **Cortisporin® Ophthalmic** *see* Neomycin, Polymyxin B, and Hydrocortisone *on page 1069*
- **Cortisporin® Otic** *see* Neomycin, Polymyxin B, and Hydrocortisone *on page 1069*
- **Cortisporin®-TC** *see* Neomycin, Colistin, Hydrocortisone, and Thonzonium *on page 1069*
- **Cortizone®-10 Maximum Strength [OTC]** *see* Hydrocortisone *on page 760*
- **Cortizone®-10 Plus Maximum Strength [OTC]** *see* Hydrocortisone *on page 760*
- **Cortizone® 10 Quick Shot [OTC]** *see* Hydrocortisone *on page 760*
- **Cortrosyn® Injection** *see page 1625*
- **Corvert®** *see* Ibutilide *on page 780*

- **Cosmegen®** *see* Dactinomycin *on page 397*
- **Cosyntropin** *see page 1625*
- **Co-Trimoxazole** *see* Sulfamethoxazole and Trimethoprim *on page 1407*
- **Coughtuss** *see* Phenylephrine, Hydrocodone, and Chlorpheniramine *on page 1202*
- **Coumadin®** *see* Warfarin *on page 1573*
- **Covera-HS®** *see* Verapamil *on page 1560*
- **Co-Vidarabine** *see* Pentostatin *on page 1184*
- **Coviracil** *see* Emtricitabine *on page 514*
- **Cozaar®** *see* Losartan *on page 922*
- **CP358774** *see* Erlotinib *on page 540*
- **CPM** *see* Cyclophosphamide *on page 380*
- **CPT-11** *see* Irinotecan *on page 829*
- **CPZ** *see* ChlorproMAZINE *on page 312*
- **Crantex HC** *see* Hydrocodone, Phenylephrine, and Guaifenesin *on page 760*
- **Creatinine Clearance Estimating Methods in Patients With Stable Renal Function** *see page 1686*
- **Creon®** *see* Pancrelipase *on page 1151*
- **Crestor®** *see* Rosuvastatin *on page 1349*
- **Crinone®** *see* Progesterone *on page 1262*
- **Crixivan®** *see* Indinavir *on page 799*
- **Crolom®** *see* Cromolyn *on page 374*
- **Cromoglycic Acid** *see* Cromolyn *on page 374*

Cromolyn (KROE moe lin)

U.S. Brand Names Crolom®; Gastrocrom®; Intal®; NasalCrom® [OTC]; Opticrom®
Synonyms Cromoglycic Acid; Cromolyn Sodium; Disodium Cromoglycate; DSCG
Generic Available Yes: Excludes aerosol, oral solution
Pharmacologic Category Mast Cell Stabilizer
Medication Safety Issues
Sound-alike/look-alike issues:
Intal® may be confused with Endal®
NasalCrom® may be confused with Nasacort®, Nasalide®
Use
Inhalation: May be used as an adjunct in the prophylaxis of allergic disorders, including asthma; prevention of exercise-induced bronchospasm
Nasal: Prevention and treatment of seasonal and perennial allergic rhinitis
Oral: Systemic mastocytosis
Ophthalmic: Treatment of vernal keratoconjunctivitis, vernal conjunctivitis, and vernal keratitis
Unlabeled/Investigational Use Oral: Food allergy, treatment of inflammatory bowel disease
Mechanism of Action/Effect Prevents the mast cell release of histamine, leukotrienes and slow-reacting substance of anaphylaxis
Contraindications Hypersensitivity to cromolyn or any component of the formulation; acute asthma attacks
Warnings/Precautions Severe anaphylactic reactions may occur rarely; cromolyn is a prophylactic drug with no benefit for acute situations; caution should be used when withdrawing the drug or tapering the dose as symptoms may reoccur; use with caution in patients with a history of cardiac arrhythmias. Transient burning or stinging may occur with ophthalmic use. Dosage of oral product should be decreased with hepatic or renal dysfunction.
Adverse Reactions
Inhalation: >10%: Gastrointestinal: Unpleasant taste in mouth
Nasal:
>10%: Respiratory: Increase in sneezing, burning, stinging, or irritation inside of nose
1% to 10%:
Central nervous system: Headache
Gastrointestinal: Unpleasant taste
Respiratory: Hoarseness, cough, postnasal drip
<1% (Limited to important or life-threatening): Anaphylactic reactions, epistaxis
Ophthalmic: Frequency not defined:
Ocular: Conjunctival injection, dryness around the eye, edema, eye irritation, immediate hypersensitivity reactions, itchy eyes, puffy eyes, styes, rash, watery eyes
Respiratory: Dyspnea
Systemic: Frequency not defined:
Cardiovascular: Angioedema, chest pain, edema, flushing, palpitation, premature ventricular contractions, tachycardia
Central nervous system: Anxiety, behavior changes, convulsions, depression, dizziness, fatigue, hallucinations, headache, irritability, insomnia, lethargy, migraine, nervousness, hypoesthesia, postprandial lightheadedness, psychosis
Dermatologic: Erythema, photosensitivity, pruritus, purpura, rash, urticaria
Gastrointestinal: Abdominal pain, constipation, diarrhea, dyspepsia, dysphagia, esophagospasm, flatulence, glossitis, nausea, stomatitis, unpleasant taste, vomiting
Genitourinary: Dysuria, urinary frequency
Hematologic: Neutropenia, pancytopenia, polycythemia
Hepatic: Liver function test abnormal
Local: Burning
Neuromuscular & skeletal: Arthralgia, leg stiffness, leg weakness, myalgia, paresthesia
Otic: Tinnitus
Respiratory: Dyspnea, pharyngitis
Miscellaneous: Lupus erythematosus
Overdosage/Toxicology Symptoms of overdose include bronchospasm, laryngeal edema, and dysuria. Treat symptomatically.

Pharmacodynamics/Kinetics

Onset of Action: Onset: Response to treatment:
Nasal spray: May occur at 1-2 weeks
Ophthalmic: May be seen within a few days; treatment for up to 6 weeks is often required
Oral: May occur within 2-6 weeks

Absorption:
Inhalation: ~8% reaches lungs upon inhalation; well absorbed
Oral: <1% of dose absorbed

Time to Peak: Serum: Inhalation: ~15 minutes

Half-Life Elimination: 80-90 minutes

Excretion: Urine and feces (equal amounts as unchanged drug); exhaled gases (small amounts)

Dosing

Adults & Elderly:

Allergic rhinitis (treatment and prophylaxis): Nasal: Instill 1 spray in each nostril 3-4 times/day

Asthma:
Note: Not effective for immediate relief of symptoms in acute asthmatic attacks; must be used at regular intervals for 2-4 weeks to be effective.
Inhalation: Metered spray: 2 inhalations 4 times/day
Nebulization solution: Inhalation: Single dose of 20 mg

Prophylaxis of bronchospasm (allergen- or exercise-induced):
Note: Administer 10-15 minutes prior to exercise or allergen exposure but no longer than 1 hour before:
Nebulization solution: Single dose of 20 mg
Metered spray: Single dose of 2 inhalations

Conjunctivitis and keratitis: Ophthalmic: 1-2 drops in each eye 4-6 times/day

Mastocytosis: Oral: 200 mg 4 times/day; given $^1/_2$ hour prior to meals and at bedtime. If control of symptoms is not seen within 2-3 weeks, dose may be increased to a maximum 40 mg/kg/day

Food allergy and inflammatory bowel disease (unlabeled use): Oral: Initial dose: 200 mg 4 times/day; may double the dose if effect is not satisfactory within 2-3 weeks; up to 400 mg 4 times/day

Pediatrics:

Allergic rhinitis (treatment and prophylaxis): Nasal: Children ≥2 years: Refer to adult dosing.

Asthma: Inhalation:
Note: For chronic control of asthma, taper frequency to the lowest effective dose (ie, 4 times/day to 3 times/day to twice daily):
Nebulization solution: Children >2 years: Initial: 20 mg 4 times/day; usual dose: 20 mg 3-4 times/day
Metered spray:
Children 5-12 years: Initial: 2 inhalations 4 times/day; usual dose: 1-2 inhalations 3-4 times/day
Children ≥12 years: Refer to adult dosing.

Prevention of allergen- or exercise-induced bronchospasm:
Note: Administer 10-15 minutes prior to exercise or allergen exposure but no longer than 1 hour before:
Nebulization solution: Children >2 years: Refer to adult dosing.
Metered spray: Children >5 years: Single dose of 2 inhalations

Systemic mastocytosis: Oral:
Children 2-12 years: 100 mg 4 times/day; not to exceed 40 mg/kg/day; given $^1/_2$ hour prior to meals and at bedtime
Children >12 years: Refer to adult dosing.

Food allergy and inflammatory bowel disease (unlabeled use): Oral:
Children <2 years: Not recommended
Children 2-12 years: Initial dose: 100 mg 4 times/day; may double the dose if effect is not satisfactory within 2-3 weeks; not to exceed 40 mg/kg/day
Children >12 years: Refer to adult dosing.
Note: Once desired effect is achieved, dose may be tapered to lowest effective dose

Renal Impairment: Specific guidelines not available; consider lower dose of oral product.

Hepatic Impairment: Specific guidelines not available; consider lower dose of oral product.

Available Dosage Forms

Aerosol, for oral inhalation, as sodium (Intal®): 800 mcg/inhalation (8.1 g) [112 metered inhalations; 56 doses], (14.2 g) [200 metered inhalations; 100 doses]

Solution for nebulization, as sodium (Intal®): 20 mg/2 mL (60s, 120s)

Solution, intranasal spray, as sodium (NasalCrom®): 40 mg/mL (13 mL, 26 mL) [5.2 mg/inhalation; contains benzalkonium chloride]

Solution, ophthalmic, as sodium (Crolom®, Opticrom®): 4% (10 mL) [contains benzalkonium chloride]

Solution, oral, as sodium (Gastrocrom®): 100 mg/5 mL (96s)

Monitoring and Teaching Issues

Physical Assessment: This is prophylactic therapy, not to be used for acute situations. Assess results of laboratory tests (long-term use) and adverse reactions. Assess knowledge/teach patient appropriate use, interventions to reduce side effects, and adverse symptoms to report.

Monitoring Laboratory Tests: Periodic pulmonary function

Patient Education: Oral: Use as directed; do not increase dosage or discontinue abruptly without consulting prescriber. Take at least 30 minutes before meals. You may experience dizziness or nervousness (use caution when driving or engaging in tasks requiring alertness until response to drug is known); diarrhea (boiled milk, yogurt, or buttermilk may help); or headache or muscle pain (mild analgesic may offer relief). Report persistent insomnia; skin rash or irritation; abdominal pain or difficulty swallowing; unusual cough, (Continued)

Cromolyn (Continued)

bronchospasm, or respiratory difficulty; decreased urination; or if condition worsens or fails to improve. **Breast-feeding precaution:** Consult prescriber if breast-feeding.

Nebulizer: Store nebulizer solution away from light. Prepare nebulizer according to package instructions. Clear as much mucus as possible before use. Rinse mouth following each use to prevent opportunistic infection and reduce unpleasant aftertaste. Report if symptoms worsen or condition fails to improve.

Nasal: Instill 1 spray into each nostril 3-4 times a day. You may experience unpleasant taste (rinsing mouth and frequent oral care may help); or headache (mild analgesic may help). Report increased sneezing, burning, stinging, or irritation inside of nose; sore throat, hoarseness, nosebleed; anaphylactic reaction (skin rash, fever, chills, backache, respiratory difficulty, chest pain); or worsening of condition or lack of improvement.

Ophthalmic: For ophthalmic use only. Wash hands before using. Tilt head back and look upward. Put drops of suspension inside lower eyelid. Close eye and roll eyeball in all directions. Do not blink for $1/2$ minute. Apply gentle pressure to inner corner of eye for 30 seconds. Do not let tip of applicator touch eye; do not contaminate tip of applicator (may cause eye infection, eye damage, or vision loss). Do not share medication with anyone else. Temporary stinging or blurred vision may occur. Inform prescriber if condition worsens or fails to improve or if you experience eye pain, redness, burning, watering, dryness, double vision, puffiness around eye, vision changes, or other adverse eye response; or worsening of condition or lack of improvement. Do not wear contact lenses during treatment.

Dietary Considerations: Oral: Should be taken at least 30 minutes before meals.

Geriatric Considerations: Assess the patient's ability to empty capsules via the Spinhaler®. Older persons often have difficulty with inhaled and ophthalmic dosage forms.

Pregnancy Risk Factor: B

Pregnancy Issues: Available evidence suggests safe use during pregnancy.

Lactation: Excretion in breast milk unknown/use caution

Breast-Feeding Issues: No data available on whether cromolyn enters into breast milk or clinical effects on the infant.

Administration

Oral: Oral solution: Open ampul and squeeze contents into glass of water; stir well. Administer at least 30 minutes before meals and at bedtime.

Inhalation: Oral inhalation: Shake canister gently before use; do not immerse canister in water.

Other: Nasal inhalation: Clear nasal passages by blowing nose prior to use.

Compatibility: Nebulizer solution is **compatible** with metaproterenol sulfate, isoproterenol hydrochloride, 0.25% isoetharine hydrochloride, epinephrine hydrochloride, terbutaline sulfate, and 20% acetylcysteine solution for at least 1 hour after their admixture.

Storage: Store at room temperature of 15°C to 30°C (59°F to 86°F); protect from light. Do not use oral solution if solution becomes discolored or forms a precipitate.

Related Information
Inhalant Agents *on page 1734*

♦ **Cromolyn Sodium** *see* Cromolyn *on page 374*

Crotamiton (kroe TAM i tonn)

U.S. Brand Names Eurax®

Generic Available No

Pharmacologic Category Scabicidal Agent

Medication Safety Issues
Sound-alike/look-alike issues:
Eurax® may be confused with Efudex®, Eulexin®, Evoxac™, Serax®, Urex®

Use Treatment of scabies (*Sarcoptes scabiei*) and symptomatic treatment of pruritus

Mechanism of Action/Effect Mechanism of action unknown

Contraindications Hypersensitivity to crotamiton or any component of the formulation; patients who manifest a primary irritation response to topical medications

Warnings/Precautions Avoid contact with face, eyes, mucous membranes, and urethral meatus. Do not apply to acutely inflamed or raw skin. For external use only.

Adverse Reactions Frequency not defined. Topical:
Dermatologic: Pruritus, contact dermatitis, rash
Local: Local irritation
Miscellaneous: Allergic sensitivity reactions, warm sensation

Overdosage/Toxicology Symptoms of ingestion include burning sensation in mouth, irritation of the buccal, esophageal and gastric mucosa, nausea, vomiting, and abdominal pain. There is no specific antidote. General measures to eliminate the drug and reduce its absorption, combined with symptomatic treatment, are recommended.

Dosing
Adults & Elderly:
Scabies: Topical: Wash thoroughly and scrub away loose scales, then towel dry; apply a thin layer and massage drug onto skin of the entire body from the neck to the toes (with special attention to skin folds, creases, and interdigital spaces). Repeat application in 24 hours. Take a cleansing bath 48 hours after the final application. Treatment may be repeated after 7-10 days if live mites are still present.

Pruritus: Topical: Massage into affected areas until medication is completely absorbed; repeat as necessary

Pediatrics: Refer to adult dosing.

Available Dosage Forms
Cream: 10% (60 g)
Lotion: 10% (60 mL, 480 mL)

Monitoring and Teaching Issues

Physical Assessment: Assess knowledge/teach patient appropriate application and use and adverse symptoms to report.

Patient Education: For topical use only. Apply lotion to whole body from the chin down being sure to cover all skin folds and creases. Apply a second application 24 hours later. Avoid eyes. Take a bath 48 hours after application. All contaminated clothing and bed linen should be washed to avoid reinfestation. If cure is not achieved after 2 doses, use alternative therapy. **Pregnancy/breast-feeding precautions:** Inform prescriber if you are or intend to become pregnant. Consult prescriber if breast-feeding.

Pregnancy Risk Factor: C

Lactation: Excretion in breast milk unknown

Administration

Topical: For external use only. Shake lotion well before using. Avoid contact with face, eyes, mucous membranes, and urethral meatus.

Storage: Store at room temperature.

- **Cruex® Cream [OTC]** see Clotrimazole on page 360
- **Crystalline Penicillin** see Penicillin G (Parenteral/Aqueous) on page 1174
- **CsA** see CycloSPORINE on page 383
- **CTX** see Cyclophosphamide on page 380
- **Cubicin™** see Daptomycin on page 404
- **Cutivate®** see Fluticasone on page 660
- **CyA** see CycloSPORINE on page 383

Cyanocobalamin (sye an oh koe BAL a min)

U.S. Brand Names Nascobal®; Twelve Resin-K

Synonyms Vitamin B_{12}

Generic Available Yes

Pharmacologic Category Vitamin, Water Soluble

Use Treatment of pernicious anemia; vitamin B_{12} deficiency; increased B_{12} requirements due to pregnancy, thyrotoxicosis, hemorrhage, malignancy, liver or kidney disease

Mechanism of Action/Effect Coenzyme for various metabolic functions, including fat and carbohydrate metabolism and protein synthesis, used in cell replication and hematopoiesis

Contraindications Hypersensitivity to cyanocobalamin or any component of the formulation; cobalt; hereditary optic nerve atrophy (Leber's disease)

Warnings/Precautions I.M. route used to treat pernicious anemia; vitamin B_{12} deficiency for >3 months results in irreversible degenerative CNS lesions; treatment of vitamin B_{12} megaloblastic anemia may result in severe hypokalemia, sometimes fatal, due to intracellular potassium shift upon anemia resolution. B_{12} deficiency masks signs of polycythemia vera; vegetarian diets may result in B_{12} deficiency; pernicious anemia occurs more often in gastric carcinoma than in general population. Patients with Leber's disease may suffer rapid optic atrophy when treated with vitamin B_{12}; an intradermal test dose of parenteral B_{12} is recommended prior to administration of intranasal product in patients suspected of cyanocobalamin sensitivity; do not use folic acid as substitute for vitamin B_{12} in preventing anemia, as progression of spinal cord degeneration may occur; some parenteral products contain aluminum: use caution in neonates and patients with renal impairment.

Drug Interactions

Decreased Effect: Ethanol and metformin may decrease B_{12} absorption. Chloramphenicol, cholestyramine, cimetidine, colchicine, neomycin, PAS, and potassium may reduce absorption and/or effect of cyanocobalamin.

Nutritional/Ethanol Interactions Ethanol: Heavy consumption may impair vitamin B_{12} absorption.

Lab Interactions Methotrexate, pyrimethamine, and most antibiotics invalidate folic acid and vitamin B_{12} diagnostic microbiological blood assays

Adverse Reactions

>10%:
  Cardiovascular: Peripheral vascular disease
  Central nervous system: Headache (2% to 11%)

1% to 10%:
  Central nervous system: Anxiety, dizziness, pain, nervousness, hypoesthesia
  Dermatologic: Itching
  Gastrointestinal: Sore throat, nausea and vomiting, dyspepsia, diarrhea
  Neuromuscular & skeletal: Weakness (1% to 4%), back pain, arthritis, myalgia, paresthesia, abnormal gait, incoordination
  Respiratory: Dyspnea, rhinitis
  Miscellaneous: Infection

Frequency not defined: Peripheral vascular thrombosis, urticaria, anaphylaxis, CHF, pulmonary edema, polycythemia vera, transient exanthema

Pharmacodynamics/Kinetics

Absorption: Oral: Variable from the terminal ileum; requires the presence of calcium and gastric "intrinsic factor" to transfer the compound across the intestinal mucosa

Bioavailability: Intranasal:
  Gel: 8.9% (relative to I.M.)
  Solution: 6.1% (relative to I.M.)

Protein Binding: To transcobalamin II

Metabolism: Converted in tissues to active coenzymes, methylcobalamin and deoxyadenosylcobalamin

Dosing

Adults & Elderly:
  Recommended daily allowance (RDA): 2.4 mcg/day
    Pregnancy: 2.6 mcg/day
    Lactation: 2.8 mcg/day

(Continued)

Cyanocobalamin (Continued)

Vitamin B$_{12}$ deficiency:
Intranasal: 500 mcg in one nostril once weekly
Oral: 250 mcg/day
I.M., deep SubQ: Initial: 30 mcg/day for 5-10 days; maintenance: 100-200 mcg/month
Pernicious anemia: I.M., deep SubQ (administer concomitantly with folic acid if needed, 1 mg/day for 1 month): 100 mcg/day for 6-7 days; if improvement, administer same dose on alternate days for 7 doses, then every 3-4 days for 2-3 weeks; once hematologic values have returned to normal, maintenance dosage: 100 mcg/month. **Note:** Alternative dosing of 1000 mcg/day for 5 days (followed by 500-1000 mcg/month) has been used.
Hematologic remission (without evidence of nervous system involvement):
Intranasal gel: 500 mcg in one nostril once weekly
Oral: 1000-2000 mcg/day
I.M., SubQ: 100-1000 mcg/month
Schilling test: I.M.: 1000 mcg

Pediatrics:
Recommended daily allowance (RDA): 0.9-2.4 mcg/day
Vitamin B$_{12}$ deficiency:
Intranasal: 500 mcg in one nostril once weekly
Oral: 250 mcg/day
I.M., deep SubQ: Dosage in children not well established: 0.2 mcg/kg for 2 days, followed by 1000 mcg/day for 2-7 days, followed by 100 mcg/week for one month; for malabsorptive causes of B$_{12}$ deficiency, monthly maintenance doses of 100 mcg have been recommended **or** as an alternative 100 mcg/day for 10-15 days, then once or twice weekly for several months
Pernicious anemia: I.M., deep SubQ (administer concomitantly with folic acid if needed, 1 mg/day for 1 month): 30-50 mcg/day for 2 or more weeks (to a total dose of 1000-5000 mcg), then follow with 100 mcg/month as maintenance dosage

Available Dosage Forms
Gel, intranasal (Nascobal®): 500 mcg/0.1 mL (2.3 mL) [contains benzalkonium chloride; delivers 8 doses]
Injection, solution: 1000 mcg/mL (1 mL, 10 mL, 30 mL) [may contain benzyl alcohol and/or aluminum]
Lozenge [OTC]: 100 mcg, 250 mcg, 500 mcg
Solution, intranasal spray (Nascobal®): 500 mcg/0.1 mL actuation (2.3 mL) [contains benzalkonium chloride; delivers 8 doses]
Tablet [OTC]: 50 mcg, 100 mcg, 250 mcg, 500 mcg, 1000 mcg, 5000 mcg
Twelve Resin-K: 1000 mcg [may be used as oral, sublingual, or buccal]
Tablet, extended release [OTC]: 1500 mcg
Tablet, sublingual [OTC]: 2500 mcg

Monitoring and Teaching Issues
Physical Assessment: Assess effectiveness and interactions of other medications patient may be taking. Assess results of laboratory tests at beginning of therapy and periodically with long-term therapy. Teach patient proper use (injection technique and needle disposal), appropriate nutritional counseling, and adverse symptoms to report.
Monitoring Laboratory Tests: Erythrocyte and reticulocyte count, hemoglobin, hematocrit; monitor potassium concentrations during early therapy.
Patient Education: Use exactly as directed. Pernicious anemia may require monthly injections for life. Report skin rash; swelling, pain, or redness of extremities; or acute persistent diarrhea. **Pregnancy precaution:** Inform prescriber if you are pregnant.
Dietary Considerations: Vegetarian diets may result in vitamin B$_{12}$ deficiency; use intranasal product at least 1 hour before or after ingestion of hot foods or liquids due to increased nasal secretions
Geriatric Considerations: There exists evidence that people, particularly elderly whose serum cobalamin concentrations <500 pg/mL, should receive replacement parenteral therapy.
Pregnancy Risk Factor: A/C (dose exceeding RDA recommendation); C (intranasal)
Lactation: Enters breast milk/compatible

Administration
Oral: Not recommended due to variable absorption; however, oral therapy of 1000-2000 mcg/day has been effective for anemia if I.M./SubQ routes refused or not tolerated.
I.M.: I.M. or deep SubQ are preferred routes of administration.
I.V.: Not recommended
Other: Intranasal: Nasal spray: Prior to initial dose, activate (prime) spray nozzle by pumping unit quickly and firmly until first appearance of spray, then prime twice more. The unit must be reprimed once immediately before each use.
Compatibility: Stable in dextran 6% in dextrose, dextran 6% in NS, D$_5$LR, D$_5$¼NS, D$_5$½NS, D$_5$NS, D$_5$W, D$_{10}$W, D$_{10}$NS, LR, ½NS, NS
Compatibility when admixed: Incompatible with chlorpromazine, phytonadione, prochlorperazine edisylate, warfarin
Storage: Injection: Clear pink to red solutions are stable at room temperature. Protect from light.

♦ **Cyclessa®** *see Ethinyl Estradiol and Desogestrel on page 578*

Cyclobenzaprine (sye kloe BEN za preen)
U.S. Brand Names Flexeril®
Synonyms Cyclobenzaprine Hydrochloride
Generic Available Yes
Pharmacologic Category Skeletal Muscle Relaxant
Medication Safety Issues
Sound-alike/look-alike issues:
Cyclobenzaprine may be confused with cycloSERINE, cyproheptadine

Flexeril® may be confused with Floxin®

Use Treatment of muscle spasm associated with acute painful musculoskeletal conditions

Mechanism of Action/Effect Centrally-acting skeletal muscle relaxant pharmacologically related to tricyclic antidepressants; reduces tonic somatic motor activity influencing both alpha and gamma motor neurons

Contraindications Hypersensitivity to cyclobenzaprine or any component of the formulation; do not use concomitantly or within 14 days of MAO inhibitors; hyperthyroidism; congestive heart failure; arrhythmias; acute recovery phase of MI

Warnings/Precautions Cyclobenzaprine shares the toxic potentials of the tricyclic antidepressants and the usual precautions of tricyclic antidepressant therapy should be observed; use with caution in patients with urinary hesitancy, angle-closure glaucoma, hepatic impairment, or in the elderly. Do not use concomitantly or within 14 days after MAO inhibitors; combination may cause hypertensive crisis, severe convulsions. Safety and efficacy have not been established in patients <15 years of age.

Drug Interactions

Cytochrome P450 Effect: Substrate of CYP1A2 (major), 2D6 (minor), 3A4 (minor)

Decreased Effect: Cyclobenzaprine may decrease effect of guanethidine; effect seen with tricyclic antidepressants and guanethidine

Increased Effect/Toxicity: CYP1A2 inhibitors may increase the levels/effects of cyclobenzaprine; example inhibitors include amiodarone, ciprofloxacin, fluvoxamine, ketoconazole, norfloxacin, ofloxacin, and rofecoxib. Because of cyclobenzaprine's similarities to the tricyclic antidepressants, there may be additive toxicities and side effects similar to tricyclic antidepressants. Cyclobenzaprine's toxicity may also be additive with other agents with anticholinergic properties. Cyclobenzaprine may enhance effects of CNS depressants. Do not use concomitantly or within 14 days of MAO inhibitors. Tramadol may increase risk of seizure; effect seen with tricyclic antidepressants and tramadol.

Nutritional/Ethanol Interactions

Ethanol: Avoid ethanol (may increase CNS depression).

Herb/Nutraceutical: Avoid valerian, kava kava, gotu kola (may increase CNS depression).

Adverse Reactions

>10%:

Central nervous system: Drowsiness (29% to 39%), dizziness (1% to 11%)

Gastrointestinal: Xerostomia (21% to 32%)

1% to 10%:

Central nervous system: Fatigue (1% to 6%), confusion (1% to 3%), headache (1% to 3%), irritability (1% to 3%), mental acuity decreased (1% to 3%), nervousness (1% to 3%)

Gastrointestinal: Abdominal pain (1% to 3%), constipation (1% to 3%), diarrhea (1% to 3%), dyspepsia (1% to 3%), nausea (1% to 3%)

Neuromuscular & skeletal: Muscle weakness (1% to 3%)

Ocular: Blurred vision (1% to 3%)

Respiratory: Pharyngitis (1% to 3%)

Overdosage/Toxicology Symptoms of overdose include troubled breathing, drowsiness, syncope, seizures, tachycardia, hallucinations, and vomiting. Following initiation of essential overdose management, treatment is supportive and symptomatic.

Pharmacodynamics/Kinetics

Onset of Action: ~1 hour

Duration of Action: 12-24 hours

Absorption: Complete

Bioavailability: 33% to 55%

Time to Peak: Serum: 3-8 hours

Half-Life Elimination: 18 hours (range: 8-37 hours)

Metabolism: Hepatic via CYP3A4, 1A2, and 2D6; may undergo enterohepatic recirculation

Excretion: Urine (as inactive metabolites); feces (as unchanged drug)

Dosing

Adults: Muscle spasm (including spasms associated with acute temporomandibular joint pain): Oral: Initial: 5 mg 3 times/day; may increase to 10 mg 3 times/day if needed. Do not use longer than 2-3 weeks.

Elderly: Plasma concentrations and adverse effects are increased in older patients. See Geriatric Considerations.

Hepatic Impairment:

Mild: 5 mg 3 times/day; use with caution and titrate slowly.

Moderate to severe: Use not recommended.

Available Dosage Forms

Tablet, as hydrochloride: 10 mg

Flexeril®: 5 mg, 10 mg [film coated]

Monitoring and Teaching Issues

Physical Assessment: Assess effectiveness and interactions of other medications patient may be taking. Monitor effectiveness of therapy (according to rationale for therapy) and adverse reactions at beginning and periodically during therapy. Assess knowledge/teach patient appropriate use, interventions to reduce side effects (postural hypotension precautions), and adverse symptoms to report.

Patient Education: Take exactly as directed. Do not increase dose or discontinue without consulting prescriber. Do not use alcohol, prescriptive or OTC antidepressants, sedatives, or pain medications without consulting prescriber. You may experience drowsiness, dizziness, lightheadedness (avoid driving or engaging in tasks that require alertness until response to drug is known); or urinary retention (void before taking medication). Report excessive drowsiness or mental agitation, chest pain, skin rash, swelling of mouth/face, difficulty speaking, ringing in ears, or blurred vision. **Breast-feeding precaution:** Breast-feeding is not recommended.

Geriatric Considerations: High doses in the elderly caused drowsiness and dizziness; therefore, use the lowest dose possible. Because cyclobenzaprine causes anticholinergic effects, it may not be the skeletal muscle relaxant of choice in the elderly.

(Continued)

Cyclobenzaprine *(Continued)*

Pregnancy Risk Factor: B

Lactation: Excretion in breast milk unknown/not recommended

Administration

    Storage: Store at room temperature 25°C (77°F); excursions permitted to 15°C to 30°C (59°F to 86°F).

♦ **Cyclobenzaprine Hydrochloride** *see Cyclobenzaprine on page 378*

♦ **Cyclogyl®** *see page 1625*

♦ **Cyclomydril® Ophthalmic** *see page 1625*

♦ **Cyclopentolate** *see page 1625*

♦ **Cyclopentolate and Phenylephrine** *see page 1625*

Cyclophosphamide *(sye kloe FOS fa mide)*

U.S. Brand Names Cytoxan®

Synonyms CPM; CTX; CYT; NSC-26271

Generic Available Yes: Tablet

Pharmacologic Category Antineoplastic Agent, Alkylating Agent

Medication Safety Issues

    Sound-alike/look-alike issues:

        Cyclophosphamide may be confused with cycloSPORINE

        Cytoxan® may be confused with cefoxitin, Centoxin®, Ciloxan®, cytarabine, CytoGam®, Cytosar®, Cytosar-U®, Cytotec®

Use

    Oncologic: Treatment of Hodgkin's and non-Hodgkin's lymphoma, Burkitt's lymphoma, chronic lymphocytic leukemia (CLL), chronic myelocytic leukemia (CML), acute myelocytic leukemia (AML), acute lymphocytic leukemia (ALL), mycosis fungoides, multiple myeloma, neuroblastoma, retinoblastoma, rhabdomyosarcoma, Ewing's sarcoma; breast, testicular, endometrial, ovarian, and lung cancers, and in conditioning regimens for bone marrow transplantation

    Nononcologic: Prophylaxis of rejection for kidney, heart, liver, and bone marrow transplants, severe rheumatoid disorders, nephrotic syndrome, Wegener's granulomatosis, idiopathic pulmonary hemosideroses, myasthenia gravis, multiple sclerosis, systemic lupus erythematosus, lupus nephritis, autoimmune hemolytic anemia, idiopathic thrombocytic purpura (ITP), macroglobulinemia, and antibody-induced pure red cell aplasia

Mechanism of Action/Effect Interferes with the normal function of DNA by alkylation and cross-linking the strands of DNA, and by possible protein modification; cyclophosphamide also possesses potent immunosuppressive activity; note that cyclophosphamide must be metabolized to its active form in the liver

Contraindications Hypersensitivity to cyclophosphamide or any component of the formulation; pregnancy

Warnings/Precautions The U.S. Food and Drug Administration (FDA) currently recommends that procedures for proper handling and disposal of antineoplastic agents be considered. Dosage adjustment needed for renal or hepatic failure. Use with caution in patients with bone marrow depression. If cyclophosphamide contacts the skin, wash and flush thoroughly with water.

Drug Interactions

    Cytochrome P450 Effect: Substrate of CYP2A6 (minor), 2B6 (major), 2C8/9 (minor), 2C19 (minor), 3A4 (major); **Inhibits** CYP3A4 (weak); **Induces** CYP2B6 (weak), 2C8/9 (weak)

    Decreased Effect: Cyclophosphamide may decrease digoxin serum levels. CYP2B6 inhibitors may decrease the levels/effects of acrolein (the active metabolite of cyclophosphamide); example inhibitors include desipramine, paroxetine, and sertraline. CYP3A4 inhibitors may decrease the levels/effects of acrolein (the active metabolite of cyclophosphamide); example inhibitors include azole antifungals, ciprofloxacin, clarithromycin, diclofenac, doxycycline, erythromycin, imatinib, isoniazid, nefazodone, nicardipine, propofol, protease inhibitors, quinidine, and verapamil.

    Increased Effect/Toxicity: Allopurinol may cause an increase in bone marrow depression and may result in significant elevations of cyclophosphamide cytotoxic metabolites.

    Anesthetic agents: Cyclophosphamide reduces serum pseudocholinesterase concentrations and may prolong the neuromuscular blocking activity of succinylcholine. Use with caution with halothane, nitrous oxide, and succinylcholine.

    Chloramphenicol causes prolonged cyclophosphamide half-life and increased toxicity.

    CYP2B6 inducers: CYP2B6 inducers may increase the levels/effects of acrolein (the active metabolite of cyclophosphamide). Example inducers include carbamazepine, nevirapine, phenobarbital, phenytoin, and rifampin.

    CYP3A4 inducers: CYP3A4 inducers may increase the levels/effects of acrolein (the active metabolite of cyclophosphamide). Example inducers include aminoglutethimide, carbamazepine, nafcillin, nevirapine, phenobarbital, phenytoin, and rifamycins.

    Doxorubicin: Cyclophosphamide may enhance cardiac toxicity of anthracyclines.

    Tetrahydrocannabinol results in enhanced immunosuppression in animal studies.

    Thiazide diuretics: Leukopenia may be prolonged.

Nutritional/Ethanol Interactions Herb/Nutraceutical: Avoid black cohosh, dong quai in estrogen-dependent tumors.

Lab Interactions Increased uric acid in serum and urine; false-positive Pap test; suppression of some skin tests

Adverse Reactions

    >10%:

        Dermatologic: Alopecia (40% to 60%) but hair will usually regrow although it may be a different color and/or texture. Hair loss usually begins 3-6 weeks after the start of therapy.

Endocrine & metabolic: Fertility: May cause sterility; interferes with oogenesis and spermatogenesis; may be irreversible in some patients; gonadal suppression (amenorrhea)

Gastrointestinal: Nausea and vomiting occur more frequently with larger doses, usually beginning 6-10 hours after administration; anorexia, diarrhea, mucositis, and stomatitis are also seen

Genitourinary: Severe, potentially fatal acute hemorrhagic cystitis, believed to be a result of chemical irritation of the bladder by acrolein, a cyclophosphamide metabolite, occurs in 7% to 12% of patients and has been reported in up to 40% of patients in some series. Patients should be encouraged to drink plenty of fluids during therapy (most adults will require at least 2 L/day), void frequently, and avoid taking the drug at night. With large I.V. doses, I.V. hydration is usually recommended. The use of mesna and/or continuous bladder irrigation is rarely needed for doses <2 g/m^2.

Hematologic: Thrombocytopenia and anemia are less common than leukopenia
Onset: 7 days
Nadir: 10-14 days
Recovery: 21 days

1% to 10%:
Cardiovascular: Facial flushing
Central nervous system: Headache
Dermatologic: Skin rash
Renal: SIADH may occur, usually with doses >50 mg/kg (or 1 g/m^2); renal tubular necrosis, which usually resolves with discontinuation of the drug, is also reported
Respiratory: Nasal congestion occurs when I.V. doses are administered too rapidly (large doses via 30-60 minute infusion); patients experience runny eyes, rhinorrhea, sinus congestion, and sneezing during or immediately after the infusion. If needed, a decongestant or decongestant/antihistamine (eg, pseudoephedrine or pseudoephedrine/triprolidine) can be used to prevent or relieve these symptoms.

Overdosage/Toxicology Symptoms of overdose include myelosuppression, alopecia, nausea, and vomiting. Treatment is supportive.

Pharmacodynamics/Kinetics
Absorption: Oral: Well absorbed
Bioavailability: >75%
Time to Peak: Serum: Oral: ~1 hour
Protein Binding: 10% to 56%
Half-Life Elimination: 4-8 hours
Metabolism: Hepatic to active metabolites acrolein, 4-aldophosphamide, 4-hydroperoxy-cyclophosphamide, and nor-nitrogen mustard
Excretion: Urine (<30% as unchanged drug, 85% to 90% as metabolites)

Dosing
Adults: Refer to individual protocols. Patients who are heavily pretreated with cytotoxic radiation or chemotherapy, or who have compromised bone marrow function may require a 33% to 50% reduction in initial dose.
Usual dose:
Oral: 50-100 mg/m^2/day as continuous therapy or 400-1000 mg/m^2 in divided doses over 4-5 days as intermittent therapy
I.V.:
Single doses: 400-1800 mg/m^2 (30-50 mg/kg) per treatment course (1-5 days) which can be repeated at 2- to 4-week intervals
Continuous daily doses: 60-120 mg/m^2 (1-2.5 mg/kg) per day
JRA/vasculitis: I.V.: 10 mg/kg every 2 weeks
High dose BMT:
I.V.:
60 mg/kg/day for 2 days (total dose: 120 mg/kg)
50 mg/kg/day for 4 days (total dose: 200 mg/kg)
1.8 g/m^2/day for 4 days (total dose: 7.2 g/m^2)
Continuous I.V.:
1.5 g/m^2/24 hours for 96 hours (total dose: 6 g/m^2)
1875 mg/m^2/24 hours for 72 hours (total dose: 5625 mg/m^2)
Note: Duration of infusion is 1-24 hours; generally combined with other high-dose chemotherapeutic drugs, lymphocyte immune globulin, or total body irradiation (TBI).
Nephrotic syndrome: Oral: 2-3 mg/kg/day every day for up to 12 weeks when corticosteroids are unsuccessful
Elderly: Refer to individual protocols: Initial and maintenance for induction: 1-2 mg/kg/day; adjust for renal clearance.
Pediatrics: Refer to individual protocols. Patients with compromised bone marrow function may require a 33% to 50% reduction in initial loading dose. Children:
Chemotherapy: Refer to adult dosing.
SLE: I.V.: 500-750 mg/m^2 every month; maximum dose: 1 g/m^2
JRA/vasculitis: I.V.: Refer to adult dosing.
Nephrotic syndrome: Refer to adult dosing.
Renal Impairment: A large fraction of cyclophosphamide is eliminated by hepatic metabolism; some authors recommend no dose adjustment unless severe renal insufficiency (Cl$_{cr}$ <20 mL/minute).
Cl$_{cr}$ >10 mL/minute: Administer 100% of normal dose.
Cl$_{cr}$ <10 mL/minute: Administer 75% of normal dose.
Hemodialysis effects: Moderately dialyzable (20% to 50%)
Administer dose posthemodialysis
CAPD effects: Unknown
CAVH effects: Unknown
Hepatic Impairment: The pharmacokinetics of cyclophosphamide are not significantly altered in the presence of hepatic insufficiency. No dosage adjustments are recommended.
(Continued)

Cyclophosphamide *(Continued)*

Available Dosage Forms
Injection, powder for reconstitution:
Cytoxan®: 500 mg, 1 g, 2 g [contains mannitol 75 mg per cyclophosphamide 100 mg]
Tablet (Cytoxan®): 25 mg, 50 mg

Monitoring and Teaching Issues
Physical Assessment: See Warnings/Precautions for use cautions. Assess potential for interactions with other pharmacological agents or herbal products patient may be taking (eg, potential for increased or prolonged adverse effects [nephrotoxicity, cardiotoxicity]; see Drug Interactions). See infusion specifics in Administration, including recommendations for pre- and posthydration. Infusion site should be monitored to prevent extravasation. Assess results of laboratory tests (eg, UA, BUN, Cr; detect nephrotoxicity; CBC with differential, platelet count; detect myelosuppression; see Monitoring Laboratory Tests). Monitor therapeutic effectiveness (according to purpose for use) and adverse response (hemorrhagic cystitis, leukopenia, renal tubular necrosis; see Adverse Reactions) prior to each infusion and regularly during therapy. Teach patient (or caregiver) proper use (oral), possible side effects/appropriate interventions (eg, importance of adequate hydration), and adverse symptoms to report (see Patient Education).

Monitoring Laboratory Tests: CBC with differential, platelet count, ESR, BUN, UA, serum electrolytes, serum creatinine

Patient Education: Do not take any new medication during therapy unless approved by prescriber. **I.V.:** Report immediately pain or swelling at infusion site; sudden difficulty breathing or swallowing, chest pain, rash. **Oral:** Take exactly as directed, during or after meals; do not take at night. It is very important to maintain adequate hydration (2-3 L/day of fluids) unless instructed to restrict fluid intake; void frequently to reduce incidence of bladder irritation. You will be more susceptible to infection (avoid crowds and exposure to infection and do not have any vaccinations without consulting prescriber). May cause loss of hair (reversible, although regrowth hair may be different color or texture); fertility or amenorrhea; nausea or vomiting (small frequent meals, good mouth care, chewing gum, or sucking lozenges may help; if persistent consult prescriber for antiemetic); headache (consult prescriber for analgesic); nasal congestion or cold symptoms (consult prescriber for decongestant); or mouth sores (use soft toothbrush or cotton swab for oral care). May cause sterility (possibly reversible) or amenorrhea. Report immediately any difficulty or pain with urination, blood in urine, change in urinary pattern; chest pain, rapid heartbeat, or palpitations; easy bruising or bleeding; unusual rash; persistent nausea or vomiting; swelling of extremities; respiratory difficulty; or unusual fatigue. **Pregnancy/breast-feeding precautions:** Inform prescriber if you are pregnant. Do not get pregnant during therapy. Consult prescriber for instruction on appropriate barrier contraceptive measures. This drug may cause severe fetal defects. Do not breast-feed.

Dietary Considerations: Tablets should be administered during or after meals.

Geriatric Considerations: Toxicity to immunosuppressives is increased in the elderly. Start with lowest recommended adult doses. Signs of infection, such as fever and WBC rise, may not occur. Lethargy and confusion may be more prominent signs of infection; adjust dose for renal function in the elderly.

Pregnancy Risk Factor: D

Lactation: Enters breast milk/contraindicated

Administration
Oral: Tablets are not scored and should not be cut or crushed; should be administered during or after meals.

I.V.: May be administered I.P., intrapleurally, IVPB, or continuous intravenous infusion. I.V. infusions may be administered over 1-24 hours. Doses >500 mg to approximately 2 g may be administered over 20-30 minutes.
To minimize bladder toxicity, increase normal fluid intake during and for 1-2 days after cyclophosphamide dose. Most adult patients will require a fluid intake of at least 2 L/day. High-dose regimens should be accompanied by vigorous hydration with or without mesna therapy.

Reconstitution: Reconstitute vials with SWI, NS, or D_5W to a concentration of 20 mg/mL.

Compatibility: Stable in D_5LR, D_5NS, D_5W, LR, ½NS, NS

Y-site administration: Incompatible with amphotericin B cholesteryl sulfate complex

Storage: Store intact vials of powder at room temperature of (25°C to 35°C). Reconstituted solutions are stable for 24 hours at room temperature (25°C) and 6 days under refrigeration (5°C). Further dilutions in D_5W or NS are stable for 24 hours at room temperature (25°C) and 6 days at refrigeration (5°C).

Additional Information May be used in combination with mesna to prevent hemorrhagic cystitis. Rarely required for doses <1.5-2 g/m^2.

Related Information
Maternal / Fetal Toxicology *on page 1762*

CycloSERINE *(sye kloe SER een)*

U.S. Brand Names Seromycin®

Generic Available No

Pharmacologic Category Antibiotic, Miscellaneous; Antitubercular Agent

Medication Safety Issues
Sound-alike/look-alike issues:
CycloSERINE may be confused with cyclobenzaprine, cycloSPORINE

Use Adjunctive treatment in pulmonary or extrapulmonary tuberculosis

Unlabeled/Investigational Use Treatment of Gaucher's disease

Mechanism of Action/Effect Inhibits bacterial cell wall synthesis by competing with amino acid (D-alanine) for incorporation into the bacterial cell wall; bacteriostatic or bactericidal

Contraindications Hypersensitivity to cycloserine or any component of the formulation

Warnings/Precautions Epilepsy, depression, severe anxiety, psychosis, severe renal insufficiency, chronic alcoholism.

Drug Interactions

Increased Effect/Toxicity: Alcohol, isoniazid, and ethionamide increase toxicity of cycloserine. Cycloserine inhibits the hepatic metabolism of phenytoin and may increase risk of epileptic seizures.

Nutritional/Ethanol Interactions

Ethanol: Avoid ethanol (may increase CNS depression).

Food: May increase vitamin B_{12} and folic acid dietary requirements.

Adverse Reactions Frequency not defined.

Cardiovascular: Cardiac arrhythmia

Central nervous system: Drowsiness, headache, dizziness, vertigo, seizure, confusion, psychosis, paresis, coma

Dermatologic: Rash

Endocrine & metabolic: Vitamin B_{12} deficiency

Hematologic: Folate deficiency

Hepatic: Liver enzymes increased

Neuromuscular & skeletal: Tremor

Overdosage/Toxicology

Symptoms of overdose include confusion, CNS depression, psychosis, coma, and seizures. Decontaminate with activated charcoal. Can be hemodialyzed. Management is supportive. Administer 100-300 mg/day of pyridoxine to reduce neurotoxic effects. Acute toxicity can occur with ingestion >1 g.

Pharmacodynamics/Kinetics

Absorption: ~70% to 90%

Time to Peak: Serum: 3-4 hours

Half-Life Elimination: Normal renal function: 10 hours

Metabolism: Hepatic

Excretion: Urine (60% to 70% as unchanged drug) within 72 hours; feces (small amounts); remainder metabolized

Dosing

Adults & Elderly: Note: Some of the neurotoxic effects may be relieved or prevented by the concomitant administration of pyridoxine.

Tuberculosis: Oral: Initial: 250 mg every 12 hours for 14 days, then give 500 mg to 1 g/day in 2 divided doses for 18-24 months (maximum daily dose: 1 g)

Pediatrics: Note: Some of the neurotoxic effects may be relieved or prevented by the concomitant administration of pyridoxine.

Tuberculosis: Oral: Children: 10-20 mg/kg/day in 2 divided doses up to 1000 mg/day for 18-24 months

Renal Impairment:

Cl_{cr} 10-50 mL/minute: Administer every 12-24 hours.

Cl_{cr} <10 mL/minute: Administer every 24 hours.

Available Dosage Forms Capsule: 250 mg

Monitoring and Teaching Issues

Physical Assessment: Use with caution in presence of epilepsy, depression, psychosis, severe renal insufficiency, chronic alcoholism (see Warnings/Precautions). Assess potential for interactions with other pharmacological agents patient may be taking (see Drug Interactions). Assess results of laboratory tests, therapeutic effectiveness, and adverse response (eg, CNS changes, arrhythmias, vitamin B_{12} deficiency, folate deficiency; see Adverse Reactions) regularly during therapy. Teach patient proper use, possible side effects/appropriate interventions (eg, importance of adequate hydration), and adverse symptoms to report (see Patient Education).

Monitoring Laboratory Tests: Periodic renal, hepatic, hematological tests, plasma cycloserine concentrations

Patient Education: Take as prescribed; do not discontinue without consulting prescriber. Avoid alcohol. Maintain recommended diet and adequate hydration (2-3 L/day of fluids) unless instructed to restrict fluid intake. May cause drowsiness or restlessness (use caution when driving or engaging in tasks that require alertness until response to drug is known). Report skin rash, acute headache, muscle pain; changes in mentation (confusion, nightmares, depression, or suicide ideation), or fluid retention (respiratory difficulty, swelling of extremities, unusual weight gain). **Pregnancy precaution:** Inform prescriber if you are or intend to become pregnant.

Dietary Considerations: May be taken with food; may increase vitamin B_{12} and folic acid dietary requirements.

Geriatric Considerations: Adjust dose for renal function.

Pregnancy Risk Factor: C

Lactation: Enters breast milk/compatible

Related Information

Antimicrobial Drugs of Choice on page 1792

FDA Name Differentiation Project: The Use of Tall-Man Letters on page 15

Tuberculosis on page 1864

♦ **Cyclosporin A** see CycloSPORINE on page 383

CycloSPORINE (SYE kloe spor een)

U.S. Brand Names Gengraf®; Neoral®; Restasis™; Sandimmune®

Synonyms CsA; CyA; Cyclosporin A

Generic Available Yes

Pharmacologic Category Immunosuppressant Agent

Medication Safety Issues

Sound-alike/look-alike issues:

CycloSPORINE may be confused with cyclophosphamide, Cyklokapron®, cycloSERINE

Gengraf® may be confused with Prograf®

Neoral® may be confused with Neurontin®, Nizoral®

Sandimmune® may be confused with Sandostatin®

(Continued)

CycloSPORINE *(Continued)*

Use Prophylaxis of organ rejection in kidney, liver, and heart transplants, has been used with azathioprine and/or corticosteroids; severe, active rheumatoid arthritis (RA) not responsive to methotrexate alone; severe, recalcitrant plaque psoriasis in nonimmunocompromised adults unresponsive to or unable to tolerate other systemic therapy

Ophthalmic emulsion (Restasis™): Increase tear production when suppressed tear production is presumed to be due to keratoconjunctivitis sicca-associated ocular inflammation (in patients not already using topical anti-inflammatory drugs or punctal plugs)

Unlabeled/Investigational Use Short-term, high-dose cyclosporine as a modulator of multi-drug resistance in cancer treatment; allogenic bone marrow transplants for prevention and treatment of graft-versus-host disease; also used in some cases of severe autoimmune disease (ie, SLE, myasthenia gravis) that are resistant to corticosteroids and other therapy; focal segmental glomerulosclerosis

Mechanism of Action/Effect Inhibits T-lymphocytes and lymphokine production and release in a reversible manner.

Contraindications Hypersensitivity to cyclosporine or any component of the formulation. Rheumatoid arthritis and psoriasis: Abnormal renal function, uncontrolled hypertension, malignancies. Concomitant treatment with PUVA or UVB therapy, methotrexate, other immunosuppressive agents, coal tar, or radiation therapy are also contraindications for use in patients with psoriasis. Ophthalmic emulsion is contraindicated in patients with active ocular infections.

Warnings/Precautions Dose-related risk of nephrotoxicity and hepatotoxicity; monitor. Use caution with other potentially nephrotoxic drugs. Increased risk of lymphomas and other malignancies. Increased risk of infection. May cause hypertension. Use caution when changing dosage forms. Monitor cyclosporine concentrations closely following the addition, modification, or deletion of other medications; live, attenuated vaccines may be less effective; use should be avoided.

Transplant patients: May cause significant hyperkalemia and hyperuricemia, seizures (particularly if used with high dose corticosteroids), and encephalopathy. To avoid toxicity or possible organ rejection, make dose adjustments based on cyclosporine blood concentrations. Anaphylaxis has been reported with I.V. use; reserve for patients who cannot take oral form.

Psoriasis: Patients should avoid excessive sun exposure. Safety and efficacy in children <18 have not been established.

Rheumatoid arthritis: Safety and efficacy for use in juvenile rheumatoid arthritis have not been established. If receiving other immunosuppressive agents, radiation or UV therapy, concurrent use of cyclosporine is not recommended.

Ophthalmic emulsion: Has not been studied in patients with a history of herpes keratitis. Safety and efficacy have not been established in patients <16 years of age.

Products may contain corn oil, castor oil, ethanol, or propylene glycol; injection also contains Cremophor® EL (polyoxyethylated castor oil).

Drug Interactions

Cytochrome P450 Effect: Substrate of CYP3A4 (major); **Inhibits** CYP2C8/9 (weak), 3A4 (moderate)

Decreased Effect: Isoniazid and ticlopidine decrease cyclosporine concentrations. The levels/effects of cyclosporine may be decreased by aminoglutethimide, carbamazepine, nafcillin, nevirapine, phenobarbital, phenytoin, rifamycins, and other CYP3A4 inducers. Orlistat may decrease absorption of cyclosporine; avoid concomitant use. Vaccination may be less effective; avoid use of live vaccines during therapy.

Increased Effect/Toxicity: The levels/effects of cyclosporine may be increased by allopurinol, azole antifungals, ciprofloxacin, clarithromycin, diclofenac, doxycycline, erythromycin, imatinib, isoniazid, metoclopramide, nefazodone, nicardipine, octreotide, propofol, protease inhibitors, quinidine, telithromycin, verapamil, and other CYP3A4 inhibitors. Cyclosporine may increase the levels/effects of selected benzodiazepines, calcium channel blockers, cisapride, cyclosporine, ergot alkaloids, selected HMG-CoA reductase inhibitors, mesoridazine, mirtazapine, nateglinide, nefazodone, pimozide, prednisolone (dosage adjustment may be required), quinidine, sildenafil (and other PDE-5 inhibitors), tacrolimus, thioridazine, venlafaxine, and other CYP3A4 substrates. Drugs that enhance nephrotoxicity of cyclosporine include aminoglycosides, amphotericin B, acyclovir, cimetidine, ketoconazole, lovastatin, melphalan, NSAIDs, ranitidine, and trimethoprim and sulfamethoxazole, Cyclosporine increases toxicity of digoxin, diuretics, methotrexate, nifedipine.

Nutritional/Ethanol Interactions

Food: Grapefruit juice increases absorption; unsupervised use should be avoided.

Herb/Nutraceutical: Avoid St John's wort; as an enzyme inducer, it may increase the metabolism of and decrease plasma levels of cyclosporine; organ rejection and graft loss have been reported. Avoid cat's claw, echinacea (have immunostimulant properties).

Lab Interactions Specific whole blood, HPLC assay for cyclosporine may be falsely elevated if sample is drawn from the same line through which dose was administered (even if flush has been administered and/or dose was given hours before).

Adverse Reactions Note: Adverse reactions reported with kidney, liver, and heart transplantation, unless otherwise noted. Although percentage is reported for specific condition, reaction may occur in anyone taking cyclosporine. [Reactions reported for rheumatoid arthritis (RA) are based on cyclosporine (modified) 2.5 mg/kg/day versus placebo.]

>10%:
Cardiovascular: Hypertension (13% to 53%; psoriasis 25% to 27%)
Central nervous system: Headache (2% to 15%; RA 17%, psoriasis 14% to 16%)
Dermatologic: Hirsutism (21% to 45%), hypertrichosis (RA 19%)
Endocrine & metabolic: Increased triglycerides (psoriasis 15%), female reproductive disorder (psoriasis 8% to 11%)

Gastrointestinal: Nausea (RA 23%), diarrhea (RA 12%), gum hyperplasia (4% to 16%), abdominal discomfort (RA 15%), dyspepsia (RA 12%)

Neuromuscular & skeletal: Tremor (12% to 55%)

Renal: Renal dysfunction/nephropathy (25% to 38%; RA 10%, psoriasis 21%), creatinine elevation ≥50% (RA 24%), increased creatinine (psoriasis 16% to 20%)

Respiratory: Upper respiratory infection (psoriasis 8% to 11%)

Miscellaneous: Infection (psoriasis 24% to 25%)

Kidney, liver, and heart transplant only (≤2% unless otherwise noted):

Cardiovascular: Flushes (<1% to 4%), MI

Central nervous system: Convulsions (1% to 5%), anxiety, confusion, fever, lethargy

Dermatologic: Acne (1% to 6%), brittle fingernails, hair breaking, pruritus

Endocrine & metabolic: Gynecomastia (<1% to 4%), hyperglycemia

Gastrointestinal: Nausea (2% to 10%), vomiting (2% to 10%), diarrhea (3% to 8%), abdominal discomfort (<1% to 7%), cramps (0% to 4%), anorexia, constipation, gastritis, mouth sores, pancreatitis, swallowing difficulty, upper GI bleed, weight loss

Hematologic: Leukopenia (<1% to 6%), anemia, thrombocytopenia

Hepatic: Hepatotoxicity (<1% to 7%)

Neuromuscular & skeletal: Paresthesia (1% to 3%), joint pain, muscle pain, tingling, weakness

Ocular: Conjunctivitis, visual disturbance

Otic: Hearing loss, tinnitus

Renal: Hematuria

Respiratory: Sinusitis (<1% to 7%)

Miscellaneous: Lymphoma (<1% to 6%), allergic reactions, hiccups, night sweats

Rheumatoid arthritis only (1% to <3% unless otherwise noted):

Cardiovascular: Hypertension (8%), edema (5%), chest pain (4%), arrhythmia (2%), abnormal heart sounds, cardiac failure, MI, peripheral ischemia

Central nervous system: Dizziness (8%), pain (6%), insomnia (4%), depression (3%), migraine (2%), anxiety, hypoesthesia, emotional lability, impaired concentration, malaise, nervousness, paranoia, somnolence, vertigo

Dermatologic: Purpura (3%), abnormal pigmentation, angioedema, cellulitis, dermatitis, dry skin, eczema, folliculitis, nail disorder, pruritus, skin disorder, urticaria

Endocrine & metabolic: Menstrual disorder (3%), breast fibroadenosis, breast pain, diabetes mellitus, goiter, hot flashes, hyperkalemia, hyperuricemia, hypoglycemia, libido increased/decreased

Gastrointestinal: Vomiting (9%), flatulence (5%), gingivitis (4%), gum hyperplasia (2%), constipation, dry mouth, dysphagia, enanthema, eructation, esophagitis, gastric ulcer, gastritis, gastroenteritis, gingival bleeding, glossitis, peptic ulcer, salivary gland enlargement, taste perversion, tongue disorder, tooth disorder, weight loss/gain

Genitourinary: Leukorrhea (1%), abnormal urine, micturition urgency, nocturia, polyuria, pyelonephritis, urinary incontinence, uterine hemorrhage

Hematologic: Anemia, leukopenia

Hepatic: Bilirubinemia

Neuromuscular & skeletal: Paresthesia (8%), tremor (8%), leg cramps/muscle contractions (2%), arthralgia, bone fracture, joint dislocation, myalgia, neuropathy, stiffness, synovial cyst, tendon disorder, weakness

Ocular: Abnormal vision, cataract, conjunctivitis, eye pain

Otic: Tinnitus, deafness, vestibular disorder

Renal: Increased BUN, hematuria, renal abscess

Respiratory: Cough (5%), dyspnea (5%), sinusitis (4%), abnormal chest sounds, bronchospasm, epistaxis

Miscellaneous: Infection (9%), abscess, allergy, bacterial infection, carcinoma, fungal infection, herpes simplex, herpes zoster, lymphadenopathy, moniliasis, diaphoresis increased, tonsillitis, viral infection

Psoriasis only (1% to <3% unless otherwise noted):

Cardiovascular: Chest pain, flushes

Central nervous system: Psychiatric events (4% to 5%), pain (3% to 4%), dizziness, fever, insomnia, nervousness, vertigo

Dermatologic: Hypertrichosis (5% to 7%), acne, dry skin, folliculitis, keratosis, pruritus, rash, skin malignancies

Endocrine & metabolic: Hot flashes

Gastrointestinal: Nausea (5% to 6%), diarrhea (5% to 6%), gum hyperplasia (4% to 6%), abdominal discomfort (3% to 6%), dyspepsia (2% to 3%), abdominal distention, appetite increased, constipation, gingival bleeding

Genitourinary: Micturition increased

Hematologic: Bleeding disorder, clotting disorder, platelet disorder, red blood cell disorder

Hepatic: Hyperbilirubinemia

Neuromuscular & skeletal: Paresthesia (5% to 7%), arthralgia (1% to 6%)

Ocular: Abnormal vision

Respiratory: Bronchospasm (5%), cough (5%), dyspnea (5%), rhinitis (5%), respiratory infection

Miscellaneous: Flu-like symptoms (8% to 10%)

Ophthalmic emulsion (Restasis™):

>10%: Ocular: Burning (17%)

1% to 10%: Ocular: Hyperemia (conjunctival 5%), eye pain, pruritus, stinging

Overdosage/Toxicology Symptoms of overdose include hepatotoxicity, nephrotoxicity, nausea, vomiting, tremor. CNS secondary to direct action of the drug may not be reflected in serum concentrations, may be more predictable by renal magnesium loss. Forced emesis may be beneficial if done within 2 hours of ingestion of cyclosporine capsules (modified). Treatment is symptomatic and supportive. Cyclosporine is not dialyzable.

Pharmacodynamics/Kinetics

Absorption:

Ophthalmic emulsion: Serum concentrations not detectable.

(Continued)

CycloSPORINE (Continued)

Oral:

Cyclosporine (non-modified): Erratic and incomplete; dependent on presence of food, bile acids, and GI motility; larger oral doses are needed in pediatrics due to shorter bowel length and limited intestinal absorption

Cyclosporine (modified): Erratic and incomplete; increased absorption, up to 30% when compared to cyclosporine (non-modified); less dependent on food, bile acids, or GI motility when compared to cyclosporine (non-modified)

Bioavailability: Oral:

Cyclosporine (non-modified): Dependent on patient population and transplant type (<10% in adult liver transplant patients and as high as 89% in renal transplant patients); bioavailability of Sandimmune® capsules and oral solution are equivalent; bioavailability of oral solution is ~30% of the I.V. solution

Children: 28% (range: 17% to 42%); gut dysfunction common in BMT patients and oral bioavailability is further reduced

Cyclosporine (modified): Bioavailability of Neoral® capsules and oral solution are equivalent:

Children: 43% (range: 30% to 68%)

Adults: 23% greater than with cyclosporine (non-modified) in renal transplant patients; 50% greater in liver transplant patients

Time to Peak: Serum: Oral:

Cyclosporine (non-modified): 2-6 hours; some patients have a second peak at 5-6 hours

Cyclosporine (modified): Renal transplant: 1.5-2 hours

Protein Binding: 90% to 98% to lipoproteins

Half-Life Elimination: Oral: May be prolonged with hepatic impairment and shorter in pediatric patients due to the higher metabolism rate

Cyclosporine (non-modified): Biphasic: Alpha: 1.4 hours; Terminal: 19 hours (range: 10-27 hours)

Cyclosporine (modified): Biphasic: Terminal: 8.4 hours (range: 5-18 hours)

Metabolism: Extensively hepatic via CYP; forms at least 25 metabolites; extensive first-pass effect following oral administration

Excretion: Primarily feces; urine (6%, 0.1% as unchanged drug and metabolites)

Dosing

Adults: Note: Neoral® and Sandimmune® are not bioequivalent and cannot be used interchangeably

Newly-transplanted patients: Adjunct therapy with corticosteroids is recommended. Initial dose should be given 4-12 hours prior to transplant or may be given postoperatively; adjust initial dose to achieve desired plasma concentration.

Oral: Dose is dependent upon type of transplant and formulation:

Cyclosporine (modified):

Renal: 9 ± 3 mg/kg/day, divided twice daily

Liver: 8 ± 4 mg/kg/day, divided twice daily

Heart: 7 ± 3 mg/kg/day, divided twice daily

Cyclosporine (non-modified): Initial dose: 15 mg/kg/day as a single dose (range 14-18 mg/kg); lower doses of 10-14 mg/kg/day have been used for renal transplants. Continue initial dose daily for 1-2 weeks; taper by 5% per week to a maintenance dose of 5-10 mg/kg/day; some renal transplant patients may be dosed as low as 3 mg/kg/day

Note: When using the non-modified formulation, cyclosporine levels may increase in liver transplant patients when the T-tube is closed; dose may need decreased

I.V.: Cyclosporine (non-modified): Initial dose: 5-6 mg/kg/day as a single dose ($\frac{1}{3}$ the oral dose), infused over 2-6 hours; use should be limited to patients unable to take capsules or oral solution; patients should be switched to an oral dosage form as soon as possible

Note: Conversion to cyclosporine (modified) from cyclosporine (non-modified): Start with daily dose previously used and adjust to obtain preconversion cyclosporine trough concentration. Plasma concentrations should be monitored every 4-7 days and dose adjusted as necessary, until desired trough level is obtained. When transferring patients with previously poor absorption of cyclosporine (non-modified), monitor trough levels at least twice weekly (especially if initial dose exceeds 10 mg/kg/day); high plasma levels are likely to occur.

Rheumatoid arthritis: Oral: Cyclosporine (modified): Initial dose: 2.5 mg/kg/day, divided twice daily; salicylates, NSAIDs, and oral glucocorticoids may be continued (refer to Drug Interactions); dose may be increased by 0.5-0.75 mg/kg/day if insufficient response is seen after 8 weeks of treatment; additional dosage increases may be made again at 12 weeks (maximum dose: 4 mg/kg/day). Discontinue if no benefit is seen by 16 weeks of therapy.

Note: Increase the frequency of blood pressure monitoring after each alteration in dosage of cyclosporine. Cyclosporine dosage should be decreased by 25% to 50% in patients with no history of hypertension who develop sustained hypertension during therapy and, if hypertension persists, treatment with cyclosporine should be discontinued.

Psoriasis: Oral: Cyclosporine (modified): Initial dose: 2.5 mg/kg/day, divided twice daily; dose may be increased by 0.5 mg/kg/day if insufficient response is seen after 4 weeks of treatment; additional dosage increases may be made every 2 weeks if needed (maximum dose: 4 mg/kg/day). Discontinue if no benefit is seen by 6 weeks of therapy. Once patients are adequately controlled, the dose should be decreased to the lowest effective dose. Doses <2.5 mg/kg/day may be effective. Treatment longer than 1 year is not recommended.

Note: Increase the frequency of blood pressure monitoring after each alteration in dosage of cyclosporine. Cyclosporine dosage should be decreased by 25% to 50% in patients with no history of hypertension who develop sustained hypertension during therapy and, if hypertension persists, treatment with cyclosporine should be discontinued.

Focal segmental glomerulosclerosis: Initial: 3 mg/kg/day divided every 12 hours
Autoimmune diseases: 1-3 mg/kg/day
Keratoconjunctivitis sicca: Ophthalmic: Instill 1 drop in each eye every 12 hours

Elderly: Refer to adult dosing (**Note:** Sandimmune® and Neoral® are not bioequivalent and cannot be used interchangeably without physician supervision).

Pediatrics: Transplant: Refer to adult dosing; children may require, and are able to tolerate, larger doses than adults.

Renal Impairment: For severe psoriasis:

Serum creatinine levels ≥25% above pretreatment levels: Take another sample within 2 weeks; if the level remains ≥25% above pretreatment levels, decrease dosage of cyclosporine (modified) by 25% to 50%. If two dosage adjustments do not reverse the increase in serum creatinine levels, treatment should be discontinued.

Serum creatinine levels ≥50% above pretreatment levels: Decrease cyclosporine dosage by 25% to 50%. If two dosage adjustments do not reverse the increase in serum creatinine levels, treatment should be discontinued.

Hemodialysis: Supplemental dose is not necessary.
Peritoneal dialysis: Supplemental dose is not necessary.

Hepatic Impairment: Dosage adjustment is probably necessary; monitor levels closely

Available Dosage Forms

Capsule, soft gel, modified: 25 mg, 100 mg [contains castor oil, ethanol]

Gengraf®: 25 mg, 100 mg [contains ethanol, castor oil, propylene glycol]

Neoral®: 25 mg, 100 mg [contains dehydrated ethanol, corn oil, castor oil, propylene glycol]

Capsule, soft gel, non-modified (Sandimmune®): 25 mg, 100 mg [contains dehydrated ethanol, corn oil]

Emulsion, ophthalmic [preservative free, single-use vial] (Restasis™): 0.05% (0.4 mL) [contains glycerin, castor oil, polysorbate 80, carbomer 1342; 32 vials/box]

Injection, solution, non-modified (Sandimmune®): 50 mg/mL (5 mL) [contains Cremophor® EL (polyoxyethylated castor oil), ethanol]

Solution, oral, modified:

Gengraf®: 100 mg/mL (50 mL) [contains castor oil, propylene glycol]

Neoral®: 100 mg/mL (50 mL) [contains dehydrated ethanol, corn oil, castor oil, propylene glycol]

Solution, oral, non-modified (Sandimmune®): 100 mg/mL (50 mL) [contains olive oil, ethanol]

Monitoring and Teaching Issues

Physical Assessment: Assess effectiveness and interactions of other medications patient may be taking. Monitor kidney and hepatic function closely. Assess results of laboratory tests, therapeutic effectiveness, and adverse reactions at beginning of therapy and periodically throughout therapy. **I.V.:** Monitor closely for first 30-60 minutes of infusion and frequently thereafter to assess for adverse reactions. **Oral:** Teach patient appropriate administration, possible side effects, and symptoms to report.

Monitoring Laboratory Tests: Cyclosporine levels, serum electrolytes, renal function, hepatic function

Patient Education: Oral: Take dose at the same time each day. You will be susceptible to infection (avoid crowds and exposure to infection and do not have any vaccinations without consulting prescriber). Practice good oral hygiene to reduce gum inflammation; see a dentist regularly during treatment. Report severe headache; unusual hair growth or deepening of voice; mouth sores or swollen gums; persistent nausea, vomiting, or abdominal pain; muscle pain or cramping; unusual swelling of extremities, weight gain, or change in urination; or chest pain or rapid heartbeat. Increase in blood pressure or damage to the kidney is possible. Your prescriber will need to monitor you closely. Do not change one brand of cyclosporine for another; any changes must be done by your prescriber. If you are taking this medication for psoriasis, your risk of cancer may be increased when taking additional medications. **Solution:** Diluting oral solution improves flavor. Dilute Neoral® with orange juice or apple juice. Dilute Sandimmune® with milk, chocolate milk, or orange juice. Avoid changing what you mix with your cyclosporine. Mix thoroughly and drink at once. Use syringe provided to measure dose. Mix in a glass container (do not use plastic or styrofoam) and rinse container with more juice/milk to ensure total dose is taken. Do not rinse syringe before or after use (may cause dose variation). **Pregnancy/breast-feeding precautions:** Inform prescriber if you are or intend to become pregnant. Do not breast-feed.

Dietary Considerations: Administer this medication consistently with relation to time of day and meals.

Pregnancy Risk Factor: C

Pregnancy Issues: Cyclosporine crosses the placenta. Based on clinical use, premature births and low birth weight were consistently observed. Use only if the benefit to the mother outweighs the possible risks to the fetus.

Lactation: Enters breast milk/contraindicated

Administration

Oral: Oral solution: Do not administer liquid from plastic or styrofoam cup. May dilute Neoral® oral solution with orange juice or apple juice. May dilute Sandimmune® oral solution with milk, chocolate milk, or orange juice. Avoid changing diluents frequently. Mix thoroughly and drink at once. Use syringe provided to measure dose. Mix in a glass container and rinse container with more diluent to ensure total dose is taken. Do not rinse syringe before or after use (may cause dose variation).

I.V.: Following dilution, intravenous admixture should be administered over 2-6 hours. Patients should be under continuous observation for at least the first 30 minutes of the infusion, and should be monitored frequently thereafter.

Other: Ophthalmic emulsion: Prior to use, invert vial several times to obtain a uniform emulsion. Remove contact lenses prior to instillation of drops; may be reinserted 15 minutes after administration. May be used with artificial tears; allow 15 minute interval between products.

(Continued)

CycloSPORINE *(Continued)*

Reconstitution:

Sandimmune® injection: Injection should be further diluted [1 mL (50 mg) of concentrate in 20-100 mL of D₅W or NS] for administration by intravenous infusion. Light protection is not required for intravenous admixtures of cyclosporine.

Stability of injection of parenteral admixture at room temperature (25°C) is 6 hours in PVC; 24 hours in Excel®, PAB® containers, or glass.

Polyoxyethylated castor oil (Cremophor® EL) surfactant in cyclosporine injection may leach phthalate from PVC containers such as bags and tubing. The actual amount of diethylhexyl phthalate (DEHP) plasticizer leached from PVC containers and administration sets may vary in clinical situations, depending on surfactant concentration, bag size, and contact time.

Compatibility: Stable in D₅W, fat emulsion 10%, fat emulsion 20%, NS

Y-site administration: Incompatible with amphotericin B cholesteryl sulfate complex

Compatibility when admixed: Incompatible with magnesium sulfate

Storage:

Capsule: Store at controlled room temperature

Injection: Store at controlled room temperature; do not refrigerate. Ampuls should be protected from light.

Ophthalmic emulsion: Store at 15°C to 25°C (59°F to 77°F). Vials are single-use; discard immediately following administration.

Oral solution: Store at controlled room temperature; do not refrigerate. Use within 2 months after opening; should be mixed in glass containers.

Additional Information Cyclosporine (modified): Refers to the capsule dosage formulation of cyclosporine in an aqueous dispersion (previously referred to as "microemulsion"). Cyclosporine (modified) has increased bioavailability as compared to cyclosporine (non-modified) and cannot be used interchangeably without close monitoring.

Related Information

FDA Name Differentiation Project: The Use of Tall-Man Letters *on page 15*
Peak and Trough Guidelines *on page 1694*

♦ **Cylert®** *see Pemoline on page 1170*
♦ **Cylex® [OTC]** *see Benzocaine on page 181*
♦ **Cymbalta®** *see Duloxetine on page 503*

Cyproheptadine *(si proe HEP ta deen)*

Synonyms Cyproheptadine Hydrochloride; Periactin

Generic Available Yes

Pharmacologic Category Antihistamine

Medication Safety Issues

Sound-alike/look-alike issues:

Cyproheptadine may be confused with cyclobenzaprine

Periactin may be confused with Perative®, Percodan®, Persantine®

Use Perennial and seasonal allergic rhinitis and other allergic symptoms including urticaria

Unlabeled/Investigational Use Appetite stimulation, blepharospasm, cluster headaches, migraine headaches, Nelson's syndrome, pruritus, schizophrenia, spinal cord damage associated spasticity, and tardive dyskinesia

Mechanism of Action/Effect A potent antihistamine and serotonin antagonist

Contraindications Hypersensitivity to cyproheptadine or any component of the formulation; narrow-angle glaucoma; bladder neck obstruction; acute asthmatic attack; stenosing peptic ulcer; GI tract obstruction; concurrent use of MAO inhibitors; avoid use in premature and term newborns due to potential association with SIDS

Warnings/Precautions Do not use in the presence of symptomatic prostate hypertrophy. Antihistamines are more likely to cause dizziness, excessive sedation, syncope, toxic confusion states, and hypotension in the elderly. In case reports, cyproheptadine has promoted weight gain in anorexic adults, though it has not been specifically studied in the elderly. All cases of weight loss or decreased appetite should be adequately assessed.

Drug Interactions

Increased Effect/Toxicity: Cyproheptadine may potentiate the effect of CNS depressants. MAO inhibitors may cause hallucinations when taken with cyproheptadine.

Nutritional/Ethanol Interactions Ethanol: Avoid ethanol (may increase CNS sedation).

Lab Interactions Diagnostic antigen skin tests; increased amylases (S); decreased fasting glucose (S)

Adverse Reactions

>10%:

Central nervous system: Slight to moderate drowsiness

Respiratory: Thickening of bronchial secretions

1% to 10%:

Central nervous system: Headache, fatigue, nervousness, dizziness

Gastrointestinal: Appetite stimulation, nausea, diarrhea, abdominal pain, xerostomia

Neuromuscular & skeletal: Arthralgia

Respiratory: Pharyngitis

Overdosage/Toxicology Symptoms of overdose include CNS depression or stimulation, dry mouth, flushed skin, fixed and dilated pupils, and apnea. There is no specific treatment for antihistamine overdose. Clinical toxicity is due to blockade of cholinergic receptors. For anticholinergic overdose with severe life-threatening symptoms, physostigmine 1-2 mg I.V. slowly, may be given to reverse these effects.

Pharmacodynamics/Kinetics
Absorption: Completely
Metabolism: Almost completely hepatic
Excretion: Urine (>50% primarily as metabolites); feces (~25%)
Dosing
Adults:
Appetite stimulation (including anorexia nervosa): Oral: 2 mg 4 times/day; may be increased gradually over a 3-week period to 8 mg 4 times/day
Allergic conditions: Oral: 4-20 mg/day divided every 8 hours (not to exceed 0.5 mg/kg/day)
Cluster headaches: Oral: 4 mg 4 times/day
Migraine headaches: Oral: 4-8 mg 3 times/day
Spasticity associated with spinal cord damage: Oral: 4 mg at bedtime; increase by a 4 mg dose every 3-4 days; average daily dose: 16 mg in divided doses; not to exceed 36 mg/day
Elderly: Oral: Initial: 4 mg twice daily
Pediatrics:
Allergic conditions: Oral: Children: 0.25 mg/kg/day or 8 mg/m²/day in 2-3 divided doses **or**
2-6 years: 2 mg every 8-12 hours (not to exceed 12 mg/day)
7-14 years: 4 mg every 8-12 hours (not to exceed 16 mg/day)
Migraine headaches: 4 mg 2-3 times/day
Spasticity associated with spinal cord damage: Oral: Children ≥12 years: Refer to adult dosing.
Appetite stimulation (Including anorexia nervosa): Children >13 years: Refer to adult dosing.
Hepatic Impairment: Dosage should be reduced in patients with significant hepatic dysfunction.
Available Dosage Forms
Syrup, as hydrochloride: 2 mg/5 mL (473 mL) [contains alcohol 5%; mint flavor]
Tablet, as hydrochloride: 4 mg
Monitoring and Teaching Issues
Physical Assessment: Assess effectiveness and interactions of other medications patient may be taking. Monitor weight periodically. Monitor effectiveness of therapy and adverse reactions (eg, excess anticholinergic effects) at beginning of therapy and periodically with long-term use. Assess knowledge/teach patient appropriate use, interventions to reduce side effects, and adverse symptoms to report.
Patient Education: Take as directed; do not exceed recommended dose. Avoid use of other depressants, alcohol, or sleep-inducing medications unless approved by prescriber. You may experience drowsiness or dizziness (use caution when driving or engaging in tasks requiring alertness until response to drug is known); or dry mouth, nausea, or abdominal pain (small frequent meals, frequent mouth care, chewing gum, or sucking hard candy may help). Report persistent sedation, confusion, or agitation; changes in urinary pattern; blurred vision; chest pain or palpitations; sore throat respiratory difficulty or expectorating (thick secretions); significant change in weight; or lack of improvement or worsening of condition. **Breast-feeding precaution:** Do not breast-feed.
Geriatric Considerations: Elderly may not tolerate anticholinergic effects.
Pregnancy Risk Factor: B
Lactation: Excretion in breast milk unknown/contraindicated
Additional Information May stimulate appetite; in case reports, cyproheptadine has promoted weight gain in anorexic adults.

- **Cyproheptadine Hydrochloride** *see* Cyproheptadine *on page 388*
- **Cystospaz®** *see* Hyoscyamine *on page 775*
- **Cystospaz-M® [DSC]** *see* Hyoscyamine *on page 775*
- **CYT** *see* Cyclophosphamide *on page 380*
- **Cytadren®** *see* Aminoglutethimide *on page 91*

Cytarabine (sye TARE a been)
U.S. Brand Names Cytosar-U®
Synonyms Arabinosylcytosine; Ara-C; Cytarabine Hydrochloride; Cytosine Arabinosine Hydrochloride; NSC-63878
Generic Available Yes
Pharmacologic Category Antineoplastic Agent, Antimetabolite
Medication Safety Issues
Sound-alike/look-alike issues:
Cytarabine may be confused with Cytadren®, Cytosar®, Cytoxan®, vidarabine
Cytosar-U® may be confused with cytarabine, Cytovene®, Cytoxan®, Neosar®
Use Cytarabine is one of the most active agents in leukemia; also active against lymphoma, meningeal leukemia, and meningeal lymphoma; has little use in the treatment of solid tumors
Mechanism of Action/Effect Inhibition of DNA synthesis in S Phase of cell division; degree of its cytotoxicity correlates linearly with its incorporation into DNA, therefore, incorporation into the DNA is responsible for drug activity and toxicity
Contraindications Hypersensitivity to cytarabine or any component of the formulation
Warnings/Precautions The U.S. Food and Drug Administration (FDA) currently recommends that procedures for proper handling and disposal of antineoplastic agents be considered. Use with caution in patients with impaired renal and hepatic function.
Drug Interactions
Decreased Effect: Decreased effect of gentamicin, flucytosine. Decreased digoxin oral tablet absorption.
Increased Effect/Toxicity: Alkylating agents and radiation and purine analogs when coadministered with cytarabine may result in increased toxic effects. Methotrexate, when administered prior to cytarabine, may enhance the efficacy and toxicity of cytarabine; some
(Continued)

Cytarabine *(Continued)*

combination treatment regimens (eg, hyper-CVAD) have been designed to take advantage of this interaction.

Adverse Reactions

>10%:

Central nervous system: Fever (>80%)

Dermatologic: Alopecia

Gastrointestinal: Nausea, vomiting, diarrhea, and mucositis which subside quickly after discontinuing the drug; GI effects may be more pronounced with divided I.V. bolus doses than with continuous infusion

Hematologic: Myelosuppression; neutropenia and thrombocytopenia are severe, anemia may also occur

Onset: 4-7 days

Nadir: 14-18 days

Recovery: 21-28 days

Hepatic: Hepatic dysfunction, mild jaundice, transaminases increased (acute)

Ocular: Tearing, ocular pain, foreign body sensation, photophobia, and blurred vision may occur with high-dose therapy; ophthalmic corticosteroids usually prevent or relieve the condition

1% to 10%:

Cardiovascular: Thrombophlebitis, cardiomegaly

Central nervous system: Dizziness, headache, somnolence, confusion, malaise; a severe cerebellar toxicity occurs in about 8% of patients receiving a high dose (>36-48 g/m^2/cycle); it is irreversible or fatal in about 1%

Dermatologic: Skin freckling, itching, cellulitis at injection site; rash, pain, erythema, and skin sloughing of the palmar and plantar surfaces may occur with high-dose therapy. Prophylactic topical steroids and/or skin moisturizers may be useful.

Genitourinary: Urinary retention

Neuromuscular & skeletal: Myalgia, bone pain

Respiratory: Syndrome of sudden respiratory distress, including tachypnea, hypoxemia, interstitial and alveolar infiltrates progressing to pulmonary edema, pneumonia

Overdosage/Toxicology

Symptoms of overdose include myelosuppression, megaloblastosis, nausea, vomiting, respiratory distress, and pulmonary edema. A syndrome of sudden respiratory distress progressing to pulmonary edema and cardiomegaly has been reported following high doses. Treatment is symptomatic and supportive.

Pharmacodynamics/Kinetics

Half-Life Elimination: Initial: 7-20 minutes; Terminal: 0.5-2.6 hours

Metabolism: Primarily hepatic; aracitidine triphosphate is the active moiety; about 86% to 96% of dose is metabolized to inactive uracil arabinoside

Excretion: Urine (~80% as metabolites) within 24-36 hours

Dosing

Adults & Elderly: I.V. bolus, IVPB, and continuous intravenous infusion doses of cytarabine are very different. Bolus doses are relatively well tolerated since the drug is rapidly metabolized. Continuous infusion uniformly results in myelosuppression. Refer to individual protocols.

Induction remission:

I.V.: 200 mg/m^2/day for 5 days at 2-week intervals

100-200 mg/m^2/day for 5- to 10-day therapy course or every day until remission

I.T.: 5-75 mg/m^2 every 2-7 days until CNS findings normalize

Maintenance remission:

I.V.: 70-200 mg/m^2/day for 2-5 days at monthly intervals

I.M., SubQ: 1-1.5 mg/kg single dose for maintenance at 1- to 4-week intervals

High-dose therapies for leukemia/lymphoma:

Doses as high as 1-3 g/m^2 have been used for refractory or secondary leukemias or refractory non-Hodgkin's lymphoma.

Doses of 1-3 g/m^2 every 12 hours for up to 12 doses have been used

Bone marrow transplant: 1.5 g/m^2 continuous infusion over 48 hours

Pediatrics: I.V. bolus, IVPB, and CIV doses of cytarabine are very different. Bolus doses are relatively well tolerated since the drug is rapidly metabolized; bolus doses are associated with greater gastrointestinal and neurotoxicity; continuous infusion uniformly results in myelosuppression. Refer to individual protocols.

Induction remission:

I.V.: 200 mg/m^2/day for 5 days at 2-week intervals

100-200 mg/m^2/day for 5- to 10-day therapy course or every day until remission

I.T.: 5-75 mg/m^2 every 4 days until CNS findings normalize

or

<1 year: 20 mg

1-2 years: 30 mg

2-3 years: 50 mg

>3 years: 70 mg

Maintenance remission: Refer to adult dosing.

Renal Impairment: In one study, 76% of patients with a Cl$_{cr}$ <60 mL/minute experienced neurotoxicity. Dosage adjustment of high-dose therapy should be considered in patients with renal insufficiency.

Hepatic Impairment: Dose may need to be adjusted in patients with liver failure since cytarabine is partially detoxified in the liver.

Available Dosage Forms

Injection, powder for reconstitution: 100 mg, 500 mg, 1 g, 2 g

Injection, solution: 20 mg/mL (5 mL, 25 mL, 50 mL); 100 mg/mL (20 mL)

Monitoring and Teaching Issues

Physical Assessment: Use with caution in presence of impaired renal and hepatic function (see Warnings/Precautions). Assess potential for interactions with other pharmacological agents patient may be taking (eg, additive myelosuppression, increased risk of cardiomyopathy, pancreatitis; see Drug Interactions). See Administration for I.V. specifics. Premedicate with antiemetic, especially with larger doses. Patient should be monitored closely for anaphylaxis, sudden onset respiratory distress, (especially with high doses). Ocular pain, conjunctivitis, or dermatologic reactions may be reduced with premedication (see Adverse Reactions). Assess results of laboratory tests (BUN, UA, Cr; hepatic function; CBC, platelet count; myelosuppression; see Monitoring Laboratory Tests) prior to therapy and on a regular basis throughout therapy. Teach patient possible side effects/appropriate interventions (eg, importance of adequate hydration) and adverse symptoms to report (see Patient Education).

Monitoring Laboratory Tests: Liver function, CBC with differential and platelet count, serum creatinine, BUN, serum uric acid

Patient Education: Do not take any new medication during therapy unless approved by prescriber. This drug is administered in infusion. You will be monitored closely during infusion; report immediately any redness, swelling, burning, or pain at injection/infusion site, sudden difficulty breathing or swallowing, chest pain, or chills. Maintain adequate hydration (2-3 L/day of fluids) unless instructed to restrict fluid intake. You will be more susceptible to infection (avoid crowds and exposure to infection and do not have any vaccinations without consulting prescriber). May cause nausea, vomiting or loss of appetite (small frequent meals, frequent mouth care, sucking lozenges, or chewing gum may help; if ineffective, consult prescriber for antiemetic medication); diarrhea (buttermilk, boiled milk, or yogurt may help; if persistent, consult with prescriber); mouth sores (use soft toothbrush or cotton swabs for oral care); or dizziness, headache, or confusion (use caution when driving or engaging in potentially hazardous tasks until response to drug is known). Report immediately any signs of CNS changes; change in gait; respiratory distress or respiratory difficulty; easy bruising or bleeding; persistent GI upset; yellowing of eyes or skin; change in color of urine or blackened stool; or any other persistent adverse effects. **Pregnancy/breast-feeding precautions:** Inform prescriber if you are pregnant. Consult prescriber for instruction on appropriate contraceptive measures. This drug may cause severe fetal defects. Breast-feeding is not recommended.

Pregnancy Risk Factor: D

Pregnancy Issues: Cytarabine is teratogenic in animal studies. Limb and ear defects have been noted in case reports when cytarabine has been used during pregnancy. The following have also been noted in the neonate: Pancytopenia, WBC depression, electrolyte abnormalities, prematurity, low birth weight, decreased hematocrit or platelets. Risk to the fetus is decreased if therapy is avoided during the 1st trimester; however, women of childbearing potential should be advised of the potential risks.

Lactation: Excretion in breast milk unknown/not recommended

Administration

I.V.: Can be administered I.M., I.V. infusion, I.T., or SubQ at a concentration not to exceed 100 mg/mL. I.V. may be administered either as a bolus, IVPB (high doses of >500 mg/m²), or continuous intravenous infusion (doses of 100-200 mg/m²). High-dose regimens are usually administered by I.V. infusion over 1-3 hours or as I.V. continuous infusion.

Other: Can be administered intrathecally.

Reconstitution: Reconstitute powder with bacteriostatic water for injection. High-dose regimens are usually administered by I.V. infusion over 1-3 hours or as I.V. continuous infusion; for I.T. use, reconstitute with preservative free saline or preservative free lactated Ringer's solution

Standard I.V. infusion dilution: Dose/250-1000 mL D_5W or NS.

Standard intrathecal dilutions: Dose/3-5 mL lactated Ringer's ± methotrexate (12 mg) ± hydrocortisone (15-50 mg)

Note: Solutions containing bacteriostatic agents should not be used for the preparation of either high doses or intrathecal doses of cytarabine; may be used for I.M., SubQ, and low-dose (100-200 mg/m²) I.V. solution.

Compatibility: Stable in D_5LR, $D_51/4NS$, D_5NS, $D_{10}NS$, D_5W, LR, NS

Y-site administration: Incompatible with allopurinol, amphotericin B cholesteryl sulfate complex, ganciclovir

Compatibility when admixed: Incompatible with fluorouracil, gentamicin, heparin, insulin (regular), nafcillin, oxacillin, penicillin G sodium

Storage:

Powder for reconstitution: Store intact vials of powder at room temperature 15°C to 30°C (59°F to 86°F). Reconstituted solutions are for up to 8 days at room temperature.

Solution: Prior to dilution, store at room temperature, 15°C to 30°C (59°F to 86°F); protect from light.

Additional Information Latex-free products: 100 mg, 500 mg, 1 g, 2 g vials (Cytosar-U®) by Pharmacia-Upjohn

Pyridoxine has been administered on days of high-dose Ara-C therapy for prophylaxis of CNS toxicity.

Related Information

Maternal / Fetal Toxicology on page 1762

♦ **Cytarabine Hydrochloride** see Cytarabine on page 389

Cytarabine (Liposomal) (sye TARE a been lip po SOE mal)

U.S. Brand Names DepoCyt™

Generic Available No

Pharmacologic Category Antineoplastic Agent, Antimetabolite

Medication Safety Issues

Sound-alike/look-alike issues:

Cytarabine may be confused with Cytadren®, Cytosar®, Cytoxan®, vidarabine

DepoCyt™ may be confused with Depoject®

(Continued)

Cytarabine (Liposomal) *(Continued)*

Use Treatment of neoplastic (lymphomatous) meningitis

Mechanism of Action/Effect This is a sustained-release formulation of the active ingredient cytarabine. Acts to inhibit DNA polymerase which decreases DNA synthesis and repair.

Contraindications Hypersensitivity to cytarabine or any component of the formulation; active meningeal infection; pregnancy

Warnings/Precautions The U.S. Food and Drug Administration (FDA) currently recommends that procedures for proper handling and disposal of antineoplastic agents be considered. The incidence and severity of chemical arachnoiditis is reduced by coadministration with dexamethasone. May cause neurotoxicity. Blockage to CSF flow may increase the risk of neurotoxicity.

Drug Interactions

Decreased Effect: No formal studies of interactions with other medications have been conducted. The limited systemic exposure minimizes the potential for interaction between liposomal cytarabine and other medications.

Increased Effect/Toxicity: No formal studies of interactions with other medications have been conducted. The limited systemic exposure minimizes the potential for interaction between liposomal cytarabine and other medications.

Lab Interactions Since cytarabine liposomes are similar in appearance to WBCs, care must be taken in interpreting CSF examinations in patients receiving liposomal cytarabine

Adverse Reactions Chemical arachnoiditis is commonly observed, and may include neck pain, neck rigidity, headache, fever, nausea, vomiting, and back pain. It may occur in up to 100% of cycles without dexamethasone prophylaxis. The incidence is reduced to 33% when dexamethasone is used concurrently.

>10%:
    Central nervous system: Headache (28%), confusion (14%), somnolence (12%), fever (11%), pain (11%)
    Gastrointestinal: Vomiting (12%), nausea (11%)
1% to 10%:
    Cardiovascular: Peripheral edema (7%)
    Gastrointestinal: Constipation (7%)
    Genitourinary: Incontinence (3%)
    Hematologic: Neutropenia (9%), thrombocytopenia (8%), anemia (1%)
    Neuromuscular & skeletal: Back pain (7%), weakness (19%), abnormal gait (4%)

Overdosage/Toxicology No overdosage with liposomal cytarabine has been reported. See Cytarabine *on page 389* for toxicology related to systemic administration.

Pharmacodynamics/Kinetics

Absorption: Systemic exposure following intrathecal administration is negligible since transfer rate from CSF to plasma is slow

Time to Peak: CSF: Intrathecal: ~5 hours

Half-Life Elimination: CSF: 100-263 hours

Metabolism: In plasma to ara-U (inactive)

Excretion: Primarily urine (as metabolites - ara-U)

Dosing

Adults & Elderly:

Lymphomatous meningitis: I.T.:
    Induction: 50 mg intrathecally every 14 days for a total of 2 doses (weeks 1 and 3)
    Consolidation: 50 mg intrathecally every 14 days for 3 doses (weeks 5, 7, and 9), followed by an additional dose at week 13
    Maintenance: 50 mg intrathecally every 28 days for 4 doses (weeks 17, 21, 25, and 29)

Dosage adjustment for toxicity: If drug-related neurotoxicity develops, dose should be reduced to 25 mg. If toxicity persists, treatment with liposomal cytarabine should be discontinued.

Note: Patients should be started on dexamethasone 4 mg twice daily (oral or I.V.) for 5 days, beginning on the day of liposomal cytarabine injection.

Available Dosage Forms Injection, suspension: 10 mg/mL (5 mL) [preservative free]

Monitoring and Teaching Issues

Physical Assessment: This medication if only for intrathecal administration. See Contraindications and Warnings/Precautions for use cautions. Patient must be monitored continuously for adverse reactions (eg, neurotoxicity [myelopathy, ataxia, confusion, coma] and chemical arachnoiditis [neck pain, neck rigidity, headache, fever, nausea, vomiting, and back pain]; see Adverse Reactions). Incidence and severity of chemical arachnoiditis may be reduced by coadministration with dexamethasone (see Adverse Reactions). Provide patient teaching according to patient condition (see Patient Education).

Monitoring Laboratory Tests: Since cytarabine liposomes are similar in appearance to WBCs, care must be taken in interpreting CSF examinations in patients receiving liposomal cytarabine

Patient Education: Patient instruction will be according to mental status. This medication can only be given by infusion into the spinal cord. You will be monitored closely during and after each infusion. Report immediately any neck pain or rigidity; headache; fever; nausea or vomiting. Report any swelling of extremities; acute weakness; unusual gait pattern; incontinence; CNS changes (confusion, speech difficulty); or other adverse effects. **Pregnancy/breast-feeding precautions:** Inform prescriber if you are pregnant. Do not get pregnant during or for 1 month following therapy. Consult prescriber for instruction on appropriate contraceptive measures. Breast-feeding is not recommended.

Pregnancy Risk Factor: D

Pregnancy Issues: Cytarabine may cause fetal harm if a pregnant woman is exposed systemically.

Lactation: Excretion in breast milk unknown/not recommended

Administration

Other: For intrathecal use only. Dose should be removed from vial immediately before administration (must be administered within 4 hours of removal). An in-line filter should **not**

be used. Vials are intended for a single use and contain no preservative. Administer directly into the CSF via an intraventricular reservoir or by direct injection into the lumbar sac. Injection should be made slowly (over 1-5 minutes). Patients should lie flat for 1 hour after lumbar puncture. Patients should be monitored closely for immediate toxic reactions.

Storage: Store under refrigeration (2°C to 8°C); protect from freezing and avoid aggressive agitation. Solutions should be used within 4 hours of withdrawal from the vial. Particles may settle in diluent over time, and may be resuspended by gentle agitation or inversion of the vial.

♦ Cytochrome P450 Enzymes: Substrates, Inhibitors, and Inducers *see page 1744*

♦ CytoGam® *see* Cytomegalovirus Immune Globulin (Intravenous-Human) *on page 393*

Cytomegalovirus Immune Globulin (Intravenous-Human)
(sye toe meg a low VYE rus i MYUN GLOB yoo lin in tra VEE nus HYU man)

U.S. Brand Names CytoGam®

Synonyms CMV-IGIV

Generic Available No

Pharmacologic Category Immune Globulin

Medication Safety Issues
Sound-alike/look-alike issues:
CytoGam® may be confused with Cytoxan®, Gamimune® N

Use Prophylaxis of cytomegalovirus (CMV) disease associated with kidney, lung, liver, pancreas, and heart transplants; concomitant use with ganciclovir should be considered in organ transplants (other than kidney) from CMV seropositive donors to CMV seronegative recipients

Unlabeled/Investigational Use Adjunct therapy in the treatment of CMV disease in immunocompromised patients

Mechanism of Action/Effect CMV-IGIV is a preparation of immunoglobulin G (as well as trace amounts of IgA and IgM) derived from pooled healthy blood donors with a high titer of CMV antibodies; administration provides a passive source of antibodies against cytomegalovirus

Contraindications Hypersensitivity to CMV-IGIV, other immunoglobulins, or any component of the formulation; immunoglobulin A deficiency

Warnings/Precautions Monitor for anaphylactic reactions during infusion. May theoretically transmit blood-borne viruses. Use with caution in patients with renal insufficiency, diabetes mellitus, patients >65 years of age, volume depletion, sepsis, paraproteinemia, or patients on concomitant nephrotoxic drugs. Stabilized with sucrose and albumin, contains no preservative.

Drug Interactions
Decreased Effect: Decreased effect of live vaccines may be seen if given within 3 months of IGIV administration. Defer vaccination or revaccinate.

Adverse Reactions <6%:
Cardiovascular: Flushing
Central nervous system: Fever, chills
Gastrointestinal: Nausea, vomiting
Neuromuscular & skeletal: Arthralgia, back pain, muscle cramps
Respiratory: Wheezing

Overdosage/Toxicology Symptoms related to volume overload would be expected to occur with overdose; treatment is symptom-directed and supportive.

Dosing
Adults:
Kidney transplant: I.V.:
Initial dose (within 72 hours of transplant): 150 mg/kg/dose
2-, 4-, 6-, and 8 weeks after transplant: 100 mg/kg/dose
12 and 16 weeks after transplant: 50 mg/kg/dose

Liver, lung, pancreas, or heart transplant: I.V.:
Initial dose (within 72 hours of transplant): 150 mg/kg/dose
2-, 4-, 6-, and 8 weeks after transplant: 150 mg/kg/dose
12 and 16 weeks after transplant: 100 mg/kg/dose

Severe CMV pneumonia: I.V.: Various regimens have been used, including 400 mg/kg CMV-IGIV in combination with ganciclovir on days 1, 2, 7, or 8, followed by 200 mg/kg CMV-IGIV on days 14 and 21

Elderly: Use with caution in patients >65 years of age; elderly may be at increased risk of renal insufficiency.

Renal Impairment: Use with caution; specific dosing adjustments are not available. Infusion rate should be the minimum practical; do not exceed 180 mg/kg/hour.

Available Dosage Forms Injection, solution [preservative free]: 50 mg ± 10 mg/mL (50 mL) [contains human albumin and sucrose]

Monitoring and Teaching Issues
Physical Assessment: Assess for history of previous allergic reactions. Monitor vital signs during infusion and observe for adverse or allergic reactions. Teach patient adverse symptoms to report.

Patient Education: This medication can only be administered by infusion. You will be monitored closely during the infusion. If you experience nausea ask for assistance, do not get up alone. Do not have any vaccinations for the next 3 months without consulting prescriber. Immediately report chills, muscle cramping, low back pain, chest pain or tightness, or respiratory difficulty. **Pregnancy/breast-feeding precautions:** Inform prescriber if you are or intend to become pregnant. Consult prescriber if breast-feeding.

Pregnancy Risk Factor: C

Lactation: Excretion in breast milk unknown

Administration
I.V.: For I.V. use only. Administer as separate infusion. Infuse beginning at 15 mg/kg/hour, then increase to 30 mg/kg/hour after 30 minutes if no untoward reactions. May titrate up to
(Continued)

Cytomegalovirus Immune Globulin (Intravenous-Human)
(Continued)

60 mg/kg/hour. Do not administer faster than 75 mL/hour. Begin infusion within 6 hours of entering vial, complete infusion within 12 hours.

Reconstitution: Dilution is not recommended. Do not shake vials. Do not use if turbid.

Compatibility: Infusion with other products is not recommended. If unavoidable, may be piggybacked into an I.V. line of sodium chloride, $2.D_5W$, D_5W, $D_{10}W$, or $D_{20}W$; do not dilute more than 1:2

Storage: Store between 2°C and 8°C (35.6°F and 46.4°F)

- ♦ **Cytosar-U®** *see Cytarabine on page 389*
- ♦ **Cytosine Arabinosine Hydrochloride** *see Cytarabine on page 389*
- ♦ **Cytotec®** *see Misoprostol on page 1015*
- ♦ **Cytovene®** *see Ganciclovir on page 695*
- ♦ **Cytoxan®** *see Cyclophosphamide on page 380*
- ♦ **Cytra-2** *see Sodium Citrate and Citric Acid on page 1382*
- ♦ **Cytra-K** *see Potassium Citrate and Citric Acid on page 1236*
- ♦ **Cytuss HC** *see Phenylephrine, Hydrocodone, and Chlorpheniramine on page 1202*
- ♦ **D2E7** *see Adalimumab on page 51*
- ♦ **d4T** *see Stavudine on page 1393*

Dacarbazine *(da KAR ba zeen)*
U.S. Brand Names DTIC-Dome®

Synonyms DIC; Dimethyl Triazeno Imidazole Carboxamide; DTIC; Imidazole Carboxamide; Imidazole Carboxamide Dimethyltriazene; WR-139007

Generic Available Yes

Pharmacologic Category Antineoplastic Agent, Alkylating Agent (Triazene)

Medication Safety Issues
Sound-alike/look-alike issues:
Dacarbazine may be confused with Dicarbosil®, procarbazine

Use Treatment of malignant melanoma, Hodgkin's disease, soft-tissue sarcomas, fibrosarcomas, rhabdomyosarcoma, islet cell carcinoma, medullary carcinoma of the thyroid, and neuroblastoma

Mechanism of Action/Effect Inhibits DNA/RNA and protein synthesis; alkylating agent

Contraindications Hypersensitivity to dacarbazine or any component of the formulation

Warnings/Precautions The U.S. Food and Drug Administration (FDA) currently recommends that procedures for proper handling and disposal of antineoplastic agents be considered. Use with caution in patients with bone marrow depression. In patients with renal and/or hepatic impairment, dosage reduction may be necessary.

Drug Interactions

Cytochrome P450 Effect: Substrate (major) of CYP1A2, 2E1

Decreased Effect: CYP1A2 inducers may decrease the levels/effects of dacarbazine; example inducers include aminoglutethimide, carbamazepine, phenobarbital, and rifampin. Patients may experience impaired immune response to vaccines; possible infection after administration of live vaccines in patients receiving immunosuppressants.

Increased Effect/Toxicity: CYP1A2 inhibitors may increase the levels/effects of dacarbazine; example inhibitors include amiodarone, ciprofloxacin, fluvoxamine, ketoconazole, norfloxacin, ofloxacin, and rofecoxib. CYP2E1 inhibitors may increase the levels/effects of dacarbazine; example inhibitors include disulfiram, isoniazid, and miconazole.

Nutritional/Ethanol Interactions
Ethanol: Avoid ethanol (due to GI irritation).
Herb/Nutraceutical: Avoid dong quai, St John's wort (may also cause photosensitization).

Adverse Reactions
>10%:
Gastrointestinal: Nausea and vomiting (>90%), can be severe and dose-limiting; nausea and vomiting decrease on successive days when dacarbazine is given daily for 5 days; diarrhea
Hematologic: Myelosuppression, leukopenia, thrombocytopenia - dose-limiting
Onset: 5-7 days
Nadir: 7-10 days
Recovery: 21-28 days
Local: Pain on infusion, may be minimized by administration through a central line, or by administration as a short infusion (eg, 1-2 hours as opposed to bolus injection)
1% to 10%:
Dermatologic: Alopecia, rash, photosensitivity
Gastrointestinal: Anorexia, metallic taste
Miscellaneous: Flu-like syndrome (fever, myalgia, malaise)

Overdosage/Toxicology Symptoms of overdose include myelosuppression and diarrhea. There are no known antidotes and treatment is symptomatic and supportive.

Pharmacodynamics/Kinetics
Onset of Action: I.V.: 18-24 days
Protein Binding: 5%
Half-Life Elimination: Biphasic: Initial: 20-40 minutes; Terminal: 5 hours
Metabolism: Extensively hepatic; hepatobiliary excretion is probably of some importance; metabolites may also have an antineoplastic effect
Excretion: Urine (~30% to 50% as unchanged drug)

Dosing
Adults & Elderly: Refer to individual protocols. Some dosage regimens include:
Intra-arterial: 50-400 mg/m² for 5-10 days
Hodgkin's disease, ABVD: 375 mg/m² days 1 and 15 every 4 weeks **or** 100 mg/m²/day for 5 days

Metastatic melanoma (alone or in combination with other agents): I.V.: 150-250 mg/m² days 1-5 every 3-4 weeks

Metastatic melanoma: I.V.: 850 mg/m² every 3 weeks

High dose: Bone marrow/blood cell transplantation: I.V.: 1-3 g/m²; maximum dose as a single agent: 3.38 g/m²; generally combined with other high-dose chemotherapeutic drugs

Pediatrics: Refer to individual protocols.

Pediatric solid tumors: I.V.: 200-470 mg/m²/day over 5 days every 21-28 days

Pediatric neuroblastoma: I.V.: 800-900 mg/m² as a single dose on day 1 of therapy every 3-4 weeks in combination therapy

Hodgkin's disease, ABVD: I.V.: 375 mg/m² on days 1 and 15 of treatment course, repeat every 28 days

Renal Impairment: Adjustment is warranted.

Hepatic Impairment: Monitor closely for signs of toxicity.

Available Dosage Forms Injection, powder for reconstitution: 100 mg, 200 mg, 500 mg

DTIC-Dome®: 200 mg

Monitoring and Teaching Issues

Physical Assessment: Use caution in presence of bone marrow depression, renal and/or hepatic impairment (see Warnings/Precautions). Assess potential for interactions with other pharmacological agents or herbal products patient may be taking (may increase or decrease effects; see Drug Interactions). See Administration for infusion specifics. Premedicate with antiemetic (emetic potential is moderately high). See Administration for infusion specifics. Infusion site must be closely monitored; extravasation can cause severe cellulitis or tissue necrosis. Assess results of laboratory tests (CBC with differential, LFTs) and patient response (see Adverse Reactions) prior to each treatment and on a regular basis throughout therapy. Teach patient possible side effects/appropriate interventions and adverse symptoms to report (see Patient Education).

Monitoring Laboratory Tests: CBC with differential, liver function

Patient Education: Do not take any new medication during therapy unless approved by prescriber. This drug can only be given by infusion. Report immediately any pain, burning, or swelling at infusion site, sudden chest pain, difficulty breathing or swallowing, or chills. Limit oral intake for 4-6 hours before infusion. Between infusions, maintain adequate hydration (2-3 L/day of fluids) unless instructed to restrict fluid intake and nutrition (small frequent meals). You will be more susceptible to infection (avoid crowds and exposure to infection and do not have any vaccinations without consulting prescriber). May cause nausea, vomiting, loss of appetite, or diarrhea (small frequent meals, good mouth care may help; consult prescriber for medication if gastrointestinal reactions are persistent); hair loss (reversible); or headache, fever, sinus congestion, or muscles aches (consult prescriber for analgesic). Report immediately any numbness in extremities or change in gait, respiratory distress or respiratory difficulty; rash; easy bruising or bleeding; yellowing of eyes or skin, change in color of urine or blackened stool; or any other persistent adverse effects.

Pregnancy/breast-feeding precautions: Inform prescriber if you are pregnant. Consult prescriber for instruction on appropriate barrier contraceptive measures. Breast-feeding is not recommended.

Pregnancy Risk Factor: C

Lactation: Excretion in breast milk unknown/not recommended

Administration

I.V.: Irritant. Infuse over 30-60 minutes.

Reconstitution: Reconstitute with a minimum of 2 mL (100 mg vial) or 4 mL (200 mg vial) of SWI, D₅W, or NS. Dilute to a concentration of 10 mg/mL.

Standard I.V. dilution: 250-500 mL D₅W or NS

Compatibility: Stable in NS, SWFI

Y-site administration: Incompatible with allopurinol, cefepime, piperacillin/tazobactam

Compatibility when admixed: Incompatible with hydrocortisone sodium succinate

Storage: Store intact vials under refrigeration (2°C to 8°C) and protect from light. Vials are stable for 4 weeks at room temperature. Reconstituted solution is stable for 24 hours at room temperature (20°C) and 96 hours under refrigeration (4°C). Solutions for infusion (in D₅W or NS) are stable for 24 hours at room temperature and protected from light. Decomposed drug turns pink.

Daclizumab (dac KLYE zue mab)

U.S. Brand Names Zenapax®

Generic Available No

Pharmacologic Category Immunosuppressant Agent

Use Part of an immunosuppressive regimen (including cyclosporine and corticosteroids) for the prophylaxis of acute organ rejection in patients receiving renal transplant

Unlabeled/Investigational Use Graft-versus-host disease

Contraindications Hypersensitivity to daclizumab or any component of the formulation

Warnings/Precautions Patients on immunosuppressive therapy are at increased risk for infectious complications and secondary malignancies. Long-term effects of daclizumab on immune function are unknown. Severe hypersensitivity reactions have been rarely reported; anaphylaxis has been observed on initial exposure and following re-exposure; medications for the management of severe allergic reaction should be available for immediate use. Anti-idiotype antibodies have been measured in patients that have received daclizumab (adults 14%; children 34%); detection of antibodies may be influenced by multiple factors and may therefore be misleading.

In cardiac transplant patients, the combined use of daclizumab, cyclosporine, mycophenolate mofetil, and corticosteroids has been associated with an increased mortality. Higher mortality may be associated with the use of antilymphocyte globulin and a higher incidence of severe infections.

Drug Interactions

Increased Effect/Toxicity: The combined use of daclizumab, cyclosporine, mycophenolate mofetil, and corticosteroids has been associated with an increased mortality in a

(Continued)

Daclizumab *(Continued)*

population of cardiac transplant recipients, particularly in patients who received antilymphocyte globulin and in patients with severe infections.

Adverse Reactions Although reported adverse events are frequent, when daclizumab is compared with placebo the incidence of adverse effects is similar between the two groups. Many of the adverse effects reported during clinical trial use of daclizumab may be related to the patient population, transplant procedure, and concurrent transplant medications. Diarrhea, fever, postoperative pain, pruritus, respiratory tract infection, urinary tract infection, and vomiting occurred more often in children than adults.

≥5%:
Cardiovascular: Chest pain, edema, hyper-/hypotension, tachycardia, thrombosis
Central nervous system: Dizziness, fatigue, fever, headache, insomnia, pain, post-traumatic pain, tremor
Dermatologic: Acne, cellulitis, wound healing impaired
Gastrointestinal: Abdominal distention, abdominal pain, constipation, diarrhea, dyspepsia, epigastric pain, nausea, pyrosis, vomiting
Genitourinary: Dysuria
Hematologic: Bleeding
Neuromuscular & skeletal: Back pain, musculoskeletal pain
Renal: Oliguria, renal tubular necrosis
Respiratory: Cough, dyspnea, pulmonary edema,
Miscellaneous: Lymphocele, wound infection

≥2% to <5%:
Central nervous system: Anxiety, depression, shivering
Dermatologic: Hirsutism, pruritus, rash
Endocrine & metabolic: Dehydration, diabetes mellitus, fluid overload
Gastrointestinal: Flatulence, gastritis, hemorrhoids
Genitourinary: Urinary retention, urinary tract bleeding
Local: Application site reaction
Neuromuscular & skeletal: Arthralgia, leg cramps, myalgia, weakness
Ocular: Vision blurred
Renal: Hydronephrosis, renal damage, renal insufficiency
Respiratory: Atelectasis, congestion, hypoxia, pharyngitis, pleural effusion, rales, rhinitis
Miscellaneous: Night sweats, prickly sensation, diaphoresis

Overdosage/Toxicology Overdose has not been reported.

Pharmacodynamics/Kinetics
Half-Life Elimination: Estimated: Adults: Terminal: 20 days; Children: 13 days

Dosing
Adults:
Note: Daclizumab is used adjunctively with other immunosuppressants (eg, cyclosporine, corticosteroids, mycophenolate mofetil, and azathioprine).
Immunoprophylaxis against acute renal allograft rejection: I.V.: 1 mg/kg infused over 15 minutes within 24 hours before transplantation (day 0), then every 14 days for 4 additional doses
Treatment of graft-versus-host disease (unlabeled use, limited data): I.V.: 0.5-1.5 mg/kg, repeat same dosage for transient response. Repeat doses have been administered 11-48 days following the initial dose.
Elderly: Refer to adult dosing. Use with caution.
Pediatrics: Refer to adult dosing.
Renal Impairment: No dosage adjustment needed.
Hepatic Impairment: No data available for patients with severe impairment.

Available Dosage Forms Injection, solution [preservative free]: 5 mg/mL (5 mL)

Monitoring and Teaching Issues
Physical Assessment: Assess potential for interactions with other prescriptions, OTC medications, or herbal products patient may be taking. Assess cardiorespiratory and renal function (fluid overload) and adverse reactions during infusion and periodically between infusions. Be alert to the possibility of the development of infection or malignancies. **Note:** Hypersensitivity reactions can occur; medications for immediate treatment of severe allergic reactions should be available for immediate use. Teach patient possible side effects/appropriate interventions and adverse symptoms to report.
Patient Education: This medication, which may help transplant rejection, can only be administered by infusion. You will be monitored closely during infusion. Report immediately any respiratory or swallowing difficulty; tightness in jaw or throat; chest pain; or rash, pain, burning, redness, or swelling at infusion site. You will be more susceptible to infection (avoid crowds and exposure to infection and do not have any vaccinations without consulting prescriber). Maintain adequate hydration (2-3 L/day of fluids) unless instructed to restrict fluid intake and nutrition (small frequent meals may be advisable). May cause headache, dizziness, fatigue (use caution when driving or engaged in tasks that require alertness until response to drug is known): back pain, leg cramps, or musculoskeletal pain (consult prescriber for approved analgesic); or nausea, vomiting, dyspepsia, or abdominal discomfort (good mouth care, small frequent meals, chewing gum, or sucking lozenges may help). Report changes in urinary pattern; unusual bleeding or bruising; chest pain or palpitations; persistent dizziness, tremors, or headache; respiratory difficulty or unusual cough; rash; opportunistic infection (vaginal itching or drainage, sores in mouth, unusual fever or chills); or other persistent adverse effects. **Pregnancy/breast-feeding precautions:** Inform prescriber if you are or intend to become pregnant. Consult prescriber if breast-feeding.

Pregnancy Risk Factor: C
Pregnancy Issues: Animal reproduction studies have not been conducted. Generally, IgG molecules cross the placenta. Do not use during pregnancy unless the potential benefit to the mother outweighs the possible risk to the fetus. Women of childbearing potential should use effective contraception before, during, and for 4 months following treatment.

Lactation: Excretion in breast milk unknown/use caution

Administration

I.V.: For I.V. administration following dilution. Daclizumab solution should be administered within 4 hours of preparation if stored at room temperature; infuse over a 15-minute period via a peripheral or central vein.

Reconstitution: Dose should be further diluted in 50 mL 0.9% sodium chloride solution. When mixing, gently invert bag to avoid foaming; do not shake. Do not use if solution is discolored. Diluted solution is stable for 24 hours at 4°C or for 4 hours at room temperature.

Compatibility: Do not mix with other medications or infuse other medications through same I.V. line.

Storage: Refrigerate vials at 2°C to 8°C (36°F to 46°F). Do not shake or freeze; protect undiluted solution against direct sunlight.

♦ DACT see Dactinomycin on page 397

Dactinomycin (dak ti noe MYE sin)

U.S. Brand Names Cosmegen®

Synonyms ACT; Act-D; Actinomycin; Actinomycin Cl; Actinomycin D; DACT; NSC-3053

Generic Available No

Pharmacologic Category Antineoplastic Agent, Antibiotic

Medication Safety Issues

Sound-alike/look-alike issues:

Dactinomycin may be confused with DAUNOrubicin

Actinomycin may be confused with Achromycin

Use Treatment of testicular tumors, melanoma, choriocarcinoma, Wilms' tumor, neuroblastoma, retinoblastoma, rhabdomyosarcoma, uterine sarcomas, Ewing's sarcoma, Kaposi's sarcoma, sarcoma botryoides, and soft tissue sarcoma

Mechanism of Action/Effect Causes cell death by inhibiting messenger RNA

Contraindications Hypersensitivity to dactinomycin or any component of the formulation; patients with concurrent or recent chickenpox or herpes zoster; avoid in infants <6 months of age

Warnings/Precautions The U.S. Food and Drug Administration (FDA) currently recommends that procedures for proper handling and disposal of antineoplastic agents be considered. Drug is extremely irritating to tissues and must be administered I.V. If extravasation occurs during I.V. use, severe damage to soft tissues will occur. Use with caution in patients who have received radiation therapy or in the presence of hepatobiliary dysfunction. Reduce dosage in patients who are receiving radiation therapy simultaneously. Toxic effects may be delayed in onset (2-4 days following a course of treatment). Effects may require 1-2 weeks to reach maximum severity.

Drug Interactions

Increased Effect/Toxicity: Dactinomycin potentiates the effects of radiation therapy.

Lab Interactions May interfere with bioassays of antibacterial drug levels

Adverse Reactions

>10%:

Central nervous system: Fatigue, malaise, fever, lethargy

Dermatologic: Alopecia (reversible), skin eruptions, acne, increased pigmentation or sloughing of previously irradiated skin, maculopapular rash

Endocrine & metabolic: Hypocalcemia

Gastrointestinal: Severe nausea, vomiting, anorexia

Hematologic: Myelosuppression, anemia

Onset: 7 days

Nadir: 14-21 days

Recovery: 21-28 days

Local: Extravasation: An irritant and should be administered through a rapidly running I.V. line; extravasation can lead to tissue necrosis, pain, and ulceration

1% to 10%: Gastrointestinal: Mucositis, stomatitis, diarrhea, abdominal pain

Overdosage/Toxicology Symptoms of overdose include myelosuppression, nausea, vomiting, glossitis, and oral ulceration. There are no known antidotes and treatment is symptomatic and supportive. Toxic effects may not be apparent until 2-4 days after a treatment course (peak after 1-2 weeks).

Pharmacodynamics/Kinetics

Time to Peak: Serum: I.V.: 2-5 minutes

Half-Life Elimination: 36 hours

Metabolism: Hepatic, minimal

Excretion: Bile (50%); feces (14%); urine (~10% as unchanged drug)

Dosing

Adults & Elderly: Refer to individual protocols.

Note: Medication orders for dactinomycin are commonly written in MICROgrams (eg, 150 mcg) although many regimens list the dose in MILLIgrams (eg, mg/kg or mg/m^2). One-time doses for >1000 mcg, or multiple-day doses for >500 mcg/day are not common. Some practitioners recommend calculation of the dosage for obese or edematous patients on the basis of body surface area in an effort to relate dosage to lean body mass.

I.V.: 2.5 mg/m^2 in divided doses over 1 week, repeated every 2 weeks **or**

0.75-2 mg/m^2 every 1-4 weeks **or**

400-600 mcg/m^2/day for 5 days, repeated every 3-6 weeks

Pediatrics: Refer to individual protocols.

Note: Dactinomycin doses are almost ALWAYS expressed in MICROGRAMS rather than milligrams. Some practitioners recommend calculation of the dosage for obese or edematous patients on the basis of body surface area in an effort to relate dosage to lean body mass.

Usual dose: I.V.: Children >6 months: 15 mcg/kg/day **or** 400-600 mcg/m^2/day for 5 days every 3-6 weeks

(Continued)

Dactinomycin *(Continued)*

Renal Impairment: No adjustment is necessary.

Available Dosage Forms Injection, powder for reconstitution: 0.5 mg [contains mannitol 20 mg]

Monitoring and Teaching Issues

Physical Assessment: Use with caution in patients who have received or are receiving radiation therapy or in the presence of hepatobiliary dysfunction (see Warnings/Precautions). See Administration for infusion specifics. Premedicate with antiemetic (highly emetic). Infusion site must be closely monitored; extravasation can cause severe cellulitis or tissue necrosis. Assess results of laboratory tests (eg, hematological, renal, and hepatic function). Monitor patient response (eg, myelosuppression, nausea, vomiting, glossitis, and oral ulceration; see Adverse Reactions) prior to each treatment and on a regular basis throughout therapy. Teach patient possible side effects/appropriate interventions and adverse symptoms to report (see Patient Education).

Monitoring Laboratory Tests: CBC with differential and platelet count, liver and renal function

Patient Education: Do not take any new medication during therapy unless approved by prescriber. This drug can only be given by infusion; report immediately any pain, burning, or swelling at infusion site; sudden chest pain, difficulty breathing or swallowing, or chills. Limit oral intake for 4-6 hours immediately before infusion. Between infusions, maintain adequate hydration (2-3 L/day of fluids) unless instructed to restrict fluid intake and nutrition (small frequent meals). You will be more susceptible to infection (avoid crowds and exposure to infection and do not have any vaccinations without consulting prescriber). May cause fatigue or malaise (use caution when driving or engaging in potentially hazardous tasks until response to drug is known); nausea, vomiting, loss of appetite, and diarrhea (consult prescriber for medication); or hair loss (reversible). Report unresolved nausea, vomiting, diarrhea, abdominal pain; difficulty swallowing; rash; or any other persistent adverse effects. **Pregnancy/breast-feeding precautions:** Inform prescriber if you are or intend to become pregnant. Do not breast-feed.

Pregnancy Risk Factor: C

Pregnancy Issues: Malformations reported in animal studies. No controlled studies in pregnant women. Use only when potential benefit justifies potential risk to the fetus.

Lactation: Excretion in breast milk unknown/contraindicated

Breast-Feeding Issues: It is not known if dactinomycin is excreted in human breast milk. Due to the potential for serious reactions in the infant, breast-feeding is not recommended.

Administration

I.V.: Vesicant. Infuse over 10-15 minutes.

Reconstitution: Dilute with 1.1 mL of preservative-free SWI to yield a final concentration of 500 mcg/mL; do not use preservative diluent as precipitation may occur.

Compatibility: Stable in D_5W, NS, SWFI

Y-site administration: Incompatible with filgrastim

Storage: Store intact vials at controlled room temperature 15°C to 30°C (59°F to 86°F) and protect from light, humidity, and heat. Reconstituted solutions are chemically stable under refrigeration for up to 60 days. Solutions in 50 mL D_5W or NS are stable for 24 hours at room temperature.

♦ **DAD** *see Mitoxantrone on page 1019*

♦ **Dalmane®** *see Flurazepam on page 655*

♦ **d-Alpha Tocopherol** *see Vitamin E on page 1569*

Dalteparin *(dal TE pa rin)*

U.S. Brand Names Fragmin®

Generic Available No

Pharmacologic Category Low Molecular Weight Heparin

Use Prevention of deep vein thrombosis which may lead to pulmonary embolism, in patients requiring abdominal surgery who are at risk for thromboembolism complications (eg, patients >40 years of age, obesity, patients with malignancy, history of deep vein thrombosis or pulmonary embolism, and surgical procedures requiring general anesthesia and lasting >30 minutes); prevention of DVT in patients undergoing hip-replacement surgery; patients immobile during an acute illness; acute treatment of unstable angina or non-Q-wave myocardial infarction; prevention of ischemic complications in patients on concurrent aspirin therapy

Unlabeled/Investigational Use Active treatment of deep vein thrombosis

Mechanism of Action/Effect Low molecular weight heparin analog; the commercial product contains 3% to 15% heparin; has been shown to inhibit both factor Xa and factor IIa (thrombin), however, the antithrombotic effect of dalteparin is characterized by a higher ratio of antifactor Xa to antifactor IIa activity (ratio = 4)

Contraindications Hypersensitivity to dalteparin or any component of the formulation; thrombocytopenia associated with a positive *in vitro* test for antiplatelet antibodies in the presence of dalteparin; hypersensitivity to heparin or pork products; patients with active major bleeding; patients with unstable angina or non-Q-wave MI undergoing regional anesthesia; not for I.M. or I.V. use

Warnings/Precautions Patients with recent or anticipated neuraxial anesthesia (epidural or spinal anesthesia) are at risk of spinal or epidural hematoma and subsequent paralysis. Consider risk versus benefit prior to neuraxial anesthesia. Risk is increased by concomitant agents which may alter hemostasis, as well as traumatic or repeated epidural or spinal puncture. Patient should be observed closely for bleeding if dalteparin is administered during or immediately following diagnostic lumbar puncture, epidural anesthesia, or spinal anesthesia.

Not to be used interchangeably (unit for unit) with heparin or any other low molecular weight heparins. Use caution in patients with known hypersensitivity to methylparaben or propylparaben, renal failure, or a history of heparin-induced thrombocytopenia. Monitor platelet count closely. Rare thrombocytopenia may occur. Consider discontinuation of dalteparin in any patient developing significant thrombocytopenia. Monitor patient closely for signs or symptoms of bleeding. Certain patients are at increased risk of bleeding. Risk factors include bacterial endocarditis; congenital or acquired bleeding disorders; active ulcerative or angiodysplastic GI diseases; severe uncontrolled hypertension; hemorrhagic stroke; or use shortly after brain, spinal, or ophthalmology surgery; in patient treated concomitantly with platelet inhibitors; recent GI bleeding; thrombocytopenia or platelet defects; severe liver disease; hypertensive or diabetic retinopathy; or in patients undergoing invasive procedures. Rare cases of thrombocytopenia with thrombosis have occurred. Multidose vials contain benzyl alcohol and should not be used in pregnant women. Heparin can cause hyperkalemia by affecting aldosterone. Similar reactions could occur with LMWHs. Monitor for hyperkalemia. Safety and efficacy in pediatric patients have not been established.

Drug Interactions
  Increased Effect/Toxicity: The risk of bleeding with dalteparin may be increased by drugs which affect platelet function (eg, aspirin, NSAIDs, dipyridamole, ticlopidine, clopidogrel), oral anticoagulants, and thrombolytic agents. Although the risk of bleeding may be increased during concurrent warfarin therapy, dalteparin is commonly continued during the initiation of warfarin therapy to assure anticoagulation and to protect against possible transient hypercoagulability.

Nutritional/Ethanol Interactions Herb/Nutraceutical: Avoid cat's claw, dong quai, evening primrose, garlic, ginseng (all have additional antiplatelet activity).

Lab Interactions Increased AST, ALT levels

Adverse Reactions 1% to 10%:
  Hematologic: Bleeding (3% to 5%), wound hematoma (0.1% to 3%)
  Local: Pain at injection site (up to 12%), injection site hematoma (0.2% to 7%)

Pharmacodynamics/Kinetics
  Onset of Action: 1-2 hours
  Duration of Action: >12 hours
  Time to Peak: Serum: 4 hours
  Half-Life Elimination: Route dependent: 2-5 hours

Dosing
  Adults & Elderly:
    Abdominal surgery (DVT prophylaxis):
     Low-to-moderate DVT risk: SubQ: 2500 int. units 1-2 hours prior to surgery, then once daily for 5-10 days postoperatively
     High DVT risk: SubQ: 5000 int. units 1-2 hours prior to surgery and then once daily for 5-10 days postoperatively
    Total hip surgery (DVT prophylaxis): SubQ: **Note:** Three treatment options are currently available. Dose is given for 5-10 days, although up to 14 days of treatment have been tolerated in clinical trials:
     Postoperative start:
     Initial: 2500 int. units 4-8 hours* after surgery
     Maintenance: 5000 int. units once daily; start at least 6 hours after postsurgical dose
     Preoperative (starting day of surgery):
     Initial: 2500 int. units within 2 hours before surgery
     Adjustment: 2500 int. units 4-8 hours* after surgery
     Maintenance: 5000 int. units once daily; start at least 6 hours after postsurgical dose
     Preoperative (starting evening prior to surgery):
     Initial: 5000 int. units 10-14 hours before surgery
     Adjustment: 5000 int. units 4-8 hours* after surgery
     Maintenance: 5000 int. units once daily, allowing 24 hours between doses.
     *Note: Dose may be delayed if hemostasis is not yet achieved.
    Unstable angina or non-Q-wave myocardial infarction: SubQ: 120 int. units/kg body weight (maximum dose: 10,000 int. units) every 12 hours for 5-8 days with concurrent aspirin therapy. Discontinue dalteparin once patient is clinically stable.
    Immobility/acute illness (DVT prophylaxis): 5000 int. units once daily

Available Dosage Forms
Injection, solution [multidose vial]: Antifactor Xa 10,000 int. units per 1 mL (9.5 mL) [contains benzyl alcohol]; antifactor Xa 25,000 units per 1 mL (3.8 mL) [contains benzyl alcohol]
Injection, solution [preservative free; prefilled syringe]: Antifactor Xa 2500 int. units per 0.2 mL (0.2 mL); antifactor Xa 5000 int. units per 0.2 mL (0.2 mL); antifactor Xa 7500 int. units per 0.3 mL (0.3 mL); antifactor Xa 10,000 int. units per 1 mL (1 mL)

Monitoring and Teaching Issues
  Physical Assessment: Use caution in presence or history of conditions that increase risk of bleeding or other complications (see Contraindications and Warnings/Precautions). Assess potential for interactions with other pharmacological agents or herbal products patient may be taking (especially anything that will impact coagulation or platelet aggregation; see Drug Interactions). Monitor results of laboratory tests (see Monitoring Laboratory Tests), therapeutic effectiveness according to purpose for use, and adverse response (eg, thrombocytopenia; see Adverse Reactions). Teach patient possible side effects/appropriate interventions and adverse symptoms to report (see Patient Education).

  Monitoring Laboratory Tests: Periodic CBC including platelet count, stool occult blood; monitoring of PT and PTT is not necessary.

  Patient Education: Do not take any new medication during therapy unless approved by prescriber (especially anything containing aspirin). This drug can only be administered by injection. You may have a tendency to bleed easily while taking this drug (brush teeth with soft brush, use waxed dental floss, use electric razor, avoid scissors or sharp knives and potentially harmful activities). Report unusual fever; unusual bleeding or bruising (bleeding gums, nosebleed, blood in urine, dark stool); pain in joints or back; severe head pain; skin rash; or redness, swelling, or pain at injection site. **Breast-feeding precaution:** Consult prescriber if breast-feeding.

Pregnancy Risk Factor: B
Pregnancy Issues: Multiple-dose vials contain benzyl alcohol (avoid in pregnant women due to association with fetal syndrome in premature infants).
(Continued)

Dalteparin *(Continued)*

Lactation: Excretion in breast milk unknown/use caution

Administration

I.M.: Do not give I.M.

Other: For deep SubQ injection only. May be injected in a U-shape to the area surrounding the navel, the upper outer side of the thigh, or the upper outer quadrangle of the buttock. Apply pressure to injection site; do not massage. Use thumb and forefinger to lift a fold of skin when injecting dalteparin to the navel area or thigh. Insert needle at a 45- to 90-degree angle. The entire length of needle should be inserted. Do not expel air bubble from fixed-dose syringe prior to injection. Air bubble (and extra solution, if applicable) may be expelled from graduated syringes.

Administration once daily beginning prior to surgery and continuing 5-10 days after surgery prevents deep vein thrombosis in patients at risk for thromboembolic complications. For unstable angina or non-Q-wave myocardial infarction, dalteparin is administered every 12 hours until the patient is stable (5-8 days).

Storage: Store at temperatures 20°C to 25°C (68°F to 77°F).

Additional Information Multidose vial contains 14 mg/mL benzyl alcohol.

Related Information

Anticoagulants, Injectable *on page 1711*

♦ **Damason-P®** *see* Hydrocodone and Aspirin *on page 757*

Danazol *(DA na zole)*

U.S. Brand Names Danocrine® [DSC]

Generic Available Yes

Pharmacologic Category Androgen

Medication Safety Issues

Sound-alike/look-alike issues:

Danazol may be confused with Dantrium®

Danocrine® may be confused with Dacriose®

Use Treatment of endometriosis, fibrocystic breast disease, and hereditary angioedema

Mechanism of Action/Effect Suppresses pituitary output of follicle-stimulating hormone and luteinizing hormone that causes regression and atrophy of normal and ectopic endometrial tissue; decreases rate of growth of abnormal breast tissue; reduces attacks associated with hereditary angioedema by increasing levels of C4 component of complement

Contraindications Hypersensitivity to danazol or any component of the formulation; undiagnosed genital bleeding; pregnancy; breast-feeding; porphyria; markedly impaired hepatic, renal, or cardiac function

Warnings/Precautions Use with caution in patients with seizure disorders, migraine, or conditions influenced by edema. Thromboembolism, thrombotic, and thrombophlebitic events have been reported (including life-threatening or fatal strokes). Peliosis hepatis and benign hepatic adenoma have been reported with long-term use. May cause benign intracranial hypertension. Breast cancer should be ruled out prior to treatment for fibrocystic breast disease. May increase risk of atherosclerosis and coronary artery disease. May cause nonreversible androgenic effects. Pregnancy must be ruled out prior to treatment. Safety and efficacy in pediatric patients have not been established.

Drug Interactions

Cytochrome P450 Effect: Inhibits CYP3A4 (weak)

Decreased Effect: Danazol may decrease effectiveness of hormonal contraceptives. Nonhormonal birth control methods are recommended.

Increased Effect/Toxicity: Danazol may increase serum levels of carbamazepine, cyclosporine, tacrolimus, and warfarin leading to toxicity; dosage adjustment may be needed; monitor. Concomitant use of danazol and HMG-CoA reductase inhibitors may lead to severe myopathy or rhabdomyolysis. Danazol may enhance the glucose-lowering effect of hypoglycemic agents.

Nutritional/Ethanol Interactions Food: Delays time to peak; high-fat meal increases plasma concentration

Lab Interactions Testosterone, androstenedione, dehydroepiandrosterone

Adverse Reactions Frequency not defined.

Cardiovascular: Benign intracranial hypertension (rare), edema, flushing, hypertension

Central nervous system: Anxiety (rare), chills (rare), convulsions (rare), depression, dizziness, emotional lability, fainting, fever (rare), Guillain-Barré syndrome, headache, nervousness, sleep disorders, tremor

Dermatologic: Acne, hair loss, mild hirsutism, maculopapular rash, papular rash, petechial rash, pruritus, purpuric rash, seborrhea, Stevens-Johnson syndrome (rare), photosensitivity (rare), urticaria, vesicular rash

Endocrine & metabolic: Amenorrhea (which may continue post therapy), breast size reduction, clitoris hypertrophy, glucose intolerance, HDL decreased, LDL increased, libido changes, nipple discharge, menstrual disturbances (spotting, altered timing of cycle), semen abnormalities (changes in volume, viscosity, sperm count/motility), spermatogenesis reduction

Gastrointestinal: Appetite changes (rare), bleeding gums (rare), constipation, gastroenteritis, nausea, pancreatitis (rare), vomiting, weight gain

Genitourinary: Vaginal dryness, vaginal irritation, pelvic pain

Hematologic: Eosinophilia, erythrocytosis (reversible), leukocytosis, leukopenia, platelet count increased, polycythemia, RBC increased, thrombocytopenia

Hepatic: Cholestatic jaundice, hepatic adenoma, jaundice, liver enzymes (elevated), malignant tumors (after prolonged use), peliosis hepatis

Neuromuscular & skeletal: Back pain, carpal tunnel syndrome (rare), extremity pain, joint lockup, joint pain, joint swelling, muscle cramps, neck pain, paresthesia, spasms, weakness

Ocular: Cataracts (rare), visual disturbances

Renal: Hematuria

Respiratory: Nasal congestion (rare)

Miscellaneous: Voice change (hoarseness, sore throat, instability, deepening of pitch), diaphoresis

Pharmacodynamics/Kinetics

Onset of Action: Therapeutic: ~4 weeks

Time to Peak: Serum: Within 2 hours

Half-Life Elimination: Variable: 4.5 hours

Metabolism: Extensively hepatic, primarily to 2-hydroxymethylethisterone

Excretion: Urine

Dosing

Adults & Elderly:

Endometriosis: Oral: Initial: 200-400 mg/day in 2 divided doses for mild disease; individualize dosage. Usual maintenance dose: 800 mg/day in 2 divided doses to achieve amenorrhea and rapid response to painful symptoms. Continue therapy uninterrupted for 3-6 months (up to 9 months).

Fibrocystic breast disease (Female): Oral: Range: 100-400 mg/day in 2 divided doses

Hereditary angioedema (Male/Female): Oral: Initial: 200 mg 2-3 times/day; after favorable response, decrease the dosage by 50% or less at intervals of 1-3 months or longer if the frequency of attacks dictates. If an attack occurs, increase the dosage by up to 200 mg/day.

Available Dosage Forms [DSC] = Discontinued product

Capsule: 50 mg, 100 mg, 200 mg

Danocrine®: 50 mg, 100 mg, 200 mg [DSC]

Monitoring and Teaching Issues

Physical Assessment: Use caution in the presence of or history of seizure disorders, migraine headaches, cardiac disease, hepatic or renal impairment (see Warnings/Precautions). Assess potential for interactions with other pharmacological agents patient may be taking (eg, anticoagulants and hypoglycemic agents; see Drug Interactions). Assess results of laboratory tests, therapeutic effectiveness according to purpose for use, and adverse response (eg, hypertension, increased LDL, CNS changes, jaundice, hematuria; see Adverse Reactions). Caution patients with diabetes to monitor glucose levels closely (may enhance the glucose-lowering effect of hypoglycemic agents). Teach patient proper use, possible side effects/appropriate interventions (eg, good self-breast-exam technique), and adverse symptoms to report (see Patient Education). **Pregnancy risk factor X:** Determine that patient is not pregnant before starting therapy. Do not give to female patients of childbearing age unless capable of complying with barrier contraceptive use. Instruct patient in appropriate contraceptive measures.

Monitoring Laboratory Tests: Liver and renal function

Patient Education: Do not take any new medication during therapy unless approved by prescriber. Take as directed; do not discontinue without consulting prescriber. Therapy may take up to several months depending on purpose for therapy. If you have diabetes, monitor serum glucose closely and notify prescriber of changes; this medication can alter hypoglycemic requirements. Consult prescriber for appropriate self breast exam technique. May cause headache, sleeplessness, anxiety (use caution when driving or engaging in potentially hazardous tasks until response to drug is known); acne, growth of body hair, deepening of voice, loss of libido, impotence, or menstrual irregularity (usually reversible). Report changes in menstrual pattern; deepening of voice or unusual growth of body hair; persistent penile erections; fluid retention (eg, swelling of ankles, feet, or hands, respiratory difficulty, or sudden weight gain); change in color of urine or stool; yellowing of eyes or skin; unusual bruising or bleeding; or other adverse reactions. **Pregnancy/breast-feeding precautions:** Inform prescriber if you are pregnant. Consult prescriber for appropriate barrier contraceptive measures. This drug may cause severe fetal defects. Do not donate blood during or for 1 month following therapy. Do not breast-feed.

Pregnancy Risk Factor: X

Pregnancy Issues: Pregnancy should be ruled out prior to treatment using a sensitive test (beta subunit test, if available). Nonhormonal contraception should be used during therapy. May cause androgenic effects to the female fetus; clitoral hypertrophy, labial fusion, urogenital sinus defect, vaginal atresia, and ambiguous genitalia have been reported.

Lactation: Enters breast milk/contraindicated

Administration

Storage: Store at controlled room temperature of 15°C to 30°C (59°F to 86°F).

♦ **Danocrine® [DSC]** *see* Danazol *on page 400*

♦ **Dantrium®** *see* Dantrolene *on page 401*

Dantrolene (DAN troe leen)

U.S. Brand Names Dantrium®

Synonyms Dantrolene Sodium

Generic Available No

Pharmacologic Category Skeletal Muscle Relaxant

Medication Safety Issues

Sound-alike/look-alike issues:

Dantrium® may be confused with danazol, Daraprim®

Use Treatment of spasticity associated with spinal cord injury, stroke, cerebral palsy, or multiple sclerosis; treatment of malignant hyperthermia

Unlabeled/Investigational Use Neuroleptic malignant syndrome (NMS)

Mechanism of Action/Effect Acts directly on skeletal muscle by interfering with release of calcium ion from the sarcoplasmic reticulum; prevents or reduces the increase in myoplasmic calcium ion concentration that activates the acute catabolic processes associated with malignant hyperthermia

Contraindications Active hepatic disease; should not be used where spasticity is used to maintain posture or balance

(Continued)

Dantrolene *(Continued)*

Warnings/Precautions Use with caution in patients with impaired cardiac function or impaired pulmonary function. Has potential for hepatotoxicity. Overt hepatitis has been most frequently observed between the third and twelfth month of therapy. Hepatic injury appears to be greater in females and in patients >35 years of age.

Drug Interactions

Cytochrome P450 Effect: Substrate of CYP3A4 (major)

Decreased Effect: CYP3A4 inducers may decrease the levels/effects of dantrolene; example inducers include aminoglutethimide, carbamazepine, nafcillin, nevirapine, phenobarbital, phenytoin, and rifamycins.

Increased Effect/Toxicity: Increased toxicity with estrogens (hepatotoxicity), CNS depressants (sedation), MAO inhibitors, phenothiazines, clindamycin (increased neuromuscular blockade), verapamil (hyperkalemia and cardiac depression), warfarin, clofibrate, and tolbutamide. CYP3A4 inhibitors may increase the levels/effects of dantrolene; example inhibitors include azole antifungals, ciprofloxacin, clarithromycin, diclofenac, doxycycline, erythromycin, imatinib, isoniazid, nefazodone, nicardipine, propofol, protease inhibitors, quinidine, and verapamil.

Nutritional/Ethanol Interactions

Ethanol: Avoid ethanol (may increase CNS depression).

Herb/Nutraceutical: Avoid valerian, St John's wort, kava kava, gotu kola (may increase CNS depression).

Lab Interactions Increased aminotransferase [ALT (SGPT)/AST (SGOT)] (S), alkaline phosphatase, LDH, BUN, and total serum bilirubin

Adverse Reactions

>10%:

Central nervous system: Drowsiness, dizziness, lightheadedness, fatigue

Dermatologic: Rash

Gastrointestinal: Diarrhea (mild), nausea, vomiting

Neuromuscular & skeletal: Muscle weakness

1% to 10%:

Cardiovascular: Pleural effusion with pericarditis

Central nervous system: Chills, fever, headache, insomnia, nervousness, mental depression

Gastrointestinal: Diarrhea (severe), constipation, anorexia, stomach cramps

Ocular: Blurred vision

Respiratory: Respiratory depression

Overdosage/Toxicology Symptoms of overdose include CNS depression, hypotension, nausea, and vomiting. For decontamination, lavage with activated charcoal and administer a cathartic. Do not use ipecac. Other treatment is supportive and symptomatic.

Pharmacodynamics/Kinetics

Absorption: Oral: Slow and incomplete

Half-Life Elimination: 8.7 hours

Metabolism: Hepatic

Excretion: Feces (45% to 50%); urine (25% as unchanged drug and metabolites)

Dosing

Adults & Elderly:

Spasticity: Oral: 25 mg/day to start, increase frequency to 2-4 times/day, then increase dose by 25 mg every 4-7 days to a maximum of 100 mg 2-4 times/day or 400 mg/day

Malignant hyperthermia:

Preoperative prophylaxis:

Oral: 4-8 mg/kg/day in 4 divided doses, begin 1-2 days prior to surgery with last dose 3-4 hours prior to surgery

I.V.: 2.5 mg/kg ~1¼ hours prior to anesthesia and infused over 1 hour with additional doses as needed and individualized

Crisis: I.V.: 2.5 mg/kg; may repeat dose up to cumulative dose of 10 mg/kg; if physiologic and metabolic abnormalities reappear, repeat regimen

Postcrisis follow-up: Oral: 4-8 mg/kg/day in 4 divided doses for 1-3 days; I.V. dantrolene may be used when oral therapy is not practical; individualize dosage beginning with 1 mg/kg or more as the clinical situation dictates

Neuroleptic malignant syndrome (unlabeled use): I.V.: 1 mg/kg; may repeat dose up to maximum cumulative dose of 10 mg/kg, then switch to oral dosage

Pediatrics:

Spasticity: Oral: Initial: 0.5 mg/kg/dose twice daily, increase frequency to 3-4 times/day at 4- to 7-day intervals, then increase dose by 0.5 mg/kg to a maximum of 3 mg/kg/dose 2-4 times/day up to 400 mg/day

Malignant hyperthermia: Refer to adult dosing.

Available Dosage Forms

Capsule, as sodium: 25 mg, 50 mg, 100 mg

Injection, powder for reconstitution, as sodium: 20 mg [contains mannitol 3 g]

Monitoring and Teaching Issues

Physical Assessment: Assess effectiveness and interactions of other medications patient may be taking. I.V.: Monitor vital signs, cardiac function, respiratory status, and I.V. site (extravasation very irritating to tissues). Monitor effectiveness of therapy and adverse reactions at beginning and periodically during therapy. Assess knowledge/teach patient appropriate use, interventions to reduce side effects, and adverse symptoms to report.

Monitoring Laboratory Tests: Liver function for potential hepatotoxicity

Patient Education: Take exactly as directed. Do not increase dose or discontinue without consulting prescriber. Do not use alcohol, prescriptive or OTC antidepressants, sedatives, or pain medications without consulting prescriber. You may experience drowsiness, dizziness, lightheadedness (avoid driving or engaging in tasks that require alertness until response to drug is known); nausea or vomiting (small frequent meals, frequent mouth care, or sucking hard candy may help); or diarrhea (buttermilk, boiled milk, or yogurt may help). Report excessive confusion; drowsiness or mental agitation; chest pain, palpitations, or respiratory difficulty; skin rash; or vision changes. **Pregnancy/breast-feeding precautions:** Inform prescriber if you are or intend to become pregnant. Breast-feeding is not recommended.

Pregnancy Risk Factor: C

Lactation: Excretion in breast milk unknown/not recommended

Administration

I.V.: Therapeutic or emergency dose can be administered with rapid continuous I.V. push. Follow-up doses should be administered over 2-3 minutes.

Reconstitution: Reconstitute vial by adding 60 mL of sterile water for injection USP (**not bacteriostatic water for injection**). Protect from light. Use within 6 hours. Avoid glass bottles for I.V. infusion.

♦ **Dantrolene Sodium** *see Dantrolene on page 401*

♦ **Dapcin** *see Daptomycin on page 404*

♦ **Dapiprazole** *see page 1625*

Dapsone (DAP sone)

Synonyms Diaminodiphenylsulfone

Generic Available Yes

Pharmacologic Category Antibiotic, Miscellaneous

Medication Safety Issues

Sound-alike/look-alike issues:

Dapsone may be confused with Diprosone®

Use Treatment of leprosy and dermatitis herpetiformis (infections caused by *Mycobacterium leprae*)

Unlabeled/Investigational Use Prophylaxis of toxoplasmosis in severely-immunocompromised patients; alternative agent for *Pneumocystis carinii* pneumonia prophylaxis (monotherapy) and treatment (in combination with trimethoprim)

Mechanism of Action/Effect Dapsone is a sulfone antimicrobial that prevents normal bacterial utilization of PABA for the synthesis of folic acid.

Contraindications Hypersensitivity to dapsone or any component of the formulation

Warnings/Precautions Use with caution in patients with severe anemia, G6PD deficiency, hypersensitivity to other sulfonamides, or restricted hepatic function.

Drug Interactions

Cytochrome P450 Effect: Substrate of CYP2C8/9 (minor), 2C19 (minor), 2E1 (minor), 3A4 (major)

Decreased Effect: Para-aminobenzoic acid and rifampin levels are decreased when given with dapsone. CYP3A4 inducers may decrease the levels/effects of dapsone; example inducers include aminoglutethimide, carbamazepine, nafcillin, nevirapine, phenobarbital, phenytoin, and rifamycins.

Increased Effect/Toxicity: Folic acid antagonists (methotrexate) may increase the risk of hematologic reactions of dapsone; probenecid decreases dapsone excretion; trimethoprim with dapsone may increase toxic effects of both drugs. CYP3A4 inhibitors may increase the levels/effects of dapsone; example inhibitors include azole antifungals, ciprofloxacin, clarithromycin, diclofenac, doxycycline, erythromycin, imatinib, isoniazid, nefazodone, nicardipine, propofol, protease inhibitors, quinidine, and verapamil.

Nutritional/Ethanol Interactions Herb/Nutraceutical: St John's wort may decrease dapsone levels.

Adverse Reactions 1% to 10%: Hematologic: Hemolysis, methemoglobinemia

Overdosage/Toxicology Symptoms of overdose include nausea, vomiting, hyperexcitability, methemoglobin-induced depression, seizures, cyanosis, and hemolysis. Following decontamination, methylene blue 1-2 mg/kg I.V. is the treatment of choice.

Pharmacodynamics/Kinetics

Absorption: Well absorbed

Half-Life Elimination: 30 hours (range: 10-50 hours)

Metabolism: Hepatic

Excretion: Urine

Dosing

Adults & Elderly:

Leprosy: Oral: 50-100 mg/day for 3-10 years

Dermatitis herpetiformis: Oral: Initial: 50 mg/day, increase to 300. mg/day, or higher to achieve full control. Reduce dosage to minimum level as soon as possible.

Pneumonia caused by *Pneumocystis carinii* (unlabeled use): Oral:

Prophylaxis: 100 mg/day

Treatment: Adults: 100 mg/day in combination with trimethoprim (15-20 mg/kg/day) for 21 days

Pediatrics:

Leprosy: Oral: Children: 1-2 mg/kg/24 hours, up to a maximum of 100 mg/day

Prophylaxis of *Pneumocystis carinii* pneumonia (unlabeled use): Oral: Children >1 month: 2 mg/kg/day once daily (maximum dose: 100 mg/day) or 4 mg/kg/dose once weekly (maximum dose: 200 mg)

Renal Impairment: No guidelines are available.

Available Dosage Forms Tablet: 25 mg, 100 mg

Monitoring and Teaching Issues

Physical Assessment: Use with caution in patients with severe anemia, G6PD deficiency, hepatic function impairment (see Warnings/Precautions). Assess potential for interactions with other pharmacological agents or herbal products patient may be taking (see Drug Interactions). Assess results of laboratory tests (CBC and LFT), therapeutic effectiveness (according to purpose for use), and adverse response (see Adverse Reactions). Teach patient appropriate use, possible side effects/appropriate interventions, and adverse symptoms to report (see Patient Education).

(Continued)

Dapsone *(Continued)*

Monitoring Laboratory Tests: Liver function, CBC

Patient Education: Do not take any new medication during therapy unless approved by prescriber. Take as directed; do not discontinue without consulting prescriber. Do not take with antacids, alkaline foods, or other medication. Therapy may take 3-10 years for leprosy. Frequent blood tests may be required. If rash develops, discontinue and notify prescriber. Report persistent sore throat, fever, chills; constant fatigue; yellowing of skin or eyes; or easy bruising or bleeding. **Pregnancy/breast-feeding precautions:** Inform prescriber if you are or intend to become pregnant. Consult prescriber if breast-feeding.

Dietary Considerations: Do not administer with antacids, alkaline foods, or drugs.

Pregnancy Risk Factor: C

Lactation: Enters breast milk/not recommended (AAP rates "compatible")

Administration

Oral: May give with meals if GI upset occurs.

Storage: Protect from light.

♦ Daptacel™ *see page 1660*

Daptomycin *(DAP toe mye sin)*

U.S. Brand Names Cubicin™

Synonyms Cidecin; Dapcin; LY146032

Generic Available No

Pharmacologic Category Antibiotic, Cyclic Lipopeptide

Use Treatment of complicated skin and skin structure infections caused by susceptible aerobic Gram-positive organisms

Unlabeled/Investigational Use Treatment of bacteremia, endocarditis, and other severe infections caused by MRSA or VRE

Mechanism of Action/Effect Daptomycin binds to components of the cell membrane of susceptible organisms and causes rapid depolarization, inhibiting intracellular synthesis of DNA, RNA, and protein. Daptomycin is bactericidal and bacterial killing is concentration-dependent.

Contraindications Hypersensitivity to daptomycin or any component of the formulation

Warnings/Precautions May be associated with an increased incidence of myopathy; discontinue in patients with signs and symptoms of myopathy in conjunction with an increase in CPK (>5 times ULN or 1000 units/L) or in asymptomatic patients with a CPK ≥10 times ULN. Myopathy may occur more frequently at dose and/or frequency in excess of recommended dosages. Not indicated for the treatment of pneumonia (poor lung penetration). Use caution in patients receiving other drugs associated with myopathy (HMG-CoA reductase inhibitors). Use caution in renal impairment (dosage adjustment required). Superinfection by resistant strains and/or pseudomembranous colitis may be associated with use. Safety and efficacy in pediatric patients have not been established.

Drug Interactions

Increased Effect/Toxicity: No clinically-significant interactions have been identified. Theoretically, concurrent use of drugs which may cause myopathy may increase the risk of these reactions. Limited clinical studies with HMG-CoA reductase inhibitors have not demonstrated an increase in adverse effects.

Adverse Reactions

1% to 10%:

Cardiovascular: Hypotension (2%), hypertension (1%)

Central nervous system: Headache (5%), insomnia (5%), dizziness (2%), fever (2%)

Dermatologic: Rash (4%), pruritus (3%)

Gastrointestinal: Constipation (6%), nausea (6%), diarrhea (5%), vomiting (3%), dyspepsia (1%)

Genitourinary: Urinary tract infection (2%)

Hematologic: Anemia (2%)

Hepatic: Transaminases increased (3%)

Local: Injection site reaction (6%)

Neuromuscular & skeletal: CPK increased (3%), limb pain (2%), arthralgia (1%)

Renal: Renal failure (2%)

Respiratory: Dyspnea (2%)

Miscellaneous: Infection (fungal, 3%)

Overdosage/Toxicology Treatment is symptomatic and supportive; hemodialysis removes approximately 15% in 4 hours.

Pharmacodynamics/Kinetics

Protein Binding: 92%

Half-Life Elimination: 8-9 hours (up to 28 hours in renal impairment)

Excretion: Urine (78%; primarily as unchanged drug); feces (6%)

Dosing

Adults & Elderly:

Skin and/or skin structure infections (complicated): I.V.: 4 mg/kg once daily for 7-14 days

Bacteremia, endocarditis (unlabeled use): I.V.: 6 mg/kg once daily

Renal Impairment: Skin and soft tissue infections: Cl_{cr} <30 mL/minute: 4 mg/kg every 48 hours

Hemodialysis (administer after hemodialysis) and/or CAPD: Dose as in Cl_{cr} <30 mL/minute

Available Dosage Forms Injection, powder for reconstitution: 250 mg, 500 mg

Monitoring and Teaching Issues

Physical Assessment: Use caution in presence of renal impairment (see Warnings/Precautions). Assess potential for interactions with other pharmacological agents (eg, HMG-CoA reductase inhibitors; see Drug Interactions). Assess results of laboratory tests (CPK), therapeutic effectiveness (eg signs and symptoms of infection), and adverse reactions (see Adverse Reactions) at beginning of therapy and on a regular basis during therapy. Note infusion directions in Administration. Teach patient possible side effects and adverse symptoms to report (eg, rash, hypotension, CNS changes, limb pain, muscle pain or weakness, opportunistic infection; see Patient Education).

Patient Education: This medication can only be administered via intravenous infusion. You will be monitored during and after each infusion. Report immediately any burning, pain, or redness at infusion site, any throat tightness, respiratory difficulty, or chest tightness. Report unusual headache, insomnia, nausea or vomiting, limb or joint pain, alteration in urination patterns, itching or pain on urination, or other possible adverse reactions. **Pregnancy/breast-feeding precautions:** Inform prescriber if you are or intend to become pregnant or breast-feed.

Geriatric Considerations: The manufacturer reports that in studies of complicated skin and skin structure infections, elderly patients had a lower clinical success rate and a higher incidence of adverse effects (no quantitative data provided in product labeling). Refer to dosing in renal impairment.

Pregnancy Risk Factor: B

Lactation: Excretion in breast milk unknown/use caution

Administration

I.V.: Infuse over 30 minutes.

Reconstitution: Reconstitute vial with NS (5 mL for 250 mg vial, 10 mL for 500 mg vial). Should be further diluted following reconstitution in an appropriate volume of NS.

Compatibility: Incompatible in dextrose-containing solutions

Storage: Store under refrigeration at 2°C to 8°C (36°F to 46°F). Reconstituted solution (either in vial or in infusion bag) is stable for a cumulative time of 12 hours at room temperature and 48 hours if refrigerated (2°C to 8°C).

Related Information

Antimicrobial Drugs of Choice *on page 1792*

♦ **Daraprim**® *see* Pyrimethamine *on page 1290*

Darbepoetin Alfa (dar be POE e tin AL fa)

U.S. Brand Names Aranesp®

Synonyms Erythropoiesis Stimulating Protein

Generic Available No

Pharmacologic Category Colony Stimulating Factor; Growth Factor; Recombinant Human Erythropoietin

Use Treatment of anemia associated with chronic renal failure (CRF), including patients on dialysis (ESRD) and patients not on dialysis; anemia associated with chemotherapy for nonmyeloid malignancies

Mechanism of Action/Effect Stimulates production of red blood cells within the bone marrow. There is a dose response relationship with this effect. This results in an increase in red blood cell counts followed by a rise in hematocrit and hemoglobin levels. When administered SubQ or I.V., darbepoetin's half-life is ~3 times that of epoetin alfa.

Contraindications Hypersensitivity to darbepoetin or any component of the formulation (including polysorbate 80 and/or albumin); uncontrolled hypertension

Warnings/Precautions Erythropoietic therapies may be associated with an increased risk of cardiovascular and/or neurologic events in chronic renal failure. Darbepoetin alfa should be managed carefully; avoid hemoglobin increases >1 g/dL in any 2-week period, and do not exceed a target level of 12 g/dL. Prior to and during therapy, iron stores must be evaluated. Supplemental iron is recommended if serum ferritin <100 mcg/mL or serum transferrin saturation <20%. In cancer patients, the risk of thrombotic events (eg, pulmonary emboli, thrombophlebitis, thrombosis) was increased by erythropoietic therapy.

Use with caution in patients with hypertension or with a history of seizures. If hypertension is difficult to control, reduce or hold darbepoetin alpha. **Not** recommended for acute correction of severe anemia or as a substitute for transfusion. Consider discontinuing in patients who receive a renal transplant.

Prior to treatment, correct or exclude deficiencies of vitamin B_{12} and/or folate, as well as other factors which may impair erythropoiesis (aluminum toxicity, inflammatory conditions, infections). Poor response should prompt evaluation of these potential factors, as well as possible malignant processes, occult blood loss, hemolysis, and/or bone marrow fibrosis. Pure red cell aplasia (PRCA) with associated neutralizing antibodies to erythropoietin has been reported, predominantly in patients with CRF. Patients with loss of response to darbepoetin alfa should be evaluated. Discontinue treatment in patients with PRCA secondary to neutralizing antibodies to erythropoietin.

Due to the delayed onset of erythropoiesis, darbepoetin is of no value in the acute treatment of anemia. Safety and efficacy in patients with underlying hematologic diseases have not been established, including porphyria, thalassemia, hemolytic anemia, and sickle cell disease. Risk of thrombosis, including pulmonary embolism, increased in cancer patients. Safety and efficacy in pediatric patients have not been established.

Nutritional/Ethanol Interactions Ethanol: Should be avoided due to adverse effects on erythropoiesis.

Adverse Reactions Note: Frequency of adverse events cited in patients with CRF or cancer and may be, in part, a reflection of population in which the drug is used and/or associated with dialysis procedures.

>10%:
Cardiovascular: Hypertension (4% to 23%), hypotension (22%), edema (21%), peripheral edema (11%), arrhythmia (10%)
Central nervous system: Fatigue (9% to 33%), fever (9% to 19%), headache (12% to 16%), dizziness (8% to 14%)
Gastrointestinal: Diarrhea (16% to 22%), constipation (5% to 18%) vomiting (15%), nausea (14%), abdominal pain (12%)
Neuromuscular & skeletal: Myalgia (21%), arthralgia (11% to 13%), limb pain (10%)
Respiratory: Upper respiratory infection (14%), dyspnea (12%), cough (10%)
Miscellaneous: Infection (27%)

(Continued)

Darbepoetin Alfa *(Continued)*

1% to 10%:
  Cardiovascular: Angina/chest pain (6% to 8%), fluid overload (6%), CHF (6%), thrombosis (6%), MI (2%)
  Central nervous system: Seizure (<1% to 1%), stroke (1%), TIA (1%)
  Dermatologic: Pruritus (8%), rash (7%)
  Endocrine & metabolic: Dehydration (5%)
  Local: Injection site pain (7%)
  Neuromuscular & skeletal: Back pain (8%), weakness (5%)
  Respiratory: Bronchitis (6%), pulmonary embolism (1%)
  Miscellaneous: Vascular access thrombosis (8%, annualized rate 0.22 events per patient year), vascular access infection (6%), influenza-like symptoms (6%), vascular access hemorrhage (6%)

Overdosage/Toxicology The maximum amount of darbepoetin which may be safely administered has not been determined. However, cardiovascular and neurologic adverse events have been correlated to excessive and/or rapid rise in hemoglobin. Phlebotomy may be performed if clinically indicated.

Pharmacodynamics/Kinetics

Onset of Action: Increased hemoglobin levels not generally observed until 2-6 weeks after initiating treatment

Absorption: SubQ: Slow

Bioavailability: CRF: SubQ: ~37% (range: 30% to 50%)

Time to Peak: SubQ: CRF: 34 hours (range: 24-72 hours); Cancer: 90 hours (range: 71-123 hours)

Half-Life Elimination: CRF: Terminal: I.V.: 21 hours, SubQ: 49 hours; **Note:** Half-life is ~3 times as long as epoetin alfa

Dosing

Adults & Elderly:

Correction of anemia associated with CRF: I.V., SubQ:
  Manufacturer recommended dosing: Initial: 0.45 mcg/kg once weekly; titrate to response; some patients may respond to doses given once every 2 weeks
  Unlabeled dosing:
  Every 2-weeks: 0.75 mcg/kg every 2 weeks
  or
  Every 4-weeks: 0.75 mcg/kg every 2 weeks; once titrated, multiply dose by 2 and give every 4 weeks

Anemia associated with chemotherapy: SubQ:
  Manufacturer recommended dosing: Initial: 2.25 mcg/kg once weekly; with inadequate response: 4.5 mcg/kg once weekly
  Unlabeled dosing:
  Every 2-weeks:
    Initial: 200 mcg every 2 weeks; inadequate response: 300 mcg every 2 weeks
  or
    Initial: 3 mcg/kg every 2 weeks; inadequate response: 5 mcg/kg every 2 weeks
  or
  Every 3-weeks (front load): Initial: 4.5 mcg/kg every week until desired Hgb obtained; maintenance: 4.5 mcg/kg (or titrated dose) every 3 weeks
  or
    Initial: 325 mcg every week until desired Hgb obtained; maintenance: 325 mcg every 3 weeks

  Treatment goals: **Note:** Titration may be required to limit rises of Hgb to <1 g/dL over any 2-week interval and to reach a Hgb concentration not to exceed 12 g/dL.
  Inadequate response: Increase dose; refer to individual dosing regimens for adjustment when Hgb increase <1 g/dL after 4-6 weeks
  Excessive response: Hold dose and/or decrease dose by 25%
    Decrease dose by 25% when Hgb increases >1 g/dL in any 2-week period **or** Hgb increases and approaches 12 g/dL in any 2-week period
    Hold dose, then decrease dose by 25% when Hgb increases despite previous dose decrease (hold until Hgb decreases) **or** when Hgb ≥13 g/dL (hold until Hgb ≤12 g/dL)

  Conversion from epoetin alfa to darbepoetin alfa: See table.

Conversion From Epoetin Alfa to Darbepoetin Alfa

Previous Dosage of Epoetin Alfa (units/week)	Darbepoetin Alfa Dosage (mcg/week)	Darbepoetin Alfa Dosage (mcg/every 2 weeks)
<2500	6.25	12.5
2500-4999	12.5	25
5000-10,999	25	50
11,000-17,999	40	80
18,000-33,999	60	120
34,000-89,999	100	200
≥90,000	200	400

Note: In patients receiving epoetin alfa 2-3 times per week, darbepoetin alfa is administered once weekly. In patients receiving epoetin alfa once weekly, darbepoetin alfa is administered once every 2 weeks.

Renal Impairment: Dosage requirements for patients with chronic renal failure who do not require dialysis may be lower than in dialysis patients. Monitor patients closely during the time period in which a dialysis regimen is initiated, dosage requirement may increase.

Available Dosage Forms

Injection, solution, with human albumin 2.5 mg/mL [preservative free, single-dose vial]: 25 mcg/mL (1 mL); 40 mcg/mL (1 mL); 60 mcg/mL (1 mL); 100 mcg/mL (1 mL); 150 mcg/0.75 mL (0.75 mL); 200 mcg/mL (1 mL); 300 mcg/mL (1 mL)

Injection, solution, with human albumin 2.5 mg/mL [preservative free, prefilled syringe]: 25 mcg/0.42 mL (0.42 mL); 40 mcg/0.4 mL (0.4 mL); 60 mcg/0.3 mL (0.3 mL); 100 mcg/0.5 mL (0.5 mL); 200 mcg/0.4 mL (0.4 mL); 300 mcg/0.6 mL (0.6 mL); 500 mcg/mL (1 mL)

Monitoring and Teaching Issues

Physical Assessment: Assess potential for interactions with other prescriptions, OTC medications, or herbal products patient may be taking (eg, nutritional or supplemental iron). Monitor blood pressure and be alert for signs of fluid retention. Assess GI function. Assess results of laboratory tests prior to and during therapy. Assess therapeutic effectiveness and adverse response on a regular basis during therapy. Teach patient proper use if self-administered (appropriate injection technique and syringe/needle disposal), possible side effects/appropriate interventions, and adverse symptoms to report.

Monitoring Laboratory Tests: Hemoglobin (weekly); prior to and during therapy, iron stores must be evaluated (supplemental iron is recommended in any patient with a serum ferritin <100 mcg/mL or serum transferrin saturation <20%)

Patient Education: Do not take any new medication during therapy without consulting prescriber. This medication can only be administered by infusion or injection (if self-administered, follow exact directions for injection and needle disposal). You will need frequent blood tests to determine appropriate dosage. Avoid alcohol and do not make significant changes in your dietary iron without consulting prescriber. Check your blood pressure as frequently as recommended and report any significant changes. May cause nausea or vomiting (small frequent meals, frequent mouth care, sucking lozenges, or chewing gum may help); diarrhea (boiled milk, buttermilk, or yogurt may help); constipation (increased dietary fruit, fiber, fluids, and increased exercise may help); or dizziness, fatigue, or headache (use caution when driving or engaging in tasks that require alertness until response to drug is known). Report signs of edema (swollen extremities, respiratory difficulty); sudden onset of acute headache, back pain, or chest pain; muscle tremors or weakness; cough or signs of respiratory infection; or other adverse effects. **Pregnancy/breast-feeding precautions:** Inform prescriber if you are or intend to become pregnant. Consult prescriber if breast-feeding.

Dietary Considerations: Supplemental iron intake may be required in patients with low iron stores.

Pregnancy Risk Factor: C

Lactation: Excretion in breast milk unknown/use caution

Administration

I.V.: May be administered by SubQ or I.V. injection. Do not shake; vigorous shaking may denature darbepoetin alfa, rendering it biologically inactive. Do not dilute or administer in conjunction with other drug solutions. Discard any unused portion of the vial; do not pool unused portions. Discontinue immediately if signs/symptoms of anaphylaxis occur.

Compatibility: Do not dilute or administer with other solutions.

Storage: Store at 2°C to 8°C (36°F to 46°F). Do not freeze or shake. Protect from light.

Darifenacin (dar i FEN a sin)

U.S. Brand Names Enablex®

Synonyms Darifenacin Hydrochloride; UK-88,525

Generic Available No

Pharmacologic Category Anticholinergic Agent

Use Management of symptoms of bladder overactivity (urge incontinence, urgency, and frequency)

Mechanism of Action/Effect Blocks muscarinic/cholinergic receptors (M3 subtype) on the smooth muscle of the urinary bladder to limit bladder contractions, reducing the symptoms of bladder irritability/overactivity (urge incontinence, urgency and frequency).

Contraindications Hypersensitivity to darifenacin or any component of the formulation; uncontrolled narrow-angle glaucoma; paralytic ileus, GI or GU obstruction

Warnings/Precautions Use with caution with hepatic impairment; dosage limitation is required in moderate hepatic impairment (Child-Pugh Class B). Not recommended for use in severe hepatic impairment (Child-Pugh Class C). Use with caution in patients with clinically-significant bladder outlet obstruction, prostatic hyperplasia (nonobstructive), or urinary retention. Use caution in patients with decreased GI motility, constipation, hiatal hernia, reflux esophagitis, and ulcerative colitis. Use caution in patients with myasthenia gravis. In patients with controlled narrow angle glaucoma, darifenacin should be used with extreme caution and only when the potential benefit outweighs risks of treatment. Safety and efficacy have not been established in pediatric patients.

Drug Interactions

Cytochrome P450 Effect: Substrate of CYP2D6 (minor), CYP3A4 (major); **Inhibits** CYP2D6 (moderate), 3A4 (weak)

Decreased Effect: Darifenacin may decrease the levels/effects of CYP2D6 prodrug substrates; example prodrug substrates include codeine, hydrocodone, oxycodone, and tramadol. CYP3A4 inducers may decrease the levels/effects of darifenacin; example inducers include aminoglutethimide, carbamazepine, nafcillin, nevirapine, phenobarbital, phenytoin, and rifamycins.

Increased Effect/Toxicity: Adverse anticholinergic effects may be additive with other anticholinergic agents (includes tricyclic antidepressants, antihistamines, and phenothiazines). Darifenacin may increase the levels/effects of CYP2D6 substrates; example substrates include amphetamines, selected beta-blockers, dextromethorphan, fluoxetine, lidocaine, mirtazapine, nefazodone, paroxetine, risperidone, ritonavir, thioridazine, tricyclic antidepressants, and venlafaxine. CYP3A4 inhibitors may increase the levels/effects of darifenacin; example inhibitors include azole antifungals, ciprofloxacin, clarithromycin, diclofenac, doxycycline, erythromycin, imatinib, isoniazid, nefazodone, nicardipine, (Continued)

Darifenacin *(Continued)*

propofol, protease inhibitors, quinidine, and verapamil. The dosage of darifenacin should not exceed 7.5 mg daily in patients receiving potent CYP3A4 inhibitors.

Adverse Reactions
>10%: Gastrointestinal: Xerostomia (19% to 35%), constipation (15% to 21%)
1% to 10%:
Central nervous system: Headache (7%), dizziness (1% to 2%)
Gastrointestinal: Dyspepsia (3% to 8%), abdominal pain (2% to 4%), nausea (2% to 4%), diarrhea (1% to 2%)
Genitourinary: Urinary tract infection (4% to 5%)
Neuromuscular & skeletal: Asthenia (2% to 3%)
Ocular: Dry eyes (2%)
Miscellaneous: Flu-like syndrome (<1% to 3%), accidental injury (<1% to 3%)

Pharmacodynamics/Kinetics
Bioavailability: 15% to 19%
Time to Peak: Plasma: 7 hours
Protein Binding: 98%
Half-Life Elimination: 13-19 hours
Metabolism: Hepatic, via CYP3A4 (major) and CYP2D6 (minor)
Excretion: Urine (60%), feces (40%); as metabolites (inactive)

Dosing
Adults & Elderly: Symptoms of bladder overactivity: Oral: Initial: 7.5 mg once daily. If response is not adequate after a minimum of 2 weeks, dosage may be increased to 15 mg once daily. Dosage should not be increased in patients with hepatic impairment or in those receiving potent inhibitors of CYP3A4.
Renal Impairment: No adjustment required.
Hepatic Impairment:
Moderate impairment (Child-Pugh Class B): Daily dosage should not exceed 7.5 mg/day
Severe impairment (Child-Pugh Class C): Has not been evaluated; use is not recommended

Available Dosage Forms Tablet, extended release: 7.5 mg, 15 mg

Monitoring and Teaching Issues
Physical Assessment: Assess potential for interactions with other prescriptions, OTC medications, or herbal products patient may be taking. Monitor therapeutic effectiveness and adverse reactions. Teach patient appropriate use, interventions to reduce side effects, and adverse symptoms to report.
Patient Education: Take as directed. Swallow tablet hold. May cause headache (consult prescriber for a mild analgesic); dizziness, nervousness, or sleepiness (use caution when driving, climbing stairs, or engaging in tasks requiring alertness until response to drug is known); or abdominal discomfort, dry mouth (small frequent meals, frequent mouth care, chewing gum, or sucking lozenges may help), diarrhea, constipation (increasing exercise, fluids, fruit/fiber may help), nausea, or vomiting (small frequent meals, increased exercise, adequate hydration may help). Report back pain, muscle spasms, alteration in gait, or numbness of extremities; unresolved or persistent constipation, diarrhea, or vomiting; or symptoms of upper respiratory infection or flu. Report difficulty urinating, or pain on urination, or abdominal pain. **Pregnancy/breast-feeding precautions:** Inform prescriber if you are or intend to become pregnant. Breast-feeding is not recommended.
Dietary Considerations: May be taken without regard to meals, with or without food.
Geriatric Considerations: There is a trend for decreased clearance with age, though no change in dose is recommended. The selectivity of darifenacin for the M3 receptor on the bladder may offer an advantage (less CNS and cardiovascular effects) over other anticholinergic agents used in the treatment of overactive bladder.
Pregnancy Risk Factor: C
Lactation: Excretion in breast milk unknown/use caution
Breast-Feeding Issues: Although human data are not available, darifenacin is excreted in the breast milk in animals.

Administration
Oral: Tablet should be swallowed whole; may be taken without regard to food.
Storage: Store at 25°C (77°F); excursions permitted to 15°C to 30°C (59°F to 86°F). Protect from light.

♦ **Darifenacin Hydrochloride** *see* Darifenacin *on page 407*
♦ **Darvocet A500™** *see* Propoxyphene and Acetaminophen *on page 1272*
♦ **Darvocet-N® 50** *see* Propoxyphene and Acetaminophen *on page 1272*
♦ **Darvocet-N® 100** *see* Propoxyphene and Acetaminophen *on page 1272*
♦ **Darvon®** *see* Propoxyphene *on page 1271*
♦ **Darvon® Compound** *see* Propoxyphene, Aspirin, and Caffeine *on page 1273*
♦ **Darvon-N®** *see* Propoxyphene *on page 1271*
♦ **Daunomycin** *see* DAUNOrubicin Hydrochloride *on page 410*

DAUNOrubicin Citrate (Liposomal)
(daw noe ROO bi sin SI trate lip po SOE mal)

U.S. Brand Names DaunoXome®
Generic Available No
Pharmacologic Category Antineoplastic Agent, Anthracycline
Medication Safety Issues
Sound-alike/look-alike issues:
DAUNOrubicin may be confused with dactinomycin, DOXOrubicin
Liposomal formulations (DaunoXome®) may be confused with conventional formulations (Adriamycin PFS®, Adriamycin RDF®, Cerubidine®, Rubex®)
Use First-line cytotoxic therapy for advanced HIV-associated Kaposi's sarcoma
Mechanism of Action/Effect Binds to DNA and inhibits DNA synthesis causing cell death

Contraindications Hypersensitivity to daunorubicin or any component of the formulation; pregnancy

Warnings/Precautions The U.S. Food and Drug Administration (FDA) currently recommends that procedures for proper handling and disposal of antineoplastic agents be considered. Daunorubicin is associated with a dose-related cardiac toxicity. The risk of similar toxicity with liposome-encapsulated daunorubicin is not certain. Use caution in patients with previous therapy with high cumulative doses of anthracyclines, cyclophosphamide, or thoracic radiation, or who have pre-existing cardiac disease.

Drug Interactions

Decreased Effect: Patients may experience impaired immune response to vaccines; possible infection after administration of live vaccines in patients receiving immunosuppressants.

Adverse Reactions

>10%:

Central nervous system: Fatigue (51%), headache (28%), neuropathy (13%)

Hematologic: Myelosuppression, neutropenia (51%), thrombocytopenia, anemia

Onset: 7 days

Nadir: 14 days

Recovery: 21 days

Gastrointestinal: Abdominal pain, vomiting, anorexia (23%); diarrhea (38%); nausea (55%)

Respiratory: Cough (28%), dyspnea (26%), rhinitis

Miscellaneous: Allergic reactions (24%)

1% to 10%:

Cardiovascular: Hypertension, palpitation, syncope, tachycardia, chest pain, edema

Dermatologic: Alopecia (8%), pruritus (7%)

Endocrine & metabolic: Hot flashes

Gastrointestinal: Constipation (7%), stomatitis (10%)

Neuromuscular & skeletal: Arthralgia (7%), myalgia (7%)

Ocular: Conjunctivitis, eye pain (5%)

Respiratory: Sinusitis

Overdosage/Toxicology Symptoms of acute overdose are increased severity of the observed dose-limiting toxicities of therapeutic doses, myelosuppression (especially granulocytopenia), fatigue, nausea, and vomiting. Treatment is symptomatic.

Pharmacodynamics/Kinetics

Half-Life Elimination: Distribution: 4.4 hours; Terminal: 3-5 hours

Metabolism: Similar to daunorubicin, but metabolite plasma levels are low

Excretion: Primarily feces; some urine

Clearance, plasma: 17.3 mL/minute

Dosing

Adults & Elderly: Refer to individual protocols.

Advanced HIV-associated Kaposi's sarcoma: I.V.:

20-40 mg/m^2 every 2 weeks

100 mg/m^2 every 3 weeks

Renal Impairment:

S_{cr} 1.2-3 mg/dL: Reduce dose to 75% of normal.

S_{cr} >3 mg/dL: Reduce dose to 50% of normal.

Hepatic Impairment:

Serum bilirubin 1.2-3 mg/dL: Reduce to 75% of normal dose.

Serum bilirubin >3 mg/dL: Reduce to 50% of normal dose.

Available Dosage Forms Injection, solution [preservative free]: 2 mg/mL (25 mL) [contains sucrose 2125 mg/25 mL]

Monitoring and Teaching Issues

Physical Assessment: See Warnings/Precautions for use cautions (eg, pre-existing bone marrow depression, impaired hepatic or renal function, or cardiac disease). Note specific infusion directions (see Administration). Infusion site must be closely monitored; extravasation can cause severe cellulitis or tissue necrosis (note application of heat or sodium bicarbonate can be harmful and is contraindicated). Assess results of laboratory tests (see Monitoring Laboratory Tests), therapeutic response, and adverse effects (hypertension, tachycardia, cough, dyspnea, gastrointestinal upset; see Adverse Reactions) prior to each infusion and on a regular basis throughout therapy. Teach patient possible side effects/appropriate interventions and adverse symptoms to report (see Patient Education).

Monitoring Laboratory Tests: Cardiac function, CBC with differential and platelet count, liver and renal function; repeat blood counts prior to each dose and withhold if the absolute granulocyte count is <750 cells/mm^3. Monitor serum uric acid levels.

Patient Education: Do not take any new medication during therapy unless approved by prescriber. This medication can only be administered by infusion. You will be monitored closely; report immediately any swelling, pain, burning, or redness at infusion site, chest pain or tightness, difficulty breathing, or difficulty swallowing. It is important to maintain adequate hydration (2-3 L/day of fluids) unless instructed to restrict fluid intake and nutrition (small frequent meals may help). You will be more susceptible to infection (avoid crowds and exposure to infection and do not have any vaccinations without consulting prescriber). May cause nausea or vomiting (small frequent meals, frequent mouth care, sucking lozenges, or chewing gum may help); diarrhea (buttermilk, boiled milk, or yogurt may help); hair loss (reversible); or red-pink urine (normal). Report immediately chest pain, swelling of extremities, respiratory difficulty, palpitations, or rapid heartbeat. Report unresolved nausea, vomiting, or diarrhea; alterations in urinary pattern (increased or decreased); opportunistic infection (eg, fever, chills, unusual bruising or bleeding, fatigue, purulent vaginal discharge, unhealed mouth sores); abdominal pain or blood in stools; excessive fatigue; or yellowing of eyes or skin. **Pregnancy/breast-feeding precautions:** Do not get pregnant or cause a pregnancy (males) while taking this medication. Consult prescriber for appropriate contraceptive measures. Breast-feeding is not recommended.

(Continued)

DAUNOrubicin Citrate (Liposomal) (Continued)

Pregnancy Risk Factor: D

Lactation: Excretion in breast milk unknown/not recommended

Administration

I.V.: Vesicant. Infuse over 1 hour; do not mix with other drugs.

Reconstitution: Only fluid which may be mixed with DaunoXome® is D_5W. Must not be mixed with saline, bacteriostatic agents such as benzyl alcohol, or any other solution.

Compatibility: Incompatible with sodium bicarbonate and fluorouracil, heparin, dexamethasone

Storage: Store in refrigerator 2°C to 8°C (37°F to 45°F); do not freeze. Protect from light.

Related Information

FDA Name Differentiation Project: The Use of Tall-Man Letters *on page 15*

DAUNOrubicin Hydrochloride (daw noe ROO bi sin hye droe KLOR ide)

U.S. Brand Names Cerubidine®

Synonyms Daunomycin; DNR; NSC-82151; Rubidomycin Hydrochloride

Generic Available Yes

Pharmacologic Category Antineoplastic Agent, Anthracycline

Medication Safety Issues

Sound-alike/look-alike issues:

DAUNOrubicin may be confused with dactinomycin, DOXOrubicin

Conventional formulations (Cerubidine®) may be confused with liposomal formulations (DaunoXome®, Doxil®)

Use Treatment of acute lymphocytic (ALL) and nonlymphocytic (ANLL) leukemias

Mechanism of Action/Effect Inhibition of DNA and RNA synthesis by intercalation between DNA base pairs and by steric obstruction. Daunomycin intercalates at points of local uncoiling of the double helix. Although the exact mechanism is unclear, it appears that direct binding to DNA (intercalation) and inhibition of DNA repair (topoisomerase II inhibition) result in blockade of DNA and RNA synthesis and fragmentation of DNA.

Contraindications Hypersensitivity to daunorubicin or any component of the formulation; congestive heart failure or arrhythmias; previous therapy with high cumulative doses of daunorubicin and/or doxorubicin; pre-existing bone marrow suppression; pregnancy

Warnings/Precautions The U.S. Food and Drug Administration (FDA) currently recommends that procedures for proper handling and disposal of antineoplastic agents be considered. I.V. use only, severe local tissue necrosis will result if extravasation occurs. Reduce dose in patients with impaired hepatic, renal, or biliary function. Severe myelosuppression is possible when used in therapeutic doses. Total cumulative dose should take into account previous or concomitant treatment with cardiotoxic agents or irradiation of chest.

Irreversible myocardial toxicity may occur as total dosage approaches:

$550 \ mg/m^2$ in adults

$400 \ mg/m^2$ in patients receiving chest radiation

$300 \ mg/m^2$ in children >2 years of age

If daunorubicin contacts the skin, wash and flush thoroughly with water.

Drug Interactions

Decreased Effect: Patients may experience impaired immune response to vaccines; possible infection after administration of live vaccines in patients receiving immunosuppressants.

Nutritional/Ethanol Interactions Ethanol: Avoid ethanol (due to GI irritation).

Lab Interactions Increased potassium (S)

Adverse Reactions

>10%:

Cardiovascular: Transient ECG abnormalities (supraventricular tachycardia, S-T wave changes, atrial or ventricular extrasystoles); generally asymptomatic and self-limiting. CHF, dose related, may be delayed for 7-8 years after treatment. Cumulative dose, radiation therapy, age, and use of cyclophosphamide all increase the risk. Recommended maximum cumulative doses:

No risk factors: $550-600 \ mg/m^2$

Concurrent radiation: $450 \ mg/m^2$

Regardless of cumulative dose, if the left ventricular ejection fraction is <30% to 40%, the drug is usually not given

Dermatologic: Alopecia, radiation recall

Gastrointestinal: Mild nausea or vomiting, stomatitis

Genitourinary: Discoloration of urine (red)

Hematologic: Myelosuppression, primarily leukopenia; thrombocytopenia and anemia

Onset: 7 days

Nadir: 10-14 days

Recovery: 21-28 days

1% to 10%:

Dermatologic: Skin "flare" at injection site; discoloration of saliva, sweat, or tears

Endocrine & metabolic: Hyperuricemia

Gastrointestinal: GI ulceration, diarrhea

Overdosage/Toxicology Symptoms of overdose include myelosuppression, nausea, vomiting, and stomatitis. There are no known antidotes. Treatment is symptomatic and supportive.

Pharmacodynamics/Kinetics

Half-Life Elimination: Distribution: 2 minutes; Elimination: 14-20 hours; Terminal: 18.5 hours; Daunorubicinol plasma half-life: 24-48 hours

Metabolism: Primarily hepatic to daunorubicinol (active), then to inactive aglycones, conjugated sulfates, and glucuronides

Excretion: Feces (40%); urine (~25% as unchanged drug and metabolites)

Dosing

Adults & Elderly: Refer to individual protocols.

Range: I.V.: 30-60 mg/m^2/day for 3-5 days, repeat dose in 3-4 weeks

AML: I.V.:

Single agent induction: 60 mg/m^2/day for 3 days; repeat every 3-4 weeks

Combination therapy induction: 45 mg/m^2/day for 3 days of the first course of induction therapy; subsequent courses: Every day for 2 days

ALL combination therapy: I.V.: 45 mg/m^2/day for 3 days

Cumulative dose should not exceed 400-600 mg/m^2

Pediatrics: Refer to individual protocols.

ALL combination therapy: I.V.: Children: Remission induction: 25-45 mg/m^2 on day 1 every week for 4 cycles **or** 30-45 mg/m^2/day for 3 days

AML combination therapy: I.V.: Children: Induction (continuous infusion): 30-60 mg/m^2/day on days 1-3 of cycle

Note: In children <2 years or <0.5 m^2, daunorubicin should be based on weight - mg/kg: 1 mg/kg per protocol with frequency dependent on regimen employed

Cumulative dose should not exceed 300 mg/m^2 in children >2 years; maximum cumulative doses for younger children are unknown.

Renal Impairment:

Cl$_{cr}$ <10 mL/minute: Administer 75% of normal dose.

S$_{cr}$ >3 mg/dL: Administer 50% of normal dose.

Hepatic Impairment:

Serum bilirubin 1.2-3 mg/dL or AST 60-180 int. units: Reduce dose to 75%.

Serum bilirubin 3.1-5 mg/dL or AST >180 int. units: Reduce dose to 50%.

Serum bilirubin >5 mg/dL: Omit use.

Available Dosage Forms

Injection, powder for reconstitution: 20 mg, 50 mg

Cerubidine®: 20 mg

Injection, solution: 5 mg/mL (4 mL, 10 mL)

Monitoring and Teaching Issues

Physical Assessment: See Warnings/Precautions for use cautions (eg, pre-existing bone marrow depression, impaired hepatic or renal function, or cardiac disease). See Administration for infusion specifics. Infusion site must be closely monitored; extravasation can cause severe cellulitis or tissue necrosis. Assess results of laboratory tests, therapeutic response, and adverse effects (eg, ECG abnormalities, CHF; see Adverse Reactions) prior to each infusion and on a regular basis throughout therapy. Teach patient possible side effects/appropriate interventions and adverse symptoms to report (see Patient Education).

Monitoring Laboratory Tests: CBC with differential, platelet count, liver function, ECG, ventricular ejection fraction, renal function

Patient Education: Do not take any new medication during therapy unless approved by prescriber. This medication can only be administered by infusion. You will be monitored closely; report immediately any swelling, pain, burning, or redness at infusion site, chest pain or tightness, difficulty breathing, or difficulty swallowing. It is important to maintain adequate hydration (2-3 L/day of fluids) unless instructed to restrict fluid intake and nutrition (small frequent meals may help). You will be more susceptible to infection (avoid crowds and exposure to infection and do not have any vaccinations without consulting prescriber). May cause nausea or vomiting (small frequent meals, frequent mouth care, sucking lozenges, or chewing gum may help); diarrhea (buttermilk, boiled milk, or yogurt may help); loss of hair (reversible); or red-pink urine (normal). Report immediately chest pain, swelling of extremities, respiratory difficulty, palpitations, or rapid heartbeat. Report unresolved nausea, vomiting, or diarrhea; alterations in urinary pattern (increased or decreased); opportunistic infection (eg, fever, chills, unusual bruising or bleeding, fatigue, purulent vaginal discharge, unhealed mouth sores); abdominal pain or blood in stools; excessive fatigue; or yellowing of eyes or skin. **Pregnancy/breast-feeding precautions:** Do not get pregnant or cause a pregnancy (males) while taking this medication. Consult prescriber for appropriate contraceptive measures. Breast-feeding is not recommended.

Pregnancy Risk Factor: D

Pregnancy Issues: May cause fetal harm when administered to a pregnant woman. Animal studies have shown an increased incidence of fetal abnormalities.

Lactation: Excretion in breast milk unknown/not recommended

Administration

I.V.: Vesicant. **Never** administer I.M. or SubQ. Administer IVP over 1-5 minutes.

Reconstitution: Dilute vials with 4 mL SWFI for a final concentration of 5 mg/mL.

Compatibility: Stable in D$_5$W, LR, NS, SWFI

Incompatible with heparin, sodium bicarbonate, fluorouracil, and dexamethasone

Y-site administration: Incompatible with allopurinol, aztreonam, cefepime, fludarabine, piperacillin/tazobactam

Compatibility when admixed: Incompatible with dexamethasone sodium phosphate, heparin

Storage: Store intact vials at room temperature and protect from light. Reconstituted solution is stable for 4 days at 15°C to 25°C. Further dilution in D$_5$W, LR, or NS is stable at room temperature (25°C) for up to 4 weeks if protected from light.

Related Information

FDA Name Differentiation Project: The Use of Tall-Man Letters *on page 15*

- **DaunoXome®** *see* DAUNOrubicin Citrate (Liposomal) *on page 408*
- **1-Day™ [OTC]** *see* Tioconazole *on page 1484*
- **Daypro®** *see* Oxaprozin *on page 1129*
- **dCF** *see* Pentostatin *on page 1184*
- **DDAVP®** *see* Desmopressin *on page 422*
- **ddC** *see* Zalcitabine *on page 1579*
- **ddI** *see* Didanosine *on page 446*

- ♦ **1-Deamino-8-D-Arginine Vasopressin** *see Desmopressin on page 422*
- ♦ **Decadron®** *see Dexamethasone on page 424*
- ♦ **Decadron® Phosphate [DSC]** *see Dexamethasone on page 424*
- ♦ **De-Chlor G** *see Hydrocodone, Phenylephrine, and Guaifenesin on page 760*
- ♦ **De-Chlor HC** *see Phenylephrine, Hydrocodone, and Chlorpheniramine on page 1202*
- ♦ **De-Chlor HD** *see Phenylephrine, Hydrocodone, and Chlorpheniramine on page 1202*
- ♦ **Declomycin®** *see Demeclocycline on page 415*

Deferoxamine (de fer OKS a meen)

U.S. Brand Names Desferal®
Synonyms Deferoxamine Mesylate
Generic Available Yes
Pharmacologic Category Antidote
Medication Safety Issues
Sound-alike/look-alike issues:
Deferoxamine may be confused with cefuroxime
Desferal® may be confused with desflurane, Dexferrum®, Disophrol®

Use Acute iron intoxication when serum iron is >450-500 mcg/dL or when clinical signs of significant iron toxicity exist; chronic iron overload secondary to multiple transfusions; iron overload secondary to congenital anemias; hemochromatosis

Unlabeled/Investigational Use Removal of corneal rust rings following surgical removal of foreign bodies; diagnostic test for iron and aluminum overload
Investigational: Treatment of aluminum accumulation in renal failure; treatment of aluminum-induced bone disease

Mechanism of Action/Effect Complexes with trivalent ions (ferric ions) to form ferrioxamine, which are removed by the kidneys

Contraindications Hypersensitivity to deferoxamine or any component of the formulation; patients with anuria, primary hemochromatosis

Warnings/Precautions Use with caution in patients with severe renal disease, pyelonephritis. May increase susceptibility to *Yersinia enterocolitica.* Ocular and auditory disturbances, as well as growth retardation (children only), have been reported following prolonged administration. Has been associated with adult respiratory distress syndrome (ARDS) following excessively high-dose treatment of acute intoxication.

Drug Interactions
Increased Effect/Toxicity: May cause loss of consciousness when administered with prochlorperazine. Concomitant treatment with vitamin C (>500 mg/day) has been associated with cardiac impairment.

Adverse Reactions Frequency not defined.
Cardiovascular: Flushing, hypotension, tachycardia, shock, edema
Central nervous system: Convulsions, fever, dizziness, neuropathy, paresthesia, seizure, exacerbation of aluminum-related encephalopathy (dialysis), headache, CNS depression, coma, aphasia, agitation
Dermatologic: Erythema, urticaria, pruritus, rash, cutaneous wheal formation
Endocrine & metabolic: Hypocalcemia
Gastrointestinal: Abdominal discomfort, diarrhea, nausea
Genitourinary: Dysuria
Hematologic: Thrombocytopenia, leukopenia
Local: Pain and induration at injection site
Neuromuscular & skeletal: Leg cramps
Ocular: Blurred vision, visual loss, scotoma, visual field defects, impaired vision, optic neuritis, cataracts, retinal pigmentary abnormalities
Otic: Hearing loss, tinnitus
Renal: Renal impairment, acute renal failure
Respiratory: Acute respiratory distress syndrome (with dyspnea, cyanosis)
Miscellaneous: Anaphylaxis

Overdosage/Toxicology Symptoms of overdose include hypotension, blurring of vision, diarrhea, leg cramps, and tachycardia. Treatment is symptomatic and supportive.

Pharmacodynamics/Kinetics
Absorption: Oral: <15%
Half-Life Elimination: Parent drug: 6.1 hours; Ferrioxamine: 5.8 hours
Metabolism: Hepatic to ferrioxamine
Excretion: Urine (as unchanged drug and metabolites)

Dosing
Adults & Elderly:
Acute iron toxicity:
I.V.: For the first 1000 mg, in fuse at 15 mg/kg/hour (although rates up to 40-50 mg/kg/hour have been given in patients with massive iron intoxication); may be followed by 500 mg every 4 hours for up to 2 doses; subsequent doses of 500 mg have been administered every 4-12 hours
Maximum recommended dose: 6 g/day (however, doses as high as 16-37 g have been administered)
Note: I.V. route is used when severe toxicity is evidenced by systemic symptoms (coma, shock, metabolic acidosis, or severe gastrointestinal bleeding) or potentially severe intoxications (serum iron level >500 mcg/dL). When severe symptoms are not present, the I.M. route may be preferred; however, the use of deferoxamine in situations where the serum iron concentration is <500 mcg/dL or when severe toxicity is not evident is a subject of some clinical debate.
Chronic iron overload:
I.M.: 500-1000 mg daily; in addition, 2000 mg should be given with each unit of blood transfused (administer separately from blood)
I.V.: 2 g after each unit of blood infusion at 15 mg/kg/hour
SubQ: 1-2 g every day over 8-24 hours

Diagnostic aid, aluminum-associated osteodystrophy: I.V.: Has been used investigationally as a single 40 mg/kg I.V. dose over 2 hours, to promote mobilization of aluminum from tissue stores

Pediatrics:

Acute iron toxicity: Children: Refer to adult dosing.

Chronic iron overload: SubQ: 20-40 mg/kg/day over 8-12 hours (via a portable, controlled infusion device)

Aluminum-induced bone disease (investigational): 20-40 mg/kg every hemodialysis treatment; frequency dependent on clinical status of the patient.

Renal Impairment: Cl_{cr} <10 mL/minute: Administer 50% of dose.

Available Dosage Forms Injection, powder for reconstitution, as mesylate: 500 mg, 2 g

Monitoring and Teaching Issues

Physical Assessment: I.V.: Infuse slowly and monitor infusion site. Monitor for acute reactions; urticaria, hypotension and shock can occur following rapid I.V. administration. With chronic therapy, perform ophthalmologic exam (fundoscopy, slit-lamp exam) and audiometry. Monitor for adverse reactions (eg, cardiac, respiratory, or CNS symptoms) and teach patient importance of reporting adverse symptoms.

Monitoring Laboratory Tests: Serum iron, total iron-binding capacity

Patient Education: I.V.: Instructions depend on patient condition. You will be monitored closely for effects of this medication and frequent blood or urine tests may be necessary. Report chest pain, rapid heartbeat, headache, pain, swelling, or irritation at infusion site; skin rash; changes or loss of hearing or vision; or acute abdominal or leg cramps. **Pregnancy/breast-feeding precautions:** Inform prescriber if you are or intend to become pregnant. Do not breast-feed.

Pregnancy Risk Factor: C

Lactation: Excretion in breast milk unknown/contraindicated

Administration

I.M.: I.M. administration is preferred in patients not in shock. Add 2 mL sterile water to 500 mg vial. For I.M. or SubQ administration, no further dilution is required.

I.V.: Urticaria, hypotension, and shock have occurred following rapid I.V. administration; give I.M., slow SubQ, or I.V. infusion.

The manufacturer states that the I.M. route is preferred; however, the I.V. route is generally preferred in patients with severe toxicity (ie, patients in shock). Maximum I.V. rate: 15 mg/kg/hour.

Reconstitution: Reconstituted solutions (sterile water) may be stored at room temperature for 7 days.

Compatibility: Stable in D_5W, LR, NS, SWFI

Storage: Protect from light.

- ◆ **Deferoxamine Mesylate** *see* Deferoxamine *on page 412*
- ◆ **Dehydrobenzperidol** *see* Droperidol *on page 500*
- ◆ **Delatestryl®** *see* Testosterone *on page 1450*

Delavirdine (de la VIR deen)

U.S. Brand Names Rescriptor®

Synonyms U-90152S

Generic Available No

Pharmacologic Category Antiretroviral Agent, Reverse Transcriptase Inhibitor (Non-nucleoside)

Use Treatment of HIV-1 infection in combination with at least two additional antiretroviral agents

Mechanism of Action/Effect Delavirdine binds directly to reverse transcriptase, blocking RNA-dependent and DNA-dependent DNA polymerase activities

Contraindications Hypersensitivity to delavirdine or any component of the formulation; concurrent use of alprazolam, cisapride, ergot alkaloids, midazolam, pimozide, or triazolam

Warnings/Precautions Avoid use with benzodiazepines, cisapride, clarithromycin, dapsone, enzyme-inducing anticonvulsants (carbamazepine, phenytoin, phenobarbital, rifampin, rifabutin, or St John's wort); may lead to loss of efficacy or development of resistance. Concurrent use of lovastatin or simvastatin should be avoided (use caution with other statins). Use caution with amphetamines, antacids, antiarrhythmics, benzodiazepines (alprazolam, midazolam, and triazolam are contraindicated), clarithromycin, dihydropyridine, calcium channel blockers, dapsone, immunosuppressants, methadone, oral contraceptives, or sildenafil.

Use with caution in patients with hepatic or renal dysfunction; due to rapid emergence of resistance, delavirdine should not be used as monotherapy; cross-resistance may be conferred to other non-nucleoside reverse transcriptase inhibitors, although potential for cross-resistance with protease inhibitors is low. Long-term effects of delavirdine are not known. Safety and efficacy have not been established in children. Rash, which occurs frequently, may require discontinuation of therapy; usually occurs within 1-3 weeks and lasts <2 weeks. Most patients may resume therapy following a treatment interruption.

Drug Interactions

Cytochrome P450 Effect: Substrate of CYP2D6 (minor), 3A4 (major); **Inhibits** CYP1A2 (weak), 2C8/9 (strong), 2C19 (strong), 2D6 (strong), 3A4 (strong)

Decreased Effect: The levels/effects of delavirdine may be decreased by aminoglutethimide, carbamazepine, nafcillin, nevirapine, phenobarbital, phenytoin, rifamycins, and other CYP3A4 inducers; concurrent therapy may lead to resistance and/or loss of efficacy. Decreased plasma concentrations of delavirdine with amprenavir, dexamethasone, didanosine, and saquinavir. Decreased absorption of delavirdine with antacids, histamine-2 receptor antagonists, proton pump inhibitors (omeprazole, lansoprazole), and didanosine. Delavirdine decreases plasma concentrations of didanosine. Delavirdine may decrease the levels/effects of CYP2D6 prodrug substrates (eg, codeine, hydrocodone, oxycodone, tramadol).

(Continued)

Delavirdine *(Continued)*

Increased Effect/Toxicity: Concurrent therapy with selected benzodiazepines (alprazolam, midazolam, triazolam), ergot derivatives, cisapride, and pimozide is contraindicated. Concurrent therapy with lovastatin or simvastatin is not recommended (per manufacturer). Delavirdine may alter the levels/effects of lopinavir, ritonavir, and saquinavir (dosage adjustments may be required). Delavirdine may increase the levels/effects of amiodarone, amphetamines, selected benzodiazepines, selected beta-blockers, calcium channel blockers, citalopram, cyclosporine, dextromethorphan, diazepam, fluoxetine, glimepiride, glipizide, lidocaine, methsuximide, mirtazapine, nateglinide, nefazodone, paroxetine, phenytoin, pioglitazone, quinidine, risperidone, rosiglitazone, sertraline, sildenafil (and other PDE-5 inhibitors), tacrolimus, thioridazine, tricyclic antidepressants, venlafaxine, warfarin, and other CYP2C8/9, 2C19, or 2D6 substrates. When used with strong CYP3A4 inhibitors, dosage adjustment/limits are recommended for sildenafil and other PDE-5 inhibitors; refer to individual monographs. Dosage adjustment is recommended with clarithromycin.

Nutritional/Ethanol Interactions Herb/Nutraceutical: Delavirdine serum concentration may be decreased by St John's wort; avoid concurrent use.

Adverse Reactions
>10%: Dermatologic: Rash (3.2% required discontinuation)
1% to 10%:
Central nervous system: Headache, fatigue
Dermatologic: Pruritus
Gastrointestinal: Nausea, diarrhea, vomiting
Metabolic: Increased ALT (SGPT), increased AST (SGOT)

Overdosage/Toxicology Reports of human overdose with delavirdine are not available. GI decontamination and supportive measures are recommended. Dialysis is unlikely to be of benefit in removing this drug since it is extensively metabolized by the liver and is highly protein bound.

Pharmacodynamics/Kinetics
Absorption: Rapid
Bioavailability: 85%
Time to Peak: Plasma: 1 hour
Protein Binding: ~98%, primarily to albumin
Half-Life Elimination: 2-11 hours
Metabolism: Hepatic via CYP3A4 and 2D6 (**Note:** May reduce CYP3A activity and inhibit its own metabolism.)
Excretion: Urine (51%, <5% as unchanged drug); feces (44%); nonlinear kinetics exhibited

Dosing
Adults & Elderly: HIV-1 infection (part of combination): Oral: 400 mg 3 times/day
Available Dosage Forms Tablet, as mesylate: 100 mg, 200 mg

Monitoring and Teaching Issues
Physical Assessment: See Warnings/Precautions for specific use cautions (eg, hepatic or renal impairment). Assess potential for interactions with other pharmacological agents or herbal products patient may be taking (see Drug Interactions). Assess patient response (see Adverse Reactions) on a regular basis during therapy. Teach patient proper use (importance of compliance to reduce potential for resistance; see Administration), possible side effects/appropriate interventions, and adverse symptoms to report (see Patient Education).

Monitoring Laboratory Tests: Liver function tests if administered with saquinavir; viral load

Patient Education: Do not take any new medication during therapy unless approved by prescriber. This drug is not a cure for HIV, nor has it been found to reduce transmission of HIV. Take as directed, with or without food. Do not take antacids within 1 hour of delavirdine. Mix 4 tablets in 3-5 oz of water, allow to stand a few minutes, and stir; drink immediately. Rinse glass and mouth following ingestion to ensure total dose administered. May cause nausea or vomiting (small frequent meals, frequent mouth care, sucking lozenges, or chewing gum may help; consult prescriber if nausea or vomiting persists). Report mouth sores; skin rash or irritation; muscle weakness or tremors; easy bruising or bleeding, fever or chills; CNS changes (eg, hallucinations, confusion, dizziness, altered coordination); swelling of face, lips, or tongue; yellowing of eyes or skin; or dark urine or pale stools. **Pregnancy/breast-feeding precautions:** Inform prescriber if you are or intend to become pregnant. Do not breast-feed.

Dietary Considerations: May be taken without regard to food.
Pregnancy Risk Factor: C
Pregnancy Issues: It is not known if delavirdine crosses the human placenta. Delavirdine was shown to be teratogenic in some animal studies. Health professionals are encouraged to contact the antiretroviral pregnancy registry to monitor outcomes of pregnant women exposed to antiretroviral medications (1-800-258-4263 or www.APRegistry.com).
Lactation: Excretion in breast milk unknown/contraindicated
Breast-Feeding Issues: HIV-infected mothers are discouraged from breast-feeding to decrease potential transmission of HIV.

Administration
Oral: Patients with achlorhydria should take the drug with an acidic beverage. Antacids and delavirdine should be separated by 1 hour. A dispersion of delavirdine may be prepared by adding 4 tablets to at least 3 oz of water. Allow to stand for a few minutes and stir until uniform dispersion. Drink immediately. Rinse glass and mouth following ingestion to ensure total dose administered.

Additional Information Potential compliance problems, frequency of administration, and adverse effects should be discussed with patients before initiating therapy to help prevent the emergence of resistance.

Related Information
Tuberculosis *on page 1864*

♦ **Delestrogen®** *see Estradiol on page 552*

- **Delta-9-Tetrahydro-Cannabinol** *see Dronabinol on page 499*
- **Delta-9 THC** *see Dronabinol on page 499*
- **Deltacortisone** *see PredniSONE on page 1247*
- **Deltadehydrocortisone** *see PredniSONE on page 1247*
- **Deltahydrocortisone** *see PrednisoLONE on page 1245*
- **Demadex®** *see Torsemide on page 1500*

Demeclocycline (dem e kloe SYE kleen)

U.S. Brand Names Declomycin®
Synonyms Demeclocycline Hydrochloride; Demethylchlortetracycline
Generic Available Yes
Pharmacologic Category Antibiotic, Tetracycline Derivative
Use Treatment of susceptible bacterial infections (acne, gonorrhea, pertussis and urinary tract infections) caused by both gram-negative and gram-positive organisms
Unlabeled/Investigational Use Treatment of chronic syndrome of inappropriate secretion of antidiuretic hormone (SIADH)
Mechanism of Action/Effect Inhibits protein synthesis by binding with the 30S and possibly the 50S ribosomal subunit(s) of susceptible bacteria; may also cause alterations in the cytoplasmic membrane; inhibits actions of ADH in patients with SIADH
Contraindications Hypersensitivity to demeclocycline, tetracyclines, or any component of the formulation; children <8 years of age; concomitant use with methoxyflurane; pregnancy
Warnings/Precautions Photosensitivity reactions occur frequently with this drug, avoid prolonged exposure to sunlight, do not use tanning equipment. Use of tetracyclines during tooth development may cause permanent discoloration of the teeth and enamel, hypoplasia and retardation of skeletal development and bone growth with risk being the greatest for children <4 years and those receiving high doses; use caution in patients with renal or hepatic impairment (eg, elderly); dosage modification required in patients with renal impairment; may act as an antianabolic agent and increase BUN; pseudotumor cerebri has been reported with tetracycline use (usually resolves with discontinuation); outdated drug can cause nephropathy; superinfection possible
Drug Interactions
  Decreased Effect: Antacid preparations containing calcium, magnesium, aluminum bismuth, or sodium bicarbonate may decrease tetracycline absorption; bile acid sequestrants, quinapril (magnesium-containing formulation), iron, or zinc may also decrease absorption; penicillins decrease therapeutic effect of tetracyclines. Although anecdotal reports suggest oral contraceptive efficacy could be reduced by tetracyclines, this has been refuted by more rigorous scientific and clinical data.
  Increased Effect/Toxicity: Methoxyflurane anesthesia may cause fatal nephrotoxicity; retinoic acid derivatives may increase adverse and toxic effects; warfarin may result in increased anticoagulation; methotrexate levels may be increased
Nutritional/Ethanol Interactions
  Food: Demeclocycline serum levels may be decreased if taken with food.
  Herb/Nutraceutical: Avoid dong quai, St John's wort (may also cause photosensitization).
Lab Interactions May interfere with tests for urinary glucose (false-negative urine glucose using Clinistix®).
Adverse Reactions Frequency not defined.
  Cardiovascular: Pericarditis
  Central nervous system: Bulging fontanels (infants), dizziness, headache, pseudotumor cerebri (adults)
  Dermatologic: Angioneurotic edema, erythema multiforme, erythematous rash, maculopapular rash, photosensitivity, pigmentation of skin, Stevens-Johnson syndrome (rare), urticaria
  Endocrine & metabolic: Discoloration of thyroid gland (brown/black), nephrogenic diabetes insipidus
  Gastrointestinal: Anorexia, diarrhea, dysphagia, enterocolitis, esophageal ulcerations, glossitis, nausea, pancreatitis, vomiting
  Genitourinary: Balanitis
  Hematologic: Eosinophilia, neutropenia, hemolytic anemia, thrombocytopenia
  Hepatic: Hepatitis (rare), hepatotoxicity (rare), liver enzymes increased, liver failure (rare)
  Neuromuscular & skeletal: Myasthenic syndrome, polyarthralgia, tooth discoloration (children <8 years, rarely in adults)
  Ocular: Visual disturbances
  Otic: Tinnitus
  Renal: Acute renal failure
  Respiratory: Pulmonary infiltrates
  Miscellaneous: Anaphylaxis, anaphylactoid purpura, lupus-like syndrome, systemic lupus erythematosus exacerbation
Overdosage/Toxicology Treatment is supportive.
Pharmacodynamics/Kinetics
  Onset of Action: SIADH: Several days
  Absorption: ~50% to 80%; reduced by food and dairy products
  Time to Peak: Serum: 3-6 hours
  Protein Binding: 41% to 50%
  Half-Life Elimination: 10-17 hours
  Metabolism: Hepatic (small amounts) to inactive metabolites; undergoes enterohepatic recirculation
  Excretion: Urine (42% to 50% as unchanged drug)
Dosing
  Adults & Elderly:
    Susceptible infections: Oral: 150 mg 4 times/day or 300 mg twice daily
    SIADH (unlabeled use): Oral: 900-1200 mg/day or 13-15 mg/kg/day divided every 6-8 hours initially, then decrease to 600-900 mg/day
(Continued)

Demeclocycline *(Continued)*

Pediatrics: Susceptible infections: Oral: ≥8 years: 8-12 mg/kg/day divided every 6-12 hours
Renal Impairment: Should be avoided in patients with renal dysfunction.
Hepatic Impairment: Should be avoided in patients with hepatic dysfunction.
Available Dosage Forms Tablet, as hydrochloride: 150 mg, 300 mg

Monitoring and Teaching Issues

Physical Assessment: Assess results of culture and sensitivity tests and patient's allergy history prior to beginning therapy. See Warnings/Precautions for use cautions (eg, renal or hepatic impairment). Assess potential for interactions with other pharmacological agents or herbal products patient may be taking (eg, increased risk of toxicity or decreased effectiveness; see Drug Interactions). Assess results of laboratory tests, therapeutic response, and adverse effects (eg, rash, anaphylactic reactions, anemia, CNS changes; see Adverse Reactions) on a regular basis throughout therapy. Advise patients with diabetes about use of Clinitest®. Teach patient proper use, possible side effects/appropriate interventions, and adverse symptoms to report (see Patient Education).

Monitoring Laboratory Tests: CBC, renal and hepatic function; perform culture and sensitivity studies prior to initiating therapy

Patient Education: Do not take any new medication during therapy unless approved by prescriber. Take on an empty stomach (1 hour before or 2 hours after meals with plenty of fluid). Take at regularly scheduled intervals around-the-clock. Avoid antacids, iron, dairy products, and other medications within 2 hours of taking demeclocycline. If you have diabetes, drug may cause false test results with Clinistix® urine glucose monitoring; use of another form of glucose monitoring is preferable. May cause photosensitivity (use sunscreen, wear protective clothing and eyewear, and avoid direct sunlight); dizziness or lightheadedness (use caution when driving or engaging in tasks that require alertness until response to drug is known); nausea or vomiting (frequent, small meals, frequent mouth care, sucking lozenges, or chewing gum may help); or diarrhea (buttermilk, yogurt, or boiled milk may help). Report rash or intense itching, yellowing of skin or eyes, change in color of urine or stools, fever or chills, dark urine or pale stools, vaginal itching or discharge, foul-smelling stools, excessive thirst or urination, acute headache, unresolved diarrhea, or respiratory difficulty. **Pregnancy/breast-feeding precautions:** Inform prescriber if you are pregnant. Do not get pregnant while taking this medication. Consult prescriber for appropriate contraceptives. Breast-feeding is not recommended.

Dietary Considerations: Should be taken 1 hour before or 2 hours after food or milk with plenty of fluid.

Geriatric Considerations: Has not been studied exclusively in the elderly.

Pregnancy Risk Factor: D

Pregnancy Issues: Tetracyclines cross the placenta and enter fetal circulation; may cause permanent discoloration of teeth if used during the last half of pregnancy. Related antibiotics have been associated with mutagenesis, embryotoxicity, and oncogenic activity in animals.

Lactation: Enters breast milk/not recommended (AAP rates tetracycline "compatible")

Administration

Oral: Administer 1 hour before or 2 hours after food or milk with plenty of fluid.

- ♦ **Demeclocycline Hydrochloride** *see Demeclocycline on page 415*
- ♦ **Demerol®** *see Meperidine on page 950*
- ♦ **4-Demethoxydaunorubicin** *see Idarubicin on page 781*
- ♦ **Demethylchlortetracycline** *see Demeclocycline on page 415*
- ♦ **Demulen®** *see Ethinyl Estradiol and Ethynodiol Diacetate on page 583*
- ♦ **Denavir®** *see Penciclovir on page 1172*

Denileukin Diftitox *(de ni LOO kin DIF ti toks)*

U.S. Brand Names ONTAK®
Generic Available No
Pharmacologic Category Antineoplastic Agent, Miscellaneous
Use Treatment of persistent or recurrent cutaneous T-cell lymphoma whose malignant cells express the CD25 component of the IL-2 receptor
Mechanism of Action/Effect Interacts with receptors on surface of malignant cells to inhibit intracellular protein synthesis rapidly leading to cell death.
Contraindications Hypersensitivity to denileukin diftitox, diphtheria toxin, interleukin-2, or any component of the formulation
Warnings/Precautions Acute hypersensitivity reactions, including anaphylaxis, may occur; most events occur during or within 24 hours of the first dose of a treatment cycle. Has been associated with a delayed-onset vascular leak syndrome, which may be severe. Denileukin diftitox may impair immune function. Use with caution in patients with pre-existing cardiovascular disease and in patients >65 years of age.

Adverse Reactions

The occurrence of adverse events diminishes after the first two treatment courses. Infusion-related hypersensitivity reactions have been reported in 69% of patients. Reactions are variable, but may include hypotension, back pain, dyspnea, vasodilation, rash, chest pain, tachycardia, dysphagia, syncope or anaphylaxis. In addition, a flu-like syndrome, beginning several hours to days following infusion, occurred in 91% of patients.

In 27% of patients a vascular leak syndrome occurred, characterized by hypotension, edema, or hypoalbuminemia. The syndrome usually developed within the first 2 weeks of infusion. Six percent of patients who developed this syndrome required hospitalization. The symptoms may persist or even worsen despite cessation of denileukin diftitox.

Severe (Grade 3 and 4) reactions which occurred with an incidence over 10% included: Chills/fever (22%), asthenia (22%), infection (24%), pain (13%), nausea/vomiting (14%), hypoalbuminemia (14%), transaminases elevation (15%), edema (15%), dyspnea (14%), and rash (13%).

The following list of symptoms reported during treatment includes all levels of severity:

>10%:

    Cardiovascular: Edema (47%), hypotension (36%), chest pain (24%), vasodilation (22%), tachycardia (12%)

    Central nervous system: Fever/chills (81%), headache (26%), pain (48%), dizziness (22%), nervousness (11%)

    Dermatologic: Rash (34%), pruritus (20%)

    Endocrine & metabolic: Hypoalbuminemia (83%), hypocalcemia (17%), weight loss (14%)

    Gastrointestinal: Nausea/vomiting (64%), anorexia (36%), diarrhea (29%)

    Hematologic: Decreased lymphocyte count (34%), anemia (18%)

    Hepatic: Transaminases increased (61%)

    Neuromuscular & skeletal: Asthenia (66%), myalgia (17%)

    Respiratory: Dyspnea (29%), increased cough (26%), pharyngitis (17%), rhinitis (13%)

    Miscellaneous: Hypersensitivity (69%), infection (48%), vascular leak syndrome (27%), diaphoresis increased (10%), paresthesia (13%)

1% to 10%:

    Cardiovascular: Hypertension (6%), arrhythmia (6%), MI (1%)

    Central nervous system: Insomnia (9%), confusion (8%)

    Endocrine & metabolic: Dehydration (9%), hypokalemia (6%), hyperthyroidism (<5%), hypothyroidism (<5%)

    Gastrointestinal: Constipation (9%), dyspepsia (7%), dysphagia (6%), pancreatitis (<5%)

    Genitourinary: Hematuria (10%), albuminuria (10%), pyuria (10%)

    Hematologic: Thrombotic events (7%), thrombocytopenia (8%), leukopenia (6%)

    Local: Injection site reaction (8%), anaphylaxis (1%)

    Neuromuscular & skeletal: Arthralgia (8%)

    Renal: Increased creatinine (7%), acute renal insufficiency (<5%), microscopic hematuria (<5%)

    Respiratory: Lung disorder (8%)

Overdosage/Toxicology Although there is no human experience in overdose, dose-limiting toxicities include nausea, vomiting, fever, chills and persistent asthenia. Treatment is supportive and symptom-directed. Fluid balance, as well as hepatic and renal function, should be closely monitored.

Pharmacodynamics/Kinetics

    Half-Life Elimination: Distribution: 2-5 minutes; Terminal: 70-80 minutes

    Metabolism: Hepatic via proteolytic degradation (animal studies)

Dosing

    Adults & Elderly: Persistent or recurrent cutaneous T-cell lymphoma: I.V.: A treatment cycle consists of 9 or 18 mcg/kg/day for 5 consecutive days administered every 21 days. The optimal duration of therapy has not been determined. Only 2% of patients who failed to demonstrate a response (at least a 25% decrease in tumor burden) prior to the fourth cycle responded to subsequent treatment.

Available Dosage Forms Injection, solution [frozen]: 150 mcg/mL (2 mL)

Monitoring and Teaching Issues

    Physical Assessment: Use caution in presence of pre-existing cardiovascular disease and in patients >65 years of age (see Warnings/Precautions). Assess results of laboratory tests prior to therapy and weekly during therapy. Patient must be monitored closely for acute hypersensitivity reaction during and for 24 hours following first infusion (see Adverse Reactions). Following infusion, patient should be monitored or taught to monitor for delayed vascular leak syndrome (eg, hypotension, edema, or hypoalbuminemia) and other adverse reactions (see Adverse Reactions). Teach patient appropriate interventions to reduce side effects and adverse reactions to report (see Patient Education).

    Monitoring Laboratory Tests: CBC, blood chemistry panel, renal and hepatic function tests, serum albumin level; repeat at weekly intervals during therapy

    Patient Education: This medication can only be administered via intravenous infusion. During infusion, report immediately any chills; chest pain, respiratory difficulty, or tightness in throat; or redness, swelling, pain, or burning at infusion site. Maintaining adequate nutrition (frequent small meals) and hydration is important (2-3 L/day) unless instructed to restrict fluid intake. You may be more susceptible to infection (avoid crowds and exposure to infection and do not have any vaccinations without consulting prescriber). May cause nausea, vomiting, anorexia, flatulence (small frequent meals, good mouth care, chewing gum, or sucking lozenges may help); constipation (increased exercise, fluids, fruit, or fiber may help); diarrhea (buttermilk, boiled milk, or yogurt may help); headache, back or muscle pain (consult prescriber for mild analgesic); dizziness, weakness, or confusion (use caution when driving, engaging in hazardous activities, or climbing stairs until effect of medication is known). Report unresolved GI effects; headache, back or muscle pain; skin dryness, rash, or sores; altered urinary patterns; flu syndrome or infection (eg, weakness, fatigue, white plaques or sores in mouth, vaginal discharge, chills, fever); CNS disturbances (insomnia, dizziness, agitation, confusion, depression); unusual bleeding or bruising, blood in urine or stool; swelling of extremities; or any other adverse effects. **Pregnancy/breast-feeding precautions:** Inform prescriber if you are or intend to become pregnant. Do not breast-feed.

    Pregnancy Risk Factor: C

    Lactation: Excretion in breast milk unknown/contraindicated

    Breast-Feeding Issues: The excretion of denileukin diftitox in breast milk is unknown, however, it is recommended that a breast-feeding woman who is treated with denileukin diftitox should discontinue nursing.

Administration

    I.V.: For I.V. use only. Should be infused over at least 15 minutes. Should not be given as an I.V. bolus. Patients should be closely observed during the infusion for symptoms of hypersensitivity. If a patient experiences a reaction, the severity of the reaction should be evaluated, and a decision should be made to either reduce the rate or discontinue the infusion. Resuscitation equipment must be readily available. Delay therapy if serum albumin is <3 g/dL.

(Continued)

Denileukin Diftitox *(Continued)*

Reconstitution: Must be brought to room temperature (25°C or 77°F) before preparing the dose. Do **not** heat vials. Thaw in refrigerator for not more than 24 hours or at room temperature for 1-2 hours. Avoid vigorous agitation. Solution may be mixed by gentle swirling. Dilute with NS to a concentration of ≥15 mcg/mL.

Compatibility: Do **not** use glass syringes or containers.

Storage: Store frozen at or -10°C; cannot be refrozen. Solutions ≥15 mcg/mL in NS should be used within 6 hours. DO NOT use glass syringes or containers.

Additional Information Formulation includes EDTA and polysorbate 20, and has a pH of 6.9-7.2.

♦ **Dentapaine [OTC]** *see* Benzocaine *on page 181*

♦ **Dent's Extra Strength Toothache [OTC]** *see* Benzocaine *on page 181*

♦ **Dent's Maxi-Strength Toothache [OTC]** *see* Benzocaine *on page 181*

♦ **Deoxycoformycin** *see* Pentostatin *on page 1184*

♦ **2'-Deoxycoformycin** *see* Pentostatin *on page 1184*

♦ **Depacon®** *see* Valproic Acid and Derivatives *on page 1543*

♦ **Depade®** *see* Naltrexone *on page 1053*

♦ **Depakene®** *see* Valproic Acid and Derivatives *on page 1543*

♦ **Depakote® Delayed Release** *see* Valproic Acid and Derivatives *on page 1543*

♦ **Depakote® ER** *see* Valproic Acid and Derivatives *on page 1543*

♦ **Depakote® Sprinkle®** *see* Valproic Acid and Derivatives *on page 1543*

♦ **DepoCyt™** *see* Cytarabine (Liposomal) *on page 391*

♦ **DepoDur™** *see* Morphine Sulfate *on page 1031*

♦ **Depo®-Estradiol** *see* Estradiol *on page 552*

♦ **Depo-Medrol®** *see* MethylPREDNISolone *on page 986*

♦ **Depo-Provera®** *see* MedroxyPROGESTERone *on page 938*

♦ **Depo-Provera® Contraceptive** *see* MedroxyPROGESTERone *on page 938*

♦ **depo-subQ provera 104™** *see* MedroxyPROGESTERone *on page 938*

♦ **Depo®-Testosterone** *see* Testosterone *on page 1450*

♦ **Deprenyl** *see* Selegiline *on page 1364*

♦ **Depression** *see page 1817*

♦ **Dermarest Dricort® [OTC]** *see* Hydrocortisone *on page 760*

♦ **Dermarest® Skin Correction Cream Plus [OTC]** *see* Hydroquinone *on page 768*

♦ **Derma-Smoothe/FS®** *see* Fluocinolone *on page 643*

♦ **Dermatophytin® Injection** *see page 1625*

♦ **Dermatophytin-O** *see page 1625*

♦ **Dermoplast® Antibacterial [OTC]** *see* Benzocaine *on page 181*

♦ **Dermoplast® Pain Relieving [OTC]** *see* Benzocaine *on page 181*

♦ **Dermtex® HC [OTC]** *see* Hydrocortisone *on page 760*

♦ **Desferal®** *see* Deferoxamine *on page 412*

♦ **Desiccated Thyroid** *see* Thyroid *on page 1469*

Desipramine *(des IP ra meen)*

U.S. Brand Names Norpramin®

Synonyms Desipramine Hydrochloride; Desmethylimipramine Hydrochloride

Restrictions A medication guide should be dispensed with each prescription. A template for the required MedGuides can be found on the FDA website at: http://www.fda.gov/cder/drug/antidepressants/labelTemplate.pdf

Generic Available Yes

Pharmacologic Category Antidepressant, Tricyclic (Secondary Amine)

Medication Safety Issues

Sound-alike/look-alike issues:

Desipramine may be confused with clomiPRAMINE, deserpidine, diphenhydrAMINE, disopyramide, imipramine, nortriptyline

Norpramin® may be confused with clomiPRAMINE, imipramine, Norpace®, nortriptyline, Tenormin®

Use Treatment of depression

Unlabeled/Investigational Use Analgesic adjunct in chronic pain; peripheral neuropathies; substance-related disorders; attention-deficit/hyperactivity disorder (ADHD)

Mechanism of Action/Effect Traditionally believed to increase the synaptic concentration of norepinephrine (and to a lesser extent, serotonin) in the central nervous system by inhibition of its reuptake by the presynaptic neuronal membrane. However, additional receptor effects have been found including desensitization of adenyl cyclase, down regulation of beta-adrenergic receptors, and down regulation of serotonin receptors.

Contraindications Hypersensitivity to desipramine, drugs of similar chemical class, or any component of the formulation; use of MAO inhibitors within 14 days; use in a patient during the acute recovery phase of MI

Warnings/Precautions Antidepressants increase the risk of suicidal thinking and behavior in children and adolescents with major depressive disorder (MDD) and other depressive disorders; consider risk prior to prescribing. All patients must be closely monitored for clinical worsening, suicidality, or unusual changes in behavior, especially during the initiation of therapy or following an increase or decrease in dosage. When used in children, the child's family or caregiver should be instructed to closely observe the patient and communicate condition with healthcare provider. A medication guide should be dispensed with each prescription. **Desipramine is FDA approved for the treatment of depression in adolescents.**

The possibility of a suicide attempt is inherent in major depression and may persist until remission occurs. Use caution in high-risk patients. Worsening depression and severe abrupt suicidality that are not part of the presenting symptoms may require discontinuation or modification of drug therapy. The patient's family or caregiver should be alerted to monitor patients for the emergence of suicidality and associated behaviors (such as agitation, irritability, hostility, impulsivity, and hypomania) and notify healthcare provider.

May worsen psychosis in some patients or precipitate a shift to mania or hypomania in patients with bipolar disorder. Patients presenting with depressive symptoms should be screened for bipolar disorder. Monotherapy in patients with bipolar disorder should be avoided. **Desipramine is not FDA approved for the treatment of bipolar depression.**

The degree of anticholinergic blockade produced by this agent is low relative to other cyclic antidepressants - however, caution should be used in patients with urinary retention, benign prostatic hyperplasia, narrow-angle glaucoma, xerostomia, visual problems, constipation, or a history of bowel obstruction. The degree of sedation and conduction disturbances with desipramine are low relative to other antidepressants. However, desipramine may cause drowsiness/sedation, resulting in impaired performance of tasks requiring alertness (eg, operating machinery or driving). Sedative effects may be additive with other CNS depressants and/or ethanol. The risk of orthostasis is moderate relative to other antidepressants. Use with caution in patients with a history of cardiovascular disease (including previous MI, stroke, tachycardia, or conduction abnormalities).

Consider discontinuing, when possible, prior to elective surgery. Therapy should not be abruptly discontinued in patients receiving high doses for prolonged periods. May lower seizure threshold - use caution in patients with a previous seizure disorder or condition predisposing to seizures such as brain damage, alcoholism, or concurrent therapy with other drugs which lower the seizure threshold. May increase the risks associated with electroconvulsive therapy. Use with caution in hyperthyroid patients or those receiving thyroid supplementation. Use with caution in patients with hepatic or renal dysfunction and in elderly patients.

Drug Interactions

Cytochrome P450 Effect: Substrate of CYP1A2 (minor), 2D6 (major); **Inhibits** CYP2A6 (moderate), 2B6 (moderate), 2D6 (moderate), 2E1 (weak), 3A4 (moderate)

Decreased Effect: Desipramine may decrease the levels/effects of CYP2D6 prodrug substrates (eg, codeine, hydrocodone, oxycodone, tramadol). Desipramine's serum levels/ effect may be decreased by carbamazepine, cholestyramine, colestipol, phenobarbital, and rifampin. Desipramine inhibits the antihypertensive effect of to bethanidine, clonidine, debrisoquin, guanadrel, guanethidine, guanabenz, or guanfacine.

Increased Effect/Toxicity: Desipramine increases the effects of amphetamines, anticholinergics, other CNS depressants (sedatives, hypnotics, or ethanol), chlorpropamide, tolazamide, and warfarin. When used with MAO inhibitors, serotonin syndrome may occur. Serotonin syndrome has also been reported with ritonavir (rare). The levels/effects of desipramine may be increased by chlorpromazine, delavirdine, fluoxetine, miconazole, paroxetine, pergolide, quinidine, quinine, ritonavir, ropinirole, and other CYP2D6 inhibitors.

Cimetidine, grapefruit juice, indinavir, methylphenidate, diltiazem, and verapamil may increase the serum concentration of TCAs. Use of lithium with a TCA may increase the risk for neurotoxicity. Phenothiazines may increase concentration of some TCAs and TCAs may increase concentration of phenothiazines. Pressor response to I.V. epinephrine, norepinephrine, and phenylephrine may be enhanced in patients receiving TCAs (**Note:** Effect is unlikely with epinephrine or levonordefrin dosages typically administered as infiltration in combination with local anesthetics). Combined use of beta-agonists or drugs which prolong QT$_c$ (including quinidine, procainamide, disopyramide, cisapride, sparfloxacin, gatifloxacin, moxifloxacin) with TCAs may predispose patients to cardiac arrhythmias.

Desipramine may increase the levels/effects of selected benzodiazepines, bupropion, calcium channel blockers, cisapride, dexmedetomidine, dextromethorphan, ergot derivatives, ifosfamide, fluoxetine, selected HMG-CoA reductase inhibitors, lidocaine, mesoridazine, mirtazapine, nateglinide, nefazodone, paroxetine, pimozide, promethazine, propofol, quinidine, risperidone, ritonavir, selegiline, sertraline, sildenafil (and other PDE-5 inhibitors), tacrolimus, thioridazine, tricyclic antidepressants, venlafaxine, and other CYP2A6, 2B6, 2D6, or 3A4 substrates.

Nutritional/Ethanol Interactions

Ethanol: Avoid ethanol (may increase CNS depression).

Food: Grapefruit juice may inhibit the metabolism of some TCAs and clinical toxicity may result.

Herb/Nutraceutical: Avoid valerian, St John's wort, SAMe, kava kava (may increase risk of serotonin syndrome and/or excessive sedation).

Lab Interactions Increased glucose; decreased glucose has also been reported

Adverse Reactions Frequency not defined.

Cardiovascular: Arrhythmias, hyper-/hypotension, palpitation, heart block, tachycardia

Central nervous system: Dizziness, drowsiness, headache, confusion, delirium, hallucinations, nervousness, restlessness, parkinsonian syndrome, insomnia, disorientation, anxiety, agitation, hypomania, exacerbation of psychosis, incoordination, seizure, extrapyramidal symptoms

Dermatologic: Alopecia, photosensitivity, skin rash, urticaria

Endocrine & metabolic: Breast enlargement, galactorrhea, SIADH

Gastrointestinal: Xerostomia, decreased lower esophageal sphincter tone may cause GE reflux, constipation, nausea, unpleasant taste, weight gain/loss, anorexia, abdominal cramps, diarrhea, heartburn

Genitourinary: Difficult urination, sexual dysfunction, testicular edema

Hematologic: Agranulocytosis, eosinophilia, purpura, thrombocytopenia

Hepatic: Cholestatic jaundice, increased liver enzyme

Neuromuscular & skeletal: Fine muscle tremor, weakness, numbness, tingling, paresthesia of extremities, ataxia

Ocular: Blurred vision, disturbances of accommodation, mydriasis, increased intraocular pressure

Miscellaneous: Diaphoresis (excessive), allergic reactions

(Continued)

Desipramine *(Continued)*

Overdosage/Toxicology Symptoms of overdose include agitation, confusion, hallucinations, hyperthermia, urinary retention, CNS depression, cyanosis, dry mucous membranes, cardiac arrhythmias, and seizures. Treatment is supportive. Ventricular arrhythmias and ECG changes (eg, QRS widening) often respond with concurrent systemic alkalinization (sodium bicarbonate 0.5-2 mEq/kg I.V. or hyperventilation). Arrhythmias unresponsive to phenytoin 15-20 mg/kg (adults) may respond to lidocaine. Physostigmine (1-2 mg I.V. slowly for adults) may be indicated for reversing life-threatening cardiac arrhythmias.

Pharmacodynamics/Kinetics
Onset of Action: 1-3 weeks; Maximum antidepressant effect: >2 weeks
Absorption: Well absorbed
Time to Peak: Plasma: 4-6 hours
Half-Life Elimination: Adults: 7-60 hours
Metabolism: Hepatic
Excretion: Urine (70%)

Dosing
Adults:
Depression: Oral: Initial: 75 mg/day in divided doses; increase gradually to 150-200 mg/day in divided or single dose; maximum: 300 mg/day
Cocaine withdrawal (unlabeled use): 50-200 mg/day in divided or single dose

Elderly: Oral: Initial: 10-25 mg/day; increase by 10-25 mg every 3 days for inpatients and every week for outpatients if tolerated; usual maintenance dose: 75-100 mg/day, but doses up to 150 mg/day may be necessary.

Pediatrics: Depression: Oral:
Children 6-12 years (unlabeled use): 10-30 mg/day or 1-5 mg/kg/day in divided doses; do not exceed 5 mg/kg/day
Adolescents: Initial: 25-50 mg/day; gradually increase to 100 mg/day in single or divided doses; maximum: 150 mg/day

Renal Impairment: Hemodialysis/peritoneal dialysis effects: Supplemental dose is not necessary.

Available Dosage Forms Tablet, as hydrochloride: 10 mg, 25 mg, 50 mg, 75 mg, 100 mg, 150 mg

Monitoring and Teaching Issues
Physical Assessment: Assess potential for interactions with other prescriptions, OTC medications, or herbal products patient may be taking. Monitor CNS status. Assess for suicidal tendencies before beginning therapy. May cause physiological or psychological dependence, tolerance, or abuse; periodically evaluate need for continued use. Caution patients with diabetes to monitor glucose levels closely; may increase or decrease serum glucose levels. Assess therapeutic response and adverse reactions at beginning of therapy and periodically with long-term use. Taper dose slowly when discontinuing. Teach patient proper use, appropriate interventions to reduce side effects, and adverse symptoms to report.

Patient Education: Do not take any new medication during therapy unless approved by prescriber. Take exactly as directed; do not increase dose or frequency. It may take 2-3 weeks to achieve desired results. This medicine may cause physical and/or psychological dependence. Avoid alcohol and grapefruit juice. Maintain adequate hydration (2-3 L/day of fluids) unless instructed to restrict fluid intake. May cause drowsiness, lightheadedness, impaired coordination, dizziness, or blurred vision (use caution when driving or engaging in tasks requiring alertness until response to drug is known); loss of appetite or disturbed taste (small frequent meals, good mouth care, chewing gum, or sucking lozenges may help); constipation (increased exercise, fluids, fruit, or fiber may help); urinary retention (void before taking medication); postural hypotension (use caution climbing stairs or when changing position from lying or sitting to standing); altered sexual drive or ability (reversible); or photosensitivity (use sunscreen, wear protective clothing and eyewear, and avoid direct sunlight). Report chest pain, palpitations, or rapid heartbeat; persistent adverse CNS effects (eg, suicidal ideation, nervousness, restlessness, insomnia, anxiety, excitation, headache, agitation, impaired coordination, changes in cognition); muscle cramping, weakness, tremors, or rigidity; blurred vision or eye pain; breast enlargement or swelling; yellowing of skin or eyes; or worsening of condition. **Pregnancy/breast-feeding precautions:** Inform prescriber if you are or intend to become pregnant. Breast-feeding is not recommended.

Geriatric Considerations: Preferred agent because of its milder side effect profile; patients may experience excitation or stimulation, in such cases, give as a single morning dose or divided dose.

Pregnancy Risk Factor: C

Lactation: Enters breast milk/not recommended (AAP rates "of concern")

Breast-Feeding Issues: Generally, it is not recommended to breast-feed if taking antidepressants because of the long half-life, active metabolites, and the potential for side effects in the infant.

Additional Information Less sedation and anticholinergic effects than with amitriptyline or imipramine

Related Information
Antidepressant Agents *on page 1713*
Antidepressant Medication Guidelines *on page 1765*
Federal OBRA Regulations: Recommended Maximum Doses *on page 1773*
Peak and Trough Guidelines *on page 1694*
Pharmacotherapy of Urinary Incontinence *on page 1858*

♦ **Desipramine Hydrochloride** *see* Desipramine *on page 418*

Desloratadine *(des lor AT a deen)*
U.S. Brand Names Clarinex®
Generic Available No

Pharmacologic Category Antihistamine, Nonsedating

Use Relief of nasal and non-nasal symptoms of seasonal allergic rhinitis (SAR) and perennial allergic rhinitis (PAR); treatment of chronic idiopathic urticaria (CIU)

Mechanism of Action/Effect Desloratadine is a long-acting antihistamine with selective H_1 receptor antagonistic activity.

Contraindications Hypersensitivity to desloratadine, loratadine, or any component of the formulation

Warnings/Precautions Dose should be adjusted in patients with liver or renal impairment. Use with caution in patients known to be slow metabolizers of desloratadine (incidence of side effects may be increased). RediTabs® contain phenylalanine. Safety and efficacy have not been established for children <6 months of age.

Drug Interactions

Increased Effect/Toxicity: With concurrent use of desloratadine and erythromycin or ketoconazole, the C_{max} and AUC of desloratadine and its metabolite are increased; however, no clinically-significant changes in the safety profile of desloratadine were observed in clinical studies.

Nutritional/Ethanol Interactions Food: Does not affect bioavailability.

Adverse Reactions

>10%: Central nervous system: Headache (14%)

1% to 10%:

Central nervous system: Fatigue (2% to 5%), somnolence (2%), dizziness (4%)
Endocrine & metabolic: Dysmenorrhea (2%)
Gastrointestinal: Xerostomia (3%), nausea (5%), dyspepsia (3%)
Neuromuscular & skeletal: Myalgia (2% to 3%)
Respiratory: Pharyngitis (3% to 4%)

Overdosage/Toxicology Information is limited to doses studied during clinical trials (up to 45 mg/day). Symptoms included somnolence, and small increases in heart rate and QT_c interval (not clinically significant). In the event of an overdose, treatment should be symptom-directed and supportive. Desloratadine and its metabolite are not removed by hemodialysis.

Pharmacodynamics/Kinetics

Time to Peak: 3 hours

Protein Binding: Desloratadine: 82% to 87%; 3-hydroxydesloratadine: 85% to 89%

Half-Life Elimination: 27 hours

Metabolism: Hepatic to active metabolite, 3-hydroxydesloratadine (specific enzymes not identified); undergoes glucuronidation. Decreased in slow metabolizers of desloratadine. Not expected to affect or be affected by medications metabolized by CYP with normal doses.

Excretion: Urine and feces (as metabolites)

Dosing

Adults & Elderly: Seasonal or perennial allergic rhinitis, chronic idiopathic urticaria: Oral: 5 mg once daily

Pediatrics: Seasonal or perennial allergic rhinitis, chronic idiopathic urticaria: Oral:

Children:

6-11 months: 1 mg once daily
12 months to 5 years: 1.25 mg once daily
6-11 years: 2.5 mg once daily
Children ≥12 years: Refer to adult dosing.

Renal Impairment:

Children: Not established
Adults: 5 mg every other day

Hepatic Impairment: 5 mg every other day

Available Dosage Forms

Syrup (Clarinex®): 0.5 mg/mL (480 mL) [bubble gum flavor]
Tablet (Clarinex®): 5 mg
Tablet, orally-disintegrating (Clarinex® RediTabs®): 5 mg [contains phenylalanine 1.75 mg/tablet; tutti-frutti flavor]

Monitoring and Teaching Issues

Physical Assessment: Assess effectiveness and interactions of other medications patient may be taking. Monitor effectiveness of therapy and adverse reactions at beginning of therapy and periodically with long-term use. Assess knowledge/teach patient appropriate use, interventions to reduce side effects, and adverse symptoms to report.

Patient Education: Take as directed; do not exceed recommended dose. Avoid use of other depressants, alcohol, or sleep-inducing medications unless approved by prescriber. You may experience headache, drowsiness, or dizziness (use caution when driving or engaging in tasks that require alertness until response to drug is known); or dry mouth, dry throat, or nausea (small frequent meals, frequent mouth care, chewing gum, or sucking hard candy may help). Report rapid heartbeat, shortness of breath, skin rash, persistent flu-like symptoms, or muscle aches. **Pregnancy/breast-feeding precautions:** Inform prescriber if you are or intend to become pregnant. Breast-feeding is not recommended.

Dietary Considerations: May be taken with or without food. Orally-disintegrating tablets contain phenylalanine 1.75 mg/tablet.

Pregnancy Risk Factor: C

Lactation: Enters breast milk/not recommended

Administration

Oral: May be taken with or without food.

RediTabs® should be placed on the tongue; tablet will disintegrate immediately. May be taken with or without water.

Syrup: A commercially-available measuring dropper or syringe calibrated to deliver 2 mL or 2.5 mL should be used to administer age-appropriate doses in children.

Storage: Syrup, tablet, orally-disintegrating tablet: Store at 25°C (77°F); excursions permitted between 15°C to 30°C (59°F to 86°F). Protect from moisture and excessive heat (85°F). Use orally-disintegrating tablet immediately after opening blister package. Syrup should be protected from light.

♦ **Desmethylimipramine Hydrochloride** *see Desipramine on page 418*

Desmopressin (des moe PRES in)

U.S. Brand Names DDAVP®; Stimate™

Synonyms 1-Deamino-8-D-Arginine Vasopressin; Desmopressin Acetate

Generic Available Yes: Excludes tablet

Pharmacologic Category Antihemophilic Agent; Hemostatic Agent; Vasopressin Analog, Synthetic

Use Treatment of diabetes insipidus; control of bleeding in hemophilia A, and mild-to-moderate classic von Willebrand disease (type I); primary nocturnal enuresis

Mechanism of Action/Effect Enhances reabsorption of water in the kidneys by increasing cellular permeability of the collecting ducts; possibly causes smooth muscle constriction with resultant vasoconstriction; raises plasma levels of von Willebrand factor and factor VIII

Contraindications Hypersensitivity to desmopressin or any component of the formulation; hemophilia B, severe classic von Willebrand disease (type IIB); patients with ≤5% factor VIII activity level; factor VIII antibodies

Warnings/Precautions Fluid intake should be adjusted downward in the elderly and very young patients to decrease the possibility of water intoxication and hyponatremia. Avoid overhydration especially when drug is used for its hemostatic effect. Use caution with cystic fibrosis or other conditions associated with fluid and electrolyte imbalance due to potential hyponatremia. Use caution with coronary artery insufficiency or hypertensive cardiovascular disease; may increase or decrease blood pressure leading to changes in heart rate. Consider switching from nasal to intravenous solution if changes in the nasal mucosa (scarring, edema) occur leading to unreliable absorption. Use caution in patients predisposed to thrombus formation; thrombotic events (acute cerebrovascular thrombosis, acute myocardial infarction) have occurred (rare). Use may rarely lead to extreme decreases in plasma osmolality, resulting in seizures and coma.

Drug Interactions

Decreased Effect: Demeclocycline and lithium may decrease ADH response.

Increased Effect/Toxicity: Chlorpropamide, fludrocortisone may increase ADH response.

Nutritional/Ethanol Interactions Ethanol: Avoid ethanol (may decrease antidiuretic effect).

Adverse Reactions Frequency not defined (may be dose or route related).

Cardiovascular: Acute cerebrovascular thrombosis, acute MI, blood pressure increased/ decreased, chest pain, edema, facial flushing, palpitation

Central nervous system: Agitation, chills, coma, dizziness, headache, insomnia, somnolence

Endocrine & metabolic: Hyponatremia, water intoxication

Gastrointestinal: Abdominal cramps, dyspepsia, nausea, sore throat, vomiting

Genitourinary: Balanitis, vulval pain

Local: Injection: Burning pain, erythema, and swelling at the injection site

Respiratory: Cough, nasal congestion, epistaxis

Miscellaneous: Allergic reactions (rare), anaphylaxis (rare)

Overdosage/Toxicology Symptoms of overdose include drowsiness, headache, confusion, anuria, and water intoxication. In case of overdose, decrease or discontinue desmopressin.

Pharmacodynamics/Kinetics

Onset of Action:

Intranasal administration: Onset of increased factor VIII activity: 30 minutes (dose related); peak effect 1.5 hours

I.V. infusion: Onset of increased factor VIII activity: 30 minutes (dose related); peak effect: 1.5-2 hours

Oral tablets: Onset of action: ADH: ~1 hour; peak effect: 4-7 hours

Bioavailability: Tablet: 5% compared to intranasal; 0.16% compared to I.V.

Half-Life Elimination:

I.V. infusion: Terminal: 75 minutes

Tablet: 1.5-2.5 hours

Metabolism: Unknown

Dosing

Adults & Elderly:

Diabetes insipidus:

I.V., SubQ: 2-4 mcg/day (0.5-1 mL) in 2 divided doses or 1/10 of the maintenance intranasal dose

Intranasal (100 mcg/mL nasal solution): 10-40 mcg/day (0.1-0.4 mL) divided 1-3 times/ day; adjust morning and evening doses separately for an adequate diurnal rhythm of water turnover. **Note:** The nasal spray pump can only deliver doses of 10 mcg (0.1 mL) or multiples of 10 mcg (0.1 mL); if doses other than this are needed, the rhinal tube delivery system is preferred.

Oral: Initial: 0.05 mg twice daily; total daily dose should be increased or decreased as needed to obtain adequate antidiuresis (range: 0.1-1.2 mg divided 2-3 times/day)

Nocturnal enuresis:

Intranasal (using 100 mcg/mL nasal solution): Initial: 20 mcg (0.2 mL) at bedtime; range: 10-40 mcg; it is recommended that ½ of the dose be given in each nostril. **Note:** The nasal spray pump can only deliver doses of 10 mcg (0.1 mL) or multiples of 10 mcg (0.1 mL); if doses other than this are needed, the rhinal tube delivery system is preferred.

Oral: 0.2 mg at bedtime; dose may be titrated up to 0.6 mg to achieve desired response. Patients previously on intranasal therapy can begin oral tablets 24 hours after the last intranasal dose.

Hemophilia A and mild-to-moderate von Willebrand disease (type I):

I.V.: 0.3 mcg/kg by slow infusion, begin 30 minutes before procedure

Nasal spray: Using high concentration spray (1.5 mg/mL): <50 kg: 150 mcg (1 spray); >50 kg: 300 mcg (1 spray each nostril); repeat use is determined by the patient's clinical condition and laboratory work. If using preoperatively, administer 2 hours before surgery.

Pediatrics:
Diabetes insipidus:
Intranasal (using 100 mcg/mL nasal solution):
> Children 3 months to 12 years: Initial: 5 mcg/day (0.05 mL/day) divided 1-2 times/day; range: 5-30 mcg/day (0.05-0.3 mL/day) divided 1-2 times/day; adjust morning and evening doses separately for an adequate diurnal rhythm of water turnover; doses <10 mcg should be administered using the rhinal tube system
> Children >12 years: Refer to adult dosing.

Oral: Children ≥4 years: Initial: 0.05 mg twice daily; total daily dose should be increased or decreased as needed to obtain adequate antidiuresis (range: 0.1-1.2 mg divided 2-3 times/day)

Hemophilia A and von Willebrand disease (type I):
I.V.: >3 months: 0.3 mcg/kg by slow infusion; may repeat dose if needed; begin 30 minutes before procedure
Intranasal: ≥11 months: Refer to adult dosing.

Nocturnal enuresis:
Children ≥6 years:
> Intranasal (using 100 mcg/mL nasal solution): Initial: 20 mcg (0.2 mL) at bedtime; range: 10-40 mcg; it is recommended that ¹/₂ of the dose be given in each nostril. **Note:** The nasal spray pump can only deliver doses of 10 mcg (0.1 mL) or multiples of 10 mcg (0.1 mL); if doses other than this are needed, the rhinal tube delivery system is preferred.
> Oral: 0.2 mg at bedtime. Dose may be titrated up to 0.6 mg to achieve desired response. Patients previously on intranasal therapy can begin oral tablets 24 hours after the last intranasal dose.

Children >12 years: Refer to adult dosing.

Available Dosage Forms
Injection, solution, as acetate (DDAVP®): 4 mcg/mL (1 mL, 10 mL)
Solution, intranasal, as acetate (DDAVP®): 100 mcg/mL (2.5 mL) [with rhinal tube]
Solution, intranasal spray, as acetate: 100 mcg/mL (5 mL) [delivers 10 mcg/spray]
DDAVP®: 100 mcg/mL (5 mL) [delivers 10 mcg/spray]
Stimate™: 1.5 mg/mL (2.5 mL) [delivers 150 mcg/spray]
Tablet, as acetate (DDAVP®): 0.1 mg, 0.2 mg

Monitoring and Teaching Issues
Physical Assessment: Use caution in presence of cystic fibrosis, coronary artery insufficiency, or hypertensive cardiovascular disease; predisposition to thrombus formation (see Warnings/Precautions). Assess results of laboratory tests (according to purpose for use), therapeutic effectiveness, and adverse reactions (eg, thromboembolism, hyponatremia, water intoxication; see Adverse Reactions) regularly throughout therapy. Teach patient proper use (if self-administered), possible side effects/appropriate interventions, and adverse symptoms to report (see Patient Education).

Patient Education: Do not take any new medication during therapy unless approved by prescriber. Use specific product as directed. Avoid alcohol; may decrease effect of medication.

Diabetes insipidus: Avoid overhydration. Weigh yourself daily at the same time in the same clothes. Report increased weight or swelling of extremities. If using intranasal product, inspect nasal membranes regularly. Report swelling or increased nasal congestion.

All uses: Report unresolved headache, respiratory difficulty, acute heartburn or nausea, abdominal cramping, vulval pain. **Breast-feeding precaution:** Consult prescriber if breast-feeding.

Geriatric Considerations: Elderly patients should be cautioned not to increase their fluid intake beyond that sufficient to satisfy their thirst in order to avoid water intoxication and hyponatremia.

Pregnancy Risk Factor: B
Lactation: Excretion in breast milk unknown/use caution

Administration
I.V.: Dilute in 0.9% sodium chloride and infuse over 15-30 minutes; dose should be diluted in 10 mL NS for children ≤10 kg; 50 mL NS for adults and children >10 kg
Other: DDAVP®: Nasal pump spray delivers 0.1 mL (10 mcg); for other doses which are not multiples, use rhinal tube. DDAVP® Nasal spray delivers fifty 10 mcg doses. Any solution remaining after 50 doses should be discarded. Pump must be primed prior to first use.

Storage:
DDAVP®:
> Tablet, nasal spray: Store at controlled room temperature of 20°C to 25°C (68°F to 77°F). Keep nasal spray in upright position.
> Rhinal tube: Store refrigerated at 2°C to 8°C (36°F to 46°F). May store at room temperature for up to 3 weeks.
> Injection: Store refrigerated at 2°C to 8°C (36°F to 46°F).
Stimate™: Store refrigerated at 2°C to 8°C (36°F to 46°F). May store at room temperature for up to 3 weeks.

Additional Information 10 mcg of desmopressin acetate is equivalent to 40 int. units

Dexamethasone (deks a METH a sone)

U.S. Brand Names Decadron®; Decadron® Phosphate [DSC]; Dexamethasone Intensol®; DexPak® TaperPak®; Maxidex®

Synonyms Dexamethasone Sodium Phosphate

Generic Available Yes

Pharmacologic Category Antiemetic; Anti-inflammatory Agent; Anti-inflammatory Agent, Ophthalmic; Corticosteroid, Ophthalmic; Corticosteroid, Systemic; Corticosteroid, Topical

Medication Safety Issues

Sound-alike/look-alike issues:

Dexamethasone may be confused with desoximetasone

Decadron® may be confused with Percodan®

Maxidex® may be confused with Maxzide®

Use Systemically and locally for chronic swelling; allergic, hematologic, neoplastic, and autoimmune diseases; may be used in management of cerebral edema, septic shock, as a diagnostic agent, antiemetic

Unlabeled/Investigational Use General indicator consistent with depression; diagnosis of Cushing's syndrome

Mechanism of Action/Effect Decreases inflammation by suppression of neutrophil migration, decreased production of inflammatory mediators, and reversal of increased capillary permeability; suppresses normal immune response. Dexamethasone's mechanism of antiemetic activity is unknown.

Contraindications Hypersensitivity to dexamethasone or any component of the formulation; active untreated infections; ophthalmic use in viral, fungal, or tuberculosis diseases of the eye

Warnings/Precautions Use with caution in patients with hypothyroidism, cirrhosis, hypertension, CHF, ulcerative colitis, or thromboembolic disorders. Corticosteroids should be used with caution in patients with diabetes, osteoporosis, peptic ulcer, glaucoma, cataracts, or tuberculosis. Use caution following acute MI (corticosteroids have been associated with myocardial rupture). Use caution in hepatic impairment. Because of the risk of adverse effects, systemic corticosteroids should be used cautiously in the elderly in the smallest possible effective dose for the shortest duration.

May cause suppression of hypothalamic-pituitary-adrenal (HPA) axis, particularly in younger children or in patients receiving high doses for prolonged periods. Symptoms of adrenocortical insufficiency in suppressed patients may result from rapid discontinuation/withdrawal; deficits in HPA response may persist for months following discontinuation and require supplementation during metabolic stress. Patients receiving 20 mg/day of prednisone (or equivalent) may be most susceptible. Particular care is required when patients are transferred from systemic corticosteroids to inhaled products due to possible adrenal insufficiency or exacerbation of underlying disease, including an increase in allergic symptoms. Fatalities have occurred due to adrenal insufficiency in asthmatic patients during and after transfer from systemic corticosteroids to aerosol steroids; aerosol steroids do **not** provide the systemic steroid needed to treat patients having trauma, surgery, or infections. Dexamethasone does not provide adequate mineralocorticoid activity in adrenal insufficiency (may be employed as a single dose while cortisol assays are performed). Dexamethasone does not cross-react with cortisol assays.

Controlled clinical studies have shown that orally-inhaled and intranasal corticosteroids may cause a reduction in growth velocity in pediatric patients. (In studies of orally-inhaled corticosteroids, the mean reduction in growth velocity was ~1 cm per year [range 0.3-1.8 cm per year] and appears to be related to dose and duration of exposure). The growth of pediatric patients receiving inhaled corticosteroids, should be monitored routinely (eg, via stadiometry). To minimize the systemic effects of orally-inhaled and intranasal corticosteroids, each patient should be titrated to the lowest effective dose.

May suppress the immune system; patients may be more susceptible to infection. Use with caution in patients with systemic infections or ocular herpes simplex. Avoid exposure to chickenpox and measles.

Drug Interactions

Cytochrome P450 Effect: Substrate of CYP3A4 (minor); **Induces** CYP2A6 (weak), 2B6 (weak), 2C8/9 (weak), 3A4 (weak)

Decreased Effect: Bile acid sequestrants may reduce the absorption of corticosteroids; separate administration by 2 hours. Aminoglutethimide may reduce the serum levels/effects of dexamethasone.

Serum concentrations of isoniazid and phenytoin may be decreased by corticosteroids. Corticosteroids may lead to a reduction in warfarin effect. Corticosteroids may suppress the response to vaccinations. The use of live vaccines is contraindicated in immunosuppressed patients. In patients receiving high doses of systemic corticosteroids for ≥14 days, wait at least 1 month between discontinuing steroid therapy and administering immunization.

Increased Effect/Toxicity: Azole antifungals, calcium channel blockers (nondihydropyridine), cyclosporine, and estrogens may increase the serum levels of corticosteroids. Antacids may increase the absorption of corticosteroids, separate administration by 2 hours. Corticosteroids may increase the serum levels of cyclosporine.

Concurrent use of nonsteroidal anti-inflammatory drugs (NSAIDs) and salicylates with corticosteroids may lead to an increased incidence of gastrointestinal adverse effects. Concurrent use with anticholinergic agents may lead to severe weakness in patients with myasthenia gravis. Concurrent use of fluoroquinolone antibiotics may increase the risk of tendon rupture, particularly in elderly patients (overall incidence rare). Concurrent use of neuromuscular blocking agents with corticosteroids may increase the risk of myopathy. The concurrent use of thalidomide with corticosteroids may increase the risk of selected adverse effects (toxic epidermal necrolysis and DVT).

Nutritional/Ethanol Interactions

Ethanol: Avoid ethanol (may enhance gastric mucosal irritation).

Food: Dexamethasone interferes with calcium absorption. Limit caffeine.

Herb/Nutraceutical: Avoid cat's claw, echinacea (have immunostimulant properties).

Adverse Reactions Frequency not defined.

Cardiovascular: Edema, hypertension, arrhythmia, cardiomyopathy, myocardial rupture (post-MI), syncope, thromboembolism, thrombophlebitis, vasculitis

Central nervous system: Insomnia, nervousness, vertigo, seizure, psychosis, pseudotumor cerebri (usually following discontinuation), headache, mood swings, delirium, hallucinations, euphoria

Dermatologic: Hirsutism, acne, skin atrophy, bruising, hyperpigmentation, pruritus (generalized), perianal pruritus (following I.V. injection), urticaria

Endocrine & metabolic: Diabetes mellitus, adrenal suppression, hyperlipidemia, Cushing's syndrome, pituitary-adrenal axis suppression, growth suppression, glucose intolerance, gynecomastia, hypokalemia, alkalosis, amenorrhea, sodium and water retention, hyperglycemia, hypercalciuria, weight gain

Gastrointestinal: Appetite increased, indigestion, peptic ulcer, nausea, vomiting, abdominal distention, ulcerative esophagitis, pancreatitis, intestinal perforation

Genitourinary: Altered (increased or decreased) spermatogenesis

Hematologic: Transient leukocytosis

Hepatic: Transaminases increased, hepatomegaly

Neuromuscular & skeletal: Arthralgia, muscle weakness, osteoporosis, fractures, myopathy (particularly in conjunction with neuromuscular disease or neuromuscular blocking agents), tendon rupture, vertebral compression fractures, neuropathy, neuritis, parasthesia

Ocular: Cataracts, glaucoma, exophthalmos, intraocular pressure increased

Miscellaneous: Infections, anaphylactoid reaction, anaphylaxis, angioedema, avascular necrosis, secondary malignancy, Kaposi's sarcoma, intractable hiccups, impaired wound healing, abnormal fat deposition, moon face

Overdosage/Toxicology When consumed in high doses over prolonged periods, systemic hypercorticism and adrenal suppression may occur. In these cases, discontinuation of the corticosteroid should be done judiciously.

Pharmacodynamics/Kinetics

Onset of Action: Acetate: Prompt

Duration of Action: Metabolic effect: 72 hours; acetate is a long-acting repository preparation

Time to Peak: Serum: Oral: 1-2 hours; I.M.: ~8 hours

Half-Life Elimination: Normal renal function: 1.8-3.5 hours; Biological half-life: 36-54 hours

Metabolism: Hepatic

Excretion: Urine and feces

Dosing

Adults:

Anti-inflammatory:

Oral, I.M., I.V. (injections should be given as sodium phosphate): 0.75-9 mg/day in divided doses every 6-12 hours

Intra-articular, intralesional, or soft tissue (as sodium phosphate): 0.4-6 mg/day

Extubation or airway edema: Oral, I.M., I.V. (injections should be given as sodium phosphate): 0.5-2 mg/kg/day in divided doses every 6 hours beginning 24 hours prior to extubation and continuing for 4-6 doses afterwards

Antiemetic:

Prophylaxis: Oral, I.V.: 10-20 mg 15-30 minutes before treatment on each treatment day

Continuous infusion regimen: Oral or I.V.: 10 mg every 12 hours on each treatment day

Mildly emetogenic therapy: Oral, I.M., I.V.: 4 mg every 4-6 hours

Delayed nausea/vomiting: Oral: 4-10 mg 1-2 times/day for 2-4 days **or**

8 mg every 12 hours for 2 days; then

4 mg every 12 hours for 2 days **or**

20 mg 1 hour before chemotherapy; then

10 mg 12 hours after chemotherapy; then

8 mg every 12 hours for 4 doses; then

4 mg every 12 hours for 4 doses

Ophthalmic anti-inflammatory:

Ophthalmic ointment: Apply thin coating into conjunctival sac 3-4 times/day; gradually taper dose to discontinue.

Ophthalmic suspension: Instill 2 drops into conjunctival sac every hour during the day and every other hour during the night; gradually reduce dose to every 3-4 hours, then to 3-4 times/day.

Steroid-responsive dermatoses: Topical: Apply 1-4 times/day. Therapy should be discontinued when control is achieved; if no improvement is seen, reassessment of diagnosis may be necessary.

Chemotherapy: Oral, I.V.: 40 mg every day for 4 days, repeated every 4 weeks (VAD regimen)

Cerebral edema: I.V. 10 mg stat, 4 mg I.M./I.V. (should be given as sodium phosphate) every 6 hours until response is maximized, then switch to oral regimen, then taper off if appropriate; dosage may be reduced after 24 days and gradually discontinued over 5-7 days

Dexamethasone suppression test (depression indicator) (unlabeled use): Oral: 1 mg at 11 PM, draw blood at 8 AM the following day for plasma cortisol determination

Cushing's syndrome, diagnostic: Oral: 1 mg at 11 PM, draw blood at 8 AM; greater accuracy for Cushing's syndrome may be achieved by the following:

Dexamethasone 0.5 mg by mouth every 6 hours for 48 hours (with 24-hour urine collection for 17-hydroxycorticosteroid excretion)

Differentiation of Cushing's syndrome due to ACTH excess from Cushing's due to other causes: Oral: Dexamethasone 2 mg every 6 hours for 48 hours (with 24-hour urine collection for 17-hydroxycorticosteroid excretion)

Multiple sclerosis (acute exacerbation): Oral: 30 mg/day for 1 week, followed by 4-12 mg/day for 1 month

(Continued)

Dexamethasone *(Continued)*

Treatment of shock:
Addisonian crisis/shock (ie, adrenal insufficiency/responsive to steroid therapy): I.V. (given as sodium phosphate): 4-10 mg as a single dose, which may be repeated if necessary

Unresponsive shock (ie, unresponsive to steroid therapy): I.V. (given as sodium phosphate): 1-6 mg/kg as a single I.V. dose or up to 40 mg initially followed by repeat doses every 2-6 hours while shock persists

Physiological replacement: Oral, I.M., I.V. (should be given as sodium phosphate): 0.03-0.15 mg/kg/day **or** 0.6-0.75 mg/m²/day in divided doses every 6-12 hours

Elderly: Refer to adult dosing. Use cautiously in the elderly in the smallest possible dose.

Pediatrics:
Antiemetic (prior to chemotherapy): I.V. (should be given as sodium phosphate): 5-20 mg given 15-30 minutes before treatment

Anti-inflammatory and/or immunosuppressant: Oral, I.M., I.V. (injections should be given as sodium phosphate): 0.08-0.3 mg/kg/day **or** 2.5-10 mg/m²/day in divided doses every 6-12 hours

Extubation or airway edema: Oral, I.M., I.V. (injections should be given as sodium phosphate): 0.5-2 mg/kg/day in divided doses every 6 hours beginning 24 hours prior to extubation and continuing for 4-6 doses afterwards

Cerebral edema: I.V. (should be given as sodium phosphate): Loading dose: 1-2 mg/kg/dose as a single dose; maintenance: 1-1.5 mg/kg/day (maximum: 16 mg/day) in divided doses every 4-6 hours for 5 days then taper for 5 days, then discontinue

Bacterial meningitis in infants and children >2 months: I.V. (should be given as sodium phosphate): 0.6 mg/kg/day in 4 divided doses every 6 hours for the first 4 days of antibiotic treatment; start dexamethasone at the time of the first dose of antibiotic

Physiologic replacement: Oral, I.M., I.V.: 0.03-0.15 mg/kg/day or 0.6-0.75 mg/m²/day in divided doses every 6-12 hours

Ophthalmic inflammation: Refer to adult dosing.

Renal Impairment: Hemodialysis or peritoneal dialysis: Supplemental dose is not necessary.

Available Dosage Forms [DSC] = Discontinued product
Elixir, as base: 0.5 mg/5 mL (240 mL) [contains alcohol 5%; raspberry flavor]
Injection, solution, as sodium phosphate: 4 mg/mL (1 mL, 5 mL, 10 mL, 25 mL, 30 mL); 10 mg/mL (1 mL, 10 mL)
Decadron® Phosphate: 4 mg/mL (5 mL, 25 mL); 24 mg/mL (5 mL) [contains sodium bisulfite] [DSC]
Ointment, ophthalmic, as sodium phosphate: 0.05% (3.5 g)
Solution, ophthalmic, as sodium phosphate: 0.1% (5 mL)
Solution, oral: 0.5 mg/5 mL (500 mL) [cherry flavor]
Solution, oral concentrate (Dexamethasone Intensol®): 1 mg/mL (30 mL) [contains alcohol 30%]
Suspension, ophthalmic (Maxidex®): 0.1% (5 mL, 15 mL)
Tablet: 0.25 mg, 0.5 mg, 0.75 mg, 1 mg, 1.5 mg, 2 mg, 4 mg, 6 mg [some 0.5 mg tablets may contain tartrazine]
Decadron®: 0.5 mg, 0.75 mg, 4 mg
DexPak® TaperPak®: 1.5 mg [51 tablets on taper dose card]

Monitoring and Teaching Issues

Physical Assessment: Assess potential for interactions with other prescriptions, OTC medications, or herbal products patient may be taking. Assess results of laboratory tests, therapeutic response, and adverse effects, according to indications for therapy, dose, route, and duration of therapy. When used for long-term therapy (>10-14 days), do not discontinue abruptly; decrease dosage incrementally. With systemic administration, caution patients with diabetes to monitor glucose levels closely (corticosteroids may alter glucose levels). Teach patient proper use (according to formulation), side effects/appropriate interventions, and symptoms to report.

Monitoring Laboratory Tests: Hemoglobin, occult blood loss, serum potassium, glucose Dexamethasone suppression test, overnight: 8 AM cortisol <6 mg/100 mL (dexamethasone 1 mg). Plasma cortisol determination should be made on the day after giving dose.

Patient Education: Do not take any new medication during therapy unless approved by prescriber. Take exactly as directed, do not increase dose or discontinue abruptly without consulting prescriber.

Oral: Take with or after meals. Avoid alcohol and limit intake of caffeine or stimulants. Prescriber may recommend increased dietary vitamins, minerals, or iron. If you have diabetes, monitor glucose levels closely (antidiabetic medication may need to be adjusted). Inform prescriber if you are experiencing greater-than-normal levels of stress (medication may need adjustment). You may be more susceptible to infection (avoid crowds and persons with contagious or infective conditions and do not have any vaccinations unless approved by prescriber). Some forms of this medication may cause GI upset (small frequent meals and frequent mouth care may help). Report promptly excessive nervousness or sleep disturbances; signs of infection (eg, sore throat, unhealed injuries); excessive growth of body hair or loss of skin color; vision changes; excessive or sudden weight gain (>3 lb/week); swelling of face or extremities; respiratory difficulty; muscle weakness; tarry stool, persistent abdominal pain; worsening of condition or failure to improve. **Pregnancy/breast-feeding precautions:** Inform prescriber if you are or intend to become pregnant. Consult prescriber if breast-feeding.

Ophthalmic: For use in eyes only. Wash hands before using. Lie down or tilt your head back and look upward. Put drops of suspension or apply thin ribbon of ointment inside lower eyelid. Close eye and roll eyeball in all directions. Do not blink for ½ minute. Apply gentle pressure to inner corner of eye for 30 seconds. Do not use any other eye preparation for at least 10 minutes. Do not let tip of applicator touch eye; do not contaminate tip of applicator (may cause eye infection, eye damage, or vision loss). Do not share medication with anyone else. Wear sunglasses in sunlight; you may be more sensitive to bright light. Inform prescriber if condition worsens, fails to improve, or if you experience eye pain, disturbances of vision, or other adverse eye response.

Topical: For external use only. Do not use for eyes, mucous membranes, or open wounds. Use exactly as directed and for no longer than the period prescribed. Before using, wash and dry area gently. Apply in thin layer (may rub in lightly). Apply light dressing (if necessary) to area being treated. Do not use occlusive dressing unless so advised by prescriber. Avoid exposing treated area to sunlight (severe sunburn may occur). Inform prescriber if condition worsens (swelling, redness, irritation, pain, open sores) or fails to improve.

Dietary Considerations: May be taken with meals to decrease GI upset. May need diet with increased potassium, pyridoxine, vitamin C, vitamin D, folate, calcium, and phosphorus.

Geriatric Considerations: Because of the risk of adverse effects, systemic corticosteroids should be used cautiously in the elderly in the smallest possible dose, and for the shortest possible time.

Pregnancy Risk Factor: C

Pregnancy Issues: Dexamethasone has been used in patients with premature labor (26-34 weeks gestation) to stimulate fetal lung maturation. Effects on the fetus: Crosses the placenta; transient leukocytosis has been reported. Available evidence suggests safe use during pregnancy.

Lactation: Excretion in breast milk unknown

Administration
Oral: Administer oral formulation with meals to decrease GI upset.
I.M.: Acetate injection is **not** for I.V. use.
I.V.: Administer as a 5-10 minute bolus; rapid injection is associated with a high incidence of perianal discomfort.
Topical: Topical formation is for external use. Do not use on open wounds. Apply sparingly to occlusive dressings. Should not be used in the presence of open or weeping lesions.

Reconstitution: Injection should be diluted in 50-100 mL NS or D_5W.

Compatibility: Stable in D_5W, NS
  Y-site administration: Incompatible with ciprofloxacin, idarubicin, midazolam, topotecan
  Compatibility in syringe: Incompatible with doxapram, glycopyrrolate
  Compatibility when admixed: Incompatible with daunorubicin, diphenhydramine with lorazepam and metoclopramide, metaraminol, vancomycin

Storage: Injection solution: Store at room temperature; protect from light and freezing.
  Stability of injection of parenteral admixture at room temperature (25°C): 24 hours
  Stability of injection of parenteral admixture at refrigeration temperature (4°C): 2 days; protect from light and freezing

Additional Information Effects of inhaled/intranasal steroids on growth have been observed in the absence of laboratory evidence of HPA axis suppression, suggesting that growth velocity is a more sensitive indicator of systemic corticosteroid exposure in pediatric patients than some commonly used tests of HPA axis function. The long-term effects of this reduction in growth velocity associated with orally-inhaled and intranasal corticosteroids, including the impact on final adult height, are unknown. The potential for "catch up" growth following discontinuation of treatment with inhaled corticosteroids has not been adequately studied.

Withdrawal/tapering of therapy: Corticosteroid tapering following short-term use is limited primarily by the need to control the underlying disease state; tapering may be accomplished over a period of days. Following longer-term use, tapering over weeks to months may be necessary to avoid signs and symptoms of adrenal insufficiency and to allow recovery of the HPA axis. Testing of HPA axis responsiveness may be of value in selected patients. Subtle deficits in HPA response may persist for months after discontinuation of therapy, and may require supplemental dosing during periods of acute illness or surgical stress.

Related Information
Antiemetics for Chemotherapy-Induced Nausea and Vomiting *on page 1788*
Corticosteroids *on page 1731*
Inhalant Agents *on page 1734*

♦ **Dexamethasone and Ciprofloxacin** *see* Ciprofloxacin and Dexamethasone *on page 331*
♦ **Dexamethasone and Neomycin** *see* Neomycin and Dexamethasone *on page 1068*
♦ **Dexamethasone and Tobramycin** *see* Tobramycin and Dexamethasone *on page 1492*
♦ **Dexamethasone Intensol®** *see* Dexamethasone *on page 424*
♦ **Dexamethasone Sodium Phosphate** *see* Dexamethasone *on page 424*

Dexchlorpheniramine (deks klor fen EER a meen)

Synonyms Dexchlorpheniramine Maleate
Generic Available Yes
Pharmacologic Category Antihistamine
Use Perennial and seasonal allergic rhinitis and other allergic symptoms including urticaria
Mechanism of Action/Effect Competes with histamine for H_1-receptor sites on effector cells in the GI tract, blood vessels, and respiratory tract
Contraindications Hypersensitivity to dexchlorpheniramine or any component of the formulation; narrow-angle glaucoma
Warnings/Precautions Causes sedation, caution must be used in performing tasks which require alertness (eg, operating machinery or driving). Sedative effects of CNS depressants or ethanol are potentiated. Use with caution in patients with angle-closure glaucoma, pyloroduodenal obstruction (including stenotic peptic ulcer), urinary tract obstruction (including bladder neck obstruction and symptomatic prostatic hyperplasia), hyperthyroidism, increased intraocular pressure, and cardiovascular disease (including hypertension and tachycardia). High sedative and anticholinergic properties, therefore may not be considered the antihistamine of choice for prolonged use in the elderly. May cause paradoxical excitation in pediatric patients, and can result in hallucinations, coma, and death in overdose.
(Continued)

Dexchlorpheniramine *(Continued)*

Drug Interactions

Decreased Effect: May increase gastric degradation of levodopa and decrease the amount of levodopa absorbed by delaying gastric emptying. Therapeutic effects of cholinergic agents (tacrine, donepezil) and neuroleptics may be antagonized.

Increased Effect/Toxicity: CNS depressants may increase the degree of sedation and respiratory depression with antihistamines. May increase the absorption of digoxin. Central and/or peripheral anticholinergic syndrome can occur when administered with amantadine, rimantadine, narcotic analgesics, phenothiazines and other antipsychotics (especially with high anticholinergic activity), tricyclic antidepressants, quinidine, disopyramide, procainamide, and antihistamines.

Nutritional/Ethanol Interactions Ethanol: Avoid ethanol (may increase CNS depression).

Lab Interactions May interfere with a methacholine bronchial challenge.

Adverse Reactions

>10%:

Central nervous system: Slight to moderate drowsiness

Respiratory: Thickening of bronchial secretions

1% to 10%:

Central nervous system: Headache, fatigue, nervousness, dizziness

Gastrointestinal: Appetite increase, weight gain, nausea, diarrhea, abdominal pain, xerostomia

Neuromuscular & skeletal: Arthralgia

Respiratory: Pharyngitis

Overdosage/Toxicology Symptoms of overdose include dry mouth, flushed skin, dilated pupils, CNS depression. There is no specific treatment for antihistamine overdose. Clinical toxicity is due to blockade of cholinergic receptors. For anticholinergic overdose with severe life-threatening symptoms, physostigmine 1-2 mg I.V. slowly, may be given to reverse these effects.

Pharmacodynamics/Kinetics

Onset of Action: ~1 hour

Duration of Action: 3-6 hours

Absorption: Well absorbed

Metabolism: Hepatic

Dosing

Adults & Elderly: Allergy symptoms: Oral: 2 mg every 4-6 hours or 4-6 mg timed release at bedtime or every 8-10 hours

Pediatrics: Allergy symptoms: Oral:

2-5 years: 0.5 mg every 4-6 hours (do not use timed release)

6-11 years: 1 mg every 4-6 hours or 4 mg timed release at bedtime

Available Dosage Forms

Syrup, as maleate: 2 mg/5 mL (480 mL, 3840 mL) [contains alcohol 6%; orange flavor]

Tablet, sustained action, as maleate: 4 mg, 6 mg

Monitoring and Teaching Issues

Physical Assessment: Assess effectiveness and interactions of other medications patient may be taking. Monitor effectiveness of therapy and adverse reactions at beginning of therapy and periodically with long-term use. Assess knowledge/teach patient appropriate use, interventions to reduce side effects, and adverse symptoms to report.

Patient Education: Take as directed; do not exceed recommended dose. Do not chew or crush sustained release tablet. Take with food or water. Avoid use of other depressants, alcohol, or sleep-inducing medications unless approved by prescriber. You may experience drowsiness or dizziness (use caution when driving or engaging in tasks requiring alertness until response to drug is known); or dry mouth, nausea, or abdominal pain (small frequent meals, frequent mouth care, chewing gum, or sucking hard candy may help). Report persistent sedation, confusion, or agitation; changes in urinary pattern; blurred vision; sore throat, respiratory difficulty or expectorating (thick secretions); or lack of improvement or worsening or condition. **Breast-feeding precaution:** Breast-feeding is not recommended.

Dietary Considerations: May be taken with food or water.

Geriatric Considerations: Anticholinergic action may cause significant confusional symptoms, constipation, or problems voiding urine.

Pregnancy Risk Factor: B

Lactation: Excretion in breast milk unknown/not recommended

Dexchlorpheniramine and Pseudoephedrine

(deks klor fen EER a meen & soo doe e FED rin)

U.S. Brand Names Duotan PD; Tanafed DP™

Synonyms Pseudoephedrine Tannate and Dexchlorpheniramine Tannate

Generic Available Yes

Pharmacologic Category Alpha/Beta Agonist; Antihistamine

Use Relief of nasal congestion associated with the common cold, hay fever, and other allergies, sinusitis, and vasomotor and allergic rhinitis

Contraindications Hypersensitivity to dexchlorpheniramine, pseudoephedrine, or any component of the formulation; severe hypertension; severe cardiovascular disease; use with or within 2 weeks of discontinuing MAO inhibitor; narrow-angle glaucoma; urinary retention; peptic ulcer disease; breast-feeding

Warnings/Precautions Use caution with hypertension, diabetes, cardiovascular disease, hyperthyroidism, increased intraocular pressure, or prostatic hyperplasia. Causes sedation,:caution must be used in performing tasks which require alertness (eg, operating machinery or driving). Sedative effects of CNS depressants or ethanol are potentiated. Use caution in elderly patients (risk of CNS depression may be increased).

Drug Interactions

Cytochrome P450 Effect: See individual monographs for dexchlorpheniramine and pseudoephedrine.

Decreased Effect: See individual monographs for chlorpheniramine and pseudoephedrine.

Increased Effect/Toxicity: See individual monographs for dexchlorpheniramine and pseudoephedrine.

Nutritional/Ethanol Interactions Ethanol: Avoid ethanol (may increase CNS depression).

Adverse Reactions See individual monographs for dexchlorpheniramine and pseudoephedrine.

Dosing

Adults: Rhinitis/decongestant: Oral: Dexchlorpheniramine tannate 2.5 mg and pseudoephedrine tannate 75 mg per 5 mL: 10-20 mL every 12 hours (maximum: 40 mL/24 hours)

Pediatrics: Rhinitis/decongestant: Oral: Dexchlorpheniramine tannate 2.5 mg and pseudoephedrine tannate 75 mg per 5 mL:

Children:

2-6 years: 2.5-5 mL every 12 hours (maximum: 10 mL/24 hours)

6-12 years: 5-10 mL every 12 hours (maximum: 20 mL/24 hours)

Children ≥12 years: Refer to adult dosing.

Available Dosage Forms Suspension (Duotan PD, Tanafed DP™): Dexchlorpheniramine tannate 2.5 mg and pseudoephedrine tannate 75 mg per 5 mL (120 mL, 480 mL) [contains sodium benzoate; strawberry-banana flavor]

Monitoring and Teaching Issues

Physical Assessment: Assess other prescription and OTC medications the patient may be taking to avoid duplications and interactions. Assess knowledge/teach patient appropriate use, side effects, and symptoms to report.

Patient Education: Do not exceed the recommended dosage. May cause drowsiness (use caution when driving or engaging in activities requiring alertness until response to drug is known). Avoid use of alcohol, sedatives, or tranquilizers without consulting prescriber. You may experience nervousness, excitability, restlessness, headache, and insomnia. Report persistent CNS changes (nervousness, dizziness, tremor, agitation, or convulsions) increased heart rate and palpitations, or sleeplessness to prescriber. **Pregnancy/Breast-feeding precaution:** Inform prescriber if you are or intend to become pregnant. Consult prescriber if breast-feeding.

Geriatric Considerations: Elderly patients should be counseled about the proper use of over-the-counter cough and cold preparations. Elderly are more predisposed to adverse effects of sympathomimetics since they frequently have cardiovascular diseases and diabetes mellitus as well as multiple drug therapies. It may be advisable to treat with a short-acting/immediate-release formulation before initiating sustained-release/long-acting formulations. Anticholinergic action may cause significant confusional symptoms, constipation, or problems voiding urine.

Pregnancy Risk Factor: C

Lactation: Excretion in breast milk unknown/not recommended

Breast-Feeding Issues: Pseudoephedrine is excreted in breast milk. The manufacturers do not recommend its use while breast-feeding; however, the AAP considers it to be "compatible" with breast-feeding. Information for dexchlorpheniramine is not available.

Administration

Oral: Shake suspension well prior to use.

♦ **Dexchlorpheniramine Maleate** *see* Dexchlorpheniramine *on page 427*

♦ **Dexedrine®** *see* Dextroamphetamine *on page 434*

♦ **Dexferrum®** *see* Iron Dextran Complex *on page 833*

Dexmedetomidine (deks MED e toe mi deen)

U.S. Brand Names Precedex™

Synonyms Dexmedetomidine Hydrochloride

Generic Available No

Pharmacologic Category Alpha$_2$-Adrenergic Agonist; Sedative

Medication Safety Issues

Sound-alike/look-alike issues:

Precedex™ may be confused with Peridex®

Use Sedation of initially intubated and mechanically ventilated patients during treatment in an intensive care setting; duration of infusion should not exceed 24 hours

Unlabeled/Investigational Use Unlabeled uses include premedication prior to anesthesia induction with thiopental; relief of pain and reduction of opioid dose following laparoscopic tubal ligation; as an adjunct anesthetic in ophthalmic surgery; treatment of shivering; premedication to attenuate the cardiostimulatory and postanesthetic delirium of ketamine

Mechanism of Action/Effect Selective alpha$_2$-adrenoceptor agonist with sedative properties; alpha$_1$ activity was observed at high doses or after rapid infusions

Contraindications Hypersensitivity to dexmedetomidine or any component of the formulation; use outside of an intensive care setting

Warnings/Precautions Should be administered only by persons skilled in management of patients in intensive care setting. Patients should be continuously monitored. Episodes of bradycardia, hypotension, and sinus arrest have been associated with dexmedetomidine. Use caution in patients with heart block, severe ventricular dysfunction, hypovolemia, diabetes, chronic hypertension, and in the elderly. Use with caution in patients receiving vasodilators or drugs which decrease heart rate. Transient hypertension has been primarily observed during the dose in association with the initial peripheral vasoconstrictive effects of dexmedetomidine. Treatment of this is not generally necessary; however, reduction of infusion rate may be desirable.

Drug Interactions

Cytochrome P450 Effect: Substrate of CYP2A6 (major); **Inhibits** CYP1A2 (weak), 2C8/9 (weak), 2D6 (strong), 3A4 (weak)

(Continued)

Dexmedetomidine *(Continued)*

Decreased Effect: Dexmedetomidine may decrease the levels/effects of CYP2D6 prodrug substrates; example prodrug substrates include codeine, hydrocodone, oxycodone, and tramadol.

Increased Effect/Toxicity: The levels/effects of dexmedetomidine may be increased by isoniazid, methoxsalen, miconazole, and other CYP2A6 inhibitors. Dexmedetomidine may increase the levels/effects of amphetamines, selected beta-blockers, dextromethorphan, fluoxetine, lidocaine, mirtazapine, nefazodone, paroxetine, risperidone, ritonavir, thioridazine, tricyclic antidepressants, venlafaxine, and other CYP2D6 substrates. Hypotension and/or bradycardia may be increased by vasodilators and heart rate-lowering agents.

Adverse Reactions
>10%:
  Cardiovascular: Hypotension (30%)
  Gastrointestinal: Nausea (11%)
1% to 10%:
  Cardiovascular: Bradycardia (8%), atrial fibrillation (7%)
  Central nervous system: Pain (3%)
  Hematologic: Anemia (3%), leukocytosis (2%)
  Renal: Oliguria (2%)
  Respiratory: Hypoxia (6%), pulmonary edema (2%), pleural effusion (3%)
  Miscellaneous: Infection (2%), thirst (2%)

Overdosage/Toxicology In reports of overdosages where the blood concentration was 13 times the upper boundary of the therapeutic range, first-degree AV block and second degree heart block occurred. No hemodynamic compromise was noted with the AV block and the heart block resolved spontaneously within one minute. Two patients who received a 2 mcg/kg loading dose over 10 minutes experienced bradycardia and/or hypotension. One patient who received a loading dose of undiluted dexmedetomidine (19.4 mcg/kg) had cardiac arrest and was successfully resuscitated.

Pharmacodynamics/Kinetics
  Onset of Action: Rapid
  Protein Binding: 94%
  Half-Life Elimination: 6 minutes; Terminal: 2 hours
  Metabolism: Hepatic via glucuronidation and CYP2A6
  Excretion: Urine (95%); feces (4%)

Dosing
  Adults:
    ICU sedation: I.V.: Initial: Loading infusion of 1 mcg/kg over 10 minutes, followed by a maintenance infusion of 0.2-0.7 mcg/kg/hour (individualized and titrated to desired clinical effect); not indicated for infusions lasting >24 hours
    Note: Solution must be diluted prior to administration.
  Elderly: Refer to adult dosing. Dosage reduction may need to be considered. No specific guidelines available. Dose selections should be cautious, at the low end of dosage range; titration should be slower, allowing adequate time to evaluate response.
  Renal Impairment: Dosage reduction may need to be considered.
  Hepatic Impairment: Dosage reduction may need to be considered. No specific guidelines available.

Available Dosage Forms Injection, solution [preservative free]: 100 mcg/mL (2 mL)

Monitoring and Teaching Issues
  Physical Assessment: Administration should be managed by professionals experienced in anesthesia. Dosage and rate of administration should be individualized and titrated to the desired effect, according to relevant clinical factors, premedication, concomitant medications, age, and general condition of patient. Assess other medications for effectiveness and safety. Other drugs that cause CNS depression may increase CNS depression induced by dexmedetomidine (monitor and adjust dosage as necessary). Continuous monitoring of vital signs, cardiac and respiratory status, and level of sedation is mandatory during infusion and until full consciousness is regained. Safety precautions must be maintained until patient is fully alert. Dexmedetomidine is an anesthetic; pain must be treated with appropriate analgesic agents. Do not discontinue abruptly (may result in rapid awakening associated with anxiety, agitation, and resistance to mechanical ventilation). Titrate infusion rate so patient awakes slowly. Monitor fluid levels (intake and output) during and following infusion. Reposition patient and provide appropriate skin, mouth, and eye care every 2-3 hours, while sedated. Provide appropriate emotional and sensory support (auditory and environmental).
  Patient Education: This is an anesthetic. Patient education should be appropriate to individual situation. Following return of consciousness, do not attempt to change position or rise from bed without assistance. Report immediately any pounding or unusual heartbeat, respiratory difficulty, or acute dizziness. **Pregnancy/breast-feeding precautions:** Inform prescriber if you are pregnant. Consult prescriber if breast-feeding.
  Pregnancy Risk Factor: C
  Lactation: Excretion in breast milk unknown/use caution

Administration
  I.V.: Administer using a controlled infusion device. Must be diluted in 0.9% sodium chloride solution to achieve the required concentration prior to administration. Advisable to use administration components made with synthetic or coated natural rubber gaskets. Parenteral products should be inspected visually for particulate matter and discoloration prior to administration.
  Compatibility: Stable in D$_5$W, LR, 0.9% NS, 20% mannitol, plasma substitute
    May adsorb to certain types of natural rubber; use components made with synthetic or coated natural rubber gaskets whenever possible.

♦ **Dexmedetomidine Hydrochloride** *see* Dexmedetomidine *on page 429*

Dexmethylphenidate (dex meth il FEN i date)

U.S. Brand Names Focalin™

Synonyms Dexmethylphenidate Hydrochloride

Controlled Substance C-II

Generic Available No

Pharmacologic Category Central Nervous System Stimulant

Use Treatment of attention-deficit/hyperactivity disorder (ADHD)

Mechanism of Action/Effect CNS stimulant

Contraindications Hypersensitivity to dexmethylphenidate, methylphenidate, or any compo-nent of the formulation; marked anxiety, tension, and agitation; glaucoma, motor tics, family history or diagnosis of Tourette's syndrome; use during or within 14 days following MAO inhibitor therapy

Warnings/Precautions Recommended to be used as part of a comprehensive treatment program for ADHD. Use with caution in patients with bipolar disorder, diabetes mellitus, cardiovascular disease, hyperthyroidism, seizure disorders, insomnia, porphyria, or hyperten-sion. Use caution in patients with history of ethanol or drug abuse. May exacerbate symp-toms of behavior and thought disorder in psychotic patients. Do not use to treat severe depression or fatigue states. Potential for drug dependency exists - avoid abrupt discontinua-tion in patients who have received for prolonged periods. Visual disturbances have been reported with methylphenidate (rare). Stimulant use has been associated with growth suppression. Stimulants may unmask tics in individuals with coexisting Tourette's syndrome. Safety and efficacy in children <6 years of age not established.

Drug Interactions

Decreased Effect: Effectiveness of antihypertensive agents may be decreased. Carbam-azepine may decrease the effect of methylphenidate.

Increased Effect/Toxicity: Methylphenidate may cause hypertensive effects when used in combination with MAO inhibitors or drugs with MAO-inhibiting activity (linezolid). Risk may be less with selegiline (MAO type B selective at low doses); it is best to avoid this combination. NMS has been reported in a patient receiving methylphenidate and venlafaxine. Methylphenidate may increase levels of phenytoin, phenobarbital, TCAs, and warfarin. Increased toxicity with clonidine and sibutramine.

Nutritional/Ethanol Interactions

Ethanol: Avoid ethanol (may cause CNS depression).

Food: High-fat meal may increase time to peak concentration.

Herb/Nutraceutical: Avoid ephedra (may cause hypertension or arrhythmias) and yohimbe (also has CNS stimulatory activity).

Adverse Reactions

>10%: Gastrointestinal: Abdominal pain (15%)

1% to 10%:

Central nervous system: Fever (5%)

Gastrointestinal: Nausea (9%), anorexia (6%)

Adverse effects seen with **methylphenidate** (frequency not defined):

Cardiovascular: Angina, cardiac arrhythmia, cerebral arteritis, cerebral occlusion, hyper-/hypotension, palpitation, pulse increase/decrease, tachycardia

Central nervous system: Depression, dizziness, drowsiness, fever, headache, insomnia, nervousness, neuroleptic malignant syndrome (NMS), Tourette's syndrome, toxic psychosis

Dermatologic: Erythema multiforme, exfoliative dermatitis, hair loss, rash, urticaria

Endocrine & metabolic: Growth retardation

Gastrointestinal: Abdominal pain, anorexia, nausea, vomiting, weight loss

Hematologic: Anemia, leukopenia, thrombocytopenic purpura

Hepatic: Abnormal liver function tests, hepatic coma, transaminases increased

Neuromuscular & skeletal: Arthralgia, dyskinesia

Ocular: Blurred vision

Renal: Necrotizing vasculitis

Respiratory: Cough increased, pharyngitis, sinusitis, upper respiratory tract infection

Miscellaneous: Hypersensitivity reactions

Overdosage/Toxicology Signs and symptoms of overdose may include agitation, cardiac arrhythmias, coma, confusion, convulsions, delirium, dry mucous membranes, euphoria, flushing, hallucinations, headache, hyper-reflexia, hyperpyrexia, hypertension, muscle twitching, mydriasis, palpitations, sweating, tachycardia, tremors and vomiting. Treatment is symptom-directed and supportive.

Pharmacodynamics/Kinetics

Absorption: Rapid

Time to Peak: Fasting: 1-1.5 hours

Half-Life Elimination: 2.2 hours

Metabolism: Via de-esterification to inactive metabolite, d-α-phenyl-piperidine acetate (d-ritalinic acid)

Excretion: Urine (90%)

Dosing

Adults:

Treatment of ADHD: Oral: Initial: 2.5 mg twice daily in patients not currently taking methylphenidate; dosage may be adjusted in 2.5-5 mg increments at weekly intervals (maximum dose: 20 mg/day); doses should be taken at least 4 hours apart

Note: When switching from methylphenidate to dexmethylphenidate, the starting dose of dexmethylphenidate should be half that of methylphenidate (maximum dose: 20 mg/day)

Dose reduction and discontinuation: Reduce dose or discontinue in patients with para-doxical aggravation. Discontinue if no improvement is seen after one month of treatment.

Pediatrics: Children ≥6 years: Treatment of ADHD: Oral: Refer to adult dose.

Available Dosage Forms Tablet, as hydrochloride: 2.5 mg, 5 mg, 10 mg

(Continued)

Dexmethylphenidate *(Continued)*

Monitoring and Teaching Issues

Physical Assessment: This drug should be used as part of a comprehensive treatment program for ADHD. Monitor closely any other medication patient may be taking for effectiveness and possible interactions prior to beginning therapy. Assess results of laboratory for effectiveness of therapy and adverse reactions at beginning of therapy and periodically with long-term use. Taper dosage when discontinuing from long-term therapy. Assess knowledge/teach patient appropriate use, interventions to reduce side effects, and importance of reporting adverse symptoms promptly.

Patient Education: Take exactly as directed; do not change dosage or discontinue without consulting prescriber. Response may take some time. Avoid alcohol, caffeine, or other stimulants. Maintain adequate hydration (2-3 L/day of fluids) unless instructed to restrict fluid intake. You may experience decreased appetite or weight loss (small frequent meals may help maintain adequate nutrition); or restlessness, impaired judgment, or dizziness (use caution when driving or engaging in tasks requiring alertness until response to drug is known). Report unresolved rapid heartbeat; excessive agitation, nervousness, insomnia, tremors, or dizziness; blackened stool; skin rash or irritation; or altered gait or movement. **Pregnancy/breast-feeding precautions:** Inform prescriber if you are or intend to become pregnant. Consult prescriber if breast-feeding.

Dietary Considerations: May be taken with or without food.

Pregnancy Risk Factor: C

Lactation: Excretion in breast milk unknown/use caution

Administration

Oral: Doses should be taken at least 4 hours apart. May be taken with or without food.

Storage: Store at 25°C (77°F). Protect from light and moisture.

♦ **Dexmethylphenidate Hydrochloride** *see Dexmethylphenidate on page 431*

♦ **DexPak® TaperPak®** *see Dexamethasone on page 424*

Dexrazoxane *(deks ray ZOKS ane)*

U.S. Brand Names Zinecard®

Synonyms ICRF-187

Generic Available No

Pharmacologic Category Cardioprotectant

Medication Safety Issues

Sound-alike/look-alike issues:

Zinecard® may be confused with Gemzar®

Use Reduction of the incidence and severity of cardiomyopathy associated with doxorubicin administration in women with metastatic breast cancer who have received a cumulative doxorubicin dose of 300 mg/m^2 and who would benefit from continuing therapy with doxorubicin. It is not recommended for use with the initiation of doxorubicin therapy.

Mechanism of Action/Effect Derivative of EDTA; potent intracellular chelating agent. The mechanism of cardioprotectant activity is not fully understood. Appears to be converted intracellularly to a ring-opened chelating agent that interferes with iron-mediated oxygen free radical generation thought to be responsible, in part, for anthracycline-induced cardiomyopathy.

Contraindications Do not use with chemotherapy regimens that do not contain an anthracycline

Warnings/Precautions Dexrazoxane may add to the myelosuppression caused by chemotherapeutic agents. Dexrazoxane does not eliminate the potential for anthracycline-induced cardiac toxicity. Carefully monitor cardiac function.

Adverse Reactions Unless specified, frequency not defined.

Dermatologic: Alopecia, urticaria, recall skin reaction, extravasation

Endocrine & metabolic: Serum amylase increased, serum calcium decreased, serum triglycerides increased

Gastrointestinal: Nausea, vomiting (mild)

Hematologic: Myelosuppression, neutropenia (~12%), thrombocytopenia (~4%)

Hepatic: AST/ALT increased, bilirubin increased

Overdosage/Toxicology Management includes supportive care until resolution of myelosuppression and related conditions is complete. Retention of a significant dose fraction of unchanged drug in the plasma pool, minimal tissue partitioning or binding, and availability of >90% of systemic drug levels in the unbound form suggest that dexrazoxane could be removed using conventional peritoneal or hemodialysis.

Pharmacodynamics/Kinetics

Protein Binding: None

Half-Life Elimination: 2.1-2.5 hours

Excretion: Urine (42%)

Clearance, renal: 3.35 L/hour/m^2; Plasma: 6.25-7.88 L/hour/m^2

Dosing

Adults & Elderly: Prevention of doxorubicin cardiomyopathy: I.V.: A 10:1 ratio of dexrazoxane:doxorubicin (500 mg/m^2 dexrazoxane: 50 mg/m^2 doxorubicin)

Hepatic Impairment: Since doxorubicin dosage is reduced in hyperbilirubinemia, a proportional reduction in dexrazoxane dosage is recommended (maintain ratio of 10:1).

Available Dosage Forms Injection, powder for reconstitution: 250 mg, 500 mg [10 mg/mL when reconstituted]

Monitoring and Teaching Issues

Physical Assessment: Assess effectiveness and interactions of other medications patient may be taking. Monitor cardiac function closely. Assess infusion site frequently. Avoid extravasation. Monitor for effectiveness of therapy and adverse effects.

Monitoring Laboratory Tests: Frequent complete blood counts are recommended; LFTs

Patient Education: This I.V. medication is given to reduce incidence of cardiac complications with doxorubicin. Report promptly any pain at infusion site. You will be more susceptible to infections. Avoid crowds and exposure to infections whenever possible. Report shortness of breath, chest discomfort, or swelling of extremities. **Pregnancy/breast-feeding precautions:** Inform prescriber if you are pregnant. Breast-feeding is not recommended.

Pregnancy Risk Factor: C

Lactation: Excretion in breast milk unknown/not recommended

Breast-Feeding Issues: Discontinue nursing during dexrazoxane therapy.

Other Issues: Follow guidelines for handling cytotoxic agents. If drug comes in contact with skin or mucosa, wash immediately with soap and water.

Administration

I.V.: Administer by slow I.V. push or rapid (5-15 minutes) I.V. infusion from a bag. Administer doxorubicin within 30 minutes after beginning the infusion with dexrazoxane.

Reconstitution: Must be reconstituted with 0.167 Molar (M/6) sodium lactate injection to a concentration of 10 mg dexrazoxane/mL sodium lactate. Reconstituted dexrazoxane solution may be diluted with either 0.9% sodium chloride injection or 5% dextrose injection to a concentration of 1.3-5 mg/mL in intravenous infusion bags.

Storage: Store intact vials at controlled room temperature (15°C to 30°C/59°F to 86°F). Reconstituted and diluted solutions are stable for 6 hours at controlled room temperature or under refrigeration (2°C to 8°C/36°F to 46°F).

Additional Information Reimbursement Guarantee Program: 1-800-808-9111

Dextran (DEKS tran)

U.S. Brand Names Gentran®; LMD®

Synonyms Dextran 40; Dextran 70; Dextran, High Molecular Weight; Dextran, Low Molecular Weight

Generic Available Yes

Pharmacologic Category Plasma Volume Expander

Medication Safety Issues

Sound-alike/look-alike issues:

Dextran may be confused with Dexatrim®, Dexedrine®

Use Blood volume expander used in treatment of shock or impending shock when blood or blood products are not available; dextran 40 is also used as a priming fluid in cardiopulmonary bypass and for prophylaxis of venous thrombosis and pulmonary embolism in surgical procedures associated with a high risk of thromboembolic complications

Mechanism of Action/Effect Produces plasma volume expansion by virtue of its highly colloidal starch structure, similar to albumin

Contraindications Hypersensitivity to dextran or any component of the formulation; marked hemostatic defects (thrombocytopenia, hypofibrinogenemia) of all types including those caused by drugs; marked cardiac decompensation; renal disease with severe oliguria or anuria

Warnings/Precautions Hypersensitivity reactions have been reported (dextran 40 rarely causes a reaction), usually early in the infusion. Monitor closely during infusion initiation for signs or symptoms of a hypersensitivity reaction. Dextran 1 is indicated for prophylaxis of serious anaphylactic reactions to dextran infusions. Administration can cause fluid or solute overload. Use caution in patients with fluid overload. Use with caution in patients with active hemorrhage. Use caution in patients receiving corticosteroids. Renal failure has been reported. Fluid status including urine output should be monitored closely. Exercise care to prevent a depression of hematocrit <30% (can cause hemodilution). Observe for signs of bleeding.

Overdosage/Toxicology Symptoms of overdose include fluid overload, pulmonary edema, increased bleeding time, and decreased platelet function. Treatment is supportive. Blood products containing clotting factors may be necessary.

Pharmacodynamics/Kinetics

Onset of Action: Minutes to 1 hour (depending upon the molecular weight polysaccharide administered)

Excretion: Urine (~75%) within 24 hours

Dosing

Adults:

Volume expansion/shock:

Children: Total dose should not exceed 20 mL/kg during first 24 hours

Adults: 500-1000 mL at a rate of 20-40 mL/minute; maximum daily dose: 20 mL/kg for first 24 hours; 10 mL/kg/day thereafter; therapy should not be continued beyond 5 days

Pump prime (Dextran 40): Varies with the volume of the pump oxygenator; generally, the 10% solution is added in a dose of 1-2 g/kg

Prophylaxis of venous thrombosis/pulmonary embolism (Dextran 40): Begin during surgical procedure and give 50-100 g on the day of surgery; an additional 50 g (500 mL) should be administered every 2-3 days during the period of risk (up to 2 weeks postoperatively); usual maximum infusion rate for nonemergency use: 4 mL/minute

Elderly: Use with extreme caution in patients with renal or hepatic impairment.

Pediatrics: Treatment of shock or impending shock (when blood or blood products are not available): I.V. (requires an infusion pump): Children: Total dose should not be >20 mL/kg during first 24 hours

Renal Impairment: Use with extreme caution.

Hepatic Impairment: Use with extreme caution.

Available Dosage Forms

Infusion [premixed in D_5W; high molecular weight]: 6% Dextran 70 (500 mL)

Infusion [premixed in D_5W; low molecular weight] (Gentran®, LMD®): 10% Dextran 40 (500 mL)

Infusion [premixed in $D_{10}W$; high molecular weight]: 32% Dextran 70 (500 mL)

(Continued)

Dextran *(Continued)*

Infusion [premixed in NS; high molecular weight] (Gentran®): 6% Dextran 70 (500 mL)

Infusion [premixed in NS; low molecular weight] (Gentran®, LMD®): 10% Dextran (500 mL)

Monitoring and Teaching Issues

Physical Assessment: See Warning/Precautions for use cautions (eg, fluid overload, active hemorrhage). Note infusion specifics in Administration. Patient should be monitored closely for fluid overload, anaphylactoid reaction, and bleeding (eg, fluid status [oliguria/ anuria], vital signs, and CVP) during first 15 minutes of first hour and periodically thereafter. Other means of maintaining circulation (eg, with epinephrine and diphenhydramine) should be available in the event of an anaphylactoid reaction. Patient teaching should be appropriate to patient condition.

Monitoring Laboratory Tests: Hemoglobin and hematocrit, electrolytes, serum protein

Patient Education: Since this medication is generally used in emergency situations, patient education should be appropriate to patient condition.

Pregnancy Risk Factor: C

Lactation: Excretion in breast milk unknown

Administration

I.V.: For I.V. infusion only (use an infusion pump). Infuse initial 500 mL at a rate of 20-40 mL/ minute if hypervolemic. Reduce rate for additional infusion to 4 mL/minute. **Observe patients closely for anaphylactic reaction.**

Compatibility: Dextran 40 is stable in D_5W, NS

Solution **incompatible** with other drugs

To prevent coagulation of blood, flush tubing well or change I.V. tubing before infusing blood after dextran.

Compatibility when admixed: Incompatible with amoxicillin

Storage: Store at room temperature. Discard partially used containers.

Additional Information Dextran 40 is known as low molecular weight dextran (LMD®) and has an average molecular weight of 40,000; dextran 75 has an average molecular weight of 75,000. Dextran 70 has an average molecular weight of 70,000; sodium content of 500 mL is 77 mEq, with pH ranging from 3.0-7.0.

Dextran 1 (DEKS tran won)

U.S. Brand Names Promit®

Generic Available No

Pharmacologic Category Plasma Volume Expander

Medication Safety Issues

Sound-alike/look-alike issues:

Dextran may be confused with Dexatrim®, Dexedrine®

Use Prophylaxis of serious anaphylactic reactions to I.V. infusion of dextran

Mechanism of Action/Effect Binds to dextran-reactive immunoglobulin without bridge formation and no formation of large immune complexes

Contraindications Hypersensitivity to dextrans or any component of the formulation; **dextran** contraindicated

Warnings/Precautions Severe hypotension and bradycardia can occur. If any reaction occurs, do not administer dextran. Mild dextran-induced anaphylactic reactions are not prevented.

Dosing

Adults & Elderly: Prophylaxis of severe reactions to dextran infusions: I.V.: 20 mL 1-2 minutes before infusion of dextran. Administer 1 dose only prior to dextran. Give 1-2 minutes before I.V. infusion of dextran. Time between dextran 1 and dextran solution should not exceed 15 minutes.

Pediatrics: Prophylaxis of severe adverse reactions to dextran: I.V. (time between dextran 1 and dextran solution should not exceed 15 minutes): Children: 0.3 mL/kg 1-2 minutes before I.V. infusion of dextran

Available Dosage Forms Injection, solution: 150 mg/mL (20 mL)

Monitoring and Teaching Issues

Physical Assessment: Dextran 1 is indicated for prophylaxis of serious anaphylactic reactions to dextran infusions (see Dosing). Patient should be monitored closely during infusion (see Dextran monograph). Patient teaching should be appropriate to patient condition.

Patient Education: Since this medication is generally administered in emergency situations, patient education should be supportive and appropriate to patient condition.

Pregnancy Risk Factor: C

Lactation: Excretion in breast milk unknown

Administration

I.V.: Infuse over 1 minute.

Compatibility: Do not dilute or admix with dextrans.

Storage: Protect from freezing.

♦ **Dextran 40** *see Dextran on page 433*

♦ **Dextran 70** *see Dextran on page 433*

♦ **Dextran, High Molecular Weight** *see Dextran on page 433*

♦ **Dextran, Low Molecular Weight** *see Dextran on page 433*

Dextroamphetamine (deks troe am FET a meen)

U.S. Brand Names Dexedrine®; Dextrostat®

Synonyms Dextroamphetamine Sulfate

Controlled Substance C-II

Generic Available Yes

Pharmacologic Category Stimulant

Medication Safety Issues
Sound-alike/look-alike issues:
Dexedrine® may be confused with dextran, Excedrin®

Use Narcolepsy; attention-deficit/hyperactivity disorder (ADHD)

Unlabeled/Investigational Use Exogenous obesity; depression; abnormal behavioral syndrome in children (minimal brain dysfunction)

Mechanism of Action/Effect Blocks reuptake of dopamine and norepinephrine from the synapse, thus increases the amount of circulating dopamine and norepinephrine in cerebral cortex to reticular activating system; inhibits the action of monoamine oxidase and causes catecholamines to be released. Peripheral actions include elevated blood pressure, weak bronchodilator, and respiratory stimulant action.

Contraindications Hypersensitivity or idiosyncrasy to dextroamphetamine or other sympathomimetic amines. Patients with advanced arteriosclerosis, symptomatic cardiovascular disease, moderate to severe hypertension (stage II or III), hyperthyroidism, glaucoma, diabetes mellitus, agitated states, patients with a history of drug abuse, and during or within 14 days following MAO inhibitor therapy. Stimulant medications are contraindicated for use in children with attention-deficit/hyperactivity disorders and concomitant Tourette's syndrome or tics.

Warnings/Precautions Use with caution in patients with bipolar disorder, cardiovascular disease, seizure disorders, insomnia, porphyria, mild hypertension (stage I), or history of substance abuse. May exacerbate symptoms of behavior and thought disorder in psychotic patients. Potential for drug dependency exists - avoid abrupt discontinuation in patients who have received for prolonged periods. Use in weight reduction programs only when alternative therapy has been ineffective. Products may contain tartrazine - use with caution in potentially sensitive individuals. Stimulant use in children has been associated with growth suppression.

Drug Interactions
Cytochrome P450 Effect: Substrate of CYP2D6 (major)

Decreased Effect: Amphetamines inhibit the antihypertensive response to guanethidine and guanadrel. Urinary acidifiers decrease the half-life and duration of action of amphetamines.

Increased Effect/Toxicity: CYP2D6 inhibitors may increase the levels/effects of dextroamphetamine; example inhibitors include chlorpromazine, delavirdine, fluoxetine, miconazole, paroxetine, pergolide, quinidine, quinine, ritonavir, and ropinirole. Dextroamphetamine may precipitate hypertensive crisis or serotonin syndrome in patients receiving MAO inhibitors (selegiline >10 mg/day, isocarboxazid, phenelzine, tranylcypromine, furazolidone). Serotonin syndrome has also been associated with combinations of amphetamines and SSRIs; these combinations should be avoided. TCAs may enhance the effects of amphetamines. Large doses of antacids or urinary alkalinizers increase the half-life and duration of action of amphetamines. May precipitate arrhythmias in patients receiving general anesthetics.

Nutritional/Ethanol Interactions
Ethanol: Avoid ethanol (may increase CNS depression).
Food: Dextroamphetamine serum levels may be altered if taken with acidic food, juices, or vitamin C.
Herb/Nutraceutical: Avoid ephedra (may cause hypertension or arrhythmias).

Adverse Reactions Frequency not defined.
Cardiovascular: Palpitations, tachycardia, hypertension, cardiomyopathy
Central nervous system: Overstimulation, euphoria, dyskinesia, dysphoria, exacerbation of motor and phonic tics, restlessness, insomnia, dizziness, headache, psychosis, Tourette's syndrome
Dermatologic: Rash, urticaria
Endocrine & metabolic: Changes in libido
Gastrointestinal: Diarrhea, constipation, anorexia, weight loss, xerostomia, unpleasant taste
Genitourinary: Impotence
Neuromuscular & skeletal: Tremor

Overdosage/Toxicology Symptoms of overdose include restlessness, tremor, confusion, hallucinations, panic, dysrhythmias, nausea, and vomiting. There is no specific antidote for dextroamphetamine intoxication and treatment is primarily supportive. Hyperactivity and agitation usually respond to reduced sensory input; however, with extreme agitation, haloperidol (2-5 mg I.M. for adults) may be required.

Pharmacodynamics/Kinetics
Onset of Action: 1-1.5 hours
Time to Peak: Serum: T_{max}: Immediate release: 3 hours; sustained release: 8 hours
Half-Life Elimination: Adults: 10-13 hours
Metabolism: Hepatic via CYP monooxygenase and glucuronidation
Excretion: Urine (as unchanged drug and inactive metabolites)

Dosing
Adults:
Narcolepsy: Oral: Initial: 10 mg/day, may increase at 10 mg increments in weekly intervals until side effects appear; maximum: 60 mg/day
Exogenous obesity (short-term adjunct): Oral: 5-30 mg/day in divided doses of 5-10 mg 30-60 minutes before meals
Elderly: Refer to adult dosing; start at lowest dose. Use with caution.
Pediatrics:
Narcolepsy: Oral: Children 6-12 years: Initial: 5 mg/day, may increase at 5 mg increments in weekly intervals until side effects appear; maximum dose: 60 mg/day
Attention-deficit/hyperactivity disorder (ADHD): Oral:
Children 3-5 years: Initial: 2.5 mg/day given every morning; increase by 2.5 mg/day in weekly intervals until optimal response is obtained, usual range: 0.1-0.5 mg/kg/dose every morning with maximum of 40 mg/day
Children ≥6 years: 5 mg once or twice daily; increase in increments of 5 mg/day at weekly intervals until optimal response is reached, usual range: 0.1-0.5 mg/kg/dose every morning with maximum of 40 mg/day (5-20 mg/day)
(Continued)

Dextroamphetamine *(Continued)*

Available Dosage Forms
Capsule, sustained release, as sulfate: 5 mg, 10 mg, 15 mg
   Dexedrine® Spansule®: 5 mg, 10 mg, 15 mg
Tablet, as sulfate: 5 mg, 10 mg
   Dexedrine®: 5 mg [contains tartrazine]
   Dextrostat®: 5 mg, 10 mg [contains tartrazine]

Monitoring and Teaching Issues
Physical Assessment: Assess effectiveness and interactions of other medications patient may be taking. Assess for history of psychopathology, homicidal or suicidal tendencies, or addiction; long-term use can result in dependence, abuse, or tolerance. Periodically evaluate the need for continued use. Monitor therapeutic effectiveness, vital signs, and adverse reactions at start of therapy, when changing dosage, and at regular intervals during therapy. Monitor serum glucose closely in patients with diabetes (amphetamines may alter antidiabetic requirements). Taper dosage slowly when discontinuing. Assess knowledge/teach patient appropriate use, possible side effects, and symptoms to report.

Patient Education: Take exactly as directed; do not increase dose or frequency without consulting prescriber. Drug may cause physical and/or psychological dependence. Take early in day to avoid sleep disturbance, 30 minutes before meals. Avoid alcohol, caffeine, or OTC medications that act as stimulants. You may experience restlessness, false sense of euphoria, or impaired judgment (use caution when driving or engaging in tasks requiring alertness until response to drug is known); dry mouth (frequent mouth care, sucking lozenges, or chewing gum may help); nausea or vomiting (small frequent meals, frequent mouth care may help); constipation (increased exercise, fluids, fruit, or fiber may help); diarrhea (buttermilk, boiled milk, or yogurt may help); or altered libido (reversible). Patients with diabetes need to monitor serum glucose closely (may alter antidiabetic medication requirements). Report chest pain, palpitations, or irregular heartbeat; extreme fatigue or depression; CNS changes (aggressiveness, restlessness, euphoria, sleep disturbances); severe unremitting abdominal distress or cramping; blackened stool; changes in sexual activity; or blurred vision. **Pregnancy/breast-feeding precautions:** Inform prescriber if you are or intend to become pregnant. Do not breast-feed.

Dietary Considerations: Should be taken 30 minutes before meals and at least 6 hours before bedtime.

Pregnancy Risk Factor: C

Lactation: Enters breast milk/contraindicated

Administration
Oral: Do not crush sustained release drug product. Administer as single dose in morning or as divided doses with breakfast and lunch. Should be administered 30 minutes before meals and at least 6 hours before bedtime.

Storage: Protect from light.

Dextroamphetamine and Amphetamine
(deks troe am FET a meen & am FET a meen)

U.S. Brand Names Adderall®; Adderall XR™

Synonyms Amphetamine and Dextroamphetamine

Controlled Substance C-II

Generic Available Yes: Tablet

Pharmacologic Category Stimulant

Medication Safety Issues
Sound-alike/look-alike issues:
   Adderall® may be confused with Inderal®

Use Attention-deficit/hyperactivity disorder (ADHD); narcolepsy

Note: Market authorization for the treatment of ADHD was withdrawn in Canada (February, 2005)

Mechanism of Action/Effect Blocks reuptake of dopamine and norepinephrine from the synapse, thus increases the amount of circulating dopamine and norepinephrine in cerebral cortex to reticular activating system; inhibits the action of monoamine oxidase and causes catecholamines to be released. Peripheral actions include elevated blood pressure, weak bronchodilator, and respiratory stimulant action.

Contraindications Hypersensitivity to dextroamphetamine, amphetamine, or any component of the formulation; advanced arteriosclerosis; symptomatic cardiovascular disease; moderate to severe hypertension; hyperthyroidism; hypersensitivity or idiosyncrasy to the sympathomimetic amines; glaucoma; agitated states; patients with a history of drug abuse; during or within 14 days following MAO inhibitor (hypertensive crisis)

Warnings/Precautions Amphetamine has a high abuse potential; prolonged use may lead to dependency. Avoid use in patients with structural cardiac abnormalities; has been associated with sudden death. Use caution in mildly hypertensive patients; amphetamines may impair the ability to engage in potentially hazardous activities. In psychotic children, amphetamines may exacerbate symptoms of behavior disturbance and thought disorder. Stimulants may unmask tics in individuals with coexisting Tourette's syndrome. Not recommended for children <3 years of age. Avoid abrupt discontinuation.

Drug Interactions
Cytochrome P450 Effect:
Dextroamphetamine: **Substrate** of CYP2D6 (major)
Amphetamine: **Substrate** of CYP2D6 (major); **Inhibits** CYP2D6 (weak)

Decreased Effect: Amphetamines inhibit the antihypertensive response to guanethidine and guanadrel. Urinary acidifiers decrease the half-life and duration of action of amphetamines.

Increased Effect/Toxicity: CYP2D6 inhibitors may increase the levels/effects of amphetamine and dextroamphetamine; example inhibitors include chlorpromazine, delavirdine, fluoxetine, miconazole, paroxetine, pergolide, quinidine, quinine, ritonavir, and ropinirole. Dextroamphetamine and amphetamine may precipitate hypertensive crisis or serotonin syndrome in patients receiving MAO inhibitors (selegiline >10 mg/day, isocarboxazid, phenelzine, tranylcypromine, furazolidone). Serotonin syndrome has also been associated with combinations of amphetamines and SSRIs; these combinations should be avoided. TCAs may enhance the effects of amphetamines, potentially leading to hypertensive crisis. Large doses of antacids or urinary alkalinizers increase the half-life and duration of action of amphetamines. May precipitate arrhythmias in patients receiving general anesthetics.

Nutritional/Ethanol Interactions
Ethanol: Avoid ethanol (may increase CNS depression).
Food: Dextroamphetamine serum levels may be altered if taken with acidic food, juices, or vitamin C. Avoid caffeine.
Herb/Nutraceutical: Avoid ephedra (may cause hypertension or arrhythmias).

Lab Interactions Increased corticosteroid levels (greatest in evening); may interfere with urinary steroid testing

Adverse Reactions
As reported with Adderall XR™:
>10%:
Central nervous system: Insomnia (1% to 27%), headache (up to 26% in adults)
Gastrointestinal: Appetite decreased (22% to 33%), abdominal pain (14%), dry mouth (up to 33% in adults), weight loss (1% to 11%)
1% to 10%:
Cardiovascular: Palpitation (2% to 4%), tachycardia (up to 6% in adults)
Central nervous system: Emotional lability (1% to 9%), agitation (up to 8% in adults), dizziness (2% to 7%), nervousness (6%), fever (4%)
Dermatologic: Photosensitization (2% to 4%)
Endocrine & metabolic: Impotence (2% to 4%), libido decreased (2% to 4%)
Gastrointestinal: Nausea (5% to 8%), vomiting (7%), constipation (2% to 4%), anorexia (3%), diarrhea (2% to 6%), dyspepsia (2%)
Neuromuscular & skeletal: Twitching (2% to 4%), weakness (2% to 6%)
Miscellaneous: Infection (2% to 4%), speech disorder (2% to 4%)

Adverse reactions reported with other amphetamines include: Cardiomyopathy, dyskinesia, dysphoria, euphoria, exacerbation of motor and phonic tics, exacerbation of Tourette's syndrome, headache, hypertension, overstimulation, palpitation, psychosis, rash, restlessness, tachycardia, tremor, urticaria

Overdosage/Toxicology Manifestations of overdose vary widely. Symptoms of central stimulation are usually followed by fatigue and depression. Cardiovascular and gastrointestinal symptoms are also reported. Treatment is symptomatic and supportive. Chlorpromazine may be used to antagonize CNS effects.

Pharmacodynamics/Kinetics
Onset of Action: 30-60 minutes
Duration of Action: 4-6 hours
Absorption: Well-absorbed
Time to Peak: T_{max}: Adderall®: 3 hours; Adderall XR™: 7 hours
Half-Life Elimination:
Children: D-amphetamine: 9 hours; L-amphetamine: 11 hours
Adults: D-amphetamine: 10 hours; L-amphetamine: 13 hours
Metabolism: Hepatic via cytochrome P450 monooxygenase and glucuronidation
Excretion: 70% of a single dose is eliminated within 24 hours; excreted as unchanged amphetamine (30%), benzoic acid, hydroxyamphetamine, hippuric acid, norephedrine, and *p*-hydroxynorephedrine
Pharmacokinetic Note: See Dextroamphetamine monograph.

Dosing
Adults & Elderly: Note: Use lowest effective individualized dose; administer first dose as soon as awake; use intervals of 4-6 hours between additional doses.
ADHD: Oral:
Adderall®: Initial: 5 mg once or twice daily; increase daily dose in 5 mg increments at weekly intervals until optimal response is obtained; usual maximum dose: 40 mg/day given in 1-3 divided doses per day.
Adderall XR™: Initial: 20 mg once daily in the morning; higher doses (up to 60 mg once daily) have been evaluated; however, there is not adequate evidence that higher doses afforded additional benefit,
Narcolepsy: *Adderall®* : Oral: Initial: 10 mg/day; increase daily dose in 10 mg increments at weekly intervals until optimal response is obtained; maximum dose: 60 mg/day given in 1-3 divided doses per day.

Pediatrics:
Note: Use lowest effective individualized dose; administer first dose as soon as awake
ADHD: Oral:
Children: <3 years: Not recommended.
Children: 3-5 years (Adderall®): Initial 2.5 mg/day given every morning; increase daily dose in 2.5 mg increments at weekly intervals until optimal response is obtained; maximum dose: 40 mg/day given in 1-3 divided doses per day. Use intervals of 4-6 hours between additional doses.
Children: ≥6 years:
Adderall®: Initial: 5 mg once or twice daily; increase daily dose in 5 mg increments at weekly intervals until optimal response is obtained; usual maximum dose: 40 mg/day given in 1-3 divided doses per day. Use intervals of 4-6 hours between additional doses.
Adderall XR™: 5-10 mg once daily in the morning; if needed, may increase daily dose in 5-10 mg increments at weekly intervals (maximum dose: 30 mg/day)
Narcolepsy: *Adderall®* : Oral:
Children: 6-12 years: Initial: 5 mg/day; increase daily dose in 5 mg increments at weekly intervals until optimal response is obtained; maximum dose: 60 mg/day given in 1-3 divided doses per day.
Children >12 years: Refer to adult dosing.
(Continued)

Dextroamphetamine and Amphetamine *(Continued)*

Available Dosage Forms

Capsule, extended release (Adderall XR™):

5 mg [dextroamphetamine sulfate 1.25 mg, dextroamphetamine saccharate 1.25 mg, amphetamine aspartate monohydrate 1.25 mg, amphetamine sulfate 1.25 mg] (equivalent to amphetamine base 3.1 mg)

10 mg [dextroamphetamine sulfate 2.5 mg, dextroamphetamine saccharate 2.5 mg, amphetamine aspartate monohydrate 2.5 mg, amphetamine sulfate 2.5 mg] (equivalent to amphetamine base 6.3 mg)

15 mg [dextroamphetamine sulfate 3.75 mg, dextroamphetamine saccharate 3.75 mg, amphetamine aspartate monohydrate 3.75 mg, amphetamine sulfate 3.75 mg] (equivalent to amphetamine base 9.4 mg)

20 mg [dextroamphetamine sulfate 5 mg, dextroamphetamine saccharate 5 mg, amphetamine aspartate monohydrate 5 mg, amphetamine sulfate 5 mg] (equivalent to amphetamine base 12.5 mg)

25 mg [dextroamphetamine sulfate 6.25 mg, dextroamphetamine saccharate 6.25 mg, amphetamine aspartate monohydrate 6.25 mg, amphetamine sulfate 6.25 mg] (equivalent to amphetamine base 15.6 mg)

30 mg [dextroamphetamine sulfate 7.5 mg, dextroamphetamine saccharate 7.5 mg, amphetamine aspartate monohydrate 7.5 mg, amphetamine sulfate 7.5 mg] (equivalent to amphetamine base 18.8 mg)

Tablet (Adderall®):

5 mg [dextroamphetamine sulfate 1.25 mg, dextroamphetamine saccharate 1.25 mg, amphetamine aspartate 1.25 mg, amphetamine sulfate 1.25 mg] (equivalent to amphetamine base 3.13 mg)

7.5 mg [dextroamphetamine 1.875 mg, dextroamphetamine saccharate 1.875 mg, amphetamine aspartate 1.875 mg, amphetamine sulfate 1.875 mg] (equivalent to amphetamine base 4.7 mg)

10 mg [dextroamphetamine sulfate 2.5 mg, dextroamphetamine saccharate 2.5 mg, amphetamine aspartate 2.5 mg, amphetamine sulfate 2.5 mg] (equivalent to amphetamine base 6.3 mg)

12.5 mg [dextroamphetamine sulfate 3.125 mg, dextroamphetamine saccharate 3.125 mg, amphetamine aspartate 3.125 mg, amphetamine sulfate 3.125 mg] (equivalent to amphetamine base 7.8 mg)

15 mg [dextroamphetamine sulfate 3.75 mg, dextroamphetamine saccharate 3.75 mg, amphetamine aspartate 3.75 mg, amphetamine sulfate 3.75 mg] (equivalent to amphetamine base 9.4 mg)

20 mg [dextroamphetamine sulfate 5 mg, dextroamphetamine saccharate 5 mg, amphetamine aspartate 5 mg, amphetamine sulfate 5 mg] (equivalent to amphetamine base 12.6 mg)

30 mg [dextroamphetamine sulfate 7.5 mg, dextroamphetamine saccharate 7.5 mg, amphetamine aspartate 7.5 mg, amphetamine sulfate 7.5 mg] (equivalent to amphetamine base 18.8 mg)

Monitoring and Teaching Issues

Physical Assessment: Assess effectiveness and interactions of other medications patient may be taking. Assess for history of psychopathology, homicidal or suicidal tendencies, or addiction; long-term use can result in dependence, abuse, or tolerance. Periodically evaluate the need for continued use. Monitor therapeutic effectiveness, blood pressure, vital signs, and adverse reactions at start of therapy, when changing dosage, and at regular intervals during therapy. Monitor serum glucose closely in patients with diabetes (amphetamines may alter antidiabetic requirements). Taper dosage slowly when discontinuing. Assess knowledge/teach patient appropriate use, possible side effects, and symptoms to report.

Patient Education: Take exactly as directed; do not increase dose or frequency without consulting prescriber. Drug may cause physical and/or psychological dependence. Take early in the day to avoid sleep disturbance. If you miss a dose, take it as soon as you can. If it is almost time for your next dose, do not take double dose. Avoid alcohol, caffeine, or OTC medications that act as stimulants. You may experience restlessness, false sense of euphoria, or impaired judgment (use caution when driving or engaging in tasks requiring alertness until response to drug is known); dry mouth (frequent mouth care, sucking lozenges, or chewing gum may help); nausea or vomiting (small frequent meals, frequent mouth care may help); constipation (increased exercise, fluids, fruit, or fiber may help); diarrhea (buttermilk, boiled milk, or yogurt may help); altered libido (reversible); or altered acuity of taste or smell. Patients with diabetes need to monitor serum glucose closely (may alter antidiabetic medication requirements). Report chest pain, palpitations, or irregular heartbeat; extreme fatigue or depression; CNS changes (aggressiveness, restlessness, euphoria, sleep disturbances); severe unremitting abdominal distress or cramping; blackened stool; changes in sexual activity; or blurred vision. **Pregnancy/breast-feeding precautions:** Inform prescriber if you are pregnant. Do not breast-feed.

Pregnancy Risk Factor: C

Pregnancy Issues: Use during pregnancy may lead to increased risk of premature delivery and low birth weight. Infants may experience symptoms of withdrawal. Teratogenic effects were reported when taken during the 1st trimester.

Lactation: Enters breast milk/contraindicated

Administration

Oral:

Adderall®: To avoid insomnia, last daily dose should be administered no less than 6 hours before retiring.

Adderall XR™: Should be given by noon. Capsule may be swallowed whole or it may be opened and the contents sprinkled on applesauce. Applesauce should be consumed immediately without chewing. Do not divide the contents of the capsule.

Storage: Store at controlled room temperature of 15°C to 30°C (59°F to 86°F)

Additional Information Treatment of ADHD may include "drug holidays" or periodic discontinuation of medication in order to assess the patient's requirments, decrease tolerance, and limit suppression of linear growth and weight; the combination of equal parts of *d*, *l*-amphetamine aspartate, *d*, *l*-amphetamine sulfate, dextroamphetamine saccharate and dextroamphetamine sulfate results in a 75:25 ratio of the dextro and levo isomers of amphetamine.

The duration of action of Adderall® is longer than methylphenidate; behavioral effects of a single morning dose of Adderall® may last throughout the school day; a single morning dose of Adderall® has been shown in several studies to be as effective as twice daily dosing of methylphenidate for the treatment of ADHD.

Related Information
Dextroamphetamine *on page 434*

♦ **Dextroamphetamine Sulfate** *see* Dextroamphetamine *on page 434*

♦ **Dextromethorphan and Guaifenesin** *see* Guaifenesin and Dextromethorphan *on page 731*

♦ **Dextromethorphan and Promethazine** *see* Promethazine and Dextromethorphan *on page 1268*

♦ **Dextromethorphan Tannate, Pyrilamine Tannate, and Phenylephrine Tannate** *see* Phenylephrine, Pyrilamine, and Dextromethorphan *on page 1204*

♦ **Dextropropoxyphene** *see* Propoxyphene *on page 1271*

♦ **Dextrostat®** *see* Dextroamphetamine *on page 434*

♦ **DFMO** *see* Eflornithine *on page 511*

♦ **DHAD** *see* Mitoxantrone *on page 1019*

♦ **DHAQ** *see* Mitoxantrone *on page 1019*

♦ **DHE** *see* Dihydroergotamine *on page 457*

♦ **D.H.E. 45®** *see* Dihydroergotamine *on page 457*

♦ **DHPG Sodium** *see* Ganciclovir *on page 695*

♦ **Diaβeta®** *see* GlyBURIDE *on page 720*

♦ **Diabetes Mellitus Management** *see page 1819*

♦ **Diabetic Tussin C®** *see* Guaifenesin and Codeine *on page 731*

♦ **Diabetic Tussin® DM [OTC]** *see* Guaifenesin and Dextromethorphan *on page 731*

♦ **Diabetic Tussin® DM Maximum Strength [OTC]** *see* Guaifenesin and Dextromethorphan *on page 731*

♦ **Diabetic Tussin® EX [OTC]** *see* Guaifenesin *on page 729*

♦ **Diagnostics and Surgical Aids** *see page 1625*

♦ **Diaminocyclohexane Oxalatoplatinum** *see* Oxaliplatin *on page 1127*

♦ **Diaminodiphenylsulfone** *see* Dapsone *on page 403*

♦ **Diamode [OTC]** *see* Loperamide *on page 914*

♦ **Diamox® Sequels®** *see* AcetaZOLAMIDE *on page 42*

♦ **Diastat®** *see* Diazepam *on page 439*

Diazepam (dye AZ e pam)

U.S. Brand Names Diastat®; Diazepam Intensol®; Valium®
Controlled Substance C-IV
Generic Available Yes: Injection, tablet, solution only
Pharmacologic Category Benzodiazepine
Medication Safety Issues
Sound-alike/look-alike issues:
Diazepam may be confused with diazoxide, Ditropan®, lorazepam
Valium® may be confused with Valcyte™

Use Management of anxiety disorders, ethanol withdrawal symptoms; skeletal muscle relaxant; treatment of convulsive disorders
Orphan drug: Viscous solution for rectal administration: Management of selected, refractory epilepsy patients on stable regimens of antiepileptic drugs (AEDs) requiring intermittent use of diazepam to control episodes of increased seizure activity

Unlabeled/Investigational Use Panic disorders; preoperative sedation, light anesthesia, amnesia

Mechanism of Action/Effect Binds to stereospecific benzodiazepine receptors on the postsynaptic GABA neuron at several sites within the central nervous system, including the limbic system, reticular formation. Enhancement of the inhibitory effect of GABA on neuronal excitability results by increased neuronal membrane permeability to chloride ions. This shift in chloride ions results in hyperpolarization (a less excitable state) and stabilization.

Contraindications Hypersensitivity to diazepam or any component of the formulation (cross-sensitivity with other benzodiazepines may exist); narrow-angle glaucoma; not for use in children <6 months of age (oral) or <30 days of age (parenteral); pregnancy

Warnings/Precautions Diazepam has been associated with increasing the frequency of grand mal seizures. Withdrawal has also been associated with an increase in the seizure frequency. Use with caution with drugs which may decrease diazepam metabolism. Avoid use in caution in elderly or debilitated patients, patients with hepatic disease (including alcoholics), respiratory disease, impaired gag reflex, or renal impairment. Active metabolites with extended half-lives may lead to delayed accumulation and adverse effects.

Acute hypotension, muscle weakness, apnea, and cardiac arrest have occurred with parenteral administration. Acute effects may be more prevalent in patients receiving concurrent barbiturates, narcotics, or ethanol. Appropriate resuscitative equipment and qualified personnel should be available during administration and monitoring. Avoid use of the injection in patients with shock, coma, or acute ethanol intoxication. Intra-arterial injection or extravasation of the parenteral formulation should be avoided. Parenteral formulation contains propylene glycol, which has been associated with toxicity when administered in high dosages.
(Continued)

Diazepam *(Continued)*

Causes CNS depression (dose-related) resulting in sedation, dizziness, confusion, or ataxia which may impair physical and mental capabilities. Use with caution in patients receiving other CNS depressants or psychoactive agents. Effects with other sedative drugs or ethanol may be potentiated. The dosage of narcotics should be reduced by approximately $\frac{1}{3}$ when diazepam is added. Benzodiazepines have been associated with falls and traumatic injury and should be used with extreme caution in patients who are at risk of these events (especially the elderly).

Use caution in patients with depression, particularly if suicidal risk may be present, or in patients with a history of drug dependence. Benzodiazepines have been associated with dependence and acute withdrawal symptoms on discontinuation or reduction in dose. Acute withdrawal, including seizures, may be precipitated in patients after administration of flumazenil to patients receiving long-term benzodiazepine therapy.

Diazepam has been associated with anterograde amnesia. Paradoxical reactions, including hyperactive or aggressive behavior, have been reported with benzodiazepines, particularly in adolescent/pediatric or psychiatric patients. Does not have analgesic, antidepressant, or antipsychotic properties.

Drug Interactions

Cytochrome P450 Effect: Substrate of CYP1A2 (minor), 2B6 (minor), 2C8/9 (minor), 2C19 (major), 3A4 (major); **Inhibits** CYP2C19 (weak), 3A4 (weak)

Decreased Effect: CYP2C19 inducers may decrease the levels/effects of diazepam; example inducers include aminoglutethimide, carbamazepine, phenytoin, and rifampin. CYP3A4 inducers may decrease the levels/effects of diazepam; example inducers include aminoglutethimide, carbamazepine, nafcillin, nevirapine, phenobarbital, phenytoin, and rifamycins.

Increased Effect/Toxicity: Diazepam potentiates the CNS depressant effects of narcotic analgesics, barbiturates, phenothiazines, ethanol, antihistamines, MAO inhibitors, sedative-hypnotics, and cyclic antidepressants. CYP2C19 inhibitors may increase the levels/effects of diazepam; example inhibitors include delavirdine, fluconazole, fluvoxamine, gemfibrozil, isoniazid, omeprazole, and ticlopidine. CYP3A4 inhibitors may increase the levels/effects of diazepam; example inhibitors include azole antifungals, ciprofloxacin, clarithromycin, diclofenac, doxycycline, erythromycin, imatinib, isoniazid, nefazodone, nicardipine, propofol, protease inhibitors, quinidine, and verapamil.

Nutritional/Ethanol Interactions

Ethanol: Avoid ethanol (may increase CNS depression).

Food: Diazepam serum levels may be increased if taken with food. Diazepam effect/toxicity may be increased by grapefruit juice; avoid concurrent use.

Herb/Nutraceutical: St John's wort may decrease diazepam levels. Avoid valerian, St John's wort, kava kava, gotu kola (may increase CNS depression).

Lab Interactions False-negative urinary glucose determinations when using Clinistix® or Diastix®

Adverse Reactions Frequency not defined.

Cardiovascular: Hypotension

Central nervous system: Drowsiness, ataxia, amnesia, slurred speech, paradoxical excitement or rage, fatigue, insomnia, memory impairment, headache, anxiety, depression, vertigo, confusion

Dermatologic: Rash

Endocrine & metabolic: Changes in libido

Gastrointestinal: Changes in salivation, constipation, nausea

Genitourinary: Incontinence, urinary retention

Hepatic: Jaundice

Local: Phlebitis, pain with injection

Neuromuscular & skeletal: Dysarthria, tremor

Ocular: Blurred vision, diplopia

Respiratory: Decrease in respiratory rate, apnea

Overdosage/Toxicology Symptoms of overdose include somnolence, confusion, coma, hypoactive reflexes, dyspnea, hypotension, slurred speech, or impaired coordination. Treatment for benzodiazepine overdose is supportive. Flumazenil has been shown to selectively block the binding of benzodiazepines to CNS receptors, resulting in a reversal of benzodiazepine-induced CNS depression, but not respiratory depression.

Pharmacodynamics/Kinetics

Onset of Action: I.V.: Status epilepticus: Almost immediate

Duration of Action: I.V.: Status epilepticus: 20-30 minutes

Absorption: Oral: 85% to 100%, more reliable than I.M.

Protein Binding: 98%

Half-Life Elimination: Parent drug: Adults: 20-50 hours; increased half-life in neonates, elderly, and those with severe hepatic disorders; Active major metabolite (desmethyldiazepam): 50-100 hours; may be prolonged in neonates

Metabolism: Hepatic

Dosing

Adults: Note: Oral absorption is more reliable than I.M.

Anxiety/sedation/skeletal muscle relaxation:

Oral: 2-10 mg 2-4 times/day

I.M., I.V.: 2-10 mg, may repeat in 3-4 hours if needed

Sedation in the ICU patient: I.V.: 0.03-0.1 mg/kg every 30 minutes to 6 hours

Status epilepticus: I.V.: 5-10 mg every 10-20 minutes, up to 30 mg in an 8-hour period; may repeat in 2-4 hours if necessary

Rapid tranquilization of agitated patient (administer every 30-60 minutes): Oral: 5-10 mg; average total dose for tranquilization: 20-60 mg

Elderly: Oral absorption is more reliable than I.M..
Oral: Initial:
Anxiety: 1-2 mg 1-2 times/day; increase gradually as needed, rarely need to use >10 mg/day.
Skeletal muscle relaxant: 2-5 mg 2-4 times/day

Pediatrics:
Conscious sedation for procedures:
Oral:
Children: 0.2-0.3 mg/kg (maximum dose: 10 mg) 45-60 minutes prior to procedure
Adolescents: 10 mg
I.V.: Adolescents: 5 mg; may repeat with 2.5 mg if needed
Febrile seizure prophylaxis: Oral: Children: 1 mg/kg/day divided every 8 hours; initiate therapy at first sign of fever and continue for 24 hours after fever is gone
Sedation or muscle relaxation or anxiety:
Oral: Children: 0.12-0.8 mg/kg/day in divided doses every 6-8 hours
I.M., I.V.: Children: 0.04-0.3 mg/kg/dose every 2-4 hours to a maximum of 0.6 mg/kg within an 8-hour period if needed
Status epilepticus:
I.V.:
Infants >30 days and Children <5 years: 0.05-0.3 mg/kg/dose given over 3-5 minutes, every 15-30 minutes to a maximum total dose of 5 mg **or** 0.2-0.5 mg/dose every 2-5 minutes to a maximum total dose of 5 mg; repeat in 2-4 hours as needed
Children ≥5 years: 0.05-0.3 mg/kg/dose given over 3-5 minutes, every 15-30 minutes to a maximum total dose of 10 mg **or** 1 mg/dose every 2-5 minutes to a maximum of 10 mg; repeat in 2-4 hours as needed
Rectal: 0.5 mg/kg/dose then 0.25 mg/kg/dose in 10 minutes if needed
Anticonvulsant (acute treatment): Rectal gel formulation:
Infants <6 months: Not recommended
Children <2 years: Safety and efficacy have not been studied
Children 2-5 years: 0.5 mg/kg
Children 6-11 years: 0.3 mg/kg
Children ≥12 years and Adults: 0.2 mg/kg
Note: Dosage should be rounded upward to the next available dose, 2.5, 5, 10, 15, and 20 mg/dose; dose may be repeated in 4-12 hours if needed; do not use more than 5 times per month or more than once every 5 days
Muscle spasm associated with tetanus: I.V., I.M.:
Infants >30 days: 1-2 mg/dose every 3-4 hours as needed
Children ≥5 years: 5-10 mg/dose every 3-4 hours as needed
Renal Impairment: Hemodialysis effects: Not dialyzable (0% to 5%); supplemental dose is **not** necessary.
Hepatic Impairment: Reduce dose by 50% in cirrhosis and avoid in severe/acute liver disease.

Available Dosage Forms
Gel, rectal (Diastat®):
Adult rectal tip [6 cm]: 5 mg/mL (15 mg, 20 mg) [contains ethyl alcohol, sodium benzoate, benzyl alcohol; twin pack]
Pediatric rectal tip [4.4 cm]: 5 mg/mL (2.5 mg, 5 mg) [contains ethyl alcohol, sodium benzoate, benzyl alcohol; twin pack]
Universal rectal tip [for pediatric and adult use; 4.4 cm]: 5 mg/mL (10 mg) [contains ethyl alcohol, sodium benzoate, benzyl alcohol; twin pack]
Injection, solution: 5 mg/mL (2 mL, 10 mL) [may contain benzyl alcohol, sodium benzoate, benzoic acid]
Solution, oral: 5 mg/5 mL (5 mL, 500 mL) [wintergreen-spice flavor]
Solution, oral concentrate (Diazepam Intensol®): 5 mg/mL (30 mL)
Tablet (Valium®): 2 mg, 5 mg, 10 mg

Monitoring and Teaching Issues
Physical Assessment: Assess effectiveness and interactions of other medications patient may be taking. Assess for history of addiction; long-term use can result in dependence, abuse, or tolerance; periodically evaluate need for continued use. Monitor blood pressure, CNS status. For inpatient use, institute safety measures and monitor effectiveness and adverse reactions. For outpatients, monitor therapeutic effectiveness and adverse reactions at beginning of therapy and periodically with long-term use. Taper dosage slowly when discontinuing. Assess knowledge/teach patient seizure precautions (if administered for seizures), appropriate use, interventions to reduce side effects, and adverse symptoms to report.

Patient Education: Take exactly as directed; do not increase dose or frequency. Drug may cause physical and/or psychological dependence. While using this medication, do not use alcohol and other prescription or OTC medications (especially pain medications, sedatives, antihistamines, or hypnotics) without consulting prescriber. Maintain adequate hydration (2-3 L/day of fluids) unless instructed to restrict fluid intake. You may experience drowsiness, dizziness, or blurred vision (use caution when driving or engaging in tasks requiring alertness until response to drug is known); nausea, vomiting, loss of appetite, or dry mouth (small frequent meals, frequent mouth care, chewing gum, or sucking lozenges may help); constipation (increased exercise, fluids, fruit, or fiber may help). If medication is used to control seizures, wear identification that you are taking an antiepileptic medication. Report CNS changes (confusion, depression, increased sedation, excitation, headache, agitation, insomnia or nightmares, dizziness, fatigue, or impaired coordination) or changes in cognition; respiratory difficulty or shortness of breath; changes in urinary pattern; changes in sexual activity; muscle cramping, weakness, tremors, or rigidity; ringing in ears or visual disturbances; excessive perspiration; excessive GI symptoms (cramping, constipation, vomiting, anorexia); or worsening of seizure activity or loss of seizure control. **Pregnancy/breast-feeding precautions:** Do not get pregnant while taking this medication; use appropriate contraceptive measures. Do not breast-feed.
(Continued)

441

Diazepam *(Continued)*

Geriatric Considerations: Due to its long-acting metabolite, diazepam is not considered a drug of choice in the elderly. Long-acting benzodiazepines have been associated with falls in the elderly. Interpretive guidelines from the Centers for Medicare and Medicaid Services (CMS) strongly discourage the use of this agent in residents of long-term care facilities.

Pregnancy Risk Factor: D

Pregnancy Issues: Benzodiazepines cross the placenta. The association between benzodiazepine exposure and malformations remains controversial. A number of types of malformation have been reported (oral cleft, inguinal hernia, cardiac defects, spina bifida, dysmorphic facial features, skeletal defects); however, confounding factors make a clear association difficult. Overall, the risk to the fetus may be low. Nonteratogenic effects (including neonatal flaccidity, respiratory and feeding problems, and withdrawal symptoms) during the postnatal period have also been reported with benzodiazepine use.

Lactation: Enters breast milk/contraindicated (AAP rates "of concern")

Breast-Feeding Issues: Clinical effects on the infant include sedation; AAP reports that USE MAY BE OF CONCERN.

Administration

I.V.: Continuous infusion is not recommended because of precipitation in I.V. fluids and absorption of drug into infusion bags and tubing. In children, do not exceed 1-2 mg/minute IVP; in adults 5 mg/minute.

Reconstitution: Most stable at pH 4-8, hydrolysis occurs at pH <3.

Compatibility: Do not mix I.V. product with other medications.

Y-site administration: Incompatible with amphotericin B cholesteryl sulfate complex, atracurium, cefepime, diltiazem, fluconazole, foscarnet, gatifloxacin, heparin, heparin with hydrocortisone sodium succinate, hydromorphone, linezolid, meropenem, pancuronium, potassium chloride, propofol, vecuronium, vitamin B complex with C

Compatibility in syringe: Incompatible with doxapram, glycopyrrolate, heparin, hydromorphone, nalbuphine, sufentanil

Compatibility when admixed: Incompatible with bleomycin, buprenorphine, dobutamine, doxorubicin, floxacillin, fluorouracil, furosemide

Storage:

Protect parenteral dosage form from light; potency is retained for up to 3 months when kept at room temperature.

Rectal gel: Store at 25°C (77°F); excursion permitted to 15°C to 30°C (59°F to 86°F).

Additional Information Intensol® should be diluted before use; diazepam does not have any analgesic effects.

Related Information

Anxiolytic / Hypnotic Use in Long-Term Care Facilities *on page 1769*
Benzodiazepines *on page 1719*
Compatibility of Drugs *on page 1723*
Federal OBRA Regulations: Recommended Maximum Doses *on page 1773*

♦ **Diazepam Intensol®** *see Diazepam on page 439*

♦ **DIC** *see Dacarbazine on page 394*

♦ **Dichloralphenazone, Acetaminophen, and Isometheptene** *see Acetaminophen, Isometheptene, and Dichloralphenazone on page 42*

♦ **Dichloralphenazone, Isometheptene, and Acetaminophen** *see Acetaminophen, Isometheptene, and Dichloralphenazone on page 42*

Diclofenac *(dye KLOE fen ak)*

U.S. Brand Names Cataflam®; Solaraze™; Voltaren®; Voltaren Ophthalmic®; Voltaren®-XR

Synonyms Diclofenac Potassium; Diclofenac Sodium

Generic Available Yes

Pharmacologic Category Nonsteroidal Anti-inflammatory Drug (NSAID); Nonsteroidal Anti-inflammatory Drug (NSAID), Ophthalmic; Nonsteroidal Anti-inflammatory Drug (NSAID), Oral

Medication Safety Issues

Sound-alike/look-alike issues:

Diclofenac may be confused with Diflucan®, Duphalac®

Cataflam® may be confused with Catapres®

Voltaren® may be confused with tramadol, Ultram®, Verelan®

Use

Immediate release: Ankylosing spondylitis; primary dysmenorrhea; acute and chronic treatment of rheumatoid arthritis, osteoarthritis

Delayed-release tablets: Acute and chronic treatment of rheumatoid arthritis, osteoarthritis, ankylosing spondylitis

Extended-release tablets: Chronic treatment of osteoarthritis, rheumatoid arthritis

Ophthalmic solution: Postoperative inflammation following cataract extraction; temporary relief of pain and photophobia in patients undergoing corneal refractive surgery

Topical gel: Actinic keratosis (AK) in conjunction with sun avoidance

Unlabeled/Investigational Use Juvenile rheumatoid arthritis

Mechanism of Action/Effect Inhibits prostaglandin synthesis by decreasing activity of the enzyme, cyclooxygenase, which results in decreased formation of prostaglandin precursors

Contraindications Hypersensitivity to diclofenac, any component of the formulation, aspirin or other NSAIDs, including patients who experience bronchospasm, asthma, rhinitis, or urticaria following NSAID or aspirin; porphyria; pregnancy (3rd trimester)

Warnings/Precautions Fatal asthmatic and anaphylactoid reactions have occurred in patients with "aspirin triad." Use with caution in patients with CHF, hypertension, dehydration, decreased renal or hepatic function, history of GI disease (bleeding, ulcers, or previous GI symptoms with NSAID use), or those receiving anticoagulants and/or corticosteroids. Use lowest effective dose for shortest period possible; bleeding risk has been correlated to dose and duration of therapy. Gastrointestinal bleeding may occur without prior symptoms of gastrointestinal irritation. Elderly are at a high risk for adverse effects from NSAIDs. As many as 60% of elderly can develop peptic ulceration and/or hemorrhage asymptomatically.

Use of NSAIDs can compromise existing renal function especially when Cl_{cr} <30 mL/minute. CNS adverse effects such as confusion, agitation, and hallucination are generally seen in overdose or high-dose situations; however, elderly may demonstrate these adverse effects at lower doses than younger adults. Withhold for at least 4-6 half-lives prior to surgical or dental procedures.

Rare cases of severe hepatic reactions (including necrosis, jaundice, fulminant hepatitis) have been reported. Vision changes (including changes in color) have been rarely reported with oral diclofenac.

Topical gel should not be applied to the eyes, open wounds, infected areas, or to exfoliative dermatitis. Monitor patients for 1 year following application of ophthalmic drops for corneal refractive procedures. Patients using ophthalmic drops should not wear soft contact lenses. Ophthalmic drops may slow/delay healing or prolong bleeding time following surgery. Elderly are at a high risk for adverse effects from NSAIDs.

Drug Interactions

Cytochrome P450 Effect: Substrate (minor) of CYP1A2, 2B6, 2C8/9, 2C19, 2D6, 3A4; **Inhibits** CYP1A2 (moderate), 2C8/9 (weak), 2E1 (weak), 3A4 (strong)

Decreased Effect: Decreased effect of diclofenac with aspirin. Decreased effect of thiazides, furosemide.

Increased Effect/Toxicity: Increased toxicity of digoxin, methotrexate, cyclosporine, lithium, insulin, sulfonylureas, potassium-sparing diuretics, warfarin, and aspirin. Diclofenac may increase the levels/effects of aminophylline, selected benzodiazepines, calcium channel blockers, cyclosporine, fluvoxamine, mexiletine, mirtazapine, nateglinide, nefazodone, ropinirole, sildenafil (and other PDE-5 inhibitors), tacrolimus, theophylline, trifluoperazine, venlafaxine, and other CYP1A2 or 3A4 substrates. Selected benzodiazepines (midazolam and triazolam), cisapride, ergot alkaloids, selected HMG-CoA reductase inhibitors (lovastatin and simvastatin), mesoridazine, pimozide, and thioridazine are generally contraindicated with strong CYP3A4 inhibitors. When used with strong CYP3A4 inhibitors, dosage adjustment/limits are recommended for sildenafil and other PDE-5 inhibitors; refer to individual monographs.

Nutritional/Ethanol Interactions

Ethanol: Avoid ethanol (may enhance gastric mucosal irritation).

Herb/Nutraceutical: Avoid cat's claw, dong quai, evening primrose, feverfew, garlic, ginger, ginkgo, red clover, horse chestnut, green tea, ginseng (all have additional antiplatelet activity).

Adverse Reactions

>10%:

Local: Application site reactions (gel): Pruritus (31% to 52%), rash (35% to 46%), contact dermatitis (19% to 33%), dry skin (25% to 27%), pain (15% to 26%), exfoliation (6% to 24%), paresthesia (8% to 20%)

Ocular: Ophthalmic drops (incidence may be dependent upon indication): Lacrimation (30%), keratitis (28%), elevated IOP (15%), transient burning/stinging (15%)

1% to 10%:

Central nervous system: Headache (7%), dizziness (3%)

Dermatologic: Pruritus (1% to 3%), rash (1% to 3%)

Endocrine & metabolic: Fluid retention (1% to 3%)

Gastrointestinal: Abdominal cramps (3% to 9%), abdominal pain (3% to 9%), constipation (3% to 9%), diarrhea (3% to 9%), flatulence (3% to 9%), indigestion (3% to 9%), nausea (3% to 9%), abdominal distention (1% to 3%), peptic ulcer/GI bleed (0.6% to 2%)

Hepatic: Increased ALT/AST (2%)

Local: Application site reactions (gel): Edema (4%)

Ocular: Ophthalmic drops: Abnormal vision, acute elevated IOP, blurred vision, conjunctivitis, corneal deposits, corneal edema, corneal opacity, corneal lesions, discharge, eyelid swelling, injection, iritis, irritation, itching, lacrimation disorder, ocular allergy

Otic: Tinnitus (1% to 3%)

Overdosage/Toxicology Symptoms of overdose include acute renal failure, vomiting, drowsiness, and leukocytosis. Management of NSAID intoxication is supportive and symptomatic.

Pharmacodynamics/Kinetics

Onset of Action: Cataflam® is more rapid than sodium salt (Voltaren®) because it dissolves in the stomach instead of the duodenum

Absorption: Topical gel: 10%

Time to Peak: Serum: Cataflam®: ~1 hour; Voltaren®: ~2 hours

Protein Binding: 99% to albumin

Half-Life Elimination: 2 hours

Metabolism: Hepatic to several metabolites

Excretion: Urine (65%); feces (35%)

Dosing

Adults & Elderly:

Analgesia/primary dysmenorrhea: Oral: Starting dose: 50 mg 3 times/day; maximum dose: 150 mg/day

Rheumatoid arthritis: Oral: 150-200 mg/day in 2-4 divided doses (100 mg/day of sustained release product)

Osteoarthritis: Oral: 100-150 mg/day in 2-3 divided doses (100-200 mg/day of sustained release product)

Ankylosing spondylitis: Oral: 100-125 mg/day in 4-5 divided doses

Cataract surgery: Ophthalmic: Instill 1 drop into affected eye 4 times/day beginning 24 hours after cataract surgery and continuing for 2 weeks

Corneal refractive surgery: Ophthalmic: Instill 1-2 drops into affected eye within the hour prior to surgery, within 15 minutes following surgery, and then continue for 4 times/day, up to 3 days

(Continued)

Diclofenac *(Continued)*

Actinic keratosis (AK): Topical (gel): Apply gel to lesion area twice daily for 60-90 days

Renal Impairment: Monitor closely in patients with significant renal impairment.

Hepatic Impairment: No adjustment necessary.

Available Dosage Forms

Gel, as sodium (Solaraze™): 30 mg/g (50 g)

Solution, ophthalmic, as sodium (Voltaren Ophthalmic®): 0.1% (2.5 mL, 5 mL)

Tablet, as potassium (Cataflam®): 50 mg

Tablet, delayed release, enteric coated, as sodium (Voltaren®): 25 mg, 50 mg, 75 mg

Tablet, extended release, as sodium (Voltaren®-XR): 100 mg

Monitoring and Teaching Issues

Physical Assessment: Assess other medications patient may be taking for effectiveness and interactions. Assess results of laboratory tests, therapeutic effectiveness, and adverse reactions (systemic or ophthalmic) at beginning of therapy and periodically throughout therapy. Schedule ophthalmic evaluations for patients who develop eye complaints during long-term NSAID therapy. Assess knowledge/teach patient appropriate use (oral, ophthalmic, gel), interventions to reduce side effects, and adverse symptoms to report.

Monitoring Laboratory Tests: CBC, liver enzymes, urine output and BUN/serum creatinine in patients receiving diuretics, occult blood loss

Patient Education: Oral: Take this medication exactly as directed; do not increase dose without consulting prescriber. Do not crush or chew tablets. Take with 8 oz of water, along with food or milk products to reduce GI distress. Maintain adequate hydration (2-3 L/day of fluids) unless instructed to restrict fluid intake. Avoid alcohol, aspirin and aspirin-containing medication, or any other anti-inflammatory medications unless consulting prescriber. You may experience dizziness, nervousness, or headache (use caution when driving or engaging in tasks requiring alertness until response to drug is known); nausea, vomiting, dry mouth, or heartburn (small frequent meals, frequent mouth care, sucking lozenges, or chewing gum may help); or constipation (increased exercise, fluids, fruit, or fiber may help). GI bleeding, ulceration, or perforation can occur with or without pain; discontinue medication and contact prescriber if persistent abdominal pain or cramping, or blood in stool occurs. Report chest pain or palpitations; breathlessness or respiratory difficulty; unusual bruising/bleeding or blood in urine, stool, mouth, or vomitus; unusual fatigue; skin rash or itching; jaundice, unusual weight gain, or swelling of extremities; change in urinary pattern; change in vision or hearing (ringing in ears). **Pregnancy/breast-feeding precautions:** Consult prescriber if you are pregnant. This drug should not be used in the 3rd trimester of pregnancy. Consult prescriber if you are breast-feeding.

Ophthalmic: For ophthalmic use only. Apply prescribed amount as often as directed. Wash hands before using. Tilt head back and look upward. Gently pull down lower lid and put drop(s) in inner corner of eye. Do not let tip of applicator touch eye; do not contaminate tip of applicator (may cause eye infection, eye damage, or vision loss). Close eye and roll eyeball in all directions. Do not blink for ½ minute. Apply gentle pressure to inner corner of eye for 30 seconds. Wipe away excess from skin around eye. Do not use any other eye preparation for at least 10 minutes. Do not share medication with anyone else. May cause sensitivity to bright light (dark glasses may help); temporary stinging or blurred vision may occur. Inform prescriber if you experience eye pain, redness, burning, watering, dryness, double vision, puffiness around eye, vision changes, other adverse eye response, worsening of condition, or lack of improvement.

Gel: This preparation is for topical use only. Treatment may take up to 3 months. Do not use more often than recommended; use at regular intervals. Wash hands before and after use. Follow directions on prescription label. Gently apply enough of the gel to cover the lesion. Advise prescriber if you are using any other skin preparations. Avoid direct sunlight and sunlamps while using this medication. You may experience dry skin, itching, peeling, swelling, or tingling at site of application. If severe skin reaction develops, stop applications and notify your prescriber at once.

Dietary Considerations: May be taken with food to decrease GI distress.

Diclofenac potassium = Cataflam®; potassium content: 5.8 mg (0.15 mEq) per 50 mg tablet

Geriatric Considerations: Elderly are at high risk for adverse effects from NSAIDs.

Pregnancy Risk Factor: B/D (3rd trimester)

Pregnancy Issues: Safety and efficacy in pregnant women have not been established. Exposure late in pregnancy may lead to premature closure of the ductus arteriosus and may inhibit uterine contractions.

Lactation: Enters breast milk/use caution

Administration

Oral: Do not crush tablets. Administer with food or milk to avoid gastric distress. Take with full glass of water to enhance absorption.

Topical: Topical gel: Cover lesion with gel and smooth into skin gently. Do not cover lesion with occlusive dressings or apply sunscreens, cosmetics, or other medications to affected area.

Other: Ophthalmic: Wait at least 5 minutes before administering other types of eye drops.

Storage: Store above 30°C (86°F); protect from moisture, store in tight container.

Related Information

Nonsalicylate / Nonsteroidal Anti-inflammatory Agents *on page 1743*

Diclofenac and Misoprostol *(dye KLOE fen ak & mye soe PROST ole)*

U.S. Brand Names Arthrotec®

Synonyms Misoprostol and Diclofenac

Generic Available No

Pharmacologic Category Nonsteroidal Anti-inflammatory Drug (NSAID), Oral; Prostaglandin

Use The diclofenac component is indicated for the treatment of osteoarthritis and rheumatoid arthritis; the misoprostol component is indicated for the prophylaxis of NSAID-induced gastric and duodenal ulceration

Dosing
Adults & Elderly:
Osteoarthritis: Oral: Arthrotec® 50: 1 tablet 2-3 times/day

Rheumatoid arthritis: Oral: Arthrotec® 50: 1 tablet 3-4 times/day

Note: For both regimens, if not tolerated by patient, the dose may be reduced to 1 tablet twice daily. Arthrotec® 75 may be used in patients who cannot tolerate full daily Arthrotec® 50 regimens. Dose: 1 tablet twice daily. However, the use of these tablets may not be as effective at preventing GI ulceration.

Renal Impairment: In renal insufficiency, diclofenac should be used with caution due to potential detrimental effects on renal function, and misoprostol dosage reduction may be required if adverse effects occur (misoprostol is renally eliminated).

Available Dosage Forms Tablet: Diclofenac sodium 50 mg and misoprostol 200 mcg; diclofenac sodium 75 mg and misoprostol 200 mcg

Monitoring and Teaching Issues
Physical Assessment: See individual agents. **Pregnancy risk factor X: Determine** that patient is not pregnant before beginning treatment and do not give to women of childbearing age or to males who may have intercourse with women of childbearing age unless both male and female are capable of complying with contraceptive measures during therapy and for 1 month following therapy. Breast-feeding is contraindicated.

Patient Education: See individual agents. Consult your prescriber before use if you have hypertension or heart failure. **Pregnancy/breast-feeding precautions:** Inform prescriber if you are pregnant. Do not get pregnant during or for 1 month following therapy. Male: Do not cause a female to become pregnant. Male/female: Consult prescriber for instruction on appropriate contraceptive measures. The misoprostol ingredient in this drug may cause severe fetal defects, miscarriage, or abortion; do not share medication with others. Do not breast-feed.

Pregnancy Risk Factor: X

Lactation: Enters breast milk/contraindicated

Related Information
Diclofenac *on page 442*

Misoprostol *on page 1015*

♦ **Diclofenac Potassium** *see Diclofenac on page 442*

♦ **Diclofenac Sodium** *see Diclofenac on page 442*

Dicloxacillin (dye kloks a SIL in)
Synonyms Dicloxacillin Sodium

Generic Available Yes

Pharmacologic Category Antibiotic, Penicillin

Use Treatment of systemic infections such as pneumonia, skin and soft tissue infections, and osteomyelitis caused by penicillinase-producing staphylococci

Mechanism of Action/Effect Interferes with bacterial cell wall synthesis; causes cell wall death

Contraindications Hypersensitivity to dicloxacillin, penicillin, or any component of the formulation

Warnings/Precautions Monitor PT if patient concurrently on warfarin. Use with caution in patients allergic to cephalosporins.

Drug Interactions
Cytochrome P450 Effect: Induces CYP3A4 (weak)

Decreased Effect: Although anecdotal reports suggest oral contraceptive efficacy could be reduced by penicillins, this has been refuted by more rigorous scientific and clinical data. Decreased effect of (warfarin) anticoagulants.

Increased Effect/Toxicity: Disulfiram, probenecid may increase penicillin levels. Penicillins may increase the exposure to methotrexate during concurrent therapy; monitor.

Nutritional/Ethanol Interactions Food: Decreases drug absorption rate; decreases drug serum concentration.

Lab Interactions Positive Coombs' test [direct]

Adverse Reactions 1% to 10%: Gastrointestinal: Nausea, diarrhea, abdominal pain

Overdosage/Toxicology Symptoms of penicillin overdose include neuromuscular hypersensitivity (eg, agitation, hallucinations, asterixis, encephalopathy, confusion, and seizures). Electrolyte imbalance may occur if the preparation contains potassium or sodium salts, especially in renal failure. Hemodialysis may be helpful to aid in removal of the drug from blood; otherwise, treatment is supportive or symptom-directed.

Pharmacodynamics/Kinetics
Absorption: 35% to 76%; rate and extent reduced by food

Time to Peak: Serum: 0.5-2 hours

Protein Binding: 96%

Half-Life Elimination: 0.6-0.8 hour; slightly prolonged with renal impairment

Excretion: Feces; urine (56% to 70% as unchanged drug); prolonged in neonates

Dosing
Adults & Elderly: Susceptible infections: Oral: 125-500 mg every 6 hours
Pediatrics: Use in newborns is not recommended.
Susceptible infections: Oral:

Children <40 kg: 12.5-25 mg/kg/day divided every 6 hours; doses of 50-100 mg/kg/day in divided doses every 6 hours have been used for therapy of osteomyelitis

Children >40 kg: 125-250 mg every 6 hours

Renal Impairment:
Dosage adjustment is not necessary.

Not dialyzable (0% to 5%); supplemental dose is not necessary.

Peritoneal dialysis effects: Supplemental dose is not necessary.

Continuous arteriovenous or venovenous hemofiltration: Supplemental dose is not necessary.

(Continued)

Dicloxacillin (Continued)

Available Dosage Forms Capsule: 250 mg, 500 mg

Monitoring and Teaching Issues

Physical Assessment: Assess results of culture and sensitivity tests and patient's allergy history prior to beginning therapy. Assess potential for interactions with other pharmacological agents patient may be taking (see Drug Interactions). Assess therapeutic effectiveness (resolution of infection) and adverse reactions (see Adverse Reactions) on a regular basis throughout therapy. Teach patient proper use, possible side effects/appropriate interventions, and adverse symptoms to report (eg, opportunistic infection; see Patient Education).

Monitoring Laboratory Tests: Perform culture and sensitivity studies prior to initiating therapy

Patient Education: Do not take any new medication during therapy unless approved by prescriber. Take medication as directed, with a large glass of water 1 hour before or 2 hours after meals. Take at regular intervals around-the-clock and take for length of time prescribed. If you have diabetes, drug may cause false test results with Clinitest® urine glucose monitoring; use of another type of glucose monitoring is preferable. May cause some gastric distress (small frequent meals may help) and diarrhea (if this persists, consult prescriber). Report fever, vaginal itching, sores in the mouth, loose foul-smelling stools, yellowing of skin or eyes, or change in color of urine or stool. **Breast-feeding precaution:** Consult prescriber if breast-feeding.

Dietary Considerations: Administer on an empty stomach 1 hour before or 2 hours after meals. Sodium content of 250 mg capsule: 13 mg (0.6 mEq)

Pregnancy Risk Factor: B

Lactation: Excretion in breast milk unknown (probably similar to penicillin G)

Breast-Feeding Issues: No data reported; however, other penicillins may be taken while breast-feeding.

Administration

Oral: Administer 1 hour before or 2 hours after meals. Administer around-the-clock to promote less variation in peak and trough serum levels.

♦ **Dicloxacillin Sodium** *see Dicloxacillin on page 445*

Didanosine (dye DAN oh seen)

U.S. Brand Names Videx®; Videx® EC

Synonyms ddl; Dideoxyinosine

Generic Available Yes: Delayed release capsule

Pharmacologic Category Antiretroviral Agent, Reverse Transcriptase Inhibitor (Nucleoside)

Medication Safety Issues

Sound-alike/look-alike issues:

Videx® may be confused with Lidex®

Use Treatment of HIV infection; always to be used in combination with at least two other antiretroviral agents

Mechanism of Action/Effect Didanosine, a purine nucleoside (adenosine) analog and the deamination product of dideoxyadenosine (ddA), inhibits HIV replication *in vitro* in both T cells and monocytes. Didanosine is converted within the cell to the mono-, di-, and triphosphates of ddA. These ddA triphosphates act as substrate and inhibitor of HIV reverse transcriptase substrate and inhibitor of HIV reverse transcriptase thereby blocking viral DNA synthesis and suppressing HIV replication.

Contraindications Hypersensitivity to didanosine or any component of the formulation

Warnings/Precautions Pancreatitis (sometimes fatal) has been reported, incidence is dose related. Risk factors for developing pancreatitis include a previous history of the condition, concurrent cytomegalovirus or *Mycobacterium avium-intracellulare* infection, and concomitant use of stavudine, pentamidine, or co-trimoxazole. Discontinue didanosine if clinical signs of pancreatitis occur. Lactic acidosis, symptomatic hyperlactatemia, and severe hepatomegaly with steatosis (sometimes fatal) have occurred with antiretroviral nucleoside analogues, including didanosine. Hepatotoxicity may occur even in the absence of marked transaminase elevations; suspend therapy in any patient developing clinical/laboratory findings which suggest hepatotoxicity. Pregnant women may be at increased risk of lactic acidosis and liver damage.

Peripheral neuropathy occurs in ~20% of patients receiving the drug. Retinal changes (including retinal depigmentation) and optic neuritis have been reported in adults and children using didanosine. Patients should undergo retinal examination every 6-12 months. Use with caution in patients with decreased renal or hepatic function, phenylketonuria, sodium-restricted diets, or with edema, CHF, or hyperuricemia. Twice-daily dosing is the preferred dosing frequency for didanosine tablets. Didanosine delayed release capsules are indicated for once-daily use.

Drug Interactions

Decreased Effect: Didanosine buffered tablets and pediatric oral solution may decrease absorption of quinolones or tetracyclines (administer 2 hours prior to didanosine buffered formulations). Didanosine should be held during PCP treatment with pentamidine. Didanosine may decrease levels of indinavir. Drugs whose absorption depends on the level of acidity in the stomach such as ketoconazole, itraconazole, and dapsone should be administered at least 2 hours prior to the buffered formulations of didanosine (not affected by delayed release capsules). Methadone may decrease didanosine concentrations.

Increased Effect/Toxicity: Concomitant administration of other drugs which have the potential to cause peripheral neuropathy or pancreatitis may increase the risk of these toxicities Allopurinol may increase didanosine concentration; avoid concurrent use. Concomitant use of antacids with buffered tablet or pediatric didanosine solution may potentiate adverse effects of aluminum- or magnesium-containing antacids. Ganciclovir may increase didanosine concentration; monitor. Hydroxyurea may precipitate didanosine-induced pancreatitis if added to therapy; concomitant use is not recommended. Coadministration with ribavirin or tenofovir may increase exposure to didanosine and/or its active metabolite increasing the risk or severity of didanosine toxicities, including pancreatitis, lactic acidosis, and peripheral neuropathy; monitor closely and suspend therapy if signs or symptoms of toxicity are noted.

Nutritional/Ethanol Interactions
Ethanol: Avoid ethanol (increases risk of pancreatitis).
Food: Decreases AUC and C_{max}. Didanosine serum levels may be decreased by 55% if taken with food.

Adverse Reactions As reported in monotherapy studies; risk of toxicity may increase when combined with other agents.

>10%:
Gastrointestinal: Increased amylase (15% to 17%), abdominal pain (7% to 13%), diarrhea (19% to 28%)
Neuromuscular & skeletal: Peripheral neuropathy (17% to 20%)
1% to 10%:
Dermatologic: Rash, pruritus
Endocrine & metabolic: Increased uric acid
Gastrointestinal: Pancreatitis; patients >65 years of age had a higher frequency of pancreatitis than younger patients
Hepatic: Increased SGOT, increased SGPT, increased alkaline phosphatase

Overdosage/Toxicology Chronic overdose may cause pancreatitis, peripheral neuropathy, diarrhea, hyperuricemia, and hepatic impairment. There is no known antidote for didanosine overdose. Treatment is symptomatic.

Pharmacodynamics/Kinetics
Absorption: Subject to degradation by acidic pH of stomach; some formulations are buffered to resist acidic pH; ≤50% reduction in peak plasma concentration is observed in presence of food. Delayed release capsules contain enteric-coated beadlets which dissolve in the small intestine.
Bioavailability: 42%
Time to Peak: Buffered tablets: 0.67 hours; Delayed release capsules: 2 hours
Protein Binding: <5%
Half-Life Elimination:
Children and Adolescents: 0.8 hour
Adults: Normal renal function: 1.5 hours; however, active metabolite, ddATP, has an intracellular half-life >12 hours *in vitro*; Renal impairment: 2.5-5 hours
Metabolism: Has not been evaluated in humans; studies conducted in dogs, show extensive metabolism with allantoin, hypoxanthine, xanthine, and uric acid being the major metabolites found in urine
Excretion: Urine (~55% as unchanged drug)
Clearance: Total body: Averages 800 mL/minute

Dosing
Adults: Treatment of HIV infection: Oral (administer on an empty stomach): Oral:
Note: Preferred dosing frequency is twice daily for didanosine tablets
Chewable tablets, powder for oral solution:
<60 kg: 125 mg twice daily or 250 mg once daily
≥60 kg: 200 mg twice daily or 400 mg once daily
Note: Adults should receive 2-4 tablets per dose for adequate buffering and absorption; tablets should be chewed or dispersed
Delayed release capsule (Videx® EC):
<60 kg: 250 mg once daily
≥60 kg; 400 mg once daily

Dosing adjustment with tenofovir (didanosine tablets or delayed release capsules; based on tenofovir product labeling):
<60 kg: 200 mg once daily
≥60 kg: 250 mg once daily
Elderly: Refer to adult dosing. Elderly patients have a higher frequency of pancreatitis (10% versus 5% in younger patients); monitor renal function and dose accordingly.
Pediatrics:
Treatment of HIV infection: Oral (administer on an empty stomach):
Children:
2 weeks to 8 months: 100 mg/m^2 twice daily
>8 months: 120 mg/m^2 twice daily; dosing range: 90-150 mg/m^2 twice daily; patients with CNS disease may require higher dose
Children <1 year should receive 1 tablet per dose and children >1 year should receive 2-4 tablets per dose for adequate buffering and absorption; tablets should be chewed or dispersed.
Adolescents: Refer to adult dosing.

Recommended Dose (mg) of Didanosine by Body Weight

Creatinine Clearance (mL/min)	≥60 kg		<60 kg	
	Tablet[1] (mg)	Delayed Release Capsule (mg)	Tablet[1] (mg)	Delayed Release Capsule (mg)
≥60	400 daily or 200 twice daily	400 daily	250 daily or 125 twice daily	250 daily
30-59	200 daily or 100 twice daily	200 daily	150 daily or 75 twice daily	125 daily
10-29	150 daily	125 daily	100 daily	125 daily
<10	100 daily	125 daily	75 daily	See footnote 2.

[1]Chewable/dispersible buffered tablet; 2 tablets must be taken with each dose; different strengths of tablets may be combined to yield the recommended dose.

[2]Not suitable for use in patients <60 kg with Cl_{cr} <10 mL/minute; use alternate formulation.

(Continued)

Didanosine (Continued)

Renal Impairment: See table on previous page.

Patients requiring hemodialysis or CAPD: Dose per Cl$_{cr}$ 10 mL/minute

Hepatic Impairment: Should be considered; monitor for toxicity.

Available Dosage Forms

Capsule, delayed release: 200 mg, 250 mg, 400 mg

Videx® EC: 125 mg, 200 mg, 250 mg, 400 mg

Powder for oral solution, pediatric (Videx®): 2 g, 4 g [makes 10 mg/mL solution after final mixing]

Tablet, buffered, chewable/dispersible (Videx®): 25 mg, 50 mg, 100 mg, 150 mg, 200 mg [all strengths contain phenylalanine 36.5 mg/tablet; orange flavor]

Monitoring and Teaching Issues

Physical Assessment: See Warnings/Precautions for use cautions (eg, decreased renal or hepatic function, phenylketonuria, edema, CHF, gout). Assess potential for interactions with other pharmacological agents patient may be taking (eg, drugs that increase risk of peripheral neuropathy or pancreatitis; see Drug Interactions). Assess results of laboratory tests (see Monitoring Laboratory Tests), therapeutic response (viral load and CD4 count), and adverse reactions (eg, peripheral neuropathy, CNS changes, pancreatitis, opportunistic infection; see Adverse Reactions) on a regular basis throughout therapy. Teach patient proper use (see Administration, Storage, and Reconstitution), possible side effects/appropriate interventions, and adverse symptoms to report (see Patient Education).

Monitoring Laboratory Tests: Serum potassium, uric acid, creatinine, hemoglobin, CBC with neutrophil, platelet count, CD4 cells, liver function, amylase; viral load

Patient Education: Do not take any new medication during therapy unless approved by prescriber. This drug will not cure HIV; use appropriate precautions to prevent spread of HIV to other persons. Take as directed. Tablets: Take 30 minutes before or 2 hours after meals; chew well or mix with water. Extended release capsules: Take 1 hour before or 2 hours after eating; do not chew or crush. Store in tightly closed container. Maintain adequate hydration (2-3 L/day of fluids) unless instructed to restrict fluid intake. A dilated retinal eye exam is recommended every 6-12 months while on this therapy. You may be susceptible to infection (avoid crowds and exposure to infection and do not have any vaccinations without consulting prescriber). May cause dizziness or weakness (use caution when driving or engaging in tasks requiring alertness until response to drug is known); nausea or vomiting (small frequent meals, frequent mouth care, chewing gum, or sucking lozenges may help); diarrhea (boiled milk, yogurt, or buttermilk may help); or headache, back or joint pain (mild analgesics may offer relief). Report immediately any loss of sensation, numbness, or tingling in fingers, toes, or feet; persistent unresolved abdominal distress (nausea, vomiting, diarrhea); or signs of infection (burning on urination, perineal itching, white plaques in mouth, unhealed sores, persistent sore throat or cough). **Pregnancy/breast-feeding precautions:** Inform prescriber if you are or intend to become pregnant. Do not breast-feed.

Dietary Considerations:

Videx® EC: Take on an empty stomach; administer at least 1 hour before or 2 hours after eating

Chewable/dispersible tablet: Take on an empty stomach, 30 minutes before or 2 hours after eating. Chew well or mix in water; if mixed in water, may add 2 tablespoons (1 oz) apple juice for flavor. Do not use other juices. Each chewable tablet contains 36.5 mg phenylalanine and 8.6 mEq magnesium. Sodium content of buffered tablets: 264.5 mg (11.5 mEq).

Geriatric Considerations: Since the elderly often have a creatinine clearance <60 mL/minute, monitor closely for adverse reactions and adjust dose accordingly to maintain efficacy (CD4 counts).

Pregnancy Risk Factor: B

Pregnancy Issues: Cases of fatal and nonfatal lactic acidosis, with or without pancreatitis, have been reported in pregnant women. It is not known if pregnancy itself potentiates this known side effect; however, pregnant women may be at increased risk of lactic acidosis and liver damage. Hepatic enzymes and electrolytes should be monitored frequently during the 3rd trimester of pregnancy. Use during pregnancy only if the potential benefit to the mother outweighs the potential risk of this complication. Didanosine has been shown to cross the placenta. Pharmacokinetics are not significantly altered during pregnancy; dose adjustments are not needed. The Perinatal HIV Guidelines Working Group considers didanosine to be an alternative NRTI in dual nucleoside combination regimens; use with stavudine only if no other alternatives are available. Health professionals are encouraged to contact the antiretroviral pregnancy registry to monitor outcomes of pregnant women exposed to antiretroviral medications (1-800-258-4263 or www.APRegistry.com).

Lactation: Excretion in breast milk unknown/contraindicated

Breast-Feeding Issues: HIV-infected mothers are discouraged from breast-feeding to decrease potential transmission of HIV.

Administration

Oral:

Chewable/dispersible buffered tablets: The 200 mg tablet should only be used in once-daily dosing. At least 2 tablets, but no more than 4 tablets, should be taken together to allow adequate buffering. Tablets may be chewed or dispersed prior to consumption. To disperse, dissolve in 1 oz water, stir until uniform dispersion is formed, and drink immediately. May also add 1 oz of clear apple juice to initial dispersion if additional flavor is needed. The apple juice dilution is stable for 1 hour at room temperature.

Pediatric powder for oral solution: Prior to dispensing, the powder should be mixed with purified water USP to an initial concentration of 20 mg/mL and then further diluted with an appropriate antacid suspension to a final mixture of 10 mg/mL. Stable for 30 days under refrigeration. Shake well prior to use.

Reconstitution: Unbuffered powder for oral solution must be reconstituted and mixed with an equal volume of antacid at time of preparation.

Storage: Tablets and delayed release capsules should be stored in tightly closed bottles at 15°C to 30°C. Undergoes rapid degradation when exposed to an acidic environment. Tablets dispersed in water are stable for 1 hour at room temperature. Reconstituted pediatric solution is stable for 30 days if refrigerated.

Additional Information A high rate of early virologic nonresponse was observed when didanosine, lamivudine, and tenofovir were used as the initial regimen in treatment-naive patients. Use of this combination is not recommended; patients currently on this regimen should be closely monitored for modification of therapy. Early virologic failure was also observed with tenofovir and didanosine delayed release capsules, plus either efavirenz or nevirapine; use caution in treatment-naive patients with high baseline viral loads.

- ◆ **Dideoxycytidine** *see Zalcitabine on page 1579*
- ◆ **Dideoxyinosine** *see Didanosine on page 446*

Diethylpropion (dye eth il PROE pee on)

U.S. Brand Names Tenuate®; Tenuate® Dospan®

Synonyms Amfepramone; Diethylpropion Hydrochloride

Controlled Substance C-IV

Generic Available Yes

Pharmacologic Category Anorexiant

Use Short-term adjunct in a regimen of weight reduction based on exercise, behavioral modification, and caloric reduction in the management of exogenous obesity for patients with an initial body mass index ≥30 kg/m² or ≥27 kg/m² in the presence of other risk factors (diabetes, hypertension)

Unlabeled/Investigational Use Migraine

Mechanism of Action/Effect Diethylpropion is used as an anorexiant possessing pharmacological and chemical properties similar to those of amphetamines. The mechanism of action of diethylpropion in reducing appetite appears to be secondary to CNS effects, specifically stimulation of the hypothalamus to release catecholamines into the central nervous system. Anorexiant effects are mediated via norepinephrine and dopamine metabolism. An increase in physical activity and metabolic effects (inhibition of lipogenesis and enhancement of lipolysis) may also contribute to weight loss.

Contraindications Hypersensitivity or idiosyncrasy to sympathomimetic amines. Patients with advanced arteriosclerosis, symptomatic cardiovascular disease, moderate to severe hypertension (stage II or III), hyperthyroidism, glaucoma, agitated states, patients with a history of drug abuse, and during or within 14 days following MAO inhibitor therapy. Concurrent use with other anorectic agents; stimulant medications are contraindicated for use in children with attention-deficit/hyperactivity disorders and concomitant Tourette's syndrome or tics.

Warnings/Precautions Use with caution in patients with bipolar disorder, diabetes mellitus, cardiovascular disease, seizure disorders, insomnia, porphyria, or mild hypertension (stage I). May exacerbate symptoms of behavior and thought disorder in psychotic patients. Potential for drug dependency exists - avoid abrupt discontinuation in patients who have received for prolonged periods. Stimulant use in children has been associated with growth suppression. Not recommended for use in patients <12 years of age.

Serious, potentially life-threatening toxicities may occur when thyroid hormones (at dosages above usual daily hormonal requirements) are used in combination with sympathomimetic amines to induce weight loss. Treatment of obesity is not an approved use for thyroid hormone.

Drug Interactions

Decreased Effect: Diethylpropion may displace guanethidine from the neuron and antagonize its antihypertensive effects; discontinue diethylpropion or use alternative antihypertensive.

Increased Effect/Toxicity: Concurrent use or use within 14 days following the administration of a MAO inhibitor is contraindicated (hypertensive crisis). Concurrent use of sibutramine and diethylpropion is contraindicated (severe hypertension, tachycardia). Concurrent use with TCAs may result in enhanced toxicity. Concurrent use with other anorectic agents may cause serious cardiac problems and is contraindicated.

Nutritional/Ethanol Interactions Ethanol: Avoid ethanol (may increase CNS depression).

Adverse Reactions Frequency not defined.

Cardiovascular: Hypertension, palpitation, tachycardia, chest pain, T-wave changes, arrhythmia, pulmonary hypertension, valvulopathy

Central nervous system: Euphoria, nervousness, insomnia, restlessness, dizziness, anxiety, headache, agitation, confusion, mental depression, psychosis, CVA, seizure

Dermatologic: Alopecia, urticaria, skin rash, ecchymosis, erythema

Endocrine & metabolic: Changes in libido, gynecomastia, menstrual irregularities, porphyria

Gastrointestinal: Nausea, vomiting, abdominal cramps, constipation, xerostomia, metallic taste

Genitourinary: Impotence

Hematologic: Bone marrow depression, agranulocytosis, leukopenia

Neuromuscular & skeletal: Tremor

Ocular: Blurred vision, mydriasis

Overdosage/Toxicology There is no specific antidote for amphetamine intoxication and treatment is primarily supportive. Hyperactivity and agitation usually respond to reduced sensory input; however, with extreme agitation, haloperidol (2-5 mg I.M. for adults) may be required.

Pharmacodynamics/Kinetics

Onset of Action: 1 hour

Duration of Action: 12-24 hours

Dosing

Adults & Elderly: Obesity (short-term adjunct): Oral:

Tablet: 25 mg 3 times/day before meals or food

Tablet, controlled release: 75 mg at midmorning

(Continued)

Diethylpropion *(Continued)*

Available Dosage Forms
Tablet, as hydrochloride (Tenuate®): 25 mg
Tablet, controlled release, as hydrochloride (Tenuate® Dospan®): 75 mg

Monitoring and Teaching Issues
Physical Assessment: Assess effectiveness and interactions of other medications patient may be taking. Assess for history of psychopathology, homicidal or suicidal tendencies, or addiction; long-term use can result in dependence, abuse, or tolerance. Periodically evaluate the need for continued use. Monitor therapeutic effectiveness, vital signs, and adverse reactions at start of therapy, when changing dosage, and at regular intervals during therapy. Monitor serum glucose closely in patients with diabetes (amphetamines may alter antidiabetic requirements). Taper dosage slowly when discontinuing. Assess knowledge/teach patient appropriate use, possible side effects, and symptoms to report.

Patient Education: Take exactly as directed; do not increase dose or frequency without consulting prescriber. Drug may cause physical and/or psychological dependence. Do not crush or chew extended release tablets. Take early in day to avoid sleep disturbance, 1 hour before meals. Avoid alcohol, caffeine, or OTC medications that act as stimulants. You may experience restlessness, false sense of euphoria, or impaired judgment (use caution when driving or engaging in tasks requiring alertness until response to drug is known); dry mouth (frequent mouth care, sucking lozenges, or chewing gum may help); nausea or vomiting (small frequent meals, frequent mouth care may help); constipation (increased exercise, fluids, fruit, or fiber may help); or diarrhea (buttermilk, boiled milk, or yogurt may help); or altered libido (reversible). Patients with diabetes need to monitor serum glucose closely (may alter antidiabetic medication requirements). Report chest pain, palpitations, or irregular heartbeat; muscle weakness or tremors; extreme fatigue or depression; CNS changes (aggressiveness, restlessness, euphoria, sleep disturbances); severe unremitting abdominal distress or cramping; changes in sexual activity; changes in urinary pattern; or blurred vision. **Breast-feeding precaution:** Breast-feeding is not recommended.

Pregnancy Risk Factor: B
Lactation: Enters breast milk/not recommended

Administration
Oral: Do not crush 75 mg controlled release tablets. Dose should not be given in evening or at bedtime. Take tablets 1 hour before meals. Take controlled-release tablet at midmorning.

Related Information
Obesity Treatment Guidelines for Adults *on page 1850*

♦ **Diethylpropion Hydrochloride** *see* Diethylpropion *on page 449*

Difenoxin and Atropine *(dye fen OKS in & A troe peen)*
U.S. Brand Names Motofen®
Synonyms Atropine and Difenoxin
Controlled Substance C-IV
Generic Available No
Pharmacologic Category Antidiarrheal
Use Treatment of diarrhea

Dosing
Adults: Diarrhea: Oral: Initial: 2 tablets, then 1 tablet after each loose stool; 1 tablet every 3-4 hours, up to 8 tablets in a 24-hour period; if no improvement after 48 hours, continued administration is not indicated
Elderly: Refer to adult dosing; use with caution.

Available Dosage Forms
Tablet: Difenoxin hydrochloride 1 mg and atropine sulfate 0.025 mg

Monitoring and Teaching Issues
Physical Assessment: Assess effects and interactions of other prescriptions, OTC medications, or herbal products patient may be taking (see Drug Interactions). Assess therapeutic effectiveness and adverse response (see Adverse Reactions and Overdose/Toxicology). Teach patient proper use, possible side effects/appropriate interventions, and adverse effects to report (see Patient Education).

Patient Education: Inform prescriber of all prescriptions, OTC medications, or herbal products you are taking, and any allergies you have. Do not take any new medication during therapy unless approved by prescriber. Take as directed; do not exceed recommended dose. If no relief in 48 hours, contact prescriber. Avoid alcohol. Keep out of reach of children; can cause severe and fatal respiratory depression if accidentally ingested. May cause lightheadedness, depression, dizziness, or weakness (use caution when driving or engaging in tasks that require alertness until response to drug is known). Report acute dizziness, headache, or GI symptoms. **Pregnancy/breast-feeding precautions:** Inform prescriber if you are or intend to become pregnant. Do not breast-feed.

Pregnancy Risk Factor: C
Lactation: Enters breast milk/contraindicated

Related Information
Atropine *on page 158*

♦ **Differin®** *see* Adapalene *on page 52*
♦ **Diflucan®** *see* Fluconazole *on page 634*

Diflunisal *(dye FLOO ni sal)*
U.S. Brand Names Dolobid®
Generic Available Yes
Pharmacologic Category Nonsteroidal Anti-inflammatory Drug (NSAID), Oral
Medication Safety Issues
Sound-alike/look-alike issues:
Dolobid® may be confused with Slo-Bid®

Use Management of inflammatory disorders usually including rheumatoid arthritis and osteoarthritis; can be used as an analgesic for treatment of mild to moderate pain

Mechanism of Action/Effect Inhibits prostaglandin synthesis by decreasing the activity of the enzyme, cyclooxygenase, which results in decreased formation of prostaglandin precursors

Contraindications Hypersensitivity to diflunisal or any component of the formulation; may be a cross-sensitivity with other NSAIDs including aspirin; should not be used in patients with active GI bleeding; pregnancy (3rd trimester)

Warnings/Precautions Peptic ulceration and GI bleeding have been reported; platelet function and bleeding time are inhibited; ophthalmologic effects; impaired renal function, use lower dosage; dehydration; peripheral edema; possibility of Reye's syndrome; elevation in liver tests. Withhold for at least 4-6 half-lives prior to surgical or dental procedures.

Drug Interactions
Decreased Effect: Decreased effect with antacids, aspirin.

Increased Effect/Toxicity: May cause increased toxicity of cyclosporine, digoxin, methotrexate, anticoagulants, phenytoin, sulfonylureas, sulfonamides, lithium, indomethacin, hydrochlorothiazide, and acetaminophen (levels) when coadministered with diflunisal.

Nutritional/Ethanol Interactions
Ethanol: Avoid ethanol (may enhance gastric mucosal irritation).

Herb/Nutraceutical: Avoid cat's claw, dong quai, evening primrose, feverfew, garlic, ginger, ginkgo, red clover, horse chestnut, green tea, ginseng (all have additional antiplatelet activity).

Lab Interactions Increased prothrombin time (S), liver tests; decreased uric acid (S)

Adverse Reactions
>10%:

Central nervous system: Headache

Endocrine & metabolic: Fluid retention

1% to 10%:

Cardiovascular: Angina pectoris, arrhythmia

Central nervous system: Dizziness

Dermatologic: Rash

Gastrointestinal: GI ulceration

Genitourinary: Vaginal bleeding

Otic: Tinnitus

Overdosage/Toxicology Symptoms of overdose include drowsiness, nausea, vomiting, hyperventilation, tachycardia, tinnitus, stupor, coma, renal failure, and leukocytosis. Management of NSAID intoxication is supportive and symptomatic.

Pharmacodynamics/Kinetics
Onset of Action: Analgesic: ~1 hour

Duration of Action: 8-12 hours

Absorption: Well absorbed

Time to Peak: Serum: 2-3 hours

Half-Life Elimination: 8-12 hours; prolonged with renal impairment

Metabolism: Extensively hepatic

Excretion: Urine (~3% as unchanged drug, 90% as glucuronide conjugates) within 72-96 hours

Dosing
Adults & Elderly:

Osteoarthritis: Oral: 500-750 mg/day in divided doses

Pain: Oral: Initial: 500-1000 mg followed by 250-500 mg every 8-12 hours; maximum daily dose: 1.5 g

Inflammatory condition: Oral: 500-1000 mg/day in 2 divided doses; maximum daily dose: 1.5 g

Renal Impairment: Cl_{cr} <50 mL/minute: Administer 50% of normal dose.

Available Dosage Forms Tablet: 250 mg, 500 mg

Monitoring and Teaching Issues
Physical Assessment: Assess patient for allergic reaction to salicylates or other NSAIDs. Assess other medications patient may be taking for additive or adverse interactions. Monitor therapeutic effectiveness and signs of adverse reactions or overdose at beginning of therapy and periodically during long-term therapy. Schedule ophthalmic evaluations for patients who develop eye complaints during long-term NSAID therapy. Assess knowledge/teach patient appropriate use, appropriate interventions to reduce side effects, and adverse reactions to report.

Patient Education: If self-administered, use exactly as directed; do not increase dose or frequency. Adverse reactions can occur with overuse. Consult your prescriber before use if you have hypertension or heart failure. Do not take longer than 3 days for fever, or 10 days for pain without consulting medical advisor. Take with food or milk. While using this medication, do not use alcohol, excessive amounts of vitamin C, or salicylate-containing foods (curry powder, prunes, raisins, tea, or licorice), other prescription or OTC medications containing aspirin or salicylate, or other NSAIDs without consulting prescriber. Maintain adequate hydration (2-3 L/day of fluids) unless instructed to restrict fluid intake. You may experience nausea, vomiting, gastric discomfort (frequent mouth care, small frequent meals, chewing gum, or sucking lozenges may help). GI bleeding, ulceration, or perforation can occur with or without pain. Stop taking medication and report ringing in ears; persistent stomach pain; unresolved nausea or vomiting; respiratory difficulty or shortness of breath; unusual bruising or bleeding (mouth, urine, stool); skin rash; unusual swelling of extremities; chest pain; or palpitations. **Pregnancy/breast-feeding precautions:** Inform prescriber if you are or intend to become pregnant. This drug should not be used in the 3rd trimester of pregnancy. Consult prescriber if breast-feeding.

(Continued)

Diflunisal (Continued)

Dietary Considerations: Should be taken with food to decrease GI distress.

Geriatric Considerations: Elderly are at high risk for adverse effects from NSAIDs.

Pregnancy Risk Factor: C (1st and 2nd trimesters); D (3rd trimester)

Lactation: Enters breast milk/use caution

Administration

Oral: Tablet should be swallowed whole; do not crush or chew.

Additional Information Diflunisal is a salicylic acid derivative which is chemically different than aspirin and is not metabolized to salicylic acid. It is not considered a salicylate. Diflunisal 500 mg is equal in analgesic efficacy to aspirin 650 mg, acetaminophen 650 mg, and acetaminophen 650 mg/propoxyphene napsylate 100 mg, but has a longer duration of effect (8-12 hours). Not recommended as an antipyretic. Not found to be clinically useful to treat fever; at doses ≥2 g/day, platelets are reversibly inhibited in function. Diflunisal is uricosuric at 500-750 mg/day; causes less GI and renal toxicity than aspirin and other NSAIDs; fecal blood loss is $\frac{1}{2}$ that of aspirin at 2.6 g/day.

Related Information

Nonsalicylate / Nonsteroidal Anti-inflammatory Agents *on page 1743*

♦ **Digibind®** *see Digoxin Immune Fab on page 455*

♦ **DigiFab™** *see Digoxin Immune Fab on page 455*

♦ **Digitek®** *see Digoxin on page 452*

Digoxin (di JOKS in)

U.S. Brand Names Digitek®; Lanoxicaps®; Lanoxin®

Generic Available Yes; Excludes capsule

Pharmacologic Category Antiarrhythmic Agent, Class IV; Cardiac Glycoside

Medication Safety Issues

Sound-alike/look-alike issues:

Digoxin may be confused with Desoxyn®, doxepin

Lanoxin® may be confused with Lasix®, Levoxyl®, Levsinex®, Lomotil®, Lonox®, Mefoxin®, Xanax®

Use Treatment of congestive heart failure and to slow the ventricular rate in tachyarrhythmias such as atrial fibrillation, atrial flutter, and supraventricular tachycardia (paroxysmal atrial tachycardia); cardiogenic shock

Mechanism of Action/Effect

Congestive heart failure: Inhibition of the sodium/potassium ATPase pump which acts to increase the intracellular sodium-calcium exchange to increase intracellular calcium leading to increased contractility

Supraventricular arrhythmias: Direct suppression of the AV node conduction to increase effective refractory period and decrease conduction velocity - positive inotropic effect, enhanced vagal tone, and decreased ventricular rate to fast atrial arrhythmias. Atrial fibrillation may decrease sensitivity and increase tolerance to higher serum digoxin concentrations.

Contraindications Hypersensitivity to digoxin or any component of the formulation; hypersensitivity to cardiac glycosides (another may be tried); history of toxicity; ventricular tachycardia or fibrillation; idiopathic hypertrophic subaortic stenosis; constrictive pericarditis; amyloid disease; second- or third-degree heart block (except in patients with a functioning artificial pacemaker); Wolff-Parkinson-White syndrome and atrial fibrillation concurrently

Warnings/Precautions Withdrawal in CHF patients may lead to recurrence of CHF symptoms. Some arrhythmias that digoxin is used to treat may be exacerbated in digoxin toxicity. Sinus nodal disease may be worsened. Adjust doses in renal impairment and when verapamil, quinidine or amiodarone are added to a patient on digoxin. Correct hypokalemia and hypomagnesemia before initiating therapy. Calcium, especially when administered rapidly I.V., can produce serious arrhythmias. When used for rate control in atrial fibrillation, response may be better in a sedentary patients than in active/hypermetabolic patients. Use with caution in acute MI (within 6 months). Reduce or hold dose 1-2 days before elective electrical cardioversion.

Drug Interactions

Cytochrome P450 Effect: Substrate of CYP3A4 (minor)

Decreased Effect: Amiloride and spironolactone may reduce the inotropic response to digoxin. Cholestyramine, colestipol, kaolin-pectin, and metoclopramide may reduce digoxin absorption. Levothyroxine (and other thyroid supplements) may decrease digoxin blood levels. Penicillamine has been associated with reductions in digoxin blood levels The following reported interactions appear to be of limited clinical significance: Aminoglutethimide, aminosalicylic acid, aluminum-containing antacids, sucralfate, sulfasalazine, neomycin, ticlopidine.

Increased Effect/Toxicity: Beta-blocking agents (propranolol), verapamil, and diltiazem may have additive effects on heart rate. Carvedilol has additive effects on heart rate and inhibits the metabolism of digoxin. Digoxin levels may be increased by amiodarone (reduce digoxin dose 50%), bepridil, cyclosporine, diltiazem, indomethacin, itraconazole, some macrolides (erythromycin, clarithromycin), methimazole, nitrendipine, propafenone, propylthiouracil, quinidine (reduce digoxin dose 33% to 50% on initiation), tetracyclines, and verapamil. Moricizine may increase the toxicity of digoxin (mechanism undefined). Spironolactone may interfere with some digoxin assays, but may also increase blood levels directly. Succinylcholine administration to patients on digoxin has been associated with an increased risk of arrhythmias. Rare cases of acute digoxin toxicity have been associated with parenteral calcium (bolus) administration. The following medications have been associated with increased digoxin blood levels which appear to be of limited clinical significance: Famciclovir, flecainide, ibuprofen, fluoxetine, nefazodone, cimetidine, famotidine, ranitidine, omeprazole, trimethoprim.

Nutritional/Ethanol Interactions

Food: Digoxin peak serum levels may be decreased if taken with food. Meals containing increased fiber (bran) or foods high in pectin may decrease oral absorption of digoxin.

Herb/Nutraceutical: Avoid ephedra (risk of cardiac stimulation). Avoid natural licorice (causes sodium and water retention and increases potassium loss).

Adverse Reactions Incidence of reactions are not always reported.

Cardiovascular: Heart block; first-, second- (Wenckebach), or third-degree heart block; asystole; atrial tachycardia with block; AV dissociation; accelerated junctional rhythm; ventricular tachycardia or ventricular fibrillation; PR prolongation; ST segment depression

Central nervous system: Visual disturbances (blurred or yellow vision), headache (3%), dizziness (5%), apathy, confusion, mental disturbances (4%), anxiety, depression, delirium, hallucinations, fever

Dermatologic: Maculopapular rash (2%), erythematous, scarlatiniform, papular, vesicular or bullous rash, urticaria, pruritus, facial, angioneurotic or laryngeal edema, shedding of fingernails or toenails, alopecia

Gastrointestinal: Nausea (3%), vomiting (2%), diarrhea (3%), abdominal pain

Neuromuscular & skeletal: Weakness

Children are more likely to experience cardiac arrhythmia as a sign of excessive dosing. The most common are conduction disturbances or tachyarrhythmia (atrial tachycardia with or without block) and junctional tachycardia. Ventricular tachyarrhythmia are less common. In infants, sinus bradycardia may be a sign of digoxin toxicity. Any arrhythmia seen in a child on digoxin should be considered as digoxin toxicity. The gastrointestinal and central nervous system symptoms are not frequently seen in children.

Overdosage/Toxicology Manifested by a wide variety of signs and symptoms difficult to distinguish from effects associated with cardiac disease. Nausea and vomiting are common early signs of toxicity and may precede or follow evidence of cardiotoxicity. Other symptoms include anorexia, diarrhea, abdominal discomfort, headache, weakness, drowsiness, visual disturbances, mental depression, confusion, restlessness, disorientation, seizures, and hallucinations. Cardiac abnormalities include ventricular tachycardia, unifocal or multifocal PVCs (bigeminal, trigeminal), paroxysmal nodal rhythms, AV dissociation, excessive slowing of the pulse, AV block of varying degree, P-R prolongation, S-T depression, and occasional atrial fibrillation. Ventricular fibrillation is a common cause of death (alterations in cardiac rate and rhythm can result in any type of known arrhythmia).

Antidote: Life-threatening digoxin toxicity is treated with Digibind®. Administer potassium except in cases of complete heart block or renal failure. Digitalis-induced arrhythmias not responsive to potassium may be treated with phenytoin or lidocaine. Cholestyramine and colestipol may decrease absorption. Other agents to consider, based on ECG and clinical assessment, include atropine, quinidine, procainamide, and propranolol. **Note:** Other antiarrhythmics appear more dangerous to use in toxicity.

Pharmacodynamics/Kinetics

Onset of Action: Oral: 1-2 hours; I.V.: 5-30 minutes; Peak effect: Oral: 2-8 hours; I.V.: 1-4 hours

Duration of Action: Adults: 3-4 days both forms

Absorption: By passive nonsaturable diffusion in the upper small intestine; food may delay, but does not affect extent of absorption

Bioavailability: Oral (formulation dependent): Elixir: 75% to 85%; Tablet: 70% to 80%

Time to Peak: Serum: Oral: ~1 hour

Protein Binding: 30%; in uremic patients, digoxin is displaced from plasma protein binding sites

Half-Life Elimination:

Age, renal and cardiac function dependent:

Neonates: Premature: 61-170 hours; Full-term: 35-45 hours

Infants: 18-25 hours

Children: 35 hours

Adults: 38-48 hours

Adults, anephric: 4-6 days

Parent drug: 38 hours; Metabolites: Digoxigenin: 4 hours; Monodigitoxoside: 3-12 hours

Metabolism: Via sequential sugar hydrolysis in the stomach or by reduction of lactone ring by intestinal bacteria (in ~10% of population, gut bacteria may metabolize up to 40% of digoxin dose); metabolites may contribute to therapeutic and toxic effects of digoxin; metabolism is reduced with CHF

Excretion: Urine (50% to 70% as unchanged drug)

Dosing

Adults:

Note: When changing from oral (tablets or liquid) or I.M. to I.V. therapy, dosage should be reduced by 20% to 25%.

Dosage Recommendations for Digoxin

Age	Total Digitalizing Dose[2] (mcg/kg[1])		Daily Maintenance Dose[3] (mcg/kg[1])	
	P.O.	I.V. or I.M.	P.O.	I.V. or I.M.
Preterm infant[1]	20-30	15-25	5-7.5	4-6
Full-term infant[1]	25-35	20-30	6-10	5-8
1 mo - 2 y[1]	35-60	30-50	10-15	7.5-12
2-5 y[1]	30-40	25-35	7.5-10	6-9
5-10 y[1]	20-35	15-30	5-10	4-8
>10 y[1]	10-15	8-12	2.5-5	2-3

[1]Based on lean body weight and normal renal function for age. Decrease dose in patients with ↓ renal function; digitalizing dose often not recommended in infants and children.

[2]Give one-half of the total digitalizing dose (TDD) in the initial dose, then give one-quarter of the TDD in each of two subsequent doses at 8- to 12-hour intervals. Obtain ECG 6 hours after each dose to assess potential toxicity.

[3]Divided every 12 hours in infants and children <10 years of age. Given once daily to children >10 years of age and adults.

(Continued)

Digoxin *(Continued)*

Atrial dysrhythmias (rate control), CHF:

Initial: Total digitalizing dose: Give ½ of the total digitalizing dose (TDD) in the initial dose, then give ¼ of the TDD in each of two subsequent doses at 9- to 12-hour intervals. Obtain ECG 6 hours after each dose to assess potential toxicity.

Oral: 0.75-1.5 mg

I.V. or I.M.: 0.5-1 mg

Daily maintenance dose: Give once daily to children >10 years of age and adults.

Oral: 0.125-0.5 mg

I.V. or I.M.: 0.1-0.4 mg

Elderly: Dose is based on lean body weight and normal renal function for age. Decrease dose in patients with decreased renal function (see Dosing in Renal Impairment).

Pediatrics: Atrial dysrhythmias (rate control), CHF: When changing from oral (tablets or liquid) or I.M. to I.V. therapy, dosage should be reduced by 20% to 25%. See table on previous page.

Renal Impairment:

Cl_{cr} 10-50 mL/minute: Administer 25% to 75% of dose or every 36 hours.

Cl_{cr} <10 mL/minute: Administer 10% to 25% of dose or every 48 hours.

Reduce loading dose by 50% in ESRD.

Not dialyzable (0% to 5%)

Available Dosage Forms

Capsule (Lanoxicaps®): 50 mcg, 100 mcg, 200 mcg [contains ethyl alcohol]

Elixir: 50 mcg/mL (2.5 mL, 5 mL, 60 mL) [contains alcohol 10%; lime flavor]

Lanoxin® (pediatric): 50 mcg/mL (60 mL) [contains alcohol 10%; lime flavor]

Injection: 250 mcg/mL (1 mL, 2 mL) [contains alcohol 10% and propylene glycol 40%]

Lanoxin®: 250 mcg/mL (2 mL) [contains alcohol 10% and propylene glycol 40%]

Injection, pediatric: 100 mcg/mL (1 mL) [contains alcohol 10% and propylene glycol 40%]

Tablet: 125 mcg, 250 mcg, 500 mcg

Digitek®, Lanoxin®: 125 mcg, 250 mcg

Monitoring and Teaching Issues

Physical Assessment: Closely assess effects and interactions with other prescriptions, OTC medications, or herbal products patient may be taking. Assess results of laboratory tests (when beginning or changing dosage, especially with I.V. administration and when patients are receiving diuretics or amphotericin). Monitor therapeutic effectiveness and adverse reactions at beginning of therapy, periodically throughout therapy, or when changing dosage Monitor for signs of digoxin toxicity. **I.V.:** Monitor ECG continuously. **Oral:** Monitor apical pulse before administering any dose. Assess knowledge/teach patient appropriate use, adverse reactions to report, and appropriate interventions to reduce side effects.

Monitoring Laboratory Tests:

When to draw serum digoxin concentrations: Digoxin serum levels should be drawn **at least 4 hours after an intravenous dose** and **at least 6 hours after an oral dose (optimally 12-24 hours after a dose).**

Initiation of therapy:

If a loading dose is given: Digoxin serum concentration may be drawn within 12-24 hours after the initial loading dose administration. Levels drawn this early may confirm the relationship of digoxin plasma levels and response but are of little value in determining maintenance doses.

If a loading dose is not given: Digoxin serum concentration should be obtained after 3-5 days of therapy.

Maintenance monitoring:

Trough concentrations should be followed just prior to the next dose or at a minimum of 4 hours after an I.V. dose and at least 6 hours after an oral dose.

Digoxin serum concentrations should be obtained within 5-7 days (approximate time to steady-state) after any dosage changes. Continue to obtain digoxin serum concentrations 7-14 days after any change in maintenance dose. **Note:** In patients with end-stage renal disease, it may take 15-20 days to reach steady-state.

Patients who are receiving potassium-depleting medications such as diuretics, should be monitored for potassium, magnesium, and calcium levels.

Digoxin serum concentrations should be obtained whenever any of the following conditions occur:

Questionable patient compliance or to evaluate clinical deterioration following an initial good response

Changing renal function

Suspected digoxin toxicity

Initiation or discontinuation of therapy with drugs (amiodarone, quinidine, verapamil) which potentially interact with digoxin; if quinidine therapy is started; digoxin levels should be drawn within the first 24 hours after starting quinidine therapy, then 7-14 days later or empirically skip one day's digoxin dose and decrease the daily dose by 50%.

Any disease changes (hypothyroidism)

Patient Education: Take as directed; do not discontinue without consulting prescriber. Maintain adequate dietary intake of potassium (do not increase without consulting prescriber). Adequate dietary potassium will reduce risk of digoxin toxicity. Take pulse at the same time each day; follow prescriber instructions for holding medication if pulse is below 50. Notify prescriber of acute changes in pulse. Report loss of appetite, nausea, vomiting, persistent diarrhea, swelling of extremities, palpitations, "yellowing" or blurred vision, mental confusion or depression, or unusual fatigue. **Pregnancy precaution:** Inform prescriber if you are or intend to become pregnant.

Dietary Considerations: Maintain adequate amounts of potassium in diet to decrease risk of hypokalemia (hypokalemia may increase risk of digoxin toxicity).

Geriatric Considerations: Elderly may develop exaggerated serum/tissue concentrations due to age-related alterations in clearance and pharmacodynamic differences. Elderly are at risk for toxicity due to age-related changes.

Pregnancy Risk Factor: C

Lactation: Enters breast milk (small amounts)/compatible

Administration

I.M.: Inject no more than 2 mL per injection site. May cause intense pain.

I.V.: Inject slowly 1-5 minutes for undiluted form. May dilute up to fourfold with SWI, D$_5$W, or NS.

Compatibility: Stable in D$_5$½NS with KCl 20 mEq, D$_5$W, D$_{10}$W, LR, ½NS, NS, and SWFI (when diluted fourfold or greater)

Y-site administration: Incompatible with amphotericin B cholesteryl sulfate complex, fluconazole, foscarnet, propofol

Compatibility in syringe: Incompatible with doxapram

Compatibility when admixed: Incompatible with dobutamine

Storage: Protect elixir and injection from light.

Related Information

Antiarrhythmic Drugs *on page 1708*
Heart Failure *on page 1828*
Peak and Trough Guidelines *on page 1694*

Digoxin Immune Fab (di JOKS in i MYUN fab)

U.S. Brand Names Digibind®; DigiFab™

Synonyms Antidigoxin Fab Fragments, Ovine

Generic Available No

Pharmacologic Category Antidote

Use Treatment of life-threatening or potentially life-threatening digoxin intoxication, including:

- acute digoxin ingestion (ie, >10 mg in adults or >4 mg in children)
- chronic ingestions leading to steady-state digoxin concentrations > 6 ng/mL in adults or >4 ng/mL in children
- manifestations of digoxin toxicity due to overdose (life-threatening ventricular arrhythmias, progressive bradycardia, second- or third-degree heart block not responsive to atropine, serum potassium >5 mEq/L in adults or >6 mEq in children)

Mechanism of Action/Effect Binds with molecules of digoxin or digitoxin and then is excreted by the kidneys and removed from the body

Contraindications Hypersensitivity to sheep products or any component of the formulation

Warnings/Precautions Suicidal attempts often involve multiple drugs. Consider other drug toxicities as well. Hypersensitivity reactions can occur. Epinephrine should be immediately available. Serum potassium levels should be monitored, especially during the first few hours after administration. Total serum digoxin concentrations will rise precipitously following administration of this drug (has no clinical meaning - avoid monitoring serum concentrations). If digoxin was being used to treat CHF then may see exacerbation of symptoms as digoxin level is reduced. Use with caution in renal failure (experience limited) - the complex will be removed from the body more slowly. Monitor for reoccurrence of digoxin toxicity. Has reversed thrombocytopenia induced by digoxin. Failure of response to adequate treatment may call diagnosis of digitalis toxicity into question. Digoxin Immune Fab is processed with papain and may cause hypersensitivity reactions in patients allergic to papaya, other papaya extracts, papain, chymopapain, or the pineapple enzyme bromelain. There may also be cross allergy with dust mite and latex allergens.

Drug Interactions

Increased Effect/Toxicity: Digoxin: Following administration of digoxin immune Fab, serum digoxin levels are markedly increased due to bound complexes (may be clinically misleading, since bound complex cannot interact with receptors).

Lab Interactions Digibind® will interfere with digitalis immunoassay measurements - this will result in clinically misleading serum digoxin concentrations fragment is eliminated from the body (several days to >1 week after Digibind® administration).

Adverse Reactions Frequency not defined.

Cardiovascular: Effects (due to withdrawal of digitalis) include exacerbation of low cardiac output states and CHF, rapid ventricular response in patients with atrial fibrillation; postural hypotension

Endocrine & metabolic: Hypokalemia

Local: Phlebitis

Miscellaneous: Allergic reactions, serum sickness

Overdosage/Toxicology Symptoms of overdose include delayed serum sickness. Treatment of serum sickness includes acetaminophen, histamine$_1$ and possibly histamine$_2$ blockers, and corticosteroids.

Digoxin Immune Fab

Tablets Ingested (0.25 mg)	Fab Dose (vials)
5	2
10	4
25	10
50	20
75	30
100	40
150	60
200	80

(Continued)

Digoxin Immune Fab *(Continued)*

Pharmacodynamics/Kinetics

Onset of Action: I.V.: Improvement in 2-30 minutes for toxicity

Half-Life Elimination: 15-20 hours; prolonged with renal impairment

Excretion: Urine; undetectable amounts within 5-7 days

Dosing

Adults & Elderly: Each vial of Digibind® 38 mg or DigiFab™ 40 mg will bind ~0.5 mg of digoxin or digitoxin.

Estimation of the dose is based on the body burden of digitalis. This may be calculated if the amount ingested is known or the postdistribution serum drug level is known (round dose to the nearest whole vial). See table on previous page.

Fab dose based on serum drug level postdistribution:
Digoxin: No. of vials = level (ng/mL) x body weight (kg) divided by 100
Digitoxin: No. of vials = digitoxin (ng/mL) x body weight (kg) divided by 1000
If neither amount ingested nor drug level are known, dose empirically as follows:
For acute toxicity: 20 vials, administered in 2 divided doses to decrease the possibility of a febrile reaction, and to avoid fluid overload in small children.
For chronic toxicity: 6 vials; for infants and small children (≤20kg), a single vial may be sufficient.

Pediatrics:

Acute toxicity: I.V.: Refer to adult dosing.

Chronic toxicity: I.V.: If amount ingested and blood level are unknown:
Children ≤20 kg: 1 vial may be sufficient. If amount ingested or blood level is known, refer to adult dosing.
Children >20 kg: Refer to adult dosing.

Renal Impairment: Renal elimination of complexed digoxin may be decreased in renal failure. Potential "rebound" may occur when immune fragments are hepatically metabolized, leaving unbound digoxin.

Available Dosage Forms Injection, powder for reconstitution:
Digibind®: 38 mg
DigiFab™: 40 mg

Monitoring and Teaching Issues

Physical Assessment: Assess allergy history prior to administration. Assess results of laboratory tests, cardiac status, vital signs, blood pressure, and adverse reactions during and following infusion. Monitor for signs of reoccurrence of cardiac toxicity.

Monitoring Laboratory Tests: Serum potassium, serum digoxin concentration prior to first dose of digoxin immune Fab, subsequent to start of Digibind® therapy; **digoxin levels will greatly increase and are not an accurate determination of body stores.**

Patient Education: Patient education and instruction will be determined by patient condition and ability to understand. Immediately report dizziness, palpitations, cramping, respiratory difficulty, rash, or itching. **Pregnancy/breast-feeding precautions:** Inform prescriber if you are pregnant. Consult prescriber if breast-feeding.

Pregnancy Risk Factor: C

Lactation: Excretion in breast milk unknown/use caution

Administration

I.V.: Continuous I.V. infusion over ≥30 minutes is preferred. Small doses (infants/small children) may be administered using tuberculin syringe.

Reconstitution: Digoxin immune Fab is reconstituted by adding 4 mL sterile water, resulting in 10 mg/mL for I.V. infusion. The reconstituted solution may be further diluted with NS to a convenient volume (eg, 1 mg/mL). Reconstituted solutions should be used within 4 hours if refrigerated.

For very small doses, vial can be reconstituted by adding an additional 36 mL of sterile isotonic saline, to achieve a final concentration of 1 mg/mL.

Storage: Should be refrigerated at 2°C to 8°C.

♦ **Dihematoporphyrin Ether** *see Porfimer on page 1230*

Dihydrocodeine, Aspirin, and Caffeine
(dye hye droe KOE deen, AS pir in, & KAF een)

U.S. Brand Names Synalgos®-DC

Synonyms Dihydrocodeine Compound

Controlled Substance C-III

Generic Available No

Pharmacologic Category Analgesic, Narcotic

Medication Safety Issues
Sound-alike/look-alike issues:
Synalgos®-DC may be confused with Synagis®

Use Management of mild to moderate pain that requires relaxation

Dosing

Adults: Pain: Oral: 1-2 capsules every 4-6 hours as needed

Elderly: Initial dosing should be cautious (low end of adult dosing range).

Available Dosage Forms Capsule (Synalgos®-DC): Dihydrocodeine bitartrate 16 mg, aspirin 356.4 mg, and caffeine 30 mg

Monitoring and Teaching Issues

Physical Assessment: Assess for history of allergies and other medications patient may be taking for additive or adverse interactions. Monitor therapeutic effectiveness and adverse reactions at beginning of therapy and at regular intervals with long-term use. May cause physical and/or psychological dependence. Assess knowledge/teach patient appropriate use (if self-administered), appropriate interventions to reduce side effects, and adverse reactions to report.

Patient Education: If self-administered, use exactly as directed; do not increase dose or frequency. Drug may cause physical and/or psychological dependence. While using this medication, do not use alcohol and other prescription or OTC medications (especially sedatives, tranquilizers, antihistamines, or pain medications) without consulting prescriber. Maintain adequate hydration (2-3 L/day of fluids) unless instructed to restrict fluid intake. May cause dizziness, drowsiness, impaired coordination, or blurred vision (use caution when driving, climbing stairs, or changing position - rising from sitting or lying to standing or when engaging in tasks requiring alertness until response to drug is known); nausea or vomiting (frequent mouth care, small frequent meals, chewing gum, or sucking lozenges may help); or constipation (increased exercise, fluids, fruit, or fiber may help; if unresolved, consult prescriber about use of stool softeners). Report chest pain or rapid heartbeat; acute headache; swelling of extremities or unusual weight gain; changes in urinary elimination; acute headache; back or flank pain or spasms; or other adverse reactions. **Pregnancy/breast-feeding precautions:** Inform prescriber if you are or intend to become pregnant. Consult prescriber if breast-feeding.

Pregnancy Risk Factor: B/D (prolonged use or high doses at term)

Lactation: Excretion in breast milk unknown/use caution

Related Information

Aspirin on page 143

♦ **Dihydrocodeine Bitartrate, Phenylephrine Hydrochloride, and Chlorpheniramine Maleate** see Phenylephrine, Hydrocodone, and Chlorpheniramine on page 1202

♦ **Dihydrocodeine Compound** see Dihydrocodeine, Aspirin, and Caffeine on page 456

Dihydrocodeine, Pseudoephedrine, and Guaifenesin
(dye hye droe KOE, soo doe e FED rin, & gwye FEN e sin)

U.S. Brand Names DiHydro-GP; Hydro-Tussin™ EXP; Pancof®-EXP

Synonyms Guaifenesin, Dihydrocodeine, and Pseudoephedrine; Pseudoephedrine Hydrochloride, Guaifenesin, and Dihydrocodeine Bitartrate

Generic Available Yes

Pharmacologic Category Antitussive/Decongestant/Expectorant

Use Temporary relief of cough and congestion associated with upper respiratory tract infections and allergies

Dosing
Adults:
Cough/congestion: Oral (Hydro-Tussin™ EXP, Pancof®-EXP): 5-10 mL every 4-6 hours as needed
Pediatrics:
Cough/congestion: Oral (Hydro-Tussin™ EXP, Pancof®-EXP): Children:
2-6 years: 1.25-2.5 mL every 4-6 hours as needed
6-12 years 2.5-5 mL every 4-6 hours as needed
≥12 years: Refer to adult dosing.

Available Dosage Forms Syrup:
DiHydro-GP: Dihydrocodeine bitartrate 7.5 mg, pseudoephedrine hydrochloride 15 mg, and guaifenesin 100 mg per 5 mL (480 mL) [vanilla flavor]
Hydro-Tussin™ EXP, Pancof®-EXP: Dihydrocodeine bitartrate 7.5 mg, pseudoephedrine hydrochloride 15 mg, and guaifenesin 100 mg per 5 mL (480 mL) [alcohol free, dye free, sugar free]

Monitoring and Teaching Issues
Physical Assessment: See individual agents.
Pregnancy Risk Factor: C

Dihydroergotamine (dye hye droe er GOT a meen)

U.S. Brand Names D.H.E. 45®; Migranal®

Synonyms DHE; Dihydroergotamine Mesylate

Generic Available Yes: Injection

Pharmacologic Category Ergot Derivative

Use Treatment of migraine headache with or without aura; injection also indicated for treatment of cluster headaches

Unlabeled/Investigational Use Adjunct for DVT prophylaxis for hip surgery, for orthostatic hypotension, xerostomia secondary to antidepressant use, and pelvic congestion with pain

Mechanism of Action/Effect Ergot alkaloid alpha-adrenergic blocker directly stimulates vascular smooth muscle to vasoconstrict peripheral and cerebral vessels; also has effects on serotonin receptors

Contraindications Hypersensitivity to dihydroergotamine or any component of the formulation; high-dose aspirin therapy; uncontrolled hypertension; ischemic heart disease, angina pectoris, history of MI, silent ischemia, or coronary artery vasospasm including Prinzmetal's angina; hemiplegic or basilar migraine; peripheral vascular disease; sepsis; severe hepatic or renal dysfunction; following vascular surgery; avoid use within 24 hours of sumatriptan, zolmitriptan, other serotonin agonists, or ergot-like agents; avoid during or within 2 weeks of discontinuing MAO inhibitors; ergot alkaloids are contraindicated with potent inhibitors of CYP3A4 (includes protease inhibitors, azole antifungals, and some macrolide antibiotics); pregnancy

Warnings/Precautions Do not give to patients with risk factors for CAD until a cardiovascular evaluation has been performed; if evaluation is satisfactory, the healthcare provider should administer the first dose and cardiovascular status should be periodically evaluated. May cause vasospastic reactions; persistent vasospasm may lead to gangrene or death in patients with compromised circulation. Discontinue if signs of vasoconstriction develop. Rare reports of increased blood pressure in patients without history of hypertension. Rare reports of adverse cardiac events (acute MI, life-threatening arrhythmias, death) have been reported following use of the injection. Cerebral hemorrhage, subarachnoid hemorrhage, and stroke have also occurred following use of the injection. Not for prolonged use. Pleural and peritoneal fibrosis have been reported with prolonged daily use. Cardiac valvular fibrosis has also (Continued)

Dihydroergotamine *(Continued)*

been associated with ergot alkaloids. Safety and efficacy in pediatric patients have not been established.

Drug Interactions

Cytochrome P450 Effect: Substrate of CYP3A4 (major); **Inhibits** CYP3A4 (weak)

Decreased Effect: Effects of dihydroergotamine may be diminished by antipsychotics, metoclopramide. Antianginal effects of nitrates may be reduced by ergot alkaloids.

Increased Effect/Toxicity: CYP3A4 inhibitors may increase the levels/effects of dihydroergotamine; example inhibitors include azole antifungals, ciprofloxacin, clarithromycin, diclofenac, doxycycline, erythromycin, imatinib, isoniazid, nefazodone, nicardipine, propofol, protease inhibitors, quinidine, and verapamil. Ergot alkaloids are contraindicated with potent CYP3A4 inhibitors. Dihydroergotamine may increase the effects of 5-HT$_1$ agonists (eg, sumatriptan), MAO inhibitors, sibutramine, and other serotonin agonists (serotonin syndrome). Severe vasoconstriction may occur when peripheral vasoconstrictors or beta-blockers are used in patients receiving ergot alkaloids; concurrent use is contraindicated.

Adverse Reactions

>10%: Nasal spray: Respiratory: Rhinitis (26%)

1% to 10%: Nasal spray:

Central nervous system: Dizziness (4%), somnolence (3%)

Endocrine & metabolic: Hot flashes (1%)

Gastrointestinal: Nausea (10%), taste disturbance (8%), vomiting (4%), diarrhea (2%)

Local: Application site reaction (6%)

Neuromuscular & skeletal: Weakness (1%), stiffness (1%)

Respiratory: Pharyngitis (3%)

Overdosage/Toxicology Symptoms of overdose include peripheral ischemia, paresthesia, headache, nausea, and vomiting. Treatment is supportive. Activated charcoal is effective at binding ergot alkaloids.

Pharmacodynamics/Kinetics

Onset of Action: 15-30 minutes

Duration of Action: 3-4 hours

Time to Peak: Serum: I.M.: 15-30 minutes

Protein Binding: 93%

Half-Life Elimination: 1.3-3.9 hours

Metabolism: Extensively hepatic

Excretion: Primarily feces; urine (10% mostly as metabolites)

Dosing

Adults:

Migraine, cluster headache:

I.M., SubQ: 1 mg at first sign of headache; repeat hourly to a maximum dose of 3 mg total; maximum dose: 6 mg/week

I.V.: 1 mg at first sign of headache; repeat hourly up to a maximum dose of 2 mg total; maximum dose: 6 mg/week

Intranasal: 1 spray (0.5 mg) of nasal spray should be administered into each nostril; if needed, repeat after 15 minutes, up to a total of 4 sprays. **Note:** Do not exceed 3 mg (6 sprays) in a 24-hour period and no more than 8 sprays in a week.

Elderly: Refer to adult dosing. Patients >65 years of age were not included in controlled clinical studies.

Renal Impairment: Contraindicated in severe renal impairment

Hepatic Impairment: Dosage reductions are probably necessary but specific guidelines are not available; contraindicated in severe hepatic dysfunction.

Available Dosage Forms

Injection, solution, as mesylate (D.H.E. 45®): 1 mg/mL (1 mL) [contains ethanol 94%]

Solution, intranasal spray, as mesylate (Migranal®): 4 mg/mL [0.5 mg/spray] (1 mL) [contains caffeine 10 mg/mL]

Monitoring and Teaching Issues

Physical Assessment: Assess potential for interactions with other prescriptions, OTC medications, or herbal products patient may be taking. Assess therapeutic response and adverse effects on a regular basis. Teach patient proper use for either nasal spray or injection (storage, administration, injection technique, and syringe/needle disposal), possible side effects/appropriate interventions, and adverse symptoms to report. **Pregnancy risk factor X:** Determine that patient is not pregnant before starting therapy. Do not give to women of childbearing are patient is unless capable of complying with contraceptive use. Breast-feeding is contraindicated.

Patient Education: Take this drug as rapidly as possible when first symptoms occur. May cause rare feelings of numbness or tingling of fingers, toes, or face (use caution and avoid injury) or drowsiness (use caution when driving or engaging in potentially hazardous tasks until response to drug is known). Report heart palpitations, severe nausea or vomiting, and severe numbness of fingers or toes.

Nasal spray: Follow directions for use on package insert. Prime inhaler before use. Wait 15 minutes between inhalations. Use no more than 4 inhalations (2 mg) for a single administration; do not use >3 mg (6 sprays) in a 24-hour period and no more than 8 sprays in a week.

I.M.: Follow directions for injections and needle disposal.

Pregnancy/breast-feeding precautions: Inform prescriber if you are pregnant. Consult prescriber for instruction on appropriate contraceptive measures. This drug may cause severe fetal defects. Do not breast-feed.

Geriatric Considerations: Monitor cardiac and peripheral effects closely in the elderly since they often have cardiovascular disease and peripheral vascular impairment (ie, diabetes mellitus, PVD) that will complicate therapy and monitoring for adverse effects.

Pregnancy Risk Factor: X

Pregnancy Issues: Dihydroergotamine is oxytocic and should not be used during pregnancy.

Lactation: May be excreted in breast milk/contraindicated

Breast-Feeding Issues: Ergot derivatives inhibit prolactin and it is known that ergotamine is excreted in breast milk (vomiting, diarrhea, weak pulse, and unstable blood pressure have been reported in nursing infants). It is not known if dihydroergotamine would also cause these effects, however, it is likely that it is excreted in human breast milk. Do not use in nursing women.

Administration

Other: Prior to administration of nasal spray, the nasal spray applicator must be primed (pumped 4 times); in order to let the drug be absorbed through the skin in the nose, patients should not inhale deeply through the nose while spraying or immediately after spraying; for best results, treatment should be initiated at the first symptom or sign of an attack; however, nasal spray can be used at any stage of a migraine attack

Storage:

Injection: Store below 25°C (77°F), do not refrigerate or freeze; protect from heat and light

Nasal spray: Prior to use, store below 25°C (77°F), do not refrigerate or freeze; once spray applicator has been prepared, use within 8 hours; discard any unused solution

♦ **Dihydroergotamine Mesylate** *see* Dihydroergotamine *on page 457*

♦ **DiHydro-GP** *see* Dihydrocodeine, Pseudoephedrine, and Guaifenesin *on page 457*

♦ **Dihydrohydroxycodeinone** *see* Oxycodone *on page 1136*

♦ **Dihydromorphinone** *see* Hydromorphone *on page 764*

♦ **Dihydroxyanthracenedione Dihydrochloride** *see* Mitoxantrone *on page 1019*

♦ **1,25 Dihydroxycholecalciferol** *see* Calcitriol *on page 233*

♦ **Dihydroxydeoxynorvinkaleukoblastine** *see* Vinorelbine *on page 1567*

♦ **Diiodohydroxyquin** *see* Iodoquinol *on page 824*

♦ **Dilacor® XR** *see* Diltiazem *on page 459*

♦ **Dilantin®** *see* Phenytoin *on page 1204*

♦ **Dilatrate®-SR** *see* Isosorbide Dinitrate *on page 839*

♦ **Dilaudid®** *see* Hydromorphone *on page 764*

♦ **Dilaudid-HP®** *see* Hydromorphone *on page 764*

♦ **Diltia XT®** *see* Diltiazem *on page 459*

Diltiazem (dil TYE a zem)

U.S. Brand Names Cardizem®; Cardizem® CD; Cardizem® LA; Cardizem® SR [DSC]; Cartia XT™; Dilacor® XR; Diltia XT®; Taztia XT™; Tiazac®

Synonyms Diltiazem Hydrochloride

Generic Available Yes

Pharmacologic Category Calcium Channel Blocker

Medication Safety Issues

Sound-alike/look-alike issues:

Diltiazem may be confused with Dilantin®

Cardizem® may be confused with Cardene®, Cardene SR®, Cardizem CD®, Cardizem SR®, cardiem

Cartia XT™ may be confused with Procardia XL®

Tiazac® may be confused with Tigan®, Ziac®

Use

Oral: Essential hypertension; chronic stable angina or angina from coronary artery spasm

Injection: Atrial fibrillation or atrial flutter; paroxysmal supraventricular tachycardia (PSVT)

Unlabeled/Investigational Use Investigational: Therapy of Duchenne muscular dystrophy

Mechanism of Action/Effect Inhibits calcium ion from entering the "slow channels" or select voltage-sensitive areas of vascular smooth muscle and myocardium during depolarization, producing a relaxation of coronary vascular smooth muscle and coronary vasodilation; increases myocardial oxygen delivery in patients with vasospastic angina

Contraindications Hypersensitivity to diltiazem or any component of the formulation; sick sinus syndrome; second- or third-degree AV block (except in patients with a functioning artificial pacemaker); hypotension (systolic <90 mm Hg); acute MI and pulmonary congestion

Warnings/Precautions Concomitant use with beta-blockers or digoxin can result in conduction disturbances. Avoid concurrent I.V. use of diltiazem and a beta-blocker. Use caution in left ventricular dysfunction (can exacerbate condition). Symptomatic hypotension can occur. Use with caution in hepatic or renal dysfunction.

Drug Interactions

Cytochrome P450 Effect: Substrate of CYP2C8/9 (minor), 2D6 (minor), 3A4 (major); Inhibits CYP2C8/9 (weak), 2D6 (weak), 3A4 (moderate)

Decreased Effect: Levels/effects of diltiazem may be decreased by aminoglutethimide, carbamazepine, nafcillin, nevirapine, phenobarbital, phenytoin, rifamycins, and other CYP3A4 inducers.

Increased Effect/Toxicity: Diltiazem effects may be additive with amiodarone, beta-blockers, or digoxin, which may lead to bradycardia, other conduction delays, and decreased cardiac output. The levels/effects of diltiazem may be increased by azole antifungals, ciprofloxacin, clarithromycin, diclofenac, doxycycline, erythromycin, imatinib, isoniazid, nefazodone, nicardipine, propofol, protease inhibitors, quinidine, telithromycin, verapamil, and other CYP3A4 inhibitors.

Diltiazem may increase the levels/effects of selected benzodiazepines, calcium channel blockers, cisapride, cyclosporine, ergot alkaloids, selected HMG-CoA reductase inhibitors, mesoridazine, mirtazapine, nateglinide, nefazodone, pimozide, quinidine, sildenafil (and other PDE-5 inhibitors), tacrolimus, thioridazine, venlafaxine, and other CYP3A4 substrates. Blood pressure-lowering effects may be additive with sildenafil, tadalafil, and vardenafil (use caution).

(Continued)

Diltiazem *(Continued)*

Nutritional/Ethanol Interactions

Ethanol: Avoid ethanol (may increase risk of hypotension or vasodilation).

Food: Diltiazem serum levels may be elevated if taken with food. Serum concentrations were not altered by grapefruit juice in small clinical trials.

Herb/Nutraceutical: St John's wort may decrease diltiazem levels. Avoid dong quai if using for hypertension (has estrogenic activity). Avoid ephedra (may worsen arrhythmia or hypertension). Avoid yohimbe, ginseng (may worsen hypertension). Avoid garlic (may have increased antihypertensive effect).

Adverse Reactions Note: Frequencies represent ranges for various dosage forms. Patients with impaired ventricular function and/or conduction abnormalities may have higher incidence of adverse reactions.

>10%:

Cardiovascular: Edema (2% to 15%)

Central nervous system: Headache (5% to 12%)

2% to 10%:

Cardiovascular: AV block (first degree 2% to 8%), edema (lower limb 2% to 8%), pain (6%), bradycardia (2% to 6%), hypotension (<2% to 4%), vasodilation (2% to 3%), extrasystoles (2%), flushing (1% to 2%), palpitation (1% to 2%)

Central nervous system: Dizziness (3% to 10%), nervousness (2%)

Dermatologic: Rash (1% to 4%)

Endocrine & metabolic: Gout (1% to 2%)

Gastrointestinal: Dyspepsia (1% to 6%), constipation (<2% to 4%), vomiting (2%), diarrhea (1% to 2%)

Local: Injection site reactions: Burning, itching (4%)

Neuromuscular & skeletal: Weakness (1% to 4%), myalgia (2%)

Respiratory: Rhinitis (<2% to 10%), pharyngitis (2% to 6%), dyspnea (1% to 6%), bronchitis (1% to 4%), sinus congestion (1% to 2%)

Overdosage/Toxicology

Primary cardiac symptoms of calcium blocker overdose include hypotension and bradycardia. Noncardiac symptoms include confusion, stupor, nausea, vomiting, metabolic acidosis, and hyperglycemia.

Following initial gastric decontamination, if possible, repeated calcium administration may promptly reverse depressed cardiac contractility (but not sinus node depression or peripheral vasodilation). Glucagon, epinephrine, and amrinone may treat refractory hypotension. Glucagon and epinephrine also increase heart rate (outside the U.S., 4-aminopyridine may be available as an antidote). Dialysis and hemoperfusion are not effective in enhancing elimination although repeat-dose activated charcoal may serve as an adjunct with sustained-release preparations.

Pharmacodynamics/Kinetics

Onset of Action: Oral: Immediate release tablet: 30-60 minutes

Absorption: 70% to 80%

Bioavailability: Oral: ~40% to 60%

Time to Peak: Serum: Immediate release tablet: 2-3 hours

Protein Binding: 77% to 85%

Half-Life Elimination: Immediate release tablet: 3-4.5 hours, may be prolonged with renal impairment

Metabolism: Hepatic; extensive first-pass effect; following single I.V. injection, plasma concentrations of N-monodesmethyldiltiazem and desacetyldiltiazem are typically undetectable; however, these metabolites accumulate to detectable concentrations following 24-hour constant rate infusion. N-monodesmethyldiltiazem appears to have 20% of the potency of diltiazem; desacetyldiltiazem is about 50% as potent as the parent compound.

Excretion: Urine and feces (primarily as metabolites)

Dosing

Adults:

Angina: Oral:

Capsule, extended release (Cardizem® CD, Cartia XT™, Dilacor® XR, Diltia XT®, Tiazac®): Initial: 120-180 mg once daily (maximum dose: 480 mg/day)

Tablet, extended release (Cardizem® LA): 180 mg once daily; may increase at 7- to 14-day intervals (maximum recommended dose: 360 mg/day)

Tablet, immediate release (Cardizem®): Usual starting dose: 30 mg 4 times/day; usual range: 180-360 mg/day

Hypertension: Oral:

Capsule, extended release (Cardizem® CD, Cartia XT™, Dilacor® XR, Diltia XT®, Tiazac®): Initial: 180-240 mg once daily; dose adjustment may be made after 14 days; usual dose range (JNC 7): 180-420 mg/day; Tiazac®: usual dose range: 120-540 mg/day

Capsule, sustained release (Cardizem® SR): Initial: 60-120 mg twice daily; dose adjustment may be made after 14 days; usual range: 240-360 mg/day

Tablet, extended release (Cardizem® LA): Initial: 180-240 mg once daily; dose adjustment may be made after 14 days; usual dose range (JNC 7): 120-540 mg/day

Atrial fibrillation, atrial flutter, PSVT: I.V.:

Initial bolus dose: 0.25 mg/kg actual body weight over 2 minutes (average adult dose: 20 mg)

Repeat bolus dose (may be administered after 15 minutes if the response is inadequate): 0.35 mg/kg actual body weight over 2 minutes (average adult dose: 25 mg)

Continuous infusion (requires an infusion pump; infusions >24 hours or infusion rates >15 mg/hour are not recommended): Initial infusion rate of 10 mg/hour; rate may be increased in 5 mg/hour increments up to 15 mg/hour as needed; some patients may respond to an initial rate of 5 mg/hour.

If diltiazem injection is administered by continuous infusion for >24 hours, the possibility of decreased diltiazem clearance, prolonged elimination half-life, and increased diltiazem and/or diltiazem metabolite plasma concentrations should be considered.

Conversion from I.V. diltiazem to oral diltiazem: Start oral approximately 3 hours after bolus dose.

Oral dose (mg/day) is approximately equal to [rate (mg/hour) x 3 + 3] x 10.
- 3 mg/hour = 120 mg/day
- 5 mg/hour = 180 mg/day
- 7 mg/hour = 240 mg/day
- 11 mg/hour = 360 mg/day

Elderly: Refer to adult dosing. **Note:** Patients ≥60 years may respond to a lower initial dose (eg, 120 mg once daily using extended release capsule)

Pediatrics:

Children: Minimal information available; some centers use the following:
Hypertension: Oral: Initial: 1.5-2 mg/kg/day in 3-4 divided doses; maximum dose: 3.5 mg/kg/day
Note: Doses up to 8 mg/kg/day given in 4 divided doses have been used for investigational therapy of Duchenne muscular dystrophy

Adolescents: Refer to adult dosing.

Renal Impairment: Use with caution as diltiazem is extensively metabolized by the liver and excreted in the kidneys and bile. Not removed by hemo- or peritoneal dialysis; supplemental dose is not necessary.

Hepatic Impairment: Use with caution as diltiazem is extensively metabolized by the liver and excreted in the kidneys and bile.

Available Dosage Forms [DSC] = Discontinued product

Capsule, extended release, as hydrochloride [once-daily dosing]: 120 mg, 180 mg, 240 mg, 300 mg
Cardizem® CD: 120 mg, 180 mg, 240 mg, 300 mg, 360 mg
Cartia XT™: 120 mg, 180 mg, 240 mg, 300 mg
Dilacor® XR, Diltia XT®: 120 mg, 180 mg, 240 mg
Taztia XT™: 120 mg, 180 mg, 240 mg, 300 mg, 360 mg
Tiazac®: 120 mg, 180 mg, 240 mg, 300 mg, 360 mg, 420 mg
Capsule, sustained release, as hydrochloride [twice-daily dosing] (Cardizem® SR [DSC]): 60 mg, 90 mg, 120 mg
Injection, solution, as hydrochloride: 5 mg/mL (5 mL, 10 mL, 25 mL)
Injection, powder for reconstitution, as hydrochloride (Cardizem®): 25 mg
Tablet, as hydrochloride (Cardizem®): 30 mg, 60 mg, 90 mg, 120 mg
Tablet, extended release, as hydrochloride (Cardizem® LA): 120 mg, 180 mg, 240 mg, 300 mg, 360 mg, 420 mg

Monitoring and Teaching Issues

Physical Assessment: See Warnings/Precautions for use cautions (eg, impaired renal or hepatic function). Assess potential for interactions with other pharmacological agents or herbal products patient may be taking (eg, increased risk of bradycardia, conduction delays, decreased cardiac output; see Drug Interactions). I.V. requires use of infusion pump and continuous cardiac and hemodynamic monitoring. Assess therapeutic effectiveness according to purpose for use (hypertension; angina; atrial fib/flutter or PSVT) and adverse reactions (see Adverse Reactions) when beginning therapy, when changing dose, and periodically during long-term therapy. Teach patient appropriate use (oral), interventions to reduce side effects, and adverse symptoms to report (see Patient Education).

Monitoring Laboratory Tests: Liver function tests

Patient Education: Do not take any new medication during therapy unless approved by prescriber. Oral: Take as directed; do not alter dosage or discontinue therapy without consulting prescriber. Do not crush or chew extended release form. Avoid (or limit) alcohol and caffeine. May cause dizziness or lightheadedness (use caution when driving or engaging in tasks requiring alertness until response to drug is known); nausea or vomiting (small frequent meals, frequent mouth care, chewing gum, or sucking lozenges may help); constipation (increased exercise, fluids, fruit, or fiber may help); or diarrhea (buttermilk, boiled milk, or yogurt may help). Report chest pain, palpitations, irregular heartbeat; unusual cough, respiratory difficulty; swelling of extremities; muscle tremors or weakness; confusion or acute lethargy; skin rash; or other adverse reactions. **Pregnancy/breast-feeding precautions:** Inform prescriber if you are or intend to become pregnant. Consult prescriber if breast-feeding.

Geriatric Considerations: Elderly may experience a greater hypotensive response.

Pregnancy Risk Factor: C

Pregnancy Issues: Teratogenic and embryotoxic effects have been demonstrated in small animals.

Lactation: Enters breast milk/not recommended (AAP considers "compatible")

Breast-Feeding Issues: Freely diffuses into breast milk; however, the AAP considers diltiazem to be **compatible** with breast-feeding. Available evidence suggest safe use during breast-feeding.

Administration

Oral: Do not crush long acting dosage forms.
Tiazac®: Capsules may be opened and sprinkled on a spoonful of applesauce. Applesauce should be swallowed without chewing, followed by drinking a glass of water.

I.V.: Bolus doses given over 2 minutes with continuous ECG and blood pressure monitoring. Continuous infusion should be via infusion pump.

Compatibility: Stable in $D_5\frac{1}{2}NS$, D_5W, NS
Y-site administration: Incompatible with diazepam, furosemide, phenytoin, rifampin, thiopental

Storage:

Capsule, tablet: Store at controlled room temperature.
Solution for injection: Store in refrigerator at 2°C to 8°C (36°F to 46°F). May be stored at room temperature for up to one month; do not freeze. Following dilution with $D_5$1/2NS, D_5W, or NS, solution is stable for 24 hours at room temperature or under refrigeration.

Related Information

Antiarrhythmic Drugs *on page 1708*
Calcium Channel Blockers *on page 1722*

- ♦ **Diltiazem Hydrochloride** *see* Diltiazem *on page 459*
- ♦ **Dimercaprol** *see page 1625*
- ♦ **Dimetapp® 12-Hour Non-Drowsy Extentabs® [OTC]** *see* Pseudoephedrine *on page 1282*
- ♦ **Dimetapp® Children's ND [OTC]** *see* Loratadine *on page 918*

Dimethyl Sulfoxide (dye meth il sul FOKS ide)

U.S. Brand Names Rimso®-50
Synonyms DMSO
Generic Available Yes
Pharmacologic Category Urinary Tract Product
Use Symptomatic relief of interstitial cystitis
Drug Interactions
    Cytochrome P450 Effect: Inhibits CYP2C8/9 (weak), 2C19 (weak)
Adverse Reactions
    >10%: Gastrointestinal: Garlic-like breath
    1% to 10%:
        Central nervous system: Headache, sedation
        Gastrointestinal: Nausea, vomiting
        Local: Local dermatitis
        Ocular: Burning eyes
Dosing
    Adults & Elderly: Interstitial cystitis: Not for I.M. or I.V. administration; only for bladder instillation. Instill 50 mL of solution directly into bladder and allow to remain for 15 minutes. Repeat in 2 weeks or until symptoms are relieved, then increase intervals between treatments.
Available Dosage Forms Solution, intravesical: 50% [500 mg/mL] (50 mL)
Monitoring and Teaching Issues
    Physical Assessment: For bladder instillation only. Assess knowledge/teach patient interventions to reduce side effects and adverse symptoms to report.
    Patient Education: This medication is only for use as a bladder instillation. Maintain adequate hydration (2-3 L/day of fluids) unless instructed to restrict fluid intake. Report persistent adverse reactions. **Pregnancy/breast-feeding precautions:** Inform prescriber if you are or intend to become pregnant. Note breast-feeding caution.
    Pregnancy Risk Factor: C
    Lactation: Excretion in breast milk unknown

- ♦ **Dimethyl Triazeno Imidazole Carboxamide** *see* Dacarbazine *on page 394*
- ♦ **Dinoprost** *see page 1625*

Dinoprostone (dye noe PROST one)

U.S. Brand Names Cervidil®; Prepidil®; Prostin E₂®
Synonyms PGE₂; Prostaglandin E₂
Generic Available No
Pharmacologic Category Abortifacient; Prostaglandin
Medication Safety Issues
    Sound-alike/look-alike issues:
        Prepidil® may be confused with Bepridil®
Use
    Gel: Promote cervical ripening prior to labor induction; usage for gel include any patient undergoing induction of labor with an unripe cervix, most commonly for pre-eclampsia, eclampsia, postdates, diabetes, intrauterine growth retardation, and chronic hypertension
    Suppositories: Terminate pregnancy from 12th through 28th week of gestation; evacuate uterus in cases of missed abortion or intrauterine fetal death; manage benign hydatidiform mole
    Vaginal insert: Initiation and/or cervical ripening in patients at or near term in whom there is a medical or obstetrical indication for the induction of labor
Mechanism of Action/Effect A synthetic prostaglandin E₂ abortifacient that stimulates uterine contractions similar to those seen during natural labor
Contraindications
    Vaginal insert: Hypersensitivity to prostaglandins; fetal distress (suspicion or clinical evidence unless delivery is imminent); unexplained vaginal bleeding during this pregnancy; strong suspicion of marked cephalopelvic disproportion; patients in whom oxytoxic drugs are contraindicated or when prolonged contraction of the uterus may be detrimental to fetal safety or uterine integrity (including previous cesarean section or major uterine surgery); greater than 6 previous term pregnancies; patients already receiving oxytoxic drugs
    Gel: Hypersensitivity to prostaglandins or any constituents of the cervical gel, history of asthma, contracted pelvis, malpresentation of the fetus. The following are "relative" contraindications and should only be considered by the physician under these circumstances: Patients in whom vaginal delivery is not indicated (ie, herpes genitalia with a lesion at the time of delivery), prior uterine surgery, breech presentation, multiple gestation, polyhydramnios, premature rupture of membranes
    Suppository: Hypersensitivity to dinoprostone, acute pelvic inflammatory disease, uterine fibroids, cervical stenosis
Warnings/Precautions Dinoprostone should be used only by medically trained personnel in a hospital; caution in patients with cervicitis, infected endocervical lesions, acute vaginitis, compromised (scarred) uterus or history of asthma, hypertension or hypotension, epilepsy, diabetes mellitus, anemia, jaundice, or cardiovascular, renal, or hepatic disease. Oxytocin should not be used simultaneously with Prepidil® (>6 hours of the last dose of Prepidil®).
Drug Interactions
    Increased Effect/Toxicity: Dinoprostone may increase the effect of oxytocin; wait 6-12 hours after dinoprostone administration before initiating oxytocin.

Adverse Reactions
>10%:
Central nervous system: Headache
Gastrointestinal: Vomiting, diarrhea, nausea
1% to 10%:
Cardiovascular: Bradycardia
Central nervous system: Fever
Neuromuscular & skeletal: Back pain

Overdosage/Toxicology Symptoms of overdose include vomiting, bronchospasm, hypotension, chest pain, abdominal cramps, and uterine contractions. Treatment is symptomatic.

Pharmacodynamics/Kinetics
Onset of Action: Uterine contractions: Within 10 minutes
Duration of Action: Up to 2-3 hours
Absorption: Vaginal: Slow
Metabolism: In many tissues including the renal, pulmonary, and splenic systems
Excretion: Primarily urine; feces (small amounts)

Dosing
Adults & Elderly:
  Abortifacient: Insert 1 suppository high in vagina, repeat at 3- to 5-hour intervals until abortion occurs up to 240 mg (maximum); continued administration for longer than 2 days is not advisable.
  Cervical ripening:
   Gel:
    Intracervical: 0.25-1 mg
    Intravaginal: 2.5 mg
   Suppositories, intracervical: 2-3 mg
   Vaginal insert (Cervidil®): Intracervical: 10 mg; remove upon onset of active labor or after 12 hours.

Available Dosage Forms
Gel, endocervical (Prepidil®): 0.5 mg/3 g syringe [each package contains a 10 mm and 20 mm shielded catheter]
Insert, vaginal (Cervidil®): 10 mg [releases 0.3 mg/hour]
Suppository, vaginal (Prostin E₂®): 20 mg

Monitoring and Teaching Issues
Physical Assessment: Monitor temperature, uterine tone, and vaginal discharge closely throughout procedure and postprocedure. Monitor abortion for completeness (other measures may be necessary if incomplete). Assess knowledge/teach patient interventions to reduce side effects and adverse symptoms to report.
Patient Education: Nausea and vomiting, cramping or uterine pain, or fever may occur. Report acute pain, respiratory difficulty, or skin rash. Closely monitor for vaginal discharge for several days. Report vaginal bleeding, itching, malodorous or bloody discharge, or severe cramping.
Pregnancy Risk Factor: C
Lactation: Excretion in breast milk unknown/opportunity for use is minimal

Administration
Other:
  Endocervical gel: Intracervically: For cervical ripening, patient should be supine in the dorsal position
  Vaginal insert: One vaginal insert is placed transversely in the posterior fornix of the vagina immediately after removal from its foil package. Patients should remain in the recumbent position for 2 hours after insertion, but thereafter may be ambulatory
  Vaginal suppository: Bring to room temperature just prior to use. Patient should remain supine for 10 minutes following insertion.
Storage: Suppositories must be kept frozen, store in freezer not above -4°C (-20°F). Bring to room temperature just prior to use. Cervical gel should be stored under refrigeration 2°C to 8°C (36°F to 46°F).

Additional Information Commercially available suppositories should not be used for extemporaneous preparation of any other dosage form of drug.

♦ **Diocto®** [OTC] *see* Docusate *on page 474*
♦ **Dioctyl Calcium Sulfosuccinate** *see* Docusate *on page 474*
♦ **Dioctyl Sodium Sulfosuccinate** *see* Docusate *on page 474*
♦ **Diotame®** [OTC] *see* Bismuth *on page 197*
♦ **Diovan®** *see* Valsartan *on page 1547*
♦ **Diovan HCT®** *see* Valsartan and Hydrochlorothiazide *on page 1549*
♦ **Dipentum®** *see* Olsalazine *on page 1114*
♦ **Diphen®** [OTC] *see* DiphenhydrAMINE *on page 463*
♦ **Diphen® AF** [OTC] *see* DiphenhydrAMINE *on page 463*
♦ **Diphenhist** [OTC] *see* DiphenhydrAMINE *on page 463*

DiphenhydrAMINE (dye fen HYE dra meen)
U.S. Brand Names Aler-Cap [OTC]; Aler-Dryl [OTC]; Aler-Tab [OTC]; AllerMax® [OTC]; Banophen® [OTC]; Benadryl® Allergy [OTC]; Benadryl® Children's Allergy [OTC]; Benadryl® Children's Allergy Fastmelt® [OTC]; Benadryl® Dye-Free Allergy [OTC]; Benadryl® Injection; Benadryl® Itch Stopping [OTC]; Benadryl® Itch Stopping Extra Strength [OTC]; Compoz® Nighttime Sleep Aid [OTC]; Diphen® [OTC]; Diphen® AF [OTC]; Diphenhist [OTC]; Dynatan™; Genahist® [OTC]; Hydramine® [OTC]; Nytol® Quick Caps [OTC]; Nytol® Quick Gels [OTC]; Siladryl® Allergy [OTC]; Siladryl® DAS [OTC]; Silphen® [OTC]; Simply Sleep® [OTC]; Sleepinal® [OTC]; Sominex® [OTC]; Sominex® Maximum Strength [OTC]; Triaminic® Thin Strips™ Cough and Runny Nose [OTC]; Twilite® [OTC]; Unisom® Maximum Strength Sleep-Gels® [OTC]

Synonyms Diphenhydramine Citrate; Diphenhydramine Hydrochloride; Diphenhydramine Tannate
(Continued)

DiphenhydrAMINE *(Continued)*

Generic Available Yes: Excludes chewable tablet, orally-disintegrating tablet, suspension, stick, strip, topical spray

Pharmacologic Category Antihistamine

Medication Safety Issues

Sound-alike/look-alike issues:

DiphenhydrAMINE may be confused with desipramine, dicyclomine, dimenhyDRINATE

Benadryl® may be confused with benazepril, Bentyl®, Benylin®, Caladryl®

Use Symptomatic relief of allergic symptoms caused by histamine release which include nasal allergies and allergic dermatosis; can be used for mild nighttime sedation; prevention of motion sickness and as an antitussive; has antinauseant and topical anesthetic properties; treatment of antipsychotic-induced extrapyramidal symptoms

Mechanism of Action/Effect Competes with histamine for H_1-receptor sites on effector cells in the gastrointestinal tract, blood vessels, and respiratory tract; anticholinergic and sedative effects are also seen

Contraindications Hypersensitivity to diphenhydramine or any component of the formulation; acute asthma; not for use in neonates

Warnings/Precautions Causes sedation, caution must be used in performing tasks which require alertness (eg, operating machinery or driving). Sedative effects of CNS depressants or ethanol are potentiated. Use with caution in patients with angle-closure glaucoma, pyloroduodenal obstruction (including stenotic peptic ulcer), urinary tract obstruction (including bladder neck obstruction and symptomatic prostatic hyperplasia), hyperthyroidism, increased intraocular pressure, and cardiovascular disease (including hypertension and tachycardia). Diphenhydramine has high sedative and anticholinergic properties, so it may not be considered the antihistamine of choice for prolonged use in the elderly. May cause paradoxical excitation in pediatric patients, and can result in hallucinations, coma, and death in overdose. Some preparations contain sodium bisulfite; syrup formulations may contain alcohol. Some preparations contain soy protein; patients with soy protein or peanut allergies should avoid.

Drug Interactions

Cytochrome P450 Effect: Inhibits CYP2D6 (moderate)

Decreased Effect: Diphenhydramine may decrease the levels/effects of CYP2D6 prodrug substrates; example prodrug substrates include codeine, hydrocodone, oxycodone, and tramadol. May increase gastric degradation of levodopa and decrease the amount of levodopa absorbed by delaying gastric emptying. Therapeutic effects of cholinergic agents (tacrine, donepezil) and neuroleptics may be antagonized.

Increased Effect/Toxicity: Diphenhydramine may increase the levels/effects of amphetamines, selected beta-blockers, dextromethorphan, fluoxetine, lidocaine, mirtazapine, nefazodone, paroxetine, risperidone, ritonavir, thioridazine, tricyclic antidepressants, venlafaxine and other CYP2D6 substrates. CNS depressants may increase the degree of sedation and respiratory depression with diphenhydramine. May increase the absorption of digoxin. Central and/or peripheral anticholinergic syndrome can occur when administered with amantadine, rimantadine, narcotic analgesics, phenothiazines and other antipsychotics (especially with high anticholinergic activity), tricyclic antidepressants, quinidine, disopyramide, procainamide, and antihistamines. Syrup should not be given to patients taking drugs that can cause disulfiram reactions (ie, metronidazole, chlorpropamide) due to high alcohol content.

Nutritional/Ethanol Interactions

Ethanol: Avoid ethanol (may increase CNS depression).

Herb/Nutraceutical: Avoid valerian, St John's wort, kava kava, gotu kola (may increase CNS depression).

Lab Interactions May suppress the wheal and flare reactions to skin test antigens.

Adverse Reactions Frequency not defined.

Cardiovascular: Hypotension, palpitation, tachycardia

Central nervous system: Sedation, sleepiness, dizziness, disturbed coordination, headache, fatigue, nervousness, paradoxical excitement, insomnia, euphoria, confusion

Dermatologic: Photosensitivity, rash, angioedema, urticaria

Gastrointestinal: Nausea, vomiting, diarrhea, abdominal pain, xerostomia, appetite increase, weight gain, dry mucous membranes, anorexia

Genitourinary: Urinary retention, urinary frequency, difficult urination

Hematologic: Hemolytic anemia, thrombocytopenia, agranulocytosis

Neuromuscular & skeletal: Tremor, paresthesia

Ocular: blurred vision

Respiratory: Thickening of bronchial secretions

Overdosage/Toxicology Symptoms of overdose include CNS stimulation or depression; overdose may result in death in infants and children. There is no specific treatment for antihistamine overdose. Clinical toxicity is due to blockade of cholinergic receptors. For anticholinergic overdose with life-threatening symptoms, physostigmine 1-2 mg SubQ or I.V. slowly may be given to reverse these effects.

Pharmacodynamics/Kinetics

Onset of Action: Maximum sedative effect: 1-3 hours

Duration of Action: 4-7 hours

Bioavailability: Oral: 40% to 60%

Time to Peak: Serum: 2-4 hours

Protein Binding: 78%

Half-Life Elimination: 2-8 hours; Elderly: 13.5 hours

Metabolism: Extensively hepatic; smaller degrees in pulmonary and renal systems; significant first-pass effect

Excretion: Urine (as unchanged drug)

Dosing

Adults:

Minor allergic rhinitis or motion sickness: Oral: 25-50 mg every 4-6 hours; maximum: 300 mg/day

Moderate to severe allergic reactions:

Oral: 25-50 mg every 4 hours, not to exceed 400 mg/day

I.M., I.V.: 10-50 mg in a single dose every 2-4 hours, not to exceed 400 mg/day

Night-time sleep aid: Oral: 50 mg at bedtime

Dystonic reaction: I.M., I.V.: 50 mg in a single dose; may repeat in 20-30 minutes if necessary

Allergic dermatosis: Topical: For external application, not longer than 7 days

Elderly: Initial: 25 mg 2-3 times/day increasing as needed

Pediatrics:

Treatment of dystonic reactions and moderate to severe allergic reactions: Oral, I.M., I.V.: 5 mg/kg/day or 150 mg/m^2/day in divided doses every 6-8 hours, not to exceed 300 mg/day

Minor allergic rhinitis or motion sickness: Oral, I.M., I.V.:

2 to <6 years: 6.25 mg every 4-6 hours; maximum: 37.5 mg/day

6 to <12 years: 12.5-25 mg every 4-6 hours; maximum: 150 mg/day

≥12 years: 25-50 mg every 4-6 hours; maximum: 300 mg/day

Night-time sleep aid: 30 minutes before bedtime: Oral, I.M., I.V.:

2 to <12 years: 1 mg/kg/dose; maximum: 50 mg/dose

≥12 years: 50 mg

Antitussive: Oral, I.M., I.V.:

2 to <6 years: 6.25 mg every 4 hours; maximum 37.5 mg/day

6 to <12 years: 12.5 mg every 4 hours; maximum 75 mg/day

≥12 years: 25 mg every 4 hours; maximum 150 mg/day

Available Dosage Forms

Caplet, as hydrochloride: 25 mg, 50 mg

Aler-Dryl, Sominex® Maximum Strength, Twilite®: 50 mg

Simply Sleep®, Nytol® Quick Caps: 25 mg

Capsule, as hydrochloride: 25 mg, 50 mg

Aler-Cap, Banophen®, Benadryl® Allergy, Diphen®, Diphenhist, Genahist®: 25 mg

Sleepinal®: 50 mg

Capsule, softgel, as hydrochloride:

Benadryl® Dye-Free Allergy: 25 mg [dye-free]

Compoz® Nighttime Sleep Aid, Nytol® Quick Gels, Unisom® Maximum Strength Sleep-Gels®: 50 mg

Cream, as hydrochloride: 2% (30 g)

Benadryl® Itch Stopping: 1% (30 g) [contains zinc acetate 0.1%]

Benadryl® Itch Stopping Extra Strength: 2% (30 g) [contains zinc acetate 0.1%]

Elixir, as hydrochloride: 12.5 mg/5 mL (480 mL)

Banophen®: 12.5 mg/5 mL (120 mL)

Diphen AF: 12.5 mg/5 mL (120 mL, 240 mL, 480 mL) [alcohol free; cherry flavor]

Gel, topical, as hydrochloride (Benadryl® Itch Stopping Extra Strength): 2% (120 mL)

Injection, solution, as hydrochloride: 50 mg/mL (1 mL)

Benadryl®: 50 mg/mL (1 mL, 10 mL)

Liquid, as hydrochloride: 12.5 mg/5 mL (120 mL)

Benadryl® Allergy: 12.5 mg/5 mL (120 mL, 240 mL) [alcohol free; contains sodium benzoate; cherry flavor]

Benadryl® Dye-Free Allergy: 12.5 mg/5 mL (120 mL) [alcohol free, dye free, sugar free; contains sodium benzoate; bubble gum flavor]

Genahist®: 12.5 mg/5 mL (120 mL) [alcohol free, sugar free; contains sodium benzoate; cherry flavor]

Hydramine®: 12.5 mg/5 mL (120 mL, 480 mL) [alcohol free]

Siladryl® Allergy: 12.5 mg/5 mL (120 mL, 240 mL, 480 mL) [alcohol free, sugar free; black cherry flavor]

Siladryl® DAS: 12.5 mg/5 mL (120 mL) [alcohol free, dye free, sugar free; black cherry flavor]

Solution, oral, as hydrochloride:

AllerMax®: 12.5 mg/5 mL (120 mL)

Banophen®: 12.5 mg/5mL (480 mL, 3840 mL) [sugar free]

Diphenhist: 12.5 mg/5 mL (120 mL, 480 mL) [contains sodium benzoate]

Solution, topical, as hydrochloride [spray] (Benadryl® Itch Stopping Extra Strength): 2% (60 mL) [contains zinc acetate 0.1%]

Stick, topical, as hydrochloride (Benadryl® Itch Stopping Extra Strength): 2% (14 mL) [contains zinc acetate 0.1%]

Strips, oral, as hydrochloride (Triaminic® Thin Strips™ Cough and Runny Nose): 12. 5 mg (16s) [grape flavor]

Suspension, as tannate (Dynatan™): 25 mg/5 mL (120 mL) [strawberry flavor]

Syrup, as hydrochloride (Silphen® Cough): 12.5 mg/5 mL (120 mL, 240 mL, 480 mL) [contains alcohol; 5%; strawberry flavor]

Tablet, as hydrochloride: 25 mg, 50 mg

Aler-Tab, AllerMax®, Compoz® Nighttime Sleep Aid: 50 mg

Benadryl® Allergy, Genahist®, Sominex®: 25 mg

Tablet, chewable, as hydrochloride (Benadryl® Children's Allergy): 12.5 mg [contains phenyl-alanine 4.2 mg/tablet; grape flavor]

Tablet, chewable, as tannate (Dynatan™): 25 mg [contains phenylalanine 1.5 mg/tablet; strawberry flavor]

Tablet, orally-disintegrating, as citrate (Benadryl® Children's Allergy Fastmelt®): 19 mg [equivalent to diphenhydramine hydrochloride 12.5 mg; contains phenylalanine 4.5 mg/tablet and soy protein isolate; cherry flavor]

(Continued)

DiphenhydrAMINE *(Continued)*

Monitoring and Teaching Issues

Physical Assessment: Assess effectiveness and interactions of other medications patient may be taking. Monitor effectiveness of therapy and adverse reactions at beginning of therapy and periodically with long-term use. Assess knowledge/teach patient appropriate use, interventions to reduce side effects, and adverse symptoms to report.

Patient Education: Take as directed; do not exceed recommended dose. Avoid use of other depressants, alcohol, or sleep-inducing medications unless approved by prescriber. You may experience drowsiness or dizziness (use caution when driving or engaging in tasks requiring alertness until response to drug is known); or dry mouth, nausea, or vomiting (small frequent meals, frequent mouth care, chewing gum, or sucking hard candy may help). Report persistent sedation, confusion, or agitation; changes in urinary pattern; blurred vision; sore throat, respiratory difficulty, or expectorating (thick secretions); or lack of improvement or worsening or condition. **Breast-feeding precaution:** Do not breast-feed.

Dietary Considerations: Tablet:

Chewable, as hydrochloride: Contains phenylalanine 4.2 mg per 12.5 mg tablet

Chewable, as tannate: Contains phenylalanine 1.5 mg per 25 mg tablet

Orally-disintegrating: Contains phenylalanine 4.5 mg per 19 mg [equivalent to diphenhydramine hydrochloride 12.5 mg] tablet; contains soy protein isolate (contraindicated in patients with soy protein allergies; use caution in peanut allergic individuals, ~10% are estimated to also have soy protein allergies)

Geriatric Considerations: Diphenhydramine has high sedative and anticholinergic properties, so it may not be considered the antihistamine of choice for prolonged use in the elderly. Its use as a sleep aid is discouraged due to its anticholinergic effects.

Pregnancy Risk Factor: B

Lactation: Enters breast milk/contraindicated

Breast-Feeding Issues: Infants may be more sensitive to the effects of antihistamines.

Administration

Oral: Swallow whole, do not crush or chew sustained release product.

Compatibility: Stable in dextran 6% in dextrose, dextran 6% in NS, D_5LR, $D_5^1/_4NS$, $D_5^1/_2NS$, D_5NS, D_5W, $D_{10}W$, fat emulsion 10%, LR, $^1/_2NS$, NS

Y-site administration: Incompatible with allopurinol, amphotericin B cholesteryl sulfate complex, cefepime, foscarnet

Compatibility in syringe: Incompatible with diatrizoate meglumine 52% and diatrizoate sodium 8%, diatrizoate sodium 60%, haloperidol, iodipamide meglumine, iodipamide meglumine 52%, ioxaglate meglumine 39.3% and ioxaglate sodium 19.6%, pentobarbital, thiopental

Compatibility when admixed: Incompatible with amobarbital, amphotericin B, dexamethasone sodium phosphate with lorazepam and metoclopramide, iodipamide meglumine, phenytoin, phenobarbital, thiopental

Storage: Protect injection from light.

Additional Information Its use as a sleep aid is discouraged due to its anticholinergic effects.

Related Information

Anxiolytic / Hypnotic Use in Long-Term Care Facilities *on page 1769*
Compatibility of Drugs in Syringe *on page 1725*
FDA Name Differentiation Project: The Use of Tall-Man Letters *on page 15*
Federal OBRA Regulations: Recommended Maximum Doses *on page 1773*

♦ **Diphenhydramine Citrate** *see* DiphenhydrAMINE *on page 463*

♦ **Diphenhydramine Hydrochloride** *see* DiphenhydrAMINE *on page 463*

♦ **Diphenhydramine, Hydrocodone, and Phenylephrine** *see* Hydrocodone, Phenylephrine, and Diphenhydramine *on page 759*

♦ **Diphenhydramine Tannate** *see* DiphenhydrAMINE *on page 463*

Diphenoxylate and Atropine *(dye fen OKS i late & A troe peen)*

U.S. Brand Names Lomotil®; Lonox®

Synonyms Atropine and Diphenoxylate

Controlled Substance C-V

Generic Available Yes

Pharmacologic Category Antidiarrheal

Medication Safety Issues

Sound-alike/look-alike issues:

Lomotil® may be confused with Lamictal®, Lamisil®, lamotrigine, Lanoxin®, Lasix®, ludiomil

Lonox® may be confused with Lanoxin®, Loprox®

Use Treatment of diarrhea

Mechanism of Action/Effect Diphenoxylate inhibits excessive GI motility and GI propulsion; commercial preparations contain a subtherapeutic amount of atropine to discourage abuse

Contraindications Hypersensitivity to diphenoxylate, atropine, or any component of the formulation; severe liver disease; jaundice; dehydration; narrow-angle glaucoma; not for use in children <2 years of age

Warnings/Precautions High doses may cause physical and psychological dependence with prolonged use. Use with caution in patients with ulcerative colitis, dehydration, and hepatic dysfunction. Reduction of intestinal motility may be deleterious in diarrhea resulting from *Shigella*, *Salmonella*, toxigenic strains of *E. coli*, and from pseudomembranous enterocolitis associated with broad spectrum antibiotics. If there is no response within 48 hours, the drug is unlikely to be effective and should be discontinued. If chronic diarrhea is not improved symptomatically within 10 days at maximum dosage of 20 mg/day, control is unlikely with further use.

Drug Interactions

Increased Effect/Toxicity: MAO inhibitors (hypertensive crisis), CNS depressants when taken with diphenoxylate may result in increased adverse effects, antimuscarinics (paralytic ileus). May prolong half-life of drugs metabolized in liver.

Nutritional/Ethanol Interactions Ethanol: Avoid ethanol (may increase CNS depression).

Adverse Reactions 1% to 10%:

Central nervous system: Nervousness, restlessness, dizziness, drowsiness, headache, mental depression

Gastrointestinal: Paralytic ileus, xerostomia

Genitourinary: Urinary retention and dysuria

Ocular: Blurred vision

Respiratory: Respiratory depression

Overdosage/Toxicology Symptoms of overdose include drowsiness, hypotension, blurred vision, flushing, dry mouth, and miosis. Administration of activated charcoal will reduce bioavailability of diphenoxylate. Naloxone, 2 mg I.V. with repeat administration as necessary up to a total of 10 mg, can also be used to reverse toxic effects of the opiate. For anticholinergic overdose with severe life-threatening symptoms, physostigmine 1-2 mg SubQ or I.V. slowly, may be given to reverse these effects.

Pharmacodynamics/Kinetics

Onset of Action:

Diphenoxylate: Antidiarrheal: 45-60 minutes; Peak antidiarrheal effect: ~2 hours

Duration of Action:

Diphenoxylate: Antidiarrheal: 3-4 hours

Absorption:

Diphenoxylate: Well absorbed

Time to Peak:

Diphenoxylate: Serum: 2 hours

Half-Life Elimination:

Diphenoxylate: 2.5 hours

Metabolism:

Diphenoxylate: Extensively hepatic to diphenoxylic acid (active)

Excretion:

Diphenoxylate: Primarily feces (as metabolites); urine (~14%, <1% as unchanged drug)

Pharmacokinetic Note: See Atropine monograph.

Dosing

Adults & Elderly: Diarrhea: Oral: 15-20 mg/day of diphenoxylate in 3-4 divided doses; maintenance: 5-15 mg/day in 2-3 divided doses

Pediatrics: Diarrhea: Oral: Use with caution in young children due to variable responses:

Liquid: 0.3-0.4 mg of diphenoxylate/kg/day in 2-4 divided doses **or**

<2 years: Not recommended

2-5 years: 2 mg of diphenoxylate 3 times/day

5-8 years: 2 mg of diphenoxylate 4 times/day

8-12 years: 2 mg of diphenoxylate 5 times/day

Available Dosage Forms

Solution, oral: Diphenoxylate hydrochloride 2.5 mg and atropine sulfate 0.025 mg per 5 mL (5 mL, 10 mL, 60 mL)

Lomotil®: Diphenoxylate hydrochloride 2.5 mg and atropine sulfate 0.025 mg per 5 mL (60 mL) [contains alcohol 15%; cherry flavor]

Tablet (Lomotil®, Lonox®): Diphenoxylate hydrochloride 2.5 mg and atropine sulfate 0.025 mg

Monitoring and Teaching Issues

Physical Assessment: Ascertain etiology of diarrhea before beginning treatment if possible. Assess effects and interactions of other prescriptions, OTC medications, or herbal products patient may be taking (see Drug Interactions). Assess therapeutic effectiveness and response (see Adverse Reactions and Overdose/Toxicology). **Note:** There is potential for physical and psychological dependence with prolonged use. Teach patient proper use, possible side effects/appropriate interventions, and adverse effects to report (see Patient Education).

Patient Education: Inform prescriber of all prescriptions, OTC medications, or herbal products you are taking, and any allergies you have. Do not take any new medication during therapy unless approved by prescriber. Take as directed; do not exceed recommended dosage. If no response within 48 hours, notify prescriber. Avoid alcohol or other prescriptive or OTC sedatives or depressants. May cause drowsiness, blurred vision, impaired coordination (use caution when driving or engaging in tasks that require alertness until response to drug is known); dry mouth (sucking on lozenges or chewing gum may help). Report difficulty urinating, persistent unrelieved diarrhea, respiratory difficulties, fever, or palpitations. **Pregnancy/breast-feeding precautions:** Inform prescriber if you are or intend to become pregnant. Consult prescriber if breast-feeding.

Geriatric Considerations: Elderly are particularly sensitive to fluid and electrolyte loss. Maintaining hydration and electrolyte balance is vital.

Pregnancy Risk Factor: C

Lactation: Use caution

Administration

Storage: Protect from light.

Related Information

Atropine *on page 158*

- ♦ **Diprolene®** *see* Betamethasone *on page 185*
- ♦ **Diprolene® AF** *see* Betamethasone *on page 185*
- ♦ **Dipropylacetic Acid** *see* Valproic Acid and Derivatives *on page 1543*

Dipyridamole (dye peer ID a mole)
U.S. Brand Names Persantine®
Generic Available Yes
Pharmacologic Category Antiplatelet Agent; Vasodilator
Medication Safety Issues
  Sound-alike/look-alike issues:
    Dipyridamole may be confused with disopyramide
    Persantine® may be confused with Periactin®, Permitil®
Use
  Oral: Used with warfarin to decrease thrombosis in patients after artificial heart valve replacement
  I.V.: Diagnostic agent in CAD
Unlabeled/Investigational Use Treatment of proteinuria in pediatric renal disease
Mechanism of Action/Effect Inhibits platelet aggregation and may cause vasodilation. May also stimulate release of prostacyclin or PGD_2 resulting in coronary vasodilation.
Contraindications Hypersensitivity to dipyridamole or any component of the formulation
Warnings/Precautions Use caution in patients with hypotension and severe cardiac disease. Use caution in patients on other antiplatelet agents or anticoagulation. Severe adverse reactions have occurred with I.V. administration (rarely); use the I.V. form with caution in patients with bronchospastic disease or unstable angina. Aminophylline should be available in case of urgency or emergency with I.V. use.
Drug Interactions
  Decreased Effect: Decreased vasodilation from I.V. dipyridamole when given to patients taking theophylline. Theophylline may reduce the pharmacologic effects of dipyridamole (hold theophylline preparations for 36-48 hours before dipyridamole facilitated stress test). Dipyridamole may counteract effect of cholinesterase inhibitor and may aggravate myasthenia gravis.
  Increased Effect/Toxicity: Adenosine blood levels and pharmacologic effects are increased with dipyridamole; consider reduced doses of adenosine.
Nutritional/Ethanol Interactions Herb/Nutraceutical: Avoid cat's claw, dong quai, evening primrose, feverfew, garlic, ginger, ginkgo, red clover, horse chestnut, green tea, ginseng (all have additional antiplatelet activity).
Adverse Reactions
  Oral:
  >10%: Dizziness (14%)
  1% to 10%:
    Central nervous system: Headache (2%)
    Dermatologic: Rash (2%)
    Gastrointestinal: Abdominal distress (6%)
  Frequency not defined: Diarrhea, vomiting, flushing, pruritus, angina pectoris, liver dysfunction
  I.V.:
  >10%:
    Cardiovascular: Exacerbation of angina pectoris (20%)
    Central nervous system: Dizziness (12%), headache (12%)
  1% to 10%:
    Cardiovascular: Hypotension (5%), hypertension (2%), blood pressure lability (2%), ECG abnormalities (ST-T changes, extrasystoles; 5% to 8%), pain (3%), tachycardia (3%)
    Central nervous system: Flushing (3%), fatigue (1%)
    Gastrointestinal: Nausea (5%)
    Neuromuscular & skeletal: Paresthesia (1%)
    Respiratory: Dyspnea (3%)
Overdosage/Toxicology Symptoms of overdose include hypotension and peripheral vasodilation. Dialysis is not effective. Treatment is symptomatic and supportive.
Pharmacodynamics/Kinetics
  Absorption: Readily, but variable
  Time to Peak: Serum: 2-2.5 hours
  Protein Binding: 91% to 99%
  Half-Life Elimination: Terminal: 10-12 hours
  Metabolism: Hepatic
  Excretion: Feces (as glucuronide conjugates and unchanged drug)
Dosing
  Adults & Elderly:
    Adjunctive therapy for prophylaxis of thromboembolism with cardiac valve replacement: Oral: 75-100 mg 4 times/day
    Evaluation of coronary artery disease: I.V.: 0.14 mg/kg/minute for 4 minutes; maximum dose: 60 mg
  Pediatrics:
    Proteinuria (unlabeled use): Oral: Doses of 4-10 mg/kg/day have been used investigationally to treat proteinuria in pediatric renal disease.
    Mechanical prosthetic heart valves (unlabeled use): Oral: 2-5 mg/kg/day (used in combination with an oral anticoagulant in children who have systemic embolism despite adequate oral anticoagulant therapy, and used in combination with low-dose oral anticoagulation (INR 2-3) plus aspirin in children in whom full-dose oral anticoagulation is contraindicated).
Available Dosage Forms
  Injection, solution: 5 mg/mL (2 mL, 10 mL)
  Tablet (Persantine®): 25 mg, 50 mg, 75 mg

Monitoring and Teaching Issues

Physical Assessment: Monitor therapeutic effectiveness (dependent on purpose for use) and adverse reactions. Observe bleeding precautions. **I.V.:** Continuous ECG and blood pressure monitoring during infusion. Assess knowledge/teach patient appropriate use, interventions to reduce side effects, and adverse symptoms to report. **Oral:** Monitor blood pressure on a regular basis. Note breast-feeding caution.

Patient Education: Oral: Take exactly as directed, with water 1 hour before meals. You may experience mild headache, transient diarrhea, or temporary dizziness (sit or lie down when taking medication). You may have a tendency to bleed easily; use caution with sharps, needles, or razors. Report chest pain, redness around mouth, acute abdominal cramping or severe diarrhea, acute and persistent headache or dizziness, rash, respiratory difficulty, or swelling of extremities. **Breast-feeding precaution:** Consult prescriber if breast-feeding.

Dietary Considerations: Should be taken with water 1 hour before meals.

Geriatric Considerations: Since evidence suggests that clinically used doses are ineffective for prevention of platelet aggregation, consideration for low-dose aspirin (81-325 mg/day) alone may be necessary. This will decrease cost as well as inconvenience.

Pregnancy Risk Factor: B

Lactation: Enters breast milk/use caution

Breast-Feeding Issues: Excretion in breast milk is reported to be minimal.

Administration

Reconstitution: Prior to administration, dilute solution for injection to a ≥1:2 ratio in NS, 1/2NS, or D_5W. Total volume should be ~20-50 mL.

Storage: I.V.: Store between 15°C to 25°C (59°F to 77°F). Do not freeze, protect from light.

♦ **Dipyridamole and Aspirin** *see* Aspirin and Dipyridamole *on page 147*

♦ **Disalcid® [DSC]** *see* Salsalate *on page 1354*

♦ **Disalicylic Acid** *see* Salsalate *on page 1354*

♦ **Discoloration of Feces Due to Drugs** *see page 1676*

♦ **Discoloration of Urine Due to Drugs** *see page 1677*

♦ **Disodium Cromoglycate** *see* Cromolyn *on page 374*

♦ **d-Isoephedrine Hydrochloride** *see* Pseudoephedrine *on page 1282*

♦ **DisperMox™** *see* Amoxicillin *on page 102*

Disulfiram (dye SUL fi ram)

U.S. Brand Names Antabuse®

Generic Available No

Pharmacologic Category Aldehyde Dehydrogenase Inhibitor

Medication Safety Issues

Sound-alike/look-alike issues:

Disulfiram may be confused with Diflucan®

Antabuse® may be confused with Anturane®

Use Management of chronic alcoholism

Mechanism of Action/Effect Disulfiram is a thiuram derivative which interferes with aldehyde dehydrogenase. When taken concomitantly with alcohol, there is an increase in serum acetaldehyde levels. High acetaldehyde causes uncomfortable symptoms including flushing, nausea, thirst, palpitations, chest pain, vertigo, and hypotension. This reaction is the basis for disulfiram use in postwithdrawal long-term care of alcoholism.

Contraindications Hypersensitivity to disulfiram and related compounds or any component of the formulation; patients receiving or using ethanol, metronidazole, paraldehyde, or ethanol-containing preparations like cough syrup or tonics; psychosis; severe myocardial disease and coronary occlusion

Warnings/Precautions Use with caution in patients with diabetes, hypothyroidism, seizure disorders, nephritis (acute or chronic), hepatic cirrhosis or insufficiency. Should never be administered to a patient when he/she is in a state of ethanol intoxication, or without his/her knowledge. Patient must receive appropriate counseling, including information on "disguised" forms of alcohol (tonics, mouthwashes, etc) and the duration of the drug's activity (up to 14 days).

Drug Interactions

Cytochrome P450 Effect: Substrate (minor) of CYP1A2, 2A6, 2B6, 2D6, 2E1, 3A4; **Inhibits** CYP1A2 (weak), 2A6 (weak), 2B6 (weak), 2C8/9 (weak), 2D6 (weak), 2E1 (strong), 3A4 (weak)

Increased Effect/Toxicity: Disulfiram results in severe ethanol intolerance (disulfiram reaction) secondary to disulfiram's ability to inhibit aldehyde dehydrogenase; this combination should be avoided. Combined use with isoniazid, metronidazole, or MAO inhibitors may result in adverse CNS effects; this combination should be avoided. Some pharmaceutic dosage forms include ethanol, including elixirs and intravenous trimethoprim-sulfamethoxazole (contains 10% ethanol as a solubilizing agent); these may inadvertently provoke a disulfiram reaction. Disulfiram may increase the levels/effects of inhalational anesthetics, trimethadione, and other CYP2E1 substrates. Disulfiram may increase serum concentrations of benzodiazepines that undergo oxidative metabolism (all but oxazepam, lorazepam, temazepam). Disulfiram increases phenytoin and theophylline serum concentrations; toxicity may occur. Disulfiram inhibits the metabolism of warfarin resulting in an increased hypoprothrombinemic response.

Nutritional/Ethanol Interactions Ethanol: Disulfiram inhibits ethanol's usual metabolism. Avoid all ethanol. Patients can have a disulfiram reaction (headache, nausea, vomiting, chest, or abdominal pain) if they drink ethanol concurrently. Avoid cough syrups and elixirs containing ethanol. Avoid vinegars, cider, extracts, and foods containing ethanol.

Adverse Reactions Frequency not defined.

Central nervous system: Drowsiness, headache, fatigue, psychosis

Dermatologic: Rash, acneiform eruptions, allergic dermatitis

Gastrointestinal: Metallic or garlic-like aftertaste

Genitourinary: Impotence

(Continued)

Disulfiram *(Continued)*

Hepatic: Hepatitis (cholestatic and fulminant), hepatic failure (multiple case reports)
Neuromuscular & skeletal: Peripheral neuritis, polyneuritis, peripheral neuropathy
Ocular: Optic neuritis

Overdosage/Toxicology Management of disulfiram reaction: Institute support measures to restore blood pressure (vasopressors and fluids). Monitor for hypokalemia.

Pharmacodynamics/Kinetics
Onset of Action: Full effect: 12 hours
Duration of Action: ~1-2 weeks after last dose
Absorption: Rapid
Metabolism: To diethylthiocarbamate
Excretion: Feces and exhaled gases (as metabolites)

Dosing
Adults & Elderly: Note: Do not administer until the patient has abstained from ethanol for at least 12 hours.

Alcoholism: Oral: Initial: 500 mg/day as a single dose for 1-2 weeks; maximum daily dose is 500 mg. Average maintenance dose: 250 mg/day; range: 125-500 mg; duration of therapy is to continue until the patient is fully recovered socially and a basis for permanent self control has been established. Maintenance therapy may be required for months or even years.

Available Dosage Forms Tablet: 250 mg

Monitoring and Teaching Issues
Physical Assessment: Assess for adverse drug interactions with other prescription or OTC drugs. Do not administer until the patient has abstained from ethanol for 12 hours. Assess results of laboratory tests and for CNS changes at beginning of therapy and periodically with long-term therapy. Advise patient about disulfiram reaction if alcohol is ingested. Assess knowledge/teach patient appropriate use, interventions to reduce side effects, and adverse symptoms to report.

Monitoring Laboratory Tests: Monitor liver function before, 10-14 days after beginning therapy, and every 6 months during therapy.

Patient Education: Tablets can be crushed or mixed with water or juice. Metallic aftertaste may occur; this will go away. Do not drink any alcohol, including products containing alcohol (such as cough and cold syrups or some mouthwashes), or use alcohol-containing skin products for at least 3 days and preferably 14 days after stopping this medication or while taking this medication. Drowsiness, tiredness, or visual changes may occur. Use care when driving or engaging in tasks requiring alertness until response to drug is known. Notify prescriber of any respiratory difficulty, weakness, nausea, vomiting, decreased appetite, yellowing of skin or eyes, or dark-colored urine. **Pregnancy/breast-feeding precautions:** Inform prescriber if you are or intend to become pregnant. Consult prescriber if breast-feeding.

Pregnancy Risk Factor: C
Lactation: Excretion in breast milk unknown

Administration
Oral: Administration of any medications containing alcohol, including topicals, is contraindicated. Do not administer disulfiram if ethanol has been consumed within the prior 12 hours.

DOBUTamine *(doe BYOO ta meen)*

Synonyms Dobutamine Hydrochloride
Generic Available Yes
Pharmacologic Category Adrenergic Agonist Agent
Medication Safety Issues
Sound-alike/look-alike issues:
DOBUTamine may be confused with DOPamine

Use Short-term management of patients with cardiac decompensation
Unlabeled/Investigational Use Positive inotropic agent for use in myocardial dysfunction of sepsis
Mechanism of Action/Effect Stimulates beta$_1$-adrenergic receptors, causing increased contractility and heart rate, with little effect on beta$_2$- or alpha-receptors
Contraindications Hypersensitivity to dobutamine or sulfites (some contain sodium metabisulfate), or any component of the formulation; idiopathic hypertrophic subaortic stenosis (IHSS)
Warnings/Precautions May increase heart rate. Patients with atrial fibrillation may experience an increase in ventricular response. An increase in blood pressure is more common, but occasionally a patient may become hypotensive. May exacerbate ventricular ectopy. If needed, correct hypovolemia first to optimize hemodynamics. Ineffective in the presence of mechanical obstruction such as severe aortic stenosis. Use caution post-MI (can increase myocardial oxygen demand). Use cautiously in the elderly starting at lower end of the dosage range.

Drug Interactions

Decreased Effect: Beta-adrenergic blockers may decrease effect of dobutamine and increase risk of severe hypotension.

Increased Effect/Toxicity: General anesthetics (eg, halothane or cyclopropane) and usual doses of dobutamine have resulted in ventricular arrhythmias in animals. Bretylium and may potentiate dobutamine's effects. Beta-blockers (nonselective ones) may increase hypertensive effect; avoid concurrent use. Cocaine may cause malignant arrhythmias. Guanethidine, MAO inhibitors, methyldopa, reserpine, and tricyclic antidepressants can increase the pressor response to sympathomimetics.

Lab Interactions May affect serum assay of chloramphenicol.

Adverse Reactions Incidence of adverse events is not always reported.

Cardiovascular: Increased heart rate, increased blood pressure, increased ventricular ectopic activity, hypotension, premature ventricular beats (5%, dose related), anginal pain (1% to 3%), nonspecific chest pain (1% to 3%), palpitation (1% to 3%)

Central nervous system: Fever (1% to 3%), headache (1% to 3%), paresthesia

Endocrine & metabolic: Slight decrease in serum potassium

Gastrointestinal: Nausea (1% to 3%)

Hematologic: Thrombocytopenia (isolated cases)

Local: Phlebitis, local inflammatory changes and pain from infiltration, cutaneous necrosis (isolated cases)

Neuromuscular & skeletal: Mild leg cramps

Respiratory: Dyspnea (1% to 3%)

Overdosage/Toxicology Symptoms of overdose include fatigue, nervousness, tachycardia, hypertension, and arrhythmias. Reduce rate of administration or discontinue infusion until condition stabilizes.

Pharmacodynamics/Kinetics

Onset of Action: I.V.: 1-10 minutes; Peak effect: 10-20 minutes

Half-Life Elimination: 2 minutes

Metabolism: In tissues and hepatically to inactive metabolites

Excretion: Urine (as metabolites)

Dosing

Adults & Elderly: Cardiac decompensation: I.V. infusion: 2.5-20 mcg/kg/minute; maximum: 40 mcg/kg/minute, titrate to desired response; see table.

Infusion Rates of Various Dilutions of Dobutamine

Desired Delivery Rate (mcg/kg/min)	Infusion Rate (mL/kg/min)	
	500 mcg/mL[1]	1000 mcg/mL[2]
2.5	0.005	0.0025
5.0	0.01	0.005
7.5	0.015	0.0075
10.0	0.02	0.01
12.5	0.025	0.0125
15.0	0.03	0.015

[1]500 mg per liter or 250 mg per 500 mL of diluent.

[2]1000 mg per liter or 250 mg per 250 mL of diluent.

Pediatrics: Cardiac decompensation: Refer to adult dosing.

Available Dosage Forms

Infusion, as hydrochloride [premixed in dextrose]: 1 mg/mL (250 mL, 500 mL); 2 mg/mL (250 mL); 4 mg/mL (250 mL)

Injection, solution, as hydrochloride: 12.5 mg/mL (20 mL, 40 mL, 100 mL) [contains sodium bisulfite]

Monitoring and Teaching Issues

Physical Assessment: Assess other medications patient may be taking for effectiveness and interactions. Infusion pump and continuous cardiac and hemodynamic monitoring are required. Monitor therapeutic effectiveness and adverse reactions. Instruct patient on adverse symptoms to report.

Monitoring Laboratory Tests: Serum glucose, renal function

Patient Education: When administered in emergencies, patient education should be appropriate to the situation. If patient is aware, instruct to promptly report chest pain, palpitations, rapid heartbeat, headache, nervousness, or restlessness, nausea or vomiting, or respiratory difficulty. **Breast-feeding precaution:** Consult prescriber if breast-feeding.

Geriatric Considerations: Beneficial hemodynamic effects have been demonstrated in elderly patients; however, significant hypotension may occur more frequently in elderly patients; monitor closely.

Pregnancy Risk Factor: B

Pregnancy Issues: Since dobutamine has not been given to pregnant women, benefits of use should outweigh the risks.

Lactation: Excretion in breast milk unknown

Administration

I.V.: Always administer via infusion device; administer into large vein.

Reconstitution: Remix solution every 24 hours. Store reconstituted solution under refrigeration for 48 hours or 6 hours at room temperature. Pink discoloration of solution indicates slight oxidation but **no** significant loss of potency. Stability of parenteral admixture at room temperature (25°C) is 48 hours; at refrigeration (4°C) stability is 7 days.

Standard adult diluent: 250 mg/500 mL D_5W; 500 mg/500 mL D_5W

Compatibility: Do not give through same I.V. line as heparin, hydrocortisone sodium succinate, cefazolin, or penicillin. **Incompatible** with heparin, cefazolin, penicillin, and in alkaline solutions (sodium bicarbonate).

(Continued)

DOBUTamine *(Continued)*

Stable in D₅LR, D₅¹/₂NS, D₅NS, D₅W, D₁₀W, LR, ¹/₂NS, NS, mannitol 20%; **incompatible** with sodium bicarbonate 5%

Y-site administration: Incompatible with acyclovir, alatrofloxacin, alteplase, aminophylline, amphotericin B cholesteryl sulfate complex, cefepime, foscarnet, indomethacin, phytonadione, piperacillin/tazobactam, thiopental, warfarin

Compatibility in syringe: Incompatible with doxapram

Compatibility when admixed: Incompatible with acyclovir, alteplase, aminophylline, bumetanide, calcium gluconate, diazepam, digoxin, floxacillin, furosemide, insulin (regular), magnesium sulfate, phenytoin, potassium phosphates, sodium bicarbonate

Additional Information Dobutamine lowers central venous pressure and wedge pressure but has little effect on pulmonary vascular resistance.

Dobutamine therapy should be avoided in patients with stable heart failure due to an increase in mortality. In patients with intractable heart failure, dobutamine may be used as a short-term infusion to provide symptomatic benefit. It is not known whether short-term dobutamine therapy in end-stage heart failure has any outcome benefit.

Dobutamine infusion during echocardiography is used as a cardiovascular stress. Wall motion abnormalities developing with increasing doses of dobutamine may help to identify ischemic and/or hibernating myocardium.

Related Information

FDA Name Differentiation Project: The Use of Tall-Man Letters *on page 15*

Inotropic and Vasoconstrictor Comparison *on page 1736*

♦ **Dobutamine Hydrochloride** *see DOBUTamine on page 470*

Docetaxel *(doe se TAKS el)*

U.S. Brand Names Taxotere®

Synonyms NSC-628503; RP-6976

Generic Available No

Pharmacologic Category Antineoplastic Agent, Natural Source (Plant) Derivative

Medication Safety Issues

Sound-alike/look-alike issues:

Taxotere® may be confused with Taxol®

Use Treatment of locally-advanced or metastatic breast cancer; adjuvant treatment of operable node-positive breast cancer (in combination with doxorubicin and cyclophosphamide); treatment of locally-advanced or metastatic nonsmall cell lung cancer (NSCLC) in combination with cisplatin in treatment of patients who have not previously received chemotherapy for unresected NSCLC; treatment of prostate cancer (hormone refractory, metastatic)

Unlabeled/Investigational Use Investigational: Treatment of gastric, pancreatic, head and neck, and ovarian cancers, soft tissue sarcoma, and melanoma

Mechanism of Action/Effect Inhibits cancer cell division by acting on the microtubules

Contraindications Hypersensitivity to docetaxel or any component of the formulation; pre-existing bone marrow suppression (neutrophils <1500 cells/mm³); pregnancy

Warnings/Precautions Hypersensitivity, including severe reactions, may occur; incidence up to 25% in patients who did not receive premedication; incidence reduced to 2.2% in patients who receive premedication. Patients should be premedicated with a steroid to prevent hypersensitivity reactions and fluid retention. A common regimen is dexamethasone 4-8 mg orally twice daily for 3-5 days, starting the day before docetaxel administration.

Fluid retention syndrome (pleural effusions, ascites, edema, and 2-15 kg weight gain) may occur. It has not been associated with cardiac, pulmonary, renal, hepatic, or endocrine dysfunction. The incidence and severity of the syndrome increase sharply at cumulative doses ≥400 mg/m².

Neutropenia was the dose-limiting toxicity. Patients with an absolute neutrophil count <1500 cells/mm³ should not receive docetaxel. Hepatic dysfunction increases risk of neutropenia and severe infections. Should generally not be given to patients with bilirubin greater than the upper limit of normal or to patients with AST (SGOT) and/or ALT (SGPT) greater than 1.5x the upper limit of normal concomitantly with alkaline phosphatase greater than 2.5x the upper limit of normal. Obtain baseline levels prior to administration. If docetaxel contacts the skin, wash and flush thoroughly with water. Contains Polysorbate 80®; diluent contains ethanol.

When administered as sequential infusions, taxane derivatives (docetaxel, paclitaxel) should be administered before platinum derivatives (carboplatin, cisplatin) to limit myelosuppression and to enhance efficacy.

Drug Interactions

Cytochrome P450 Effect: Substrate of CYP3A4 (major); **Inhibits** CYP3A4 (weak)

Decreased Effect: CYP3A4 inducers may decrease the levels/effects of docetaxel; example inducers include aminoglutethimide, carbamazepine, nafcillin, nevirapine, phenobarbital, phenytoin, and rifamycins.

Increased Effect/Toxicity: CYP3A4 inhibitors may increase the levels/effects of docetaxel; example inhibitors include azole antifungals, ciprofloxacin, clarithromycin, diclofenac, doxycycline, erythromycin, imatinib, isoniazid, nefazodone, nicardipine, propofol, protease inhibitors, quinidine, and verapamil. When administered as sequential infusions, observational studies indicate a potential for increased toxicity when platinum derivatives (carboplatin, cisplatin) are administered before taxane derivatives (docetaxel, paclitaxel).

Nutritional/Ethanol Interactions

Ethanol: Avoid ethanol (due to GI irritation).

Herb/Nutraceutical: St John's wort may decrease docetaxel levels.

Adverse Reactions Note: Frequencies cited for nonsmall cell lung cancer and breast cancer treatment. Exact frequency may vary based on tumor type, prior and/or current treatment, premedication, and dosage of docetaxel.

>10%:

Cardiovascular: Fluid retention, including peripheral edema, pleural effusion, and ascites (33% to 47%); may be more common at cumulative doses ≥400 mg/m^2. Up to 64% in breast cancer patients with dexamethasone premedication.

Dermatologic: Alopecia (56% to 76%); nail disorder (11% to 31%, banding, onycholysis, hypo- or hyperpigmentation)

Gastrointestinal: Mucositis/stomatitis (26% to 42%, severe in 6% to 7%), may be dose-limiting (premedication may reduce frequency and severity); nausea and vomiting (40% to 80%, severe in 1% to 5%); diarrhea (33% to 43%)

Hematologic: Myelosuppression, neutropenia (75% to 85%), thrombocytopenia, anemia
Onset: 4-7 days
Nadir: 5-9 days
Recovery: 21 days

Hepatic: Transaminases increased (18%)

Neuromuscular & skeletal: Myalgia (3% to 21%); neurosensory changes (paresthesia, dysesthesia, pain) noted in 23% to 49% (severe in up to 6%). Motor neuropathy (including weakness) noted in as many as 16% of lung cancer patients (severe in up to 5%). Neuropathy may be more common at higher cumulative docetaxel dosages or with prior cisplatin therapy.

Ocular: Epiphora associated with canalicular stenosis (up to 77% with weekly administration; up to 1% with every-3-week administration)

Miscellaneous: Hypersensitivity reactions (6% to 13%; angioedema, rash, flushing, fever, hypotension); frequency substantially reduced by premedication with dexamethasone starting one day prior to docetaxel administration.

1% to 10%:

Cardiovascular: Hypotension (3%)

Dermatologic: Rash and skin eruptions (6%)

Gastrointestinal: Taste perversion (6%)

Hepatic: Bilirubin increased (9%)

Neuromuscular & skeletal: Arthralgia (3% to 9%)

Miscellaneous: Infusion site reactions (up to 4%)

Pharmacodynamics/Kinetics

Protein Binding: 94%, primarily to alpha$_1$-acid glycoprotein, albumin, and lipoproteins

Half-Life Elimination: Alpha, beta, gamma: 4 minutes, 36 minutes, and 10-18 hours, respectively

Metabolism: Hepatic; oxidation via CYP3A4 to metabolites

Excretion: Feces (75%); urine (6%); ~80% within 48 hours
Clearance: Total body: Mean: 21 L/hour/m^2

Pharmacokinetic Note: Exhibits linear pharmacokinetics at the recommended dosage range.

Dosing

Adults & Elderly: Refer to individual protocols:

Breast cancer:
Locally-advanced or metastatic: I.V.: 60-100 mg/m^2 every 3 weeks; patients initially started at 60 mg/m^2 who do not develop toxicity may tolerate higher doses
Operable, node-positive (adjuvant treatment): 75 mg/m^2 every 3 weeks for 6 courses

Nonsmall-cell lung cancer: I.V.: 75 mg/m^2 every 3 weeks

Prostate cancer:: I.V.: 75 mg/m^2 every 3 weeks; prednisone (5 mg twice daily) is administered continuously

Dosing adjustments for toxicity: I.V.:

Note: Toxicity includes febrile neutropenia, neutrophils ≤500/mm^3 for >1 week, severe or cumulative cutaneous reactions; in nonsmall cell lung cancer, this may also include other grade 3/4 nonhematologic toxicities.

Breast cancer: Patients dosed initially at 100 mg/m^2; reduce dose to 75 mg/m^2; **Note:** If the patient continues to experience these adverse reactions, the dosage should be reduced to 55 mg/m^2 or therapy should be discontinued

Breast cancer, adjuvant treatment: TAC regimen should be administered when neutrophils are ≥1500 cells/mm^3. Patients experiencing febrile neutropenia should receive G-CSF in all subsequent cycles. Patients continuing to experience febrile neutropenia or patients experiencing severe/cumulative cutaneous reactions or moderate neurosensory effects (signs/symptoms) should receive a reduced dose (60 mg/m^2) of docetaxel. Discontinue therapy in patients continuing to experience these reactions after dosage reduction.

Nonsmall cell lung cancer:
Monotherapy: Patients dosed initially at 75 mg/m^2 should have dose held until toxicity is resolved, then resume at 55 mg/m^2; discontinue patients who develop ≥ grade 3 peripheral neuropathy.
Combination therapy: Patients dosed initially at 75 mg/m^2, in combination with cisplatin, should have the docetaxel dosage reduced to 65 mg/m^2 in subsequent cycles; if further adjustment is required, dosage may be reduced to 50 mg/m^2

Prostate cancer: Reduce dose to 60 mg/m^2; discontinue therapy if adverse reactions persist at lower dose.

Pediatrics: Children ≥16 years: Refer to adult dosing.

Hepatic Impairment: Total bilirubin ≥ the upper limit of normal (ULN), or AST (SGOT)/ALT (SGPT) >1.5 times ULN concomitant with alkaline phosphatase >2.5 times ULN: Docetaxel **should not be administered.**

Available Dosage Forms Injection, solution [concentrate]: 20 mg/0.5 mL (0.5 mL, 2 mL) [contains Polysorbate 80®; diluent contains ethanol 13%]

Monitoring and Teaching Issues

Physical Assessment: See Warnings/Precautions for use cautions (eg, neutropenia, fluid retention syndrome, hypersensitivity). Assess potential for interactions with other pharmacological agents or herbal products patient may be taking (eg, drugs that may increase or decrease levels/effects of docetaxel; see Drug Interactions). **Caution:** Anaphylactoid-like reactions have been reported; premedication with dexamethasone may be advisable (see (Continued)

Docetaxel *(Continued)*

Dosing adjustments for toxicity and Administration). See infusion specifics in Administration. Assess results of laboratory tests, therapeutic response, and adverse effects (eg, severe fluid retention, pleural effusion, opportunistic infections; see Adverse Reactions) on a regular basis. Teach patient possible side effects/appropriate interventions and adverse symptoms to report (see Patient Education).

Monitoring Laboratory Tests: CBC with differential and platelet count; liver function especially bilirubin, AST, ALT, and alkaline phosphatase

Patient Education: Do not take any new medication during therapy unless approved by prescriber. This medication can only be administered by infusion; report immediately any pain, burning, swelling, or redness at infusion site, difficulty breathing or swallowing, chest pain, or sudden chills. It is important to maintain adequate hydration (2-3 L/day of fluids) unless instructed to restrict fluid intake and adequate nutrition (small frequent meals may help). You will be more susceptible to infection (avoid crowds and exposure to infection and do not have any vaccinations without consulting prescriber). May cause nausea or vomiting (small frequent meals, frequent mouth care, sucking lozenges, or chewing gum may help); loss of hair (reversible); or diarrhea (buttermilk, boiled milk, or yogurt may help; if unresolved, contact prescriber for medication relief). Report immediately swelling of extremities, respiratory difficulty, unusual weight gain, abdominal distention, chest pain, palpitations, fever, chills, unusual bruising or bleeding, signs of infection, excessive fatigue, or rash. **Pregnancy/breast-feeding precautions:** Inform prescriber if you are pregnant. Do not get pregnant while taking this drug. Consult prescriber for appropriate contraceptives. Do not breast-feed.

Pregnancy Risk Factor: D

Pregnancy Issues: Docetaxel was found to be embryotoxic and fetotoxic in animal studies. A pregnancy registry is available for all cancers diagnosed during pregnancy at Cooper Health (856-757-7876).

Lactation: Excretion in breast milk unknown/contraindicated

Breast-Feeding Issues: The manufacturer recommends discontinuing nursing prior to treatment.

Administration

I.V.: Irritant.

Premedication with corticosteroids is recommended to prevent hypersensitivity reactions and pulmonary/peripheral edema (see Additional Information).

Administer I.V. infusion over 1-hour through nonsorbing (nonpolyvinylchloride) tubing; in-line filter is not necessary. When administered as sequential infusions, taxane derivatives should be administered before platinum derivatives (cisplatin, carboplatin) to limit myelosuppression and to enhance efficacy.

Reconstitution: Intact vials of solution should be diluted with 13% (w/w) ethanol/water to a final concentration of 10 mg/mL. Mix by repeated inversions; do not shake. Docetaxel dose should then be further diluted with NS or D$_5$W to a final concentration of 0.3-0.74 mg/mL and must be prepared in a glass bottle, polypropylene, or polyolefin plastic bag to prevent leaching of plasticizers.

Compatibility: Stable in D$_5$W, NS

Y-site administration: Incompatible with amphotericin B, doxorubicin liposome, methylprednisolone sodium succinate, nalbuphine

Storage: Intact vials should be stored at 2°C to 25°C (36°F to 77°F) and protected from light. Freezing does not adversely affect the product. Vials should be stored at room temperature for approximately 5 minutes before using. Following initial dilution, solution is stable for 8 hours at room temperature or under refrigeration. Following second dilution, the manufacturer recommends using within 4 hours. According to other references, the final diluted solutions are stable for up to 4 weeks at room temperature 15°C to 25°C (59°F to 77°F) in polyolefin containers.

Additional Information Premedication with oral corticosteroids is recommended for all patients to decrease the incidence and severity of fluid retention and severity of hypersensitivity reactions. Suggested regimens include:

Breast cancer, NSCLC: Dexamethasone 8-10 mg twice daily for 3-5 days. Start 1 day prior to docetaxel.

Prostate cancer: Dexamethasone 8 mg at 12 hours, 3 hours, and 1 hour before docetaxel infusion. Prednisone is also administered as a part of combination treatment.

Docusate *(DOK yoo sate)*

U.S. Brand Names Colace® [OTC]; Diocto® [OTC]; Docusoft-S™ [OTC]; DOK™ [OTC]; DOS® [OTC]; D-S-S® [OTC]; Dulcolax® Stool Softener [OTC]; Enemeez® [OTC]; Fleet® Sof-Lax® [OTC]; Genasoft® [OTC]; Phillips'® Stool Softener Laxative [OTC]; Silace [OTC]; Surfak® [OTC]

Synonyms Dioctyl Calcium Sulfosuccinate; Dioctyl Sodium Sulfosuccinate; Docusate Calcium; Docusate Potassium; Docusate Sodium; DOSS; DSS

Generic Available Yes: Excludes gelcap

Pharmacologic Category Stool Softener

Medication Safety Issues

Sound-alike/look-alike issues:

Docusate may be confused with Doxinate®

Colace® may be confused with Calan®

Surfak® may be confused with Surbex®

Use Stool softener in patients who should avoid straining during defecation and constipation associated with hard, dry stools; prophylaxis for straining (Valsalva) following myocardial infarction. A safe agent to be used in elderly; some evidence that doses <200 mg are ineffective; stool softeners are unnecessary if stool is well hydrated or "mushy" and soft; shown to be ineffective used long-term.

Unlabeled/Investigational Use Ceruminolytic

Mechanism of Action/Effect Reduces surface tension of the oil-water interface of the stool resulting in enhanced incorporation of water and fat allowing for stool softening

Contraindications Hypersensitivity to docusate or any component of the formulation; concomitant use of mineral oil; intestinal obstruction, acute abdominal pain, nausea, or vomiting

Warnings/Precautions Prolonged, frequent, or excessive use may result in dependence or electrolyte imbalance.

Lab Interactions Decreased potassium (S), chloride (S)

Adverse Reactions 1% to 10%:

Gastrointestinal: Intestinal obstruction, diarrhea, abdominal cramping

Miscellaneous: Throat irritation

Overdosage/Toxicology Symptoms of overdose include abdominal cramps, diarrhea, fluid loss, and hypokalemia. Treatment is symptomatic.

Pharmacodynamics/Kinetics

Onset of Action: 12-72 hours

Excretion: Feces

Dosing

Adults & Elderly: Note: Docusate salts are interchangeable; the amount of sodium, calcium, or potassium per dosage unit is clinically insignificant.

Stool softener:

Oral: 50-500 mg/day in 1-4 divided doses

Rectal: Add 50-100 mg of docusate liquid to enema fluid (saline or water); give as retention or flushing enema

Pediatrics: Note: Docusate salts are interchangeable; the amount of sodium, calcium, or potassium per dosage unit is clinically insignificant.

Stool softener:

Oral:

Infants and Children <3 years: 10-40 mg/day in 1-4 divided doses

Children:

3-6 years: 20-60 mg/day in 1-4 divided doses

6-12 years: 40-150 mg/day in 1-4 divided doses

Adolescents: Refer to adult dosing.

Rectal: Older Children: Refer to adult dosing.

Available Dosage Forms

Capsule, as calcium (Surfak®): 240 mg

Capsule, as sodium: 100 mg, 250 mg

Colace®: 50 mg [contains sodium 3 mg], 100 mg [contains sodium 5 mg]

Docusoft-S™: 100 mg [contains sodium 5 mg]

DOK™, Genasoft®: 100 mg

DOS®, D-S-S®: 100 mg, 250 mg

Dulcolax® Stool Softener: 100 mg [contains sodium 5 mg]

Phillips'® Stool Softener Laxative: 100 mg [contains sodium 5.2 mg]

Enema, rectal, as sodium (Enemeez®): 283 mg/5 mL 5 mL

Gelcap, as sodium (Fleet® Sof-Lax®): 100 mg

Liquid, as sodium: 150 mg/15 mL (480 mL)

Colace®: 150 mg/15 mL (30 mL) [contains sodium 1 mg/mL]

Diocto®: 150 mg/15 mL (480 mL) [vanilla flavor]

Silace: 150 mg/15 mL (480 mL) [lemon-vanilla flavor]

Syrup, as sodium: 60 mg/15 mL (480 mL)

Colace®, Diocto®: 60 mg/15 mL (480 mL) [alcohol free, sugar free; contains sodium 36 mg/ 5 mL]

Silace: 20 mg/5 mL (480 mL) [peppermint flavor]

Monitoring and Teaching Issues

Physical Assessment: See Warnings/Precautions and Drug Interactions for use cautions. Monitor for effectiveness and instruct patient in proper use (avoid excessive or prolonged use) and adverse effects to report.

Patient Education: Docusate should be taken with a full glass of water, milk, or fruit juice. Do not use if abdominal pain, nausea, or vomiting are present. Laxative use should be used for a short period of time (<1 week). Prolonged use may result in abuse, dependence, as well as fluid and electrolyte loss. Report bleeding or constipation. **Pregnancy precaution:** Inform prescriber if you are or intend to become pregnant.

Dietary Considerations: Should be taken with a full glass of water, milk, or fruit juice.

Geriatric Considerations: A safe agent to be used in the elderly. Some evidence that doses <200 mg are ineffective.

Pregnancy Risk Factor: C

Lactation: Excretion in breast milk unknown/compatible

Administration

Oral: Docusate liquid should be given with milk, or fruit juice, to mask the bitter taste. Capsules should be administered with a full glass of water, milk, or fruit juice.

Related Information

Laxatives, Classification and Properties *on page 1737*

Docusate and Senna (DOK yoo sate & SEN na)

U.S. Brand Names Peri-Colace® *(reformulation)* [OTC]; Senokot-S® [OTC]

Synonyms Senna and Docusate; Senna-S

Generic Available Yes

Pharmacologic Category Laxative, Stimulant; Stool Softener

Medication Safety Issues

Sound-alike/look-alike issues:

Senokot® may be confused with Depakote®

Use Short-term treatment of constipation

Unlabeled/Investigational Use Evacuate the colon for bowel or rectal examinations; management/prevention of opiate-induced constipation

Mechanism of Action/Effect Docusate is a stool softener; sennosides are laxatives

(Continued)

Docusate and Senna *(Continued)*

Contraindications Hypersensitivity to any component; intestinal obstruction; acute intestinal inflammation (eg, Crohn's disease); ulcerative colitis; appendicitis; abdominal pain of unknown origin; concurrent use of mineral oil; pregnancy (per Commission E for senna)

Warnings/Precautions Not recommended for over-the-counter (OTC) use in patients experiencing stomach pain, nausea, vomiting, or a sudden change in bowel movements which lasts >2 weeks. OTC labeling does not recommend for use longer than 1 week. Not recommended for OTC use in children <2 years of age.

Adverse Reactions Frequency not defined.

Gastrointestinal: Nausea, vomiting, diarrhea, abdominal cramps

Genitourinary: Urine discoloration (red/brown)

Dosing

Adults: Constipation: OTC ranges: Oral: Initial: 2 tablets (17.2 mg sennosides plus 100 mg docusate) once daily (maximum: 4 tablets twice daily)

Elderly: Constipation: OTC ranges: Oral: Consider half the initial dose in older, debilitated patients

Pediatrics: Constipation: OTC ranges: Oral: Children:

2-6 years: Initial: 4.3 mg sennosides plus 25 mg docusate ($1/2$ tablet) once daily (maximum: 1 tablet twice daily)

6-12 years: Initial: 8.6 sennosides plus 50 mg docusate (1 tablet) once daily (maximum: 2 tablets twice daily)

≥12 years: Refer to adult dosing.

Available Dosage Forms

Tablet: Docusate sodium 50 mg and sennosides 8.6 mg

Peri-Colace® (reformulation): Docusate sodium 50 mg and sennosides 8.6 mg

Senokot-S®: Docusate sodium 50 mg and sennosides 8.6 mg [sugar free; contains sodium 3 mg/tablet]

Monitoring and Teaching Issues

Physical Assessment: Determine cause of constipation before treating. Teach patient proper use, side effects/interventions, and symptoms to report (see Patient Education).

Patient Education: Take exactly as directed. **Do not** exceed recommended dosage. Your urine may be discolored (red-brown) this is normal. Stop use and contact prescriber if you develop nausea, vomiting, persistent diarrhea, or abdominal cramps. If constipation worsens or you experience no relief contact prescriber. **Note:** Increased fluids, fruits, fiber and exercise may help relieve constipation.

Dietary Considerations: Senokot-S®: Sodium content: 3 mg per tablet

Administration

Oral: Once-daily doses should be taken at bedtime.

Additional Information Individual product labeling should be consulted prior to dosing.

Related Information

Docusate *on page 474*

Laxatives, Classification and Properties *on page 1737*

◆ **Docusate Calcium** *see Docusate on page 474*

◆ **Docusate Potassium** *see Docusate on page 474*

◆ **Docusate Sodium** *see Docusate on page 474*

◆ **Docusoft-S™ [OTC]** *see Docusate on page 474*

Dofetilide *(doe FET il ide)*

U.S. Brand Names Tikosyn™

Generic Available No

Pharmacologic Category Antiarrhythmic Agent, Class III

Use Maintenance of normal sinus rhythm in patients with chronic atrial fibrillation/atrial flutter of longer than 1-week duration who have been converted to normal sinus rhythm; conversion of atrial fibrillation and atrial flutter to normal sinus rhythm

Mechanism of Action/Effect Blocks cardiac potassium ion channels and increases action potential duration due to delayed repolarization

Contraindications Hypersensitivity to dofetilide or any component of the formulation; patients with paroxysmal atrial fibrillation; patients with congenital or acquired long QT syndromes, do not use if a baseline QT interval or QT_c is >440 msec (500 msec in patients with ventricular conduction abnormalities); severe renal impairment (estimated Cl_{cr} <20 mL/minute); concurrent use with verapamil, cimetidine, hydrochlorothiazide (alone or in combinations), trimethoprim (alone or in combination with sulfamethoxazole), ketoconazole, prochlorperazine, or megestrol; baseline heart rate <50 beats/minute; other drugs that prolong QT intervals (phenothiazines, cisapride, bepridil, tricyclic antidepressants, certain oral macrolides: sparfloxacin, gatifloxacin, moxifloxacin); hypokalemia or hypomagnesemia; concurrent amiodarone

Warnings/Precautions Note: Must be initiated (or reinitiated) by a cardiologist in a setting with continuous monitoring and staff familiar with the recognition and treatment of life-threatening arrhythmias. Patients must be monitored with continuous ECG for a minimum of 3 days, or for a minimum of 12 hours after electrical or pharmacological cardioversion to normal sinus rhythm, whichever is greater. Patients should be readmitted for continuous monitoring if dosage is later increased.

Reserve for patients who are highly symptomatic with atrial fibrillation/atrial flutter. Torsade de pointes significantly increases with doses >500 mcg twice daily. Hold class I or class III antiarrhythmics for at least three half-lives prior to starting dofetilide. Use in patients on amiodarone therapy only if serum amiodarone level is <0.3 mg/L or if amiodarone was stopped for >3 months previously. Correct hypokalemia or hypomagnesemia before starting dofetilide and maintained within normal limits during treatment. Risk of hypokalemia and/or hypomagnesemia may be increased by potassium-depleting diuretics, increasing the risk of torsade de pointes. Concurrent use with other drugs known to prolong QT_c interval is not recommended.

Patients with sick sinus syndrome or with second or third degree heart block should not receive dofetilide unless a functional pacemaker is in place. Defibrillation threshold is reduced in patients with ventricular tachycardia or ventricular fibrillation undergoing implantation of a cardioverter-defibrillator device. Safety/efficacy in children (<18 years of age) have not been established. Use with caution in renal impairment; not recommended in patients receiving drugs which may compete for renal secretion via cationic transport. Use with caution in patients with severe hepatic impairment.

Drug Interactions

Cytochrome P450 Effect: Substrate of CYP3A4 (minor)

Increased Effect/Toxicity: Dofetilide concentrations are increased by cimetidine, verapamil, ketoconazole, and trimethoprim (concurrent use of these agents is contraindicated). Dofetilide levels may also be increased by renal cationic transport inhibitors (including triamterene, metformin, amiloride, and megestrol). Diuretics and other drugs which may deplete potassium and/or magnesium (aminoglycoside antibiotics, amphotericin, cyclosporine) may increase dofetilide's toxicity (torsade de pointes); concurrent use of hydrochlorothiazide is contraindicated. Use of QT_c-prolonging agents (including bepridil, cisapride, clarithromycin, erythromycin, tricyclic antidepressants, phenothiazines, sparfloxacin, gatifloxacin, moxifloxacin) is contraindicated.

Nutritional/Ethanol Interactions Herb/Nutraceutical: St John's wort may decrease dofetilide levels. Avoid ephedra (may worsen arrhythmia).

Adverse Reactions

Supraventricular arrhythmia patients (incidence > placebo)

>10%: Central nervous system: Headache (11%)

2% to 10%:
Central nervous system: Dizziness (8%), insomnia (4%)
Cardiovascular: Ventricular tachycardia (2.6% to 3.7%), chest pain (10%), torsade de pointes (3.3% in CHF patients and 0.9% in patients with a recent MI; up to 10.5% in patients receiving doses in excess of those recommended). Torsade de pointes occurs most frequently within the first 3 days of therapy.
Dermatologic: Rash (3%)
Gastrointestinal: Nausea (5%), diarrhea (3%), abdominal pain (3%)
Neuromuscular & skeletal: Back pain (3%)
Respiratory: Dyspnea (6%), respiratory tract infection (7%)
Miscellaneous: Flu syndrome (4%)

<2%:
Central nervous system: CVA, facial paralysis, flaccid paralysis, migraine, paralysis
Cardiovascular: AV block (0.4% to 1.5%), ventricular fibrillation (0% to 0.4%), bundle branch block, heart block, edema, heart arrest, myocardial infarct, sudden death, syncope
Dermatologic: Angioedema
Gastrointestinal: Liver damage
Neuromuscular & skeletal: Paresthesia
Respiratory: Cough

>2% (incidence ≤ placebo): Anxiety, pain, angina, atrial fibrillation, hypertension, palpitation, supraventricular tachycardia, peripheral edema, urinary tract infection, weakness, arthralgia, diaphoresis

Overdosage/Toxicology The major dose-related toxicity is torsade de pointes. Treatment should be symptomatic and supportive. Watch for excessive prolongation of the QT interval in overdose situations. Continuous cardiac monitoring is necessary. A charcoal slurry is helpful when given early (15 minutes) after the overdose.

Pharmacodynamics/Kinetics

Absorption: >90%

Bioavailability: >90%

Time to Peak: Fasting: 2-3 hours

Protein Binding: 60% to 70%

Half-Life Elimination: 10 hours

Metabolism: Hepatic via CYP3A4, but low affinity for it; metabolites formed by N-dealkylation and N-oxidation

Excretion: Urine (80%, 80% as unchanged drug, 20% as inactive or minimally active metabolites); renal elimination consists of glomerular filtration and active tubular secretion via cationic transport system

Dosing

Adults: Note: QT_c must be determined prior to first dose

Antiarrhythmic: Oral:
Initial: 500 mcg orally twice daily. Initial dosage must be adjusted in patients with estimated Cl_{cr} <60 mL/minute. Dofetilide may be initiated at lower doses than recommended based on physician discretion.

Modification of dosage in response to initial dose: QT_c interval should be measured 2-3 hours after the initial dose. If the QT_c >15% of baseline, or if the QT_c is >500 msec (550 msec in patients with ventricular conduction abnormalities), dofetilide should be adjusted. If the starting dose is 500 mcg twice daily, then adjust to 250 mcg twice daily. If the starting dose was 250 mcg twice daily, then adjust to 125 mcg twice daily. If the starting dose was 125 mcg twice daily, then adjust to 125 mcg every day.

Continued monitoring for doses 2-5: QT_c interval must be determined 2-3 hours after each subsequent dose of dofetilide for in-hospital doses 2-5. If the measured QT_c is >500 msec (550 msec in patients with ventricular conduction abnormalities) dofetilide should be stopped.

Elderly: Refer to adult dosing. No specific dosage adjustments are recommended based on age; however, careful assessment of renal function is particularly important in this population. See Geriatric Considerations.

Renal Impairment:

Cl_{cr} >60 mL/minute: Administer 500 mcg twice daily.
Cl_{cr} 40-60 mL/minute: Administer 250 mcg twice daily.
Cl_{cr} 20-39 mL/minute: Administer 125 mcg twice daily.

(Continued)

Dofetilide *(Continued)*

Cl_{cr} <20 mL/minute: Contraindicated in this group

Hepatic Impairment: No dosage adjustments required in Child-Pugh class A and B; patients with severe hepatic impairment were not studied.

Available Dosage Forms Capsule: 125 mcg, 250 mcg, 500 mcg

Monitoring and Teaching Issues

Physical Assessment: Assess other medications patient may be taking for effectiveness and interactions. Must be initiated or reinitiated by a cardiologist in a setting with continuous ECG monitoring for a period of time at beginning or adjustment of therapy. Assess results of laboratory tests, therapeutic effectiveness, and adverse reactions at beginning of therapy and on a regular basis with long-term therapy. Assess knowledge/teach patient appropriate use, interventions to reduce side effects, and adverse reactions to report.

Monitoring Laboratory Tests: Serum creatinine; check serum potassium and magnesium levels if on medications where these electrolyte disturbances can occur, or if patient has a history of hypokalemia or hypomagnesemia.

Patient Education: Take exactly as directed; do not take additional doses or discontinue without consulting prescriber. Do not open capsules. If you miss a dose, take your normal amount at the next scheduled time. You will need regular cardiac checkups and blood tests when taking this medication. You may experience headache, dizziness, or difficulty sleeping (use caution when driving or engaging in tasks requiring alertness until response to drug is known); or abdominal pain, diarrhea, or nausea (small frequent meals and increased dietary bulk may help). Inform prescriber immediately if you experience fainting; severe GI discomfort or diarrhea; chest palpitations, irregular heartbeat, or chest pain; increased thirst; respiratory difficulty; skin rash; back pain; or alteration in muscle strength or gait. **Pregnancy/breast-feeding precautions:** Inform your prescriber if you are or intend to become pregnant. Breast-feeding is not recommended.

Pregnancy Risk Factor: C

Pregnancy Issues: Dofetilide has been shown to adversely affect *in utero* growth, organogenesis, and survival of rats and mice. There are no adequate and well-controlled studies in pregnant women. Dofetilide should be used with extreme caution in pregnant women and in women of childbearing age only when the benefit to the patient unequivocally justifies the potential risk to the fetus.

Lactation: Excretion in breast milk unknown/not recommended

Administration

Oral: Do not open capsules.

Related Information

Antiarrhythmic Drugs *on page 1708*

♦ **DOK™ [OTC]** *see Docusate on page 474*

Dolasetron *(dol A se tron)*

U.S. Brand Names Anzemet®

Synonyms Dolasetron Mesylate; MDL 73,147EF

Generic Available No

Pharmacologic Category Antiemetic; Selective 5-HT$_3$ Receptor Antagonist

Medication Safety Issues

Sound-alike/look-alike issues:

Anzemet® may be confused with Aldomet®

Use Prevention of nausea and vomiting associated with emetogenic cancer chemotherapy, including initial and repeat courses; prevention of postoperative nausea and vomiting and treatment of postoperative nausea and vomiting (injectable form only)

Generally **not** recommended for treatment of existing chemotherapy-induced emesis (CIE) or for prophylaxis of nausea from agents with a low emetogenic potential.

Mechanism of Action/Effect Selective 5-HT$_3$ receptor antagonist, blocking serotonin, both peripherally on vagal nerve terminals and centrally in the chemoreceptor trigger zone

Contraindications Hypersensitivity to dolasetron or any component of the formulation

Warnings/Precautions Administer with caution in patients who have or may develop prolongation of cardiac conduction intervals, particularly QT$_c$ intervals. These include patients with hypokalemia, hypomagnesemia, patients taking diuretics which may cause electrolyte disturbances, patients with congenital QT syndrome, patients taking antiarrhythmic drugs or drug which prolong QT interval, and cumulative high-dose anthracycline therapy.

Drug Interactions

Cytochrome P450 Effect: Substrate (minor) of CYP2C8/9, 3A4; **Inhibits** CYP2D6 (weak)

Decreased Effect: Blood levels of active metabolite are decreased during coadministration of rifampin.

Increased Effect/Toxicity: Increased blood levels of active metabolite may occur during concurrent administration of cimetidine and atenolol. Inhibitors of this isoenzyme may increase blood levels of active metabolite. Due to the potential to potentiate QT$_c$ prolongation, drugs which may prolong QT interval directly (eg, antiarrhythmics) or by causing alterations in electrolytes (eg, diuretics) should be used with caution.

Nutritional/Ethanol Interactions Herb/Nutraceutical: St John's wort may decrease dolasetron levels.

Adverse Reactions

>10%:

Central nervous system: Headache (31%), dizziness, lightheadedness (23%)

Gastrointestinal: Loose stools/diarrhea (50%); increased appetite (27%); taste alterations (12%)

1% to 10%:

Cardiovascular: Hypertension, hypotension (6%), ECG abnormalities, prolonged P-R, QRS, and QT$_c$ intervals

Central nervous system: Sedation (8%), slow movement (3%), nervousness (3%), fatigue (2%), listlessness, grogginess

Gastrointestinal: Nausea (6%), constipation (3%), diarrhea, abdominal pain, flatulence
Hepatic: Mild elevations of serum aminotransferases (7%)
Local: Pain at injection site (1%)
Neuromuscular & skeletal: Paresthesia
Ocular: Visual disturbances (mostly blurred vision) (9%); photosensitivity (2%)

Overdosage/Toxicology Prolongation of QT, AV block, severe hypotension, and dizziness have been reported. Treatment is supportive, and continuous ECG monitoring (telemetry) is recommended.

Pharmacodynamics/Kinetics
Half-Life Elimination: Dolasetron: 10 minutes; MDL 74,156: 8 hours
Metabolism: Hepatic to a reduced alcohol (active metabolite MDL 74,156)
Excretion: Urine (as unchanged drug)

Dosing
Adults & Elderly:
Nausea and vomiting associated with cancer chemotherapy:
Oral: 200 mg single dose
I.V.:
0.6-5 mg/kg as a single dose
50 mg 1-2 minute bolus
2.4-3 mg/kg 20-minute infusion
Postoperative nausea and vomiting:
Prevention:
Oral: 100 mg within 2 hours before surgery (doses of 25-200 mg have been used)
I.V.: 12.5 mg ~15 minutes before stopping anesthesia
Treatment: I.V. (only): 12.5 mg as soon as needed
Pediatrics:
Note: Not recommended in children <2 years
Nausea and vomiting prophylaxis, chemotherapy-induced (including initial and repeat courses): Children 2-16 years:
Oral: 1.8 mg/kg within 1 hour before chemotherapy; maximum: 100 mg/dose
I.V.: 1.8 mg/kg ~30 minutes before chemotherapy; maximum: 100 mg/dose
Postoperative nausea and vomiting: Children 2-16 years:
Prevention:
Oral: 1.2 mg/kg within 2 hours before surgery; maximum: 100 mg/dose
I.V.: 0.35 mg/kg (maximum: 12.5 mg) ~15 minutes before stopping anesthesia
Treatment: I.V. (only): 0.35 mg/kg as soon as needed

Available Dosage Forms
Injection, solution, as mesylate: 20 mg/mL (0.625 mL, 5 mL) [single-use ampuls and vial]; 20 mg/mL (25 mL) [multidose vial]
Tablet, as mesylate: 50 mg, 100 mg

Monitoring and Teaching Issues
Physical Assessment: See Warnings/Precautions for use cautions (eg presence of or potential for prolongation of cardiac conduction intervals). Assess potential for interactions with other pharmacological agents or herbal products patient may be taking (eg, antiarrhythmics, diuretics; see Drug Interactions). Assess therapeutic effectiveness and adverse reactions (eg, cardiac abnormalities; see Adverse Reactions) on a regular basis. Teach patient possible side effects/appropriate interventions and adverse symptoms to report (see Patient Education).
Patient Education: This drug is given to reduce the incidence of nausea and vomiting. May cause headache, drowsiness, or dizziness (request assistance when getting up or changing position and do not perform activities requiring alertness until response to drug is known). Report immediately any chest pain, rapid heartbeat, or palpitations; unusual pain, chills, or fever; severe headache or diarrhea; chest pain, palpitations, or tightness; swelling of throat or feeling of tightness in throat; or difficulty urinating.
Pregnancy Risk Factor: B
Lactation: Excretion in breast milk unknown

Administration
Oral: I.V. injection solution may be diluted in apple or apple-grape juice.
I.V.: I.V. injection may be given either undiluted IVP over 30 seconds or infused over 15 minutes.
Reconstitution: Dilute in 50-100 mL of a compatible solution.
Compatibility: Stable in 0.9% NS, D$_5$W, D$_5$W and 0.45% NS, D$_5$W and LR, LR, and 10% mannitol injection
Storage: Store intact vials at room temperature. Protect from light. After dilution, I.V. dolasetron is stable under normal lighting conditions at room temperature for 24 hours or under refrigeration for 48 hours with the following **compatible** intravenous fluids: 0.9% sodium chloride injection, 5% dextrose injection, 5% dextrose and 0.45% sodium chloride injection, 5% dextrose and lactated Ringer's injection, lactated Ringer's injection, and 10% mannitol injection

Additional Information Efficacy of dolasetron, for chemotherapy treatment, is enhanced with concomitant administration of dexamethasone 20 mg (increases complete response by 10% to 20%). Oral administration of the intravenous solution is equivalent to tablets. A single I.V. dose of dolasetron mesylate (1.8 or 2.4 mg/kg) has comparable safety and efficacy to a single 32 mg I.V. dose of ondansetron in patients receiving cisplatin chemotherapy.

Related Information
Antiemetics for Chemotherapy-Induced Nausea and Vomiting *on page 1788*

- **Dolasetron Mesylate** *see Dolasetron on page 478*
- **Dolgic® LQ** *see Butalbital, Acetaminophen, and Caffeine on page 225*
- **Dolgic® Plus** *see Butalbital, Acetaminophen, and Caffeine on page 225*
- **Dolobid®** *see Diflunisal on page 450*
- **Dolophine®** *see Methadone on page 967*

Donepezil (doh NEP e zil)

U.S. Brand Names Aricept®
Synonyms E2020
Generic Available No
Pharmacologic Category Acetylcholinesterase Inhibitor (Central)
Medication Safety Issues
Sound-alike/look-alike issues:
Aricept® may be confused with AcipHex®, Ascriptin®
Use Treatment of mild to moderate dementia of the Alzheimer's type
Unlabeled/Investigational Use Attention-deficit/hyperactivity disorder (ADHD), behavioral syndromes in dementia
Mechanism of Action/Effect Alzheimer's disease is characterized by cholinergic deficiency in the cortex and basal forebrain, which contributes to cognitive deficits. Donepezil reversibly and noncompetitively inhibits centrally-active acetylcholinesterase, the enzyme responsible for hydrolysis of acetylcholine. This appears to result in increased concentrations of acetylcholine available for synaptic transmission in the central nervous system.
Contraindications Hypersensitivity to donepezil, piperidine derivatives, or any component of the formulation
Warnings/Precautions May cause bradycardia and/or heart block with or without a history of cardiac disease; syncopal episodes have been associated with donepezil. Use with caution in patients with sick sinus syndrome or other supraventricular cardiac conduction abnormalities, in patients with seizures, COPD, or asthma; avoid use in nursing mothers. Use with caution in patients at risk of ulcer disease (ie, previous history or NSAID use), or in patients with bladder outlet obstruction. May cause diarrhea, nausea, and/or vomiting, which may be dose-related.
Drug Interactions
Cytochrome P450 Effect: Substrate (minor) of CYP2D6, 3A4
Decreased Effect: Anticholinergic agents (benztropine) may inhibit the effects of donepezil.
Increased Effect/Toxicity: A synergistic effect may be seen with concurrent administration of succinylcholine or cholinergic agonists (bethanechol).
Nutritional/Ethanol Interactions Herb/Nutraceutical: St John's wort may decrease donepezil levels.
Adverse Reactions
>10%:
Central nervous system: Headache
Gastrointestinal: Nausea, diarrhea
1% to 10%:
Cardiovascular: Syncope, chest pain, hyper-/hypotension, atrial fibrillation, hot flashes
Central nervous system: Abnormal dreams, depression, dizziness, fatigue, insomnia, somnolence
Dermatologic: Bruising
Gastrointestinal: Anorexia, vomiting, weight loss, fecal incontinence, GI bleeding, bloating, epigastric pain
Genitourinary: Frequent urination
Neuromuscular & skeletal: Muscle cramps, arthritis, body pain
Overdosage/Toxicology Implement general supportive measures. Donepezil can cause a cholinergic crisis characterized by severe nausea, vomiting, salivation, sweating, bradycardia, hypotension, collapse, and convulsions. Increased muscle weakness is a possibility and may result in death if respiratory muscles are involved.

Tertiary anticholinergics, such as atropine, may be used as an antidote for overdose. I.V. atropine sulfate titrated to effect is recommended with an initial dose of 1-2 mg I.V., with subsequent doses based upon clinical response. Atypical increases in blood pressure and heart rate have been reported with other cholinomimetics when coadministered with quaternary anticholinergics such as glycopyrrolate.
Pharmacodynamics/Kinetics
Absorption: Well absorbed
Bioavailability: 100%
Time to Peak: Plasma: 3-4 hours
Protein Binding: 96%, primarily to albumin (75%) and α_1-acid glycoprotein (21%)
Half-Life Elimination: 70 hours; time to steady-state: 15 days
Metabolism: Extensively to four major metabolites (two are active) via CYP2D6 and 3A4; undergoes glucuronidation
Excretion: Urine (as unchanged drug)
Dosing
Adults & Elderly: Alzheimer's disease: Oral: Initial: 5 mg/day at bedtime; may increase to 10 mg/day at bedtime after 4-6 weeks.
Pediatrics: ADHD (unlabeled use): Oral: 5 mg/day
Available Dosage Forms Tablet, as hydrochloride: 5 mg, 10 mg
Monitoring and Teaching Issues
Physical Assessment: Assess bladder adequacy prior to administering medication. Assess other medications patient may be taking for effectiveness and interactions. Assess results of laboratory tests, therapeutic effect, and adverse reactions (eg, cholinergic crisis). Monitor pulse. Assess knowledge/teach patient appropriate use, interventions to reduce side effects, and adverse symptoms to report.
Patient Education: This medication will not cure the disease, but may help reduce symptoms. Use as directed; do not increase dose or discontinue without consulting prescriber. Maintain adequate hydration (2-3 L/day of fluids) unless instructed to restrict fluid intake. May cause dizziness, sedation, or hypotension (rise slowly from sitting or lying position and use caution when driving or climbing stairs); vomiting or loss of appetite (small frequent meals, frequent mouth care, chewing gum, or sucking lozenges may help); or diarrhea (boiled milk, yogurt, or buttermilk may help). Report persistent abdominal discomfort; significantly increased salivation, sweating, tearing, or urination; flushed skin; chest pain or

palpitations; acute headache; unresolved diarrhea; excessive fatigue, insomnia, dizziness, or depression; increased muscle, joint, or body pain; vision changes or blurred vision; or shortness of breath or wheezing. **Pregnancy/breast-feeding precautions:** Inform prescriber if you are or intend to become pregnant. Breast-feeding is not recommended.

Geriatric Considerations: Donepezil is a new anticholinesterase for the treatment of Alzheimer's disease. It has been shown to cause an improvement in the ADAS-cog scores. As compared to tacrine, donepezil does **not** cause elevations in liver function tests and does not require routine laboratory monitoring. In addition, it is dosed once a day versus tacrine's four doses per day. For these reasons, donepezil may be preferred over tacrine in the treatment of mild to moderate dementia of the Alzheimer's type.

Pregnancy Risk Factor: C

Lactation: Excretion in breast milk unknown/not recommended

Additional Information Donepezil does not significantly elevate liver enzymes.

♦ **Donnatal®** *see* Hyoscyamine, Atropine, Scopolamine, and Phenobarbital *on page 777*

♦ **Donnatal Extentabs®** *see* Hyoscyamine, Atropine, Scopolamine, and Phenobarbital *on page 777*

DOPamine (DOE pa meen)

Synonyms Dopamine Hydrochloride; Intropin

Generic Available Yes

Pharmacologic Category Adrenergic Agonist Agent

Medication Safety Issues
Sound-alike/look-alike issues:
DOPamine may be confused with DOBUTamine, Dopram®

Use Adjunct in the treatment of shock (eg, MI, open heart surgery, renal failure, cardiac decompensation) which persists after adequate fluid volume replacement

Unlabeled/Investigational Use Symptomatic bradycardia or heart block unresponsive to atropine or pacing

Mechanism of Action/Effect Stimulates both adrenergic and dopaminergic receptors, lower doses are mainly dopaminergic stimulating and produce renal and mesenteric vasodilation, higher doses also are both dopaminergic and beta$_1$-adrenergic stimulating and produce cardiac stimulation and renal vasodilation; large doses stimulate alpha-adrenergic receptors

Contraindications Hypersensitivity to sulfites (commercial preparation contains sodium bisulfite); pheochromocytoma; ventricular fibrillation

Warnings/Precautions Use with caution in patients with cardiovascular disease or cardiac arrhythmias or patients with occlusive vascular disease. Correct hypovolemia and electrolytes when used in hemodynamic support. May cause increases in HR and arrhythmia. Avoid infiltration - may cause severe tissue necrosis. Use with caution in post-MI patients. Avoid sudden discontinuation.

Drug Interactions
Decreased Effect: Tricyclic antidepressants may have a decreased effect when coadministered with dopamine. Guanethidine's hypotensive effects may only be partially reversed; may need to use a direct-acting sympathomimetic.

Increased Effect/Toxicity: Dopamine's effects are prolonged and intensified by MAO inhibitors, alpha- and beta-adrenergic blockers, cocaine, general anesthetics, methyldopa, phenytoin, reserpine, and TCAs.

Adverse Reactions Frequency not defined.
Cardiovascular: Ectopic beats, tachycardia, anginal pain, palpitation, hypotension, vasoconstriction
Central nervous system: Headache
Gastrointestinal: Nausea and vomiting
Respiratory: Dyspnea

Overdosage/Toxicology Symptoms of overdose include severe hypertension, cardiac arrhythmias, acute renal failure. Treat symptomatically.

Important: Antidote for peripheral ischemia: To prevent sloughing and necrosis in ischemic areas, the area should be infiltrated as soon as possible with 10-15 mL of saline solution containing 5-10 mg of Regitine (brand of phentolamine), an adrenergic blocking agent. A syringe with a fine hypodermic needle should be used, and the solution liberally infiltrated throughout the ischemic area. Sympathetic blockade with phentolamine causes immediate and conspicuous local hyperemic changes if the area is infiltrated within 12 hours. Therefore, phentolamine should be given as soon as possible after extravasation is noted.

Pharmacodynamics/Kinetics
Onset of Action: Adults: 5 minutes
Duration of Action: Adults: <10 minutes
Half-Life Elimination: 2 minutes
Metabolism: Renal, hepatic, plasma; 75% to inactive metabolites by monoamine oxidase and 25% to norepinephrine
Excretion: Urine (as metabolites)
Clearance: Neonates: Varies and appears to be age related; prolonged clearance with combined hepatic and renal impairment
Pharmacokinetic Note: Dopamine has exhibited nonlinear kinetics in children; with medication changes, may not achieve steady-state for ~1 hour rather than 20 minutes.

Dosing
Adults & Elderly:
Hemodynamic support: I.V. infusion: 1-5 mcg/kg/minute up to 50 mcg/kg/minute, titrate to desired response; infusion may be increased by 1-4 mcg/kg/minute at 10- to 30-minute intervals until optimal response is obtained
Note: If dosages >20-30 mcg/kg/minute are needed, a more direct-acting vasopressor may be more beneficial (ie, epinephrine, norepinephrine).
Hemodynamic effects of dopamine are dose dependent:
Low-dose: 1-5 mcg/kg/minute, increased renal blood flow and urine output
(Continued)

DOPamine *(Continued)*

Intermediate-dose: 5-15 mcg/kg/minute, increased renal blood flow, heart rate, cardiac contractility, and cardiac output

High-dose: >15 mcg/kg/minute, alpha-adrenergic effects begin to predominate, vasoconstriction, increased blood pressure

Pediatrics: Hemodynamic support: I.V. infusion:

Children: 1-20 mcg/kg/minute, maximum: 50 mcg/kg/minute continuous infusion, titrate to desired response.

Available Dosage Forms

Infusion, as hydrochloride [premixed in D_5W]: 0.8 mg/mL (250 mL, 500 mL); 1.6 mg/mL (250 mL, 500 mL); 3.2 mg/mL (250 mL)

Injection, solution, as hydrochloride: 40 mg/mL (5 mL, 10 mL); 80 mg/mL (5 mL); 160 mg/mL (5 mL) [contains sodium metabisulfite]

Monitoring and Teaching Issues

Physical Assessment: Assess other medications patient may be taking for effectiveness and interactions. Infusion pump, continuous cardiac and hemodynamic monitoring, and frequent assessment of I.V. site is required for inpatient therapy. Low-dose home infusion therapy requires frequent monitoring of cardiac and renal status and adverse reactions. Monitor therapeutic effectiveness and adverse reactions. Instruct patient on adverse symptoms to report.

Monitoring Laboratory Tests: Serum glucose, renal function

Patient Education: When administered in emergencies, patient education should be appropriate to the situation. If patient is aware, instruct to promptly report chest pain, palpitations, rapid heartbeat, headache, nervousness or restlessness, nausea or vomiting, or respiratory difficulty.

Geriatric Considerations: Has not been specifically studied in the elderly.

Pregnancy Risk Factor: C

Lactation: Excretion in breast milk unknown

Administration

I.V.: Vesicant. **Must be diluted prior to use.** Do not discontinue suddenly - sudden discontinuation may lead to marked hypotension.

Compatibility: Stable in D_5LR, $D_5^{1}/_2NS$, D_5NS, D_5W, $D_{10}W$, LR, mannitol 20%, NS; **incompatible** with sodium bicarbonate 5%, and alkaline solutions or iron salts.

Y-site administration: Incompatible with acyclovir, alteplase, amphotericin B cholesteryl sulfate complex, cefepime, indomethacin, insulin (regular), thiopental

Compatibility when admixed: Incompatible with acyclovir, alteplase, amphotericin B, ampicillin, metronidazole with sodium bicarbonate, penicillin G potassium

Storage: Protect from light. Solutions that are darker than slightly yellow should not be used.

Additional Information Dopamine is most frequently used for treatment of hypotension because of its peripheral vasoconstrictor action. In this regard, dopamine is often used together with dobutamine and minimizes hypotension secondary to dobutamine-induced vasodilation. Thus, pressure is maintained by increased cardiac output (from dobutamine) and vasoconstriction (by dopamine). It is critical neither dopamine nor dobutamine be used in patients in the absence of correcting any hypovolemia as a cause of hypotension.

Low-dose dopamine is often used in the intensive care setting for presumed beneficial effects on renal function. However, there is no clear evidence that low-dose dopamine confers any renal or other benefit. Indeed, dopamine may act on dopamine receptors in the carotid bodies causing chemoreflex suppression. In patients with heart failure, dopamine may inhibit breathing and cause pulmonary shunting. Both these mechanisms would act to decrease minute ventilation and oxygen saturation. This could potentially be deleterious in patients with respiratory compromise and patients being weaned from ventilators.

Related Information

Compatibility of Drugs *on page 1723*
FDA Name Differentiation Project: The Use of Tall-Man Letters *on page 15*
Inotropic and Vasoconstrictor Comparison *on page 1736*

♦ **Dopamine Hydrochloride** *see* DOPamine *on page 481*

Dornase Alfa *(DOOR nase AL fa)*

U.S. Brand Names Pulmozyme®

Synonyms DNase; Recombinant Human Deoxyribonuclease

Generic Available No

Pharmacologic Category Enzyme

Use Management of cystic fibrosis patients to reduce the frequency of respiratory infections that require parenteral antibiotics, and to improve pulmonary function

Unlabeled/Investigational Use Treatment of chronic bronchitis

Mechanism of Action/Effect The hallmark of cystic fibrosis lung disease is the presence of abundant, purulent airway secretions composed primarily of highly polymerized DNA. Dornase selectively cleaves DNA, thus reducing mucous viscosity and as a result, airflow in the lung is improved and the risk of bacterial infection may be decreased.

Contraindications Hypersensitivity to dornase alfa, Chinese hamster ovary cell products (eg, epoetin alfa), or any component of the formulation

Warnings/Precautions No clinical trials have been conducted to demonstrate safety and effectiveness of dornase in children <5 years of age, in patients with pulmonary function <40% of normal, or in patients for longer treatment periods >12 months.

Adverse Reactions

>10%:

Respiratory: Pharyngitis

Miscellaneous: Voice alteration

1% to 10%:

Cardiovascular: Chest pain

Dermatologic: Rash

Ocular: Conjunctivitis

Respiratory: Laryngitis, cough, dyspnea, hemoptysis, rhinitis, hoarse throat, wheezing

Pharmacodynamics/Kinetics

Onset of Action: Nebulization: Enzyme levels are measured in sputum in ~15 minutes

Duration of Action: Rapidly declines

Dosing

Adults & Elderly: Mucolytic: Inhalation: 2.5 mg once daily through selected nebulizers

Pediatrics:

Mucolytic (cystic fibrosis): Inhalation:

Children >3 months to Adults: 2.5 mg once daily through selected nebulizers; experience in children <5 years is limited

Note: Patients unable to inhale or exhale orally throughout the entire treatment period may use Pari-Baby™ nebulizer. Some patients may benefit from twice daily administration.

Available Dosage Forms Solution for nebulization: 1 mg/mL (2.5 mL)

Monitoring and Teaching Issues

Physical Assessment: Assess effectiveness of therapy (reduced incidence of pulmonary infections or improved pulmonary function) and adverse reactions (see Adverse Reactions) at beginning of therapy and periodically with long-term use. Teach patient or caregiver appropriate use of nebulizer and adverse symptoms to report (see Patient Education).

Patient Education: Use exactly as directed by prescriber (see following administration information). Report any signs of adverse response, skin rash, sore throat, respiratory wheezing, cough, or respiratory difficulty. **Breast-feeding precaution:** Consult prescriber if breast-feeding.

Self-administered nebulizer: Store in refrigerator, away from light. Do not combine with any other medications in the nebulizer. Wash hands before and after treatment. Wash and dry nebulizer after each treatment. Twist open the top of one unit dose vial and squeeze contents into nebulizer reservoir. Connect nebulizer reservoir to the mouthpiece or face mask. Connect nebulizer to compressor. Sit in comfortable, upright position. Put on face mask and turn on compressor. Avoid leakage around the mask to avoid mist getting into eyes. Breathe calmly and deeply until no more mist is formed in nebulizer (about 5 minutes). At this point, treatment is finished.

Pregnancy Risk Factor: B

Lactation: Excretion in breast milk unknown

Administration

Compatibility: Should not be diluted or mixed with any other drugs in the nebulizer, this may inactivate the dornase alfa.

Storage: Must be stored in the refrigerator at 2°C to 8°C (36°F to 46°F) and protected from strong light. Should not be exposed to room temperature for a total of 24 hours.

♦ **Doryx®** *see* Doxycycline *on page 496*

Dorzolamide (dor ZOLE a mide)

U.S. Brand Names Trusopt®

Synonyms Dorzolamide Hydrochloride

Generic Available No

Pharmacologic Category Carbonic Anhydrase Inhibitor; Ophthalmic Agent, Antiglaucoma

Use Lowers intraocular pressure in patients with ocular hypertension or open-angle glaucoma

Contraindications Hypersensitivity to dorzolamide or any component of the formulation

Warnings/Precautions Although administered topically, systemic absorption occurs. Similar adverse reactions attributed to sulfonamides may occur. Chemical similarities are present among sulfonamides, sulfonylureas, carbonic anhydrase inhibitors, thiazides, and loop diuretics (except ethacrynic acid). In patients with allergy to one of these compounds, a risk of cross-reaction exists; avoid use when previous reaction has been severe. Not recommended for use in patients with severe renal impairment (Cl_{cr} <30 mL/minute); use with caution in patients with hepatic impairment. detachment has been reported after filtration procedures.

Contains benzalkonium chloride is the preservative which may be absorbed by soft contact lenses. Dorzolamide should not be administered while wearing soft contact lenses. Safety and efficacy in children <2 years of age have not been established.

Drug Interactions

Cytochrome P450 Effect: Substrate (minor) of CYP2C8/9, 3A4

Increased Effect/Toxicity: High-dose salicylate therapy may result in carbonic anhydrase inhibitor accumulation and toxicity including CNS depression and metabolic acidosis; avoid use if possible.

Adverse Reactions

>10%:

Gastrointestinal: Bitter taste following administration (25%)

Ocular: Burning, stinging or discomfort immediately following administration (33%); superficial punctate keratitis (10% to 15%); signs and symptoms of ocular allergic reaction (10%)

1% to 5%: Ocular: Blurred vision, conjunctivitis, dryness, lid reactions, photophobia, tearing

Overdosage/Toxicology Symptoms of overdose include electrolyte imbalance, development of an acidotic state and possible CNS effects. Treatment should be symptom-directed and supportive.

Pharmacodynamics/Kinetics

Onset of Action: Peak effect: 2 hours

Duration of Action: 8-12 hours

Absorption: Topical: Reaches systemic circulation where it accumulates in RBCs during chronic dosing as a result of binding to CA-11

Protein Binding: 33%

Half-Life Elimination: Terminal RBC: 147 days; washes out of RBCs nonlinearly, resulting in a rapid decline of drug concentration initially, followed by a slower elimination phase with a half-life of about 4 months

(Continued)

Dorzolamide *(Continued)*

Metabolism: To N-desethyl metabolite (less potent than parent drug)

Excretion: Urine (as unchanged drug and metabolite, N-desethyl)

Dosing

Adults & Elderly: Reduction of intraocular pressure: Ophthalmic: Instill 1 drop in the affected eye(s) 3 times/day

Pediatrics: Refer to adult dosing.

Available Dosage Forms Solution, ophthalmic, as hydrochloride: 2% (5 mL, 10 mL) [contains benzalkonium chloride]

Monitoring and Teaching Issues

Physical Assessment: Assess potential for interactions with other prescriptions, OTC medications, or herbal products patient may be taking. Assess therapeutic response and adverse effects. Teach patient proper use, side effects/appropriate interventions, and symptoms to report.

Patient Education: For use in eyes only. If serious or unusual reactions or signs of hypersensitivity occur, discontinue use of the product. If any ocular reactions, particularly conjunctivitis and lid reactions, discontinue use and notify prescriber. If an intercurrent ocular condition (eg, trauma, ocular surgery, infection) occur, immediately seek your prescriber's advice concerning the continued use of the present multidose container. Avoid allowing the tip of the dispensing container to contact the eye or surround structures. Take out contact lenses before using medicine. Lenses can be replaced 15 minutes after medicine is given. **Pregnancy precaution:** Inform prescriber if you are pregnant.

Pregnancy Risk Factor: C

Lactation: Excretion in breast milk unknown/not recommended

Administration

Other: If more than one topical ophthalmic drug is being used, administer the drugs at least 10 minutes apart. Instruct patients to avoid allowing the tip of the dispensing container to contact the eye or surrounding structures. Ocular solutions can become contaminated by common bacteria known to cause ocular infections. Serious damage to the eye and subsequent loss of vision may occur from using contaminated solutions.

Storage: Store at room temperature (25°C).

Related Information

Glaucoma Drug Therapy *on page 1827*

- **Dorzolamide Hydrochloride** *see* Dorzolamide *on page 483*
- **DOS® [OTC]** *see* Docusate *on page 474*
- **DOSS** *see* Docusate *on page 474*
- **Dovonex®** *see* Calcipotriene *on page 231*

Doxacurium *(doks a KYOO ri um)*

U.S. Brand Names Nuromax®

Synonyms Doxacurium Chloride

Generic Available No

Pharmacologic Category Neuromuscular Blocker Agent, Nondepolarizing

Medication Safety Issues

Sound-alike/look-alike issues:

Doxacurium may be confused with doxapram, DOXOrubicin

Use Adjunct to general anesthesia to facilitate endotracheal intubation and to relax skeletal muscles during surgery; to facilitate mechanical ventilation in ICU patients; does not relieve pain or produce sedation; the characteristics of this agent make it especially useful in procedures requiring careful maintenance of hemodynamic stability for prolonged periods

Mechanism of Action/Effect Prevents depolarization of muscle membrane and subsequent muscle contraction by acting as a competitive antagonist to acetylcholine at the alpha subunits of the nicotinic cholinergic receptors on the motor endplates in skeletal muscle, also interferes with the mobilization of acetylcholine presynaptically; the neuromuscular blockade can be pharmacologically reversed with an anticholinesterase agent (neostigmine, edrophonium, pyridostigmine)

Contraindications Hypersensitivity to doxacurium or any component of the formulation

Warnings/Precautions Use with caution in the elderly, effects and duration are more variable; product contains benzyl alcohol, use with caution in newborns; use with caution in patients with renal or hepatic impairment; certain clinical conditions may result in potentiation or antagonism of neuromuscular blockade

Increased sensitivity in patients with myasthenia gravis, Eaton-Lambert syndrome; resistance in burn patients (>30% of body) for period of 5-70 days postinjury; resistance in patients with muscle trauma, denervation, immobilization, infection; does not counteract bradycardia produced by anesthetics/vagal stimulation. Cross-sensitivity with other neuromuscular-blocking agents may occur; use extreme caution in patients with previous anaphylactic reactions.

Drug Interactions

Decreased Effect: Effect of nondepolarizing neuromuscular blockers may be reduced by carbamazepine (chronic use), corticosteroids (also associated with myopathy - see increased effect), phenytoin (chronic use), sympathomimetics, and theophylline.

Increased Effect/Toxicity: Increased effects are possible with aminoglycosides, beta-blockers, clindamycin, calcium channel blockers, halogenated anesthetics, imipenem, ketamine, lidocaine, loop diuretics (furosemide), macrolides (case reports), magnesium sulfate, procainamide, quinidine, quinolones, tetracyclines, and vancomycin. May increase risk of myopathy when used with high- dose corticosteroids for extended periods.

Overdosage/Toxicology

Overdosage is manifested by prolonged neuromuscular blockage.

Treatment is supportive; reverse blockade with neostigmine, pyridostigmine, or edrophonium.

Pharmacodynamics/Kinetics
Onset of Action: 5-11 minutes

Duration of Action: 30 minutes (range: 12-54 minutes)

Protein Binding: 30%

Excretion: Primarily urine and feces (as unchanged drug); recovery time prolonged in elderly

Dosing
Adults & Elderly: Administer I.V.; dose to effect; doses will vary due to interpatient variability; use ideal body weight for obese patients.

Surgery (adjunct to anesthesia): I.V.: 0.05-0.08 mg/kg with thiopental/narcotic or 0.025 mg/kg after initial dose of succinylcholine for intubation; initial maintenance dose of 0.005-0.01 mg/kg after 100-160 minutes followed by repeat doses every 30-45 minutes
Pretreatment/priming: I.V.: 10% of intubating dose given 3-5 minutes before initial dose

Neuromuscular blockade in the ICU : I.V.: 0.05 mg/kg bolus followed by 0.025 mg/kg every 2-3 hours or 0.25-0.75 mcg/kg/minute once initial recovery from bolus dose observed

Pediatrics: Note: Administer I.V.; dose to effect; doses will vary due to interpatient variability; use ideal body weight for obese patients

Surgery (adjunct to anesthesia): Children >2 years: I.V.: Initial: 0.03-0.05 mg/kg followed by maintenance doses of 0.005-0.01 mg/kg after 30-45 minutes

Renal Impairment: Reduce initial dose and titrate carefully as duration may be prolonged.

Available Dosage Forms Injection, solution, as chloride: 1 mg/mL (5 mL) [contains benzyl alcohol]

Monitoring and Teaching Issues
Physical Assessment: Only clinicians experienced in the use of neuromuscular blocking drugs should administer and/or manage the use of doxacurium. Dosage and rate of administration should be individualized and titrated to the desired effect, according to relevant clinical factors, premedication, concomitant medications, age, and general condition of the patient. Ventilatory support must be instituted and maintained until adequate respiratory muscle function and/or airway protection are assured. Assess other medications for effectiveness and safety. Other drugs that affect neuromuscular activity may increase/decrease neuromuscular block induced by doxacurium. This drug does not cause anesthesia or analgesia; pain must be treated with appropriate analgesic agents. Continuous monitoring of vital signs, cardiac status, respiratory status, and degree of neuromuscular block (objective assessment with peripheral external nerve stimulator) is mandatory during infusion and until full muscle tone has returned. Muscle tone returns in a predictable pattern, starting with diaphragm, abdomen, chest, limbs, and finally muscles of the neck, face, and eyes. Safety precautions must be maintained until full muscle tone has returned. **Note:** It may take longer for return of muscle tone in obese or elderly patients or patients with renal or hepatic disease, myasthenia gravis, myopathy, other neuromuscular disease, dehydration, electrolyte imbalance, or severe acid/base imbalance. Provide appropriate patient teaching/support prior to and following administration.

Long-term use: Monitor fluid levels (intake and output) during and following infusion. Reposition patient and provide appropriate skin care, mouth care, and care of patient's eyes every 2-3 hours while sedated. Provide appropriate emotional and sensory support (auditory and environmental).

Patient Education: Patient will usually be unconscious prior to administration. Patient education should be appropriate to individual situation. Reassurance of constant monitoring and emotional support to reduce fear and anxiety should precede and follow administration. Following return of muscle tone, do not attempt to change position or rise from bed without assistance. Report immediately any skin rash or hives, pounding heartbeat, respiratory difficulty, or muscle tremors. **Pregnancy precaution:** Inform prescriber if you are pregnant.

Pregnancy Risk Factor: C

Administration
I.V.: May be given rapid I.V. injection undiluted or via a continuous infusion using an infusion pump. Use infusion solutions within 24 hours of preparation.

Compatibility: Stable in D_5LR, D_5NS, D_5W, LR, NS

Storage: Stable for 24 hours at room temperature when diluted, up to 0.1 mg/mL in dextrose 5% or normal saline.

Additional Information Doxacurium is a long-acting nondepolarizing neuromuscular blocker with virtually no cardiovascular side effects. Characteristics of this agent make it especially useful in procedures requiring careful maintenance of hemodynamic stability for prolonged periods; reduce dosage in renal or hepatic impairment. It does not relieve pain or produce sedation. It does not appear to have a cumulative effect on duration of blockade.

♦ **Doxacurium Chloride** *see* Doxacurium *on page 484*

Doxazosin (doks AY zoe sin)
U.S. Brand Names Cardura®

Synonyms Doxazosin Mesylate

Generic Available Yes

Pharmacologic Category Alpha₁ Blocker

Medication Safety Issues
Sound-alike/look-alike issues:
Doxazosin may be confused with doxapram, doxepin, DOXOrubicin
Cardura® may be confused with Cardene®, Cordarone®, Cordran®, Coumadin®, K-Dur®, Ridaura®

Use Treatment of hypertension alone or in conjunction with diuretics, cardiac glycosides, ACE inhibitors, or calcium antagonists (particularly appropriate for those with hypertension and other cardiovascular risk factors such as hypercholesterolemia and diabetes mellitus); treatment of urinary outflow obstruction and/or obstructive and irritative symptoms associated with
(Continued)

Doxazosin *(Continued)*

benign prostatic hyperplasia (BPH), particularly useful in patients with troublesome symptoms who are unable or unwilling to undergo invasive procedures, but who require rapid symptomatic relief; can be used in combination with finasteride

Mechanism of Action/Effect Competitively inhibits postsynaptic alpha-adrenergic receptors which results in vasodilation of veins and arterioles and a decrease in total peripheral resistance and blood pressure; approximately 50% as potent on a weight by weight basis as prazosin

Contraindications Hypersensitivity to quinazolines (prazosin, terazosin), doxazosin, or any component of the formulation; concurrent use with phosphodiesterase-5 (PDE-5) inhibitors including sildenafil (>25 mg), tadalafil, or vardenafil

Warnings/Precautions Can cause significant orthostatic hypotension and syncope, especially with first dose. Prostate cancer should be ruled out before starting for BPH. May need dosage adjustment in severe hepatic dysfunction. Anticipate a similar effect if therapy is interrupted for a few days, if dosage is rapidly increased, or if another antihypertensive drug is introduced.

Drug Interactions

Decreased Effect: Decreased hypotensive effect with NSAIDs.

Increased Effect/Toxicity: Increased hypotensive effect with beta-blockers, diuretics, ACE inhibitors, calcium channel blockers, other antihypertensive medications, sildenafil (use with extreme caution at a dose ≤25 mg), tadalafil (contraindicated by the manufacturer), and vardenafil (contraindicated by the manufacturer).

Nutritional/Ethanol Interactions Herb/Nutraceutical: Avoid dong quai if using for hypertension (has estrogenic activity). Avoid ephedra, yohimbe, ginseng (may worsen hypertension). Avoid saw palmetto when used for BPH (due to limited experience with this combination). Avoid garlic (may have increased antihypertensive effect).

Lab Interactions Increased urinary VMA 17%, norepinephrine metabolite 42%

Adverse Reactions Note: "Combination therapy" refers to doxazosin and finasteride.

>10%:

Cardiovascular: Postural hypotension (combination therapy 18%)

Central nervous system: Dizziness (16% to 19%; combination therapy 23%), headache (10% to 14%)

Endocrine & metabolic: Impotence (combination therapy 23%), libido decreased (combination therapy 12%)

Genitourinary: Ejaculation disturbances (combination therapy 14%)

Neuromuscular & skeletal: Weakness (combination therapy 17%)

1% to 10%:

Cardiovascular: Orthostatic hypotension (dose related; 0.3% up to 10%), edema (3% to 4%), hypotension (2%), palpitation (1% to 2%), chest pain (1% to 2%), arrhythmia (1%), syncope (2%), flushing (1%)

Central nervous system: Fatigue (8% to 12%), somnolence (3% to 5%), nervousness (2%), pain (2%), vertigo (2%), insomnia (1%), anxiety (1%), paresthesia (1%), movement disorder (1%), ataxia (1%), hypertonia (1%), depression (1%), weakness (1%)

Dermatologic: Rash (1%), pruritus (1%)

Endocrine & metabolic: Sexual dysfunction (2%)

Gastrointestinal: Abdominal pain (2%), diarrhea (2%), dyspepsia (1% to 2%), nausea (2% to 3%), xerostomia (1% to 2%), constipation (1%), flatulence (1%)

Genitourinary: Urinary tract infection (1%), impotence (1%), polyuria (2%), incontinence (1%)

Neuromuscular & skeletal: Back pain (2%), arthritis (1%), muscle weakness (1%), myalgia (1%), muscle cramps (1%)

Ocular: Abnormal vision (1% to 2%), conjunctivitis (1%)

Otic: Tinnitus (1%)

Respiratory: Rhinitis (3%), dyspnea (1% to 3%), respiratory disorder (1%), epistaxis (1%)

Miscellaneous: Diaphoresis increased (1%), flu-like syndrome (1%)

Overdosage/Toxicology Symptoms of overdose include severe hypotension, drowsiness, and tachycardia. Treatment is supportive and symptomatic.

Pharmacodynamics/Kinetics

Duration of Action: >24 hours

Time to Peak: Serum: 2-3 hours

Half-Life Elimination: 22 hours

Metabolism: Extensively hepatic

Excretion: Feces (63%); urine (9%)

Pharmacokinetic Note: Not significantly affected by increased age.

Dosing

Adults: Hypertension or urinary outflow obstruction: Oral: 1 mg once daily in morning or evening; may be increased to 2 mg once daily; thereafter titrate upwards, if needed, over several weeks, balancing therapeutic benefit with doxazosin-induced postural hypotension; maximum dose for **hypertension** is 16 mg/day, for **BPH:** 8 mg/day (goal: 4-8 mg/day)

Elderly: Oral: Initial: 0.5 mg once daily

Available Dosage Forms Tablet: 1 mg, 2 mg, 4 mg, 8 mg

Monitoring and Teaching Issues

Physical Assessment: See Warnings/Precautions for use caution. Assess potential for interactions with other pharmacological agents or herbal products patient may be taking (see Drug Interactions). Assess results of laboratory tests, therapeutic effectiveness (blood pressure), and adverse reactions (eg, hypotension, CNS changes, urinary retention; see Adverse Reactions) at beginning of therapy and on a regular basis with long-term therapy. When discontinuing, blood pressure should be closely monitored and dose tapered slowly over 1 week or more. Teach patient proper use, possible side effects/appropriate interventions, and adverse symptoms to report (see Patient Education).

Monitoring Laboratory Tests: White blood count

Patient Education: Do not take any new medication during therapy unless approved by prescriber. Take as directed, at bedtime. Do not skip dose or discontinue without consulting prescriber. Follow recommended diet and exercise program. May cause drowsiness, dizziness, or impaired judgment (use caution when driving or engaging in tasks that require alertness until response to drug is known); postural hypotension (use caution when rising from sitting or lying position or when climbing stairs); dry mouth or nausea (frequent mouth care or sucking lozenges may help). Report increased nervousness or depression; sudden weight gain (weigh yourself in the same clothes at the same time of day once a week); unusual or persistent swelling of ankles, feet, or extremities; palpitations or rapid heartbeat; muscle weakness, fatigue, or pain; or other persistent side effects. **Pregnancy/ breast-feeding precautions:** Inform prescriber if you are or intend to become pregnant. Consult prescriber if breast-feeding.

Geriatric Considerations: Adverse reactions such as dry mouth and urinary problems can be particularly bothersome in the elderly.

Pregnancy Risk Factor: C

Lactation: Excretion in breast milk unknown

Administration

Oral: Syncope may occur usually within 90 minutes of the initial dose.

Additional Information First-dose hypotension occurs less frequently with doxazosin as compared to prazosin; this may be due to its slower onset of action.

Related Information

Pharmacotherapy of Urinary Incontinence *on page 1858*

♦ **Doxazosin Mesylate** *see* Doxazosin *on page 485*

Doxepin (DOKS e pin)

U.S. Brand Names Prudoxin™; Sinequan®; Zonalon®

Synonyms Doxepin Hydrochloride

Restrictions A medication guide should be dispensed with each prescription. A template for the required MedGuides can be found on the FDA website at: http://www.fda.gov/cder/drug/antidepressants/labelTemplate.pdf

Generic Available Yes: Capsule, solution

Pharmacologic Category Antidepressant, Tricyclic (Tertiary Amine); Topical Skin Product

Medication Safety Issues

Sound-alike/look-alike issues:

Doxepin may be confused with digoxin, doxapram, doxazosin, Doxidan®, doxycycline

Sinequan® may be confused with saquinavir, Serentil®, Seroquel®, Singulair®

Zonalon® may be confused with Zone-A Forte®

Use

Oral: Depression

Topical: Short-term (<8 days) management of moderate pruritus in adults with atopic dermatitis or lichen simplex chronicus

Unlabeled/Investigational Use Analgesic for certain chronic and neuropathic pain; anxiety

Mechanism of Action/Effect Increases the synaptic concentration of serotonin and norepinephrine in the central nervous system by inhibition of their reuptake by the presynaptic neuronal membrane

Contraindications Hypersensitivity to doxepin, drugs from similar chemical class, or any component of the formulation; narrow-angle glaucoma; urinary retention; use of MAO inhibitors within 14 days; use in a patient during acute recovery phase of MI

Warnings/Precautions Antidepressants increase the risk of suicidal thinking and behavior in children and adolescents with major depressive disorder (MDD) and other depressive disorders; consider risk prior to prescribing. All patients must be closely monitored for clinical worsening, suicidality, or unusual changes in behavior, especially during the initiation of therapy or following an increase or decrease in dosage. When used in children, the child's family or caregiver should be instructed to closely observe the patient and communicate condition with healthcare provider. A medication guide should be dispensed with each prescription. **Doxepin is approved for treatment of depression in adolescents.**

The possibility of a suicide attempt is inherent in major depression and may persist until remission occurs. Use caution in high-risk patients. Worsening depression and severe abrupt suicidality that are not part of the presenting symptoms may require discontinuation or modification of drug therapy. The patient's family or caregiver should be alerted to monitor patients for the emergence of suicidality and associated behaviors (such as agitation, irritability, hostility, impulsivity, and hypomania) and call healthcare provider.

May worsen psychosis in some patients or precipitate a shift to mania or hypomania in patients with bipolar disorder. Patients presenting with depressive symptoms should be screened for bipolar disorder. Monotherapy in patients with bipolar disorder should be avoided. **Doxepin is not FDA approved for the treatment of bipolar depression.**

The risks of sedative and anticholinergic effects are high relative to other antidepressant agents. Doxepin frequently causes sedation, which may result in impaired performance of tasks requiring alertness (eg, operating machinery or driving). Sedative effects may be additive with other CNS depressants and/or ethanol. Also use caution in patients with benign prostatic hyperplasia, xerostomia, visual problems, constipation, or history of bowel obstruction.

May cause orthostatic hypotension or conduction disturbances (risks are moderate relative to other antidepressants). Use with caution in patients with a history of cardiovascular disease (including previous MI, stroke, tachycardia, or conduction abnormalities). Consider discontinuation, when possible, prior to elective surgery. Therapy should not be abruptly discontinued in patients receiving high doses for prolonged periods.

Use caution in patients with a previous seizure disorder or condition predisposing to seizures such as brain damage, alcoholism, or concurrent therapy with other drugs which lower the
(Continued)

Doxepin (Continued)

seizure threshold. Use with caution in hyperthyroid patients or those receiving thyroid supplementation. Use with caution in patients with hepatic or renal dysfunction and in elderly patients.

Cream formulation is for external use only (not for ophthalmic, vaginal, or oral use). Do not use occlusive dressings. Use for >8 days may increase risk of contact sensitization. Doxepin is significantly absorbed following topical administration; plasma levels may be similar to those achieved with oral administration.

Drug Interactions

Cytochrome P450 Effect: Substrate (major) of CYP1A2, 2D6, 3A4

Decreased Effect: CYP1A2 inducers may decrease the levels/effects of doxepin; example inducers include aminoglutethimide, carbamazepine, phenobarbital, and rifampin. Doxepin inhibits the antihypertensive response to bethanidine, clonidine, debrisoquin, guanadrel, guanethidine, guanabenz, and guanfacine. Cholestyramine and colestipol may bind TCAs and reduce their absorption. CYP3A4 inducers may decrease the levels/effects of doxepin; example inducers include aminoglutethimide, carbamazepine, nafcillin, nevirapine, phenobarbital, phenytoin, and rifamycins.

Increased Effect/Toxicity: Doxepin increases the effects of amphetamines, anticholinergics, other CNS depressants (sedatives, hypnotics, or ethanol), chlorpropamide, tolazamide, and warfarin. When used with MAO inhibitors, hyperpyrexia, hypertension, tachycardia, confusion, seizures, and **deaths have been reported** (serotonin syndrome). Serotonin syndrome has also been reported with ritonavir (rare).

CYP1A2 inhibitors may increase the levels/effects of doxepin; example inhibitors include amiodarone, ciprofloxacin, fluvoxamine, ketoconazole, norfloxacin, ofloxacin, and rofecoxib. CYP2D6 inhibitors may increase the levels/effects of doxepin; example inhibitors include chlorpromazine, delavirdine, fluoxetine, miconazole, paroxetine, pergolide, quinidine, quinine, ritonavir, and ropinirole. CYP3A4 inhibitors may increase the levels/effects of doxepin. Example inhibitors include azole antifungals, ciprofloxacin, clarithromycin, diclofenac, doxycycline, erythromycin, imatinib, isoniazid, nefazodone, nicardipine, propofol, protease inhibitors, quinidine, and verapamil. Cimetidine, grapefruit juice, indinavir, methylphenidate, diltiazem, and verapamil may increase the serum concentrations of TCAs. Use of lithium with a TCA may increase the risk for neurotoxicity. Phenothiazines may increase concentration of some TCAs and TCAs may increase concentration of phenothiazines.

Pressor response to I.V. epinephrine, norepinephrine, and phenylephrine may be enhanced in patients receiving TCAs (**Note:** Effect is unlikely with epinephrine or levonordefrin dosages typically administered as infiltration in combination with local anesthetics). Combined use of beta-agonists or drugs which prolong QT_c (including quinidine, procainamide, disopyramide, cisapride, sparfloxacin, gatifloxacin, moxifloxacin) with TCAs may predispose patients to cardiac arrhythmias.

Nutritional/Ethanol Interactions

Ethanol: Avoid ethanol (may increase CNS depression).

Food: Grapefruit juice may inhibit the metabolism of some TCAs and clinical toxicity may result.

Herb/Nutraceutical: Avoid valerian, St John's wort, SAMe, kava kava (may increase risk of serotonin syndrome and/or excessive sedation).

Lab Interactions Increased glucose

Adverse Reactions

Oral: Frequency not defined.

Cardiovascular: Hyper-/hypotension, tachycardia

Central nervous system: Drowsiness, dizziness, headache, disorientation, ataxia, confusion, seizure

Dermatologic: Alopecia, photosensitivity, rash, pruritus

Endocrine & metabolic: Breast enlargement, galactorrhea, SIADH, increase or decrease in blood sugar, increased or decreased libido

Gastrointestinal: Xerostomia, constipation, vomiting, indigestion, anorexia, aphthous stomatitis, nausea, unpleasant taste, weight gain, diarrhea, trouble with gums, decreased lower esophageal sphincter tone may cause GE reflux

Genitourinary: Urinary retention, testicular edema

Hematologic: Agranulocytosis, leukopenia, eosinophilia, thrombocytopenia, purpura

Neuromuscular & skeletal: Weakness, tremor, numbness, paresthesia, extrapyramidal symptoms, tardive dyskinesia

Ocular: Blurred vision

Otic: Tinnitus

Miscellaneous: Diaphoresis (excessive), allergic reactions

Topical:

>10%:

Central nervous system: Drowsiness (22%)

Dermatologic: Stinging/burning (23%)

1% to 10%:

Cardiovascular: Edema (1%)

Central nervous system: Dizziness (2%), emotional changes (2%)

Gastrointestinal: Xerostomia (10%), taste alteration (2%)

Overdosage/Toxicology Symptoms of overdose include confusion, hallucinations, seizures, urinary retention, hypothermia, hypotension, tachycardia, and cyanosis. Following initiation of essential overdose management, toxic symptoms should be treated symptomatically.

Pharmacodynamics/Kinetics

Onset of Action: Peak effect: Antidepressant: Usually >2 weeks; Anxiolytic: May occur sooner

Absorption: Following topical application, plasma levels may be similar to those achieved with oral administration

Protein Binding: 80% to 85%
Half-Life Elimination: Adults: 6-8 hours
Metabolism: Hepatic; metabolites include desmethyldoxepin (active)
Excretion: Urine
Dosing
Adults:
  Depression and/or anxiety (unlabeled use): Oral: Initial: 25-150 mg/day at bedtime or in 2-3 divided doses; may gradually increase up to 300 mg/day; single dose should not exceed 150 mg; select patients may respond to 25-50 mg/day.
  Chronic urticaria, angioedema, nocturnal pruritus: Oral: 10-30 mg/day
  Pruritus: Topical: Apply a thin film 4 times/day with at least 3- to 4-hour interval between applications; not recommended for use >8 days. (Oral administration of doxepin 25-50 mg has also been used, but systemic adverse effects are increased.)
Elderly:
  Depression and/or anxiety (unlabeled use): Oral: Initial: 10-25 mg at bedtime; increase by 10-25 mg every 3 days for inpatients and weekly for outpatients if tolerated. Rarely does the maximum dose required exceed 75 mg/day; a single bedtime dose is recommended.
  Pruritus: Topical: Refer to adult dosing.
Pediatrics:
  Depression and/or anxiety: Oral:
    Children (unlabeled use): 1-3 mg/kg/day in single or divided doses
    Adolescents: Initial: 25-50 mg/day in single or divided doses; gradually increase to 100 mg/day
Hepatic Impairment: Use a lower dose and adjust gradually.
Available Dosage Forms [DSC] = Discontinued product
  Capsule, as hydrochloride: 10 mg, 25 mg, 50 mg, 75 mg, 100 mg, 150 mg
    Sinequan®: 10 mg, 25 mg, 50 mg, 75 mg, 100 mg [DSC], 150 mg [DSC]
  Cream, as hydrochloride:
    Prudoxin™: 5% (45 g) [contains benzyl alcohol]
    Zonalon®: 5% (30 g, 45 g) [contains benzyl alcohol]
  Solution, oral concentrate, as hydrochloride (Sinequan®): 10 mg/mL (120 mL)
Monitoring and Teaching Issues
  Physical Assessment: Assess other medications patient may be taking for effectiveness and interactions. Assess results of laboratory tests, therapeutic effectiveness, and adverse reactions at beginning of therapy and periodically with long-term use. Monitor CNS status. Be alert for signs of clinical worsening, suicidal ideation, or other changes in behavior. Taper dosage slowly when discontinuing. Assess knowledge/teach patient appropriate use, interventions to reduce side effects, and adverse symptoms to report.
  Patient Education: Oral: Take exactly as directed; do not increase dose or frequency. It may take several weeks to achieve desired results. Avoid alcohol, caffeine, and other prescription or OTC medications not approved by prescriber. Maintain adequate hydration (2-3 L/day of fluids) unless instructed to restrict fluid intake. You may experience drowsiness, lightheadedness, impaired coordination, dizziness, or blurred vision (use caution when driving or engaging in tasks requiring alertness until response to drug is known); constipation (increased exercise, fluids, fruit, or fiber may help); urinary retention (void before taking medication); postural hypotension (use caution climbing stairs or when changing position from lying or sitting to standing); altered sexual drive or ability (reversible); or photosensitivity (use sunscreen, wear protective clothing and eyewear, and avoid direct sunlight). Report persistent CNS effects (eg, nervousness, restlessness, insomnia, anxiety, excitation, headache, agitation, impaired coordination, changes in cognition); muscle cramping, weakness, tremors, or rigidity; chest pain, palpitations, or irregular heartbeat; blurred vision or eye pain; yellowing of skin or eyes; or worsening of condition.
  Pregnancy/breast-feeding precautions: Inform prescriber if you are or intend to become pregnant. Breast-feeding is not recommended.
  Topical: Use as directed. Apply in thin layer; do not overuse. Report increased skin irritation, worsening of condition or lack of improvement.
  Geriatric Considerations: The oral form is the preferred agent when sedation is a desired property. Less potential for anticholinergic effects than amitriptyline and less orthostatic hypotension than imipramine. However, dosing should be approached cautiously, initiated at the low end of the dosage range.
  Pregnancy Risk Factor: B (cream); C (all other forms)
  Lactation: Enters breast milk/not recommended (AAP rates "of concern")
  Breast-Feeding Issues: Generally, it is not recommended to breast-feed if taking antidepressants because of the long half-life, active metabolites, and the potential for side effects in the infant.
Administration
  Oral: Do not mix oral concentrate with carbonated beverages (physically incompatible).
  Topical: Apply thin film to affected area; use of occlusive dressings is not recommended.
  Storage: Protect from light.
Related Information
  Antidepressant Agents *on page 1713*
  Antidepressant Medication Guidelines *on page 1765*
  Federal OBRA Regulations: Recommended Maximum Doses *on page 1773*

 ◆ **Doxepin Hydrochloride** *see* Doxepin *on page 487*

Doxercalciferol (doks er kal si fe FEER ole)
U.S. Brand Names Hectorol®
Synonyms 1α-Hydroxyergocalciferol
Generic Available No
Pharmacologic Category Vitamin D Analog
Use Treatment of secondary hyperparathyroidism in patients with chronic kidney disease
Mechanism of Action/Effect Doxercalciferol is metabolized to the active form of vitamin D.
(Continued)

Doxercalciferol *(Continued)*

Contraindications Hypersensitivity to any component of the formulation; history of hypercalcemia or evidence of vitamin D toxicity

Warnings/Precautions Other forms of vitamin D should be discontinued when doxercalciferol is started. Hyperphosphatemia should be corrected before initiating therapy. Use with caution in patients with hepatic impairment. Safety and efficacy have not been established in pediatric patients.

Drug Interactions

Decreased Effect: Absorption of doxercalciferol is reduced with mineral oil and cholestyramine.

Increased Effect/Toxicity: Doxercalciferol toxicity may be increased by concurrent use of other vitamin D supplements or magnesium-containing antacids and supplements.

Adverse Reactions

Note: As reported in dialysis patients.

>10%:
Cardiovascular: Edema (34%)
Central nervous system: Headache (28%), malaise (28%), dizziness (12%)
Gastrointestinal: Nausea/vomiting (24%)
Respiratory: Dyspnea (12%)

1% to 10%:
Cardiovascular: Bradycardia (7%)
Central nervous system: Sleep disorder (3%)
Dermatologic: Pruritus (8%)
Gastrointestinal: Anorexia (5%), constipation (3%), dyspepsia (5%), weight gain (5%)
Neuromuscular & skeletal: Arthralgia (5%)
Miscellaneous: Abscess (3%)

Overdosage/Toxicology Doxercalciferol, in excess, can cause hypercalcemia, hypercalciuria, hyperphosphatemia, and oversuppression of PTH secretion. Following withdrawal of the drug and calcium supplements, hypercalcemia treatment consists of a low calcium diet and monitoring. Adjustments of calcium in the dialysis bath can also be made if necessary. When calcium levels normalize, doxercalciferol can be restarted. Reduce each dose by at least 2.5 mcg. Monitor serum calcium levels closely.

Signs and symptoms of early hypercalcemia include: Anorexia, bone pain, constipation, headache, metallic taste, muscle pain, nausea, somnolence, vomiting, weakness, xerostomia

Signs and symptoms of late hypercalcemia include: Albuminuria, anorexia, apathy, AST/ALT increased, BUN increased, cardiac arrhythmias, conjunctivitis (calcific), dehydration, ectopic calcification, growth arrested, hypercholesterolemia, hypertension, hyperthermia, libido decreased, nocturia, pancreatitis, photophobia, polydipsia, polyuria, pruritus, psychosis (rare), rhinorrhea, sensory disturbances, urinary tract infections, weight loss

Pharmacodynamics/Kinetics

Half-Life Elimination: Active metabolite: 32-37 hours; up to 96 hours

Metabolism: Hepatic via CYP27

Dosing

Adults & Elderly: Secondary hyperparathyroidism:

Oral:

Dialysis patients: Dose should be titrated to lower iPTH to 150-300 pg/mL; dose is adjusted at 8-week intervals (maximum dose: 20 mcg 3 times/week)

Initial dose: iPTH >400 pg/mL: 10 mcg 3 times/week at dialysis

Dose titration:

iPTH level decreased by 50% and >300 pg/mL: Dose can be increased to 12.5 mcg 3 times/week for 8 more weeks; this titration process can continue at 8-week intervals; each increase should be by 2.5 mcg/dose

iPTH level 150-300 pg/mL: Maintain current dose

iPTH level <100 pg/mL: Suspend doxercalciferol for 1 week; resume at a reduced dose; decrease each dose (not weekly dose) by at least 2.5 mcg

Predialysis patients: Dose should be titrated to lower iPTH to 35-70 pg/mL with stage 3 disease or to 70-110 pg/mL with stage 4 disease: Dose may be adjusted at 2-week intervals (maximum dose: 3.5 mcg/day)

Initial dose: 1 mcg/day

Dose titration:

iPTH level >70 pg/mL with stage 3 disease or >110 pg/mL with stage 4 disease: Increase dose by 0.5 mcg every 2 weeks as necessary

iPTH level 35-70 pg/mL with stage 3 disease or 70-110 pg/mL with stage 4 disease: Maintain current dose

iPTH level is <35 pg/mL with stage 3 disease or <70 pg/mL with stage 4 disease: Suspend doxercalciferol for 1 week, then resume at a reduced dose (at least 0.5 mcg lower)

I.V.:

Dialysis patients: Dose should be titrated to lower iPTH to 150-300 pg/mL; dose is adjusted at 8-week intervals (maximum dose: 18 mcg/week)

Initial dose: iPTH level >400 pg/mL: 4 mcg 3 times/week after dialysis, administered as a bolus dose

Dose titration:

iPTH level decreased by 50% and >300 pg/mL: Dose can be increased by 1-2 mcg at 8-week intervals, as necessary

iPTH level 150-300 pg/mL: Maintain the current dose

iPTH level <100 pg/mL: Suspend doxercalciferol for 1 week; resume at a reduced dose (at least 1 mcg lower)

Renal Impairment: No adjustment is required.
Hepatic Impairment: Use caution in these patients; no guidelines for dosage adjustment.
Available Dosage Forms
 Capsule: 0.5 mcg, 2.5 mcg [contains coconut oil]
 Injection, solution: 2 mcg/mL (2 mL) [contains disodium edetate]
Monitoring and Teaching Issues
 Physical Assessment: Monitor therapeutic effectiveness (laboratory results), adverse reactions. Monitor for fluid retention. Assess knowledge/teach patient appropriate use, interventions to reduce side effects, and adverse reactions to report.
 Monitoring Laboratory Tests:
  Dialysis patients: Before initiating, check iPTH, serum calcium and phosphorus. Check weekly thereafter until stable. Serum iPTH, calcium, phosphorus, and alkaline phosphatase should be monitored.
  Predialysis patients: iPTH, serum calcium and phosphorus every 2 weeks for 3 months following initiation and dose adjustments, then monthly for 3 months, then every 3 months
 Patient Education: Be clear on dose and directions for taking. Stop other vitamin D products. Do not miss doses. Avoid magnesium-containing antacids and supplements. Report headache, dizziness, weakness, sleepiness, severe nausea, vomiting, dry mouth, loss of appetite, constipation, metallic taste, muscle and/or bone pain, significant fluid retention, malaise, shortness of breath, and difficulty thinking or concentrating to your prescriber. Do not take over-the-counter medicines or supplements without first consulting your prescriber. Follow diet and calcium supplements as directed by your prescriber.
 Dietary Considerations: Based on serum levels, dietary phosphorus may be restricted and/or controlled with calcium-based phosphorus binders. The daily combined calcium intake (dietary and calcium based phosphate binder) should be 1.5-2 g. Additional vitamin D supplements and magnesium-containing antacids should be avoided. Capsules contain coconut oil.
 Pregnancy Risk Factor: B
 Lactation: Excretion in breast milk unknown/not recommended
 Breast-Feeding Issues: Excretion in breast milk is unknown. Other vitamin D derivatives are excreted in breast milk; there is a potential for adverse effects. Therefore, the manufacturer recommends that breast-feeding be discontinued or doxercalciferol discontinued, depending upon importance of the drug to the mother.
Administration
 Storage: Store at controlled room temperature of 15°C to 30°C (59°F to 86°F). The injection should be protected from light.

♦ **Doxil**® *see* DOXOrubicin (Liposomal) *on page 493*

DOXOrubicin (doks oh ROO bi sin)

U.S. Brand Names Adriamycin PFS®; Adriamycin RDF®; Rubex®
Synonyms ADR; Adria; Doxorubicin Hydrochloride; Hydroxydaunomycin Hydrochloride; Hydroxyldaunorubicin Hydrochloride; NSC-123127
Generic Available Yes
Pharmacologic Category Antineoplastic Agent, Anthracycline
Medication Safety Issues
 Sound-alike/look-alike issues:
  DOXOrubicin may be confused with dactinomycin, DAUNOrubicin, doxacurium, doxapram, doxazosin, idarubicin
  Adriamycin PFS® may be confused with achromycin, Aredia®, Idamycin®
  Rubex® may be confused with Robaxin®
  Conventional formulations (Adriamycin PFS®, Adriamycin RDF®, Rubex®) may be confused with liposomal formulations (DaunoXome®, Doxil®)
Use Treatment of leukemias, lymphomas, multiple myeloma, osseous and nonosseous sarcomas, mesotheliomas, germ cell tumors of the ovary or testis, and carcinomas of the head and neck, thyroid, lung, breast, stomach, pancreas, liver, ovary, bladder, prostate, uterus, and neuroblastoma
Mechanism of Action/Effect Inhibits DNA and RNA synthesis, active throughout cell cycle, results in cell death.
Contraindications Hypersensitivity to doxorubicin or any component of the formulation; congestive heart failure or arrhythmias; previous therapy with high cumulative doses of doxorubicin and/or daunorubicin; pre-existing bone marrow suppression; pregnancy
Warnings/Precautions The U.S. Food and Drug Administration (FDA) currently recommends that procedures for proper handling and disposal of antineoplastic agents be considered. Total dose should not exceed 550 mg/m² or 450 mg/m² in patients with previous or concomitant treatment with daunorubicin, cyclophosphamide, or irradiation of the cardiac region. Irreversible myocardial toxicity may occur as total dosage approaches 550 mg/m². I.V. use only, severe local tissue necrosis will result if extravasation occurs. Elderly and pediatric patients are at higher risk of cardiotoxicity (delayed). Reduce dose in patients with impaired hepatic function. Severe myelosuppression is also possible. Administration of live vaccines to immunosuppressed patients may be hazardous. Heart failure may occur during therapy or months to years after therapy. Treatment may increase the risk of other neoplasms. Secondary acute myelogenous leukemia may occur following treatment.
Drug Interactions
 Cytochrome P450 Effect: Substrate (major) of CYP2D6, 3A4; **Inhibits** CYP2B6 (moderate), 2D6 (weak), 3A4 (weak)
 Decreased Effect: The levels/effects of doxorubicin may be decreased by aminoglutethimide, carbamazepine, nafcillin, nevirapine, phenobarbital, phenytoin, rifamycins, and other CYP3A4 inducers. Doxorubicin may decrease plasma levels and effectiveness of digoxin. Doxorubicin may decrease the antiviral activity of zidovudine.
 Increased Effect/Toxicity: Allopurinol may enhance the antitumor activity of doxorubicin (animal data only). Cyclosporine may increase doxorubicin levels, enhancing hematologic toxicity or may induce coma or seizures. Cyclophosphamide enhances the cardiac toxicity
(Continued)

DOXOrubicin *(Continued)*

of doxorubicin by producing additional myocardial cell damage. Mercaptopurine increases doxorubicin toxicities. Streptozocin greatly enhances leukopenia and thrombocytopenia. Verapamil alters the cellular distribution of doxorubicin and may result in increased cell toxicity by inhibition of the P-glycoprotein pump. Paclitaxel reduces doxorubicin clearance and increases toxicity if administered prior to doxorubicin. High doses of progesterone enhance toxicity (neutropenia and thrombocytopenia).

Doxorubicin may increase the levels/effects of bupropion, promethazine, propofol, selegiline, sertraline, and other CYP2B6 substrates. The levels/effects of doxorubicin may be increased by azole antifungals, chlorpromazine, ciprofloxacin, clarithromycin, delavirdine, diclofenac, doxycycline, erythromycin, fluoxetine, imatinib, isoniazid, miconazole, nefazodone, nicardipine, paroxetine, pergolide, propofol, protease inhibitors, quinidine, quinine, ritonavir, ropinirole, telithromycin, verapamil and other inhibitors of CYP2D6 or 3A4. Based on mouse studies, cardiotoxicity may be enhanced by verapamil. Concurrent therapy with actinomycin-D may result in recall pneumonitis following radiation.

Nutritional/Ethanol Interactions Herb/Nutraceutical: St John's wort may decrease doxorubicin levels. Avoid black cohosh, dong quai in estrogen-dependent tumors.

Adverse Reactions

>10%:

Dermatologic: Alopecia, radiation recall

Gastrointestinal: Nausea, vomiting, stomatitis, GI ulceration, anorexia, diarrhea

Genitourinary: Discoloration of urine, mild dysuria, urinary frequency, hematuria, bladder spasms, cystitis following bladder instillation

Hematologic: Myelosuppression, primarily leukopenia (75%); thrombocytopenia and anemia

Onset: 7 days

Nadir: 10-14 days

Recovery: 21-28 days

1% to 10%:

Cardiovascular: Transient ECG abnormalities (supraventricular tachycardia, S-T wave changes, atrial or ventricular extrasystoles); generally asymptomatic and self-limiting. CHF, dose related, may be delayed for 7-8 years after treatment. Cumulative dose, mediastinal/pericardial radiation therapy, cardiovascular disease, age, and use of cyclophosphamide (or other cardiotoxic agents) all increase the risk.

Recommended maximum cumulative doses:

No risk factors: 550 mg/m^2

Concurrent radiation: 450 mg/m^2

Note: Regardless of cumulative dose, if the left ventricular ejection fraction is <30% to 40%, the drug is usually not given.

Dermatologic: Skin "flare" at injection site; discoloration of saliva, sweat, or tears

Endocrine & metabolic: Hyperuricemia

Overdosage/Toxicology Symptoms of overdose include myelosuppression, nausea, vomiting, and myocardial toxicity. Treatment of acute overdose consists of treatment of the severely myelosuppressed patient with hospitalization, antibiotics, platelet and granulocyte transfusions, and symptomatic treatment of mucositis.

Pharmacodynamics/Kinetics

Absorption: Oral: Poor (<50%)

Protein Binding: Plasma: 70%

Half-Life Elimination:

Distribution: 10 minutes

Elimination: Doxorubicin: 1-3 hours; Metabolites: 3-3.5 hours

Terminal: 17-30 hours

Male: 54 hours; Female: 35 hours

Metabolism: Primarily hepatic to doxorubicinol (active), then to inactive aglycones, conjugated sulfates, and glucuronides

Excretion: Feces (~40% to 50% as unchanged drug); urine (~3% to 10% as metabolites, 1% doxorubicinol, <1% Adriamycin aglycones, and unchanged drug)

Clearance: Male: 113 L/hour; Female: 44 L/hour

Dosing

Adults & Elderly: Refer to individual protocols.

Usual or typical dose: I.V.: 60-75 mg/m^2 as a single dose, repeat every 21 days **or** other dosage regimens like 20-30 mg/m^2/day for 2-3 days, repeat in 4 weeks **or** 20 mg/m^2 once weekly.

Note: The lower dose regimen should be given to patients with decreased bone marrow reserve, prior therapy or marrow infiltration with malignant cells.

Pediatrics: Refer to individual protocols. Usual/typical dosages: I.V.:

Children:

35-75 mg/m^2 as a single dose, repeat every 21 days **or**

20-30 mg/m^2 once weekly **or**

60-90 mg/m^2 given as a continuous infusion over 96 hours every 3-4 weeks

Renal Impairment:

Adjustments are not required.

Hemodialysis effects: Supplemental dose is not necessary.

Hepatic Impairment:

ALT/AST 2-3 times ULN: Administer 75% of dose

ALT/AST >3 times ULN **or** bilirubin 1.2-3 mg/dL (20-51 μmol/L): Administer 50% of dose

Bilirubin 3.1-5 mg/dL (51-85 μmol/L): Administer 25% of dose

Bilirubin >5 mg/dL (85 μmol/L): Do not administer

Available Dosage Forms

Injection, powder for reconstitution, as hydrochloride: 10 mg, 20 mg, 50 mg [contains lactose]

Adriamycin RDF®: 10 mg, 20 mg, 50 mg, 150 mg [contains lactose; rapid dissolution formula]

Rubex®: 50 mg, 100 mg [contains lactose]

Injection, solution, as hydrochloride [preservative free]: 2 mg/mL (5 mL, 10 mL, 25 mL, 100 mL)

Adriamycin PFS® [preservative free]: 2 mg/mL (5 mL, 10 mL, 25 mL, 37.5 mL, 100 mL)

Monitoring and Teaching Issues

Physical Assessment: Note Warnings/Precautions for use cautions (eg, impaired renal function, existing cardiovascular disease). Assess potential for interactions with other pharmacological agents or herbal products patient may be taking (eg, potential to reduce or increase levels/effects of doxorubicin; see Drug Interactions). See Administration infusion specifics. Premedication with antiemetic is recommended (especially with larger doses). Infusion site must be closely monitored; extravasation can cause sloughing or tissue necrosis (do not apply heat or sodium bicarbonate). Assess results of laboratory tests and patient response prior to each treatment and on a regular basis throughout therapy. Teach patient possible side effects/appropriate interventions (eg, importance of adequate hydration) and adverse symptoms to report (see Patient Education).

Monitoring Laboratory Tests: CBC with differential, platelet count, cardiac and liver function

Patient Education: Do not take any new medication during therapy unless approved by prescriber. This medication can only be administered intravenously. Report immediately any swelling, pain, burning, redness at infusion site, sudden difficulty breathing or swallowing, chest pains, or chills. Maintain adequate nutrition (small frequent meals may help). You will be more susceptible to infection (avoid crowds and exposure to infection and do not have any vaccinations without consulting prescriber). May cause nausea or vomiting (small frequent meals, frequent mouth care, sucking lozenges, or chewing gum may help); diarrhea (buttermilk, boiled milk, or yogurt may help); loss of hair (reversible); or darker yellow urine (normal). Report immediately chest pain, swelling of extremities, respiratory difficulty, palpitations, or rapid heartbeat. Report unresolved nausea, vomiting, or diarrhea; alterations in urinary pattern (increased or decreased); opportunistic infection (fever, chills, unusual bruising or bleeding fatigue, purulent vaginal discharge, unhealed mouth sores); abdominal pain or blood in stools; excessive fatigue; or yellowing of eyes or skin. **Pregnancy/breast-feeding precautions:** Inform prescriber if you are pregnant. Do not get pregnant while taking this medication or for 1 month following therapy. Consult prescriber for appropriate contraceptives. Do not breast-feed.

Pregnancy Risk Factor: D

Pregnancy Issues: Advise patients to avoid becoming pregnant (females) and to avoid causing pregnancy (males).

Lactation: Enters breast milk/contraindicated

Administration

I.V.: Vesicant. Administer I.V. push over 1-2 minutes or IVPB. Infusion via central venous line recommended.

Reconstitution: Reconstitute lyophilized powder with NS to a final concentration of 2 mg/mL as follows. Reconstituted solution is stable for 7 days at room temperature (25°C) and 15 days under refrigeration (5°C) when protected from light.

Further dilution in D$_5$W or NS is stable for 48 hours at room temperature (25°C) when protected from light.

Unstable in solutions with a pH <3 or >7. Avoid aluminum needles as precipitation or decomposition (darkening of solution) may occur; protect from direct sunlight.

Standard I.V. dilution:

I.V. push: Dose/syringe (concentration: 2 mg/mL)

Syringes are stable for 7 days at room temperature (25°C) and 15 days under refrigeration (5°C) when protected from light.

IVPB: Dose/50-100 mL D$_5$W or NS

IVPB solutions are stable for 48 hours at room temperature (25°C) when protected from light.

Compatibility: Stable in D$_5$W, LR, NS

Y-site administration: Incompatible with allopurinol, amphotericin B cholesteryl sulfate complex, cefepime, ganciclovir, piperacillin/tazobactam, propofol

Compatibility in syringe: Incompatible with furosemide, heparin

Compatibility when admixed: Incompatible with aminophylline, diazepam, fluorouracil

Storage: Store intact vials of solution under refrigeration at 2°C to 8°C and protected from light. Store intact vials of lyophilized powder at room temperature (15°C to 30°C).

Related Information

FDA Name Differentiation Project: The Use of Tall-Man Letters *on page 15*

♦ **Doxorubicin Hydrochloride** *see* DOXOrubicin *on page 491*

♦ **Doxorubicin Hydrochloride (Liposomal)** *see* DOXOrubicin (Liposomal) *on page 493*

DOXOrubicin (Liposomal) (doks oh ROO bi sin lip pah SOW mal)

U.S. Brand Names Doxil®

Synonyms Doxorubicin Hydrochloride (Liposomal)

Generic Available No

Pharmacologic Category Antineoplastic Agent, Anthracycline

Medication Safety Issues

Sound-alike/look-alike issues:

DOXOrubicin may be confused with dactinomycin, DAUNOrubicin, doxacurium, doxapram, doxazosin, idarubicin

Doxil® may be confused with Doxy®, Paxil®

Liposomal formulations (Doxil®) may be confused with conventional formulations (Adriamycin PFS®, Adriamycin RDF®, Cerubidine®, Rubex®).

Use Treatment of AIDS-related Kaposi's sarcoma, breast cancer, ovarian cancer, solid tumors

Mechanism of Action/Effect Inhibits DNA and RNA synthesis of susceptible bacteria, active throughout cell cycle, results in cell death

Contraindications Hypersensitivity to doxorubicin, other anthracyclines, or any component of the formulation; breast-feeding, pregnancy

(Continued)

DOXOrubicin (Liposomal) *(Continued)*

Warnings/Precautions The U.S. Food and Drug Administration (FDA) currently recommends that procedures for the proper handling and disposal of antineoplastic agents be considered.

Doxorubicin is associated with dose-related myocardial damage leading to congestive heart failure. Doxorubicin and liposomal doxorubicin should be used cautiously in patients with high cumulative doses of anthracyclines, anthracenediones, and cyclophosphamide. Caution should also be used in patients with previous thoracic radiation or who have pre-existing cardiac disease. Total cumulative doses of anthracyclines, including liposomal doxorubicin and anthracenediones should not exceed 550 mg/m^2 or 400 mg/m^2 in patients with previous or concomitant treatment (with daunorubicin, cyclophosphamide, or irradiation of the cardiac region); irreversible myocardial toxicity may occur at these doses. Symptoms of anthracycline-induced CHF and/or cardiomyopathy may be delayed in onset (up to 7-8 years in some cases). For I.V. use only; local tissue irritation will result if extravasation occurs; reduce dose in patients with impaired hepatic function; severe myelosuppression is also possible. Acute infusion reactions may occur, some may be serious/life-threatening. Liposomal formulations of doxorubicin should not be substituted for doxorubicin hydrochloride on a mg-per-mg basis.

Hand-foot syndrome (palmar-plantar erythrodysesthesia) has been reported in up to 51% of patients with ovarian cancer (and significantly lower frequency in patients with Kaposi's sarcoma). May occur early in treatment, but is usually seen after 2-3 treatment cycles. Dosage modification may be required. In severe cases, treatment discontinuation may be required.

Drug Interactions

Cytochrome P450 Effect: Substrate (major) of CYP2D6, 3A4; **Inhibits** CYP2B6 (moderate), 2D6 (weak), 3A4 (weak)

Decreased Effect: The levels/effects of doxorubicin may be decreased by aminoglutethimide, carbamazepine, nafcillin, nevirapine, phenobarbital, phenytoin, rifamycins, and other CYP3A4 inducers. Doxorubicin may decrease plasma levels and effectiveness of digoxin. Doxorubicin may decrease the antiviral activity of zidovudine.

Increased Effect/Toxicity: Allopurinol may enhance the antitumor activity of doxorubicin (animal data only). Cyclosporine may increase doxorubicin levels, enhancing hematologic toxicity or may induce coma or seizures. Cyclophosphamide enhances the cardiac toxicity of doxorubicin by producing additional myocardial cell damage. Mercaptopurine increases doxorubicin toxicities. Streptozocin greatly enhances leukopenia and thrombocytopenia. Verapamil alters the cellular distribution of doxorubicin and may result in increased cell toxicity by inhibition of the P-glycoprotein pump. Paclitaxel reduces doxorubicin clearance and increases toxicity if administered prior to doxorubicin. High doses of progesterone enhance toxicity (neutropenia and thrombocytopenia).

Doxorubicin may increase the levels/effects of bupropion, promethazine, propofol, selegiline, sertraline, and other CYP2B6 substrates. The levels/effects of doxorubicin may be increased by azole antifungals, chlorpromazine, ciprofloxacin, clarithromycin, delavirdine, diclofenac, doxycycline, erythromycin, fluoxetine, imatinib, isoniazid, miconazole, nefazodone, nicardipine, paroxetine, pergolide, propofol, protease inhibitors, quinidine, quinine, ritonavir, ropinirole, telithromycin, verapamil and other inhibitors of CYP2D6 or 3A4. Based on mouse studies, cardiotoxicity may be enhanced by verapamil. Concurrent therapy with actinomycin-D may result in recall pneumonitis following radiation.

Nutritional/Ethanol Interactions

Ethanol: Avoid ethanol (due to GI irritation).

Herb/Nutraceutical: St John's wort may decrease doxorubicin levels. Avoid black cohosh, dong quai in estrogen-dependent tumors.

Adverse Reactions

>10%:

Cardiovascular: Peripheral edema (up to 11%)

Central nervous system: Fever (8% to 12%), headache (up to 11%), pain (up to 21%)

Dermatologic: Alopecia (9% to 19%); palmar-plantar erythrodysesthesia/hand-foot syndrome (up to 51% in ovarian cancer, 4% in Kaposi's sarcoma), rash (up to 29% in ovarian cancer, up to 5% in Kaposi's sarcoma)

Gastrointestinal: Stomatitis (5% to 41%), vomiting (8% to 33%), nausea (18% to 46%), mucositis (up to 14%), constipation (up to 30%), anorexia (up to 20%), diarrhea (5% to 21%), dyspepsia (up to 12%), intestinal obstruction (up to 11%)

Hematologic: Myelosuppression, neutropenia (12% to 62%), leukopenia (36%), thrombocytopenia (13% to 65%), anemia (6% to 74%)

Onset: 7 days

Nadir: 10-14 days

Recovery: 21-28 days

Neuromuscular & skeletal: Weakness (7% to 40%), back pain (up to 12%)

Respiratory: Pharyngitis (up to 16%), dyspnea (up to 15%)

1% to 10%:

Cardiovascular: Cardiac arrest, chest pain, edema, hypotension, pallor, tachycardia, vasodilation

Central nervous system: Agitation, anxiety, chills, confusion, depression, dizziness, emotional lability, insomnia, somnolence, vertigo

Dermatologic: Acne, dry skin (6%), dermatitis, furunculosis, herpes simplex/zoster, maculopapular rash, pruritus, rash, skin discoloration, vesiculobullous rash

Endocrine & metabolic: Dehydration, hyperbilirubinemia, hyperglycemia, hypocalcemia, hypokalemia, hyponatremia

Gastrointestinal: Abdomen enlarged, ascites, cachexia, dyspepsia, dysphagia, esophagitis, flatulence, gingivitis, glossitis, ileus, mouth ulceration, rectal bleeding, taste perversion, weight loss, xerostomia

Genitourinary: Cystitis, dysuria, leukorrhea, pelvic pain, polyuria, urinary incontinence, urinary tract infection, urinary urgency, vaginal bleeding

Hematologic: Ecchymosis, hemolysis, prothrombin time increased

Hepatic: ALT increased

Local: Thrombophlebitis

Neuromuscular & skeletal: Arthralgia, hypertonia, myalgia, neuralgia, neuritis (peripheral), neuropathy, paresthesia (up to 10%), pathological fracture,

Ocular: Conjunctivitis, dry eyes, retinitis

Otic: Ear pain

Renal: Albuminuria, hematuria

Respiratory: Apnea, cough increased (up to 10%), epistaxis, pleural effusion, pneumonia, rhinitis, sinusitis

Miscellaneous: Allergic reaction; infusion-related reactions (bronchospasm, chest tightness, chills, dyspnea, facial edema, flushing, headache, hypotension, pruritus); moniliasis, diaphoresis

Overdosage/Toxicology Symptoms of overdose include increases in mucositis, leukopenia, and thrombocytopenia. For acute overdose, treatment of the severely myelosuppressed patient consists of hospitalization, antibiotics, hematopoietic growth factors, platelet and granulocyte transfusion, and symptomatic treatment of mucositis.

Pharmacodynamics/Kinetics

Protein Binding: Unknown; nonliposomal doxorubicin 70%

Half-Life Elimination: Terminal: Distribution: 4.7-5.2 hours, Elimination: 44-55 hours

Metabolism: Hepatic and in plasma to doxorubicinol and the sulfate and glucuronide conjugates of 4-demethyl,7-deoxyaglycones

Excretion: Urine (5% as doxorubicin or doxorubicinol)

Clearance: Mean: 0.041 L/hour/m^2

Dosing

Adults & Elderly: Refer to individual protocols.

AIDS-KS: I.V.: 20 mg/m^2 every 3 weeks

Breast cancer: I.V.: 20-80 mg/m^2/dose every 8 weeks

Ovarian cancer: I.V.: 50 mg/m^2/dose every 4 weeks

Solid tumors: I.V.: 50-60 mg/m^2/dose every 3-4 weeks

Hepatic Impairment:

ALT/AST 2-3 times ULN: Administer 75% of dose

ALT/AST >3 times ULN or bilirubin 1.2-3 mg/dL (20-51 μmol/L): Administer 50% of dose

Bilirubin 3.1-5 mg/dL (51-85 μmol/L): Administer 25% of dose

Bilirubin >5 mg/dL (85 μmol/L): Do not administer

Available Dosage Forms Injection, solution, as hydrochloride: 2 mg/mL (10 mL, 25 mL)

Monitoring and Teaching Issues

Physical Assessment: See Warnings/Precautions for use cautions (eg, impaired renal function, existing cardiovascular disease). Assess potential for interactions with other pharmacological agents or herbal products patient may be taking (eg, potential to reduce or increase levels/effects of doxorubicin; see Drug Interactions). See Administration infusion specifics. Premedication with antiemetic is recommended (especially with larger doses). Infusion site must be closely monitored; extravasation can cause sloughing or tissue necrosis (do not apply heat or sodium bicarbonate). Assess results of laboratory tests, and patient response prior to each treatment and on a regular basis throughout therapy. Teach patient possible side effects/appropriate interventions (eg, importance of adequate hydration) and adverse symptoms to report (see Patient Education).

Monitoring Laboratory Tests: CBC with differential, platelet count, echocardiogram, liver function

Patient Education: Do not take any new medication during therapy unless approved by prescriber. This medication can only be administered by infusion; report immediately any swelling, pain, burning, redness at infusion site, sudden difficulty breathing or swallowing, chest pain, or chills. Avoid alcohol. It is important to maintain adequate hydration (2-3 L/day of fluids) unless instructed to restrict fluid intake and adequate nutrition (small frequent meals may help). You will be more susceptible to infection (avoid crowds and exposure to infection and do not have any vaccinations without consulting prescriber). May cause nausea or vomiting (small frequent meals, frequent mouth care, sucking lozenges, or chewing gum may help); diarrhea (buttermilk, boiled milk, or yogurt may help); loss of hair (reversible); or red-pink urine (normal). Report immediately chest pain, swelling of extremities, respiratory difficulty, palpitations, or rapid heartbeat. Report unresolved nausea, vomiting, or diarrhea; alterations in urinary pattern (increased or decreased); opportunistic infection (fever, chills, unusual bruising or bleeding fatigue, purulent vaginal discharge, unhealed mouth sores); abdominal pain or blood in stools; excessive fatigue; or yellowing of eyes or skin. **Pregnancy/breast-feeding precautions:** Do not get pregnant while taking this medication or for 1 month following therapy. Consult prescriber for appropriate contraceptives. Do not breast-feed.

Pregnancy Risk Factor: D

Pregnancy Issues: Advise patients to avoid becoming pregnant (females) and to avoid causing pregnancy (males).

Lactation: Excretion in breast milk unknown/contraindicated

Administration

I.V.: Irritant. May be administered IVPB over 30 minutes; manufacturer recommends administering at initial rate of 1 mg/minute to minimize risk of infusion reactions until the absence of a reaction has been established, then increase the infusion rate for completion over 1 hour. Do not administer as a bolus injection or undiluted solution. **Do not administer intramuscular or subcutaneous. Do not use with in-line filters.**

Reconstitution: Doses Doxil® ≤90 mg must be diluted in 250 mL of D$_5$W prior to administration. Doses >90 mg should be diluted in 500 mL D$_5$W.

Compatibility: Stable in D$_5$W

Y-site administration: Incompatible with amphotericin B, amphotericin B cholesteryl sulfate complex, buprenorphine, cefoperazone, ceftazidime, docetaxel, fluorouracil, furosemide, heparin, hydroxyzine, mannitol, meperidine, metoclopramide, mitoxantrone, (Continued)

DOXOrubicin (Liposomal) *(Continued)*

morphine, ofloxacin, paclitaxel, piperacillin/tazobactam, promethazine, sodium bicarbonate

Storage: Store intact vials of solution under refrigeration (2°C to 8°C); avoid freezing. Prolonged freezing may adversely affect liposomal drug products, however, short-term freezing (<1 month) does not appear to have a deleterious effect. Diluted doxorubicin hydrochloride liposome injection may be refrigerated at 2°C to 8°C or at room temperature; administer within 24 hours. **Do not use with in-line filters.**

♦ **Doxy-100®** *see Doxycycline on page 496*

Doxycycline *(doks i SYE kleen)*

U.S. Brand Names Adoxa™; Doryx®; Doxy-100®; Monodox®; Periostat®; Vibramycin®; Vibra-Tabs®

Synonyms Doxycycline Calcium; Doxycycline Hyclate; Doxycycline Monohydrate

Generic Available Yes: Excludes powder for oral solution, syrup

Pharmacologic Category Antibiotic, Tetracycline Derivative

Medication Safety Issues

Sound-alike/look-alike issues:

Doxycycline may be confused with dicyclomine, doxepin, doxylamine

Doxy-100® may be confused with Doxil®

Monodox® may be confused with Maalox®

Use Principally in the treatment of infections caused by susceptible *Rickettsia*, *Chlamydia*, and *Mycoplasma*; alternative to mefloquine for malaria prophylaxis; treatment for syphilis, uncomplicated *Neisseria gonorrhoeae*, *Listeria*, *Actinomyces israelii*, and *Clostridium* infections in penicillin-allergic patients; used for community-acquired pneumonia and other common infections due to susceptible organisms; anthrax due to *Bacillus anthracis*, including inhalational anthrax (postexposure); treatment of infections caused by uncommon susceptible gram-negative and gram-positive organisms including *Borrelia recurrentis*, *Ureaplasma urealyticum*, *Haemophilus ducreyi*, *Yersinia pestis*, *Francisella tularensis*, *Vibrio cholerae*, *Campylobacter fetus*, *Brucella* spp, *Bartonella bacilliformis*, and *Calymmatobacterium granulomatis*

Unlabeled/Investigational Use Sclerosing agent for pleural effusion injection; vancomycin-resistant enterococci (VRE)

Mechanism of Action/Effect Inhibits protein synthesis by binding with the 30S and possibly the 50S ribosomal subunit(s) of susceptible bacteria; may also cause alterations in the cytoplasmic membrane

Doxycycline inhibits collagenase *in vitro* and has been shown to inhibit collagenase in the gingival crevicular fluid in adults with periodontitis

Contraindications Hypersensitivity to doxycycline, tetracycline or any component of the formulation; children <8 years of age, except in treatment of anthrax (including inhalational anthrax postexposure prophylaxis); severe hepatic dysfunction; pregnancy

Warnings/Precautions Do not use during pregnancy - use of tetracyclines during tooth development may cause permanent discoloration of the teeth and enamel hypoplasia. Prolonged use may result in superinfection, including oral or vaginal candidiasis. Photosensitivity reaction may occur with this drug; avoid prolonged exposure to sunlight or tanning equipment.

Drug Interactions

Cytochrome P450 Effect: Substrate of CYP3A4 (major); **Inhibits** CYP3A4 (moderate)

Decreased Effect: Decreased levels of doxycycline may occur when taken with antacids containing aluminum, calcium, or magnesium. Decreased levels when taken with iron, bismuth subsalicylate, barbiturates, sucralfate, didanosine, and quinapril. Concurrent use of tetracycline and Penthrane® has been reported to result in fatal renal toxicity. Although anecdotal reports suggest oral contraceptive efficacy could be reduced by tetracyclines, this has been refuted by more rigorous scientific and clinical data. The levels/effects of doxycycline may be decreased by include aminoglutethimide, carbamazepine, nafcillin, nevirapine, phenobarbital, phenytoin, rifamycins, and other CYP3A4 inducers.

Increased Effect/Toxicity: Increased digoxin toxicity when taken with digoxin. Increased prothrombin time with warfarin. Doxycycline may increase the levels/effects of selected benzodiazepines, calcium channel blockers, cyclosporine, mirtazapine, nateglinide, nefazodone, quinidine, sildenafil (and other PDE-5 inhibitors), tacrolimus, venlafaxine, and other CYP3A4 substrates. Selected benzodiazepines (midazolam, triazolam), cisapride, ergot alkaloids, selected HMG-CoA reductase inhibitors (lovastatin and simvastatin), mesoridazine, pimozide, and thioridazine are generally contraindicated with strong CYP3A4 inhibitors. When used with strong CYP3A4 inhibitors, dosage adjustment/limits are recommended

Nutritional/Ethanol Interactions

Ethanol: Chronic ethanol ingestion may reduce the serum concentration of doxycycline.

Food: Doxycycline serum levels may be slightly decreased if taken with food or milk. Administration with iron or calcium may decrease doxycycline absorption. May decrease absorption of calcium, iron, magnesium, zinc, and amino acids.

Herb/Nutraceutical: St John's wort may decrease doxycycline levels. Avoid dong quai, St John's wort (may also cause photosensitization).

Lab Interactions False-negative urine glucose using Clinistix®

Adverse Reactions Frequency not defined.

Cardiovascular: Intracranial hypertension, pericarditis

Dermatologic: Angioneurotic edema, exfoliative dermatitis (rare), photosensitivity, rash, urticaria

Endocrine & metabolic: Brown/black discoloration of thyroid gland (no dysfunction reported)

Gastrointestinal: Anorexia, diarrhea, dysphagia, enterocolitis, esophagitis (rare), esophageal ulcerations (rare), glossitis, inflammatory lesions in anogenital region, tooth discoloration (children)

Hematologic: Eosinophilia, hemolytic anemia, neutropenia, thrombocytopenia

Renal: Increased BUN

Miscellaneous: Anaphylactoid purpura, anaphylaxis, bulging fontanels (infants), SLE exacerbation

Note: Adverse effects in clinical trials with Periostat® occurring at a frequency more than 1% greater than placebo included nausea, dyspepsia, joint pain, diarrhea, menstrual cramp, and pain.

Overdosage/Toxicology Symptoms of overdose include nausea, anorexia, and diarrhea. Treatment is supportive.

Pharmacodynamics/Kinetics

Absorption: Oral: Almost complete; reduced by food or milk by 20%

Time to Peak: Serum: 1.5-4 hours

Protein Binding: 90%

Half-Life Elimination: 12-15 hours (usually increases to 22-24 hours with multiple doses); End-stage renal disease: 18-25 hours

Metabolism: Not hepatic; partially inactivated in GI tract by chelate formation

Excretion: Feces (30%); urine (23%)

Dosing

Adults & Elderly:

Susceptible infections: Oral, I.V.: 100-200 mg/day in 1-2 divided doses

Acute gonococcal infection (PID) in combination with another antibiotic: 100 mg every 12 hours until improved, followed by 100 mg orally twice daily to complete 14 days

Community-acquired pneumonia, bronchitis: Oral, I.V.: 100 mg twice daily

Uncomplicated chlamydial infections: Oral: 100 mg twice daily for ≥7 days

Endometritis, salpingitis, parametritis, or peritonitis: 100 mg I.V. twice daily with cefoxitin 2 g every 6 hours for 4 days and for ≥48 hours after patient improves; then continue with oral therapy 100 mg twice daily to complete a 10- to 14-day course of therapy

Sclerosing agent for pleural effusion injection (unlabeled use): 500 mg as a single dose in 30-50 mL of NS or SWI

Lyme disease: Oral: 100 mg twice daily for 14-21 days

Syphilis:

Early syphilis: Oral, I.V.: 200 mg/day in divided doses for 14 days

Late syphilis: Oral, I.V.: 200 mg/day in divided doses for 28 days

Periodontitis: Oral (Periostat®): 20 mg twice daily as an adjunct following scaling and root planing; may be administered for up to 9 months. Safety beyond 12 months of treatment and efficacy beyond 9 months of treatment have not been established.

Anthrax:

Inhalational (postexposure prophylaxis): Oral, I.V. (use oral route when possible): 100 mg every 12 hours for 60 days; **Note:** Preliminary recommendation, FDA review and update is anticipated.

Cutaneous (treatment): Oral: 100 mg every 12 hours for 60 days. **Note:** In the presence of systemic involvement, extensive edema, lesions on head/neck, refer to I.V. dosing for treatment of inhalational/gastrointestinal/oropharyngeal anthrax

Inhalational/gastrointestinal/oropharyngeal (treatment): I.V.: Initial: 100 mg every 12 hours; switch to oral therapy when clinically appropriate; some recommend initial loading dose of 200 mg, followed by 100 mg every 8-12 hours

Note: Initial treatment should include two or more agents predicted to be effective (per CDC recommendations). Agents suggested for use in conjunction with doxycycline or ciprofloxacin include rifampin, vancomycin, imipenem, penicillin, ampicillin, chloramphenicol, clindamycin, and clarithromycin. May switch to oral antimicrobial therapy when clinically appropriate. Continue combined therapy for 60 days.

Pediatrics:

Susceptible infections:

Children ≥8 years (<45 kg): Oral, I.V.: 2-5 mg/kg/day in 1-2 divided doses, not to exceed 200 mg/day

Children >8 years (>45 kg): Oral, I.V.: Refer to adult dosing.

Anthrax:

Inhalational (postexposure prophylaxis): Oral, I.V. (use oral route when possible):

≤8 years: 2.2 mg/kg every 12 hours for 60 days

>8 years and ≤45 kg: 2.2 mg/kg every 12 hours for 60 days

>8 years and >45 kg: 100 mg every 12 hours for 60 days

Cutaneous (treatment): Oral: See dosing for "Inhalational (postexposure prophylaxis)"

Note: In the presence of systemic involvement, extensive edema, and/or lesions on head/neck, doxycycline should initially be administered I.V.

Inhalational/gastrointestinal/oropharyngeal (treatment): I.V.: Refer to dosing for inhalational anthrax (postexposure prophylaxis); switch to oral therapy when clinically appropriate.

Note: Initial treatment should include two or more agents predicted to be effective (per CDC recommendations). Agents suggested for use in conjunction with doxycycline or ciprofloxacin include rifampin, vancomycin, imipenem, penicillin, ampicillin, chloramphenicol, clindamycin, and clarithromycin. May switch to oral antimicrobial therapy when clinically appropriate. Continue combined therapy for 60 days

Renal Impairment: No adjustment necessary.

Not dialyzable; 0% to 5% by hemo- and peritoneal methods or by continuous arteriovenous or venovenous hemofiltration; supplemental dose is not necessary.

Available Dosage Forms

Capsule, as hyclate: 50 mg, 100 mg

Vibramycin®: 100 mg

Capsule, as monohydrate (Monodox®): 50 mg, 100 mg

Capsule, coated pellets, as hyclate (Doryx®): 75 mg, 100 mg

Injection, powder for reconstitution, as hyclate (Doxy-100®): 100 mg

Powder for oral suspension, as monohydrate (Vibramycin®): 25 mg/5 mL (60 mL) [raspberry flavor]

(Continued)

Doxycycline *(Continued)*

Syrup, as calcium (Vibramycin®): 50 mg/5 mL (480 mL) [contains sodium metabisulfite; raspberry-apple flavor]
Tablet, as hyclate: 100 mg
  Periostat®: 20 mg
  Vibra-Tabs®: 100 mg
Tablet, as monohydrate (Adoxa™): 50 mg, 75 mg, 100 mg

Monitoring and Teaching Issues

Physical Assessment: Assess results of culture and sensitivity test and patient's allergy history prior to beginning therapy. Assess potential for interactions with other pharmacological agents or herbal products patient may be taking (see Drug Interactions). See Administration for intravenous infusion specifics. Infusion site must be closely monitored; extravasation can be very irritating to veins (use of central line is preferable). Assess therapeutic effectiveness (resolution of infections) and adverse response (see Adverse Reactions) on a regular basis throughout therapy. Advise patients with diabetes about use of Clinistix®. Teach patient appropriate use/administration (oral), possible side effects, interventions to reduce side effects (eg, importance of adequate hydration) and adverse symptoms to report (see Patient Education).

Monitoring Laboratory Tests: Perform culture and sensitivity testing prior to initiating therapy.

Patient Education: If administered by infusion, report immediately any acute back pain, difficulty breathing or swallowing, chest tightness, pain, redness, or swelling at infusion site. **Oral:** Do not take any new medication during therapy unless approved by prescriber. Take entire prescription as directed, even if you are feeling better. Take each oral dose with food or a full glass of water to reduce stomach upset. Avoid alcohol and maintain adequate hydration (2-3 L/day of fluids) unless instructed to restrict fluid intake. If you have diabetes, drug may cause false test results with Clinistix® urine glucose monitoring; use of another form of glucose monitoring is preferable. You may be very sensitive to sunlight (use sunblock, wear protective clothing and eyewear, or avoid exposure to direct sunlight). May cause lightheadedness, dizziness, or drowsiness (use caution when driving or engaging in tasks that require alertness until response to drug is known); nausea or vomiting (small frequent meals, frequent mouth care, sucking lozenges, or chewing gum may help); or diarrhea (buttermilk, boiled milk, or yogurt may help). Report skin rash or itching; easy bruising or bleeding; yellowing of skin or eyes; pale stool or dark urine; unhealed mouth sores; vaginal itching or discharge; fever, chills, or unusual cough. **Pregnancy/breast-feeding precautions:** Inform prescriber if you are pregnant. Do not get pregnant while taking this medication. Consult prescriber for appropriate contraceptive measures. Breast-feeding is not recommended.

Dietary Considerations: Take with food if gastric irritation occurs. While administration with food may decrease GI absorption of doxycycline by up to 20%, administration on an empty stomach is not recommended due to GI intolerance. Of currently available tetracyclines, doxycycline has the least affinity for calcium.

Pregnancy Risk Factor: D

Pregnancy Issues: Exposure during the last half or pregnancy causes permanent yellow-gray-brown discoloration of the teeth. Tetracyclines also form a complex in bone-forming tissue, leading to a decreased fibula growth rate when given to premature infants. According to the FDA, the Teratogen Information System concluded that therapeutic doses during pregnancy are unlikely to produce substantial teratogenic risk, but data are insufficient to say that there is no risk. In general, reports of exposure have been limited to short durations of therapy in the first trimester. When considering treatment for life-threatening infection and/or prolonged duration of therapy (such as in anthrax), the potential risk to the fetus must be balanced against the severity of the potential illness.

Lactation: Enters breast milk/not recommended

Administration

Oral: Administer with adequate fluid to reduce risk of esophageal irritation and ulceration. May give with meals to decrease GI upset.

  Doryx®: Capsules may be opened and contents sprinkled on applesauce. Applesauce should be swallowed immediately; do not chew. Follow with 8 ounces of water. Applesauce should not be hot and should be soft enough to swallow without chewing.

I.V.: Infuse slowly, usually over 1-4 hours. Avoid extravasation.

Reconstitution: I.V. infusion: Following reconstitution with sterile water for injection, dilute to a final concentration of 0.1-1 mg/mL using a compatible solution. Protect from light. Stability varies based on solution.

Compatibility: Stable in NS, D₅W, LR, D₅LR

Y-site administration: Incompatible with allopurinol, heparin, piperacillin/tazobactam

Storage: Capsules/tablets: Store at controlled room temperature; protect from light

Related Information

Antimicrobial Drugs of Choice *on page 1792*
Community-Acquired Pneumonia in Adults *on page 1807*
I.V. to Oral Conversion *on page 1688*
Prophylaxis for Exposure to Communicable Diseases *on page 1859*

◆ **Doxycycline Calcium** *see Doxycycline on page 496*
◆ **Doxycycline Hyclate** *see Doxycycline on page 496*
◆ **Doxycycline Monohydrate** *see Doxycycline on page 496*
◆ **DPA** *see Valproic Acid and Derivatives on page 1543*
◆ **DPH** *see Phenytoin on page 1204*
◆ **Dramamine® Less Drowsy Formula [OTC]** *see Meclizine on page 937*
◆ **Drisdol®** *see Ergocalciferol on page 538*
◆ **Drithocreme®** *see Anthralin on page 123*
◆ **Dritho-Scalp®** *see Anthralin on page 123*

Dronabinol (droe NAB i nol)

U.S. Brand Names Marinol®

Synonyms Delta-9-Tetrahydro-Cannabinol; Delta-9 THC; Tetrahydrocannabinol; THC

Controlled Substance C-III

Generic Available No

Pharmacologic Category Antiemetic; Appetite Stimulant

Medication Safety Issues

Sound-alike/look-alike issues:

Dronabinol may be confused with droperidol

Use Chemotherapy-associated nausea and vomiting refractory to other antiemetic; AIDS- and cancer-related anorexia

Mechanism of Action/Effect Unknown, may inhibit endorphins in the emetic center, suppress prostaglandin synthesis, and/or inhibit medullary activity through an unspecified cortical action

Contraindications Hypersensitivity to dronabinol or any component of the formulation, or marijuana; should be avoided in patients with a history of schizophrenia

Warnings/Precautions Use with caution in patients with heart disease, hepatic disease, or seizure disorders. Reduce dosage in patients with severe hepatic impairment. May have potential for abuse; drug is psychoactive substance in marijuana. Monitor for possible psychotic reaction with first dose.

Drug Interactions

Increased Effect/Toxicity: Increased toxicity (drowsiness) with alcohol, barbiturates, and benzodiazepines.

Nutritional/Ethanol Interactions

Ethanol: Avoid ethanol (may increase CNS depression).

Food: Administration with high-lipid meals may increase absorption.

Herb/Nutraceutical: St John's wort may decrease dronabinol levels.

Lab Interactions Decreased FSH, LH, growth hormone, testosterone

Adverse Reactions

>10%:

Central nervous system: Drowsiness (48%), sedation (53%), confusion (30%), dizziness (21%), detachment, anxiety, difficulty concentrating, mood change

Gastrointestinal: Appetite increased (when used as an antiemetic), xerostomia (38% to 50%)

1% to 10%:

Cardiovascular: Orthostatic hypotension, tachycardia

Central nervous system: Ataxia (4%), depression (7%), headache, vertigo, hallucinations (5%), memory lapse (4%)

Neuromuscular & skeletal: Paresthesia, weakness

Overdosage/Toxicology Symptoms of overdose include tachycardia, hyper- and hypotension. Treatment is symptomatic.

Pharmacodynamics/Kinetics

Onset of Action: Within 1 hour

Absorption: Oral: 90% to 95%; ~5% to 10% of dose gets into systemic circulation

Time to Peak: Serum: 2-3 hours

Protein Binding: 97% to 99%

Half-Life Elimination: THC: 19-24 hours; THC metabolites: 49-53 hours

Metabolism: Hepatic to at least 50 metabolites, some of which are active; 11-hydroxy-trahydrocannabinol (11-OH-THC) is the major metabolite; extensive first-pass effect

Excretion: Feces (35% as unconjugated metabolites); urine (10% to 15% as acid metabolites and conjugates)

Dosing

Adults & Elderly:

Antiemetic: Oral: 5 mg/m^2 1-3 hours before chemotherapy, then give 5 mg/m^2/dose every 2-4 hours after chemotherapy for a total of 4-6 doses/day; dose may be increased up to a maximum of 15 mg/m^2/dose if needed (dosage may be increased by 2.5 mg/m^2 increments).

Appetite stimulant (AIDS-related): Oral: Initial: 2.5 mg twice daily (before lunch and dinner); titrate up to a maximum of 20 mg/day.

Pediatrics: Antiemetic: Oral: NCI protocol recommends 5 mg/m^2 starting 6-8 hours before chemotherapy and every 4-6 hours after to be continued for 12 hours after chemotherapy is discontinued.

Hepatic Impairment: Usual dose should be reduced in patients with severe liver failure.

Available Dosage Forms Capsule, gelatin: 2.5 mg, 5 mg, 10 mg [contains sesame oil]

Monitoring and Teaching Issues

Physical Assessment: Use caution in the presence of heart disease, hepatic disease, or seizure disorders (see Warnings/Precautions). Assess potential for interactions with other pharmacological agents or herbal products patient may be taking (see Drug Interactions). Assess effectiveness of therapy according to purpose for use. Monitor closely for adverse psychotic reactions; this drug is the psychoactive substance in marijuana (see Adverse Reactions). Teach patient appropriate use, possible side effects/appropriate interventions, and adverse symptoms to report (see Patient Education).

Patient Education: Do not take any new medication during therapy unless approved by prescriber (especially barbiturates, and benzodiazepines). Take exactly as directed; do not increase dose or take more often than prescribed. Avoid alcohol. May cause psychotic reaction, impaired coordination or judgment, faintness, dizziness, or drowsiness (do not drive or engage in activities that require alertness and coordination until response to drug is known); or clumsiness, unsteadiness, or muscular weakness (change position slowly and use caution when climbing stairs). Report excessive or persistent CNS changes (euphoria, anxiety, depression, memory lapse, bizarre thought patterns, excitability, inability to control thoughts or behavior, fainting); respiratory difficulties; rapid heartbeat; or other adverse (Continued)

Dronabinol *(Continued)*

reactions. **Pregnancy/breast-feeding precautions:** Inform prescriber if you are or intend to become pregnant. Do not breast-feed.

Pregnancy Risk Factor: C

Lactation: Enters breast milk/contraindicated

Administration
  Storage: Store in a cool place.

Droperidol (droe PER i dole)

U.S. Brand Names Inapsine®

Synonyms Dehydrobenzperidol

Generic Available Yes

Pharmacologic Category Antiemetic; Antipsychotic Agent, Typical

Medication Safety Issues
  Sound-alike/look-alike issues:
    Droperidol may be confused with dronabinol
    Inapsine® may be confused with Nebcin®

Use Antiemetic in surgical and diagnostic procedures; preoperative medication in patients when other treatments are ineffective or inappropriate

Mechanism of Action/Effect Droperidol is a butyrophenone antipsychotic; antiemetic effect is a result of blockade of dopamine stimulation of the chemoreceptor trigger zone. Other effects include alpha-adrenergic blockade, peripheral vascular dilation, and reduction of the pressor effect of epinephrine resulting in hypotension and decreased peripheral vascular resistance; may also reduce pulmonary artery pressure

Contraindications Hypersensitivity to droperidol or any component of the formulation; known or suspected QT prolongation, including congenital long QT syndrome (prolonged QT_c is defined as >440 msec in males or >450 msec in females)

Warnings/Precautions May alter cardiac conduction. Cases of QT prolongation and torsade de pointes, including some fatal cases, have been reported. Use extreme caution in patients with bradycardia (<50 bpm), cardiac disease, concurrent MAOI therapy, Class I and Class III antiarrhythmics or other drugs known to prolong QT interval, and electrolyte disturbances (hypokalemia or hypomagnesemia), including concomitant drugs which may alter electrolytes (diuretics).

Use with caution in patients with seizures, bone marrow suppression, or severe liver disease. May be sedating, use with caution in disorders where CNS depression is a feature. Caution in patients with hemodynamic instability, predisposition to seizures, subcortical brain damage, renal or respiratory disease. Esophageal dysmotility and aspiration have been associated with antipsychotic use. Caution in breast cancer or other prolactin-dependent tumors. May cause orthostatic hypotension - use with caution in patients at risk of this effect. Significant hypotension may occur; injection contains benzyl alcohol; injection also contains sulfites which may cause allergic reaction.

Relative to other neuroleptics, droperidol has a low potency of cholinergic blockade. Use with caution in patients with decreased gastrointestinal motility, urinary retention, BPH, xerostomia, or visual problems. May worsen myasthenia gravis.

May cause extrapyramidal symptoms, including tardive dyskinesia. May be associated with neuroleptic malignant syndrome (NMS) or pigmentary retinopathy. Safety in children <6 months of age has not been established.

Drug Interactions
  Increased Effect/Toxicity: Droperidol in combination with certain forms of conduction anesthesia may produce peripheral vasodilitation and hypotension. Droperidol and CNS depressants will likely have additive CNS effects. Droperidol and cyclobenzaprine may have an additive effect on prolonging the QT interval. Use caution with other agents known to prolong QT interval (Class I or Class III antiarrhythmics, some quinolone antibiotics, cisapride, some phenothiazines, pimozide, tricyclic antidepressants). Potassium- or magnesium-depleting agents (diuretics, aminoglycosides, amphotericin B, cyclosporine) may increase risk of arrhythmias. Metoclopramide may increase risk of extrapyramidal symptoms (EPS).

Adverse Reactions
  >10%:
    Cardiovascular: QT_c prolongation (dose dependent)
    Central nervous system: Restlessness, anxiety, extrapyramidal symptoms, dystonic reactions, pseudoparkinsonian signs and symptoms, tardive dyskinesia, seizure, altered central temperature regulation, sedation, drowsiness
    Endocrine & metabolic: Swelling of breasts
    Gastrointestinal: Weight gain, constipation
  1% to 10%:
    Cardiovascular: Hypotension (especially orthostatic), tachycardia, abnormal T waves with prolonged ventricular repolarization, hypertension
    Central nervous system: Hallucinations, persistent tardive dyskinesia, akathisia
    Gastrointestinal: Nausea, vomiting
    Genitourinary: Dysuria

Overdosage/Toxicology Symptoms of overdose include hypotension, tachycardia, hallucinations, and extrapyramidal symptoms. Following initiation of essential overdose management, toxic symptom treatment and supportive treatment should be initiated. Prolonged QT interval, seizures, and arrhythmias have been reported.

Pharmacodynamics/Kinetics

Onset of Action: Peak effect: Parenteral: Within 30 minutes

Duration of Action: Parenteral: 2-4 hours, may extend to 12 hours

Absorption: I.M.: Rapid

Protein Binding: Extensive

Half-Life Elimination: Adults: 2.3 hours

Metabolism: Hepatic, to *p*-fluorophenylacetic acid, benzimidazolone, *p*-hydroxypiperidine

Excretion: Urine (75%, <1% as unchanged drug); feces (22%, 11% to 50% as unchanged drug)

Dosing

Adults & Elderly: Titrate carefully to desired effect: Nausea and vomiting: I.M., I.V.: Initial: 2.5 mg; additional doses of 1.25 mg may be administered to achieve desired effect; administer additional doses with caution

Pediatrics: Titrate carefully to desired effect: Children 2-12 years: Nausea and vomiting: I.M., I.V.: 0.05-0.06 mg/kg (maximum initial dose: 0.1 mg/kg); additional doses may be repeated to achieve effect; administer additional doses with caution

Available Dosage Forms Injection, solution: 2.5 mg/mL (1 mL, 2 mL)

Monitoring and Teaching Issues

Physical Assessment: Assess other medications the patient may be taking for effectiveness and interactions. Monitor vital signs; cardiac and respiratory status on a frequent basis and especially immediately following administration and for several hours afterward. Monitor for extrapyramidal symptoms for 24-48 hours after therapy. Teach and use safety precautions until the patient is stable. Teach adverse reactions to report.

Monitoring Laboratory Tests: To identify QT prolongation, a 12-lead ECG prior to use is recommended; ECG monitoring for 2-3 hours following administration is recommended. Lipid profile, fasting blood glucose/Hgb A_{1c}, serum magnesium and potassium; BMI

Patient Education: This drug may cause you to feel very sleepy; do not attempt to get up without assistance. May cause orthostatic hypotension (use caution when changing position from lying or sitting to standing). You may experience constipation, (increasing exercise, fluids, fruit/fiber may help). Immediately report any respiratory difficulty, confusion, loss of thought processes, or palpitations. **Pregnancy/breast-feeding precautions:** Inform prescriber if you are pregnant. Consult prescriber if breast-feeding.

Geriatric Considerations: Use of droperidol in the elderly may result in severe and often irreversible undesirable effects. Before initiating antipsychotic therapy, the clinician should investigate possible reversible causes.

Pregnancy Risk Factor: C

Lactation: Excretion in breast milk unknown

Administration

I.V.: Administer I.M. or I.V.; I.V. should be administered as a rapid IVP (over 30-60 seconds); for I.V. infusion, dilute in 50-100 mL NS or D_5W. ECG monitoring for 2-3 hours after administration is recommended.

Compatibility: Stable in D_5W, LR, NS

Y-site administration: Incompatible with allopurinol, amphotericin B cholesteryl sulfate complex, cefepime, fluorouracil, foscarnet, furosemide, leucovorin, nafcillin, piperacillin/tazobactam

Compatibility in syringe: Incompatible with fluorouracil, furosemide, heparin, leucovorin, methotrexate, ondansetron, pentobarbital

Storage: Droperidol ampuls/vials should be stored at room temperature and protected from light. Solutions diluted in NS or D_5W are stable at room temperature for up to 7 days.

Additional Information Does not possess analgesic effects; has little or no amnesic properties.

Related Information

Antiemetics for Chemotherapy-Induced Nausea and Vomiting *on page 1788*

♦ **Drospirenone and Ethinyl Estradiol** *see* Ethinyl Estradiol and Drospirenone *on page 581*

Drotrecogin Alfa (dro TRE coe jin AL fa)

U.S. Brand Names Xigris®

Synonyms Activated Protein C, Human, Recombinant; Drotrecogin Alfa, Activated; Protein C (Activated), Human, Recombinant

Generic Available No

Pharmacologic Category Protein C (Activated)

Use Reduction of mortality from severe sepsis (associated with organ dysfunction) in adults at high risk of death (eg, APACHE II score ≥25)

Unlabeled/Investigational Use Purpura fulminans

Mechanism of Action/Effect Decreases mortality from severe sepsis by blocking thrombotic activity. Blocks factor Va and VIIIa. In addition, may have other anti-inflammatory effects.

Contraindications Hypersensitivity to drotrecogin alfa or any component of the formulation; active internal bleeding; recent hemorrhagic stroke (within 3 months); severe head trauma (within 2 months); recent intracranial or intraspinal surgery (within 2 months); intracranial neoplasm or mass lesion; evidence of cerebral herniation; presence of an epidural catheter; trauma with an increased risk of life-threatening bleeding

Warnings/Precautions Increases risk of bleeding; careful evaluation of risks and benefit is required prior to initiation (see Contraindications). Bleeding risk is increased in patients receiving concurrent therapeutic heparin, oral anticoagulants, glycoprotein IIb/IIIa antagonists, platelet aggregation inhibitors, or aspirin at a dosage of >650 mg/day (within 7 days). In addition, an increased bleeding risk is associated with prolonged INR (>3.0), gastrointestinal bleeding (within 6 weeks), decreased platelet count (<30,000/mm³), thrombolytic therapy (within 3 days), recent ischemic stroke (within 3 months), intracranial AV malformation or aneurysm, known bleeding diathesis, severe hepatic disease (chronic), or other condition where bleeding is a significant hazard or difficult to manage due to its location. Discontinue if (Continued)

Drotrecogin Alfa *(Continued)*

significant bleeding occurs (may consider continued use after stabilization). Treatment interruption required for invasive procedures. During treatment, aPTT cannot be used to assess coagulopathy (PT/INR not affected).

Efficacy not established in adult patients at a low risk of death. Patients with pre-existing nonsepsis-related medical conditions with a poor prognosis (anticipated survival <28 days), patients with acute pancreatitis (no established source of infection), HIV-infected patients with a CD4 count ≤50 cells/mm^3, chronic dialysis patients, pre-existing hypercoagulable conditions, and patients who had received bone marrow, liver, lung, pancreas, or small bowel transplants were excluded from the clinical trial which established benefit. In addition, patients with a high body weight (>135 kg) were not evaluated. Safety and efficacy have not been established in pediatric patients.

Drug Interactions

Increased Effect/Toxicity: Concurrent use of antiplatelet agents, including aspirin (>650 mg/day, recent use within 7 days), cilostazol, clopidogrel, dipyridamole, ticlopidine, NSAIDs, or glycoprotein IIb/IIIa antagonists (recent use within 7 days) may increase risk of bleeding. Concurrent use of low molecular weight heparins or heparin at therapeutic rates of infusion may increase the risk of bleeding. However, the use of low-dose prophylactic heparin does not appear to affect safety. Recent use of thrombolytic agents (within 3 days) may increase the risk of bleeding. Recent use of warfarin (within 7 days or elevation of INR ≥3) may increase the risk of bleeding. Other drugs which interfere with coagulation may increase risk of bleeding (including antithrombin III, danaparoid, direct thrombin inhibitors)

Nutritional/Ethanol Interactions Herb/Nutraceutical: Recent use/intake of herbs with anticoagulant or antiplatelet activity (including cat's claw, feverfew, garlic, ginkgo, ginseng, and horse chestnut seed) may increase the risk of bleeding.

Lab Interactions May interfere with one-stage coagulation assays based on the aPTT (such as factor VIII, IX, and XI assays).

Adverse Reactions As with all drugs which may affect hemostasis, bleeding is the major adverse effect associated with drotrecogin alfa. Hemorrhage may occur at virtually any site. Risk is dependent on multiple variables, including the dosage administered, concurrent use of multiple agents which alter hemostasis, and patient predisposition.

>10%
  Dermatologic: Bruising
  Gastrointestinal: Gastrointestinal bleeding
1% to 10%: Hematologic: Bleeding (serious 2.4% during infusion vs 3.5% during 28-day study period; individual events listed as <1%)

Overdosage/Toxicology No reported experience with overdose. Hemorrhagic complications are likely consequence of overdose. Treatment is supportive, including immediate interruption of the infusion and monitoring for hemorrhagic complications. No known antidote.

Pharmacodynamics/Kinetics

Duration of Action: Plasma nondetectable within 2 hours of discontinuation

Half-Life Elimination: 1.6 hours

Metabolism: Inactivated by endogenous plasma protease inhibitors; mean clearance: 40 L/hour; increased with severe sepsis (~50%)

Dosing

Adults:
  Purpura fulminans (unlabeled use): 24 mcg/kg/hour
  Severe sepsis: I.V.: 24 mcg/kg/hour for a total of 96 hours; stop infusion **immediately** if clinically-important bleeding is identified.

Pediatrics: Purpura fulminans (unlabeled use): Refer to adult dosing.

Renal Impairment: No specific adjustment recommended.

Available Dosage Forms Injection, powder for reconstitution [preservative free]: 5 mg [contains sucrose 31.8 mg], 20 mg [contains sucrose 124.9 mg]

Monitoring and Teaching Issues

Physical Assessment: Assess potential for interactions with other prescriptions, OTC medications, or herbal products patient may be taking (especially drugs affecting coagulation or platelet activity). Assess results of laboratory tests prior to, during, and following therapy. Patient must be monitored very closely for bleeding during and following infusion (hemorrhage may occur at virtually any site). If significant bleeding occurs, infusion should be stopped and prescriber notified immediately. Bleeding precautions must be observed. Patient instruction should be according to patient condition.

Monitoring Laboratory Tests: Hemoglobin/hematocrit, PT/INR, platelet count

Patient Education: Inform prescriber of all prescriptions, OTC medications, or herbal products you are taking, and any allergies you have. This medication can only be administered by infusion. You will be monitored closely. Report immediately any unusual or acute abdominal pain or headache, or respiratory difficulty. You will be more susceptible to bleeding and bruising; remain in bed and ring for assistance to avoid falling or injuring yourself. Avoid sharps of any kind (knives, scissors, needles, nail clippers, etc; shave with a safety razor). **Pregnancy/breast-feeding precautions:** Inform prescriber if you are pregnant. Breast-feeding is not recommended.

Pregnancy Risk Factor: C

Lactation: Excretion in breast milk unknown/not recommended

Administration

I.V.: Administer via infusion pump. Administration must be completed within 12 hours of solution preparation. Suspend administration for 2 hours prior to invasive procedures or other procedure with significant bleeding risk; may continue treatment immediately following uncomplicated, minimally-invasive procedures, but delay for 12 hours after major invasive procedures/surgery.

Reconstitution: Reconstitute 5 mg vials with 2.5 mL and 20 mg vials with 10 mL sterile water for injection (resultant solution ~2 mg/mL). Must be further diluted (within 3 hours of reconstitution) in 0.9% sodium chloride, typically to a concentration between 100 mcg/mL and 200 mcg/mL when using infusion pump and between 100 mcg/mL and 1000 mcg/mL when infused via syringe pump. Although product information states administration must be completed within 12 hours of preparation, additional studies (data on file, Lilly Research Laboratories) show that the final solution is stable for 14 hours at 15°C to 30°C (59°F to 86°F). If not used immediately, a prepared solution may be stored in the refrigerator for up to 12 hours. The total expiration time (refrigeration and administration) should be ≤24 hours from time of preparation.

Compatibility: Stable in NS; only NS, dextrose, LR, or dextrose/saline mixtures may be infused through the same line.

Y-site administration: Incompatible: Amiodarone, ampicillin/sulbactam sodium, ceftazidime, ciprofloxacin, clindamycin, cyclosporine, dobutamine hydrochloride, dopamine hydrochloride, epinephrine hydrochloride, fosphenytoin, furosemide, gentamicin sulfate, heparin sodium, human serum albumin, imipenem/cilastatin sodium, insulin human (regular), levofloxacin, magnesium sulfate, metronidazole, midazolam hydrochloride, nitroprusside sodium, norepinephrine bitartrate, piperacillin/tazobactam sodium, potassium phosphate, ranitidine hydrochloride, ticarcillin/clavulanate, tobramycin sulfate, vancomycin hydrochloride

Storage: Store vials under refrigeration at 2°C to 8°C (36°F to 46°F). Protect from light. Do not freeze.

Additional Information Prepared by recombinant DNA technology in human cell line

- **Drotrecogin Alfa, Activated** *see* Drotrecogin Alfa *on page 501*
- **Droxia™** *see* Hydroxyurea *on page 771*
- **Dryvax®** *see page 1660*
- **DSCG** *see* Cromolyn *on page 374*
- **D-Ser(Bu^t)⁶,Azgly¹⁰-LHRH** *see* Goserelin *on page 725*
- **D-S-S® [OTC]** *see* Docusate *on page 474*
- **DTIC** *see* Dacarbazine *on page 394*
- **DTIC-Dome®** *see* Dacarbazine *on page 394*
- **DTO** *see* Opium Tincture *on page 1122*
- **D-Trp(6)-LHRH** *see* Triptorelin *on page 1533*
- **Dulcolax® Milk of Magnesia [OTC]** *see* Magnesium Hydroxide *on page 930*
- **Dulcolax® Stool Softener [OTC]** *see* Docusate *on page 474*

Duloxetine (doo LOX e teen)

U.S. Brand Names Cymbalta®

Synonyms Duloxetine Hydrochloride; LY248686; (+)-(S)-N-Methyl-γ-(1-Naphthyloxy)-2-Thiophenepropylamine Hydrochloride

Restrictions A medication guide should be dispensed with each prescription. A template for the required MedGuides can be found on the FDA website at: http://www.fda.gov/cder/drug/antidepressants/labelTemplate.pdf

Generic Available No

Pharmacologic Category Antidepressant, Serotonin/Norepinephrine Reuptake Inhibitor

Medication Safety Issues
Sound-alike/look-alike issues:
Duloxetine may be confused with fluoxetine.

Use Treatment of major depressive disorder; management of pain associated with diabetic neuropathy

Unlabeled/Investigational Use Treatment of stress incontinence; management of chronic pain syndromes; management of fibromyalgia

Mechanism of Action/Effect Inhibits reuptake of both norepinephrine and serotonin (SNRI); improves symptoms of depression.

Contraindications Hypersensitivity to duloxetine or any component of the formulation; concomitant use or within 2 weeks of MAO inhibitors; uncontrolled narrow angle glaucoma

Warnings/Precautions Antidepressants increase the risk of suicidal thinking and behavior in children and adolescents with major depressive disorder (MDD) and other depressive disorders; consider risk prior to prescribing. All patients must be closely monitored for clinical worsening, suicidality, or unusual changes in behavior, especially during the initiation of therapy or following an increase or decrease in dosage. When used in children, the child's family or caregiver should be instructed to closely observe the patient and communicate condition with healthcare provider. A medication guide should be dispensed with each prescription. **Duloxetine is not FDA approved for use in children.**

The possibility of a suicide attempt is inherent in major depression and may persist until remission occurs. Use caution in high-risk patients. Worsening depression and severe abrupt suicidality that are not part of the presenting symptoms may require discontinuation or modification of drug therapy. The patient's family or caregiver should be alerted to monitor patients for the emergence of suicidality and associated behaviors (such as agitation, irritability, hostility, impulsivity, and hypomania) and call healthcare provider.

May worsen psychosis in some patients or precipitate a shift to mania or hypomania in patients with bipolar disorder. Patients presenting with depressive symptoms should be screened for bipolar disorder. Monotherapy in patients with bipolar disorder should be avoided. **Duloxetine is not FDA approved for the treatment of bipolar depression.**

Duloxetine may cause increased urinary resistance; advise patient to report symptoms of urinary hesitation/difficulty. Has a low potential to impair cognitive or motor performance. Use caution with a previous seizure disorder or condition predisposing to seizures such as brain damage or alcoholism. Avoid use in patients with hepatic impairment or in patients with substantial alcohol intake; may cause hepatotoxicity. Use with caution in patients with controlled narrow angle glaucoma. May cause or exacerbate sexual dysfunction. Use caution with renal impairment or with concomitant CNS depressants.

A potential exists for severe reactions when used with MAO inhibitors; serotonin syndrome (hyperthermia, muscular rigidity, mental status changes/agitation, autonomic instability) may
(Continued)

Duloxetine *(Continued)*

occur. Use caution during concurrent therapy with other drugs which lower the seizure threshold.

Upon discontinuation of duloxetine therapy, gradually taper dose. If intolerable symptoms occur following a decrease in dosage or upon discontinuation of therapy, then resuming the previous dose with a more gradual taper should be considered. May increase the risks associated with electroconvulsive therapy. Consider discontinuing, when possible, prior to elective surgery.

Drug Interactions

Cytochrome P450 Effect: Substrate (major) of CYP1A2, 2D6; **inhibits** CYP2D6 (moderate)

Decreased Effect: CYP1A2 inducers may decrease the levels/effects of duloxetine. Example inducers include aminoglutethimide, carbamazepine, phenobarbital, and rifampin.

Increased Effect/Toxicity: Hyperpyrexia, hypertension, tachycardia, confusion, seizures, and deaths have been reported with MAO inhibitors (serotonin syndrome); this combination is contraindicated. Avoid use of linezolid (due to MAO activity). Duloxetine may increase serum concentrations of thioridazine, which has been associated with the development of malignant ventricular arrhythmias. Serum levels/effects of tricyclic antidepressants may be increased by duloxetine.

Concurrent use of duloxetine with buspirone, meperidine, moclobemide, nefazodone, SSRIs, sibutramine, tramadol and trazodone and venlafaxine may cause serotonin syndrome; avoid concurrent use. Concurrent use of selegiline with SSRIs has been reported to cause serotonin syndrome (less than with nonselective MAO inhibitors). Concurrent use of sumatriptan and similar drugs (serotonin agonists) may result in weakness, hyper-reflexia, and incoordination.

CYP1A2 and CYP2D6 inhibitors may increase the levels/effects of duloxetine. Example inhibitors include amiodarone, chlorpromazine, ciprofloxacin, delavirdine, fluvoxamine, fluoxetine, ketoconazole, miconazole, norfloxacin, ofloxacin, paroxetine, pergolide, quinidine, quinine, rofecoxib, ritonavir, and ropinirole.

Nutritional/Ethanol Interactions

Ethanol: Avoid ethanol (may increase CNS depression and/or hepatotoxic potential of duloxetine).

Herb/Nutraceutical: Avoid valerian, St John's wort, SAMe, kava kava, and gotu kola (may increase CNS depression).

Adverse Reactions

>10%:

Central nervous system: Insomnia (8% to 11%%), somnolence (7% to 12%), dizziness (9% to 17%), headache (up to 15%)

Gastrointestinal: Nausea (20% to 22%), xerostomia (5% to 7%), constipation (5% to 11%), appetite decreased (8% to 11%)

1% to 10%:

Central nervous system: Fatigue (8% to 10%), anxiety (3%), fever (up to 1%), irritability, lethargy, nervousness, restlessness, sleep disorder, nightmares

Dermatologic: Pruritus, rash

Endocrine & metabolic: Libido decreased (3% to 6%), orgasm abnormality (3% to 4%), hot flushes (2%), hypoglycemia (1%), hypoesthesia (1%)

Gastrointestinal: Diarrhea (7% to 11%), appetite decreased (5% to 8%), vomiting (5%), dyspepsia (4%), loose stools (3%), anorexia (3%), weight loss (2%), gastritis (1%), weight gain (1%)

Genitourinary: Erectile dysfunction (1%), ejaculation delayed (3%), ejaculatory dysfunction (3%), urinary symptoms (hesitancy, obstructive symptoms; 1%), dysuria

Hepatic: Transaminases increased: Occasionally associated with hyperbilirubinemia and/or increased alkaline phosphatase (1%)

Neuromuscular & skeletal: Myalgia (4%), muscle cramp (4%), tremor (3% to 5%), rigors (1%)

Ocular: Blurred vision (4%)

Respiratory: Cough (up to 3%), pharyngolaryngeal pain (1%)

Miscellaneous: Diaphoresis increased (6%), night sweats

Overdosage/Toxicology Treatment is symptomatic and supportive.

Pharmacodynamics/Kinetics

Absorption: Well absorbed, 2-hour delay in absorption after ingestion

Time to Peak: 6 hours

Protein Binding: >90%

Half-Life Elimination: 12 hours (range 8-17 hours)

Metabolism: Hepatic, via CYP1A2 and CYP2D6; forms multiple metabolites (inactive)

Excretion: As metabolites; urine (70%), feces (20%)

Dosing

Adults:

Treatment of depression: Oral: Initial: 40-60 mg/day; dose may be divided (ie, 20 or 30 mg twice daily) or given as a single daily dose of 60 mg; maximum dose: 60 mg/day

Management of diabetic neuropathy: Oral: 60 mg once daily. Lower initial doses may be considered in patients where tolerability is a concern and/or renal impairment is present.

Management of chronic pain syndromes (unlabeled use): Oral: 60 mg once daily

Management of fibromyalgia (unlabeled use): 60 mg twice daily

Management of stress incontinence (unlabeled use): Oral: 40 mg twice daily

Elderly:

Treatment of major depressive disorder: Oral: Initial dose: 20 mg 1-2 times/day; increase to 40-60 mg/day as a single daily dose or in divided doses

Other indications: Refer to adult dosing.

Renal Impairment: Not recommended for use in Cl$_{cr}$ <30 mL/minute or ESRD. In mild-moderate impairment, lower initial doses may be considered with titration guided by response and tolerability.

Hepatic Impairment: Not recommended for use in hepatic impairment.

Available Dosage Forms Capsule: 20 mg, 30 mg, 60 mg [contains enteric coated pellets]

Monitoring and Teaching Issues

Physical Assessment: Assess other medications patient may be taking for effectiveness and potential interactions (See Drug Interactions). Can cause increase in blood pressure. Monitor blood pressure at the beginning of treatment and periodically throughout treatment. Monitor for worsening of depression and suicide ideation. Taper dosage slowly when discontinuing. Do not discontinue abruptly. Assess knowledge/teach appropriate use of this medication, interventions to reduce side effects and adverse reactions.

Patient Education: Take exactly as directed; swallow capsule whole. Do not open or crush. It may take 2-3 weeks to achieve desired results. Inform prescriber of all prescription medications, OTC medications, or herbal products you are taking. Maintain adequate hydration (2-3 L/day of fluid) unless instructed to restrict fluid intake by prescriber. Avoid alcohol use. Can cause drowsiness, dizziness, fatigue, insomnia (use caution when driving or engaging in activities requiring alertness until response to drug is known). You may experience headache, nausea, diarrhea (buttermilk, yogurt, or boiled milk may help), constipation (increased exercise, fluids, fruit, or fiber may help), appetite decrease, or xerostomia. Report persistent insomnia, dizziness, headache, thoughts of suicide, worsening of anxiety, panic attacks, agitation, irritability, akathisia, hostility, hypomania, mania. **Pregnancy/breast-feeding precautions:** Inform prescriber if you are or intend to become pregnant. Consult prescriber before breast-feeding.

Dietary Considerations: May be taken without regard to meals.

Geriatric Considerations: Has not been studied exclusively in the elderly, however, its low anticholinergic activity, minimal sedation, and hypotension makes this a potentially valuable antidepressant in treating elderly with depression. No dose adjustment is necessary for age alone, additional studies are necessary; adjust dose for renal function in the elderly. Higher doses required for the treatment of the urinary stress incontinence and neuropathic pain.

Pregnancy Risk Factor: C

Pregnancy Issues: Nonteratogenic effects including respiratory distress, cyanosis, apnea, seizures, temperature instability, feeding difficulty, vomiting, hypoglycemia, hypo- or hypertonia, hyper-reflexia, jitteriness, irritability, constant crying, and tremor have been reported in the neonate immediately following delivery after exposure late in the third trimester. Adverse effects may be due to toxic effects of SNRI or drug discontinuation. There are no adequate and well-controlled studies in pregnant women. Use during pregnancy only if the potential benefit to the mother outweighs the possible risk to the fetus. If treatment during pregnancy is required, consider tapering therapy during the third trimester.

Lactation: Excretion in breast milk unknown/not recommended

Breast-Feeding Issues: In animals, duloxetine is excreted in breast milk. No studies have been conducted in humans. SSRIs have been associated with excessive somnolence, decreased feeding, and weight loss in nursing infants (relevance to SNRIs is not clearly established).

Administration

Oral: Capsule should be swallowed whole; do not break open or crush.

Storage: Store at 25°C (77°F), excursions permitted to 15°C to 30°C (59°F to 86°F)

Related Information

Antidepressant Agents *on page 1713*

- ◆ **Duloxetine Hydrochloride** *see* Duloxetine *on page 503*
- ◆ **DuoNeb™** *see* Ipratropium and Albuterol *on page 827*
- ◆ **Duotan PD** *see* Dexchlorpheniramine and Pseudoephedrine *on page 428*
- ◆ **DuP 753** *see* Losartan *on page 922*
- ◆ **Duraclon™** *see* Clonidine *on page 354*
- ◆ **Duradrin®** *see* Acetaminophen, Isometheptene, and Dichloralphenazone *on page 42*
- ◆ **Duragesic®** *see* Fentanyl *on page 618*
- ◆ **Duramorph®** *see* Morphine Sulfate *on page 1031*
- ◆ **Duratuss® DM** *see* Guaifenesin and Dextromethorphan *on page 731*
- ◆ **Duricef®** *see* Cefadroxil *on page 267*
- ◆ **DW286** *see* Gemifloxacin *on page 706*
- ◆ **Dyazide®** *see* Hydrochlorothiazide and Triamterene *on page 754*

Dyclonine (DYE kloe neen)

U.S. Brand Names Cēpacol® Maximum Strength [OTC]; Sucrets® [OTC]

Synonyms Dyclonine Hydrochloride

Generic Available No

Pharmacologic Category Local Anesthetic; Local Anesthetic, Oral

Medication Safety Issues

Sound-alike/look-alike issues:

Dyclonine may be confused with dicyclomine

Use Local anesthetic prior to laryngoscopy, bronchoscopy, or endotracheal intubation; use topically for temporary relief of pain associated with oral mucosa or anogenital lesions

Mechanism of Action/Effect Blocks impulses at peripheral nerve endings in skin and mucous membranes by altering cell membrane permeability to ionic transfer

Contraindications Contraindicated in patients allergic to chlorobutanol (preservative used in dyclonine) or dyclonine

Warnings/Precautions Use with caution in patients with sepsis or traumatized mucosa in the area of application to avoid rapid systemic absorption. May impair swallowing and enhance the danger of aspiration. Use with caution in patients with shock or heart block. Resuscitative equipment, oxygen, and resuscitative drugs should be immediately available when dyclonine topical solution is administered to mucous membranes. **Not for injection or ophthalmic use.**

(Continued)

Dyclonine *(Continued)*

Overdosage/Toxicology Symptoms of overdose are CNS (seizures, excitation) and cardio-vascular (hypotension, myocardial depression). Treatment is supportive and symptomatic.

Pharmacodynamics/Kinetics
Onset of Action: Local anesthetic: 2-10 minutes
Duration of Action: 30-60 minutes

Dosing
Adults & Elderly: Note: Administered as topical solution, use lowest dose needed to provide effective anesthesia:

Mouth sores: Topical: 5-10 mL of 0.5% or 1% to oral mucosa (swab or swish and then spit) 3-4 times/day as needed; maximum single dose: 200 mg (40 mL of 0.5% solution or 20 mL of 1% solution)

Bronchoscopy: Topical: Use 2 mL of the 1% solution or 4 mL of the 0.5% solution sprayed onto the larynx and trachea every 5 minutes until the reflex has been abolished.

Pediatrics: Refer to adult dosing.

Available Dosage Forms
Lozenge, as hydrochloride (Sucrets®): 1.2 mg, 2 mg, 3 mg [cherry, lemon, wintergreen, and assorted flavors]
Spray, oral, as hydrochloride (Cēpacol® Maximum Strength): 0.1% (120 mL) [cherry and menthol flavors]

Monitoring and Teaching Issues
Physical Assessment: Monitor for effectiveness of anesthesia and for adverse or toxic reactions. Monitor for return of sensation. Teach patient adverse reactions to report; use and teach appropriate interventions to promote safety.
Patient Education: This medication is given to reduce sensation in the injected area. When used in mouth or throat; do not eat or drink anything for at least 1 hour following treatment. Take small sips of water at first to ensure that you can swallow without difficulty. Your tongue and mouth may be numb, use caution to avoid biting yourself. Immediately report swelling of face, lips, tongue; chest pain or palpitations; increased restlessness, confusion, anxiety, or dizziness. **Pregnancy/breast-feeding precautions:** Inform prescriber if you are or intend to become pregnant. Consult prescriber if breast-feeding.
Dietary Considerations: Food should not be ingested for 60 minutes following application in the mouth or throat area.
Pregnancy Risk Factor: C
Lactation: Excretion in breast milk unknown
Administration
Storage: Store in tight, light-resistant containers.

* **Dyclonine Hydrochloride** *see Dyclonine on page 505*
* **Dynacin®** *see Minocycline on page 1012*
* **DynaCirc®** *see Isradipine on page 845*
* **DynaCirc® CR** *see Isradipine on page 845*
* **Dynatan™** *see DiphenhydrAMINE on page 463*
* **Dynex** *see Guaifenesin and Pseudoephedrine on page 733*
* **E2020** *see Donepezil on page 480*
* **EarSol® HC** *see Hydrocortisone on page 760*
* **Easprin®** *see Aspirin on page 143*
* **EC-Naprosyn®** *see Naproxen on page 1056*
* *E. coli* **Asparaginase** *see Asparaginase on page 141*
* **Econopred® Plus** *see PrednisoLONE on page 1245*
* **Ecotrin® [OTC]** *see Aspirin on page 143*
* **Ecotrin® Low Strength [OTC]** *see Aspirin on page 143*
* **Ecotrin® Maximum Strength [OTC]** *see Aspirin on page 143*
* **Edecrin®** *see Ethacrynic Acid on page 575*
* **Edex®** *see Alprostadil on page 76*

Edrophonium *(ed roe FOE nee um)*

U.S. Brand Names Enlon®; Reversol®
Synonyms Edrophonium Chloride
Generic Available No
Pharmacologic Category Antidote; Cholinergic Agonist; Diagnostic Agent
Use Diagnosis of myasthenia gravis; differentiation of cholinergic crises from myasthenia crises; reversal of nondepolarizing neuromuscular blockers; adjunct treatment of respiratory depression caused by curare overdose
Mechanism of Action/Effect Inhibits destruction of acetylcholine by acetylcholinesterase. This facilitates transmission of impulses across myoneural junction and results in increased cholinergic responses such as miosis, increased tonus of intestinal and skeletal muscles, bronchial and ureteral constriction, bradycardia, and increased salivary and sweat gland secretions.
Contraindications Hypersensitivity to edrophonium, sulfites, or any component of the formulation; GI or GU obstruction
Warnings/Precautions Use with caution in patients with bronchial asthma and those receiving a cardiac glycoside. Atropine sulfate should always be readily available as an antagonist. Overdosage can cause cholinergic crisis which may be fatal (DUMBELS - **d**iarrhea, **u**rination, **m**iosis, **b**ronchospasm/**b**radycardia, **e**xcitation, **l**acrimation, **s**alivation/excessive **s**weating), and acute muscle weakness. I.V. atropine should be readily available for treatment of cholinergic reactions.
Drug Interactions
Decreased Effect: Atropine, nondepolarizing muscle relaxants, procainamide, and quinidine may antagonize the effects of edrophonium.

Increased Effect/Toxicity: Digoxin may enhance bradycardia potential of edrophonium. Effects of succinylcholine, decamethonium, nondepolarizing muscle relaxants (eg, pancuronium, vecuronium) are prolonged by edrophonium. I.V. acetazolamide, neostigmine, physostigmine, and acute muscle weakness may increase the effects of edrophonium.

Lab Interactions Increased aminotransferase [ALT (SGPT)/AST (SGOT)] (S), amylase (S)

Adverse Reactions Frequency not defined.

Cardiovascular: Arrhythmias (especially bradycardia), hypotension, decreased carbon monoxide, tachycardia, AV block, nodal rhythm, nonspecific ECG changes, cardiac arrest, syncope, flushing

Central nervous system: Convulsions, dysarthria, dysphonia, dizziness, loss of consciousness, drowsiness, headache

Dermatologic: Skin rash, thrombophlebitis (I.V.), urticaria

Gastrointestinal: Hyperperistalsis, nausea, vomiting, salivation, diarrhea, stomach cramps, dysphagia, flatulence

Genitourinary: Urinary urgency

Neuromuscular & skeletal: Weakness, fasciculations, muscle cramps, spasms, arthralgia

Ocular: Small pupils, lacrimation

Respiratory: Increased bronchial secretions, laryngospasm, bronchiolar constriction, respiratory muscle paralysis, dyspnea, respiratory depression, respiratory arrest, bronchospasm

Miscellaneous: Diaphoresis (increased), anaphylaxis, allergic reactions

Overdosage/Toxicology Symptoms of overdose include muscle weakness, nausea, vomiting, miosis, bronchospasm, and respiratory paralysis. Maintain an adequate airway. For muscarinic symptoms, the antidote is atropine 0.4-0.5 mg I.V. repeated every 3-10 minutes (initial doses as high as 1.2 mg have been administered). Skeletal muscle effects of edrophonium are not alleviated by atropine.

Pharmacodynamics/Kinetics

Onset of Action: I.M.: 2-10 minutes; I.V.: 30-60 seconds

Duration of Action: I.M.: 5-30 minutes: I.V.: 10 minutes

Half-Life Elimination: 1.8 hours

Dosing

Adults & Elderly: Usually administered I.V., however, if not possible, I.M. or SubQ may be used.

Diagnosis of Myasthenia gravis:

I.V.: 2 mg test dose administered over 15-30 seconds; 8 mg given 45 seconds later if no response is seen. Test dose may be repeated after 30 minutes.

I.M.: Initial: 10 mg; if no cholinergic reaction occurs, give 2 mg 30 minutes later to rule out false-negative reaction.

Titration of oral anticholinesterase therapy: 1-2 mg given 1 hour after oral dose of anticholinesterase; if strength improves, an increase in neostigmine or pyridostigmine dose is indicated.

Differentiation of cholinergic from myasthenic crisis: I.V.: 1 mg; may repeat after 1 minute. **Note:** Intubation and controlled ventilation may be required if patient has cholinergic crisis.

Reversal of nondepolarizing neuromuscular blocking agents (neostigmine with atropine usually preferred): I.V.: 10 mg over 30-45 seconds; may repeat every 5-10 minutes up to 40 mg.

Termination of paroxysmal atrial tachycardia: I.V. rapid injection: 5-10 mg

Pediatrics: Usually administered I.V., however, if not possible, I.M. or SubQ may be used:

Infants:

I.M.: 0.5-1 mg

I.V.: Initial: 0.1 mg, followed by 0.4 mg if no response; total dose = 0.5 mg

Children:

Diagnosis: Initial: 0.04 mg/kg over 1 minute followed by 0.16 mg/kg if no response, to a maximum total dose of 5 mg for children <34 kg, or 10 mg for children >34 kg **or**

Alternative dosing (manufacturer's recommendation):

≤34 kg: 1 mg; if no response after 45 seconds, repeat dosage in 1 mg increments every 30-45 seconds, up to a total of 5 mg

>34 kg: 2 mg; if no response after 45 seconds, repeat dosage in 1 mg increments every 30-45 seconds, up to a total of 10 mg

I.M.:

<34 kg: 1 mg

>34 kg: 5 mg

Titration of oral anticholinesterase therapy: 0.04 mg/kg once given 1 hour after oral intake of the drug being used in treatment. If strength improves, an increase in neostigmine or pyridostigmine dose is indicated.

Renal Impairment: Dose may need to be reduced in patients with chronic renal failure.

Available Dosage Forms Injection, solution, as chloride:

Enlon®: 10 mg/mL (15 mL) [contains sodium sulfite]

Reversol®: 10 mg/mL (10 mL) [contains sodium sulfite]

Monitoring and Teaching Issues

Physical Assessment: Administration of edrophonium for MG diagnosis is supervised by a neurologist and use as a neuromuscular blocking agent is supervised by an anesthesiologist. Patient must be monitored closely during and following procedure, especially for cholinergic crisis; keep atropine at hand for antidote. Patients receiving the medication for MG testing will have been advised by their neurologist about drug effects. Those patients receiving medication for neuromuscular block will be unaware of drug effects. Patient should never be left alone until all drug effects and the possibility of cholinergic crisis have passed.

Patient Education: Pregnancy/breast-feeding precautions: Inform prescriber if you are or intend to become pregnant. Consult prescriber if breast-feeding.

(Continued)

Edrophonium (Continued)

Geriatric Considerations: Many elderly will have diseases which may influence the use of edrophonium. Also, many elderly will need doses reduced 50% due to creatinine clearances in the 10-50 mL/minute range (common in the aged). Side effects or concomitant disease may warrant use of pyridostigmine.

Pregnancy Risk Factor: C

Lactation: Excretion in breast milk unknown

Additional Information Atropine should be administered along with edrophonium when reversing the effects of nondepolarizing agents to antagonize the cholinergic effects at the muscarinic receptors, especially bradycardia. It is important to recognize the difference in dose for diagnosis of myasthenia gravis versus reversal of muscle relaxant, a much larger dose is needed for desired effect of reversal of muscle paralysis.

♦ **Edrophonium Chloride** see Edrophonium on page 506

♦ **E.E.S.®** see Erythromycin on page 543

Efalizumab (e fa li ZOO mab)

U.S. Brand Names Raptiva™

Synonyms Anti-CD11a; hu1124

Generic Available No

Pharmacologic Category Immunosuppressant Agent; Monoclonal Antibody

Use Treatment of chronic moderate-to-severe plaque psoriasis in patients who are candidates for systemic therapy or phototherapy

Mechanism of Action/Effect Efalizumab is a recombinant monoclonal antibody; efalizumab blocks multiple T-cell mediated responses involved in the pathogenesis of psoriatic plaques.

Contraindications Hypersensitivity to efalizumab or any component of the formulation

Warnings/Precautions May result in increased susceptibility to infections; use caution with chronic infections, history of recurrent infection, or the elderly. Discontinue therapy if serious infection develops. Use caution in patients at high risk for malignancy or history of malignancy; effects of efalizumab on the development of malignancies is unknown. Psoriasis may worsen with efalizumab treatment or following discontinuation (rare). First-dose reactions have been reported; a lower, conditioning dose is recommended to reduce the incidence and severity of reactions. Concomitant use with other immunosuppressant agents is not recommended. Produced in a Chinese hamster cell medium. Safety and efficacy in pediatric patients or patients with renal or hepatic impairment have not been established.

Drug Interactions

Decreased Effect: Note: Formal drug interaction studies have not been conducted. Acellular, live, and live-attenuated vaccines should not be administered during therapy.

Adverse Reactions

>10%:

Central nervous system: Headache (32%), chills (13%)

Gastrointestinal: Nausea (11%)

Hematologic: Lymphocytosis (40%), leukocytosis (26%)

Miscellaneous: First-dose reaction (29%, described as chills, fever, headache, myalgia, and nausea occurring within 2 days of the first injection; percent reported in patients receiving a 1 mg/kg dose; severity decreased with 0.7 mg/kg dose); infection (29%, serious infection <1%)

1% to 10%:

Cardiovascular: Peripheral edema (1% to 2%)

Central nervous system: Pain (10%), fever (7%)

Dermatologic: Acne (4%), psoriasis (1% to 2%), urticaria (1%)

Hepatic: Alkaline phosphatase elevated (4%)

Neuromuscular & skeletal: Myalgia (8%), back pain (4%), arthralgia (1% to 2%), weakness (1% to 2%)

Miscellaneous: Antibodies to efalizumab (6%), hypersensitivity reaction (8%), flu-like syndrome (7%)

Overdosage/Toxicology Limited data. Severe vomiting reported in one patient receiving 10 mg/kg intravenously. In case of overdose, monitor for 24-48 hours.

Pharmacodynamics/Kinetics

Onset of Action: Reduction of CD11a expression and free CD11a-binding sites seen 1-2 days after the first dose; time to steady state serum concentration: 4 weeks

Response to therapy (75% reduction from baseline of PASI score): Observed after 12 weeks

Duration of Action: CD11a expression was ~74% of baseline at 5-13 weeks after discontinuing dose; free CD11a binding sites were at ~85% of baseline at 8-13 weeks following discontinuation; response to therapy (75% reduction from baseline PASI score) continued 1-2 months after discontinuation

Bioavailability: SubQ: 50%

Excretion: Time to eliminate (at steady state): 25 days

Dosing

Adults: Psoriasis: SubQ: Initial: 0.7 mg/kg, followed by weekly dose of 1 mg/kg (maximum: 200 mg/dose)

Available Dosage Forms Injection, powder for reconstitution: 150 mg [contains sucrose 123.2 mg/vial; delivers 125 mg/1.25 mL; packaged with prefilled syringe containing sterile water for injection]

Monitoring and Teaching Issues

Physical Assessment: Assess results of laboratory tests. Be alert to the possibility of the development of infection or malignancy. Assess therapeutic effectiveness and adverse reactions on a regular basis throughout therapy. Do not administer any immunizations with acellular, live, or live-attenuated vaccines during therapy with efalizumab. Teach patient possible side effects/appropriate interventions and adverse symptoms to report.

Monitoring Laboratory Tests: Platelet counts (at least monthly at the start of treatment, every 3 months as therapy continues)

Patient Education: This medication can only be given by injection. Do not take any new medications during therapy without consulting prescriber. You may be more susceptible to infection while on this therapy; avoid crowds and exposure to infections, and do not have any immunizations while on this therapy. Notify prescriber of any allergic response (headache, chills, muscle pain, rash, difficulty breathing, or swelling around mouth within 3 days of first dose). May cause mild edema in extremities; back or muscle pain or flu-like syndrome (consult prescriber for appropriate analgesic). Report unusual infection; weight gain >5 pounds in 1 week; persistent muscle or joint pain or weakness; infection; other persistent reactions or worsening of psoriasis. **Pregnancy/breast-feeding precautions:** Inform prescriber if you are or intend to be pregnant. Do not breast-feed.

Pregnancy Risk Factor: C

Lactation: Excretion in breast milk unknown/not recommended

Breast-Feeding Issues: A decrease in the ability to mount an antibody response was observed in the offspring of lactating mice. It is not known if efalizumab is excreted in human milk. However, since maternal immunoglobulins are present, and animal data suggest possible adverse effects in the nursing infant, it is recommended to discontinue nursing or discontinue efalizumab.

Administration

Other: For SubQ injection in the abdomen, buttocks, thigh, or upper arm

Reconstitution: Slowly inject 1.3 mL of the provided diluent into vial; gently swirl to mix, do not shake.

Storage: Powder should be stored under refrigeration at 2°C to 8°C (36°F to 46°F) and protected from light. Following reconstitution, solution should be stored at room temperature and used within 8 hours. Discard unused solution.

Efavirenz (e FAV e renz)

U.S. Brand Names Sustiva®

Generic Available No

Pharmacologic Category Antiretroviral Agent, Reverse Transcriptase Inhibitor (Non-nucleoside)

Use Treatment of HIV-1 infections in combination with at least two other antiretroviral agents

Mechanism of Action/Effect As a non-nucleoside reverse transcriptase inhibitor, efavirenz has activity against HIV-1 by binding to reverse transcriptase. It consequently blocks the RNA-dependent and DNA-dependent DNA polymerase activities including HIV-1 replication. It does not require intracellular phosphorylation for antiviral activity.

Contraindications Clinically-significant hypersensitivity to efavirenz or any component of the formulation; concurrent use of cisapride, midazolam, triazolam, voriconazole, or ergot alkaloids (includes dihydroergotamine, ergotamine, ergonovine, methylergonovine); pregnancy

Warnings/Precautions Do not use as single-agent therapy; avoid pregnancy; women of childbearing potential should undergo pregnancy testing prior to initiation of therapy; use caution with other agents metabolized by cytochrome P450 isoenzyme 3A4 (see Contraindications); use caution with history of mental illness/drug abuse (predisposition to psychological reactions); may cause CNS and psychiatric symptoms, which include impaired concentration, dizziness or drowsiness (avoid potentially hazardous tasks such as driving or operating machinery if these effects are noted); serious psychiatric side effects have been associated with efavirenz, including severe depression, suicide, paranoia, and mania; discontinue if severe rash (involving blistering, desquamation, mucosal involvement or fever) develops. Children are more susceptible to development of rash; prophylactic antihistamines may be used. Caution in patients with known or suspected hepatitis B or C infection (monitoring of liver function is recommended); hepatic impairment. Persistent elevations of serum transaminases >5 times the upper limit of normal should prompt evaluation - benefit of continued therapy should be weighed against possible risk of hepatotoxicity. Concomitant use with St John's wort is not recommended.

Drug Interactions

Cytochrome P450 Effect: Substrate (major) of CYP2B6, 3A4; **Inhibits** CYP2C8/9 (weak), 2C19 (weak), 3A4 (weak); **Induces** CYP2B6 (weak), 3A4 (weak)

Decreased Effect: CYP2B6 inducers may decrease the levels/effects of efavirenz; example inducers include carbamazepine, nevirapine, phenobarbital, phenytoin, and rifampin. St John's wort may decrease serum concentrations of efavirenz. Concentrations of atazanavir, indinavir, and/or lopinavir may be reduced; dosage adjustments required. Concentrations of saquinavir may be decreased (use as sole protease inhibitor is not recommended). Serum concentrations of methadone may be decreased; monitor for withdrawal. May decrease (or increase) effect of warfarin. Serum concentrations of sertraline may be decreased by efavirenz. CYP3A4 inducers may decrease the levels/effects of efavirenz; example inducers include aminoglutethimide, carbamazepine, nafcillin, nevirapine, phenobarbital, phenytoin, and rifamycins. Voriconazole serum levels may be reduced by efavirenz (concurrent use is contraindicated).

Increased Effect/Toxicity: Coadministration with medications metabolized by these enzymes may lead to increased concentration-related effects. Cisapride, midazolam, triazolam, and ergot alkaloids may result in life-threatening toxicities; concurrent use is contraindicated. May increase (or decrease) effect of warfarin.

Nutritional/Ethanol Interactions

Ethanol: Avoid ethanol (hepatic and CNS adverse effects).

Food: Avoid high-fat meals (increase the absorption of efavirenz).

Herb/Nutraceutical: St John's wort may decrease efavirenz serum levels. Avoid concurrent use.

Lab Interactions False-positive test for cannabinoids have been reported when the CEDIA DAU Multilevel THC assay is used. False-positive results with other assays for cannabinoids have not been observed.

Adverse Reactions

>10%:

Central nervous system: Dizziness* (2% to 28%), depression (1% to 16%), insomnia (6% to 16%), anxiety (1% to 11%), pain* (1% to 13%)

(Continued)

Efavirenz *(Continued)*

    Dermatologic: Rash* (NCI grade 1: 9% to 11%, NCI grade 2: 15% to 32%, NCI grade 3 or 4: <1%); 26% experienced new rash vs 17% in control groups; up to 46% of pediatric patients experience rash (median onset: 8 days)

    Endocrine & metabolic: HDL increased (25% to 35%), total cholesterol increased (20% to 40%)

    Gastrointestinal: Diarrhea* (3% to 14%), nausea* (2% to 12%)

1% to 10%:

    Central nervous system: Impaired concentration (2% to 8%), headache* (2% to 7%), somnolence (2% to 7%), fatigue (2% to 7%), abnormal dreams (1% to 6%), nervousness (2% to 6%), severe depression (2%), hallucinations (1%)

    Dermatologic: Pruritus (1% to 9%)

    Gastrointestinal: Vomiting* (6% to 7%), dyspepsia (3%), abdominal pain (1% to 3%), anorexia (1% to 2%)

    Miscellaneous: Diaphoresis increased (1% to 2%)

*Adverse effect reported in ≥10% of patients 3-16 years of age

Overdosage/Toxicology Increased central nervous system symptoms and involuntary muscle contractions have been reported in accidental overdose. Treatment is supportive. Activated charcoal may enhance elimination; dialysis is unlikely to remove the drug.

Pharmacodynamics/Kinetics

Absorption: Increased by fatty meals

Time to Peak: 3-8 hours

Protein Binding: >99%, primarily to albumin

Half-Life Elimination: Single dose: 52-76 hours; Multiple doses: 40-55 hours

Metabolism: Hepatic via CYP3A4 and 2B6; may induce its own metabolism

Excretion: Feces (16% to 41% primarily as unchanged drug); urine (14% to 34% as metabolites)

Dosing

Adults & Elderly: Dosing at bedtime is recommended to limit central nervous system effects; should not be used as single-agent therapy.

    HIV infection (as part of combination): Oral: 600 mg once daily

Pediatrics: Dosing at bedtime is recommended to limit central nervous system effects; should not be used as single-agent therapy. Dosage is based on body weight.

    HIV infection (as part of combination): Oral:
      10 kg to <15 kg: 200 mg once daily
      15 kg to <20 kg: 250 mg once daily
      20 kg to <25 kg: 300 mg once daily
      25 kg to <32.5 kg: 350 mg once daily
      32.5 kg to <40 kg: 400 mg once daily
      ≥40 kg: 600 mg once daily

Renal Impairment: No adjustment is necessary.

Hepatic Impairment: Limited clinical experience - use with caution.

Available Dosage Forms

Capsule: 50 mg, 100 mg, 200 mg

Tablet: 600 mg

Monitoring and Teaching Issues

Physical Assessment: Do not use as single-agent therapy. See Warnings/Precautions for use cautions (eg, mental illness, hepatic disease or impairment). Assess potential for interactions with other pharmacological agents or herbal products patient may be taking (eg, increased risk for CNS depression, or toxicities; see Drug Interactions). Assess results of laboratory test, therapeutic effectiveness (CD4 counts and viral load), and adverse reactions (CNS changes, rash, increased lipid levels; see Adverse Reactions) on a regular basis throughout therapy. Teach patient proper use, possible side effects/appropriate interventions, and adverse symptoms to report (see Patient Education).

Monitoring Laboratory Tests: Monitor serum transaminases (discontinuation of treatment should be considered for persistent elevations greater than five times the upper limit of normal), cholesterol, and triglycerides.

Patient Education: Do not take any new medication during therapy unless approved by prescriber. This drug is not a cure for HIV nor has it been found to reduce transmission of HIV. Take as directed, on an empty stomach (1 hour before or 2 hours after eating). This drug is usually used in combination with other medications; maintain recommended schedule of all medications. Maintain adequate hydration (2-3 L/day of fluids) unless instructed to restrict fluid intake. Avoid alcohol (may cause undesirable reactions). May cause dizziness, anxiety, tremor, impaired coordination, inability to concentrate (use caution when driving or engaging in tasks requiring alertness until response to drug is known); nausea or vomiting (small frequent meals, good mouth care, chewing gum, or sucking lozenges may help; consult prescriber if nausea or vomiting persists); or diarrhea (buttermilk, boiled milk, or yogurt may help). Report CNS changes (acute headache, abnormal dreams, sleepiness or fatigue, seizures, hallucinations, amnesia, emotional lability, confusion); muscle pain, weakness, tremors, numbness; rash; or other unusual effects. **Pregnancy/breast-feeding precautions:** Inform prescriber if you are or intend to become pregnant. Do not breast-feed.

Dietary Considerations: Should be taken on an empty stomach.

Pregnancy Risk Factor: D

Pregnancy Issues: Teratogenic effects have been observed in Primates receiving efavirenz. Severe CNS defects have been reported in infants following efavirenz exposure in the first trimester. Pregnancy should be avoided and alternate therapy should be considered in women of childbearing potential. Women of childbearing potential should undergo pregnancy testing prior to initiation of efavirenz. Barrier contraception should be used in combination with other (hormonal) methods of contraception. If therapy with efavirenz is administered during pregnancy, avoid use during the first trimester. Health professionals are encouraged to contact the antiretroviral pregnancy registry to monitor outcomes of pregnant women exposed to antiretroviral medications (1-800-258-4263 or www.APRegistry.com).

Lactation: Excretion is breast milk unknown/contraindicated

Breast-Feeding Issues: HIV-infected mothers are discouraged from breast-feeding to decrease potential transmission of HIV.

Administration
Oral: Administer on an empty stomach.
Storage: Store below 25°C (77°F).

Additional Information Efavirenz oral solution is available only through an expanded access (compassionate use) program. Enrollment information may be obtained by calling 1-877-372-7097.

Early virologic failure was observed with tenofovir and didanosine delayed release capsules, plus either efavirenz or nevirapine; use caution in treatment-naive patients with high baseline viral loads.

Related Information
Tuberculosis *on page 1864*

Eflornithine (ee FLOR ni theen)

U.S. Brand Names Vaniqa™
Synonyms DFMO; Eflornithine Hydrochloride
Generic Available No
Pharmacologic Category Antiprotozoal; Topical Skin Product
Medication Safety Issues
Sound-alike/look-alike issues:
Vaniqa™ may be confused with Viagra®

Use Cream: Females ≥12 years: Reduce unwanted hair from face and adjacent areas under the chin
Orphan status: Injection: Treatment of meningoencephalitic stage of *Trypanosoma brucei gambiense* infection (sleeping sickness)

Mechanism of Action/Effect Eflornithine exerts antitumor and antiprotozoal effects through specific, irreversible ("suicide") inhibition of the enzyme ornithine decarboxylase (ODC). ODC is the rate-limiting enzyme in the biosynthesis of putrescine, spermine, and spermidine, the major polyamines in nucleated cells. Polyamines are necessary for the synthesis of DNA, RNA, and proteins and are, therefore, necessary for cell growth and differentiation. Although many microorganisms and higher plants are able to produce polyamines from alternate biochemical pathways, all mammalian cells depend on ornithine decarboxylase to produce polyamines. Eflornithine inhibits ODC and rapidly depletes animal cells of putrescine and spermidine; the concentration of spermine remains the same or may even increase. Rapidly dividing cells appear to be most susceptible to the effects of eflornithine. Topically, the inhibition of ODC in the skin leads to a decreased rate of hair growth.

Contraindications Hypersensitivity to eflornithine or any component of the formulation

Warnings/Precautions
Injection: Must be diluted before use. Frequent monitoring for myelosuppression should be done. Use with caution in patients with a history of seizures and in patients with renal impairment. Serial audiograms should be obtained. Due to the potential for relapse, patients should be followed up for at least 24 months.

Cream: For topical use by females only. Discontinue if hypersensitivity occurs. Safety and efficacy in children <12 years has not been studied.

Drug Interactions
Decreased Effect: Cream: Possible interactions with other topical products have not been studied.
Increased Effect/Toxicity: Cream: Possible interactions with other topical products have not been studied.

Adverse Reactions
Injection:
>10%: Hematologic (reversible): Anemia (55%), leukopenia (37%), thrombocytopenia (14%)
1% to 10%:
Central nervous system: Seizures (may be due to the disease) (8%), dizziness
Dermatologic: Alopecia
Gastrointestinal: Vomiting, diarrhea
Hematologic: Eosinophilia
Otic: Hearing impairment
Topical:
>10%: Dermatologic: Acne (11% to 21%), pseudofolliculitis barbae (5% to 15%)
1% to 10%:
Central nervous system: Headache (4% to 5%), dizziness (1%), vertigo (0.3% to 1%)
Dermatologic: Pruritus (3% to 4%), burning skin (2% to 4%), tingling skin (1% to 4%), dry skin (2% to 3%), rash (1% to 3%), facial edema (0.3% to 3%), alopecia (1% to 2%), skin irritation (1% to 2%), erythema (0% to 2%), ingrown hair (0.3% to 2%), folliculitis (0% to 1%)
Gastrointestinal: Dyspepsia (2%), anorexia (0.7% to 2%)

Overdosage/Toxicology No known antidote; treatment is supportive. In mice and rats, CNS depression, seizures, death have occurred. Overdose with topical product is not expected due to low percutaneous penetration.
(Continued)

Eflornithine *(Continued)*

Pharmacodynamics/Kinetics
Absorption: Topical: <1%
Half-Life Elimination: I.V.: 3-3.5 hours; Topical: 8 hours
Excretion: Primarily urine (as unchanged drug)

Dosing
Adults & Elderly:
Unwanted facial hair (Females): Topical: Apply thin layer of cream to affected areas of face and adjacent chin twice daily, at least 8 hours apart.
Treatment of infections caused by *Trypanosoma*: I.V. infusion (orphan drug): 100 mg/kg/dose given every 6 hours (over at least 45 minutes) for 14 days.
Pediatrics: Unwanted facial hair (females): Children ≥12 years: Refer to adult dosing.
Renal Impairment: Injection: Dose should be adjusted although no specific guidelines are available.

Available Dosage Forms
Cream, topical, as hydrochloride: 13.9% (30 g)
Injection, solution, as hydrochloride: 200 mg/mL (100 mL) [orphan drug status]

Monitoring and Teaching Issues
Physical Assessment: Laboratory tests and results should be monitored on regular basis during therapy. Serial audiograms are recommended. Monitor effectiveness according to purpose for use. Patient should be monitored for adverse reactions, especially with infusion administration. Assess knowledge/teach patient appropriate use, adverse reactions and possible interventions, and adverse reactions to report.
Monitoring Laboratory Tests: CBC with platelet counts
Patient Education: I.V.: This medication can only be administered I.V.; you will be closely monitored during therapy. Report immediately any sings of acute GI upset, seizures, altered hearing. You may lose your hair, however, it will grow back when therapy is discontinued.

Cream: This medication is for external use only. It will not prevent hair growth, but may decrease rate of growth. You will still need to use hair removal techniques while using eflornithine cream. Use only as directed; do not use more often or discontinue without consulting prescriber. Wait at least 5 minutes after removing hair to apply cream. Wash hands thoroughly prior to using cream. Apply thin lay of cream to affected areas of face and chin twice daily (at least 8 hours apart). Rub in thoroughly. Wash hands thoroughly after rubbing cream in. Do not wash area for 8 hours following application. Once cream has dried you may apply make-up over the affected area. Improvement may be seen in 4-8 weeks. Following discontinuation of therapy you may see hair growth return in about 8 weeks. You may be required to have blood tests if used for extended period of time. Report any skin irritation, rash, tingling, or skin eruptions; persistent headache, dizziness; or GI disturbances.

Pregnancy/breast-feeding precautions: Inform prescriber if you are or intend to become pregnant. Consult prescriber if breast-feeding.
Pregnancy Risk Factor: C
Lactation: Excretion in breast milk unknown/use caution

Administration
Storage:
Injection: Must be diluted before use and used within 24 hours of preparation.
Cream: Store at controlled room temperature 25°C (77°F); do not freeze.

* **Eflornithine Hydrochloride** *see Eflornithine on page 511*
* **Efudex®** *see Fluorouracil on page 647*
* **E-Gems® [OTC]** *see Vitamin E on page 1569*
* **Elavil® [DSC]** *see Amitriptyline on page 96*
* **Eldepryl®** *see Selegiline on page 1364*
* **Eldopaque® [OTC]** *see Hydroquinone on page 768*
* **Eldopaque Forte®** *see Hydroquinone on page 768*
* **Eldoquin® [OTC]** *see Hydroquinone on page 768*
* **Eldoquin Forte®** *see Hydroquinone on page 768*
* **Electrolyte Lavage Solution** *see Polyethylene Glycol-Electrolyte Solution on page 1226*
* **Electrolyte Lavage Solution** *see Polyethylene Glycol-Electrolyte Solution and Bisacodyl on page 1228*
* **Elestat™** *see Epinastine on page 524*

Eletriptan *(el e TRIP tan)*
U.S. Brand Names Relpax®
Synonyms Eletriptan Hydrobromide
Generic Available No
Pharmacologic Category Serotonin 5-HT$_{1B, 1D}$ Receptor Agonist
Use Acute treatment of migraine, with or without aura
Mechanism of Action/Effect The therapeutic effect for migraine is due to serotonin agonist activity causing vasoconstriction in cranial arteries.
Contraindications Hypersensitivity to eletriptan or any component of the formulation; ischemic heart disease or signs or symptoms of ischemic heart disease (including Prinzmetal's angina, angina pectoris, MI, silent myocardial ischemia); cerebrovascular syndromes (including strokes, transient ischemic attacks); peripheral vascular syndromes (including ischemic bowel disease); uncontrolled hypertension; use within 24 hours of ergotamine derivatives; use within 24 hours of another 5-HT$_1$ agonist; use within 72 hours of potent CYP3A4 inhibitors; management of hemiplegic or basilar migraine; prophylactic treatment of migraine; severe hepatic impairment
Warnings/Precautions Eletriptan is indicated only in patients ≥18 years of age with a clear diagnosis of migraine headache. If a patient does not respond to the first dose, the diagnosis

of migraine should be reconsidered. Do not give to patients with risk factors for CAD until a cardiovascular evaluation has been performed; if evaluation is satisfactory, the healthcare provider should administer the first dose and cardiovascular status should be periodically evaluated. Cardiac events (coronary artery vasospasm, transient ischemia, MI, ventricular tachycardia/fibrillation, cardiac arrest, and death), cerebral/subarachnoid hemorrhage, stroke, peripheral vascular ischemia, and colonic ischemia have been reported with 5-HT$_1$ agonist administration. Significant elevation in blood pressure, including hypertensive crisis, has also been reported on rare occasions in patients with and without a history of hypertension. Use with caution with renal or mild to moderate hepatic impairment. Safety and efficacy in pediatric patients have not been established.

Drug Interactions
Cytochrome P450 Effect: Substrate of CYP3A4 (major)
Increased Effect/Toxicity: CYP3A4 inhibitors increase serum concentration and half-life of eletriptan; do not use eletriptan within 72 hours of potent CYP3A4 inhibitors (eg, azole antifungals, ciprofloxacin, clarithromycin, diclofenac, doxycycline, erythromycin, imatinib, isoniazid, nefazodone, nicardipine, propofol, protease inhibitors, quinidine, verapamil). Ergot-containing drugs prolong vasospastic reactions; do not use within 24 hours of eletriptan.

Nutritional/Ethanol Interactions Food: High-fat meal increases bioavailability.

Adverse Reactions 1% to 10%:
Cardiovascular: Chest pain/tightness (1% to 4%; placebo 1%), palpitation
Central nervous system: Dizziness (3% to 7%; placebo 3%), somnolence (3% to 7%; placebo 4%), headache (3% to 4%; placebo 3%), chills, pain, vertigo
Gastrointestinal: Nausea (4% to 8%; placebo 5%), xerostomia (2% to 4%, placebo 2%), dysphagia (1% to 2%), abdominal pain/discomfort (1% to 2%; placebo 1%), dyspepsia (1% to 2%; placebo 1%)
Neuromuscular & skeletal: Weakness (4% to 10%), paresthesia (3% to 4%), back pain, hypertonia, hypoesthesia
Respiratory: Pharyngitis
Miscellaneous: Diaphoresis

Overdosage/Toxicology Hypertension or more serious cardiovascular symptoms may occur. Clinical and electrocardiographic monitoring needed for at least 20 hours even if patient is asymptomatic. Treatment is symptom-directed and supportive.

Pharmacodynamics/Kinetics
Absorption: Well absorbed
Bioavailability: ~50%, increased with high-fat meal
Time to Peak: Plasma: 1.5-2 hours
Protein Binding: ~85%
Half-Life Elimination: 4 hours (Elderly: 4.4-5.7 hours); Metabolite: ~13 hours
Metabolism: Hepatic via CYP3A4; forms one metabolite (active)

Dosing
Adults: Acute migraine: Oral: 20-40 mg; if the headache improves but returns, dose may be repeated after 2 hours have elapsed since first dose; maximum 80 mg/day
Note: If the first dose is ineffective, diagnosis needs to be re-evaluated. Safety of treating >3 headaches/month has not been established.
Renal Impairment: No dosing adjustment needed; monitor for increased blood pressure.
Hepatic Impairment:
Mild to moderate impairment: No adjustment necessary.
Severe impairment: Use is contraindicated.

Available Dosage Forms Tablet, as hydrobromide [film coated]: 20 mg, 40 mg [as base]

Monitoring and Teaching Issues
Physical Assessment: See Warnings/Precautions for use cautions (eg, >18 years of age, clear diagnosis of migraine, hypertension, cardiovascular status). Assess potential for interactions with other pharmacological agents patient may be taking (eg, ergot-containing drugs; other 5-HT$_1$ agonists; see Drug Interactions). Assess therapeutic effectiveness (relief of migraine) and adverse response (hypertension, cardiac events; see Adverse Reactions). Teach patient proper use, possible side effects/appropriate interventions and adverse symptoms to report (see Patient Education).
Patient Education: This drug is to be used to reduce your migraine, not to prevent the number of attacks. Follow exact instructions for use. Do not crush, break, or chew tablet. Do not take within 24 hours of any other medication (especially any other migraine medications) without first consulting prescriber. If headache improves but returns, dose may be repeated after 2 hours. Do not exceed two doses in 24 hours (may take either 20 mg or 40 mg twice daily). If you have no relief with the first dose, do not take a second dose without consulting prescriber. May cause dizziness or drowsiness (use caution when driving or engaging in tasks requiring alertness until response to drug is known); nausea, vomiting, or abdominal pain. Report immediately any chest pain, tightness, or palpitations; muscle weakness or tremors; back pain; difficulty breathing; changes in CNS (abnormal thought processes, depression, insomnia, confusion, agitation); swelling of eyelids, face, lips, throat; rash, hives, or any other adverse reactions. **Pregnancy/breast-feeding precautions:** Inform prescriber if you are or intend to become pregnant. Consult prescriber if breast-feeding.
Pregnancy Risk Factor: C
Lactation: Enters breast milk/use caution

Administration
Storage: Store at 25°C (77°F). Excursions permitted to 15°C to 30°C (59°F to 86°F).

Related Information
Antimigraine Drugs: 5-HT$_1$ Receptor Agonists *on page 1716*

- **Elipten** *see Aminoglutethimide on page 91*
- **Elitek™** *see Rasburicase on page 1309*
- **Elixophyllin®** *see Theophylline on page 1457*
- **ElixSure® Congestion [OTC]** *see Pseudoephedrine on page 1282*
- **ElixSure™ Fever/Pain [OTC]** *see Acetaminophen on page 38*
- **Ellence®** *see Epirubicin on page 527*
- **Elocon®** *see Mometasone Furoate on page 1026*
- **Eloxatin™** *see Oxaliplatin on page 1127*
- **Elspar®** *see Asparaginase on page 141*
- **Emcyt®** *see Estramustine on page 559*
- **Emend®** *see Aprepitant on page 133*

Emtricitabine (em trye SYE ta been)

U.S. Brand Names Emtriva™
Synonyms BW524W91; Coviracil; FTC
Generic Available No
Pharmacologic Category Antiretroviral Agent, Reverse Transcriptase Inhibitor (Nucleoside)
Use Treatment of HIV infection in combination with at least two other antiretroviral agents
Unlabeled/Investigational Use Investigational: Hepatitis B
Mechanism of Action/Effect Nucleoside reverse transcriptase inhibitor which interferes with viral RNA-dependent DNA synthesis, resulting in inhibition of viral replication.
Contraindications Hypersensitivity to emtricitabine or any component of the formulation
Warnings/Precautions Lactic acidosis, severe hepatomegaly, and hepatic failure have occurred rarely with emtricitabine (similar to other nucleoside analogues). Some cases have been fatal; stop treatment if lactic acidosis or hepatotoxicity occur. Prior liver disease, obesity, extended duration of therapy, and female gender may represent risk factors for severe hepatic reactions. Testing for hepatitis B is recommended prior to the initiation of therapy; hepatitis B may be exacerbated following discontinuation of emtricitabine. Use caution in patients with renal impairment (dosage adjustment required).
Drug Interactions
    Increased Effect/Toxicity: Concomitant use of ribavirin and nucleoside analogues may increase the risk of developing lactic acidosis.
Nutritional/Ethanol Interactions Food: Food decreases peak plasma concentrations, but does not alter the extent of absorption or overall systemic exposure.
Adverse Reactions Clinical trials were conducted in patients receiving other antiretroviral agents, and it is not possible to correlate frequency of adverse events with emtricitabine alone. The range of frequencies of adverse events is generally comparable to comparator groups, with the exception of hyperpigmentation, which occurred more frequently in patients receiving emtricitabine.
    >10%:
        Central nervous system: Headache (13% to 22%), dizziness (4% to 25%), insomnia (7% to 16%)
        Dermatologic: Rash (17% to 30%; includes rash, pruritus, maculopapular rash, vesiculobullous rash, pustular rash, and allergic reaction)
        Gastrointestinal: Diarrhea (23%), nausea (13% to 18%), abdominal pain (8% to 14%)
        Neuromuscular & skeletal: Weakness (12% to 16%), CPK increased (11% to 12%)
        Respiratory: Cough (14%), rhinitis (12% to 18%)
    1% to 10%:
        Central nervous system: Abnormal dreams (2% to 11%), depression (6% to 9%), neuropathy/neuritis (4%)
        Dermatologic: Hyperpigmentation (2% to 6%; primarily of palms and/or soles but may include tongue, arms, lip and nails; generally mild and nonprogressive without associated local reactions such as pruritus or rash)
        Endocrine & metabolic: Serum triglycerides increased (9% to 10%), disordered glucose homeostasis (2% to 3%), serum amylase increased (2% to 5%)
        Gastrointestinal: Dyspepsia (4% to 8%), vomiting (9%)
        Hepatic: Transaminases increased (2% to 6%), bilirubin increased (1%)
        Neuromuscular & skeletal: Myalgia (4% to 6%), arthralgia (3% to 5%), paresthesia (5% to 6%)
Overdosage/Toxicology Treatment is supportive and symptom-directed. Approximately 30% of a dose is removed by hemodialysis.
Pharmacodynamics/Kinetics
    Absorption: Rapid, extensive
    Bioavailability: 93%
    Protein Binding: <4%
    Half-Life Elimination: Normal renal function: 10 hours
    Metabolism: Limited, via oxidation and conjugation (not via CYP isoenzymes)
    Excretion: Urine (86% primarily as unchanged drug, 13% as metabolites); feces (14%)
Dosing
    Adults & Elderly: HIV infection: Oral: 200 mg once daily
    Renal Impairment:
        Cl$_{cr}$ 30-49 mL/minute: 200 mg every 48 hours
        Cl$_{cr}$ 15-29 mL/minute: 200 mg every 72 hours
        Cl$_{cr}$ <15 mL/minute (including hemodialysis patients): 200 mg every 96 hours
    Hepatic Impairment: No adjustment required.
Available Dosage Forms Capsule: 200 mg
Monitoring and Teaching Issues
    Physical Assessment: Use caution in presence of hepatic disease or renal impairment, obesity, and female gender (see Warnings/Precautions). Assess results of laboratory tests, effectiveness of therapy (viral load and CD4 count), and adverse reactions on regular basis during therapy (eg, lactic acidosis, hepatomegaly, hepatic failure; Adverse Reactions).

Encourage patient to enroll in antiretroviral registry if pregnant. Teach patient use, possible side effects/appropriate interventions, and adverse symptoms to report (see Patient Education).

Monitoring Laboratory Tests: Viral load, CD4, liver function tests; hepatitis B testing is recommended prior to initiation of therapy

Patient Education: Do not take any new medication during therapy without consulting prescriber (you will be provided with a list of specific medications that should not be used). This is not a cure for HIV, nor has it been found to reduce transmission of HIV. Take as directed. Maintain adequate hydration (2-3 L/day of fluids) unless instructed to restrict fluid intake. Emtricitabine is prescribed with a combination of other medications; time these medications as directed by prescriber. May cause hyperpigmentation of hands, soles, or lips (normal). May cause headache, dizziness, or insomnia (use caution when driving or engaging in hazardous tasks until response to drug is known); nausea, vomiting, or abdominal discomfort (small frequent meals, frequent mouth care, chewing gum, or sucking lozenges may help); diarrhea (consult prescriber if persistent); or muscle or skeletal pain (consult prescriber for approved analgesic). Report respiratory difficulty, rash, CNS changes, or any persistent adverse effects. **Pregnancy/breast-feeding precautions:** Inform prescriber if you are or intend to become pregnant. Breast-feeding is not recommended.

Dietary Considerations: May be taken with or without food.

Pregnancy Risk Factor: B

Pregnancy Issues: Cases of fatal and nonfatal lactic acidosis, with or without pancreatitis, have been reported in pregnant women receiving reverse transcriptase inhibitors. It is not known if pregnancy itself potentiates this known side effect; however, pregnant women may be at increased risk of lactic acidosis and liver damage. Hepatic enzymes and electrolytes should be monitored frequently during the 3rd trimester of pregnancy. There are no studies of emtricitabine during pregnancy. The Perinatal HIV Guidelines Working Group considers emtricitabine to be an alternative NRTI in dual nucleoside combination regimens. Health professionals are encouraged to contact the antiretroviral pregnancy registry to monitor outcomes of pregnant women exposed to antiretroviral medications (1-800-258-4263 or www.APRegistry.com).

Lactation: Excretion in breast milk unknown/not recommended

Breast-Feeding Issues: HIV-infected women are discouraged from breast-feeding to decrease the potential transmission of HIV.

Administration

Oral: May be administered with or without food.

Storage: Store capsules at 25°C (77°F); excursions permitted to 15°C to 30°C (59°F to 86°F).

Emtricitabine and Tenofovir (em trye SYE ta been & te NOE fo veer)

U.S. Brand Names Truvada™

Synonyms Tenofovir and Emtricitabine

Generic Available No

Pharmacologic Category Antiretroviral Agent, Reverse Transcriptase Inhibitor (Nucleoside); Antiretroviral Agent, Reverse Transcriptase Inhibitor (Nucleotide)

Use Treatment of HIV infection in combination with other antiretroviral agents

Dosing

Adults: HIV: Oral: One tablet (emtricitabine 200 mg and tenofovir 300 mg) once daily

Elderly: See adult dosing.

Renal Impairment:

Cl_{cr} 30-49 mL/minute: Increase interval to every 48 hours.

Cl_{cr} <30 mL/minute or hemodialysis: Not recommended.

Available Dosage Forms Tablet, film coated: Emtricitabine 200 mg and tenofovir disoproxil fumarate 300 mg

Monitoring and Teaching Issues

Physical Assessment: See individual agents.

Pregnancy Risk Factor: B

Lactation: Excretion in breast milk unknown/not recommended

- **Emtriva™** see Emtricitabine on page 514
- **ENA 713** see Rivastigmine on page 1340
- **Enablex®** see Darifenacin on page 407

Enalapril (e NAL a pril)

U.S. Brand Names Vasotec®

Synonyms Enalaprilat; Enalapril Maleate

Generic Available Yes

Pharmacologic Category Angiotensin-Converting Enzyme (ACE) Inhibitor

Medication Safety Issues

Sound-alike/look-alike issues:

Enalapril may be confused with Anafranil®, Elavil®, Eldepryl®, nafarelin, ramipril

Use Management of mild to severe hypertension; treatment of congestive heart failure, left ventricular dysfunction after myocardial infarction

Unlabeled/Investigational Use

Unlabeled: Hypertensive crisis, diabetic nephropathy, rheumatoid arthritis, diagnosis of anatomic renal artery stenosis, hypertension secondary to scleroderma renal crisis, diagnosis of aldosteronism, idiopathic edema, Bartter's syndrome, postmyocardial infarction for prevention of ventricular failure

Investigational: Severe congestive heart failure in infants, neonatal hypertension, acute pulmonary edema

Mechanism of Action/Effect Competitive inhibitor of angiotensin-converting enzyme (ACE); prevents conversion of angiotensin I to angiotensin II, a potent vasoconstrictor; results in (Continued)

Enalapril *(Continued)*

lower levels of angiotensin II which causes an increase in plasma renin activity and a reduction in aldosterone secretion

Contraindications Hypersensitivity to enalapril or enalaprilat; angioedema related to previous treatment with an ACE inhibitor; patients with idiopathic or hereditary angioedema; bilateral renal artery stenosis; pregnancy (2nd and 3rd trimesters)

Warnings/Precautions Anaphylactic reactions can occur. Angioedema can occur at any time during treatment (especially following first dose). Angioedema may involve head and neck (potentially affecting the airway) or the intestine (presenting with abdominal pain). Careful blood pressure monitoring with first dose (hypotension can occur especially in volume depleted patients). Dosage adjustment needed in renal impairment. Use with caution in hypovolemia; collagen vascular diseases; valvular stenosis (particularly aortic stenosis); hyperkalemia; or before, during, or immediately after anesthesia. Avoid rapid dosage escalation which may lead to renal insufficiency.

Rare toxicities associated with ACE inhibitors include cholestatic jaundice (which may progress to hepatic necrosis) and neutropenia/agranulocytosis with myeloid hyperplasia. Hypersensitivity reactions may be seen during hemodialysis with high-flux dialysis membranes (eg, AN69). Hyperkalemia may rarely occur. Use with caution in unilateral renal artery stenosis and pre-existing renal insufficiency.

Drug Interactions

Cytochrome P450 Effect: Substrate of CYP3A4 (major)

Decreased Effect: Aspirin (high dose) may reduce the therapeutic effects of ACE inhibitors; at low dosages this does not appear to be significant. Antacids may decrease the bioavailability of ACE inhibitors (may be more likely to occur with captopril); separate administration times by 1-2 hours. NSAIDs may reduce the hypotensive effects of ACE inhibitors. More likely to occur in low renin or volume-dependent hypertensive patients. CYP3A4 inducers may decrease the levels/effects of enalapril; example inducers include aminoglutethimide, carbamazepine, nafcillin, nevirapine, phenobarbital, phenytoin, and rifamycins.

Increased Effect/Toxicity: Potassium supplements, co-trimoxazole (high dose), angiotensin II receptor antagonists (eg, candesartan, losartan, irbesartan), or potassium-sparing diuretics (amiloride, spironolactone, triamterene) may result in elevated serum potassium levels when combined with enalapril. ACE inhibitor effects may be increased by phenothiazines or probenecid (increases levels of captopril). ACE inhibitors may increase serum concentrations/effects of digoxin, lithium, and sulfonlyureas.

Diuretics have additive hypotensive effects with ACE inhibitors, and hypovolemia increases the potential for adverse renal effects of ACE inhibitors. In patients with compromised renal function, coadministration with NSAIDs may result in further deterioration of renal function. Allopurinol and ACE inhibitors may cause a higher risk of hypersensitivity reaction when taken concurrently.

Nutritional/Ethanol Interactions Herb/Nutraceutical: St John's wort may decrease enalapril levels. Avoid dong quai if using for hypertension (has estrogenic activity). Avoid ephedra, yohimbe, ginseng (may worsen hypertension). Avoid natural licorice (causes sodium and water retention and increases potassium loss). Avoid garlic (may have increased antihypertensive effect).

Lab Interactions Positive Coombs' [direct]; may cause false-positive results in urine acetone determinations using sodium nitroprusside reagent

Adverse Reactions Note: Frequency ranges include data from hypertension and heart failure trials. Higher rates of adverse reactions have generally been noted in patients with CHF. However, the frequency of adverse effects associated with placebo is also increased in this population.

1% to 10%:

Cardiovascular: Hypotension (0.9% to 7%), chest pain (2%), syncope (0.5% to 2%), orthostasis (2%), orthostatic hypotension (2%)

Central nervous system: Headache (2% to 5%), dizziness (4% to 8%), fatigue (2% to 3%)

Dermatologic: Rash (2%)

Gastrointestinal: Abnormal taste, abdominal pain, vomiting, nausea, diarrhea, anorexia, constipation

Neuromuscular & skeletal: Weakness

Renal: Increased serum creatinine (0.2% to 20%), worsening of renal function (in patients with bilateral renal artery stenosis or hypovolemia)

Respiratory (1% to 2%): Bronchitis, cough, dyspnea

Overdosage/Toxicology Mild hypotension was the primary toxic effect seen with acute overdose. Bradycardia may also occur. Hyperkalemia occurs even with therapeutic doses, especially in patients with renal insufficiency and those taking NSAIDs. Following initiation of essential overdose management, toxic symptom treatment and supportive treatment should be initiated.

Pharmacodynamics/Kinetics

Onset of Action: Oral: ~1 hour

Duration of Action: Oral: 12-24 hours

Absorption: Oral: 55% to 75%

Time to Peak: Serum: Oral: Enalapril: 0.5-1.5 hours; Enalaprilat (active): 3-4.5 hours

Protein Binding: 50% to 60%

Half-Life Elimination:

Enalapril: Adults: Healthy: 2 hours; Congestive heart failure: 3.4-5.8 hours

Enalaprilat: Infants 6 weeks to 8 months old: 6-10 hours; Adults: 35-38 hours

Metabolism: Prodrug, undergoes hepatic biotransformation to enalaprilat

Excretion: Urine (60% to 80%); some feces

Dosing

Adults & Elderly: Use lower listed initial dose in patients with hyponatremia, hypovolemia, severe congestive heart failure, decreased renal function, or in those receiving diuretics.

Asymptomatic left ventricular dysfunction: Oral: 2.5 mg twice daily, titrated as tolerated to 20 mg/day

Hypertension:

Oral: 2.5-5 mg/day then increase as required, usually at 1- to 2-week intervals; usual dose range (JNC 7): 2.5-40 mg/day in 1-2 divided doses. **Note:** Initiate with 2.5 mg if patient is taking a diuretic which cannot be discontinued. May add a diuretic if blood pressure cannot be controlled with enalapril alone.

I.V. (Enalaprilat): 1.25 mg/dose, given over 5 minutes every 6 hours; doses as high as 5 mg/dose every 6 hours have been tolerated for up to 36 hours. If patients are concomitantly receiving diuretic therapy, begin with 0.625 mg I.V. over 5 minutes; if the effect is not adequate after 1 hour, repeat the dose and administer 1.25 mg at 6-hour intervals thereafter; if adequate, administer 0.625 mg I.V. every 6 hours.

Heart failure:

Oral: As standard therapy alone or with diuretics, beta-blockers, and digoxin, initiate with 2.5 mg once or twice daily (usual range: 5-20 mg/day in 2 divided doses; target: 40 mg). Titrate slowly at 1- to 2-week intervals.

I.V.: Avoid I.V. administration in patients with unstable heart failure or those suffering acute myocardial infarction.

Conversion from I.V. to oral therapy if not concurrently on diuretics: 5 mg once daily; subsequent titration as needed; if concurrently receiving diuretics and responding to 0.625 mg I.V. every 6 hours, initiate with 2.5 mg/day.

Pediatrics:

Hypertension: Oral: Children 1 month to 16 years: Initial: 0.08 mg/kg (up to 5 mg) once daily; adjust dosage based on patient response; doses >0.58 mg/kg (40 mg) have not been evaluated in pediatric patients

Heart failure (non-FDA approved):

Infants and Children:

Oral (Enalapril): Initial: 0.1 mg/kg/day in 1-2 divided doses; increase as required over 2 weeks to maximum of 0.5 mg/kg/day; mean dose required for CHF improvement in 39 children (9 days to 17 years) was 0.36 mg/kg/day; investigationally, select individuals have been treated with doses up to 0.94 mg/kg/day

I.V. (Enalaprilat): 5-10 mcg/kg/dose administered every 8-24 hours (as determined by blood pressure readings); monitor patients carefully; select patients may require higher doses

Adolescents: Refer to adult dosing.

Renal Impairment:

Oral: Enalapril: Hypertension:

Cl$_{cr}$ 30-80 mL/minute: Administer 5 mg/day titrated upwards to maximum of 40 mg.

Cl$_{cr}$ <30 mL/minute: Administer 2.5 mg day titrated upward until blood pressure is controlled up to a maximum of 40 mg.

For heart failure patients with sodium <130 mEq/L or serum creatinine >1.6 mg/dL, initiate dosage with 2.5 mg/day, increasing to twice daily as needed; increase further in increments of 2.5 mg/dose at >4-day intervals to a maximum daily dose of 40 mg.

I.V.: Enalaprilat:

Cl$_{cr}$ >30 mL/minute: Initiate with 1.25 mg every 6 hours and increase dose based on response.

Cl$_{cr}$ <30 mL/minute: Initiate with 0.625 mg every 6 hours and increase dose based on response.

Moderately dialyzable (20% to 50%)

Administer dose postdialysis (eg, 0.625 mg I.V. every 6 hours) or administer 20% to 25% supplemental dose following dialysis; Clearance: 62 mL/minute

Peritoneal dialysis effects: Supplemental dose is not necessary, although some removal of drug occurs.

Hepatic Impairment: Hydrolysis of enalapril to enalaprilat may be delayed and/or impaired in patients with severe hepatic impairment, but the pharmacodynamic effects of the drug do not appear to be significantly altered. No dosage adjustment is necessary.

Available Dosage Forms

Injection, solution, as enalaprilat: 1.25 mg/mL (1 mL, 2 mL) [contains benzyl alcohol]

Tablet, as maleate (Vasotec®): 2.5 mg, 5 mg, 10 mg, 20 mg

Monitoring and Teaching Issues

Physical Assessment: See Warnings/Precautions for use cautions (eg, renal impairment, hypovolemia, aortic stenosis, post anesthesia). Assess potential for interactions with other pharmacological agents or herbal products patient may be taking (especially anything that may impact fluid balance or cardiac status; see Drug Interactions). **Infusion:** See Administration details. Blood pressure should be closely monitored with first dose or change in dose. Assess results of laboratory tests closely during first 3 months of therapy and regularly thereafter. Assess therapeutic effectiveness according to purpose for use and adverse response on a regular basis during therapy (eg, anaphylactic reaction, hypovolemia, angioedema, postural hypotension; see Adverse Reactions). Teach patient appropriate use, possible side effects/appropriate interventions, and adverse symptoms to report (see Patient Education).

Monitoring Laboratory Tests: CBC, renal function tests, electrolytes. If patient has renal impairment then a baseline WBC with differential and serum creatinine should be evaluated and monitored closely during the first 3 months of therapy.

Patient Education: Do not take any new medication during therapy unless approved by prescriber. Do not use potassium supplement or salt substitutes without consulting prescriber. Take exactly as directed; do not discontinue without consulting prescriber. Take first dose at bedtime. Take all doses on an empty stomach, 1 hour before or 2 hours after meals. This drug does not eliminate need for diet or exercise regimen as recommended by prescriber. May cause dizziness, fainting, or lightheadedness (use caution when driving or engaging in tasks that require alertness until response to drug is known); postural hypotension (use caution when rising from lying or sitting position or climbing stairs); or nausea, vomiting, abdominal pain, dry mouth, or transient loss of appetite (small frequent meals, frequent mouth care, sucking lozenges, or chewing gum may help). Report persistent (Continued)

Enalapril *(Continued)*

nausea and vomiting; chest pain or palpitations; mouth sores; fever or chills; swelling of extremities, face, mouth, or tongue; skin rash; numbness, tingling, or pain in muscles; respiratory difficulty or unusual cough; or other persistent adverse reactions. **Pregnancy precaution:** Inform prescriber if you are or intend to become pregnant. This drug should not be used in the 2nd or 3rd trimester of pregnancy. Consult prescriber for appropriate contraceptive measures if necessary.

Dietary Considerations: Limit salt substitutes or potassium-rich diet.

Geriatric Considerations: Due to frequent decreases in glomerular filtration (also creatinine clearance) with aging, elderly patients may have exaggerated responses to ACE inhibitors.

Pregnancy Risk Factor: C/D (2nd and 3rd trimesters)

Pregnancy Issues: ACE inhibitors can cause fetal injury or death if taken during the 2nd or 3rd trimester. Discontinue ACE inhibitors as soon as pregnancy is detected.

Lactation: Enters breast milk/compatible

Breast-Feeding Issues: Crosses into breast milk. Detectable levels but appears clinically insignificant. AAP considers **compatible** with breast-feeding.

Administration

I.V.: Give direct IVP over at least 5 minutes or dilute up to 50 mL and infuse.

Reconstitution: Enalaprilat: I.V. is stable for 24 hours at room temperature in D_5W or NS.

Compatibility: Stable in dextran 40 10% in dextrose, D_5LR, D_5NS, D_5W, hetastarch 6%, NS

Y-site administration: Incompatible with amphotericin B, amphotericin B cholesteryl sulfate complex, cefepime, phenytoin

Storage: Enalaprilat: Clear, colorless solution which should be stored at <30°C.

Related Information

Angiotensin Agents *on page 1704*
Heart Failure *on page 1828*

Enalapril and Felodipine *(e NAL a pril & fe LOE di peen)*

U.S. Brand Names Lexxel®
Synonyms Felodipine and Enalapril
Generic Available No
Pharmacologic Category Antihypertensive Agent, Combination
Use Treatment of hypertension, however, not indicated for initial treatment of hypertension; replacement therapy in patients receiving separate dosage forms (for patient convenience); when monotherapy with one component fails to achieve desired antihypertensive effect, or when dose-limiting adverse effects limit upward titration of monotherapy

Dosing

Adults: Hypertension: Oral: 1 tablet/day, individualize dose to achieve optimal effect. In some patients, the effect of enalapril may diminish toward the end of the dosing interval. Twice daily dosing may be considered.

Elderly: Recommended initial dose of felodipine is 2.5 mg daily. Titration of individual components is preferred.

Renal Impairment: Cl_{cr} <30 mL/minute: Recommended initial dose of enalapril is 2.5 mg/day. Titration of individual components is preferred.

Hepatic Impairment: Recommended initial dose of felodipine is 2.5 mg daily. Titration of individual components is preferred.

Available Dosage Forms Tablet, extended release:
Enalapril maleate 5 mg and felodipine 2.5 mg
Enalapril maleate 5 mg and felodipine 5 mg

Monitoring and Teaching Issues

Physical Assessment: See individual agents.

Patient Education: See individual agents. **Pregnancy/breast-feeding precautions:** Inform prescriber if you are or intend to become pregnant. Consult prescriber if breast-feeding.

Pregnancy Risk Factor: C/D (2nd and 3rd trimesters)

Lactation: Enters breast milk/use caution

Related Information

Enalapril *on page 515*
Felodipine *on page 613*

Enalapril and Hydrochlorothiazide

(e NAL a pril & hye droe klor oh THYE a zide)

U.S. Brand Names Vaseretic®
Synonyms Hydrochlorothiazide and Enalapril
Generic Available Yes
Pharmacologic Category Antihypertensive Agent, Combination
Use Treatment of hypertension

Dosing

Adults: Hypertension: Dose is individualized based on components.

Elderly: Refer to dosing in individual monographs; adjust for renal impairment.

Renal Impairment:
Cl_{cr} >30 mL/minute: Administer usual dose.
Severe renal failure: Avoid; loop diuretics are recommended.

Available Dosage Forms Tablet:
5-12.5: Enalapril maleate 5 mg and hydrochlorothiazide 12.5 mg
10-25: Enalapril maleate 10 mg and hydrochlorothiazide 25 mg

Monitoring and Teaching Issues

Physical Assessment: See individual agents.

Patient Education: See individual agents. **Pregnancy precaution:** Inform prescriber if you are or intend to become pregnant.

Pregnancy Risk Factor: C/D (2nd and 3rd trimesters)
Lactation: Enters breast milk (both ingredients)/compatible
Related Information
  Enalapril *on page 515*
  Hydrochlorothiazide *on page 751*

♦ **Enalaprilat** *see Enalapril on page 515*
♦ **Enalapril Maleate** *see Enalapril on page 515*
♦ **Enbrel®** *see Etanercept on page 573*
♦ **Endagen™-HD** *see Phenylephrine, Hydrocodone, and Chlorpheniramine on page 1202*
♦ **Endal® HD** *see Hydrocodone, Phenylephrine, and Diphenhydramine on page 759*
♦ **Endal® HD Plus** *see Phenylephrine, Hydrocodone, and Chlorpheniramine on page 1202*
♦ **Endocet®** *see Oxycodone and Acetaminophen on page 1138*
♦ **Endodan®** *see Oxycodone and Aspirin on page 1139*
♦ **Enemeez® [OTC]** *see Docusate on page 474*
♦ **Enerjets [OTC]** *see Caffeine on page 229*

Enfuvirtide (en FYOO vir tide)

U.S. Brand Names Fuzeon™
Synonyms T-20
Generic Available No
Pharmacologic Category Antiretroviral Agent, Fusion Protein Inhibitor
Use Treatment of HIV-1 infection in combination with other antiretroviral agents in treatment-experienced patients with evidence of HIV-1 replication despite ongoing antiretroviral therapy
Mechanism of Action/Effect Inhibits the fusion of HIV-1 virus with CD4 cells
Contraindications Hypersensitivity to enfuvirtide or any component of the formulation
Warnings/Precautions Monitor closely for signs/symptoms of pneumonia; associated with an increased incidence during clinical trials, particularly in patients with a low CD4 cell count, high initial viral load, I.V. drug use, smoking, or a history of lung disease. May cause hypersensitivity reactions (symptoms may include rash, fever, nausea, vomiting, hypotension, and elevated transaminases). In addition, local injection site reactions may occur. Safety and efficacy have not been established in children <6 years of age.
Drug Interactions
  Decreased Effect: No significant interactions identified.
  Increased Effect/Toxicity: No significant interactions identified.
Adverse Reactions
  >10%:
    Central nervous system: Insomnia (11%)
    Local: Injection site reactions (98%; may include pain, erythema, induration, pruritus, ecchymosis, nodule or cyst formation)
  1% to 10%:
    Central nervous system: Depression (9%), anxiety (6%)
    Dermatologic: Pruritus (5%)
    Endocrine & metabolic: Weight loss (7%), anorexia (3%)
    Gastrointestinal: Triglycerides increased (9%), appetite decreased (6%), constipation (4%), abdominal pain (3%), pancreatitis (2%), taste disturbance (2%), serum amylase increased (6%)
    Hematologic: Eosinophilia (8%), anemia (2%)
    Hepatic: Transaminases increased (4%)
    Local: Injection site infection (1%)
    Neuromuscular & skeletal: Neuropathy (9%), weakness (6%), myalgia (5%)
    Ocular: Conjunctivitis (2%)
    Respiratory: Cough (7%), pneumonia (4.7 events per 100 patient years vs 0.61 events per 100 patient years in control group), sinusitis (6%)
    Miscellaneous: Infections (4% to 6%), flu-like symptoms (2%), lymphadenopathy (2%)
Overdosage/Toxicology No clinical experience in overdosage. Treatment is supportive.
Pharmacodynamics/Kinetics
  Time to Peak: 8 hours
  Protein Binding: 92%
  Half-Life Elimination: 3.8 hours
  Metabolism: Proteolytic hydrolysis (CYP isoenzymes do not appear to contribute to metabolism); clearance: 24.8 mL/hour/kg
Dosing
  Adults: HIV Treatment: SubQ: 90 mg twice daily
  Elderly: See adults dosing.
  Pediatrics: HIV treatment: SubQ: Children ≥6 years: 2 mg/kg twice daily (maximum dose: 90 mg twice daily)
  Renal Impairment: No dosage adjustment required.
Available Dosage Forms Injection, powder for reconstitution [single-use vial]: 108 mg [90 mg/mL following reconstitution; available in convenience kit of 60 vials, SWFI, syringes, alcohol wipes, patient instructions]
Monitoring and Teaching Issues
  Physical Assessment: Use caution and monitor closely for symptoms of pneumonia with history of I.V. drug use, smoking, or lung disease (see Warnings/Precautions). See Administration for infusion specifics. Assess therapeutic response (CD4 level and viral load) and adverse reactions (pneumonia, neuropathy, CNS changes; see Adverse Reactions) on a regular basis throughout therapy. Teach patient or caregiver proper reconstitution, injection procedure, and needle/syringe disposal. Teach patient possible side effects/appropriate interventions and adverse symptoms to report (eg, hypersensitivity reactions, injection site infection; see Patient Education).
  (Continued)

Enfuvirtide (Continued)

Patient Education: Do not take any new medication during therapy unless approved by prescriber. Food does not affect timing of injection, however, this drug will be prescribed with other anti-HIV medications; follow exact instructions for timing (spacing) all medications. This drug can only be administered by injection, follow exact injection instructions that come with your medication. Do not mix any other medications in the same syringe. Inject into the upper arm, abdomen, or anterior thigh; do not inject in the same area you did the time before and do not inject around the naval, into scar tissues, a bruise, a mole, or where there is an injection site reaction. Make sure you have adequate supply of on hand; do not allow supply to run out. Do not miss or skip a dose; if you miss a dose, take the missed dose as soon as you can and take the next dose as scheduled. If it is close to the time for the next dose, wait and take the next dose as regularly scheduled. Do not take two doses at the same time. May cause injection site reactions such as itching, swelling, redness, pain, hardened skin, or bumps (usually last for <7 days). May cause insomnia, anorexia (small frequent meals may help), constipation (increased dietary fiber, fruit, fluids, or exercise may help). Notify prescriber immediately if you experience a hypersensitivity reaction (rash, fever, nausea, vomiting, hypotension, blood in urine) or injection site becomes infected (red, painful, swollen, drainage). Report CNS disturbances (depression, anxiety); weakness, loss of feeling, or muscle pain; respiratory infections, difficulty breathing, flu-like symptoms, unusual cough, fever, alteration in urinary pattern; swelling of legs or feet; or any other persistent adverse reactions. **Pregnancy/breast-feeding precautions:** Notify prescriber if you are or intend to become pregnant. Do not breast-feed.

Pregnancy Risk Factor: B

Pregnancy Issues: Teratogenic effects were not observed in animal studies, however there are no studies in pregnant women. An antiretroviral registry has been established to monitor maternal and fetal outcomes in women receiving antiretroviral drugs. Physicians are encouraged to register patients at 1-800-258-4263 or www.APRegistry.com.

Lactation: Excretion in breast milk unknown/contraindicated

Breast-Feeding Issues: HIV-infected mothers are discouraged from breast-feeding to decrease potential transmission of HIV.

Administration

Other: Inject subcutaneously into upper arm, abdomen, or anterior thigh. Do not inject into moles, scar tissue, bruises, or the navel. Rotate injection site, give injections at a site different from the preceding injection site; do not inject into any site where an injection site reaction is evident.

Reconstitution: Reconstitute with 1.1 mL SWFI; tap vial for 10 seconds and roll gently to ensure contact with diluent; then allow to stand until solution is completed; may require up to 45 minutes to form solution. Reconstituted solutions should be refrigerated and must be used within 24 hours.

Storage: Store powder at 25 °C (77°F). Excursions permitted to 15°C to 30°C (59 to 86°F).

♦ Engerix-B® *see page 1660*

♦ Enlon® *see Edrophonium on page 506*

Enoxaparin (ee noks a PA rin)

U.S. Brand Names Lovenox®

Synonyms Enoxaparin Sodium

Generic Available No

Pharmacologic Category Low Molecular Weight Heparin

Medication Safety Issues

Sound-alike/look-alike issues:

Lovenox® may be confused with Lotronex®, Protonix®

High alert medication: The Institute for Safe Medication Practices (ISMP) includes this medication among its list of drugs which have a heightened risk of causing significant patient harm when used in error.

Use

DVT Treatment (acute): Inpatient treatment (patients with and without pulmonary embolism) and outpatient treatment (patients without pulmonary embolism)

DVT prophylaxis: Following hip or knee replacement surgery, abdominal surgery, or in medical patients with severely-restricted mobility during acute illness in patients at risk of thromboembolic complications

Note: High-risk patients include those with one or more of the following risk factors: >40 years of age, obesity, general anesthesia lasting >30 minutes, malignancy, history of deep vein thrombosis or pulmonary embolism

Unstable angina and non-Q-wave myocardial infarction (to prevent ischemic complications)

Unlabeled/Investigational Use Prophylaxis and treatment of thromboembolism in children

Mechanism of Action/Effect Low molecular weight heparin that blocks factor Xa and IIa to prevent thrombus and clot formation

Contraindications Hypersensitivity to enoxaparin, heparin, or any component of the formulation; thrombocytopenia associated with a positive *in vitro* test for antiplatelet antibodies in the presence of enoxaparin; hypersensitivity to pork products; active major bleeding; not for I.M. or I.V. use

Warnings/Precautions Patients with recent or anticipated neuraxial anesthesia (epidural or spinal anesthesia) are at risk of spinal or epidural hematoma and subsequent paralysis. Consider risk versus benefit prior to neuraxial anesthesia; risk is increased by concomitant agents which may alter hemostasis, as well as traumatic or repeated epidural or spinal puncture. Patient should be observed closely for bleeding if enoxaparin is administered during or immediately following diagnostic lumbar puncture, epidural anesthesia, or spinal anesthesia.

Not recommended for thromboprophylaxis in patients with prosthetic heart valves (especially pregnant women). Not to be used interchangeably (unit for unit) with heparin or any other low molecular weight heparins. Use caution in patients with history of heparin-induced thrombocytopenia. Monitor patient closely for signs or symptoms of bleeding. Certain patients are at increased risk of bleeding. Risk factors include bacterial endocarditis; congenital or acquired bleeding disorders; active ulcerative or angioplastic GI diseases; severe uncontrolled hypertension; hemorrhagic stroke; use shortly after brain, spinal, or ophthalmology surgery; patients treated concomitantly with platelet inhibitors; recent GI bleeding; thrombocytopenia or platelet defects; severe liver disease; hypertensive or diabetic retinopathy; or in patients undergoing invasive procedures. Monitor platelet count closely. Rare cases of thrombocytopenia have occurred. Manufacturer recommends discontinuation of therapy if platelets are <100,000/mm^3. Risk of bleeding may be increased in women <45 kg and in men <57 kg. Use caution in patients with renal failure; dosage adjustment needed if Cl_{cr} <30 mL/minute. Safety and efficacy in pediatric patients have not been established. Use with caution in the elderly (delayed elimination may occur). Heparin can cause hyperkalemia by affecting aldosterone. Similar reactions could occur with LMWHs. Monitor for hyperkalemia. Multiple-dose vials contain benzyl alcohol (use caution in pregnant women).

Drug Interactions

Increased Effect/Toxicity: Risk of bleeding with enoxaparin may be increased with thrombolytic agents, oral anticoagulants (warfarin), drugs which affect platelet function (eg, aspirin, NSAIDs, dipyridamole, ticlopidine, clopidogrel, and IIb/IIIa antagonists). Although the risk of bleeding may be increased during concurrent therapy with warfarin, enoxaparin is commonly continued during the initiation of warfarin therapy to assure anticoagulation and to protect against possible transient hypercoagulability. Some cephalosporins and penicillins may block platelet aggregation, theoretically increasing the risk of bleeding.

Nutritional/Ethanol Interactions Herb/Nutraceutical: Avoid cat's claw, dong quai, evening primrose, feverfew, garlic, ginger, ginkgo, red clover, horse chestnut, green tea, ginseng (all have additional antiplatelet activity).

Lab Interactions Increased AST, ALT levels

Adverse Reactions As with all anticoagulants, bleeding is the major adverse effect of enoxaparin. Hemorrhage may occur at virtually any site. Risk is dependent on multiple variables. At the recommended doses, single injections of enoxaparin do not significantly influence platelet aggregation or affect global clotting time (ie, PT or aPTT).

1% to 10%:
Central nervous system: Fever (5% to 8%), confusion, pain
Dermatologic: Erythema, bruising
Gastrointestinal: Nausea (3%), diarrhea
Hematologic: Hemorrhage (5% to 13%), thrombocytopenia (2%), hypochromic anemia (2%)
Hepatic: Increased ALT/AST
Local: Injection site hematoma (9%), local reactions (irritation, pain, ecchymosis, erythema)
Thrombocytopenia with thrombosis: Cases of heparin-induced thrombocytopenia (some complicated by organ infarction, limb ischemia, or death) have been reported.

Overdosage/Toxicology Symptoms of overdose include hemorrhage. Protamine sulfate has been used to reverse effects (protamine 1 mg neutralizes enoxaparin 1 mg). Monitor aPTT 2-4 hours after first infusion; consider readministration of protamine (50% of original dose). Note: anti-Xa activity is never completely neutralized (maximum of 60% to 75%). Avoid overdose of protamine.

Pharmacodynamics/Kinetics

Onset of Action: Peak effect: SubQ: Antifactor Xa and antithrombin (antifactor IIa): 3-5 hours

Duration of Action: 40 mg dose: Antifactor Xa activity: ~12 hours

Protein Binding: Does not bind to heparin binding proteins

Half-Life Elimination: Plasma: 2-4 times longer than standard heparin, independent of dose; based on anti-Xa activity: 4.5-7 hours

Metabolism: Hepatic, to lower molecular weight fragments (little activity)

Excretion: Urine (40% of dose; 10% as active fragments)

Dosing

Adults:

DVT prophylaxis: SubQ:
Hip replacement surgery:
Twice-daily dosing: 30 mg twice daily, with initial dose within 12-24 hours after surgery, and every 12 hours until risk of DVT has diminished or the patient is adequately anticoagulated on warfarin.
Once-daily dosing: 40 mg once daily, with initial dose within 9-15 hours before surgery, and daily until risk of DVT has diminished or the patient is adequately anticoagulated on warfarin.
Knee replacement surgery: 30 mg twice daily, with initial dose within 12-24 hours after surgery, and every 12 hours until risk of DVT has diminished (usually 7-10 days).
Abdominal surgery: 40 mg once daily, with initial dose given 2 hours prior to surgery; continue until risk of DVT has diminished (usual 7-10 days).
Medical patients with severely-restricted mobility during acute illness: 40 mg once daily; continue until risk of DVT has diminished

DVT treatment (acute): SubQ: **Note:** Start warfarin within 72 hours and continue enoxaparin until INR is between 2.0 and 3.0 (usually 7 days).
Inpatient treatment (with or without pulmonary embolism): 1 mg/kg/dose every 12 hours or 1.5 mg/kg once daily.
Outpatient treatment (without pulmonary embolism): 1 mg/kg/dose every 12 hours.

Unstable angina or non-Q-wave MI: SubQ: 1 mg/kg twice daily in conjunction with oral aspirin therapy (100-325 mg once daily); continue until clinical stabilization (a minimum of at least 2 days)

Elderly: SubQ: Increased incidence of bleeding with doses of 1.5 mg/kg/day or 1 mg/kg every 12 hours. Injection-associated bleeding and serious adverse reactions are also increased in the elderly. Careful attention should be paid to elderly patients <45 kg.
(Continued)

Enoxaparin *(Continued)*

Pediatrics: Thromboembolism (unlabeled use): SubQ:
Infants <2 months: Initial:
   Prophylaxis: 0.75 mg/kg every 12 hours
   Treatment: 1.5 mg/kg every 12 hours
Infants >2 months and Children ≤18 years: Initial:
   Prophylaxis: 0.5 mg/kg every 12 hours
   Treatment: 1 mg/kg every 12 hours
Maintenance: See **Dosage Titration** table:

Enoxaparin Pediatric Dosage Titration

Antifactor Xa	Dose Titration	Time to Repeat Antifactor Xa Level
<0.35 units/mL	Increase dose by 25%	4 h after next dose
0.35-0.49 units/mL	Increase dose by 10%	4 h after next dose
0.5-1 unit/mL	Keep same dosage	Next day, then 1 wk later, then monthly (4 h after dose)
1.1-1.5 units/mL	Decrease dose by 20%	Before next dose
1.6-2 units/mL	Hold dose for 3 h and decrease dose by 30%	Before next dose, then 4 h after next dose
>2 units/mL	Hold all doses until antifactor Xa is 0.5 units/mL, then decrease dose by 40%	Before next dose and every 12 h until antifactor Xa <0.5 units/mL

Modified from Monagle P, Michelson AD, Bovill E, et al, "Antithrombotic Therapy in Children," *Chest*, 2001, 119:344S-70S.

Renal Impairment:
Cl_{cr} ≥30 mL/minute: No specific adjustment recommended (per manufacturer); monitor closely for bleeding.
Cl_{cr} <30 mL/minute:
   DVT prophylaxis in abdominal surgery, hip replacement, knee replacement, or in medical patients during acute illness: SubQ: 30 mg once daily
   DVT treatment (inpatient or outpatient treatment in conjunction with warfarin): SubQ: 1 mg/kg once daily
   Unstable angina, non-Q-wave MI (with ASA): SubQ: 1 mg/kg once daily
   Dialysis: Enoxaparin has not been FDA approved for use in dialysis patients. It's elimination is primarily via the renal route. Serious bleeding complications have been reported with use in patients who are dialysis dependent or have severe renal failure. LMWH administration at fixed doses without monitoring has greater unpredictable anticoagulant effects in patients with chronic kidney disease. If used, dosages should be reduced and anti-Xa activity frequently monitored, as accumulation may occur with repeated doses. Many clinicians would not use enoxaparin in this population especially without timely anti-Xa activity assay results.
   Hemodialysis: Supplemental dose is not necessary.
   Peritoneal dialysis: Significant drug removal is unlikely based on physiochemical characteristics.

Available Dosage Forms
Injection, solution, as sodium [graduated prefilled syringe; preservative free]: 60 mg/0.6 mL (0.6 mL); 80 mg/0.8 mL (0.8 mL); 100 mg/mL (1 mL); 120 mg/0.8 mL (0.8 mL); 150 mg/mL (1 mL)
Injection, solution, as sodium [multidose vial]: 100 mg/mL (3 mL) [contains benzyl alcohol]
Injection, solution, as sodium [prefilled syringe; preservative free]: 30 mg/0.3 mL (0.3 mL); 40 mg/0.4 mL (0.4 mL)

Monitoring and Teaching Issues
Physical Assessment: Use caution in presence or history of conditions that increase risk of bleeding or other complications (see Contraindications and Warnings/Precautions). Assess potential for interactions with other pharmaceutical agents or herbal products patient may be taking (especially anything that will impact coagulation or platelet aggregation; see Drug Interactions). Note specific injection directions. Monitor results of laboratory tests, therapeutic effectiveness according to purpose for use, and adverse response (eg, bleeding, thrombosis; see Adverse Reactions). Teach patient possible side effects/appropriate interventions and adverse symptoms to report (see Patient Education). See Pregnancy Issues.
Monitoring Laboratory Tests: Platelets, occult blood, anti-Xa activity, if available; the monitoring of PT and/or aPTT is not necessary.
Patient Education: Do not take any new medication during therapy without consulting prescriber. This drug can only be administered by injection. If self-administered, follow exact directions for injection and needle disposal. You may have a tendency to bleed easily while taking this drug (brush teeth with soft brush, use waxed dental floss, use electric razor, avoid scissors or sharp knives, and potentially harmful activities). Report chest pain; persistent constipation; persistent erection; unusual bleeding or bruising (bleeding gums, nosebleed, blood in urine, dark stool); pain in joints or back; or redness, swelling, burning, or pain at injection site. **Pregnancy/breast-feeding precautions:** Inform prescriber if you are pregnant. Consult prescriber if breast-feeding.
Geriatric Considerations: No specific recommendations.
Pregnancy Risk Factor: B
Pregnancy Issues: There are no adequate and well-controlled studies using enoxaparin in pregnant women. Postmarketing reports include congenital abnormalities (cause and effect not established) and also fetal death when used in pregnant women. In addition, prosthetic valve thrombosis, including fatal cases, has been reported in pregnant women receiving enoxaparin as thromboprophylaxis. Multiple-dose vials contain benzyl alcohol; use caution in pregnant women.

Lactation: Excretion in breast milk unknown/use caution

Breast-Feeding Issues: This drug has a high molecular weight that would minimize excretion in breast milk and is inactivated by the GI tract which further reduces the risk to the infant.

Administration

Other: Should be administered by deep SubQ injection to the left or right anterolateral and left or right posterolateral abdominal wall. To avoid loss of drug from the 30 mg and 40 mg syringes, do not expel the air bubble from the syringe prior to injection. In order to minimize bruising, do not rub injection site. An automatic injector (Lovenox EasyInjector™) is available with the 30 mg and 40 mg syringes to aid the patient with self-injections. **Note:** Enoxaparin is available in 100 mg/mL and 150 mg/mL concentrations.

Compatibility: Stable in NS

Storage: Store at 15°C to 25°C (59°F to 77°F). Do not freeze. Do not mix with other injections or infusions.

Related Information

Anticoagulants, Injectable *on page 1711*

♦ **Enoxaparin Sodium** *see* Enoxaparin *on page 520*

♦ **Enpresse™** *see* Ethinyl Estradiol and Levonorgestrel *on page 585*

Entacapone (en TA ka pone)

U.S. Brand Names Comtan®

Generic Available No

Pharmacologic Category Anti-Parkinson's Agent, COMT Inhibitor

Use Adjunct to levodopa/carbidopa therapy in patients with idiopathic Parkinson's disease who experience "wearing-off" symptoms at the end of a dosing interval

Mechanism of Action/Effect Entacapone inhibits COMT peripherally and alters the pharmacokinetics of levodopa so serum levels of levodopa become more sustained when used with levodopa/carbidopa combinations.

Contraindications Hypersensitivity to entacapone or any of component of the formulation

Warnings/Precautions May increase risk of orthostatic hypotension and syncope. May cause diarrhea, hallucinations; may cause or exacerbate dyskinesia. This drug should be slowly withdrawn if discontinuation is needed. Use caution in patients with hepatic impairment and renal impairment. Other drugs metabolized by COMT (see drug interactions) may cause increases in heart rate, arrhythmias, and changes in blood pressure when used concurrently.

Drug Interactions

Cytochrome P450 Effect: Inhibits CYP1A2 (weak), 2A6 (weak), 2C8/9 (weak), 2C19 (weak), 2D6 (weak), 2E1 (weak), 3A4 (weak)

Increased Effect/Toxicity: Entacapone may decrease the metabolism and increase the side effects of COMT substrates (eg, apomorphine, bitolterol, dobutamine, dopamine, epinephrine, norepinephrine, isoproterenol, isoetharine, and methyldopa). Effects on mental status may be additive with other CNS depressants; includes barbiturates, benzodiazepines, TCAs, antipsychotics, ethanol, narcotic analgesics, and other sedative-hypnotics. Concurrent use of nonselective MAO inhibitors with entacapone may increase the risk of cardiovascular side effects; selective MAO inhibitors (eg, selegiline) appear to pose limited risk.

Nutritional/Ethanol Interactions Ethanol: Avoid ethanol (may increase CNS adverse effects).

Adverse Reactions

>10%:
  Gastrointestinal: Nausea (14%)
  Neuromuscular & skeletal: Dyskinesia (25%), placebo (15%)

1% to 10%:
  Cardiovascular: Orthostatic hypotension (4%), syncope (1%)
  Central nervous system: Dizziness (8%), fatigue (6%), hallucinations (4%), anxiety (2%), somnolence (2%), agitation (1%)
  Dermatologic: Purpura (2%)
  Gastrointestinal: Diarrhea (10%), abdominal pain (8%), constipation (6%), vomiting (4%), dry mouth (3%), dyspepsia (2%), flatulence (2%), gastritis (1%), taste perversion (1%)
  Genitourinary: Brown-orange urine discoloration (10%)
  Neuromuscular & skeletal: Hyperkinesia (10%), hypokinesia (9%), back pain (4%), weakness (2%)
  Respiratory: Dyspnea (3%)
  Miscellaneous: Diaphoresis increased (2%), bacterial infection (1%)

Overdosage/Toxicology There have been no reported cases of overdose with this drug.

Pharmacodynamics/Kinetics

Onset of Action: Rapid; Peak effect: 1 hour

Absorption: Rapid

Bioavailability: 35%

Time to Peak: Serum: 1 hour

Protein Binding: 98%, primarily to albumin

Half-Life Elimination: B phase: 0.4-0.7 hours; Y phase: 2.4 hours

Metabolism: Isomerization to the *cis*-isomer, followed by direct glucuronidation of the parent and *cis*-isomer

Excretion: Feces (90%); urine (10%)

Dosing

Adults & Elderly: Parkinson's disease: Oral: 200 mg with each dose of levodopa/carbidopa, up to a maximum of 8 times/day (maximum daily dose: 1600 mg/day). To optimize therapy, the dosage of levodopa may need reduced or the dosing interval may need extended. Patients taking levodopa ≥800mg/day or who had moderate-to-severe dyskinesias prior to therapy required an average decrease of 25% in the daily levodopa dose.
(Continued)

Entacapone *(Continued)*

Renal Impairment: No adjustment is required; dialysis patients were not studied.

Hepatic Impairment: Dosage adjustment in chronic therapy with standard treatment has not been studied.

Available Dosage Forms Tablet: 200 mg

Monitoring and Teaching Issues

Physical Assessment: Assess other medications patient may be taking for effectiveness and interactions. Monitor therapeudic effectiveness and adverse reactions. Monitor blood pressure. Taper dosage when discontinuing. Assess knowledge/teach patient appropriate use, interventions to reduce side effects, and adverse reactions to report.

Patient Education: Take exactly as directed; do not alter dosage or discontinue without consulting prescriber. May be taken with food. Notify prescriber if any other prescription medications you are taking. Avoid all alcohol or OTC medications unless approved by your prescriber. Orange-brown urine is normal with this medication. You may experience dizziness, fatigue, or sleepiness (use caution when driving or engaging in tasks requiring alertness until response to drug is known); postural hypotension (rise slowly when getting up from chair or bed, when climbing stairs); or unusual taste, nausea, vomiting, flatulence, or upset stomach (small frequent meals, good mouth care, chewing gum, or sucking hard candy may help). Report any increased or abnormal skeletal movements or pain; unresolved sedation, nausea, diarrhea, constipation, or GI distress; signs of infection; persistent dizziness or sleepiness; or other unusual responses. **Pregnancy/breast-feeding precautions:** Inform prescriber if you are or intend to become pregnant. Consult prescriber if breast-feeding.

Dietary Considerations: May be taken with or without food.

Pregnancy Risk Factor: C

Lactation: Excretion in breast milk unknown/use caution

♦ **Entacapone, Carbidopa, and Levodopa** *see* Levodopa, Carbidopa, and Entacapone *on page 888*

♦ **Enterex® Glutapak-10® [OTC]** *see* Glutamine *on page 719*

♦ **Entex® PSE** *see* Guaifenesin and Pseudoephedrine *on page 733*

♦ **Entocort™ EC** *see* Budesonide *on page 210*

♦ **Enulose®** *see* Lactulose *on page 860*

♦ **Epaxal Berna®** *see page 1660*

♦ **Epidermal Thymocyte Activating Factor** *see* Aldesleukin *on page 62*

♦ **Epifrin® [DSC]** *see* Epinephrine *on page 525*

Epinastine *(ep i NAS teen)*

U.S. Brand Names Elestat™

Synonyms Epinastine Hydrochloride

Generic Available No

Pharmacologic Category Antihistamine, H_1 Blocker, Ophthalmic

Use Treatment of allergic conjunctivitis

Mechanism of Action/Effect Selective H_1-receptor antagonist; inhibits release of histamine from the mast cell

Contraindications Hypersensitivity to epinastine or any component of the formulation

Warnings/Precautions Contains benzalkonium chloride; contact lenses should be removed prior to use. Not for the treatment of contact lens irritation. Safety and efficacy in children <3 years of age have not been established.

Adverse Reactions 1% to 10%:

Central nervous system: Headache (1% to 3%)

Ocular: Burning sensation, folliculosis, hyperemia, pruritus

Respiratory: Cough (1% to 3%), pharyngitis (1% to 3%), rhinitis (1% to 3%), sinusitis (1% to 3%)

Miscellaneous: Infection (10%; defined as cold symptoms and upper respiratory infection)

Pharmacodynamics/Kinetics

Onset of Action: 3-5 minutes

Duration of Action: 8 hours

Absorption: Low systemic absorption following topical application

Protein Binding: 64%

Half-Life Elimination: 12 hours

Metabolism: <10% metabolized

Excretion: I.V.: Urine (55%); feces (30%)

Dosing

Adults & Elderly: Allergic conjunctivitis: Ophthalmic: Instill 1 drop into each eye twice daily. Continue throughout period of exposure, even in the absence of symptoms.

Pediatrics: Allergic conjunctivitis: Ophthalmic: Children ≥3 years: Refer to adult dosing.

Available Dosage Forms Solution, ophthalmic, as hydrochloride: 0.05% (5 mL) [contains benzalkonium chloride]

Monitoring and Teaching Issues

Physical Assessment: For ophthalmic use only. Assess therapeutic effectiveness and adverse reactions on a regular basis throughout therapy. Teach patient possible side effects/appropriate interventions and adverse symptoms to report.

Patient Education: For ophthalmic use only. Use exactly as directed. Do not wear contact lenses if eyes are red. May cause headache (consult prescriber for analgesic if persistent). Report unusual or persistent cough of cold symptoms related to use, or if condition does not improve.

Ophthalmic: Wash hands before using. Remove contact lenses before application (may be reinserted after 10 minutes). Gently pull lower eyelid forward and instill prescribed amount in lower eyelid. Avoid touching tip of dropper to eye. Close eye and roll eyeball in all directions. May cause blurred vision, temporary stinging or burning sensation.

Geriatric Considerations: No difference in safety and efficacy was observed between elderly and younger patients.

Pregnancy Risk Factor: C

Lactation: Excretion in breast milk unknown/use caution

Administration

Other: For ophthalmic use only; avoid touching tip of applicator to eye or other surfaces. Contact lenses should be removed prior to application, may be reinserted after 10 minutes. Do not wear contact lenses if eyes are red.

Storage: Store at controlled room temperature of 15°C to 25°C (59°F to 77°F). Keep tightly closed.

♦ **Epinastine Hydrochloride** *see* Epinastine *on page 524*

Epinephrine (ep i NEF rin)

U.S. Brand Names Adrenalin®; Epifrin® [DSC]; EpiPen®; EpiPen® Jr; Primatene® Mist [OTC]

Synonyms Adrenaline; Epinephrine Bitartrate; Epinephrine Hydrochloride

Generic Available Yes: Solution for injection

Pharmacologic Category Alpha/Beta Agonist; Antidote; Ophthalmic Agent, Antiglaucoma

Medication Safety Issues

Sound-alike/look-alike issues:

Epinephrine may be confused with ephedrine

Epifrin® may be confused with ephedrine, EpiPen®

EpiPen® may be confused with Epifrin®

Medication errors have occurred due to confusion with epinephrine products expressed as ratio strengths (eg, 1:1000 vs 1:10,000).

Epinephrine 1:1000 = 1 mg/mL and is most commonly used SubQ.

Epinephrine 1:10,000 = 0.1 mg/mL and is used I.V.

Use Treatment of bronchospasms, anaphylactic reactions, cardiac arrest, management of open-angle (chronic simple) glaucoma; added to local anesthetics to decrease systemic absorption, increase duration of action, and decrease toxicity of the local anesthetic

Unlabeled/Investigational Use ACLS guidelines: Ventricular fibrillation (VF) or pulseless ventricular tachycardia (VT) unresponsive to initial defibrillatory shocks; pulseless electrical activity, asystole, hypotension unresponsive to volume resuscitation; symptomatic bradycardia or heart block unresponsive to atropine or pacing

Mechanism of Action/Effect Stimulates alpha-, beta$_1$-, and beta$_2$-adrenergic receptors resulting in relaxation of smooth muscle of the bronchial tree, cardiac stimulation, and dilation of skeletal muscle vasculature; small doses can cause vasodilation via beta$_2$-vascular receptors; large doses may produce constriction of skeletal and vascular smooth muscle; decreases production of aqueous humor and increases aqueous outflow; dilates the pupil by contracting the dilator muscle

Contraindications Hypersensitivity to epinephrine or any component of the formulation; cardiac arrhythmias; angle-closure glaucoma

Warnings/Precautions Use with caution in elderly patients, patients with diabetes mellitus, cardiovascular diseases (angina, tachycardia, prostatic hyperplasia, history of seizures, renal dysfunction, myocardial infarction), thyroid disease, cerebral arteriosclerosis, or Parkinson's. Some products contain sulfites as preservatives. Rapid I.V. infusion may cause death from cerebrovascular hemorrhage or cardiac arrhythmias. Oral inhalation of epinephrine is **not** the preferred route of administration.

Drug Interactions

Decreased Effect: Decreased bronchodilation with β-blockers. Decreases antihypertensive effects of methyldopa or guanethidine.

Increased Effect/Toxicity: Increased cardiac irritability if administered concurrently with halogenated inhalation anesthetics, beta-blocking agents, or alpha-blocking agents.

Nutritional/Ethanol Interactions Herb/Nutraceutical: Avoid ephedra, yohimbe (may cause CNS stimulation).

Lab Interactions Increased bilirubin (S), catecholamines (U), glucose, uric acid (S)

Adverse Reactions Frequency not defined.

Cardiovascular: Tachycardia (parenteral), pounding heartbeat, flushing, hypertension, pallor, chest pain, increased myocardial oxygen consumption, cardiac arrhythmia, sudden death, angina, vasoconstriction

Central nervous system: Nervousness, anxiety, restlessness, headache, dizziness, lightheadedness, insomnia

Gastrointestinal: Nausea, vomiting, xerostomia, dry throat

Genitourinary: Acute urinary retention in patients with bladder outflow obstruction

Neuromuscular & skeletal: Weakness, trembling

Ocular: Precipitation of or exacerbation of narrow-angle glaucoma, transient stinging, burning, eye pain, allergic lid reaction, ocular irritation

Renal: Decreased renal and splanchnic blood flow

Respiratory: Wheezing, dyspnea

Miscellaneous: Diaphoresis (increased)

Overdosage/Toxicology Symptoms of overdose include hypertension, which may result in subarachnoid hemorrhage and hemiplegia; arrhythmias; unusually large pupils; pulmonary edema; renal failure; and metabolic acidosis. There is no specific antidote for epinephrine intoxication and treatment is primarily supportive.

Pharmacodynamics/Kinetics

Onset of Action: Bronchodilation: SubQ: ~5-10 minutes; Inhalation: ~1 minute; Conjunctival instillation: IOP declines ~1 hour

Peak effect: Conjunctival instillation: 4-8 hours

Duration of Action: Conjunctival instillation: Ocular effect: 12-24 hours

Metabolism: Taken up into the adrenergic neuron and metabolized by monoamine oxidase and catechol-o-methyltransferase; circulating drug hepatically metabolized

Excretion: Urine (as inactive metabolites, metanephrine, and sulfate and hydroxy derivatives of mandelic acid; small amounts as unchanged drug)

(Continued)

Epinephrine *(Continued)*

Dosing

Adults & Elderly:

Asystole:

I.V.: 1 mg every 3-5 minutes; if this approach fails, higher doses of epinephrine (up to 0.2 mg/kg) may be used, but are not recommended (Class Indeterminate; 2000 ACLS guidelines)

Intratracheal: Administer 2-2.5 times the recommended I.V. dose; dilute in 10 mL NS or distilled water. **Note:** Absorption is greater with distilled water, but causes more adverse effects on PaO$_2$.

Bronchospasm:

I.M., SubQ (1:1000): 0.1-0.5 mg every 10-15 minutes to 4 hours

Suspension (1:200) SubQ: 0.1-0.3 mL (0.5-1.5 mg)

I.V.: 0.1-0.25 mg (single dose maximum: 1 mg)

Nebulization: Instill 8-15 drops into nebulizer reservoirs; administer 1-3 inhalations 4-6 times/day.

Hypotension (refractory to dopamine/dobutamine): Continuous I.V. infusion: Initial: 1 mcg/minute (range: 1-10 mcg/minute); titrate to desired effect; severe cardiac dysfunction may require doses >10 mcg/minute (up to 0.1 mcg/kg/minute)

Hypersensitivity reaction: I.M., SubQ: 0.2-0.5 mg every 20 minutes to 4 hours (single dose maximum: 1 mg)

Glaucoma: Ophthalmic: Instill 1-2 drops in eye(s) once or twice daily.

Nasal congestion: Intranasal: Apply locally as drops or spray or with sterile swab.

Pediatrics:

Bronchodilator:

SubQ: Infants and Children: 10 mcg/kg (0.01 mL/kg of **1:1000**) (single doses not to exceed 0.5 mg) **or** suspension (1:200): 0.005 mL/kg/dose (0.025 mg/kg/dose) to a maximum of 0.15 mL (0.75 mg for single dose) every 8-12 hours

Nebulization: Infants and Children: 0.25-0.5 mL of 2.25% **racemic epinephrine** solution diluted in 3 mL normal saline, or L-epinephrine at an equivalent dose; racemic epinephrine 10 mg = 5 mg L-epinephrine; use lower end of dosing range for younger infants.

Bradycardia:

I.V.: 0.01 mg/kg (0.1 mL/kg of **1:10,000** solution) every 3-5 minutes as needed (maximum: 1 mg/10 mL)

Intratracheal: 0.1 mg/kg (0.1 mL/kg of **1:1000** solution every 3-5 minutes); doses as high as 0.2 mg/kg may be effective

Asystole or pulseless arrest:

I.V. or intraosseous: Initial dose: 0.01 mg/kg (0.1 mL/kg of a **1:10,000** solution). Subsequent doses: 0.1 mg/kg (0.1 mL/kg of a **1:1000** solution); doses as high as 0.2 mg/kg may be effective; repeat every 3-5 minutes.

Intratracheal: 0.1 mg/kg (0.1 mL/kg of a **1:1000** solution); doses as high as 0.2 mg/kg may be effective.

Hypersensitivity reaction: SubQ: 0.01 mg/kg every 15 minutes for 2 doses then every 4 hours as needed (single doses not to exceed 0.5 mg)

Refractory hypotension (refractory to dopamine/dobutamine): Continuous I.V. infusions of 0.1-1 mcg/kg/minute; titrate dosage to desired effect.

Nasal congestion: Intranasal: Children ≥6 years: Apply locally as drops or spray or with sterile swab.

Available Dosage Forms

Aerosol for oral inhalation (Primatene® Mist): 0.22 mg/inhalation (15 mL, 22.5 mL) [contains CFCs]

Injection, solution [prefilled auto injector]:

EpiPen®: 0.3 mg/0.3 mL [1:1000] (2 mL) [contains sodium metabisulfite; available as single unit or in double-unit pack with training unit]

EpiPen® Jr: 0.15 mg/0.3 mL [1:2000] (2 mL) [contains sodium metabisulfite; available as single unit or in double-unit pack with training unit]

Injection, solution, as hydrochloride: 0.1 mg/mL [1:10,000] (10 mL); 1 mg/mL [1:1000] (1 mL) [products may contain sodium metabisulfite]

Adrenalin®: 1 mg/mL [1:1000] (1 mL, 30 mL) [contains sodium bisulfite]

Solution for oral inhalation, as hydrochloride: Adrenalin®: 1% [10 mg/mL, 1:100] (7.5 mL) [contains sodium bisulfite]

Solution, ophthalmic, as hydrochloride (Epifrin®): 0.5% (15 mL); 1% (15 mL); 2% (15 mL) [contains benzalkonium chloride and sodium metabisulfite] [DSC]

Monitoring and Teaching Issues

Physical Assessment: Assess other medications patient may be taking for effectiveness and interactions. Monitor therapeutic effectiveness (according to purpose for use) and adverse reactions. Monitor vital signs. Assess knowledge/teach patient appropriate use, interventions to reduce side effects, and adverse symptoms to report. I.V. central line with infusion pump and continuous cardiac/hemodynamic monitoring is necessary.

Patient Education: Use this medication exactly as directed; do not take more than recommended dosage. Avoid other stimulant prescriptive or OTC medications to avoid serious overdose reactions. You may experience dizziness, blurred vision, restlessness (use caution when driving or engaging in tasks requiring alertness until response to drug is known); or difficulty urinating (empty bladder immediately before taking this medication). Report excessive nervousness or excitation, inability to sleep, facial flushing, pounding heartbeat, muscle tremors or weakness, chest pain or palpitations, bronchial irritation or coughing, or increased sweating.

Ophthalmic: Wash hands before instilling. Sit or lie down to instill. Open eye, look at ceiling, and instill prescribed amount of medication. Close eye and roll eye in all directions, and apply gentle pressure to inner corner of eye. Do not let tip of applicator touch eye; do not contaminate tip of applicator (may cause eye infection, eye damage, or vision loss).

Temporary stinging or burning may occur. Report persistent pain, burning, vision changes, swelling, itching, or worsening of condition.

Aerosol: Use aerosol or nebulizer as per instructions. Clear as much mucus as possible before use. Rinse mouth following each use. If more than one inhalation is necessary, wait 1 minute between inhalations. May cause restlessness or nervousness; use caution when driving or engaging in hazardous activities until response to medication is known. Report persistent nervousness, restlessness, sleeplessness, palpitations, tachycardia, chest pain, muscle tremors, dizziness, flushing, or if breathing difficulty persists.

Nasal: Instill 1 spray into each nostril 3-4 times a day. Report if symptoms worsen or nasal passages become irritated.

Pregnancy/breast-feeding precautions: Inform prescriber if you are or intend to become pregnant. Consult prescriber if breast-feeding.

Geriatric Considerations: The use of epinephrine in the treatment of acute exacerbations of asthma was studied in older adults. A dose of 0.3 mg SubQ every 20 minutes for three doses was well tolerated in older patients with no history of angina or recent myocardial infarction. There was no significant difference in the incidence of ventricular arrhythmias in older adults versus younger adults.

Pregnancy Risk Factor: C

Pregnancy Issues: Crosses the placenta. Reported association with malformations in 1 study; may be secondary to severe maternal disease.

Lactation: Excretion in breast milk unknown

Administration

I.M.: I.M. administration into the buttocks should be avoided.

I.V.: Central line administration only. I.V. infusions require an infusion pump.

Endotracheal: Doses (2-2.5 times the I.V. dose) should be diluted to 10 mL with NS or distilled water prior to administration.

Epinephrine can be administered SubQ, I.M. (Sus-Phrine®), I.V.

Other: Intratracheal: Dilute in NS or distilled water. Absorption is greater with distilled water, but causes more adverse effects on PaO_2. Pass catheter beyond tip of tracheal tube, stop compressions, spray drug quickly down tube. Follow immediately with several quick insufflations and continue chest compressions.

Reconstitution:

Standard diluent: 1 mg/250 mL NS

Preparation of adult I.V. infusion: Dilute 1 mg in 250 mL of D_5W or NS (4 mcg/mL). Administer at an initial rate of 1 mcg/minute and increase to desired effects. At 20 mcg/minute pure alpha effects occur.

1 mcg/minute: 15 mL/hour

2 mcg/minute: 30 mL/hour

3 mcg/minute: 45 mL/hour, etc

Stability of injection of parenteral admixture at room temperature (25°C) or refrigeration (4°C) is 24 hours.

Compatibility: Stable in dextran 6% in dextrose, dextran 6% in NS, D_5LR, $D_5^{1}/_4NS$, $D_5^{1}/_2NS$, D_5NS, D_5W, $D_{10}W$, $D_{10}NS$, LR, NS; **incompatible** with sodium bicarbonate 5%

Y-site administration: Incompatible with ampicillin, thiopental

Compatibility when admixed: Incompatible with aminophylline, hyaluronidase, mephentermine, sodium bicarbonate

Storage: Epinephrine is sensitive to light and air. Protection from light is recommended. Oxidation turns drug pink, then a brown color. **Solutions should not be used if they are discolored or contain a precipitate.**

Related Information

Compatibility of Drugs *on page 1723*

Glaucoma Drug Therapy *on page 1827*

Inhalant Agents *on page 1734*

Inotropic and Vasoconstrictor Comparison *on page 1736*

♦ **Epinephrine and Lidocaine** *see* Lidocaine and Epinephrine *on page 901*

♦ **Epinephrine Bitartrate** *see* Epinephrine *on page 525*

♦ **Epinephrine Hydrochloride** *see* Epinephrine *on page 525*

♦ **EpiPen®** *see* Epinephrine *on page 525*

♦ **EpiPen® Jr** *see* Epinephrine *on page 525*

♦ **Epipodophyllotoxin** *see* Etoposide *on page 599*

♦ **EpiQuin™ Micro** *see* Hydroquinone *on page 768*

Epirubicin (ep i ROO bi sin)

U.S. Brand Names Ellence®

Synonyms Pidorubicin; Pidorubicin Hydrochloride

Generic Available No

Pharmacologic Category Antineoplastic Agent, Anthracycline

Medication Safety Issues

Sound-alike/look-alike issues:

Ellence® may be confused with Elase®

Use Adjuvant therapy for primary breast cancer

Mechanism of Action/Effect Epirubicin inhibits DNA and RNA synthesis throughout the cell cycle.

Contraindications Hypersensitivity to epirubicin, other anthracyclines, or anthracenediones; severe myocardial insufficiency, severe arrhythmias; recent myocardial infarction; severe hepatic dysfunction; baseline neutrophil count 1500 cells/mm³; previous anthracycline treatment up to maximum cumulative dose; pregnancy

Warnings/Precautions The U.S. Food and Drug Administration (FDA) currently recommends that procedures for proper handling and disposal of antineoplastic agents be considered. The primary toxicity is myelosuppression; severe thrombocytopenia or anemia may

(Continued)

Epirubicin *(Continued)*

occur. Thrombophlebitis and thromboembolic phenomena (including pulmonary embolism) have occurred.

Potential cardiotoxicity, particularly in patients who have received prior anthracyclines, prior radiotherapy to the mediastinal/pericardial area, or who have pre-existing cardiac disease, may occur. Acute toxicity (primarily arrhythmias) and delayed toxicity (CHF) have been described. Delayed toxicity usually develops late in the course of therapy or within 2-3 months after completion, however, events with an onset of several months to years after termination of treatment have been described. The risk of delayed cardiotoxicity increases more steeply at dosages above 900 mg/m^2, and this dose should be exceeded only with extreme caution. Toxicity may be additive with other anthracyclines or anthracenediones, and may be increased in pediatric patients. Regular monitoring of LVEF and discontinuation at the first sign of impairment is recommended especially in patients with risk factors or impaired cardiac function.

Reduce dosage and use with caution in mild to moderate hepatic impairment or in severe renal dysfunction (serum creatinine >5 mg/dL). May cause tumor lysis syndrome or radiation recall. Treatment with anthracyclines may increase the risk of secondary leukemias. For I.V. administration only, severe local tissue necrosis will result if extravasation occurs. Epirubicin is emetogenic. Women ≥70 years of age should be especially monitored for toxicity; women of childbearing age should be advised to avoid becoming pregnant.

Drug Interactions
Increased Effect/Toxicity: Cimetidine increased the blood levels of epirubicin (AUC increased by 50%).

Nutritional/Ethanol Interactions
Ethanol: Avoid ethanol (due to GI irritation).

Herb/Nutraceutical: St John's wort may decrease doxorubicin levels. Avoid black cohosh, dong quai in estrogen-dependent tumors.

Adverse Reactions
>10%:
  Central nervous system: Lethargy (1% to 46%)
  Dermatologic: Alopecia (69% to 95%)
  Endocrine & metabolic: Amenorrhea (69% to 72%), hot flashes (5% to 39%)
  Gastrointestinal: Nausea, vomiting (83% to 92%), mucositis (9% to 59%), diarrhea (7% to 25%)
  Hematologic: Leukopenia (49% to 80%; Grade 3 and 4: 1.5% to 58.6%), neutropenia (54% to 80%), anemia (13% to 72%), thrombocytopenia (5% to 49%)
  Local: Injection site reactions (3% to 20%)
  Ocular: Conjunctivitis (1% to 15%)
  Miscellaneous: Infection (15% to 21%)
1% to 10%:
  Cardiovascular: CHF (0.4% to 1.5%), decreased LVEF (asymptomatic) (1.4% to 1.8%); recommended maximum cumulative dose: 900 mg/m^2
  Central nervous system: Fever (1% to 5%)
  Dermatologic: Rash (1% to 9%), skin changes (0.7% to 5%)
  Gastrointestinal: Anorexia (2% to 3%)
Other reactions (percentage not specified): Acute lymphoid leukemia, acute myelogenous leukemia (0.2% at 3 years), anaphylaxis, hypersensitivity, photosensitivity reaction, premature menopause in women, pulmonary embolism, radiation recall, skin and nail hyperpigmentation, thromboembolic phenomena, thrombophlebitis, transaminases increased, urticaria

Overdosage/Toxicology
Symptoms of overdose are generally extensions of known cytotoxic effects, including myelosuppression, mucositis, gastrointestinal bleeding, lactic acidosis, multiple organ failure, and death. Treatment is supportive.

Pharmacodynamics/Kinetics
Protein Binding: 77% to albumin
Half-Life Elimination: Triphasic; Mean terminal: 33 hours
Metabolism: Extensive via hepatic and extrahepatic (including RBCs) routes
Excretion: Feces; urine (lesser extent)

Dosing
Adults: I.V.: 100-120 mg/m^2 once weekly every 3-4 weeks **or** 50-60 mg/m^2 days 1 and 8 every 3-4 weeks
  Breast cancer:
    CEF-120: 60 mg/m^2 on days 1 and 8 every 28 days for 6 cycles
    FEC-100: 100 mg/m^2 on day 1 every 21 days for 6 cycles
    Note: Note: Patients receiving 120 mg/m^2/cycle as part of combination therapy should also receive prophylactic therapy with sulfamethoxazole/trimethoprim or a fluoroquinolone.
  Dosage modifications:
    Delay day 1 dose until platelets are ≥100,000/mm^3, ANC ≥1500/mm^3, and nonhematologic toxicities have recovered to ≤grade 1
    Reduce day 1 dose in subsequent cycles to 75% of previous day 1 dose if patient experiences nadir platelet counts <50,000/mm^3, ANC <250/mm^3, neutropenic fever, or grade 3/4 nonhematologic toxicity during the previous cycle
    For divided doses (day 1 and day 8), reduce day 8 dose to 75% of day 1 dose if platelet counts are 75,000-100,000/mm^3 and ANC is 1000-1499/mm^3; omit day 8 dose if platelets are <75,000/mm^3, ANC <1000/mm^3, or grade 3/4 nonhematologic toxicity
    Dosage adjustment in bone marrow dysfunction: Heavily-treated patients, patients with pre-existing bone marrow depression or neoplastic bone marrow infiltration: Lower starting doses (75-90 mg/mm^2) should be considered.
  Elderly: Plasma clearance of epirubicin in elderly female patients was noted to be reduced by 35%. Although no initial dosage reduction is specifically recommended, particular care

should be exercised in monitoring toxicity and adjusting subsequent dosage in elderly patients (particularly females >70 years of age).

Renal Impairment: Severe renal impairment (serum creatinine >5 mg/dL): Lower doses should be considered.

Hepatic Impairment:

Bilirubin 1.2-3 mg/dL or AST 2-4 times the upper limit of normal: 50% of recommended starting dose.

Bilirubin >3 mg/dL or AST >4 times the upper limit of normal: 25% of recommended starting dose.

Available Dosage Forms Injection, solution [preservative free]: 2 mg/mL (25 mL, 100 mL)

Monitoring and Teaching Issues

Physical Assessment: See Warnings/Precautions for use cautions (eg, renal or hepatic impairment). Assess potential for interactions with herbal products patient may be taking (see Nutritional/Ethanol Interactions). Note infusion specifics in Administration. Premedication with an antiemetic may be useful (emetogenic). Infusion site must be monitored closely to prevent extravasation; severe local tissue necrosis will result if extravasation occurs. Assess results of laboratory tests (see Monitoring Laboratory Tests) and patient response prior to each treatment and on a regular basis throughout therapy (eg, acute nausea and vomiting, anemia, cardiotoxicity, infection, bleeding; see Adverse Reactions). Teach patient possible side effects/appropriate interventions (eg, importance of adequate hydration) and adverse symptoms to report (see Patient Education).

Monitoring Laboratory Tests: CBC with differential and platelet count, liver function tests, renal function, ECG, and left ventricular ejection fraction (baseline and repeated measurement). The method used for assessment of LVEF (echocardiogram or MUGA) should be consistent during routine monitoring.

Patient Education: Do not take any new medication during therapy unless approved by prescriber. This medication can only be administered by infusion. Report immediately any swelling, pain, burning, redness at infusion site; sudden difficulty breathing or swallowing, chest pain, or chills. Maintain adequate hydration (2-3 L/day of fluids) unless instructed to restrict fluid intake and adequate nutrition (small frequent meals may help). You will be more susceptible to infection (avoid crowds and exposure to infection and do not have any vaccinations without consulting prescriber). May cause nausea or vomiting (small frequent meals, frequent mouth care, sucking lozenges, or chewing gum may help); diarrhea (buttermilk, boiled milk, or yogurt may help); loss of hair (reversible); hyperpigmentation of skin or nails; mouth sores (frequent mouth care, soft toothbrush may help); or changes in menstrual cycle (consult prescriber). Report chest pain, swelling of extremities, palpitations, or rapid heartbeat; respiratory difficulty or unusual cough; unresolved nausea, vomiting, or diarrhea; alterations in urinary pattern (increased or decreased); opportunistic infection (fever, chills, unusual bruising or bleeding, fatigue, purulent vaginal discharge, unhealed mouth sores); skin rash; abdominal pain; blood in urine or stool; or other unresolved reactions. **Pregnancy/breast-feeding precautions:** Do not get pregnant while taking this medication and for 1 month following therapy. Consult prescriber for appropriate barrier contraceptives. Do not breast-feed.

Pregnancy Risk Factor: D

Pregnancy Issues: Epirubicin is mutagenic and carcinogenic. If a pregnant woman is treated with epirubicin, or if a woman becomes pregnant while receiving this drug, she should be informed of the potential hazard to the fetus. Women of childbearing potential should be advised to avoid becoming pregnant.

Lactation: Excretion in breast milk unknown/contraindicated

Breast-Feeding Issues: Excretion in human breast milk is unknown, however, other anthracyclines are excreted. Breast-feeding is contraindicated.

Administration

I.V.: Administer I.V. into the tubing of a freely-flowing intravenous infusion (0.9% sodium chloride or 5% glucose solution) over 3-5 minutes.

Compatibility: Stable in D₅W, LR, NS; **incompatible** with any solution of alkaline pH

Incompatible with heparin, fluorouracil

Compatibility in syringe: Incompatible with fluorouracil, ifosfamide with mesna, any solution of alkaline pH

Storage: Store refrigerated (2°C to 8°C/36°F to 46°F). Protect from light. Solution should be used within 24 hours of penetrating the rubber stopper.

♦ **Epitol®** *see* Carbamazepine *on page 249*

♦ **Epivir®** *see* Lamivudine *on page 861*

♦ **Epivir-HBV®** *see* Lamivudine *on page 861*

Eplerenone (e PLER en one)

U.S. Brand Names Inspra™

Generic Available No

Pharmacologic Category Antihypertensive; Selective Aldosterone Blocker

Medication Safety Issues

Sound-alike/look-alike issues:

Inspra™ may be confused with Spiriva®

Use Treatment of hypertension (may be used alone or in combination with other antihypertensive agents); treatment of CHF following acute MI

Mechanism of Action/Effect Aldosterone increases blood pressure primarily by inducing sodium reabsorption. Eplerenone reduces blood pressure by blocking aldosterone binding at mineralocorticoid receptors found in the kidney, heart, blood vessels and brain.

Contraindications Hypersensitivity to eplerenone or any component of the formulation; serum potassium >5.5 mEq/L; Cl_cr ≤30 mL/minute; concomitant use of strong CYP3A4 inhibitors (see Drug Interactions for details)

The following additional contraindications apply to patients with hypertension: Type 2 diabetes mellitus (noninsulin dependent, NIDDM) with microalbuminuria; serum creatinine (Continued)

Eplerenone *(Continued)*

>2.0 mg/dL in males or >1.8 mg/dL in females; Cl_{cr} <50 mL/minute; concomitant use with potassium supplements or potassium-sparing diuretics

Warnings/Precautions Dosage adjustment needed for patients on moderate CYP3A4 inhibitors (see drug interactions for details). Monitor closely for hyperkalemia; increases in serum potassium were dose related during clinical trials and rates of hyperkalemia also increased with declining renal function. Safety and efficacy have not been established in pediatric patients or in patients with severe hepatic impairment. Use with caution in CHF patients post-MI with diabetes.

Drug Interactions

Cytochrome P450 Effect: Substrate of CYP3A4 (major)

Decreased Effect: NSAIDs may decrease the antihypertensive effects of eplerenone. CYP3A4 inducers may decrease the levels/effects of eplerenone; example inducers include aminoglutethimide, carbamazepine, nafcillin, nevirapine, phenobarbital, phenytoin, and rifamycins.

Increased Effect/Toxicity: ACE inhibitors, angiotensin II receptor antagonists, NSAIDs, potassium supplements, and potassium-sparing diuretics increase the risk of hyperkalemia; concomitant use with potassium supplements and potassium-sparing diuretics is contraindicated; monitor potassium levels with ACE inhibitors and angiotensin II receptor antagonists. Potent CYP3A4 inhibitors (eg, itraconazole, ketoconazole) lead to fivefold increase in eplerenone; concurrent use is contraindicated. Less potent CYP3A4 inhibitors (eg, erythromycin, fluconazole, saquinavir, verapamil) lead to approximately twofold increase in eplerenone; starting dose should be decreased to 25 mg/day. Although interaction studies have not been conducted, monitoring of lithium levels is recommended.

Nutritional/Ethanol Interactions

Food: Grapefruit juice increases eplerenone AUC ~25%.

Herb/Nutraceutical: St John's wort decreases eplerenone AUC ~30%.

Adverse Reactions

>10%: Endocrine & metabolic: Hypertriglyceridemia (1% to 15%, dose related)

1% to 10%:

Central nervous system: Dizziness (3%), fatigue (2%)

Endocrine & metabolic: Breast pain (males <1% to 1%), serum creatinine increased (6% in CHF), gynecomastia (males <1% to 1%), hyponatremia (2%, dose related), hypercholesterolemia (<1% to 1%); hyperkalemia (mild-to-moderate hypertension <1%; left ventricular dysfunction ~6% had serum potassium ≥6 mEq/L)

Gastrointestinal: Diarrhea (2%), abdominal pain (1%)

Genitourinary: Abnormal vaginal bleeding (<1% to 2%)

Renal: Albuminuria (1%)

Respiratory: Cough (2%)

Miscellaneous: Flu-like syndrome (2%)

Overdosage/Toxicology Cases of human overdose have not been reported; hypotension or hyperkalemia would be expected. Treatment should be symptom-directed and supportive. Eplerenone is not removed by hemodialysis; binds extensively to charcoal.

Pharmacodynamics/Kinetics

Time to Peak: Plasma: 1.5 hours; may take up to 4 weeks for full therapeutic effect

Protein Binding: ~50%; primarily to alpha$_1$-acid glycoproteins

Half-Life Elimination: 4-6 hours

Metabolism: Primarily hepatic via CYP3A4; metabolites inactive

Excretion: Urine (67%; <5% as unchanged drug), feces (32%)

Dosing

Adults:

Hypertension: Oral: Initial: 50 mg once daily; may increase to 50 mg twice daily if response is not adequate; may take up to 4 weeks for full therapeutic response. Doses >100 mg/day are associated with increased risk of hyperkalemia and no greater therapeutic effect.

Dose modification during concurrent use with moderate CYP3A4 inhibitors: Initial: 25 mg once daily

Congestive heart failure (post-MI): Oral: Initial: 25 mg once daily; dosage goal: titrate to 50 mg once daily within 4 weeks, as tolerated

Dosage adjustment per serum potassium concentrations for CHF:

Serum level <5.0 mEq/L:

Increase dose from 25 mg every other day to 25 mg daily **or**

Increase dose from 25 mg daily to 50 mg daily

5.0-5.4 mEq/L: No adjustment needed

5.5-5.9 mEq/L:

Decrease dose from 50 mg daily to 25 mg daily **or**

Decrease dose from 25 mg daily to 25 mg every other day **or**

Decrease does from 25 mg every other day to withhold medication

Potassium level ≥6.0 mEq/L: Withhold medication until potassium <5.5 mEq/L, then restart at 25 mg every other day

Elderly: See Geriatric Considerations.

Renal Impairment:

Patients with hypertension with Cl_{cr} <50 mL/minute or serum creatinine >2.0 mg/dL in males or >1.8 mg/dL in females: Use is contraindicated; risk of hyperkalemia increases with declining renal function.

Patients with CHF post-MI: Use with caution.

Hepatic Impairment: No dosage adjustment needed for mild-to-moderate impairment. Safety and efficacy not established for severe impairment.

Available Dosage Forms Tablet [film coated]: 25 mg, 50 mg

Monitoring and Teaching Issues

Physical Assessment: See Contraindications and Warnings/Precautions for use cautions. Assess potential for interactions with other pharmacological agents or herbal products patient may be taking (eg, increased risk of toxicity; see Drug Interactions). Assess results of laboratory tests prior to and periodically during therapy (eg, potassium levels, renal function), therapeutic effectiveness (blood pressure), and adverse response at beginning of and at regular intervals during therapy (eg, hypotension, hyperkalemia; see Adverse Reactions). Teach patient proper use, possible side effects/appropriate interventions, and adverse reactions to report (see Patient Education).

Monitoring Laboratory Tests: Serum potassium (levels monitored every 2 weeks for the first 1-2 months, then monthly in clinical trials); renal function

Patient Education: Do not take any new medication during therapy without consulting prescriber. Take exactly as directed at the same time of day, without regard for meals. Do not alter dose or discontinue without consulting prescriber; it may take up to 4 weeks to achieve desired results. Do not use potassium supplement or salt substitutes without consulting prescriber. This drug does not eliminate need for diet or exercise regimen as recommended by prescriber. May cause dizziness, fainting, lightheadedness (use caution when driving or engaging in tasks that require alertness until response to drug is known); postural hypotension (use caution when rising from lying or sitting position or climbing stairs); diarrhea (boiled milk, buttermilk, or yogurt may help); breast pain (males); or abnormal vaginal bleeding. Report chest pain, palpitations; unusual cough or flu-like symptoms; or other persistent or severe adverse effects. **Breast-feeding precaution:** Breast-feeding is not recommended.

Dietary Considerations: May be taken with or without food. Do not use salt substitutes containing potassium.

Geriatric Considerations: Since this medication is contraindicated in patients with a Cl_{cr} <50 mL/minute, it will have limited use in older adults. Due to physiologic changes older adults may be at increased risk of hyperkalemia when using this medication.

Pregnancy Risk Factor: B

Lactation: Excretion in breast milk unknown/not recommended

Administration

Oral: May be administered with or without food.

Storage: Store at controlled room temperature of 25°C (77°F).

♦ **EPO** *see Epoetin Alfa on page 531*

Epoetin Alfa (e POE e tin AL fa)

U.S. Brand Names Epogen®; Procrit®

Synonyms EPO; Erythropoietin; rHuEPO-α

Generic Available No

Pharmacologic Category Colony Stimulating Factor

Medication Safety Issues

Sound-alike/look-alike issues:

Epogen® may be confused with Neupogen®

Use

Treatment of anemia related to zidovudine therapy in HIV-infected patients; in patients when the endogenous erythropoietin level is ≤500 mU/mL and the dose of zidovudine is ≤4200 mg/week

Treatment of anemia associated with chronic renal failure (CRF) including dialysis (end-stage renal disease, ESRD) and nondialysis patients. Prior to therapy, serum ferritin should be >100 ng/dL and transferrin saturation (serum iron/iron binding capacity x 100) of 20% to 30%; nondialysis patients should have a hematocrit <30%

Treatment of anemia in cancer patients on chemotherapy; in patients with nonmyeloid malignancies where anemia is caused by the effect of the concomitantly administered chemotherapy; to decrease the need for transfusions in patients who will be receiving chemotherapy for a minimum of 2 months

Reduction of allogeneic blood transfusion in surgery patients (with hemoglobin >10 g/dL up to 13 g/dL) scheduled to undergo elective, noncardiac, nonvascular surgery

Unlabeled/Investigational Use Anemia associated with rheumatic disease; hypogenerative anemia of Rh hemolytic disease; sickle cell anemia; acute renal failure; Gaucher's disease; Castleman's disease; paroxysmal nocturnal hemoglobinuria; anemia of critical illness (limited documentation); anemia of prematurity

Mechanism of Action/Effect Induces red blood cell production in the bone marrow to be released into the blood stream where they mature to erythrocytes; results in rise in hematocrit and hemoglobin levels

Contraindications Hypersensitivity to albumin (human) or mammalian cell-derived products; uncontrolled hypertension

Warnings/Precautions Use caution with history of seizures or hypertension; blood pressure should be controlled prior to start of therapy and monitored closely throughout treatment. Excessive rate of rise of hematocrit may be possibly associated with the exacerbation of hypertension or seizures; decrease the epoetin dose if the hemoglobin increase exceeds 1 g/dL in any 2-week period. Use caution in patients at risk for thrombosis or with history of cardiovascular disease. Increased mortality has occurred when aggressive dosing is used in CHF or anginal patients undergoing hemodialysis.

Pure red cell aplasia (PRCA) with neutralizing antibodies to erythropoietin has been reported in limited patients treated with recombinant products; may occur more in patients with CRF.

Prior to and during therapy iron stores must be evaluated. Iron supplementation should be given during therapy to provide for increased requirements during expansion of the red cell mass secondary to marrow stimulation by EPO unless iron stores are already in excess.

Use caution with porphyria. Not recommended for acute correction of severe anemia or as a substitute for transfusion. For patients receiving renal transplant, consider discontinuing at transplant or within 2 weeks of successful engraftment.

For patients with endogenous serum EPO levels which are inappropriately low for hemoglobin level, documentation of the serum EPO level will help indicate which patients may benefit from EPO therapy.

(Continued)

Epoetin Alfa (Continued)

Adverse Reactions

>10%:
    Cardiovascular: Hypertension
    Central nervous system: Headache, fever
    Gastrointestinal: Nausea
    Neuromuscular & skeletal: Arthralgias

1% to 10%:
    Cardiovascular: Edema, chest pain
    Central nervous system: Fatigue, seizure
    Gastrointestinal: Vomiting, diarrhea
    Hematologic: Clotted access
    Neuromuscular & skeletal: Asthenia

Overdosage/Toxicology Symptoms of overdose include erythrocytosis. Maintain adequate airway and provide other supportive measures and agents for treating anaphylaxis when the I.V. drug is given.

Pharmacodynamics/Kinetics

Onset of Action: Several days; Peak effect: 2-3 weeks

Bioavailability: SubQ: ~21% to 31%; Intraperitoneal epoetin: 3% (a few patients)

Time to Peak: Serum: SubQ: Chronic renal failure: 5-24 hours

Half-Life Elimination: Circulating: Chronic renal failure: 4-13 hours; Healthy volunteers: 20% shorter

Metabolism: Some degradation does occur

Excretion: Feces (majority); urine (small amounts, 10% unchanged in normal volunteers)

Dosing

Adults & Elderly: Individuals with anemia due to iron deficiency, sickle cell disease, autoimmune hemolytic anemia, and bleeding, generally have appropriate endogenous EPO levels to drive erythropoiesis and would not ordinarily be candidates for EPO therapy.

  Chronic renal failure patients: I.V., SubQ: Initial dose: 50-100 units/kg 3 times/week
    Titration: Reduce dose by 25% when hemoglobin approaches 12 g/dL **or** when hemoglobin increases 1 g/dL in any 2-week period. Increase dose by 25% if hemoglobin does not increase by 2 g/dL after 8 weeks of therapy and hemoglobin is below suggested target range; suggested target hematocrit range: 10-12 g/dL.
    Maintenance dose: Individualize to target range; limit additional dosage increases to every 4 weeks (or longer)
    Dialysis patients: Median dose: 75 units/kg 3 times/week
    Nondialysis patients: Median dose: 75-150 units/kg

  Zidovudine-treated, HIV-infected patients (patient with erythropoietin levels >500 mU/mL is unlikely to respond): I.V., SubQ: 100 units/kg 3 times/week for 8 weeks
    Increase dose by 50-100 units/kg 3 times/week if response is not satisfactory in terms of reducing transfusion requirements or increasing hemoglobin after 8 weeks of therapy. Evaluate response every 4-8 weeks thereafter and adjust the dose accordingly by 50-100 units/kg increments 3 times/week. If patient has not responded satisfactorily to a 300 unit/kg dose 3 times/week, a response to higher doses is unlikely. Stop dose if hemoglobin exceeds 13 g/dL and resume treatment at a 25% dose reduction when hemoglobin drops to 12 g/dL.

  Cancer patients on chemotherapy: Treatment of patients with erythropoietin levels >200 mU/mL is **not recommended**. SubQ:
    150 units/kg 3 times/week or 40,000 units once weekly; commonly used doses range from 10,000 units 3 times/week to 40,000-60,000 units once weekly.
    Dose adjustment: If response is not satisfactory after a sufficient period of evaluation (8 weeks of 3 times/week and 4 weeks of once-weekly therapy), the dose may be increased every 4 weeks (or longer) up to 300 units/kg 3 times/week, **or** when dosed weekly, increased all at once to 60,000 units weekly. If patient does not respond, a response to higher doses is unlikely. Stop dose when hemoglobin drops to 12 g/dL; reduce dose by 25% if hemoglobin increases by 1 g/dL in any 2-week period.
    Alternative dose (unlabeled dosing): Initial dose: 60,000 units once weekly for 8 weeks.
    Dose adjustment: If patient does not respond, a response to higher doses is unlikely. If response is adequate (hemoglobin increases >2 g/dL after 8 weeks), begin maintenance dose of 120,000 units, to be given once every 3 weeks. During any point of initial or maintenance therapy, if the hemoglobin increases 1.3 g/dL in a 2-week period, decrease dose to 40,000 units once weekly. Stop dose if hemoglobin exceeds 15 g/dL and resume treatment at 20,000 units once-weekly when hemoglobin drops to 13 g/dL.

  Surgery patients: Prior to initiating treatment, obtain a hemoglobin to establish that is >10 mg/dL or ≤13 mg/dL: SubQ: Initial dose: 300 units/kg/day for 10 days before surgery, on the day of surgery, and for 4 days after surgery
    Alternative dose: 600 units/kg in once weekly doses (21, 14, and 7 days before surgery) plus a fourth dose on the day of surgery

  Anemia of critical illness (unlabeled use): SubQ: 40,000 units once weekly

Pediatrics:

  Anemia of prematurity (unlabeled use): Infants: I.V., SubQ: Dosing range: 500-1250 units/kg/week; commonly used dose: 250 units/kg 3 times/week; supplement with oral iron therapy 3-8 mg/kg/day

  Chronic renal failure patients: I.V., SubQ: Initial dose: 50 units/kg 3 times/week
    Dosage adjustment: Reduce dose by 25% when hemoglobin approaches 12 g/dL **or** when hemoglobin increases 1 g/dL in any 2-week period. Increase dose by 25% if hemoglobin does not increase by 2 g/dL after 8 weeks of therapy and hemoglobin is below suggested target range; suggested target hemoglobin range: 10-12 g/dL
    Maintenance dose: Individualize to target range; limit additional dosage increases to every 4 weeks (or longer)
    Dialysis patients: Median dose: 167 units/kg/week **or** 76 units/kg 2-3 times/week
    Nondialysis patients: Dosing range: 50-250 units/kg 1-3 times/week

Zidovudine-treated, HIV-infected patients (patient with erythropoietin levels >500 mU/mL is unlikely to respond): I.V., SubQ: Initial dose: Reported dosing range: 50-400 units/kg 2-3 times/week

Cancer patients on chemotherapy: Treatment of patients with erythropoietin levels >200 mU/mL is **not recommended**: I.V., SubQ: Dosing range: 25-300 units/kg 3-7 times/ week; commonly reported initial dose: 150 units/kg

Dosage adjustment: If response is not satisfactory after a sufficient period of evaluation (8 weeks), the dose may be increased every 4 weeks (or longer) up to 300 units/kg 3 times/week. If patient does not respond, a response to higher doses is unlikely. Stop dose if hemoglobin exceeds 13 g/dL and resume treatment at a 25% dose reduction when hemoglobin drops to 12 g/dL; reduce dose by 25% if hemoglobin increases by 1 g/dL in any 2-week period, or if hemoglobin approaches 12 g/dL.

Renal Impairment:

Dialysis patient: Usually administered as I.V. bolus 3 times/week. While administration is independent of the dialysis procedure, it may be administered into the venous line at the end of the dialysis procedure to obviate the need for additional venous access.

Chronic renal failure patients not on dialysis: May be given either as an I.V. or SubQ injection.

Hemodialysis: Supplemental dose is not necessary.

Peritoneal dialysis: Supplemental dose is not necessary.

Available Dosage Forms

Injection, solution [preservative free]: 2000 units/mL (1 mL); 3000 units/mL (1 mL); 4000 units/mL (1 mL); 10,000 units/mL (1 mL); 40,000 units/mL (1 mL) [contains human albumin]

Injection, solution [with preservative]: 10,000 units/mL (2 mL); 20,000 units/mL (1 mL) [contains human albumin and benzyl alcohol]

Monitoring and Teaching Issues

Physical Assessment: Use caution in presence of seizure history, hypertension, risk for thrombosis, cardiovascular disease (see Warning/Precautions). See Administration specifics. I.V. lines should be monitored closely for possible clotting. Assess results of laboratory tests (eg, hematocrit determination twice weekly), therapeutic effectiveness (correction of anemia), and adverse response on a regular basis during therapy (eg, hypovolemia, angioedema, postural hypotension; see Adverse Reactions). Teach patient proper use if self-administered (appropriate SubQ injection technique and syringe/needle disposal), possible side effects/appropriate interventions, and adverse symptoms to report (see Patient Education).

Monitoring Laboratory Tests: Hematocrit should be determined twice weekly until stabilization within the target range (30% to 36%), and twice weekly for at least 2-6 weeks after a dose increase. See table.

Test	Initial Phase Frequency	Maintenance Phase Frequency
Hematocrit/hemoglobin	2 x/week	2-4 x/month
Blood pressure	3 x/week	3 x/week
Serum ferritin	Monthly	Quarterly
Transferrin saturation	Monthly	Quarterly
Serum chemistries including CBC with differential, creatinine, blood urea nitrogen, potassium, phosphorous	Regularly per routine	Regularly per routine

Patient Education: Do not take any new medication during therapy without consulting prescriber. If self-administered, follow exact directions for injection and needle disposal. You will require frequent blood tests to determine appropriate dosage. Do not make significant changes in your dietary iron without consulting prescriber. Report signs or symptoms of edema (eg, swollen extremities, respiratory difficulty, rapid weight gain); onset of severe headache; acute back pain; chest pain; or muscular tremors or seizure activity. **Pregnancy/breast-feeding precautions:** Inform prescriber if you are or intend to become pregnant. Consult prescriber if breast-feeding.

Geriatric Considerations: There is limited information about the use of epoetin alfa in the elderly. Endogenous erythropoietin secretion has been reported to be decreased in older adults with normocytic or iron-deficiency anemias or those with a serum hemoglobin concentration <12 g/dL; one study did not find such a relationship in the elderly with chronic anemia. A blunted erythropoietin response to anemia has been reported in patients with cancer, rheumatoid arthritis, and AIDS.

Pregnancy Risk Factor: C

Pregnancy Issues: Epoetin alpha has been shown to have adverse effects in rats when given in doses 5 times the human dose. Use only if potential benefit justifies the potential risk to the fetus.

Lactation: Excretion in breast milk unknown/use caution

Breast-Feeding Issues: When administered enterally to neonates (mixed with human milk or infant formula), rHuEPO-α did not significantly increase serum EPO concentrations. If passage via breast milk does occur, risk to a nursing infant appears low.

Administration

I.V.:

Patients with CRF on dialysis: May be administered I.V. bolus into the venous line after dialysis.

Patients with CRF not on dialysis: May be administered I.V. or SubQ

Reconstitution: For minimal dilution, mix with bacteriostatic 0.9% sodium chloride, containing 20 mL of 0.9% sodium chloride and benzyl alcohol as the bacteriostatic agent. Dilutions of 1:10 and 1:20 (1 part epoetin:19 parts sodium chloride) are stable for 18 hours at room temperature. Results showed no loss of epoetin alfa after a 1:20 dilution. 250 mcg/ mL albumin remaining after a 1:10 dilution of formulated epoetin alfa should be sufficient to prevent it from binding to commonly encountered containers. Prior to SubQ administration, (Continued)

Epoetin Alfa *(Continued)*

preservative free solutions may be mixed with bacteriostatic NS containing benzyl alcohol 0.9% in a 1:1 ratio.

Compatibility: Stable in $D_{10}W$ with albumin 0.05%, $D_{10}W$ with albumin 0.1%; **incompatible** with $D_{10}W$ with albumin 0.01%, $D_{10}W$, NS

Storage: Vials should be stored at 2°C to 8°C (36°F to 46°F); **do not freeze or shake**.

> **Single-dose 1 mL vial** contains no preservative: Use one dose per vial; do not re-enter vial; discard unused portions.
>
> Single-use vials (except 40,000 units/mL vial) are stable for 2 weeks at room temperature; single-dose 40,000 units/mL vial is stable for 1 week at room temperature.
>
> **Multidose 1 mL or 2 mL vial** contains preservative; store at 2°C to 8°C after initial entry and between doses; discard 21 days after initial entry. Multidose vials (with preservative) are stable for 1 week at room temperature.

Additional Information Due to the delayed onset of erythropoiesis (7-10 days to increase reticulocyte count; 2-6 weeks to increase hemoglobin), erythropoietin is of no value in the acute treatment of anemia. Emergency/stat orders for erythropoietin are inappropriate.

Factors Limiting Response to Epoetin Alfa

Factor	Mechanism
Iron deficiency	Limits hemoglobin synthesis
Blood loss/hemolysis	Counteracts epoetin alfa-stimulated erythropoiesis
Infection/inflammation	Inhibits iron transfer from storage to bone marrow
	Suppresses erythropoiesis through activated macrophages
Aluminum overload	Inhibits iron incorporation into heme protein
Bone marrow replacement Hyperparathyroidism Metastatic, neoplastic	Limits bone marrow volume
Folic acid/vitamin B_{12} deficiency	Limits hemoglobin synthesis
Patient compliance	Self-administered epoetin alfa or iron therapy

Professional Services:
Amgen (Epogen®): 1-800-772-6436
Ortho Biotech (Procrit®): 1-800-325-7504
Reimbursement Assistance:
Amgen: 1-800-272-9376
Ortho Biotech: 1-800-553-3851

♦ **Epogen**® *see* Epoetin Alfa *on page 531*

Epoprostenol (e poe PROST en ole)

U.S. Brand Names Flolan®

Synonyms Epoprostenol Sodium; PGI_2; PGX; Prostacyclin

Restrictions Orders for epoprostenol are distributed by two sources in the United States. Information on orders or reimbursement assistance may be obtained from either Accredo Health, Inc (1-800-935-6526) or TheraCom, Inc (1-877-356-5264).

Generic Available No

Pharmacologic Category Prostaglandin

Use Orphan drug: Treatment of primary pulmonary hypertension; treatment of secondary pulmonary hypertension due to intrinsic precapillary pulmonary vascular disease

Unlabeled/Investigational Use Other potential uses include pulmonary hypertension associated with ARDS, SLE, or CHF; neonatal pulmonary hypertension; cardiopulmonary bypass surgery; hemodialysis; atherosclerosis; peripheral vascular disorders; and neonatal purpura fulminans

Mechanism of Action/Effect Naturally occur ring prostacyclin (PGI_2) which acts as a strong vasodilator in all vascular beds; inhibits platelet aggregation

Contraindications Hypersensitivity to epoprostenol or to structurally-related compounds; chronic use in patients with CHF due to severe left ventricular systolic dysfunction

Warnings/Precautions Abrupt interruptions or large sudden reductions in dosage may result in rebound pulmonary hypertension. Some patients with primary pulmonary hypertension have developed pulmonary edema during dose ranging, which may be associated with pulmonary veno-occlusive disease. During chronic use, unless contraindicated, anticoagulants should be coadministered to reduce the risk of thromboembolism. Use cautiously in patients who have bleeding tendencies (inhibits platelet aggregation).

Drug Interactions

> **Increased Effect/Toxicity:** The hypotensive effects of epoprostenol may be exacerbated by other vasodilators, diuretics, or by using acetate in dialysis fluids. Patients treated with anticoagulants (heparins, warfarin, thrombin inhibitors) or antiplatelet agents (ticlopidine, clopidogrel, IIb/IIIa antagonists, aspirin) and epoprostenol should be monitored for increased bleeding risk.

Adverse Reactions

> \>10%:
> Cardiovascular: Flushing, tachycardia, shock, syncope, heart failure
> Central nervous system: Fever, chills, anxiety, nervousness, dizziness, headache, hyperesthesia, pain
> Gastrointestinal: Diarrhea, nausea, vomiting
> Neuromuscular & skeletal: Jaw pain, myalgia, tremor, paresthesia
> Respiratory: Hypoxia
> Miscellaneous: Sepsis, flu-like symptoms

1% to 10%:
  Cardiovascular: Bradycardia, hypotension, angina pectoris, edema, arrhythmia, pallor, cyanosis, palpitation, cerebrovascular accident, myocardial ischemia, chest pain
  Central nervous system: Seizures, confusion, depression, insomnia
  Dermatologic: Pruritus, rash
  Endocrine & metabolic: Hypokalemia
  Gastrointestinal: Abdominal pain, anorexia, constipation, weight change
  Hematologic: Hemorrhage, disseminated intravascular coagulation
  Hepatic: Ascites
  Neuromuscular & skeletal: Arthralgias, bone pain, weakness
  Ocular: Amblyopia
  Respiratory: Cough increase, dyspnea, epistaxis, pleural effusion
  Miscellaneous: Diaphoresis

Overdosage/Toxicology Symptoms of overdose include headache, hypotension, tachycardia, nausea, vomiting, diarrhea, and flushing. If any of these symptoms occur, reduce the infusion rate until symptoms subside. If symptoms do not subside, consider drug discontinuation. No fatal events have been reported following overdose with epoprostenol.

Pharmacodynamics/Kinetics
  Half-Life Elimination: 2.7-6 minutes; Continuous infusion: ~15 minutes
  Metabolism: Rapidly hydrolyzed at neutral pH in blood and subject to some enzymatic degradation to one active metabolite and 13 inactive metabolites
  Excretion: Urine (12% as unchanged drug)

Dosing
  Adults & Elderly: Pulmonary hypertension associated with scleroderma: I.V.:
    Acute dose ranging: The initial infusion rate should be 2 ng/kg/minute by continuous I.V. and increased in increments of 2 ng/kg/minute every 15 minutes or longer until dose-limiting effects are elicited (such as chest pain, anxiety, dizziness, changes in heart rate, dyspnea, nausea, vomiting, headache, hypotension and/or flushing).
    Continuous chronic infusion: Initial: 4 ng/kg/minute **less** than the maximum-tolerated infusion rate determined during acute dose ranging.
    If maximum-tolerated infusion rate is <5 ng/kg/minute the chronic infusion rate should be ¹/₂ the maximum-tolerated acute infusion rate.
    Dosage adjustments: Dose adjustments in the chronic infusion rate should be based on persistence, recurrence, or worsening of patient symptoms of pulmonary hypertension. If symptoms persist or reoccur after improving, the infusion rate should be increased by 1-2 ng/kg/minute increments, every 15 minutes or more. Following establishment of a new chronic infusion rate, the patient should be observed and vital signs monitored.

Available Dosage Forms Injection, powder for reconstitution, as sodium: 0.5 mg, 1.5 mg [provided with 50 mL sterile diluent]

Monitoring and Teaching Issues
  Physical Assessment: Institutional: Continuous pulmonary and hemodynamic arterial monitoring, protimes. **Noninstitutional:** Avoid sudden rate reduction or abrupt withdrawal or interruption of therapy. When adjustment in rate is made, monitor blood pressure (standing and supine) and pulse for several hours to ensure tolerance to new rate. Monitor for bleeding. Monitor (or teach appropriate caregiver or patient to monitor) vital signs on 3 times/day basis. Monitor for improved pulmonary function and improved quality of life. Be alert for any infusion pump malfunction. Assess for signs of overdose (eg, hypoxia, flushing, tachycardia, fever, chills, anxiety, acute headache, tremor, vomiting, diarrhea).

  Patient Education: Therapy on this drug will probably be prolonged, possibly for years. You may experience mild headache, nausea or vomiting, and some muscular pains (use of a mild analgesia may be recommended by your prescriber). Report immediately any signs or symptoms of acute or severe headache, back pain, increased difficult breathing, flushing, fever or chills, any unusual bleeding or bruising, or any onset of unresolved diarrhea. **Breast-feeding precaution:** Consult prescriber if breast-feeding.

Pregnancy Risk Factor: B
Lactation: Excretion in breast milk unknown

Administration
  Reconstitution: Prepare fresh solutions every 24 hours. Reconstitute with sterile diluent for epoprostenol. See table.

Preparation of Epoprostenol Infusion

To make 100 mL of solution with concentration:	Directions
3000 ng/mL	Dissolve one 0.5 mg vial with 5 mL supplied diluent, withdraw 3 mL, and add to sufficient diluent to make a total of 100 mL.
5000 ng/mL	Dissolve one 0.5 mg vial with 5 mL supplied diluent, withdraw entire vial contents, and add a sufficient volume of diluent to make a total of 100 mL.
10,000 ng/mL	Dissolve two 0.5 mg vials each with 5 mL supplied diluent, withdraw entire vial contents, and add a sufficient volume of diluent to make a total of 100 mL.
15,000 ng/mL	Dissolve one 1.5 mg vial with 5 mL supplied diluent, withdraw entire vial contents, and add a sufficient volume of diluent to make a total of 100 mL.

  Compatibility: Stable in D_5W, $D_{10}W$, NS
  Do not mix or administer with any other drugs prior to or during administration. Stable for 8 hours at room temperature.
  Storage: Refrigerate ampuls. Protect from freezing. Prepare fresh solutions every 24 hours.

♦ **Epoprostenol Sodium** *see* Epoprostenol *on page 534*

Eprosartan (ep roe SAR tan)

U.S. Brand Names Teveten®

Generic Available No

Pharmacologic Category Angiotensin II Receptor Blocker

Use Treatment of hypertension; may be used alone or in combination with other antihypertensives

Mechanism of Action/Effect Eprosartan is an angiotensin receptor antagonist which blocks the vasoconstriction and aldosterone-secreting effects of angiotensin II.

Contraindications Hypersensitivity to eprosartan or any component of the formulation; sensitivity to other A-II receptor antagonists; bilateral renal artery stenosis; pregnancy (2nd and 3rd trimesters)

Warnings/Precautions Avoid use or use a smaller dose in patients who are volume depleted; correct depletion first. Deterioration in renal function can occur with initiation. Use with caution in unilateral renal artery stenosis and pre-existing renal insufficiency; significant aortic/mitral stenosis. Safety and efficacy in pediatric patients has not established.

Drug Interactions

Cytochrome P450 Effect: Inhibits CYP2C8/9 (weak)

Increased Effect/Toxicity: Eprosartan may increase risk of lithium toxicity. May increase risk of hyperkalemia with potassium-sparing diuretics (eg, amiloride, potassium, spironolactone, triamterene), potassium supplements, or high doses of trimethoprim.

Nutritional/Ethanol Interactions Herb/Nutraceutical: Avoid dong quai if using for hypertension (has estrogenic activity). Avoid ephedra, yohimbe, ginseng (may worsen hypertension). Avoid garlic (may have increased antihypertensive effect).

Adverse Reactions 1% to 10%:

Central nervous system: Fatigue (2%), depression (1%)

Endocrine & metabolic: Hypertriglyceridemia (1%)

Gastrointestinal: Abdominal pain (2%)

Genitourinary: Urinary tract infection (1%)

Respiratory: Upper respiratory tract infection (8%), rhinitis (4%), pharyngitis (4%), cough (4%)

Miscellaneous: Viral infection (2%), injury (2%)

Overdosage/Toxicology The most likely manifestations of overdose would be hypotension and tachycardia. Initiate supportive care for symptomatic hypotension.

Pharmacodynamics/Kinetics

Bioavailability: 300 mg dose: 13%

Time to Peak: Serum: Fasting: 1-2 hours

Protein Binding: 98%

Half-Life Elimination: Terminal: 5-9 hours

Metabolism: Minimally hepatic

Excretion: Feces (90%); urine (7% primarily as unchanged drug)

Clearance: 7.9 L/hour

Dosing

Adults & Elderly: Hypertension: Oral: Dosage must be individualized. Can administer once or twice daily with total daily doses of 400-800 mg. Usual starting dose is 600 mg once daily as monotherapy in patients who are euvolemic. Limited clinical experience with doses >800 mg.

Renal Impairment: No starting dosage adjustment is necessary; however, carefully monitor the patient.

Hepatic Impairment: No starting dosage adjustment is necessary; however, carefully monitor the patient.

Available Dosage Forms Tablet: 400 mg, 600 mg

Monitoring and Teaching Issues

Physical Assessment: See Warnings/Precautions for use cautions (eg, renal impairment). Assess potential for interactions with other pharmacological agents or herbal products patient may be taking (especially anything that may impact blood pressure; see Drug Interactions). Assess results of laboratory tests, therapeutic effectiveness, and adverse response on a regular basis during therapy (eg, hypotension; see Adverse Reactions). Teach patient appropriate use, possible side effects/appropriate interventions, and adverse symptoms to report (see Patient Education).

Monitoring Laboratory Tests: Electrolytes, serum creatinine, BUN, urinalysis

Patient Education: Do not take any new medication during therapy unless approved by prescriber. Take exactly as directed and do not discontinue without consulting prescriber. This drug does not eliminate need for diet or exercise regimen as recommended by prescriber. May cause dizziness, fainting, or lightheadedness (use caution when driving or engaging in tasks that require alertness until response to drug is known); or postural hypotension (use caution when rising from lying or sitting position or climbing stairs). Report chest pain or palpitations; respiratory infection or cold symptoms; unusual cough; swelling of face, tongue, lips, or extremities; changes in urinary pattern; extreme fatigue; or other adverse response. **Pregnancy/breast-feeding precautions:** Inform prescriber if you are or intend to become pregnant. This drug should not be used in the 2nd or 3rd trimester of pregnancy. Consult prescriber for appropriate contraceptive measures if necessary. Breast-feeding is not recommended.

Pregnancy Risk Factor: C (1st trimester); D (2nd and 3rd trimesters)

Pregnancy Issues: Discontinue as soon as possible when pregnancy is detected. Drugs that act directly on renin-angiotensin can cause fetal and neonatal morbidity and death. Adverse effects to the fetus appear to be limited to the 2nd and 3rd trimesters.

Lactation: Not recommended

Related Information

Angiotensin Agents on page 1704

♦ **Eprosartan and HCTZ** see Eprosartan and Hydrochlorothiazide on page 537

Eprosartan and Hydrochlorothiazide
(ep roe SAR tan & hye droe klor oh THYE a zide)

U.S. Brand Names Teveten® HCT

Synonyms Eprosartan and HCTZ; Eprosartan Mesylate and Hydrochlorothiazide; Hydrochlorothiazide and Eprosartan

Generic Available No

Pharmacologic Category Angiotensin II Receptor Blocker Combination; Antihypertensive Agent, Combination; Diuretic, Thiazide

Use Treatment of hypertension (not indicated for initial treatment)

Dosing
  Adults & Elderly: Hypertension: Oral: Dose is individualized (combination substituted for individual components)
    Usual recommended dose: Eprosartan 600 mg/hydrochlorothiazide 12.5 mg once daily (maximum dose: Eprosartan 600 mg/hydrochlorothiazide 25 mg once daily)
  Renal Impairment: Initial dose adjustments not recommended by manufacturer; carefully monitor patient. Hydrochlorothiazide is ineffective in patients with Cl$_{cr}$ <30 mL/minute.
  Hepatic Impairment: Initial dose adjustments not recommended by manufacturer; carefully monitor patient.

Available Dosage Forms
  Tablet:
    600 mg/12.5 mg: Eprosartan 600 mg and hydrochlorothiazide 12.5 mg
    600 mg/25 mg: Eprosartan 600 mg and hydrochlorothiazide 25 mg

Monitoring and Teaching Issues
  Physical Assessment: See individual components.
  Patient Education: See individual agents. **Pregnancy/breast-feeding precautions:** Inform prescriber if you are or intend to become pregnant. Breast-feeding is not recommended.
  Pregnancy Risk Factor: C/D (2nd and 3rd trimesters)
  Lactation: Excretion in breast milk unknown/not recommended

Related Information
  Eprosartan *on page 536*
  Hydrochlorothiazide *on page 751*

♦ **Eprosartan Mesylate and Hydrochlorothiazide** *see* Eprosartan and Hydrochlorothiazide *on page 537*

♦ **Epsom Salts** *see* Magnesium Sulfate *on page 931*

♦ **EPT** *see* Teniposide *on page 1439*

♦ **Eptacog Alfa (Activated)** *see* Factor VIIa (Recombinant) *on page 606*

Eptifibatide (ep TIF i ba tide)

U.S. Brand Names Integrilin®

Synonyms Intrifiban

Generic Available No

Pharmacologic Category Antiplatelet Agent, Glycoprotein IIb/IIIa Inhibitor

Use Treatment of patients with acute coronary syndrome (UA/NQMI), including patients who are to be managed medically and those undergoing percutaneous coronary intervention (PCI including PTCA; intracoronary stenting)

Mechanism of Action/Effect Eptifibatide is a IIb/IIa antagonist that reversibly blocks platelet aggregation and prevents thrombosis.

Contraindications Hypersensitivity to eptifibatide or any component of the product; active abnormal bleeding or a history of bleeding diathesis within the previous 30 days; history of CVA within 30 days or a history of hemorrhagic stroke; severe hypertension (systolic blood pressure >200 mm Hg or diastolic blood pressure >110 mm Hg) not adequately controlled on antihypertensive therapy; major surgery within the preceding 6 weeks; current or planned administration of another parenteral GP IIb/IIIa inhibitor; thrombocytopenia; dependency on renal dialysis

Warnings/Precautions Bleeding is the most common complication. Most major bleeding occurs at the arterial access site where the cardiac catheterization was done. When bleeding can not be controlled with pressure, discontinue infusion and heparin. Use caution in patients with hemorrhagic retinopathy or with other drugs that affect hemostasis. Concurrent use with thrombolytics has not been established as safe. Minimize other procedures including arterial and venous punctures, I.M. injections, nasogastric tubes, etc. Prior to sheath removal, the aPTT or ACT should be checked (do not remove unless aPTT is <45 seconds or the ACT <150 seconds).

Drug Interactions
  Increased Effect/Toxicity: Eptifibatide effect may be increased by other drugs which affect hemostasis include thrombolytics, oral anticoagulants, NSAIDs, dipyridamole, heparin, low molecular weight heparins, ticlopidine, and clopidogrel. Avoid concomitant use of other IIb/IIIa inhibitors. Cephalosporins which contain the MTT side chain may theoretically increase the risk of hemorrhage. Use with aspirin and heparin may increase bleeding over aspirin and heparin alone. However, aspirin and heparin were used concurrently in the majority of patients in the major clinical studies of eptifibatide.

Adverse Reactions Bleeding is the major drug-related adverse effect. Major bleeding was reported in 4.4% to 10.8%; minor bleeding was reported in 10.5% to 14.2%; requirement for transfusion was reported in 5.5% to 12.8%. Incidence of bleeding is also related to heparin intensity (aPTT goal 50-70 seconds). Patients weighing <70 kg may have an increased risk of major bleeding.

Cardiovascular: Hypotension
Local: Injection site reaction
Neuromuscular & skeletal: Back pain

1% to 10%: Hematologic: Thrombocytopenia (1.2% to 3.2%)
(Continued)

Eptifibatide *(Continued)*

Overdosage/Toxicology Two cases of human overdose have been reported; neither case was eventful or associated with major bleeding. Symptoms of overdose in animal studies include loss of righting reflex, dyspnea, ptosis, decreased muscle tone, and petechial hemorrhage. Treatment is supportive.

Pharmacodynamics/Kinetics

Onset of Action: Within 1 hour

Duration of Action: Platelet function restored ~4 hours following discontinuation

Protein Binding: ~25%

Half-Life Elimination: 2.5 hours

Excretion: Primarily urine (as eptifibatide and metabolites); significant renal impairment may alter disposition of this compound

Clearance: Total body: 55-58 mL/kg/hour; Renal: ~50% of total in healthy subjects

Dosing

Adults & Elderly:

Acute coronary syndrome: I.V.: Bolus of 180 mcg/kg (maximum: 22.6 mg) over 1-2 minutes, begun as soon as possible following diagnosis, followed by a continuous infusion of 2 mcg/kg/minute (maximum: 15 mg/hour) until hospital discharge or initiation of CABG surgery, up to 72 hours. Concurrent aspirin (160-325 mg initially and daily thereafter) and heparin therapy (target aPTT 50-70 seconds) are recommended.

Percutaneous coronary intervention (PCI) with or without stenting: I.V.: Bolus of 180 mcg/kg (maximum: 22.6 mg) administered immediately before the initiation of PCI, followed by a continuous infusion of 2 mcg/kg/minute (maximum: 15 mg/hour). A second 180 mcg/kg bolus (maximum: 22.6 mg) should be administered 10 minutes after the first bolus. Infusion should be continued until hospital discharge or for up to 18-24 hours, whichever comes first. Concurrent aspirin (160-325 mg 1-24 hours before PCI and daily thereafter) and heparin therapy (ACT 200-300 seconds during PCI) are recommended. Heparin infusion after PCI is discouraged. In patients who undergo coronary artery bypass graft surgery, discontinue infusion prior to surgery.

Renal Impairment: Dialysis is a contraindication to use.

Acute coronary syndrome: I.V.: Cl_{cr} <50 mL/minute or S_{cr} >2 mg/dL: Use 180 mcg/kg bolus (maximum: 22.6 mg) and 1 mcg/kg/minute infusion (maximum: 7.5 mg/hour)

Percutaneous coronary intervention (PCI) with or without stenting: I.V.: Cl_{cr} <50 mL/minute or S_{cr} >2 mg/dL: Use 180 mcg/kg bolus (maximum: 22.6 mg) administered immediately before the initiation of PCI and followed by a continuous infusion of 1 mcg/kg/minute (maximum: 7.5 mg/hour). A second 180 mcg/kg (maximum: 22.6 mg) bolus should be administered 10 minutes after the first bolus.

Available Dosage Forms Injection, solution: 0.75 mg/mL (100 mL); 2 mg/mL (10 mL, 100 mL)

Monitoring and Teaching Issues

Physical Assessment: Assess other medications for possible interactions or additive effects. Monitor vital signs and laboratory results prior to, during, and after therapy. Monitor closely for signs of excessive/unusual bleeding. Observe and teach patient bleeding precautions and adverse reactions to report.

Monitoring Laboratory Tests: Laboratory tests at baseline and monitoring during therapy: hematocrit and hemoglobin, platelet count, serum creatinine, PT/aPTT (maintain aPTT between 50-70 seconds unless PCI is to be performed), and ACT with PCI (maintain ACT between 200-300 seconds during PCI). Prior to sheath removal, the aPTT or ACT should be checked (do not remove unless aPTT is <45 seconds or the ACT <150 seconds).

Patient Education: Emergency use may dictate depth of patient education. This medication can only be administered I.V. You will have a tendency to bleed easily following this medication. Use caution to prevent injury (use electric razor, use soft toothbrush, use caution with sharps). If bleeding occurs, apply pressure to bleeding spot until bleeding stops completely. Report unusual bruising or bleeding (eg, blood in urine, stool, or vomitus, bleeding gums), dizziness or vision changes, or back pain. **Breast-feeding precaution:** Breast-feeding is not recommended.

Pregnancy Risk Factor: B

Lactation: Excretion in breast milk unknown/not recommended

Administration

I.V.: Do not shake vial. Administer bolus doses by I.V. push over 1-2 minutes. Begin continuous infusion immediately following bolus administration; administer directly from the 100 mL vial.

Compatibility: Stable in NS (infusion may contain up to 60 mEq/L KCl), NS/D_5W (infusion may contain up to 60 mEq/L KCl)

Storage: Vials should be stored refrigerated at 2°C to 8°C (36°F to 46°F). Vials can be kept at room temperature for 2 months. Protect from light until administration. Do not use beyond the expiration date. Discard any unused portion left in the vial.

- ◆ **Epzicom™** *see Abacavir and Lamivudine on page 33*
- ◆ **Equagesic®** *see Aspirin and Meprobamate on page 147*
- ◆ **Equanil** *see Meprobamate on page 952*
- ◆ **Equetro™** *see Carbamazepine on page 249*
- ◆ **Erbitux™** *see Cetuximab on page 299*

Ergocalciferol *(er goe kal SIF e role)*

U.S. Brand Names Calciferol™; Drisdol®

Synonyms Activated Ergosterol; Viosterol; Vitamin D_2

Generic Available Yes: Capsule

Pharmacologic Category Vitamin D Analog

Medication Safety Issues
Sound-alike/look-alike issues:
Calciferol™ may be confused with calcitriol
Drisdol® may be confused with Drysol™

Use Treatment of refractory rickets, hypophosphatemia, hypoparathyroidism; dietary supplement

Mechanism of Action/Effect Stimulates calcium and phosphate absorption from the small intestine, promotes secretion of calcium from bone to blood; promotes renal tubule phosphate resorption

Contraindications Hypersensitivity to ergocalciferol or any component of the formulation; hypercalcemia; malabsorption syndrome; evidence of vitamin D toxicity

Warnings/Precautions Administer with extreme caution in patients with impaired renal function, heart disease, renal stones, or arteriosclerosis. Must give concomitant calcium supplementation. Maintain adequate fluid intake. Avoid hypercalcemia. Renal function impairment with secondary hyperparathyroidism. Use as a dietary supplement is recommended for all breast-fed or nonbreast-fed infants receiving <500 mL/day of vitamin D-fortified formula, and in adults and children receiving <500 mL/day of vitamin D-fortified milk and who do not get regular sun exposure.

Drug Interactions
Decreased Effect: Cholestyramine, colestipol, mineral oil may decrease oral absorption.
Increased Effect/Toxicity: Thiazide diuretics may increase vitamin D effects. Cardiac glycosides may increase toxicity.

Adverse Reactions Generally well tolerated
Frequency not defined: Cardiac arrhythmia, hypertension (late), irritability, headache, psychosis (rare), somnolence, hyperthermia (late), pruritus, decreased libido (late), hypercholesterolemia, mild acidosis (late), polydipsia (late), nausea, vomiting, anorexia, pancreatitis, metallic taste, weight loss (rare), xerostomia, constipation, polyuria (late), increased BUN (late), increased LFTs (late), bone pain, myalgia, weakness, conjunctivitis, photophobia (late), vascular/nephrocalcinosis (rare)

Overdosage/Toxicology Symptoms of chronic overdose include hypercalcemia, weakness, fatigue, lethargy, and anorexia. Following withdrawal of the drug and oral decontamination, treatment consists of bedrest, liberal intake of fluids, reduced calcium intake, and cathartic administration. Severe hypercalcemia requires I.V. hydration and forced diuresis with I.V. furosemide. Urine output should be monitored and maintained at >3 mL/kg/hour during the acute treatment phase. I.V. saline can quickly and significantly increase excretion of calcium into urine. Calcitonin, mithramycin, and bisphosphonates have all been used successfully to treat the more resistant cases of vitamin D-induced hypercalcemia.

Pharmacodynamics/Kinetics
Onset of Action: Peak effect: ~1 month following daily doses
Absorption: Readily; requires bile
Metabolism: Inactive until hydroxylated hepatically and renally to calcifediol and then to calcitriol (most active form)

Dosing
Adults: Oral dosing is preferred; I.M. therapy is required with GI, liver, or biliary disease associated with malabsorption.

Dietary supplement (each 1 mcg = 40 int. units): Oral:
18-50 years: 5 mcg/day (200 int. units/day)
51-70 years: 10 mcg/day (400 int. units/day)
Familial phosphatemia: 10,000-80,000 int. units/day and phosphorus 1-2 g/day
Renal failure: Oral: 500 mcg/day (20,000 int. units)
Hypoparathyroidism: Oral: 625 mcg to 5 mg/day (25,000-200,000 int. units) and calcium supplements
Vitamin D-dependent rickets: Oral: 250 mcg to 1.5 mg/day (10,000-60,000 int. units)
Nutritional rickets and osteomalacia: Oral:
With normal absorption: 25-125 mcg/day (1000-5000 int. units)
With malabsorption: 250-7500 mcg/day (10,000-300,000 int. units)
Vitamin D-resistant rickets: Oral: 250-1500 mcg/day (10,000-60,000 int. units) with phosphate supplements

Elderly: Refer to adult dosing (see Geriatric Considerations and Additional Information).
Dietary supplement (each 1 mcg = 40 int. units): >70 years: Oral: 15 mcg/day (600 int. units/day)

Pediatrics: Oral dosing is preferred; I.M. therapy is required with GI, liver, or biliary disease associated with malabsorption.
Dietary supplement (each mcg = 40 int. units): Infants and Children: 5 mcg/day (200 int. units/day)
Renal failure: Children: 100-1000 mcg/day (4000-40,000 int. units)
Hypoparathyroidism: Children: 1.25-5 mg/day (50,000-200,000 int. units) and calcium supplements
Vitamin D-dependent rickets: Children: 75-125 mcg/day (3000-5000 int. units); maximum: 1500 mcg/day
Nutritional rickets and osteomalacia:
Children with normal absorption: 25-125 mcg/day (1000-5000 int. units)
Children with malabsorption: 250-625 mcg/day (10,000-25,000 int. units)
Vitamin D-resistant rickets: Children: Initial: 1000-2000 mcg/day (40,000-80,000 int. units) with phosphate supplements; daily dosage is increased at 3- to 4-month intervals in 250-500 mcg (10,000-20,000 int. units) increments
Familial hypophosphatemia: 10,000-80,000 units daily plus 1-2 g/day elemental phosphorus

Available Dosage Forms [DSC] = Discontinued product
Capsule (Drisdol®): 50,000 int. units [1.25 mg; contains tartrazine and soybean oil]
Injection, solution (Calciferol™): 500,000 int. units/mL [12.5 mg/mL] (1 mL) [contains sesame oil] [DSC]
Liquid, drops (Calciferol™, Drisdol®): 8000 int. units/mL [200 mcg/mL] (60 mL) [OTC]
(Continued)

Ergocalciferol (Continued)

Monitoring and Teaching Issues

Physical Assessment: Assess effectiveness and interactions of other medications patient may be taking. Assess results of laboratory tests, therapeutic effectiveness, and adverse effects at beginning of therapy and regularly with long-term use. Teach patient proper use if self-administered (appropriate injection technique and syringe/needle disposal), appropriate nutritional counseling, possible side effects/interventions, and adverse symptoms to report.

Monitoring Laboratory Tests: Serum calcium, BUN, phosphorus every 1-2 weeks

Patient Education: Take exact dose prescribed; do not take more than recommended. Your prescriber may recommend a special diet; do not increase calcium intake without consulting prescriber. Avoid magnesium supplements or magnesium-containing antacids. You may experience nausea, vomiting, or metallic taste (small frequent meals, frequent mouth care, or sucking hard candy may help). Report chest pain or palpitations; acute headache, dizziness, or feeling of weakness; unresolved nausea or vomiting; persistent metallic taste; unrelieved muscle or bone pain; or CNS irritability. **Pregnancy precaution:** Inform prescriber if you are pregnant.

Geriatric Considerations: Recommended daily allowances (RDA) have not been developed for persons >65 years of age. Vitamin D, folate, and B_{12} (cyanocobalamin) have decreased absorption with age, but the clinical significance is yet unknown. Calorie requirements decrease with age and therefore, nutrient density must be increased to ensure adequate nutrient intake, including vitamins and minerals. Therefore, the use of a daily supplement with a multiple vitamin with minerals is recommended. Elderly consume less vitamin D, absorption may be decreased and many elderly have decreased sun exposure; therefore, elderly >70 years of age should receive supplementation with 600 units (15 mcg)/day. This is a recommendation of particular need to those with high risk for osteoporosis.

Pregnancy Risk Factor: A/C (dose exceeding RDA recommendation)

Lactation: Enters breast milk/compatible

Administration

I.M.: Parenteral injection is for I.M. use only.

Storage: Protect from light.

Additional Information Ergocalciferol 1.25 mg provides 50,000 int. units of vitamin D activity.

Erlotinib (er LOE tye nib)

U.S. Brand Names Tarceva™

Synonyms CP358774; Erlotinib Hydrochloride; NSC-718781; OSI-774; R 14-15

Generic Available No

Pharmacologic Category Antineoplastic Agent, Tyrosine Kinase Inhibitor; Epidermal Growth Factor Receptor (EGFR) Inhibitor

Use Salvage therapy of advanced or metastatic nonsmall-cell lung cancer

Unlabeled/Investigational Use Salvage therapy of advanced or metastatic breast, colorectal, and head and neck tumors

Mechanism of Action/Effect Inhibits the intracellular phosphorylation of tyrosine kinase associated with epidermal growth factor receptor (EGFR) which is located on both normal and cancer cells causing cell death.

Contraindications Hypersensitivity to erlotinib or any component of the formulation; pregnancy

Warnings/Precautions Rare, sometimes fatal, pulmonary toxicity (interstitial pneumonia, interstitial lung disease, obliterative bronchiolitis, pulmonary fibrosis) has occurred; an interruption of therapy should occur with unexplained pulmonary symptoms (dyspnea, cough, and fever); use caution in hepatic or severe renal impairment. Safety and efficacy in pediatric patients have not been established.

Drug Interactions

Cytochrome P450 Effect: Substrate of CYP1A2 (minor), 3A4 (major)

Decreased Effect: Rifamycins and CYP3A4 inducers may decrease erlotinib levels/effects; example inducers include aminoglutethimide, carbamazepine, nafcillin, nevirapine, phenobarbital, and phenytoin.

Increased Effect/Toxicity: Ketoconazole and CYP3A4 inhibitors may increase erlotinib levels/effects; example inhibitors include azole antifungals, ciprofloxacin, clarithromycin, diclofenac, doxycycline, erythromycin, imatinib, isoniazid, nefazodone, nicardipine, propofol, protease inhibitors, quinidine, and verapamil.

Nutritional/Ethanol Interactions

Herb/Nutraceutical: Avoid St John's wort (may increase metabolism and decrease erlotinib concentrations).

Adverse Reactions

>10%:

Central nervous system: Fatigue (14% to 55%), anxiety (21%), headache (17%), depression (16%), insomnia (12%)

Dermatologic: Acneiform rash (50% to 88%), pruritus (13% to 55%), dry skin (12% to 35%), erythema (18%)

Gastrointestinal: Diarrhea (30% to 56%), anorexia (23% to 52%), nausea (11% to 33%), vomiting (23%), mucositis (17% to 18%), glossodynia (18%), xerostomia (17%), pain (14%), constipation (12%), dyspepsia (12%), dysphagia (12%), weight loss (12%), abnormal taste (11%), abdominal pain (11%)

Hepatic: Hyperbilirubinemia (20%)

Neuromuscular & Skeletal: Arthralgia (14%), paresthesia (11%)

Ocular: Conjunctivitis (12%), keratoconjunctivitis sicca (12%)

Respiratory: Dyspnea (21% to 41%), cough (16% to 33%)

Miscellaneous: Infection (24%)

1% to 10%:
  Hepatic: Liver function test abnormalities (4%)
  Ocular: Keratitis (6%)
  Respiratory: Pneumonitis (6%)

Overdosage/Toxicology Specific overdose-related toxicities include diarrhea, rash, and liver transaminase elevation. Overdose management should include withdrawal of erlotinib, and symptom-based and supportive treatment.

Pharmacodynamics/Kinetics
  Absorption: Oral: 60% on an empty stomach; ~100% on a full stomach
  Bioavailability: 100% when given with food
  Time to Peak: Plasma: 1-7 hours
  Protein Binding: 92% to 95%, albumin and α_1-acid glycoprotein
  Half-Life Elimination: 24-36 hours
  Metabolism: Hepatic, CYP3A4 (major), CYP1A1 (minor), CYP1A2 (minor), and CYP1C (minor)
  Excretion: Primarily as metabolites: Feces (83%); urine (8%)

Dosing
  Adults: Locally advanced or metastatic nonsmall cell lung cancer: Oral: 150 mg/day until disease progression or unacceptable toxicity occurs; dose reduction (if required) should be done in increments of 50 mg
    Note: Dose reductions are more likely to be needed when erlotinib is administered concomitantly with strong CYP3A4 inhibitors. Likewise, the CYP3A4 inducers may require increased doses; doses of >150 mg/day should be considered with rifampin. (Note: See drug interaction information for examples of CYP3A4 inhibitors and inducers).
    Dosage adjustment for toxicity: Patients experiencing poorly-tolerated diarrhea or a severe skin reaction may benefit from a brief therapy interruption. Patients experiencing acute onset (or worsening) of pulmonary symptoms should have therapy interrupted and be evaluated for drug-induced interstitial lung disease.
  Elderly: See adult dosing.
  Hepatic Impairment: Dose reduction or interruption should be considered if liver function changes are severe.

Available Dosage Forms Tablet: 25 mg, 100 mg, 150 mg

Monitoring and Teaching Issues
  Physical Assessment: Assess potential for interactions with other prescriptions, OTCs, or biologicals patient is taking; especially CYP3A4 inhibitors or inducers (see Drug Interactions). Assess laboratory test results (LFTs), patient response, and adverse reactions (see Adverse Reactions). Teach patient/caregiver possible side effects, appropriate interventions, and adverse symptoms to report (see Patient Education).
  Monitoring Laboratory Tests: Periodic liver function tests (asymptomatic increases in liver enzymes have occurred)
  Patient Education: Take exactly as directed; 1 hour before or 2 hours after food. Maintain adequate nutrition and fluid intake (small frequent meals may help). May cause fatigue (adequate rest periods may help); rash or dry skin (use nonirritating skin lotion that does not contain alcohol or other irritants); nausea or anorexia (small frequent meals, good mouth care, or sucking lozenges may help), or diarrhea (boiled milk, yogurt). Report persistent gastrointestinal changes (including abdominal pain, diarrhea, nausea); conjunctivitis or visual changes; difficulty breathing or unusual cough; signs of infection or other persistent adverse effects. **Pregnancy/breast-feeding precautions:** Inform prescriber if you are pregnant. Do not get pregnant while taking this medication or for two weeks after discontinuing. This drug may cause fetal deformities or loss of pregnancy; see prescriber for appropriate contraceptives. Consult prescriber if breast-feeding.
  Geriatric Considerations: In clinical trials, there was no significant difference between older and younger adults in survival benefit, safety, or pharmacokinetics. No dosage adjustment necessary in elderly patients.
  Pregnancy Risk Factor: D
  Lactation: Excretion in breast milk unknown/not recommended

Administration
  Oral: The manufacturer recommends administration on an empty stomach (at least 1 hour before or 2 hours after the ingestion of food) even though this reduces drug absorption by approximately 40%. Administration after a meal results in nearly 100% absorption.
  Storage: Store at room temperature between 15°C and 30°C (59°F and 86°F).

♦ Erlotinib Hydrochloride *see* Erlotinib *on page 540*
♦ Errin™ *see* Norethindrone *on page 1096*
♦ Ertaczo™ *see* Sertaconazole *on page 1367*

Ertapenem (er ta PEN em)

U.S. Brand Names Invanz®
Synonyms Ertapenem Sodium; L-749,345; MK0826
Generic Available No
Pharmacologic Category Antibiotic, Carbapenem
Medication Safety Issues
  Sound-alike/look-alike issues:
    Invanz® may be confused with Avinza™

Use Treatment of moderate-severe, complicated intra-abdominal infections, skin and skin structure infections, pyelonephritis, acute pelvic infections, and community-acquired pneumonia. Antibacterial coverage includes aerobic gram-positive organisms, aerobic gram-negative organisms, anaerobic organisms.

  Note: Methicillin-resistant *Staphylococcus*, *Enterococcus* spp, penicillin-resistant strains of *Streptococcus pneumoniae*, beta-lactamase-positive strains of *Haemophilus influenzae* are **resistant** to ertapenem, as are most *Pseudomonas aeruginosa*.
  (Continued)

Ertapenem *(Continued)*

Mechanism of Action/Effect Inhibits cell wall biosynthesis; cell wall assembly is arrested and the bacteria eventually lyse.

Contraindications Hypersensitivity to ertapenem, other carbapenems, or any other component of the formulation; anaphylactic reactions to beta-lactam antibiotics. If using intramuscularly, known hypersensitivity to local anesthetics of the amide type (lidocaine is the diluent).

Warnings/Precautions Dosage adjustment required with impaired renal function; prolonged use may result in superinfection; use with caution in patients with CNS disorder (eg, brain lesions, history of seizures), compromised renal function, hypersensitivity to beta-lactams, the elderly; safety and efficacy in patients <18 years of age have not been established.

Drug Interactions
Decreased Effect: Ertapenem may decrease valproic acid serum concentrations to subtherapeutic levels; monitor.

Adverse Reactions
1% to 10%:
Cardiovascular: Swelling/edema (3%), chest pain (1%), hypertension (0.7% to 2%), hypotension (1% to 2%), tachycardia (1% to 2%)
Central nervous system: Headache (6% to 7%), altered mental status (ie, agitation, confusion, disorientation, decreased mental acuity, changed mental status, somnolence, stupor) (3% to 5%), fever (2% to 5%), insomnia (3%), dizziness (2%), fatigue (1%), anxiety (0.8% to 1%)
Dermatologic: Rash (2% to 3%), pruritus (1% to 2%), erythema (1% to 2%)
Gastrointestinal: Diarrhea (9% to 10%), nausea (6% to 9%), abdominal pain (4%), vomiting (4%), constipation (3% to 4%), acid regurgitation (1% to 2%), dyspepsia (1%), oral candidiasis (0.1% to 1%)
Genitourinary: Vaginitis (1% to 3%)
Hematologic: Platelet count increased (4% to 7%), eosinophils increased (1% to 2%)
Hepatic: Hepatic enzyme elevations (7% to 9%), alkaline phosphatase increase (4% to 7%)
Local: Infused vein complications (5% to 7%), phlebitis/thrombophlebitis (1.5% to 2%), extravasation (0.7% to 2%)
Neuromuscular & skeletal: Leg pain (0.4% to 1%)
Respiratory: Dyspnea (1% to 3%), cough (1% to 2%), pharyngitis (0.7% to 1%), rales/rhonchi (0.5% to 1%), respiratory distress (0.2% to 1%)

Overdosage/Toxicology Treatment is symptom-directed and supportive. Removed by hemodialysis.

Pharmacodynamics/Kinetics
Absorption: I.M.: Almost complete
Bioavailability: I.M.: 90%
Time to Peak: I.M.: 2.3 hours
Protein Binding: Concentration dependent: 85% at 300 mcg/mL, 95% at <100 mcg/mL
Half-Life Elimination: 4 hours
Metabolism: Hydrolysis to inactive metabolite
Excretion: Urine (80% as unchanged drug and metabolite); feces (10%)

Dosing
Adults & Elderly: Note: I.V. therapy may be administered for up to 14 days; I.M. for up to 7 days
Intra-abdominal infection: I.M., I.V.: 1 g/day for 5-14 days
Skin and skin structure infections: I.M., I.V.: 1 g/day for 7-14 days
Community-acquired pneumonia: I.M., I.V.: 1 g/day; duration of total antibiotic treatment: 10-14 days
Urinary tract infections/pyelonephritis: I.M., I.V.: 1 g/day; duration of total antibiotic treatment: 10-14 days
Acute pelvic infections: I.M., I.V.: 1 g/day for 3-10 days
Pediatrics: Safety and efficacy have not been established for pediatric patients.
Renal Impairment: Cl_{cr} <30 mL/minute: 500 mg/day
Hemodialysis: When the daily dose is given within 6 hours prior to hemodialysis, a supplementary dose of 150 mg is required following hemodialysis.
Hepatic Impairment: Adjustments cannot be recommended (lack of experience and research in this patient population).

Available Dosage Forms Injection, powder for reconstitution: 1 g [contains sodium 137 mg/g]

Monitoring and Teaching Issues
Physical Assessment: Assess results of culture and sensitivity tests and patient history of previous allergies or adverse drug reactions. See Contraindications and Warnings/Precautions for use cautions (eg, impaired renal function; CNS disorder, compromised renal function). See Administration for specific infusion/injection directions. Monitor closely for adverse reactions, especially CNS adverse effects (history of seizures, head injuries, or other CNS events increases risk; see Adverse Reactions). Teach patient appropriate use, interventions to reduce side effects, and adverse symptoms to report (see Patient Education).

Patient Education: This medication can only be administered intravenously or by intramuscular injections; report redness, warmth, swelling, irritation at infusion/injection site; sudden difficulty breathing or swallowing, chest pain, or chills. Maintain adequate hydration (2-3 L/day of fluids) unless instructed to restrict fluid intake and nutrition. Report unresolved nausea or vomiting (small frequent meals, frequent mouth care, and sucking hard candy may help). Report immediately any CNS changes (eg, dizziness, disorientation, visual disturbances, headaches, confusion, or seizures). Report prolonged GI effects, diarrhea, vomiting, abdominal pain; change in respirations or respiratory difficulty; chest pain or palpitations; skin rash; foul-smelling vaginal discharge; or white plaques in mouth. **Breast-feeding precaution:** Consult prescriber if breast-feeding.

Dietary Considerations: Sodium content: 137 mg (~6 mEq) per gram of ertapenem
Pregnancy Risk Factor: B
Lactation: Enters breast milk/use caution
Breast-Feeding Issues: The concentration in human breast milk within 24 hours of last dose (1 g I.V. for 3-10 days) ranged from <0.13 mcg/mL (lower limit of quantitation) to 0.38 mcg/mL. Five days after discontinuation of therapy, the ertapenem level was undetectable in 80% (4 of 5 women) and below the lower limit of quantitation in 20% (1 of 5 women).

Administration

I.M.: Avoid injection into a blood vessel. Make sure patient does not have an allergy to lidocaine or another anesthetic of the amide type. Administer by deep I.M. injection into a large muscle mass (eg, gluteal muscle or lateral part of the thigh). Do not administer I.M. preparation or drug reconstituted for I.M. administration intravenously.

I.V.: Infuse over 30 minutes

Reconstitution:

I.M.: Reconstitute 1 g vial with 3.2 mL of 1% lidocaine HCl injection (without epinephrine). Shake well. Use within 1 hour after preparation.

I.V.: Reconstitute 1 g vial with 10 mL of water for injection, 0.9% sodium chloride injection, or bacteriostatic water for injection. Shake well. Transfer to 50 mL of 0.9% sodium chloride injection.

Compatibility: Do not mix with other medications or use diluents containing dextrose.

Storage: Before reconstitution store at ≤25°C (77°F). Reconstituted I.V. solution may be stored at room temperature and used within 6 hours **or** refrigerated, stored for up to 24 hours and used within 4 hours after removal from refrigerator. Do not freeze.

Related Information

Antimicrobial Drugs of Choice *on page 1792*
Community-Acquired Pneumonia in Adults *on page 1807*

♦ **Ertapenem Sodium** *see* Ertapenem *on page 541*
♦ *Erwinia* **Asparaginase** *see* Asparaginase *on page 141*
♦ **Eryc**® *see* Erythromycin *on page 543*
♦ **Eryderm**® *see* Erythromycin *on page 543*
♦ **Erygel**® *see* Erythromycin *on page 543*
♦ **EryPed**® *see* Erythromycin *on page 543*
♦ **Ery-Tab**® *see* Erythromycin *on page 543*
♦ **Erythrocin**® *see* Erythromycin *on page 543*

Erythromycin (er ith roe MYE sin)

U.S. Brand Names Akne-Mycin®; A/T/S®; E.E.S.®; Eryc®; Eryderm®; Erygel®; EryPed®; Ery-Tab®; Erythrocin®; PCE®; Romycin®; Staticin® [DSC]; Theramycin Z®; T-Stat® [DSC]

Synonyms Erythromycin Base; Erythromycin Estolate; Erythromycin Ethylsuccinate; Erythromycin Gluceptate; Erythromycin Lactobionate; Erythromycin Stearate

Generic Available Yes

Pharmacologic Category Antibiotic, Macrolide; Antibiotic, Ophthalmic; Antibiotic, Topical; Topical Skin Product; Topical Skin Product, Acne

Medication Safety Issues

Sound-alike/look-alike issues:

Erythromycin may be confused with azithromycin, clarithromycin, Ethmozine®
Akne-Mycin® may be confused with AK-Mycin®
E.E.S.® may be confused with DES
Eryc® may be confused with Emcyt®, Ery-Tab®
Ery-Tab® may be confused with Eryc®
Erythrocin® may be confused with Ethmozine®

Use

Systemic: Treatment of susceptible bacterial infections including *S. pyogenes*, some *S. pneumoniae*, some *S. aureus*, *M. pneumoniae*, *Legionella pneumophila*, diphtheria, pertussis, chancroid, *Chlamydia*, erythrasma, *N. gonorrhoeae*, *E. histolytica*, syphilis and nongonococcal urethritis, and *Campylobacter* gastroenteritis; used in conjunction with neomycin for decontaminating the bowel

Ophthalmic: Treatment of superficial eye infections involving the conjunctiva or cornea; neonatal ophthalmia

Topical: Treatment of acne vulgaris

Unlabeled/Investigational Use Systemic: Treatment of gastroparesis

Mechanism of Action/Effect Inhibits RNA-dependent protein synthesis

Contraindications Hypersensitivity to erythromycin or any component of the formulation

Systemic: Pre-existing liver disease (erythromycin estolate); concomitant use with ergot derivatives, pimozide, or cisapride

Warnings/Precautions Systemic: Use caution with hepatic impairment with or without jaundice has occurred, it may be accompanied by malaise, nausea, vomiting, abdominal colic, and fever; discontinue use if these occur; avoid using erythromycin lactobionate in neonates since formulations may contain benzyl alcohol which is associated with toxicity in neonates; observe for superinfections. Use in infants has been associated with infantile hypertrophic pyloric stenosis (IHPS). Macrolides have been associated with rare QT prolongation and ventricular arrhythmias, including torsade de pointes.

Drug Interactions

Cytochrome P450 Effect: Substrate of CYP2B6 (minor), 3A4 (major); **Inhibits** CYP1A2 (weak), 3A4 (moderate)

Decreased Effect: Erythromycin may decrease the serum concentrations of zafirlukast. Erythromycin may antagonize the therapeutic effects of clindamycin and lincomycin. The levels/effects of erythromycin may be decreased by aminoglutethimide, carbamazepine, nafcillin, nevirapine, phenobarbital, phenytoin, rifamycins, and other CYP3A4 inducers.

Increased Effect/Toxicity: Avoid concomitant use of the following with erythromycin due to increased risk of malignant arrhythmias: Cisapride, gatifloxacin, moxifloxacin, pimozide, sparfloxacin, thioridazine. Other agents that prolong the QT_c interval, including type Ia (eg, (Continued)

Erythromycin *(Continued)*

quinidine) and type III antiarrhythmic agents, and selected antipsychotic agents (eg, mesoridazine, thioridazine) should be used with extreme caution. Concurrent use of ergot alkaloids with erythromycin is also contraindicated.

Erythromycin is a moderate CYP3A4 inhibitor, and may increase the levels/effects of selected benzodiazepines, calcium channel blockers, cyclosporine, mirtazapine, nateglinide, nefazodone, quinidine, sildenafil (and other PDE-5 inhibitors), tacrolimus, venlafaxine, and other CYP3A4 substrates. Selected benzodiazepines (midazolam, triazolam), cisapride, ergot alkaloids, selected HMG-CoA reductase inhibitors (lovastatin and simvastatin), and pimozide are generally contraindicated with strong CYP3A4 inhibitors. When used with strong CYP3A4 inhibitors, dosage adjustment/limits are recommended for sildenafil and other PDE-5 inhibitors; refer to individual monographs. The effects of neuromuscular-blocking agents and warfarin have been potentiated by erythromycin.

The levels/effects of erythromycin may be increased by azole antifungals, ciprofloxacin, clarithromycin, diclofenac, doxycycline, imatinib, isoniazid, nefazodone, nicardipine, propofol, protease inhibitors, quinidine, telithromycin, verapamil, and other CYP3A4 inhibitors.

Nutritional/Ethanol Interactions
Ethanol: Avoid ethanol (may decrease absorption of erythromycin or enhance ethanol effects).

Food: Increased drug absorption with meals; erythromycin serum levels may be altered if taken with food.

Herb/Nutraceutical: St John's wort may decrease erythromycin levels.

Lab Interactions False-positive urinary catecholamines

Adverse Reactions
Systemic:
Cardiovascular: Ventricular arrhythmia, QT_c prolongation, torsade de pointes (rare), ventricular tachycardia (rare)

Central nervous system: Headache (8%), pain (2%), fever, seizure

Dermatitis: Rash (3%), pruritus (1%)

Gastrointestinal: Abdominal pain (8%), cramping, nausea (8%), oral candidiasis, vomiting (3%), diarrhea (7%), dyspepsia (2%), flatulence (2%), anorexia, pseudomembranous colitis, hypertrophic pyloric stenosis (including cases in infants or IHPS), pancreatitis

Hematologic: Eosinophilia (1%)

Hepatic: Cholestatic jaundice (most common with estolate), increased liver function tests (2%)

Local: Phlebitis at the injection site, thrombophlebitis

Neuromuscular & skeletal: Weakness (2%)

Respiratory: Dyspnea (1%), cough (3%)

Miscellaneous: Hypersensitivity reactions, allergic reactions

Topical: 1% to 10%: Dermatologic: Erythema, desquamation, dryness, pruritus

Overdosage/Toxicology Symptoms of overdose include nausea, vomiting, diarrhea, prostration, reversible pancreatitis, hearing loss with or without tinnitus or vertigo. Care is general and supportive only.

Pharmacodynamics/Kinetics
Absorption: Oral: Variable but better with salt forms than with base form; 18% to 45%; ethylsuccinate may be better absorbed with food

Time to Peak: Serum: Base: 4 hours; Ethylsuccinate: 0.5-2.5 hours; delayed with food due to differences in absorption

Protein Binding: 75% to 90%

Half-Life Elimination: Peak: 1.5-2 hours; End-stage renal disease: 5-6 hours

Metabolism: Hepatic via demethylation

Excretion: Primarily feces; urine (2% to 15% as unchanged drug)

Dosing
Adults & Elderly:
Susceptible infections (usual dose):
Oral: (Note: Due to differences in absorption, 400 mg erythromycin ethylsuccinate produces the same serum levels as 250 mg erythromycin base, sterate or estolate)
Base: 30-50 mg/kg/day in 2-4 divided doses; do not exceed 2 g/day
Estolate: 30-50 mg/kg/day in 2-4 divided doses; do not exceed 2 g/day
Ethylsuccinate: 30-50 mg/kg/day in 2-4 divided doses; do not exceed 3.2 g/day
Stearate: 30-50 mg/kg/day in 2-4 divided doses; do not exceed 2 g/day
I.V.: Lactobionate: 15-20 mg/kg/day divided every 6 hours or 500 mg to 1 g every 6 hours, or given as a continuous infusion over 24 hours (maximum: 4 g/24 hours)

Ophthalmic infection: Ophthalmic: Instill ½" (1.25 cm) 2-6 times/day depending on the severity of the infection

Dermatologic infection: Topical: Apply over the affected area twice daily after the skin has been thoroughly washed and patted dry

Preop bowel preparation: 1 g erythromycin base at 1, 2, and 11 PM on the day before surgery combined with mechanical cleansing of the large intestine and oral neomycin

Gastrointestinal prokinetic (unlabeled use): I.V., Oral: Erythromycin has been used as a prokinetic agent to improve gastric emptying time and intestinal motility. In adults, 200 mg was infused I.V. initially followed by 250 mg orally 3 times/day 30 minutes before meals. Lower dosages have been used in some trials.

Pediatrics:
Prophylaxis of neonatal gonococcal or chlamydial conjunctivitis: Neonates: Ophthalmic: 0.5-1 cm ribbon of ointment should be instilled into each conjunctival sac

Susceptible infections (systemic): Infants and Children:
Oral: **Note:** Due to differences in absorption, 400 mg erythromycin ethylsuccinate produces the same serum levels as 250 mg erythromycin base, stearate or estolate).
Base: 30-50 mg/kg/day in 2-4 divided doses; do not exceed 2 g/day
Estolate: 30-50 mg/kg/day in 2-4 divided doses; do not exceed 2 g/day

Ethylsuccinate: 30-50 mg/kg/day in 2-4 divided doses; do not exceed 3.2 g/day

Stearate: 30-50 mg/kg/day in 2-4 divided doses; do not exceed 2 g/day

I.V. (as lactobionate): 15-50 mg/kg/day divided every 6 hours, not to exceed 4 g/day

Preop bowel preparation: Oral: 20 mg/kg erythromycin base at 1, 2, and 11 PM on the day before surgery combined with mechanical cleansing of the large intestine and oral neomycin

Ophthalmic infection: Ophthalmic: Refer to adult dosing.

Topical: Refer to adult dosing.

Renal Impairment: Slightly dialyzable (5% to 20%); supplemental dose is not necessary in hemo- or peritoneal dialysis or in continuous arteriovenous or venovenous hemofiltration.

Available Dosage Forms [CAN] = Canadian brand name

Capsule, delayed release, enteric-coated pellets, as base (Eryc®): 250 mg

Gel, topical: 2% (30 g, 60 g)

A/T/S®: 2% (30 g) [contains alcohol 92%]

Erygel®: 2% (30 g, 60 g) [contains alcohol 92%]

Granules for oral suspension, as ethylsuccinate (E.E.S.®): 200 mg/5 mL (100 mL, 200 mL) [cherry flavor]

Injection, powder for reconstitution, as lactobionate (Erythrocin®): 500 mg, 1 g

Ointment, ophthalmic: 0.5% [5 mg/g] (1 g, 3.5 g)

Romycin®: 0.5% [5 mg/g] (3.5 g)

Ointment, topical (Akne-Mycin®): 2% (25 g)

Powder for oral suspension, as ethylsuccinate (EryPed®): 200 mg/5 mL (100 mL, 200 mL) [fruit flavor]; 400 mg/5 mL (100 mL, 200 mL) [banana flavor]

Powder for oral suspension, as ethylsuccinate [drops] (EryPed®): 100 mg/2.5 mL (50 mL) [fruit flavor]

Solution, topical: 2% (60 mL)

A/T/S®: 2% (60 mL) [contains alcohol 66%]

Eryderm®, T-Stat® [DSC], Theramycin Z®: 2% (60 mL) [contain alcohol]

Sans Acne® [CAN]: 2% (60 mL) [contains ethyl alcohol 44%; not available in U.S.]

Staticin®: 1.5% (60 mL) [DSC]

Suspension, oral, as estolate: 125 mg/5 mL (480 mL); 250 mg/5 mL (480 mL)

Suspension, oral, as ethylsuccinate: 200 mg/5 mL (480 mL); 400 mg/5 mL (480 mL)

E.E.S.®: 200 mg/5 mL (100 mL, 480 mL) [fruit flavor]; 400 mg/5 mL (100 mL, 480 mL) [orange flavor]

Swab (T-Stat® [DSC]): 2% (60s)

Tablet, chewable, as ethylsuccinate (EryPed®): 200 mg [fruit flavor] [DSC]

Tablet, delayed release, enteric coated, as base (Ery-Tab®): 250 mg, 333 mg, 500 mg

Tablet [film coated], as base: 250 mg, 500 mg

Tablet [film coated], as ethylsuccinate (E.E.S.®): 400 mg

Tablet [film coated], as stearate: 250 mg

Erythrocin®: 250 mg, 500 mg

Tablet [polymer-coated particles], as base (PCE®): 333 mg, 500 mg

Monitoring and Teaching Issues

Physical Assessment: Assess results of culture and sensitivity tests and patient's previous allergy history prior to therapy. See Warnings/Precautions for use cautions. Assess potential for interactions with other pharmacological agents or herbal products patient may be taking (see Drug Interactions). See Administration specifics. Assess therapeutic effectiveness and adverse reactions (see Adverse Reactions). Teach patient proper use (according to formulation and purpose for use), possible side effects/appropriate interventions, and adverse symptoms to report (see Patient Education).

Monitoring Laboratory Tests: Perform culture and sensitivity studies prior to initiating drug therapy.

Patient Education: Do not take any new medication during therapy unless approved by prescriber

Oral: Take as directed, around-the-clock, with a full glass of water (not juice or milk); may take with food to reduce GI upset. Do not chew or crush extended release capsules or tablets. Take complete prescription even if you are feeling better. Avoid alcohol (may cause adverse response). May cause nausea, vomiting, or mouth sores (small frequent meals, frequent mouth care may help). Report immediately any unusual malaise, nausea, vomiting, abdominal colic, or fever; skin rash or itching; easy bruising or bleeding; vaginal itching or discharge; watery or bloody diarrhea; yellowing of skin or eyes, pale stool or dark urine; white plaques, sores, or fuzziness in mouth; or any change in hearing.

Ophthalmic: Instill as many times per day as directed. Wash hands before using. Gently pull lower eyelid forward, instill prescribed amount of ointment into lower eyelid. Close eye and roll eyeball in all directions. May cause blurred vision; use caution when driving or engaging in tasks that require clear vision until vision clears. Report any adverse reactions such as rash or itching, swelling, burning or pain in eye, worsening of condition, or if condition does not improve.

Topical: Wash and dry area thoroughly. Apply a thin film as many times a day as prescribed to the affected area. May cover with porous sterile bandage.

Dietary Considerations: Systemic: Drug may cause GI upset; may take with food.

Geriatric Considerations: Dose of erythromycin does not need to be adjusted in the elderly unless there is severe renal impairment or hepatic dysfunction. Elderly patients may be at an increased risk for torsade de pointes. Risk of ototoxicity may be increased in elderly, particularly when dose is ≥4 g/day in conjunction with renal or hepatic impairment.

Pregnancy Risk Factor: B

Lactation: Enters breast milk/use caution (AAP considers "compatible")

Administration

Oral: Do not crush enteric coated drug product. GI upset, including diarrhea, is common. May be administered with food to decrease GI upset. Do not give with milk or acidic beverages.

(Continued)

Erythromycin *(Continued)*

I.V.: Infuse 1 g over 20-60 minutes.

Other: Avoid contact of tip of ophthalmic ointment tube with affected eye.

Reconstitution: Erythromycin lactobionate should be reconstituted with sterile water for injection without preservatives to avoid gel formation. I.V. form has the longest stability in NS and should be prepared in this base solution whenever possible. Do not use D_5W as a diluent unless sodium bicarbonate is added to solution. If I.V. must be prepared in D_5W, 0.5 mL of the 8.4% sodium bicarbonate solution should be added per each 100 mL of D_5W.

Stability of parenteral admixture at room temperature (25°C) and at refrigeration temperature (4°C) is 24 hours.

Standard diluent: 500 mg/250 mL D_5W/NS; 750 mg/250 mL D_5W/NS; 1 g/250 mL D_5W/NS.

Compatibility: Erythromycin lactobionate: Stable in NS; **incompatible** with D_5LR, $D_{10}W$

Y-site administration: Incompatible with fluconazole

Compatibility in syringe: Incompatible with ampicillin, heparin

Compatibility when admixed: Incompatible with colistimethate, floxacillin, furosemide, heparin, metaraminol, metoclopramide, riboflavin, vitamin B complex with C

Storage:

Injection: Reconstituted solution is stable for 2 weeks when refrigerated or for 24 hours at room temperature. Erythromycin I.V. infusion solution is stable at pH 6-8; stability of lactobionate is pH dependent; I.V. form has longest stability in NS. Stability of parenteral admixture at room temperature (25°C) and at refrigeration temperature (4°C) is 24 hours.

Granules for oral suspension: After mixing, store under refrigeration and use within 10 days.

Powder for oral suspension: Refrigerate to preserve taste. Erythromycin ethylsuccinate may be stored at room temperature if used within 14 days. EryPed® drops should be used within 35 days following reconstitution; may store at room temperature or under refrigeration.

Topical and ophthalmic formulations: Store at room temperature.

Additional Information Due to differences in absorption, 400 mg erythromycin ethylsuccinate produces the same serum levels as 250 mg erythromycin base, stearate, or estolate. Do not use D_5W as a diluent unless sodium bicarbonate is added to solution; infuse over 20-60 minutes.

Related Information

Antimicrobial Drugs of Choice *on page 1792*
Community-Acquired Pneumonia in Adults *on page 1807*
Compatibility of Drugs *on page 1723*
I.V. to Oral Conversion *on page 1688*
Prophylaxis for Exposure to Communicable Diseases *on page 1859*

Erythromycin and Benzoyl Peroxide

(er ith roe MYE sin & BEN zoe il per OKS ide)

U.S. Brand Names Benzamycin®; Benzamycin® Pak

Synonyms Benzoyl Peroxide and Erythromycin

Generic Available No

Pharmacologic Category Topical Skin Product; Topical Skin Product, Acne

Use Topical control of acne vulgaris

Dosing

Adults & Elderly: Acne: Topical: Apply twice daily, morning and evening.

Pediatrics: Adolescents: Refer to adult dosing.

Available Dosage Forms

Gel, topical:

Benzamycin®: Erythromycin 30 mg and benzoyl peroxide 50 mg per g (47 g)

Benzamycin® Pak: Erythromycin 30 mg and benzoyl peroxide 50 mg per 0.8 g packet (60s) [supplied with diluent containing alcohol]

Monitoring and Teaching Issues

Physical Assessment: See individual agents.

Patient Education: See individual agents. This product contains benzoyl peroxide which may bleach or stain clothing. **Pregnancy/breast-feeding precautions:** Inform prescriber if you are or intend to become pregnant. Consult prescriber if breast-feeding.

Pregnancy Risk Factor: C

Lactation: Excretion in breast milk unknown/use caution

Related Information

Erythromycin *on page 543*

Erythromycin and Sulfisoxazole (er ith roe MYE sin & sul fi SOKS a zole)

U.S. Brand Names Pediazole®

Synonyms Sulfisoxazole and Erythromycin

Generic Available Yes

Pharmacologic Category Antibiotic, Macrolide; Antibiotic, Macrolide Combination; Antibiotic, Sulfonamide Derivative

Medication Safety Issues

Sound-alike/look-alike issues:

Pediazole® may be confused with Pediapred®

Use Treatment of susceptible bacterial infections of the upper and lower respiratory tract, otitis media in children caused by susceptible strains of *Haemophilus influenzae*, and many other infections in patients allergic to penicillin

Dosing

Adults: Susceptible infections: Oral (dosage recommendation is based on the product's erythromycin content): 400 mg erythromycin and 1200 mg sulfisoxazole every 6 hours

Elderly: Not recommended for use in the elderly.

Pediatrics: Susceptible infections: Oral (dosage recommendation is based on the product's erythromycin content): ≥2 months: 50 mg/kg/day erythromycin and 150 mg/kg/day sulfisoxazole in divided doses every 6 hours; not to exceed 2 g erythromycin/day or 6 g sulfisoxazole/day for 10 days

Renal Impairment: Sulfisoxazole must be adjusted in renal impairment.

Cl$_{cr}$ 10-50 mL/minute: Administer every 8-12 hours.

Cl$_{cr}$ <10 mL/minute: Administer every 12-24 hours.

Available Dosage Forms Powder for oral suspension: Erythromycin ethylsuccinate 200 mg and sulfisoxazole acetyl 600 mg per 5 mL (100 mL, 150 mL, 200 mL) [strawberry-banana flavor]

Monitoring and Teaching Issues

Physical Assessment: See individual agents.

Patient Education: See individual agents. **Pregnancy precaution:** Inform prescriber if you are or intend to become pregnant.

Pregnancy Risk Factor: C

Lactation: Enters breast milk/compatible

Related Information

Erythromycin *on page 543*

SulfiSOXAZOLE *on page 1412*

♦ **Erythromycin Base** *see Erythromycin on page 543*

♦ **Erythromycin Estolate** *see Erythromycin on page 543*

♦ **Erythromycin Ethylsuccinate** *see Erythromycin on page 543*

♦ **Erythromycin Gluceptate** *see Erythromycin on page 543*

♦ **Erythromycin Lactobionate** *see Erythromycin on page 543*

♦ **Erythromycin Stearate** *see Erythromycin on page 543*

♦ **Erythropoiesis Stimulating Protein** *see Darbepoetin Alfa on page 405*

♦ **Erythropoietin** *see Epoetin Alfa on page 531*

Escitalopram (es sye TAL oh pram)

U.S. Brand Names Lexapro™

Synonyms Escitalopram Oxalate; Lu-26-054; S-Citalopram

Restrictions A medication guide should be dispensed with each prescription. A template for the required MedGuides can be found on the FDA website at: http://www.fda.gov/cder/drug/antidepressants/labelTemplate.pdf

Generic Available No

Pharmacologic Category Antidepressant, Selective Serotonin Reuptake Inhibitor

Use Treatment of major depressive disorder; generalized anxiety disorders (GAD)

Mechanism of Action/Effect Escitalopram is the S-enantiomer of the racemic derivative citalopram, which selectively inhibits the reuptake of serotonin with little to no effect on norepinephrine or dopamine reuptake. It has no or very low affinity for 5-HT$_{1-7}$, alpha- and beta-adrenergic, D$_{1-5}$, H$_{1-3}$, M$_{1-5}$, and benzodiazepine receptors. Escitalopram does not bind or has low affinity for Na$^+$, K$^+$, Cl$^-$, and Ca^{++} ion channels.

Contraindications Hypersensitivity to escitalopram, citalopram, or any component of the formulation; concomitant use or within 2 weeks of MAO inhibitors

Warnings/Precautions Antidepressants increase the risk of suicidal thinking and behavior in children and adolescents with major depressive disorder (MDD) and other depressive disorders; consider risk prior to prescribing. All patients must be closely monitored for clinical worsening, suicidality, or unusual changes in behavior, especially during the initiation of therapy or following an increase or decrease in dosage. When used in children, the child's family or caregiver should be instructed to closely observe the patient and communicate condition with healthcare provider. A medication guide should be dispensed with each prescription. **Escitalopram is not FDA approved for use in children.**

The possibility of a suicide attempt is inherent in major depression and may persist until remission occurs. Use caution in high-risk patients. Worsening depression and severe abrupt suicidality that are not part of the presenting symptoms may require discontinuation or modification of drug therapy. The patient's family or caregiver should be alerted to monitor patients for the emergence of suicidality and associated behaviors (such as agitation, irritability, hostility, impulsivity, and hypomania) and call healthcare provider.

May worsen psychosis in some patients or precipitate a shift to mania or hypomania in patients with bipolar disorder. Patients presenting with depressive symptoms should be screened for bipolar disorder. Monotherapy in patients with bipolar disorder should be avoided. **Escitalopram is not FDA approved for the treatment of bipolar depression.**

The potential for a severe reaction exists when used with MAO inhibitors; serotonin syndrome (hyperthermia, muscular rigidity, mental status changes/agitation, autonomic instability) may occur. May increase the risks associated with electroconvulsive therapy. Has a low potential to impair cognitive or motor performance; caution operating hazardous machinery or driving.

Use caution with a previous seizure disorder or condition predisposing to seizures such as brain damage, alcoholism, or concurrent therapy with other drugs which lower the seizure threshold. May cause hyponatremia/SIADH. May cause or exacerbate sexual dysfunction. Use caution with renal or liver impairment; concomitant CNS depressants; pregnancy (high doses of citalopram has been associated with teratogenicity in animals). Use caution with concomitant use of NSAIDs, ASA, or other drugs that affect coagulation; the risk of bleeding is potentiated.

Upon discontinuation of escitalopram therapy, gradually taper dose. If intolerable symptoms occur following a decrease in dosage or upon discontinuation of therapy, then resuming the previous dose with a more gradual taper should be considered.
(Continued)

Escitalopram *(Continued)*

Drug Interactions

Cytochrome P450 Effect: Substrate (major) of CYP2C19, 3A4; **Inhibits** CYP2D6 (weak)

Decreased Effect: CYP2C19 inducers may decrease the levels/effects of imipramine; example inducers include aminoglutethimide, carbamazepine, phenytoin, and rifampin. CYP3A4 inducers may decrease the levels/effects of escitalopram; example inducers include aminoglutethimide, carbamazepine, nafcillin, nevirapine, phenobarbital, phenytoin, and rifamycins.

Increased Effect/Toxicity: Escitalopram should not be used with nonselective MAO inhibitors (phenelzine, isocarboxazid) or other drugs with MAO inhibition (linezolid); fatal reactions have been reported. Wait 5 weeks after stopping escitalopram before starting a nonselective MAO inhibitor and 2 weeks after stopping an MAO inhibitor before starting escitalopram. Concurrent selegiline has been associated with mania, hypertension, or serotonin syndrome (risk may be reduced relative to nonselective MAO inhibitors).

CYP2C19 inhibitors may increase the levels/effects of imipramine; example inhibitors include delavirdine, fluconazole, fluvoxamine, gemfibrozil, isoniazid, omeprazole, and ticlopidine. CYP3A4 inhibitors may increase the levels/effects of escitalopram; example inhibitors include azole antifungals, ciprofloxacin, clarithromycin, diclofenac, doxycycline, erythromycin, imatinib, isoniazid, nefazodone, nicardipine, propofol, protease inhibitors, quinidine, and verapamil.

Combined use of SSRIs and buspirone, meperidine, moclobemide, nefazodone, other SSRIs, tramadol, trazodone, and venlafaxine may increase the risk of serotonin syndrome. Escitalopram increases serum levels/effects of CYP2D6 substrates (tricyclic antidepressants). Escitalopram may increase desipramine levels.

Combined use of sumatriptan (and other serotonin agonists) may result in toxicity; weakness, hyper-reflexia, and incoordination have been observed with sumatriptan and SSRIs. In addition, concurrent use may theoretically increase the risk of serotonin syndrome; includes sumatriptan, naratriptan, rizatriptan, and zolmitriptan.

Concomitant use of escitalopram and NSAIDs, aspirin, or other drugs affecting coagulation has been associated with an increased risk of bleeding; monitor.

Nutritional/Ethanol Interactions

Ethanol: Avoid ethanol (may increase CNS depression).

Herb/Nutraceutical: Avoid valerian, St John's wort, SAMe, kava kava, and gotu kola (may increase CNS depression).

Adverse Reactions

>10%:

Central nervous system: Headache (24%), somnolence (6% to 13%), insomnia (9% to 12%)

Gastrointestinal: Nausea (15%)

Genitourinary: Ejaculation disorder (9% to 14%)

1% to 10%:

Cardiovascular: Chest pain, hypertension, palpitation

Central nervous system: Dizziness (5%), fatigue (5% to 8%), dreaming abnormal, concentration impaired, fever, irritability, lethargy, lightheadedness, migraine, vertigo, yawning

Dermatologic: Rash

Endocrine & metabolic: Libido decreased (3% to 7%), anorgasmia (2% to 6%), hot flashes, menstrual cramps, menstrual disorder

Gastrointestinal: Diarrhea (8%), xerostomia (6% to 9%), appetite decreased (3%), constipation (3% to 5%), indigestion (3%), abdominal pain (2%), abdominal cramps, appetite increased, flatulence, gastroenteritis, gastroesophageal reflux, heartburn, toothache, vomiting, weight gain/loss

Genitourinary: Impotence (3%), urinary tract infection, urinary frequency

Neuromuscular & skeletal: Arthralgia, limb pain, muscle cramp, myalgia, neck/shoulder pain, paresthesia, tremor

Ocular: Blurred vision

Otic: Earache, tinnitus

Respiratory: Rhinitis (5%), sinusitis (3%), bronchitis, cough, nasal or sinus congestion, sinus headache

Miscellaneous: Diaphoresis (4% to 5%), flu-like syndrome (5%), allergy

Overdosage/Toxicology Treatment should be symptom-directed and supportive.

Pharmacodynamics/Kinetics

Time to Peak: Escitalopram: 5 ± 1.5 hours; S-desmethylcitalopram: 14 hours

Protein Binding: 56% to plasma proteins

Half-Life Elimination: Escitalopram: 27-32 hours; S-desmethylcitalopram: 59 hours

Metabolism: Hepatic via CYP2C19 and 3A4 to an active metabolite, S-desmethylcitalopram (S-DCT; 1/7 the activity); S-DCT is metabolized to S-didesmethylcitalopram (S-DDCT; active; 1/27 the activity) via CYP2D6

Excretion: Urine (Escitalopram: 8%; S-DCT: 10%)

Clearance: Total body: 37-40 L/hour; Renal: Escitalopram: 2.7 L/hour; S-desmethylcitalopram: 6.9 L/hour

Dosing

Adults: Depression, GAD: Oral: Initial: 10 mg/day; dose may be increased to 20 mg/day after at least 1 week

Elderly: Depression: Oral: 5-10 mg/day; doses may be increased by 5-10 mg/day after at least 1 week.

Renal Impairment:

Mild to moderate impairment: No dosage adjustment needed.

Severe impairment: Cl_{cr} <20 mL/minute: Use caution.

Hepatic Impairment: 10 mg/day

Available Dosage Forms

Solution, oral: 1 mg/mL (240 mL) [peppermint flavor]

Tablet: 5 mg, 10 mg, 20 mg

Monitoring and Teaching Issues

Physical Assessment: Assess potential for interactions with other prescriptions, OTC medications, or herbal products patient may be taking (eg, MAO inhibitors and other SSRIs). Assess therapeutic effectiveness and adverse reactions at the beginning of therapy and on a regular basis throughout therapy (eg, suicidal ideation, mania, hypomania, anxiety, or panic attacks). Teach patient proper use, possible side effects, interventions to reduce side effects, and adverse symptoms to report.

Patient Education: Do not take any new medication during therapy without consulting prescriber. Take exactly as directed; do not alter dose or discontinue without consulting prescriber (effects of medication may take up to 3 weeks to occur). Avoid other stimulants: caffeine or alcohol. May cause dizziness, lightheadedness, insomnia, impaired concentration, headache (use caution when driving or engaging in tasks requiring alertness until response to drug is known); nausea, vomiting, loss or increase of appetite, indigestion, or heartburn (small frequent meals, frequent mouth care, sucking lozenges, or chewing gum may help); constipation (increased dietary fluid, fruit, fiber, and increased exercise may help); sexual dysfunction (reversible when drug is discontinued); hot flashes or menstrual cramps; or muscle pain, cramps, or tremor (consult prescriber for approved analgesia). Report immediately any CNS changes such as increased depression, confusion, impaired concentration, severe headache, insomnia, nightmares, irritability, acute anxiety, panic attacks, or thoughts of suicide; persistent GI changes; chest pain or palpitations; blurred vision or vision changes; ringing in ears; unusual cough; or other persistent adverse effects. **Pregnancy/breast-feeding precautions:** Inform prescriber if you are or intend to become pregnant. Breast-feeding is not recommended.

Dietary Considerations: May be taken with or without food.

Pregnancy Risk Factor: C

Pregnancy Issues: Teratogenic effects have been reported in animal studies. Nonteratogenic effects including respiratory distress, cyanosis, apnea, seizures, temperature instability, feeding difficulty, vomiting, hypoglycemia, hypo- or hypertonia, hyper-reflexia, jitteriness, irritability, constant crying, and tremor have been reported in the neonate immediately following delivery after exposure late in the third trimester. Adverse effects may be due to toxic effects of SSRI or drug discontinuation. In some cases, may present clinically as serotonin syndrome. There are no adequate and well-controlled studies in pregnant women. Use during pregnancy only if the potential benefit to the mother outweighs the possible risk to the fetus. If treatment during pregnancy is required, consider tapering therapy during the third trimester.

Lactation: Enters breast milk/not recommended

Breast-Feeding Issues: Escitalopram is excreted in human milk. Excessive somnolence, decreased feeding and weight loss have been reported in breast-fed infants. A decision should be made whether to continue or discontinue nursing or discontinue the drug.

Administration

Oral: Administer once daily (morning or evening), with or without food.

Storage: Store at 25°C (77°F).

Additional Information The tablet and oral solution dosage forms are bioequivalent. Clinically, escitalopram 20 mg is equipotent to citalopram 40 mg. Do not coadminister with citalopram.

Related Information

Antidepressant Agents *on page 1713*

- ◆ **Escitalopram Oxalate** *see* Escitalopram *on page 547*
- ◆ **Esclim®** *see* Estradiol *on page 552*
- ◆ **Eserine Salicylate** *see* Physostigmine *on page 1208*
- ◆ **Esgic®** *see* Butalbital, Acetaminophen, and Caffeine *on page 225*
- ◆ **Esgic-Plus™** *see* Butalbital, Acetaminophen, and Caffeine *on page 225*
- ◆ **Eskalith®** *see* Lithium *on page 908*
- ◆ **Eskalith CR®** *see* Lithium *on page 908*

Esmolol *(ES moe lol)*

U.S. Brand Names Brevibloc®

Synonyms Esmolol Hydrochloride

Generic Available Yes: Excludes infusion

Pharmacologic Category Antiarrhythmic Agent, Class II; Beta Blocker, Beta₁ Selective

Medication Safety Issues

Sound-alike/look-alike issues:

Esmolol may be confused with Osmitrol®

Brevibloc® may be confused with bretylium, Brevital®, Bumex®, Buprenex®

Use Treatment of supraventricular tachycardia and atrial fibrillation/flutter (primarily to control ventricular rate); treatment of tachycardia and/or hypertension (especially intraoperative or postoperative)

Mechanism of Action/Effect Class II antiarrhythmic: Beta₁ adrenergic receptor blocking agent that competes with beta₁ adrenergic agonists for available beta receptor sites; it is a selective beta₁ antagonist with a very short duration of action; has little if any intrinsic sympathomimetic activity; and lacks membrane stabilizing action; it is administered intravenously and is used when beta blockade of short duration is desired or in critically-ill patients in whom adverse effects of bradycardia, heart failure or hypotension may necessitate rapid withdrawal of the drug

Contraindications Hypersensitivity to esmolol or any component of the formulation; sinus bradycardia; heart block greater than first degree (except in patients with a functioning artificial pacemaker); cardiogenic shock; bronchial asthma (relative); uncompensated cardiac failure; hypotension; pregnancy (2nd and 3rd trimesters)

Warnings/Precautions Hypotension is common; patients need close blood pressure monitoring. Administer cautiously in compensated heart failure and monitor for a worsening of the condition. Use caution in patients with PVD (can aggravate arterial insufficiency). Use caution *(Continued)*

Esmolol *(Continued)*

with concurrent use of beta-blockers and either verapamil or diltiazem; bradycardia or heart block can occur. Avoid concurrent I.V. use of both agents. Use beta-blockers cautiously in patients with bronchospastic disease; monitor pulmonary status closely. Use with caution in patients with diabetes - may mask prominent hypoglycemic symptoms. May mask signs of thyrotoxicosis. May cause fetal bradycardia when administered in the 3rd trimester of pregnancy or at delivery. Use caution in patients with renal dysfunction (active metabolite retained). Do not use in the treatment of hypertension associated with vasoconstriction related to hypothermia. Extravasation can lead to skin necrosis and sloughing.

Drug Interactions

Decreased Effect: Decreased effect of beta-blockers with aluminum salts, barbiturates, calcium salts, cholestyramine, colestipol, NSAIDs, penicillins (ampicillin), rifampin, salicylates, and sulfinpyrazone due to decreased bioavailability and plasma levels. Beta-blockers may decrease the effect of sulfonylureas. Xanthines (eg, theophylline, caffeine) may decrease effects of esmolol.

Increased Effect/Toxicity: Esmolol may increase the effect/toxicity of verapamil, and may increase potential for hypertensive crisis after or during withdrawal of either agent when combined with clonidine. Esmolol may extend the effect of neuromuscular blocking agents (succinylcholine). Esmolol may increase digoxin serum levels by 10% to 20% and may increase theophylline concentrations. Morphine may increase esmolol blood concentrations.

Lab Interactions Increased cholesterol (S), glucose

Adverse Reactions

>10%:
Cardiovascular: Asymptomatic hypotension (25%), symptomatic hypotension (12%)
Miscellaneous: Diaphoresis (10%)

1% to 10%:
Cardiovascular: Peripheral ischemia (1%)
Central nervous system: Dizziness (3%), somnolence (3%), confusion (2%), headache (2%), agitation (2%), fatigue (1%)
Gastrointestinal: Nausea (7%), vomiting (1%)
Local: Pain on injection (8%)

Overdosage/Toxicology Symptoms of overdose include hypotension, bradycardia, and heart block. Initially, fluids may be the best treatment for hypotension. Sympathomimetics (eg, epinephrine or dopamine), glucagon, or a pacemaker can be used to treat the toxic bradycardia, asystole, and/or hypotension.

Pharmacodynamics/Kinetics

Onset of Action: Beta-blockade: I.V.: 2-10 minutes (quickest when loading doses are administered)

Duration of Action: 10-30 minutes; prolonged following higher cumulative doses, extended duration of use

Protein Binding: 55%

Half-Life Elimination: Adults: 9 minutes

Metabolism: In blood by esterases

Excretion: Urine (~69% as metabolites, 2% unchanged drug)

Dosing

Adults & Elderly: Infusion requires an infusion pump (must be adjusted to individual response and tolerance):

Intraoperative tachycardia and/or hypertension (immediate control): I.V.: Initial bolus: 80 mg (~1 mg/kg) over 30 seconds, followed by a 150 mcg/kg/minute infusion, if necessary. Adjust infusion rate as needed to maintain desired heart rate and/or blood pressure, up to 300 mcg/kg/minute.

Supraventricular tachycardia or gradual control of postoperative tachycardia/hypertension: I.V.: Loading dose: 500 mcg/kg over 1 minute; follow with a 50 mcg/kg/minute infusion for 4 minutes; response to this initial infusion rate may be a rough indication of the responsiveness of the ventricular rate.

Infusion may be continued at 50 mcg/kg/minute or, if the response is inadequate, titrated upward in 50 mcg/kg/minute increments (increased no more frequently than every 4 minutes) to a maximum of 200 mcg/kg/minute.

Note: To achieve more rapid response, following the initial loading dose and 50 mcg/kg/minute infusion, rebolus with a second 500 mcg/kg loading dose over 1 minute, and increase the maintenance infusion to 100 mcg/kg/minute for 4 minutes. If necessary, a third (and final) 500 mcg/kg loading dose may be administered, prior to increasing to an infusion rate of 150 mcg/kg/minute. After 4 minutes of the 150 mcg/kg/minute infusion, the infusion rate may be increased to a maximum rate of 200 mcg/kg/minute (without a bolus dose).

Supraventricular tachycardias (SVT); usual dose range: 50-200 mcg/kg/minute with average dose of 100 mcg/kg/minute. For control of postoperative hypertension, as many as one-third of patients may require higher doses (250-300 mcg/kg/minute) to control blood pressure; the safety of doses >300 mcg/kg/minute has not been studied.

Guidelines for withdrawal of therapy:
Transfer to alternative antiarrhythmic drug (propranolol, digoxin, verapamil).
Infusion should be reduced by 50% 30 minutes following the first dose of the alternative agent.
Following the second dose of the alternative drug, patient's response should be monitored and if control is adequate for the first hours, esmolol may be discontinued.

Pediatrics:

Supraventricular tachycardias: I.V.: Children: A limited amount of information regarding esmolol use in pediatric patients is currently available. Some centers have utilized doses of 100-500 mcg/kg given over 1 minute for control of supraventricular tachycardias.

Postoperative hypertension: I.V.: Loading doses of 500 mcg/kg/minute over 1 minute with maximal doses of 50-250 mcg/kg/minute (mean = 173) have been used in addition to nitroprusside to treat postoperative hypertension after coarctation of aorta repair.

Renal Impairment: Not removed by hemo- or peritoneal dialysis. Supplemental dose is not necessary.

Available Dosage Forms

Infusion [premixed in sodium chloride; preservative free] (Brevibloc®): 2000 mg (100 mL) [20 mg/mL; double strength]; 2500 mg (250 mL) [10 mg/mL]

Injection, solution, as hydrochloride: 10 mg/mL (10 mL) [premixed in sodium chloride]

Brevibloc®: 10 mg/mL (10 mL) [alcohol free; premixed in sodium chloride]; 20 mg/mL (5 mL) [alcohol free; double strength; premixed in sodium chloride]; 250 mg/mL (10 mL) [contains alcohol 25%; concentrate]

Monitoring and Teaching Issues

Physical Assessment: Assess other medications patient may be taking for effectiveness and interactions. Requires continuous cardiac, hemodynamic, and infusion site monitoring (extravasation). If diabetic, may mask signs of hypoglycemia. Monitor blood sugars closely. Monitor therapeutic effectiveness and adverse reactions.

Patient Education: Esmolol is administered in emergencies, patient education should be appropriate to the situation. **Pregnancy/breast-feeding precautions:** Inform prescriber if you are pregnant. Consult prescriber if breast-feeding.

Geriatric Considerations: Due to alterations in the beta-adrenergic autonomic nervous system, beta-adrenergic blockade may result in less hemodynamic response than seen in younger adults.

Pregnancy Risk Factor: C (manufacturer); D (2nd and 3rd trimesters - expert analysis)

Lactation: Excretion in breast milk unknown

Administration

I.V.: The 250 mg/mL ampul is **not** for direct I.V. injection, but rather must first be diluted to a final concentration of 10 mg/mL (ie, 2.5 g in 250 mL or 5 g in 500 mL). Concentrations >10 mg/mL or infusion into small veins or through a butterfly catheter should be avoided (can cause thrombophlebitis).

Reconstitution: Stability of parenteral admixture at room temperature (25°C) and at refrigeration temperature (4°C) is 24 hours.

Standard diluent: 5 g/500 mL NS

Compatibility: Stable in D$_5$LR, D$_5$^{1}/$_2$NS, D$_5$NS, D$_5$W, D$_5$W with KCl 40 mEq/L, LR, ^{1}/$_2$NS, NS, sodium bicarbonate 5%

Y-site administration: Incompatible with amphotericin B cholesteryl sulfate complex, furosemide, warfarin

Compatibility when admixed: Incompatible with diazepam, procainamide, sodium bicarbonate, thiopental

Storage: Clear, colorless to light yellow solution should be stored at room temperature and protected from temperatures >40°C.

Related Information

Antiarrhythmic Drugs *on page 1708*
Beta-Blockers *on page 1720*

♦ **Esmolol Hydrochloride** *see* Esmolol *on page 549*

Esomeprazole (es oh ME pray zol)

U.S. Brand Names Nexium®

Synonyms Esomeprazole Magnesium

Generic Available No

Pharmacologic Category Proton Pump Inhibitor; Substituted Benzimidazole

Use Short-term (4-8 weeks) treatment of erosive esophagitis; maintaining symptom resolution and healing of erosive esophagitis; treatment of symptomatic gastroesophageal reflux disease; as part of a multidrug regimen for *Helicobacter pylori* eradication in patients with duodenal ulcer disease (active or history of within the past 5 years); prevention of gastric ulcers associated with continuous NSAID therapy

Mechanism of Action/Effect Prevents gastric acid secretion

Contraindications Hypersensitivity to esomeprazole, substituted benzimidazoles (ie, lansoprazole, omeprazole, pantoprazole, rabeprazole), or any component of the formulation

Warnings/Precautions Relief of symptoms does not preclude the presence of a gastric malignancy. Atrophic gastritis (by biopsy) has been noted with long-term omeprazole therapy; this may also occur with esomeprazole. No reports of enterochromaffin-like (ECL) cell carcinoids, dysplasia, or neoplasia has occurred. Safety and efficacy in pediatric patients have not been established.

Drug Interactions

Cytochrome P450 Effect: Substrate of CYP2C19 (major), 3A4 (minor)

Decreased Effect: CYP2C19 inducers may decrease the levels/effects of esomeprazole; example inducers include aminoglutethimide, carbamazepine, phenytoin, and rifampin. Proton pump inhibitors may decrease the absorption of atazanavir, indinavir, iron salts, itraconazole, and ketoconazole.

Increased Effect/Toxicity: Esomeprazole and omeprazole may increase the levels of benzodiazepines metabolized by oxidation (eg, diazepam, midazolam, triazolam) and carbamazepine.

Nutritional/Ethanol Interactions Food: Absorption is decreased by 43% to 53% when taken with food.

Adverse Reactions 1% to 10%:

Central nervous system: Headache (4% to 6%)

Gastrointestinal: Diarrhea (4%), nausea, flatulence, abdominal pain (4%), constipation, xerostomia

Overdosage/Toxicology Symptoms of overdose may include confusion, drowsiness, blurred vision, tachycardia, nausea, sweating, headache or dry mouth. Treatment is symptom-directed and supportive; not dialyzable.

(Continued)

Esomeprazole (Continued)

Pharmacodynamics/Kinetics
Bioavailability: 90% with repeat dosing
Time to Peak: 1.5 hours
Protein Binding: 97%
Half-Life Elimination: 1-1.5 hours
Metabolism: Hepatic via CYP2C19 and 3A4 enzymes to hydroxy, desmethyl, and sulfone metabolites (all inactive)
Excretion: Urine (80%); feces (20%)

Dosing
Adults & Elderly:
  Healing of erosive esophagitis: Oral: 20-40 mg once daily for 4-8 weeks; may consider an additional 4-8 weeks of treatment if patient is not healed
  Maintenance of healing of erosive esophagitis: Oral: 20 mg once daily; clinical trials evaluated therapy for ≤6 months
  Symptomatic gastroesophageal reflux: Oral: 20 mg once daily for 4 weeks; may consider an additional 4 weeks of treatment if symptoms do not resolve
  Peptic ulcer disease: Eradication of *Helicobacter pylori*: Oral: 40 mg once daily; requires combination therapy
  Prevention of NSAID-induced gastric ulcers: 20-40 mg once daily for up to 6 months
Renal Impairment: No adjustment is necessary.
Hepatic Impairment:
  Mild-to-moderate hepatic impairment (Child-Pugh Class A or B): No dosage adjustment needed.
  Severe hepatic impairment (Child-Pugh Class C): Dose should not exceed 20 mg/day.

Available Dosage Forms Capsule, delayed release: 20 mg, 40 mg

Monitoring and Teaching Issues
Physical Assessment: Assess other medications patient may be taking for effectiveness and interactions (especially those dependent on cytochrome P450 metabolism or those dependent on a acid environment for absorption). Monitor effectiveness of therapeutic effectiveness and adverse reactions at beginning of therapy and periodically throughout therapy. Assess knowledge/teach appropriate use of this medication, interventions to reduce side effects, and adverse symptoms to report.
Monitoring Laboratory Tests: Susceptibility testing is recommended in patients who fail *H. pylori* eradication regimen (esomeprazole, clarithromycin, and amoxicillin).
Patient Education: Take as directed, 1 hour before eating at same time each day. Swallow capsule whole; do not crush or chew. If you cannot swallow capsule whole, open capsule, mix contents with 1 tablespoon of applesauce, and swallow immediately; do not chew mixture. Do not store for future use. You may experience headache; constipation (increased exercise, fluids, fruit, or fiber may help); diarrhea (boiled milk, yogurt, or butter-milk may help); or abdominal pain (should diminish with use). Report persistent headache, diarrhea, constipation, abdominal pain, changes in urination or pain on urination, chest pain or palpitations, changes in respiratory status, CNS changes, persistent muscular aches or pain, ringing in ears or visual changes, or other adverse reactions.
Breast-feeding precaution: Breast-feeding is not recommended.
Dietary Considerations: Take at least 1 hour before meals; best if taken before breakfast.
Pregnancy Risk Factor: B
Lactation: Excretion in breast milk unknown/not recommended
Breast-Feeding Issues: Omeprazole is excreted in breast milk; breast-feeding is not recommended.

Administration
Oral: Capsule should be swallowed whole and taken at least 1 hour before eating (best if taken before breakfast). For patients with difficulty swallowing, open capsule and mix contents with 1 tablespoon of applesauce. Swallow immediately; mixture should not be chewed or warmed. The mixture should not be stored for future use.
Other: Nasogastric tube: Open capsule and place intact granules into a 60 mL syringe; mix with 50 mL of water. Replace plunger and shake vigorously for 15 seconds. Ensure that no granules remain in syringe tip. Do not administer if pellets dissolve or disintegrate. After administration, flush nasogastric tube with additional water. Use suspension immediately after preparation.
Compatibility: The contents of the capsule may be mixed in applesauce or water; pellets also remain intact when exposed to orange juice, apple juice, and yogurt.
Storage: Store at 15°C to 30°C (59°F to 86°F). Keep container tightly closed.
Additional Information Esomeprazole is the S-isomer of omeprazole.

Related Information
Helicobacter pylori Treatment *on page 1835*

- **Esomeprazole Magnesium** *see* Esomeprazole *on page 551*
- **Esoterica® Regular [OTC]** *see* Hydroquinone *on page 768*
- **Esterified Estrogens** *see* Estrogens (Esterified) *on page 569*
- **Estrace®** *see* Estradiol *on page 552*
- **Estraderm®** *see* Estradiol *on page 552*

Estradiol (es tra DYE ole)

U.S. Brand Names Alora®; Climara®; Delestrogen®; Depo®-Estradiol; Esclim®; Estrace®; Estraderm®; Estrasorb™; Estring®; EstroGel®; Femring™; Femtrace®; Gynodiol®; Menostar™; Vagifem®; Vivelle®; Vivelle-Dot®
Synonyms Estradiol Acetate; Estradiol Cypionate; Estradiol Hemihydrate; Estradiol Trans-dermal; Estradiol Valerate
Generic Available Yes: Oral tablet, patch
Pharmacologic Category Estrogen Derivative

Medication Safety Issues

Sound-alike/look-alike issues:

Alora® may be confused with Aldara™

Estraderm® may be confused with Testoderm®

Transdermal patch may contain conducting metal (eg, aluminum); remove patch prior to MRI.

Use Treatment of moderate-to-severe vasomotor symptoms associated with menopause; treatment of vulvar and vaginal atrophy; hypoestrogenism (due to hypogonadism, castration, or primary ovarian failure); prostatic cancer (palliation), breast cancer (palliation); osteoporosis (prophylaxis); abnormal uterine bleeding due to hormonal imbalance; postmenopausal urogenital symptoms of the lower urinary tract (urinary urgency, dysuria)

Mechanism of Action/Effect Estrogens modulate the pituitary secretion of gonadotropins, luteinizing hormone, and follicle-stimulating hormone through a negative feedback system; estrogen replacement reduces elevated levels of these hormones in postmenopausal women.

Contraindications Hypersensitivity to estradiol or any component of the formulation; undiagnosed abnormal vaginal bleeding; history of or current thrombophlebitis or venous thromboembolic disorders (including DVT, PE); active or recent (within 1 year) arterial thromboembolic disease (eg, stroke, MI); carcinoma of the breast, except in appropriately selected patients being treated for metastatic disease; estrogen-dependent tumor; hepatic dysfunction or disease; porphyria; pregnancy

Warnings/Precautions

Cardiovascular-related considerations: Estrogens with or without progestin should not be used to prevent coronary heart disease. Use caution with cardiovascular disease or dysfunction. May increase the risks of hypertension, myocardial infarction (MI), stroke, pulmonary emboli (PE), and deep vein thrombosis; incidence of these effects was shown to be significantly increased in postmenopausal women using conjugated equine estrogens (CEE) in combination with medroxyprogesterone acetate (MPA). Nonfatal MI, PE, and thrombophlebitis have also been reported in males taking high doses of CEE (eg, for prostate cancer). Estrogen compounds are generally associated with lipid effects such as increased HDL-cholesterol and decreased LDL-cholesterol. Triglycerides may also be increased; use with caution in patients with familial defects of lipoprotein metabolism. Whenever possible, estrogens should be discontinued at least 4-6 weeks prior to surgeries associated with an increased risk of thromboembolism or during periods of prolonged immobilization.

Neurological considerations: The risk of dementia may be increased in postmenopausal women; increased incidence was observed in women ≥65 years of age taking CEE in combination with MPA.

Cancer-related considerations: Unopposed estrogens may increase the risk of endometrial carcinoma in postmenopausal women. Estrogens may increase the risk of breast cancer. An increased risk of invasive breast cancer was observed in postmenopausal women using CEE in combination with MPA; a smaller increase in risk was seen with estrogen therapy alone in observational studies. An increase in abnormal mammograms has also been reported with estrogen and progestin therapy. Estrogen use may lead to severe hypercalcemia in patients with breast cancer and bone metastases; discontinue estrogen if hypercalcemia occurs.

Estrogens may cause retinal vascular thrombosis; discontinue permanently if papilledema or retinal vascular lesions are observed on examination. Use with caution in patients with diseases which may be exacerbated by fluid retention, including asthma, epilepsy, migraine, diabetes or renal dysfunction. Use with caution in patients with a history of severe hypocalcemia, SLE, hepatic hemangiomas, endometriosis, and gallbladder disease. Use caution with history of cholestatic jaundice associated with past estrogen use or pregnancy. Safety and efficacy in pediatric patients have not been established. Prior to puberty, estrogens may cause premature closure of the epiphyses, premature breast development in girls or gynecomastia in boys. Vaginal bleeding and vaginal cornification may also be induced in girls.

Before prescribing estrogen therapy to postmenopausal women, the risks and benefits must be weighed for each patient. Women should be informed of these risks and benefits, as well as possible effects of progestin when added to estrogen therapy. Estrogens with or without progestin should be used for shortest duration possible consistent with treatment goals. Conduct periodic risk:benefit assessments.

When used solely for prevention of osteoporosis in women at significant risk, nonestrogen treatment options should be considered. When used solely for the treatment of vulvar and vaginal atrophy, topical vaginal products should be considered. Use caution applying topical products to severely atrophic vaginal mucosa. Absorption of topical emulsion is increased by application of sunscreen; do not apply both products within close proximity of each other. Application of gel formulation with sunscreen has not been evaluated. Transdermal patch may contain conducting metal (eg, aluminum); remove patch prior to MRI.

Drug Interactions

Cytochrome P450 Effect: Substrate of CYP1A2 (major), 2A6 (minor), 2B6 (minor), 2C8/9 (minor), 2C19 (minor), 2D6 (minor), 2E1 (minor), 3A4 (major); **Inhibits** CYP1A2 (weak); **Induces** CYP3A4 (weak)

Decreased Effect: CYP1A2 inducers may decrease the levels/effects of estradiol; example inducers include aminoglutethimide, carbamazepine, phenobarbital, and rifampin. CYP3A4 inducers may decrease the levels/effects of estradiol; example inducers include aminoglutethimide, carbamazepine, nafcillin, nevirapine, phenobarbital, phenytoin, and rifamycins.

Increased Effect/Toxicity: Estradiol with hydrocortisone increases corticosteroid toxic potential. Anticoagulants and estradiol increase the potential for thromboembolic events.

Nutritional/Ethanol Interactions

Ethanol: Avoid ethanol (routine use increases estrogen level and risk of breast cancer). Ethanol may also increase the risk of osteoporosis.

Food: Folic acid absorption may be decreased

Herb/Nutraceutical: St John's wort may decrease estradiol levels. Avoid black cohosh, dong quai (has estrogenic activity). Avoid red clover, saw palmetto, ginseng.

(Continued)

Estradiol (Continued)

Lab Interactions Increased Prothrombin and factors VII, VIII, IX, X; increased platelet aggregability, thyroid-binding globulin, total thyroid hormone (T_4), serum triglycerides/phospholipids; decreased antithrombin III, serum folate concentration

Adverse Reactions Frequency not defined.

Cardiovascular: Edema, hypertension, MI, venous thromboembolism

Central nervous system: Anxiety, dizziness, epilepsy exacerbation, headache, irritability, mental depression, migraine, mood disturbances, nervousness

Dermatologic: Chloasma, erythema multiforme, erythema nodosum, hemorrhagic eruption, hirsutism, loss of scalp hair, melasma, rash, pruritus

Endocrine & metabolic: Breast enlargement, breast tenderness, libido (changes in), increased thyroid-binding globulin, increased total thyroid hormone (T_4), increased serum triglycerides/phospholipids, increased HDL-cholesterol, decreased LDL-cholesterol, impaired glucose tolerance, hypercalcemia

Gastrointestinal: Abdominal cramps, abdominal pain, bloating, cholecystitis, cholelithiasis, diarrhea, flatulence, gallbladder disease, nausea, pancreatitis, vomiting, weight gain/loss

Genitourinary: Alterations in frequency and flow of menses, changes in cervical secretions, endometrial cancer, increased size of uterine leiomyomata, Pap smear suspicious, vaginal candidiasis

Vaginal: Trauma from applicator insertion may occur in women with severely atrophic vaginal mucosa

Hematologic: Aggravation of porphyria, antithrombin III and antifactor Xa decreased, levels of fibrinogen increased, platelet aggregability increased and platelet count; increased prothrombin and factors VII, VIII, IX, X

Hepatic: Cholestatic jaundice

Local: Transdermal patches: Burning, erythema, irritation, thrombophlebitis

Neuromuscular & skeletal: Chorea, back pain

Ocular: Intolerance to contact lenses, steeping of corneal curvature

Respiratory: Pulmonary thromboembolism

Miscellaneous: Anaphylactoid/anaphylactic reactions, carbohydrate intolerance

Overdosage/Toxicology Symptoms of overdose include fluid retention, jaundice, thrombophlebitis, nausea, and vomiting. Toxicity is unlikely following single exposure of excessive doses. Treatment following emesis and charcoal administration should be supportive and symptomatic.

Pharmacodynamics/Kinetics

Absorption: Oral, topical: Well absorbed

Protein Binding: 37% to sex hormone-binding globulin; 61% to albumin

Metabolism: Hepatic via oxidation and conjugation in GI tract; hydroxylated via CYP3A4 to metabolites; first-pass effect; enterohepatic recirculation; reversibly converted to estrone and estriol

Excretion: Primarily urine (as metabolites estrone and estriol); feces (small amounts)

Dosing

Adults & Elderly: All dosage needs to be adjusted based upon the patient's response:

Atrophic vaginitis, vulvar/vaginal atrophy:

Intravaginal:

Vaginal cream: Atrophic vaginitis, kraurosis vulvae: Insert 2-4 g/day for 2 weeks then gradually reduce to ¹/₂ the initial dose for 2 weeks followed by a maintenance dose of 1 g 1-3 times/week

Vaginal ring:

Postmenopausal vaginal atrophy, urogenital symptoms (Estring®): 2 mg intravaginally; following insertion, ring should remain in place for 90 days

Vulvar/vaginal atrophy (Femring™): 0.05 mg intravaginally; following insertion, ring should remain in place for 3 months; dose may be increased to 0.1 mg if needed

Vaginal tablets (Vagifem®): Atrophic vaginitis: Initial: Insert 1 tablet once daily for 2 weeks; maintenance: Insert 1 tablet twice weekly. Attempts to discontinue or taper medication should be made at 3- to 6-month intervals

Topical gel: Vulvar/vaginal atrophy: 1.25 g/day applied at the same time each day

Transdermal: Refer to product-specific dosing (below)

Breast cancer (females; inoperable, progressing): Oral: 10 mg 3 times/day for at least 3 months

Hypogonadism:

Oral: 1-2 mg/day in a cyclic regimen for 3 weeks on drug, then 1 week off drug

I.M.: Cypionate: 1.5-2 mg monthly; Valerate: 10-20 mg every 4 weeks

Transdermal: Refer to product-specific dosing (below)

Osteoporosis prevention (females):

Oral: 0.5 mg/day in a cyclic regimen (3 weeks on and 1 week off of drug)

Transdermal: Refer to product-specific dosing (below)

Prostate cancer:

I.M. (valerate): ≥30 mg or more every 1-2 weeks

Oral (androgen-dependent, inoperable, progressing): 10 mg 3 times/day for at least 3 months

Vasomotor symptoms (moderate-severe) associated with menopause:

Oral (in addition to I.M. dosing): 1-2 mg daily, adjusted as necessary to limit symptoms. Administrations should be cyclic (3 weeks on, 1 week off). Patients should be re-evaluated at 3-6 month intervals to determine if treatment is still necessary

I.M.: Cypionate: 1-5 mg every 3-4 weeks; Valerate: 10-20 mg every 4 weeks

Topical emulsion: 3.84 g applied once daily in the morning

Topical gel: 1.25 g/day applied at the same time each day

Vaginal ring (Femring™): 0.05 mg intravaginally; following insertion, ring should remain in place for 3 months; dose may be increased to 0.1 mg if needed

Transdermal: See product-specific dosing (below)

Transdermal product-specific dosing:

Note: Indicated dose may be used continuously in patients without an intact uterus. May be given continuously or cyclically (3 weeks on, 1 week off) in patients with an intact uterus **(exception - Menostar™, see specific dosing instructions).** When changing patients from oral to transdermal therapy, start transdermal patch 1 week after discontinuing oral hormone (may begin sooner if symptoms reappear within 1 week):

Transdermal once-weekly patch:

Moderate to severe vasomotor symptoms associated with menopause (Climara®): Apply 0.025 mg/day patch once weekly. Adjust dose as necessary to control symptoms. Patients should be re-evaluated at 3- to 6-month intervals to determine if treatment is still necessary.

Prevention of osteoporosis in postmenopausal women:

Climara®: Apply patch once weekly; minimum effective dose 0.025 mg/day; adjust dosage based on response to therapy as indicated by biological markers and bone mineral density.

Menostar™: Apply patch once weekly. In women with a uterus, also administer a progestin for 14 days every 6-12 months.

Transdermal twice-weekly patch (Alora®, Esclim®, Estraderm®, Vivelle®):

Moderate to severe vasomotor symptoms associated with menopause, vulvar/vaginal atrophy, female hypogonadism: Titrate to lowest dose possible to control symptoms, adjusting initial dose after the first month of therapy; re-evaluate therapy at 3- to 6-month intervals to taper or discontinue medication:

Alora®, Esclim®, Estraderm®, Vivelle-Dot®: Apply 0.05 mg patch twice weekly

Vivelle®: Apply 0.0375 mg patch twice weekly

Prevention of osteoporosis in postmenopausal women:

Alora®, Vivelle®, Vivelle-Dot®: Apply 0.025 mg patch twice weekly, increase dose as necessary

Estraderm®: Apply 0.05 mg patch twice weekly

Available Dosage Forms

Cream, vaginal (Estrace®): 0.1 mg/g (12 g) [refill tube]; 0.1 mg/g (42.5 g) [tube with applicator]

Emulsion, topical, as hemihydrate (Estrasorb™): 2.5 mg/g (56s) [each pouch contains 4.35 mg estradiol hemihydrate; contents of two pouches delivers estradiol 0.05 mg/day]

Gel, topical (EstroGel®): 0.06% (93 g) [pump; delivers estradiol 0.75 mg/1.25 g; 64 doses]

Injection, oil, as cypionate (Depo®-Estradiol): 5 mg/mL (5 mL) [contains chlorobutanol; in cottonseed oil]

Injection, oil, as valerate (Delestrogen®):

10 mg/mL (5 mL) [contains chlorobutanol; in sesame oil]

20 mg/mL (5 mL) [contains benzyl alcohol; in castor oil]

40 mg/mL (5 mL) [contains benzyl alcohol; in castor oil]

Ring, vaginal, as base (Estring®): 2 mg [total estradiol 2 mg; releases 7.5 mcg/day over 90 days] (1s)

Ring, vaginal, as acetate (Femring™): 0.05 mg [total estradiol 12.4 mg; releases 0.05 mg/day over 3 months] (1s); 0.1 mg [total estradiol 24.8 mg; releases 0.1 mg/day over 3 months] (1s)

Tablet, oral, as acetate (Femtrace®): 0.45 mg, 0.9 mg, 1.8 mg

Tablet, oral, micronized: 0.5 mg, 1 mg, 2 mg

Estrace®: 0.5 mg, 1 mg, 2 mg [2 mg tablets contain tartrazine]

Gynodiol®: 0.5 mg, 1 mg, 1.5 mg, 2 mg

Tablet, vaginal, as base (Vagifem®): 25 mcg [contains lactose]

Transdermal system: 0.05 mg/24 hours (4s) [once-weekly patch]; 0.1 mg/24 hours (4s) [once-weekly patch]

Alora® [twice-weekly patch]:

0.025 mg/24 hours [9 cm², total estradiol 0.77 mg] (8s)

0.05 mg/24 hours [18 cm², total estradiol 1.5 mg] (8s, 24s)

0.075 mg/24 hours [27 cm², total estradiol 2.3 mg] (8s)

0.1 mg/24 hours [36 cm², total estradiol 3.1 mg] (8s)

Climara® [once-weekly patch]:

0.025 mg/24 hours [6.5 cm², total estradiol 2.04 mg] (4s)

0.0375 mg/24 hours [9.375 cm², total estradiol 2.85 mg] (4s)

0.05 mg/24 hours [12.5 cm², total estradiol 3.8 mg] (4s)

0.06 mg/24 hours [15 cm², total estradiol 4.55 mg] (4s)

0.075 mg/24 hours [18.75 cm², total estradiol 5.7 mg] (4s)

0.1 mg/24 hours [25 cm², total estradiol 7.6 mg] (4s)

Esclim® [twice-weekly patch]:

0.025 mg/day [11 cm², total estradiol 5 mg] (8s)

0.0375 mg/day [16.5 cm², total estradiol 7.5 mg] (8s)

0.05 mg/day [22 cm², total estradiol 10 mg] (8s)

0.075 mg/day [33 cm², total estradiol 15 mg] (8s)

0.1 mg/day [44 cm², total estradiol 20 mg] (8s)

Estraderm® [twice-weekly patch]:

0.05 mg/24 hours [10 cm², total estradiol 4 mg] (8s)

0.1 mg/24 hours [20 cm², total estradiol 8 mg] (8s)

Menostar™ [once-weekly patch]: 0.014 mg/24 hours [3.25 cm², total estradiol 1 mg] (4s)

Vivelle® [twice-weekly patch]:

0.05 mg/24 hours [14.5 cm², total estradiol 4.33 mg] (8s)

0.1 mg/24 hours [29 cm², total estradiol 8.66 mg] (8s)

Vivelle-Dot® [twice-weekly patch]:

0.025 mg/day [2.5 cm², total estradiol 0.39 mg] (8s)

0.0375 mg/day [3.75 cm², total estradiol 0.585 mg] (8s)

0.05 mg/day [5 cm², total estradiol 0.78 mg] (8s)

0.075 mg/day [7.5 cm², total estradiol 1.17 mg] (8s)

0.1 mg/day [10 cm², total estradiol 1.56 mg] (8s)

Monitoring and Teaching Issues

Physical Assessment: See Warnings/Precautions for specific use cautions. Assess potential for interactions with other pharmacological agents or herbal products patient may

(Continued)

Estradiol *(Continued)*

be taking (eg, may increase or decrease levels/effects of estradiol or increase potential for toxicity or thrombolic events; see Drug Interactions). Assess results of annual gynecological exam, therapeutic effectiveness (dependent on rationale for use), and adverse effects (eg, thromboembolism, hypertension, edema, CNS changes; see Adverse Reactions) on a regular basis during therapy. Note: Before prescribing estrogen therapy to postmenopausal women, the risks and benefits must be weighed for each patient. Women should be informed of these risks and benefits, as well as possible effects of progestin when added to estrogen therapy. Estrogens with or without progestin should be used for shortest duration possible consistent with treatment goals and periodic assessment of risk:benefit should be made. Caution patients with diabetes to monitor glucose levels closely (may impair glucose tolerance). Teach patient appropriate administration/use according to formulation (eg, vaginal, oral, topical; see Administration), possible side effects/appropriate interventions, and adverse symptoms to report, importance of frequent self-breast exams, and need for annual gynecological exam (see Patient Education). **Pregnancy risk factor X:** Determine that patient is not pregnant before starting therapy. Do not give to females of childbearing age unless patient is capable of complying with contraceptive use. Advise patient about contraceptive measures as appropriate.

Monitoring Laboratory Tests: Yearly Papanicolaou smear, mammogram. Adequate diagnostic measures, including endometrial sampling, if indicated, should be performed to rule out malignancy in all cases of undiagnosed abnormal vaginal bleeding.

Patient Education: Do not take any new medication during therapy without consulting prescriber. Use/apply exactly as directed and maintain prescribed cycles or term as prescribed. Avoid routine use of excessive alcohol (ethanol may increase the risk of breast cancer). Annual gynecologic and regular self-breast exams are important. If you have diabetes, monitor glucose levels closely (may impair glucose tolerance). You may experience nausea, vomiting or abdominal pain (small frequent meals may help); dizziness or mental depression (use caution when driving); rash; hair loss; headache; or breast pain, increased/decreased libido, or enlargement/tenderness of breasts; or difficult/painful menstrual cycles. Report unusual swelling of extremities; sudden acute pain in legs or calves, chest, or abdomen; shortness of breath; severe headache or vomiting; sudden blindness; weakness or numbness of arm or leg; unusual vaginal bleeding; yellowing of skin or eyes; unusual bruising or bleeding; or other persistent adverse reactions. You may become intolerant to wearing contact lenses, notify prescriber if this occurs. **Pregnancy/breast-feeding precautions:** Inform prescriber if you are pregnant. Do not get pregnant while taking this medication. Consult prescriber for appropriate contraceptive measures. This medication may cause fetal defects and should not be used during pregnancy. Consult prescriber if breast-feeding.

Transdermal patch: Apply to clean dry skin. Do not apply transdermal patch to breasts. Apply to trunk of body (preferably abdomen). Rotate application sites. Aerosol topical corticosteroids may reduce allergic skin reaction; report persistent skin reaction.

Intravaginal cream: Insert high in vagina. Wash hands and applicator before and after use.

Topical emulsion: Contents of two pouches are applied one at time to each thigh and rubbed into thigh and calf. Excess on hands should be applied to buttocks. Wash hands with soap and water after application. Allow skin to dry before covering legs with clothes. Do not apply sunscreen soon after or before applying emulsion. Do not apply to red or irritated skin.

Topical gel: Apply dose to one arm at the same time each day. Allow to dry for 5 minutes prior to dressing. Wash hands with soap and water after application. Do not apply to red or irritated skin. Do not apply to breast.

Dietary Considerations: Ensure adequate calcium and vitamin D intake when used for the prevention of osteoporosis.

Geriatric Considerations: Before prescribing estrogen therapy to postmenopausal women, the risks and benefits must be weighed for each patient. Data in women 80 years and older is minimal and it is unclear if reduced risk is applicable to women in this age group. Women should be informed of risks and benefits, as well as possible side effects and the return of menstrual bleeding (when cycled with a progestin), and should be involved in the prescribing options. Oral therapy may be more convenient for vaginal atrophy and urinary incontinence.

Pregnancy Risk Factor: X

Pregnancy Issues: Estrogens are not indicated for use during pregnancy or immediately postpartum. Increased risk of fetal reproductive tract disorders and other birth defects have been observed with diethylstilbestrol (DES); do not use during pregnancy.

Lactation: Enters breast milk/use caution

Breast-Feeding Issues: The AAP considers ethinyl estradiol, an estrogen derivative, to be "usually compatible" with breast-feeding. Estrogen has been shown to decrease the quantity and quality of human milk; use only if clearly needed; monitor the growth of the infant closely.

Administration

I.M.: Injection for intramuscular administration only.

Topical:

Emulsion: Apply to clean dry skin while in a sitting position. Contents of two pouches (total 3.48 g) are to be applied individually, once daily in the morning. Apply contents of first pouch to left thigh, massage into skin of left thigh and calf until thoroughly absorbed (~3 minutes). Apply excess from both hands to the buttocks. Apply contents of second pouch to the right thigh, massage into skin of right thigh and calf until thoroughly absorbed (~3 minutes). Apply excess from both hands to buttocks. Wash hands with soap and water. Allow skin to dry before covering legs with clothing. Do not apply to other areas of body. Do not apply to red or irritated skin.

Gel: Apply to clean, dry, unbroken skin at the same time each day. Apply gel to the arm, from the wrist to the shoulder. Spread gel as thinly as possible over one arm. Allow to dry for 5 minutes prior to dressing. Gel is flammable; avoid fire or flame until dry. After application, wash hands with soap and water. Prior to the first use, pump must be primed. Do not apply gel to breast.

Transdermal patch: Aerosol topical corticosteroids applied under the patch may reduce allergic reactions. Do not apply transdermal system to breasts, but place on trunk of body (preferably abdomen). Rotate application sites allowing a 1-week interval between applications at a particular site. Do not apply to oily, damaged or irritated skin; avoid waistline or other areas where tight clothing may rub the patch off. Apply patch immediately after removing from protective pouch. In general, if patch falls off, the same patch may be reapplied or a new system may be used for the remainder of the dosing interval. Swimming, bathing, or showering are not expected to affect use of the patch. Note the following exceptions:

Estraderm®: Do not apply to an area exposed to direct sunlight.

Menostar™: Swimming, bathing, or wearing patch while in a sauna have not been studied; adhesion of patch may be decreased or delivery of estradiol may be affected. Remove patch slowly after use to avoid skin irritation. If any adhesive remains on the skin after removal, first allow skin to dry for 15 minutes, then gently rub area with an oil-based cream or lotion. If patch falls off, a new patch should be applied for the remainder of the dosing interval.

Other: Vaginal ring: Exact positioning is not critical for efficacy, however, patient should not feel anything once inserted. In case of discomfort, ring should be pushed further into vagina. If ring is expelled prior to 90 days, it may be rinsed off and reinserted.

♦ **Estradiol Acetate** *see* Estradiol *on page 552*

Estradiol and Norethindrone (es tra DYE ole & nor eth IN drone)

U.S. Brand Names Activella®; CombiPatch®

Synonyms Norethindrone and Estradiol

Generic Available No

Pharmacologic Category Estrogen and Progestin Combination

Medication Safety Issues

Transdermal patch may contain conducting metal (eg, aluminum); remove patch prior to MRI.

Use Women with an intact uterus:

Tablet: Treatment of moderate-to-severe vasomotor symptoms associated with menopause; treatment of vulvar and vaginal atrophy; prophylaxis for postmenopausal osteoporosis

Transdermal patch: Treatment of moderate-to-severe vasomotor symptoms associated with menopause; treatment of vulvar and vaginal atrophy; treatment of hypoestrogenism due to hypogonadism, castration, or primary ovarian failure

Contraindications Hypersensitivity to estrogens, progestins, or any components; carcinoma of the breast; estrogen-dependent tumor; undiagnosed abnormal vaginal bleeding; history of or current thrombophlebitis or venous thromboembolic disorders (including DVT, PE); active or recent (within 1 year) arterial thromboembolic disease (eg, stroke, MI); hysterectomy; hepatic dysfunction or disease; pregnancy

Warnings/Precautions

Cardiovascular-related considerations: Estrogens with or without progestin should not be used to prevent coronary heart disease. Use caution with cardiovascular disease or dysfunction. May increase the risks of hypertension, myocardial infarction (MI), stroke, pulmonary emboli (PE), and deep vein thrombosis; incidence of these effects was shown to be significantly increased in postmenopausal women using conjugated equine estrogens (CEE) in combination with medroxyprogesterone acetate (MPA). Nonfatal MI, PE, and thrombophlebitis have also been reported in males taking high doses of CEE (eg, for prostate cancer). Estrogen compounds are generally associated with lipid effects such as increased HDL-cholesterol and decreased LDL-cholesterol. Triglycerides may also be increased; use with caution in patients with familial defects of lipoprotein metabolism. Whenever possible, estrogens should be discontinued at least 4-6 weeks prior to surgeries associated with an increased risk of thromboembolism or during periods of prolonged immobilization.

Neurological considerations: The risk of dementia may be increased in postmenopausal women; increased incidence was observed in women ≥65 years of age taking CEE in combination with MPA.

Cancer-related considerations: Unopposed estrogens may increase the risk of endometrial carcinoma in postmenopausal women. Estrogens may increase the risk of breast cancer. An increased risk of invasive breast cancer was observed in postmenopausal women using CEE in combination with MPA; a smaller increase in risk was seen with estrogen therapy alone in observational studies. An increase in abnormal mammograms has also been reported with estrogen and progestin therapy. Estrogen use may lead to severe hypercalcemia in patients with breast cancer and bone metastases; discontinue estrogen if hypercalcemia occurs.

Estrogens may cause retinal vascular thrombosis; discontinue permanently if papilledema or retinal vascular lesions are observed on examination. Use with caution in patients with diseases which may be exacerbated by fluid retention, including asthma, epilepsy, migraine, diabetes or renal dysfunction. Use with caution in patients with a history of severe hypocalcemia, SLE, hepatic hemangiomas, porphyria, endometriosis, and gallbladder disease. Use caution with history of cholestatic jaundice associated with past estrogen use or pregnancy. Safety and efficacy in pediatric patients have not been established.

Before prescribing estrogen therapy to postmenopausal women, the risks and benefits must be weighed for each patient. Women should be informed of these risks and benefits, as well as possible effects of progestin when added to estrogen therapy. Estrogens with or without progestin should be used for shortest duration possible consistent with treatment goals. Conduct periodic risk:benefit assessments.

When used solely for prevention of osteoporosis in women at significant risk, nonestrogen treatment options should be considered. When used solely for the treatment of vulvar and vaginal atrophy, topical vaginal products should be considered.

Transdermal patch may contain conducting metal (eg, aluminum); remove patch prior to MRI. (Continued)

Estradiol and Norethindrone *(Continued)*

Drug Interactions

Cytochrome P450 Effect:

Estradiol: **Substrate** of CYP1A2 (major), 2A6 (minor), 2B6 (minor), 2C8/9 (minor), 2C19 (minor), 2D6 (minor), 2E1 (minor), 3A4 (major); **Inhibits** CYP1A2 (weak); **Induces** CYP3A4 (weak)

Norethindrone: **Substrate** of CYP3A4 (major); **Induces** CYP2C19 (weak)

Nutritional/Ethanol Interactions

Ethanol: Avoid ethanol (routine use increases estrogen level and risk of breast cancer). Ethanol may also increase the risk of osteoporosis.

Food: Folic acid absorption may be decreased

Herb/Nutraceutical: St John's wort may decrease estradiol levels. Avoid black cohosh, dong quai (has estrogenic activity). Avoid red clover, saw palmetto, ginseng.

Adverse Reactions Frequency not defined.

Cardiovascular: Altered blood pressure, cardiovascular accident, edema, venous thromboembolism

Central nervous system: Dizziness, fatigue, headache, insomnia, mental depression, migraine, nervousness

Dermatologic: Chloasma, erythema multiforme, erythema nodosum, hemorrhagic eruption, hirsutism, itching, loss of scalp hair, melasma, pruritus, skin rash

Endocrine & metabolic: Breast enlargement, breast tenderness, breast pain, libido (changes in)

Gastrointestinal: Abdominal pain, bloating, changes in appetite, flatulence, gallbladder disease, nausea, pancreatitis, vomiting, weight gain/loss

Genitourinary: Alterations in frequency and flow of menses, changes in cervical secretions, cystitis-like syndrome, increased size of uterine leiomyomata, premenstrual-like syndrome, vaginal candidiasis, vaginitis

Hematologic: Aggravation of porphyria

Hepatic: Cholestatic jaundice

Local: Application site reaction (transdermal patch)

Neuromuscular & skeletal: Arthralgia, back pain, chorea, myalgia, weakness

Ocular: Intolerance to contact lenses, steeping of corneal curvature

Respiratory: Pharyngitis, pulmonary thromboembolism, rhinitis

Miscellaneous: Allergic reactions, carbohydrate intolerance, flu-like syndrome

Pharmacodynamics/Kinetics

Bioavailability: Activella®: Estradiol: 50%; Norethindrone: 100%

Time to Peak: Activella®: Estradiol: 5-8 hours

Half-Life Elimination:

Activella®: Estradiol: 12-14 hours; Norethindrone: 8-11 hours

Pharmacokinetic Note: See individual agents.

Dosing

Adults & Elderly:

Hypoestrogenism: Transdermal (patch):

Continuous combined regimen: Apply one patch twice weekly

Continuous sequential regimen: Apply estradiol-only patch for first 14 days of cycle, followed by one CombiPatch® applied twice weekly for the remaining 14 days of a 28-day cycle.

Osteoporosis, prevention in postmenopausal females (Activella®): Oral: 1 tablet daily

Menopause (moderate to severe vasomotor symptoms); vulvar and vaginal atrophy:

Oral (Activella®): 1 tablet daily

Transdermal (patch):

Continuous combined regimen: Apply one patch twice weekly

Continuous sequential regimen: Apply estradiol-only patch for first 14 days of cycle, followed by one CombiPatch® applied twice weekly for the remaining 14 days of a 28-day cycle.

Transdermal patch, combination pack (product-specific dosing for Canadian formulation):

Estalis®: Continuous combined regimen: Apply a new patch twice weekly during a 28-day cycle

Estalis-Sequi®: Continuous sequential regimen: Apply estradiol-only patch (Vivelle®) for first 14 days, followed by one Estalis® patch applied twice weekly during the last 14 days of a 28-day cycle

Note: In women previously receiving oral estrogens, initiate upon reappearance of menopausal symptoms following discontinuation of oral therapy.

Available Dosage Forms [CAN] = Canadian brand name

Combination pack (Estalis-Sequi® [CAN; not available in U.S.]):

140/50:

Transdermal system (Vivelle®): Estradiol 50 mcg per day (4s) [14.5 sq cm; total estradiol 4.33 mg]

Transdermal system (Estalis®): Norethindrone acetate 140 mcg and estradiol 50 mcg per day (4s) [9 sq cm; total norethindrone acetate 2.7 mg, total estradiol 0.62 mg; not available in U.S.]

250/50:

Transdermal system (Vivelle®): Estradiol 50 mcg per day (4s) [14.5 sq cm; total estradiol 4.33 mg]

Transdermal system (Estalis®): Norethindrone acetate 250 mcg and estradiol 50 mcg per day (4s) [16 sq cm; total norethindrone acetate 4.8 mg, total estradiol 0.51 mg; not available in U.S.]

Tablet (Activella®): Estradiol 1 mg and norethindrone acetate 0.5 mg (28s)

Transdermal system:

CombiPatch®:

0.05/0.14: Estradiol 0.05 mg and norethindrone acetate 0.14 mg per day (8s) [9 sq cm]

0.05/0.25: Estradiol 0.05 mg and norethindrone acetate 0.25 mg per day (8s) [16 sq cm]

Estalis® [CAN]:

140/50: Norethindrone acetate 140 mcg and estradiol 50 mcg per day (8s) [9 sq cm; total norethindrone acetate 2.7 mg, total estradiol 0.62 mg; not available in U.S.]

250/50 Norethindrone acetate 250 mcg and estradiol 50 mcg per day (8s) [16 sq cm; total norethindrone acetate 4.8 mg, total estradiol 0.51 mg; not available in U.S.]

Monitoring and Teaching Issues

Physical Assessment: Assess potential for interactions with other prescriptions, OTC medications, or herbal products patient may be taking. Assess results of annual gynecological exam (eg, Pap smear, mammogram), therapeutic effectiveness (dependent on rationale for use), and adverse effects (eg, thromboembolism, hypertension, edema, CNS changes) on a regular basis during therapy. **Note:** Before prescribing estrogen therapy to postmenopausal women, the risks and benefits must be weighed for each patient. Women should be informed of these risks and benefits, as well as possible effects of progestin when added to estrogen therapy. Caution patients with diabetes to monitor glucose levels closely (may impair glucose tolerance). Teach patient appropriate administration/use according to formulation, possible side effects, interventions to reduce side effects, adverse symptoms to report, importance of frequent self-breast exams, and need for annual gynecological exam. **Pregnancy risk factor X:** Determine that patient is not pregnant before starting therapy.

Patient Education: Do not take any new medication during therapy without consulting prescriber. Use/apply exactly as directed and maintain prescribed cycles or term as prescribed. Avoid routine use of alcohol (ethanol may increase the risk of breast cancer or osteoporosis). Annual gynecologic and regular self-breast exams are important. If you have diabetes, monitor glucose levels closely (may impair glucose tolerance). You may experience nausea, vomiting or abdominal pain (small frequent meals may help); dizziness or mental depression (use caution when driving); rash; hair loss; headache; or breast pain, increased/decreased libido, or enlargement/tenderness of breasts. difficult/painful menstrual cycles. Report significant swelling of extremities; sudden acute pain in legs or calves, chest, or abdomen; shortness of breath; severe headache or vomiting; sudden blindness; weakness or numbness of arm or leg; unusual vaginal bleeding; yellowing of skin or eyes; unusual bruising or bleeding, or other persistent adverse reactions. You may become intolerant to wearing contact lenses, notify prescriber if this occurs. **Pregnancy/breast-feeding precautions:** Inform prescriber if you are pregnant. Do not get pregnant while taking this medication. This medication may cause fetal defects and should not be used during pregnancy. Consult prescriber if breast-feeding.

Pregnancy Risk Factor: X

Pregnancy Issues: Estrogens/progestins should not be used during pregnancy.

Estrogens: Increased risk of fetal reproductive tract disorders and other birth defects; do not use during pregnancy.

Progestins: Associated with fetal genital abnormalities when used during the 1st trimester; not recommended for use during pregnancy.

Lactation: Enters breast milk/use caution

Administration

Other: Transdermal patch: Apply to clean dry skin. Do not apply transdermal patch to breasts; apply to lower abdomen, avoiding waistline. Rotate application sites.

Related Information

Estradiol *on page 552*

Norethindrone *on page 1096*

♦ **Estradiol Cypionate** *see* Estradiol *on page 552*

♦ **Estradiol Hemihydrate** *see* Estradiol *on page 552*

♦ **Estradiol Transdermal** *see* Estradiol *on page 552*

♦ **Estradiol Valerate** *see* Estradiol *on page 552*

Estramustine (es tra MUS teen)

U.S. Brand Names Emcyt®

Synonyms Estramustine Phosphate Sodium; NSC-89199

Generic Available No

Pharmacologic Category Antineoplastic Agent, Alkylating Agent; Antineoplastic Agent, Hormone; Antineoplastic Agent, Hormone (Estrogen/Nitrogen Mustard)

Medication Safety Issues

Sound-alike/look-alike issues:

Emcyt® may be confused with Eryc®

Use Palliative treatment of prostatic carcinoma (progressive or metastatic)

Mechanism of Action/Effect Mechanism is not completely clear. It appears to bind to microtubule proteins, preventing normal tubulin function. The antitumor effect may be due solely to an estrogenic effect. Estramustine causes a marked decrease in plasma testosterone and an increase in estrogen levels.

Contraindications Hypersensitivity to estramustine or any component, estradiol or nitrogen mustard; active thrombophlebitis or thromboembolic disorders

Warnings/Precautions The U.S. Food and Drug Administration (FDA) currently recommends that procedures for proper handling and disposal of antineoplastic agents be considered. Glucose tolerance may be decreased; elevated blood pressure may occur. Exacerbation of peripheral edema or congestive heart disease may occur. Use with caution in patients with impaired liver function, renal insufficiency, metabolic bone diseases, or history of cardiovascular disease (eg, thrombophlebitis, thrombosis, or thromboembolic disease). Use caution in patients with prostate cancer and osteoblastic metastases due to increased risk of hypocalcemia.

Drug Interactions

Decreased Effect: Milk products and calcium-rich foods/drugs may impair the oral absorption of estramustine phosphate sodium.

Nutritional/Ethanol Interactions Food: Estramustine serum levels may be decreased if taken with dairy products.

(Continued)

Estramustine (Continued)

Adverse Reactions
>10%:

Cardiovascular: Impaired arterial circulation; ischemic heart disease; venous thromboembolism; cardiac decompensation (58%), about 50% of complications occur within the first 2 months of therapy, 85% occur within the first year; edema

Endocrine & metabolic: Sodium and water retention, gynecomastia, breast tenderness, libido decreased

Gastrointestinal: Nausea, vomiting, may be dose-limiting

Hematologic: Thrombocytopenia

Local: Thrombophlebitis (nearly 100% with I.V. administration)

Respiratory: Dyspnea

1% to 10%:

Cardiovascular: Myocardial infarction

Central nervous system: Insomnia, lethargy

Gastrointestinal: Diarrhea, anorexia, flatulence

Hematologic: Leukopenia

Hepatic: Serum transaminases increased, jaundice

Neuromuscular & skeletal: Leg cramps

Respiratory: Pulmonary embolism

Overdosage/Toxicology Symptoms of overdose include nausea, vomiting, and myelosuppression. There are no known antidotes; treatment is symptomatic and supportive.

Pharmacodynamics/Kinetics
Absorption: Oral: 75%

Time to Peak: Serum: 2-3 hours

Half-Life Elimination: Terminal: 20-24 hours

Metabolism: GI tract: Initial dephosphorylation; Hepatic: Oxidation and hydrolysis; metabolites include estramustine, estrone, estradiol, nitrogen mustard

Excretion: Feces (2.9% to 4.8% as unchanged drug)

Dosing
Adults & Elderly: Refer to individual protocols.

Prostate carcinoma: Oral: 10-16 mg/kg/day (14 mg/kg/day is most common) or 140 mg 4 times/day (some patients have been maintained for >3 years on therapy) Refer to individual protocols.

Available Dosage Forms Capsule, as phosphate sodium: 140 mg

Monitoring and Teaching Issues
Physical Assessment: See Warnings/Precautions for use cautions (eg, impaired renal or hepatic function, history of CV disease, CHD). Assess potential for interactions with other pharmacological agents patient may be taking (see Drug Interactions). Assess results of laboratory tests, therapeutic effectiveness, and adverse response on a regular basis during therapy (eg, hypertension, CNS changes, thromboembolism; see Adverse Reactions). Teach patient appropriate use, possible side effects/appropriate interventions, and adverse symptoms to report (see Patient Education).

Monitoring Laboratory Tests: Serum calcium, liver function tests

Patient Education: Do not take any new medication during therapy without consulting prescriber. It may take several weeks to manifest effects of this medication. Store capsules in refrigerator. Do not take with milk or milk products. Preferable to take on empty stomach, 1 hour before or 2 hours after meals. May cause nausea or vomiting (small frequent meals, frequent mouth care, chewing gum, or sucking lozenges may help); flatulence; diarrhea (buttermilk, boiled milk, or yogurt); decreased libido (reversible); or breast tenderness or enlargement. Report sudden acute pain or cramping in legs or calves, chest pain, shortness of breath, weakness or numbness of arms or legs, respiratory difficulty, or edema (increased weight, swelling of legs or feet). **Pregnancy/breast-feeding precautions:** Male: Do not cause a female to become pregnant. Male/female: Consult prescriber for instruction on appropriate barrier contraceptive measures. This drug may cause severe fetal defects. Do not breast-feed.

Dietary Considerations: Should be taken at least 1 hour before or 2 hours after eating.

Pregnancy Risk Factor: C

Lactation: Excretion in breast milk unknown/contraindicated

Administration
Oral: Administer at least 1 hour before or 2 hours after eating.

Storage: Refrigerate at 2°C to 8°C (36°F to 46°F). Capsules may be stored outside of refrigerator for up to 24-48 hours without affecting potency.

- ◆ **Estramustine Phosphate Sodium** see Estramustine on page 559
- ◆ **Estrasorb™** see Estradiol on page 552
- ◆ **Estring®** see Estradiol on page 552
- ◆ **EstroGel®** see Estradiol on page 552
- ◆ **Estrogenic Substances, Conjugated** see Estrogens (Conjugated/Equine) on page 563

Estrogens (Conjugated A/Synthetic)
(ES troe jenz, KON joo gate ed, aye, sin THET ik)

U.S. Brand Names Cenestin®

Generic Available No

Pharmacologic Category Estrogen Derivative

Medication Safety Issues

Sound-alike/look-alike issues:

Cenestin® may be confused with Senexon®

Use Treatment of moderate to severe vasomotor symptoms of menopause; treatment of vulvar and vaginal atrophy

Mechanism of Action/Effect Estrogens modulate the pituitary secretion of gonadotropins, luteinizing hormone, and follicle-stimulating hormone through a negative feedback system; estrogen replacement reduces elevated levels of these hormones in postmenopausal women

Contraindications Hypersensitivity to estrogens or any component of the formulation; undiagnosed abnormal vaginal bleeding; history of or current thrombophlebitis or venous thromboembolic disorders (including DVT, PE); active or recent (within 1 year) arterial thromboembolic disease (eg, stroke, MI); carcinoma of the breast; estrogen-dependent tumor; hepatic dysfunction or disease; pregnancy

Warnings/Precautions

Cardiovascular-related considerations: Estrogens with or without progestin should not be used to prevent coronary heart disease. Use caution with cardiovascular disease or dysfunction. May increase the risks of hypertension, myocardial infarction (MI), stroke, pulmonary emboli (PE), and deep vein thrombosis; incidence of these effects was shown to be significantly increased in postmenopausal women using conjugated equine estrogens (CEE) in combination with medroxyprogesterone acetate (MPA). Nonfatal MI, PE, and thrombophlebitis have also been reported in males taking high doses of CEE (eg, for prostate cancer). Estrogen compounds are generally associated with lipid effects such as increased HDL-cholesterol and decreased LDL-cholesterol. Triglycerides may also be increased; use with caution in patients with familial defects of lipoprotein metabolism. Whenever possible, estrogens should be discontinued at least 4-6 weeks prior to surgeries associated with an increased risk of thromboembolism or during periods of prolonged immobilization.

Neurological considerations: The risk of dementia may be increased in postmenopausal women; increased incidence was observed in women ≥65 years of age taking CEE in combination with MPA.

Cancer-related considerations: Unopposed estrogens may increase the risk of endometrial carcinoma in postmenopausal women. Estrogens may increase the risk of breast cancer. An increased risk of invasive breast cancer was observed in postmenopausal women using CEE in combination with MPA; a smaller increase in risk was seen with estrogen therapy alone in observational studies. An increase in abnormal mammograms has also been reported with estrogen and progestin therapy. Estrogen use may lead to severe hypercalcemia in patients with breast cancer and bone metastases; discontinue estrogen if hypercalcemia occurs.

Estrogens may cause retinal vascular thrombosis; discontinue permanently if papilledema or retinal vascular lesions are observed on examination. Use with caution in patients with diseases which may be exacerbated by fluid retention, including asthma, epilepsy, migraine, diabetes or renal dysfunction. Use with caution in patients with a history of severe hypocalcemia, SLE, hepatic hemangiomas, porphyria, endometriosis, and gallbladder disease. Use caution with history of cholestatic jaundice associated with past estrogen use or pregnancy. Safety and efficacy in pediatric patients have not been established. Prior to puberty, estrogens may cause premature closure of the epiphyses, premature breast development in girls or gynecomastia in boys. Vaginal bleeding and vaginal cornification may also be induced in girls.

Before prescribing estrogen therapy to postmenopausal women, the risks and benefits must be weighed for each patient. Women should be informed of these risks and benefits, as well as possible effects of progestin when added to estrogen therapy. Estrogens with or without progestin should be used for shortest duration possible consistent with treatment goals. Conduct periodic risk:benefit assessments.

When used solely for prevention of osteoporosis in women at significant risk, nonestrogen treatment options should be considered. When used solely for the treatment of vulvar and vaginal atrophy, topical vaginal products should be considered.

Drug Interactions

Cytochrome P450 Effect:

Based on estradiol and estrone: **Substrate** of CYP1A2 (major), 2A6 (minor), 2B6 (minor), 2C8/9 (minor), 2C19 (minor), 2D6 (minor), 2E1 (minor), 3A4 (major); **Inhibits** CYP1A2 (weak); **Induces** CYP3A4 (weak)

Decreased Effect: CYP1A2 inducers may decrease the levels/effects of estrogens; example inducers include aminoglutethimide, carbamazepine, phenobarbital, and rifampin. CYP3A4 inducers may decrease the levels/effects of estrogen; example inducers include aminoglutethimide, carbamazepine, nafcillin, nevirapine, phenobarbital, phenytoin, and rifamycins.

Increased Effect/Toxicity: CYP3A4 enzyme inhibitors may increase estrogen plasma concentrations leading to increased incidence of adverse effects; examples of CYP3A4 enzyme inhibitors include clarithromycin, erythromycin, itraconazole, ketoconazole, and ritonavir. Anticoagulants increase the potential for thromboembolic events Estrogens may enhance the effects of hydrocortisone and prednisone

Nutritional/Ethanol Interactions

Ethanol: Avoid ethanol (routine use increases estrogen level and risk of breast cancer).

Food: Grapefruit juice may increase estrogen levels, leading to increased adverse effects.

Herb/Nutraceutical: St John's wort may decrease levels. Avoid black cohosh, dong quai (has estrogenic activity). Avoid red clover, saw palmetto, ginseng (due to potential hormonal effects).

Lab Interactions Pathologist should be advised of estrogen/progesterone therapy when specimens are submitted. Reduced response to metyrapone test observed with conjugated estrogens (equine).

Adverse Reactions Adverse effects associated with estrogen therapy; frequency not defined

Cardiovascular: Edema, hypertension, venous thromboembolism

Central nervous system: Dizziness, headache, mental depression, migraine

Dermatologic: Chloasma, erythema multiforme, erythema nodosum, hemorrhagic eruption, hirsutism, loss of scalp hair, melasma

Endocrine & metabolic: Breast enlargement, breast tenderness, libido (changes in), thyroid-binding globulin increased, total thyroid hormone (T_4) increased, serum triglycerides/phospholipids increased, HDL-cholesterol increased, LDL-cholesterol decreased, impaired glucose tolerance, hypercalcemia

(Continued)

Estrogens (Conjugated A/Synthetic) *(Continued)*

Gastrointestinal: Abdominal cramps, bloating, cholecystitis, cholelithiasis, gallbladder disease, nausea, pancreatitis, vomiting, weight gain/loss

Genitourinary: Alterations in frequency and flow of menses, changes in cervical secretions, endometrial cancer, increased size of uterine leiomyomata, vaginal candidiasis

Hematologic: Aggravation of porphyria, antithrombin III and antifactor Xa decreased, levels of fibrinogen decreased, platelet aggregability and platelet count increased; prothrombin and factors VII, VIII, IX, X increased

Hepatic: Cholestatic jaundice

Neuromuscular & skeletal: Chorea

Ocular: Intolerance to contact lenses, steeping of corneal curvature

Respiratory: Pulmonary thromboembolism

Miscellaneous: Carbohydrate intolerance

Overdosage/Toxicology Symptoms of overdose include nausea and vomiting; withdrawal bleeding may occur in females. Toxicity is unlikely following single exposures of excessive doses, any treatment following emesis and charcoal administration should be supportive and symptomatic.

Pharmacodynamics/Kinetics

Absorption: Readily absorbed

Time to Peak: 4-16 hours

Protein Binding: Sex hormone-binding globulin (SHBG) and albumin

Metabolism: Hepatic to metabolites

Excretion: Urine

Dosing

Adults: The lowest dose that will control symptoms should be used. Medication should be discontinued as soon as possible.

Menopause, moderate to severe vasomotor symptoms: Oral: 0.45 mg/day; may be titrated up to 1.25 mg/day; attempts to discontinue medication should be made at 3- to 6-month intervals

Vulvar and vaginal atrophy: Oral: 0.3 mg/day

Elderly: Refer to adult dosing. A higher incidence of stroke and invasive breast cancer were observed in women >75 years in a WHI substudy using conjugated equine estrogen.

Available Dosage Forms Tablet: 0.3 mg, 0.45 mg, 0.625 mg, 0.9 mg, 1.25 mg

Monitoring and Teaching Issues

Physical Assessment: See Warnings/Precautions for specific use cautions. Assess potential for interactions with other pharmacological agents or herbal products patient may be taking (eg, increased potential for decreased levels/effects or increased potential for toxicity or thrombotic events; see Drug Interactions). Assess results of annual gynecological exam, therapeutic effectiveness (dependent on rationale for use), and adverse effects (eg, thromboembolism, hypertension, edema, CNS changes; see Adverse Reactions) on a regular basis during therapy. **Note:** Before prescribing estrogen therapy to postmenopausal women, the risks and benefits must be weighed for each patient. Women should be informed of these risks and benefits, as well as possible effects of progestin when added to estrogen therapy. Estrogens with or without progestin should be used for shortest duration possible consistent with treatment goals and periodic assessment of risk:benefit should be made. Caution patients with diabetes to monitor glucose levels closely (may impair glucose tolerance). Teach patient appropriate use, possible side effects/appropriate interventions, and adverse symptoms to report, importance of frequent self-breast exams, and need for annual gynecological exam (see Patient Education). **Pregnancy risk factor X:** Determine that patient is not pregnant before starting therapy. Do not give to females of childbearing age unless patient is capable of complying with contraceptive use. Advise patient about contraceptive measures as appropriate.

Monitoring Laboratory Tests: Yearly Papanicolaou smear, mammogram. Adequate diagnostic measures, including endometrial sampling, if indicated, should be performed to rule out malignancy in all cases of undiagnosed abnormal vaginal bleeding.

Patient Education: Do not take any new medication during therapy without consulting prescriber. Take exactly as directed and maintain prescribed cycles or term as prescribed. Avoid routine use of alcohol (ethanol may increase the risk of breast cancer). Annual gynecologic and regular self-breast exams are important. If you have diabetes, monitor glucose levels closely (may impair glucose tolerance). You may experience nausea, vomiting or abdominal pain (small frequent meals may help); dizziness or mental depression (use caution when driving); rash; hair loss; headache; breast pain, increased/decreased libido, or enlargement/tenderness of breasts; or difficult/painful menstrual cycles. Report significant swelling of extremities; sudden acute pain in legs, calves, chest, or abdomen; shortness of breath; severe headache or vomiting; sudden blindness; weakness or numbness of arm or leg; unusual vaginal bleeding; yellowing of skin or eyes; unusual bruising or bleeding, or other persistent adverse reactions. You may become intolerant to wearing contact lenses, notify prescriber if this occurs. **Pregnancy/breast-feeding precautions:** Inform prescriber if you are pregnant. Do not get pregnant while taking this medication. Consult prescriber for appropriate contraceptive measures. This medication may cause fetal defects and should not be used during pregnancy. Consult prescriber if breast-feeding.

Pregnancy Risk Factor: X

Lactation: Enters breast milk/use caution

Administration

Storage: Store at room temperature of 25°C (77°F).

Additional Information Not biologically equivalent to conjugated estrogens from equine source. Contains 9 unique estrogenic compounds (equine source contains at least 10 active estrogenic compounds).

The use of estrogens for the prevention of other chronic diseases, as well as their potential negative effects on women's health, has been debated. Data published from the Women's Health Initiative (WHI) has provided some additional insight on this controversial topic. In the

WHI, one arm of the study compared postmenopausal women with an intact uterus using CEE 0.625 mg in combination with MPA 2.5 mg daily, versus placebo. This arm of the study was stopped in 2002. In March, 2004, it was announced that the arm of the study comparing placebo to CEE alone in postmenopausal women without a uterus was ended.

Based on preliminary findings, the FDA has requested labeling changes be made to estrogen products used in postmenopausal women. The updates include information from the Women's Health Initiative Memory Study (WHIMS) as well as information collected from the completed CEE/MPA arm of the WHI study. Complete analysis of the WHI data is forthcoming, and will include all information collected through February, 2004.

Related Information

Pharmacotherapy of Urinary Incontinence on page 1858

Estrogens (Conjugated/Equine) (ES troe jenz KON joo gate ed, EE kwine)

U.S. Brand Names Premarin®

Synonyms CEE; C.E.S.; Estrogenic Substances, Conjugated

Generic Available No

Pharmacologic Category Estrogen Derivative

Medication Safety Issues

Sound-alike/look-alike issues:

Premarin® may be confused with Primaxin®, Provera®, Remeron®

Use Treatment of moderate to severe vasomotor symptoms associated with menopause; treatment of vulvar and vaginal atrophy; hypoestrogenism (due to hypogonadism, castration, or primary ovarian failure); prostatic cancer (palliation); breast cancer (palliation); osteoporosis (prophylaxis, postmenopausal women at significant risk only); abnormal uterine bleeding

Unlabeled/Investigational Use Uremic bleeding

Mechanism of Action/Effect Estrogens modulate the pituitary secretion of gonadotropins, luteinizing hormone, and follicle-stimulating hormone through a negative feedback system; estrogen replacement reduces elevated levels of these hormones in postmenopausal women

Contraindications Hypersensitivity to estrogens or any component of the formulation; undiagnosed abnormal vaginal bleeding; history of or current thrombophlebitis or venous thromboembolic disorders (including DVT, PE); active or recent (within 1 year) arterial thromboembolic disease (eg, stroke, MI); carcinoma of the breast (except in appropriately selected patients being treated for metastatic disease); estrogen-dependent tumor; hepatic dysfunction or disease; pregnancy

Warnings/Precautions

Cardiovascular-related considerations: Estrogens with or without progestin should not be used to prevent coronary heart disease. Use caution with cardiovascular disease or dysfunction. May increase the risks of hypertension, myocardial infarction (MI), stroke, pulmonary emboli (PE), and deep vein thrombosis; incidence of these effects was shown to be significantly increased in postmenopausal women using conjugated equine estrogens (CEE) in combination with medroxyprogesterone acetate (MPA). Nonfatal MI, PE, and thrombophlebitis have also been reported in males taking high doses of CEE (eg, for prostate cancer). Estrogen compounds are generally associated with lipid effects such as increased HDL-cholesterol and decreased LDL-cholesterol. Triglycerides may also be increased; use with caution in patients with familial defects of lipoprotein metabolism. Whenever possible, estrogens should be discontinued at least 4-6 weeks prior to surgeries associated with an increased risk of thromboembolism or during periods of prolonged immobilization.

Neurological considerations: The risk of dementia may be increased in postmenopausal women; increased incidence was observed in women ≥65 years of age taking CEE in combination with MPA.

Cancer-related considerations: Unopposed estrogens may increase the risk of endometrial carcinoma in postmenopausal women. Estrogens may increase the risk of breast cancer. An increased risk of invasive breast cancer was observed in postmenopausal women using CEE in combination with MPA; a smaller increase in risk was seen with estrogen therapy alone in observational studies. An increase in abnormal mammograms has also been reported with estrogen and progestin therapy. Estrogen use may lead to severe hypercalcemia in patients with breast cancer and bone metastases; discontinue estrogen if hypercalcemia occurs.

Estrogens may cause retinal vascular thrombosis; discontinue permanently if papilledema or retinal vascular lesions are observed on examination. Use with caution in patients with diseases which may be exacerbated by fluid retention, including asthma, epilepsy, migraine, diabetes or renal dysfunction. Use with caution in patients with a history of severe hypocalcemia, SLE, hepatic hemangiomas, porphyria, endometriosis, and gallbladder disease. Use caution with history of cholestatic jaundice associated with past estrogen use or pregnancy. Safety and efficacy in pediatric patients have not been established. Prior to puberty, estrogens may cause premature closure of the epiphyses, premature breast development in girls or gynecomastia in boys. Vaginal bleeding and vaginal cornification may also be induced in girls.

Before prescribing estrogen therapy to postmenopausal women, the risks and benefits must be weighed for each patient. Women should be informed of these risks and benefits, as well as possible effects of progestin when added to estrogen therapy. Estrogens with or without progestin should be used for shortest duration possible consistent with treatment goals. Conduct periodic risk:benefit assessments.

When used solely for prevention of osteoporosis in women at significant risk, nonestrogen treatment options should be considered. When used solely for the treatment of vulvar and vaginal atrophy, topical vaginal products should be considered. Use caution applying topical products to severely atrophic vaginal mucosa.
(Continued)

Estrogens (Conjugated/Equine) *(Continued)*

Drug Interactions

Cytochrome P450 Effect:
Based on estradiol and estrone: **Substrate** of CYP1A2 (major), 2A6 (minor), 2B6 (minor), 2C8/9 (minor), 2C19 (minor), 2D6 (minor), 2E1 (minor), 3A4 (major); Inhibits CYP1A2 (weak); Induces CYP3A4 (weak)

Decreased Effect: CYP1A2 inducers may decrease the levels/effects of estrogens; example inducers include aminoglutethimide, carbamazepine, phenobarbital, and rifampin. CYP3A4 inducers may decrease the levels/effects of estrogens; example inducers include aminoglutethimide, carbamazepine, nafcillin, nevirapine, phenobarbital, phenytoin, and rifamycins.

Increased Effect/Toxicity: Hydrocortisone taken with estrogen may cause corticosteroid-induced toxicity. Increased potential for thromboembolic events with anticoagulants.

Nutritional/Ethanol Interactions
Ethanol: Avoid ethanol (routine use increases estrogen level and risk of breast cancer). Ethanol may also increase the risk of osteoporosis.

Food: Folic acid absorption may be decreased.

Herb/Nutraceutical: St John's wort may decrease levels. Avoid black cohosh, dong quai (has estrogenic activity). Avoid red clover, saw palmetto, ginseng (due to potential hormonal effects).

Lab Interactions Increased Prothrombin and factors VII, VIII, IX, X; increased platelet aggregability, thyroid-binding globulin, total thyroid hormone (T_4), serum triglycerides/phospholipids; decreased antithrombin III, serum folate concentration

Adverse Reactions
Note: Percentages reported in postmenopausal women.

>10%:
Central nervous system: Headache (26% to 32%; placebo 28%)
Endocrine & metabolic: Breast pain (7% to 12%; placebo 9%)
Gastrointestinal: Abdominal pain (15% to 17%)
Genitourinary: Vaginal hemorrhage (2% to 14%)
Neuromuscular & skeletal: Back pain (13% to 14%)

1% to 10%:
Central nervous system: Nervousness (2% to 5%)
Endocrine & metabolic: Leukorrhea (4% to 7%)
Gastrointestinal: Flatulence (6% to 7%)
Genitourinary: Vaginitis (5% to 7%), vaginal moniliasis (5% to 6%)
Neuromuscular & skeletal: Weakness (7% to 8%), leg cramps (3% to 7%)

In addition, the following have been reported with estrogen and/or progestin therapy:
Cardiovascular: Edema, hypertension, MI, stroke, venous thromboembolism
Central nervous system: Dizziness, epilepsy exacerbation, headache, irritability, mental depression, migraine, mood disturbances, nervousness
Dermatologic: Angioedema, chloasma, erythema multiforme, erythema nodosum, hemorrhagic eruption, hirsutism, loss of scalp hair, melasma, pruritus, rash, urticaria
Endocrine & metabolic: Breast cancer, breast enlargement, breast tenderness, libido (changes in), increased thyroid-binding globulin, increased total thyroid hormone (T_4), increased serum triglycerides/phospholipids, increased HDL-cholesterol, decreased LDL-cholesterol, impaired glucose tolerance, hypercalcemia, hypocalcemia
Gastrointestinal: Abdominal cramps, bloating, cholecystitis, cholelithiasis, gallbladder disease, nausea, pancreatitis, vomiting, weight gain/loss
Genitourinary: Alterations in frequency and flow of menses, changes in cervical secretions, endometrial cancer, endometrial hyperplasia, increased size of uterine leiomyomata, vaginal candidiasis
Hematologic: Aggravation of porphyria, decreased antithrombin III and antifactor Xa, increased levels of fibrinogen, increased platelet aggregability and platelet count; increased prothrombin and factors VII, VIII, IX, X
Hepatic: Cholestatic jaundice, hepatic hemangiomas enlarged
Neuromuscular & skeletal: Arthralgias, chorea, leg cramps
Local: Thrombophlebitis
Ocular: Intolerance to contact lenses, retinal vascular thrombosis, steeping of corneal curvature
Respiratory: Asthma exacerbation, pulmonary thromboembolism
Miscellaneous: Anaphylactoid/anaphylactic reactions, carbohydrate intolerance

Overdosage/Toxicology Toxicity is unlikely following single exposures of excessive doses, any treatment following emesis and charcoal administration should be supportive and symptomatic. Effects noted after large doses include headache, nausea, and vomiting. Bleeding may occur in females.

Pharmacodynamics/Kinetics

Absorption: Well absorbed

Metabolism: Hepatic via CYP3A4; estradiol is converted to estrone and estriol; also undergoes enterohepatic recirculation; estrone sulfite is the main metabolite in postmenopausal women

Excretion: Urine (primarily estrone, also as estradiol, estriol and conjugates)

Dosing

Adults:

Breast cancer palliation, metastatic disease in selected patients (male and female): Oral: 10 mg 3 times/day for at least 3 months

Uremic bleeding (unlabeled use): I.V.: 0.6 mg/kg/day for 5 days

Androgen-dependent prostate cancer (males): Oral: 1.25-2.5 mg 3 times/day

Prevention of osteoporosis in postmenopausal women: Oral: Initial: 0.3 mg/day, cyclically* or daily, depending on medical assessment of patient. Dose may be adjusted based on bone mineral density and clinical response. The lowest effective dose should be used.

Menopause (moderate to severe vasomotor symptoms): Oral: Initial: 0.3 mg/day. May be given cyclically* or daily, depending on medical assessment of patient. The lowest dose that will control symptoms should be used. Medication should be discontinued as soon as possible.

Vulvar and vaginal atrophy: Oral: Initial: 0.3 mg/day. The lowest dose that will control symptoms should be used. May be given cyclically* or daily, depending on medical assessment of patient. Medication should be discontinued as soon as possible.
Vaginal cream: Intravaginal: $^1/_2$ to 2 g/day given cyclically*

Female hypogonadism: Oral: 0.3-0.625 mg/day given cyclically*; dose may be titrated in 6- to 12-month intervals; progestin treatment should be added to maintain bone mineral density once skeletal maturity is achieved.

Female castration, primary ovarian failure: Oral: 1.25 mg/day given cyclically*; adjust according to severity of symptoms and patient response. For maintenance, adjust to the lowest effective dose.

Abnormal uterine bleeding:
Acute/heavy bleeding:
  Oral (unlabeled route): 1.25 mg, may repeat every 4 hours for 24 hours, followed by 1.25 mg once daily for 7-10 days
  I.M., I.V.: 25 mg, may repeat in 6-12 hours if needed
  Note: Treatment should be followed by a low-dose oral contraceptive; medroxyprogesterone acetate along with or following estrogen therapy can also be given
Nonacute/lesser bleeding: Oral (unlabeled route): 1.25 mg once daily for 7-10 days

*Cyclic administration: Either 3 weeks on, 1 week off or 25 days on, 5 days off
Elderly: Refer to adult dosing. A higher incidence of stroke and breast cancer was observed in women >75 years in a WHI substudy.
Pediatrics: Adolescents: Refer to adult dosing.
Hepatic Impairment:
  Mild to moderate liver impairment: Dosage reduction of estrogens is recommended.
  Severe liver impairment: **Not recommended.**
Available Dosage Forms
Cream, vaginal: 0.625 mg/g (42.5 g)
Injection, powder for reconstitution: 25 mg [contains lactose 200 mg; diluent contains benzyl alcohol]
Tablet: 0.3 mg, 0.45 mg, 0.625 mg, 0.9 mg, 1.25 mg
Monitoring and Teaching Issues
Physical Assessment: See Warnings/Precautions for specific use cautions. Assess potential for interactions with other pharmacological agents or herbal products patient may be taking (eg, increased potential for decreased levels/effects or increased potential for toxicity or thrombolic events; see Drug Interactions). Assess results of annual gynecological exam, therapeutic effectiveness (dependent on rationale for use), and adverse effects (eg, thromboembolism, hypertension, edema, CNS changes; see Adverse Reactions) on a regular basis during therapy. **Note:** Before prescribing estrogen therapy to postmenopausal women, the risks and benefits must be weighed for each patient. Women should be informed of these risks and benefits, as well as possible effects of progestin when added to estrogen therapy. Estrogens with or without progestin should be used for shortest duration possible consistent with treatment goals and periodic assessment of risk:benefit should be made. Caution patients with diabetes to monitor glucose levels closely (may impair glucose tolerance). Teach patient appropriate administration/use according to formulation (eg, oral, vaginal; see Administration), possible side effects/appropriate interventions, and adverse symptoms to report, importance of frequent self-breast exams, and need for annual gynecological exam (see Patient Education). **Pregnancy risk factor X:** Determine that patient is not pregnant before starting therapy. Do not give to females of childbearing age unless patient is capable of complying with contraceptive use. Advise patient about contraceptive measures as appropriate.

Monitoring Laboratory Tests: Yearly physical examination that includes blood pressure and Papanicolaou smear. Adequate diagnostic measures, including endometrial sampling, if indicated, should be performed to rule out malignancy in all cases of undiagnosed abnormal vaginal bleeding.

Patient Education: Do not take any new medication during therapy without consulting prescriber. Use/apply exactly as directed and maintain prescribed cycles or term as prescribed. Avoid routine use of alcohol (ethanol may increase the risk of breast cancer). Annual gynecologic and regular self-breast exams are important. If you have diabetes, monitor glucose levels closely (may impair glucose tolerance). You may experience nausea, vomiting or abdominal pain (small frequent meals may help); dizziness or mental depression (use caution when driving); rash; hair loss; headache; breast pain, increased/decreased libido, or enlargement/tenderness of breasts; or difficult/painful menstrual cycles. Report significant swelling of extremities; sudden acute pain in legs, calves, chest, or abdomen; shortness of breath; severe headache or vomiting; sudden blindness; weakness or numbness of arm or leg; unusual vaginal bleeding; yellowing of skin or eyes; unusual bruising or bleeding, or other persistent adverse reactions. You may become intolerant to wearing contact lenses, notify prescriber if this occurs. **Pregnancy/breast-feeding precautions:** Inform prescriber if you are pregnant. Do not get pregnant while taking this medication. Consult prescriber for appropriate contraceptive measures. This medication may cause fetal defects and should not be used during pregnancy. Consult prescriber if breast-feeding.

Dietary Considerations: Ensure adequate calcium and vitamin D intake when used for the prevention of osteoporosis. Powder for reconstitution for injection (25 mg) contains lactose 200 mg.

Geriatric Considerations: Before prescribing estrogen therapy to postmenopausal women, the risks and benefits must be weighed for each patient. Data in women 80 years and older is minimal and it is unclear if reduced risk is applicable to women in this age group. Women should be informed of risks and benefits, as well as possible side effects and the return of menstrual bleeding (when cycled with a progestin), and should be
(Continued)

Estrogens (Conjugated/Equine) (Continued)

involved in prescribing options. Oral therapy may be more convenient for vaginal atrophy and urinary incontinence.

Pregnancy Risk Factor: X

Pregnancy Issues: Increased risk of fetal reproductive tract disorders and other birth defects; do not use during pregnancy.

Lactation: Enters breast milk/use caution

Breast-Feeding Issues: The AAP considers ethinyl estradiol, an estrogen derivative, to be "usually compatible" with breast-feeding. Estrogen has been shown to decrease the quantity and quality of human milk. Use only if clearly needed. Monitor the growth of the infant closely.

Administration

Oral: Give at bedtime to minimize adverse effects.

I.M.: May be administered intramuscularly.

I.V.: Administer I.V. doses slowly to avoid a flushing reaction.

Other: Vaginal cream: Administer at bedtime to minimize adverse effects.

Reconstitution: Injection: Reconstitute using provided diluent; do not shake violently.

Compatibility: Stable in D_5W and NS

Compatibility when admixed: Incompatible with ascorbic acid

Storage:

Injection: Refrigerate at 2°C to 8°C (36°F to 46°F) prior to reconstitution. Following reconstitution, solution may be stored under refrigeration for up to 60 days. Do not use if darkening or precipitation occurs.

Tablets, vaginal cream: Store at room temperature (25°C).

Additional Information The use of estrogens for the prevention of other chronic diseases, as well as their potential negative effects on women's health, has been debated. Data published from the Women's Health Initiative (WHI) has provided some additional insight on this controversial topic. In the WHI, one arm of the study compared postmenopausal women with an intact uterus using CEE 0.625 mg in combination with MPA 2.5 mg daily, versus placebo. This arm of the study was stopped in 2002. In March, 2004, it was announced that the arm of the study comparing placebo to CEE alone in postmenopausal women without a uterus was ended.

Based on preliminary findings, the FDA has requested labeling changes be made to estrogen products used in postmenopausal women. The updates include information from the Women's Health Initiative Memory Study (WHIMS) as well as information collected from the completed CEE/MPA arm of the WHI study. Complete analysis of the WHI data is forthcoming, and will include all information collected through February, 2004.

Related Information

Pharmacotherapy of Urinary Incontinence *on page 1858*

Estrogens (Conjugated/Equine) and Medroxyprogesterone

(ES troe jenz KON joo gate ed/EE kwine & me DROKS ee proe JES te rone)

U.S. Brand Names Premphase®; Prempro™

Synonyms Medroxyprogesterone and Estrogens (Conjugated); MPA and Estrogens (Conjugated)

Generic Available No

Pharmacologic Category Estrogen and Progestin Combination

Medication Safety Issues

Sound-alike/look-alike issues:

Premphase® may be confused with Prempro™

Prempro™ may be confused with Premphase®

Use Women with an intact uterus: Treatment of moderate to severe vasomotor symptoms associated with menopause; treatment of atrophic vaginitis; osteoporosis (prophylaxis)

Mechanism of Action/Effect

Estrogens modulate the pituitary secretion of gonadotropins, luteinizing hormone, and follicle-stimulating hormone through a negative feedback system; estrogen replacement reduces elevated levels of these hormones in postmenopausal women.

In women with adequate estrogen, MPA transforms a proliferative endometrium into a secretory endometrium; when administered with conjugated estrogens, reduces the incidence of endometrial hyperplasia and risk of adenocarcinoma.

Contraindications Hypersensitivity to conjugated estrogens, medroxyprogesterone (MPA), or any component of the formulation; undiagnosed abnormal vaginal bleeding; history of or current thrombophlebitis or venous thromboembolic disorders (including DVT, PE); active or recent (within 1 year) arterial thromboembolic disease (eg, stroke, MI); carcinoma of the breast; estrogen-dependent tumor; hepatic dysfunction or disease; pregnancy

Warnings/Precautions

Cardiovascular-related considerations: Estrogens with or without progestin should not be used to prevent coronary heart disease. Use caution with cardiovascular disease or dysfunction. May increase the risks of hypertension, myocardial infarction (MI), stroke, pulmonary emboli (PE), and deep vein thrombosis; incidence of these effects was shown to be significantly increased in postmenopausal women using conjugated equine estrogens (CEE) in combination with medroxyprogesterone acetate (MPA). Nonfatal MI, PE, and thrombophlebitis have also been reported in males taking high doses of CEE (eg, for prostate cancer). Estrogen compounds are generally associated with lipid effects such as increased HDL-cholesterol and decreased LDL-cholesterol. Triglycerides may also be increased; use with caution in patients with familial defects of lipoprotein metabolism. Whenever possible, estrogens should be discontinued at least 4-6 weeks prior to surgeries associated with an increased risk of thromboembolism or during periods of prolonged immobilization.

Neurological considerations: The risk of dementia may be increased in postmenopausal women; increased incidence was observed in women ≥65 years of age taking CEE in combination with MPA.

Cancer-related considerations: Unopposed estrogens may increase the risk of endometrial carcinoma in postmenopausal women. Estrogens may increase the risk of breast cancer. An increased risk of invasive breast cancer was observed in postmenopausal women using CEE in combination with MPA; a smaller increase in risk was seen with estrogen therapy alone in observational studies. An increase in abnormal mammograms has also been reported with estrogen and progestin therapy. Estrogen use may lead to severe hypercalcemia in patients with breast cancer and bone metastases; discontinue estrogen if hypercalcemia occurs.

Estrogens may cause retinal vascular thrombosis; discontinue permanently if papilledema or retinal vascular lesions are observed on examination. Use with caution in patients with diseases which may be exacerbated by fluid retention, including asthma, epilepsy, migraine, diabetes or renal dysfunction. Use with caution in patients with a history of severe hypocalcemia, SLE, hepatic hemangiomas, porphyria, endometriosis, and gallbladder disease. Use caution with history of cholestatic jaundice associated with past estrogen use or pregnancy. Safety and efficacy in pediatric patients have not been established. Prior to puberty, estrogens may cause premature closure of the epiphyses, premature breast development in girls or gynecomastia in boys. Vaginal bleeding and vaginal cornification may also be induced in girls.

Before prescribing estrogen therapy to postmenopausal women, the risks and benefits must be weighed for each patient. Women should be informed of these risks and benefits, as well as possible effects of progestin when added to estrogen therapy. Estrogens with or without progestin should be used for shortest duration possible consistent with treatment goals. Conduct periodic risk:benefit assessments.

When used solely for prevention of osteoporosis in women at significant risk, nonestrogen treatment options should be considered. When used solely for the treatment of vulvar and vaginal atrophy, topical vaginal products should be considered.

Drug Interactions
Cytochrome P450 Effect:
Based on estradiol and estrone: **Substrate** of CYP1A2 (major), 2A6 (minor), 2B6 (minor), 2C8/9 (minor), 2C19 (minor), 2D6 (minor), 2E1 (minor), 3A4 (major); **Inhibits** CYP1A2 (weak); **Induces** CYP3A4 (weak)

Medroxyprogesterone: **Substrate** of CYP3A4 (major); **Induces** CYP3A4 (weak)
Decreased Effect:
Conjugated estrogens:

Anticonvulsants which are enzyme inducers (barbiturates, carbamazepine, phenobarbital, phenytoin, primidone) may potentially decrease estrogen levels.

Rifampin, nelfinavir, and ritonavir decrease estradiol serum concentrations

MPA: Aminoglutethimide: May decrease effects by increasing hepatic metabolism
Increased Effect/Toxicity:
Hydrocortisone taken with estrogen may cause corticosteroid-induced toxicity. Increased potential for thromboembolic events with anticoagulants.

Nutritional/Ethanol Interactions
Ethanol: Avoid ethanol (routine use increases estrogen level and risk of breast cancer). Ethanol may also increase the risk of osteoporosis.

Food: Folic acid absorption may be decreased.

Herb/Nutraceutical: St John's wort may decrease levels. Avoid black cohosh, dong quai (has estrogenic activity). Avoid red clover, saw palmetto, ginseng (due to potential hormonal effects).

Lab Interactions Accelerated PT, partial thromboplastin time, and platelet aggregation time; increased platelet count; increased HDL; increased factors II, VII antigen, VIII coagulant activity, IX, X, XII, XII-X complex, II-VII-X complex, and beta-thromboglobulin; increased levels of fibrinogen and fibrinogen activity; increased plasminogen antigen and activity; increased thyroid-binding globulin; increased triglycerides; impaired glucose tolerance; reduced response to metyrapone test; reduced serum folate concentration; other binding proteins may be elevated; decreased LDL; decreased levels of antifactor Xa and antithrombin III; decreased antithrombin III activity

Adverse Reactions
>10%:

Central nervous system: Headache (28% to 37%), pain (11% to 13%), depression (6% to 11%)

Endocrine & metabolic: Breast pain (32% to 38%), dysmenorrhea (8% to 13%)

Gastrointestinal: Abdominal pain (16% to 23%), nausea (9% to 11%)

Neuromuscular & skeletal: Back pain (13% to 16%)

Respiratory: Pharyngitis (11% to 13%)

Miscellaneous: Infection (16% to 18%), flu-like syndrome (10% to 13%)

1% to 10%:

Cardiovascular: Peripheral edema (3% to 4%)

Central nervous system: Dizziness (3% to 5%)

Dermatologic: Pruritus (5% to 10%), rash (4% to 6%)

Endocrine & metabolic: Leukorrhea (5% to 9%)

Gastrointestinal: Flatulence (8% to 9%), diarrhea (5% to 6%), dyspepsia (5% to 6%)

Genitourinary: Vaginitis (5% to 7%), cervical changes (4% to 5%), vaginal hemorrhage (1% to 3%)

Neuromuscular & skeletal: Weakness (6% to 10%), arthralgia (7% to 9%), leg cramps (3% to 5%), hypertonia (3% to 4%)

Respiratory: Sinusitis (7% to 8%), rhinitis (6% to 8%)

Additional adverse effects reported with conjugated estrogens and/or progestins: Abdominal cramps, acne, abnormal uterine bleeding, aggravation of porphyria, amenorrhea, anaphylactoid reactions, anaphylaxis, antifactor Xa decreased, antithrombin III decreased, appetite changes, bloating, breast enlargement, breast tenderness, cerebral embolism, cerebral thrombosis, chloasma, cholestatic jaundice, cholecystitis, cholelithiasis, chorea, contact lens intolerance, cystitis-like syndrome, decreased carbohydrate tolerance, dizziness; factors VII, VIII, IX, X, XII, VII-X complex, and II-VII-X complex increased; endometrial hyperplasia, erythema multiforme, erythema nodosum, galactorrhea, hemorrhagic eruption, fatigue, fibrinogen increased, impaired glucose tolerance, HDL-cholesterol increased, (Continued)

Estrogens (Conjugated/Equine) and Medroxyprogesterone
(Continued)

hirsutism, hypertension, increase in size of uterine leiomyomata, gallbladder disease, insomnia, LDL-cholesterol decreased, libido changes, loss of scalp hair, melasma, migraine, nervousness, optic neuritis, pancreatitis, platelet aggregability and platelet count increased, premenstrual like syndrome, PT and PTT accelerated, pulmonary embolism, pyrexia, retinal thrombosis, somnolence, steepening of corneal curvature, thrombophlebitis, thyroid-binding globulin increased, total thyroid hormone (T_4) increased, triglycerides increased, urticaria, vaginal candidiasis, vomiting, weight gain/loss

Overdosage/Toxicology Effects noted after large doses include nausea, vomiting; withdrawal bleeding may occur in females. Treatment should be supportive and symptomatic.

Pharmacodynamics/Kinetics
Pharmacokinetic Note: See individual agents.

Dosing
Adults:
Treatment of moderate to severe vasomotor symptoms associated with menopause or treatment of atrophic vaginitis in females with an intact uterus: (Note: The lowest dose that will control symptoms should be used; medication should be discontinued as soon as possible): Oral:

Premphase®: One maroon conjugated estrogen 0.625 mg tablet daily on days 1 through 14 and one light blue conjugated estrogen 0.625 mg/MPA 5 mg tablet daily on days 15 through 28; re-evaluate patients at 3- and 6-month intervals to determine if treatment is still necessary; monitor patients for signs of endometrial cancer; rule out malignancy if unexplained vaginal bleeding occurs

Prempro™: One conjugated estrogen 0.3 mg/MPA 1.5 mg tablet daily; re-evaluate at 3-and 6-month intervals to determine if therapy is still needed; dose may be increased to a maximum of one conjugated estrogen 0.625 mg/MPA 5 mg tablet daily in patients with bleeding or spotting, once malignancy has been ruled out

Osteoporosis prophylaxis in females with an intact uterus: Oral:

Premphase®: One maroon conjugated estrogen 0.625 tablet daily on days 1 through 14 and one light blue conjugated estrogen 0.625 mg/MPA 5 mg tablet daily on days 15 through 28; monitor patients for signs of endometrial cancer; rule out malignancy if unexplained vaginal bleeding occurs

Prempro™: One conjugated estrogen 0.3 mg/MPA 1.5 mg tablet daily; dose may be increased to one conjugated estrogen 0.625 mg/MPA 5 mg tablet daily; in patients with bleeding or spotting, once malignancy has been ruled out

Elderly: Refer to adult dosing. A higher incidence of stroke and breast cancer was observed in women >75 years in a WHI substudy.

Available Dosage Forms Tablet:
Premphase® [therapy pack contains 2 separate tablet formulations]: Conjugated estrogens 0.625 mg [14 maroon tablets] and conjugated estrogen 0.625 mg/medroxyprogesterone acetate 5 mg [14 light blue tablets] (28s)

Prempro™:
0.3/1.5: Conjugated estrogens 0.3 mg and medroxyprogesterone acetate 1.5 mg (28s)
0.45/1.5: Conjugated estrogens 0.45 mg and medroxyprogesterone acetate 1.5 mg (28s)
0.625/2.5: Conjugated estrogens 0.625 mg and medroxyprogesterone acetate 2.5 mg (28s)
0.625/5: Conjugated estrogens 0.625 mg and medroxyprogesterone acetate 5 mg (28s)

Monitoring and Teaching Issues
Physical Assessment: Assess potential for interactions with other prescriptions, OTC medications, or herbal products patient may be taking. Assess results of annual gynecological exam (eg, Pap smear and mammogram), therapeutic effectiveness (dependent on rationale for use), and adverse effects (eg, thromboembolism, hypertension, edema, CNS changes) on a regular basis during therapy. **Note:** Before prescribing estrogen therapy to postmenopausal women, the risks and benefits must be weighed for each patient. Women should be informed of these risks and benefits, as well as possible effects of progestin when added to estrogen therapy. Caution patients with diabetes to monitor glucose levels closely (may impair glucose tolerance). Teach patient appropriate administration/use according to formulation, possible side effects, interventions to reduce side effects, adverse reactions to report, importance of frequent self-breast exams, and need for annual gynecological exam. **Pregnancy risk factor X:** Determine that patient is not pregnant before starting therapy.

Monitoring Laboratory Tests: Serum cholesterol, HDL, LDL triglycerides

Patient Education: Do not take any new medication during therapy without consulting prescriber. Take exactly as directed and maintain prescribed cycles or term as prescribed. Avoid routine use of alcohol (ethanol may increase the risk of breast cancer or osteoporosis). Annual gynecologic and regular self-breast exams are important. If you have diabetes, monitor glucose levels closely (may impair glucose tolerance). You may experience nausea, vomiting or abdominal pain (small frequent meals may help); dizziness or mental depression (use caution when driving); rash; hair loss; headache; or breast pain, increased/decreased libido, or enlargement/tenderness of breasts. difficult/painful menstrual cycles. Report significant swelling of extremities; sudden acute pain in legs or calves, chest, or abdomen; shortness of breath; severe headache or vomiting; sudden blindness; weakness or numbness of arm or leg; unusual vaginal bleeding; yellowing of skin or eyes; unusual bruising or bleeding, or other persistent adverse reactions. You may become intolerant to wearing contact lenses, notify prescriber if this occurs. **Pregnancy/breast-feeding precautions:** Inform prescriber if you are pregnant. Do not get pregnant while taking this medication. This medication may cause fetal defects and should not be used during pregnancy.

Dietary Considerations: Administration with food decreases nausea, administer with food. Ensure adequate calcium and vitamin D intake when used for the prevention of osteoporosis.

Pregnancy Risk Factor: X
Pregnancy Issues:
Estrogens: Increased risk of fetal reproductive tract disorders and other birth defects; do not use during pregnancy.
Progestins: Associated with fetal genital abnormalities when used during the 1st trimester; not recommended for use during pregnancy.
Lactation:
Estrogens: Enters breast milk/use caution
Progestins: Enters breast milk/use caution
Breast-Feeding Issues: The AAP considers ethinyl estradiol, an estrogen derivative, to be "usually compatible" with breast-feeding. Estrogen has been shown to decrease the quantity and quality of human milk. Monitor the growth of the infant closely. The AAP considers medroxyprogesterone to be "usually compatible" with breast-feeding.

Administration
Storage: Store at room temperature 20°C to 25°C (68°F to 77°F).

Additional Information The use of estrogens for the prevention of other chronic diseases, as well as their potential negative effects on women's health, has been debated. Data published from the Women's Health Initiative (WHI) has provided some additional insight on this controversial topic. In the WHI, one arm of the study compared postmenopausal women with an intact uterus using CEE 0.625 mg in combination with MPA 2.5 mg daily, versus placebo. This arm of the study was stopped in 2002. In March, 2004, it was announced that the arm of the study comparing placebo to CEE alone in postmenopausal women without a uterus was ended.

Based on preliminary findings, the FDA has requested labeling changes be made to estrogen products used in postmenopausal women. The updates include information from the Women's Health Initiative Memory Study (WHIMS) as well as information collected from the completed CEE/MPA arm of the WHI study. Complete analysis of the WHI data is forthcoming, and will include all information collected through February, 2004.

Related Information
Estrogens (Conjugated/Equine) *on page 563*
MedroxyPROGESTERone *on page 938*

Estrogens (Esterified) (ES troe jenz, es TER i fied)

U.S. Brand Names Menest®
Synonyms Esterified Estrogens
Generic Available No
Pharmacologic Category Estrogen Derivative
Medication Safety Issues
Sound-alike/look-alike issues:
Estratab® may be confused with Estratest®, Estratest® H.S.
Use Treatment of moderate to severe vasomotor symptoms associated with menopause; treatment of vulvar and vaginal atrophy; hypoestrogenism (due to hypogonadism, castration, or primary ovarian failure); prostatic cancer (palliation); breast cancer (palliation); osteoporosis (prophylaxis, in women at significant risk only)
Mechanism of Action/Effect Esterified estrogens contain a mixture of estrogenic substances; the principle component is estrone. Estrogens modulate the pituitary secretion of gonadotropins, luteinizing hormone, and follicle-stimulating hormone through a negative feedback system; estrogen replacement reduces elevated levels of these hormones.
Contraindications Hypersensitivity to estrogens or any component of the formulation; undiagnosed abnormal vaginal bleeding; history of or current thrombophlebitis or venous thromboembolic disorders (including DVT, PE); active or recent (within 1 year) arterial thromboembolic disease (eg, stroke, MI); carcinoma of the breast, except in appropriately selected patients being treated for metastatic disease; estrogen-dependent tumor; hepatic dysfunction or disease; pregnancy
Warnings/Precautions
Cardiovascular-related considerations: Estrogens with or without progestin should not be used to prevent coronary heart disease. Use caution with cardiovascular disease or dysfunction. May increase the risks of hypertension, myocardial infarction (MI), stroke, pulmonary emboli (PE), and deep vein thrombosis; incidence of these effects was shown to be significantly increased in postmenopausal women using conjugated equine estrogens (CEE) in combination with medroxyprogesterone acetate (MPA). Nonfatal MI, PE, and thrombophlebitis have also been reported in males taking high doses of CEE (eg, for prostate cancer). Estrogen compounds are generally associated with lipid effects such as increased HDL-cholesterol and decreased LDL-cholesterol. Triglycerides may also be increased; use with caution in patients with familial defects of lipoprotein metabolism. Whenever possible, estrogens should be discontinued at least 4-6 weeks prior to surgeries associated with an increased risk of thromboembolism or during periods of prolonged immobilization.

Neurological considerations: The risk of dementia may be increased in postmenopausal women; increased incidence was observed in women ≥65 years of age taking CEE in combination with MPA.

Cancer-related considerations: Unopposed estrogens may increase the risk of endometrial carcinoma in postmenopausal women. Estrogens may increase the risk of breast cancer. An increased risk of invasive breast cancer was observed in postmenopausal women using CEE in combination with MPA; a smaller increase in risk was seen with estrogen therapy alone in observational studies. An increase in abnormal mammograms has also been reported with estrogen and progestin therapy. Estrogen use may lead to severe hypercalcemia in patients with breast cancer and bone metastases; discontinue estrogen if hypercalcemia occurs.

Estrogens may cause retinal vascular thrombosis; discontinue permanently if papilledema or retinal vascular lesions are observed on examination. Use with caution in patients with diseases which may be exacerbated by fluid retention, including asthma, epilepsy, migraine, diabetes or renal dysfunction. Use with caution in patients with a history of severe hypocalcemia, SLE, hepatic hemangiomas, porphyria, endometriosis, and gallbladder disease. Use
(Continued)

Estrogens (Esterified) *(Continued)*

caution with history of cholestatic jaundice associated with past estrogen use or pregnancy. Safety and efficacy in pediatric patients have not been established. Prior to puberty, estrogens may cause premature closure of the epiphyses, premature breast development in girls or gynecomastia in boys. Vaginal bleeding and vaginal cornification may also be induced in girls.

Before prescribing estrogen therapy to postmenopausal women, the risks and benefits must be weighed for each patient. Women should be informed of these risks and benefits, as well as possible effects of progestin when added to estrogen therapy. Estrogens with or without progestin should be used for shortest duration possible consistent with treatment goals. Conduct periodic risk:benefit assessments.

When used solely for prevention of osteoporosis in women at significant risk, nonestrogen treatment options should be considered. When used solely for the treatment of vulvar and vaginal atrophy, topical vaginal products should be considered.

Drug Interactions

Cytochrome P450 Effect: Based on estrone: **Substrate** of CYP1A2 (major), 2B6 (minor), 2C8/9 (minor), 2E1 (minor), 3A4 (major)

Decreased Effect: CYP1A2 inducers may decrease the levels/effects of estrogens; example inducers include aminoglutethimide, carbamazepine, phenobarbital, and rifampin. CYP3A4 inducers may decrease the levels/effects of estrogens; example inducers include aminoglutethimide, carbamazepine, nafcillin, nevirapine, phenobarbital, phenytoin, and rifamycins.

Increased Effect/Toxicity: Hydrocortisone taken with estrogen may cause corticosteroid-induced toxicity. Increased potential for thromboembolic events with anticoagulants.

Nutritional/Ethanol Interactions

Ethanol: Avoid ethanol (routine use increases estrogen level and risk of breast cancer). Ethanol may also increase the risk of osteoporosis.

Food: Folic acid absorption may be decreased.

Herb/Nutraceutical: St John's wort may decrease levels. Avoid black cohosh, dong quai (has estrogenic activity). Avoid red clover, saw palmetto, ginseng (due to potential hormonal effects).

Lab Interactions Endocrine function test may be altered; increased prothrombin and factors VII, VIII, IX, X; increased platelet aggregability, thyroid-binding globulin, total thyroid hormone (T_4), serum triglycerides/phospholipids; decreased antithrombin III, serum folate concentration

Adverse Reactions Frequency not defined.

Cardiovascular: Edema, hypertension, venous thromboembolism

Central nervous system: Dizziness, headache, mental depression, migraine

Dermatologic: Chloasma, erythema multiforme, erythema nodosum, hemorrhagic eruption, hirsutism, loss of scalp hair, melasma

Endocrine & metabolic: Breast enlargement, breast tenderness, libido (changes in), increased thyroid-binding globulin, increased total thyroid hormone (T_4), increased serum triglycerides/phospholipids, increased HDL-cholesterol, decreased LDL-cholesterol, impaired glucose tolerance, hypercalcemia

Gastrointestinal: Abdominal cramps, bloating, cholecystitis, cholelithiasis, gallbladder disease, nausea, pancreatitis, vomiting, weight gain/loss

Genitourinary: Alterations in frequency and flow of menses, changes in cervical secretions, endometrial cancer, increased size of uterine leiomyomata, vaginal candidiasis

Hematologic: Aggravation of porphyria, decreased antithrombin III and antifactor Xa, increased levels of fibrinogen, increased platelet aggregability and platelet count; increased prothrombin and factors VII, VIII, IX, X

Hepatic: Cholestatic jaundice

Neuromuscular & skeletal: Chorea

Ocular: Intolerance to contact lenses, steeping of corneal curvature

Respiratory: Pulmonary thromboembolism

Miscellaneous: Carbohydrate intolerance

Overdosage/Toxicology Toxicity is unlikely following single exposures of excessive doses, any treatment following emesis and charcoal administration should be supportive and symptomatic. Effects noted after large doses include headache, nausea, and vomiting. Bleeding may occur in females.

Pharmacodynamics/Kinetics

Absorption: Readily

Metabolism: Rapidly hepatic to estrone sulfate, conjugated and unconjugated metabolites; first-pass effect

Excretion: Urine (as unchanged drug and as glucuronide and sulfate conjugates)

Dosing

Adults:

Prostate cancer (palliation): Oral: 1.25-2.5 mg 3 times/day

Female hypogonadism: Oral: 2.5-7.5 mg of estrogen daily for 20 days followed by a 10-day rest period. Administer cyclically (3 weeks on and 1 week off). If bleeding does not occur by the end of the 10-day period, repeat the same dosing schedule; the number of courses dependent upon the responsiveness of the endometrium. If bleeding occurs before the end of the 10-day period, begin an estrogen-progestin cyclic regimen of 2.5-7.5 mg esterified estrogens daily for 20 days. During the last 5 days of estrogen therapy, give an oral progestin. If bleeding occurs before regimen is concluded, discontinue therapy and resume on the fifth day of bleeding.

Menopause, moderate to severe vasomotor symptoms: Oral: 1.25 mg/day administered cyclically (3 weeks on and 1 week off). If patient has not menstruated within the last 2 months or more, cyclic administration is started arbitrary. If the patient is menstruating, cyclical administration is started on day 5 of the bleeding. For short-term use only and should be discontinued as soon as possible. Re-evaluate at 3- to 6-month intervals for tapering or discontinuation of therapy.

Atopic vaginitis and kraurosis vulvae: Oral: 0.3 to ≥1.25 mg/day, depending on the tissue response of the individual patient. Administer cyclically. For short-term use only and should be discontinued as soon as possible. Re-evaluate at 3- to 6-month intervals for tapering or discontinuation of therapy.

Breast cancer (palliation): Oral: 10 mg 3 times/day for at least 3 months

Osteoporosis in postmenopausal women: Oral: Initial: 0.3 mg/day and increase to a maximum daily dose of 1.25 mg/day; initiate therapy as soon as possible after menopause; cyclically or daily, depending on medical assessment of patient. Monitor patients with an intact uterus for signs of endometrial cancer; rule out malignancy if unexplained vaginal bleeding occurs

Female castration and primary ovarian failure: Oral: 1.25 mg/day, cyclically. Adjust dosage upward or downward, according to the severity of symptoms and patient response. For maintenance, adjust dosage to lowest level that will provide effective control.

Elderly: Refer to adult dosing. A higher incidence of stroke and invasive breast cancer were observed in women >75 years in a WHI substudy using conjugated equine estrogen.

Hepatic Impairment:

Mild to moderate liver impairment: Dosage reduction of estrogens is recommended.
Severe liver impairment: **Not recommended**.

Available Dosage Forms Tablet: 0.3 mg, 0.625 mg, 1.25 mg, 2.5 mg

Monitoring and Teaching Issues

Physical Assessment: See Warnings/Precautions for specific use cautions. Assess potential for interactions with other pharmacological agents or herbal products patient may be taking (eg, increased potential for decreased levels/effects or increased potential for toxicity or thrombotic events; see Drug Interactions). Assess results of annual gynecological exam, therapeutic effectiveness (dependent on rationale for use), and adverse effects (eg, thromboembolism, hypertension, edema, CNS changes; see Adverse Reactions) on a regular basis during therapy. **Note:** Before prescribing estrogen therapy to postmenopausal women, the risks and benefits must be weighed for each patient. Women should be informed of these risks and benefits, as well as possible effects of progestin when added to estrogen therapy. Estrogens with or without progestin should be used for shortest duration possible consistent with treatment goals and periodic assessment of risk:benefit should be made. Caution patients with diabetes to monitor glucose levels closely (may impair glucose tolerance). Teach patient appropriate use, possible side effects/appropriate interventions, adverse symptoms to report, importance of frequent self-breast exams, and need for annual gynecological exam (see Patient Education). **Pregnancy risk factor X:** Determine that patient is not pregnant before starting therapy. Do not give to females of childbearing age unless patient is capable of complying with contraceptive use. Advise patient about contraceptive measures as appropriate.

Monitoring Laboratory Tests: Yearly Papanicolaou smear, mammogram. Adequate diagnostic measures, including endometrial sampling, if indicated, should be performed to rule out malignancy in all cases of undiagnosed abnormal vaginal bleeding.

Patient Education: Do not take any new medication during therapy without consulting prescriber. Take exactly as directed and maintain prescribed cycles or term as prescribed. Avoid routine use of alcohol (ethanol may increase the risk of breast cancer). Annual gynecologic and regular self-breast exams are important. If you have diabetes, monitor glucose levels closely (may impair glucose tolerance). You may experience nausea, vomiting or abdominal pain (small frequent meals may help); dizziness or mental depression (use caution when driving); rash; hair loss; headache; breast pain, increased/decreased libido, or enlargement/tenderness of breasts; or difficult/painful menstrual cycles. Report significant swelling of extremities; sudden acute pain in legs, calves, chest, or abdomen; shortness of breath; severe headache or vomiting; sudden blindness; weakness or numbness of arm or leg; unusual vaginal bleeding; yellowing of skin or eyes; unusual bruising or bleeding, or other persistent adverse reactions. You may become intolerant to wearing contact lenses, notify prescriber if this occurs. **Pregnancy/breast-feeding precautions:** Inform prescriber if you are pregnant. Do not get pregnant while taking this medication. Consult prescriber for appropriate contraceptive measures. This medication may cause fetal defects and should not be used during pregnancy. Consult prescriber if breast-feeding.

Dietary Considerations: Should be taken with food at same time each day. Ensure adequate calcium and vitamin D intake when used for the prevention of osteoporosis.

Pregnancy Risk Factor: X

Pregnancy Issues: Increased risk of fetal reproductive tract disorders and other birth defects; do not use during pregnancy.

Lactation: Enters breast milk/use caution

Breast-Feeding Issues: The AAP considers ethinyl estradiol, an estrogen derivative, to be "usually compatible" with breast-feeding. Estrogen has been shown to decrease the quantity and quality of human milk; use only if clearly needed; monitor the growth of the infant closely.

Administration

Storage: Store below 30°C (86°F); protect from moisture

Additional Information The use of estrogens for the prevention of other chronic diseases, as well as their potential negative effects on women's health, has been debated. Data published from the Women's Health Initiative (WHI) has provided some additional insight on this controversial topic. In the WHI, one arm of the study compared postmenopausal women with an intact uterus using CEE 0.625 mg in combination with MPA 2.5 mg daily, versus placebo. This arm of the study was stopped in 2002. In March, 2004, it was announced that the arm of the study comparing placebo to CEE alone in postmenopausal women without a uterus was ended.

Based on preliminary findings, the FDA has requested labeling changes be made to estrogen products used in postmenopausal women. The updates include information from the Women's Health Initiative Memory Study (WHIMS) as well as information collected from the (Continued)

Estrogens (Esterified) *(Continued)*

completed CEE/MPA arm of the WHI study. Complete analysis of the WHI data is forth-coming, and will include all information collected through February, 2004.

♦ **Estrostep® Fe** *see Ethinyl Estradiol and Norethindrone on page 589*

Eszopiclone *(es zoe PIK lone)*

U.S. Brand Names Lunesta™
Controlled Substance C-IV
Generic Available No
Pharmacologic Category Hypnotic, Nonbenzodiazepine
Use Treatment of insomnia
Mechanism of Action/Effect Interact with the GABA-receptor complex to promote sleep.
Contraindications Hypersensitivity to eszopiclone or any component of the formulation
Warnings/Precautions Symptomatic treatment of insomnia should be initiated only after careful evaluation of potential causes of sleep disturbance. Tolerance did not develop over 6 months of use. Use with caution in patients with depression or a history of drug dependence. Abrupt discontinuance may lead to withdrawal symptoms. Use with caution in patients receiving other CNS depressants or psychoactive medications. May impair physical and mental capabilities. Use caution in patients with respiratory compromise or liver dysfunction. Safety and efficacy in children have not been established.
Drug Interactions
   Cytochrome P450 Effect: Substrate of CYP2E1 (minor), 3A4 (major)
   Decreased Effect: CYP3A4 inducers may decrease the levels/effects of eszopiclone; example inducers include aminoglutethimide, carbamazepine, nafcillin, nevirapine, pheno-barbital, phenytoin, and rifamycins.
   Increased Effect/Toxicity: CYP3A4 inhibitors may increase the levels/effects of eszopiclone; example inhibitors include azole antifungals, ciprofloxacin, clarithromycin, diclofenac, doxycycline, erythromycin, imatinib, isoniazid, nefazodone, nicardipine, propofol, protease inhibitors, quinidine, and verapamil. Concurrent use with olanzapine may lead to decreased psychomotor function.
Nutritional/Ethanol Interactions
   Ethanol: Use caution with concurrent use. Effects are additive and may decrease psycho-motor function.
   Food: Onset of action may be reduced if taken with or immediately after a heavy meal.
   Herb/Nutraceutical: Avoid valerian, St John's wort, kava kava, gotu kola (may increase CNS depression).
Adverse Reactions
   >10%:
      Central nervous system: Headache (15% to 21%)
      Gastrointestinal: Unpleasant taste (8% to 34%)
   1% to 10%:
      Cardiovascular: Chest pain, peripheral edema
      Central nervous system: Somnolence (8% to 10%), dizziness (5% to 7%), hallucinations (1% to 3%), anxiety (1% to 3%), nervousness (up to 5%), confusion (up to 3%), depres-sion (1% to 4%), abnormal dreams (1% to 3%), migraine
      Dermatologic: Rash (3% to 4%), pruritus (1% to 4%)
      Endocrine & metabolic: Libido decreased (up to 3%), dysmenorrhea (up to 3%), gyneco-mastia (males up to 3%)
      Gastrointestinal: Xerostomia (3% to 7%), dyspepsia (5% to 6%), nausea (5%), diarrhea (2% to 4%), vomiting (up to 3%)
      Genitourinary: Urinary tract infection (up to 3%)
      Neuromuscular & skeletal: Neuralgia (up to 3%)
      Miscellaneous: Infection (5% to 10%), viral infection (3%)
Overdosage/Toxicology Overdose symptoms range from somnolence to coma. Treatment is symptom-directed and supportive. Flumazenil may be useful.
Pharmacodynamics/Kinetics
   Absorption: Rapid; high-fat/heavy meal may delay absorption
   Time to Peak: 1 hour
   Protein Binding: 52% to 59%
   Half-Life Elimination: 6 hours; Elderly (≥65 years): ~9 hours
   Metabolism: Hepatic via oxidation and demethylation (CYP2E1, 3A4); 2 primary metabo-lites; one with activity less than parent
   Excretion: Urine (75%, primarily as metabolites; <10% as parent drug)
Dosing
   Adults:
      Insomnia: Oral: Initial: 2 mg before bedtime (maximum dose: 3 mg)
         Concurrent use with strong CYP3A4 inhibitor: 1 mg before bedtime; if needed, dose may be increased to 2 mg
   Elderly:
      Difficulty **falling** asleep: Initial: 1 mg before bedtime; maximum dose: 2 mg.
      Difficulty **staying** asleep: 2 mg before bedtime.
   Renal Impairment: No adjustment required.
   Hepatic Impairment:
      Mild-to-moderate: Use with caution; dosage adjustment unnecessary
      Severe: Maximum dose: 2 mg
Available Dosage Forms Tablet [film coated]: 1 mg, 2 mg, 3 mg
Monitoring and Teaching Issues
   Physical Assessment: Evaluate potential causes of insomnia prior to initiating medication. Assess effectiveness and interactions of other medications patient may be taking Assess for history of addiction; long-term use can result in dependence, abuse, or tolerance. After long-term use, taper dosage slowly when discontinuing. Monitor for CNS depression. For inpatient use, institute safety measures and monitor effectiveness and adverse reactions.

For outpatients, monitor for effectiveness of therapy and adverse reactions at beginning of therapy and periodically with long-term use. Assess knowledge/teach patient appropriate use, interventions to reduce side effects, and adverse symptoms to report.

Patient Education: Use exactly as directed; do not increase dose or frequency or discontinue without consulting prescriber. Drug may cause physical and/or psychological dependence. While using this medication, do not use alcohol or other prescription or OTC medications (especially, pain medications, sedatives, antihistamines, or hypnotics) without consulting prescriber. Take immediately prior to bedtime (quick onset) or when having difficulty falling asleep. Do not use unless you are able to get 8 or more hours of sleep before you must be active again. Swallow whole, do not crush or break tablet. Maintain adequate hydration (2-3 L/day of fluids) unless instructed to restrict fluid intake. You may experience drowsiness, dizziness, lightheadedness, or difficulty with coordination (use caution when driving or engaging in tasks requiring alertness until response to drug is known); headache, or unpleasant taste. Report CNS changes (confusion, depression, increased sedation, excitation, severe headache, abnormal thinking, insomnia, or nightmares). **Pregnancy/breast-feeding precautions:** Inform prescriber if you are or intend to become pregnant. Consult prescriber if breast-feeding.

Dietary Considerations: Avoid taking after a heavy meal; may delay onset.

Geriatric Considerations: In subjects >65 years of age, the AUC was increased by 41%. The manufacturer reports that in studies, the pattern of adverse reactions in elderly subjects was not different from that seen in younger adults. See Pharmacodynamics/kinetics, Dosing, and Adverse Reactions.

Pregnancy Risk Factor: C

Lactation: Excretion in breast milk unknown/use caution

Administration

Oral: Because of the rapid onset of action, eszopiclone should be administered immediately prior to bedtime or after the patient has gone to bed and is having difficulty falling asleep. Do not take with, or immediately following, a high-fat meal. Do not crush or break tablet.

Storage: Store at 15°C to 30°C (59°F to 86°F).

♦ **ETAF** *see* Aldesleukin *on page 62*

Etanercept (et a NER sept)

U.S. Brand Names Enbrel®

Generic Available No

Pharmacologic Category Antirheumatic, Disease Modifying; Tumor Necrosis Factor (TNF) Blocking Agent

Use Treatment of moderately- to severely-active rheumatoid arthritis, moderately- to severely-active polyarticular juvenile arthritis, or psoriatic arthritis in patients who have had an inadequate response to one or more disease-modifying antirheumatic drugs (DMARDs); reduction in signs and symptoms of active ankylosing spondylitis (AS); treatment of chronic plaque psoriasis (moderate-to-severe)

Unlabeled/Investigational Use Crohn's disease

Mechanism of Action/Effect Etanercept is a recombinant DNA-derived protein composed of tumor necrosis factor receptor (TNFR) linked to the Fc portion of human IgG1. Etanercept binds tumor necrosis factor (TNF) and blocks its interaction with cell surface receptors. TNF plays an important role in the inflammatory processes of rheumatoid arthritis (RA) and the resulting joint pathology.

Contraindications Hypersensitivity to etanercept or any component of the formulation; patients with sepsis (mortality may be increased); active infections (including chronic or local infection)

Warnings/Precautions Etanercept may affect defenses against infections and malignancies. Safety and efficacy in patients with immunosuppression or chronic infections have not been evaluated. Rare cases of tuberculosis have been reported. Discontinue administration if patient develops a serious infection. Do not start drug administration in patients with an active infection. Use caution in patients predisposed to infection, such as poorly-controlled diabetes.

Use caution in patients with pre-existing or recent-onset demyelinating CNS disorders, CHF, or a history of significant hematologic abnormalities. Discontinue if significant hematologic abnormalities are confirmed.

The long-term immunogenicity, carcinogenic potential, or effect on fertility are unknown. The safety of etanercept has not been studied in children <4 years of age.

Allergic reactions may occur (<2%), but anaphylaxis has not been observed. If an anaphylactic reaction or other serious allergic reaction occurs, administration of etanercept should be discontinued immediately.

Patients should be brought up to date with all immunizations before initiating therapy. Live vaccines should not be given concurrently. Patients with a significant exposure to varicella virus should temporarily discontinue etanercept. Treatment with varicella zoster immune globulin should be considered.

Drug Interactions

Decreased Effect: Specific drug interaction studies have not been conducted with etanercept. Live vaccines should not be given during therapy.

Increased Effect/Toxicity: Specific drug interaction studies have not been conducted with etanercept. An increased rate of serious infections has been noted with concurrent anakinra therapy, without additional improvement in American College of Rheumatology (ACR) response criteria.

Adverse Reactions Events reported include those >3% with incidence higher than placebo.

>10%:
Central nervous system: Headache (17%):
Local: Injection site reaction (37%)
Respiratory: Respiratory tract infection (upper, 29%; other than upper, 38%), rhinitis (12%)
Miscellaneous: Infection (35%), positive ANA (11%), positive antidouble-stranded DNA antibodies (15% by RIA, 3% by *Crithidia luciliae* assay)

(Continued)

Etanercept *(Continued)*

≥3% to 10%:
  Central nervous system: Dizziness (7%)
  Dermatologic: Rash (5%)
  Gastrointestinal: Abdominal pain (5%), dyspepsia (4%), nausea (9%), vomiting (3%)
  Neuromuscular & skeletal: Weakness (5%)
  Respiratory: Pharyngitis (7%), respiratory disorder (5%), sinusitis (3%), cough (6%)
  Pediatric patients (JRA): The percentages of patients reporting abdominal pain (17%) and vomiting (13%) were higher than in adult RA. Two patients developed varicella infection associated with aseptic meningitis which resolved without complications (see Warnings/Precautions).

Overdosage/Toxicology No dose-limiting toxicities have been observed during clinical trials. Single I.V. doses up to 60 mg/m^2 have been administered to healthy volunteers in an endotoxemia study without evidence of dose-limiting toxicities.

Pharmacodynamics/Kinetics
Onset of Action: ~2-3 weeks
Time to Peak: 72 hours (range: 48-96 hours)
Half-Life Elimination: 115 hours (range: 98-300 hours)
Excretion: Clearance: Children: 45.9 mL/hour/m^2; Adults: 89 mL/hour (52 mL/hour/m^2)

Dosing
Adults:
  Rheumatoid arthritis, psoriatic arthritis, ankylosing spondylitis: SubQ:
    Once-weekly dosing: 50 mg once weekly
    Twice-weekly dosing: 25 mg given twice weekly (individual doses should be separated by 72-96 hours)
  Note: If the physician determines that it is appropriate, patients may self-inject after proper training in injection technique.
Elderly: SubQ: Although greater sensitivity of some elderly patients cannot be ruled out, no overall differences in safety or effectiveness were observed.
Pediatrics:
  Juvenile rheumatoid arthritis: Children 4-17 years: SubQ:
    Once-weekly dosing: 0.8 mg/kg (maximum: 50 mg/dose) once weekly
    Twice-weekly dosing: 0.4 mg/kg (maximum: 25 mg/dose) twice weekly (individual doses should be separated by 72-96 hours)

Available Dosage Forms
Injection, powder for reconstitution: 25 mg [diluent contains benzyl alcohol; packaging may contain dry natural rubber (latex)]
Injection, solution: 50 mg/mL (0.98 mL) [prefilled syringe with 27-gauge $^1/_2$ inch needle]

Monitoring and Teaching Issues
Physical Assessment: Monitor for signs and symptoms of infection. Assess for liver dysfunction. Monitor effectiveness of therapy (eg, pain, range of motion, mobility, ADL function, inflammation). Assess knowledge/teach patient appropriate administration (injection technique and needle disposal if self-administered), possible side effects/interventions, and adverse symptoms to report.
Patient Education: If self-injecting, follow instructions for injection and disposal of needles exactly. If redness, swelling, or irritation appears at the injection site, contact prescriber. Do not have any vaccinations while using this medication without consulting prescriber first. You may experience headache or dizziness (use caution when driving or engaging in tasks requiring alertness until response to drug is known). If stomach pain or cramping; unusual bleeding or bruising; persistent fever; paleness; blood in vomitus, stool, or urine occurs, stop medication and contact prescriber **immediately**. Also immediately report skin rash, unusual muscle or bone weakness, or signs of respiratory flu or other infection (eg, chills, fever, sore throat, easy bruising or bleeding, mouth sores, unhealed sores).
Breast-feeding precaution: Breast-feeding is not recommended.
Pregnancy Risk Factor: B
Lactation: Excretion in breast milk unknown/not recommended
Breast-Feeding Issues: It is not known whether etanercept is excreted in human milk or absorbed systemically after ingestion. Because many immunoglobulins are excreted in human milk, and because of the potential for serious adverse reactions in nursing infants from Enbrel®, a decision should be made whether to discontinue nursing or to discontinue the drug.

Administration
Other: Administer subcutaneously. Rotate injection sites. New injections should be given at least one inch from an old site and never into areas where the skin is tender, bruised, red, or hard.
  Powder for reconstitution: Follow package instructions carefully for reconstitution. **Note:** The needle cover of the diluent syringe (multidose vial) may contain dry natural rubber (latex) which should not be handled by persons sensitive to this substance. The maximum amount injected at any single site should not exceed 25 mg.
  Prefilled syringe: May be allowed to reach room temperature prior to injection.
Reconstitution: Reconstitute aseptically with 1 mL sterile bacteriostatic water for injection, USP (supplied). Do not filter reconstituted solution during preparation or administration. **Note:** The needle cover of the diluent syringe may contain dry natural rubber (latex), which should not be handled by persons sensitive to this substance. Swirl to mix; do not shake or vigorously agitate.
Storage: The prefilled syringe or dose tray containing etanercept (sterile powder) must be refrigerated at 2°C to 8°C (36°F to 46°F). Do not freeze. Reconstituted solutions of etanercept should be administered as soon as possible after reconstitution. If not administered immediately after reconstitution, etanercept may be stored in the vial at 2°C to 8°C (36°F to 46°F) for up to 14 days.

♦ **Ethacrynate Sodium** *see* Ethacrynic Acid *on page 575*

Ethacrynic Acid (eth a KRIN ik AS id)

U.S. Brand Names Edecrin®

Synonyms Ethacrynate Sodium

Generic Available No

Pharmacologic Category Diuretic, Loop

Medication Safety Issues
Sound-alike/look-alike issues:
Edecrin® may be confused with Eulexin®, Ecotrin®

Use Management of edema associated with congestive heart failure; hepatic cirrhosis or renal disease; short-term management of ascites due to malignancy, idiopathic edema, and lymphedema

Mechanism of Action/Effect Inhibits reabsorption of sodium and chloride in the ascending loop of Henle and distal renal tubule, interfering with the chloride-binding cotransport system, thus causing increased excretion of water, sodium, chloride, magnesium, and calcium

Contraindications Hypersensitivity to ethacrynic acid or any component of the formulation; anuria; history of severe watery diarrhea caused by this product; infants

Warnings/Precautions Adjust dose to avoid dehydration. In cirrhosis, avoid electrolyte and acid/base imbalances that might lead to hepatic encephalopathy. Ototoxicity is associated with rapid I.V. administration, renal impairment, excessive doses, and concurrent use of other ototoxins. Has been associated with a higher incidence of ototoxicity than other loop diuretics. Hypersensitivity reactions can rarely occur, however, ethacrynic acid has no cross-reactivity to sulfonamides or sulfonylureas. Monitor fluid status and renal function in an attempt to prevent oliguria, azotemia, and reversible increases in BUN and creatinine. Close medical supervision of aggressive diuresis required. Watch for and correct electrolyte disturbances. Coadministration of antihypertensives may increase the risk of hypotension.

Drug Interactions
Decreased Effect: Probenecid decreases diuretic effects of ethacrynic acid. Glucose tolerance may be decreased by loop diuretics, requiring adjustment of hypoglycemic agents. Cholestyramine or colestipol may reduce bioavailability of ethacrynic acid. Indomethacin (and other NSAIDs) may reduce natriuretic and hypotensive effects of diuretics.

Increased Effect/Toxicity: Ethacrynic acid-induced hypokalemia may predispose to digoxin toxicity and may increase the risk of arrhythmia with drugs which may prolong QT interval, including type Ia and type III antiarrhythmic agents, cisapride, and some quinolones (sparfloxacin, gatifloxacin, and moxifloxacin). The risk of toxicity from lithium and salicylates (high dose) may be increased by loop diuretics. Hypotensive effects and/or adverse renal effects of ACE inhibitors and NSAIDs are potentiated by ethacrynic acid-induced hypovolemia. The effects of peripheral adrenergic-blocking drugs or ganglionic blockers may be increased by ethacrynic acid.

Ethacrynic acid may increase the risk of ototoxicity with other ototoxic agents (aminoglycosides, cis-platinum), especially in patients with renal dysfunction. Synergistic diuretic effects occur with thiazide-type diuretics. Diuretics tend to be synergistic with other antihypertensive agents, and hypotension may occur. Nephrotoxicity has been associated with concomitant use of cephaloridine or cephalexin.

Adverse Reactions Frequency not defined.
Central nervous system: Headache, fatigue, apprehension, confusion, fever, chills, encephalopathy (patients with pre-existing liver disease); vertigo
Dermatologic: Skin rash, Henoch-Schönlein purpura (in patient with rheumatic heart disease)
Endocrine & metabolic: Hyponatremia, hyperglycemia, variations in phosphorus, CO_2 content, bicarbonate, and calcium; reversible hyperuricemia, gout, hyperglycemia, hypoglycemia (occurred in two uremic patients who received doses above those recommended)
Gastrointestinal: Anorexia, malaise, abdominal discomfort or pain, dysphagia, nausea, vomiting, diarrhea, gastrointestinal bleeding, acute pancreatitis (rare)
Genitourinary: Hematuria
Hepatic: Jaundice, abnormal liver function tests
Hematology: Agranulocytosis, severe neutropenia, thrombocytopenia
Local: Thrombophlebitis (with intravenous use), local irritation and pain,
Ocular: Blurred vision
Otic: Tinnitus, temporary or permanent deafness
Renal: Serum creatinine increased

Overdosage/Toxicology Symptoms of overdose include electrolyte depletion, volume depletion, dehydration, and circulatory collapse. Treatment is supportive.

Pharmacodynamics/Kinetics
Onset of Action: Diuresis: Oral: ~30 minutes; I.V.: 5 minutes; Peak effect: Oral: 2 hours; I.V.: 30 minutes
Duration of Action: Oral: 12 hours; I.V.: 2 hours
Absorption: Oral: Rapid
Protein Binding: >90%
Half-Life Elimination: Normal renal function: 2-4 hours
Metabolism: Hepatic (35% to 40%) to active cysteine conjugate
Excretion: Feces and urine (30% to 60% as unchanged drug)

Dosing
Adults: I.V. formulation should be diluted in D_5W or NS (1 mg/mL) and infused over several minutes.

Edema:
Oral: 50-100 mg/day in 1-2 divided doses; may increase in increments of 25-50 mg at intervals of several days to a maximum of 400 mg/24 hours.
I.V.: 0.5-1 mg/kg/dose (maximum: 100 mg/dose); repeat doses not routinely recommended; however, if indicated, repeat doses every 8-12 hours.

Elderly: Oral: Initial: 25-50 mg/day

Pediatrics:
Edema: Oral: Children: 1 mg/kg/dose once daily; increase at intervals of 2-3 days as needed, to a maximum of 3 mg/kg/day.

(Continued)

Ethacrynic Acid *(Continued)*

Renal Impairment:
Cl$_{cr}$ <10 mL/minute: Avoid use.

Not removed by hemo- or peritoneal dialysis; supplemental dose is not necessary.

Available Dosage Forms
Injection, powder for reconstitution, as ethacrynate sodium: 50 mg

Tablet: 25 mg

Monitoring and Teaching Issues
Physical Assessment: See Warnings/Precautions for use cautions (eg, impaired hepatic function, dehydration, electrolyte imbalance). Assess potential for interactions with other pharmacological agents or herbal products patient may be taking (especially anything that would impact blood pressure or add to risk of ototoxicity; see Drug Interactions). **Infusion:** See Administration. Assess results of laboratory tests, therapeutic effectiveness (according to purpose for use), and adverse response (eg, dehydration, electrolyte imbalance, CNS changes; see Adverse Reactions) on a regular basis during therapy. Caution patients with diabetes to monitor glucose levels closely (may cause hyper/hypoglycemia). Teach patient appropriate use, possible side effects/appropriate interventions, and adverse symptoms to report (see Patient Education).

Monitoring Laboratory Tests: Renal function, serum electrolytes

Patient Education: Do not take any new medication during therapy without consulting prescriber. Take prescribed dose with food early in day. Include orange juice or bananas (or other potassium-rich foods) in your diet, but do not take potassium supplements without consulting prescriber. If you have diabetes, monitor serum glucose closely (this medication may alter glucose levels). May cause postural hypotension (use caution when rising from lying or sitting position, when climbing stairs, or when driving); lightheadedness, dizziness, or drowsiness (use caution driving or when engaging in hazardous activities); diarrhea (buttermilk, boiled milk, or yogurt may help); or decreased accommodation to heat (avoid excessive exercise in hot weather). Report hearing changes (ringing in ears); persistent headache; unusual confusion or nervousness; abdominal pain or blood in stool (black stool); palpitations, chest pain, rapid heartbeat; flu-like symptoms; skin rash or itching; blurred vision; swelling of ankles or feet; weight changes of more than 3 lb/day; increased fatigue; joint/muscle swelling, pain, cramping, or trembling; or other persistent adverse reactions. **Breast-feeding precaution:** Do not breast-feed.

Dietary Considerations: This product may cause a potassium loss. Your healthcare provider may prescribe a potassium supplement, another medication to help prevent the potassium loss, or recommend that you eat foods high in potassium, especially citrus fruits. Do not change your diet on your own while taking this medication, especially if you are taking potassium supplements or medications to reduce potassium loss. Too much potassium can be as harmful as too little.

Geriatric Considerations: Ethacrynic acid is rarely used because of its increased incidence of ototoxicity as compared to the other loop diuretics (see Additional Information).

Pregnancy Risk Factor: B

Lactation: Contraindicated

Administration
I.V.: Injection should **not** be given SubQ or I.M. due to local pain and irritation. Single I.V. doses should not exceed 100 mg. Administer each 10 mg over a minute.

Compatibility: Stable in D$_5$NS, D$_5$W, LR, NS

Incompatible whole blood or its derivatives

Compatibility when admixed: Incompatible with hydralazine, procainamide, ranitidine, tolazoline, triflupromazine

Ethambutol (e THAM byoo tole)

U.S. Brand Names Myambutol®

Synonyms Ethambutol Hydrochloride

Generic Available Yes

Pharmacologic Category Antitubercular Agent

Medication Safety Issues
Sound-alike/look-alike issues:
Myambutol® may be confused with Nembutal®

Use Treatment of tuberculosis and other mycobacterial diseases in conjunction with other antituberculosis agents

Mechanism of Action/Effect Suppresses mycobacteria multiplication by interfering with RNA synthesis

Contraindications Hypersensitivity to ethambutol or any component of the formulation; optic neuritis; use in children, unconscious patients, or any other patient who may be unable to discern and report visual changes

Warnings/Precautions May cause optic neuritis, resulting in decreased visual acuity or other vision changes. Discontinue promptly in patients with changes in vision, color blindness, or visual defects (effects normally reversible, but reversal may require up to a year). Use only in children whose visual acuity can accurately be determined and monitored (not recommended for use in children <13 years of age). Dosage modification is required in patients with renal insufficiency. Hepatic toxicity has been reported, possibly due to concurrent therapy.

Drug Interactions
Decreased Effect: Decreased absorption with aluminum hydroxide. Avoid concurrent administration of aluminum-containing antacids for at least 4 hours following ethambutol.

Lab Interactions Increased uric acid (S)

Adverse Reactions Frequency not defined.
Cardiovascular: Myocarditis, pericarditis

Central nervous system: Headache, confusion, disorientation, malaise, mental confusion, fever, dizziness, hallucinations

Dermatologic: Rash, pruritus, dermatitis, exfoliative dermatitis

Endocrine & metabolic: Acute gout or hyperuricemia

Gastrointestinal: Abdominal pain, anorexia, nausea, vomiting

Hematologic: Leukopenia, thrombocytopenia, eosinophilia, neutropenia, lymphadenopathy

Hepatic: Abnormal LFTs, hepatotoxicity (possibly related to concurrent therapy), hepatitis

Neuromuscular & skeletal: Peripheral neuritis, arthralgia

Ocular: Optic neuritis; symptoms may include decreased acuity, scotoma, color blindness, or visual defects (usually reversible with discontinuation, irreversible blindness has been described)

Renal: Nephritis

Respiratory: Infiltrates (with or without eosinophilia), pneumonitis

Miscellaneous: Anaphylaxis, anaphylactoid reaction; hypersensitivity syndrome (rash, eosinophilia, and organ-specific inflammation)

Overdosage/Toxicology Symptoms of overdose include decrease in visual acuity, anorexia, joint pain, and numbness of extremities. Treatment is supportive.

Pharmacodynamics/Kinetics

Absorption: ~80%

Time to Peak: Serum: 2-4 hours

Protein Binding: 20% to 30%

Half-Life Elimination: 2.5-3.6 hours; End-stage renal disease: 7-15 hours

Metabolism: Hepatic (20%) to inactive metabolite

Excretion: Urine (~50%) and feces (20%) as unchanged drug

Dosing

Adults & Elderly:

Treatment of tuberculosis (suggested doses by lean body weight):

Daily therapy: 15-25 mg/kg

  40-55 kg: 800 mg

  56-75 kg: 1200 mg

  76-90 kg: 1600 mg (maximum dose regardless of weight)

Twice weekly directly observed therapy (DOT): 50 mg/kg

  40-55 kg: 2000 mg

  56-75 kg: 2800 mg

  76-90 kg: 4000 mg (maximum dose regardless of weight)

Three times/week DOT: 25-30 mg/kg (maximum: 2.5 g)

  40-55 kg: 1200 mg

  56-75 kg: 2000 mg

  76-90 kg: 2400 mg (maximum dose regardless of weight)

Note: Used as part of a multidrug regimen. Treatment regimens consist of an initial 2 month phase, followed by a continuation phase of 4 or 7 additional months; frequency of dosing may differ depending on phase of therapy.

Disseminated *Mycobacterium avium* complex (MAC) in patients with advanced HIV infection: 15 mg/kg ethambutol in combination with azithromycin 600 mg daily

Pediatrics:

Treatment of tuberculosis Oral:

Daily therapy: 15-20 mg/kg/day (maximum: 1 g/day)

Twice weekly directly observed therapy (DOT): 50 mg/kg (maximum: 4 g/dose)

See "Note" in adult dosing.

Renal Impairment:

Cl$_{cr}$ 10-50 mL/minute: Administer every 24-36 hours.

Cl$_{cr}$ <10 mL/minute: Administer every 48 hours.

Slightly dialyzable (5% to 20%); administer dose postdialysis.

Peritoneal dialysis: Dose as for Cl$_{cr}$ <10 mL/minute.

Continuous arteriovenous or venovenous hemofiltration: Administer every 24-36 hours.

Available Dosage Forms Tablet, as hydrochloride: 100 mg, 400 mg

Monitoring and Teaching Issues

Physical Assessment: Assess results of baseline and periodic laboratory tests (see Monitoring Laboratory tests), therapeutic effectiveness, and adverse response (eg, CNS changes, neuritis, and ocular changes; see Adverse Reactions) on a regular basis during therapy. Teach patient appropriate use (need to adhere to dosing program), possible side effects/appropriate interventions, and adverse symptoms to report (see Patient Education).

Monitoring Laboratory Tests: Baseline and periodic (monthly) visual testing (each eye individually, as well as both eyes tested together) in patients receiving >15 mg/kg/day; baseline and periodic renal, hepatic, and hematopoietic tests

Patient Education: Take as scheduled, with meals. Avoid missing doses and do not discontinue without consulting prescriber. Avoid aluminum-containing antacids for at least 4 hours following ethambutol. May cause GI distress (small frequent meals and good oral care may help), dizziness, disorientation, drowsiness (avoid driving or engaging in tasks that require alertness until response to drug is known). You will need to have frequent ophthalmic exams and periodic medical check-ups to evaluate drug effects. Report vision changes, numbness or tingling of extremities, or persistent loss of appetite. **Pregnancy precaution:** Inform prescriber if you are or intend to become pregnant.

Dietary Considerations: May be taken with food as absorption is not affected, may cause gastric irritation.

Geriatric Considerations: Since most elderly patients acquired their tuberculosis before current antituberculin regimens were available, ethambutol is only indicated when patients are from areas where drug resistant *M. tuberculosis* is endemic, in HIV-infected elderly patients, and when drug resistant *M. tuberculosis* is suspected (see dose adjustments for renal impairment).

Pregnancy Risk Factor: C

Pregnancy Issues: There are no adequate and well-controlled studies in pregnant women; teratogenic effects have been seen in animals. Ethambutol has been used safely during pregnancy.

Lactation: Enters breast milk/use caution (AAP considers "compatible")

Breast-Feeding Issues: The manufacturer suggests use during breast-feeding only if benefits to the mother outweigh the possible risk to the infant. Some references suggest

(Continued)

Ethambutol *(Continued)*

that exposure to the infant is low and does not produce toxicity, and breast-feeding should not be discouraged. Other references recommend if breast-feeding, monitor the infant for rash, malaise, nausea, or vomiting.

Administration
Storage: Store at controlled room temperature of 20°C to 25°C (68°F to 77°F).
Related Information
Tuberculosis *on page 1864*

♦ **Ethambutol Hydrochloride** *see* Ethambutol *on page 576*

Ethinyl Estradiol and Desogestrel
(ETH in il es tra DYE ole & des oh JES trel)

U.S. Brand Names Apri®; Cyclessa®; Desogen®; Kariva™; Mircette®; Ortho-Cept®; Solia™; Velivet™

Synonyms Desogestrel and Ethinyl Estradiol; Ortho Cept

Generic Available Yes

Pharmacologic Category Contraceptive; Estrogen and Progestin Combination

Medication Safety Issues
Sound-alike/look-alike issues:
Ortho-Cept® may be confused with Ortho-Cyclen®

Use Prevention of pregnancy

Unlabeled/Investigational Use Treatment of hypermenorrhea (menorrhagia); pain associated with endometriosis; dysmenorrhea; dysfunctional uterine bleeding

Mechanism of Action/Effect Combination hormonal contraceptives inhibit ovulation and also produce changes in the cervical mucus and endometrium creating an unfavorable environment for sperm penetration and nidation.

Contraindications Hypersensitivity to ethinyl estradiol, etonogestrel, desogestrel, or any component of the formulation; history of or current thrombophlebitis or venous thromboembolic disorders (including DVT, PE); active or recent (within 1 year) arterial thromboembolic disease (eg, stroke, MI); cerebral vascular disease, coronary artery disease, valvular heart disease with complications, severe hypertension; diabetes mellitus with vascular involvement; severe headache with focal neurological symptoms; known or suspected breast carcinoma, endometrial cancer, estrogen-dependent neoplasms, undiagnosed abnormal genital bleeding; hepatic dysfunction or tumor, cholestatic jaundice of pregnancy, jaundice with prior combination hormonal contraceptive use; major surgery with prolonged immobilization; heavy smoking (≥15 cigarettes/day) in patients >35 years of age; pregnancy

Warnings/Precautions Combination hormonal contraceptives do not protect against HIV infection or other sexually-transmitted diseases. The risk of cardiovascular side effects increases in women who smoke cigarettes, especially those who are >35 years of age; women who use combination hormonal contraceptives should be strongly advised not to smoke. Combination hormonal contraceptives may lead to increased risk of myocardial infarction, use with caution in patients with risk factors for coronary artery disease. May increase the risk of thromboembolism. Combination hormonal contraceptives may have a dose-related risk of vascular disease, hypertension, and gallbladder disease. Women with hypertension should be encouraged to use another form of contraception. The use of combination hormonal contraceptives has been associated with a slight increase in frequency of breast cancer, however, studies are not consistent. Combination hormonal contraceptives may cause glucose intolerance. Retinal thrombosis has been reported (rarely). Use with caution in patients with renal disease, conditions that may be aggravated by fluid retention, depression, or history of migraine. Not for use prior to menarche.

The minimum dosage combination of estrogen/progestin that will effectively treat the individual patient should be used. New patients should be started on products containing <50 mcg of estrogen per tablet.

Drug Interactions
Cytochrome P450 Effect:
Ethinyl estradiol: **Substrate** of CYP2C8/9 (minor), 3A4 (major), 3A5-7 (minor); **Inhibits** CYP1A2 (weak), 2B6 (weak), 2C19 (weak), 3A4 (weak)
Desogestrel: **Substrate** of CYP2C19 (major)
Decreased Effect: CYP2C19 inducers may decrease the levels/effects of desogestrel; example inducers include aminoglutethimide, carbamazepine, phenytoin, and rifampin. CYP3A4 inducers may decrease the levels/effects of ethinyl estradiol; example inducers include aminoglutethimide, carbamazepine, nafcillin, phenobarbital, phenytoin, and rifamycins. Combination hormonal contraceptives may decrease plasma levels of acetaminophen, clofibric acid, lorazepam, morphine, oxazepam, salicylic acid, temazepam. Contraceptive effect decreased by acitretin, amprenavir, griseofulvin, lopinavir, nelfinavir, nevirapine, penicillins (effect not consistent), ritonavir, tetracyclines (effect not consistent), troglitazone. Combination hormonal contraceptives may decrease (or increase) the effects of coumarin derivatives.
Increased Effect/Toxicity: Acetaminophen, ascorbic acid, and repaglinide may increase plasma levels of estrogen component. Atorvastatin and indinavir increase plasma levels of combination hormonal contraceptives. Combination hormonal contraceptives increase the plasma levels of alprazolam, chlordiazepoxide, cyclosporine, diazepam, prednisolone, selegiline, theophylline, tricyclic antidepressants. Combination hormonal contraceptives may increase (or decrease) the effects of coumarin derivatives.

Nutritional/Ethanol Interactions
Food: CNS effects of caffeine may be enhanced if combination hormonal contraceptives are used concurrently with caffeine. Grapefruit juice increases ethinyl estradiol concentrations and would be expected to increase progesterone serum levels as well; clinical implications are unclear.
Herb/Nutraceutical: St John's wort may decrease the effectiveness of combination hormonal contraceptives by inducing hepatic enzymes. Avoid dong quai and black cohosh (have estrogen activity). Avoid saw palmetto, red clover, ginseng.

Lab Interactions Increased platelet aggregation, thyroid-binding globulin, total thyroid hormone (T_4), serum triglycerides/phospholipids; decreased antithrombin III, serum folate concentration

Adverse Reactions Frequency not defined.

Cardiovascular: Arterial thromboembolism, cerebral hemorrhage, cerebral thrombosis, edema, hypertension, mesenteric thrombosis, MI

Central nervous system: Depression, dizziness, headache, migraine, nervousness, premenstrual syndrome, stroke

Dermatologic: Acne, erythema multiforme, erythema nodosum, hirsutism, loss of scalp hair, melasma (may persist), rash (allergic)

Endocrine & metabolic: Amenorrhea, breakthrough bleeding, breast enlargement, breast secretion, breast tenderness, carbohydrate intolerance, lactation decreased (postpartum), glucose tolerance decreased, libido changes, menstrual flow changes, sex hormone-binding globulins (SHBG) increased, spotting, temporary infertility (following discontinuation), thyroid-binding globulin increased, triglycerides increased

Gastrointestinal: Abdominal cramps, appetite changes, bloating, cholestasis, colitis, gallbladder disease, jaundice, nausea, vomiting, weight gain/loss

Genitourinary: Cervical erosion changes, cervical secretion changes, cystitis-like syndrome, vaginal candidiasis, vaginitis

Hematologic: Antithrombin III decreased, folate levels decreased, hemolytic uremic syndrome, norepinephrine induced platelet aggregability increased, porphyria, prothrombin increased; factors VII, VIII, IX, and X

Hepatic: Benign liver tumors, Budd-Chiari syndrome, cholestatic jaundice, hepatic adenomas

Local: Thrombophlebitis

Ocular: Cataracts, change in corneal curvature (steepening), contact lens intolerance, optic neuritis, retinal thrombosis

Renal: Impaired renal function

Respiratory: Pulmonary thromboembolism

Miscellaneous: Hemorrhagic eruption

Overdosage/Toxicology Toxicity is unlikely following single exposures of excessive doses. May cause withdrawal bleeding in females. Any treatment following emesis and charcoal administration should be supportive and symptomatic.

Pharmacodynamics/Kinetics

Absorption:

Desogestrel: Rapid and complete

Protein Binding:

Desogestrel: Etonogestrel (active metabolite): 98%, primarily to sex hormone-binding globulin

Half-Life Elimination:

Desogestrel: 37.1 hours

Metabolism:

Desogestrel: Hepatic via CYP2C9 to active metabolite etonogestrel (3-keto-desogestrel); etonogestrel metabolized via CYP3A4

Excretion:

Desogestrel: Urine and feces (as metabolites)

Dosing

Adults: Female: Contraception: Oral:

Schedule 1 (Sunday starter): Dose begins on first Sunday after onset of menstruation; if the menstrual period starts on Sunday, take first tablet that very same day. **With a Sunday start, an additional method of contraception should be used until after the first 7 days of consecutive administration.**

For 21-tablet package: Dosage is 1 tablet daily for 21 consecutive days, followed by 7 days off of the medication; a new course begins on the 8th day after the last tablet is taken.

For 28-tablet package: Dosage is 1 tablet daily without interruption.

Schedule 2 (Day 1 starter): Dose starts on first day of menstrual cycle taking 1 tablet daily.

For 21-tablet package: Dosage is 1 tablet daily for 21 consecutive days, followed by 7 days off of the medication; a new course begins on the 8th day after the last tablet is taken.

For 28-tablet package: Dosage is 1 tablet daily without interruption.

If all doses have been taken on schedule and one menstrual period is missed, continue dosing cycle. If two consecutive menstrual periods are missed, pregnancy test is required before new dosing cycle is started.

Missed doses **monophasic formulations** (refer to package insert for complete information):

One dose missed: Take as soon as remembered or take 2 tablets next day

Two consecutive doses missed in the first 2 weeks: Take 2 tablets as soon as remembered or 2 tablets next 2 days. **An additional method of contraception should be used for 7 days after missed dose.**

Two consecutive doses missed in week 3 or three consecutive doses missed at any time: Schedule 1 (Sunday starter): Continue to take 1 tablet daily until Sunday, then discard the rest of the pack, and a new pack is started that same day. Schedule 2 (Day 1 starter): Current pack should be discarded, and a new pack started that same day. **An additional method of contraception should be used for 7 days after missed dose.**

Missed doses **biphasic/triphasic formulations** (refer to package insert for complete information):

One dose missed: Take as soon as remembered or take 2 tablets next day.

Two consecutive doses missed in week 1 or week 2 of the pack: Take 2 tablets as soon as remembered and 2 tablets the next day. Resume taking 1 tablet daily until the pack is empty. **An additional method of contraception should be used for 7 days after a missed dose.**

(Continued)

Ethinyl Estradiol and Desogestrel *(Continued)*

Two consecutive doses missed in week 3 of the pack; **an additional method of contraception must be used for 7 days after a missed dose:**

Schedule 1 (Sunday starter): Take 1 tablet every day until Sunday. Discard the remaining pack and start a new pack of pills on the same day.

Schedule 2 (Day 1 starter): Discard the remaining pack and start a new pack the same day.

Three or more consecutive doses missed; **an additional method of contraception must be used for 7 days after a missed dose:**

Schedule 1 (Sunday starter): Take 1 tablet every day until Sunday; on Sunday, discard the pack and start a new pack.

Schedule 2 (Day 1 starter): Discard the remaining pack and begin new pack of tablets starting on the same day.

Pediatrics: Female: Contraception: Oral: See adult dosing; not to be used prior to menarche.

Renal Impairment: Specific guidelines not available; use with caution.

Hepatic Impairment: Contraindicated in patients with hepatic impairment.

Available Dosage Forms Tablet:

Low-dose formulation:

Kariva™:

Day 1-21: Ethinyl estradiol 0.02 mg and desogestrel 0.15 mg [21 white tablets]

Day 22-23: 2 inactive light green tablets

Day 24-28: Ethinyl estradiol 0.01 mg [5 light blue tablets] (28s)

Mircette®:

Day 1-21: Ethinyl estradiol 0.02 mg and desogestrel 0.15 mg [21 white tablets]

Day 22-23: 2 inactive green tablets

Day 24-28: Ethinyl estradiol 0.01 mg [5 yellow tablets] (28s)

Monophasic formulations:

Apri® 28: Ethinyl estradiol 0.03 mg and desogestrel 0.15 mg [21 rose tablets and 7 white inactive tablets] (28s)

Desogen®, Solia™: Ethinyl estradiol 0.03 mg and desogestrel 0.15 mg [21 white tablets and 7 green inactive tablets] (28s)

Ortho-Cept® 28: Ethinyl estradiol 0.03 mg and desogestrel 0.15 mg [21 orange tablets and 7 green inactive tablets] (28s)

Triphasic formulation:

Cyclessa®:

Day 1-7: Ethinyl estradiol 0.025 mg and desogestrel 0.1 mg [7 light yellow tablets]

Day 8-14: Ethinyl estradiol 0.025 mg and desogestrel 0.125 mg [7 orange tablets]

Day 14-21: Ethinyl estradiol 0.025 mg and desogestrel 0.15 mg [7 red tablets]

Day 21-28: 7 green inactive tablets (28s)

Velivet™:

Day 1-7: Ethinyl estradiol 0.025 mg and desogestrel 0.1 mg [7 beige tablets]

Day 8-14: Ethinyl estradiol 0.025 mg and desogestrel 0.125 mg [7 orange tablets]

Day 14-21: Ethinyl estradiol 0.025 mg and desogestrel 0.15 mg [7 pink tablets]

Day 21-28: 7 white inactive tablets (28s)

Monitoring and Teaching Issues

Physical Assessment: Monitor blood pressure on a regular basis. Assess for adverse reactions and potential drug interactions. Assess knowledge/teach importance of regular (monthly) blood pressure checks and annual physical assessment, Pap smear, and vision assessment. Teach importance of maintaining prescribed schedule of dosing. **Pregnancy risk factor X:** Do not use if patient is pregnant.

Patient Education: Oral contraceptives do not protect against HIV infection or other sexually-transmitted diseases. Take exactly as directed by prescriber (see package insert). You are at risk of becoming pregnant if doses are missed. Detailed and complete information on dosing and missed doses can be found in the package insert. Be aware that some medications may reduce the effectiveness of oral contraceptives; an alternate form of contraception may be needed. Check all medicines (prescription and over-the-counter), herbal and alternative products with prescriber. It is important that you check your blood pressure monthly (same day each month) and that you have an annual physical assessment, Pap smear, and vision exam while taking this medication. Avoid smoking while taking this medication; smoking increases risk of adverse effects, including thromboembolic events and heart attacks. You may experience loss of appetite (small frequent meals will help); or constipation (increased exercise, fluids, fruit, fiber, or stool softeners may help). If you have diabetes, use accurate serum glucose testing to identify any changes in glucose tolerance; notify prescriber of significant changes so antidiabetic medication can be adjusted if necessary. Report immediately pain or muscle soreness; warmth, swelling, pain, or redness in calves; shortness of breath; sudden loss of vision; unresolved leg/foot swelling; change in menstrual pattern (unusual bleeding, amenorrhea, breakthrough spotting); breast tenderness that does not go away; acute abdominal cramping; signs of vaginal infection (drainage, pain, itching); CNS changes (blurred vision, confusion, acute anxiety, or unresolved depression); or significant weight gain (>5 lb/week). Notify prescriber of changes in contact lens tolerance. **Pregnancy/breast-feeding precautions:** This medication should not be used during pregnancy. If you suspect you may become pregnant, contact prescriber immediately.

Dietary Considerations: Should be taken at same time each day.

Pregnancy Risk Factor: X

Pregnancy Issues: Pregnancy should be ruled out prior to treatment and discontinued if pregnancy occurs. In general, the use of combination hormonal contraceptives when inadvertently taken early in pregnancy have not been associated with teratogenic effects. Due to increased risk of thromboembolism postpartum, combination hormonal contraceptives should not be started earlier than 4-6 weeks following delivery.

Lactation: Enters breast milk/not recommended (AAP rates "compatible")

Breast-Feeding Issues: Jaundice and breast enlargement in the nursing infant have been reported following the use of combination hormonal contraceptives. May decrease the quality and quantity of breast milk; a nonhormonal form of contraception is recommended.

Administration

Oral: Administer at the same time each day.

Storage: Store at controlled room temperature of 25°C (77°F).

Ethinyl Estradiol and Drospirenone
(ETH in il es tra DYE ole & droh SPYE re none)

U.S. Brand Names Yasmin®

Synonyms Drospirenone and Ethinyl Estradiol

Generic Available No

Pharmacologic Category Contraceptive; Estrogen and Progestin Combination

Use Prevention of pregnancy

Unlabeled/Investigational Use Treatment of hypermenorrhea (menorrhagia); pain associated with endometriosis; dysmenorrhea; dysfunctional uterine bleeding

Mechanism of Action/Effect Combination oral contraceptives inhibit ovulation and also produce changes in the cervical mucus and endometrium creating an unfavorable environment for sperm penetration and nidation.

Contraindications Hypersensitivity to ethinyl estradiol, drospirenone, or to any component of the formulation; history of or current thrombophlebitis or venous thromboembolic disorders (including DVT, PE); active or recent (within 1 year) arterial thromboembolic disease (eg, stroke, MI); cerebral vascular disease, coronary artery disease, severe hypertension; diabetes with vascular involvement; headache with focal neurological symptoms; known or suspected breast carcinoma, endometrial cancer, estrogen-dependent neoplasms, undiagnosed abnormal genital bleeding; renal insufficiency, hepatic dysfunction or tumor, adrenal insufficiency, cholestatic jaundice of pregnancy, jaundice with prior oral contraceptive use; heavy smoking (≥15 cigarettes/day) in patients >35 years of age; pregnancy

Warnings/Precautions Oral contraceptives do not protect against HIV infection or other sexually-transmitted diseases. The risk of cardiovascular side effects increases in women who smoke cigarettes, especially those who are >35 years of age; women who use oral contraceptives should be strongly advised not to smoke. Oral contraceptives may lead to increased risk of myocardial infarction, use with caution in patients with risk factors for coronary artery disease. May increase the risk of thromboembolism. Oral contraceptives may have a dose-related risk of vascular disease (decreases HDL), hypertension, and gallbladder disease; a preparation with the lowest effective estrogen/progesterone combination should be used. Women with high blood pressure should be encouraged to use another form of contraception. Oral contraceptives may cause glucose intolerance. Retinal thrombosis has been reported (rarely) with oral contraceptive use. Use with caution in patients with conditions that may be aggravated by fluid retention, depression, or patients with history of migraine. Not for use prior to menarche.

Drospirenone has antimineralocorticoid activity that may lead to hyperkalemia in patients with renal insufficiency, hepatic dysfunction, or adrenal insufficiency. Use caution with medications that may increase serum potassium.

Drug Interactions

Cytochrome P450 Effect:

Ethinyl estradiol: **Substrate** of CYP2C8/9 (minor), 3A4 (major), 3A5-7 (minor); **Inhibits** CYP1A2 (weak), 2B6 (weak), 2C19 (weak), 3A4 (weak)

Drospirenone: **Substrate** of CYP3A4 (minor); **Inhibits** CYP1A2 (weak), 2C8/9 (weak), 2C19 (weak), 3A4 (weak)

Decreased Effect: Oral contraceptives may decrease the plasma concentration of acetaminophen, clofibric acid, morphine, salicylic acid, and temazepam. Aminoglutethimide, anticonvulsants (carbamazepine, felbamate, phenobarbital, phenytoin, topiramate), phenylbutazone, rifampin, and ritonavir may increase metabolism leading to decreased effect of oral contraceptives. Oral contraceptives may decrease (or increase) the effects of coumarin derivatives.

Increased Effect/Toxicity: ACE inhibitors, aldosterone antagonists, angiotensin II receptor antagonists, heparin, NSAIDs (when taken daily, long term), and potassium-sparing diuretics increase risk of hyperkalemia with concomitant use. Acetaminophen, ascorbic acid, and atorvastatin may increase plasma concentrations of oral contraceptives. Ethinyl estradiol may increase plasma concentrations of cyclosporine, prednisolone, selegiline, and theophylline. Oral contraceptives may increase (or decrease) the effects of coumarin derivatives.

Nutritional/Ethanol Interactions

Food: CNS effects of caffeine may be enhanced if oral contraceptives are used concurrently with caffeine. Grapefruit juice increases ethinyl estradiol concentrations; clinical implications are unclear.

Herb/Nutraceutical: St John's wort may decrease the effectiveness of oral contraceptives by inducing hepatic enzymes; may also result in breakthrough bleeding.

Adverse Reactions

>1%:

Central nervous system: Depression, dizziness, emotional lability, headache, migraine, nervousness

Dermatologic: Acne, pruritus, rash

Endocrine & metabolic: Amenorrhea, dysmenorrhea, intermenstrual bleeding, menstrual irregularities

Gastrointestinal: Abdominal pain, diarrhea, gastroenteritis, nausea, vomiting

Genitourinary: Cystitis, leukorrhea, vaginal moniliasis, vaginitis

Neuromuscular & skeletal: Back pain, weakness

Respiratory: Bronchitis, pharyngitis, sinusitis, upper respiratory infection

Miscellaneous: Allergic reaction, flu-like syndrome, infection

(Continued)

Ethinyl Estradiol and Drospirenone *(Continued)*

Adverse reactions reported with other oral contraceptives: Appetite changes, antithrombin III decreased, arterial thromboembolism, benign liver tumors, breast changes, Budd-Chiari syndrome, carbohydrate intolerance, cataracts, cerebral hemorrhage, cerebral thrombosis, cervical changes, change in corneal curvature (steepening), cholestatic jaundice, colitis, contact lens intolerance, decreased lactation (postpartum), deep vein thrombosis, diplopia, edema, erythema multiforme, erythema nodosum; factors VII, VIII, IX, X increased; folate serum concentrations decreased, gallbladder disease, glucose intolerance, hemorrhagic eruption, hemolytic uremic syndrome, hepatic adenomas, hirsutism, hypercalcemia, hypertension, hyperglycemia, libido changes, melasma, mesenteric thrombosis, MI, papilledema, platelet aggregability increased, porphyria, premenstrual syndrome, proptosis, prothrombin increased, pulmonary thromboembolism, renal function impairment, retinal thrombosis, sex hormone-binding globulin increased, thrombophlebitis, thyroid-binding globulin increased, total thyroid hormone (T_4) increased, triglycerides/phospholipids increased, vaginal candidiasis, weight changes

Overdosage/Toxicology May cause nausea; withdrawal bleeding may occur in females. Due to antimineralocorticoid properties of drospirenone, monitor potassium and sodium serum concentrations and evidence of metabolic acidosis.

Pharmacodynamics/Kinetics

Bioavailability:
> **Drospirenone:** 76%

Time to Peak:
> **Drospirenone:** 1-3 hours

Protein Binding:
> **Drospirenone:** Serum proteins (excluding sex hormone-binding globulin and corticosteroid binding globulin): 97%

Half-Life Elimination:
> **Drospirenone:** 30 hours

Metabolism:
> **Drospirenone:** To inactive metabolites; minor metabolism hepatically via CYP3A4

Excretion:
> **Drospirenone:** Urine and feces

Dosing

Adults: Female: Contraception: Oral: Dosage is 1 tablet daily for 28 consecutive days. Dose should be taken at the same time each day, either after the evening meal or at bedtime. Dosing may be started on the first day of menstrual period (Day 1 starter) or on the first Sunday after the onset of the menstrual period (Sunday starter).

Day 1 starter: Dose starts on first day of menstrual cycle taking 1 tablet daily.

Sunday starter: Dose begins on first Sunday after onset of menstruation; if the menstrual period starts on Sunday, take first tablet that very same day. **With a Sunday start, an additional method of contraception should be used until after the first 7 days of consecutive administration.**

If all doses have been taken on schedule and one menstrual period is missed, continue dosing cycle. If two consecutive menstrual periods are missed, pregnancy test is required before new dosing cycle is started.

If doses have been missed during the first 3 weeks and the menstrual period is missed, pregnancy should be ruled out prior to continuing treatment.

> **Missed doses (monophasic formulations)** (refer to package insert for complete information):
>
> One dose missed: Take as soon as remembered or take 2 tablets next day
>
> Two consecutive doses missed in the first 2 weeks: Take 2 tablets as soon as remembered or 2 tablets next 2 days. **An additional method of contraception should be used for 7 days after missed dose.**
>
> Two consecutive doses missed in week 3 or three consecutive doses missed at any time: **An additional method of contraception must be used for 7 days after a missed dose.**
>
> > Day 1 starter: Current pack should be discarded, and a new pack should be started that same day.
> >
> > Sunday starter: Continue dose of 1 tablet daily until Sunday, then discard the rest of the pack, and a new pack should be started that same day.
>
> Any number of doses missed in week 4: Continue taking one pill each day until pack is empty; no back-up method of contraception is needed

Pediatrics: Female: Contraception: Oral: Refer to adult dosing; not to be used prior to menarche.

Renal Impairment: Contraindicated in patients with renal dysfunction (Cl_{cr} ≤50 mL/minute).

Hepatic Impairment: Contraindicated in patients with hepatic dysfunction.

Available Dosage Forms Tablet: Ethinyl estradiol 0.03 mg and drospirenone 3 mg [21 yellow active tablets and 7 white inactive tablets] (28s)

Monitoring and Teaching Issues

Physical Assessment: Monitor or teach patient to monitor blood pressure on a regular (monthly) basis, and the importance of annual physical examinations (including Pap smear and vision exam). Assess knowledge/teach patient the importance of maintaining prescribed schedule of dosing, possible side effects, appropriate interventions, and adverse reactions to report. **Pregnancy risk factor X:** Determine patient is not pregnant prior to prescribing.

Patient Education: Take exactly as directed by prescriber (see package insert). An additional form of contraception should be used until after the first 7 consecutive days of administration. You are at risk of becoming pregnant if doses are missed. If you miss a dose, take as soon as possible or double the dose the next day. If two or more consecutive doses are missed, contact prescriber for restarting directions. Detailed and complete information on dosing and missed doses can be found in the package insert. If any number of doses are missed in week 4, continue taking one pill each day until pack is empty; no back-up method of contraception is needed. Be aware that some medications may reduce the effectiveness of oral contraceptives; an alternate form of contraception may be needed (see Drug Interactions). It is important that you check your blood pressure monthly (on same day each month) and report any increased blood pressure to prescriber. Have an annual physical assessment, Pap smear, and vision exam while taking this medication. Avoid smoking while taking this medication; smoking increases risk of adverse effects, including thromboembolic events and heart attacks. You may experience loss of appetite (small frequent meals will help); or constipation (increased exercise, fluids, fruit, fiber, or stool softeners may help). If you have diabetes, you should use accurate serum glucose testing to identify any changes in glucose tolerance; notify prescriber of significant changes so antidiabetic medication can be adjusted if necessary. Report immediately pain or muscle soreness; warmth, swelling, pain, or redness in calves; shortness of breath; sudden loss of vision; unresolved leg/foot swelling or weight gain (>5 lb); change in menstrual pattern (unusual bleeding, amenorrhea, breakthrough spotting); breast tenderness that does not go away; acute abdominal cramping; signs of vaginal infection (drainage, pain, itching); CNS changes (blurred vision, confusion, acute anxiety, or unresolved depression); or other persistent adverse effects. **Pregnancy/breast-feeding precautions:** Inform prescriber if you are pregnant. Breast-feeding is not recommended.

Pregnancy Risk Factor: X

Pregnancy Issues: In general, the use of oral contraceptives when inadvertently taken early in pregnancy have not been associated with teratogenic effects. Esophageal atresia was reported in one infant with a single-cycle exposure to ethinyl estradiol and drospirenone *in utero* (association not known). Pregnancy should be ruled out prior to treatment and discontinued if pregnancy occurs. Due to increased risk of thromboembolism postpartum, do not start oral contraceptives earlier than 4-6 weeks following delivery.

Lactation: Enters breast milk/not recommended

Breast-Feeding Issues: The amount of drospirenone excreted in breast milk is ~0.02%, resulting in a maximum of ~3 mcg/day drospirenone to the infant. Jaundice and breast enlargement in the nursing infant have been reported following the use of other oral contraceptives. In addition, may decrease the quality and quantity of breast milk. Other forms of contraception are recommended while breast-feeding.

Administration
Oral: To be taken at the same time each day, either after the evening meal or at bedtime

Storage: Store at 25°C (77°F).

Ethinyl Estradiol and Ethynodiol Diacetate
(ETH in il es tra DYE ole & e thye noe DYE ole dye AS e tate)

U.S. Brand Names Demulen®; Zovia™

Synonyms Ethynodiol Diacetate and Ethinyl Estradiol

Generic Available Yes

Pharmacologic Category Contraceptive; Estrogen and Progestin Combination

Medication Safety Issues
Sound-alike/look-alike issues:
Demulen® may be confused with Dalmane®, Demerol®

Use Prevention of pregnancy

Unlabeled/Investigational Use Treatment of hypermenorrhea (menorrhagia); pain associated with endometriosis; dysmenorrhea; dysfunctional uterine bleeding

Mechanism of Action/Effect Combination hormonal contraceptives inhibit ovulation and also produce changes in the cervical mucus and endometrium creating an unfavorable environment for sperm penetration and nidation.

Contraindications Hypersensitivity to ethinyl estradiol, ethynodiol diacetate, or any component of the formulation; history of or current thrombophlebitis or venous thromboembolic disorders (including DVT, PE); active or recent (within 1 year) arterial thromboembolic disease (eg, stroke, MI); cerebral vascular disease, coronary artery disease, valvular heart disease with complications, severe hypertension; diabetes mellitus with vascular involvement; severe headache with focal neurological symptoms; known or suspected breast carcinoma, endometrial cancer, estrogen-dependent neoplasms, undiagnosed abnormal genital bleeding; hepatic dysfunction or tumor, cholestatic jaundice of pregnancy, jaundice with prior combination hormonal contraceptive use; major surgery with prolonged immobilization; heavy smoking (≥15 cigarettes/day) in patients >35 years of age; pregnancy

Warnings/Precautions Combination hormonal contraceptives do not protect against HIV infection or other sexually-transmitted diseases. The risk of cardiovascular side effects increases in women who smoke cigarettes, especially those who are >35 years of age; women who use combination hormonal contraceptives should be strongly advised not to smoke. Combination hormonal contraceptives may lead to increased risk of myocardial infarction, use with caution in patients with risk factors for coronary artery disease. May increase the risk of thromboembolism. Combination hormonal contraceptives may have a dose-related risk of vascular disease, hypertension, and gallbladder disease. Women with hypertension should be encouraged to use a nonhormonal form of contraception. The use of combination hormonal contraceptives has been associated with a slight increase in frequency of breast cancer, however, studies are not consistent. Combination hormonal contraceptives may cause glucose intolerance. Retinal thrombosis has been reported (rarely). Use with caution in patients with renal disease, conditions that may be aggravated by fluid retention, depression, or history of migraine. Not for use prior to menarche.

The minimum dosage combination of estrogen/progestin that will effectively treat the individual patient should be used. New patients should be started on products containing <50 mcg of estrogen per tablet.

Drug Interactions
Cytochrome P450 Effect: Ethinyl estradiol: **Substrate** of CYP2C8/9 (minor), 3A4 (major), 3A5-7 (minor); **Inhibits** CYP1A2 (weak), 2B6 (weak), 2C19 (weak), 3A4 (weak)

Decreased Effect: CYP3A4 inducers may decrease the levels/effects of ethinyl estradiol; example inducers include aminoglutethimide, carbamazepine, nafcillin, nevirapine, phenobarbital, phenytoin, and rifamycins. Combination hormonal contraceptives may decrease plasma levels of acetaminophen, clofibric acid, lorazepam, morphine, oxazepam, salicylic
(Continued)

Ethinyl Estradiol and Ethynodiol Diacetate *(Continued)*

acid, temazepam. Contraceptive effect decreased by acitretin, aminoglutethimide, amprenavir, anticonvulsants, griseofulvin, lopinavir, nelfinavir, penicillins (effect not consistent), rifampin, ritonavir, tetracyclines (effect not consistent). Combination hormonal contraceptives may decrease (or increase) the effects of coumarin derivatives.

Increased Effect/Toxicity: Acetaminophen and ascorbic acid may increase plasma levels of estrogen component. Atorvastatin and indinavir increase plasma levels of combination hormonal contraceptives. Combination hormonal contraceptives increase the plasma levels of alprazolam, chlordiazepoxide, cyclosporine, diazepam, prednisolone, selegiline, theophylline, tricyclic antidepressants. Combination hormonal contraceptives may increase (or decrease) the effects of coumarin derivatives.

Nutritional/Ethanol Interactions

Food: CNS effects of caffeine may be enhanced if combination hormonal contraceptives are used concurrently with caffeine. Grapefruit juice increases ethinyl estradiol concentrations and would be expected to increase progesterone serum levels as well; clinical implications are unclear.

Herb/Nutraceutical: St John's wort may decrease the effectiveness of combination hormonal contraceptives by inducing hepatic enzymes. Avoid dong quai and black cohosh (have estrogen activity). Avoid saw palmetto, red clover, ginseng.

Lab Interactions Increased platelet aggregation, thyroid-binding globulin, total thyroid hormone (T_4), serum triglycerides/phospholipids; decreased antithrombin III, serum folate concentration

Adverse Reactions Frequency not defined.

Cardiovascular: Arterial thromboembolism, cerebral hemorrhage, cerebral thrombosis, edema, hypertension, mesenteric thrombosis, MI

Central nervous system: Depression, dizziness, headache, migraine, nervousness, premenstrual syndrome, stroke

Dermatologic: Acne, erythema multiforme, erythema nodosum, hirsutism, loss of scalp hair, melasma (may persist), rash (allergic)

Endocrine & metabolic: Amenorrhea, breakthrough bleeding, breast enlargement, breast secretion, breast tenderness, carbohydrate intolerance, lactation decreased (postpartum), glucose tolerance decreased, libido changes, menstrual flow changes, sex hormone-binding globulins (SHBG) increased, spotting, temporary infertility (following discontinuation), thyroid-binding globulin increased, triglycerides increased

Gastrointestinal: Abdominal cramps, appetite changes, bloating, cholestasis, colitis, gallbladder disease, jaundice, nausea, vomiting, weight gain/loss

Genitourinary: Cervical erosion changes, cervical secretion changes, cystitis-like syndrome, vaginal candidiasis, vaginitis

Hematologic: Antithrombin III decreased, folate levels decreased, hemolytic uremic syndrome, norepinephrine induced platelet aggregability increased, porphyria, prothrombin increased; factors VII, VIII, IX, and X increased

Hepatic: Benign liver tumors, Budd-Chiari syndrome, cholestatic jaundice, hepatic adenomas

Local: Thrombophlebitis

Ocular: Cataracts, change in corneal curvature (steepening), contact lens intolerance, optic neuritis, retinal thrombosis

Renal: Impaired renal function

Respiratory: Pulmonary thromboembolism

Miscellaneous: Hemorrhagic eruption

Overdosage/Toxicology Toxicity is unlikely following single exposures of excessive doses. May cause withdrawal bleeding in females. Any treatment following emesis and charcoal administration should be supportive and symptomatic.

Pharmacodynamics/Kinetics

Half-Life Elimination:

Ethynodiol diacetate (converted to norethindrone) Terminal: 5-14 hours

Metabolism:

Ethynodiol diacetate (converted to norethindrone): Hepatic conjugation

Dosing

Adults:

Female: Contraception: Oral:

Schedule 1 (Sunday starter): Dose begins on first Sunday after onset of menstruation; if the menstrual period starts on Sunday, take first tablet that very same day. **With a Sunday start, an additional method of contraception should be used until after the first 7 days of consecutive administration:**

For 21-tablet package: 1 tablet/day for 21 consecutive days, followed by 7 days off of the medication; a new course begins on the 8th day after the last tablet is taken

For 28-tablet package: 1 tablet/day without interruption

Schedule 2 (Day-1 starter): Dose starts on first day of menstrual cycle taking 1 tablet/day:

For 21-tablet package: 1 tablet/day for 21 consecutive days, followed by 7 days off of the medication; a new course begins on the 8th day after the last tablet is taken

For 28-tablet package: 1 tablet/day without interruption

If all doses have been taken on schedule and one menstrual period is missed, continue dosing cycle. If two consecutive menstrual periods are missed, pregnancy test is required before new dosing cycle is started.

Missed doses **monophasic formulations** (refer to package insert for complete information):

One dose missed: Take as soon as remembered or take 2 tablets next day

Two consecutive doses missed in the first 2 weeks: Take 2 tablets as soon as remembered or 2 tablets next 2 days. **An additional method of contraception should be used for 7 days after missed dose.**

Two consecutive doses missed in week 3 or three consecutive doses missed at any time: **An additional method of contraception must be used for 7 days after a missed dose:**

Schedule 1 (Sunday starter): Continue dose of 1 tablet daily until Sunday, then discard the rest of the pack, and a new pack should be started that same day.

Schedule 2 (Day-1 starter): Current pack should be discarded, and a new pack should be started that same day.

Pediatrics: Female: Contraception: Oral: Refer to adult dosing; not to be used prior to menarche.

Renal Impairment: Specific guidelines not available; use with caution.

Hepatic Impairment: Contraindicated in patients with hepatic impairment.

Available Dosage Forms [DSC] = Discontinued product

Tablet, monophasic formulations:

Demulen® 1/35-28: Ethinyl estradiol 0.035 mg and ethynodiol diacetate 1 mg [21 white tablets and 7 blue inactive tablets] (28s)

Demulen® 1/50-21: Ethinyl estradiol 0.05 mg and ethynodiol diacetate 1 mg [white tablets] (21s) [DSC]

Demulen® 1/50-28: Ethinyl estradiol 0.05 mg and ethynodiol diacetate 1 mg [21 white tablets and 7 pink inactive tablets] (28s) [DSC]

Zovia™ 1/35-28: Ethinyl estradiol 0.035 mg and ethynodiol diacetate 1 mg [21 light pink tablets and 7 white inactive tablets] (28s)

Zovia™ 1/50-28: Ethinyl estradiol 0.05 mg and ethynodiol diacetate 1 mg [21 pink tablets and 7 white inactive tablets] (28s)

Monitoring and Teaching Issues

Physical Assessment: Monitor or teach patient to monitor blood pressure on a regular basis. Monitor or teach patient to monitor for occurrence of adverse effects and symptoms to report. Assess knowledge/teach importance of regular (monthly) blood pressure checks and annual physical assessment, Pap smear, and vision assessment. Teach importance of maintaining prescribed schedule of dosing. **Pregnancy risk factor X:** Do not use if patient is pregnant.

Patient Education: Oral contraceptives do not protect against HIV or other sexually-transmitted diseases. Take exactly as directed by prescriber (also see package insert). You are at risk of becoming pregnant if doses are missed. Detailed and complete information on dosing and missed doses can be found in the package insert. Be aware that some medications may reduce the effectiveness of oral contraceptives; an alternate form of contraception may be needed. Check all medicines (prescription and OTC), herbal, and alternative products with prescriber. It is important that you check your blood pressure monthly (on same day each month) and that you have an annual physical assessment, Pap smear, and vision assessment while taking this medication. Avoid smoking while taking this medication; smoking increases risk of adverse effects, including thromboembolic events and heart attacks. You may experience loss of appetite (small frequent meals will help); or constipation (increased exercise, fluids, fruit, fiber, or stool softeners may help). If you have diabetes, use accurate serum glucose testing to identify any changes in glucose tolerance; notify prescriber of significant changes so antidiabetic medication can be adjusted if necessary. Report immediately pain or muscle soreness; warmth, swelling, pain, or redness in calves; shortness of breath; sudden loss of vision; unresolved leg/foot swelling; change in menstrual pattern (unusual bleeding, amenorrhea, breakthrough spotting); breast tenderness that does not go away; acute abdominal cramping; signs of vaginal infection (drainage, pain, itching); CNS changes (blurred vision, confusion, acute anxiety, or unresolved depression); or significant weight gain (>5 lb/week). Notify prescriber of changes in contact lens tolerance. **Pregnancy/breast-feeding precautions:** This medication should not be used during pregnancy. If you suspect you may become pregnant, contact prescriber immediately. Consult prescriber if breast-feeding.

Dietary Considerations: Should be taken with food at same time each day.

Pregnancy Risk Factor: X

Pregnancy Issues: Pregnancy should be ruled out prior to treatment and discontinued if pregnancy occurs. In general, the use of combination hormonal contraceptives when inadvertently taken early in pregnancy have not been associated with teratogenic effects. Due to increased risk of thromboembolism postpartum, combination hormonal contraceptives should not be started earlier than 4-6 weeks following delivery.

Lactation: Enters breast milk/not recommended (AAP rates "compatible")

Breast-Feeding Issues: Jaundice and breast enlargement in the nursing infant have been reported following the use of combination hormonal contraceptives. May decrease the quality and quantity of breast milk; a nonhormonal form of contraception is recommended.

Administration

Oral: Administer at the same time each day.

Storage: Store at controlled room temperature of 25°C (77°F).

Ethinyl Estradiol and Levonorgestrel

(ETH in il es tra DYE ole & LEE voe nor jes trel)

U.S. Brand Names Alesse®; Aviane™; Enpresse™; Lessina™; Levlen®; Levlite™; Levora®; Lutera™; Nordette®; Portia™; PREVEN®; Seasonale®; Tri-Levlen®; Triphasil®; Trivora®

Synonyms Levonorgestrel and Ethinyl Estradiol

Generic Available Yes

Pharmacologic Category Contraceptive; Estrogen and Progestin Combination

Medication Safety Issues

Sound-alike/look-alike issues:

Alesse® may be confused with Aleve®

Nordette® may be confused with Nicorette®

PREVEN® may be confused with Prevnar®

Tri-Levlen® may be confused with Trilafon®

Triphasil® may be confused with Tri-Norinyl®

Use Prevention of pregnancy; postcoital contraception

(Continued)

Ethinyl Estradiol and Levonorgestrel *(Continued)*

Unlabeled/Investigational Use Treatment of hypermenorrhea (menorrhagia); pain associated with endometriosis; dysmenorrhea; dysfunctional uterine bleeding

Mechanism of Action/Effect Combination oral contraceptives inhibit ovulation and also produce changes in the cervical mucus and endometrium creating an unfavorable environment for sperm penetration and nidation

Contraindications Hypersensitivity to ethinyl estradiol, levonorgestrel, or any component of the formulation; history of or current thrombophlebitis or venous thromboembolic disorders (including DVT, PE); active or recent (within 1 year) arterial thromboembolic disease (eg, stroke, MI); cerebral vascular disease, coronary artery disease, valvular heart disease with complications, severe hypertension; diabetes mellitus with vascular involvement; severe headache with focal neurological symptoms; known or suspected breast carcinoma, endometrial cancer, estrogen-dependent neoplasms, undiagnosed abnormal genital bleeding; hepatic dysfunction or tumor, cholestatic jaundice of pregnancy, jaundice with prior combination hormonal contraceptive use; major surgery with prolonged immobilization; heavy smoking (≥15 cigarettes/day) in patients >35 years of age; pregnancy

Warnings/Precautions Combination hormonal contraceptives do not protect against HIV infection or other sexually-transmitted diseases. The risk of cardiovascular side effects increases in women who smoke cigarettes, especially those who are >35 years of age; women who use combination hormonal contraceptives should be strongly advised not to smoke. Combination hormonal contraceptives may lead to increased risk of myocardial infarction, use with caution in patients with risk factors for coronary artery disease. May increase the risk of thromboembolism. Combination hormonal contraceptives may have a dose-related risk of vascular disease, hypertension, and gallbladder disease. Women with hypertension should be encouraged to use another form of contraception. The use of combination hormonal contraceptives has been associated with a slight increase in frequency of breast cancer, however, studies are not consistent. Combination hormonal contraceptives may cause glucose intolerance. Retinal thrombosis has been reported (rarely). Use with caution in patients with renal disease, conditions that may be aggravated by fluid retention, depression, or history of migraine. Not for use prior to menarche.

The minimum dosage combination of estrogen/progestin that will effectively treat the individual patient should be used. New patients should be started on products containing <50 mcg of estrogen per tablet.

Drug Interactions

Cytochrome P450 Effect:

Ethinyl estradiol: **Substrate** of CYP2C8/9 (minor), 3A4 (major), 3A5-7 (minor); **Inhibits** CYP1A2 (weak), 2B6 (weak), 2C19 (weak), 3A4 (weak)

Levonorgestrel: **Substrate** of CYP3A4 (major)

Decreased Effect: CYP3A4 inducers may decrease the levels/effects of ethinyl estradiol and/or levonorgestrel; example inducers include aminoglutethimide, carbamazepine, nafcillin, nevirapine, phenobarbital, phenytoin, and rifamycins. Combination hormonal contraceptives may decrease plasma levels of acetaminophen, clofibric acid, lorazepam, morphine, oxazepam, salicylic acid, temazepam. Contraceptive effect decreased by acitretin, aminoglutethimide, amprenavir, anticonvulsants, griseofulvin, lopinavir, nelfinavir, penicillins (effect not consistent), rifampin, ritonavir, tetracyclines (effect not consistent). Combination hormonal contraceptives may decrease (or increase) the effects of coumarin derivatives.

Increased Effect/Toxicity: Acetaminophen and ascorbic acid may increase plasma levels of estrogen component. Atorvastatin and indinavir increase plasma levels of combination hormonal contraceptives. Combination hormonal contraceptives increase the plasma levels of alprazolam, chlordiazepoxide, cyclosporine, diazepam, prednisolone, selegiline, theophylline, tricyclic antidepressants. Combination hormonal contraceptives may increase (or decrease) the effects of coumarin derivatives.

Nutritional/Ethanol Interactions

Food: CNS effects of caffeine may be enhanced if combination hormonal contraceptives are used concurrently with caffeine. Grapefruit juice increases ethinyl estradiol concentrations and would be expected to increase progesterone serum levels as well; clinical implications are unclear.

Herb/Nutraceutical: St John's wort may decrease the effectiveness of combination hormonal contraceptives by inducing hepatic enzymes. Avoid dong quai and black cohosh (have estrogen activity). Avoid saw palmetto, red clover, ginseng.

Lab Interactions Increased prothrombin and factors VII, VIII, IX, X; increased platelet aggregability, thyroid-binding globulin, total thyroid hormone (T_4), serum triglycerides/phospholipids; decreased antithrombin III, serum folate concentration

Adverse Reactions Frequency not defined.

Cardiovascular: Arterial thromboembolism, cerebral hemorrhage, cerebral thrombosis, edema, hypertension, mesenteric thrombosis, MI

Central nervous system: Depression, dizziness, headache, migraine, nervousness, premenstrual syndrome, stroke

Dermatologic: Acne, erythema multiforme, erythema nodosum, hirsutism, loss of scalp hair, melasma (may persist), rash (allergic)

Endocrine & metabolic: Amenorrhea, breakthrough bleeding, breast enlargement, breast secretion, breast tenderness, carbohydrate intolerance, lactation decreased (postpartum), glucose tolerance decreased, libido changes, menstrual flow changes, sex hormone-binding globulins (SHBG) increased, spotting, temporary infertility (following discontinuation), thyroid-binding globulin increased, triglycerides increased

Gastrointestinal: Abdominal cramps, appetite changes, bloating, cholestasis, colitis, gallbladder disease, jaundice, nausea, vomiting, weight gain/loss

Genitourinary: Cervical erosion changes, cervical secretion changes, cystitis-like syndrome, vaginal candidiasis, vaginitis

Hematologic: Antithrombin III decreased, folate levels decreased, hemolytic uremic syndrome, norepinephrine induced platelet aggregability increased, porphyria, prothrombin increased; factors VII, VIII, IX, and X increased

Hepatic: Benign liver tumors, Budd-Chiari syndrome, cholestatic jaundice, hepatic adenomas

Local: Thrombophlebitis

Ocular: Cataracts, change in corneal curvature (steepening), contact lens intolerance, optic neuritis, retinal thrombosis

Renal: Impaired renal function

Respiratory: Pulmonary thromboembolism

Miscellaneous: Hemorrhagic eruption

Overdosage/Toxicology Toxicity is unlikely following single exposures of excessive doses. May cause withdrawal bleeding in females. Any treatment following emesis and charcoal administration should be supportive and symptomatic.

Pharmacodynamics/Kinetics

Pharmacokinetic Note: See individual agents.

Dosing

Adults: Female:

Contraception, 28-day cycle: Oral:

Schedule 1 (Sunday starter): Dose begins on first Sunday after onset of menstruation; if the menstrual period starts on Sunday, take first tablet that very same day. With a Sunday start, an additional method of contraception should be used until after the first 7 days of consecutive administration:

For 21-tablet package: 1 tablet/day for 21 consecutive days, followed by 7 days off of the medication; a new course begins on the 8th day after the last tablet is taken

For 28-tablet package: 1 tablet/day without interruption

Schedule 2 (Day-1 starter): Dose starts on first day of menstrual cycle taking 1 tablet/day:

For 21-tablet package: 1 tablet/day for 21 consecutive days, followed by 7 days off of the medication; a new course begins on the 8th day after the last tablet is taken

For 28-tablet package: 1 tablet/day without interruption

If all doses have been taken on schedule and one menstrual period is missed, continue dosing cycle. If two consecutive menstrual periods are missed, pregnancy test is required before new dosing cycle is started.

Missed doses **monophasic formulations** (refer to package insert for complete information):

One dose missed: Take as soon as remembered or take 2 tablets next day

Two consecutive doses missed in the first 2 weeks: Take 2 tablets as soon as remembered or 2 tablets next 2 days. An additional method of contraception should be used for 7 days after missed dose.

Two consecutive doses missed in week 3 or three consecutive doses missed at any time: An additional method of contraception must be used for 7 days after a missed dose:

Schedule 1 (Sunday starter): Continue dose of 1 tablet daily until Sunday, then discard the rest of the pack, and a new pack should be started that same day.

Schedule 2 (Day-1 starter): Current pack should be discarded, and a new pack should be started that same day.

Missed doses **biphasic/triphasic formulations** (refer to package insert for complete information):

One dose missed: Take as soon as remembered or take 2 tablets next day.

Two consecutive doses missed in week 1 or week 2 of the pack: Take 2 tablets as soon as remembered and 2 tablets the next day. Resume taking 1 tablet daily until the pack is empty. An additional method of contraception should be used for 7 days after a missed dose.

Two consecutive doses missed in week 3 of the pack: An additional method of contraception must be used for 7 days after a missed dose.

Schedule 1 (Sunday starter): Take 1 tablet every day until Sunday. Discard the remaining pack and start a new pack of pills on the same day.

Schedule 2 (Day-1 starter): Discard the remaining pack and start a new pack the same day.

Three or more consecutive doses missed: An additional method of contraception must be used for 7 days after a missed dose.

Schedule 1 (Sunday starter): Take 1 tablet every day until Sunday; on Sunday, discard the pack and start a new pack.

Schedule 2 (Day-1 starter): Discard the remaining pack and begin new pack of tablets starting on the same day.

Contraception, 91-day cycle (Seasonale®): Oral: One active tablet/day for 84 consecutive days, followed by 1 inactive tablet/day for 7 days; if all doses have been taken on schedule and one menstrual period is missed, pregnancy should be ruled out prior to continuing therapy.

Missed doses:

One dose missed: Take as soon as remembered or take 2 tablets the next day

Two consecutive doses missed: Take 2 tablets as soon as remembered or 2 tablets the next 2 days. An additional nonhormonal method of contraception should be used for 7 consecutive days after the missed dose.

Three or more consecutive doses missed: Do not take the missed doses; continue taking 1 tablet/day until pack is complete. Bleeding may occur during the following week. An additional nonhormonal method of contraception should be used for 7 consecutive days after the missed dose.

Emergency contraception (PREVEN®): Oral: Initial: 2 tablets as soon as possible (but within 72 hours of unprotected intercourse), followed by a second dose of 2 tablets 12 hours later. Repeat dose or use antiemetic if vomiting occurs within 1 hour of dose.

Pediatrics: Female: Contraception or emergency contraception: Oral: Refer to adult dosing; not to be used prior to menarche.

(Continued)

Ethinyl Estradiol and Levonorgestrel *(Continued)*

Renal Impairment: Specific guidelines not available; use with caution.

Hepatic Impairment: Contraindicated in patients with hepatic impairment.

Available Dosage Forms Tablet: Note: [DSC] = Discontinued product

PREVEN®: Ethinyl estradiol 0.05 mg and levonorgestrel 0.25 mg (4s) [also available as a kit containing 4 tablets and a pregnancy test]

Low-dose formulations:

Alesse® 28: Ethinyl estradiol 0.02 mg and levonorgestrel 0.1 mg [21 pink tablets and 7 light green inactive tablets] (28s)

Aviane™ 28: Ethinyl estradiol 0.02 mg and levonorgestrel 0.1 mg [21 orange tablets and 7 light green inactive tablets] (28s)

Lessina™ 28, Levlite™ 28: Ethinyl estradiol 0.02 mg and levonorgestrel 0.1 mg [21 pink tablets and 7 white inactive tablets] (28s)

Lutera™: Ethinyl estradiol 0.02 mg and levonorgestrel 0.1 mg [21 white tablets and 7 peach inactive tablets] (28s)

Monophasic formulations:

Levlen® 28: Ethinyl estradiol 0.03 mg and levonorgestrel 0.15 mg [21 light orange tablets and 7 pink inactive tablets] (28s)

Levora® 28: Ethinyl estradiol 0.03 mg and levonorgestrel 0.15 mg [21 white tablets and 7 peach inactive tablets] (28s)

Nordette® 21: Ethinyl estradiol 0.03 mg and levonorgestrel 0.15 mg [light orange tablets] (21s)

Nordette® 28: Ethinyl estradiol 0.03 mg and levonorgestrel 0.15 mg [21 light orange tablets and 7 pink inactive tablets] (28s)

Portia™ 28: Ethinyl estradiol 0.03 mg and levonorgestrel 0.15 mg [21 pink tablets and 7 white inactive tablets] (28s)

Seasonale®: Ethinyl estradiol 0.03 mg and levonorgestrel 0.15 mg [84 pink tablets and 7 white inactive tablets; extended cycle regimen]

Triphasic formulations:

Enpresse™:

Day 1-6: Ethinyl estradiol 0.03 mg and levonorgestrel 0.05 mg [6 pink tablets]

Day 7-11: Ethinyl estradiol 0.04 mg and levonorgestrel 0.075 mg [5 white tablets]

Day 12-21: Ethinyl estradiol 0.03 mg and levonorgestrel 0.125 mg [10 orange tablets]

Day 22-28: 7 light green inactive tablets (28s)

Triphasil® 21 [DSC]:

Day 1-6: Ethinyl estradiol 0.03 mg and levonorgestrel 0.05 mg [6 brown tablets]

Day 7-11: Ethinyl estradiol 0.04 mg and levonorgestrel 0.075 mg [5 white tablets]

Day 12-21: Ethinyl estradiol 0.03 mg and levonorgestrel 0.125 mg [10 light yellow tablets] (21s)

Tri-Levlen® 28, Triphasil® 28:

Day 1-6: Ethinyl estradiol 0.03 mg and levonorgestrel 0.05 mg [6 brown tablets]

Day 7-11: Ethinyl estradiol 0.04 mg and levonorgestrel 0.075 mg [5 white tablets]

Day 12-21: Ethinyl estradiol 0.03 mg and levonorgestrel 0.125 mg [10 light yellow tablets]

Day 22-28: 7 light green inactive tablets (28s)

Trivora® 28:

Day 1-6: Ethinyl estradiol 0.03 mg and levonorgestrel 0.05 mg [6 blue tablets]

Day 7-11: Ethinyl estradiol 0.04 mg and levonorgestrel 0.075 mg [5 white tablets]

Day 12-21: Ethinyl estradiol 0.03 mg and levonorgestrel 0.125 mg [10 pink tablets]

Day 22-28: 7 peach inactive tablets (28s)

Monitoring and Teaching Issues

Physical Assessment: Monitor blood pressure on a regular basis. Assess for adverse reactions and potential drug interactions. Assess knowledge/teach importance of regular (monthly) blood pressure checks and annual physical assessment, Pap smear, and vision assessment. Teach importance of maintaining prescribed schedule of dosing (see Dosing for dosing and missed dose information). **Pregnancy risk factor X:** Do not use if patient is pregnant. Breast-feeding is not recommended.

Patient Education: Oral contraceptives do not protect against HIV or other sexually-transmitted diseases. Take exactly as directed by prescriber (also see package insert). You are at risk of becoming pregnant if doses are missed. Detailed and complete information on dosing and missed doses can be found in the package insert. Be aware that some medications may reduce the effectiveness of oral contraceptives; an alternate form of contraception may be needed. It is important that you check your blood pressure monthly (on same day each month) and that you have an annual physical assessment, Pap smear, and vision assessment while taking this medication. Avoid smoking while taking this medication; smoking increases risk of adverse effects, including thromboembolic events and heart attacks. You may experience loss of appetite (small frequent meals will help); or constipation (increased exercise, fluids, fruit, fiber, or stool softeners may help). If you have diabetes, use accurate serum glucose testing to identify any changes in glucose tolerance; notify prescriber of significant changes so antidiabetic medication can be adjusted if necessary. Report immediately pain or muscle soreness; warmth, swelling, pain, or redness in calves; shortness of breath; sudden loss of vision; unresolved leg/foot swelling; change in menstrual pattern (unusual bleeding, amenorrhea, breakthrough spotting); breast tenderness that does not go away; acute abdominal cramping; signs of vaginal infection (drainage, pain, itching); CNS changes (blurred vision, confusion, acute anxiety, or unresolved depression); or significant weight gain (>5 lb/week). Notify prescriber of changes in contact lens tolerance. **Pregnancy/breast-feeding precautions:** This medication should not be used during pregnancy. If you suspect you may become pregnant, contact prescriber immediately. Breast-feeding is not recommended.

Emergency contraceptive kit (PREVEN®) is **not** recommended for ongoing pregnancy protection or as a routine form of contraception. PREVEN® emergency contraceptive kit contains a pregnancy test. This test can be used to verify an existing pregnancy resulting from intercourse that occurred earlier in the concurrent menstrual cycle or the previous cycle. If a positive pregnancy result is obtained, the patient should **not** take the pills in the PREVEN® kit. The patient should be instructed that if she vomits within 1 hour of taking either dose of the medication, she should contact her healthcare professional to discuss whether to repeat that dose or to take an antiemetic.

Dietary Considerations: Should be taken at the same time each day.

Pregnancy Risk Factor: X

Pregnancy Issues: Pregnancy should be ruled out prior to treatment and discontinued if pregnancy occurs. In general, the use of combination hormonal contraceptives when inadvertently taken early in pregnancy have not been associated with teratogenic effects. Due to increased risk of thromboembolism postpartum, combination hormonal contraceptives should not be started earlier than 4-6 weeks following delivery.

Lactation: Enters breast milk/not recommended

Breast-Feeding Issues: Jaundice and breast enlargement in the nursing infant have been reported following the use of combination hormonal contraceptives. May decrease the quality and quantity of breast milk; alternative form of contraception is recommended.

Administration
Oral: Administer at the same time each day.

Storage: Store at controlled room temperature of 25°C (77°F).

Related Information
Levonorgestrel *on page 891*

♦ **Ethinyl Estradiol and NGM** *see* Ethinyl Estradiol and Norgestimate *on page 593*

Ethinyl Estradiol and Norethindrone
(ETH in il es tra DYE ole & nor eth IN drone)

U.S. Brand Names Aranelle™; Brevicon®; Estrostep® Fe; femhrt®; Junel™; Junel™ Fe; Loestrin®; Loestrin® Fe; Microgestin™; Microgestin™ Fe; Modicon®; Necon® 0.5/35; Necon® 1/35; Necon® 7/7/7; Necon® 10/11; Norinyl® 1+35; Nortrel™; Nortrel™ 7/7/7; Ortho-Novum®; Ovcon®; Tri-Norinyl®

Synonyms Norethindrone Acetate and Ethinyl Estradiol; Ortho Novum

Generic Available Yes

Pharmacologic Category Contraceptive; Estrogen and Progestin Combination

Medication Safety Issues
Sound-alike/look-alike issues:
femhrt® may be confused with Femara®
Modicon® may be confused with Mylicon®
Norinyl® may be confused with Nardil®
Tri-Norinyl® may be confused with Triphasil®

Use Prevention of pregnancy; treatment of acne; moderate to severe vasomotor symptoms associated with menopause; prevention of osteoporosis (in women at significant risk only)

Unlabeled/Investigational Use Treatment of hypermenorrhea (menorrhagia); pain associated with endometriosis, dysmenorrhea; dysfunctional uterine bleeding

Mechanism of Action/Effect Combination oral contraceptives inhibit ovulation, and also produce changes in the cervical mucus and the endometrium, creating an unfavorable environment for sperm penetration and nidation. In postmenopausal women, exogenous estrogen is used to replace decreased endogenous production. The addition of progestin reduces the incidence of endometrial hyperplasia and risk of endometrial cancer in women with an intact uterus.

Contraindications Hypersensitivity to ethinyl estradiol, norethindrone, norethindrone acetate, or any component of the formulation; history of or current thrombophlebitis or venous thromboembolic disorders (including DVT, PE); active or recent (within 1 year) arterial thromboembolic disease (eg, stroke, MI); cerebral vascular disease, coronary artery disease, severe hypertension; diabetes mellitus with vascular involvement; severe headache with focal neurological symptoms; known or suspected breast carcinoma, endometrial cancer, estrogen-dependent neoplasms, undiagnosed abnormal genital bleeding; hepatic dysfunction or tumor, cholestatic jaundice of pregnancy, jaundice with prior combination hormonal contraceptive use; major surgery with prolonged immobilization; heavy smoking (≥15 cigarettes/day) in patients >35 years of age; pregnancy

Warnings/Precautions
Cardiovascular-related considerations: Use caution with cardiovascular disease or dysfunction. Combination estrogen/progestin therapy has been associated with an increased risk of cardiovascular disease, which may be dose related. May increase the risks of hypertension, myocardial infarction (MI), stroke, pulmonary emboli (PE), and deep vein thrombosis; incidence of these effects was shown to be significantly increased in postmenopausal women using conjugated equine estrogens (CEE) in combination with medroxyprogesterone acetate (MPA). Nonfatal MI, PE, and thrombophlebitis have also been reported in males taking high doses of CEE (eg, for prostate cancer). An increased risk of MI has been noted with use of combination hormonal contraceptives, primarily in women with underlying risk factors. The risk of cardiovascular events increases in women who smoke cigarettes, especially those who are >35 years of age; women who use combination hormonal contraceptives should be strongly advised not to smoke. Women with hypertension should be encouraged to use another form of contraception. Estrogen compounds are generally associated with lipid effects such as increased HDL-cholesterol and decreased LDL-cholesterol. Triglycerides may also be increased; use with caution in patients with familial defects of lipoprotein metabolism. Estrogens with or without progestin should not be used to prevent coronary heart disease in postmenopausal women. Whenever possible, estrogens should be discontinued at least 4-6 weeks prior to surgeries associated with an increased risk of thromboembolism or during periods of prolonged immobilization. Estrogens may cause retinal vascular thrombosis. Discontinue pending examination in cases of sudden partial or complete vision loss, sudden onset of proptosis, diplopia, or migraine; discontinue permanently if papilledema or retinal vascular lesions are observed on examination.

Cancer-related considerations: Estrogens may increase the risk of breast cancer. The use of combination hormonal contraceptives has been associated with a slight increase in
(Continued)

Ethinyl Estradiol and Norethindrone *(Continued)*

frequency of breast cancer, however studies are not consistent. An increased risk of invasive breast cancer was observed in postmenopausal women using CEE in combination with MPA; a smaller increase in risk was seen with estrogen therapy alone in observational studies. An increase in abnormal mammograms has also been reported with estrogen and progestin therapy in postmenopausal women. Unopposed estrogens may increase the risk of endometrial carcinoma in postmenopausal women. Estrogen use may lead to severe hypercalcemia in postmenopausal patients with breast cancer and bone metastases; discontinue estrogen if hypercalcemia occurs.

Use with caution in patients with diseases which may be exacerbated by fluid retention, including asthma, epilepsy, migraine, diabetes or renal dysfunction. Use with caution in patients with a history of severe hypocalcemia, SLE, hepatic hemangiomas, porphyria, endometriosis, and gallbladder disease. Use caution with history of cholestatic jaundice associated with past estrogen use or pregnancy.

Combination hormonal contraceptives do not protect against HIV infection or other sexually-transmitted diseases. The minimum dosage combination of estrogen/progestin that will effectively treat the individual patient should be used. New patients should be started on products containing <50 mcg of estrogen per tablet. When used for acne, use only in females ≥15 years, who also desire combination hormonal contraceptive therapy, are unresponsive to topical treatments, and have no contraindications to combination hormonal contraceptive use; treatment must continue for at least 6 months. Not for use prior to menarche.

The risk of dementia may be increased in postmenopausal women; increased incidence was observed in women ≥65 years of age taking CEE in combination with MPA. Before prescribing estrogen therapy to postmenopausal women, the risks and benefits must be weighed for each patient. Women should be informed of these risks and benefits, as well as possible effects of progestin when added to estrogen therapy. Estrogens with or without progestin should be used for shortest duration possible consistent with treatment goals. Conduct periodic risk:benefit assessments. When used solely for prevention of osteoporosis in women at significant risk, nonestrogen treatment options should be considered.

Drug Interactions

Cytochrome P450 Effect:

Ethinyl estradiol: **Substrate** of CYP2C8/9 (minor), 3A4 (major), 3A5-7 (minor); **Inhibits** CYP1A2 (weak), 2B6 (weak), 2C19 (weak), 3A4 (weak)

Norethindrone: **Substrate** of CYP3A4 (major); **Induces** CYP2C19 (weak)

Decreased Effect: CYP3A4 inducers may decrease the levels/effects of ethinyl estradiol and norethindrone; example inducers include aminoglutethimide, carbamazepine, nafcillin, nevirapine, phenobarbital, phenytoin, and rifamycins. Combination hormonal contraceptives may decrease plasma levels of acetaminophen, clofibric acid, lorazepam, morphine, oxazepam, salicylic acid, temazepam. Contraceptive effect decreased by acitretin, aminoglutethimide, amprenavir, anticonvulsants, griseofulvin, lopinavir, nelfinavir, penicillins (effect not consistent), rifampin, ritonavir, tetracyclines (effect not consistent), troglitazone. Oral contraceptives may decrease (or increase) the effects of coumarin derivatives.

Increased Effect/Toxicity: Acetaminophen and ascorbic acid may increase plasma levels of estrogen component. Atorvastatin and indinavir increase plasma levels of combination hormonal contraceptives. Combination hormonal contraceptives increase the plasma levels of alprazolam, chlordiazepoxide, cyclosporine, diazepam, prednisolone, selegiline, theophylline, tricyclic antidepressants. Combination hormonal contraceptives may increase (or decrease) the effects of coumarin derivatives.

Nutritional/Ethanol Interactions

Ethanol: Routine use increases estrogen level and risk of breast cancer; avoid ethanol. Ethanol may also increase the risk of osteoporosis.

Food: CNS effects of caffeine may be enhanced if combination hormonal contraceptives are used concurrently with caffeine. Grapefruit juice increases ethinyl estradiol concentrations and would be expected to increase progesterone serum levels as well; clinical implications are unclear. Norethindrone absorption is increased by 27% following administration with food.

Herb/Nutraceutical: St John's wort may decrease the effectiveness of combination hormonal contraceptives by inducing hepatic enzymes. Avoid dong quai and black cohosh (have estrogen activity). Avoid saw palmetto, red clover, ginseng.

Lab Interactions Increased prothrombin and factors VII, VIII, IX, X; increased platelet aggregability, thyroid-binding globulin, total thyroid hormone (T_4), serum triglycerides/phospholipids; decreased antithrombin III, serum folate concentration; pathologist should be advised of estrogen/progesterone therapy when specimens are submitted

Adverse Reactions As reported with oral contraceptive agents. Frequency not defined.

Cardiovascular: Arterial thromboembolism, cerebral hemorrhage, cerebral thrombosis, edema, hypertension, mesenteric thrombosis, MI

Central nervous system: Depression, dizziness, headache, migraine, nervousness, premenstrual syndrome, stroke

Dermatologic: Acne, erythema multiforme, erythema nodosum, hirsutism, loss of scalp hair, melasma (may persist), rash (allergic)

Endocrine & metabolic: Amenorrhea, breakthrough bleeding, breast enlargement, breast secretion, breast tenderness, carbohydrate intolerance, lactation decreased (postpartum), glucose tolerance decreased, libido changes, menstrual flow changes, sex hormone-binding globulins (SHBG) increased, spotting, temporary infertility (following discontinuation), thyroid-binding globulin increased, triglycerides increased

Gastrointestinal: Abdominal cramps, appetite changes, bloating, cholestasis, colitis, gallbladder disease, jaundice, nausea, vomiting, weight gain/loss

Genitourinary: Cervical erosion changes, cervical secretion changes, cystitis-like syndrome, vaginal candidiasis, vaginitis

Hematologic: Antithrombin III decreased, folate levels decreased, hemolytic uremic syndrome, norepinephrine induced platelet aggregability increased, porphyria, prothrombin increased; factors VII, VIII, IX, and X

Hepatic: Benign liver tumors, Budd-Chiari syndrome, cholestatic jaundice, hepatic adenomas

Local: Thrombophlebitis

Ocular: Cataracts, change in corneal curvature (steepening), contact lens intolerance, optic neuritis, retinal thrombosis

Renal: Impaired renal function

Respiratory: Pulmonary thromboembolism

Miscellaneous: Hemorrhagic eruption

Overdosage/Toxicology Toxicity is unlikely following single exposures of excessive doses. May cause withdrawal bleeding in females. Any treatment following emesis and charcoal administration should be supportive and symptomatic.

Pharmacodynamics/Kinetics

Absorption: Ethinyl estradiol: Rapid

Bioavailability: Ethinyl estradiol: 43% to 55%

Protein Binding: Ethinyl estradiol: >95% to albumin

Half-Life Elimination: Ethinyl estradiol: 19-24 hours

Metabolism: Ethinyl estradiol: Hepatic via oxidation and conjugation in GI tract; hydroxylated via CYP3A4 to metabolites; first-pass effect; enterohepatic recirculation; reversibly converted to estrone and estriol

Excretion: Ethinyl estradiol: Urine (as estradiol, estrone, and estriol); feces

Pharmacokinetic Note: Norethindrone: See individual monograph.

Dosing

Adults:

Adolescents ≥15 years and Adults: Female: Acne: Estrostep®: Oral: Refer to dosing for contraception

Moderate-to-severe vasomotor symptoms associated with menopause: Initial: femhrt® 0.5/2.5: Oral: 1 tablet daily; patient should be re-evaluated at 3- to 6-month intervals to determine if treatment is still necessary; patient should be maintained on lowest effective dose

Prevention of osteoporosis: Initial: femhrt® 0.5/2.5: Oral: 1 tablet daily; patient should be maintained on lowest effective dose

Contraception: Oral:

Schedule 1 (Sunday starter): Dose begins on first Sunday after onset of menstruation; if the menstrual period starts on Sunday, take first tablet that very same day. With a Sunday start, an additional method of contraception should be used until after the first 7 days of consecutive administration.

For 21-tablet package: Dosage is 1 tablet daily for 21 consecutive days, followed by 7 days off of the medication; a new course begins on the 8th day after the last tablet is taken.

For 28-tablet package: Dosage is 1 tablet daily without interruption.

Schedule 2 (Day 1 starter): Dose starts on first day of menstrual cycle taking 1 tablet daily.

For 21-tablet package: Dosage is 1 tablet daily for 21 consecutive days, followed by 7 days off of the medication; a new course begins on the 8th day after the last tablet is taken.

For 28-tablet package: Dosage is 1 tablet daily without interruption.

If all doses have been taken on schedule and one menstrual period is missed, continue dosing cycle. If two consecutive menstrual periods are missed, pregnancy test is required before new dosing cycle is started.

Missed doses **monophasic formulations** (refer to package insert for complete information):

One dose missed: Take as soon as remembered or take 2 tablets next day Two consecutive doses missed in the first 2 weeks: Take 2 tablets as soon as remembered or 2 tablets next 2 days. An additional method of contraception should be used for 7 days after missed dose.

Two consecutive doses missed in week 3 or three consecutive doses missed at any time: An additional method of contraception must be used for 7 days after a missed dose.

Schedule 1 (Sunday starter): Continue dose of 1 tablet daily until Sunday, then discard the rest of the pack, and a new pack should be started that same day.

Schedule 2 (Day 1 starter): Current pack should be discarded, and a new pack should be started that same day.

Missed doses **biphasic/triphasic formulations** (refer to package insert for complete information):

One dose missed: Take as soon as remembered or take 2 tablets next day.

Two consecutive doses missed in week 1 or week 2 of the pack: Take 2 tablets as soon as remembered and 2 tablets the next day. Resume taking 1 tablet daily until the pack is empty. An additional method of contraception should be used for 7 days after a missed dose.

Two consecutive doses missed in week 3 of the pack: An additional method of contraception must be used for 7 days after a missed dose.

Schedule 1 (Sunday Starter): Take 1 tablet every day until Sunday. Discard the remaining pack and start a new pack of pills on the same day.

Schedule 2 (Day 1 starter): Discard the remaining pack and start a new pack the same day.

Three or more consecutive doses missed: An additional method of contraception must be used for 7 days after a missed dose.

Schedule 1 (Sunday Starter): Take 1 tablet every day until Sunday; on Sunday, discard the pack and start a new pack.

Schedule 2 (Day 1 Starter): Discard the remaining pack and begin new pack of tablets starting on the same day.

Pediatrics: Female:

Acne: Oral (Estrostep®): For use in females ≥15 years; refer to adult dosing for contraception

Contraception: Oral: Refer to adult dosing; not to be used prior to menarche.

(Continued)

Ethinyl Estradiol and Norethindrone *(Continued)*

Renal Impairment: Specific guidelines not available; use with caution.
Hepatic Impairment: Contraindicated in patients with hepatic impairment.

Available Dosage Forms

Tablet: femhrt®:
  1/5: Ethinyl estradiol 5 mcg and norethindrone acetate 1 mg [white tablets]
  0.5/2.5: Ethinyl estradiol 2.5 mcg and norethindrone acetate 0.5 mg [white tablets]

Tablet, monophasic formulations:
  Brevicon®: Ethinyl estradiol 0.035 mg and norethindrone 0.5 mg [21 blue tablets and 7 orange inactive tablets] (28s)
  Junel™ 21 1/20: Ethinyl estradiol 0.02 mg and norethindrone acetate 1 mg [yellow tablets] (21s)
  Junel™ 21 1.5/30: Ethinyl estradiol 0.03 mg and norethindrone acetate 1.5 mg [pink tablets] (21s)
  Junel™ Fe 1/20: Ethinyl estradiol 0.02 mg and norethindrone acetate 1 mg [21 yellow tablets] and ferrous fumarate 75 mg [7 brown tablets] (28s)
  Junel™ Fe 1.5/30: Ethinyl estradiol 0.03 mg and norethindrone acetate 1.5 mg [21 pink tablets] and ferrous fumarate 75 mg [7 brown tablets] (28s)
  Loestrin® 21 1/20, Microgestin™ 1/20: Ethinyl estradiol 0.02 mg and norethindrone acetate 1 mg [white tablets] (21s)
  Loestrin® 21 1.5/30, Microgestin™ 1.5/30: Ethinyl estradiol 0.03 mg and norethindrone acetate 1.5 mg [green tablets] (21s)
  Loestrin® Fe 1/20, Microgestin™ Fe 1/20: Ethinyl estradiol 0.02 mg and norethindrone acetate 1 mg [21 white tablets] and ferrous fumarate 75 mg [7 brown tablets] (28s)
  Loestrin® Fe 1.5/30, Microgestin™ Fe 1.5/30: Ethinyl estradiol 0.03 mg and norethindrone acetate 1.5 mg [21 green tablets] and ferrous fumarate 75 mg [7 brown tablets] (28s)
  Modicon® 28: Ethinyl estradiol 0.035 mg and norethindrone 0.5 mg [21 white tablets and 7 green inactive tablets] (28s)
  Necon® 0.5/35-28: Ethinyl estradiol 0.035 mg and norethindrone 0.5 mg [21 light yellow tablets and 7 white inactive tablets] (28s)
  Necon® 1/35-28: Ethinyl estradiol 0.035 mg and norethindrone 1 mg [21 dark yellow tablets and 7 white inactive tablets] (28s)
  Norinyl® 1+35: Ethinyl estradiol 0.035 mg and norethindrone 1 mg [21 yellow-green tablets and 7 orange inactive tablets] (28s)
  Nortrel™ 0.5/35 mg:
    Ethinyl estradiol 0.035 mg and norethindrone 0.5 mg [light yellow tablets] (21s)
    Ethinyl estradiol 0.035 mg and norethindrone 0.5 mg [21 light yellow tablets and 7 white inactive tablets] (28s)
  Nortrel™ 1/35 mg:
    Ethinyl estradiol 0.035 mg and norethindrone 1 mg [yellow tablets] (21s)
    Ethinyl estradiol 0.035 mg and norethindrone 1 mg [21 yellow tablets and 7 white inactive tablets] (28s)
  Ortho-Novum® 1/35 28: Ethinyl estradiol 0.035 mg and norethindrone 1 mg [21 peach tablets and 7 green inactive tablets] (28s)
  Ovcon® 35 21-day: Ethinyl estradiol 0.035 mg and norethindrone 0.4 mg [peach tablets] (21s)
  Ovcon® 35 28-day: Ethinyl estradiol 0.035 mg and norethindrone 0.4 mg [21 peach tablets and 7 green inactive tablets] (28s)
  Ovcon® 50: Ethinyl estradiol 0.05 mg and norethindrone 1 mg [21 yellow tablets and 7 green inactive tablets] (28s)

Tablet, biphasic formulations:
  Necon® 10/11-28:
    Day 1-10: Ethinyl estradiol 0.035 mg and norethindrone 0.5 mg [10 light yellow tablets]
    Day 11-21: Ethinyl estradiol 0.035 mg and norethindrone 1 mg [11 dark yellow tablets]
    Day 22-28: 7 white inactive tablets (28s)
  Ortho-Novum® 10/11-28:
    Day 1-10: Ethinyl estradiol 0.035 mg and norethindrone 0.5 mg [10 white tablets]
    Day 11-21: Ethinyl estradiol 0.035 mg and norethindrone 1 mg [11 peach tablets]
    Day 22-28: 7 green inactive tablets (28s)

Tablet, triphasic formulations:
  Aranelle™:
    Day 1-7: Ethinyl estradiol 0.035 mg and norethindrone 0.5 mg [7 light yellow tablets]
    Day 8-16: Ethinyl estradiol 0.035 mg and norethindrone 1 mg [9 white tablets]
    Day 17-21: Ethinyl estradiol 0.035 mg and norethindrone 0.5 mg [5 light yellow tablets]
    Day 22-28: 7 peach inactive tablets (28s)
  Estrostep® Fe:
    Day 1-5: Ethinyl estradiol 0.02 mg and norethindrone acetate 1 mg [5 white triangular tablets]
    Day 6-12: Ethinyl estradiol 0.03 mg and norethindrone acetate 1 mg [7 white square tablets]
    Day 13-21: Ethinyl estradiol 0.035 mg and norethindrone acetate 1 mg [9 white round tablets]
    Day 22-28: Ferrous fumarate 75 mg [7 brown tablets] (28s)
  Necon® 7/7/7, Ortho-Novum® 7/7/7 28:
    Day 1-7: Ethinyl estradiol 0.035 mg and norethindrone 0.5 mg [7 white tablets]
    Day 8-14: Ethinyl estradiol 0.035 mg and norethindrone 0.75 mg [7 light peach tablets]
    Day 15-21: Ethinyl estradiol 0.035 mg and norethindrone 1 mg [7 peach tablets]
    Day 22-28: 7 green inactive tablets (28s)
  Nortrel™ 7/7/7 28:
    Day 1-7: Ethinyl estradiol 0.035 mg and norethindrone 0.5 mg [7 light yellow tablets]
    Day 8-14: Ethinyl estradiol 0.035 mg and norethindrone 0.75 mg [7 blue tablets]
    Day 15-21: Ethinyl estradiol 0.035 mg and norethindrone 1 mg [7 peach tablets]
    Day 22-28: 7 white inactive tablets (28s)

Ortho-Novum® 7/7/7 28:
>Day 1-7: Ethinyl estradiol 0.035 mg and norethindrone 0.5 mg [7 white tablets]
>Day 8-14: Ethinyl estradiol 0.035 mg and norethindrone 0.75 mg [7 light peach tablets]
>Day 15-21: Ethinyl estradiol 0.035 mg and norethindrone 1 mg [7 peach tablets]
>Day 22-28: 7 green inactive tablets (28s)

Tri-Norinyl® 28:
>Day 1-7: Ethinyl estradiol 0.035 mg and norethindrone 0.5 mg [7 blue tablets]
>Day 8-16: Ethinyl estradiol 0.035 mg and norethindrone 1 mg [9 yellow-green tablets]
>Day 17-21: Ethinyl estradiol 0.035 mg and norethindrone 0.5 mg [5 blue tablets]
>Day 22-28: 7 orange inactive tablets (28s)

Monitoring and Teaching Issues

Physical Assessment: Assess other medications patient may be taking for effectiveness and interactions. Teach patient importance of monthly blood pressure checks, annual physical assessment, Pap smear, vision assessment; and appropriate use (eg, maintaining prescribed schedule of dosing), interventions to reduce side effects (eg, alcohol and smoking cessation), and adverse symptoms to report. **Pregnancy risk factor X:** Do not use if patient is pregnant.

Patient Education: Oral contraceptives do not protect against HIV infection or other sexually-transmitted diseases. Take exactly as directed by prescriber (detailed and complete information on dosing and missed doses can also be found in the package insert). You are at risk of becoming pregnant if doses are missed. Do not take any new medication during therapy without consulting prescriber. Avoid ethanol (routine use increases estrogen level and risk of breast cancer; may also increase risk of osteoporosis). Avoid smoking while taking this medication; smoking increases risk of adverse effects, including thromboembolic events and heart attacks. If you have diabetes, use accurate serum glucose testing to identify any changes in glucose tolerance (notify prescriber of significant changes). It is important that you check your blood pressure on the same day of each month (notify prescriber of significant changes) and that you have an annual physical assessment, Pap smear, and vision assessment while taking this medication. May cause loss of appetite (small frequent meals will help); or constipation (increased exercise, fluids, fruit, fiber, or stool softeners may help). Report immediately pain or muscle soreness; warmth, swelling, pain, or redness in calves; shortness of breath; sudden loss of vision; unresolved leg/foot swelling; change in menstrual pattern (unusual bleeding, amenorrhea, breakthrough spotting); breast tenderness that does not go away; acute abdominal cramping; signs of vaginal infection (drainage, pain, itching); CNS changes (blurred vision, confusion, acute anxiety, or unresolved depression); or significant weight gain (>5 lb/week). Notify prescriber of changes in contact lens tolerance. **Pregnancy/breast-feeding precautions:** This medication should not be used during pregnancy. Consult prescriber for appropriate form of contraception. If you suspect you may become pregnant, contact prescriber immediately. Breast-feeding is not recommended.

Dietary Considerations: Should be taken at same time each day. May be taken with or without food. Ensure adequate calcium and vitamin D intake when used for the prevention of osteoporosis.

Pregnancy Risk Factor: X

Pregnancy Issues: Pregnancy should be ruled out prior to treatment and discontinued if pregnancy occurs. In general, the use of combination hormonal contraceptives when inadvertently taken early in pregnancy have not been associated with teratogenic effects. Due to increased risk of thromboembolism postpartum, combination hormonal contraceptives should not be started earlier than 4-6 weeks following delivery.

Lactation: Enters breast milk/not recommended

Breast-Feeding Issues: Jaundice and breast enlargement in the nursing infant have been reported following the use of combination hormonal contraceptives. May decrease the quality and quantity of breast milk; alternative form of contraception is recommended.

Administration

Oral: Administer at the same time each day.

Storage: Store at controlled room temperature of 25°C (77°F).
Estrostep®: Protect from light.

Additional Information Norethindrone acetate 1 mg is equivalent to ethinyl estradiol 2.8 mcg.

Related Information

Norethindrone *on page 1096*

Ethinyl Estradiol and Norgestimate

(ETH in il es tra DYE ole & nor JES ti mate)

U.S. Brand Names MonoNessa™; Ortho-Cyclen®; Ortho Tri-Cyclen®; Ortho Tri-Cyclen® Lo; Previfem™; Sprintec™; TriNessa™; Tri-Previfem™; Tri-Sprintec™

Synonyms Ethinyl Estradiol and NGM; Norgestimate and Ethinyl Estradiol; Ortho Cyclen; Ortho Tri Cyclen

Generic Available Yes

Pharmacologic Category Contraceptive; Estrogen and Progestin Combination

Medication Safety Issues
Sound-alike/look-alike issues:
>Ortho-Cyclen® may be confused with Ortho-Cept®

Use Prevention of pregnancy; treatment of acne

Unlabeled/Investigational Use Treatment of hypermenorrhea (menorrhagia); pain associated with endometriosis; dysmenorrhea; dysfunctional uterine bleeding

Mechanism of Action/Effect Combination hormonal contraceptives inhibit ovulation and also produce changes in the cervical mucus and endometrium creating an unfavorable environment for sperm penetration and nidation.

Contraindications Hypersensitivity to ethinyl estradiol, norgestimate, or any component of the formulation; history of or current thrombophlebitis or venous thromboembolic disorders (including DVT, PE); active or recent (within 1 year) arterial thromboembolic disease (eg, stroke, MI); cerebral vascular disease, coronary artery disease, valvular heart disease with
(Continued)

Ethinyl Estradiol and Norgestimate *(Continued)*

complications, severe hypertension; severe headache with focal neurological symptoms; known or suspected breast carcinoma, endometrial cancer, estrogen-dependent neoplasms, undiagnosed abnormal genital bleeding; hepatic dysfunction or tumor, cholestatic jaundice of pregnancy, jaundice with prior combination hormonal contraceptive use; heavy smoking (≥15 cigarettes/day) in patients >35 years of age; pregnancy

Warnings/Precautions Combination hormonal contraceptives do not protect against HIV infection or other sexually-transmitted diseases. The risk of cardiovascular side effects increases in women who smoke cigarettes, especially those who are >35 years of age; women who use combination hormonal contraceptives should be strongly advised not to smoke. Combination hormonal contraceptives may lead to increased risk of myocardial infarction, use with caution in patients with risk factors for coronary artery disease. May increase the risk of thromboembolism. Combination hormonal contraceptives may have a dose-related risk of vascular disease, hypertension, and gallbladder disease. Women with hypertension should be encouraged to use a nonhormonal form of contraception. The use of combination hormonal contraceptives has been associated with a slight increase in frequency of breast cancer, however, studies are not consistent. Combination hormonal contraceptives may cause glucose intolerance. Retinal thrombosis has been reported (rarely). Use with caution in patients with renal disease, conditions that may be aggravated by fluid retention, depression, or history of migraine. Not for use prior to menarche.

The minimum dosage combination of estrogen/progestin that will effectively treat the individual patient should be used. New patients should be started on products containing <50 mcg of estrogen per tablet.

Acne: For use only in females ≥15 years, who also desire combination hormonal contraceptive therapy, are unresponsive to topical treatments, and have no contraindications to combination hormonal contraceptive use; treatment must continue for at least 6 months.

Drug Interactions

Cytochrome P450 Effect: Ethinyl estradiol: **Substrate** of CYP2C8/9 (minor), 3A4 (major), 3A5-7 (minor); **Inhibits** CYP1A2 (weak), 2B6 (weak), 2C19 (weak), 3A4 (weak)

Decreased Effect: CYP3A4 inducers may decrease the levels/effects of ethinyl estradiol; example inducers include aminoglutethimide, carbamazepine, nafcillin, nevirapine, phenobarbital, phenytoin, and rifamycins. Combination hormonal contraceptives may decrease plasma levels of acetaminophen, clofibric acid, lorazepam, morphine, oxazepam, salicylic acid, temazepam. Contraceptive effect decreased by acitretin, aminoglutethimide, amprenavir, anticonvulsants, griseofulvin, lopinavir, nelfinavir, nevirapine, penicillins (effect not consistent), rifampin, ritonavir, tetracyclines (effect not consistent). Combination hormonal contraceptives may decrease (or increase) the effects of coumarin derivatives.

Increased Effect/Toxicity: Acetaminophen and ascorbic acid may increase plasma levels of estrogen component. Atorvastatin and indinavir increase plasma levels of combination hormonal contraceptives. Combination hormonal contraceptives increase the plasma levels of alprazolam, chlordiazepoxide, cyclosporine, diazepam, prednisolone, selegiline, theophylline, tricyclic antidepressants. Combination hormonal contraceptives may increase (or decrease) the effects of coumarin derivatives.

Nutritional/Ethanol Interactions

Food: CNS effects of caffeine may be enhanced if combination hormonal contraceptives are used concurrently with caffeine. Grapefruit juice increases ethinyl estradiol concentrations and would be expected to increase progesterone serum levels as well; clinical implications are unclear.

Herb/Nutraceutical: St John's wort may decrease the effectiveness of combination hormonal contraceptives by inducing hepatic enzymes. Avoid dong quai and black cohosh (have estrogen activity). Avoid saw palmetto, red clover, ginseng.

Lab Interactions Increased amylase (S), cholesterol (S), iron (B), sodium (S), thyroxine (S); decreased calcium (S), protein, prothrombin time

Adverse Reactions Frequency not defined.

Cardiovascular: Arterial thromboembolism, cerebral hemorrhage, cerebral thrombosis, edema, hypertension, mesenteric thrombosis, MI

Central nervous system: Depression, dizziness, headache, migraine, nervousness, premenstrual syndrome, stroke

Dermatologic: Acne, erythema multiforme, erythema nodosum, hirsutism, loss of scalp hair, melasma (may persist), rash (allergic)

Endocrine & metabolic: Amenorrhea, breakthrough bleeding, breast enlargement, breast secretion, breast tenderness, carbohydrate intolerance, lactation decreased (postpartum), glucose tolerance decreased, libido changes, menstrual flow changes, sex hormone-binding globulins (SHBG) increased, spotting, temporary infertility (following discontinuation), thyroid-binding globulin increased, triglycerides increased

Gastrointestinal: Abdominal cramps, appetite changes, bloating, cholestasis, colitis, gallbladder disease, jaundice, nausea, vomiting, weight gain/loss

Genitourinary: Cervical erosion changes, cervical secretion changes, cystitis-like syndrome, vaginal candidiasis, vaginitis

Hematologic: Antithrombin III decreased, folate levels decreased, hemolytic uremic syndrome, norepinephrine induced platelet aggregability increased, porphyria, prothrombin increased; factors VII, VIII, IX, and X increased

Hepatic: Benign liver tumors, Budd-Chiari syndrome, cholestatic jaundice, hepatic adenomas

Local: Thrombophlebitis

Ocular: Cataracts, change in corneal curvature (steepening), contact lens intolerance, optic neuritis, retinal thrombosis

Renal: Impaired renal function

Respiratory: Pulmonary thromboembolism

Miscellaneous: Hemorrhagic eruption

Overdosage/Toxicology Toxicity is unlikely following single exposures of excessive doses. May cause withdrawal bleeding in females. Any treatment following emesis and charcoal administration should be supportive and symptomatic.

Pharmacodynamics/Kinetics

Absorption:

Norgestimate: Well absorbed

Protein Binding:

Norgestimate: To albumin and sex hormone-binding globulin (SHBG); SHBG capacity is affected by plasma ethinyl estradiol levels

Half-Life Elimination:

Norgestimate: 17-deacetylnorgestimate: 12-30 hours

Metabolism:

Norgestimate: Hepatic; forms 17-deacetylnorgestimate (major active metabolite) and other metabolites

Excretion:

Norgestimate: Urine and feces

Dosing

Adults: Female:

Acne (Ortho Tri-Cyclen®): Oral: Refer to dosing for contraception

Contraception: Oral:

Schedule 1 (Sunday starter): Dose begins on first Sunday after onset of menstruation; if the menstrual period starts on Sunday, take first tablet that very same day. **With a Sunday start, an additional method of contraception should be used until after the first 7 days of consecutive administration.**

For 21-tablet package: Dosage is 1 tablet daily for 21 consecutive days, followed by 7 days off of the medication; a new course begins on the 8th day after the last tablet is taken.

For 28-tablet package: Dosage is 1 tablet daily without interruption.

Schedule 2 (Day 1 starter): Dose starts on first day of menstrual cycle taking 1 tablet daily.

For 21-tablet package: Dosage is 1 tablet daily for 21 consecutive days, followed by 7 days off of the medication; a new course begins on the 8th day after the last tablet is taken.

For 28-tablet package: Dosage is 1 tablet daily without interruption.

If all doses have been taken on schedule and one menstrual period is missed, continue dosing cycle. If two consecutive menstrual periods are missed, pregnancy test is required before new dosing cycle is started.

Missed doses **monophasic formulations** (refer to package insert for complete information):

One dose missed: Take as soon as remembered or take 2 tablets next day

Two consecutive doses missed in the first 2 weeks: Take 2 tablets as soon as remembered or 2 tablets next 2 days. **An additional method of contraception should be used for 7 days after missed dose.**

Two consecutive doses missed in week 3 or three consecutive doses missed at any time: **An additional method of contraception must be used for 7 days after a missed dose:**

Schedule 1 (Sunday starter): Continue dose of 1 tablet daily until Sunday, then discard the rest of the pack, and a new pack should be started that same day.

Schedule 2 (Day 1 starter): Current pack should be discarded, and a new pack should be started that same day.

Missed doses **biphasic/triphasic formulations** (refer to package insert for complete information):

One dose missed: Take as soon as remembered or take 2 tablets next day.

Two consecutive doses missed in week 1 or week 2 of the pack: Take 2 tablets as soon as remembered and 2 tablets the next day. Resume taking 1 tablet daily until the pack is empty. **An additional method of contraception must be used for 7 days after a missed dose.**

Two consecutive doses missed in week 3 of the pack. **An additional method of contraception must be used for 7 days after a missed dose.**

Schedule 1 (Sunday starter): Take 1 tablet every day until Sunday. Discard the remaining pack and start a new pack of pills on the same day.

Schedule 2 (Day 1 starter): Discard the remaining pack and start a new pack the same day.

Three or more consecutive doses missed. **An additional method of contraception must be used for 7 days after a missed dose.**

Schedule 1 (Sunday starter): Take 1 tablet every day until Sunday; on Sunday, discard the pack and start a new pack.

Schedule 2 (Day 1 starter): Discard the remaining pack and begin new pack of tablets starting on the same day.

Pediatrics: Female:

Acne: Oral: Children ≥15 years; refer to adult dosing for contraception

Contraception: Oral: Refer to adult dosing; not to be used prior to menarche.

Renal Impairment: Specific guidelines not available; use with caution.

Hepatic Impairment: Contraindicated in patients with hepatic impairment.

Available Dosage Forms Tablet:

Monophasic formulations:

MonoNessa™, Ortho-Cyclen®: Ethinyl estradiol 0.035 mg and norgestimate 0.25 mg [21 blue tablets and 7 green inactive tablets] (28s)

Previfem™: Ethinyl estradiol 0.035 mg and norgestimate 0.25 mg [21 blue tablets and 7 teal inactive tablets] (28s)

Sprintec™: Ethinyl estradiol 0.035 mg and norgestimate 0.25 mg [21 blue tablets and 7 white inactive tablets] (28s)

Triphasic formulations:

Ortho Tri-Cyclen®, TriNessa™:

Day 1-7: Ethinyl estradiol 0.035 mg and norgestimate 0.18 mg [7 white tablets]

Day 8-14: Ethinyl estradiol 0.035 mg and norgestimate 0.215 mg [7 light blue tablets]

Day 15-21: Ethinyl estradiol 0.035 mg and norgestimate 0.25 mg [7 blue tablets]

(Continued)

Ethinyl Estradiol and Norgestimate *(Continued)*

Day 22-28: 7 green inactive tablets (28s)

Tri-Previfem™:
  Day 1-7: Ethinyl estradiol 0.035 mg and norgestimate 0.18 mg [7 white tablets]
  Day 8-14: Ethinyl estradiol 0.035 mg and norgestimate 0.215 mg [7 light blue tablets]
  Day 15-21: Ethinyl estradiol 0.035 mg and norgestimate 0.25 mg [7 blue tablets]
  Day 22-28: 7 teal inactive tablets (28s)

Tri-Sprintec™:
  Day 1-7: Ethinyl estradiol 0.035 mg and norgestimate 0.18 mg [7 gray tablets]
  Day 8-14: Ethinyl estradiol 0.035 mg and norgestimate 0.215 mg [7 light blue tablets]
  Day 15-21: Ethinyl estradiol 0.035 mg and norgestimate 0.25 mg [7 blue tablets]
  Day 22-28: 7 white inactive tablets (28s)

Ortho Tri-Cyclen® Lo:
  Day 1-7: Ethinyl estradiol 0.025 mg and norgestimate 0.18 mg [7 white tablets]
  Day 8-14: Ethinyl estradiol 0.025 mg and norgestimate 0.215 mg [7 light blue tablets]
  Day 15-21: Ethinyl estradiol 0.025 mg and norgestimate 0.25 mg [7 dark blue tablets]
  Day 22-28: 7 green inactive tablets (28s)

Monitoring and Teaching Issues

Physical Assessment: Assess for adverse reactions and potential drug interactions. Emphasize importance of regular (monthly) blood pressure checks and annual physical assessment, Pap smear, and vision assessment. Teach importance of maintaining prescribed schedule of dosing. **Pregnancy risk factor X:** Do not use if patient is pregnant.

Patient Education: Oral contraceptives do not protect against HIV or other sexually-transmitted diseases. Take exactly as directed by prescriber (also see package insert). You are at risk of becoming pregnant if doses are missed. Detailed and complete information on dosing and missed doses can be found in the package insert. Be aware that some medications may reduce the effectiveness of oral contraceptives; an alternate form of contraception may be needed. Check all medicines (prescription and OTC), herbal, and alternative products with prescriber. It is important that you check your blood pressure monthly (on same day each month) and that you have an annual physical assessment, Pap smear, and vision assessment while taking this medication. Avoid smoking while taking this medication; smoking increases risk of adverse effects, including thromboembolic events and heart attacks. You may experience loss of appetite (small frequent meals will help); or constipation (increased exercise, fluids, fruit, fiber, or stool softeners may help). If you have diabetes, use accurate serum glucose testing to identify any changes in glucose tolerance; notify prescriber of significant changes so antidiabetic medication can be adjusted if necessary. Report immediately pain or muscle soreness; warmth, swelling, pain, or redness in calves; shortness of breath; sudden loss of vision; unresolved leg/ foot swelling; change in menstrual pattern (unusual bleeding, amenorrhea, breakthrough spotting); breast tenderness that does not go away; acute abdominal cramping; signs of vaginal infection (drainage, pain, itching); CNS changes (blurred vision, confusion, acute anxiety, or unresolved depression); or significant weight gain (>5 lb/week). Notify prescriber of changes in contact lens tolerance. **Pregnancy/breast-feeding precautions:** This medication should not be used during pregnancy. If you suspect you may become pregnant, contact prescriber immediately. Consult prescriber if breast-feeding.

Dietary Considerations: Should be taken at same time each day.

Pregnancy Risk Factor: X

Pregnancy Issues: Pregnancy should be ruled out prior to treatment and discontinued if pregnancy occurs. In general, the use of combination hormonal contraceptives when inadvertently taken early in pregnancy have not been associated with teratogenic effects. Due to increased risk of thromboembolism postpartum, combination hormonal contraceptives should not be started earlier than 4-6 weeks following delivery.

Lactation: Enters breast milk/not recommended (AAP rates "compatible")

Breast-Feeding Issues: Jaundice and breast enlargement in the nursing infant have been reported following the use of combination hormonal contraceptives. May decrease the quality and quantity of breast milk; a nonhormonal form of contraception is recommended.

Administration

Oral: Administer at the same time each day.

Storage: Store at controlled room temperature of 25°C (77°F).

♦ **Ethiofos** *see* Amifostine *on page 86*

♦ **Ethmozine®** *see* Moricizine *on page 1030*

Ethosuximide *(eth oh SUKS i mide)*

U.S. Brand Names Zarontin®

Generic Available Yes

Pharmacologic Category Anticonvulsant, Succinimide

Medication Safety Issues
  Sound-alike/look-alike issues:
    Ethosuximide may be confused with methsuximide
    Zarontin® may be confused with Xalatan®, Zantac®, Zaroxolyn®

Use Management of absence (petit mal) seizures

Mechanism of Action/Effect Increases the seizure threshold and suppresses paroxysmal spike-and-wave pattern in absence seizures; depresses nerve transmission in the motor cortex

Contraindications Hypersensitivity to succinimides or any component of the formulation

Warnings/Precautions Use with caution in patients with hepatic or renal disease; abrupt withdrawal of the drug may precipitate absence status; ethosuximide may increase tonic-clonic seizures in patients with mixed seizure disorders; ethosuximide must be used in combination with other anticonvulsants in patients with both absence and tonic-clonic seizures. Succinimides have been associated with severe blood dyscrasias and cases of systemic lupus erythematosus. Consider evaluation of blood counts in patients with signs/

symptoms of infection. Safety and efficacy in patients <3 years of age have not been established.

Drug Interactions

Cytochrome P450 Effect: Substrate of CYP3A4 (major)

Decreased Effect: CYP3A4 inducers may decrease the levels/effects of ethosuximide; example inducers include aminoglutethimide, carbamazepine, nafcillin, nevirapine, phenobarbital, phenytoin, and rifamycins.

Increased Effect/Toxicity: Ethosuximide may elevate phenytoin levels. Valproate acid has been reported to both increase and decrease ethosuximide levels. CYP3A4 inhibitors may increase the levels/effects of ethosuximide; example inhibitors include azole antifungals, ciprofloxacin, clarithromycin, diclofenac, doxycycline, erythromycin, imatinib, isoniazid, nefazodone, nicardipine, propofol, protease inhibitors, quinidine, and verapamil.

Nutritional/Ethanol Interactions

Ethanol: Avoid ethanol (may increase CNS depression).

Herb/Nutraceutical: St John's wort may decrease ethosuximide levels.

Lab Interactions Increased alkaline phosphatase (S); positive Coombs' [direct]; decreased calcium (S)

Adverse Reactions Frequency not defined.

Central nervous system: Ataxia, drowsiness, sedation, dizziness, lethargy, euphoria, headache, irritability, hyperactivity, fatigue, night terrors, disturbance in sleep, inability to concentrate, aggressiveness, mental depression (with cases of overt suicidal intentions), paranoid psychosis

Dermatologic: Stevens-Johnson syndrome, SLE, rash, hirsutism

Endocrine & metabolic: Increased libido

Gastrointestinal: Weight loss, gastric upset, cramps, epigastric pain, diarrhea, nausea, vomiting, anorexia, abdominal pain, gum hypertrophy, tongue swelling

Genitourinary: Vaginal bleeding, microscopic hematuria

Hematologic: Leukopenia, agranulocytosis, pancytopenia, eosinophilia

Ocular: Myopia

Miscellaneous: Hiccups

Overdosage/Toxicology Acute overdose can cause CNS depression, ataxia, stupor, coma, hypotension. Chronic overdose can cause skin rash, confusion, ataxia, proteinuria, hepatic dysfunction, and hematuria. Treatment is supportive. Hemoperfusion and hemodialysis may be useful.

Pharmacodynamics/Kinetics

Time to Peak: Serum: Capsule: ~2-4 hours; Syrup: <2-4 hours

Half-Life Elimination: Serum: Children: 30 hours; Adults: 50-60 hours

Metabolism: Hepatic (~80% to 3 inactive metabolites)

Excretion: Urine, slowly (50% as metabolites, 10% to 20% as unchanged drug); feces (small amounts)

Dosing

Adults & Elderly: Management of absence (petit mal) seizures: Oral: Initial: 250 mg twice daily; increase by 250 mg as needed every 4-7 days up to 1.5 g/day in 2 divided doses; usual maintenance dose: 20-40 mg/kg/day in 2 divided doses

Pediatrics:

Absence (petit mal) seizures: Oral:

Children 3-6 years: Initial: 250 mg/day (or 15 mg/kg/day) in 2 divided doses; increase every 4-7 days; usual maintenance dose: 15-40 mg/kg/day in 2 divided doses.

Children >6 years: Refer to adult dosing.

Renal Impairment: Use with caution.

Hepatic Impairment: Use with caution.

Available Dosage Forms

Capsule: 250 mg

Syrup: 250 mg/5 mL (473 mL) [contains sodium benzoate; raspberry flavor]

Monitoring and Teaching Issues

Physical Assessment: Assess effectiveness and interactions of other medications patient may be taking. Monitor therapeutic effectiveness, laboratory values, and adverse reactions at beginning of therapy and periodically with long-term use. Observe and teach seizure/safety precautions. Taper dosage slowly when discontinuing. Assess knowledge/teach patient appropriate use, interventions to reduce side effects, and adverse symptoms to report.

Monitoring Laboratory Tests: Trough serum concentrations, CBC, platelets, liver enzymes, urinalysis

Patient Education: Take exactly as directed; do not increase dose or frequency or discontinue without consulting prescriber. While using this medication, do not use alcohol and other prescription or OTC medications (especially pain medications, sedatives, antihistamines, or hypnotics) without consulting prescriber. Maintain adequate hydration (2-3 L/day of fluids) unless instructed to restrict fluid intake. You may experience drowsiness, dizziness, or blurred vision (use caution when driving or engaging in tasks requiring alertness until response to drug is known); nausea, vomiting, loss of appetite, or dry mouth (small frequent meals, frequent mouth care, chewing gum, or sucking lozenges may help); or constipation (increased exercise, fluids, fruit, or fiber may help). Wear identification of epileptic status and medications. Report CNS changes, mentation changes, or changes in cognition; muscle cramping, weakness, tremors, or changes in gait; persistent GI symptoms (cramping, constipation, vomiting, anorexia); rash or skin irritations; unusual bruising or bleeding (mouth, urine, stool); or worsening of seizure activity or loss of seizure control.

Pregnancy precaution: Inform prescriber if you are or intend to become pregnant.

Dietary Considerations: Increase dietary intake of folate; may be administered with food or milk.

Geriatric Considerations: No specific studies with the use of this medication in the elderly. Consider renal function and proceed slowly with dosing increases; monitor closely.

(Continued)

597

Ethosuximide *(Continued)*

Pregnancy Risk Factor: C

Lactation: Enters breast milk/compatible

Administration

Oral: Administer with food or milk to avoid GI upset.

Related Information

Anticonvulsants By Seizure Type *on page 1712*

Peak and Trough Guidelines *on page 1694*

♦ **Ethoxynaphthamido Penicillin Sodium** *see* Nafcillin *on page 1048*

♦ **Ethyl Aminobenzoate** *see* Benzocaine *on page 181*

♦ **Ethyl Esters of Omega-3 Fatty Acids** *see* Omega-3-Acid Ethyl Esters *on page 1117*

♦ **Ethynodiol Diacetate and Ethinyl Estradiol** *see* Ethinyl Estradiol and Ethynodiol Diacetate *on page 583*

♦ **Ethyol®** *see* Amifostine *on page 86*

Etodolac *(ee toe DOE lak)*

U.S. Brand Names Lodine®; Lodine® XL

Synonyms Etodolic Acid

Generic Available Yes

Pharmacologic Category Nonsteroidal Anti-inflammatory Drug (NSAID), Oral

Medication Safety Issues

Sound-alike/look-alike issues:

Lodine® may be confused with codeine, iodine, Iopidine®, Lopid®

Use Acute and long-term use in the management of signs and symptoms of osteoarthritis and management of pain; rheumatoid arthritis; juvenile rheumatoid arthritis

Mechanism of Action/Effect Inhibits prostaglandin synthesis which results in decreased formation of prostaglandin precursors

Contraindications Hypersensitivity to etodolac, aspirin, other NSAIDs, or any component of the formulation; active gastric/duodenal ulcer disease; patients with "aspirin triad" (bronchial asthma, aspirin intolerance, rhinitis); pregnancy (3rd trimester)

Warnings/Precautions Fatal asthmatic and anaphylactoid reactions have occurred in patients with "aspirin triad." Use with caution in patients with CHF, hypertension, dehydration, decreased renal or hepatic function, history of GI disease (bleeding, ulcers, or previous GI symptoms with NSAID use), or those receiving anticoagulants and/or corticosteroids. Use lowest effective dose for shortest period possible; bleeding risk has been correlated to dose and duration of therapy. Gastrointestinal bleeding may occur without prior symptoms of gastrointestinal irritation. Elderly are at a high risk for adverse effects from NSAIDs. As many as 60% of elderly can develop peptic ulceration and/or hemorrhage asymptomatically.

Use of NSAIDs can compromise existing renal function especially when Cl_{cr} <30 mL/minute. CNS adverse effects such as confusion, agitation, and hallucination are generally seen in overdose or high-dose situations; however, elderly may demonstrate these adverse effects at lower doses than younger adults. Withhold for at least 4-6 half-lives prior to surgical or dental procedures.

The extended release formulation consists of drug within a nondeformable matrix; following drug release/absorption, the matrix/shell is expelled in the stool. The use of nondeformable products in patients with known stricture/narrowing of the GI tract has been associated with symptoms of obstruction.

Drug Interactions

Decreased Effect: Decreased effect with aspirin. May reduce effect of some diuretics and antihypertensive effect of β-blockers.

Increased Effect/Toxicity: Etodolac may increase effect/toxicity of aspirin (GI irritation), lithium, methotrexate, digoxin, cyclosporine (nephrotoxicity), and warfarin (bleeding).

Nutritional/Ethanol Interactions

Ethanol: Avoid ethanol (may enhance gastric mucosal irritation).

Food: Etodolac peak serum levels may be decreased if taken with food.

Herb/Nutraceutical: Avoid cat's claw, dong quai, evening primrose, feverfew, garlic, ginger, ginkgo, red clover, horse chestnut, green tea, ginseng (all have additional antiplatelet activity)

Lab Interactions False-positive for urinary bilirubin and ketone increase bleeding time. Etodolac may cause a lowering of serum uric acid levels.

Adverse Reactions 1% to 10%:

Central nervous system: Depression (1% to 3%)

Dermatologic: Rash (1% to 3%), pruritus (1% to 3%)

Gastrointestinal: Abdominal cramps (3% to 9%), nausea (3% to 9%), vomiting (1% to 3%), dyspepsia (10%), diarrhea (3% to 9%), constipation (1% to 3%), flatulence (3% to 9%), melena (1% to 3%), gastritis (1% to 3%)

Genitourinary: Polyuria (1% to 3%)

Neuromuscular & skeletal: Weakness (3% to 9%)

Ocular: Blurred vision (1% to 3%)

Otic: Tinnitus (1% to 3%)

Overdosage/Toxicology Symptoms of overdose include acute renal failure, vomiting, drowsiness, leukocytosis. Management of NSAID intoxication is supportive and symptomatic.

Pharmacodynamics/Kinetics
Onset of Action: Analgesic: 2-4 hours; Maximum anti-inflammatory effect: A few days
Absorption: Well absorbed
Time to Peak: Serum: 1 hour
Protein Binding: High
Half-Life Elimination: 7 hours
Metabolism: Hepatic
Excretion: Urine

Dosing
Adults & Elderly:
Acute pain: Oral: 200-400 mg every 6-8 hours, as needed, not to exceed total daily doses of 1200 mg; for patients weighing <60 kg, total daily dose should not exceed 20 mg/kg/day.
Rheumatoid arthritis, osteoarthritis:
Regular release: Initial: 600-1200 mg/day given in divided doses: 400 mg 2 times/day; 300 mg 2 or 3 times/day; 500 mg 2 times/day; total daily dose should not exceed 1200 mg; for patients weighing <60 kg, total daily dose should not exceed 20 mg/kg/day
Extended release (Lodine® XL): 400-1000 mg once daily
Note: A single dose of 76-100 mg is comparable to the analgesic effect of aspirin 650 mg
Pediatrics:
Juvenile rheumatoid arthritis (Lodine® XL): Oral: Children 6-16 years:
20-30 kg: 400 mg once daily
31-45 kg: 600 mg once daily
46-60 kg: 800 mg once daily
Children >60 kg: 1000 mg once daily

Available Dosage Forms [DSC] = Discontinued product
Capsule (Lodine®): 200 mg, 300 mg
Tablet: 400 mg, 500 mg
Lodine®: 400 mg, 500 mg [DSC]
Tablet, extended release (Lodine® XL): 400 mg, 500 mg, 600 mg

Monitoring and Teaching Issues
Physical Assessment: Systemic: Assess effectiveness and interactions of other medications patient may be taking. Assess results of laboratory tests and therapeutic and adverse reactions at beginning of therapy and periodically throughout therapy. Assess knowledge/teach patient appropriate use, interventions to reduce side effects, and adverse symptoms to report.

Monitoring Laboratory Tests: CBC, liver enzymes; in patients receiving diuretics, monitor BUN/serum creatinine.

Patient Education: Take this medication exactly as directed; do not increase dose without consulting prescriber. Do not crush tablets or break capsules. Take with food or milk to reduce GI distress. Maintain adequate hydration (2-3 L/day of fluids) unless instructed to restrict fluid intake. Do not use alcohol, aspirin or aspirin-containing medication, or any other anti-inflammatory medications without consulting prescriber. You may experience anorexia, nausea, vomiting, or heartburn (small frequent meals, frequent mouth care, sucking lozenges, or chewing gum may help); drowsiness, dizziness, nervousness, or headache (use caution when driving or engaging in tasks requiring alertness until response to drug is known); or fluid retention (weigh yourself weekly and report unusual (3-5 lb/week) weight gain). GI bleeding, ulceration, or perforation can occur with or without pain; discontinue medication and contact prescriber if persistent abdominal pain or cramping, or blood in stool occurs. Report breathlessness, respiratory difficulty, or unusual cough; chest pain, rapid heartbeat, palpitations; unusual bruising/bleeding; blood in urine, stool, mouth, or vomitus; swollen extremities; skin rash or itching; acute fatigue; or hearing changes (ringing in ears). **Pregnancy/breast-feeding precautions:** Inform prescriber if you are or intend to become pregnant. This drug should not be used in the 3rd trimester of pregnancy. Do not breast-feed.

Dietary Considerations: May be taken with food to decrease GI distress.

Geriatric Considerations: Elderly are at high risk for adverse effects from NSAIDs. As much as 60% of elderly who experience GI side effects can develop peptic ulceration and/or hemorrhage asymptomatically.

Pregnancy Risk Factor: C/D (3rd trimester)
Lactation: Excretion in breast milk unknown/contraindicated

Administration
Storage: Protect from moisture.

Related Information
Nonsalicylate / Nonsteroidal Anti-inflammatory Agents *on page 1743*

♦ **Etodolic Acid** *see* Etodolac *on page 598*
♦ **Etopophos®** *see* Etoposide Phosphate *on page 602*

Etoposide (e toe POE side)
U.S. Brand Names Toposar®; VePesid®
Synonyms Epipodophyllotoxin; VP-16; VP-16-213
Generic Available Yes
Pharmacologic Category Antineoplastic Agent, Podophyllotoxin Derivative
Medication Safety Issues
Sound-alike/look-alike issues:
VePesid® may be confused with Versed
Use Treatment of lymphomas, ANLL, lung, testicular, bladder, and prostate carcinoma, hepatoma, rhabdomyosarcoma, uterine carcinoma, neuroblastoma, mycosis fungoides, Kaposi's sarcoma, histiocytosis, gestational trophoblastic disease, Ewing's sarcoma, Wilms' tumor, and brain tumors
Mechanism of Action/Effect Inhibits DNA synthesis leading to cell death.
(Continued)

Etoposide *(Continued)*

Contraindications Hypersensitivity to etoposide or any component of the formulation; **intrathecal administration**; pregnancy

Warnings/Precautions The U.S. Food and Drug Administration (FDA) currently recommends that procedures for proper handling and disposal of antineoplastic agents be considered. Severe myelosuppression with resulting infection or bleeding may occur. Administer I.V. infusions over a period of at least 30-60 minutes. **Must be diluted - do not give IVP.** Dosage should be adjusted in patients with hepatic or renal impairment.

If etoposide contacts the skin, wash and flush thoroughly with water.

Drug Interactions

Cytochrome P450 Effect: Substrate of CYP1A2 (minor), 2E1 (minor), 3A4 (major); **Inhibits** CYP2C8/9 (weak), 3A4 (weak)

Decreased Effect: CYP3A4 inducers may decrease the levels/effects of etoposide; example inducers include aminoglutethimide, carbamazepine, nafcillin, nevirapine, phenobarbital, phenytoin, and rifamycins.

Increased Effect/Toxicity: The effects of etoposide may be increased by calcium antagonists (increased effects noted *in vitro*). Cyclosporine may increase the levels of etoposide. Etoposide may increase the effects/toxicity of methotrexate and warfarin. There have been reports of frequent hepatic dysfunction with hyperbilirubinemia, ascites, and thrombocytopenia when etoposide is combined with carmustine. CYP3A4 inhibitors may increase the levels/effects of etoposide; example inhibitors include azole antifungals, ciprofloxacin, clarithromycin, diclofenac, doxycycline, erythromycin, imatinib, isoniazid, nefazodone, nicardipine, propofol, protease inhibitors, quinidine, and verapamil.

Nutritional/Ethanol Interactions

Ethanol: Avoid ethanol (may increase GI irritation).

Food: Administration of food does not affect GI absorption with doses ≤200 mg of injection.

Herb/Nutraceutical: St John's wort may decrease etoposide levels.

Adverse Reactions

>10%:

Cardiovascular: Hypotension if the drug is infused too fast

Dermatologic: Alopecia (22% to 93%)

Endocrine & metabolic: Ovarian failure (38%), amenorrhea

Gastrointestinal: Mild to moderate nausea and vomiting; mucositis, especially at high doses; anorexia (10% to 13%)

Hematologic: Myelosuppression, leukopenia (91%), thrombocytopenia (41%), anemia

Onset: 5-7 days

Nadir: 7-14 days

Recovery: 21-28 days

1% to 10%:

Gastrointestinal: Stomatitis (1% to 6%), diarrhea (1% to 13%), abdominal pain

Neuromuscular & skeletal: Peripheral neuropathies (0.7% to 2%)

Overdosage/Toxicology Symptoms of overdose include bone marrow suppression, leukopenia, thrombocytopenia, nausea, and vomiting. Treatment is supportive.

Pharmacodynamics/Kinetics

Absorption: Oral: 25% to 75%; significant inter- and intrapatient variation

Time to Peak: Serum: Oral: 1-1.5 hours

Protein Binding: 94% to 97%

Half-Life Elimination: Terminal: 4-15 hours; Children: Normal renal/hepatic function: 6-8 hours

Metabolism: Hepatic to hydroxy acid and cislactone metabolites

Excretion:

Children: Urine (≤55% as unchanged drug)

Adults: Urine (42% to 67%; 8% to 35% as unchanged drug) within 24 hours; feces (up to 16%)

Dosing

Adults & Elderly: Refer to individual protocols.

Small cell lung cancer:

Oral: Twice the I.V. dose rounded to the nearest 50 mg given once daily if total dose ≤400 mg or in divided doses if >400 mg

I.V.: 35 mg/m²/day for 4 days or 50 mg/m²/day for 5 days every 3-4 weeks total dose ≤400 mg/day or in divided doses if >400 mg/day

IVPB: 200-250 mg/m² repeated every 7 weeks

Continuous intravenous infusion: 500 mg/m² over 24 hours every 3 weeks

Testicular cancer:

IVPB: 50-100 mg/m²/day for 5 days repeated every 3-4 weeks

I.V.: 100 mg/m² every other day for 3 doses repeated every 3-4 weeks

BMT/relapsed leukemia: I.V.: 2.4-3.5 g/m² or 25-70 mg/kg administered over 4-36 hours

BMT high dose: I.V.: 750-2400 mg/m²; 10-60 mg/kg; duration of infusion is 1-4 hours to 24 hours; generally combined with other high-dose chemotherapeutic drugs or total body irradiation (TBI).

Pediatrics: Refer to individual protocols.

Children: I.V.: 60-120 mg/m²/day for 3-5 days every 3-6 weeks

AML: I.V.:

Remission induction: 150 mg/m²/day for 2-3 days for 2-3 cycles

Intensification or consolidation: 250 mg/m²/day for 3 days, courses 2-5

Brain tumor: I.V.: 150 mg/m²/day on days 2 and 3 of treatment course

Neuroblastoma: I.V.: 100 mg/m²/day over 1 hour on days 1-5 of cycle; repeat cycle every 4 weeks

BMT conditioning regimen used in patients with rhabdomyosarcoma or neuroblastoma: I.V. continuous infusion: 160 mg/m²/day for 4 days

Conditioning regimen for allogenic BMT: I.V.: 60 mg/kg/dose as a single dose

Renal Impairment:
Cl_{cr} 10-50 mL/minute: Administer 75% of normal dose.
Cl_{cr} <10 mL minute: Administer 50% of normal dose.
Hemodialysis effects: Supplemental dose is not necessary.
CAPD effects: Unknown
CAVH effects: Unknown

Hepatic Impairment:
Bilirubin 1.5-3 mg/dL or AST 60-180 units: Reduce dose by 50%.
Bilirubin >3 mg/dL or AST >180 units: Reduce by 75%.

Available Dosage Forms
Capsule, softgel (VePesid®): 50 mg
Injection, solution: 20 mg/mL (5 mL, 25 mL, 50 mL) [may contain benzyl alcohol or alcohol]
Toposar®: 20 mg/mL (5 mL, 10 mL, 25 mL) [contains benzyl alcohol]
VePesid®: 20 mg/mL (5 mL, 7.5 mL, 25 mL, 50 mL) [contains benzyl alcohol and alcohol 30%]

Monitoring and Teaching Issues
Physical Assessment: See Warnings/Precautions for use cautions. Assess potential for interactions with other pharmacological agents and herbal products patient may be taking (eg, potential for increasing/decreasing levels or effects of etoposide; see Drug Interactions). Specific Administration directions should be noted prior to beginning treatment. Infusion site should be monitored closely to prevent extravasation (application of cold or hydrocortisone is contraindicated). Assess results of laboratory tests, therapeutic effectiveness, and adverse response prior to each treatment and on a regular basis throughout therapy (hypotension, myelosuppression [infection, bleeding]; see Adverse Reactions). Teach patient possible side effects/appropriate interventions and adverse symptoms to report (see Patient Education).

Monitoring Laboratory Tests: CBC with differential, platelet count, bilirubin, renal function

Patient Education: Do not take any new medication during therapy unless approved by prescriber. This medication may be administered by infusion. Report immediately any swelling, pain, burning, or redness at infusion site. Avoid alcohol. It is important to maintain adequate hydration (2-3 L/day of fluids) unless instructed to restrict fluid intake and adequate nutrition (small frequent meals may help). You will be more susceptible to infection (avoid crowds and exposure to infection and do not have any vaccinations without consulting prescriber). May cause nausea or vomiting (small frequent meals, frequent mouth care, sucking lozenges, or chewing gum may help); diarrhea (buttermilk, boiled milk, or yogurt may help); loss of hair (reversible); or mouth sores (use soft toothbrush or cotton swabs for oral care and rinse mouth frequently). Report immediately chest pain, swelling of extremities, respiratory difficulty, palpitations, or rapid heartbeat. Report extreme fatigue, pain or numbness in extremities, severe GI upset or diarrhea, bleeding or bruising, fever, chills, sore throat, vaginal discharge, respiratory difficulty, yellowing of eyes or skin, or any changes in color of urine or stool. **Pregnancy/breast-feeding precautions:** Do not get pregnant while taking this medication. Consult prescriber for appropriate contraceptive measures to use during and for 1 month following therapy. Do not breast-feed.

Pregnancy Risk Factor: D

Lactation: Enters breast milk/contraindicated

Administration
Oral: If necessary, the injection may be used for oral administration. Mix with orange juice, apple juice, or lemonade to a concentration of 0.4 mg/mL or less, and use within a 3-hour period.

I.M.: Do not administer I.M. or SubQ (severe tissue necrosis).

I.V.: Irritant. Administer lower doses IVPB over at least 30 minutes to minimize the risk of hypotensive reactions.

Reconstitution: VP-16 should be further diluted in D_5W or NS for administration. Diluted solutions have concentration-dependent stability: More concentrated solutions have shorter stability times.

At room temperature in D_5W or NS in polyvinyl chloride, the concentration is stable as follows:
0.2 mg/mL: 96 hours
0.4 mg/mL: 48 hours
0.6 mg/mL: 8 hours
1 mg/mL: 2 hours
2 mg/mL: 1 hour
20 mg/mL (undiluted): 24 hours

Standard I.V. dilution:
Lower dose regimens (<1 g/dose):
Doses may be diluted in 100-1000 mL of D_5W or NS
If the concentration is less than or equal to 0.6 mg/mL, the bag should be mixed with the appropriate expiration dating.
If the concentration is >0.6 mg/mL, the concentration is highly unstable and a syringe of undiluted etoposide accompanied with the appropriate volume of diluent will be sent to the nursing unit to be mixed at the bedside just prior to administration.

High-dose regimens (>1g/dose):
Total dose should be drawn into an empty Viaflex® container and the appropriate amount of diluent (for a final concentration of 1 mg/mL) will be sent.
Use the **2-Channel Pump Method**: Instill all of the etoposide dose into one Viaflex® container (concentration = 20 mg/mL). Infuse this into one channel (Baxter Flow-Guard 6300 Dual Channel Volumetric Infusion Pump - or any 2-channel infusion pump that does not require a "hard" plastic cassette). Infuse the indicated diluent (ie, D_5W or NS) at a rate of at least 20 times the infusion rate of the etoposide to simulate a 1 mg/mL concentration in the line. The etoposide should be Y-sited into the port most proximal to the patient. A 0.22 micron filter should be attached to the line after the Y-site and before entry into the patient.

(Continued)

Etoposide *(Continued)*

Compatibility: Stable in D$_5$W, LR

Y-site administration: Incompatible with cefepime, filgrastim, idarubicin

Storage: Store intact vials of injection at room temperature and protected from light. Injection solution contains polyethylene glycol vehicle with absolute alcohol. Store oral capsules under refrigeration. Capsules are stable for 3 months at room temperature.

Etoposide Phosphate *(e toe POE side FOS fate)*

U.S. Brand Names Etopophos®

Generic Available No

Pharmacologic Category Antineoplastic Agent, Podophyllotoxin Derivative

Use Treatment of refractory testicular tumors and small cell lung cancer

Mechanism of Action/Effect Etoposide phosphate is converted *in vivo* to the active moiety, etoposide, by dephosphorylation. Etoposide inhibits mitotic activity; inhibits cells from entering prophase; inhibits DNA synthesis. Initially thought to be mitotic inhibitors similar to podophyllotoxin, but actually have no effect on microtubule assembly. However, later shown to induce DNA strand breakage and inhibition of topoisomerase II (an enzyme which breaks and repairs DNA); etoposide acts in late S or early G2 phases.

Contraindications Hypersensitivity to etoposide, etoposide phosphate, or any component of the formulation; **intrathecal administration**; pregnancy

Warnings/Precautions The U.S. Food and Drug Administration (FDA) currently recommends that procedures for proper handling and disposal of antineoplastic agents be considered. Severe myelosuppression with resulting infection or bleeding may occur. Dosage should be adjusted in patients with hepatic or renal impairment. Use caution in elderly patients (may be more likely to develop severe myelosuppression, GI effects, and/or alopecia).

If etoposide phosphate contacts the skin, wash and flush thoroughly with water.

Drug Interactions

Cytochrome P450 Effect: Substrate of CYP1A2 (minor), 2E1 (minor), 3A4 (major); **Inhibits** CYP2C8/9 (weak), 3A4 (weak)

Decreased Effect: CYP3A4 inducers may decrease the levels/effects of etoposide; example inducers include aminoglutethimide, carbamazepine, nafcillin, nevirapine, phenobarbital, phenytoin, and rifamycins.

Increased Effect/Toxicity: Etoposide taken with warfarin may result in prolongation of bleeding times. Alteration of methotrexate transport has been found as a slow efflux of methotrexate and its polyglutamated form out of the cell, leading to intercellular accumulation of methotrexate. Calcium antagonists increase the rate of VP-16-induced DNA damage and cytotoxicity *in vitro*. Use with carmustine has shown reports of frequent hepatic dysfunction with hyperbilirubinemia, ascites, and thrombocytopenia. Cyclosporine may cause additive cytotoxic effects on tumor cells. CYP3A4 inhibitors may increase the levels/effects of etoposide; example inhibitors include azole antifungals, ciprofloxacin, clarithromycin, diclofenac, doxycycline, erythromycin, imatinib, isoniazid, nefazodone, nicardipine, propofol, protease inhibitors, quinidine, and verapamil.

Nutritional/Ethanol Interactions

Ethanol: Avoid ethanol (may increase GI irritation).

Food: Administration of food does not affect GI absorption with doses ≤200 mg of injection.

Herb/Nutraceutical: St John's wort may decrease etoposide levels.

Adverse Reactions Based on **etoposide**:

>10%:

Cardiovascular: Hypotension if the drug is infused too fast

Dermatologic: Alopecia (22% to 93%)

Endocrine & metabolic: Ovarian failure (38%), amenorrhea

Gastrointestinal: Mild to moderate nausea and vomiting; mucositis, especially at high doses; anorexia (10% to 13%)

Hematologic: Myelosuppression, leukopenia (91%), thrombocytopenia (41%), anemia

Onset: 5-7 days

Nadir: 7-14 days

Recovery: 21-28 days

1% to 10%:

Gastrointestinal: Stomatitis (1% to 6%), diarrhea (1% to 13%), abdominal pain

Neuromuscular & skeletal: Peripheral neuropathies (0.7% to 2%)

Overdosage/Toxicology Symptoms of overdose include bone marrow suppression, leukopenia, thrombocytopenia, nausea, and vomiting. Treatment is supportive.

Pharmacodynamics/Kinetics

Protein Binding: 94% to 97%

Half-Life Elimination: Terminal: 4-15 hours; Children: Normal renal/hepatic function: 6-8 hours

Metabolism: Hepatic (with a biphasic decay)

Excretion: Urine (as unchanged drug and metabolites), feces (2% to 16%); Children: I.V.: Urine (≤55% as unchanged drug)

Dosing

Adults & Elderly: Refer to individual protocols.

Small cell lung cancer: I.V. (in combination with other approved chemotherapeutic drugs): **Equivalent doses of etoposide phosphate to an etoposide dosage** range of 35 mg/m²/day for 4 days to 50 mg/m²/day for 5 days. Courses are repeated at 3- to 4-week intervals after adequate recovery from any toxicity.

Testicular cancer: I.V. (in combination with other approved chemotherapeutic agents): **Equivalent doses of etoposide phosphate to an etoposide dosage** range of 50-100 mg/m²/day on days 1-5 to 100 mg/m²/day on days 1, 3, and 5. Courses are repeated at 3- to 4-week intervals after adequate recovery from any toxicity.

BMT high dose: I.V.: 0.5-2 g/m² divided into 2 daily doses; maximum single-dose agent: 3.2 g/m²; generally combined with other high-dose chemotherapeutic drugs.

Renal Impairment:
Cl$_{cr}$ 15-50 mL/minute: Administer 75% of normal dose.
Cl$_{cr}$ <15 mL minute: Data is not available and further dose reduction should be considered in these patients.
Hemodialysis: Supplemental dose is not necessary.
Peritoneal dialysis: Supplemental dose is not necessary.
CAPD effects: Unknown
CAVH effects: Unknown

Hepatic Impairment:
Bilirubin 1.5-3 mg/dL or AST 60-180 units: Reduce dose by 50%.
Bilirubin 3-5 mg/dL or AST >180 units: Reduce dose by 75%.
Bilirubin >5 mg/dL: Do not administer.

Available Dosage Forms Injection, powder for reconstitution, as base: 100 mg

Monitoring and Teaching Issues
Physical Assessment: See Contraindications, Warnings/Precautions for use cautions (eg, hepatic or renal impairment). Assess potential for interactions with other pharmacological agents and herbal products patient may be taking (eg, potential for increasing/decreasing levels or effects of etoposide; see Drug Interactions). See Reconstitution for specific directions. Assess results of laboratory tests, therapeutic effectiveness, and adverse response (see Adverse Reactions) prior to each treatment and on a regular basis throughout therapy. Teach patient possible side effects/appropriate interventions and adverse symptoms to report (see Patient Education).

Monitoring Laboratory Tests: CBC with differential, platelet count, bilirubin, renal function

Patient Education: Do not take any new medication during therapy unless approved by prescriber. This medication is administered by infusion; report immediately any swelling, pain, burning, redness at infusion site; sudden difficulty breathing or swallowing, chest pain, or chills. It is important to maintain adequate hydration (2-3 L/day of fluids) unless instructed to restrict fluid intake and adequate nutrition (small frequent meals may help). You will be more susceptible to infection (avoid crowds and exposure to infection and do not have any vaccinations without consulting prescriber). May cause nausea or vomiting (small frequent meals, frequent mouth care, sucking lozenges, or chewing gum may help); diarrhea (buttermilk, boiled milk, or yogurt may help); loss of hair (reversible); or mouth sores (use soft toothbrush or cotton swabs for oral care and rinse mouth frequently). Report immediately chest pain, swelling of extremities, respiratory difficulty, palpitations, or rapid heartbeat. Report extreme fatigue, pain or numbness in extremities, severe GI upset or diarrhea, bleeding or bruising, fever, chills, sore throat, vaginal discharge, respiratory difficulty, yellowing of eyes or skin, or changes in color of urine or stool. **Pregnancy/breast-feeding precautions:** Do not get pregnant while taking this medication. Consult prescriber for appropriate contraceptive measures to use during and for 1 month following therapy. Do not breast-feed.

Geriatric Considerations: Elderly patients may be more susceptible to severe myelosuppression. Other adverse effects including GI toxicity, infectious complications, weakness, and alopecia may occur more frequently in elderly.

Pregnancy Risk Factor: D
Lactation: Enters breast milk/contraindicated

Administration
I.V.: Etoposide phosphate solutions should be administered over 5-210 minutes.
Reconstitution: Reconstituted vials with 5 mL or 10 mL SWI, D$_5$W, NS, bacteriostatic SWI, or bacteriostatic NS to a concentration of 20 mg/mL or 10 mg/mL etoposide (22.7 mg/mL or 11.4 mg/mL etoposide phosphate), respectively. These solutions may be administered without further dilution or may be further diluted to a concentration as low as 0.1 mg/mL etoposide with either D$_5$W or NS. Solutions are stable in glass or plastic containers at room temperature 20°C to 25°C (68°F to 77°F) or under refrigeration 2°C to 8°C (36°F to 47°F) for up to 24 hours.
Compatibility: Stable in D$_5$W, NS, SWFI
Y-site administration: Incompatible with amphotericin B, cefepime, chlorpromazine, imipenem/cilastatin, methylprednisolone sodium succinate, mitomycin, prochlorperazine edisylate
Storage: Store intact vials of injection under refrigeration 2°C to 8°C (36°F to 46°F). Protect from light. Store capsules in refrigerator.

Exemestane (ex e MES tane)

U.S. Brand Names Aromasin®
Generic Available No
Pharmacologic Category Antineoplastic Agent, Aromatase Inactivator
Use Treatment of advanced breast cancer in postmenopausal women whose disease has progressed following tamoxifen therapy
Mechanism of Action/Effect Exemestane prevents conversion of androgens to estrogens (Aromatase inhibitor) and lowers circulating estrogen levels.
Contraindications Hypersensitivity to exemestane or any component of the formulation; pregnancy
Warnings/Precautions Not indicated for premenopausal women; not to be given with estrogen-containing agents. Use with caution in hepatic impairment or renal insufficiency. (Continued)

Exemestane *(Continued)*

Drug Interactions
Cytochrome P450 Effect: Substrate of CYP3A4 (major)

Decreased Effect: CYP3A4 inducers may decrease the levels/effects of exemestane (example inducers include aminoglutethimide, carbamazepine, nafcillin, nevirapine, phenobarbital, phenytoin, and rifamycins). Rifampin may decrease exemestane levels; increased dosage recommended.

Nutritional/Ethanol Interactions
Food: Plasma levels increased by 40% when exemestane was taken with a fatty meal.

Herb/Nutraceutical: St John's wort may decrease exemestane levels. Avoid black cohosh, dong quai in estrogen-dependent tumors.

Adverse Reactions
>10%:
Central nervous system: Fatigue (22%), pain (13%), depression (13%), insomnia (11%), anxiety (10%)
Endocrine & metabolic: Hot flashes (13%)
Gastrointestinal: Nausea (18%)

1% to 10%:
Cardiovascular: Edema (7%), hypertension (5%), chest pain
Central nervous system: Dizziness (8%), headache (8%), fever (5%), hypoesthesia, confusion
Dermatologic: Rash, itching, alopecia
Gastrointestinal: Vomiting (7%), abdominal pain (6%), anorexia (6%), constipation (5%), diarrhea (4%), increased appetite (3%), dyspepsia
Genitourinary: Urinary tract infection
Neuromuscular & skeletal: Weakness, paresthesia, pathological fracture, arthralgia
Respiratory: Dyspnea (10%), cough (6%), bronchitis, sinusitis, pharyngitis, rhinitis
Miscellaneous: Influenza-like symptoms (6%), diaphoresis (6%), lymphedema, infection

A dose-dependent decrease in sex hormone-binding globulin has been observed with daily doses of 25 mg or more. Serum luteinizing hormone and follicle-stimulating hormone levels have increased with this medicine.

Overdosage/Toxicology If an overdose should occur, general supportive care would be indicated.

Pharmacodynamics/Kinetics
Absorption: Rapid and moderate (~42%) following oral administration; absorption increases ~40% following high-fat meal

Time to Peak: Women with breast cancer: 1.2 hours

Protein Binding: 90%, primarily to albumin and α_1-acid glycoprotein

Half-Life Elimination: 24 hours

Metabolism: Extensively hepatic; oxidation (CYP3A4) of methylene group, reduction of 17-keto group with formation of many secondary metabolites; metabolites are inactive

Excretion: Urine (<1% as unchanged drug, 39% to 45% as metabolites); feces (36% to 48%)

Dosing
Adults & Elderly: Breast cancer: Oral: 25 mg once daily after a meal

Dosage adjustment with CYP3A4 inducers: 50 mg once daily when used with potent inducers (eg, rifampin, phenytoin)

Renal Impairment: Safety of chronic dosing in renal impairment has not been established.

Hepatic Impairment: Safety of chronic dosing in hepatic impairment has not been established.

Available Dosage Forms Tablet: 25 mg

Monitoring and Teaching Issues
Physical Assessment: Use caution in presence of hepatic or renal impairment (see Warnings/Precautions). Assess patient response (see Adverse Reactions) prior to each treatment and on a regular basis throughout therapy. Teach patient proper use, possible side effects/appropriate interventions (eg, importance of adequate hydration), and adverse symptoms to report (refer to Patient Education). **For use in postmenopausal women only.**

Patient Education: Do not take any new medication during therapy unless approved by prescriber. Take after meals at approximately the same time each day. You may be more susceptible to infection (avoid crowds or exposure to infection and do not have any vaccinations unless approved by prescriber). May cause headache, dizziness, confusion, fatigue, anxiety, insomnia (use caution when driving or engaging in tasks requiring alertness until response to medication is known); indigestion, nausea, vomiting, loss of appetite (small frequent meals, good mouth care, chewing gum, or sucking hard candy may help); or hot flashes (cool dark room or cold compresses may help). Report chest pain, palpitations; acute headache, visual disturbances; unresolved GI problems; itching or burning on urination, vaginal discharge; acute joint, back, bone, or muscle pain; respiratory difficulty, unusual cough, respiratory infection; or other adverse reactions. **For use in postmenopausal women only.**

Pregnancy Risk Factor: D

Pregnancy Issues: Exemestane has been associated with prolonged gestation, abnormal or difficult labor, increased resorption, reduced number of live fetuses, decreased fetal weight, and retarded ossification in rats. It is not indicated for premenopausal women, but if exposure occurred during pregnancy, risk to the fetus and potential risk for loss of the pregnancy should be discussed.

Lactation: Excretion in breast milk unknown/use caution

Administration
Storage: Store at 25°C (77°F)

◆ ex-lax® [OTC] *see* Senna *on page 1365*
◆ ex-lax® Maximum Strength [OTC] *see* Senna *on page 1365*
◆ EZ-Char™ [OTC] *see* Charcoal *on page 302*

Ezetimibe (ez ET i mibe)

U.S. Brand Names Zetia™

Generic Available No

Pharmacologic Category Antilipemic Agent, 2-Azetidinone

Medication Safety Issues

Sound-alike/look-alike issues:

Zetia™ may be confused with Zestril®

Use Use in combination with dietary therapy for the treatment of primary hypercholesterolemia (as monotherapy or in combination with HMG-CoA reductase inhibitors); homozygous sitosterolemia; homozygous familial hypercholesterolemia (in combination with atorvastatin or simvastatin)

Mechanism of Action/Effect Inhibits absorption of cholesterol at the brush border of the small intestine, leading to a decreased delivery of cholesterol to the liver, reduction of hepatic cholesterol stores and an increased clearance of cholesterol from the blood; decreases total C, LDL-C, ApoB, and triglycerides while increasing HDL-C

Contraindications Hypersensitivity to ezetimibe or any component of the formulation

Warnings/Precautions Secondary causes of hyperlipidemia should be ruled out prior to therapy. Use caution with renal or mild hepatic impairment; not recommended for use with moderate or severe hepatic impairment. Safety and efficacy have not been established in patients <10 years of age.

Drug Interactions

Decreased Effect: Bile acid sequestrants may decrease ezetimibe bioavailability; administer ezetimibe ≥2 hours before or ≥4 hours after bile acid sequestrants.

Increased Effect/Toxicity: Cyclosporine may increase plasma levels of ezetimibe. Fibric acid derivatives may increase bioavailability of ezetimibe (safety and efficacy of concomitant use not established). Ezetimibe may increase serum levels of cyclosporine.

Adverse Reactions 1% to 10%:

Cardiovascular: Chest pain (3%), dizziness (3%), fatigue (2%)

Central nervous system: Headache (8%)

Gastrointestinal: Diarrhea (3% to 4%), abdominal pain (3%)

Neuromuscular & skeletal: Arthralgia (4%)

Respiratory: Sinusitis (4% to 5%), pharyngitis (2% to 3%, placebo 2%)

Overdosage/Toxicology Doses of up to 50 mg/day were well-tolerated. Treatment should be symptom-directed and supportive.

Pharmacodynamics/Kinetics

Bioavailability: Variable

Time to Peak: Plasma: 4-12 hours

Protein Binding: >90% to plasma proteins

Half-Life Elimination: 22 hours (ezetimibe and metabolite)

Metabolism: Undergoes conjugation in the small intestine and liver; forms metabolite (active); may undergo enterohepatic recycling

Excretion: Feces (78%, 69% as ezetimibe); urine (11%, 9% as metabolite)

Dosing

Adults & Elderly:

Hyperlipidemias: Oral: 10 mg/day

Sitosterolemia: Oral: 10 mg/day

Pediatrics: Hyperlipidemias: Children ≥10 years: Refer to adult dosing.

Renal Impairment: Bioavailability increased with severe impairment; no dosing adjustment recommended.

Hepatic Impairment: Bioavailability increased with hepatic impairment

Mild impairment (Child-Pugh score 5-6): No dosing adjustment necessary.

Moderate to severe impairment (Child-Pugh score 7-15): Use of ezetimibe not recommended.

Available Dosage Forms Tablet: 10 mg [capsule shaped]

Monitoring and Teaching Issues

Physical Assessment: Use caution in presence of renal or hepatic impairment (see Warnings/Precautions). Assess potential for interactions with other pharmacological agent prescriptions patient may be taking (eg, timing of concurrent medication; see Drug Interactions). Assess results of laboratory tests prior to and periodically during therapy, therapeutic effectiveness, and adverse response at beginning of and at regular intervals during therapy (see Adverse Reactions). Teach patient proper use, possible side effects/appropriate interventions, and adverse reactions to report (see Patient Education).

Monitoring Laboratory Tests: Total cholesterol profile prior to therapy, and when clinically indicated and/or periodically thereafter

Patient Education: Do not take any new medication during therapy without consulting prescriber. Take at the same time of day, without regard for meals. Take 2 hours before or 4 hours after bile acid binding agents (ie, Questran®). This medication does not replace the need for dietary and exercise recommendations of prescriber. May cause headache, dizziness, or fatigue (use caution when driving or engaged in potentially hazardous tasks until response to drug is known); diarrhea (boiled milk, buttermilk, or yogurt may help); or abdominal pain. Report any severe or persistent side effects (eg, chest pain; muscle, skeletal, or joint pain; increased perspiration). **Pregnancy/breast-feeding precautions:** Inform prescriber if you are or intend to become pregnant. Breast-feeding is not recommended.

Dietary Considerations: May be taken without regard to meals. Before initiation of therapy, patients should be placed on a standard cholesterol-lowering diet for 6 weeks and the diet should be continued during drug therapy.

(Continued)

Ezetimibe *(Continued)*

Pregnancy Risk Factor: C

Lactation: Excretion in breast milk unknown/not recommended

Administration

Oral: May be administered without regard to meals. May be taken at the same time as HMG-CoA reductase inhibitors. Administer ≥2 hours before or ≥4 hours after bile acid sequestrants.

Storage: Store at controlled room temperature of 15°C to 30°C (59°F to 86°F). Protect from moisture.

Related Information

Hyperlipidemia Management *on page 1836*

Lipid-Lowering Agents *on page 1738*

Ezetimibe and Simvastatin *(ez ET i mibe & SIM va stat in)*

U.S. Brand Names Vytorin™

Generic Available No

Pharmacologic Category Antilipemic Agent, 2-Azetidinone; Antilipemic Agent, HMG-CoA Reductase Inhibitor

Use Used in combination with dietary therapy for the treatment of primary hypercholesterolemia and homozygous familial hypercholesterolemia

Dosing

Adults & Elderly:

Homozygous familial hypercholesterolemia: Oral: Ezetimibe 10 mg and simvastatin 40 mg once daily or ezetimibe 10 mg and simvastatin 80 mg once daily in the evening

Hyperlipidemias: Oral: Initial: Ezetimibe 10 mg and simvastatin 20 mg once daily in the evening

Patients who require >55% reduction in LDL-C: Initial: Ezetimibe 10 mg and simvastatin 40 mg once daily

Dosage adjustment with concomitant medications: Oral:

Cyclosporine: Patient must demonstrate tolerance to simvastatin ≥5 mg once daily. Dose should **not** exceed ezetimibe 10 mg and simvastatin 10 mg once daily.

Fibrates or niacin: Simvastatin dose should **not** exceed 10 mg/day.

Amiodarone or verapamil: Simvastatin dose should **not** exceed 20 mg/day.

Renal Impairment: Dosage adjustment unnecessary in mild to moderate renal dysfunction. In severe dysfunction, start only if patient tolerates 5 mg daily of simvastatin; monitor closely.

Hepatic Impairment: Dosage adjustment unnecessary in mild hepatic dysfunction.

Available Dosage Forms Tablet:

10/10: Ezetimibe 10 mg and simvastatin 10 mg

10/20: Ezetimibe 10 mg and simvastatin 20 mg

10/40: Ezetimibe 10 mg and simvastatin 40 mg

10/80: Ezetimibe 10 mg and simvastatin 80 mg

Monitoring and Teaching Issues

Physical Assessment: See individual agents. **Pregnancy risk factor X: Determine** that patient is not pregnant before starting therapy. Do not give to females of childbearing age unless patient is capable of complying with contraceptive use. Breast-feeding is contraindicated.

Pregnancy Risk Factor: X

Lactation: Excretion in breast milk unknown/contraindicated

♦ **F₃T** *see* Trifluridine *on page 1525*
♦ **Factive®** *see* Gemifloxacin *on page 706*

Factor VIIa (Recombinant) *(FAK ter SEV en ree KOM be nant)*

U.S. Brand Names NovoSeven®

Synonyms Coagulation Factor VIIa; Eptacog Alfa (Activated); rFVIIa

Generic Available No

Pharmacologic Category Antihemophilic Agent; Blood Product Derivative

Medication Safety Issues

Sound-alike/look-alike issues:

NovoSeven® may be confused with Novacet®

Use Treatment of bleeding episodes in patients with hemophilia A or B when inhibitors to factor VIII or factor IX are present

Mechanism of Action/Effect Promotes hemostasis by activating the extrinsic pathway of the coagulation cascade to promote formation of a fibrin-platelet hemostatic plug.

Contraindications Hypersensitivity to factor VII or any component of the formulation; hypersensitivity to mouse, hamster, or bovine proteins

Warnings/Precautions Patients should be monitored for signs and symptoms of activation of the coagulation system or thrombosis. Thrombotic events may be increased in patients with disseminated intravascular coagulation (DIC), advanced atherosclerotic disease, sepsis or crush injury. Decreased dosage or discontinuation is warranted in confirmed DIC. Efficacy with prolonged infusions and data evaluating this agent's long-term adverse effects are limited.

Adverse Reactions 1% to 10%:

Cardiovascular: Hypertension

Hematologic: Hemorrhage, decreased plasma fibrinogen

Musculoskeletal: Hemarthrosis

Overdosage/Toxicology Experience with overdose in humans is limited; an increased risk of thrombotic events may occur in overdosage. Treatment is symptomatic and supportive.

Pharmacodynamics/Kinetics
Half-Life Elimination: 2.3 hours (1.7-2.7)
Excretion: Clearance: 33 mL/kg/hour (27-49)

Dosing
Adults & Elderly: Hemophilia A or B (when inhibitors to Factor VIII or Factor IX are present): I.V. administration only: 90 mcg/kg every 2 hours until hemostasis is achieved or until the treatment is judged ineffective. The dose and interval may be adjusted based upon the severity of bleeding and the degree of hemostasis achieved. The duration of therapy following hemostasis has not been fully established; for patients experiencing severe bleeds, dosing should be continued at 3- to 6-hour intervals after hemostasis has been achieved and the duration of dosing should be minimized.

In clinical trials, dosages have ranged from 35-120 mcg/kg and a decision on the final therapeutic dosages was reached within 8 hours in the majority of patients.

Pediatrics: Refer to adult dosing.

Available Dosage Forms Injection, powder for reconstitution [preservative free]: 1.2 mg, 2.4 mg, 4.8 mg [latex free; contains sodium 0.44 mEq/mg rFVIIa, polysorbate 80]

Monitoring and Teaching Issues
Physical Assessment: See Warnings/Precautions for use cautions. Assess potential for interactions with other pharmacological agents or herbal products the patient may be taking that may affect coagulation or platelet function. Assess results of laboratory tests. Patient should be monitored closely during and after therapy (eg, vital signs, cardiac and CNS status, hemolytic status, hypersensitivity). Provide patient education according to patient condition.

Monitoring Laboratory Tests: Although the prothrombin time, aPTT, and factor VII clotting activity have no correlation with achieving hemostasis, these parameters may be useful as adjunct tests to evaluate efficacy and guide dose or interval adjustments

Patient Education: This medication can only be administered by infusion; report immediately any swelling, pain, burning, or itching at infusion site. Report acute headache, visual changes, pain in joints or muscles, respiratory difficulty, chills, back pain, dizziness, nausea, or other unusual effects. **Pregnancy precaution:** Inform prescriber if you are or intend to become pregnant.

Dietary Considerations: Contains sodium 0.44 mEq/mg rFVIIa

Pregnancy Risk Factor: C

Lactation: Excretion in breast milk unknown/compatible

Administration
I.V.: I.V. administration only; reconstitute only with the specified volume of sterile water for injection, USP; administer within 3 hours after reconstitution.

Storage: Store under refrigeration (2°C to 8°C/36°F to 46°F). Reconstituted solutions may be stored at room temperature or under refrigeration, but must be infused within 3 hours of reconstitution.

- ♦ **Factor VIII (Human)** see Antihemophilic Factor (Human) on page 124
- ♦ **Factor VIII (Porcine)** see Antihemophilic Factor (Porcine) on page 126
- ♦ **Factor VIII (Recombinant)** see Antihemophilic Factor (Recombinant) on page 127
- ♦ **Factrel®** see Gonadorelin on page 724

Famciclovir (fam SYE kloe veer)

U.S. Brand Names Famvir®

Generic Available No

Pharmacologic Category Antiviral Agent

Use Management of acute herpes zoster (shingles) and recurrent episodes of genital herpes; treatment of recurrent herpes simplex in immunocompetent patients

Mechanism of Action/Effect The prodrug famciclovir undergoes rapid biotransformation to the active compound, penciclovir, then intracellular conversion to triphosphate which is active against HSV-1, HSV-2, VZV, and EBV infected cells.

Contraindications Hypersensitivity to famciclovir or any component of the formulation

Warnings/Precautions Has not been studied in immunocompromised patients or patients with ophthalmic or disseminated zoster. Dosage adjustment is required in patients with renal insufficiency (Cl_{cr} <60 mL/minute) and in patients with noncompensated hepatic disease. Safety and efficacy have not been established in children <18 years of age. May be carcinogenic/mutagenic.

Drug Interactions
Increased Effect/Toxicity:
Cimetidine: Penciclovir AUC may increase due to impaired metabolism.
Digoxin: C_{max} of digoxin increases by ~19%.
Probenecid: Penciclovir serum levels significantly increase.
Theophylline: Penciclovir AUC/C_{max} may increase and renal clearance decrease, although not clinically significant.

Nutritional/Ethanol Interactions Food: Rate of absorption and/or conversion to penciclovir and peak concentration are reduced with food, but bioavailability is not affected.

Adverse Reactions 1% to 10%:
Central nervous system: Fatigue (4% to 6%), fever (1% to 3%), dizziness (3% to 5%), somnolence (1% to 2%), headache
Dermatologic: Pruritus (1% to 4%)
Gastrointestinal: Diarrhea (4% to 8%), vomiting (1% to 5%), constipation (1% to 5%), anorexia (1% to 3%), abdominal pain (1% to 4%), nausea
Neuromuscular & skeletal: Paresthesia (1% to 3%)
Respiratory: Sinusitis/pharyngitis (2%)

Overdosage/Toxicology Supportive and symptomatic care is recommended. Hemodialysis may enhance elimination.

Pharmacodynamics/Kinetics
Absorption: Food decreases maximum peak concentration and delays time to peak; AUC remains the same
(Continued)

Famciclovir *(Continued)*

Bioavailability: 77%

Time to Peak: 0.9 hours; C_{max} and T_{max} are decreased and prolonged with noncompensated hepatic impairment

Protein Binding: 20%

Half-Life Elimination: Penciclovir: 2-3 hours (10, 20, and 7 hours in HSV-1, HSV-2, and VZV-infected cells respectively); prolonged with renal impairment

Metabolism: Rapidly deacetylated and oxidized to penciclovir; not via CYP

Excretion: Urine (>90% as unchanged drug)

Dosing

Adults & Elderly: Initiate therapy as soon as herpes zoster is diagnosed:

Acute herpes zoster: Oral: 500 mg every 8 hours for 7 days

Genital herpes: Oral:

First episode: 250 mg 3 times/day for 7-10 days

Recurrent episodes: 125 mg twice daily for 5 days (500 mg twice daily for 7 days in HIV infected patients)

Prophylaxis: 250 mg twice daily

Severe (hospitalized patients): 250 mg twice daily

Recurrent herpes simplex in immunocompetent patients: Oral: 125 mg twice daily for 5 days

Recurrent orolabial herpes or genital herpes in HIV-infected patients: Oral: 500 mg twice daily for 7 days

Renal Impairment:

Herpes zoster:

Cl_{cr} ≥60 mL/minute: Administer 500 mg every 8 hours.

Cl_{cr} 40-59 mL/minute: Administer 500 mg every 12 hours.

Cl_{cr} 20-39 mL/minute: Administer 500 mg every 24 hours.

Cl_{cr} <20 mL/minute: Administer 250 mg every 24 hours.

Recurrent genital herpes:

Cl_{cr} ≥40 mL/minute: Administer 125 mg every 12 hours.

Cl_{cr} 20-39 mL/minute: Administer 125 mg every 24 hours.

Cl_{cr} <20 mL/minute: Administer 125 mg every 24 hours.

Suppression of recurrent genital herpes

Cl_{cr} ≥40 mL/minute: Administer 250 mg every 12 hours.

Cl_{cr} 20-39 mL/minute: Administer 125 mg every 12 hours.

Cl_{cr} <20 mL/minute: Administer 125 mg every 24 hours.

Recurrent orolabial or genital herpes in HIV-infected patients:

Cl_{cr} ≥40 mL/minute: Administer 500 mg every 12 hours.

Cl_{cr} 20-39 mL/minute: Administer 500 mg every 24 hours.

Cl_{cr} <20 mL/minute: Administer 250 mg every 24 hours.

Available Dosage Forms Tablet: 125 mg, 250 mg, 500 mg

Monitoring and Teaching Issues

Physical Assessment: See Warnings/Precautions for use cautions (eg, hepatic or renal impairment). Assess periodic CBC during long-term therapy. Assess potential for interactions with other pharmacological agents the patient may be taking (see Drug Interactions). Assess results of laboratory tests, therapeutic effectiveness according to purpose for use, and adverse response (eg, persistent fatigue, gastrointestinal upset; see Adverse Reactions). Teach patient proper use, possible side effects/appropriate interventions, and adverse symptoms to report (see Patient Education).

Monitoring Laboratory Tests: Periodic CBC during long-term therapy

Patient Education: Take for prescribed length of time, even if condition improves. Do not discontinue without consulting prescriber. This is not a cure for genital herpes nor does it prevent the spread of infection to others. Avoid sexual contact while lesions are present. May cause mild GI disturbances (eg, nausea, vomiting, constipation, diarrhea), fatigue, headache, or muscle aches and pains. If these are severe, contact prescriber. **Breast-feeding precaution:** Do not breast-feed.

Dietary Considerations: May be taken with food or on an empty stomach.

Geriatric Considerations: For herpes zoster (shingles) infections, famciclovir should be started within 72 hours of the appearance of the rash to be effective. Famciclovir has been shown to accelerate healing, reduce the duration of viral shedding, and resolve posthepatic neuralgia faster than placebo. Comparison trials to acyclovir or valacyclovir are not available. Adjust dose for estimated renal function.

Pregnancy Risk Factor: B

Lactation: Excretion in breast milk unknown/contraindicated

Breast-Feeding Issues: There is no specific data describing the excretion of famciclovir in breast milk and for its associated tumorigenicity. Discontinue nursing or the drug during lactation; however, acyclovir is a possible alternative for the nursing mother.

Additional Information Most effective if therapy is initiated within 72 hours of initial lesion.

Famotidine *(fa MOE ti deen)*

U.S. Brand Names Fluxid™; Pepcid®; Pepcid® AC [OTC]

Generic Available Yes: Injection, tablet

Pharmacologic Category Histamine H_2 Antagonist

Use Therapy and treatment of duodenal ulcer, gastric ulcer, control gastric pH in critically-ill patients, symptomatic relief in gastritis, gastroesophageal reflux, active benign ulcer, and pathological hypersecretory conditions

OTC labeling: Relief of heartburn, acid indigestion, and sour stomach

Unlabeled/Investigational Use Part of a multidrug regimen for *H. pylori* eradication to reduce the risk of duodenal ulcer recurrence

Mechanism of Action/Effect Competitive inhibition of histamine at H_2 receptors of the gastric parietal cells, which inhibits gastric acid secretion

Contraindications Hypersensitivity to famotidine, other H₂ antagonists, or any component of the formulation

Warnings/Precautions Modify dose in patients with renal impairment; chewable tablets contain phenylalanine; multidose vials contain benzyl alcohol

OTC labeling: When used for self-medication, patients should be instructed not to use if they have difficulty swallowing, have vomiting with blood, or bloody or black stools. Not for use with other acid reducers.

Drug Interactions

Decreased Effect: Decreased serum levels of ketoconazole and itraconazole (reduced absorption).

Nutritional/Ethanol Interactions

Ethanol: Avoid ethanol (may cause gastric mucosal irritation).

Food: Famotidine bioavailability may be increased if taken with food.

Adverse Reactions

Note: Agitation and vomiting have been reported in up to 14% of pediatric patients <1 year of age.

1% to 10%:

Central nervous system: Dizziness (1%), headache (5%)

Gastrointestinal: Constipation (1%), diarrhea (2%)

Overdosage/Toxicology Symptoms of overdose include hypotension, tachycardia, vomiting, and drowsiness. Treatment is symptomatic and supportive.

Pharmacodynamics/Kinetics

Onset of Action: GI: Oral: Within 1-3 hour

Duration of Action: 10-12 hours

Bioavailability: Oral: 40% to 50%

Time to Peak: Serum: Oral: ~1-3 hours

Protein Binding: 15% to 20%

Half-Life Elimination:

Injection, oral suspension, tablet: 2.5-3.5 hours; prolonged with renal impairment; Oliguria: 20 hours

Orally-disintegrating tablet: 2.5-5 hours

Excretion: Urine (as unchanged drug)

Dosing

Adults & Elderly:

Duodenal ulcer: Oral: Acute therapy: 40 mg/day at bedtime for 4-8 weeks; maintenance therapy: 20 mg/day at bedtime

Gastric ulcer: Oral: Acute therapy: 40 mg/day at bedtime

Hypersecretory conditions: Oral: Initial: 20 mg every 6 hours, may increase in increments up to 160 mg every 6 hours

GERD: Oral: 20 mg twice daily for 6 weeks

Esophagitis and accompanying symptoms due to GERD: Oral: 20 mg or 40 mg twice daily for up to 12 weeks

Peptic ulcer disease: Eradication of *Helicobacter pylori* (unlabeled use): Oral: 40 mg once daily; requires combination therapy with antibiotics

Patients unable to take oral medication: I.V.: 20 mg every 12 hours

Heartburn, indigestion, sour stomach: OTC labeling: Oral: 10-20 mg every 12 hours; dose may be taken 15-60 minutes before eating foods known to cause heartburn

Pediatrics: Treatment duration and dose should be individualized

Peptic ulcer: 1-16 years:

Oral: 0.5 mg/kg/day at bedtime or divided twice daily (maximum dose: 40 mg/day); doses of up to 1 mg/kg/day have been used in clinical studies

I.V.: 0.25 mg/kg every 12 hours (maximum dose: 40 mg/day); doses of up to 0.5 mg/kg have been used in clinical studies

GERD: Oral:

<3 months: 0.5 mg/kg once daily

3-12 months: 0.5 mg/kg twice daily

1-16 years: 1 mg/kg/day divided twice daily (maximum dose: 40 mg twice daily); doses of up to 2 mg/kg/day have been used in clinical studies

Heartburn, indigestion, sour stomach: OTC labeling: Oral: Children ≥12 years: Refer to adult dosing.

Renal Impairment: Cl_cr <50 mL/minute: Manufacturer recommendation: Administer 50% of dose **or** increase the dosing interval to every 36-48 hours (to limit potential CNS adverse effects).

Available Dosage Forms [DSC] = Discontinued product

Gelcap (Pepcid® AC): 10 mg

Infusion [premixed in NS] (Pepcid®): 20 mg (50 mL)

Injection, solution: 10 mg/mL (4 mL, 20 mL, 50 mL) [contains benzyl alcohol]

Pepcid®: 10 mg/mL (4 mL [DSC], 20 mL)

Injection, solution [preservative free] (Pepcid®): 10 mg/mL (2 mL)

Powder for oral suspension (Pepcid®): 40 mg/5 mL (50 mL) [contains sodium benzoate; cherry-banana-mint flavor]

Tablet: 10 mg [OTC], 20 mg, 40 mg

Pepcid®: 20 mg, 40 mg [film coated]

Pepcid® AC: 10 mg, 20 mg

Tablet, chewable (Pepcid® AC): 10 mg [contains phenylalanine 1.4 mg/tablet; mint flavor]

Tablet, orally-disintegrating (Fluxid™): 20 mg, 40 mg [cherry flavor]

Monitoring and Teaching Issues

Physical Assessment: See Warnings/Precautions for use cautions (eg, renal impairment). Assess patient response (see Adverse Reactions) on a regular basis throughout therapy.

I.V.: See Administration specifics. Teach patient proper use, possible side effects/appropriate interventions, and adverse symptoms to report (see Patient Education).

Patient Education: Do not take any new medication during therapy without consulting prescriber. Take as directed; do not alter dose or frequency or discontinue without

(Continued)

Famotidine *(Continued)*

consulting prescriber. May cause some drowsiness or dizziness (use caution when driving or engaging in tasks that require alertness until response to drug is known); constipation (increased exercise, fluids, fruit, or fiber may help); or diarrhea (buttermilk, boiled milk, or yogurt may help). Report acute headache, unresolved constipation or diarrhea, palpitations, black tarry stools, abdominal pain, rash, worsening of condition being treated, or recurrence of symptoms after therapy is completed.

Oral-disintegrating tablet: Place tablet on tongue and let it disintegrate. Do not break or chew tablet.

Oral suspension: Shake well before use.

OTC: Do not use for more than 14 days unless recommended by prescriber.

Breast-feeding precaution: Breast-feeding is not recommended.

Dietary Considerations: Phenylalanine content: Pepcid® AC chewable: Each 10 mg tablet contains phenylalanine 1.4 mg

Geriatric Considerations: H_2 blockers are the preferred drugs for treating PUD in the elderly due to cost and ease of administration. They are no less or more effective than any other therapy. Famotidine is one of the preferred agents (due to side effects, drug interaction profile, and pharmacokinetics). Treatment for PUD in the elderly is recommended for 12 weeks since their lesions are typically larger; therefore, take longer to heal. Always adjust dose based upon creatinine clearance, since slight accumulation may result in CNS side effects, mainly confusion.

Pregnancy Risk Factor: B

Lactation: Enters breast milk/not recommended

Breast-Feeding Issues: Famotidine is concentrated in breast milk, but to a lesser degree than cimetidine or ranitidine; some sources prefer its use if one of these agents is needed.

Administration
Oral:
Suspension: Shake vigorously before use. May be taken with or without food.
Tablet: May be taken with or without food.
Orally-disintegrating tablet: Place tablet on tongue with dry hands; tablet dissolves rapidly in saliva. May be taken with or without liquid or food. Do not break tablet.
I.V.:
I.V. push: Inject over at least 2 minutes
Solution for infusion: Administer over 15-30 minutes

Reconstitution: Solution for injection:
I.V. push: Dilute famotidine with NS (or another compatible solution) to a total of 5-10 mL (some centers also administer undiluted).
Infusion: Dilute with D_5W 100 mL or another compatible solution.

Compatibility: Stable in D_5W, $D_{10}W$, LR, fat emulsion 10%, NS, sodium bicarbonate 5%
Y-site administration: Incompatible with alatrofloxacin, amphotericin B cholesteryl sulfate complex, cefepime, piperacillin/tazobactam

Storage:
Oral:
Powder for oral suspension: Prior to mixing, dry powder should be stored at room temperature of 25°C (77°F). Reconstituted oral suspension is stable for 30-days at room temperature. Do not freeze.
Tablet: Store at 20°C (77°F); excursions permitted between 15°C to 30°C (59°F to 86°F). Protect from moisture.
Orally-disintegrating tablet: Store at 20°C to 25°C (68°F to 77°F); excursions permitted between 15°C to 30°C (59°F to 86°F). Protect from moisture.
I.V.:
Solution for injection: Prior to use, store at 2°C to 8°C (36°F to 46°F). If solution freezes, allow to solubilize at room temperature.
I.V. push: Following reconstitution, solutions for I.V. push should be used immediately, or may be stored in refrigerator and used within 48 hours.
Infusion: Following reconstitution, solutions for infusion are stable for 7 days at room temperature.
Solution for injection, premixed bags: Store at room temperature of 25°C (77°F). Avoid excessive heat.

♦ **Famvir®** *see Famciclovir on page 607*
♦ **Fareston®** *see Toremifene on page 1498*
♦ **Faslodex®** *see Fulvestrant on page 687*

Fat Emulsion *(fat e MUL shun)*

U.S. Brand Names Intralipid®; Liposyn® III
Synonyms Intravenous Fat Emulsion
Generic Available No
Pharmacologic Category Caloric Agent
Use Source of calories and essential fatty acids for patients requiring parenteral nutrition of extended duration
Mechanism of Action/Effect Essential for normal structure and function of cell membranes
Contraindications Hypersensitivity to fat emulsion or any component of the formulation; severe egg or legume (soybean) allergies; pathologic hyperlipidemia, lipoid nephrosis pancreatitis with hyperlipemia
Warnings/Precautions Use caution in patients with severe liver damage, pulmonary disease, anemia, or blood coagulation disorder; use with caution in jaundiced, premature, and low birth weight children. Some formulations may contain aluminum which may accumulate following prolonged administration in renally-impaired patients. Premature neonates are particularly at risk of accumulation/toxicity from aluminum. To avoid hyperlipidemia and/or fat deposition, do not exceed recommended daily doses.

Adverse Reactions Frequency not defined.
Cardiovascular: Cyanosis, flushing, chest pain
Central nervous system: Headache, dizziness
Endocrine & metabolic: Hyperlipemia, hypertriglyceridemia
Gastrointestinal: Nausea, vomiting, diarrhea
Hematologic: Hypercoagulability, thrombocytopenia in neonates (rare)
Hepatic: Hepatomegaly, pancreatitis
Local: Thrombophlebitis
Respiratory: Dyspnea
Miscellaneous: Sepsis, diaphoresis, brown pigment deposition in the reticuloendothelial system (significance unknown)

Overdosage/Toxicology Rapid administration results in fluid or fat overload causing dilution of serum electrolytes, overhydration, pulmonary edema, impaired pulmonary diffusion capacity, and metabolic acidosis. Treatment is supportive.

Pharmacodynamics/Kinetics
Half-Life Elimination: 0.5-1 hour
Metabolism: Undergoes lipolysis to free fatty acids which are utilized by reticuloendothelial cells

Dosing
Adults & Elderly:
Caloric source: I.V. (fat emulsion should not exceed 60% of the total daily calories): Initial: 1 g/kg/day, increase by 0.5-1 g/kg/day to a maximum of 2.5 g/kg/day of 10% and 3 g/kg/day of 20%; maximum rate of infusion: 0.25 g/kg/hour (1.25 mL/hour of 20% solution); do not exceed 50 mL/hour (20%) or 100 mL/hour (10%)
Prevention of fatty acid deficiency (8% to 10% of total caloric intake): I.V.: 0.5-1 g/kg/24 hours
500 mL twice weekly at rate of 1 mL/minute for 30 minutes, then increase to 500 mL over 4-6 hours
Note: May be used on a daily basis as a caloric source in TPN
Pediatrics:
Caloric source: I.V. (fat emulsion should not exceed 60% of the total daily calories):
Premature Infants: Initial dose: 0.25-0.5 g/kg/day, increase by 0.25-0.5 g/kg/day to a maximum of 3 g/kg/day depending on needs/nutritional goals; limit to 1 g/kg/day if on phototherapy; maximum rate of infusion: 0.15 g/kg/hour (0.75 mL/kg/hour of 20% solution)
Infants and Children: Initial dose: 0.5-1 g/kg/day, increase by 0.5 g/kg/day to a maximum of 3 g/kg/day depending on needs/nutritional goals; maximum rate of infusion: 0.25 g/kg/hour (1.25 mL/kg/hour of 20% solution)
Adolescents: Refer to adult dosing.
Prevention of essential fatty acid deficiency (8% to 10% of total caloric intake): I.V.: 0.5-1 g/kg/24 hours
Children: 5-10 mL/kg/day at 0.1 mL/minute then up to 100 mL/hour

Available Dosage Forms Injection, emulsion [soybean oil]:
Intralipid®: 10% [100 mg/mL] (100 mL, 250 mL, 500 mL); 20% [200 mg/mL] (50 mL, 100 mL, 250 mL, 500 mL, 1000 mL); 30% [300 mg/mL] (500 mL)
Liposyn® III: 10% [100 mg/mL] (200 mL, 500 mL); 20% [200 mg/mL] (200 mL, 500 mL); 30% [300 mg/mL] (500 mL)

Monitoring and Teaching Issues
Physical Assessment: Assess for allergy to eggs prior to initiating therapy (pruritic urticaria can occur in patients allergic to eggs). Inspect emulsion before administering. Do not administer if oil separation or oiliness is noted. Monitor closely for allergic reactions, fluid overload, thrombosis or sepsis.
Monitoring Laboratory Tests: Serum triglycerides before initiation of therapy and at least weekly during therapy. Frequent (some advise daily) platelet counts should be performed in neonatal patients receiving parenteral lipids.
Patient Education: Report pain at infusion site, respiratory difficulty, chest pain, calf pain, or excessive sweating. **Pregnancy precaution:** Inform prescriber if you are pregnant.
Pregnancy Risk Factor: C
Lactation: Excretion in breast milk unknown/compatible

Administration
I.V.: At the onset of therapy, the patient should be observed for any immediate allergic reactions such as dyspnea, cyanosis, and fever. Infuse for 10-15 minutes at a slower rate. Infuse 10% at 1 mL/minute. If no untoward effects, may increase rate to 500 mL over 4-6 hours. Infuse 20% at 0.5 mL/minute initially; increase to rate of 250 mL over 4-6 hours.
Storage: May be stored at room temperature. Do not store partly used bottles for later use. Do not use if emulsion appears to be oiling out.

♦ **Fazaclo**™ *see* Clozapine *on page 362*
♦ **5-FC** *see* Flucytosine *on page 636*
♦ **FC1157a** *see* Toremifene *on page 1498*
♦ **FDA Name Differentiation Project: The Use of Tall-Man Letters** *see page 15*
♦ **FDA Pregnancy Categories** *see page 16*
♦ **Federal OBRA Regulations: Recommended Maximum Doses** *see page 1773*
♦ **Feiba VH®** *see* Anti-inhibitor Coagulant Complex *on page 128*

Felbamate (FEL ba mate)
U.S. Brand Names Felbatol®
Restrictions A patient "informed consent" form should be completed and signed by the patient and physician. Copies are available from Wallace Pharmaceuticals by calling 609-655-6147.
Generic Available No
Pharmacologic Category Anticonvulsant, Miscellaneous
(Continued)

Felbamate *(Continued)*

Use Not as a first-line antiepileptic treatment; only in those patients who respond inadequately to alternative treatments and whose epilepsy is so severe that a substantial risk of aplastic anemia and/or liver failure is deemed acceptable in light of the benefits conferred by its use. Patient must be fully advised of risk and provide signed written informed consent. Felbamate can be used as either monotherapy or adjunctive therapy in the treatment of partial seizures (with and without generalization) and in adults with epilepsy.

Orphan drug: Adjunctive therapy in the treatment of partial and generalized seizures associated with Lennox-Gastaut syndrome in children

Mechanism of Action/Effect Mechanism of action is unknown but has properties in common with other marketed anticonvulsants. Has weak inhibitory effects on GABA-receptor binding, benzodiazepine receptor binding, and is devoid of activity at the MK-801 receptor binding site of the NMDA receptor-ionophore complex.

Contraindications Hypersensitivity to felbamate or any component of the formulation; use with caution in those patients who have demonstrated hypersensitivity reactions to other carbamates

Warnings/Precautions Use with caution in patients allergic to other carbamates (eg, meprobamate). Antiepileptic drugs should not be suddenly discontinued because of the possibility of increasing seizure frequency. **Reported 10 cases of aplastic anemia in the U.S. after $2\frac{1}{2}$ to 6 months of therapy.** Carter Wallace and the FDA recommended the use of this agent be suspended unless withdrawal of the product would place a patient at greater risk as compared to the frequently fatal form of anemia. Felbamate has also been associated with rare cases of hepatic failure (estimated >6 cases per 75,000 patients per year). Use caution in renal impairment (dose adjustment recommended). "Informed consent" (concerning hematological/hepatic risks) should be documented prior to initiation of therapy.

Drug Interactions

Cytochrome P450 Effect: Substrate of CYP2E1 (minor), 3A4 (major); **Inhibits** CYP2C19 (weak); **Induces** CYP3A4 (weak)

Decreased Effect: Felbamate may decrease carbamazepine levels and increase levels of the active metabolite of carbamazepine (10,11-epoxide) resulting in carbamazepine toxicity; monitor for signs of carbamazepine toxicity (dizziness, ataxia, nystagmus, drowsiness). CYP3A4 inducers may decrease the levels/effects of felbamate; example inducers include aminoglutethimide, carbamazepine, nafcillin, nevirapine, phenobarbital, phenytoin, and rifamycins.

Increased Effect/Toxicity: Felbamate increases serum phenytoin, phenobarbital, and valproic acid concentrations which may result in toxicity; consider decreasing phenytoin or phenobarbital dosage by 25%. A decrease in valproic acid dosage may also be necessary. CYP3A4 inhibitors may increase the levels/effects of felbamate; example inhibitors include azole antifungals, ciprofloxacin, clarithromycin, diclofenac, doxycycline, erythromycin, imatinib, isoniazid, nefazodone, nicardipine, propofol, protease inhibitors, quinidine, and verapamil.

Nutritional/Ethanol Interactions

Ethanol: Avoid ethanol (may increase CNS depression).

Food: Food does not affect absorption.

Herb/Nutraceutical: Avoid evening primrose (seizure threshold decreased).

Lab Interactions Blood urea nitrogen is slightly lower (1.25 mg/dL). May cause slightly elevated serum cholesterol level (about 7 mg/dL) in patients receiving about 2.6 g/day.

Adverse Reactions

>10%:

Central nervous system: Somnolence, headache, fatigue, dizziness

Gastrointestinal: Nausea, anorexia, vomiting, constipation

1% to 10%:

Cardiovascular: Chest pain, palpitation, tachycardia

Central nervous system: Depression or behavior changes, nervousness, anxiety, ataxia, stupor, malaise, agitation, psychological disturbances, aggressive reaction

Dermatologic: Skin rash, acne, pruritus

Gastrointestinal: Xerostomia, diarrhea, abdominal pain, weight gain, taste perversion

Neuromuscular & skeletal: Tremor, abnormal gait, paresthesia, myalgia

Ocular: Diplopia, abnormal vision

Respiratory: Sinusitis, pharyngitis

Miscellaneous: ALT increase

Overdosage/Toxicology Symptoms of overdose include sedation, gastrointestinal upset, and tachycardia. Provide general supportive care.

Pharmacodynamics/Kinetics

Absorption: Rapid and almost complete; food has no effect upon the tablet's absorption

Time to Peak: Serum: ~3 hours

Protein Binding: 22% to 25%, primarily to albumin

Half-Life Elimination: 20-23 hours (average); prolonged in renal dysfunction

Excretion: Urine (40% to 50% as unchanged drug, 40% as inactive metabolites)

Dosing

Adults & Elderly:

Anticonvulsant, monotherapy: Oral:

Initial: 1200 mg/day in divided doses 3 or 4 times/day; titrate previously untreated patients under close clinical supervision, increasing the dosage in 600 mg increments every 2 weeks to 2400 mg/day based on clinical response and thereafter to 3600 mg/day as clinically indicated

Conversion to monotherapy: Initiate at 1200 mg/day in divided doses 3 or 4 times/day, reduce the dosage of the concomitant anticonvulsant(s) by 20% to 33% at the initiation of felbamate therapy; at week 2, increase the felbamate dosage to 2400 mg/day while reducing the dosage of the other anticonvulsant(s) up to an additional 33% of their original dosage; at week 3, increase the felbamate dosage up to 3600 mg/day and continue to reduce the dosage of the other anticonvulsant(s) as clinically indicated

Pediatrics:
  Anticonvulsant, monotherapy: Oral: Children >14 years: Refer to adult dosing.
  Adjunctive therapy, Lennox-Gastaut (ages 2-14 years): Oral:
    Week 1: Felbamate: 15 mg/kg/day divided 3-4 times/day
      Concomitant anticonvulsant(s): Reduce original dosage by 20% to 30%.
    Week 2: Felbamate: 30 mg/kg/day divided 3-4 times/day
      Concomitant anticonvulsant(s): Reduce original dosage up to an additional 33%.
    Week 3: Felbamate: 45 mg//kg/day divided 3-4 times/day
      Concomitant anticonvulsant(s): Reduce dosage as clinically indicated.
  Adjunctive therapy: Children >14 years and Adults:
    Week 1: Felbamate: 1200 mg/day initial dose
      Concomitant anticonvulsant(s): Reduce original dosage by 20% to 33%.
    Week 2: Felbamate: 2400 mg/day (therapeutic range)
      Concomitant anticonvulsant(s): Reduce original dosage by up to an additional 33%.
    Week 3: Felbamate: 3600 mg/day (therapeutic range)
      Concomitant anticonvulsant(s): Reduce original dosage as clinically indicated.
  Renal Impairment: Use caution; reduce initial and maintenance doses by 50% (half-life prolonged by 9-15 hours)
Available Dosage Forms
  Suspension, oral: 600 mg/5 mL (240 mL, 960 mL)
  Tablet: 400 mg, 600 mg
Monitoring and Teaching Issues
  Physical Assessment: Assess effectiveness and interactions of other medications patient may be taking. Monitor therapeutic effectiveness (seizure activity, force, type, duration), laboratory values, and adverse reactions at beginning of therapy and periodically with long-term use. Taper dosage slowly when discontinuing. Assess knowledge/teach patient safety and seizure precautions, appropriate use, interventions to reduce side effects, and adverse symptoms to report.
  Monitoring Laboratory Tests: Monitor serum levels of concomitant anticonvulsant therapy; monitor AST, ALT, and bilirubin on a weekly basis. Hematologic evaluations before therapy begins, frequently during therapy, and for a significant period after discontinuation.
  Patient Education: Take exactly as directed; do not increase dose or frequency or discontinue without consulting prescriber. While using this medication, do not use alcohol and other prescription or OTC medications (especially pain medications, sedatives, antihistamines, or hypnotics) without consulting prescriber. Maintain adequate hydration (2-3 L/day of fluids) unless instructed to restrict fluid intake. You may experience drowsiness, dizziness, or blurred vision (use caution when driving or engaging in tasks requiring alertness until response to drug is known); or nausea, vomiting, loss of appetite, or dry mouth (small frequent meals, frequent mouth care, chewing gum, or sucking lozenges may help). Wear identification of epileptic status and medications. Report CNS changes, mentation changes, or changes in cognition; muscle cramping, weakness, tremors, changes in gait; persistent GI symptoms (cramping, constipation, vomiting, anorexia); rash or skin irritations; unusual bruising or bleeding (mouth, urine, stool); cough, runny nose, sore throat, or respiratory difficulty; or worsening of seizure activity or loss of seizure control. **Pregnancy/breast-feeding precautions:** Inform prescriber if you are or intend to become pregnant. Breast-feeding is not recommended.
  Dietary Considerations: May be taken without regard to meals.
  Geriatric Considerations: Clinical studies have not included large numbers of patients >65 years of age. Due to decreased hepatic and renal function, dosing should start at the lower end of the dosage range.
  Pregnancy Risk Factor: C
  Lactation: Enters breast milk/not recommended
Administration
  Oral: Administer on an empty stomach for best absorption.
  Storage: Store medication in tightly closed container at room temperature away from excessive heat.
  Additional Information Monotherapy has not been associated with gingival hyperplasia, impaired concentration, weight gain, or abnormal thinking. Because felbamate is the only drug shown effective in Lennox-Gastaut syndrome, it is considered an orphan drug for this indication.

♦ **Felbatol®** *see* Felbamate *on page 611*
♦ **Feldene®** *see* Piroxicam *on page 1224*

Felodipine (fe LOE di peen)

U.S. Brand Names Plendil®
Generic Available No
Pharmacologic Category Calcium Channel Blocker
Medication Safety Issues
  Sound-alike/look-alike issues:
    Plendil® may be confused with Isordil®, pindolol, Pletal®, Prilosec®, Prinivil®
Use Treatment of hypertension
Mechanism of Action/Effect Inhibits calcium ions from entering the "slow channels" or select voltage-sensitive areas of vascular smooth muscle and myocardium during depolarization
Contraindications Hypersensitivity to felodipine, any component of the formulation, or other calcium channel blocker
Warnings/Precautions Use caution in patients with heart failure particularly with concurrent beta-blocker use. Elderly patients and patients with hepatic impairment should start off with a lower dose. Peripheral edema is the most common side effect (occurs within 2-3 weeks of starting therapy). May cause reflex tachycardia, hypotension, or syncope (rare). Use caution in hepatic impairment. Safety and efficacy in children have not been established. Dosage titration should occur after 14 days on a given dose.
(Continued)

Felodipine *(Continued)*

Drug Interactions

Cytochrome P450 Effect: Substrate of CYP3A4 (major); **Inhibits** CYP2C8/9 (weak), 2D6 (weak), 3A4 (weak)

Decreased Effect: Felodipine may decrease pharmacologic actions of theophylline. Calcium may reduce the calcium channel blocker's effects, particularly hypotension. Felodipine may decrease pharmacologic actions of theophylline. CYP3A4 inducers may decrease the levels/effects of felodipine; example inducers include aminoglutethimide, carbamazepine, nafcillin, nevirapine, phenobarbital, phenytoin, and rifamycins.

Increased Effect/Toxicity: CYP3A4 inhibitors may increase the levels/effects of felodipine; example inhibitors include azole antifungals, ciprofloxacin, clarithromycin, diclofenac, doxycycline, erythromycin, imatinib, isoniazid, nefazodone, nicardipine, propofol, protease inhibitors, quinidine, and verapamil. Beta-blockers may have increased pharmacokinetic or pharmacodynamic interactions with felodipine. Cyclosporine increases felodipine's serum concentration. Blood pressure-lowering effects may be additive with sildenafil, tadalafil, and vardenafil (use caution). Felodipine may increase tacrolimus serum levels (monitor).

Nutritional/Ethanol Interactions

Ethanol: Increases felodipine's absorption; watch for a greater hypotensive effect.

Food: Increased therapeutic and vasodilator side effects, including severe hypotension and myocardial ischemia, may occur if felodipine is taken with grapefruit juice; avoid concurrent use. High-fat/carbohydrate meals will increase C_{max} by 60%; grapefruit juice will increase C_{max} by twofold.

Herb/Nutraceutical: St John's wort may decrease felodipine levels. Avoid dong quai if using for hypertension (has estrogenic activity). Avoid ephedra, yohimbe, ginseng (may worsen hypertension). Avoid garlic (may have increased antihypertensive effect).

Adverse Reactions

>10%: Central nervous system: Headache (11% to 15%)

2% to 10%: Cardiovascular: Peripheral edema (2% to 17%), tachycardia (0.4% to 2.5%), flushing (4% to 7%)

Overdosage/Toxicology

Primary cardiac symptoms of calcium blocker overdose include hypotension and bradycardia. Noncardiac symptoms include confusion, stupor, nausea, vomiting, metabolic acidosis, and hyperglycemia. Treat symptomatically.

Pharmacodynamics/Kinetics

Onset of Action: 2-5 hours

Duration of Action: 16-24 hours

Absorption: 100%; absolute: 20% due to first-pass effect

Protein Binding: >99%

Half-Life Elimination: 11-16 hours

Metabolism: Hepatic; extensive first-pass effect

Excretion: Urine (as metabolites)

Dosing

Adults: Hypertension: Oral: 5-10 mg once daily; increase by 5 mg at 2-week intervals, as needed, to a maximum of 20 mg/day; usual dose range (JNC 7): 2.5-20 mg once daily.

Elderly: Oral: Initial 2.5 mg/day

Hepatic Impairment: Initial: 2.5 mg/day; monitor blood pressure

Available Dosage Forms Tablet, extended release: 2.5 mg, 5 mg, 10 mg

Monitoring and Teaching Issues

Physical Assessment: See Warnings/Precautions for use cautions (eg, hepatic impairment, heart failure). Assess potential for interactions with pharmacological agents or herbal products the patient may be taking (eg, beta blockers or other drugs that affect blood pressure; see Drug Interactions). Assess for therapeutic effectiveness and signs/symptoms of adverse reactions at beginning of therapy, when changing dosage, and periodically throughout long-term therapy (see Adverse Reactions). When discontinuing, taper gradually (over 2 weeks). Teach patient proper use, possible side effects/interventions, and adverse symptoms to report (see Patient Education).

Patient Education: Do not take any new medication during therapy unless approved by prescriber. Take exactly as directed, without food. Avoid concurrent grapefruit juice and alcohol (may cause hypotension). Swallow whole, do not crush or chew. Do not alter dose or stop taking without consulting prescriber. Monitor blood pressure and/or pulse as instructed by prescriber. May cause headache (consult prescriber for analgesic); nausea or vomiting (small frequent meals, frequent mouth care, chewing gum, or sucking lozenges may help); constipation (increased dietary bulk and fluids may help); or drowsiness (use caution when driving or engaging in tasks that require alertness until response to drug is known). Report irregular heartbeat, chest pain or palpitations; persistent headache; vomiting; constipation; peripheral or facial swelling; weight gain >5 lb/week; dyspnea or respiratory changes; persistent dizziness; or other adverse reactions. **Pregnancy/breast-feeding precautions:** Inform prescriber if you are or intend to become pregnant. Consult prescriber if breast-feeding.

Dietary Considerations: Should be taken without food.

Geriatric Considerations: Elderly may experience a greater hypotensive response. Theoretically, constipation may be more of a problem in the elderly.

Pregnancy Risk Factor: C

Pregnancy Issues: Potentially, calcium channel blockers may prolong labor. There are no adequate or well-controlled studies in pregnant women.

Lactation: Excretion in breast milk unknown/not recommended

Administration

Oral: Do not crush or chew extended release tablets; swallow whole.

Additional Information Felodipine maintains renal and mesenteric blood flow during hemorrhagic shock in animals.

Related Information

Calcium Channel Blockers *on page 1722*

- **Felodipine and Enalapril** *see* Enalapril and Felodipine *on page 518*
- **Femara**® *see* Letrozole *on page 874*
- **femhrt**® *see* Ethinyl Estradiol and Norethindrone *on page 589*
- **Femiron**® [OTC] *see* Ferrous Fumarate *on page 623*
- **Femizol-M**™ [OTC] *see* Miconazole *on page 999*
- **Femring**™ *see* Estradiol *on page 552*
- **Femtrace**® *see* Estradiol *on page 552*

Fenofibrate (fen oh FYE brate)

U.S. Brand Names Antara™; Lofibra™; TriCor®
Synonyms Procetofene; Proctofene
Generic Available No
Pharmacologic Category Antilipemic Agent, Fibric Acid
Use Adjunct to dietary therapy for the treatment of adults with very high elevations of serum triglyceride levels (types IV and V hyperlipidemia) who are at risk of pancreatitis and who do not respond adequately to a determined dietary effort; adjunct to dietary therapy for the reduction of low density lipoprotein cholesterol (LDL-C), total cholesterol (total-C), triglycerides, and apolipoprotein B (apo B) in adult patients with primary hypercholesterolemia or mixed dyslipidemia (Fredrickson types IIa and IIb)
Mechanism of Action/Effect Fenofibric acid is believed to increase VLDL catabolism by enhancing the synthesis of lipoprotein lipase; as a result of a decrease in VLDL levels, total plasma triglycerides are reduced by 30% to 60%. Modest increase in HDL occurs in some hypertriglyceridemic patients.
Contraindications Hypersensitivity to fenofibrate or any component of the formulation; hepatic or severe renal dysfunction including primary biliary cirrhosis and unexplained persistent liver function abnormalities; pre-existing gallbladder disease
Warnings/Precautions Hepatic transaminases can become significantly elevated (dose-related). Regular monitoring of liver function tests is required. May cause cholelithiasis. Use caution with warfarin; adjustments in warfarin therapy may be required. Use caution with HMG-CoA reductase inhibitors (may lead to myopathy, rhabdomyolysis). The effect of fenofibrate on coronary artery disease morbidity and mortality has not been established. Therapy should be withdrawn if an adequate response is not obtained after 2 months of therapy at the maximal daily dose. Rare hypersensitivity reactions may occur. Dose adjustment is required for renal impairment and elderly patients. Safety and efficacy in children have not been established.

Drug Interactions

Cytochrome P450 Effect: Substrate of CYP3A4 (minor); **Inhibits** (weak) CYP1A6, 2C9, 2C19
Decreased Effect: Bile acid sequestrants may decrease absorption of fenofibrate (separate administration).
Increased Effect/Toxicity: Fenofibrate may increase the effects of sulfonylureas and warfarin. Concurrent use of fenofibrate with HMG-CoA reductase inhibitors may increase the risk of myopathy and rhabdomyolysis. Ezetimibe's serum concentration may be increased with concurrent use.

Adverse Reactions

1% to 10%:
  Gastrointestinal: Abdominal pain (5%), constipation (2%)
  Hepatic: ALT increased (3%), AST increased (3%), creatine phosphokinase increased (3%), liver function tests abnormal (7%)
  Neuromuscular & skeletal: Back pain (3%)
  Respiratory: Respiratory disorder (6%), rhinitis (2%)

Frequency not defined:
  Cardiovascular: Angina pectoris, arrhythmia, atrial fibrillation, cardiovascular disorder, chest pain, coronary artery disorder, edema, electrocardiogram abnormality, extrasystoles, hyper-/hypotension, migraine, MI, palpitation, peripheral edema, peripheral vascular disorder, phlebitis, tachycardia, varicose veins, vasodilatation
  Central nervous system: Anxiety, depression, dizziness, fever, insomnia, malaise, nervousness, neuralgia, pain, somnolence, vertigo
  Dermatologic: Acne, alopecia, bruising, contact dermatitis, eczema, fungal dermatitis, maculopapular rash, nail disorder, photosensitivity reaction, pruritus, skin ulcer, Stevens-Johnson syndrome, toxic epidermal necrolysis, urticaria
  Endocrine & metabolic: Diabetes mellitus, gout, gynecomastia, hypoglycemia, hyperuricemia
  Gastrointestinal: Anorexia, appetite increased, colitis, diarrhea, dry mouth, duodenal ulcer, dyspepsia, eructation, esophagitis, flatulence, gastroenteritis, gastritis, gastrointestinal disorder, nausea, peptic ulcer, rectal disorder, rectal hemorrhage, tooth disorder, vomiting, weight gain/loss
  Genitourinary: Cystitis, dysuria, prostatic disorder, libido decreased, pregnancy (unintended), urinary frequency, urolithiasis, vaginal moniliasis
  Hematologic: Agranulocytosis, anemia, eosinophilia, leukopenia, lymphadenopathy, thrombocytopenia
  Hepatic: Cholelithiasis, cholecystitis, fatty liver deposits
  Neuromuscular & skeletal: Arthralgia, arthritis, arthrosis, bursitis, hypertonia, joint disorder, leg cramps, muscle pain, myalgia, myasthenia, myopathy, myositis, paresthesia, rhabdomyolysis, tenderness, tenosynovitis, weakness
  Ocular: Abnormal vision, amblyopia, cataract, conjunctivitis, eye disorder, refraction disorder
  Otic: Ear pain, otitis media
  Renal: Creatinine increased, kidney function abnormality
  Respiratory: Asthma, bronchitis, cough increased, dyspnea, laryngitis, pharyngitis, pneumonia, sinusitis
  Miscellaneous: Allergic reaction, cyst, diaphoresis, herpes simplex, herpes zoster, hypersensitivity reaction, infection

(Continued)

Fenofibrate *(Continued)*

Overdosage/Toxicology Symptoms of overdose include nausea, vomiting, diarrhea, and GI distress. Treatment is supportive. Hemodialysis has no effect on removal of fenofibric acid from the plasma.

Pharmacodynamics/Kinetics
Absorption: Increased when taken with meals

Time to Peak: 4-8 hours

Protein Binding: >99%

Half-Life Elimination: 20-23 hours

Metabolism: Tissue and plasma via esterases to active form, fenofibric acid; undergoes inactivation by glucuronidation hepatically or renally

Excretion: Urine (60% as metabolites); feces (25%); hemodialysis has no effect on removal of fenofibric acid from plasma

Dosing
Adults:
Hypertriglyceridemia: Oral: Initial:
Antara™: 43-130 mg/day
Lofibra™: 67 mg/day with meals, up to 200 mg/day
TriCor®: 48 mg/day, up to 145 mg/day
Previously dosed as 54 mg/day with meals (up to 160 mg/day) using the old tablet formulation

Hypercholesterolemia or mixed hyperlipidemia: Oral: Early:
Antara™: 130 mg/day
Lofibra™: 200 mg/day with meals
TriCor®: 145 mg/day
Previously dosed as 160 mg/day with meals using the old tablet formulation

Elderly: Initial: 43 mg/day (Antara™) or 67 mg/day (Lofibra™) or 48 mg/day (TriCor®)

Renal Impairment: Use caution in dosage adjustment. Monitor renal function and lipid panel before adjusting. Decrease dose or increase dosing interval for patients with renal failure: Initial: 43 mg/day(Antara™) or 67 mg/day (Lofibra™) or 48 mg/day (TriCor®) Hemodialysis has no effect on removal of fenofibric acid from the plasma.

Available Dosage Forms
Capsule [micronized]
Antara™: 43 mg, 87 mg, 130 mg
Lofibra™: 67 mg, 134 mg, 200 mg
Tablet
TriCor®: 54 mg [DSC], 160 mg [DSC]
TriCor® [new formulation]: 48 mg, 145 mg

Monitoring and Teaching Issues
Physical Assessment: See Warnings/Precautions for use cautions (eg, hepatic or renal dysfunction, gallbladder disease). Assess potential for interactions with other pharmacological agents the patient may be taking (eg, increased risk of myopathy and rhabdomyolysis; see Drug Interactions). Assess result of laboratory tests (see Monitoring Laboratory Tests) and patient response on a regular basis throughout therapy (see Adverse Reactions; eg, arrhythmias, gastrointestinal upset, CNS changes, hypoglycemia, myalgia). Teach patient possible side effects/appropriate interventions and adverse symptoms to report (see Patient Education).

Monitoring Laboratory Tests: Total serum cholesterol and triglyceride concentration and CLDL, LDL, and HDL levels should be measured periodically; if only marginal changes are noted in 6-8 weeks, the drug should be discontinued. Serum transaminases should be measured every 3 months; if ALT values increase >100 units/L, therapy should be discontinued. Monitor LFTs prior to initiation, at 6 and 12 weeks after initiation or first dose, then periodically thereafter.

Patient Education: Do not take any new medication during therapy without consulting prescriber. Take as directed with food. Do not change dosage or dosage form or frequency without consulting prescriber. Maintain diet and exercise program as prescribed. May cause mild GI disturbances (eg, gas, diarrhea, constipation, nausea); inform prescriber if these are severe. Report immediately unusual muscle pain or weakness, skin rash or irritation, insomnia, persistent dizziness; chest pain or palpitations; difficult respirations; or any other persistent adverse effects; **Pregnancy/breast-feeding precautions:** Inform prescriber if you are or intend to become pregnant. Breast-feeding is not recommended.

Dietary Considerations: Capsule should be taken with food. Tablet may be taken with or without food.

Pregnancy Risk Factor: C

Pregnancy Issues: Although teratogenicity and mutagenicity tests in animals have been negative, significant risk has been identified with clofibrate. Use should be avoided, if possible, in pregnant women since the neonatal glucuronide conjugation pathways are immature.

Lactation: Excretion in breast milk unknown/not recommended

Breast-Feeding Issues: Tumor formation was observed in animal studies; nursing is not recommended if the medication cannot be discontinued.

Administration
Oral: 6-8 weeks of therapy is required to determine efficacy.
Capsule: Administer with meals.
Tablet: May be administered with or without food.

Related Information
Hyperlipidemia Management *on page 1836*
Lipid-Lowering Agents *on page 1738*

Fenoprofen *(fen oh PROE fen)*
U.S. Brand Names Nalfon®
Synonyms Fenoprofen Calcium

Generic Available Yes: Tablet

Pharmacologic Category Nonsteroidal Anti-inflammatory Drug (NSAID), Oral

Medication Safety Issues
Sound-alike/look-alike issues:
Fenoprofen may be confused with flurbiprofen
Nalfon® may be confused with Naldecon®

Use Symptomatic treatment of acute and chronic rheumatoid arthritis and osteoarthritis; relief of mild to moderate pain

Mechanism of Action/Effect Inhibits prostaglandin synthesis by decreasing the activity of the enzyme, cyclooxygenase, which results in decreased formation of prostaglandin precursors

Contraindications Hypersensitivity to fenoprofen, aspirin, or other NSAIDs; pregnancy (3rd trimester)

Warnings/Precautions Fatal asthmatic and anaphylactoid reactions have occurred in patients with "aspirin triad." Use with caution in patients with CHF, hypertension, dehydration, decreased renal or hepatic function, history of GI disease (bleeding, ulcers, or previous GI symptoms with NSAID use), or those receiving anticoagulants and/or corticosteroids. Use lowest effective dose for shortest period possible; bleeding risk has been correlated to dose and duration of therapy. Gastrointestinal bleeding may occur without prior symptoms of gastrointestinal irritation. Elderly are at a high risk for adverse effects from NSAIDs. As many as 60% of elderly can develop peptic ulceration and/or hemorrhage asymptomatically.

Use of NSAIDs can compromise existing renal function especially when Cl_{cr} <30 mL/minute. CNS side effects such as confusion, agitation, and hallucination are generally seen in overdose or high-dose situations; however, elderly may demonstrate these adverse effects at lower doses than younger adults. Do not exceed 3200 mg/day. Withhold for at least 4-6 half-lives prior to surgical or dental procedures.

Drug Interactions
Decreased Effect: Decreased effect with phenobarbital.
Increased Effect/Toxicity: Increased effect/toxicity of phenytoin, sulfonamides, sulfonylureas, salicylates, and oral anticoagulants. Serum concentration/toxicity of methotrexate may be increased.

Nutritional/Ethanol Interactions
Ethanol: Avoid ethanol (may enhance gastric mucosal irritation).
Food: Fenoprofen peak serum levels may be decreased if taken with food.
Herb/Nutraceutical: Avoid cat's claw, dong quai, evening primrose, feverfew, garlic, ginger, ginkgo, red clover, horse chestnut, green tea, ginseng (all have additional antiplatelet activity).

Lab Interactions Increased chloride (S), sodium (S)

Adverse Reactions
>10%:
Central nervous system: Dizziness (7% to 15%), somnolence (9% to 15%)
Gastrointestinal: Abdominal cramps (2% to 4%), heartburn, indigestion, nausea (8% to 14%), dyspepsia (10% to 14%), flatulence (14%), anorexia (14%), constipation (7% to 14%), occult blood in stool (14%), vomiting (3% to 14%), diarrhea (2% to 14%)
1% to 10%:
Central nervous system: Headache (9%)
Dermatologic: Itching
Endocrine & metabolic: Fluid retention

Overdosage/Toxicology Symptoms of overdose include acute renal failure, vomiting, drowsiness, and leukocytosis. Management of NSAID intoxication is supportive and symptomatic.

Pharmacodynamics/Kinetics
Onset of Action: A few days
Absorption: Rapid, 80%
Time to Peak: Serum: ~2 hours
Protein Binding: 99%
Half-Life Elimination: 2.5-3 hours
Metabolism: Extensively hepatic
Excretion: Urine (2% to 5% as unchanged drug); feces (small amounts)

Dosing
Adults & Elderly:
Rheumatoid arthritis and osteoarthritis: Oral: 300-600 mg 3-4 times/day up to 3.2 g/day
Mild to moderate pain: Oral: 200 mg every 4-6 hours as needed

Available Dosage Forms
Capsule, as calcium (Nalfon®): 200 mg, 300 mg
Tablet, as calcium: 600 mg

Monitoring and Teaching Issues
Physical Assessment: Assess effectiveness and interactions of other medications patient may be taking. Assess results of laboratory tests, therapeutic effectiveness, and adverse reactions at beginning of therapy and periodically throughout therapy. Assess knowledge/teach patient appropriate use, interventions to reduce side effects, and adverse symptoms to report.

Monitoring Laboratory Tests: CBC, liver enzymes; urine output and BUN/serum creatinine in patients receiving diuretics

Patient Education: Take this medication exactly as directed; do not increase dose without consulting prescriber. Do not crush tablets or break capsules. Take with food or milk to reduce GI distress. Maintain adequate hydration (2-3 L/day of fluids) unless instructed to restrict fluid intake. Do not use alcohol, aspirin, or aspirin-containing medication, or any other anti-inflammatory medications without consulting prescriber. You may experience drowsiness, dizziness, nervousness, or headache (use caution when driving or engaging in tasks requiring alertness until response to drug is known); anorexia, nausea, vomiting, or heartburn (small frequent meals, frequent mouth care, sucking lozenges, or chewing gum (Continued)

Fenoprofen (Continued)

may help); or fluid retention (weigh yourself weekly and report unusual (3-5 lb/week) weight gain). GI bleeding, ulceration, or perforation can occur with or without pain; discontinue medication and contact prescriber if persistent abdominal pain or cramping, or blood in stool occurs. Report breathlessness, respiratory difficulty, or unusual cough; chest pain, rapid heartbeat, palpitations; unusual bruising/bleeding; blood in urine, stool, mouth, or vomitus; swollen extremities; skin rash or itching; acute fatigue; or hearing changes (ringing in ears). **Pregnancy/breast-feeding precautions:** Inform prescriber if you are or intend to become pregnant. This drug should not be used in the 3rd trimester of pregnancy. Breast-feeding is not recommended.

Dietary Considerations: May be taken with food to decrease GI distress.

Geriatric Considerations: Elderly are at high risk for adverse effects from NSAIDs. As much as 60% of elderly can develop peptic ulceration and/or hemorrhage asymptomatically. The concomitant use of H_2 blockers, omeprazole, and sucralfate is not effective as prophylaxis with the exception of NSAID-induced duodenal ulcers which may be prevented by the use of ranitidine. Misoprostol is the only prophylactic agent proven effective. Also, concomitant disease and drug use contribute to the risk for GI adverse effects. Use lowest effective dose for shortest period possible. Consider renal function decline with age. Use of NSAIDs can compromise existing renal function especially when Cl_{cr} is ≤30 mL/minute. Tinnitus may be a difficult and unreliable indication of toxicity due to age-related hearing loss or eighth cranial nerve damage. CNS adverse effects such as confusion, agitation, and hallucination are generally seen in overdose or high-dose situations, but elderly may demonstrate these adverse effects at lower doses than younger adults.

Pregnancy Risk Factor: B/D (3rd trimester)

Lactation: Enters breast milk/not recommended

Administration

Oral: Do not crush tablets. Swallow whole with a full glass of water. Take with food to minimize stomach upset.

Related Information

Nonsalicylate / Nonsteroidal Anti-inflammatory Agents *on page 1743*

♦ **Fenoprofen Calcium** *see Fenoprofen on page 616*

Fentanyl (FEN ta nil)

U.S. Brand Names Actiq®; Duragesic®; Sublimaze®

Synonyms Fentanyl Citrate

Controlled Substance C-II

Generic Available Yes: Excludes lozenge

Pharmacologic Category Analgesic, Narcotic; General Anesthetic

Medication Safety Issues

Sound-alike/look-alike issues:

Fentanyl may be confused with alfentanil, sufentanil

Transdermal patch may contain conducting metal (eg, aluminum); remove patch prior to MRI.

Use

Injection: Sedation, relief of pain, preoperative medication, adjunct to general or regional anesthesia

Transdermal: Management of moderate-to-severe chronic pain

Transmucosal (Actiq®): Management of breakthrough cancer pain

Mechanism of Action/Effect Binds with stereospecific receptors at many sites within the CNS, increases pain threshold, alters pain reception, inhibits ascending pain pathways

Contraindications Hypersensitivity to fentanyl or any component of the formulation; increased intracranial pressure; severe respiratory disease or depression including acute asthma (unless patient is mechanically ventilated); paralytic ileus; severe liver or renal insufficiency; pregnancy (prolonged use or high doses near term)

Transmucosal lozenges (Actiq®) or transdermal patches must not be used in patients who are intolerant to opioids. Patients are considered opioid-tolerant if they are taking at least 60 mg morphine/day, 30 mg oral oxycodone/day, 8 mg oral hydromorphone/day, 50 mcg transdermal fentanyl/hour, or an equivalent dose of another opioid for ≥1 week. Transdermal patches are not for use in acute pain, mild pain, or postoperative pain management.

Warnings/Precautions An opioid-containing analgesic regimen should be tailored to each patient's needs and based upon the type of pain being treated (acute versus chronic), the route of administration, degree of tolerance for opioids (naive versus chronic user), age, weight, and medical condition. The optimal analgesic dose varies widely among patients. Doses should be titrated to pain relief/prevention. Fentanyl shares the toxic potentials of opiate agonists, and precautions of opiate agonist therapy should be observed. Use with caution in patients with bradycardia. Rapid I.V. infusion may result in skeletal muscle and chest wall rigidity leading to respiratory distress and/or apnea, bronchoconstriction, laryngospasm. Inject slowly over 3-5 minutes. Nondepolarizing skeletal muscle relaxant may be required. Tolerance or drug dependence may result from extended use. Use caution in patients with a history of drug dependence or abuse. The elderly may be particularly susceptible to the CNS depressant and constipating effects of narcotics.

Topical patches: Serious or life-threatening hypoventilation may occur, even in opioid-tolerant patients. Serum fentanyl concentrations may increase approximately 33% for patients with a body temperature of 40°C secondary to a temperature-dependent increase in fentanyl release from the system and increased skin permeability. Patients who experience adverse reactions should be monitored for at least 24 hours after removal of the patch. Transdermal patch may contain conducting metal (eg, aluminum); remove patch prior to MRI. Safety and efficacy of transdermal system have been limited to children >2 years of age who are opioid tolerant.

Drug Interactions

Cytochrome P450 Effect: Substrate of CYP3A4 (major); **Inhibits** CYP3A4 (weak)

Decreased Effect: CYP3A4 inducers (including carbamazepine, phenytoin, phenobarbital, rifampin) may decrease serum levels of fentanyl by increasing metabolism.

Increased Effect/Toxicity: Increased sedation with CNS depressants, phenothiazines. Tricyclic antidepressants may potentiate fentanyl's adverse effects. Potential for serotonin syndrome if combined with other serotonergic drugs. CYP3A4 inhibitors may increase the levels/effects of fentanyl; potentially fatal respiratory depression may occur when a potent inhibitor is used in a patient receiving chronic fentanyl (eg, transdermal); example inhibitors include azole antifungals, ciprofloxacin, clarithromycin, diclofenac, doxycycline, erythromycin, imatinib, isoniazid, nefazodone, nicardipine, propofol, protease inhibitors, quinidine, and verapamil.

Nutritional/Ethanol Interactions

Ethanol: Avoid ethanol (may increase CNS depression).

Food: Glucose may cause hyperglycemia.

Herb/Nutraceutical: St John's wort may decrease fentanyl levels. Avoid valerian, St John's wort, kava kava, gotu kola (may increase CNS depression).

Adverse Reactions

>10%:

Cardiovascular: Hypotension, bradycardia

Central nervous system: CNS depression, confusion, drowsiness, sedation

Gastrointestinal: Nausea, vomiting, constipation, xerostomia

Neuromuscular & skeletal: Chest wall rigidity (high dose I.V.), weakness

Ocular: Miosis

Respiratory: Respiratory depression

Miscellaneous: Diaphoresis

1% to 10%:

Cardiovascular: Cardiac arrhythmia, edema, orthostatic hypotension, hypertension, syncope

Central nervous system: Abnormal dreams, abnormal thinking, agitation, amnesia, dizziness, euphoria, fatigue, fever, hallucinations, headache, insomnia, nervousness, paranoid reaction

Dermatologic: Erythema, papules, pruritus, rash

Gastrointestinal: Abdominal pain, anorexia, biliary tract spasm, diarrhea, dyspepsia, flatulence

Local: Application site reaction

Neuromuscular & skeletal: Abnormal coordination, abnormal gait, back pain, paresthesia, rigors, tremor

Respiratory: Apnea, bronchitis, dyspnea, hemoptysis, pharyngitis, rhinitis, sinusitis, upper respiratory infection

Miscellaneous: Hiccups, flu-like syndrome, speech disorder

Overdosage/Toxicology Symptoms of overdose include CNS depression, respiratory depression, and miosis. Treatment is supportive. Naloxone, 2 mg I.V. with repeat administration as necessary up to a total of 10 mg, can also be used to reverse toxic effects of the opiate. Patients who experience adverse reactions during use of transdermal fentanyl should be monitored for at least 24 hours after removal of the patch.

Pharmacodynamics/Kinetics

Onset of Action: Analgesic: I.M.: 7-15 minutes; I.V.: Almost immediate; Transmucosal: 5-15 minutes

Peak effect: Transmucosal: Analgesic: 20-30 minutes

Duration of Action: I.M.: 1-2 hours; I.V.: 0.5-1 hour; Transmucosal: Related to blood level; respiratory depressant effect may last longer than analgesic effect

Absorption: Transmucosal: Rapid, ~25% from the buccal mucosa; 75% swallowed with saliva and slowly absorbed from GI tract

Bioavailability: Transmucosal: ~50% (range: 36% to 71%)

Half-Life Elimination: 2-4 hours; Transmucosal: 6.6 hours (range: 5-15 hours); Transdermal: 17 hours (half-life is influenced by absorption rate)

Metabolism: Hepatic, primarily via CYP3A4

Excretion: Urine (primarily as metabolites, 10% as unchanged drug)

Dosing

Adults: Note: These are guidelines and do not represent the maximum doses that may be required in all patients. Doses should be titrated to pain relief/prevention. Monitor vital signs routinely. Single I.M. doses have a duration of 1-2 hours, single I.V. doses last 0.5-1 hour.

Premedication: I.M., slow I.V.: 50-100 mcg/dose 30-60 minutes prior to surgery

Adjunct to regional anesthesia: I.M., slow I.V.: 50-100 mcg /dose; if I.V. used give over 1-2 minutes

Severe pain: I.M.: 50-100 mcg/dose every 1-2 hours as needed; patients with prior opiate exposure may tolerate higher initial doses

Adjunct to general anesthesia: Slow I.V.:

Low dose: Initial: 2 mcg/kg/dose; Maintenance: Additional doses infrequently needed

Moderate dose: Initial: 2-20 mcg/kg/dose; Maintenance: 25-100 mcg/dose may be given slow I.V. or I.M. as needed

High dose: Initial: 20-50 mcg/kg/dose; Maintenance: 25 mcg to one-half the initial loading dose may be given as needed

General anesthesia without additional anesthetic agents: Slow I.V.: 50-100 mcg/kg with O_2 and skeletal muscle relaxant

Mechanically-ventilated patients (based on 70 kg patient): Slow I.V.: 0.35-1.5 mcg/kg every 30-60 minutes as needed; infusion: 0.7-10 mcg/kg/hour

Patient-controlled analgesia (PCA): I.V.: Usual concentration: 50 mcg/mL

Demand dose: Usual: 10 mcg; range: 10-50 mcg

Lockout interval: 5-8 minutes

(Continued)

Fentanyl (Continued)

Breakthrough cancer pain: Transmucosal: Actiq® dosing should be individually titrated to provide adequate analgesia with minimal side effects. It is indicated only for management of breakthrough cancer pain in patients who are tolerant to and currently receiving opioid therapy for persistent cancer pain. An initial starting dose of 200 mcg should be used for the treatment of breakthrough cancer pain. Patients should be monitored closely in order to determine the proper dose. If redosing for the same episode is necessary, the second dose may be started 15 minutes after completion of the first dose. Dosing should be titrated so that the patient's pain can be treated with one single dose. Generally, 1-2 days is required to determine the proper dose of analgesia with limited side effects. Once the dose has been determined, consumption should be limited to 4 units/day or less. Patients needing more than 4 units/day should have the dose of their long-term opioid re-evaluated. If signs of excessive opioid effects occur before a dose is complete, the unit should be removed from the patient's mouth immediately, and subsequent doses decreased.

Opioid Analgesics
Initial Oral Dosing Commonly Used for Severe Pain

Drug	Equianalgesic Dose (mg)		Initial Oral Dose	
	Oral[1]	Parenteral[2]	Children (mg/kg)	Adults (mg)
Buprenorphine	—	0.4	—	—
Butorphanol	—	2	—	—
Hydromorphone	7.5	1.5	0.06	4-8
Levorphanol	4 (acute) 1 (chronic)	2 (acute) 1 (chronic)	0.04	2-4
Meperidine	300	75	Not Recommended	
Methadone	10	5	0.2	0.2
Morphine	30	10	0.3	15-30
Nalbuphine	—	10	—	—
Pentazocine	50	30	—	—
Oxycodone	20	—	0.3	10.20
Oxymorphone	1	—	—	—

From "Principles of Analgesic Use in the Treatment of Acute Pain and Cancer Pain," *Am Pain Soc*, Fifth Ed.

[1]Elderly: Starting dose should be lower for this population group

[2]Standard parenteral doses for acute pain in adults; can be used to doses for I.V. infusions and repeated small I.V. bolus. Single I.V. boluses, use half the I.M. dose.
Children >6 months: I.V. dose = parenteral equianalgesic dose x weight (kg)/100

Recommended Initial Duragesic® Dose Based Upon Daily Oral Morphine Dose[1]

Oral 24-Hour Morphine (mg/d)	Duragesic® Dose (mcg/h)
60-134[2]	25
135-224	50
225-314	75
315-404	100
405-494	125
495-584	150
585-674	175
675-764	200
765-854	225
855-944	250
945-1034	275
1035-1124	300

Product information, Duragesic® — Janssen Pharmaceutica

[1]Should not be used to convert from Duragesic® to other therapies because this conversion to Duragesic® is conservative. Use of this table for conversion to other analgesic therapies can overestimate the dose of the new agent; overdosage of the new analgesic agent is possible (see dosage for discontinuation of Duragesic®).

[2]Pediatric patients initiating therapy on a 25 mcg/hour Duragesic® system should be opioid-tolerant and receiving at least 60 mg oral morphine equivalents per day.

Pain management (chronic): Transdermal:

Initial: To convert patients from oral or parenteral opioids to transdermal formulation, a 24-hour analgesic requirement should be calculated (based on prior opiate use). This analgesic requirement should be converted to the equianalgesic oral morphine dose (see equianalgesic dosage table). The initial fentanyl dosage may be approximated from the 24-hour morphine dosage (see table) and titrated to minimize adverse effects and provide analgesia. Change patch every 72 hours.

Titration: Short-acting agents may be required until analgesic efficacy is established and/or as supplements for "breakthrough" pain. The amount of supplemental doses should be closely monitored. Appropriate dosage increases may be based on daily supplemental dosage using the ratio of 45 mg/24 hours of oral morphine to a 12.5 mcg/hour increase in fentanyl dosage. See tables on previous page.

Frequency of adjustment: The dosage should not be titrated more frequently than every 3 days after the initial dose or every 6 days thereafter. Patients should wear a consistent fentanyl dosage through 2 applications (6 days) before dosage increase based on supplemental opiate dosages can be estimated.

Frequency of application: The majority of patients may be controlled on every 72-hour administration, however, a small number of patients require every 48-hour administration.

Elderly: Elderly have been found to be twice as sensitive as younger patients to the effects of fentanyl. A wide range of doses may be used. When choosing a dose, take into consideration the following patient factors: age, weight, physical status, underlying disease states, other drugs used, type of anesthesia used, and the surgical procedure to be performed.

Transmucosal: Dose should be reduced to 2.5-5 mcg/kg. Suck on lozenge vigorously approximately 20-40 minutes before the start of procedure.

Pediatrics: Note: These are guidelines and do not represent the maximum doses that may be required in all patients. Doses should be titrated to pain relief/prevention. Monitor vital signs routinely.

Sedation for minor procedures/analgesia: Children 1-12 years: I.M., I.V.: 1-2 mcg/kg/ dose; may repeat at 30- to 60-minute intervals. **Note:** Children 18-36 months of age may require 2-3 mcg/kg/dose

Continuous sedation/analgesia: Children 1-12 years: I.V.: Initial I.V. bolus: 1-2 mcg/kg then 1 mcg/kg/hour; titrate upward; usual: 1-3 mcg/kg/hour

Pain management: Transdermal:

Children >2 years who are opioid tolerant: Initial dose: 25 mcg/hour system (higher doses have been used based on equianalgesic conversion); change patch every 72 hours

Children >12 years: Refer to adult dosing.

Hepatic Impairment: Actiq®: Although fentanyl kinetics may be altered in hepatic disease, Actiq® can be used successfully in the management of breakthrough cancer pain. Doses should be titrated to reach clinical effect with careful monitoring of patients with severe hepatic disease.

Available Dosage Forms

Infusion [premixed in NS]: 0.05 mg (10 mL); 1 mg (100 mL); 1.25 mg (250 mL); 2 mg (100 mL); 2.5 mg (250 mL)

Injection, solution, as citrate [preservative free]: 0.05 mg/mL (2 mL, 5 mL, 10 mL, 20 mL, 30 mL, 50 mL)

Sublimaze®: 0.05 mg/mL (2 mL, 5 mL, 10 mL, 20 mL)

Lozenge, oral transmucosal, as citrate (Actiq®): 200 mcg, 400 mcg, 600 mcg, 800 mcg, 1200 mcg, 1600 mcg [mounted on a plastic radiopaque handle; raspberry flavor]

Transdermal system: 25 mcg/hour [6.25 cm²] (5s); 50 mcg/hour [12.5 cm²] (5s); 75 mcg/hour [18.75 cm²]; 100 mcg/hour [25 cm²] (5s)

Duragesic®: 12 mcg/hour [5 cm²] (5s); 25 mcg/hour [10 cm²] (5s); 50 mcg/hour [20 cm²] (5s); 75 mcg/hour [30 cm²] (5s); 100 mcg/hour [40 cm²] (5s)

Monitoring and Teaching Issues

Physical Assessment: Assess other medications patient may be taking for additive or adverse interactions. Monitor therapeutic effectiveness and signs of adverse or overdose reactions. Monitor blood pressure, CNS and respiratory status, and degree of sedation at beginning of therapy and at regular intervals with long-term use. Monitor closely for 12 hours after transdermal product is removed. Order safety precautions for inpatient use. May cause physical and/or psychological dependence. Assess knowledge/teach patient appropriate use (if self-administered), adverse reactions to report, and appropriate interventions to reduce side effects.

Patient Education: While using this medication, do not use alcohol and other prescription or OTC medications (especially sedatives, tranquilizers, antihistamines, or pain medications) without consulting prescriber. If using Actiq® Oral Transmucosal, you may be at risk for dental caries due to the sugar content. Maintain good oral hygiene. Maintain adequate hydration (2-3 L/day of fluids) unless instructed to restrict fluid intake. May cause hypotension, dizziness, drowsiness, impaired coordination, or blurred vision (use caution when driving, climbing stairs, or changing position - rising from sitting or lying to standing, or when engaging in tasks requiring alertness until response to drug is known); nausea or vomiting (frequent mouth care, small frequent meals, chewing gum, or sucking lozenges may help); or constipation (increased exercise, fluids, fruit, or fiber may help; if unresolved, consult prescriber about use of stool softeners). Report acute dizziness, chest pain, slow or rapid heartbeat, acute headache; confusion or changes in mentation; changes in voiding frequency or amount; swelling of extremities or unusual weight gain; shortness of breath or respiratory difficulty; or vision changes. **Pregnancy/breast-feeding precautions:** Inform prescriber if you are or intend to become pregnant. Consult prescriber if breast-feeding.

Administration:

Transdermal: Apply to clean, dry skin, immediately after removing from package. Firmly press in place and hold for 30 seconds.

Actiq® transmucosal: Actiq® preparations contain an amount of medication that can be fatal to children. Keep all units out of the reach of children and discard any open units properly. Actiq® Welcome Kits are available which contain educational materials, safe storage, and disposal instructions.

Dietary Considerations: Actiq® contains 2 g sugar per unit.

Geriatric Considerations: The elderly may be particularly susceptible to the CNS depressant and constipating effects of narcotics; therefore, use with caution.

Pregnancy Risk Factor: C/D (prolonged use or high doses at term)

Pregnancy Issues: Fentanyl crosses the placenta and has been used safely during labor. Chronic use during pregnancy has shown detectable serum levels in the newborn with mild opioid withdrawal (case report).

(Continued)

Fentanyl *(Continued)*

Lactation: Enters breast milk/not recommended (AAP rates "compatible")

Breast-Feeding Issues: Fentanyl is excreted in low concentrations into breast milk. Breast-feeding is considered acceptable following single doses to the mother; however, no information is available when used long-term.

Administration

I.V.: Muscular rigidity may occur with rapid I.V. administration. During prolonged administration, dosage requirements may decrease.

Topical: Transdermal: Apply to nonirritated and nonirradiated skin, such as chest, back, flank, or upper arm. Upper back is preferred location in children. Do not shave skin; hair at application site should be clipped. Prior to application, clean site with clear water and allow to dry completely. Do not cut patch. Apply patch immediately after removing from package. Firmly press in place and hold for 30 seconds. Change patch every 72 hours. Keep transdermal product (both used and unused) out of the reach of children. Do **not** use soap, alcohol, or other solvents to remove transdermal gel if it accidentally touches skin, as they may increase transdermal absorption; use copious amounts of water. Avoid exposing application site to external heat sources (eg, heating pad, electric blanket, heat lamp, hot tub).

Other: Transmucosal: Foil overwrap should be removed just prior to administration. Once removed, patient should place the unit in mouth and allow it to dissolve. Do **not** chew. Actiq® units may be occasionally moved from one side of the mouth to the other. The unit should be consumed over a period of 15 minutes. Unit should be removed after it is consumed or if patient has achieved an adequate response and/or shows signs of respiratory depression. For patients who have received transmucosal product within 6-12 hours, it is recommended that if other narcotics are required, they should be used at starting doses $^1/_4$ to $^1/_3$ those usually recommended.

Compatibility: Stable in D_5W, NS

Compatibility in syringe: Incompatible with pentobarbital

Compatibility when admixed: Incompatible with fluorouracil, methohexital, pentobarbital, thiopental

Storage:

Injection formulation: Store at controlled room temperature of 15°C to 25°C (59°F to 86°F). Protect from light.

Transdermal: Do not store above 25°C (77°F).

Transmucosal: Store at controlled room temperature of 15°C to 30°C (59°F to 86°F).

Additional Information Fentanyl is 50-100 times as potent as morphine; morphine 10 mg I.M. is equivalent to fentanyl 0.1-0.2 mg I.M.; fentanyl has less hypotensive effects than morphine due to lack of histamine release. However, fentanyl may cause rigidity with high doses. If the patient has required high-dose analgesia or has used for a prolonged period (~7 days), taper dose to prevent withdrawal; monitor for signs and symptoms of withdrawal.

Transmucosal (oral lozenge): Disposal of Actiq® units: After consumption of a complete unit, the handle may be disposed of in a trash container that is out of the reach of children. For a partially-consumed unit, or a unit that still has any drug matrix remaining on the handle, the handle should be placed under hot running tap water until the drug matrix has dissolved. Special child-resistant containers are available to temporarily store partially consumed units that cannot be disposed of immediately.

Transdermal system (Duragesic®): Upon removal of the patch, ~17 hours are required before serum concentrations fall to 50% of their original values. Opioid withdrawal symptoms are possible. Gradual downward titration (potentially by the sequential use of lower-dose patches) is recommended. Keep transdermal product (both used and unused) out of the reach of children. Do **not** use soap, alcohol, or other solvents to remove transdermal gel if it accidentally touches skin as they may increase transdermal absorption, use copious amounts of water.

Related Information

Compatibility of Drugs *on page 1723*
Compatibility of Drugs in Syringe *on page 1725*
Narcotic / Opioid Analgesic Comparison *on page 1739*

◆ **Fentanyl Citrate** *see Fentanyl on page 618*
◆ **Feosol® [OTC]** *see Ferrous Sulfate on page 624*
◆ **Feostat® [OTC]** *see Ferrous Fumarate on page 623*
◆ **Feratab® [OTC]** *see Ferrous Sulfate on page 624*
◆ **Fer-Gen-Sol [OTC]** *see Ferrous Sulfate on page 624*
◆ **Fergon® [OTC]** *see Ferrous Gluconate on page 624*
◆ **Fer-In-Sol® [OTC]** *see Ferrous Sulfate on page 624*
◆ **Fer-Iron® [OTC]** *see Ferrous Sulfate on page 624*
◆ **Ferretts [OTC]** *see Ferrous Fumarate on page 623*

Ferric Gluconate *(FER ik GLOO koe nate)*

U.S. Brand Names Ferrlecit®

Synonyms Sodium Ferric Gluconate

Generic Available No

Pharmacologic Category Iron Salt

Medication Safety Issues

Sound-alike/look-alike issues:

Ferrlecit® may be confused with Ferralet®

Use Repletion of total body iron content in patients with iron-deficiency anemia who are undergoing hemodialysis in conjunction with erythropoietin therapy

Mechanism of Action/Effect Supplies a source to elemental iron necessary to the function of hemoglobin, myoglobin and specific enzyme systems; allows transport of oxygen via hemoglobin

Contraindications Hypersensitivity to ferric gluconate or any component of the formulation; use in any anemia not caused by iron deficiency; heart failure (of any severity); iron overload

Warnings/Precautions Potentially serious hypersensitivity reactions may occur. Fatal immediate hypersensitivity reactions have occurred with other iron carbohydrate complexes. Avoid rapid administration. Flushing and transient hypotension may occur. May augment hemodialysis-induced hypotension. Use with caution in elderly patients. Safety and efficacy in children <6 years of age have not been established. Contains benzyl alcohol; do not use in neonates.

Drug Interactions

Decreased Effect: Chloramphenicol may decrease effect of ferric gluconate injection; ferric gluconate injection may decrease the absorption of oral iron

Adverse Reactions Major adverse reactions include hypotension and hypersensitivity reactions. Hypersensitivity reactions have included pruritus, chest pain, hypotension, nausea, abdominal pain, flank pain, fatigue and rash.

Cardiovascular: Hypotension (serious hypotension in 1%), chest pain, hypertension, syncope, tachycardia, angina, MI, pulmonary edema, hypovolemia, peripheral edema

Central nervous system: Headache, fatigue, fever, malaise, dizziness, paresthesia, insomnia, agitation, somnolence, pain

Dermatologic: Pruritus, rash

Endocrine & metabolic: Hyperkalemia, hypoglycemia, hypokalemia

Gastrointestinal: Abdominal pain, nausea, vomiting, diarrhea, rectal disorder, dyspepsia, flatulence, melena, epigastric pain

Genitourinary: Urinary tract infection

Hematologic: Anemia, abnormal erythrocytes, lymphadenopathy

Local: Injection site reactions, pain

Neuromuscular & skeletal: Weakness, back pain, leg cramps, myalgia, arthralgia, paresthesia, groin pain

Ocular: Blurred vision, conjunctivitis

Respiratory: Dyspnea, cough, rhinitis, upper respiratory infection, pneumonia

Miscellaneous: Hypersensitivity reactions, infection, rigors, chills, flu-like syndrome, sepsis, carcinoma, diaphoresis increased

Overdosage/Toxicology Symptoms of iron overdose include CNS toxicity, acidosis, hepatic and renal impairment, hematemesis, and lethargy. A serum iron level ≥300 mcg/mL requires treatment due to severe toxicity. Treatment is generally symptomatic and supportive, but severe overdoses may be treated with deferoxamine. Deferoxamine may be administered I.V. (80 mg/kg over 24 hours) or I.M. (40-90 mg/kg every 8 hours). Usual toxic dose of elemental iron: ≥35 mg/kg.

Pharmacodynamics/Kinetics

Half-Life Elimination: Bound: 1 hour

Dosing

Adults & Elderly: Note: A test dose of 2 mL diluted in 50 mL 0.9% sodium chloride over 60 minutes was previously recommended (not in current manufacturer labeling).

Repletion of iron in hemodialysis patients: I.V.: 125 mg elemental iron per 10 mL (either by I.V. infusion or slow I.V. injection). Most patients will require a cumulative dose of 1 g elemental iron over approximately 8 sequential dialysis treatments to achieve a favorable response.

Pediatrics: Repletion of iron in hemodialysis patients: I.V.: Children ≥6 years: 1.5 mg/kg (maximum: 125 mg/dose) diluted in NS 25 mL, administered over 60 minutes at 8 sequential dialysis sessions

Available Dosage Forms Injection, solution: Elemental iron 12.5 mg/mL (5 mL) [contains benzyl alcohol and sucrose 20%]

Monitoring and Teaching Issues

Physical Assessment: Assess results of test dose, infusion rate, effectiveness of therapy (laboratory results), and adverse reactions at beginning of therapy and periodically during therapy. Monitor blood pressure during infusion. Hypotension can occur. Be alert to the potential for hypersensitivity reactions. Assess knowledge/teach patient adverse symptoms to report.

Monitoring Laboratory Tests: Hemoglobin and hematocrit, serum ferritin, iron saturation

Patient Education: This medication will be administered by I.V. in conjunction with your dialysis treatment. Report chest pain, rapid heartbeat, or palpitations; respiratory difficulty; headache, dizziness, agitation, or inability to sleep; nausea, vomiting, abdominal or flank pain; or skin rash, itching, or redness. **Breast-feeding precaution:** Consult prescriber if breast-feeding.

Pregnancy Risk Factor: B

Lactation: Excretion in breast milk unknown/use caution

Administration

I.V.: Adults: May be diluted prior to administration; avoid rapid administration. Infusion rate should not exceed 2.1 mg/minute. If administered undiluted, infuse slowly at a rate of up to 12.5 mg/minute.

Reconstitution: For I.V. infusion, dilute 10 mL ferric gluconate in 0.9% sodium chloride (children: 25 mL NS, adults: 100 mL NS); use immediately after dilution. Do **not** mix with parenteral nutrition solutions or other medications.

Compatibility: Stable in NS

Do not mix with parenteral nutrition solutions or other medications.

Storage: Store at 20°C to 25°C (68°F to 77°F).

♦ Ferrlecit® *see* Ferric Gluconate *on page 622*

♦ Ferro-Sequels® [OTC] *see* Ferrous Fumarate *on page 623*

Ferrous Fumarate (FER us FYOO ma rate)

U.S. Brand Names Femiron® [OTC]; Feostat® [OTC]; Ferretts [OTC]; Ferro-Sequels® [OTC]; Hemocyte® [OTC]; Ircon® [OTC]; Nephro-Fer® [OTC]

Synonyms Iron Fumarate

Generic Available Yes: Tablet

(Continued)

Ferrous Fumarate *(Continued)*

Pharmacologic Category Iron Salt

Medication Safety Issues
Sound-alike/look-alike issues:
Feostat® may be confused with Feosol®

Use Prevention and treatment of iron-deficiency anemias

Dosing
Adults & Elderly: (Dose expressed in terms of elemental iron):
Treatment of iron deficiency: Oral: 60-100 mg twice daily up to 60 mg 2 times/day
Prophylaxis of iron deficiency: Oral: 60-100 mg/day
Note: To avoid GI upset, start with a single daily dose and increase by 1 tablet/day each week or as tolerated until desired daily dose is achieved
Pediatrics: (Dose expressed in terms of elemental iron):
Treatment of severe iron-deficiency anemia: Oral: 4-6 mg Fe/kg/day in 3 divided doses
Treatment of mild-to-moderate iron-deficiency anemia: Oral: 3 mg Fe/kg/day in 1-2 divided doses
Prophylaxis of iron deficiency: Oral: 1-2 mg Fe/kg/day

Available Dosage Forms
Tablet: 324 mg [elemental iron 106 mg]
Femiron®: 63 mg [elemental iron 20 mg]
Ferretts: 325 mg [elemental iron 106 mg]
Hemocyte®: 324 mg [elemental iron 106 mg]
Ircon®: 200 mg [elemental iron 66 mg]
Nephro-Fer®: 350 mg [elemental iron 115 mg; contains tartrazine]
Tablet, chewable (Feostat®): 100 mg [elemental iron 33 mg; chocolate flavor]
Tablet, timed release (Ferro-Sequels®): 150 mg [elemental iron 50 mg; contains docusate sodium and sodium benzoate]

Monitoring and Teaching Issues
Patient Education: May color stool black. Take between meals for maximum absorption; take with food if GI upset occurs. Do not take with milk or antacids. Keep out of reach of children.
Pregnancy Risk Factor: A

Ferrous Gluconate *(FER us GLOO koe nate)*

U.S. Brand Names Fergon® [OTC]

Synonyms Iron Gluconate

Generic Available Yes

Pharmacologic Category Iron Salt

Use Prevention and treatment of iron-deficiency anemias

Dosing
Adults & Elderly: (Dose expressed in terms of elemental iron):
Treatment of iron deficiency anemia: Oral: 60 mg twice daily up to 60 mg 4 times/day
Prophylaxis of iron deficiency: Oral: 60 mg/day
Pediatrics: (Dose expressed in terms of elemental iron):
Treatment of severe iron-deficiency anemia: Oral: 4-6 mg Fe/kg/day in 3 divided doses
Treatment of mild-to-moderate iron-deficiency anemia: Oral: 3 mg Fe/kg/day in 1-2 divided doses
Prophylaxis: Oral: 1-2 mg Fe/kg/day

Available Dosage Forms
Tablet: 246 mg [elemental iron 28 mg]; 300 mg [elemental iron 34 mg]; 325 mg [elemental iron 36 mg]
Fergon®: 240 mg [elemental iron 27 mg]

Monitoring and Teaching Issues
Patient Education: May color stool black. Take between meals for maximum absorption; take with food if GI upset occurs. Do not take with milk or antacids. Keep out of reach of children.
Pregnancy Risk Factor: A

Ferrous Sulfate *(FER us SUL fate)*

U.S. Brand Names Feosol® [OTC]; Feratab® [OTC]; Fer-Gen-Sol [OTC]; Fer-In-Sol® [OTC]; Fer-Iron® [OTC]; Slow FE® [OTC]

Synonyms FeSO₄; Iron Sulfate

Generic Available Yes

Pharmacologic Category Iron Salt

Medication Safety Issues
Sound-alike/look-alike issues:
Feosol® may be confused with Feostat®, Fer-In-Sol®
Fer-In-Sol® may be confused with Feosol®
Slow FE® may be confused with Slow-K®

Use Prevention and treatment of iron-deficiency anemias

Contraindications Hypersensitivity to iron salts or any component of the formulation; hemochromatosis, hemolytic anemia

Warnings/Precautions Administration of iron for >6 months should be avoided except in patients with continued bleeding, menorrhagia, or repeated pregnancies; avoid in patients with peptic ulcer, enteritis, or ulcerative colitis. Anemia in the elderly is often caused by "anemia of chronic disease" or associated with inflammation rather than blood loss. Iron stores are usually normal or increased, with a serum ferritin >50 ng/mL and a decreased total iron binding capacity. Hence, the "anemia of chronic disease" is not secondary to iron deficiency but the inability of the reticuloendothelial system to reclaim available iron stores.

Drug Interactions
Decreased Effect: Absorption of oral preparation of iron and tetracyclines are decreased when both of these drugs are given together. Absorption of fluoroquinolones, levodopa,

methyldopa, and penicillamine may be decreased due to formation of a ferric ion-quinolone complex. Concurrent administration of antacids, H_2 blockers (cimetidine), or proton pump inhibitors may decrease iron absorption. Response to iron therapy may be delayed by chloramphenicol.

Increased Effect/Toxicity: Concurrent administration of ≥200 mg vitamin C per 30 mg elemental iron increases absorption of oral iron.

Nutritional/Ethanol Interactions Food: Cereals, dietary fiber, tea, coffee, eggs, and milk may decrease absorption.

Lab Interactions False-positive for blood in stool by the guaiac test

Adverse Reactions

>10%: Gastrointestinal: GI irritation, epigastric pain, nausea, dark stools, vomiting, stomach cramping, constipation

1% to 10%:

Gastrointestinal: Heartburn, diarrhea

Genitourinary: Discoloration of urine

Miscellaneous: Liquid preparations may temporarily stain the teeth

Overdosage/Toxicology

Symptoms of overdose include acute GI irritation; erosion of GI mucosa, hepatic and renal impairment, coma, hematemesis, lethargy, acidosis

Following treatment for fluid losses, metabolic acidosis, and shock, a severe iron overdose may be treated with deferoxamine. Deferoxamine may be administered I.V. (80 mg/kg over 24 hours) or I.M. (40-90 mg/kg every 8 hours). Usual toxic dose of elemental iron: ≥35 mg/kg.

Pharmacodynamics/Kinetics

Onset of Action: Hematologic response: Oral: ~3-10 days

Peak effect: Reticulocytosis: 5-10 days; hemoglobin increases within 2-4 weeks

Absorption: Iron is absorbed in the duodenum and upper jejunum; in persons with normal serum iron stores, 10% of an oral dose is absorbed; this is increased to 20% to 30% in persons with inadequate iron stores. Food and achlorhydria will decrease absorption

Protein Binding: To transferrin

Excretion: Urine, sweat, sloughing of the intestinal mucosa, and menses

Dosing

Adults & Elderly: Dose expressed in terms of ferrous sulfate:

Treatment of iron deficiency anemia: Oral: 300 mg twice daily up to 300 mg 4 times/day or 250 mg (extended release) 1-2 times/day

Prophylaxis of iron deficiency: Oral: 300 mg/day

Pediatrics: Dosage expressed in terms of elemental iron:

Treatment of severe iron-deficiency anemia: Oral: 4-6 mg Fe/kg/day in 3 divided doses

Treatment of mild-to-moderate iron-deficiency anemia: Oral: 3 mg Fe/kg/day in 1-2 divided doses

Prophylaxis: Oral: 1-2 mg Fe/kg/day up to a maximum of 15 mg/day

Available Dosage Forms

Elixir: 220 mg/5 mL (480 mL) [elemental iron 44 mg/5 mL; contains alcohol]

Liquid, oral drops: 75 mg/0.6 mL (50 mL) [elemental iron 15 mg/0.6 mL]

Fer-Gen-Sol: 75 mg/0.6 mL (50 mL) [elemental iron 15 mg/0.6 mL]

Fer-In-Sol®: 75 mg/0.6 mL (50 mL) [elemental iron 15 mg/0.6 mL; contains alcohol 0.2% and sodium bisulfite]

Fer-Iron®: 75 mg/0.6 mL (50 mL) [elemental iron 15 mg/0.6 mL]

Tablet: 324 mg [elemental iron 65 mg]; 325 mg [elemental iron 65 mg]

Feratab®: 300 mg [elemental iron 60 mg]

Tablet, exsiccated (Feosol): 200 mg [elemental iron 65 mg]

Tablet, exsiccated, timed release (Slow FE®): 160 mg [elemental iron 50 mg]

Monitoring and Teaching Issues

Physical Assessment: Assess therapeutic response and adverse effects. May cause GI irritation. Monitor GI function (observe for epigastric pain, nausea, dark stools, vomiting, stomach cramping, constipation).

Monitoring Laboratory Tests: Serum iron, total iron binding capacity, reticulocyte count, hemoglobin

Patient Education: May color stool black. Take between meals for maximum absorption; take with food if GI upset occurs. Do not take with milk or antacids. You may experience constipation; increasing exercise, fluids, fruit/fiber may help. Keep out of reach of children.

Dietary Considerations: Should be taken with water or juice on an empty stomach; may be administered with food to prevent irritation; however, do not take with cereals, dietary fiber, tea, coffee, eggs, or milk.

Elemental iron content of iron salts in ferrous sulfate is 20% (ie, 300 mg ferrous sulfate is equivalent to 60 mg ferrous iron)

Pregnancy Risk Factor: A

♦ **FeSO₄** see Ferrous Sulfate on page 624

♦ **FeverALL® [OTC]** see Acetaminophen on page 38

♦ **Fever Due to Drugs** see page 1679

Fexofenadine (feks oh FEN a deen)

U.S. Brand Names Allegra®

Synonyms Fexofenadine Hydrochloride

Generic Available No

Pharmacologic Category Antihistamine, Nonsedating

Medication Safety Issues

Sound-alike/look-alike issues:

Allegra® may be confused with Viagra®

Use Relief of symptoms associated with seasonal allergic rhinitis; treatment of chronic idiopathic urticaria

(Continued)

Fexofenadine *(Continued)*

Mechanism of Action/Effect Fexofenadine is an active metabolite of terfenadine and like terfenadine it competes with histamine for H_1-receptor sites on effector cells in the GI tract, blood vessels, and respiratory tract; binds to lung receptors significantly greater than it binds to cerebellar receptors, resulting in a greatly reduced sedative potential

Contraindications Hypersensitivity to fexofenadine or any component of the formulation

Warnings/Precautions Safety and efficacy in children <6 years of age have not been established.

Drug Interactions

Cytochrome P450 Effect: Substrate of CYP3A4 (minor); **Inhibits** CYP2D6 (weak)

Decreased Effect: Aluminum- and magnesium-containing antacids decrease plasma levels of fexofenadine; separate administration is recommended.

Increased Effect/Toxicity: Erythromycin and ketoconazole increased the levels of fexofenadine; however, no increase in adverse events or QT_c intervals was noted. The effect of other macrolide agents or azoles has not been investigated.

Nutritional/Ethanol Interactions

Ethanol: Avoid ethanol (although limited with fexofenadine, may increase risk of sedation).

Food: Fruit juice (apple, grapefruit, orange, pineapple) may decrease bioavailability of fexofenadine by ~36%.

Herb/Nutraceutical: St John's wort may decrease fexofenadine levels.

Adverse Reactions

>10%: Central nervous system: Headache (7% to 11%)

1% to 10%:

Central nervous system: Fever (2%), dizziness (2%), pain (2%), drowsiness (1% to 2%), fatigue (1%)

Endocrine & metabolic: Dysmenorrhea (2%)

Gastrointestinal: Nausea (2%), dyspepsia (1%)

Neuromuscular & skeletal: Back pain (2% to 3%)

Otic: Otitis media (2%)

Respiratory: Cough (4%), upper respiratory tract infection (3% to 4%), sinusitis (2%)

Miscellaneous: Viral infection (3%)

Overdosage/Toxicology Limited information from overdose describes dizziness, drowsiness, and dry mouth. Not effectively removed by hemodialysis. Doses up to 690 mg twice daily were administered for 1 month without significant adverse effects. Treatment is supportive.

Pharmacodynamics/Kinetics

Onset of Action: 60 minutes

Duration of Action: Antihistaminic effect: ≥12 hours

Time to Peak: Serum: ~2.6 hours

Protein Binding: 60% to 70%, primarily albumin and alpha$_1$-acid glycoprotein

Half-Life Elimination: 14.4 hours

Metabolism: ~5% mostly by gut flora; 0.5% to 1.5% by CYP

Excretion: Feces (~80%) and urine (~11%) as unchanged drug

Dosing

Adults:

Seasonal allergic rhinitis: Oral: 60 mg twice daily **or** 180 mg once daily

Chronic idiopathic urticaria: Oral: 60 mg twice daily

Elderly: Starting dose: 60 mg once daily; adjust for renal impairment.

Pediatrics: Allergic rhinitis, idiopathic urticaria:

Children 6-11 years: Oral: 30 mg twice daily

Children ≥12 years: Refer to adult dosing.

Renal Impairment: Cl_{cr} <80 mL/minute:

Children 6-11 years: Initial: 30 mg once daily

Children ≥12 years and Adults: Initial: 60 mg once daily

Not effectively removed by hemodialysis

Available Dosage Forms Tablet, as hydrochloride: 30 mg, 60 mg, 180 mg

Monitoring and Teaching Issues

Physical Assessment: Assess effectiveness and interactions of other medications patient may be taking. Monitor effectiveness of therapy and adverse reactions at beginning of therapy and periodically with long-term use. Assess knowledge/teach patient appropriate use, interventions to reduce side effects, and adverse symptoms to report.

Patient Education: Take as directed; do not exceed recommended dose. Store at room temperature in a dry place. If taking antacids, separate administration of antacid and this medication. Avoid use of other depressants, alcohol, or sleep-inducing medications unless approved by prescriber. You may experience mild drowsiness or dizziness (use caution when driving or engaging in tasks requiring alertness until response to drug is known); or nausea (small frequent meals, frequent mouth care, chewing gum, or sucking hard candy may help). Report persistent sedation or drowsiness, menstrual irregularities, or lack of improvement or worsening or condition. **Pregnancy/breast-feeding precautions:** Inform prescriber if you are or intend to become pregnant. Consult prescriber if breast-feeding.

Geriatric Considerations: Plasma levels in the elderly are generally higher than those observed in other age groups. Once daily dosing is recommended when starting therapy in elderly patients or patients with decreased renal function.

Pregnancy Risk Factor: C

Lactation: Excretion in breast milk unknown/use caution (AAP rates "compatible")

Administration

Oral: Administer with water.

Storage: Store at controlled room temperature of 20°C to 25°C (68°F to 77°F). Protect from excessive moisture.

Fexofenadine and Pseudoephedrine
(feks oh FEN a deen & soo doe e FED rin)

U.S. Brand Names Allegra-D® 12 Hour; Allegra-D® 24 Hour

Synonyms Pseudoephedrine and Fexofenadine

Generic Available No

Pharmacologic Category Antihistamine/Decongestant Combination

Medication Safety Issues
Sound-alike/look-alike issues:
Allegra-D® may be confused with Viagra®

Use Relief of symptoms associated with seasonal allergic rhinitis in adults and children ≥12 years of age

Dosing
Adults & Elderly: Allergic symptoms and nasal congestion: Oral:
Allegra-D® 12 Hour: One tablet twice daily
Allegra-D® 24 Hour: One tablet once daily

Pediatrics: Children ≥12 years: Refer to adult dosing.

Renal Impairment:
Allegra-D® 12 Hour: Cl$_{cr}$ <80 mL/minute (based on fexofenadine component): One tablet once daily.
Allegra-D® 24 Hour: Avoid use.

Available Dosage Forms Tablet, extended release:
Allegra-D® 12 Hour: Fexofenadine hydrochloride 60 mg [immediate release] and pseudoephedrine hydrochloride 120 mg [extended release]
Allegra-D® 24 Hour: Fexofenadine hydrochloride 180 mg [immediate release] and pseudoephedrine hydrochloride 240 mg [extended release]

Monitoring and Teaching Issues
Physical Assessment: See individual agents.

Patient Education: Patients should be instructed to take tablets only as prescribed. Do not exceed the recommended dose. If nervousness, dizziness, or sleeplessness occur, discontinue use and consult the physician. Patients should also be advised against the concurrent use of the tablets with over-the-counter antihistamines and decongestants. The product should not be used by patients who are hypersensitive to it or to any of its ingredients. Due to its pseudoephedrine component, this product should not be used by patients with narrow-angle glaucoma, urinary retention, or by patients receiving a monoamine oxidase (MAO) inhibitor or within 14 days of stopping use of MAO inhibitor. It also should not be used by patients with severe hypertension or severe coronary artery disease. Patients should be told that this product should be used in pregnancy or lactation only if the potential benefit justifies the potential risk to the fetus or nursing infant. Patients should be cautioned not to break or chew the tablet. Patients should be directed to swallow the tablet whole. Patients should be instructed not to take the tablet with food. Patients should also be instructed to store the medication in a tightly closed container in a cool, dry place, away from children. **Pregnancy/breast-feeding precautions:** Inform prescriber if you are pregnant. Consult prescriber if breast-feeding.

Pregnancy Risk Factor: C

Lactation: Enters breast milk/use caution (AAP rates "compatible")

Related Information
Fexofenadine *on page 625*
Pseudoephedrine *on page 1282*

♦ **Fexofenadine Hydrochloride** *see* Fexofenadine *on page 625*
♦ **Fiberall®** *see* Psyllium *on page 1284*

Filgrastim (fil GRA stim)

U.S. Brand Names Neupogen®

Synonyms G-CSF; Granulocyte Colony Stimulating Factor

Generic Available No

Pharmacologic Category Colony Stimulating Factor

Medication Safety Issues
Sound-alike/look-alike issues:
Neupogen® may be confused with Epogen®, Neumega®, Nutramigen®

Use Stimulation of granulocyte production in patients with malignancies, including myeloid malignancies; receiving myelosuppressive therapy associated with a significant risk of neutropenia; severe chronic neutropenia (SCN); receiving bone marrow transplantation (BMT); undergoing peripheral blood progenitor cell (PBPC) collection

Mechanism of Action/Effect Stimulates the production, maturation, and activation of neutrophils, G-CSF activates neutrophils to increase both their migration and cytotoxicity. Natural proteins which stimulate hematopoietic stem cells to proliferate, prolong cell survival, stimulate cell differentiation, and stimulate functional activity of mature cells. CSFs are produced by a wide variety of cell types. Specific mechanisms of action are not yet fully understood, but possibly work by a second-messenger pathway with resultant protein production. See table.

Comparative Effects — G-CSF vs GM-CSF

Proliferation/Differentiation	G-CSF (Filgrastim)	GM-CSF (Sargramostim)
Neutrophils	Yes	Yes
Eosinophils	No	Yes
Macrophages	No	Yes
Neutrophil migration	Enhanced	Inhibited

(Continued)

Filgrastim *(Continued)*

Contraindications Hypersensitivity to filgrastim, *E. coli*-derived proteins, or any component of the formulation; concurrent myelosuppressive chemotherapy or radiation therapy

Warnings/Precautions Complete blood count and platelet count should be obtained prior to chemotherapy. Do not use G-CSF in the period 24 hours before to 24 hours after administration of cytotoxic chemotherapy because of the potential sensitivity of rapidly dividing myeloid cells to cytotoxic chemotherapy. Precaution should be exercised in the usage of G-CSF in any malignancy with myeloid characteristics. G-CSF can potentially act as a growth factor for any tumor type, particularly myeloid malignancies. Tumors of nonhematopoietic origin may have surface receptors for G-CSF.

Allergic-type reactions have occurred in patients receiving the parent compound, filgrastim (G-CSF) with first or later doses. Reactions tended to occur more frequently with intravenous administration and within 30 minutes of infusion. Rare cases of splenic rupture or adult respiratory distress syndrome have been reported in association with filgrastim; patients must be instructed to report left upper quadrant pain or shoulder tip pain or respiratory distress. Use caution in patients with sickle cell diseases; sickle cell crises have been reported following filgrastim therapy.

Drug Interactions
Increased Effect/Toxicity: Drugs which may potentiate the release of neutrophils (eg, lithium) should be used with caution.

Adverse Reactions
>10%:
Cardiovascular: Chest pain
Central nervous system: Fever
Dermatologic: Alopecia
Endocrine & metabolic: Fluid retention
Gastrointestinal: Nausea, vomiting, diarrhea, mucositis; splenomegaly - up to 33% of patients with cyclic neutropenia/congenital agranulocytosis receiving filgrastim for ≥14 days; rare in other patients
Neuromuscular & skeletal: Bone pain (24%), commonly in the lower back, posterior iliac crest, and sternum
1% to 10%:
Cardiovascular: S-T segment depression (3%)
Central nervous system: Headache
Dermatologic: Rash
Gastrointestinal: Anorexia, constipation, sore throat
Hematologic: Leukocytosis
Local: Pain at injection site
Neuromuscular & skeletal: Weakness
Respiratory: Dyspnea, cough

Overdosage/Toxicology No clinical adverse effects have been seen with high doses producing ANC >10,000/mm^3. After discontinuing the drug there is a 50% decrease in circulating levels of neutrophils within 1-2 days, and return to pretreatment levels within 1-7 days.

Pharmacodynamics/Kinetics
Onset of Action: ~24 hours; plateaus in 3-5 days
Duration of Action: ANC decreases by 50% within 2 days after discontinuing G-CSF; white counts return to the normal range in 4-7 days; peak plasma levels can be maintained for up to 12 hours
Absorption: SubQ: 100%
Time to Peak: Serum: SubQ: 2-6 hours
Half-Life Elimination: 1.8-3.5 hours
Metabolism: Systemically degraded

Dosing
Adults & Elderly: Refer to individual protocols.
Note: Dosing should be based on actual body weight (even in morbidly obese patients). Rounding doses to the nearest vial size often enhances patient convenience and reduces costs without compromising clinical response.

Myelosuppressive therapy: I.V., SubQ: 5 mcg/kg/day - doses may be increased by 5 mcg/kg according to the duration and severity of the neutropenia.
Bone marrow transplantation: I.V., SubQ: 5-10 mcg/kg/day - doses may be increased by 5 mcg/kg according to the duration and severity of neutropenia; recommended steps based on neutrophil response:
When ANC >1000/mm^3 for 3 consecutive days: Reduce filgrastim dose to 5 mcg/kg/day.
If ANC remains >1000/mm^3 for 3 more consecutive days: Discontinue filgrastim.
If ANC decreases to <1000/mm^3: Resume at 5 mcg/kg/day.
If ANC decreases <1000/mm^3 during the 5 mcg/kg/day dose: Increase filgrastim to 10 mcg/kg/day and follow the above steps.
Peripheral blood progenitor cell (PBPC) collection: I.V., SubQ: 10 mcg/kg/day **or** 5-8 mcg/kg twice daily in donors. The optimal timing and duration of growth factor stimulation has not been determined.
Severe chronic neutropenia: SubQ:
Congenital: 6 mcg/kg twice daily
Idiopathic/cyclic: 5 mcg/kg/day
Pediatrics: Children: Refer to adult dosing.

Available Dosage Forms
Injection, solution [preservative free]: 300 mcg/mL (1 mL, 1.6 mL) [vial; contains sodium 0.035 mg/mL and sorbitol]
Injection, solution [preservative free]: 600 mcg/mL (0.5 mL, 0.8 mL) [prefilled Singleject® syringe; contains sodium 0.035 mg/mL and sorbitol]

Monitoring and Teaching Issues

Physical Assessment: Assess for hypersensitivity to *E. coli* products prior to beginning therapy. See Warnings/Precautions for use cautions. Assess potential for interactions with pharmacological agents the patient may be taking that may potentiate the release of neutrophils. Assess results of CBC and platelet counts twice weekly during therapy (see Monitoring Laboratory Tests). Monitor therapeutic effectiveness and signs/symptoms of adverse reactions at beginning of therapy and periodically throughout therapy (eg, allergic-type reactions have occurred in patients receiving G-CSF with first or later doses; see Warnings/Precautions and Adverse Reactions). If self-administered, teach patient (or caregiver) proper storage, administration, and syringe/needle disposal. Teach patient (or caregiver) possible side effects/appropriate interventions and adverse symptoms to report (see Patient Education).

Monitoring Laboratory Tests: CBC and platelet count should be obtained twice weekly. Leukocytosis (white blood cell counts $\geq 100,000/mm^3$) has been observed in ~2% of patients receiving G-CSF at doses >5 mcg/kg/day. Monitor platelets and hematocrit regularly.

Patient Education: Do not take any new medication during therapy unless approved by prescriber. If self-administered, follow directions for proper storage and administration of SubQ medication. Never reuse syringes or needles. May cause bone pain (request analgesic); nausea or vomiting (small frequent meals may help); hair loss (reversible); or sore mouth (frequent mouth care with soft toothbrush or cotton swab may help). Report unusual fever or chills; unhealed sores; severe bone pain; pain, redness, or swelling at injection site; unusual swelling of extremities or respiratory difficulty; or chest pain and palpitations.
Pregnancy/breast-feeding precautions: Inform prescriber if you are or intend to become pregnant. Consult prescriber if breast-feeding.

Dietary Considerations: Injection solution contains sodium 0.035 mg/mL and sorbitol.

Pregnancy Risk Factor: C

Lactation: Excretion in breast milk unknown/use caution

Administration

I.V.: May be administered undiluted by SubQ or IVP administration. May also be administered by I.V. infusion over 15-60 minutes in D_5W.

Reconstitution: Filgrastim may be diluted in dextrose 5% in water to a concentration ≥ 15 mcg/mL for I.V. infusion administration. Minimum concentration is 15 mcg/mL. Concentrations <15 mcg/mL require addition of albumin (1 mL of 5%) to the bag to prevent absorption to plastics/PVC.

Compatibility: Standard diluent: ≥ 375 mcg/25 mL D_5W. Stable in D_5W; **incompatible** with NS

Y-site administration: Incompatible with amphotericin B, cefepime, cefoperazone, cefotaxime, cefoxitin, ceftizoxime, ceftriaxone, cefuroxime, clindamycin, dactinomycin, etoposide, fluorouracil, furosemide, heparin, mannitol, methylprednisolone sodium succinate, metronidazole, mitomycin, piperacillin, prochlorperazine edisylate, thiotepa

Storage: Intact vials and prefilled syringes should be stored under refrigeration at 2°C to 8°C (36°F to 46°F) and protected from direct sunlight. Filgrastim should be protected from freezing and temperatures >30°C to avoid aggregation. If inadvertently frozen, thaw in a refrigerator and use within 24 hours; do not use if frozen >24 hours or frozen more than once. The solution should not be shaken since bubbles and/or foam may form. If foaming occurs, the solution should be left undisturbed for a few minutes until bubbles dissipate.

Filgrastim vials and prefilled syringes are stable for 7 days at 9°C to 30°C (47°F to 86°F), however, the manufacturer recommends discarding after 24 hours because of microbiological concerns. The product is packaged without a preservative.

Undiluted filgrastim is stable for 24 hours at 15°C to 30°C and for 2 weeks at 2°C to 8°C (36°F to 46°F) in tuberculin syringes. However, the manufacturer recommends to use immediately because of concern for bacterial contamination.

Filgrastim diluted for I.V. infusion (≥ 15 mcg/mL) is stable for 7 days at 2°C to 8°C (36°F to 46°F).

Additional Information

Reimbursement Hotline: 1-800-272-9376
Professional Services [Amgen]: 1-800-77-AMGEN

Finasteride (fi NAS teer ide)

U.S. Brand Names Propecia®; Proscar®

Generic Available No

Pharmacologic Category 5 Alpha-Reductase Inhibitor

Medication Safety Issues

Sound-alike/look-alike issues:
Proscar® may be confused with ProSom®, Prozac®, Psorcon®

Use

Propecia®: Treatment of male pattern hair loss in **men only**. Safety and efficacy were demonstrated in men between 18-41 years of age.

Proscar®: Treatment of symptomatic benign prostatic hyperplasia (BPH); can be used in combination with an alpha blocker, doxazosin

Unlabeled/Investigational Use Adjuvant monotherapy after radical prostatectomy in the treatment of prostatic cancer; female hirsutism

Mechanism of Action/Effect Finasteride inhibits conversion of testosterone to dihydrotestosterone and markedly suppresses serum dihydrotestosterone levels

Contraindications Hypersensitivity to finasteride or any component of the formulation; pregnancy; not for use in children

Warnings/Precautions A minimum of 6 months of treatment may be necessary to determine whether an individual will respond to finasteride. Use with caution in those patients with hepatic dysfunction. Carefully monitor patients with a large residual urinary volume or severely diminished urinary flow for obstructive uropathy. These patients may not be candidates for finasteride therapy.

(Continued)

Finasteride *(Continued)*

Drug Interactions

Cytochrome P450 Effect: Substrate of CYP3A4 (minor)

Nutritional/Ethanol Interactions

Herb/Nutraceutical: St John's wort may decrease finasteride levels. Avoid saw palmetto (concurrent use has not been adequately studied).

Adverse Reactions Note: "Combination therapy" refers to finasteride and doxazosin.

>10%:

Endocrine & metabolic: Impotence (19%; combination therapy 23%), libido decreased (10%; combination therapy 12%)

Genitourinary: Neuromuscular & skeletal: Weakness (5%; combination therapy 17%)

1% to 10%:

Cardiovascular: Postural hypotension (9%; combination therapy 18%), edema (1%, combination therapy 3%)

Central nervous system: Dizziness (7%; combination therapy 23%), somnolence (2%; combination therapy 3%)

Genitourinary: Ejaculation disturbances (7%; combination therapy 14%), decreased volume of ejaculate

Endocrine & metabolic: Gynecomastia (2%)

Respiratory: Dyspnea (1%; combination therapy 2%), rhinitis (1%; combination therapy 2%)

Pharmacodynamics/Kinetics

Onset of Action: 3-6 months of ongoing therapy

Duration of Action:

After a single oral dose as small as 0.5 mg: 65% depression of plasma dihydrotestosterone levels persists 5-7 days

After 6 months of treatment with 5 mg/day: Circulating dihydrotestosterone levels are reduced to castrate levels without significant effects on circulating testosterone; levels return to normal within 14 days of discontinuation of treatment

Bioavailability: Mean: 63%

Time to Peak: Serum: 2-6 hours

Protein Binding: 90%

Half-Life Elimination: Elderly: 8 hours; Adults: 6 hours (3-16)

Metabolism: Hepatic via CYP3A4; two active metabolites (<20% activity of finasteride)

Excretion: Feces (57%) and urine (39%) as metabolites

Dosing

Adults & Elderly:

Benign prostatic hyperplasia (Proscar®): Oral: 5 mg/day as a single dose; clinical responses occur within 12 weeks to 6 months of initiation of therapy; long-term administration is recommended for maximal response

Male pattern baldness (Propecia®): Oral: 1 mg daily

Female hirsutism (unlabeled use): Oral: 5 mg/day

Renal Impairment: No adjustment is necessary.

Hepatic Impairment: Use with caution in patients with liver function abnormalities because finasteride is metabolized extensively in the liver

Available Dosage Forms

Tablet [film coated]:

Propecia®: 1 mg

Proscar®: 5 mg

Monitoring and Teaching Issues

Physical Assessment: See Warnings/Precautions for use cautions (eg, hepatic impairment). Assess potential for interactions with herbal products patient may be taking (see Nutritional/Ethanol Interactions). Assess therapeutic effectiveness and signs/symptoms of adverse reactions (see Adverse Reactions). Teach patient proper use, possible side effects/appropriate interventions and adverse symptoms to report (see Patient Education).

Pregnancy risk factor X: Instruct patient on absolute need for contraceptives. Women of childbearing age should not touch or handle broken tablets.

Monitoring Laboratory Tests: Finasteride does not interfere with free PSA levels.

Patient Education: Inform prescriber of all prescriptions, OTC medications, or herbal products you are taking, and any allergies you have. Do not take any new medication during therapy unless approved by prescriber. Results of therapy may take several months. Take with or without meals. May cause decreased libido or impotence during therapy. Report any increase in urinary volume or voiding patterns. Report changes in breast condition (pain, lumps, or nipple discharge) in male and female patients. **Pregnancy precaution:** This drug will cause fetal abnormalities; use contraceptives and do not allow women of childbearing age to touch or handle broken or crushed tablets.

Geriatric Considerations: Clearance of finasteride is decreased in the elderly, but no dosage reductions are necessary.

Pregnancy Risk Factor: X

Lactation: Excretion in breast milk unknown/contraindicated

Breast-Feeding Issues: Not indicated for use in women.

Administration

Oral: Administration with food may delay the rate and reduce the extent of oral absorption. Women of childbearing age should not touch or handle broken tablets.

Storage: Store below 30°C (86°F). Protect from light.

♦ Fioricet® *see* Butalbital, Acetaminophen, and Caffeine *on page 225*

♦ Fioricet® with Codeine *see* Butalbital, Acetaminophen, Caffeine, and Codeine *on page 226*

♦ Fiorinal® *see* Butalbital, Aspirin, and Caffeine *on page 226*

♦ Fiorinal® With Codeine *see* Butalbital, Aspirin, Caffeine, and Codeine *on page 227*

♦ Fisalamine *see* Mesalamine *on page 957*

♦ Fish Oil *see* Omega-3-Acid Ethyl Esters *on page 1117*

♦ **FK506** *see* Tacrolimus *on page 1419*

♦ **Flagyl®** *see* Metronidazole *on page 995*

♦ **Flagyl ER®** *see* Metronidazole *on page 995*

♦ **Flagyl® I.V. RTU™** *see* Metronidazole *on page 995*

♦ **Flarex®** *see* Fluorometholone *on page 646*

♦ **Flebogamma®** *see* Immune Globulin (Intravenous) *on page 793*

Flecainide (fle KAY nide)

U.S. Brand Names Tambocor™

Synonyms Flecainide Acetate

Generic Available Yes

Pharmacologic Category Antiarrhythmic Agent, Class Ic

Medication Safety Issues

Sound-alike/look-alike issues:

Flecainide may be confused with fluconazole

Tambocor™ may be confused with tamoxifen

Use Prevention and suppression of documented life-threatening ventricular arrhythmias (eg, sustained ventricular tachycardia); controlling symptomatic, disabling supraventricular tachycardias in patients without structural heart disease in whom other agents fail

Mechanism of Action/Effect Class Ic antiarrhythmic; slows conduction in cardiac tissue by altering transport of ions across cell membranes; causes slight prolongation of refractory periods; decreases the rate of rise of the action potential without affecting its duration; increases electrical stimulation threshold of ventricle, His-Purkinje system; possesses local anesthetic and moderate negative inotropic effects

Contraindications Hypersensitivity to flecainide or any component of the formulation; pre-existing second- or third-degree AV block or with right bundle branch block when associated with a left hemiblock (bifascicular block) (except in patients with a functioning artificial pacemaker); cardiogenic shock; coronary artery disease (based on CAST study results); concurrent use of ritonavir or amprenavir

Warnings/Precautions Not recommend for patients with chronic atrial fibrillation. A worsening or new arrhythmia may occur (proarrhythmic effect). Use caution in heart failure (may precipitate or exacerbate CHF). Dose-related increases in PR, QRS, and QT intervals occur. Use with caution in sick sinus syndrome or with permanent pacemakers or temporary pacing wires (can increase endocardial pacing thresholds). Due to potential to exacerbate toxicity, pre-existing hypokalemia or hyperkalemia should be corrected before initiation of flecainide. Use caution in patients with significant hepatic impairment.

Drug Interactions

Cytochrome P450 Effect: Substrate of CYP1A2 (minor), 2D6 (major); **Inhibits** CYP2D6 (weak)

Decreased Effect: Smoking and acid urine increase flecainide clearance.

Increased Effect/Toxicity: CYP2D6 inhibitors may increase the levels/effects of flecainide; example inhibitors include chlorpromazine, delavirdine, fluoxetine, miconazole, paroxetine, pergolide, quinidine, quinine, ritonavir, and ropinirole. Flecainide concentrations may be increased by amiodarone (reduce flecainide 25% to 33%), and propranolol. Beta-adrenergic blockers, disopyramide, verapamil may enhance flecainide's negative inotropic effects. Alkalinizing agents (ie, high-dose antacids, cimetidine, carbonic anhydrase inhibitors, sodium bicarbonate) may decrease flecainide clearance, potentially increasing toxicity. Propranolol blood levels are increased by flecainide.

Nutritional/Ethanol Interactions Food: Clearance may be decreased in patients following strict vegetarian diets due to urinary pH ≥8. Dairy products (milk, infant formula, yogurt) may interfere with the absorption of flecainide in infants; there is one case report of a neonate (GA 34 weeks PNA >6 days) who required extremely large doses of oral flecainide when administered every 8 hours with feedings ("milk feeds"); changing the feedings from "milk feeds" to 5% glucose feeds alone resulted in a doubling of the flecainide serum concentration and toxicity.

Adverse Reactions

>10%:

Central nervous system: Dizziness (19% to 30%)

Ocular: Visual disturbances (16%)

Respiratory: Dyspnea (~10%)

1% to 10%:

Cardiovascular: Palpitations (6%), chest pain (5%), edema (3.5%), tachycardia (1% to 3%), proarrhythmic (4% to 12%), sinus node dysfunction (1.2%)

Central nervous system: Headache (4% to 10%), fatigue (8%), nervousness (5%) additional symptoms occurring at a frequency between 1% and 3%: fever, malaise, hypoesthesia, paresis, ataxia, vertigo, syncope, somnolence, tinnitus, anxiety, insomnia, depression

Dermatologic: Rash (1% to 3%)

Gastrointestinal: Nausea (9%), constipation (1%), abdominal pain (3%), anorexia (1% to 3%), diarrhea (0.7% to 3%)

Neuromuscular & skeletal: Tremor (5%), weakness (5%), paresthesia (1%)

Ocular: Diplopia (1% to 3%), blurred vision

Overdosage/Toxicology Flecainide has a narrow therapeutic index and severe toxicity may occur slightly above the therapeutic range, especially if combined with other antiarrhythmic drugs. (Acute single ingestion of twice the daily therapeutic dose is life-threatening). Symptoms of overdose include increase in P-R, QRS, or QT intervals and amplitude of the T wave, AV block, bradycardia, hypotension, ventricular arrhythmias (monomorphic or polymorphic ventricular tachycardia), and asystole. Other symptoms include dizziness, blurred vision, headache, and GI upset. Treatment is supportive.

(Continued)

Flecainide *(Continued)*

Pharmacodynamics/Kinetics
Absorption: Oral: Rapid
Bioavailability: 85% to 90%
Time to Peak: Serum: ~1.5-3 hours
Protein Binding: Alpha$_1$ glycoprotein: 40% to 50%
Half-Life Elimination: Infants: 11-12 hours; Children: 8 hours; Adults: 7-22 hours, increased with congestive heart failure or renal dysfunction; End-stage renal disease: 19-26 hours
Metabolism: Hepatic
Excretion: Urine (80% to 90%, 10% to 50% as unchanged drug and metabolites)

Dosing
Adults & Elderly:
Life-threatening ventricular arrhythmias: Oral:
Initial: 100 mg every 12 hours; increase by 50-100 mg/day (given in 2 doses/day) every 4 days; maximum: 400 mg/day
For patients receiving 400 mg/day who are not controlled and have trough concentrations <0.6 mcg/mL, dosage may be increased to 600 mg/day.
Prevention of paroxysmal supraventricular arrhythmias: Oral:
Note: In patients with disabling symptoms but no structural heart disease
Initial: 50 mg every 12 hours; increase by 50 mg twice daily at 4-day intervals; maximum: 300 mg/day

Pediatrics:
Life-threatening ventricular arrhythmias: Oral: Children:
Initial: 3 mg/kg/day or 50-100 mg/m^2/day in 3 divided doses
Usual maintenance: 3-6 mg/kg/day or 100-150 mg/m^2/day in 3 divided doses; up to 11 mg/kg/day or 200 mg/m^2/day for uncontrolled patients with subtherapeutic levels

Renal Impairment:
Cl$_{cr}$ <10 mL/minute: Decrease usual dose by 25% to 50% in severe renal impairment. Not dialyzable (0% to 5%) via hemo- or peritoneal dialysis; no supplemental dose is necessary.

Hepatic Impairment: Monitoring of plasma levels is recommended because half-life is significantly increased. When transferring from another antiarrhythmic agent, allow for 2-4 half-lives of the agent to pass before initiating flecainide therapy.

Available Dosage Forms Tablet, as acetate: 50 mg, 100 mg, 150 mg

Monitoring and Teaching Issues
Physical Assessment: Assess other medications patient may be taking for effectiveness and interactions. Monitor cardiac status. Assess results of laboratory tests, therapeutic effectiveness, and adverse reactions when beginning therapy, when titrating dosage, and periodically during long-term therapy. **Note:** Flecainide has a low toxic:therapeutic ratio and overdose may easily produce severe and life-threatening reactions. Assess knowledge/teach patient appropriate use, interventions to reduce side effects, and adverse symptoms to report.

Monitoring Laboratory Tests: Periodic serum concentrations, especially in patients with renal or hepatic impairment

Patient Education: Take exactly as directed, around-the-clock. Do not discontinue without consulting prescriber. You will require frequent monitoring while taking this medication. You may experience lightheadedness, nervousness, dizziness, visual disturbances (use caution when driving or engaging in tasks requiring alertness until response to drug is known); or nausea, vomiting, or loss of appetite (small frequent meals may help). Report palpitations, chest pain, excessively slow or rapid heartbeat; acute nervousness, headache, or fatigue; unusual weight gain; unusual cough; respiratory difficulty; swelling of hands or ankles; or muscle tremor, numbness, or weakness. **Pregnancy precaution:** Inform prescriber if you are or intend to become pregnant.

Pregnancy Risk Factor: C
Lactation: Enters breast milk/compatible

Administration
Oral: Administer around-the-clock to promote less variation in peak and trough serum levels.

Related Information
Antiarrhythmic Drugs *on page 1708*

- Flecainide Acetate *see* Flecainide *on page 631*
- Fleet® Sof-Lax® [OTC] *see* Docusate *on page 474*
- Fletcher's® Castoria® [OTC] *see* Senna *on page 1365*
- Flexeril® *see* Cyclobenzaprine *on page 378*
- Flolan® *see* Epoprostenol *on page 534*
- Flomax® *see* Tamsulosin *on page 1426*
- Flonase® *see* Fluticasone *on page 660*
- Florical® [OTC] *see* Calcium Carbonate *on page 235*
- Florinef® *see* Fludrocortisone *on page 639*
- Flovent® [DSC] *see* Fluticasone *on page 660*
- Flovent® HFA *see* Fluticasone *on page 660*
- Flovent® Rotadisk® [DSC] *see* Fluticasone *on page 660*
- Floxin® *see* Ofloxacin *on page 1107*
- Floxin Otic Singles *see* Ofloxacin *on page 1107*

Floxuridine *(floks YOOR i deen)*
U.S. Brand Names FUDR®
Synonyms Fluorodeoxyuridine; FUDR; 5-FUDR; NSC-27640
Generic Available Yes
Pharmacologic Category Antineoplastic Agent, Antimetabolite (Pyrimidine Antagonist)

Medication Safety Issues
Sound-alike/look-alike issues:
FUDR® may be confused with Fludara®

Use Management of hepatic metastases of colorectal and gastric cancers

Mechanism of Action/Effect Mechanism of action and pharmacokinetics are very similar to fluorouracil; floxuridine is the deoxyribonucleotide of fluorouracil. Floxuridine is a fluorinated pyrimidine antagonist which inhibits DNA and RNA synthesis and methylation of deoxy-uridylic acid to thymidylic acid.

Contraindications Hypersensitivity to floxuridine, fluorouracil, or any component of the formulation; pregnancy

Warnings/Precautions The U.S. Food and Drug Administration (FDA) currently recommends that procedures for proper handling and disposal of antineoplastic agents be considered.

Use caution in impaired kidney or liver function. Discontinue if intractable vomiting or diarrhea, precipitous fall in leukocyte or platelet counts, or myocardial ischemia occur. Use with caution in patients who have had high-dose pelvic radiation or previous use of alkylating agents. Use of floxuridine with pentostatin has been associated with a high incidence of fatal pulmonary toxicity; this combination is not recommended.

If floxuridine contacts the skin, wash and flush thoroughly with water.

Drug Interactions
Decreased Effect: Patients may experience impaired immune response to vaccines; possible infection after administration of live vaccines in patients receiving immunosuppressants.

Increased Effect/Toxicity: Any form of therapy which adds to the stress of the patient, interferes with nutrition, or depresses bone marrow function will increase the toxicity of floxuridine. Pentostatin and floxuridine administered together has resulted in fatal pulmonary toxicity.

Nutritional/Ethanol Interactions Ethanol: Avoid ethanol (due to GI irritation).

Lab Interactions Increased potassium (S)

Adverse Reactions
>10%:
Gastrointestinal: Stomatitis, diarrhea; may be dose-limiting
Hematologic: Myelosuppression, may be dose-limiting; leukopenia, thrombocytopenia, anemia
Onset: 4-7 days
Nadir: 5-9 days
Recovery: 21 days

1% to 10%:
Dermatologic: Alopecia, photosensitivity, hyperpigmentation of the skin, localized erythema, dermatitis
Gastrointestinal: Anorexia
Hepatic: Biliary sclerosis, cholecystitis, jaundice

Pharmacodynamics/Kinetics
Metabolism: Hepatic; Active metabolites: Floxuridine monophosphate (FUDR-MP) and fluorouracil; Inactive metabolites: Urea, CO_2, α-fluoro-β-alanine, α-fluoro-β-guanidopropionic acid, α-fluoro-β-ureidopropionic acid, and dihydrofluorouracil

Excretion: Urine: Fluorouracil, urea, α-fluoro-β-alanine, α-fluoro-β-guanidopropionic acid, α-fluoro-β-ureidopropionic acid, and dihydrofluorouracil; exhaled gases (CO_2)

Dosing
Adults: Refer to individual protocols.
Colorectal or gastric metastases:
Intra-arterial: Primarily by an implantable pump: 0.1-0.6 mg/kg/day continuous intra-arterial administration for 14 days then heparinized saline is given for 14 days; toxicity requires dose reduction.
I.V.: Many regimens in use, examples:
0.15 mg/kg/day for 7-14 days
0.5-1 mg/kg/day for 6-15 days
30 mg/kg/day for 5 days, then 15 mg/kg/day every other day, up to 11 days

Elderly: Adjust dose since elderly patients are prone to toxicity.

Renal Impairment: Adjust dose relative to toxicity; patients with renal insufficiency are prone to toxicity.

Available Dosage Forms Injection, powder for reconstitution: 500 mg

Monitoring and Teaching Issues
Physical Assessment: See Warnings/Precautions for use cautions (eg, impaired renal or hepatic function). Assess potential for interactions with other pharmacological agents the patient may be taking (see Drug Interactions). See Administration for infusion specifics. Assess results of laboratory tests, therapeutic effectiveness, and adverse response (eg, CNS changes, acute gastrointestinal reactions; see Adverse Reactions) on a regular basis throughout therapy. Teach patient (caregiver) use and care of implantable pump, possible side effects/appropriate interventions and adverse symptoms to report (see Patient Education).

Monitoring Laboratory Tests: CBC, platelet count, liver function

Patient Education: Do not take any new medication during therapy unless approved by prescriber. This drug is administered by infusion; follow instructions of prescriber for use and care of implantable pump. Avoid alcohol. It is important to maintain adequate hydration (2-3 L/day of fluids) unless instructed to restrict fluid intake and nutrition (small frequent meals may help). You will be more susceptible to infection (avoid crowds and exposure to infection and do not have any vaccinations without consulting prescriber). May cause nausea or vomiting (small frequent meals, frequent mouth care, sucking lozenges, or chewing gum may help); loss of hair (reversible); diarrhea (buttermilk, boiled milk, or yogurt may help reduce diarrhea); mouth sores (use a soft toothbrush or cotton swabs for oral care); or sterility. Increased emotional or physical stress will adversely affect the response
(Continued)

Floxuridine *(Continued)*

to this medication. Notify prescriber if you are experiencing unusual or elevated levels of stress. Report extreme fatigue; pain or numbness in extremities; severe GI upset or diarrhea; bleeding or bruising; fever, chills, or sore throat; vaginal discharge; or signs of fluid retention (eg, swelling extremities, respiratory difficulty, unusual weight gain). **Pregnancy/breast-feeding precautions:** Do not get pregnant while taking this medication and for 1 month following therapy. Consult prescriber for appropriate contraceptives. Do not breast-feed.

Pregnancy Risk Factor: D

Lactation: Excretion in breast milk unknown/contraindicated

Administration

I.V.: For intra-arterial use, use infusion pump, either external or implanted.

Reconstitution: Reconstitute with 5 mL SWI for a final concentration of 100 mg/mL; further dilute in 500-1000 mL D$_5$W or NS for I.V. infusion.

Compatibility: Stable in D$_5$W, NS, SWFI

Y-site administration: Incompatible with allopurinol, cefepime

Storage: Store intact vials at room temperature of 15°C to 30°C (59°F to 86°F). Reconstituted vials are stable for up to 2 weeks under refrigeration at 2°C to 8°C (36°C to 46°C). Further dilution in 500-1000 mL D$_5$W or NS is stable for 2 weeks at room temperature. Solutions in 0.9% sodium chloride are stable in some ambulatory infusion pumps for up to 21 days.

♦ **Flubenisolone** *see Betamethasone on page 185*

Fluconazole *(floo KOE na zole)*

U.S. Brand Names Diflucan®

Generic Available Yes

Pharmacologic Category Antifungal Agent, Oral; Antifungal Agent, Parenteral

Medication Safety Issues

Sound-alike/look-alike issues:

Fluconazole may be confused with flecainide

Diflucan® may be confused with diclofenac, Diprivan®, disulfiram

Use Treatment of candidiasis (vaginal, oropharyngeal, esophageal, urinary tract infections, peritonitis, pneumonia, and systemic infections); cryptococcal meningitis; antifungal prophylaxis in allogeneic bone marrow transplant recipients

Mechanism of Action/Effect Interferes with cytochrome P450 activity, decreasing ergosterol synthesis (principal sterol in fungal cell membrane) and inhibiting cell membrane formation

Contraindications Hypersensitivity to fluconazole, other azoles, or any component of the formulation; concomitant administration with cisapride

Warnings/Precautions Should be used with caution in patients with renal and hepatic dysfunction or previous hepatotoxicity from other azole derivatives. Patients who develop abnormal liver function tests during fluconazole therapy should be monitored closely and discontinued if symptoms consistent with liver disease develop. Use caution in patients at risk of proarrhythmias.

Drug Interactions

Cytochrome P450 Effect: Inhibits CYP1A2 (weak), 2C8/9 (strong), 2C19 (strong), 3A4 (moderate)

Decreased Effect: Rifampin decreases concentrations of fluconazole.

Increased Effect/Toxicity: Concurrent use of fluconazole with cisapride is contraindicated due to the potential for malignant arrhythmias. Fluconazole may increase the levels/effects of amiodarone, selected benzodiazepines, calcium channel blockers, cisapride, citalopram, cyclosporine, diazepam, ergot derivatives, fluoxetine, glimepiride, glipizide, HMG-CoA reductase inhibitors, methsuximide, mirtazapine, nateglinide, nefazodone, phenytoin, pioglitazone, propranolol, rosiglitazone, sertraline, sildenafil (and other PDE-5 inhibitors), tacrolimus, venlafaxine, warfarin, and other substrates of CYP2C8/9, 2C19, and 3A4.

Adverse Reactions Frequency not always defined.

Cardiovascular: Angioedema, pallor, QT prolongation, torsade de pointes

Central nervous system: Headache (2% to 13%), seizure, dizziness

Dermatologic: Rash (2%), alopecia, toxic epidermal necrolysis, Stevens-Johnson syndrome

Endocrine & metabolic: Hypercholesterolemia, hypertriglyceridemia, hypokalemia

Gastrointestinal: Nausea (4% to 7%), vomiting (2%), abdominal pain (2% to 6%), diarrhea (2% to 3%), taste perversion, dyspepsia

Hematologic: Agranulocytosis, leukopenia, neutropenia, thrombocytopenia

Hepatic: Hepatic failure (rare), hepatitis, cholestasis, jaundice, increased ALT/AST, increased alkaline phosphatase

Respiratory: Dyspnea

Miscellaneous: Anaphylactic reactions (rare)

Overdosage/Toxicology Symptoms of overdose include decreased lacrimation, salivation, respiration and motility, urinary incontinence, and cyanosis. Treatment includes supportive measures. A 3-hour hemodialysis will remove 50%.

Pharmacodynamics/Kinetics

Bioavailability: Oral: >90%

Time to Peak: Oral: 1-2 hours

Protein Binding: Plasma: 11% to 12%

Half-Life Elimination: Normal renal function: ~30 hours

Excretion: Urine (80% as unchanged drug)

Dosing

Adults & Elderly: The daily dose of fluconazole is the same for both oral and I.V. administration

Fungal infections: Oral, I.V.: **Note:** Susceptibility for *Candida* is divided into susceptible, susceptible-dose dependent (SDD), and resistant. Increased dose (up to 400 mg/day)

may be used to treat SDD strains, especially when there has been treatment failure at lower doses.

Once-daily dosing by indication: See table.

Fluconazole Once-Daily Dosing – Adults

Indication	Day 1	Daily Therapy	Minimum Duration of Therapy
Oropharyngeal candidiasis (OPC) (long-term suppression)	200 mg	200 mg	Chronic therapy in AIDS patients with history of OPC
Esophageal candidiasis	200 mg	100-200 mg	14-21 d after clinical improvement
Prevention of candidiasis in bone marrow transplant	400 mg	400 mg	3 d before neutropenia, 7 d after neutrophils >1000 cells/mm^3
Urinary candidiasis	--	200 mg	14 d
Candidemia, primary therapy, non-neutropenic	--	400-800 mg	14 d after last positive blood culture and resolution of signs/symptoms
Candidemia, alternative therapy, non-neutropenic	--	800 mg with AmB for 4-7 d, followed by 800 mg/day	14 d after last positive blood culture and resolution of signs/symptoms
Candidemia, secondary, neutropenic	--	6-12 mg/kg/day	14 d after last positive blood culture and resolution of signs/symptoms
Cryptococcal meningitis consolidation (after induction with amphotericin plus flucytosine)	--	400 mg	10 wk
relapse suppression (maintenance)	--	200-400 mg	N/A
Vaginal candidiasis	150 mg	Single dose	N/A

N/A = not applicable. AmB = conventional deoxycholate amphotericin B.

Pediatrics: Fungal infections: Oral, I.V.: Once-daily dosing by indication: See table.

Fluconazole Once-Daily Dosing – Children

Indication	Day 1	Daily Therapy	Minimum Duration of Therapy
Oropharyngeal candidiasis	6 mg/kg	3 mg/kg	14 d
Esophageal candidiasis	6 mg/kg	3-12 mg/kg	21 d and for at least 2 wk following resolution of symptoms
Systemic candidiasis	—	6 mg/kg every 12 hours	28 d
Cryptococcal meningitis acute	12 mg/kg	6-12 mg/kg	10-12 wk after CSF culture becomes negative
relapse suppression	6 mg/kg	6 mg/kg	N/A

N/A = Not applicable.

Renal Impairment:

No adjustment for vaginal candidiasis single-dose therapy

For multiple dosing, administer usual load then adjust daily doses

Cl$_{cr}$ ≤50 mL/minute (no dialysis): Administer 50% of recommended dose or administer every 48 hours.

Hemodialysis: 50% is removed by hemodialysis; administer 100% of daily dose (according to indication) after each dialysis treatment.

Continuous arteriovenous or venovenous hemofiltration: Dose as for Cl$_{cr}$ 10-50 mL/minute.

Available Dosage Forms

Infusion [premixed in sodium chloride]: 2 mg/mL (100 mL, 200 mL)

Diflucan® [premixed in sodium chloride or dextrose] 2 mg/mL (100 mL, 200 mL)

Powder for oral suspension (Diflucan®): 10 mg/mL (35 mL); 40 mg/mL (35 mL) [contains sodium benzoate; orange flavor]

Tablet (Diflucan®): 50 mg, 100 mg, 150 mg, 200 mg

Monitoring and Teaching Issues

Physical Assessment: Obtain cultures and assess allergy history prior to beginning therapy. See Warnings/Precautions for use cautions (eg, renal and hepatic dysfunction). Assess potential for interactions with other pharmacological agents the patient may be taking (eg, potential for toxicities; see Drug Interactions). See Administration specifics for I.V. use. Assess results of laboratory tests (renal and hepatic function) therapeutic effectiveness (resolution of fungal infection), and adverse response (eg, hepatotoxicity [jaundice], skin disorders, abdominal pain; see Adverse Reactions) on a regular basis throughout therapy. Teach patient use (full course of therapy may require weeks or months after symptoms resolve), possible side effects/appropriate interventions, and adverse symptoms to report (see Patient Education).

Monitoring Laboratory Tests: Culture prior to beginning therapy, periodic liver function (AST, ALT, alkaline phosphatase) and renal function, potassium

(Continued)

Fluconazole *(Continued)*

Patient Education: Do not take any new medication during therapy unless approved by prescriber. Take as directed, around-the-clock. It is very important to take full course of medication as ordered even if symptoms resolve. Take with or without food. Follow good hygiene measures to prevent reinfection. Frequent blood tests may be required. Maintain adequate hydration (2-3 L/day of fluids) unless instructed to restrict fluid intake. May cause headache, dizziness, drowsiness (use caution when driving or engaging in tasks that require alertness until response to drug is known); or nausea, vomiting, or diarrhea (small frequent meals, frequent mouth care, sucking lozenges, or chewing gum may help). Report skin rash, redness, or irritation; persistent GI upset; urinary pattern changes; excessively dry eyes or mouth; or changes in color of stool or urine. **Pregnancy/breast-feeding precautions:** Inform prescriber if you are or intend to become pregnant. Consult prescriber if breast-feeding.

Dietary Considerations: Take with or without regard to food.

Geriatric Considerations: Dose may need adjustment based on changes of renal function.

Pregnancy Risk Factor: C

Pregnancy Issues: When used in high doses, fluconazole is teratogenic in animal studies. Following exposure during the first trimester, case reports have noted similar malformations in humans when used in higher doses (400 mg/day) over extended periods of time. Use of lower doses (150 mg as a single dose or 200 mg/day) may have less risk; however, additional data is needed. Use during pregnancy only if the potential benefit to the mother outweighs any potential risk to the fetus.

Lactation: Enters breast/not recommended (AAP rates "compatible")

Breast-Feeding Issues: Fluconazole is found in breast milk at concentration similar to plasma.

Administration

I.M.: For I.V. only; do not administer I.M. or SubQ

I.V.: Do not exceed 200 mg/hour when giving I.V. infusion

Compatibility: Stable in D_5W, LR, NS

Y-site administration: Incompatible with amphotericin B, amphotericin B cholesteryl sulfate complex, ampicillin, calcium gluconate, cefotaxime, ceftazidime, ceftriaxone, cefuroxime, chloramphenicol, clindamycin, co-trimoxazole, diazepam, digoxin, erythromycin lactobionate, furosemide, haloperidol, hydroxyzine, imipenem/cilastatin, pentamidine, piperacillin, ticarcillin

Compatibility when admixed: Incompatible with co-trimoxazole

Storage:
Powder for oral suspension: Store dry powder at ≤30°C (86°F). Following reconstitution, store at 5°C to 30°C (41°F to 86°F). Discard unused portion after 2 weeks. Do not freeze.
Injection: Store injection in glass at 5°C to 30°C (41°F to 86°F). Store injection in Viaflex® at 5°C to 25°C (41°F to 77°F). Protect from freezing. Do not unwrap unit until ready for use.

Related Information
I.V. to Oral Conversion *on page 1688*

Flucytosine *(floo SYE toe seen)*

U.S. Brand Names Ancobon®

Synonyms 5-FC; 5-Flurocytosine

Generic Available No

Pharmacologic Category Antifungal Agent, Oral

Medication Safety Issues
Sound-alike/look-alike issues:
Flucytosine may be confused with fluorouracil
Ancobon® may be confused with Oncovin®

Use Adjunctive treatment of susceptible fungal infections (usually *Candida* or *Cryptococcus*); synergy with amphotericin B for certain fungal infections (*Cryptococcus* spp., *Candida* spp.)

Mechanism of Action/Effect Penetrates fungal cells and interferes with fungal RNA and protein synthesis

Contraindications Hypersensitivity to flucytosine or any component of the formulation

Warnings/Precautions Use with extreme caution in patients with renal dysfunction; dosage adjustment required. Avoid use as monotherapy; resistance rapidly develops. Use with caution in patients with bone marrow depression; patients with hematologic disease or who have been treated with radiation or drugs that suppress the bone marrow may be at greatest risk. Bone marrow toxicity can be irreversible.

Drug Interactions

Decreased Effect: Cytarabine may inactivate flucytosine activity.

Increased Effect/Toxicity: Increased effect with amphotericin B. Amphotericin B-induced renal dysfunction may predispose patient to flucytosine accumulation and myelosuppression.

Nutritional/Ethanol Interactions Food: Food decreases the rate, but not the extent of absorption.

Lab Interactions Flucytosine causes markedly false elevations in serum creatinine values when the Ektachem® analyzer is used.

Adverse Reactions Frequency not defined.
Cardiovascular: Cardiac arrest, myocardial toxicity, ventricular dysfunction, chest pain
Central nervous system: Confusion, headache, hallucinations, dizziness, drowsiness, psychosis, parkinsonism, ataxia, sedation, pyrexia, seizure, fatigue
Dermatologic: Rash, photosensitivity, pruritus, urticaria, Lyell's syndrome
Endocrine & metabolic: Temporary growth failure, hypoglycemia, hypokalemia
Gastrointestinal: Nausea, vomiting, diarrhea, abdominal pain, loss of appetite, dry mouth, hemorrhage, ulcerative colitis
Hematologic: Bone marrow suppression, anemia, leukopenia, thrombocytopenia, agranulocytosis, aplastic anemia, eosinophilia, pancytopenia

Hepatic: Liver enzymes increased, hepatitis, jaundice, azotemia, bilirubin increased

Neuromuscular & skeletal: Peripheral neuropathy, paresthesia, weakness

Otic: Hearing loss

Renal: BUN and serum creatinine increased, renal failure, azotemia, crystalluria

Respiratory: Respiratory arrest, dyspnea

Miscellaneous: Anaphylaxis, allergic reaction

Overdosage/Toxicology Symptoms of overdose include nausea, vomiting, diarrhea, hepatitis, and bone marrow suppression. Treatment is supportive. Removed by hemodialysis.

Pharmacodynamics/Kinetics

Absorption: 75% to 90%

Time to Peak: Serum: ~2-6 hours

Protein Binding: 2% to 4%

Half-Life Elimination: Normal renal function: 2-5 hours; Anuria: 85 hours (range: 30-250); End stage renal disease: 75-200 hours

Metabolism: Minimally hepatic; deaminated, possibly via gut bacteria, to 5-fluorouracil

Excretion: Urine (>90% as unchanged drug)

Dosing

Adults & Elderly: Fungal infections (adjunct): Oral: 50-150 mg/kg/day in divided doses every 6 hours

Pediatrics: Refer to adult dosing.

Renal Impairment: Use lower initial dose:

Cl_{cr} 20-40 mL/minute: Dose every 12 hours

Cl_{cr} 10-20 mL/minute: Dose every 24 hours

Cl_{cr} <10 mL/minute: Dose every 24-48 hours

Hemodialysis: Dialyzable (50% to 100%); administer dose posthemodialysis

Peritoneal dialysis: Adults: Administer 0.5-1 g every 24 hours

Continuous arteriovenous or venovenous hemodiafiltration effects: Dose as for Cl_{cr} 10-50 mL/minute

Available Dosage Forms Capsule: 250 mg, 500 mg

Monitoring and Teaching Issues

Physical Assessment: See Warnings/Precautions for use cautions (eg, renal dysfunction, bone marrow depression, hematologic disease). Assess potential for interactions with other pharmacological agents the patient may be taking (see Drug Interactions). Assess results of laboratory tests prior to and during treatment (see Monitoring Laboratory Tests). Monitor therapeutic effectiveness (resolution of fungal infection) and adverse response (eg, cardiac incidents, CNS changes, bone marrow suppression, jaundice, skin reactions, hearing loss; see Adverse Reactions) on a regular basis throughout therapy. Teach patient use (full course of therapy may require some time after symptoms resolve), possible side effects/appropriate interventions, and adverse symptoms to report (see Patient Education).

Monitoring Laboratory Tests:

Pretreatment: Electrolytes, CBC, BUN, renal function, blood culture

During treatment: CBC and LFTs frequently, serum flucytosine concentration, renal function

Patient Education: Do not take any new medication during therapy unless approved by prescriber. Take capsules one at a time over a few minutes with food to reduce GI upset. It is very important to take full course of medication as ordered even if symptoms resolve. Practice good hygiene measures to prevent reinfection. Frequent blood tests may be required. May cause nausea and vomiting (small frequent meals may help). Report rash; respiratory difficulty; CNS changes (eg, confusion, hallucinations, ataxia, acute headache); yellowing of skin or eyes; changes in color of stool or urine; unresolved diarrhea or anorexia; unusual bleeding, fatigue, or weakness; or other persistent adverse reactions. **Pregnancy/breast-feeding precautions:** Inform prescriber if you are or intend to become pregnant. Breast-feeding is not recommended.

Geriatric Considerations: Adjust for renal function.

Pregnancy Risk Factor: C

Lactation: Excretion in breast milk unknown/not recommended

Administration

Oral: Administer around-the-clock to promote less variation in peak and trough serum levels. To avoid nausea and vomiting, administer a few capsules at a time over 15 minutes until full dose is taken.

Storage: Store at 25°C (77°F). Protect from light.

♦ **Fludara®** see Fludarabine on page 637

Fludarabine (floo DARE a been)

U.S. Brand Names Fludara®

Synonyms Fludarabine Phosphate

Generic Available Yes

Pharmacologic Category Antineoplastic Agent, Antimetabolite (Purine Antagonist)

Medication Safety Issues

Sound-alike/look-alike issues:

Fludarabine may be confused with Flumadine®

Fludara® may be confused with FUDR®

Use Treatment of chronic lymphocytic leukemia (CLL) (including refractory CLL); non-Hodgkin's lymphoma in adults

Unlabeled/Investigational Use Treatment of non-Hodgkin's lymphoma and acute leukemias in pediatric patients; reduced-intensity conditioning regimens prior to allogeneic hematopoietic stem cell transplantation (generally administered in combination with busulfan and antithymocyte globulin or lymphocyte immune globulin, or in combination with melphalan and alemtuzumab)

Mechanism of Action/Effect Inhibits DNA synthesis by inhibition of DNA polymerase and ribonucleotide reductase.

(Continued)

Fludarabine (Continued)

Contraindications Hypersensitivity of fludarabine or any component of the formulation; pregnancy

Warnings/Precautions The U.S. Food and Drug Administration (FDA) currently recommends that procedures for proper handling and disposal of antineoplastic agents be considered. Use with caution with renal insufficiency, patients with a fever, documented infection, or pre-existing hematological disorders (particularly granulocytopenia) or in patients with pre-existing central nervous system disorder (epilepsy), spasticity, or peripheral neuropathy. Life-threatening and sometimes fatal autoimmune hemolytic anemia have occurred. Severe myelosuppression (trilineage bone marrow hypoplasia/aplasia) has been reported (rare); the duration of significant cytopenias in these cases may be prolonged (up to 1 year).

Drug Interactions

Increased Effect/Toxicity: Combined use with pentostatin may lead to severe, even fatal, pulmonary toxicity.

Nutritional/Ethanol Interactions Ethanol: Avoid ethanol (due to GI irritation).

Adverse Reactions

>10%:

Cardiovascular: Edema

Central nervous system: Fatigue, somnolence (30%), chills, pain

Dermatologic: Rash

Hematologic: Myelosuppression, common, dose-limiting toxicity, primarily leukopenia and thrombocytopenia

Nadir: 10-14 days

Recovery: 5-7 weeks

Neuromuscular & skeletal: Paresthesia, myalgia, weakness

1% to 10%:

Cardiovascular: CHF

Central nervous system: Malaise, headache

Dermatologic: Alopecia

Endocrine & metabolic: Hyperglycemia

Gastrointestinal: Anorexia, stomatitis (1.5%), diarrhea (1.8%), mild nausea/vomiting (3% to 10%)

Hematologic: Eosinophilia, hemolytic anemia, may be dose-limiting, possibly fatal in some patients

Overdosage/Toxicology There are clear dose-dependent toxic neurologic effects associated with fludarabine. Doses of 96 mg/m^2/day for 5-7 days are associated with a syndrome characterized by delayed blindness, coma, and death. Symptoms have appeared from 21-60 days following the last dose. Central nervous system toxicity has distinctive features of delayed onset and progressive encephalopathy resulting in fatality. CNS toxicity is reported at an incidence rate of 36% at high doses (≥96 mg/m^2/day for 5-7 days) and <0.2% for low doses (≤125 mg/m^2/course).

Pharmacodynamics/Kinetics

Bioavailability: 75%

Half-Life Elimination: 2-fluoro-vidarabine: 9 hours

Metabolism: I.V.: Fludarabine phosphate is rapidly dephosphorylated to 2-fluoro-vidarabine, which subsequently enters tumor cells and is phosphorylated to the active triphosphate derivative; rapidly dephosphorylated in the serum

Excretion: Urine (60%, 23% as 2-fluoro-vidarabine) within 24 hours

Dosing

Adults & Elderly:

Chronic lymphocytic leukemia: 25 mg/m^2/day for 5 days every 28 days

Non-Hodgkin's lymphoma: Loading dose: 20 mg/m^2 followed by 30 mg/m^2/day for 48 hours

Reduced-intensity conditioning regimens prior to allogeneic hematopoietic stem cell transplantation (unlabeled use): 120-150 mg/m^2 administered in divided doses over 4-5 days

Pediatrics:

Acute leukemia (unlabeled use): 10 mg/m^2 bolus over 15 minutes followed by continuous infusion of 30.5 mg/m^2/day for 5 days **or**

10.5 mg/m^2 bolus over 15 minutes followed by 30.5 mg/m^2/day for 48 hours

Solid tumors (unlabeled use): 9 mg/m^2 bolus followed by 27 mg/m^2/day continuous infusion for 5 days

Renal Impairment:

Cl$_{cr}$ 30-70 mL/minute: Reduce dose by 20%

Cl$_{cr}$ <30 mL/minute: Not recommended

Available Dosage Forms Injection, powder for reconstitution, as phosphate: 50 mg

Monitoring and Teaching Issues

Physical Assessment: Use caution in the presence of renal insufficiency, fever, infection, hematological disorders, central nervous system disorders or peripheral neuropathy (see Warnings/Precautions). See Administration for infusion specifics. Assess results of laboratory tests prior to each treatment and on a regular basis throughout therapy. Monitor patient response closely (especially CNS and neuromuscular effects; see Adverse Reactions and Overdose/Toxicology). Teach patient possible side effects/appropriate interventions and adverse symptoms to report (see Patient Education).

Monitoring Laboratory Tests: CBC with differential, platelet count, AST, ALT, creatinine, serum albumin, uric acid

Patient Education: Do not take any new medication during therapy unless approved by prescriber. This drug can only be administered by infusion. Avoid excessive alcohol during treatment (may increase gastrointestinal irritation). It is important to maintain adequate hydration (2-3 L/day of fluids) unless instructed to restrict fluid intake and nutrition (small frequent meals may help). You will be more susceptible to infection (avoid crowds and exposure to infection and do not have any vaccinations without consulting prescriber). May cause mild nausea or vomiting (small frequent meals, frequent mouth care, sucking lozenges, or chewing gum may help); loss of hair (reversible); diarrhea (buttermilk, boiled milk, or yogurt may help); or mouth sores (use soft toothbrush or cotton swabs for oral care). Report changes in vision; changes in mental alertness; extreme fatigue; pain or numbness in extremities; severe GI upset or diarrhea; bleeding or bruising; fever, chills, or sore throat; vaginal discharge; difficulty or pain on urination; muscle pain or weakness; unusual cough or respiratory difficulty; or other persistent side effects. **Pregnancy/breast-feeding precautions:** Inform prescriber if you are pregnant. Do not get pregnant while taking this medication and for 1 month following therapy. Consult prescriber for appropriate contraceptives. Do not breast-feed.

Pregnancy Risk Factor: D

Lactation: Excretion in breast milk unknown/contraindicated

Administration

I.V.: Administer I.V. over 15-30 minutes or continuous infusion.

Reconstitution: Reconstitute vials with SWI, NS, or D_5W to a concentration of 10-25 mg/mL. Standard I.V. dilution: 50-100 mL D_5W or NS.

Compatibility: Stable in D_5W, NS, SWFI

    Y-site administration: Incompatible Acyclovir, amphotericin B, chlorpromazine, daunorubicin, ganciclovir, hydroxyzine, prochlorperazine edisylate

Storage: Store intact vials under refrigeration (2°C to 8°C). Reconstituted solution is stable for 16 days at room temperature (22°C to 25°C) and under refrigeration (2°C to 8°C). Further dilution in 100 mL D_5W or NS is stable for 48 hours at room temperature or refrigeration.

◆ **Fludarabine Phosphate** *see Fludarabine on page 637*

Fludarocortisone (floo droe KOR ti sone)

U.S. Brand Names Florinef®

Synonyms Fludrocortisone Acetate; Fluohydrisone Acetate; Fluohydrocortisone Acetate; 9α-Fluorohydrocortisone Acetate

Generic Available Yes

Pharmacologic Category Corticosteroid, Systemic

Medication Safety Issues

    Sound-alike/look-alike issues:

        Florinef® may be confused with Fiorinal®

Use Partial replacement therapy for primary and secondary adrenocortical insufficiency in Addison's disease; treatment of salt-losing adrenogenital syndrome

Mechanism of Action/Effect Promotes increased reabsorption of sodium and loss of potassium from renal distal tubules

Contraindications Hypersensitivity to fludrocortisone or any component of the formulation; systemic fungal infections

Warnings/Precautions Taper dose gradually when therapy is discontinued. Patients with Addison's disease are more sensitive to the action of the hormone and may exhibit side effects in an exaggerated degree.

Drug Interactions

    Decreased Effect: Anticholinesterases effects are antagonized. Decreased corticosteroid effects by rifampin, barbiturates, and hydantoins. May decrease salicylate levels.

Adverse Reactions Frequency not defined.

    Cardiovascular: Hypertension, edema, CHF

    Central nervous system: Convulsions, headache, dizziness

    Dermatologic: Acne, rash, bruising

    Endocrine & metabolic: Hypokalemic alkalosis, suppression of growth, hyperglycemia, HPA suppression

    Gastrointestinal: Peptic ulcer

    Neuromuscular & skeletal: Muscle weakness

    Ocular: Cataracts

    Miscellaneous: Diaphoresis, anaphylaxis (generalized)

Overdosage/Toxicology Symptoms of overdose include hypertension, edema, hypokalemia, excessive weight gain. When consumed in excessive quantities, systemic hypercorticism and adrenal suppression may occur. In those cases, discontinuation of the corticosteroid should be done judiciously.

Pharmacodynamics/Kinetics

    Absorption: Rapid and complete

    Time to Peak: Serum: ~1.7 hours

    Protein Binding: 42%

    Half-Life Elimination: Plasma: 30-35 minutes; Biological: 18-36 hours

    Metabolism: Hepatic

Dosing

    Adults & Elderly: Mineralocorticoid deficiency: Oral: 0.05-0.2 mg/day with ranges of 0.1 mg 3 times/week to 0.2 mg/day

    Pediatrics: Mineralocorticoid deficiency: Oral: Infants and Children: 0.05-0.1 mg/day

Available Dosage Forms Tablet, as acetate: 0.1 mg

Monitoring and Teaching Issues

    Physical Assessment: Assess effectiveness and interactions of other medications patient may be taking. Monitor for effectiveness of therapy and adverse reactions according to dose and length of therapy. Assess knowledge/teach patient appropriate use, possible side effects/interventions, and adverse symptoms to report (ie, opportunistic infection, adrenal suppression). Instruct patients with diabetes to monitor serum glucose levels closely; corticosteroids can alter glycemic response. Dose may need to be increased if patient is experiencing higher than normal levels of stress. When discontinuing, taper dose and frequency slowly.

    Monitoring Laboratory Tests: Serum electrolytes, serum renin activity

    Patient Education: Take exactly as directed. Do not take more than prescribed dose and do not discontinue abruptly; consult prescriber. Take with or after meals. Take once-a-day (Continued)

Fludrocortisone *(Continued)*

dose with food in the morning. Limit intake of caffeine or stimulants. Maintain adequate nutrition; consult prescriber for possibility of special dietary recommendations. If you have diabetes, monitor serum glucose closely and notify prescriber of changes; this medication can alter glycemic response. Notify prescriber if you are experiencing higher than normal levels of stress; medication may need adjustment. Periodic ophthalmic examinations will be necessary with long-term use. You will be susceptible to infection (avoid crowds and exposure to infection). You may experience insomnia or nervousness; use caution when driving or engaging in tasks requiring alertness until response to drug is known. Report weakness, change in menstrual pattern, vision changes, signs of hyperglycemia, signs of infection (eg, fever, chills, mouth sores, perianal itching, vaginal discharge), other persistent side effects, or worsening of condition. **Pregnancy/breast-feeding precautions:** Inform prescriber if you are or intend to become pregnant. Consult prescriber if breast-feeding.

Dietary Considerations: Systemic use of mineralocorticoids/corticosteroids may require a diet with increased potassium, vitamins A, B$_6$, C, D, folate, calcium, zinc, and phosphorus, and decreased sodium. With fludrocortisone, a decrease in dietary sodium is often not required as the increased retention of sodium is usually the desired therapeutic effect.

Geriatric Considerations: The most common use of fludrocortisone in the elderly is orthostatic hypotension that is unresponsive to more conservative measures. Attempt nonpharmacologic measures (hydration, support stockings etc) before starting drug therapy.

Pregnancy Risk Factor: C

Lactation: Excretion in breast milk unknown

Administration

Oral: Administration in conjunction with a glucocorticoid is preferable.

Additional Information In patients with salt-losing forms of congenital adrenogenital syndrome, use along with cortisone or hydrocortisone. Fludrocortisone 0.1 mg has sodium retention activity equal to DOCA® 1 mg.

Related Information

Corticosteroids *on page 1731*

♦ **Fludrocortisone Acetate** *see* Fludrocortisone *on page 639*

♦ **Flumadine**® *see* Rimantadine *on page 1329*

Flumazenil *(FLOO may ze nil)*

U.S. Brand Names Romazicon®

Generic Available Yes

Pharmacologic Category Antidote

Use Benzodiazepine antagonist; reverses sedative effects of benzodiazepines used in conscious sedation and general anesthesia; treatment of benzodiazepine overdose

Mechanism of Action/Effect Competitively inhibits the activity at the benzodiazepine recognition site on the GABA/benzodiazepine receptor complex. Flumazenil does not antagonize the CNS effect of drugs affecting GABA-ergic neurons by means other than the benzodiazepine receptor (ethanol, barbiturates, general anesthetics) and does not reverse the effects of opioids.

Contraindications Hypersensitivity to flumazenil, benzodiazepines, or any component of the formulation; patients given benzodiazepines for control of potentially life-threatening conditions (eg, control of intracranial pressure or status epilepticus); patients who are showing signs of serious cyclic-antidepressant overdosage

Warnings/Precautions Benzodiazepine reversal may result in seizures in some patients. Patients who may develop seizures include patients on benzodiazepines for long-term sedation, tricyclic antidepressant overdose patients, concurrent major sedative-hypnotic drug withdrawal, recent therapy with repeated doses of parenteral benzodiazepines, myoclonic jerking or seizure activity prior to flumazenil administration. Flumazenil does not reverse respiratory depression/hypoventilation or cardiac depression. Resedation occurs more frequently in patients where a large single dose or cumulative dose of a benzodiazepine is administered along with a neuromuscular blocking agent and multiple anesthetic agents. Flumazenil should be used with caution in the intensive care unit because of increased risk of unrecognized benzodiazepine dependence in such settings. Should not be used to diagnose benzodiazepine-induced sedation. Reverse neuromuscular blockade before considering use. Flumazenil does not antagonize the CNS effects of other GABA agonists (such as ethanol, barbiturates, or general anesthetics); nor does it reverse narcotics. Use with caution in patients with a history of panic disorder; may provoke panic attacks. Use caution in drug and ethanol-dependent patients; these patients may also be dependent on benzodiazepines. Not recommended for treatment of benzodiazepine dependence. Use with caution in head injury patients. Use caution in patients with mixed drug overdoses; toxic effects of other drugs taken may emerge once benzodiazepine effects are reversed. Flumazenil does not consistently reverse amnesia; patient may not recall verbal instructions after procedure. Use caution in severe hepatic dysfunction and in patients relying on a benzodiazepine for seizure control. Safety and efficacy have not been established in children >1 year of age.

Drug Interactions

Increased Effect/Toxicity: Flumazenil reverses the effects of these nonbenzodiazepine hypnotics (zaleplon, zolpidem, zopiclone).

Adverse Reactions

>10%: Gastrointestinal: Vomiting, nausea

1% to 10%:

Cardiovascular: Palpitations

Central nervous system: Headache, anxiety, nervousness, insomnia, abnormal crying, euphoria, depression, agitation, dizziness, emotional lability, ataxia, depersonalization, increased tears, dysphoria, paranoia, fatigue, vertigo

Endocrine & metabolic: Hot flashes

Gastrointestinal: Xerostomia

Local: Pain at injection site

Neuromuscular & skeletal: Tremor, weakness, paresthesia

Ocular: Abnormal vision, blurred vision

Respiratory: Dyspnea, hyperventilation

Miscellaneous: Diaphoresis

Overdosage/Toxicology Excessively high doses may cause anxiety, agitation, increased muscle tone, hyperesthesia and seizures.

Pharmacodynamics/Kinetics

Onset of Action: 1-3 minutes; 80% response within 3 minutes; Peak effect: 6-10 minutes

Duration of Action: Resedation: ~1 hour; duration related to dose given and benzodiazepine plasma concentrations; reversal effects of flumazenil may wear off before effects of benzodiazepine

Protein Binding: 40% to 50%

Half-Life Elimination: Adults: Alpha: 7-15 minutes; Terminal: 41-79 minutes

Metabolism: Hepatic; dependent upon hepatic blood flow

Excretion: Feces; urine (0.2% as unchanged drug)

Dosing

Adults: See table.

Flumazenil

Adult dosage for **reversal of conscious sedation and general anesthesia:**	
Initial dose	0.2 mg intravenously over 15 seconds
Repeat doses	If desired level of consciousness is not obtained, 0.2 mg may be repeated at 1-minute intervals.
Maximum total cumulative dose	1 mg (usual dose: 0.6-1 mg) **In the event of resedation:** Repeat doses may be given at 20-minute intervals with maximum of 1 mg/dose and 3 mg/hour.
Adult dosage for **suspected benzodiazepine overdose:**	
Initial dose	0.2 mg intravenously over 30 seconds; if the desired level of consciousness is not obtained, 0.3 mg can be given over 30 seconds
Repeat doses	0.5 mg over 30 seconds repeated at 1-minute intervals
Maximum total cumulative dose	3 mg (usual dose: 1-3 mg) Patients with a partial response at 3 mg may require additional titration up to a total dose of 5 mg. If a patient has not responded 5 minutes after cumulative dose of 5 mg, the major cause of sedation is not likely due to benzodiazepines. **In the event of resedation:** May repeat doses at 20-minute intervals with maximum of 1 mg/dose and 3 mg/hour.

Resedation: Repeated doses may be given at 20-minute intervals as needed; repeat treatment doses of 1 mg (at a rate of 0.5 mg/minute) should be given at any time and no more than 3 mg should be given in any hour. After intoxication with high doses of benzodiazepines, the duration of a single dose of flumazenil is not expected to exceed 1 hour; if desired, the period of wakefulness may be prolonged with repeated low intravenous doses of flumazenil, or by an infusion of 0.1-0.4 mg/hour. Most patients with benzodiazepine overdose will respond to a cumulative dose of 1-3 mg and doses >3 mg do not reliably produce additional effects. Rarely, patients with a partial response at 3 mg may require additional titration up to a total dose of 5 mg. **If a patient has not responded 5 minutes after receiving a cumulative dose of 5 mg, the major cause of sedation is not likely to be due to benzodiazepines.**

Elderly: Refer to adult dosing. No differences in safety or efficacy have been reported; however, increased sensitivity may occur in some elderly patients.

Pediatrics:

Reversal of benzodiazepine when used in conscious sedation or general anesthesia:
I.V.: Initial dose: 0.01 mg/kg (maximum dose: 0.2 mg) given over 15 seconds; may repeat 0.01 mg/kg (maximum dose: 0.2 mg) after 45 seconds, and then every minute (maximum: 4 doses) to a maximum of total cumulative dose of 0.05 mg/kg or 1 mg, whichever is lower; usual total dose: 0.08-1 mg (mean: 0.65 mg).

Renal Impairment: Not significantly affected by renal failure (Cl$_{cr}$ <10 mL/minute) or hemodialysis beginning 1 hour after drug administration.

Hepatic Impairment: Initial dose of flumazenil used for initial reversal of benzodiazepine effects is not changed; however, subsequent doses in liver disease patients should be reduced in amount or frequency.

Available Dosage Forms Injection, solution: 0.1 mg/mL (5 mL, 10 mL) [contains edetate sodium]

Monitoring and Teaching Issues

Physical Assessment: Assess level of consciousness frequently. Monitor vital signs and airway closely. ECG monitoring and oxygenation via pulse oximetry is highly recommended. Observe continually for resedation, respiratory depression, preseizure activity, or other residual benzodiazepine effects. May require pain medication sooner after reversal. Assess for nausea and vomiting.

Patient Education: Flumazenil does not consistently reverse amnesia. Do not engage in activities requiring alertness for 18-24 hours after discharge. Avoid alcohol or OTC medications for 24 hours after receiving this medication, unless approved by prescriber. Resedation may occur in patients on long-acting benzodiazepines (such as diazepam). **Pregnancy/breast-feeding precautions:** Inform prescriber if you are or intend to become pregnant. Consult prescriber if breast-feeding.

(Continued)

Flumazenil (Continued)

Pregnancy Risk Factor: C
Lactation: Excretion in breast milk unknown/use caution
Administration
    I.V.: Administer in freely-running I.V. into large vein. Inject over 15 seconds for conscious sedation and general anesthesia and over 30 seconds for overdose.
    Reconstitution: For I.V. use only. Once drawn up in the syringe or mixed with solution use within 24 hours. Discard any unused solution after 24 hours.
    Compatibility: Stable in D_5W, LR, NS
    Storage: Store at 15°C to 30°C (59°F to 86°F).

♦ FluMist™ *see page 1660*

Flunisolide (floo NISS oh lide)

U.S. Brand Names AeroBid®; AeroBid®-M; Nasarel®
Generic Available Yes: Nasal spray
Pharmacologic Category Corticosteroid, Inhalant (Oral); Corticosteroid, Nasal
Medication Safety Issues
    Sound-alike/look-alike issues:
        Flunisolide may be confused with Flumadine®, fluocinonide
        Nasarel® may be confused with Nizoral®
Use Steroid-dependent asthma; nasal solution is used for seasonal or perennial rhinitis
Mechanism of Action/Effect Decreases inflammation by suppression of migration of polymorphonuclear leukocytes and reversal of increased capillary permeability; does not depress hypothalamus
Contraindications Hypersensitivity to flunisolide or any component of the formulation; acute status asthmaticus; viral, tuberculosis, fungal, or bacterial respiratory infections; infections of the nasal mucosa
Warnings/Precautions Not to be used in status asthmaticus or for the relief of acute bronchospasm. May cause suppression of hypothalamic-pituitary-adrenal (HPA) axis, particularly in younger children or in patients receiving high doses for prolonged periods. Fatalities have occurred due to adrenal insufficiency in asthmatic patients during and after transfer from systemic corticosteroids to aerosol steroids; aerosol steroids do **not** provide the systemic steroid needed to treat patients having trauma, surgery, or infections. Withdrawal and discontinuation of the corticosteroid should be done slowly and carefully.

Controlled clinical studies have shown that orally-inhaled and intranasal corticosteroids may cause a reduction in growth velocity in pediatric patients, which appears to be related to dose and duration of exposure.

May suppress the immune system, patients may be more susceptible to infection. Use with caution in patients with systemic infections or ocular herpes simplex. Avoid exposure to chickenpox and measles.
Drug Interactions
    Increased Effect/Toxicity: Expected interactions similar to other corticosteroids
        Salmeterol: The addition of salmeterol has been demonstrated to improve response to inhaled corticosteroids (as compared to increasing steroid dosage).
Adverse Reactions
    >10%:
        Cardiovascular: Pounding heartbeat
        Central nervous system: Dizziness, headache, nervousness
        Dermatologic: Itching, rash
        Endocrine & metabolic: Adrenal suppression, menstrual problems
        Gastrointestinal: GI irritation, anorexia, sore throat, bitter taste
        Local: Nasal burning, *Candida* infection of the nose or pharynx, atrophic rhinitis
        Respiratory: Sneezing, cough, upper respiratory tract infection, bronchitis, nasal congestion, nasal dryness
        Miscellaneous: Increased susceptibility to infection
    1% to 10%:
        Central nervous system: Insomnia, psychic changes
        Dermatologic: Acne, urticaria
        Gastrointestinal: Increase in appetite, xerostomia, dry throat, loss of taste perception
        Ocular: Cataracts
        Respiratory: Epistaxis
        Miscellaneous: Diaphoresis, loss of smell
Overdosage/Toxicology When consumed in high doses over prolonged periods, systemic hypercorticism and adrenal suppression may occur. In those cases, discontinuation of the corticosteroid should be done judiciously.
Pharmacodynamics/Kinetics
    Absorption: Nasal inhalation: ~50%
    Bioavailability: 40% to 50%
    Half-Life Elimination: 1.8 hours
    Metabolism: Rapidly hepatic to active metabolites
    Excretion: Urine and feces (equal amounts)
Dosing
    Adults & Elderly:
        Asthma: Oral inhalation: 2 inhalations twice daily (morning and evening) up to 8 inhalations/day maximum
        Seasonal allergic rhinitis: Nasal: 2 sprays in each nostril twice daily (morning and evening); maximum: 8 sprays/day in each nostril
    Pediatrics:
        Asthma (Children >6 years): Oral inhalation: 2 inhalations twice daily (morning and evening) up to 4 inhalations/day

Seasonal allergic rhinitis (Children >6 years): Intranasal: 1 spray each nostril twice daily (morning and evening), not to exceed 4 sprays/day each nostril

Available Dosage Forms

Aerosol for oral inhalation:
AeroBid®: 250 mcg/actuation (7 g) [100 metered doses; contains CFCs]
AeroBid®-M: 250 mcg/actuation (7 g) [100 metered doses; contains CFCs; menthol flavor]
Solution, intranasal spray (Nasarel®): 25 mcg/actuation (25 mL) [200 sprays; contains benzalkonium chloride]

Monitoring and Teaching Issues

Physical Assessment: Not to be used to treat status asthmaticus or fungal infections of nasal passages. Monitor therapeutic effectiveness and adverse reactions. When changing from systemic steroids to inhalational steroid, taper reduction of systemic medication slowly. Assess knowledge/teach patient appropriate use, interventions to reduce side effects, and adverse symptoms to report.

Patient Education: Use as directed; do not use nasal preparations for oral inhalation. Do not increase dosage or discontinue abruptly without consulting prescriber. Review use of inhaler or spray with prescriber or follow package insert for directions. Keep oral inhaler clean and unobstructed. Always rinse mouth and throat after use of inhaler to prevent opportunistic infection. If you are also using an inhaled bronchodilator, wait 10 minutes before using this steroid aerosol. You may experience dizziness, anxiety, or blurred vision (rise slowly from sitting or lying position and use caution when driving or engaging in tasks requiring alertness until response to drug is known); or taste disturbance or aftertaste (frequent mouth care and mouth rinses may help). Report pounding heartbeat or chest pain; acute nervousness or inability to sleep; severe sneezing or nosebleed; respiratory difficulty, sore throat, hoarseness, or bronchitis; respiratory difficulty or bronchospasms; disturbed menstrual pattern; vision changes; loss of taste or smell perception; or worsening of condition or lack of improvement. **Pregnancy/breast-feeding precautions:** Inform prescriber if you are or intend to become pregnant. Consult prescriber if breast-feeding.

Inhaler: Sit when using. Take deep breaths for 3-5 minutes, and clear nasal passages before administration (use decongestant as needed). Hold breath for 5-10 seconds after use, and wait 1-3 minutes between inhalations. Follow package insert instructions for use. Do not exceed maximum dosage. If also using inhaled bronchodilator, use before flunisolide. Rinse mouth and throat after use to reduce aftertaste and prevent candidiasis.

Geriatric Considerations: Many elderly patients have difficulty using metered dose inhalers, which can limit their effectiveness. Assess technique in all older patients. A spacer device may be beneficial for the oral inhaler.

Pregnancy Risk Factor: C

Lactation: Excretion in breast milk unknown/use caution

Administration

Inhalation: Shake well before using. Do not use Nasalide® or Nasarel® orally. Throw out product after it has been opened for 3 months.

Additional Information Does not contain fluorocarbons; contains polyethylene glycol vehicle.

Effects of inhaled/intranasal steroids on growth have been observed in the absence of laboratory evidence of HPA axis suppression, suggesting that growth velocity is a more sensitive indicator of systemic corticosteroid exposure in pediatric patients than some commonly used tests of HPA axis function. The long-term effects of this reduction in growth velocity associated with orally-inhaled and intranasal corticosteroids, including the impact on final adult height, are unknown. The potential for "catch up" growth following discontinuation of treatment with inhaled corticosteroids has not been adequately studied.

Related Information

Asthma *on page 1799*
Inhalant Agents *on page 1734*

Fluocinolone (floo oh SIN oh lone)

U.S. Brand Names Capex™; Derma-Smoothe/FS®; Synalar®

Synonyms Fluocinolone Acetonide

Generic Available Yes; Excludes oil, shampoo

Pharmacologic Category Corticosteroid, Topical

Medication Safety Issues

Sound-alike/look-alike issues:
Fluocinolone may be confused with fluocinonide

Use Relief of susceptible inflammatory dermatosis [low, medium, high potency topical corticosteroid]; psoriasis of the scalp; atopic dermatitis in children ≥2 years of age

Mechanism of Action/Effect Topical corticosteroid with anti-inflammatory, antipruritic, and vasoconstrictive properties.

Contraindications Hypersensitivity to fluocinolone or any component of the formulation; TB of skin, herpes (including varicella)

Warnings/Precautions Adverse systemic effects may occur when used on large areas of the body, denuded areas, for prolonged periods of time, with an occlusive dressing, and/or in infants or small children. Infants and small children may be more susceptible to adrenal axis suppression from topical corticosteroid therapy. Derma-Smoothe/FS® contains peanut oil; use caution in peanut-sensitive children.

Adverse Reactions Frequency not defined.

Dermatologic: Acneiform eruptions, allergic contact dermatitis, burning, dryness, folliculitis, irritation, itching, hypertrichosis, hypopigmentation, miliaria, perioral dermatitis, skin atrophy, striae

Endocrine & metabolic: Cushing's syndrome, HPA axis suppression

Miscellaneous: Secondary infection

Overdosage/Toxicology Topically-applied products may be absorbed in sufficient amounts to produce systemic effects, particularly if applied to large surface area or to inflamed/
(Continued)

Fluocinolone *(Continued)*

damaged skin. Systemic hypercorticism and adrenal suppression may occur; in those cases, discontinuation and withdrawal of the corticosteroid should be done judiciously.

Pharmacodynamics/Kinetics

Absorption: Dependent on strength of preparation, amount applied, nature of skin at application site, vehicle, and use of occlusive dressing; increased in areas of skin damage, inflammation, or occlusion

Metabolism: Primarily in skin; small amount absorbed into systemic circulation is primarily hepatic to inactive compounds

Excretion: Urine (primarily as glucuronide and sulfate, also as unconjugated products); feces (small amounts)

Dosing

Adults & Elderly:

Corticosteroid-responsive dermatoses: Topical: Cream, ointment, solution: Apply a thin layer to affected area 2-4 times/day; may use occlusive dressings to manage psoriasis or recalcitrant conditions

Atopic dermatitis (Derma-Smoothe/FS®): Topical: Apply thin film to affected area 3 times/day

Scalp psoriasis (Derma-Smoothe/FS®): Topical: Massage thoroughly into wet or damp-ened hair/scalp; cover with shower cap. Leave on overnight (or for at least 4 hours). Remove by washing hair with shampoo and rinsing thoroughly.

Seborrheic dermatitis of the scalp (Capex™): Topical: Apply no more than 1 ounce to scalp once daily; work into lather and allow to remain on scalp for ~5 minutes. Remove from hair and scalp by rinsing thoroughly with water.

Pediatrics: Children ≥2 years:

Atopic dermatitis (Derma-Smoothe/FS®): Topical: Moisten skin; apply to affected area twice daily; do not use for longer than 4 weeks

Corticosteroid-responsive dermatoses: Refer to adult dosing.

Available Dosage Forms

Cream, as acetonide: 0.01% (15 g, 60 g); 0.025% (15 g, 60 g)
  Synalar®: 0.025% (15 g, 60 g)

Oil, as acetonide:
  Derma-Smoothe/FS® [eczema oil]: 0.01% (120 mL) [contains peanut oil]
  Derma-Smoothe/FS® [scalp oil]: 0.01% (120 mL) [contains peanut oil; packaged with shower caps]

Ointment, as acetonide (Synalar®): 0.025% (15 g, 60 g)

Shampoo, as acetonide (Capex™): 0.01% (120 mL)

Solution, as acetonide: 0.01% (60 mL)
  Synalar®: 0.01% (20 mL, 60 mL)

Monitoring and Teaching Issues

Physical Assessment: Assess potential for interactions with other prescriptions, OTC medications, or herbal products patient may be taking. Assess patient response. Teach patient proper use (according to formulation), side effects/appropriate interventions, and symptoms to report.

Patient Education: For external use only. Do not use for eyes, mucous membranes, or open wounds. Use exactly as directed and for no longer than the period prescribed. Before using, wash and dry area gently. Apply in a thin layer (may rub in lightly). Apply light dressing (if necessary) to area being treated. Do not use occlusive dressing unless so advised by prescriber. Avoid prolonged or excessive use around sensitive tissues, genital, or rectal areas. Avoid exposing treated area to direct sunlight. Inform prescriber if condition worsens (redness, swelling, irritation, signs of infection, or open sores) or fails to improve. **Pregnancy/breast-feeding precautions:** Inform prescriber if you are or intend to become pregnant. Consult prescriber if breast-feeding.

Pregnancy Risk Factor: C

Pregnancy Issues: In general, the use of topical corticosteroids during pregnancy is not considered to have significant risk, however, intrauterine growth retardation in the infant has been reported (rare). The use of large amounts or for prolonged periods of time should be avoided.

Lactation: Excretion in breast milk unknown/use caution

Breast-Feeding Issues: Systemic corticosteroids are excreted in human milk. It is not known if sufficient quantities of fluocinolone are absorbed following topical administration to produce detectable amounts in breast milk. Hypertension in the nursing infant has been reported following corticosteroid ointment applied to the nipples. Use with caution.

Administration

Topical: Apply thin film to affected area; avoid eyes.

Reconstitution: Capex™: Prior to dispensing, the contents of the capsule should be emptied into the liquid shampoo; shake well. Discard after 3 months.

Storage: Store at controlled room temperature in tightly-closed container.

Related Information

Corticosteroids *on page 1731*

♦ **Fluocinolone Acetonide** *see* Fluocinolone *on page 643*

Fluocinolone, Hydroquinone, and Tretinoin

(floo oh SIN oh lone, HYE droe kwin one, & TRET i noyn)

U.S. Brand Names Tri-Luma™

Synonyms Hydroquinone, Fluocinolone Acetonide, and Tretinoin; Tretinoin, Fluocinolone Acetonide, and Hydroquinone

Generic Available No

Pharmacologic Category Corticosteroid, Topical; Depigmenting Agent; Retinoic Acid Derivative

Use Short-term treatment of moderate to severe melasma of the face

Dosing

Adults & Elderly: Melasma: Topical: Apply a thin film once daily to hyperpigmented areas of melasma (including ¹/₂ inch of normal-appearing surrounding skin). Apply 30 minutes prior to bedtime; not indicated for use beyond 8 weeks. Do not use occlusive dressings.

Renal Impairment: No dosage adjustment required.

Available Dosage Forms Cream, topical: Hydroquinone 4%, tretinoin 0.05%, fluocinolone acetonide 0.01% (30 g) [contains sodium metabisulfite]

Monitoring and Teaching Issues

Physical Assessment: Assess potential for interactions with other prescriptions, OTC medications, or herbal products patient may be taking (eg, anything with photosensitizing effect). Assess therapeutic effectiveness and adverse response. Teach patient use, possible side effects/interventions, and adverse symptoms to report.

Patient Education: This medication is for topical (skin) use only. Use exactly as directed (see below). Do not overuse or use for a longer period of time than prescribed. You will be sensitive to sunlight (avoid sunlight, wear sunscreen with SPF 30, and wear protective clothing); and sensitive to irritating skin products or cosmetics (avoid medicated preparations or agents with irritating or drying effects, you may use moisturizers and/or nonirritating cosmetics during the day). You may experience irritation and sensitivity to temperature changes, or excess bleaching effects. Report persistent burning, irritation, or eruptions on the skin; or if the condition being treated worsens or does not improve.

Application: Wash hands before beginning. Wash face with mild cleanser, rinse, and pat dry. Apply medication sparingly, in a very light film, rub in lightly. Avoid any contact with open or abraded skin, mucous membranes, eyes, mouth, or nose.

Pregnancy/breast-feeding precautions: Inform prescriber if you are or intend to become pregnant. Consult prescriber if breast-feeding.

Pregnancy Risk Factor: C

Lactation: Excretion in breast milk unknown/use caution

Related Information

Fluocinolone *on page 643*
Hydroquinone *on page 768*
Tretinoin (Oral) *on page 1514*
Tretinoin (Topical) *on page 1516*

Fluocinonide (floo oh SIN oh nide)

U.S. Brand Names Lidex®; Lidex-E®; Vanos™

Generic Available Yes

Pharmacologic Category Corticosteroid, Topical

Medication Safety Issues

Sound-alike/look-alike issues:

Fluocinonide may be confused with flunisolide, fluocinolone

Lidex® may be confused with Lasix®, Videx®, Wydase®

Use Anti-inflammatory, antipruritic; treatment of plaque-type psoriasis (up to 10% of body surface area) [high-potency topical corticosteroid]

Contraindications Hypersensitivity to fluocinonide or any component of the formulation; viral, fungal, or tubercular skin lesions; herpes simplex

Warnings/Precautions Adverse systemic effects may occur when used on large areas of the body, denuded areas, for prolonged periods of time, with an occlusive dressing, and/or in infants or small children. Pediatric patients may be more susceptible to HPA axis suppression. Lower-strength cream (0.05%) may be used cautiously on face or opposing skin surfaces that may rub or touch (eg, skin folds of the groin, axilla, and breasts); higher-strength (0.1%) should not be used on the face, groin, or axillae. Use of the 0.1% cream for >2 weeks or in patients <18 years of age is not recommended.

Drug Interactions

Increased Effect/Toxicity: No data reported. Concomitant use with other corticosteroids (by any route) may increase the risk of HPA axis suppression.

Adverse Reactions Frequency not defined.

Cardiovascular: Intracranial hypertension

Dermatologic: Acne, allergic dermatitis, contact dermatitis, dry skin, folliculitis, hypertrichosis, hypopigmentation, maceration of the skin, miliaria, perioral dermatitis, pruritus, skin atrophy, striae, telangiectasia

Endocrine & metabolic: Cushing's syndrome, growth retardation, HPA suppression, hyperglycemia

Local: Burning, irritation

Renal: Glycosuria

Miscellaneous: Secondary infection

Pharmacodynamics/Kinetics

Absorption: Dependent on strength of product, amount applied, and nature of skin at application site; ranges from ~1% in areas of thick stratum corneum (palms, soles, elbows, etc) to 36% in areas of thin stratum corneum (face, eyelids, etc); increased in areas of skin damage, inflammation, or occlusion

Metabolism: Primarily in skin; small amount absorbed into systemic circulation is primarily hepatic to inactive compounds

Excretion: Urine (primarily as glucuronide and sulfate, also as unconjugated products); feces (small amounts as metabolites)

Dosing

Adults & Elderly:

Pruritus and inflammation: Topical (0.5% cream): Apply thin layer to affected area 2-4 times/day depending on the severity of the condition. Therapy should be discontinued when control is achieved; if no improvement is seen, reassessment of diagnosis may be necessary.

Plaque-type psoriasis (Vanos™): Topical (0.1% cream): Apply a thin layer once or twice daily to affected areas (limited to <10% of body surface area). **Note:** Not recommended
(Continued)

Fluocinonide (Continued)

for use >2 consecutive weeks or >60 g/week total exposure. Discontinue when control is achieved.

Pediatrics: Refer to adult dosing.

Available Dosage Forms
Cream, anhydrous, emollient (Lidex®): 0.05% (15 g, 30 g, 60 g)
Cream, aqueous, emollient (Lidex-E®): 0.05% (15 g, 30 g, 60 g)
Cream (Vanos™): 0.01% (30 g, 60 g)
Gel (Lidex®): 0.05% (15 g, 30 g, 60 g)
Ointment (Lidex®): 0.05% (15 g, 30 g, 60 g)
Solution (Lidex®): 0.05% (60 mL) [contains alcohol 35%]

Monitoring and Teaching Issues
Physical Assessment: Assess potential for interactions with other prescriptions, OTC medications, or herbal products patient may be taking. Assess patient response. Teach patient proper use (according to formulation), side effects/appropriate interventions, and symptoms to report.

Patient Education: For external use only. Do not use for eyes, mucous membranes, or open wounds. Use exactly as directed and for no longer than the period prescribed. Before using, wash and dry area gently. Apply in a thin layer (may rub in lightly). Apply light dressing (if necessary) to area being treated. Do not use occlusive dressing unless so advised by prescriber. Avoid prolonged or excessive use around sensitive tissues, genital, or rectal areas. Avoid exposing treated area to direct sunlight. Inform prescriber if condition worsens (redness, swelling, irritation, signs of infection, or open sores) or fails to improve.

Pregnancy precaution: Inform prescriber if you are or intend to become pregnant.

Pregnancy Risk Factor: C

Related Information
Corticosteroids *on page 1731*

- ◆ **Fluohydrisone Acetate** *see* Fludrocortisone *on page 639*
- ◆ **Fluohydrocortisone Acetate** *see* Fludrocortisone *on page 639*
- ◆ **Fluoracaine® Ophthalmic** *see page 1625*
- ◆ **Fluorescein Sodium** *see page 1625*
- ◆ **Fluorets® Ophthalmic Strips** *see page 1625*
- ◆ **Fluor-I-Strip®** *see page 1625*
- ◆ **Fluor-I-Strip-AT®** *see page 1625*
- ◆ **Fluorodeoxyuridine** *see* Floxuridine *on page 632*
- ◆ **9α-Fluorohydrocortisone Acetate** *see* Fludrocortisone *on page 639*

Fluorometholone (flure oh METH oh lone)

U.S. Brand Names Eflone® [DSC]; Flarex®; Fluor-Op® [DSC]; FML®; FML® Forte

Generic Available Yes: Suspension (as base)

Pharmacologic Category Corticosteroid, Ophthalmic

Use Treatment of steroid-responsive inflammatory conditions of the eye

Mechanism of Action/Effect Decreases inflammation by suppression of migration of polymorphonuclear leukocytes and reversal of increased capillary permeability

Contraindications Hypersensitivity to fluorometholone or any component of the formulation; viral diseases of the cornea and conjunctiva (including epithelial herpes simplex keratitis, vaccinia and varicella); mycobacterial or fungal infections of the eye; untreated eye infections which may be masked/enhanced by a steroid

Warnings/Precautions Not recommended in children <2 years of age. Prolonged use may result in glaucoma, elevated intraocular pressure, or other ocular damage. May exacerbate severity of viral infections, use caution in patients with history of herpes simplex. Re-evaluate after 2 days if symptoms have not improved. May delay healing following cataract surgery. Some products contain sulfites.

Adverse Reactions Frequency not defined.
Ocular: Anterior uveitis, burning upon application, cataract formation, conjunctival hyperemia, conjunctivitis, corneal ulcers, glaucoma with optic nerve damage, perforation of the globe, secondary ocular infection (bacterial, fungal, viral), intraocular pressure elevation, visual acuity and field defects, keratitis, mydriasis, stinging upon application, delayed wound healing
Miscellaneous: Systemic hypercorticoidism (rare) and taste perversion have also been reported

Overdosage/Toxicology When consumed in high doses over prolonged periods, systemic hypercorticism and adrenal suppression may occur. In those cases, discontinuation of the corticosteroid should be done judiciously.

Pharmacodynamics/Kinetics
Absorption: Into aqueous humor with slight systemic absorption

Dosing
Adults & Elderly:
Ocular inflammation: Ophthalmic:
Ointment: Apply small amount (~½ inch ribbon) to conjunctival sac every 4 hours in severe cases; 1-3 times/day in mild to moderate cases.
Solution: Instill 1-2 drops into conjunctival sac every hour during day, every 2 hours at night until favorable response is obtained, then use 1 drop every 4 hours; for mild to moderate inflammation, instill 1-2 drops into conjunctival sac 2-4 times/day.
Note: Re-evaluate therapy if improvement is not seen within 2 days; use care not to discontinue prematurely; in chronic conditions, gradually decrease dosing frequency prior to discontinuing treatment.
Pediatrics: Children >2 years: Refer to adult dosing.

Available Dosage Forms [DSC] = Discontinued product
Ointment, ophthalmic, as base (FML®): 0.1% (3.5 g)
Suspension, ophthalmic, as base: (5 mL, 10 mL, 15 mL)

Fluor-Op®: 0.1% (5 mL, 10 mL, 15 mL) [contains benzalkonium chloride and polyvinyl alcohol] [DSC]

FML®: 0.1% (5 mL, 10 mL, 15 mL) [contains benzalkonium chloride]

FML® Forte: 0.25% (2 mL, 5 mL, 10 mL, 15 mL) [contains benzalkonium chloride]

Suspension, ophthalmic, as acetate:

Eflone®: 0.1% (5 mL, 10 mL) [DSC]

Flarex®: 0.1% (5 mL, 10 mL) [contains benzalkonium chloride]

Monitoring and Teaching Issues

Physical Assessment: Monitor intraocular pressure in patients with glaucoma or when used for ≥10 days; monitor for presence of secondary infections (including the development of fungal infections and exacerbation of viral infections). Assess knowledge/teach patient appropriate use, interventions to reduce side effects, and adverse symptoms to report.

Patient Education: For ophthalmic use only. Apply prescribed amount as often as directed. Wash hands before using. Wipe away excess from skin around eye. Do not use any other eye preparation for at least 10 minutes. Do not touch tip of applicator to eye or any other surface. Do not share medication with anyone else. May cause sensitivity to bright light (dark glasses may help); temporary stinging or blurred vision may occur. Do not wear contacts during administration and for 15 minutes after. Inform prescriber if you experience eye pain, redness, burning, watering, dryness, double vision, puffiness around eye, vision changes, or other adverse eye response; worsening of condition or lack of improvement.

Ointment: Gently squeeze the tube to apply to inside of lower lid. Close eye for 1-2 minutes and roll eyeball in all directions.

Suspension: Shake well before using. Tilt head back and look upward. Gently pull down lower lid and put drop(s) in inner corner of eye. Close eye and roll eyeball in all directions. Do not blink for 30 seconds. Apply gentle pressure to inner corner of eye for 30 seconds.

Pregnancy/breast-feeding precautions: Inform prescriber if you are pregnant. Consult prescriber if breast-feeding.

Pregnancy Risk Factor: C

Lactation: Excretion in breast milk unknown/use caution

Administration

Storage: Store at room temperature.

♦ **Fluorometholone and Sulfacetamide** *see* Sulfacetamide Sodium and Fluorometholone *on page 1405*

♦ **Fluor-Op® [DSC]** *see* Fluorometholone *on page 646*

♦ **Fluoroplex®** *see* Fluorouracil *on page 647*

Fluorouracil (flure oh YOOR a sil)

U.S. Brand Names Adrucil®; Carac™; Efudex®; Fluoroplex®

Synonyms 5-Fluorouracil; FU; 5-FU

Generic Available Yes: Injection, topical solution

Pharmacologic Category Antineoplastic Agent, Antimetabolite

Medication Safety Issues

Sound-alike/look-alike issues:

Fluorouracil may be confused with flucytosine

Efudex® may be confused with Efidac (Efidac 24®), Eurax®

Use Treatment of carcinomas of the breast, colon, head and neck, pancreas, rectum, or stomach; topically for the management of actinic or solar keratoses and superficial basal cell carcinomas

Mechanism of Action/Effect Interferes with DNA synthesis by blocking the methylation of deoxyuricytic acid.

Contraindications Hypersensitivity to fluorouracil or any component of the formulation; poor nutritional status; depressed bone marrow function; thrombocytopenia; potentially serious infections; major surgery within the previous month; dihydropyrimidine dehydrogenase (DPD) enzyme deficiency; pregnancy

Warnings/Precautions The U.S. Food and Drug Administration (FDA) currently recommends that procedures for proper handling and disposal of antineoplastic agents be considered. Use with caution in patients who have had high-dose pelvic radiation or previous use of alkylating agents. Use with caution in patients with impaired kidney or liver function. The drug should be discontinued if intractable vomiting or diarrhea, precipitous fall in leukocyte or platelet counts or myocardial ischemia occurs. Systemic toxicity normally associated with parenteral administration (including neutropenia, neurotoxicity, and gastrointestinal toxicity) has been associated with topical use particularly in patients with a genetic deficiency of dihydropyrimidine dehydrogenase (DPD).

Drug Interactions

Increased Effect/Toxicity: Fluorouracil may increase effects of warfarin.

Nutritional/Ethanol Interactions

Ethanol: Avoid ethanol (due to GI irritation).

Herb/Nutraceutical: Avoid black cohosh, dong quai in estrogen-dependent tumors.

Adverse Reactions Toxicity depends on route and duration of treatment

I.V.:

Cardiovascular: Angina, myocardial ischemia, nail changes

Central nervous system: Acute cerebellar syndrome, confusion, disorientation, euphoria, headache, nystagmus

Dermatologic: Alopecia, dermatitis, dry skin, fissuring, palmar-plantar erythrodysesthesia syndrome, pruritic maculopapular rash, photosensitivity, vein pigmentations

Gastrointestinal: Anorexia, bleeding, diarrhea, esophagopharyngitis, nausea, sloughing, stomatitis, ulceration, vomiting

Hematologic: Agranulocytosis, anemia, leukopenia, pancytopenia, thrombocytopenia

Myelosuppression:

Onset: 7-10 days

Nadir: 9-14 days

(Continued)

Fluorouracil *(Continued)*

    Recovery: 21-28 days
    Local: Thrombophlebitis
    Ocular: Lacrimation, lacrimal duct stenosis, photophobia, visual changes
    Respiratory: Epistaxis
    Miscellaneous: Anaphylaxis, generalized allergic reactions, loss of nails

Topical: Note: Systemic toxicity normally associated with parenteral administration (including neutropenia, neurotoxicity, and gastrointestinal toxicity) has been associated with topical use particularly in patients with a genetic deficiency of dihydropyrimidine dehydrogenase (DPD).
    Central nervous system: Headache, telangiectasia
    Dermatologic: Photosensitivity, pruritus, rash, scarring
    Hematologic: Leukocytosis
    Local: Allergic contact dermatitis, burning, crusting, dryness, edema, erosion, erythema, hyperpigmentation, irritation, pain, soreness, ulceration
    Ocular: Eye irritation (burning, watering, sensitivity, stinging, itching)
    Miscellaneous: Birth defects, miscarriage

Overdosage/Toxicology Symptoms of overdose include myelosuppression, nausea, vomiting, diarrhea, and alopecia. No specific antidote exists. Monitor hematologically for at least 4 weeks. Treatment is supportive.

Pharmacodynamics/Kinetics

Duration of Action: ~3 weeks

Bioavailability: <75%, erratic and undependable

Half-Life Elimination: Biphasic: Initial: 6-20 minutes; two metabolites, FdUMP and FUTP, have prolonged half-lives depending on the type of tissue

Metabolism: Hepatic (90%) via dehydrogenase enzyme; FU must be metabolized to be active

Excretion: Lung (large amounts as CO_2); urine (5% as unchanged drug) in 6 hours

Dosing

Adults & Elderly:
Refer to individual protocols.
    I.V. bolus: 500-600 mg/m² every 3-4 weeks **or**
    425 mg/m² on days 1-5 every 4 weeks
    Continuous I.V. infusion: 1000 mg/m²/day for 4-5 days every 3-4 weeks **or**
    2300-2600 mg/m² on day 1 every week **or**
    300-400 mg/m²/day **or**
    225 mg/m²/day for 5-8 weeks (with radiation therapy)
Actinic keratoses: Topical:
    Carac™: Apply thin film to lesions once daily for up to 4 weeks, as tolerated
    Efudex®: Apply to lesions twice daily for 2-4 weeks; complete healing may not be evident for 1-2 months following treatment
    Fluoroplex®: Apply to lesions twice daily for 2-6 weeks
Basal cell carcinoma: Topical: Efudex®: Apply to affected lesions twice daily for 3-6 weeks; treatment may be continued for up to 10-12 weeks
Pediatrics: Refer to adult dosing.
Renal Impairment: Hemodialysis: Administer dose following hemodialysis.
Hepatic Impairment: Bilirubin >5 mg/dL: Omit use.

Available Dosage Forms

Cream, topical:
    Carac™: 0.5% (30 g)
    Efudex®: 5% (25 g, 40 g)
    Fluoroplex®: 1% (30 g) [contains benzyl alcohol]
Injection, solution: 50 mg/mL (10 mL, 20 mL, 50 mL, 100 mL)
    Adrucil®: 50 mg/mL (10 mL, 50 mL, 100 mL)
Solution, topical (Efudex®): 2% (10 mL); 5% (10 mL)

Monitoring and Teaching Issues

Physical Assessment: Note specific Warnings/Precautions for use cautions. Assess potential for interactions with other pharmacological agents or herbal products the patient may be taking (see Drug Interactions). Assess results of laboratory tests prior to each infusion and regularly with all formulations, including topical use. Assess patient response (eg, cardiovascular, respiratory, and renal function; see Adverse Reactions and Overdose/Toxicology) prior to each infusion and on a regular basis throughout therapy. **Note:** The drug should be discontinued if intractable vomiting or diarrhea, precipitous fall in leukocyte or platelet counts, or myocardial ischemia occurs. Teach patient proper use (oral or topical application), possible side effects/appropriate interventions (eg, importance of adequate hydration), and adverse symptoms to report (see Patient Education). **Pregnancy risk factor D/X:** Determine that patient is not pregnant before starting therapy. Do not give to females of childbearing age unless patient is capable of complying with contraceptive use. Male/female: Advise patient about contraceptive measures as appropriate.

Monitoring Laboratory Tests: CBC with differential, platelet count, renal and liver function

Patient Education: Do not take any new medication during therapy without consulting prescriber. Avoid excessive alcohol (may increase gastrointestinal irritation). Maintain adequate hydration (2-3 L/day of fluids) unless instructed to restrict fluid intake and nutrition (small frequent meals may help). May cause sensitivity to sunlight (use sunblock, wear protective clothing, and avoid direct sunlight); susceptibility to infection (avoid crowds and exposure to infection); nausea, vomiting, diarrhea, or loss of appetite (small frequent meals may help; request medication); weakness, lethargy, dizziness, decreased vision (use caution when driving or engaging in tasks requiring alertness until response to drug is known); or headache (request medication). Report signs and symptoms of infection (eg, fever, chills, sore throat, burning urination, vaginal itching or discharge, fatigue, mouth sores); bleeding (eg, black or tarry stools, easy bruising, unusual bleeding); vision changes; unremitting nausea, vomiting, or abdominal pain; CNS changes; respiratory difficulty; chest pain or palpitations; severe skin reactions to topical application; or any other adverse reactions.

Topical: Use as directed; do not overuse. Wash hands thoroughly before and after applying medication. Avoid contact with eyes, nostrils, and mouth. Avoid occlusive dressings; use a porous dressing. May cause local reaction (pain, burning, or swelling), if severe contact prescriber.

Oral solution: may be mixed in water, grape juice, or carbonated beverage. It is generally best to drink undiluted solution, then rinse the mouth. CocaCola® has been recommended as the "best chaser" for oral fluorouracil.

Pregnancy/breast-feeding precautions: Inform prescriber if you are pregnant. Do not get pregnant during or for 1 month following therapy. Male: Do not cause a pregnancy. Male/female: Consult prescriber for instruction on appropriate contraceptive measures. This drug may cause severe fetal defects. Breast-feeding is not recommended.

Dietary Considerations: Increase dietary intake of thiamine.

Pregnancy Risk Factor: D (injection); X (topical)

Pregnancy Issues: There are no adequate and well-controlled studies in pregnant women, however, fetal defects and miscarriages have been reported following use of topical and intravenous products. Use is contraindicated during pregnancy.

Lactation: Excretion in breast milk unknown/not recommended

Administration

Oral: I.V. formulation may be given orally mixed in water, grape juice, or carbonated beverage. It is generally best to drink undiluted solution, then rinse the mouth. CocaCola® has been recommended as the "best chaser" for oral fluorouracil.

I.V.: Irritant. Direct I.V. push injection (50 mg/mL solution needs no further dilution) or by I.V. infusion. Toxicity may be reduced by giving the drug as a constant infusion. Bolus doses may be administered by slow IVP or IVPB.

Topical: Wash hands immediately after topical application of the 5% cream; for external use only.

Reconstitution: Further dilution in D$_5$W or NS at concentrations of 0.5-10 mg/mL are stable for 72 hours at 4°C to 25°C.

Compatibility: Stable in D$_5$LR, D$_5$W, NS

Incompatible with concentrations >25 mg/mL of fluorouracil and >2 mg/mL of leucovorin (precipitation occurs)

Y-site administration: Incompatible with amphotericin B cholesteryl sulfate complex, droperidol, filgrastim, ondansetron, topotecan, vinorelbine

Compatibility in syringe: Incompatible with droperidol, epirubicin

Compatibility when admixed: Incompatible with carboplatin, cisplatin, cytarabine, diazepam, doxorubicin, fentanyl, leucovorin, metoclopramide, morphine

Storage:

Injection: Store intact vials at room temperature and protect from light; slight discoloration does not usually denote decomposition. If exposed to cold, a precipitate may form; **gentle** heating to 60°C will dissolve the precipitate without impairing the potency; solutions in 50-1000 mL NS or D$_5$W, or undiluted solutions in syringes are stable for 72 hours at room temperature.

Topical: Store at controlled room temperature.

♦ **5-Fluorouracil** *see Fluorouracil on page 647*

Fluoxetine (floo OKS e teen)

U.S. Brand Names Prozac®; Prozac® Weekly™; Sarafem™

Synonyms Fluoxetine Hydrochloride

Restrictions A medication guide should be dispensed with each prescription. A template for the required MedGuides can be found on the FDA website at: http://www.fda.gov/cder/drug/antidepressants/labelTemplate.pdf

Generic Available Yes; Excludes delayed release capsule

Pharmacologic Category Antidepressant, Selective Serotonin Reuptake Inhibitor

Medication Safety Issues

Sound-alike/look-alike issues:

Fluoxetine may be confused with duloxetine, fluvastatin

Prozac® may be confused with Prilosec®, Proscar®, ProSom®, ProStep®

Sarafem™ may be confused with Serophene®

Use Treatment of major depressive disorder; treatment of binge-eating and vomiting in patients with moderate-to-severe bulimia nervosa; obsessive-compulsive disorder (OCD); premenstrual dysphoric disorder (PMDD); panic disorder with or without agoraphobia

Unlabeled/Investigational Use Selective mutism

Mechanism of Action/Effect Inhibits CNS neuron serotonin reuptake; minimal or no effect on reuptake of norepinephrine or dopamine; does not significantly bind to alpha-adrenergic, histamine or cholinergic receptors

Contraindications Hypersensitivity to fluoxetine or any component of the formulation; patients currently receiving MAO inhibitors, thioridazine, or mesoridazine

Note: MAO inhibitor therapy must be stopped for 14 days before fluoxetine is initiated. Treatment with MAO inhibitors, thioridazine, or mesoridazine should not be initiated until 5 weeks after the discontinuation of fluoxetine.

Warnings/Precautions Antidepressants increase the risk of suicidal thinking and behavior in children and adolescents with major depressive disorder (MDD) and other depressive disorders; consider risk prior to prescribing. All patients must be closely monitored for clinical worsening, suicidality, or unusual changes in behavior, especially during the initiation of therapy or following an increase or decrease in dosage. When used in children, the child's family or caregiver should be instructed to closely observe the patient and communicate condition with healthcare provider. A medication guide should be dispensed with each prescription. **Fluoxetine is FDA approved for the treatment of OCD in children ≥7 years of age and MDD in children ≥8 years of age.**

(Continued)

Fluoxetine *(Continued)*

The possibility of a suicide attempt is inherent in major depression and may persist until remission occurs. Use caution in high-risk patients. Worsening depression and severe abrupt suicidality that are not part of the presenting symptoms may require discontinuation or modification of drug therapy. The patient's family or caregiver should be alerted to monitor patients for the emergence of suicidality and associated behaviors (such as agitation, irritability, hostility, impulsivity, and hypomania) and call healthcare provider.

May worsen psychosis in some patients or precipitate a shift to mania or hypomania in patients with bipolar disorder. Patients presenting with depressive symptoms should be screened for bipolar disorder. Monotherapy in patients with bipolar disorder should be avoided. **Fluoxetine is not FDA approved for the treatment of bipolar depression.** May cause insomnia, anxiety, nervousness or anorexia. Use with caution in patients where weight loss is undesirable. May impair cognitive or motor performance; caution operating hazardous machinery or driving.

The potential for severe reactions exists when used with MAO inhibitors; serotonin syndrome (hyperthermia, muscular rigidity, mental status changes/agitation, autonomic instability) may occur. Fluoxetine may elevate plasma levels of thioridazine and increase the risk of QT_c interval prolongation. This may lead to serious ventricular arrhythmias such as torsade de pointes-type arrhythmias and sudden death. Fluoxetine use has been associated with occurrences of significant rash and allergic events, including vasculitis, lupus-like syndrome, laryngospasm, anaphylactoid reactions, and pulmonary inflammatory disease.

Use caution in patients with a previous seizure disorder or condition predisposing to seizures such as brain damage, alcoholism, or concurrent therapy with other drugs which lower the seizure threshold. Use with caution in patients with hepatic or renal dysfunction and in elderly patients. May cause hyponatremia/SIADH. May increase the risks associated with electroconvulsive treatment. Use with caution in patients at risk of bleeding or receiving concurrent anticoagulant therapy - may cause impairment in platelet function. May alter glycemic control in patients with diabetes. Due to the long half-life of fluoxetine and its metabolites, the effects and interactions noted may persist for prolonged periods following discontinuation. May cause or exacerbate sexual dysfunction. Discontinuation symptoms (eg, dysphoric mood, irritability, agitation, confusion, anxiety, insomnia, hypomania) may occur upon abrupt discontinuation. Taper dose when discontinuing therapy.

Drug Interactions

Cytochrome P450 Effect: Substrate of CYP1A2 (minor), 2B6 (minor), 2C8/9 (major), 2C19 (minor), 2D6 (major), 2E1 (minor), 3A4 (minor); **Inhibits** CYP1A2 (moderate), 2B6 (weak), 2C8/9 (weak), 2C19 (moderate), 2D6 (strong), 3A4 (weak)

Decreased Effect: The levels/effects of fluoxetine may be decreased by carbamazepine, phenobarbital, phenytoin, rifampin, rifapentine, secobarbital and other CYP2C8/9 inducers. Fluoxetine may decrease the levels/effects of CYP2D6 prodrug substrates (eg, codeine, hydrocodone, oxycodone, tramadol). Cyproheptadine may inhibit the effects of serotonin reuptake inhibitors. Lithium levels may be decreased by fluoxetine (in addition to reports of increased lithium levels).

Increased Effect/Toxicity: Fluoxetine should not be used with nonselective MAO inhibitors (phenelzine, isocarboxazid) or other drugs with MAO inhibition (linezolid); fatal reactions have been reported. Wait 5 weeks after stopping fluoxetine before starting a nonselective MAO inhibitor and 2 weeks after stopping an MAO inhibitor before starting fluoxetine. Concurrent selegiline has been associated with mania, hypertension, or serotonin syndrome (risk may be reduced relative to nonselective MAO inhibitors).

Fluoxetine may inhibit the metabolism of thioridazine or mesoridazine, resulting in increased plasma levels and increasing the risk of QT_c interval prolongation. This may lead to serious ventricular arrhythmias, such as torsade de pointes-type arrhythmias and sudden death. Do not use together. Wait at least 5 weeks after discontinuing fluoxetine prior to starting thioridazine.

Fluoxetine may increase the levels/effects of aminophylline, amphetamines, selected beta-blockers, citalopram, dextromethorphan, diazepam, fluvoxamine, lidocaine, mexiletine, methsuximide, mirtazapine, nefazodone, paroxetine, phenytoin, propranolol, risperidone, ritonavir, ropinirole, sertraline, theophylline, thioridazine, tricyclic antidepressants, trifluoperazine, venlafaxine, and other substrates of CYP1A2, 2C19, or 2D6.

Combined use of SSRIs and amphetamines, buspirone, meperidine, nefazodone, serotonin agonists (such as sumatriptan), sibutramine, other SSRIs, sympathomimetics, ritonavir, tramadol, and venlafaxine may increase the risk of serotonin syndrome. Combined use of sumatriptan (and other serotonin agonists) may result in toxicity; weakness, hyper-reflexia, and incoordination have been observed with sumatriptan and SSRIs. In addition, concurrent use may theoretically increase the risk of serotonin syndrome.

Concurrent lithium may increase risk of neurotoxicity, and lithium levels may be increased. Risk of hyponatremia may increase with concurrent use of loop diuretics (bumetanide, furosemide, torsemide). Fluoxetine may increase the hypoprothrombinemic response to warfarin. Concomitant use of fluoxetine and NSAIDs, aspirin, or other drugs affecting coagulation has been associated with an increased risk of bleeding; monitor.

The levels/effects of fluoxetine may be increased by chlorpromazine, delavirdine, fluconazole, gemfibrozil, ketoconazole, miconazole, nicardipine, NSAIDs, paroxetine, pergolide, pioglitazone, quinidine, quinine, ritonavir, ropinirole, sulfonamides, and other CYP2C8/9 or 2D6 inhibitors.

Nutritional/Ethanol Interactions

Ethanol: Avoid ethanol (may increase CNS depression). Depressed patients should avoid/limit intake.

Herb/Nutraceutical: Avoid valerian, St John's wort, kava kava, gotu kola (may increase CNS depression).

Lab Interactions Increased albumin in urine

Adverse Reactions Percentages listed for adverse effects as reported in placebo-controlled trials and were generally similar in adults and children; actual frequency may be dependent upon diagnosis and in some cases the range presented may be lower than or equal to placebo for a particular disorder.

>10%:

Central nervous system: Insomnia (10% to 33%), headache (21%), anxiety (6% to 15%), nervousness (8% to 14%), somnolence (5% to 17%)

Endocrine & metabolic: Libido decreased (1% to 11%)

Gastrointestinal: Nausea (12% to 29%), diarrhea (8% to 18%), anorexia (4% to 11%), xerostomia (4% to 12%)

Neuromuscular & skeletal: Weakness (7% to 21%), tremor (3% to 13%)

Respiratory: Pharyngitis (3% to 11%), yawn (<1% to 11%)

1% to 10%:

Cardiovascular: Vasodilation (1% to 5%), fever (2%), chest pain, hemorrhage, hypertension, palpitation

Central nervous system: Dizziness (9%), dream abnormality (1% to 5%), thinking abnormality (2%), agitation, amnesia, chills, confusion, emotional lability, sleep disorder

Dermatologic: Rash (2% to 6%), pruritus (4%)

Endocrine & metabolic: Ejaculation abnormal (<1% to 7%), impotence (<1% to 7%)

Gastrointestinal: Dyspepsia (6% to 10%), constipation (5%), flatulence (3%), vomiting (3%), weight loss (2%), appetite increased, taste perversion, weight gain

Genitourinary: Urinary frequency

Ocular: Vision abnormal (2%)

Otic: Ear pain, tinnitus

Respiratory: Sinusitis (1% to 6%)

Miscellaneous: Flu-like syndrome (3% to 10%), diaphoresis (2% to 8%)

Overdosage/Toxicology Among 633 adult patients who overdosed on fluoxetine alone, 34 resulted in a fatal outcome. Symptoms of overdose include ataxia, sedation, coma, and ECG abnormalities (QT prolongation, torsade de pointes). Respiratory depression may occur, especially with coingestion of ethanol or other drugs. Seizures rarely occur. Treatment is supportive.

Pharmacodynamics/Kinetics

Absorption: Well absorbed; delayed 1-2 hours with weekly formulation

Time to Peak: 6-8 hours

Protein Binding: 95%

Half-Life Elimination: Adults:

Parent drug: 1-3 days (acute), 4-6 days (chronic), 7.6 days (cirrhosis); Metabolite (norfluoxetine): 9.3 days (range: 4-16 days), 12 days (cirrhosis)

Due to long half-life, resolution of adverse reactions after discontinuation may be slow

Metabolism: Hepatic to norfluoxetine (active; equal to fluoxetine)

Excretion: Urine (10% as norfluoxetine, 2.5% to 5% as fluoxetine)

Pharmacokinetic Note: Weekly formulation results in greater fluctuations between peak and trough concentrations of fluoxetine and norfluoxetine compared to once-daily dosing (24% daily/164% weekly; 17% daily/43% weekly, respectively). Trough concentrations are 76% lower for fluoxetine and 47% lower for norfluoxetine than the concentrations maintained by 20 mg once-daily dosing. Steady-state fluoxetine concentrations are ~50% lower following the once-weekly regimen compared to 20 mg once daily. Average steady-state concentrations of once-daily dosing were highest in children ages 6 to <13 (fluoxetine 171 ng/mL; norfluoxetine 195 ng/mL), followed by adolescents ages 13 to <18 (fluoxetine 86 ng/mL; norfluoxetine 113 ng/mL); concentrations were considered to be within the ranges reported in adults (fluoxetine 91-302 ng/mL; norfluoxetine 72-258 ng/mL).

Dosing

Adults:

Depression, OCD, PMDD, bulimia: 20 mg/day in the morning; may increase after several weeks by 20 mg/day increments; maximum: 80 mg/day; doses >20 mg may be given once daily or divided twice daily. **Note:** Lower doses of 5-10 mg/day have been used for initial treatment.

Usual dosage range:

Depression: 20-40 mg/day; patients maintained on Prozac® 20 mg/day may be changed to Prozac® Weekly™ 90 mg/week, starting dose 7 days after the last 20 mg/day dose

Obsessive compulsive disorder (OCD): 40-80 mg/day

Premenstrual dysphoric disorder (Sarafem™): 20 mg/day continuously, **or** 20 mg/day starting 14 days prior to menstruation and through first full day of menses (repeat with each cycle)

Bulimia nervosa: 60-80 mg/day

Panic disorder: Initial: 10 mg/day; after 1 week, increase to 20 mg/day; may increase after several weeks; doses >60 mg/day have not been evaluated

Elderly: Oral: Some patients may require an initial dose of 10 mg/day with dosage increases of 10 mg and 20 mg every several weeks as tolerated; should not be taken at night unless patient experiences sedation.

Pediatrics:

Depression: Oral: 8-18 years: 10-20 mg/day; lower-weight children can be started at 10 mg/day, may increase to 20 mg/day after 1 week if needed

OCD: Oral: 7-18 years: Initial: 10 mg/day; in adolescents and higher-weight children, dose may be increased to 20 mg/day after 2 weeks. Range: 10-60 mg/day

Selective mutism (unlabeled use): Oral:

<5 years: No dosing information available

5-18 years: Initial: 5-10 mg/day; titrate upwards as needed (usual maximum dose: 60 mg/day)

Renal Impairment:

Single dose studies: Pharmacokinetics of fluoxetine and norfluoxetine were similar among subjects with all levels of impaired renal function, including anephric patients on chronic hemodialysis.

(Continued)

Fluoxetine *(Continued)*

Chronic administration: Additional accumulation of fluoxetine or norfluoxetine may occur in patients with severely impaired renal function.

Not removed by hemodialysis; use of lower dose or less frequent dosing is not usually necessary.

Hepatic Impairment: Elimination half-life of fluoxetine is prolonged in patients with hepatic impairment. A lower dose or less frequent dosing of fluoxetine should be used in these patients.

Cirrhosis patient: Administer a lower dose or less frequent dosing interval.
Compensated cirrhosis without ascites: Administer 50% of normal dose.

Available Dosage Forms

Capsule, as hydrochloride: 10 mg, 20 mg, 40 mg
  Prozac®: 10 mg, 20 mg, 40 mg
  Sarafem™: 10 mg, 20 mg
Capsule, delayed release, as hydrochloride (Prozac® Weekly™): 90 mg
Solution, oral, as hydrochloride (Prozac®): 20 mg/5 mL (120 mL) [contains alcohol 0.23% and benzoic acid; mint flavor]
Tablet, as hydrochloride: 10 mg, 20 mg
  Prozac® [scored]: 10 mg

Monitoring and Teaching Issues

Physical Assessment: Assess other medications patient may be taking for effectiveness and interactions. Assess results of laboratory tests, therapeutic effectiveness, and adverse reactions at beginning of therapy and periodically with long-term use. Taper dosage slowly when discontinuing. Assess mental status for depression, suicidal ideation, anxiety, social functioning, mania, or panic attack. Assess knowledge/teach patient appropriate use, interventions to reduce side effects and adverse symptoms to report.

Monitoring Laboratory Tests: Baseline liver and renal function before beginning drug therapy

Patient Education: Take exactly as directed; do not increase dose or frequency. It may take 2-3 weeks to achieve desired results. Take once-a-day dose in the morning to reduce incidence of insomnia. Avoid alcohol, caffeine, and other prescription or OTC medications not approved by prescriber. Maintain adequate hydration (2-3 L/day of fluids) unless instructed to restrict fluid intake. You may experience drowsiness, lightheadedness, impaired coordination, dizziness, or blurred vision (use caution when driving or engaging in tasks requiring alertness until response to drug is known); constipation (increased exercise, fluids, fruit, or fiber may help); anorexia (maintain regular dietary intake to avoid excessive weight loss); or postural hypotension (use caution when climbing stairs or changing position from lying or sitting to standing). If you have diabetes, monitor serum glucose closely (may cause hypoglycemia). Report persistent CNS effects (nervousness, restlessness, insomnia, anxiety, excitation, headache, sedation); thoughts of suicide; rash or skin irritation; muscle cramping, tremors, or change in gait; respiratory depression or respiratory difficulty; or worsening of condition. **Pregnancy/breast-feeding precautions:** Inform prescriber if you are pregnant. Breast-feeding is not recommended.

Dietary Considerations: May be taken with or without food.

Geriatric Considerations: Fluoxetine's favorable side effect profile makes it a useful alternative to the traditional tricyclic antidepressants. Its potential stimulating and anorexic effects may be bothersome to some patients. Has not been shown to be superior in efficacy to the traditional tricyclic antidepressants or other SSRIs. The long half-life in the elderly makes it less attractive compared to other SSRIs. Data from a clinical trial comparing fluoxetine to tricyclics suggests that fluoxetine is significantly less effective than nortriptyline in hospitalized elderly patients with unipolar major affective disorder, especially those with melancholia and concurrent cardiovascular diseases. As with other SSRIs, fluoxetine has been associated with hyponatremia in elderly patients.

Pregnancy Risk Factor: C

Pregnancy Issues: Fluoxetine crosses the placenta. Nonteratogenic effects including respiratory distress, cyanosis, apnea, seizures, temperature instability, feeding difficulty, vomiting, hypoglycemia, hypo- or hypertonia, hyper-reflexia, jitteriness, irritability, constant crying, and tremor have been reported in the neonate immediately following delivery after exposure to other SSRIs late in the third trimester. Adverse effects may be due to toxic effects of SSRI or drug discontinuation. In some cases, may present clinically as serotonin syndrome. There are no adequate and well-controlled studies in pregnant women. Use during pregnancy only if the potential benefit to the mother outweighs the possible risk to the fetus. If treatment during pregnancy is required, consider tapering SSRI therapy during the third trimester.

Lactation: Enters breast milk/not recommended (AAP rates "of concern")

Breast-Feeding Issues: Colic, irritability, slow weight gain, feeding and sleep disorders have been reported in nursing infants.

Administration

Storage: All dosage forms should be stored at controlled room temperature of 15°C to 30°C (50°F to 86°F); oral liquid should be dispensed in a light-resistant container

Additional Information ECG may reveal S-T segment depression; not shown to be teratogenic in rodents; 15-60 mg/day, buspirone and cyproheptadine, may be useful in treatment of sexual dysfunction during treatment with a selective serotonin reuptake inhibitor.

Weekly capsules are a delayed release formulation containing enteric-coated pellets of fluoxetine hydrochloride, equivalent to 90 mg fluoxetine. Therapeutic equivalence of weekly formulation with daily formulation for delaying time to relapse has not been established.

Related Information

Antidepressant Agents *on page 1713*
Antidepressant Medication Guidelines *on page 1765*

♦ **Fluoxetine and Olanzapine** *see* Olanzapine and Fluoxetine *on page 1112*
♦ **Fluoxetine Hydrochloride** *see* Fluoxetine *on page 649*

Fluphenazine (floo FEN a zeen)

U.S. Brand Names Prolixin® [DSC]; Prolixin Decanoate®
Synonyms Fluphenazine Decanoate
Generic Available Yes: Injection, tablet
Pharmacologic Category Antipsychotic Agent, Typical, Phenothiazine
Medication Safety Issues
Sound-alike/look-alike issues:
Prolixin® may be confused with Proloprim®

Use Management of manifestations of psychotic disorders and schizophrenia; depot formulation may offer improved outcome in individuals with psychosis who are nonadherent with oral antipsychotics

Unlabeled/Investigational Use Pervasive developmental disorder

Mechanism of Action/Effect Fluphenazine is a piperazine phenothiazine antipsychotic which blocks postsynaptic mesolimbic dopaminergic D_1 and D_2 receptors in the brain; depresses the release of hypothalamic and hypophyseal hormones; believed to depress the reticular activating system thus affecting basal metabolism, body temperature, wakefulness, vasomotor tone, and emesis

Contraindications Hypersensitivity to fluphenazine or any component of the formulation (cross-reactivity between phenothiazines may occur); severe CNS depression; coma; subcortical brain damage; blood dyscrasias; hepatic disease

Warnings/Precautions May be sedating, use with caution in disorders where CNS depression is a feature. Use with caution in Parkinson's disease. Caution in patients with hemodynamic instability; bone marrow suppression; predisposition to seizures; severe cardiac, renal, or respiratory disease. Esophageal dysmotility and aspiration have been associated with antipsychotic use - use with caution in patients at risk of pneumonia (ie, Alzheimer's disease). Caution in breast cancer or other prolactin-dependent tumors (may elevate prolactin levels). May alter temperature regulation or mask toxicity of other drugs due to antiemetic effects. May alter cardiac conduction; life-threatening arrhythmias have occurred with therapeutic doses of phenothiazines. Hypotension may occur, particularly with I.M. administration. May cause orthostatic hypotension - use with caution in patients at risk of this effect or those who would tolerate transient hypotensive episodes (cerebrovascular disease, cardiovascular disease, or other medications which may predispose). Adverse effects of depot injections may be prolonged.

Due to anticholinergic effects, use caution in patients with decreased gastrointestinal motility, urinary retention, BPH, xerostomia, visual problems, narrow-angle glaucoma (screening is recommended), and myasthenia gravis. Relative to other antipsychotics, fluphenazine has a low potency of cholinergic blockade.

May cause extrapyramidal symptoms, including pseudoparkinsonism, acute dystonic reactions, akathisia and tardive dyskinesia (risk of these reactions is high relative to other antipsychotics). May be associated with neuroleptic malignant syndrome (NMS) or pigmentary retinopathy.

Drug Interactions
Cytochrome P450 Effect: Substrate of CYP2D6 (major); **Inhibits** CYP1A2 (weak), 2C8/9 (weak), 2D6 (weak), 2E1 (weak)
Decreased Effect: Phenothiazines inhibit the activity of guanethidine, guanadrel, levodopa, and bromocriptine. Barbiturates and cigarette smoking may enhance the hepatic metabolism of fluphenazine. Fluphenazine and possibly other low potency antipsychotics may reverse the pressor effects of epinephrine.
Increased Effect/Toxicity: CYP2D6 inhibitors may increase the levels/effects of fluphenazine; example inhibitors include chlorpromazine, delavirdine, fluoxetine, miconazole, paroxetine, pergolide, quinidine, quinine, ritonavir, and ropinirole. Effects on CNS depression may be additive when fluphenazine is combined with CNS depressants (narcotic analgesics, ethanol, barbiturates, cyclic antidepressants, antihistamines, sedative-hypnotics). Fluphenazine may increase the effects/toxicity of anticholinergics, antihypertensives, lithium (rare neurotoxicity), trazodone, or valproic acid. Concurrent use with TCA may produce increased toxicity or altered therapeutic response. Chloroquine and propranolol may increase chlorpromazine concentrations. Hypotension may occur when fluphenazine is combined with epinephrine. May increase the risk of arrhythmia when combined with antiarrhythmics, cisapride, pimozide, sparfloxacin, or other drugs which prolong QT interval. Metoclopramide may increase risk of extrapyramidal symptoms (EPS).

Nutritional/Ethanol Interactions
Ethanol: Avoid ethanol (may increase CNS depression).
Herb/Nutraceutical: Avoid dong quai, St John's wort (may also cause photosensitization). Avoid kava kava, gotu kola, valerian, St John's wort (may increase CNS depression).

Lab Interactions Increased cholesterol (S), glucose; decreased uric acid (S)

Adverse Reactions Frequency not defined.
Cardiovascular: Hyper-/hypotension, tachycardia, fluctuations in blood pressure, arrhythmia, edema
Central nervous system: Parkinsonian symptoms, akathisia, dystonias, tardive dyskinesia, dizziness, hyper-reflexia, headache, cerebral edema, drowsiness, lethargy, restlessness, excitement, bizarre dreams, EEG changes, depression, seizure, NMS, altered central temperature regulation
Dermatologic: Dermatitis, eczema, erythema, itching, photosensitivity, rash, seborrhea, skin pigmentation, urticaria
Endocrine & metabolic: Changes in menstrual cycle, breast pain, amenorrhea, galactorrhea, gynecomastia, libido (changes in), elevated prolactin, SIADH
Gastrointestinal: Weight gain, loss of appetite, salivation, xerostomia, constipation, paralytic ileus, laryngeal edema
Genitourinary: Ejaculatory disturbances, impotence, polyuria, bladder paralysis, enuresis
Hematologic: Agranulocytosis, leukopenia, thrombocytopenia, nonthrombocytopenic purpura, eosinophilia, pancytopenia
Hepatic: Cholestatic jaundice, hepatotoxicity
(Continued)

Fluphenazine *(Continued)*

Neuromuscular & skeletal: Trembling of fingers, SLE, facial hemispasm
Ocular: Pigmentary retinopathy, cornea and lens changes, blurred vision, glaucoma
Respiratory: Nasal congestion, asthma

Overdosage/Toxicology Symptoms of overdose include deep sleep, hypo- or hypertension, dystonia, seizures, extrapyramidal symptoms, and respiratory failure. Following initiation of essential overdose management, toxic symptom treatment and supportive treatment should be initiated.

Pharmacodynamics/Kinetics

Onset of Action: I.M., SubQ (derivative dependent): Hydrochloride salt: ~1 hour
Peak effect: Neuroleptic: Decanoate: 48-96 hours

Duration of Action: Hydrochloride salt: 6-8 hours; Decanoate: 24-72 hours

Absorption: Oral: Erratic and variable

Protein Binding: 91% and 99%

Half-Life Elimination: Derivative dependent: Hydrochloride: 33 hours; Decanoate: 163-232 hours

Metabolism: Hepatic

Excretion: Urine (as metabolites)

Dosing

Adults:

Psychosis:

Oral: 0.5-10 mg/day in divided doses at 6- to 8-hour intervals; some patients may require up to 40 mg/day

I.M.: 2.5-10 mg/day in divided doses at 6- to 8-hour intervals (parenteral dose is $^1/_3$ to $^1/_2$ the oral dose for the hydrochloride salts)

Long-acting maintenance injections (Depot):

I.M., SubQ (decanoate): 12.5 mg every 3 weeks

Conversion from hydrochloride to decanoate I.M.: 0.5 mL (12.5 mg) decanoate every 3 weeks is approximately equivalent to 10 mg hydrochloride/day

Elderly: Initial (nonpsychotic patient, dementia behavior): 1-2.5 mg/day; increase dose at 4- to 7-day intervals by 1-2.5 mg/day. Increase dosing intervals (bid, tid) as necessary to control response or side effects. Maximum daily dose: 20 mg; gradual increases (titration) may prevent some side effects or decrease their severity.

Pediatrics: Childhood-onset pervasive developmental disorder (unlabeled use): Oral: 0.04 mg/kg/day

Renal Impairment: Use with caution; not dialyzable (0% to 5%).

Hepatic Impairment: Use with caution.

Available Dosage Forms [DSC] = Discontinued product

Elixir, as hydrochloride (Prolixin®): 2.5 mg/5 mL (60 mL) [contains alcohol 14% and sodium benzoate] [DSC]

Injection, oil, as decanoate: 25 mg/mL (5 mL) [may contain benzyl alcohol, sesame oil]
Prolixin Decanoate®: 25 mg/mL (5 mL) [contains benzyl alcohol, sesame oil]

Injection, solution, as hydrochloride (Prolixin® [DSC]): 2.5 mg/mL (10 mL)

Solution, oral concentrate, as hydrochloride (Prolixin®): 5 mg/mL (120 mL) [contains alcohol 14%] [DSC]

Tablet, as hydrochloride: 1 mg, 2.5 mg, 5 mg, 10 mg
Prolixin®: 1 mg, 2.5 mg, 5 mg [contains tartrazine], 10 mg [DSC]

Monitoring and Teaching Issues

Physical Assessment: Assess other medications patient is taking for effectiveness and interactions. Review ophthalmic screening and assess results of laboratory tests, therapeutic effectiveness, and adverse reactions at beginning of therapy and periodically with long-term use. With I.M. or SubQ use, monitor closely for hypotension. Initiate at lower doses and taper dosage slowly when discontinuing. Assess knowledge/teach patient appropriate use, interventions to reduce side effects, and adverse symptoms to report.

Monitoring Laboratory Tests: CBC prior to and regularly during therapy, lipid profile, liver and kidney function, fasting blood glucose/Hgb A_{1c}; BMI

Patient Education: Use exactly as directed; do not increase dose or frequency. Do not discontinue without consulting prescriber. Dilute with water, milk, orange or grapefruit juice; do not dilute with beverages containing caffeine, tannin, or pectinate (eg, coffee, colas, tea, or apple juice). Do not take within 2 hours of any antacid. Avoid alcohol or caffeine and other prescription or OTC medications not approved by prescriber. Avoid skin contact with medication; may cause contact dermatitis (wash immediately with warm, soapy water). Maintain adequate hydration (2-3 L/day of fluids) unless instructed to restrict fluid intake. You may experience excess drowsiness, lightheadedness, dizziness, or blurred vision (use caution driving or when engaging in tasks requiring alertness until response to drug is known); dry mouth, upset stomach, nausea, vomiting (small frequent meals, frequent mouth care, chewing gum, or sucking lozenges may help); constipation (increased exercise, fluids, fruits, or fiber may help); postural hypotension (use caution climbing stairs or when changing position from lying or sitting to standing); urinary retention (void before taking medication); ejaculatory dysfunction (reversible); decreased perspiration (avoid strenuous exercise in hot environments); or photosensitivity (use sunscreen, wear protective clothing and eyewear, and avoid direct sunlight). Report persistent CNS effects (eg, trembling fingers, altered gait or balance, excessive sedation, seizures, unusual movements, anxiety, abnormal thoughts, confusion, personality changes); chest pain, palpitations, rapid heartbeat, severe dizziness; unresolved urinary retention or changes in urinary pattern; altered menstrual pattern, change in libido, swelling or pain in breasts (male or female); vision changes; skin rash or irritation or yellowing of skin; or worsening of condition. **Pregnancy/breast-feeding precautions:** Inform prescriber if you are or intend to become pregnant. Breast-feeding is not recommended.

Geriatric Considerations: (See Warnings/Precautions, Adverse Reactions, and Overdose/Toxicology.) Elderly patients have an increased risk of adverse response to side effects or adverse reactions to antipsychotics.

Pregnancy Risk Factor: C
Lactation: Enters breast milk/not recommended
Administration
    Oral: Avoid contact of oral solution or injection with skin (contact dermatitis). Oral liquid should be diluted in the following **only**: Water, saline, homogenized milk, carbonated orange beverages, pineapple, apricot, prune, orange, tomato, and grapefruit juices. Do **not** dilute in beverages containing caffeine, tannics, or pectinate.
    I.M.: Watch for hypotension when administering I.M.
Additional Information Less sedative and hypotensive effects than chlorpromazine.
Related Information
    Antipsychotic Agents *on page 1717*
    Antipsychotic Medication Guidelines *on page 1766*
    Federal OBRA Regulations: Recommended Maximum Doses *on page 1773*

♦ **Fluphenazine Decanoate** *see Fluphenazine on page 653*

Flurazepam (flure AZ e pam)
U.S. Brand Names Dalmane®
Synonyms Flurazepam Hydrochloride
Controlled Substance C-IV
Generic Available Yes
Pharmacologic Category Benzodiazepine
Medication Safety Issues
    Sound-alike/look-alike issues:
    Flurazepam may be confused with temazepam
    Dalmane® may be confused with Demulen®, Dialume®
Use Short-term treatment of insomnia
Mechanism of Action/Effect Binds to stereospecific benzodiazepine receptors on the postsynaptic GABA neuron at several sites within the central nervous system, including the limbic system, reticular formation. Enhancement of the inhibitory effect of GABA on neuronal excitability results by increased neuronal membrane permeability to chloride ions. This shift in chloride ions results in hyperpolarization (a less excitable state) and stabilization.
Contraindications Hypersensitivity to flurazepam or any component of the formulation (cross-sensitivity with other benzodiazepines may exist); narrow-angle glaucoma; pregnancy
Warnings/Precautions As a hypnotic, should be used only after evaluation of potential causes of sleep disturbance. Failure of sleep disturbance to resolve after 7-10 days may indicate psychiatric or medical illness. Use is not recommended in patients with depressive disorders or psychoses. Avoid use in patients with sleep apnea. Use with caution in patients receiving concurrent CYP3A4 inhibitors, particularly when these agents are added to therapy. Use with caution in elderly or debilitated patients, patients with hepatic disease (including alcoholics), renal impairment, respiratory disease, impaired gag reflex, or obese patients.

Causes CNS depression (dose-related) which may impair physical and mental capabilities. Use with caution in patients receiving other CNS depressants or psychoactive agents. Benzodiazepines have been associated with falls and traumatic injury and should be used with extreme caution in patients who are at risk of these events (especially the elderly). May cause physical or psychological dependence - use with caution in patients with a history of drug dependence.

Benzodiazepines have been associated with anterograde amnesia. Paradoxical reactions, including hyperactive or aggressive behavior, have been reported with benzodiazepines, particularly in adolescent/pediatric or psychiatric patients. Does not have analgesic, antidepressant, or antipsychotic properties.
Drug Interactions
    Cytochrome P450 Effect: Substrate of CYP3A4 (major); **Inhibits** CYP2E1 (weak)
    Decreased Effect: CYP3A4 inducers may decrease the levels/effects of flurazepam; example inducers include aminoglutethimide, carbamazepine, nafcillin, nevirapine, phenobarbital, phenytoin, and rifamycins.
    Increased Effect/Toxicity: CYP3A4 inhibitors may increase the levels/effects of flurazepam; example inhibitors include azole antifungals, ciprofloxacin, clarithromycin, diclofenac, doxycycline, erythromycin, imatinib, isoniazid, nefazodone, nicardipine, propofol, protease inhibitors, quinidine, and verapamil. Serum levels and response to flurazepam may be increased by cimetidine, clozapine, CNS depressants, diltiazem, disulfiram, digoxin, ethanol, fluconazole, fluoxetine, fluvoxamine, grapefruit juice, labetalol, levodopa, loxapine, metoprolol, metronidazole, nelfinavir, omeprazole, and valproic acid.
Nutritional/Ethanol Interactions
    Ethanol: Avoid ethanol (may increase CNS depression).
    Food: Serum levels and response to flurazepam may be increased by grapefruit juice, but unlikely because of flurazepam's high oral bioavailability.
    Herb/Nutraceutical: Avoid valerian, St John's wort, kava kava, gotu kola (may increase CNS depression).
Lab Interactions Elevated alkaline phosphatase, AST, ALT, and bilirubin (total and direct)
Adverse Reactions Frequency not defined.
    Cardiovascular: Palpitations, chest pain
    Central nervous system: Drowsiness, ataxia, lightheadedness, memory impairment, depression, headache, hangover effect, confusion, nervousness, dizziness, falling, apprehension, irritability, euphoria, slurred speech, restlessness, hallucinations, paradoxical reactions, talkativeness
    Dermatologic: Rash, pruritus
    Gastrointestinal: Xerostomia, constipation, increased/excessive salivation, heartburn, upset stomach, nausea, vomiting, diarrhea, increased or decreased appetite, bitter taste, weight gain/loss
    Hematologic: Granulocytopenia
    Hepatic: Elevated AST/ALT, total bilirubin, alkaline phosphatase, cholestatic jaundice
    Neuromuscular & skeletal: Dysarthria, body/joint pain, reflex slowing, weakness
(Continued)

Flurazepam *(Continued)*

Ocular: Blurred vision, burning eyes, difficulty focusing

Otic: Tinnitus

Respiratory: Apnea, dyspnea

Miscellaneous: Diaphoresis, drug dependence

Overdosage/Toxicology Symptoms of overdose include respiratory depression, hypoactive reflexes, unsteady gait, and hypotension. Treatment for benzodiazepine overdose is supportive. Flumazenil has been shown to selectively block the binding of benzodiazepines to CNS receptors, resulting in a reversal of benzodiazepine-induced CNS depression. Respiratory depression may not be reversed.

Pharmacodynamics/Kinetics

Onset of Action: Hypnotic: 15-20 minutes; Peak effect: 3-6 hours

Duration of Action: 7-8 hours

Half-Life Elimination: Desalkylflurazepam:

Adults: Single dose: 74-90 hours; Multiple doses: 111-113 hours

Elderly (61-85 years): Single dose: 120-160 hours; Multiple doses: 126-158 hours

Metabolism: Hepatic to N-desalkylflurazepam (active)

Dosing

Adults: Insomnia (short-term treatment): Oral: 15-30 mg at bedtime

Elderly: Oral: 15 mg at bedtime. Avoid use if possible.

Pediatrics: Hypnotic: Oral:

≤15 years: Dose not established

>15 years: 15 mg at bedtime

Available Dosage Forms Capsule, as hydrochloride: 15 mg, 30 mg

Monitoring and Teaching Issues

Physical Assessment: For short-term use. Assess effectiveness and interactions of other medications patient may be taking. Assess for history of addiction; long-term use can result in dependence, abuse, or tolerance. Evaluate periodically for need for continued use. Monitor for CNS changes. After long-term use, taper dosage slowly when discontinuing. For inpatient use, institute safety measures and monitor effectiveness and adverse reactions. For outpatients, monitor therapeutic effectiveness and adverse reactions at beginning of therapy and periodically with long-term use. Assess knowledge/teach patient appropriate use, interventions to reduce side effects, and adverse symptoms to report. **Pregnancy risk factor X:** Determine that patient is not pregnant before starting therapy. Do not give to sexually-active female patients unless capable of complying with contraceptive use.

Patient Education: Use exactly as directed; do not increase dose or frequency or discontinue without consulting prescriber. Drug may cause physical and/or psychological dependence. May take with food to decrease GI upset. While using this medication, do not use alcohol or other prescription or OTC medications (especially, pain medications, sedatives, antihistamines, or hypnotics) without consulting prescriber. Maintain adequate hydration (2-3 L/day of fluids) unless instructed to restrict fluid intake. You may experience drowsiness, dizziness, lightheadedness, or blurred vision (use caution when driving or engaging in tasks requiring alertness until response to drug is known); dry mouth, nausea, or vomiting (small frequent meals, frequent mouth care, chewing gum, or sucking lozenges may help); difficulty urinating (void before taking medication); or altered libido (resolves when medication is discontinued). Report CNS changes (confusion, depression, increased sedation, excitation, headache, abnormal thinking, insomnia, or nightmares, memory impairment, impaired coordination); muscle pain or weakness; respiratory difficulty; persistent dizziness, chest pain, or palpitations; alterations in normal gait; vision changes; ringing in ears; or ineffectiveness of medication. **Pregnancy/breast-feeding precautions:** Inform prescriber if you are pregnant. Do not get pregnant during or for 1 month following therapy. Consult prescriber for instruction on appropriate contraceptive measures. This drug may cause severe fetal defects. Breast-feeding is not recommended.

Geriatric Considerations: Due to its long-acting metabolite, flurazepam is not considered a drug of choice in the elderly. Long-acting benzodiazepines have been associated with falls in the elderly. Interpretive guidelines from the Centers for Medicare and Medicaid Services (CMS) discourage the use of this agent in residents of long-term care facilities.

Pregnancy Risk Factor: X

Pregnancy Issues: Benzodiazepines cross the placenta. The association between benzodiazepine exposure and malformations remains controversial. A number of types of malformation have been reported (oral cleft, inguinal hernia, cardiac defects, spina bifida, dysmorphic facial features, skeletal defects); however, confounding factors make a clear association difficult. Overall, the risk to the fetus may be low. Nonteratogenic effects (including neonatal flaccidity, respiratory and feeding problems, and withdrawal symptoms) during the postnatal period have also been reported with benzodiazepine use.

Lactation: Excretion in breast milk unknown/not recommended

Administration

Oral: Give 30 minutes to 1 hour before bedtime on an empty stomach with full glass of water. Can be taken with food if GI distress occurs.

Storage: Store in light-resistant containers.

Related Information

Anxiolytic / Hypnotic Use in Long-Term Care Facilities *on page 1769*

Benzodiazepines *on page 1719*

Federal OBRA Regulations: Recommended Maximum Doses *on page 1773*

♦ **Flurazepam Hydrochloride** *see* Flurazepam *on page 655*

Flurbiprofen *(flure BI proe fen)*

U.S. Brand Names Ansaid®; Ocufen®

Synonyms Flurbiprofen Sodium

Generic Available Yes

Pharmacologic Category Nonsteroidal Anti-inflammatory Drug (NSAID), Ophthalmic; Nonsteroidal Anti-inflammatory Drug (NSAID), Oral

Medication Safety Issues
Sound-alike/look-alike issues:
Flurbiprofen may be confused with fenoprofen
Ansaid® may be confused with Asacol®, Axid®
Ocufen® may be confused with Ocuflox®, Ocupress®

Use
Oral: Treatment of rheumatoid arthritis and osteoarthritis
Ophthalmic: Inhibition of intraoperative miosis

Mechanism of Action/Effect Inhibits prostaglandin synthesis by decreasing the activity of the enzyme, cyclooxygenase, which results in decreased formation of prostaglandin precursors

Contraindications Hypersensitivity to flurbiprofen or any component of the formulation; dendritic keratitis; pregnancy (3rd trimester); patients with "aspirin triad" (bronchial asthma, aspirin intolerance, rhinitis)

Warnings/Precautions Fatal asthmatic and anaphylactoid reactions have occurred in patients with "aspirin triad." Use with caution in patients with CHF, hypertension, dehydration, decreased renal or hepatic function, history of GI disease (bleeding, ulcers, or previous GI symptoms with NSAID use), or those receiving anticoagulants and/or corticosteroids. Use lowest effective dose for shortest period possible; bleeding risk has been correlated to dose and duration of therapy. Gastrointestinal bleeding may occur without prior symptoms of gastrointestinal irritation. Elderly are at a high risk for adverse effects from NSAIDs. As many as 60% of elderly can develop peptic ulceration and/or hemorrhage asymptomatically.

Use of NSAIDs can compromise existing renal function especially when Cl_{cr} <30 mL/minute. CNS adverse effects such as confusion, agitation, and hallucination are generally seen in overdose or high-dose situations; however, elderly may demonstrate these adverse effects at lower doses than younger adults. Do not exceed 300 mg/day. Withhold for at least 4-6 half-lives prior to surgical or dental procedures.

Drug Interactions
Cytochrome P450 Effect: Substrate of CYP2C8/9 (minor); **Inhibits** CYP2C8/9 (strong)
Decreased Effect: Ophthalmic: When used with concurrent administration of flurbiprofen, acetylcholine chloride and carbachol have been shown to be ineffective. Reports of acetylcholine chloride and carbachol being ineffective when used with flurbiprofen.
Increased Effect/Toxicity: Flurbiprofen may increase cyclosporine, digoxin, lithium, and methotrexate serum concentrations. The renal adverse effects of ACE inhibitors may be potentiated by NSAIDs. Corticosteroids may increase the risk of GI ulceration. Flurbiprofen may increase the levels/effects amiodarone, fluoxetine, glimepiride, glipizide, nateglinide, phenytoin, pioglitazone, rosiglitazone, sertraline, warfarin, and other CYP2C8/9 substrates.

Nutritional/Ethanol Interactions
Ethanol: Avoid ethanol (may enhance gastric mucosal irritation).
Food: Food may decrease the rate but not the extent of absorption.
Herb/Nutraceutical: Avoid cat's claw, dong quai, evening primrose, feverfew, garlic, ginger, ginkgo, red clover, horse chestnut, green tea, ginseng (all have additional antiplatelet activity).

Adverse Reactions
Ophthalmic: Frequency not defined: Ocular: Slowing of corneal wound healing, mild ocular stinging, itching and burning, ocular irritation, fibrosis, miosis, mydriasis, bleeding tendency increased
Oral:
>1%:
Cardiovascular: Edema
Central nervous system: Amnesia, anxiety, depression, dizziness, headache, insomnia, malaise, nervousness, somnolence
Dermatologic: Rash
Gastrointestinal: Abdominal pain, constipation, diarrhea, dyspepsia, flatulence, GI bleeding, nausea, vomiting, weight changes
Hepatic: Liver enzymes elevated
Neuromuscular & skeletal: Reflexes increased, tremor, vertigo, weakness
Ocular: Vision changes
Otic: Tinnitus
Respiratory: Rhinitis

Overdosage/Toxicology Symptoms of overdose include apnea, metabolic acidosis, coma, nystagmus, leukocytosis, and renal failure. Management of NSAID intoxication is supportive and symptomatic. Since many NSAIDs undergo enterohepatic cycling, multiple doses of charcoal may be needed to reduce the potential for delayed toxicities.

Pharmacodynamics/Kinetics
Onset of Action: ~1-2 hours
Time to Peak: 1.5 hours
Protein Binding: 99%, primarily albumin
Half-Life Elimination: 5.7 hours
Metabolism: Hepatic via CYP2C9; forms metabolites
Excretion: Urine

Dosing
Adults & Elderly:
Rheumatoid arthritis and osteoarthritis: Oral: 200-300 mg/day in 2-, 3-, or 4 divided doses; do not administer more than 100 mg for any single dose; maximum: 300 mg/day
Management of postoperative dental pain: 100 mg every 12 hours
Ophthalmic anti-inflammatory/surgical aid: Ophthalmic: Instill 1 drop every 30 minutes, beginning 2 hours prior to surgery (total of 4 drops in each affected eye)

Available Dosage Forms
Solution, ophthalmic, as sodium (Ocufen®): 0.03% (2.5 mL) [contains thimerosal]
Tablet (Ansaid®): 50 mg, 100 mg
(Continued)

Flurbiprofen (Continued)

Monitoring and Teaching Issues

Physical Assessment: Assess for allergic reaction to salicylate or other NSAIDs. Assess effectiveness and interactions of other medications patient may be taking. Monitor therapeutic response and adverse reactions at beginning of therapy and periodically throughout therapy. Assess knowledge/teach patient proper use, appropriate interventions to reduce side effects, and adverse symptoms to report.

Patient Education: Oral: Take this medication exactly as directed; do not increase dose without consulting prescriber. Do not crush tablets. Take with food or milk to reduce GI distress. Maintain adequate hydration (2-3 L/day of fluids) unless instructed to restrict fluid intake. Do not use alcohol, aspirin or aspirin-containing medication, or any other anti-inflammatory medications without consulting prescriber. You may experience drowsiness, dizziness, nervousness, or headache (use caution when driving or engaging in tasks requiring alertness until response to drug is known); anorexia, nausea, vomiting, or heartburn (small frequent meals, frequent mouth care, sucking lozenges, or chewing gum may help); fluid retention (weigh yourself weekly and report unusual (3-5 lb/week) weight gain). GI bleeding, ulceration, or perforation can occur with or without pain; discontinue medication and contact prescriber if persistent abdominal pain or cramping, or blood in stool occurs. Report breathlessness, respiratory difficulty, or unusual cough; chest pain, rapid heartbeat, palpitations; unusual bruising/bleeding; blood in urine, stool, mouth, or vomitus; swollen extremities; skin rash or itching; acute fatigue; or hearing changes (ringing in ears). **Pregnancy/breast-feeding precautions:** Inform prescriber if you are or intend to become pregnant. This drug should not be used in the 3rd trimester of pregnancy. Breast-feeding is not recommended.

Ophthalmic: Wash hands before instilling. Sit or lie down to instill. Open eye, look at ceiling, and instill prescribed amount of medication. Close eye and roll eye in all directions, and apply gentle pressure to inner corner of eye. Do not let tip of applicator touch eye; do not contaminate tip of applicator (may cause eye infection, eye damage, or vision loss). Use protective dark eyewear until healed; avoid direct sunlight. Temporary stinging or burning may occur. Report persistent pain, burning, redness, vision changes, swelling, itching, or worsening of condition.

Dietary Considerations: Tablet may be taken with food, milk, or antacid to decrease GI effects.

Geriatric Considerations: Elderly are at high risk for adverse effects from NSAIDs. As much as 60% of elderly can develop peptic ulceration and/or hemorrhage asymptomatically. The concomitant use of H_2 blockers, omeprazole, and sucralfate is not effective as prophylaxis with the exception of NSAID-induced duodenal ulcers which may be prevented by the use of ranitidine. Misoprostol is the only prophylactic agent proven effective. Also, concomitant disease and drug use contribute to the risk for GI adverse effects. Use lowest effective dose for shortest period possible. Consider renal function decline with age. Use of NSAIDs can compromise existing renal function especially when Cl_{cr} is $\leq$30 mL/minute. Tinnitus may be a difficult and unreliable indication of toxicity due to age-related hearing loss or eighth cranial nerve damage. CNS adverse effects such as confusion, agitation, and hallucination are generally seen in overdose or high-dose situations, but elderly may demonstrate these adverse effects at lower doses than younger adults.

Pregnancy Risk Factor: C/D (3rd trimester)

Lactation: Enters breast milk/not recommended

Administration

Oral: Take with a full glass of water.

Related Information

Nonsalicylate / Nonsteroidal Anti-inflammatory Agents *on page 1743*

- ◆ **Flurbiprofen Sodium** *see* Flurbiprofen *on page 656*
- ◆ **5-Flurocytosine** *see* Flucytosine *on page 636*

Flutamide (FLOO ta mide)

U.S. Brand Names Eulexin®

Synonyms Niftolid; 4′-Nitro-3′-Trifluoromethylisobutyrantide; NSC-147834; SCH 13521

Generic Available Yes

Pharmacologic Category Antineoplastic Agent, Antiandrogen

Medication Safety Issues

Sound-alike/look-alike issues:

Flutamide may be confused with Flumadine®, thalidomide

Eulexin® may be confused with Edecrin®, Eurax®

Use Treatment of metastatic prostatic carcinoma in combination therapy with LHRH agonist analogues

Unlabeled/Investigational Use Female hirsutism

Mechanism of Action/Effect Nonsteroidal antiandrogen that inhibits androgen uptake or inhibits binding of androgen in target tissues

Contraindications Hypersensitivity to flutamide or any component of the formulation; severe hepatic impairment; pregnancy

Warnings/Precautions Product labeling states flutamide is not for use in women, particularly for nonlife-threatening conditions. Patients with glucose-6 phosphate dehydrogenase deficiency or hemoglobin M disease or smokers are at risk of toxicities associated with aniline exposure, including methemoglobinemia, hemolytic anemia, and cholestatic jaundice. Monitor methemoglobin levels. Severe and potentially fatal hepatic injury may occur (50% of cases within first 3 months of therapy). Serum transaminases should be monitored at baseline and monthly for the first four months of therapy, and periodically thereafter. These should also be repeated at the first sign and symptom of liver dysfunction. Use of flutamide is not recommended in patients with baseline elevation of transaminase levels (>2 times the upper limit of normal). Flutamide should be discontinued immediately at any time if the patient develops jaundice or elevation in serum transaminase levels (>2 times upper limit of normal).

Drug Interactions

Cytochrome P450 Effect: Substrate (major) of CYP1A2, 3A4; **Inhibits** CYP1A2 (weak)

Decreased Effect: CYP1A2 inducers may decrease the levels/effects of flutamide; example inducers include aminoglutethimide, carbamazepine, phenobarbital, and rifampin. CYP3A4 inducers may decrease the levels/effects of flutamide; example inducers include aminoglutethimide, carbamazepine, nafcillin, nevirapine, phenobarbital, phenytoin, and rifamycins.

Increased Effect/Toxicity: CYP1A2 inhibitors may increase the levels/effects of flutamide; example inhibitors include amiodarone, ciprofloxacin, fluvoxamine, ketoconazole, lomeflox-acin, ofloxacin, and rofecoxib. CYP3A4 inhibitors may increase the levels/effects of flutamide; example inhibitors include azole antifungals, ciprofloxacin, clarithromycin, diclo-fenac, doxycycline, erythromycin, imatinib, isoniazid, nefazodone, nicardipine, propofol, protease inhibitors, quinidine, and verapamil. Warfarin effects may be increased.

Nutritional/Ethanol Interactions

Food: No effect on bioavailability of flutamide.

Herb/Nutraceutical: St John's wort may decrease flutamide levels.

Adverse Reactions

>10%:
Endocrine & metabolic: Gynecomastia, hot flashes, breast tenderness, galactorrhea (9% to 42%); impotence; decreased libido; tumor flare
Gastrointestinal: Nausea, vomiting (11% to 12%)
Hepatic: Increased AST (SGOT) and LDH levels, transient, mild

1% to 10%:
Cardiovascular: Hypertension (1%), edema
Central nervous system: Drowsiness, confusion, depression, anxiety, nervousness, head-ache, dizziness, insomnia
Dermatologic: Pruritus, ecchymosis, photosensitivity, herpes zoster
Gastrointestinal: Anorexia, increased appetite, constipation, indigestion, upset stomach (4% to 6%); diarrhea
Hematologic: Anemia (6%), leukopenia (3%), thrombocytopenia (1%)
Neuromuscular & skeletal: Weakness (1%)

Overdosage/Toxicology Symptoms of overdose include hypoactivity, ataxia, anorexia, vomiting, slow respiration, and lacrimation. Induce vomiting. Management is supportive. Dialysis is of no benefit.

Pharmacodynamics/Kinetics

Absorption: Oral: Rapid and complete

Protein Binding: Parent drug: 94% to 96%; 2-hydroxyflutamide: 92% to 94%

Half-Life Elimination: 5-6 hours (2-hydroxyflutamide)

Metabolism: Extensively hepatic to more than 10 metabolites, primarily 2-hydroxyflutamide (active)

Excretion: Primarily urine (as metabolites)

Dosing

Adults & Elderly: Refer to individual protocols.

Prostate carcinoma: Oral: 250 mg 3 times/day; alternatively, once-daily doses of 0.5-1.5 g have been used (unlabeled dosing)

Female hirsutism (unlabeled use): Oral: 250 mg daily

Available Dosage Forms Capsule: 125 mg

Monitoring and Teaching Issues

Physical Assessment: Note specific Warnings/Precautions for use cautions (eg, risk of fatality). Assess potential for interactions with other pharmacological agents or herbal products the patient may be taking (risk for increased or decreased levels/effects of flutamide; see Drug Interactions). Assess results of laboratory tests prior to and periodically during therapy (see Monitoring Laboratory Tests). Therapeutic effectiveness (eg, reduction of tumor) and adverse response should be assessed on a regular basis throughout therapy (eg, galactorrhea, CNS changes, ataxia, anorexia, vomiting, lacrimation, anemia; see Adverse Reactions). Teach patient proper use, possible side effects/appropriate interven-tions, and adverse symptoms to report (eg, chest pain, respiratory difficulty, abdominal pain; see Patient Education).

Monitoring Laboratory Tests: Serum transaminase levels should be obtained at baseline and repeated monthly for the first 4 months of therapy, and periodically thereafter. LFTs should be checked at the first sign or symptom of liver dysfunction. Other parameters include tumor reduction, testosterone/estrogen, prostate specific antigen, and phosphatase serum levels.

Patient Education: Do not take any new medication during therapy unless approved by prescriber. Take as directed; do not discontinue without consulting prescriber. May cause decreased libido, impotence, swelling of breasts, or decreased appetite (small frequent meals may help). Report chest pain or palpitation; acute abdominal pain; pain, tingling, or numbness of extremities; swelling of extremities or unusual weight gain; respiratory diffi-culty; or other persistent adverse effects. **Pregnancy/breast-feeding precautions:** Inform prescriber if you are pregnant and do not get pregnant during or for 1 month following therapy. Consult prescriber for instruction on appropriate contraceptive measures. This drug may cause severe fetal defects. Breast-feeding is not recommended.

Geriatric Considerations: A study has shown that the addition of flutamide to leuprolide therapy in patients with advanced prostatic cancer increased median actuarial survival time to 34.9 months versus 27.9 months with leuprolide alone. No specific dose alterations are necessary in the elderly.

Pregnancy Risk Factor: D

Lactation: Excretion in breast milk unknown/not recommended

Administration

Oral: Usually administered orally in 3 divided doses; contents of capsule may be opened and mixed with applesauce, pudding, or other soft foods. Mixing with a beverage is not recom-mended.

Storage: Store at room temperature.

Fluticasone (floo TIK a sone)

U.S. Brand Names Cutivate®; Flonase®; Flovent® [DSC]; Flovent® HFA; Flovent® Rotadisk® [DSC]

Synonyms Fluticasone Propionate

Generic Available Yes: Cream, ointment

Pharmacologic Category Corticosteroid, Inhalant (Oral); Corticosteroid, Nasal; Corticosteroid, Topical; Corticosteroid, Topical (Medium Potency)

Medication Safety Issues
Sound-alike/look-alike issues:
Cutivate® may be confused with Ultravate®

Use
Inhalation: Maintenance treatment of asthma as prophylactic therapy. It is also indicated for patients requiring oral corticosteroid therapy for asthma to assist in total discontinuation or reduction of total oral dose. NOT indicated for the relief of acute bronchospasm.
Intranasal: Management of seasonal and perennial allergic rhinitis and nonallergic rhinitis in patients ≥4 years of age
Topical: Relief of inflammation and pruritus associated with corticosteroid-responsive dermatoses in patients ≥3 months of age

Mechanism of Action/Effect Fluticasone belongs to a new group of corticosteroids which utilizes a fluorocarbothioate ester linkage at the 17 carbon position; extremely potent vasoconstrictive and anti-inflammatory activity; has a weak HPA inhibitory potency when applied topically, which gives the drug a high therapeutic index. The effectiveness of inhaled fluticasone is due to its direct local effect. The mechanism of action for all topical corticosteroids is believed to be a combination of three important properties: anti-inflammatory activity, immunosuppressive properties, and antiproliferative actions.

Contraindications Hypersensitivity to fluticasone or any component of the formulation; primary treatment of status asthmaticus
Topical: Do not use if infection is present at treatment site, in the presence of skin atrophy, or for the treatment of rosacea or perioral dermatitis

Warnings/Precautions May cause hypercorticism or suppression of hypothalamic-pituitary-adrenal (HPA) axis, particularly in younger children or in patients receiving high doses for prolonged periods. HPA axis suppression may lead to adrenal crisis. Fluticasone may cause less HPA axis suppression than therapeutically equivalent oral doses of prednisone. Particular care is required when patients are transferred from systemic corticosteroids to inhaled products due to possible adrenal insufficiency or withdrawal from steroids, including an increase in allergic symptoms. Patients receiving 20 mg per day of prednisone (or equivalent) may be most susceptible. Concurrent use of ritonavir (and potentially other strong inhibitors of CYP3A4) may increase fluticasone levels and effects on HPA suppression.

Controlled clinical studies have shown that orally-inhaled and intranasal corticosteroids may cause a reduction in growth velocity in pediatric patients. (In studies of orally-inhaled corticosteroids, the mean reduction in growth velocity was approximately 1 centimeter per year [range 0.3-1.8 cm per year] and appears to be related to dose and duration of exposure.) To minimize the systemic effects of orally-inhaled and intranasal corticosteroids, each patient should be titrated to the lowest effective dose. The risk of growth velocity reduction with intranasal administration of fluticasone may be very low.

May suppress the immune system, patients may be more susceptible to infection. Use with caution, if at all, in patients with systemic infections, active or quiescent tuberculosis infection, or ocular herpes simplex. Avoid exposure to chickenpox and measles.

Supplemental steroids (oral or parenteral) may be needed during stress or severe asthma attacks. Rare cases of vasculitis (Churg-Strauss syndrome) or other eosinophilic conditions can occur.

Inhalation: Not to be used in status asthmaticus or for the relief of acute bronchospasm. Flovent® Rotadisk® and Flovent® Diskus® [CAN] contain lactose; very rare anaphylactic reactions have been reported in patients with severe milk protein allergy.

Topical: May also cause suppression of HPA axis, especially when used on large areas of the body, denuded areas, for prolonged periods of time or with an occlusive dressing. Pediatric patients may be more susceptible to systemic toxicity. Safety and efficacy in pediatric patients <3 months of age have not been established.

Drug Interactions
Cytochrome P450 Effect: Substrate of CYP3A4 (major)
Increased Effect/Toxicity:
CYP3A4 inhibitors: Serum level and/or toxicity of fluticasone may be increased; this effect was shown with ketoconazole, but not erythromycin. Other potential inhibitors include amiodarone, cimetidine, clarithromycin, delavirdine, diltiazem, dirithromycin, disulfiram, fluoxetine, fluvoxamine, grapefruit juice, indinavir, itraconazole, ketoconazole, nefazodone, nevirapine, propoxyphene, quinupristin-dalfopristin, ritonavir, saquinavir, verapamil, zafirlukast, zileuton. Ritonavir may increase serum levels (due to CYP3A4 inhibition) and the potential for steroid-related adverse effects (eg, Cushing syndrome, adrenal suppression).
Salmeterol: The addition of salmeterol has been demonstrated to improve response to inhaled corticosteroids (as compared to increasing steroid dosage).

Nutritional/Ethanol Interactions Herb/Nutraceutical: In theory, St John's wort may decrease serum levels of fluticasone by inducing CYP3A4 isoenzymes.

Adverse Reactions
Oral inhalation:
>10%:
Central nervous system: Headache (5% to 11%)

Respiratory: Upper respiratory tract infection (16% to 18%)

3% to 10%:

Respiratory: Throat irritation (8% to 10%), sinusitis/sinus infection (4% to 7%), cough (4% to 6%; placebo: 5%), bronchitis (2% to 6%; placebo 5%), hoarseness/dysphonia (2% to 6%), upper respiratory tract inflammation (2% to 5%)

Miscellaneous: Candidiasis (2% to 5%)

1% to 3%:

Cardiovascular: Chest symptoms

Central nervous system: Dizziness, fever, migraine, pain

Gastrointestinal: Diarrhea, dyspepsia, gastrointestinal infection (viral), gastrointestinal discomfort/pain, hyposalivation

Genitourinary: Urinary tract infection

Neuromuscular & skeletal: Musculoskeletal pain, muscle pain, muscle stiffness/tightness/rigidity

Respiratory: rhinitis, pharyngitis/throat infection, rhinorrhea/postnasal drip, nasal sinus disorder, laryngitis

Miscellaneous: Viral infection, injuries (including muscle, soft tissue)

Nasal inhalation:

>10%: Headache (7% to 16%), pharyngitis (6% to 8%)

1% to 10%:

Central nervous system: Dizziness (1% to 3%), fever (1% to 3%)

Gastrointestinal: Nausea/vomiting (3% to 5%), abdominal pain (1% to 3%), diarrhea (1% to 3%)

Respiratory: Epistaxis (6% to 7%), asthma symptoms (3% to 7%), cough (4%), blood in nasal mucous (1% to 3%), runny nose (1% to 3%), bronchitis (1% to 3%)

Miscellaneous: Aches and pains (1% to 3%), flu-like symptoms (1% to 3%)

Topical: Pruritus (3%), skin irritation (3%), exacerbation of eczema (2%), dryness (1%), numbness of fingers (1%)

Reported with other topical corticosteroids (in decreasing order of occurrence): Irritation, folliculitis, acneiform eruptions, hypopigmentation, perioral dermatitis, allergic contact dermatitis, secondary infection, skin atrophy, striae, miliaria, pustular psoriasis from chronic plaque psoriasis

Overdosage/Toxicology When consumed in high doses over prolonged periods, systemic hypercorticism and adrenal suppression may occur. In those cases, discontinuation of the corticosteroid should be done judiciously.

Pharmacodynamics/Kinetics

Absorption:

Topical cream: 5% (increased with inflammation)

Oral inhalation: Absorbed systemically primarily via lungs; minimal GI absorption due to presystemic metabolism

Bioavailability: Oral inhalation: Flovent®: 30%; decreased with Flovent® HFA (30% lower)

Protein Binding: 91%

Metabolism: Hepatic via CYP3A4 to 17β-carboxylic acid (negligible activity)

Excretion: Feces (as parent drug and metabolites); urine (<5% as metabolites)

Dosing

Adults & Elderly:

Asthma: Inhalation, oral: Note: Titrate to the lowest effective dose once asthma stability is achieved

Flovent®, Flovent® HFA: Manufacturers labeling: Dosing based on previous therapy

Bronchodilator alone: Recommended starting dose: 88 mcg twice daily; highest recommended dose: 440 mcg twice daily

Inhaled corticosteroids: Recommended starting dose: 88-220 mcg twice daily; highest recommended dose: 440 mcg twice daily; a higher starting dose may be considered in patients previously requiring higher doses of inhaled corticosteroids

Oral corticosteroids:

Recommended starting dose:

Flovent®: 880 mcg twice daily

Flovent® HFA: 440 mcg twice daily

Highest recommended dose: 880 mcg twice daily; starting dose is patient dependent. In patients on chronic oral corticosteroids therapy, reduce prednisone dose no faster than 2.5-5 mg/day on a weekly basis; begin taper after 1 week of fluticasone therapy

NIH Asthma Guidelines (administer in divided doses twice daily).

"Low" dose: 88-264 mcg/day

"Medium" dose: 264-660 mcg/day

"High" dose: >660 mcg/day

Flovent® Rotadisk®: Dosing based on previous therapy

Bronchodilator alone: Recommended starting dose 100 mcg twice daily; highest recommended dose: 500 mcg twice daily

Inhaled corticosteroids: 100-250 mcg twice daily; highest recommended dose: 500 mcg twice daily; a higher starting dose may be considered in patients previously requiring higher doses of inhaled corticosteroids

Oral corticosteroids: 1000 mcg twice daily; highest recommended dose: 1000 mcg twice daily; starting dose is patient dependent. In patients on chronic oral corticosteroids therapy, reduce prednisone dose no faster than 2.5 mg/day on a weekly basis; begin taper after ≥1 week of fluticasone therapy

Flovent® Diskus® [CAN]:

Mild asthma: 100-250 mcg twice daily

Moderate asthma: 250-500 mcg twice daily

Severe asthma: 500 mcg twice daily; may increase to 1000 mcg twice daily in very severe patients requiring high doses of corticosteroids

Inflammation/pruritus associated with corticosteroid-responsive dermatoses:

Topical: Apply sparingly in a thin film twice daily; therapy should be discontinued when

(Continued)

Fluticasone *(Continued)*

control is achieved. If no improvement is seen within 2 weeks, reassessment of diagnosis may be necessary.

Rhinitis: Intranasal: Initial: 2 sprays (50 mcg/spray) per nostril once daily; may also be divided into 100 mcg twice a day. After the first few days, dosage may be reduced to 1 spray per nostril once daily for maintenance therapy. Dosing should be at regular intervals.

Pediatrics:

Asthma: Inhalation, oral:

Flovent®, Flovent® HFA:
  Children <12 years (unlabeled use): NIH Asthma Guidelines (administer in divided doses twice daily):
    "Low" dose: 88-176 mcg/day
    "Medium" dose: 176-440 mcg/day
    "High" dose: >440 mcg/day
  Children ≥12 years: Refer to adult dosing.

Flovent® Rotadisk®: **Note:** Titrate to the lowest effective dose once asthma stability is achieved.
  Children ≥4-11 years: Dosing based on previous therapy
    Bronchodilator alone: Recommended starting dose: 50 mcg twice daily; highest recommended dose: 100 mcg twice daily
    Inhaled corticosteroids: Recommended starting dose: 50 mcg twice daily; highest recommended dose: 100 mcg twice daily; a higher starting dose may be considered in patients previously requiring higher doses of inhaled corticosteroids
  Children ≥11 years: Refer to adult dosing.

Flovent® Diskus® [CAN]:
  Children 4-16 years: Usual starting dose: 50-100 mcg twice daily; may increase to 200 mcg twice daily in patients not adequately controlled; titrate to the lowest effective dose once asthma stability is achieved
  Children ≥16 years: Refer to adult dosing.

Inflammation/pruritus associated with corticosteroid-responsive dermatoses:
Topical: Children ≥3 months: Apply sparingly in a thin film twice daily; therapy should be discontinued when control is achieved. If no improvement is seen within 2 weeks, reassessment of diagnosis may be necessary. Safety and efficacy for use in pediatric patients <3 months have not been established.

Rhinitis: Intranasal: Children ≥4 years and Adolescents: Initial: 1 spray (50 mcg/spray) per nostril once daily; patients not adequately responding or patients with more severe symptoms may use 2 sprays (100 mcg) per nostril. Depending on response, dosage may be reduced to 100 mcg daily. Total daily dosage should not exceed 2 sprays in each nostril (200 mcg)/day. Dosing should be at regular intervals.

Hepatic Impairment: Fluticasone is primarily cleared in the liver. Fluticasone plasma levels may be increased in patients with hepatic impairment, use with caution; monitor.

Available Dosage Forms [DSC] = Discontinued product; [CAN] = Canadian brand name
Aerosol for oral inhalation, as propionate [contains CFCs] (Flovent®):
  44 mcg/inhalation (7.9 g) [60 metered doses], (13 g) [120 metered doses] [DSC]
  110 mcg/inhalation (7.9 g) [60 metered doses], (13 g) [120 metered doses] [DSC]
  220 mcg/inhalation (7.9 g) [60 metered doses], (13 g) [120 metered doses] [DSC]
Aerosol for oral inhalation, as propionate [CFC free] (Flovent® HFA)
  44 mcg/inhalation (10.6 g) [120 metered doses]
  110 mcg/inhalation (12 g) [120 metered doses]
  220 mcg/inhalation (12 g) [120 metered doses]
Cream, as propionate (Cutivate®): 0.05% (15 g, 30 g, 60 g)
Ointment, as propionate (Cutivate®): 0.005% (15 g, 30 g, 60 g)
Powder for oral inhalation, as propionate [prefilled blister pack] (Flovent® Diskus®) [CAN; not available in the United States]:
  50 mcg (28s, 60s) [contains lactose]
  100 mcg (28s, 60s) [contains lactose]
  250 mcg (28s, 60s) [contains lactose]
  500 mcg (28s, 60s) [contains lactose]
Powder for oral inhalation, as propionate [4 blisters of the drug per Rotadisk®, 15 Rotadisks® per pack] (Flovent® Rotadisk®):
  50 mcg (60s) [delivers 44 mcg/inhalation, contains lactose/milk protein] [DSC]
  100 mcg (60s) [delivers 88 mcg/inhalation, contains lactose/milk protein] [DSC]
  250 mcg (60s) [delivers 220 mcg/inhalation, contains lactose/milk protein] [DSC]
Suspension, intranasal spray, as propionate (Flonase®): 50 mcg/inhalation (16 g) [120 metered doses]

Monitoring and Teaching Issues
Physical Assessment: Monitor effectiveness of therapy and adverse reactions at beginning of therapy and periodically with long-term use. May take as long as 2 weeks before full benefit of medication is known. Assess knowledge/teach patient appropriate use, interventions to reduce side effects, and adverse symptoms to report. Monitor for possible eosinophilic conditions (including Churg-Strauss syndrome); growth (adolescents and children); and signs/symptoms of HPA axis suppression/adrenal insufficiency.

Patient Education: Use as directed; do not overuse and use only for length of time prescribed. Although you may see improvement within a few hours of use, the full benefit of the medication may not be achieved for several days. Do not change the prescribed dosage without consulting prescriber. Avoid exposure to chickenpox or measles. If exposed, inform your prescriber as soon as possible. **Pregnancy/breast-feeding precautions:** Inform prescriber if you are or intend to become pregnant. Consult prescriber if breast-feeding.

Metered-dose inhalation: Sit when using. Take deep breaths for 3-5 minutes, and clear nasal passages before administration (use decongestant as needed). Hold breath for 5-10 seconds after use, and wait 1-3 minutes between inhalations. Follow package insert instructions for use. Do not exceed maximum dosage. If also using inhaled bronchodilator, use before fluticasone. Rinse mouth and throat after use to reduce aftertaste and prevent candidiasis.

Nasal spray: Shake gently before use. Use at regular intervals, no more frequently than directed. Report unusual cough or spasm; persistent nasal bleeding, burning, or irritation; or worsening of condition.

Powder for oral inhalation: Flovent® Diskus®: Do not attempt to take device apart. Do not use with a spacer device. Do not exhale into the Diskus®, use in a level horizontal position. Do not wash the mouthpiece.

Topical: For external use only. Apply thin film of cream to affected area only; rub in lightly. Do not apply occlusive covering unless advised by prescriber. Wash hand thoroughly after use; avoid contact with eyes. Notify prescriber if skin condition persists or worsens. Do not use for treatment of diaper dermatitis or under diapers or plastic pants.

Dietary Considerations: Flovent® Rotadisk® and Flovent® Diskus® [CAN] contains lactose; very rare anaphylactic reactions have been reported with Flovent® Rotadisk® in patients with severe milk protein allergy.

Geriatric Considerations: No specific information for the elderly patient is available.

Pregnancy Risk Factor: C

Pregnancy Issues: There are no adequate and well-controlled studies using inhaled fluticasone in pregnant women. Oral corticosteroid use has shown animals to be more prone to teratogenic effects than humans. Due to the natural increase in corticosteroid production during pregnancy, most women may require a lower steroid dose; use with caution.

Lactation: Excretion in breast milk unknown/use caution

Breast-Feeding Issues: Systemic corticosteroids are excreted in human milk. The extent of topical absorption is variable. Use with caution while breast-feeding; do not apply to nipples.

Administration
Inhalation:
Aerosol inhalation: Shake container thoroughly before using. Take 3-5 deep breaths. Use inhaler on inspiration. Allow 1 full minute between inhalations. Rinse mouth with water after use to reduce aftertaste and incidence of candidiasis. Flovent® HFA inhaler must be primed before first use, when not used for 7 days, or if dropped. To prime the first time, release 4 sprays into air; shake well before each spray and spray away from face. If dropped or not used for 7 days, prime by releasing a single test spray.

Nasal spray: Shake bottle gently before using. Prime pump prior to first use (press 6 times until fine spray appears). Blow nose to clear nostrils. Insert applicator into nostril, keeping bottle upright, and close off the other nostril. Breathe in through nose. While inhaling, press pump to release spray. Nasal applicator may be removed and rinsed with warm water to clean.

Powder for oral inhalation:
Flovent® Rotadisk®: Prior to use, one foil disk containing 4 blisters of medication must be inserted into Diskhaler®. After 4 inhalations have been taken from the Diskhaler®, a new foil disk should be inserted. Do not use with a spacer device. Do not exhale into Diskhaler®. Use in horizontal position. At least weekly, Diskhaler® should be cleaned.

Flovent® Diskus® [CAN]: Do not use with a spacer device. Do not exhale into Diskus®. Do not wash or take apart. Use in horizontal position.

Topical: Apply sparingly in a thin film of cream or ointment. Rub in lightly. Do not use for diaper dermatitis.

Storage:
Aerosol (oral inhalation), cream: Store between 2°C to 30°C (36°F to 86°F). Store aerosol with nozzle end down, protect from freezing and direct sunlight. Discard aerosol after labeled number of doses has been used.

Flovent® HFA: Store at 25°C (77°F); excursions permitted to 15°C to 30°C (59°F to 86°F). Store with mouthpiece down.

Nasal spray: Store between 4°C to 30°C (39°F to 86°F). Discard after labeled number of doses has been used, even if bottle is not completely empty.

Powder for oral inhalation:
Flovent® Diskus® [CAN]: Store between 2°C to 30°C in a dry place away from direct frost, heat, or sunlight. Do not store in a damp environment (eg, bathroom). Protect from temperatures >30°C (>86°F).

Flovent® Rotadisk®: Store at controlled room temperature of 20°C to 25°C (68°F to 77°F). Use blisters within 2 months of opening protective pouch.

Additional Information Effects of inhaled/intranasal steroids on growth have been observed in the absence of laboratory evidence of HPA axis suppression, suggesting that growth velocity is a more sensitive indicator of systemic corticosteroid exposure in pediatric patients than some commonly used tests of HPA axis function. The long-term effects of this reduction in growth velocity associated with orally-inhaled and intranasal corticosteroids, including the impact on final adult height, are unknown. The potential for "catch up" growth following discontinuation of treatment with inhaled corticosteroids has not been adequately studied. The product labeling notes that intranasal administration was not associated with a statistically-significant reduction in growth velocity (based on a small study conducted over 1 year).

In the United States, dosage for the metered dose inhaler (Flovent®, Flovent® HFA) is expressed as the amount of drug which leaves the actuater and is delivered to the patient. This differs from other countries, which express the dosage as the amount of drug which leaves the valve.

Related Information
Asthma *on page 1799*
Corticosteroids *on page 1731*
Inhalant Agents *on page 1734*

Fluticasone and Salmeterol (floo TIK a sone & sal ME te role)

U.S. Brand Names Advair Diskus®

Synonyms Salmeterol and Fluticasone

Generic Available No

Pharmacologic Category Beta$_2$-Adrenergic Agonist; Corticosteroid, Inhalant (Oral)

Medication Safety Issues

Sound-alike/look-alike issues:

Advair may be confused with Advicor®

Use Maintenance treatment of asthma in adults and children ≥4 years; **not** for use for relief of acute bronchospasm; maintenance treatment of COPD associated with chronic bronchitis

Dosing

Adults & Elderly: Do not use to transfer patients from systemic corticosteroid therapy

COPD: Oral inhalation: Fluticasone 250 mcg/salmeterol 50 mcg twice daily, 12 hours apart

Asthma (maintenance): Oral inhalation: One inhalation twice daily, morning and evening, 12 hours apart

Note: Advair Diskus® is available in 3 strengths, initial dose prescribed should be based upon previous asthma therapy. Dose should be increased after 2 weeks if adequate response is not achieved. Patients should be titrated to lowest effective dose once stable. (Because each strength contains salmeterol 50 mcg/inhalation, dose adjustments should be made by changing inhaler strength. No more than 1 inhalation of any strength should be taken more than twice a day). Maximum dose: Fluticasone 500 mcg/salmeterol 50 mcg, one inhalation twice daily.

Patients not currently on inhaled corticosteroids: Fluticasone 100 mcg/salmeterol 50 mcg

Patients currently using inhaled beclomethasone dipropionate:

≤420 mcg/day: Fluticasone 100 mcg/salmeterol 50 mcg

462-840 mcg/day: Fluticasone 250 mcg/salmeterol 50 mcg

Patients currently using inhaled budesonide:

≤400 mcg/day: Fluticasone 100 mcg/salmeterol 50 mcg

800-1200 mcg/day: Fluticasone 250 mcg/salmeterol 50 mcg

1600 mcg/day: Fluticasone 500 mcg/salmeterol 50 mcg

Patients currently using inhaled flunisolide:

≤1000 mcg/day: Fluticasone 100 mcg/salmeterol 50 mcg

1250-2000 mcg/day: Fluticasone 250 mcg/salmeterol 50 mcg

Patients currently using inhaled fluticasone propionate aerosol:

≤176 mcg/day: Fluticasone 100 mcg/salmeterol 50 mcg

440 mcg/day: Fluticasone 250 mcg/salmeterol 50 mcg

660-880 mcg/day: Fluticasone 500 mcg/salmeterol 50 mcg

Patients currently using inhaled fluticasone propionate powder:

≤200 mcg/day: Fluticasone 100 mcg/salmeterol 50 mcg

500 mcg/day: Fluticasone 250 mcg/salmeterol 50 mcg

1000 mcg/day: Fluticasone 500 mcg/salmeterol 50 mcg

Patients currently using inhaled triamcinolone acetonide:

≤1000 mcg/day: Fluticasone 100 mcg/salmeterol 50 mcg

1100-1600 mcg/day: Fluticasone 250 mcg/salmeterol 50 mcg

Pediatrics: Asthma: Oral inhalation:

Children 4-11 years: Fluticasone 100 mg/salmeterol 50 mg twice daily, 12 hours apart

Children ≥12 years: Refer to adult dosing.

Hepatic Impairment: Fluticasone is cleared by hepatic metabolism. No dosing adjustment suggested. Use with caution in patients with impaired liver function.

Available Dosage Forms Powder for oral inhalation:

100/50: Fluticasone propionate 100 mcg and salmeterol xinafoate 50 mcg (28s, 60s) [contains lactose]

250/50: Fluticasone propionate 250 mcg and salmeterol xinafoate 50 mcg (28s, 60s) [contains lactose]

500/50: Fluticasone propionate 500 mcg and salmeterol xinafoate 50 mcg (28s, 60s) [contains lactose]

Monitoring and Teaching Issues

Physical Assessment: See individual agents.

Patient Education: See individual agents. **Pregnancy/breast-feeding precautions:** Inform prescriber if you are or intend to become pregnant. Consult prescriber if breast-feeding.

Pregnancy Risk Factor: C

Lactation:

Fluticasone: Excretion in breast milk unknown/use caution

Salmeterol: Enters breast milk/use caution

Related Information

Fluticasone *on page 660*

Salmeterol *on page 1352*

♦ **Fluticasone Propionate** *see* Fluticasone *on page 660*

Fluvastatin (FLOO va sta tin)

U.S. Brand Names Lescol®; Lescol® XL

Generic Available No

Pharmacologic Category Antilipemic Agent, HMG-CoA Reductase Inhibitor

Medication Safety Issues

Sound-alike/look-alike issues:

Fluvastatin may be confused with fluoxetine

Use To be used as a component of multiple risk factor intervention in patients at risk for atherosclerosis vascular disease due to hypercholesterolemia

Adjunct to dietary therapy to reduce elevated total cholesterol (total-C), LDL-C, triglyceride, and apolipoprotein B (apo-B) levels and to increase HDL-C in primary hypercholesterolemia and mixed dyslipidemia (Fredrickson types IIa and IIb); to slow the progression of coronary atherosclerosis in patients with coronary heart disease; reduce risk of coronary revascularization procedures in patients with coronary heart disease

Mechanism of Action/Effect Acts by competitively inhibiting 3-hydroxyl-3-methyl-glutaryl-coenzyme A (HMG-CoA) reductase, the enzyme that catalyzes the reduction of HMG-CoA to mevalonate; this is an early rate-limiting step in cholesterol biosynthesis. HDL is increased while total, LDL and VLDL cholesterols, apolipoprotein B, and plasma triglycerides are decreased.

Contraindications Hypersensitivity to fluvastatin or any component of the formulation; active liver disease; unexplained persistent elevations of serum transaminases; pregnancy; breast-feeding

Warnings/Precautions Secondary causes of hyperlipidemia should be ruled out prior to therapy. Liver function must be monitored by periodic laboratory assessment. Rhabdomyolysis with acute renal failure has occurred with fluvastatin and other HMG-CoA reductase inhibitors. Risk may be increased with concurrent use of other drugs which may cause rhabdomyolysis (including gemfibrozil, fibric acid derivatives, or niacin at doses ≥ 1 g/day). Temporarily discontinue in any patient experiencing an acute or serious condition predisposing to renal failure secondary to rhabdomyolysis. Use caution in patients with previous liver disease or heavy ethanol use. Treatment in patients <18 years of age is not recommended.

Drug Interactions

Cytochrome P450 Effect: Substrate (minor) of CYP2C8/9, 2D6, 3A4; **Inhibits** CYP1A2 (weak), 2C8/9 (moderate), 2D6 (weak), 3A4 (weak)

Decreased Effect: Administration of cholestyramine at the same time with fluvastatin reduces absorption and clinical effect of fluvastatin. Separate administration times by at least 4 hours. Rifampin and rifabutin may decrease fluvastatin blood levels.

Increased Effect/Toxicity: Cimetidine, omeprazole, ranitidine, and ritonavir may increase fluvastatin blood levels. Clofibrate, erythromycin, gemfibrozil, fenofibrate, and niacin may increase the risk of myopathy and rhabdomyolysis. Anticoagulant effect of warfarin may be increased by fluvastatin. Cholestyramine effect will be additive with fluvastatin if administration times are separated. Fluvastatin may increase C_{max} and decrease clearance of digoxin. Fluvastatin may increase the levels/effects of amiodarone, fluoxetine, glimepiride, glipizide, nateglinide, phenytoin, pioglitazone, rosiglitazone, sertraline, warfarin, and other CYP2C8/9 substrates.

Nutritional/Ethanol Interactions

Ethanol: Avoid excessive ethanol consumption (due to potential hepatic effects).

Food: Reduces rate but not the extent of absorption.

Lab Interactions Increased serum transaminases, CPK, alkaline phosphatase, and bilirubin and thyroid function tests

Adverse Reactions As reported with fluvastatin capsules; in general, adverse reactions reported with fluvastatin extended release tablet were similar, but the incidence was less.

1% to 10%:

Central nervous system: Headache (9%), fatigue (3%), insomnia (3%)

Gastrointestinal: Dyspepsia (8%), diarrhea (5%), abdominal pain (5%), nausea (3%)

Genitourinary: Urinary tract infection (2%)

Neuromuscular & skeletal: Myalgia (5%)

Respiratory: Sinusitis (3%), bronchitis (2%)

Overdosage/Toxicology GI complaints and elevated SGOT and SGPT have been reported following large doses of the extended release tablets. In case of overdose, supportive measure should be instituted, as required; dialyzability is not known.

Pharmacodynamics/Kinetics

Bioavailability: Absolute: Capsule: 24%; Extended release tablet: 29%

Protein Binding: >98%

Half-Life Elimination: Capsule: <3 hours; Extended release tablet: 9 hours

Metabolism: To inactive and active metabolites [oxidative metabolism via CYP2C9 (75%), 2C8 (~5%), and 3A4 (~20%) isoenzymes]; active forms do not circulate systemically; extensive first-pass hepatic extraction

Excretion: Feces (90%): urine (5%)

Dosing

Adults & Elderly:

Dyslipidemia (also delay in progression of CAD): Oral:

Patients requiring $\geq 25\%$ decrease in LDL-C: 40 mg capsule or 80 mg extended release tablet once daily in the evening; may also use 40 mg capsule twice daily

Patients requiring <25% decrease in LDL-C: 20 mg capsule once daily in the evening

Dosing range: 20-80 mg/day; adjust dose based on response to therapy; maximum response occurs within 4-6 weeks

Renal Impairment: Less than 6% is excreted renally. No dosage adjustment needed with mild to moderate renal impairment; use with caution in severe impairment.

Hepatic Impairment: Levels may accumulate in patients with liver disease (increased AUC and C_{max}). Use caution with severe hepatic impairment or heavy ethanol ingestion. Contraindicated in active liver disease or unexplained transaminase elevations. Decrease dose and monitor effects carefully in patients with hepatic insufficiency.

Available Dosage Forms

Capsule (Lescol®): 20 mg, 40 mg

Tablet, extended release (Lescol® XL): 80 mg

Monitoring and Teaching Issues

Physical Assessment: See Warnings/Precautions for use cautions (liver or kidney impairment, rhabdomyolysis). Assess potential for interactions with other pharmacological agents or herbal products the patient may be taking (eg, increased risk of rhabdomyolysis; see Drug Interactions). Assess results of baseline and periodic laboratory tests. Monitor therapeutic effectiveness (reduced hyperlipidemia) and adverse response on a regular basis throughout therapy (eg, myalgia, gastrointestinal disturbances; see Adverse Reactions). Teach patient proper use, possible side effects/appropriate interventions, and adverse symptoms to report (see Patient Education). **Pregnancy risk factor X:** Determine that

(Continued)

Fluvastatin *(Continued)*

patient is not pregnant before starting therapy. Do not give to sexually active female patients unless capable of complying with effective contraceptive use. Instruct patient in appropriate contraceptive measures.

Monitoring Laboratory Tests: Obtain baseline LFTs and total cholesterol profile. Repeat tests at 12 weeks after initiation of therapy or elevation in dose, and periodically thereafter. Monitor LDL-C at intervals no less than 4 weeks.

Patient Education: Do not take any new medication during therapy unless approved by prescriber. Take as directed, with or without food. Follow diet and exercise regimen as prescribed. You may experience nausea or dyspepsia (small frequent meals, frequent mouth care, chewing gum, or sucking lozenges may help); diarrhea (buttermilk, boiled milk, or yogurt may help); or headache (consult prescriber for approved analgesic). Report immediately any muscle pain or cramping; tremor; or CNS changes (eg, memory loss, depression, personality changes; numbness, weakness, tingling or pain in extremities). **Pregnancy/breast-feeding precautions:** Inform prescriber if you are pregnant. Consult prescriber for instruction on appropriate contraceptive measures. This drug may cause severe fetal defects. Do not donate blood during or for 1 month following therapy. Do not breast-feed.

Dietary Considerations: Before initiation of therapy, patients should be placed on a standard cholesterol-lowering diet for 3-6 months and the diet should be continued during drug therapy. May be taken without regard to meals.

Geriatric Considerations: The definition of and, therefore, when to treat hyperlipidemia in the elderly is a controversial issue. The National Cholesterol Education Program recommends that all adults maintain a plasma cholesterol <160 mg/dL. In elderly patients with one additional risk factor, goal LDL would decrease to <130 mg/dL. Pharmacologic treatment should be reserved for those who are unable to obtain a desirable plasma cholesterol concentration by diet alone and for whom the benefits of treatment are believed to outweigh the potential adverse effects, drug interactions, and cost of treatment.

Pregnancy Risk Factor: X

Pregnancy Issues: Animal studies have shown delays in fetal skeletal development and fetal, neonatal, and maternal mortality. Congenital anomalies following use of other HMG-CoA reductase inhibitors in humans have been reported (rare). Use in women of childbearing potential only if they are highly unlikely to conceive; discontinue if pregnancy occurs.

Lactation: Enters breast milk/contraindicated

Breast-Feeding Issues: Fluvastatin is excreted in human breast milk (milk plasma ratio 2:1); do not use in breast-feeding women.

Administration

Oral: Patient should be placed on a standard cholesterol-lowering diet before and during treatment; fluvastatin may be taken without regard to meals; adjust dosage as needed in response to periodic lipid determinations during the first 4 weeks after a dosage change; lipid-lowering effects are additive when fluvastatin is combined with a bile-acid binding resin or niacin, however, it must be administered at least 2 hours following these drugs.

Storage: Store at 25°C (77°F); protect from light.

Related Information

Hyperlipidemia Management *on page 1836*
Lipid-Lowering Agents *on page 1738*

♦ Fluvirin® *see page 1660*

Fluvoxamine *(floo VOKS a meen)*

Synonyms Luvox

Restrictons A medication guide should be dispensed with each prescription. A template for the required MedGuides can be found on the FDA website at: http://www.fda.gov/cder/drug/antidepressants/labelTemplate.pdf

Generic Available Yes

Pharmacologic Category Antidepressant, Selective Serotonin Reuptake Inhibitor

Medication Safety Issues

Sound-alike/look-alike issues:
Fluvoxamine may be confused with flavoxate
Luvox may be confused with Lasix®, Levoxyl®

Use Treatment of obsessive-compulsive disorder (OCD) in children ≥8 years of age and adults

Unlabeled/Investigational Use Treatment of major depression; panic disorder; anxiety disorders in children

Mechanism of Action/Effect Inhibits CNS neuron serotonin uptake; minimal or no effect on reuptake of norepinephrine or dopamine; does not significantly bind to alpha-adrenergic, histamine or cholinergic receptors

Contraindications Hypersensitivity to fluvoxamine or any component of the formulation; concurrent use with pimozide, thioridazine, mesoridazine, or cisapride; use of MAO inhibitors within 14 days

Warnings/Precautions Antidepressants increase the risk of suicidal thinking and behavior in children and adolescents with major depressive disorder (MDD) and other depressive disorders; consider risk prior to prescribing. All patients must be closely monitored for clinical worsening, suicidality, or unusual changes in behavior, especially during the initiation of therapy or following an increase or decrease in dosage. When used in children, the child's family or caregiver should be instructed to closely observe the patient and communicate condition with healthcare provider. A medication guide should be dispensed with each prescription. **Fluvoxamine is FDA approved for the treatment of OCD in children ≥8 years of age.**

The possibility of a suicide attempt is inherent in major depression and may persist until remission occurs. Use caution in high-risk patients. Worsening depression and severe abrupt suicidality that are not part of the presenting symptoms may require discontinuation or modification of drug therapy. The patient's family or caregiver should be alerted to monitor patients for the emergence of suicidality and associated behaviors (such as agitation, irritability, hostility, impulsivity, and hypomania) and call healthcare provider.

May worsen psychosis in some patients or precipitate a shift to mania or hypomania in patients with bipolar disorder. Patients presenting with depressive symptoms should be screened for bipolar disorder. Monotherapy in patients with bipolar disorder should be avoided. **Fluvoxamine is not FDA approved for the treatment of bipolar depression.**

The potential for severe reaction exits when used with MAO inhibitors - serotonin syndrome (hyperthermia, muscular rigidity, mental status changes/agitation, autonomic instability) may occur. Fluvoxamine has a low potential to impair cognitive or motor performance; caution operating hazardous machinery or driving. Use caution in patients with a previous seizure disorder or condition predisposing to seizures such as brain damage, alcoholism, or concurrent therapy with other drugs which lower the seizure threshold.

May increase the risks associated with electroconvulsive therapy. Use with caution in patients with hepatic or renal dysfunction and in elderly patients. May cause hyponatremia/SIADH. Use with caution in patients with renal insufficiency or other concurrent illness (cardiovascular disease). Use with caution in patients at risk of bleeding or receiving concurrent anticoagulant therapy, although not consistently noted, fluvoxamine may cause impairment in platelet function. May cause or exacerbate sexual dysfunction.

Drug Interactions
Cytochrome P450 Effect: Substrate (major) of CYP1A2, 2D6; **Inhibits** CYP1A2 (strong), 2B6 (weak), 2C8/9 (weak), 2C19 (strong), 2D6 (weak), 3A4 (weak)

Decreased Effect: The levels/effects of fluvoxamine may be decreased by aminoglutethimide, carbamazepine, phenobarbital, rifampin, and other CYP1A2 inducers. Cyproheptadine, a serotonin antagonist, may inhibit the effects of serotonin reuptake inhibitors (fluvoxamine); monitor for altered antidepressant response.

Increased Effect/Toxicity: Fluvoxamine should not be used with nonselective MAO inhibitors (phenelzine, isocarboxazid) and drugs with MAO inhibitor properties (linezolid); fatal reactions have been reported. Wait 5 weeks after stopping fluvoxamine before starting a nonselective MAO inhibitor and 2 weeks after stopping an MAO inhibitor before starting fluvoxamine. Concurrent selegiline has been associated with mania, hypertension, or serotonin syndrome (risk may be reduced relative to nonselective MAO inhibitors).

Fluvoxamine may inhibit the metabolism of thioridazine or mesoridazine, resulting in increased plasma levels and increasing the risk of QT_c interval prolongation. This may lead to serious ventricular arrhythmias, such as torsade de pointes-type arrhythmias and sudden death. Do not use together. Wait at least 5 weeks after discontinuing fluvoxamine prior to starting thioridazine. Fluvoxamine may increase the levels/effects of aminophylline, citalopram, diazepam, mexiletine, mirtazapine, methsuximide, phenytoin, propranolol, ropinirole, sertraline, theophylline, trifluoperazine and other substrates of CYP1A2 or 2C19.

The levels/effects of fluvoxamine may be increased by amiodarone, amphetamines, selected beta-blockers, chlorpromazine, ciprofloxacin, delavirdine, fluoxetine, ketoconazole, miconazole, norfloxacin, ofloxacin, paroxetine, pergolide, quinidine, quinine, ritonavir, rofecoxib, ropinirole, and other CYP1A2 or 2D6 inhibitors.

Combined use of SSRIs and amphetamines, buspirone, meperidine, nefazodone, serotonin agonists (such as sumatriptan), sibutramine, other SSRIs, sympathomimetics, ritonavir, tramadol, and venlafaxine may increase the risk of serotonin syndrome. Combined use of sumatriptan (and other serotonin agonists) may result in toxicity; weakness, hyper-reflexia, and incoordination have been observed with sumatriptan and SSRIs. In addition, concurrent use may theoretically increase the risk of serotonin syndrome; includes sumatriptan, naratriptan, rizatriptan, and zolmitriptan.

Concurrent lithium may increase risk of nephrotoxicity. Risk of hyponatremia may increase with concurrent use of loop diuretics (bumetanide, furosemide, torsemide). Fluvoxamine may increase the hypoprothrombinemic response to warfarin. Concomitant use of fluvoxamine and NSAIDs, aspirin, or other drugs affecting coagulation has been associated with an increased risk of bleeding; monitor.

Nutritional/Ethanol Interactions
Ethanol: Avoid ethanol. Depressed patients should avoid/limit intake.

Food: The bioavailability of melatonin has been reported to be increased by fluvoxamine.

Herb/Nutraceutical: Avoid valerian, St John's wort, SAMe, kava kava (may increase risk of serotonin syndrome and/or excessive sedation).

Adverse Reactions
>10%:
Central nervous system: Headache (22%), somnolence (22%), insomnia (21%), nervousness (12%), dizziness (11%)
Gastrointestinal: Nausea (40%), diarrhea (11%), xerostomia (14%)
Neuromuscular & skeletal: Weakness (14%)

1% to 10%:
Cardiovascular: Palpitations
Central nervous system: Somnolence, mania, hypomania, vertigo, abnormal thinking, agitation, anxiety, malaise, amnesia, yawning, hypertonia, CNS stimulation, depression
Endocrine & metabolic: Decreased libido
Gastrointestinal: Abdominal pain, vomiting, dyspepsia, constipation, abnormal taste, anorexia, flatulence, weight gain
Genitourinary: Delayed ejaculation, impotence, anorgasmia, urinary frequency, urinary retention
Neuromuscular & skeletal: Tremors
Ocular: Blurred vision
Respiratory: Dyspnea
Miscellaneous: Diaphoresis

Overdosage/Toxicology
Symptoms of overdose include drowsiness, nausea, vomiting, abdominal pain, tremor, sinus bradycardia, and seizures. A specific antidote does not exist. Treatment is supportive.

(Continued)

Fluvoxamine (Continued)

Pharmacodynamics/Kinetics

Absorption: Steady-state plasma concentrations have been noted to be 2-3 times higher in children than those in adolescents; female children demonstrated a significantly higher AUC than males

Bioavailability: 53%; not significantly affected by food

Time to Peak: Plasma: 3-8 hours

Protein Binding: ~80%, primarily to albumin

Half-Life Elimination: ~15 hours

Metabolism: Hepatic

Excretion: Urine

Dosing

Adults: Obsessive-compulsive disorder: Oral: Initial: 50 mg at bedtime; adjust in 50 mg increments at 4- to 7-day intervals; usual dose range: 100-300 mg/day; divide total daily dose into 2 doses. Administer larger portion at bedtime.

Note: When total daily dose exceeds 50 mg, the dose should be given in 2 divided doses.

Elderly: Reduce dose, titrate slowly. See Geriatric Considerations.

Pediatrics: Obsessive-compulsive disorder: Oral: Children 8-17 years: Initial: 25 mg at bedtime; adjust in 25 mg increments at 4- to 7-day intervals, as tolerated, to maximum therapeutic benefit: Range: 50-200 mg/day

Maximum dose: Children: 8-11 years: 200 mg/day; Adolescents: 300 mg/day; lower doses may be effective in female versus male patients

Note: When total daily dose exceeds 50 mg, the dose should be given in 2 divided doses.

Hepatic Impairment: Reduce dose, titrate slowly.

Available Dosage Forms Tablet: 25 mg, 50 mg, 100 mg

Monitoring and Teaching Issues

Physical Assessment: Assess other medications patient may be taking for effectiveness and interactions. Assess results of laboratory tests, therapeutic effectiveness, and adverse reactions at beginning of therapy and periodically with long-term use. Taper dosage slowly when discontinuing (allow 3-4 weeks between discontinuing Luvox® and starting another antidepressant). Assess mental status for depression, suicidal ideation, anxiety, social functioning, mania, or panic attack. Assess knowledge/teach patient appropriate use, interventions to reduce side effects, and adverse symptoms to report.

Monitoring Laboratory Tests: Liver and kidney function assessment prior to beginning drug therapy

Patient Education: Take exactly as directed; do not increase dose or frequency. It may take 2-3 weeks to achieve desired results. Avoid alcohol, caffeine, and other prescription or OTC medications unless approved by prescriber. Maintain adequate hydration (2-3 L/day of fluids) unless instructed to restrict fluid intake. You may experience drowsiness, lightheadedness, impaired coordination, dizziness, or blurred vision (use caution when driving or engaging in tasks requiring alertness until response to drug is known); nausea, vomiting, or anorexia (small frequent meals, frequent mouth care, chewing gum, or sucking lozenges may help); constipation (increased exercise, fluids, fruits, or fiber may help); diarrhea (buttermilk, yogurt, or boiled milk may help); postural hypotension (use caution when climbing stairs or changing position from lying or sitting to standing); or decreased sexual function or libido (reversible). Report persistent CNS effects (nervousness, restlessness, insomnia, anxiety, excitation, headache, sedation, seizures, mania, abnormal thinking); rash or skin irritation; muscle cramping, tremors, or change in gait; chest pain or palpitations; change in urinary pattern; or worsening of condition. **Pregnancy/breast-feeding precautions:** Inform prescriber if you are or intend to become pregnant. Breast-feeding is not recommended.

Geriatric Considerations: Modify the initial dose and the subsequent dose titration in the elderly. It may be best to select a different agent when treating depression in the elderly.

Pregnancy Risk Factor: C

Pregnancy Issues: Nonteratogenic effects including respiratory distress, cyanosis, apnea, seizures, temperature instability, feeding difficulty, vomiting, hypoglycemia, hypo- or hypertonia, hyper-reflexia, jitteriness, irritability, constant crying, and tremor have been reported in the neonate immediately following delivery after exposure to other SSRIs late in the third trimester. Adverse effects may be due to toxic effects of SSRI or drug discontinuation. In some cases, may present clinically as serotonin syndrome. There are no adequate and well-controlled studies in pregnant women. Use during pregnancy only if the potential benefit to the mother outweighs the possible risk to the fetus. If treatment during pregnancy is required, consider tapering therapy during the third trimester.

Lactation: Enters breast milk/not recommended (AAP rates "of concern")

Administration

Storage: Protect from high humidity and store at controlled room temperature 15°C to 30°C (59°F to 86°F); dispense in tight containers

Related Information

Antidepressant Agents *on page 1713*

Antidepressant Medication Guidelines *on page 1765*

♦ Fluxid™ *see Famotidine on page 608*

♦ Fluzone® *see page 1660*

♦ FML® *see Fluorometholone on page 646*

♦ FML® Forte *see Fluorometholone on page 646*

♦ FML-S® *see Sulfacetamide Sodium and Fluorometholone on page 1405*

♦ Focalin™ *see Dexmethylphenidate on page 431*

♦ Foille® [OTC] *see Benzocaine on page 181*

♦ Folacin *see Folic Acid on page 669*

♦ Folate *see Folic Acid on page 669*

Folic Acid (FOE lik AS id)

Synonyms Folacin; Folate; Pteroylglutamic Acid

Generic Available Yes

Pharmacologic Category Vitamin, Water Soluble

Medication Safety Issues
Sound-alike/look-alike issues:
Folic acid may be confused with folinic acid

Use Treatment of megaloblastic and macrocytic anemias due to folate deficiency; dietary supplement to prevent neural tube defects

Mechanism of Action/Effect Folic acid is necessary for formation of a number of coenzymes in many metabolic systems, particularly for purine and pyrimidine synthesis; required for nucleoprotein synthesis and maintenance in erythropoiesis; stimulates WBC and platelet production in folate deficiency anemia

Contraindications Hypersensitivity to folic acid or any component of the formulation

Warnings/Precautions Not appropriate for monotherapy with pernicious, aplastic, or normocytic anemias when anemia is present with vitamin D deficiency. Doses >0.1 mg/day may obscure pernicious anemia with continuing irreversible nerve damage progression. Resistance to treatment may occur with depressed hematopoiesis, alcoholism, deficiencies of other vitamins. Injection contains benzyl alcohol (1.5%) as preservative (use care in administration to neonates).

Drug Interactions
Decreased Effect: Folic acid may decrease phenytoin concentrations. Folic acid may diminish the therapeutic effect of raltitrexed.

Lab Interactions Falsely low serum concentrations may occur with the *Lactobacillus casei* assay method in patients on anti-infectives (eg, tetracycline).

Adverse Reactions Frequency not defined.
Allergic reaction, bronchospasm, flushing (slight), malaise (general), pruritus, rash

Pharmacodynamics/Kinetics
Onset of Action: Peak effect: Oral: 0.5-1 hour
Absorption: Proximal part of small intestine

Dosing
Adults:
Anemia: Oral, I.M., I.V., SubQ: 0.4 mg/day
Pregnant and lactating women: 0.8 mg/day
RDA: Expressed as dietary folate equivalents: 400 mcg/day
Prevention of neural tube defects: Oral:
Females of childbearing potential: 400 mcg/day
Females at high risk or with family history of neural tube defects: 4 mg/day
Elderly: Refer to adults dosing. Vitamin B_{12} deficiency must be ruled out before initiating folate therapy due to frequency of combined nutritional deficiencies: RDA requirements (1999): 400 mcg/day (0.4 mg) minimum.
Pediatrics:
Anemia: Oral, I.M., I.V., SubQ:
Infants: 0.1 mg/day
Children <4 years: Up to 0.3 mg/day
Children >4 years and Adults: Refer to adult dosing.
RDA: Expressed as dietary folate equivalents: Oral: Children:
1-3 years: 150 mcg/day
4-8 years: 200 mcg/day
9-13 years: 300 mcg/day
≥14 years: Refer to adult dosing.

Available Dosage Forms
Injection, solution, as sodium folate: 5 mg/mL (10 mL) [contains benzyl alcohol]
Tablet: 0.4 mg, 0.8 mg, 1 mg

Monitoring and Teaching Issues
Physical Assessment: Assess potential for interactions with other prescriptions, OTC medications, or herbal products patient may be taking. Assess therapeutic effectiveness and adverse response on a regular basis throughout therapy. Teach patient proper use, possible side effects/appropriate interventions, and adverse symptoms to report.
Patient Education: Do not take any new medication during therapy unless approved by prescriber. Take exactly as prescribed. Toxicity can occur from elevated doses. Increased intake of foods high in folic acid (eg, dried beans, nuts, bran, vegetables, fruits) may be recommended by prescriber. Excessive use of alcohol increases requirement for folic acid. May turn urine more intensely yellow. Report skin rash. **Pregnancy precaution:** Inform prescriber if you are pregnant.
Dietary Considerations: As of January 1998, the FDA has required manufacturers of enriched flour, bread, corn meal, pasta, rice and other grain products to add folic acid to their products. The intent is to help decrease the risk of neural tube defects by increasing folic acid intake. Other foods which contain folic acid include dark green leafy vegetables, citrus fruits and juices, and lentils.
Geriatric Considerations: Elderly frequently have combined nutritional deficiencies. Must rule out vitamin B_{12} deficiency before initiating folate therapy. Elderly RDA requirements from 1999 RDA are 400 mcg minimum (0.4 mg). Elderly, due to decreased nutrient intake, may benefit from daily intake of a multiple vitamin with minerals.
Pregnancy Risk Factor: A
Lactation: Enters breast milk/compatible

Administration
Oral: A diluted solution for oral administration may be prepared by diluting 1 mL of folic acid injection (5 mg/mL), with 49 mL sterile water for injection. Resulting solution is 0.1 mg folic acid per 1 mL.
(Continued)

Folic Acid (Continued)

I.M.: May also be administered by deep I.M. injection.

I.V.: May also be administered by I.V. injection by diluting 1 mL of folic acid injection (5 mg/mL), with 49 mL sterile water for injection. Resulting solution is 0.1 mg folic acid per 1 mL.

Compatibility: Stable in D_5W, $D_{20}W$, NS, fat emulsion 10%; **incompatible** with $D_{40}W$, $D_{50}W$

Compatibility in syringe: **Incompatible** with doxapram

Compatibility when admixed: **Incompatible** with calcium gluconate

Additional Information The RDA for folic acid is presented as dietary folate equivalents (DFE). DFE adjusts for the difference in bioavailability of folic acid from food as compared to dietary supplements.

- ♦ **Folinic Acid** *see* Leucovorin *on page 875*
- ♦ **Follistim® [DSC]** *see* Follitropins *on page 670*
- ♦ **Follistim® AQ** *see* Follitropins *on page 670*
- ♦ **Follitropin Alfa** *see* Follitropins *on page 670*
- ♦ **Follitropin Alpha** *see* Follitropins *on page 670*
- ♦ **Follitropin Beta** *see* Follitropins *on page 670*

Follitropins (foe li TRO pins)

U.S. Brand Names Bravelle™; Follistim® [DSC]; Follistim® AQ; Gonal-f®; Gonal-f™ RFF

Synonyms Follitropin Alfa; Follitropin Alpha; Follitropin Beta; Recombinant Human Follicle Stimulating Hormone; rFSH-alpha; rFSH-beta; rhFSH-alpha; rhFSH-beta; Urofollitropin

Generic Available No

Pharmacologic Category Gonadotropin; Ovulation Stimulator

Use

Urofollitropin (Bravelle™): Ovulation induction in patients who previously received pituitary suppression; Assisted Reproductive Technologies (ART) ART

Follitropin alfa (Gonal-f®), Follitropin beta (Follistim®): Ovulation induction in patients in whom the cause of infertility is functional and not caused by primary ovarian failure; ART; spermatogenesis induction

Follitropin beta (Follistim® AQ): Ovulation induction in patients in whom the cause of infertility is functional and not caused by primary ovarian failure; ART

Mechanism of Action/Effect Urofollitropin is a preparation of highly purified follicle-stimulating hormone (FSH) extracted from the urine of postmenopausal women. Follitropin alfa and follitropin beta are human FSH preparations of recombinant DNA origin. Follitropins stimulate ovarian follicular growth in women who do not have primary ovarian failure. FSH is required for normal follicular growth, maturation, and gonadal steroid production.

Contraindications Hypersensitivity to follitropins or any component of the formulation; high levels of FSH indicating primary gonadal failure (ovarian or testicular); uncontrolled thyroid or adrenal dysfunction; the presence of any cause of infertility other than anovulation; tumor of the ovary, breast, uterus, hypothalamus, testis, or pituitary gland; abnormal vaginal bleeding of undetermined origin; ovarian cysts or enlargement not due to polycystic ovary syndrome; pregnancy

Warnings/Precautions These medications should only be used by physicians who are thoroughly familiar with infertility problems and their management. To minimize risks, use only at the lowest effective dose. Monitor ovarian response with serum estradiol and vaginal ultrasound on a regular basis.

Ovarian enlargement which may be accompanied by abdominal distention or abdominal pain, occurs in ~20% of those treated with urofollitropin and hCG, and generally regresses without treatment within 2-3 weeks. Ovarian hyperstimulation syndrome, characterized by severe ovarian enlargement, abdominal pain/distention, nausea, vomiting, diarrhea, dyspnea, and oliguria, and may be accompanied by ascites, pleural effusion, hypovolemia, electrolyte imbalance, hemoperitoneum, and thromboembolic events is reported in about 6% of patients. If hyperstimulation occurs, stop treatment and hospitalize patient. This syndrome develops rapidly within 24 hours to several days and generally occurs during the 7-10 days immediately following treatment. Hemoconcentration associated with fluid loss into the abdominal cavity has occurred and should be assessed by fluid intake & output, weight, hematocrit, serum & urinary electrolytes, urine specific gravity, BUN and creatinine, and abdominal girth. Determinations should be performed daily or more often if the need arises. Treatment is primarily symptomatic and consists of bed rest, fluid and electrolyte replacement and analgesics. The ascitic, pleural and pericardial fluids should never be removed because of the potential danger of injury.

Serious pulmonary conditions (atelectasis, acute respiratory distress syndrome and exacerbation of asthma) have been reported. Thromboembolic events, both in association with and separate from ovarian hyperstimulation syndrome, have been reported.

Multiple pregnancies have been associated with these medications, including triplet and quintuplet gestations. Advise patient of the potential risk of multiple births before starting the treatment.

Follistim® AQ: Contains trace amounts of neomycin and streptomycin. Must be administered using the Follistim Pen™; dose adjustment required when switching from powder for injection to solution for injection due to accuracy of pen device.

Adverse Reactions Frequency varies by specific product and route of administration.

>10%:

Central nervous system: Headache (up to 27%)

Gastrointestinal: Abdominal pain (up to 23%)

2% to 10%:

Central nervous system: Dizziness, fever

Dermatologic: Acne (male), dermoid cyst (male), dry skin, body rash, hair loss, hives

Endocrine & metabolic: Ovarian hyperstimulation syndrome, adnexal torsion, mild-to-moderate ovarian enlargement, ovarian cysts, breast tenderness, gynecomastia (male)

Gastrointestinal: Nausea, vomiting, diarrhea, abdominal cramps, bloating, flatulence, dyspepsia

Genitourinary: Urinary tract infection, menstrual disorder, intermenstrual bleeding, dysmenorrhea, cervical lesion

Local: Pain, rash, swelling, or irritation at the site of injection

Neuromuscular & skeletal: Back pain, varicose veins (male)

Respiratory: Exacerbation of asthma, sinusitis, pharyngitis

Miscellaneous: Febrile reactions accompanied by chills, musculoskeletal, joint pains, malaise, headache, and fatigue; flu-like symptoms

Overdosage/Toxicology Aside from possible ovarian hyperstimulation and multiple gestations, little is known concerning the consequences of an acute overdose. Treatment is symptomatic.

Pharmacodynamics/Kinetics
Onset of Action: Peak effect: Spermatogenesis, median: 165 days (range: 25-327 days); Follicle development: Within cycle

Absorption: Rate limited: I.M., SubQ: Slower than elimination rate

Bioavailability: Ranges from ~66% to 82% depending on agent

Time to Peak:
Follitropin alfa: SubQ: 16 hours; I.M.: 25 hours
Follitropin beta: I.M.: 27 hours
Urofollitropin: Single dose: SubQ: 15-20 hours, I.M.: 10-17 hours; Multiple doses: I.M., SubQ: 10 hours

Half-Life Elimination:
Mean: SubQ: Follitropin alfa: 24-32 hours; Follitropin beta: ~30 hours; Urofollitropin: 32-37 hours
Mean terminal: Multiple doses: I.M. follitropin alfa, SubQ follitropin beta: ~30 hours; I.M. urofollitropin: 15 hours, SubQ urofollitropin: 21 hours

Metabolism: Total clearance of follitropin alfa was 0.6 L/hour following I.V. administration

Excretion: Clearance: Follitropin alfa: I.V.: 0.6 L/hour

Dosing
Adults: Note: Use the lowest dose consistent with the expectation of good results. Over the course of treatment, doses may vary depending on individual patient response. When used for ovulation induction, if response to follitropin is appropriate, hCG is given 1 day following the last dose. Withhold hCG if serum estradiol is >2000 pg/mL, if the ovaries are abnormally enlarged, or if abdominal pain occurs.

Urofollitropin: Bravelle™:
Ovulation induction: Female: I.M., SubQ: Initial: 150 int. units daily for the first 5 days of treatment. Dose adjustments of ≤75-150 int. units can be made every ≥2 days; maximum daily dose: 450 int. units; treatment >12 days is not recommended
ART: Female: SubQ: 225 int. units for the first 5 days; dose may be adjusted based on patient response, but adjustments should not be made more frequently than once every 2 days; maximum adjustment: 75-150 int. units; maximum daily dose: 450 int. units; maximum duration of treatment: 12 days

Follitropin alfa: Gonal-f®: SubQ:
Ovulation induction: Female: Initial: 75 int. units/day; consider dose adjustment after 5-7 days; additional dose adjustments of up to 37.5 int. units may be considered after 14 days; further dose increases of the same magnitude can be made, if necessary, every 7 days (maximum dose: 300 int. units)
ART: Female: Initiate therapy with follitropin alfa in the early follicular phase (cycle day 2 or day 3) at a dose of 150 int. units/day, until sufficient follicular development is attained. In most cases, therapy should not exceed 10 days. In patients whose endogenous gonadotropin levels are suppressed, initiate follitropin alfa at a dose of 225 int. units/day. Continue treatment until adequate follicular development is indicated as determined by ultrasound in combination with measurement of serum estradiol levels. Consider adjustments to dose after 5 days based on the patient's response; adjust subsequent dosage every 3-5 days by ≤75-150 int. units additionally at each adjustment. Doses >450 int. units/day are not recommended. Once adequate follicular development is evident, administer hCG (5000-10,000 units) to induce final follicular maturation in preparation for oocyte.
Spermatogenesis induction: Male: Therapy should begin with hCG pretreatment until serum testosterone is in normal range, then 150 int. units 3 times/week with hCG 3 times/week; continue with lowest dose needed to induce spermatogenesis (maximum dose: 300 int. units 3 times/week); may be given for up to 18 months

Follitropin beta:
Follistim®: I.M., SubQ:
Ovulation induction: Female: Stepwise approach: Initiate therapy with 75 int. units/day for up to 14 days. Increase by 37.5 int. units at weekly intervals until follicular growth or serum estradiol levels indicate an adequate response. The maximum, individualized, daily dose that has been safely used for ovulation induction in patients during clinical trials is 300 int. units.
ART: Female: A starting dose of 150-225 int. units of follitropin beta is recommended for at least the first 4 days of treatment. The dose may be adjusted for the individual patient based upon their ovarian response. Daily maintenance doses ranging from 75-300 int. units for 6-12 days are usually sufficient, although longer treatment may be necessary. Maintenance doses of up to 375-600 int. units may be necessary according to individual response. The maximum daily dose used in clinical studies is 600 int. units. When a sufficient number of follicles of adequate size are present, the final maturation of the follicles is induced by administering hCG at a dose of 5000-10,000 int. units. Oocyte retrieval is performed 34-36 hours later. Withhold

(Continued)

Follitropins *(Continued)*

hCG in cases where the ovaries are abnormally enlarged on the last day of follitropin beta therapy.

Follistim®: Male: SubQ: **Spermatogenesis induction:**

Note: Begin therapy with hCG pretreatment to normalize serum testosterone levels. Once normal levels are reached, follitropin beta therapy is initiated, and must be administered concurrently with hCG treatment.

450 int. units/week given as 225 int. units twice weekly or 150 int. units 3 times/week with hCG; treatment response was noted at up to 12 months

Follistim® AQ: SubQ:

Ovulation induction: Female: Stepwise approach: Initiate therapy with 75 int. units/ day for up to 7 days. A lower dose should be given if previous doses were administered using the powder for injection (see dosing conversion). Increase by 25 or 50 int. units at weekly intervals until follicular growth or serum estradiol levels indicate an adequate response. The maximum (individualized) daily dose that has been safely used for ovulation induction in patients during clinical trials is 175 int. units.

ART: Female: A starting dose of 150-225 int. units of follitropin beta is recommended for at least the first 5 days of treatment. The dose may be adjusted for the individual patient based upon their ovarian response. A lower dose should be given if previous doses were administered using the powder for injection (see dosing conversion). The maximum daily dose used in clinical studies is 450 int. units. When a sufficient number of follicles of adequate size are present, the final maturation of the follicles is induced by administering hCG at a dose of 5000-10,000 int. units. Oocyte retrieval is performed 34-36 hours later. Withhold hCG in cases where the ovaries are abnormally enlarged on the last day of follitropin beta therapy.

Follistim® AQ Dosing Conversion guidelines: See table.

Follistim® AQ Dosing Conversion

Dose Administered Using Powder for Solution/Conventional Syringe	Follistim® AQ Dose Administered Using Follistim Pen™
75 int. units	50 int. units
150 int. units	125 int. units
225 int. units	175 int. units
300 int. units	250 int. units
375 int. units	300 int. units
450 int. units	375 int. units

Elderly: Refer to adult dosing. Clinical studies did not include patients >65 years of age.

Available Dosage Forms [DSC] = Discontinued product

Injection, powder for reconstitution [packaged with diluent]:

Follitropin alfa [rDNA origin, single-dose ampul] (Gonal-f®): 75 int. units, 150 int. units [DSC]

Follitropin alfa [rDNA origin, multidose vial] (Gonal-f®): 450 int. units [contains sucrose 30 mg; packaged with calibrated syringes]

Follitropin alfa [rDNA origin, single-dose vial] (Gonal-f™ RFF): 75 int. units [packaged with diluent in prefilled syringe]

Follitropin beta [rDNA origin] (Follistim®): 75 int. units [DSC]

Urofollitropin [urine derived] (Bravelle™): 75 int. units

Injection, solution:

Follitropin alfa [rDNA origin, prefilled multidose pen] (Gonal-f™ RFF Pen): 300 int. units/0.5 mL (0.5 mL) [contains sucrose 60 mg/mL]; 450 int. units/0.7 mL (0.7 mL) [contains sucrose 60 mg/mL]; 900 int. units/1.5 mL (1.5 mL) [contains sucrose 60 mg/mL]

Follitropin beta [rDNA origin, prefilled cartridge] (Follistim® AQ) 437.5 int. units/0.525 mL (0.525 mL) [delivers 300 int. units]; 737.5 int. units/0.885 mL (0.885 mL) [delivers 600 int. units]

Monitoring and Teaching Issues

Physical Assessment: This medication should only be prescribed by a fertility specialist. Assess results of laboratory tests and therapeutic effectiveness on a regular basis. Assess knowledge/teach patient appropriate use (injection technique and syringe disposal), interventions to reduce side effects, and adverse symptoms to report. **Pregnancy risk factor X:** Pregnancy must be excluded before starting medication.

Monitoring Laboratory Tests: Monitor sufficient follicular maturation. This may be directly estimated by sonographic visualization of the ovaries and endometrial lining or measuring serum estradiol levels. The combination of both ultrasonography and measurement of estradiol levels is useful for monitoring for the growth and development of follicles and timing hCG administration.

Spermatogenesis: Monitor serum testosterone levels, sperm count

Patient Education: This medication can only be administered by injection. If you are using this medication at home, follow exact instruction for administering injections and disposal of syringes. Administer exact amount as instructed; do not alter dosage or miss a dose. If dose is missed, notify prescriber. Frequent laboratory tests will be required while you are on this therapy; do not miss appointments for laboratory tests or ultrasound. You may experience headache, dizziness, or fever (use caution when driving or engaging in tasks requiring alertness until response to drug is known); or nausea or vomiting (small frequent meals, frequent oral care, sucking lozenges, or chewing gum may help). Report immediately abdominal pain/distension, bloating, persistent nausea, vomiting, diarrhea; dyspnea; respiratory difficulty, exacerbation of asthma; swelling, pain, or redness of extremities; itching or burning on urination; menstrual irregularity, acute backache; rash, pain, or inflammation at injection site; or other adverse response. **Pregnancy/breast-feeding precautions:** Inform your prescriber if you are pregnant.

Pregnancy Risk Factor: X

Pregnancy Issues: Ectopic pregnancy, congenital abnormalities, and multiple births have been reported. The incidence of congenital abnormality is similar during natural conception.

Lactation: Excretion in breast milk unknown/not recommended

Administration

I.M.:

Urofollitropin: Bravelle™: Administer I.M. or SubQ; gently massage site after administration. For I.M. injection, administer in upper quadrant of buttock near hip.

Follitropin beta: Follistim®: Administer I.M. or SubQ to female patients; administer SubQ only to males. The best site for I.M. injection is the upper outer quadrant of the buttock muscle.

Other:

Urofollitropin: Bravelle™: Administer SubQ or I.M.; gently massage site after administration. For SubQ injection, administer on lower abdomen; thigh is not recommended unless abdomen cannot be used.

Follitropin alpha: Gonal-f®: Administer SubQ. Contents of multidose vials should be administered using the calibrated syringes provided by the manufacturer. Do not shake solution; allow any bubbles to settle prior to administration.

Follitropin beta:

Follistim®: Administer SubQ or I.M. to female patients; administer SubQ only to males. The most convenient sites for SubQ injection are either in the abdomen around the navel or in the upper thigh.

Follistim® AQ: Administer SubQ only. Prefilled cartridges must be administered using the Follistim Pen™ which can be set to deliver the appropriate dose.

Reconstitution:

Urofollitropin: Bravelle™: Dissolve contents of vial in 1 mL **sterile saline**; gently swirl (do not shake); do not use if solution is not clear or contains particles. If more than 1 vial is required for a single dose, up to 6 vials can be reconstituted with 1 mL sterile saline and administered as a single injection. This is done by first reconstituting 1 vial with sterile saline as previously described, withdrawing the entire contents of the reconstituted vial and (using this as the diluent for the second vial) injecting into the second vial, etc. Use immediately after reconstitution.

Follitropin alfa: Gonal-f®:

Single-dose ampul: Dissolve the contents of one or more ampuls in 0.5-1 mL of sterile water for injection (concentration should not exceed 225 int. units/0.5 mL)

Multidose vial: Dissolve the contents of vial by slowly injecting bacteriostatic water for injection; do not shake. If bubbles appear, allow to settle prior to use. Final concentration: 600 int. units/mL.

Follitropin beta: Follistim®: Inject 1 mL of 0.45% sodium chloride injection into vial of follitropin beta. **Do not shake**, but gently swirl until solution is clear; generally the follitropin beta dissolves immediately. Use immediately after reconstitution.

Storage:

Urofollitropin (Bravelle™): Lyophilized powder may be stored in the refrigerator or at room temperature of 3°C to 25°C (37°F to 77°F). Protect from light; use immediately after reconstitution.

Follitropin alfa

Gonal-f®: Store powder refrigerated or at room temperature of 2°C to 25°C (36°F to 77°F). Protect from light. Following reconstitution, multidose vials may be stored under refrigeration or at room temperature for up to 28 days; protect from light.

Gonal-f™ RFF:

Pen: Prior to dispensing, store under refrigeration at 2°C to 8°C (36°F to 46°F). Upon dispensing, patient may store under refrigeration until product expiration date or at room temperature of 20°C to 25°C (68°F to 77°F) for up to 1 month. Protect from light; do not freeze. After first use, use within 28 days.

Vial: Store at room temperature or under refrigeration; use immediately after reconstitution.

Follitropin beta:

Follistim®: Store powder refrigerated or at room temperature of 2°C to 25°C (36°F to 77°F). Protect from light.

Follistim® AQ: Prior to dispensing, store refrigerated at 2°C to 8°C (36°F to 46°F). After dispensed, may be stored under refrigeration or at room temperature for up to 3 months. Once cartridge is pierced, must be stored in refrigerator and used within 28 days. Protect from light. Do not freeze.

Fondaparinux (fon da PARE i nuks)

U.S. Brand Names Arixtra®

Synonyms Fondaparinux Sodium

Generic Available No

Pharmacologic Category Factor Xa Inhibitor

Use Prophylaxis of deep vein thrombosis (DVT) in patients undergoing surgery for hip replacement, knee replacement, or hip fracture surgery (including extended prophylaxis following hip fracture surgery); treatment of acute pulmonary embolism (PE); treatment of acute DVT without PE

Mechanism of Action/Effect Fondaparinux prevents factor Xa from binding with antithrombin III and inhibits thrombin formation and thrombus development.

Contraindications Hypersensitivity to fondaparinux or any component of the formulation; severe renal impairment (Cl$_{cr}$ <30 mL/minute); body weight <50 kg (prophylaxis); active major bleeding; bacterial endocarditis; thrombocytopenia associated with a positive *in vitro* test for antiplatelet antibody in the presence of fondaparinux

Warnings/Precautions Patients with recent or anticipated neuraxial anesthesia (epidural or spinal anesthesia) are at risk of spinal or epidural hematoma and subsequent paralysis. Not to be used interchangeably (unit-for-unit) with heparin, low molecular weight heparins (Continued)

Fondaparinux *(Continued)*

(LMWHs), or heparinoids. Use caution in patients with moderate renal dysfunction (Cl_{cr} 30-50 mL/minute). Discontinue if severe dysfunction or labile function develops.

Use caution in congenital or acquired bleeding disorders; active ulcerative or angiodysplastic gastrointestinal disease; hemorrhagic stroke; shortly after brain, spinal, or ophthalmologic surgery; or in patients taking platelet inhibitors. Risk of major bleeding may be increased if initial dose is administered earlier then recommended (initiation recommended at 6-8 hours following surgery). Discontinue agents that may enhance the risk of hemorrhage if possible. If thrombocytopenia occurs discontinue fondaparinux. Use caution in the elderly, patients with a history of heparin-induced thrombocytopenia, patients with a bleeding diathesis, uncontrolled hypertension, recent gastrointestinal ulceration, diabetic retinopathy, and hemorrhage. Use caution in patients <50 kg who are being treated for DVT/PE; fondaparinux clearance may be decreased. Safety and efficacy in pediatric patients have not been established.

Drug Interactions
Increased Effect/Toxicity: Anticoagulants, antiplatelet agents, drotrecogin alfa, NSAIDs, salicylates, and thrombolytic agents may enhance the anticoagulant effect and/or increase the risk of bleeding.

Nutritional/Ethanol Interactions Herb/Nutraceutical: Avoid alfalfa, anise, bilberry, bladderwrack, bromelain, cat's claw, celery, coleus, cordyceps, dong quai, evening primrose oil, fenugreek, feverfew, garlic, ginger, ginkgo biloba, ginseng (American/Panax/Siberian), grape seed, green tea, guggul, horse chestnut seed, horseradish, licorice, prickly ash, red clover, reishi, sweet clover, turmeric, white willow (all possess anticoagulant or antiplatelet activity and as such, may enhance the anticoagulant effects of fondaparinux).

Lab Interactions International standards of heparin or LMWH are not the appropriate calibrators for antifactor Xa activity of fondaparinux.

Adverse Reactions As with all anticoagulants, bleeding is the major adverse effect. Hemorrhage may occur at any site. Risk appears increased by a number of factors including renal dysfunction, age (>75 years), and weight (<50 kg).
>10%:
  Central nervous system: Fever (4% to 14%)
  Gastrointestinal: Nausea (11%)
  Hematologic: Anemia (20%)
1% to 10%:
  Cardiovascular: Edema (9%), hypotension (4%), confusion (3%)
  Central nervous system: Insomnia (5%), dizziness (4%), headache (2% to 5%), pain (2%)
  Dermatologic: Rash (8%), purpura (4%), bullous eruption (3%)
  Endocrine & metabolic: Hypokalemia (1% to 4%)
  Gastrointestinal: Constipation (5% to 9%), nausea (3%), vomiting (6%), diarrhea (3%), dyspepsia (2%)
  Genitourinary: Urinary tract infection (4%), urinary retention (3%)
  Hematologic: Moderate thrombocytopenia (50,000-100,000/mm^3: 3%), major bleeding (1% to 3%), minor bleeding (3% to 4%), hematoma (3%); risk of major bleeding increased as high as 5% in patients receiving initial dose <6 hours following surgery
  Hepatic: SGOT increased (2%), SGPT increased (3%)
  Local: Injection site reaction (bleeding, rash, pruritus)
  Miscellaneous: Wound drainage increased (5%)

Overdosage/Toxicology Treatment is symptom-directed and supportive. Hemodialysis may increase clearance by 20%.

Pharmacodynamics/Kinetics
Absorption: Rapid and complete
Bioavailability: 100%
Time to Peak: 2-3 hours
Protein Binding: ≥94% to antithrombin III
Half-Life Elimination: 17-21 hours; prolonged with worsening renal impairment
Excretion: Urine (as unchanged drug)

Dosing
Adults & Elderly:
  DVT prophylaxis: SubQ: Adults ≥50 kg: 2.5 mg once daily. **Note:** Initiate dose after hemostasis has been established, 6-8 hours postoperatively.
    Usual duration: 5-9 days (up to 11 days) following hip replacement or knee replacement. Extended prophylaxis is recommended following hip fracture surgery (has been tolerated for up to 32 days).
  Acute DVT/PE treatment: SubQ: Adults:
    <50 kg: 5 mg once daily
    50-100 kg: 7.5 mg once daily
    >100 kg: 10 mg once daily
Renal Impairment:
  Cl_{cr} 30-50 mL/minute: Use caution
  Cl_{cr} <30 mL/minute: Contraindicated

Available Dosage Forms Injection, solution, as sodium: 2.5 mg/0.5 mL (0.5 mL) [prefilled syringe]

Monitoring and Teaching Issues
Physical Assessment: Assess potential for interactions with other prescriptions, OTC medications, or herbal products patient may be taking (especially anything that will affect coagulation or platelet function). Bleeding precautions should be observed. Assess results of laboratory tests, therapeutic effectiveness, and adverse response regularly during therapy. Teach patient possible side effects/appropriate interventions (eg, bleeding precautions) and adverse symptoms to report.

Monitoring Laboratory Tests: CBC with platelets, serum creatinine; stool occult blood tests

Patient Education: Do not take any new medication during therapy without consulting prescriber. This drug can only be administered by injection. Report pain, burning, redness, or swelling at injection site. You may have a tendency to bleed easily while taking this drug (brush teeth with soft brush, floss with waxed floss, use electric razor, avoid scissors or sharp knives, and avoid potentially harmful activities). May cause nausea or vomiting (small frequent meals, frequent mouth care, chewing gum, or sucking lozenges may help); or dizziness, headache, insomnia (use caution when driving or engaging in tasks that require alertness until response to drug is known). Report unusual bleeding or bruising (bleeding gums, nosebleed, blood in urine, dark stool); pain in joints or back; CNS changes (fever, confusion); unusual fever; persistent nausea or GI upset; changes in urinary pattern; or other persistent adverse response. **Breast-feeding precaution:** Consult prescriber if breast-feeding.

Geriatric Considerations: Patients studied for DVT prophylaxis following elective knee or hip fracture surgery averaged 67.5 and 77 years of age, respectively. Use with caution in patients with estimated or actual creatinine clearance between 30-50 mL/minute. Contraindicated in patients whose Cl_{cr} <30 mL/minute.

Pregnancy Risk Factor: B

Pregnancy Issues: Reproductive animal studies have not shown fetal harm. Based on case reports, small amounts of fondaparinux have been detected in the umbilical cord following multiple doses during pregnancy. There are no adequate and well-controlled studies in pregnant women; use only if clearly needed.

Lactation: Excretion in breast milk unknown/use caution

Administration

I.M.: Do not administer I.M.

Other: For SubQ administration only. Do not mix with other injections or infusions. Do not expel air bubble from syringe before injection. Administer according to recommended regimen; early initiation (before 6 hours after surgery) has been associated with increased bleeding.

Compatibility: Do not mix with other injections or infusions.

Storage: Store at 15°C to 30°C (59°F to 86°F).

Related Information

Anticoagulants, Injectable *on page 1711*

♦ **Fondaparinux Sodium** *see* Fondaparinux *on page 673*
♦ **Foradil® Aerolizer™** *see* Formoterol *on page 675*

Formoterol (for MOH te rol)

U.S. Brand Names Foradil® Aerolizer™
Synonyms Formoterol Fumarate
Generic Available No
Pharmacologic Category Beta$_2$-Adrenergic Agonist
Medication Safety Issues
Sound-alike/look-alike issues:
Foradil® may be confused with Toradol®
Foradil® capsules for inhalation are for administration via Aerolizer™ inhaler and are not for oral use.

Use Maintenance treatment of asthma and prevention of bronchospasm in patients ≥5 years of age with reversible obstructive airway disease, including patients with symptoms of nocturnal asthma, who require regular treatment with inhaled, short-acting beta$_2$ agonists; maintenance treatment of bronchoconstriction in patients with COPD; prevention of exercise-induced bronchospasm in patients ≥5 years of age

Note: Oxeze® is also approved in Canada for acute relief of symptoms ("on demand" treatment) in patients ≥6 years of age.

Mechanism of Action/Effect Relaxes bronchial smooth muscle

Contraindications Hypersensitivity to adrenergic amines, formoterol, or any component of the formulation

Note: The approved U.S. labeling lists the need for acute bronchodilation as a contraindication; however, a formulation (Oxeze®) is approved for acute treatment in other countries (ie, Canada).

Warnings/Precautions Optimize anti-inflammatory treatment before initiating maintenance treatment with formoterol. Do not use as a component of chronic therapy without an anti-inflammatory agent. Patient must be instructed to seek medical attention in cases where acute symptoms are not relieved by rapid-onset beta-agonist or when a previous level of response is diminished. Treatment must not be delayed. Rarely, paradoxical bronchospasm may occur with use of inhaled bronchodilating agents; this should be distinguished from inadequate response.

Acute episodes should be treated with rapid-onset beta$_2$ agonist. The approved U.S. labeling states that formoterol is not meant to relieve acute asthmatic symptoms. Although, a formulation of formoterol (Oxeze®) is approved for acute treatment outside the U.S. (ie, Canada).

Do not exceed recommended dose; serious adverse events (including fatalities) have been associated with excessive use of inhaled sympathomimetics. Beta$_2$ agonists may increase risk of arrhythmias, decrease serum potassium, prolong QT$_c$ interval, or increase serum glucose. These effects may be exacerbated in hypoxemia. Use caution in patients with cardiovascular disease (arrhythmia or hypertension or CHF), convulsive disorders, diabetes, glaucoma, hyperthyroidism, or hypokalemia. Beta agonists may cause elevation in blood pressure, heart rate, and result in CNS stimulation/excitation. Safety and efficacy have not been established in children <5 years of age.

Drug Interactions

Cytochrome P450 Effect: Substrate (minor) of CYP2A6, 2C8/9, 2C19, 2D6

Increased Effect/Toxicity: Adrenergic agonists, antidepressants (tricyclic), beta-blockers, corticosteroids, diuretics, drugs that prolong QT$_c$ interval, MAO inhibitors, theophylline derivatives

Adverse Reactions Children are more likely to have infection, inflammation, abdominal pain, nausea, and dyspepsia.

(Continued)

Formoterol *(Continued)*

>10%:

Endocrine & metabolic: Serum glucose increased, serum potassium decreased

Miscellaneous: Viral infection (17%)

1% to 10%:

Cardiovascular: Chest pain (2%)

Central nervous system: Tremor (2%), dizziness (2%), insomnia (2%), dysphonia (1%)

Dermatologic: Rash (1%)

Respiratory: Bronchitis (5%), infection (3%), dyspnea (2%), tonsillitis (1%)

Overdosage/Toxicology Symptoms of overdose include tachycardia, tremor, hypertension, angina, and seizures. Hypokalemia also may occur. Cardiac arrest and death may be associated with abuse of beta-agonist bronchodilators. Treatment includes immediate discontinuation and symptomatic and supportive therapies. Cautious use of beta-adrenergic blocking agents may be considered in severe cases.

Pharmacodynamics/Kinetics

Onset of Action: Within 3 minutes; 80% of peak effect within 15 minutes

Duration of Action: Improvement in FEV_1 observed for 12 hours in most patients

Absorption: Rapidly into plasma

Time to Peak: Maximum improvement in FEV_1 in 1-3 hours

Protein Binding: 61% to 64% *in vitro* at higher concentrations than achieved with usual dosing

Half-Life Elimination: ~10-14 hours

Metabolism: Hepatic via direct glucuronidation and O-demethylation; CYP2D6, CYP2C19, CYP2C8/9, CYP2A6 involved in O-demethylation

Excretion:

Children 5-12 years: Urine (6% as unchanged drug, 7% to 9% as direct glucuronide metabolites)

Adults: Urine (15% to 18% as direct glucuronide metabolites, 10% as unchanged drug)

Dosing

Adults & Elderly:

Asthma (maintenance): Inhalation: 12 mcg capsule every 12 hours

Oxeze® (CAN): **Note:** Not labeled for use in the U.S.: Inhalation: 6 mcg or 12 mcg every 12 hours. Maximum dose: Children: 24 mcg/day; Adults: 48 mcg/day

Exercise-induced bronchospasm: Inhalation: 12 mcg capsule at least 15 minutes before exercise on an "as needed" basis; additional doses should not be used for another 12 hours. **Note:** If already using for asthma maintenance then should not use additional doses for exercise-induced bronchospasm.

Oxeze® (CAN): **Note:** Not labeled for use in the U.S.: Children ≥6 years and Adults: Inhalation: 6 mcg or 12 mcg at least 15 minutes before exercise.

COPD (maintenance): Inhalation: 12 mcg capsule every 12 hours

Acute ("on demand") relief of bronchoconstriction: *Indication for Oxeze® approved in Canada:* 6 mcg or 12 mcg as a single dose (maximum dose: 72 mcg in any 24-hour period). The prolonged use of high dosages (48 mcg/day for ≥3 consecutive days) may be a sign of suboptimal control, and should prompt the re-evaluation of therapy.

Pediatrics:

Asthma maintenance: Inhalation: Children ≥5 years: Refer to adult dosing.

Exercise-induced bronchospasm: Inhalation: Children ≥5 years: Refer to adult dosing.

Acute "on demand" treatment of bronchospasm (Oxeze® [CAN]): Inhalation: Refer to adult dosing.

Renal Impairment: Not studied

Available Dosage Forms [CAN] = Canadian brand name

Aerosol, oral (Oxeze® [CAN]): 6 mcg/dose (60 doses), 12 mcg/dose (60 doses) [contains lactose 600 mcg/dose]

Powder for oral inhalation, as fumarate [capsule]: 12 mcg (12s, 60s) [contains lactose 25 mg]

Monitoring and Teaching Issues

Physical Assessment: Assess other medications patient may be taking for effectiveness and interactions. Monitor therapeutic effectiveness and adverse reactions at beginning of therapy and periodically throughout period of therapy. Assess knowledge/teach appropriate use of medication, interventions to reduce side effects, and adverse symptoms to report.

Monitoring Laboratory Tests: FEV_1, peak flow, and/or other pulmonary function tests; serum potassium, serum glucose (in selected patients)

Patient Education: Do not swallow capsules; this medication can only be used in the Aerolizer™ Inhaler. Use exactly as directed and do not use more often than recommended. Store capsules in blister and do not remove from blister until ready for treatment. Maintain adequate hydration (2-3 L/day of fluids) unless instructed to restrict fluid intake. It is recommended that you wear identification (Med-Alert bracelet) if you have an asthmatic condition. You may experience nervousness, dizziness, or insomnia (use caution when driving or engaging in hazardous activities until response to medication is known); dry mouth, nausea, or GI discomfort (small frequent meals, good mouth care, sucking lozenges, or chewing gum may help); or difficulty voiding (always void before treatment). Report any unresolved GI upset, nervousness or dizziness, muscle cramping, chest pain or palpitations, skin rash, signs of infection, unusual cough, or worsening of condition. **Pregnancy/breast-feeding precautions:** Inform prescriber if you are or intend to become pregnant. Consult prescriber if breast-feeding.

Administration: Follow directions for use and storage of inhaler exactly. Wash hands prior to treatment and sit in comfortable position for treatment. Remove capsule from foil blister immediately before treatment and place capsule in the capsule-chamber in the base of the Aerolizer™ Inhaler. Press both buttons once only and then release. Hold inhaler in a level, horizontal position, exhale fully (do not exhale into inhaler). Tilt head slightly back and inhale from inhaler rapidly, steadily, and deeply. Hold breath as long as possible. If any powder remains in capsule, exhale and inhale again. Repeat until capsule is empty. Throw away empty capsule. Do not use a spacer with Aerolizer™. Do not wash inhaler; store in dry place.

Pregnancy Risk Factor: C

Pregnancy Issues: There are no adequate and well-controlled studies in pregnant women. Use only if benefit outweighs risk to the fetus. Beta agonists interfere with uterine contractility so use during labor only if benefit outweighs risk to the fetus.

Lactation: Excretion in breast milk unknown/use caution

Administration

Inhalation: Remove capsule from foil blister **immediately** before use. Place capsule in the capsule-chamber in the base of the Aerolizer™ Inhaler. Must only use the Aerolizer™ Inhaler. Press both buttons **once only** and then release. Keep inhaler in a level, horizontal position. Exhale fully. Do not exhale into inhaler. Tilt head slightly back and inhale (rapidly, steadily and deeply). Hold breath as long as possible. If any powder remains in capsule, exhale and inhale again. Repeat until capsule is empty. Throw away empty capsule; do not leave in inhaler. Do not use a spacer with the Aerolizer™ Inhaler. Always keep capsules and inhaler dry.

Storage: Prior to dispensing, store in refrigerator at 2°C to 8°C (36°F to 46°F); after dispensing, store at room temperature at 20°C to 25°C (68°F to 77°F). Protect from heat and moisture. Capsules should always be stored in the blister and only removed immediately before use. Always check expiration date. Use within 4 months of purchase date or product expiration date, whichever comes first.

Related Information

Inhalant Agents *on page 1734*

- ◆ **Formoterol Fumarate** *see Formoterol on page 675*
- ◆ **Formulation R™ [OTC]** *see Phenylephrine on page 1200*
- ◆ **5-Formyl Tetrahydrofolate** *see Leucovorin on page 875*
- ◆ **Fortamet™** *see Metformin on page 965*
- ◆ **Fortaz®** *see Ceftazidime on page 283*
- ◆ **Forteo™** *see Teriparatide on page 1448*
- ◆ **Fortovase®** *see Saquinavir on page 1355*
- ◆ **Fosamax®** *see Alendronate on page 66*

Fosamprenavir (FOS am pren a veer)

U.S. Brand Names Lexiva™

Synonyms Fosamprenavir Calcium; GW433908G

Generic Available No

Pharmacologic Category Antiretroviral Agent, Protease Inhibitor

Medication Safety Issues

Sound-alike/look-alike issues:

Lexiva™ may be confused with Levitra®

Use Treatment of HIV infections in combination with at least two other antiretroviral agents

Mechanism of Action/Effect Fosamprenavir is rapidly and almost completely converted to amprenavir *in vivo*. Amprenavir binds to the protease activity site and inhibits the activity of the enzyme. HIV protease is required for the cleavage of viral polyprotein precursors into individual functional proteins found in infectious HIV. Inhibition prevents cleavage of these polyproteins, resulting in the formation of immature, noninfectious viral particles.

Contraindications Hypersensitivity to amprenavir or any component of the formulation; concurrent therapy with cisapride, ergot derivatives, midazolam, pimozide, and triazolam; severe previous allergic reaction to sulfonamides

Warnings/Precautions Because of hepatic metabolism and effect on cytochrome P450 enzymes, amprenavir should be used with caution in combination with other agents metabolized by this system (see Contraindications and Drug Interactions). Avoid concurrent administration of lovastatin or simvastatin (may increase the risk of rhabdomyolysis). Avoid use of hormonal contraceptives, rifampin, and/or St John's wort (may lead to loss of virologic response and/or resistance). Use with caution in patients with diabetes mellitus, sulfonamide allergy, hepatic impairment, or hemophilia. Redistribution of fat may occur (eg, buffalo hump, peripheral wasting, cushingoid appearance). Dosage adjustment is required for combination therapies (ritonavir and/or efavirenz); in addition, the risk of hyperlipidemia may be increased during concurrent therapy. Discontinue therapy in severe or dermatologic reactions or when a moderate rash is accompanied by systemic symptoms.

Drug Interactions

Cytochrome P450 Effect: As amprenavir: **Substrate** of CYP2C8/9 (minor), 3A4 (major); **Inhibits** CYP2C19 (weak), 3A4 (strong)

Decreased Effect: CYP3A4 inducers may decrease the levels/effects of amprenavir; example inducers include aminoglutethimide, carbamazepine, nafcillin, nevirapine, phenobarbital, phenytoin, and rifamycins. The administration of didanosine (buffered formulation) should be separated from amprenavir by 1 hour to limit interaction between formulations. Serum concentrations of estrogen (oral contraceptives) may be decreased, use alternative (nonhormonal) forms of contraception. Dexamethasone may decrease the therapeutic effect of amprenavir. Serum concentrations of delavirdine may be decreased; may lead to loss of virologic response and possible resistance to delavirdine; concomitant use is not recommended. Efavirenz and nevirapine may decrease serum concentrations of amprenavir (dosing for combinations not established). Avoid St John's wort (may lead to subtherapeutic concentrations of amprenavir). Effect of amprenavir may be diminished when administered with methadone (consider alternative antiretroviral); in addition, effect of methadone may be reduced (dosage increase may be required).

Increased Effect/Toxicity: Concurrent use of cisapride, midazolam, pimozide, quinidine, or triazolam is contraindicated. Concurrent use of ergot alkaloids (dihydroergotamine, ergotamine, ergonovine, methylergonovine) with amprenavir is also contraindicated (may cause vasospasm and peripheral ischemia). Concurrent use of oral solution with disulfiram or metronidazole is contraindicated, due to the risk of propylene glycol toxicity.

(Continued)

Fosamprenavir *(Continued)*

Serum concentrations of amiodarone, bepridil, lidocaine, quinidine and other antiarrhythmics may be increased, potentially leading to toxicity; when amprenavir is coadministered with ritonavir, flecainide and propafenone are contraindicated. HMG-CoA reductase inhibitors serum concentrations may be increased by amprenavir, increasing the risk of myopathy/rhabdomyolysis; lovastatin and simvastatin are not recommended; fluvastatin and pravastatin may be safer alternatives.

Amprenavir may increase the levels/effects of selected benzodiazepines (midazolam and triazolam are contraindicated), calcium channel blockers, cyclosporine, mirtazapine, nateglinide, nefazodone, quinidine, sildenafil (and other PDE-5 inhibitors), tacrolimus, venlafaxine, and other CYP3A4 substrates. When used with strong CYP3A4 inhibitors, dosage adjustment/limits are recommended for sildenafil and other PDE-5 inhibitors; refer to individual monographs.

Concurrent therapy with ritonavir may result in increased serum concentrations: dosage adjustment is recommended. Clarithromycin, indinavir, nelfinavir may increase serum concentrations of amprenavir.

Nutritional/Ethanol Interactions Herb/Nutraceutical: Amprenavir serum concentration may be decreased by St John's wort; avoid concurrent use.

Adverse Reactions

>10%:
Central nervous system: Headache (19% to 21%), fatigue (10% to 18%)
Dermatologic: Rash (17% to 35%; moderate to severe reactions 3% to 8%)
Gastrointestinal: Nausea (37% to 39%), diarrhea (34% to 52%), vomiting (16% to 20%), abdominal pain (5% to 11%)

1% to 10%:
Central nervous system: Depression (8%), fatigue, headache, paresthesia
Dermatologic: Pruritus (3% to 8%)
Endocrine & metabolic: Hypertriglyceridemia (0% to 11%), serum lipase increased (6% to 8%), hyperglycemia (<1% to 2%)
Hematologic: Neutropenia (3%)
Hepatic: Transaminases increased (4% to 8%)
Miscellaneous: Perioral tingling/numbness (2% to 10%)

Overdosage/Toxicology Treatment is symptomatic and supportive.

Pharmacodynamics/Kinetics

Absorption: 63%
Bioavailability: Not established; food does not have a significant effect on absorption
Time to Peak: 1.5-4 hours
Protein Binding: 90%
Half-Life Elimination: 7.7 hours
Metabolism: Fosamprenavir is rapidly and almost completely converted to amprenavir by cellular phosphatases; amprenavir is hepatically metabolized via CYP isoenzymes (primarily CYP3A4)
Excretion: Feces (75%); urine (14% as metabolites; <1% as unchanged drug)

Dosing

Adults:

HIV infection, therapy-naive patients: Oral: 1400 mg twice daily (without ritonavir)
Dosage adjustments when administered in combination therapy:
Concurrent therapy with ritonavir: Adjustments necessary for both agents:
Fosamprenavir 1400 mg plus ritonavir 200 mg once daily **or**
Fosamprenavir 700 mg plus ritonavir 100 mg twice daily
Concurrent therapy with efavirenz and ritonavir: Fosamprenavir 1400 mg daily plus ritonavir 300 mg once daily; no dosage adjustment recommended for twice-daily regimen

HIV infection, protease inhibitor-experienced patients: Oral: Fosamprenavir 700 mg plus ritonavir 100 mg twice daily. **Note:** Once-daily administration is not recommended in protease inhibitor-experienced patients.

Renal Impairment: No dosage adjustment required.

Hepatic Impairment:
Note: No recommendations are available for dosage adjustment in patients receiving ritonavir and fosamprenavir.
Mild-moderate impairment (Child-Pugh score 5-8): Reduce dosage of fosamprenavir to 700 mg twice daily (without concurrent ritonavir)
Severe impairment: Use is not recommended.

Available Dosage Forms Tablet, as calcium: 700 mg

Monitoring and Teaching Issues

Physical Assessment: Use caution in presence of diabetes mellitus, sulfonamide allergy, hepatic impairment, hemophilia (see Warnings/Precautions). Assess potential for adverse interactions with other pharmacological agents or herbal products the patient may be taking (eg, statins, hormonal contraceptives, St. John's wort, methadone, benzodiazepines, midazolam, calcium channel blockers; see Drug Interactions for extensive list). A list of medications that should not be used is available with each bottle and patients should be provided with this information. Assess results of laboratory tests and patient response at regular intervals during therapy (eg, headache, gastrointestinal disturbances, rash, hyperlipidemia; see Adverse Reactions). Teach patient proper use, drugs that should not be used, possible side effects/ appropriate interventions, and adverse symptoms to report (see Patient Education).

Monitoring Laboratory Tests: Viral load

Patient Education: You will be provided with a list of specific medications that should not be used during therapy. However, do not take any new prescriptions, over-the-counter medications, or herbal products during therapy (even if they are not on the list) without consulting prescriber. This is not a cure for HIV, nor has it been found to reduce transmission of HIV. Take as directed, with meals. Maintain adequate hydration (2-3 L/day of fluids) unless instructed to restrict fluid intake. This medication will be prescribed with a combination of other medications; time these medications as directed by prescriber. You may be advised to check your glucose levels; this class of drugs can cause exacerbation or new-onset diabetes. May cause body changes due to redistribution of body fat, facial atrophy, or breast enlargement (normal effects of drug); headache, dizziness, or fatigue (use caution when driving or engaged in potentially hazardous tasks until response to drug is known); nausea or vomiting (small frequent meals, frequent mouth care, chewing gum, or sucking lozenges may help); diarrhea (buttermilk, boiled milk, or yogurt may help); back pain, or arthralgia (consult prescriber for approved analgesic). Report rash, tingling or numbness in or around mouth, or any persistent adverse effects. **Pregnancy/breast-feeding precautions:** Inform prescriber if you are or intend to become pregnant. Effectiveness of oral contraceptives may be decreased, use of alternative (nonhormonal) forms of contraception is recommended; consult prescriber for appropriate contraceptives. Do not breast-feed.

Dietary Considerations: May be taken with or without food.

Pregnancy Risk Factor: C

Pregnancy Issues: It is not known if amprenavir crosses the human placenta and there are no clinical studies currently underway to evaluate its use in pregnant women. Pregnancy and protease inhibitors are both associated with an increased risk of hyperglycemia. Glucose levels should be closely monitored. Health professionals are encouraged to contact the antiretroviral pregnancy registry to monitor outcomes of pregnant women exposed to antiretroviral medications (1-800-258-4263 or www.APRegistry.com).

Lactation: Excretion in breast milk unknown/contraindicated

Breast-Feeding Issues: HIV-infected mothers are discouraged from breast-feeding to decrease potential transmission of HIV.

Administration

Storage: Store at 25°C (77°F); excursions permitted to 15°C to 30°C (59°F to 86°F).

♦ **Fosamprenavir Calcium** see Fosamprenavir on page 677

Foscarnet (fos KAR net)

U.S. Brand Names Foscavir®

Synonyms PFA; Phosphonoformate; Phosphonoformic Acid

Generic Available No

Pharmacologic Category Antiviral Agent

Use

Treatment of herpes virus infections suspected to be caused by acyclovir-resistant (HSV, VZV) or ganciclovir-resistant (CMV) strains; this occurs almost exclusively in immunocompromised persons (eg, with advanced AIDS) who have received prolonged treatment for a herpes virus infection

Treatment of CMV retinitis in persons with AIDS

Unlabeled/Investigational Use Other CMV infections in persons unable to tolerate ganciclovir; may be given in combination with ganciclovir in patients who relapse after monotherapy with either drug

Mechanism of Action/Effect Pyrophosphate analogue which acts as a noncompetitive inhibitor of many viral RNA and DNA polymerases as well as HIV reverse transcriptase. Inhibitory effects occur at concentrations which do not affect host cellular DNA polymerases; however, some human cell growth suppression has been observed with high in vitro concentrations. Similar to ganciclovir, foscarnet is a virostatic agent. Foscarnet does not require activation by thymidine kinase.

Contraindications Hypersensitivity to foscarnet or any component of the formulation; Cl_{cr} <0.4 mL/minute/kg during therapy

Warnings/Precautions Renal impairment occurs to some degree in the majority of patients treated with foscarnet. Renal impairment may occur at any time (usually reversible within 1 week following dose adjustment or discontinuation, but some severe cases). Renal function should be closely monitored. Foscarnet may cause tooth disorders. Safety and effectiveness in children have not been studied. Monitor electrolytes carefully, particularly calcium, magnesium, phosphate, and potassium. Seizures have been experienced by up to 10% of AIDS patients. Risk factors for seizures include a low baseline absolute neutrophil count (ANC), impaired baseline renal function and low total serum calcium. Some patients who have experienced seizures have died, while others have been able to continue or resume foscarnet treatment after their mineral or electrolyte abnormality has been corrected, their underlying disease state treated, or their dose decreased. Foscarnet has been shown to be mutagenic in vitro and in mice at very high doses.

Drug Interactions

Increased Effect/Toxicity: Concurrent use with ciprofloxacin (or other fluoroquinolone) increases seizure potential. Acute renal failure (reversible) has been reported with cyclosporine due most likely to a synergistic toxic effect. Nephrotoxic drugs (amphotericin B, I.V. pentamidine, aminoglycosides, etc) should be avoided, if possible, to minimize additive renal risk with foscarnet. Concurrent use of pentamidine also increases the potential for hypocalcemia. Protease inhibitors (ritonavir, saquinavir) have been associated with an increased risk of renal impairment during concurrent use of foscarnet

Adverse Reactions

>10%:

Central nervous system: Fever (65%), headache (26%), seizure (10%)

Gastrointestinal: Nausea (47%), diarrhea (30%), vomiting

Hematologic: Anemia (33%)

Renal: Abnormal renal function/decreased creatinine clearance (27%)

1% to 10%:

Central nervous system: Fatigue, malaise, dizziness, hypoesthesia, depression/confusion/anxiety (≥5%)

Dermatologic: Rash

Endocrine & metabolic: Electrolyte imbalance (especially potassium, calcium, magnesium, and phosphorus)

(Continued)

Foscarnet *(Continued)*

Gastrointestinal: Anorexia
Hematologic: Granulocytopenia, leukopenia (≥5%), thrombocytopenia, thrombosis
Local: Injection site pain
Neuromuscular & skeletal: Paresthesia, involuntary muscle contractions, rigors, neuropathy (peripheral), weakness
Ocular: Vision abnormalities
Respiratory: Coughing, dyspnea (≥5%)
Miscellaneous: Sepsis, diaphoresis (increased)

Overdosage/Toxicology Symptoms of overdose include seizures, renal dysfunction, perioral or limb paresthesia, and hypocalcemia. Treatment is supportive.

Pharmacodynamics/Kinetics
Half-Life Elimination: ~3 hours
Metabolism: Biotransformation does not occur
Excretion: Urine (≤28% as unchanged drug)

Dosing
Adults & Elderly:
CMV retinitis: I.V.:
Induction treatment: 60 mg/kg/dose every 8 hours for 14-21 days
Maintenance therapy: 90-120 mg/kg/day as a single infusion
Acyclovir-resistant HSV induction treatment: I.V.: 40 mg/kg/dose every 8-12 hours for 14-21 days
Pediatrics: Adolescents: Refer to adult dosing.
Renal Impairment: See tables.

Induction Dosing of Foscarnet in Patients With Abnormal Renal Function

Cl_cr (mL/min/kg)	HSV Equivalent to 40 mg/kg q12h	HSV Equivalent to 40 mg/kg q8h	CMV Equivalent to 60 mg/kg q8h	CMV Equivalent to 90 mg/kg q12h
<0.4	Not recommended	Not recommended	Not recommended	Not recommended
≥0.4-0.5	20 mg/kg every 24 hours	35 mg/kg every 24 hours	50 mg/kg every 24 hours	50 mg/kg every 24 hours
>0.5-0.6	25 mg/kg every 24 hours	40 mg/kg every 24 hours	60 mg/kg every 24 hours	60 mg/kg every 24 hours
>0.6-0.8	35 mg/kg every 24 hours	25 mg/kg every 12 hours	40 mg/kg every 12 hours	80 mg/kg every 24 hours
>0.8-1.0	20 mg/kg every 12 hours	35 mg/kg every 12 hours	50 mg/kg every 12 hours	50 mg/kg every 12 hours
>1.0-1.4	30 mg/kg every 12 hours	30 mg/kg every 8 hours	45 mg/kg every 8 hours	70 mg/kg every 12 hours
>1.4	40 mg/kg every 12 hours	40 mg/kg every 8 hours	60 mg/kg every 8 hours	90 mg/kg every 12 hours

Maintenance Dosing of Foscarnet in Patients With Abnormal Renal Function

Cl_cr (mL/min/kg)	CMV Equivalent to 90 mg/kg q24h	CMV Equivalent to 120 mg/kg q24h
<0.4	Not recommended	Not recommended
≥0.4-0.5	50 mg/kg every 48 hours	65 mg/kg every 48 hours
>0.5-0.6	60 mg/kg every 48 hours	80 mg/kg every 48 hours
>0.6-0.8	80 mg/kg every 48 hours	105 mg/kg every 48 hours
>0.8-1.0	50 mg/kg every 24 hours	65 mg/kg every 24 hours
>1.0-1.4	70 mg/kg every 24 hours	90 mg/kg every 24 hours
>1.4	90 mg/kg every 24 hours	120 mg/kg every 24 hours

Available Dosage Forms Injection, solution: 24 mg/mL (250 mL, 500 mL)

Monitoring and Teaching Issues
Physical Assessment: See Warnings/Precautions for use cautions (eg, electrolyte imbalance, renal impairment, dental status). Assess potential for interactions with other pharmacological agents the patient may be taking (eg, increased risk of seizures, renal failure, electrolyte imbalance; see Drug Interactions). See Administration for infusion specifics. Assess results of laboratory tests, therapeutic effectiveness (resolution of viral infection), and adverse response (eg, nephrotoxicity, electrolyte imbalance, seizures; see Adverse Reactions). Teach patient possible side effects/appropriate interventions and adverse symptoms to report (see Patient Education).

Monitoring Laboratory Tests: Renal function, CBC, electrolytes, calcium, magnesium

Patient Education: Do not take any new medication during therapy unless approved by prescriber. Foscarnet is not a cure for the disease; progression may occur during or following therapy. While on therapy, it is important to maintain adequate hydration (2-3 L/day of fluids) unless instructed to restrict fluid intake and nutrition (small frequent meals may help). Regular dental check-ups are recommended. May cause dizziness or confusion (use caution when driving or engaging in tasks that require alertness until response to drug is known); nausea and vomiting (small frequent meals, frequent mouth care, chewing gum or sucking lozenges may help); or diarrhea (buttermilk, boiled milk, or yogurt may help). Report any change in sensorium or seizures; unresolved diarrhea or vomiting; unusual fever, chills, sore throat, unhealed sores, swollen lymph glands; or malaise. **Pregnancy/breast-feeding precautions:** Inform prescriber if you are pregnant. Contraceptives are recommended to reduce transmission of disease. Do not breast-feed.

Geriatric Considerations: Information on the use of foscarnet is lacking in the elderly. Dose adjustments and proper monitoring must be performed because of the decreased renal function common in older patients.

Pregnancy Risk Factor: C

Lactation: Excretion in breast milk unknown/contraindicated

Breast-Feeding Issues: The CDC recommends **not** to breast-feed if diagnosed with HIV to avoid postnatal transmission of the virus.

Administration

I.V.: Use an infusion pump, at a rate not exceeding 1 mg/kg/minute. Adult induction doses of 60 mg/kg are administered over 1 hour. Adult maintenance doses of 90-120 mg/kg are infused over 2 hours.

Reconstitution: Foscarnet should be diluted in D_5W or NS and transferred to PVC containers. It is stable for 24 hours at room temperature or refrigeration. For peripheral line administration, foscarnet **must** be diluted to 12 mg/mL with D_5W or NS. For central line administration, foscarnet may be administered undiluted.

Compatibility: Stable in D_5W, NS; **incompatible** with LR, dextrose 30%, TPN, I.V. solutions containing calcium, magnesium, or vancomycin

Y-site administration: Incompatible with acyclovir, amphotericin B, diazepam, digoxin, diphenhydramine, dobutamine, droperidol, ganciclovir, haloperidol, leucovorin, midazolam, pentamidine, prochlorperazine edisylate, promethazine, trimetrexate

Storage: Foscarnet injection is a clear, colorless solution. It should be stored at room temperature and protected from temperatures >40°C and from freezing.

Additional Information Sodium loading with 500 mL of 0.9% sodium chloride solution before and after foscarnet infusion helps to minimize the risk of nephrotoxicity.

♦ **Foscavir**® see Foscarnet on page 679

Fosinopril (foe SIN oh pril)

U.S. Brand Names Monopril®

Synonyms Fosinopril Sodium

Generic Available Yes

Pharmacologic Category Angiotensin-Converting Enzyme (ACE) Inhibitor

Medication Safety Issues

Sound-alike/look-alike issues:

Fosinopril may be confused with lisinopril

Monopril® may be confused with Accupril®, minoxidil, moexipril, Monoket®, Monurol™, ramipril

Use Treatment of hypertension, either alone or in combination with other antihypertensive agents; treatment of congestive heart failure, left ventricular dysfunction after myocardial infarction

Mechanism of Action/Effect Competitive inhibitor of angiotensin-converting enzyme (ACE); prevents conversion of angiotensin I to angiotensin II, a potent vasoconstrictor; results in lower levels of angiotensin II which causes an increase in plasma renin activity and a reduction in aldosterone secretion; a CNS mechanism may also be involved in hypotensive effect as angiotensin II increases adrenergic outflow from CNS; vasoactive kallikreins may be decreased in conversion to active hormones by ACE inhibitors, thus reducing blood pressure

Contraindications Hypersensitivity to fosinopril or any component of the formulation; angioedema related to previous treatment with an ACE inhibitor; idiopathic or hereditary angioedema; bilateral renal artery stenosis; pregnancy (2nd and 3rd trimesters)

Warnings/Precautions Anaphylactic reactions can occur. Angioedema can occur at any time during treatment (especially following first dose). Angioedema may involve head and neck (potentially affecting the airway) or the intestine (presenting with abdominal pain). Careful blood pressure monitoring (hypotension can occur especially in volume depleted patients). Dosage adjustment needed in severe renal impairment (Cl_{cr} <10 mL/minute). Use with caution in hypovolemia; collagen vascular diseases; valvular stenosis (particularly aortic stenosis); hyperkalemia; or before, during, or immediately after anesthesia. Avoid rapid dosage escalation which may lead to renal insufficiency. Rare toxicities associated with ACE inhibitors include cholestatic jaundice (which may progress to hepatic necrosis) and neutropenia/agranulocytosis with myeloid hyperplasia. Hypersensitivity reactions may be seen during hemodialysis with high-flux dialysis membranes (eg, AN69). Hyperkalemia may rarely occur. Use with caution in unilateral renal artery stenosis and pre-existing renal insufficiency.

Drug Interactions

Decreased Effect: Aspirin (high dose) may reduce the therapeutic effects of ACE inhibitors; at low dosages this does not appear to be significant. Rifampin may decrease the effect of ACE inhibitors. Antacids may decrease the bioavailability of ACE inhibitors (may be more likely to occur with captopril); separate administration times by 1-2 hours. NSAIDs, specifically indomethacin, may reduce the hypotensive effects of ACE inhibitors. More likely to occur in low renin or volume dependent hypertensive patients.

Increased Effect/Toxicity: Potassium supplements, co-trimoxazole (high dose), angiotensin II receptor antagonists (eg, candesartan, losartan, irbesartan), or potassium-sparing diuretics (amiloride, spironolactone, triamterene) may result in elevated serum potassium levels when combined with fosinopril. ACE inhibitor effects may be increased by phenothiazines or probenecid (increases levels of captopril). ACE inhibitors may increase serum concentrations/effects of digoxin, lithium, and sulfonlyureas.

Diuretics have additive hypotensive effects with ACE inhibitors, and hypovolemia increases the potential for adverse renal effects of ACE inhibitors. In patients with compromised renal function, coadministration with NSAIDs may result in further deterioration of renal function. Allopurinol and ACE inhibitors may cause a higher risk of hypersensitivity reaction when taken concurrently.

Nutritional/Ethanol Interactions Herb/Nutraceutical: Avoid dong quai if using for hypertension (has estrogenic activity). Avoid ephedra, garlic, yohimbe, ginseng (may worsen hypertension).

(Continued)

Fosinopril *(Continued)*

Lab Interactions Positive Coombs' (direct); may cause false-positive results in urine acetone determinations using sodium nitroprusside reagent; may cause false low serum digoxin levels with the Digi-Tab RIA kit for digoxin.

Adverse Reactions Note: Frequency ranges include data from hypertension and heart failure trials. Higher rates of adverse reactions have generally been noted in patients with CHF. However, the frequency of adverse effects associated with placebo is also increased in this population.

>10%: Central nervous system: Dizziness (2% to 12%)

1% to 10%:
   Cardiovascular: Orthostatic hypotension (1% to 2%), palpitation (1%)
   Central nervous system: Dizziness (1% to 2%; up to 12% in CHF patients), headache (3%), fatigue (1% to 2%)
   Endocrine & metabolic: Hyperkalemia (2.6%)
   Gastrointestinal: Diarrhea (2%), nausea/vomiting (1.2% to 2.2%)
   Hepatic: Transaminases increased
   Neuromuscular & skeletal: Musculoskeletal pain (<1% to 3%), noncardiac chest pain (<1% to 2%), weakness (1%)
   Renal: Increased serum creatinine, worsening of renal function (in patients with bilateral renal artery stenosis or hypovolemia)
   Respiratory: Cough (2% to 10%)
   Miscellaneous: Upper respiratory infection (2%)

>1% but ≤ frequency in patients receiving placebo: Sexual dysfunction, fever, flu-like syndrome, dyspnea, rash, headache, insomnia

Other events reported with ACE inhibitors: Neutropenia, agranulocytosis, eosinophilic pneumonitis, cardiac arrest, pancytopenia, hemolytic anemia, anemia, aplastic anemia, thrombocytopenia, acute renal failure, hepatic failure, jaundice, symptomatic hyponatremia, bullous pemphigus, exfoliative dermatitis, Stevens-Johnson syndrome. In addition, a syndrome which may include fever, myalgia, arthralgia, interstitial nephritis, vasculitis, rash, eosinophilia and positive ANA, and elevated ESR has been reported for other ACE inhibitors.

Overdosage/Toxicology Mild hypotension has been the primary toxic effect seen with acute overdose. Bradycardia may also occur; hyperkalemia occurs even with therapeutic doses, especially in patients with renal insufficiency and those taking NSAIDs. Treatment is symptom-directed and supportive.

Pharmacodynamics/Kinetics
Onset of Action: 1 hour
Duration of Action: 24 hours
Absorption: 36%
Bioavailability: 36%
Time to Peak: Serum: ~3 hours
Protein Binding: 95%
Half-Life Elimination: Serum (fosinoprilat): 12 hours
Metabolism: Prodrug, hydrolyzed to its active metabolite fosinoprilat by intestinal wall and hepatic esterases
Excretion: Urine and feces (as fosinoprilat and other metabolites in roughly equal proportions, 45% to 50%)

Dosing
Adults & Elderly:
   Hypertension: Oral: Initial: 10 mg/day; increase to a maximum dose of 80 mg/day. Most patients are maintained on 20-40 mg/day. May need to divide the dose into two if trough effect is inadequate. Discontinue the diuretic, if possible 2-3 days before initiation of therapy. Resume diuretic therapy carefully, if needed.
   Heart failure: Oral: Initial: 10 mg/day (5 mg if renal dysfunction present) and increase, as needed, to a maximum of 40 mg once daily over several weeks. Usual dose: 20-40 mg/day. If hypotension, orthostasis, or azotemia occurs during titration, consider decreasing concomitant diuretic dose, if any.
Pediatrics: Hypertension: Children >50 kg: Oral: Initial: 5-10 mg once daily
Renal Impairment: None needed since hepatobiliary elimination compensates adequately diminished renal elimination.
   Hemodialysis: Moderately dialyzable (20% to 50%)
Hepatic Impairment: Decrease dose and monitor effects

Available Dosage Forms Tablet, as sodium: 10 mg, 20 mg, 40 mg

Monitoring and Teaching Issues
Physical Assessment: See Warnings/Precautions for use cautions (eg, renal impairment, hypovolemia, aortic stenosis, post anesthesia). Assess potential for interactions with other pharmacological agents or herbal products patient may be taking (especially anything that may impact fluid balance or cardiac status; see Drug Interactions). Assess results of laboratory tests, therapeutic effectiveness according to purpose for use, and adverse response on a regular basis during therapy (eg, anaphylactic reactions, hypovolemia, angioedema, postural hypotension; see Adverse Reactions). Teach patient appropriate use, possible side effects/appropriate interventions, and adverse symptoms to report (refer Patient Education).

Monitoring Laboratory Tests: CBC, renal function tests, electrolytes. If patient has renal impairment, a baseline WBC with differential and serum creatinine should be evaluated and monitored closely during initial therapy.

Patient Education: Inform prescriber of all prescriptions, OTC medications, or herbal products you are taking, and any allergies you have. Do not take any new medication during therapy unless approved by prescriber. Do not use potassium supplement or salt substitutes without consulting prescriber. Take exactly as directed; do not discontinue without consulting prescriber. This drug does not eliminate need for diet or exercise regimen as recommended by prescriber. May cause dizziness, fainting, or lightheadedness (use caution when driving or engaging in tasks that require alertness until response to drug is known); postural hypotension (use caution when rising from lying or sitting position or climbing stairs); or nausea, vomiting, abdominal pain, dry mouth, or loss of appetite (small frequent meals, frequent mouth care, sucking lozenges, or chewing gum may help), report if these persist. Report chest pain or palpitations; mouth sores; fever or chills; swelling of extremities, face, mouth, or tongue; skin rash; numbness, tingling, or pain in muscles; respiratory difficulty; unusual cough; or other persistent adverse reactions. **Pregnancy/breast-feeding precautions:** Inform prescriber if you are or intend to become pregnant. This drug should not be used in the 2nd or 3rd trimester of pregnancy. Consult prescriber for appropriate contraceptive measures if necessary. Breast-feeding is not recommended.

Dietary Considerations: Should not take a potassium salt supplement without the advice of healthcare provider.

Geriatric Considerations: Due to frequent decreases in glomerular filtration (also creatinine clearance) with aging, elderly patients may have exaggerated responses to ACE inhibitors. Differences in clinical response due to hepatic changes are not observed. ACE inhibitors may be preferred agents in elderly patients with congestive heart failure and diabetes mellitus. Diabetic proteinuria is reduced and insulin sensitivity is enhanced. In general, the side effect profile is favorable in the elderly and causes little or no CNS confusion; use lowest dose recommendations initially.

Pregnancy Risk Factor: C/D (2nd and 3rd trimesters)

Pregnancy Issues: ACE inhibitors can cause fetal injury or death if taken during the 2nd or 3rd trimester. Discontinue ACE inhibitors as soon as pregnancy is detected.

Lactation: Enters breast milk/not recommended

Administration

Storage: Store at 25°C (77°F); excursions permitted to 15°C to 30°C (59°F to 86°F). Protect from moisture by keeping bottle tightly closed.

Related Information

Angiotensin Agents *on page 1704*
Heart Failure *on page 1828*

♦ **Fosinopril Sodium** *see* Fosinopril *on page 681*

Fosphenytoin (FOS fen i toyn)

U.S. Brand Names Cerebyx®
Synonyms Fosphenytoin Sodium
Generic Available No
Pharmacologic Category Anticonvulsant, Hydantoin
Medication Safety Issues
Sound-alike/look-alike issues:
Cerebyx® may be confused with Celebrex®, Celexa™, Cerezyme®

Use Used for the control of generalized convulsive status epilepticus and prevention and treatment of seizures occurring during neurosurgery; indicated for short-term parenteral administration when other means of phenytoin administration are unavailable, inappropriate or deemed less advantageous (the safety and effectiveness of fosphenytoin in this use has not been systematically evaluated for more than 5 days)

Mechanism of Action/Effect Diphosphate ester salt of phenytoin which acts as a water soluble prodrug of phenytoin; after administration, plasma esterases convert fosphenytoin to phosphate, formaldehyde and phenytoin as the active moiety; phenytoin works by stabilizing neuronal membranes and decreasing seizure activity by increasing efflux or decreasing influx of sodium ions across cell membranes in the motor cortex during generation of nerve impulses

Contraindications Hypersensitivity to phenytoin, other hydantoins, or any component of the formulation; patients with sinus bradycardia, sinoatrial block, second- and third-degree AV block, or Adams-Stokes syndrome; occurrence of rash during treatment (should not be resumed if rash is exfoliative, purpuric, or bullous); treatment of absence seizures

Warnings/Precautions Doses of fosphenytoin are expressed as their phenytoin sodium equivalent (PE). Antiepileptic drugs should not be abruptly discontinued. Hypotension may occur, especially after I.V. administration at high doses and high rates of administration. Administration of phenytoin has been associated with atrial and ventricular conduction depression and ventricular fibrillation. Careful cardiac monitoring is needed when administering I.V. loading doses of fosphenytoin. Acute hepatotoxicity associated with a hypersensitivity syndrome characterized by fever, skin eruptions, and lymphadenopathy has been reported to occur within the first 2 months of treatment. Discontinue if skin rash or lymphadenopathy occurs. Use with caution in patients with hypotension, severe myocardial insufficiency, diabetes mellitus, porphyria, hypoalbuminemia, hypothyroidism, fever, or hepatic or renal dysfunction.

Drug Interactions

Cytochrome P450 Effect: As phenytoin: **Substrate** of CYP2C8/9 (major), 2C19 (major), 3A4 (minor); **Induces** CYP2B6 (strong), 2C8/9 (strong), 2C19 (strong), 3A4 (strong)

Decreased Effect: Phenytoin may enhance the metabolism of estrogen and/or oral contraceptives, decreasing their clinical effect; an alternative method of contraception should be considered. Phenytoin may increase the metabolism of anticonvulsants including barbiturates, carbamazepine, ethosuximide, felbamate, lamotrigine, tiagabine, topiramate, and zonisamide. Valproic acid may increase, decrease, or have no effect on phenytoin serum concentrations. Phenytoin may also decrease the serum concentrations/effects of some antiarrhythmics (disopyramide, propafenone, quinidine, quetiapine) and tricyclic antidepressants may be reduced by phenytoin. Phenytoin may enhance the metabolism of doxycycline, decreasing its clinical effect; higher dosages may be required. Phenytoin may increase the metabolism of chloramphenicol or itraconazole.

Phenytoin may decrease the levels/effects of amiodarone, benzodiazepines, bupropion, calcium channel blockers, carbamazepine, citalopram, clarithromycin, cyclosporine, efavirenz, erythromycin, estrogens, fluoxetine, glimepiride, glipizide, losartan, methsuximide, mirtazapine, nateglinide, nefazodone, nevirapine, phenytoin, pioglitazone, promethazine, propranolol, protease inhibitors, proton pump inhibitors, rosiglitazone, selegiline, (Continued)

Fosphenytoin (Continued)

sertraline, sulfonamides, tacrolimus, venlafaxine. voriconazole, warfarin, zafirlukast, and other CYP2B6, 2C8/9, 2C19, or 3A4 substrates.

The levels/effects of phenytoin may be decreased by aminoglutethimide, carbamazepine, phenobarbital, rifampin, rifapentine, secobarbital, and other CYP2C8/9 or 2C19 inducers. Clozapine and vigabatrin may reduce phenytoin serum concentrations. Case reports indicate ciprofloxacin may increase or decrease serum phenytoin concentrations. Dexamethasone may decrease serum phenytoin concentrations. Replacement of folic acid has been reported to increase the metabolism of phenytoin, decreasing its serum concentrations and/or increasing seizures.

Initially, phenytoin increases the response to warfarin; this is followed by a decrease in response to warfarin. Phenytoin may inhibit the anti-Parkinson effect of levodopa. The duration of neuromuscular blockade from neuromuscular-blocking agents may be decreased by phenytoin. Phenytoin may enhance the metabolism of methadone resulting in methadone withdrawal. Phenytoin may decrease serum levels/effects of digitalis glycosides, theophylline, and thyroid hormones.

Several chemotherapeutic agents have been associated with a decrease in serum phenytoin levels; includes cisplatin, bleomycin, carmustine, methotrexate, and vinblastine. Enzyme-inducing anticonvulsant therapy may reduce the effectiveness of some chemotherapy regimens (specifically in ALL). Teniposide and methotrexate may be cleared more rapidly in these patients.

Increased Effect/Toxicity: The sedative effects of phenytoin may be additive with other CNS depressants including ethanol, barbiturates, sedatives, antidepressants, narcotic analgesics, and benzodiazepines. Selected anticonvulsants (felbamate, gabapentin, and topiramate) have been reported to increase phenytoin levels/effects. In addition, serum phenytoin concentrations may be increased by allopurinol, amiodarone, calcium channel blockers (including diltiazem and nifedipine), cimetidine, disulfiram, methylphenidate, metronidazole, omeprazole, selective serotonin reuptake inhibitors (SSRIs), ticlopidine, tricyclic antidepressants, trazodone, and trimethoprim. Case reports indicate ciprofloxacin may increase or decrease serum phenytoin concentrations.

The levels/effects of phenytoin may be increased by delavirdine, fluconazole, fluvoxamine, gemfibrozil, isoniazid, ketoconazole, nicardipine, NSAIDs, omeprazole, pioglitazone, sulfonamides, ticlopidine, and other CYP2C8/9 or 2C19 inhibitors.

Phenytoin enhances the conversion of primidone to phenobarbital resulting in elevated phenobarbital serum concentrations. Concurrent use of acetazolamide with phenytoin may result in an increased risk of osteomalacia. Concurrent use of phenytoin and lithium has resulted in lithium intoxication. Valproic acid (and sulfisoxazole) may displace phenytoin from binding sites; valproic acid may increase, decrease, or have no effect on phenytoin serum concentrations. Phenytoin transiently increased the response to warfarin initially; this is followed by an inhibition of the hypoprothrombinemic response. Phenytoin may enhance the hepatotoxic potential of acetaminophen overdoses. Concurrent use of dopamine and intravenous phenytoin may lead to an increased risk of hypotension.

Nutritional/Ethanol Interactions

Ethanol:

Acute use: Avoid or limit ethanol (inhibits metabolism of phenytoin); watch for sedation.

Chronic use: Avoid or limit ethanol (stimulates metabolism of phenytoin).

Lab Interactions May decrease serum concentrations of thyroxine; may produce artifactually low results in dexamethasone or metyrapone tests; may cause increase serum concentrations of glucose, alkaline phosphatase, and gamma glutamyl transpeptidase (GGT)

Adverse Reactions The more important adverse clinical events caused by the I.V. use of fosphenytoin or phenytoin are cardiovascular collapse and/or central nervous system depression. Hypotension can occur when either drug is administered rapidly by the I.V. route. Do not exceed a rate of 150 mg phenytoin equivalent/minute when administering fosphenytoin.

The adverse clinical events most commonly observed with the use of fosphenytoin in clinical trials were nystagmus, dizziness, pruritus, paresthesia, headache, somnolence, and ataxia. Paresthesia and pruritus were seen more often following fosphenytoin (versus phenytoin) administration and occurred more often with I.V. fosphenytoin than with I.M. administration. These events were dose- and rate-related (doses ≥15 mg/kg at a rate of 150 mg/minute). These sensations, generally described as itching, burning, or tingling are usually not at the infusion site. The location of the discomfort varied with the groin mentioned most frequently. The paresthesia and pruritus were transient events that occurred within several minutes of the start of infusion and generally resolved within 10 minutes after completion of infusion.

Transient pruritus, tinnitus, nystagmus, somnolence, and ataxia occurred 2-3 times more often at doses ≥15 mg/kg and rates ≥150 mg/minute.

I.V. administration (maximum dose/rate):

>10%:

Central nervous system: Nystagmus, dizziness, somnolence, ataxia

Dermatologic: Pruritus

1% to 10%:

Cardiovascular: Hypotension, vasodilation, tachycardia

Central nervous system: Stupor, incoordination, paresthesia, extrapyramidal syndrome, tremor, agitation, hypoesthesia, dysarthria, vertigo, brain edema, headache

Gastrointestinal: Nausea, tongue disorder, dry mouth, vomiting

Neuromuscular & skeletal: Pelvic pain, muscle weakness, back pain

Ocular: Diplopia, amblyopia

Otic: Tinnitus, deafness

Miscellaneous: Taste perversion

I.M. administration (substitute for oral phenytoin):
1% to 10%:
Central nervous system: Nystagmus, tremor, ataxia, headache, incoordination, somnolence, dizziness, paresthesia, reflexes decreased
Dermatologic: Pruritus
Gastrointestinal: Nausea, vomiting
Hematologic/lymphatic: Ecchymosis
Neuromuscular & skeletal: Muscle weakness

Overdosage/Toxicology Symptoms of fosphenytoin overdose include bradycardia, asystole, cardiac arrest, hypotension, vomiting, metabolic acidosis, and lethargy. Treatment is supportive for hypotension.

Pharmacodynamics/Kinetics
Bioavailability: I.M.: Fosphenytoin: 100%
Time to Peak: Conversion to phenytoin: Following I.V. administration (maximum rate of administration): 15 minutes; following I.M. administration, peak phenytoin levels are reached in 3 hours
Protein Binding: Fosphenytoin: 95% to 99% to albumin; can displace phenytoin and increase free fraction (up to 30% unbound) during the period required for conversion of fosphenytoin to phenytoin
Half-Life Elimination: Fosphenytoin: 15 minutes; Phenytoin: Variable (mean: 12-29 hours); kinetics of phenytoin are saturable
Metabolism: Fosphenytoin is rapidly converted via hydrolysis to phenytoin; phenytoin is metabolized in the liver and forms metabolites
Excretion: Phenytoin: Urine (as inactive metabolites)
Pharmacokinetic Note: Refer to Phenytoin monograph for additional information.

Dosing
Adults:
The dose, concentration in solutions, and infusion rates for fosphenytoin are expressed as phenytoin sodium equivalents (PE); fosphenytoin should always be prescribed and dispensed in phenytoin sodium equivalents (PE)

Status epilepticus: I.V.: Loading dose: 15-20 mg PE/kg I.V. administered at 100-150 mg PE/minute
Nonemergent loading and maintenance dosing: I.V. or I.M.:
Loading dose: 10-20 mg PE/kg I.V. or I.M. (maximum I.V. rate: 150 mg PE/minute)
Initial daily maintenance dose: 4-6 mg PE/kg/day I.V. or I.M.

Substitution for oral phenytoin therapy: I.M. or I.V.: May be substituted for oral phenytoin sodium at the same total daily dose; however, Dilantin® capsules are ~90% bioavailable by the oral route; phenytoin, supplied as fosphenytoin, is 100% bioavailable by both the I.M. and I.V. routes; for this reason, plasma phenytoin concentrations may increase when I.M. or I.V. fosphenytoin is substituted for oral phenytoin sodium therapy; in clinical trials I.M. fosphenytoin was administered as a single daily dose utilizing either 1 or 2 injection sites; some patients may require more frequent dosing
Elderly: Phenytoin clearance is decreased in geriatric patients; lower doses may be required. In addition, older adults may have lower serum albumin which may increase the free fraction and, therefore, pharmacologic response. Refer to adult dosing.

Pediatrics:
Note: The dose, concentration in solutions, and infusion rates for fosphenytoin are expressed as phenytoin sodium equivalents (PE); fosphenytoin should always be prescribed and dispensed in phenytoin sodium equivalents (PE).

Infants and Children (unlabeled use): I.V.:
Loading dose: 10-20 mg PE/kg for the treatment of generalized convulsive status epilepticus.
Maintenance dosing: Phenytoin dosing guidelines in pediatric patients are used when dosing fosphenytoin using doses in PE equal to the phenytoin doses (ie, phenytoin 1 mg = fosphenytoin 1 PE); maintenance doses may be started 8-12 hours after a loading dose

Renal Impairment: Free phenytoin levels should be monitored closely in patients with renal disease or in those with hypoalbuminemia; furthermore, fosphenytoin clearance to phenytoin may be increased without a similar increase in phenytoin clearance in these patients leading to increase frequency and severity of adverse events.
Hepatic Impairment: Phenytoin clearance may be substantially reduced in cirrhosis and plasma level monitoring with dose adjustment advisable. Free phenytoin levels should be monitored closely in patients with hepatic disease or in those with hypoalbuminemia; furthermore, fosphenytoin clearance to phenytoin may be increased without a similar increase in phenytoin clearance in these patients leading to increase frequency and severity of adverse events.

Available Dosage Forms Injection, solution, as sodium: 75 mg/mL [equivalent to phenytoin sodium 50 mg/mL] (2 mL, 10 mL)

Monitoring and Teaching Issues
Physical Assessment: Assess all other medications patient may be taking. Continuous monitoring is essential during infusion and for 30 minutes following infusion. Monitor closely for adverse or overdose reactions during and following infusion.
Monitoring Laboratory Tests: Serum phenytoin, renal function, albumin
Patient Education: Patients may not be in a position to evaluate their response. If conscious or alert, advise patient to report signs or symptoms of palpitations, racing or falling heartbeat, respiratory difficulty, acute faintness, or CNS disturbances (eg, somnolence, ataxia), and visual disturbances. **Pregnancy precaution:** Inform prescriber if you are pregnant.
Dietary Considerations: Provides phosphate 0.0037 mmol/mg PE fosphenytoin
Geriatric Considerations: No significant changes in fosphenytoin pharmacokinetics with age have been noted. Phenytoin clearance is decreased in the elderly and lower doses may be needed. Elderly may have reduced hepatic clearance due to age decline in Phase I (Continued)

Fosphenytoin *(Continued)*

metabolism. Elderly may have low albumin which will increase free fraction and, therefore, pharmacologic response. Monitor closely in those who are hypoalbuminemic. Free fraction measurements advised, also elderly may display a higher incidence of adverse effects (cardiovascular) when using the I.V. loading regimen; therefore, recommended to decrease loading I.V. dose to 25 mg/minute.

Pregnancy Risk Factor: D

Pregnancy Issues: Fosphenytoin is the prodrug of phenytoin. Refer to Phenytoin monograph for additional information.

Lactation: Excretion in breast milk unknown/not recommended

Breast-Feeding Issues: Fosphenytoin is the prodrug of phenytoin. It is not known if fosphenytoin is excreted in breast milk prior to conversion to phenytoin. Refer to Phenytoin monograph for additional information.

Administration

I.M.: I.M. may be administered as a single daily dose using either 1 or 2 injection sites.

I.V.: Rates of infusion:
Children: 1-3 mg PE/kg/minute
Adults: Should not exceed 150 mg PE/minute

Reconstitution: Must be diluted to concentrations 1.5-25 mg PE/mL, in normal saline or D_5W, for I.V. infusion

Compatibility: Stable in D_5LR, $D_5^{1}/_2NS$, D_5W, $D_{10}W$, hetastarch 6% in NS, mannitol 20%, LR, NS

Y-site administration: Incompatible with midazolam

Storage: Refrigerate at 2°C to 8°C (36°F to 46°F). Do not store at room temperature for more than 48 hours. Do not use vials that develop particulate matter.

Additional Information 1.5 mg fosphenytoin is approximately equivalent to 1 mg phenytoin. Equimolar fosphenytoin dose is 375 mg (75 mg/mL solution) to phenytoin 250 mg (50 mg/mL).

♦ **Fosphenytoin Sodium** *see* Fosphenytoin *on page 683*
♦ **Fragmin®** *see* Dalteparin *on page 398*
♦ **Frova®** *see* Frovatriptan *on page 686*

Frovatriptan *(froe va TRIP tan)*

U.S. Brand Names Frova®

Synonyms Frovatriptan Succinate

Generic Available No

Pharmacologic Category Antimigraine Agent; Serotonin 5-HT$_{1B, 1D}$ Receptor Agonist

Use Acute treatment of migraine with or without aura in adults

Mechanism of Action/Effect Blocks 5-HT$_{1B}$ and 5-HT$_{1D}$ receptors. Relieves symptoms of migraine by blocking vasoconstrictive and other effects of serotonin.

Contraindications Hypersensitivity to frovatriptan or any component of the formulation; patients with ischemic heart disease or signs or symptoms of ischemic heart disease (including Prinzmetal's angina, angina pectoris, myocardial infarction, silent myocardial ischemia); cerebrovascular syndromes (including strokes, transient ischemic attacks); peripheral vascular syndromes (including ischemic bowel disease); uncontrolled hypertension; use within 24 hours of ergotamine derivatives; use within 24 hours of another 5-HT$_1$ agonist; management of hemiplegic or basilar migraine; prophylactic treatment of migraine; severe hepatic impairment

Warnings/Precautions Not intended for migraine prophylaxis, or treatment of cluster headaches, hemiplegic or basilar migraines. Cardiac events, cerebral/subarachnoid hemorrhage, and stroke have been reported with 5-HT$_1$ agonist administration. May cause vasospastic reactions resulting in colonic, peripheral, or coronary ischemia. Do not give to patients with risk factors for CAD until a cardiovascular evaluation has been performed. If the evaluation is satisfactory, the healthcare provider should administer the first dose and cardiovascular status should be periodically evaluated. Significant elevation in blood pressure has been reported on rare occasions in patients using other 5-HT$_{1D}$ agonists with and without a history of hypertension. Peripheral vascular ischemia and colonic ischemia with abdominal pain and bloody diarrhea have occurred. Use with caution in patients with a history of seizure disorder. Safety and efficacy in pediatric patients have not been established.

Drug Interactions

Cytochrome P450 Effect: Substrate of CYP1A2 (minor)

Increased Effect/Toxicity: The effects of frovatriptan may be increased by estrogen derivatives and propranolol. Ergot derivatives may increase the effects of frovatriptan (do not use within 24 hours of each other). SSRIs may exhibit additive toxicity with frovatriptan or other serotonin agonists (eg, antidepressants, dextromethorphan, tramadol) leading to serotonin syndrome.

Nutritional/Ethanol Interactions Food: Food does not affect frovatriptan bioavailability.

Adverse Reactions 1% to 10%:
Cardiovascular: Chest pain (2%), flushing (4%), palpitation (1%)
Central nervous system: Dizziness (8%), fatigue (5%), headache (4%), hot or cold sensation (3%), anxiety (1%), dysesthesia (1%), hypoesthesia (1%), insomnia (1%), pain (1%)
Gastrointestinal: Hyposalivation (3%), dyspepsia (2%), abdominal pain (1%), diarrhea (1%), vomiting (1%)
Neuromuscular & skeletal: Paresthesia (4%), skeletal pain (3%)
Ocular: Visual abnormalities (1%)
Otic: Tinnitus (1%)
Respiratory: Rhinitis (1%), sinusitis (1%)
Miscellaneous: Diaphoresis (1%)

Overdosage/Toxicology Single oral doses of up to 100 mg have been reported without adverse effects. Treatment of overdose should be supportive and symptomatic. Monitor for at least 48 hours or until signs and symptoms subside. It is not known if hemodialysis or peritoneal dialysis is effective.

Pharmacodynamics/Kinetics
Bioavailability: 20% to 30%
Time to Peak: 2-4 hours
Protein Binding: 15%
Half-Life Elimination: 26 hours
Metabolism: Primarily hepatic via CYP1A2
Excretion: Feces (62%); urine (32%)
Dosing
Adults & Elderly: Migraine: Oral: 2.5 mg; if headache recurs, a second dose may be given if first dose provided some relief and at least 2 hours have elapsed since the first dose (maximum daily dose: 7.5 mg)
Renal Impairment: No adjustment necessary.
Hepatic Impairment: No adjustment necessary in mild to moderate hepatic impairment; use with caution in severe impairment
Available Dosage Forms Tablet, as base: 2.5 mg
Monitoring and Teaching Issues
Physical Assessment: Assess potential for interactions with other prescriptions, OTC medications, or herbal products patient may be taking (eg, ergot derivatives). Cardiovascular status should be evaluated prior to initiating medication and periodically thereafter. Assess effectiveness and adverse response. Teach patient proper use, possible side effects/appropriate interventions, and adverse symptoms to report.
Patient Education: This drug is to be used to reduce your migraine, not to prevent or reduce the number of attacks. Follow exact instructions for use. Do not take within 24 hours of any other migraine medication without first consulting prescriber. If first dose brings relief, a second dose may be taken anytime after 2 hours if migraine returns. Do not take more than three tablets (7.5 mg) in 24 hours without consulting prescriber. May cause dizziness, fatigue, insomnia, or drowsiness (use caution when driving or engaging in tasks requiring alertness until response to drug is known); dry mouth (frequent mouth care and sucking on lozenges may help); skin flushing or hot flashes (cool clothes or a cool environment may help); or mild abdominal discomfort or vomiting (small frequent meals, good mouth care, chewing gum, or sucking lozenges may help). Report immediately any chest pain, palpitations, or irregular heartbeat; severe dizziness, acute headache, stiff or painful neck, facial swelling, muscle weakness or pain, changes in mental acuity, blurred vision, eye pain, or ringing in ears; changes in urinary pattern; respiratory difficulty; or other persistent adverse effects. **Pregnancy/breast-feeding precautions:** Inform prescriber if you are or intend to become pregnant. Consult prescriber if breast-feeding.
Pregnancy Risk Factor: C
Lactation: Excretion in breast milk unknown/use caution
Administration
Oral: Administer with fluids.
Storage: Store at room temperature of 25°C (77°F); protect from moisture and light.
Related Information
Antimigraine Drugs: 5-HT$_1$ Receptor Agonists *on page 1716*

Fulvestrant (fool VES trant)
U.S. Brand Names Faslodex®
Synonyms ICI-182,780; Zeneca 182,780; ZM-182,780
Generic Available No
Pharmacologic Category Antineoplastic Agent, Estrogen Receptor Antagonist
Use Treatment of hormone receptor positive metastatic breast cancer in postmenopausal women with disease progression following antiestrogen therapy.
Unlabeled/Investigational Use Endometriosis; uterine bleeding
Mechanism of Action/Effect Steroidal compound which competitively binds to estrogen receptors on tumors and other tissue targets; inhibits estrogen effects. Fulvestrant has no estrogen-receptor agonist activity. Causes down-regulation of estrogen receptors and inhibits tumor growth.
Contraindications Hypersensitivity to fulvestrant or any component of the formulation; contraindications to I.M. injections (bleeding diatheses, thrombocytopenia, or therapeutic anticoagulation); pregnancy
Warnings/Precautions Use caution in hepatic impairment.
Drug Interactions
Cytochrome P450 Effect: Substrate of CYP3A4 (minor)
Adverse Reactions
>10%:
Cardiovascular: Vasodilation (18%)
Central nervous system: Pain (19%), headache (15%)
Endocrine & metabolic: Hot flushes (19% to 24%)
Gastrointestinal: Nausea (26%), vomiting (13%), constipation (13%), diarrhea (12%), abdominal pain (12%)
Local: Injection site reaction (11%)
Neuromuscular & skeletal: Weakness (23%), bone pain (16%), back pain (14%)
Respiratory: Pharyngitis (16%), dyspnea (15%)
(Continued)

Fulvestrant *(Continued)*

1% to 10%:
Cardiovascular: Edema (9%), chest pain (7%)
Central nervous system: Dizziness (7%), insomnia (7%), paresthesia (6%), fever (6%), depression (6%), anxiety (5%)
Dermatologic: Rash (7%)
Gastrointestinal: Anorexia (9%), weight gain (1% to 2%)
Genitourinary: Pelvic pain (10%), urinary tract infection (6%), vaginitis (2% to 3%)
Hematologic: Anemia (5%)
Neuromuscular and skeletal: Arthritis (3%)
Respiratory: Cough (10%)
Miscellaneous: Diaphoresis increased (5%)

Overdosage/Toxicology No specific experience in overdose. Treatment is supportive.

Pharmacodynamics/Kinetics
Duration of Action: I.M.: Plasma levels maintained for at least 1 month
Bioavailability: Oral: Poor
Time to Peak: Plasma: I.M.: 7-9 days
Protein Binding: 99%
Half-Life Elimination: ~40 days
Metabolism: Hepatic via multiple pathways (CYP3A4 substrate, relative contribution to metabolism unknown)
Excretion: Feces (>90%); urine (<1%)

Dosing
Adults: Metastatic breast cancer (postmenopausal women): I.M.: 250 mg at 1-month intervals
Renal Impairment: No dosage adjustment required.
Hepatic Impairment: Use in moderate to severe hepatic impairment has not been evaluated; use caution

Available Dosage Forms Injection, solution: 50 mg/mL (2.5 mL, 5 mL) [[prefilled syringe; contains alcohol, benzyl alcohol, benzyl stearate, castor oil]

Monitoring and Teaching Issues
Physical Assessment: Use caution in hepatic impairment. See Administration for injection specifics. Assess therapeutic effectiveness and adverse response (eg, vasodilation, edema, gastrointestinal disturbances, dyspnea, pain; see Adverse Reactions) on a regular basis throughout therapy. Teach patient use (if self-administered, injection technique and syringe/needle disposal), possible side effects/appropriate interventions, and adverse symptoms to report (see Patient Education).
Patient Education: Do not take any new medication during therapy unless approved by prescriber. If self-administered, follow directions for injection and syringe/needle disposal. You may experience bone pain, back pain, or headache (consult prescriber for approved analgesic); nausea, vomiting, or loss of appetite (small frequent meals, frequent mouth care, sucking lozenges, or chewing gum may help); dizziness (use caution when driving or engaging in tasks requiring alertness until response to drug is known); or increased perspiration. Report persistent pain; chest pain or palpitations; swelling of extremities or unusual weight gain (>5 lb/week); cough or respiratory difficulty; burning on urination or changes in urinary pattern; or other persistent, unrelieved adverse effects. **Pregnancy/breast-feeding precautions:** Approved only for postmenopausal women. Severe fetal damage can occur with this drug. Do not breast-feed.
Pregnancy Risk Factor: D
Pregnancy Issues: Antiestrogenic compounds have been associated with embryotoxicity, abnormalities in fetal development, and failure to maintain pregnancy in animal models. Approved for use only in postmenopausal women.
Lactation: Excretion in breast milk unknown/contraindicated
Breast-Feeding Issues: Approved for use only in postmenopausal women

Administration
I.M.: I.M. injection into a relatively large muscle (ie, buttock); do not administer I.V., SubQ, or intra-arterially. May be administered as a single 5 mL injection or two concurrent 2.5 mL injections.
Storage: Store under refrigeration at 2°C to 8°C (36°F to 46°F).

♦ Fungizone® *see* Amphotericin B (Conventional) *on page 109*
♦ Fungoid® Tincture [OTC] *see* Miconazole *on page 999*
♦ Furadantin® *see* Nitrofurantoin *on page 1088*
♦ Furazosin *see* Prazosin *on page 1243*

Furosemide *(fyoor OH se mide)*

U.S. Brand Names Lasix®
Synonyms Frusemide
Generic Available Yes
Pharmacologic Category Diuretic, Loop
Medication Safety Issues
Sound-alike/look-alike issues:
Furosemide may be confused with torsemide
Lasix® may be confused with Esidrix®, Lanoxin®, Lidex®, Lomotil®, Luvox®, Luxiq®

Use Management of edema associated with congestive heart failure and hepatic or renal disease; alone or in combination with antihypertensives in treatment of hypertension
Mechanism of Action/Effect Inhibits reabsorption of sodium and chloride in the ascending loop of Henle and distal renal tubule, interfering with the chloride-binding cotransport system, thus causing increased excretion of water, sodium, chloride, magnesium, and calcium
Contraindications Hypersensitivity to furosemide, any component, or sulfonylureas; anuria; patients with hepatic coma or in states of severe electrolyte depletion until the condition improves or is corrected

Warnings/Precautions In cirrhosis, avoid electrolyte and acid/base imbalances that might lead to hepatic encephalopathy. Ototoxicity is associated with rapid I.V. administration, renal impairment, excessive doses, and concurrent use of other ototoxins. Hypersensitivity reactions can rarely occur. Monitor fluid status and renal function in an attempt to prevent oliguria, azotemia, electrolyte disturbances, dehydration, and reversible increases in BUN and creatinine. Coadministration of antihypertensives may increase the risk of hypotension. Avoid use of medications in which the toxicity is enhanced by hypokalemia (including quinolones with QT prolongation).

Chemical similarities are present among sulfonamides, sulfonylureas, carbonic anhydrase inhibitors, thiazides, and loop diuretics (except ethacrynic acid). Use in patients with sulfonylurea allergy is specifically contraindicated in product labeling, however, a risk of cross-reaction exists in patients with allergy to any of these compounds; avoid use when previous reaction has been severe.

Drug Interactions

Decreased Effect: Indomethacin, aspirin, phenobarbital, phenytoin, and NSAIDs may reduce natriuretic and hypotensive effects of furosemide. Colestipol, cholestyramine, and sucralfate may reduce the effect of furosemide; separate administration by 2 hours. Furosemide may antagonize the effect of skeletal muscle relaxants (tubocurarine). Glucose tolerance may be decreased by furosemide, requiring an adjustment in the dose of hypoglycemic agents. Metformin may decrease furosemide concentrations.

Increased Effect/Toxicity: Furosemide-induced hypokalemia may predispose to digoxin toxicity and may increase the risk of arrhythmia with drugs which may prolong QT interval, including type Ia and type III antiarrhythmic agents, cisapride, and some quinolones (sparfloxacin, gatifloxacin, and moxifloxacin). The risk of toxicity from lithium and salicylates (high dose) may be increased by loop diuretics. Hypotensive effects and/or adverse renal effects of ACE inhibitors and NSAIDs are potentiated by furosemide-induced hypovolemia. The effects of peripheral adrenergic-blocking drugs or ganglionic blockers may be increased by furosemide.

Furosemide may increase the risk of ototoxicity with other ototoxic agents (aminoglycosides, cis-platinum), especially in patients with renal dysfunction. Synergistic diuretic effects occur with thiazide-type diuretics. Diuretics tend to be synergistic with other antihypertensive agents, and hypotension may occur.

Nutritional/Ethanol Interactions

Food: Furosemide serum levels may be decreased if taken with food.

Herb/Nutraceutical: Avoid dong quai if using for hypertension (has estrogenic activity). Avoid ephedra, yohimbe, ginseng (may worsen hypertension). Limit intake of natural licorice. Avoid garlic (may have increased antihypertensive effect).

Adverse Reactions Frequency not defined.

Cardiovascular: Orthostatic hypotension, necrotizing angiitis, thrombophlebitis, chronic aortitis, acute hypotension, sudden death from cardiac arrest (with I.V. or I.M. administration)

Central nervous system: Paresthesias, vertigo, dizziness, lightheadedness, headache, blurred vision, xanthopsia , fever, restlessness

Dermatologic: Exfoliative dermatitis, erythema multiforme, purpura, photosensitivity, urticaria, rash, pruritus, cutaneous vasculitis

Endocrine & metabolic: Hyperglycemia, hyperuricemia, hypokalemia, hypochloremia, metabolic alkalosis, hypocalcemia, hypomagnesemia, gout, hyponatremia

Gastrointestinal: Nausea, vomiting, anorexia, oral and gastric irritation, cramping, diarrhea, constipation, pancreatitis, intrahepatic cholestatic jaundice, ischemia hepatitis

Genitourinary: Urinary bladder spasm, urinary frequency

Hematological: Aplastic anemia (rare), thrombocytopenia, agranulocytosis (rare), hemolytic anemia, leukopenia, anemia, purpura

Neuromuscular & skeletal: Muscle spasm, weakness

Otic: Hearing impairment (reversible or permanent with rapid I.V. or I.M. administration), tinnitus, reversible deafness (with rapid I.V. or I.M. administration)

Renal: Vasculitis, allergic interstitial nephritis, glycosuria, fall in glomerular filtration rate and renal blood flow (due to overdiuresis), transient rise in BUN

Miscellaneous: Anaphylaxis (rare), exacerbate or activate systemic lupus erythematosus

Overdosage/Toxicology Symptoms of overdose include electrolyte depletion, volume depletion, hypotension, dehydration, and circulatory collapse. Treatment is supportive.

Pharmacodynamics/Kinetics

Onset of Action: Diuresis: Oral: 30-60 minutes; I.M.: 30 minutes; I.V.: ~5 minutes; Peak effect: Oral: 1-2 hours

Duration of Action: Oral: 6-8 hours; I.V.: 2 hours

Absorption: Oral: 60% to 67%

Protein Binding: >98%

Half-Life Elimination: Normal renal function: 0.5-1.1 hours; End-stage renal disease: 9 hours

Metabolism: Minimally hepatic

Excretion: Urine (Oral: 50%, I.V.: 80%) within 24 hours; feces (as unchanged drug); nonrenal clearance prolonged with renal impairment

Dosing

Adults:

Edema, CHF, or hypertension (diuresis):

Oral: 20-80 mg/dose initially increased in increments of 20-40 mg/dose at intervals of 6-8 hours; usual maintenance dose interval is twice daily or every day

Usual dosage range for hypertension (JNC 7): 20-80 mg/day in 2 divided doses

I.M., I.V.: 20-40 mg/dose, may be repeated in 1-2 hours as needed and increased by 20 mg/dose with each succeeding dose up to 1000 mg/day; usual dosing interval: 6-12 hours

Continuous I.V. infusion: Initial I.V. bolus dose of 0.1 mg/kg followed by continuous I.V. infusion doses of 0.1 mg/kg/hour doubled every 2 hours to a maximum of 0.4 mg/kg/hour if urine output is <1 mL/kg/hour have been found to be effective and result in a

(Continued)

Furosemide *(Continued)*

lower daily requirement of furosemide than with intermittent dosing. Other studies have used 20-160 mg/hour continuous I.V. infusion.

Refractory heart failure: Oral, I.V.: Doses up to 8 g/day have been used.

Elderly: Oral, I.M., I.V.: Initial: 20 mg/day; increase slowly to desired response.

Pediatrics:

Edema, CHF, or hypertension (diuresis): Infants and Children:

Oral: 1-2 mg/kg/dose increased in increments of 1 mg/kg/dose with each succeeding dose until a satisfactory effect is achieved to a maximum of 6 mg/kg/dose no more frequently than 6 hours

I.M., I.V.: 1 mg/kg/dose, increasing by each succeeding dose at 1 mg/kg/dose at intervals of 6-12 hours until a satisfactory response up to 6 mg/kg/dose

Renal Impairment:

Acute renal failure: Doses up to 1-3 g/day may be necessary to initiate desired response; avoid use in oliguric states.

Not removed by hemo- or peritoneal dialysis; supplemental dose is not necessary.

Hepatic Impairment: Diminished natriuretic effect with increased sensitivity to hypokalemia and volume depletion in cirrhosis. Monitor effects, particularly with high doses.

Available Dosage Forms

Injection, solution: 10 mg/mL (2 mL, 4 mL, 8 mL, 10 mL)

Solution, oral: 10 mg/mL (60 mL, 120 mL) [orange flavor]; 40 mg/5 mL (5 mL, 500 mL) [pineapple-peach flavor]

Tablet (Lasix®): 20 mg, 40 mg, 80 mg

Monitoring and Teaching Issues

Physical Assessment: Assess for allergy to sulfonylurea before beginning therapy. See Warnings/Precautions for use cautions. Assess potential for interactions with other pharmacological agents or herbal products the patient may be taking (especially anything that may impact fluid balance or increase potential for ototoxicity or hypotension; see Drug Interactions). For intravenous use see Administration specifics. Assess results of laboratory tests (electrolytes), therapeutic effectiveness, and adverse response on a regular basis during therapy (eg, dehydration, electrolyte imbalance, postural hypotension; see Adverse Reactions). Caution patients with diabetes about closely monitoring glucose levels (glucose tolerance may be decreased). Teach patient appropriate use, possible side effects/appropriate interventions, and adverse symptoms to report (see Patient Education).

Monitoring Laboratory Tests: Serum electrolytes, renal function

Patient Education: Do not take any new medication during therapy unless approved by prescriber. Take as directed with food or milk (to reduce GI distress) early in the day (daily), or if twice daily, take last dose in late afternoon in order to avoid sleep disturbance and achieve maximum therapeutic effect. Keep medication in original container, away from light; do not use discolored medication. Follow dietary advice of prescriber; include bananas or orange juice or other potassium-rich foods in daily diet, but do not take potassium supplements without advice of prescriber. Weigh yourself each day, at the same time, in the same clothes when beginning therapy and weekly with long-term therapy. Report unusual or unanticipated weight gain or loss. May cause dizziness, blurred vision, or drowsiness (use caution when driving or engaging in tasks that require alertness until response to drug is known); postural hypotension (use caution when rising from lying or sitting position or when climbing stairs); or sensitivity to sunlight (use sunblock or wear protective clothing and sunglasses). Report signs of edema (eg, weight gain, swollen ankles, feet, or hands); trembling, numbness or unusual fatigue, cramping or muscle weakness, palpitations, unresolved nausea or vomiting, change in hearing, or other persistent adverse reactions. **Pregnancy/breast-feeding precautions:** Inform prescriber if you are or intend to become pregnant. Consult prescriber if breast-feeding.

Dietary Considerations: This product may cause a potassium loss; your healthcare provider may prescribe a potassium supplement, another medication to help prevent the potassium loss, or recommend that you eat foods high in potassium, especially citrus fruits; do not change your diet on your own while taking this medication, especially if you are taking potassium supplements or medications to reduce potassium loss; too much potassium can be as harmful as too little; ideally, should be administered on an empty stomach; however, may be administered with food or milk if GI distress; do not mix with acidic solutions. Sodium content of 1 mL (injection): 0.162 mEq

Geriatric Considerations: Severe loss of sodium and/or increase in BUN can cause confusion. For any change in mental status in patients on furosemide, monitor electrolytes and renal function.

Pregnancy Risk Factor: C

Pregnancy Issues: Crosses the placenta. Increased fetal urine production, electrolyte disturbances reported. Generally, use of diuretics during pregnancy is avoided due to risk of decreased placental perfusion.

Lactation: Enters breast milk/use caution

Breast-Feeding Issues: Crosses into breast milk; may suppress lactation. AAP has NO RECOMMENDATION.

Administration

I.V.: Replace parenteral therapy with oral therapy as soon as possible. I.V. injections should be given slowly may be administered undiluted direct I.V. at a maximum rate of 0.5 mg/kg/minute for doses <120 mg and 4 mg/minute for doses >120 mg; maximum rate of administration for IVPB or infusion: 4 mg/minute. For continuous infusion furosemide in patients with severely-impaired renal function, do not exceed 4 mg/minute.

Reconstitution: I.V. infusion solution mixed in NS or D_5W solution is stable for 24 hours at room temperature. May also be diluted for infusion 1-2 mg/mL (maximum: 10 mg/mL) over 10-15 minutes (following infusion rate parameters).

Compatibility: Stable in D_5LR, D_5NS, D_5W, $D_{10}W$, $D_{20}W$, mannitol 20%, LR, NS

Y-site administration: Incompatible with alatrofloxacin, amiodarone, amsacrine, chlorpromazine, ciprofloxacin, clarithromycin, diltiazem, droperidol, esmolol, filgrastim, fluconazole, gatifloxacin, gemcitabine, gentamicin, hydralazine, idarubicin, levofloxacin, metoclopramide, midazolam, milrinone, netilmicin, nicardipine, ondansetron, quinidine gluconate, thiopental, vecuronium, vinblastine, vincristine, vinorelbine

Compatibility in syringe: Incompatible with doxapram, doxorubicin, droperidol, metoclopramide, milrinone, vinblastine, vincristine

Compatibility when admixed: Incompatible with buprenorphine, chlorpromazine, diazepam, dobutamine, erythromycin lactobionate, isoproterenol, meperidine, metoclopramide, netilmicin, prochlorperazine edisylate, promethazine

Storage: Furosemide injection should be stored at controlled room temperature and protected from light. Exposure to light may cause discoloration. Do not use furosemide solutions if they have a yellow color. Refrigeration may result in precipitation or crystallization, however, resolubilization at room temperature or warming may be performed without affecting the drugs stability.

Related Information
Compatibility of Drugs *on page 1723*
Heart Failure *on page 1828*

♦ **Fuzeon**™   *see* Enfuvirtide *on page 519*

Gabapentin (GA ba pen tin)

U.S. Brand Names Neurontin®
Generic Available Yes: Capsule, tablet
Pharmacologic Category Anticonvulsant, Miscellaneous
Medication Safety Issues
Sound-alike/look-alike issues:
Neurontin® may be confused with Neoral®, Noroxin®

Use Adjunct for treatment of partial seizures with and without secondary generalized seizures in patients >12 years of age with epilepsy; adjunct for treatment of partial seizures in pediatric patients 3-12 years of age; management of postherpetic neuralgia (PHN) in adults

Unlabeled/Investigational Use Social phobia; chronic pain

Mechanism of Action/Effect Exact mechanism of action is not known, but does have properties in common with other anticonvulsants; although structurally related to GABA, it does not interact with GABA receptors

Contraindications Hypersensitivity to gabapentin or any component of the formulation

Warnings/Precautions Avoid abrupt withdrawal, may precipitate seizures; use cautiously in patients with severe renal dysfunction; male rat studies demonstrated an association with pancreatic adenocarcinoma (clinical implication unknown). May cause CNS depression, which may impair physical or mental abilities. Patients must be cautioned about performing tasks which require mental alertness (eg, operating machinery or driving). Effects with other sedative drugs or ethanol may be potentiated. Pediatric patients (3-12 years of age) have shown increased incidence of CNS-related adverse effects, including emotional lability, hostility, thought disorder, and hyperkinesia. Safety and efficacy in children <3 years of age have not been established.

Drug Interactions
Increased Effect/Toxicity: Sedative effects may be additive with CNS depressants; includes ethanol, barbiturates, narcotic analgesics, and other sedative agents; monitor for increased effect

Nutritional/Ethanol Interactions
Ethanol: Avoid ethanol (may increase CNS depression).
Food: Does not change rate or extent of absorption.
Herb/Nutraceutical: Avoid evening primrose (seizure threshold decreased). Avoid valerian, St John's wort, kava kava, gotu kola (may increase CNS depression).

Lab Interactions False positives have been reported with the Ames N-Multistix SG® dipstick test for urine protein

Adverse Reactions As reported in patients >12 years of age, unless otherwise noted in children (3-12 years)
>10%:
Central nervous system: Somnolence (20%; children 8%), dizziness (17% to 28%; children 3%), ataxia (13%), fatigue (11%)
Miscellaneous: Viral infection (children 11%)
1% to 10%:
Cardiovascular: Peripheral edema (2% to 8%), vasodilatation (1%)
Central nervous system: Fever (children 10%), hostility (children 8%), emotional lability (children 4%), fatigue (children 3%), headache (3%), ataxia (3%), abnormal thinking (2% to 3%; children 2%), amnesia (2%), depression (2%), dysarthria (2%), nervousness (2%), abnormal coordination (1% to 2%), twitching (1%), hyperesthesia (1%)
Dermatologic: Pruritus (1%), rash (1%)
Endocrine & metabolic: Hyperglycemia (1%)
Gastrointestinal: Diarrhea (6%), Nausea/vomiting (3% to 4%; children 8%), abdominal pain (3%), weight gain (adults and children 2% to 3%), dyspepsia (2%), flatulence (2%), dry throat (2%), xerostomia (2% to 5%), constipation (2% to 4%), dental abnormalities (2%), appetite stimulation (1%)
Genitourinary: Impotence (2%)
Hematologic: Leukopenia (1%), decreased WBC (1%)
Neuromuscular & skeletal: Tremor (7%), weakness (6%), hyperkinesia (children 3%), abnormal gait (2%), back pain (2%), myalgia (2%), fracture (1%)
Ocular: Nystagmus (8%), diplopia (1% to 6%), blurred vision (3% to 4%), conjunctivitis (1%)
Otic: Otitis media (1%)
Respiratory: Rhinitis (4%), bronchitis (children 3%), respiratory infection (children 3%), pharyngitis (1% to 3%), cough (2%)
Miscellaneous: Infection (5%)

Overdosage/Toxicology Acute oral overdoses of up to 49 g have been reported; double vision, slurred speech, drowsiness, lethargy, and diarrhea were observed. Patients recovered
(Continued)

Gabapentin *(Continued)*

with supportive care. Decontaminate using lavage/activated charcoal with cathartic. Multiple dosing of activated charcoal may be useful; hemodialysis may be useful.

Pharmacodynamics/Kinetics

Absorption: 50% to 60% from proximal small bowel by L-amino transport system

Bioavailability: Inversely proportional to dose due to saturable absorption:

900 mg/day: 60%
1200 mg/day: 47%
2400 mg/day: 34%
3600 mg/day: 33%
4800 mg/day: 27%

Protein Binding: 0%

Half-Life Elimination: 5-7 hours; anuria 132 hours; during dialysis 3.8 hours

Excretion: Proportional to renal function; urine (as unchanged drug)

Dosing

Adults:

Anticonvulsant: Oral:

Initial: 300 mg 3 times/day, if necessary the dose may be increased up to 1800 mg/day

Maintenance: 900-1800 mg/day administered in 3 divided doses; doses of up to 2400 mg/day have been tolerated in long-term clinical studies; up to 3600 mg/day has been tolerated in short-term studies

Note: If gabapentin is discontinued or if another anticonvulsant is added to therapy, it should be done slowly over a minimum of 1 week.

Chronic pain (unlabeled use): Oral: 300-1800 mg/day given in 3 divided doses has been the most common dosage range

Postoperative pain (unlabeled use): 300-1200 mg 1-2 hours before surgery

Postherpetic neuralgia: Day 1: 300 mg, Day 2: 300 mg twice daily, Day 3: 300 mg 3 times/day; dose may be titrated as needed for pain relief (range: 1800-3600 mg/day, daily doses >1800 mg do not generally show greater benefit)

Elderly: Studies in elderly patients have shown a decrease in clearance as age increases. This is most likely due to age-related decreases in renal function; dose reductions may be needed.

Pediatrics:

Anticonvulsant: Oral

Children 3-12 years: Initial: 10-15 mg/kg/day in 3 divided doses; titrate to effective dose over ~3 days; dosages of up to 50 mg/kg/day have been tolerated in clinical studies

Children 3-4 years: Effective dose: 40 mg/kg/day in 3 divided doses

Children ≥5-12 years: Effective dose: 25-35 mg/kg/day in 3 divided doses

Children >12 years: Refer to adult dosing.

Note: If gabapentin is discontinued or if another anticonvulsant is added to therapy, it should be done slowly over a minimum of 1 week

Renal Impairment: Children ≥12 years and Adults: See table.

Hemodialysis: Dialyzable

Gabapentin Dosing Adjustments in Renal Impairment

Creatinine Clearance (mL/min)	Daily Dose Range
≥60	300-1200 mg tid
>30-59	200-700 mg bid
>15-29	200-700 mg daily
15[1]	100-300 mg daily
Hemodialysis[2]	125-350 mg

[1]Cl$_{cr}$<15 mL/minute: Reduce daily dose in proportion to creatinine clearance.

[2]Single supplemental dose administered after each 4 hours of hemodialysis

Available Dosage Forms

Capsule (Neurontin®): 100 mg, 300 mg, 400 mg

Solution, oral (Neurontin®): 250 mg/5 mL (480 mL) [cool strawberry anise flavor]

Tablet: 100 mg, 300 mg, 400 mg

Neurontin®: 600 mg, 800 mg

Monitoring and Teaching Issues

Physical Assessment: Assess effectiveness and interactions of other medications patient may be taking. Monitor therapeutic effectiveness, laboratory values, and adverse reactions at beginning of therapy and periodically with long-term use. Assess for CNS depression. Taper dosage slowly when discontinuing. Assess knowledge/teach patient safety and seizure precautions, appropriate use, interventions to reduce side effects, and adverse symptoms to report.

Monitoring Laboratory Tests: Monitor serum levels of concomitant anticonvulsant therapy. Routine monitoring of gabapentin levels is not mandatory.

Patient Education: Take exactly as directed; do not increase dose or frequency. It may take 2-3 weeks to achieve desired results; may cause physical and/or psychological dependence. If prescribed once-a-day, take dose at bedtime. If taking antacids, take at least 2 hours after antacids. Do not stop medication abruptly, may lead to increased seizure activity. Avoid alcohol, caffeine, and other prescription or OTC medications not approved by prescriber. Maintain adequate hydration (2-3 L/day of fluids) unless instructed to restrict fluid intake. You may experience drowsiness, lightheadedness, impaired coordination, dizziness, or blurred vision (use caution when driving or engaging in tasks requiring alertness until response to drug is known); nausea, vomiting, or anorexia (small frequent meals, frequent mouth care, chewing gum, or sucking lozenges may help); constipation (increased exercise, fluids, fruit, or fiber may help); diarrhea (buttermilk, yogurt, or boiled milk may help); postural hypotension (use caution when climbing stairs or changing position from lying or sitting to standing); or decreased sexual function or libido (reversible).

Report persistent CNS effects (nervousness, restlessness, insomnia, anxiety, excitation, headache, sedation, seizures, mania, abnormal thinking); rash or skin irritation; muscle cramping, tremors, or change in gait; chest pain or palpitations; change in urinary pattern; or worsening of condition. **Pregnancy/breast-feeding precautions:** Inform prescriber if you are or intend to become pregnant. Breast-feeding is not recommended.

Dietary Considerations: May be taken without regard to meals.

Geriatric Considerations: No clinical studies to specifically evaluate this drug in the elderly have been performed; however, in premarketing studies, patients >65 years of age did not demonstrate any difference in side effect profiles from younger adults. Since gabapentin is eliminated renally, dose **must** be adjusted for creatinine clearance in the elderly patient.

Pregnancy Risk Factor: C

Pregnancy Issues: No data on crossing the placenta; there have been reports of normal pregnancy outcomes, as well as respiratory distress, pyloric stenosis, and inguinal hernia following 1st trimester exposure to gabapentin plus carbamazepine; epilepsy itself, number of medications, genetic factors, or a combination of these probably influence the teratogenicity of anticonvulsant therapy. Use during pregnancy only if the potential benefit to the mother outweighs the potential risk to the fetus.

Lactation: Enters breast milk/use caution

Breast-Feeding Issues: Gabapentin is excreted in human breast milk. A nursed infant could be exposed to ~1 mg/kg/day of gabapentin; the effect on the child is not known. Use in breast-feeding women only if the benefits to the mother outweigh the potential risk to the infant.

Administration

Oral: Administer first dose on first day at bedtime to avoid somnolence and dizziness. Dosage must be adjusted for renal function; when given 3 times daily, the maximum time between doses should not exceed 12 hours.

Storage: Store at 25°C (77°F); excursions permitted to 15°C to 30°C (59°F to 86°F).

Related Information

Anticonvulsants By Seizure Type *on page 1712*

♦ **Gabitril®** *see* Tiagabine *on page 1471*

Galantamine (ga LAN ta meen)

U.S. Brand Names Reminyl®
Synonyms Galantamine Hydrobromide
Generic Available No
Pharmacologic Category Acetylcholinesterase Inhibitor (Central)
Medication Safety Issues
Sound-alike/look-alike issues:
Reminyl® may be confused with Amaryl®
Use Treatment of mild-to-moderate dementia of Alzheimer's disease
Mechanism of Action/Effect Increases the concentration of acetylcholine in the brain by slowing its metabolism.
Contraindications Hypersensitivity to galantamine or any component of the formulation; severe liver dysfunction (Child-Pugh score 10-15); severe renal dysfunction (Cl$_{cr}$ <9 mL/minute)
Warnings/Precautions May exaggerate neuromuscular blockade effects of depolarizing neuromuscular-blocking agents like succinylcholine. Vagotonic effects on the SA and AV nodes may lead to bradycardia or AV block. Use caution in patients with supraventricular cardiac conduction delays (without a functional pacemaker in place) or patients taking concurrent medications that slow conduction through the SA or AV node. Use caution in peptic ulcer disease (or in patients at risk); seizure disorder; asthma; COPD; mild to moderate liver dysfunction; moderate renal dysfunction. May cause bladder outflow obstruction. Safety and efficacy in children have not been established.

Drug Interactions

Cytochrome P450 Effect: Substrate (minor) of CYP2D6, 3A4
Decreased Effect: Anticholinergic agents are antagonized by galantamine. CYP inducers may decrease galantamine levels.
Increased Effect/Toxicity: Succinylcholine: increased neuromuscular blockade. Amiodarone, beta-blockers without ISA activity, diltiazem, verapamil may increase bradycardia. NSAIDs increase risk of peptic ulcer. Cimetidine, ketoconazole, paroxetine, other CYP3A4 inhibitors, other CYP2D6 inhibitors increase levels of galantamine. Concurrent cholinergic agents may have synergistic effects. Digoxin may lead to AV block.

Nutritional/Ethanol Interactions

Ethanol: Avoid ethanol (may increase CNS adverse events).
Herb/Nutraceutical: St John's wort may decrease galantamine serum levels; avoid concurrent use.

Adverse Reactions

>10%: Gastrointestinal: Nausea (6% to 24%), vomiting (4% to 13%), diarrhea (6% to 12%)
1% to 10%:
Cardiovascular: Bradycardia (2% to 3%), syncope (0.4% to 2.2%: dose related), chest pain (≥1%)
Central nervous system: Dizziness (9%), headache (8%), depression (7%), fatigue (5%), insomnia (5%), somnolence (4%), tremor (3%)
Gastrointestinal: Anorexia (7% to 9%), weight loss (5% to 7%), abdominal pain (5%), dyspepsia (5%), flatulence (≥1%)
Genitourinary: Urinary tract infection (8%), hematuria (<1% to 3%), incontinence (≥1%)
Hematologic: Anemia (3%)
Respiratory: Rhinitis (4%)
Overdosage/Toxicology Symptoms of overdose may include bradycardia, collapse, convulsions, defecation, gastrointestinal cramping, hypotension, lacrimation, muscle fasciculations, muscle weakness, QT prolongation, respiratory depression, salivation, severe nausea, sweating, torsade de pointes, urination, ventricular tachycardia, vomiting. Treatment is (Continued)

Galantamine *(Continued)*

symptom-directed and supportive. Atropine may be used as an antidote; initial dose 0.5-1 mg I.V. and titrate to effect. An atypical response in blood pressure and heart rate has been reported. Effects of hemodialysis are unknown.

Pharmacodynamics/Kinetics

Duration of Action: 3 hours; maximum inhibition of erythrocyte acetylcholinesterase ~40% at 1 hour post 10 mg oral dose; levels return to baseline at 30 hours

Absorption: Rapid and complete

Bioavailability: 80% to 100%

Time to Peak: 1 hour

Protein Binding: 18%

Half-Life Elimination: 6-8 hours

Metabolism: Hepatic; linear, CYP2D6 and 3A4; metabolized to epigalanthaminone and galanthaminone both of which have acetylcholinesterase inhibitory activity 130 times less than galantamine

Excretion: Urine (25%)

Dosing

Adults & Elderly:

Alzheimer's dementia (mild-to-moderate): Oral: Initial: 4 mg twice a day for 4 weeks

If 8 mg per day tolerated, increase to 8 mg twice daily for ≥4 weeks

If 16 mg per day tolerated, increase to 12 mg twice daily; range: 16-24 mg/day in 2 divided doses

Note: Doses should be taken with breakfast and dinner. If therapy is interrupted for ≥3 days, restart at the lowest dose and increase to current dose.

Renal Impairment:

Moderate renal impairment: Maximum dose: 16 mg/day.

Severe renal dysfunction (Cl$_{cr}$ <9 mL/minute): Use is not recommended

Hepatic Impairment:

Moderate liver dysfunction (Child-Pugh score 7-9): Maximum dose: 16 mg/day

Severe liver dysfunction (Child-Pugh score 10-15): Use is not recommended

Available Dosage Forms

Solution, oral, as hydrobromide: 4 mg/mL (100 mL) [with calibrated pipette]

Tablet, as hydrobromide: 4 mg, 8 mg, 12 mg

Monitoring and Teaching Issues

Physical Assessment: Assess bladder and sphincter adequacy prior to starting therapy. Assess other medications patient may be taking for effectiveness and interactions (especially those dependent on cytochrome P450 metabolism). Monitor therapeutic effectiveness and adverse reactions at beginning of therapy and periodically throughout therapy (eg, cholinergic crisis). Assess knowledge/teach appropriate use, interventions to reduce side effects, and adverse symptoms to report.

Patient Education: This medication will not cure Alzheimer's disease, but may help reduce symptoms. Use exactly as directed; do not increase dose or discontinue without consulting prescriber. Maintain adequate hydration (2-3 L/day of fluids) unless instructed to restrict fluid intake. May cause dizziness, sedation, hypotension, or tremor (use caution when driving or engaging in hazardous tasks, rise slowly from sitting or lying position, and use caution when climbing stairs until response to drug is known); diarrhea (boiled milk, yogurt, or buttermilk may help); or nausea or vomiting (small frequent meals, good mouth care, sucking lozenges, or chewing gum may help). Report persistent GI disturbances; significantly increased salivation, sweating, or tearing; excessive fatigue, insomnia, dizziness, or depression; increased muscle, joint, or body pain or spasms; vision changes; respiratory changes, wheezing, or signs of dyspnea; chest pain or palpitations; or other adverse reactions. **Breast-feeding precaution:** Breast-feeding is not recommended.

Dietary Considerations: Take with breakfast and dinner.

Pregnancy Risk Factor: B

Lactation: Excretion in breast milk unknown/not recommended

Administration

Oral: Take with breakfast and dinner. If therapy is interrupted for ≥3 days, restart at the lowest dose and increase to current dose as patient tolerates. If using oral solution, mix dose with 3-4 ounces of any nonalcoholic beverage; mix well and drink immediately.

Storage: Store at 15°C to 30°C (59°F to 86°F). Do not freeze oral solution; protect from light.

♦ **Galantamine Hydrobromide** *see Galantamine on page 693*

Gallium Nitrate *(GAL ee um NYE trate)*

U.S. Brand Names Ganite™

Synonyms NSC-15200

Generic Available No

Pharmacologic Category Calcium-Lowering Agent

Use Treatment of hypercalcemia

Mechanism of Action/Effect Inhibits bone resorption by inhibiting osteoclast function

Contraindications Hypersensitivity to gallium nitrate or any component of the formulation; severe renal dysfunction (creatinine >2.5 mg/dL)

Warnings/Precautions Use caution with renal impairment or when administering other nephrotoxic drugs (eg, aminoglycosides, amphotericin B); consider discontinuing gallium nitrate during treatment with nephrotoxic drugs. Maintain adequate hydration. Use intended for the treatment of symptomatic cancer-related hypercalcemia not responding to hydration. Safety and efficacy in pediatric patients have not been established.

Drug Interactions

Increased Effect/Toxicity: Concurrent use of low-dose gallium nitrate with cyclophosphamide has been associated with dyspnea, stomatitis, asthenia, and rarely interstitial pneumonitis. Concurrent use nephrotoxic drugs (eg, aminoglycosides, amphotericin B) with gallium nitrate may increase nephrotoxic effects.

Adverse Reactions Not all frequencies defined.

Cardiovascular: Hypotension, tachycardia, edema of lower extremities

Central nervous system: Lethargy, confusion, dreams, hallucinations, hypothermia, fever

Dermatologic: Rash

Endocrine & metabolic: Hypophosphatemia (>50%, usually asymptomatic); hypocalcemia; mild respiratory alkalosis with hyperchloremia

Hematologic: Anemia, leukopenia

Gastrointestinal: Nausea (14%, generally mild), vomiting, diarrhea, constipation

Neuromuscular & skeletal: Paresthesia

Renal: Nephrotoxicity (>10%, generally reversible and reported to be minimized with adequate hydration and urine output)

Respiratory: Dyspnea, rales, rhonchi, pleural effusion, pulmonary infiltrates

Note: Toxicities reported with doses higher than those used to treat hypercalcemia (ie, in trials evaluating anticancer effect): Optic neuritis, tinnitus, hearing acuity decreased, metallic taste, hypomagnesemia, encephalopathy

Overdosage/Toxicology Symptoms of overdose include nausea, vomiting, and increased risk of nephrotoxicity.

Pharmacodynamics/Kinetics

Onset of Action: Onset of calcium lowering: Seen within 24-48 hours of beginning therapy, with normocalcemia achieved within 4-7 days of beginning therapy

Bioavailability: Oral: 5%

Half-Life Elimination: Alpha: 1.25 hours; Beta: ~24 hours

Elimination half-life varies with method of administration (72-115 hours with prolonged intravenous infusion versus 24 hours with bolus administration); long elimination half-life may be related to slow release from tissue such as bone

Excretion: Primarily renal with no prior metabolism in the liver or kidney; long elimination half-life may be related to slow release from tissue such as bone; elimination half-life varies with method of administration (72-115 hours with prolonged intravenous infusion versus 24 hours with bolus administration)

Dosing

Adults: Hypercalcemia: I.V.: 200 mg/m^2/day for 5 days; duration may be shortened during a course if normocalcemia is achieved. If hypercalcemia is mild and with very few symptoms, 100 mg/m^2/day may be used.

Renal Impairment:

Serum creatinine >2.5 mg/dL: Contraindicated

Serum creatinine 2 to <2.5 mg/dL: No guidelines exist; frequent monitoring is recommended.

Available Dosage Forms Injection, solution [preservative free]: 25 mg/mL (20 mL)

Monitoring and Teaching Issues

Physical Assessment: See Warnings/Precautions for use cautions (eg, renal impairment). Assess potential for interactions with other pharmacological agents patient may be taking (eg, risk of nephrotoxicity; see Drug Interactions). Assess results of laboratory tests, therapeutic effectiveness (calcium levels), and adverse response on a regular basis throughout therapy (eg, hypotension, tachycardia, gastrointestinal upset, hypocalcemia; see Adverse Reactions). Teach patient possible side effects/appropriate interventions and adverse symptoms to report (see Patient Education).

Monitoring Laboratory Tests: Renal function, serum calcium (daily), serum phosphorus (twice weekly)

Patient Education: This medication is given by intravenous infusion; report immediately any redness, swelling, or pain at infusion site. Report chest pain or palpitations, difficulty breathing, rash, CNS changes (confusion, dreams, hallucinations); numbness, pain, or tingling in extremities; unusual and persistent fatigue or lethargy; changes in urinary pattern or output; or other adverse reactions. **Pregnancy/breast-feeding precautions:** Inform prescriber if you are or intend to be pregnant or breast-feed.

Pregnancy Risk Factor: C

Lactation: Excretion in breast milk unknown/not recommended

Breast-Feeding Issues: Due to the potential for adverse reactions in the nursing infant, it is recommended to discontinue nursing during treatment or discontinue gallium nitrate.

Administration

I.V.: Continuous I.V. infusion; daily dose is administered in 1000 mL of 0.9% NaCl or D$_5$W.

Storage: Store unopened vials (25 mg/mL) at room temperature of 15°C to 30°C (59°F to 86°F); not light sensitive. Solutions in 0.9% NaCl or D$_5$W are stable for 48 hours at room temperature or for 7 days under refrigeration at 2°C to 8°C (36°F to 46°F).

- Gamimune® N *see* Immune Globulin (Intravenous) *on page 793*
- Gamma Benzene Hexachloride *see* Lindane *on page 902*
- Gammagard® S/D *see* Immune Globulin (Intravenous) *on page 793*
- Gammaphos *see* Amifostine *on page 86*
- Gammar®-P I.V. *see* Immune Globulin (Intravenous) *on page 793*
- Gamunex® *see* Immune Globulin (Intravenous) *on page 793*

Ganciclovir (gan SYE kloe veer)

U.S. Brand Names Cytovene®; Vitrasert®

Synonyms DHPG Sodium; GCV Sodium; Nordeoxyguanosine

Generic Available Yes: Capsule

Pharmacologic Category Antiviral Agent

Medication Safety Issues

Sound-alike/look-alike issues:

Cytovene® may be confused with Cytosar®, Cytosar-U®

Use

Parenteral: Treatment of CMV retinitis in immunocompromised individuals, including patients with acquired immunodeficiency syndrome; prophylaxis of CMV infection in transplant patients

(Continued)

Ganciclovir *(Continued)*

Oral: Alternative to the I.V. formulation for maintenance treatment of CMV retinitis in immuno-compromised patients, including patients with AIDS, in whom retinitis is stable following appropriate induction therapy and for whom the risk of more rapid progression is balanced by the benefit associated with avoiding daily I.V. infusions.

Implant: Treatment of CMV retinitis

Unlabeled/Investigational Use May be given in combination with foscarnet in patients who relapse after monotherapy with either drug

Mechanism of Action/Effect Ganciclovir is phosphorylated to a substrate which competitively inhibits the binding of deoxyguanosine triphosphate to DNA polymerase resulting in inhibition of viral DNA synthesis.

Contraindications Hypersensitivity to ganciclovir, acyclovir, or any component of the formulation; absolute neutrophil count <500/mm^3; platelet count <25,000/mm^3

Warnings/Precautions Dosage adjustment or interruption of ganciclovir therapy may be necessary in patients with neutropenia and/or thrombocytopenia and patients with impaired renal function. Use with extreme caution in children since long-term safety has not been determined and due to ganciclovir's potential for long-term carcinogenic and adverse reproductive effects. Ganciclovir may adversely affect spermatogenesis and fertility. Due to its mutagenic potential, contraceptive precautions for female and male patients need to be followed during and for at least 90 days after therapy with the drug. Take care to administer only into veins with good blood flow.

Drug Interactions

Decreased Effect: A decrease in blood levels of ganciclovir AUC may occur when used with didanosine.

Increased Effect/Toxicity: Immunosuppressive agents may increase hematologic toxicity of ganciclovir. Imipenem/cilastatin may increase seizure potential. Oral ganciclovir increases blood levels of zidovudine, although zidovudine decreases steady-state levels of ganciclovir. Since both drugs have the potential to cause neutropenia and anemia, some patients may not tolerate concomitant therapy with these drugs at full dosage. Didanosine levels are increased with concurrent ganciclovir. Other nephrotoxic drugs (eg, amphotericin and cyclosporine) may have additive nephrotoxicity with ganciclovir.

Adverse Reactions

>10%:

Central nervous system: Fever (38% to 48%)

Dermatologic: Rash (15% oral, 10% I.V.)

Gastrointestinal: Abdominal pain (17% to 19%), diarrhea (40%), nausea (25%), anorexia (15%), vomiting (13%)

Hematologic: Anemia (20% to 25%), leukopenia (30% to 40%)

1% to 10%:

Central nervous system: Confusion, neuropathy (8% to 9%), headache (4%)

Dermatologic: Pruritus (5%)

Hematologic: Thrombocytopenia (6%), neutropenia with ANC <500/mm^3 (5% oral, 14% I.V.)

Neuromuscular & skeletal: Paresthesia (6% to 10%), weakness (6%)

Ocular: Retinal detachment (8% oral, 11% I.V.; relationship to ganciclovir not established)

Miscellaneous: Sepsis (4% oral, 15% I.V.)

Overdosage/Toxicology Symptoms of overdose include neutropenia, vomiting, hypersalivation, bloody diarrhea, cytopenia, and testicular atrophy. Treatment is supportive. Hemodialysis removes 50% of the drug. Hydration may be of some benefit.

Pharmacodynamics/Kinetics

Bioavailability: Oral: Fasting: 5%; Following food: 6% to 9%; Following fatty meal: 28% to 31%

Protein Binding: 1% to 2%

Half-Life Elimination: 1.7-5.8 hours; prolonged with renal impairment; End-stage renal disease: 5-28 hours

Excretion: Urine (80% to 99% as unchanged drug)

Dosing

Adults & Elderly: Dosing is based on total body weight.

CMV retinitis:

I.V. (slow infusion):

Induction therapy: 5 mg/kg/dose every 12 hours for 14-21 days followed by maintenance therapy

Maintenance therapy: 5 mg/kg/day as a single daily dose for 7 days/week or 6 mg/kg/day for 5 days/week

Oral: 1000 mg 3 times/day with food **or** 500 mg 6 times/day with food

Ocular implant: Intravitreally: One implant for 5- to 8-month period; following depletion of ganciclovir, as evidenced by progression of retinitis, implant may be removed and replaced

Prevention of CMV disease in patients with advanced HIV infection and normal renal function: Oral: 1000 mg 3 times/day with food

Prevention of CMV disease in transplant patients: Same initial and maintenance dose as CMV retinitis except duration of initial course is 7-14 days, duration of maintenance therapy is dependent on clinical condition and degree of immunosuppression

Pediatrics: CMV retinitis: Children >3 months: Refer to adult dosing.

Renal Impairment:

I.V. (Induction):

Cl_{cr} 50-69 mL/minute: Administer 2.5 mg/kg/dose every 12 hours.

Cl_{cr} 25-49 mL/minute: Administer 2.5 mg/kg/dose every 24 hours.

Cl_{cr} 10-24 mL/minute: Administer 1.25 mg/kg/dose every 24 hours.

Cl_{cr} <10 mL/minute: Administer 1.25 mg/kg/dose 3 times/week following hemodialysis.

I.V. (Maintenance):

Cl_{cr} 50-69 mL/minute: Administer 2.5 mg/kg/dose every 24 hours.

Cl_{cr} 25-49 mL/minute: Administer 1.25 mg/kg/dose every 24 hours.

Cl_{cr} 10-24 mL/minute: Administer 0.625 mg/kg/dose every 24 hours

Cl_{cr} <10 mL/minute: Administer 0.625 mg/kg/dose 3 times/week following hemodialysis.

Oral:

Cl_{cr} 50-69 mL/minute: Administer 1500 mg/day or 500 mg 3 times/day.

Cl_{cr} 25-49 mL/minute: Administer 1000 mg/day or 500 mg twice daily.

Cl_{cr} 10-24 mL/minute: Administer 500 mg/day.

Cl_{cr} <10 mL/minute: Administer 500 mg 3 times/week following hemodialysis.

Hemodialysis effects: Dialyzable (50%) following hemodialysis; administer dose postdialysis. During peritoneal dialysis, dose as for Cl_{cr} <10 mL/minute. During continuous arteriovenous or venovenous hemofiltration, administer 2.5 mg/kg/dose every 24 hours.

Available Dosage Forms

Capsule (Cytovene®): 250 mg, 500 mg

Implant, intravitreal (Vitrasert®): 4.5 mg [released gradually over 5-8 months]

Injection, powder for reconstitution, as sodium (Cytovene®): 500 mg

Monitoring and Teaching Issues

Physical Assessment: See Warnings/Precautions for use cautions (eg, impaired renal function, contraceptive precautions during and for 90 days following therapy). Assess potential for interactions with other pharmacological agents patient may be taking (increased risk for neutropenia, hematologic toxicity, nephrotoxicity; see Drug Interactions). **I.V.:** See Administration for infusion specifics. Assess results of laboratory tests prior to therapy and on a regular basis during therapy. Monitor therapeutic effectiveness and adverse response throughout therapy (eg, paresthesia, neutropenia, anemia, nephrotoxicity, retinal detachment; see Adverse Reactions). Teach possible side effects/appropriate interventions and adverse symptoms to report (see Patient Education).

Monitoring Laboratory Tests: CBC with differential and platelet count, serum creatinine before beginning therapy and on a regular basis thereafter; liver function tests

Patient Education: Do not take any new medication during therapy unless approved by prescriber. Ganciclovir is not a cure for CMV retinitis. For oral administration, take as directed and maintain adequate hydration (2-3 L/day of fluids) unless instructed to restrict fluid intake. You will need frequent blood tests and regular ophthalmic exams while taking this drug. You may experience increased susceptibility to infection (avoid crowds and exposure to infection and do not have any vaccinations without consulting prescriber). You may experience confusion or headache (use cautions when driving or engaging in potentially hazardous tasks until response to drug is known); nausea, vomiting, or anorexia (small frequent meals, frequent mouth care, chewing gum, or sucking lozenges may help); diarrhea (buttermilk, boiled milk, or yogurt may help); or photosensitivity (use sunscreen, wear protective clothing and eyewear, and avoid direct sunlight). Report rash; infection (fever, chills, unusual bleeding or bruising, infection, or unhealed sores or white plaques in mouth); abdominal pain; tingling, weakness, or pain in extremities; any vision changes; or pain, redness, or swelling at injection site. **Pregnancy/breast-feeding precautions:** Inform prescriber if you are pregnant. Males and females should use appropriate contraceptive measures during and for 60-90 days following end of therapy. Consult prescriber for appropriate contraceptive measures. Do not breast-feed.

Dietary Considerations: Sodium content of 500 mg vial: 46 mg

Geriatric Considerations: Adjust dose based upon renal function.

Pregnancy Risk Factor: C

Lactation: Excretion in breast milk unknown/contraindicated

Breast-Feeding Issues: The CDC recommends **not** to breast-feed if diagnosed with HIV to avoid postnatal transmission of the virus.

Administration

Oral: Oral ganciclovir should be administered with food.

I.V.: The same precautions utilized with antineoplastic agents should be followed with ganciclovir administration. Ganciclovir should not be administered by I.M., SubQ, or rapid IVP. Administer by slow I.V. infusion over at least 1 hour at a final concentration for administration not to exceed 10 mg/mL. Too rapid infusion can cause increased toxicity and excessive plasma levels.

Reconstitution: Preparation should take place in a vertical laminar flow hood with the same precautions as antineoplastic agents. Drug product should be reconstituted immediately before use and any unused portion should be discarded appropriately. Reconstitute powder with sterile water **not** bacteriostatic water because parabens may cause precipitation. Reconstituted solution is stable for 12 hours at room temperature, however, conflicting data indicates that reconstituted solution is stable for 60 days under refrigeration (4°C). Stability of parenteral admixture at room temperature (25°C) and at refrigeration temperature (4°C) is 5 days.

Compatibility: Stable in D₅W, LR, NS; **incompatible** with bacteriostatic water for injection (contains parabens and may cause precipitation)

Y-site administration: Incompatible with aldesleukin, amifostine, amsacrine, aztreonam, cefepime, cytarabine, doxorubicin, fludarabine, foscarnet, gemcitabine, ondansetron, piperacillin/tazobactam, sargramostim, vinorelbine

Storage: Intact vials should be stored at room temperature and protected from temperatures >40°C.

♦ **Ganidin NR** see Guaifenesin *on page 729*

Ganirelix (ga ni REL ix)

U.S. Brand Names Antagon®

Synonyms Ganirelix Acetate

Generic Available No

Pharmacologic Category Gonadotropin Releasing Hormone Antagonist

Use Inhibits premature luteinizing hormone (LH) surges in women undergoing controlled ovarian hyperstimulation in fertility clinics.

Mechanism of Action/Effect Suppresses gonadotropin secretion and luteinizing hormone secretion to prevent ovulation until the follicles are of adequate size.

(Continued)

Ganirelix *(Continued)*

Contraindications Hypersensitivity to ganirelix or any component of the formulation; hypersensitivity to gonadotropin-releasing hormone or any other analog; known or suspected pregnancy

Warnings/Precautions Should only be prescribed by fertility specialists. The packaging contains natural rubber latex (may cause allergic reactions). Pregnancy must be excluded before starting medication.

Drug Interactions

Decreased Effect: No formal studies have been performed.

Increased Effect/Toxicity: No formal studies have been performed.

Adverse Reactions 1% to 10%:

Central nervous system: Headache (3%)

Endocrine & metabolic: Ovarian hyperstimulation syndrome (2%)

Gastrointestinal: Abdominal pain (5%), nausea (1%), and abdominal pain (1%)

Genitourinary: Vaginal bleeding (2%)

Local: Injection site reaction (1%)

Pharmacodynamics/Kinetics

Absorption: SubQ: Rapid

Bioavailability: 91.1%

Time to Peak: 1.1 hours

Protein Binding: 81.9%

Half-Life Elimination: 16.2 hours

Metabolism: Hepatic to two primary metabolites (1-4 and 1-6 peptide)

Excretion: Feces (75%) within 288 hours; urine (22%) within 24 hours

Dosing

Adults & Elderly: Adjunct to controlled ovarian hyperstimulation: SubQ: 250 mcg/day during the mid-to-late phase after initiating follicle-stimulating hormone on day 2 or 3 of cycle. Treatment should be continued daily until the day of chorionic gonadotropin administration.

Available Dosage Forms Injection, solution, as acetate: 250 mcg/0.5 mL [prefilled glass syringe with 27-gauge x ½ inch needle]

Monitoring and Teaching Issues

Physical Assessment: This medication should only be prescribed by a fertility specialist. Assess/teach patient use (demonstrate injection procedures, syringe disposal), interventions to reduce side-effects, and adverse reactions to report. **Pregnancy risk factor X:** Pregnancy must be excluded before starting medication.

Monitoring Laboratory Tests: Ultrasound to assess the follicle's size

Patient Education: This drug can only be given by injection as demonstrated. Use this and any other medications as directed by prescriber; do not skip any doses. You must keep all scheduled ultrasound appointments. You may experience headache (use of mild analgesic may help); or nausea (small frequent meals, good mouth care, chewing gum, or sucking hard candy may help). Report immediately any sudden or acute abdominal pain; vaginal bleeding; or pain, itching, or signs of infection at injection site. **Note:** Packaging contains natural rubber latex; if you have a known latex allergy advise prescriber. **Pregnancy/breast-feeding precautions:** Do not get pregnant while taking this drug. Breast-feeding is not recommended.

Pregnancy Risk Factor: X

Pregnancy Issues: Fetal resorption occurred in pregnant rats and rabbits. These effects are results of hormonal alterations and could result in fetal loss in humans. The drug should not be used in pregnant women.

Lactation: Excretion in breast milk unknown/not recommended

Administration

Storage: Store at controlled room temperature of 15°C to 30°C (59°F to 86°F).

♦ **Ganirelix Acetate** *see* Ganirelix *on page 697*

♦ **Ganite™** *see* Gallium Nitrate *on page 694*

♦ **Gani-Tuss DM NR** *see* Guaifenesin and Dextromethorphan *on page 731*

♦ **Gani-Tuss® NR** *see* Guaifenesin and Codeine *on page 731*

♦ **Gantrisin®** *see* SulfiSOXAZOLE *on page 1412*

♦ **Gastrocrom®** *see* Cromolyn *on page 374*

Gatifloxacin *(gat i FLOKS a sin)*

U.S. Brand Names Tequin®; Zymar™

Generic Available No

Pharmacologic Category Antibiotic, Ophthalmic; Antibiotic, Quinolone

Use

Oral, I.V.: Treatment of the following infections when caused by susceptible bacteria: Acute bacterial exacerbation of chronic bronchitis; acute sinusitis; community-acquired pneumonia including pneumonia caused by multidrug-resistant *S. pneumoniae* (MDRSP); uncomplicated skin and skin structure infection; uncomplicated urinary tract infections (cystitis); complicated urinary tract infections; pyelonephritis; uncomplicated urethral and cervical gonorrhea; acute, uncomplicated rectal infections in women

Ophthalmic: Bacterial conjunctivitis

Mechanism of Action/Effect Inhibits bacterial DNA

Contraindications Hypersensitivity to gatifloxacin, other quinolone antibiotics, or any component of the formulation

Warnings/Precautions Use with caution in patients with significant bradycardia (or receiving drugs which may cause bradycardia), acute myocardial ischemia, cardiovascular disease (especially with conduction disturbances), or individuals at risk of seizures (CNS disorders or concurrent therapy with medications which may lower seizure threshold). May cause increased CNS stimulation, increased intracranial pressure, convulsions, or psychosis.

Discontinue in patients who experience significant CNS adverse effects (dizziness, hallucinations, suicidal ideation or actions), cardiovascular adverse effects (QT prolongation [concentration dependent], arrhythmia) or hypersensitivity reactions. Use caution in patients with known prolongation of QT interval, uncorrected hypokalemia, or concurrent administration of other medications known to prolong the QT interval (including Class Ia and Class III antiarrhythmics, cisapride, erythromycin, antipsychotics, and tricyclic antidepressants). Use caution in renal dysfunction and severe hepatic insufficiency. Serious disruptions in glucose regulation (including hyperglycemia and severe hypoglycemia) may occur, generally in patients with diabetes and typically within 1-3 days of initiation. Monitor closely and discontinue if hyper- or hypoglycemia occur. Quinolones may exacerbate myasthenia gravis. May cause peripheral neuropathy (rare); discontinue if symptoms of sensory or sensorimotor neuropathy occur.

Pseudomembranous colitis should be considered in all patients with diarrhea. Tendon inflammation and/or rupture has been reported with this and other quinolone antibiotics. Risk may be increased with concurrent corticosteroids, particularly in the elderly. Discontinue at first sign of tendon inflammation or pain. Safety and efficacy for ophthalmic use have not been established in children <1 year of age. Safety and efficacy for systemic use have not been established in patients <18 years of age.

Drug Interactions
Decreased Effect: Concurrent administration of metal cations, including most antacids (not calcium carbonate), oral electrolyte supplements, quinapril, sucralfate, and some didanosine formulations (chewable/buffered tablets and pediatric powder for oral suspension) may decrease quinolone levels; separate doses.

Increased Effect/Toxicity: Gatifloxacin may increase the effects/toxicity of hypoglycemic agents and warfarin. Concomitant use with corticosteroids may increase the risk of tendon rupture. Concomitant use with other QT_c-prolonging agents (eg, Class Ia and Class III antiarrhythmics, erythromycin, cisapride, antipsychotics, and cyclic antidepressants) may result in arrhythmias, such as torsade de pointes. Probenecid may increase gatifloxacin levels.

Nutritional/Ethanol Interactions Herb/Nutraceutical: Avoid dong quai, St John's wort (may also cause photosensitization).

Adverse Reactions
Systemic therapy:
3% to 10%:
Central nervous system: Headache (3%), dizziness (3%)
Gastrointestinal: Nausea (8%), diarrhea (4%)
Genitourinary: Vaginitis (6%)
Local: Injection site reactions (5%)
0.1% to 3%: Abdominal pain, abnormal dreams, abnormal vision, agitation, alkaline phosphatase increased, allergic reaction, anorexia, anxiety, arthralgia, back pain, chest pain, chills, confusion, constipation, diaphoresis, dry skin, dyspepsia, dyspnea, dysuria, facial edema, fever, flatulence, gastritis, glossitis, hematuria, hyperglycemia, hypertension, insomnia, leg cramps, mouth ulceration, nervousness, oral candidiasis, palpitation, paresthesia, peripheral edema, pharyngitis, pruritus, rash, serum amylase increased, serum bilirubin increased, serum transaminases increased, somnolence, stomatitis, taste perversion, thirst, tinnitus, tremor, weakness, vasodilation, vertigo, vomiting

Ophthalmic therapy:
5% to 10%: Ocular: Conjunctival irritation, keratitis, lacrimation increased, papillary conjunctivitis
1% to 4%:
Central nervous system: Headache
Gastrointestinal: Taste disturbance
Ocular: Chemosis, conjunctival hemorrhage, discharge, dry eye, edema, irritation, pain, visual acuity decreased

Overdosage/Toxicology Potential symptoms of overdose may include CNS excitation, seizures, QT prolongation, and arrhythmias (including torsade de pointes). Patients should be monitored by continuous ECG in the event of an overdose. Management is supportive and symptomatic. Not removed by dialysis.

Pharmacodynamics/Kinetics
Absorption: Oral: Well absorbed; Ophthalmic: Not measurable
Bioavailability: 96%
Time to Peak: Oral: 1 hour
Protein Binding: 20%
Half-Life Elimination: 7.1-13.9 hours; ESRD/CAPD: 30-40 hours
Metabolism: Only 1%; no interaction with CYP
Excretion: Excretion: Urine (70% as unchanged drug, <1% as metabolites); feces (5%)

Dosing
Adults & Elderly:
Acute sinusitis: Oral, I.V.: 400 mg every 24 hours for 10 days
Bacterial conjunctivitis: Ophthalmic:
Days 1 and 2: Instill 1 drop into affected eye(s) every 2 hours while awake (maximum: 8 times/day)
Days 3-7: Instill 1 drop into affected eye(s) up to 4 times/day while awake
Community-acquired pneumonia: Oral, I.V.: 400 mg every 24 hours for 7-14 days
COPD (acute bacterial exacerbation): Oral, I.V.: 400 mg every 24 hours for 5 days
Uncomplicated skin/skin structure infections: Oral, I.V.: 400 mg every 24 hours for 7-10 days
Urinary tract infections (uncomplicated or cystitis): Oral, I.V.: 400 mg single dose or 200 mg every 24 hours for 3 days
Urinary tract infections (complicated): Oral, I.V.: 400 mg every 24 hours for 7-10 days
Pyelonephritis: Oral, I.V.: 400 mg every 24 hours for 7-10 days
Gonorrhea (uncomplicated urethral infection in men, cervical or rectal gonorrhea in women): Oral, I.V.: 400 mg single dose
(Continued)

Gatifloxacin *(Continued)*

Pediatrics: Bacterial conjunctivitis: Children ≥1 year: Ophthalmic: Refer to adult dosing.

Renal Impairment: Creatinine clearance <40 mL/minute (or patients on hemodialysis/ CAPD) should receive an initial dose of 400 mg, followed by a subsequent dose of 200 mg every 24 hours. Patients receiving single-dose or 3-day therapy for appropriate indications do not require dosage adjustment. Administer after hemodialysis.

Hepatic Impairment: No dosage adjustment is required in mild-moderate hepatic disease. No data are available in severe hepatic impairment (Child-Pugh Class C).

Available Dosage Forms

Injection, infusion [premixed in D_5W] (Tequin®): 200 mg (100 mL); 400 mg (200 mL)

Injection, solution [preservative free] (Tequin®): 10 mg/mL (40 mL)

Powder for oral suspension (Tequin®): 200 mg/5 mL (25 mL, 50 mL, 75 mL, 100 mL) [contains phenylalanine 168 mg/5 mL; fruit flavor]

Solution, ophthalmic (Zymar™): 0.3% (5 mL) [contains benzalkonium chloride]

Tablet (Tequin®): 200 mg, 400 mg

Monitoring and Teaching Issues

Physical Assessment: Assess allergy history before initiating therapy. See Warnings/ Precautions for specific use cautions (eg, bradycardia, history of seizures, renal or hepatic dysfunction). Assess potential for interactions with other pharmacological agents or herbal products patient may be taking (eg, increased risk of tendon rupture, arrhythmias, toxicity; see Drug Interactions). For intravenous use see Administration. Patient must be monitored closely during and after infusion for immediate allergic reaction. Assess CBC, therapeutic effectiveness resolution of infection, and adverse effects regularly during therapy (eg, hyper/hypoglycemia, changes in CNS [especially in elderly patients]; see Adverse Reactions). Caution patients with diabetes to monitor glucose closely (serious disruptions in glucose regulation [hyperglycemia and hypoglycemia] may occur). Teach patient appropriate use (oral/ophthalmic), possible side effects/appropriate interventions, and adverse symptoms to report (eg, hyper or hypoglycemia, tendon pain, adverse CNS changes; see Patient Education).

Monitoring Laboratory Tests: WBC

Patient Education: Do not take any new medication during therapy without consulting prescriber. **Pregnancy/breast-feeding precautions:** Inform prescriber if you are or intend to be pregnant. Do not breast-feed while taking this medication.

I.V.: Report any redness, pain, itching, burning, or signs of irritation at infusion site; swelling of mouth, lips, or tongue, back pain, tendon pain; dizziness, abnormal thinking, or anxiety

Ophthalmic: Tilt head back and instill drops in affected eye as often as directed for length of time prescribed. Do not allow dropper to touch any surface, including the eyes or hands. Apply light pressure to the inside corner of the eye (near the nose) after each drop. Do not wear contact lenses if being treated for a bacterial eye infection. May cause some temporary stinging, burning, itching, redness or tearing; eyelid swelling or itching, or a bad taste in you mouth after instillation. Report persistent pain, burning, swelling, or visual disturbances.

Oral: Take exactly as directed with or without food. Avoid alcohol. Take 4 hours before antacids or mineral supplements (iron, magnesium, or zinc). Do not miss a dose (take a missed dose as soon as possible unless it is almost time for your next dose). Take entire prescription even if feeling better. If you have diabetes, monitor glucose closely and notify prescriber of any significant changes (the medication may disrupt glucose management). Maintain adequate hydration (2-3 L/day of fluids) unless instructed to restrict fluids. May cause nausea, vomiting, taste perversion (small frequent meals, good mouth care, chewing gum, or sucking hard candy may help); headache, dizziness, insomnia, anxiety (use caution when driving or engaging in tasks requiring alertness until response is known). Report immediately any CNS changes (dizziness, insomnia, hallucinations, suicidal ideation or actions); rash or itching; respiratory or swallowing difficulty; tendon pain; swelling of mouth, lips, tongue, or throat; chest pain or tightness; or back pain. Report changes in voiding pattern, vaginal itching, burning, or discharge; vision changes or hearing; abnormal bruising or bleeding or blood in urine; or other adverse reactions.

Dietary Considerations: May take tablets with or without food, milk, or calcium supplements. Gatifloxacin should be taken 4 hours before supplements (including multivitamins) containing iron, zinc, or magnesium. Oral suspension contains phenylalanine 168 mg/5 mL.

Pregnancy Risk Factor: C

Pregnancy Issues: Reports of arthropathy (observed in immature animals and reported rarely in humans) have limited the use of fluoroquinolones during pregnancy. Gatifloxacin has been show to be fetotoxic in animal studies. There are no adequate and well-controlled studies in pregnant women. Based on limited data, quinolones are not expected to be a major human teratogen. Although quinolone antibiotics should not be used as first-line agents during pregnancy, when considering treatment for life-threatening infection and/or prolonged duration of therapy, the potential risk to the fetus must be balanced against the severity of the potential illness.

Lactation: Excretion in breast milk unknown/use caution

Breast-Feeding Issues: Other quinolones are known to be excreted in breast milk. The manufacturer recommends using caution if gatifloxacin is administered while nursing.

Administration

Oral: May be administered with or without food, milk, or calcium supplements. Gatifloxacin should be taken 4 hours before supplements (including multivitamins) containing iron, zinc, or magnesium. Suspension may be administered through a gastric feeding tube.

I.V.: For I.V. infusion only. Concentrated injection (10 mg/mL) must be diluted to 2 mg/mL prior to administration. No further dilution is required for premixed 100 mL and 200 mL solutions. Infuse over 60 minutes. Avoid rapid or bolus infusions.

Reconstitution:

Powder for oral suspension: Reconstitute with appropriate amount of water as specified on bottle. Shake vigorously until suspended. Discard any unused portion after 14 days.

Solution for injection: Single-use vials must be diluted to a concentration of 2 mg/mL prior to administration; do not dilute with SWFI (a hypertonic solution results).

Compatibility: Stable in D$_5$LR, D$_5$W, D$_5$NS, 5% dextrose or 0.45% sodium chloride containing up to 20 mEq/L potassium chloride, M/6 sodium lactate, NS, Plasma-Lyte® 56/ 5% dextrose injection, 5% sodium bicarbonate injection; **incompatible** with SWFI (results in a hypertonic solution)

Y-site administration: Incompatible with amphotericin B, amphotericin B cholesteryl sulfate complex, cefoperazone, cefoxitin, diazepam, furosemide, heparin, phenytoin, piperacillin, piperacillin/tazobactam, potassium phosphates, vancomycin

Storage:

Ophthalmic solution: Store between 15°C to 25°C (59°F to 77°F). Do not freeze.

Powder for oral suspension: Prior to reconstitution, store at 25°C (77°F); do not freeze. Following reconstitution, store under refrigeration at 2°C to 8°C (36°F to 46°F); do not freeze.

Solution for injection: Store at 25°C (77°F). Do not freeze. Following dilution, stable for 14 days.

Tablet: Store at 25°C (77°F).

Related Information

Antimicrobial Drugs of Choice *on page 1792*

Community-Acquired Pneumonia in Adults *on page 1807*

I.V. to Oral Conversion *on page 1688*

Tuberculosis *on page 1864*

♦ **G-CSF** *see* Filgrastim *on page 627*

♦ **GCV Sodium** *see* Ganciclovir *on page 695*

Gefitinib (ge FI tye nib)

U.S. Brand Names Iressa™

Synonyms NSC-715055; ZD1839

Generic Available No

Pharmacologic Category Antineoplastic Agent, Tyrosine Kinase Inhibitor

Use Second-line treatment of nonsmall cell lung cancer (**Note:** In response to the lack of improved survival data from the ISEL trial, AstraZeneca has temporarily suspended promotion of this drug.)

Unlabeled/Investigational Use Brain cancer, breast cancer, colon cancer, head and neck cancer, ovarian cancer

Mechanism of Action/Effect The mechanism of gefitinib is not fully understood. Gefitinib inhibits tyrosine kinase activity, particularly in the epidermal growth factor receptor (EGFR), resulting in inhibition of cell growth and reproduction. It might also inhibit angiogenesis in the tumor.

Contraindications Hypersensitivity to gefitinib or any component of the formulation; pregnancy

Warnings/Precautions Rare, sometimes fatal, pulmonary toxicity (alveolitis, interstitial pneumonia, pneumonitis) has occurred; use caution in hepatic or severe renal impairment; safety and efficacy in pediatric patients have not been established

Drug Interactions

Cytochrome P450 Effect: Substrate of CYP3A4 (major); **Inhibits** CYP2C19 (weak), 2D6 (weak)

Decreased Effect: Gefitinib effects may be decreased by H$_2$-receptor blockers and sodium bicarbonate. CYP3A4 inducers may decrease the levels/effects of gefitinib; example inducers include aminoglutethimide, carbamazepine, nafcillin, nevirapine, phenobarbital, phenytoin, and rifamycins.

Increased Effect/Toxicity: Gefitinib may increase the effects of warfarin. CYP3A4 inhibitors may increase the levels/effects of gefitinib; example inhibitors include azole antifungals, ciprofloxacin, clarithromycin, diclofenac, doxycycline, erythromycin, imatinib, isoniazid, nefazodone, nicardipine, propofol, protease inhibitors, quinidine, and verapamil.

Nutritional/Ethanol Interactions Food: Grapefruit juice may increase serum gefitinib concentrations; St John's wort may decrease serum gefitinib concentrations.

Adverse Reactions Based on 250 mg/day:

>10%:

Dermatologic: Rash (43%), acne (25%), dry skin (13%)

Gastrointestinal: Diarrhea (48%), nausea (13%), vomiting (12%)

1% to 10%:

Cardiovascular: Peripheral edema (2%)

Dermatologic: Pruritus (8%)

Gastrointestinal: Anorexia (7%), weight loss (3%), mouth ulceration (1%)

Neuromuscular & skeletal: Weakness (6%)

Ocular: Amblyopia (2%), conjunctivitis (1%)

Respiratory: Dyspnea (2%), interstitial lung disease (1%)

Overdosage/Toxicology No specific overdose-related toxicities reported; Overdose management should be symptom-based and supportive.

Pharmacodynamics/Kinetics

Absorption: Oral: slow

Bioavailability: 60%

Time to Peak: Plasma: Oral: 3-7 hours

Protein Binding: 90%, albumin and alpha$_1$-acid glycoprotein

Half-Life Elimination: I.V.: 48 hours

Metabolism: Hepatic, primarily via CYP3A4; forms metabolites

Excretion: Feces (86%); urine (<4%)

Dosing

Adults: Note: In response to the lack of improved survival data from the ISEL trial, AstraZeneca has temporarily suspended promotion of this drug.

(Continued)

Gefitinib (Continued)

Nonsmall cell lung cancer: Oral: 250 mg/day; consider 500 mg/day in patients receiving effective CYP3A4 inducers (eg, rifampin, phenytoin)

Dosage adjustment for toxicity: Patients experiencing poorly-tolerated diarrhea may benefit from a brief (up to 14 days) therapy interruption. Patients experiencing acute onset (or worsening) of pulmonary symptoms should have therapy interrupted and be evaluated for drug-induced interstitial lung disease. Patients experiencing new eye symptoms should consider therapy interruption until situation resolved.

Elderly: No adjustment necessary. Refer to adult dosing.

Renal Impairment: No adjustment necessary.

Hepatic Impairment: No adjustment necessary.

Available Dosage Forms Tablet: 250 mg

Monitoring and Teaching Issues

Physical Assessment: Use caution in presence of hepatic or renal impairment (see Warnings/Precautions). Assess potential for interactions with other pharmacological agents or herbal products patient may be taking (eg, may increase or decrease levels/effects of gefitinib; see Drug Interactions). Assess results of liver function tests on a regular basis. Teach patient proper use, possible side effects/appropriate interventions, and adverse symptoms to report (see Patient Education).

Monitoring Laboratory Tests: Periodic liver function tests (asymptomatic increases in liver enzymes have occurred)

Patient Education: Do not take any new medication during therapy without consulting prescriber. Take exactly as directed with or without food. Do not take with grapefruit juice and do not take antacids 2 hours before or 2 hours after taking this mediation. You will need periodic laboratory tests while taking this medication. Maintain adequate hydration (2-3 L/day of fluids) unless instructed to restrict fluid intake. You may experience loss of appetite, nausea and vomiting (small frequent meals and frequent mouth care may help), or diarrhea (buttermilk, boiled milk, or yogurt may help). Report immediately persistent diarrhea; skin rash; unusual or persistent respiratory difficulty or wheezing; chest pain or cough; any change in vision, eye pain, or signs of eye infection; unusual weakness or joint pain; or other persistent adverse reactions. **Pregnancy/breast-feeding precautions:** Inform prescriber if you are pregnant. Do not get pregnant. Consult prescriber for appropriate contraceptive measures while on this medication. Breast-feeding is not recommended.

Dietary Considerations: Food does not affect gefitinib absorption.

Pregnancy Risk Factor: D

Pregnancy Issues: Animal studies have demonstrated fetal harm; there are no well-controlled studies in pregnant women. The risk of fetal harm should be carefully weighed. Women of childbearing potential should be advised to avoid pregnancy.

Lactation: Excretion in breast milk unknown/not recommended

Administration

Oral: May administer with or without food.

For patients unable to swallow tablets or for administration via NG tube: Tablets may be dispersed in noncarbonated drinking water. Drop whole tablet (do not crush) into $\frac{1}{2}$ glass of water; stir until tablet is dispersed (~10 minutes). Drink immediately. Rinse with $\frac{1}{2}$ glass of water and drink.

Storage: Store tablets at controlled room temperature of 20°C to 25°C (68°F to 77°F).

- ♦ **Gelatin, Absorbable** *see page 1625*
- ♦ **Gelfilm® Ophthalmic** *see page 1625*
- ♦ **Gelfoam® Topical** *see page 1625*

Gemcitabine (jem SITE a been)

U.S. Brand Names Gemzar®

Synonyms Gemcitabine Hydrochloride

Generic Available No

Pharmacologic Category Antineoplastic Agent, Antimetabolite (Pyrimidine Antagonist)

Medication Safety Issues

Sound-alike/look-alike issues:

Gemzar® may be confused with Zinecard®

Use

Adenocarcinoma of the pancreas; first-line therapy in locally-advanced (nonresectable stage II or stage III) or metastatic (stage IV) adenocarcinoma of the pancreas (indicated for patients previously treated with fluorouracil)

Breast cancer: First-line therapy in metastatic breast cancer after failure of an anthra-cycline-containing adjuvant therapy (unless contraindicated); used in combination with paclitaxel

Nonsmall-cell lung cancer: First-line therapy in locally-advanced (stage IIIA or IIIB) or metastatic (stage IV) nonsmall-cell lung cancer; used in combination with cisplatin

Unlabeled/Investigational Use Bladder cancer, ovarian cancer

Mechanism of Action/Effect A pyrimidine antimetabolite that inhibits DNA synthesis by inhibition of DNA polymerase and ribonucleotide reductase, specific for the S-phase of the cycle.

Contraindications Hypersensitivity to gemcitabine or any component of the formulation; pregnancy

Warnings/Precautions The U.S. Food & Drug Administration (FDA) recommends that procedures for proper handling and disposal of antineoplastic agents be considered. Prolongation of the infusion time >60 minutes and more frequent than weekly dosing have been shown to increase toxicity. Gemcitabine can suppress bone marrow function manifested by leukopenia, thrombocytopenia and anemia, and myelosuppression is usually the dose-limiting toxicity. Gemcitabine may cause fever in the absence of clinical infection. Gemcitabine should be used with caution in patients with pre-existing renal impairment and hepatic impairment. Safety and efficacy have not been established with radiation therapy or in pediatric patients.

Drug Interactions

Decreased Effect: No confirmed interactions have been reported. No specific drug interaction studies have been conducted.

Nutritional/Ethanol Interactions Ethanol: Avoid ethanol (due to GI irritation).

Adverse Reactions Percentages reported with single-agent therapy for pancreatic cancer and other malignancies.

>10%:

Central nervous system: Pain (42% to 48%; grades 3 and 4: <1% to 9%), fever (38% to 41%; grades 3 and 4: ≤2%), somnolence (11%; grades 3 and 4: <1%). Fever was reported to occur in the absence of infection in pancreatic cancer treatment.

Dermatologic: Rash (28% to 30%; grades 3 and 4: <1%), alopecia (15% to 16%; grades 3 and 4: <1%). Rash in pancreatic cancer treatment was typically a macular or finely-granular maculopapular pruritic eruption of mild-to-moderate severity involving the trunk and extremities.

Gastrointestinal: Nausea and vomiting (69% to 71%; grades 3 and 4: 1% to 13%), constipation (23% to 31%; grades 3 and 4: <1% to 3%), diarrhea (19% to 30%; grades 3 and 4: ≤3%), stomatitis (10% to 11%; grades 3 and 4: <1%)

Hematologic: Anemia (73% to 68%; grades 3 and 4: 1% to 8%), leukopenia (62% to 64%; grades 3 and 4: <1% to 9%), neutropenia (61% to 63%; grades 3 and 4: 6% to 19%), thrombocytopenia (24% to 36%; grades 3 and 4: <1% to 7%), hemorrhage (4% to 17%; grades 3 or 4: <1%). Myelosuppression may be the dose-limiting toxicity with pancreatic cancer

Hepatic: Transaminases increased (68% to 78%; grades 3 and 4: 1% to 12%), alkaline phosphatase increased (55% to 77%; grades 3 and 4: 2% to 16%), bilirubin increased (13% to 26%; grades 3 or 4: <1% to 6%). Serious hepatotoxicity was reported rarely in pancreatic cancer treatment.

Renal: Proteinuria (32% to 45%; grades 3 and 4: <1%), hematuria (23% to 35%; grades 3 and 4: <1%), BUN increased (15% to 16%; grades 3 and 4: 0%)

Respiratory: Dyspnea (10% to 23%; grades 3 and 4: <1% to 3%)

Miscellaneous: Infection (10% to 16%; grades 3 or 4: <1% to 2%)

1% to 10%:

Local: Injection site reactions (4%)

Neuromuscular & skeletal: Paresthesias (10%)

Renal: Creatinine increased (6% to 8%)

Respiratory: Bronchospasm (<2%)

Overdosage/Toxicology Symptoms of overdose include myelosuppression, paresthesia, and severe rash. The principle toxicities were seen when a single dose as high as 5700 mg/m^2 was administered by I.V. infusion over 30 minutes every 2 weeks. Monitor blood counts and administer supportive therapy as needed.

Pharmacodynamics/Kinetics

Time to Peak: 30 minutes

Protein Binding: Low

Half-Life Elimination: Infusion time: ≤1 hour: 32-94 minutes; Infusion time: 3-4 hours: 4-10.5 hours

Metabolism: Hepatic, metabolites: di- and triphosphates (active); uridine derivative (inactive)

Excretion: Urine (99%, 92% to 98% as intact drug or inactive uridine metabolite); feces (<1%)

Dosing

Adults & Elderly: Refer to individual protocols. Note: Prolongation of the infusion time >60 minutes has been shown to increase toxicity. I.V.:

Pancreatic cancer: Initial: 1000 mg/m^2 over 30 minutes once weekly for up to 7 weeks followed by 1 week rest; subsequent cycles once weekly for 3 consecutive weeks out of every 4 weeks. Patients who complete an entire cycle of therapy may have the dose in subsequent cycles increased by 25% as long as the absolute granulocyte count (AGC) nadir is >1500 x 10^6/L, platelet nadir is >100,000 x 10^6/L, and nonhematologic toxicity is less than WHO Grade 1. If the increased dose is tolerated (with the same parameters) the dose in subsequent cycles may again be increased by 20%.

Nonsmall cell lung cancer in combination with cisplatin:

28-day cycle: 1000 mg/m^2 over 30 minutes on days 1, 8, 15; repeat every 28 days

or

21-day cycle: 1250 mg/m^2 over 30 minutes on days 1, 8; repeat every 21 days

Breast cancer in combination with paclitaxel: 1250 mg/m^2 over 30 minutes on days 1 and 8 of each 21-day cycle

Bladder cancer (unlabeled use): 1000 mg/m^2 once weekly for 3 weeks; repeat cycle every 4 weeks

Ovarian cancer (unlabeled use): 1000 mg/m^2 once weekly for 3 weeks; repeat cycle every 4 weeks

Dosing adjustment for toxicity:

Pancreatic cancer: Hematologic toxicity:

AGC ≥1000 x 10^6/L and platelet count ≥100,000 x 10^6/L: Administer 100% of full dose

AGC 500-999 x 10^6/L or platelet count 50,000-90,000 x 10^6/L: Administer 75% of full dose

AGC <500 x 10^6/L or platelet count <50,000 x 10^6/L: Hold dose

Nonsmall-cell lung cancer:

Hematologic toxicity: Refer to guidelines for pancreatic cancer. Cisplatin dosage may also need adjusted.

Severe (grades 3 or 4) nonhematologic toxicity (except alopecia, nausea, and vomiting): Hold or decrease dose by 50%.

Breast cancer:

Hematologic toxicity: Adjustments based on granulocyte and platelet counts on day 8:

AGC ≥1200 x 10^6/L and platelet count ≥75,000 x 10^6/L: Administer 100% of full dose

(Continued)

Gemcitabine *(Continued)*

AGC 1000-1199 x 10⁶/L or platelet count ≥50,000-75,000 x 10⁶/L: Administer 75% of full dose

AGC 700-999 x 10⁶/L and platelet count ≥50,000 x 10⁶/L: Administer 50% of full dose

AGC <700 x 10⁶/L or platelet count <50,000 x 10⁶/L: Hold dose

Severe (grades 3 or 4) nonhematologic toxicity (except alopecia, nausea, and vomiting): Hold or decrease dose by 50%. Paclitaxel dose may also need adjusted.

Renal Impairment: Use with caution; has not been studied in patients with significant renal dysfunction.

Hepatic Impairment: Use with caution; gemcitabine has not been studied in patients with significant hepatic dysfunction.

Available Dosage Forms Injection, powder for reconstitution, as hydrochloride: 200 mg, 1 g

Monitoring and Teaching Issues

Physical Assessment: See Warnings/Precautions for use cautions (eg, renal or hepatic impairment). See specific Administration directions (adverse reactions increase when infused >60 minutes). Assess results of laboratory tests (eg, CBC with differential and platelet count) prior to each dose. Monitor patient response (symptom relief) and adverse reactions prior to each treatment and on a regular basis throughout therapy (eg, CNS changes, rash, gastrointestinal upset, anemia, myelosuppression, anemia, dyspnea; see Adverse Reactions). Teach patient possible side effects/appropriate interventions and adverse symptoms to report (see Patient Education).

Monitoring Laboratory Tests: Monitor CBC, including differential and platelet count, prior to each dose. Renal and hepatic function should be performed prior to initiation of therapy and periodically thereafter.

Patient Education: Do not take any new medication during therapy unless approved by prescriber. This drug is administered by infusion; report any redness, pain, or swelling at infusion site. During therapy, do not use alcohol. Maintain adequate hydration (2-3 L/day of fluids) unless instructed to restrict fluid intake and nutrition (small frequent meals may help). You will be more susceptible to infection (avoid crowds and exposure to infection and do not have any vaccinations without consulting prescriber). You may experience fatigue, lethargy, somnolence (use caution when driving or engaging in potentially hazardous tasks until response to drug is known); nausea or vomiting (small frequent meals, frequent mouth care, sucking lozenges, or chewing gum may help); loss of hair (reversible); mouth sores (frequent mouth care and use of a soft toothbrush or cotton swabs may help); or diarrhea (buttermilk, boiled milk, or yogurt may help reduce diarrhea). This drug may cause sterility. Report extreme fatigue; severe GI upset or diarrhea; bleeding or bruising; fever, chills, sore throat; vaginal discharge; signs of fluid retention (swelling extremities, respiratory difficulty, unusual weight gain); yellowing of skin or eyes; change in color of urine or stool; or muscle or skeletal pain or weakness, or other persistent adverse effects. **Pregnancy/breast-feeding precautions:** Inform prescriber if you are pregnant. Do not get pregnant while taking this medication. Consult prescriber for appropriate contraceptives measures. This drug may cause severe fetal birth defects. Do not breast-feed.

Geriatric Considerations: Clearance is affected by age. There is no evidence; however, that unusual dose adjustment was necessary in patients older than 65 years of age. In general, adverse reaction rates were similar to patients older and younger than 65 years. Grade 3/4 thrombocytopenia was more common in the elderly.

Pregnancy Risk Factor: D

Pregnancy Issues: It is embryotoxic causing fetal malformations (cleft palate, incomplete ossification, fused pulmonary artery, absence of gallbladder) in animals. There are no studies in pregnant women. If patient becomes pregnant she should be informed of risks.

Lactation: Excretion in breast milk unknown/contraindicated

Administration

I.V.: Administer over 30 minutes. **Note**: Prolongation of the infusion time >60 minutes has been shown to increase toxicity.

Reconstitution: Reconstitute the 200 mg vial with preservative free 0.9% NaCl 5 mL or the 1000 mg vial with preservative free 25 mL 0.9% NaCl 25 mL.

Resulting solution is approximately 38 mg/mL, but is variable. A suggestion is to withdraw the entire solution into a syringe in order to determine the final concentration. The appropriate dose may be further diluted with 0.9% sodium chloride injection to concentrations as low as 0.1 mg/mL.

Compatibility: Stable in D₅W, NS

Y-site administration: Incompatible with acyclovir, amphotericin B, cefoperazone, cefotaxime, furosemide, ganciclovir, imipenem/cilastatin, irinotecan, methotrexate, methylprednisolone sodium succinate, mitomycin, piperacillin, piperacillin/tazobactam, prochlorperazine edisylate

Storage: Store intact vials at room temperature (20°C to 25°C/68°F to 77°F). Reconstituted vials and infusion solutions diluted in 0.9% sodium chloride are stable up to 24 hours. Do not refrigerate.

♦ **Gemcitabine Hydrochloride** *see Gemcitabine on page 702*

Gemfibrozil *(jem FI broe zil)*

U.S. Brand Names Lopid®

Synonyms CI-719

Generic Available Yes

Pharmacologic Category Antilipemic Agent, Fibric Acid

Medication Safety Issues

Sound-alike/look-alike issues:

Lopid® may be confused with Levbid®, Lodine®, Lorabid®, Slo-bid™

Use Treatment of hypertriglyceridemia in types IV and V hyperlipidemia for patients who are at greater risk for pancreatitis and who have not responded to dietary intervention

Mechanism of Action/Effect Inhibits lipolysis and decreases subsequent hepatic fatty acid uptake and hepatic secretion of VLDL; decreases serum levels of VLDL and increases HDL levels

Contraindications Hypersensitivity to gemfibrozil or any component of the formulation; significant hepatic or renal dysfunction; primary biliary cirrhosis; pre-existing gallbladder disease

Warnings/Precautions Possible increased risk of malignancy and cholelithiasis. No evidence of cardiovascular mortality benefit. Anemia and leukopenia have been reported. Elevations in serum transaminases can be seen. Discontinue if lipid response not seen. Be careful in patient selection; this is not a first- or second-line choice. Other agents may be more suitable. Adjustments in warfarin therapy may be required with concurrent use. Use caution when combining gemfibrozil with HMG-CoA reductase inhibitors (may lead to myopathy, rhabdomyolysis). Renal function deterioration has been seen when used in patients with a serum creatinine >2.0 mg/dL. Safety and efficacy in pediatric patients have not been established.

Drug Interactions

Cytochrome P450 Effect: Substrate of CYP3A4 (minor); **Inhibits** CYP1A2 (moderate), 2C8/9 (strong), 2C19 (strong)

Decreased Effect: Cyclosporine's blood levels may be reduced during concurrent therapy. Rifampin may decrease gemfibrozil blood levels.

Increased Effect/Toxicity: Gemfibrozil may potentiate the effects of bexarotene (avoid concurrent use), sulfonylureas (including glyburide, chlorpropamide), and warfarin. HMG-CoA reductase inhibitors (atorvastatin, fluvastatin, lovastatin, pravastatin, simvastatin) may increase the risk of myopathy and rhabdomyolysis. The manufacturer warns against the concurrent use of lovastatin (if unavoidable, limit lovastatin to <20 mg/day). Combination therapy with statins has been used in some patients with resistant hyperlipidemias (with great caution). Gemfibrozil may increase the serum concentration of repaglinide (resulting in severe, prolonged hypoglycemia); the addition of itraconazole may augment the effects of gemfibrozil on repaglinide (consider alternative therapy). Gemfibrozil may increase the levels/effects of aminophylline, amiodarone, citalopram, diazepam, fluoxetine, fluvoxamine, glimepiride, glipizide, methsuximide, mexiletine, mirtazapine, nateglinide, phenytoin, pioglitazone, propranolol, ropinirole, rosiglitazone, sertraline, theophylline, trifluoperazine, warfarin, and other substrates of CYP1A2, 2C8/9, or 2C19.

Nutritional/Ethanol Interactions Ethanol: Avoid ethanol to decrease triglycerides.

Adverse Reactions

>10% Gastrointestinal: Dyspepsia (20%)

1% to 10%:

Central nervous system: Fatigue (4%), vertigo (2%), headache (1%)

Dermatologic: Eczema (2%), rash (2%)

Gastrointestinal: Abdominal pain (10%), diarrhea (7%), nausea/vomiting (3%), constipation (1%)

Reports where causal relationship has not been established: Weight loss, extrasystoles, pancreatitis, hepatoma, colitis, confusion, seizure, syncope, retinal edema, decreased fertility (male), renal dysfunction, positive ANA, drug-induced lupus-like syndrome, thrombocytopenia, anaphylaxis, vasculitis, alopecia, photosensitivity

Overdosage/Toxicology Symptoms of overdose include abdominal pain, diarrhea, nausea, and vomiting. Treatment is supportive.

Pharmacodynamics/Kinetics

Onset of Action: May require several days

Absorption: Well absorbed

Time to Peak: Serum: 1-2 hours

Protein Binding: 99%

Half-Life Elimination: 1.4 hours

Metabolism: Hepatic via oxidation to two inactive metabolites; undergoes enterohepatic recycling

Excretion: Urine (70% primarily as unchanged drug)

Dosing

Adults & Elderly: Hyperlipidemia/hypertriglyceridemia: Oral: 1200 mg/day in 2 divided doses, 30 minutes before breakfast and dinner

Renal Impairment: Hemodialysis effects: Not removed by hemodialysis; supplemental dose is not necessary.

Available Dosage Forms Tablet [film coated]: 600 mg

Monitoring and Teaching Issues

Physical Assessment: See Warnings/Precautions for use cautions. Assess potential for interactions with other pharmacological agents patient may be taking (eg, increased risk of myopathy, rhabdomyolysis, hypoglycemia and toxicity; see Drug Interactions). Assess results of laboratory tests (serum cholesterol and LFTs), therapeutic effectiveness (decreased lipid levels), and patient response periodically during therapy (eg, see Adverse Reactions). Teach possible proper use, side effects/appropriate interventions, and adverse symptoms to report (see Patient Education).

Monitoring Laboratory Tests: Serum cholesterol, LFTs

Patient Education: Do not take any new medication during therapy unless approved by prescriber. Should be taken 30 minutes before meals. Take with milk or meals if GI upset occurs. Avoid alcohol to reduce triglycerides. Follow dietary recommendations of prescriber. You will need check-ups and blood work to assess effectiveness of therapy. You may experience loss of appetite and flatulence (small frequent meals may help); or diarrhea (buttermilk, boiled milk, or yogurt may help). Report severe stomach pain, nausea, vomiting; headache; persistent diarrhea; or vision changes. **Pregnancy/breast-feeding precautions:** Inform prescriber if you are or intend to become pregnant. Do not breast-feed.

Dietary Considerations: Before initiation of therapy, patients should be placed on a standard cholesterol-lowering diet for 3-6 months and the diet should be continued during drug therapy.

(Continued)

Gemfibrozil *(Continued)*

Geriatric Considerations: Gemfibrozil is the drug of choice for the treatment of hypertri-glyceridemia and hypoalphaproteinemia in the elderly; it is usually well tolerated; myositis may be more common in patients with poor renal function.

Pregnancy Risk Factor: C

Lactation: Excretion in breast milk unknown/contraindicated

Related Information

Hyperlipidemia Management *on page 1836*

Lipid-Lowering Agents *on page 1738*

Gemifloxacin *(je mi FLOKS a sin)*

U.S. Brand Names Factive®

Synonyms DW286; Gemifloxacin Mesylate; LA 20304a; SB-265805

Generic Available No

Pharmacologic Category Antibiotic, Quinolone

Use Treatment of acute exacerbation of chronic bronchitis; treatment of community-acquired pneumonia, including pneumonia caused by multidrug-resistant strains of *S. pneumoniae* (MDRSP)

Unlabeled/Investigational Use Acute sinusitis, uncomplicated urinary tract infection

Mechanism of Action/Effect Gemifloxacin is a DNA gyrase inhibitor and also inhibits topoisomerase IV. These enzymes are required for DNA replication and transcription, DNA repair, recombination, and transposition; quinolones are bactericidal

Contraindications Hypersensitivity to gemifloxacin, other fluoroquinolones, or any compo-nent of the formulation

Warnings/Precautions Fluoroquinolones may prolong QT_c interval; avoid use of gemiflox-acin in patients with uncorrected hypokalemia, hypomagnesemia, or concurrent administra-tion of other medications known to prolong the QT interval (including class Ia and class III antiarrhythmics, cisapride, erythromycin, antipsychotics, and tricyclic antidepressants). Use with caution in patients with significant bradycardia or acute myocardial ischemia. Use with caution in individuals at risk of seizures (CNS disorders or concurrent therapy with medica-tions which may lower seizure threshold). Discontinue in patients who experience significant CNS adverse effects (dizziness, hallucinations, suicidal ideation or actions). Use caution in renal dysfunction (dosage adjustment required).

Severe hypersensitivity reactions, including anaphylaxis, have occurred with quinolone therapy. If an allergic reaction occurs (itching, urticaria, dyspnea or facial edema, loss of consciousness, tingling, cardiovascular collapse), discontinue drug immediately. Prolonged use may result in superinfection; pseudomembranous colitis may occur and should be considered in all patients who present with diarrhea. Tendon inflammation and/or rupture has been reported with other quinolone antibiotics; risk may increase with concurrent corticoste-roids, particularly in the elderly. Discontinue at first sign of tendon inflammation or pain. Peripheral neuropathy has been linked to the use of quinolones; these cases were rare. Experience with quinolones in immature animals has resulted in permanent arthropathy. Safety and effectiveness in pediatric patients (<18 years of age) have not been established.

Drug Interactions

Decreased Effect: Concurrent administration of metal cations, including most antacids, oral electrolyte supplements, quinapril, sucralfate, and some didanosine formulations (chewable/buffered tablets and pediatric powder for oral suspension), may decrease quinolone levels; separate doses.

Increased Effect/Toxicity: Gemifloxacin may increase the effects/toxicity of glyburide and warfarin. Concomitant use with corticosteroids may increase the risk of tendon rupture. Concomitant use with other QT_c-prolonging agents (eg, Class Ia and Class III antiar-rhythmics, erythromycin, cisapride, antipsychotics, and cyclic antidepressants) may result in arrhythmias, such as torsade de pointes. Probenecid may increase gemifloxacin levels.

Nutritional/Ethanol Interactions Herb/Nutraceutical: Avoid dong quai, St John's wort (may also cause photosensitization).

Adverse Reactions

1% to 10%:

Central nervous system: Headache (1%), dizziness (1%)

Dermatologic: Rash (3%)

Gastrointestinal: Diarrhea (4%), nausea (3%), abdominal pain (1%), vomiting (1%)

Hepatic: Transaminases increased (1% to 2%)

Important adverse effects reported with other agents in this drug class include (not reported for gemifloxacin): Allergic reactions, CNS stimulation, hepatitis, jaundice, peripheral neuropathy, pneumonitis (eosinophilic), seizure; sensorimotor-axonal neuropathy (pares-thesia, hypoesthesias, dysesthesias, weakness); severe dermatologic reactions (toxic epidermal necrolysis, Stevens-Johnson syndrome); tendon rupture, torsade de pointes, vasculitis

Overdosage/Toxicology Treatment should be symptom-directed and supportive; 20% to 30% removed by hemodialysis.

Pharmacodynamics/Kinetics

Absorption: Well absorbed from the GI tract

Bioavailability: 71%

Time to Peak: Plasma: 1-2 hours

Protein Binding: 60% to 70%

Half-Life Elimination: 7 hours (range 4-12 hours)

Metabolism: Hepatic (minor); forms metabolites (CYP isoenzymes are not involved)

Excretion: Urine (30% to 40%); feces (60%)

Dosing

Adults & Elderly:

Susceptible infections: Oral: 320 mg once daily

Duration of therapy:

Acute exacerbations of chronic bronchitis: 5 days

Community-acquired pneumonia (mild to moderate severity): 7 days

Renal Impairment: Cl$_{cr}$ ≤40 mL/minute (or patients on hemodialysis/CAPD): 160 mg once daily (administer dose following hemodialysis)

Hepatic Impairment: No adjustment required.

Available Dosage Forms Tablet, as mesylate: 320 mg

Monitoring and Teaching Issues

Physical Assessment: Assess allergy history before initiating therapy. See Warnings/Precautions for use cautions (eg, bradycardia, CNS disorders, renal dysfunction, colitis). Assess potential for interactions with other pharmacological agents or herbal products patient may be taking (eg, increased risk of tendon rupture or arrhythmias; see Drug Interactions). Assess WBC results, therapeutic effectiveness (resolution of infection), and adverse effects regularly during therapy (eg, hypersensitivity, opportunistic infection, pseudomembranous colitis, tendon inflammation; see Warnings/Precautions and Adverse Reactions). Teach patient proper use, possible side effects/appropriate interventions, and adverse symptoms to report (see Patient Education).

Monitoring Laboratory Tests: WBC

Patient Education: Do not take any new medications during therapy without consulting prescriber. Take exactly as directed (with or without food). Should be taken at least 3 hours before or 2 hours after antacids or other drug products containing calcium, iron, magnesium, or zinc (including multivitamins). Take entire prescription, even if feeling better. Maintain adequate hydration (2-3 L/day of fluids) unless instructed to restrict fluid intake. May cause headache or dizziness (use caution when driving or engaging in hazardous tasks until response to drug is known); nausea, vomiting, or abdominal discomfort (small frequent meals, frequent mouth care, chewing gum, or sucking lozenges may help); or diarrhea (consult prescriber if persistent). If signs of inflammation or tendon pain occur, discontinue use immediately and report to prescriber. Discontinue use immediately and report to prescriber if you experience signs of allergic reaction (eg, itching, rash, respiratory difficulty, facial edema, or difficulty swallowing), chest pain, or palpitations. Report CNS changes (eg, hallucinations, suicidal ideation, seizures) or signs of opportunistic infection (unusual fever or chills; vaginal itching or foul-smelling vaginal discharge; easy bruising or bleeding; tendon or muscle pain). **Pregnancy/breast-feeding precautions:** Inform prescriber if you are or intend to become pregnant. Breast-feeding is not recommended.

Dietary Considerations: May take tablets with or without food, milk, or calcium supplements. Gemifloxacin should be taken 3 hours before or 2 hours after supplements (including multivitamins) containing iron, zinc, or magnesium.

Geriatric Considerations: The risk of torsade de pointes and tendon inflammation and/or rupture associated with the concomitant use of corticosteroids and quinolones is increased in the elderly population. Adjust dose for renal function.

Pregnancy Risk Factor: C

Pregnancy Issues: There are no adequate and well-controlled studies in pregnant women. Reports of arthropathy (observed in immature animals and reported rarely in humans) have limited the use of fluoroquinolones in pregnancy. Reversible fetal growth retardation was observed with gemifloxacin in some animal studies. Based on limited data, quinolones are not expected to be a major human teratogen. Although quinolone antibiotics should not be used as first-line agents during pregnancy, when considering treatment for life-threatening infection and/or prolonged duration of therapy, the potential risk to the fetus must be balanced against the severity of the potential illness.

Lactation: Excretion in breast milk unknown/not recommended

Breast-Feeding Issues: Other quinolones are known to be excreted in breast milk. The manufacturer recommends using gemifloxacin while breast-feeding only if the possible benefit to the mother outweighs the possible risk to the infant.

Administration

Oral: May be administered with or without food, milk, or calcium supplements. Gemifloxacin should be taken 3 hours before or 2 hours after supplements (including multivitamins) containing iron, zinc, or magnesium.

Storage: Store at 25°C (77°F); excursions permitted to 15°C to 30°C (59°F to 86°F). Protect from light.

♦ **Gemifloxacin Mesylate** *see* Gemifloxacin *on page 706*

Gemtuzumab Ozogamicin (gem TOO zoo mab oh zog a MY sin)

U.S. Brand Names Mylotarg®

Generic Available No

Pharmacologic Category Antineoplastic Agent, Monoclonal Antibody

Use Treatment of acute myeloid leukemia (CD33 positive) in first relapse in patients who are ≥60 years of age and who are not considered candidates for cytotoxic chemotherapy.

Mechanism of Action/Effect Antibody to CD33 antigen, which is expressed on leukemic blasts in 80% of patients with acute myeloid leukemia (AML), as well as normal myeloid cells. Binding results in internalization of the antibody-antigen complex. Following internalization, the calicheamicin derivative is released inside the myeloid cell. The calicheamicin derivative binds to DNA resulting in double strand breaks and cell death. Pluripotent stem cells and nonhematopoietic cells are not affected.

Contraindications Hypersensitivity to gemtuzumab ozogamicin, calicheamicin derivatives, or any component of the formulation; patients with anti-CD33 antibody; pregnancy

Warnings/Precautions The U.S. Food and Drug Administration (FDA) currently recommends that procedures for proper handling and disposal of antineoplastic agents be considered. Gemtuzumab has been associated with severe veno-occlusive disease or hepatotoxicity. Risk may be increased by combination chemotherapy, previous hepatic disease, or hematopoietic stem cell transplant.

Infusion-related events are common, generally reported to occur with the first dose at the end of the 2-hour intravenous infusion. These symptoms usually resolved after 2-4 hours with a supportive therapy of acetaminophen, diphenhydramine, and intravenous fluids. Fewer infusion-related events were observed after the second dose. **Infusion-related reactions may** (Continued)

Gemtuzumab Ozogamicin *(Continued)*

be severe (including anaphylaxis, pulmonary edema, or ARDS). Symptomatic intrinsic lung disease or high peripheral blast counts may increase the risk of severe reactions. Consider discontinuation in patients who develop severe infusion-related reactions.

Severe myelosuppression occurs in all patients at recommended dosages. Use caution in patients with renal impairment (no clinical experience) and hepatic impairment (no clinical experience in patients with bilirubin >2 mg/dL). Tumor lysis syndrome may occur as a consequence of leukemia treatment, adequate hydration and prophylactic allopurinol must be instituted prior to use. Other methods to lower WBC <30,000 cells/mm^3 may be considered (hydroxyurea or leukapheresis) to minimize the risk of tumor lysis syndrome, and/or severe infusion reactions. Postinfusion reactions, which may include fever, chills, hypotension, or dyspnea, may occur during the first 24 hours after administration. Safety and efficacy have not been established in pediatric patients or in patients with poor performance status and organ dysfunction have not been established.

Drug Interactions
Decreased Effect: No formal drug interaction studies have been conducted.
Increased Effect/Toxicity: No formal drug interaction studies have been conducted.
Nutritional/Ethanol Interactions Ethanol: Avoid ethanol (due to GI irritation).
Lab Interactions None known
Adverse Reactions Percentages established in adults >60 years of age. **Note:** A postinfusion symptom complex (fever, chills, less commonly hypertension, and/or dyspnea) may occur within 24 hours of administration.

>10%:
Cardiovascular: Peripheral edema (21%), hypertension (16%), hypotension (20%)
Central nervous system: Chills (66%), fever (82%), headache (37%), pain (25%), dizziness (11%), insomnia (18%)
Dermatologic: Rash (23%), petechiae (21%), ecchymosis (15%), cutaneous herpes simplex (21%)
Endocrine & metabolic: Hypokalemia (30%)
Gastrointestinal: Nausea (68%), vomiting (58%), diarrhea (38%), anorexia (31%), abdominal pain (29%), constipation (28%), stomatitis/mucositis (25%), abdominal distention (11%), dyspepsia (11%)
Hematologic: Neutropenia (98%; median recovery 40.5 days), thrombocytopenia (99%; median recovery 39 days); anemia (52%), bleeding (15%), lymphopenia
Hepatic: Hyperbilirubinemia (29%), LDH increased (18%), transaminases increased (9% to 18%)
Local: Local reaction (25%)
Neuromuscular & skeletal: Weakness (45%), back pain (18%)
Respiratory: Dyspnea (26%), epistaxis (29%; severe 3%), cough (19%), pharyngitis (14%)
Miscellaneous: Infection (30%), sepsis (24%), neutropenic fever (20%)
1% to 10%:
Cardiovascular: Tachycardia (10%)
Central nervous system: Depression (10%), cerebral hemorrhage (2%), intracranial hemorrhage (2%)
Dermatologic: Pruritus (6%)
Endocrine & metabolic: Hypomagnesemia (4%), hyperglycemia (10%)
Genitourinary: Hematuria (10%; severe 1%), vaginal hemorrhage (7%)
Hematologic: Hemorrhage (8%), disseminated intravascular coagulation (DIC) (2%)
Hepatic: PT increased, veno-occlusive disease (range: 1% to 20% in relapsed patients; higher frequency in patients with prior history of subsequent hematopoietic stem cell transplant)
Neuromuscular & skeletal: Arthralgia (10%)
Respiratory: Rhinitis (10%), hypoxia (6%), pneumonia (10%)
Overdosage/Toxicology Symptoms are unknown. General supportive measures should be instituted. Gemtuzumab ozogamicin is not dialyzable.
Pharmacodynamics/Kinetics
Half-Life Elimination: Calicheamicin: Total: Initial: 45 hours, Repeat dose: 60 hours; Unconjugated: 100 hours (no change noted in repeat dosing)
Dosing
Adults & Elderly: Refer to individual protocols.
AML (CD33 positive in patients ≥60 years): I.V.: 9 mg/m^2, infused over 2 hours. A full treatment course is a total of two doses administered with 14 days between doses. Full hematologic recovery is not necessary for administration of the second dose. There has been only limited experience with repeat courses of gemtuzumab ozogamicin.
Note: The patient should receive diphenhydramine 50 mg orally and acetaminophen 650-1000 mg orally 1 hour prior to administration of each dose. Acetaminophen dosage should be repeated as needed every 4 hours for two additional doses. Pretreatment with methylprednisolone may ameliorate infusion-related symptoms.
Available Dosage Forms Injection, powder for reconstitution: 5 mg
Monitoring and Teaching Issues
Physical Assessment: See Warnings/Precautions for use cautions. Premedication with acetaminophen and diphenhydramine should be administered prior to each infusion; see Dosing and Administration for specific pretreatment and infusion specifics. Patient must be monitored closely during and for 4 hours following treatment for infusion-related reactions which can be severe (anaphylaxis, pulmonary edema, or ARDS). Assess results of laboratory tests, patient response and adverse reactions frequently during therapy (eg, tachycardia, hyper or hypotension, CNS changes, gastrointestinal disturbance, hepatic reaction; see Adverse Reactions). Teach patient purpose for use, possible side effects/appropriate interventions, and adverse symptoms to report (see Patient Education).
Monitoring Laboratory Tests: Monitor electrolytes, LFTs, CBC with differential, and platelet counts frequently.

Patient Education: This medication can only be administered intravenously. During infusion you will be closely monitored; report immediately any burning, pain, swelling at infusion site; difficulty breathing or swallowing, chest pain, or chills. You will need frequent laboratory tests during course of therapy. Do not use alcohol, aspirin-containing medications, or any prescription or OTC medications without consulting your prescriber. It is important to maintain adequate hydration (2-3 L/day of fluids) unless instructed to restrict fluid intake and nutrition (small frequent meals will help). You will be susceptible to infection (avoid crowds and exposure to infection). You may experience nausea or vomiting (small frequent meals, good mouth care, sucking lozenges or chewing gum may help); contact prescriber if nausea and vomiting persists. Frequent mouth care with a soft toothbrush or soft swabs and avoidance of spicy or salty foods may reduce mouth sores. Report immediately, fever, chills; unusual bleeding or bruising; signs of infection (eg, sore throat, cough, white plaques in mouth or perianal area, burning on urination); respiratory difficulties; chest pain or palpitations; yellowing of the eyes or skin; swelling of extremities; rapid weight gain; right upper quadrant pain; or other persistent adverse effects. **Pregnancy/breast-feeding precautions:** Inform prescriber if you are or intend to become pregnant. Breast-feeding is not recommended.

Pregnancy Risk Factor: D

Pregnancy Issues: May cause fetal harm when administered to a pregnant woman. Women of childbearing potential should avoid becoming pregnant while receiving treatment. If used in pregnancy or if patient becomes pregnant during treatment, the patients should be apprised of potential hazard to the fetus.

Lactation: Excretion in breast milk unknown/not recommended

Administration

I.V.: Administer as infusion only, over at least 2 hours. Do not administer I.V. push (bolus). Infuse through a separate line equipped with a low protein-binding 1.2 micron terminal filter. May be infused peripherally or through a central line. Cover with UV protective bag during infusion. Premedication with acetaminophen and diphenhydramine should be administered prior to each infusion.

Reconstitution: Prepare in biologic safety hood with the fluorescent light turned **off**. Allow to warm to room temperature prior to reconstitution. Reconstitute vial with 5 mL sterile water for injection, USP. Final concentration in vial is 1 mg/mL. Dilute desired dose in 100 mL of 0.9% sodium chloride injection. The resulting I.V. bag should be placed in a UV protectant bag and infused immediately. Reconstituted vials may be stored under refrigeration for up to 8 hours.

Compatibility: No information; infuse via separate line

Storage: Light sensitive; protect from light. Store vials under refrigeration 2°C to 8°C or 36°F to 46°F.

Gentamicin (jen ta MYE sin)

U.S. Brand Names Genoptic®; Gentacidin® [DSC]; Gentak®

Synonyms Gentamicin Sulfate

Generic Available Yes

Pharmacologic Category Antibiotic, Aminoglycoside; Antibiotic, Ophthalmic; Antibiotic, Topical

Medication Safety Issues

Sound-alike/look-alike issues:

Gentamicin may be confused with kanamycin

Garamycin® may be confused with kanamycin, Terramycin®

Use Treatment of susceptible bacterial infections, normally gram-negative organisms including *Pseudomonas*, *Proteus*, *Serratia*, and gram-positive *Staphylococcus*; treatment of bone infections, respiratory tract infections, skin and soft tissue infections, as well as abdominal and urinary tract infections, endocarditis, and septicemia; used topically to treat superficial infections of the skin or ophthalmic infections caused by susceptible bacteria; prevention of bacterial endocarditis prior to dental or surgical procedures

Mechanism of Action/Effect Bactericidal; interferes with bacterial protein synthesis resulting in cell death

Contraindications Hypersensitivity to gentamicin or other aminoglycosides

(Continued)

Gentamicin *(Continued)*

Warnings/Precautions Not intended for long-term therapy due to toxic hazards associated with extended administration. Pre-existing renal insufficiency, vestibular or cochlear impairment, myasthenia gravis, hypocalcemia, conditions which depress neuromuscular transmission.

Parenteral aminoglycosides have been associated with significant nephrotoxicity or ototoxicity. Ototoxicity may be directly proportional to the amount of drug given and the duration of treatment and may not be reversible. Tinnitus or vertigo are indications of vestibular injury and impending hearing loss. Renal damage is usually reversible.

Drug Interactions

Increased Effect/Toxicity: Penicillins, cephalosporins, amphotericin B, loop diuretics may increase nephrotoxic potential. Aminoglycosides may potentiate the effects of neuromuscular blocking agents.

Lab Interactions Increased protein, BUN, AST, GPT, alkaline phosphatase, serum creatinine; decreased magnesium potassium, sodium, calcium

Adverse Reactions

>10%:

Central nervous system: Neurotoxicity (vertigo, ataxia)

Neuromuscular & skeletal: Gait instability

Otic: Ototoxicity (auditory), ototoxicity (vestibular)

Renal: Nephrotoxicity, decreased creatinine clearance

1% to 10%:

Cardiovascular: Edema

Dermatologic: Skin itching, reddening of skin, rash

Overdosage/Toxicology Symptoms of overdose include ototoxicity, nephrotoxicity, and neuromuscular toxicity. Serum level monitoring is recommended. The treatment of choice, following a single acute overdose, appears to be maintenance of urine output of at least 3 mL/kg/hour during the acute treatment phase. Dialysis is of questionable value in enhancing aminoglycoside elimination.

Pharmacodynamics/Kinetics

Absorption: Oral: None

Time to Peak: Serum: I.M.: 30-90 minutes; I.V.: 30 minutes after 30-minute infusion

Protein Binding: <30%

Half-Life Elimination:

Infants: <1 week old: 3-11.5 hours; 1 week to 6 months old: 3-3.5 hours

Adults: 1.5-3 hours; End-stage renal disease: 36-70 hours

Excretion: Urine (as unchanged drug)

Clearance: Directly related to renal function

Dosing

Adults & Elderly: Individualization is **critical** because of the low therapeutic index.

Use of ideal body weight (IBW) for determining the mg/kg/dose appears to be more accurate than dosing on the basis of total body weight (TBW). In morbid obesity, dosage requirement may best be estimated using a dosing weight of IBW + 0.4 (TBW - IBW).

Initial and periodic plasma drug levels (eg, peak and trough with conventional dosing) should be determined, particularly in critically-ill patients with serious infections or in disease states known to significantly alter aminoglycoside pharmacokinetics (eg, cystic fibrosis, burns, or major surgery).

Systemic infections: I.M., I.V.:

Severe, life-threatening infections:

Conventional dosing: 2-2.5 mg/kg/dose every 8-12 hours; to ensure adequate peak concentrations early in therapy, higher initial dosages (eg, loading doses up to 3 mg/kg) may be considered in selected patients when extracellular water is increased (edema, septic shock, postsurgical, or trauma)

Once-daily dosing: Some clinicians suggest a daily dose of 4-7 mg/kg once daily for all patients with normal renal function; this dose is at least as efficacious with similar, if not less, toxicity than conventional dosing.

Urinary tract infections: 1.5 mg/kg/dose every 8 hours

Synergy (for gram-positive infections): 1 mg/kg/dose

Prevention of bacterial endocarditis:

Dental, oral, or upper respiratory procedures: 1.5 mg/kg (not to exceed 80 mg) with ampicillin (1-2 g) 30 minutes prior to procedure

GI/GU surgery: 1.5 mg/kg (not to exceed 80 mg) with ampicillin (2 g) 30 minutes prior to procedure

CNS infections: Intrathecal: 4-8 mg/day

Ocular infections: Ophthalmic:

Ointment: Instill 1/2" (1.25 cm) 2-3 times/day to every 3-4 hours

Solution: Instill 1-2 drops every 2-4 hours, up to 2 drops every hour for severe infections

Superficial dermatologic infections: Topical: Apply 3-4 times/day to affected area

Pediatrics: Individualization is **critical** because of the low therapeutic index.

Use of ideal body weight (IBW) for determining the mg/kg/dose appears to be more accurate than dosing on the basis of total body weight (TBW). In morbid obesity, dosage requirement may best be estimated using a dosing weight of IBW + 0.4 (TBW - IBW).

Initial and periodic plasma drug levels (eg, peak and trough with conventional dosing) should be determined, particularly in critically-ill patients with serious infections or in disease states known to significantly alter aminoglycoside pharmacokinetics (eg, cystic fibrosis, burns, or major surgery).

Susceptible systemic infections: I.M., I.V.:

Infants and Children <5 years: 2.5 mg/kg/dose every 8 hours*

Children ≥5 years: 2-2.5 mg/kg/dose every 8 hours*

*Note: Higher individual doses and/or more frequent intervals (eg, every 6 hours) may be required in selected clinical situations (cystic fibrosis) or serum levels document the need

Prevention of bacterial endocarditis: Dental, oral, upper respiratory procedures, GI/GU procedures: Children >5 years: 1.5 mg/kg with ampicillin (50 mg/kg) 30 minutes prior to procedure

CNS infections: Intrathecal: See adult dosing.

Ophthalmic, Dermatologic infections: See adult dosing.

Renal Impairment:

Conventional dosing:

Cl_{cr} ≥60 mL/minute: Administer every 8 hours

Cl_{cr} 40-60 mL/minute: Administer every 12 hours

Cl_{cr} 20-40 mL/minute: Administer every 24 hours

Cl_{cr} <20 mL/minute: Loading dose, then monitor levels

High-dose therapy: Interval may be extended (eg, every 48 hours) in patients with moderate renal impairment (Cl_{cr} 30-59 mL/minute) and/or adjusted based on serum level determinations.

Hemodialysis: Dialyzable; removal by hemodialysis: 30% removal of aminoglycosides occurs during 4 hours of HD; administer dose after dialysis and follow levels

Removal by continuous ambulatory peritoneal dialysis (CAPD):

Administration via CAPD fluid:

Gram-negative infection: 4-8 mg/L (4-8 mcg/mL) of CAPD fluid

Gram-positive infection (eg, synergy): 3-4 mg/L (3-4 mcg/mL) of CAPD fluid

Administration via I.V., I.M. route during CAPD: Dose as for Cl_{cr} <10 mL/minute and follow levels

Removal via continuous arteriovenous or venovenous hemofiltration: Dose as for Cl_{cr} 10-40 mL/minute and follow levels

Hepatic Impairment: Monitor plasma concentrations.

Available Dosage Forms [DSC] = Discontinued product

Cream, topical, as sulfate: 0.1% (15 g, 30 g)

Infusion, as sulfate [premixed in NS]: 40 mg (50 mL); 60 mg (50 mL, 100 mL); 70 mg (50 mL); 80 mg (50 mL, 100 mL); 90 mg (100 mL); 100 mg (50 mL, 100 mL); 120 mg (100 mL)

Injection, solution, as sulfate [ADD-Vantage® vial]: 10 mg/mL (6 mL, 8 mL, 10 mL)

Injection, solution, as sulfate: 40 mg/mL (2 mL, 20 mL) [may contain sodium metabisulfite]

Injection, solution, pediatric, as sulfate: 10 mg/mL (2 mL) [may contain sodium metabisulfite]

Injection, solution, pediatric, as sulfate [preservative free]: 10 mg/mL (2 mL)

Ointment, ophthalmic, as sulfate (Gentak®): 0.3% [3 mg/g] (3.5 g)

Ointment, topical, as sulfate: 0.1% (15 g, 30 g)

Solution, ophthalmic, as sulfate: 0.3% (5 mL, 15 mL) [contains benzalkonium chloride]

Genoptic®: 0.3% (1 mL) [contains benzalkonium chloride]

Gentacidin®: 0.3% (5 mL) [contains benzalkonium chloride] [DSC]

Gentak®: 0.3% (5 mL, 15 mL) [contains benzalkonium chloride]

Monitoring and Teaching Issues

Physical Assessment: Assess effectiveness and interactions of other medications patient may be taking. Assess kidney function and hearing before, during, and following therapy. **Note:** This medication has a very low TI. Monitor for decreased renal function, ototoxicity, and neurotoxicity. Perform hearing tests prior to initiating treatment and periodically during therapy (>2 weeks) if at high risk. Monitor therapeutic effectiveness, laboratory values and adverse reactions at beginning of therapy and periodically throughout therapy. Assess knowledge/teach patient appropriate use, interventions to reduce side effects, and adverse symptoms to report.

Monitoring Laboratory Tests: Urinalysis, BUN, serum creatinine, plasma gentamicin levels (as appropriate to dosing method). Peak levels are drawn 30 minutes after the end of a 30-minute infusion or 1 hour after initiation of infusion or I.M. injection. The trough is drawn just before the next dose. Levels are typically obtained after the third dose in conventional dosing. Perform culture and sensitivity studies prior to initiating therapy to determine the causative organism and its susceptibility to gentamicin.

Patient Education: Take exactly as directed and when prescribed. Drink adequate amounts of water (2-3 L/day) unless instructed to restrict fluid intake. You may experience headaches, ringing in ears, dizziness, blurred vision (use caution when driving or engaging in tasks requiring alertness until response to drug is known); GI upset, loss of appetite (small frequent meals and frequent mouth care may help); or photosensitivity (use sunscreen wear protective clothing and eyewear, and avoid direct sunlight). Report severe headache, changes in hearing acuity, ringing in ears, change in balance, changes in urine pattern, respiratory difficulty, rash, fever, unhealed sores, sores in mouth, vaginal drainage, muscle or bone pain, change in gait, or worsening of condition. **Pregnancy/breast-feeding precautions:** Inform prescriber if you are or intend to become pregnant. Consult prescriber if breast-feeding.

Ophthalmic: Wash hands before instilling. Sit or lie down to instill. Open eye, look at ceiling, and instill prescribed amount of solution (Ointment: Pull lower lid down gently, instill thin ribbon of ointment inside lid.) Close eye and roll eye in all directions, and apply gentle pressure to inner corner of eye. Do not let tip of applicator touch eye; do not contaminate tip of applicator (may cause eye infection, eye damage, or vision loss). Temporary stinging or blurred vision may occur. Report persistent pain, burning, vision changes, swelling, itching, or worsening of condition.

Topical: Apply thin film of ointment to affected area as often as recommended. May apply porous dressing. Report persistent burning, swelling, itching, worsening of condition, or lack of response to therapy.

Dietary Considerations: Calcium, magnesium, potassium: Renal wasting may cause hypocalcemia, hypomagnesemia, and/or hypokalemia.

Geriatric Considerations: Aminoglycosides are important therapeutic interventions for susceptible organisms and as empiric therapy in seriously ill patients. Their use is not without risk of toxicity, however. Additional studies comparing high-dose, once-daily

(Continued)

Gentamicin *(Continued)*

aminoglycosides to traditional dosing regimens in the elderly are needed before once-daily aminoglycoside dosing can be routinely adopted to this patient population.

Pregnancy Risk Factor: C

Lactation: Enters breast milk (small amounts)/use caution (AAP rates "compatible")

Breast-Feeding Issues: No data reported; however, gentamicin is not absorbed orally and other aminoglycosides may be taken while breast-feeding.

Administration

I.M.: Administer by deep I.M. route if possible. Slower absorption and lower peak concentrations, probably due to poor circulation in the atrophic muscle, may occur following I.M. injection; in paralyzed patients, suggest I.V. route.

I.V.: Administer other antibiotics at least 1 hour before or 1 hour after gentamicin.

Other: Administer any other ophthalmics 10 minutes before or after gentamicin preparations.

Reconstitution: I.V. infusion solutions mixed in NS or D_5W solution are stable for 24 hours at room temperature and refrigeration.

Premixed bag: Manufacturer expiration date; remove from overwrap stability: 30 days

Compatibility: Stable in dextran 40, D_5W, $D_{10}W$, mannitol 20%, LR, NS; **incompatible** with fat emulsion 10%

Y-site administration: Incompatible with allopurinol, amphotericin B cholesteryl sulfate complex, cefamandole, furosemide, heparin, hetastarch, idarubicin, indomethacin, iodipamide meglumine, phenytoin, propofol, warfarin

Compatibility in syringe: Incompatible with ampicillin, cefamandole, heparin

Compatibility when admixed: Incompatible with amphotericin B, ampicillin, cefamandole, cefazolin with clindamycin, cefepime, heparin, nafcillin, ticarcillin

Storage: Gentamicin is a colorless to slightly yellow solution which should be stored between 2°C to 30°C, but refrigeration is not recommended.

Related Information

Antimicrobial Drugs of Choice *on page 1792*
Compatibility of Drugs *on page 1723*
Peak and Trough Guidelines *on page 1694*

♦ Gentamicin Sulfate *see* Gentamicin *on page 709*
♦ Gentran® *see* Dextran *on page 433*
♦ Geocillin® *see* Carbenicillin *on page 252*
♦ Geodon® *see* Ziprasidone *on page 1589*
♦ Geref® Diagnostic *see page 1625*
♦ Geref® Injection *see page 1625*
♦ GF196960 *see* Tadalafil *on page 1422*
♦ GG *see* Guaifenesin *on page 729*
♦ Giltuss HC® *see* Hydrocodone, Phenylephrine, and Guaifenesin *on page 760*
♦ Glargine, Insulin *see* Insulin Preparations *on page 805*

Glatiramer Acetate *(gla TIR a mer AS e tate)*

U.S. Brand Names Copaxone®

Synonyms Copolymer-1

Generic Available No

Pharmacologic Category Biological, Miscellaneous

Medication Safety Issues

Sound-alike/look-alike issues:

Copaxone® may be confused with Compazine®

Use Treatment of relapsing-remitting type multiple sclerosis; studies indicate that it reduces the frequency of attacks and the severity of disability; appears to be most effective for patients with minimal disability

Contraindications Previous hypersensitivity to any component of the copolymer formulation, glatiramer acetate, or mannitol

Warnings/Precautions For SubQ use only, **not for I.V. administration**. Glatiramer acetate is antigenic, and may possibly lead to the induction of untoward host responses. Systemic postinjection reactions occur in a substantial percentage of patients (~10% in premarketing studies). Safety and efficacy have not been established in patients <18 years of age.

Adverse Reactions Reported in >2% of patients in placebo-controlled trials:

>10%:

Cardiovascular: Chest pain (21%), vasodilation (27%), palpitation (17%)

Central nervous system: Pain (28%), anxiety (23%)

Dermatologic: Pruritus (18%), rash (18%), diaphoresis (15%)

Gastrointestinal: Nausea (22%), diarrhea (12%)

Local: Injection site reactions: Pain (73%), erythema (66%), inflammation (49%), pruritus (40%), mass (27%), induration (13%), welt (11%)

Neuromuscular & skeletal: Weakness (41%), arthralgia (24%), hypertonia (22%), back pain (16%)

Respiratory: Dyspnea (19%), rhinitis (14%)

Miscellaneous: Infection (50%), flu-like syndrome (19%), lymphadenopathy (12%)

1% to 10%:

Cardiovascular: Peripheral edema (7%), facial edema (6%), edema (3%), tachycardia (5%)

Central nervous system: Fever (8%), vertigo (6%), migraine (5%), syncope (5%), agitation (4%), chills (4%), confusion (2%), nervousness (2%), speech disorder (2%)

Dermatologic: Bruising (8%), erythema (4%), urticaria (4%), skin nodule (2%)

Endocrine & metabolic: Dysmenorrhea (6%)

Gastrointestinal: Anorexia (8%), vomiting (6%), gastrointestinal disorder (5%), gastroenteritis (3%), weight gain (3%)

Genitourinary: Urinary urgency (10%), vaginal moniliasis (8%)

Local: Injection site reactions: Hemorrhage (8%), urticaria (5%)

Neuromuscular & skeletal: Tremor (7%), foot drop (3%)

Ocular: Eye disorder (4%), nystagmus (2%)

Otic: Ear pain (7%)

Respiratory: Bronchitis (9%), laryngismus (5%)

Miscellaneous: Neck pain (8%), bacterial infection (5%), herpes simplex (4%), cyst (2%)

Overdosage/Toxicology Well tolerated; no serious toxicities can be anticipated

Pharmacodynamics/Kinetics

Metabolism: SubQ: Large percentage hydrolyzed locally

Dosing

Adults & Elderly: Multiple sclerosis (relapsing-remitting): SubQ: 20 mg daily

Available Dosage Forms Injection, solution [preservative free]: 20 mg/mL (1 mL) [prefilled syringe; contains mannitol; packaged with alcohol pads]

Monitoring and Teaching Issues

Physical Assessment: Assess potential for interactions with other prescriptions, OTC medications, or herbal products patient may be taking. Assess effectiveness and adverse response (eg, postinjection reactions: Self-resolving flushing, chest tightness, dyspnea, palpitations). Teach patient proper use (reconstitution, injection technique, and syringe/needle disposal), possible side effects/appropriate interventions, and adverse symptoms to report.

Patient Education: This drug will not cure MS, but may help relieve the severity and frequency of attacks. This drug can only be given by subcutaneous injection; your prescriber will instruct you in how to prepare the medication, proper injection technique, and syringe/needle disposal. If using prefilled glass syringe, use **only** the auto*ject*® 2 *for glass syringe* device (not the original Copaxone® autoject). Do not stop or change doses without consulting your prescriber. May cause a transient reaction after injection, including flushing, chest tightness, dyspnea, or palpitations (usually last 30 minutes or less). May cause weakness, dizziness, confusion, nervousness, or anxiety (use caution when driving or engaging in tasks requiring alertness until response to drug is known); or nausea or vomiting (frequent mouth care and sucking on lozenges may help). Report chest pain or pounding heartbeat; persistent diarrhea or GI upset; infection (vaginal itching or drainage, sores in mouth, unusual fever or chills) or flu-like symptoms (swollen glands, chills, excessive sweating); bruising, rash, or skin irritation; joint pain or neck pain; swelling of puffiness of face; vision changes or ear pain; unusual cough or respiratory difficulty; alterations in menstrual pattern; skin depression, hard lump, redness, pain, or swelling at injection site; or any other persistent adverse reactions. **Breast-feeding precaution:** Consult prescriber if breast-feeding.

Pregnancy Risk Factor: B

Lactation: Excretion in breast milk unknown/use caution

Administration

Other: For SubQ administration in the arms, abdomen, hips or thighs. Bring to room temperature prior to use.

Storage: Store in refrigerator at 2°C to 8°C (36°F to 46°F); excursions to room temperature for up to 1 week do not have a negative impact on potency.

♦ **Glaucoma Drug Therapy** *see page 1827*

♦ **Gleevec**® *see Imatinib on page 785*

♦ **Gliadel**® *see Carmustine on page 260*

♦ **Glibenclamide** *see GlyBURIDE on page 720*

Glimepiride (GLYE me pye ride)

U.S. Brand Names Amaryl®

Generic Available No

Pharmacologic Category Antidiabetic Agent, Sulfonylurea

Medication Safety Issues

Sound-alike/look-alike issues:

Glimepiride may be confused with glipiZIDE

Amaryl® may be confused with Altace®, Amerge®, Reminyl®

Use Management of type 2 diabetes mellitus (noninsulin dependent, NIDDM) as an adjunct to diet and exercise to lower blood glucose or in combination with metformin; use in combination with insulin to lower blood glucose in patients whose hyperglycemia cannot be controlled by diet and exercise in conjunction with an oral hypoglycemic agent

Mechanism of Action/Effect Stimulates insulin release from the pancreatic beta cells; reduces glucose output from the liver; insulin sensitivity is increased at peripheral target sites

Contraindications Hypersensitivity to glimepiride, any component of the formulation, or sulfonamides; diabetic ketoacidosis (with or without coma)

Warnings/Precautions The administration of oral hypoglycemic drugs (eg, tolbutamide) has been reported to be associated with increased cardiovascular mortality as compared to treatment with diet alone or diet plus insulin. All sulfonylurea drugs are capable of producing severe hypoglycemia. Hypoglycemia is more likely to occur when caloric intake is deficient, after severe or prolonged exercise, when ethanol is ingested, or when more than one glucose-lowering drug is used.

Chemical similarities are present among sulfonamides, sulfonylureas, carbonic anhydrase inhibitors, thiazides, and loop diuretics (except ethacrynic acid). Use in patients with sulfonamide allergy is specifically contraindicated in product labeling, however, a risk of cross-reaction exists in patients with allergy to any of these compounds; avoid use when previous reaction has been severe.

Product labeling states oral hypoglycemic drugs may be associated with an increased cardiovascular mortality. Data to support this association are limited, and several studies (UKPDS) have not supported an association.

Drug Interactions

Cytochrome P450 Effect: Substrate of CYP2C8/9 (major)

Decreased Effect: CYP2C8/9 inducers may decrease the levels/effects of glimepiride; example inducers include carbamazepine, phenobarbital, phenytoin, rifampin, rifapentine, (Continued)

Glimepiride (Continued)

and secobarbital. There may be a decreased effect of glimepiride with corticosteroids, estrogens, oral contraceptives, thiazide and other diuretics, phenothiazines, NSAIDs, thyroid products, nicotinic acid, isoniazid, sympathomimetics, urinary alkalinizers, and charcoal. **Note:** However, pooled data did **not** demonstrate drug interactions with calcium channel blockers, estrogens, NSAIDs, HMG-CoA reductase inhibitors, sulfonamides, or thyroid hormone.

Increased Effect/Toxicity: CYP2C8/9 inhibitors may increase the levels/effects of glimepiride; example inhibitors include delavirdine, ketoconazole, nicardipine, NSAIDs, and pioglitazone. Beta-blockers, chloramphenicol, cimetidine, clofibrate, fluconazole, gemfibrozil, pegvisomant, salicylates, sulfonamides, and tricyclic antidepressants may increase the hypoglycemic effects of glimepiride. Glimepiride may increase effects of coumarins and cyclosporine.

Nutritional/Ethanol Interactions
Ethanol: Caution with ethanol (may cause hypoglycemia).
Herb/Nutraceutical: Caution with chromium, garlic, gymnema (may cause hypoglycemia).

Adverse Reactions 1% to 10%: Central nervous system: Headache

Overdosage/Toxicology Symptoms of overdose include low blood sugar, tingling of lips and tongue, nausea, yawning, confusion, agitation, tachycardia, sweating, convulsions, stupor, and coma. Intoxication with sulfonylureas can cause hypoglycemia and are best managed with glucose administration (oral for milder hypoglycemia or by injection in more severe forms). Patients should be monitored for a minimum of 24-48 hours after ingestion.

Pharmacodynamics/Kinetics
Onset of Action: Peak effect: Blood glucose reductions: 2-3 hours
Duration of Action: 24 hours
Absorption: 100%; delayed when given with food
Protein Binding: >99.5%
Half-Life Elimination: 5-9 hours
Metabolism: Completely hepatic
Excretion: Urine and feces (as metabolites)

Dosing
Adults:
Type 2 diabetes: Oral:
Initial: 1-2 mg once daily, administered with breakfast or the first main meal
Adjustment: Allow several days between dose titrations: usual maintenance dose: 1-4 mg once daily; after a dose of 2 mg once daily, increase in increments of 2 mg at 1- to 2-week intervals based upon the patient's blood glucose response to a maximum of 8 mg once daily

Combination with insulin therapy:
Note: Fasting glucose level for instituting combination therapy is in the range of >150 mg/dL in plasma or serum depending on the patient)
Initial: 8 mg once daily with the first main meal
Adjustment: After starting with low-dose insulin, upward adjustments of insulin can be done approximately weekly as guided by frequent measurements of fasting blood glucose. Once stable, combination-therapy patients should monitor their capillary blood glucose on an ongoing basis, preferably daily.

Elderly: Initial: 1 mg/day; dose titration and maintenance dosing should be conservative to avoid hypoglycemia

Renal Impairment: Cl_{cr} <22 mL/minute: Initial starting dose should be 1 mg and dosage increments should be based on fasting blood glucose levels.

Available Dosage Forms Tablet: 1 mg, 2 mg, 4 mg

Monitoring and Teaching Issues
Physical Assessment: Assess any allergies prior to beginning therapy. Assess potential for interactions with other prescriptions, OTC medications, or herbal products patient may be taking. Assess results of laboratory tests, therapeutic effectiveness, and adverse response at regular intervals during therapy. Teach patient proper use (or refer patient to diabetic educator for instruction), possible side effects/appropriate interventions, and adverse symptoms to report.

Monitoring Laboratory Tests: Urine for glucose and ketones, fasting blood glucose, hemoglobin A_{1c}, fructosamine

Patient Education: Do not take any new medication during therapy unless approved by prescriber. This medication is used to control diabetes; it is not a cure. Monitor glucose as recommended by prescriber. Other important components of treatment plan may include prescribed diet and exercise regimen (consult prescriber or diabetic educator). Always carry quick source of sugar with you. Take exactly as directed with breakfast or the first main meal of the day. Do not change dose or discontinue without consulting prescriber. Avoid alcohol while taking this medication; could cause severe reaction. Do not take other medication within 2 hours of this medication unless advised by prescriber. If you experience hypoglycemic reaction, contact prescriber immediately. You may experience side effects during first weeks of therapy (eg, headache, nausea); consult prescriber if these persist. Report severe or persistent side effects (eg, hypoglycemia: palpitations, sweaty palms, lightheadedness; extended vomiting or flu-like symptoms; skin rash; easy bruising or bleeding; or change in color of urine or stool). **Pregnancy/breast-feeding precautions:** Inform prescriber if you are or intend to become pregnant. Do not breast-feed.

Dietary Considerations: Administer with breakfast or the first main meal of the day. Dietary modification based on ADA recommendations is a part of therapy. Decreases blood glucose concentration. Hypoglycemia may occur. Must be able to recognize symptoms of hypoglycemia (palpitations, sweaty palms, lightheadedness).

Geriatric Considerations: Rapid and prolonged hypoglycemia (>12 hours) despite hypertonic glucose injections have been reported; age, hepatic, and renal impairment are independent risk factors for hypoglycemia; dosage titration should be made at weekly intervals. How "tightly" a geriatric patient's blood glucose should be controlled is controversial; however, a fasting blood sugar <150 mg/dL is now an acceptable end point. Such a decision should be based on the patient's functional and cognitive status, how well they recognize hypoglycemic or hyperglycemic symptoms, and how to respond to them and their other disease states.

Pregnancy Risk Factor: C

Pregnancy Issues: Abnormal blood glucose levels are associated with a higher incidence of congenital abnormalities. Insulin is the drug of choice for the control of diabetes mellitus during pregnancy.

Lactation: Excretion in breast milk unknown/contraindicated

Administration

Oral: May be taken with a meal or food. Patients who are NPO may need to have their dose held to avoid hypoglycemia.

Related Information

Diabetes Mellitus Management *on page 1819*

GlipiZIDE (GLIP i zide)

U.S. Brand Names Glucotrol®; Glucotrol® XL

Synonyms Glydiazinamide

Generic Available Yes

Pharmacologic Category Antidiabetic Agent, Sulfonylurea

Medication Safety Issues

Sound-alike/look-alike issues:

GlipiZIDE may be confused with glimepiride, glyBURIDE

Glucotrol® may be confused with Glucophage®, Glucotrol® XL, glyBURIDE

Glucotrol® XL may be confused with Glucotrol®

Use Management of type 2 diabetes mellitus (noninsulin dependent, NIDDM)

Mechanism of Action/Effect Stimulates insulin release from the pancreatic beta cells; reduces glucose output from the liver; insulin sensitivity is increased at peripheral target sites

Contraindications Hypersensitivity to glipizide or any component of the formulation, other sulfonamides; type 1 diabetes mellitus (insulin dependent, IDDM)

Warnings/Precautions Use with caution in patients with severe hepatic disease.

Chemical similarities are present among sulfonamides, sulfonylureas, carbonic anhydrase inhibitors, thiazides, and loop diuretics (except ethacrynic acid). Use in patients with sulfonamide allergy is specifically contraindicated in product labeling, however, a risk of cross-reaction exists in patients with allergy to any of these compounds; avoid use when previous reaction has been severe.

Avoid use of extended release tablets (Glucotrol® XL) in patients with known stricture/narrowing of the GI tract.

Product labeling states oral hypoglycemic drugs may be associated with an increased cardiovascular mortality as compared to treatment with diet alone or diet plus insulin. Data to support this association are limited, and several studies, including a large prospective trial (UKPDS) have not supported an association.

Drug Interactions

Cytochrome P450 Effect: Substrate of 2C8/9 (major)

Decreased Effect: CYP2C8/9 inducers may decrease the levels/effects of glipizide; example inducers include carbamazepine, phenobarbital, phenytoin, rifampin, rifapentine, and secobarbital. Decreased effect of glipizide with beta-blockers, cholestyramine, hydantoins, thiazide diuretics, urinary alkalinizers, and charcoal.

Increased Effect/Toxicity: CYP2C8/9 inhibitors may increase the levels/effects of glipizide; example inhibitors include delavirdine, fluconazole, gemfibrozil, ketoconazole, nicardipine, NSAIDs, pioglitazone, and sulfonamides. Increased effects/hypoglycemic effects of glipizide with H_2 antagonists, anticoagulants, androgens, cimetidine, salicylates, tricyclic antidepressants, probenecid, MAO inhibitors, methyldopa, digitalis glycosides, and urinary acidifiers.

Nutritional/Ethanol Interactions

Ethanol: Caution with ethanol (may cause hypoglycemia or rare disulfiram reaction).

Food: A delayed release of insulin may occur if glipizide is taken with food. Immediate release tablets should be administered 30 minutes before meals to avoid erratic absorption.

Herb/Nutraceutical: Caution with chromium, garlic, gymnema (may cause hypoglycemia).

Adverse Reactions Frequency not defined.

Cardiovascular: Edema, syncope

Central nervous system: Anxiety, depression, dizziness, headache, insomnia, nervousness

Dermatologic: Rash, urticaria, photosensitivity, pruritus

Endocrine & metabolic: Hypoglycemia, hyponatremia, SIADH (rare)

Gastrointestinal: Anorexia, nausea, vomiting, diarrhea, epigastric fullness, constipation, heartburn, flatulence

Hematologic: Blood dyscrasias, aplastic anemia, hemolytic anemia, bone marrow suppression, thrombocytopenia, agranulocytosis

Hepatic: Cholestatic jaundice, hepatic porphyria

Neuromuscular & skeletal: Arthralgia, leg cramps, myalgia, tremor

Ocular: Blurred vision

Renal: Diuretic effect (minor)

Miscellaneous: Diaphoresis, disulfiram-like reaction

Overdosage/Toxicology Symptoms of overdose include low blood sugar, tingling of lips and tongue, nausea, yawning, confusion, agitation, tachycardia, sweating, convulsions, stupor, and coma. Intoxication with sulfonylureas can cause hypoglycemia and are best managed with glucose administration (oral for milder hypoglycemia or by injection in more severe forms).

(Continued)

GlipiZIDE *(Continued)*

Pharmacodynamics/Kinetics
Onset of Action: Peak effect: Blood glucose reductions: 1.5-2 hours
Duration of Action: 12-24 hours
Absorption: Delayed with food
Protein Binding: 92% to 99%
Half-Life Elimination: 2-4 hours
Metabolism: Hepatic with metabolites
Excretion: Urine (60% to 80%, 91% to 97% as metabolites); feces (11%)

Dosing
Adults:
Type 2 diabetes: Oral (allow several days between dose titrations): Initial: 5 mg/day; adjust dosage at 2.5-5 mg daily increments as determined by blood glucose response at intervals of several days.
Immediate release tablet: Maximum recommended once-daily dose: 15 mg; maximum recommended total daily dose: 40 mg
Extended release tablet (Glucotrol® XL): Maximum recommended dose: 20 mg
When transferring from insulin to glipizide:
Current insulin requirement ≤20 units: Discontinue insulin and initiate glipizide at usual dose
Current insulin requirement >20 units: Decrease insulin by 50% and initiate glipizide at usual dose; gradually decrease insulin dose based on patient response. Several days should elapse between dosage changes.
Elderly: Initial: 2.5 mg/day; increase by 2.5-5 mg/day at 1- to 2-week intervals.
Renal Impairment: Cl_{cr} <10 mL/minute: Some investigators recommend not using.
Hepatic Impairment: Initial dosage should be 2.5 mg/day.

Available Dosage Forms
Tablet (Glucotrol®): 5 mg, 10 mg
Tablet, extended release: 5 mg, 10 mg
(Glucotrol® XL): 2.5 mg, 5 mg, 10 mg

Monitoring and Teaching Issues
Physical Assessment: Assess potential for interactions with other prescriptions, OTC medications, or herbal products patient may be taking, and any allergies they may have. Assess results of laboratory tests, therapeutic effects, and adverse response (eg, hypoglycemia) at regular intervals during therapy. Teach patient proper use (or refer patient to diabetic educator for instruction), possible side effects/appropriate interventions, and adverse symptoms to report.
Monitoring Laboratory Tests: Urine for glucose and ketones, fasting blood glucose, hemoglobin A_{1c}, fructosamine
Patient Education: Do not take any new medication during therapy unless approved by prescriber. This medication is used to control diabetes; it is not a cure. Monitor glucose as recommended by prescriber. Other important components of treatment plan may include prescribed diet and exercise regimen (consult prescriber or diabetic educator). Always carry quick source of sugar with you. Take exactly as directed. Immediate release tablets should be taken 30 minutes before meals, at the same time each day. Extended release tablets should be taken with breakfast. Do not chew or crush extended release tablets. Do not change dose or discontinue without consulting prescriber. Avoid alcohol while taking this medication; could cause severe reaction. Do not take other medication within 2 hours of this medication unless advised by prescriber. If you experience hypoglycemic reaction, contact prescriber immediately. You may experience more sensitivity to sunlight (use sunscreen, wear protective clothing and eyewear, and avoid direct sunlight); or headache or nausea (consult prescriber if these persist). Report severe or persistent side effects (eg, hypoglycemia: palpitations, sweaty palms, lightheadedness; extended vomiting; diarrhea or constipation; flu-like symptoms; skin rash; easy bruising or bleeding; or change in color of urine or stool). **Pregnancy/breast-feeding precautions:** Inform prescriber if you are or intend to become pregnant. Breast-feeding is not recommended.
Dietary Considerations: Take immediate release tablets 30 minutes before meals; extended release tablets should be taken with breakfast. Dietary modification based on ADA recommendations is a part of therapy. Decreases blood glucose concentration. Hypoglycemia may occur. Must be able to recognize symptoms of hypoglycemia (palpitations, sweaty palms, lightheadedness).
Geriatric Considerations: Glipizide is a useful agent since there are few drug to drug interactions and elimination of the active drug is not dependent upon renal function. How "tightly" a geriatric patient's blood glucose should be controlled is controversial; however, a fasting blood sugar <150 mg/dL is now an acceptable end point. Such a decision should be based on the patient's functional and cognitive status, how well they recognize hypoglycemic or hyperglycemic symptoms, and how to respond to them and their other disease states.
Pregnancy Risk Factor: C
Pregnancy Issues: Crosses the placenta. Abnormal blood glucose levels are associated with a higher incidence of congenital abnormalities. Insulin is the drug of choice for the control of diabetes mellitus during pregnancy. If glipizide is used during pregnancy, discontinue and change to insulin at least 1 month prior to delivery to decrease prolonged hypoglycemia in the neonate.
Lactation: Excretion in breast milk unknown/not recommended
Breast-Feeding Issues: Due to risk of neonatal hypoglycemia, breast-feeding is not recommended. Discontinue nursing or consider switching to insulin if diet alone does not control blood glucose.

Administration
Oral: Administer immediate release tablets 30 minutes before a meal to achieve greatest reduction in postprandial hyperglycemia. Extended release tablets should be given with breakfast. Patients who are NPO may need to have their dose held to avoid hypoglycemia.

Related Information
Diabetes Mellitus Management *on page 1819*
FDA Name Differentiation Project: The Use of Tall-Man Letters *on page 15*

Glipizide and Metformin (GLIP i zide & met FOR min)
U.S. Brand Names Metaglip™
Synonyms Glipizide and Metformin Hydrochloride; Metformin and Glipizide
Generic Available No
Pharmacologic Category Antidiabetic Agent, Biguanide; Antidiabetic Agent, Sulfonylurea
Use Initial therapy for management of type 2 diabetes mellitus (noninsulin dependent, NIDDM) when hyperglycemia cannot be managed with diet and exercise alone. Second-line therapy for management of type 2 diabetes (NIDDM) when hyperglycemia cannot be managed with a sulfonylurea or metformin along with diet and exercise.
Dosing
Adults:
Type 2 diabetes, first-line therapy: Oral: Initial: Glipizide 2.5 mg/metformin 250 mg once daily with a meal. Dose adjustment: Increase dose by 1 tablet/day every 2 weeks, up to a maximum of glipizide 10 mg/metformin 1000 mg daily
Patients with fasting plasma glucose (FPG) 280-320 mg/dL: Oral: Consider glipizide 2.5 mg/metformin 500 mg twice daily. Dose adjustment: Increase dose by 1 tablet/day every 2 weeks, up to a maximum of glipizide 10 mg/metformin 2000 mg daily in divided doses
Type 2 diabetes, second-line therapy: Oral: Glipizide 2.5 mg/metformin 500 mg **or** glipizide 5 mg/metformin 500 mg twice daily with morning and evening meals; starting dose should not exceed current daily dose of glipizide (or sulfonylurea equivalent) or metformin. Dose adjustment: Titrate dose in increments of no more than glipizide 5 mg/metformin 500 mg, up to a maximum dose of glipizide 20 mg/metformin 2000 mg daily.
Elderly: Conservative doses are recommended in the elderly due to potentially decreased renal function; **do not titrate to maximum dose**; should not be used in patients ≥80 years unless renal function is verified as normal
Renal Impairment: Risk of lactic acidosis increases with degree of renal impairment; contraindicated in renal disease or renal dysfunction (see Contraindications).
Hepatic Impairment: Use should be avoided; liver disease is a risk factor for the development of lactic acidosis during metformin therapy.
Available Dosage Forms Tablet [film coated]:
2.5/250: Glipizide 2.5 mg and metformin 250 mg
2.5/500: Glipizide 2.5 mg and metformin 500 mg
5/500: Glipizide 5 mg and metformin 500 mg
Monitoring and Teaching Issues
Physical Assessment: See Contraindications, Warnings/Precautions, and Dosing for use cautions. Assess potential for interactions with other prescriptions, OTC medications, or herbal products patient may be taking, and any allergies they may have (see Drug Interactions). Assess results of laboratory tests (see Monitoring Laboratory Tests), therapeutic effects, and adverse response (eg, hypoglycemia; see Adverse Reactions and Overdose/Toxicology) at regular intervals during therapy. Teach patient proper use (or refer patient to diabetic educator for instruction), possible side effects, interventions to reduce side effects, and adverse symptoms to report (see Patient Education).
Patient Education: Inform prescriber of all prescriptions, OTC medications, or herbal products you are taking, and any allergies you have. Do not take any new medication during therapy unless approved by prescriber. This medication is used to control diabetes; it is not a cure. Monitor glucose as recommended by prescriber. Other important components of treatment plan may include prescribed diet and exercise regimen (consult prescriber or diabetic educator). Always carry quick source of sugar with you. Take exactly as directed. All doses should be administered with a meal. Twice-daily dosing should be taken with the morning and evening meals. Do not change dose or discontinue without consulting prescriber. Avoid overuse of alcohol while taking this medication (could cause severe reaction). Do not take other medication within 2 hours of this medication unless advised by prescriber. If you experience hypoglycemic reaction, contact prescriber immediately. You may experience more sensitivity to sunlight (use sunscreen, wear protective clothing and eyewear, and avoid direct sunlight); drowsiness, dizziness, or headache (use caution driving or engaging in potentially hazardous tasks until response to drug is known); nausea or vomiting (taking with meals, eating small frequent meals, frequent mouth care, or sucking lozenges may help). Report severe or persistent side effects (eg, hypoglycemia); palpitations, sweaty palms, lightheadedness; extended vomiting; diarrhea or constipation; flu-like symptoms; skin rash; easy bruising or bleeding; or change in color of urine or stool, sudden chest discomfort, slow or irregular heartbeat, or other adverse reactions). **Pregnancy/breast-feeding precautions:** Inform prescriber if you are or intend to become pregnant. Breast-feeding is not recommended.
Pregnancy Risk Factor: C
Lactation: Excretion in breast milk unknown/not recommended
Related Information
GlipiZIDE *on page 715*
Metformin *on page 965*

- **Glipizide and Metformin Hydrochloride** *see Glipizide and Metformin on page 717*
- **Glivec** *see Imatinib on page 785*
- **Gln** *see Glutamine on page 719*
- **GlucaGen®** *see Glucagon on page 717*
- **GlucaGen® Diagnostic Kit** *see Glucagon on page 717*

Glucagon (GLOO ka gon)
U.S. Brand Names GlucaGen®; GlucaGen® Diagnostic Kit; Glucagon Diagnostic Kit; Glucagon Emergency Kit
Synonyms Glucagon Hydrochloride
(Continued)

Glucagon (Continued)

Generic Available No

Pharmacologic Category Antidote; Diagnostic Agent

Medication Safety Issues
Sound-alike/look-alike issues:
Glucagon may be confused with Glaucon®

Use Management of hypoglycemia; diagnostic aid in radiologic examinations to temporarily inhibit GI tract movement

Unlabeled/Investigational Use Used with some success as a cardiac stimulant in management of severe cases of beta-adrenergic blocking agent overdosage; treatment of myocardial depression due to calcium channel blocker overdose

Mechanism of Action/Effect Stimulates adenylate cyclase to produce increased cyclic AMP, which promotes hepatic glycogenolysis and gluconeogenesis, causing a raise in blood glucose levels

Contraindications Hypersensitivity to glucagon or any component of the formulation; insulinoma; pheochromocytoma

Warnings/Precautions Use caution with prolonged fasting, starvation, adrenal insufficiency or chronic hypoglycemia; levels of glucose stores in liver may be decreased. Following response to therapy, oral carbohydrates should be administered to prevent hypoglycemia.

Drug Interactions
Increased Effect/Toxicity: Oral anticoagulant: Hypoprothrombinemic effects may be increased possibly with bleeding; effect seen with glucagon doses of 50 mg administered over 1-2 days

Nutritional/Ethanol Interactions Glucagon depletes glycogen stores.

Adverse Reactions Frequency not defined.
Cardiovascular: Hypotension (up to 2 hours after GI procedures), hypertension, tachycardia
Gastrointestinal: Nausea, vomiting (high incidence with rapid administration of high doses)
Miscellaneous: Hypersensitivity reactions, anaphylaxis

Overdosage/Toxicology Symptoms include hypokalemia, nausea and vomiting, inhibition of GI tract motility, decreased blood pressure, tachycardia

Pharmacodynamics/Kinetics
Onset of Action: Peak effect: Blood glucose levels: Parenteral: I.V.: 5-20 minutes; I.M.: 30 minutes; SubQ: 30-45 minutes

Duration of Action: Hyperglycemia: 60-90 minutes

Half-Life Elimination: Plasma: 3-10 minutes

Metabolism: Primarily hepatic; some inactivation occurring renally and in plasma

Dosing
Adults & Elderly:
Hypoglycemia or insulin shock therapy: I.M., I.V., SubQ: 1 mg; may repeat in 20 minutes as needed
Note: If patient fails to respond to glucagon, I.V. dextrose must be given.
Beta-blocker overdose, calcium channel blocker overdose (unlabeled use): I.V.: 5-10 mg over 1 minutes followed by an infusion of 1-10 mg/hour. The following has also been reported for beta-blocker overdose: 3-10 mg or initially 0.5-5 mg bolus followed by continuous infusion 1-5 mg/hour
Diagnostic aid: I.M., I.V.: 0.25-2 mg 10 minutes prior to procedure

Pediatrics:
Hypoglycemia or insulin shock therapy: I.M., I.V., SubQ:
Children <20 kg: 0.5 mg or 20-30 mcg/kg/dose; repeated in 20 minutes as needed
Children ≥20 kg: Refer to adult dosing.
Note: If patient fails to respond to glucagon, I.V. dextrose must be given.

Available Dosage Forms
Injection, powder for reconstitution, as hydrochloride:
GlucaGen®: 1 mg [equivalent to 1 unit; contains lactose 107 mg]
GlucaGen® Diagnostic Kit: 1 mg [equivalent to 1 unit; contains lactose 107 mg; packaged with sterile water]
Glucagon®: 1 mg [equivalent to 1 unit; contains lactose 49 mg]
Glucagon Diagnostic Kit, Glucagon Emergency Kit: 1 mg [equivalent to 1 unit; contains lactose 49 mg; packaged with diluent syringe containing glycerin 12 mg/mL and water for injection]

Monitoring and Teaching Issues
Physical Assessment: Arouse patient from hypoglycemic or insulin shock as soon as possible and administer carbohydrates. Evaluate insulin dosage and patient's ability to administer appropriate dose. Instruct patient (or significant other) in appropriate administration procedures for emergency use of glucagon. If home glucose monitoring device is available, check blood sugar as soon as possible.

Monitoring Laboratory Tests: Blood glucose

Patient Education: Identify appropriate support person to administer glucagon if necessary. Follow prescribers instructions for administering glucagon. Review diet, insulin administration, and testing procedures with prescriber or diabetic educator.

Dietary Considerations: Administer carbohydrates to patient as soon as possible after response to treatment.

Pregnancy Risk Factor: B

Lactation: Excretion in breast milk unknown/compatible

Administration
I.V.: Bolus may be associated with nausea and vomiting. Continuous infusions may be used in beta-blocker overdose/toxicity.

Reconstitution: Reconstitute powder for injection by adding 1 mL of sterile diluent to a vial containing 1 unit of the drug, to provide solutions containing 1 mg of glucagon/mL. Gently roll vial to dissolve. If dose to be administered is <2 mg of the drug, then use only the diluent provided by the manufacturer. If >2 mg, use sterile water for injection. Use immediately after reconstitution. May be kept at 5°C for up to 48 hours if necessary.

Storage: Prior to reconstitution, store at controlled room temperature of 20°C to 25° (69°F to 77°F). Do not freeze.

Additional Information 1 unit = 1 mg

♦ **Glucagon Diagnostic Kit** *see* Glucagon *on page 717*

♦ **Glucagon Emergency Kit** *see* Glucagon *on page 717*

♦ **Glucagon Hydrochloride** *see* Glucagon *on page 717*

♦ **Glucocerebrosidase** *see* Alglucerase *on page 69*

♦ **Glucophage®** *see* Metformin *on page 965*

♦ **Glucophage® XR** *see* Metformin *on page 965*

♦ **Glucotrol®** *see* GlipiZIDE *on page 715*

♦ **Glucotrol® XL** *see* GlipiZIDE *on page 715*

♦ **Glucovance®** *see* Glyburide and Metformin *on page 721*

♦ **Glu-K® [OTC]** *see* Potassium Gluconate *on page 1236*

♦ **Glulisine, Insulin** *see* Insulin Preparations *on page 805*

Glutamine (GLOO ta meen)

U.S. Brand Names Enterex® Glutapak-10® [OTC]; NutreStore™; Resource® GlutaSolve® [OTC]; Sympt-X [OTC]; Sympt-X G.I. [OTC]

Synonyms Gln; L-Glutamine

Pharmacologic Category Amino Acid

Use Treatment of short bowel syndrome when used in combination with nutritional support and growth hormone therapy; a medical food used to promote GI tract healing and nutritional supplementation with GI disorders, HIV/AIDS, cancer, and other critical illnesses

Mechanism of Action/Effect Glutamine regulates gastrointestinal cell growth, function, and regeneration. Considered a "conditionally essential" amino acid during metabolic stress and injury.

Warnings/Precautions Use caution with hepatic or renal impairment. NutreStore™ should be used with nutritional support based on individual patient requirements. Medical foods are intended to be used under the direction of a healthcare provider.

Adverse Reactions Frequency not defined.

Cardiovascular: Facial edema, peripheral edema

Central nervous system: Dizziness, fever, headache, pain

Dermatologic: Pruritus, rash

Gastrointestinal: Abdominal pain, flatulence, nausea, pancreatitis, tenesmus, vomiting

Neuromuscular & skeletal: Arthralgia, back pain, hypoesthesia

Otic: Ear or hearing symptoms

Respiratory: Rhinitis

Miscellaneous: Flu-like syndrome, infection, sepsis

Pharmacodynamics/Kinetics

Half-Life Elimination: I.V.: 1 hour

Metabolism: Via splanchnic tissue, lymphocytes, kidney, and liver to glutamate and ammonia

Pharmacokinetic Note: As reported in healthy adults; parameters may vary following oral administration in patients with short bowel syndrome.

Dosing

Adults:

Nutritional supplement (Enterex® Glutapak-10®, Resource® GlutaSolve®, Sympt-X, Sympt-X G.I.): Oral: Average dose: 10 g 3 times/day; dosing range: 5-30 g/day

Short bowel syndrome (NutreStore™): Oral: 30 g/day administered as 5 g 6 times/day (every 2-3 hours while awake) for up to 16 weeks; to be used in combination with growth hormone and nutritional support

Available Dosage Forms

Powder for oral solution:

Enterex® Glutapak-10®: 10 g/packet (50s)

NutreStore™: 5 g/packet

Resource® GlutaSolve®: 15 g/packet (56s)

Sympt-X, Sympt-X G.I.: 10 g/packet (60s)

Monitoring and Teaching Issues

Physical Assessment: See Contraindications, Warnings/Precautions, and Dosing for cautious use. Assess therapeutic effectiveness according to purpose for use and adverse response (see Adverse Reactions). Teach patient proper use (reconstitution and storage), possible side effects/appropriate interventions, and adverse symptoms to report (see Patient Education).

Monitoring Laboratory Tests: BUN

Patient Education: Prepare, store, and use exactly as directed. Do not exceed recommended dosage. May case increased flatulence, nausea or vomiting or abdominal pain; if persistent or severe contact prescriber. Report facial or peripheral swelling, rash; unusual back pain; or other persistent adverse reactions. **Pregnancy/breast-feeding precautions:** Inform prescriber if you are or intent to become pregnant or breast-feed.

Dietary Considerations: NutreStore™: To be used in combination with a specialized diet. May be taken with food or a snack.

Pregnancy Risk Factor: C

Lactation: Excretion in breast milk unknown/use caution

Breast-Feeding Issues: The amount of total protein and free amino acids found in breast milk varies during lactation. Effects of the suggested oral dose of glutamine are unknown.

Administration

Oral:

Enterex® Glutapak-10®: Prior to use, mix with clear liquids or semisolid food. If administering via feeding tube, mix each 10 g packet with ≥60 mL water. Use immediately after preparation. May also be added directly to enteral formula if used within 24 hours.

(Continued)

Glutamine (Continued)

Resource® GlutaSolve®: Mix each 15 g packet with 120-240 mL of water. May also be mixed in hot or cold beverages, applesauce, or pudding. If administering via feeding tube, mix with 60-120 mL water. Use immediately after preparation.

NutreStore™: Mix each packet (5 g) with ~240 mL of water prior to administration. May be given with meals or snacks

Sympt-X, Sympt-X G.I.: Mix dose with 6-8 ounces of juice or another beverage, may also be mixed with applesauce or pudding. Administer with meals. If administering via feeding tube, mix with ≥60 mL water; do not add directly to feeding bag. Use immediately after preparation.

Storage: Store at controlled room temperature.

♦ **Glybenclamide** *see* GlyBURIDE *on page 720*

♦ **Glybenzcyclamide** *see* GlyBURIDE *on page 720*

GlyBURIDE (GLYE byoor ide)

U.S. Brand Names Diaβeta®; Glynase® PresTab®; Micronase®

Synonyms Diabeta; Glibenclamide; Glybenclamide; Glybenzcyclamide

Generic Available Yes

Pharmacologic Category Antidiabetic Agent, Sulfonylurea

Medication Safety Issues

Sound-alike/look-alike issues:

GlyBURIDE may be confused with glipiZIDE, Glucotrol®

Diaβeta® may be confused with Diabinese®, Zebeta®

Micronase® may be confused with microK®, miconazole, Micronor®

Use Management of type 2 diabetes mellitus (noninsulin dependent, NIDDM)

Unlabeled/Investigational Use Alternative to insulin in women for the treatment of gestational diabetes (11-33 weeks gestation)

Mechanism of Action/Effect Stimulates insulin release from the pancreatic beta cells; reduces glucose output from the liver; insulin sensitivity is increased at peripheral target sites

Contraindications Hypersensitivity to glyburide, any component of the formulation, or other sulfonamides; type 1 diabetes mellitus (insulin dependent, IDDM), diabetic ketoacidosis with or without coma

Warnings/Precautions Elderly: Rapid and prolonged hypoglycemia (>12 hours) despite hypertonic glucose injections have been reported; age and hepatic and renal impairment are independent risk factors for hypoglycemia; dosage titration should be made at weekly intervals. Use with caution in patients with renal and hepatic impairment, malnourished or debilitated conditions, or adrenal or pituitary insufficiency.

Chemical similarities are present among sulfonamides, sulfonylureas, carbonic anhydrase inhibitors, thiazides, and loop diuretics (except ethacrynic acid). Use in patients with sulfonamide allergy is specifically contraindicated in product labeling, however, a risk of cross-reaction exists in patients with allergy to any of these compounds; avoid use when previous reaction has been severe.

Product labeling states oral hypoglycemic drugs may be associated with an increased cardiovascular mortality as compared to treatment with diet alone or diet plus insulin. Data to support this association are limited, and several studies, including a large prospective trial (UKPDS) have not supported an association.

Drug Interactions

Cytochrome P450 Effect: Inhibits CYP3A4 (weak)

Decreased Effect: Thiazides and other diuretics, corticosteroids may decrease effectiveness of glyburide.

Increased Effect/Toxicity: Increased hypoglycemic effects of glyburide may occur with oral anticoagulants (warfarin), phenytoin, other hydantoins, salicylates, NSAIDs, sulfonamides, and beta-blockers. Ethanol ingestion may cause disulfiram reactions.

Nutritional/Ethanol Interactions

Ethanol: Caution with ethanol (may cause hypoglycemia).

Herb/Nutraceutical: Caution with chromium, garlic, gymnema (may cause hypoglycemia).

Adverse Reactions Frequency not defined.

Central nervous system: Headache, dizziness

Dermatologic: Pruritus, rash, urticaria, photosensitivity reaction

Endocrine & metabolic: Hypoglycemia, hyponatremia (SIADH reported with other sulfonylureas)

Gastrointestinal: Nausea, epigastric fullness, heartburn, constipation, diarrhea, anorexia

Genitourinary: Nocturia

Hematologic: Leukopenia, thrombocytopenia, hemolytic anemia, aplastic anemia, bone marrow suppression, agranulocytosis

Hepatic: Cholestatic jaundice, hepatitis

Neuromuscular & skeletal: Arthralgia, paresthesia

Ocular: Blurred vision

Renal: Diuretic effect (minor)

Overdosage/Toxicology Symptoms of overdose include severe hypoglycemia, seizures, cerebral damage, tingling of lips and tongue, nausea, yawning, confusion, agitation, tachycardia, sweating, convulsions, stupor, and coma. Intoxication with sulfonylureas can cause hypoglycemia and is best managed with glucose administration (oral for milder hypoglycemia or by injection in more severe forms).

Pharmacodynamics/Kinetics

Onset of Action: Serum insulin levels begin to increase 15-60 minutes after a single dose

Duration of Action: ≤24 hours

Time to Peak: Serum: Adults: 2-4 hours

Protein Binding: Plasma: >99%

Half-Life Elimination: 5-16 hours; may be prolonged with renal or hepatic impairment

Metabolism: To one moderately active and several inactive metabolites

Excretion: Feces (50%) and urine (50%) as metabolites

Dosing

Adults:

Type 2 diabetes: Oral:

Note: Regular tablets cannot be used interchangeably with micronized tablet formulations

Regular tablets (Diaβeta®, Micronase®):

Initial: 2.5-5 mg/day, administered with breakfast or the first main meal of the day. In patients who are more sensitive to hypoglycemic drugs, start at 1.25 mg/day.

Adjustment: Increase in increments of no more than 2.5 mg/day at weekly intervals based on the patient's blood glucose response

Maintenance: 1.25-20 mg/day given as single or divided doses; maximum: 20 mg/day

Micronized tablets (Glynase® PresTab®):

Initial: 1.5-3 mg/day, administered with breakfast or the first main meal of the day in patients who are more sensitive to hypoglycemic drugs, start at 0.75 mg/day. Increase in increments of no more than 1.5 mg/day in weekly intervals based on the patient's blood glucose response.

Maintenance: 0.75-12 mg/day given as a single dose or in divided doses. Some patients (especially those receiving >6 mg/day) may have a more satisfactory response with twice-daily dosing.

Elderly: Regular tablets (Diaβeta®, Micronase®): Oral: Initial: 1.25-2.5 mg/day, increase by 1.25-2.5 mg/day every 1-3 weeks. Refer to adult dosing.

Renal Impairment: Cl$_{cr}$ <50 mL/minute: Not recommended

Hepatic Impairment: Use conservative initial and maintenance doses and avoid use in severe disease.

Available Dosage Forms

Tablet (Diaβeta®, Micronase®): 1.25 mg, 2.5 mg, 5 mg

Tablet, micronized (Glynase® PresTab®): 1.5 mg, 3 mg, 6 mg

Monitoring and Teaching Issues

Physical Assessment: Assess allergy history prior to beginning therapy. Assess potential for interactions with other prescriptions, OTC medications, or herbal products patient may be taking. Assess results of laboratory tests, therapeutic effectiveness, and adverse response (eg, hypoglycemia) at regular intervals during therapy. Teach patient proper use (or refer patient to diabetic educator) for instruction, possible side effects/appropriate interventions, and adverse symptoms to report.

Monitoring Laboratory Tests: Fasting blood glucose, hemoglobin A$_{1c}$, fructosamine

Patient Education: Do not take any new medication during therapy unless approved by prescriber. This medication is used to control diabetes; it is not a cure. Monitor glucose as recommended by prescriber. Other important components of treatment plan may include prescribed diet and exercise regimen (consult prescriber or diabetic educator). If you experience hypoglycemic reaction, contact prescriber immediately. Always carry quick source of sugar with you. Take exactly as directed, 30 minutes before meal(s) at the same time each day. Do not change dose or discontinue without consulting prescriber. Avoid alcohol while taking this medication; could cause severe reaction. Do not take other medication within 2 hours of this medication unless advised by prescriber. You may experience more sensitivity to sunlight (use sunscreen, wear protective clothing and eyewear, and avoid direct sunlight); headache; or nausea (consult prescriber if these persist). Report severe or persistent side effects; hypoglycemia (palpitations, sweaty palms, lightheadedness); extended vomiting, diarrhea, or constipation; flu-like symptoms; skin rash; easy bruising or bleeding; or change in color of urine or stool. **Pregnancy/breast-feeding precautions:** Inform prescriber if you are or intend to become pregnant. Do not breast-feed.

Dietary Considerations: Should be taken with meals at the same time each day. Dietary modification based on ADA recommendations is a part of therapy. Decreases blood glucose concentration. Hypoglycemia may occur. Must be able to recognize symptoms of hypoglycemia (palpitations, sweaty palms, lightheadedness).

Geriatric Considerations: Rapid and prolonged hypoglycemia (>12 hours) despite hypertonic glucose injections have been reported; age, hepatic, and renal impairment are independent risk factors for hypoglycemia; conservative initial dosing and slow titration are required to avoid hypoglycemic reactions; dosage titration should be made at weekly intervals.

Pregnancy Risk Factor: C

Pregnancy Issues: Crosses the placenta. Hypoglycemia; ear defects reported; other malformations reported but may have been secondary to poor maternal glucose control/diabetes. Insulin is the drug of choice for the control of diabetes mellitus during pregnancy.

Lactation: Excretion in breast milk unknown/contraindicated

Administration

Oral: Administer with meals at the same time each day. Patients who are anorexic or NPO may need to have their dose held to avoid hypoglycemia.

Related Information

Diabetes Mellitus Management *on page 1819*

FDA Name Differentiation Project: The Use of Tall-Man Letters *on page 15*

Glyburide and Metformin (GLYE byoor ide & met FOR min)

U.S. Brand Names Glucovance®

Synonyms Glyburide and Metformin Hydrochloride; Metformin and Glyburide

(Continued)

Glyburide and Metformin *(Continued)*

Generic Available Yes

Pharmacologic Category Antidiabetic Agent, Biguanide; Antidiabetic Agent, Sulfonylurea

Use Initial therapy for management of type 2 diabetes mellitus (noninsulin dependent, NIDDM). Second-line therapy for management of type 2 diabetes (NIDDM) when hyperglycemia cannot be managed with a sulfonylurea or metformin; combination therapy with a thiazolidinedione may be required to achieve additional control.

Dosing

Adults: Note: Dose must be individualized. All doses should be taken with a meal. Twice daily dosage should be taken with the morning and evening meals. Dosages expressed as glyburide/metformin components.

Type 2 diabetes: Oral:

No prior treatment with sulfonylurea or metformin: Initial: 1.25 mg/250 mg once daily with a meal; patients with Hb A$_{1c}$ >9% or fasting plasma glucose (FPG) >200 mg/dL may start with 1.25 mg/250 mg twice daily. Adjustment: Dosage may be increased in increments of 1.25 mg/250 mg, at intervals of not less than 2 weeks; maximum daily dose: 10 mg/2000 mg (limited experience with higher doses)

Previously treated with a sulfonylurea or metformin alone: Initial: 2.5 mg/500 mg or 5 mg/500 mg twice daily; increase in increments no greater than 5 mg/500 mg; maximum daily dose: 20 mg/2000 mg

Note: When switching patients previously on a sulfonylurea and metformin together, do not exceed the daily dose of glyburide (or glyburide equivalent) or metformin.

Combination with thiazolidinedione: May be combined with a thiazolidinedione in patients with an inadequate response to glyburide/metformin therapy, however the risk of hypoglycemia may be increased.

Elderly: Refer to adult dosing. Adjust carefully to renal function. Should not be used in patients ≥80 years of age unless renal function is verified as normal.

Available Dosage Forms

Tablet [film coated]:

1.25 mg/250 mg: Glyburide 1.25 mg and metformin hydrochloride 250 mg

2.5 mg/500 mg: Glyburide 2.5 mg and metformin hydrochloride 500 mg

5 mg/500 mg: Glyburide 5 mg and metformin hydrochloride 500 mg

Monitoring and Teaching Issues

Physical Assessment: See individual agents.

Patient Education: See individual agents. **Pregnancy/breast-feeding precautions:** Inform prescriber if you are or intend to become pregnant. Consult prescriber if breast-feeding.

Pregnancy Risk Factor: B (manufacturer); C (expert analysis)

Lactation: No data available/use caution

Related Information

GlyBURIDE *on page 720*

Metformin *on page 965*

♦ **Glyburide and Metformin Hydrochloride** *see* Glyburide and Metformin *on page 721*

♦ **Glycerol Guaiacolate** *see* Guaifenesin *on page 729*

♦ **Glyceryl Trinitrate** *see* Nitroglycerin *on page 1090*

♦ **GlycoLax™** *see* Polyethylene Glycol-Electrolyte Solution *on page 1226*

Glycopyrrolate *(glye koe PYE roe late)*

U.S. Brand Names Robinul®; Robinul® Forte

Synonyms Glycopyrronium Bromide

Generic Available Yes: Injection

Pharmacologic Category Anticholinergic Agent

Use Inhibit salivation and excessive secretions of the respiratory tract preoperatively; reversal of neuromuscular blockade; control of upper airway secretions; adjunct in treatment of peptic ulcer

Mechanism of Action/Effect Blocks the action of acetylcholine at parasympathetic sites in smooth muscle, secretory glands, and the CNS

Contraindications Hypersensitivity to glycopyrrolate or any component of the formulation; severe ulcerative colitis, toxic megacolon complicating ulcerative colitis, paralytic ileus, obstructive disease of GI tract, intestinal atony in the elderly or debilitated patient; narrow-angle glaucoma; acute hemorrhage; tachycardia; obstructive uropathy; myasthenia gravis

Warnings/Precautions Not recommended in children <12 years of age for the management of peptic ulcer and <16 years for preanesthetic use. Infants, patients with Down syndrome, and children with spastic paralysis or brain damage may be hypersensitive to antimuscarine effects. Use caution in elderly, patients with autonomic neuropathy, hepatic or renal disease, ulcerative colitis may precipitate/aggravate toxic megacolon, hyperthyroidism, CAD, CHF, arrhythmias, tachycardia, BPH, or hiatal hernia with reflux. Caution should be used in individuals demonstrating decreased pigmentation (skin and iris coloration, dark versus light) since there has been some evidence that these individuals have an enhanced sensitivity to the anticholinergic response. May cause drowsiness, eye sensitivity to light, or blurred vision; caution should be used when performing tasks which require mental alertness, such as driving. The risk of heat stroke with this medication may be increased during exercise or hot weather. Product packaging may contain latex. Injection contains benzyl alcohol (associated with gasping syndrome in neonates).

Drug Interactions

Increased Effect/Toxicity: Effects of other anticholinergic agents or medications with anticholinergic activity may be increased by glycopyrrolate. Severity of potassium chloride-induced gastrointestinal lesions (when potassium is given in a wax matrix formulation) may be increased by glycopyrrolate.

Adverse Reactions Frequency not defined.

Cardiovascular: Arrhythmias, cardiac arrest, heart block, hyper-/hypotension, malignant hyperthermia, palpitation, QT_c interval prolongation, tachycardia

Central nervous system: Confusion, dizziness, drowsiness, excitement, headache, insomnia, nervousness, seizures

Dermatologic: Dry skin, pruritus, sensitivity to light increased

Endocrine & metabolic: Lactation suppression

Gastrointestinal: Bloated feeling, constipation, dry throat, dysphagia, loss of taste, nausea, vomiting, xerostomia

Genitourinary: Impotence, urinary hesitancy, urinary retention

Local: Irritation at injection site

Neuromuscular & skeletal: Weakness

Ocular: Blurred vision, cycloplegia, mydriasis, ocular tension increased, photophobia, sensitivity to light increased

Respiratory: Respiratory depression

Miscellaneous: Anaphylactoid reactions, diaphoresis decreased, hypersensitivity reactions

Overdosage/Toxicology Symptoms of overdose include blurred vision, urinary retention, tachycardia, and absent bowel sounds. For anticholinergic overdose with severe life-threatening symptoms, physostigmine 1-2 mg SubQ or I.V. slowly, may be given to reverse these effects.

Pharmacodynamics/Kinetics

Onset of Action: Oral: 50 minutes; I.M.: 15-30 minutes; I.V.: ~1 minute

Peak effect: Oral: ~1 hour; I.M.: 30-45 minutes

Duration of Action: Vagal effect: 2-3 hours; Inhibition of salivation: Up to 7 hours; Anticholinergic: Oral 8-12 hours

Absorption: Oral: Poor and erratic

Bioavailability: ~10%

Half-Life Elimination: ~30-75 minutes

Metabolism: Hepatic (minimal)

Excretion: Urine

Dosing

Adults & Elderly:

Reduction of secretions: I.M.:

Preoperative: I.M.: 4.4 mcg/kg 30-60 minutes before procedure

Intraoperative: I.V.: 0.1 mg repeated as needed at 2- to 3-minute intervals

Reversal of neuromuscular blockade: I.V.: 0.2 mg for each 1 mg of neostigmine or 5 mg of pyridostigmine administered or 5-15 mcg/kg glycopyrrolate with 25-70 mcg/kg of neostigmine or 0.1-0.3 mg/kg of pyridostigmine (agents usually administered simultaneously, but glycopyrrolate may be administered first if bradycardia is present)

Peptic ulcer:

Oral: 1-2 mg 2-3 times/day

I.M., I.V.: 0.1-0.2 mg 3-4 times/day

Pediatrics:

Reduction of secretions:

Preoperative: I.M.:

<2 years: 4.4-8.8 mcg/kg 30-60 minutes before procedure

>2 years: 4.4 mcg/kg 30-60 minutes before procedure

Intraoperative: I.V.: 4 mcg/kg not to exceed 0.1 mg; repeat at 2- to 3-minute intervals as needed.

Chronic:

Oral: 40-100 mcg/kg/dose 3-4 times/day

I.M., I.V.: 4-10 mcg/kg/dose every 3-4 hours; maximum: 0.2 mg/dose or 0.8 mg/24 hours

Reversal of neuromuscular blockade: Refer to adult dosing.

Available Dosage Forms

Injection, solution (Robinul®): 0.2 mg/mL (1 mL, 2 mL, 5 mL, 20 mL) [contains benzyl alcohol]

Tablet:

Robinul®: 1 mg

Robinul® Forte: 2 mg

Monitoring and Teaching Issues

Physical Assessment: Assess potential for interactions with other prescriptions, OTC medications, or herbal products patient may be taking (eg, anything that may add to anticholinergic effects). Assess therapeutic effectiveness and adverse response (eg, excessive dryness: Eyes, nose, mouth, throat). Teach patient proper use (self-administered), possible side effects/appropriate interventions, and adverse symptoms to report.

Patient Education: Do not take any new medication during therapy unless approved by prescriber. Take as directed before meals; do not increase dose and do not discontinue without consulting prescriber. Void before taking medication. You may experience dizziness or blurred vision (use caution when driving or engaging in tasks that require alertness until response to drug is known); dry mouth (sucking on lozenges may help); photosensitivity (wear dark glasses in bright sunlight); decreased ability to sweat (use caution in hot weather or hot rooms or engaging in strenuous activity); or impotence (temporary). Report excessive and persistent anticholinergic effects (blurred vision, headache, flushing, tachycardia, nervousness, constipation, dizziness, insomnia, mental confusion or excitement, dry mouth, altered taste perception, dysphagia, palpitations, bradycardia, urinary hesitancy or retention, impotence, decreased sweating). **Breast-feeding precaution:** Consult prescriber if breast-feeding.

Geriatric Considerations: Anticholinergic agents are generally not well tolerated in the elderly and their use should be avoided when possible.

(Continued)

Glycopyrrolate *(Continued)*

Pregnancy Risk Factor: B
Lactation: Excretion in breast milk unknown
Administration
  I.V.: Administer at a rate of 0.2 mg over 1-2 minutes.
  Compatibility: Stable in $D_5^1/_2NS$, D_5W, $D_{10}W$, LR, NS
    Compatibility in syringe: Incompatible with chloramphenicol, dexamethasone sodium phosphate, diazepam, dimenhydrinate, methohexital, pentazocine, pentobarbital, secobarbital, sodium bicarbonate, thiopental
    Compatibility when admixed: Incompatible with methylprednisolone sodium succinate
  Storage: Store at 20°C to 25°C (68°F to 77°F).
Related Information
  Compatibility of Drugs *on page 1723*
  Compatibility of Drugs in Syringe *on page 1725*

- **Glycopyrronium Bromide** *see* Glycopyrrolate *on page 722*
- **Glydiazinamide** *see* GlipiZIDE *on page 715*
- **Glynase® PresTab®** *see* GlyBURIDE *on page 720*
- **Glyquin®** *see* Hydroquinone *on page 768*
- **Glyquin-XM™** *see* Hydroquinone *on page 768*
- **Glyset®** *see* Miglitol *on page 1008*
- **GM-CSF** *see* Sargramostim *on page 1358*
- **GnRH** *see* Gonadorelin *on page 724*
- **GoLYTELY®** *see* Polyethylene Glycol-Electrolyte Solution *on page 1226*

Gonadorelin *(goe nad oh RELL in)*

U.S. Brand Names Factrel®
Synonyms GnRH; Gonadorelin Acetate; Gonadorelin Hydrochloride; Gonadotropin Releasing Hormone; LHRH; LRH; Luteinizing Hormone Releasing Hormone
Generic Available No
Pharmacologic Category Diagnostic Agent; Gonadotropin
Medication Safety Issues
  Sound-alike/look-alike issues:
    Gonadorelin may be confused with gonadotropin, guanadrel
    Factrel® may be confused with Sectral®
    Gonadotropin may be confused with gonadorelin
Use Evaluation of functional capacity and response of gonadotrophic hormones; evaluate abnormal gonadotropin regulation as in precocious puberty and delayed puberty.
  Orphan drug: Lutrepulse®: Induction of ovulation in females with hypothalamic amenorrhea
Mechanism of Action/Effect Stimulates the release of luteinizing hormone (LH) from the anterior pituitary gland
Contraindications Hypersensitivity to gonadorelin or any component of the formulation; women with any condition that could be exacerbated by pregnancy; patients who have ovarian cysts or causes of anovulation other than those of hypothalamic origin; any condition that may worsened by reproductive hormones
Warnings/Precautions Hypersensitivity and anaphylactic reactions have occurred following multiple-dose administration. Use with caution in women in whom pregnancy could worsen pre-existing conditions (eg, pituitary prolactinemia). Multiple pregnancy is a possibility with gonadorelin.
Drug Interactions
  Decreased Effect: Decreased levels/effect with oral contraceptives, digoxin, phenothiazines, and dopamine antagonists.
  Increased Effect/Toxicity: Increased levels/effect with androgens, estrogens, progestins, glucocorticoids, spironolactone, and levodopa.
Adverse Reactions 1% to 10%: Local: Pain at injection site
Overdosage/Toxicology Symptoms of overdose include abdominal discomfort, nausea, headache, and flushing. Treatment is symptomatic.
Pharmacodynamics/Kinetics
  Onset of Action: Peak effect: Maximal LH release: ~20 minutes
  Duration of Action: 3-5 hours
  Half-Life Elimination: 4 minutes
Dosing
  Adults:
    Diagnostic test: I.V., SubQ (hydrochloride salt): 100 mcg administered in women during early phase of menstrual cycle (day 1-7)
    Primary hypothalamic amenorrhea: I.V. (acetate): 5 mcg every 90 minutes via Lutrepulse® pump kit at treatment intervals of 21 days (pump will pulsate every 90 minutes for 7 days)
  Pediatrics: Diagnostic test: Children >12 years: Refer to adult dosing.
Available Dosage Forms Injection, powder for reconstitution, as hydrochloride (Factrel®): 100 mcg [diluent contains benzyl alcohol]
Monitoring and Teaching Issues
  Physical Assessment: Assess other medications patient may be taking for effectiveness and interactions. When used for induction of ovulation, assess results of laboratory tests and therapeutic effectiveness. Assess knowledge/teach patient appropriate use (use of pulsating pump if applicable), interventions to reduce side effects, and adverse symptoms to report.
  Monitoring Laboratory Tests: LH, FSH
  Patient Education: If receiving this drug via pulsating pump, check all procedures with prescriber, and use exactly as prescribed. Report any rash, pain, or inflammation at

injection site, and any change in respiratory status. **Breast-feeding precaution:** Consult prescriber if breast-feeding.

Pregnancy Risk Factor: B

Lactation: Excretion in breast milk unknown

Administration

I.V.:

Factrel®: Give I.V. push over 30 seconds.

Lutrepulse®: A presterilized reservoir bag with the infusion catheter set supplied with the kit should be filled with the reconstituted solution and administered I.V. using the Lutrepulse® pump. Set the pump to deliver 25-50 mL of solution, based upon the dose, over a pulse period of 1 minute and at a pulse frequency of 90 minutes.

Reconstitution:

Factrel®: Prepare immediately prior to use. After reconstitution, store at room temperature and use within 1 day. Discard unused portion.

Lutrepulse®: Reconstitute with diluent immediately prior to use and transfer to plastic reservoir. The solution will supply 90-minute pulsatile doses for 7 consecutive days (Lutrepulse® pump).

♦ **Gonadorelin Acetate** *see* Gonadorelin *on page 724*

♦ **Gonadorelin Hydrochloride** *see* Gonadorelin *on page 724*

♦ **Gonadotropin Releasing Hormone** *see* Gonadorelin *on page 724*

♦ **Gonak**™ *see page 1625*

♦ **Gonal-f**® *see* Follitropins *on page 670*

♦ **Gonal-f**™ **RFF** *see* Follitropins *on page 670*

♦ **Goniosol**® *see page 1625*

Goserelin (GOE se rel in)

U.S. Brand Names Zoladex®

Synonyms D-Ser(Buᵗ)⁶,Azgly¹⁰-LHRH; Goserelin Acetate; ICI-118630; NSC-606864

Generic Available No

Pharmacologic Category Gonadotropin Releasing Hormone Agonist

Use Palliative treatment of advanced breast cancer and carcinoma of the prostate; treatment of endometriosis, including pain relief and reduction of endometriotic lesions; endometrial thinning agent as part of treatment for dysfunctional uterine bleeding

Mechanism of Action/Effect LHRH synthetic analog of luteinizing hormone-releasing hormone also known as gonadotropin-releasing hormone (GnRH)

Contraindications Hypersensitivity to goserelin or any component of the formulation; pregnancy (or potential to become pregnant); breast-feeding

Warnings/Precautions Transient worsening of signs and symptoms, usually manifested by an increase in cancer-related pain, may develop during the first few weeks of treatment. Urinary tract obstruction or spinal cord compression have been reported when used for prostate cancer; closely observe patients for weakness, paresthesias, and urinary tract obstruction in first few weeks of therapy. Decreased bone density has been reported in women and may be irreversible; use caution if other risk factors are present; evaluate and institute preventative treatment if necessary. Safety and efficacy have not been established in pediatric patients.

Lab Interactions Serum alkaline phosphatase, serum acid phosphatase, serum testosterone, serum LH and FSH, serum estradiol

Adverse Reactions Percentages reported in males with prostatic carcinoma and females with endometriosis using the 1-month implant:

>10%:

Central nervous system: Headache (female 75%, male 1% to 5%), emotional lability (female 60%), depression (female 54%, male 1% to 5%), pain (female 17%, male 8%), insomnia (female 11%, male 5%)

Endocrine & metabolic: Hot flashes (female 96%, male 62%), sexual dysfunction (21%), erections decreased (18%), libido decreased (female 61%), breast enlargement (female 18%)

Genitourinary: Lower urinary symptoms (male 13%), vaginitis (75%), dyspareunia (female 14%)

Miscellaneous: Diaphoresis (female 45%, male 6%); infection (female 13%)

1% to 10%:

Cardiovascular: CHF (male 5%), arrhythmia, cerebrovascular accident, hypertension, MI, peripheral vascular disorder, chest pain, palpitation, tachycardia, edema

Central nervous system: Lethargy (male 8%), dizziness (female 6%, male 5%), abnormal thinking, anxiety, chills, fever, malaise, migraine, somnolence

Dermatologic: Rash (female >1%, male 6%), alopecia, bruising, dry skin, skin discoloration

Endocrine & metabolic: Breast pain (female 7%), breast swelling/tenderness (male 1% to 5%), dysmenorrhea, gout, hyperglycemia

Gastrointestinal: Anorexia (female >1%, male 5%), nausea (male 5%), constipation, diarrhea, flatulence, dyspepsia, ulcer, vomiting, weight increased, xerostomia

Genitourinary: Renal insufficiency, urinary frequency, urinary obstruction, urinary tract infection, vaginal hemorrhage

Hematologic: Anemia, hemorrhage

Neuromuscular & skeletal: Arthralgia, bone mineral density decreased (female; ~4% decrease in 6 months), joint disorder, paresthesia

Ocular: Amblyopia, dry eyes

Respiratory: Upper respiratory tract infection (male 7%), COPD (male 5%), pharyngitis (female 5%), bronchitis, cough, epistaxis, rhinitis, sinusitis

Miscellaneous: Allergic reaction

Overdosage/Toxicology Symptomatic management

(Continued)

Goserelin (Continued)

Pharmacodynamics/Kinetics
Absorption: SubQ: Rapid and can be detected in serum in 10 minutes

Time to Peak: SubQ: Male: 12-15 days, Female: 8-22 days

Half-Life Elimination: SubQ: Male: ~4 hours, Female: ~2 hours; Renal impairment: Male: 12 hours

Excretion: Urine (90%)

Pharmacokinetic Note: Data reported using the 1-month implant.

Dosing
Adults & Elderly:
Prostate cancer: SubQ:

Monthly implant: 3.6 mg injected into upper abdomen every 28 days

3-month implant: 10.8 mg injected into the upper abdominal wall every 12 weeks

Note: Treatment should begin 8 weeks prior to radiotherapy in Stage B2-C prostate cancer; treatment may continue indefinitely

Breast cancer, endometriosis, endometrial thinning: SubQ: Monthly implant: 3.6 mg injected into upper abdomen every 28 days

Note: For breast cancer, treatment may continue indefinitely; for endometriosis, it is recommended that duration of treatment not exceed 6 months. Only 1-2 doses are recommended for endometrial thinning.

Available Dosage Forms
Injection, solution, 1-month implant [disposable syringe; single-dose]: 3.6 mg [with 16-gauge hypodermic needle]

Injection, solution, 3-month implant [disposable syringe; single-dose]: 10.8 mg [with 14-gauge hypodermic needle]

Monitoring and Teaching Issues
Physical Assessment: Assess potential for interactions with other prescriptions, OTC medications, or herbal products patient may be taking. Assess therapeutic effectiveness and adverse response periodically during therapy. Teach patient proper use, possible side effects/appropriate interventions, and adverse symptoms to report. **Pregnancy risk factor X:** Determine that patient is not pregnant before beginning treatment. Do not give to women of childbearing age unless female is capable of complying with contraceptive measures 1 month prior to therapy, during therapy, and at least 12 weeks following therapy. Instruct patient in appropriate contraceptive measures.

Patient Education: Do not take any new medication during therapy unless approved by prescriber. This drug must be implanted under the skin of your abdomen every 28 days; it is important to maintain appointment schedule. Males or females, you may experience systemic hot flashes (layered, cool clothes may help); headache (consult prescriber for approved analgesic); constipation (increased bulk and water in diet or stool softener may help); sexual dysfunction (decreased libido, males: decreased erection, females: vaginal dryness); or bone pain (consult prescriber for approved analgesic). Symptoms may worsen temporarily during first weeks of therapy. Report chest pain, palpitations, or respiratory difficulty; swelling of extremities; unusual persistent nausea, vomiting, or constipation; chest pain or respiratory difficulty; unresolved dizziness; or skin rash. **Pregnancy/breast-feeding precautions:** Inform prescriber if you are pregnant; do not get pregnant 1 month before, during, or for 1 month following therapy. Consult prescriber for instruction on appropriate contraceptive measures. This drug may cause severe fetal defects. Do not donate blood during or for 1 month following therapy (same reason). Do not breast-feed.

Pregnancy Risk Factor: X (endometriosis, endometrial thinning); D (advanced breast cancer)

Pregnancy Issues: Goserelin has been found to be teratogenic and increases pregnancy loss in animal studies. Women of childbearing potential should avoid pregnancy. Pregnancy must be ruled out prior to treatment. Use of nonhormonal contraception should be used during therapy and following discontinuation until the return of menses (or for at least 12 weeks).

Lactation: Enters breast milk/contraindicated

Administration
Other: Subcutaneous implant: Insert the hypodermic needle into the subcutaneous fat. Do not try to aspirate with the goserelin syringe. If the needle is in a large vessel, blood will immediately appear in the syringe chamber. Change the direction of the needle so it parallels the abdominal wall. Push the needle in until the barrel hub touches the patient's skin. Fully depress the plunger to discharge. Withdraw needle and bandage the site. Confirm discharge by ensuring tip of the plunger is visible within the tip of the needle.

Storage: Zoladex® should be stored at room temperature not to exceed 25°C (77°F). Protect from light. Should be dispensed in a lightproof bag.

♦ **Goserelin Acetate** *see Goserelin on page 725*

♦ **GP 47680** *see Oxcarbazepine on page 1132*

♦ **G-Phed** *see Guaifenesin and Pseudoephedrine on page 733*

♦ **GR38032R** *see Ondansetron on page 1119*

Granisetron (gra NI se tron)
U.S. Brand Names Kytril®

Synonyms BRL 43694

Generic Available No

Pharmacologic Category Antiemetic; Selective 5-HT$_3$ Receptor Antagonist

Use Prophylaxis of chemotherapy-related emesis; prophylaxis of nausea and vomiting associated with radiation therapy, including total body irradiation and fractionated abdominal radiation; prophylaxis of postoperative nausea and vomiting (PONV)

Generally **not** recommended for treatment of existing chemotherapy-induced emesis (CIE) or for prophylaxis of nausea from agents with a low emetogenic potential.

Mechanism of Action/Effect Selective 5-HT$_3$ receptor antagonist, blocking serotonin, both peripherally on vagal nerve terminals and centrally in the chemoreceptor trigger zone.

Contraindications Previous hypersensitivity to granisetron, other 5-HT$_3$ receptor antagonists, or any component of the formulation

Warnings/Precautions Chemotherapy-related emesis: **Granisetron should be used on a scheduled basis, not on an "as needed" (PRN) basis**, since data support the use of this drug in the prevention of nausea and vomiting and not in the rescue of nausea and vomiting. Granisetron should be used only in the first 24-48 hours of receiving chemotherapy or radiation. Data do not support any increased efficacy of granisetron in delayed nausea and vomiting. May be prescribed for patients who are refractory to or have severe adverse reactions to standard antiemetic therapy or young patients (ie, <45 years of age who are more likely to develop extrapyramidal symptoms to high-dose metoclopramide) who are to receive highly emetogenic chemotherapeutic agents. Should not be prescribed for chemotherapeutic agents with a low emetogenic potential (eg, bleomycin, busulfan, etoposide, 5-fluorouracil, vinblastine, vincristine).

Routine prophylaxis for PONV is not recommended. In patients where nausea and vomiting must be avoided postoperatively, administer to all patients even when expected incidence of nausea and vomiting is low. Use caution following abdominal surgery or in chemotherapy-induced nausea and vomiting; may mask progressive ileus or gastric distention. Use caution in patients with liver disease or in pregnancy. Safety and efficacy in children <2 years of age have not been established. Injection contains benzyl alcohol and should not be used in neonates.

Drug Interactions
  Cytochrome P450 Effect: Substrate of CYP3A4 (minor)

Nutritional/Ethanol Interactions Herb/Nutraceutical: St John's wort may decrease granisetron levels.

Adverse Reactions
  >10%:
    Central nervous system: Headache (8% to 21%)
    Gastrointestinal: Constipation (3% to 18%)
  1% to 10%:
    Cardiovascular: Hypertension (1% to 2%)
    Central nervous system: Dizziness, insomnia, anxiety, somnolence, fever (3% to 8%), pain (10%)
    Gastrointestinal: Abdominal pain, diarrhea (1% to 9%), dyspepsia
    Hepatic: Elevated liver enzymes (5% to 6%)
    Neuromuscular & skeletal: Weakness (5% to 18%)

Overdosage/Toxicology Treatment should be symptomatic and supportive.

Pharmacodynamics/Kinetics
  Duration of Action: Generally up to 24 hours
  Protein Binding: 65%
  Half-Life Elimination: Cancer patients: 10-12 hours; Healthy volunteers: 4-5 hours; PONV: 9 hours
  Metabolism: Hepatic via N-demethylation, oxidation, and conjugation; some metabolites may have 5-HT$_3$ antagonist activity
  Excretion: Urine (12% as unchanged drug, 49% as metabolites); feces (34% as metabolites)

Dosing
  Adults & Elderly:
    Prophylaxis of chemotherapy-related emesis:
      Oral: 2 mg once daily up to 1 hour before chemotherapy or 1 mg twice daily; the first 1 mg dose should be given up to 1 hour before chemotherapy.
      I.V.:
        Within U.S.: 10 mcg/kg/dose (or 1 mg/dose) administered IVPB over 5 minutes given within 30 minutes of chemotherapy: for some drugs (eg, carboplatin, cyclophosphamide) with a later onset of emetic action, 10 mcg/kg every 12 hours may be necessary.
        Outside U.S.: 40 mcg/kg/dose (or 3 mg/dose); maximum: 9 mg/24 hours
        Breakthrough: Repeat the dose 2-3 times within the first 24 hours as necessary **(not based on controlled trials, or generally recommended)**
    Prophylaxis of radiation therapy-associated emesis: Oral: 2 mg once daily given 1 hour before radiation therapy.
    Postoperative nausea and vomiting (PONV): I.V.:
      Prevention: 1 mg given undiluted over 30 seconds; administer before induction of anesthesia or before reversal of anesthesia
      Treatment: 1 mg given undiluted over 30 seconds
  Pediatrics: Prophylaxis associated with cancer chemotherapy: Children >2 years: Refer to adult dosing.
  Renal Impairment: No dosage adjustment required.
  Hepatic Impairment: Kinetic studies in patients with hepatic impairment showed that total clearance was approximately halved; however, standard doses were very well tolerated.

Available Dosage Forms
  Injection, solution: 1 mg/mL (4 mL) [contains benzyl alcohol]
  Injection, solution [preservative free]: 0.1 mg/mL (1 mL); 1 mg/mL (1 mL)
  Solution, oral: 2 mg/10 mL (30 mL) [contains sodium benzoate; orange flavor]
  Tablet: 1 mg

Monitoring and Teaching Issues
  Physical Assessment: See Warnings/Precautions for specific use cautions. Blood pressure and cardiac status should be monitored. Assess therapeutic effectiveness (antiemetic) and adverse response (eg, acute headache, CNS changes; see Adverse Reactions) periodically during therapy. Teach patient proper use (self-administered oral) possible side effects/appropriate interventions and adverse symptoms to report (see Patient Education).
  (Continued)

Granisetron *(Continued)*

Patient Education: This drug will be administered on days when you receive chemotherapy to reduce nausea and vomiting. If outpatient chemotherapy, you may be given oral medication to take after return home; take as directed. May also be given to prevent or treat nausea and vomiting after surgery; take as directed. You may experience drowsiness (use caution when driving); persistent or acute headache (request analgesic from prescriber); or nausea (frequent mouth care, chewing gum, or sucking on lozenges may help). Report unrelieved headache, fever, diarrhea, constipation, or abdominal pain. **Breast-feeding precaution:** Consult prescriber if breast-feeding.

Geriatric Considerations: Clinical trials with patients older than 65 years of age are limited; however, the data indicates that safety and efficacy are similar to that observed in younger adults. No adjustment in dose necessary for elderly.

Pregnancy Risk Factor: B

Lactation: Excretion in breast milk unknown/use caution

Administration

Oral: Doses should be given up to 1 hour prior to initiation of chemotherapy/radiation

I.V.: Administer as rapid (30 second) I.V. push or a short (5-10 minutes) infusion.
> For prevention of PONV, administer before induction of anesthesia or before reversal of anesthesia.
> For PONV, administer undiluted over 30 seconds.

Compatibility: Stable in $D_5\frac{1}{2}NS$, D_5NS, D_5W, NS, bacteriostatic water

Y-site administration: Incompatible with amphotericin B

Storage:
> I.V.: Store at 25°C (77°F); excursions permitted to 15°C to 30°C (59°F to 86°F). Protect from light. Do not freeze vials. Stable when mixed in NS or D_5W for 7 days under refrigeration and for 3 days at room temperature.
> Oral: Store tablet or oral solution at 15°C to 30°C (59°F to 86°F). Protect from light.

Related Information

Antiemetics for Chemotherapy-Induced Nausea and Vomiting *on page 1788*

- **Granulocyte Colony Stimulating Factor** *see Filgrastim on page 627*
- **Granulocyte-Macrophage Colony Stimulating Factor** *see Sargramostim on page 1358*
- **Grifulvin® V** *see Griseofulvin on page 728*

Griseofulvin *(gri see oh FUL vin)*

U.S. Brand Names Grifulvin® V; Gris-PEG®

Synonyms Griseofulvin Microsize; Griseofulvin Ultramicrosize

Generic Available Yes: Ultramicrosized product

Pharmacologic Category Antifungal Agent, Oral

Medication Safety Issues
Sound-alike/look-alike issues:
> Fulvicin® may be confused with Furacin®

Use Treatment of susceptible tinea infections of the skin, hair, and nails

Mechanism of Action/Effect Inhibits fungal cell mitosis at metaphase; binds to human keratin making it resistant to fungal invasion

Contraindications Hypersensitivity to griseofulvin or any component of the formulation; severe liver disease; porphyria (interferes with porphyrin metabolism)

Warnings/Precautions Safe use in children ≤2 years of age has not been established; during long-term therapy, periodic assessment of hepatic, renal, and hematopoietic functions should be performed; may cause fetal harm when administered to pregnant women; avoid exposure to intense sunlight to prevent photosensitivity reactions; hypersensitivity cross reaction between penicillins and griseofulvin is possible.

Drug Interactions

Cytochrome P450 Effect: Induces CYP1A2 (weak), 2C8/9 (weak), 3A4 (weak)

Decreased Effect: Barbiturates may decrease levels. Decreased warfarin activity. Decreased oral contraceptive effectiveness.

Increased Effect/Toxicity: Increased toxicity with ethanol, may cause tachycardia and flushing.

Nutritional/Ethanol Interactions
Ethanol: Avoid ethanol (may increase CNS depression). Ethanol will cause "disulfiram"-type reaction consisting of flushing, headache, nausea, and in some patients, vomiting and chest and/or abdominal pain.
Food: Griseofulvin concentrations may be increased if taken with food, especially with high-fat meals.

Lab Interactions False-positive urinary VMA levels

Adverse Reactions Frequency not defined.
Central nervous system: Headache, fatigue, dizziness, insomnia, mental confusion
Dermatologic: Rash (most common), urticaria (most common), photosensitivity, erythema multiforme, angioneurotic edema (rare)
Gastrointestinal: Nausea, vomiting, epigastric distress, diarrhea, GI bleeding
Genitourinary: Menstrual irregularities (rare)
Hematologic: Leukopenia, granulocytopenia
Neuromuscular & skeletal: Paresthesia (rare)
Renal: Hepatotoxicity, proteinuria, nephrosis
Miscellaneous: Oral thrush, drug-induced lupus-like syndrome (rare)

Overdosage/Toxicology Symptoms of overdose include lethargy, vertigo, blurred vision, nausea, vomiting, and diarrhea. Treatment is supportive.

Pharmacodynamics/Kinetics

Absorption: Ultramicrosize griseofulvin absorption is almost complete; absorption of microsize griseofulvin is variable (25% to 70% of an oral dose); enhanced by ingestion of a fatty meal (GI absorption of ultramicrosize is ~1.5 times that of microsize)

Half-Life Elimination: 9-22 hours
Metabolism: Extensively hepatic
Excretion: Urine (<1% as unchanged drug); feces; perspiration
Dosing
Adults & Elderly:
Tinea infections: Oral:
Microsize: 500-1000 mg/day in single or divided doses
Ultramicrosize: 330-375 mg/day in single or divided doses; doses up to 750 mg/day have been used for infections more difficult to eradicate such as tinea unguium and tinea pedis.
Note: Duration of therapy depends on the site of infection:
Tinea corporis: 2-4 weeks
Tinea capitis: 4-6 weeks or longer (up to 8-12 weeks)
Tinea pedis: 4-8 weeks
Tinea unguium: 4-6 months
Pediatrics:
Tinea infections: Oral: Children >2 years:
Microsize: 10-15 mg/kg/day in single or divided doses. In the treatment of tinea capitis, higher dosages (20-25 mg/kg/day for 8-12 weeks) have been recommended by some authors (unlabeled).
Ultramicrosize: 5.5-7.3 mg/kg/day in single or divided doses. In the treatment of tinea capitis, higher dosages (15 mg/kg/day for 8-12 weeks) have been recommended by some authors (unlabeled).
Available Dosage Forms
Suspension, oral, microsize (Grifulvin® V): 125 mg/5 mL (120 mL) [contains alcohol 0.2%]
Tablet, microsize (Grifulvin® V): 500 mg
Tablet, ultramicrosize: 125 mg, 250 mg, 330 mg
Gris-PEG®: 125 mg, 250 mg
Monitoring and Teaching Issues
Physical Assessment: Assess allergic history prior to beginning treatment (see Warnings/Precautions). Assess potential for interactions with other pharmacological agents or herbal products patient may be taking (eg, decreased effectiveness of oral contraceptives; see Drug Interactions). Monitor results of laboratory tests, therapeutic effectiveness (resolution of viral infection), and adverse response periodically during therapy (eg, CNS changes, gastrointestinal upset, rash, opportunistic infection; see Adverse Reactions). Teach patient proper use, possible side effects/appropriate interventions and adverse symptoms to report (see Patient Education).
Monitoring Laboratory Tests: Periodic renal, hepatic, and hematopoietic function especially with long-term use
Patient Education: Take as directed, around-the-clock with food. Take full course of medication even if symptoms abate; do not discontinue without consulting prescriber. Avoid alcohol while taking this drug (may cause adverse reactions). Practice good hygiene measures to prevent reinfection. Frequent blood tests may be required with prolonged therapy. You may experience nausea, vomiting, or diarrhea (small frequent meals, frequent mouth care, sucking lozenges, or chewing gum may help); confusion, dizziness, drowsiness (use caution when driving or engaging in tasks that require alertness until response to drug is known); or increased sensitivity to sun (use sunscreen, wear protective clothing and eyewear, and avoid excessive exposure to direct sunlight). Report skin rash; respiratory difficulty; CNS changes (confusion, dizziness, acute headache); changes in color of stool or urine; white plaques in mouth; or worsening of condition. **Pregnancy/breast-feeding precautions:** Inform prescriber if you are or intend to become pregnant. This medication may interfere with oral contraceptives; consult prescriber for appropriate contraceptive. Consult prescriber if breast-feeding.
Pregnancy Risk Factor: C
Lactation: Excretion in breast milk unknown
Administration
Oral: Oral: Administer with a fatty meal (peanuts or ice cream) to increase absorption, or with food or milk to avoid GI upset

◆ **Griseofulvin Microsize** *see* Griseofulvin *on page 728*
◆ **Griseofulvin Ultramicrosize** *see* Griseofulvin *on page 728*
◆ **Gris-PEG®** *see* Griseofulvin *on page 728*
◆ **Growth Hormone** *see* Human Growth Hormone *on page 745*
◆ **Guaifen-C** *see* Guaifenesin and Codeine *on page 731*

Guaifenesin (gwye FEN e sin)
U.S. Brand Names Allfen Jr; Diabetic Tussin® EX [OTC]; Ganidin NR; Guiatuss™ [OTC]; Humibid® e [OTC]; Iophen NR; Mucinex® [OTC]; Naldecon Senior EX® [OTC]; Organ-1 NR; Organidin® NR; Phanasin [OTC]; Phanasin® Diabetic Choice [OTC]; Q-Tussin [OTC]; Robitussin® [OTC]; Scot-Tussin® Expectorant [OTC]; Siltussin DAS [OTC]; Siltussin SA [OTC]; Tussin [OTC]
Synonyms GG; Glycerol Guaiacolate
Generic Available Yes: Excludes extended release
Pharmacologic Category Expectorant
Medication Safety Issues
Sound-alike/look-alike issues:
Guaifenesin may be confused with guanfacine
Mucinex® may be confused with Mucomyst®
Naldecon® may be confused with Nalfon®
Use Help loosen phlegm and thin bronchial secretions to make coughs more productive
Mechanism of Action/Effect Thought to act as an expectorant by irritating the gastric mucosa and stimulating respiratory tract secretions, thereby increasing respiratory fluid volumes and decreasing mucus viscosity
(Continued)

Guaifenesin *(Continued)*

Contraindications Hypersensitivity to guaifenesin or any component of the formulation

Warnings/Precautions Not for persistent cough such as occurs with smoking, asthma, chronic bronchitis, or emphysema or cough accompanied by excessive secretions. When used for self-medication (OTC), contact healthcare provider if needed for >7 days or for a cough with a fever, rash, or persistent headache.

Lab Interactions Possible color interference with determination of 5-HIAA and VMA; discontinue 48 hours prior to test

Adverse Reactions Frequency not defined.

Central nervous system: Dizziness, drowsiness, headache

Dermatologic: Rash

Endocrine & metabolic: Uric acid levels decreased

Gastrointestinal: Nausea, vomiting, stomach pain

Postmarketing and/or case reports: Kidney stone formation (with consumption of large quantities)

Overdosage/Toxicology Symptoms of overdose include vomiting, lethargy, coma, and respiratory depression. Treatment is supportive.

Pharmacodynamics/Kinetics

Absorption: Well absorbed

Half-Life Elimination: ~1 hour

Excretion: Urine (as unchanged drug and metabolites)

Dosing

Adults & Elderly:

Cough (expectorant): Oral: 200-400 mg every 4 hours to a maximum of 2.4 g/day

Extended release tablet: 600-1200 mg every 12 hours, not to exceed 2.4 g/day

Pediatrics:

Cough (expectorant): Oral: Children:

6 months to 2 years: 25-50 mg every 4 hours, not to exceed 300 mg/day

2-5 years: 50-100 mg every 4 hours, not to exceed 600 mg/day

6-11 years: 100-200 mg every 4 hours, not to exceed 1.2 g/day

>12 years: Refer to adult dosing.

Available Dosage Forms

Liquid: 100 mg/5 mL (120 mL, 480 mL)

Diabetic Tussin EX®: 100 mg/5 mL (120 mL) [alcohol free, sugar free, dye free; contains phenylalanine 8.4 mg/5 mL]

Ganidin NR: 100 mg/5 mL (480 mL) [raspberry flavor]

Iophen NR: 100 mg/5 mL (480 mL)

Naldecon Senior EX®: 200 mg/5 mL (120 mL) [alcohol free, sugar free; contains sodium benzoate]

Organidin® NR: 100 mg/5 mL (480 mL) [contains sodium benzoate; raspberry flavor]

Q-Tussin: 100 mg/5 mL (120 mL, 240 mL, 480 mL, 3840 mL) [alcohol free; cherry flavor]

Siltussin DAS: 100 mg/5 mL (120 mL) [alcohol free, dye free, sugar free; strawberry flavor]

Syrup: 100 mg/5 mL (120 mL, 480 mL)

Guiatuss™: 100 mg/5 mL (120 mL, 480 mL) [alcohol free; fruit-mint flavor]

Phanasin: 100 mg/5 mL (120 mL, 240 mL) [alcohol free, sugar free; mint flavor]

Phanasin® Diabetic Choice: 100 mg/5 mL (120 mL) [alcohol free, sugar free; mint flavor]

Robitussin®: 100 mg/5 mL (5 mL, 10 mL, 15 mL, 30 mL, 120 mL, 240 mL, 480 mL) [alcohol free; contains sodium benzoate]

Scot-Tussin® Expectorant: 100 mg/5 mL (120 mL) [alcohol free, dye free, sugar free; contains benzoic acid; grape flavor]

Siltussin SA: 100 mg/5 mL (120 mL, 240 mL, 480 mL) [alcohol free, sugar free; strawberry flavor]

Tussin: 100 mg/5 mL (120 mL, 240 mL)

Syrup, oral drops (Phanasin®): 50 mg/mL (50 mL) [alcohol free, sugar free; fruit flavor]

Tablet: 200 mg

Allfen Jr: 400 mg [dye free]

Humibid® *e*: 400 mg

Organ-1 NR, Organidin® NR: 200 mg

Tablet, extended release (Mucinex®): 600 mg

Monitoring and Teaching Issues

Physical Assessment: Assess effectiveness of therapy and adverse reactions (see Adverse Reactions) at beginning of therapy and periodically with long-term use. Teach patient appropriate use, interventions to reduce side effects, and adverse symptoms to report (see Patient Education).

Patient Education: Take as prescribed; do not exceed prescribed dose or frequency. Do not chew or crush extended release tablet. Maintain adequate hydration (2-3 L/day of fluids) unless instructed to restrict fluid intake. You may experience some drowsiness (use caution when driving or engaging in tasks requiring alertness until response to drug is known). Report excessive drowsiness, respiratory difficulty, or lack of improvement or worsening of condition. **Pregnancy/breast-feeding precautions:** Inform prescriber if you are or intend to become pregnant. Consult prescriber if breast-feeding.

Dietary Considerations: Diabetic Tussin® EX contains phenylalanine 8.4 mg/5 mL.

Pregnancy Risk Factor: C

Lactation: Excretion in breast milk unknown/use caution

Administration

Oral: Do not crush, chew, or break extended release tablets. Administer with a full glass of water.

◆ Guaifenesin AC *see* Guaifenesin and Codeine *on page 731*

Guaifenesin and Codeine (gwye FEN e sin & KOE deen)

U.S. Brand Names Brontex®; Cheracol®; Cheratussin AC; Diabetic Tussin C®; Gani-Tuss® NR; Guaifen-C; Guaifenesin AC; Guaituss AC®; Iophen-C NR; Kolephrin® #1; Mytussin® AC; Robafen® AC; Romilar® AC; Tussi-Organidin® NR; Tussi-Organidin® S-NR

Synonyms Codeine and Guaifenesin

Controlled Substance C-V

Generic Available Yes

Pharmacologic Category Antitussive; Cough Preparation; Expectorant

Medication Safety Issues
Sound-alike/look-alike issues:
Halotussin® may be confused with Halotestin®

Use Temporary control of cough due to minor throat and bronchial irritation

Dosing
Adults & Elderly: Cough (antitussive/expectorant): Oral: 5-10 mL every 4-8 hours not to exceed 60 mL/24 hours

Pediatrics: Cough (antitussive/expectorant): Oral:
2-6 years: 1-1.5 mg/kg codeine/day divided into 4 doses administered every 4-6 hours (maximum: 30 mg/24 hours)
6-12 years: 5 mL every 4 hours, not to exceed 30 mL/24 hours
>12 years: 10 mL every 4 hours, up to 60 mL/24 hours

Available Dosage Forms
Liquid:
Brontex®: Guaifenesin 75 mg and codeine phosphate 2.5 mg per 5 mL (480 mL) [alcohol free; strawberry mint flavor]
Diabetic Tussin C®: Guaifenesin 200 mg and codeine phosphate 10 mg per 5 mL (480 mL) [contains phenylalanine 0.03 mcg/5 mL; cherry vanilla flavor]
Gani-Tuss® NR: Guaifenesin 100 mg and codeine phosphate 10 mg per 5 mL (480 mL) [raspberry flavor]
Guaifen-C: Guaifenesin 75 mg and codeine phosphate 2.5 mg per 5 mL (480 mL) [cherry flavor]
Guaifenesin AC: Guaifenesin 100 mg and codeine phosphate 10 mg per 5 mL (120 mL, 480 mL) [alcohol free, sugar free; raspberry flavor]
Iophen-C NR: Guaifenesin 100 mg and codeine phosphate 10 mg per 5 mL (480 mL) [raspberry flavor]
Kolephrin® #1: Guaifenesin 100 mg and codeine phosphate 10 mg per 5 mL (120 mL) [contains sodium 1.1 mg/5 mL and sodium benzoate]
Tussi-Organidin® NR: Guaifenesin 100 mg and codeine phosphate 10 mg per 5 mL (480 mL) [contains sodium benzoate; raspberry flavor]
Tussi-Organidin® S-NR: Guaifenesin 100 mg and codeine phosphate 10 mg per 5 mL (120 mL) [contains sodium benzoate; raspberry flavor]
Syrup:
Cheracol®: Guaifenesin 100 mg and codeine phosphate 10 mg per 5 mL (120 mL) [contains alcohol 4.75% and benzoic acid]
Cheratussin AC: Guaifenesin 100 mg and codeine phosphate 10 mg per 5 mL (120 mL, 240 mL, 480 mL)
Guaituss AC®: Guaifenesin 100 mg and codeine phosphate 10 mg per 5 mL (120 mL, 480 mL) [contains alcohol; sugar free; fruit-mint flavor]
Mytussin® AC: Guaifenesin 100 mg and codeine phosphate 10 mg per 5 mL (120 mL, 480 mL) [contains alcohol; sugar free; fruit flavor]
Robafen® AC: Guaifenesin 100 mg and codeine phosphate 10 mg per 5 mL (120 mL, 480 mL)
Romilar® AC: Guaifenesin 100 mg and codeine phosphate 10 mg per 5 mL (480 mL) [contains benzoic acid and phenylalanine; alcohol free, sugar free, dye free; grape flavor]
Tablet (Brontex®): Guaifenesin 300 mg and codeine phosphate 10 mg

Monitoring and Teaching Issues
Physical Assessment: See individual agents.
Patient Education: See individual agents. **Pregnancy/breast-feeding precautions:** Inform prescriber if you are or intend to become pregnant. Consult prescriber if breast-feeding.
Pregnancy Risk Factor: C
Lactation: Excretion in breast milk unknown/use caution

Related Information
Codeine *on page 366*
Guaifenesin *on page 729*

Guaifenesin and Dextromethorphan
(gwye FEN e sin & deks troe meth OR fan)

U.S. Brand Names Altarussin DM [OTC]; Amibid DM; Aquatab® DM [DSC]; Benylin® Expectorant [OTC]; Cheracol® D [OTC]; Cheracol® Plus [OTC]; Diabetic Tussin® DM [OTC]; Diabetic Tussin® DM Maximum Strength [OTC]; Duratuss® DM; Gani-Tuss DM NR; Genatuss DM® [OTC]; Guaifenex® DM; Guaituss-DM® [OTC]; Humibid® CS [OTC]; Humibid® DM [DSC]; Hydro-Tussin™ DM; Kolephrin® GG/DM [OTC]; Mucinex® DM [OTC]; Respa-DM®; Robafen DM [OTC]; Robitussin® DM [OTC]; Robitussin® DM Infant [OTC]; Robitussin® Sugar Free Cough [OTC]; Safe Tussin® 30 [OTC]; Scot-Tussin® Senior [OTC]; Silexin® [OTC]; Siltussin DM [OTC]; Siltussin DM DAS [OTC]; Touro® DM; Tussi-Organidin® DM NR [DSC]; Vicks® 44E [OTC]; Vicks® Pediatric Formula 44E [OTC]; Z-Cof LA™

Synonyms Dextromethorphan and Guaifenesin

Generic Available Yes

Pharmacologic Category Antitussive; Cough Preparation; Expectorant

Medication Safety Issues
Sound-alike/look-alike issues:
Benylin® may be confused with Benadryl®, Ventolin®

Use Temporary control of cough due to minor throat and bronchial irritation
(Continued)

731

Guaifenesin and Dextromethorphan *(Continued)*

Dosing
Adults & Elderly: Cough (antitussive/expectorant): Oral:

General dosing guidelines: Guaifenesin 200-400 mg and dextromethorphan 10-20 mg every 4 hours (maximum dose: Guaifenesin 2400 mg and dextromethorphan 120 mg per day)

Product-specific labeling:

Benylin®: 20 mL every 4 hours (maximum: 6 doses/24 hours)

Guaifenex® DM, Mucinex® DM, Touro® DM: 1-2 tablets every 12 hours (maximum: 4 tablets/24 hours)

Humibid® CD: 1 tablet every 4 hours (maximum: 6 tablets/24 hours)

Robitussin® DM, Robitussin® Sugar Free Cough: 10 mL every 4 hours (maximum: 6 doses/24 hours)

Vicks® 44E: 15 mL every 4 hours (maximum: 6 doses/24 hours)

Vicks® Pediatric Formula 44E: 30 mL every 4 hours (maximum: 6 doses/24 hours)

Z-Cof LA™: 1 tablet every 12 hours

Pediatrics: Cough (antitussive/expectorant): Oral: Children:

2-6 years:

General dosing guidelines: Guaifenesin 50-100 mg and dextromethorphan 2.5-5 mg every 4 hours (maximum dose: Guaifenesin 600 mg and dextromethorphan 30 mg per day)

Product-specific labeling:

Benylin®: 5 mL every 4 hour (maximum: 6 doses/24 hours)

Guaifenex® DM, Touro® DM: 1/2 tablet every 12 hours (maximum: 1 tablet/24 hour)

Robitussin® DM, Robitussin® DM Infant, Robitussin® Sugar Free Cough: 2.5 mL every 4 hours (maximum: 6 doses/24 hours)

Vicks® Pediatric Formula 44E: 7.5 mL every 4 hours (maximum: 6 doses/24 hours)

6-12 years:

General dosing guidelines: Guaifenesin 100-200 mg and dextromethorphan 5-10 mg every 4 hours (maximum dose: Guaifenesin 1200 mg and dextromethorphan 60 mg per day)

Product-specific labeling:

Benylin®: 10 mL every 4 hours (maximum: 6 doses/24 hours)

Guaifenex® DM, Touro® DM: 1 tablet every 12 hours (maximum: 2 tablets/24 hours)

Humibid® CS: 1/2 tablet every 4 hours (maximum: 6 doses/24 hours)

Robitussin® DM, Robitussin® Sugar Free Cough: 5 mL every 4 hours (maximum: 6 doses/24 hours)

Vicks® 44E: 7.5 mL every 4 hours (maximum: 6 doses/24 hours)

Vicks® Pediatric Formula 44E: 15 mL every 4 hours (maximum: 6 doses/24 hours)

Z-Cof LA™: 1/2 tablet very 12 hours

≥12 years: Refer to adult dosing.

Available Dosage Forms [DSC] = Discontinued product
Liquid: Guaifenesin 100 mg and dextromethorphan hydrobromide 10 mg per 5 mL (480 mL)

Diabetic Tussin® DM: Guaifenesin 100 mg and dextromethorphan hydrobromide 10 mg per 5 mL (120 mL) [alcohol free, sugar free, dye free; contains phenylalanine 8.4 mg/5 mL]

Diabetic Tussin® DM Maximum Strength: Guaifenesin 200 mg and dextromethorphan hydrobromide 10 mg per 5 mL (120 mL) [alcohol free, sugar free, dye free; contains phenylalanine 8.4 mg/5 mL]

Duratuss® DM: Guaifenesin 200 mg and dextromethorphan hydrobromide 20 mg per 5 mL (480 mL) [contains alcohol 5%, sodium benzoate; fruit flavor]

Gani-Tuss® DM NR: Guaifenesin 100 mg and dextromethorphan hydrobromide 10 mg per 5 mL (480 mL) [raspberry flavor]

Hydro-Tussin™ DM: Guaifenesin 200 mg and dextromethorphan hydrobromide 20 mg per 5 mL (480 mL) [alcohol free, sugar free]

Kolephrin® GG/DM: Guaifenesin 150 mg and dextromethorphan hydrobromide 10 mg per 5 mL (120 mL) [alcohol free; cherry flavor]

Safe Tussin®: Guaifenesin 100 mg and dextromethorphan hydrobromide 15 mg per 5 mL (120 mL) [alcohol free, sodium free, sugar free, dye free; mint flavor]

Scot-Tussin® Senior: Guaifenesin 200 mg and dextromethorphan hydrobromide 15 mg per 5 mL (120 mL) [alcohol free, sodium free, sugar free]

Tussi-Organidin® DM NR: Guaifenesin 100 mg and dextromethorphan hydrobromide 10 mg per 5 mL (120 mL, 480 mL) [contains sodium benzoate; raspberry flavor] [DSC]

Vicks® 44E: Guaifenesin 200 mg and dextromethorphan hydrobromide 20 mg per 15 mL (120 mL, 235 mL) [contains sodium 31 mg/15 mL, alcohol, sodium benzoate]

Vicks® Pediatric Formula 44E: Guaifenesin 100 mg and dextromethorphan hydrobromide 10 mg per 15 mL (120 mL) [alcohol free; contains sodium 30 mg/15 mL, sodium benzoate; cherry flavor]

Liquid, oral drops (Robitussin® DM Infant): Guaifenesin 100 mg and dextromethorphan hydrobromide 5 mg per 2.5 mL (30 mL) [alcohol free; contains sodium benzoate; fruit punch flavor]

Syrup: Guaifenesin 100 mg and dextromethorphan hydrobromide 10 mg per 5 mL (120 mL, 480 mL)

Altarussin DM: Guaifenesin 100 mg and dextromethorphan hydrobromide 10 mg per 5 mL (120 mL, 240 mL, 480 mL, 3840 mL)

Benylin® Expectorant: Guaifenesin 100 mg and dextromethorphan hydrobromide 5 mg per 5 mL (120 mL) [alcohol free, sugar free; contains sodium benzoate; raspberry flavor]

Cheracol® D: Guaifenesin 100 mg and dextromethorphan hydrobromide 10 mg per 5 mL (120 mL, 180 mL) [contains alcohol, benzoic acid]

Cheracol® Plus: Guaifenesin 100 mg and dextromethorphan hydrobromide 10 mg per 5 mL (120 mL)

Genatuss DM®: Guaifenesin 100 mg and dextromethorphan hydrobromide 10 mg per 5 mL (120 mL) [cherry flavor]

Guiatuss® DM: Guaifenesin 100 mg and dextromethorphan hydrobromide 10 mg per 5 mL (120 mL, 480 mL, 3840 mL) [alcohol free; fruit-mint flavor]

Robafen® DM: Guaifenesin 100 mg and dextromethorphan hydrobromide 10 mg per 5 mL (120 mL)

Robitussin®-DM: Guaifenesin 100 mg and dextromethorphan hydrobromide 10 mg per 5 mL (5 mL, 120 mL, 360 mL, 480 mL) [alcohol free; contains sodium benzoate]

Robitussin® Sugar Free Cough: Guaifenesin 100 mg and dextromethorphan hydrobromide 10 mg per 5 mL (120 mL) [alcohol free, sugar free; contains sodium benzoate]

Silexin®: Guaifenesin 100 mg and dextromethorphan hydrobromide 10 mg per 5 mL (45 mL, 480 mL) [alcohol free, sugar free)]

Siltussin DM: Guaifenesin 100 mg and dextromethorphan hydrobromide 10 mg per 5 mL (120 mL, 240 mL, 480 mL) [strawberry flavor]

Siltussin DM DAS: Guaifenesin 100 mg and dextromethorphan hydrobromide 10 mg per 5 mL (120 mL) [alcohol free, dye free, sugar free; strawberry flavor]

Tablet:
Humibid® CS: Guaifenesin 400 mg and dextromethorphan hydrobromide 20 mg
Silexin®: Guaifenesin 100 mg and dextromethorphan hydrobromide 10 mg

Tablet, extended release: Guaifenesin 500 mg and dextromethorphan hydrobromide 30 mg; Guaifenesin 600 mg and dextromethorphan hydrobromide 30 mg; Guaifenesin 1000 mg and dextromethorphan hydrobromide 60 mg

Amidbid DM, Guaifenex® DM, Humibid® DM [DSC], Mucinex® DM, Respa-DM®: Guaifenesin 600 mg and dextromethorphan hydrobromide 30 mg

Aquatab® DM: Guaifenesin 1200 mg and dextromethorphan hydrobromide 60 mg [DSC]
Touro® DM: Guaifenesin 575 mg and dextromethorphan hydrobromide 30 mg

Tablet, long acting [scored] (Z-Cof LA): Guaifenesin 650 mg and dextromethorphan hydrobromide 30 mg

Monitoring and Teaching Issues
Physical Assessment: See individual agents.
Patient Education: Also see Guaifenesin.
Based on Dextromethorphan component: Do not exceed recommended dosage; take with a large glass of water; if cough lasts more than 1 week or is accompanied by a rash, fever, or headache, notify physician.
Pregnancy/breast-feeding precautions: Inform prescriber if you are or intend to become pregnant. Consult prescriber if breast-feeding.
Pregnancy Risk Factor: C
Lactation: Excretion in breast milk unknown/use caution
Related Information
Guaifenesin *on page 729*

Guaifenesin and Pseudoephedrine (gwye FEN e sin & soo doe e FED rin)
U.S. Brand Names Ambifed-G; Ami-Tex PSE; Aquatab® D [DSC]; Congestac® [OTC]; Dynex; Entex® PSE; Eudal®-SR; G-Phed; Guaifenex® GP; Guaifenex® PSE; Guaifenex™-Rx [DSC]; Guaimax-D®; Levall G; Maxifed®; Maxifed-G®; Miraphen PSE; Mucinex®-D [OTC]; Nasatab® LA; PanMist®-JR; PanMist®-LA; PanMist®-S; Profen Forte®; Profen II®; Pseudo GG TR; Pseudovent™; Pseudovent™ 400; Pseudovent™-Ped; Refenesen Plus [OTC]; Respaire®-60 SR; Respaire®-120 SR; Robitussin-PE® [OTC]; Robitussin® Severe Congestion [OTC]; Sudafed® Non-Drying Sinus [OTC]; Touro LA®; Zephrex®; Zephrex LA®
Synonyms Pseudoephedrine and Guaifenesin
Generic Available Yes
Pharmacologic Category Alpha/Beta Agonist; Expectorant
Medication Safety Issues
Sound-alike/look-alike issues:
Entex® may be confused with Tenex®
Profen II® may be confused with Profen II DM®, Profen Forte®, Profen Forte™ DM
Profen Forte® may be confused with Profen II®, Profen II DM®, Profen Forte™ DM
Use Temporary relief of nasal congestion and to help loosen phlegm and thin bronchial secretions in the treatment of cough
Dosing
Adults: Expectorant/decongestant: Oral:
Ambifed-G, Aquatab® D, Dynex, Entex® PSE, Eudal®-SR, G-Phed, Guaifenex® GP, Guaifenex® PSE 120, Guaimax-D®, Levall G, Miraphen PSE, Mucinex®-D 1200/120, Nasatab® LA, PanMist®-LA, Profen Forte®, Pseudovent™, Respaire®-120 SR, Touro LA, Zephrex® LA: One tablet or capsule every 12 hours (maximum: 2 tablets or capsules in 24 hours)
Congestac®: One caplet every 4-6 hours (maximum: 4 caplets in 24 hours)
Guaifenex® PSE 60, Maxifed-G®, Mucinex®-D 600/60, PanMist®-JR, Pseudovent™-Ped, Respaire®-60 SR: 1-2 tablets or capsules every 12 hours (maximum: 4 tablets or capsules/24 hours)
Guaifenex® PSE 80, PanMist®-LA: One tablet every twelve hours (maximum: 3 tablets/24 hours)
Guaifenex™ RX: 1-2 of the AM tablets every morning and 1-2 of the PM tablets 12 hours following morning dose
Maxifed®, Profen II®: One to 1½ tablets every 12 hours (maximum: 3 tablets/24 hours)
PanMist®-S: Up to 10 mL 4 times/day
Robitussin® PE: 10 mL every 4-6 hours (maximum: 4 doses/24 hours)
Robitussin® Severe Congestion, Sudafed® Non-Drying Sinus: Two capsules every 4 hours (maximum: 4 doses/24 hours)
Zephrex®: One tablet every 6 hours
Elderly: Refer to adult dosing; use with caution.
Pediatrics: Expectorant/decongestant: Oral:
Children 2-6 years:
Guaifenex® PSE 60: One-half tablet every 12 hours (maximum: 1 tablet/12 hours)
Maxifed-G®: One-third to ½ tablet every 12 hours (maximum: 1 tablet/12 hours)
PanMist® S: 2.5 mL 4 times/day (maximum: Pseudoephedrine 4 mg/kg/day)
Robitussin® PE: 2.5 mL every 4-6 hours (maximum: 4 doses/24 hours)
(Continued)

Guaifenesin and Pseudoephedrine *(Continued)*

Children 6-12 years:
Ambifed-G, Dynex, Eudal-SR®, Guaimax-D®, Guaifenex® PSE 80, Guaifenex® PSE 120, Maxifed®, Miraphen PSE, Nasatab® LA, PanMist® LA, Profen II®, Profen Forte®, Zephrex® LA: One-half caplet or tablet every 12 hours (maximum: 1 tablet/24 hours)
Congestac®: One-half caplet every 4-6 hours (maximum: 2 caplets/24 hours)
Guaifenex® PSE 60, PanMist®-JR, Pseudovent™-Ped, Respaire®-60 SR: One tablet or capsule every 12 hours (maximum: 2 tablets or capsules every 24 hours)
Levall G: One capsule every 24 hours
Maxifed-G®: One-half to 1 tablet every 12 hours (maximum: 2 tablets/24 hours)
PanMist® S: 5 mL 4 times/day (maximum: Pseudoephedrine 4 mg/kg/day)
Robitussin® PE: 5 mL every 4-6 hours (maximum: 4 doses/24 hours)
Robitussin® Severe Congestion: One capsule every 4 hours (maximum: 4 doses/24 hours)
Zephrex®: One-half tablet every 6 hours
>12 years: Refer to adult dosing.

Available Dosage Forms [DSC] = Discontinued product
Caplet (Congestac®, Refenesen Plus): Guaifenesin 400 mg and pseudoephedrine hydrochloride 60 mg
Caplet, long acting (Touro LA®): Guaifenesin 500 mg and pseudoephedrine hydrochloride 120 mg
Caplet, prolonged release (Ambifed-G): Guaifenesin 1000 mg and pseudoephedrine hydrochloride 60 mg
Capsule, extended release:
Respaire®-60 SR: Guaifenesin 200 mg and pseudoephedrine hydrochloride 60 mg
Respaire®-120 SR: Guaifenesin 250 mg and pseudoephedrine hydrochloride 120 mg
Capsule, liquicap (Sudafed® Non-Drying Sinus): Guaifenesin 200 mg and pseudoephedrine hydrochloride 30 mg
Capsule, softgel (Robitussin® Severe Congestion): Guaifenesin 200 mg and pseudoephedrine hydrochloride 30 mg
Capsule, variable release:
Entex® PSE: Guaifenesin 400 mg [immediate release] and pseudoephedrine hydrochloride 120 mg [extended release]
G-Phed: Guaifenesin 250 mg [immediate release] and pseudoephedrine hydrochloride 120 mg [prolonged release]
Levall G: Guaifenesin 400 mg [immediate release] and pseudoephedrine hydrochloride 90 mg [extended release]
Pseudovent™: Guaifenesin 250 mg [immediate release] and pseudoephedrine hydrochloride 120 mg [prolonged release]
Pseudovent™-Ped: Guaifenesin 300 mg [immediate release] and pseudoephedrine hydrochloride 60 mg [prolonged release]
Pseudovent™ 400: Guaifenesin 400 mg [immediate release] and pseudoephedrine hydrochloride 1200 mg [extended release]
Combination package (Guaifenex™-Rx) [14-day treatment package; each package contains] [DSC]:
Tablet, extended release: Guaifenesin 600 mg and pseudoephedrine hydrochloride 60 mg (28s) [for AM dose]
Tablet, extended release: Guaifenesin 600 mg (28s) [for PM dose]
Syrup: Guaifenesin 200 mg and pseudoephedrine hydrochloride 40 mg per 5 mL (480 mL)
PanMist®-S: Guaifenesin 200 mg and pseudoephedrine hydrochloride 40 mg per 5 mL (480 mL) [alcohol free; grape flavor]
Robitussin-PE®: Guaifenesin 100 mg and pseudoephedrine hydrochloride 30 mg per 5 mL (120 mL, 240 mL) [alcohol free; contains sodium benzoate]
Tablet: Zephrex®: Guaifenesin 400 mg and pseudoephedrine hydrochloride 60 mg
Tablet, extended release: Guaifenesin 550 mg and pseudoephedrine hydrochloride 60 mg; guaifenesin 595 mg and pseudoephedrine hydrochloride 48 mg; guaifenesin 600 mg and pseudoephedrine hydrochloride 60 mg; guaifenesin 600 mg and pseudoephedrine hydrochloride 120 mg; guaifenesin 795 mg and pseudoephedrine hydrochloride 85 mg; guaifenesin 800 mg and pseudoephedrine hydrochloride 45 mg; guaifenesin 800 mg and pseudoephedrine hydrochloride 60 mg; guaifenesin 800 mg and pseudoephedrine hydrochloride 90 mg; guaifenesin 1200 mg and pseudoephedrine hydrochloride 50 mg; guaifenesin 1200 mg and pseudoephedrine hydrochloride 60 mg; guaifenesin 1200 mg and pseudoephedrine hydrochloride 75 mg; guaifenesin 1200 mg and pseudoephedrine hydrochloride 90 mg; guaifenesin 1200 mg and pseudoephedrine hydrochloride 120 mg
Ami-Tex PSE, Guaimax-D®, Zephrex LA®: Guaifenesin 600 mg and pseudoephedrine hydrochloride 120 mg
Aquatab® D: Guaifenesin 1200 mg and pseudoephedrine hydrochloride 75 mg [DSC]
Guaifenex® GP: Guaifenesin 1200 mg and pseudoephedrine hydrochloride 120 mg [dye free]
Guaifenex® PSE 60: Guaifenesin 600 mg and pseudoephedrine hydrochloride 60 mg
Guaifenex® PSE 80: Guaifenesin 800 mg and pseudoephedrine hydrochloride 80 mg
Maxifed®: Guaifenesin 700 mg and pseudoephedrine hydrochloride 80 mg
Maxifed-G®: Guaifenesin 550 mg and pseudoephedrine hydrochloride 60 mg
Mucinex®-D 600/60: Guaifenesin 600 mg and pseudoephedrine hydrochloride 60 mg
Mucinex®-D 1200/120: Guaifenesin 1200 mg and pseudoephedrine hydrochloride 120 mg
PanMist®-JR, Pseudo GG TR: Guaifenesin 595 mg and pseudoephedrine hydrochloride 48 mg
PanMist®-LA: Guaifenesin 795 mg and pseudoephedrine hydrochloride 85 mg
Profen II®: Guaifenesin 800 mg and pseudoephedrine hydrochloride 45 mg
Profen Forte®: Guaifenesin 800 mg and pseudoephedrine hydrochloride 90 mg
Tablet, long acting:
Dynex: Guaifenesin 1200 mg and pseudoephedrine hydrochloride 90 mg
Guaifenex® PSE 120: Guaifenesin 600 mg and pseudoephedrine hydrochloride 120 mg [dye free]

Miraphen PSE: Guaifenesin 600 mg and pseudoephedrine hydrochloride 120 mg

Tablet, sustained release (Nasatab® LA): Guaifenesin 500 mg and pseudoephedrine hydrochloride 120 mg

Monitoring and Teaching Issues

Physical Assessment: See individual agents.

Patient Education: See individual agents. **Pregnancy/breast-feeding precautions:** Inform prescriber if you are or intend to become pregnant. Consult prescriber if breast-feeding.

Pregnancy Risk Factor: C

Lactation: Enters breast milk/contraindicated (by some manufacturers)

Related Information

Guaifenesin *on page 729*

Pseudoephedrine *on page 1282*

♦ **Guaifenesin, Dihydrocodeine, and Pseudoephedrine** *see* Dihydrocodeine, Pseudoephedrine, and Guaifenesin *on page 457*

♦ **Guaifenesin, Hydrocodone Bitartrate, and Phenylephrine Hydrochloride** *see* Hydrocodone, Phenylephrine, and Guaifenesin *on page 760*

Guaifenesin, Pseudoephedrine, and Codeine

(gwye FEN e sin, soo doe e FED rin, & KOE deen)

U.S. Brand Names Cheratussin DAC; Codafed® Expectorant; Codafed® Pediatric Expectorant; Guiatuss™ DAC®; Mytussin® DAC; Nucofed® Expectorant; Nucofed® Pediatric Expectorant; Nucotuss® [DSC]

Synonyms Codeine, Guaifenesin, and Pseudoephedrine; Pseudoephedrine, Guaifenesin, and Codeine

Controlled Substance C-III; C-V

Generic Available Yes

Pharmacologic Category Antitussive/Decongestant/Expectorant

Medication Safety Issues

Sound-alike/look-alike issues:

Halotussin® may be confused with Halotestin®

Use Temporarily relieves nasal congestion and controls cough due to minor throat and bronchial irritation; helps loosen phlegm and thin bronchial secretions to make coughs more productive

Dosing

Adults: Expectorant/decongestant/cough suppressant: Oral: 10 mL syrup every 4 hours

Elderly: Refer to adult dosing; use with caution.

Pediatrics: Expectorant/decongestant/cough suppressant: Oral:

Children 6-12 years: 5 mL every 4 hours, not to exceed 40 mL/24 hours

Children >12 years: Refer to adult dosing.

Available Dosage Forms [DSC] = Discontinued product

Liquid (Cheratussin DAC): Guaifenesin 100 mg, pseudoephedrine hydrochloride 30 mg, and codeine phosphate 10 mg per 5 mL (480 mL) [sugar free]

Syrup:

Codafed® Expectorant: Guaifenesin 200 mg, pseudoephedrine hydrochloride 60 mg, and codeine phosphate 20 mg per 5 mL (480 mL) [wintergreen flavor]

Codafed® Pediatric Expectorant: Guaifenesin 100 mg, pseudoephedrine hydrochloride 30 mg, and codeine phosphate 10 mg per 5 mL (480 mL) [strawberry flavor]

Guiatuss™ DAC: Guaifenesin 100 mg, pseudoephedrine hydrochloride 30 mg, and codeine phosphate 10 mg per 5 mL (480 mL)

Mytussin® DAC: Guaifenesin 100 mg, pseudoephedrine hydrochloride 30 mg, and codeine phosphate 10 mg per 5 mL (120 mL, 480 mL) [sugar free; contains alcohol 1.7%; strawberry-raspberry flavor]

Nucofed® Expectorant, Nucotuss® Expectorant [DSC]: Guaifenesin 200 mg, pseudoephedrine hydrochloride 60 mg, and codeine phosphate 20 mg per 5 mL (480 mL) [contains alcohol 12.5%; cherry flavor]

Nucofed® Pediatric Expectorant: Guaifenesin 100 mg, pseudoephedrine hydrochloride 30 mg, and codeine phosphate 10 mg per 5 mL (480 mL) [contains alcohol 6%; strawberry flavor]

Monitoring and Teaching Issues

Physical Assessment: See individual agents.

Patient Education: See individual agents. **Pregnancy/breast-feeding precautions:** Inform prescriber if you are or intend to become pregnant. Consult prescriber if breast-feeding.

Pregnancy Risk Factor: C

Lactation: Excretion in breast milk unknown/use caution

Related Information

Codeine *on page 366*

Guaifenesin *on page 729*

Pseudoephedrine *on page 1282*

♦ **Guaifenex® DM** *see* Guaifenesin and Dextromethorphan *on page 731*

♦ **Guaifenex® GP** *see* Guaifenesin and Pseudoephedrine *on page 733*

♦ **Guaifenex® PSE** *see* Guaifenesin and Pseudoephedrine *on page 733*

♦ **Guaifenex™-Rx [DSC]** *see* Guaifenesin and Pseudoephedrine *on page 733*

♦ **Guaimax-D®** *see* Guaifenesin and Pseudoephedrine *on page 733*

♦ **Guaituss AC®** *see* Guaifenesin and Codeine *on page 731*

♦ **Guiatuss™ [OTC]** *see* Guaifenesin *on page 729*

♦ **Guiatuss™ DAC®** *see* Guaifenesin, Pseudoephedrine, and Codeine *on page 735*

♦ **Guiatuss-DM® [OTC]** *see* Guaifenesin and Dextromethorphan *on page 731*

♦ **GW433908G** *see* Fosamprenavir *on page 677*

♦ **Gyne-Lotrimin® 3 [OTC]** *see* Clotrimazole *on page 360*

♦ **Gynodiol®** *see* Estradiol *on page 552*
♦ **Habitrol** *see* Nicotine *on page 1079*
♦ **Haemophilus** B Conjugate Vaccine *see page 1660*

Halcinonide (hal SIN oh nide)

U.S. Brand Names Halog®; Halog®-E [DSC]
Generic Available No
Pharmacologic Category Corticosteroid, Topical
Medication Safety Issues
Sound-alike/look-alike issues:
Halcinonide may be confused with Halcion®
Halog® may be confused with Haldol®, Mycolog®

Use Inflammation of corticosteroid-responsive dermatoses [high potency topical corticosteroid]
Contraindications Hypersensitivity to halcinonide or any component of the formulation; viral, fungal, or tubercular skin lesions
Warnings/Precautions Adverse systemic effects may occur when used on large areas of the body, denuded areas, for prolonged periods of time, with an occlusive dressing, and/or in infants or small children.
Adverse Reactions Frequency not defined: Itching; dry skin; folliculitis; hypertrichosis; acneiform eruptions; hypopigmentation; perioral dermatitis; allergic contact dermatitis; skin maceration; skin atrophy; striae; local burning, irritation, miliaria; secondary infection
Overdosage/Toxicology When consumed in excessive quantities, systemic hypercorticism and adrenal suppression may occur; in those cases, discontinuation and withdrawal of the corticosteroid should be done judiciously
Pharmacodynamics/Kinetics
Absorption: Percutaneous absorption varies by location of topical application and use of occlusive dressings
Metabolism: Primarily hepatic
Excretion: Urine
Dosing
Adults & Elderly: Steroid-responsive dermatoses: Topical: Apply sparingly 1-3 times/day; occlusive dressing may be used for severe or resistant dermatoses; a thin film is effective; do not overuse. Therapy should be discontinued when control is achieved; if no improvement is seen, reassessment of diagnosis may be necessary.
Pediatrics: Refer to adult dosing.
Available Dosage Forms [DSC] = Discontinued product
Cream (Halog®): 0.1% (15 g, 30 g, 60 g, 240 g)
Cream, emollient base (Halog®-E): 0.1% (30 g, 60 g) [DSC]
Ointment (Halog®): 0.1% (15 g, 30 g, 60 g, 240 g)
Solution, topical (Halog®): 0.1% (20 mL, 60 mL)
Monitoring and Teaching Issues
Physical Assessment: Assess potential for interactions with other prescriptions, OTC medications, or herbal products patient may be taking. Assess patient response. Teach patient proper use (according to formulation), side effects/appropriate interventions, and symptoms to report.
Patient Education: For external use only. Do not use for eyes, mucous membranes, or open wounds. Use exactly as directed and for no longer than the period prescribed. Before using, wash and dry area gently. Apply in a thin layer (may rub in lightly). Apply light dressing (if necessary) to area being treated. Do not use occlusive dressing unless so advised by prescriber. Avoid prolonged or excessive use around sensitive tissues, genital, or rectal areas. Avoid exposing treated area to direct sunlight. Inform prescriber if condition worsens (redness, swelling, irritation, signs of infection, or open sores) or fails to improve.
Pregnancy precaution: Inform prescriber if you are or intend to become pregnant.
Pregnancy Risk Factor: C

♦ **Halcion®** *see* Triazolam *on page 1522*
♦ **Haldol®** *see* Haloperidol *on page 736*
♦ **Haldol® Decanoate** *see* Haloperidol *on page 736*
♦ **HalfLytely® and Bisacodyl** *see* Polyethylene Glycol-Electrolyte Solution and Bisacodyl *on page 1228*
♦ **Halfprin® [OTC]** *see* Aspirin *on page 143*
♦ **Halog®** *see* Halcinonide *on page 736*
♦ **Halog®-E [DSC]** *see* Halcinonide *on page 736*

Haloperidol (ha loe PER i dole)

U.S. Brand Names Haldol®; Haldol® Decanoate
Synonyms Haloperidol Decanoate; Haloperidol Lactate
Generic Available Yes
Pharmacologic Category Antipsychotic Agent, Typical
Medication Safety Issues
Sound-alike/look-alike issues:
Haloperidol may be confused Halotestin®
Haldol® may be confused with Halcion®, Halenol®, Halog®, Halotestin®, Stadol®

Use Management of schizophrenia; control of tics and vocal utterances of Tourette's disorder in children and adults; severe behavioral problems in children
Unlabeled/Investigational Use Treatment of psychosis; may be used for the emergency sedation of severely-agitated or delirious patients; adjunctive treatment of ethanol dependence; antiemetic
Mechanism of Action/Effect Haloperidol is a butyrophenone antipsychotic which blocks postsynaptic mesolimbic dopaminergic D_1 and D_2 receptors in the brain; depresses the

release of hypothalamic and hypophyseal hormones; believed to depress the reticular activating system thus affecting basal metabolism, body temperature, wakefulness, vasomotor tone, and emesis

Contraindications Hypersensitivity to haloperidol or any component of the formulation; Parkinson's disease; severe CNS depression; bone marrow suppression; severe cardiac or hepatic disease; coma

Warnings/Precautions May be sedating, use with caution in disorders where CNS depression is a feature. Caution in patients with hemodynamic instability, predisposition to seizures, subcortical brain damage, renal or respiratory disease. Esophageal dysmotility and aspiration have been associated with antipsychotic use - use with caution in patients at risk of pneumonia (ie, Alzheimer's disease). Caution in breast cancer or other prolactin-dependent tumors (may elevate prolactin levels). May alter temperature regulation or mask toxicity of other drugs due to antiemetic effects. Hypotension may occur, particularly with parenteral administration. Decanoate form should never be administered I.V. Adverse effects of decanoate may be prolonged. Avoid in thyrotoxicosis.

May alter cardiac conduction - life-threatening arrhythmias have occurred with therapeutic doses of antipsychotics. Use with caution in patients at risk of hypotension (orthostasis) or those who would tolerate transient hypotensive episodes (cerebrovascular disease, cardiovascular disease, or other medications which may predispose).

Use with caution in patients with decreased gastrointestinal motility, urinary retention, BPH, xerostomia, or visual problems. May exacerbate narrow-angle glaucoma (screening is recommended) or worsen myasthenia gravis. Relative to other neuroleptics, haloperidol has a low potency of cholinergic blockade.

May cause extrapyramidal symptoms, including pseudoparkinsonism, acute dystonic reactions, akathisia, and tardive dyskinesia (risk of these reactions is high relative to other neuroleptics). May be associated with neuroleptic malignant syndrome (NMS) or pigmentary retinopathy. Some tablets contain tartrazine.

Drug Interactions

Cytochrome P450 Effect: Substrate of CYP1A2 (minor), 2D6 (major), 3A4 (major); **Inhibits** CYP2D6 (moderate), 3A4 (moderate)

Decreased Effect: Haloperidol may inhibit the ability of bromocriptine to lower serum prolactin concentrations. Benztropine (and other anticholinergics) may inhibit the therapeutic response to haloperidol and excess anticholinergic effects may occur. Barbiturates, carbamazepine, and cigarette smoking may enhance the hepatic metabolism of haloperidol. Haloperidol may inhibit the antiparkinsonian effect of levodopa; avoid this combination. The levels/effects of haloperidol may be decreased by aminoglutethimide, carbamazepine, nafcillin, nevirapine, phenobarbital, phenytoin, rifamycins, and other CYP3A4 inducers. Haloperidol may decrease the levels/effects of CYP2D6 prodrug substrates (eg, codeine, hydrocodone, oxycodone, tramadol).

Increased Effect/Toxicity: Haloperidol concentrations/effects may be increased by chloroquine, propranolol, and sulfadoxine-pyridoxine. The levels/effects of haloperidol may be increased by azole antifungals, chlorpromazine, ciprofloxacin, clarithromycin, delavirdine, diclofenac, doxycycline, erythromycin, fluoxetine, imatinib, isoniazid, miconazole, nefazodone, nicardipine, paroxetine, pergolide, propofol, protease inhibitors, quinidine, quinine, ritonavir, ropinirole, telithromycin, verapamil, and other CYP2D6 or 3A4 inhibitors.

Haloperidol may increase the levels/effects of amphetamines, selected beta-blockers, selected benzodiazepines, calcium channel blockers, cisapride, cyclosporine, dextromethorphan, ergot alkaloids, fluoxetine, selected HMG-CoA reductase inhibitors, lidocaine, mesoridazine, mirtazapine, nateglinide, nefazodone, paroxetine, risperidone, ritonavir, sildenafil (and other PDE-5 inhibitors), tacrolimus, thioridazine, tricyclic antidepressants, venlafaxine, and other substrates of CYP2D6 or 3A4.

Haloperidol may increase the effects of antihypertensives, CNS depressants (ethanol, narcotics, sedative-hypnotics), lithium, trazodone, and TCAs. Haloperidol in combination with indomethacin may result in drowsiness, tiredness, and confusion. Metoclopramide may increase risk of extrapyramidal symptoms (EPS).

Nutritional/Ethanol Interactions

Ethanol: Avoid ethanol (may increase CNS depression).

Herb/Nutraceutical: Avoid valerian, St John's wort, kava kava, gotu kola (may increase CNS depression).

Lab Interactions decreased cholesterol (S)

Adverse Reactions Frequency not defined.

Cardiovascular: Hyper-/hypotension, tachycardia, arrhythmia, abnormal T waves with prolonged ventricular repolarization, torsade de pointes (case-control study ~4%)

Central nervous system: Restlessness, anxiety, extrapyramidal symptoms, dystonic reactions, pseudoparkinsonian signs and symptoms, tardive dyskinesia, neuroleptic malignant syndrome (NMS), altered central temperature regulation, akathisia, tardive dystonia, insomnia, euphoria, agitation, drowsiness, depression, lethargy, headache, confusion, vertigo, seizure

Dermatologic: Hyperpigmentation, pruritus, rash, contact dermatitis, alopecia, photosensitivity (rare)

Endocrine & metabolic: Amenorrhea, galactorrhea, gynecomastia, sexual dysfunction, lactation, breast engorgement, mastalgia, menstrual irregularities, hyperglycemia, hypoglycemia, hyponatremia

Gastrointestinal: Nausea, vomiting, anorexia, constipation, diarrhea, hypersalivation, dyspepsia, xerostomia

Genitourinary: Urinary retention, priapism

Hematologic: Cholestatic jaundice, obstructive jaundice

Ocular: Blurred vision

Respiratory: Laryngospasm, bronchospasm

Miscellaneous: Heat stroke, diaphoresis

Overdosage/Toxicology Symptoms of overdose include deep sleep, dystonia, agitation, dysrhythmias, and extrapyramidal symptoms. Treatment is supportive and symptomatic. (Continued)

Haloperidol *(Continued)*

Pharmacodynamics/Kinetics
Onset of Action: Sedation: I.V.: ~1 hour
Duration of Action: Decanoate: ~3 weeks
Bioavailability: Oral: 60%
Time to Peak: Serum: 20 minutes
Protein Binding: 90%
Half-Life Elimination: 20 hours
Metabolism: Hepatic to inactive compounds
Excretion: Urine (33% to 40% as metabolites) within 5 days; feces (15%)

Dosing
Adults:
Psychosis:
Oral: 0.5-5 mg 2-3 times/day; usual maximum: 30 mg/day
I.M. (as lactate): 2-5 mg every 4-8 hours as needed
I.M. (as decanoate): Initial: 10-20 times the daily oral dose administered at 4-week intervals. Maintenance dose: 10-15 times initial oral dose; used to stabilize psychiatric symptoms

Delirium in the intensive care unit (unlabeled use, unlabeled route):
I.V.: 2-10 mg; may repeat bolus doses every 20-30 minutes until calm achieved then administer 25% of the maximum dose every 6 hours; monitor ECG and QT_c interval
Intermittent I.V.: 0.03-0.15 mg/kg every 30 minutes to 6 hours
Oral: Agitation: 5-10 mg
Continuous I.V. infusion (100 mg/100 mL D_5W): Rates of 3-25 mg/hour have been used
Rapid tranquilization of severely-agitated patient (unlabeled use; administer every 30-60 minutes):
Oral: 5-10 mg
I.M.: 5 mg
Average total dose (oral or I.M.) for tranquilization: 10-20 mg

Elderly: Nonpsychotic patients, dementia behavior: Initial: Oral: 0.25-0.5 mg 1-2 times/day; increase dose at 4- to 7-day intervals by 0.25-0.5 mg/day. Increase dosing intervals (twice daily, 3 times/day, etc) as necessary to control response or side effects.

Pediatrics:
Sedation/psychotic disorders: Oral:
Children: 3-12 years (15-40 kg): Initial: 0.05 mg/kg/day or 0.25-0.5 mg/day given in 2-3 divided doses; increase by 0.25-0.5 mg every 5-7 days; maximum: 0.15 mg/kg/day
Usual maintenance:
Agitation or hyperkinesia: 0.01-0.03 mg/kg/day once daily
Nonpsychotic disorders: 0.05-0.075 mg/kg/day in 2-3 divided doses
Psychotic disorders: 0.05-0.15 mg/kg/day in 2-3 divided doses
Children 6-12 years: Sedation/psychotic disorders: I.M. (as lactate): 1-3 mg/dose every 4-8 hours to a maximum of 0.15 mg/kg/day; change over to oral therapy as soon as able.

Renal Impairment: Hemodialysis/peritoneal dialysis: Supplemental dose is not necessary.

Available Dosage Forms Note: Strength expressed as base:
Injection, oil, as decanoate (Haldol® Decanoate): 50 mg/mL (1 mL, 5 mL); 100 mg/mL (1 mL, 5 mL) [contains benzyl alcohol, sesame oil]
Injection, solution, as lactate (Haldol®): 5 mg/mL (1 mL, 10 mL)
Solution, oral concentrate, as lactate (Haldol®): 2 mg/mL (15 mL, 120 mL)
Tablet: 0.5 mg, 1 mg, 2 mg, 5 mg, 10 mg, 20 mg

Monitoring and Teaching Issues
Physical Assessment: Assess other medications patient is taking for effectiveness and interactions (especially drugs metabolized by P450 enzymes). Review ophthalmic screening. Monitor therapeutic effectiveness and adverse reactions at beginning of therapy and periodically with long-term use. With I.M. or I.V. use, monitor for hypotension. Initiate at lower doses and taper dosage slowly when discontinuing. Assess knowledge/teach patient appropriate use, interventions to reduce side effects, and adverse symptoms to report.

Monitoring Laboratory Tests: Lipid profile, fasting blood glucose/Hgb A_{1c}; BMI

Patient Education: Use exactly as directed; do not increase dose or frequency. It may take 2-3 weeks to achieve desired results; do not discontinue without consulting prescriber. Dilute oral concentration with water or juice. Do not take within 2 hours of any antacid. Store away from light. Avoid alcohol or caffeine and other prescription or OTC medications not approved by prescriber. Maintain adequate hydration (2-3 L/day of fluids) unless instructed to restrict fluid intake. Avoid skin contact with medication; may cause contact dermatitis (wash immediately with warm, soapy water). You may experience excess drowsiness, restlessness, dizziness, or blurred vision (use caution driving or when engaging in tasks requiring alertness until response to drug is known); nausea or vomiting (small frequent meals, frequent mouth care, chewing gum, or sucking lozenges may help); constipation (increased exercise, fluids, fruit, or fiber may help); postural hypotension (use caution climbing stairs or when changing position from lying or sitting to standing); urinary retention (void before taking medication); or decreased perspiration (avoid strenuous exercise in hot environments). Report persistent CNS effects (eg, trembling fingers, altered gait or balance, excessive sedation, seizures, unusual movements, anxiety, abnormal thoughts, confusion, personality changes); chest pain, palpitations, rapid heartbeat, severe dizziness; unresolved urinary retention or changes in urinary pattern; vision changes; skin rash or yellowing of skin; respiratory difficulty; or worsening of condition. **Pregnancy/breast-feeding precautions:** Inform prescriber if you are or intend to become pregnant. Breast-feeding is not recommended.

Geriatric Considerations: (See Warnings/Precautions, Adverse Reactions, and Overdose/Toxicology.) Elderly patients have an increased risk of adverse response to side effects or adverse reactions to antipsychotics.

Pregnancy Risk Factor: C

Lactation: Enters breast milk/not recommended (AAP rates "of concern")

Breast-Feeding Issues: Decline in developmental scores may be seen in nursing infants.

Administration

Oral: Dilute the oral concentrate with water or juice before administration. **Note:** Avoid skin contact with oral medication; may cause contact dermatitis.

I.M.: The decanoate injectable formulation should be administered I.M. only; **do not give decanoate I.V.**

I.V.:

Decanoate: Do **not** administer I.V.

Lactate: Although not an FDA-approved route of administration, Haldol® has been administered by this route in many acute care settings.

Reconstitution: Haloperidol lactate may be administered IVPB or I.V. infusion in D$_5$W solutions. NS solutions should not be used due to reports of decreased stability and incompatibility.

Standardized dose: 0.5-100 mg/50-100 mL D$_5$W

Stability of standardized solutions is 38 days at room temperature (24°C).

Compatibility: Stable in D$_5$W

Y-site administration: Incompatible with allopurinol, amphotericin B cholesteryl sulfate complex, cefepime, fluconazole, foscarnet, heparin, piperacillin/tazobactam, sargramostim

Compatibility in syringe: Incompatible with diphenhydramine, heparin, hydroxyzine, ketorolac

Storage: Protect oral dosage forms from light. Haloperidol lactate injection should be stored at controlled room temperature and protected from light, freezing, and temperatures >40°C. Exposure to light may cause discoloration and the development of a grayish-red precipitate over several weeks.

Related Information

Antiemetics for Chemotherapy-Induced Nausea and Vomiting *on page 1788*

Antipsychotic Agents *on page 1717*

Antipsychotic Medication Guidelines *on page 1766*

Federal OBRA Regulations: Recommended Maximum Doses *on page 1773*

♦ **Haloperidol Decanoate** *see* Haloperidol *on page 736*

♦ **Haloperidol Lactate** *see* Haloperidol *on page 736*

♦ **Haltran® [OTC] [DSC]** *see* Ibuprofen *on page 777*

♦ **Havrix®** *see page 1660*

♦ **hBNP** *see* Nesiritide *on page 1071*

♦ **hCG** *see* Chorionic Gonadotropin (Human) *on page 319*

♦ **H-C Tussive** *see* Phenylephrine, Hydrocodone, and Chlorpheniramine *on page 1202*

♦ **HCTZ** *see* Hydrochlorothiazide *on page 751*

♦ **HCTZ and Telmisartan** *see* Telmisartan and Hydrochlorothiazide *on page 1433*

♦ **HDA® Toothache [OTC]** *see* Benzocaine *on page 181*

♦ **Healon®** *see page 1625*

♦ **Healon® GV** *see page 1625*

♦ **Heart Failure** *see page 1828*

♦ **Hectorol®** *see* Doxercalciferol *on page 489*

♦ **Helicobacter pylori Treatment** *see page 1835*

♦ **Helidac®** *see* Bismuth Subsalicylate, Metronidazole, and Tetracycline *on page 199*

♦ **Helistat®** *see page 1625*

♦ **Helixate® FS** *see* Antihemophilic Factor (Recombinant) *on page 127*

♦ **Hemabate®** *see* Carboprost Tromethamine *on page 257*

♦ **Hemocyte® [OTC]** *see* Ferrous Fumarate *on page 623*

♦ **Hemofil® M** *see* Antihemophilic Factor (Human) *on page 124*

♦ **Hemorrhoidal HC** *see* Hydrocortisone *on page 760*

♦ **Hemotene®** *see page 1625*

♦ **Hemril®-30** *see* Hydrocortisone *on page 760*

Heparin (HEP a rin)

U.S. Brand Names HepFlush®-10; Hep-Lock®

Synonyms Heparin Calcium; Heparin Lock Flush; Heparin Sodium

Generic Available Yes

Pharmacologic Category Anticoagulant

Medication Safety Issues

Sound-alike/look-alike issues:

Heparin may be confused with Hespan®

High alert medication: The Institute for Safe Medication Practices (ISMP) includes this medication among its list of drugs which have a heightened risk of causing significant patient harm when used in error.

Heparin lock flush solution is intended only to maintain patency of I.V. devices and is **not** to be used for anticoagulant therapy.

Use Prophylaxis and treatment of thromboembolic disorders

Note: Heparin lock flush solution is intended only to maintain patency of I.V. devices and is **not** to be used for anticoagulant therapy.

Mechanism of Action/Effect Potentiates the action of antithrombin III and thereby inactivates thrombin (as well as activated coagulation factors IX, X, XI, XII, and plasmin) and prevents the conversion of fibrinogen to fibrin; heparin also stimulates release of lipoprotein lipase (lipoprotein lipase hydrolyzes triglycerides to glycerol and free fatty acids) (Continued)

Heparin *(Continued)*

Contraindications Hypersensitivity to heparin or any component of the formulation; severe thrombocytopenia; uncontrolled active bleeding except when due to DIC; suspected intracranial hemorrhage; not for I.M. use; not for use when appropriate monitoring parameters cannot be obtained

Warnings/Precautions Hemorrhage is the most common complication. Risk factors for bleeding include bacterial endocarditis; congenital or acquired bleeding disorders; active ulcerative or angiodysplastic GI diseases; severe uncontrolled hypertension; hemorrhagic stroke; or use shortly after brain, spinal, or ophthalmology surgery; patient treated concomitantly with platelet inhibitors; conditions associated with increased bleeding tendencies (hemophilia, vascular purpura); recent GI bleeding; thrombocytopenia or platelet defects; severe liver disease; hypertensive or diabetic retinopathy; or in patients undergoing invasive procedures. A higher incidence of bleeding has been reported in women >60 years of age.

Patients who develop thrombocytopenia on heparin may be at risk of developing a new thrombus ("White-clot syndrome"). Hypersensitivity reactions can occur. Heparin should be used cautiously in patients with a documented hypersensitivity reaction and only in life-threatening situations. Osteoporosis can occur following long-term use (>6 months). May cause hyperkalemia due to effects on aldosterone. Discontinue therapy and consider alternatives if platelets are <100,000/mm^3. Patients >60 years of age may require lower doses of heparin.

Heparin does not possess fibrinolytic activity and, therefore, cannot lyse established thrombi; discontinue heparin if hemorrhage occurs; severe hemorrhage or overdosage may require protamine

Drug Interactions

Decreased Effect: Nitroglycerin (I.V.) may decrease heparin's anticoagulant effect. This interaction has not been validated in some studies, and may only occur at high nitroglycerin dosages.

Increased Effect/Toxicity: The risk of hemorrhage associated with heparin may be increased by oral anticoagulants (warfarin), thrombolytics, dextran, and drugs which affect platelet function (eg, aspirin, NSAIDs, dipyridamole, ticlopidine, clopidogrel, IIb/IIIa antagonists). However, heparin is often used in conjunction with thrombolytic therapy or during the initiation of warfarin therapy to assure anticoagulation and to protect against possible transient hypercoagulability. Cephalosporins which contain the MTT side chain and parenteral penicillins (may inhibit platelet aggregation) may increase the risk of hemorrhage. Other drugs reported to increase heparin's anticoagulant effect include antihistamines, tetracycline, quinine, nicotine, and cardiac glycosides (digoxin).

Nutritional/Ethanol Interactions

Food: When taking for >6 months, may interfere with calcium absorption.

Herb/Nutraceutical: Avoid cat's claw, dong quai, evening primrose, feverfew, red clover, horse chestnut, garlic, green tea, ginseng, ginkgo (all have additional antiplatelet activity).

Lab Interactions Increased thyroxine (S) (competitive protein binding methods), PT, PTT, bleeding time. A volume of at least 10 mL of blood should be removed and discarded from a heparinized line before blood samples are sent for coagulation testing.

Adverse Reactions

Cardiovascular: Chest pain, vasospasm (possibly related to thrombosis), hemorrhagic shock

Central nervous system: Fever, headache, chills

Dermatologic: Unexplained bruising, urticaria, alopecia, dysesthesia pedis, purpura, eczema, cutaneous necrosis (following deep SubQ injection), erythematous plaques (case reports)

Endocrine & metabolic: Hyperkalemia (supression of aldosterone), rebound hyperlipidemia on discontinuation

Gastrointestinal: Nausea, vomiting, constipation, hematemesis

Genitourinary: Frequent or persistent erection

Hematologic: Hemorrhage, blood in urine, bleeding from gums, epistaxis, adrenal hemorrhage, ovarian hemorrhage, retroperitoneal hemorrhage, thrombocytopenia (see note)

Hepatic: Elevated liver enzymes (AST/ALT)

Local: Irritation, ulceration, cutaneous necrosis have been rarely reported with deep SubQ injections, I.M. injection (not recommended) is associated with a high incidence of these effects

Neuromuscular & skeletal: Peripheral neuropathy, osteoporosis (chronic therapy effect)

Ocular: Conjunctivitis (allergic reaction)

Respiratory: Hemoptysis, pulmonary hemorrhage, asthma, rhinitis, bronchospasm (case reports)

Miscellaneous: Allergic reactions, anaphylactoid reactions

Note: Thrombocytopenia has been reported to occur at an incidence between 0% and 30%. It is often of no clinical significance. However, immunologically mediated heparin-induced thrombocytopenia has been estimated to occur in 1% to 2% of patients, and is marked by a progressive fall in platelet counts and, in some cases, thromboembolic complications (skin necrosis, pulmonary embolism, gangrene of the extremities, stroke or MI). For recommendations regarding platelet monitoring during heparin therapy, consult "Seventh ACCP Consensus Conference on Antithrombotic and Thrombolytic Therapy."

Overdosage/Toxicology The primary symptom of overdose is bleeding. Antidote is protamine; dose 1 mg neutralizes 1 mg (100 units) of heparin. Discontinue all heparin if evidence of progressive immune thrombocytopenia occurs.

Pharmacodynamics/Kinetics

Onset of Action: Anticoagulation: I.V.: Immediate; SubQ: ~20-30 minutes

Absorption: Oral, rectal, I.M.: Erratic at best from all these routes of administration; SubQ absorption is also erratic, but considered acceptable for prophylactic use

Half-Life Elimination: Mean: 1.5 hours; Range: 1-2 hours; affected by obesity, renal function, hepatic function, malignancy, presence of pulmonary embolism, and infections

Metabolism: Hepatic; may be partially metabolized in the reticuloendothelial system

Excretion: Urine (small amounts as unchanged drug)

Dosing

Adults:

DVT Prophylaxis (low-dose heparin): SubQ: 5000 units every 8-12 hours

Systemic anticoagulation: I.V. infusion (weight-based dosing per institutional nomogram recommended):

Acute coronary syndromes or MI: Fibrinolytic therapy: I.V. infusion:

Alteplase, reteplase, or tenecteplase with dosing as follows: Concurrent bolus of 60 units/kg (maximum: 4000 units), then 12 units/kg/hour (maximum: 1000 units/hour) as continuous infusion. Check aPTT every 4-6 hours; adjust to target of 1.5-2 times the upper limit of control (50-70 seconds in clinical trials); usual range 10-30 units/kg/hour. Duration of heparin therapy depends on concurrent therapy and the specific patient risks for systemic or venous thromboembolism.

Streptokinase: Heparin use optional depending on concurrent therapy and specific patient risks for systemic or venous thromboembolism (anterior MI, CHF, previous embolus, atrial fibrillation, LV thrombus): If heparin is administered, start when aPTT <2 times the upper limit of control; do not use a bolus, but initiate infusion adjusted to a target aPTT of 1.5-2 times the upper limit of control (50-70 seconds in clinical trials). If heparin is not administered by infusion, 7500-12,500 units SubQ every 12 hours (when aPTT <2 times the upper limit of control) is recommended.

Percutaneous coronary intervention: Heparin bolus and infusion may be administered to an activated clotting time (ACT) of 300-350 seconds if no concurrent GPIIb/IIIa receptor antagonist is administered or 200-250 seconds if a GPIIb/IIIa receptor antagonist is administered.

Unstable angina (high-risk and some intermediate-risk patients): Initial bolus of 60-70 units/kg (maximum: 5000 units), followed by an initial infusion of 12-15 units/kg/hour (maximum: 1000 units/hour). The American College of Chest Physicians consensus conference has recommended dosage adjustments to correspond to a therapeutic range equivalent to heparin levels of 0.3-0.7 units/mL by antifactor Xa determinations.

Venous thromboembolism :

DVT/PE: I.V. push: 80 units/kg followed by continuous infusion of 18 units/kg/hour

DVT: SubQ: 17,500 units every 12 hours

Intermittent I.V. Anticoagulation: Intermittent I.V.: Initial: 10,000 units, then 50-70 units/kg (5000-10,000 units) every 4-6 hours

Maintenance of line patency (line flushing): When using daily flushes of heparin to maintain patency of single and double lumen central catheters, 10 units/mL is commonly used for younger infants (eg, <10 kg) while 100 units/mL is used for older infants, children, and adults. Capped PVC catheters and peripheral heparin locks require flushing more frequently (eg, every 6-8 hours). Volume of heparin flush is usually similar to volume of catheter (or slightly greater). Additional flushes should be given when stagnant blood is observed in catheter, after catheter is used for drug or blood administration, and after blood withdrawal from catheter.

Parenteral nutrition: Addition of heparin (0.5-3 unit/mL) to peripheral and central parenteral nutrition has not been shown to decrease catheter-related thrombosis. The final concentration of heparin used for TPN solutions may need to be decreased to 0.5 units/mL in small infants receiving larger amounts of volume in order to avoid approaching therapeutic amounts. Arterial lines are heparinized with a final concentration of 1 unit/mL.

Elderly: Patients >60 years of age may have higher serum levels and clinical response (longer aPTTs) as compared to younger patients receiving similar dosages. Lower dosages may be required.

Pediatrics:

Anticoagulation: Intermittent I.V.: Initial: 50-100 units/kg, then 50-100 units/kg every 4 hours

Anticoagulation: I.V. infusion: Initial: 50 units/kg, then 15-25 units/kg/hour; increase dose by 2-4 units/kg/hour every 6-8 hours as required

Note: Refer to adult dosing for notes on line flushing and TPN.

Available Dosage Forms [DSC] = Discontinued product

Infusion, as sodium [premixed in NaCl 0.45%; porcine intestinal mucosa source]: 12,500 units (250 mL); 25,000 units (250 mL, 500 mL)

Infusion, as sodium [preservative free; premixed in D₅W; porcine intestinal mucosa source]: 10,000 units (100 mL) [contains sodium metabisulfite]; 12,500 units (250 mL) [contains sodium metabisulfite]; 20,000 units (500 mL) [contains sodium metabisulfite]; 25,000 units (250 mL, 500 mL) [contains sodium metabisulfite]

Infusion, as sodium [preservative free; premixed in NaCl 0.9%; porcine intestinal mucosa source]: 1000 units (500 mL); 2000 units (1000 mL)

Injection, solution, as sodium [beef lung source; multidose vial]: 1000 units/mL (10 mL, 30 mL); 5000 units/mL (10 mL), 10,000 units/mL (1 mL, 4 mL) [contains benzyl alcohol] [DSC]

Injection, solution, as sodium [lock flush preparation; porcine intestinal mucosa source; multidose vial]: 10 units/mL (1 mL, 10 mL, 30 mL) [contains parabens]; 100 units/mL (1 mL, 5 mL) [contains parabens]

Injection, solution, as sodium [lock flush preparation; porcine intestinal mucosa source; multidose vial]: 10 units/mL (10 mL, 30 mL); 100 units/mL (10 mL, 30 mL) [contains benzyl alcohol]

Hep-Lock®: 10 units/mL (1 mL, 2 mL, 10 mL, 30 mL); 100 units/mL (1 mL, 2 mL, 10 mL, 30 mL) [contains benzyl alcohol]

Injection, solution, as sodium [lock flush preparation; porcine intestinal mucosa source; prefilled syringe]: 10 units/mL (1 mL, 2 mL, 3 mL, 5 mL); 100 units/mL (1 mL, 2 mL, 3 mL, 5 mL) [contains benzyl alcohol]

Injection, solution, as sodium [preservative free; lock flush preparation; porcine intestinal mucosa source; prefilled syringe]: 100 units/mL (5 mL)

Injection, solution, as sodium [preservative free; lock flush preparation; porcine intestinal mucosa source; vial] (HepFlush®-10): 10 units/mL (10 mL)

(Continued)

Heparin *(Continued)*

Injection, solution, as sodium [porcine intestinal mucosa source; multidose vial]: 1000 units/mL (1 mL, 10 mL, 30 mL) [contains benzyl alcohol]; 1000 units/mL (1 mL, 10 mL, 30 mL) [contains methylparabens]; 5000 units/mL (1 mL, 10 mL) [contains benzyl alcohol]; 5000 units/mL (1 mL) [contains methylparabens]; 10,000 units/mL (1 mL, 4 mL) [contains benzyl alcohol]; 10,000 units/mL (1 mL, 5 mL) [contains methylparabens]; 20,000 units/mL (1 mL) [contains methylparabens]

Injection, solution, as sodium [porcine intestinal mucosa source; prefilled syringe]: 5000 units/mL (1 mL) [contains benzyl alcohol]

Injection, solution, as sodium [preservative free; porcine intestinal mucosa source; prefilled syringe]: 10,000 units/mL (0.5 mL)

Injection, solution, as sodium [preservative free; porcine intestinal mucosa source; vial]: 1000 units/mL (2 mL); 2000 units/mL (5 mL); 2500 units/mL (10 mL)

Monitoring and Teaching Issues

Physical Assessment: See Warnings/Precautions for use cautions (eg, risk factors for increased bleeding). Assess potential for interactions with other pharmacological agents or herbal products patient may be taking (especially anything that will affect coagulation or platelet function; see Drug Interactions). Note specific infusion directions in Administration. Bleeding precautions should be observed at all times during heparin therapy. Assess results of laboratory tests regularly (see Monitoring Laboratory Tests) for dosing adjustments and therapeutic effectiveness. Patient response should be assessed regularly during therapy (eg, hypersensitivity reaction, bleeding, chest pain, hyperkalemia, peripheral neuropathy; see Adverse Reactions). Teach possible side effects/appropriate interventions (eg, bleeding precautions) and adverse symptoms to report (see Patient Education).

Monitoring Laboratory Tests: Platelet counts, hemoglobin, hematocrit, signs of bleeding; aPTT or ACT depending upon indication. For intermittent I.V. injections, PTT is measured 3.5-4 hours after I.V. injection. **Note:** Continuous I.V. infusion is preferred vs I.V. intermittent injections. For full-dose heparin (ie, nonlow-dose), the dose should be titrated according to PTT results. For anticoagulation, an aPTT 1.5-2.5 times normal is usually desired; aPTT is usually measured prior to heparin therapy, 6-8 hours after initiation of a continuous infusion (following a loading dose), and 6-8 hours after changes in the infusion rate; increase or decrease infusion by 2-4 units/kg/hour dependent on PTT.

Heparin infusion dose adjustment:

aPTT >3x control: Decrease infusion rate 50%.

aPTT 2-3x control: Decrease infusion rate 25%.

aPTT 1.5-2x control: No change.

aPTT <1.5x control: Increase rate of infusion 25%; max 2500 units/hour.

Patient Education: Do not take any new medication, including over-the-counter and biological products, during therapy unless approved by prescriber. This drug can only be administered by infusion or injection. You may have a tendency to bleed easily while taking this drug (brush teeth with soft brush, floss with waxed floss, use electric razor, avoid scissors or sharp knives, and potentially harmful activities). Report immediately any chest pain; difficulty breathing or unusual cough; bleeding or bruising (bleeding gums, nosebleed, blood in urine, dark stool); pain in joints or back; CNS changes (fever, confusion); unusual fever; persistent nausea or GI upset; change in vision, or swelling, pain, or redness at injection site. **Pregnancy precaution:** Inform prescriber if you are pregnant.

Geriatric Considerations: At similar dosages, heparin levels tend to be higher in elderly patients (>60 years of age). In the clinical setting, age has not been shown to be a reliable predictor of a patient's anticoagulant response to heparin. However, it is common for older patients to have a "standard" response for the first 24-48 hours after a loading dose (5000 units) and a maintenance infusion of 800-1000 units/hour. After this period, they then have an exaggerated response (eg, elevated PTT), requiring a lower infusion rate. Hence, monitor closely during this period of therapy. Older women (>60 years of age) are more likely to have bleeding complications and osteoporosis may be a problem when used >3 months or total daily dose exceeds 30,000 units.

Pregnancy Risk Factor: C

Lactation: Does not enter breast milk/compatible

Administration

I.M.: Do not administer I.M. due to pain, irritation, and hematoma formation.

I.V.:

Continuous infusion: Infuse via infusion pump.

Heparin lock: Inject via injection cap using positive pressure flushing technique. Heparin lock flush solution is intended only to maintain patency of I.V. devices and is **not** to be used for anticoagulant therapy.

Other: SubQ: Inject in subcutaneous tissue only (not muscle tissue). Injection sites should be rotated (usually left and right portions of the abdomen, above iliac crest).

Reconstitution: Stability at room temperature and refrigeration:

Prepared bag: 24 hours

Premixed bag: After seal is broken 4 days

Out of overwrap stability: 30 days

Standard diluent: 25,000 units/500 mL D_5W (premixed)

Minimum volume: 250 mL D_5W

Compatibility: Stable in dextran 6% in dextrose, dextran 6% in NS, D_5LR, $D_5^1/_4NS$, $D_5^1/_2NS$, $D_{25}W$, fat emulsion 10%, $^1/_2NS$, NS

Y-site administration: Incompatible with alatrofloxacin, alteplase, amiodarone, amphotericin B cholesteryl sulfate complex, amsacrine, ciprofloxacin, clarithromycin, diazepam, doxycycline, ergotamine, filgrastim, gatifloxacin, gentamicin, haloperidol, idarubicin, isosorbide dinitrate, levofloxacin, methotrimeprazine, nicardipine, phenytoin, tobramycin, triflupromazine, vancomycin

Compatibility in syringe: Incompatible with amikacin, amiodarone, chlorpromazine, diazepam, doxorubicin, droperidol, droperidol and fentanyl, erythromycin, erythromycin lactobionate, gentamicin, haloperidol, kanamycin, meperidine, methotrimeprazine, pentazocine, promethazine, streptomycin, tobramycin, triflupromazine, vancomycin, warfarin

Compatibility when admixed: Incompatible with alteplase, amikacin, atracurium, ciprofloxacin, cytarabine, daunorubicin, erythromycin lactobionate, gentamicin, hyaluronidase, kanamycin, levorphanol, meperidine, morphine, polymyxin B sulfate, promethazine, streptomycin

Storage: Heparin solutions are colorless to slightly yellow. Minor color variations do not affect therapeutic efficacy. Heparin should be stored at controlled room temperature and protected from freezing and temperatures >40°C.

Additional Information Heparin lock flush solution is intended only to maintain patency of I.V. devices and is **not** to be used for anticoagulant therapy.

Related Information
Anticoagulants, Injectable *on page 1711*
Anticoagulant Therapy Guidelines *on page 1784*
Compatibility of Drugs *on page 1723*
Compatibility of Drugs in Syringe *on page 1725*
Overdose and Toxicology *on page 1775*

Hetastarch (HET a starch)

U.S. Brand Names Hespan®; Hextend®
Synonyms HES; Hydroxyethyl Starch
Generic Available Yes: Sodium chloride infusion
Pharmacologic Category Plasma Volume Expander, Colloid
Medication Safety Issues
Sound-alike/look-alike issues:
Hespan® may be confused with heparin
Use Blood volume expander used in treatment of hypovolemia
Hespan®: Adjunct in leukapheresis to improve harvesting and increasing the yield of granulocytes by centrifugal means
Unlabeled/Investigational Use Hextend®: Priming fluid in pump oxygenators during cardiopulmonary bypass, and as a plasma volume expander during cardiopulmonary bypass
Mechanism of Action/Effect Produces plasma volume expansion by virtue of its highly colloidal starch structure, similar to albumin
Contraindications Hypersensitivity to hydroxyethyl starch or any component of the formulation; severe bleeding disorders, renal failure with oliguria or anuria, or severe congestive heart failure; per the manufacturer, Hextend® is also contraindicated in the treatment of lactic acidosis and in leukapheresis
Warnings/Precautions Anaphylactoid reactions have occurred; use caution in patients allergic to corn (may have cross allergy to hetastarch); use with caution in patients with thrombocytopenia (may interfere with platelet function); large volume may cause drops in hemoglobin concentrations; use with caution in patients at risk from overexpansion of blood volume, including the very young or aged patients, those with CHF or pulmonary edema; volumes >1500 mL may interfere with platelet function and prolong PT and PTT times; use with caution in patients with history of liver disease; note electrolyte content of Hextend® including calcium, lactate, and potassium; use caution in situations where electrolyte and/or acid-base disturbances may be exacerbated (renal impairment, respiratory alkalosis). Safety and efficacy in pediatric patients have not been established, but limited data available.
Adverse Reactions Frequency not defined.
Cardiovascular: Circulatory overload, heart failure, peripheral edema
Central nervous system: Chills, fever, headache, intracranial bleeding
Dermatologic: Itching, pruritus, rash
Endocrine & metabolic: Amylase levels increased, parotid gland enlargement, indirect bilirubin increased, metabolic acidosis
Gastrointestinal: Vomiting
Hematologic: Bleeding, factor VIII:C plasma levels decreased, decreased plasma aggregation decreased, von Willebrand factor decreased, dilutional coagulopathy; prolongation of PT, PTT, clotting time, and bleeding time; thrombocytopenia, anemia, disseminated intravascular coagulopathy (rare), hemolysis (rare)
Neuromuscular & skeletal: Myalgia
Miscellaneous: Anaphylactoid reactions, hypersensitivity, flu-like symptoms (mild)
Overdosage/Toxicology Symptoms of overdose include heart failure, nausea, vomiting, circulatory overload, and bleeding. Treatment is supportive. Hetastarch is not eliminated by hemodialysis.
(Continued)

Hetastarch (Continued)

Pharmacodynamics/Kinetics
Onset of Action: Volume expansion: I.V.: ~30 minutes

Duration of Action: 24-36 hours

Metabolism: Molecules >50,000 daltons require enzymatic degradation by the reticuloendothelial system or amylases in the blood

Excretion: Urine (~40%) within 24 hours; smaller molecular weight molecules readily excreted

Dosing
Adults & Elderly:

Volume expansion: 500-1000 mL (up to 1500 mL/day) or 20 mL/kg/day (up to 1500 mL/day); larger volumes (15,000 mL/24 hours) have been used safely in small numbers of patients

Leukapheresis: 250-700 mL; **Note:** Citrate anticoagulant is added before use.

Pediatrics: Safety and efficacy have not been established.

Renal Impairment: Cl_{cr} <10 mL/minute: Initial dose is the same but subsequent doses should be reduced by 20% to 50% of normal.

Available Dosage Forms
Infusion [premixed in lactated electrolyte injection] (Hextend®): 6% (500 mL)

Infusion, solution [premixed in NaCl 0.9%] (Hespan®): 6% (500 mL)

Monitoring and Teaching Issues
Physical Assessment: See Warnings/Precautions for use cautions (eg, allergy to corn, CHF, pulmonary edema). Patient must be monitored closely for hypersensitivity (anaphylactic reaction) and other major adverse reactions (eg, circulatory overload, cranial bleed, pulmonary edema; see Adverse Reactions). Blood pressure, pulse, central venous pressure, and urine output should be monitored every 5-15 minutes for the first hour and closely thereafter (if pulmonary artery catheter in place, monitor PCWP, SVR, and PVR). Patient teaching should be appropriate to patient condition (see Patient Education).

Monitoring Laboratory Tests: Leukapheresis: CBC, total leukocyte and platelet counts, leukocyte differential count, hemoglobin, hematocrit, PT, PTT

Patient Education: Report immediately any respiratory difficulty, acute headache, muscle pain, or abdominal cramping. **Pregnancy/breast-feeding precautions:** Inform prescriber if you are pregnant. Consult prescriber if breast-feeding.

Pregnancy Risk Factor: C

Lactation: Excretion in breast milk unknown/use caution

Administration
I.V.: Administer I.V. only; infusion pump is required. May administer up to 1.2 g/kg/hour (20 mL/kg/hour). Change I.V. tubing or flush copiously with normal saline before administering blood through the same line. Change I.V. tubing at least every 24 hours. Do not administer Hextend® with blood through the same administration set. Anaphylactoid reactions can occur, have epinephrine and resuscitative equipment available.

Other: Leukapheresis: Mix Hespan® and citrate well. Administer to the input line of the centrifuge apparatus at a ration of 1:8 to 1:13 to venous whole blood.

Reconstitution: Do not use if crystalline precipitate forms or is turbid deep brown.

Compatibility: Stable in NS

Y-site administration: Incompatible with amikacin, cefamandole, cefoperazone, cefotaxime, cefoxitin, gentamicin, ranitidine, theophylline, tobramycin

Storage: Store at room temperature; do not freeze. In leukapheresis, admixtures of 500-560 mL of Hespan® with citrate concentrations up to 2.5% are compatible for 24 hours.

Additional Information
Hetastarch is a synthetic polymer derived from a waxy starch composed of amylopectin.

Hespan®: 6% hetastarch in 0.9% sodium chloride
Molecular weight: 450,000
Sodium: 154 mEq/L
Chloride: 154 mEq/L

Hextend®: 6% hetastarch in lactated electrolyte injection
Molecular weight: 670,000
Sodium: 143 mEq/L
Chloride: 124 mEq/L
Calcium: 5 mEq/L
Potassium: 3 mEq/L
Magnesium: 0.9 mEq/L
Lactate: 28 mEq/L
Dextrose: 0.99 g/L

♦ **HMM** *see* Altretamine *on page 82*

♦ **HMR 3647** *see* Telithromycin *on page 1430*

♦ **HMS Liquifilm**® *see* Medrysone *on page 940*

♦ **HN₂** *see* Mechlorethamine *on page 935*

♦ **Horse Antihuman Thymocyte Gamma Globulin** *see* Antithymocyte Globulin (Equine) *on page 129*

♦ **H.P. Acthar**® **Gel** *see page 1625*

♦ **HTF919** *see* Tegaserod *on page 1429*

♦ **hu1124** *see* Efalizumab *on page 508*

♦ **Humalog**® *see* Insulin Preparations *on page 805*

♦ **Humalog**® **Mix 75/25**™ *see* Insulin Preparations *on page 805*

♦ **Human Antitumor Necrosis Factor-Alpha** *see* Adalimumab *on page 51*

Human Growth Hormone (HYU man grothe HOR mone)

U.S. Brand Names Genotropin®; Genotropin Miniquick®; Humatrope®; Norditropin®; Norditropin® NordiFlex®; Nutropin®; Nutropin AQ®; Nutropin Depot® [DSC]; Protropin® [DSC]; Saizen®; Serostim®; Tev-Tropin™; Zorbtive™

Synonyms Growth Hormone; Somatrem; Somatropin

Generic Available No

Pharmacologic Category Growth Hormone

Medication Safety Issues

Sound-alike/look-alike issues:

Protropin® may be confused with Proloprim®, protamine, Protopam®

Somatrem may be confused with somatropin

Somatropin may be confused with somatrem, sumatriptan

Use

Children:

Long-term treatment of growth failure due to inadequate endogenous growth hormone secretion (Genotropin®, Humatrope®, Norditropin®, Nutropin®, Nutropin AQ®, Nutropin Depot®, Protropin®, Saizen®, Tev-Tropin™)

Long-term treatment of short stature associated with Turner syndrome (Humatrope®, Nutropin®, Nutropin AQ®)

Treatment of Prader-Willi syndrome (Genotropin®)

Treatment of growth failure associated with chronic renal insufficiency (CRI) up until the time of renal transplantation (Nutropin®, Nutropin AQ®)

Long-term treatment of growth failure in children born small for gestational age who fail to manifest catch-up growth by 2 years of age (Genotropin®)

Long-term treatment of idiopathic short stature (nongrowth hormone-deficient short stature) defined by height standard deviation score (SDS) less than or equal to -2.25 and growth rate not likely to attain normal adult height (Humatrope®)

Adults:

AIDS-wasting or cachexia with concomitant antiviral therapy (Serostim®)

Replacement of endogenous growth hormone in patients with adult growth hormone deficiency who meet both of the following criteria (Genotropin®, Humatrope®, Norditropin®, Nutropin®, Nutropin AQ®, Saizen®):

Biochemical diagnosis of adult growth hormone deficiency by means of a subnormal response to a standard growth hormone stimulation test (peak growth hormone ≤5 mcg/L)

and

Adult-onset: Patients who have adult growth hormone deficiency whether alone or with multiple hormone deficiencies (hypopituitarism) as a result of pituitary disease, hypothalamic disease, surgery, radiation therapy, or trauma

or

Childhood-onset: Patients who were growth hormone deficient during childhood, confirmed as an adult before replacement therapy is initiated

Treatment of short-bowel syndrome (Zorbtive™)

Unlabeled/Investigational Use Investigational: Congestive heart failure; AIDS-wasting/cachexia in children (Serostim®)

Mechanism of Action/Effect Human growth hormone stimulates growth of linear bone, skeletal muscle, and organs; stimulates erythropoietin which increases red blood cell mass; exerts both insulin-like and diabetogenic effects; enhances transmucosal transport of water, electrolytes, and nutrients across the gut

Contraindications Hypersensitivity to growth hormone or any component of the formulation; growth promotion in pediatric patients with closed epiphyses; progression of any underlying intracranial lesion or actively growing intracranial tumor; acute critical illness due to complications following open heart or abdominal surgery; multiple accidental trauma or acute respiratory failure; evidence of active malignancy; use in patients with Prader-Willi syndrome **without** growth hormone deficiency (except Genotropin®) or in patients with Prader-Willi syndrome **with** growth hormone deficiency who are severely obese or have severe respiratory impairment. Saizen® and Norditropin® are contraindicated with proliferative or preproliferative retinopathy.

Warnings/Precautions Use with caution in patients with diabetes or with risk factors for glucose intolerance. Intracranial hypertension has been reported with growth hormone product, funduscopic examinations are recommended; progression of scoliosis may occur in children experiencing rapid growth; patients with growth hormone deficiency may develop slipped capital epiphyses more frequently, evaluate any child with new onset of a limp or with complaints of hip or knee pain; patients with Turner syndrome are at increased risk for otitis media and other ear/hearing disorders, cardiovascular disorders (including stroke, aortic aneurysm, hypertension), and thyroid disease, monitor carefully. Concurrent glucocorticoid therapy may inhibit growth promotion effects; may require dosage adjustment or replacement glucocorticoid therapy in patients with ACTH deficiency. Products may contain benzyl alcohol, m-Cresol or glycerin, some products may be manufactured by recombinant DNA (Continued)

Human Growth Hormone *(Continued)*

technology using *E. coli* as a host, consult specific product labeling. When administering to newborns, reconstitute with sterile water or saline for injection. Not for I.V. injection.

Fatalities have been reported in pediatric patients with Prader-Willi syndrome following the use of growth hormone. The reported fatalities occurred in patients with one or more risk factors, including severe obesity, sleep apnea, respiratory impairment, or unidentified respiratory infection; male patients with one or more of these factors may be at greater risk. Treatment interruption is recommended in patients who show signs of upper airway obstruction, including the onset of, or increased, snoring. In addition, evaluation of and/or monitoring for sleep apnea and respiratory infections are recommended.

Drug Interactions

Decreased Effect: Glucocorticoid therapy may inhibit growth-promoting effects. Growth hormone may induce insulin resistance in patients with diabetes mellitus; monitor glucose and adjust insulin dose as necessary.

Adverse Reactions

Growth hormone deficiency: Antigrowth hormone antibodies, carpal tunnel syndrome (rare), fluid balance disturbances, glucosuria, gynecomastia (rare), headache, hematuria, hyperglycemia (mild), hypoglycemia, hypothyroidism, leukemia, lipoatrophy, muscle pain, increased growth of pre-existing nevi (rare), pain/ local reactions at the injection site, pancreatitis (rare), peripheral edema, exacerbation of psoriasis, rash, seizure, weakness

Idiopathic short stature: Humatrope®: Myalgia (24%), scoliosis (19%), otitis media (16%), arthralgia (11%), arthrosis (11%), hyperlipidemia (8%), gynecomastia (5%), hip pain (3%), hypertension (3%)

Prader-Willi syndrome: Genotropin®: Aggressiveness, arthralgia, edema, hair loss, headache, benign intracranial hypertension, myalgia; fatalities associated with use in this population have been reported

Turner syndrome: Humatrope®: Surgical procedures (45%), otitis media (43%), ear disorders (18%), hypothyroidism (13%), increased nevi (11%), peripheral edema (7%)

Adult growth hormone replacement: Increased ALT, increased AST, arthralgia, back pain, carpal tunnel syndrome, diabetes mellitus, fatigue, flu-like syndrome, gastritis, gastroenteritis, generalized edema, glucose intolerance, gynecomastia (rare), headache, hypertension, hypoesthesia, hypothyroidism, infection (nonviral), insomnia, joint disorder, laryngitis, myalgia, nausea, increased growth of pre-existing nevi, pain, pancreatitis (rare), paresthesia, peripheral edema, pharyngitis, rhinitis, stiffness in extremities, weakness

AIDS wasting or cachexia (limited): Serostim®: Musculoskeletal discomfort (54%), increased tissue turgor (27%), diarrhea (26%), neuropathy (26%), nausea (26%), fatigue (17%), albuminuria (15%), increased diaphoresis (14%), anorexia (12%), anemia (12%), increased AST (12%), insomnia (11%), tachycardia (11%), hyperglycemia (10%), increased ALT (10%)

Short-bowel syndrome: Zorbtive™: Peripheral edema (69% to 81%), edema (facial: 44% to 50%; peripheral 13%), arthralgia (13% to 44%), injection site reaction (19% to 31%), flatulence (25%), abdominal pain (20% to 25%), vomiting (19%), malaise (13%), nausea (13%), diaphoresis increased (13%), rhinitis (7%), dizziness (6%)

Small for gestational age: Genotropin®: Mild, transient hyperglycemia; benign intracranial hypertension (rare); central precocious puberty; jaw prominence (rare); aggravation of pre-existing scoliosis (rare); injection site reactions; progression of pigmented nevi

Overdosage/Toxicology Symptoms of acute overdose may include initial hypoglycemia (with subsequent hyperglycemia), fluid retention, headache, nausea, and vomiting. Long-term overdose may result in signs and symptoms of acromegaly.

Pharmacodynamics/Kinetics

Duration of Action: Maintains supraphysiologic levels for 18-20 hours

Absorption: I.M., SubQ: Well absorbed

Half-Life Elimination: Preparation and route of administration dependent

Metabolism: Hepatic and renal (~90%)

Excretion: Urine

Pharmacokinetic Note: Somatrem and somatropin have equivalent pharmacokinetic properties.

Dosing

Adults:

Growth hormone deficiency: To minimize adverse events in older or overweight patients, reduced dosages may be necessary. During therapy, dosage should be decreased if required by the occurrence of side effects or excessive IGF-I levels.

Somatropin:

Norditropin®: SubQ: Initial dose ≤0.004 mg/kg/day; after 6 weeks of therapy, may increase dose to 0.016 mg/kg/day

Nutropin®, Nutropin® AQ: SubQ: ≤0.006 mg/kg/day; dose may be increased according to individual requirements, up to a maximum of 0.025 mg/kg/day in patients <35 years of age, or up to a maximum of 0.0125 mg/kg/day in patients ≥35 years of age

Humatrope®: SubQ: ≤0.006 mg/kg/day; dose may be increased according to individual requirements, up to a maximum of 0.0125 mg/kg/day

Genotropin®: SubQ: Weekly dosage: ≤0.04 mg/kg divided into 6-7 doses; dose may be increased at 4- to 8-week intervals according to individual requirements, to a maximum of 0.08 mg/kg/week

Saizen®: SubQ: ≤0.005 mg/kg/day; dose may be increased to not more than 0.01 mg/ kg/day after 4 weeks, based on individual requirements.

AIDS-wasting or cachexia:

Serostim®: SubQ: Dose should be given once daily at bedtime; patients who continue to lose weight after 2 weeks should be re-evaluated for opportunistic infections or other clinical events; rotate injection sites to avoid lipodystrophy

Daily dose based on body weight:

<35 kg: 0.1 mg/kg

35-45 kg: 4 mg

45-55 kg: 5 mg

>55 kg: 6 mg

Short-bowel syndrome (Zorbtive™): SubQ: 0.1 mg/kg once daily for 4 weeks (maximum: 8 mg/day)

Fluid retention (moderate) or arthralgias: Treat symptomatically or reduce dose by 50%

Severe toxicity: Discontinue therapy for up to 5 days; when symptoms resolve, restart at 50% of dose. If severe toxicity recurs or does not disappear within 5 days after discontinuation, permanently discontinue treatment.

Elderly: Patients ≥65 years of age may be more sensitive to the action of growth hormone and more prone to adverse effects; in general, dosing should be cautious, beginning at low end of dosing range.

Pediatrics:

Growth hormone deficiency:

Somatrem: *Protropin®:* I.M., SubQ: Weekly dosage: 0.3 mg/kg divided into daily doses

Somatropin:

Genotropin®: SubQ: Weekly dosage: 0.16-0.24 mg/kg divided into 6-7 doses

Humatrope®: I.M., SubQ: Weekly dosage: 0.18 mg/kg; maximum replacement dose: 0.3 mg/kg/week; dosing should be divided into equal doses given 3 times/week on alternating days, 6 times/week, or daily

Norditropin®: SubQ: Weekly dosage: 0.024-0.034 mg/kg administered in the evening, divided into doses 6-7 times/week; cartridge and vial formulations are bioequivalent; cartridge formulation does not need to be reconstituted prior to use

Nutropin Depot®: SubQ:

Once-monthly injection: 1.5 mg/kg administered on the same day of each month; patients >15 kg will require more than 1 injection per dose

Twice-monthly injection: 0.75 mg/kg administered twice each month on the same days of each month (eg, days 1 and 15 of each month); patients >30 kg will require more than 1 injection per dose

Nutropin®, Nutropin® AQ: SubQ: Weekly dosage: 0.3 mg/kg divided into daily doses; pubertal patients: ≤0.7 mg/kg/week divided daily

Tev-Tropin™: SubQ: Up to 0.1 mg/kg administered 3 times/week

Saizen®: I.M., SubQ: 0.06 mg/kg/dose administered 3 times/week

Note: Therapy should be discontinued when patient has reached satisfactory adult height, when epiphyses have fused, or when the patient ceases to respond. Growth of 5 cm/year or more is expected, if growth rate does not exceed 2.5 cm in a 6-month period, double the dose for the next 6 months; if there is still no satisfactory response, discontinue therapy

Chronic renal insufficiency (CRI): *Nutropin®, Nutropin® AQ:* SubQ: Weekly dosage: 0.35 mg/kg divided into daily injections; continue until the time of renal transplantation

Dosage recommendations in patients treated for CRI who require dialysis:

Hemodialysis: Administer dose at night prior to bedtime or at least 3-4 hours after hemodialysis to prevent hematoma formation from heparin

CCPD: Administer dose in the morning following dialysis

CAPD: Administer dose in the evening at the time of overnight exchange

Turner syndrome: *Humatrope®, Nutropin®, Nutropin® AQ:* SubQ: Weekly dosage: ≤0.375 mg/kg divided into equal doses 3-7 times per week

Prader-Willi syndrome: *Genotropin®:* SubQ: Weekly dosage: 0.24 mg/kg divided into 6-7 doses

Small for gestational age: *Genotropin®:* SubQ: Weekly dosage: 0.48 mg/kg divided into 6-7 doses

Idiopathic short stature: *Humatrope®:* SubQ: Weekly dosage: 0.37 mg/kg divided into equal doses 6-7 times/week

AIDS-wasting or cachexia (unlabeled use): *Serostim®:* SubQ: Limited data; doses of 0.04 mg/kg/day were reported in five children, 6-17 years of age; doses of 0.07 mg/kg/day were reported in six children, 8-14 years of age

Renal Impairment: Reports indicate patients with chronic renal failure tend to have decreased clearance; specific dosing suggestions not available

Hepatic Impairment: Clearance may be reduced in patients with severe hepatic dysfunction; specific dosing suggestions are not available.

Available Dosage Forms [DSC] = Discontinued product

Injection, powder for reconstitution [rDNA origin]:

Somatrem: Protropin® [diluent contains benzyl alcohol]: 10 mg [~30 int. units] [DSC]

Somatropin:

Genotropin® [preservative free]: 1.5 mg [4 int. units/mL] [delivers 1.3 mg/mL]

Genotropin® [with preservative]:

5.8 mg [15 int. units/mL] [delivers 5 mg/mL]

13.8 mg [36 int. units/mL] [delivers 12 mg/mL]

Genotropin Miniquick® [preservative free]: 0.2 mg, 0.4 mg, 0.6 mg, 0.8 mg, 1 mg, 1.2 mg, 1.4 mg, 1.6 mg, 1.8 mg, 2 mg [each strength delivers 0.25 mL]

Humatrope®: 5 mg [~15 int. units], 6 mg [18 int. units], 12 mg [36 int. units], 24 mg [72 int. units]

Nutropin® [diluent contains benzyl alcohol]: 5 mg [~15 int. units]; 10 mg [~30 int. units]

Nutropin Depot® [preservative free]: 13.5 mg, 18 mg, 22.5 mg [DSC]

Tev-Tropin™ 5 mg [15 int. units] [diluent contains benzyl alcohol]

Saizen® [diluent contains benzyl alcohol]: 5 mg [~15 int. units; contains sucrose 34.2 mg]; 8.8 mg [~26.4 int. units; contains sucrose 60.2 mg]

Serostim®: 4 mg [12 int. units; contains sucrose 27.3 mg]; 5 mg [15 int. units; contains sucrose 34.2 mg]; 6 mg [18 int. units; contains sucrose 41 mg]

Zorbtive™: 8.8 mg [~26.4 int. units; contains sucrose 60.19 mg; packaged with diluent containing benzyl alcohol]

Injection, solution [rDNA origin]: Somatropin:

Norditropin®: 5 mg/1.5 mL (1.5 mL); 15 mg/1.5 mL (1.5 mL) [cartridge]

Norditropin® NordiFlex®: 5 mg/1.5 mL (1.5 mL); 15 mg/1.5 mL (1.5 mL) [prefilled pen]

Nutropin AQ®: 5 mg/mL [~15 int. units/mL] (2 mL) [vial or cartridge]

(Continued)

Human Growth Hormone *(Continued)*

Monitoring and Teaching Issues

Physical Assessment: Assess potential for interactions with other prescriptions, OTC medications, or herbal products patient may be taking. Assess results of laboratory tests, therapeutic effectiveness (according to purpose for use), and adverse reactions Perform funduscopic examinations at initiation of therapy and periodically during treatment; Instruct patients with diabetes to monitor glucose levels closely (may induce insulin intolerance). Instruct patient in proper use if self-administered (storage, reconstitution, injection techniques, and syringe/needle disposal), possible side effects/appropriate interventions, and adverse symptoms to report. Pediatrics: Monitor growth curve: annually determine bone age.

Monitoring Laboratory Tests: Periodic thyroid function tests, periodical urine testing for glucose, somatomedin C (IGF-I) levels; serum phosphorus, alkaline phosphatase and parathyroid hormone. If growth deceleration is observed in children treated for growth hormone deficiency, and not due to other causes, evaluate for presence of antibody formation. Strict blood glucose monitoring in diabetic patients.

Somatrem (Protropin®): Consider changing to somatropin if antibody binding capacity is >2 mg/L

Patient Education: This drug can only be administered by injection. If self-administered, you will be instructed by prescriber on proper storage, reconstitution, injection technique, and syringe/needle disposal. Use exactly as prescribed; do not discontinue or alter dose without consulting prescriber. Report immediately any pain, redness, burning, drainage, or swelling at injection site. If you have diabetes, monitor glucose levels closely; this medication may cause an alteration in your insulin levels. May cause side effects which are particular to purpose for use and formulation prescribed; your prescriber will instruct you in particular side effects for your medication. Report immediately unusual or persistent bleeding, excessive fatigue or swelling (edema) of extremities, joint or muscle pain or headache, nausea or vomiting, personality changes, or other persistent adverse effects. **Pregnancy/breast-feeding precaution:** Inform prescriber if you are or intend to become pregnant. Breast-feeding is not recommended.

Dietary Considerations:

Prader-Willi syndrome: All patients should have effective weight control (use is contraindicated in severely-obese patients).

Short-bowel syndrome: Intravenous parenteral nutrition requirements may need reassessment as gastrointestinal absorption improves.

Pregnancy Risk Factor: B/C (depending upon manufacturer)

Lactation: Excretion in breast milk unknown/not recommended

Administration

I.M.: Do not shake; administer SubQ or I.M. (rotate administration sites to avoid tissue atrophy); refer to product labeling. When administering to newborns, reconstitute with sterile water for injection. Cartridge must be administered using the corresponding color-coded NordiPen® injection pen.

Reconstitution:

Somatrem: Protropin®: Vial:

5 mg: Reconstitute with 1-5 mL bacteriostatic water for injection.

10 mg: Reconstitute with 1-10 mL bacteriostatic water for injection.

Somatropin:

Genotropin®: Reconstitute with diluent provided.

Genotropin MiniQuick®: Reconstitute with diluent provided. Consult the instructions provided with the reconstitution device.

Humatrope®:

Cartridge: Consult HumatroPen™ User Guide for complete instructions for reconstitution. **Do not use diluent provided with vials.**

Vial: 5 mg: Reconstitute with 1.5-5 mL diluent provided.

Norditropin®: Vial: Reconstitute with 2 mL of diluent provided.

Nutropin®: Vial:

5 mg: Reconstitute with 1-5 mL bacteriostatic water for injection.

10 mg: Reconstitute with 1-10 mL bacteriostatic water for injection.

Nutropin Depot®: Reconstitute with diluent provided **only**.

Saizen®: Vial:

5 mg: Reconstitute with 1-3 mL bacteriostatic water for injection or sterile water for injection; gently swirl; do not shake.

8.8 mg: Reconstitute with 2-3 mL bacteriostatic water for injection or sterile water for injection; gently swirl; do not shake.

Serostim®: Vial: Reconstitute with 0.5-1 mL sterile water for injection.

Tev-Tropin™: Reconstitute with 1-5 mL of diluent provided. Gently swirl; do not shake. May use preservative-free NS for use in newborns.

Zorbtive™: 8.8 mg vial: Reconstitute with 1-2 mL bacteriostatic water for injection; use within 14 days

Storage:

Somatrem: Protropin®: Before and after reconstitution, store at 2°C to 8°C (36°F to 46°F), avoid freezing; when reconstituted with bacteriostatic water for injection; use within 14 days; when reconstituted with sterile water for injection, use immediately (only one dose per vial) and discard unused portion

Somatropin:

Genotropin®: Store at 2°C to 8°C (36°F to 46°F), do not freeze, protect from light

1.5 mg cartridge: Following reconstitution, store under refrigeration and use within 24 hours; discard unused portion

5.8 mg and 13.8 mg cartridge: Following reconstitution, store under refrigeration and use within 21 days

Miniquick®: Store in refrigerator prior to dispensing, but may be stored ≤25°C (77°F) for up to 3 months after dispensing; once reconstituted, solution must be refrigerated and used within 24 hours; discard unused portion

Humatrope®:
  Vial: Before and after reconstitution, store at 2°C to 8°C (36°F to 46°F), avoid freezing; when reconstituted with bacteriostatic water for injection, use within 14 days; when reconstituted with sterile water for injection, use within 24 hours and discard unused portion
  Cartridge: Before and after reconstitution, store at 2°C to 8°C (36°F to 46°F), avoid freezing; following reconstitution, stable for 14 days under refrigeration. Dilute with solution provided with cartridges **ONLY**; do not use diluent provided with vials
Norditropin®: Store at 2°C to 8°C (36°F to 46°F), do not freeze; avoid direct light
  Cartridge: Must be used within 4 weeks once inserted into pen
  Prefilled pen: Must be used within 4 weeks after initial injection
Nutropin®: Before and after reconstitution, store at 2°C to 8°C (36°F to 46°F), avoid freezing
  Vial: Reconstitute with bacteriostatic water for injection; use reconstituted vials within 14 days; when reconstituted with sterile water for injection, use immediately and discard unused portion
  AQ formulation: Use within 28 days following initial use
  Depot formulation: Before suspension, store at 2°C to 8°C (36°F to 46°F), avoid freezing; use suspended solution immediately; dilute only with diluent provided
Saizen®: Prior to reconstitution, store at room temperature 15°C to 30°C (59°F to 86°F); following reconstitution with bacteriostatic water for injection, reconstituted solution should be refrigerated and used within 14 days; when reconstituted with sterile water for injection, use immediately and discard unused portion
Serostim®: Prior to reconstitution, store at room temperature 15°C to 30°C (59°F to 86°F); reconstitute with sterile water for injection; store reconstituted solution under refrigeration and use within 24 hours, avoid freezing. Do not use if cloudy
Tev-Tropin™: Prior to reconstitution, store at 2°C to 8°C (36°F to 46°F). Following reconstitution with bacteriostatic NS, solution should be refrigerated and used within 14 days. Some cloudiness may occur; do not use if cloudiness persists after warming to room temperature.
Zorbtive™: Store unopened vials and diluent at room temperature of 15°C to 30°C (59°F to 86°F). Store reconstituted 8.8 mg vial under refrigeration at 2°C to 8°C (36°F to 46°F); avoid freezing.

- ◆ **Human LFA-3/IgG(1) Fusion Protein** *see* Alefacept *on page 64*
- ◆ **Humate-P®** *see* Antihemophilic Factor (Human) *on page 124*
- ◆ **Humatrope®** *see* Human Growth Hormone *on page 745*
- ◆ **Humibid® CS [OTC]** *see* Guaifenesin and Dextromethorphan *on page 731*
- ◆ **Humibid® DM [DSC]** *see* Guaifenesin and Dextromethorphan *on page 731*
- ◆ **Humibid® e [OTC]** *see* Guaifenesin *on page 729*
- ◆ **Humira®** *see* Adalimumab *on page 51*
- ◆ **Humulin® 50/50** *see* Insulin Preparations *on page 805*
- ◆ **Humulin® 70/30** *see* Insulin Preparations *on page 805*
- ◆ **Humulin® L** *see* Insulin Preparations *on page 805*
- ◆ **Humulin® N** *see* Insulin Preparations *on page 805*
- ◆ **Humulin® R** *see* Insulin Preparations *on page 805*
- ◆ **Humulin® R (Concentrated) U-500** *see* Insulin Preparations *on page 805*
- ◆ **Humulin® U** *see* Insulin Preparations *on page 805*
- ◆ **Hurricaine®** *see* Benzocaine *on page 181*
- ◆ **HXM** *see* Altretamine *on page 82*
- ◆ **Hyate:C®** *see* Antihemophilic Factor (Porcine) *on page 126*
- ◆ **Hycamptamine** *see* Topotecan *on page 1497*
- ◆ **Hycamtin®** *see* Topotecan *on page 1497*
- ◆ **hycet™** *see* Hydrocodone and Acetaminophen *on page 754*

HydrALAZINE (hye DRAL a zeen)

Synonyms Apresoline [DSC]; Hydralazine Hydrochloride
Generic Available Yes
Pharmacologic Category Vasodilator
Medication Safety Issues
  Sound-alike/look-alike issues:
    HydrALAZINE may be confused with hydrOXYzine
Use Management of moderate to severe hypertension, congestive heart failure, hypertension secondary to pre-eclampsia/eclampsia; treatment of primary pulmonary hypertension
Mechanism of Action/Effect Direct vasodilation of arterioles (with little effect on veins) with decreased systemic resistance
Contraindications Hypersensitivity to hydralazine or any component of the formulation; mitral valve rheumatic heart disease
Warnings/Precautions May cause a drug-induced lupus-like syndrome (more likely on larger doses, longer duration). Adjust dose in severe renal dysfunction. Use with caution in CAD (increase in tachycardia may increase myocardial oxygen demand). Use with caution in pulmonary hypertension (may cause hypotension). Titrate cautiously to response. Hypotensive effect after I.V. administration may be delayed and unpredictable in some patients. Hydralazine-induced fluid and sodium retention may require addition or increased dosage of a diuretics.
Drug Interactions
  Cytochrome P450 Effect: Inhibits CYP3A4 (weak)
  Decreased Effect: NSAIDs (eg, indomethacin) may decrease the hemodynamic effects of hydralazine.
  Increased Effect/Toxicity: Hydralazine may increase levels of beta-blockers (metoprolol, propranolol). Some beta-blockers (acebutolol, atenolol, and nadolol) are unlikely to be affected due to limited hepatic metabolism. Concurrent use of hydralazine with MAO
(Continued)

HydrALAZINE *(Continued)*

inhibitors may cause a significant decrease in blood pressure. Propranolol may increase hydralazine serum concentrations.

Nutritional/Ethanol Interactions
Ethanol: Avoid ethanol (may increase CNS depression).
Food: Food enhances bioavailability of hydralazine.
Herb/Nutraceutical: Avoid dong quai if using for hypertension (has estrogenic activity). Avoid ephedra, yohimbe, ginseng (may worsen hypertension). Avoid garlic (may have increased antihypertensive effect).

Adverse Reactions Frequency not defined.
Cardiovascular: Tachycardia, angina pectoris, orthostatic hypotension (rare), dizziness (rare), paradoxical hypertension, peripheral edema, vascular collapse (rare), flushing
Central nervous system: Increased intracranial pressure (I.V., in patient with pre-existing increased intracranial pressure), fever (rare), chills (rare), anxiety*, disorientation*, depression*, coma*
Dermatologic: Rash (rare), urticaria (rash), pruritus (rash)
Gastrointestinal: Anorexia, nausea, vomiting, diarrhea, constipation, adynamic ileus
Genitourinary: Difficulty in micturition, impotence
Hematologic: Hemolytic anemia (rare), eosinophilia (rare), decreased hemoglobin concentration (rare), reduced erythrocyte count (rare), leukopenia (rare), agranulocytosis (rare), thrombocytopenia (rare)
Neuromuscular & skeletal: Rheumatoid arthritis, muscle cramps, weakness, tremor, peripheral neuritis (rare)
Ocular: Lacrimation, conjunctivitis
Respiratory: Nasal congestion, dyspnea
Miscellaneous: Drug-induced lupus-like syndrome (dose related; fever, arthralgia, splenomegaly, lymphadenopathy, asthenia, myalgia, malaise, pleuritic chest pain, edema, positive ANA, positive LE cells, maculopapular facial rash, positive direct Coombs' test, pericarditis, pericardial tamponade), diaphoresis
*Seen in uremic patients and severe hypertension where rapidly escalating doses may have caused hypotension leading to these effects.

Overdosage/Toxicology Symptoms of overdose include hypotension, tachycardia, and shock. Treatment is supportive and symptomatic.

Pharmacodynamics/Kinetics
Onset of Action: Oral: 20-30 minutes; I.V.: 5-20 minutes
Duration of Action: Oral: Up to 8 hours; I.V.: 1-4 hours; **Note:** May vary depending on acetylator status of patient
Bioavailability: 30% to 50%; increased with food
Protein Binding: 85% to 90%
Half-Life Elimination: Normal renal function: 2-8 hours; End-stage renal disease: 7-16 hours
Metabolism: Hepatically acetylated; extensive first-pass effect (oral)
Excretion: Urine (14% as unchanged drug)

Dosing
Adults:
Hypertension: Oral:
Initial: 10 mg 4 times/day; increase by 10-25 mg/dose every 2-5 days (maximum: 300 mg/day); usual dose range (JNC 7): 25-100 mg/day in 2 divided doses
Acute hypertension: I.M., I.V.: Initial: 10-20 mg/dose every 4-6 hours as needed, may increase to 40 mg/dose; change to oral therapy as soon as possible.
Pre-eclampsia/eclampsia: I.M., I.V.: 5 mg/dose then 5-10 mg every 20-30 minutes as needed
Congestive heart failure: Oral:
Initial dose: 10-25 mg 3-4 times/day
Adjustment: Dosage must be adjusted based on individual response.
Target dose: 75 mg 4 times/day in combination with isosorbide dinitrate (40 mg 4 times a day)
Range: Typically 200-600 mg daily in 2-4 divided doses. Dosages as high as 3 g/day have been used in some patients for symptomatic and hemodynamic improvement. Hydralazine 75 mg 4 times a day combined with isosorbide dinitrate 40 mg 4 times a day were shown in clinical trials to provide a mortality benefit in the treatment of CHF. Higher doses may be used for symptomatic and hemodynamic improvement following optimization of standard therapy.
Elderly: Oral: Initial: 10 mg 2-3 times/day; increase by 10-25 mg/day every 2-5 days.
Pediatrics:
Hypertension: Oral: Initial: 0.75-1 mg/kg/day in 2-4 divided doses; increase over 3-4 weeks to maximum of 7.5 mg/kg/day in 2-4 divided doses; maximum daily dose: 200 mg/day
Acute hypertension: I.M., I.V.: 0.1-0.2 mg/kg/dose (not to exceed 20 mg) every 4-6 hours as needed, up to 1.7-3.5 mg/kg/day in 4-6 divided doses
Renal Impairment:
Cl$_{cr}$ 10-50 mL/minute: Administer every 8 hours.
Cl$_{cr}$ <10 mL/minute: Administer every 8-16 hours in fast acetylators and every 12-24 hours in slow acetylators.
Hemodialysis effects: Supplemental dose is not necessary.
Peritoneal dialysis effects: Supplemental dose is not necessary.

Available Dosage Forms
Injection, solution, as hydrochloride: 20 mg/mL (1 mL)
Tablet, as hydrochloride: 10 mg, 25 mg, 50 mg, 100 mg

Monitoring and Teaching Issues
Physical Assessment: Use caution in presence of renal dysfunction, CAD, orpulmonary hypertension (see Warnings/Precautions). Assess potential for interactions with other pharmacological agents or herbalproducts patient may be taking (especially anything that may

impact blood pressure; see Drug Interactions). For infusion seeAdministration specifics. Orthostatic precautions should be observed and patient monitored closely during and following infusion.Assess results of laboratory tests, therapeutic effectiveness (decreased blood pressure), and adverse response (eg, hypotension,fluid retention; see Adverse Reactions) periodically during therapy. Teach patient proper use (oral), possible side-effects/appropriate interventions, and adverse symptoms to report (see Patient Education).

Monitoring Laboratory Tests: ANA titer

Patient Education: Do not take any new medication during therapy unless approved by prescriber. Take as directed, with meals. Avoid alcohol. This medication does not replace other antihypertensive interventions; follow prescriber's instructions for diet and lifestyle changes. Weigh daily at the same time, in the same clothes for the first 2 weeks and weekly thereafter. Report weight gain >5 lb/week or swelling of feet or ankles. May cause postural hypotension, dizziness, or weakness (change position slowly when rising from sitting or lying position, climbing stairs, and avoid driving or activities requiring alertness until response to drug is known); nausea or vomiting (small frequent meals, frequent mouth care, chewing gum, or sucking lozenges may help); impotence (reversible); diarrhea (boiled milk, buttermilk, or yogurt may help); or constipation (increased exercise, fluids, fruit, or fiber may help). Report chest pain, rapid heartbeat, or palpitations; flu-like symptoms; respiratory difficulty; skin rash; numbness and tingling of extremities; muscle cramps, weakness, or tremors; persistent GI problems; or other adverse reactions. **Pregnancy precaution:** Inform prescriber if you are or intend to become pregnant.

Dietary Considerations: Administer with meals.

Pregnancy Risk Factor: C

Pregnancy Issues: Crosses the placenta. One report of fetal arrhythmia; transient neonatal thrombocytopenia and fetal distress reported following late 3rd trimester use. A large amount of clinical experience with the use of this drug for management of hypertension during pregnancy is available.

Lactation: Enters breast milk/compatible

Breast-Feeding Issues: Crosses into breast milk in extremely small amounts. Available evidence suggests safe use during breast-feeding. AAP considers **compatible** with breast-feeding.

Administration

I.V.: Inject over 1 minute. Hypotensive effect may be delayed and unpredictable in some patients.

Reconstitution: Hydralazine should be diluted in NS for IVPB administration due to decreased stability in D_5W. Stability of IVPB solution in NS is 4 days at room temperature.

Compatibility: Stable in dextran 6% in dextrose, dextran 6% in NS, D_5LR, $D_5^{1}/_4NS$, $D_5^{1}/_2NS$, D_5NS, $D_{10}W$, LR, $^{1}/_2NS$, NS; **incompatible** with D_5W

Y-site administration: Incompatible with aminophylline, ampicillin, diazoxide, furosemide **Compatibility when admixed: Incompatible** with aminophylline, ampicillin, chlorothiazide, edetate calcium disodium, ethacrynate, hydrocortisone sodium succinate, mephentermine, methohexital, nitroglycerin, phenobarbital, verapamil

Storage: Intact ampuls/vials of hydralazine should not be stored under refrigeration because of possible precipitation or crystallization.

Related Information

FDA Name Differentiation Project: The Use of Tall-Man Letters *on page 15*
Heart Failure *on page 1828*

Hydralazine and Hydrochlorothiazide (hye DRAL a zeen & hye droe klor oh THYE a zide)

Synonyms Apresazide [DSC]; Hydrochlorothiazide and Hydralazine

Generic Available Yes

Pharmacologic Category Antihypertensive Agent, Combination

Use Management of moderate to severe hypertension and treatment of congestive heart failure

Dosing

Adults: Hypertension: Oral: 1 capsule twice daily

Elderly: Refer to dosing in individual monographs.

Available Dosage Forms

Capsule:

25/25: Hydralazine hydrochloride 25 mg and hydrochlorothiazide 25 mg
50/50: Hydralazine hydrochloride 50 mg and hydrochlorothiazide 50 mg
100/50: Hydralazine hydrochloride 100 mg and hydrochlorothiazide 50 mg

Monitoring and Teaching Issues

Physical Assessment: See individual agents.

Patient Education: See individual agents. **Pregnancy precaution:** Inform prescriber if you are or intend to become pregnant.

Pregnancy Risk Factor: C

Lactation: Enters breast milk/compatible

Related Information

HydrALAZINE *on page 749*
Hydrochlorothiazide *on page 751*

♦ **Hydralazine Hydrochloride** *see* HydrALAZINE *on page 749*

♦ **Hydramine® [OTC]** *see* DiphenhydrAMINE *on page 463*

♦ **Hydrated Chloral** *see* Chloral Hydrate *on page 303*

♦ **Hydrea®** *see* Hydroxyurea *on page 771*

Hydrochlorothiazide (hye droe klor oh THYE a zide)

U.S. Brand Names Microzide™

Synonyms HCTZ

Generic Available Yes

Pharmacologic Category Diuretic, Thiazide

(Continued)

Hydrochlorothiazide *(Continued)*

Medication Safety Issues

Sound-alike/look-alike issues:

Hydrochlorothiazide may be confused with hydrocortisone, hydroflumethiazide

Esidrix may be confused with Lasix®

Use Management of mild to moderate hypertension; treatment of edema in congestive heart failure and nephrotic syndrome

Unlabeled/Investigational Use Treatment of lithium-induced diabetes insipidus

Mechanism of Action/Effect Inhibits sodium reabsorption in the distal tubules causing increased excretion of sodium and water as well as potassium and hydrogen ions

Contraindications Hypersensitivity to hydrochlorothiazide or any component of the formulation, thiazides, or sulfonamide-derived drugs; anuria; renal decompensation; pregnancy

Warnings/Precautions Avoid in severe renal disease (ineffective as a diuretic). Electrolyte disturbances (hypokalemia, hypochloremic alkalosis, hyponatremia) can occur. Use with caution in severe hepatic dysfunction; hepatic encephalopathy can be caused by electrolyte disturbances. Gout may be precipitated in patients with a history of gout, a familial predisposition to gout, or chronic renal failure. Use caution in patients with diabetes; may alter glucose control. May cause SLE exacerbation or activation. Use with caution in patients with moderate or high cholesterol concentrations. Photosensitization may occur. Correct hypokalemia before initiating therapy.

Chemical similarities are present among sulfonamides, sulfonylureas, carbonic anhydrase inhibitors, thiazides, and loop diuretics (except ethacrynic acid). Use in patients with sulfonamide allergy is specifically contraindicated in product labeling, however, a risk of cross-reaction exists in patients with allergy to any of these compounds; avoid use when previous reaction has been severe.

Drug Interactions

Decreased Effect: Effects of oral hypoglycemics may be decreased. Decreased absorption of hydrochlorothiazide with cholestyramine and colestipol. NSAIDs can decrease the efficacy of thiazides, reducing the diuretic and antihypertensive effects.

Increased Effect/Toxicity: Increased effect of hydrochlorothiazide with furosemide and other loop diuretics. Increased hypotension and/or renal adverse effects of ACE inhibitors may result in aggressively diuresed patients. Beta-blockers increase hyperglycemic effects of thiazides in type 2 diabetes mellitus. Cyclosporine and thiazides can increase the risk of gout or renal toxicity. Digoxin toxicity can be exacerbated if a thiazide induces hypokalemia or hypomagnesemia. Lithium toxicity can occur with thiazides due to reduced renal excretion of lithium. Thiazides may prolong the duration of action with neuromuscular blocking agents.

Nutritional/Ethanol Interactions

Food: Hydrochlorothiazide peak serum levels may be decreased if taken with food. This product may deplete potassium, sodium, and magnesium.

Herb/Nutraceutical: Avoid dong quai if using for hypertension (has estrogenic activity). Dong quai may also cause photosensitization. Avoid ephedra, ginseng, yohimbe (may worsen hypertension). Avoid garlic (may have increased antihypertensive effect).

Lab Interactions Increased creatine phosphokinase [CPK] (S), ammonia (B), amylase (S), calcium (S), chloride (S), cholesterol (S), glucose, acid (S); decreased chloride (S), magnesium, potassium (S), sodium (S); tyramine and phentolamine tests; histamine tests for pheochromocytoma

Adverse Reactions

1% to 10%:

Cardiovascular: Orthostatic hypotension, hypotension

Dermatologic: Photosensitivity

Endocrine & metabolic: Hypokalemia

Gastrointestinal: Anorexia, epigastric distress

Overdosage/Toxicology Symptoms of overdose include hypermotility, diuresis, lethargy, confusion, and muscle weakness. Treatment is supportive.

Pharmacodynamics/Kinetics

Onset of Action: Diuresis: ~2 hours; Peak effect: 4-6 hours

Duration of Action: 6-12 hours

Absorption: ~50% to 80%

Bioavailability: 50% to 80%

Time to Peak: 1-2.5 hours

Protein Binding: 68%

Half-Life Elimination: 5.6-14.8 hours

Metabolism: Not metabolized

Excretion: Urine (as unchanged drug)

Dosing

Adults:

Edema (diuresis): Oral: 25-100 mg/day in 1-2 doses; maximum: 200 mg/day

Hypertension: Oral: 12.5-50 mg/day; minimal increase in response and more electrolyte disturbances are seen with doses >50 mg/day

Elderly: Oral: 12.5-25 mg once daily; minimal increase in response and more electrolyte disturbances are seen with doses >50 mg/day (see Geriatric Considerations).

Pediatrics: Hypertension, edema (diuretic): Oral (effect of drug may be decreased when used every day):

Children <6 months: 2-3 mg/kg/day in 2 divided doses

Children >6 months: 2 mg/kg/day in 2 divided doses

Note: In pediatric patients, chlorothiazide may be preferred over hydrochlorothiazide as there are more dosage formulations (eg, suspension) available.

Renal Impairment: Cl$_{cr}$ <30 mL/minute: Dosing adjustment not effective, therefore not generally recommended.

Available Dosage Forms

Capsule (Microzide™): 12.5 mg

Tablet: 25 mg, 50 mg

Monitoring and Teaching Issues

Physical Assessment: Assess allergy history prior to beginning therapy (sulfonamides). See Warnings/Precautions for specific use cautions (renal or hepatic disease, diabetes, SLE, hyperlipidemia). Assess potential for interactions with other pharmacological or herbal products patient may be taking (altered effect of oral hypoglycemics, increased risk of hypotension or toxicity; see Drug Interactions). Assess results of laboratory tests, therapeutic effectiveness (according to purpose for use), and adverse response regularly during therapy (eg, hypotension, hypokalemia, confusion; see Adverse Reactions). Caution patients with diabetes to monitor glucose levels closely; may alter glucose control. Teach proper use, possible side effects/appropriate interventions, and adverse symptoms to report (see Patient Education). **Note:** See Pregnancy Issues.

Monitoring Laboratory Tests: Serum electrolytes, BUN, creatinine

Patient Education: Do not take any new medication during therapy unless approved by prescriber. This medication does not replace other antihypertensive interventions; follow prescriber's instructions for diet and lifestyle changes. Take as directed, with meals, early in the day to avoid nocturia. Your prescriber may prescribe a potassium supplement or recommend that you eat foods high in potassium (include bananas and/or orange juice in daily diet). Do not change your diet on your own while taking this medication, especially if you are taking potassium supplements or medications to reduce potassium loss; too much potassium can be as harmful as too little. If you have diabetes, monitor serum glucose closely; this medication may increase serum glucose levels. May cause dizziness or postural hypotension (use caution when rising from sitting or lying position, when driving, climbing stairs, or engaging in tasks that require alertness until response to drug is known); nausea or vomiting (small frequent meals, frequent mouth care, sucking lozenges, or chewing gum may help); impotence (reversible); constipation (increased exercise, fluids, fruit, or fiber may help); or photosensitivity (use sunscreen, wear protective clothing and eyewear, and avoid direct sunlight). Report persistent flu-like symptoms, chest pain, palpitations, muscle cramping, respiratory difficulty, skin rash or itching, unusual bruising or easy bleeding, or excessive fatigue. **Pregnancy/breast-feeding precautions:** Inform prescriber if you are pregnant. Consult prescriber if breast-feeding.

Geriatric Considerations: Hydrochlorothiazide is not effective in patients with a Cl$_{cr}$ <30 mL/minute, therefore, it may not be a useful agent in many elderly patients.

Pregnancy Risk Factor: B (manufacturer); D (expert analysis)

Pregnancy Issues: Although there are no adequate and well-controlled studies using hydrochlorothiazide in pregnancy, thiazide diuretics may cause an increased risk of congenital defects. Hypoglycemia, hypokalemia, hyponatremia, jaundice, and thrombocytopenia are also reported as possible complications to the fetus or newborn.

Lactation: Enters breast milk/use caution (AAP rates "compatible")

Administration

Oral: May be taken with food or milk. Take early in day to avoid nocturia. Take the last dose of multiple doses no later than 6 PM unless instructed otherwise.

Additional Information If given the morning of surgery it may render the patient volume depleted and blood pressure may be labile during general anesthesia. Effect of drug may be decreased when used every day.

Related Information

Heart Failure *on page 1828*

♦ **Hydrochlorothiazide and Amiloride** *see* Amiloride and Hydrochlorothiazide *on page 90*
♦ **Hydrochlorothiazide and Benazepril** *see* Benazepril and Hydrochlorothiazide *on page 180*
♦ **Hydrochlorothiazide and Bisoprolol** *see* Bisoprolol and Hydrochlorothiazide *on page 201*
♦ **Hydrochlorothiazide and Captopril** *see* Captopril and Hydrochlorothiazide *on page 248*
♦ **Hydrochlorothiazide and Enalapril** *see* Enalapril and Hydrochlorothiazide *on page 518*
♦ **Hydrochlorothiazide and Eprosartan** *see* Eprosartan and Hydrochlorothiazide *on page 537*
♦ **Hydrochlorothiazide and Hydralazine** *see* Hydralazine and Hydrochlorothiazide *on page 751*
♦ **Hydrochlorothiazide and Irbesartan** *see* Irbesartan and Hydrochlorothiazide *on page 829*
♦ **Hydrochlorothiazide and Lisinopril** *see* Lisinopril and Hydrochlorothiazide *on page 908*
♦ **Hydrochlorothiazide and Losartan** *see* Losartan and Hydrochlorothiazide *on page 924*
♦ **Hydrochlorothiazide and Methyldopa** *see* Methyldopa and Hydrochlorothiazide *on page 981*
♦ **Hydrochlorothiazide and Moexipril** *see* Moexipril and Hydrochlorothiazide *on page 1026*
♦ **Hydrochlorothiazide and Olmesartan Medoxomil** *see* Olmesartan and Hydrochlorothiazide *on page 1113*
♦ **Hydrochlorothiazide and Propranolol** *see* Propranolol and Hydrochlorothiazide *on page 1276*
♦ **Hydrochlorothiazide and Quinapril** *see* Quinapril and Hydrochlorothiazide *on page 1296*

Hydrochlorothiazide and Spironolactone

(hye droe klor oh THYE a zide & speer on oh LAK tone)

U.S. Brand Names Aldactazide®

Synonyms Spironolactone and Hydrochlorothiazide

Generic Available Yes

Pharmacologic Category Antihypertensive Agent, Combination

Medication Safety Issues
Sound-alike/look-alike issues:
Aldactazide® may be confused with Aldactone®

Use Management of mild to moderate hypertension; treatment of edema in congestive heart failure and nephrotic syndrome, and cirrhosis of the liver accompanied by edema and/or ascites

(Continued)

Hydrochlorothiazide and Spironolactone *(Continued)*

Dosing
  Adults: Hypertension, edema: Oral:
    Hydrochlorothiazide 25 mg and spironolactone 25 mg: $^1/_2$-8 tablets daily
    Hydrochlorothiazide 50 mg and spironolactone 50 mg: $^1/_2$-4 tablets daily in 1-2 doses
  Elderly: Oral: Initial: 1 tablet/day; increase as necessary.
  Renal Impairment: Efficacy of hydrochlorothiazide is limited in patients with Cl_{cr} <30 mL/minute.

Available Dosage Forms Tablet: Hydrochlorothiazide 25 mg and spironolactone 25 mg
  Aldactazide®:
    25/25: Hydrochlorothiazide 25 mg and spironolactone 25 mg
    50/50: Hydrochlorothiazide 50 mg and spironolactone 50 mg

Monitoring and Teaching Issues
  Physical Assessment: See individual agents.
  Patient Education: See individual agents. **Pregnancy/breast-feeding precautions:** Inform prescriber if you are or intend to become pregnant. Consult prescriber if breast-feeding.
  Pregnancy Risk Factor: C
  Lactation: Enters breast milk/use caution

Related Information
  Hydrochlorothiazide *on page 751*
  Spironolactone *on page 1391*

♦ **Hydrochlorothiazide and Telmisartan** *see* Telmisartan and Hydrochlorothiazide *on page 1433*

Hydrochlorothiazide and Triamterene
  (hye droe klor oh THYE a zide & trye AM ter een)
  U.S. Brand Names Dyazide®; Maxzide®; Maxzide®-25
  Synonyms Triamterene and Hydrochlorothiazide
  Generic Available Yes
  Pharmacologic Category Antihypertensive Agent, Combination; Diuretic, Potassium-Sparing; Diuretic, Thiazide

Medication Safety Issues
  Sound-alike/look-alike issues:
    Dyazide® may be confused with diazoxide, Dynacin®
    Maxzide® may be confused with Maxidex®

Use Management of mild to moderate hypertension; treatment of edema in congestive heart failure and nephrotic syndrome

Dosing
  Adults & Elderly: Hypertension, edema: Oral:
    Triamterene 37.5 mg and hydrochlorothiazide 25 mg: 1-2 tablets/capsules once daily
    Triamterene 75 mg and hydrochlorothiazide 50 mg: $^1/_2$-1 tablet daily

Available Dosage Forms
  Capsule (Dyazide®): Hydrochlorothiazide 25 mg and triamterene 37.5 mg
  Tablet:
    Maxzide®: Hydrochlorothiazide 50 mg and triamterene 75 mg
    Maxzide®-25: Hydrochlorothiazide 25 mg and triamterene 37.5 mg

Monitoring and Teaching Issues
  Physical Assessment: See individual agents.
  Patient Education: See individual agents. **Pregnancy/breast-feeding precautions:** Inform prescriber if you are or intend to become pregnant. Consult prescriber if breast-feeding.
  Pregnancy Risk Factor: C (per manufacturer)
  Lactation: Excretion in breast milk unknown/use caution

Related Information
  Hydrochlorothiazide *on page 751*

♦ **Hydrochlorothiazide and Valsartan** *see* Valsartan and Hydrochlorothiazide *on page 1549*
♦ **Hydrocil® [OTC]** *see* Psyllium *on page 1284*

Hydrocodone and Acetaminophen
  (hye droe KOE done & a seet a MIN oh fen)
  U.S. Brand Names Anexsia®; Bancap HC®; Ceta-Plus®; Co-Gesic®; hycet™; Lorcet® 10/650; Lorcet®-HD; Lorcet® Plus; Lortab®; Margesic® H; Maxidone™; Norco®; Stagesic®; Vicodin®; Vicodin® ES; Vicodin® HP; Zydone®
  Synonyms Acetaminophen and Hydrocodone
  Controlled Substance C-III
  Generic Available Yes
  Pharmacologic Category Analgesic Combination (Narcotic)

Medication Safety Issues
  Sound-alike/look-alike issues:
    Lorcet® may be confused with Fioricet®
    Lortab® may be confused with Cortef®, Lorabid®, Luride®
    Vicodin® may be confused with Hycodan®, Hycomine®, Indocin®, Uridon®
    Zydone® may be confused with Vytone®

Use Relief of moderate to severe pain
Contraindications Hypersensitivity to hydrocodone, acetaminophen, or any component of the formulation; CNS depression; severe respiratory depression
Warnings/Precautions Use with caution in patients with hypersensitivity reactions to other phenanthrene derivative opioid agonists (morphine, hydromorphone, levorphanol, oxycodone, oxymorphone); tolerance or drug dependence may result from extended use.

Respiratory depressant effects may be increased with head injuries. Use caution with acute abdominal conditions; clinical course may be obscured. Use caution with thyroid dysfunction, prostatic hyperplasia, hepatic or renal disease naive, and in the elderly. Causes sedation; caution must be used in performing tasks which require alertness (eg, operating machinery or driving).

Limit acetaminophen to <4 g/day. May cause severe hepatic toxicity in acute overdose; in addition, chronic daily dosing in adults has resulted in liver damage in some patients. Use with caution in patients with alcoholic liver disease; consuming ≥3 alcoholic drinks/day may increase the risk of liver damage. Use caution in patients with known G6PD deficiency.

Drug Interactions
Cytochrome P450 Effect:
Hydrocodone: **Substrate** of CYP2D6 (major)

Acetaminophen: **Substrate** (minor) of CYP1A2, 2A6, 2C8/9, 2D6, 2E1, 3A4; **Inhibits** CYP3A4 (weak)

Increased Effect/Toxicity: Also see Acetaminophen monograph. Hydrocodone with other narcotic analgesics, CNS depressants, antianxiety agents, or antipsychotics may cause enhanced CNS depression. MAO inhibitors or tricyclic antidepressants with hydrocodone may increase the effect of either agent.

Nutritional/Ethanol Interactions
Ethanol: Avoid ethanol (may increase CNS depression); consuming ≥3 alcoholic drinks/day may increase the risk of liver damage

Herb/Nutraceutical: Avoid valerian, St John's wort, SAMe, kava kava (may increase risk of excessive sedation).

Adverse Reactions Frequency not defined.
Cardiovascular: Bradycardia, cardiac arrest, circulatory collapse, coma, hypotension

Central nervous system: anxiety, dizziness, drowsiness, dysphoria, euphoria, fear, lethargy, lightheadedness, malaise, mental clouding, mental impairment, mood changes, physiological dependence, sedation, somnolence, stupor

Dermatologic: Pruritus, rash

Endocrine & metabolic: Hypoglycemic coma

Gastrointestinal: Abdominal pain, constipation, gastric distress, heartburn, nausea, peptic ulcer, vomiting

Genitourinary: Ureteral spasm, urinary retention, vesical sphincter spasm

Hematologic: Agranulocytosis, bleeding time prolonged, hemolytic anemia, iron deficiency anemia, occult blood loss, thrombocytopenia

Hepatic: Hepatic necrosis, hepatitis

Neuromuscular & skeletal: Skeletal muscle rigidity

Otic: Hearing impairment or loss (chronic overdose)

Renal: Renal toxicity, renal tubular necrosis

Respiratory: Acute airway obstruction, apnea, dyspnea, respiratory depression (dose related)

Miscellaneous: Allergic reactions, clamminess, diaphoresis

Overdosage/Toxicology Symptoms of overdose include hepatic necrosis, blood dyscrasias, and respiratory depression. Treatment consists of acetylcysteine 140 mg/kg orally (loading) followed by 70 mg/kg every 4 hours for 17 doses; therapy should be initiated based upon laboratory analysis suggesting a high probability for hepatotoxic potential. Naloxone, 2 mg I.V. with repeat administration as necessary up to a total of 10 mg, can also be used to reverse toxic effects of the opiate. Activated charcoal is effective at binding certain chemicals, and this is especially true for acetaminophen.

Pharmacodynamics/Kinetics
Onset of Action:
Hydrocodone: Narcotic analgesic: 10-20 minutes

Duration of Action:
Hydrocodone: 4-8 hours

Half-Life Elimination:
Hydrocodone: 3.3-4.4 hours

Metabolism:
Hydrocodone: Hepatic; O-demethylation; N-demethylation and 6-ketosteroid reduction

Excretion:
Hydrocodone: Urine

Pharmacokinetic Note: See Acetaminophen monograph.

Dosing
Adults:
Pain management (analgesic): Oral (doses should be titrated to appropriate analgesic effect): Average starting dose in opioid naive patients: Hydrocodone 5-10 mg 4 times/day; the dosage of acetaminophen should be limited to ≤4 g/day (and possibly less in patients with hepatic impairment or ethanol use).

Dosage ranges (based on specific product labeling): Hydrocodone 2.5-10 mg every 4-6 hours; maximum: 60 mg hydrocodone/day (maximum dose of hydrocodone may be limited by the acetaminophen content of specific product)

Elderly: Doses should be titrated to appropriate analgesic effect; 2.5-5 mg of the hydrocodone component every 4-6 hours. Do not exceed 4 g/day of acetaminophen.

Pediatrics:
Pain management (analgesic): Oral (doses should be titrated to appropriate analgesic effect):

Children 2-13 years or <50 kg: Hydrocodone 0.135 mg/kg/dose every 4-6 hours; do not exceed 6 doses/day or the maximum recommended dose of acetaminophen

Children ≥50 kg: Refer to adult dosing.

Hepatic Impairment: Use with caution. Limited, low-dose therapy usually well tolerated in hepatic disease/cirrhosis; however, cases of hepatotoxicity at daily acetaminophen dosages <4 g/day have been reported. Avoid chronic use in hepatic impairment.

Available Dosage Forms
Capsule (Bancap HC®, Ceta-Plus®, Lorcet®-HD, Margesic® H, Stagesic®): Hydrocodone bitartrate 5 mg and acetaminophen 500 mg

(Continued)

Hydrocodone and Acetaminophen *(Continued)*

Elixir: Hydrocodone bitartrate 7.5 mg and acetaminophen 500 mg per 15 mL (480 mL)
  Lortab®: Hydrocodone bitartrate 7.5 mg and acetaminophen 500 mg per 15 mL (480 mL)
    [contains alcohol 7%; tropical fruit punch flavor]
Solution, oral (hycet™): Hydrocodone bitartrate 7.5 mg and acetaminophen 325 mg per 15
  mL (480 mL) [contains alcohol 7%; tropical fruit punch flavor]
Tablet:
  Hydrocodone bitartrate 2.5 mg and acetaminophen 500 mg
  Hydrocodone bitartrate 5 mg and acetaminophen 325 mg
  Hydrocodone bitartrate 5 mg and acetaminophen 500 mg
  Hydrocodone bitartrate 7.5 mg and acetaminophen 325 mg
  Hydrocodone bitartrate 7.5 mg and acetaminophen 500 mg
  Hydrocodone bitartrate 7.5 mg and acetaminophen 650 mg
  Hydrocodone bitartrate 7.5 mg and acetaminophen 750 mg
  Hydrocodone bitartrate 10 mg and acetaminophen 325 mg
  Hydrocodone bitartrate 10 mg and acetaminophen 500 mg
  Hydrocodone bitartrate 10 mg and acetaminophen 650 mg
  Hydrocodone bitartrate 10 mg and acetaminophen 660 mg
  Anexsia®:
    5/500: Hydrocodone bitartrate 5 mg and acetaminophen 500 mg
    7.5/650: Hydrocodone bitartrate 7.5 mg and acetaminophen 650 mg
  Co-Gesic® 5/500: Hydrocodone bitartrate 5 mg and acetaminophen 500 mg
  Lorcet® 10/650: Hydrocodone bitartrate 10 mg and acetaminophen 650 mg
  Lorcet® Plus: Hydrocodone bitartrate 7.5 mg and acetaminophen 650 mg
  Lortab®:
    2.5/500: Hydrocodone bitartrate 2.5 mg and acetaminophen 500 mg
    5/500: Hydrocodone bitartrate 5 mg and acetaminophen 500 mg
    7.5/500: Hydrocodone bitartrate 7.5 mg and acetaminophen 500 mg
    10/500: Hydrocodone bitartrate 10 mg and acetaminophen 500 mg
  Maxidone™: Hydrocodone bitartrate 10 mg and acetaminophen 750 mg
  Norco®:
    Hydrocodone bitartrate 5 mg and acetaminophen 325 mg
    Hydrocodone bitartrate 7.5 mg and acetaminophen 325 mg
    Hydrocodone bitartrate 10 mg and acetaminophen 325 mg
  Vicodin®: Hydrocodone bitartrate 5 mg and acetaminophen 500 mg
  Vicodin® ES: Hydrocodone bitartrate 7.5 mg and acetaminophen 750 mg
  Vicodin® HP: Hydrocodone bitartrate 10 mg and acetaminophen 660 mg
  Zydone®:
    Hydrocodone bitartrate 5 mg and acetaminophen 400 mg
    Hydrocodone bitartrate 7.5 mg and acetaminophen 400 mg
    Hydrocodone bitartrate 10 mg and acetaminophen 400 mg

Monitoring and Teaching Issues

Physical Assessment: Assess patient for history of liver disease or ethanol abuse
(acetaminophen and excessive ethanol may have adverse liver effects). Assess other
medications patient may be taking for additive or adverse interactions. Monitor therapeutic
effectiveness and signs of adverse reactions at beginning of therapy and at regular intervals with long-term use. Order safety precautions for inpatient use. May cause physical
and/or psychological dependence. Discontinue slowly after long-term use. Assess knowl-
edge/teach patient appropriate use, adverse reactions to report, and appropriate interventions to reduce side effects.

Patient Education: If self-administered, use exactly as directed; do not increase dose or
frequency. Drug may cause physical and/or psychological dependence. Take with food or
milk. While using this medication, do not use alcohol and other prescription or OTC
medications (especially sedatives, tranquilizers, antihistamines, or pain medications)
without consulting prescriber. Maintain adequate hydration (2-3 L/day of fluids) unless
instructed to restrict fluid intake. May cause dizziness, lightheadedness, confusion, or
drowsiness (use caution when driving, climbing stairs, or changing position - rising from
sitting or lying to standing, or when engaging in tasks requiring alertness until response to
drug is known); or nausea or vomiting (frequent mouth care, frequent sips of fluids,
chewing gum, or sucking lozenges may help). Report chest pain or palpitations; persistent
dizziness, shortness of breath, or respiratory difficulty; unusual bleeding or bruising; or
unusual fatigue and weakness. **Pregnancy/breast-feeding precautions:** Inform
prescriber if you are or intend to become pregnant. Do not breast-feed.

Geriatric Considerations: The elderly may be particularly susceptible to the CNS depressant action (sedation, confusion) and constipating effects of narcotics. If 1 tablet/dose is
used, it may be useful to add an additional 325 mg of acetaminophen to maximize analgesic effect and minimize additional risk of narcotic related adverse effects.

Pregnancy Risk Factor: C/D (prolonged use or high doses near term)

Pregnancy Issues: Animal reproduction studies have not been conducted with this combination product. Opioid analgesics are considered FDA risk category D if used for prolonged
periods or in large doses near term. Withdrawal symptoms may be observed in babies born
to mothers taking opioids regularly during pregnancy. Respiratory depression may be
observed in the newborn if opioids are given close to delivery.

Lactation: Excretion in breast milk unknown/contraindicated

Breast-Feeding Issues: Acetaminophen is excreted in breast milk. The AAP considers it
to be "compatible" with breast-feeding. Information is not available for hydrocodone;
codeine and other opioids are excreted in breast milk and the AAP considers codeine to be
"compatible" with breast-feeding. The manufacturers recommend discontinuing the medication or to discontinue nursing during therapy.

Related Information

Acetaminophen *on page 38*

Hydrocodone and Aspirin (hye droe KOE done & AS pir in)

U.S. Brand Names Damason-P®

Synonyms Aspirin and Hydrocodone

Controlled Substance C-III

Generic Available No

Pharmacologic Category Analgesic Combination (Narcotic)

Use Relief of moderate to moderately severe pain

Mechanism of Action/Effect

Based on **hydrocodone** component: Binds to opiate receptors in the CNS, altering the perception of and response to pain; suppresses cough in medullary center; produces generalized CNS depression

Based on **aspirin** component: Inhibits prostaglandin synthesis, acts on the hypothalamus heat-regulating center to reduce fever, blocks prostaglandin synthetase action which prevents formation of the platelet-aggregating substance thromboxane A_2

Contraindications

Based on **hydrocodone** component: Hypersensitivity to hydrocodone or any component of the formulation

Based on **aspirin** component: Hypersensitivity to salicylates, other NSAIDs, or any component of the formulation; asthma; rhinitis; nasal polyps; inherited or acquired bleeding disorders (including factor VII and factor IX deficiency); pregnancy (in 3rd trimester especially); do not use in children (<16 years) for viral infections (chickenpox or flu symptoms), with or without fever, due to a potential association with Reye's syndrome

Warnings/Precautions Use with caution in patients with impaired renal function, erosive gastritis, or peptic ulcer disease. Children and teenagers should not use for chickenpox or flu symptoms before a physician is consulted about Reye's syndrome.

Drug Interactions

Cytochrome P450 Effect:

Hydrocodone: **Substrate** of CYP2D6 (major)

Aspirin: **Substrate** of CYP2C8/9 (minor)

Decreased Effect: Based on **aspirin** component: The effects of ACE inhibitors may be blunted by aspirin administration (may be significant only at higher aspirin dosages). Aspirin may decrease the effects of beta-blockers, loop diuretics (furosemide), thiazide diuretics, and probenecid. Aspirin may cause a decrease in NSAIDs serum concentration and decrease the effects of probenecid. Increased serum salicylate levels when taken with with urine acidifiers (ammonium chloride, methionine).

Increased Effect/Toxicity:

Based on **hydrocodone** component: CNS depressants, MAO inhibitors, general anesthetics, and tricyclic antidepressants may potentiate the effects of opiate agonists; dextroamphetamine may enhance the analgesic effect of opiate agonists.

Based on **aspirin** component: May increase methotrexate serum levels/toxicity and may displace valproic acid from binding sites which can result in toxicity. NSAIDs and aspirin increase GI adverse effects (ulceration). Aspirin with oral anticoagulants (warfarin), thrombolytic agents, heparin, low molecular weight heparins, and antiplatelet agents (ticlopidine, clopidogrel, dipyridamole, NSAIDs, and IIb/IIIa antagonists) may increase risk of bleeding. Bleeding times may be additionally prolonged with verapamil. The effects of older sulfonylurea agents (tolazamide, tolbutamide) may be potentiated due to displacement from plasma proteins. This effect does not appear to be clinically significant for newer sulfonylurea agents (glyburide, glipizide, glimepiride).

Nutritional/Ethanol Interactions

Based on **hydrocodone** component: Ethanol: Avoid or limit ethanol (may increase CNS depression). Watch for sedation.

Based on **aspirin** component:

Ethanol: Avoid ethanol (may enhance gastric mucosal damage).

Food: Food may decrease the rate but not the extent of oral absorption. Take with food or large volume of water or milk to minimize GI upset.

Herb/Nutraceutical: Avoid cat's claw, dong quai, evening primrose, feverfew, garlic, ginger, ginkgo, red clover, horse chestnut, green tea, ginseng (all have additional antiplatelet activity).

Lab Interactions Urine glucose, urinary 5-HIAA, serum uric acid

Adverse Reactions

>10%:

Cardiovascular: Hypotension

Central nervous system: Lightheadedness, dizziness, sedation, drowsiness, fatigue

Gastrointestinal: Nausea, heartburn, stomach pain, dyspepsia, epigastric discomfort

Neuromuscular & skeletal: Weakness

1% to 10%:

Cardiovascular: Bradycardia

Central nervous system: Confusion

Dermatologic: Rash

Gastrointestinal: Vomiting, gastrointestinal ulceration

Genitourinary: Decreased urination

Hematologic: Hemolytic anemia

Respiratory: Dyspnea

Miscellaneous: Anaphylactic shock

Overdosage/Toxicology Naloxone is the antidote for hydrocodone. Naloxone, 2 mg I.V. with repeat administration as necessary up to a total of 10 mg, can also be used to reverse toxic effects of the opiate. Nomograms, such as the "Done" nomogram, can be very helpful for estimating the severity of aspirin poisoning and for directing treatment using serum salicylate levels. Treatment can also be based upon symptomatology; symptoms of aspirin overdose include tinnitus, headache, dizziness, confusion, metabolic acidosis, hyperpyrexia, hypoglycemia, and coma.

(Continued)

Hydrocodone and Aspirin *(Continued)*

Pharmacodynamics/Kinetics
Onset of Action:
Hydrocodone: Narcotic analgesic: 10-20 minutes
Duration of Action:
Hydrocodone: 4-8 hours
Half-Life Elimination:
Hydrocodone: 3.3-4.4 hours
Metabolism:
Hydrocodone: Hepatic; O-demethylation; N-demethylation and 6-ketosteroid reduction
Excretion:
Hydrocodone: Urine
Pharmacokinetic Note: See Aspirin monograph.

Dosing
Adults: Pain management (analgesic): Oral: 1-2 tablets every 4-6 hours as needed for pain
Elderly: Refer to dosing in individual monographs.

Available Dosage Forms Tablet: Hydrocodone bitartrate 5 mg and aspirin 500 mg

Monitoring and Teaching Issues
Physical Assessment: Do not use for persons with allergic reaction to aspirin or aspirin-containing medications. Assess other medications patient may be taking for additive or adverse interactions. Monitor therapeutic effectiveness and adverse reactions at beginning of therapy and at regular intervals with long-term use. May cause physical and/or psychological dependence. Discontinue slowly after long-term use. Assess knowledge/teach patient appropriate use if self-administered. Teach patient to monitor for adverse reactions, adverse reactions to report, and appropriate interventions to reduce side effects.

Patient Education: If self-administered, use exactly as directed; do not increase dose or frequency. Drug may cause physical and/or psychological dependence. Take with food or milk. While using this medication, do not use alcohol, excessive amounts of vitamin C, or salicylate-containing foods (curry powder, prunes, raisins, tea, or licorice), other aspirin- or salicylate-containing medications, and other prescription or OTC medications (especially sedatives, tranquilizers, antihistamines, or pain medications) without consulting prescriber. Maintain adequate hydration (2-3 L/day of fluids) unless instructed to restrict fluid intake. May cause hypotension, dizziness, drowsiness, impaired coordination, or blurred vision (use caution when driving, climbing stairs, or changing position - rising from sitting or lying to standing, or when engaging in tasks requiring alertness until response to drug is known); nausea, vomiting, or dry mouth (frequent mouth care, small frequent meals, chewing gum, or sucking lozenges may help); or constipation (increased exercise, fluids, fruit, or fiber may help; if unresolved, consult prescriber about use of stool softeners). Report ringing in ears; persistent stomach pain; unresolved nausea or vomiting; respiratory difficulty or shortness of breath; yellowing of skin or eyes; changes in color of stool or urine; or unusual bruising or bleeding. **Pregnancy/breast-feeding precautions:** Use appropriate contraceptive measures; do not get pregnant while taking this drug. Do not breast-feed.

Pregnancy Risk Factor: D
Lactation: Enters breast milk/contraindicated
Breast-Feeding Issues:
Hydrocodone: No data reported.
Aspirin: Cautious use due to potential adverse effects in nursing infants.

Administration
Oral: Administer with food or a full glass of water to minimize GI distress.

Related Information
Aspirin *on page 143*

Hydrocodone and Ibuprofen *(hye droe KOE done & eye byoo PROE fen)*

U.S. Brand Names Vicoprofen®
Synonyms Ibuprofen and Hydrocodone
Controlled Substance C-III
Generic Available Yes
Pharmacologic Category Analgesic, Narcotic
Use Short-term (generally <10 days) management of moderate to severe acute pain; is not indicated for treatment of such conditions as osteoarthritis or rheumatoid arthritis

Dosing
Adults: Analgesic: Oral (Short-term use is recommended, not to exceed 10 days): 1 tablet every 4-6 hours, do not exceed 5 tablets during a 24-hour period.
Elderly: Refer to dosing in individual monographs.

Available Dosage Forms
Tablet: Hydrocodone bitartrate 5 mg and ibuprofen 200 mg; hydrocodone bitartrate 7.5 mg and ibuprofen 200 mg
Vicoprofen®: Hydrocodone bitartrate 7.5 mg and ibuprofen 200 mg

Monitoring and Teaching Issues
Physical Assessment: Assess other medications patient may be taking for additive or adverse interactions. Monitor for effectiveness of pain relief and monitor for signs of overdose. Monitor vital signs and signs of adverse reactions at beginning of therapy and at regular intervals with long-term use. May cause physical and/or psychological dependence. Discontinue slowly after long-term use. For inpatients, implement safety measures (eg, side rails up, call light within reach, instructions to call for assistance). Assess knowledge/teach patient appropriate use if self-administered. Teach patient to monitor for adverse reactions, adverse reactions to report, and appropriate interventions to reduce side effects.

Patient Education: If self-administered, use exactly as directed; do not increase dose or frequency. Drug may cause physical and/or psychological dependence. Take with food or milk. While using this medication, do not use alcohol and other prescription or OTC medications (especially sedatives, tranquilizers, antihistamines, or pain medications) without consulting prescriber. Maintain adequate hydration (2-3 L/day of fluids) unless instructed to restrict fluid intake. May cause dizziness, drowsiness, confusion, nervousness, or anxiety (use caution when driving, climbing stairs, or changing position - rising from sitting or lying to standing, or when engaging in tasks requiring alertness until response to drug is known); nausea, dry mouth, decreased appetite, or gastric distress (frequent mouth care, frequent sips of fluids, chewing gum, or sucking lozenges may help); or constipation (increased exercise, fluids, fruit, or fiber may help; if unresolved, consult prescriber about use of stool softeners). Report chest pain or palpitations; persistent dizziness, shortness of breath, or respiratory difficulty; unusual bleeding (stool, mouth, urine) or bruising; unusual fatigue and weakness; change in elimination patterns; or change in color of urine or stool. **Pregnancy/breast-feeding precautions:** Inform prescriber if you are or intend to become pregnant. Do not breast-feed.

Pregnancy Risk Factor: C/D (3rd trimester)

Lactation: Excretion in breast milk unknown/contraindicated

Related Information

Ibuprofen *on page 777*

♦ **Hydrocodone Bitartrate, Carbinoxamine Maleate, and Pseudoephedrine Hydrochloride** *see* Hydrocodone, Carbinoxamine, and Pseudoephedrine *on page 759*

♦ **Hydrocodone Bitartrate, Phenylephrine Hydrochloride, and Diphenhydramine Hydrochloride** *see* Hydrocodone, Phenylephrine, and Diphenhydramine *on page 759*

Hydrocodone, Carbinoxamine, and Pseudoephedrine

(hye droe KOE done, kar bi NOKS a meen, & soo doe e FED rin)

U.S. Brand Names Histex™ HC; Tri-Vent™ HC

Synonyms Carbinoxamine, Pseudoephedrine, and Hydrocodone; Hydrocodone Bitartrate, Carbinoxamine Maleate, and Pseudoephedrine Hydrochloride; Pseudoephedrine, Hydrocodone, and Carbinoxamine

Controlled Substance C-III

Generic Available Yes

Pharmacologic Category Antihistamine/Decongestant/Antitussive

Use Symptomatic relief of cough, congestion, and rhinorrhea associated with the common cold, influenza, bronchitis, or sinusitis

Dosing

Adults: Relief of cough, congestion, and runny nose: Oral: 5-10 mL every 4-6 hours; maximum dose: 30 mL/24 hours

Pediatrics: Relief of cough, congestion, and runny nose: Oral:

Children *2-10 years:* Dosing based on hydrocodone content: 0.6 mg/kg/day given in 4 divided doses. Alternately, the following dosing may be used based on age:

2-4 years: 1.25 mL every 4-6 hours; maximum dose: 7.5 mL/24 hours

4-10 years: 2.5 mL every 4-6 hours; maximum dose: 15 mL/24 hours

Children >10 years: Refer to adult dosing.

Available Dosage Forms Liquid: Hydrocodone bitartrate 5 mg, carbinoxamine maleate 2 mg, and pseudoephedrine hydrochloride 30 mg per 5 mL (480 mL)

Histex™ HC, Tri-Vent™ HC: Hydrocodone bitartrate 5 mg, carbinoxamine maleate 2 mg, and pseudoephedrine hydrochloride 30 mg per 5 mL (480 mL) [alcohol free, sugar free; peach flavor]

Monitoring and Teaching Issues

Pregnancy Risk Factor: C

Lactation: Excretion in breast milk unknown/use caution

Related Information

Pseudoephedrine *on page 1282*

♦ **Hydrocodone, Chlorpheniramine, and Pseudoephedrine** *see* Pseudoephedrine, Hydrocodone, and Chlorpheniramine *on page 1283*

♦ **Hydrocodone, Phenylephrine, and Chlorpheniramine** *see* Phenylephrine, Hydrocodone, and Chlorpheniramine *on page 1202*

Hydrocodone, Phenylephrine, and Diphenhydramine

(hye droe KOE done, fen il EF rin, & dye fen HYE dra meen)

U.S. Brand Names Endal® HD; Hydro DP; TussiNate™

Synonyms Diphenhydramine, Hydrocodone, and Phenylephrine; Hydrocodone Bitartrate, Phenylephrine Hydrochloride, and Diphenhydramine Hydrochloride; Phenylephrine, Diphenhydramine, and Hydrocodone

Controlled Substance C-III

Generic Available Yes

Pharmacologic Category Antihistamine/Decongestant/Antitussive; Antitussive; Decongestant; Histamine H_1 Antagonist

Medication Safety Issues

Sound-alike/look-alike issues:

Endal® may be confused with Depen®, Intal®

Use Symptomatic relief of cough and congestion associated with the common cold, sinusitis, or acute upper respiratory tract infections

Dosing

Adults: Relief of cough, congestion: Oral: 10 mL every 4 hours (maximum: 40 mL/24 hours)

Pediatrics: Relief of cough, congestion: Oral:

Children 6-12 years: 5 mL every 4 hours (maximum: 20 mL/24 hours)

Children >12 years: Refer to adult dosing.

Available Dosage Forms

Syrup:

Endal® HD: Hydrocodone bitartrate 2 mg, phenylephrine hydrochloride 7.5 mg, and diphenhydramine hydrochloride 12.5 mg per 5 mL (480 mL) [alcohol free, sugar free; contains sodium benzoate; cherry flavor]

(Continued)

Hydrocodone, Phenylephrine, and Diphenhydramine
(Continued)

Hydro DP: Hydrocodone bitartrate 2 mg, phenylephrine hydrochloride 7.5 mg, and diphenhydramine hydrochloride 12.5 mg per 5 mL (480 mL) [cherry flavor]

TussiNate™: Hydrocodone bitartrate 3.5 mg, phenylephrine hydrochloride 5 mg, and diphenhydramine hydrochloride 12.5 mg per 5 mL (480 mL) [alcohol free; contains sodium benzoate; black raspberry flavor]

Monitoring and Teaching Issues
Pregnancy Risk Factor: C
Lactation: Excretion in breast milk unknown/contraindicated
Related Information
DiphenhydrAMINE on page 463
Phenylephrine on page 1200

Hydrocodone, Phenylephrine, and Guaifenesin
(hye droe KOE done, fen il EF rin, & gwye FEN e sin)

U.S. Brand Names Crantex HC; De-Chlor G; Giltuss HC®; Hydro-GP; Levall 5.0; Quintex HC; Tussafed® HC

Synonyms Guaifenesin, Hydrocodone Bitartrate, and Phenylephrine Hydrochloride; Phenylephrine, Guaifenesin, and Hydrocodone

Controlled Substance C-III

Generic Available Yes

Pharmacologic Category Antitussive/Decongestant/Expectorant

Use Temporary relief of cough, congestion, and other symptoms associated with colds or allergies

Dosing
Adults: Cough/congestion: Oral:
Crantex HC: 5-10 mL every 4-6 hours (maximum: 40 mL/24 hours)
Giltuss HC®: 5 mL every 6 hours (maximum: 6 doses/24 hours)
Tussafed® HC: 10 mL every 4-6 hours as needed (maximum: 6 doses/24 hours)
Pediatrics: Cough/congestion: Oral: Children:
2-6 years (Crantex HC): 2.5 mL every 4-6 hours (maximum: 10 mL/24 hours)
3-6 years:
Giltuss HC®: 1.25 mL every 6 hours (maximum: 6 doses/24 hours)
Tussafed® HC: 2.5 mL every 4-6 hours as needed (maximum: 6 doses/24 hours)
6-12 years:
Crantex HC: 5 mL every 4-6 hours (maximum: 4 doses/24 hours)
Giltuss HC®: 2.5 mL every 6 hours (maximum: 6 doses/24 hours)
Tussafed® HC: 5 mL every 4-6 hours as needed (maximum: 6 doses/24 hours)
≥12 years: Refer to adult dosing.

Available Dosage Forms
Liquid: Hydrocodone bitartrate 2mg, phenylephrine hydrochloride 10 mg, and guaifenesin 100 mg per 5 mL (120 mL, 480 mL)
Crantex HC: Hydrocodone bitartrate 5 mg, phenylephrine hydrochloride 7.5 mg, and guaifenesin 100 mg per 5 mL (480 mL) [alcohol free, dye free, sugar free; black cherry flavor]
De-Chlor G: Hydrocodone bitartrate 2 mg, phenylephrine hydrochloride 10 mg, and guaifenesin 100 mg per 5 mL (480 mL) [grape-menthol mint flavor]
Giltuss HC®: Hydrocodone bitartrate 5 mg, phenylephrine hydrochloride 10 mg, and guaifenesin 300 mg per 5 mL (480 mL) [alcohol free, dye free, sugar free; strawberry banana flavor]
Hydro-GP: Hydrocodone bitartrate 2.5 mg, phenylephrine hydrochloride 7.5 mg, and guaifenesin 50 mg per 5 mL (480 mL) [cherry flavor]
Levall 5.0: Hydrocodone bitartrate 5 mg, phenylephrine hydrochloride 15 mg, and guaifenesin 100 mg per 5 mL (480 mL) [grape flavor]
Quintex HC: Hydrocodone bitartrate 5 mg, phenylephrine hydrochloride 7.5 mg, and guaifenesin 100 mg per 5 mL (480 mL) [black cherry flavor]
Syrup (Tussafed® HC): Hydrocodone bitartrate 2.5 mg, phenylephrine hydrochloride 7.5 mg, and guaifenesin 50 mg per 5 mL (480 mL) [alcohol free]

Monitoring and Teaching Issues
Physical Assessment: See individual agents.
Pregnancy Risk Factor: C
Lactation: Excretion in breast milk unknown/use caution

Hydrocortisone (hye droe KOR ti sone)
U.S. Brand Names Anucort-HC®; Anusol-HC®; Anusol® HC-1 [OTC]; Aquanil™ HC [OTC]; Beta-HC®; Caldecort® [OTC]; Cetacort®; Colocort®; CortaGel® Maximum Strength [OTC] [DSC]; Cortaid® Intensive Therapy [OTC]; Cortaid® Maximum Strength [OTC]; Cortaid® Sensitive Skin [OTC]; Cortef®; Corticool® [OTC]; Cortifoam®; Cortizone®-10 Maximum Strength [OTC]; Cortizone®-10 Plus Maximum Strength [OTC]; Cortizone® 10 Quick Shot [OTC]; Dermarest Dricort® [OTC]; Dermtex® HC [OTC]; EarSol® HC; Hemril®-30; Hydrocortone® [DSC]; HydroZone Plus [OTC]; Hytone®; IvySoothe® [OTC]; LactiCare-HC® [DSC]; Locoid®; Locoid Lipocream®; Nupercainal® Hydrocortisone Cream [OTC]; Nutracort®; Pandel®; Post Peel Healing Balm [OTC]; Preparation H® Hydrocortisone [OTC]; Proctocort®; ProctoCream® HC; Procto-Kit™; Procto-Pak™; Proctosert; Proctosol-HC®; Proctozone-HC™; Sarnol®-HC [OTC]; Solu-Cortef®; Summer's Eve® SpecialCare™ Medicated Anti-Itch Cream [OTC]; Texacort®; Westcort®

Synonyms A-hydroCort; Compound F; Cortisol; Hemorrhoidal HC; Hydrocortisone Acetate; Hydrocortisone Butyrate; Hydrocortisone Probutate; Hydrocortisone Sodium Succinate; Hydrocortisone Valerate

Generic Available Yes: Excludes acetate foam, butyrate cream and ointment, gel as base, otic drops as base, probutate cream, sodium succinate injection

Pharmacologic Category Corticosteroid, Rectal; Corticosteroid, Systemic; Corticosteroid, Topical

Medication Safety Issues

Sound-alike/look-alike issues:

Hydrocortisone may be confused with hydrocodone, hydroxychloroquine, hydrochlorothiazide

Anusol® may be confused with Anusol-HC®, Aplisol®, Aquasol®

Anusol-HC® may be confused with Anusol®

Cortef® may be confused with Lortab®

Cortizone® may be confused with cortisone

Hytone® may be confused with Vytone®

Proctocort® may be confused with ProctoCream®

ProctoCream® may be confused with Proctocort®

Use Management of adrenocortical insufficiency; relief of inflammation of corticosteroid-responsive dermatoses (low and medium potency topical corticosteroid); adjunctive treatment of ulcerative colitis

Mechanism of Action/Effect Decreases inflammation by suppression of migration of polymorphonuclear leukocytes and reversal of increased capillary permeability

Contraindications Hypersensitivity to hydrocortisone or any component of the formulation; serious infections, except septic shock or tuberculous meningitis; viral, fungal, or tubercular skin lesions

Warnings/Precautions Use with caution in patients with hyperthyroidism, cirrhosis, nonspecific ulcerative colitis, hypertension, osteoporosis, thromboembolic tendencies, CHF, convulsive disorders, myasthenia gravis, thrombophlebitis, peptic ulcer, diabetes, glaucoma, cataracts, or tuberculosis. Use caution in hepatic impairment. May cause HPA axis suppression. Acute adrenal insufficiency may occur with abrupt withdrawal after long-term therapy or with stress. Young pediatric patients may be more susceptible to adrenal axis suppression from topical therapy. Avoid use of topical preparations with occlusive dressings or on weeping or exudative lesions. Because of the risk of adverse effects, systemic corticosteroids should be used cautiously in the elderly, in the smallest possible dose, and for the shortest possible time.

Drug Interactions

Cytochrome P450 Effect: Substrate of CYP3A4 (minor); **Induces** CYP3A4 (weak)

Decreased Effect: Hydrocortisone may decrease the hypoglycemic effect of insulin. Phenytoin, phenobarbital, ephedrine, and rifampin increase metabolism of hydrocortisone resulting in a decreased steroid blood level.

Increased Effect/Toxicity: Hydrocortisone in combination with oral anticoagulants may increase prothrombin time. Potassium-depleting diuretics increase risk of hypokalemia. Cardiac glycosides increase risk of arrhythmias or digitalis toxicity secondary to hypokalemia.

Nutritional/Ethanol Interactions

Ethanol: Avoid ethanol (may enhance gastric mucosal irritation).

Food: Hydrocortisone interferes with calcium absorption.

Herb/Nutraceutical: St John's wort may decrease hydrocortisone levels. Avoid cat's claw, echinacea (have immunostimulant properties).

Adverse Reactions

Systemic:

>10%:

Central nervous system: Insomnia, nervousness

Gastrointestinal: Increased appetite, indigestion

1% to 10%:

Dermatologic: Hirsutism

Endocrine & metabolic: Diabetes mellitus

Neuromuscular & skeletal: Arthralgia

Ocular: Cataracts

Respiratory: Epistaxis

Topical:

>10%: Dermatologic: Eczema (12.5%)

1% to 10%: Dermatologic: Pruritus (6%), stinging (2%), dry skin (2%)

Overdosage/Toxicology When consumed in high doses for prolonged periods, systemic hypercorticism and adrenal suppression may occur. In those cases, discontinuation of the corticosteroid should be done judiciously.

Pharmacodynamics/Kinetics

Onset of Action:

Hydrocortisone acetate: Slow

Hydrocortisone sodium succinate (water soluble): Rapid

Duration of Action: Hydrocortisone acetate: Long

Absorption: Rapid by all routes, except rectally

Half-Life Elimination: Biologic: 8-12 hours

Metabolism: Hepatic

Excretion: Urine (primarily as 17-hydroxysteroids and 17-ketosteroids)

Dosing

Adults & Elderly: Dose should be based on severity of disease and patient response.

Acute adrenal insufficiency: I.M., I.V.: Succinate: 100 mg I.V. bolus, then 300 mg/day in divided doses every 8 hours or as a continuous infusion for 48 hours. Once patient is stable change to oral, 50 mg every 8 hours for 6 doses, then taper to 30-50 mg/day in divided doses.

Chronic adrenal corticoid insufficiency/physiologic replacement: Oral: 20-30 mg/day

Anti-inflammatory or immunosuppressive: Oral, I.M., I.V.: Succinate: 15-240 mg every 12 hours

Congenital adrenal hyperplasia: Oral: Initial: 10-20 mg/m^2/day in 3 divided doses; a variety of dosing schedules have been used. **Note:** Inconsistencies have occurred with

(Continued)

Hydrocortisone *(Continued)*

liquid formulations; tablets may provide more reliable levels. Doses must be individualized by monitoring growth, bone age, and hormonal levels. Mineralocorticoid and sodium supplementation may be required based upon electrolyte regulation and plasma renin activity.

Shock: I.M., I.V.: Succinate: 500 mg to 2 g every 2-6 hours

Status asthmaticus: I.V.: Succinate: 1-2 mg/kg/dose every 6 hours for 24 hours, then maintenance of 0.5-1 mg/kg every 6 hours

Stress dosing (surgery) in patients known to be adrenally-suppressed or on chronic systemic steroids: I.V.:

Minor stress (ie, inguinal herniorrhaphy): 25 mg/day for 1 day

Moderate stress (ie, joint replacement, cholecystectomy): 50-75 mg/day (25 mg every 8-12 hours) for 1-2 days

Major stress (pancreatoduodenectomy, esophagogastrectomy, cardiac surgery): 100-150 mg/day (50 mg every 8-12 hours) for 2-3 days

Rheumatic diseases:

Intralesional, intra-articular, soft tissue injection: Acetate:

Large joints: 25 mg (up to 37.5 mg)

Small joints: 10-25 mg

Tendon sheaths: 5-12.5 mg

Soft tissue infiltration: 25-50 mg (up to 75 mg)

Bursae: 25-37.5 mg

Ganglia: 12.5-25 mg

Dermatosis: Topical: Apply to affected area 2-4 times/day.

Ulcerative colitis: Rectal: 10-100 mg 1-2 times/day for 2-3 weeks

Pediatrics: Dose should be based on severity of disease and patient response.

Acute adrenal insufficiency: I.M., I.V.:

Infants and young Children: Succinate: 1-2 mg/kg/dose bolus, then 25-150 mg/day in divided doses every 6-8 hours

Older Children: Succinate: 1-2 mg/kg bolus then 150-250 mg/day in divided doses every 6-8 hours

Anti-inflammatory or immunosuppressive:

Infants and Children:

Oral: 2.5-10 mg/kg/day **or** 75-300 mg/m^2/day every 6-8 hours

I.M., I.V.: Succinate: 1-5 mg/kg/day **or** 30-150 mg/m^2/day divided every 12-24 hours

Adolescents: Oral, I.M., I.V.: Succinate: 15-240 mg every 12 hours

Congenital adrenal hyperplasia: Oral: Initial: 10-20 mg/m^2/day in 3 divided doses; a variety of dosing schedules have been used. **Note:** Inconsistencies have occurred with liquid formulations; tablets may provide more reliable levels. Doses must be individualized by monitoring growth, bone age, and hormonal levels. Mineralocorticoid and sodium supplementation may be required based upon electrolyte regulation and plasma renin activity

Physiologic replacement: Children:

Oral: 0.5-0.75 mg/kg/day **or** 20-25 mg/m^2/day every 8 hours

I.M.: Succinate: 0.25-0.35 mg/kg/day **or** 12-15 mg/m^2/day once daily

Shock: I.M., I.V.: Succinate:

Children: Initial: 50 mg/kg, then repeated in 4 hours and/or every 24 hours as needed

Adolescents: 500 mg to 2 g every 2-6 hours

Status asthmaticus: Children: I.V.: Succinate: 1-2 mg/kg/dose every 6 hours for 24 hours, then maintenance of 0.5-1 mg/kg every 6 hours.

Dermatosis: Topical: Children >2 years: Apply to affected area 2-4 times/day (Buteprate: Apply once or twice daily).

Available Dosage Forms [DSC] = Discontinued product

Aerosol, rectal, as acetate (Cortifoam®): 10% (15 g) [90 mg/applicator]

Cream, rectal, as acetate (Nupercainal® Hydrocortisone Cream): 1% (30 g) [strength expressed as base]

Cream, rectal, as base:

Cortizone®-10: 1% (30g) [contains aloe]

Preparation H® Hydrocortisone: 1% (27 g)

Cream, topical, as acetate: 0.5% (9 g, 30 g, 60 g) [available with aloe]; 1% (30 g, 454 g) [available with aloe]

Cream, topical, as base: 0.5% (30 g); 1% (1.5 g, 30 g, 114 g, 454 g); 2.5% (20 g, 30 g, 454 g)

Anusol-HC®: 2.5% (30 g) [contains benzyl alcohol]

Caldecort®: 1% (30 g) [contains aloe vera gel]

Cortaid® Intensive Therapy: 1% (60 g)

Cortaid® Maximum Strength: 1% (15 g, 30 g, 40 g, 60 g) [contains aloe vera gel and benzyl alcohol]

Cortaid® Sensitive Skin: 0.5% (15 g) [contains aloe vera gel]

Cortizone®-10 Maximum Strength: 1% (15 g, 30 g, 60 g) [contains aloe]

Cortizone®-10 Plus Maximum Strength: 1% (30 g, 60 g) [contains vitamins A, D, E and aloe]

Dermarest® Dricort®: 1% (15 g, 30 g)

HydroZone Plus, Proctocort®, Procto-Pak™: 1% (30 g)

Hytone®: 2.5% (30 g, 60 g)

IvySoothe®: 1% (30 g) [contains aloe]

Post Peel Healing Balm: 1% (23 g)

ProctoCream® HC: 2.5% (30 g) [contains benzyl alcohol]

Procto-Kit™: 1% (30 g) [packaged with applicator tips and finger cots]; 2.5% (30g) [packaged with applicator tips and finger cots]

Proctosol-HC®, Proctozone-HC™: 2.5% (30 g)

Summer's Eve® SpecialCare™ Medicated Anti-Itch Cream: 1% (30 g)

Cream, topical, as butyrate (Locoid®, Locoid Lipocream®): 0.1% (15 g, 45 g)

Cream, topical, as probutate (Pandel®): 0.1% (15 g, 45 g, 80 g)

Cream, topical, as valerate (Westcort®): 0.2% (15 g, 45 g, 60 g)

Gel, topical, as base:
Corticool® 1% (45 g)
CortaGel® Maximum Strength: 1% (15 g, 30 g) [contains aloe vera gel] [DSC]
Injection, powder for reconstitution, as sodium succinate (Solu-Cortef®): 100 mg, 250 mg,
500 mg, 1 g [diluent contains benzyl alcohol; strength expressed as base]
Lotion, topical, as base: 1% (120 mL); 2.5% (60 mL)
Aquanil™ HC: 1% (120 mL)
Beta-HC®, Cetacort®, Sarnol®-HC: 1% (60 mL)
HydroZone Plus: 1% (120 mL)
Hytone®: 2.5% (60 mL)
LactiCare-HC®: 1% (120 mL); 2.5% (60 mL, 120 mL) [DSC]
Nutracort®: 1% (60 mL, 120 mL); 2.5% (60 mL, 120 mL)
Ointment, topical, as acetate: 1% (30 g) [strength expressed as base; available with aloe]
Anusol® HC-1: 1% (21 g) [strength expressed as base]
Cortaid® Maximum Strength: 1% (15 g, 30 g) [strength expressed as base]
Ointment, topical, as base: 0.5% (30 g); 1% (30 g, 454 g); 2.5% (20 g, 30 g, 454 g)
Cortizone®-10 Maximum Strength: 1% (30 g, 60 g)
Hytone®: 2.5% (30 g)
Ointment, topical, as butyrate (Locoid®): 0.1% (15 g, 45 g)
Ointment, topical, as valerate (Westcort®): 0.2% (15 g, 45 g, 60 g)
Solution, otic, as base (EarSol® HC): 1% (30 mL) [contains alcohol 44%, benzyl benzoate,
yerba santa]
Solution, topical, as base (Texacort®): 2.5% (30 mL) [contains alcohol]
Solution, topical, as butyrate (Locoid®): 0.1% (20 mL, 60 mL) [contains alcohol 50%]
Solution, topical spray, as base:
Cortaid® Intensive Therapy: 1% (60 mL) [contains alcohol]
Cortizone® 10 Quick Shot: 1% (44 mL) [contains benzyl alcohol]
Dermtex® HC: 1% (52 mL) [contains menthol 1%]
Suppository, rectal, as acetate: 25 mg (12s, 24s, 100s)
Anucort-HC®: 25 mg (12s, 24s, 100s)
Anusol-HC®, Proctosol-HC®: 25 mg (12s, 24s)
Encort™: 30 mg (12s)
Hemril®-30, Proctocort®, Proctosert: 30 mg (12s, 24s)
Suspension, rectal, as base: 100 mg/60 mL (7s)
Colocort®: 100 mg/60 mL (1s, 7s)
Tablet, as base: 20 mg
Cortef®: 5 mg, 10 mg, 20 mg
Hydrocortone®: 10 mg [DSC]

Monitoring and Teaching Issues

Physical Assessment: Monitor laboratory results, effects and interactions of other medications patient may be taking, response to therapy and adverse effects according to diagnosis, formulation of hydrocortisone, dosage, and extent of time used. Systemic administration and long-term use will require close and frequent monitoring, especially for Cushing's syndrome. Assess for signs of fluid retention. Taper dosage when discontinuing. Assess/teach patient appropriate use, interventions for possible adverse reactions, and symptoms to report. Topical absorption may be minimal.

Monitoring Laboratory Tests: Serum glucose, electrolytes

Patient Education: Systemic: Take as directed; do not increase doses and do not stop abruptly without consulting prescribed. Dosage of systemic hydrocortisone is usually tapered off gradually. Take oral dose with food to reduce GI upset. Avoid alcohol. Hydrocortisone may cause immunosuppression and mask symptoms of infection; avoid exposure to contagion and notify prescriber of any signs of infection (eg, fever, chills, sore throat, injury) and notify dentist or surgeon (if necessary) that you are taking this medication. You may experience increased appetite, indigestion, or increased nervousness. Report any sudden weight gain (>5 lb/week), swelling of extremities or respiratory difficulty, abdominal pain, severe vomiting, black or tarry stools, fatigue, anorexia, weakness, or unusual mood swings. **Pregnancy/breast-feeding precautions:** Inform prescriber if you are or intend to become pregnant. Consult prescriber if breast-feeding.

Topical: Before applying, wash area gently and thoroughly. Apply a thin film to cleansed area and rub in gently until medication vanishes. Avoid use of occlusive dressings over topical application unless directed by a physician. Avoid use on weeping or exudative lesions. Avoid exposing affected area to sunlight; you will be more sensitive and severe sunburn may occur. Consult prescriber if breast-feeding.

Rectal: Gently insert suppository as high as possible with gloved finger while lying down. Avoid injury with long or sharp fingernails. Remain in resting position for 10 minutes after insertion.

Dietary Considerations: Systemic use of corticosteroids may require a diet with increased potassium, vitamins A, B₆, C, D, folate, calcium, zinc, phosphorus, and decreased sodium. Sodium content of 1 g (sodium succinate injection): 47.5 mg (2.07 mEq)

Pregnancy Risk Factor: C

Pregnancy Issues: There are no adequate and well-controlled studies in pregnant women. Corticosteroid use has been associated with cleft palate, neonatal adrenal suppression, low birth weight, and cataracts in the infant; including cases associated with topical administration. Use only if potential benefit to the mother exceeds the potential risk to the fetus. Avoid high doses or prolonged use.

Lactation: Excretion in breast milk unknown/use caution

Breast-Feeding Issues: It is not known if hydrocortisone is excreted in breast milk, however, other corticosteroids are excreted. Prednisone and prednisolone are excreted in breast milk; the AAP considers them to be "usually compatible" with breast-feeding. Hypertension was reported in a nursing infant when a topical corticosteroid was applied to the nipples of the mother.

(Continued)

Hydrocortisone *(Continued)*

Administration
Oral: Administer with food or milk to decrease GI upset.

I.V.:
Parenteral: Hydrocortisone sodium succinate may be administered by I.M. or I.V. routes.

I.V. bolus: Dilute to 50 mg/mL and give over 30 seconds to several minutes (depending on the dose).

I.V. intermittent infusion: Dilute to 1 mg/mL and give over 20-30 minutes.

Note: Should be administered in a 0.1-1 mg/mL concentration due to stability problems.

Topical: Apply a thin film sparingly to clean, dry skin and rub in gently.

Reconstitution:
Sodium succinate: Reconstitute 100 mg vials with bacteriostatic water (not >2 mL). Act-O-Vial (self-contained powder for injection plus diluent) may be reconstituted by pressing the activator to force diluent into the powder compartment. Following gentle agitation, solution may be withdrawn via syringe through a needle inserted into the center of the stopper. May be administered (I.V. or I.M.) without further dilution.

Solutions for I.V. infusion: Reconstituted solutions may be added to an appropriate volume of compatible solution for infusion. Concentration should generally not exceed 1 mg/mL. However, in cases where administration of a small volume of fluid is desirable, 100-3000 mg may be added to 50 mL of D_5W or NS (stability limited to 4 hours).

Compatibility:
Hydrocortisone sodium phosphate: Stable in D_5W, NS, fat emulsion 10%

Y-site administration: Incompatible with sargramostim

Compatibility in syringe: Incompatible with doxapram

Hydrocortisone sodium succinate: Stable in dextran 6% in dextrose, dextran 6% in NS, D_5LR, $D_5^1/_4NS$, $D_5^1/_2NS$, D_5NS, D_5W, $D_{10}W$, $D_{20}W$, LR, $^1/_2NS$, NS, fat emulsion 10%

Y-site administration: Incompatible with ciprofloxacin, diazepam, ergotamine, idarubicin, midazolam, phenytoin, sargramostim

Compatibility in syringe: Incompatible with doxapram

Compatibility when admixed: Incompatible with aminophylline with cephalothin, bleomycin, colistimethate, ephedrine, hydralazine, nafcillin, pentobarbital, phenobarbital, prochlorperazine edisylate, promethazine

Storage: Store at controlled room temperature 20°C to 25°C (59°F to 86°F). Hydrocortisone sodium phosphate and hydrocortisone sodium succinate are clear, light yellow solutions which are heat labile.

Sodium succinate: After initial reconstitution, hydrocortisone sodium succinate solutions are stable for 3 days at room temperature or under refrigeration when protected from light. Stability of parenteral admixture (Solu-Cortef®) at room temperature (25°C) and at refrigeration temperature (4°C) is concentration-dependent:

Stability of concentration 1 mg/mL: 24 hours

Stability of concentration 2 mg/mL to 60 mg/mL: At least 4 hours

Solutions for I.V. infusion: Reconstituted solutions may be added to an appropriate volume of compatible solution for infusion. Concentration should generally not exceed 1 mg/mL. However, in cases where administration of a small volume of fluid is desirable, 100-3000 mg may be added to 50 mL of D_5W or NS (stability limited to 4 hours).

Additional Information Hydrocortisone base topical cream, lotion, and ointments in concentrations of 0.25%, 0.5%, and 1% may be OTC or prescription depending on the product labeling.

Related Information
Compatibility of Drugs *on page 1723*
Corticosteroids *on page 1731*

♦ **Hydrocortisone Acetate** *see* Hydrocortisone *on page 760*

♦ **Hydrocortisone, Acetic Acid, and Propylene Glycol Diacetate** *see* Acetic Acid, Propylene Glycol Diacetate, and Hydrocortisone *on page 44*

♦ **Hydrocortisone and Benzoyl Peroxide** *see* Benzoyl Peroxide and Hydrocortisone *on page 183*

♦ **Hydrocortisone and Ciprofloxacin** *see* Ciprofloxacin and Hydrocortisone *on page 331*

♦ **Hydrocortisone, Bacitracin, Neomycin, and Polymyxin B** *see* Bacitracin, Neomycin, Polymyxin B, and Hydrocortisone *on page 172*

♦ **Hydrocortisone Butyrate** *see* Hydrocortisone *on page 760*

♦ **Hydrocortisone, Neomycin, and Polymyxin B** *see* Neomycin, Polymyxin B, and Hydrocortisone *on page 1069*

♦ **Hydrocortisone, Neomycin, Colistin, and Thonzonium** *see* Neomycin, Colistin, Hydrocortisone, and Thonzonium *on page 1069*

♦ **Hydrocortisone Probutate** *see* Hydrocortisone *on page 760*

♦ **Hydrocortisone, Propylene Glycol Diacetate, and Acetic Acid** *see* Acetic Acid, Propylene Glycol Diacetate, and Hydrocortisone *on page 44*

♦ **Hydrocortisone Sodium Succinate** *see* Hydrocortisone *on page 760*

♦ **Hydrocortisone Valerate** *see* Hydrocortisone *on page 760*

♦ **Hydrocortone® [DSC]** *see* Hydrocortisone *on page 760*

♦ **Hydro DP** *see* Hydrocodone, Phenylephrine, and Diphenhydramine *on page 759*

♦ **Hydro-GP** *see* Hydrocodone, Phenylephrine, and Guaifenesin *on page 760*

Hydromorphone *(hye droe MOR fone)*

U.S. Brand Names Dilaudid®; Dilaudid-HP®; Palladone™

Synonyms Dihydromorphinone; Hydromorphone Hydrochloride

Controlled Substance C-II; An FDA-approved medication guide is available at www.fda.gov/cder/Offices/ODS/labeling.htm; distribute to each patient to whom this medication is dispensed.

Generic Available Yes: Excludes capsule, liquid, powder for injection

Pharmacologic Category Analgesic, Narcotic

Medication Safety Issues

Sound-alike/look-alike issues:

Dilaudid® may be confused with Demerol®, Dilantin®

Hydromorphone may be confused with morphine; significant overdoses have occurred when hydromorphone products have been inadvertently administered instead of morphine sulfate. Commercially available prefilled syringes of both products looks similar and are often stored in close proximity to each other. **Note:** Hydromorphone 1 mg oral is approximately equal to morphine 4 mg oral; hydromorphone 1 mg I.V. is approximately equal to morphine 5 mg I.V..

Dilaudid®, Dilaudid-HP®: Extreme caution should be taken to avoid confusing the highly-concentrated (Dilaudid-HP®) injection with the less-concentrated (Dilaudid®) injectable product.

Use Management of moderate-to-severe pain

Unlabeled/Investigational Use Antitussive

Mechanism of Action/Effect Binds to opiate receptors in the CNS, causing inhibition of ascending pain pathways, altering the perception of and response to pain; causes cough supression by direct central action in the medulla; produces generalized CNS depression

Contraindications Hypersensitivity to hydromorphone, any component of the formulation, or other phenanthrene derivative; increased intracranial pressure; acute or severe asthma, severe respiratory depression (in absence of resuscitative equipment or ventilatory support); severe CNS depression; pregnancy (prolonged use or high doses at term)

Palladone™ is also contraindicated with known or suspected paralytic ileus.

Warnings/Precautions Controlled release capsules should only be used when continuous analgesia is required over an extended period of time. Palladone™ should only be used in opioid tolerant patients requiring doses of hydromorphone >12 mg/day (or equianalgesic dose of another opioid) and who have been at that dose for >7 days. Controlled release products are not to be used on an as needed basis. Hydromorphone shares toxic potential of opiate agonists, and precaution of opiate agonist therapy should be observed; use with caution in patients with hypersensitivity to other phenanthrene opiates, respiratory disease, biliary tract disease, acute pancreatitis, or severe liver or renal failure; tolerance or drug dependence may result from extended use. Those at risk for opioid abuse include patients with a history of substance abuse or mental illness.

An opioid-containing analgesic regimen should be tailored to each patient's needs and based upon the type of pain being treated (acute versus chronic), the route of administration, degree of tolerance for opioids (naive versus chronic user), age, weight, and medical condition. The optimal analgesic dose varies widely among patients. Doses should be titrated to pain relief/prevention. I.M. use may result in variable absorption and a lag time to peak effect.

Some dosage forms contain trace amounts of sodium bisulfite which may cause allergic reactions in susceptible individuals.

Drug Interactions

Decreased Effect: Hydromorphone may diminish the effects of pegvisomant.

Increased Effect/Toxicity: Effects may be additive with CNS depressants; hypotensive effects may be increased with phenothiazines; serotonergic effects may be additive with SSRIs

Nutritional/Ethanol Interactions

Ethanol: Avoid ethanol (may increase CNS depression).

Herb/Nutraceutical: Avoid valerian, St John's wort, kava kava, gotu kola (may increase CNS depression).

Lab Interactions Increased aminotransferase [ALT (SGPT)/AST (SGOT)] (S)

Adverse Reactions Frequency not defined.

Cardiovascular: Palpitations, hypotension, peripheral vasodilation, tachycardia, bradycardia, flushing of face

Central nervous system: CNS depression, increased intracranial pressure, fatigue, headache, nervousness, restlessness, dizziness, lightheadedness, drowsiness, hallucinations, mental depression, seizure

Dermatologic: Pruritus, rash, urticaria

Endocrine & metabolic: Antidiuretic hormone release

Gastrointestinal: Nausea, vomiting, constipation, stomach cramps, xerostomia, anorexia, biliary tract spasm, paralytic ileus

Genitourinary: Decreased urination, ureteral spasm, urinary tract spasm

Hepatic: LFTs increased, AST increased, ALT increased

Local: Pain at injection site (I.M.)

Neuromuscular & skeletal: Trembling, weakness, myoclonus

Ocular: Miosis

Respiratory: Respiratory depression, dyspnea

Miscellaneous: Histamine release, physical and psychological dependence

Overdosage/Toxicology Symptoms of overdose include CNS depression, respiratory depression, miosis, apnea, pulmonary edema, and convulsions. Along with supportive measures, naloxone, 2 mg I.V. with repeat administration as necessary up to a total of 10 mg, can also be used to reverse toxic effects of the opiate.

Pharmacodynamics/Kinetics

Onset of Action: Analgesic: Immediate release formulations: Oral: 15-30 minutes; Peak effect: Oral: 30-60 minutes
(Continued)

Hydromorphone *(Continued)*

Duration of Action: Immediate release formulations: 4-5 hours
Absorption: I.M.: Variable and delayed; Palladone™: Biphasic
Bioavailability: 62%
Protein Binding: ~20%
Half-Life Elimination: Immediate release formulations: 1-3 hours; Palladone™: 18.6 hours
Metabolism: Hepatic; to inactive metabolites
Excretion: Urine (primarily as glucuronide conjugates)

Dosing

Adults:

Antitussive (unlabeled use): Oral: 1 mg every 3-4 hours as needed

Acute pain (moderate to severe): Note: These are guidelines and do not represent the maximum doses that may be required in all patients. Doses should be titrated to pain relief/prevention. Doses should be titrated to appropriate analgesic effects; when changing routes of administration, note that oral doses are <50% as effective as parenteral doses (may be only one-fifth as effective).

Oral:
Initial: Opiate-naive: 2-4 mg every 3-4 hours as needed; patients with prior opiate exposure may require higher initial doses
Usual dosage range: 2-8 mg every 3-4 hours as needed

I.V.: Initial: Opiate-naive: 0.2-0.6 mg every 2-3 hours as needed; patients with prior opiate exposure may tolerate higher initial doses
Note: More frequent dosing may be needed.
Mechanically-ventilated patients (based on 70 kg patient): 0.7-2 mg every 1-2 hours as needed; infusion (based on 70 kg patient): 0.5-1 mg/hour

Patient-controlled analgesia (PCA): (Opiate-naive: Consider lower end of dosing range)
Usual concentration: 0.2 mg/mL
Demand dose: Usual: 0.1-0.2 mg; range: 0.05-0.5 mg
Lockout interval: 5-15 minutes
4-hour limit: 4-6 mg

Epidural:
Bolus dose: 1-1.5 mg
Infusion concentration: 0.05-0.075 mg/mL
Infusion rate: 0.04-0.4 mg/hour
Demand dose: 0.15 mg
Lockout interval: 30 minutes

I.M., SubQ: **Note:** I.M. use may result in variable absorption and a lag time to peak effect.
Initial: Opiate-naive: 0.8-1 mg every 4-6 hours as needed; patients with prior opiate exposure may require higher initial doses
Usual dosage range: 1-2 mg every 3-6 hours as needed

Rectal: 3 mg every 4-8 hours as needed

Chronic pain: Note: Patients taking opioids chronically may become tolerant and require doses higher than the usual dosage range to maintain the desired effect. Tolerance can be managed by appropriate dose titration. There is no optimal or maximal dose for hydromorphone in chronic pain. The appropriate dose is one that relieves pain throughout its dosing interval without causing unmanageable side effects.

Controlled release formulation (Hydromorph Contin®, not available in U.S.): Oral: 3-30 mg every 12 hours. **Note:** A patient's hydromorphone requirement should be established using prompt release formulations; conversion to long acting products may be considered when chronic, continuous treatment is required. Higher dosages should be reserved for use only in opioid-tolerant patients.

Extended release formulation (Palladone™): Oral: For use only in opioid-tolerant patients requiring extended treatment of pain. Initial Palladone™ dose should be calculated using standard conversion estimates based on previous total daily opioid dose, rounding off to the most appropriate strength available. Doses should be administered once every 24 hours. Discontinue all previous around-the-clock opioids when treatment is initiated. Dose may be adjusted every 2 days as needed.
Conversion from transdermal fentanyl to oral Palladone™ (limited clinical experience): Initiate Palladone™ 18 hours after removal of patch; substitute Palladone™ 12 mg/day for each fentanyl 50 mcg/hour patch; monitor closely
Conversion from opioid combination drugs: Initial dose: Palladone™ 12 mg/day in patients receiving around-the-clock fixed combination-opioid analgesics with a total dose greater than or equal to oxycodone 45 mg/day, hydrocodone 45 mg/day, or codeine 300 mg/day

Elderly: Doses should be titrated to appropriate analgesic effects. When changing routes of administration, note that oral doses are less than half as effective as parenteral doses (may be only 20% as effective).

Pain: Oral: 1-2 mg every 4-6 hours
Antitussive: Refer to adult dosing.

Pediatrics:

Acute pain (moderate to severe): Note: These are guidelines and do not represent the maximum doses that may be required in all patients. Doses should be titrated to pain relief/prevention.
Young Children ≥6 months and <50 kg:
Oral: 0.03-0.08 mg/kg/dose every 3-4 hours as needed
I.V.: 0.015 mg/kg/dose every 3-6 hours as needed
Older Children >50 kg: Refer to adult dosing.

Antitussive: Oral:
Children 6-12 years: 0.5 mg every 3-4 hours as needed
Children >12 years: 1 mg every 3-4 hours as needed

Hepatic Impairment: Dose adjustment should be considered.

Available Dosage Forms [CAN] = Canadian brand name

Capsule, controlled release (Hydromorph Contin®) [CAN]: 3 mg, 6 mg, 12 mg, 18 mg, 24 mg, 30 mg [not available in U.S.]

Capsule, extended release, as hydrochloride (Palladone™): 12 mg, 16 mg, 24 mg, 32 mg

Injection, powder for reconstitution, as hydrochloride (Dilaudid-HP®): 250 mg

Injection, solution, as hydrochloride: 1 mg/mL (1 mL); 2 mg/mL (1 mL, 20 mL); 4 mg/mL (1 mL); 10 mg/mL (1 mL, 5 mL, 10 mL)

Dilaudid®: 1 mg/mL (1 mL); 2 mg/mL (1 mL, 20 mL) [20 mL size contains edetate sodium; vial stopper contains latex]; 4 mg/mL (1 mL)

Dilaudid-HP®: 10 mg/mL (1 mL, 5 mL, 50 mL)

Liquid, oral, as hydrochloride (Dilaudid®): 1 mg/mL (480 mL) [may contain trace amounts of sodium bisulfite]

Suppository, rectal, as hydrochloride (Dilaudid®): 3 mg (6s)

Tablet, as hydrochloride (Dilaudid®): 2 mg, 4 mg, 8 mg (8 mg tablets may contain trace amounts of sodium bisulfite)

Monitoring and Teaching Issues

Physical Assessment: Assess other medications patient may be taking for additive or adverse interactions. Monitor for effectiveness of pain relief, adverse reactions, and signs of overdose at beginning of therapy and periodically during long-term use. May cause physical and/or psychological dependence. Monitor blood pressure, CNS and respiratory status, and degree of sedation at beginning of therapy and at regular intervals with long-term use. For inpatients, implement safety measures. Assess knowledge/teach patient appropriate use (if self-administered). Teach patient to monitor for adverse reactions, adverse reactions to report, and appropriate interventions to reduce side effects. Discontinue slowly after prolonged use.

Patient Education: If self-administered, use exactly as directed; do not increase dose or frequency. Drug may cause physical and/or psychological dependence. Palladone™ must be swallowed whole. While using this medication, do not use alcohol and other prescription or OTC medications (especially sedatives, tranquilizers, antihistamines, or pain medications) without consulting prescriber. Maintain adequate hydration (2-3 L/day of fluids) unless instructed to restrict fluid intake. May cause dizziness, drowsiness, impaired coordination, or blurred vision (use caution when driving, climbing stairs, or changing position - rising from sitting or lying to standing, or when engaging in tasks requiring alertness until response to drug is known); loss of appetite, nausea, or vomiting (frequent mouth care, small frequent meals, chewing gum, or sucking lozenges may help); or constipation (increased exercise, fluids, fruit, or fiber may help; if unresolved, consult prescriber about use of stool softeners). Report chest pain, slow or rapid heartbeat, acute dizziness, or persistent headache; swelling of extremities or unusual weight gain; changes in urinary elimination; acute headache; back or flank pain or spasms; or other adverse reactions. **Pregnancy/breast-feeding precautions:** Inform prescriber if you are or intend to become pregnant. Breast-feeding is not recommended.

Geriatric Considerations: Elderly may be particularly susceptible to the CNS depressant and constipating effects of narcotics.

Pregnancy Risk Factor: C/D (prolonged use or high doses at term)

Pregnancy Issues: Hydromorphone was teratogenic in some, but not all, animal studies; however, maternal toxicity was also reported. Hydromorphone crosses the placenta. Chronic opioid use during pregnancy may lead to a withdrawal syndrome in the neonate. Symptoms include irritability, hyperactivity, loss of sleep pattern, abnormal crying, tremor, vomiting, diarrhea, weight loss, or failure to gain weight.

Lactation: Excretion in breast milk unknown/not recommended

Breast-Feeding Issues: Other opioid analgesics can be found in breast milk; specific data for hydromorphone is not available. The possibility of sedation or respiratory depression in the nursing infant should be considered.

Administration

Oral:

Hydromorph Contin®: Capsule should be swallowed whole; do not crush or chew; contents may be sprinkled on soft food and swallowed

Palladone™: Capsule must be swallowed whole; do not break open, crush, chew, dissolve, or sprinkle on food.

I.M.: May be given SubQ or I.M.; vial stopper contains latex

I.V.: For IVP, must be given slowly over 2-3 minutes (rapid IVP has been associated with an increase in side effects, especially respiratory depression and hypotension)

Other: May be given SubQ or I.M.

Compatibility: Stable in D_5LR, D_5W, $D_5{}^{1}/_2NS$, D_5NS, LR, $^{1}/_2NS$, NS

Y-site administration: Incompatible with amphotericin B cholesteryl sulfate complex, diazepam, minocycline, phenobarbital, phenytoin, sargramostim, tetracycline, thiopental

Compatibility in syringe: Incompatible with ampicillin, diazepam, hyaluronidase, phenobarbital, phenytoin

Compatibility when admixed: Incompatible with sodium bicarbonate, thiopental

Storage: Store injection and oral dosage forms at 25°C (77°F). Protect tablets from light. A slightly yellowish discoloration has not been associated with a loss of potency.

Additional Information Equianalgesic doses: Morphine 10 mg I.M. = hydromorphone 1.5 mg I.M.

Related Information

Narcotic / Opioid Analgesic Comparison *on page 1739*

- ◆ **Hydromorphone Hydrochloride** *see* Hydromorphone *on page 764*
- ◆ **Hydron CP** *see* Phenylephrine, Hydrocodone, and Chlorpheniramine *on page 1202*
- ◆ **Hydron PSC** *see* Pseudoephedrine, Hydrocodone, and Chlorpheniramine *on page 1283*
- ◆ **Hydro-PC II** *see* Phenylephrine, Hydrocodone, and Chlorpheniramine *on page 1202*
- ◆ **Hydro PC II Plus** *see* Phenylephrine, Hydrocodone, and Chlorpheniramine *on page 1202*
- ◆ **Hydroquinol** *see* Hydroquinone *on page 768*

Hydroquinone (HYE droe kwin one)

U.S. Brand Names Alphaquin HP; Claripel™; Dermarest® Skin Correction Cream Plus [OTC]; Eldopaque® [OTC]; Eldopaque Forte®; Eldoquin® [OTC]; Eldoquin Forte®; EpiQuin™ Micro; Esoterica® Regular [OTC]; Glyquin®; Glyquin-XM™; Lustra®; Lustra-AF™; Melanex®; Melpaque HP®; Melquin-3®; Melquin HP®; NeoStrata AHA [OTC]; Nuquin HP®; Palmer's® Skin Success Eventone® Fade Cream [OTC]; Solaquin® [OTC]; Solaquin Forte®

Synonyms Hydroquinol; Quinol

Generic Available Yes

Pharmacologic Category Depigmenting Agent

Medication Safety Issues

Sound-alike/look-alike issues:

Eldopaque® may be confused with Eldoquin®

Eldoquin® may be confused with Eldopaque®

Eldopaque Forte® may be confused with Eldoquin Forte®

Eldoquin Forte® may be confused with Eldopaque Forte®

Use Gradual bleaching of hyperpigmented skin conditions

Mechanism of Action/Effect Produces reversible depigmentation of the skin by suppression of melanocyte metabolic processes, in particular the inhibition of the enzymatic oxidation of tyrosine to DOPA (3,4-dihydroxyphenylalanine); sun exposure reverses this effect and will cause repigmentation.

Contraindications Hypersensitivity to hydroquinone or any component of the formulation; sunburn, depilatory usage

Warnings/Precautions Limit application to area no larger than face and neck or hands and arms.

Adverse Reactions Frequency not defined.

Dermatologic: Dermatitis, dryness, erythema, stinging, inflammatory reaction, sensitization

Local: Irritation

Pharmacodynamics/Kinetics

Onset of Action: Onset of depigmentation produced by hydroquinone varies among individuals

Duration of Action: Onset and duration of depigmentation produced by hydroquinone varies among individuals

Dosing

Adults & Elderly: Bleaching: Topical: Apply a thin layer and rub in twice daily.

Pediatrics: Refer to adult dosing.

Available Dosage Forms

Cream, topical: 4% (30 g) [may contain sodium metabisulfite]

Alphaquin HP: 4% (30 g, 60 g)

Eldoquin®: 2% (15 g, 30 g)

Eldoquin Forte®: 4% (30 g) [contains sodium metabisulfite]

EpiQuin™ Micro: 4% (30 g) [contains benzyl alcohol and sodium metabisulfite]

Esoterica® Regular: 2% (85 g) [contains sodium bisulfite]

Lustra®: 4% (30 g) [contains sodium metabisulfite]

Melquin HP®: 4% (15 g, 30 g) [contains sodium metabisulfite]

Cream, topical [with sunscreen]: 4% (30 g) [may contain sodium metabisulfite]

Claripel™: 4% (30 g, 45 g) [contains sodium metabisulfite]

Dermarest® Skin Correcting Cream Plus: 2% (85 g) [contains aloe vera, sodium bisulfite]

Eldopaque®: 2% (15 g, 30 g)

Eldopaque Forte®: 4% (30 g) [contains sodium metabisulfite]

Glyquin®: 4% (30 g)

Glyquin-XM™: 4% (30 g)

Lustra-AF™: 4% (30 g, 60 g) [contains sodium metabisulfite]

Melpaque HP®: 4% (15 g, 30 g) [contains sodium metabisulfite; sunblocking cream base]

Nuquin HP®: 4% (15 g, 30 g, 60 g) [contains sodium metabisulfite]

Palmer's® Skin Success Eventone® Fade Cream: 2% (81 g, 132 g) [contains sodium sulfite; available in regular, oily skin, and dry skin formulas]

Solaquin®: 2% (30 g)

Solaquin Forte®: 4% (30 g) [contains sodium metabisulfite]

Gel, topical (NeoStrata AHA): 2% (45 g) [contains glycolic acid 10%, sodium bisulfite, and sodium sulfite]

Gel, topical [with sunscreen]: 4% (30 g)

Nuquin HP: 4% (15 g, 30 g) [contains sodium bisulfite]

Solaquin Forte®: 4% (30 g) [contains sodium metabisulfite]

Solution, topical (Melanex®, Melquin-3®): 3% (30 mL) [contains alcohol]

Monitoring and Teaching Issues

Physical Assessment: See application directions above. When applied to large areas or for extensive periods of time, monitor for adverse reactions. Assess knowledge/teach patient appropriate application and use and adverse symptoms to report.

Patient Education: Use exactly as directed; do not overuse. Therapeutic effect may take several weeks. Test response by applying to small area of unbroken skin and check in 24 hours; if irritation or blistering occurs do not use. Avoid contact with eyes. Do not apply to open wounds or weeping areas. Before using, wash and dry area gently. Apply a thin film to affected area and rub in gently. Avoid direct sunlight or use sunblock or protective clothing to prevent repigmentation. Report swelling, redness, rash, itching, signs of infection, worsening of condition, or lack of healing. **Pregnancy/breast-feeding precautions:** Inform prescriber if you are or intend to become pregnant. Consult prescriber if breast-feeding.

Pregnancy Risk Factor: C
Lactation: Excretion in breast milk unknown
Administration
Topical: For external use only; avoid contact with eyes

- ◆ **Hydroquinone, Fluocinolone Acetonide, and Tretinoin** *see* Fluocinolone, Hydroquinone, and Tretinoin *on page 644*
- ◆ **Hydro-Tussin™-CBX** *see* Carbinoxamine and Pseudoephedrine *on page 254*
- ◆ **Hydro-Tussin™ DM** *see* Guaifenesin and Dextromethorphan *on page 731*
- ◆ **Hydro-Tussin™ EXP** *see* Dihydrocodeine, Pseudoephedrine, and Guaifenesin *on page 457*
- ◆ **Hydro-Tussin™ HC** *see* Pseudoephedrine, Hydrocodone, and Chlorpheniramine *on page 1283*

Hydroxocobalamin (hye droks oh koe BAL a min)

Synonyms Vitamin B$_{12}$
Generic Available Yes
Pharmacologic Category Vitamin, Water Soluble
Use Treatment of pernicious anemia, vitamin B$_{12}$ deficiency, increased B$_{12}$ requirements due to pregnancy, thyrotoxicosis, hemorrhage, malignancy, liver or kidney disease
Unlabeled/Investigational Use Neuropathies, multiple sclerosis
Mechanism of Action/Effect Coenzyme for various metabolic functions, including fat and carbohydrate metabolism and protein synthesis, used in cell replication and hematopoiesis
Contraindications Hypersensitivity to cyanocobalamin or any component of the formulation, cobalt; patients with hereditary optic nerve atrophy
Warnings/Precautions Some products contain benzoyl alcohol. Avoid use in premature infants. An intradermal test dose should be performed for hypersensitivity. Use only if oral supplementation not possible or when treating pernicious anemia.
Adverse Reactions Frequency not defined.
Cardiovascular: Peripheral vascular thrombosis
Dermatologic: Itching, urticaria
Gastrointestinal: Diarrhea
Miscellaneous: Hypersensitivity reactions
Dosing
Adults & Elderly: Vitamin B$_{12}$ deficiency: I.M.: 30 mcg/day for 5-10 days, followed by 100-200 mcg/month
Pediatrics: Vitamin B$_{12}$ deficiency: I.M.: 1-5 mg given in single doses of 100 mcg over 2 or more weeks, followed by 30-50 mcg/month.
Available Dosage Forms Injection, solution: 1000 mcg/mL (30 mL)
Monitoring and Teaching Issues
Physical Assessment: Assess results of laboratory tests at beginning of therapy and periodically with long-term therapy. Assess knowledge/teach patient appropriate administration (injection technique and needle disposal), appropriate nutrition, and adverse symptoms to report.
Monitoring Laboratory Tests: Reticulocyte count, Hct, iron and folic acid, and serum levels before treatment, after first week of treatment, and routinely thereafter
Patient Education: Use exactly as directed. Pernicious anemia may require monthly injections for life. Report skin rash; swelling, pain, or redness in extremities; or acute persistent diarrhea. **Pregnancy precaution:** Inform prescriber if you are pregnant.
Geriatric Considerations: Evidence exists that people, particularly elderly, whose serum cobalamin concentrations are <500 pg/mL, should receive replacement parenteral therapy. This recommendation is based upon neuropsychiatric disorders and cardiovascular disorders associated with lower sodium cobalamin concentrations.
Pregnancy Risk Factor: A/C (dose exceeding RDA recommendation)
Lactation: Enters breast milk/compatible
Administration
I.M.: Administer I.M. only. May require coadministration of folic acid.
Storage: Clear pink to red solutions are stable at room temperature; protect from light; incompatible with chlorpromazine, phytonadione, prochlorperazine, warfarin, ascorbic acid, dextrose, heavy metals, oxidizing or reducing agents; avoid freezing

- ◆ **Hydroxyamphetamine and Tropicamide** *see page 1625*
- ◆ **Hydroxycarbamide** *see* Hydroxyurea *on page 771*

Hydroxychloroquine (hye droks ee KLOR oh kwin)

U.S. Brand Names Plaquenil®
Synonyms Hydroxychloroquine Sulfate
Generic Available Yes
Pharmacologic Category Aminoquinoline (Antimalarial)
Medication Safety Issues
Sound-alike/look-alike issues:
Hydroxychloroquine may be confused with hydrocortisone
Plaquenil® may be confused with Platinol®
Use Suppression and treatment of acute attacks of malaria; treatment of systemic lupus erythematosus and rheumatoid arthritis
Unlabeled/Investigational Use Porphyria cutanea tarda, polymorphous light eruptions
Mechanism of Action/Effect Interferes with digestive vacuole function within sensitive malarial parasites by increasing the pH and interfering with lysosomal degradation of hemoglobin; inhibits locomotion of neutrophils and chemotaxis of eosinophils; impairs complement-dependent antigen-antibody reactions
Contraindications Hypersensitivity to hydroxychloroquine, 4-aminoquinoline derivatives, or any component of the formulation; retinal or visual field changes attributable to 4-aminoquinolines
(Continued)

Hydroxychloroquine *(Continued)*

Warnings/Precautions Use with caution in patients with hepatic disease, G6PD deficiency, psoriasis, and porphyria. Long-term use in children is not recommended. Perform baseline and periodic (6 months) ophthalmologic examinations. Test periodically for muscle weakness.

Drug Interactions

Decreased Effect: Chloroquine and other 4-aminoquinolones absorption may be decreased due to GI binding with kaolin or magnesium trisilicate.

Increased Effect/Toxicity: Cimetidine increases levels of chloroquine and probably other 4-aminoquinolones.

Nutritional/Ethanol Interactions Ethanol: Avoid ethanol (due to GI irritation).

Adverse Reactions Frequency not defined.

Cardiovascular: Cardiomyopathy (rare, relationship to hydroxychloroquine unclear)

Central nervous system: Irritability, nervousness, emotional changes, nightmares, psychosis, headache, dizziness, vertigo, seizure, ataxia, lassitude

Dermatologic: Bleaching of hair, alopecia, pigmentation changes (skin and mucosal; black-blue color), rash (urticarial, morbilliform, lichenoid, maculopapular, purpuric, erythema annulare centrifugum, Stevens-Johnson syndrome, acute generalized exanthematous pustulosis, and exfoliative dermatitis)

Endocrine & metabolic: Weight loss

Gastrointestinal: Anorexia, nausea, vomiting, diarrhea, abdominal cramping

Hematologic: Aplastic anemia, agranulocytosis, leukopenia, thrombocytopenia, hemolysis (in patients with glucose-6-phosphate deficiency)

Hepatic: Abnormal liver function/hepatic failure (isolated cases)

Neuromuscular & skeletal: Myopathy, palsy, or neuromyopathy leading to progressive weakness and atrophy of proximal muscle groups (may be associated with mild sensory changes, loss of deep tendon reflexes, and abnormal nerve conduction)

Ocular: Disturbance in accommodation, keratopathy, corneal changes/deposits (visual disturbances, blurred vision, photophobia - reversible on discontinuation), macular edema, atrophy, abnormal pigmentation, retinopathy (early changes reversible - may progress despite discontinuation if advanced), optic disc pallor/atrophy, attenuation of retinal arterioles, pigmentary retinopathy, scotoma, decreased visual acuity, nystagmus

Otic: Tinnitus, deafness

Miscellaneous: Exacerbation of porphyria and nonlight sensitive psoriasis

Overdosage/Toxicology Symptoms of overdose include headache, drowsiness, visual changes, cardiovascular collapse, and seizures followed by respiratory and cardiac arrest. Treatment is symptomatic. Urinary alkalinization will enhance renal elimination.

Pharmacodynamics/Kinetics

Onset of Action: Rheumatic disease: May require 4-6 weeks to respond

Absorption: Complete

Time to Peak: Rheumatic disease: Several months

Protein Binding: 55%

Half-Life Elimination: 32-50 days

Metabolism: Hepatic

Excretion: Urine (as metabolites and unchanged drug); may be enhanced by urinary acidification

Dosing

Adults & Elderly:

Note: Hydroxychloroquine sulfate 200 mg is equivalent to 155 mg hydroxychloroquine base and 250 mg chloroquine phosphate.

Chemoprophylaxis of malaria: 310 mg base weekly on same day each week; begin 2 weeks before exposure. Continue for 4-6 weeks after leaving endemic area; if suppressive therapy is not begun prior to the exposure, double the initial dose and give in 2 doses, 6 hours apart.

Malaria, acute attack: 620 mg first dose day 1; 310 mg in 6 hours day 1; 310 mg in 1 dose day 2; and 310 mg in 1 dose on day 3

Rheumatoid arthritis: 310-465 mg/day to start taken with food or milk; increase dose until optimum response level is reached; usually after 4-12 weeks dose should be reduced by $1/2$ and a maintenance dose of 155-310 mg/day given

Lupus erythematosus: 310 mg every day or twice daily for several weeks depending on response; 155-310 mg/day for prolonged maintenance therapy

Pediatrics:

Note: Hydroxychloroquine sulfate 200 mg is equivalent to 155 mg hydroxychloroquine base and 250 mg chloroquine phosphate.

Chemoprophylaxis of malaria: Oral: 5 mg/kg (base) once weekly; should not exceed the recommended adult dose. Begin 2 weeks before exposure and continue for 4-6 weeks after leaving endemic area. If suppressive therapy is not begun prior to the exposure, double the initial dose and give in 2 doses, 6 hours apart.

Malaria, acute attack: Oral: 10 mg/kg (base) initial dose; followed by 5 mg/kg at 6, 24, and 48 hours.

Juvenile rheumatoid arthritis (JRA) or SLE: Oral: 3-5 mg/kg/day divided 1-2 times/day; avoid exceeding 7 mg/kg/day.

Hepatic Impairment: Use with caution; dosage adjustment may be necessary.

Available Dosage Forms Tablet, as sulfate: 200 mg [equivalent to 155 mg base]

Monitoring and Teaching Issues

Physical Assessment: Use caution in presence of hepatic disease, G6PD deficiency, psoriasis, and porphyria (see Warnings/Precautions). Assess potential for interactions with other pharmacological agents patient may be taking (see Drug Interactions). Assess results of periodic CBC and liver function tests, therapeutic effectiveness (according to purpose for therapy), and adverse response (eg, deep tendon reflexes, muscle weakness; see Adverse Reactions). Teach patient appropriate use, possible side effects/interventions, and adverse symptoms to report (see Patient Education).

Monitoring Laboratory Tests: CBC, liver function

Patient Education: Do not take any new medication during therapy unless approved by prescriber. It is important to complete full course of therapy, which may take up to 6 months for full effect. May be taken with meals to decrease GI upset and bitter aftertaste. Avoid alcohol. You should have regular ophthalmic exams (every 4-6 months) if using this medication over extended periods. You may experience skin discoloration (blue/black), hair bleaching, or skin rash. If you have psoriasis, you may experience exacerbation. You may experience dizziness, headache, nervousness, or lightheadedness (use caution when driving or engaging in tasks requiring alertness until response to drug is known); nausea, vomiting, or loss of appetite (small frequent meals, frequent mouth care, sucking lozenges, or chewing gum may help); or increased sensitivity to sunlight (wear dark glasses and protective clothing, use sunblock, and avoid direct exposure to sunlight). Report weakness, numbness, tingling or tremors in muscles; vision changes; rash or itching; persistent diarrhea or GI disturbances; change in hearing acuity or ringing in the ears; chest pain or palpitation; CNS changes; unusual fatigue; easy bruising or bleeding, or any other persistent adverse reactions. **Pregnancy precaution:** Inform prescriber if you are or intend to become pregnant.

Dietary Considerations: May be taken with food or milk.

Pregnancy Risk Factor: C

Lactation: Enters breast milk/compatible

Administration
    Oral: Take with food or milk.

♦ **Hydroxychloroquine Sulfate** *see* Hydroxychloroquine *on page 769*

♦ **Hydroxydaunomycin Hydrochloride** *see* DOXOrubicin *on page 491*

♦ **1α-Hydroxyergocalciferol** *see* Doxercalciferol *on page 489*

♦ **Hydroxyethyl Starch** *see* Hetastarch *on page 743*

♦ **Hydroxyldaunorubicin Hydrochloride** *see* DOXOrubicin *on page 491*

♦ **Hydroxypropyl Methylcellulose** *see page 1625*

Hydroxyurea (hye droks ee yoor EE a)

U.S. Brand Names Droxia™; Hydrea®; Mylocel™

Synonyms Hydroxycarbamide

Generic Available Yes: Capsule

Pharmacologic Category Antineoplastic Agent, Antimetabolite

Medication Safety Issues
    Sound-alike/look-alike issues:
        Hydroxyurea may be confused with hydrOXYzine

Use CML in chronic phase; radiosensitizing agent in the treatment of primary brain tumors, head and neck tumors, uterine cervix and nonsmall cell lung cancer, and psoriasis; treatment of hematologic conditions such as essential thrombocytosis, polycythemia vera, hypereosinophilia, and hyperleukocytosis due to acute leukemia. Has shown activity against renal cell cancer, melanoma, ovarian cancer, head and neck cancer (excluding lip cancer), and prostate cancer.

    Orphan drug: Droxia™: Sickle cell anemia: Specifically for patients >18 years of age who have had at least three "painful crises" in the previous year - to reduce frequency of these crises and the need for blood transfusions

Unlabeled/Investigational Use Treatment of HIV; treatment of psoriasis

Mechanism of Action/Effect Interferes with synthesis of DNA, without interfering with RNA synthesis

Contraindications Hypersensitivity to hydroxyurea or any component of the formulation; severe anemia; severe bone marrow suppression; WBC <2500/mm^3 or platelet count <100,000/mm^3; pregnancy

Warnings/Precautions Use with caution in patients with renal impairment, in patients who have received prior irradiation therapy with exacerbation of postirradiation erythema, bone marrow suppression, erythrocytic abnormalities, mucositis, and in the elderly. The U.S. Food and Drug Administration (FDA) currently recommends that procedures for proper handling and disposal of antineoplastic agents be considered. May cause pancreatitis, neuropathy, or hepatotoxicity; risk is increased in HIV-infected patients receiving didanosine and/or stavudine. Secondary leukemias have been reported with long-term use.

Drug Interactions
    Increased Effect/Toxicity: Zidovudine, zalcitabine, didanosine may increase synergy. The potential for neurotoxicity may increase with concomitant administration with fluorouracil. Hydroxyurea modulates the metabolism and cytotoxicity of cytarabine; dose reduction is recommended. Hydroxyurea may precipitate didanosine- or stavudine-induced pancreatitis, hepatotoxicity, or neuropathy; concomitant use is not recommended.

Adverse Reactions Frequency not defined.
    Cardiovascular: Edema
    Central nervous system: Drowsiness (with high doses), hallucinations, headache, dizziness, disorientation, seizure, fever, chills
    Dermatologic: Erythema of the hands and face, maculopapular rash, pruritus, dry skin, dermatomyositis-like skin changes, hyperpigmentation, atrophy of skin and nails, scaling and violet papules (long-term use), nail banding, skin cancer
    Endocrine & metabolic: Hyperuricemia
    Gastrointestinal: Nausea, vomiting, stomatitis, anorexia, diarrhea, constipation, mucositis (potentiated in patients receiving radiation), pancreatitis, ulceration of buccal mucosa and GI epithelium (severe intoxication)
        Emetic potential: Low (10% to 30%)
    Genitourinary: Dysuria
    Hematologic: Myelosuppression (primarily leukopenia); Dose-limiting toxicity, causes a rapid drop in leukocyte count (seen in 4-5 days in nonhematologic malignancy and more rapidly in leukemia); thrombocytopenia and anemia occur less often
        Onset: 24-48 hours
(Continued)

Hydroxyurea *(Continued)*

Nadir: 10 days

Recovery: 7 days after stopping drug (reversal of WBC count occurs rapidly but the platelet count may take 7-10 days to recover)

Other hematologic effects include megaloblastic erythropoiesis, macrocytosis, hemolysis, decreased serum iron, persistent cytopenias, secondary leukemias (long-term use)

Hepatic: Elevation of hepatic enzymes, hepatotoxicity, hyperbilirubinemia (polycythemia vera)

Neuromuscular & skeletal: Weakness, peripheral neuropathy

Renal: Increased creatinine and BUN due to impairment of renal tubular function

Respiratory: Acute diffuse pulmonary infiltrates (rare), dyspnea, pulmonary fibrosis

Overdosage/Toxicology Symptoms of overdose include myelosuppression, facial swelling, hallucinations, and disorientation. Treatment is supportive.

Pharmacodynamics/Kinetics

Absorption: Readily ($\geq$80%)

Time to Peak: ~2 hours

Half-Life Elimination: 3-4 hours

Metabolism: Hepatic and via GI tract; 50% degradation by enzymes of intestinal bacteria

Excretion: Urine (80%, 50% as unchanged drug, 30% as urea); exhaled gases (as CO_2)

Dosing

Adults & Elderly: Refer to individual protocols.

Note: Dose should always be titrated to patient response and WBC counts; usual oral doses range from 10-30 mg/kg/day or 500-3000 mg/day; if WBC count falls to <2500 cells/mm^3, or the platelet count to <100,000/mm^3, therapy should be stopped for at least 3 days and resumed when values rise toward normal.

Solid tumors: Oral:

Intermittent therapy: 80 mg/kg as a single dose every third day

Continuous therapy: 20-30 mg/kg/day given as a single dose/day

Concomitant therapy with irradiation: 80 mg/kg as a single dose every third day starting at least 7 days before initiation of irradiation

Resistant chronic myelocytic leukemia: Oral: Continuous therapy: 20-30 mg/kg as a single daily dose

HIV (unlabeled use; in combination with antiretroviral agents): 1000-1500 mg daily in single or divided doses

Psoriasis: 1000-1500 mg daily in single or divided doses

Sickle cell anemia (moderate/severe disease): Initial: 15 mg/kg/day, increased by 5 mg/kg every 12 weeks if blood counts are in an acceptable range until the maximum tolerated dose of 35 mg/kg/day is achieved or the dose that does not produce toxic effects

Pediatrics: Refer to individual protocols. All dosage should be based on ideal or actual body weight, whichever is less: Children:

Note: No FDA-approved dosage regimens have been established; dosages of 1500-3000 mg/m^2 as a single dose in combination with other agents every 4-6 weeks have been used in the treatment of pediatric astrocytoma, medulloblastoma, and primitive neuroectodermal tumors

CML: Oral: Initial: 10-20 mg/kg/day once daily; adjust dose according to hematologic response

Renal Impairment:

Sickle cell anemia: Cl$_{cr}$ <60 mL/minute or ESRD: Reduce initial dose to 7.5 mg/kg; titrate to response/avoidance of toxicity (refer to usual dosing).

Other indications:

Cl$_{cr}$ 10-50 mL/minute: Administer 50% of normal dose.

Cl$_{cr}$ <10 mL/minute: Administer 20% of normal dose.

Hemodialysis effects: Supplemental dose is not necessary.

CAPD effects: Unknown

CAVH effects: Dose for GFR 10-50 mL/minute.

Available Dosage Forms

Capsule: 500 mg

Droxia™: 200 mg, 300 mg, 400 mg

Hydrea®: 500 mg

Tablet (Mylocel™): 1000 mg

Monitoring and Teaching Issues

Physical Assessment: Use with caution in presence of renal impairment, radiation therapy, or bone marrow suppression (see Warnings/Precautions for use cautions). Assess potential for interactions with other pharmacological agents patient may be taking (eg, potential for increased neurotoxicity or hepatotoxicity; see Drug Interactions for specifics). Hydroxyurea therapy requires close supervision to assess results of laboratory tests, therapeutic effectiveness, and adverse response (see Adverse Reactions). Teach proper use and need for frequent monitoring, possible side effects/appropriate interventions, and adverse symptoms to report (see Patient Education).

Monitoring Laboratory Tests: CBC with differential, platelets, renal and liver function, serum uric acid

Sickle cell disease: Monitor for toxicity every 2 weeks. If toxicity occurs, stop treatment until the bone marrow recovers; restart at 2.5 mg/kg/day less than the dose at which toxicity occurs. If no toxicity occurs over the next 12 weeks, then the subsequent dose should be increased by 2.5 mg/kg/day. Reduced dosage of hydroxyurea alternating with erythropoietin may decrease myelotoxicity and increase levels of fetal hemoglobin in patients who have not been helped by hydroxyurea alone.

Acceptable range: Neutrophils $\geq$2500 cells/mm^3, platelets $\geq$95,000/mm^3, hemoglobin >5.3 g/dL, and reticulocytes $\geq$95,000/mm^3 if the hemoglobin concentration is <9 g/dL

Toxic range: Neutrophils <2000 cells/mm^3, platelets <80,000/mm^3, hemoglobin <4.5 g/dL, and reticulocytes <80,000/mm^3 if the hemoglobin concentration is <9 g/dL

Patient Education: Do not take any new medication during therapy unless approved by prescriber. Take capsules exactly as directed by prescriber (dosage and timing will be specific to purpose of therapy). Contents of capsule may be emptied into a glass of water and taken immediately. You will require frequent monitoring and blood tests while taking this medication to assess effectiveness and monitor adverse reactions. You will be susceptible to infection (avoid crowds and exposure to infection and do not have any vaccinations without consulting prescriber). May cause nausea, vomiting, or loss of appetite (small frequent meals, frequent mouth care, sucking lozenges, or chewing gum may help); constipation (increased exercise, fluid, fruit, or fiber may help); diarrhea (buttermilk, boiled milk, or yogurt may help); or mouth sores (frequent mouth care will help). Report persistent vomiting, diarrhea, constipation, stomach pain, or mouth sores; skin rash, redness, irritation, or sores; painful or difficult urination; CNS changes (increased confusion, depression, hallucinations, lethargy, or seizures); opportunistic infection (persistent fever or chills, unusual fatigue, white plaques in mouth, vaginal discharge, or unhealed sores); unusual lassitude, weakness, or muscle tremors; easy bruising/bleeding; or blood in vomitus, stool, or urine. Note: People not taking hydroxyurea should not be exposed to it. If powder from capsule is spilled, wipe up with damp, disposable towel immediately, and discard the towel in a closed container, such as a plastic bag. Wash hands thoroughly. **Pregnancy/breast-feeding precautions:** Do not get pregnant while taking this medication. Consult prescriber for appropriate contraceptive measures. Do not breast-feed.

Geriatric Considerations: Elderly may be more sensitive to the effects of this drug. Advance dose slowly and adjust dose for renal function with careful monitoring.

Pregnancy Risk Factor: D

Pregnancy Issues: Hydroxyurea is teratogenic and fetotoxic in animals; data on use during human pregnancy is limited. Effective contraception is recommended in women of child-bearing potential.

Lactation: Enters breast milk/contraindicated

Administration

Oral: Capsules may be opened and emptied into water (will not dissolve completely).

Storage: Store capsules at room temperature. Capsules may be opened and emptied into water (will not dissolve completely).

Additional Information Although I.V. use is reported, no parenteral product is commercially available in the U.S.

If WBC decreases to <2500/mm^3 or platelet count to <100,000/mm^3, interrupt therapy until values rise significantly toward normal. Treat anemia with whole blood replacement; do not interrupt therapy. Adequate trial period to determine effectiveness is 6 weeks. Almost all patients receiving hydroxyurea in clinical trials needed to have their medication stopped for a time to allow their low blood count to return to acceptable levels.

HydrOXYzine (hye DROKS i zeen)

U.S. Brand Names Atarax®; Vistaril®

Synonyms Hydroxyzine Hydrochloride; Hydroxyzine Pamoate

Generic Available Yes

Pharmacologic Category Antiemetic; Antihistamine

Medication Safety Issues

Sound-alike/look-alike issues:

HydrOXYzine may be confused with hydrALAZINE, hydroxyurea

Atarax® may be confused with amoxicillin, Ativan®

Vistaril® may be confused with Restoril®, Versed, Zestril®

Use Treatment of anxiety; preoperative sedative; antipruritic

Unlabeled/Investigational Use Antiemetic; ethanol withdrawal symptoms

Mechanism of Action/Effect Competes with histamine for H$_1$-receptor sites on effector cells in the gastrointestinal tract, blood vessels, and respiratory tract. Possesses skeletal muscle relaxing, bronchodilator, antihistamine, antiemetic, and analgesic properties.

Contraindications Hypersensitivity to hydroxyzine or any component of the formulation; early pregnancy

Warnings/Precautions Causes sedation, caution must be used in performing tasks which require alertness (eg, operating machinery or driving). Sedative effects of CNS depressants or ethanol are potentiated. SubQ, intra-arterial, and I.V. administration are not recommended since thrombosis and digital gangrene can occur; extravasation can result in sterile abscess and marked tissue induration; should be used with caution in patients with narrow-angle glaucoma, prostatic hyperplasia, and bladder neck obstruction; should also be used with caution in patients with asthma or COPD. Not recommended for use as a sedative or anxiolytic in the elderly.

Drug Interactions

Cytochrome P450 Effect: Inhibits CYP2D6 (weak)

Increased Effect/Toxicity: CNS depressants, anticholinergics, used in combination with hydroxyzine may result in additive effects.

Nutritional/Ethanol Interactions

Ethanol: Avoid ethanol (may increase CNS depression).

Herb/Nutraceutical: Avoid valerian, St John's wort, kava kava, gotu kola (may increase CNS depression).

Adverse Reactions Frequency not defined.

Central nervous system: Drowsiness, headache, fatigue, nervousness, dizziness, hallucination

Dermatologic: Pruritus, rash, urticaria

Gastrointestinal: Xerostomia

Neuromuscular & skeletal: Tremor, paresthesia, seizure, involuntary movements

Ocular: Blurred vision

Respiratory: Thickening of bronchial secretions

Miscellaneous: Allergic reaction

Overdosage/Toxicology Symptoms of overdose include seizures, sedation, and hypotension. There is no specific treatment for antihistamine overdose. Clinical toxicity is due to (Continued)

HydrOXYzine *(Continued)*

blockade of cholinergic receptors. For anticholinergic overdose with severe life-threatening symptoms, physostigmine 1-2 mg I.V. slowly, may be given to reverse these effects.

Pharmacodynamics/Kinetics
Onset of Action: 15-30 minutes
Duration of Action: 4-6 hours
Absorption: Oral: Rapid
Time to Peak: ~2 hours
Half-Life Elimination: 3-7 hours
Metabolism: Exact fate unknown

Dosing
Adults:
Antiemetic: I.M.: 25-100 mg/dose every 4-6 hours as needed
Anxiety: Oral: 25-100 mg 4 times/day; maximum: 600 mg/day
Preoperative sedation:
Oral: 50-100 mg
I.M.: 25-100 mg
Management of pruritus: Oral: 25 mg 3-4 times/day
Elderly: Management of pruritus: 10 mg 3-4 times/day; increase to 25 mg 3-4 times/day if necessary.
Pediatrics:
Preoperative sedation:
Oral: 0.6 mg/kg/dose every 6 hours
I.M.: 0.5-1.1 mg/kg/dose every 4-6 hours as needed
Pruritus, anxiety: Manufacturer labeling:
<6 years: 50 mg daily in divided doses
≥6 years: 50-100 mg daily in divided doses
Hepatic Impairment: Change dosing interval to every 24 hours in patients with primary biliary cirrhosis.

Available Dosage Forms [DSC] = Discontinued product
Capsule, as pamoate (Vistaril®): 25 mg, 50 mg, 100 mg
Injection, solution, as hydrochloride: 25 mg/mL (1 mL); 50 mg/mL (1 mL, 2 mL, 10 mL)
Suspension, oral, as pamoate (Vistaril®): 25 mg/5 mL (120 mL, 480 mL) [lemon flavor]
Syrup, as hydrochloride: 10 mg/5 mL (120 mL, 480 mL)
Atarax®: 10 mg/5 mL (480 mL) [contains alcohol, sodium benzoate; mint flavor] [DSC]
Tablet, as hydrochloride: 10 mg, 25 mg, 50 mg
Atarax®: 10 mg, 25 mg, 50 mg, 100 mg [DSC]

Monitoring and Teaching Issues
Physical Assessment: Assess other medications patient may be taking for effectiveness and possible interactions. **Systemic:** Monitor therapeutic effectiveness and adverse reactions; ensure patient safety (institute safety precautions), have patient void prior to administration; and ensure adequate hydration and environmental temperature control. **Oral:** Monitor therapeutic effectiveness according to purpose for use, adverse reactions. Assess knowledge/teach patient appropriate use, interventions to reduce side effects, and adverse symptoms to report.

Patient Education: Will cause drowsiness. While using this medication, do not use alcohol and other prescription or OTC medications (especially sedatives, tranquilizers, antihistamines, or pain medications) without consulting prescriber. Use caution when driving or engaging in activities requiring alertness until response to drug is known. **Pregnancy/breast-feeding precautions:** Inform prescriber if you are or intend to become pregnant. Breast-feeding is contraindicated.

Geriatric Considerations: Anticholinergic effects are not well tolerated in the elderly. Hydroxyzine may be useful as a short-term antipruritic, but it is not recommended for use as a sedative or anxiolytic in the elderly.

Pregnancy Risk Factor: C

Pregnancy Issues: Hydroxyzine-induced fetal abnormalities at high dosages in animal studies. Use in early pregnancy is contraindicated by the manufacturer.

Lactation: Enters breast milk/contraindicated

Administration
I.M.: Administer deep in large muscle.
I.V.: Irritant. Use caution when administering I.V.
Compatibility:
Y-site administration: Incompatible with allopurinol, amifostine, amphotericin B cholesteryl sulfate complex, cefepime, doxorubicin liposome, fluconazole, fludarabine, paclitaxel, piperacillin/tazobactam, sargramostim
Compatibility in syringe: Incompatible with dimenhydrinate, haloperidol, ketorolac, pentobarbital, ranitidine
Compatibility when admixed: Incompatible with aminophylline, amobarbital, chloramphenicol, penicillin G potassium, penicillin G sodium, pentobarbital, phenobarbital
Storage: Protect from light. Store at 15°C to 30°C and protected from freezing.

Additional Information
Hydroxyzine hydrochloride: Atarax®, Vistaril® injection
Hydroxyzine pamoate: Vistaril® capsule and suspension

Related Information
Anxiolytic / Hypnotic Use in Long-Term Care Facilities *on page 1769*
Compatibility of Drugs *on page 1723*
Compatibility of Drugs in Syringe *on page 1725*
FDA Name Differentiation Project: The Use of Tall-Man Letters *on page 15*
Federal OBRA Regulations: Recommended Maximum Doses *on page 1773*

♦ **Hydroxyzine Hydrochloride** *see* HydrOXYzine *on page 773*
♦ **Hydroxyzine Pamoate** *see* HydrOXYzine *on page 773*
♦ **HydroZone Plus [OTC]** *see* Hydrocortisone *on page 760*

♦ **Hygroton** *see Chlorthalidone on page 314*
♦ **Hyoscine Butylbromide** *see Scopolamine Derivatives on page 1360*
♦ **Hyoscine Hydrobromide** *see Scopolamine Derivatives on page 1360*

Hyoscamine (hye oh SYE a meen)

U.S. Brand Names Anaspaz®; Cystospaz®; Cystospaz-M® [DSC]; Hyosine; Levbid®; Levsin®; Levsinex®; Levsin/SL®; NuLev™; Spacol [DSC]; Spacol T/S [DSC]; Symax SL; Symax SR

Synonyms Hyoscyamine Sulfate; *l*-Hyoscyamine Sulfate

Generic Available Yes

Pharmacologic Category Anticholinergic Agent

Medication Safety Issues
Sound-alike/look-alike issues:
Anaspaz® may be confused with Anaprox®, Antispas®
Levbid® may be confused with Lithobid®, Lopid®, Lorabid®
Levsinex® may be confused with Lanoxin®

Use
Oral: Adjunctive therapy for peptic ulcers, irritable bowel, neurogenic bladder/bowel; treatment of infant colic, GI tract disorders caused by spasm; to reduce rigidity, tremors, sialorrhea, and hyperhidrosis associated with parkinsonism; as a drying agent in acute rhinitis

Injection: Preoperative antimuscarinic to reduce secretions and block cardiac vagal inhibitory reflexes; to improve radiologic visibility of the kidneys; symptomatic relief of biliary and renal colic; reduce GI motility to facilitate diagnostic procedures (ie, endoscopy, hypotonic duodenography); reduce pain and hypersecretion in pancreatitis, certain cases of partial heart block associated with vagal activity; reversal of neuromuscular blockade

Mechanism of Action/Effect Blocks the action of acetylcholine at parasympathetic sites in smooth muscle, secretory glands, and the CNS; increases cardiac output, dries secretions, antagonizes histamine and serotonin

Contraindications Hypersensitivity to belladonna alkaloids or any component of the formulation; glaucoma; obstructive uropathy; myasthenia gravis; obstructive GI tract disease, paralytic ileus, intestinal atony of elderly or debilitated patients; severe ulcerative colitis, toxic megacolon complicating ulcerative colitis; unstable cardiovascular status in acute hemorrhage, myocardial ischemia

Warnings/Precautions Heat prostration may occur in hot weather. Diarrhea may be a sign of incomplete intestinal obstruction, treatment should be discontinued if this occurs. May produce side effects as seen with other anticholinergic medications including drowsiness, dizziness, blurred vision, or psychosis. Children and the elderly may be more susceptible to these effects. Use with caution in children with spastic paralysis. Use with caution in patients with autonomic neuropathy, coronary heart disease, CHF, cardiac arrhythmias, prostatic hyperplasia, hyperthyroidism, hypertension, chronic lung disease, renal disease, and hiatal hernia associated with reflux esophagitis. Use with caution in the elderly, may precipitate undiagnosed glaucoma and/or severely impair memory function (especially in those patients with previous memory problems). NuLev™ contains phenylalanine.

Drug Interactions
Decreased Effect: Decreased effect with antacids.
Increased Effect/Toxicity: Increased toxicity with amantadine, antihistamines, antimuscarinics, haloperidol, phenothiazines, tricyclic antidepressants, and MAO inhibitors.

Adverse Reactions Frequency not defined.
Cardiovascular: Palpitations, tachycardia
Central nervous system: Ataxia, dizziness, drowsiness, headache, insomnia, mental confusion/excitement, nervousness, speech disorder
Dermatologic: Urticaria
Endocrine & metabolic: Lactation suppression
Gastrointestinal: Bloating, constipation, dry mouth, loss of taste, nausea, vomiting
Genitourinary: Impotence, urinary hesitancy, urinary retention
Neuromuscular & skeletal: Weakness
Ocular: Blurred vision, cycloplegia, increased ocular tension, mydriasis
Miscellaneous: Allergic reactions, sweating decreased

Overdosage/Toxicology Symptoms of overdose include dilated, unreactive pupils; blurred vision; hot, dry flushed skin; CNS stimulation; dryness of mucous membranes; difficulty swallowing; foul breath; diminished or absent bowel sounds; urinary retention; tachycardia; hyperthermia; hypertension; and increased respiratory rate. For anticholinergic overdose with severe life-threatening symptoms, physostigmine 0.5-2 mg SubQ or I.V. slowly, may be given to reverse these effects; may repeat as necessary to reverse the effects, up to total of 5 mg. Hyoscyamine sulfate is dialyzable.

Pharmacodynamics/Kinetics
Onset of Action: 2-3 minutes
Duration of Action: 4-6 hours
Absorption: Well absorbed
Protein Binding: 50%
Half-Life Elimination: 3-5 hours
Metabolism: Hepatic
Excretion: Urine

Dosing
Adults & Elderly:
Gastrointestinal spasms:
Oral or S.L.: 0.125-0.25 mg every 4 hours or as needed (before meals or food); maximum: 1.5 mg/24 hours
Product-specific dosing: Cystospaz®: 0.15-0.3 mg up to 4 times/day
Oral, timed release: 0.375-0.75 mg every 12 hours; maximum: 1.5 mg/24 hours
I.M., I.V., SubQ: 0.25-0.5 mg; may repeat as needed up to 4 times/day, at 4-hour intervals
Diagnostic procedures: I.V.: 0.25-0.5 mg given 5-10 minutes prior to procedure
(Continued)

Hyoscyamine *(Continued)*

Preanesthesia: I.V.: 5 mcg/kg given 30-60 minutes prior to induction of anesthesia or at the time preoperative narcotics or sedatives are administered

To reduce drug-induced bradycardia during surgery: I.V.: 0.125 mg; repeat as needed

Reverse neuromuscular blockade: I.V.: 0.2 mg for every 1 mg neostigmine (or the physostigmine/pyridostigmine equivalent)

Pediatrics:

Gastrointestinal disorders:

Children <2 years: Oral: Dose as listed, based on age and weight (kg) using the 0.125 mg/mL drops. Repeat dose every 4 hours as needed:

3.4 kg: 4 drops; maximum: 24 drops/24 hours

5 kg: 5 drops; maximum: 30 drops/24 hours

7 kg: 6 drops; maximum: 36 drops/24 hours

10 kg: 8 drops; maximum: 48 drops/24 hours

Children 2-12 years: Oral or S.L.: Dose as listed, based on age and weight (kg); repeat dose every 4 hours as needed:

10 kg: 0.031-0.033 mg; maximum: 0.75 mg/24 hours

20 kg: 0.0625 mg; maximum: 0.75 mg/24 hours

40 kg: 0.0938 mg; maximum: 0.75 mg/24 hours

50 kg: 0.125 mg; maximum: 0.75 mg/24 hours

Preanesthesia: Children >2 years: I.V.: Refer to adult dosing.

Available Dosage Forms [DSC] = Discontinued product

Capsule, timed release, as sulfate (Cystospaz-M® [DSC], Levsinex®): 0.375 mg

Elixir, as sulfate: 0.125 mg/5 mL (480 mL)

Hyosine: 0.125 mg/5 mL (480 mL) [contains alcohol 20% and sodium benzoate; orange flavor]

Levsin®: 0.125 mg/5 mL (480 mL) [contains alcohol 20%; orange flavor]

Injection, solution, as sulfate (Levsin®): 0.5 mg/mL (1 mL)

Liquid, as sulfate (Spacol [DSC]): 0.125 mg/5 mL (120 mL) [sugar free, alcohol free, simethicone based, bubble gum flavor]

Solution, oral drops, as sulfate: 0.125 mg/mL (15 mL)

Hyosine: 0.125 mg/mL (15 mL) [contains alcohol 5% and sodium benzoate; orange flavor]

Levsin®: 0.125 mg/mL (15 mL) [contains alcohol 5%; orange flavor]

Tablet (Cystospaz®): 0.15 mg

Tablet, as sulfate (Anaspaz®, Levsin®, Spacol [DSC]): 0.125 mg

Tablet, extended release, as sulfate (Levbid®, Symax SR, Spacol T/S [DSC]): 0.375 mg

Tablet, orally-disintegrating, as sulfate (NuLev™): 0.125 mg [contains phenylalanine 1.7 mg/tablet, mint flavor]

Tablet, sublingual, as sulfate: 0.125 mg

Levsin/SL®: 0.125 mg [peppermint flavor]

Symax SL: 0.125 mg

Monitoring and Teaching Issues

Physical Assessment: Assess potential for interactions with other prescriptions, OTC medications, or herbal products patient may be taking (eg, anything that may add to anticholinergic effects). **I.V./I.M.:** Have patient void before administration. Assess therapeutic effectiveness and adverse response (eg, excessive dryness of eyes, nose, mouth, or throat). Teach patient proper use (according to formulations prescribed), possible side effects/appropriate interventions, and adverse symptoms to report.

Patient Education: Do not take any new medication during therapy unless approved by prescriber. Take as directed before meals; do not increase dose and do not discontinue without consulting prescriber. Void immediately before taking medication. Do not crush or chew (swallow whole) extended release form. Levbid® and Levsinex® may not completely disintegrate and may be excreted. You may experience dizziness or blurred vision (use caution when driving or engaging in tasks that require alertness until response to drug is known); dry mouth (sucking on lozenges may help); photosensitivity (wear dark glasses in bright sunlight); decreased ability to sweat (use caution in hot weather or hot rooms or when engaging in strenuous activity); or impotence (temporary). Report excessive and persistent anticholinergic effects (blurred vision, headache, flushing, tachycardia, nervousness, constipation, dizziness, insomnia, mental confusion or excitement, dry mouth, altered taste perception, dysphagia, palpitations, bradycardia, urinary hesitancy or retention, impotence, decreased sweating). **Pregnancy/breast-feeding precautions:** Inform prescriber if you are or intend to become pregnant. Breast-feeding is not recommended.

Sublingual tablets: Place tablet under tongue and allow to dissolve.

Orally-disintegrating tablet: Place tablet on tongue and allow to disintegrate before swallowing. Take with or without food.

Dietary Considerations: Should be taken before meals or food; NuLev™ contains phenylalanine

Geriatric Considerations: Avoid long-term use. The potential for toxic reactions is higher than the potential benefit, elderly are particularly prone to CNS side effects of anticholinergics (eg, confusion, delirium, hallucinations). Side effects often occur before clinical response is obtained. Generally not recommended because of the side effects.

Pregnancy Risk Factor: C

Lactation: Enters breast milk/not recommended

Breast-Feeding Issues: Excreted in breast milk in trace amounts. May also suppress lactation. Breast-feeding is not recommended.

Administration

Oral: Oral: Tablets should be administered before meals or food.

Levbid®: Tablets are scored and may be broken in half for dose titration; do not crush or chew.

Levsin/SL®: Tablets may be used sublingually, chewed, or swallowed whole.

NuLev™: Tablet is placed on tongue and allowed to disintegrate before swallowing; may take with or without water.

Symax SL: Tablets may be used sublingually or swallowed whole.

I.M.: May be administered without dilution.

I.V.: Inject over at least 1 minute. May be administered without dilution.

Storage: Store at controlled room temperature. Protect NuLev™ from moisture.

Hyoscyamine, Atropine, Scopolamine, and Phenobarbital

(hye oh SYE a meen, A troe peen, skoe POL a meen, & fee noe BAR bi tal)

U.S. Brand Names Donnatal®; Donnatal Extentabs®

Synonyms Atropine, Hyoscyamine, Scopolamine, and Phenobarbital; Belladonna Alkaloids With Phenobarbital; Phenobarbital, Hyoscyamine, Atropine, and Scopolamine; Scopolamine, Hyoscyamine, Atropine, and Phenobarbital

Generic Available Yes: Elixir, tablet

Pharmacologic Category Anticholinergic Agent; Antispasmodic Agent, Gastrointestinal

Medication Safety Issues

Sound-alike/look-alike issues:

Donnatal® may be confused with Donnagel®

Use Adjunct in treatment of irritable bowel syndrome, acute enterocolitis, duodenal ulcer

Dosing

Adults & Elderly: Spasmolytic: Oral:

Donnatal®: 1-2 tablets or 5-10 mL of elixir 3-4 times/day

Donnatal Extentabs®: 1 tablet every 12 hours; may increase to 1 tablet every 8 hours if needed

Pediatrics: Oral: Donnatal® elixir: To be given every 4-6 hours; initial dose based on weight:

4.5 kg: 0.5 mL every 4 hours **or** 0.75 mL every 6 hours

10 kg: 1 mL every 4 hours **or** 1.5 mL every 6 hours

14 kg: 1.5 mL every 4 hours **or** 2 mL every 6 hours

23 kg: 2.5 mL every 4 hours **or** 3.8 mL every 6 hours

34 kg: 3.8 mL every 4 hours **or** 5 mL every 6 hours

≥45 kg: 5 mL every 4 hours **or** 7.5 mL every 6 hours

Available Dosage Forms

Elixir (Donnatal®): Hyoscyamine sulfate 0.1037 mg, atropine sulfate 0.0194 mg, scopolamine hydrobromide 0.0065 mg, and phenobarbital 16.2 mg per 5 mL (120 mL, 480 mL) [contains alcohol 23%; citrus flavor]

Tablet (Donnatal®): Hyoscyamine sulfate 0.1037 mg, atropine sulfate 0.0194 mg, scopolamine hydrobromide 0.0065 mg, and phenobarbital 16.2 mg

Tablet, extended release (Donnatal Extentabs®): Hyoscyamine sulfate 0.3111 mg, atropine sulfate 0.0582 mg, scopolamine hydrobromide 0.0195 mg, and phenobarbital 48.6 mg

Monitoring and Teaching Issues

Physical Assessment: See individual agents.

Patient Education: See individual agents. **Pregnancy/breast-feeding precautions:** Inform prescriber if you are or intend to become pregnant. Consult prescriber if breast-feeding.

Pregnancy Risk Factor: C

Lactation: Excretion in breast milk unknown/use caution

Related Information

Atropine *on page 158*

Hyoscyamine *on page 775*

Phenobarbital *on page 1196*

Scopolamine Derivatives *on page 1360*

♦ **Hyoscyamine Sulfate** *see* Hyoscyamine *on page 775*

♦ **Hyosine** *see* Hyoscyamine *on page 775*

♦ **Hyperlipidemia Management** *see page 1836*

♦ **Hypertension** *see page 1841*

♦ **Hyphed** *see* Pseudoephedrine, Hydrocodone, and Chlorpheniramine *on page 1283*

♦ **Hytone®** *see* Hydrocortisone *on page 760*

♦ **Hytrin®** *see* Terazosin *on page 1442*

♦ **Hyzaar®** *see* Losartan and Hydrochlorothiazide *on page 924*

♦ **131 I Anti-B1 Antibody** *see* Tositumomab and Iodine I 131 Tositumomab *on page 1501*

♦ **131 I-Anti-B1 Monoclonal Antibody** *see* Tositumomab and Iodine I 131 Tositumomab *on page 1501*

♦ **Ibidomide Hydrochloride** *see* Labetalol *on page 857*

♦ **Ibu-200 [OTC]** *see* Ibuprofen *on page 777*

Ibuprofen (eye byoo PROE fen)

U.S. Brand Names Advil® [OTC]; Advil® Children's [OTC]; Advil® Infants' [OTC]; Advil® Junior [OTC]; Advil® Migraine [OTC]; Genpril® [OTC]; Haltran® [OTC] [DSC]; Ibu-200 [OTC]; I-Prin [OTC]; Menadol® [OTC]; Midol® Maximum Strength Cramp Formula [OTC]; Motrin®; Motrin® Children's [OTC]; Motrin® IB [OTC]; Motrin® Infants' [OTC]; Motrin® Junior Strength [OTC]; Motrin® Migraine Pain [OTC]; Proprinal [OTC]; Ultraprin [OTC]

Synonyms *p*-Isobutylhydratropic Acid

Generic Available Yes: Caplet, suspension, tablet

Pharmacologic Category Nonsteroidal Anti-inflammatory Drug (NSAID), Oral

Medication Safety Issues

Sound-alike/look-alike issues:

Haltran® may be confused with Halfprin®

Use Inflammatory diseases and rheumatoid disorders including juvenile rheumatoid arthritis, mild to moderate pain, fever, dysmenorrhea

Unlabeled/Investigational Use Cystic fibrosis, gout, ankylosing spondylitis, acute migraine headache

(Continued)

Ibuprofen *(Continued)*

Mechanism of Action/Effect Inhibits prostaglandin synthesis by decreasing the activity of the enzyme, cyclooxygenase, which results in decreased formation of prostaglandin precursors

Contraindications Hypersensitivity to ibuprofen, any component of the formulation, aspirin, or other NSAIDs; patients with "aspirin triad" (bronchial asthma, aspirin intolerance, rhinitis); pregnancy (3rd trimester)

Warnings/Precautions Fatal asthmatic and anaphylactoid reactions have occurred in patients with "aspirin triad." Use with caution in patients with CHF, hypertension, dehydration, decreased renal or hepatic function, history of GI disease (bleeding, ulcers, or previous GI symptoms with NSAID use), or those receiving anticoagulants and/or corticosteroids. Use lowest effective dose for shortest period possible; bleeding risk has been correlated to dose and duration of therapy. Gastrointestinal bleeding may occur without prior symptoms of gastrointestinal irritation. Elderly are at a high risk for adverse effects from NSAIDs. As many as 60% of elderly can develop peptic ulceration and/or hemorrhage asymptomatically.

Use of NSAIDs can compromise existing renal function especially when Cl_{cr} <30 mL/minute. CNS adverse effects such as confusion, agitation, and hallucination are generally seen in overdose or high-dose situations; however, elderly may demonstrate these adverse effects at lower doses than younger adults. Do not exceed 3200 mg/day. Withhold for at least 4-6 half-lives prior to surgical or dental procedures.

OTC labeling: Recommended dosages should not be exceeded, due to an increased risk of GI bleeding. Consuming ≥3 alcoholic beverages/day may increase the risk of GI bleeding. When used for self-medication, patients should be instructed to contact healthcare provider if used for fever lasting >3 days or for pain lasting >10 days in adults or >3 days in children. Do not use for >2 days or administer to children <3 years of age unless instructed by healthcare provider. Consult healthcare provider when sore throat pain is severe, persistent, or accompanied by fever, headache, nausea, and/or vomiting.

Drug Interactions

Cytochrome P450 Effect: Substrate (minor) of CYP2C8/9, 2C19; **Inhibits** CYP2C8/9 (strong)

Decreased Effect: Aspirin may decrease ibuprofen serum concentrations. Ibuprofen may decrease the effect of some antihypertensive agents (including ACE inhibitors and angiotensin antagonists) and diuretics.

Increased Effect/Toxicity: Ibuprofen may increase cyclosporine, digoxin, lithium, and methotrexate serum concentrations. The renal adverse effects of ACE inhibitors may be potentiated by NSAIDs. Corticosteroids may increase the risk of GI ulceration. Ibuprofen may increase the levels/effects of amiodarone, fluoxetine, glimepiride, glipizide, nateglinide, phenytoin, pioglitazone, rosiglitazone, sertraline, warfarin, and other CYP2C8/9 substrates.

Nutritional/Ethanol Interactions

Ethanol: Avoid ethanol (may enhance gastric mucosal irritation).

Food: Ibuprofen peak serum levels may be decreased if taken with food.

Herb/Nutraceutical: Avoid cat's claw, dong quai, evening primrose, feverfew, garlic, ginger, ginkgo, red clover, horse chestnut, green tea, ginseng (all have additional antiplatelet activity).

Lab Interactions Increased chloride (S), sodium (S), bleeding time

Adverse Reactions

1% to 10%:

Cardiovascular: Edema (1% to 3%)

Central nervous system: Dizziness (3% to 9%), headache (1% to 3%), nervousness (1% to 3%)

Dermatologic: Itching (1% to 3%), rash (3% to 9%)

Endocrine & metabolic: Fluid retention (1% to 3%)

Gastrointestinal: Dyspepsia (1% to 3%), vomiting (1% to 3%), abdominal pain/cramps/distress (1% to 3%), heartburn (3% to 9%), nausea (3% to 9%), diarrhea (1% to 3%), constipation (1% to 3%), flatulence (1% to 3%), epigastric pain (3% to 9%), appetite decreased (1% to 3%)

Otic: Tinnitus (3% to 9%)

Overdosage/Toxicology Symptoms of overdose include apnea, metabolic acidosis, coma, nystagmus, seizures, leukocytosis, and renal failure. Management of NSAID intoxication is supportive and symptomatic. Since many NSAIDs undergo enterohepatic cycling, multiple doses of charcoal may be needed to reduce the potential for delayed toxicities.

Pharmacodynamics/Kinetics

Onset of Action: Analgesic: 30-60 minutes; Anti-inflammatory: ≤7 days; Peak effect: 1-2 weeks

Duration of Action: 4-6 hours

Absorption: Oral: Rapid (85%)

Time to Peak: ~1-2 hours

Protein Binding: 90% to 99%

Half-Life Elimination: 2-4 hours; End-stage renal disease: Unchanged

Metabolism: Hepatic via oxidation

Excretion: Urine (1% as free drug); some feces

Dosing

Adults & Elderly:

Inflammatory disease: Oral: 400-800 mg/dose 3-4 times/day (maximum: 3.2 g/day)

Analgesia/pain/fever/dysmenorrhea: Oral: 200-400 mg/dose every 4-6 hours (maximum daily dose: 1.2 g, unless directed by physician)

OTC labeling (analgesic, antipyretic): Oral: 200 mg every 4-6 hours as needed (maximum: 1200 mg/24 hours)

Pediatrics:

Antipyretic: Oral: 6 months to 12 years: Temperature <102.5°F (39°C): 5 mg/kg/dose; temperature >102.5°F: 10 mg/kg/dose given every 6-8 hours; maximum daily dose: 40 mg/kg/day

Juvenile rheumatoid arthritis: Oral: 30-50 mg/kg/24 hours divided every 8 hours; start at lower end of dosing range and titrate upward (maximum: 2.4 g/day)

Analgesic: Oral: 4-10 mg/kg/dose every 6-8 hours

Cystic fibrosis (unlabeled use): Oral: Chronic (>4 years) twice daily dosing adjusted to maintain serum levels of 50-100 mcg/mL has been associated with slowing of disease progression in younger patients with mild lung disease

OTC labeling (analgesic, antipyretic): Oral:

Children 6 months to 11 years: See table; use of weight to select dose is preferred; doses may be repeated every 6-8 hours (maximum: 4 doses/day)

Children ≥12 years: Refer to adult dosing.

Ibuprofen Dosing

Weight (lb)	Age	Dosage (mg)
12-17	6-11 mo	50
18-23	12-23 mo	75
24-35	2-3 y	100
35-47	4-5 y	150
48-59	6-8 y	200
60-71	9-10 y	250
72-95	11 y	300

Hepatic Impairment: Avoid use in severe hepatic impairment.

Available Dosage Forms [DSC] = Discontinued product

Caplet: 200 mg [OTC]
Advil®: 200 mg [contains sodium benzoate]
Ibu-200, Menadol®, Motrin® IB, Motrin® Migraine Pain: 200 mg
Motrin® Junior Strength: 100 mg [contains tartrazine]

Capsule, liqui-gel:
Advil®: 200 mg
Advil® Migraine: 200 mg [solubilized ibuprofen]

Gelcap:
Advil®: 200 mg
Motrin® IB: 200 mg [contains benzyl alcohol]

Suspension, oral: 100 mg/5 mL (5 mL, 120 mL, 480 mL)
Advil® Children's: 100 mg/5 mL (60 mL, 120 mL) [contains sodium benzoate; blue raspberry, fruit, and grape flavors]
Motrin® Children's: 100 mg/5 mL (60 mL, 120 mL) [contains sodium benzoate; berry, dye free berry, bubble gum, and grape flavors]

Suspension, oral drops: 40 mg/mL (15 mL)
Advil® Infants': 40 mg/mL (15 mL) [contains sodium benzoate; fruit and grape flavors]
Motrin® Infants': 40 mg/mL (15 mL, 30 mL) [contains sodium benzoate; berry and dye-free berry flavors]

Tablet: 200 mg [OTC], 400 mg, 600 mg, 800 mg
Advil®: 200 mg [contains sodium benzoate]
Advil® Junior: 100 mg [contains sodium benzoate; coated tablets]
Genpril®, Haltran® [DSC], I-Prin, Midol® Maximum Strength Cramp Formula, Motrin® IB, Proprinal, Ultraprin: 200 mg
Motrin®: 400 mg, 600 mg, 800 mg

Tablet, chewable:
Advil® Children's: 50 mg [contains phenylalanine 2.1 mg; fruit and grape flavors]
Advil® Junior: 100 mg [contains phenylalanine 2.1 mg; fruit and grape flavors]
Motrin® Children's: 50 mg [contains phenylalanine 1.4 mg; orange flavor]
Motrin® Junior Strength: 100 mg [contains phenylalanine 2.1 mg; grape and orange flavors]

Monitoring and Teaching Issues

Physical Assessment: Assess patient for allergic reaction to salicylates or other NSAIDs. Assess other medications patient may be taking for additive or adverse interactions. Monitor therapeutic effectiveness and signs of adverse reactions or overdose at beginning of therapy and periodically during long-term therapy. With long-term therapy, periodic ophthalmic exams are recommended. Assess knowledge/teach patient appropriate use. Teach patient to monitor for adverse reactions, adverse reactions to report, and appropriate interventions to reduce side effects.

Monitoring Laboratory Tests: CBC, periodic liver function, renal function (serum BUN, creatinine)

Patient Education: If self-administered, use exactly as directed; do not increase dose or frequency. Adverse reactions can occur with overuse. Consult your prescriber before use if you have hypertension or heart failure. Do not take longer than 3 days for fever, or 10 days for pain without consulting medical advisor. Take with food or milk. While using this medication, do not use alcohol, excessive amounts of vitamin C, or salicylate containing foods (curry powder, prunes, raisins, tea, or licorice), other prescription or OTC medications containing aspirin or salicylate, or other NSAIDs without consulting prescriber. Maintain adequate hydration (2-3 L/day of fluids) unless instructed to restrict fluid intake. You may experience nausea, vomiting, gastric discomfort (frequent mouth care, small frequent meals, chewing gum, sucking lozenges may help). GI bleeding, ulceration, or perforation can occur with or without pain. Stop taking medication and report ringing in ears; persistent cramping or stomach pain; unresolved nausea or vomiting; respiratory difficulty or shortness of breath; unusual bruising or bleeding (mouth, urine, stool); skin rash; unusual

(Continued)

Ibuprofen *(Continued)*

swelling of extremities; chest pain; or palpitations. **Pregnancy/breast-feeding precautions:** Inform prescriber if you are or intend to become pregnant. This drug should not be used in the 3rd trimester of pregnancy. Consult prescriber if breast-feeding.

Dietary Considerations: Should be taken with food. Chewable tablets may contain phenylalanine; amount varies by product, consult manufacturers labeling.

Geriatric Considerations: Elderly are at a high risk for adverse effects from NSAIDs. As much as 60% of elderly can develop peptic ulceration and/or hemorrhage asymptomatically. The concomitant use of H_2 blockers, omeprazole, and sucralfate is not effective as prophylaxis with the exception of NSAID-induced duodenal ulcers which may be prevented by the use of ranitidine. Misoprostol is the only prophylactic agent proven effective. Also, concomitant disease and drug use contribute to the risk for GI adverse effects. Use lowest effective dose for shortest period possible. Consider renal function decline with age. Use of NSAIDs can compromise existing renal function especially when Cl_{cr} is ≤30 mL/minute. Tinnitus may be a difficult and unreliable indication of toxicity due to age-related hearing loss or eighth cranial nerve damage. CNS adverse effects such as confusion, agitation, and hallucination are generally seen in overdose or high-dose situations, but elderly may demonstrate these adverse effects at lower doses than younger adults.

Pregnancy Risk Factor: B/D (3rd trimester)

Lactation: Enters breast milk/use caution (AAP rates "compatible")

Breast-Feeding Issues: Limited data suggests minimal excretion in breast milk.

Administration

Oral: Administer with food.

Related Information

Nonsalicylate / Nonsteroidal Anti-inflammatory Agents *on page 1743*

- ◆ **Ibuprofen and Hydrocodone** *see* Hydrocodone and Ibuprofen *on page 758*
- ◆ **Ibuprofen and Oxycodone** *see* Oxycodone and Ibuprofen *on page 1140*

Ibutilide *(i BYOO ti lide)*

U.S. Brand Names Corvert®

Synonyms Ibutilide Fumarate

Generic Available No

Pharmacologic Category Antiarrhythmic Agent, Class III

Use Acute termination of atrial fibrillation or flutter of recent onset; the effectiveness of ibutilide has not been determined in patients with arrhythmias >90 days in duration

Mechanism of Action/Effect Exact mechanism of action is unknown; prolongs the action potential in cardiac tissue

Contraindications Hypersensitivity to ibutilide or any component of the formulation; QT_c >440 msec

Warnings/Precautions Potentially fatal arrhythmias (eg, polymorphic ventricular tachycardia) can occur with ibutilide, **usually** in association with torsade de pointes (QT prolongation). The drug should be given in a setting of continuous ECG monitoring and by personnel trained in treating arrhythmias particularly polymorphic ventricular tachycardia. Patients with chronic atrial fibrillation often revert after conversion; the risks of treatment may not be justified when compared to alternative management. Safety and efficacy in children have not been established. Use caution in elderly patients. Avoid concurrent use of any drug that can prolong QT interval. Correct hyperkalemia and hypomagnesemia before using. Monitor for heart block.

Drug Interactions

Increased Effect/Toxicity: Class Ia antiarrhythmic drugs (disopyramide, quinidine, and procainamide) and other class III drugs such as amiodarone and sotalol should not be given concomitantly with ibutilide due to their potential to prolong refractoriness. Signs of digoxin toxicity may be masked when coadministered with ibutilide. Toxicity of ibutilide is potentiated by concurrent administration of other drugs which may prolong QT interval: phenothiazines, tricyclic and tetracyclic antidepressants, cisapride, sparfloxacin, gatifloxacin, moxifloxacin, and erythromycin.

Adverse Reactions 1% to 10%:

Cardiovascular: Sustained polymorphic ventricular tachycardia (ie, torsade de pointes) (1.7%, often requiring cardioversion), nonsustained polymorphic ventricular tachycardia (2.7%), nonsustained monomorphic ventricular tachycardia (4.9%), ventricular extrasystoles (5.1%), nonsustained monomorphic VT (4.9%), tachycardia/supraventricular tachycardia (2.7%), hypotension (2%), bundle branch block (1.9%), AV block (1.5%), bradycardia (1.2%), QT segment prolongation, hypertension (1.2%), palpitation (1%)

Central nervous system: Headache (3.6%)

Gastrointestinal: Nausea (>1%)

Overdosage/Toxicology Symptoms of overdose include CNS depression, rapid gasping breathing, and convulsions. Arrhythmias occur. Treatment is supportive. Antiarrhythmics are generally avoided.

Pharmacodynamics/Kinetics

Onset of Action: ~90 minutes after start of infusion ($^1/_2$ of conversions to sinus rhythm occur during infusion)

Protein Binding: 40%

Half-Life Elimination: 2-12 hours (average: 6 hours)

Metabolism: Extensively hepatic; oxidation

Excretion: Urine (82%, 7% as unchanged drug and metabolites); feces (19%)

Dosing

Adults:

Atrial fibrillation/flutter: I.V.:

<60 kg: 0.01 mg/kg over 10 minutes

≥60 kg: 1 mg over 10 minutes

If the arrhythmia does not terminate within 10 minutes after the end of the initial infusion, a second infusion of equal strength may be infused over a 10-minute period.

Elderly: Refer to adult dosing. Dose selection should be cautious, usually starting at the lower end of the dosing range.

Available Dosage Forms Injection, solution, as fumarate: 0.1 mg/mL (10 mL)

Monitoring and Teaching Issues

Physical Assessment: Assess other medications patient may be taking for effectiveness and interactions. Requires infusion pump and continuous cardiac and hemodynamic monitoring during and for 4 hours following infusion. Assess results of laboratory tests, therapeutic effectiveness, and adverse reactions. Teach patient adverse symptoms to report.

Monitoring Laboratory Tests: Electrolytes

Patient Education: This drug is only given I.V. and you will be on continuous cardiac monitoring during and for several hours following administration. You may experience headache or irregular heartbeat during infusion. Report chest pain or respiratory difficulty immediately. **Pregnancy/breast-feeding precautions:** Inform prescriber if you are or intend to become pregnant. Do not breast-feed.

Pregnancy Risk Factor: C

Pregnancy Issues: Teratogenic and embryocidal in rats; avoid use in pregnancy.

Lactation: Enters breast milk/contraindicated

Administration

I.V.: May be administered undiluted or diluted in 50 mL diluent (0.9% NS or D_5W). Infuse over 10 minutes.

Reconstitution: May be administered undiluted or diluted in 50 mL diluent (0.9% NS or D_5W). Admixtures are chemically and physically stable for 24 hours at room temperature and for 48 hours at refrigerated temperatures.

Related Information

Antiarrhythmic Drugs *on page 1708*

♦ **Ibutilide Fumarate** *see* Ibutilide *on page 780*

♦ **ICI-182,780** *see* Fulvestrant *on page 687*

♦ **ICI-204,219** *see* Zafirlukast *on page 1577*

♦ **ICI-46474** *see* Tamoxifen *on page 1424*

♦ **ICI-118630** *see* Goserelin *on page 725*

♦ **ICI-176334** *see* Bicalutamide *on page 195*

♦ **ICI-D1033** *see* Anastrozole *on page 121*

♦ **ICRF-187** *see* Dexrazoxane *on page 432*

♦ **Idamycin PFS®** *see* Idarubicin *on page 781*

Idarubicin *(eye da ROO bi sin)*

U.S. Brand Names Idamycin PFS®

Synonyms 4-Demethoxydaunorubicin; 4-DMDR; Idarubicin Hydrochloride; IDR; IMI 30; NSC-256439; SC 33428

Generic Available Yes

Pharmacologic Category Antineoplastic Agent, Anthracycline; Antineoplastic Agent, Antibiotic

Medication Safety Issues

Sound-alike/look-alike issues:

Idarubicin may be confused with DOXOrubicin

Idamycin PFS® may be confused with Adriamycin

Use Treatment of acute leukemias (AML, ANLL, ALL), accelerated phase or blast crisis of chronic myelogenous leukemia (CML), breast cancer

Unlabeled/Investigational Use Autologous hematopoietic stem cell transplantation (in combination with busulfan)

Mechanism of Action/Effect Similar to daunorubicin, idarubicin exhibits inhibitory effects on DNA and RNA polymerase.

Contraindications Hypersensitivity to idarubicin, other anthracyclines, or any component of the formulation; bilirubin >5 mg/dL; pregnancy

Warnings/Precautions The U.S. Food and Drug Administration (FDA) currently recommends that procedures for proper handling and disposal of antineoplastic agents be considered. Can cause myocardial toxicity and is more common in patients who have previously received anthracyclines or have pre-existing cardiac disease; reduce dose in patients with impaired hepatic function.

Idarubicin preparation should be performed in a Class II laminar flow biologic safety cabinet. Personnel should be wearing surgical gloves and a closed front surgical gown with knit cuffs. Appropriate safety equipment is recommended for preparation, administration, and disposal of antineoplastics. If idarubicin contacts the skin, wash and flush thoroughly with water.

Drug Interactions

Decreased Effect: Patients may experience impaired immune response to vaccines; possible infection after administration of live vaccines in patients receiving immunosuppressants.

Adverse Reactions

>10%:

Cardiovascular: Transient ECG abnormalities (supraventricular tachycardia, S-T wave changes, atrial or ventricular extrasystoles); generally asymptomatic and self-limiting. CHF, dose related. The relative cardiotoxicity of idarubicin compared to doxorubicin is unclear. Some investigators report no increase in cardiac toxicity at cumulative oral idarubicin doses up to 540 mg/m²; other reports suggest a maximum cumulative intravenous dose of 150 mg/m².

Central nervous system: Headache

Dermatologic: Alopecia (25% to 30%), radiation recall, skin rash (11%), urticaria

Gastrointestinal: Nausea, vomiting (30% to 60%); diarrhea (9% to 22%); stomatitis (11%); GI hemorrhage (30%)

Genitourinary: Discoloration of urine (darker yellow)

(Continued)

Idarubicin *(Continued)*

Hematologic: Myelosuppression, primarily leukopenia; thrombocytopenia and anemia. Effects are generally less severe with oral dosing.

Nadir: 10-15 days

Recovery: 21-28 days

Hepatic: Bilirubin and transaminases increased (44%)

1% to 10%:

Central nervous system: Seizures

Neuromuscular & skeletal: Peripheral neuropathy

Overdosage/Toxicology Symptoms of overdose include severe myelosuppression and increased GI toxicity. Treatment is supportive. It is unlikely that therapeutic efficacy or toxicity would be altered by conventional peritoneal or hemodialysis.

Pharmacodynamics/Kinetics

Absorption: Oral: Variable (4% to 77%; mean: ~30%)

Time to Peak: Serum: 1-5 hours

Protein Binding: 94% to 97%

Half-Life Elimination: Oral: 14-35 hours; I.V.: 12-27 hours

Metabolism: Hepatic to idarubicinol (pharmacologically active)

Excretion:

Oral: Urine (~5% of dose; 0.5% to 0.7% as unchanged drug, 4% as idarubicinol); hepatic (8%)

I.V.: Urine (13% as idarubicinol, 3% as unchanged drug); hepatic (17%)

Dosing

Adults & Elderly: Refer to individual protocols.

Leukemia: I.V.:

Induction: 12 mg/m^2/day for 3 days

Consolidation: 10-12 mg/m^2/day for 2 days

Stem cell transplantation (unlabeled use): 20 mg/m^2/24 hours continuous I.V. infusion (with high-dose oral busulfan)

Pediatrics:

Leukemia: I.V.: 10-12 mg/m^2 once daily for 3 days every 3 weeks.

Solid tumors: I.V.: 5 mg/m^2 once daily for 3 days every 3 weeks.

Renal Impairment: Dose reduction is recommended.

Serum creatinine ≥2 mg/dL: Reduce dose by 25%.

Hepatic Impairment:

Bilirubin 1.5-5 mg/dL or AST 60-180 units: Reduce dose 50%.

Bilirubin >5 mg/dL or AST >180 units: Do not administer.

Available Dosage Forms Injection, solution, as hydrochloride [preservative free] (Idamycin PFS®): 1 mg/mL (5 mL, 10 mL, 20 mL)

Monitoring and Teaching Issues

Physical Assessment: See Warnings/Precautions for use cautions. See Administration for specific infusion directions. Infusion site must be closely monitored; extravasation can cause severe cellulitis or tissue necrosis (eg, do not apply heat). Assess results of laboratory tests prior to each infusion and on a regular basis throughout therapy. Monitor therapeutic effectiveness (symptom relief) and adverse response frequently for full course of therapy (eg, cardiac toxicity, myelosuppression, peripheral neuropathy; see Adverse Reactions). Teach patient possible side effects/appropriate interventions and adverse symptoms to report (see Patient Education).

Monitoring Laboratory Tests: CBC with differential, platelet count, cardiac function, serum electrolytes, creatinine, uric acid, ALT, AST, bilirubin

Patient Education: Do not take any new medication during therapy unless approved by prescriber. This medication is only administered by intravenous infusion; report immediately any swelling, pain, burning, redness at infusion site or sudden onset of chest pain, breathing or swallowing difficulty or chills. It is important to maintain adequate hydration (2-3 L/day of fluids) unless instructed to restrict fluid intake and nutrition (small frequent meals). You will be more susceptible to infection (avoid crowds and exposure to infection and do not have any vaccinations without consulting prescriber). You may experience nausea or vomiting (small frequent meals, frequent mouth care, sucking lozenges, or chewing gum may help); diarrhea (buttermilk, boiled milk, or yogurt may help); or loss of hair (reversible). Urine may turn darker (normal). Report immediately chest pain, swelling of extremities, respiratory difficulty, palpitations, or rapid heartbeat. Report unresolved nausea, vomiting, or diarrhea; alterations in urinary pattern (increased or decreased); opportunistic infection (eg, fever, chills, unusual bruising or bleeding, signs of infection fatigue, purulent vaginal discharge, unhealed mouth sores); abdominal pain or blood in stools; excessive fatigue; yellowing of eyes or skin; swelling of extremities; respiratory difficulty; or unresolved diarrhea. **Pregnancy/breast-feeding precautions:** Do not get pregnant while taking this medication. Consult prescriber for appropriate contraceptive measures. Consult prescriber if breast-feeding.

Geriatric Considerations: During induction therapy, patients >60 years of age experience CHF, arrhythmias, MI, and decline in LVEF more frequently than younger populations.

Pregnancy Risk Factor: D

Lactation: Excretion in breast milk unknown

Administration

I.V.: Do not administer I.M. or SubQ; administer as slow push over 3-5 minutes, preferably into the side of a freely-running saline or dextrose infusion **or** as intermittent infusion over 10-15 minutes into a free-flowing I.V. solution of NS or D$_5$W; also occasionally administered as a bladder lavage.

Compatibility: Stable in D$_5$NS, D$_5$W, LR, NS, SWFI; **incompatible** with bacteriostatic water

Y-site administration: **Incompatible** with acyclovir, allopurinol, ampicillin/sulbactam, cefazolin, cefepime, ceftazidime, clindamycin, dexamethasone sodium phosphate, etoposide, fluorouracil, furosemide, gentamicin, heparin, hydrocortisone sodium succinate, lorazepam, meperidine, methotrexate, piperacillin/tazobactam, sodium bicarbonate, teniposide, vancomycin, vincristine

Compatibility when admixed: Incompatible with heparin

Storage: Store intact vials of solution under refrigeration (2°C to 8°C/36°F to 46°F). Protect from light. Solutions diluted in D_5W or NS for infusion are stable for 4 weeks at room temperature, protected from light. Syringe and IVPB solutions are stable for 72 hours at room temperature and 7 days under refrigeration.

♦ **Idarubicin Hydrochloride** *see* Idarubicin *on page 781*
♦ **IDEC-C2B8** *see* Rituximab *on page 1338*
♦ **IDR** *see* Idarubicin *on page 781*
♦ **Ifex®** *see* Ifosfamide *on page 783*
♦ **IFLrA** *see* Interferon Alfa-2a *on page 809*

Ifosfamide (eye FOSS fa mide)

U.S. Brand Names Ifex®
Synonyms Isophosphamide; NSC-109724; Z4942
Generic Available Yes
Pharmacologic Category Antineoplastic Agent, Alkylating Agent; Antineoplastic Agent, Alkylating Agent (Nitrogen Mustard)
Use Treatment of lung cancer, Hodgkin's and non-Hodgkin's lymphoma, breast cancer, acute and chronic lymphocytic leukemias, ovarian cancer, sarcomas, pancreatic and gastric carcinomas

Orphan drug: Treatment of testicular cancer
Mechanism of Action/Effect Inhibits protein synthesis and DNA synthesis
Contraindications Hypersensitivity to ifosfamide or any component of the formulation; patients with severely depressed bone marrow function; pregnancy
Warnings/Precautions The U.S. Food and Drug Administration (FDA) currently recommends that procedures for proper handling and disposal of antineoplastic agents be considered. Used in combination with mesna as a prophylactic agent to protect against hemorrhagic cystitis. Use with caution in patients with impaired renal function or those with compromised bone marrow reserve. Carcinogenic in rats.

Preparation of ifosfamide should be performed in a Class II laminar flow biologic safety cabinet. Personnel should be wearing surgical gloves and a closed front surgical gown with knit cuffs. Appropriate safety equipment is recommended for preparation, administration, and disposal of antineoplastics. If ifosfamide contacts the skin, wash and flush thoroughly with water.

Drug Interactions
Cytochrome P450 Effect: Substrate of CYP2A6 (minor), 2B6 (minor), 2C8/9 (minor), 2C19 (minor), 3A4 (major); **Inhibits** CYP3A4 (weak); **Induces** CYP2C8/9 (weak)
Decreased Effect: CYP3A4 inhibitors may decrease the levels/effects of acrolein (the active metabolite of ifosfamide); example inhibitors include azole antifungals, ciprofloxacin, clarithromycin, diclofenac, doxycycline, erythromycin, imatinib, isoniazid, nefazodone, nicardipine, propofol, protease inhibitors, quinidine, and verapamil.
Increased Effect/Toxicity: CYP3A4 inducers may increase the levels/effects of acrolein (the active metabolite of ifosfamide); example inducers include aminoglutethimide, carbamazepine, nafcillin, nevirapine, phenobarbital, phenytoin, and rifamycins.
Nutritional/Ethanol Interactions Herb/Nutraceutical: St John's wort may decrease ifosfamide levels.
Adverse Reactions
>10%:
  Central nervous system: Somnolence, confusion, hallucinations (12%)
  Dermatologic: Alopecia (75% to 100%)
  Endocrine & metabolic: Metabolic acidosis (31%)
  Gastrointestinal: Nausea and vomiting (58%), may be more common with higher doses or bolus infusions; constipation
  Genitourinary: Hemorrhagic cystitis (40% to 50%), patients should be vigorously hydrated (at least 2 L/day) and receive mesna
  Hematologic: Myelosuppression, leukopenia (65% to 100%), thrombocytopenia (10%) - dose related
    Onset: 7-14 days
    Nadir: 21-28 days
    Recovery: 21-28 days
  Renal: Hematuria (6% to 92%)
1% to 10%:
  Central nervous system: Hallucinations, depressive psychoses, polyneuropathy
  Dermatologic: Dermatitis, nail banding/ridging, hyperpigmentation
  Endocrine & metabolic: SIADH, sterility
  Hematologic: Anemia
  Hepatic: Transaminases increased (3%)
  Local: Phlebitis
  Renal: BUN/creatinine increased (6%)
  Respiratory: Nasal stuffiness
Overdosage/Toxicology Symptoms of overdose include myelosuppression, nausea, vomiting, diarrhea, and alopecia; direct extensions of the drug's pharmacologic effect. Treatment is supportive.
Pharmacodynamics/Kinetics
  Bioavailability: Estimated at 100%
  Time to Peak: Plasma: Oral: Within 1 hour
  Protein Binding: Negligible
  Half-Life Elimination: Beta: High dose: 11-15 hours (3800-5000 mg/m²); Lower dose: 4-7 hours (1800 mg/m²)
  (Continued)

Ifosfamide *(Continued)*

Metabolism: Hepatic to active metabolites phosphoramide mustard, acrolein, and inactive dichloroethylated and carboxy metabolites; acrolein is the agent implicated in development of hemorrhagic cystitis

Excretion: Urine (15% to 50% as unchanged drug, 41% as metabolites)

Pharmacokinetic Note: Pharmacokinetics are dose dependent.

Dosing

Adults & Elderly: Refer to individual protocols.

Antineoplastic: I.V.:

50 mg/kg/day or 700-2000 mg/m^2 for 5 days every 3-4 weeks

Alternatives: 2400 mg/m^2/day for 3 days or 5000 mg/m^2 as a single dose every 3-4 weeks

Note: To prevent bladder toxicity, ifosfamide should be given with extensive hydration consisting of at least 2 L of oral or I.V. fluid per day. The dose-limiting toxicity is hemorrhagic cystitis and, therefore, ifosfamide should be used in conjunction with a uroprotective agent, such as mesna.

Pediatrics: Refer to individual protocols.

Antineoplastic: I.V.:

1200-1800 mg/m^2/day for 3-5 days every 21-28 days **or**

5 g/m^2 once every 21-28 days **or**

3 g/m^2/day for 2 days every 21-28 days

See "Note" in adult dosing.

Renal Impairment: Limited experience in renal impairment; manufacturer does not provide adjustment. Several published recommendations include dose reductions between 20% and 30% in significant renal impairment. Consult individual protocols.

Hepatic Impairment: Although no specific guidelines are available, it is possible that adjusted doses are indicated in hepatic disease. Falkson G, et al (*Invest New Drugs*, 1992, 10:337-43) recommended the following dosage adjustments:

AST >300 or bilirubin >3.0 mg/dL: Decrease ifosfamide dose by 75%

Available Dosage Forms Injection, powder for reconstitution: 1 g, 3 g [packaged with Mesnex® (mesna) 1 g]

Monitoring and Teaching Issues

Physical Assessment: Use caution in presence of impaired renal function or compromised bone marrow reserve (see Warnings/Precautions for use cautions). Assess potential for interactions with other pharmacological agents or herbal products patient may be taking (eg, may increase or decrease levels/effects of ifosfamide; see Drug Interactions). See Administration for infusion specifics. To prevent bladder toxicity, maintain adequate hydration for 72 hours prior to infusion to minimize risk of hemorrhagic cystitis (2-3 L/day). Premedicate with antiemetic may be advisable prior to each infusion. Assess vital signs and results of laboratory tests prior to each infusion and regularly during therapy. Monitor therapeutic effectiveness (according to purpose for use) and adverse response throughout therapy (eg, CNS depression or psychoses, hematuria, [hemorrhagic cystitis], myelosuppression [anemia]; see Adverse Reactions). Teach patient (or caregiver) possible side effects/appropriate interventions (eg, importance of adequate hydration) and adverse symptoms to report (see Patient Education).

Monitoring Laboratory Tests: CBC with differential, platelet count, urinalysis, liver and renal function

Patient Education: Do not take any new medication during therapy unless approved by prescriber. This drug can only be administered by infusion. Report immediately any swelling, redness, or pain at infusion site. Maintain adequate hydration (2-3 L/day of fluids) unless instructed to restrict fluid intake, for at least 3 days prior to infusion and each day of therapy. You will be more susceptible to infection (avoid crowds and exposure to infection and do not have any vaccinations without consulting prescriber). May cause loss of hair (reversible, although regrowth hair may be different color or texture); fertility or amenorrhea; nausea or vomiting (small frequent meals, good mouth care, chewing gum, or sucking lozenges may help; if persistent consult prescriber for antiemetic); headache (consult prescriber for analgesic); or mouth sores (use soft toothbrush or cotton swab for oral care). Report any difficulty or pain with urination; chest pain, rapid heartbeat, or palpitations; CNS changes (eg, hallucinations, confusion, somnolence); unusual rash; persistent nausea or vomiting; swelling of extremities; respiratory difficulty; unusual fatigue; or opportunistic infection (eg, fever, chills, easy bruising or unusual bleeding). **Pregnancy/breast-feeding precautions:** Inform prescriber if you are pregnant. Do not get pregnant during or for 1 month following therapy. Male: Do not cause a female to become pregnant. Male/female: Consult prescriber for instruction on appropriate barrier contraceptive measures. This drug may cause severe fetal defects. Do not breast-feed.

Pregnancy Risk Factor: D

Lactation: Enters breast milk/contraindicated

Administration

I.V.: Administer slow I.V. push, IVPB over 30 minutes to several hours or continuous intravenous infusion over 5 days.

Reconstitution: Dilute powder with SWI or NS to a concentration of 50 mg/mL. Further dilution in 50-1000 mL D$_5$W or NS is recommended for I.V. infusion.

Compatibility: Stable in D$_5$LR, D$_5$NS, D$_5$W, LR, ^{1}/$_2$NS, NS; **incompatible** with bacteriostatic SWI or bacteriostatic NS

Y-site administration: Incompatible with cefepime, methotrexate

Compatibility in syringe: Incompatible with mesna with epirubicin

Compatibility when admixed: Incompatible with mesna with epirubicin

Storage: Store intact vials at room temperature. Reconstituted solutions may be stored under refrigeration for up to 21 days. Solutions diluted for administration are stable for 7 days at room temperature and for 6 weeks under refrigeration.

♦ **IgG4-Kappa Monoclonal Antibody** *see* Natalizumab *on page 1059*

♦ **IL-2** *see* Aldesleukin *on page 62*

Imatinib (eye MAT eh nib)

U.S. Brand Names Gleevec®

Synonyms CGP 57148B; Glivec; Imatinib Mesylate; STI571

Generic Available No

Pharmacologic Category Antineoplastic Agent, Tyrosine Kinase Inhibitor

Use Treatment of adult patients with Philadelphia chromosome-positive (Ph+) chronic myeloid leukemia (CML), including newly-diagnosed patients as well as patients in blast crisis, accelerated phase, or in chronic phase after failure of interferon-alpha therapy; treatment of pediatric patients with Ph+ CML (chronic phase) recurring following stem cell transplant or who are resistant to interferon-alpha therapy; treatment of Kit-positive (CD117) unresectable and/or (metastatic) malignant gastrointestinal stromal tumors (GIST)

Mechanism of Action/Effect Inhibits a specific enzyme (Bcr-Abl tyrosine kinase) produced by the Philadelphia chromosome found in many patients with chronic myeloid leukemia (CML). Inhibition of this enzyme blocks proliferation and induces cell death in leukemic cells. Also inhibits tyrosine kinase for platelet-derived growth factor (SCF), c-kit, and events mediated by PDGF and SCF.

Contraindications Hypersensitivity to imatinib or any component of the formulation; pregnancy

Warnings/Precautions Often associated with fluid retention, weight gain, and edema; occasionally leading to significant complications, including pleural effusion, pericardial effusion, pulmonary edema, and ascites. Use caution in patients where fluid accumulation may be poorly tolerated, such as in cardiovascular disease (CHF or hypertension) and pulmonary disease. Severe dermatologic reactions have been reported; reintroduction has been attempted following resolution. Successful resumption at a lower dose (with corticosteroids and/or antihistamine) has been described; however, some patients may experience recurrent reactions.

Use with caution in renal impairment, hematologic impairment, or hepatic disease. May cause GI irritation, hematologic toxicity (neutropenia, or thrombocytopenia), or hepatotoxicity. Hepatotoxic reactions may be severe. Has been associated with development of opportunistic infections. Use with caution in patients receiving concurrent therapy with drugs which alter cytochrome P450 activity or require metabolism by these isoenzymes. Safety and efficacy in patients <3 years of age have not been established.

Drug Interactions

Cytochrome P450 Effect: Substrate of CYP1A2 (minor), 2D6 (minor), 2C8/9 (minor), 2C19 (minor), 3A4 (major), **Inhibits** CYP2C8/9 (weak), 2D6 (weak), 3A4 (strong)

Decreased Effect: The levels/effects of imatinib may be decreased by aminoglutethimide, carbamazepine, nafcillin, nevirapine, phenobarbital, phenytoin, rifamycins, and other CYP3A4 inducers. Dosage of imatinib should be increased by at least 50% (with careful monitoring) when used concurrently with a strong inducer.

Increased Effect/Toxicity: Note: Drug interaction data are limited. Few clinical studies have been conducted. Many interactions listed here are derived by extrapolation from *in vitro* inhibition of cytochrome P450 isoenzymes. Chronic use of acetaminophen may increase potential for hepatotoxic reaction with imatinib (case report of hepatic failure with concurrent therapy).

Imatinib may increase the levels/effects of amiodarone, selected benzodiazepines, calcium channel blockers, cisapride, cyclosporine, ergot derivatives, fluoxetine, glimepiride, glipizide, HMG-CoA reductase inhibitors, nateglinide, phenytoin, phenytoin, propranolol, sertraline, mirtazapine, nateglinide, nefazodone, pioglitazone, rosiglitazone, sertraline, sildenafil (and other PDE-5 inhibitors), tacrolimus, venlafaxine, warfarin, and other substrates of CYP2C8/9 or 3A4. Selected benzodiazepines (midazolam and triazolam), cisapride, ergot alkaloids, selected HMG-CoA reductase inhibitors (lovastatin and simvastatin), mesoridazine, pimozide, and thioridazine are generally contraindicated with strong CYP3A4 inhibitors. When used with strong CYP3A4 inhibitors, dosage adjustment/limits are recommended for sildenafil and other PDE-5 inhibitors; consult individual monographs.

The levels/effects of imatinib may be increased by azole antifungals, ciprofloxacin, clarithromycin, diclofenac, doxycycline, erythromycin, isoniazid, nefazodone, nicardipine, propofol, protease inhibitors, quinidine, telithromycin, verapamil, and other CYP3A4 inhibitors.

Nutritional/Ethanol Interactions

Ethanol: Avoid ethanol.

Food: Food may reduce gastrointestinal irritation.

Herb/Nutraceutical: Avoid St John's wort (may increase metabolism and decrease imatinib plasma concentration).

Adverse Reactions Adverse reactions listed were established in patients with a wide variation in level of illness or specific diagnosis. In many cases, other medications were used concurrently (relationship to imatinib not specific). Effects reported in children were similar to adults, except that musculoskeletal pain was less frequent and peripheral edema was not reported.

>10%:

Central nervous system: Fatigue (29% to 41%), pyrexia (5% to 41%), headache (25% to 35%), dizziness (11% to 13%), insomnia (10% to 13%)

Dermatologic: Rash (26% to 44%), pruritus (8% to 13%), bruising (2% to 11%)

Endocrine & metabolic: Fluid retention (3% to 22% includes aggravated edema, anasarca, ascites, pericardial effusion, pleural effusion, pulmonary edema, excludes GIST); hypokalemia (5% to 13%)

Gastrointestinal: Nausea (42% to 71%), diarrhea (30% to 60%), vomiting (15% to 56%), abdominal pain (23% to 37%), weight increased (3% to 30%), dyspepsia (11% to 24%), flatulence (16% to 23%), anorexia (6% to 17%), constipation (6% to 15%), taste disturbance (1% to 14%)

Hematologic: Hemorrhage (18% to 52%), neutropenia (grade 3 or 4: 2% to 48%), thrombocytopenia (grade 3 or 4: <1% to 31%)

(Continued)

Imatinib *(Continued)*

Neuromuscular & skeletal: Muscle cramps (27% to 55%), musculoskeletal pain (11% to 46%), arthralgia (25% to 36%), joint pain (27%), myalgia (8% to 25%), weakness (5% to 12%), back pain (10% to 11%), rigors (8% to 11%)

Ocular: Lacrimation (6% to 11%)

Respiratory: Cough (12% to 26%), dyspnea (9% to 20%), nasopharyngitis (8% to 19%), upper respiratory tract infection (3% to 15%), pharyngolaryngeal pain (14%), epistaxis (5% to 13%), pneumonia (3% to 12%), sore throat (8% to 11%)

Miscellaneous: Superficial edema (53% to 76%), night sweats (10% to 14%)

1% to 10%:

Central nervous system: Paresthesia (1% to 10%)

Hematologic: Anemia (grade 3 or 4: <1% to 4%)

Hepatic: Ascites or pleural effusion (GIST: 4% to 6%), alkaline phosphatase increased (grade 3 or 4: <1% to 5%), ALT increased (grade 3 or 4: <1% to 4%), bilirubin increased (grade 3 or 4: <1% to 4%), AST increased (grade 3 or 4: <1% to 3%)

Renal: Albumin decreased (grade 3 or 4: 3% to 4%), creatine increased (grade 3 or 4: <1% to 3%)

Miscellaneous: Flu-like syndrome (<1% to 10%)

Overdosage/Toxicology Experience with overdose is limited (>800 mg/day). Hematologic adverse effects are more common at dosages >750 mg/day. Treatment is symptomatic and supportive.

Pharmacodynamics/Kinetics

Bioavailability: 98%

Time to Peak: 2-4 hours

Protein Binding: 95% to albumin and alpha$_1$-acid glycoprotein

Half-Life Elimination: Parent drug: 18 hours; N-demethyl metabolite: 40 hours

Metabolism: Hepatic via CYP3A4 (minor metabolism via CYP1A2, CYP2D6, CYP2C9, CYP2C19); primary metabolite (active): N-demethylated piperazine derivative

Excretion: Feces (68% primarily as metabolites, 20% as unchanged drug); urine (13% primarily as metabolites, 5% as unchanged drug)

Clearance: Highly variable; Mean: 8-14 L/hour (for 50 kg and 100 kg male, respectively)

Dosing

Adults & Elderly:

CML:

Chronic phase: Oral: 400 mg once daily; may be increased to 600 mg daily in the event of disease progression, loss of previously achieved response, or failure to achieve response after at least 3 months of therapy and in the absence of severe adverse reaction

Accelerated phase or blast crisis: 600 mg once daily; may be increased to 800 mg daily (400 mg twice daily) in the event of disease progression, loss of previously achieved response, or failure to achieve response after at least 3 months of therapy and in the absence of severe adverse reaction

Gastrointestinal stromal tumors: 400-600 mg/day.

Note: Dosage should be increased by at least 50% when used concurrently with a potent enzyme-inducing agent (ie, rifampin, phenytoin).

Dosage adjustment for hepatotoxicity or other nonhematologic adverse reactions: Refer to "Hepatic Impairment" dosing.

Dosage adjustment for hematologic adverse reactions:

Chronic phase (initial dose 400 mg/day in adults or 260 mg/m^2/day in children) or GIST (initial dose 400 mg or 600 mg): If ANC <1.0 x 10^9/L and/or platelets <50 x 10^9/L: Discontinue until ANC ≥1.5 x 10^9/L and platelets ≥75 x 10^9/L; resume treatment at original initial dose of 400 or 600 mg/day (260 mg/m^2/day in children). If depression in neutrophils or platelets recurs, withhold until recovery, and reinstitute treatment at a reduced dose:

Children:

If initial dose 260 mg/m^2/day, reduce dose to 200 mg/m^2/day

If initial dose 340 mg/m^2/day, reduce dose to 260 mg/m^2/day

Adults:

If initial dose 400 mg, reduce dose to 300 mg

If initial dose 600 mg, reduce dose to 400 mg

Accelerated phase or blast crisis: Adults: Check to establish whether cytopenia is related to leukemia (bone marrow aspirate). If unrelated to leukemia, reduce dose of imatinib by 25%. If cytopenia persists for an additional 2 weeks, further reduce dose to 50% of original dose. If cytopenia persists for 4 weeks and is still unrelated to leukemia, stop treatment until ANC ≥1.0 x 10^9/L and platelets ≥20 x 10^9/L, resume treatment at 50% of original dose.

Pediatrics:

CML (chronic phase): Oral: 260 mg/m^2/day; may be increased to 340 mg/m^2/day in the event of disease progression, loss of previously achieved response, or failure to achieve response after at least 3 months of therapy and in the absence of severe adverse reaction. Dose may be given once daily or in 2 divided doses.

Note: Dosage should be increased by at least 50% when used concurrently with a potent enzyme-inducing agent (ie, rifampin, phenytoin).

Dosage adjustment for hepatotoxicity or other nonhematologic adverse reactions: Refer to "Hepatic Impairment" dosing.

Dosage adjustment for hematologic adverse reactions: Refer to adult dosing.

Hepatic Impairment: Hepatotoxicity or other nonhematologic adverse reactions: If elevations of bilirubin >3 times upper limit of normal (ULN) or transaminases (ALT/AST) >5 times ULN occur, withhold until bilirubin <1.5 times ULN or transaminases <2.5 times ULN. Resume treatment at a reduced dose:

Children:

If initial dose 260 mg/m^2/day, reduce dose to 200 mg/m^2/day

If initial dose 340 mg/m^2/day, reduce dose to 260 mg/m^2/day

Adults:

If initial dose 400 mg, reduce dose to 300 mg

If initial dose 600 mg, reduce dose to 400 mg

Available Dosage Forms Tablet: 100 mg, 400 mg

Monitoring and Teaching Issues

Physical Assessment: Use caution when fluid accumulation may be poorly tolerated (CHF, hypertension), renal or hepatic impairment (see Warnings/Precautions for specific use cautions). Monitor closely any other pharmacological agents or herbal products patient may be taking for effectiveness and possible interactions prior to beginning therapy (especially those drugs affected by cytochrome P450 actions; see Drug Interactions). Assess results of laboratory tests on a regular basis (see Monitoring Laboratory Tests). Monitor therapeutic effectiveness and adverse reactions at beginning of therapy and periodically during therapy (eg, weight and fluid status, hemorrhage, paresthesia, respiratory or CNS changes; see Adverse Reactions). Teach appropriate use, interventions to reduce side effects, and symptoms to report (see Patient Education).

Monitoring Laboratory Tests: CBC (weekly for first month, biweekly for second month, then periodically thereafter), liver function tests (at baseline and monthly or as clinically indicated), and renal function.

Patient Education: Take with food or a large glass of water. Avoid alcohol, chronic use of acetaminophen or aspirin, OTC or prescription medications, or herbal products unless approved by prescriber. Maintain adequate hydration (2-3 L/day of fluids) unless instructed to restrict fluid intake. You will be required to have regularly scheduled laboratory tests while on this medication. You will be more susceptible to infection (avoid crowds and exposure to infection and do not receive any vaccination unless approved by prescriber). You may experience headache or fatigue (use caution when driving or engaging in tasks requiring alertness until response to drug in known); loss of appetite, nausea, vomiting, or mouth sores (small frequent meals, frequent mouth care, chewing gum, or sucking lozenges may help); constipation (increased exercise, fluids, fruit, or fiber may help); or diarrhea (buttermilk, boiled milk, or yogurt may reduce diarrhea). Report chest pain, palpitations, or swelling of extremities; cough, respiratory difficulty, or wheezing; weight gain >5 lb; skin rash; muscle or bone pain, tremors, or cramping; persistent fatigue or weakness; easy bruising or unusual bleeding (eg, tarry stools, blood in vomitus, stool, urine, or mouth); persistent GI problems or pain; or other adverse effects. **Pregnancy/breast-feeding precautions:** Inform prescriber if you are pregnant. Do not get pregnant. Use appropriate contraception while on this medication. Breast-feeding is not recommended.

Dietary Considerations: Should be taken with food and a large glass of water to decrease gastrointestinal irritation.

Geriatric Considerations: Incidence of edema and edema-related adverse effects is increased in elderly patients.

Pregnancy Risk Factor: D

Lactation: Excretion in breast milk unknown/not recommended

Administration

Oral: Should be administered with food and a large glass of water. Tablets may be dispersed in water or apple juice, stir until dissolved and use immediately.

Storage: Store at 25°C (77°F); excursions permitted to 15°C to 30°C (59°F to 86°F).

Additional Information Median time to hematologic response was one month; only short-term studies have been completed. Follow-up is insufficient to estimate duration of cytogenic response.

♦ **Imatinib Mesylate** see Imatinib on page 785

♦ **IMC-C225** see Cetuximab on page 299

♦ **Imdur®** see Isosorbide Mononitrate on page 841

♦ **IMI 30** see Idarubicin on page 781

♦ **Imidazole Carboxamide** see Dacarbazine on page 394

♦ **Imidazole Carboxamide Dimethyltriazene** see Dacarbazine on page 394

♦ **Imipemide** see Imipenem and Cilastatin on page 787

Imipenem and Cilastatin (i mi PEN em & sye la STAT in)

U.S. Brand Names Primaxin®

Synonyms Imipemide

Generic Available No

Pharmacologic Category Antibiotic, Carbapenem

Medication Safety Issues

Sound-alike/look-alike issues:

Primaxin® may be confused with Premarin®, Primacor®

Use Treatment of respiratory tract, urinary tract, intra-abdominal, gynecologic, bone and joint, skin structure, and polymicrobic infections as well as bacterial septicemia and endocarditis. Antibacterial activity includes resistant gram-negative bacilli (*Pseudomonas aeruginosa* and *Enterobacter* sp), gram-positive bacteria (methicillin-sensitive *Staphylococcus aureus* and *Streptococcus* sp) and anaerobes.

Note: I.M. administration is not intended for severe or life-threatening infections (eg, septicemia, endocarditis, shock).

Mechanism of Action/Effect A carbapenem with broad-spectrum antibacterial activity including resistant gram-negative bacilli (*Pseudomonas aeruginosa* and *Enterococcus* sp), gram-positive bacteria (methicillin-sensitive *Staphylococcus aureus* and *Enterococcus* sp) and anaerobes; inhibits cell wall synthesis; cilastatin prevents renal metabolism of imipenem

Contraindications Hypersensitivity to imipenem/cilastatin or any component of the formulation; consult information on Lidocaine for contraindications associated with I.M. dosing

Warnings/Precautions Dosage adjustment is required in patients with impaired renal function. Prolonged use may result in superinfection. Has been associated with CNS adverse events. Use with caution in patients with a history of seizures or hypersensitivity to

(Continued)

Imipenem and Cilastatin *(Continued)*

beta-lactams. Elderly patients often require lower doses (adjust carefully to renal function). Doses for I.M. administration are mixed with lidocaine, consult information on lidocaine for associated warnings/precautions.

Drug Interactions

Decreased Effect: Imipenem may decrease valproic acid concentrations to subtherapeutic levels; monitor.

Lab Interactions Interferes with urinary glucose determination using Clinitest®

Adverse Reactions 1% to 10%:

Gastrointestinal: Nausea/diarrhea/vomiting (1% to 2%)

Local: Phlebitis (3%), pain at I.M. injection site (1.2%)

Overdosage/Toxicology Symptoms of overdose include neuromuscular hypersensitivity and seizures. Hemodialysis may be helpful to aid in removal of the drug from blood; otherwise, treatment is supportive or symptom-directed.

Pharmacodynamics/Kinetics

Absorption: I.M.: Imipenem: 60% to 75%; cilastatin: 95% to 100%

Half-Life Elimination: Both drugs: 60 minutes; prolonged with renal impairment

Metabolism: Renally by dehydropeptidase; activity is blocked by cilastatin; cilastatin is partially metabolized renally

Excretion: Both drugs: Urine (~70% as unchanged drug)

Dosing

Adults & Elderly: Dosage based on **imipenem** content:

Moderate infections:

I.M.: 750 mg every 12 hours

I.V.:

Fully-susceptible organisms: 500 mg every 6-8 hours (1.5-2 g/day)

Moderately-susceptible organisms: 500 mg every 6 hours or 1 g every 8 hours (2-3 g/day)

Severe infections: I.V.: Note: I.M. administration is not intended for severe or life-threatening infections (eg, septicemia, endocarditis, shock):

Fully-susceptible organisms: 500 mg every 6 hours (2 g/day)

Moderately-susceptible organisms: 1 g every 6-8 hours (3-4 g/day)

Maximum daily dose should not exceed 50 mg/kg or 4 g/day, whichever is lower

Urinary tract infection, uncomplicated: I.V.: 250 mg every 6 hours (1 g/day)

Urinary tract infection, complicated: I.V.: 500 mg every 6 hours (2 g/day)

Mild infections: Note: Rarely a suitable option in mild infections; normally reserved for moderate-severe cases:

I.M.: 500 mg every 12 hours; intra-abdominal infections: 750 mg every 12 hours

Imipenem and Cilastatin Dosage in Renal Impairment

Reduced I.V. Dosage Regimen Based on Creatinine Clearance (mL/minute/1.73 m²) and Body Weight (kg)					
	Body Weight (kg)				
	≥70	**60**	**50**	**40**	**30**
Total daily dose for normal renal function: 1 g/day					
Cl_cr ≥71	250 mg q6h	250 mg q8h	125 mg q6h	125 mg q6h	125 mg q8h
Cl_cr 41-70	250 mg q8h	125 mg q6h	125 mg q6h	125 mg q8h	125 mg q8h
Cl_cr 21-40	250 mg q12h	250 mg q12h	125 mg q8h	125 mg q12h	125 mg q12h
Cl_cr 6-20	250 mg q12h	125 mg q12h	125 mg q12h	125 mg q12h	125 mg q12h
Total daily dose for normal renal function: 1.5 g/day					
Cl_cr ≥71	500 mg q8h	250 mg q6h	250 mg q6h	250 mg q8h	125 mg q6h
Cl_cr 41-70	250 mg q6h	250 mg q8h	250 mg q8h	125 mg q6h	125 mg q8h
Cl_cr 21-40	250 mg q8h	250 mg q8h	250 mg q12h	125 mg q8h	125 mg q12h
Cl_cr 6-20	250 mg q12h	250 mg q12h	250 mg q12h	125 mg q12h	125 mg q12h
Total daily dose for normal renal function: 2 g/day					
Cl_cr ≥71	500 mg q6h	500 mg q8h	250 mg q6h	250 mg q6h	250 mg q8h
Cl_cr 41-70	500 mg q8h	250 mg q6h	250 mg q6h	250 mg q8h	125 mg q6h
Cl_cr 21-40	250 mg q6h	250 mg q8h	250 mg q8h	250 mg q12h	125 mg q8h
Cl_cr 6-20	250 mg q12h	250 mg q12h	250 mg q12h	250 mg q12h	125 mg q12h
Total daily dose for normal renal function: 3 g/day					
Cl_cr ≥71	1000 mg q8h	750 mg q8h	500 mg q6h	500 mg q8h	250 mg q6h
Cl_cr 41-70	500 mg q6h	500 mg q8h	500 mg q8h	250 mg q6h	250 mg q8h
Cl_cr 21-40	500 mg q8h	500 mg q8h	250 mg q6h	250 mg q8h	250 mg q8h
Cl_cr 6-20	500 mg q12h	500 mg q12h	250 mg q12h	250 mg q12h	250 mg q12h
Total daily dose for normal renal function: 4 g/day					
Cl_cr ≥71	1000 mg q6h	1000 mg q8h	750 mg q8h	500 mg q6h	500 mg q8h
Cl_cr 41-70	750 mg q8h	750 mg q8h	500 mg q6h	500 mg q8h	250 mg q6h
Cl_cr 21-40	500 mg q6h	500 mg q8h	500 mg q8h	250 mg q6h	250 mg q8h
Cl_cr 6-20	500 mg q12h	500 mg q12h	500 mg q12h	250 mg q12h	250 mg q12h

I.V.:
Fully-susceptible organisms: 250 mg every 6 hours (1g/day)
Moderately-susceptible organisms: 500 mg every 6 hours (2 g/day)
Pediatrics: Dosage based on **imipenem** content:
Non-CNS infections: I.V.:
Neonates:
<1 week: 25 mg/kg every 12 hours
1-4 weeks: 25 mg/kg every 8 hours
4 weeks to 3 months: 25 mg/kg every 6 hours
Children: >3 months: 15-25 mg/kg every 6 hours
Maximum dosage: Susceptible infections: 2 g/day; moderately susceptible organisms: 4 g/day
Cystic fibrosis: I.V.: Children: Doses up to 90 mg/kg/day have been used
Renal Impairment: I.V.: **Note:** Adjustments have not been established for I.M. dosing:
Patients with a Cl_{cr} <5 mL/minute/1.73 m^2 should not receive imipenem/cilastatin unless hemodialysis is instituted within 48 hours.
Patients weighing <30 kg with impaired renal function should not receive imipenem/cilastatin.
Hemodialysis: Use the dosing recommendation for patients with a Cl_{cr} 6-20 mL/minute.
Peritoneal dialysis: Dose as for Cl_{cr} <10 mL/minute.
Continuous arteriovenous or venovenous hemofiltration: Dose as for Cl_{cr} 20-30 mL/minute; monitor for seizure activity. Imipenem is well removed by CAVH but cilastatin is not; removes 20 mg of imipenem per liter of filtrate per day.

See table on previous page.
Available Dosage Forms
Injection, powder for reconstitution [I.M.]: Imipenem 500 mg and cilastatin 500 mg [contains sodium 32 mg (1.4 mEq)]
Injection, powder for reconstitution [I.V.]: Imipenem 250 mg and cilastatin 250 mg [contains sodium 18.8 mg (0.8 mEq)]; imipenem 500 mg and cilastatin 500 mg [contains sodium 37.5 mg (1.6 mEq)]
Monitoring and Teaching Issues
Physical Assessment: Assess results of culture and sensitivity tests and patient's allergy history prior to beginning therapy. See Warnings/Precautions for use cautions (eg, impaired renal function, history of CNS events). See Administration for I.M. and I.V. specifics. Assess results of laboratory tests, therapeutic effectiveness (resolution of infection), and adverse response (see Adverse Reactions) periodically during therapy. Advise patients with diabetes about use of Clinitest®. Teach patient possible side effects/appropriate interventions and adverse symptoms to report (see Patient Education).
Monitoring Laboratory Tests: Perform culture and sensitivity studies prior to initiating therapy. Periodically monitor renal, hepatic, and hematologic function.
Patient Education: Do not take any new medication during therapy unless approved by prescriber. This medication can only be administered by injection or infusion. Report immediately any warmth, swelling, pain, or redness at infusion or injection site. Maintain adequate hydration (2-3 L/day of fluids) unless instructed to restrict fluid intake and nutrition (small frequent meals). May cause false test results with Clinitest®; use of another type of glucose testing is preferable. Report immediately any CNS changes (dizziness, hallucinations, anxiety, visual disturbances); swelling of throat, tongue, lips, or face; chills or fever; or unusual discharge or foul-smelling urine. **Pregnancy/breast-feeding precautions:** Inform prescriber if you are or intend to become pregnant. Consult prescriber if breast-feeding.
Dietary Considerations: Sodium content of 1 g injection:
I.M.: 64.4 mg (2.8 mEq)
I.V.: 73.6 mg (3.2 mEq)
Geriatric Considerations: Many of the seizures attributed to imipenem/cilastatin were in elderly patients. Dose must be carefully adjusted for creatinine clearance.
Pregnancy Risk Factor: C
Lactation: Enters breast milk (small amounts)/use caution
Administration
I.M.: Prepare 500 mg vial with 2 mL 1% lidocaine; prepare 750 mg vial with 3 mL 1% lidocaine **(do not use lidocaine with epinephrine)**. Administer by deep injection into a large muscle (gluteal or lateral thigh). Aspiration is necessary to avoid inadvertent injection into a blood vessel.
I.V.: Do not administer I.V. push. Final concentration should not exceed 5 mg/mL. Infuse over 30-60 minutes.
Reconstitution: All IVPB should be prepared fresh. Do not use dextrose as a diluent due to limited stability. Reconstituted solutions are stable 10 hours at room temperature and 48 hours at refrigeration (4°C) with NS. If reconstituted with 5% or 10% dextrose injection, 5% dextrose and sodium bicarbonate, 5% dextrose and 0.9% sodium chloride, is stable for 4 hours at room temperature and 24 hours when refrigerated. Imipenem is inactivated at acidic or alkaline pH.
Standard diluent: 500 mg/100 mL NS; 1 g/250 mL NS
Compatibility: Y-site administration: Incompatible with allopurinol, amphotericin B cholesteryl sulfate complex, etoposide phosphate, fluconazole, gemcitabine, lorazepam, meperidine, midazolam, sargramostim, sodium bicarbonate
Storage: Imipenem/cilastatin powder for injection should be stored at <30°C.
Related Information
Antimicrobial Drugs of Choice *on page 1792*
Community-Acquired Pneumonia in Adults *on page 1807*

Imipramine *(im IP ra meen)*
U.S. Brand Names Tofranil®; Tofranil-PM®
Synonyms Imipramine Hydrochloride; Imipramine Pamoate
(Continued)

Imipramine *(Continued)*

Restrictions A medication guide should be dispensed with each prescription. A template for the required MedGuides can be found on the FDA website at: http://www.fda.gov/cder/drug/antidepressants/labelTemplate.pdf

Generic Available Yes: Tablet

Pharmacologic Category Antidepressant, Tricyclic (Tertiary Amine)

Medication Safety Issues

Sound-alike/look-alike issues:

Imipramine may be confused with amitriptyline, desipramine, Norpramin®

Use Treatment of depression; treatment of nocturnal enuresis in children

Unlabeled/Investigational Use Analgesic for certain chronic and neuropathic pain; panic disorder; attention-deficit/hyperactivity disorder (ADHD)

Mechanism of Action/Effect Traditionally believed to increase the synaptic concentration of serotonin and/or norepinephrine in the central nervous system by inhibition of their reuptake by the presynaptic neuronal membrane. However, additional receptor effects have been found including desensitization of adenyl cyclase, down regulation of beta-adrenergic receptors, and down regulation of serotonin receptors.

Contraindications Hypersensitivity to imipramine (cross-reactivity with other dibenzodiazepines may occur) or any component of the formulation; concurrent use of MAO inhibitors (within 14 days); in a patient during acute recovery phase of MI; pregnancy

Warnings/Precautions Antidepressants increase the risk of suicidal thinking and behavior in children and adolescents with major depressive disorder (MDD) and other depressive disorders; consider risk prior to prescribing. All patients must be closely monitored for clinical worsening, suicidality, or unusual changes in behavior, especially during the initiation of therapy or following an increase or decrease in dosage. When used in children, the child's family or caregiver should be instructed to closely observe the patient and communicate condition with healthcare provider. A medication guide should be dispensed with each prescription. **Imipramine is FDA approved for the treatment of nocturnal enuresis in children ≥6 years of age.**

The possibility of a suicide attempt is inherent in major depression and may persist until remission occurs. Use caution in high-risk patients. Worsening depression and severe abrupt suicidality that are not part of the presenting symptoms may require discontinuation or modification of drug therapy. The patient's family or caregiver should be alerted to monitor patients for the emergence of suicidality and associated behaviors (such as agitation, irritability, hostility, impulsivity, and hypomania) and notify healthcare provider.

May worsen psychosis in some patients or precipitate a shift to mania or hypomania in patients with bipolar disorder. Patients presenting with depressive symptoms should be screened for bipolar disorder. Monotherapy in patients with bipolar disorder should be avoided. **Imipramine is not FDA approved for the treatment of bipolar depression.**

The degree of sedation, anticholinergic effects, orthostasis, and conduction abnormalities are high relative to other antidepressants. Imipramine often causes drowsiness/sedation, resulting in impaired performance of tasks requiring alertness (eg, operating machinery or driving). Sedative effects may be additive with other CNS depressants and/or ethanol. Use with caution in patients with a history of cardiovascular disease (including previous MI, stroke, tachycardia, or conduction abnormalities). Use with caution in patients with urinary retention, benign prostatic hyperplasia, narrow-angle glaucoma, xerostomia, visual problems, constipation, or a history of bowel obstruction.

Consider discontinuing, when possible, prior to elective surgery. Therapy should not be abruptly discontinued in patients receiving high doses for prolonged periods. May lower seizure threshold - use caution in patients with a previous seizure disorder or condition predisposing to seizures such as brain damage, alcoholism, or concurrent therapy with other drugs which lower the seizure threshold. May increase the risks associated with electroconvulsive therapy. Use with caution in hyperthyroid patients or those receiving thyroid supplementation. Use with caution in patients with hepatic or renal dysfunction and in elderly patients. Has been associated with photosensitization.

Drug Interactions

Cytochrome P450 Effect: Substrate of CYP1A2 (minor), 2B6 (minor), 2C19 (major), 2D6 (major), 3A4 (minor); **Inhibits** CYP1A2 (weak), 2C19 (weak), 2D6 (moderate), 2E1 (weak)

Decreased Effect: CYP2C19 inducers may decrease the levels/effects of imipramine; example inducers include aminoglutethimide, carbamazepine, phenytoin, and rifampin. Imipramine inhibits the antihypertensive response to bethanidine, clonidine, debrisoquin, guanadrel, guanethidine, guanabenz, and guanfacine. Cholestyramine and colestipol may bind TCAs and reduce their absorption; monitor for altered response.

Increased Effect/Toxicity: When used with MAO inhibitors, hyperpyrexia, hypertension, tachycardia, confusion, seizures, and **deaths have been reported** (serotonin syndrome). Serotonin syndrome has also been reported with ritonavir (rare). Use of lithium with a TCA may increase the risk for neurotoxicity.

CYP2C19 inhibitors may increase the levels/effects of imipramine; example inhibitors include delavirdine, fluconazole, fluvoxamine, gemfibrozil, isoniazid, omeprazole, and ticlopidine. Imipramine increases the effects of amphetamines, anticholinergics, other CNS depressants (sedatives, hypnotics, or ethanol), chlorpropamide, tolazamide, and warfarin. CYP2D6 inhibitors may increase the levels/effects of imipramine; example inhibitors include chlorpromazine, delavirdine, fluoxetine, miconazole, paroxetine, pergolide, quinidine, quinine, ritonavir, and ropinirole.

Phenothiazines may increase concentration of some TCAs and TCAs may increase concentration of phenothiazines. Pressor response to I.V. epinephrine, norepinephrine, and phenylephrine may be enhanced in patients receiving TCAs (**Note:** Effect is unlikely with epinephrine or levonordefrin dosages typically administered as infiltration in combination with local anesthetics).

Combined use of beta-agonists or drugs which prolong QT_c (including quinidine, procainamide, disopyramide, cisapride, sparfloxacin, gatifloxacin, moxifloxacin) with TCAs may predispose patients to cardiac arrhythmias.

Nutritional/Ethanol Interactions

Ethanol: Avoid ethanol (may increase CNS depression).

Food: Grapefruit juice may inhibit the metabolism of some TCAs and clinical toxicity may result.

Herb/Nutraceutical: St John's wort may decrease imipramine levels. Avoid valerian, St John's wort, SAMe, kava kava (may increase risk of serotonin syndrome and/or excessive sedation).

Lab Interactions Increased glucose

Adverse Reactions Frequency not defined.

Cardiovascular: Orthostatic hypotension, arrhythmia, tachycardia, hypertension, palpitation, MI, heart block, ECG changes, CHF, stroke

Central nervous system: Dizziness, drowsiness, headache, agitation, insomnia, nightmares, hypomania, psychosis, fatigue, confusion, hallucinations, disorientation, delusions, anxiety, restlessness, seizure

Endocrine & metabolic: Gynecomastia, breast enlargement, galactorrhea, increase or decrease in libido, increase or decrease in blood sugar, SIADH

Gastrointestinal: Nausea, unpleasant taste, weight gain, xerostomia, constipation, ileus, stomatitis, abdominal cramps, vomiting, anorexia, epigastric disorders, diarrhea, black tongue, weight loss

Genitourinary: Urinary retention, impotence

Neuromuscular & skeletal: Weakness, numbness, tingling, paresthesia, incoordination, ataxia, tremor, peripheral neuropathy, extrapyramidal symptoms

Ocular: Blurred vision, disturbances of accommodation, mydriasis

Otic: Tinnitus

Miscellaneous: Diaphoresis

Overdosage/Toxicology

Symptoms of overdose include confusion, hallucinations, constipation, cyanosis, tachycardia, urinary retention, ventricular tachycardia, and seizures. Following initiation of essential overdose management, toxic symptoms should be treated. Ventricular arrhythmias often respond to concurrent systemic alkalinization (sodium bicarbonate 0.5-2 mEq/kg I.V.) Physostigmine (1-2 mg I.V. slowly for adults) may be indicated to reverse life-threatening cardiac arrhythmias.

Pharmacodynamics/Kinetics

Onset of Action: Peak antidepressant effect: Usually after ≥2 weeks

Absorption: Well absorbed

Half-Life Elimination: 6-18 hours

Metabolism: Hepatic via CYP to desipramine (active) and other metabolites; significant first-pass effect

Excretion: Urine (as metabolites)

Dosing

Adults: Antidepressant:

Oral: Initial: 25 mg 3-4 times/day; increase dose gradually, total dose may be given at bedtime; maximum: 300 mg/day.

Note: Maximum antidepressant effect may not be seen for 2 or more weeks after initiation of therapy.

Elderly:

Antidepressant: Initial: 10-25 mg at bedtime; increase by 10-25 mg every 3 days for inpatients and weekly for outpatients if tolerated. Average daily dose to achieve a therapeutic concentration: 100 mg/day; range: 50-150 mg/day.

Urinary incontinence (urge or mixed type): 10-50 mg at bedtime or twice daily

Pediatrics:

Depression: Oral:

Children (unlabeled use): 1.5 mg/kg/day with dosage increments of 1 mg/kg every 3-4

Adolescents: Initial: 30-40 mg/day; increase gradually; maximum: 100 mg/day in single or divided doses. days to a maximum dose of 5 mg/kg/day in 1-4 divided doses; monitor carefully especially with doses ≥3.5 mg/kg/day.

Enuresis: Oral: Children ≥6 years: Initial: 25 mg at bedtime, if inadequate response still seen after 1 week of therapy, increase by 25 mg/day; dose should not exceed 2.5 mg/kg/day or 50 mg at bedtime if 6-12 years of age or 75 mg at bedtime if ≥12 years of age.

Adjunct in the treatment of cancer pain (unlabeled use): Oral: Children: Initial: 0.2-0.4 mg/kg at bedtime; dose may be increased by 50% every 2-3 days up to 1-3 mg/kg/dose at bedtime.

Available Dosage Forms

Capsule, as pamoate (Tofranil-PM®): 75 mg, 100 mg, 125 mg, 150 mg

Tablet, as hydrochloride (Tofranil®): 10 mg, 25 mg, 50 mg [generic tablets may contain sodium benzoate]

Monitoring and Teaching Issues

Physical Assessment: Assess other medications patient may be taking for effectiveness and interactions. Assess results of laboratory tests, therapeutic effectiveness, and adverse reactions at beginning of therapy and periodically with long-term use. Assess CNS status and be alert for suicidal ideation. Taper dosage slowly when discontinuing (allow 3-4 weeks between discontinuing Tofranil® and starting another antidepressant). Assess knowledge/teach patient appropriate use, interventions to reduce side effects, and adverse symptoms to report.

Monitoring Laboratory Tests: ECG, CBC

Patient Education: Take exactly as directed; do not increase dose or frequency. It may take 2-3 weeks to achieve desired results. Take in the evening. Avoid alcohol, caffeine, and other prescription or OTC medications not approved by prescriber. Maintain adequate hydration (2-3 L/day of fluids) unless instructed to restrict fluid intake. You may experience drowsiness, lightheadedness, impaired coordination, dizziness, or blurred vision (use caution when driving or engaging in tasks requiring alertness until response to drug is known); nausea, vomiting, altered taste, dry mouth (small frequent meals, frequent mouth (Continued)

Imipramine (Continued)

care, chewing gum, or sucking lozenges may help); constipation (increased exercise, fluids, fruit, or fiber may help); diarrhea (buttermilk, yogurt, or boiled milk may help); postural hypotension (use caution when climbing stairs or changing position from lying or sitting to standing); or urinary retention (void before taking medication). Report persistent insomnia; muscle cramping or tremors; chest pain, palpitations, rapid heartbeat, swelling of extremities, or severe dizziness; unresolved urinary retention; rash or skin irritation; yellowing of eyes or skin; pale stools/dark urine; or worsening of condition. **Pregnancy/breast-feeding precautions:** Do not get pregnant while taking this medication; use appropriate contraceptive measures. Breast-feeding is not recommended.

Geriatric Considerations: Orthostatic hypotension is a concern with this agent, especially in patients taking other medications that may affect blood pressure. May precipitate arrhythmias in predisposed patients; may aggravate seizures. A less anticholinergic antidepressant may be a better choice. Data from a clinical trial comparing fluoxetine to tricyclics suggests that fluoxetine is significantly less effective than nortriptyline in hospitalized elderly patients with unipolar major affective disorder, especially those with melancholia and concurrent cardiovascular diseases.

Pregnancy Risk Factor: D

Lactation: Enters breast milk/not recommended (AAP rates "of concern")

Related Information

Antidepressant Agents on page 1713
Antidepressant Medication Guidelines on page 1765
Federal OBRA Regulations: Recommended Maximum Doses on page 1773
Peak and Trough Guidelines on page 1694
Pharmacotherapy of Urinary Incontinence on page 1858

♦ **Imipramine Hydrochloride** see Imipramine on page 789

♦ **Imipramine Pamoate** see Imipramine on page 789

Imiquimod (i mi KWI mod)

U.S. Brand Names Aldara™

Generic Available No

Pharmacologic Category Skin and Mucous Membrane Agent; Topical Skin Product

Medication Safety Issues

Sound-alike/look-alike issues:
Aldara™ may be confused with Alora®

Use Treatment of external genital and perianal warts/condyloma acuminata in children ≥12 years of age and adults; nonhyperkeratotic, nonhypertrophic actinic keratosis; superficial basal cell carcinoma (SBCC)

Unlabeled/Investigational Use Treatment of common warts

Mechanism of Action/Effect Mechanism of action is unknown; however, induces cytokines, including interferon-alfa and others

Contraindications Hypersensitivity to imiquimod or any component of the formulation

Warnings/Precautions Imiquimod has not been evaluated for the treatment of urethral, intravaginal, cervical, rectal, or intra-anal human papilloma viral disease and is not recommended for these conditions. Topical imiquimod is not intended for ophthalmic use. Topical imiquimod administration is not recommended until genital/perianal tissue is healed from any previous drug or surgical treatment. Imiquimod has the potential to exacerbate inflammatory conditions of the skin. May increase sunburn susceptibility; patients should protect themselves from the sun. Use in basal cell carcinoma should be limited to superficial carcinomas with a maximum diameter of 2 cm. Efficacy in treatment of SBCC lesions of the face, head, and anogenital area, or other subtypes of basal cell carcinoma, have not been established. Safety and efficacy in immunosuppressed patients have not been established. Safety and efficacy in patients <12 years of age have not been established.

Drug Interactions

Cytochrome P450 Effect: Substrate (minor) of CYP1A2, 3A4

Adverse Reactions

>10%:
Local, mild/moderate: Erythema (54% to 61%), itching (22% to 32%), erosion (21% to 32%), burning (9% to 26%), excoriation/flaking (18% to 25%), edema (12% to 17%), scabbing (9% to 13%), fungal infection (2% to 11%)
Respiratory: Upper respiratory infection (15%)

1% to 10%:
Cardiovascular: Atrial fibrillation (1%)
Central nervous system: Pain (2% to 8%), headache (4% to 5%), fatigue (actinic keratosis 1%), fever (actinic keratosis 1%), dizziness (1%)
Endocrine & metabolic: Hypercholesterolemia (2%)
Gastrointestinal: Diarrhea (3%), dyspepsia (3%)
Local:
Severe: Hyperkeratosis (actinic keratosis 9%), erythema (4%), eczema (2%), erosion (1%), edema (1%), alopecia (actinic keratosis 1%)
Mild/moderate: Pain, induration, ulceration (5% to 7%), vesicles (2% to 3%), soreness (<1% to 3%)
Neuromuscular & skeletal: Myalgia (1%), back pain (actinic keratosis 1%)
Respiratory: Sinusitis (7%), pharyngitis (2%)
Miscellaneous: Influenza-like symptoms (1% to 3%), squamous cell carcinoma (4%)

Overdosage/Toxicology Overdosage is unlikely because of minimal percutaneous absorption. Persistent topical overdosing of imiquimod could result in severe local skin reactions. The most clinically serious adverse event reported following multiple oral imiquimod doses of ≥200 mg was hypotension that resolved following oral or I.V. fluid administration. Treat symptomatically

Pharmacodynamics/Kinetics
Absorption: Minimal

Excretion: Urine and feces (<0.9%)

Dosing
Adults & Elderly:
Perianal warts/condyloma acuminata: Topical: Apply 3 times/week on alternative days prior to bedtime and leave on skin for 6-10 hours. Remove by washing with mild soap and water. Continue imiquimod treatment until there is total clearance of the genital/perianal warts for ≤16 weeks. A rest period of several days may be taken if required by the patient's discomfort or severity of the local skin reaction. Treatment may resume once the reaction subsides.

Actinic keratosis: Topical: Apply twice weekly for 16 weeks to a treatment area on face or scalp; apply prior to bedtime and leave on skin for 8 hours. Remove with mild soap and water.

Common warts (unlabeled use): Topical: Apply once daily prior to bedtime.

Superficial basal cell carcinoma: Topical: Apply once daily prior to bedtime, 5 days/week for 6 weeks. Treatment area should include a 1 cm margin of skin around the tumor. Leave on skin for 8 hours.

Pediatrics: Perianal warts/condyloma acuminata: Topical: Children ≥12 years: Refer to adult dosing.

Available Dosage Forms Cream: 5% (12s) [contains benzyl alcohol; single-dose packets]

Monitoring and Teaching Issues
Physical Assessment: Teach patient appropriate use, possible side effects/appropriate interventions, and adverse symptoms to report.

Patient Education: This medication will not eliminate nor prevent the transmission of the virus. For external use only; avoid contact with eyes, mouth, or vagina. Use only as frequently as directed and apply as instructed. Exposure to sun should be avoided or minimized. Use sunscreen or wear protective clothing if sun exposure is unavoidable. Sexual contact (vaginal, anal, or oral) should be avoided while cream is on skin. May cause pain, itching, redness, burning, flaking, swelling, or scabbing in treated area. If these effects persist or become severe or open sores develop, stop treatment and notify prescriber. Prescriber may recommend a rest period of several days before resuming treatment. **Pregnancy/breast-feeding precautions:** Inform prescriber if you are or intend to become pregnant. This medication may weaken condoms or vaginal diaphragms; consult prescriber for appropriate forms of protection. Consult prescriber if breast-feeding.

Apply treatment just prior to sleeping and leave on 6-10 hours. Wash hands thoroughly before and after application. Wash and dry area to be treated before applying cream. After treatment period, remove cream with mild soap and water. Apply a thin layer to external warts and rub in until cream is no longer visible. Avoid use of excessive cream. May cover area with light gauze dressing or cotton underwear; do not apply occlusive dressing.

Pregnancy Risk Factor: C

Lactation: Excretion in breast milk unknown/consult prescriber

Administration
Topical: Nonocclusive dressings such as cotton gauze or cotton underwear may be used in the management of skin reactions. Handwashing before and after cream application is recommended. Imiquimod is packaged in single-use packets that contain sufficient cream to cover a wart area of up to 20 cm²; avoid use of excessive amounts of cream. Instruct patients to apply imiquimod to external or perianal warts; not for vaginal use. Apply a thin layer to the wart area and rub in until the cream is no longer visible. Do not occlude the application site.

Storage: Do not store at <25°C (7°F); avoid freezing.

♦ Imitrex® see Sumatriptan on page 1415
♦ Immune Globulin (Intramuscular) see page 1660

Immune Globulin (Intravenous) (i MYUN GLOB yoo lin, IN tra VEE nus)

U.S. Brand Names Carimune™ [DSC]; Carimune™ NF; Flebogamma®; Gamimune® N; Gammagard® S/D; Gammar®-P I.V.; Gamunex®; Iveegam EN; Octagam®; Panglobulin®; Panglobulin® NF; Polygam® S/D; Venoglobulin®-S [DSC]

Synonyms IVIG

Generic Available No

Pharmacologic Category Immune Globulin

Medication Safety Issues

Sound-alike/look-alike issues:

Gamimune® N may be confused with CytoGam®

Use

Treatment of primary immunodeficiency syndromes (congenital agammaglobulinemia, severe combined immunodeficiency syndromes [SCIDS], common variable immunodeficiency, X-linked immunodeficiency, Wiskott-Aldrich syndrome); idiopathic thrombocytopenic purpura (ITP); Kawasaki disease (in combination with aspirin)

Prevention of bacterial infection in B-cell chronic lymphocytic leukemia (CLL); pediatric HIV infection; bone marrow transplant (BMT)

Unlabeled/Investigational Use Autoimmune diseases (myasthenia gravis, SLE, bullous pemphigoid, severe rheumatoid arthritis), Guillain-Barré syndrome; used in conjunction with appropriate anti-infective therapy to prevent or modify acute bacterial or viral infections in patients with iatrogenically-induced or disease-associated immunodepression; autoimmune hemolytic anemia or neutropenia, refractory dermatomyositis/polymyositis

Mechanism of Action/Effect Replacement therapy for primary and secondary immunodeficiencies; interference with F_c receptors on the cells of the reticuloendothelial system for autoimmune cytopenias and ITP; possible role of contained antiviral-type antibodies

Contraindications Hypersensitivity to immune globulin or any component of the formulation; selective IgA deficiency

(Continued)

Immune Globulin (Intravenous) *(Continued)*

Warnings/Precautions Anaphylactic hypersensitivity reactions can occur, especially in IgA-deficient patients; studies indicate that the currently available products have no discernible risk of transmitting HIV or hepatitis B; aseptic meningitis may occur with high doses (≥2 g/kg). Use with caution in the elderly, patients with renal disease, diabetes mellitus, volume depletion, sepsis, paraproteinemia, and nephrotoxic medications due to risk of renal dysfunction. Patients should be adequately hydrated prior to therapy. Acute renal dysfunction (increased serum creatinine, oliguria, acute renal failure) can rarely occur; usually within 7 days of use (more likely with products stabilized with sucrose). Use caution in patients with a history of thrombotic events or cardiovascular disease; there is clinical evidence of a possible association between thrombotic events and administration of intravenous immune globulin. For intravenous administration only.

Drug Interactions

Decreased Effect: Decreased effect of live virus vaccines (eg, measles, mumps, rubella); separate administration by at least 3 months

Lab Interactions Octagam® contains maltose which may interfere with blood and urine glucose tests.

Adverse Reactions Frequency not defined.

Cardiovascular: Flushing of the face, tachycardia, hyper-/hypotension, chest tightness, angioedema, lightheadedness, chest pain, MI, CHF, pulmonary embolism

Central nervous system: Anxiety, chills, dizziness, drowsiness, fatigue, fever, headache, irritability, lethargy, malaise, aseptic meningitis syndrome

Dermatologic: Pruritus, rash, urticaria

Gastrointestinal: Abdominal cramps, diarrhea, nausea, sore throat, vomiting

Hematologic: Autoimmune hemolytic anemia, mild hemolysis

Hepatic: Liver function test increased

Local: Pain or irritation at the infusion site

Neuromuscular & skeletal: Arthralgia, back or hip pain, myalgia, nuchal rigidity

Ocular: Photophobia, painful eye movements

Renal: Acute renal failure, acute tubular necrosis, anuria, BUN increased, creatinine increased, nephrotic syndrome, oliguria, proximal tubular nephropathy, osmotic nephrosis

Respiratory: Cough, dyspnea, wheezing, nasal congestion, rhinorrhea, sinusitis

Miscellaneous: Diaphoresis, hypersensitivity reactions, anaphylaxis

Pharmacodynamics/Kinetics

Onset of Action: I.V.: Provides immediate antibody levels

Duration of Action: Immune effects: 3-4 weeks (variable)

Half-Life Elimination: IgG (variable among patients): Healthy subjects: 14-24 days; Patients with congenital humoral immunodeficiencies: 26-40 days; hypermetabolism associated with fever and infection have coincided with a shortened half-life

Dosing

Adults & Elderly: Approved doses and regimens may vary between brands; check manufacturer guidelines. **Note:** Some clinicians dose IVIG on ideal body weight or an adjusted ideal body weight in morbidly obese patients. The volume of distribution of IVIG preparations in healthy subjects is similar to that observed with endogenous IgG. IVIG remains primarily in the intravascular space. Patients with congenital humoral immunodeficiencies appear to have about 70% of the IVIG available in the intravascular space.

Primary immunodeficiency disorders: I.V.: 200-400 mg/kg every 4 weeks or as per monitored serum IgG concentrations

Flebogamma®, Gamunex®, Octagam®: 300-600 mg/kg every 3-4 weeks; adjusted based on dosage and interval in conjunction with monitored serum IgG concentrations.

B-cell chronic lymphocytic leukemia (CLL): I.V.: 400 mg/kg/dose every 3 weeks

Idiopathic thrombocytopenic purpura (ITP): I.V.:

Acute: 400 mg/kg/day for 5 days or 1000 mg/kg/day for 1-2 days

Chronic: 400 mg/kg as needed to maintain platelet count >30,000/mm³; may increase dose to 800 mg/kg (1000 mg/kg if needed)

Kawasaki disease: Initiate therapy within 10 days of disease onset: I.V.: 2 g/kg as a single dose administered over 10 hours, or 400 mg/kg/day for 4 days. **Note:** Must be used in combination with aspirin: 80-100 mg/kg/day in 4 divided doses for 14 days; when fever subsides, dose aspirin at 3-5 mg/kg once daily for ≥6-8 weeks

Acquired immunodeficiency syndrome (patients must be symptomatic) (unlabeled use): I.V.: Various regimens have been used, including:

200-250 mg/kg/dose every 2 weeks

or

400-500 mg/kg every month or every 4 weeks

Autoimmune hemolytic anemia and neutropenia (unlabeled use): I.V.: 1000 mg/kg/dose for 2-3 days

Autoimmune diseases (unlabeled use): I.V.: 400 mg/kg/day for 4 days

Bone marrow transplant: I.V.: 500 mg/kg beginning on days 7 and 2 pretransplant, then 500 mg/kg/week for 90 days post-transplant

Adjuvant to severe cytomegalovirus infections (unlabeled use): I.V.: 500 mg/kg/dose every other day for 7 doses

Guillain-Barré syndrome (unlabeled use): I.V.: Various regimens have been used, including:

400 mg/kg/day for 4 days

or

1000 mg/kg/day for 2 days

or

2000 mg/kg/day for one day

Refractory dermatomyositis (unlabeled use): I.V.: 2 g/kg/dose every month x 3-4 doses

Refractory polymyositis (unlabeled use): I.V.: 1 g/kg/day x 2 days every month x 4 doses

Chronic inflammatory demyelinating polyneuropathy (unlabeled use): I.V.: Various regimens have been used, including:

400 mg/kg/day for 5 doses once each month

or

800 mg/kg/day for 3 doses once each month

or

1000 mg/kg/day for 2 days once each month

Pediatrics: Approved doses and regimens may vary between brands; check manufacturer guidelines. **Note:** Some clinicians dose IVIG on ideal body weight or an adjusted ideal body weight in morbidly obese patients. The volume of distribution of IVIG preparations in healthy subjects is similar to that observed with endogenous IgG. IVIG remains primarily in the intravascular space. Patients with congenital humoral immunodeficiencies appear to have about 70% of the IVIG available in the intravascular space.

Pediatric HIV: I.V.: 400 mg/kg every 28 days

Severe systemic viral and bacterial infections: Children: I.V.: 500-1000 mg/kg/week

Prevention of gastroenteritis: Infants and Children: Oral: 50 mg/kg/day divided every 6 hours

For additional indications, refer to adult dosing.

Renal Impairment: Cl_{cr} <10 mL/minute: Avoid use; in patients at risk of renal dysfunction, consider infusion at a rate less than maximum.

Available Dosage Forms [DSC] = Discontinued product

Injection, powder for reconstitution [preservative free]:

Carimune™: 1 g, 3 g, 6 g, 12 g [contains sucrose] [DSC]

Gammar®-P I.V.: 1 g [DSC], 2.5 g [DSC], 5 g, 10 g [stabilized with human albumin and sucrose]

Iveegam EN: 0.5 g [DSC], 1 g [DSC], 2.5 g [DSC], 5 g [stabilized with glucose]

Panglobulin®: 6 g, 12 g [contains sucrose]

Injection, powder for reconstitution [preservative free, nanofiltered]:

Carimune™ NF: 3 g, 6 g, 12 g [contains sucrose]

Panglobulin® NF: 6 g, 12 g [contains sucrose]

Injection, powder for reconstitution [preservative free, solvent detergent treated]:

Gammagard® S/D: 2.5 g, 5 g, 10 g [stabilized with human albumin, glycine, glucose, and polyethylene glycol]

Polygam® S/D: 5 g, 10 g [stabilized with human albumin, glycine, glucose, and polyethylene glycol]

Injection, solution [preservative free; solvent detergent-treated]:

Gamimune® N: 10% [100 mg/mL] (10 mL, 25 mL, 50 mL, 100 mL, 200 mL)

Octagam®: 5% [50 mg/mL] (20 mL, 50 mL, 100 mL, 200 mL) [sucrose free; contains sodium 30 mmol/L and maltose]

Venoglobulin®-S: 5% [50 mg/mL] (50 mL, 100 mL, 200 mL); 10% [100 mg/mL] (50 mL, 100 mL, 200 mL) [stabilized with human albumin] [DSC]

Injection, solution [preservative free]:

Flebogamma®: 5% (10 mL, 50 mL, 100 mL, 200 mL) [PEG precipitated/chromatography purified]

Gamunex®: 10% (10 mL, 25 mL, 50 mL, 100 mL, 200 mL) [caprylate/chromatography purified]

Monitoring and Teaching Issues

Physical Assessment: Assess for history of previous allergic reactions. Patient should be monitored during infusion for vital sign changes and adverse or allergic reactions. Teach patient adverse symptoms to report.

Patient Education: This medication can only be administered by infusion. You will be monitored closely during the infusion. If you experience nausea ask for assistance, do not get up alone. Do not have any vaccinations for the next 3 months without consulting prescriber. Immediately report chills; chest pain, tightness, or rapid heartbeat; acute back pain; or respiratory difficulty. **Pregnancy/breast-feeding precautions:** Inform prescriber if you are or intend to become pregnant. Consult prescriber if breast-feeding.

Dietary Considerations: Octagam® contains sodium 30 mmol/L

Pregnancy Risk Factor: C

Lactation: Excretion in breast milk unknown

Administration

I.V.: For I.V. use only. For initial treatment, a lower concentration and/or a slower rate of infusion should be used.

Reconstitution: Dilution is dependent upon the manufacturer and brand; do not shake, avoid foaming; discard unused portion:

Carimune™ NF, Panglobulin® NF: Reconstitute with NS, D_5W, or SWFI.

Iveegam EN: Reconstitute with SWFI; use immediately after reconstitution

Gammagard® S/D, Polygam® S/D: Reconstitute with sterile water for injection; when diluted aseptically in a sterile laminar air flow hood, may store diluted solution under refrigeration for up to 24 hours. If reconstituted outside of laminar flow hood, use within 2 hours

Panglobulin®: Reconstitute with NS, D_5W, or SWFI; when diluted aseptically in a sterile laminar flow hood, may store diluted solution under refrigeration for up to 24 hours.

Gammar®-P I.V.: Reconstitute with SWFI.

Gamunex®: Dilute in D_5W only.

Compatibility: Stable in D_5W, $D_{15}W$, $D_5\frac{1}{4}NS$

Storage: Stability and dilution is dependent upon the manufacturer and brand; do not freeze:

Carimune™ NF, Panglobulin® NF: Prior to reconstitution, store at or below 30°C (86°F). Following reconstitution, store under refrigeration; use within 24 hours. Do not freeze.

Flebogamma®: Store at 2°C to 25°C (36°F to 77°F).

Gamimune® N, Iveegam EN: Store at 2°C to 8°C (36°F to 46°F).

(Continued)

Immune Globulin (Intravenous) *(Continued)*

Gammar®-P I.V., Gammagard® S/D, Polygam® S/D, Venoglobulin®-S: Store below 25°C (77°F).

Gamunex®: May be stored for up to 5 months at room temperature up to 25°C (up to 77°F) within 18 months of manufacture date.

Octagam®: Store at 2°C to 8°C (36°F to 46°F) for 24 months or ≤25°C (77°F) for 18 months.

Panglobulin®: Store at room temperature, below 30°C (86°F).

Polygam® S/D: Store at room temperature at or below 25°C (77°F); do not freeze.

Additional Information

Intravenous Immune Globulin Product Comparison:

Carimune™ NF, Panglobulin® NF:

FDA indication: Primary immunodeficiency, ITP
Contraindication: IgA deficiency
IgA content: 720 mcg/mL
Plasma source: Pooled donors
Half-life: 23 days
IgG subclass (%):
   IgG1 (60-70): 60.5
   IgG2 (19-31): 30.2
   IgG3 (5-8.4): 6.6
   IgG4 (0.7-4): 2.8
Storage: Room temperature at or below 30°C (86°F); refrigerate after reconstitution
Recommendations for **initial** infusion rate: 0.5-1 mL/minute
Maximum infusion rate: 2 mg/kg/minute

Flebogamma®:

FDA indication: Primary immunodeficiency
Contraindication: IgA deficiency, intolerance to fructose/sorbitol, history of anaphylaxis with blood products
IgA content: <50 mcg/mL
Plasma source: Pooled donors
Half-life: 30-45 days
IgG subclass (%):
   IgG_1 (60-70): 70
   IgG_2 (19-31): 25
   IgG_3 (5-8.4): 3
   IgG_4 (0.7-4): 2
Storage: 2°C to 25°C
Recommendations for **initial** infusion rate: 0.01 mL/kg/minute
Maximum infusion rate: 0.1 mL/kg/minute (0.06 mL/kg/minute in renal impairment)

Gamimune® N:

FDA indication: Primary immunodeficiency, ITP
Contraindication: IgA deficiency
IgA content: 270 mcg/mL
Adverse reactions (%): 5.2
Plasma source: >2000 paid donors
Half-life: 21 days
IgG subclass (%):
   IgG_1 (60-70): 60
   IgG_2 (19-31): 29.4
   IgG_3 (5-8.4): 6.5
   IgG_4 (0.7-4): 4.1
Monomers (%): >95
Gamma globulin (%): >98
Storage: Refrigerate
Recommendations for **initial** infusion rate: 0.01-0.02 mL/kg/minute
Maximum infusion rate: 0.08 mL/kg/minute
Maximum concentration for infusion (%): 10

Gammagard® SD:

FDA indication: Primary immunodeficiency, ITP, CLL prophylaxis
Contraindication: None (caution with IgA deficiency)
IgA content: 0.92-1.6 mcg/mL
Adverse reactions (%): 6
Plasma source: 4000-5000 paid donors
Half-life: 24 days
IgG subclass (%):
   IgG_1 (60-70): 67 (66.8)*
   IgG_2 (19-31): 25 (25.4)
   IgG_3 (5-8.4): 5 (7.4)
   IgG_4 (0.7-4): 3 (0.3)
Monomers (%): >95
Gamma globulin (%): >90
Storage: Room temperature
Recommendations for **initial** infusion rate: 0.5 mL/kg/hour
Maximum infusion rate: 4 mL/kg/hour
Maximum concentration for infusion (%): 5

Gammar®-P I.V.:

FDA indication: Primary immunodeficiency
Contraindication: IgA deficiency
IgA content: <20 mcg/mL
Adverse reactions (%): 15
Plasma source: >8000 paid donors

Half-life: 21-24 days
IgG subclass (%):
  IgG$_1$ (60-70): 69
  IgG$_2$ (19-31): 23
  IgG$_3$ (5-8.4): 6
  IgG$_4$ (0.7-4): 2
Monomers (%): >98
Gamma globulin (%): >98
Storage: Room temperature
Recommendations for **initial** infusion rate: 0.01-0.02 mL/kg/minute
Maximum infusion rate: 0.06 mL/kg/minute
Maximum concentration for infusion (%): 5

Gamunex®:
FDA indication: Primary immunodeficiency, ITP
Contraindication: Caution in severe, selective IgA deficiency
IgA content: 40 mcg/mL
IgM content: <2 mcg/mL
Plasma source: Pooled donors
Half-life: 36 days
IgG subclass (%):
  IgG$_1$ (60-70): 65
  IgG$_2$ (19-31): 26
  IgG$_3$ (5-8.4): 5.6
  IgG$_4$ (0.7-4): 2.6
Monomer + dimer (%): 100
Gamma globulin (%): >98
Storage: 2°C to 8°C; may be stored at room temperature for 5 months (only during first 18 months after manufacture)
Recommendations for **initial** infusion rate: 0.01 mL/kg/minute
Maximum infusion rate: 0.08 mL/kg/minute
Maximum concentration for infusion (%): 10

Octagam®:
FDA indication: Primary immunodeficiency
Contraindications: IgA deficiency
IgA content: 100 mcg/mL
Half-life: Immunodeficiency: 40 days
IgG subclass (%):
  IgG$_1$ (60-70): 65
  IgG$_2$ (19-31): 30
  IgG$_3$ (5-8.4): 3
  IgG$_4$ (0.7-4): 2
Monomers (%): ≥90
Gamma globulin (%): 96
Storage: Refrigerated or room temperature
Recommendations for initial infusion rate: 0.6 mL/kg/hour
Maximum infusion rate: 4 mL/kg/hour
Maximum concentration for infusion: 5%

Polygam®:
FDA indication: Primary immunodeficiency, ITP, CLL
Contraindication: None (caution with IgA deficiency)
IgA content: 0.74 ± 0.33 mcg/mL
Adverse reactions (%): 6
Plasma source: 50,000 voluntary donors
Half-life: 21-25 days
IgG subclass (%):
  IgG$_1$ (60-70): 67
  IgG$_2$ (19-31): 25
  IgG$_3$ (5-8.4): 5
  IgG$_4$ (0.7-4): 3
Monomers (%): >95
Gamma globulin (%): >90
Storage: Room temperature
Recommendations for **initial** infusion rate: 0.5 mL/kg/hour
Maximum infusion rate: 4 mL/kg/hour
Maximum concentration for infusion (%): 10

Venoglobulin®-S:
FDA indication: Primary immunodeficiency, ITP
Contraindication: IgA deficiency
IgA content: 20-24 mcg/mL
Adverse reactions (%): 6
Plasma source: 6000-9000 paid donors
Half-life: 29 days
IgG subclass (%):
  IgG$_1$ (60-70): 62.3**
  IgG$_2$ (19-31): 32.8
  IgG$_3$ (5-8.4): 2.9
  IgG$_4$ (0.7-4): 2
Monomers (%): >98
Gamma globulin (%): >98
Storage: Room temperature
Recommendations for **initial** infusion rate: 0.01-0.02 mL/kg/minute
Maximum infusion rate: 0.04 mL/kg/minute
Maximum concentration for infusion (%): 10
(Continued)

Immune Globulin (Intravenous) *(Continued)*

*Skvaril F and Gardi A, "Differences Among Available Immunoglobulin Preparations for Intravenous Use," *Pediatr Infect Dis J*, 1988, 7:543-48.

**Roomer J, Morgenthaler JJ, Scherz R, et al, "Characterization of Various Immunoglobulin Preparations for Intravenous Application," *Vox Sang*, 1982, 42:62-73.

♦ **Immunization Recommendations** *see page 1645*

♦ **Immunizations (Vaccines)** *see page 1660*

♦ **Imodium® A-D [OTC]** *see Loperamide on page 914*

♦ **Imogam®** *see page 1660*

♦ **Imovax® Rabies** *see page 1660*

♦ **Imuran®** *see Azathioprine on page 164*

♦ **Inapsine®** *see Droperidol on page 500*

Indapamide *(in DAP a mide)*

U.S. Brand Names Lozol®

Generic Available Yes

Pharmacologic Category Diuretic, Thiazide-Related

Medication Safety Issues

Sound-alike/look-alike issues:

Indapamide may be confused with Iopidine®

Use Management of mild to moderate hypertension; treatment of edema in congestive heart failure and nephrotic syndrome

Mechanism of Action/Effect Enhances sodium, chloride, and water excretion by interfering with the transport of sodium ions across the renal tubular epithelium

Contraindications Hypersensitivity to indapamide or any component of the formulation, thiazides, or sulfonamide-derived drugs; anuria; renal decompensation; pregnancy (based on expert analysis)

Warnings/Precautions Use with caution in severe renal disease. Use with caution in severe hepatic dysfunction; hepatic encephalopathy can be caused by electrolyte disturbances. Gout may be precipitated in patients with a history of gout, a familial predisposition to gout, or chronic renal failure. Use caution in patients with diabetes; may alter glucose control. May cause SLE exacerbation or activation. Use with caution in patients with moderate or high cholesterol concentrations. Photosensitization may occur. Correct hypokalemia before initiating therapy. Electrolyte disturbances (hypokalemia, hypochloremic alkalosis, hyponatremia) may occur with use.

Chemical similarities are present among sulfonamides, sulfonylureas, carbonic anhydrase inhibitors, thiazides, and loop diuretics (except ethacrynic acid). Use in patients with thiazide or sulfonamide allergy is specifically contraindicated in product labeling, however, a risk of cross-reaction exists in patients with allergy to any of these compounds; avoid use when previous reaction has been severe.

Drug Interactions

Decreased Effect: Effects of oral hypoglycemics may be decreased. Decreased absorption of indapamide with cholestyramine and colestipol. NSAIDs can decrease the efficacy of thiazide-type diuretics, reducing the diuretic and antihypertensive effects.

Increased Effect/Toxicity: The diuretic effect of indapamide is synergistic with furosemide and other loop diuretics. Increased hypotension and/or renal adverse effects of ACE inhibitors may result in aggressively diuresed patients. Cyclosporine and thiazide-type diuretics can increase the risk of gout or renal toxicity. Digoxin toxicity can be exacerbated if a diuretic induces hypokalemia or hypomagnesemia. Lithium toxicity can occur with thiazide-type diuretics due to reduced renal excretion of lithium. Thiazide-type diuretics may prolong the duration of action of neuromuscular blocking agents.

Nutritional/Ethanol Interactions Herb/Nutraceutical: Avoid dong quai if using for hypertension (has estrogenic activity). Avoid ephedra, yohimbe, ginseng (may worsen hypertension). Avoid garlic (may have increased antihypertensive effect).

Adverse Reactions 1% to 10%:

Cardiovascular: Orthostatic hypotension, palpitation (<5%), flushing

Central nervous system: Dizziness (<5%), lightheadedness (<5%), vertigo (<5%), headache (≥5%), restlessness (<5%), drowsiness (<5%), fatigue, lethargy, malaise, lassitude, anxiety, agitation, depression, nervousness (≥5%)

Dermatologic: Rash (<5%), pruritus (<5%), hives (<5%)

Endocrine & metabolic: Hyperglycemia (<5%), hyperuricemia (<5%)

Gastrointestinal: Anorexia, gastric irritation, nausea, vomiting, abdominal pain, cramping, bloating, diarrhea, constipation, dry mouth, weight loss

Genitourinary: Nocturia, frequent urination, polyuria, impotence (<5%), reduced libido (<5%), glycosuria (<5%)

Neuromuscular & skeletal: Muscle cramps, spasm, weakness (≥5%)

Ocular: Blurred vision (<5%)

Renal: Necrotizing angiitis, vasculitis, cutaneous vasculitis (<5%)

Respiratory: Rhinorrhea (<5%)

Overdosage/Toxicology Symptoms of overdose include lethargy, diuresis, hypermotility, confusion, and muscle weakness. Treatment is supportive.

Pharmacodynamics/Kinetics
Onset of Action: 1-2 hours
Duration of Action: ≤36 hours
Absorption: Complete
Time to Peak: 2-2.5 hours
Protein Binding: Plasma: 71% to 79%
Half-Life Elimination: 14-18 hours
Metabolism: Extensively hepatic
Excretion: Urine (~60%) within 48 hours; feces (~16% to 23%)

Dosing
Adults & Elderly:
Edema (diuretic): Oral: 2.5-5 mg/day. **Note:** There is little therapeutic benefit to increasing the dose >5 mg/day; there is, however, an increased risk of electrolyte disturbances.
Hypertension: Oral: 1.25 mg in the morning, may increase to 5 mg/day by increments of 1.25-2.5 mg; consider adding another antihypertensive and decreasing the dose if response is not adequate.

Available Dosage Forms
Tablet: 1.25 mg, 2.5 mg
Lozol®: 1.25 mg

Monitoring and Teaching Issues
Physical Assessment: Assess allergy history prior to beginning therapy (sulfonamides, thiazides). See Warnings/Precautions for specific use cautions (eg, renal or hepatic disease, diabetes, SLE, hyperlipidemia). Assess potential for interactions with other pharmacological agents or herbal products patient may be taking (eg, altered effect of oral hypoglycemics increased risk of hypotension or toxicity; see Drug Interactions). Assess results of laboratory tests, therapeutic effectiveness according to purpose for use, and adverse response at regular intervals during therapy (hypotension, hypokalemia, confusion; see Adverse Reactions). Instruct patients with diabetes to monitor glucose levels closely; may interfere with oral hypoglycemic medications. Teach patient proper use, possible side effects (eg, orthostatic hypotension, photosensitivity) and appropriate interventions, and adverse symptoms to report (see Patient Education).
Monitoring Laboratory Tests: Serum electrolytes, renal function
Patient Education: Do not take any new medication during therapy unless approved by prescriber. Take as directed, early in the day with food or milk. Do not exceed recommended dosage. This medication does not replace other antihypertensive interventions; follow prescriber's instructions for diet and lifestyle changes. If you have diabetes, monitor serum glucose closely (medication may decrease effect of oral hypoglycemics). Monitor weight on a regular basis. Report sudden or excessive weight gain (>5 lb/week), swelling of ankles or hands, or respiratory difficulty. You may experience dizziness, weakness, or drowsiness (use caution when rising from sitting or lying position, when climbing stairs and when driving or engaging in tasks that require alertness until response to drug is known); sensitivity to sunlight (use sunblock, wear protective clothing or sunglasses); impotence (reversible); or dry mouth or thirst (frequent mouth care, chewing gum, or sucking lozenges may help). Report any changes in visual acuity; unusual bleeding; chest pain or palpitations; or numbness, tingling, or cramping of muscles. **Pregnancy/breast-feeding precaution:** Inform prescriber if you are pregnant. Consult prescriber if breast-feeding.
Dietary Considerations: May be taken with food or milk to decrease GI adverse effects.
Geriatric Considerations: Thiazide diuretics lose efficacy when Cl_{cr} is <30-35 mL/minute. Many elderly may have Cl_{cr} below this limit. Calculate Cl_{cr} for elderly before initiating therapy. Indapamide has the advantage over thiazide diuretics in that it is effective when Cl_{cr} is <30 mL/minute.
Pregnancy Risk Factor: B (manufacturer); D (expert analysis)
Lactation: Excretion in breast milk unknown

Administration
Oral: May be taken with food or milk. Take early in day to avoid nocturia. Take the last dose of multiple doses no later than 6 PM unless instructed otherwise.

♦ **Inderal®** *see Propranolol on page 1273*
♦ **Inderal® LA** *see Propranolol on page 1273*
♦ **Inderide®** *see Propranolol and Hydrochlorothiazide on page 1276*

Indinavir (in DIN a veer)
U.S. Brand Names Crixivan®
Synonyms Indinavir Sulfate
Generic Available No
Pharmacologic Category Antiretroviral Agent, Protease Inhibitor
Medication Safety Issues
Sound-alike/look-alike issues:
Indinavir may be confused with Denavir™
Use Treatment of HIV infection; should always be used as part of a multidrug regimen (at least three antiretroviral agents)
Mechanism of Action/Effect Indinavir is a protease inhibitor which prevents cleavage of protein precursors essential for HIV infection of new cells and viral replication.
Contraindications Hypersensitivity to indinavir or any component of the formulation; concurrent use of amiodarone, cisapride, triazolam, midazolam, pimozide, or ergot alkaloids
Warnings/Precautions Because indinavir may cause nephrolithiasis/urolithiasis the drug should be discontinued if signs and symptoms occur. Adequate hydration is recommended. May cause tubulointerstitial nephritis (rare); severe asymptomatic leukocyturia may warrant evaluation. Indinavir should not be administered concurrently with lovastatin or simvastatin (caution with atorvastatin and cerivastatin) because of competition for metabolism of these drugs through the CYP3A4 system, and potential serious or life-threatening events. Use caution with other drugs metabolized by this enzyme (particular caution with phosphodiesterase-5 inhibitors, including sildenafil). Avoid concurrent use of St John's wort. Patients with (Continued)

Indinavir *(Continued)*

hepatic insufficiency due to cirrhosis should have dose reduction. Warn patients about fat redistribution that can occur. Indinavir has been associated with hemolytic anemia (discontinue if diagnosed), hepatitis, and hyperglycemia (exacerbation or new-onset diabetes). Treatment may result in immune reconstitution syndrome (acute inflammatory response to indolent or residual opportunistic infections). Use caution in patients with hemophilia; spontaneous bleeding has been reported.

Drug Interactions

Cytochrome P450 Effect: Substrate of CYP2D6 (minor), 3A4 (major); **Inhibits** CYP2C8/9 (weak), 2C19 (weak), 2D6 (weak), 3A4 (strong)

Decreased Effect: The levels/effects of indinavir may be decreased by aminoglutethimide, carbamazepine, nafcillin, nevirapine, phenobarbital, phenytoin, rifamycins, and other CYP3A4 inducers; dosage adjustment may be recommended (see individual agents). Rifampin and/or St John's wort (*Hypericum perforatum*); should not be used with indinavir.

Increased Effect/Toxicity: Indinavir may increase the levels/effects of selected benzodiazepines, calcium channel blockers, cyclosporine, mirtazapine, nateglinide, nefazodone, quinidine, sildenafil (and other PDE-5 inhibitors), tacrolimus, venlafaxine, and other CYP3A4 substrates. Selected benzodiazepines (midazolam, triazolam), cisapride, ergot alkaloids, selected HMG-CoA reductase inhibitors (lovastatin and simvastatin), mesoridazine, pimozide, and thioridazine are generally contraindicated with strong CYP3A4 inhibitors. When used with strong CYP3A4 inhibitors, dosage adjustment/limits are recommended for sildenafil and other PDE-5 inhibitors; refer to individual monographs.

Itraconazole or ketoconazole may increase the serum concentrations of indinavir; dosage adjustment is recommended. The levels/effects of indinavir may be increased by azole antifungals, ciprofloxacin, clarithromycin, diclofenac, doxycycline, erythromycin, imatinib, isoniazid, nefazodone, nicardipine, propofol, protease inhibitors, quinidine, verapamil, and other CYP3A4 inhibitors.

When used with delavirdine, serum levels of indinavir are increased; dosage adjustment of indinavir may be required for this combination. Serum levels of both nelfinavir and indinavir are increased with concurrent use. Serum concentrations of indinavir may be increased by ritonavir; serum levels of ritonavir and saquinavir may be increased; dosage adjustments of indinavir are required during concurrent therapy. Rifabutin serum concentrations has been increased when coadministered with indinavir; dosage adjustments of both agents required. Concurrent use or atazanavir with indinavir may increase the risk of hyperbilirubinemia.

Nutritional/Ethanol Interactions

Food: Indinavir bioavailability may be decreased if taken with food. Meals high in calories, fat, and protein result in a significant decrease in drug levels. Indinavir serum concentrations may be decreased by grapefruit juice.

Herb/Nutraceutical: St John's wort *(Hypericum)* appears to induce CYP3A enzymes and has lead to 57% reductions in indinavir AUCs and 81% reductions in trough serum concentrations, which may lead to treatment failures; should not be used concurrently with indinavir.

Adverse Reactions

Protease inhibitors cause dyslipidemia which includes elevated cholesterol and triglycerides and a redistribution of body fat centrally to cause increased abdominal girth, buffalo hump, facial atrophy, and breast enlargement. These agents also cause hyperglycemia (exacerbation or new-onset diabetes).

10%:

Gastrointestinal: Nausea (12%)
Hepatic: Hyperbilirubinemia (14%)
Renal: Nephrolithiasis/urolithiasis (29%, pediatric patients; 12% adult patients)

1% to 10%:

Central nervous system: Headache (6%), insomnia (3%)
Gastrointestinal: Abdominal pain (9%), diarrhea/vomiting (4% to 5%), taste perversion (3%)
Neuromuscular & skeletal: Weakness (4%), flank pain (3%)
Renal: Hematuria

Pharmacodynamics/Kinetics

Absorption: Administration with a high fat, high calorie diet resulted in a reduction in AUC and in maximum serum concentration (77% and 84% respectively); lighter meal resulted in little or no change in these parameters.

Bioavailability: Good

Time to Peak: 0.8 ± 0.3 hour

Protein Binding: Plasma: 60%

Half-Life Elimination: 1.8 ± 0.4 hour

Metabolism: Hepatic via CYP3A4 enzymes; seven metabolites of indinavir identified

Excretion: Urine and feces

Dosing

Adults & Elderly: HIV: Oral: 800 mg every 8 hours

Note: Dosage adjustments for indinavir when administered in combination therapy:

Delavirdine, itraconazole, or ketoconazole: Reduce indinavir dose to 600 mg every 8 hours

Efavirenz: Increase indinavir dose to 1000 mg every 8 hours

Lopinavir and ritonavir (Kaletra™): Indinavir 600 mg twice daily

Nevirapine: Increase indinavir dose to 1000 mg every 8 hours

Rifabutin: Reduce rifabutin to $1/2$ the standard dose plus increase indinavir to 1000 mg every 8 hours

Ritonavir: Adjustments necessary for both agents:

Ritonavir 100-200 mg twice daily plus indinavir 800 mg twice daily **or**

Ritonavir 400 mg twice daily plus indinavir 400 mg twice daily

Pediatrics: HIV: Investigational: 500 mg/m^2 every 8 hours (patients with smaller BSA may require lower doses of 300-400 mg/m^2 every 8 hours)

Hepatic Impairment: 600 mg every 8 hours with mild/medium impairment due to cirrhosis or with ketoconazole coadministration

Available Dosage Forms Capsule: 100 mg, 200 mg, 333 mg, 400 mg

Monitoring and Teaching Issues

Physical Assessment: See Warnings/Precautions for specific use cautions (hepatic insufficiency, hemophilia). Assess potential for interactions with other pharmacological agents or herbal products patient may be taking (see Drug Interactions for specific interaction warnings). Assess results of laboratory tests, therapeutic effectiveness (CD4 count and viral load), and adverse response at regular intervals during treatment (eg, dyslipidemia, nephrolithiasis, hyperglycemia, leukocyturia; see Adverse Reactions). Teach patient proper use (importance of following multidrug regimen), possible side effects/appropriate interventions (eg, glucose testing; protease inhibitors may cause hyperglycemia [exacerbation or new-onset diabetes]), and adverse symptoms to report (see Patient Education).

Monitoring Laboratory Tests: Monitor viral load, CD4 count, triglycerides, cholesterol, glucose, liver function tests, CBC, urinalysis (severe leukocyturia should be monitored frequently).

Patient Education: Do not take any new medication during therapy unless approved by prescriber. Indinavir is not a cure for AIDS, nor will it prevent transmission of HIV. Take as directed, around-the-clock, with a large glass of water, preferably 1 hour before or 2 hours after meals. May take with light meal (eg, dry toast, skim milk, corn flakes) to reduce GI upset. Capsules are sensitive to moisture medication should be stored and used in the original container and the desiccant should remain in the bottle. Maintain adequate hydration (2-3 L/day of fluids) unless instructed to restrict fluid intake. Indinavir may be prescribed with a combination of other medications; time these medications as directed by prescriber. You may be advised to check your glucose levels (this drug can cause exacerbation of diabetes or new-onset diabetes). May cause body changes due to redistribution of body fat, facial atrophy, or breast enlargement (normal effects of drug); nausea or vomiting (small frequent meals, frequent mouth care, chewing gum, or sucking lozenges may help); muscle weakness or flank pain (consult prescriber for approved analgesic); or headache or insomnia (consult prescriber for medication). Report chest pain or palpitations, difficult or painful urination, persistent diarrhea or vomiting, or other persistent adverse effects. **Pregnancy/breast-feeding precautions:** Inform prescriber if you are or intend to become pregnant. Do not breast-feed.

Dietary Considerations: Should be taken without food but with water 1 hour before or 2 hours after a meal. Administration with lighter meals (eg, dry toast, skim milk, corn flakes) resulted in little/no change in indinavir concentration. If taking with ritonavir, may take with food. Patient should drink at least 48 oz of water daily.

Pregnancy Risk Factor: C

Pregnancy Issues: Safety and pharmacokinetic studies are currently underway in pregnant women; hyperbilirubinemia may be exacerbated in neonates and indinavir plasma levels may be lower in pregnant women. Pregnancy and protease inhibitors are both associated with an increased risk of hyperglycemia. Glucose levels should be closely monitored. The Perinatal HIV Guidelines Working Group considers indinavir to be an alternative PI if nelfinavir or saquinavir/ritonavir are not able to be used. Healthcare professionals are encouraged to contact the antiretroviral pregnancy registry to monitor outcomes of pregnant women exposed to antiretroviral medications (1-800-258-4263 or www.APRegistry.com).

Lactation: Enters breast milk/contraindicated

Breast-Feeding Issues: Indinavir is minimally excreted in breast milk. HIV-infected mothers are discouraged from breast-feeding to decrease potential transmission of HIV.

Administration

Oral: Drink at least 48 oz of water daily. Administer with water, 1 hour before or 2 hours after a meal. Administer around-the-clock to avoid significant fluctuation in serum levels.

Storage: Capsules are sensitive to moisture; medication should be stored and used in the original container and the desiccant should remain in the bottle

Related Information
Tuberculosis *on page 1864*

Indomethacin (in doe METH a sin)

U.S. Brand Names Indocin®; Indocin® I.V.; Indocin® SR

Synonyms Indometacin; Indomethacin Sodium Trihydrate

Generic Available Yes: Capsule, suspension

Pharmacologic Category Nonsteroidal Anti-inflammatory Drug (NSAID), Oral; Nonsteroidal Anti-inflammatory Drug (NSAID), Parenteral

Medication Safety Issues
Sound-alike/look-alike issues:
Indocin® may be confused with Imodium®, Lincocin®, Minocin®, Vicodin®

Use Management of inflammatory diseases and rheumatoid disorders; moderate pain; acute gouty arthritis, acute bursitis/tendonitis, moderate to severe osteoarthritis, rheumatoid arthritis, ankylosing spondylitis; I.V. form used as alternative to surgery for closure of patent ductus arteriosus in neonates

Mechanism of Action/Effect Inhibits prostaglandin synthesis by decreasing the activity of the enzyme, cyclooxygenase, which results in decreased formation of prostaglandin precursors

Contraindications Hypersensitivity to indomethacin, any component of the formulation, aspirin, or other NSAIDs; patients in whom asthma, urticaria, or rhinitis are precipitated by
(Continued)

Indomethacin *(Continued)*

NSAIDs/aspirin; active GI bleeding or ulcer disease; premature neonates with necrotizing enterocolitis; impaired renal function; active bleeding; thrombocytopenia; pregnancy (3rd trimester)

Warnings/Precautions Fatal asthmatic and anaphylactoid reactions have occurred in patients with "aspirin triad." Use with caution in patients with CHF, hypertension, dehydration, decreased renal or hepatic function, history of GI disease (bleeding, ulcers, or previous GI symptoms with NSAID use), or those receiving anticoagulants and/or corticosteroids. Use lowest effective dose for shortest period possible; bleeding risk has been correlated to dose and duration of therapy. Gastrointestinal bleeding may occur without prior symptoms of gastrointestinal irritation. Elderly are at a high risk for adverse effects from NSAIDs. As many as 60% of elderly can develop peptic ulceration and/or hemorrhage asymptomatically.

Use of NSAIDs can compromise existing renal function especially when Cl_{cr} <30 mL/minute. CNS adverse effects such as confusion, agitation, and hallucination are generally seen in overdose or high-dose situations; however, elderly may demonstrate these adverse effects at lower doses than younger adults. Withhold for at least 4-6 half-lives prior to surgical or dental procedures.

Drug Interactions

Cytochrome P450 Effect: Substrate (minor) of CYP2C8/9, 2C19; **Inhibits** CYP2C8/9 (strong), 2C19 (weak)

Decreased Effect: May decrease antihypertensive effects of beta-blockers, hydralazine, ACE inhibitors, and angiotensin II antagonists. Indomethacin may decrease the antihypertensive and diuretic effect of thiazides (eg, hydrochlorothiazide) and loop diuretics (furosemide, bumetanide).

Increased Effect/Toxicity: Indomethacin may increase serum potassium with potassium-sparing diuretics. Probenecid may increase indomethacin serum concentrations. Other NSAIDs may increase GI adverse effects. May increase nephrotoxicity of cyclosporine and increase renal adverse effects of ACE inhibitors. Indomethacin may increase serum concentrations of digoxin, methotrexate, lithium, and aminoglycosides (reported with I.V. use in neonates). Indomethacin may increase the levels/effects of amiodarone, fluoxetine, glimepiride, glipizide, nateglinide, phenytoin, pioglitazone, rosiglitazone, sertraline, warfarin, and other CYP2C8/9 substrates.

Nutritional/Ethanol Interactions

Ethanol: Avoid ethanol (may enhance gastric mucosal irritation).

Food: Food may decrease the rate but not the extent of absorption. Indomethacin peak serum levels may be delayed if taken with food.

Herb/Nutraceutical: Avoid cat's claw, dong quai, evening primrose, feverfew, garlic, ginger, ginkgo, red clover, horse chestnut, green tea, ginseng (all have additional antiplatelet activity).

Lab Interactions Positive Coombs' [direct]; increased sodium, chloride, bleeding time

Adverse Reactions

>10%: Central nervous system: Headache (12%)

1% to 10%:

Central nervous system: Dizziness (3% to 9%), drowsiness (<1%), fatigue (<3%), vertigo (<3%), depression (<3%), malaise (<3%), somnolence (<3%)

Gastrointestinal: Nausea (3% to 9%), epigastric pain (3% to 9%), abdominal pain/cramps/distress (<3%), anorexia (<1%), GI bleeding (<1%), ulcers (<1%), perforation (<1%), heartburn (<3%), indigestion (3% to 9%), constipation (<3%), diarrhea (<3%), dyspepsia (3% to 9%)

Hematologic: Inhibition of platelet aggregation (3% to 9%)

Otic: Tinnitus (<3%)

Overdosage/Toxicology Symptoms of overdose include drowsiness, lethargy, nausea, vomiting, seizures, paresthesia, headache, dizziness, GI bleeding, cerebral edema, tinnitus, leukocytosis, and renal failure. Management of NSAID intoxication is supportive and symptomatic.

Pharmacodynamics/Kinetics

Onset of Action: ~30 minutes

Duration of Action: 4-6 hours

Absorption: Prompt and extensive

Time to Peak: Oral: ~3-4 hours

Protein Binding: 90%

Half-Life Elimination: 4.5 hours; prolonged with neonates

Metabolism: Hepatic; significant enterohepatic recirculation

Excretion: Urine (primarily as glucuronide conjugates)

Dosing

Adults & Elderly: Inflammatory/rheumatoid disorders: Oral: 25-50 mg/dose 2-3 times/day; maximum dose: 200 mg/day; extended release capsule should be given on a 1-2 times/day schedule; maximum dose for sustained release is 150 mg/day; best to start older adults on 25 mg dose given 2-3 times/day

Pediatrics:

Patent ductus arteriosus:

Neonates: I.V.: Initial: 0.2 mg/kg, followed by 2 doses depending on postnatal age (PNA):

PNA at time of FIRST dose <48 hours: 0.1 mg/kg at 12- to 24-hour intervals

PNA at time of FIRST dose 2-7 days: 0.2 mg/kg at 12- to 24-hour intervals

PNA at time of FIRST dose >7 days: 0.25 mg/kg at 12- to 24-hour intervals

Note: In general, may use 12-hour dosing interval if urine output >1 mL/kg/hour after prior dose; use 24-hour dosing interval if urine output is <1 mL/kg/hour but >0.6 mL/kg/hour; doses should be withheld if patient has oliguria (urine output <0.6 mL/kg/hour) or anuria

Inflammatory/rheumatoid disorders: Children: Oral: 1-2 mg/kg/day in 2-4 divided doses; maximum dose: 4 mg/kg/day; not to exceed 150-200 mg/day

Available Dosage Forms

Capsule (Indocin®): 25 mg, 50 mg

Capsule, sustained release (Indocin® SR): 75 mg

Injection, powder for reconstitution, as sodium trihydrate (Indocin® I.V.): 1 mg

Suspension, oral (Indocin®): 25 mg/5 mL (237 mL) [contains alcohol 1%; pineapple-coconut-mint flavor]

Monitoring and Teaching Issues

Physical Assessment: Assess potential for interactions with other prescriptions, OTC medications, or herbal products patient may be taking. Assess results of laboratory tests, therapeutic effectiveness (according to rationale for use), and adverse response when beginning therapy and at regular intervals during treatment. Teach patient proper use, side effects/appropriate interventions (regular ophthalmic evaluations with long-term use), and adverse symptoms to report.

Monitoring Laboratory Tests: Renal function (serum creatinine, BUN), CBC, liver function

Patient Education: Do not take any new medication during therapy without consulting prescriber. Use exactly as directed; do not increase dose without consulting prescriber. Do not crush, break, or chew capsules. Take with food or milk to reduce GI distress. Maintain adequate hydration (2-3 L/day of fluids) unless instructed to restrict fluid intake. May cause drowsiness, dizziness, nervousness, or headache (use caution when driving or engaging in tasks that require alertness until response to drug is known); anorexia, nausea, vomiting, or heartburn (small frequent meals, frequent mouth care, chewing gum, or sucking lozenges may help): fluid retention (weigh yourself weekly and report unusually weight gain >3-5 lb/week); or may turn urine green (normal). GI bleeding, ulceration, or perforation can occur with or without pain; discontinue medication and contact prescriber if persistent abdominal pain or cramping or blood in stool occurs. Report difficult breathing or unusual cough; chest pain, rapid heartbeat, or palpitations; unusual bruising or bleeding; blood in urine, gums, or vomitus; swollen extremities; skin rash, irritation, or itching; acute persistent fatigue; or vision changes or ringing in ears. **Pregnancy/breast-feeding precautions:** Inform prescriber if you are or intend to become pregnant. This drug should not be used in the 3rd trimester of pregnancy. Consult prescriber if breast-feeding.

Dietary Considerations: May cause GI upset, bleeding, ulceration, perforation; take with food or milk to minimize GI upset.

Geriatric Considerations: Elderly are at high risk for adverse effects from NSAIDs. As much as 60% of elderly can develop peptic ulceration and/or hemorrhage asymptomatically. The concomitant use of H_2 blockers, omeprazole, and sucralfate is not effective as prophylaxis with the exception of NSAID-induced duodenal ulcers which may be prevented by the use of ranitidine. Misoprostol is the only prophylactic agent proven effective. Also, concomitant disease and drug use contribute to the risk for GI adverse effects. Use lowest effective dose for shortest period possible. Consider renal function decline with age. Use of NSAIDs can compromise existing renal function especially when Cl_{cr} is ≤30 mL/minute. Tinnitus may be a difficult and unreliable indication of toxicity due to age-related hearing loss or eighth cranial nerve damage. CNS adverse effects such as confusion, agitation, and hallucination are generally seen in overdose or high-dose situations, but elderly may demonstrate these adverse effects at lower doses than younger adults. Indomethacin frequently causes confusion at recommended doses in the elderly.

Pregnancy Risk Factor: B/D (3rd trimester)

Lactation: Enters breast milk/use caution (AAP rates "compatible")

Administration

Oral: Administer with food, milk, or antacids to decrease GI adverse effects. Extended release capsules must be swallowed whole, do not crush.

I.V.: Administer over 20-30 minutes at a concentration of 0.5-1 mg/mL in preservative-free sterile water for injection or normal saline. Reconstitute I.V. formulation just prior to administration; discard any unused portion; avoid I.V. bolus administration or infusion via an umbilical catheter into vessels near the superior mesenteric artery as these may cause vasoconstriction and can compromise blood flow to the intestines. Do not administer intra-arterially.

Reconstitution: Reconstitute just prior to administration; discard any unused portion. Do not use preservative-containing diluents for reconstitution.

Compatibility: Stable in NS

Y-site administration: Incompatible with amino acid injection, calcium gluconate, cimetidine, dobutamine, dopamine, gentamicin, levofloxacin, tobramycin, tolazoline

Storage: I.V.: Store below 30°C (86°F). Protect from light.

Related Information

Nonsalicylate / Nonsteroidal Anti-inflammatory Agents *on page 1743*

- ♦ **Indomethacin Sodium Trihydrate** *see* Indomethacin *on page 801*
- ♦ **INF-alpha 2** *see* Interferon Alfa-2b *on page 811*
- ♦ **Infanrix®** *see page 1660*
- ♦ **INFeD®** *see* Iron Dextran Complex *on page 833*
- ♦ **Infergen®** *see* Interferon Alfacon-1 *on page 817*

Infliximab (in FLIKS e mab)

U.S. Brand Names Remicade®

Synonyms Infliximab, Recombinant

Generic Available No

Pharmacologic Category Antirheumatic, Disease Modifying; Gastrointestinal Agent, Miscellaneous; Monoclonal Antibody; Tumor Necrosis Factor (TNF) Blocking Agent

Medication Safety Issues

Sound-alike/look-alike issues:

Remicade® may be confused with Renacidin®, Rituxan®

Use

Ankylosing spondylitis: Improving signs and symptoms of disease

(Continued)

Infliximab (Continued)

Crohn's disease: Induction and maintenance of remission in patients with moderate to severe disease who have an inadequate response to conventional therapy; to reduce the number of draining enterocutaneous and rectovaginal fistulas and to maintain fistula closure

Rheumatoid arthritis: Inhibits the progression of structural damage and improves physical function in patients with moderate to severe disease; used with methotrexate

Mechanism of Action/Effect Infliximab is a monoclonal antibody that binds to human tumor necrosis factor alpha (TNFα), thereby decreasing inflammatory and other responses.

Contraindications Hypersensitivity to murine proteins or any component of the formulation; doses >5 mg/kg in patients with moderate or severe congestive heart failure (NYHA Class III/IV)

Warnings/Precautions Serious infections (including sepsis, pneumonia, and fatal infections) have been reported in patients receiving TNF-blocking agents. Many of the serious infections in patients treated with infliximab have occurred in patients on concomitant immunosuppressive therapy. Caution should be exercised when considering the use of infliximab in patients with a chronic infection or history of recurrent infection. Infliximab should not be given to patients with a clinically important, active infection. Patients who develop a new infection while undergoing treatment with infliximab should be monitored closely. If a patient develops a serious infection or sepsis, infliximab should be discontinued. Reactivation of hepatitis B has occurred in chronic virus carriers; evaluate prior to initiation and during treatment. Patients should be evaluated for latent tuberculosis infection with a tuberculin skin test prior to infliximab therapy. Treatment of latent tuberculosis should be initiated before infliximab is used. Tuberculosis (may be disseminated or extrapulmonary) has been reactivated in patients previously exposed to TB while on infliximab. Most cases have been reported within the first 3-6 months of treatment. Other opportunistic infections (eg, invasive fungal infections, listeriosis, *Pneumocystis*) have occurred during therapy. The risk/benefit ratio should be weighed in patients who have resided in regions where histoplasmosis is endemic.

Impact on the development and course of malignancies is not fully defined. As compared to the general population, an increased risk of lymphoma has been noted in clinical trials; however, rheumatoid arthritis has been previously associated with an increased rate of lymphoma.

Severe hepatic reactions have been reported during treatment. Use caution with CHF; if a decision is made to use with CHF, monitor closely and discontinue if exacerbated or new symptoms occur. Use caution with history of hematologic abnormalities; hematologic toxicities (eg, leukopenia, neutropenia, thrombocytopenia, pancytopenia) have been reported; discontinue if significant abnormalities occur. Autoimmune antibodies and a lupus-like syndrome have been reported. If antibodies to double-stranded DNA are confirmed in a patient with lupus-like symptoms, infliximab should be discontinued. Rare cases of demyelinating disease have been reported, use with caution in patients with pre-existing or recent onset CNS demyelinating disorders, or seizures; discontinue if significant CNS adverse reactions develop.

Medications for the treatment of hypersensitivity reactions should be available for immediate use. Safety and efficacy for use in juvenile rheumatoid arthritis and in pediatric patients with Crohn's disease have not been established.

Drug Interactions
Decreased Effect: Specific drug interaction studies have not been conducted.

Decreased toxicity: Immunosuppressants: When used with infliximab, may decrease the risk of infusion related reactions, and may decrease development of antidouble-stranded DNA antibodies

Increased Effect/Toxicity: Specific drug interaction studies have not been conducted. Infliximab may be associated with increased risk of serious infection when used in combination with anakinra.

Adverse Reactions Note: Although profile is similar, frequency of effects may be different in specific populations (Crohn's disease vs rheumatoid arthritis). Percentages reported with rheumatoid arthritis:

>10%:

Central nervous system: Headache (18%)

Dermatologic: Rash (10%)

Gastrointestinal: Nausea (21%), diarrhea (12%), abdominal pain (12%)

Genitourinary: Urinary tract infection (8%)

Local: Infusion reactions (20%)

Neuromuscular & skeletal: Arthralgia (8%), back pain (8%)

Respiratory: Upper respiratory tract infection (32%), cough (12%), sinusitis (14%), pharyngitis (12%)

Miscellaneous: Development of antinuclear antibodies (~50%), infection (36%), development of antibodies to double-stranded DNA (17%); Crohn's patients with fistulizing disease: Development of new abscess (15%)

5% to 10%:

Cardiovascular: Hypertension (7%)

Central nervous system: Pain (8%), fatigue (9%), fever (7%)

Dermatologic: Pruritus (7%)

Gastrointestinal: Dyspepsia (10%)

Respiratory: Bronchitis (10%), dyspnea (6%), rhinitis (8%)

Miscellaneous: Moniliasis (5%)

Overdosage/Toxicology Doses of up to 20 mg/kg have been given without toxic effects. In case of overdose, treatment should be symptom-directed and supportive.

Pharmacodynamics/Kinetics
Onset of Action: Crohn's disease: ~2 weeks
Half-Life Elimination: 8-9.5 days

Dosing
Adults & Elderly:
Crohn's disease: I.V.:
Induction regimen: 5 mg/kg at 0, 2, and 6 weeks, followed by 5 mg/kg every 8 weeks; dose may be increased to 10 mg/kg in patients who respond but then lose their response. If no response by week 14, consider discontinuing therapy.
Rheumatoid arthritis: I.V. (in combination with methotrexate therapy): 3 mg/kg at 0, 2, and 6 weeks then every 8 weeks thereafter; doses have ranged from 3-10 mg/kg intravenous infusion repeated at 4- to 8-week intervals
Ankylosing spondylitis: I.V.: 5 mg/kg at 0, 2, and 6 weeks, followed by 5 mg/kg every 6 weeks thereafter
Dosage adjustment with CHF: Weigh risk versus benefits for individual patient:
NYHA Class III or IV: ≤5 mg/kg
Pediatrics: Safety and efficacy have not been established
Renal Impairment: No adjustment is recommended.
Hepatic Impairment: No adjustment necessary.
Available Dosage Forms Injection, powder for reconstitution [preservative free]: 100 mg

Monitoring and Teaching Issues
Physical Assessment: Monitor therapeutic effectiveness, adverse reactions. Place and read PPD before initiation. Treatment of latent TB infection should be initiated prior to treatment with infliximab. Teach patient appropriate interventions to reduce side effects and adverse symptoms to report.
Patient Education: This drug can only be administered by infusion. Avoid receiving immunizations unless approved by prescriber. Report headache or unusual fatigue; increased nausea or abdominal pain; cough, runny nose, respiratory difficulty; chest pain or persistent dizziness; fatigue, muscle pain or weakness, back pain; fever or chills; mouth sores; vaginal itching or discharge; sore throat; unhealed sores; or frequent infections. **Breast-feeding precaution:** Breast-feeding is not recommended.
Pregnancy Risk Factor: B (manufacturer)
Pregnancy Issues: Reproduction studies have not been conducted. Use during pregnancy only if clearly needed. A Rheumatoid Arthritis and Pregnancy Registry has been established for women exposed to infliximab during pregnancy (Organization of Teratology Information Services, 877-311-8972).
Lactation: Excretion in breast milk unknown/not recommended
Breast-Feeding Issues: It is not known whether infliximab is secreted in human milk. Because many immunoglobulins are secreted in milk and the potential for serious adverse reactions exists, a decision should be made whether to discontinue nursing or discontinue the drug, taking into account the importance of the drug to the mother.

Administration
I.V.: Infuse over at least 2 hours.
Reconstitution: Reconstitute vials with 10 mL sterile water for injection; swirl vial gently to dissolve powder, do not shake, allow solution to stand for 5 minutes; total dose of reconstituted product should be further diluted to 250 mL of 0.9% sodium chloride injection; infusion of dose should begin within 3 hours of preparation
Compatibility: Do not infuse with other agents.
Storage: Store vials at 2°C to 8°C (36°F to 46°F). Do not freeze.

- ◆ **Infliximab, Recombinant** *see* Infliximab *on page 803*
- ◆ **Influenza Virus Vaccine** *see page 1660*
- ◆ **Infumorph®** *see* Morphine Sulfate *on page 1031*
- ◆ **INH** *see* Isoniazid *on page 836*
- ◆ **Inhalant Agents** *see page 1734*
- ◆ **Innohep®** *see* Tinzaparin *on page 1482*
- ◆ **InnoPran XL™** *see* Propranolol *on page 1273*
- ◆ **Inotropic and Vasoconstrictor Comparison** *see page 1736*
- ◆ **Inspra™** *see* Eplerenone *on page 529*

Insulin Preparations (IN su lin prep a RAY shuns)
U.S. Brand Names Apidra™; Humalog®; Humalog® Mix 75/25™; Humulin® 50/50; Humulin® 70/30; Humulin® L; Humulin® N; Humulin® R; Humulin® R (Concentrated) U-500; Humulin® U; Lantus®; Lente® Iletin® II [DSC]; Novolin® 70/30; Novolin® L [DSC]; Novolin® N; Novolin® R; NovoLog®; NovoLog® Mix 70/30; NPH Iletin® II; Regular Iletin® II; Velosulin® BR (Buffered) [DSC]
Synonyms Aspart, Insulin; Glargine, Insulin; Glulisine, Insulin; Lente, Insulin; Lispro, Insulin; NPH, Insulin; Regular, Insulin
Generic Available No
Pharmacologic Category Antidiabetic Agent, Insulin; Antidote

Medication Safety Issues
Sound-alike/look-alike issues:
Humalog® may be confused with Humulin®
Humalog® Mix 75/25™ may be confused with Humulin® 70/30.
Humulin® may be confused with Humalog®, Humira®
Lantus® may be confused with Lente®
Lente® may be confused with Lantus®
Novolin® may be confused with NovoLog®
Novolin® 70/30 may be confused with NovoLog® Mix 70/30
NovoLog® may be confused with Novolin®
NovoLog® Mix 70/30 may be confused with Novolin® 70/30
(Continued)

Insulin Preparations *(Continued)*

High alert medication: The Institute for Safe Medication Practices (ISMP) includes this medication among its list of drugs which have a heightened risk of causing significant patient harm when used in error.

Concentrated solutions (eg, U-500) should not be available in patient care areas.

Use Treatment of type 1 diabetes mellitus (insulin dependent, IDDM); type 2 diabetes mellitus (noninsulin dependent, NIDDM) unresponsive to treatment with diet and/or oral hypoglycemics; adjunct to parenteral nutrition

Unlabeled/Investigational Use Hyperkalemia (regular insulin only; use with glucose to shift potassium into cells to lower serum potassium levels)

Mechanism of Action/Effect The principal hormone required for proper glucose utilization in normal metabolic processes; it is obtained from beef or pork pancreas or a biosynthetic process converting pork insulin to human insulin; insulins are categorized into 3 groups related to promptness, duration, and intensity of action

Contraindications Hypersensitivity to any component of the formulation

Warnings/Precautions Hypoglycemia is the most common adverse effect of insulin. The timing of hypoglycemia differs among various insulin formulations. Any change of insulin should be made cautiously; changing manufacturers, type and/or method of manufacture, may result in the need for a change of dosage; human insulin differs from animal-source insulin; regular insulin is the only insulin to be used I.V.; hypoglycemia may result from increased work or exercise without eating; use of long-acting insulin preparations (insulin glargine, Ultralente®, insulin U) may delay recovery from hypoglycemia; use with caution in renal or hepatic impairment

In type 1 diabetes mellitus (insulin dependent, IDDM), insulin lispro (Humalog®) and insulin glulisine (Apidra™) should be used in combination with a long-acting insulin. However, in type 2 diabetes mellitus (noninsulin dependent, NIDDM), insulin lispro (Humalog®) may be used without a long-acting insulin when used in combination with a sulfonylurea.

Insulin aspart (Apidra™, NovoLog®, NovoLog® Mix 70/30): Safety and efficacy of use in children have not been established

Drug Interactions

Cytochrome P450 Effect: Induces CYP1A2 (weak)

Decreased Effect: Decreased hypoglycemic effect of insulin with corticosteroids, dextrothyroxine, diltiazem, dobutamine, epinephrine, niacin, oral contraceptives, thiazide diuretics, thyroid hormone, and smoking.

Increased Effect/Toxicity: Increased hypoglycemic effect of insulin with alcohol, alpha-blockers, anabolic steroids, beta-blockers (nonselective beta-blockers may delay recovery from hypoglycemic episodes and mask signs/symptoms of hypoglycemia; cardioselective beta-blocker agents may be alternatives), clofibrate, guanethidine, MAO inhibitors, pentamidine, phenylbutazone, salicylates, sulfinpyrazone, and tetracyclines.

Insulin increases the risk of hypoglycemia associated with oral hypoglycemic agents (including sulfonylureas, metformin, pioglitazone, rosiglitazone, and troglitazone).

Nutritional/Ethanol Interactions

Ethanol: Caution with ethanol (may increase hypoglycemia).

Food: Insulin shifts potassium from extracellular to intracellular space. Decreases potassium serum concentration.

Herb/Nutraceutical: Use caution with chromium, garlic, gymnema (may increase hypoglycemia).

Adverse Reactions Frequency not defined.

Cardiovascular: Palpitation, tachycardia, pallor

Central nervous system: Fatigue, mental confusion, loss of consciousness, headache, hypothermia

Dermatologic: Urticaria, redness

Endocrine & metabolic: Hypoglycemia

Gastrointestinal: Hunger, nausea, numbness of mouth

Local: Itching, edema, stinging, pain or warmth at injection site; atrophy or hypertrophy of SubQ fat tissue

Neuromuscular & skeletal: Muscle weakness, paresthesia, tremor

Ocular: Transient presbyopia or blurred vision

Miscellaneous: Diaphoresis, anaphylaxis, local allergy, systemic allergic symptoms

Overdosage/Toxicology Symptoms of overdose include tachycardia, anxiety, hunger, tremor, pallor, headache, motor dysfunction, speech disturbances, sweating, palpitations, coma, and death. Antidote is glucose and glucagon, if necessary.

Pharmacodynamics/Kinetics

Onset of Action: Biosynthetic NPH human insulin is more rapid than corresponding porcine insulins; human insulin and purified porcine regular insulin are similarly efficacious following SubQ administration. Medium-acting SubQ Lente®-type human insulins did not differ from the corresponding porcine insulins

Insulin aspart (NovoLog®): 0.17-0.33 hours; Peak effect: 1-3 hours

Inulin lispro (Humalog®), insulin glulisine (Apidra™): 0.25 hours; Peak effect: 0.5-1.5 hours

Insulin aspart (NovoLog®): 0.5 hours; Peak effect: 1-3 hours

Insulin, regular (Novolin® R): 0.5-1 hours; Peak effect: 2-3 hours

Isophane insulin suspension (NPH) (Novolin® N): 1-1.5 hours; Peak effect: 4-12 hours

Insulin zinc suspension (Lente®): 1-2.5 hours; Peak effect: 8-12 hours

Isophane insulin suspension and regular insulin injection (Novolin® 70/30): 0.5 hours; Peak effect: 2-12 hours

Extended insulin zinc suspension (Ultralente®): 4-8 hours; Peak effect: 16-18 hours

Duration of Action: Biosynthetic NPH human insulin shows a shorter duration of action than corresponding porcine insulins; human insulin and purified porcine regular insulin are similarly efficacious following SubQ administration. The duration of action of highly purified porcine insulins is shorter than that of conventional insulin equivalents. Duration depends on type of preparation and route of administration as well as patient-related variables. In general, the larger the dose of insulin, the longer the duration of activity.

Insulin aspart (NovoLog®): 3-5 hours

Lispro (Humalog®): 6-8 hours

Insulin, regular (Novolin® R): 8-12 hours

Isophane insulin suspension (NPH) (Novolin® N): 24 hours

Insulin zinc suspension (Lente®): 18-24 hours

Isophane insulin suspension and regular insulin injection (Novolin® 70/30): 24 hours

Extended insulin zinc suspension (Ultralente®): >36 hours

Insulin glargine (Lantus®): 24 hours

Absorption: Biosynthetic regular human insulin is absorbed from the SubQ injection site more rapidly than insulins of animal origin (60-90 minutes peak vs 120-150 minutes peak respectively) and lowers the initial blood glucose much faster. Human Ultralente® insulin is absorbed about twice as quickly as its bovine equivalent, and bioavailability is also improved. Human Lente® insulin preparations are also absorbed more quickly than their animal equivalents. Insulin glargine (Lantus®) is designed to form microprecipitates when injected subcutaneously. Small amounts of insulin glargine are then released over a 24-hour period, with no pronounced peak. Insulin glargine (Lantus®) for the treatment of type 1 diabetes (insulin dependent, IDDM) and type 2 diabetes mellitus (noninsulin dependent, NIDDM) in patients who require basal (long-acting) insulin.

Bioavailability: Medium-acting SubQ Lente®-type human insulins did not differ from the corresponding porcine insulins

Dosing

Adults & Elderly: Dose requires continuous medical supervision; may administer I.M., or SubQ; regular insulin may also be administered I.V.

Diabetes mellitus: The number and size of daily doses, time of administration, and diet and exercise require continuous medical supervision. In addition, specific formulations may require distinct administration procedures (see Administration).

Usual initial dose: 0.5-1 unit/kg/day in divided doses

Adjust dose to maintain premeal and bedtime blood glucose of 80-140 mg/dL (children <5 years: 100-200 mg/dL)

Insulin glargine (Lantus®): SubQ:

Type 2 diabetes (patient not already on insulin): 10 units once daily, adjusted according to patient response (range in clinical study 2-100 units/day)

Patients already receiving insulin: In clinical studies, when changing to insulin glargine from once-daily NPH or Ultralente® insulin, the initial dose was not changed; when changing from twice-daily NPH to once-daily insulin glargine, the total daily dose was reduced by 20% and adjusted according to patient response

Hyperkalemia (unlabeled use): Administer dextrose at 0.5-1 mL/kg and regular insulin 1 unit for every 4-5 g dextrose given

Diabetic ketoacidosis: Children and Adults: Regular insulin: I.V. loading dose: 0.1 unit/kg, then maintenance continuous infusion: 0.1 unit/kg/hour (range: 0.05-0.2 units/kg/hour depending upon the rate of decrease of serum glucose - too rapid decrease of serum glucose may lead to cerebral edema).

Optimum rate of decrease (serum glucose): 80-100 mg/dL/hour

Note: Newly-diagnosed patients with IDDM presenting in DKA and patients with blood sugars <800 mg/dL may be relatively "sensitive" to insulin and should receive loading and initial maintenance doses approximately $1/2$ of those indicated above.

Infusion should continue until reversal of acid-base derangement/ketonemia. Serum glucose is not a direct indicator of these abnormalities, and may decrease more rapidly than correction of the range of metabolic abnormalities.

Pediatrics: Refer to adult dosing. Adolescents (growth spurts): 0.8-1.2 units/kg/day in divided doses.

Renal Impairment: Insulin requirements are reduced due to changes in insulin clearance or metabolism.

Cl_{cr} 10-50 mL/minute: Administer 75% of normal dose.

Cl_{cr} <10 mL/minute: Administer 25% to 50% of normal dose and monitor glucose closely.

Hemodialysis: Because of a large molecular weight (6000 daltons), insulin is not significantly removed by either peritoneal or hemodialysis.

Supplemental dose is not necessary.

Peritoneal dialysis: Supplemental dose is not necessary.

Continuous arteriovenous or venovenous hemofiltration effects: Supplemental dose is not necessary.

Available Dosage Forms [DSC] = Discontinued product

RAPID-ACTING:

Injection, solution, aspart, human:

NovoLog®: 100 units/mL (10 mL vial)

NovoLog® [InnoLet®]: 100 units/mL (3 mL prefilled syringe)

NovoLog® [PenFill®]: 100 units/mL (3 mL cartridge)

Injection, solution, lispro, human (Humalog®): 100 units/mL (1.5 mL cartridge [DSC], 3 mL disposable pen, 10 mL vial)

Injection, solution, glulisine (Apidra™): 100 units/mL (10 mL vial)

SHORT-ACTING:

Injection, solution, regular, human:

Humulin® R: 100 units/mL (10 mL vial)

Novolin® R: 100 units/mL (1.5 mL prefilled syringe, 10 mL vial)

Novolin® R [PenFill®]: 100 units/mL (1.5 mL cartridge, 3 mL cartridge)

Injection, solution, regular, human, buffered (Velosulin® BR) [DSC]: 100 units/mL (10 mL vial)

Injection, solution, regular, human, concentrate (Humulin® R U-500): 500 units/mL (20 mL vial)

Injection, solution, regular, purified pork (Regular Iletin® II): 100 units/mL (10 mL vial)

(Continued)

Insulin Preparations *(Continued)*

INTERMEDIATE-ACTING:

Injection, suspension, lente, human [zinc] (Humulin® L, Novolin® L [DSC]): 100 units/mL (10 mL vial)

Injection, suspension, lente, purified pork [zinc] (Lente® Iletin® II): 100 units/mL (10 mL vial) [DSC]

Injection, suspension, NPH, human [isophane]:

Humulin® N: 100 units/mL (3 mL disposable pen, 10 mL vial)

Novolin® N: 100 units/mL (1.5 mL prefilled syringe, 10 mL vial)

Novolin® N [PenFill®]: 100 units/mL (1.5 mL cartridge, 3 mL cartridge)

Injection, suspension, NPH, purified pork [isophane] (NPH Iletin® II): 100 units/mL (10 mL vial)

LONG-ACTING:

Injection, suspension, Ultralente®, human [zinc] (Humulin® U Ultralente®): 100 units/mL (10 mL vial)

Injection, solution, glargine, human (Lantus®): 100 unit/mL (10 mL vial)

COMBINATION, INTERMEDIATE-ACTING:

Injection, aspart protamine human suspension 70% and rapid-acting aspart human solution 30% (NovoLog® Mix 70/30): 100 units/mL (3 mL cartridge, 3 mL prefilled syringe)

Injection, lispro protamine human suspension 75% and rapid-acting lispro human solution 25% (Humalog® Mix 75/25™): 100 units/mL (3 mL disposable pen, 10 mL vial)

Injection, NPH human insulin suspension 50% and short-acting regular human insulin solution 50% (Humulin® 50/50): 100 units/mL (10 mL vial)

Injection, NPH human insulin suspension 70% and short-acting regular human insulin solution 30%:

Humulin® 70/30: 100 units/mL (3 mL disposable pen, 10 mL vial)

Novolin® 70/30: 100 units/mL (1.5 mL prefilled syringe, 10 mL vial)

Novolin® 70/30 [PenFill®]: 100 units/mL (1.5 mL cartridge, 3 mL cartridge)

Monitoring and Teaching Issues

Physical Assessment: Assess potential for interactions with other prescriptions, OTC medications, or herbal products patient may be taking. Assess results of laboratory tests, therapeutic effectiveness, and adverse response (eg, hypoglycemia) at regular intervals during therapy. Teach patient proper use, including appropriate injection technique and syringe/needle disposal and monitoring requirements (or refer to diabetic educator), possible side effects/appropriate interventions, and adverse symptoms to report.

Monitoring Laboratory Tests: Urine sugar and acetone, serum glucose, electrolytes, Hb A$_{1c}$, lipid profile

Patient Education: Do not take any new medication during therapy unless approved by prescriber. This medication is used to control diabetes; it is not a cure. It is imperative to follow other components of prescribed treatment (eg, diet and exercise regimen). Take exactly as directed. Do not change dose or discontinue unless advised by prescriber. With insulin aspart (NovoLog®), you must start eating within 5-10 minutes after injection. Insulin glulisine (Apidra™) should be administered within 15 minutes before or within 20 minutes after start of meal. If you experience hypoglycemic reaction, contact prescriber immediately. Always carry quick source of sugar with you. Monitor glucose levels as directed by prescriber. Report adverse side effects, including chest pain or palpitations; persistent fatigue, confusion, headache; skin rash or redness; numbness of mouth, lips, or tongue; muscle weakness or tremors; vision changes; respiratory difficulty; or nausea, vomiting, or flu-like symptoms. **Pregnancy precaution:** Inform prescriber if you are or intend to become pregnant.

Dietary Considerations: Dietary modification based on ADA recommendations is a part of therapy. Monitor potassium serum concentration.

Geriatric Considerations: How "tightly" a geriatric patient's blood glucose should be controlled is controversial; however, a fasting blood sugar <150 mg/dL is now an acceptable end point. Such a decision should be based on the patient's functional and cognitive status, how well they recognize hypoglycemic or hyperglycemic symptoms, and how to respond to them and their other disease states. Patients who are unable to accurately draw up their dose will need assistance such as prefilled syringes. Initial doses may require considerations for renal function in the elderly with dosing adjusted subsequently based on blood glucose monitoring.

Pregnancy Risk Factor: B; C (insulin glargine [Lantus®]; insulin aspart [NovoLog®])

Pregnancy Issues: Does not cross the placenta. Insulin is the drug of choice for the control of diabetes mellitus during pregnancy.

Lactation: Does not enter breast milk/compatible

Breast-Feeding Issues: The gastrointestinal tract destroys insulin when administered orally and therefore would not be expected to be absorbed intact by the breast-feeding infant.

Administration

I.V.: Regular insulin may be administered by SubQ, I.M., or I.V. routes. Buffered insulin (Velosulin® BR) should not be administered with any other form of insulin.

I.V. administration (requires use of an infusion pump): **Only regular insulin** may be administered I.V.

To be ordered as units/hour: Example: Standard diluent of regular insulin only: 100 units/100 mL NS (can be given as a more diluted solution, ie, 100 units/250 mL NS)

Other: SubQ administration: Cold injections should be avoided. SubQ administration is usually made into the thighs, arms, buttocks, or abdomen, with sites rotated. When mixing regular insulin with other preparations of insulin, regular insulin should be drawn into syringe first. Buffered insulin (Velosulin® BR) should not be mixed with any other form of insulin.

Insulin lispro (Humalog®): May be administered within 15 minutes before or immediately after a meal.

Insulin glulisine (Apidra™): Should be administered within 15 minutes before or within 20 minutes after start of meal. Can be infused SubQ by external insulin pump; do not dilute or mix with other insulins when used in an external pump for SubQ infusion; should replace insulin in reservoir every 48 hours.

Insulin aspart (NovoLog®): Should be administered immediately before a meal (within 5-10 minutes of the start of a meal). Can be infused SubQ by external insulin pump; do not dilute or mix with other insulins when used in an external pump for SubQ infusion; should replace insulin in reservoir every 48 hours.

Human regular insulin: Should be administered within 30-60 minutes before a meal.

Intermediate-acting insulins (such as NPH): May be administered 1-2 times/day.

Long-acting insulins (such as Ultralente®, Lantus®): May be administered once daily.

Insulin glargine (Lantus®): Should be administered once daily, at any time of day, but should be administered at the same time each day. Cannot be diluted or mixed with any other insulin or solution.

Regular insulin may be administered by SubQ, I.M., or I.V. routes

Reconstitution: Standard diluent for regular insulin: 100 units/100 mL NS; **Note:** All bags should be prepared fresh; tubing should be flushed 30 minutes prior to administration to allow adsorption as time permits

Compatibility: Buffered insulin (Velosulin® BR) should not be mixed with any other form of insulin. Isophane insulin suspension (NPH) is **compatible** with regular insulin. Protamine zinc insulin suspension is **compatible** with regular insulin. Insulin glulisine (Apidra™) may be mixed with NPH insulin in the same syringe (glulisine should be withdrawn first).

Y-site administration: Incompatible with dopamine, nafcillin, norepinephrine, ranitidine

Compatibility when admixed: Incompatible with aminophylline, amobarbital, chlorothiazide, cytarabine, dobutamine, methylprednisolone sodium succinate, octreotide, pentobarbital, phenobarbital, phenytoin, thiopental

Storage:

Newer neutral formulation of regular insulin is stable at room temperature up to one month (studies indicate up to 24-30 months)

Insulin aspart (NovoLog®) and insulin glulisine (Apidra™): Can be infused SubQ by external insulin pump; do not dilute or mix with other insulins when used in an external pump for SubQ infusion; insulin in reservoir should be replaced every 48 hours. Do not expose to temperatures ≥37°C (98.6°F).

Insulin glargine (Lantus®): When refrigeration is unavailable, 10 mL vials may be stored at room temperature for up to 28 days; solution not used within this time must be discarded

Insulin lispro (Humalog®): Prior to use, store in refrigerator; do not use if it has been frozen. If not refrigerated, use within 28 days and protect from heat and light. Once opened (in-use), vials may be stored in refrigerator or for up to 28 days at room temperature. Cartridges/pens should be stored at room temperature and used within 28 days.

Freezing causes more damage to insulin than room temperatures up to 100°F. Avoid direct sunlight.

Additional Information The term "purified" refers to insulin preparations containing no more than 10 ppm proinsulin (purified and human insulins are less immunogenic). Buffering agent in Velosulin® BR may alter the activity of other insulin products.

Related Information

Diabetes Mellitus Management *on page 1819*

♦ **Intal**® *see* Cromolyn *on page 374*

♦ **Integrilin**® *see* Eptifibatide *on page 537*

♦ **α-2-Interferon** *see* Interferon Alfa-2b *on page 811*

Interferon Alfa-2a (in ter FEER on AL fa too aye)

U.S. Brand Names Roferon-A®

Synonyms IFLrA; rIFN-A

Restrictions An FDA-approved medication guide is available at www.fda.gov/cder/Offices/ODS/labeling.htm; distribute to each patient to whom this medication is dispensed.

Generic Available No

Pharmacologic Category Interferon

Medication Safety Issues

Sound-alike/look-alike issues:

Interferon alfa-2a may be confused with interferon alfa-2b

Roferon-A® may be confused with Rocephin®

Use

Patients >18 years of age: Hairy cell leukemia, AIDS-related Kaposi's sarcoma, chronic hepatitis C

Children and Adults: Chronic myelogenous leukemia (CML), Philadelphia chromosome positive, within 1 year of diagnosis (limited experience in children)

Unlabeled/Investigational Use Adjuvant therapy for malignant melanoma, AIDS-related thrombocytopenia, cutaneous ulcerations of Behçet's disease, brain tumors, metastatic ileal carcinoid tumors, cervical and colorectal cancers, genital warts, idiopathic mixed cryoglobulinemia, hemangioma, hepatitis D, hepatocellular carcinoma, idiopathic hypereosinophilic syndrome, mycosis fungoides, Sézary syndrome, low-grade non-Hodgkin's lymphoma, macular degeneration, multiple myeloma, renal cell carcinoma, basal and squamous cell skin cancer, essential thrombocythemia, cutaneous T-cell lymphoma

Mechanism of Action/Effect Alpha interferons are a family of proteins that have antiviral, antiproliferative, and immune-regulating activity. Inhibits cell growth and proliferation and enhances immune response.

Contraindications Hypersensitivity to alfa interferon, benzyl alcohol, or any component of the formulation; autoimmune hepatitis; visceral AIDS-related Kaposi's sarcoma associated with rapidly-progressing or life-threatening disease; hepatic decompensation (Child-Pugh Class B or C)

(Continued)

Interferon Alfa-2a *(Continued)*

Warnings/Precautions Use caution in patients with a history of depression. May cause severe psychiatric adverse events (psychosis, mania, depression, suicidal behavior/ideation) in patients with and without previous psychiatric symptoms; careful neuropsychiatric monitoring is required during therapy. Use with caution in patients with seizure disorders, brain metastases, or compromised CNS function. Higher doses in the elderly or in malignancies other than hairy cell leukemia may result in severe obtundation.

Use caution in patients with autoimmune diseases, pre-existing cardiac disease (ischemic or thromboembolic), arrhythmias, renal impairment (Cl_{cr} <50 mL/minute), mild hepatic impairment, or myelosuppression. Also use caution in patients receiving therapeutic immunosuppression. Use caution in patients with diabetes or pre-existing thyroid disease. Discontinue if persistent unexplained pulmonary infiltrates are noted. Gastrointestinal ischemia, ulcerative colitis and hemorrhage have been associated rarely with alpha interferons; some cases are severe and life-threatening. Ophthalmologic disorders have occurred in patients receiving alpha interferons; close monitoring is warranted.

Treatment should be discontinued in patients with worsening or persistently severe signs/symptoms of autoimmune, infectious, ischemic, or neuropsychiatric disorders (including depression and/or suicidal thoughts/behavior). Discontinue treatment if neutrophils <0.5 x 10^9/L or platelets <25 x 10^9/L. **Due to differences in dosage, patients should not change brands of interferons.** Injection solution contains benzyl alcohol; do not use in neonates or infants. Safety and efficacy in children <18 years of age have not been established.

Drug Interactions

Cytochrome P450 Effect: Inhibits CYP1A2 (weak)

Decreased Effect: Prednisone may decrease the therapeutic effects of interferon alpha. A decreased response to erythropoietin has been reported (case reports) in patients receiving interferons. Interferon alpha may decrease the serum concentrations of melphalan (may or may not decrease toxicity of melphalan).

Increased Effect/Toxicity: Note: May exacerbate the toxicity of other agents with respect to CNS, myelotoxicity, or cardiotoxicity. Theophylline clearance has been reported to be decreased in hepatitis patients receiving interferon. Interferons may increase the adverse/toxic effects of ACE inhibitors, specifically the development of granulocytopenia. Agranulocytosis has been reported with concurrent use of clozapine (case report). Interferons may increase the anticoagulant effects of warfarin, and interferons may increase serum levels of zidovudine.

Adverse Reactions Note: A flu-like syndrome (fever, chills, tachycardia, malaise, myalgia, arthralgia, headache) occurs within 1-2 hours of administration; may last up to 24 hours and may be dose-limiting (symptoms in up to 92% of patients). For the listing below, the percentage of incidence noted generally corresponds to highest reported ranges. Incidence depends upon dosage and indication.

>10%:
Cardiovascular: Chest pain (4% to 11%), edema (11%), hypertension (11%)
Central nervous system: Psychiatric disturbances (including depression and suicidal behavior/ideation; reported incidence highly variable, generally >15%), fatigue (90%), headache (52%), dizziness (21%), irritability (15%), insomnia (14%), somnolence, lethargy, confusion, mental impairment, and motor weakness (most frequently seen at high doses [>100 million units], usually reverses within a few days); vertigo (19%); mental status changes (12%)
Dermatologic: Rash (usually maculopapular) on the trunk and extremities (7% to 18%), alopecia (19% to 22%), pruritus (13%), dry skin
Endocrine & metabolic: Hypocalcemia (10% to 51%), hyperglycemia (33% to 39%), transaminases increased (25% to 30%), alkaline phosphatase increased (48%)
Gastrointestinal: Loss of taste, anorexia (30% to 70%), nausea (28% to 53%), vomiting (10% to 30%, usually mild), diarrhea (22% to 34%, may be severe), taste change (13%), dry throat, xerostomia, abdominal cramps, abdominal pain
Hematologic: (often due to underlying disease): Myelosuppression; neutropenia (32% to 70%); thrombocytopenia (22% to 70%); anemia (24% to 65%, may be dose-limiting, usually seen only during the first 6 months of therapy)
Onset: 7-10 days
Nadir: 14 days, may be delayed 20-40 days in hairy cell leukemia
Recovery: 21 days
Hepatic: Elevation of AST (SGOT) (77% to 80%), LDH (47%), bilirubin (31%)
Local: Injection site reaction (29%)
Neuromuscular & skeletal: Weakness (may be severe at doses >20,000,000 units/day); arthralgia and myalgia (5% to 73%, usually during the first 72 hours of treatment); rigors
Renal: Proteinuria (15% to 25%)
Respiratory: Cough (27%), irritation of oropharynx (14%)
Miscellaneous: Flu-like syndrome (up to 92% of patients), diaphoresis (15%)
1% to 10%:
Cardiovascular: Hypotension (6%), supraventricular tachyarrhythmia, palpitation (<3%), acute MI (<1% to 1%)
Central nervous system: Confusion (10%), delirium
Dermatologic: Erythema (diffuse), urticaria
Endocrine & metabolic: Hyperphosphatemia (2%)
Gastrointestinal: Stomatitis, pancreatitis (<5%), flatulence, liver pain
Genitourinary: Impotence (6%), menstrual irregularities
Neuromuscular & skeletal: Leg cramps; peripheral neuropathy, paresthesia (7%), and numbness (4%) are more common in patients previously treated with vinca alkaloids or receiving concurrent vinblastine
Ocular: Conjunctivitis (4%)
Respiratory: Dyspnea (7.5%), epistaxis (4%), rhinitis (3%)
Miscellaneous: Antibody production to interferon (10%)

Overdosage/Toxicology Symptoms of overdose include CNS depression, obtundation, flu-like symptoms, and myelosuppression. Treatment is supportive.

Pharmacodynamics/Kinetics

Absorption: Filtered and absorbed at the renal tubule

Bioavailability: I.M.: 83%; SubQ: 90%

Time to Peak: Serum: I.M., SubQ: ~6-8 hours

Half-Life Elimination: I.V.: 3.7-8.5 hours (mean: ~5 hours)

Metabolism: Primarily renal; filtered through glomeruli and undergoes rapid proteolytic degradation during tubular reabsorption

Dosing

Adults & Elderly: Refer to individual protocols.

Hairy cell leukemia: SubQ, I.M.: 3 million units/day for 16-24 weeks, then 3 million units 3 times/week for up to 6-24 months

Chronic myelogenous leukemia (CML): SubQ, I.M.: 9 million units/day, continue treatment until disease progression

AIDS-related Kaposi's sarcoma: SubQ, I.M.: 36 million units/day for 10-12 weeks, then 36 million units 3 times/week; to minimize adverse reactions, can use escalating dose (3-, 9-, then 18 million units each day for 3 days, then 36 million units daily thereafter).

Hepatitis C: SubQ, I.M.: 3 million units 3 times/week for 12 months

Pediatrics: Refer to individual protocols. Children (limited data):

Chronic myelogenous leukemia (CML): I.M.: 2.5-5 million units/m^2/day. **Note:** In juveniles, higher dosages (30 million units/m^2/day) have been associated with severe adverse events, including death.

Renal Impairment: Not removed by hemodialysis

Available Dosage Forms Injection, solution, [single-dose prefilled syringe; SubQ use only]: 3 million units/0.5 mL (0.5 mL); 6 million units/0.5 mL (0.5 mL); 9 million units/0.5 mL (0.5 mL) [contains benzyl alcohol]

Monitoring and Teaching Issues

Physical Assessment: Assess results of laboratory results on a regular basis. Monitor for effectiveness of therapy and possible adverse reactions. Monitor for neuropsychiatric changes. Patients with pre-existing cardiac abnormalities or advanced stages of cancer should have ECG before and during treatment. Assess knowledge/instruct patient/caregiver on appropriate reconstitution, injection and needle disposal, possible side effects, and symptoms to report.

Monitoring Laboratory Tests: Baseline chest x-ray, ECG, CBC with differential, liver function, electrolytes, platelets

Patient Education: Use as directed; do not change dosage or schedule of administration without consulting prescriber. Maintain adequate hydration (2-3 L/day of fluids) unless instructed to restrict fluid intake. You may experience flu-like syndrome (acetaminophen may help); nausea, vomiting, dry mouth, or metallic taste (small frequent meals, frequent mouth care, sucking lozenges, or chewing gum may help); or drowsiness, dizziness, agitation, abnormal thinking (use caution when driving or engaging in tasks requiring alertness until response to drug is known). Inform prescriber **immediately** if you feel depressed or have any thoughts of suicide. Report unusual bruising or bleeding; persistent abdominal disturbances; unusual fatigue; muscle pain or tremors; chest pain or palpitation; swelling of extremities or unusual weight gain; respiratory difficulty; pain, swelling, or redness at injection site; or other unusual symptoms. **Pregnancy/breast-feeding precautions:** Inform prescriber if you are or intend to become pregnant. Consult prescriber if breast-feeding.

Geriatric Considerations: No specific data is available for the elderly; however, pay close attention to Warnings/Precautions since the elderly often have reduced Cl$_{cr}$ (<50 mL/minute), diabetes, and hyper-/hypothyroidism.

Pregnancy Risk Factor: C

Pregnancy Issues: Safety and efficacy for use during pregnancy have not been established. Interferon alpha has been shown to decrease serum estradiol and progesterone levels in humans. Menstrual irregularities and abortion have been reported in animals. Effective contraception is recommended during treatment.

Lactation: Enters breast milk/contraindicated (AAP rates "compatible")

Breast-Feeding Issues: Women with hepatitis C should be instructed that there is a theoretical risk the virus may be transmitted in breast milk. HIV-infected mothers are discouraged from breast-feeding to decrease potential transmission of HIV.

Administration

I.M.: Reconstitute with recommended amount of bacteriostatic water and agitate gently; do not shake. **Note:** Different vial strengths require different amounts of diluent.

Other: SubQ administration is suggested for those who are at risk for bleeding or are thrombocytopenic. Rotate SubQ injection site. Patient should be well hydrated. Reconstitute with recommended amount of bacteriostatic water and agitate gently; do not shake. **Note:** Different vial strengths require different amounts of diluent.

Reconstitution: Reconstitute vial with the diluent provided, or SWFI, NS, or D$_5$W; concentrations ≥3 x 10^6 units/mL are hypertonic.

Storage: Refrigerate (2°C to 8°C/36°F to 46°F); do not freeze; do not shake. After reconstitution, the solution is stable for 24 hours at room temperature and for 1 month when refrigerated.

♦ **Interferon Alfa-2a (PEG Conjugate)** see Peginterferon Alfa-2a on page 1165

Interferon Alfa-2b (in ter FEER on AL fa too bee)

U.S. Brand Names Intron® A

Synonyms INF-alpha 2; α-2-Interferon; rLFN-α2

Generic Available No

Pharmacologic Category Interferon

(Continued)

Interferon Alfa-2b *(Continued)*

Medication Safety Issues
Sound-alike/look-alike issues:
Interferon alfa-2b may be confused with interferon alfa-2a

Use
Patients ≥1 year of age: Chronic hepatitis B

Patients ≥18 years of age: Condyloma acuminata, chronic hepatitis C, hairy cell leukemia, malignant melanoma, AIDS-related Kaposi's sarcoma, follicular non-Hodgkin's lymphoma

Unlabeled/Investigational Use AIDS-related thrombocytopenia, cutaneous ulcerations of Behçet's disease, carcinoid syndrome, cervical cancer, lymphomatoid granulomatosis, genital herpes, hepatitis D, chronic myelogenous leukemia (CML), non-Hodgkin's lymphomas (other than follicular lymphoma, see approved use), polycythemia vera, medullary thyroid carcinoma, multiple myeloma, renal cell carcinoma, basal and squamous cell skin cancers, essential thrombocytopenia, thrombocytopenic purpura

Investigational: West Nile virus

Mechanism of Action/Effect Alpha interferons are a family of proteins that have antiviral, antiproliferative, and immune-regulating activity. Inhibits cell growth and proliferation and enhances immune response.

Contraindications Hypersensitivity to interferon alfa or any component of the formulation; patients with visceral AIDS-related Kaposi's sarcoma associated with rapidly-progressing or life-threatening disease; decompensated liver disease; autoimmune hepatitis; history of autoimmune disease; immunosuppressed transplant patients

Warnings/Precautions Suicidal ideation or attempts may occur more frequently in pediatric patients when compared to adults. May cause severe psychiatric adverse events (psychosis, mania, depression, suicidal behavior/ideation) in patients with and without previous psychiatric symptoms, avoid use in severe psychiatric disorders or in patients with a history of depression; careful neuropsychiatric monitoring is required during therapy. Use with caution in patients with a history of seizures, brain metastases, multiple sclerosis, cardiac disease (ischemic or thromboembolic), arrhythmias, myelosuppression, hepatic impairment, or renal dysfunction (use is not recommended if Cl$_{cr}$<50 mL/minute). Use caution in patients with a history of pulmonary disease, coagulopathy, thyroid disease (monitor thyroid function), hypertension, or diabetes mellitus (particularly if prone to DKA). Caution in patients receiving drugs that may cause lactic acidosis (eg, nucleoside analogues).

Avoid use in patients with autoimmune disorders; worsening of psoriasis and/or development of autoimmune disorders has been associated with alpha interferons. Higher doses in elderly patients, or diseases other than hairy cell leukemia, may result in increased CNS toxicity. Treatment should be discontinued in patients who develop severe pulmonary symptoms with chest x-ray changes, autoimmune disorders, worsening of hepatic function, psychiatric symptoms (including depression and/or suicidal thoughts/behaviors), ischemic and/or infectious disorders. Ophthalmologic disorders (including retinal hemorrhages, cotton wool spots and retinal artery or vein obstruction) have occurred in patients receiving alpha interferons. Hypertriglyceridemia has been reported (discontinue if severe).

Safety and efficacy in children <1 year of age have not been established. Do not treat patients with visceral AIDS-related Kaposi's sarcoma associated with rapidly-progressing or life-threatening disease. A transient increase in SGOT (>2x baseline) is common in patients treated with interferon alfa-2b for chronic hepatitis. Therapy generally may continue, however, functional indicators (albumin, prothrombin time, bilirubin) should be monitored at 2-week intervals. **Due to differences in dosage, patients should not change brands of interferons.**

Intron® A may cause bone marrow suppression, including very rarely, aplastic anemia. Hemolytic anemia (hemoglobin <10 g/dL) was observed in 10% of treated patients in clinical trials; anemia occurred within 1-2 weeks of initiation of therapy.

Drug Interactions
Cytochrome P450 Effect: Inhibits CYP1A2 (weak)

Increased Effect/Toxicity: Theophylline clearance has been reported to be decreased in hepatitis patients receiving interferon. Interferons may increase the adverse/toxic effects of ACE inhibitors, specifically the development of granulocytopenia. Agranulocytosis has been reported with concurrent use of clozapine (case report). Interferons may increase the anticoagulant effects of warfarin, and interferons may increase serum levels of zidovudine.

Adverse Reactions Note: In a majority of patients, a flu-like syndrome (fever, chills, tachycardia, malaise, myalgia, headache), occurs within 1-2 hours of administration; may last up to 24 hours and may be dose-limiting.

>10%:

Cardiovascular: Chest pain (2% to 28%)

Central nervous system: Fatigue (8% to 96%), headache (21% to 62%), fever (34% to 94%), depression (4% to 40%), somnolence (1% to 33%), irritability (1% to 22%), paresthesia (1% to 21%, more common in patients previously treated with vinca alkaloids or receiving concurrent vinblastine), dizziness (7% to 23%), confusion (1% to 12%), malaise (3% to 14%), pain (3% to 15%), insomnia (1% to 12%), impaired concentration (1% to 14%, usually reverses within a few days), amnesia (1% to 14%), chills (45% to 54%)

Dermatologic: Alopecia (8% to 38%), rash (usually maculopapular) on the trunk and extremities (1% to 25%), pruritus (3% to 11%), dry skin (1% to 10%)

Endocrine & metabolic: Alkaline phosphatase increased (48%), hypocalcemia (10% to 51%), hyperglycemia (33% to 39%), amenorrhea (up to 12% in lymphoma)

Gastrointestinal: Anorexia (1% to 69%), nausea (19% to 66%), vomiting (2% to 32%, usually mild), diarrhea (2% to 45%, may be severe), taste change (2% to 24%), xerostomia (1% to 28%), abdominal pain (2% to 23%), gingivitis (2% to 14%), constipation (1% to 14%)

Hematologic: Myelosuppression; neutropenia (30% to 66%); thrombocytopenia (5% to 15%); anemia (15% to 32%, may be dose-limiting, usually seen only during the first 6 months of therapy)

Onset: 7-10 days

Nadir: 14 days, may be delayed 20-40 days in hairy cell leukemia

Recovery: 21 days

Hepatic: Right upper quadrant pain (15% in hepatitis C), transaminases increased (increased SGOT in up to 63%)

Local: Injection site reaction (1% to 20%)

Neuromuscular & skeletal: Weakness (5% to 63%) may be severe at doses >20,000,000 units/day; mild arthralgia and myalgia (5% to 75% - usually during the first 72 hours of treatment), rigors (2% to 42%), back pain (1% to 19%), musculoskeletal pain (1% to 21%), paresthesia (1% to 21%)

Renal: Urinary tract infection (up to 5% in hepatitis C)

Respiratory: Dyspnea (1% to 34%), cough (1% to 31%), pharyngitis (1% to 31%),

Miscellaneous: Loss of smell, flu-like symptoms (5% to 79%), diaphoresis (2% to 21%)

5% to 10%:

Cardiovascular: Hypertension (9% in hepatitis C)

Central nervous system: Anxiety (1% to 9%), nervousness (1% to 3%), vertigo (up to 8% in lymphoma)

Dermatologic: Dermatitis (1% to 8%)

Endocrine & metabolic: Decreased libido (1% to 5%)

Gastrointestinal: Loose stools (1% to 21%), dyspepsia (2% to 8%)

Neuromuscular & skeletal: Hypoesthesia (1% to 10%)

Respiratory: Nasal congestion (1% to 10%)

Overdosage/Toxicology Symptoms of overdose include CNS depression, obtundation, flu-like symptoms, and myelosuppression. Treatment is supportive.

Pharmacodynamics/Kinetics

Bioavailability: I.M.: 83%; SubQ: 90%

Time to Peak: Serum: I.M., SubQ: ~3-12 hours

Half-Life Elimination: I.M., I.V.: 2 hours; SubQ: 3 hours

Metabolism: Primarily renal

Dosing

Adults & Elderly: Refer to individual protocols.

Hairy cell leukemia: I.M., SubQ: 2 million units/m^2 3 times/week for 2-6 months

Lymphoma (follicular): SubQ: 5 million units 3 times/week for up to 18 months

Malignant melanoma: 20 million units/m^2 I.V. for 5 consecutive days per week for 4 weeks, then 10 million units/m^2 SubQ 3 times/week for 48 weeks

AIDS-related Kaposi's sarcoma: I.M., SubQ: 30 million units/m^2 3 times/week

Chronic hepatitis B: I.M., SubQ: 5 million units/day or 10 million units 3 times/week for 16 weeks

Chronic hepatitis C: I.M., SubQ: 3 million units 3 times/week for 16 weeks. In patients with normalization of ALT at 16 weeks, continue treatment for 18-24 months; consider discontinuation if normalization does not occur at 16 weeks. **Note:** May be used in combination therapy with ribavirin in previously untreated patients or in patients who relapse following alpha interferon therapy; refer to Interferon Alfa-2b and Ribavirin Combination Pack monograph.

Condyloma acuminata: Intralesionally: 1 million units/lesion (maximum: 5 lesions/treatment) 3 times/week (on alternate days) for 3 weeks. May administer a second course at 12-16 weeks.

Dosage adjustment for toxicity: Manufacturer-recommended adjustments, listed according to indication:

Lymphoma (follicular):

Severe toxicity (neutrophils <1000 cells/mm^3 or platelets <50,000 cells/mm^3): Reduce dose by 50% or temporarily discontinue

AST/ALT >5 times ULN: Permanently discontinue

Hairy cell leukemia:

Severe toxicity: Reduce dose by 50% or temporarily discontinue; permanently discontinue if persistent or recurrent severe toxicity is noted

Hepatitis B or C:

WBC <1500 cells/mm^3, granulocytes <750 cells/mm^3, or platelet count <50,000 cells/mm^3: Reduce dose by 50%

WBC <1000 cells/mm^3, granulocytes <500 cells/mm^3, or platelet count <25,000 cells/mm^3: Permanently discontinue

Kaposi sarcoma: Severe toxicity: Reduce dose by 50% or temporarily discontinue

Malignant melanoma:

Severe toxicity (neutrophils <500 cells/mm^3 or AST/ALT >5 times ULN): Reduce dose by 50% or temporarily discontinue

Neutrophils <250 cells/mm^3 or AST/ALT >10 times ULN: Permanently discontinue

Pediatrics: Refer to individual protocols.

Chronic hepatitis B: SubQ: Children 1-17 years: 3 million units/m^2 3 times/week for 1 week; then 6 million units/m^2 3 times/week; maximum: 10 million units 3 times/week; total duration of therapy 16-24 weeks

Renal Impairment: Combination therapy with ribavirin (hepatitis C) should not be used in patients with reduced renal function (Cl$_{cr}$ <50 mL/minute).

Available Dosage Forms

Injection, powder for reconstitution: 10 million units; 18 million units; 50 million units [contains human albumin]

Injection, solution [multidose prefilled pen]:

Delivers 3 million units/0.2 mL (1.5 mL) [delivers 6 doses; 18 million units]

Delivers 5 million units/0.2 mL (1.5 mL) [delivers 6 doses; 30 million units]

Delivers 10 million units/0.2 mL (1.5 mL) [delivers 6 doses; 60 million units]

Injection, solution [multidose vial]: 6 million units/mL (3 mL); 10 million units/mL (2.5 mL)

Injection, solution [single-dose vial]: 10 million units/ mL (1 mL)

(Continued)

Interferon Alfa-2b *(Continued)*

See also Interferon Alfa-2b and Ribavirin Combination Pack monograph.

Monitoring and Teaching Issues

Physical Assessment: Assess results of laboratory tests on a regular basis, therapeutic effectiveness, and adverse reactions. Patients with pre-existing cardiac abnormalities, or in advanced stages of cancer should have ECGs taken before and during treatment. Monitor for neuropsychiatric changes.

Assess knowledge/instruct patient/caregiver on appropriate reconstitution, injection and needle disposal, possible side effects, and symptoms to report.

Monitoring Laboratory Tests: Baseline chest x-ray, ECG, CBC with differential, liver function, electrolytes, platelets

Patient Education: Use as directed; do not change dosage or schedule of administration without consulting prescriber. Maintain adequate hydration (2-3 L/day of fluids) unless instructed to restrict fluid intake. You may experience flu-like syndrome (acetaminophen may help); nausea, vomiting, dry mouth, or metallic taste (small frequent meals, frequent mouth care, sucking lozenges, or chewing gum may help); fatigue, drowsiness, insomnia, dizziness, agitation, abnormal thinking (use caution when driving or engaging in tasks requiring alertness until response to drug is known). Inform prescriber **immediately** if you feel depressed or have any thoughts of suicide. Report unusual bruising or bleeding; persistent abdominal disturbances; unusual fatigue; muscle pain or tremors; chest pain or palpitation; swelling of extremities or unusual weight gain; respiratory difficulty; pain, swelling, or redness at injection site; or other unusual symptoms. **Pregnancy/breast-feeding precautions:** Inform prescriber if you are or intend to become pregnant. Consult prescriber if breast-feeding.

Pregnancy Risk Factor: C

Pregnancy Issues: Safety and efficacy for use during pregnancy have not been established. Interferon alpha has been shown to decrease serum estradiol and progesterone levels in humans. Menstrual irregularities and abortion have been reported in animals. Effective contraception is recommended during treatment.

Lactation: Enters breast milk/not recommended (AAP rates "compatible")

Breast-Feeding Issues: Women with hepatitis C should be instructed that there is a theoretical risk the virus may be transmitted in breast milk. HIV-infected mothers are discouraged from breast-feeding to decrease potential transmission of HIV.

Administration

Other: SubQ administration is suggested for those who are at risk for bleeding or are thrombocytopenic. Rotate SubQ injection site. Patient should be well hydrated. Reconstitute with recommended amount of SWFI and agitate gently; do not shake. **Note:** Different vial strengths require different amounts of diluent. Not every dosage form is appropriate for every indication; refer to manufacturer's labeling.

Reconstitution: The manufacturer recommends reconstituting vial with the diluent provided (SWFI). To prepare solution for infusion, further dilute appropriate dose in NS 100 mL. Final concentration should not be <10 million units/100 mL.

Compatibility: Stable in LR, NS; **incompatible** with D_5W

Storage: Store powder and solution for injection (vials and pens) under refrigeration (2°C to 8°C).

Powder for injection: Following reconstitution, should be used immediately, but may be stored under refrigeration for up to 24 hours.

Prefilled pens: After first use, discard unused portion after 1 month.

Interferon Alfa-2b and Ribavirin

(in ter FEER on AL fa too bee & rye ba VYE rin)

U.S. Brand Names Rebetron®

Synonyms Interferon Alfa-2b and Ribavirin Combination Pack; Ribavirin and Interferon Alfa-2b Combination Pack

Restrictions An FDA-approved medication guide is available at www.fda.gov/cder/Offices/ODS/labeling.htm; distribute to each patient to whom this medication is dispensed.

Generic Available No

Pharmacologic Category Antiviral Agent; Interferon

Use Combination therapy for the treatment of chronic hepatitis C in patients with compensated liver disease previously untreated with alpha interferon or who have relapsed after alpha interferon therapy

Mechanism of Action/Effect

Interferon Alfa-2b: Alpha interferons are a family of proteins, produced by nucleated cells, that have antiviral, antiproliferative, and immune-regulating activity. There are 16 known subtypes of alpha interferons. Interferons interact with cells through high affinity cell surface receptors. Following activation, multiple effects can be detected including induction of gene transcription. Inhibits cellular growth, alters the state of cellular differentiation, interferes with oncogene expression, alters cell surface antigen expression, increases phagocytic activity of macrophages, and augments cytotoxicity of lymphocytes for target cells

Ribavirin: Inhibits replication of RNA and DNA viruses; inhibits influenza virus RNA polymerase activity and inhibits the initiation and elongation of RNA fragments resulting in inhibition of viral protein synthesis

Contraindications Hypersensitivity to interferon alfa-2b, ribavirin, or any component of the formulation; autoimmune hepatitis; males with a pregnant female partner; pregnancy

Warnings/Precautions

Interferon alfa-2b: Suicidal ideation or attempts may occur more frequently in pediatric patients when compared to adults. May cause severe psychiatric adverse events (psychosis, mania, depression, suicidal behavior/ideation) in patients with and without previous psychiatric symptoms, avoid use in severe psychiatric disorders or in patients with a history of depression; careful neuropsychiatric monitoring is required during therapy. Use with caution in patients with a history of seizures, brain metastases, multiple sclerosis, cardiac disease (ischemic or thromboembolic), arrhythmias, myelosuppression, hepatic impairment, or renal dysfunction (use is not recommended if Cl$_{cr}$<50 mL/minute). Use caution in patients with a history of pulmonary disease, coagulopathy, thyroid disease (monitor thyroid function), hypertension, or diabetes mellitus (particularly if prone to DKA). Caution in patients receiving drugs that may cause lactic acidosis (eg, nucleoside analogues). Avoid use in patients with autoimmune disorders; worsening of psoriasis and/or development of autoimmune disorders has been associated with alpha interferons. Higher doses in elderly patients, or diseases other than hairy cell leukemia, may result in increased CNS toxicity. Treatment should be discontinued in patients who develop severe pulmonary symptoms with chest x-ray changes, autoimmune disorders, worsening of hepatic function, psychiatric symptoms (including depression and/or suicidal thoughts/behaviors), ischemic and/or infectious disorders. Ophthalmologic disorders (including retinal hemorrhages, cotton wool spots and retinal artery or vein obstruction) have occurred in patients receiving alpha interferons. Hypertriglyceridemia has been reported (discontinue if severe).

Safety and efficacy in children <3 years of age have not been established. Do not treat patients with visceral AIDS-related Kaposi's sarcoma associated with rapidly-progressing or life-threatening disease. A transient increase in SGOT (>2x baseline) is common in patients treated with interferon alfa-2b for chronic hepatitis. Therapy generally may continue, however, functional indicators (albumin, prothrombin time, bilirubin) should be monitored at 2-week intervals. **Due to differences in dosage, patients should not change brands of interferons.**

Intron® A may cause bone marrow suppression, including very rarely, aplastic anemia. Hemolytic anemia (hemoglobin <10 g/dL) was observed in 10% of treated patients in clinical trials; anemia occurred within 1-2 weeks of initiation of therapy.

Ribavirin: Oral: Anemia has been observed in patients receiving the interferon/ribavirin combination. Severe psychiatric events have also occurred including depression and suicidal behavior during combination therapy; avoid use in patients with a psychiatric history. Hemolytic anemia is a significant toxicity; usually occurring within 1-2 weeks. Assess cardiac disease before initiation. Anemia may worsen underlying cardiac disease; use caution. If any deterioration in cardiovascular status occurs, discontinue therapy. Use caution in pulmonary disease; pulmonary symptoms have been associated with administration. Use caution in patients with sarcoidosis (exacerbation reported). Negative pregnancy test is required before initiation and monthly thereafter. Avoid pregnancy in female patients and female partners of patients during therapy. Discontinue therapy in suspected/confirmed pancreatitis. Use caution in elderly patients; higher frequency of anemia; take renal function into consideration before initiating. Safety and efficacy have not been established in organ transplant patients, decompensated liver disease, concurrent hepatitis B virus or HIV exposure, or pediatric patients <3 years of age. Use caution in patients receiving concurrent medications which may cause lactic acidosis (eg, nucleoside analogues).

Drug Interactions

Cytochrome P450 Effect: Interferon Alfa-2b: **Inhibits** CYP1A2 (weak)

Decreased Effect:
Interferon alpha: Prednisone may decrease the therapeutic effects of interferon alpha. A decreased response to erythropoietin has been reported (case reports) in patients receiving interferons. Interferon alpha may decrease the serum concentrations of melphalan (may or may not decrease toxicity of melphalan). Thyroid dysfunction has been reported during treatment; monitor response to thyroid hormones.
Ribavirin: Decreased effect of stavudine and zidovudine.

Increased Effect/Toxicity: Interferon alpha: Cimetidine may augment the antitumor effects of interferon in melanoma. Theophylline clearance has been reported to be decreased in hepatitis patients receiving interferon. Vinblastine enhances interferon toxicity in several patients; increased incidence of paresthesia has also been noted. Interferons may increase the adverse/toxic effects of ACE inhibitors, specifically the development of granulocytopenia. Agranulocytosis has been reported with concurrent use of clozapine (case report). Interferons may increase the anticoagulant effects of warfarin, and interferons may increase serum levels of zidovudine. Concomitant use of ribavirin and nucleoside analogues may increase the risk of developing lactic acidosis.

Adverse Reactions Note: Adverse reactions listed are specific to combination regimen in previously untreated hepatitis patients. See individual agents for additional adverse reactions reported with each agent during therapy for other diseases.

>10%:
Central nervous system: Fatigue (children 61%; adults 68%), headache (63%), insomnia (children 14%; adults 39%), fever (children 61%; adults 37%), depression (children 13%; adults 32% to 36%), irritability (children 10%; adults 23% to 32%), dizziness (17% to 23%), emotional lability (children 16%; adults 7% to 11%), impaired concentration (5% to 14%)
Dermatologic: Alopecia (23% to 32%), pruritus (children 12%; adults 19% to 21%), rash (17% to 28%)
Gastrointestinal: Nausea (33% to 46%), anorexia (children 51%; adults 25% to 27%), dyspepsia (children <1%; adults 14% to 16%), vomiting (children 42%; adults 9% to 11%)
Hematologic: Leukopenia, neutropenia (usually recovers within 4 weeks of treatment discontinuation), anemia
Hepatic: Hyperbilirubinemia (27%; only 0.9% to 2% >3.0-6 mg/dL)
Local: Injection site inflammation (13%)
Neuromuscular & skeletal: Myalgia (children 32%; adults 61% to 64%), rigors (40%), arthralgia (children 15%; adults 30% to 33%), musculoskeletal pain (20% to 28%)
Respiratory: Dyspnea (children 5%; adults 18% to 19%)
Miscellaneous: Flu-like syndrome (children 31%; adults 14% to 18%)

1% to 10%:
Cardiovascular: Chest pain (5% to 9%)
Central nervous system: Nervousness (3% to 4%)
Endocrine & metabolic: Thyroid abnormalities (hyper- or hypothyroidism), serum uric acid increased, hyperglycemia

(Continued)

Interferon Alfa-2b and Ribavirin *(Continued)*

Gastrointestinal: Taste perversion (children <1%; adults 7% to 8%)
Hematologic: Hemolytic anemia (10%), thrombocytopenia, anemia
Local: Injection site reaction (7%)
Neuromuscular & skeletal: Weakness (5% to 9%)
Respiratory: Sinusitis (children <1%; adults 9% to 10%)

Overdosage/Toxicology Interferon Alfa-2b: Signs and symptoms of overdose include CNS depression, obtundation, flu-like symptoms, myelosuppression; treatment is supportive.

Pharmacodynamics/Kinetics
Pharmacokinetic Note: See individual agents.

Dosing
Adults & Elderly:
Chronic hepatitis C: Recommended dosage of combination therapy:
Intron® A: SubQ: 3 million int. units 3 times/week **and**
Rebetol® capsule: Oral:
≤75 kg (165 pounds): 1000 mg/day (two 200 mg capsules in the morning and three 200 mg capsules in the evening)
>75 kg: 1200 mg/day (three 200 mg capsules in the morning and three 200 mg capsules in the evening)

Pediatrics: Chronic hepatitis C:
Children ≥3 years: **Note:** Duration of therapy: genotype 1: 48 weeks; genotype 2 or 3: 24 weeks. Discontinue treatment in any patient if HCV-RNA is not below the limits of detection of the assay after 24 weeks of therapy. Combination therapy:
Intron® A: SubQ:
25-61 kg: 3 million int. units/m^2 3 times/week
>61 kg: Refer to Adults dosing
Rebetol®: Oral: **Note:** Oral solution should be used in children 3-5 years of age, children ≤25 kg, or those unable to swallow capsules.
Capsule/solution: 15 mg/kg/day in 2 divided doses (morning and evening)
Capsule dosing recommendations:
25-36 kg: 400 mg/day (200 mg morning and evening)
37-49 kg: 600 mg/day (200 mg in the morning and two 200 mg capsules in the evening)
50-61 kg: 800 mg/day (two 200 mg capsules morning and evening)
>61 kg: Refer to adult dosing.

Renal Impairment: Patients with Cl$_{cr}$ <50 mL/minutes should not receive ribavirin.

Available Dosage Forms Combination package:
For patients ≤75 kg [contains single-dose vials]:
Injection, solution: Interferon alfa-2b (Intron® A): 3 million int. units/0.5 mL (0.5 mL) [6 vials (3 million int. units/vial), 6 syringes, and alcohol swabs]
Capsules: Ribavirin (Rebetol®): 200 mg (70s)
For patients ≤75 kg [contains multidose vials]:
Injection, solution: Interferon alfa-2b (Intron® A): 3 million int. units/0.5 mL (3.8 mL) [1 multidose vial (18 million int. units/vial), 6 syringes, and alcohol swabs]
Capsules: Ribavirin (Rebetol®): 200 mg (70s)
For patients ≤75 kg [contains multidose pen]:
Injection, solution: Interferon alfa-2b (Intron® A): 3 million int. units/0.2 mL (1.5 mL) [1 multidose pen (18 million int. units/pen), 6 needles, and alcohol swabs]
Capsules: Ribavirin (Rebetol®): 200 mg (70s)
For patients >75 kg [contains single-dose vials]:
Injection, solution: Interferon alfa-2b (Intron® A): 3 million int. units/0.5 mL (0.5 mL) [6 vials (3 million int. units/vial), 6 syringes, and alcohol swabs]
Capsules: Ribavirin (Rebetol®): 200 mg (84s)
For patients >75 kg [contains multidose vials]:
Injection, solution: Interferon alfa-2b (Intron® A): 3 million int. units/0.5 mL (3.8 mL) [1 multidose vial (18 million int. units/vial), 6 syringes, and alcohol swabs]
Capsules: Ribavirin (Rebetol®): 200 mg (84s)
For patients >75 kg [contains multidose pen]:
Injection, solution: Interferon alfa-2b (Intron® A): 3 million int. units/0.2 mL (1.5 mL) [1 multidose pen (18 million int. units/pen), 6 needles, and alcohol swabs]
Capsules: Ribavirin (Rebetol®): 200 mg (84s)
For Rebetol® dose reduction [contains single-dose vials]:
Injection, solution: Interferon alfa-2b (Intron® A): 3 million int. units/0.5 mL (0.5 mL) [6 vials (3 million int. units/vial), 6 syringes, and alcohol swabs]
Capsules: Ribavirin (Rebetol®): 200 mg (42s)
For Rebetol® dose reduction [contains multidose vials]:
Injection, solution: Interferon alfa-2b (Intron® A): 3 million int. units/0.5 mL (3.8 mL) [1 multidose vial (18 million int. units/vial), 6 syringes, and alcohol swabs]
Capsules: Ribavirin (Rebetol®): 200 mg (42s)
For Rebetol® dose reduction [contains multidose pen]:
Injection, solution: Interferon alfa-2b (Intron® A): 3 million int. units/0.2 mL (1.5 mL) [1 multidose pen (18 million int. units/pen), 6 needles, and alcohol swabs]
Capsules: Ribavirin (Rebetol®): 200 mg (42s)

Monitoring and Teaching Issues
Physical Assessment: Assess other medications patient may be taking for increased risk of drug/drug interactions. Baseline chest x-rays and ECGs are recommended. Patients with pre-existing cardiac abnormalities, or in advanced stages of cancer should have ECGs taken before and during treatment. Monitor for neuropsychiatric changes. Monitor laboratory results and adverse reactions on a frequent and regular basis during therapy (see monographs for Interferon Alfa-2b and Ribavirin). Assess knowledge/teach patient appropriate use (including appropriate injection technique and needle disposal), interventions to reduce side effects, and adverse symptoms to report. **Pregnancy risk factor X:** Determine that patient is not pregnant before beginning treatment and do not give to women of childbearing age or to males who may have intercourse with women of childbearing ages

unless both male and female are capable of complying with contraceptive measures for 6 months prior to therapy and for 1 month following therapy.

Monitoring Laboratory Tests: Obtain pretreatment CBC, liver function tests, TSH, and electrolytes and monitor routinely throughout therapy (at 2 weeks and 4 weeks, more frequently if indicated); discontinue if WBC <1.0 x 10^9/L, neutrophils <0.5 x 10^9/L, platelets <25 x 10^9/L, or if hemoglobin <8.5 g/dL (in cardiac patients, discontinue if hemoglobin <12 g/dL after 4 weeks of dosage reduction). Pretreatment and monthly pregnancy test for women of childbearing age. Reticulocyte count, serum HCV RNA levels

Patient Education: This a combination therapy. Both the injections and the oral capsules are necessary for effective therapy. Follow administration directions exactly and dispose of needles as instructed. Do not discontinue, alter dose or frequency without consulting prescriber. Do not crush, chew, or open capsules. Take at the same times each day. Maintain adequate hydration (2-3 L/day of fluids) unless instructed to restrict fluid intake. You may experience flu-like symptoms (consult prescriber for relief); nausea, vomiting, or GI upset (small frequent meals, frequent mouth care, sucking lozenges, or chewing gum may help); or insomnia, drowsiness, lethargy, fatigue, dizziness, abnormal thinking (use caution when driving or engaging in tasks that require alertness until response to drug is known). Report unusual bruising or bleeding, inflammation or pain at injection site, persistent GI disturbances, muscle pain or tremors, chest pain or palpitations, swelling of extremities, unusual weight gain, or rash. Contact prescriber immediately if you experience unusual agitation, nervousness, feelings of depression, or have thoughts of suicide. **Pregnancy/breast-feeding precautions:** This drug will cause severe fetal defects. Inform prescriber if you are pregnant. Females must not get pregnant or males must not cause a pregnancy during therapy, and for 6 months after therapy is completed. Pregnancy tests are required for females. Consult prescriber for instruction on appropriate contraceptive measures. Breast-feeding is not recommended.

Dietary Considerations: Take oral formulation without regard to food, but always in a consistent manner with respect to food intake (ie, always take with food or always take on an empty stomach).

Pregnancy Risk Factor: X

Pregnancy Issues: Abortifacient and teratogenic effects have been reported. Women of childbearing potential should not be treated unless 2 reliable forms of contraception are used. In addition, male patients and their female partners must also use 2 reliable forms of contraception. Pregnancy must be avoided for 6 months following therapy.

Lactation: Excretion in breast milk unknown/not recommended

Breast-Feeding Issues: Women with hepatitis C should be instructed that there is a theoretical risk the virus may be transmitted in breast milk.

Administration

Oral: Capsule should not be opened, crushed, chewed, or broken. Capsules are not for use in children <5 years of age. Use oral solution for children 3-5 years, those ≤25 kg, or those who cannot swallow capsules.

Other: See individual agents.

Storage: Store the Rebetol® capsules plus Intron® A injection combination package refrigerated between 2°C and 8°C (36°F and 46°F)

When separated, the individual carton of Rebetol® capsules should be stored refrigerated between 2°C and 8°C (36°F and 46°F) or at 25°C (77°F); excursions are permitted between 15°C and 30°C (59°F and 86°F)

When separated, the individual carton or vial of Intron® A injection and the Intron® A multidose pen should be stored refrigerated between 2°C and 8°C (36°F and 46°F)

Related Information

Interferon Alfa-2b *on page 811*
Ribavirin *on page 1318*

♦ **Interferon Alfa-2b and Ribavirin Combination Pack** *see* Interferon Alfa-2b and Ribavirin *on page 814*

Interferon Alfacon-1 (in ter FEER on AL fa con one)

U.S. Brand Names Infergen®

Restrictions An FDA-approved medication guide is available at www.fda.gov/cder/Offices/ODS/labeling.htm; distribute to each patient to whom this medication is dispensed.

Generic Available No

Pharmacologic Category Interferon

Use Treatment of chronic hepatitis C virus (HCV) infection in patients ≥18 years of age with compensated liver disease and anti-HCV serum antibodies or HCV RNA.

Mechanism of Action/Effect Alpha interferons are a family of proteins, produced by nucleated cells, that have antiviral, antiproliferative, and immune-regulating activity. There are at least 25 alpha interferons identified. Interferons interact with cells through high affinity cell surface receptors. Following activation, multiple effects can be detected. Interferons induce gene transcription, inhibit cellular growth, alter the state of cellular differentiation, interfere with oncogene expression, alter cell surface antigen expression, increase phagocytic activity of macrophages, and augment cytotoxicity of lymphocytes for target cells. Although all alpha interferons share similar properties, the actual biological effects vary between subtypes.

Contraindications Hypersensitivity to interferon alfacon-1 or any component of the formulation, other alpha interferons, or *E. coli*-derived products

Warnings/Precautions Severe psychiatric adverse effects, including depression, suicidal ideation, and suicide attempt, may occur. Avoid use in severe psychiatric disorders. Use with caution in patients with a history of depression. Use with caution in patients with prior cardiac disease (ischemic or thromboembolic), arrhythmias, patients who are chronically immunosuppressed, and patients with endocrine disorders. Do not use in patients with hepatic decompensation. Ophthalmologic disorders (including retinal hemorrhages, cotton wool spots and retinal artery or vein obstruction) have occurred in patients using other alpha interferons. Prior to start of therapy, visual exams are recommended for patients with diabetes mellitus or hypertension. Treatment should be discontinued in patients with worsening or persistently severe signs/symptoms of autoimmune, infectious, ischemic (including (Continued)

Interferon Alfacon-1 *(Continued)*

radiographic changes or worsening hepatic function), or neuropsychiatric disorders (including depression and/or suicidal thoughts/behavior). Use caution in patients with autoimmune disorders; type-1 interferon therapy has been reported to exacerbate autoimmune diseases. Do not use interferon alfacon-1 in patients with autoimmune hepatitis. Use caution in patients with low peripheral blood counts or myelosuppression, including concurrent use of myelosuppressive therapy. Safety and efficacy have not been determined for patients <18 years of age.

Drug Interactions

Decreased Effect: Prednisone may decrease the therapeutic effects of interferon alpha. A decreased response to erythropoietin has been reported (case reports) in patients receiving interferons. Interferon alpha may decrease the serum concentrations of melphalan (may or may not decrease toxicity of melphalan).

Increased Effect/Toxicity: Cimetidine may augment the antitumor effects of interferon in melanoma. Theophylline clearance has been reported to be decreased in hepatitis patients receiving interferon. Vinblastine enhances interferon toxicity in several patients; increased incidence of paresthesia has also been noted. Interferons may increase the adverse/toxic effects of ACE inhibitors, specifically the development of granulocytopenia. Agranulocytosis has been reported with concurrent use of clozapine (case report). Interferons may increase the anticoagulant effects of warfarin, and interferons may increase serum levels of zidovudine.

Adverse Reactions Adverse reactions reported using 9 mcg/dose interferon alfacon-1 3 times/week. Reactions listed were reported in ≥5% of patients treated.

>10%:

Central nervous system: Headache (82%), fatigue (69%), fever (61%), insomnia (39%), nervousness (31%), depression (26%), dizziness (22%), anxiety (19%), noncardiac chest pain (13%), emotional lability (12%), malaise (11%)

Dermatologic: Alopecia (14%), pruritus (14%), rash (13%)

Endocrine & metabolic: Hot flashes (13%)

Gastrointestinal: Abdominal pain (41%), nausea (40%), diarrhea (29%), anorexia (24%), dyspepsia (21%), vomiting (12%)

Hematologic: Granulocytopenia (23%), thrombocytopenia (19%), leukopenia (15%)

Local: Injection site erythema (23%)

Neuromuscular & skeletal: Myalgia (58%), body pain (54%), arthralgia (51%), back pain (42%), limb pain (26%), neck pain (14%), skeletal pain (14%), paresthesia (13%)

Respiratory: Pharyngitis (34%), upper respiratory tract infection (31%), cough (22%), sinusitis (17%), rhinitis (13%), respiratory tract congestion (12%)

Miscellaneous: Flu-like syndrome (15%), diaphoresis increased (12%)

1% to 10%:

Cardiovascular: Peripheral edema (9%), hypertension (5%), tachycardia (4%), palpitation (3%)

Central nervous system: Amnesia (10%), hypoesthesia (10%), abnormal thinking (8%), agitation (6%), confusion (4%), somnolence (4%)

Dermatologic: Bruising (6%), erythema (6%), dry skin (6%), wound (4%)

Endocrine & metabolic: Thyroid test abnormalities (9%), dysmenorrhea (9%), increased triglycerides (6%), menstrual disorder (6%), decreased libido (5%), hypothyroidism (4%)

Gastrointestinal: Constipation (9%), flatulence (8%), toothache (7%), decreased salivation (6%), hemorrhoids (6%), weight loss (5%), taste perversion (3%)

Genitourinary: Vaginitis (8%), genital moniliasis (2%)

Hepatic: Hepatomegaly (5%), liver tenderness (5%), increased prothrombin time (3%)

Local: Injection site pain (9%), access pain (8%), injection site bruising (6%)

Neuromuscular & skeletal: Weakness (9%), hypertonia (7%), musculoskeletal disorder (4%)

Ocular: Conjunctivitis (8%), eye pain (5%), vision abnormalities (3%)

Otic: Tinnitus (6%), earache (5%), otitis (2%)

Respiratory: Upper respiratory tract congestion (10%), epistaxis (8%), dyspnea (7%), bronchitis (6%)

Miscellaneous: Allergic reaction (7%), lymphadenopathy (6%), lymphocytosis (5%), infection (3%)

Flu-like symptoms (which included headache, fatigue, fever, myalgia, rigors, arthralgia, and increased diaphoresis) were the most commonly reported adverse reaction. This was reported separately from flu-like syndrome. Most patients were treated symptomatically.

Other adverse reactions associated with interferon therapy include arrhythmia, autoimmune disorders, chest pain, hepatotoxic reactions, lupus erythematosus, MI, neuropsychiatric disorders (including suicidal thoughts/behavior), pneumonia, pneumonitis, severe hypersensitivity reactions (rare), vasculitis

Overdosage/Toxicology One overdose has been reported. A patient received ten times the prescribed dose (150 mcg) for 3 days. In addition to an increase in anorexia, chills, fever, and myalgia, there was also an increase in ALT, AST, and LDH. Laboratory values reportedly returned to baseline within 30 days.

Pharmacodynamics/Kinetics

Time to Peak: Healthy volunteers: 24-36 hours

Pharmacokinetic Note: Pharmacokinetic studies have not been conducted on patients with chronic hepatitis C.

Dosing

Adults & Elderly:

Chronic HCV infection: SubQ: 9 mcg 3 times/week for 24 weeks; allow 48 hours between doses.

Patients who have previously tolerated interferon therapy but did not respond or relapsed: SubQ: 15 mcg 3 times/week for 6 months

Dose reduction for toxicity: Dose should be held in patients who experience a severe adverse reaction, and treatment should be stopped or decreased if the reaction does not become tolerable.

Doses were reduced from 9 mcg to 7.5 mcg in the pivotal study.
For patients receiving 15 mcg/dose, doses were reduced in 3 mcg increments. Efficacy is decreased with doses <7.5 mcg.

Pediatrics: Not indicated for patients <18 years of age.

Hepatic Impairment: Avoid use in decompensated hepatic disease.

Available Dosage Forms Injection, solution [preservative free]: 30 mcg/mL (0.3 mL, 0.5 mL)

Monitoring and Teaching Issues

Physical Assessment: Assess other medications patient may be taking for effectiveness and interactions. Monitor for signs of depression and suicidal ideation. Assess results of laboratory tests on a regular basis during therapy. Patient with pre-existing diabetes mellitus or hypertension should have an ophthalmic exam prior to beginning treatment. Patient must be monitored closely for adverse reactions. If self-administered, instruct patient in appropriate storage, injection technique, and syringe disposal. Assess knowledge/teach patient purpose for use, adverse reactions and interventions, and adverse reactions to report.

Monitoring Laboratory Tests: Hemoglobin and hematocrit, white blood cell count, platelets, triglycerides, and thyroid function. Laboratory tests should be taken 2 weeks prior to therapy, after therapy has begun, and periodically during treatment. HCV RNA, and ALT to determine success/response to therapy.

The following guidelines were used during the clinical studies as acceptable baseline values:

Platelet count $\geq$75 x 10^9/L
Hemoglobin $\geq$100 g/L
ANC $\geq$1500 x 10^6/L
S_{cr} <180 μmol/L (<2 mg/dL) or Cl_{cr} >0.83 mL/second (>50 mL/minute)
Serum albumin $\geq$25 g/L
Bilirubin WNL
TSH and T_4 WNL

Patient Education: Use exactly as directed (if self-administered, follow exact instructions for injection and syringe disposal). Do not alter dosage or brand of medication without consulting prescriber. You will need frequent laboratory tests during course of therapy. If you have diabetes or hypertension you should have ophthalmic exam prior to beginning therapy. You may experience headache, dizziness, nervousness, anxiety (use caution when driving or engaging in dangerous tasks until response to medication is known); nausea, vomiting, diarrhea, or loss of appetite (small frequent meals, frequent mouth care, sucking hard candy or chewing gum may help); flu-like symptoms such as headache, fatigue, muscle or joint pain, increased perspiration (mild non-narcotic analgesic may help); or hair lose (will probably grow back when treatment is completed). Promptly report any persistent GI upset; insomnia, depression, anxiety, nervousness; chest pain or palpitations; muscle, bone, or joint pain; respiratory difficulties or congestion; vision changes; or other persistent adverse effects. **Pregnancy/breast-feeding precautions:** Inform prescriber if you are or intend to become pregnant. Consult prescriber if breast-feeding.

Pregnancy Risk Factor: C

Pregnancy Issues: There have been no well-controlled studies in pregnant women. Animal studies have shown embryolethal or abortifacient effects. Males and females who are being treated with interferon alfacon-1 should use effective contraception.

Lactation: Excretion in breast milk unknown/use caution (AAP rates "compatible")

Breast-Feeding Issues: Women with hepatitis C should be instructed that there is a theoretical risk the virus may be transmitted in breast milk.

Administration

I.V.: Interferon alfacon-1 is given by SubQ injection, 3 times/week, with at least 48 hours between doses.

Storage: Store in refrigerator 2°C to 8°C (36°F to 46°F). Do not freeze. Avoid exposure to direct sunlight. Do not shake vigorously.

Interferon Beta-1a (in ter FEER on BAY ta won aye)

U.S. Brand Names Avonex®; Rebif®

Synonyms rIFN beta-1a

Restrictions An FDA-approved medication guide is available at www.fda.gov/cder/Offices/ODS/labeling.htm; distribute to each patient to whom this medication is dispensed.

Generic Available No

Pharmacologic Category Interferon

Medication Safety Issues
Sound-alike/look-alike issues:
Avonex® may be confused with Avelox®

Use Treatment of relapsing forms of multiple sclerosis (MS)

Mechanism of Action/Effect Mechanism in the treatment of MS is unknown; slows the accumulation of physical disability and decreases frequency of clinical MS exacerbations

Contraindications Hypersensitivity to natural or recombinant interferons, human albumin, or any other component of the formulation

Warnings/Precautions Interferons have been associated with severe psychiatric adverse events (psychosis, mania, depression, suicidal behavior/ideation) in patients with and without previous psychiatric symptoms, avoid use in severe psychiatric disorders and use caution in patients with a history of depression; patients exhibiting depressive symptoms should be closely monitored and discontinuation of therapy should be considered.

Allergic reactions, including anaphylaxis, have been reported. Caution should be used in patients with hepatic impairment or in those who abuse alcohol. Rare cases of severe hepatic injury, including hepatic failure, have been reported in patients receiving interferon beta-1a; risk may be increased by ethanol use or concurrent therapy with hepatotoxic drugs. Treatment should be suspended if jaundice or symptoms of hepatic dysfunction occur. Hematologic effects, including pancytopenia (rare) and thrombocytopenia, have been reported. (Continued)

Interferon Beta-1a *(Continued)*

Associated with a high incidence of flu-like adverse effects; use of analgesics and/or antipyretics on treatment days may be helpful. Use caution in patients with pre-existing cardiovascular disease, pulmonary disease, seizure disorders, myelosuppression, or renal impairment. Safety and efficacy in patients <18 years of age have not been established.

Drug Interactions

Increased Effect/Toxicity: Interferons may increase the adverse/toxic effects of ACE inhibitors, specifically the development of granulocytopenia. Agranulocytosis has been reported with concurrent use of clozapine (case report). Interferons may increase the anticoagulant effects of warfarin, and interferons may increase serum levels of zidovudine. Concurrent use of hepatotoxic drugs may increase the risk of hepatic injury in patients receiving interferon beta-1a.

Adverse Reactions

>10%:

Central nervous system: Headache (Avonex® 58%; Rebif® 65% to 70%), fatigue (Rebif® 33% to 41%), fever (Avonex® 20%; Rebif® 25% to 28%), pain (Avonex® 23%), chills (Avonex® 19%), depression (Avonex® 18%), dizziness (Avonex® 14%)

Gastrointestinal: Nausea (Avonex® 23%), abdominal pain (Avonex® 8%; Rebif® 20% to 22%)

Genitourinary: Urinary tract infection (Avonex® 17%)

Hematologic: Leukopenia (Rebif® 28% to 36%)

Hepatic: ALT increased (Rebif® 20% to 27%), AST increased (Rebif® 10% to 17%)

Local: Injection site reaction (Avonex® 3%; Rebif® 89% to 92%)

Neuromuscular & skeletal: Myalgia (Avonex® 29%; Rebif® 25%), back pain (Rebif® 23% to 25%), weakness (Avonex® 24%), skeletal pain (Rebif® 10% to 15%), rigors (Rebif® 6% to 13%)

Ocular: Vision abnormal (Rebif® 7% to 13%)

Respiratory: Sinusitis (Avonex® 14%), upper respiratory tract infection (Avonex® 14%)

Miscellaneous: Flu-like symptoms (Avonex® 49%; Rebif® 56% to 59%), neutralizing antibodies (significance not known; Avonex® 5%; Rebif® 24%), lymphadenopathy (Rebif® 11% to 12%)

1% to 10% (reported with one or both products):

Cardiovascular: Chest pain, vasodilation

Central nervous system: Convulsions, malaise, migraine, somnolence

Dermatologic: Alopecia, erythematous rash, maculopapular rash, urticaria

Endocrine & metabolic: Thyroid disorder

Gastrointestinal: Toothache, xerostomia

Genitourinary: Micturition frequency, urinary incontinence

Hematologic: Anemia, thrombocytopenia

Hepatic: Bilirubinemia, hepatic function abnormal

Local: Injection site bruising, injection site inflammation, injection site necrosis, injection site pain

Neuromuscular & skeletal: Arthralgia, coordination abnormal, hypertonia

Ocular: Eye disorder, xerophthalmia

Respiratory: Bronchitis

Miscellaneous: Infection

Overdosage/Toxicology Symptoms of overdose include CNS depression, obtundation, flu-like symptoms, myelosuppression. Treatment is supportive.

Pharmacodynamics/Kinetics

Time to Peak: Serum: Avonex® (I.M.): 3-15 hours; Rebif® (SubQ): 16 hours

Half-Life Elimination: Avonex®: 10 hours; Rebif®: 69 hours

Pharmacokinetic Note: Limited data due to small doses used.

Dosing

Adults & Elderly: Multiple sclerosis: **Note:** Analgesics and/or antipyretics may help decrease flu-like symptoms on treatment days:

I.M. (Avonex®): 30 mcg once weekly

SubQ (Rebif®): Doses should be separated by at least 48 hours:

Target dose 44 mcg 3 times/week: 11

Initial: 8.8 mcg (20 % of final dose) 3 times/week for 8 weeks

Titration: 22 mcg (50% of final dose) 3 times/week for 8 weeks

Final dose: 44 mcg 3 times/week

Target dose 22 mcg 3 times/week:

Initial: 4.4 mcg (20 % of final dose) 3 times/week for 8 weeks

Titration: 11 mcg (50% of final dose) 3 times/week for 8 weeks

Final dose: 22 mcg 3 times/week

Hepatic Impairment: Rebif®: If liver function tests increase or in case of leukopenia: Decrease dose 20% to 50% until toxicity resolves

Available Dosage Forms

Combination package [preservative free] (Rebif® Titration Pack):

Injection, solution: 8.8 mcg/0.2 mL (0.2 mL) [6 prefilled syringes; contains albumin]

Injection, solution: 22 mcg/0.5 mL (0.5 mL) [6 prefilled syringes; contains albumin]

Injection, powder for reconstitution (Avonex®): 33 mcg [6.6 million units; provides 30 mcg/mL following reconstitution] [contains albumin; packaged with SWFI, alcohol wipes, and access pin and needle]

Injection, solution (Avonex®): 30 mcg/0.5 mL (0.5 mL) [albumin free; prefilled syringe; syringe cap contains latex; packaged with alcohol wipes, gauze pad, and adhesive bandages]

Injection, solution [preservative free] (Rebif®): 22 mcg/0.5 mL (0.5 mL) [prefilled syringe; contains albumin]; 44 mcg/0.5 mL (0.5 mL) [prefilled syringe; contains albumin]

Monitoring and Teaching Issues

Physical Assessment: Assess results of laboratory tests on a regular a basis, therapeutic effectiveness, and adverse reactions. Monitor for signs of depression and suicidal ideation. Assess knowledge/instruct patient/caregiver on appropriate reconstitution, injection and needle disposal, possible side effects, and symptoms to report.

Monitoring Laboratory Tests: Liver function, blood chemistries, complete blood count and differential, BUN, creatinine

Avonex®: Frequency of monitoring for patients receiving Avonex® has not been specifically defined; in clinical trials, monitoring was at 6-month intervals.

Rebif®: CBC and liver function testing at 1-, 3-, and 6-month, then periodically thereafter. Thyroid function every 6 months (in patients with pre-existing abnormalities and/or clinical indications)

Patient Education: This is not a cure for MS; you will continue to receive regular treatment and follow-up for MS. Use as directed; do not change dosage or schedule of administration without consulting prescriber. If self-injecting and you miss a dose, take it as soon as you remember, but two injections should not be given within 48 hours of each other. Maintain adequate hydration (2-3 L/day of fluids) unless instructed to restrict fluid intake. You may experience flu-like syndrome (analgesics and/or antipyretics may help); nausea, vomiting, or loss of appetite (small frequent meals, frequent mouth care, sucking lozenges, or chewing gum may help); or drowsiness, sleep disturbances, dizziness, agitation, or abnormal thinking (use caution when driving or engaging in tasks requiring alertness until response to drug is known). Inform prescriber **immediately** if you feel depressed or have any thoughts of suicide. Report unusual bruising or bleeding; persistent abdominal disturbances; unusual fatigue; muscle pain or tremors; chest pain or palpitations; swelling of extremities; visual disturbances; pain, swelling, or redness at injection site; or other unusual symptoms. **Pregnancy/breast-feeding precautions:** Inform prescriber if you are or intend to become pregnant. Breast-feeding is not recommended.

Pregnancy Risk Factor: C

Pregnancy Issues: Safety and efficacy in pregnant women have not been established. Treatment should be discontinued if a woman becomes pregnant, or plans to become pregnant during therapy. A dose-related abortifacient activity was reported in Rhesus monkeys.

Lactation: Excretion in breast milk unknown/not recommended

Breast-Feeding Issues: Potential for serious adverse reactions. Because its use has not been evaluated during lactation, a decision should be made to either discontinue breast-feeding or discontinue the drug.

Administration

I.M.: Avonex®: Must be given by I.M. injection.

Other: Rebif®: Administer SubQ at the same time of day on the same 3 days each week (ie, late afternoon/evening Mon, Wed, Fri). Rotate injection sites.

Reconstitution: Avonex®: Reconstitute with 1.1 mL of diluent and swirl gently to dissolve. Do not shake. The reconstituted product contains no preservative and is for single-use only; discard unused portion.

Storage:

Avonex®:

Prefilled syringe: Store at 2°C to 8°C (36°F to 46°F); do not freeze, protect from light. Allow to warm to room temperature prior to use. Use within 12 hours after removing from refrigerator.

Vial: Store unreconstituted vial at 2°C to 8°C (36°F to 46°F). If refrigeration is not available, may be stored at 25°C (77°F) for up to 30 days. Do not freeze, protect from light. Following reconstitution, use immediately, but may be stored up to 6 hours at 2°C to 8°C (36°F to 46°F); do not freeze.

Rebif®: Store at 2°C to 8°C (36°F to 46°F). Do not freeze, protect from light. May also be stored ≤25°C (77°F) for up to 30 days if protected from heat and light.

Interferon Beta-1b (in ter FEER on BAY ta won bee)

U.S. Brand Names Betaseron®

Synonyms rIFN beta-1b

Generic Available No

Pharmacologic Category Interferon

Use Treatment of relapsing forms of multiple sclerosis (MS)

Mechanism of Action/Effect Alters the expression and response to cell surface antigens and can enhance immune cell activities; mechanism in MS in unknown

Contraindications Hypersensitivity to E. coli-derived products, natural or recombinant interferon beta, albumin human or any other component of the formulation

Warnings/Precautions Interferons have been associated with severe psychiatric adverse events (psychosis, mania, depression, suicidal behavior/ideation) in patients with and without previous psychiatric symptoms, avoid use in severe psychiatric disorders and use caution in patients with a history of depression; patients exhibiting symptoms of depression should be closely monitored and discontinuation of therapy should be considered. Due to high incidence of flu-like adverse effects, use caution in patients with pre-existing cardiovascular disease, pulmonary disease, seizure disorders, myelosuppression, renal impairment or hepatic impairment. Severe injection site reactions (necrosis) may occur; patient and/or caregiver competency in injection technique should be confirmed and periodically re-evaluated. Safety and efficacy in patients <18 years of age have not been established.

Drug Interactions

Increased Effect/Toxicity: Interferons may increase the adverse/toxic effects of ACE inhibitors, specifically the development of granulocytopenia. Risk: Monitor A case report of agranulocytosis has been reported with concurrent use of clozapine. Case reports of decreased hematopoietic effect with erythropoietin. Interferon alpha may decrease the P450 isoenzyme metabolism of theophylline. Interferons may increase the anticoagulant effects of warfarin. Interferons may decrease the metabolism of zidovudine.

Adverse Reactions Note: Flu-like symptoms (including at least two of the following - headache, fever, chills, malaise, diaphoresis, and myalgia) are reported in the majority of patients (60%) and decrease over time (average duration ~1 week).

>10%:

Cardiovascular: Peripheral edema (15%), chest pain (11%)

(Continued)

Interferon Beta-1b *(Continued)*

Central nervous system: Headache (57%), fever (36%), pain (51%), chills (25%), dizziness (24%), insomnia (24%)

Dermatologic: Rash (24%), skin disorder (12%)

Endocrine & metabolic: Metrorrhagia (11%)

Gastrointestinal: Nausea (27%), diarrhea (19%), abdominal pain (19%), constipation (20%), dyspepsia (14%)

Genitourinary: Urinary urgency (13%)

Hematologic: Lymphopenia (88%), neutropenia (14%), leukopenia (14%)

Local: Injection site reaction (85%), inflammation (53%), pain (18%)

Neuromuscular & skeletal: Weakness (61%), myalgia (27%), hypertonia (50%), myasthenia (46%), arthralgia (31%), incoordination (21%)

Miscellaneous: Flu-like symptoms (60%)

1% to 10%:

Cardiovascular: Palpitation (4%), vasodilation (8%), hypertension (7%), tachycardia (4%), peripheral vascular disorder (6%)

Central nervous system: Anxiety (10%), malaise (8%), nervousness (7%)

Dermatologic: Alopecia (4%)

Endocrine & metabolic: Menorrhagia (8%), dysmenorrhea (7%)

Genitourinary: Impotence (9%), pelvic pain (6%), cystitis (8%), urinary frequency (7%), weight gain (7%), prostatic disorder (3%)

Hematologic: Lymphadenopathy (8%)

Hepatic: SGPT increased >5x baseline (10%), SGOT increased >5x baseline (3%)

Local: Injection site necrosis (5%), edema (3%), mass (2%)

Neuromuscular & skeletal: Leg cramps (4%)

Respiratory: Dyspnea (7%)

Miscellaneous: Diaphoresis (4%), hypersensitivity (3%)

Overdosage/Toxicology Symptoms of overdose include CNS depression, obtundation, flu-like symptoms, and myelosuppression. Treatment is supportive.

Pharmacodynamics/Kinetics

Time to Peak: 1-8 hours

Half-Life Elimination: 8 minutes to 4.3 hours

Pharmacokinetic Note: Limited data due to small doses used.

Dosing

Adults & Elderly: Multiple sclerosis (relapsing-remitting): SubQ: 0.25 mg (8 million units) every other day

Pediatrics: Not recommended in children <18 years of age

Available Dosage Forms Injection, powder for reconstitution [preservative free]: 0.3 mg [9.6 million units] [contains albumin; packaged with prefilled syringe containing diluent]

Monitoring and Teaching Issues

Physical Assessment: Monitor laboratory results. Monitor closely for adverse reactions, especially patients with psychiatric or suicidal histories. Assess patient/caregiver knowledge and teach proper administration for SubQ injections and disposal of needles if appropriate. Teach the need for adequate hydration. Monitor for opportunistic infection.

Monitoring Laboratory Tests: Hemoglobin, liver function, blood chemistries

Patient Education: This is not a cure for MS; you will continue to receive regular treatment and follow-up for MS. Use as directed; do not change dosage or schedule of administration without consulting prescriber. Maintain adequate hydration (2-3 L/day of fluids) unless instructed to restrict fluid intake. You may experience flu-like syndrome (acetaminophen may help); nausea, vomiting, or loss of appetite (small frequent meals, frequent mouth care, sucking lozenges, or chewing gum may help); or drowsiness, sleep disturbances, dizziness, agitation, or abnormal thinking (use caution when driving or engaging in tasks requiring alertness until response to drug is known). Inform prescriber **immediately** if you feel depressed or have any thoughts of suicide. Report any broken skin or black-blue discoloration around the injection site. Report unusual bruising or bleeding; persistent abdominal disturbances; unusual fatigue; muscle pain or tremors; chest pain or palpitations, swelling of extremities; visual disturbances; pain, swelling, or redness at injection site; or other unusual symptoms. **Pregnancy/breast-feeding precautions:** Inform prescriber if you are or intend to become pregnant. Do not breast-feed.

Pregnancy Risk Factor: C

Pregnancy Issues: Safety and efficacy in pregnant women has not been established. Treatment should be discontinued if a woman becomes pregnant, or plans to become pregnant during therapy. A dose-related abortifacient activity was reported in Rhesus monkeys.

Lactation: Excretion in breast milk unknown/contraindicated

Breast-Feeding Issues: Because its use has not been evaluated during lactation, breast-feeding is not recommended

Administration

Other: SubQ: Withdraw 1 mL of reconstituted solution from the vial into a sterile syringe fitted with a 27-gauge needle and inject the solution subcutaneously. Sites for self-injection include arms, abdomen, hips, and thighs. SubQ administration is suggested for those who are at risk for bleeding or are thrombocytopenic. Rotate SubQ injection site. Patient should be well hydrated.

Reconstitution: To reconstitute solution, inject 1.2 mL of diluent (provided); gently swirl to dissolve, do not shake. Reconstituted solution provides 0.25 mg/mL. Use product within 3 hours of reconstitution.

Storage: Store at room temperature of 25°C (77°F); excursions permitted to 15°C to 30°C (59°F to 86°F). If not used immediately following reconstitution, refrigerate solution at 2°C to 8°C (36°F to 46°F); do not freeze or shake solution.

Additional Information May be available only in small supplies; for information on availability and distribution, call the patient information line at 800-580-3837.

Interferon Gamma-1b (in ter FEER on GAM ah won bee)

U.S. Brand Names Actimmune®

Generic Available No

Pharmacologic Category Interferon

Use Reduce frequency and severity of serious infections associated with chronic granulomatous disease; delay time to disease progression in patients with severe, malignant osteopetrosis

Contraindications Hypersensitivity to interferon gamma, *E. coli* derived proteins, or any component of the formulation

Warnings/Precautions Patients with pre-existing cardiac disease, seizure disorders, CNS disturbances, or myelosuppression should be carefully monitored; long-term effects on growth and development are unknown; safety and efficacy in children <1 year of age have not been established.

Drug Interactions

Cytochrome P450 Effect: Inhibits CYP1A2 (weak), 2E1 (weak)

Increased Effect/Toxicity: Interferon gamma-1b may increase hepatic enzymes or enhance myelosuppression when taken with other myelosuppressive agents. May decrease cytochrome P450 concentrations leading to increased serum concentrations of drugs metabolized by this pathway.

Nutritional/Ethanol Interactions Herb/Nutraceutical: Dietary supplements containing aristolochic acid (found most often in Chinese medicines/herbal therapies); cases of nephropathy and ESRD associated with their use.

Adverse Reactions Based on 50 mcg/m^2 dose administered 3 times weekly for chronic granulomatous disease

>10%:

Central nervous system: Fever (52%), headache (33%), chills (14%), fatigue (14%)

Dermatologic: Rash (17%)

Gastrointestinal: Diarrhea (14%), vomiting (13%)

Local: Injection site erythema or tenderness (14%)

1% to 10%:

Central nervous system: Depression (3%)

Gastrointestinal: Nausea (10%), abdominal pain (8%)

Neuromuscular & skeletal: Myalgia (6%), arthralgia (2%), back pain (2%)

Pharmacodynamics/Kinetics

Absorption: I.M., SubQ: Slowly

Time to Peak: Plasma: I.M.: 4 hours (1.5 ng/mL); SubQ: 7 hours (0.6 ng/mL)

Half-Life Elimination: I.V.: 38 minutes; I.M., SubQ: 3-6 hours

Dosing

Adults & Elderly: If severe reactions occur, modify dose (50% reduction) or therapy should be discontinued until adverse reactions abate.

Chronic granulomatous disease: SubQ:

BSA ≤0.5 m^2: 1.5 mcg/kg/dose 3 times/week

BSA >0.5 m^2: 50 mcg/m^2 (1 million int. units/m^2) 3 times/week

Severe, malignant osteopetrosis: Children >1 year: SubQ:

BSA ≤0.5 m^2: 1.5 mcg/kg/dose 3 times/week

BSA >0.5 m^2: 50 mcg/m^2 (1 million int. units/m^2) 3 times/week

Note: Previously expressed as 1.5 million units/m^2; 50 mcg is equivalent to 1 million int. units/m^2.

Pediatrics: Children >1 year: Refer to adult dosing.

Available Dosage Forms Injection, solution [preservative free]: 100 mcg [2 million int. units] (0.5 mL)

Previously, 100 mcg was expressed as 3 million units. This is equivalent to 2 million int. units.

Monitoring and Teaching Issues

Physical Assessment: Monitor closely for effectiveness and/or interactions. Assess results of laboratory tests on a regular basis, therapeutic effectiveness, and adverse reactions. Assess knowledge and instruct patient/caregiver on appropriate reconstitution, injection and needle disposal, possible side effects, and symptoms to report.

Monitoring Laboratory Tests: CBC, platelet counts, renal and liver function, urinalysis (at 3-month intervals during treatment)

Patient Education: This is not a cure for MS; you will continue to receive regular treatment and follow-up for MS. Use as directed; do not change the dosage or schedule of administration without consulting prescriber. Maintain adequate hydration (2-3 L/day of fluids) unless instructed to restrict fluid intake. You may experience flu-like syndrome (acetaminophen may help); nausea, vomiting, or loss of appetite (small frequent meals, frequent mouth care, sucking lozenges, or chewing gum may help); or drowsiness, dizziness, agitation, or abnormal thinking (use caution when driving or engaging in tasks requiring alertness until response to drug is known). Report unusual bruising or bleeding; persistent abdominal disturbances; unusual fatigue; muscle pain or tremors; chest pain or palpitations; swelling of extremities; visual disturbances; pain, swelling, or redness at injection site; or other unusual symptoms. **Pregnancy/breast-feeding precautions:** Inform prescriber if you are or intend to become pregnant. Do not breast-feed.

Pregnancy Risk Factor: C

Pregnancy Issues: Safety and efficacy in pregnant women has not been established. Treatment should be discontinued if a woman becomes pregnant, or plans to become pregnant during therapy. A dose-related abortifacient activity was reported in Rhesus monkeys.

Lactation: Excretion in breast milk unknown/contraindicated

Breast-Feeding Issues: Potential for serious adverse reactions. Because its use has not been evaluated during lactation, breast-feeding is not recommended

Administration

Storage: Store in refrigerator. Do not freeze. Do not shake. Discard if left unrefrigerated for >12 hours.

- **Interleukin-2** *see* Aldesleukin *on page 62*
- **Intralipid®** *see* Fat Emulsion *on page 610*
- **Intravenous Fat Emulsion** *see* Fat Emulsion *on page 610*
- **Intrifiban** *see* Eptifibatide *on page 537*
- **Intron® A** *see* Interferon Alfa-2b *on page 811*
- **Intropin** *see* DOPamine *on page 481*
- **Invanz®** *see* Ertapenem *on page 541*
- **Invirase®** *see* Saquinavir *on page 1355*
- **Iodine I 131 Tositumomab and Tositumomab** *see* Tositumomab and Iodine I 131 Tositumomab *on page 1501*

Iodoquinol (eye oh doe KWIN ole)

U.S. Brand Names Yodoxin®
Synonyms Diiodohydroxyquin
Generic Available No
Pharmacologic Category Amebicide
Use Treatment of acute and chronic intestinal amebiasis; asymptomatic cyst passers; *Blastocystis hominis* infections; ineffective for amebic hepatitis or hepatic abscess
Mechanism of Action/Effect Contact amebicide that works in the lumen of the intestine by an unknown mechanism
Contraindications Hypersensitivity to iodine or iodoquinol or any component of the formulation; hepatic damage; pre-existing optic neuropathy
Warnings/Precautions Optic neuritis, optic atrophy, and peripheral neuropathy have occurred following prolonged use. Avoid long-term therapy. Use with caution in patients with thyroid disease.
Lab Interactions May increase protein-bound serum iodine concentrations reflecting a decrease in ^{131}I uptake; false-positive ferric chloride test for phenylketonuria
Adverse Reactions Frequency not defined.
Central nervous system: Fever, chills, agitation, retrograde amnesia, headache
Dermatologic: Rash, urticaria, pruritus
Endocrine & metabolic: Thyroid gland enlargement
Gastrointestinal: Diarrhea, nausea, vomiting, stomach pain, abdominal cramps
Neuromuscular & skeletal: Peripheral neuropathy, weakness
Ocular: Optic neuritis, optic atrophy, visual impairment
Miscellaneous: Itching of rectal area
Overdosage/Toxicology Chronic overdose can result in vomiting, diarrhea, abdominal pain, metallic taste, paresthesia, paraplegia, and loss of vision. Can lead to destruction of long fibers of the spinal cord and optic nerve. Acute overdose may cause delirium, stupor, coma, and amnesia. Treatment is symptomatic.
Pharmacodynamics/Kinetics
Absorption: Poor and erratic
Metabolism: Hepatic
Excretion: Feces (high percentage)
Dosing
Adults: Treatment of susceptible infections: Oral: 650 mg 3 times/day after meals for 20 days; not to exceed 2 g/day
Elderly: This agent is no longer a drug of choice; use only if other therapy is contraindicated or has failed. Due to optic nerve damage, use cautiously in the elderly.
Pediatrics: Treatment of susceptible infections: Oral: Children: 30-40 mg/kg/day (maximum: 650 mg/dose) in 3 divided doses for 20 days; not to exceed 1.95 g/day
Available Dosage Forms Tablet: 210 mg, 650 mg
Monitoring and Teaching Issues
Physical Assessment: Check allergy history (iodine) prior to beginning therapy. Perform ophthalmological exams with long-term therapy. Teach patient appropriate use, reinfection prevention, possible side effects/interventions, and adverse symptoms to report.
Monitoring Laboratory Tests: Ophthalmologic exam
Patient Education: Do not take any new medication during therapy unless approved by prescriber. Take as directed; complete full course of therapy. Maintain adequate hydration (2-3 L/day of fluids) unless instructed to restrict fluid intake and nutrition (small frequent meals may help). You may experience GI upset (small frequent meals, frequent mouth care, sucking lozenges, or chewing gum may help). Report unresolved or severe nausea or vomiting, skin rash, fever, or fatigue. **Pregnancy/breast-feeding precautions:** Inform prescriber if you are or intend to become pregnant. Consult prescriber if breast-feeding.
Dietary Considerations: Should be taken after meals.
Pregnancy Risk Factor: C
Lactation: Excretion in breast milk unknown
Administration
Oral: Tablets may be crushed and mixed with applesauce or chocolate syrup. May take with food or milk to reduce stomach upset. Complete full course of therapy.

- **Iophen-C NR** *see* Guaifenesin and Codeine *on page 731*
- **Iophen NR** *see* Guaifenesin *on page 729*
- **Iopidine®** *see page 1625*
- **Iopidine®** *see* Apraclonidine *on page 132*
- **Iosat™ [OTC]** *see* Potassium Iodide *on page 1237*
- **I-Paracaine®** *see page 1625*

Ipecac Syrup (IP e kak SIR up)

Synonyms Syrup of Ipecac
Generic Available Yes
Pharmacologic Category Antidote

Use Treatment of acute oral drug overdosage and in certain poisonings

Mechanism of Action/Effect Irritates the gastric mucosa and stimulates the medullary chemoreceptor trigger zone to induce vomiting

Contraindications Hypersensitivity to ipecac or any component of the formulation; do not use in unconscious patients; patients with no gag reflex; following ingestion of strong bases, acids, or volatile oils; when seizures are likely

Warnings/Precautions Do not confuse ipecac syrup with ipecac fluid extract, which is 14 times more potent. Use with caution in patients with cardiovascular disease and bulimics. May not be effective in antiemetic overdose.

Drug Interactions

  Decreased Effect: Activated charcoal, milk, carbonated beverages decrease the effect of ipecac syrup.

  Increased Effect/Toxicity: Phenothiazines (chlorpromazine has been associated with serious dystonic reactions).

Nutritional/Ethanol Interactions Food: Milk, carbonated beverages may decrease effectiveness.

Adverse Reactions Frequency not defined.

  Cardiovascular: Cardiotoxicity

  Central nervous system: Lethargy

  Gastrointestinal: Protracted vomiting, diarrhea

  Neuromuscular & skeletal: Myopathy

Overdosage/Toxicology Contains cardiotoxin. Symptoms of overdose include tachycardia, CHF, atrial fibrillation, depressed myocardial contractility, myocarditis, diarrhea, persistent vomiting, and hypotension. Treatment is activated charcoal and gastric lavage.

Pharmacodynamics/Kinetics

  Onset of Action: 15-30 minutes

  Duration of Action: 20-25 minutes; 60 minutes in some cases

  Absorption: Significant amounts, mainly when it does not produce emesis

  Excretion: Urine; emetine (alkaloid component) may be detected in urine 60 days after excess dose or chronic use

Dosing

  Adults & Elderly: Emetic: Oral: 15-30 mL followed by 200-300 mL of water; repeat dose one time if vomiting does not occur within 20 minutes.

  Pediatrics: Emetic: Oral:

    6-12 months: 5-10 mL followed by 10-20 mL/kg of water; repeat dose one time if vomiting does not occur within 20 minutes.

    1-12 years: 15 mL followed by 10-20 mL/kg of water; repeat dose one time if vomiting does not occur within 20 minutes.

    Note: If emesis does not occur within 30 minutes after second dose, ipecac must be removed from stomach by gastric lavage.

Available Dosage Forms Syrup: 70 mg/mL (30 mL) [contains alcohol]

Monitoring and Teaching Issues

  Physical Assessment: The Poison Control Center should be contacted before administration. Administer only to conscious patients. If vomiting does not occur within 30 minutes, contact the Poison Control Center (or prescriber) again. Assess patient's knowledge for home use.

  Patient Education: The Poison Control Center should be contacted before administration. Take only as directed; do not take more than recommended or more often than recommended. Follow with 8 oz of water. If vomiting does not occur within 30 minutes, contact the Poison Control Center or emergency services again. Do not administer if vomiting. If vomiting occurs after taking, do not eat or drink until vomiting subsides. **Breast-feeding precaution:** Consult prescriber if breast-feeding.

  Pregnancy Risk Factor: C

  Lactation: Excretion in breast milk unknown/use caution

Administration

  Oral: Do **not** administer to unconscious patients. Patients should be kept active and moving following administration of ipecac. If vomiting does not occur after second dose, gastric lavage may be considered to remove ingested substance.

Additional Information The benefit of ipecac syrup to treat poisoning in children has been questioned. In November 2003, the American Academy of Pediatrics recommended that syrup of ipecac no longer be used routinely for the management of poisonings in the home. They advised parents to dispose of existing supplies of ipecac to help prevent inappropriate use.

♦ **I-Pentolate**® *see page 1625*

♦ **IPOL**® *see page 1660*

Ipratropium (i pra TROE pee um)

U.S. Brand Names Atrovent®; Atrovent® HFA

Synonyms Ipratropium Bromide

Generic Available Yes: Excludes solution for oral inhalation

Pharmacologic Category Anticholinergic Agent

Medication Safety Issues

  Sound-alike/look-alike issues:

    Atrovent® may be confused with Alupent®

Use Anticholinergic bronchodilator used in bronchospasm associated with COPD, bronchitis, and emphysema; symptomatic relief of rhinorrhea associated with the common cold and allergic and nonallergic rhinitis

Mechanism of Action/Effect Blocks the action of acetylcholine at parasympathetic sites in bronchial smooth muscle causing bronchodilation

Contraindications Hypersensitivity to ipratropium, atropine, its derivatives, or any component of the formulation

(Continued)

Ipratropium *(Continued)*

In addition, Atrovent® inhalation aerosol is contraindicated in patients with hypersensitivity to soya lecithin or related food products (eg, soybean and peanut). **Note:** Other formulations may include these components; refer to product-specific labeling.

Warnings/Precautions Not indicated for the initial treatment of acute episodes of broncho-spasm. Use with caution in patients with myasthenia gravis, narrow-angle glaucoma, benign prostatic hyperplasia (BPH), or bladder neck obstruction.

Drug Interactions
Increased Effect/Toxicity: Increased toxicity with anticholinergics or drugs with anticholin-ergic properties.

Adverse Reactions
Inhalation aerosol and inhalation solution:
>10%: Bronchitis (10% to 23%), upper respiratory tract infection (13%)
1% to 10%:
Cardiovascular: Palpitation
Central nervous system: Dizziness (2% to 3%)
Dermatologic: Rash (1%)
Gastrointestinal: Nausea, xerostomia, stomach upset, dry mucous membranes
Renal: Urinary tract infection
Respiratory: Nasal congestion, dyspnea (10%), sputum increased (1%), bronchospasm (2%), pharyngitis (3%), rhinitis (2%), sinusitis (5%)
Miscellaneous: Flu-like syndrome

Nasal spray: Respiratory: Epistaxis (8%), nasal dryness (5%), nausea (2%)

Overdosage/Toxicology Symptoms of overdose include dry mouth, drying of respiratory secretions, cough, nausea, GI distress, blurred vision or impaired visual accommodation, headache, and nervousness. Acute overdose with ipratropium by inhalation is unlikely since it is so poorly absorbed. However, if poisoning occurs, it can be treated like any other anticho-linergic toxicity. An anticholinergic overdose with severe life-threatening symptoms may be treated with physostigmine 1-2 mg SubQ or I.V. slowly.

Pharmacodynamics/Kinetics
Onset of Action: Bronchodilation: 1-3 minutes; Peak effect: 1.5-2 hours
Duration of Action: ≤4 hours
Absorption: Negligible

Dosing
Adults & Elderly:
Bronchospasm:
Nebulization: 500 mcg (one unit-dose vial) 3-4 times/day with doses 6-8 hours apart
Metered dose inhaler: 2 inhalations 4 times/day, up to 12 inhalations/24 hours
Colds (symptomatic relief of rhinorrhea): Safety and efficacy of use beyond 4 days not established: Nasal spray (0.06%): 2 sprays in each nostril 3-4 times/day
Allergic/nonallergic rhinitis: Nasal spray (0.03%): 2 sprays in each nostril 2-3 times/day

Pediatrics:
Bronchospasm:
Nebulization:
Infants and Children ≤12 years: 125-250 mcg 3 times/day
Children >12 years: Refer to adult dosing.
Metered dose inhaler:
Children 3-12 years: 1-2 inhalations 3 times/day, up to 6 inhalations/24 hours
Children >12 years: Refer to adult dosing.
Colds (symptomatic relief of rhinorrhea): Intranasal: Safety and efficacy of use beyond 4 days in patients with the common cold have not been established:
Children 5-11 years: 0.06%: 2 sprays in each nostril 3 times/day
Children ≥5 years and Adults: 0.06%: 2 sprays in each nostril 3-4 times/day
Allergic/nonallergic rhinitis: Intranasal: Children ≥6 years: Refer to adult dosing.

Available Dosage Forms
Solution for nebulization, as bromide: 0.02% (2.5 mL)
Solution for oral inhalation, as bromide (Atrovent®): 18 mcg/actuation (14 g) [contains soya lecithin and chlorofluorocarbons]
Solution for oral inhalation, as bromide (Atrovent® HFA): 17 mcg/actuation (12.9 g)
Solution, intranasal spray, as bromide (Atrovent®): 0.03% (30 mL); 0.06% (15 mL)

Monitoring and Teaching Issues
Physical Assessment: Assess potential for interactions with other prescriptions, OTC medications, or herbal products patient may be taking (especially anything that may have anticholinergic properties). Assess patient response on a regular basis throughout therapy. Teach patient proper use, possible side effects/appropriate interventions (eg, importance of adequate hydration), and adverse symptoms to report.

Patient Education: Do not take any new medication during therapy without consulting prescriber. Use exactly as directed (see below). Do not use more often than recom-mended. Store solution away from light. Maintain adequate hydration (2-3 L/day of fluids) unless instructed to restrict fluid intake. May cause sensitivity to heat (avoid extremes in temperature); nervousness, dizziness, or fatigue (use caution when driving or engaging in tasks requiring alertness until response to drug is known); dry mouth, unpleasant taste, stomach upset (small frequent meals, frequent mouth care, chewing gum, or sucking hard candy may help); or difficulty urinating (always void before treatment). Report unresolved GI upset, dizziness or fatigue, vision changes, palpitations, persistent inability to void, nervousness, or insomnia. **Breast-feeding precaution:** Consult prescriber if breast-feeding.

Inhaler: Follow instructions for use accompanying the product. Close eyes when adminis-tering ipratropium; blurred vision may result if sprayed into eyes. Effects are enhanced by holding breath 10 seconds after inhalation; wait at least 1 full minute between inhalations.

Nebulizer: Wash hands before and after treatment. Wash and dry nebulizer after each treatment. Twist open the top of one unit dose vial and squeeze the contents into the nebulizer reservoir. Connect the nebulizer reservoir to the mouthpiece or face mask. Connect nebulizer to compressor. Sit in a comfortable, upright position. Place mouthpiece in your mouth or put on the face mask and turn on the compressor. If a face mask is used, avoid leakage around the mask (temporary blurring of vision, worsening of narrow-angle glaucoma, or eye pain may occur if mist gets into eyes). Breathe calmly and deeply until no more mist is formed in the nebulizer (about 5 minutes). At this point, treatment is finished.

Dietary Considerations: Some dosage forms may contain soya lecithin. Do not use in patients allergic to soya lecithin or related food products such as soybean and peanut.

Geriatric Considerations: Older patients may find it difficult to use the metered dose inhaler. A spacer device may be useful. Ipratropium has not been specifically studied in the elderly, but it is poorly absorbed from the airways and appears to be safe in this population.

Pregnancy Risk Factor: B

Lactation: Excretion in breast milk unknown/use caution

Administration
  Inhalation:
    Atrovent®: Shake inhaler before each use; rinsing mouth after each use decreases dry mouth side effect
    Atrovent® HFA: Prime inhaler by releasing 2 test sprays into the air. If the inhaler has not been used for >3 days, reprime.
  Compatibility: Compatible for 1 hour when mixed with albuterol in a nebulizer
  Storage: Store at 15°C to 30°C (59°F to 86°F). Do not store near heat or open flame.

Related Information
  Inhalant Agents *on page 1734*

Ipratropium and Albuterol (i pra TROE pee um & al BYOO ter ole)

U.S. Brand Names Combivent®; DuoNeb™

Synonyms Albuterol and Ipratropium

Generic Available No

Pharmacologic Category Bronchodilator

Medication Safety Issues
  Sound-alike/look-alike issues:
    Combivent® may be confused with Combivir®

Use Treatment of COPD in those patients that are currently on a regular bronchodilator who continue to have bronchospasms and require a second bronchodilator

Dosing
  Adults & Elderly:
    COPD:
      Inhalation: 2 metered-dose inhalations 4 times/day; may receive additional doses as necessary, but total number of doses in 24 hours should not exceed 12 inhalations.
      Inhalation via nebulization: Initial: 3 mL every 6 hours (maximum: 3 mL every 4 hours)

Available Dosage Forms
  Aerosol for oral inhalation (Combivent®): Ipratropium bromide 18 mcg and albuterol sulfate 103 mcg per actuation [200 doses] (14.7 g) [contains soya lecithin]
  Solution for oral inhalation (DuoNeb™): Ipratropium bromide 0.5 mg [0.017%] and albuterol base 2.5 mg [0.083%] per 3 mL vial (30s, 60s)

Monitoring and Teaching Issues
  Physical Assessment: See individual agents.
  Patient Education: See individual agents. **Pregnancy/breast-feeding precautions:** Inform prescriber if you are or intend to become pregnant. Consult prescriber if breast-feeding.

Pregnancy Risk Factor: C

Lactation: Excretion in breast milk unknown

Related Information
  Albuterol *on page 59*
  Ipratropium *on page 825*

♦ **Ipratropium Bromide** *see* Ipratropium *on page 825*

♦ **I-Prin [OTC]** *see* Ibuprofen *on page 777*

♦ **Iproveratril Hydrochloride** *see* Verapamil *on page 1560*

♦ **Iquix®** *see* Levofloxacin *on page 888*

Irbesartan (ir be SAR tan)

U.S. Brand Names Avapro®

Generic Available No

Pharmacologic Category Angiotensin II Receptor Blocker

Medication Safety Issues
  Sound-alike/look-alike issues:
    Avapro® may be confused with Anaprox®

Use Treatment of hypertension alone or in combination with other antihypertensives; treatment of diabetic nephropathy in patients with type 2 diabetes mellitus (noninsulin dependent, NIDDM) and hypertension

Mechanism of Action/Effect Irbesartan is an angiotensin receptor antagonist. Angiotensin II acts as a vasoconstrictor and stimulates the release of aldosterone, which results in reabsorption of sodium and water. These effects result in an elevation in blood pressure. Irbesartan blocks the AT1 angiotensin II receptor, thereby blocking the vasoconstriction and the aldosterone secreting effects of angiotensin II.

Contraindications Hypersensitivity to irbesartan or any component of the formulation; hypersensitivity to other A-II receptor antagonists; bilateral renal artery stenosis; pregnancy (2nd and 3rd trimesters)

Warnings/Precautions Avoid use or use smaller doses in patients who are volume depleted; correct depletion first. Deterioration in renal function can occur with initiation. Use with caution in unilateral renal artery stenosis and pre-existing renal insufficiency; significant
(Continued)

Irbesartan *(Continued)*

aortic/mitral stenosis. Safety and efficacy have not been established in pediatric patients <6 years of age.

Drug Interactions

Cytochrome P450 Effect: **Substrate** of CYP2C8/9 (minor); **Inhibits** CYP2C8/9 (moderate), 2D6 (weak), 3A4 (weak)

Increased Effect/Toxicity: Potassium salts/supplements, co-trimoxazole (high dose), ACE inhibitors, and potassium-sparing diuretics (amiloride, spironolactone, triamterene) may increase the risk of hyperkalemia. Irbesartan may increase the levels/effects of amiodarone, fluoxetine, glimepiride, glipizide, nateglinide, phenytoin, pioglitazone, rosiglitazone, sertraline, warfarin, and other CYP2C8/9 substrates.

Nutritional/Ethanol Interactions Herb/Nutraceutical: Avoid dong quai if using for hypertension (has estrogenic activity). Avoid ephedra, yohimbe, ginseng (may worsen hypertension). Avoid garlic (may have increased antihypertensive effect).

Adverse Reactions Unless otherwise indicated, percentage of incidence is reported for patients with hypertension.

>10%: Endocrine & metabolic: Hyperkalemia (19%, diabetic nephropathy)

1% to 10%:
Cardiovascular: Orthostatic hypotension (5%, diabetic nephropathy)
Central nervous system: Fatigue (4%), dizziness (10%, diabetic nephropathy)
Gastrointestinal: Diarrhea (3%), dyspepsia (2%)
Respiratory: Upper respiratory infection (9%), cough (2.8% versus 2.7% in placebo)

>1% but frequency ≤ placebo: Abdominal pain, anxiety, chest pain, edema, headache, influenza, musculoskeletal pain, nausea, nervousness, pharyngitis, rash, rhinitis, sinus abnormality, syncope, tachycardia, urinary tract infection, vertigo, vomiting

Overdosage/Toxicology Likely manifestations of overdose include hypotension and tachycardia. Treatment is supportive. Not removed by hemodialysis.

Pharmacodynamics/Kinetics

Onset of Action: Peak levels in 1-2 hours

Duration of Action: >24 hours

Bioavailability: 60% to 80%

Time to Peak: Serum: 1.5-2 hours

Protein Binding: Plasma: 90%

Half-Life Elimination: Terminal: 11-15 hours

Metabolism: Hepatic, primarily CYP2C9

Excretion: Feces (80%); urine (20%)

Dosing

Adults & Elderly:

Hypertension: Oral: 150 mg once daily; patients may be titrated to 300 mg once daily. **Note:** Starting dose in volume-depleted patients should be 75 mg.

Nephropathy in patients with type 2 diabetes and hypertension: Oral: Target dose: 300 mg once daily

Pediatrics: Hypertension: Oral:
<6 years: Safety and efficacy have not been established.
≥6-12 years: Initial: 75 mg once daily; may be titrated to a maximum of 150 mg once daily
13-16 years: Refer to adult dosing.

Renal Impairment: No dosage adjustment necessary with mild to severe impairment unless the patient is also volume depleted.

Available Dosage Forms Tablet: 75 mg, 150 mg, 300 mg

Monitoring and Teaching Issues

Physical Assessment: Use caution in presence of renal insufficiency or aortic/mitral stenosis (see Warnings/Precautions for specific use cautions). Assess potential for interactions with other pharmacological agents or herbal products patient may be taking (risk of hyperkalemia or toxicity; see Drug Interactions). Assess results of laboratory tests, therapeutic effectiveness, and adverse response at regular intervals during therapy (eg, hypotension; see Adverse Reactions). Teach patient proper use, possible side effects/ appropriate interventions, and adverse symptoms to report (see Patient Education).

Monitoring Laboratory Tests: Electrolytes, serum creatinine, BUN, urinalysis

Patient Education: Do not take any new medication during therapy unless approved by prescriber. Take exactly as directed; do not discontinue without consulting prescriber. May be taken with or without food. Take first dose at bedtime. This medication does not replace other antihypertensive interventions; follow prescriber's instructions for diet and lifestyle changes. May cause dizziness, fainting, or lightheadedness (use caution when driving or engaging in tasks that require alertness until response to drug is known); nausea, vomiting, or abdominal pain (small frequent meals, frequent mouth care, sucking lozenges, or chewing gum may help); or diarrhea (buttermilk, boiled milk, yogurt may help). Report chest pain or palpitations, skin rash, fluid retention (swelling of extremities), respiratory difficulty or unusual cough, or other persistent adverse reactions. **Pregnancy/ breast-feeding precautions:** Inform prescriber if you are or intend to become pregnant. This drug should not be used in the 2nd or 3rd trimester of pregnancy. Consult prescriber for appropriate contraceptive measures if necessary. Do not breast-feed.

Dietary Considerations: May be taken with or without food.

Pregnancy Risk Factor: C/D (2nd and 3rd trimesters)

Pregnancy Issues: The drug should be discontinued as soon as possible after detection of pregnancy. Drugs which act directly on the renin-angiotensin system can cause fetal and neonatal morbidity and death.

Lactation: Excretion in breast milk unknown/contraindicated

Administration

Storage: Store at room temperature of 15°C to 30°C (59°F to 86°F).

Related Information

Angiotensin Agents *on page 1704*

Irbesartan and Hydrochlorothiazide
(ir be SAR tan & hye droe klor oh THYE a zide)

U.S. Brand Names Avalide®

Synonyms Avapro® HCT; Hydrochlorothiazide and Irbesartan

Generic Available No

Pharmacologic Category Antihypertensive Agent, Combination

Medication Safety Issues
Sound-alike/look-alike issues:
Avalide® may be confused with Avandia®

Use Combination therapy for the management of hypertension

Dosing
Adults & Elderly:
Hypertension: Oral: Dose must be individualized. A patient who is not controlled with either agent alone may be switched to the combination product. Mean effect increases with the dose of each component. The lowest dosage available is irbesartan 150 mg/hydrochlorothiazide 12.5 mg. Dose increases should be made not more frequently than every 2-4 weeks.
Pediatrics: Refer to adult dosing.

Available Dosage Forms
Tablet:
Irbesartan 150 mg and hydrochlorothiazide 12.5 mg
Irbesartan 300 mg and hydrochlorothiazide 12.5 mg

Monitoring and Teaching Issues
Physical Assessment: See individual agents.
Patient Education: See individual agents. **Pregnancy/breast-feeding precautions:** Inform prescriber if you are or intend to become pregnant. Do not breast-feed.
Pregnancy Risk Factor: C/D (2nd and 3rd trimesters)
Lactation: Enters breast milk/contraindicated

Related Information
Hydrochlorothiazide *on page 751*
Irbesartan *on page 827*

♦ **Ircon® [OTC]** *see* Ferrous Fumarate *on page 623*

♦ **Iressa™** *see* Gefitinib *on page 701*

Irinotecan (eye rye no TEE kan)

U.S. Brand Names Camptosar®

Synonyms Camptothecin-11; CPT-11; NSC-616348

Generic Available No

Pharmacologic Category Antineoplastic Agent, Natural Source (Plant) Derivative

Use Treatment of metastatic carcinoma of the colon or rectum

Unlabeled/Investigational Use Lung cancer (small cell and nonsmall cell), cervical cancer, gastric cancer, pancreatic cancer, leukemia, lymphoma, breast cancer

Mechanism of Action/Effect Irinotecan and its active metabolite (SN-38) bind reversibly to topoisomerase I and stabilize the cleavable complex so that religation of the cleaved DNA strand cannot occur. This results in the accumulation of cleavable complexes and single-strand DNA breaks. This interaction results in single-stranded DNA breaks and cell death consistent with S-phase cell cycle specificity.

Contraindications Hypersensitivity to irinotecan or any component of the formulation; concurrent use of atazanavir, ketoconazole, St John's wort; pregnancy

Warnings/Precautions The U.S. Food and Drug Administration (FDA) currently recommends that procedures for proper handling and disposal of antineoplastic agents be considered. Irinotecan can induce both early and late forms of diarrhea (mediated by different mechanisms). The administration of irinotecan should be delayed until the patient recovers and subsequent doses should be decreased. Premedication with loperamide is not recommended.

Deaths due to sepsis following severe myelosuppression have been reported. Therapy should be discontinued if neutropenic fever occurs or if the absolute neutrophil count is <500/mm³. The dose of irinotecan should be reduced if there is a clinically significant decrease in the total WBC (<200/mm³), neutrophil count (<1000/mm³), hemoglobin (<8 g/dL), or platelet count (<100,000/mm³). Routine administration of a colony-stimulating factor is generally not necessary. Avoid extravasation.

Patients with even modest elevations in total serum bilirubin levels (1.0-2.0 mg/dL) have a significantly greater likelihood of experiencing first-course grade 3 or 4 neutropenia than those with bilirubin levels that were <1.0 mg/dL. Patients with abnormal glucuronidation of bilirubin, such as those with Gilbert's syndrome, may also be at greater risk of myelosuppression when receiving therapy with irinotecan. Hold diuretics during dosing due to potential risk of dehydration secondary to vomiting and/or diarrhea induced by irinotecan.

One report describes three patients who developed akathisia after receiving prochlorperazine pretreatment and irinotecan. As the patients had received prochlorperazine previously, without developing akathisia, it was suggested that the akathisia resulted from an interaction between prochlorperazine and irinotecan. There are no further supporting data for such an interaction.

Use caution in patients who previously received pelvic/abdominal radiation, elderly patients with comorbid conditions, or baseline performance status of 2; close monitoring is recommended.

Drug Interactions
Cytochrome P450 Effect: Substrate (major) of CYP2B6, 3A4
Decreased Effect: CYP2B6 inducers may decrease the levels/effects of irinotecan; example inducers include carbamazepine, nevirapine, phenobarbital, phenytoin, and rifampin. CYP3A4 inducers may decrease the levels/effects of irinotecan; example (Continued)

829

Irinotecan *(Continued)*

inducers include aminoglutethimide, carbamazepine, nafcillin, nevirapine, phenobarbital, phenytoin, and rifamycins. St John's wort decreases therapeutic effect of irinotecan; discontinue ≥2 weeks prior to irinotecan therapy; **concurrent use during irinotecan therapy is contraindicated.**

Increased Effect/Toxicity: CYP2B6 inhibitors may increase the levels/effects of irinotecan; example inhibitors include desipramine, paroxetine, and sertraline. CYP3A4 inhibitors may increase the levels/effects of irinotecan; example inhibitors include azole antifungals, ciprofloxacin, clarithromycin, diclofenac, doxycycline, erythromycin, imatinib, isoniazid, nefazodone, nicardipine, propofol, protease inhibitors, quinidine, and verapamil. Bevacizumab may increase the adverse effects of irinotecan (eg, diarrhea, neutropenia). Ketoconazole increases the levels/effects of irinotecan and active metabolite; discontinue ketoconazole 1 week prior to irinotecan therapy; **concurrent use during irinotecan therapy is contraindicated.**

Nutritional/Ethanol Interactions Herb/Nutraceutical: St John's wort decreases the efficacy of irinotecan.

Adverse Reactions

>10%:

Cardiovascular: Vasodilation

Central nervous system: Insomnia, dizziness, fever (45.4%)

Dermatologic: Alopecia (60.5%), rash

Gastrointestinal: Irinotecan therapy may induce two different forms of diarrhea. Onset, symptoms, proposed mechanisms and treatment are different. Overall, 56.9% of patients treated experience abdominal pain and/or cramping during therapy. Anorexia, constipation, flatulence, stomatitis, and dyspepsia have also been reported.

Diarrhea: Dose-limiting toxicity with weekly dosing regimen

Early diarrhea (50.7% incidence, grade 3/4 8%) usually occurs during or within 24 hours of administration. May be accompanied by symptoms of cramping, vomiting, flushing, and diaphoresis. It is thought to be mediated by cholinergic effects which can be successfully managed with atropine (refer to Warnings/Precautions).

Late diarrhea (87.8% incidence) usually occurs >24 hours after treatment. National Cancer Institute (NCI) grade 3 or 4 diarrhea (31%) occurs in 30.6% of patients. Late diarrhea generally occurs with a median of 11 days after therapy and lasts approximately 3 days. Patients experiencing grade 3 or 4 diarrhea were noted to have symptoms a total of 7 days. Correlated with irinotecan or SN-38 levels in plasma and bile. Due to the duration, dehydration and electrolyte imbalances are significant clinical concerns. Loperamide therapy is recommended. The incidence of grade 3 or 4 late diarrhea is significantly higher in patients ≥65 years of age; close monitoring and prompt initiation of high-dose loperamide therapy is prudent (refer to Warnings/Precautions).

Emetic potential: Moderately high (86.2% incidence, however, only 12.5% grade 3 or 4 vomiting)

Hematologic: Myelosuppressive: Dose-limiting toxicity with 3 week dosing regimen

Grade 1-4 neutropenia occurred in 53.9% of patients. Patients who had previously received pelvic or abdominal radiation therapy were noted to have a significantly increased incidence of grade 3 or 4 neutropenia. White blood cell count nadir is 15 days after administration and is more frequent than thrombocytopenia. Recovery is usually within 24-28 days and cumulative toxicity has not been observed.

WBC: Mild to severe

Platelets: Mild

Onset (days): 10

Nadir (days): 14-16

Recovery (days): 21-28

Neuromuscular & skeletal: Weakness (75.7%)

Respiratory: Dyspnea (22%), cough, rhinitis, decreased DLCO (in a few patients)

Miscellaneous: Diaphoresis

1% to 10%: **Irritant chemotherapy**; thrombophlebitis has been reported

Note: In limited pediatric experience, dehydration (often associated with severe hypokalemia and hyponatremia) was among the most significant grade 3/4 adverse events, with a frequency up to 29%. In addition, grade 3/4 infection was reported in 24%.

Overdosage/Toxicology Symptoms of overdose include bone marrow suppression, leukopenia, thrombocytopenia, nausea, and vomiting. Treatment is supportive.

Pharmacodynamics/Kinetics

Time to Peak: SN-38: 30-minute infusion: ~1 hour

Protein Binding: Plasma: Parent drug: 30% to 68%; SN-38 (active drug): 95%

Half-Life Elimination: Parent drug: Alpha: 0.2 hours, Beta: 2.5 hours, Gamma: 14.2 hours; SN-38: 3-23.9 hours

Metabolism: Via intestinal mucosa, plasma, hepatic, and perhaps in some tumors; converted to SN-38 by carboxylesterase enzymes; undergoes glucuronidation, the metabolites having much less activity than SN-38. Enterohepatic recirculation results in a second peak in the concentration of SN-38. The lactones of both irinotecan and SN-38 undergo hydrolysis to inactive hydroxy acid forms.

Excretion: Urine (~20% of dose) within 24 hours; SN-38 excretion in 24 hours accounted for 0.25% of administered dose

Dosing

Adults & Elderly: Refer to individual protocols.

Single-agent therapy:

I.V.: Weekly regimen: 125 mg/m^2 over 90 minutes on days 1, 8, 15, and 22, followed by a 2-week rest

Adjusted dose level -1: 100 mg/m^2

Adjusted dose level -2: 75 mg/m^2

I.V.: Once-every-3-week regimen: 350 mg/m^2 over 90 minutes, once every 3 weeks

Adjusted dose level -1: 300 mg/m^2

Adjusted dose level -2: 250 mg/m^2

Note: A reduction in the starting dose by one dose level may be considered for patients ≥65 years of age, prior pelvic/abdominal radiotherapy, performance status of 2, or increased bilirubin (dosing for patients with a bilirubin >2 mg/dL cannot be recommended based on lack of data per manufacturer)

Depending on the patient's ability to tolerate therapy, doses should be adjusted in increments of 25-50 mg/m^2. Irinotecan doses may from 50-150 mg/m^2 for the weekly regimen; from 50-200 mg/m^2 for the once-every-3-week regimen.

Combination therapy with fluorouracil and leucovorin: Six-week (42-day) cycle:

Regimen 1: I.V.: 125 mg/m^2 over 90 minutes on days 1, 8, 15, and 22; to be given in combination with bolus leucovorin and fluorouracil (leucovorin administered immediately following irinotecan; fluorouracil immediately following leucovorin)

Adjusted dose level -1: 100 mg/m^2
Adjusted dose level -2: 75 mg/m^2

Regimen 2: 180 mg/m^2 over 90 minutes on days 1, 15, and 22; to be given in combination with infusional leucovorin and bolus/infusion fluorouracil (leucovorin administered immediately following irinotecan; fluorouracil immediately following leucovorin)

Adjusted dose level -1: 150 mg/m^2
Adjusted dose level -2: 120 mg/m^2

Note: For all regimens: It is recommended that new courses begin only after the granulocyte count recovers to ≥1500/mm^3, the platelet count recovers to ≥100,000/mm^3, and treatment-related diarrhea has fully resolved. Treatment should be delayed 1-2 weeks to allow for recovery from treatment-related toxicities. If the patient has not recovered after a 2-week delay, consideration should be given to discontinuing irinotecan.

Dosing adjustment for toxicities: A decrease in dose level corresponds to a decrease in irinotecan dosage by 25-50 mg/m^2; specific dose levels corresponding to individual protocols should be consulted. Single-agent schedules and combination schedules: See tables on next page.

Hepatic Impairment: AUC of irinotecan and SN-38 have been reported to be higher in patients with known hepatic tumor involvement. The manufacturer recommends that no change in dosage or administration be made for patients with liver metastases and normal hepatic function. In patients with a combined history of prior pelvic/abdominal irradiation and modestly elevated total serum bilirubin levels (1.0-2.0 mg/dL) prior to treatment with irinotecan, there may be substantially increased likelihood of grade 3 or 4 neutropenia. Consideration may be given to starting irinotecan at a lower dose (eg, 100 mg/m^2) in such patients. Definite recommendations regarding the most appropriate starting dose in patients who have pretreatment total serum bilirubin elevations >2.0 mg/dL are not available, but it is likely that lower starting doses will need to be considered in such patients.

Available Dosage Forms Injection, solution, as hydrochloride: 20 mg/mL (2 mL, 5 mL)

Monitoring and Teaching Issues

Physical Assessment: See Warnings/Precautions for specific use cautions (eg, previous pelvic or abdominal radiation). Assess potential for interactions with other pharmacological agents prescriptions or herbal products patient may be taking (eg, potential for increased or decreased levels/effects of irinotecan; see Drug Interactions). Premedicate with antiemetic (emetic potential moderately high). Infusion site must be monitored to prevent extravasation. Assess results of laboratory tests, therapeutic effectiveness, and adverse response at regular intervals during therapy (eg, acute diarrhea, neutropenia, sepsis, mucositis and/or stomatitis; see Adverse Reactions and Dosing). Teach patient possible side effects/appropriate interventions, and adverse symptoms to report (see Patient Education).

Monitoring Laboratory Tests: CBC with differential and platelet count

Patient Education: Do not take any new medication during therapy unless approved by prescriber. This drug is administered by intravenous infusion; report immediately any burning, pain, redness, swelling at infusion site or sudden chest pain, difficulty breathing or swallowing, or chills. Maintain adequate hydration (3-4 L/day of fluids) unless instructed to restrict fluid intake during therapy. May cause severe diarrhea; report immediately any diarrhea or signs of dehydration (eg, fainting, dizziness, lightheadedness). You will be more susceptible to infection (avoid crowds and exposure to infection and do not have any vaccinations without consulting prescriber). You may experience nausea or vomiting (small frequent meals, frequent mouth care, sucking lozenges, or chewing gum may help); hair loss (will regrow after treatment is completed). Report unresolved nausea, or vomiting, alterations in urinary pattern (increased or decreased); opportunistic infection (fever, chills, unusual bruising or bleeding, fatigue, purulent vaginal discharge, unhealed mouth sores), chest pain, respiratory difficulty, unexplained weakness or fatigue; or other persistent effects. **Pregnancy/breast-feeding precautions:** Inform prescriber if you are pregnant. Do not get pregnant or cause a pregnancy (males) while taking this medication. Consult prescriber for use appropriate contraceptive measures (may cause severe fetal defects). Do not breast-feed.

Pregnancy Risk Factor: D

Pregnancy Issues: Has shown to be teratogenic in animals. Teratogenic effects include a variety of external, visceral, and skeletal abnormalities. The patient should be warned of potential hazards to the fetus.

Lactation: Enters breast milk/contraindicated

Administration

I.V.: Administer by I.V. infusion, usually over 90 minutes.

Reconstitution: Dilute in D$_5$W or NS to a final concentration of 0.12-2.8 mg/mL. Due to the relatively acidic pH, irinotecan appears to be more stable in D$_5$W than NS. D$_5$W (500 mL) is the preferred diluent for most doses.

Compatibility: Stable in D$_5$W, NS

Y-site administration: Incompatible with gemcitabine

Compatibility when admixed: Incompatible with methylprednisolone sodium succinate

Storage: Store intact vials of injection at room temperature; protect from light. D$_5$W (500 mL) is the preferred diluent for most doses. Solutions diluted in NS may precipitate if refrigerated. Solutions diluted in 250-500 mL D$_5$W are stable for 24 hours at room temperature or 48 hours under refrigeration.

(Continued)

Irinotecan *(Continued)*

Single-Agent Schedule: Recommended Dosage Modifications[1]

Toxicity NCI Grade[2] (Value)	During a Cycle of Therapy	At Start of Subsequent Cycles of Therapy (After Adequate Recovery), Compared to Starting Dose in Previous Cycle[1]	
	Weekly	Weekly	Once Every 3 Weeks
No toxicity	Maintain dose level	↑ 25 mg/m² up to a maximum dose of 150 mg/m²	Maintain dose level
Neutropenia			
1 (1500-1999/mm³)	Maintain dose level	Maintain dose level	Maintain dose level
2 (1000-1499/mm³)	↓ 25 mg/m²	Maintain dose level	Maintain dose level
3 (500-999/mm³)	Omit dose until resolved to ≤ grade 2, then ↓ 25 mg/m²	↓ 25 mg/m²	↓ 50 mg/m²
4 (<500/mm³)	Omit dose until resolved to ≤ grade 2, then ↓ 50 mg/m²	↓ 50 mg/m²	↓ 50 mg/m²
Neutropenic Fever (grade 4 neutropenia and ≥ grade 2 fever)	Omit dose until resolved, then ↓ 50 mg/m²	↓ 50 mg/m²	↓ 50 mg/m²
Other Hematologic Toxicities	Dose modifications for leukopenia, thrombocytopenia, and anemia during a course of therapy and at the start of subsequent courses of therapy are also based on NCI toxicity criteria and are the same as recommended for neutropenia above.		
Diarrhea			
1 (2-3 stools/day > pretreatment)	Maintain dose level	Maintain dose level	Maintain dose level
2 (4-6 stools/day > pretreatment)	↓ 25 mg/m²	Maintain dose level	Maintain dose level
3 (7-9 stools/day > pretreatment)	Omit dose until resolved to ≤ grade 2, then ↓ 25 mg/m²	↓ 25 mg/m²	↓ 50 mg/m²
4 (≥10 stools/day > pretreatment)	Omit dose until resolved to ≤ grade 2, then ↓ 50 mg/m²	↓ 50 mg/m²	↓ 50 mg/m²
Other Nonhematologic Toxicities[3]			
1	Maintain dose level	Maintain dose level	Maintain dose level
2	↓ 25 mg/m²	↓ 25 mg/m²	↓ 50 mg/m²
3	Omit dose until resolved to ≤ grade 2, then ↓ 25 mg/m²	↓ 25 mg/m²	↓ 50 mg/m²
4	Omit dose until resolved to ≤ grade 2, then ↓ 50 mg/m²	↓ 50 mg/m²	↓ 50 mg/m²

[1]All dose modifications should be based on the worst preceding toxicity.
[2]National Cancer Institute Common Toxicity Criteria (version 1.0).
[3]Excludes alopecia, anorexia, asthenia.

Combination Schedules: Recommended Dosage Modifications[1]

Toxicity NCI[2]Grade (Value)	During a Cycle of Therapy	At the Start of Subsequent Cycles of Therapy (After Adequate Recovery), Compared to the Starting Dose in the Previous Cycle[1]
No toxicity	Maintain dose level	Maintain dose level
Neutropenia		
1 (1500-1999/mm³)	Maintain dose level	Maintain dose level
2 (1000-1499/mm³)	↓ 1 dose level	Maintain dose level
3 (500-999/mm³)	Omit dose until resolved to ≤ grade 2, then ↓ 1 dose level	↓ 1 dose level
4 (<500/mm³)	Omit dose until resolved to ≤ grade 2, then ↓ 2 dose levels	↓ 2 dose levels
Neutropenic Fever (grade 4 neutropenia and ≥ grade 2 fever)	Omit dose until resolved, then ↓ 2 dose levels	
Other Hematologic Toxicities	Dose modifications for leukopenia or thrombocytopenia during a course of therapy and at the start of subsequent courses of therapy are also based on NCI toxicity criteria and are the same as recommended for neutropenia above.	
Diarrhea		
1 (2-3 stools/day > pretreatment)	Delay dose until resolved to baseline, then give same dose	Maintain dose level
2 (4-6 stools/day > pretreatment)	Omit dose until resolved to baseline, then ↓ 1 dose level	Maintain dose level
3 (7-9 stools/day > pretreatment)	Omit dose until resolved to baseline, then ↓ by 1 dose level	↓ 1 dose level
4 (≥10 stools/day > pretreatment)	Omit dose until resolved to baseline, then ↓ 2 dose levels	↓ 2 dose levels
Other Nonhematologic Toxicities[3]		
1	Maintain dose level	Maintain dose level
2	Omit dose until resolved to ≤ grade 1, then ↓ 1 dose level	Maintain dose level
3	Omit dose until resolved to ≤ grade 2, then ↓ 1 dose level	↓ 1 dose level
4	Omit dose until resolved to ≤ grade 2, then ↓ 2 dose levels	↓ 2 dose levels
Mucositis and/or stomatitis	Decrease only 5-FU, not irinotecan	Decrease only 5-FU, not irinotecan

[1]All dose modifications should be based on the worst preceding toxicity.
[2]National Cancer Institute Common Toxicity Criteria (version 1.0).
[3]Excludes alopecia, anorexia, asthenia.

Iron Dextran Complex (EYE ern DEKS tran KOM pleks)
U.S. Brand Names Dexferrum®; INFeD®
Generic Available No
Pharmacologic Category Iron Salt
Medication Safety Issues
Sound-alike/look-alike issues:
Dexferrum® may be confused with Desferal®

Use Treatment of microcytic hypochromic anemia resulting from iron deficiency in patients in whom oral administration is infeasible or ineffective

Mechanism of Action/Effect The released iron, from the plasma, eventually replenishes the depleted iron stores in the bone marrow where it is incorporated into hemoglobin

Contraindications Hypersensitivity to iron dextran or any component of the formulation; all anemias that are not involved with iron deficiency; hemochromatosis; hemolytic anemia

Warnings/Precautions Use with caution in patients with history of asthma, hepatic impairment, or rheumatoid arthritis. Not recommended in children <4 months of age. Deaths associated with parenteral administration following anaphylactic-type reactions have been reported. Use only in patients where the iron deficient state is not amenable to oral iron therapy. A test dose of 0.5 mL I.V. or I.M. should be given to observe for adverse reactions. I.V. administration of iron dextran is often preferred.

Drug Interactions
Decreased Effect: Decreased effect with chloramphenicol.
Nutritional/Ethanol Interactions Food: Iron bioavailability may be decreased if taken with dairy products.
Lab Interactions May cause falsely elevated values of serum bilirubin and falsely decreased values of serum calcium.

Adverse Reactions
>10%:
Cardiovascular: Flushing
Central nervous system: Dizziness, fever, headache, pain
Gastrointestinal: Nausea, vomiting, metallic taste
Local: Staining of skin at the site of I.M. injection
Miscellaneous: Diaphoresis
1% to 10%:
Cardiovascular: Hypotension (1% to 2%)
Dermatologic: Urticaria (1% to 2%), phlebitis (1% to 2%)
Gastrointestinal: Diarrhea
Genitourinary: Discoloration of urine
Note: Diaphoresis, urticaria, arthralgia, fever, chills, dizziness, headache, and nausea may be delayed 24-48 hours after I.V. administration or 3-4 days after I.M. administration.
Anaphylactoid reactions: Respiratory difficulties and cardiovascular collapse have been reported and occur most frequently within the first several minutes of administration.

Overdosage/Toxicology Symptoms of overdose include erosion of GI mucosa, pulmonary edema, hyperthermia, convulsions, tachycardia, hepatic and renal impairment, coma, hematemesis, lethargy, tachycardia, and acidosis. Serum iron level >300 mcg/mL requires treatment of overdose due to severe toxicity. If severe iron overdose (when the serum iron concentration exceeds the total iron-binding capacity) occurs, it may be treated with deferoxamine. Deferoxamine may be administered I.V. (80 mg/kg over 24 hours) or I.M. (40-90 mg/kg every 8 hours).

Milliliters of Iron Dextran (50 mg/mL) Required for Hemoglobin Restoration and Replacement of Iron Stores

Patient's IBW (kg)	Observed Hemoglobin							
	3 g/dL	4 g/dL	5 g/dL	6 g/dL	7 g/dL	8 g/dL	9 g/dL	10 g/dL
5	3	3	3	3	2	2	2	2
10	7	6	6	5	5	4	4	3
15	10	9	9	8	7	7	6	5
20	16	15	14	13	12	11	10	9
25	20	18	17	16	15	14	13	12
30	23	22	21	19	18	17	15	14
35	27	26	24	23	21	20	18	17
40	31	29	28	26	24	22	21	19
45	35	33	31	29	27	25	23	21
50	39	37	35	32	30	28	26	24
55	43	41	38	36	33	31	28	26
60	47	44	42	39	36	34	31	28
65	51	48	45	42	39	36	34	31
70	55	52	49	45	42	39	36	33
75	59	55	52	49	45	42	39	35
80	63	59	55	52	48	45	41	38
85	66	63	59	55	51	48	44	40
90	70	66	62	58	54	50	46	42
95	74	70	66	62	57	53	49	45
100	78	74	69	65	60	56	52	47

Iron dextran doses calculated for normal adult hemoglobin of 14.8 g/dL for IBW >15 kg, and normal hemoglobin of 12.0 g/dL for IBW ≤15 kg.

Pharmacodynamics/Kinetics
Absorption:
I.M.: 50% to 90% promptly absorbed; balance slowly absorbed over month
(Continued)

Iron Dextran Complex *(Continued)*

I.V.: Uptake of iron by the reticuloendothelial system appears to be constant at about 10-20 mg/hour

Excretion: Urine and feces via reticuloendothelial system

Dosing

Adults & Elderly:

Note: A 0.5 mL test dose should be given prior to starting iron dextran therapy.

Iron-deficiency anemia: I.M., I.V.:

Dose (mL) = 0.0476 x LBW (kg) x (normal Hgb - observed Hgb) + (1 mL/5 kg) of LBW to a maximum of 14 mL for iron stores (LBW = lean body weight)

Adults and children >15 kg: Dose (mL) = 0.0442 (desired Hgb - observed Hgb) x IBW + [0.26 x IBW (kg)]; see table on previous page.

IBW (male) = 50 kg + (2.3 kg x inches over 60")

IBW (female) = 45.5 kg + (2.3 kg x inches over 60")

Iron replacement therapy for blood loss: I.M., I.V.: Replacement iron (mg) = blood loss (mL) x Hct

Maximum daily dosage:

Manufacturer's labeling: **Note:** Replacement of larger estimated iron deficits may be achieved by serial administration of smaller incremental dosages. Daily dosages should be limited to: Adults >50 kg: 100 mg iron (2 mL)

Total dose infusion (unlabeled): The entire dose (estimated iron deficit) may be diluted and administered as a one-time I.V. infusion.

Pediatrics: Note: A 0.5 mL test dose (0.25 mL in infants) should be given prior to starting iron dextran therapy.

Iron-deficiency anemia: Refer to adult dosing.

Iron replacement therapy for blood loss: Refer to adult dosing.

Maximum daily dose:

5-10 kg: 50 mg iron (1 mL)

10-50 kg: 100 mg iron (2 mL)

Available Dosage Forms Note: Strength expressed as elemental iron

Injection, solution:

Dexferrum®: 50 mg/mL (1 mL, 2 mL)

INFeD®: 50 mg/mL (2 mL)

Monitoring and Teaching Issues

Physical Assessment: Assess results of laboratory tests regularly and patient for adverse reactions. Note that adverse response may occur some time (1-4 days) after administration. Assess patients with rheumatoid arthritis for exacerbated swelling and joint pain; adjust medications as needed.

Monitoring Laboratory Tests: Hemoglobin, hematocrit, reticulocyte count, serum ferritin

Patient Education: You will need frequent blood tests while on this therapy. If you have rheumatoid arthritis you may experience increased swelling or joint pain; consult prescriber for medication adjustment. If you experience dizziness or severe headache, use caution when driving or engaging in tasks that require alertness until response to drug is known. Small frequent meals, frequent mouth care, sucking lozenges, or chewing gum may relieve nausea and metallic taste. You may experience increased sweating. Report acute GI problems, fever, respiratory difficulty, rapid heartbeat, yellowing of skin or eyes, or swelling of hands and feet. **Pregnancy/breast-feeding precautions:** Inform prescriber if you are or intend to become pregnant. Do not breast-feed.

Geriatric Considerations: Anemia in the elderly is most often caused by "anemia of chronic disease", a result of aging effect in bone marrow, or associated with inflammation rather than blood loss. Iron stores are usually normal or increased, with a serum ferritin >50 ng/mL and a decreased total iron binding capacity. Hence, the anemia is not secondary to iron deficiency but the inability of the reticuloendothelial system to use available iron stores. I.V. administration of iron dextran is often preferred over I.M. in the elderly secondary to a decreased muscle mass and the need for daily injections.

Pregnancy Risk Factor: C

Lactation: Enters breast milk/contraindicated

Administration

I.M.: Note: Test dose: A test dose should be given on the first day of therapy; patient should be observed for 1 hour for hypersensitivity reaction, then the remaining dose (dose minus test dose) should be given. Epinephrine should be available.

I.M.: Use Z-track technique (displacement of the skin laterally prior to injection); injection should be deep into the upper outer quadrant of buttock; subsequent injections should be given into alternate buttock.

I.V.: A test dose should be given on the first day of therapy and administer gradually over at least 5 minutes. Subsequent dose(s) may be administered by I.V. bolus at rate of ≤50 mg/minute or diluted in 250-1000 mL NS and infused over 1-6 hours (initial 25 mL should be given slowly and patient should be observed for allergic reactions); avoid dilutions with dextrose (increased incidence of local pain and phlebitis)

Reconstitution: Stability of parenteral admixture at room temperature (25°C) is 3 months.

Standard diluent: Dose/250-1000 mL NS

Minimum volume: 250 mL NS

Compatibility: Stable in D_5W, NS

Storage: Store at room temperature.

♦ **Iron Fumarate** *see Ferrous Fumarate on page 623*

♦ **Iron Gluconate** *see Ferrous Gluconate on page 624*

Iron Sucrose *(EYE ern SOO krose)*

U.S. Brand Names Venofer®

Generic Available No

Pharmacologic Category Iron Salt

Use Treatment of iron-deficiency anemia in patients undergoing chronic hemodialysis who are receiving supplemental erythropoietin therapy

Mechanism of Action/Effect Iron sucrose is dissociated by the reticuloendothelial system into iron and sucrose. The released iron increases serum iron concentrations and is incorporated into hemoglobin.

Contraindications Hypersensitivity to iron sucrose or any component of the formulation; evidence of iron overload; anemia not caused by iron deficiency

Warnings/Precautions Rare, potentially life-threatening anaphylactic and anaphylactoid reactions have been reported. Facilities for cardiopulmonary resuscitation should be available during administration. Hypotension has been reported frequently in patients receiving intravenous iron, may be related to total dose or rate of administration (avoid rapid I.V. injection), follow recommended guidelines. Withhold iron in the presence of tissue iron overload; periodic monitoring of hemoglobin, hematocrit, serum ferritin, and transferrin saturation is recommended. Safety and efficacy in children have not been established.

Drug Interactions
Decreased Effect: Chloramphenicol may diminish the therapeutic effects of iron sucrose injection. Iron sucrose injection may reduce the absorption of oral iron preparations.

Adverse Reactions
>5%:
Cardiovascular: Hypotension (36%; may be related to total dose or rate of administration)
Central nervous system: Headache
Gastrointestinal: Diarrhea, nausea, vomiting
Neuromuscular & skeletal: Leg cramps (23%)
1% to 5%:
Cardiovascular: Chest pain, CHF, hypertension, hypervolemia
Central nervous system: Fever, dizziness, malaise
Dermatologic: Pruritus
Gastrointestinal: Abdominal pain, taste perversion
Hepatic: Hepatic enzymes increased
Local: Application site reaction
Neuromuscular & skeletal: Musculoskeletal pain, weakness
Respiratory: Cough, dyspnea, pneumonia
Miscellaneous: Sepsis

Overdosage/Toxicology Symptoms associated with overdose or rapid infusion include hypotension, headache, vomiting, nausea, dizziness, joint aches, paresthesia, abdominal and muscle pain, edema, and cardiovascular collapse. Reducing rate of infusion can alleviate some symptoms. Most symptoms can be treated with I.V. fluids, hydrocortisone, and/or antihistamines.

Although rare, if a severe iron overdose (serum iron concentration exceeds TIBC) occurs, deferoxamine may be administered intravenously.

Pharmacodynamics/Kinetics
Half-Life Elimination: Healthy adults: 6 hours
Metabolism: Dissociated into iron and sucrose by the reticuloendothelial system
Excretion: Healthy adults: Urine (5%) within 24 hours

Dosing
Adults: Doses expressed in mg of **elemental** iron.
Iron-deficiency anemia: I.V.: 100 mg (5 mL of iron sucrose injection) administered 1-3 times/week during dialysis, to a total dose of 1000 mg (10 doses); administer no more than 3 times/week; may continue to administer at lowest dose necessary to maintain target hemoglobin, hematocrit, and iron storage parameters
Test dose: Product labeling does not indicate need for a test dose in product-naive patients; test doses were administered in some clinical trials as 50 mg (2.5 mL) in 50 mL 0.9% NaCl administered over 3-10 minutes
Elderly: Insufficient data to identify differences between elderly and other adults; use caution.

Available Dosage Forms Injection, solution [preservative free]: 20 mg of elemental iron/mL (5 mL)

Monitoring and Teaching Issues
Physical Assessment: Assess other medications patient may be taking for effectiveness and interactions. Facilities for cardiopulmonary resuscitation must be available during administration. Monitor blood pressure closely during infusion. Assess results of laboratory tests, therapeutic effectiveness, and adverse reactions at beginning of therapy and periodically throughout therapy. Assess knowledge/teach patient appropriate use according to product and purpose (dangers of iron overdosing), interventions to reduce side effects, and adverse symptoms to report.

Monitoring Laboratory Tests: Hematocrit, hemoglobin, serum ferritin, transferrin, percent transferrin saturation, TIBC; takes about 4 weeks of treatment to see increased serum iron and ferritin, and decreased TIBC. Serum iron concentrations should be drawn 48 hours after last dose.

Patient Education: I.V.: You will be watched closely during infusion. You will need frequent blood tests while on this therapy. You may experience hypotension (use caution when driving or climbing stairs or engaging in tasks requiring alertness until response to drug is known); black tarry stools (normal), nausea, vomiting (taking with meals will reduce this), constipation (adequate fluids and exercise may help, may need a stool softener); or diarrhea (buttermilk, boiled milk, or yogurt may help). Report immediately severe unresolved GI irritation (cramping, nausea, vomiting, diarrhea, constipation); headache, lethargy, fatigue, dizziness, or other CNS changes; rapid respiration; leg cramps; chest pain or palpations; vision changes; choking sensation; loss of consciousness; or convulsions.
Breast-feeding precaution: Consult prescriber if breast-feeding.

(Continued)

Iron Sucrose *(Continued)*

Pregnancy Risk Factor: B

Lactation: Excretion in breast milk unknown/use caution

Administration

I.V.: Not for rapid (bolus) I.V. injection; can be administered through dialysis line. Do not mix with other medications or parenteral nutrient solutions.

Slow I.V. injection: 1 mL (20 mg iron) of undiluted solution per minute (5 minutes/vial)

Infusion: Dilute 1 vial (5 mL) in maximum of 100 mL 0.9% NaCl; infuse over at least 15 minutes.

Reconstitution: May be administered via the dialysis line as an undiluted solution or by diluting 100 mg (5 mL) in 100 mL normal saline. Solution is stable for 48 hours at room temperature or under refrigeration. Do not mix with other medications.

Storage: Store vials at room temperature.

♦ **Iron Sulfate** *see* Ferrous Sulfate *on page 624*

♦ **ISD** *see* Isosorbide Dinitrate *on page 839*

♦ **ISDN** *see* Isosorbide Dinitrate *on page 839*

♦ **ISMN** *see* Isosorbide Mononitrate *on page 841*

♦ **Ismo®** *see* Isosorbide Mononitrate *on page 841*

♦ **Isobamate** *see* Carisoprodol *on page 258*

♦ **Isochron™** *see* Isosorbide Dinitrate *on page 839*

♦ **Isometheptene, Acetaminophen, and Dichloralphenazone** *see* Acetaminophen, Isometheptene, and Dichloralphenazone *on page 42*

♦ **Isometheptene, Dichloralphenazone, and Acetaminophen** *see* Acetaminophen, Isometheptene, and Dichloralphenazone *on page 42*

Isoniazid *(eye soe NYE a zid)*

U.S. Brand Names Nydrazid® [DSC]

Synonyms INH; Isonicotinic Acid Hydrazide

Generic Available Yes

Pharmacologic Category Antitubercular Agent

Use Treatment of susceptible tuberculosis infections; treatment of latent tuberculosis infection (LTBI)

Mechanism of Action/Effect Unknown, but may include the inhibition of myocolic acid synthesis resulting in disruption of the bacterial cell wall

Contraindications Hypersensitivity to isoniazid or any component of the formulation; acute liver disease; previous history of hepatic damage during isoniazid therapy

Warnings/Precautions Use with caution in patients with renal impairment and chronic liver disease. Severe and sometimes fatal hepatitis may occur or develop even after many months of treatment. Patients must report any prodromal symptoms of hepatitis, such as fatigue, weakness, malaise, anorexia, nausea, or vomiting. Periodic ophthalmic examinations are recommended even when usual symptoms do not occur. Pyridoxine (10-50 mg/day) is recommended in individuals likely to develop peripheral neuropathies.

Drug Interactions

Cytochrome P450 Effect: Substrate of CYP2E1 (major); **Inhibits** CYP1A2 (weak), 2A6 (moderate), 2C8/9 (moderate), 2C19 (strong), 2D6 (moderate), 2E1 (moderate), 3A4 (strong); **Induces** CYP2E1 (after discontinuation) (weak)

Decreased Effect: Decreased effect/levels of isoniazid with aluminum salts or antacids. Isoniazid may decrease the levels/effects of CYP2D6 prodrug substrates (eg, codeine, hydrocodone, oxycodone, tramadol).

Increased Effect/Toxicity: Concurrent use of disulfiram may result in acute intolerance reactions. Isoniazid may increase the levels/effects of amiodarone, amphetamines, benzo-diazepines, beta-blockers, calcium channel blockers, citalopram, dexmedetomidine, dextromethorphan, diazepam, fluoxetine, glimepiride, glipizide, ifosfamide, inhalational anesthetics, lidocaine, mesoridazine, methsuximide, mirtazapine, nateglinide, nefazodone, paroxetine, phenytoin, pioglitazone, propranolol, risperidone, ritonavir, rosiglitazone, sertraline, sildenafil (and other PDE-5 inhibitors) tacrolimus, theophylline, thioridazine, tricyclic antidepressants, trimethadione, venlafaxine, warfarin, and other substrates of CYP2A6, 2C8/9, 2C19, 2D6, 2E1, or 3A4. Selected benzodiazepines (midazolam and triazolam), cisapride, ergot alkaloids, selected HMG-CoA reductase inhibitors (lovastatin and simvastatin), and pimozide are generally contraindicated with strong CYP3A4 inhibitors. Mesoridazine and thioridazine are generally contraindicated with strong CYP2D6 inhibitors. When used with strong CYP3A4 inhibitors, dosage adjustment/limits are recommended for sildenafil and other PDE-5 inhibitors; consult individual monographs.

Nutritional/Ethanol Interactions

Ethanol: Avoid ethanol (increases the risk of hepatitis).

Food: Isoniazid serum levels may be decreased if taken with food. Has some ability to inhibit tyramine metabolism; several case reports of mild reactions (flushing, palpitations) after ingestion of cheese with or without wine. Isoniazid decreases folic acid absorption. Isoniazid alters pyridoxine metabolism.

Lab Interactions False-positive urinary glucose with Clinitest®

Adverse Reactions Frequency not defined.

Cardiovascular: Hypertension, palpitation, tachycardia, vasculitis

Central nervous system: Dizziness, slurred speech, lethargy, fever, depression, psychosis, seizure

Dermatologic: Rash (morbilliform, maculopapular, pruritic, or exfoliative), flushing

Endocrine & metabolic: Hyperglycemia, metabolic acidosis, gynecomastia, pellagra, pyridoxine deficiency

Gastrointestinal: Anorexia, nausea, vomiting, stomach pain

Hematologic: Agranulocytosis, anemia (sideroblastic, hemolytic, or aplastic), thrombocytopenia, eosinophilia, lymphadenopathy

Hepatic: LFTs mildly increased (10% to 20%); hyperbilirubinemia, jaundice, hepatitis (may involve progressive liver damage; risk increases with age; 2.3% in patients >50 years)

Neuromuscular & skeletal: Weakness, peripheral neuropathy (dose-related incidence, 10% to 20% incidence with 10 mg/kg/day), hyper-reflexia, arthralgia, lupus-like syndrome

Ocular: Blurred vision, loss of vision

Overdosage/Toxicology Symptoms of overdose include nausea, vomiting, slurred speech, dizziness, blurred vision, hallucinations, stupor, coma, and intractable seizures. The onset of metabolic acidosis is within 30 minutes to 3 hours. Because of high morbidity and mortality rates with isoniazid overdose, patients who are asymptomatic after an overdose should be monitored for 4-6 hours. Pyridoxine has been shown to be effective in the treatment of intoxication, especially when seizures occur. Pyridoxine I.V. is administered on a milligram to milligram dose. If the amount of isoniazid ingested is unknown, 5 g of pyridoxine should be given over 3-5 minutes and may be followed by an additional 5 g in 30 minutes. Treatment is supportive. Forced diuresis and hemodialysis can result in more rapid removal.

Pharmacodynamics/Kinetics

Absorption: Rapid and complete; rate can be slowed with food

Time to Peak: Serum: 1-2 hours

Protein Binding: 10% to 15%

Half-Life Elimination: Fast acetylators: 30-100 minutes; Slow acetylators: 2-5 hours; may be prolonged with hepatic or severe renal impairment

Metabolism: Hepatic with decay rate determined genetically by acetylation phenotype

Excretion: Urine (75% to 95%); feces; saliva

Dosing

Adults & Elderly: Recommendations often change due to resistant strains and newly-developed information; consult *MMWR* for current CDC recommendations. Intramuscular is available in patients who are unable to either take or absorb oral therapy.

Treatment of latent tuberculosis infection (LTBI): 300 mg/day or 900 mg twice weekly for 6-9 months in patients who do not have HIV infection (9 months is optimal, 6 months may be considered to reduce costs of therapy) and 9 months in patients who have HIV infection. Extend to 12 months of therapy if interruptions in treatment occur.

Treatment of active TB infection (drug susceptible):
Daily therapy: 5 mg/kg/day given daily (usual dose: 300 mg/day); 10 mg/kg/day in 1-2 divided doses in patients with disseminated disease
Twice weekly directly observed therapy (DOT): 15 mg/kg (maximum: 900 mg); 3 times/ week therapy: 15 mg/kg (maximum: 900 mg)

Note: Treatment may be defined by the number of doses administered (eg, "six-month" therapy involves 192 doses of INH and rifampin, and 56 doses of pyrazinamide). Six months is the shortest interval of time over which these doses may be administered, assuming no interruption of therapy.

Note: Concomitant administration of 6-50 mg/day pyridoxine is recommended in malnourished patients or those prone to neuropathy (eg, alcoholics, diabetics)

Pediatrics: Recommendations often change due to resistant strains and newly-developed information; consult *MMWR* for current CDC recommendations. Intramuscular is available in patients who are unable to either take or absorb oral therapy.

Treatment of latent TB infection (LTBI): Infants and Children: Oral: 10-20 mg/kg/day in 1-2 divided doses (maximum: 300 mg/day) or 20-40 mg/kg (maximum: 900 mg/dose) twice weekly for 9 months

Treatment of active TB infection: Infants and Children: Oral:
Daily therapy: 10-15 mg/kg/day in 1-2 divided doses (maximum: 300 mg/day)
Twice weekly directly observed therapy (DOT): 20-30 mg/kg (maximum: 900 mg)

Renal Impairment:
Cl_{cr} <10 mL/minute: Administer 50% of normal dose
Hemodialysis: Dialyzable (50% to 100%)
Administer dose postdialysis
Peritoneal dialysis, continuous arteriovenous or venovenous hemofiltration: Dose for Cl_{cr} <10 mL/minute

Hepatic Impairment: Dose should be reduced in severe hepatic disease.

Available Dosage Forms

Injection, solution (Nydrazid®): 100 mg/mL (10 mL) [DSC]
Syrup: 50 mg/5 mL (473 mL) [orange flavor]
Tablet: 100 mg, 300 mg

Monitoring and Teaching Issues

Physical Assessment: Use caution in presence of hepatic or renal impairment (see Warnings/Precautions for specific use cautions). Assess potential for interactions with other pharmacological agents patient may be taking (eg, risk of toxicity or decreased effects; see Drug Interactions). Assess results of laboratory tests, therapeutic effectiveness, and adverse response at regular intervals during therapy (eg, nausea, vomiting, peripheral neuropathy, liver damage, CNS changes; see Adverse Reactions and Overdose/Toxicology). Advise patients with diabetes about use of Clinitest®. Teach patient proper use, possible side effects/appropriate interventions (eg, diet [see Tyramine Content of Foods list *on page 1758*] and ophthalmic examinations), and adverse symptoms to report (see Patient Education).

Monitoring Laboratory Tests: Transaminase levels at baseline 1, 3, 6, and 9 months

Patient Education: Do not take any new medication during therapy unless approved by prescriber. Best if taken on an empty stomach, 1 hour before or 2 hours after meals. Avoid missing any dose and do not discontinue without notifying prescriber. Avoid excessive alcohol and tyramine-containing foods (eg, aged cheese, broad beans, dry sausage, preserved meats or sausages, liver pate, fish, soy bean, protein supplements, wine) and increase dietary intake of folate, niacin, and magnesium. May cause false test results with Clinitest®; use of another type of glucose testing is preferable. You will need to have frequent ophthalmic exams and periodic medical check-ups to evaluate drug effects. You may experience nausea or vomiting (small frequent meals, frequent mouth care, chewing gum, or sucking lozenges may help). Report tingling or numbness in hands or feet, loss of sensation, unusual weakness, fatigue, nausea or vomiting, dark colored urine, change in
(Continued)

Isoniazid *(Continued)*

urinary pattern, yellowing skin or eyes, or change in color of stool; prodromal hepatitis, such as fatigue, weakness, malaise, anorexia, nausea, or vomiting. **Pregnancy precaution:** Inform prescriber if you are or intend to become pregnant.

Dietary Considerations: Should be taken 1 hour before or 2 hours after meals on an empty stomach; increase dietary intake of folate, niacin, magnesium. No need to restrict tyramine-containing foods.

Geriatric Considerations: Age has not been shown to affect the pharmacokinetics of INH since acetylation phenotype determines clearance and half-life, acetylation rate does not change significantly with age. Most strains of *M. tuberculosis* found the elderly should be susceptible to INH since most acquired their initial infection prior to INH's introduction.

Pregnancy Risk Factor: C

Lactation: Enters breast milk/compatible

Breast-Feeding Issues: Small amounts of isoniazid are excreted in breast milk. However, women with tuberculosis should not be discouraged from breast-feeding. Pyridoxine supplementation is recommended for the mother and infant.

Administration

Oral: Should be administered 1 hour before or 2 hours after meals on an empty stomach.

Storage: Protect oral dosage forms from light.

Additional Information The AAP recommends that pyridoxine supplementation (1-2 mg/kg/day) should be administered to malnourished patients, children or adolescents on meat or milk-deficient diets, breast-feeding infants, and those predisposed to neuritis to prevent peripheral neuropathy; administration of isoniazid syrup has been associated with diarrhea

Related Information

Overdose and Toxicology *on page 1775*

Tuberculosis *on page 1864*

Tyramine Content of Foods *on page 1758*

♦ **Isoniazid and Rifampin** *see* Rifampin and Isoniazid *on page 1326*

♦ **Isoniazid, Rifampin, and Pyrazinamide** *see* Rifampin, Isoniazid, and Pyrazinamide *on page 1326*

♦ **Isonicotinic Acid Hydrazide** *see* Isoniazid *on page 836*

♦ **Isonipecaine Hydrochloride** *see* Meperidine *on page 950*

♦ **Isophosphamide** *see* Ifosfamide *on page 783*

Isoproterenol (eye soe proe TER e nole)

U.S. Brand Names Isuprel®

Synonyms Isoproterenol Hydrochloride

Generic Available Yes

Pharmacologic Category Beta$_1$- & Beta$_2$-Adrenergic Agonist Agent

Medication Safety Issues

Sound-alike/look-alike issues:

Isuprel® may be confused with Disophrol®, Ismelin®, Isordil®

Use Ventricular arrhythmias due to AV nodal block; hemodynamically compromised bradyrrhythmias or atropine- and dopamine-resistant bradyarrhythmias (when transcutaneous/venous pacing is not available); temporary use in third-degree AV block until pacemaker insertion

Unlabeled/Investigational Use Temporizing measure before transvenous pacing for torsade de pointes; diagnostic aid (vasovagal syncope)

Mechanism of Action/Effect Stimulates beta$_1$- and beta$_2$-receptors resulting in relaxation of bronchial, GI, and uterine smooth muscle, increased heart rate and contractility, vasodilation of peripheral vasculature

Contraindications Hypersensitivity to sulfites or isoproterenol, any component of the formulation, or other sympathomimetic amines; angina, pre-existing cardiac arrhythmias (ventricular); tachycardia or AV block caused by cardiac glycoside intoxication

Warnings/Precautions Use with extreme caution; not currently a treatment of choice; use with caution in elderly patients, patients with diabetes, renal or cardiovascular disease, seizure disorder, or hyperthyroidism; excessive or prolonged use may result in decreased effectiveness.

Drug Interactions

Increased Effect/Toxicity: Sympathomimetic agents may cause headaches and elevate blood pressure. General anesthetics may cause arrhythmias.

Nutritional/Ethanol Interactions Herb/Nutraceutical: Avoid ephedra, yohimbe (may cause CNS stimulation).

Adverse Reactions Frequency not defined.

Cardiovascular: Premature ventricular beats, bradycardia, hyper-/hypotension, chest pain, palpitation, tachycardia, ventricular arrhythmia, MI size increased

Central nervous system: Headache, nervousness or restlessness

Endocrine & metabolic: Serum glucose increased, serum potassium decreased, hypokalemia

Gastrointestinal: Nausea, vomiting

Respiratory: Dyspnea

Overdosage/Toxicology Symptoms of overdose include tachycardia, tremor, hypertension or hypotension, angina, and seizures. Hypokalemia also may occur. Cardiac arrest and death may be associated with abuse of beta-agonist bronchodilators. Treatment includes immediate discontinuation and symptomatic and supportive therapies. Cautious use of beta-adrenergic blocking agents may be considered in severe cases.

Pharmacodynamics/Kinetics
Onset of Action: Bronchodilation: I.V.: Immediate
Duration of Action: I.V.: 10-15 minutes
Half-Life Elimination: 2.5-5 minutes
Metabolism: Via conjugation in many tissues including hepatic and pulmonary
Excretion: Urine (primarily as sulfate conjugates)

Dosing
Adults & Elderly: Cardiac arrhythmias: I.V.: Initial: 2 mcg/minute; titrate to patient response (2-10 mcg/minute)
Pediatrics: Cardiac arrhythmias: I.V.: Start 0.1 mcg/kg/minute (usual effective dose 0.2-2 mcg/kg/minute)

Available Dosage Forms Injection, solution, as hydrochloride: 0.02 mg/mL (10 mL); 0.2 mg/mL (1:5000) (1 mL, 5 mL) [contains sodium metabisulfite]

Monitoring and Teaching Issues
Physical Assessment: Assess results of laboratory tests, cardiac, respiratory, and hemodynamic status when used in acute or emergency situations. Assess knowledge/teach patient appropriate use and administration procedures and adverse reactions to report.
Monitoring Laboratory Tests: ECG, arterial blood gas, serum magnesium, serum potassium, serum glucose (in selected patients)
Patient Education: You may experience nervousness, dizziness, or fatigue (use caution when driving or engaging in tasks requiring alertness until response to drug is known); or dry mouth, nausea, or vomiting (small frequent meals may reduce the incidence of nausea or vomiting). If you have diabetes, check blood sugar; blood glucose level may be increased. Report chest pain, rapid heartbeat or palpitations, unresolved/persistent GI upset, dizziness, fatigue, trembling, increased anxiety, sleeplessness, or respiratory difficulty. **Pregnancy/breast-feeding precautions:** Inform prescriber if you are pregnant. Consult prescriber if breast-feeding.
Pregnancy Risk Factor: C
Lactation: Excretion in breast milk unknown

Administration
I.V.: I.V. infusion administration requires the use of an infusion pump. To prepare for infusion: 1 mg isoproterenol to 500 mL D_5W, final concentration 2 mcg/mL
Reconstitution: Stability of parenteral admixture at room temperature (25°C) or at refrigeration (4°C) is 24 hours.

Standard diluent: 2 mg/500 mL D_5W; 4 mg/500 mL D_5W
Minimum volume: 1 mg/100 mL D_5W

Compatibility: Stable in dextran 6% in dextrose, dextran 6% in NS, D_5LR, $D_5^1/_4$ NS, $D_5^1/_2NS$, D_5NS, D_5W, $D_{10}W$, LR, $^1/_2NS$, NS; **incompatible** with sodium bicarbonate 5%, and alkaline solutions
Compatibility when admixed: Incompatible with aminophylline, furosemide, sodium bicarbonate
Storage: Isoproterenol solution should be stored at room temperature. It should not be used if a color or precipitate is present. Exposure to air, light, or increased temperature may cause a pink to brownish pink color to develop.

Related Information
Inotropic and Vasoconstrictor Comparison *on page 1736*

♦ **Isoproterenol Hydrochloride** *see* Isoproterenol *on page 838*

♦ **Isoptin® SR** *see* Verapamil *on page 1560*

♦ **Isopto® Atropine** *see* Atropine *on page 158*

♦ **Isopto® Carpine** *see* Pilocarpine *on page 1210*

♦ **Isopto® Hyoscine** *see* Scopolamine Derivatives *on page 1360*

♦ **Isordil®** *see* Isosorbide Dinitrate *on page 839*

Isosorbide Dinitrate (eye soe SOR bide dye NYE trate)
U.S. Brand Names Dilatrate®-SR; Isochron™; Isordil®
Synonyms ISD; ISDN
Generic Available Yes: Tablet, sublingual tablet
Pharmacologic Category Vasodilator
Medication Safety Issues
Sound-alike/look-alike issues:
Isordil® may be confused with Inderal®, Isuprel®
Use Prevention and treatment of angina pectoris; for congestive heart failure; to relieve pain, dysphagia, and spasm in esophageal spasm with GE reflux
Unlabeled/Investigational Use Esophageal spastic disorders
Mechanism of Action/Effect Relaxes vascular smooth muscles, decreases arterial resistance and venous return which reduces cardiac oxygen demand. Additionally, coronary artery dilation improves collateral flow to ischemic regions; esophageal smooth muscle is relaxed via the same mechanism.
Contraindications Hypersensitivity to isosorbide dinitrate or any component of the formulation; hypersensitivity to organic nitrates; concurrent use with phosphodiesterase-5 (PDE-5) inhibitors (sildenafil, tadalafil, or vardenafil); angle-closure glaucoma (intraocular pressure may be increased); head trauma or cerebral hemorrhage (increase intracranial pressure); severe anemia
Warnings/Precautions Use with caution in volume depletion, hypotension, and right ventricular infarctions. Paradoxical bradycardia and increased angina pectoris can accompany hypotension. Postural hypotension may also occur; ethanol may potentiate this effect. Tolerance does develop to nitrates and appropriate dosing is needed to minimize this. Safety and efficacy have not been established in pediatric patients. Nitrate may aggravate angina caused by hypertrophic cardiomyopathy.
(Continued)

Isosorbide Dinitrate *(Continued)*

Drug Interactions

Cytochrome P450 Effect: Substrate of CYP3A4 (major)

Decreased Effect: CYP3A4 inducers may decrease the levels/effects of isosorbide dinitrate; example inducers include aminoglutethimide, carbamazepine, nafcillin, nevirapine, phenobarbital, phenytoin, and rifamycins.

Increased Effect/Toxicity: CYP3A4 inhibitors may increase the levels/effects of isosorbide dinitrate; example inhibitors include azole antifungals, ciprofloxacin, clarithromycin, diclofenac, doxycycline, erythromycin, imatinib, isoniazid, nefazodone, nicardipine, propofol, protease inhibitors, quinidine, and verapamil. Significant reduction of systolic and diastolic blood pressure with concurrent use of sildenafil, tadalafil, or vardenafil (contraindicated). Do not administer sildenafil, tadalafil, or vardenafil within 24 hours of a nitrate preparation.

Nutritional/Ethanol Interactions
Ethanol: Caution with ethanol (may increase risk of hypotension).

Lab Interactions
Decreased cholesterol (S)

Adverse Reactions
Frequency not defined.

Cardiovascular: Hypotension (infrequent), postural hypotension, crescendo angina (uncommon), rebound hypertension (uncommon), pallor, cardiovascular collapse, tachycardia, shock, flushing, peripheral edema

Central nervous system: Headache (most common), lightheadedness (related to blood pressure changes), syncope (uncommon), dizziness, restlessness

Gastrointestinal: Nausea, vomiting, bowel incontinence, xerostomia

Genitourinary: Urinary incontinence

Hematologic: Methemoglobinemia (rare, overdose)

Neuromuscular & skeletal: Weakness

Ocular: Blurred vision

Miscellaneous: Cold sweat

The incidence of hypotension and adverse cardiovascular events may be increased when used in combination with sildenafil (Viagra®).

Overdosage/Toxicology
Symptoms of overdose include hypotension, throbbing headache, palpitations, visual disturbances, tachycardia, methemoglobinemia, flushing, diaphoresis, metabolic acidosis, and coma. High levels or methemoglobinemia can cause signs or symptoms of hypoxemia. Treat symptomatically.

Pharmacodynamics/Kinetics

Onset of Action: Sublingual tablet: 2-10 minutes; Chewable tablet: 3 minutes; Oral tablet: 45-60 minutes

Duration of Action: Sublingual tablet: 1-2 hours; Chewable tablet: 0.5-2 hours; Oral tablet: 4-6 hours

Half-Life Elimination: Parent drug: 1-4 hours; Metabolite (5-mononitrate): 4 hours

Metabolism: Extensively hepatic to conjugated metabolites, including isosorbide 5-mononitrate (active) and 2-mononitrate (active)

Excretion: Urine and feces

Dosing

Adults:

Angina: Oral: 5-40 mg 4 times/day or 40 mg every 8-12 hours in sustained released dosage form

Congestive heart failure:

Oral:

Initial: 10 mg 3 times/day

Target: 40 mg 3 times/day

Maximum: 80 mg 3 times/day

Sublingual: 2.5-10 mg every 4-6 hours

Chewable tablet: 5-10 mg every 2-3 hours

Esophageal spastic disorders (unlabeled use):

Oral: 5-10 mg before meals

Sublingual: 2.5 mg after meals

Note: Tolerance to nitrate effects develops with chronic exposure. Dose escalation does not overcome this effect. Tolerance can only be overcome by short periods of nitrate absence from the body. Short periods (10-12 hours) of nitrate withdrawal help minimize tolerance. General recommendations are to take the last dose of short-acting agents no later than 7 PM; administer 2-3 times/day rather than 4 times/day. Sustained release preparations could be administered at times to allow a 15- to 17-hour interval between first and last daily dose. Example: Administer sustained release at 8 AM and 2 PM for a twice daily regimen.

Elderly: Elderly patients should be given lowest recommended adult daily doses initially and titrate upward.

Renal Impairment: Hemodialysis: During hemodialysis, administer dose postdialysis or administer supplemental 10-20 mg dose. During peritoneal dialysis, supplemental dose is not necessary.

Available Dosage Forms
[DSC] = Discontinued product

Capsule, sustained release (Dilatrate®-SR): 40 mg

Tablet: 5 mg, 10 mg, 20 mg, 30 mg,

Isordil®: 5 mg, 10 mg [DSC], 20 mg [DSC], 30 mg [DSC], 40 mg

Tablet, extended release (Isochron™): 40 mg

Tablet, sublingual: 2.5 mg, 5 mg

Isordil®: 2.5 mg, 5 mg, 10 mg [DSC]

Monitoring and Teaching Issues

Physical Assessment: Use caution in presence of volume depletion, hypotension, and right ventricular infarctions (see Warnings/Precautions for specific use cautions). Assess potential for interactions with other pharmacological agents patient may be taking (potential for decreased or increased levels/effects of isosorbide; see Drug Interactions). See Dosing

"Note" and Administration for specific directions. Assess therapeutic effectiveness and adverse response at regular intervals during therapy (eg, hypotension; see Adverse Reactions). When discontinuing, reduce dosage gradually. Teach patient proper use, possible side effects/appropriate interventions, and adverse symptoms to report (see Patient Education).

Patient Education: Do not take any new medication during therapy unless approved by prescriber. Take exactly as directed, at the same time each day. Do not chew or swallow sublingual tablets; allow them to dissolve under your tongue. Do not crush or chew sustained release capsules, swallow whole with 8 oz water. Do not change brands without consulting prescriber. Do not discontinue abruptly. Keep medication in original container, tightly closed. Avoid alcohol; combination may cause severe hypotension. May cause postural hypotension (take medication while sitting down and use caution when rising from sitting or lying position or climbing stairs); dizziness, weakness, or blurred vision (use caution when driving or engaging in hazardous activities until response to drug is known); or nausea or vomiting (small frequent meals, frequent mouth care, chewing gum, or sucking lozenges may help). If chest pain occurs, seek emergency medical help at once. Report acute headache, rapid heartbeat, unusual restlessness or dizziness, muscular weakness, or blurring vision. **Pregnancy/breast-feeding precautions:** Inform prescriber if you are or intend to become pregnant. Consult prescriber if breast-feeding.

Pregnancy Risk Factor: C

Lactation: Excretion in breast milk unknown

Administration

Oral: Do not administer around-the-clock; the first dose of nitrates should be administered in a physician's office to observe for maximal cardiovascular dynamic effects and adverse effects (orthostatic blood pressure drop, headache); when immediate release products are prescribed twice daily (recommend 7 AM and noon); for 3 times/day dosing (recommend 7 AM, noon, and 5 PM); when sustained-release products are indicated, suggest once a day in morning or via twice daily dosing at 8 AM and 2 PM. Do not crush sublingual tablets.

Related Information

Heart Failure *on page 1828*

Isosorbide Mononitrate (eye soe SOR bide mon oh NYE trate)

U.S. Brand Names Imdur®; Ismo®; Monoket®

Synonyms ISMN

Generic Available Yes

Pharmacologic Category Vasodilator

Medication Safety Issues

Sound-alike/look-alike issues:

Imdur® may be confused with Imuran®, Inderal LA®, K-Dur®

Monoket® may be confused with Monopril®

Use Long-acting metabolite of the vasodilator isosorbide dinitrate used for the prophylactic treatment of angina pectoris

Mechanism of Action/Effect Systemic venodilation, decreasing preload and increasing ejection fractions; improves congestive symptoms in heart failure and improves the myocardial perfusion in patients with coronary artery disease

Contraindications Hypersensitivity to isosorbide or any component of the formulation; hypersensitivity to organic nitrates; concurrent use with phosphodiesterase-5 (PDE-5) inhibitors (sildenafil, tadalafil, or vardenafil); angle-closure glaucoma (intraocular pressure may be increased); head trauma or cerebral hemorrhage (increase intracranial pressure); severe anemia

Warnings/Precautions Use with caution in volume depletion, hypotension, and right ventricular infarctions. Paradoxical bradycardia and increased angina pectoris can accompany hypotension. Orthostatic hypotension can also occur; ethanol can accentuate this. Tolerance does develop to nitrates and appropriate dosing is needed to minimize this (drug-free interval). Safety and efficacy have not been established in pediatric patients. Nitrates may aggravate angina caused by hypertrophic cardiomyopathy.

Drug Interactions

Cytochrome P450 Effect: Substrate of CYP3A4 (major)

Increased Effect/Toxicity: CYP3A4 inhibitors may increase the levels/effects of isosorbide dinitrate; example inhibitors include azole antifungals, ciprofloxacin, clarithromycin, diclofenac, doxycycline, erythromycin, imatinib, isoniazid, nefazodone, nicardipine, propofol, protease inhibitors, quinidine, and verapamil. Significant reduction of systolic and diastolic blood pressure with concurrent use of sildenafil, tadalafil, or vardenafil (contraindicated). Do not administer sildenafil, tadalafil, or vardenafil within 24 hours of a nitrate preparation.

Nutritional/Ethanol Interactions Ethanol: Caution with ethanol (may increase risk of hypotension).

Adverse Reactions

>10%: Central nervous system: Headache (19% to 38%)

1% to 10%:

Central nervous system: Dizziness (3% to 5%)

Gastrointestinal: Nausea/vomiting (2% to 4%)

The incidence of hypotension and adverse cardiovascular events may be increased when used in combination with sildenafil (Viagra®).

Overdosage/Toxicology Symptoms of overdose include hypotension, throbbing headache, palpitations, visual disturbances, tachycardia, methemoglobinemia, flushing, diaphoresis, metabolic acidosis, and coma. High levels or methemoglobinemia can cause signs or symptoms of hypoxemia. Treat symptomatically.

Pharmacodynamics/Kinetics

Onset of Action: 30-60 minutes

Absorption: Nearly complete and low intersubject variability in its pharmacokinetic parameters and plasma concentrations

(Continued)

Isosorbide Mononitrate *(Continued)*

Half-Life Elimination: Mononitrate: ~4 hours

Metabolism: Hepatic

Excretion: Urine and feces

Dosing

Adults:

Angina: Oral:

Regular tablet: 5-10 mg twice daily with the two doses given 7 hours apart (eg, 8 AM and 3 PM) to decrease tolerance development; then titrate to 10 mg twice daily in first 2-3 days.

Extended release tablet: Initial: 30-60 mg given in morning as a single dose; titrate upward as needed, giving at least 3 days between increases; maximum daily single dose: 240 mg

Note: Tolerance to nitrate effects develops with chronic exposure. Dose escalation does not overcome this effect. Tolerance can only be overcome by short periods of nitrate absence from the body. Short periods (10-12 hours) of nitrate withdrawal help minimize tolerance. Recommended dosage regimens incorporate this interval. General recommendations are to take the last dose of short-acting agents no later than 7 PM; administer 2 times/day rather than 4 times/day. Administer sustained release tablet once daily in the morning.

Elderly: Start with lowest recommended adult dose.

Renal Impairment: Not necessary for elderly or patients with altered renal or hepatic function. Tolerance to nitrate effects develops with chronic exposure.

Available Dosage Forms

Tablet: 10 mg, 20 mg

Ismo®: 20 mg

Monoket®: 10 mg, 20 mg

Tablet, extended release (Imdur®): 30 mg, 60 mg, 120 mg

Monitoring and Teaching Issues

Physical Assessment: Use cautions in presence of volume depletion, hypotension, and right ventricular infarctions (see Warnings/Precautions for specific use cautions). Assess potential for interactions with other pharmacological agents patient may be taking (potential for decreased or increased levels/effects of isosorbide; see Drug Interactions). See Dosing "Note" and Administration for specific directions. Assess therapeutic effectiveness and adverse response at regular intervals during therapy (eg, hypotension; see Adverse Reactions). When discontinuing, reduce dosage gradually. Teach patient proper use, possible side effects/appropriate interventions, and adverse symptoms to report (see Patient Education).

Patient Education: Do not take any new medication during therapy unless approved by prescriber. Take exactly as directed, at the same time each day. Do not crush or chew sustained release capsules, swallow whole with 8 oz water. Do not change brands without consulting prescriber. Do not discontinue abruptly. Keep medication in original container, tightly closed. Avoid alcohol; combination may cause severe hypotension. May cause postural hypotension (take medication while sitting down and use caution when rising from sitting or lying position or climbing stairs); dizziness, weakness, or blurred vision (use caution when driving or engaging in hazardous activities until response to drug is known); or nausea or vomiting (small frequent meals, frequent mouth care, chewing gum, or sucking lozenges may help). If chest pain occurs, seek emergency medical help at once. Report acute headache, rapid heartbeat, unusual restlessness or dizziness, muscular weakness, or blurring vision. **Pregnancy/breast-feeding precautions:** Inform prescriber if you are or intend to become pregnant. Consult prescriber if breast-feeding.

Geriatric Considerations: The first dose of nitrates (sublingual, chewable, oral) should be taken in a physician's office to observe for maximal cardiovascular dynamic effects and adverse effects (orthostatic blood pressure drop, headache). The use of nitrates for angina may occasionally promote reflux esophagitis. This may require dose adjustments or changing therapeutic agents to correct this adverse effect.

Pregnancy Risk Factor: C

Lactation: Excretion in breast milk unknown

Administration

Oral: Do not administer around-the-clock; Monoket® and Ismo® should be scheduled twice daily with doses 7 hours apart (8 AM and 3 PM); Imdur® may be administered once daily. Extended release tablets should not be chewed or crushed. Should be swallowed with a half-glassful of fluid.

Storage: Tablets should be stored in a tight container at room temperature of 15°C to 30°C (59°F to 86°F).

Isotretinoin *(eye soe TRET i noyn)*

U.S. Brand Names Accutane®; Amnesteem™; Claravis™; Sotret®

Synonyms 13-*cis*-Retinoic Acid

Restrictions A new program for risk minimization (RiskMAP) is being designed by the FDA and the manufacturers of isotretinoin. Details may be found on the FDA website at http://www.fda.gov/bbs/topics/ANSWERS/2004/ANS01328.html. When implemented, RiskMAP will strengthen the current prescribing and dispensing requirements. Under the current guidelines, prescriptions for isotretinoin may not be dispensed unless they are affixed with a yellow, self-adhesive, qualification sticker filled out by the prescriber. Telephone, fax, or computer-generated prescriptions are no longer valid. Prescriptions may not be written for more than a 1-month supply and must be dispensed with a patient education guide every month. In addition, prescriptions for females must be filled within 7 days of the qualification date noted on the yellow sticker; prescriptions filled after 7 days of the noted date are considered to be expired and cannot be honored. Pharmacists may call the manufacturer to confirm the prescriber's authority to write for this medication; however, this is not mandatory.

Prescribers will be provided with qualification stickers after they have read the details of the program and have signed (and mailed to the manufacturer) their agreement to participate. Audits of pharmacies will be conducted to monitor program compliance.

An FDA-approved medication guide is available at www.fda.gov/cder/Offices/ODS/labeling.htm; distribute to each patient to whom this medication is dispensed.

Generic Available Yes

Pharmacologic Category Retinoic Acid Derivative

Medication Safety Issues
Sound-alike/look-alike issues:
Accutane® may be confused with Accolate®, Accupril®

Use Treatment of severe recalcitrant nodular acne unresponsive to conventional therapy

Unlabeled/Investigational Use Investigational: Treatment of children with metastatic neuroblastoma or leukemia that does not respond to conventional therapy

Mechanism of Action/Effect Reduces sebaceous gland size and reduces sebum production; regulates cell proliferation and differentiation

Contraindications Hypersensitivity to isotretinoin or any component of the formulation; sensitivity to parabens, vitamin A, or other retinoids; pregnancy

Warnings/Precautions This medication should only be prescribed by prescribers competent in treating severe recalcitrant nodular acne, are experienced in the use of systemic retinoids and are participating in the pregnancy prevention programs authorized by the FDA and product manufacturer. Use with caution in patients with diabetes mellitus, hypertriglyceridemia; acute pancreatitis and fatal hemorrhagic pancreatitis (rare) have been reported. Not to be used in women of childbearing potential unless woman is capable of complying with effective contraceptive measures. Patients must select and commit to two forms of contraception. Therapy is begun after two negative pregnancy tests; effective contraception must be used for at least 1 month before beginning therapy, during therapy, and for 1 month after discontinuation of therapy. Prescriptions should be written for no more than a 1-month supply, and pregnancy testing and counseling should be repeated monthly. Because of the high likelihood of teratogenic effects (~20%), do not prescribe isotretinoin for women who are or who are likely to become pregnant while using the drug (see Additional Information for details). Male and female patients must be enrolled in the manufacturer sponsored and FDA approved monitoring programs.

Depression, psychosis, aggressive or violent behavior, and rarely suicidal thoughts and actions have been reported during isotretinoin usage. Discontinuation of treatment alone may not be sufficient, further evaluation may be necessary. Cases of pseudotumor cerebri (benign intracranial hypertension) have been reported, some with concomitant use of tetracycline (avoid using together). Patients with papilledema, headache, nausea, vomiting, and visual disturbances should be referred to a neurologist and treatment with isotretinoin discontinued. Hearing impairment, which can continue after therapy is discontinued, may occur. Clinical hepatitis, elevated liver enzymes, inflammatory bowel disease, skeletal hyperostosis, premature epiphyseal closure, vision impairment, corneal opacities, and decreased night vision have also been reported with the use of isotretinoin. Bone mineral density may decrease; use caution in patients with a genetic predisposition to bone disorders (ie osteoporosis, osteomalacia) and with disease states or concomitant medications that can induce bone disorders. Patients may be at risk when participating in activities with repetitive impact (such as sports). Safety of long-term use is not established and is not recommended.

Drug Interactions
Decreased Effect: Isotretinoin may increase clearance of carbamazepine resulting in reduced carbamazepine levels. Retinoic acid derivatives may diminish the therapeutic effect of oral contraceptives (two forms of contraception are recommended in females of childbearing potential during retinoic acid therapy).

Increased Effect/Toxicity: Increased toxicity: Corticosteroids may cause osteoporosis; interactive effect with isotretinoin unknown; use with caution. Phenytoin may cause osteomalacia; interactive effect with isotretinoin unknown; use with caution. Cases of pseudotumor cerebri have been reported in concurrent use with tetracycline; avoid combination.

Nutritional/Ethanol Interactions
Ethanol: Avoid or limit ethanol (may increase triglyceride levels if taken in excess).
Food: Isotretinoin bioavailability increased if taken with food or milk.
Herb/Nutraceutical: Avoid dong quai, St John's wort (may also cause photosensitization and may decrease the effectiveness of oral contraceptives). Additional vitamin A supplements may lead to vitamin A toxicity (dry skin, irritation, arthralgias, myalgias, abdominal pain, hepatic changes); avoid use.

Adverse Reactions Frequency not defined.
Cardiovascular: Palpitation, tachycardia, vascular thrombotic disease, stroke, chest pain, syncope, flushing
Central nervous system: Edema, fatigue, pseudotumor cerebri, dizziness, drowsiness, headache, insomnia, lethargy, malaise, nervousness, paresthesia, seizure, stroke, suicidal ideation, suicide attempts, suicide, depression, psychosis, aggressive or violent behavior, emotional instability
Dermatologic: Cutaneous allergic reactions, purpura, acne fulminans, alopecia, bruising, cheilitis, dry mouth, dry nose, dry skin, epistaxis, eruptive xanthomas, fragility of skin, hair abnormalities, hirsutism, hyperpigmentation, hypopigmentation, peeling of palms, peeling of soles, photoallergic reactions, photosensitizing reactions, pruritus, rash, dystrophy, paronychia, facial erythema, seborrhea, eczema, increased sunburn susceptibility, diaphoresis, urticaria, abnormal wound healing
Endocrine & metabolic: Increased triglycerides (25%), elevated blood glucose, increased HDL, increased cholesterol, abnormal menses
Gastrointestinal: Weight loss, inflammatory bowel disease, regional ileitis, pancreatitis, bleeding and inflammation of the gums, colitis, nausea, nonspecific gastrointestinal symptoms
Genitourinary: Nonspecific urogenital findings
Hematologic: Anemia, thrombocytopenia, neutropenia, agranulocytosis, pyogenic granuloma
Hepatic: Hepatitis
(Continued)

Isotretinoin *(Continued)*

Neuromuscular & skeletal: Skeletal hyperostosis, calcification of tendons and ligaments, premature epiphyseal closure, arthralgia, CPK elevations, arthritis, tendonitis, bone abnormalities, weakness, back pain (29% in pediatric patients), rhabdomyolysis (rare), bone mineral density decreased

Ocular: Corneal opacities, decreased night vision, cataracts, color vision disorder, conjunctivitis, dry eyes, eyelid inflammation, keratitis, optic neuritis, photophobia, visual disturbances

Otic: Hearing impairment, tinnitus

Renal: Vasculitis, glomerulonephritis,

Respiratory: Bronchospasms, respiratory infection, voice alteration, Wegener's granulomatosis

Miscellaneous: Allergic reactions, anaphylactic reactions, lymphadenopathy, infection, disseminated herpes simplex, diaphoresis

Overdosage/Toxicology Symptoms of overdose include headache, vomiting, flushing, abdominal pain, cheilosis, dizziness, and ataxia. All signs or symptoms have been transient. Patients should not donate blood for at least 30 days following overdose. Male patients should use a condom or avoid sexual activity for 30 days following overdose.

Pharmacodynamics/Kinetics

Time to Peak: Serum: 3-5 hours

Protein Binding: 99% to 100%; primarily albumin

Half-Life Elimination: Terminal: Parent drug: 21 hours; Metabolite: 21-24 hours

Metabolism: Hepatic via CYP2B6, 2C8, 2C9, 2D6, 3A4; forms metabolites; major metabolite: 4-oxo-isotretinoin (active)

Excretion: Urine and feces (equal amounts)

Dosing

Adults & Elderly: Severe recalcitrant nodular acne: Oral: 0.5-2 mg/kg/day in 2 divided doses (dosages as low as 0.05 mg/kg/day have been reported to be beneficial) for 15-20 weeks or until the total cyst count decreases by 70%, whichever is sooner. A second course of therapy may be initiated after a period of ≥2 months off therapy.

Pediatrics:

Neuroblastoma (investigational): Oral: Children: Maintenance therapy for neuroblastoma: 100-250 mg/m²/day in 2 divided doses

Acne (severe recalcitrant nodular): Children: Refer to adult dosing.

Hepatic Impairment: Empiric dose reductions are recommended in patient with hepatitis.

Available Dosage Forms

Capsule:

Accutane®: 10 mg, 20 mg, 40 mg [contains soybean oil and parabens]

Amnesteem™: 10 mg, 20 mg, 40 mg [contains soybean oil]

Claravis™: 10 mg, 20 mg, 40 mg

Sotret®: 10 mg, 20 mg, 30 mg, 40 mg [contains soybean oil]

Monitoring and Teaching Issues

Physical Assessment: Assess effectiveness and interactions of other medications patient may be taking. Assess results of laboratory tests, therapeutic effectiveness, and adverse reactions at beginning of therapy and regularly with long-term use. Monitor patients with diabetes closely. Assess knowledge/teach patient appropriate use, possible side effects/interventions, and adverse symptoms to report. **Pregnancy risk factor X:** Determine that patient is not pregnant before beginning treatment and do not give to women of childbearing age unless female is capable of complying with contraceptive measures 1 month prior to therapy, during therapy, and 1 month following therapy.

Monitoring Laboratory Tests: Must have pregnancy test prior to beginning therapy, CBC with differential and platelet count, baseline sedimentation rate, serum triglycerides, liver enzymes

Patient Education: A patient information/consent form must be signed before this medication is prescribed. Do not sign (and do not take this medication) if you do not understand any information on the form. Use exactly as directed; do not take more than recommended. Prescriptions will be written for a 1-month supply and must be filled within 7 days; they will not be honored if filled after that time or if they do not have the appropriate yellow qualification sticker attached. Capsule can be chewed and swallowed, swallowed, or opened with a large needle and contents sprinkled on applesauce or ice cream. Whole capsules should be swallowed with a full glass of liquid. Do not take any other vitamin A products, limit vitamin A intake, and increase exercise during therapy. Limit or avoid alcohol intake. Exacerbations of acne may occur during first weeks of therapy. You may experience headache, loss of night vision, lethargy, or visual disturbances (use caution when driving or engaging in tasks requiring alertness until response to drug is known); photosensitivity (use sunscreen, wear protective clothing and eyewear, and avoid direct sunlight); dry mouth or nausea (small frequent meals, sucking hard candy, or chewing gum may may help); or dryness, redness, or itching of skin, eye irritation, or increased sensitivity to contact lenses (wear regular glasses). Discontinue therapy and report acute vision changes, ringing in the ears or changes in hearing, rectal bleeding, abdominal cramping, or unresolved diarrhea. **Pregnancy/breast-feeding precautions:** Inform prescriber if you are pregnant. Do not get pregnant 1 month before, during, or for 1 month following therapy. This drug may cause severe fetal defects. Two forms of contraception and monthly tests to rule out pregnancy are required during therapy. It is important to note that any type of contraception may fail, it is the responsibility of the patient to be compliant with contraceptive therapy. Do not donate blood during or for 1 month following therapy (same reason). Do not breast-feed.

Dietary Considerations: Should be taken with food. Limit intake of vitamin A; avoid use of other vitamin A products. Some formulations may contain soybean oil.

Pregnancy Risk Factor: X

Pregnancy Issues: Major fetal abnormalities (both internal and external), spontaneous abortion, premature births and low IQ scores in surviving infants have been reported. This medication is contraindicated in females of childbearing potential unless they are able to comply with the guidelines of pregnancy prevention programs put in place by the FDA and the manufacturer of Accutane®.

Lactation: Excretion in breast milk unknown/contraindicated

Administration

Oral: Administer with food. Capsules can be swallowed, or chewed and swallowed. The capsule may be opened with a large needle and the contents placed on applesauce or ice cream for patients unable to swallow the capsule. Whole capsules should be swallowed with a full glass of liquid.

Storage: Store at room temperature and protect from light.

Additional Information Females of childbearing potential must receive oral and written information reviewing the hazards of therapy and the effects that isotretinoin can have on a fetus. Therapy should not begin without two negative pregnancy tests, one to be performed in the physician's office when qualifying the patient for treatment, the second test performed on the second day of the next normal menstrual period or 11 days after the last unprotected intercourse, whichever is last. Two forms of contraception (a primary and secondary form as described in the pregnancy prevention program materials) must be used during treatment and limitations to their use must be explained. Prescriptions should be written for no more than a 1-month supply, and pregnancy testing and counseling should be repeated monthly. Urine pregnancy test kits (for monthly pregnancy testing) and a Pregnancy Prevention Program kit (to be given to the patient prior to therapy) are provided by the manufacturer. Any cases of accidental pregnancy should be reported to the manufacturer or the FDA MedWatch Program. All patients (male and female) must read and sign the informed consent material provided in the pregnancy prevention program. Prescriptions will not be honored unless they have the yellow qualification sticker affixed.

The manufacturers of isotretinoin have developed comprehensive educational programs for healthcare providers and patients. Prior to prescribing isotretinoin, healthcare providers must be registered in one of these programs. Additional information for Accutane® and the corresponding S.M.A.R.T. (System To Manage Accutane®-Related Teratogenicity) program may be obtained from Roche Laboratories. Additional information for Amnesteem™ and the S.P.I.R.I.T.™ program (System To Prevent Isotretinoin-Related Issues of Teratogenicity) program maybe obtained from Bertek Pharmaceuticals. Additional information for Sotret® and I.M.P.A.R.T.™ (Isotretinoin Medication Program: Alerting you to the Risks of Teratogenicity) may be obtained from Ranbaxy Pharmaceuticals.

Note: In November 2004, the Food and Drug Administration (FDA) announced an update to the monitoring programs currently implemented to decrease fetal exposures to isotretinoin. The strengthened program, risk minimization action plan (RiskMAP), will include Accutane® as well as all the generic equivalents. When implemented, RiskMAP will replace the SMART program, which is managed by Roche, as well as programs supported by other isotretinoin manufacturers such as S.P.I.R.I.T.™ (Bertek Pharmaceuticals) and I.M.P.A.R.T.™ (Ranbaxy Pharmaceuticals).

Related Information
Maternal / Fetal Toxicology on page 1762

Isradipine (iz RA di peen)

U.S. Brand Names DynaCirc®; DynaCirc® CR

Generic Available No

Pharmacologic Category Calcium Channel Blocker

Medication Safety Issues
Sound-alike/look-alike issues:
DynaCirc® may be confused with Dynabac®, Dynacin®

Use Treatment of hypertension

Mechanism of Action/Effect Inhibits calcium ion from entering the "slow channels" or select voltage-sensitive areas of vascular smooth muscle and myocardium during depolarization

Contraindications Hypersensitivity to isradipine or any component of the formulation; hypotension (<90 mm Hg systolic)

Warnings/Precautions Use cautiously in CHF, hypertropic cardiomyopathy (IHSS), and in hepatic dysfunction. Safety and efficacy have not been established in pediatric patients. Adjust doses at 2- to 4-week intervals.

Drug Interactions
Cytochrome P450 Effect: Substrate of CYP3A4 (major); **Inhibits** CYP3A4 (weak)

Decreased Effect: NSAIDs (diclofenac) may decrease the antihypertensive response of isradipine. Isradipine may cause a decrease in lovastatin effect. CYP3A4 inducers may decrease the levels/effects of isradipine; example inducers include aminoglutethimide, carbamazepine, nafcillin, nevirapine, phenobarbital, phenytoin, and rifamycins.

Increased Effect/Toxicity: Isradipine may increase cardiovascular adverse effects of beta-blockers. Isradipine may minimally increase cyclosporine levels. CYP3A4 inhibitors may increase the levels/effects of isradipine; example inhibitors include azole antifungals, ciprofloxacin, clarithromycin, diclofenac, doxycycline, erythromycin, imatinib, isoniazid, nefazodone, nicardipine, propofol, protease inhibitors, quinidine, and verapamil. Blood pressure-lowering effects may be additive with sildenafil, tadalafil, and vardenafil (use caution).

Nutritional/Ethanol Interactions
Food: Administration with food delays absorption, but does not affect availability

Herb/Nutraceutical: St John's wort may decrease isradipine levels. Avoid dong quai if using for hypertension (has estrogenic activity). Avoid ephedra, yohimbe, ginseng (may worsen hypertension). Avoid garlic (may have increased antihypertensive effect).

Adverse Reactions
>10%: Central nervous system: Headache (dose related 2% to 22%)

1% to 10%:
Cardiovascular: Edema (dose related 1% to 9%), palpitation (dose related 1% to 5%), flushing (dose related 1% to 5%), tachycardia (1% to 3%), chest pain (2% to 3%)
Central nervous system: Dizziness (2% to 8%), fatigue (dose related 1% to 9%), flushing (9%)

(Continued)

Isradipine *(Continued)*

Dermatologic: Rash (1.5% to 2%)

Gastrointestinal: Nausea (1% to 5%), abdominal discomfort (≤3%), vomiting (≤1%), diarrhea (≤3%)

Renal: Urinary frequency (1% to 3%)

Respiratory: Dyspnea (1% to 3%)

Overdosage/Toxicology Primary cardiac symptoms of calcium blocker overdose include hypotension and bradycardia. Hypotension is caused by peripheral vasodilation, myocardial depression, and bradycardia. Bradycardia results from sinus bradycardia, second- or third-degree atrioventricular block, or sinus arrest with junctional rhythm. Intraventricular conduction is usually not affected so QRS duration is normal (verapamil does prolong the PR interval and bepridil prolongs the QT interval and may cause ventricular arrhythmias, including torsade de pointes).

Noncardiac symptoms include confusion, stupor, nausea, vomiting, metabolic acidosis and hyperglycemia. Repeated calcium administration may promptly reverse the depressed cardiac contractility (but not sinus node depression or peripheral vasodilation).

Pharmacodynamics/Kinetics

Duration of Action: 8-16 hours

Absorption: 90% to 95%

Bioavailability: 15% to 24%

Time to Peak: Serum: 1-1.5 hours

Protein Binding: 95%

Half-Life Elimination: 8 hours

Metabolism: Hepatic; extensive first-pass effect

Excretion: Urine (as metabolites)

Dosing

Adults & Elderly: Hypertension: Oral: 2.5 mg twice daily; antihypertensive response is seen in 2-3 hours; maximal response in 2-4 weeks; increase dose at 2- to 4-week intervals at 2.5-5 mg increments; usual dose range (JNC 7): 2.5-10 mg/day in 2 divided doses. **Note:** Most patients show no improvement with doses >10 mg/day except adverse reaction rate increases. Therefore, maximal dose in older adults should be 10 mg/day.

Available Dosage Forms

Capsule (DynaCirc®): 2.5 mg, 5 mg

Tablet, controlled release (DynaCirc® CR): 5 mg, 10 mg

Monitoring and Teaching Issues

Physical Assessment: Use caution in presence of CHF, hypertropic cardiomyopathy (IHSS), and hepatic dysfunction (see Warnings/Precautions for specific use cautions). Assess potential for interactions with other pharmacological agents or herbal products patient may be taking (eg, potential to increase or decrease levels/effects of isradipine; see Drug Interactions). Assess therapeutic effectiveness (normotensive) and adverse response at regular intervals during therapy (eg, tachycardia, hypotension, edema, dyspnea; see Adverse Reactions). Teach patient proper use, possible side effects/appropriate interventions, and adverse symptoms to report (see Patient Education).

Patient Education: Do not take any new medication during therapy unless approved by prescriber. Take as prescribed, with or without food. Do not stop abruptly without consulting prescriber. Do not crush extended release tablets. This medication does not replace other antihypertensive interventions; follow prescriber's instructions for diet and lifestyle changes. You may experience headache (if unrelieved, consult prescriber for approved analgesic); nausea or vomiting (small frequent meals, frequent mouth care, chewing gum, or sucking lozenges may help); constipation (increased dietary bulk and fluids may help); or dizziness, fatigue, confusion (use caution when driving or engaging in potentially hazardous tasks until response to drug is known). Report unrelieved headache, vomiting, or constipation; chest pain, palpitations, or rapid heartbeat; swelling of hands or feet or sudden weight gain (>5 lb/week); or unusual cramps in legs or feet. **Pregnancy/breast-feeding precautions:** Inform prescriber if you are or intend to become pregnant. Breast-feeding is not recommended.

Dietary Considerations: May be taken without regard to meals.

Geriatric Considerations: Elderly may experience a greater hypotensive response. Constipation may be more of a problem in the elderly.

Pregnancy Risk Factor: C

Lactation: Excretion in breast milk unknown/not recommended

Administration

Oral: May open capsule; avoid crushing contents

Related Information

Calcium Channel Blockers *on page 1722*

♦ Istalol™ *see* Timolol *on page 1478*

♦ Isuprel® *see* Isoproterenol *on page 838*

Itraconazole *(i tra KOE na zole)*

U.S. Brand Names Sporanox®

Generic Available No

Pharmacologic Category Antifungal Agent, Oral

Medication Safety Issues

Sound-alike/look-alike issues:

Sporanox® may be confused with Suprax®

Use Treatment of susceptible fungal infections in immunocompromised and immunocompetent patients including blastomycosis and histoplasmosis; indicated for aspergillosis, and onychomycosis of the toenail; treatment of onychomycosis of the fingernail without concomitant toenail infection via a pulse-type dosing regimen; has activity against *Aspergillus*, *Candida*, *Coccidioides*, *Cryptococcus*, *Sporothrix*, tinea unguium

Oral: Useful in superficial mycoses including dermatophytoses (eg, tinea capitis), pityriasis versicolor, sebopsoriasis, vaginal and chronic mucocutaneous candidiases; systemic mycoses including candidiasis, meningeal and disseminated cryptococcal infections, paracoccidioidomycosis, coccidioidomycoses; miscellaneous mycoses such as sporotrichosis, chromomycosis, leishmaniasis, fungal keratitis, alternariosis, zygomycosis

Oral solution: Treatment of oral and esophageal candidiasis

Intravenous solution: Indicated in the treatment of blastomycosis, histoplasmosis (nonmeningeal), and aspergillosis (in patients intolerant or refractory to amphotericin B therapy); empiric therapy of febrile neutropenic fever

Mechanism of Action/Effect Interferes with cytochrome P450 activity, decreasing ergosterol synthesis (principal sterol in fungal cell membrane) and inhibiting cell membrane formation

Contraindications Hypersensitivity to itraconazole, any component of the formulation, or to other azoles; concurrent administration with cisapride, dofetilide, ergot derivatives, levomethadyl, lovastatin, midazolam, pimozide, quinidine, simvastatin, or triazolam; treatment of onychomycosis in patients with evidence of left ventricular dysfunction, CHF, or a history of CHF

Warnings/Precautions Discontinue if signs or symptoms of CHF or neuropathy occur during treatment. Rare cases of serious cardiovascular adverse events (including death), ventricular tachycardia, and torsade de pointes have been observed due to increased cisapride concentrations induced by itraconazole. Use with caution in patients with left ventricular dysfunction or a history of CHF. Not recommended for use in patients with active liver disease, elevated liver enzymes, or prior hepatotoxic reactions to other drugs. Itraconazole has been associated with rare cases of serious hepatotoxicity (including fatal cases and cases within the first week of treatment); treatment should be discontinued in patients who develop clinical symptoms of liver dysfunction or abnormal liver function tests during itraconazole therapy except in cases where expected benefit exceeds risk. Large differences in itraconazole pharmacokinetic parameters have been observed in cystic fibrosis patients receiving the solution; if a patient with cystic fibrosis does not respond to therapy, alternate therapies should be considered. Due to differences in bioavailability, oral capsules and oral solution **cannot** be used interchangeably. Intravenous formulation should be used with caution in renal impairment; consider conversion to oral therapy if renal dysfunction/toxicity is noted. Initiation of treatment with oral solution is not recommended in patients at immediate risk for systemic candidiasis (eg, patients with severe neutropenia).

Drug Interactions

Cytochrome P450 Effect: Substrate of CYP3A4 (major); **Inhibits** CYP3A4 (strong)

Decreased Effect: Absorption of itraconazole requires gastric acidity; therefore, antacids, H_2 antagonists (cimetidine, famotidine, nizatidine, and ranitidine), proton pump inhibitors (omeprazole, lansoprazole, rabeprazole), and sucralfate may significantly reduce bioavailability resulting in treatment failures and should not be administered concomitantly. Antacids may decrease serum concentration of itraconazole; administer antacids 1 hour before or 2 hours after itraconazole capsules. Serum levels of itraconazole may be decreased with didanosine, isoniazid, and nevirapine. The levels/effects of itraconazole may be reduced by aminoglutethimide, carbamazepine, nafcillin, phenobarbital, phenytoin, rifamycins, and other CYP3A4 inducers. Oral contraceptive efficacy may be reduced (limited data).

Increased Effect/Toxicity: Itraconazole is a strong inhibitor of CYP3A4, and is contraindicated with cisapride, dofetilide, ergot derivatives, lovastatin, midazolam, pimozide, quinidine, simvastatin, and triazolam. Itraconazole may also increase the levels of alfentanil, benzodiazepines (alprazolam, diazepam, and others), buspirone, busulfan, calcium channel blockers (felodipine, nifedipine, verapamil), carbamazepine, corticosteroids, cyclosporine, digoxin, docetaxel, eletriptan, HMG-CoA reductase inhibitors (except fluvastatin, pravastatin), indinavir, oral hypoglycemics (sulfonylureas), phenytoin, rifabutin, ritonavir, saquinavir, sirolimus, tacrolimus, trimetrexate, vincristine, vinblastine, warfarin, and zolpidem. Other medications metabolized by CYP3A4 should be used with caution. Serum concentrations of itraconazole may be increased by strong CYP3A4 inhibitors. Serum concentrations of PDE-5 inhibitors (sildenafil, tadalafil, and vardenafil) are increased by itraconazole; specific dosage reductions/limitations are recommended.

Nutritional/Ethanol Interactions

Food:

Capsules: Enhanced by food and possibly by gastric acidity. cola drinks have been shown to increase the absorption of the capsules in patients with achlorhydria or those taking H_2-receptor antagonists or other gastric acid suppressors. Avoid grapefruit juice.

Solution: Decreased by food, time to peak concentration prolonged by food.

Herb/Nutraceutical: St John's wort may decrease itraconazole levels.

Adverse Reactions Listed incidences are for higher doses appropriate for systemic fungal infection.

>10%: Gastrointestinal: Nausea (11%)

1% to 10%:

Cardiovascular: Edema (4%), hypertension (3%)

Central nervous system: Headache (4%), fatigue (2% to 3%), malaise (1%), fever (3%), dizziness (2%)

Dermatologic: Rash (9%), pruritus (3%)

Endocrine & metabolic: Decreased libido (1%), hypertriglyceridemia, hypokalemia (2%)

Gastrointestinal: Abdominal pain (2%), anorexia (1%), vomiting (5%), diarrhea (3%)

Hepatic: Abnormal LFTs (3%), hepatitis

Renal: Albuminuria (1%)

Overdosage/Toxicology Overdoses are well tolerated. Treatment is supportive. Dialysis is not effective.

Pharmacodynamics/Kinetics

Absorption: Requires gastric acidity; capsule better absorbed with food, solution better absorbed on empty stomach; hypochlorhydria has been reported in HIV-infected patients; therefore, oral absorption in these patients may be decreased

(Continued)

Itraconazole *(Continued)*

Bioavailability: Variable, ~ 55% (oral solution) in 1 small study; **Note:** Oral solution has a higher degree of bioavailability (149% ± 68%) relative to oral capsules; should not be interchanged

Protein Binding: Plasma: 99.9%; metabolite hydroxy-itraconazole: 99.5%

Half-Life Elimination: Oral: After single 200 mg dose: 21 ± 5 hours; 64 hours at steady-state; I.V.: steady-state: 35 hours; steady-state concentrations are achieved in 13 days with multiple administration of itraconazole 100-400 mg/day.

Metabolism: Extensively hepatic via CYP3A4 into >30 metabolites including hydroxy-itraconazole (major metabolite); appears to have *in vitro* antifungal activity. Main metabolic pathway is oxidation; may undergo saturation metabolism with multiple dosing.

Excretion: Feces (~3% to 18%); urine (~0.03% as parent drug, 40% as metabolites)

Dosing

Adults & Elderly:

Blastomycosis/histoplasmosis:

Oral: 200 mg once daily, if no obvious improvement or there is evidence of progressive fungal disease, increase the dose in 100 mg increments to a maximum of 400 mg/day. Doses >200 mg/day are given in 2 divided doses. Length of therapy varies from 1 day to >6 months depending on the condition and mycological response.

I.V.: 200 mg twice daily for 4 doses, followed by 200 mg daily

Aspergillosis:

Oral: 200-400 mg/day

I.V.: 200 mg twice daily for 4 doses, followed by 200 mg daily

Onychomycosis: Oral: 200 mg once daily for 12 consecutive weeks

Life-threatening infections:

Oral: Loading dose: 200 mg 3 times/day (600 mg/day) should be given for the first 3 days of therapy.

I.V.: 200 mg twice daily for 4 doses, followed by 200 mg daily

Oropharyngeal candidiasis: Oral (solution): 200 mg once daily for 1-2 weeks; in patients unresponsive or refractory to fluconazole: 100 mg twice daily (clinical response expected in 1-2 weeks)

Esophageal candidiasis: Oral (solution): 100-200 mg once daily for a minimum of 3 weeks; continue dosing for 2 weeks after resolution of symptoms

Pediatrics: Efficacy and safety have not been established; a small number of patients 3-16 years of age have been treated with 100 mg/day for systemic fungal infections with no serious adverse effects reported. A dose of 5 mg/kg once daily was used in a pharmacokinetic study using the oral solution in patients 6 months-12 years; duration of study was 2 weeks.

Renal Impairment: Not necessary. Itraconazole injection is not recommended in patients with a creatinine clearance <30 mL/minute; hydroxypropyl-β-cyclodextrin (the excipient) is eliminated primarily by the kidneys.

Not dialyzable

Hepatic Impairment: May be necessary, but specific guidelines are not available. Risk-to-benefit evaluation should be undertaken in patients who develop liver function abnormalities during treatment.

Available Dosage Forms

Capsule: 100 mg

Injection, solution: 10 mg/mL (25 mL) [packaged in a kit containing sodium chloride 0.9% (50 mL); filtered infusion set (1)]

Solution, oral: 100 mg/10 mL (150 mL) [cherry flavor]

Monitoring and Teaching Issues

Physical Assessment: Use caution with left ventricular dysfunction, renal impairment, CHF, hepatic impairment (see Warnings/Precautions for use cautions). Assess potential for interactions with other pharmacological or herbal products patient may be taking (eg, anything that reduces gastric acidity may result in treatment failure of itraconazole; see Drug Interactions). See Administration for oral solution and infusion (specific oral capsules and oral solution cannot be used interchangeably). Assess results of laboratory tests, therapeutic effectiveness (resolution of fungal infection), and adverse reactions at regular intervals during therapy (see Adverse Reactions). Teach patient proper use (eg, necessity of taking full course of therapy), possible side effects/appropriate interventions, and adverse symptoms to report (see Patient Education). See Pregnancy Issues.

Monitoring Laboratory Tests: Liver function in patients with pre-existing hepatic dysfunction, and in all patients being treated for longer than 1 month.

Patient Education: Do not take any new medication during therapy unless approved by prescriber. Use exactly as directed. Take full course of medication even if infection appears to be resolved, do not discontinue without consulting prescriber (treatment for some fungal infections may take several weeks or months). Take capsule with food; solution on empty stomach, 1 hour before or 2 hours after meals. Do not take antacids of other medications within 1 hour before or 2 hours after itraconazole. Avoid grapefruit juice while taking this medication. Observe good hygiene measures to prevent reinfection. If you have diabetes, test serum glucose regularly (may affect response to oral hypoglycemics). Frequent blood tests may be required with prolonged therapy. May cause dizziness or drowsiness (use caution when driving or engaging in tasks that require alertness until response to drug is known); nausea, vomiting, or anorexia (small frequent meals, frequent mouth care, sucking lozenges, or chewing gum may help). Stop therapy and report any signs and symptoms that may suggest liver dysfunction (eg, unusual fatigue, anorexia, nausea and/or vomiting, jaundice, dark urine, or pale stool) immediately so that the appropriate laboratory testing can be done. **Pregnancy/breast-feeding precautions:** Inform prescriber if you are or intend to become pregnant. Consult prescriber about appropriate contraceptive use; efficacy of oral contraceptives may be reduced. Breast-feeding is not recommended.

Dietary Considerations:

Capsule: Administer with food.

Solution: Take without food, if possible.

Pregnancy Risk Factor: C

Pregnancy Issues: Should not be used to treat onychomycosis during pregnancy. Effective contraception should be used during treatment and for 2 months following treatment. Congenital abnormalities have been reported during postmarketing surveillance, but a causal relationship has not been established.

Lactation: Enters breast milk/not recommended

Administration

Oral: Doses >200 mg/day are given in 2 divided doses; do not administer with antacids. Capsule absorption is best if taken with food, therefore, it is best to administer itraconazole after meals; solution should be taken on an empty stomach. When treating oropharyngeal and esophageal candidiasis, solution should be swished vigorously in mouth, then swallowed.

I.V.: Using a flow control device, infuse 60 mL of the dilute solution (3.33 mg/mL = 200 mg itraconazole, pH ~4.8) intravenously over 60 minutes, using an extension line and the infusion set provided. After administration, flush the infusion set with 15-20 mL of 0.9% sodium chloride over 30 seconds to 15 minutes, via the two-way stopcock. Do not use bacteriostatic sodium chloride injection, USP. The compatibility of Sporanox® injection with flush solutions other than 0.9% sodium chloride (normal saline) is not known. Discard the entire infusion line.

Reconstitution: Dilute with 0.9% sodium chloride only. Do not use dextrose or lactated Ringer's. A precise mixing ratio is required to maintain stability (3.33:1) and avoid precipitate formation. Add 25 mL (1 ampul) to 50 mL 0.9% sodium chloride. Mix and withdraw 15 mL of solution before infusing.

Storage:

Capsule: Store at room temperature, 15°C to 25°C (59°F to 77°F); protect from light and moisture

Oral solution: Store at ≤25°C (77°F); do not freeze

Solution for injection: Store at ≤25°C (77°F); protect from light; do not freeze. Stable for 48 hours at room temperature or under refrigeration.

Additional Information Due to potential toxicity, the manufacturer recommends confirmation of diagnosis testing of nail specimens prior to treatment of onychomycosis.

Ketoconazole (kee toe KOE na zole)

U.S. Brand Names Nizoral®; Nizoral® A-D [OTC]

Generic Available Yes

Pharmacologic Category Antifungal Agent, Oral; Antifungal Agent, Topical

(Continued)

Ketoconazole *(Continued)*

Medication Safety Issues
Sound-alike/look-alike issues:

Nizoral® may be confused with Nasarel®, Neoral®, Nitrol®

Use Treatment of susceptible fungal infections, including candidiasis, oral thrush, blastomycosis, histoplasmosis, paracoccidioidomycosis, coccidioidomycosis, chromomycosis, candiduria, chronic mucocutaneous candidiasis, as well as certain recalcitrant cutaneous dermatophytoses; used topically for treatment of tinea corporis, tinea cruris, tinea versicolor, and cutaneous candidiasis, seborrheic dermatitis

Unlabeled/Investigational Use Treatment of prostate cancer (androgen synthesis inhibitor)

Mechanism of Action/Effect Inhibits several fungal enzymes that results in a build-up of toxic concentrations of hydrogen peroxide resulting in cell death; inhibits androgen synthesis

Contraindications Hypersensitivity to ketoconazole or any component of the formulation; CNS fungal infections (due to poor CNS penetration); coadministration with ergot derivatives or cisapride is contraindicated due to risk of potentially fatal cardiac arrhythmias

Warnings/Precautions Use with caution in patients with impaired hepatic function; has been associated with hepatotoxicity, including some fatalities; perform periodic liver function tests; high doses of ketoconazole may depress adrenocortical function.

Drug Interactions
Cytochrome P450 Effect: Substrate of CYP3A4 (major); **Inhibits** CYP1A2 (strong), 2A6 (moderate), 2B6 (weak), 2C8/9 (strong), 2C19 (moderate), 2D6 (moderate), 3A4 (strong)

Decreased Effect: Oral: Absorption requires gastric acidity; therefore, antacids, H_2 antagonists (cimetidine, famotidine, nizatidine, and ranitidine), proton pump inhibitors (omeprazole, lansoprazole, rabeprazole), and sucralfate may significantly reduce bioavailability resulting in treatment failures and should not be administered concomitantly. Decreased serum levels with didanosine and isoniazid. The levels/effects of ketoconazole may be decreased by aminoglutethimide, carbamazepine, nafcillin, nevirapine, phenobarbital, phenytoin, rifamycins, or other CYP3A4 inducers. **Should not be administered concomitantly with rifampin.** Oral contraceptive efficacy may be reduced (limited data). Ketoconazole may decrease the levels/effects of CYP2D6 prodrug substrates (eg, codeine, hydrocodone, oxycodone, tramadol).

Increased Effect/Toxicity: Due to inhibition of hepatic CYP3A4, ketoconazole use is contraindicated with cisapride, lovastatin, midazolam, simvastatin, and triazolam due to large substantial increases in the toxicity of these agents. Ketoconazole may increase the serum levels/effects of amiodarone, amphetamines, benzodiazepines, beta-blockers, buspirone, busulfan, calcium channel blockers, citalopram, dexmedetomidine, dextromethorphan, diazepam, digoxin, docetaxel, fluoxetine, fluvoxamine, glimepiride, glipizide, ifosfamide, inhalational anesthetics, lidocaine, mesoridazine, methsuximide, mexiletine, mirtazapine, nateglinide, nefazodone, paroxetine, phenytoin, pioglitazone, propranolol, risperidone, ritonavir, ropinirole, rosiglitazone, sertraline, sirolimus, tacrolimus, theophylline, thioridazine, tricyclic antidepressants, trifluoperazine, trimetrexate, venlafaxine, vincristine, vinblastine, warfarin, zolpidem, and other substrates of CYP1A2, 2A6, 2C8/9, 2C19, 2D6, or 3A4. Selected benzodiazepines (midazolam and triazolam), cisapride, ergot alkaloids, selected HMG-CoA reductase inhibitors (lovastatin and simvastatin), and pimozide are generally contraindicated with strong CYP3A4 inhibitors. Mesoridazine and thioridazine are generally contraindicated with strong CYP2D6 inhibitors. When used with strong CYP3A4 inhibitors, dosage adjustment/limits are recommended for sildenafil and other PDE-5 inhibitors; consult individual monographs.

Nutritional/Ethanol Interactions
Food: Ketoconazole peak serum levels may be prolonged if taken with food.

Herb/Nutraceutical: St John's wort may decrease ketoconazole levels.

Adverse Reactions
Oral: 1% to 10%:

Dermatologic: Pruritus (2%)

Gastrointestinal: Nausea/vomiting (3% to 10%), abdominal pain (1%)

Cream: Severe irritation, pruritus, stinging (~5%)

Shampoo: Increases in normal hair loss, irritation (<1%), abnormal hair texture, scalp pustules, mild dryness of skin, itching, oiliness/dryness of hair

Overdosage/Toxicology Oral: Symptoms of overdose include dizziness, headache, nausea, vomiting, diarrhea. Overdoses are well tolerated. Treatment includes supportive measures and gastric decontamination.

Pharmacodynamics/Kinetics
Absorption: Oral: Rapid (~75%); Shampoo: None

Bioavailability: Decreases as gastric pH increases

Time to Peak: Serum: 1-2 hours

Protein Binding: 93% to 96%

Half-Life Elimination: Biphasic: Initial: 2 hours; Terminal: 8 hours

Metabolism: Partially hepatic via CYP3A4 to inactive compounds

Excretion: Feces (57%); urine (13%)

Dosing
Adults & Elderly:

Fungal infections:

Oral: 200-400 mg/day as a single daily dose

Shampoo: Apply twice weekly for 4 weeks with at least 3 days between each shampoo.

Topical: Rub gently into the affected area once daily to twice daily.

Prostate cancer (unlabeled use): Oral: Adults: 400 mg 3 times/day

Pediatrics:

Fungal infections: Oral:

Children ≥2 years: 3.3-6.6 mg/kg/day as a single dose for 1-2 weeks for candidiasis, for at least 4 weeks in recalcitrant dermatophyte infections, and for up to 6 months for other systemic mycoses

Renal Impairment: Not dialyzable (0% to 5%)
Hepatic Impairment: Dose reductions should be considered in patients with severe liver disease.

Available Dosage Forms
Cream, topical: 2% (15 g, 30 g, 60 g)
Shampoo, topical (Nizoral® A-D): 1% (6 mL, 120 mL, 210 mL)
Tablet (Nizoral®): 200 mg

Monitoring and Teaching Issues
Physical Assessment: See Warnings/Precautions for specific use cautions (eg, impaired liver function). Assess potential for interactions with other pharmacological agents or herbal products patient may be taking (eg, anything that reduces gastric acidity may result in treatment failures with ketoconazole, concurrent use of ergot derivatives or cisapride increases the risk of potentially fatal cardiac arrhythmias, oral contraceptive efficacy may be reduced; see Drug Interactions). Assess liver function periodically. Monitor therapeutic effect (resolution of viral infection) and adverse reactions on a regular basis (see Adverse Reactions). Instruct patients with diabetes to monitor glucose levels closely; may impact effectiveness of oral hypoglycemics. Teach patient proper use (necessity of completely full therapy), possible side effects/appropriate interventions (eg, importance of adequate hydration), and adverse symptoms to report (see Patient Education).
Monitoring Laboratory Tests: Liver function
Patient Education: Do not take any new medication during therapy without consulting prescriber. Oral formulation may be taken with food, at least 2 hours before any antacids. Take full course of medication as directed; some infections may require long periods of therapy. If you have diabetes, test serum glucose regularly; may impact effectiveness of oral hypoglycemics. May cause nausea and vomiting (small frequent meals, frequent mouth care, sucking lozenges, or chewing gum may help); headache (mild analgesic may be necessary); or dizziness (use caution when driving). Report unresolved headache, rash or itching, yellowing of eyes or skin, changes in color of urine or stool, chest pain or palpitations, or sense of fullness or ringing in ears. **Pregnancy/breast-feeding precautions:** Inform prescriber if you are or intend to become pregnant. Breast-feeding is not recommended.

Topical: Wash and dry area before applying medication thinly. Do not cover with occlusive dressing. Report severe skin irritation or if condition does not improve.

Shampoo: Allow 3 days between shampoos. You may experience some hair loss, scalp irritations, itching change in hair texture, or scalp pustules. Report severe side effects or if infestation persists.

Dietary Considerations: May be taken with food or milk to decrease GI adverse effects.
Pregnancy Risk Factor: C
Lactation: Enters breast milk/not recommended

Administration
Oral: Do not take with antacids; take at least 2 hours before antacids.
Topical: Cream and shampoo: External use only.

Ketoprofen (kee toe PROE fen)
U.S. Brand Names Orudis® KT [OTC]; Oruvail®
Generic Available Yes: Capsule
Pharmacologic Category Nonsteroidal Anti-inflammatory Drug (NSAID), Oral
Medication Safety Issues
Sound-alike/look-alike issues:
Oruvail® may be confused with Clinoril®, Elavil®
Use Acute and long-term treatment of rheumatoid arthritis and osteoarthritis; primary dysmenorrhea; mild to moderate pain
Mechanism of Action/Effect Inhibits prostaglandin synthesis by decreasing the activity of the enzyme, cyclooxygenase, which results in decreased formation of prostaglandin precursors
Contraindications Hypersensitivity to ketoprofen, any component of the formulation, or other NSAIDs/aspirin; pregnancy (3rd trimester)
Warnings/Precautions Fatal asthmatic and anaphylactoid reactions have occurred in patients with "aspirin triad." Use with caution in patients with CHF, hypertension, dehydration, decreased renal or hepatic function, history of GI disease (bleeding, ulcers, or previous GI symptoms with NSAID use), or those receiving anticoagulants and/or corticosteroids. Use lowest effective dose for shortest period possible; bleeding risk has been correlated to dose and duration of therapy. Gastrointestinal bleeding may occur without prior symptoms of gastrointestinal irritation. Elderly are at a high risk for adverse effects from NSAIDs. As many as 60% of elderly can develop peptic ulceration and/or hemorrhage asymptomatically.

Use of NSAIDs can compromise existing renal function especially when Cl_{cr} <30 mL/minute. CNS adverse effects such as confusion, agitation, and hallucination are generally seen in overdose or high-dose situations; however, elderly may demonstrate these adverse effects at lower doses than younger adults. Do not exceed 300 mg/day. Withhold for at least 4-6 half-lives prior to surgical or dental procedures.

Drug Interactions
Cytochrome P450 Effect: Inhibits CYP2C8/9 (weak)
Decreased Effect: Decreased effect of diuretics (loop and thiazides). May decrease effects of antihypertensives.
Increased Effect/Toxicity: Increased effect/toxicity with antiplatelet agents, corticosteroids, cyclosporine, probenecid, lithium, anticoagulants, and methotrexate.
Nutritional/Ethanol Interactions
Ethanol: Avoid ethanol (due to GI irritation).
Food: Although food affects the bioavailability of ketoprofen, analgesic efficacy is not significantly diminished; food slows rate of absorption resulting in delayed and reduced peak serum concentrations.
Lab Interactions Increased chloride (S), sodium (S), bleeding time
(Continued)

Ketoprofen *(Continued)*

Adverse Reactions
>10%: Gastrointestinal: Dyspepsia (11%)

1% to 10%:
- Central nervous system: Headache (3% to 9%), nervousness, dizziness, somnolence, insomnia, malaise, depression
- Dermatologic: Rash, itching
- Endocrine & metabolic: Fluid retention
- Gastrointestinal: Vomiting (>1%), diarrhea (3% to 9%), nausea (3% to 9%), constipation (3% to 9%), abdominal distress/cramping/pain (3% to 9%), flatulence (3% to 9%), anorexia (>1%), stomatitis (>1%)
- Genitourinary: Urinary tract infection (>1%)
- Ocular: Visual disturbances
- Otic: Tinnitus
- Renal: Renal function impairment

Overdosage/Toxicology
Symptoms of overdose include apnea, metabolic acidosis, coma, nystagmus, seizures, leukocytosis, and renal failure. Management of NSAID intoxication is supportive and symptomatic. Since many NSAIDs undergo enterohepatic cycling, multiple doses of charcoal may be needed to reduce the potential for delayed toxicities.

Pharmacodynamics/Kinetics
Absorption: Almost complete

Time to Peak: Capsule: 0.5-2 hours; Capsule, extended release: 6-7 hours

Protein Binding: >99%, primarily albumin

Half-Life Elimination: Capsule: 2.5 hours; Capsule, extended release: 5.4 hours

Metabolism: Hepatic

Excretion: Urine (~80%, primarily as glucuronide conjugates)

Dosing
Adults:

Rheumatoid arthritis or osteoarthritis: Oral:
- *Capsule:* 50-75 mg 3-4 times/day up to a maximum of 300 mg/day
- *Capsule, extended release:* 200 mg once daily

Mild to moderate pain: Oral: Capsule: 25-50 mg every 6-8 hours up to a maximum of 300 mg/day
- *OTC labeling:* 12.5 mg every 4-6 hours, up to a maximum of 6 tablets/24 hours

Elderly: Initial: 25-50 mg 3-4 times/day; increase up to 150-300 mg/day (maximum daily dose: 300 mg)

Pediatrics:

Mild to moderate pain, rheumatoid arthritis: Children ≥16 years: Refer to adult dosing.

Renal Impairment:
- Mild impairment: Maximum dose: 150 mg/day
- Severe impairment: Maximum dose: 100 mg/day

Hepatic Impairment: Hepatic impairment and serum albumin <3.5 g/dL: Maximum dose: 100 mg/day

Available Dosage Forms
Capsule: 50 mg, 75 mg

Capsule, extended release (Oruvail®): 100 mg, 150 mg, 200 mg

Tablet (Orudis® KT): 12.5 mg [contains tartrazine and sodium benzoate]

Monitoring and Teaching Issues
Physical Assessment: Assess effectiveness and interactions of other medications patient may be taking. Assess results of laboratory tests, therapeutic effectiveness, and adverse or overdose reactions at beginning of therapy and periodically throughout therapy. Schedule ophthalmic evaluations for patients who develop eye complaints during long-term NSAID therapy. Assess knowledge/teach patient appropriate use, interventions to reduce side effects, and adverse symptoms to report.

Monitoring Laboratory Tests: CBC, occult blood loss, periodic liver function; renal function (urine output, serum BUN, creatinine)

Patient Education: Take this medication exactly as directed; do not increase dose without consulting prescriber. Do not crush tablets or break capsules. Take with food or milk to reduce GI distress. Maintain adequate hydration (2-3 L/day of fluids) unless instructed to restrict fluid intake. Do not use alcohol, aspirin or aspirin-containing medication, or any other anti-inflammatory medications without consulting prescriber. You may experience drowsiness, dizziness, nervousness, or headache (use caution when driving or engaging in tasks requiring alertness until response to drug is known); anorexia, nausea, vomiting, or heartburn (small frequent meals, frequent mouth care, sucking lozenges, or chewing gum may help); fluid retention (weigh yourself weekly and report unusual (3-5 lb/week) weight gain). GI bleeding, ulceration, or perforation can occur with or without pain; discontinue medication and contact prescriber if persistent abdominal pain or cramping, or blood in stool occurs. Report breathlessness, respiratory difficulty, or unusual cough; chest pain, rapid heartbeat, palpitations; unusual bruising/bleeding; blood in urine, stool, mouth, or vomitus; swollen extremities; skin rash or itching; acute fatigue; or hearing changes (ringing in ears). **Pregnancy/breast-feeding precautions:** Inform prescriber if you are or intend to become pregnant. This drug should not be used in the 3rd trimester of pregnancy. Breast-feeding is not recommended.

Dietary Considerations: In order to minimize gastrointestinal effects, ketoprofen can be prescribed to be taken with food or milk.

Geriatric Considerations: Elderly are at high risk for adverse effects from NSAIDs. As much as 60% of elderly can develop peptic ulceration and/or hemorrhage asymptomatically. The concomitant use of H_2 blockers, omeprazole, and sucralfate is not effective as prophylaxis with the exception of NSAID-induced duodenal ulcers which may be prevented by the use of ranitidine. Misoprostol is the only prophylactic agent proven effective. Also, concomitant disease and drug use contribute to the risk for GI adverse effects. Use lowest effective dose for shortest period possible. Consider renal function decline with age. Use of NSAIDs can compromise existing renal function especially when Cl_{cr} is ≤30 mL/minute.

Tinnitus may be a difficult and unreliable indication of toxicity due to age-related hearing loss or eighth cranial nerve damage. CNS adverse effects such as confusion, agitation, and hallucination are generally seen in overdose or high-dose situations, but elderly may demonstrate these adverse effects at lower doses than younger adults.

Pregnancy Risk Factor: B/D (3rd trimester)

Pregnancy Issues: Exposure to NSAIDs late in pregnancy may lead to premature closure of the ductus arteriosus and may inhibit uterine contractions.

Lactation: Excretion in breast milk unknown/not recommended

Administration

Oral: May take with food to reduce GI upset. Do not crush or break extended release capsules.

Related Information

Nonsalicylate / Nonsteroidal Anti-inflammatory Agents *on page 1743*

Ketorolac (KEE toe role ak)

U.S. Brand Names Acular®; Acular LS™; Acular® PF; Toradol®

Synonyms Ketorolac Tromethamine

Generic Available Yes: Injection, tablet

Pharmacologic Category Nonsteroidal Anti-inflammatory Drug (NSAID), Ophthalmic; Nonsteroidal Anti-inflammatory Drug (NSAID), Oral; Nonsteroidal Anti-inflammatory Drug (NSAID), Parenteral

Medication Safety Issues

Sound-alike/look-alike issues:

Acular® may be confused with Acthar®, Ocular®

Toradol® may be confused with Foradil®, Inderal®, Tegretol®, Torecan®, tramadol

Use

Oral, injection: Short-term (≤5 days) management of moderately-severe acute pain requiring analgesia at the opioid level

Ophthalmic: Temporary relief of ocular itching due to seasonal allergic conjunctivitis; postoperative inflammation following cataract extraction; reduction of ocular pain and photophobia following incisional refractive surgery, reduction of ocular pain, burning and stinging following corneal refractive surgery

Mechanism of Action/Effect A potent NSAID; provides analgesia by inhibiting the synthesis of prostaglandin

Contraindications Hypersensitivity to ketorolac, aspirin, other NSAIDs, or any component of the formulation; patients who have developed nasal polyps, angioedema, or bronchospastic reactions to other NSAIDs; active or history of peptic ulcer disease; recent or history of GI bleeding or perforation; patients with advanced renal disease or risk of renal failure; labor and delivery; nursing mothers; prophylaxis before major surgery; suspected or confirmed cerebrovascular bleeding; hemorrhagic diathesis; concurrent ASA or other NSAIDs; epidural or intrathecal administration; concomitant probenecid; pregnancy (3rd trimester)

Warnings/Precautions

Systemic: Treatment should be started with I.V./I.M. administration then changed to oral only as a continuation of treatment. Total therapy is not to exceed 5 days. Should not be used for minor or chronic pain. Hypersensitivity reactions have occurred flowing the first dose of ketorolac injection, including patients without prior exposure to ketorolac, aspirin, or other NSAIDs. Fatal asthmatic and anaphylactoid reactions have occurred in patients with "aspirin triad." Use with caution in patients with CHF, hypertension, dehydration, decreased renal or hepatic function, history of GI disease (bleeding, ulcers, or previous GI symptoms with NSAID use), or those receiving anticoagulants and/or corticosteroids. Use lowest effective dose for shortest period possible; bleeding risk has been correlated to dose and duration of therapy. Gastrointestinal bleeding may occur without prior symptoms of gastrointestinal irritation. Use extra caution and increase dosages in the elderly because it is cleared renally somewhat slower the elderly are also more sensitive to the renal effects of NSAIDs and have a greater risk of GI perforation and bleeding. As many as 60% of elderly may develop peptic ulceration and/or hemorrhage asymptomatically. CNS adverse effects such as confusion, agitation, and hallucination are generally seen in overdose or high-dose situations; however, elderly may demonstrate these adverse effects at lower doses than younger adults.

Use of NSAIDs can compromise existing renal function especially when Cl_{cr} <30 mL/minute. May prolong bleeding time; do not use when hemostasis is critical. Patients should be euvolemic prior to treatment. Low doses of narcotics may be needed for breakthrough pain. Withhold for at least 4-6 half-lives prior to surgical or dental procedures.

Ophthalmic: May increase bleeding time associated with ocular surgery. Use with caution in patients with known bleeding tendencies or those receiving anticoagulants. Healing time may be slowed or delayed. Corneal thinning, erosion, or ulceration have been reported with topical NSAIDs; discontinue if corneal epithelial breakdown occurs. Use caution with complicated ocular surgery, corneal denervation, corneal epithelial defects, diabetes, rheumatoid arthritis, ocular surface disease, or ocular surgeries repeated within short periods of time; risk of corneal epithelial breakdown may be increased. Use for >24 hours prior to or for >14 days following surgery also increases risk of corneal adverse effects. Do not administer while wearing soft contact lenses. Safety and efficacy in pediatric patients <3 years of age have not been established.

Drug Interactions

Decreased Effect: Decreased effect: Decreased antihypertensive effect seen with ACE inhibitors and angiotensin II antagonists; decreased antiepileptic effect seen with carbamazepine, phenytoin

Increased Effect/Toxicity: Increased toxicity: Lithium, methotrexate, probenecid increased drug level; increased effect/toxicity with salicylates, probenecid, anticoagulants, nondepolarizing muscle relaxants, alprazolam, fluoxetine, thiothixene

Nutritional/Ethanol Interactions

Ethanol: Avoid ethanol (may enhance gastric mucosal irritation).

(Continued)

Ketorolac *(Continued)*

Food: Oral: High-fat meals may delay time to peak (by ~1 hour) and decrease peak concentrations.

Herb/Nutraceutical: Avoid cat's claw, dong quai, evening primrose, feverfew, garlic, ginger, ginkgo, red clover, horse chestnut, green tea, ginseng (all have additional antiplatelet activity).

Lab Interactions Increased chloride (S), sodium (S), bleeding time

Adverse Reactions

Systemic:

>10%:

Central nervous system: Headache (17%)

Gastrointestinal: Gastrointestinal pain (13%), dyspepsia (12%), nausea (12%)

>1% to 10%:

Cardiovascular: Edema (4%), hypertension

Central nervous system: Dizziness (7%), drowsiness (6%)

Dermatologic: Pruritus, purpura, rash

Gastrointestinal: Diarrhea (7%), constipation, flatulence, gastrointestinal fullness, vomiting, stomatitis

Local: Injection site pain (2%)

Miscellaneous: Diaphoresis

Ophthalmic solution:

>10%: Ocular: Transient burning/stinging (Acular®: 40%; Acular® PF: 20%)

>1% to 10%:

Central nervous system: Headache

Ocular: Conjunctival hyperemia, corneal infiltrates, iritis, ocular edema, ocular inflammation, ocular irritation, ocular pain, superficial keratitis, superficial ocular infection

Miscellaneous: Allergic reactions

Overdosage/Toxicology Symptoms of overdose include abdominal pain, peptic ulcers, and metabolic acidosis. Management of NSAID intoxication is supportive and symptomatic. Dialysis is not effective.

Pharmacodynamics/Kinetics

Onset of Action: Analgesic: I.M.: ~10 minutes; Peak effect: Analgesic: 2-3 hours

Duration of Action: Analgesic: 6-8 hours

Absorption: Oral: Well absorbed

Time to Peak: Serum: I.M.: 30-60 minutes

Protein Binding: 99%

Half-Life Elimination: 2-8 hours; increased 30% to 50% in elderly

Metabolism: Hepatic

Excretion: Urine (61% as unchanged drug)

Dosing

Adults:

Pain management (acute; moderately-severe): Children ≥16 years and Adults:

Note: The maximum combined duration of treatment (for parenteral and oral) is 5 days; do not increase dose or frequency; supplement with low dose opioids if needed for breakthrough pain. For patients <50 kg and/or ≥65 years of age, see Elderly dosing.

I.M.: 60 mg as a single dose or 30 mg every 6 hours (maximum daily dose: 120 mg)

I.V.: 30 mg as a single dose or 30 mg every 6 hours (maximum daily dose: 120 mg)

Oral: 20 mg, followed by 10 mg every 4-6 hours; do not exceed 40 mg/day; oral dosing is intended to be a continuation of I.M. or I.V. therapy only

Ophthalmic uses:

Seasonal allergic conjunctivitis (relief of ocular itching) (Acular®): Ophthalmic: Instill 1 drop (0.25 mg) 4 times/day for seasonal allergic conjunctivitis

Inflammation following cataract extraction (Acular®): Ophthalmic: Instill 1 drop (0.25 mg) to affected eye(s) 4 times/day beginning 24 hours after surgery; continue for 2 weeks

Pain and photophobia following incisional refractive surgery (Acular® PF): Ophthalmic: Instill 1 drop (0.25 mg) 4 times/day to affected eye for up to 3 days

Pain following corneal refractive surgery (Acular LS™): Ophthalmic: Instill 1 drop 4 times/day as needed to affected eye for up to 4 days

Elderly: Elderly >65 years: Renal insufficiency or weight <50 kg: **Note:** Ketorolac has decreased clearance and increased half-life in the elderly. In addition, the elderly have reported increased incidence of GI bleeding, ulceration, and perforation. The maximum combined duration of treatment (for parenteral and oral) is 5 days.

I.M.: 30 mg as a single dose or 15 mg every 6 hours (maximum daily dose: 60 mg)

I.V.: 15 mg as a single dose or 15 mg every 6 hours (maximum daily dose: 60 mg)

Oral: 10 mg every 4-6 hours; do not exceed 40 mg/day; oral dosing is intended to be a continuation of I.M. or I.V. therapy only

Pediatrics: Note: Do not exceed adult doses.

Anti-inflammatory, single-dose treatment: Children 2-16 years:

I.M.: 1 mg/kg (maximum: 30 mg)

I.V.: 0.5 mg/kg (maximum: 15 mg)

Oral (unlabeled): 1 mg/kg as a single dose reported in one study

Anti-inflammatory, multiple-dose treatment (unlabeled): Children 2-16 years: Limited pediatric studies. The maximum combined duration of treatment (for parenteral and oral) is 5 days.

I.V.: Initial dose: 0.5 mg/kg followed by 0.25-1 mg/kg every 6 hours for up to 48 hours; maximum daily dose: 90 mg

Oral: 0.25 mg/kg every 6 hours

Ophthalmic uses: Children ≥3 years: Refer to adult dosing.

Renal Impairment: Do not use in patients with advanced renal impairment. Patients with moderately-elevated serum creatinine should use half the recommended dose, not to exceed 60 mg/day I.M./I.V.

Hepatic Impairment: Use with caution, may cause elevation of liver enzymes

Available Dosage Forms

Injection, solution, as tromethamine: 15 mg/mL (1 mL); 30 mg/mL (1 mL, 2 mL, 30 mL) [contains alcohol]

Solution, ophthalmic, as tromethamine:

Acular®: 0.5% (3 mL, 5 mL, 10 mL) [contains benzalkonium chloride]

Acular LS™: 0.4% (5 mL) [contains benzalkonium chloride]

Acular® P.F. [preservative free]: 0.5% (0.4 mL)

Tablet, as tromethamine (Toradol®): 10 mg

Monitoring and Teaching Issues

Physical Assessment: Assess allergy history prior to beginning therapy. Assess potential for interactions with other prescriptions, OTC medications, or herbal products patient may be taking. **I.V./I.M.:** Vital signs should be monitored on a regular basis during infusion or following injection. Assess results of laboratory tests, therapeutic effectiveness, and adverse response on a regular basis throughout therapy. Teach patient proper use, possible side effects/appropriate interventions (eg, importance of adequate hydration), and adverse symptoms to report.

Monitoring Laboratory Tests: Renal function (serum creatinine, BUN, urine output), CBC, liver function, platelets

Patient Education: Do not take any new medication during therapy without consulting prescriber (especially aspirin-containing products or other NSAIDs or any other NSAIDs). Use exactly as directed; do not increase dose or frequency. Adverse reactions can occur with overuse. Oral doses may be taken with food or milk. Avoid alcohol. Maintain adequate hydration (2-3 L/day of fluids) unless instructed to restrict fluid intake. May cause nausea or vomiting (frequent mouth care, small frequent meals, chewing gum, or sucking lozenges may help). Report GI bleeding, ulceration or perforation with or without pain (stop medication and report abdominal pain or blood in urine or stool); ringing in ears; unresolved nausea or vomiting; respiratory difficulty or shortness of breath; skin rash; unusual swelling of extremities; chest pain; or palpitations. **Pregnancy/breast-feeding precautions:** Inform prescriber if you are or intend to become pregnant. This drug should not be used in the 2nd or 3rd trimester of pregnancy. Consult prescriber for appropriate contraceptive measures if necessary. Consult prescriber if breast-feeding.

Ophthalmic: Instill drops as often as recommended. Wash hands before instilling. Sit or lie down to instill. Open eye, look at ceiling, and instill prescribed amount of solution. Close eye and roll eye in all directions. Apply gentle pressure to inner corner of eye for 1-2 minutes after instillation. Do not let tip of applicator touch eye; do not contaminate tip of applicator (may cause eye infection, eye damage, or vision loss). Temporary stinging or blurred vision may occur. Do not wear soft contact lenses. Report persistent pain, burning, double vision, swelling, itching, or worsening of condition.

Dietary Considerations: Administer tablet with food or milk to decrease gastrointestinal distress.

Geriatric Considerations: Ketorolac is eliminated more slowly in the elderly. It is recommended to use lower doses in the elderly. The elderly are at high risk for adverse effects from NSAIDs. As much as 60% of elderly can develop peptic ulceration and/or hemorrhage asymptomatically. The concomitant use of H_2 blockers, omeprazole, and sucralfate is not effective as prophylaxis with the exception of NSAID-induced duodenal ulcers which may be prevented by the use of ranitidine. Misoprostol is the only prophylactic agent proven effective. Also, concomitant disease and drug use contribute to the risk for GI adverse effects. Use lowest effective dose for shortest period possible. Consider renal function decline with age. Use of NSAIDs can compromise existing renal function especially when Cl_{cr} is ≤30 mL/minute. Tinnitus may be a difficult and unreliable indication of toxicity due to age-related hearing loss or eighth cranial nerve damage. CNS adverse effects such as confusion, agitation, and hallucination are generally seen in overdose or high-dose situations, but elderly may demonstrate these adverse effects at lower doses than younger adults.

Pregnancy Risk Factor: C/D (3rd trimester); ophthalmic: C

Pregnancy Issues: Ketorolac is contraindicated during labor and delivery (may inhibit uterine contractions and adversely affect fetal circulation). Avoid use of ketorolac ophthalmic solution during late pregnancy.

Lactation: Enters breast milk/contraindicated (AAP rates "compatible")

Administration

Oral: May take with food to reduce GI upset.

I.M.: Administer slowly and deeply into the muscle. Analgesia begins in 30 minutes and maximum effect within 2 hours.

I.V.: Administer I.V. bolus over a minimum of 15 seconds; onset within 30 minutes; peak analgesia within 2 hours.

Other: Ophthalmic solution: Contact lenses should be removed before instillation.

Compatibility: Stable in D_5NS, D_5W, LR, NS

Compatibility when admixed: Incompatible with hydroxyzine, meperidine, morphine, promethazine

Storage: Ketorolac injection and ophthalmic solution should be stored at controlled room temperature and protected from light. Injection is clear and has a slight yellow color. Precipitation may occur at relatively low pH values. Store tablets at controlled room temperature.

Additional Information First parenteral NSAID for analgesia; 30 mg provides the analgesia comparable to 12 mg of morphine or 100 mg of meperidine.

Related Information

Nonsalicylate / Nonsteroidal Anti-inflammatory Agents *on page 1743*

♦ **Ketorolac Tromethamine** *see* Ketorolac *on page 853*

Ketotifen (kee toe TYE fen)

U.S. Brand Names Zaditor™

Synonyms Ketotifen Fumarate

(Continued)

Ketotifen *(Continued)*

Generic Available No

Pharmacologic Category Antihistamine, H_1 Blocker, Ophthalmic

Use Temporary prevention of eye itching due to allergic conjunctivitis

Contraindications Hypersensitivity to ketotifen or any component of the formulation (the preservative is benzalkonium chloride)

Adverse Reactions 1% to 10%:

Ocular: Allergic reactions, burning or stinging, conjunctivitis, discharge, dry eyes, eye pain, eyelid disorder, itching, keratitis, lacrimation disorder, mydriasis, photophobia, rash

Respiratory: Pharyngitis

Miscellaneous: Flu syndrome

Overdosage/Toxicology No serious signs or symptoms seen after ingestion of up to 20 mg of ketotifen

Pharmacodynamics/Kinetics

Onset of Action: Minutes

Duration of Action: 8-12 hours

Absorption: Minimally systemic

Dosing

Adults & Elderly: Allergic conjunctivitis: Ophthalmic: Instill 1 drop into the affected eye(s) twice daily, every 8-12 hours

Pediatrics: Children ≥3 years: Refer to adult dosing.

Available Dosage Forms Solution, ophthalmic, as fumarate: 0.025% (5 mL) [contains benzalkonium chloride]

Monitoring and Teaching Issues

Physical Assessment: Assess potential for interactions with other prescriptions, OTC medications, or herbal products patient may be taking. Assess therapeutic response and adverse effects. Teach patient proper use, side effects/appropriate interventions, and symptoms to report.

Patient Education: For use in eyes only. Do not let tip of applicator touch eye; do not contaminate tip of applicator (may cause eye infection, eye damage, or vision loss). Not to be used to treat contact lens-related irritation. Wait at least 10 minutes before putting soft contact lenses in. Do not wear contact lenses if eyes are red. Store at room temperature.

Pregnancy/breast-feeding precautions: Inform prescriber if you are pregnant or breast-feeding.

Pregnancy Risk Factor: C

Pregnancy Issues: Oral treatment administered to pregnant animals have resulted in retarded ossification of the sternebrae, slight increase in postnatal mortality, and a decrease in weight gain in the first 4 days of life. Topical ocular administration has not been studied.

Lactation: Use caution

Administration

Storage: Stable at room temperature.

- ◆ Kristalose™ *see* Lactulose *on page 860*
- ◆ K-Tab® *see* Potassium Chloride *on page 1233*
- ◆ Ku-Zyme® HP *see* Pancrelipase *on page 1151*
- ◆ Kytril® *see* Granisetron *on page 726*
- ◆ L-749,345 *see* Ertapenem *on page 541*
- ◆ L 754030 *see* Aprepitant *on page 133*
- ◆ LA 20304a *see* Gemifloxacin *on page 706*

Labetalol (la BET a lole)

U.S. Brand Names Normodyne®; Trandate®
Synonyms Ibidomide Hydrochloride; Labetalol Hydrochloride
Generic Available Yes
Pharmacologic Category Beta Blocker With Alpha-Blocking Activity
Medication Safety Issues
Sound-alike/look-alike issues:
Labetalol may be confused with betaxolol, Hexadrol®, lamotrigine
Trandate® may be confused with tramadol, Trandar®, Trental®, Tridrate®
Use Treatment of mild to severe hypertension; I.V. for hypertensive emergencies
Mechanism of Action/Effect Blocks alpha-, beta$_1$-, and beta$_2$-adrenergic receptor sites; elevated renins are reduced
Contraindications Hypersensitivity to labetalol or any component of the formulation; sinus bradycardia; heart block greater than first degree (except in patients with a functioning artificial pacemaker); cardiogenic shock; bronchial asthma; uncompensated cardiac failure; pregnancy (2nd and 3rd trimesters)
Warnings/Precautions Use only with extreme caution in compensated heart failure and monitor for a worsening of the condition. Use caution with concurrent use of beta-blockers and either verapamil or diltiazem; bradycardia or heart block can occur. Avoid concurrent I.V. use of both agents. Patients with bronchospastic disease should not receive beta-blockers. Labetalol may be used with caution in patients with nonallergic bronchospasm (chronic bronchitis, emphysema). Use cautiously in patients with diabetes because it can mask prominent hypoglycemic symptoms. Can mask signs of thyrotoxicosis. Can cause fetal harm when administered in pregnancy. Use cautiously in hepatic impairment. Use caution when using I.V. labetalol and inhalational anesthetics concurrently (significant myocardial depression). Avoid abrupt discontinuation in patients with a history of CAD.
Drug Interactions
Cytochrome P450 Effect: Substrate of CYP2D6 (major); **Inhibits** CYP2D6 (weak)
Decreased Effect: Decreased effect of beta-blockers with aluminum salts, barbiturates, calcium salts, cholestyramine, colestipol, NSAIDs, penicillins (ampicillin), rifampin, salicylates, and sulfinpyrazone due to decreased bioavailability and plasma levels. Beta-blockers may decrease the effect of sulfonylureas.
Increased Effect/Toxicity: CYP2D6 inhibitors may increase the levels/effects of labetalol; example inhibitors include chlorpromazine, delavirdine, fluoxetine, miconazole, paroxetine, pergolide, quinidine, quinine, ritonavir, and ropinirole. Cimetidine increases the bioavailability of labetalol. Labetalol has additive hypotensive effects with other antihypertensive agents. Concurrent use with alpha-blockers (prazosin, terazosin) and beta-blockers increases the risk of orthostasis. Concurrent use with diltiazem, verapamil, or digoxin may increase the risk of bradycardia with beta-blocking agents. Halothane, enflurane, isoflurane, and potentially other inhalation anesthetics may cause synergistic hypotension. Beta-blockers may affect the action or levels of ethanol, disopyramide, nondepolarizing muscle relaxants, and theophylline although the effects are difficult to predict.
Nutritional/Ethanol Interactions
Food: Labetalol serum concentrations may be increased if taken with food.
Herb/Nutraceutical: Avoid dong quai if using for hypertension (has estrogenic activity). Avoid ephedra, yohimbe, ginseng (may worsen hypertension). Avoid natural licorice (causes sodium and water retention and increases potassium loss). Avoid garlic (may have increased antihypertensive effect).
Lab Interactions False-positive urine catecholamines, VMA if measured by fluorometric or photometric methods; use HPLC or specific catecholamine radioenzymatic technique
Adverse Reactions
>10%:
Central nervous system: Dizziness (1% to 16%)
Gastrointestinal: Nausea (0% to 19%)
1% to 10%:
Cardiovascular: Edema (0% to 2%), hypotension (1% to 5%); with IV use, hypotension may occur in up to 58%
Central nervous system: Fatigue (1% to 10%), paresthesia (1% to 5%), headache (2%), vertigo (2%)
Dermatologic: Rash (1%), scalp tingling (1% to 5%)
Gastrointestinal: Vomiting (<1% to 3%), dyspepsia (1% to 4%)
Genitourinary: Ejaculatory failure (0% to 5%), impotence (1% to 4%)
Hepatic: Transaminases increased (4%)
Neuromuscular & skeletal: Weakness (1%)
Respiratory: Nasal congestion (1% to 6%), dyspnea (2%)
Miscellaneous: Taste disorder (1%), abnormal vision (1%)
Other adverse reactions noted with beta-adrenergic blocking agents include mental depression, catatonia, disorientation, short-term memory loss, emotional lability, clouded sensorium, intensification of pre-existing AV block, laryngospasm, respiratory distress, agranulocytosis, thrombocytopenic purpura, nonthrombocytopenic purpura, mesenteric artery thrombosis, and ischemic colitis.
Overdosage/Toxicology Symptoms of intoxication include cardiac disturbances, CNS toxicity, bronchospasm, hypoglycemia, and hyperkalemia. The most common cardiac symptoms include hypotension and bradycardia. Atrioventricular block, intraventricular conduction disturbances, cardiogenic shock, and asystole may occur with severe overdose, especially
(Continued)

Labetalol *(Continued)*

with membrane-depressant drugs (eg, propranolol). CNS effects include convulsions, coma, and respiratory arrest and are commonly seen with propranolol and other membrane-depressant and lipid-soluble drugs. Treatment is symptomatic. Glucagon may be administered to improve cardiac function.

Pharmacodynamics/Kinetics

Onset of Action: Oral: 20 minutes to 2 hours; I.V.: 2-5 minutes; Peak effect: Oral: 1-4 hours; I.V.: 5-15 minutes

Duration of Action: Oral (dose dependent): 8-24 hours; I.V.: 2-4 hours

Bioavailability: Oral: 25%; increased with liver disease, elderly, and concurrent cimetidine

Protein Binding: 50%

Half-Life Elimination: Normal renal function: 2.5-8 hours

Metabolism: Hepatic, primarily via glucuronide conjugation; extensive first-pass effect

Excretion: Urine (<5% as unchanged drug)

Clearance: Possibly decreased in neonates/infants

Dosing

Adults:

Hypertension: Oral: Initial: 100 mg twice daily, may increase as needed every 2-3 days by 100 mg until desired response is obtained; usual dose: 200-400 mg twice daily; not to exceed 2.4 g/day

Usual dose range (JNC 7): 200-800 mg/day in 2 divided doses

Acute hypertension (hypertensive urgency/emergency):

I.V. bolus: 20 mg or 1-2 mg/kg whichever is lower, IVP over 2 minutes, may give 40-80 mg at 10-minute intervals, up to 300 mg total dose

I.V. infusion: Initial: 2 mg/minute; titrate to response up to 300 mg total dose. Administration requires the use of an infusion pump.

Note: Continuous infusion at low rates (2-4 mg/hour) have been used in some settings for patients unable to transition rapidly to oral medication.

Elderly: Oral: Initial: 100 mg 1-2 times/day increasing as needed

Pediatrics: Note: Due to limited documentation of its use, labetalol should be initiated cautiously in pediatric patients with careful dosage adjustment and blood pressure monitoring.

Hypertension:

Oral: Limited information regarding labetalol use in pediatric patients is currently available in literature. Some centers recommend initial oral doses of 4 mg/kg/day in 2 divided doses. Reported oral doses have started at 3 mg/kg/day and 20 mg/kg/day and have increased up to 40 mg/kg/day.

I.V.: Intermittent bolus doses of 0.3-1 mg/kg/dose have been reported.

Pediatric hypertensive emergencies: Initial continuous infusions of 0.4-1 mg/kg/hour with a maximum of 3 mg/kg/hour have been used; administration requires the use of an infusion pump.

Renal Impairment: Not removed by hemo- or peritoneal dialysis; supplemental dose is not necessary.

Hepatic Impairment: Dosage reduction may be necessary.

Available Dosage Forms

Injection, solution, as hydrochloride (Normodyne®): 5 mg/mL (20 mL, 40 mL)

Injection, solution, as hydrochloride [prefilled syringe]: 5 mg/mL (4 mL)

Normodyne®: 5 mg/mL (4 mL, 8 mL)

Tablet, as hydrochloride: 100 mg, 200 mg, 300 mg

Normodyne®: 100 mg, 200 mg, 300 mg

Trandate®: 100 mg, 200 mg [contains sodium benzoate], 300 mg

Monitoring and Teaching Issues

Physical Assessment: Assess potential for interactions with other prescriptions, OTC medications, or herbal products patient may be taking (especially anything that will effect blood pressure). Blood pressure and heart rate should be assessed prior to and following first dose and any change in dosage. Caution patients with diabetes to monitor glucose levels closely; beta-blockers may alter glucose tolerance. Assess results of laboratory tests, therapeutic effectiveness, and adverse response (eg, CHF). Teach patient proper use, possible side effects/appropriate interventions, and adverse symptoms to report.

Patient Education: Do not take any new medication during therapy unless approved by prescriber. Take as directed, with meals. Do not skip dose or discontinue without consulting prescriber. This medication does not replace other antihypertensive interventions; follow prescriber's instructions for diet and lifestyle changes. If you have diabetes, monitor serum glucose closely and notify prescriber of changes (this medication can alter hypoglycemic requirements). You may experience drowsiness, dizziness, or impaired judgment (use caution when driving or engaging in tasks that require alertness until response to drug is known); postural hypotension (use caution when rising from sitting or lying position or when climbing stairs); dry mouth, nausea, or loss of appetite (frequent mouth care or sucking lozenges may help); or sexual dysfunction (reversible, may resolve with continued use). Report altered CNS status (eg, fatigue, depression, numbness or tingling of fingers, toes, or skin); palpitations or slowed heartbeat; respiratory difficulty; edema or cold extremities; or other persistent side effects. **Pregnancy/breast-feeding precautions:** Inform prescriber if you are or intend to become pregnant. Consult prescriber if breast-feeding.

Geriatric Considerations: Due to alterations in the beta-adrenergic autonomic nervous system, beta-adrenergic blockade may result in less hemodynamic response than seen in younger adults.

Pregnancy Risk Factor: C (manufacturer); D (2nd and 3rd trimesters - expert analysis)

Pregnancy Issues: Labetalol crosses the placenta. Beta-blockers have been associated with persistent bradycardia, hypotension, and IUGR; IUGR is probably related to maternal hypertension. Available evidence suggests beta-blockers are generally safe during pregnancy (JNC 7). Cases of neonatal hypoglycemia have been reported following maternal use of beta-blockers at parturition or during breast-feeding. Monitor breast-fed infant for symptoms of beta-blockade.

Lactation: Enters breast milk/use caution (AAP rates "compatible")

Breast-Feeding Issues: Available evidence suggests safe use during breast-feeding. Monitor breast-fed infant for symptoms of beta-blockade.

Administration

I.V.: Bolus administered over 2 minutes.

Reconstitution: Stability of parenteral admixture at room temperature (25°C) and refrigeration temperature (4°C) is 3 days.

Standard diluent: 500 mg/250 mL D_5W
Minimum volume: 250 mL D_5W

Compatibility: Stable in D_5LR, $D_5{}^1/_4NS$, $D_5{}^1/_3NS$, D_5NS, D_5W, LR, NS; most stable at pH of 2-4. **Incompatible** with sodium bicarbonate 5% and alkaline solutions.

Y-site administration: Incompatible with amphotericin B cholesteryl sulfate complex, cefoperazone, ceftriaxone, nafcillin, thiopental, warfarin

Compatibility when admixed: Incompatible with sodium bicarbonate

Storage: Labetalol should be stored at room temperature or under refrigeration and should be protected from light and freezing. The solution is clear to slightly yellow.

Related Information

Beta-Blockers *on page 1720*

- ◆ **Labetalol Hydrochloride** *see Labetalol on page 857*
- ◆ **Laboratory Reference Values for Adults** *see page 1698*
- ◆ **Laboratory Reference Values for Children** *see page 1702*
- ◆ **LactiCare-HC® [DSC]** *see Hydrocortisone on page 760*
- ◆ **Lactinex® [OTC]** *see Lactobacillus on page 859*

Lactobacillus (lak toe ba SIL us)

U.S. Brand Names Bacid® [OTC]; Kala® [OTC]; Lactinex® [OTC]; Megadophilus® [OTC]; MoreDophilus® [OTC]; Probiotica® [OTC]; Superdophilus® [OTC]

Synonyms *Lactobacillus acidophilus*; *Lactobacillus acidophilus* and *Lactobacillus bulgaricus*; *Lactobacillus reuteri*

Generic Available Yes

Pharmacologic Category Antidiarrheal

Use Treatment of uncomplicated diarrhea particularly that caused by antibiotic therapy; re-establish normal physiologic and bacterial flora of the intestinal tract

Mechanism of Action/Effect Creates an environment unfavorable to potentially pathogenic fungi or bacteria through the production of lactic acid, and favors establishment of an aciduric flora, thereby suppressing the growth of pathogenic microorganisms; helps re-establish normal intestinal flora

Contraindications Allergy to milk or lactose

Warnings/Precautions Discontinue if high fever is present. Do not use in children <2 years of age.

Adverse Reactions No data reported

Pharmacodynamics/Kinetics

Absorption: Oral: None

Excretion: Feces

Dosing

Adults & Elderly: Diarrhea: Oral:

Capsules: 2 capsules 2-4 times/day

Granules: 1 packet added to or taken with cereal, food, milk, fruit juice, or water, 3-4 times/day

Powder: 1 teaspoonful daily with liquid

Tablet, chewable: 4 tablets 3-4 times/day; may follow each dose with a small amount of milk, fruit juice, or water

Pediatrics: Children >2 years: Refer to adult dosing.

Available Dosage Forms

Capsule: *Lactobacillus acidophilus* 100 million units

Bacid®: *Lactobacillus acidophilus* 500 million units

Megadophilus®, Superdophilus®: *Lactobacillus acidophilus* 2 billion units [available in dairy based or dairy free formulations]

Granules (Lactinex®): Mixed culture *L. acidophilus*, *L. bulgaricus* per 1 g packet (12s)

Powder:

Megadophilus®, Superdophilus®: *Lactobacillus acidophilus* 2 billion units per half-teaspoon (49 g) [available in dairy based or dairy free formulations]

MoreDophilus®: *Lactobacillus acidophilus* 12.4 billion units per teaspoon [carrot derived] (30 g, 120 g)

Tablet (Kala®): *Lactobacillus acidophilus* 200 million units [soy based]

Tablet, chewable:

Lactinex®: Mixed culture *L. acidophilus*, *L. bulgaricus*

Probiotica®: *L. reuteri* 100 million units (30s, 60s) [lemon flavor]

Monitoring and Teaching Issues

Physical Assessment: See Warnings/Precautions for use cautions. Teach patient proper use and adverse symptoms to report (eg, discontinue and notify prescriber if high fever develops; see Patient Education).

Patient Education: Use exactly as directed; do not take more than prescribed. Granules in capsules may be added to or taken with cereal, food, milk, fruit juice, or water. You may experience increased flatus while taking this medication. Discontinue and notify prescriber if a high fever develops. Refrigerate Lactinex® and Bacid®. **Breast-feeding precaution:** Consult prescriber if breast-feeding.

Dietary Considerations: Granules or contents of capsules may be added to or administered with cereal, food, milk, fruit juice, or water.

(Continued)

Lactobacillus (Continued)

Pregnancy Risk Factor: Not available

Lactation: Excretion in breast milk unknown/use caution

Administration

Storage: Store in refrigerator.

♦ *Lactobacillus acidophilus* *see Lactobacillus on page 859*

♦ *Lactobacillus acidophilus* and *Lactobacillus bulgaricus* *see Lactobacillus on page 859*

♦ *Lactobacillus reuteri* *see Lactobacillus on page 859*

♦ *Lactoflavin* *see Riboflavin on page 1321*

Lactulose (LAK tyoo lose)

U.S. Brand Names Constulose®; Enulose®; Generlac; Kristalose™

Generic Available Yes

Pharmacologic Category Ammonium Detoxicant; Laxative, Miscellaneous

Medication Safety Issues

Sound-alike/look-alike issues:

Lactulose may be confused with lactose

Use Adjunct in the prevention and treatment of portal-systemic encephalopathy; treatment of chronic constipation

Mechanism of Action/Effect The bacterial degradation of lactulose resulting in an acidic pH inhibits the diffusion of NH_3 into the blood by causing the conversion of NH_3 to NH_4+; also enhances the diffusion of NH_3 from the blood into the gut where conversion to NH_4+ occurs; produces an osmotic effect in the colon with resultant distention promoting peristalsis

Contraindications Hypersensitivity to lactulose or any component of the formulation; galactosemia (or patients requiring a low galactose diet)

Warnings/Precautions Use with caution in patients with diabetes mellitus; monitor periodically for electrolyte imbalance when lactulose is used >6 months or in patients predisposed to electrolyte abnormalities (eg, elderly); patients receiving lactulose and an oral anti-infective agent should be monitored for possible inadequate response to lactulose

Drug Interactions

Decreased Effect: Oral neomycin, laxatives, antacids

Adverse Reactions Frequency not defined: Gastrointestinal: Flatulence, diarrhea (excessive dose), abdominal discomfort, nausea, vomiting, cramping

Overdosage/Toxicology Symptoms of overdose include diarrhea, abdominal pain, hypochloremic alkalosis, dehydration, hypotension, and hypokalemia. Treatment includes supportive care.

Pharmacodynamics/Kinetics

Absorption: Not appreciable

Metabolism: Via colonic flora to lactic acid and acetic acid; requires colonic flora for drug activation

Excretion: Primarily feces and urine (~3%)

Dosing

Adults & Elderly:

Note: Diarrhea may indicate overdosage and responds to dose reduction.

Acute portal-systemic encephalopathy (PSE):

Oral: 20-30 g (30-45 mL) every 1-2 hours to induce rapid laxation; adjust dosage daily to produce 2-3 soft stools; doses of 30-45 mL may be given hourly to cause rapid laxation, then reduce to recommended dose; usual daily dose: 60-100 g (90-150 mL) daily

Rectal: 200 g (300 mL) diluted with 700 mL of H_2O or NS; administer rectally via rectal balloon catheter and retain 30-60 minutes every 4-6 hours.

Constipation: Oral: 10-20 g/day (15-30 mL/day) increased to 60 mL/day in 1-2 divided doses if necessary

Pediatrics: Diarrhea may indicate overdosage and responds to dose reduction.

Prevention of portal systemic encephalopathy (PSE): Oral:

Infants: 2.5-10 mL/day divided 3-4 times/day; adjust dosage to produce 2-3 stools/day.

Older Children: Daily dose of 40-90 mL divided 3-4 times/day; if initial dose causes diarrhea, then reduce it immediately; adjust dosage to produce 2-3 stools/day.

Constipation: Oral: 5 g/day (7.5 mL) after breakfast

Available Dosage Forms

Crystals for reconstitution (Kristalose™): 10 g/packet (30s), 20 g/packet (30s)

Syrup: 10 g/15 mL (15 mL, 30 mL, 237 mL, 473 mL, 946 mL, 1890 mL)

Constulose®: 10 g/15 mL (240 mL, 960 mL)

Enulose®: 10 g/15 mL (480 mL)

Generlac: 10 g/15 mL (480 mL, 1920 mL)

Monitoring and Teaching Issues

Physical Assessment: See Warnings/Precautions for specific use cautions (eg, diabetes mellitus). Assess results of laboratory tests, therapeutic effectiveness (soft formed stools or resolution of CNS status in PSE), and adverse response (eg, CHF; see Adverse Reactions). Monitor frequency/consistency of stools; diarrhea may indicate overdose. Teach patient proper use, possible side effects/appropriate interventions, and adverse symptoms to report (see Patient Education).

Monitoring Laboratory Tests: Serum potassium, serum ammonia

Patient Education: Not for long-term use. Take as directed, alone, or diluted with water, juice or milk, or take with food. Laxative results may not occur for 24-48 hours; do not take more often than recommended or for a longer time than recommended. Do not use any other laxatives while taking lactulose. Increased fiber, fluids, and exercise may also help reduce constipation. Do not use if experiencing abdominal pain, nausea, or vomiting. Diarrhea may indicate overdose. May cause flatulence, belching, or abdominal cramping.

Report persistent or severe diarrhea or abdominal cramping. **Breast-feeding precaution:** Consult prescriber if breast-feeding.

Dietary Considerations: Contraindicated in patients on galactose-restricted diet; may be mixed with fruit juice, milk, water, or citrus-flavored carbonated beverages.

Geriatric Considerations: Elderly are more likely to show CNS signs of dehydration and electrolyte loss than younger adults. Therefore, monitor closely for fluid and electrolyte loss with chronic use. Sorbitol is equally effective as a laxative and less expensive. However, sorbitol **cannot be substituted** in the treatment of hepatic encephalopathy.

Pregnancy Risk Factor: B

Lactation: Excretion in breast milk unknown

Administration

Oral: Dilute lactulose in water, usually 60-120 mL, prior to administering through a gastric or feeding tube.

Other: Syrup formulation has been used in preparation of rectal solution.

Storage: Keep solution at room temperature to reduce viscosity. Discard solution if cloudy or very dark.

Related Information

Laxatives, Classification and Properties *on page 1737*

♦ **Ladakamycin** *see Azacitidine on page 161*

♦ **L-AmB** *see Amphotericin B (Liposomal) on page 113*

♦ **Lamictal®** *see Lamotrigine on page 863*

♦ **Lamisil®** *see Terbinafine on page 1444*

♦ **Lamisil® AT™ [OTC]** *see Terbinafine on page 1444*

Lamivudine (la MI vyoo deen)

U.S. Brand Names Epivir®; Epivir-HBV®

Synonyms 3TC

Generic Available No

Pharmacologic Category Antiretroviral Agent, Reverse Transcriptase Inhibitor (Nucleoside)

Medication Safety Issues

Sound-alike/look-alike issues:
Lamivudine may be confused with lamotrigine
Epivir® may be confused with Combivir®

Use

Epivir®: Treatment of HIV infection when antiretroviral therapy is warranted; should always be used as part of a multidrug regimen (at least three antiretroviral agents)

Epivir-HBV®: Treatment of chronic hepatitis B associated with evidence of hepatitis B viral replication and active liver inflammation

Unlabeled/Investigational Use Prevention of HIV following needlesticks (with or without protease inhibitor)

Mechanism of Action/Effect Lamivudine is a cytosine analog. *In vitro*, lamivudine is phosphorylated to its active 5'-triphosphate metabolite (L-TP), which inhibits HIV reverse transcription via viral DNA chain termination; L-TP also inhibits the RNA- and DNA-dependent DNA polymerase activities of reverse transcriptase. The monophosphate form is incorporated into viral DNA by hepatitis B polymerase, resulting in DNA chain termination.

Contraindications Hypersensitivity to lamivudine or any component of the formulation

Warnings/Precautions A decreased dosage is recommended in patients with renal dysfunction since AUC, C_{max}, and half-life increased with diminishing renal function; use with extreme caution in children with history of pancreatitis or risk factors for development of pancreatitis. Do not use as monotherapy in treatment of HIV. Treatment of HBV in patients with unrecognized/untreated HIV may lead to rapid HIV resistance. In addition, treatment of HIV in patients with unrecognized/untreated HBV may lead to rapid HBV resistance. Patients with HIV infection should receive only dosage forms appropriate for treatment of HIV.

Lactic acidosis and severe hepatomegaly with steatosis have been reported, including fatal cases. Use caution in hepatic impairment. Pregnancy, obesity, and/or prolonged therapy may increase the risk of lactic acidosis and liver damage.

Monitor patients closely for several months following discontinuation of therapy for chronic hepatitis B; clinical exacerbations may occur.

Drug Interactions

Decreased Effect: Zalcitabine and lamivudine may inhibit the intracellular phosphorylation of each other; concomitant use should be avoided.

Increased Effect/Toxicity: Zidovudine concentrations increase significantly (~39%) with lamivudine coadministration. sulfamethoxazole/trimethoprim increases lamivudine's blood levels. Concomitant use of ribavirin and nucleoside analogues may increase the risk of developing lactic acidosis (includes adefovir, didanosine, lamivudine, stavudine, zalcitabine, zidovudine). Trimethoprim (and other drugs excreted by organic cation transport) may increase serum levels/effects of lamivudine.

Nutritional/Ethanol Interactions Food: Food decreases the rate of absorption and C_{max}; however, there is no change in the systemic AUC. Therefore, may be taken with or without food.

Adverse Reactions (As reported in adults treated for HIV infection)

>10%:
Central nervous system: Headache, fatigue
Gastrointestinal: Nausea, diarrhea, vomiting, pancreatitis (range: 0.5% to 18%; higher percentage in pediatric patients)
Neuromuscular & skeletal: Peripheral neuropathy, paresthesia, musculoskeletal pain

1% to 10%:
Central nervous system: Dizziness, depression, fever, chills, insomnia
Dermatologic: Rash
Gastrointestinal: Anorexia, abdominal pain, heartburn, elevated amylase
Hematologic: Neutropenia

(Continued)

Lamivudine *(Continued)*

Hepatic: Elevated AST, ALT

Neuromuscular & skeletal: Myalgia, arthralgia

Respiratory: Nasal signs and symptoms, cough

Overdosage/Toxicology Limited information is available, although there have been no clinical signs or symptoms noted, and hematologic tests remained normal in overdose. No antidote is available. Limited (negligible) removal following 4-hour hemodialysis. It is not known if continuous 24-hour hemodialysis would be effective.

Pharmacodynamics/Kinetics

Absorption: Rapid

Bioavailability: Absolute: Cp_{max} decreased with food although AUC not significantly affected

Children: 66%

Adults: 87%

Protein Binding: Plasma: <36%

Half-Life Elimination: Children: 2 hours; Adults: 5-7 hours

Metabolism: 5.6% to trans-sulfoxide metabolite

Excretion: Primarily urine (as unchanged drug)

Dosing

Adults & Elderly: Note: The formulation and dosage of Epivir-HBV® are not appropriate for patients infected with both HBV and HIV.

HIV: Oral (use with at least two other antiretroviral agents): 150 mg twice daily **or** 300 mg once daily

Prevention of HIV following needlesticks (unlabeled use): Oral: 150 mg twice daily (with zidovudine with or without a protease inhibitor, depending on risk)

Treatment of hepatitis B (Epivir-HBV®): Oral: 100 mg/day

Pediatrics: Note: The formulation and dosage of Epivir-HBV® are not appropriate for patients infected with both HBV and HIV.

HIV: Oral (use with at least two other antiretroviral agents)

3 months to 16 years: 4 mg/kg twice daily (maximum: 150 mg twice daily)

>16 years: Refer to adult dosing.

Treatment of hepatitis B: Oral: Children 2-17 years: 3 mg/kg once daily (maximum: 100 mg/day)

Renal Impairment: Oral:

Pediatric patients: Insufficient data; however, dose reduction should be considered.

Treatment of HIV patients >16 years:

Cl_{cr} 30-49 mL/minute: Administer 150 mg once daily.

Cl_{cr} 15-29 mL/minute: Administer 150 mg first dose, then 100 mg once daily.

Cl_{cr} 5-14 mL/minute: Administer 150 mg first dose, then 50 mg once daily.

Cl_{cr} <5 mL/minute: Administer 50 mg first dose, then 25 mg once daily.

Dialysis: No data available.

Treatment of hepatitis B patients: Adults:

Cl_{cr} 30-49 mL/minute: Administer 100 mg first dose, then 50 mg once daily.

Cl_{cr} 15-29 mL/minute: Administer 100 mg first dose, then 25 mg once daily.

Cl_{cr} 5-14 mL/minute: Administer 35 mg first dose, then 15 mg once daily.

Cl_{cr} <5 mL/minute: Administer 35 mg first dose, then 25 mg once daily.

Dialysis: Negligible amounts are removed by 4-hour hemodialysis or peritoneal dialysis. Supplemental dosing is not required.

Available Dosage Forms

Solution, oral:

Epivir®: 10 mg/mL (240 mL) [strawberry-banana flavor]

Epivir-HBV®: 5 mg/mL (240 mL) [strawberry-banana flavor]

Tablet:

Epivir®: 150 mg, 300 mg

Epivir-HBV®: 100 mg

Monitoring and Teaching Issues

Physical Assessment: Use caution in presence of impaired hepatic or renal function (see Warnings/Precautions for specific use cautions). Assess potential for interactions with other pharmacological agents patient may be taking (eg, increased risk of toxicity; see Drug Interactions). Assess results of laboratory tests, therapeutic effectiveness, and adverse reactions on a regular basis throughout therapy (eg, nausea/vomiting [dehydration], peripheral neuropathy, hepatitis B [jaundice, fatigue, anorexia]; see Adverse Reactions) Monitor patients closely for several months following discontinuation of therapy for chronic hepatitis B and clinical exacerbations. Teach patient proper use (importance of adhering to full treatment regimen), possible side effects/appropriate interventions, and adverse symptoms to report (see Patient Education).

Monitoring Laboratory Tests: Amylase, bilirubin, liver enzymes, CBC

Patient Education: Do not take any new medication during therapy unless approved by prescriber. Lamivudine is not a cure for HIV or hepatitis B, nor has it been found to reduce transmission. You will need frequent blood tests to adjust dosage for maximum therapeutic effect. Take as directed for full course of therapy; do not discontinue (even if feeling better). Take with or without food. Do not take antacids within 1 hour of lamivudine. Mix four tablets in 3-5 oz water, allow to stand a few minutes, stir, and drink immediately. This may be prescribed as part of a multidrug regimen; it is vital that you maintain that regimen and time medications as instructed. May cause loss of appetite or change in taste (sucking on lozenges, chewing gum, or small frequent meals may help); dizziness or numbness (use caution when driving or engaging in tasks that require alertness until response to drug is known); or headache, fever, and muscle pain (an analgesic may be recommended). Report persistent lethargy or unusual fatigue, yellowing of eyes, pale stool and dark urine; acute headache, severe nausea or vomiting, respiratory difficulty, loss of sensation, rash; or other persistent adverse effects. **Pregnancy/breast-feeding precautions:** Inform prescriber if you are or intend to become pregnant. Do not breast-feed.

Dietary Considerations: May be taken with or without food. Each 5 mL of oral solution contains 1 g of sucrose.

Pregnancy Risk Factor: C

Pregnancy Issues: Lamivudine crosses the placenta. The pharmacokinetics of lamivudine during pregnancy are not significantly altered and dosage adjustment is not required. The Perinatal HIV Guidelines Working Group recommends lamivudine for use during pregnancy; the combination of lamivudine with zidovudine is the recommended dual combination NRTI in pregnancy. It may also be used in combination with zidovudine in HIV-infected women who are in labor, but have had no prior antiretroviral therapy, in order to reduce the maternal-fetal transmission of HIV. Cases of lactic acidosis/hepatic steatosis syndrome have been reported in pregnant women receiving nucleoside analogues. It is not known if pregnancy itself potentiates this known side effect; however, pregnant women may be at increased risk of lactic acidosis and liver damage. Hepatic enzymes and electrolytes should be monitored frequently during the 3rd trimester of pregnancy in women receiving nucleoside analogues. Health professionals are encouraged to contact the antiretroviral pregnancy registry to monitor outcomes of pregnant women exposed to antiretroviral medications (1-800-258-4263 or www.APRegistry.com).

Lactation: Enters breast milk/contraindicated

Breast-Feeding Issues: HIV-infected mothers are discouraged from breast-feeding to decrease potential transmission of HIV.

Administration

Oral: May be taken with or without food. Adjust dosage in renal failure.

Storage: Store at 2°C to 25°C (68°F to 77°F) tightly closed.

Additional Information Lamivudine has been well studied in the treatment of chronic hepatitis B infection. Potential compliance problems, frequency of administration, and adverse effects should be discussed with patients before initiating therapy to help prevent the emergence of resistance.

A high rate of early virologic nonresponse was observed when abacavir, lamivudine and tenofovir were used as the initial regimen in treatment-naive patients. A high rate of early virologic nonresponse was also observed when didanosine, lamivudine, and tenofovir were used as the initial regimen in treatment-naive patients. Use of either of these combinations is not recommended; patients currently on either of these regimens should be closely monitored for modification of therapy.

♦ **Lamivudine, Abacavir, and Zidovudine** see Abacavir, Lamivudine, and Zidovudine on page 34
♦ **Lamivudine and Abacavir** see Abacavir and Lamivudine on page 33
♦ **Lamivudine and Zidovudine** see Zidovudine and Lamivudine on page 1587

Lamotrigine (la MOE tri jeen)

U.S. Brand Names Lamictal®

Synonyms BW-430C; LTG

Generic Available No

Pharmacologic Category Anticonvulsant, Miscellaneous

Medication Safety Issues

Sound-alike/look-alike issues:

Lamotrigine may be confused with labetalol, Lamisil®, lamivudine, Lomotil®, ludiomil

Lamictal® may be confused with Lamisil®, Lomotil®, ludiomil

Use Adjunctive therapy in the treatment of generalized seizures of Lennox-Gastaut syndrome and partial seizures in adults and children ≥2 years of age; conversion to monotherapy in adults with partial seizures who are receiving treatment with valproate or a single enzyme-inducing antiepileptic drug; maintenance treatment of bipolar disorder

Mechanism of Action/Effect A triazine derivative which inhibits release of glutamate (an excitatory amino acid) and inhibits voltage-sensitive sodium channels, which stabilizes neuronal membranes. Lamotrigine has weak inhibitory effect on the $5HT_3$ receptor; in vitro inhibits dihydrofolate reductase.

Contraindications Hypersensitivity to lamotrigine or any component of the formulation

Warnings/Precautions Severe and potentially life-threatening skin rashes requiring hospitalization have been reported (children 0.8%; adults 0.3%); risk may be increased by coadministration with valproic acid, higher than recommended starting doses, and rapid dose titration. The majority of cases occur in the first 8 weeks; however, isolated cases may occur after prolonged treatment. Discontinue at first sign of rash unless rash is clearly not drug related. Use with caution in patients with impaired renal, hepatic, or cardiac function. Avoid abrupt cessation, taper over at least 2 weeks if possible. May cause CNS depression, which may impair physical or mental abilities. Patients must be cautioned about performing tasks which require mental alertness (eg, operating machinery or driving). Effects with other sedative drugs or ethanol may be potentiated. **Use caution in writing and/or interpreting prescriptions/orders; medication dispensing errors have occurred with similar-sounding medications (Lamisil®, ludiomil, lamivudine, labetalol, and Lomotil®).**

Drug Interactions

Decreased Effect: Acetaminophen (chronic administration), carbamazepine, oral contraceptives (estrogens), phenytoin, phenobarbital may decrease concentrations of lamotrigine; dosage adjustments may be needed when adding or withdrawing agent; monitor

Increased Effect/Toxicity: Lamotrigine may increase the epoxide metabolite of carbamazepine resulting in toxicity. Valproic acid increases blood levels of lamotrigine. Valproic acid inhibits the clearance of lamotrigine, dosage adjustment required when adding or withdrawing valproic acid; inhibition appears maximal at valproic acid 250-500 mg/day; the incidence of serious rash may be increased by valproic acid. Toxicity has been reported following addition of sertraline (limited documentation).

Nutritional/Ethanol Interactions

Ethanol: Avoid ethanol (may increase CNS depression).

Food: Has no effect on absorption.

Herb/Nutraceutical: Avoid evening primrose (seizure threshold decreased).

(Continued)

Lamotrigine *(Continued)*

Adverse Reactions Percentages reported in adults receiving adjunctive therapy:

>10%:

Central nervous system: Headache (29%), dizziness (38%), ataxia (22%), somnolence (14%)

Gastrointestinal: Nausea (19%)

Ocular: Diplopia (28%), blurred vision (16%)

Respiratory: Rhinitis (14%)

1% to 10%:

Cardiovascular: Peripheral edema

Central nervous system: Depression (4%), anxiety (4%), irritability (3%), confusion, speech disorder (3%), difficulty concentrating (2%), malaise, seizure (includes exacerbations) (2% to 3%), incoordination (6%), insomnia (6%), pain, amnesia, hostility, memory decreased, nervousness, vertigo

Dermatologic: Hypersensitivity rash (10%; serious rash requiring hospitalization - adults 0.3%, children 0.8%), pruritus (3%)

Gastrointestinal: Abdominal pain (5%), vomiting (9%), diarrhea (6%), dyspepsia (5%), xerostomia, constipation (4%), anorexia (2%), tooth disorder (3%)

Genitourinary: Vaginitis (4%), dysmenorrhea (7%), amenorrhea (2%)

Neuromuscular & skeletal: Tremor (4%), arthralgia (2%), neck pain (2%)

Ocular: Nystagmus (2%), visual abnormality

Respiratory: Epistaxis, bronchitis, dyspnea

Miscellaneous: Flu syndrome (7%), fever (6%)

Overdosage/Toxicology Symptoms of overdose include QRS prolongation, AV block, dizziness, drowsiness, sedation, and ataxia. Enhancement of elimination: Multiple dosing of activated charcoal may be useful.

Pharmacodynamics/Kinetics

Bioavailability: 98%

Time to Peak: Plasma: 1-4 hours

Protein Binding: 55%

Half-Life Elimination: Adults: 25-33 hours; Concomitant valproic acid therapy: 59-70 hours; Concomitant phenytoin or carbamazepine therapy: 13-14 hours

Metabolism: Hepatic and renal; metabolized by glucuronic acid conjugation to inactive metabolites

Excretion: Urine (94%, ~90% as glucuronide conjugates and ~10% unchanged); feces (2%)

Dosing

Adults & Elderly: Note: Only whole tablets should be used for dosing, round calculated dose down to the nearest whole tablet:

Lennox-Gastaut (adjunctive) or treatment of partial seizures (adjunctive): Oral:

Patients receiving AED regimens containing valproic acid: Initial dose: 25 mg every other day for 2 weeks, then 25 mg every day for 2 weeks; dose may be increased by 25-50 mg every day for 1-2 weeks in order to achieve maintenance dose. Maintenance dose: 100-400 mg/day in 1-2 divided doses (usual range 100-200 mg/day).

Patients receiving enzyme-inducing AED regimens without valproic acid: Initial dose: 50 mg/day for 2 weeks, then 100 mg in 2 doses for 2 weeks; thereafter, daily dose can be increased by 100 mg every 1-2 weeks to be given in 2 divided doses. Usual maintenance dose: 300-500 mg/day in 2 divided doses; doses as high as 700 mg/day have been reported

Conversion to monotherapy (partial seizures in patients ≥16 years of age):

Adjunctive therapy with valproate: Initiate and titrate as per recommendations to a lamotrigine dose of 200 mg/day. Then taper valproate dose in decrements of not more than 500 mg/day at intervals of one week (or longer) to a valproate dosage of 500 mg/day; this dosage should be maintained for one week. The lamotrigine dosage should then be increased to 300 mg/day while valproate is decreased to 250 mg/day; this dosage should be maintained for one week. Valproate may then be discontinued, while the lamotrigine dose is increased by 100 mg/day at weekly intervals to achieve a lamotrigine maintenance dose of 500 mg/day.

Adjunctive therapy with enzyme-inducing AED: Initiate and titrate as per recommendations to a lamotrigine dose of 500 mg/day. Concomitant enzyme-inducing AED should then be withdrawn by 20% decrements each week over a 4-week period. Patients should be monitored for rash.

Adjunctive therapy with nonenzyme-inducing AED: No specific guidelines available

Bipolar disorder: 25 mg/day for 2 weeks, followed by 50 mg/day for 2 weeks, followed by 100 mg/day for 1 week; thereafter, daily dosage may be increased to 200 mg/day

Patients receiving valproic acid: Initial: 25 mg every other day for 2 weeks, followed by 25 mg/day for 2 weeks, followed by 50 mg/day for 1 week, followed by 100 mg/day (target dose) thereafter. **Note:** If valproate is discontinued, increase daily lamotrigine dose in 50 mg increments at weekly intervals until daily dosage of 200 mg is attained.

Patients receiving enzyme-inducing drugs (eg, carbamazepine): Initial: 50 mg/day for 2 weeks, followed by 100 mg/day (in divided doses) for 2 weeks, followed by 200 mg/day (in divided doses) for 1 week, followed by 300 mg/day (in divided doses) for 1 week. May increase to 400 mg/day (in divided doses) during week 7 and thereafter. **Note:** If carbamazepine (or other enzyme-inducing drug) is discontinued, decrease daily lamotrigine dose in 100 mg increments at weekly intervals until daily dosage of 200 mg is attained.

Discontinuing therapy: Decrease dose by ~50% per week, over at least 2 weeks unless safety concerns require a more rapid withdrawal.

Restarting therapy after discontinuation: If lamotrigine has been withheld for >5 half-lives, consider restarting according to initial dosing recommendations.

Pediatrics: Note: Only whole tablets should be used for dosing, rounded down to the nearest whole tablet.

Lennox-Gastaut (adjunctive) or partial seizures (adjunctive): Oral:

Children 2-12 years: **Note:** Children 2-6 years will likely require maintenance doses at the higher end of recommended range

Patients receiving AED regimens containing valproic acid:

Weeks 1 and 2: 0.15 mg/kg/day in 1-2 divided doses; round dose down to the nearest whole tablet. For patients >6.7 kg and <14 kg, dosing should be 2 mg every other day.

Weeks 3 and 4: 0.3 mg/kg/day in 1-2 divided doses; round dose down to the nearest whole tablet

Maintenance dose: Titrate dose to effect; after week 4, increase dose every 1-2 weeks by a calculated increment; calculate increment as 0.3 mg/kg/day rounded down to the nearest whole tablet; add this amount to the previously administered daily dose; usual maintenance: 1-5 mg/kg/day in 1-2 divided doses; maximum: 200 mg/day

Patients receiving enzyme-inducing AED regimens without valproic acid:

Weeks 1 and 2: 0.6 mg/kg/day in 2 divided doses; round dose down to the nearest whole tablet

Weeks 3 and 4: 1.2 mg/kg/day in 2 divided doses; round dose down to the nearest whole tablet

Maintenance dose: Titrate dose to effect; after week 4, increase dose every 1-2 weeks by a calculated increment; calculate increment as 1.2 mg/kg/day rounded down to the nearest whole tablet; add this amount to the previously administered daily dose; usual maintenance: 5-15 mg/kg/day in 2 divided doses; maximum: 400 mg/day

Children >12 years: Refer to adult dosing.

Conversion from single enzyme-inducing AED regimen to monotherapy: Children ≥16 years: Refer to adult dosing.

Discontinuing therapy: Decrease dose by ~50% per week, over at least 2 weeks unless safety concerns require a more rapid withdrawal.

Restarting therapy after discontinuation: If lamotrigine has been withheld for >5 half-lives, consider restarting according to initial dosing recommendations.

Renal Impairment: Decreased dosage may be effective in patients with significant renal impairment; use with caution.

Hepatic Impairment:

Child-Pugh Grade B: Reduce initial, escalation, and maintenance doses by 50%.

Child-Pugh Grade C: Reduce initial, escalation, and maintenance doses by 75%.

Available Dosage Forms

Tablet: 25 mg, 100 mg, 150 mg, 200 mg [contains lactose]

Tablet, combination package [each unit-dose starter kit contains]:

Lamictal® (blue kit; for patients taking valproate):

Tablet: Lamotrigine 25 mg (35s)

Lamictal® (green kit; for patients taking carbamazepine, phenytoin, phenobarbital, primidone or rifampin and **not** taking valproate):

Tablet: Lamotrigine 25 mg (84s)

Tablet: Lamotrigine 100 mg (10s)

Lamictal® (orange kit; for patients **not** taking carbamazepine, phenytoin, phenobarbital, primidone, rifampin, or valproate; for use in bipolar patients only):

Tablet: Lamotrigine 25 mg (42s)

Tablet: Lamotrigine 100 mg (7s)

Tablet, dispersible/chewable: 2 mg, 5 mg, 25 mg [black currant flavor]

Monitoring and Teaching Issues

Physical Assessment: Assess effectiveness and interactions of other medications patient may be taking. Monitor therapeutic effectiveness, laboratory values, and adverse reactions at beginning of therapy and periodically with long-term use. Taper dosage slowly when discontinuing. Observe and teach seizure/safety precautions. Use caution in writing and/or interpreting prescriptions/orders. Confusion between Lamictal® (lamotrigine) and Lamisil® (terbinafine) has occurred. Assess knowledge/teach patient appropriate use, interventions to reduce side effects, and adverse symptoms to report.

Monitoring Laboratory Tests: Serum levels of concurrent anticonvulsants, LFTs, renal function

Patient Education: Take exactly as directed; do not increase dose or frequency or discontinue without consulting prescriber. Only whole tablets should be used for dosing, rounded down to the nearest whole tablet. When having the prescription refilled, contact the prescriber if the medicine looks different or the label name has changed. While using this medication, do not use alcohol and other prescription or OTC medications (especially pain medications, sedatives, antihistamines, or hypnotics) without consulting prescriber. Maintain adequate hydration (2-3 L/day of fluids) unless instructed to restrict fluid intake. You may experience drowsiness, dizziness, or blurred vision (use caution when driving or engaging in tasks requiring alertness until response to drug is known); or nausea, vomiting, loss of appetite, heartburn, or dry mouth (small frequent meals, frequent mouth care, chewing gum, or sucking lozenges may help). Wear identification of epileptic status and medications. Report CNS changes, mentation changes, or changes in cognition; persistent GI symptoms (cramping, constipation, vomiting, anorexia); skin rash; swelling of face, lips, or tongue; easy bruising or bleeding (mouth, urine, stool); vision changes; worsening of seizure activity, or loss of seizure control. **Pregnancy/breast-feeding precautions:** Inform prescriber if you are or intend to become pregnant. Breast-feeding is not recommended.

Dietary Considerations: Take without regard to meals; drug may cause GI upset.

Geriatric Considerations: Use with caution in the elderly with significant renal impairment.

Pregnancy Risk Factor: C

Pregnancy Issues: Safety and efficacy in pregnant women have not been established. Healthcare providers may enroll patients in the Lamotrigine Pregnancy Registry by calling (800) 336-2176. Patients may enroll themselves in the North American Antiepileptic Drug Pregnancy Registry by calling (888) 233-2334. Dose of lamotrigine may need adjustment

(Continued)

Lamotrigine *(Continued)*

during pregnancy to maintain clinical response; lamotrigine serum levels may decrease during pregnancy and return to prepartum levels following delivery.

Lactation: Enters breast milk/not recommended (AAP rates "of concern")

Administration

Oral: Doses should be rounded down to the nearest whole tablet. Dispersible tablets may be chewed, dispersed in water, or swallowed whole. To disperse tablets, add to a small amount of liquid (just enough to cover tablet); let sit ~1 minute until dispersed; swirl solution and consume immediately. Do not administer partial amounts of liquid. If tablets are chewed, a small amount of water or diluted fruit juice should be used to aid in swallowing.

Storage: Store at 25°C (77°F). Excursions are permitted to 15°C to 30°C (59°F to 86°F). Protect from light.

Related Information

Anticonvulsants By Seizure Type *on page 1712*

♦ **Lamprene® [DSC]** *see* Clofazimine *on page 347*

♦ **Lanacane® [OTC]** *see* Benzocaine *on page 181*

♦ **Lanacane® Maximum Strength [OTC]** *see* Benzocaine *on page 181*

♦ **Lanoxicaps®** *see* Digoxin *on page 452*

♦ **Lanoxin®** *see* Digoxin *on page 452*

Lansoprazole *(lan SOE pra zole)*

U.S. Brand Names Prevacid®; Prevacid® SoluTab™

Generic Available No

Pharmacologic Category Proton Pump Inhibitor; Substituted Benzimidazole

Medication Safety Issues

Sound-alike/look-alike issues:

Prevacid® may be confused with Pravachol®, Prevpac®, Prilosec®, Prinivil®

Use

Oral: Short-term treatment of active duodenal ulcers; maintenance treatment of healed duodenal ulcers; as part of a multidrug regimen for *H. pylori* eradication to reduce the risk of duodenal ulcer recurrence; short-term treatment of active benign gastric ulcer; treatment of NSAID-associated gastric ulcer; to reduce the risk of NSAID-associated gastric ulcer in patients with a history of gastric ulcer who require an NSAID; short-term treatment of symptomatic GERD; short-term treatment for all grades of erosive esophagitis; to maintain healing of erosive esophagitis; long-term treatment of pathological hypersecretory conditions, including Zollinger-Ellison syndrome

I.V.: Short-term treatment (≤7 days) of erosive esophagitis in adults unable to take oral medications

Unlabeled/Investigational Use Active ulcer bleeding (parenteral formulation)

Mechanism of Action/Effect A proton pump inhibitor which decreases acid secretion in gastric parietal cells

Contraindications Hypersensitivity to lansoprazole, substituted benzimidazoles (ie, esomeprazole, omeprazole, pantoprazole, rabeprazole), or any component of the formulation

Warnings/Precautions Severe liver dysfunction may require dosage reductions. Symptomatic response does not exclude malignancy. Safety and efficacy have not been established in children <1 year of age.

Drug Interactions

Cytochrome P450 Effect: Substrate of CYP2C8/9 (minor), 2C19 (major), 3A4 (major); **Inhibits** CYP2C8/9 (weak), 2C19 (moderate), 2D6 (weak), 3A4 (weak); **Induces** CYP1A2 (weak)

Decreased Effect: Proton pump inhibitors may decrease the absorption of atazanavir, indinavir, itraconazole, and ketoconazole. The levels/effects of lansoprazole may be decreased by aminoglutethimide, carbamazepine, nafcillin, nevirapine, phenobarbital, phenytoin, rifamycins, and other CYP2C19 or 3A4 inducers.

Increased Effect/Toxicity: Lansoprazole may increase the levels/effects of citalopram, diazepam, methsuximide, phenytoin, propranolol, sertraline, and other CYP2C19 substrates.

Nutritional/Ethanol Interactions

Ethanol: Avoid ethanol (may cause gastric mucosal irritation).

Food: Lansoprazole serum concentrations may be decreased if taken with food.

Adverse Reactions 1% to 10%:

Central nervous system: Headache (children 1-11 years 3%, 12-17 years 7%)

Gastrointestinal: Abdominal pain (children 12-17 years 5%; adults 2%), constipation (children 1-11 years 5%; adults 1%), diarrhea (4%; 4% to 7% at doses of 30-60 mg/day), nausea (children 12-17 years 3%; adults 1%)

Overdosage/Toxicology No symptoms of toxicity were observed in animal studies; limited human experience in overdose. Treatment is symptomatic and supportive. Lansoprazole is not removed by hemodialysis.

Pharmacodynamics/Kinetics

Duration of Action: >1 day

Absorption: Rapid

Bioavailability: 80%; decreased 50% to 70% if given 30 minutes after food

Time to Peak: Plasma: 1.7 hours

Protein Binding: 97%

Half-Life Elimination: 2 hours; Elderly: 2-3 hours; Hepatic impairment: ≤7 hours

Metabolism: Hepatic via CYP2C19 and 3A4, and in parietal cells to two inactive metabolites

Excretion: Feces (67%); urine (33%)

Dosing

Adults & Elderly:

Symptomatic GERD: Oral: Short-term treatment: 15 mg once daily for up to 8 weeks

Erosive esophagitis:

Oral: Short-term treatment: 30 mg once daily for up to 8 weeks; continued treatment for an additional 8 weeks may be considered for recurrence or for patients that do not heal after the first 8 weeks of therapy; maintenance therapy: 15 mg once daily

I.V.: 30 mg once daily for up to 7 days; patients should be switched to an oral formulation as soon as they can take oral medications.

Hypersecretory conditions: Oral: Initial: 60 mg once daily; adjust dose based upon patient response and to reduce acid secretion to <10 mEq/hour (5 mEq/hour in patients with prior gastric surgery); doses of 90 mg twice daily have been used; administer doses >120 mg/day in divided doses

Duodenal ulcer: Oral: Short-term treatment: 15 mg once daily for 4 weeks; maintenance therapy: 15 mg once daily

Peptic ulcer disease: Eradication of *Helicobacter pylori*: Currently accepted recommendations (may differ from product labeling): Oral: Dose varies with regimen: 30 mg once daily or 60 mg/day in 2 divided doses; requires combination therapy with antibiotics

Gastric ulcer: Oral: Short-term treatment: 30 mg once daily for up to 8 weeks

NSAID-associated gastric ulcer (healing): Oral: 30 mg once daily for 8 weeks; controlled studies did not extend past 8 weeks

NSAID-associated gastric ulcer (to reduce risk): Oral: 15 mg once daily for up to 12 weeks; controlled studies did not extend past 12 weeks

Prevention of rebleeding in peptic ulcer bleed (unlabeled use): I.V.: 60 mg, followed by 6 mg/hour infusion for 72 hours

Pediatrics:

GERD, erosive esophagitis: Oral: Children 1-11 years:

≤30 kg: 15 mg once daily

>30 kg: 30 mg once daily

Note: Doses were increased in some pediatric patients if still symptomatic after 2 or more weeks of treatment (maximum dose: 30 mg twice daily)

Erosive esophagitis: Children 12-17 years: Oral: 30 mg once daily for up to 8 weeks

Nonerosive GERD: Children 12-17 years: Oral: 15 mg once daily for up to 8 weeks

Renal Impairment: No adjustment is necessary.

Hepatic Impairment: May require a dose reduction.

Available Dosage Forms

Capsule, delayed release (Prevacid®): 15 mg, 30 mg

Granules, for oral suspension, delayed release (Prevacid®): 15 mg/packet (30s), 30 mg/packet (30s) [strawberry flavor]

Injection, powder for reconstitution (Prevacid®): 30 mg

Tablet, orally-disintegrating (Prevacid® SoluTab™): 15 mg [contains phenylalanine 2.5 mg; strawberry flavor]; 30 mg [contains phenylalanine 5.1 mg; strawberry flavor]

Monitoring and Teaching Issues

Physical Assessment: Assess periodic laboratory results and assess effectiveness of medications that require an acid medium for absorption (eg, ketoconazole, itraconazole). Monitor effectiveness of ulcer symptom relief.

Monitoring Laboratory Tests: CBC, liver function, renal function, and serum gastrin levels. Patients with Zollinger-Ellison syndrome should be monitored for gastric acid output, which should be maintained at ≤10 mEq/hour during the last hour before the next lansoprazole dose.

Patient Education: Take as directed, before eating. Do not crush or chew granules. Patients who may have difficulty swallowing capsules may open the delayed-release capsules and sprinkle the contents on applesauce, pudding, cottage cheese, or yogurt. Avoid alcohol. Report unresolved diarrhea. **Breast-feeding precaution:** Breast-feeding is not recommended.

Dietary Considerations: Should be taken before eating; best if taken before breakfast. Prevacid® SoluTab™ contains phenylalanine 2.5 mg per 15 mg tablet; phenylalanine 5.1 mg per 30 mg tablet.

Geriatric Considerations: The clearance of lansoprazole is decreased in the elderly; however, the half-life is only increased by 50% to 100%. This still results in a short half-life and no accumulation is seen in the elderly. The rate of healing and side effects is similar to younger adults; no dosage adjustment is necessary.

Pregnancy Risk Factor: B

Lactation: Excretion in breast milk unknown/not recommended

Administration

Oral: Administer before food; best if taken before breakfast. The intact granules should not be chewed or crushed; however, in addition to oral suspension, several options are available for those patients unable to swallow capsules:

Capsules may be opened and the intact granules sprinkled on 1 tablespoon of applesauce, Ensure® pudding, cottage cheese, yogurt, or strained pears. The granules should then be swallowed immediately.

Capsules may be opened and emptied into ~60 mL orange juice, apple juice, or tomato juice; mix and swallow immediately. Rinse the glass with additional juice and swallow to assure complete delivery of the dose.

Capsule granules may be mixed with apple, cranberry, grape, orange, pineapple, prune, tomato and V-8® juice and stored for up to 30 minutes.

Delayed release oral suspension granules should be mixed with 2 tablespoonfuls (30 mL) of water; no other liquid should be used. Stir well and drink immediately. Should not be administered through enteral administration tubes.

Orally-disintegrating tablets: Should not be swallowed whole or chewed. Place tablet on tongue; allow to dissolve (with or without water) until particles can be swallowed. Orally-disintegrating tablets may also be administered via an oral syringe: Place the 15 mg tablet in an oral syringe and draw up ~4 mL water, or place the 30 mg tablet in an

(Continued)

Lansoprazole *(Continued)*

oral syringe and draw up ~10 mL water. After tablet has dispersed, administer within 15 minutes. Refill the syringe with water (2 mL for the 15 mg tablet; 4 mL for the 30 mg tablet), shake gently, then administer any remaining contents.

I.V.: Administer over 30 minutes. Use of an in-line filter is required. Before and after administration, flush I.V. line with NS, LR, or D_5W. Do not administer with other medications.

Other: Nasogastric tube administration:

Capsule: Capsule can be opened, the granules mixed (not crushed) with 40 mL of apple juice and then injected through the NG tube into the stomach, then flush tube with additional apple juice. Granules for oral suspension should not be administered through enteral administration tubes.

Orally-disintegrating tablet: Nasogastric tube (≥8 French): Place a 15 mg tablet in a syringe and draw up ~4 mL water, or place the 30 mg tablet in a syringe and draw up ~10 mL water. After tablet has dispersed, administer within 15 minutes. Refill the syringe with ~5 mL water, shake gently, and then flush the nasogastric tube.

Reconstitution:

Oral suspension: Empty packet into container with 2 tablespoons of water. Do **not** mix with other liquids or food. Stir well and drink immediately.

Powder for injection: Reconstitute with sterile water 5 mL; mix gently until dissolved. Prior to administration, further dilute with 50 mL of NS, LR, or D_5W.

Storage: Store at 15°C to 30°C (59°F to 86°F); protect from light and moisture.

Powder for injection: After reconstitution, the solution may be stored for up to 1 hour at room temperature prior to final dilution. Following final dilution, solutions mixed with NS or LR are stable at room temperature for 24 hours; solutions mixed with D_5W are stable for 12 hours

Related Information
Helicobacter pylori Treatment *on page 1835*

Lansoprazole, Amoxicillin, and Clarithromycin
(lan SOE pra zole, a moks i SIL in, & kla RITH roe mye sin)

U.S. Brand Names Prevpac®

Synonyms Amoxicillin, Lansoprazole, and Clarithromycin; Clarithromycin, Lansoprazole, and Amoxicillin

Generic Available No

Pharmacologic Category Antibiotic, Macrolide Combination; Antibiotic, Penicillin; Gastrointestinal Agent, Miscellaneous

Medication Safety Issues
Sound-alike/look-alike issues:
Prevpac® may be confused with Prevacid®

Use Eradication of *H. pylori* to reduce the risk of recurrent duodenal ulcer

Dosing
Adults & Elderly: *H. pylori* eradication: Oral: Lansoprazole 30 mg, amoxicillin 1 g, and clarithromycin 500 mg taken together twice daily for 10 or 14 days

Available Dosage Forms Combination package (Prevpac®) [each administration card contains]:
Capsule (Trimox®): Amoxicillin 500 mg (4 capsules/day)
Capsule, delayed release (Prevacid®): Lansoprazole 30 mg (2 capsules/day)
Tablet (Biaxin®): Clarithromycin 500 mg (2 tablets/day)

Monitoring and Teaching Issues
Physical Assessment: See individual agents.
Patient Education: See individual agents. **Pregnancy/breast-feeding precautions:** Inform prescriber if you are or intend to become pregnant. Do not breast-feed.

Pregnancy Risk Factor: C (clarithromycin)
Lactation: Excretion in breast milk unknown/not recommended

Related Information
Amoxicillin *on page 102*
Clarithromycin *on page 342*
Lansoprazole *on page 866*

Lansoprazole and Naproxen (lan SOE pra zole & na PROKS en)

U.S. Brand Names Prevacid® NapraPAC™

Synonyms NapraPAC™; Naproxen and Lansoprazole

Generic Available No

Pharmacologic Category Nonsteroidal Anti-inflammatory Drug (NSAID), Oral; Proton Pump Inhibitor

Medication Safety Issues Note: Differences in the frequency of some adverse events may be related to use for a specific indication.

>10%:
Cardiovascular: Flushing (33%)
Central nervous system: Mood changes (up to 12%)
Dermatologic: Skin changes (19%)
Endocrine & metabolic: Hot flashes (3% to 80%), fluid retention (32%), altered menses (13% to 25%), amenorrhea (16%)
Gastrointestinal: Nausea (26%), weight loss (23%)
Genitourinary: Vaginal bleeding (up to 23%), vaginal discharge (30% to 55%)
Neuromuscular & skeletal: Bone pain, tumor pain, and local disease flare (including increase in lesion size and erythema) during treatment of metastatic breast cancer (generally resolves with continuation)
1% to 10%:
Cardiovascular : Edema (4%)
Central nervous system: Fatigue(4%), depression (2%)
Dermatologic: Alopecia (<1% to 5%)

Endocrine & metabolic: Oligomenorrhea (9%), menstrual disorder (6%)
Gastrointestinal: Constipation (up to 4%), abdominal cramps (1%), anorexia (1%)
Genitourinary: Ovarian cyst (3%)
Hematologic: Thrombocytopenia (<1% to 10%)
Hepatic: SGOT increased (5%), serum bilirubin increased (2%)
Neuromuscular & skeletal: Bone pain (6%), musculoskeletal pain (3%), pain (3%)
Renal: Serum creatinine increased (up to 2%)
Respiratory: Cough (4%)
Miscellaneous: Infection/sepsis (up to 6%), allergic reaction (up to 3%)
<1%, infrequent, or frequency not defined: Cataract, cholestasis, corneal changes, deep vein thrombosis, dizziness, endometriosis, endometrial cancer, endometrial hyperplasia, endometrial polyps, , fatty liver, hepatic necrosis, hepatitis, hypercalcemia, hyperlipidemias, lightheadedness, pancreatitis, peripheral edema, phlebitis, pruritus vulvae, pulmonary embolism, retinal vein thrombosis, retinopathy, second primary tumors, stroke, taste disturbances, tumor pain and local disease flare (including increase in lesion size and erythema) during treatment of metastatic breast cancer (generally resolves with continuation), uterine fibroids, vaginal dryness
Postmarketing and/or case reports: Angioedema, bullous pemphigoid, erythema multiforme, hypersensitivity reactions, headache, hypertriglyceridemia, interstitial pneumonitis, impotence (males), loss of libido (males), rash, Stevens-Johnson syndrome
Sound-alike/look-alike issues:
Prevacid® may be confused with Pravachol®, Prevpac®, Prilosec®, Prinivil®
Use Reduction of the risk of NSAID-associated gastric ulcers in patients with history of gastric ulcer who require an NSAID for the treatment of rheumatoid arthritis, osteoarthritis, and ankylosing spondylitis
Dosing
Adults: Reduce NSAID-associated gastric ulcers during treatment for arthritis: Oral: Lansoprazole 15 mg once daily in the morning; naproxen 375 mg or 500 mg twice daily
Elderly: Naproxen: Dosing adjustment should be considered.
Renal Impairment: Naproxen: Dosing adjustment should be considered.
Hepatic Impairment: Naproxen: Dosing adjustment should be considered.
Available Dosage Forms Combination package:
Prevacid® NapraPAC™ 375 [each administration card contains]:
Capsule, delayed release (Prevacid®): Lansoprazole 15 mg (7 capsules per card)
Tablet (Naprosyn®): Naproxen 375 mg (14 tablets per card)
Prevacid® NapraPAC™ 500 [each administration card contains]:
Capsule, delayed release (Prevacid®): Lansoprazole 15 mg (7 capsules per card)
Tablet (Naprosyn®): Naproxen 500 mg (14 tablets per card)
Monitoring and Teaching Issues
Pregnancy Risk Factor: B (naproxen: D/third trimester)
Lactation: Enters breast milk/not recommended
Related Information
Lansoprazole *on page 866*
Naproxen *on page 1056*

Latanoprost (la TA noe prost)

U.S. Brand Names Xalatan®
Generic Available No
Pharmacologic Category Ophthalmic Agent, Antiglaucoma; Prostaglandin, Ophthalmic
Medication Safety Issues
Sound-alike/look-alike issues:
Xalatan® may be confused with Travatan®, Zarontin®
Use Reduction of elevated intraocular pressure in patients with open-angle glaucoma or ocular hypertension
Contraindications Hypersensitivity to latanoprost or any component of the formulation
Warnings/Precautions Latanoprost may gradually change eye color, increasing the amount of brown pigment in the iris by increasing the number of melanosome in melanocytes. The long-term effects on the melanocytes and the consequences of potential injury to the melanocytes or deposition of pigment granules to other areas of the eye is currently unknown. Patients should be examined regularly, and depending on the clinical situation, treatment may be stopped if increased pigmentation ensues.

There have been reports of bacterial keratitis associated with the use of multiple-dose containers of topical ophthalmic products. Do not administer while wearing contact lenses.
Drug Interactions
Decreased Effect: *In vitro* studies have shown that precipitation occurs when eye drops containing thimerosal are mixed with latanoprost. If such drugs are used, administer with an interval of at least 5 minutes between applications. May be used concomitantly with other topical ophthalmic drugs if administration is separated by at least 5 minutes.
Adverse Reactions
>10%: Ocular: Blurred vision, burning and stinging, conjunctival hyperemia, foreign body sensation, itching, increased pigmentation of the iris, and punctate epithelial keratopathy
1% to 10%:
Cardiovascular: Chest pain, angina pectoris
Dermatologic: Rash, allergic skin reaction
Neuromuscular & skeletal: Myalgia, arthralgia, back pain
Ocular: Dry eye, excessive tearing, eye pain, lid crusting, lid edema, lid erythema, lid discomfort/pain, photophobia
Respiratory: Upper respiratory tract infection, cold, flu
(Continued)

Latanoprost *(Continued)*

Overdosage/Toxicology
Symptoms include ocular irritation and conjunctival or episcleral hyperemia
Treatment should be symptomatic

Pharmacodynamics/Kinetics
Onset of Action: 3-4 hours; Peak effect: Maximum: 8-12 hours

Absorption: Through the cornea where the isopropyl ester prodrug is hydrolyzed by ester-ases to the biologically active acid. Peak concentration is reached in 2 hours after topical administration in the aqueous humor.

Half-Life Elimination: 17 minutes

Metabolism: Primarily hepatic via fatty acid beta-oxidation

Excretion: Urine (as metabolites)

Dosing
Adults & Elderly: Glaucoma: Ophthalmic: 1 drop (1.5 mcg) in the affected eye(s) once daily in the evening; do not exceed the once daily dosage because it has been shown that more frequent administration may decrease the IOP lowering effect

Note: A medication delivery device (Xal-Ease™) is available for use with Xalatan®.

Available Dosage Forms Solution, ophthalmic: 0.005% (2.5 mL) [contains benzalkonium chloride]

Monitoring and Teaching Issues
Physical Assessment: Assess potential for interactions with other prescriptions, OTC medications, or herbal products patient may be taking. Assess therapeutic response and adverse effects (eg, blurred vision, burning and stinging, conjunctival hyperemia, foreign body sensation, itching, increased pigmentation of the iris, and punctate epithelial keratop-athy). Teach patient proper use, side effects/appropriate interventions, and symptoms to report.

Patient Education: For use in eyes only. Iris color may change because of an increase of the brown pigment (cosmetically different eye coloration that may occur). Iris pigmentation changes may be more noticeable in patients with green-brown, blue/gray-brown, or yellow-brown irides. If any ocular reaction develops, particularly conjunctivitis and lid reac-tions, immediately notify prescriber. If more than one topical ophthalmic drug is being used, administer the drugs at least 5 minutes apart. Latanoprost contains benzalkonium chloride, which may be absorbed by contact lenses. Remove contact lenses prior to administration; lenses may be reinserted after 15 minutes. Do not let tip of applicator touch eye; do not contaminate tip of applicator (may cause eye infection, eye damage, or vision loss). Serious damage to the eye and subsequent loss of vision may result from using contami-nated solutions. A delivery aid, Xal-Ease™, is available for administering Xalatan®. **Preg-nancy precaution:** Inform prescriber if you are pregnant.

Pregnancy Risk Factor: C

Administration
Other: If more than one topical ophthalmic drug is being used, administer the drugs at least 5 minutes apart. A delivery aid, Xal-Ease™, is available for administering Xalatan®.

Storage: Protect from light; store intact bottles under refrigeration (2°C to 8°C/36°F to 46°F). Once opened, the container may be stored at room temperature up to 25°C (77°F) for 6 weeks.

Related Information
Glaucoma Drug Therapy *on page 1827*

♦ **Laxatives, Classification and Properties** *see page 1737*
♦ **L-Carnitine** *see Levocarnitine on page 884*
♦ **LCR** *see VinCRIStine on page 1564*
♦ **L-Deprenyl** *see Selegiline on page 1364*
♦ **LDP-341** *see Bortezomib on page 203*

Leflunomide *(le FLOO noh mide)*
U.S. Brand Names Arava®

Generic Available No

Pharmacologic Category Antirheumatic, Disease Modifying

Use Treatment of active rheumatoid arthritis; indicated to reduce signs and symptoms, and to retard structural damage and improve physical function

Mechanism of Action/Effect Inhibits pyrimidine synthesis, resulting in antiproliferative and anti-inflammatory effects

Contraindications Hypersensitivity to leflunomide or any component of the formulation; pregnancy

Warnings/Precautions Leflunomide has been associated with rare reports of hepatotoxicity, hepatic failure, and death. Hepatic disease (including seropositive hepatitis B or C patients) and/or concurrent exposure to other hepatotoxins may increase the risk of hepatotoxicity. Monitoring of hepatic function is required.

Not recommended for patients with severe immune deficiency, bone marrow dysplasia, or uncontrolled infection. Has been associated with rare pancytopenia, agranulocytosis, and thrombocytopenia, particularly when given in combination with methotrexate or other immu-nosuppressive agents. Monitoring of hematologic function is required. Use with caution in patients with a prior history of significant hematologic abnormalities. Discontinue if evidence of bone marrow suppression or severe dermatologic reaction occurs, and begin procedure to accelerate elimination (cholestyramine or activated charcoal, see Overdosage/Toxicology). Interstitial lung disease has been associated (rarely) with leflunomide use. Discontinue in patients who develop new onset or worsening of pulmonary symptoms; accelerated elimina-tion procedures should be considered if interstitial lung disease occurs; fatal outcomes have been reported. Consider interruption of therapy and accelerated elimination in patients who develop serious infections. The use of live vaccines is not recommended.

Women of childbearing potential should not receive leflunomide until pregnancy has been excluded; patients have been counseled concerning fetal risk and reliable contraceptive measures have been confirmed. Caution in renal impairment. Leflunomide will increase uric acid excretion. Immunosuppression may increase the risk of lymphoproliferative disorders or other malignancies.

Drug Interactions

Cytochrome P450 Effect: Inhibits CYP2C8/9 (weak)

Decreased Effect: Administration of cholestyramine and activated charcoal enhance the elimination of leflunomide's active metabolite.

Increased Effect/Toxicity: Theoretically, concomitant use of drugs metabolized by this enzyme, including many NSAIDs, may result in increased serum concentrations and possible toxic effects. Coadministration with methotrexate increases the risk of hepatotoxicity. Leflunomide may also enhance the hepatotoxicity of other drugs. Tolbutamide free fraction may be increased. Rifampin may increase serum concentrations of leflunomide. Leflunomide has uricosuric activity and may enhance activity of other uricosuric agents.

Nutritional/Ethanol Interactions Food: No interactions with food have been noted.

Adverse Reactions

>10%:
  Gastrointestinal: Diarrhea (17%)
  Respiratory: Respiratory tract infection (15%)

1% to 10%:
  Cardiovascular: Hypertension (10%), chest pain (2%), palpitation, tachycardia, vasculitis, vasodilation, varicose vein, edema (peripheral)
  Central nervous system: Headache (7%), dizziness (4%), pain (2%), fever, malaise, migraine, anxiety, depression, insomnia, sleep disorder
  Dermatologic: Alopecia (10%), rash (10%), pruritus (4%), dry skin (2%), eczema (2%), acne, dermatitis, hair discoloration, hematoma, herpes infection, nail disorder, subcutaneous nodule, skin disorder/discoloration, skin ulcer, bruising
  Endocrine & metabolic: Hypokalemia (1%), diabetes mellitus, hyperglycemia, hyperlipidemia, hyperthyroidism, menstrual disorder
  Gastrointestinal: Nausea (9%), abdominal pain (5%), dyspepsia (5%), weight loss (4%), anorexia (3%), gastroenteritis (3%), stomatitis (3%), vomiting (3%), cholelithiasis, colitis, constipation, esophagitis, flatulence, gastritis, gingivitis, melena, candidiasis (oral), enlarged salivary gland, tooth disorder, xerostomia, taste disturbance
  Genitourinary: Urinary tract infection (5%), albuminuria, cystitis, dysuria, hematuria, vaginal candidiasis, prostate disorder, urinary frequency
  Hematologic: Anemia
  Hepatic: Abnormal LFTs (5%)
  Neuromuscular & skeletal: Back pain (5%), joint disorder (4%), weakness (3%), tenosynovitis (3%), synovitis (2%), arthralgia (1%), paresthesia (2%), muscle cramps (1%), neck pain, pelvic pain, increased CPK, arthrosis, bursitis, myalgia, bone necrosis, bone pain, tendon rupture, neuralgia, neuritis
  Ocular: Blurred vision, cataract, conjunctivitis, eye disorder
  Respiratory: Bronchitis (7%), cough (3%), pharyngitis (3%), pneumonia (2%), rhinitis (2%), sinusitis (2%), asthma, dyspnea, epistaxis
  Miscellaneous: Infection (4%), accidental injury (5%), allergic reactions (2%), diaphoresis

Overdosage/Toxicology There is no human experience with overdose. Leflunomide is not dialyzable. Cholestyramine and/or activated charcoal enhance elimination of leflunomide's active metabolite (M1). In cases of significant overdose or toxicity, cholestyramine 8 g every 8 hours for 1-3 days or activated charcoal 50 g every 6 hours for 24 hours may be administered to enhance elimination. Plasma levels are reduced by ~40% in 24 hours and 49% to 65% after 48 hours of cholestyramine dosing. Activated charcoal reduces plasma levels by 37% after 24 hours and 48% after 48 hours of continuous dosing. Activated charcoal without sorbitol should be used.

To reach undetectable levels (recommended in women of childbearing potential who wish to become pregnant), an extended protocol is necessary. Without this procedure, it may take up to 2 years to reach plasma concentrations <0.02 mg/L (a concentration expected to have minimal risk of teratogenicity based on animal models). The procedure consists of the following steps: Administer cholestyramine 8 g 3 times/day for 11 days (the 11 days do not need to be consecutive). Plasma levels <0.02 mg/L should be verified by two separate tests performed at least 14 days apart. If plasma levels are >0.02 mg/L, additional cholestyramine treatment should be considered.

Pharmacodynamics/Kinetics

Bioavailability: 80%

Time to Peak: 6-12 hours

Half-Life Elimination: Mean: 14-15 days; enterohepatic recycling appears to contribute to the long half-life of this agent, since activated charcoal and cholestyramine substantially reduce plasma half-life

Metabolism: Hepatic to A77 1726 (MI) which accounts for nearly all pharmacologic activity; further metabolism to multiple inactive metabolites; undergoes enterohepatic recirculation

Excretion: Feces (48%); urine (43%)

Dosing

Adults & Elderly: Rheumatoid arthritis: Oral: Initial: 100 mg/day for 3 days, followed by 20 mg/day; dosage may be decreased to 10 mg/day in patients who have difficulty tolerating the 20 mg dose. Due to the long half-life of the active metabolite, plasma levels may require a prolonged period to decline after dosage reduction.

Renal Impairment: No specific dosage adjustment is recommended. There is no clinical experience in the use of leflunomide in patients with renal impairment. The free fraction of MI is doubled in dialysis patients. Patients should be monitored closely for adverse effects requiring dosage adjustment.

Hepatic Impairment: No specific dosage adjustment is recommended. Since the liver is involved in metabolic activation and subsequent metabolism/elimination of leflunomide, patients with hepatic impairment should be monitored closely for adverse effects requiring dosage adjustment.

(Continued)

Leflunomide *(Continued)*

Dosing adjustment in hepatic toxicity: Guidelines for dosage adjustment or discontinuation based on the severity and persistence of ALT elevation secondary to leflunomide have been developed. If ALT elevations >2 times but ≤3 times ULN are noted, reduce dose to 10 mg/day, and monitor closely. If elevations persist or if elevations >3 times ULN are observed, discontinue leflunomide and initiate protocol to accelerate elimination. Cholestyramine (8 g 3 times/day for 1-3 days) or activated charcoal (50 g every 6 hours for 24 hours) may be administered to decrease leflunomide concentrations rapidly. If elevations >3 times ULN persist additional cholestyramine and/or activated charcoal may be required.

Available Dosage Forms Tablet: 10 mg, 20 mg

Monitoring and Teaching Issues

Physical Assessment: Assess other medications patient may be taking for effectiveness and interactions. Assess results of laboratory tests, therapeutic effectiveness, and adverse reactions. Monitor for signs and symptoms of severe infection or hepatic dysfunction. Monitor for new onset or worsening of pulmonary symptoms. **Pregnancy risk factor X:** Determine that patient is not pregnant before starting therapy. Do not give to sexually-active female patients unless capable of complying with contraceptive use. Breast-feeding is contraindicated.

Monitoring Laboratory Tests: A complete blood count (WBC, hemoglobin, hematocrit, and platelet count) as well as serum transaminase determinations should be monitored at baseline and monthly during the initial 6 months of treatment; if stable, monitoring frequency may be decreased to every 6-8 weeks thereafter (continue monthly when used in combination with other immunosuppressive agents).

Patient Education: Take as directed; do not increase dose without consulting prescriber. Maintain adequate hydration (2-3 L/day of fluids) unless instructed to restrict fluid intake. Store medication away from light. You may experience diarrhea (buttermilk, boiled milk, or yogurt may help); nausea, vomiting, loss of appetite, and flatulence (small frequent meals, frequent mouth care, chewing gum, or sucking lozenges may help); or dizziness (use caution when driving or engaging in tasks requiring alertness until response to drug is known). If you have diabetes, monitor blood sugars closely; this medication may alter glucose levels. If you experience symptoms such as nausea, vomiting, stomach pain or swelling, jaundice, dark urine, or unusual tiredness, report these to your prescriber **immediately.** Report chest pain, palpitations, rapid heartbeat, or swelling of extremities; persistent GI problems; skin rash, mucus membrane lesions, redness, irritation, acne, ulcers; frequent, painful, or difficult urination; or genital itching or irritation; depression, acute headache, anxiety, or difficulty sleeping; muscle tremors, cramping or weakness, back pain, or altered gait; cough, cold symptoms, wheezing, or respiratory difficulty; easy bruising/bleeding; blood in vomitus, stool, urine; or other unusual effects related to this medication. **Pregnancy/breast-feeding precautions:** Inform prescriber if you are pregnant. Do not get pregnant or have sex unless using appropriate contraception while on this medication. This drug may cause severe fetal defects. Do not breast-feed.

Dietary Considerations: Administer without regard to meals.

Pregnancy Risk Factor: X

Pregnancy Issues: Leflunomide is contraindicated in pregnant women or women of childbearing potential who are not using reliable contraception. Pregnancy must be excluded prior to initiating treatment. Following treatment, pregnancy should be avoided until undetectable plasma levels (< 0.02 mcg/mL) are verified. This may be accomplished by an extended drug elimination procedure: Administer cholestyramine 8 g 3 times/day for 11 days (the 11 days do not need to be consecutive). Plasma levels <0.02 mg/L should be verified by two separate tests performed at least 14 days apart. If plasma levels are >0.02 mg/L, additional cholestyramine treatment should be considered.

Lactation: Excretion in breast milk unknown/contraindicated

Breast-Feeding Issues: It is not known whether leflunomide is secreted in human milk. Because many immunoglobulins are secreted in milk, and the potential for serious adverse reactions exists, a decision should be made whether to discontinue nursing or discontinue the drug, taking into account the importance of the drug to the mother.

Administration

Storage: Protect from light; store at 25°C (77°F).

♦ **Lente® Iletin® II [DSC]** *see* Insulin Preparations *on page 805*

♦ **Lente, Insulin** *see* Insulin Preparations *on page 805*

Lepirudin *(leh puh ROO din)*

U.S. Brand Names Refludan®

Synonyms Lepirudin (rDNA); Recombinant Hirudin

Generic Available No

Pharmacologic Category Anticoagulant, Thrombin Inhibitor

Use Indicated for anticoagulation in patients with heparin-induced thrombocytopenia (HIT) and associated thromboembolic disease in order to prevent further thromboembolic complications

Unlabeled/Investigational Use Investigational: Prevention or reduction of ischemic complications associated with unstable angina

Mechanism of Action/Effect Lepirudin is a highly specific direct thrombin inhibitor. Each molecule is capable of binding one molecule of thrombin and inhibiting its thrombogenic activity.

Contraindications Hypersensitivity to hirudins or any component of the formulation

Warnings/Precautions Cautiously administer after a thrombolytic episode; risk of intracranial bleeding. Hemorrhage is the most common complication. Patients at increased risk of bleeding include: bacterial endocarditis; congenital or acquired bleeding disorders; recent puncture of large vessels or organ biopsy; recent CVA, stroke, intracerebral surgery, or other neuraxial procedure; severe uncontrolled hypertension; renal impairment; recent major surgery; recent major bleeding (intracranial, GI, intraocular, or pulmonary). With renal impairment, relative overdose might occur even with standard dosage regimen. The bolus dose and rate of infusion must be reduced in patients with known or suspected renal insufficiency.

Strict monitoring of aPTT is required; formation of antihirudin antibodies can increase the anticoagulant effect of lepirudin. Use cautiously in cirrhosis. Allergic reactions may occur frequently in patients treated concomitantly with streptokinase; caution is warranted during re-exposure (anaphylaxis has been reported). Potentially may cause hyperkalemia by affecting aldosterone (similar to heparin).

Drug Interactions

Increased Effect/Toxicity: Thrombolytics may enhance anticoagulant properties of lepirudin on aPTT and can increase the risk of bleeding complications. Bleeding risk may also be increased by oral anticoagulants (warfarin) and platelet function inhibitors (NSAIDs, dipyridamole, ticlopidine, clopidogrel, IIb/IIIa antagonists, and aspirin).

Nutritional/Ethanol Interactions Herb/Nutraceutical: Avoid cat's claw, dong quai, evening primrose, feverfew, garlic, ginger, ginkgo, red clover, horse chestnut, green tea, ginseng (all have additional antiplatelet activity).

Adverse Reactions As with all anticoagulants, bleeding is the most common adverse event associated with lepirudin. Hemorrhage may occur at virtually any site. Risk is dependent on multiple variables.

HIT patients:

>10%: Hematologic: Anemia (12%), bleeding from puncture sites (11%), hematoma (11%)

1% to 10%:

Cardiovascular: Heart failure (3%), pericardial effusion (1%), ventricular fibrillation (1%)

Central nervous system: Fever (7%)

Dermatologic: Eczema (3%), maculopapular rash (4%)

Gastrointestinal: GI bleeding/rectal bleeding (5%)

Genitourinary: Vaginal bleeding (2%)

Hepatic: Transaminases increased (6%)

Renal: Hematuria (4%)

Respiratory: Epistaxis (4%)

Non-HIT populations (including those receiving thrombolytics and/or contrast media):

1% to 10%: Respiratory: Bronchospasm/stridor/dyspnea/cough

Overdosage/Toxicology Risk of bleeding is increased, and therefore management is directed towards control of bleeding.

Pharmacodynamics/Kinetics

Half-Life Elimination: Initial: ~10 minutes: Terminal: Healthy volunteers: 1.3 hours; Significant renal impairment (Cl_{cr} <15 mL/minute and on hemodialysis): ≤2 days

Metabolism: Via release of amino acids via catabolic hydrolysis of parent drug

Excretion: Urine (~48%, 35% as unchanged drug and unchanged drug fragments of parent drug); systemic clearance is proportional to glomerular filtration rate or creatinine clearance

Dosing

Adults & Elderly: Note: Maximum dose: Do not exceed 0.21 mg/kg/hour unless an evaluation of coagulation abnormalities limiting response has been completed. **Dosing is weight-based, however, patients weighing >110 kg should not receive doses greater than the recommended dose for a patient weighing 110 kg (44 mg bolus and initial maximal infusion rate of 16.5 mg/hour).**

Heparin-induced thrombocytopenia: I.V.: Bolus dose: 0.4 mg/kg IVP (over 15-20 seconds), followed by continuous infusion at 0.15 mg/kg/hour; bolus and infusion must be reduced in renal insufficiency

Concomitant use with thrombolytic therapy: I.V.: Bolus dose: 0.2 mg/kg IVP (over 15-20 seconds), followed by continuous infusion at 0.1 mg/kg/hour

Dosing adjustments during infusions: Monitor first aPTT 4 hours after the start of the infusion. Subsequent determinations of aPTT should be obtained at least once daily during treatment. More frequent monitoring is recommended in renally impaired patients. Any aPTT ratio measurement out of range (1.5-2.5) should be confirmed prior to adjusting dose, unless a clinical need for immediate reaction exists. If the aPTT is below target range, increase infusion by 20%. If the aPTT is in excess of the target range, decrease infusion rate by 50%. A repeat aPTT should be obtained 4 hours after any dosing change.

Transition to oral anticoagulants: Reduce lepirudin dose gradually to reach aPTT ratio just above 1.5 before starting warfarin therapy; as soon as INR reaches 2.0, lepirudin therapy should be discontinued.

Renal Impairment: All patients with Cl_{cr} <60 or serum creatinine >1.5 mg/dL require dosage reduction.

Initial: Bolus dose: 0.2 mg/kg IVP (over 15-20 seconds); see table. Additional bolus doses of 0.1 mg/kg may be administered every other day (only if aPTT falls below lower therapeutic limit).

Lepirudin Infusion Rates in Patients With Renal Impairment

Creatinine Clearance (mL/min)	Serum Creatinine (mg/dL)	Adjusted Infusion Rate	
		% of Standard Initial Infusion Rate	mg/kg/h
45-60	1.6-2.0	50%	0.075
30-44	2.1-3.0	30%	0.045
15-29	3.1-6.0	15%	0.0225
<15	>6.0	Avoid or STOP infusion	

Available Dosage Forms Injection, powder for reconstitution: 50 mg

(Continued)

Lepirudin (Continued)

Monitoring and Teaching Issues

Physical Assessment: Use caution in presence of any bleeding, renal or hepatic impairment (see Warnings/Precautions for specific use cautions). Assess potential for interactions with other pharmacological agents or herbal products patient may be taking (especially anything that will affect coagulation or platelet function; see Drug Interactions). See Administration for infusion specifics. Bleeding precautions should be observed. Assess results of laboratory tests, therapeutic effectiveness, and adverse response regularly during therapy (eg, hypersensitivity reaction, bleeding, chest pain, rash; see Adverse Reactions). Teach possible side effects/appropriate interventions (eg, bleeding precautions) and adverse symptoms to report (see Patient Education).

Monitoring Laboratory Tests: The aPTT ratio should be maintained between 1.5 and 2.5.

Patient Education: Do not take any new medication during therapy unless approved by prescriber. This drug can only be administered by infusion. Report immediately any pain, swelling, burning, or bleeding at infusion site. You may have a tendency to bleed easily while taking this drug (brush teeth with soft brush, floss with waxed floss, use electric razor, avoid scissors or sharp knives, and avoid potentially harmful activities). Report immediately any unusual bleeding or bruising (bleeding gums, nosebleed, blood in urine, dark stool); pain in joints or back; unusual fever; persistent nausea or GI upset; or swelling or pain at injection site. **Breast-feeding precaution:** Consult prescriber if breast-feeding.

Pregnancy Risk Factor: B

Lactation: Enters breast milk/consult prescriber

Administration

Oral: Administer **only** intravenously

I.V.: I.V. bolus: Inject slowly for continuous infusion; solutions with 0.2 or 0.4 mg/mL may be used.

Reconstitution: Reconstitute 50 mg vials with 1 mL water for injection or 0.9% sodium chloride injection. Bolus dose: Prepare 5 mg/mL solution by transferring contents of 1 reconstituted vial to single use, sterile syringe. Dilute to total volume of 10 mL with 0.9 sodium chloride or 5% dextrose injection. To prepare continuous infusion solutions, either 0.9% sodium chloride or 5% dextrose may be used. Add contents of two reconstituted vials to either 250 mL (to prepare 0.4 mg/mL solution) or 500 mL (to prepare 0.2 mg/mL solution). Once reconstituted, use immediately. Reconstituted solutions remain stable for 24 hours (duration of infusion).

♦ **Lepirudin (rDNA)** *see Lepirudin on page 872*

♦ **Lescol®** *see Fluvastatin on page 664*

♦ **Lescol® XL** *see Fluvastatin on page 664*

♦ **Lessina™** *see Ethinyl Estradiol and Levonorgestrel on page 585*

Letrozole (LET roe zole)

U.S. Brand Names Femara®

Generic Available No

Pharmacologic Category Antineoplastic Agent, Aromatase Inhibitor

Medication Safety Issues

Sound-alike/look-alike issues:

Femara® may be confused with femhrt®

Use First-line treatment of hormone receptor positive or hormone receptor unknown, locally advanced, or metastatic breast cancer in postmenopausal women; treatment of advanced breast cancer in postmenopausal women with disease progression following antiestrogen therapy; extended adjuvant treatment of early breast cancer in postmenopausal women who have received 5 years of adjuvant tamoxifen therapy

Mechanism of Action/Effect Competitive inhibitor of the aromatase enzyme system, which catalyzes conversion of androgens to estrogens. Inhibition leads to a significant reduction in plasma estrogen levels. Does not affect synthesis of adrenal or thyroid hormones, aldosterone, or androgens.

Contraindications Hypersensitivity to letrozole or any component of the formulation; pregnancy

Warnings/Precautions Dose-related effects on hematologic or chemistry parameters have not been observed. Increases in transaminases ≥5 times the upper limit of normal and of bilirubin ≥1.5 times the upper limit of normal were most often, but not always, associated with metastatic liver disease. For use in postmenopausal women only.

Drug Interactions

Cytochrome P450 Effect: Substrate (minor) of CYP2A6, 3A4; **Inhibits** CYP2A6 (strong), 2C19 (weak)

Increased Effect/Toxicity: Letrozole may increase the levels/effects of CYP2A6 substrates; example substrates include dexmedetomidine and ifosfamide.

Adverse Reactions

>10%:

Cardiovascular: Hot flushes (5% to 19%)

Central nervous system: Headache (8% to 12%), fatigue (6% to 13%)

Gastrointestinal: Nausea (13% to 17%)

Neuromuscular & skeletal: Musculoskeletal pain, bone pain (22%), back pain (18%), arthralgia (8% to 16%)

Respiratory: Dyspnea (7% to 18%), cough (5% to 13%)

2% to 10%:

Cardiovascular: Chest pain (3% to 8%), peripheral edema (5%), hypertension (5% to 8%)

Central nervous system: Pain (5%), insomnia (7%), dizziness (3% to 5%), somnolence (2% to 3%), depression (<5%), anxiety (<5%), vertigo (<5%)

Dermatologic: Rash (4% to 5%), alopecia (<5%), pruritus (1% to 2%)

Endocrine & metabolic: Breast pain (7%), hypercholesterolemia (3%), hypercalcemia (<5%)

Gastrointestinal: Vomiting (7%), constipation (6% to 10%), diarrhea (5% to 8%), abdominal pain (5% to 6%), anorexia (3% to 5%), dyspepsia (3% to 4%), weight loss (7%), weight gain (2%)

Neuromuscular & skeletal: Weakness (4% to 6%)

Miscellaneous: Flu (6%)

Overdosage/Toxicology Firm recommendations for treatment are not possible; emesis could be induced if the patient is alert. In general, supportive care and frequent monitoring of vital signs are appropriate.

Pharmacodynamics/Kinetics

Absorption: Well absorbed; not affected by food

Time to Peak: Steady state, plasma: 2-6 weeks

Protein Binding: Plasma: Weak

Half-Life Elimination: Terminal: ~2 days

Metabolism: Hepatic via CYP3A4 and CYP2A6 to an inactive carbinol metabolite

Excretion: Urine (75% as glucuronide carbinol metabolite, 6% as unchanged drug)

Dosing

Adults & Elderly: Refer to individual protocols.

Breast cancer: Oral: 2.5 mg once daily

Renal Impairment: No dosage adjustment is required in patients with renal impairment if Cl_{cr} is ≥10 mL/minute.

Hepatic Impairment:

Mild-to-moderate impairment: No adjustment recommended

Severe impairment: Child-Pugh class C: 2.5 mg every other day

Available Dosage Forms Tablet: 2.5 mg

Monitoring and Teaching Issues

Physical Assessment: See Warnings/Precautions for use cautions. Assess results of laboratory tests, therapeutic effectiveness (slowing of disease process), and adverse reactions on a regular basis throughout therapy (see Adverse Reactions). Teach patient proper use, possible side effects/appropriate interventions, and adverse symptoms to report (see Patient Education).

Monitoring Laboratory Tests: CBC, thyroid function tests, serum electrolytes, serum transaminases, serum creatinine

Patient Education: Do not take any new medication during therapy unless approved by prescriber. Take as directed, without regard to food. You may experience nausea, vomiting, hot flashes, or loss of appetite (frequent mouth care, small frequent meals, chewing gum, or sucking lozenges may help); musculoskeletal pain or headache (mild analgesics may offer relief); sleepiness, fatigue, or dizziness (use caution when driving, climbing stairs, or engaging in tasks that require alertness until response to drug is known); constipation (increased exercise, or dietary fruit or fluids may help); diarrhea (buttermilk, boiled milk, or yogurt may help); or loss of hair (will grow back). Report chest pain, pressure, palpitations, or swollen extremities; weakness, severe headache, numbness, or loss of strength in any part of the body; difficulty speaking; vaginal bleeding; unusual signs of bleeding or bruising; respiratory difficulty; severe nausea; muscle pain; or skin rash. For use in postmenopausal women only.

Dietary Considerations: May be taken without regard to meals. Calcium and vitamin D supplementation are recommended.

Pregnancy Risk Factor: D

Pregnancy Issues: Letrozole may cause fetal harm when administered to pregnant women. Letrozole is embryotoxic and fetotoxic when administered to rats. There are no studies in pregnant women and letrozole is indicated for postmenopausal women.

Lactation: Excretion in breast milk unknown/not recommended

Administration

Storage: Store at 15°C to 30°C (59°F to 86°F)

Leucovorin (loo koe VOR in)

Synonyms Calcium Leucovorin; Citrovorum Factor; Folinic Acid; 5-Formyl Tetrahydrofolate; Leucovorin Calcium

Generic Available Yes

Pharmacologic Category Antidote; Vitamin, Water Soluble

Medication Safety Issues

Sound-alike/look-alike issues:

Leucovorin may be confused with Leukeran®, Leukine®

Folinic acid may be confused with folic acid

Use Antidote for folic acid antagonists (methotrexate, trimethoprim, pyrimethamine); treatment of megaloblastic anemias when folate is deficient as in infancy, sprue, pregnancy, and nutritional deficiency when oral folate therapy is not possible; in combination with fluorouracil in the treatment of colon cancer

Mechanism of Action/Effect A reduced form of folic acid, leucovorin supplies the necessary cofactor blocked by methotrexate, enters the cells via the same active transport system as methotrexate. Stabilizes the binding of 5-dUMP and thymidylate synthetase, enhancing the activity of fluorouracil.

Contraindications Hypersensitivity to leucovorin or any component of the formulation; pernicious anemia or vitamin B_{12} deficient megaloblastic anemias; should **NOT** be administered intrathecally/intraventricularly

Drug Interactions

Decreased Effect: May decrease efficacy of co-trimoxazole against *Pneumocystis carinii* pneumonitis

Adverse Reactions Frequency not defined.

Dermatologic: Rash, pruritus, erythema, urticaria

Hematologic: Thrombocytosis

Respiratory: Wheezing

Miscellaneous: Anaphylactoid reactions

(Continued)

Leucovorin (Continued)

Pharmacodynamics/Kinetics

Onset of Action: Oral: ~30 minutes; I.V.: ~5 minutes

Absorption: Oral, I.M.: Rapid and well absorbed

Bioavailability: 31% following 200 mg dose; 98% following doses ≤25 mg

Half-Life Elimination: Leucovorin: 15 minutes; 5MTHF: 33-35 minutes

Metabolism: Intestinal mucosa and hepatically to 5-methyl-tetrahydrofolate (5MTHF; active)

Excretion: Urine (80% to 90%); feces (5% to 8%)

Dosing

Adults & Elderly: Note: This drug should be given parenterally instead of orally in patients with GI toxicity, nausea, vomiting, and when individual doses are >25 mg.

Treatment of folic acid antagonist overdosage: Oral: 2-15 mg/day for 3 days or until blood counts are normal, **or** 5 mg every 3 days; doses of 6 mg/day are needed for patients with platelet counts <100,000/mm^3.

Folate-deficient megaloblastic anemia: I.M.: 1 mg/day

Megaloblastic anemia secondary to congenital deficiency of dihydrofolate reductase: I.M.: 3-6 mg/day

Rescue dose: Initial: I.V.: 10 mg/m^2, then:

Oral, I.M., I.V., SubQ: 10-15 10 mg/m^2 every 6 hours until methotrexate level <0.05 μmol/mL; if methotrexate level remains >5 μmol/mL at 48-72 hours after the end of the methotrexate infusion, increase to 20-100 mg/m^2 every 6 hours until methotrexate level <0.05 μmol/mL

Investigational: Post I.T. methotrexate: Oral, I.V.: 12 mg/m^2 as a single dose

Pediatrics: Refer to adult dosing.

Available Dosage Forms

Injection, powder for reconstitution, as calcium: 50 mg, 100 mg, 200 mg, 350 mg, 500 mg

Injection, solution, as calcium: 10 mg/mL (50 mL)

Tablet, as calcium: 5 mg, 10 mg, 15 mg, 25 mg

Monitoring and Teaching Issues

Physical Assessment: Monitor for adverse reactions.

Monitoring Laboratory Tests: Plasma methotrexate concentration as a therapeutic guide to high-dose methotrexate therapy with leucovorin factor rescue. Leucovorin is continued until the plasma methotrexate level is <0.05 μmol/mL. Each dose of leucovorin is increased if the plasma methotrexate concentration is excessively high. With 4- to 6-hour high-dose methotrexate infusions, plasma drug values in excess of 50 and 1 μmol at 24 and 48 hours after starting the infusion, respectively, are often predictive of delayed methotrexate clearance.

Patient Education: Take as directed, at evenly spaced intervals around-the-clock. Maintain hydration (2-3 L of water/day while taking for rescue therapy). For folic acid deficiency, eat foods high in folic acid (eg, meat proteins, bran, dried beans, asparagus, green leafy vegetables). Report respiratory difficulty, lethargy, or rash or itching. **Pregnancy precaution:** Inform prescriber if you are or intend to become pregnant.

Pregnancy Risk Factor: C

Lactation: Enters breast milk/compatible

Administration

Oral: Doses >25 mg should be administered parenterally.

I.V.: Refer to individual protocols. Leucovorin calcium should be administered I.M. or I.V. I.V. infusion should not exceed 160 mg/minute of leucovorin. Leucovorin should not be administered concurrently with methotrexate. It is commonly initiated 24 hours after the start of methotrexate. Toxicity to normal tissues may be irreversible if leucovorin is not initiated by ~40 hours after the start of methotrexate.

As a rescue after folate antagonists: Leucovorin may be administered by I.V. bolus injection, I.M. injection, or orally. Doses >25 mg should be administered parenterally.

In combination with fluorouracil: When leucovorin is used to modulate fluorouracil activity, the fluorouracil is usually given after, or at the midpoint, of the leucovorin infusion. Leucovorin is usually administered by I.V. bolus injection or short (10-15 minutes) I.V. infusion. Other administration schedules have been used; refer to individual protocols.

Reconstitution: Reconstitute with SWFI, bacteriostatic NS, BWFI, NS, or D$_5$W.

Compatibility: Stable in D$_{10}$NS, D$_5$W, D$_{10}$W, LR, SWFI, bacteriostatic water, NS, bacteriostatic NS

Y-site administration: Incompatible with amphotericin B cholesteryl sulfate complex, droperidol, foscarnet, sodium bicarbonate

Compatibility in syringe: Incompatible with droperidol

Compatibility when admixed: Incompatible with concentrations >2 mg/mL of leucovorin and >25 mg/mL of fluorouracil

Storage: Store at room temperature; protect from light. Reconstituted solution is chemically stable for 7 days; reconstitutions with bacteriostatic water for injection, U.S.P., must be used within 7 days. Parenteral admixture is stable for 24 hours stored at room temperature (25°C) and for 4 days when stored under refrigeration (4°C).

- ◆ **Leucovorin Calcium** see Leucovorin on page 875
- ◆ **Leukeran®** see Chlorambucil on page 305
- ◆ **Leukine®** see Sargramostim on page 1358

Leuprolide (loo PROE lide)

U.S. Brand Names Eligard®; Lupron®; Lupron Depot®; Lupron Depot-Ped®; Viadur®

Synonyms Abbott-43818; Leuprolide Acetate; Leuprorelin Acetate; NSC-377526; TAP-144

Generic Available Yes: Injection (solution)

Pharmacologic Category Gonadotropin Releasing Hormone Agonist

Medication Safety Issues

Sound-alike/look-alike issues:

Lupron® may be confused with Nuprin®

Use Palliative treatment of advanced prostate carcinoma; management of endometriosis as initial treatment and/or treatment of recurrent symptoms; preoperative treatment of anemia caused by uterine leiomyomata (fibroids); central precocious puberty

Unlabeled/Investigational Use Treatment of breast, ovarian, and endometrial cancer; infertility; prostatic hyperplasia

Mechanism of Action/Effect Potent inhibitor of gonadotropin secretion; continuous daily administration results in suppression of ovarian and testicular steroidogenesis due to decreased levels of LH and FSH with subsequent decrease in testosterone (male) and estrogen (female) levels. Leuprolide may also have a direct inhibitory effect on the testes, and act by a different mechanism not directly related to reduction in serum testosterone.

Contraindications Hypersensitivity to leuprolide, GnRH, GnRH-agonist analogs, or any component of the formulation; spinal cord compression (orchiectomy suggested); undiagnosed abnormal vaginal bleeding; pregnancy; breast-feeding

Warnings/Precautions Transient increases in testosterone serum levels occur at the start of treatment. Tumor flare, bone pain, neuropathy, urinary tract obstruction, and spinal cord compression have been reported when used for prostate cancer; closely observe patients for weakness, paresthesias, hematuria, and urinary tract obstruction in first few weeks of therapy. Observe patients with metastatic vertebral lesions or urinary obstruction closely. Exacerbation of endometriosis or uterine leiomyomata may occur initially. Decreased bone density has been reported when used for ≥6 months. Use caution in patients with a history of psychiatric illness; alteration in mood, memory impairment, and depression have been associated with use.

Lab Interactions Interferes with pituitary gonadotropic and gonadal function tests during and up to 3 months after therapy

Adverse Reactions

Children: 1% to 10%

Central nervous system: Pain (2%)

Dermatologic: Acne (2%), rash (2%), seborrhea (2%)

Genitourinary: Vaginitis (2%), vaginal bleeding (2%), vaginal discharge (2%)

Local: Injection site reaction (5%)

Adults (frequency dependent upon formulation and indication):

Cardiovascular: Angina, atrial fibrillation, CHF, deep vein thrombosis, edema, hot flashes, hypertension, MI, tachycardia

Central nervous system: Abnormal thinking, agitation, amnesia, confusion, convulsion, dementia, depression, dizziness, fatigue, fever, headache, insomnia, pain, vertigo

Dermatologic: Alopecia, bruising, cellulitis

Endocrine & metabolic: Bone density decreased, breast enlargement, breast tenderness, dehydration, hyperglycemia, hyperlipidemia, hyperphosphatemia, libido decreased, menstrual disorders, potassium decreased

Gastrointestinal: Anorexia, appetite increased, diarrhea, dysphagia, eructation, GI hemorrhage, gingivitis, gum hemorrhage, intestinal obstruction, nausea, peptic ulcer

Genitourinary: Balanitis, impotence, nocturia, penile shrinkage, testicular atrophy, urinary disorder, vaginitis

Hematologic: Platelets decreased, PT prolonged, WBC increased

Hepatic: Hepatomegaly, liver function tests abnormal

Local: Abscess, injection site reaction

Neuromuscular & skeletal: Leg cramps, myalgia, paresthesia, weakness

Renal: BUN increased

Respiratory: Allergic reaction, emphysema, hemoptysis, hypoxia, lung edema, pulmonary embolism

Miscellaneous: Body odor, flu-like syndrome, neoplasm, night sweats, voice alteration

Overdosage/Toxicology Treatment is supportive.

Pharmacodynamics/Kinetics

Onset of Action: Following transient increase, testosterone suppression occurs in ~2-4 weeks of continued therapy

Bioavailability: Oral: None; SubQ: 94%

Protein Binding: 43% to 49%

Half-Life Elimination: 3 hours

Metabolism: Major metabolite, pentapeptide (M-1)

Excretion: Urine (<5% as parent and major metabolite)

Dosing

Adults & Elderly:

Advanced prostatic carcinoma:

SubQ:

Eligard®: 7.5 mg monthly **or** 22.5 mg every 3 months **or** 30 mg every 4 months **or** 45 mg every 6 months

Lupron®: 1 mg/day

Viadur®: 65 mg implanted subcutaneously every 12 months

I.M.:

Lupron Depot®: 7.5 mg/dose given monthly (every 28-33 days) **or**

Lupron Depot-3®: 22.5 mg every 3 months **or**

Lupron Depot-4®: 30 mg every 4 months

Endometriosis: I.M.: Initial therapy may be with leuprolide alone or in combination with norethindrone; if retreatment for an additional 6 months is necessary, norethindrone should be used. Retreatment is not recommended for longer than one additional 6-month course.

Lupron Depot®: 3.75 mg/month for up to 6 months **or**

Lupron Depot-3®: 11.25 mg every 3 months for up to 2 doses (6 months total duration of treatment)

Uterine leiomyomata (fibroids): I.M. (in combination with iron):

Lupron Depot®: 3.75 mg/month for up to 3 months **or**

Lupron Depot-3®: 11.25 mg as a single injection

(Continued)

Leuprolide *(Continued)*

Pediatrics:
Precocious puberty (consider discontinuing by age 11 for females and by age 12 for males):

SubQ (Lupron®): 20-45 mcg/kg/day; titrate dose upward by 10 mcg/kg/day if down-regulation is not achieved

I.M. (Lupron Depot-Ped®): 0.3 mg/kg/dose given every 28 days (minimum dose: 7.5 mg)
≤25 kg: 7.5 mg
>25-37.5 kg: 11.25 mg
>37.5 kg: 15 mg
Titrate dose upward in 3.75 mg every 4 weeks if down-regulation is not achieved.

Available Dosage Forms
Implant (Viadur®): 65 mg [released over 12 months; packaged with administration kit]

Injection, solution, as acetate (Lupron®): 5 mg/mL (2.8 mL) [contains benzyl alcohol; packaged with syringes and alcohol swabs]

Injection, powder for reconstitution, as acetate [depot formulation; prefilled syringe]:
Eligard®:
7.5 mg [released over 1 month]
22.5 mg [released over 3 months]
30 mg [released over 4 months]
45 mg [released over 6 months]
Lupron Depot®: 3.75 mg, 7.5 mg [released over 1 month; contains polysorbate 80]
Lupron Depot®-3 Month: 11.25 mg, 22.5 mg [released over 3 months; contains polysorbate 80]
Lupron Depot®-4 Month: 30 mg [released over 4 months; contains polysorbate 80]
Lupron Depot-Ped®: 7.5 mg, 11.25 mg, 15 mg [released over 1 month; contains polysorbate 80]

Monitoring and Teaching Issues
Physical Assessment: Assess results of laboratory tests, therapeutic effectiveness, and adverse reactions (eg, urinary tract obstruction, weakness, paresthesias, and urinary tract obstruction in first few weeks of therapy) on a regular basis throughout therapy. Teach patient (or caregiver) proper use (eg, storage, injection technique, syringe/needle disposal), possible side effects/appropriate interventions, and adverse symptoms to report.

Pregnancy risk factor X: Determine that patient is not pregnant before beginning treatment and do not give to females of childbearing age unless capable of complying with contraceptive measures 1 month prior to therapy, during therapy, and 1 month following therapy. Instruct patient in appropriate contraceptive measures.

Monitoring Laboratory Tests: Precocious puberty: GnRH testing (blood LH and FSH levels), testosterone in males and estradiol in females

Patient Education: Use as directed. Do not discontinue without consulting prescriber. You may experience disease flare (increased bone pain) and urinary retention during early treatment (usually resolves); dizziness, headache, lethargy, or faintness (use caution when driving or engaging in tasks that require alertness until response to drug is known); nausea or vomiting (small frequent meals or analgesics may help); hot flashes, flushing, or redness (cold clothes and cool environment may help); breast swelling or tenderness; or decreased libido. Report irregular or rapid heartbeat, palpitations, chest pain; inability to void or changes in urinary pattern; unresolved nausea or vomiting; numbness of extremities; breast swelling or pain, respiratory difficulty, or redness, swelling or pain at injection sites. **Pregnancy/breast-feeding precautions:** Inform prescriber if you are pregnant. Do not get pregnant. Consult prescriber for appropriate contraceptive use during and for a time following therapy. Do not breast-feed.

Geriatric Considerations: Leuprolide has the advantage of not increasing risk of atherosclerotic vascular disease, causing swelling of breasts, fluid retention, and thromboembolism as compared to estrogen therapy.

Pregnancy Risk Factor: X

Pregnancy Issues: Pregnancy must be excluded prior to the start of treatment. Although leuprolide usually inhibits ovulation and stops menstruation, contraception is not ensured and a nonhormonal contraceptive should be used. May cause fetal harm if administered to a pregnant woman.

Lactation: Excretion in breast milk unknown/contraindicated

Administration
I.M.:
Eligard®: Packaged in two syringes; one contains the Atrigel® polymer system, and the second contains leuprolide acetate powder; follow instructions for mixing; must be administered within 30 minutes of mixing

Lupron Depot®: Do not use needles smaller than 22 gauge; reconstitute only with diluent provided

Other: Viadur® implant: Requires surgical implantation (subcutaneous) and removal at 12-month intervals

Storage:
Lupron®: Store unopened vials of injection in refrigerator, vial in use can be kept at room temperature of ≤30°C (86°F) for several months with minimal loss of potency. Protect from light and store vial in carton until use. Do not freeze.

Eligard®: Store at 2°C to 8°C (36°F to 46°F). Allow to reach room temperature prior to using; once mixed, must be administered within 30 minutes.

Lupron Depot® may be stored at room temperature of 25°C, excursions permitted to 15°C to 30°C (59°F to 86°F). Upon reconstitution, the suspension does not contain a preservative and should be used immediately.

Viadur® may be stored at room temperature of 15°C to 30°C (59°F and 86°F).

Additional Information
Eligard® Atrigel®: A nongelatin-based, biodegradable, polymer matrix

Viadur®: Leuprolide acetate implant containing 72 mg of leuprolide acetate, equivalent to 65 mg leuprolide free base. One Viadur® implant delivers 120 mcg of leuprolide/day over 12 months.

♦ **Leuprolide Acetate** *see* Leuprolide *on page 876*
♦ **Leuprorelin Acetate** *see* Leuprolide *on page 876*
♦ **Leurocristine Sulfate** *see* VinCRIStine *on page 1564*
♦ **Leustatin®** *see* Cladribine *on page 340*

Levalbuterol (leve al BYOO ter ole)

U.S. Brand Names Xopenex®; Xopenex HFA™
Synonyms Levalbuterol Tartrate, Levalbuterol Hydrochloride; R-Albuterol
Generic Available No
Pharmacologic Category Beta$_2$-Adrenergic Agonist
Medication Safety Issues
Sound-alike/look-alike issues:
Xopenex® may be confused with Xanax®
Use Treatment or prevention of bronchospasm in adults and children with reversible obstructive airway disease
Mechanism of Action/Effect Relaxes bronchial smooth muscle by action on beta-2 receptors with little effect on heart rate
Contraindications Hypersensitivity to levalbuterol, albuterol, or any component of the formulation
Warnings/Precautions Optimize anti-inflammatory treatment before initiating maintenance treatment with levalbuterol. Do not use as a component of chronic therapy without an anti-inflammatory agent. Only the mildest form of asthma (Step 1 and/or exercise-induced) would not require concurrent use based upon asthma guidelines. Patient must be instructed to seek medical attention in cases where acute symptoms are not relieved or a previous level of response is diminished. The need to increase frequency of use may indicate deterioration of asthma, and treatment must not be delayed.

Use caution in patients with cardiovascular disease (arrhythmia or hypertension or CHF), convulsive disorders, diabetes, glaucoma, hyperthyroidism, or hypokalemia. Beta agonists may cause elevation in blood pressure, heart rate, and result in CNS stimulation/excitation. Beta$_2$ agonists may increase risk of arrhythmia, increase serum glucose, or decrease serum potassium.

Do not exceed recommended dose; serious adverse events including fatalities, have been associated with excessive use of inhaled sympathomimetics. Rarely, paradoxical bronchospasm may occur with use of inhaled bronchodilating agents; this should be distinguished from inadequate response. Use with caution during labor and delivery. Safety and efficacy have not been established in patients <4 years of age.

Drug Interactions
Decreased Effect: Beta-blockers (particularly nonselective agents) block the effect of levalbuterol. Digoxin levels may be decreased.
Increased Effect/Toxicity: May add to effects of medications which deplete potassium (eg, loop or thiazide diuretics). Cardiac effects of levalbuterol may be potentiated in patients receiving MAO inhibitors, tricyclic antidepressants, sympathomimetics (eg, amphetamine, dobutamine), or inhaled anesthetics (eg, enflurane).

Adverse Reactions
>10%:
Endocrine & metabolic: Serum glucose increased, serum potassium decreased
Respiratory: Viral infection (7% to 12%), rhinitis (3% to 11%)
>2% to 10%:
Central nervous system: Nervousness (3% to 10%), tremor (≤7%), anxiety (≤3%), dizziness (1% to 3%), migraine (≤3%), pain (1% to 3%)
Cardiovascular: Tachycardia (~3%)
Gastrointestinal: Dyspepsia (1% to 3%)
Neuromuscular & skeletal: Leg cramps (≤3%)
Respiratory: Asthma (9%), pharyngitis (8%), cough (1% to 4%), nasal edema (1% to 3%), sinusitis (1% to 4%)
Miscellaneous: Flu-like syndrome (1% to 4%), accidental injury (≤3%)
Overdosage/Toxicology Symptoms of overdose include tachycardia, tremor, hypertension, angina, and seizures. Hypokalemia also may occur. Cardiac arrest and death may be associated with abuse of beta-agonist bronchodilators. Treatment includes immediate discontinuation and symptomatic and supportive therapies. Cautious use of beta-adrenergic blocking agents may be considered in severe cases.

Pharmacodynamics/Kinetics
Onset of Action:
Aerosol: 5.5-10.2 minutes; Peak effect: ~77 minutes
Nebulization: 10-17 minutes (measured as a 15% increase in FEV$_1$); Peak effect: 1.5 hours
Duration of Action:
Aerosol: 3-4 hours (up to 6 hours in some patients)
Nebulization: 5-6 hours (up to 8 hours in some patients)
Absorption: A portion of inhaled dose is absorbed to systemic circulation
Time to Peak: Aerosol: 0.5 hours; Nebulization: 0.2 hours
Half-Life Elimination: 3.3-4 hours
Dosing
Adults: Bronchospasm:
Metered-dose inhalation: Aerosol: 1-2 puffs every 4-6 hours.
Nebulization: 0.63 mg 3 times/day at intervals of 6-8 hours; dosage may be increased to 1.25 mg 3 times/day with close monitoring for adverse effects. Most patients gain optimal benefit from regular use
(Continued)

Levalbuterol *(Continued)*

Elderly: Only a small number of patients have been studied. Although greater sensitivity of some elderly patients cannot be ruled out, no overall differences in safety or effectiveness were observed. An initial dose of 0.63 mg should be used in all patients >65 years of age.

Pediatrics: Bronchospasm:

Metered-dose inhalation: Aerosol: Children ≥4 years: Refer to adult dosing.

Nebulization:

Children 6-11 years: 0.31 mg 3 times/day (maximum dose: 0.63 mg 3 times/day)

Children >12 years: Refer to adult dosing.

Available Dosage Forms Note: Strength expressed as base

Aerosol, oral, as tartrate: 45 mcg/actuation (15 g) [200 doses; chlorofluorocarbon free]

Solution for nebulization, as hydrochloride: 0.31 mg/3 mL (24s); 0.63 mg/3 mL (24s); 1.25 mg/3 mL (24s)

Solution for nebulization, concentrate, as hydrochloride: 1.25 mg/0.5 mL (30s)

Monitoring and Teaching Issues

Physical Assessment: Assess effectiveness and interactions of other medications patient may be taking. Monitor therapeutic effectiveness (patient response and lab values), adverse reactions (eg, anaphylaxis or hypertension, first dose administered under supervision), or overdose. Patients with diabetes should monitor serum glucose on a regular basis (possibility of hyperglycemia). Assess knowledge/teach patient appropriate use (safe use of nebulizer), interventions to reduce side effects, and adverse reactions to report.

Monitoring Laboratory Tests: FEV_1 and/or peak expiratory flow rate, arterial blood gases (if condition warrants); serum potassium, serum glucose (in selected patients)

Patient Education: Use only when necessary or as prescribed; tolerance may develop with overuse. Do not administer more frequently than prescribed. First dose should not be used when you are alone. Avoid OTC medications without consulting prescriber. Maintain adequate hydration (2-3 L/day of fluids) unless instructed to restrict fluid intake. Stress or excessive exercising may exacerbate wheezing or bronchospasm (controlled breathing or relaxation techniques may help). If you have diabetes, you will need to monitor serum glucose levels closely until response is known; notify diabetic advisor if hyperglycemia occurs. You may experience tremor, anxiety, dizziness (use caution when driving or engaging in hazardous activities until response to drug is known); or temporarily upset stomach, nausea, or vomiting (small frequent meals, frequent mouth care, chewing gum, or sucking hard candy may help). Paradoxical bronchospasm can occur. Stop drug immediately and notify prescriber if any of the following occur: chest pain, tightness, palpitations; severe headache; respiratory difficulty; increased nervousness, restlessness, or trembling; muscle cramps or weakness; or seizures. Report unusual signs of flu or infection, leg or muscle cramps, unusual cough, persistent GI problems, vision changes, or other adverse effects. **Pregnancy/breast-feeding precautions:** Inform prescriber if you are or intend to become pregnant. Consult prescriber if breast-feeding.

Pregnancy Risk Factor: C

Pregnancy Issues: Teratogenic effects were not observed in animal studies; however, racemic albuterol was teratogenic in some species. There are no adequate and well-controlled studies in pregnant women. This drug should be used during pregnancy only if benefit exceeds risk. Use caution if needed for bronchospasm during labor and delivery; has potential to interfere with uterine contractions.

Lactation: Excretion in breast milk unknown/use caution

Breast-Feeding Issues: It is not known whether levalbuterol is excreted in human milk. Plasma levels following oral inhalation are low. Racemic albuterol was shown to be tumorigenic in animal studies.

Administration

Inhalation:

Aerosol: Shake well before use; prime with 4 test sprays prior to first use or if inhaler has not been use of more than 3 days. Clean actuator (mouthpiece) weekly.

Inhalation: Safety and efficacy were established when administered with the following nebulizers: PARI LC Jet™, PARI LC Plus™, as well as the following compressors: PARI Master®, Dura-Neb® 2000, and Dura-Neb® 3000. Concentrated solution should be diluted prior to use.

Reconstitution: Concentrated solution should be diluted with 2.5 mL NS prior to use.

Storage:

Aerosol: Store at 20°C to 25°C (68°F to 77°F); protect from freezing and direct sunlight. Store with mouthpiece down. Discard after 200 actuations.

Solution for nebulization: Store in protective foil pouch at room temperature of 20°C to 25°C (68°F to 77°F). Protect from light and excessive heat. Vials should be used within 2 weeks after opening protective pouch. Use within 1 week and protect from light if removed from pouch. Vials of concentrated solution should be used immediately after removing from protective pouch.

Related Information

Inhalant Agents *on page 1734*

♦ **Levalbuterol Tartrate, Levalbuterol Hydrochloride** *see* Levalbuterol *on page 879*

♦ **Levall 5.0** *see* Hydrocodone, Phenylephrine, and Guaifenesin *on page 760*

♦ **Levall G** *see* Guaifenesin and Pseudoephedrine *on page 733*

♦ **Levaquin®** *see* Levofloxacin *on page 888*

♦ **Levarterenol Bitartrate** *see* Norepinephrine *on page 1095*

♦ **Levbid®** *see* Hyoscyamine *on page 775*

Levetiracetam *(lee va tye RA se tam)*

U.S. Brand Names Keppra®

Generic Available No

Pharmacologic Category Anticonvulsant, Miscellaneous

Medication Safety Issues
Sound-alike/look-alike issues:
Potential for dispensing errors between Keppra® and Kaletra™ (lopinavir/ritonavir)

Use Indicated as adjunctive therapy in the treatment of partial onset seizures in adults with epilepsy

Unlabeled/Investigational Use Bipolar disorder; partial onset seizures in children with epilepsy

Mechanism of Action/Effect Precise mechanism has not been defined. Does not appear to bind receptors or increase second messengers currently known to be involved in inhibitory or excitatory neurotransmission. Anticonvulsant activity is related to protection from secondary generalization from focal seizure activity. May selectively prevent hypersynchronization of epileptiform activity, inhibiting propagation of seizure activity.

Contraindications Hypersensitivity to levetiracetam or any component of the formulation

Warnings/Precautions May cause CNS adverse events, including somnolence and fatigue (treated by discontinuation, reduction, or hospitalization) or coordination difficulty (usually treated by reduction). Behavioral abnormalities, such as psychosis, hallucinations, psychotic depression and other behavioral symptoms (agitation, anger, aggression, irritability, hostility, anxiety, apathy, emotional lability, depersonalization, and depression) have been treated by reduction of dose and in some cases hospitalization. Levetiracetam should be withdrawn gradually to minimize the potential of increased seizure frequency. There is a potential for dispensing errors between Keppra® and Kaletra™ (lopinavir/ritonavir); use caution when prescribing, dispensing, or administering. Use caution with renal impairment (dosage adjustment may be necessary).

Drug Interactions
Increased Effect/Toxicity: No interaction was observed in pharmacokinetic trials with other anticonvulsants, including phenytoin, carbamazepine, valproic acid, phenobarbital, lamotrigine, gabapentin, and primidone.

Nutritional/Ethanol Interactions
Ethanol: Avoid ethanol (may increase CNS depression).
Food: Food may delay, but does not affect the extent of absorption.

Adverse Reactions
>10%:
Central nervous system: Somnolence (15%), headache (14%)
Neuromuscular & skeletal: Weakness (15%)
Miscellaneous: Infection (13%)
<10%:
Cardiovascular: Chest pain
Central nervous system: Pain (7%), psychotic symptoms (1%), amnesia (2%), ataxia (3%), depression (4%), dizziness (9%), emotional lability (2%), nervousness (4%), vertigo (3%), agitation, anger, aggression, irritability, hostility (2%), anxiety (2%), apathy, depersonalization, confusion, convulsion, fever, insomnia, thinking abnormal
Dermatologic: Bruising, rash
Gastrointestinal: Anorexia (3%), abdominal pain, constipation, diarrhea, dyspepsia, gastroenteritis, gingivitis, nausea, vomiting, weight gain
Hematologic: Decreased erythrocyte counts (3%), decreased leukocytes (2% to 3%)
Neuromuscular & skeletal: Ataxia and other coordination difficulties (3%), paresthesia (2%), arthralgia, back pain, tremor
Ocular: Diplopia (2%), amblyopia, otitis media
Respiratory: Pharyngitis (6%), rhinitis (4%), cough (2%), sinusitis (2%), bronchitis
Miscellaneous: Flu-like symptoms

Overdosage/Toxicology Limited experience. Symptoms would be expected to include drowsiness, somnolence and ataxia. Treatment is symptomatic and supportive. Hemodialysis may be effective.

Pharmacodynamics/Kinetics
Onset of Action: Peak effect: 1 hour
Absorption: Rapid and complete
Bioavailability: 100%
Protein Binding: <10%
Half-Life Elimination: 6-8 hours
Metabolism: Not extensive; primarily by enzymatic hydrolysis; forms metabolites (inactive)
Excretion: Urine (66%)
Dialyzable: ~50% of pooled levetiracetam removed during standard 4-hour hemodialysis

Dosing
Adults & Elderly:
Partial onset seizures (adjunctive): Oral: Initial: 500 mg twice daily; additional dosing increments may be given (1000 mg/day additional every 2 weeks) to a maximum recommended daily dose of 3000 mg
Bipolar disorder (unlabeled use): Initial: 500 mg twice daily; if tolerated, increase to 500 mg twice daily; dose may be increased every 3 days until target dose of 3000 mg/day is reached; maximum: 4000 mg/day

Pediatrics:
Partial onset seizures: Oral:
Children 4-16 years (unlabeled use): 10-20 mg/kg/day in 2 divided doses; may increase weekly by 10-20 mg/kg, up to a maximum of 60 mg/kg
Children ≥16 years: Refer to adult dosing.
Bipolar disorder (unlabeled use): Oral: Children ≥16 years: Refer to adult dosing.

Renal Impairment:
Cl_{cr} >80 mL/minute: 500-1500 mg every 12 hours
Cl_{cr} 50-80 mL/minute: 500-1000 mg every 12 hours
Cl_{cr} 30-50 mL/minute: 250-750 mg every 12 hours
Cl_{cr} <30 mL/minute: 250-500 mg every 12 hours
End-stage renal disease patients using dialysis: 500-1000 mg every 24 hours; a supplemental dose of 250-500 mg following dialysis is recommended

(Continued)

Levetiracetam (Continued)

Hepatic Impairment: No adjustment necessary.

Available Dosage Forms

Solution, oral: 100 mg/mL (480 mL) [dye free; grape flavor]

Tablet: 250 mg, 500 mg, 750 mg

Monitoring and Teaching Issues

Physical Assessment: Assess effectiveness and interactions of other medications patient may be taking. Monitor therapeutic effectiveness, laboratory values, and adverse reactions at beginning of therapy and periodically with long-term use. Monitor for CNS depression (somnolence and fatigue), behavioral abnormalities (psychosis, hallucinations, psychotic depression), and other behavioral symptoms (agitation, anger, aggression, irritability, hostility, anxiety, apathy, emotional lability, depersonalization, and depression). Taper dosage slowly when discontinuing. Observe and teach seizure/safety precautions. Assess knowledge/teach patient appropriate use, interventions to reduce side effects, and adverse symptoms to report.

Patient Education: Take exactly as directed; do not increase dose or frequency or discontinue without consulting prescriber. While using this medication, do not use alcohol and other prescription or OTC medications (especially pain medications, sedatives, antihistamines, or hypnotics) without consulting prescriber. Maintain adequate hydration (2-3 L/day of fluids) unless instructed to restrict fluid intake. You may experience drowsiness, dizziness, or blurred vision (use caution when driving or engaging in tasks requiring alertness until response to drug is known); or nausea, vomiting, loss of appetite, or dry mouth (small frequent meals, frequent mouth care, chewing gum, or sucking lozenges may help). Wear identification of epileptic status and medications. Report CNS changes, mentation changes, or changes in cognition; muscle cramping, weakness, tremors, changes in gait; persistent GI symptoms (cramping, constipation, vomiting, anorexia); rash or skin irritations; unusual bruising or bleeding (mouth, urine, stool); or worsening of seizure activity or loss of seizure control. **Pregnancy/breast-feeding precautions:** Inform prescriber if you are or intend to become pregnant. Breast-feeding is not recommended.

Dietary Considerations: May be taken with or without food.

Pregnancy Risk Factor: C

Pregnancy Issues: Developmental toxicities were observed in animal studies. There are no adequate and well-controlled studies in pregnant women. Two registries are available for women exposed to levetiracetam during pregnancy:

Antiepileptic Drug Pregnancy Registry (888-233-2334 or http://www.mgh.harvard.edu/aed/)

Keppra® pregnancy registry (888-537-7734 or http://www.keppra.com)

Lactation: Enters breast milk/not recommended

Administration

Oral: Tablets may be crushed and placed in food if unable to swallow whole (bitter taste may be expected).

Storage: Store at 25°C (77°F).

Related Information

Anticonvulsants By Seizure Type *on page 1712*

♦ **Levitra®** *see* Vardenafil *on page 1552*

♦ **Levlen®** *see* Ethinyl Estradiol and Levonorgestrel *on page 585*

♦ **Levlite™** *see* Ethinyl Estradiol and Levonorgestrel *on page 585*

Levobupivacaine (LEE voe byoo PIV a kane)

U.S. Brand Names Chirocaine® [DSC]

Generic Available No

Pharmacologic Category Local Anesthetic

Use Production of local or regional anesthesia for surgery and obstetrics, and for postoperative pain management

Mechanism of Action/Effect Blocks both the initiation and transmission of nerve impulses

Contraindications Hypersensitivity to levobupivacaine, any component of the formulation, bupivacaine, or any local anesthetic of the amide type

Warnings/Precautions Local anesthetics should be administered only by clinicians familiar with the use of local anesthetic agents, procedures, and management of drug-related toxicity and other acute emergencies. Resuscitative equipment and medications should be readily available. Not for intravenous injection (cardiac arrest may occur) or obstetrical paracervical block. Risk of cardiac toxicity increases with higher concentration solutions. Avoid use of 0.75% solution with obstetrical patients. Use with caution in patients with hypotension, hypovolemia, heart block, hepatic impairment, cardiac impairment, or those receiving other local anesthetics or structurally-related agents.

Drug Interactions

Cytochrome P450 Effect: Substrate (minor) of CYP1A2, 3A4

Nutritional/Ethanol Interactions Herb/Nutraceutical: St John's wort may decrease levobupivacaine levels.

Adverse Reactions

>10%:

Cardiovascular: Hypotension (20% to 31%)

Central nervous system: Pain (postoperative) (7% to 18%), fever (7% to 17%)

Gastrointestinal: Nausea (12% to 21%), vomiting (8% to 14%)

Hematologic: Anemia (10% to 12%)

1% to 10%:

Cardiovascular: Abnormal ECG (3%), bradycardia (2%), tachycardia (2%), hypertension (1%)

Central nervous system: Pain (4% to 8%), headache (5% to 7%), dizziness (5% to 6%), hypoesthesia (3%), somnolence (1%), anxiety (1%), hypothermia (2%)

Dermatologic: Pruritus (4% to 9%), purpura (1%)

Endocrine & metabolic: Breast pain - female (1%)

Gastrointestinal: Constipation (3% to 7%), enlarged abdomen (3%), flatulence (2%), abdominal pain (2%), dyspepsia (2%), diarrhea (1%)

Genitourinary: Urinary incontinence (1%), urine flow decreased (1%), urinary tract infection (1%)

Hematologic: Leukocytosis (1%)

Local: Anesthesia (1%)

Neuromuscular & skeletal: Back pain (6%), rigors (3%), paresthesia (2%)

Ocular: Diplopia (3%)

Renal: Albuminuria (3%), hematuria (2%)

Respiratory: Cough (1%)

Miscellaneous: Fetal distress (5% to 10%), delayed delivery (6%), hemorrhage in pregnancy (2%), uterine abnormality (2%), increased wound drainage (1%)

Overdosage/Toxicology Related to local concentration or due to unintended intrathecal or intravenous injection. Symptoms may include restlessness, anxiety, incoherent speech, lightheadedness, numbness and tingling of the mouth and lips, metallic taste, tinnitus, dizziness, blurred vision, tremors, respiratory arrest, twitching, depression or drowsiness. In addition, cardiac toxicity, including AV block, bradycardia, arrhythmia, and hypotension may occur. Treatment is symptomatic.

Pharmacodynamics/Kinetics

Onset of Action: Epidural: 10-14 minutes

Duration of Action: Dose dependent: 1-8 hours

Absorption: Dependent on route of administration and dose

Time to Peak: Epidural: 30 minutes

Protein Binding: Plasma: >97%

Half-Life Elimination: 1.3 hours

Metabolism: Extensively hepatic via CYP3A4 and CYP1A2

Excretion: Urine (71%) and feces (24%) as metabolites

Dosing

Adults & Elderly: Note: Rapid injection of a large volume of local anesthetic solution should be avoided. Fractional (incremental) doses are recommended.

Guidelines (individual response varies): See table.

	Concentration	Volume	Dose	Motor Block
Surgical Anesthesia				
Epidural for surgery	0.5%-0.75%	10-20 mL	50-150 mg	Moderate to complete
Epidural for C-section	0.5%	20-30 mL	100-150 mg	Moderate to complete
Peripheral nerve	0.25%-0.5%	0.4 mL/kg (30 mL)	1-2 mg/kg (75-150 mg)	Moderate to complete
Ophthalmic	0.75%	5-15 mL	37.5-112.5 mg	Moderate to complete
Local infiltration	0.25%	60 mL	150 mg	Not applicable
Pain Management				
Levobupivacaine can be used epidurally with fentanyl or clonidine; dilutions for epidural administration should be made with preservative free 0.9% saline according to standard hospital procedures for sterility				
Labor analgesia (epidural bolus)	0.25%	10-20 mL	25-50 mg	Minimal to moderate
Postoperative pain (epidural infusion)	0.125%[1]-0.25%	4-10 mL/h	5-25 mg/h	Minimal to moderate

[1]0.125%: Adjunct therapy with fentanyl or clonidine.

Maximum dosage: Epidural doses up to 375 mg have been administered incrementally to patients during a surgical procedure.

Intraoperative block and postoperative pain: 695 mg in 24 hours

Postoperative epidural infusion over 24 hours: 570 mg

Single-fractionated injection for brachial plexus block: 300 mg

Available Dosage Forms [DSC] = Discontinued product

Injection, solution [preservative free]: 2.5 mg/mL (10 mL, 30 mL); 5 mg/mL (10 mL, 30 mL); 7.5 mg/mL (10 mL, 30 mL) [DSC]

Monitoring and Teaching Issues

Physical Assessment: Monitor for effectiveness of anesthesia according to purpose for use. Monitor closely during and after injection for symptoms of CNS, cardiac toxicity, or hypotension. Monitor for return of sensation. Use appropriate patient safety measures until full return of sensation. Teach patient adverse symptoms to report.

Patient Education: This medication is given to reduce sensation and pain. You will experience decreased sensation to pain, heat, or cold in the area and/or decreased muscle strength (depending on area of application). Until sensation returns, use caution to prevent injury (eg, avoid extremes of heat or cold to area, do not use sharp objects, avoid driving, climbing stairs, or sudden moves if muscle strength is affected). Immediately report chest pain or palpitations; increased restlessness, anxiety, dizziness or lightheadedness; sensation of sudden muscle weakness; swelling or tingling of mouth or lips; metallic taste; vision changes or hearing. **Breast-feeding precaution:** Consult prescriber if breast-feeding.

Pregnancy Risk Factor: B

Pregnancy Issues: Local anesthetics rapidly cross the placenta and may cause varying degrees of maternal, fetal, and neonatal toxicity. Close maternal and fetal monitoring (heart rate and electronic fetal monitoring advised) are required during obstetrical use.

Lactation: Excretion in breast milk unknown/use caution

Administration

Other: Isopropyl or ethyl alcohol are recommended to disinfect the surface of the vial. Disinfectants containing heavy metals should not be used for mucous membrane disinfection since they have been related to incidents of swelling and edema. Prior to administration, it is essential that aspiration for blood or cerebrospinal fluid (where applicable) be performed prior to injecting any local anesthetic, both before the original dosage and at all subsequent doses (to avoid intravascular or intrathecal injection). A negative aspiration does not ensure against intrathecal or intravascular injection. Rapid injection of a large

(Continued)

Levobupivacaine (Continued)

volume of local anesthetic solution should be avoided. Fractional (incremental) doses are recommended. Monitor patient during and after injection for symptoms of CNS or cardiac toxicity.

Compatibility: Stable in 0.9% NS USP. Stable for 24 hours in PVC bags at room temperature when diluted to 0.625-2.5 mg levobupivacaine per mL.

Incompatible with alkaline pH solutions (pH >8.5)

Storage: Store at room temperature (20°C to 25°C/68°F to 77°F). Disinfectants containing heavy metals should not be used for mucous membrane disinfection since they have been related to incidents of swelling and edema. Isopropyl or ethyl alcohol is recommended. Stability of solution in vial has been demonstrated following an autoclave cycle at 121°C for 15 minutes.

Levocabastine (LEE voe kab as teen)

U.S. Brand Names Livostin® [DSC]

Synonyms Levocabastine Hydrochloride

Generic Available No

Pharmacologic Category Antihistamine, H_1 Blocker, Ophthalmic

Medication Safety Issues

Sound-alike/look-alike issues:

Levocabastine may be confused with levobunolol, levocarnitine

Livostin® may be confused with lovastatin

Use Treatment of allergic conjunctivitis

Contraindications Hypersensitivity to levocabastine any component of product; use while soft contact lenses are being worn

Warnings/Precautions Safety and efficacy in children <12 years of age have not been established. Not for injection. Not for use in patients wearing soft contact lenses during treatment.

Adverse Reactions

>10%: Local: Transient burning, stinging, discomfort

1% to 10%:

Central nervous system: Headache, somnolence, fatigue

Dermatologic: Rash

Gastrointestinal: Xerostomia

Ocular: Blurred vision, eye pain, somnolence, red eyes, eyelid edema

Respiratory: Dyspnea

Pharmacodynamics/Kinetics

Absorption: Topical: Systemic

Dosing

Adults & Elderly: Allergic conjunctivitis: Ophthalmic: Instill 1 drop in affected eye(s) 4 times/day for up to 2 weeks

Pediatrics: Children ≥12 years: Refer to adult dosing.

Available Dosage Forms [DSC] = Discontinued product

Suspension, ophthalmic: 0.05% (5 mL, 10 mL) [contains benzalkonium chloride] [DSC]

Monitoring and Teaching Issues

Physical Assessment: Assess potential for interactions with other prescriptions, OTC medications, or herbal products patient may be taking. Assess therapeutic response and adverse effects. Teach patient proper use, side effects/appropriate interventions, and symptoms to report.

Patient Education: For use in eyes only. Shake well before using. Do not let tip of applicator touch eye; do not contaminate tip of applicator (may cause eye infection, eye damage, or vision loss). Do not wear contact lenses during treatment. This medication may cause drowsiness in some patients. **Pregnancy precaution:** Inform prescriber if you are pregnant.

Pregnancy Risk Factor: C

♦ **Levocabastine Hydrochloride** see Levocabastine on page 884

Levocarnitine (lee voe KAR ni teen)

U.S. Brand Names Carnitor®

Synonyms L-Carnitine

Generic Available Yes

Pharmacologic Category Dietary Supplement

Medication Safety Issues

Sound-alike/look-alike issues:

Levocarnitine may be confused with levocabastine

Use Orphan drug:

Oral: Primary systemic carnitine deficiency; acute and chronic treatment of patients with an inborn error of metabolism which results in secondary carnitine deficiency

I.V.: Acute and chronic treatment of patients with an inborn error of metabolism which results in secondary carnitine deficiency; prevention and treatment of carnitine deficiency in patients with end-stage renal disease (ESRD) who are undergoing hemodialysis.

Mechanism of Action/Effect Carnitine is a naturally occurring metabolic compound which facilitates energy production

Warnings/Precautions Caution in patients with seizure disorders or in those at risk of seizures (CNS mass or medications which may lower seizure threshold). Both new-onset seizure activity as well as an increased frequency of seizures has been observed. Safety and efficacy of oral carnitine have not been established in ESRD. Chronic administration of high oral doses to patients with severely compromised renal function or ESRD patients on dialysis may result in accumulation of metabolites.

Lab Interactions Normal carnitine levels are 40-50 µmol/L; levels should be maintained on therapy between 35-60 µmol/L. therapy between 35-60 µmol/L.

Adverse Reactions Frequencies noted with I.V. therapy (hemodialysis patients):
Cardiovascular: Hypertension (18% to 21%), peripheral edema (3% to 6%)
Central nervous system: Dizziness (10% to 18%), fever (5% to 12%), paresthesia (3% to 12%), depression (5% to 6%)
Endocrine & metabolic: Hypercalcemia (6% to 15%)
Gastrointestinal: Diarrhea (9% to 35%), abdominal pain (5% to 21%), vomiting (9% to 21%), nausea (5% to 12%)
Neuromuscular & skeletal: Weakness (9% to 12%)
Miscellaneous: Allergic reaction (2% to 6%)

Overdosage/Toxicology No reports of overdose. Easily removed by dialysis.

Pharmacodynamics/Kinetics
  Bioavailability: Tablet/solution: 15% to 16%
  Time to Peak: Tablet/solution: 3.3 hours
  Half-Life Elimination: 17.4 hours
  Metabolism: Hepatic (limited with moderate renal impairment), to trimethylamine (TMA) and trimethylamine N-oxide (TMAO)
  Excretion: Urine (4% to 9% as unchanged drug); metabolites also eliminated in urine

Dosing
  Adults & Elderly:
    Carnitine supplementation: Oral: 990 mg (oral tablets) 2-3 times/day or 1-3 g/day (oral solution)
    Metabolic disorders: I.V.: 50 mg/kg as a slow 2- to 3-minute I.V. bolus or by I.V. infusion
    Severe metabolic crisis: I.V.:
      Initial: A loading dose of 50 mg/kg over 2-3 minutes followed by an equivalent dose over the following 24 hours administered as every 3 hours or every 4 hours (never less than every 6 hours either by infusion or by intravenous injection)
      Subsequent dosing: All subsequent daily doses are recommended to be in the range of 50 mg/kg or as therapy may require.
      Maximum: The highest dose administered has been 300 mg/kg.
      It is recommended that a plasma carnitine concentration be obtained prior to beginning parenteral therapy accompanied by weekly and monthly monitoring.
    ESRD patients on hemodialysis: I.V.:
      Predialysis levocarnitine concentrations below normal (40-50 μmol/L): 10-20 mg/kg dry body weight as a slow 2- to 3-minute bolus after each dialysis session
      Adjustment: Dosage adjustments should be guided by predialysis trough levocarnitine concentrations and downward dose adjustments (to 5 mg/kg after dialysis) may be made as early as every 3rd or 4th week of therapy.
  Pediatrics:
    Carnitine supplementation:
      Oral: Infants/Children: Initial: 50 mg/kg/day; titrate to 50-100 mg/kg/day in divided doses with a maximum dose of 3 g/day
      I.V.: Refer to adult dosing.

Available Dosage Forms
  Capsule: 250 mg
  Injection, solution (Carnitor®): 200 mg/mL (5 mL)
  Solution, oral (Carnitor®): 100 mg/mL (118 mL) [cherry flavor]
  Tablet: 500 mg
  Carnitor®: 330 mg

Monitoring and Teaching Issues
  Physical Assessment: Monitor therapeutic effectiveness according to rational for therapy and adverse reactions (eg, CNS, hypertension). **Oral:** Monitor therapeutic effectiveness and assess severity. Assess knowledge and teach patient appropriate use, interventions to reduce side effects, and adverse reactions to report.
  Monitoring Laboratory Tests: Plasma concentrations should be obtained prior to beginning parenteral therapy, and should be monitored weekly to monthly. In metabolic disorders: monitor blood chemistry and plasma carnitine levels (maintain between 35-60 μmol/L). In ESRD patients on dialysis: Plasma levels below the normal range should prompt initiation of therapy. Monitor predialysis (trough) plasma carnitine levels.
  Patient Education: I.V.: Report immediately any dizziness, loss of feeling, acute headache, tremors, or nausea.

  Oral: Take exactly as directed; do not alter dose or frequency except as directed by prescriber. Dissolve solution in any liquid and drink with or following meals. The oral solution should be consumed slowly and spaced evenly throughout the day to improve tolerance. You may experience abdominal pain, nausea, or vomiting (small frequent meals, chewing gum, or sucking hard candy); diarrhea (yogurt, boiled milk, or buttermilk may help); or dizziness (use caution driving or engaging in hazardous activities until response to drug is known). Report acute headache, chest pain, tremors, or visual changes; muscle or skeletal weakness; skin rash; swelling of extremities; or other adverse effects.
  Breast-feeding precaution: Consult prescriber if breast-feeding.

Pregnancy Risk Factor: B
Lactation: Excretion in breast milk unknown/use caution
Breast-Feeding Issues: In breast-feeding women, use must be weighed against the potential exposure of the infant to increased carnitine intake. Use caution in breast-feeding women.

Administration
  Oral: Solution may be dissolved in either drink or liquid food. The oral solution should be consumed slowly and spaced evenly throughout the day to improve tolerance. Doses should be spaced every 3 to 4 hours throughout the day, preferably during or following meals.
  I.V.: Hemodialysis patients: Injection should be given over 2-3 minutes into the venous return line after each dialysis session.
  Storage: Store at 25°C (77°F). Compatible at concentrations between 0.5-8 mg/mL in 0.9% sodium chloride or lactated Ringer's solution. Stable in PVC bags for 24 hours.
(Continued)

Levocarnitine *(Continued)*

Additional Information Although supplemental carnitine has been shown to increase carnitine concentrations, effects on the signs and symptoms of carnitine deficiency have not been determined.

Levodopa and Carbidopa *(lee voe DOE pa & kar bi DOE pa)*

U.S. Brand Names Parcopa™; Sinemet®; Sinemet® CR

Synonyms Carbidopa and Levodopa

Generic Available Yes: Excludes orally-disintegrating tablet

Pharmacologic Category Anti-Parkinson's Agent, Dopamine Agonist

Use Idiopathic Parkinson's disease; postencephalitic parkinsonism; symptomatic parkinsonism

Unlabeled/Investigational Use Restless leg syndrome

Mechanism of Action/Effect Parkinson's symptoms are due to a lack of striatal dopamine; levodopa circulates in the plasma to the blood-brain-barrier (BBB), where it crosses, to be converted by striatal enzymes to dopamine; carbidopa inhibits the peripheral plasma breakdown of levodopa by inhibiting its decarboxylation, and thereby increases available levodopa at the BBB

Contraindications Hypersensitivity to levodopa, carbidopa, or any component of the formulation; narrow-angle glaucoma; use of MAO inhibitors within prior 14 days (however, may be administered concomitantly with the manufacturer's recommended dose of an MAO inhibitor with selectivity for MAO type B); history of melanoma or undiagnosed skin lesions

Warnings/Precautions Use with caution in patients with history of cardiovascular disease (including myocardial infarction and arrhythmias); pulmonary diseases such as asthma, psychosis, wide-angle glaucoma, peptic ulcer disease; as well as in renal, hepatic, or endocrine disease. Sudden discontinuation of levodopa may cause a worsening of Parkinson's disease. Elderly may be more sensitive to CNS effects of levodopa. May cause or exacerbate dyskinesias. May cause orthostatic hypotension; Parkinson's disease patients appear to have an impaired capacity to respond to a postural challenge; use with caution in patients at risk of hypotension (such as those receiving antihypertensive drugs) or where transient hypotensive episodes would be poorly tolerated (cardiovascular disease or cerebrovascular disease). Observe patients closely for development of depression with concomitant suicidal tendencies. Has been associated with a syndrome resembling neuroleptic malignant syndrome on withdrawal or significant dosage reduction after long-term use. Protein in the diet should be distributed throughout the day to avoid fluctuations in levodopa absorption.

Drug Interactions

Decreased Effect: Antipsychotics, benzodiazepines, L-methionine, phenytoin, pyridoxine, spiramycin, and tacrine may inhibit the antiparkinsonian effects of levodopa; monitor for reduced effect. Antipsychotics may inhibit the antiparkinsonian effects of levodopa via dopamine receptor blockade. Use antipsychotics with low dopamine blockade (clozapine, olanzapine, quetiapine). High-protein diets may inhibit levodopa's efficacy; avoid high protein foods. Iron binds levodopa and reduces its bioavailability; separate doses of iron and levodopa.

Increased Effect/Toxicity: Concurrent use of levodopa with nonselective MAO inhibitors may result in hypertensive reactions via an increased storage and release of dopamine, norepinephrine, or both. Use with carbidopa to minimize reactions if combination is necessary; otherwise avoid combination.

Nutritional/Ethanol Interactions

Ethanol: Avoid ethanol (due to CNS depression).

Food: Avoid high protein diets and high intakes of vitamin B_6.

Herb/Nutraceutical: Avoid kava kava (may decrease effects). Pyridoxine in doses >10-25 mg (for levodopa alone) or higher doses >200 mg/day (for levodopa/carbidopa) may decrease efficacy.

Lab Interactions False-positive reaction for urinary glucose with Clinitest®; false-negative reaction using Clinistix®; false-positive urine ketones with Acetest®, Ketostix®, Labstix®

Adverse Reactions Frequency not defined.

Cardiovascular: Orthostatic hypotension, arrhythmia, chest pain, hypertension, syncope, palpitation, phlebitis

Central nervous system: Dizziness, anxiety, confusion, nightmares, headache, hallucinations, on-off phenomenon, decreased mental acuity, memory impairment, disorientation, delusions, euphoria, agitation, somnolence, insomnia, gait abnormalities, nervousness, ataxia, EPS, falling, psychosis, peripheral neuropathy, seizure (causal relationship not established)

Dermatologic: Rash, alopecia, malignant melanoma, hypersensitivity (angioedema, urticaria, pruritus, bullous lesions, Henoch-Schönlein purpura)

Endocrine & metabolic: Increased libido

Gastrointestinal: Anorexia, nausea, vomiting, constipation, GI bleeding, duodenal ulcer, diarrhea, dyspepsia, taste alterations, sialorrhea, heartburn

Genitourinary: Discoloration of urine, urinary frequency

Hematologic: Hemolytic anemia, agranulocytosis, thrombocytopenia, leukopenia; decreased hemoglobin and hematocrit; abnormalities in AST and ALT, LDH, bilirubin, BUN, Coombs' test

Neuromuscular & skeletal: Choreiform and involuntary movements, paresthesia, bone pain, shoulder pain, muscle cramps, weakness

Ocular: Blepharospasm, oculogyric crises (may be associated with acute dystonic reactions)

Renal: Difficult urination

Respiratory: Dyspnea, cough

Miscellaneous: Hiccups, discoloration of sweat, diaphoresis (increased)

Overdosage/Toxicology Symptoms of overdose include palpitations, arrhythmias, spasms; may cause hypertension or hypotension. Treatment is supportive. ECG monitoring is warranted. May precipitate a variety of arrhythmias.

Pharmacodynamics/Kinetics
Pharmacokinetic Note: See individual agents.

Dosing

Adults:

Parkinson's disease: Oral: Initial:

Immediate release tablet:

Initial: Carbidopa 25 mg/levodopa 100 mg 3 times/day

Dosage adjustment: Alternate tablet strengths may be substituted according to individual carbidopa/levodopa requirements. Increase by 1 tablet every other day as necessary, except when using the carbidopa 25 mg/levodopa 250 mg tablets where increases should be made using $1/_2$-1 tablet every 1-2 days. Use of more than 1 dosage strength or dosing 4 times/day may be required (maximum: 8 tablets of any strength/day or 200 mg of carbidopa and 2000 mg of levodopa)

Sustained release tablet:

Initial: Carbidopa 50 mg/levodopa 200 mg 2 times/day, at intervals not <6 hours

Dosage adjustment: May adjust every 3 days; intervals should be between 4-8 hours during the waking day (maximum: 8 tablets/day)

Restless leg syndrome (unlabeled use): Oral: Carbidopa 25 mg/levodopa 100 mg given 30-60 minutes before bedtime; may repeat dose once

Elderly: Initial dose: 25/100 twice daily, increase as necessary. Sinemet® CR may be used as initial therapy.

Available Dosage Forms

Tablet immediate release (Sinemet®):

10/100: Carbidopa 10 mg and levodopa 100 mg

25/100: Carbidopa 25 mg and levodopa 100 mg

25/250: Carbidopa 25 mg and levodopa 250 mg

Tablet, immediate release, orally-disintegrating (Parcopa™):

10/100: Carbidopa 10 mg and levodopa 100 mg [contains phenylalanine 3.4 mg/tablet; mint flavor]

25/100: Carbidopa 25 mg and levodopa 100 mg [contains phenylalanine 3.4 mg/tablet; mint flavor]

25/250: Carbidopa 25 mg and levodopa 250 mg [contains phenylalanine 8.4 mg/tablet; mint flavor]

Tablet, sustained release (Sinemet® CR):

Carbidopa 25 mg and levodopa 100 mg

Carbidopa 50 mg and levodopa 200 mg

Monitoring and Teaching Issues

Physical Assessment: Assess effectiveness and interactions of other medications patient may be taking. Monitor therapeutic effectiveness and adverse reactions (including levodopa toxicity) at beginning of therapy and periodically throughout therapy. Assess knowledge/teach patient appropriate use, interventions to reduce side effects, and adverse symptoms to report.

Patient Education: Take exactly as directed; do not change dosage or discontinue without consulting prescriber. Do not crush sustained release form. Therapeutic effects may take several weeks or months to achieve and you may need frequent monitoring during first weeks of therapy. Take with meals if GI upset occurs, before meals if dry mouth occurs, after eating if drooling or if nausea occurs. Take at the same time each day. Maintain adequate hydration (2-3 L/day of fluids) unless instructed to restrict fluid intake; void before taking medication. Do not use alcohol and prescription or OTC sedatives or CNS depressants without consulting prescriber. Urine or perspiration may appear darker. You may experience drowsiness, dizziness, confusion, or vision changes (use caution when driving, climbing stairs, or engaging in tasks requiring alertness until response to drug is known); orthostatic hypotension (use caution when changing position - rising to standing from sitting or lying); increased susceptibility to heat stroke, decreased perspiration (use caution in hot weather - maintain adequate fluids and reduce exercise activity); constipation (increased exercise, fluids, fruit, or fiber may help); dry skin or nasal passages (consult prescriber for appropriate relief); or nausea, vomiting, loss of appetite, or stomach discomfort (small frequent meals, frequent mouth care, chewing gum, or sucking lozenges may help). Report unresolved constipation or vomiting; chest pain or irregular heartbeat; respiratory difficulty; acute headache or dizziness; CNS changes (hallucination, loss of memory, nervousness, etc); painful or difficult urination; abdominal pain or blood in stool; increased muscle spasticity or rigidity; skin rash; or significant worsening of condition. **Pregnancy/breast-feeding precautions:** Inform prescriber if you are or intend to become pregnant. Consult prescriber if breast-feeding.

Dietary Considerations: Levodopa peak serum concentrations may be decreased if taken with food. High protein diets (>2 g/kg) may decrease the efficacy of levodopa via competition with amino acids in crossing the blood-brain barrier.

Parcopa™: Contains phenylalanine 3.4 mg per 10/100 mg and 25/100 mg strengths; phenylalanine 8.4 mg in 25/250 mg strength

Geriatric Considerations: The elderly may be more sensitive to the CNS effects of levodopa.

Pregnancy Risk Factor: C

Lactation: Excretion in breast milk unknown/use caution

Administration

Oral: Space doses evenly over the waking hours. Give with meals to decrease GI upset. Sustained release product should not be crushed. Orally-disintegrating tablets do not require water; the tablet should disintegrate on the tongue's surface before swallowing.

Storage: Store at 20°C to 25°C (68°F to 77°F); excursions are allowed between 15°C to 30°C (59°F to 86°F). Protect from light and moisture.

Additional Information 50-100 mg/day of carbidopa is needed to block the peripheral conversion of levodopa to dopamine. "On-off" (a clinical syndrome characterized by sudden periods of drug activity/inactivity), can be managed by giving smaller, more frequent doses of Sinemet® or adding a dopamine agonist or selegiline; when adding a new agent, doses of Sinemet® can usually be decreased. Protein in the diet should be distributed throughout the (Continued)

Levodopa and Carbidopa *(Continued)*

day to avoid fluctuations in levodopa absorption. Levodopa is the drug of choice when rigidity is the predominant presenting symptom.

Conversion from levodopa to carbidopa/levodopa: **Note:** Levodopa must be discontinued at least 12 hours prior to initiation of levodopa/carbidopa:

Initial dose: Levodopa portion of carbidopa/levodopa should be at least 25% of previous levodopa therapy.

Levodopa <1500 mg/day: Sinemet® or Parcopa™ (levodopa 25 mg/carbidopa 100 mg) 3-4 times/day

Levodopa ≥1500 mg/day: Sinemet® or Parcopa™ (levodopa 25 mg/carbidopa 250 mg) 3-4 times/day

Conversion from immediate release carbidopa/levodopa (Sinemet® or Parcopa™) to Sinemet® CR (50/200):

Sinemet® or Parcopa™ [total daily dose of levodopa]/Sinemet® CR:

Sinemet® or Parcopa™ (levodopa 300-400 mg/day): Sinemet® CR (50/200) 1 tablet twice daily

Sinemet® or Parcopa™ (levodopa 500-600 mg/day): Sinemet® CR (50/200) 1 1/2 tablets twice daily or 1 tablet 3 times/day

Sinemet® or Parcopa™ (levodopa 700-800 mg/day): Sinemet® CR (50/200) 4 tablets in 3 or more divided doses

Sinemet® or Parcopa™ (levodopa 900-1000 mg/day): Sinemet® CR (50/200) 5 tablets in 3 or more divided doses

Intervals between doses of Sinemet® CR should be 4-8 hours while awake; when divided doses are not equal, smaller doses should be given toward the end of the day,

Levodopa, Carbidopa, and Entacapone
(lee voe DOE pa, kar bi DOE pa, & en TA ka pone)

U.S. Brand Names Stalevo™

Synonyms Carbidopa, Levodopa, and Entacapone; Entacapone, Carbidopa, and Levodopa

Generic Available No

Pharmacologic Category Anti-Parkinson's Agent, COMT Inhibitor; Anti-Parkinson's Agent, Dopamine Agonist

Use Treatment of idiopathic Parkinson's disease

Dosing

Adults & Elderly:

Note: All strengths of Stalevo™ contain a carbidopa/levodopa ratio of 1:4 plus entacapone 200 mg.

Parkinson's disease: Oral: Dose should be individualized based on therapeutic response; doses may be adjusted by changing strength or adjusting interval. Fractionated doses are not recommended and only 1 tablet should be given at each dosing interval; maximum dose: 8 tablets/day (equivalent to entacapone 1600 mg/day)

Patients previously treated with carbidopa/levodopa immediate release tablets (ratio of 1:4):

With current entacapone therapy: May switch directly to corresponding strength of combination tablet. No data available on transferring patients from controlled release preparations or products with a 1:10 ratio of carbidopa/levodopa.

Without entacapone therapy:

If current levodopa dose is >600 mg/day: Levodopa dose reduction may be required when adding entacapone to therapy; therefore, titrate dose using individual products first (carbidopa/levodopa immediate release with a ratio of 1:4 plus entacapone 200 mg); then transfer to combination product once stabilized.

If current levodopa dose is <600 mg without dyskinesias: May transfer to corresponding dose of combination product; monitor, dose reduction of levodopa may be required.

Renal Impairment: Use caution with severe renal impairment; specific dosing recommendations not available.

Hepatic Impairment: Use with caution; specific dosing recommendations not available.

Available Dosage Forms

Tablet [film coated]:

50: Carbidopa 12.5 mg, levodopa 50 mg, and entacapone 200 mg

100: Carbidopa 25 mg, levodopa 100 mg, and entacapone 200 mg

150: Carbidopa 37.5 mg, levodopa 150 mg, and entacapone 200 mg

Monitoring and Teaching Issues

Physical Assessment: See individual agents.

Patient Education: See individual agents. **Pregnancy/breast-feeding precautions:** Inform prescriber if you are or intend to become pregnant. Consult prescriber if breast-feeding.

Pregnancy Risk Factor: C

Lactation: Excretion in breast milk unknown/use caution

Related Information

Entacapone *on page 523*

♦ **Levo-Dromoran®** *see Levorphanol on page 893*

Levofloxacin *(lee voe FLOKS a sin)*

U.S. Brand Names Iquix®; Levaquin®; Quixin™

Generic Available No

Pharmacologic Category Antibiotic, Quinolone

Use

Systemic: Treatment of mild, moderate, or severe infections caused by susceptible organisms. Includes the treatment of community-acquired pneumonia, including multidrug resistant strains of *S. pneumoniae* (MDRSP); nosocomial pneumonia; chronic bronchitis (acute bacterial exacerbation); acute maxillary sinusitis; urinary tract infection (uncompli-cated or complicated), including acute pyelonephritis caused by *E. coli*; prostatitis (chronic bacterial); skin or skin structure infections (uncomplicated or complicated); prevention of inhalational anthrax (postexposure)

Ophthalmic: Treatment of bacterial conjunctivitis caused by susceptible organisms (Quixin™ 0.5% ophthalmic solution); treatment of corneal ulcer caused by susceptible organisms (Iquix® 1.5% ophthalmic solution)

Mechanism of Action/Effect Levofloxacin, a fluorinated quinolone, is a pyridine carboxylic acid derivative which exerts a broad spectrum bactericidal effect. It inhibits DNA gyrase inhibitor, an essential bacterial enzyme that maintains the superhelical structure of DNA. DNA gyrase is required for DNA replication and transcription, DNA repair, recombination, and transposition within the bacteria.

Contraindications Hypersensitivity to levofloxacin, any component of the formulation, or other quinolones

Warnings/Precautions Systemic: Not recommended in children <18 years of age; CNS stimulation may occur (tremor, restlessness, confusion, and very rarely hallucinations or seizures); use with caution in patients with known or suspected CNS disorders or renal dysfunction; use caution to avoid possible photosensitivity reactions during and for several days following fluoroquinolone therapy

Rare cases of torsade de pointes have been reported in patients receiving levofloxacin. Risk may be minimized by avoiding use in patients with known prolongation of QT interval, bradycardia, hypokalemia, hypomagnesemia, cardiomyopathy, or in those receiving concur-rent therapy with Class Ia or Class III antiarrhythmics.

Severe hypersensitivity reactions, including anaphylaxis, have occurred with quinolone therapy. If an allergic reaction occurs (itching, urticaria, dyspnea or facial edema, loss of consciousness, tingling, cardiovascular collapse), discontinue drug immediately. Prolonged use may result in superinfection; pseudomembranous colitis may occur and should be considered in all patients who present with diarrhea. Tendon inflammation and/or rupture has been reported; risk may be increased with concurrent corticosteroids, particularly in the elderly. Discontinue at first sign of tendon inflammation or pain. Peripheral neuropathies have been linked to levofloxacin use; discontinue if numbness, tingling, or weakness develops. Quinolones may exacerbate myasthenia gravis.

Ophthalmic solution: For topical use only. Do not inject subconjunctivally or introduce into anterior chamber of the eye. Contact lenses should not be worn during treatment for bacterial conjunctivitis. Safety and efficacy in children <1 year of age (Quixin™) or <6 years of age (Iquix®) have not been established. **Note:** Indications for ophthalmic solutions are product concentration-specific and should not be used interchangeably.

Drug Interactions

Decreased Effect: Concurrent administration of metal cations, including most antacids, oral electrolyte supplements, quinapril, sucralfate, and some didanosine formulations (chewable/buffered tablets and pediatric powder for oral suspension), may decrease quinolone levels; separate doses.

Increased Effect/Toxicity: Levofloxacin may increase the effects/toxicity of glyburide and warfarin. Concomitant use with corticosteroids may increase the risk of tendon rupture. Concomitant use with other QT_c-prolonging agents (eg, Class Ia and Class III antiar-rhythmics, erythromycin, cisapride, antipsychotics, and cyclic antidepressants) may result in arrhythmias, such as torsade de pointes. Probenecid may increase levofloxacin levels.

Adverse Reactions

Central nervous system: Dizziness, fever, headache, insomnia

Gastrointestinal: Abdominal pain, constipation, diarrhea, dyspepsia, nausea, vomiting

Ocular (with ophthalmic solution use): Decreased vision (transient), foreign body sensation, transient ocular burning, ocular pain or discomfort, photophobia

Respiratory: Dyspnea, pharyngitis

Overdosage/Toxicology

Symptoms of overdose include acute renal failure, seizures

Treatment should include GI decontamination and supportive care; not removed by perito-neal or hemodialysis

Pharmacodynamics/Kinetics

Absorption: Rapid and complete

Bioavailability: 99%

Time to Peak: 1-2 hours

Protein Binding: 50%

Half-Life Elimination: 6-8 hours

Metabolism: Minimally hepatic

Excretion: Primarily urine (as unchanged drug)

Dosing

Adults & Elderly: Note: Sequential therapy (intravenous to oral) may be instituted based on prescriber's discretion.

Chronic bronchitis (acute bacterial exacerbation): Oral, I.V.: 500 mg every 24 hours for at least 7 days

Inhalational anthrax: 500 mg every 24 hours for 60 days, beginning as soon as possible after exposure

Maxillary sinusitis (acute): Oral, I.V.: 500 mg every 24 hours for 10-14 days

Pneumonia: Oral, I.V.:

Community-acquired: 500 mg every 24 hours for 7-14 days or 750 mg every 24 hours for 5 days (efficacy of 5-day regimen for MDRSP not established)

Nosocomial: 750 mg every 24 hours for 7-14 days

Prostatitis (chronic bacterial): Oral, I.V.: 500 mg every 24 hours for 28 days

Skin infections: Oral, I.V.:

Uncomplicated: 500 mg every 24 hours for 7-10 days

Complicated: 750 mg every 24 hours for 7-14 days

(Continued)

Levofloxacin *(Continued)*

Urinary tract infections: Oral, I.V.:
Uncomplicated: 250 mg once daily for 3 days
Complicated, including acute pyelonephritis: 250 mg every 24 hours for 10 days

Bacterial conjunctivitis: Ophthalmic (0.5% ophthalmic solution):
Treatment day 1 and day 2: Instill 1-2 drops into affected eye(s) every 2 hours while awake, up to 8 times/day
Treatment day 3 through day 7: Instill 1-2 drops into affected eye(s) every 4 hours while awake, up to 4 times/day

Corneal ulceration: Ophthalmic (1.5% ophthalmic solution):
Treatment day 1 through day 3: Instill 1-2 drops into affected eye(s) every 30 minutes to 2 hours while awake and ~4-6 hours after retiring.
Treatment day 4 to treatment completion: Instill 1-2 drops into affected eye(s) every 1-4 hours while awake.

Pediatrics: Not approved for systemic use in children.
Conjunctivitis (bacterial): Ophthalmic: Children ≥1 year: Refer to adult dosing.
Corneal ulceration: Ophthalmic: Children ≥6 years: Refer to adult dosing.

Renal Impairment: Administer first dose as indicated in patients with normal renal function, then adjust dose as follows:

Chronic bronchitis, acute maxillary sinusitis, uncomplicated skin infection, community-acquired pneumonia, chronic bacterial prostatitis, or inhalational anthrax:
Cl_{cr} 20-49 mL/minute: 250 mg every 24 hours
Cl_{cr} 10-19 mL/minute: 250 mg every 48 hours
Hemodialysis/CAPD: 250 mg every 48 hours
Uncomplicated UTI: No dosage adjustment required
Complicated UTI, acute pyelonephritis: Cl_{cr} 10-19 mL/minute: 250 mg every 48 hours
Complicated skin infection, community-acquired pneumonia, or nosocomial pneumonia:
Cl_{cr} 20-49 mL/minute: Administer 750 mg every 48 hours
Cl_{cr} 10-19 mL/minute: Administer 500 mg every 48 hours
Hemodialysis/CAPD: 250 mg every 48 hours

Available Dosage Forms

Infusion [premixed in D_5W] (Levaquin®): 250 mg (50 mL); 500 mg (100 mL); 750 mg (150 mL)
Injection, solution [preservative free] (Levaquin®): 25 mg/mL (20 mL, 30 mL)
Solution, ophthalmic:
Iquix®: 1.5% (5 mL)
Quixin™: 0.5% (5 mL) [contains benzalkonium chloride]
Solution, oral (Levaquin®): 25 mg/mL (480 mL) [contains benzyl alcohol]
Tablet (Levaquin®): 250 mg, 500 mg, 750 mg
Levaquin® Leva-Pak: 750 mg (5s)

Monitoring and Teaching Issues

Physical Assessment: Assess results of culture and sensitivity tests and patient's allergy history before initiating therapy. Use caution with known CNS disorders or renal impairment (see Warnings/Precautions for use cautions). Assess potential for interactions with other prescriptions, OTC medications, or herbal products patient may be taking (eg, increased risk of tendon rupture or arrhythmias; see Drug Interactions). See Administration for infusion specifics; if an allergic reaction occurs (itching, urticaria, dyspnea or facial edema, loss of consciousness, tingling, cardiovascular collapse), drug should be discontinued immediately and prescriber notified. Assess results of laboratory tests, therapeutic effectiveness (resolution of infection), and adverse reactions regularly during therapy (eg, hypersensitivity reactions, diarrhea, opportunistic infection, tendon rupture; see Adverse Reactions). Teach patient proper use (according to formulation), possible side effects/appropriate interventions, and adverse symptoms to report (see Patient Education).

Monitoring Laboratory Tests: Perform culture and sensitivity studies prior to initiating drug therapy. Monitor CBC periodically during therapy. Monitor renal or hepatic function if therapy is prolonged.

Patient Education: Do not take any new medication during therapy unless approved by prescriber. If administered by infusion, report immediately any chest or back pain, tightness in chest, difficulty swallowing, swelling of face or mouth, or redness, swelling or pain at infusion site. **Pregnancy/breast-feeding precautions:** Inform prescriber if you are or intend to become pregnant. Breast-feeding is not recommended.

Oral: Take exactly as directed; at least 1 hour before or 2 hours after antacids or other drug products containing calcium, iron, or zinc. Take entire prescription even if feeling better. Maintain adequate hydration (2-3 L/day of fluids) unless advised by prescriber to restrict fluid intake. May cause dizziness, lightheadedness, or confusion (use caution when driving or engaging in tasks that require alertness until response to drug is known); nausea or vomiting (small frequent meals, frequent mouth care, sucking lozenges, or chewing gum may help); or photosensitivity (use sunscreen, wear protective clothing and eyewear, and avoid direct sunlight). Discontinue use immediately and report to prescriber if inflammation, tendon pain, or allergic reaction occurs (itching urticaria, respiratory difficulty, facial edema, difficulty swallowing, loss of consciousness, tingling, chest pain, palpitations). Report persistent diarrhea or constipation; signs of infection (unusual fever or chills); vaginal itching or foul-smelling vaginal discharge; or easy bruising or bleeding.

Ophthalmic: Wash hands before instilling solution. Sit or lie down to instill. Open eye, look at ceiling, and instill prescribed amount of solution. Close eye and roll eye in all directions, and apply gentle pressure to inner corner of eye. Do not let tip of applicator touch eye; do not contaminate tip of applicator (may cause eye infection, eye damage, or vision loss). Temporary stinging or blurred vision may occur. Report persistent pain, burning, vision changes, swelling, itching, or worsening of condition. Discontinue medication and contact prescriber immediately if you develop a rash or allergic reaction. Do not wear contact lenses.

Dietary Considerations: Tablets may be taken without regard to meals. Oral solution should be administered on an empty stomach (1 hour before or 2 hours after a meal).

Geriatric Considerations: The risk of torsade de pointes and tendon inflammation and/or rupture associated with the concomitant use of corticosteroids and quinolones is increased in the elderly population. Adjust dose for renal function.

Pregnancy Risk Factor: C

Pregnancy Issues: Reports of arthropathy (observed in immature animals and reported rarely in humans) have limited the use of fluoroquinolones in pregnancy. Teratogenic effects were not observed with levofloxacin in animal studies; however, decreased body weight and increased fetal mortality were reported. Based on limited data, quinolones are not expected to be a major human teratogen. Although quinolone antibiotics should not be used as first-line agents during pregnancy, when considering treatment for life-threatening infection and/or prolonged duration of therapy, the potential risk to the fetus must be balanced against the severity of the potential illness.

Lactation: Excretion in breast milk unknown/not recommended

Breast-Feeding Issues: Other quinolones are known to be excreted in breast milk. Based on data from ofloxacin, excretion of levofloxacin would be expected. The manufacturer recommends to discontinue nursing or to discontinue levofloxacin.

Administration

Oral: Tablets may be administered without regard to meals. Oral solution should be administered 1 hour before or 2 hours after meals.

I.V.: Infuse 250-500 mg I.V. solution over 60 minutes; infuse 750 mg I.V. solution over 90 minutes. Too rapid of infusion can lead to hypotension. Avoid administration through an intravenous line with a solution containing multivalent cations (eg, magnesium, calcium).

Reconstitution: Solution for injection: Single-use vials must be further diluted in compatible solution to a final concentration of 5 mg/mL prior to infusion.

Compatibility: Stable in D$_5$LR, D$_5$NS, D$_5$W, NS; **incompatible** with mannitol 20%, sodium bicarbonate 5%

Y-site administration: Incompatible with acyclovir, alprostadil, furosemide, heparin, indomethacin, nitroglycerin, sodium nitroprusside

Storage:

Solution for injection:

Vial: Store at room temperature; protect from light. Diluted solution is stable for 72 hours when stored at room temperature; stable for 14 days when stored under refrigeration. When frozen, stable for 6 months; do not refreeze. Do not thaw in microwave or by bath immersion.

Premixed: Store at ≤25°C (77°F); protect from freezing and light.

Tablet, oral solution: Store at 25°C (77°F); excursions permitted to 15°C to 25°C (59°F to 77°F).

Ophthalmic solution: Store at 15°C to 25°C (59°F to 77°F).

Related Information

Antimicrobial Drugs of Choice *on page 1792*
I.V. to Oral Conversion *on page 1688*
Tuberculosis *on page 1864*

Levonorgestrel (LEE voe nor jes trel)

U.S. Brand Names Mirena®; Plan B®

Synonyms LNg 20

Generic Available No

Pharmacologic Category Contraceptive; Progestin

Use Prevention of pregnancy

Mechanism of Action/Effect Ovulation is inhibited and an insufficient luteal phase has also been demonstrated with levonorgestrel administration.

Contraindications Hypersensitivity to levonorgestrel or any component of the formulation; undiagnosed abnormal uterine bleeding, active hepatic disease or malignant tumors, active thrombophlebitis, or thromboembolic disorders (current or history of), known or suspected carcinoma of the breast; history of intracranial hypertension; renal impairment; pregnancy

Additional product-specific contraindications: Intrauterine system: Congenital or acquired uterine anomaly, acute pelvic inflammatory disease, history of pelvic inflammatory disease (unless there has been a subsequent intrauterine pregnancy), postpartum endometritis, infected abortion within past 3 months, known or suspected uterine or cervical neoplasia, unresolved/abnormal Pap smear, untreated acute cervicitis or vaginitis, patient or partner with multiple sexual partners, conditions which increase susceptibility to infections (ie, leukemia, AIDS, I.V. drug abuse), unremoved IUD, history of ectopic pregnancy, conditions which predispose to ectopic pregnancy

Warnings/Precautions Menstrual bleeding patterns may be altered, missed menstrual periods should not be used to identify early pregnancy. These products do not protect against HIV infection or other sexually-transmitted diseases. Patients presenting with lower abdominal pain should be evaluated for follicular atresia and ectopic pregnancy. Patients receiving enzyme-inducing medications should be evaluated for an alternative method of contraception. Levonorgestrel may affect glucose tolerance, monitor serum glucose in patients with diabetes. Safety and efficacy for use in renal or hepatic impairment have not been established. Use with caution in conditions that may be aggravated by fluid retention, depression, or history of migraine. Only for use in women of reproductive age.

Use of combination hormonal contraceptives increases the risk of cardiovascular side effects in women who smoke cigarettes, especially those who are >35 years of age; although this may be an estrogen-related effect, the risk with progestin-only contraceptives is not known and women should be strongly advised not to smoke. Combination hormonal contraceptives may lead to increased risk of myocardial infarction and should be used with caution in patients with risk factors for coronary artery disease; the actual risk with progestin-only contraceptives is not known, however, there have been postmarketing reports of myocardial infarction in women using levonorgestrel-only contraception. May increase the risk of thromboembolism; discontinue therapy if this occurs. Combination hormonal contraceptives may have a dose-related risk of vascular disease and hypertension; strokes have also been (Continued)

Levonorgestrel (Continued)

reported with postmarketing use of levonorgestrel-only contraception. Women with hypertension should be encouraged to use a nonhormonal form of contraception. The use of combination hormonal contraceptives has been associated with a slight increase in frequency of breast cancer (studies are not consistent); studies with progestin only contraceptives have been similar. Retinal thrombosis has been reported (rarely) with combination hormonal contraceptives and may be related to the estrogen component, however, progestin-only therapy should also be discontinued with unexplained partial or complete loss of vision.

Additional formulation-specific warnings:

Intrauterine system: Increased incidence of group A streptococcal sepsis and pelvic inflammatory disease (may be asymptomatic); may perforate uterus or cervix; risk of perforation is increased in lactating women; partial penetration or embedment in the myometrium may decrease effectiveness and lead to difficult removal; postpartum insertion should be delayed until uterine involution is complete; use caution in patients with coagulopathy or receiving anticoagulants

Oral tablet: Not intended to be used for routine contraception and will not terminate an existing pregnancy

Drug Interactions

Cytochrome P450 Effect: Substrate of CYP3A4 (major)

Decreased Effect: CYP3A4 inducers may decrease the levels/effects of levonorgestrel; example inducers include aminoglutethimide, carbamazepine, nafcillin, nevirapine, phenobarbital, phenytoin, and rifamycins.

Nutritional/Ethanol Interactions Herb/Nutraceutical: St John's wort (an enzyme inducer) may decrease serum levels of levonorgestrel.

Lab Interactions Increased triiodothyronine uptake; decreased concentrations of sex hormone-binding globulin, thyroxine concentrations (slight)

Adverse Reactions

Intrauterine system:

>5%:

Cardiovascular: Hypertension

Central nervous system: Headache, depression, nervousness

Dermatologic: Acne

Endocrine & metabolic: Breast pain, dysmenorrhea, decreased libido, abnormal Pap smear, amenorrhea (20% at 1 year), enlarged follicles (12%)

Gastrointestinal: Abdominal pain, nausea, weight gain

Genitourinary: Leukorrhea, vaginitis

Neuromuscular & skeletal: Back pain

Respiratory: Upper respiratory tract infection, sinusitis

<3% and postmarketing reports: Alopecia, anemia, cervicitis, dyspareunia, eczema, failed insertion, migraine, sepsis, vomiting

Oral tablets:

>10%:

Central nervous system: Fatigue (17%), headache (17%), dizziness (11%)

Endocrine & metabolic: Heavier menstrual bleeding (14%), lighter menstrual bleeding (12%), breast tenderness (11%)

Gastrointestinal: Nausea (23%), abdominal pain (18%)

1% to 10%: Gastrointestinal: Vomiting (6%), diarrhea (5%)

Overdosage/Toxicology Can result if >6 capsules are *in situ*. Symptoms include uterine bleeding irregularities and fluid retention.

Pharmacodynamics/Kinetics

Duration of Action: Intrauterine system: Up to 5 years

Absorption: Rapid and complete

Bioavailability: 100%

Protein Binding: Highly bound to albumin and sex hormone-binding globulin

Half-Life Elimination: Oral tablet: ~24 hours

Metabolism: To inactive metabolites

Excretion: Primarily urine

Dosing

Adults & Elderly: Females:

Long-term prevention of pregnancy: Intrauterine system (Mirena®): To be inserted into uterine cavity; should be inserted within 7 days of onset of menstruation or immediately after 1st trimester abortion. Releases 20 mcg levonorgestrel/day over 5 years. May be removed and replaced with a new unit at anytime during menstrual cycle. Do not leave any one system in place for >5 years.

Emergency contraception: Oral tablet (Plan B™): One 0.75 mg tablet as soon as possible within 72 hours of unprotected sexual intercourse. A second 0.75 mg tablet should be taken 12 hours after the first dose; may be used at any time during menstrual cycle.

Available Dosage Forms

Intrauterine device (Mirena®): 52 mg levonorgestrel/unit [releases levonorgestrel 20 mcg/day]

Tablet (Plan B®): 0.75 mg

Monitoring and Teaching Issues

Physical Assessment: Monitor for prolonged menstrual bleeding, amenorrhea, irregularity of menses, and other adverse effects. Caution patient about need for annual medical exams. **Pregnancy risk factor X.**

Patient Education: This drug does not protect against HIV infection or other sexually-transmitted diseases. Cigarette smoking is not recommended. You may experience cramping, headache, abdominal discomfort, hair loss, weight changes, or unusual menses (breakthrough bleeding, irregularity, excessive bleeding). Report sudden acute headache or visual disturbance, unusual nausea or vomiting, any loss of feeling in arms or legs, or lower abdominal pain. **Pregnancy/breast-feeding precautions:** Inform prescriber if you are pregnant. Consult prescriber if breast-feeding.

Intrauterine system: This method provides up to 5 years of birth control from a T-shaped device inserted into the uterus. It will be inserted and removed by your prescriber. Notify your prescriber if the system comes out by itself, if you have long-lasting or heavy bleeding, unusual vaginal discharge, low abdominal pain, painful sexual intercourse, chills or fever. There is an increased risk of ectopic pregnancy with this product. Thread placement should be checked following each menstrual cycle; do not pull thread.

Tablet: This method provides emergency contraception. It is used after your normal form of birth control has failed, or following unprotected sexual intercourse. It should be used within 72 hours. Contact prescriber if you vomit within 1 hour of taking either dose.

Pregnancy Risk Factor: X

Pregnancy Issues: Epidemiologic studies have not shown an increased risk of birth defects when used prior to pregnancy or inadvertently during early pregnancy, although rare reports of congenital anomalies have been reported.

Intrauterine system: Women who become pregnant with an IUD in place risk septic abortion (septic shock and death may occur), removal of IUD may result in pregnancy loss. In addition, miscarriage, premature labor, and premature delivery may occur if pregnancy is continued with IUD in place.

Lactation: Enters breast milk/use caution (AAP rates "compatible")

Breast-Feeding Issues: Enters breast milk (infant serum levels of ~7% have been found when using the intrauterine system, 1% to 6% with the oral tablets), use caution; not considered contraception method of first choice for breast-feeding women (AAP considers **compatible** with breast-feeding)

Administration

Other: Intrauterine system: Inserted in the uterine cavity, to a depth of 6-9 cm, with the provided insertion device; should not be forced into the uterus

Storage: Store at room temperature of 25°C (77°F).

Additional Information Intrauterine system: The cumulative 5-year pregnancy rate is ~0.7 pregnancies/100 users. Over 70% of women in the trials had previously used IUDs. The reported pregnancy rate after 12 months was ≤0.2 pregnancies/100 users. Approximately 80% of women who wish to conceive have become pregnant within 12 months of device removal. The recommended patient profile for this product: A woman who has at least one child, is in a stable and mutually-monogamous relationship, no history of pelvic inflammatory disease, and no history of ectopic pregnancy or predisposition to ectopic pregnancy.

Oral tablet: When used as directed for emergency contraception, the expected pregnancy rate is decreased from 8% to 1%. Approximately 87% of women have their next menstrual period at approximately the expected time. A rapid return to fertility following use is expected.

♦ **Levonorgestrel and Ethinyl Estradiol** see Ethinyl Estradiol and Levonorgestrel on page 585

♦ **Levophed**® see Norepinephrine on page 1095

♦ **Levora**® see Ethinyl Estradiol and Levonorgestrel on page 585

Levorphanol (lee VOR fa nole)

U.S. Brand Names Levo-Dromoran®

Synonyms Levorphanol Tartrate; Levorphan Tartrate

Controlled Substance C-II

Generic Available Yes: Tablet

Pharmacologic Category Analgesic, Narcotic

Use Relief of moderate to severe pain; also used parenterally for preoperative sedation and an adjunct to nitrous oxide/oxygen anesthesia; 2 mg levorphanol produces analgesia comparable to that produced by 10 mg of morphine

Mechanism of Action/Effect Levorphanol tartrate is a synthetic opioid agonist that is classified as a morphinan derivative. Opioids interact with stereospecific opioid receptors in various parts of the central nervous system and other tissues.

Contraindications Hypersensitivity to levorphanol or any component of the formulation; pregnancy (prolonged use or high doses at term)

Warnings/Precautions An opioid-containing analgesic regimen should be tailored to each patient's needs and based upon the type of pain being treated (acute versus chronic), the route of administration, degree of tolerance for opioids (naive versus chronic user), age, weight, and medical condition. The optimal analgesic dose varies widely among patients. Doses should be titrated to pain relief/prevention.

Use with caution in patients with hypersensitivity reactions to other phenanthrene derivative opioid agonists (morphine, hydrocodone, hydromorphone, levorphanol, oxycodone, oxymorphone); respiratory diseases including asthma, emphysema, COPD, or severe liver or renal insufficiency. Some preparations contain sulfites which may cause allergic reactions. May be habit-forming. Dextromethorphan has equivalent antitussive activity but has much lower toxicity in accidental overdose. Elderly may be particularly susceptible to the CNS depressant and constipating effects of narcotics.

Drug Interactions

Increased Effect/Toxicity: CNS depression is enhanced with coadministration of other CNS depressants.

Nutritional/Ethanol Interactions

Ethanol: Avoid or limit ethanol (may increase CNS depression). Watch for sedation.

Herb/Nutraceutical: Avoid valerian, St John's wort, kava kava, gotu kola (may increase CNS depression).

Adverse Reactions Frequency not defined.

Cardiovascular: Palpitations, hypotension, bradycardia, peripheral vasodilation, cardiac arrest, shock, tachycardia

Central nervous system: CNS depression, fatigue, drowsiness, dizziness, nervousness, headache, restlessness, anorexia, malaise, confusion, coma, convulsion, insomnia, amnesia, mental depression, hallucinations, paradoxical CNS stimulation, intracranial pressure (increased)

(Continued)

Levorphanol *(Continued)*

Dermatologic: Pruritus, urticaria, rash

Endocrine & metabolic: Antidiuretic hormone release

Gastrointestinal: Nausea, vomiting, dyspepsia, stomach cramps, xerostomia, constipation, abdominal pain, dry mouth, biliary tract spasm, paralytic ileus

Genitourinary: Decreased urination, urinary tract spasm, urinary retention

Local: Pain at injection site

Neuromuscular & skeletal: Weakness

Ocular: Miosis, diplopia

Respiratory: Respiratory depression, apnea, hypoventilation, cyanosis

Miscellaneous: Histamine release, physical and psychological dependence

Overdosage/Toxicology Symptoms of overdose include CNS depression, respiratory depression, miosis, apnea, pulmonary edema, and convulsions. Naloxone, 2 mg I.V. with repeat administration as necessary up to a total dose of 10 mg, can be used to reverse opiate effects.

Pharmacodynamics/Kinetics

Onset of Action: Oral: 10-60 minutes

Duration of Action: 4-8 hours

Half-Life Elimination: 11-16 hours

Metabolism: Hepatic

Excretion: Urine (as inactive metabolite)

Dosing

Adults & Elderly: Note: These are guidelines and do not represent the maximum doses that may be required in all patients. Doses should be titrated to pain relief/prevention.

Acute pain (moderate to severe):

Oral: Initial: Opiate-naive: 2 mg every 6-8 hours as needed; patients with prior opiate exposure may require higher initial doses; usual dosage range: 2-4 mg every 6-8 hours as needed

I.M., SubQ: Initial: Opiate-naive: 1 mg every 6-8 hours as needed; patients with prior opiate exposure may require higher initial doses; usual dosage range: 1-2 mg every 6-8 hours as needed

I.V. (slow): Initial: Opiate-naive: Up to 1 mg/dose every 3-6 hours as needed; patients with prior opiate exposure may require higher initial doses

Chronic pain: Patients taking opioids chronically may become tolerant and require doses higher than the usual dosage range to maintain the desired effect. Tolerance can be managed by appropriate dose titration. There is no optimal or maximal dose for levorphanol in chronic pain. The appropriate dose is one that relieves pain throughout its dosing interval without causing unmanageable side effects.

Premedication: I.M., SubQ: 1-2 mg/dose 60-90 minutes prior to surgery; older or debilitated patients usually require less drug

Hepatic Impairment: Reduce dose in patients with liver disease.

Available Dosage Forms

Injection, solution, as tartrate: 2 mg/mL (1 mL, 10 mL)

Tablet, as tartrate: 2 mg

Monitoring and Teaching Issues

Physical Assessment: Assess other medications patient may be taking for additive or adverse interactions. Monitor therapeutic effectiveness, adverse reactions and signs of overdose. Monitor vital signs, CNS and respiratory status, at beginning of therapy and at regular intervals with long-term use. May cause physical and/or psychological dependence. Safety measures required for inpatients. Assess knowledge/teach patient appropriate use (if self-administered). Teach patient to monitor for adverse reactions, adverse reactions to report, and appropriate interventions to reduce side effects. Discontinue slowly after prolonged use.

Patient Education: If self-administered, use exactly as directed; do not increase dose or frequency. Drug may cause physical and/or psychological dependence. While using this medication, do not use alcohol and other prescription or OTC medications (especially sedatives, tranquilizers, antihistamines, or pain medications) without consulting prescriber. Maintain adequate hydration (2-3 L/day of fluids) unless instructed to restrict fluid intake. May cause hypotension, dizziness, drowsiness, impaired coordination, or blurred vision (use caution when driving, climbing stairs, or changing position - rising from sitting or lying to standing, or when engaging in tasks requiring alertness until response to drug is known); loss of appetite, nausea, or vomiting (frequent mouth care, small frequent meals, chewing gum, or sucking lozenges may help); or constipation (increased exercise, fluids, fruit, or fiber may help; if unresolved, consult prescriber about use of stool softeners). Report chest pain, slow or rapid heartbeat, acute dizziness, or persistent headache; swelling of extremities or unusual weight gain; changes in urinary elimination; acute headache; back or flank pain or spasms; blurred vision; skin rash; or shortness of breath. **Pregnancy/breast-feeding precautions:** Inform prescriber if you are or intend to become pregnant. Breast-feeding is not recommended.

Geriatric Considerations: The elderly may be particularly susceptible to the CNS depressant and constipating effects of narcotics.

Pregnancy Risk Factor: B/D (prolonged use or high doses at term)

Lactation: Excretion in breast milk unknown/not recommended

Administration

Oral: For lactating women, administer 4-6 hours prior to breast-feeding.

I.V.: Inject 3 mg over 4-5 minutes

Compatibility: when admixed: Incompatible with aminophylline, ammonium chloride, amobarbital, chlorothiazide, heparin, pentobarbital, phenobarbital, phenytoin, sodium bicarbonate, thiopental

Storage: Store at room temperature. Protect from freezing.

Related Information

Narcotic / Opioid Analgesic Comparison *on page 1739*

♦ **Levorphanol Tartrate** *see* Levorphanol *on page 893*
♦ **Levorphan Tartrate** *see* Levorphanol *on page 893*
♦ **Levothroid®** *see* Levothyroxine *on page 895*

Levothyroxine (lee voe thye ROKS een)

U.S. Brand Names Levothroid®; Levoxyl®; Synthroid®; Unithroid®
Synonyms Levothyroxine Sodium; *L*-Thyroxine Sodium; T_4
Generic Available Yes
Pharmacologic Category Thyroid Product
Medication Safety Issues
  Sound-alike/look-alike issues:
    Levothyroxine may be confused with liothyronine
    Levoxyl® may be confused with Lanoxin®, Luvox®
    Synthroid® may be confused with Symmetrel®

  To avoid errors due to misinterpretation of a decimal point, always express dosage in mcg (**not** mg).

Use Replacement or supplemental therapy in hypothyroidism; pituitary TSH suppression

Mechanism of Action/Effect It is believed the thyroid hormone exerts its many metabolic effects through control of DNA transcription and protein synthesis

Contraindications Hypersensitivity to levothyroxine sodium or any component of the formulation; recent MI or thyrotoxicosis; uncorrected adrenal insufficiency

Warnings/Precautions Ineffective and potentially toxic for weight reduction. High doses may produce serious or even life-threatening toxic effects particularly when used with some anorectic drugs. Use with caution and reduce dosage in patients with angina pectoris or other cardiovascular disease. Use cautiously in the elderly since they may be more likely to have compromised cardiovascular functions. Patients with adrenal insufficiency, myxedema, diabetes mellitus and insipidus may have symptoms exaggerated or aggravated. Thyroid replacement requires periodic assessment of thyroid status. Chronic hypothyroidism predisposes patients to coronary artery disease. Levoxyl® may rapidly swell and disintegrate causing choking or gagging (should be administered with a full glass of water); use caution in patients with dysphagia or other swallowing disorders.

Drug Interactions
  Decreased Effect: Also refer to Additional Information. Some medications may decrease absorption of levothyroxine: Cholestyramine, colestipol (separate administration by at least 2 hours); aluminum- and magnesium-containing antacids, iron preparations, sucralfate, Kayexalate® (separate administration by at least 4 hours). Enzyme inducers (phenytoin, phenobarbital, carbamazepine, and rifampin/rifabutin) may decrease levothyroxine levels. Levothyroxine may decrease effect of oral sulfonylureas. Serum levels of digoxin and theophylline may be altered by thyroid function. Estrogens may decrease serum free-thyroxine concentrations.

  Increased Effect/Toxicity: Also refer to Additional Information. Levothyroxine may potentiate the hypoprothrombinemic effect of warfarin (and other oral anticoagulants). Tricyclic antidepressants (TCAs) coadministered with levothyroxine may increase potential for toxicity of both drugs. Coadministration with ketamine may lead to hypertension and tachycardia.

Nutritional/Ethanol Interactions Food: Taking levothyroxine with enteral nutrition may cause reduced bioavailability and may lower serum thyroxine levels leading to signs or symptoms of hypothyroidism. Limit intake of goitrogenic foods (eg, asparagus, cabbage, peas, turnip greens, broccoli, spinach, Brussels sprouts, lettuce, soybeans). Soybean flour (infant formula), cottonseed meal, walnuts, and dietary fiber may decrease absorption of levothyroxine from the GI tract.

Lab Interactions Many drugs may have effects on thyroid function tests: para-aminosalicylic acid, aminoglutethimide, amiodarone, barbiturates, carbamazepine, chloral hydrate, clofibrate, colestipol, corticosteroids, danazol, diazepam, estrogens, ethionamide, fluorouracil, I.V. heparin, insulin, lithium, methadone, methimazole, mitotane, nitroprusside, oxyphenbutazone, phenylbutazone, PTU, perphenazine, phenytoin, propranolol, salicylates, sulfonylureas, and thiazides.

Adverse Reactions Frequency not defined.
  Cardiovascular: Angina, arrhythmia, blood pressure increased, cardiac arrest, flushing, heart failure, MI, palpitation, pulse increased, tachycardia
  Central nervous system: Anxiety, emotional lability, fatigue, fever, headache, hyperactivity, insomnia, irritability, nervousness, pseudotumor cerebri (children), seizure (rare)
  Dermatologic: Alopecia
  Endocrine & metabolic: Fertility impaired, menstrual irregularities
  Gastrointestinal: Abdominal cramps, appetite increased, diarrhea, vomiting, weight loss
  Hepatic: Liver function tests increased
  Neuromuscular & skeletal: Bone mineral density decreased, muscle weakness, tremor, slipped capital femoral epiphysis (children)
  Respiratory: Dyspnea
  Miscellaneous: Diaphoresis, heat intolerance, hypersensitivity (to inactive ingredients, symptoms include urticaria, pruritus, rash, flushing, angioedema, GI symptoms, fever, arthralgia, serum sickness, wheezing)
    Levoxyl®: Choking, dysphagia, gagging

Overdosage/Toxicology
  Chronic: Chronic overdose may cause hyperthyroidism, weight loss, nervousness, sweating, tachycardia, insomnia, heat intolerance, menstrual irregularities, palpitations, psychosis, and fever. Overtreatment of children may result in premature closure of epiphyses or craniosynostosis (infants). Reduce dose or temporarily discontinue therapy. Hypothalamic-pituitary-thyroid axis will return to normal in 6-8 weeks. Serum T_4 levels do not correlate well with toxicity. Provide general supportive care
  (Continued)

Levothyroxine *(Continued)*

Acute: Acute overdose may cause fever, hypoglycemia, CHF, and unrecognized adrenal insufficiency. Acute massive overdose may be life-threatening; treatment should be symptomatic and supportive. Massive overdose may be a require beta-blockers for increased sympathomimetic activity.

Pharmacodynamics/Kinetics

Onset of Action: Therapeutic: Oral: 3-5 days; I.V. 6-8 hours; Peak effect: I.V.: ~24 hours

Absorption: Oral: Erratic (40% to 80%); decreases with age

Time to Peak: Serum: 2-4 hours

Protein Binding: >99%

Half-Life Elimination: Euthyroid: 6-7 days; Hypothyroid: 9-10 days; Hyperthyroid: 3-4 days

Metabolism: Hepatic to triiodothyronine (active)

Excretion: Urine and feces; decreases with age

Dosing

Adults: Doses should be adjusted based on clinical response and laboratory parameters.

Hypothyroidism:

Oral: 1.7 mcg/kg/day in otherwise healthy adults <50 years old, children in whom growth and puberty are complete, and older adults who have been recently treated for hyperthyroidism or who have been hypothyroid for only a few months. Titrate dose every 6 weeks. Average starting dose ~100 mcg; usual doses are ≤200 mcg/day; doses ≥300 mcg/day are rare (consider poor compliance, malabsorption, and/or drug interactions).

Note: For patients >50 years or patients with cardiac disease, refer to elderly dosing.

I.M., I.V.: 50% of the oral dose

Severe hypothyroidism: Oral: Initial: 12.5-25 mcg/day; adjust dose by 25 mcg/day every 2-4 weeks as appropriate

Subclinical hypothyroidism (if treated): Oral: 1 mcg/kg/day

TSH suppression: Oral:

Well-differentiated thyroid cancer: Highly individualized; Doses >2 mcg/kg/day may be needed to suppress TSH to <0.1 mU/L.

Benign nodules and nontoxic multinodular goiter: Goal TSH suppression: 0.1-0.3 mU/L

Myxedema coma or stupor: I.V.: 200-500 mcg, then 100-300 mcg the next day if necessary; smaller doses should be considered in patients with cardiovascular disease

Elderly: Doses should be adjusted based on clinical response and laboratory parameters.

Hypothyroidism:

Oral:

>50 years without cardiac disease **or** <50 years with cardiac disease: Initial: 25-50 mcg/day; adjust dose at 6- to 8-week intervals as needed

>50 years with cardiac disease: Initial: 12.5-25 mcg/day; adjust dose by 12.5-25 mcg increments in 4- to 6-week intervals

Note: Elderly patients may require <1 mcg/kg/day

I.M., I.V.: 50% of the oral dose

Myxedema coma: I.V.: Refer to adult dosing; lower doses may be needed

Pediatrics: Doses should be adjusted based on clinical response and laboratory parameters.

Hypothyroidism:

Oral:

Newborns: Initial: 10-15 mcg/kg/day. Lower doses of 25 mcg/day should be considered in newborns at risk for cardiac failure. Newborns with T_4 levels <5 mcg/dL should be started at 50 mcg/day. Adjust dose at 4- to 6-week intervals.

Infants and Children: Dose based on body weight and age as listed below. Children with severe or chronic hypothyroidism should be started at 25 mcg/day; adjust dose by 25 mcg every 2-4 weeks. In older children, hyperactivity may be decreased by starting with $\frac{1}{4}$ of the recommended dose and increasing by $\frac{1}{4}$ dose each week until the full replacement dose is reached. Refer to adult dosing once growth and puberty are complete.

0-3 months: 10-15 mcg/kg/day

3-6 months: 8-10 mcg/kg/day

6-12 months: 6-8 mcg/kg/day

1-5 years: 5-6 mcg/kg/day

6-12 years: 4-5 mcg/kg/day

12 years: 2-3 mcg/kg/day

I.M., I.V.: 50% of the oral dose

Available Dosage Forms

Injection, powder for reconstitution, as sodium: 0.2 mg, 0.5 mg

Synthroid® 0.2 mg

Tablet, as sodium: 25 mcg, 50 mcg, 75 mcg, 88 mcg, 100 mcg, 112 mcg, 125 mcg, 150 mcg, 175 mcg, 200 mcg, 300 mcg

Levothroid®: 25 mcg, 50 mcg, 75 mcg, 88 mcg, 100 mcg, 112 mcg, 125 mcg, 137 mcg [DSC], 150 mcg, 175 mcg, 200 mcg, 300 mcg

Levoxyl®, Synthroid®: 25 mcg, 50 mcg, 75 mcg, 88 mcg, 100 mcg, 112 mcg, 125 mcg, 137 mcg, 150 mcg, 175 mcg, 200 mcg, 300 mcg

Unithroid®: 25 mcg, 50 mcg, 75 mcg, 88 mcg, 100 mcg, 112 mcg, 125 mcg, 150 mcg, 175 mcg, 200 mcg, 300 mcg

Monitoring and Teaching Issues

Physical Assessment: Use with caution in presence of cardiovascular disease, adrenal insufficiency, or diabetes mellitus (see Warnings/Precautions for specific use cautions). Assess potential for interactions with other pharmacological agents patient may be taking (eg, toxic effects with some anorectic drugs, decreased effect of oral hypoglycemics, decreased or increased effect of levothyroxine; see Drug Interactions). See Administration for I.V. specifics. Assess results of laboratory tests, therapeutic benefits, and adverse effects on a regular basis during therapy (eg, hypo- or hyperthyroidism; see Adverse Reactions). **Important:** Many drugs may have effects on thyroid function tests. Teach patient proper use, possible side effects/appropriate interventions (eg, goitrogenic foods), and adverse symptoms to report (see Patient Education).

Monitoring Laboratory Tests: Thyroid function (serum thyroxine, thyrotropin concentrations), resin triiodothyronine uptake (rT_3U), free thyroxine index (FTI), T_4, TSH, TSH may be elevated during the first few months of thyroid replacement despite patients being clinically euthyroid. In cases where T_4 remains low and TSH is within normal limits, an evaluation of "free" (unbound) T_4 is needed to evaluate further increase in dosage.

Patient Education: Consult prescriber before taking new medication or herbal products during therapy; some other medications or herbals may cause adverse effects with levothyroxine. Thyroid replacement therapy is generally for life. Take as directed, in the morning 30 minutes before breakfast. Do not take antacids or iron preparations within 8 hours of thyroid medication. Do not change brands and do not discontinue without consulting prescriber. Do not eat excessive amounts of goitrogenic foods (eg, asparagus, cabbage, peas, turnip greens, broccoli, spinach, brussel sprouts, lettuce, soybeans). Report chest pain, rapid heart rate, palpitations, heat intolerance, excessive sweating, increased nervousness, agitation, or lethargy.

Dietary Considerations: Should be taken on an empty stomach, at least 30 minutes before food.

Geriatric Considerations: The elderly do not have a change in serum thyroxine (T_4) associated with aging; however, plasma T_3 concentrations are decreased 25% to 40% in the elderly. There is no compensatory rise in thyrotropin suggesting that lower T_3 is not reacted upon as a deficiency by the pituitary. This indicates a slightly lower than normal dosage of thyroid hormone replacement is usually sufficient in older patients than in younger adult patients. TSH must be monitored since insufficient thyroid replacement (elevated TSH) is a risk for coronary artery disease and excessive replacement (low TSH) may cause signs of hyperthyroidism and excessive bone loss. Some clinicians suggest levothyroxine is the drug of choice for replacement therapy.

Pregnancy Risk Factor: A

Pregnancy Issues: Untreated maternal hypothyroidism may have adverse effects on fetal growth and development and is associated with higher rate of complications (spontaneous abortion, pre-eclampsia, stillbirth, premature delivery). Treatment should not be discontinued during pregnancy. TSH levels should be monitored during each trimester and 6-8 weeks postpartum. Increased doses may be needed during pregnancy.

Lactation: Enters breast milk/compatible

Breast-Feeding Issues: Minimally excreted in human milk; adequate levels are needed to maintain normal lactation

Administration

Oral: Administer in the morning on an empty stomach, at least 30 minutes before food. Tablets may be crushed and suspended in 1-2 teaspoonfuls of water; suspension should be used immediately. Levoxyl® should be administered with a full glass of water to prevent gagging (due to tablet swelling).

I.V.: Dilute vial with 5 mL normal saline; use immediately after reconstitution; do not mix with other IV fluids

Reconstitution: Dilute vial with 5 mL normal saline. Shake well and use immediately after reconstitution; discard any unused portions.

Compatibility: Do not mix I.V. solution with other I.V. infusion solutions.

Storage: Store tablets and injection at room temperature of 15°C to 30°C (59°F to 86°F). Protect tablets from light and moisture.

Additional Information Equivalent doses: Thyroid USP 60 mg ~ levothyroxine 0.05-0.06 mg ~ liothyronine 0.015-0.0375 mg
50-60 mg thyroid ~ 50-60 mcg levothyroxine and 12.5-15 mcg liothyronine

Note: Several medications have effects on thyroid production or conversion. The impact in thyroid replacement has not been specifically evaluated, but patient response should be monitored:

Methimazole: Decreases thyroid hormone secretion, while propylthiouracil decrease thyroid hormone secretion and decreases conversion of T_4 to T_3.

Beta-adrenergic antagonists: Decrease conversion of T_4 to T_3 (dose related, propranolol ≥160 mg/day); patients may be clinically euthyroid.

Iodide, iodine-containing radiographic contrast agents may decrease thyroid hormone secretion; may also increase thyroid hormone secretion, especially in patients with Graves' disease.

Other agents reported to impact on thyroid production/conversion include aminoglutethimide, amiodarone, chloral hydrate, diazepam, ethionamide, interferon-alpha, interleukin-2, lithium, lovastatin (case report), glucocorticoids (dose-related), mercaptopurine, sulfonamides, thiazide diuretics, and tolbutamide.

In addition, a number of medications have been noted to cause transient depression in TSH secretion, which may complicate interpretation of monitoring tests for levothyroxine, including corticosteroids, octreotide, and dopamine. Metoclopramide may increase TSH secretion

♦ **Librium**® *see* Chlordiazepoxide *on page 308*

♦ **LidaMantle**® *see* Lidocaine *on page 898*

♦ **Lidex**® *see* Fluocinonide *on page 645*

♦ **Lidex-E**® *see* Fluocinonide *on page 645*

Lidocaine (LYE doe kane)

U.S. Brand Names Anestacon®; Band-Aid® Hurt-Free™ Antiseptic Wash [OTC]; Burnamycin [OTC]; Burn Jel [OTC]; Burn-O-Jel [OTC]; LidaMantle®; Lidoderm®; L-M-X™ 4 [OTC]; L-M-X™ 5 [OTC]; Premjact® [OTC]; Solarcaine® Aloe Extra Burn Relief [OTC]; Topicaine® [OTC]; Xylocaine®; Xylocaine® MPF; Xylocaine® Viscous; Zilactin-L® [OTC]

Synonyms Lidocaine Hydrochloride; Lignocaine Hydrochloride

Generic Available Yes: Cream, gel, injection, lotion, ointment, solution

Pharmacologic Category Analgesic, Topical; Antiarrhythmic Agent, Class Ib; Local Anesthetic

Medication Safety Issues

High alert medication: The Institute for Safe Medication Practices (ISMP) includes this medication (I.V. formulation) among its list of drugs which have a heightened risk of causing significant patient harm when used in error.

Transdermal patch may contain conducting metal (eg, aluminum); remove patch prior to MRI.

Use Local anesthetic and acute treatment of ventricular arrhythmias from myocardial infarction, cardiac manipulation, digitalis intoxication; drug of choice for ventricular ectopy, ventricular tachycardia (VT), ventricular fibrillation (VF); for pulseless VT or VF preferably administer **after** defibrillation and epinephrine; control of premature ventricular contractions, wide-complex paroxysmal supraventricular tachycardia (PSVT); control of hemodynamically compromising PVCs; hemodynamically stable VT

Rectal: Temporary relief of pain and itching due to anorectal disorders

Topical: Local anesthetic for use in laser, cosmetic, and outpatient surgeries; minor burns, cuts, and abrasions of the skin

Orphan drug: Lidoderm® Patch: Relief of allodynia (painful hypersensitivity) and chronic pain in postherpetic neuralgia

Mechanism of Action/Effect Class Ib antiarrhythmic; suppresses automaticity of conduction tissue by increasing electrical stimulation threshold of ventricles, His-Purkinje system, and spontaneous depolarization of ventricles during diastole by direct action on tissues; blocks both initiation and conduction of nerve impulses by decreasing the neuronal membrane's permeability to sodium ions, which results in inhibition of depolarization with resultant blockade of conduction

Contraindications Hypersensitivity to lidocaine or any component of the formulation; hypersensitivity to another local anesthetic of the amide type; Adam-Stokes syndrome; severe degrees of SA, AV, or intraventricular heart block (except in patients with a functioning artificial pacemaker); premixed injection may contain corn-derived dextrose and its use is contraindicated in patients with allergy to corn-related products

Warnings/Precautions

Intravenous: Constant ECG monitoring is necessary during I.V. administration. Use cautiously in hepatic impairment, any degree of heart block, Wolff-Parkinson-White syndrome, CHF, marked hypoxia, severe respiratory depression, hypovolemia, history of malignant hyperthermia, or shock. Increased ventricular rate may be seen when administered to a patient with atrial fibrillation. Correct any underlying causes of ventricular arrhythmias. Monitor closely for signs and symptoms of CNS toxicity. The elderly may be prone to increased CNS and cardiovascular side effects. Reduce dose in hepatic dysfunction and CHF.

Injectable anesthetic: Follow appropriate administration techniques so as not to administer any intravascularly. Solutions containing antimicrobial preservatives should not be used for epidural or spinal anesthesia. Some solutions contain a bisulfite; avoid in patients who are allergic to bisulfite. Resuscitative equipment, medicine and oxygen should be available in case of emergency. Use products containing epinephrine cautiously in patients with significant vascular disease, compromised blood flow, or during or following general anesthesia (increased risk of arrhythmias). Adjust the dose for the elderly, pediatric, acutely ill, and debilitated patients.

Topical: L-M-X™ 4 cream: Do not leave on large body areas for >2 hours. Observe young children closely to prevent accidental ingestion. Not for use ophthalmic use or for use on mucous membranes.

Transdermal patch: May contain conducting metal (eg, aluminum); remove patch prior to MRI.

Drug Interactions

Cytochrome P450 Effect: Substrate of CYP1A2 (minor), 2A6 (minor), 2B6 (minor), 2C8/9 (minor), 2D6 (major), 3A4 (major); **Inhibits** CYP1A2 (strong), 2D6 (moderate), 3A4 (moderate)

Decreased Effect: The levels/effects of lidocaine may be decreased by aminoglutethimide, carbamazepine, nafcillin, nevirapine, phenobarbital, phenytoin, rifamycins and other CYP3A4 inducers. Lidocaine may decrease the levels/effects of CYP2D6 prodrug substrates (eg, codeine, hydrocodone, oxycodone, tramadol).

Increased Effect/Toxicity: The levels/effects of lidocaine may be increased by amphetamines, amiodarone, azole antifungals, beta-blockers, chlorpromazine, ciprofloxacin, clarithromycin, delavirdine, diclofenac, doxycycline, erythromycin, fluoxetine, imatinib, isoniazid, miconazole, nefazodone, nicardipine, paroxetine, pergolide, propofol, protease inhibitors, quinidine, quinine, ritonavir, ropinirole, verapamil, and other CYP2D6 or 3A4 inhibitors. Concomitant cimetidine or propranolol may result in increased serum concentrations of lidocaine resulting in toxicity.

Lidocaine may increase the levels/effects of aminophylline, amphetamines, selected beta-blockers, selected benzodiazepines, calcium channel blockers, cisapride, cyclosporine, dextromethorphan, ergot alkaloids, fluoxetine, fluvoxamine, selected HMG-CoA reductase inhibitors, lidocaine, mesoridazine, mexiletine, mirtazapine, nateglinide, nefazodone, paroxetine, risperidone, ritonavir, ropinirole, sildenafil (and other PDE-5 inhibitors), tacrolimus, theophylline, thioridazine, tricyclic antidepressants, trifluoperazine, venlafaxine, and other substrates of CYP1A2, 2D6 or 3A4. The effect of succinylcholine may be enhanced by lidocaine.

Nutritional/Ethanol Interactions Herb/Nutraceutical: St John's wort may decrease lidocaine levels; avoid concurrent use.

Adverse Reactions Effects vary with route of administration. Many effects are dose related.

Frequency not defined:
Cardiovascular: Bradycardia, hypotension, heart block, arrhythmia, cardiovascular collapse, sinus node supression, increase defibrillator threshold, vascular insufficiency (periarticular injections), arterial spasms
Central nervous system: Drowsiness after administration is usually a sign of a high blood level. Other effects may include lightheadedness, dizziness, tinnitus, blurred vision, vomiting, twitching, tremor, lethargy, coma, agitation, slurred speech, seizure, anxiety, euphoria, hallucinations, paresthesia, psychosis
Dermatologic: Itching, rash, edema of the skin, contact dermatitis
Gastrointestinal: Nausea, vomiting, taste disorder
Local: Thrombophlebitis
Neuromuscular & skeletal: Transient radicular pain (subarachnoid administration; up to 1.9%)
Ocular: Blurred vision, diplopia
Respiratory: Dyspnea, respiratory depression or arrest, bronchospasm
Miscellaneous: Allergic reactions, urticaria, edema, anaphylactoid reaction

Following spinal anesthesia positional headache (3%), shivering (2%) nausea, peripheral nerve symptoms, respiratory inadequacy and double vision

Overdosage/Toxicology Lidocaine has a narrow therapeutic index. Severe toxicity may occur at doses slightly above the therapeutic range, especially in conjunction with other antiarrhythmic drugs. Symptoms of overdose include sedation, confusion, coma, seizures, respiratory arrest, and cardiac toxicity (sinus arrest, AV block, asystole, and hypotension). QRS and QT intervals are usually normal, although they may be prolonged after massive overdose. Other effects include dizziness, paresthesia, tremor, ataxia, and GI disturbance. Treatment is supportive.

Pharmacodynamics/Kinetics
Onset of Action: Single bolus dose: 45-90 seconds
Duration of Action: 10-20 minutes
Protein Binding: 60% to 80% to alpha$_1$ acid glycoprotein
Half-Life Elimination: Biphasic: Prolonged with congestive heart failure, liver disease, shock, severe renal disease; Initial: 7-30 minutes; Terminal: Infants, premature: 3.2 hours, Adults: 1.5-2 hours
Metabolism: 90% hepatic; active metabolites monoethylglycinexylidide (MEGX) and glycinexylidide (GX) can accumulate and may cause CNS toxicity

Dosing
Adults & Elderly:
Antiarrhythmic:
I.V.: 1-1.5 mg/kg bolus over 2-3 minutes; may repeat doses of 0.5-0.75 mg/kg in 5-10 minutes up to a total of 3 mg/kg; continuous infusion: 1-4 mg/minute
Infusion rates: 2 g/250 mL D$_5$W (infusion pump should be used):
1 mg/minute: 7 mL/hour
2 mg/minute: 15 mL/hour
3 mg/minute: 21 mL/hour
4 mg/minute: 30 mL/hour
Ventricular fibrillation (after defibrillation and epinephrine):
I.V.: Initial: 1.5 mg/kg, may repeat boluses as above; follow with continuous infusion after return of perfusion.
Intratracheal: 2-2.5 times the recommended I.V. dose; dilute in 10 mL NS or distilled water. **Note:** Absorption is greater with distilled water, but causes more adverse effects on PaO$_2$.
Prevention of ventricular fibrillation: Initial bolus: 0.5 mg/kg; repeat every 5-10 minutes to a total dose of 2 mg/kg
Refractory ventricular fibrillation: Repeat 1.5 mg/kg bolus may be given 3-5 minutes after initial dose.
E.T. (loading dose only): 2-2.5 times the I.V. dose
Note: Decrease dose in patients with CHF, shock, or hepatic disease.

Anesthetic, topical:
Cream:
LidaMantle®: Skin irritation: Apply to affected area 2-3 times/day as needed
L-M-X™ 4: Apply ¼ inch thick layer to intact skin. Leave on until adequate anesthetic effect is obtained. Remove cream and cleanse area before beginning procedure.
L-M-X™ 5: Relief of anorectal pain and itching: Rectal: Apply topically to clean, dry area **or** using applicator, insert rectally, up to 6 times/day
Gel, ointment, solution: Apply to affected area ≤3 times/day as needed (maximum dose: 4.5 mg/kg, not to exceed 300 mg)
Jelly: Maximum dose: 30 mL (600 mg) in any 12-hour period:
Anesthesia of male urethra: 5-30 mL (100-600 mg)
Anesthesia of female urethra: 3-5 mL (60-100 mg)
Lubrication of endotracheal tube: Apply a moderate amount to external surface only
Liquid: Cold sores and fever blisters: Apply to affected area every 6 hours as needed
Patch: Postherpetic neuralgia: Apply patch to most painful area. Up to 3 patches may be applied in a single application. Patch may remain in place for up to 12 hours in any 24-hour period.
(Continued)

Lidocaine *(Continued)*

Anesthetic, local injectable: Varies with procedure, degree of anesthesia needed, vascularity of tissue, duration of anesthesia required, and physical condition of patient; maximum: 4.5 mg/kg/dose; do not repeat within 2 hours.

Pediatrics:

Antiarrhythmic:

I.V., I.O.: **(Note:** For use in pulseless VT or VF, give after defibrillation and epinephrine): Loading dose: 1 mg/kg; follow with continuous infusion; may administer second bolus of 0.5-1 mg/kg if delay between bolus and start of infusion is >15 minutes; continuous infusion: 20-50 mcg/kg/minute. Use 20 mcg/kg/minute in patients with shock, hepatic disease, cardiac arrest, mild CHF; moderate to severe CHF may require ½ loading dose and lower infusion rates to avoid toxicity.

E.T. (loading dose only): 2-10 times the I.V. bolus dose

Anesthetic, topical:

Cream:

LidaMantle®: Skin irritation: Refer to adult dosing.

L-M-X™ 4: Children ≥2 years: Refer to adult dosing.

L-M-X™ 5: Relief of anorectal pain and itching: Rectal: Children ≥12 years: Refer to adult dosing.

Jelly: Children ≥10 years: Dose varies with age and weight (maximum dose: 4.5 mg/kg)

Liquid: Cold sores and fever blisters: Children ≥5 years: Refer to adult dosing.

Injectable local anesthetic: Refer to adult dosing.

Renal Impairment: Not dialyzable (0% to 5%) by hemo- or peritoneal dialysis; supplemental dose is not necessary.

Hepatic Impairment: Reduce dose in acute hepatitis and decompensated cirrhosis by 50%.

Available Dosage Forms

Cream, rectal (L-M-X™ 5): 5% (15 g, 30 g) [contains benzyl alcohol]

Cream, topical (L-M-X™ 4): 4% (5 g, 15 g, 30 g) [contains benzyl alcohol]

Cream, topical, as hydrochloride: 3% (30 g)

LidaMantle®: 3% (30 g, 85 g)

Gel, topical:

Burn-O-Jel: 0.5% (90 g)

Topicaine®: 4% (10 g, 30 g, 113 g) [contains benzyl alcohol, aloe vera, and jojoba]

Gel, topical, as hydrochloride: 2% (30 g)

Burn Jel: 2% (3.5 g, 120 g)

Solarcaine® Aloe Extra Burn Relief: 0.5% (226 g) [contains aloe vera gel and tartrazine]

Infusion, as hydrochloride [premixed in D_5W]: 0.4% [4 mg/mL] (250 mL, 500 mL); 0.8% [8 mg/mL] (250 mL, 500 mL)

Injection, solution, as hydrochloride: 0.5% [5 mg/mL] (50 mL); 1% [10 mg/mL] (5 mL, 20 mL, 30 mL, 50 mL); 1.5% [15 mg/mL] (20 mL); 2% [20 mg/mL] (2 mL, 5 mL, 10 mL, 20 mL, 50 mL)

Xylocaine®: 0.5% [5 mg/mL] (50 mL); 1% [10 mg/mL] (10 mL, 20 mL, 50 mL); 2% [20 mg/mL] (1.8 mL, 10 mL, 20 mL, 50 mL)

Injection, solution, as hydrochloride [preservative free]: 0.5% [5 mg/mL] (50 mL); 1% [10 mg/mL] (2 mL, 5 mL, 30 mL); 1.5% [15 mg/mL] (20 mL); 2% [20 mg/mL] (5 mL, 10 mL); 4% [40 mg/mL] (5 mL); 10% [100 mg/mL] (10 mL); 20% [200 mg/mL] (10 mL)

Xylocaine®: 10% [100 mg/mL] (5 mL) [for ventricular arrhythmias]

Xylocaine® MPF: 0.5% [5 mg/mL] (50 mL); 1% [10 mg/mL] (2 mL, 5 mL, 10 mL, 30 mL); 1.5% [15 mg/mL] (10 mL, 20 mL); 2% [20 mg/mL] (2 mL, 5 mL, 10 mL); 4% [40 mg/mL] (5 mL)

Injection, solution, as hydrochloride [premixed in $D_{7.5}W$, preservative free]: 5% (2 mL)

Xylocaine® MPF: 1.5% (2 mL)

Jelly, topical, as hydrochloride:

Anestacon®: 2% (15 mL) [contains benzalkonium chloride]

Xylocaine®: 2% (5 mL, 30 mL)

Liquid, topical (Zilactin®-L): 2.5% (7.5 mL)

Lotion, topical, as hydrochloride (LidMantle®): 3% (177 mL)

Ointment, topical: 5% (37 g)

Patch, transdermal (Lidoderm®): 5% (30s)

Solution, topical, as hydrochloride: 4% [40 mg/mL] (50 mL)

Band-Aid® Hurt-Free™ Antiseptic Wash: 2% (180 mL)

Xylocaine®: 4% [40 mg/mL] (50 mL)

Solution, viscous, as hydrochloride: 2% [20 mg/mL] (20 mL, 100 mL)

Xylocaine® Viscous: 2% [20 mg/mL] (100 mL, 450 mL)

Spray, topical:

Burnamycin: 0.5% (60 mL) [contains aloe vera gel and menthol]

Premjact®: 9.6% (13 mL)

Solarcaine® Aloe Extra Burn Relief: 0.5% (127 g) [contains aloe vera]

Monitoring and Teaching Issues

Physical Assessment: Assess other medications patient may be taking for adverse interactions. **Local anesthetic:** Monitor for effectiveness of anesthesia, and adverse reactions. **Dental/local anesthetic:** Use caution to prevent gagging or choking. Avoid food or drink for 1 hour. Teach patient adverse reactions to report; use and teach appropriate interventions to promote safety. **Antiarrhythmic: I.V.:** ECG and vital signs must be closely and continually monitored. Keep patient supine to reduce hypotensive effects. Assess frequently for adverse reactions or signs of CNS toxicity. Teach patient adverse reactions to report and appropriate interventions to promote safety.

Monitoring Laboratory Tests: I.V.: Serum lidocaine levels. Therapeutic levels range from 1.5-5 mcg/mL; >6 mcg/mL is associated with toxicity.

Patient Education: I.V.: You will be monitored during infusion. Do not get up without assistance. Report dizziness, numbness, double vision, nausea, pain or burning at infusion site, nightmares, hearing strange noises, seeing unusual visions, or respiratory difficulty.

Dermatologic: You will experience decreased sensation to pain, heat, or cold in the area and/or decreased muscle strength (depending on area of application) until effects wear off; use necessary caution to reduce incidence of possible injury until full sensation returns. Report irritation, pain, persistent numbness, tingling, swelling; restlessness, dizziness, acute weakness; blurred vision; ringing in ears; or respiratory difficulty.

Dental/local anesthetic: Lidocaine can cause numbness of tongue, cheeks, and throat. Do not eat or drink for 1 hour after use. Take small sips of water at first to ensure that you can swallow without difficulty. Your tongue and mouth may be numb; use caution avoid biting yourself. Immediately report swelling of face, lips, or tongue.

Transdermal patch: Patch may be cut to appropriate size. Apply patch to most painful area. Up to 3 patches may be applied in a single application. Patch may remain in place for up to 12 hours in any 24-hour period. Remove immediately if burning sensation occurs. Wash hands after application.

Pregnancy precaution: Inform prescriber if you are pregnant.

Dietary Considerations: Premixed injection may contain corn-derived dextrose and its use is contraindicated in patients with allergy to corn-related products.

Geriatric Considerations: Due to decreases in Phase I metabolism and possibly decrease in splanchnic perfusion with age, there may be a decreased clearance or increased half-life in the elderly and increased risk for CNS side effects and cardiac effects.

Pregnancy Risk Factor: B

Lactation: Enters breast milk (small amounts)/use caution (AAP rates "compatible")

Administration

I.V.: Use microdrip (60 drops/mL) or infusion pump to administer an accurate dose.

Topical:

Patch: May be cut to appropriate size. Remove immediately if burning sensation occurs. Wash hands after application.

Gel (Topicaine®): Avoid mucous membranes; remove prior to laser treatment.

Other: Intratracheal: Dilute in NS or distilled water. Absorption is greater with distilled water, but causes more adverse effects on PaO_2. Pass catheter beyond tip of tracheal tube, stop compressions, spray drug quickly down tube. Follow immediately with several quick insufflations and continue chest compressions.

Reconstitution: Standard diluent: 2 g/250 mL D_5W

Compatibility: Stable in D_5LR, $D_5\frac{1}{2}NS$, D_5NS, D_5W, LR, $\frac{1}{4}NS$, NS

Y-site administration: Incompatible with amphotericin B cholesteryl sulfate complex, thiopental

Compatibility in syringe: Incompatible with cefazolin

Compatibility when admixed: Incompatible with amphotericin B, dacarbazine, methohexital, phenytoin

Storage: Lidocaine injection is stable at room temperature. Stability of parenteral admixture at room temperature (25°C) is the expiration date on premixed bag; out of overwrap stability is 30 days.

Related Information

Antiarrhythmic Drugs *on page 1708*
Compatibility of Drugs *on page 1723*
Peak and Trough Guidelines *on page 1694*

Lidocaine and Epinephrine (LYE doe kane & ep i NEF rin)

U.S. Brand Names LidoSite™; Xylocaine® MPF With Epinephrine; Xylocaine® With Epinephrine

Synonyms Epinephrine and Lidocaine

Generic Available Yes

Pharmacologic Category Local Anesthetic

Medication Safety Issues

Transdermal patch may contain conducting metal (eg, aluminum); remove patch prior to MRI.

Use Local infiltration anesthesia; AVS for nerve block; topical local analgesia for superficial dermatologic procedures

Dosing

Adults & Elderly: Dosage varies with the anesthetic procedure, degree of anesthesia needed, vascularity of tissue, duration of anesthesia required, and physical condition of patient.

Dental anesthesia, infiltration, or conduction block:

Children <10 years: 20-30 mg (1-1.5 mL) of lidocaine hydrochloride as a 2% solution with epinephrine 1:100,000; maximum: 4-5 mg of lidocaine hydrochloride/kg of body weight or 100-150 mg as a single dose

# of Cartridges (1.8 mL)	Lidocaine HCl (2%) (mg)	Epinephrine 1:100,000 (mg)
1	36	0.018
2	72	0.036
3	108	0.054
4	144	0.072
5	180	0.090
6	216	0.108
7	252	0.126
8	288	0.144
9	324	0.162
10	360	0.180

(Continued)

Lidocaine and Epinephrine (Continued)

Children >10 years and Adults: Do not exceed 6.6 mg/kg body weight or 300 mg of lidocaine hydrochloride and 3 mcg (0.003 mg) of epinephrine/kg of body weight or 0.2 mg epinephrine per dental appointment. The effective anesthetic dose varies with procedure, intensity of anesthesia needed, duration of anesthesia required, and physical condition of the patient. Always use the lowest effective dose along with careful aspiration.

The following numbers of dental carpules (1.8 mL) provide the indicated amounts of lidocaine hydrochloride 2% and epinephrine 1:100,000 (see table on previous page):

For most routine dental procedures, lidocaine hydrochloride 2% with epinephrine 1:100,000 is preferred. When a more pronounced hemostasis is required, a 1:50,000 epinephrine concentration should be used. The following numbers of dental carpules (1.8 mL) provide the indicated amounts of lidocaine hydrochloride 2% and epinephrine 1:50,000 (see table):

# of Cartridges (1.8 mL)	Lidocaine HCl (2%) (mg)	Epinephrine 1:50,000 (mg)
1	36	0.036
2	72	0.072
3	108	0.108
4	144	0.144
5	180	0.180
6	216	0.216

Dermatologic procedure: Topical: Place 1 transdermal patch over area requiring analgesia; attach patch to iontophoretic controller and leave on for 10 minutes. Remove patch and perform procedure within 10-20 minutes of patch removal. Do not use another patch for 30 minutes.

Pediatrics: Local anesthetic:

Infiltration: Use lidocaine concentrations of 0.5% to 1% (or even more diluted) to decrease possibility of toxicity. Lidocaine dose should not exceed 7 mg/kg/dose; do not repeat within 2 hours.

Dermatologic procedure: Topical: Children ≥5 years: Refer to adult dosing.

Available Dosage Forms

Injection, solution, as hydrochloride, with epinephrine 1:50,000 (Xylocaine® with Epinephrine): Lidocaine 2% [20 mg/mL] (1.8 mL) [contains sodium metabisulfite]

Injection, solution, as hydrochloride, with epinephrine 1:100,000: Lidocaine 1% [10 mg/mL] (20 mL, 30 mL, 50 mL); Lidocaine 2% (20 mL, 30 mL, 50 mL)

Xylocaine® with Epinephrine: Lidocaine 1% [10 mg/mL] (10 mL, 20 mL, 50 mL); Lidocaine 2% (1.8 mL, 10 mL, 20 mL, 50 mL) [contains sodium metabisulfite]

Injection, solution, as hydrochloride, with epinephrine 1:200,000: Lidocaine 0.5% [5 mg/mL] (50 mL)

Xylocaine® with Epinephrine: Lidocaine 0.5% [5 mg/mL] (50 mL) [contains sodium metabisulfite]

Injection, solution, as hydrochloride, with epinephrine 1:200,000 [methylparaben free]: Lidocaine 1% [10 mg/mL] (30 mL); Lidocaine 1.5% (5 mL, 30 mL); Lidocaine 2% (20 mL) [contains sodium metabisulfite]

Xylocaine® MPF with Epinephrine: Lidocaine 1% [10 mg/mL] (5 mL, 10 mL, 30 mL); 1.5% [15 mg/mL] (5 mL, 10 mL, 30 mL); Lidocaine 2% [20 mg/mL] (5 mL, 10 mL, 20 mL) [contains sodium metabisulfite]

Transdermal system (LidoSite™): Lidocaine 10%, epinephrine 0.1% (25s) [contains sodium metabisulfite; for use only with LidoSite™ controller]

Monitoring and Teaching Issues

Physical Assessment: See individual agents.

Patient Education: See individual agents.

Pregnancy Risk Factor: B

Lactation: Enters breast milk/compatible

Related Information

Epinephrine on page 525

Lidocaine on page 898

♦ **Lidocaine Hydrochloride** see Lidocaine on page 898

♦ **Lidoderm®** see Lidocaine on page 898

♦ **LidoSite™** see Lidocaine and Epinephrine on page 901

♦ **Lignocaine Hydrochloride** see Lidocaine on page 898

Lindane (LIN dane)

Synonyms Benzene Hexachloride; Gamma Benzene Hexachloride; Hexachlorocyclohexane

Restrictions An FDA-approved medication guide is available at www.fda.gov/cder/Offices/ODS/labeling.htm; distribute to each patient to whom this medication is dispensed.

Generic Available Yes

Pharmacologic Category Antiparasitic Agent, Topical; Pediculocide; Scabicidal Agent

Use Treatment of *Sarcoptes scabiei* (scabies), *Pediculus capitis* (head lice), and *Phthirus pubis* (crab lice); FDA recommends reserving lindane as a second-line agent or with inadequate response to other therapies

Mechanism of Action/Effect Directly absorbed by parasites and ova through the exoskeleton; stimulates the nervous system resulting in seizures and death of parasitic arthropods

Contraindications Hypersensitivity to lindane or any component of the formulation; uncontrolled seizure disorders; crusted (Norwegian) scabies, acutely-inflamed skin or raw, weeping surfaces or other skin conditions which may increase systemic absorption

Warnings/Precautions Not considered a drug of first choice; seizures and death have been reported with use; use with caution in infants, small children, patients <50 kg, or patients with a history of seizures; use caution with conditions which may increase risk of seizures or medications which decrease seizure threshold; use caution with hepatic impairment; avoid contact with face, eyes, mucous membranes, and urethral meatus. Because of the potential for systemic absorption and CNS side effects, lindane should be used with caution; consider permethrin or crotamiton agent first. Oil-based hair dressing may increase toxic potential. A lindane medication use guide must be given to all patients along with instructions for proper use. Should be used as a part of an overall lice management program.

Drug Interactions

Increased Effect/Toxicity: Increased toxicity: Drugs which lower seizure threshold

Adverse Reactions Frequency not defined (includes postmarketing and/or case reports).

Cardiovascular: Cardiac arrhythmia

Central nervous system: Ataxia, dizziness, headache, restlessness, seizure, pain

Dermatologic: Alopecia, contact dermatitis, skin and adipose tissue may act as repositories, eczematous eruptions, pruritus, urticaria

Gastrointestinal: Nausea, vomiting

Hematologic: Aplastic anemia

Hepatic: Hepatitis

Local: Burning and stinging

Neuromuscular & skeletal: Paresthesias

Renal: Hematuria

Respiratory: Pulmonary edema

Overdosage/Toxicology Symptoms of overdose include vomiting, restlessness, ataxia, seizures, arrhythmias, pulmonary edema, hematuria, and hepatitis. The drug is absorbed through the skin, mucous membranes, and GI tract, and has occasionally caused serious CNS, hepatic, and renal toxicity when used excessively for prolonged periods, or with accidental ingestion. If ingested, perform gastric lavage and general supportive measures.

Pharmacodynamics/Kinetics

Absorption: ≤13% systemically

Time to Peak: Serum: Children: 6 hours

Half-Life Elimination: Children: 17-22 hours

Metabolism: Hepatic

Excretion: Urine and feces

Dosing

Adults & Elderly:

Scabies: Topical: Apply a thin layer of lotion and massage it on skin from the neck to the toes; after 8-12 hours, bathe and remove the drug

Head lice, crab lice: Topical: Apply shampoo to dry hair and massage into hair for 4 minutes; add small quantities of water to hair until lather forms, then rinse hair thoroughly and comb with a fine tooth comb to remove nits. Amount of shampoo needed is based on length and density of hair; most patients will require 30 mL (maximum: 60 mL).

Pediatrics: Refer to adult dosing.

Available Dosage Forms

Lotion, topical: 1% (60 mL)

Shampoo, topical: 1% (60 mL) [contains alcohol 0.5%]

Monitoring and Teaching Issues

Physical Assessment: Assess head, hair, and skin surfaces for presence of lice and nits. Assess knowledge/teach patient appropriate application, use, and adverse symptoms to report.

Patient Education: For external use only. Do not apply to face and avoid getting in eyes. Do not apply immediately after hot soapy bath. For scabies, Apply from neck to toes. Bathe to remove drug after 8-12 hours. For head lice or crab lice, massage into dry hair for 4 minutes; add water to hair to form lather, then rinse thoroughly. Clothing and bedding must be washed in hot water or dry cleaned to kill nits. Wash combs and brushes with lindane shampoo and thoroughly rinse. May need to treat all members of household and all sexual contacts concurrently. Report if condition persists or infection occurs. **Pregnancy/breast-feeding precautions:** Inform prescriber if you are pregnant. Do not breast-feed.

Geriatric Considerations: Safety and efficacy have not been studied in the elderly; deaths following use have been reported.

Pregnancy Risk Factor: C

Pregnancy Issues: There are no adequate and well-controlled studies in pregnant women. CDC recommends alternative treatment in pregnant women (pyrethrins with piperonyl butoxide or permethrin for lice, permethrin for scabies). Per manufacturer, should be used no more than twice in a pregnancy. Reapplication of lindane is **not** the appropriate treatment if itching continues after the single treatment.

Lactation: Enters breast milk/contraindicated

Breast-Feeding Issues: Nursing mothers should interrupt breast-feeding, express and discard milk for at least 24 hours following use.

Administration

Oral: Never administer orally.

Topical: For topical use only. Caregivers should apply with gloves (avoid natural latex, may be permeable to lindane). Rinse off with warm (not hot) water.

Lotion: Apply to dry, cool skin; do not apply to face or eyes. Wait at least 1 hour after bathing or showering (wet or warm skin increases absorption). Skin should be clean and free of any other lotions, creams, or oil prior to lindane application.

Shampoo: Apply to clean, dry hair. Wait at least 1 hour after washing hair before applying lindane shampoo. Hair should be washed with a shampoo not containing a conditioner; hair and skin of head and neck should be free of any lotions, oils, or creams prior to lindane application.

Linezolid (li NE zoh lid)

U.S. Brand Names Zyvox™
Generic Available No
Pharmacologic Category Antibiotic, Oxazolidinone
Medication Safety Issues
Sound-alike/look-alike issues:
Zyvox™ may be confused with Vioxx®, Zosyn®, Zovirax®

Use Treatment of vancomycin-resistant *Enterococcus faecium* (VRE) infections, nosocomial pneumonia caused by *Staphylococcus aureus* including MRSA or *Streptococcus pneumoniae* (including multidrug-resistant strains [MDRSP]), complicated and uncomplicated skin and skin structure infections (including diabetic foot infections without concomitant osteomyelitis), and community-acquired pneumonia caused by susceptible gram-positive organisms

Mechanism of Action/Effect Inhibits bacterial protein synthesis by binding to bacterial 23S ribosomal RNA of the 50S subunit. This prevents the formation of a functional 70S initiation complex that is essential for the bacterial translation process. Linezolid is bacteriostatic against enterococci and staphylococci and bactericidal against most strains of streptococci.

Contraindications Hypersensitivity to linezolid or any other component of the formulation

Warnings/Precautions Myelosuppression has been reported and may be dependent on duration of therapy (generally >2 weeks of treatment); use with caution in patients with pre-existing myelosuppression, in patients receiving other drugs which may cause bone marrow suppression, or in chronic infection (previous or concurrent antibiotic therapy). Weekly CBC monitoring is recommended. Discontinue linezolid in patients developing myelosuppression (or in whom myelosuppression worsens during treatment).

Lactic acidosis has been reported with use. Patients who develop recurrent nausea and vomiting, unexplained acidosis, or low bicarbonate levels need immediate evaluation.

Linezolid has mild MAO inhibitor properties and has the potential to have the same interactions as other MAO inhibitors; use with caution in uncontrolled hypertension, pheochromocytoma, carcinoid syndrome, or untreated hyperthyroidism; avoid use with serotonergic agents such as TCAs, venlafaxine, trazodone, sibutramine, meperidine, dextromethorphan, and SSRIs; consider alternatives before initiating outpatient treatment (unnecessary use may lead the development of resistance to linezolid).

Drug Interactions
Increased Effect/Toxicity: Linezolid is a reversible, nonselective inhibitor of MAO. Serotonergic agents (eg, TCAs, venlafaxine, trazodone, sibutramine, meperidine, dextromethorphan, and SSRIs) may cause a serotonin syndrome (eg, hyperpyrexia, cognitive dysfunction) when used concomitantly. Adrenergic agents (eg, phenylpropanolamine, pseudoephedrine, sympathomimetic agents, vasopressor or dopaminergic agents) may cause hypertension. Tramadol may increase the risk of seizures when used concurrently with linezolid. Myelosuppressive medications may increase risk of myelosuppression when used concurrently with linezolid.

Nutritional/Ethanol Interactions
Ethanol: Avoid ethanol (may contain tyramine, hypertensive crisis may result).
Food: Avoid foods (eg, cheese) and beverages containing tyramine in patients receiving linezolid (hypertensive crisis may result).

Adverse Reactions Percentages as reported in adults; frequency similar in pediatric patients
1% to 10%:
Cardiovascular: Hypertension (1% to 3%)
Central nervous system: Headache (0.5% to 11%), insomnia (3%), dizziness (0.4% to 2%), fever (2%)
Dermatologic: Rash (2%)
Gastrointestinal: Nausea (3% to 10%), diarrhea (3% to 11%), vomiting (1% to 4%), constipation (2%), taste alteration (1% to 2%), tongue discoloration (0.2% to 1%), oral moniliasis (0.4% to 1%), pancreatitis
Genitourinary: Vaginal moniliasis (1% to 2%)
Hematologic: Thrombocytopenia (0.3% to 10%), anemia, leukopenia, neutropenia; **Note:** Myelosuppression (including anemia, leukopenia, pancytopenia, and thrombocytopenia; may be more common in patients receiving linezolid for >2 weeks)
Hepatic: Abnormal LFTs (0.4% to 1%)
Miscellaneous: Fungal infection (0.1% to 2%)

Overdosage/Toxicology Treatment includes supportive care. Hemodialysis may improve elimination (30% of a dose is removed during a 3-hour hemodialysis session).

Pharmacodynamics/Kinetics
Absorption: Rapid and extensive
Bioavailability: 100%
Time to Peak: Adults: Oral: 1-2 hours
Protein Binding: Adults: 31%
Half-Life Elimination: Children ≥1 week (full-term) to 11 years: 1.5-3 hours; Adults: 4-5 hours
Metabolism: Hepatic via oxidation of the morpholine ring, resulting in two inactive metabolites (aminoethoxyacetic acid, hydroxyethyl glycine); does not involve CYP
Excretion: Urine (30% as parent drug, 50% as metabolites); feces (9% as metabolites)
Nonrenal clearance: 65%; increased in children ≥1 week to 11 years

Dosing
Adults & Elderly:
VRE infections: Oral, I.V.: 600 mg every 12 hours for 14-28 days
Nosocomial pneumonia, complicated skin and skin structure infections, community-acquired pneumonia including concurrent bacteremia: Oral, I.V.: 600 mg every 12 hours for 10-14 days
Uncomplicated skin and skin structure infections: Oral: 400 mg every 12 hours for 10-14 days

Pediatrics:

VRE infections: Oral, I.V.:

Preterm neonates (<34 weeks gestational age): 10 mg/kg every 12 hours; neonates with a suboptimal clinical response can be advanced to 10 mg/kg every 8 hours. By day 7 of life, all neonates should receive 10 mg/kg every 8 hours.

Infants (excluding preterm neonates <1 week) and Children ≤11 years: 10 mg/kg every 8 hours for 14-28 days

Children ≥12 years: Refer to adult dosing.

Nosocomial pneumonia, complicated skin and skin structure infections, community acquired pneumonia including concurrent bacteremia: Oral, I.V.:

Infants (excluding preterm neonates <1 week) and Children ≤11 years: 10 mg/kg every 8 hours for 10-14 days

Children ≥12 years: Refer to adult dosing.

Uncomplicated skin and skin structure infections: Oral:

Infants (excluding preterm neonates <1 week) and Children <5 years: 10 mg/kg every 8 hours for 10-14 days

Children 5-11 years: 10 mg/kg every 12 hours for 10-14 days

Children ≥12-18 years: 600 mg every 12 hours for 10-14 days

Renal Impairment: No adjustment is recommended. The two primary metabolites may accumulate in patients with renal impairment but the clinical significance is unknown. Weigh the risk of accumulation of metabolites versus the benefit of therapy. Both linezolid and the two metabolites are eliminated by dialysis. Linezolid should be given after hemodialysis.

Hepatic Impairment: No dosage adjustment required for mild to moderate hepatic insufficiency (Child-Pugh class A or B). Use in severe hepatic insufficiency has not been adequately evaluated.

Available Dosage Forms

Infusion [premixed]: 200 mg (100 mL) [contains sodium 1.7 mEq]; 400 mg (200 mL) [contains sodium 3.3 mEq]; 600 mg (300 mL) [contains sodium 5 mEq]

Powder for oral suspension: 20 mg/mL (150 mL) [contains phenylalanine 20 mg/5 mL, sodium benzoate, and sodium 0.4 mEq/5 mL; orange flavor]

Tablet: 400 mg, 600 mg [each strength contains sodium 0.1 mEq/tablet]

Monitoring and Teaching Issues

Physical Assessment: Assess for previous drug allergies before administering first dose. See Warnings/Precautions for use cautions (eg, myelosuppression, uncontrolled hypertension). Assess other pharmacological agents patient may be taking for effectiveness and interactions (eg, serotonergic agents may increase resistance to linezolid and increase risk of serotonin syndrome, increased risk of hypertension with adrenergic agents; see Drug Interactions). Assess results of laboratory tests, therapeutic effectiveness (resolution of infection), and adverse reactions on a regular basis (see Adverse Reactions). Teach patient proper use (oral), possible side effects/appropriate interventions (eg, tyramine free diet; see Tyramine Content of Foods list *on page 1758*), and adverse symptoms to report (see Patient Education).

Monitoring Laboratory Tests: Weekly CBC and platelet counts, particularly in patients at increased risk of bleeding, with pre-existing myelosuppression, on concomitant medications that cause bone marrow suppression, in those who require >2 weeks of therapy, or in those with chronic infection who have received previous or concomitant antibiotic therapy.

Patient Education:

Oral: Take exactly as directed; with or without food. Do not alter dosage without consulting prescriber. Complete full course of therapy even if condition appears controlled. Maintain adequate hydration (2-3 L/day of fluids) unless instructed to restrict fluid intake. Avoid alcohol. Avoid tyramine-containing foods (eg, pickles, aged cheese, wine).

Oral/I.V.: You may experience GI discomfort, nausea, vomiting, taste alteration (small frequent meals, frequent mouth care, sucking lozenges, or chewing gum may help); mild headache (analgesic may help); or constipation (increase exercise, fluids, fruit, or fiber may help). Report immediately unresolved, liquid diarrhea; white plaques in mouth; skin rash or irritation; acute headache, dizziness, blurred vision; or other persistent adverse reactions. **Pregnancy/breast-feeding precautions:** Inform prescriber if you are or intend to become pregnant. Consult prescriber if breast-feeding.

Dietary Considerations: Take with or without food. Suspension contains 20 mg phenylalanine per teaspoonful. Sodium content: 0.1 mEq/tablet; 0.4 mEq/5 mL; 1.7 mEq/100 mL infusion; 3.3 mEq/200 mL infusion; 5 mEq/300 mL infusion

Pregnancy Risk Factor: C

Lactation: Excretion in breast milk unknown/use caution

Administration

Oral: Oral suspension: Invert gently to mix prior to administration, do not shake

I.V.: Administer intravenous infusion over 30-120 minutes. Do not mix or infuse with other medications. When the same intravenous line is used for sequential infusion of other medications, flush line with D_5W, NS, or LR before and after infusing linezolid. The yellow color of the injection may intensify over time without affecting potency.

Compatibility:

Y-site administration: Incompatible with amphotericin B, chlorpromazine, diazepam, erythromycin, pentamidine, phenytoin, sulfamethoxazole/trimethoprim

Compatibility when admixed: Incompatible with ceftriaxone

Storage:

Infusion: Store at 25°C (77°F). Protect from light. Keep infusion bags in overwrap until ready for use. Protect infusion bags from freezing.

Oral suspension: Following reconstitution, store at room temperature; use reconstituted suspension within 21 days

Related Information

Antimicrobial Drugs of Choice *on page 1792*

Community-Acquired Pneumonia in Adults *on page 1807*

♦ **Lioresal®** *see* Baclofen *on page 172*

- ◆ **Lipancreatin** *see* Pancrelipase *on page 1151*
- ◆ **Lipid-Lowering Agents** *see page 1738*
- ◆ **Lipitor®** *see* Atorvastatin *on page 152*
- ◆ **Liposyn® III** *see* Fat Emulsion *on page 610*
- ◆ **Lipram 4500** *see* Pancrelipase *on page 1151*
- ◆ **Lipram-CR** *see* Pancrelipase *on page 1151*
- ◆ **Lipram-PN** *see* Pancrelipase *on page 1151*
- ◆ **Lipram-UL** *see* Pancrelipase *on page 1151*
- ◆ **Liquid Antidote** *see* Charcoal *on page 302*

Lisinopril (lyse IN oh pril)

U.S. Brand Names Prinivil®; Zestril®

Generic Available Yes

Pharmacologic Category Angiotensin-Converting Enzyme (ACE) Inhibitor

Medication Safety Issues

Sound-alike/look-alike issues:

Lisinopril may be confused with fosinopril, Lioresal®, Risperdal®

Prinivil® may be confused with Plendil®, Pravachol®, Prevacid®, Prilosec®, Proventil®

Zestril® may be confused with Desyrel®, Restoril®, Vistaril®, Zetia™, Zostrix®

Use Treatment of hypertension, either alone or in combination with other antihypertensive agents; adjunctive therapy in treatment of CHF (afterload reduction); treatment of acute myocardial infarction within 24 hours in hemodynamically-stable patients to improve survival; treatment of left ventricular dysfunction after myocardial infarction

Mechanism of Action/Effect Competitive inhibitor of angiotensin-converting enzyme (ACE); prevents conversion of angiotensin I to angiotensin II, a potent vasoconstrictor; results in lower levels of angiotensin II which causes an increase in plasma renin activity and a reduction in aldosterone secretion

Contraindications Hypersensitivity to lisinopril or any component of the formulation; angioedema related to previous treatment with an ACE inhibitor; bilateral renal artery stenosis; pregnancy (2nd and 3rd trimesters)

Warnings/Precautions Anaphylactic reactions can occur. Angioedema can occur at any time during treatment (especially following first dose). Angioedema may involve head and neck (potentially affecting the airway) or the intestine (presenting with abdominal pain). Careful blood pressure monitoring with first dose (hypotension can occur especially in volume depleted patients). Dosage adjustment needed in renal impairment. Use with caution in hypovolemia; collagen vascular diseases; valvular stenosis (particularly aortic stenosis); hyperkalemia; or before, during, or immediately after anesthesia. Avoid rapid dosage escalation, which may lead to renal insufficiency. Rare toxicities associated with ACE inhibitors include cholestatic jaundice (which may progress to hepatic necrosis) and neutropenia/agranulocytosis with myeloid hyperplasia. If patient has renal impairment then a baseline WBC with differential and serum creatinine should be evaluated and monitored closely during the first 3 months of therapy. Hypersensitivity reactions may be seen during hemodialysis with high-flux dialysis membranes (eg, AN69). Deterioration in renal function can occur with initiation. Use with caution in unilateral renal artery stenosis and pre-existing renal insufficiency. Safety and efficacy have not been established in children <6 years of age.

Drug Interactions

Decreased Effect: Aspirin (high dose) may reduce the therapeutic effects of ACE inhibitors; at low dosages this does not appear to be significant. Rifampin may decrease the effect of ACE inhibitors. Antacids may decrease the bioavailability of ACE inhibitors (may be more likely to occur with captopril); separate administration times by 1-2 hours. NSAIDs, specifically indomethacin, may reduce the hypotensive effects of ACE inhibitors. More likely to occur in low renin or volume dependent hypertensive patients.

Increased Effect/Toxicity: Potassium supplements, co-trimoxazole (high dose), angiotensin II receptor antagonists (eg, candesartan, losartan, irbesartan), or potassium-sparing diuretics (amiloride, spironolactone, triamterene) may result in elevated serum potassium levels when combined with lisinopril. ACE inhibitor effects may be increased by phenothiazines or probenecid (increases levels of captopril). ACE inhibitors may increase serum concentrations/effects of digoxin, lithium, and sulfonlyureas.

Diuretics have additive hypotensive effects with ACE inhibitors, and hypovolemia increases the potential for adverse renal effects of ACE inhibitors. In patients with compromised renal function, coadministration with NSAIDs may result in further deterioration of renal function. Allopurinol and ACE inhibitors may cause a higher risk of hypersensitivity reaction when taken concurrently.

Nutritional/Ethanol Interactions Herb/Nutraceutical: Avoid dong quai if using for hypertension (has estrogenic activity). Avoid ephedra, yohimbe, ginseng (may worsen hypertension). Avoid garlic (may have increased antihypertensive effect).

Lab Interactions May cause false-positive results in urine acetone determinations using sodium nitroprusside reagent; increased potassium (S), serum creatinine/BUN

Adverse Reactions Note: Frequency ranges include data from hypertension and heart failure trials. Higher rates of adverse reactions have generally been noted in patients with CHF. However, the frequency of adverse effects associated with placebo is also increased in this population.

1% to 10%:

Cardiovascular: Orthostatic effects (1%), hypotension (1% to 4%)

Central nervous system: Headache (4% to 6%), dizziness (5% to 12%), fatigue (3%)

Dermatologic: Rash (1% to 2%)

Endocrine & metabolic: Hyperkalemia (2% to 5%)

Gastrointestinal: Diarrhea (3% to 4%), nausea (2%), vomiting (1%), abdominal pain (2%)

Genitourinary: Impotence (1%)

Hematologic: Decreased hemoglobin (small)

Neuromuscular & skeletal: Chest pain (3%), weakness (1%)

Renal: BUN increased (2%); deterioration in renal function (in patients with bilateral renal artery stenosis or hypovolemia); serum creatinine increased (often transient)

Respiratory: Cough (4% to 9%), upper respiratory infection (2% to 2%)

Overdosage/Toxicology Mild hypotension may be the primary toxic effect seen with acute overdose. Bradycardia may also occur; hyperkalemia occurs even with therapeutic doses, especially in patients with renal insufficiency and those taking NSAIDs. Treatment and is symptomatic and supportive.

Pharmacodynamics/Kinetics

Onset of Action: 1 hour; Peak effect: Hypotensive: Oral: ~6 hours

Duration of Action: 24 hours

Absorption: Well absorbed; unaffected by food

Protein Binding: 25%

Half-Life Elimination: 11-12 hours

Excretion: Primarily urine (as unchanged drug)

Dosing

Adults:

Hypertension: Oral: Initial: 10 mg/day; increase doses 5-10 mg/day at 1- to 2-week intervals; maximum daily dose: 40 mg

Note: Patients taking diuretics should have them discontinued 2-3 days prior to initiating lisinopril if possible. Restart diuretic after blood pressure is stable if needed. If diuretic cannot be discontinued prior to therapy, begin with 5 mg with close supervision until stable blood pressure. In patients with hyponatremia (<130 mEq/L), start dose at 2.5 mg/day.

Congestive heart failure: Oral: Initial: 5 mg; then increase by no more than 10 mg increments at intervals no less than 2 weeks to a maximum daily dose of 40 mg. Usual maintenance: 5-40 mg/day as a single dose. Patients should start/continue standard therapy, including diuretics, beta-blockers, and digoxin, as indicated.

Acute myocardial infarction (within 24 hours in hemodynamically stable patients): Oral: 5 mg immediately, then 5 mg at 24 hours, 10 mg at 48 hours, and 10 mg every day thereafter for 6 weeks. Patients should continue to receive standard treatments such as thrombolytics, aspirin, and beta-blockers.

Elderly: Oral:

Initial: 2.5-5 mg/day; increase doses 2.5-5 mg/day at 1- to 2-week intervals; maximum daily dose: 40 mg

Patients taking diuretics should have them discontinued 2-3 days prior to initiating lisinopril if possible. Restart diuretic after blood pressure is stable if needed. In patients with hyponatremia (<130 mEq/L), start dose at 2.5 mg/day (see Renal Impairment).

Pediatrics:

Hypertension: Children ≥6 years: Oral: Initial: 0.07 mg/kg once daily (up to 5 mg); increase dose at 1- to 2-week intervals; doses >0.61 mg/kg or >40 mg have not been evaluated.

Renal Impairment:

Adults: Initial doses should be modified and upward titration should be cautious, based on response (maximum: 40 mg/day)

Cl_{cr} >30 mL/minute: Initial: 10 mg/day

Cl_{cr} 10-30 mL/minute: Initial: 5 mg/day

Hemodialysis: Initial: 2.5 mg/day; dialyzable (50%)

Children: Use in not recommended in pediatric patients with GFR <30 mL/minute/1.73 m^2

Available Dosage Forms [DSC] = Discontinued product

Tablet: 2.5 mg, 5 mg, 10 mg, 20 mg, 30 mg, 40 mg

Prinivil®: 2.5 mg [DSC], 5 mg, 10 mg, 20 mg, 30 mg, 40 mg

Zestril®: 2.5 mg, 5 mg, 10 mg, 20 mg, 30 mg, 40 mg

Monitoring and Teaching Issues

Physical Assessment: Use caution in presence of renal impairment; hypovolemia; collagen vascular diseases; valvular stenosis; hyperkalemia; or before, during, or immediately after anesthesia (see Warnings/Precautions for specific use cautions). Assess potential for interactions with other pharmacological agents or herbal products patient may be taking (especially anything that may impact fluid balance or cardiac status; see Drug Interactions). Assess results of laboratory tests, therapeutic effectiveness, and adverse response on a regular basis during therapy (eg, hypovolemia, angioedema, postural hypotension; see Adverse Reactions). Teach patient proper use, possible side effects/appropriate interventions, and adverse symptoms to report (see Patient Education).

Monitoring Laboratory Tests: CBC, renal function tests, electrolytes. If patient has renal impairment, a baseline WBC with differential and serum creatinine should be evaluated and monitored closely during the first 3 months of therapy.

Patient Education: Do not take any new medication during therapy unless approved by prescriber. Do not use potassium supplement or salt substitutes without consulting prescriber. Take exactly as directed; do not discontinue without consulting prescriber. Take first dose at bedtime. Take all doses on an empty stomach, 1 hour before or 2 hours after meals. This drug does not eliminate need for diet or exercise regimen as recommended by prescriber. May cause dizziness, fainting, or lightheadedness (use caution when driving or engaging in tasks that require alertness until response to drug is known); postural hypotension (use caution when rising from lying or sitting position or climbing stairs); or nausea, vomiting, abdominal pain, dry mouth, or transient loss of appetite (small frequent meals, frequent mouth care, sucking lozenges, or chewing gum may help) report if these persist. Report chest pain or palpitations; mouth sores; fever or chills; swelling of extremities, face, mouth, or tongue; skin rash; numbness, tingling, or pain in muscles; respiratory difficulty or unusual cough; or other persistent adverse reactions. **Pregnancy/breast-feeding precautions:** Inform prescriber if you are or intend to become pregnant. This drug should not be used in the 2nd or 3rd trimester of pregnancy. Consult prescriber for appropriate contraceptive measures. Breast-feeding is not recommended.

Geriatric Considerations: Due to frequent decreases in glomerular filtration (also creatinine clearance) with aging, elderly patients may have exaggerated responses to ACE inhibitors. Differences in clinical response due to hepatic changes are not observed. ACE

(Continued)

Lisinopril *(Continued)*

inhibitors may be preferred agents in elderly patients with congestive heart failure and diabetes mellitus. Diabetic proteinuria is reduced and insulin sensitivity is enhanced. In general, the side effect profile is favorable in the elderly and causes little or no CNS confusion. Use lowest dose recommendations initially.

Pregnancy Risk Factor: C/D (2nd and 3rd trimesters)

Pregnancy Issues: ACE inhibitors can cause fetal injury or death if taken during the 2nd or 3rd trimester. Discontinue ACE inhibitors as soon as pregnancy is detected.

Lactation: Excretion in breast milk unknown/not recommended

Breast-Feeding Issues: Lisinopril is not recommended (per manufacturer) in breast-feeding women. A similar drug, captopril, has been rated as compatible.

Administration

Oral: Watch for hypotensive effects within 1-3 hours of first dose or new higher dose.

Related Information

Angiotensin Agents *on page 1704*
Heart Failure *on page 1828*

Lisinopril and Hydrochlorothiazide

(lyse IN oh pril & hye droe klor oh THYE a zide)

U.S. Brand Names Prinzide®; Zestoretic®

Synonyms Hydrochlorothiazide and Lisinopril

Generic Available Yes

Pharmacologic Category Antihypertensive Agent, Combination

Use Treatment of hypertension

Dosing

Adults & Elderly: Hypertension: Oral: Initial: Lisinopril 10 mg/hydrochlorothiazide 12.5 mg or lisinopril 20 mg/hydrochlorothiazide 12.5 mg with further increases of either or both components could depend on clinical response. Doses >80 mg/day lisinopril or >50 mg/day hydrochlorothiazide are not recommended.

Renal Impairment: Dosage adjustments should be made with caution. Usual regimens of therapy need not be adjusted as long as patient's Cl_{cr} >30 mL/minute. In patients with more severe renal impairment, loop diuretics are preferred.

Available Dosage Forms Tablet:
Lisinopril 10 mg and hydrochlorothiazide 12.5 mg
Lisinopril 20 mg and hydrochlorothiazide 12.5 mg
Lisinopril 20 mg and hydrochlorothiazide 25 mg

Monitoring and Teaching Issues

Physical Assessment: See individual agents.

Patient Education: See individual agents. **Pregnancy/breast-feeding precautions:** Inform prescriber if you are or intend to become pregnant. Consult prescriber if breast-feeding.

Pregnancy Risk Factor: C/D (2nd and 3rd trimesters)

Lactation:
Hydrochlorothiazide: Compatible
Lisinopril: Excretion in breast milk unknown

Related Information

Hydrochlorothiazide *on page 751*
Lisinopril *on page 906*

♦ **Lispro, Insulin** *see* Insulin Preparations *on page 805*

Lithium (LITH ee um)

U.S. Brand Names Eskalith®; Eskalith CR®; Lithobid®

Synonyms Lithium Carbonate; Lithium Citrate

Generic Available Yes

Pharmacologic Category Lithium

Medication Safety Issues
Sound-alike/look-alike issues:
Eskalith® may be confused with Estratest®
Lithobid® may be confused with Levbid®, Lithostat®

Use Management of bipolar disorders; treatment of mania in individuals with bipolar disorder (maintenance treatment prevents or diminishes intensity of subsequent episodes)

Unlabeled/Investigational Use Potential augmenting agent for antidepressants; aggression, post-traumatic stress disorder, conduct disorder in children

Mechanism of Action/Effect Stabilizes mood by actions on nerve cells of the central nervous system; involves serotonin, phosphatidylinositol cycle, and dopamine receptor sensitivity

Contraindications Hypersensitivity to lithium or any component of the formulation; avoid use in patients with severe cardiovascular or renal disease, or with severe debilitation, dehydration, or sodium depletion; pregnancy

Warnings/Precautions Lithium toxicity is closely related to serum levels and can occur at therapeutic doses; serum lithium determinations are required to monitor therapy. Use with caution in patients with thyroid disease, mild-moderate renal impairment, or mild-moderate cardiovascular disease. Use caution in patients receiving medications which alter sodium excretion (eg, diuretics, ACE inhibitors, NSAIDs), or in patients with significant fluid loss (protracted sweating, diarrhea, or prolonged fever); temporary reduction or cessation of therapy may be warranted. Some elderly patients may be extremely sensitive to the effects of lithium, see Dosing. Chronic therapy results in diminished renal concentrating ability (nephrogenic DI); this is usually reversible when lithium is discontinued. Changes in renal function should be monitored, and re-evaluation of treatment may be necessary. Use caution in patients at risk of suicide (suicidal thoughts or behavior).

Use with caution in patients receiving neuroleptic medications - a syndrome resembling NMS has been associated with concurrent therapy. Lithium may impair the patient's alertness, affecting the ability to operate machinery or driving a vehicle. Neuromuscular-blocking agents should be administered with caution; the response may be prolonged.

Higher serum concentrations may be required and tolerated during an acute manic phase; however, the tolerance decreases when symptoms subside. Normal fluid and salt intake must be maintained during therapy.

Safety and efficacy have not been established in children <12 years of age.

Drug Interactions

Decreased Effect: Combined use of lithium and chlorpromazine may lower serum concentrations of both drugs. Lithium may blunt the pressor response to sympathomimetics (epinephrine, norepinephrine). Caffeine (xanthine derivatives) may lower lithium serum concentrations by increasing urinary lithium excretion (monitor).

Increased Effect/Toxicity: Concurrent use of lithium with carbamazepine, diltiazem, SSRIs (fluoxetine, fluvoxamine), haloperidol, methyldopa, metronidazole (rare), phenothiazines, phenytoin, TCAs, and verapamil may increase the risk for neurotoxicity. A rare encephalopathic syndrome has been reported in association with haloperidol (causal relationship not established). Lithium concentrations/toxicity may be increased by diuretics, NSAIDs (sulindac and aspirin may be exceptions), ACE inhibitors, angiotensin receptor antagonists (losartan), tetracyclines, or COX-2 inhibitors (celecoxib).

Lithium and MAO inhibitors should generally be avoided due to use reports of fatal malignant hyperpyrexia; risk with selective MAO type B inhibitors (selegiline) appears to be lower. Potassium iodide may enhance the hypothyroid effects of lithium. Combined use of lithium with tricyclic antidepressants or sibutramine may increase the risk of serotonin syndrome; this combination is best avoided. Lithium may potentiate effect of neuromuscular blockers.

Nutritional/Ethanol Interactions Food: Lithium serum concentrations may be increased if taken with food. Limit caffeine.

Lab Interactions Increased calcium (S), glucose, magnesium, potassium (S); decreased thyroxine (S)

Adverse Reactions Frequency not defined.

Cardiovascular: Cardiac arrhythmia, hypotension, sinus node dysfunction, flattened or inverted T waves (reversible), edema, bradycardia, syncope

Central nervous system: Dizziness, vertigo, slurred speech, blackout spells, seizure, sedation, restlessness, confusion, psychomotor retardation, stupor, coma, dystonia, fatigue, lethargy, headache, pseudotumor cerebri, slowed intellectual functioning, tics

Dermatologic: Dry or thinning of hair, folliculitis, alopecia, exacerbation of psoriasis, rash

Endocrine & metabolic: Euthyroid goiter and/or hypothyroidism, hyperthyroidism, hyperglycemia, diabetes insipidus

Gastrointestinal: Polydipsia, anorexia, nausea, vomiting, diarrhea, xerostomia, metallic taste, weight gain, salivary gland swelling, excessive salivation

Genitourinary: Incontinence, polyuria, glycosuria, oliguria, albuminuria

Hematologic: Leukocytosis

Neuromuscular & skeletal: Tremor, muscle hyperirritability, ataxia, choreoathetoid movements, hyperactive deep tendon reflexes, myasthenia gravis (rare)

Ocular: Nystagmus, blurred vision, transient scotoma

Miscellaneous: Coldness and painful discoloration of fingers and toes

Overdosage/Toxicology Symptoms include sedation, confusion, tremors, joint pain, visual changes, seizures, and coma. There is no specific antidote for lithium poisoning. For acute ingestion, following initiation of essential overdose management, discontinue lithium and remove any unabsorbed lithium via gastric lavage (activated charcoal is ineffective as it does not bind lithium). Correct fluid and electrolyte imbalances, provide supportive care. In severe cases, patient should be dialyzed. Hemodialysis is preferred (and more effective) than peritoneal dialysis. The goal is to decrease serum lithium level to <1 mEq/L on a serum sample drawn 6-8 hours after completion of dialysis. Agents that increase the excretion of lithium are of questionable value.

Pharmacodynamics/Kinetics

Absorption: Rapid and complete

Bioavailability: Not affected by food; Capsule, immediate release tablet: 95% to 100%; Extended release tablet: 60% to 90%; Syrup: 100%

Time to Peak: Serum: Nonsustained release: ~0.5-2 hours; slow release: 4-12 hours; syrup: 15-60 minutes

Protein Binding: Not protein bound

Half-Life Elimination: 18-24 hours; can increase to more than 36 hours in elderly or with renal impairment

Metabolism: Not metabolized

Excretion: Urine (90% to 98% as unchanged drug); sweat (4% to 5%); feces (1%)

Clearance: 80% of filtered lithium is reabsorbed in the proximal convoluted tubules; therefore, clearance approximates 20% of GFR or 20-40 mL/minute

Dosing

Adults:

Bipolar disorders: Oral: 900-2400 mg/day in 3-4 divided doses or 900-1800 mg/day in two divided doses of sustained release

Note: Monitor serum concentrations and clinical response (efficacy and toxicity) to determine proper dose

Elderly: Bipolar disorders: Oral: Initial: 300 mg twice daily; increase weekly in increments of 300 mg/day, monitoring levels; rarely need to go >900-1200 mg/day.

Pediatrics:

Bipolar disorders: Oral: Children 6-12 years: 15-60 mg/kg/day in 3-4 divided doses; dose not to exceed usual adult dosage. **Note:** Monitor serum concentrations and clinical response (efficacy and toxicity) to determine proper dose.

(Continued)

Lithium (Continued)

Conduct disorder (unlabeled use): Oral: Children 6-12 years: 15-30 mg/kg/day in 3-4 divided doses; dose not to exceed usual adult dosage

Renal Impairment:

Cl_{cr} 10-50 mL/minute: Administer 50% to 75% of normal dose.

Cl_{cr} <10 mL/minute: Administer 25% to 50% of normal dose.

Dialyzable (50% to 100%); 4-7 times more efficient than peritoneal dialysis

Available Dosage Forms

Capsule, as carbonate: 150 mg, 300 mg, 600 mg

Eskalith®: 300 mg [contains benzyl alcohol]

Syrup, as citrate: 300 mg/5 mL (5 mL, 10 mL, 480 mL) [contains alcohol]

Tablet, as carbonate: 300 mg

Tablet, controlled release, as carbonate (Eskalith CR®): 450 mg

Tablet, slow release, as carbonate (Lithobid®): 300 mg

Monitoring and Teaching Issues

Physical Assessment: Assess effectiveness and interactions of other medications patient may be taking. Monitor cardiovascular status; assess for fluid retention. Monitor laboratory results at beginning of therapy, when adjusting dose, and periodically thereafter. Monitor effectiveness of therapy and adverse reactions at beginning of therapy and periodically with long-term use. **Note:** Lithium has a very small window of safety (TI). Assess knowledge/teach patient appropriate use, interventions to reduce side effects, and importance of reporting adverse symptoms promptly.

Monitoring Laboratory Tests: Serum lithium every 4-5 days during initial therapy. Monitor renal and thyroid; serum electrolytes; CBC with differential, urinalysis.

Levels should be obtained twice weekly until both patient's clinical status and levels are stable then levels may be obtained every 1-3 months.

Timing of serum samples: Draw trough just before next dose (8-12 hours after previous dose).

Therapeutic levels:

Acute mania: 0.6-1.2 mEq/L (SI: 0.6-1.2 mmol/L)

Protection against future episodes in most patients with bipolar disorder: 0.8-1 mEq/L (SI: 0.8-1.0 mmol/L); a higher rate of relapse is described in subjects who are maintained at <0.4 mEq/L (SI: 0.4 mmol/L).

Elderly patients can usually be maintained at lower end of therapeutic range (0.6-0.8 mEq/L).

Toxic concentration: >1.5 mEq/L (SI: >2 mmol/L)

Adverse effect levels:

GI complaints/tremor: 1.5-2 mEq/L

Confusion/somnolence: 2-2.5 mEq/L

Seizures/death: >2.5 mEq/L

Patient Education: Take exactly as directed; do not change dosage without consulting prescriber. Do not crush or chew extended or slow release tablets or capsules. Maintain adequate hydration (2-3 L/day of fluids) unless instructed to restrict fluid intake (especially in summer). Avoid changes in sodium content (eg, low sodium diets); reduction of sodium can increase lithium toxicity. Limit caffeine intake (diuresis can increase lithium toxicity). Frequent blood test and monitoring will be necessary. You may experience decreased appetite or altered taste sensation (small frequent meals may help maintain nutrition); or drowsiness or dizziness, especially during early therapy (use caution when driving or engaging in tasks requiring alertness until response to drug is known). Immediately report unresolved diarrhea, abrupt changes in weight, muscular tremors or lack of coordination, fever, or changes in urinary volume. **Pregnancy/breast-feeding precautions:** Do not get pregnant while taking this medication; use appropriate contraceptive measures. Do not breast-feed.

Dietary Considerations: May be taken with meals to avoid GI upset; have patient drink 2-3 L of water daily.

Geriatric Considerations: Some elderly patients may be extremely sensitive to the effects of lithium. Initial doses need to be adjusted for renal function in the elderly; thereafter, adjust doses based upon serum concentrations and response.

Pregnancy Risk Factor: D

Pregnancy Issues: Cardiac malformations in the infant, including Ebstein's anomaly, are associated with use of lithium during the first trimester of pregnancy. Nontoxic effects to the newborn include shallow respiration, hypotonia, lethargy, cyanosis, diabetes insipidus, thyroid depression, and nontoxic goiter when lithium is used near term. Efforts should be made to avoid lithium use during the first trimester; if an alternative therapy is not appropriate, the lowest possible dose of lithium should be used throughout the pregnancy. Fetal echocardiography and ultrasound to screen for anomalies should be conducted between 16-20 weeks of gestation. Lithium levels should be monitored in the mother and may need adjusted following delivery.

Lactation: Enters breast milk/contraindicated

Administration

Oral: Administer with meals to decrease GI upset. Slow release tablets must be swallowed whole; do not crush or chew.

Related Information

Maternal / Fetal Toxicology on page 1762

Peak and Trough Guidelines on page 1694

- ♦ **Lithium Carbonate** see Lithium on page 908
- ♦ **Lithium Citrate** see Lithium on page 908
- ♦ **Lithobid®** see Lithium on page 908
- ♦ **Livostin®** [DSC] see Levocabastine on page 884
- ♦ **LMD®** see Dextran on page 433
- ♦ **L-M-X™ 4** [OTC] see Lidocaine on page 898

♦ **L-M-X™ 5 [OTC]** *see* Lidocaine *on page 898*
♦ **LNg 20** *see* Levonorgestrel *on page 891*
♦ **Locoid®** *see* Hydrocortisone *on page 760*
♦ **Locoid Lipocream®** *see* Hydrocortisone *on page 760*
♦ **Lodine®** *see* Etodolac *on page 598*
♦ **Lodine® XL** *see* Etodolac *on page 598*

Lodoxamide (loe DOKS a mide)

U.S. Brand Names Alomide®
Synonyms Lodoxamide Tromethamine
Generic Available No
Pharmacologic Category Mast Cell Stabilizer
Use Treatment of vernal keratoconjunctivitis, vernal conjunctivitis, and vernal keratitis
Contraindications Hypersensitivity to lodoxamide tromethamine or any component of the formulation
Warnings/Precautions Safety and efficacy in children <2 years of age have not been established. Not for injection. Not for use in patients wearing soft contact lenses during treatment.
Adverse Reactions
>10%: Local: Transient burning, stinging, discomfort
1% to 10%:
Central nervous system: Headache
Ocular: Blurred vision, corneal erosion/ulcer, eye pain, corneal abrasion, blepharitis
Overdosage/Toxicology Symptoms include feeling of warmth of flushing, headache, dizziness, fatigue, sweating, nausea, loose stools, and urinary frequency/urgency; consider emesis in the event of accidental ingestion
Pharmacodynamics/Kinetics
Absorption: Topical: Negligible
Dosing
Adults & Elderly: Vernal conjunctivitis, keratitis: Ophthalmic: Children ≥2 years and Adults: Instill 1-2 drops in eye(s) 4 times/day for up to 3 months
Pediatrics: Children ≥2 years: Refer to adult dosing.
Available Dosage Forms Solution, ophthalmic: 0.1% (10 mL) [contains benzalkonium chloride]
Monitoring and Teaching Issues
Physical Assessment: Assess potential for interactions with other prescriptions, OTC medications, or herbal products patient may be taking. Assess patient response. Teach patient proper use, side effects/appropriate interventions, and symptoms to report.
Patient Education: For use in eyes only. Avoid wearing soft contact lenses while using this medication. Wash hands before using. Lie down or tilt your head back and look upward. Hold dropper tip as near as possible to your eyelid without touching it. Pull the lower lid of eye down to form a pocket. Drop the prescribed number of drops into the pocket made by the lower lid and the eye. (Placing drops on the surface of the eyeball can cause stinging.) Do not blink or rub eye. Close your eye and press lightly against the inside corner of your eye for about 1 minute. Repeat in other eye if directed by prescriber. Replace and tighten cap right away, do not allow tip of dropper to become contaminated. Wipe off any excess liquid from cheek. Wash your hands again. Do not use any other eye medication without consulting prescriber. Do not share mediation with anyone else. You may experience temporary stinging or burning in the eyes, headache, increased eye tearing or dry eye, sneezing, or blurred vision. Inform prescriber if you experience eye pain, disturbance of vision; skin rash; swelling in or around the eyes; any other adverse response; or if condition worsens or fails to improve. Store medication at room temperature, away from excess heat and moisture. Do not use if solution has changed color, is cloudy, or contains particles.
Pregnancy Risk Factor: B

♦ **Lodoxamide Tromethamine** *see* Lodoxamide *on page 911*
♦ **Loestrin®** *see* Ethinyl Estradiol and Norethindrone *on page 589*
♦ **Loestrin® Fe** *see* Ethinyl Estradiol and Norethindrone *on page 589*
♦ **Lofibra™** *see* Fenofibrate *on page 615*
♦ **L-OHP** *see* Oxaliplatin *on page 1127*

Lomefloxacin (loe me FLOKS a sin)

U.S. Brand Names Maxaquin®
Synonyms Lomefloxacin Hydrochloride
Generic Available No
Pharmacologic Category Antibiotic, Quinolone
Use Acute bacterial exacerbation of chronic bronchitis caused by susceptible gram-negative organisms; urinary tract infections (uncomplicated and complicated) caused by susceptible organisms; surgical prophylaxis (transrectal prostate biopsy or transurethral procedures)
Mechanism of Action/Effect Inhibits DNA-gyrase in susceptible organisms thereby inhibits relaxation of supercoiled DNA and promotes breakage of DNA strands. DNA gyrase (topoisomerase II), is an essential bacterial enzyme that maintains the superhelical structure of DNA and is required for DNA replication and transcription, DNA repair, recombination, and transposition.
Contraindications Hypersensitivity to lomefloxacin, any component of the formulation, or other members of the quinolone group (such as, nalidixic acid, oxolinic acid, cinoxacin, norfloxacin, and ciprofloxacin); avoid use in children <18 years of age due to association of other quinolones with transient arthropathies
Warnings/Precautions CNS stimulation may occur (tremor, restlessness, confusion, and very rarely hallucinations or seizures); use with caution in patients with known or suspected CNS disorders; use caution to avoid possible photosensitivity reactions during and for several days following fluoroquinolone therapy. Use caution in renal impairment; may require dosage
(Continued)

Lomefloxacin *(Continued)*

adjustment. Severe hypersensitivity reactions, including anaphylaxis, have occurred with quinolone therapy. If an allergic reaction occurs (itching, urticaria, dyspnea or facial edema, loss of consciousness, tingling, cardiovascular collapse), discontinue drug immediately. Prolonged use may result in superinfection; pseudomembranous colitis may occur and should be considered in all patients who present with diarrhea.

Rare incidence of peripheral neuropathy has been documented; discontinue if patient experiences symptoms of neuropathy including pain, burning, tingling, weakness or other sensory abnormalities. Tendon inflammation and/or rupture has been reported. Risk may be increased with concurrent corticosteroids, particularly in the elderly. Discontinue at first sign of tendon inflammation or pain. Quinolones may exacerbate myasthenia gravis; use with caution (rare, potentially life-threatening weakness of respiratory muscles may occur); avoid use in children <18 years of age due to association of other quinolones with transient arthropathies. Safety and efficacy has not been established in pediatric patients and adolescents <18 years of age, pregnant or lactating women.

Drug Interactions
Cytochrome P450 Effect: Inhibits CYP1A2 (weak)

Decreased Effect: Concurrent administration of metal cations, including most antacids, oral electrolyte supplements, quinapril, sucralfate, and some didanosine formulations (chewable/buffered tablets and pediatric powder for oral suspension), may decrease quinolone level; separate doses.

Increased Effect/Toxicity: Concomitant use with corticosteroids may increase the risk of tendon rupture. Probenecid may increase lomefloxacin levels.

Nutritional/Ethanol Interactions
Food: Lomefloxacin peak serum levels may be prolonged if taken with food.
Herb/Nutraceutical: Avoid dong quai, St John's wort (may cause photosensitization).

Adverse Reactions 1% to 10%:
Central nervous system: Headache (4%), dizziness (2%)
Dermatologic: Photosensitivity (2%)
Gastrointestinal: Nausea (4%), abdominal pain (1%), diarrhea (1%)

Overdosage/Toxicology Symptoms of overdose include acute renal failure and seizures. Treatment is supportive; not removed by peritoneal or hemodialysis.

Pharmacodynamics/Kinetics
Absorption: Well absorbed (95% to 98%)
Time to Peak: 1.5 hours
Protein Binding: 10%
Half-Life Elimination: 7.8 hours
Excretion: Urine (65% as unchanged drug, 9% as metabolite); feces (10% as unchanged drug)

Dosing
Adults & Elderly:
Acute bacterial exacerbation of chronic bronchitis: Oral: 400 mg once daily for 10 days
Urinary tract infection (UTI) due to susceptible organisms: Oral:
Uncomplicated cystitis caused by Escherichia coli: 400 mg once daily for 3 successive days
Uncomplicated cystitis caused by Klebsiella pneumoniae, Proteus mirabilis, **or** *Staphylococcus saprophyticus:* 400 mg once daily for 10 successive days
Complicated UTI caused by Escherichia coli, Klebsiella pneumoniae, Proteus mirabilis, or Pseudomonas aeruginosa: 400 mg once daily for 14 successive days
Urologic surgical prophylaxis: Oral:
Transrectal prostate biopsy: 400 mg as a single dose, 1-6 hours before procedure
Transurethral surgical procedure: 400 mg as a single dose, 2-6 hours before procedure

Renal Impairment:
Cl_{cr} 10-40 mL/minute: Initial loading dose = 400 mg; followed by 200 mg once daily maintenance dose
Hemodialysis: Same as for renal impairment.

Available Dosage Forms Tablet: 400 mg

Monitoring and Teaching Issues
Physical Assessment: Assess results of culture and sensitivity tests and allergy history before initiating therapy. Use caution with known CNS disorders or renal impairment (see Warnings/Precautions for use cautions). Assess potential for interactions with other prescriptions, OTC medications, or herbal products patient may be taking (eg, increased risk of tendon rupture or arrhythmias; see Drug Interactions). Assess results of laboratory tests, therapeutic effectiveness (resolution of infection), and adverse reactions regularly during therapy (eg, hypersensitivity reactions [itching, urticaria, dyspnea or facial edema, loss of consciousness, tingling, cardiovascular collapse; can occur days after therapy has started], diarrhea, opportunistic infection, pseudomembraneous colitis, tendon rupture; see Adverse Reactions). Teach patient proper use (according to formulation), possible side effects/appropriate interventions, and adverse symptoms to report (see Patient Education).

Monitoring Laboratory Tests: Perform culture and sensitivity studies prior to initiating therapy to determine the causative organism and its susceptibility to lomefloxacin. Monitor CBC, renal and hepatic function periodically if therapy is prolonged.

Patient Education: Do not take any new medication during therapy unless approved by prescriber. Take exactly as directed (with or without food) at least 1 hour before or 2 hours after antacids or other drug products containing calcium, iron, or zinc (including multivitamins). Take entire prescription even if feeling better. Maintain adequate hydration (2-3 L/day of fluids) unless instructed to restrict fluid intake. May cause dizziness, lightheadedness, or confusion (use caution when driving or engaging in tasks that require alertness until response to drug is known); nausea or vomiting (small frequent meals, frequent mouth care, sucking lozenges, or chewing gum may help); or photosensitivity (use sunscreen, wear protective clothing and eyewear, and avoid direct sunlight). Discontinue use immediately and report to prescriber if inflammation, tendon pain, or allergic reaction occurs (itching urticaria, respiratory difficulty, facial edema, difficulty swallowing, loss of consciousness, tingling, chest pain, palpitations). Report palpitations or chest pain; CNS changes (hallucinations, suicidal ideation, excitability, seizures); persistent diarrhea or constipation; signs of opportunistic infection (unusual fever or chills, vaginal itching or foul-smelling vaginal discharge, easy bruising or bleeding). **Pregnancy/breast-feeding precautions:** Inform prescriber if you are or intend to become pregnant. Do not breast-feed.

Dietary Considerations: May be taken without regard to meals.

Geriatric Considerations: Dosage adjustment is not necessary in patients with normal renal function, $Cl_{cr} \geq 40$ mL/minute; otherwise, follow dosage guidelines for renal impairment. Age-associated increase in half-life and decrease in clearance are thought to be secondary to age-related changes in renal function.

Pregnancy Risk Factor: C

Pregnancy Issues: Reports of arthropathy (observed in immature animals and reported rarely in humans) have limited the use of fluoroquinolones in pregnancy. Teratogenic effects were not observed with lomefloxacin in animal studies; however, an increase in fetal loss was observed in one species. Based on limited data, quinolones are not expected to be a major human teratogen. Although quinolone antibiotics should not be used as first-line agents during pregnancy, when considering treatment for life-threatening infection and/or prolonged duration of therapy, the potential risk to the fetus must be balanced against the severity of the potential illness.

Lactation: Excretion in breast milk unknown/not recommended

Breast-Feeding Issues: Other quinolones are known to be excreted in breast milk. The manufacturer recommends to discontinue nursing or to discontinue the lomefloxacin.

Administration
Oral: Take 1 hour before or 2 hours after meals.

- **Lomefloxacin Hydrochloride** see Lomefloxacin on page 911
- **Lomotil**® see Diphenoxylate and Atropine on page 466

Lomustine (loe MUS teen)

U.S. Brand Names CeeNU®

Synonyms CCNU

Generic Available No

Pharmacologic Category Antineoplastic Agent, Alkylating Agent

Use Treatment of brain tumors and Hodgkin's disease, non-Hodgkin's lymphoma, melanoma, renal carcinoma, lung cancer, colon cancer

Mechanism of Action/Effect Inhibits DNA and RNA synthesis via carbamylation of DNA polymerase, alkylation of DNA, and alteration of RNA, proteins, and enzymes

Contraindications Hypersensitivity to lomustine, any component of the formulation, or other nitrosoureas; pregnancy

Warnings/Precautions The U.S. Food and Drug Administration (FDA) currently recommends that procedures for proper handling and disposal for antineoplastic agents be considered. Use with caution in patients with depressed platelet, leukocyte or erythrocyte counts. Bone marrow depression, notably thrombocytopenia and leukopenia, may lead to bleeding and overwhelming infections in an already compromised patient; will last for at least 6 weeks after a dose, do not give courses more frequently than every 6 weeks because the toxicity is cumulative. Use with caution in patients with liver function abnormalities.

Drug Interactions
Cytochrome P450 Effect: Substrate of CYP2D6 (major); **Inhibits** CYP2D6 (weak), 3A4 (weak)

Decreased Effect: Decreased effect with phenobarbital, resulting in reduced efficacy of both drugs.

Increased Effect/Toxicity: CYP2D6 inhibitors may increase the levels/effects of lomustine; example inhibitors include chlorpromazine, delavirdine, fluoxetine, miconazole, paroxetine, pergolide, quinidine, quinine, ritonavir, and ropinirole. Increased toxicity with cimetidine, reported to cause bone marrow depression or to potentiate the myelosuppressive effects of lomustine.

Nutritional/Ethanol Interactions Ethanol: Avoid ethanol (due to GI irritation).

Lab Interactions Liver function tests

Adverse Reactions
>10%:
Gastrointestinal: Nausea and vomiting, usually within 3-6 hours after oral administration. Administration of the dose at bedtime, with an antiemetic, significantly reduces both the incidence and severity of nausea.
Hematologic: Myelosuppression, common, dose-limiting, may be cumulative and irreversible
Onset: 10-14 days
Nadir: Leukopenia: 6 weeks
Thrombocytopenia: 4 weeks
Recovery: 6-8 weeks
1% to 10%:
Dermatologic: Rash
Gastrointestinal: Anorexia, stomatitis, diarrhea
Genitourinary: Progressive azotemia, renal failure, decrease in kidney size
Hematologic: Anemia
Hepatic: Elevated liver enzymes, transient, reversible

Overdosage/Toxicology Symptoms of overdose include nausea, vomiting, and leukopenia. There are no known antidotes. Treatment is symptomatic and supportive.
(Continued)

Lomustine *(Continued)*

Pharmacodynamics/Kinetics

Duration of Action: Marrow recovery: ≤6 weeks

Absorption: Complete; appears in plasma within 3 minutes after administration

Time to Peak: Serum: Active metabolite: ~3 hours

Protein Binding: 50%

Half-Life Elimination: Parent drug: 16-72 hours; Active metabolite: Terminal: 1.3-2 days

Metabolism: Rapidly hepatic via hydroxylation producing at least two active metabolites; enterohepatically recycled

Excretion: Urine; feces (<5%); expired air (<10%)

Dosing

Adults & Elderly: Refer to individual protocols.

Chemotherapy: Oral: 100-130 mg/m^2 as a single dose every 6 weeks; readjust after initial treatment according to platelet and leukocyte counts

With compromised marrow function: Initial dose: 100 mg/m^2 as a single dose every 6 weeks

Note: Repeat courses should only be administered after adequate recovery: WBC >4000 and platelet counts >100,000

Subsequent dosing adjustment based on nadir:

Leukocytes 2000-2900/mm^3, platelets 25,000-74,999/mm^3: Administer 70% of prior dose

Leukocytes <2000/mm^3, platelets <25,000/mm^3: Administer 50% of prior dose

Pediatrics: Chemotherapy: Oral (refer to individual protocols): Children: 75-150 mg/m^2 as a single dose every 6 weeks; subsequent doses are readjusted after initial treatment according to platelet and leukocyte counts.

Renal Impairment:

Cl_{cr} 10-50 mL/minute: Administer 75% of normal dose.

Cl_{cr} <10 mL/minute: Administer 50% of normal dose.

Hemodialysis effects: Supplemental dose is not necessary.

Available Dosage Forms

Capsule: 10 mg, 40 mg, 100 mg

Capsule [dose pack]: 10 mg (2s); 40 mg (2s); 100 mg (2s)

Monitoring and Teaching Issues

Physical Assessment: Use caution in presence of depressed platelet, leukocyte or erythrocyte counts, bone marrow depression (see Warnings/Precautions for specific use cautions). Assess potential for interactions with other pharmacological agents patient may be taking (eg, decreased levels/effects of lomustine, increased toxicity; see Drug Interactions). Assess results of laboratory tests, therapeutic effectiveness, and adverse reactions prior to each treatment and on a regular basis throughout therapy (see Adverse Reactions). Teach patient possible side effects/appropriate interventions and adverse symptoms to report (see Patient Education).

Monitoring Laboratory Tests: CBC with differential, platelet count, hepatic and renal function, pulmonary function

Patient Education: Do not take any new medication during therapy unless approved by prescriber. Take with fluids on an empty stomach; do not eat or drink for 2 hours prior to or following administration to reduce nausea and vomiting. Your prescriber may recommend that you take your medication at bedtime with an prescribed antiemetic to reduce the severity of nausea. During therapy, do not use alcohol. It is important to maintain adequate hydration (2-3 L/day of fluids) unless instructed to restrict fluid intake and nutrition (small frequent meals may help). You will be more susceptible to infection (avoid crowds and exposure to infection; do not have any vaccinations without consulting prescriber). You may experience hair loss (reversible); nausea or vomiting (small frequent meals, frequent mouth care, sucking lozenges, or chewing gum may help or consult prescriber for approved antiemetic); mouth sores (frequent mouth care and use of a soft toothbrush or cotton swabs may help); or diarrhea (buttermilk, boiled milk, or yogurt may help reduce diarrhea; consult prescriber for approved medication). Report persistent nausea, vomiting, or diarrhea; bleeding or bruising; fever, chills, sore throat; vaginal discharge; rash; blood in urine, stool, or vomitus; delayed healing of any wounds; yellowing of skin or eyes; or changes in color of urine of stool. **Pregnancy/breast-feeding precautions:** Do not get pregnant while taking this medication and for 1 month following therapy. Consult prescriber for appropriate barrier contraceptives measures. This drug may cause severe fetal birth defects. Do not breast-feed.

Dietary Considerations: Should be taken with fluids on an empty stomach; no food or drink for 2 hours after administration to decrease nausea.

Pregnancy Risk Factor: D

Pregnancy Issues: May cause fetal harm when administered to a pregnant woman. Women of childbearing potential should be advised to avoid pregnancy and should be advised of the potential harm to the fetus.

Lactation: Enters breast milk/contraindicated

Administration

Oral: Take with fluids on an empty stomach; no food or drink for 2 hours after administration.

Storage: Refrigerate (<40°C/<104°F).

♦ **Lonox®** *see* Diphenoxylate and Atropine *on page 466*

Loperamide *(loe PER a mide)*

U.S. Brand Names Diamode [OTC]; Imodium® A-D [OTC]; Kao-Paverin® [OTC]; K-Pek II [OTC]

Synonyms Loperamide Hydrochloride

Generic Available Yes

Pharmacologic Category Antidiarrheal

Medication Safety Issues

Sound-alike/look-alike issues:

Imodium® A-D may be confused with Indocin®, Ionamin®

Use Treatment of acute diarrhea and chronic diarrhea associated with inflammatory bowel disease; chronic functional diarrhea (idiopathic), chronic diarrhea caused by bowel resection or organic lesions; to decrease the volume of ileostomy discharge

Unlabeled/Investigational Use Treatment of traveler's diarrhea in combination with trimethoprim-sulfamethoxazole (co-trimoxazole) (3-day therapy)

Mechanism of Action/Effect Acts directly on intestinal muscles to inhibit peristalsis and prolongs transit time enhancing fluid and electrolyte movement through intestinal mucosa; reduces fecal volume, increases viscosity, and diminishes fluid and electrolyte loss; demonstrates antisecretory activity; exhibits peripheral action

Contraindications Hypersensitivity to loperamide or any component of the formulation; bloody diarrhea; patients who must avoid constipation; diarrhea resulting from some infections; pseudomembranous colitis

Warnings/Precautions Large first-pass metabolism, use with caution in hepatic dysfunction; should not be used if diarrhea accompanied by high fever, blood in stool; use with caution in patients with a history of penicillin allergy, especially IgE-mediated reactions (eg, anaphylaxis, urticaria)

Drug Interactions

Increased Effect/Toxicity: Loperamide may potentiate the adverse effects of CNS depressants, phenothiazines, tricyclic antidepressants.

Adverse Reactions Frequency not defined.

Cardiovascular: Shock

Central nervous system: Dizziness, drowsiness, fatigue, sedation

Dermatologic: Rash, toxic epidermal necrolysis

Gastrointestinal: Abdominal cramping, abdominal distention, constipation, dry mouth, nausea, paralytic ileus, vomiting

Miscellaneous: Anaphylaxis

Overdosage/Toxicology Symptoms of overdose include CNS and respiratory depression, GI cramping, constipation, GI irritation, nausea, and vomiting. Overdose is noted when daily doses approximate 60 mg of loperamide. Treatment of overdose includes gastric lavage followed by 100 g activated charcoal through a nasogastric tube. Naloxone, 2 mg I.V. with repeat administration as necessary up to a total dose of 10 mg, can be used to reverse opiate effects.

Pharmacodynamics/Kinetics

Onset of Action: 0.5-1 hour

Absorption: <40%

Protein Binding: 97%

Half-Life Elimination: 7-14 hours

Metabolism: Hepatic (>50%) to inactive compounds

Excretion: Urine and feces (1% as metabolites, 30% to 40% as unchanged drug)

Dosing

Adults & Elderly:

Acute diarrhea: Oral: Initial: 4 mg (2 capsules), followed by 2 mg after each loose stool, up to 16 mg/day (8 capsules)

Chronic diarrhea: Oral: Initial: Follow acute diarrhea; maintenance dose should be slowly titrated downward to minimum required to control symptoms (typically, 4-8 mg/day in divided doses)

Traveler's diarrhea: Oral: Treat for no more than 2 days: 4 mg after first loose stool followed by 2 mg after each subsequent stool; maximum dose: 8 mg/day

Pediatrics:

Acute diarrhea: Oral:

Initial doses (in first 24 hours):

2-6 years: 1 mg 3 times/day

6-8 years: 2 mg twice daily

8-12 years: 2 mg 3 times/day

Maintenance: After initial dosing, 0.1 mg/kg doses after each loose stool, but not exceeding initial dosage

Chronic diarrhea: Oral: 0.08-0.24 mg/kg/day divided 2-3 times/day, maximum: 2 mg/dose

Traveler's diarrhea: Treat for no more than 2 days

Children 6-8 years: 1 mg after first loose stool followed by 1 mg after each subsequent stool; maximum dose: 4 mg/day

Children 9-11 years: 2 mg after first loose stool followed by 1 mg after each subsequent stool; maximum dose: 6 mg/day

Children ≥12 years: Refer to adult dosing.

Available Dosage Forms

Caplet, as hydrochloride: 2 mg

Diamode, Imodium® A-D, Kao-Paverin®: 2 mg

Capsule, as hydrochloride: 2 mg

Liquid, oral, as hydrochloride: 1 mg/5 mL (5 mL, 10 mL, 120 mL)

Imodium® A-D: 1 mg/5 mL (60 mL, 120 mL) [contains sodium benzoate, benzoic acid; cherry mint flavor]

Tablet, as hydrochloride: 2 mg

K-Pek II: 2 mg

Monitoring and Teaching Issues

Physical Assessment: Assess for cause of diarrhea before administering first dose. See Warnings/Precautions for use cautions. Assess potential for adverse interactions with other pharmaceutical agents patient may be taking (eg, loperamide may potentiate the adverse effects of CNS depressants, phenothiazines, tricyclic antidepressants; see Drug Interactions). Teach patient proper use, possible side effects/appropriate interventions, and adverse symptoms to report (see Patient Education).

Patient Education: Take exactly as directed. Do not exceed recommended or prescribed dose. May cause drowsiness (use caution when driving or engaged in hazardous tasks until response to medication is known). Increased exercise, identifying and avoiding foods that cause diarrhea, safe food preparation and storage, use of buttermilk, yogurt, or boiled (Continued)

Loperamide *(Continued)*

milk may help reduce diarrhea. If acute diarrhea lasts longer than 48 hours, consult prescriber. Report rash, abdominal pain, bloody diarrhea, or other adverse reactions.

Geriatric Considerations: Elderly are particularly sensitive to fluid and electrolyte loss. This generally results in lethargy, weakness, and confusion. Repletion and maintenance of electrolytes and water are essential in the treatment of diarrhea. Drug therapy must be limited in order to avoid toxicity with this agent.

Pregnancy Risk Factor: B

Lactation: Enters breast milk/compatible

Administration

Oral: Therapy for chronic diarrhea should not exceed 10 days.

♦ **Loperamide Hydrochloride** *see* Loperamide *on page 914*

♦ **Lopid**® *see* Gemfibrozil *on page 704*

Lopinavir and Ritonavir (loe PIN a veer & rit ON uh veer)

U.S. Brand Names Kaletra™

Synonyms Ritonavir and Lopinavir

Generic Available No

Pharmacologic Category Antiretroviral Agent, Protease Inhibitor

Medication Safety Issues

Sound-alike/look-alike issues:

Potential for dispensing errors between Kaletra™ and Keppra® (levetiracetam)

Use Treatment of HIV infection in combination with other antiretroviral agents

Dosing

Adults: HIV infection (as a component of combination therapy): Oral (take with food): Lopinavir 400 mg/ritonavir 100 mg twice daily

Dosage adjustment when taken with amprenavir, efavirenz. nelfinavir, or nevirapine: Oral (take with food): Lopinavir 533 mg/ritonavir 133 mg twice daily

Elderly: Initial studies did not include enough elderly patients to determine effects based on age. Use with caution due to possible decreased hepatic, renal, and cardiac function.

Pediatrics: HIV infection (component of combination therapy): Oral (take with food):

Children 6 months to 12 years: Dosage based on weight, presented based on mg of lopinavir (maximum dose: Lopinavir 400 mg/ritonavir 100 mg)

7-<15 kg: 12 mg/kg twice daily

15-40 kg: 10 mg/kg twice daily

>40 kg: Refer to adult dosing.

Children >12 years: Refer to adult dosing.

Dosage adjustment when taken with efavirenz or nevirapine:

Children 6 months to 12 years:

7-<15 kg: 13 mg/kg twice daily

15-45 kg: 11 mg/kg twice daily

>45 kg: Refer to adult dosing

Note: In the USHHS guidelines, the cutoff for adult dosing is 50 kg. (Pediatric Guidelines - December 14, 2001, are available at http://www.aidsinfo.nih.gov, last accessed January 22, 2003.)

Children >12 years: Refer to adult dosing.

Renal Impairment: Has not been studied in patients with renal impairment; however, a decrease in clearance is not expected.

Hepatic Impairment: No specific guidelines available - plasma levels may be increased in patients with mild-to-moderate hepatic impairment. Lopinavir's AUC may be increased by 30%.

Available Dosage Forms

Capsule: Lopinavir 133.3 mg and ritonavir 33.3 mg

Solution, oral: Lopinavir 80 mg and ritonavir 20 mg per mL (160 mL) [contains alcohol 42.4%]

Monitoring and Teaching Issues

Physical Assessment: See Contraindications, Warnings/Precautions, and Dosing for use cautions. Assess potential for interactions with other prescriptions, OTC medications, or herbal products patient may be taking (see Drug Interactions). Assess patient response at regular intervals during therapy (see Adverse Reactions and Overdose/Toxicology). Teach patient proper use, possible side effects/appropriate interventions (eg, glucose testing; protease inhibitors may cause hyperglycemia [exacerbation or new-onset diabetes]), and adverse symptoms to report (see Patient Education).

Patient Education: Inform prescriber of all prescriptions, OTC medications, or herbal products you are taking, and any allergies you have. Do not take any new medication during therapy unless approved by prescriber. This is not a cure for HIV, nor has it been shown to reduce transmission of HIV. Take as directed, with meals. Maintain adequate hydration (2-3 L/day of fluids) unless instructed to restrict fluid intake. This drug may be prescribed with a combination of other medications; time these medications as directed by prescriber. You may be advised to check your glucose levels (this drug can cause exacerbation or new-onset diabetes). May cause body changes due to redistribution of body fat, facial atrophy, or breast enlargement (normal effects of drug); dizziness, insomnia, abnormal thinking (use caution when driving or engaging in potentially hazardous tasks until response to drug is known); nausea, vomiting, or taste perversion (small frequent meals, frequent mouth care, chewing gum, or sucking lozenges may help); muscle weakness (consult prescriber for approved analgesic); headache or insomnia (consult prescriber for medication); gynecomastia, hypogonadism (male), decreased libido, or abnormal ejaculation; muscle weakness; or hair loss. Report chest pain, calf pain, redness or swelling, facial edema, palpitations; respiratory difficulty; unresolved and persistent GI effects; rash or skin breakdown or discoloration; or any other persistent adverse effects. **Pregnancy/breast-feeding precautions:** Inform prescriber if you are or intend to become pregnant. May reduce effectiveness of some contraceptives. Consult prescriber for appropriate contraceptive measures. Do not breast-feed.

Pregnancy Risk Factor: C
Lactation: Excretion in breast milk unknown/contraindicated
Related Information
Ritonavir *on page 1335*

♦ **Lopressor**® *see* Metoprolol *on page 993*
♦ **Lorabid**® *see* Loracarbef *on page 917*

Loracarbef (lor a KAR bef)

U.S. Brand Names Lorabid®
Generic Available No
Pharmacologic Category Antibiotic, Carbacephem
Medication Safety Issues
Sound-alike/look-alike issues:
Lorabid® may be confused with Levbid®, Lopid®, Lortab®, Slo-bid™
Use Infections caused by susceptible organisms involving the respiratory tract, acute otitis media, sinusitis, skin and skin structure, bone and joint, and urinary tract and gynecologic
Mechanism of Action/Effect Inhibits bacterial cell wall synthesis by binding to one or more of the penicillin binding proteins (PBPs); inhibits the final transpeptidation step of peptidoglycan synthesis in bacterial cell walls, thus inhibiting cell wall biosynthesis.
Contraindications Hypersensitivity to loracarbef, any component of the formulation, or cephalosporins
Warnings/Precautions Modify dosage in patients with severe renal impairment; prolonged use may result in superinfection; use with caution in patients with a previous history of hypersensitivity to other beta-lactam antibiotics (eg, penicillins, cephalosporins)
Drug Interactions
Increased Effect/Toxicity: Loracarbef serum levels are increased with coadministered probenecid.
Nutritional/Ethanol Interactions Food: Administration with food decreases and delays the peak plasma concentration.
Adverse Reactions ≥1%:
Central nervous system: Headache (1% to 3%), somnolence (<2%)
Dermatologic: Rash (1% to 3%)
Gastrointestinal: Diarrhea (4% to 6%), nausea (2%), vomiting (1% to 3%), anorexia (<2%), abdominal pain (1%)
Genitourinary: Vaginitis (1%)
Respiratory: Rhinitis (2% to 6%)
Overdosage/Toxicology Symptoms of overdose include abdominal discomfort and diarrhea. Treatment is supportive.
Pharmacodynamics/Kinetics
Absorption: Rapid
Time to Peak: Serum: ~1 hour
Half-Life Elimination: ~1 hour
Excretion: Clearance: Plasma: ~200-300 mL/minute
Dosing
Adults & Elderly:
Uncomplicated urinary tract infections: Oral: 200 mg once daily for 7 days
Skin and soft tissue infections: Oral: 200 mg every 12 hours for 7 days
Uncomplicated pyelonephritis: Oral: 400 mg every 12 hours for 14 days
Pharyngitis/tonsillitis: Oral: 200 mg every 12 hours for 10 days
Sinusitis: Oral: 400 mg every 12 hours for 10 days
Upper/lower respiratory tract infection: Oral: 400 mg every 12 hours for 7-14 days
Pediatrics:
Acute otitis media: Oral: Children: 15 mg/kg twice daily for 10 days
Pharyngitis and impetigo: Oral: Children: 7.5-15 mg/kg twice daily for 10 days
Renal Impairment:
Cl_{cr} ≥50 mL/minute: Administer usual dose.
Cl_{cr} 10-49 mL/minute: Administer 50% of usual dose at usual interval or usual dose given half as often.
Cl_{cr} <10 mL/minute: Administer usual dose every 3-5 days.
Hemodialysis: Doses should be administered after dialysis sessions.
Available Dosage Forms
Capsule: 200 mg, 400 mg
Powder for oral suspension: 100 mg/5 mL (100 mL); 200 mg/5 mL (100 mL) [strawberry bubble gum flavor]
Monitoring and Teaching Issues
Physical Assessment: Assess results of culture and sensitivity tests and patient's allergy history prior to starting treatment. Use with caution in presence of renal impairment (see Warnings/Precautions for use cautions). Assess therapeutic effectiveness (resolution of infection) and adverse response on a regular basis during therapy (eg, rash, diarrhea, nausea, vomiting, opportunistic infection; see Adverse Reactions). Teach patient proper use, possible side effects/appropriate interventions, and adverse symptoms to report (see Patient Education).
Monitoring Laboratory Tests: Perform culture and sensitivity studies prior to initiating therapy.
Patient Education: Do not take any new medication during therapy unless approved by prescriber. Take as directed, preferably on an empty stomach, 1 hour before or 2 hours after meals. Take entire prescription even if feeling better. Shake suspension well before using. Maintain adequate hydration (2-3 L/day of fluids) unless instructed to restrict fluid intake. May cause nausea, vomiting, or anorexia (small frequent meals, frequent mouth care, sucking lozenges, or chewing gum may help). Report immediately any signs of skin rash, joint or back pain, or respiratory difficulty; signs of opportunistic infection (unusual fever, chills, vaginal itching or foul-smelling vaginal discharge, easy bruising or bleeding); (Continued)

Loracarbef *(Continued)*

or other persistent adverse reactions. **Breast-feeding precaution:** Consult prescriber if breast-feeding.

Dietary Considerations: Should be taken on an empty stomach at least 1 hour before or 2 hours after meals.

Geriatric Considerations: Half-life is slightly prolonged with age, presumably due to the reduced creatinine clearance related to aging. Adjust dose for renal function.

Pregnancy Risk Factor: B

Lactation: Excretion in breast milk unknown/use caution

Administration

Oral: Take on an empty stomach at least 1 hour before or 2 hours after meals. Finish all medication. Shake suspension well before using.

Storage: Suspension may be kept at room temperature for 14 days.

Loratadine (lor AT a deen)

U.S. Brand Names Alavert™ [OTC]; Claritin® [OTC]; Claritin® Hives Relief [OTC]; Dimetapp® Children's ND [OTC]; Tavist® ND [OTC]

Generic Available Yes

Pharmacologic Category Antihistamine, Nonsedating

Medication Safety Issues

Sound-alike/look-alike issues:

Dimetapp® may be confused with Dermatop®, Dimetabs®, Dimetane®

Use Relief of nasal and non-nasal symptoms of seasonal allergic rhinitis; treatment of chronic idiopathic urticaria

Mechanism of Action/Effect Long-acting tricyclic antihistamine with selective peripheral histamine H_1 receptor antagonistic properties; management of idiopathic chronic urticaria

Contraindications Hypersensitivity to loratadine or any component of the formulation

Warnings/Precautions Patients with liver or renal impairment should start with a lower dose (10 mg every other day), since their ability to clear the drug will be reduced. Safety in children <6 years of age has not been established.

Drug Interactions

Cytochrome P450 Effect: Substrate (minor) of CYP2D6, 3A4; **Inhibits** CYP2C19 (moderate), 2D6 (weak)

Increased Effect/Toxicity: Increased toxicity with procarbazine, other antihistamines. Protease inhibitors (amprenavir, ritonavir, nelfinavir) may increase the serum levels of loratadine. Loratadine may increase the levels/effects of citalopram, diazepam, methsuximide, phenytoin, propranolol, sertraline, and other CYP2C19 substrates.

Nutritional/Ethanol Interactions

Ethanol: Avoid ethanol (although sedation is limited with loratadine, may increase risk of CNS depression).

Food: Increases bioavailability and delays peak.

Herb/Nutraceutical: St John's wort may decrease loratadine levels.

Adverse Reactions

Adults:

Central nervous system: Headache (12%), somnolence (8%), fatigue (4%)

Gastrointestinal: Xerostomia (3%)

Children:

Central nervous system: Nervousness (4% ages 6-12 years), fatigue (3% ages 6-12 years, 2% to 3% ages 2-5 years), malaise (2% ages 6-12 years)

Dermatologic: Rash (2% to 3% ages 2-5 years)

Gastrointestinal: Abdominal pain (2% ages 6-12 years), stomatitis (2% to 3% ages 2-5 years)

Neuromuscular & skeletal: Hyperkinesia (3% ages 6-12 years)

Ocular: Conjunctivitis (2% ages 6-12 years)

Respiratory: Wheezing (4% ages 6-12 years), dysphonia (2% ages 6-12 years), upper respiratory infection (2% ages 6-12 years), epistaxis (2% to 3% ages 2-5 years), pharyngitis (2% to 3% ages 2-5 years), flu-like symptoms (2% to 3% ages 2-5 years)

Miscellaneous: Viral infection (2% to 3% ages 2-5 years)

Overdosage/Toxicology Symptoms of overdose include somnolence, tachycardia, and headache. No specific antidote is available. Treatment is symptomatic and supportive. Loratadine is not eliminated by dialysis.

Pharmacodynamics/Kinetics

Onset of Action: 1-3 hours; Peak effect: 8-12 hours

Duration of Action: >24 hours

Absorption: Rapid

Half-Life Elimination: 12-15 hours

Metabolism: Extensively hepatic via CYP2D6 and 3A4 to active metabolite

Excretion: Urine (40%) and feces (40%) as metabolites

Dosing

Adults & Elderly: Seasonal allergic rhinitis, chronic idiopathic urticaria: Oral: 10 mg/day

Pediatrics:

Children 2-5 years: Seasonal allergic rhinitis, chronic idiopathic urticaria: Oral: 5 mg once daily

Children ≥6 years: Refer to adult dosing.

Renal Impairment:

Cl$_{cr}$ ≤30 mL/minute:

Children 2-5 years: 5 mg every other day

Children ≥6 years and Adults: 10 mg every other day

Hepatic Impairment:

Elimination half-life increases with severity of disease.

Children 2-5 years: 5 mg every other day

Children ≥6 years and Adults: 10 mg every other day

Available Dosage Forms

Syrup (Claritin®): 1 mg/mL (120 mL) [contains sodium benzoate; fruit flavor]

Tablet (Alavert™, Claritin®, Claritin® Hives Relief; Tavist® ND): 10 mg

Tablet, rapidly-disintegrating: 10 mg

Alavert™: 10 mg [contains phenylalanine 8.4 mg/tablet]

Claritin® RediTabs: 10 mg [mint flavor]

Dimetapp® Children's ND: 10 mg [contains phenylalanine 8.4 mg/tablet]

Monitoring and Teaching Issues

Physical Assessment: Assess effectiveness and interactions of other medications patient may be taking. Monitor effectiveness of therapy and adverse reactions at beginning of therapy and periodically with long-term use. Assess knowledge/teach patient appropriate use, interventions to reduce side effects, and adverse symptoms to report.

Patient Education: Take as directed; do not exceed recommended dose. Avoid use of other depressants, alcohol, or sleep-inducing medications unless approved by prescriber. You may experience drowsiness or dizziness (use caution when driving or engaging in tasks requiring alertness until response to drug is known); or dry mouth or nausea (small frequent meals, frequent mouth care, chewing gum, or sucking hard candy may help). Report persistent dizziness, sedation, or seizures; chest pain, rapid heartbeat, or palpitations; swelling of face, mouth, lips, or tongue; respiratory difficulty; changes in urinary pattern; yellowing of skin or eyes; dark urine or pale stool; or lack of improvement or worsening or condition. **Breast-feeding precaution:** Consult prescriber if breast-feeding.

Rapidly-disintegrating tablets: Place tablet on tongue; it dissolves rapidly. May be used with or without water. Use within 6 months of opening foil pouch, and immediately after opening individual tablet blister.

Dietary Considerations: Take on an empty stomach. Alavert™ and Dimetapp® Children's ND contain phenylalanine 8.4 mg per 10 mg tablet.

Geriatric Considerations: Loratadine is one of the newer, nonsedating antihistamines. Because of its low incidence of side effects, it seems to be a good choice in the elderly. However, there is a wide variation in loratadine half-life reported in the elderly and this should be kept in mind when initiating dosing.

Pregnancy Risk Factor: B

Lactation: Enters breast milk/not recommended (AAP rates "compatible")

Administration

Oral: Take on an empty stomach.

Storage: Store at 2°C to 25°C (36°F to 77°F).

Rapidly-disintegrating tablets: Use within 6 months of opening foil pouch, and immediately after opening individual tablet blister. Store in a dry place.

Loratadine and Pseudoephedrine (lor AT a deen & soo doe e FED rin)

U.S. Brand Names Alavert™ Allergy and Sinus [OTC]; Claritin-D® 12-Hour [OTC]; Claritin-D® 24-Hour [OTC]

Synonyms Pseudoephedrine and Loratadine

Generic Available Yes

Pharmacologic Category Antihistamine/Decongestant Combination

Use Temporary relief of symptoms of seasonal allergic rhinitis, other upper respiratory allergies, or the common cold

Dosing

Adults & Elderly: Seasonal allergic rhinitis/nasal congestion:

Oral: 1 tablet every 12 hours

Extended release: 1 tablet daily

Pediatrics: Seasonal allergic rhinitis/nasal congestion: Children ≥12 years: Refer to adult dosing.

Renal Impairment: Cl_{cr} <30 mL/minute:

Claritin-D® 12-Hour: 1 tablet daily

Claritin-D® 24-Hour: 1 tablet every other day

Hepatic Impairment: Should be avoided.

Available Dosage Forms

Tablet, extended release: Loratadine 10 mg and pseudoephedrine sulfate 240 mg

Alavert™ Allergy and Sinus, Claritin-D® 12-hour: Loratadine 5 mg and pseudoephedrine sulfate 120 mg

Claritin-D® 24-hour: Loratadine 10 mg and pseudoephedrine sulfate 240 mg

Monitoring and Teaching Issues

Physical Assessment: See individual agents.

Patient Education: See individual agents. Do not crush, break, or chew tablet. Take with a full glass of water. **Breast-feeding precaution:** Breast-feeding is not recommended.

Pregnancy Risk Factor: B

Lactation: Enters breast milk/not recommended

Related Information

Loratadine on page 918
Pseudoephedrine on page 1282

Lorazepam (lor A ze pam)

U.S. Brand Names Ativan®; Lorazepam Intensol®

Controlled Substance C-IV

Generic Available Yes

Pharmacologic Category Benzodiazepine

Medication Safety Issues

Sound-alike/look-alike issues:

Lorazepam may be confused with alprazolam, clonazepam, diazepam, temazepam

Ativan® may be confused with Atarax®, Atgam®, Avitene®

(Continued)

Lorazepam *(Continued)*

Use

Oral: Management of anxiety disorders or short-term relief of the symptoms of anxiety or anxiety associated with depressive symptoms

I.V.: Status epilepticus, preanesthesia for desired amnesia, antiemetic adjunct

Unlabeled/Investigational Use Ethanol detoxification; insomnia; psychogenic catatonia; partial complex seizures; agitation (I.V.)

Mechanism of Action/Effect Binds to stereospecific benzodiazepine receptors on the post-synaptic GABA neuron at several sites within the central nervous system, including the limbic system, reticular formation. Enhancement of the inhibitory effect of GABA on neuronal excitability results by increased neuronal membrane permeability to chloride ions. This shift in chloride ions results in hyperpolarization (a less excitable state) and stabilization.

Contraindications Hypersensitivity to lorazepam or any component of the formulation (cross-sensitivity with other benzodiazepines may exist); acute narrow-angle glaucoma; sleep apnea (parenteral); intra-arterial injection of parenteral formulation; severe respiratory insufficiency (except during mechanical ventilation); pregnancy

Warnings/Precautions Causes CNS depression (dose-related) which may impair physical and mental capabilities. Use with caution in patients receiving other CNS depressants or psychoactive agents. Benzodiazepines have been associated with falls and traumatic injury and should be used with extreme caution in patients who are at risk of these events (especially the elderly). Use with caution in patients with a history of drug dependence.

Use with caution in elderly or debilitated patients, patients with hepatic disease (including alcoholics), renal impairment, respiratory disease, impaired gag reflex, or obese patients. Prolonged lorazepam use may have a possible relationship to GI disease, including esophageal dilation. Use is not recommended in patients with depressive disorders or psychoses. Avoid use in patients with sleep apnea.

The parenteral formulation of lorazepam contains polyethylene glycol and propylene glycol. Toxicity reported with prolonged infusion. Also contains benzyl alcohol - avoid rapid injection in neonates or prolonged infusions. Intra-arterial injection or extravasation should be avoided.

Benzodiazepines have been associated with anterograde amnesia. Paradoxical reactions, including hyperactive or aggressive behavior, have been reported with benzodiazepines, particularly in adolescent/pediatric or psychiatric patients. Does not have analgesic, antidepressant, or antipsychotic properties.

Drug Interactions

Decreased Effect: Oral contraceptives may increase the clearance of lorazepam. Lorazepam may decrease the antiparkinsonian efficacy of levodopa. Theophylline and other CNS stimulants may antagonize the sedative effects of lorazepam.

Increased Effect/Toxicity: Ethanol and other CNS depressants may increase the CNS effects of lorazepam. Scopolamine in combination with parenteral lorazepam may increase the incidence of sedation, hallucinations, and irrational behavior. There are rare reports of significant respiratory depression, stupor, and/or hypotension with concomitant use of loxapine and lorazepam. Use caution if concomitant administration of loxapine and CNS drugs is required.

Nutritional/Ethanol Interactions

Ethanol: Avoid or limit ethanol (may increase CNS depression).

Herb/Nutraceutical: Avoid valerian, St John's wort, kava kava, gotu kola (may increase CNS depression).

Lab Interactions May result in elevated liver function tests

Adverse Reactions

>10%:

Central nervous system: Sedation

Respiratory: Respiratory depression

1% to 10%:

Cardiovascular: Hypotension

Central nervous system: Confusion, dizziness, akathisia, unsteadiness, headache, depression, disorientation, amnesia

Dermatologic: Dermatitis, rash

Gastrointestinal: Weight gain/loss, nausea, changes in appetite

Neuromuscular & skeletal: Weakness

Respiratory: Nasal congestion, hyperventilation, apnea

Overdosage/Toxicology Symptoms of overdose include confusion, coma, hypoactive reflexes, dyspnea, labored breathing. **Note:** Prolonged infusions have been associated with toxicity from propylene glycol and/or polyethylene glycol. Treatment for benzodiazepine overdose is supportive. Flumazenil has been shown to selectively block the binding of benzodiazepines to CNS receptors, resulting in a reversal of benzodiazepine-induced CNS depression but not respiratory depression

Pharmacodynamics/Kinetics

Onset of Action: Hypnosis: I.M.: 20-30 minutes; Sedation: I.V.: 5-20 minutes; Anticonvulsant: I.V.: 5 minutes, oral: 30-60 minutes

Duration of Action: 6-8 hours

Absorption: Oral, I.M.: Prompt

Protein Binding: 85%; free fraction may be significantly higher in elderly

Half-Life Elimination: Neonates: 40.2 hours; Older children: 10.5 hours; Adults: 12.9 hours; Elderly: 15.9 hours; End-stage renal disease: 32-70 hours

Metabolism: Hepatic to inactive compounds

Excretion: Urine; feces (minimal)

Dosing

Adults:

Antiemetic: Oral, I.V. (**Note:** May be administered sublingually; not a labeled route): 0.5-2 mg every 4-6 hours as needed

Anxiety and sedation: Oral: 1-10 mg/day in 2-3 divided doses; usual dose: 2-6 mg/day in divided doses; initial dose should not exceed 2 mg in debilitated patients

Insomnia: Oral: 2-4 mg at bedtime

Preoperative:
I.M.: 0.05 mg/kg administered 2 hours before surgery; maximum: 4 mg/dose
I.V.: 0.044 mg/kg 15-20 minutes before surgery; usual maximum: 2 mg/dose

Operative amnesia: I.V.: Up to 0.05 mg/kg; maximum: 4 mg/dose

Status epilepticus: I.V.: 4 mg/dose given slowly over 2-5 minutes; may repeat in 10-15 minutes; usual maximum dose: 8 mg

Rapid tranquilization of agitated patient (administer every 30-60 minutes):
Oral: 1-2 mg
I.M.: 0.5-1 mg
Average total dose for tranquilization: 4-8 mg

Agitation in the ICU patient (unlabeled):
I.V.: 0.02-0.06 mg/kg every 2-6 hours
I.V. infusion: 0.01-0.1 mg/kg/hour

Elderly: Anxiety and sedation: Oral, I.V.: 0.5-4 mg/day; refer to adult dosing for other indications. Dose selection should generally be on the low end of the dosage range (ie, initial dose not to exceed 2 mg)

Pediatrics:

Antiemetic: Children 2-15 years: I.V.: 0.05 mg/kg (up to 2 mg/dose) prior to chemotherapy

Anxiety and sedation: Infants and Children: Oral, I.V.: Usual: 0.05 mg/kg/dose (range: 0.02-0.09 mg/kg) every 4-8 hours

Sedation (preprocedure): Infants and Children:
Oral, I.M., I.V.: Usual: 0.05 mg/kg; range: 0.02-0.09 mg/kg
I.V.: May use smaller doses (eg, 0.01-0.03 mg/kg) and repeat every 20 minutes, as needed to titrate to effect

Status epilepticus: I.V.:
Infants and Children: 0.1 mg/kg slow I.V. over 2-5 minutes, do not exceed 4 mg/single dose; may repeat second dose of 0.05 mg/kg slow I.V. in 10-15 minutes if needed
Adolescents: 0.07 mg/kg slow I.V. over 2-5 minutes; maximum: 4 mg/dose; may repeat in 10-15 minutes

Available Dosage Forms

Injection, solution (Ativan®): 2 mg/mL (1 mL, 10 mL); 4 mg/mL (1 mL, 10 mL) [contains benzyl alcohol]

Solution, oral concentrate (Lorazepam Intensol®): 2 mg/mL (30 mL) [alcohol free, dye free]

Tablet (Ativan®): 0.5 mg, 1 mg, 2 mg

Monitoring and Teaching Issues

Physical Assessment: Assess other medications the patient may be taking for effectiveness and interactions. **Oral:** Assess for history of addiction; long-term use can result in dependence, abuse, or tolerance; periodically evaluate need for continued use. For inpatient use, institute safety measures and monitor effectiveness and adverse reactions. For outpatients, monitor therapeutic effectiveness and adverse reactions at beginning of therapy and periodically with long-term use. Taper dosage slowly when discontinuing. Assess knowledge/teach patient appropriate use, interventions to reduce side effects, and adverse symptoms to report. **I.V./I.M.:** Monitor vital signs and CNS status (possible retrograde amnesia I.V.), and ability to void. Maintain bedrest for 2-3 hours, and observe when up.

Patient Education: Oral: Take exactly as directed; do not increase dose or frequency. Drug may cause physical and/or psychological dependence. Do not use alcohol or other prescription or OTC medications (especially pain medications, sedatives, antihistamines, or hypnotics) without consulting prescriber. Maintain adequate hydration (2-3 L/day of fluids) unless instructed to restrict fluid intake. You may experience drowsiness, lightheadedness, impaired coordination, dizziness, or blurred vision (use caution when driving or engaging in tasks requiring alertness until response to drug is known); nausea, vomiting, or dry mouth (small frequent meals, frequent mouth care, chewing gum, or sucking lozenges may help); constipation (increased exercise, fluids, fruit, or fiber may help); altered sexual drive or ability (reversible); or photosensitivity (use sunscreen, wear protective clothing and eyewear, and avoid direct sunlight). Report persistent CNS effects (eg, confusion, depression, increased sedation, excitation, headache, agitation, insomnia or nightmares, dizziness, fatigue, impaired coordination, changes in personality, or changes in cognition); changes in urinary pattern; chest pain, palpitations, or rapid heartbeat; muscle cramping, weakness, tremors, or rigidity; ringing in ears or visual disturbances; excessive perspiration; excessive GI symptoms (cramping, constipation, vomiting, anorexia); or worsening of condition. **Pregnancy/breast-feeding precautions:** Do not get pregnant while taking this medication; use appropriate contraceptive measures. Do not breast-feed.

Geriatric Considerations: Because lorazepam is relatively short-acting with an inactive metabolite, it is a preferred agent to use in elderly patients when a benzodiazepine is indicated. Use with caution since elderly patients have decreased pulmonary reserve and are more prone to hypoxia.

Pregnancy Risk Factor: D

Pregnancy Issues: Benzodiazepines cross the placenta. The association between benzodiazepine exposure and malformations remains controversial. A number of types of malformation have been reported (oral cleft, inguinal hernia, cardiac defects, spina bifida, dysmorphic facial features, skeletal defects); however, confounding factors make a clear association difficult. Overall, the risk to the fetus may be low. Nonteratogenic effects (including neonatal flaccidity, respiratory and feeding problems, and withdrawal symptoms) during the postnatal period have also been reported with benzodiazepine use.

Lactation: Enters breast milk/contraindicated (AAP rates "of concern")

Breast-Feeding Issues: Crosses into breast milk and no data on clinical effects on the infant. AAP states MAY BE OF CONCERN.

Other Issues: Taper dosage gradually after long-term therapy, especially in epileptic patients. Abrupt withdrawal may cause tremors, nausea, vomiting, abdominal and/or muscle cramps.

(Continued)

Lorazepam *(Continued)*

Administration
I.M.: Should be administered deep into the muscle mass.

I.V.: Inadvertent intra-arterial injection may produce arteriospasm resulting in gangrene which may require amputation.

Reconstitution: Infusion: Use 2 mg/mL injectable solution to prepare; dilute ≤1 mg/mL and mix in glass bottle; precipitation may develop; can also be administered undiluted via infusion

Compatibility:

Y-site administration: Incompatible with aldesleukin, aztreonam, floxacillin, foscarnet, idarubicin, imipenem/cilastatin, omeprazole, ondansetron, sargramostim, sufentanil

Compatibility in syringe: Incompatible with sufentanil

Compatibility when admixed: Incompatible with buprenorphine, dexamethasone sodium phosphate with diphenhydramine and metoclopramide

Storage: Intact vials should be refrigerated and protected from light. Do not use discolored or precipitate-containing solutions. Injectable vials may be stored at room temperature for up to 60 days. Parenteral admixture is stable at room temperature (25°C) for 24 hours.

Additional Information Oral doses >0.09 mg/kg produced increased ataxia without increased sedative benefit vs lower doses; preferred anxiolytic when I.M. route needed. Abrupt discontinuation after sustained use (generally >10 days) may cause withdrawal symptoms.

Related Information
Anxiolytic / Hypnotic Use in Long-Term Care Facilities *on page 1769*

Benzodiazepines *on page 1719*

Federal OBRA Regulations: Recommended Maximum Doses *on page 1773*

♦ **Lorazepam Intensol®** *see Lorazepam on page 919*

♦ **Lorcet® 10/650** *see Hydrocodone and Acetaminophen on page 754*

♦ **Lorcet®-HD** *see Hydrocodone and Acetaminophen on page 754*

♦ **Lorcet® Plus** *see Hydrocodone and Acetaminophen on page 754*

♦ **Lortab®** *see Hydrocodone and Acetaminophen on page 754*

Losartan *(loe SAR tan)*

U.S. Brand Names Cozaar®

Synonyms DuP 753; Losartan Potassium; MK594

Generic Available No

Pharmacologic Category Angiotensin II Receptor Blocker

Medication Safety Issues

Sound-alike/look-alike issues:

Losartan may be confused with valsartan

Cozaar® may be confused with Hyzaar®, Zocor®

Use Treatment of hypertension (HTN); treatment of diabetic nephropathy in patients with type 2 diabetes mellitus (noninsulin dependent, NIDDM) and a history of hypertension; stroke risk reduction in patients with HTN and left ventricular hypertrophy (LVH)

Mechanism of Action/Effect As a selective and competitive, nonpeptide angiotensin II receptor antagonist, losartan blocks the vasoconstrictor and aldosterone-secreting effects of angiotensin II. Losartan increases urinary flow rate and in addition to being natriuretic and kaliuretic, increases excretion of chloride, magnesium, uric acid, calcium, and phosphate.

Contraindications Hypersensitivity to losartan or any component of the formulation; hypersensitivity to other A-II receptor antagonists; bilateral renal artery stenosis; pregnancy (2nd and 3rd trimesters)

Warnings/Precautions Avoid use or use a smaller dose in patients who are volume depleted. Deterioration in renal function can occur with initiation. Use with caution in unilateral renal artery stenosis and pre-existing renal insufficiency; significant aortic/mitral stenosis. When used to reduce the risk of stroke in patients with HTN and LVH, may not be effective in African-American population. Use caution with hepatic dysfunction, dose adjustment may be needed.

Drug Interactions
Cytochrome P450 Effect: Substrate (major) of CYP2C8/9, 3A4; **Inhibits** CYP1A2 (weak), 2C8/9 (moderate), 2C19 (weak), 3A4 (weak)

Decreased Effect: The levels/effects of losartan may be decreased by aminoglutethimide, carbamazepine, nafcillin, nevirapine, phenobarbital, phenytoin, rifampin, rifapentine, secobarbital, and other CYP2C8/9 or 3A4 inducers. NSAIDs may decrease the efficacy of losartan.

Increased Effect/Toxicity: Cimetidine may increase the absorption of losartan by 18% (clinical effect is unknown). Potassium salts/supplements, co-trimoxazole (high dose), ACE inhibitors, and potassium-sparing diuretics (amiloride, spironolactone, triamterene) may increase the risk of hyperkalemia. Risk of lithium toxicity may be increased by losartan. Losartan may increase the levels/effects of amiodarone, fluoxetine, glimepiride, glipizide, nateglinide, phenytoin, pioglitazone, rosiglitazone, sertraline, warfarin, and other CYP2C8/9 substrates. Fluconazole may increase the levels/effects of losartan.

Nutritional/Ethanol Interactions Herb/Nutraceutical: St John's wort may decrease levels. Avoid dong quai if using for hypertension (has estrogenic activity). Avoid ephedra, yohimbe, ginseng (may worsen hypertension). Avoid garlic (may have increased antihypertensive effect).

Adverse Reactions
>10%:

Cardiovascular: Chest pain (12% diabetic nephropathy)

Central nervous system: Fatigue (14% diabetic nephropathy)

Endocrine: Hypoglycemia (14% diabetic nephropathy)

Gastrointestinal: Diarrhea (2% to 15% diabetic nephropathy)

Genitourinary: Urinary tract infection (13% diabetic nephropathy)

Hematologic: Anemia (14% diabetic nephropathy)

Neuromuscular & skeletal: Weakness (14% diabetic nephropathy), back pain (2% hypertension to 12% diabetic nephropathy)

Respiratory: Cough (11% diabetic nephropathy; 17% to 29% hypertension but similar to that associated with hydrochlorothiazide or placebo therapy)

1% to 10%:

Cardiovascular: Hypotension (7% diabetic nephropathy), orthostatic hypotension (4% hypertension to 4% diabetic nephropathy), first-dose hypotension (dose related: <1% with 50 mg, 2% with 100 mg)

Central nervous system: Dizziness (4%), hypoesthesia (5% diabetic nephropathy), fever (4% diabetic nephropathy), insomnia (1%)

Dermatology: Cellulitis (7% diabetic nephropathy)

Endocrine: Hyperkalemia (<1% hypertension to 7% diabetic nephropathy)

Gastrointestinal: Gastritis (5% diabetic nephropathy), weight gain (4% diabetic nephropathy), dyspepsia (1% to 4%), abdominal pain (2%), nausea (2%)

Neuromuscular & skeletal: Muscular weakness (7% diabetic nephropathy), knee pain (5% diabetic nephropathy), leg pain (1% to 5%), muscle cramps (1%), myalgia (1%)

Respiratory: Bronchitis (10% diabetic nephropathy), upper respiratory infection (8%), nasal congestion (2%), sinusitis (1% hypertension to 6% diabetic nephropathy)

Miscellaneous: Infection (5% diabetic nephropathy), flu-like syndrome (10% diabetic nephropathy)

Overdosage/Toxicology Hypotension and tachycardia may occur with significant overdose. Treatment should be supportive. Not removed via hemodialysis.

Pharmacodynamics/Kinetics

Onset of Action: 6 hours

Bioavailability: 25% to 33%; AUC of E-3174 is four times greater than that of losartan

Time to Peak: Serum: Losartan: 1 hour; E-3174: 3-4 hours

Protein Binding: Plasma: High

Half-Life Elimination: Losartan: 1.5-2 hours; E-3174: 6-9 hours

Metabolism: Hepatic (14%) via CYP2C9 and 3A4 to an active metabolite E-3174 (40 times more potent than losartan); extensive first-pass effect

Excretion: Excretion: Urine (4% as unchanged drug, 6% as active metabolite)

Clearance: Plasma: Losartan: 600 mL/minute; Active metabolite: 50 mL/minute

Dosing

Adults & Elderly:

Hypertension: Oral: Initial: 25-50 mg once daily; can be administered once or twice daily with total daily doses ranging from 25-100 mg

Usual initial doses in patients receiving diuretics or those with intravascular volume depletion: 25 mg

Nephropathy in patients with type 2 diabetes and hypertension: Oral: Initial: 50 mg once daily; can be increased to 100 mg once daily based on blood pressure response

Stroke reduction (HTN with LVH): Oral: 50 mg once daily (maximum daily dose: 100 mg); may be used in combination with a thiazide diuretic

Pediatrics:

Hypertension: Oral: Children 6-16 years: 0.7 mg/kg once daily (maximum: 50 mg/day); adjust dose based on response; doses >1.4 mg/kg (maximum: 100 mg) have not been studied.

Renal Impairment:

Children: Use is not recommended if Cl_{cr} <30 mL/minute.

Adults: No adjustment necessary.

Hepatic Impairment: Reduce the initial dose to 25 mg/day; divide dosage intervals into two.

Available Dosage Forms Tablet [film coated], as potassium: 25 mg, 50 mg, 100 mg

Monitoring and Teaching Issues

Physical Assessment: Use caution in presence of impaired renal function, significant aortic/mitral stenosis (see Warnings/Precautions for specific use cautions). Assess potential for interactions with other pharmacological agents or herbal products patient may be taking (eg, decreased of increased levels/effects of losartan, risk of toxicities; see Drug Interactions). Assess results of laboratory tests, therapeutic effectiveness (normotensive), and adverse response on a regular basis during therapy (eg, hypotension; see Adverse Reactions). Teach patient proper use, possible side effects/appropriate interventions, and adverse symptoms to report (see Patient Education).

Monitoring Laboratory Tests: Electrolytes, serum creatinine, BUN, urinalysis, CBC

Patient Education: Do not take any new medication during therapy unless approved by prescriber. Do not use potassium supplement or salt substitutes without consulting prescriber. Take exactly as directed and do not discontinue without consulting prescriber. Preferable to take at same time each day; without regard to meals. This drug does not eliminate need for diet or exercise as recommended by your prescriber. May cause dizziness, fainting, or lightheadedness (use caution when driving or engaging in tasks that require alertness until response to drug is known); postural hypotension (use caution when rising from lying or sitting position or climbing stairs); diarrhea (boiled milk, buttermilk, or yogurt may help). Report chest pain or palpitations; unrelenting headache; back or muscle pain or weakness; CNS changes (delusions or depression); swelling of face mouth, tongue or throat; or other persistent adverse reactions. **Pregnancy/breast-feeding precautions:** Inform prescriber if you are or intend to become pregnant. This drug should not be used in the 2nd or 3rd trimester of pregnancy. Consult prescriber for appropriate contraceptive measures. Breast-feeding is not recommended.

Dietary Considerations: May be taken with or without food.

Geriatric Considerations: Serum concentrations of losartan and its metabolites are not significantly different in the elderly patient and no initial dose adjustment is necessary even in low creatinine clearance states (<30 mL/minute).

Pregnancy Risk Factor: C/D (2nd and 3rd trimesters)

Pregnancy Issues: Discontinue as soon as possible when pregnancy is detected. Drugs which act directly on renin-angiotensin can cause fetal and neonatal morbidity and death. (Continued)

Losartan *(Continued)*

Lactation: Excretion in breast milk unknown/not recommended

Breast-Feeding Issues: Avoid use in the nursing mother, if possible, since it is postulated that losartan is excreted in breast milk. Recommend discontinuing drug or discontinuing nursing based on the importance of the drug to the mother.

Administration

Oral: May be administered with or without food.

Storage: Store at 15°C to 30°C (59°F to 86°F). Protect from light.

Related Information

Angiotensin Agents *on page 1704*

Losartan and Hydrochlorothiazide

(loe SAR tan & hye droe klor oh THYE a zide)

U.S. Brand Names Hyzaar®

Synonyms Hydrochlorothiazide and Losartan

Generic Available No

Pharmacologic Category Angiotensin II Receptor Blocker Combination; Antihypertensive Agent, Combination; Diuretic, Thiazide

Medication Safety Issues

Sound-alike/look-alike issues:

Hyzaar® may be confused with Cozaar®

Use Treatment of hypertension

Dosing

Adults: Hypertension (dosage must be individualized): Oral: 1 tablet/day

Elderly: Refer to dosing in individual monographs.

Renal Impairment: Usual regimens may be followed as long as Cl$_{cr}$ is ≥30 mL/minute. In patients with more severe renal impairment, loop diuretics are preferred.

Hepatic Impairment: Not recommended for titration in patients with hepatic impairment.

Available Dosage Forms Tablet [film coated]:

50-12.5: Losartan potassium 50 mg and hydrochlorothiazide 12.5 mg

100-25: Losartan potassium 100 mg and hydrochlorothiazide 25 mg

Monitoring and Teaching Issues

Physical Assessment: See individual agents.

Patient Education: See individual agents. **Pregnancy/breast-feeding precautions:** Inform prescriber if you are or intend to become pregnant. Do not breast-feed.

Pregnancy Risk Factor: C/D (2nd and 3rd trimesters)

Lactation: Enters breast milk/contraindicated

Related Information

Hydrochlorothiazide *on page 751*

Losartan *on page 922*

♦ **Losartan Potassium** *see* Losartan *on page 922*

♦ **Lotemax®** *see* Loteprednol *on page 924*

♦ **Lotensin®** *see* Benazepril *on page 178*

♦ **Lotensin® HCT** *see* Benazepril and Hydrochlorothiazide *on page 180*

Loteprednol (loe te PRED nol)

U.S. Brand Names Alrex®; Lotemax®

Synonyms Loteprednol Etabonate

Generic Available No

Pharmacologic Category Corticosteroid, Ophthalmic

Use

Suspension, 0.2% (Alrex®): Temporary relief of signs and symptoms of seasonal allergic conjunctivitis

Suspension, 0.5% (Lotemax®): Inflammatory conditions (treatment of steroid-responsive inflammatory conditions of the palpebral and bulbar conjunctiva, cornea, and anterior segment of the globe such as allergic conjunctivitis, acne rosacea, superficial punctate keratitis, herpes zoster keratitis, iritis, cyclitis, selected infective conjunctivitis, when the inherent hazard of steroid use is accepted to obtain an advisable diminution in edema and inflammation) and treatment of postoperative inflammation following ocular surgery

Contraindications Hypersensitivity to loteprednol, other corticosteroids, and any component of the formulation; viral diseases of the cornea and conjunctiva; mycobacterial infection of the eye; fungal diseases of ocular structures

Warnings/Precautions For ophthalmic use only; patients should be re-evaluated if symptoms fail to improve after 2 days. Intraocular pressure should be monitored if this product is used >10 days. Prolonged use may result in glaucoma and injury to the optic nerve. Visual defects in acuity and field of vision may occur. Posterior subcapsular cataracts may form after long-term use. Use with caution in presence of glaucoma (steroids increase intraocular pressure). Perforation may occur with topical steroids in diseases which thin the cornea or sclera. Steroids may mask infection or enhance existing infection. Steroid use may delay healing after cataract surgery.

Adverse Reactions

>10%:

Central nervous system: Headache

Respiratory: Rhinitis, pharyngitis

1% to 10%: Ocular: Abnormal vision/blurring, burning on instillation, chemosis, dry eyes, itching, injection, conjunctivitis/irritation, corneal abnormalities, eyelid erythema, papillae uveitis

Pharmacodynamics/Kinetics
Absorption: None

Dosing
Adults & Elderly:

Seasonal allergic conjunctivitis: Ophthalmic: 0.2% suspension (Alrex®): Instill 1 drop into affected eye(s) 4 times/day.

Inflammatory conditions: Ophthalmic: 0.5% suspension (Lotemax®): Apply 1-2 drops into the conjunctival sac of the affected eye(s) 4 times/day. During the initial treatment within the first week, the dosing may be increased up to 1 drop every hour. Advise patients not to discontinue therapy prematurely. If signs and symptoms fail to improve after 2 days, re-evaluate the patient.

Postoperative inflammation: Ophthalmic: 0.5% suspension (Lotemax®): Apply 1-2 drops into the conjunctival sac of the operated eye(s) 4 times/day beginning 24 hours after surgery and continuing throughout the first 2 weeks of the postoperative period.

Available Dosage Forms Suspension, ophthalmic, as etabonate:
Alrex®: 0.2% (5 mL, 10 mL) [contains benzalkonium chloride]
Lotemax®: 0.5% (2.5 mL, 5 mL, 10 mL, 15 mL) [contains benzalkonium chloride]

Monitoring and Teaching Issues
Physical Assessment: Assess potential for interactions with other prescriptions, OTC medications, or herbal products patient may be taking. Assess therapeutic response and adverse effects. Teach patient proper use, side effects/appropriate interventions, and symptoms to report.

Patient Education: For use in eyes only. Store in a cool place. Shake well before using. Do not let tip of applicator touch eye; do not contaminate tip of applicator (may cause eye infection, eye damage, or vision loss). Tilt head back, place medication in conjunctival sac, and close eyes. Apply finger pressure at corner of eye for 1 minute following application. May cause temporary sensitivity to bright light, blurring or stinging, changes in visual acuity, headache, runny nose, or sore throat. Do not discontinue therapy prematurely. If improvement is not noted within 2 days, notify prescriber. Report persistent vision changes, signs of increased infection, swollen eyelids, extreme itching, or if inflammation does not improve. **Pregnancy precaution:** Inform prescriber if you are pregnant.

Pregnancy Risk Factor: C
Lactation: Excretion in breast milk unknown/use caution

Loteprednol and Tobramycin (loe te PRED nol & toe bra MYE sin)
U.S. Brand Names Zylet™
Synonyms Loteprednol Etabonate and Tobramycin; Tobramycin and Loteprednol Etabonate
Generic Available No
Pharmacologic Category Antibiotic/Corticosteroid, Ophthalmic
Use Treatment of steroid-responsive ocular inflammatory conditions where either a superficial bacterial ocular infection or the risk of a superficial bacterial ocular infection exists

Dosing
Adults & Elderly: Ophthalmic: Instill 1-2 drops into the affected eye(s) every 4-6 hours; may increase frequency during the first 24-48 hours to every 1-2 hours. Interval should increase as signs and symptoms improve. Further evaluation should occur for use of greater than 20 mL.

Available Dosage Forms Suspension, ophthalmic: Loteprednol 0.5% and tobramycin 0.3% (2.5 mL, 5 mL, 10 mL) [contains benzalkonium chloride]

Monitoring and Teaching Issues
Pregnancy Risk Factor: C
Lactation: Excretion in breast milk unknown/use caution

Lovastatin (LOE va sta tin)
U.S. Brand Names Altocor™ [DSC]; Altoprev™; Mevacor®
Synonyms Mevinolin; Monacolin K
Generic Available Yes: Immediate release tablet
Pharmacologic Category Antilipemic Agent, HMG-CoA Reductase Inhibitor
Medication Safety Issues
Sound-alike/look-alike issues:
Lovastatin may be confused with Leustatin®, Livostin®, Lotensin®
Altocor™ may be confused with Advicor®
Mevacor® may be confused with Mivacron®

Use
Adjunct to dietary therapy to decrease elevated serum total and LDL-cholesterol concentrations in primary hypercholesterolemia

Primary prevention of coronary artery disease (patients without symptomatic disease with average to moderately elevated total and LDL-cholesterol and below average HDL-cholesterol); slow progression of coronary atherosclerosis in patients with coronary heart disease

Adjunct to dietary therapy in adolescent patients (10-17 years of age, females >1 year postmenarche) with heterozygous familial hypercholesterolemia having LDL >189 mg/dL, **or** LDL >160 mg/dL with positive family history of premature cardiovascular disease (CVD), **or** LDL >160 mg/dL with the presence of at least two other CVD risk factors
(Continued)

Lovastatin *(Continued)*

Mechanism of Action/Effect Lovastatin acts by competitively inhibiting 3-hydroxyl-3-methylglutaryl-coenzyme A (HMG-CoA) reductase, the enzyme that catalyzes the rate-limiting step in cholesterol biosynthesis.

Contraindications Hypersensitivity to lovastatin or any component of the formulation; active liver disease; unexplained persistent elevations of serum transaminases; pregnancy; breast-feeding

Warnings/Precautions Liver function must be monitored by periodic laboratory assessment. Rhabdomyolysis with acute renal failure has occurred. Risk is dose-related and is increased with concurrent use of lipid-lowering agents which may cause rhabdomyolysis (gemfibrozil, fibric acid derivatives, or niacin at doses ≥1 g/day) or during concurrent use with potent CYP3A4 inhibitors (including amiodarone, clarithromycin, cyclosporine, erythromycin, itraconazole, ketoconazole, nefazodone, grapefruit juice in large quantities, verapamil, or protease inhibitors such as indinavir, nelfinavir, or ritonavir). Weigh the risk versus benefit when combining any of these drugs with lovastatin. Temporarily discontinue in any patient experiencing an acute or serious condition predisposing to renal failure secondary to rhabdomyolysis. Use with caution in patients who consume large amounts of ethanol or have a history of liver disease. Safety and efficacy of the immediate release tablet have not been evaluated in prepubertal patients, patients <10 years of age, or doses >40 mg/day in appropriately-selected adolescents; extended release tablets have not been studied in patients <20 years of age.

Drug Interactions

Cytochrome P450 Effect: Substrate of CYP3A4 (major); **Inhibits** CYP2C8/9 (weak), 2D6 (weak), 3A4 (weak)

Decreased Effect: Cholestyramine taken with lovastatin reduces lovastatin absorption and effect.

Increased Effect/Toxicity: CYP3A4 inhibitors may increase the levels/effects of lovastatin; example inhibitors include azole antifungals, ciprofloxacin, clarithromycin, diclofenac, doxycycline, erythromycin, imatinib, isoniazid, nefazodone, nicardipine, propofol, protease inhibitors, quinidine, and verapamil. Suspend lovastatin therapy during concurrent clarithromycin, erythromycin, itraconazole, or ketoconazole therapy. Cyclosporine, clofibrate, fenofibrate, gemfibrozil, and niacin also may increase the risk of myopathy and rhabdomyolysis. The effect/toxicity of warfarin (elevated PT) and levothyroxine may be increased by lovastatin. Digoxin, norethindrone, and ethinyl estradiol levels may be increased. Effects are additive with other lipid-lowering therapies.

Nutritional/Ethanol Interactions

Ethanol: Avoid excessive ethanol consumption (due to potential hepatic effects).

Food: Food **decreases** the bioavailability of lovastatin extended release tablets and **increases** the bioavailibity of lovastatin immediate release tablets. Lovastatin serum concentrations may be increased if taken with grapefruit juice; avoid concurrent intake of large quantities (>1 quart/day).

Herb/Nutraceutical: St John's wort may decrease lovastatin levels.

Lab Interactions Increased liver transaminases (S), altered thyroid function tests

Adverse Reactions Percentages as reported with immediate release tablets; similar adverse reactions seen with extended release tablets.

>10%: Neuromuscular & skeletal: Increased CPK (>2x normal) (11%)

1% to 10%:

Central nervous system: Headache (2% to 3%), dizziness (0.5% to 1%)

Dermatologic: Rash (0.8% to 1%)

Gastrointestinal: Abdominal pain (2% to 3%), constipation (2% to 4%), diarrhea (2% to 3%), dyspepsia (1% to 2%), flatulence (4% to 5%), nausea (2% to 3%)

Neuromuscular & skeletal: Myalgia (2% to 3%), weakness (1% to 2%), muscle cramps (0.6% to 1%)

Ocular: Blurred vision (0.8% to 1%)

Overdosage/Toxicology Few adverse events have been reported. Treatment is symptomatic.

Pharmacodynamics/Kinetics

Onset of Action: LDL-cholesterol reductions: 3 days

Absorption: 30%; increased with extended release tablets when taken in the fasting state

Bioavailability: Increased with extended release tablets

Time to Peak: Serum: 2-4 hours

Protein Binding: 95%

Half-Life Elimination: 1.1-1.7 hours

Metabolism: Hepatic; extensive first-pass effect; hydrolyzed to B-hydroxy acid (active)

Excretion: Feces (~80% to 85%); urine (10%)

Dosing

Adults & Elderly:

Dyslipidemia and primary prevention of CAD: Oral: Initial: 20 mg with evening meal, then adjust at 4-week intervals; maximum: 80 mg/day immediate release tablet **or** 60 mg/day extended release tablet.

Dosage modification/limits based on concurrent therapy:

Cyclosporine and other immunosuppressant drugs: Initial dose: 10 mg/day with a maximum recommended dose of 20 mg/day

Concurrent therapy with fibrates and/or lipid-lowering doses of niacin (>1 g/day): Maximum recommended dose: 20 mg/day. Concurrent use with fibrates should be avoided unless risk to benefit favors use.

Concurrent therapy with amiodarone or verapamil: Maximum recommended dose: 40 mg/day of regular release or 20 mg/day with extended release.

Dosage adjustment in renal impairment: Cl_{cr} <30 mL/minute: Use doses >20 mg/day with caution.

Pediatrics:

Heterozygous familial hypercholesterolemia: Oral (immediate release tablet): Adolescents 10-17 years:

LDL reduction <20%: Initial: 10 mg/day with evening meal

LDL reduction ≥20%: Initial: 20 mg/day with evening meal

Usual range: 10-40 mg with evening meal, then adjust dose at 4-week intervals

Renal Impairment: Cl$_{cr}$ <30 mL/minute: Use with caution and carefully consider doses >20 mg/day.

Available Dosage Forms [DSC] = Discontinued product

Tablet: 10 mg, 20 mg, 40 mg

Mevacor®: 20 mg, 40 mg

Tablet, extended release (Altocor™ [DSC], Altoprev™): 10 mg, 20 mg, 40 mg, 60 mg

Monitoring and Teaching Issues

Physical Assessment: See Warnings/Precautions for use cautions (eg, impaired liver function). Assess potential for interactions with other pharmacological agents or herbal products patient may be taking (eg, increased risk of myopathy or rhabdomyolysis; see Drug Interactions). Assess results of laboratory tests (see Monitoring Laboratory Tests) and patient response on a regular basis throughout therapy (eg, rash, myalgia, blurred vision, abdominal pain; see Adverse Reactions). Teach patient proper use, possible side effects/appropriate interventions, and adverse symptoms to report (see Patient Education). **Pregnancy risk factor X:** Determine that patient is not pregnant before starting therapy. Do not give to women of childbearing age unless they are capable of complying with effective contraceptive use. Instruct patient in appropriate contraceptive measures.

Monitoring Laboratory Tests: Obtain baseline LFTs and total cholesterol profile. LFTs should be performed before initiation of therapy, at 6 and 12 weeks after initiation or first dose, and periodically thereafter.

Patient Education: Inform prescriber of all prescriptions, OTC medications, or herbal products you are taking, and any allergies you have. Do not take any new medication during therapy unless approved by prescriber. Take as directed, with food at evening meal. Follow diet and exercise regimen as prescribed. You will have periodic blood tests to assess effectiveness. You may experience nausea or dyspepsia (small frequent meals, frequent mouth care, sucking lozenges may help); diarrhea (buttermilk, boiled milk, or yogurt may help); or headache (see prescriber for analgesic). Report muscle pain or cramping; tremor; CNS changes (eg, memory loss, depression, personality changes; numbness, weakness, tingling or pain in extremities); any blurred visions or changes in visual acuity; or other adverse reactions. **Pregnancy/breast-feeding precautions:** Inform prescriber if you are pregnant. Consult prescriber for appropriate contraceptive measures to use during and for 1 month following therapy. This drug may cause severe fetal defects. Do not donate blood during or for 1 month following therapy. Do not breast-feed.

Dietary Considerations: Before initiation of therapy, patients should be placed on a standard cholesterol-lowering diet for 6 weeks and the diet should be continued during drug therapy. Avoid intake of large quantities of grapefruit juice (≥1 quart/day); may increase toxicity.

Geriatric Considerations: The definition of and, therefore, when to treat hyperlipidemia in the elderly is a controversial issue. The National Cholesterol Education Program recommends that all adults maintain a plasma cholesterol <160 mg/dL. In elderly patients with one additional risk factor, goal LDL would decrease to <130 mg/dL. Pharmacologic treatment should be reserved for those who are unable to obtain a desirable plasma cholesterol concentration by diet alone and for whom the benefits of treatment are believed to outweigh the potential adverse effects, drug interactions, and cost of treatment.

Pregnancy Risk Factor: X

Pregnancy Issues: Safety and efficacy have not been established for use during pregnancy (treatment should be discontinued if pregnancy is recognized). Administer to women of childbearing potential only if conception is unlikely; females should be counseled on appropriate contraceptive methods.

Lactation: Excretion unknown/contraindicated

Administration

Oral: Administer immediate release tablet with meals. Administer extended release tablet at bedtime; do not crush or chew.

Storage:

Tablet, immediate release: Store between 5°C to 30°C (41°F to 86°F). Protect from light.

Tablet, extended release: Store between 20°C to 25°C (68°F to 77°F). Avoid excessive heat and humidity.

Related Information

Hyperlipidemia Management *on page 1836*

Lipid-Lowering Agents *on page 1738*

Lutropin Alfa (LOO troe pin AL fa)

U.S. Brand Names Luveris®

Synonyms Recombinant Human Luteinizing Hormone; r-hLH

Generic Available No

Pharmacologic Category Gonadotropin; Ovulation Stimulator

Use Stimulation of follicular development in infertile hypogonadotropic hypogonadal (HH) women with profound luteinizing hormone (LH) deficiency; to be used in combination with follitropin alfa

Mechanism of Action/Effect Replaces endogenously secreted luteinizing hormone. Stimulates development of the follicle and prepares reproductive tract for implantation and pregnancy.

Contraindications Hypersensitivity to lutropin alfa or any component of the formulation; primary ovarian failure; uncontrolled thyroid or adrenal dysfunction; uncontrolled organic intracranial lesion; abnormal uterine bleeding of undetermined origin; ovarian cyst or enlargement of undetermined origin; sex hormone-dependent tumors of the reproductive tract and accessory organs; pregnancy

Warnings/Precautions For use by infertility specialists. May cause ovarian hyperstimulation syndrome (OHSS); if severe, treatment should be discontinued and patient should be hospitalized. OHSS results in a rapid (<24 hours to 7 days) accumulation of fluid in the peritoneal cavity, thorax, and possibly the pericardium, which may become more severe if pregnancy occurs; monitor for ovarian enlargement. Patients should be advised of the potential risk for multiple births before beginning therapy. Safety and efficacy have not been established with hepatic or renal dysfunction. Not for use in children or postmenopausal women.

Adverse Reactions

1% to 10%:

Central nervous system: Headache (10%), fatigue (2% to 3%)

Endocrine & metabolic: Ovarian hyperstimulation (6%)

Gastrointestinal: Nausea (7%), constipation (2% to 3%), diarrhea (2% to 3%)

Adverse events reported with gonadotropin or menotropin therapy: Adnexal torsion, arterial thromboembolism, congenital abnormalities, ectopic pregnancy, hemoperitoneum, ovarian enlargement (mild-to-moderate), ovarian neoplasms (infrequent), postpartum fever, premature labor, pulmonary complications, spontaneous abortion, vascular complications

Overdosage/Toxicology Multiple gestations and ovarian hyperstimulation may occur following overdose.

Pharmacodynamics/Kinetics

Bioavailability: 56% ± 23%

Time to Peak: 4-16 hours

Half-Life Elimination: Terminal: ~18 hours

Excretion: Urine (<5% unchanged)

Dosing

Adults: Infertility: Female: SubQ: 75 units daily until adequate follicular development is noted; maximum duration of treatment: 14 days; to be used concomitantly with follitropin alfa

Available Dosage Forms Injection, powder for reconstitution: 75 int. units [contains sucrose; packaged with SWFI]

Monitoring and Teaching Issues

Physical Assessment: This medication should only be prescribed by a fertility specialist. For subcutaneous use only. Administer around navel area. Instruct patient in appropriate administration technique and disposal of used needles and syringes. **Pregnancy risk factor X:** Pregnancy must be excluded before starting medication. Consult prescriber if breast-feeding.

Patient Education: For subcutaneous injection only. Follow administration schedule as directed by prescriber. Do not alter dosage or miss dose. If dose missed, notify prescriber. You may experience headache, nausea (small frequent meals, frequent oral care, sucking lozenges, or chewing gum may help), fatigue, constipation, or diarrhea. Report immediately abdominal pain/distension, persistent nausea. **Pregnancy/breast-feeding precautions:** Pregnancy must be excluded before starting medication. Consult prescriber if breast-feeding.

Pregnancy Risk Factor: X

Lactation: Excretion in breast milk unknown/use caution

Administration

Other: SubQ: Administer on the stomach, a few inches above or below the navel.

Reconstitution: Reconstitute with SWFI; mix gently, do not shake.

Storage: Store under refrigeration or at room temperature of 2°C to 25°C (36°F to 77°F). Protect from light. Use immediately after reconstitution.

- **Lymphocyte Mitogenic Factor** *see* Aldesleukin *on page 62*
- **Lysodren®** *see* Mitotane *on page 1018*
- **Macrobid®** *see* Nitrofurantoin *on page 1088*
- **Macrodantin®** *see* Nitrofurantoin *on page 1088*

Magaldrate and Simethicone (MAG al drate & sye METH i kone)
U.S. Brand Names Riopan Plus® [OTC] [DSC]; Riopan Plus® Double Strength [OTC] [DSC]
Synonyms Simethicone and Magaldrate
Generic Available Yes
Pharmacologic Category Antacid; Antiflatulent
Medication Safety Issues
 Sound-alike/look-alike issues:
  Riopan Plus® may be confused with Repan®
Use Relief of hyperacidity associated with peptic ulcer, gastritis, peptic esophagitis and hiatal hernia which are accompanied by symptoms of gas
Dosing
 Adults & Elderly: Hyperacidity/gas: Oral: 5-10 mL between meals and at bedtime
Available Dosage Forms [DSC] = Discontinued product
 Suspension, oral: Magaldrate 540 mg and simethicone 20 mg per 5 mL (360 mL)
  Riopan Plus®: Magaldrate 540 mg and simethicone 20 mg per 5 mL (360 mL) [DSC]
  Riopan Plus® Double Strength: Magaldrate 1080 mg and simethicone 40 mg per 5 mL (360 mL) [DSC]
Monitoring and Teaching Issues
 Patient Education: See individual agents. **Pregnancy precaution:** Inform prescriber if you are or intend to become pregnant.
 Pregnancy Risk Factor: C
 Lactation: Excretion in breast milk unknown/compatible

- **Mag Delay® [OTC]** *see* Magnesium Chloride *on page 929*
- **Mag G® [OTC]** *see* Magnesium Gluconate *on page 930*
- **Magnesia Magma** *see* Magnesium Hydroxide *on page 930*

Magnesium Chloride (mag NEE zhum KLOR ide)
U.S. Brand Names Chloromag®; Mag Delay® [OTC]; Mag-SR® [OTC]; Slow-Mag® [OTC]
Generic Available Yes: Injection
Pharmacologic Category Magnesium Salt
Use Correction or prevention of hypomagnesemia
Dosing
 Adults & Elderly: Dietary supplement: Oral: Dietary supplement: 54-283 mg/day in divided doses
  In TPN: I.V.: 8-24 mEq/day
 Pediatrics:
  In TPN: I.V.: Children: 2-10 mEq/day
   Note: The usual recommended pediatric maintenance intake of magnesium ranges from 0.2-0.6 mEq/kg/day. The dose of magnesium may also be based on the caloric intake; on that basis, 3-10 mEq/day of magnesium are needed; maximum maintenance dose: 8-16 mEq/day
 Renal Impairment: Patients in severe renal failure should not receive magnesium due to toxicity from accumulation. Patients with a Cl_{cr} <25 mL/minute should be monitored by serum magnesium levels.
Available Dosage Forms
 Injection, solution (Chloromag®): 200 mg/mL [1.97 mEq/mL] (50 mL)
 Tablet [enteric coated] (Slow-Mag®): Elemental magnesium 64 mg [contains elemental calcium 106 mg]
 Tablet, extended release (Mag Delay®, Mag-SR®): Magnesium chloride hexahydrate 535 mg [equivalent to elemental magnesium 64 mg]
Monitoring and Teaching Issues
 Pregnancy Risk Factor: D

Magnesium Citrate (mag NEE zhum SIT rate)
Synonyms Citrate of Magnesia
Generic Available Yes
Pharmacologic Category Laxative, Saline; Magnesium Salt
Use Evacuation of bowel prior to certain surgical and diagnostic procedures or overdose situations
Contraindications Renal failure, appendicitis, abdominal pain, intestinal impaction, obstruction or perforation, diabetes mellitus, complications in gastrointestinal tract, patients with colostomy or ileostomy, ulcerative colitis or diverticulitis
Lab Interactions Increased magnesium; decreased protein, decreased calcium (S), decreased potassium (S)
Adverse Reactions 1% to 10%:
 Cardiovascular: Hypotension
 Endocrine & metabolic: Hypermagnesemia
 Gastrointestinal: Abdominal cramps, diarrhea, gas formation
 Respiratory: Respiratory depression
Overdosage/Toxicology
 Serious, potentially life-threatening electrolyte disturbances may occur with long-term use or overdosage due to diarrhea; hypermagnesemia may occur. CNS depression, confusion, hypotension, muscle weakness, blockage of peripheral neuromuscular transmission.
 Serum level >4 mEq/L (4.8 mg/dL): Deep tendon reflexes may be depressed
 Serum level ≥10 mEq/L (12 mg/dL): Deep tendon reflexes may disappear, respiratory paralysis may occur, heart block may occur
 (Continued)

Magnesium Citrate *(Continued)*

I.V. calcium (5-10 mEq) will reverse respiratory depression or heart block; in extreme cases, peritoneal dialysis or hemodialysis may be required.

Serum level >12 mEq/L may be fatal, serum level ≥10 mEq/L may cause complete heart block

Pharmacodynamics/Kinetics
Absorption: Oral: 15% to 30%
Excretion: Urine

Dosing
Adults & Elderly: Cathartic: Oral: Adults: $1/2$ to 1 full bottle (120-300 mL)
Pediatrics: Cathartic: Oral: Children:
<6 years: 0.5 mL/kg up to a maximum of 200 mL repeated every 4-6 hours until stools are clear
6-12 years: 100-150 mL
≥12 years: Refer to adult dosing.
Renal Impairment: Patients in severe renal failure should not receive magnesium due to toxicity from accumulation. Patients with a Cl_{cr} <25 mL/minute should be monitored by serum magnesium levels.

Available Dosage Forms
Solution, oral: 290 mg/5 mL (300 mL) [cherry and lemon flavors]
Tablets: 100 mg [as elemental magnesium]

Monitoring and Teaching Issues
Physical Assessment: Assess therapeutic response and adverse effects.
Patient Education: Take with a glass of water, fruit juice, or citrus flavored carbonated beverage to improve taste. Chill before using. Report severe abdominal pain to physician.
Dietary Considerations: Magnesium content of 5 mL: 3.85-4.71 mEq
Pregnancy Risk Factor: B

Administration
Oral: To increase palatability, chill the solution prior to administration.

Related Information
Laxatives, Classification and Properties *on page 1737*

Magnesium Gluconate *(mag NEE zhum GLOO koe nate)*
U.S. Brand Names Almora® [OTC]; Mag G® [OTC]; Magonate® [OTC]; Magonate® Sport [OTC] [DSC]; Magtrate® [OTC]
Generic Available Yes: Tablet
Pharmacologic Category Magnesium Salt
Use Dietary supplement for treatment of magnesium deficiencies

Dosing
Adults & Elderly: The recommended dietary allowance (RDA) of magnesium is 4.5 mg/kg which is a total daily allowance of 350-400 mg for adult men and 280-300 mg for adult women. During pregnancy the RDA is 300 mg and during lactation the RDA is 355 mg. Dietary supplement: Oral: 54-483 mg/day in divided doses; refer to product labeling
Pediatrics: Dietary supplement: Oral: Children: 3-6 mg/kg/day in divided doses 3-4 times/day; maximum: 400 mg/day
Renal Impairment: Patients in severe renal failure should not receive magnesium due to toxicity from accumulation. Patients with a Cl_{cr} <25 mL/minute should be monitored by serum magnesium levels.

Available Dosage Forms [DSC] = Discontinued product
Solution:
Magonate®: 1000 mg/5 mL (480 mL) [magnesium 4.8 mEq/5 mL; equivalent to elemental magnesium 54 mg/5 mL; contains sodium benzoate]
Magonate® Sport: 1000 mg/5 mL (30 mL) [magnesium 4.8 mEq/5 mL; equivalent to elemental magnesium 54 mg/5 mL; contains sodium benzoate; fruit flavor] [DSC]
Tablet (Almora®, Mag G®, Magonate®, Magtrate®): 500 mg [magnesium 2.4 mEq; equivalent to elemental magnesium 27 mg]

Magnesium Hydroxide *(mag NEE zhum hye DROKS ide)*
U.S. Brand Names Dulcolax® Milk of Magnesia [OTC]; Phillips'® Milk of Magnesia [OTC]
Synonyms Magnesia Magma; Milk of Magnesia; MOM
Generic Available Yes: Liquid
Pharmacologic Category Antacid; Magnesium Salt
Use Short-term treatment of occasional constipation and symptoms of hyperacidity, magnesium replacement therapy

Dosing
Adults & Elderly:
Laxative: Oral: ≥12 years: 30-60 mL/day or in divided doses
Antacid: Oral: 5-15 mL up to 4 times/day as needed
Pediatrics:
Laxative: Oral:
<2 years: 0.5 mL/kg/dose
2-5 years: 5-15 mL/day or in divided doses
6-12 years: 15-30 mL/day or in divided doses
≥12 years: 30-60 mL/day or in divided doses
Antacid: Oral:
Children: 2.5-5 mL as needed up to 4 times/day
Renal Impairment: Patients in severe renal failure should not receive magnesium due to toxicity from accumulation. Patients with a Cl_{cr} <25 mL/minute should be monitored by serum magnesium levels.

Available Dosage Forms
Liquid, oral: 400 mg/5 mL (360 mL, 480 mL, 960 mL, 3780 mL)
Dulcolax® Milk of Magnesia: 400 mg/5 mL (360 mL, 780 mL) [regular and mint flavors]

Phillips'® Milk of Magnesia: 400 mg/5 mL (120 mL, 360 mL, 780 mL) [original, French vanilla, cherry, and mint flavors]

Liquid, oral concentrate: 800 mg/5 mL (100 mL, 400 mL)

Phillips'® Milk of Magnesia [concentrate]: 800 mg/5 mL (240 mL) [strawberry créme flavor]

Tablet, chewable (Phillips'® Milk of Magnesia): 311 mg [mint flavor]

Monitoring and Teaching Issues

Pregnancy Risk Factor: B

Related Information

Laxatives, Classification and Properties *on page 1737*

Magnesium Oxide (mag NEE zhum OKS ide)

U.S. Brand Names Mag-Ox® 400 [OTC]; Uro-Mag® [OTC]

Generic Available Yes: Tablet

Pharmacologic Category Electrolyte Supplement, Oral

Use Electrolyte replacement

Contraindications Patients with colostomy or an ileostomy, appendicitis, ulcerative colitis, diverticulitis, heart block, myocardial damage, serious renal impairment, hepatitis, Addison's disease, hypersensitivity to any component

Warnings/Precautions Hypermagnesemia and toxicity may occur due to decreased renal clearance (Cl_{cr} <30 mL/minute) of absorbed magnesium. Use with caution in digitalized patients (may alter cardiac conduction leading heart block). Use with caution in patients with lithium administration. Elderly patients, due to disease or drug therapy, may be predisposed to diarrhea; diarrhea may result in electrolyte imbalance; monitor for toxicity.

Drug Interactions

Decreased Effect: Decreased absorption of aminoquinolones, digoxin, nitrofurantoin, penicillamine, and tetracyclines may occur with magnesium salts

Increased Effect/Toxicity: Nondepolarizing neuromuscular blockers

Lab Interactions Increased magnesium; decreased protein, calcium (S), decreased potassium (S)

Adverse Reactions

>10%: Gastrointestinal: Diarrhea

1% to 10%:

Cardiovascular: Hypotension, ECG changes

Central nervous system: Mental depression, coma

Gastrointestinal: Nausea, vomiting

Respiratory: Respiratory depression

Overdosage/Toxicology

Magnesium antacids are also laxative and may cause diarrhea and hypokalemia. In patients with renal failure, magnesium may accumulate to toxic levels.

Serious, potentially life-threatening electrolyte disturbances may occur with long-term use or overdosage due to diarrhea; hypermagnesemia may occur. CNS depression, confusion, hypotension, muscle weakness, blockage of peripheral neuromuscular transmission.

Serum level >4 mEq/L (4.8 mg/dL): Deep tendon reflexes may be depressed

Serum level ≥10 mEq/L (12 mg/dL): Deep tendon reflexes may disappear, respiratory paralysis may occur, heart block may occur

I.V. calcium (5-10 mEq) will reverse respiratory depression or heart block; in extreme cases, peritoneal dialysis or hemodialysis may be required.

Serum level >12 mEq/L may be fatal, serum level ≥10 mEq/L may cause complete heart block

Pharmacodynamics/Kinetics

Onset of Action: Laxative: 4-8 hours

Excretion: Urine (up to 30% as absorbed magnesium ions); feces (as unabsorbed drug)

Dosing

Adults & Elderly:

Dietary supplement: Oral: 20-40 mEq (1-2 tablets) 2-3 times/day

Product labeling:

Mag-Ox 400®: 1-2 tablets daily with food

Uro-Mag®: 1-2 tablets 3 times/day with food

Note: Oral magnesium is not generally adequate for repletion in patients with serum magnesium concentrations <1.5 mEq/L

Renal Impairment: Patients in severe renal failure should not receive magnesium due to toxicity from accumulation. Patients with a Cl_{cr} <25 mL/minute should be monitored by serum magnesium levels.

Available Dosage Forms

Capsule (Uro-Mag®): 140 mg [magnesium 7 mEq; equivalent to elemental magnesium 84 mg]

Tablet (Mag-Ox® 400): 400 mg [magnesium 20 mEq; equivalent to elemental magnesium 242 mg]

Monitoring and Teaching Issues

Physical Assessment: Assess therapeutic response and adverse effects.

Dietary Considerations: Should be taken with food. Contains 60% elemental magnesium; 49.6 mEq magnesium/g; 25 mmol magnesium/g.

Pregnancy Risk Factor: B

Magnesium Sulfate (mag NEE zhum SUL fate)

Synonyms Epsom Salts

Generic Available Yes

Pharmacologic Category Antacid; Anticonvulsant, Miscellaneous; Electrolyte Supplement, Parenteral; Laxative, Saline; Magnesium Salt

Medication Safety Issues

Sound-alike/look-alike issues:

Magnesium sulfate may be confused with manganese sulfate, morphine sulfate

Avoid use of $MgSO_4$ abbreviation; errors have occurred with its use.

(Continued)

Magnesium Sulfate *(Continued)*

High alert medication: The Institute for Safe Medication Practices (ISMP) includes this medication (I.V. formulation) among its list of drugs which have a heightened risk of causing significant patient harm when used in error.

Use Treatment and prevention of hypomagnesemia; seizure prevention in severe pre-eclampsia or eclampsia, pediatric acute nephritis; short-term treatment torsade de pointes; treatment of cardiac arrhythmias (VT/VF) caused by hypomagnesemia; short-term treatment of constipation or soaking aid

Dosing

Adults & Elderly:

Daily allowance: The recommended dietary allowance (RDA) of magnesium is 4.5 mg/kg which is a total daily allowance of 350-400 mg for adult men and 280-300 mg for adult women. During pregnancy the RDA is 300 mg and during lactation the RDA is 355 mg. Average daily intakes of dietary magnesium have declined in recent years due to processing of food. The latest estimate of the average American dietary intake was 349 mg/day. Dose represented as magnesium sulfate unless stated otherwise.

Note: Serum magnesium is poor reflection of repletional status as the majority of magnesium is intracellular; serum levels may be transiently normal for a few hours after a dose is given, therefore, aim for consistently high normal serum levels in patients with normal renal function for most efficient repletion

Hypomagnesemia:
Oral: 3 g every 6 hours for 4 doses as needed
I.M., I.V.: 1 g every 6 hours for 4 doses; for severe hypomagnesemia: 8-12 g magnesium sulfate/day in divided doses has been used

Eclampsia, pre-eclampsia:
I.M.: 1-4 g every 4 hours
I.V.: Initial: 4 g, then switch to I.M. or 1-4 g/hour by continuous infusion
Note: Maximum dose not to exceed 30-40 g/day; maximum rate of infusion: 1-2 g/hour

Life-threatening arrhythmia: I.V.: 1-2 g (8-16 mEq) in 100 mL D$_5$W, administered over 5-60 minutes followed by an infusion of 0.5-1 g/hour, **or**
1-6 g administered over several minutes, followed by (in some cases) I.V. infusion of 3-20 mg/minute for 5-48 hours (depending on patient response and serum magnesium levels)

Maintenance electrolyte requirements:
Daily requirements: 0.2-0.5 mEq/kg/24 hours or 3-10 mEq/1000 kcal/24 hours
Maximum: 8-16 mEq/24 hours
Cathartic: Oral: 10-30 g/day in a single or divided doses
Soaking aid: Topical: Dissolve 2 capfuls of powder per gallon of warm water

Pediatrics:

Note: Serum magnesium is poor reflection of repletional status as the majority of magnesium is intracellular; serum levels may be transiently normal for a few hours after a dose is given, therefore, aim for consistently high normal serum levels in patients with normal renal function for most efficient repletion

Hypomagnesemia:
Children: I.M., I.V.: 25-50 mg/kg/dose (0.2-0.4 mEq/kg/dose) every 4-6 hours for 3-4 doses, maximum single dose: 2000 mg (16 mEq), may repeat if hypomagnesemia persists (higher dosage up to 100 mg/dose magnesium sulfate I.V. has been used)
Maintenance: I.V.: 30-60 mg/kg/day (0.25-0.5 mEq/kg/day)

Management of seizures and hypertension: I.M., I.V.: 20-100 mg/kg/dose every 4-6 hours as needed; in severe cases doses as high as 200 mg/kg/dose have been used

Cathartic: Oral: Children:
2-5 years: 2.5-5 g/kg/day in a single or divided doses
6-11 years: 5-10 g/day in a single or divided doses
≥12 years: Refer to adult dosing.

Renal Impairment: Patients in severe renal failure should not receive magnesium due to toxicity from accumulation. Patients with a Cl$_{cr}$ <25 mL/minute should be monitored by serum magnesium levels.

Available Dosage Forms

Infusion [premixed in D$_5$W]: 10 mg/mL (100 mL); 20 mg/mL (500 mL, 1000 mL)
Infusion [premixed in water for injection]: 40 mg/mL (100 mL, 500 mL, 1000 mL); 80 mg/mL (50 mL)
Injection, solution: 125 mg/mL (8 mL); 500 mg/mL (2 mL, 5 mL, 10 mL, 20 mL, 50 mL)
Powder: Magnesium sulfate USP (480 g, 1810 g, 1920 g)

Monitoring and Teaching Issues

Patient Education: Take in divided doses. Report diarrhea (>5 stools/day) or changes in mental function to prescriber.

Pregnancy Risk Factor: B

- **Magonate® [OTC]** *see* Magnesium Gluconate *on page 930*
- **Magonate® Sport [OTC] [DSC]** *see* Magnesium Gluconate *on page 930*
- **Mag-Ox® 400 [OTC]** *see* Magnesium Oxide *on page 931*
- **Mag-SR® [OTC]** *see* Magnesium Chloride *on page 929*
- **Magtrate® [OTC]** *see* Magnesium Gluconate *on page 930*
- **Malarone®** *see* Atovaquone and Proguanil *on page 155*
- **Mandelamine®** *see* Methenamine *on page 970*
- **Mandrake** *see* Podophyllum Resin *on page 1226*

Mannitol *(MAN i tole)*

U.S. Brand Names Osmitrol®; Resectisol®
Synonyms D-Mannitol
Generic Available Yes
Pharmacologic Category Diuretic, Osmotic

Medication Safety Issues

Sound-alike/look-alike issues:

Osmitrol® may be confused with esmolol

Use Reduction of increased intracranial pressure associated with cerebral edema; promotion of diuresis in the prevention and/or treatment of oliguria or anuria due to acute renal failure; reduction of increased intraocular pressure; promoting urinary excretion of toxic substances; genitourinary irrigant in transurethral prostatic resection or other transurethral surgical procedures

Mechanism of Action/Effect Increases the osmotic pressure of glomerular filtrate, which inhibits tubular reabsorption of water and electrolytes and increases urinary output

Contraindications Hypersensitivity to mannitol or any component or the formulation; severe renal disease (anuria); dehydration; active intracranial bleeding; severe pulmonary edema or congestion

Warnings/Precautions Should not be administered until adequacy of renal function and urine flow is established. Cardiovascular status should also be evaluated. Do not administer electrolyte-free mannitol solutions with blood.

Drug Interactions

Increased Effect/Toxicity: Lithium toxicity (with diuretic-induced hyponatremia).

Adverse Reactions Frequency not defined.

Cardiovascular: Circulatory overload, CHF

Central nervous system: Headache, convulsions, headache, chills, dizziness

Dermatologic: Rash

Endocrine & metabolic: Fluid and electrolyte imbalance, water intoxication, dehydration and hypovolemia secondary to rapid diuresis, hyponatremia

Gastrointestinal: Nausea, vomiting, xerostomia

Genitourinary: Polyuria, dysuria

Local: Tissue necrosis

Ocular: Blurred vision

Respiratory: Pulmonary edema

Miscellaneous: Allergic reactions

Overdosage/Toxicology Symptoms of overdose include polyuria, hypotension, cardiovascular collapse, pulmonary edema, hyponatremia, hypokalemia, oliguria, and seizures. Increased electrolyte excretion and fluid overload can occur. Hemodialysis will clear mannitol and reduce osmolality.

Pharmacodynamics/Kinetics

Onset of Action: Diuresis: Injection: 1-3 hours; Reduction in intracerebral pressure: ~15 minutes

Duration of Action: Reduction in intracerebral pressure: 3-6 hours

Half-Life Elimination: 1.1-1.6 hours

Metabolism: Minimally hepatic to glycogen

Excretion: Primarily urine (as unchanged drug)

Dosing

Adults & Elderly:

Test dose (to assess adequate renal function): I.V.: 12.5 g (200 mg/kg) over 3-5 minutes to produce a urine flow of at least 30-50 mL of urine per hour over the next 2-3 hours.

Edema (osmotic diuretic): Initial: 0.5-1 g/kg; Maintenance: 0.25-0.5 g/kg every 4-6 hours; usual adult dose: 20-200 g/24 hours

Intracranial pressure/Cerebral edema: I.V.: 1.5-2 g/kg/dose as a 15% to 20% solution over ≥30 minutes; maintain serum osmolality 310-320 mOsm/kg.

Preoperative for neurosurgery: I.V.: 1.5-2 g/kg administered 1-1.5 hours prior to surgery.

Transurethral: Irrigation: Use urogenital solution as required for irrigation.

Pediatrics:

Test dose (to assess adequate renal function): I.V.: Children: 200 mg/kg over 3-5 minutes to produce a urine flow of at least 1 mL/kg for 1-3 hours

Edema (osmotic diuretic): I.V.: Children: Initial: 0.5-1 g/kg; Maintenance: 0.25-0.5 g/kg given every 4-6 hours

Available Dosage Forms

Injection, solution: 5% [50 mg/mL] (1000 mL); 10% [100 mg/mL] (500 mL, 1000 mL); 15% [150 mg/mL] (500 mL); 20% [200 mg/mL] (150 mL, 250 mL, 500 mL); 25% [250 mg/mL] (50 mL)

Osmitrol®: 5% [50 mg/mL] (1000 mL); 10% [100 mg/mL] (500 mL, 1000 mL); 15% [150 mg/mL] (500 mL); 20% [200 mg/mL] (250 mL, 500 mL)

Solution, urogenital (Resectisol®): 5% [50 mg/mL] (2000 mL, 4000 mL)

Monitoring and Teaching Issues

Physical Assessment: See Warnings/Precautions for use cautions. Lithium toxicity is increased with concurrent use. See Administration for infusion specifics. Infusion site must be monitored for extravasation. Assess results of laboratory tests, therapeutic effectiveness (according to purpose for use), and adverse response (eg, circulatory overload, CHF, rash, water intoxication; see Adverse Reactions). Patient teaching should be appropriate to patient condition (see Patient Education).

Monitoring Laboratory Tests: Renal function, serum electrolytes, serum and urine osmolality. For treatment of elevated intracranial pressure, maintain serum osmolality 310-320 mOsm/kg

Patient Education: This medication can only be given by infusion. Report immediately any muscle weakness, numbness, tingling, acute headache, nausea, dizziness, blurred vision, eye pain, respiratory difficulty, chest pain, or pain at infusion site. **Pregnancy/breast-feeding precautions:** Inform prescriber if you are pregnant. Consult prescriber if breast-feeding.

(Continued)

Mannitol (Continued)

Pregnancy Risk Factor: C

Lactation: Excretion in breast milk unknown

Administration

I.V.: Vesicant. Do not administer with blood. Crenation and agglutination of red blood cells may occur if administered with whole blood.

Compatibility:

Y-site administration: Incompatible with cefepime, doxorubicin liposome, filgrastim

Compatibility when admixed: Incompatible with imipenem/cilastatin, meropenem

Storage: Should be stored at room temperature (15°C to 30°C) and protected from freezing. Crystallization may occur at low temperatures. Do not use solutions that contain crystals, heating in a hot water bath and vigorous shaking may be utilized for resolubilization. Cool solutions to body temperature before using.

Additional Information May autoclave or heat to redissolve crystals; mannitol 20% has an approximate osmolarity of 1100 mOsm/L and mannitol 25% has an approximate osmolarity of 1375 mOsm/L

Mebendazole (me BEN da zole)

U.S. Brand Names Vermox®

Generic Available Yes

Pharmacologic Category Anthelmintic

Use Treatment of pinworms (*Enterobius vermicularis*), whipworms (*Trichuris trichiura*), roundworms (*Ascaris lumbricoides*), and hookworms (*Ancylostoma duodenale*)

Mechanism of Action/Effect Selectively and irreversibly blocks glucose uptake and other nutrients in susceptible adult intestine-dwelling helminths

Contraindications Hypersensitivity to mebendazole or any component of the formulation

Warnings/Precautions Pregnancy and children <2 years of age are relative contraindications since safety has not been established. Not effective for hydatid disease.

Drug Interactions

Decreased Effect: Anticonvulsants such as carbamazepine and phenytoin may increase metabolism of mebendazole

Nutritional/Ethanol Interactions Food: Mebendazole serum levels may be increased if taken with food.

Lab Interactions Increased LFTs

Adverse Reactions Frequency not defined.

Cardiovascular: Angioedema

Central nervous system: Fever, dizziness, headache, seizure

Dermatologic: Rash, itching, alopecia (with high doses)

Gastrointestinal: Abdominal pain, diarrhea, nausea, vomiting

Hematologic: Neutropenia (sore throat, unusual fatigue)

Neuromuscular & skeletal: Unusual weakness

Overdosage/Toxicology Symptoms of overdose include abdominal pain and altered mental status. Treatment is supportive.

Pharmacodynamics/Kinetics
Absorption: 2% to 10%
Time to Peak: Serum: 2-4 hours
Protein Binding: 95%
Half-Life Elimination: 1-11.5 hours
Metabolism: Extensively hepatic
Excretion: Primarily feces; urine (5% to 10%)

Dosing
Adults & Elderly:
Pinworms: Oral: 100 mg as a single dose; may need to repeat after 2 weeks; treatment should include family members in close contact with patient.
Whipworms, roundworms, hookworms: Oral: 1 tablet twice daily, morning and evening on 3 consecutive days; if patient is not cured within 3-4 weeks, a second course of treatment may be administered.
Capillariasis: Oral: 200 mg twice daily for 20 days
Pediatrics: Refer to adult dosing.
Renal Impairment: Not dialyzable (0% to 5%)
Hepatic Impairment: Dosage reduction may be necessary in patients with liver dysfunction.

Available Dosage Forms Tablet, chewable: 100 mg

Monitoring and Teaching Issues
Physical Assessment: Since worm infestations are easily transmitted, all persons sharing same household should be treated. Teach proper use, transmission prevention, side effects/appropriate interventions, and adverse reactions to report (see Patient Education).
Monitoring Laboratory Tests: Check for helminth ova in feces within 3-4 weeks following the initial therapy. Periodically assess hematologic and hepatic function.
Patient Education: Take exactly as directed for full course of medication. Tablets may be chewed, swallowed whole, or crushed and mixed with food. Increase dietary intake of fruit juices. All family members and close friends should also be treated. To reduce possibility of reinfection, wash hands and scrub nails carefully with soap and hot water before handling food, before eating, and before and after toileting. Keep hands out of mouth. Disinfect toilet daily and launder bed linens, undergarments, and nightclothes daily with hot water and soap. Do not go barefoot and do not sit directly on grass or ground. May cause abdominal pain, nausea, or vomiting (small frequent meals, frequent mouth care, sucking lozenges, or chewing gum may help); or hair loss (reversible). Report skin rash or itching, unusual fatigue or sore throat, unresolved diarrhea or vomiting, or CNS changes. **Pregnancy/breast-feeding precautions:** Inform prescriber if you are or intend to become pregnant. Consult prescriber if breast-feeding.
Dietary Considerations: Tablet can be crushed and mixed with food, swallowed whole, or chewed.
Pregnancy Risk Factor: C
Lactation: Excretion in breast milk unknown/use caution
Breast-Feeding Issues: Since only 2% to 10% of mebendazole is absorbed, it is unlikely that it is excreted in breast milk in significant quantities.

Administration
Oral: Tablets may be chewed, swallowed whole, or crushed and mixed with food.

Mechlorethamine (me klor ETH a meen)

U.S. Brand Names Mustargen®
Synonyms Chlorethazine; Chlorethazine Mustard; HN_2; Mechlorethamine Hydrochloride; Mustine; Nitrogen Mustard; NSC-762
Generic Available No
Pharmacologic Category Antineoplastic Agent, Alkylating Agent (Nitrogen Mustard)
Use Combination therapy of Hodgkin's disease and malignant lymphomas; non-Hodgkin's lymphoma; may be used by intracavitary injection for treatment of metastatic tumors; pleural and other malignant effusions; topical treatment of mycosis fungoides
Mechanism of Action/Effect Bifunctional alkylating agent that inhibits DNA and RNA synthesis via formation of carbonium ions; produces interstrand and intrastrand cross-links in DNA resulting in miscoding, breakage, and failure of replication. Although not cell phase-specific *per se*, mechlorethamine effect is most pronounced in the S phase, and cell proliferation is arrested in the G_2 phase.
Contraindications Hypersensitivity to mechlorethamine or any component of the formulation; pre-existing profound myelosuppression or infection; pregnancy
Warnings/Precautions The U.S. Food and Drug Administration (FDA) currently recommends that procedures for proper handling and disposal of antineoplastic agents be considered. Appropriate safety equipment is recommended for preparation, administration, and disposal of antineoplastics. If mechlorethamine contacts the skin, wash and flush thoroughly with water. Mechlorethamine is a potent vesicant; if extravasation occurs, severe tissue damage (leading to ulceration and necrosis) and pain may occur. Patients with lymphomas should receive prophylactic allopurinol 2-3 days prior to therapy to prevent complications resulting from tumor lysis.

Drug Interactions
Decreased Effect: Patients may experience impaired immune response to vaccines; possible infection after administration of live vaccines in patients receiving immunosuppressants.
Nutritional/Ethanol Interactions Ethanol: Avoid ethanol (due to GI irritation).

Adverse Reactions
>10%:
Dermatologic: Alopecia; hyperpigmentation of veins; contact and allergic dermatitis (50% with topical use)
Endocrine & metabolic: Chromosomal abnormalities, delayed menses, oligomenorrhea, amenorrhea, impaired spermatogenesis
(Continued)

935

Mechlorethamine *(Continued)*

Gastrointestinal: Nausea and vomiting (almost 100%), onset may be within minutes of drug administration

Genitourinary: Azoospermia

Hematologic: Myelosuppression, leukopenia, and thrombocytopenia

Onset: 4-7 days

Nadir: 14 days

Recovery: 21 days

1% to 10%:

Central nervous system: Fever

Gastrointestinal: Diarrhea, anorexia, metallic taste

Otic: Tinnitus

Overdosage/Toxicology Suppression of all formed elements of blood, uric acid crystals, nausea, vomiting, and diarrhea. Sodium thiosulfate is the specific antidote for nitrogen mustard extravasations. Treatment of systemic overdose is supportive.

Pharmacodynamics/Kinetics

Duration of Action: Unchanged drug is undetectable in blood within a few minutes

Absorption: Intracavitary administration: Incomplete secondary to rapid deactivation by body fluids

Half-Life Elimination: <1 minute

Metabolism: Rapid hydrolysis and demethylation, possibly in plasma

Excretion: Urine (50% as metabolites, <0.01% as unchanged drug)

Dosing

Adults & Elderly: Refer to individual protocols. Dosage should be based on ideal dry weight. The presence of edema or ascites must be considered so that dosage will be based on actual weight unaugmented by these conditions.

MOPP: I.V.: 6 mg/m^2 on days 1 and 8 of a 28-day cycle

Typical dose: I.V.: 0.4 mg/kg **or** 12-16 mg/m^2 for one dose **or** divided into 0.1 mg/kg/day for 4 days, repeated at 4- to 6-week intervals

Intracavitary: 10-20 mg diluted in 10 mL of SWI or 0.9% sodium chloride

Intrapericardially: 0.2-0.4 mg/kg diluted in up to 100 mL of 0.9% sodium chloride

Mycosis fungoides: Topical mechlorethamine has been used in the treatment of cutaneous lesions of mycosis fungoides. A skin test should be performed prior to treatment with the topical preparation to detect sensitivity and possible irritation (use fresh mechlorethamine 0.1 mg/mL and apply over a 3 x 5 cm area of normal skin).

Pediatrics: Refer to individual protocols. Dosage should be based on ideal dry weight; the presence of edema or ascites must be considered so that dosage will be based on actual weight unaugmented by these conditions.

MOPP: Children: I.V.: 6 mg/m^2 on days 1 and 8 of a 28-day cycle

Renal Impairment:

Hemodialysis: Not removed; supplemental dosing is not necessary.

Peritoneal dialysis: Not removed; supplemental dosing is not necessary.

Available Dosage Forms Injection, powder for reconstitution, as hydrochloride: 10 mg

Monitoring and Teaching Issues

Physical Assessment: See Warnings/Precautions for use cautions. See Administration for infusion specifics. Premedication with antiemetic recommended (highly emetogenic; may begin within minutes). Infusion site must be closely monitored; extravasation can cause severe sloughing or tissue necrosis. Assess results of laboratory tests prior to each treatment and on a regular basis throughout therapy. Monitor closely during infusion and between treatments (eg, adverse reactions can be severe and involve systems; see Adverse Reactions). Teach patient possible side effects/appropriate interventions (eg, importance of adequate hydration) and adverse symptoms to report (see Patient Education).

Monitoring Laboratory Tests: CBC with differential and platelet count

Patient Education: This medication can only be given by infusion. Report immediately any swelling, redness, pain, or burning at infusion site. Do not use alcohol during treatment; may increase gastric irritation. Maintain adequate fluid balance (2-3 L/day) unless instructed to restrict fluid intake and adequate nutrition (small frequent meals, frequent mouth care, sucking lozenges, or chewing gum may reduce anorexia and nausea). May cause discoloration (brown color) of veins used for infusion; hair loss (reversible); easy bleeding or bruising (use soft toothbrush or cotton swabs and frequent mouth care, use electric razor, avoid sharp knives or scissors); or increased susceptibility to infection (avoid crowds and exposure to infection and do not have any vaccinations unless approved by prescriber). This drug may cause menstrual irregularities, permanent sterility, and birth defects. Report changes in auditory or visual acuity; unusual bleeding or bruising or persistent fever or sore throat; blood in urine, stool, or vomitus; delayed healing of any wounds; skin rash; yellowing of skin or eyes; changes in color of urine or stool; acute or unresolved nausea or vomiting; diarrhea; or loss of appetite. **Pregnancy/breast-feeding precautions:** Inform prescriber if you are pregnant. Do not get pregnant while taking this medication and for 1 month following therapy; consult prescriber for appropriate barrier contraceptives. Breast-feeding is not recommended.

Pregnancy Risk Factor: D

Lactation: Excretion in breast milk unknown/not recommended

Administration

I.V.: Vesicant. Margin of error is very slight. Check dosage carefully before administration. Administer with caution. Administer I.V. push through a free-flowing I.V. over 1-3 minutes at a concentration not to exceed 1 mg/mL.

Reconstitution: Must be prepared immediately before use; solution is stable for only 15-60 minutes after dilution. Dilute powder with 10 mL SWI to a final concentration of 1 mg/mL. May be diluted in up to 100 mL NS for intracavitary administration.

Compatibility: Stable in sterile water for injection; **incompatible** with D$_5$W

Y-site administration: Incompatible with allopurinol, cefepime

Compatibility when admixed: Incompatible with methohexital
Storage: Store intact vials at room temperature.

♦ **Mechlorethamine Hydrochloride** *see Mechlorethamine on page 935*

Meclizine (MEK li zeen)

U.S. Brand Names Antivert®; Bonine® [OTC]; Dramamine® Less Drowsy Formula [OTC]
Synonyms Meclizine Hydrochloride; Meclozine Hydrochloride
Generic Available Yes
Pharmacologic Category Antiemetic; Antihistamine
Medication Safety Issues
Sound-alike/look-alike issues:
Antivert® may be confused with Axert™
Use Prevention and treatment of symptoms of motion sickness; management of vertigo with diseases affecting the vestibular system
Mechanism of Action/Effect Has central anticholinergic action by blocking chemoreceptor trigger zone; decreases excitability of the middle ear labyrinth and blocks conduction in the middle ear vestibular-cerebellar pathways
Contraindications Hypersensitivity to meclizine or any component of the formulation
Warnings/Precautions Use with caution in patients with angle-closure glaucoma, prostatic hyperplasia, pyloric or duodenal obstruction, or bladder neck obstruction. Use with caution in hot weather, and during exercise. Elderly may be at risk for anticholinergic side effects such as glaucoma, prostatic hyperplasia, constipation, GI obstructive disease. If vertigo does not respond in 1-2 weeks, it is advised to discontinue use.
Drug Interactions
Increased Effect/Toxicity: Increased toxicity with CNS depressants, neuroleptics, and anticholinergics.
Nutritional/Ethanol Interactions Ethanol: Avoid ethanol (may increase CNS depression).
Adverse Reactions
>10%:
Central nervous system: Slight to moderate drowsiness
Respiratory: Thickening of bronchial secretions
1% to 10%:
Central nervous system: Headache, fatigue, nervousness, dizziness
Gastrointestinal: Appetite increase, weight gain, nausea, diarrhea, abdominal pain, xerostomia
Neuromuscular & skeletal: Arthralgia
Respiratory: Pharyngitis
Overdosage/Toxicology Symptoms of overdose include CNS depression, confusion, nervousness, hallucinations, dizziness, blurred vision, nausea, vomiting, and hyperthermia. There is no specific treatment for antihistamine overdose. Clinical toxicity is due to blockade of cholinergic receptors. For anticholinergic overdose with severe life-threatening symptoms, physostigmine 1-2 mg I.V. slowly, may be given to reverse these effects.
Pharmacodynamics/Kinetics
Onset of Action: ~1 hour
Duration of Action: 8-24 hours
Half-Life Elimination: 6 hours
Metabolism: Hepatic
Excretion: Urine (as metabolites); feces (as unchanged drug)
Dosing
Adults & Elderly:
Motion sickness: Oral: 12.5-25 mg 1 hour before travel, repeat dose every 12-24 hours if needed; doses up to 50 mg may be needed
Vertigo: Oral: 25-100 mg/day in divided doses
Pediatrics: Children >12 years: Refer to adult dosing.
Available Dosage Forms
Tablet, as hydrochloride: 12.5 mg, 25 mg
Antivert®: 12.5 mg, 25 mg, 50 mg
Dramamine® Less Drowsy Formula: 25 mg
Tablet, chewable, as hydrochloride (Bonine®): 25 mg
Monitoring and Teaching Issues
Physical Assessment: Determine cause of vomiting before beginning therapy. Assess effectiveness and interactions of other medications patient may be taking. Monitor effectiveness of therapy and adverse response. Assess knowledge/teach patient possible side effects/appropriate interventions and adverse symptoms to report.
Patient Education: Take exactly as prescribed; do not increase dose. Avoid alcohol, other CNS depressants, sleeping aids without consulting prescriber. You may experience dizziness, drowsiness, or blurred vision (use caution when driving or engaging in tasks that require alertness until response to drug is known); dry mouth (frequent mouth care, sucking lozenges, or chewing gum may help); constipation (increased exercise, fluids, fruit, or may help); or heat intolerance (avoid excessive exercise, hot environments, maintain adequate hydration). Report CNS change (hallucination, confusion, nervousness); sudden or unusual weight gain; unresolved nausea or diarrhea; chest pain or palpitations; muscle pain; or changes in urinary pattern. **Breast-feeding precaution:** Breast-feeding is not recommended.
Geriatric Considerations: Due to anticholinergic action, use lowest dose in divided doses to avoid side effects and their inconvenience. Limit use if possible. May cause confusion or aggravate symptoms of confusion in those with dementia.
Pregnancy Risk Factor: B
Lactation: Excretion in breast milk unknown/not recommended

♦ **Meclizine Hydrochloride** *see Meclizine on page 937*
♦ **Meclozine Hydrochloride** *see Meclizine on page 937*
♦ **Medicinal Carbon** *see Charcoal on page 302*

+ **Medicinal Charcoal** *see Charcoal on page 302*
+ **Medicone®** **[OTC]** *see Phenylephrine on page 1200*
+ **Medigesic®** *see Butalbital, Acetaminophen, and Caffeine on page 225*
+ **Medrol®** *see MethylPREDNISolone on page 986*

MedroxyPROGESTERone (me DROKS ee proe JES te rone)

U.S. Brand Names Depo-Provera®; Depo-Provera® Contraceptive; depo-subQ provera 104™; Provera®

Synonyms Acetoxymethylprogesterone; Medroxyprogesterone Acetate; Methylacetoxyprogesterone; MPA

Generic Available Yes

Pharmacologic Category Contraceptive; Progestin

Medication Safety Issues

Sound-alike/look-alike issues:

MedroxyPROGESTERone may be confused with hydroxyprogesterone, methylPREDNISolone, methylTESTOSTERone

Provera® may be confused with Covera®, Parlodel®, Premarin®

Use Endometrial carcinoma or renal carcinoma; secondary amenorrhea or abnormal uterine bleeding due to hormonal imbalance; reduction of endometrial hyperplasia in nonhysterectomized postmenopausal women receiving conjugated estrogens; prevention of pregnancy; management of endometriosis-associated pain

Mechanism of Action/Effect Inhibits secretion of pituitary gonadotropins, which prevents follicular maturation and ovulation; causes endometrial thinning

Contraindications Hypersensitivity to medroxyprogesterone or any component of the formulation; history of or current thrombophlebitis or venous thromboembolic disorders (including DVT, PE); cerebral vascular disease; severe hepatic dysfunction or disease; carcinoma of the breast or genital organs, undiagnosed vaginal bleeding; missed abortion, diagnostic test for pregnancy; pregnancy

Warnings/Precautions Prolonged use of medroxyprogesterone contraceptive injection may result in a loss of bone mineral density (BMD). Loss is related to the duration of use, and may not be completely reversible on discontinuation of the drug. The impact on peak bone mass in adolescents should be considered in treatment decisions. Long-term use (ie, >2 years) should be limited to situations where other birth control methods are inadequate.

Use caution with cardiovascular disease or dysfunction. MPA used in combination with estrogen may increase the risks of hypertension, myocardial infarction (MI), stroke, pulmonary emboli (PE), and deep vein thrombosis; incidence of these effects was shown to be significantly increased in postmenopausal women using conjugated equine estrogens (CEE) in combination with MPA. MPA in combination with estrogens should not be used to prevent coronary heart disease.

The risk of dementia may be increased in postmenopausal women; increased incidence was observed in women ≥65 years of age taking MPA in combination with CEE. An increased risk of invasive breast cancer was observed in postmenopausal women using MPA in combination with CEE. An increase in abnormal mammograms has also been reported with estrogen and progestin therapy.

Discontinue pending examination in cases of sudden partial or complete vision loss, sudden onset of proptosis, diplopia, or migraine; discontinue permanently if papilledema or retinal vascular lesions are observed on examination. Use with caution in patients with diseases that may be exacerbated by fluid retention (including asthma, epilepsy, migraine, diabetes, or renal dysfunction). Use caution with history of depression. Whenever possible, progestins in combination with estrogens should be discontinued at least 4-6 weeks prior to surgeries associated with an increased risk of thromboembolism or during periods of prolonged immobilization. Progestins used in combination with estrogen should be used for shortest duration possible consistent with treatment goals. Conduct periodic risk:benefit assessments.

Drug Interactions

Cytochrome P450 Effect: Substrate of CYP3A4 (major); **Induces** CYP3A4 (weak)

Decreased Effect: CYP3A4 inducers may decrease the levels/effects of medroxyprogesterone; example inducers include aminoglutethimide, carbamazepine, nafcillin, nevirapine, phenobarbital, phenytoin, and rifamycins.

Nutritional/Ethanol Interactions

Food: Bioavailability of the oral tablet is increased when taken with food; half-life is unchanged

Lab Interactions

The following tests may be decreased: Steroid levels (plasma and urinary), gonadotropin levels, SHBG concentration, T_3 uptake

The following tests may be increased: Protein-bound iodine, butanol extractable protein-bound iodine, Factors II, VII, VIII, IX, X

Pathologist should be advised of estrogen/progesterone therapy when specimens are submitted.

Adverse Reactions Adverse effects as reported with any dosage form; percent ranges presented are noted with the MPA contraceptive injection:

>5%:

Central nervous system: Dizziness, headache, nervousness

Endocrine & metabolic: Libido decreased, menstrual irregularities (includes bleeding, amenorrhea, or both)

Gastrointestinal: Abdominal pain/discomfort, weight changes (average 3-5 pounds after 1 year, 8 pounds after 2 years)

Neuromuscular & skeletal: Weakness

1% to 5%:

Cardiovascular: Edema

Central nervous system: Depression, fatigue, insomnia, irritability, pain

Dermatologic: Acne, alopecia, rash

Endocrine & metabolic: Anorgasmia, breast pain, hot flashes

Gastrointestinal: Bloating, nausea
Genitourinary: Cervical smear abnormal, leukorrhea, menometrorrhagia, menorrhagia, pelvic pain, urinary tract infection, vaginitis, vaginal infection, vaginal hemorrhage
Local: Injection site atrophy, injection site reaction, injection site pain
Neuromuscular & skeletal: Arthralgia, backache, leg cramp
Respiratory: Respiratory tract infections

Overdosage/Toxicology Toxicity is unlikely following single exposure of excessive doses. Supportive treatment is adequate in most cases.

Pharmacodynamics/Kinetics
Absorption: Oral: Well absorbed; I.M.: Slow
Time to Peak: Oral: 2-4 hours
Protein Binding: 86% to 90% primarily to albumin; does not bind to sex hormone-binding globulin
Half-Life Elimination: Oral: 12-17 hours; I.M. (Depo-Provera® Contraceptive): 50 days; SubQ: ~40 days
Metabolism: Extensively hepatic via hydroxylation and conjugation; forms metabolites
Excretion: Urine

Dosing
Adults & Elderly:
Amenorrhea: Oral: 5-10 mg/day for 5-10 days
Abnormal uterine bleeding: Oral: 5-10 mg for 5-10 days starting on day 16 or 21 of cycle
Contraception:
Depo-Provera® Contraceptive: I.M.: 150 mg every 3 months
depo-subQ provera 104™: SubQ: 104 mg every 3 months (every 12-14 weeks)
Endometriosis: depo-subQ provera 104™: SubQ: 104 mg every 3 months (every 12-14 weeks)
Endometrial or renal carcinoma (Depo-Provera®): I.M.: 400-1000 mg/week
Accompanying cyclic estrogen therapy, postmenopausal: Oral: 5-10 mg for 12-14 consecutive days each month, starting on day 1 or day 16 of the cycle; lower doses may be used if given with estrogen continuously throughout the cycle
Pediatrics: Adolescents:
Abnormal uterine bleeding: Refer to adult dosing.
Amenorrhea: Refer to adult dosing.
Contraception: Refer to adult dosing.
Endometriosis: Refer to adult dosing.
Hepatic Impairment: Use is contraindicated with severe impairment. Consider lower dose or less frequent administration with mild-to-moderate impairment. Use of the contraceptive injection has not been studied in patients with hepatic impairment; consideration should be given to not readminister if jaundice develops

Available Dosage Forms
Injection, suspension, as acetate: 150 mg/mL (1 mL)
Depo-Provera®: 400 mg/mL (2.5 mL)
Depo-Provera® Contraceptive: 150 mg/mL (1 mL) [prefilled syringe or vial]
depo-subQ provera 104™: 104 mg/0.65 mL (0.65 mL) [prefilled syringe]
Tablet, as acetate (Provera®): 2.5 mg, 5 mg, 10 mg

Monitoring and Teaching Issues
Physical Assessment: Monitor for effectiveness of therapy and adverse effects. Instruct patient on appropriate dose scheduling (according to purpose of therapy), possible side effects, and symptoms to report. **Pregnancy risk factor X:** Determine that patient is not pregnant before starting therapy. Do not give to sexually-active female patients unless capable of complying with contraceptive use.

Monitoring Laboratory Tests: Must have pregnancy test prior to beginning therapy.

Patient Education: Follow dosage schedule and do not take more than prescribed. You may experience sensitivity to sunlight (use sunblock, wear protective clothing and eyewear, and avoid extensive exposure to direct sunlight); dizziness, anxiety, depression (use caution when driving or engaging in tasks that require alertness until response to drug is known); changes in appetite (maintain adequate hydration 2-3 L/day of fluids unless instructed to restrict fluid intake and diet); decreased libido or increased body hair (reversible when drug is discontinued); hot flashes (cool clothes and environment may help). May cause discoloration of stool (green). Report swelling of face, lips, or mouth; absence or altered menses; abdominal pain; vaginal itching, irritation, or discharge; heat, warmth, redness, or swelling of extremities; or sudden onset change in vision. **Pregnancy precaution:** Inform prescriber if you are pregnant. Consult prescriber for instruction on appropriate contraceptive measures.

Injection for contraception: This product does not protect against HIV or other sexually-transmitted diseases.
Dietary Considerations: Ensure adequate calcium and vitamin D intake when used for the prevention of pregnancy
Geriatric Considerations: No specific recommendations for dosage adjustments. Monitor closely for adverse effects when starting therapy.
Pregnancy Risk Factor: X
Pregnancy Issues: There is an increased risk of minor birth defects in children whose mothers take progesterones during the first 4 months of pregnancy. Hypospadias has been reported in male and mild masculinization of the external genitalia has been reported in female babies exposed during the first trimester. High doses are used to impair fertility. Low birth weight has been reported in neonates from unexpected pregnancies which occurred 1-2 months following injection of medroxyprogesterone (MPA) contraceptive. Ectopic pregnancies have been reported with use of the MPA contraceptive injection. When therapy is discontinued, fertility returns sooner in women of lower body weight. Median time to conception/return to ovulation following discontinuation of MPA contraceptive injection is 10 months following the last injection.
(Continued)

MedroxyPROGESTERone (Continued)

Lactation: Enters breast milk/compatible

Breast-Feeding Issues: Composition, quality and quantity of breast milk are not affected; adverse developmental and behavioral effects have not been noted following exposure of infant to MPA while breast-feeding.

Administration

I.M.: Depo-Provera® Contraceptive: Administer first dose during the first 5 days of menstrual period, or within the first 5 days postpartum if not breast-feeding, or at the sixth week postpartum if breast feeding exclusively. Shake vigorously prior to administration. Administer by deep I.M. injection in the gluteal or deltoid muscle.

Other: SubQ: depo-subQ provera 104™: Administer first dose during the first 5 days of menstrual period, or at the sixth week postpartum if breast-feeding. Shake vigorously prior to administration. Administer by SubQ injection in the upper thigh or abdomen; avoid boney areas and the umbilicus. Administer over 5-7 seconds. Do not rub the injection area. When switching from combined hormonal contraceptives (estrogen plus progestin), the first injection should be within 7 days after the last active pill, or removal of patch or ring. If switching from the I.M. to SubQ formulation, the next dose should be given within the prescribed dosing period for the I.M. injection.

Related Information

FDA Name Differentiation Project: The Use of Tall-Man Letters *on page 15*

♦ **Medroxyprogesterone Acetate** *see* MedroxyPROGESTERone *on page 938*

♦ **Medroxyprogesterone and Estrogens (Conjugated)** *see* Estrogens (Conjugated/Equine) and Medroxyprogesterone *on page 566*

Medrysone (ME dri sone)

U.S. Brand Names HMS Liquifilm®

Generic Available No

Pharmacologic Category Corticosteroid, Ophthalmic

Use Treatment of allergic conjunctivitis, vernal conjunctivitis, episcleritis, ophthalmic epinephrine sensitivity reaction

Mechanism of Action/Effect Decreases inflammation by suppression of migration of polymorphonuclear leukocytes and reversal of increased capillary permeability

Contraindications Hypersensitivity to medrysone or any component of the formulation; fungal, viral, or untreated pus-forming bacterial ocular infections; not for use in iritis and uveitis

Warnings/Precautions Prolonged use has been associated with the development of corneal or scleral perforation and posterior subcapsular cataracts. May mask or enhance the establishment of acute purulent untreated infections of the eye. Use caution in patients with glaucoma. Medrysone is a synthetic corticosteroid; structurally related to progesterone; if no improvement after several days of treatment, discontinue medrysone and institute other therapy. Duration of therapy: 3-4 days to several weeks dependent on type and severity of disease. Taper dose to avoid disease exacerbation. Safety and efficacy have not been established in children <3 years of age.

Adverse Reactions Frequency not defined: Ocular: Acute anterior uveitis, allergic reactions, blurred vision (mild, temporary), burning, cataracts, conjunctivitis, corneal thinning, corneal ulcers, delayed wound healing, foreign body sensation, glaucoma, IOP increased, keratitis, mydriasis, optic nerve damage, ptosis, secondary ocular infection stinging, visual activity defects

Overdosage/Toxicology Systemic toxicity is unlikely from the ophthalmic preparation.

Pharmacodynamics/Kinetics

Absorption: Through aqueous humor

Metabolism: Hepatic if absorbed

Excretion: Urine and feces

Dosing

Adults & Elderly: Conjunctivitis: Ophthalmic: Instill 1 drop in conjunctival sac 2-4 times/day up to every 4 hours; may use every 1-2 hours during first 1-2 days.

Pediatrics: Children ≥3 years: Refer to adult dosing.

Available Dosage Forms Solution, ophthalmic: 1% (5 mL, 10 mL) [contains benzalkonium chloride]

Monitoring and Teaching Issues

Physical Assessment: Assess knowledge/teach patient appropriate use, possible side effects/appropriate interventions, and adverse symptoms to report.

Patient Education: This medication is only for use in your eyes. Use exactly as directed (see below). May cause sensitivity to light (dark glasses may help); or temporary stinging, burning, or blurred vision. Report pain, swelling, scratchiness, itching, watering, or dryness of eye; drainage, redness, or sign of eye infection; change in vision (eg, double vision, reduced visual field, halo around lights); or worsening of condition or lack of improvement in 3-4 days. **Pregnancy/breast-feeding precautions:** Inform prescriber if you are pregnant. Consult prescriber if breast-feeding.

Wash hands thoroughly before using. Shake well before using. Do not allow applicator tip to touch eye. Gently pull down lower lid and put drop(s) into inner corner of eye. Close eye and roll eyeball in all directions. Do not blink for 30 seconds. Apply gentle pressure to inner corner of eye for 30 seconds. Gently wipe away any excess from skin around eye. Do not use any other eye medication for 10-15 minutes.

Pregnancy Risk Factor: C
Lactation: Excretion in breast milk unknown/use caution
Administration
Other: Ophthalmic: Shake well before using. Do not touch dropper to the eye.
Storage: Store at room temperature of 25°C (77°F). Protect from freezing.

Mefloquine (ME floe kwin)

U.S. Brand Names Lariam®

Synonyms Mefloquine Hydrochloride

Restrictions A medication guide and wallet card must be provided to patients when mefloquine is dispensed for malaria. An FDA-approved medication guide is available at www.fda.gov/cder/Offices/ODS/labeling.htm.

Generic Available Yes

Pharmacologic Category Antimalarial Agent

Use Treatment of acute malarial infections and prevention of malaria

Mechanism of Action/Effect Mefloquine is a quinoline-methanol compound structurally similar to quinine; mefloquine's effectiveness in the treatment and prophylaxis of malaria is due to the destruction of the asexual blood forms of the malarial pathogens that affect humans, Plasmodium falciparum, P. vivax, P. malariae, P. ovale

Contraindications Hypersensitivity mefloquine, related compounds (such as quinine and quinidine), or any component of the formulation; history of convulsions; cardiac conduction abnormalities; severe psychiatric disorder (including active or recent history of depression, generalized anxiety disorder, psychosis, or schizophrenia); use with halofantrine

Warnings/Precautions Use with caution in patients with a previous history of depression (see Contraindications regarding severe psychiatric illness, including active/recent depression). May cause a range of psychiatric symptoms (anxiety, paranoia, depression, hallucinations and psychosis). Occasionally, symptoms have been reported to persist long after mefloquine has been discontinued. Rare cases of suicidal ideation and suicide have been reported (no causal relationship established). The appearance of psychiatric symptoms such as acute anxiety, depression, restlessness or confusion may be considered a prodrome to more serious events. When used as prophylaxis, substitute an alternative medication. Discontinue if unexplained neuropsychiatric disturbances occur. Use caution in patients with significant cardiac disease. If mefloquine is to be used for a prolonged period, periodic evaluations including liver function tests and ophthalmic examinations should be performed. (Retinal abnormalities have not been observed with mefloquine in humans; however, it has with long-term administration to rats.) In cases of life-threatening, serious, or overwhelming malaria infections due to Plasmodium falciparum, patients should be treated with intravenous antimalarial drug. Mefloquine may be given orally to complete the course. Dizziness, loss of balance, and other CNS disorders have been reported; due to long half-life, effects may persist after mefloquine is discontinued. Use caution in activities requiring alertness and fine motor coordination (driving, piloting planes, operating machinery, deep sea diving, etc).

Drug Interactions
Cytochrome P450 Effect: Substrate of CYP3A4 (major); Inhibits CYP2D6 (weak), 3A4 (weak)

Decreased Effect: Mefloquine may decrease the effect of valproic acid, carbamazepine, phenobarbital, and phenytoin. CYP3A4 inducers may decrease the levels/effects of mefloquine; example inducers include aminoglutethimide, carbamazepine, nafcillin, nevirapine, phenobarbital, phenytoin, and rifamycins.

Increased Effect/Toxicity: Use caution with drugs that alter cardiac conduction; increased toxicity with chloroquine, quinine, and quinidine (hold treatment until at least 12 hours after these later drugs); increased toxicity with halofantrine (concurrent use is contraindicated). CYP3A4 inhibitors may increase the levels/effects of mefloquine; example inhibitors include azole antifungals, ciprofloxacin, clarithromycin, diclofenac, doxycycline, erythromycin, imatinib, isoniazid, nefazodone, nicardipine, propofol, protease inhibitors, quinidine, and verapamil.

Nutritional/Ethanol Interactions Food: Food increases bioavailability by ~40%.

Adverse Reactions
Frequency not defined: Neuropsychiatric events
1% to 10%:
Central nervous system: Headache, fever, chills, fatigue
Dermatologic: Rash
Gastrointestinal: Vomiting (3%), diarrhea, stomach pain, nausea, appetite decreased
Neuromuscular & skeletal: Myalgia
Otic: Tinnitus

Overdosage/Toxicology Treatment is supportive. Monitor cardiac function and psychiatric status for at least 24 hours.

Pharmacodynamics/Kinetics
Absorption: Well absorbed
Bioavailability: Increased by food
Time to Peak: Plasma: 6-24 hours (median: ~17 hours)
Protein Binding: 98%
Half-Life Elimination: 21-22 days
Metabolism: Extensively hepatic; main metabolite is inactive
Excretion: Primarily bile and feces; urine (9% as unchanged drug, 4% as primary metabolite)

Dosing
Adults & Elderly: Dose expressed as mg of mefloquine hydrochloride:
Malaria treatment (mild to moderate infection): Oral: 5 tablets (1250 mg) as a single dose. Take with food and at least 8 oz of water. If clinical improvement is not seen within 48-72 hours, an alternative therapy should be used for retreatment.
Malaria prophylaxis: Oral: 1 tablet (250 mg) weekly starting 1 week before, arrival in endemic area, continuing weekly during travel and for 4 weeks after leaving endemic area. Take with food and at least 8 oz of water.
(Continued)

Mefloquine (Continued)

Pediatrics: Dose expressed as mg of mefloquine hydrochloride: Children ≥6 months and >5 kg:

Malaria treatment: Oral: 20-25 mg/kg in 2 divided doses, taken 6-8 hours apart (maximum: 1250 mg) Take with food and an ample amount of water. If clinical improvement is not seen within 48-72 hours, an alternative therapy should be used for retreatment.

Malaria prophylaxis: Oral: 5 mg/kg/once weekly (maximum dose: 250 mg) starting 1 week before, arrival in endemic area, continuing weekly during travel and for 4 weeks after leaving endemic area. Take with food and an ample amount of water.

Renal Impairment: No dosage adjustment needed in patients with renal impairment or on dialysis.

Hepatic Impairment: Half-life may be prolonged and plasma levels may be higher.

Available Dosage Forms Tablet, as hydrochloride: 250 mg [equivalent to 228 mg base]

Monitoring and Teaching Issues

Physical Assessment: Use caution in patients with thrombophlebitis (see Warnings/Precautions for specific use cautions). Assess therapeutic effects and adverse reactions on a regular basis throughout therapy (eg, hypertension, cardiomyopathy, hyperglycemia, hepatotoxicity; see Adverse Reactions). Teach patient proper use, possible side effects/appropriate interventions (eg, importance of adequate hydration), and adverse symptoms to report (see Patient Education).

Monitoring Laboratory Tests: When use is prolonged, periodically monitor liver function tests.

Patient Education: Do not take any new medication during therapy unless approved by prescriber. Follow dosage schedule and do not take more than prescribed. May cause sensitivity to sunlight (use sunblock, wear protective clothing, and avoid extended exposure to direct sunlight); dizziness, anxiety, depression (use caution when driving or engaging in tasks that require alertness until response to drug is known); or change in appetite. Maintain adequate nutrition and maintain adequate hydration (2-3 L/day of fluids) unless instructed to restrict fluid intake; decreased libido or increased body hair (reversible when drug is discontinued); or hot flashes (cool clothes and environment may help). Report swelling of face, lips, or mouth; absent or altered menses; abdominal pain; vaginal itching, irritation, or discharge; heat, warmth, redness, or swelling of extremities; or sudden onset change in vision. **Pregnancy/breast-feeding precautions:** Do not get pregnant while taking this medication and for 1 month following therapy; consult prescriber for appropriate contraceptives. This drug may cause fetal defects. Do not donate blood during or for 1 month following therapy. Do not breast-feed.

Dietary Considerations: Take with food and with at least 8 oz of water.

Pregnancy Risk Factor: C

Lactation: Enters breast milk/not recommended

Breast-Feeding Issues: Excreted in small quantities; effect to nursing infant is unknown. Breast-feeding is not recommended during therapy and the long half-life of mefloquine should also be considered once therapy is complete.

Administration

Oral: Administer with food and with at least 8 oz of water. When used for malaria prophylaxis, dose should be taken once weekly on the same day each week. If vomiting occurs within 30-60 minutes after dose, an additional half-dose may be given. Tablets may be crushed and suspended in a small amount of water, milk, or another beverage for persons unable to swallow tablets.

Storage: Store at 25°C (77°F); excursions permitted to 15°C to 30°C (59°F to 86°F)

◆ **Mefloquine Hydrochloride** *see* Mefloquine *on page 941*

◆ **Mefoxin®** *see* Cefoxitin *on page 279*

◆ **Megace®** *see* Megestrol *on page 942*

◆ **Megadophilus® [OTC]** *see* Lactobacillus *on page 859*

Megestrol (me JES trole)

U.S. Brand Names Megace®

Synonyms 5071-1DL(6); Megestrol Acetate; NSC-10363

Generic Available Yes

Pharmacologic Category Antineoplastic Agent, Hormone; Appetite Stimulant; Progestin

Medication Safety Issues

Sound-alike/look-alike issues:

Megace® may be confused with Reglan®

Use Palliative treatment of breast and endometrial carcinoma

Orphan drug: Treatment of anorexia, cachexia, or significant weight loss (≥10% baseline body weight) and confirmed diagnosis of AIDS

Unlabeled/Investigational Use Uterine bleeding

Mechanism of Action/Effect A synthetic progestin with antiestrogenic properties which disrupt the estrogen receptor cycle. May also have a direct effect on the endometrium. Megestrol is an antineoplastic progestin thought to act through an antileutenizing effect mediated via the pituitary.

Contraindications Hypersensitivity to megestrol or any component of the formulation; pregnancy

Warnings/Precautions Use with caution in patients with a history of thrombophlebitis. Elderly females may have vaginal bleeding or discharge. May suppress hypothalamic-pituitary-adrenal (HPA) axis during chronic administration. Consider the possibility of adrenal suppression in any patient receiving or being withdrawn from chronic therapy when signs/symptoms suggestive of hypoadrenalism are noted (during stress or in unstressed state). Laboratory evaluation and replacement/stress doses of rapid-acting glucocorticoid should be considered.

Nutritional/Ethanol Interactions Herb/Nutraceutical: Avoid black cohosh, dong quai in estrogen-dependent tumors.

Lab Interactions Altered thyroid and liver function tests

Adverse Reactions

Cardiovascular: Edema, hypertension (≤8%), cardiomyopathy, palpitation

Central nervous system: Insomnia, fever (2% to 6%), headache (≤10%), pain (≤6%, similar to placebo), confusion (1% to 3%), convulsions (1% to 3%), depression (1% to 3%)

Dermatologic: Allergic rash (2% to 12%) with or without pruritus, alopecia

Endocrine & metabolic: Breakthrough bleeding and amenorrhea, spotting, changes in menstrual flow, changes in cervical erosion and secretions, increased breast tenderness, changes in vaginal bleeding pattern, edema, fluid retention, hyperglycemia (≤6%), diabetes, HPA axis suppression, adrenal insufficiency, Cushing's syndrome

Gastrointestinal: Weight gain (not attributed to edema or fluid retention), nausea, vomiting (7%), diarrhea (8% to 15%, similar to placebo), constipation (1% to 3%)

Genitourinary: Impotence (4% to 14%), decreased libido (≤5%)

Hepatic: Cholestatic jaundice, hepatotoxicity, hepatomegaly (1% to 3%)

Local: Thrombophlebitis

Neuromuscular & skeletal: Carpal tunnel syndrome, weakness, paresthesia (1% to 3%)

Respiratory: Hyperpnea, dyspnea (1% to 3%), cough (1% to 3%)

Miscellaneous: Diaphoresis

Overdosage/Toxicology Toxicity is unlikely following single exposure of excessive doses.

Pharmacodynamics/Kinetics

Absorption: Well absorbed orally

Time to Peak: Serum: 1-3 hours

Half-Life Elimination: 15-100 hours

Metabolism: Completely hepatic to free steroids and glucuronide conjugates

Excretion: Urine (57% to 78% as steroid metabolites and inactive compound); feces (8% to 30%)

Dosing

Adults & Elderly: Refer to individual protocols.

Breast carcinoma (female): Oral: 40 mg 4 times/day

Endometrial carcinoma: Oral: 40-320 mg/day in divided doses; use for 2 months to determine efficacy; maximum doses used have been up to 800 mg/day.

Uterine bleeding (unlabeled use): Oral: 40 mg 2-4 times/day

HIV-related cachexia (male/female): Oral: Initial: 800 mg/day; daily doses of 400 and 800 mg/day were found to be clinically effective.

Renal Impairment: No data available; however, the urinary excretion of megestrol acetate administered in doses of 4-90 mg ranged from 56% to 78% within 10 days.

Hemodialysis: Megestrol acetate has not been tested for dialyzability; however, due to its low solubility, it is postulated that dialysis would not be an effective means of treating an overdose.

Available Dosage Forms

Suspension, oral, as acetate: 40 mg/mL (240 mL) [contains alcohol 0.06% and sodium benzoate; lemon-lime flavor]

Tablet, as acetate: 20 mg, 40 mg

Monitoring and Teaching Issues

Physical Assessment: Use caution in presence of thrombophlebitis (see Warnings/Precautions for use cautions). Assess potential for interactions with herbal products patient may be taking. Assess therapeutic effects according to purpose for use and adverse reactions regularly during therapy (eg, hypertension, CNS changes (confusion, convulsions, insomnia), rash, changes in menses, gastrointestinal upset, jaundice, thrombophlebitis; see Adverse Reactions). Teach patient proper use, possible side effects/appropriate interventions (eg, importance of adequate hydration), and adverse symptoms to report (see Patient Education). **Pregnancy risk factor X:** Determine that patient is not pregnant before beginning treatment. Instruct patients of childbearing age about using appropriate contraceptive measures during therapy and for 1 month following therapy.

Patient Education: Inform prescriber of all prescriptions, OTC medications, or herbal products you are taking, and any allergies you have. Do not take any new medication during therapy unless approved by prescriber. Follow dosage schedule and do not take more than prescribed. May cause sensitivity to sunlight (use sunblock, wear protective clothing, and avoid extended exposure to direct sunlight); dizziness, anxiety, depression (use caution when driving or engaging in tasks that require alertness until response to drug is known); change in appetite (maintain adequate hydration [2-3 L/day of fluids, unless instructed to restrict fluid intake] and diet); decreased libido or increased body hair (reversible when drug is discontinued); or hot flashes (cool clothes and environment may help). Report swelling of face, lips, or mouth; absent or altered menses; abdominal pain; vaginal itching, irritation, or discharge; heat, warmth, redness, or swelling of extremities; or sudden onset change in vision. **Pregnancy/breast-feeding precautions:** Do not get pregnant while taking this medication and for 1 month following therapy; consult prescriber for appropriate contraceptives. This drug may cause fetal defects. Do not donate blood during or for 1 month following therapy. Do not breast-feed.

Geriatric Considerations: Elderly females may have vaginal bleeding or discharge and need to be forewarned of this side effect and inconvenience. No specific changes in dose are required for elderly. Megestrol has been used in the treatment of the failure to thrive syndrome in cachectic elderly in addition to proper nutrition.

Pregnancy Risk Factor: X

Lactation: Enters breast milk/contraindicated

Administration

Oral: Megestrol acetate (Megace®) oral suspension is compatible with water, orange juice, apple juice, or Sustacal H.C. for immediate consumption.

Storage: Store at 25°C (77°F); excursions permitted at 15°C to 30°C (59°F to 86°F)

♦ Megestrol Acetate *see* Megestrol *on page 942*

♦ Melanex® *see* Hydroquinone *on page 768*

♦ Mellaril® [DSC] *see* Thioridazine *on page 1463*

Meloxicam (mel OKS i kam)

U.S. Brand Names Mobic®

Generic Available No

Pharmacologic Category Nonsteroidal Anti-inflammatory Drug (NSAID), Oral

Use Relief of signs and symptoms of osteoarthritis and rheumatoid arthritis

Mechanism of Action/Effect Inhibits prostaglandin synthesis by decreasing the activity of the enzyme, cyclooxygenase, which results in decreased formation of prostaglandin precursors

Contraindications Hypersensitivity to meloxicam or any component of the formulation, aspirin, or other NSAIDs; pregnancy C/D (3rd trimester)

Warnings/Precautions Fatal asthmatic and anaphylactoid reactions have occurred in patients with "aspirin triad." Use with caution in patients with CHF, hypertension, dehydration, decreased renal or hepatic function, history of GI disease (bleeding, ulcers, or previous GI symptoms with NSAID use), or those receiving anticoagulants and/or corticosteroids. Use lowest effective dose for shortest period possible; bleeding risk has been correlated to dose and duration of therapy. Gastrointestinal bleeding may occur without prior symptoms of gastrointestinal irritation. Elderly are at a high risk for adverse effects from NSAIDs. As many as 60% of elderly can develop peptic ulceration and/or hemorrhage asymptomatically.

Use of NSAIDs can compromise existing renal function especially when Cl_{cr} <30 mL/minute. CNS adverse effects such as confusion, agitation, and hallucination are generally seen in overdose or high-dose situations; however, elderly may demonstrate these adverse effects at lower doses than younger adults. Do not exceed 15 mg/day. Withhold for at least 4-6 half-lives prior to surgical or dental procedures.

Drug Interactions

Cytochrome P450 Effect: Substrate (minor) of CYP2C8/9, 3A4; **Inhibits** CYP2C8/9 (weak)

Decreased Effect: Cholestyramine (and possibly colestipol) increases the clearance of meloxicam. Hydralazine's antihypertensive effect is decreased; avoid concurrent use. Loop diuretic efficacy (diuretic and antihypertensive effect) may be reduced by NSAIDs. Antihypertensive effects of thiazide diuretics are decreased; avoid concurrent use.

Increased Effect/Toxicity: Anticoagulants (warfarin, heparin, LMWHs) in combination with NSAIDs can cause increased risk of bleeding. Antiplatelet drugs (ticlopidine, clopidogrel, aspirin, abciximab, dipyridamole, eptifibatide, tirofiban) can cause an increased risk of bleeding. Aspirin increases serum concentrations (AUC) of meloxicam (in addition to potential for additive adverse effects); concurrent use is not recommended. Corticosteroids may increase the risk of GI ulceration; avoid concurrent use. NSAIDs may increase serum creatinine, potassium, blood pressure, and cyclosporine levels; monitor cyclosporine levels and renal function carefully. Lithium levels can be increased; avoid concurrent use if possible or monitor lithium levels and adjust dose. When NSAID is stopped, lithium will need adjustment again. Serum concentration/toxicity of methotrexate may be increased. Warfarin INRs may be increased by meloxicam. Monitor INR closely, particularly during initiation or change in dose. May increase risk of bleeding. Use lowest possible dose for shortest duration possible.

Nutritional/Ethanol Interactions Ethanol: Avoid ethanol (may enhance gastric mucosal irritation).

Adverse Reactions 2% to 10%:

Cardiovascular: Edema (2% to 3%)

Central nervous system: Headache and dizziness occurred in 2% to 8% of patients, but occurred less frequently than placebo in controlled trials

Dermatologic: Pruritus (<1% to 2%), rash (1% to 3%)

Gastrointestinal: Diarrhea (3% to 6%), dyspepsia (4% to 9%), nausea (3% to 7%), flatulence (3%), abdominal pain (2% to 5%)

Respiratory: Cough (<1% to 2%), pharyngitis (1% to 3%), upper respiratory infection (2% to 3%)

Miscellaneous: Flu-like symptoms (5% to 6%), falls (3%)

Overdosage/Toxicology Symptoms of overdose include lethargy, drowsiness, nausea, vomiting, and epigastric pain. Rarely, severe symptoms have been associated with NSAID overdose including apnea, metabolic acidosis, coma, nystagmus, seizures, leukocytosis, and renal failure. Management of NSAID intoxication is supportive and symptomatic. Since meloxicam undergoes enterohepatic cycling, multiple doses of charcoal may be needed to reduce the potential for delayed toxicities. Cholestyramine has been shown to increase meloxicam clearance. Meloxicam is not dialyzable.

Pharmacodynamics/Kinetics

Bioavailability: 89%

Time to Peak: 5-10 hours

Protein Binding: 99.4%

Half-Life Elimination: 15-20 hours

Metabolism: Hepatic via CYP2C9 and CYP3A4 (minor)

Excretion: Urine and feces (as inactive metabolites)

Dosing

Adults & Elderly: Osteoarthritis, rheumatoid arthritis: Oral: Initial: 7.5 mg once daily; some patients may receive additional benefit from an increased dose of 15 mg once daily.

Renal Impairment:

Mild to moderate impairment: No specific dosage recommendations

Significant impairment (Cl_{cr} ≤15 mL/minute): Avoid use

Hepatic Impairment:

Mild (Child-Pugh class A) to moderate (Child-Pugh class B) hepatic dysfunction: No dosage adjustment is necessary

Severe hepatic impairment: Patients with severe hepatic impairment have not been adequately studied

Available Dosage Forms

Suspension: 7.5 mg/5 mL (100 mL) [contains sodium benzoate; raspberry flavor]

Tablet: 7.5 mg, 15 mg

Monitoring and Teaching Issues

Physical Assessment: Assess effectiveness and interactions of other medications patient may be taking. Assess results of laboratory tests, therapeutic effectiveness, and adverse reactions at beginning of therapy and periodically throughout therapy. Assess knowledge/ teach patient appropriate use, interventions to reduce side effects, and adverse symptoms to report.

Monitoring Laboratory Tests: CBC, periodic liver function, renal function (serum BUN, and creatinine)

Patient Education: Take this medication exactly as directed; do not increase dose without consulting prescriber. Take with food or milk to reduce GI distress. Maintain adequate hydration (2-3 L/day of fluids) unless instructed to restrict fluid intake. Avoid alcohol, excessive vitamin C intake, or salicylate-containing foods (eg, curry powder, prunes, raisins, tea, or licorice). Do not use aspirin or aspirin-containing medication, or any other anti-inflammatory medications without consulting prescriber. You may experience anorexia, nausea, vomiting, or heartburn (small frequent meals, frequent mouth care, sucking lozenges, or chewing gum may help); drowsiness, dizziness, nervousness, or headache (use caution when driving or engaging in tasks requiring alertness until response to drug is known); or fluid retention (weigh yourself weekly and report unusual (3-5 lb/week) weight gain). GI bleeding, ulceration, or perforation can occur with or without pain; discontinue medication and contact prescriber if persistent abdominal pain or cramping, or blood in stool occurs. Report breathlessness, respiratory difficulty, or unusual cough; chest pain, rapid heartbeat, palpitations; unusual bruising/bleeding; blood in urine, stool, mouth, or vomitus; swollen extremities; skin rash or itching; acute fatigue, hearing changes (ringing in ears); or other adverse reactions. **Pregnancy/breast-feeding precautions:** Inform prescriber if you are or intend to become pregnant. This drug should not be used in the 3rd trimester of pregnancy. Do not breast-feed.

Dietary Considerations: Should be taken with food or milk to minimize gastrointestinal irritation.

Pregnancy Risk Factor: C/D (3rd trimester)

Pregnancy Issues: May cause premature closure of the ductus arteriosus in the 3rd trimester of pregnancy.

Lactation: Excretion in breast milk unknown/contraindicated

Breast-Feeding Issues: It is not known whether meloxicam is excreted in human milk. Due to a potential for serious adverse reactions, the manufacturer recommends that a decision be made whether to discontinue nursing or discontinue the drug, taking into account the importance of the drug to the mother.

Administration

Storage: Store at 25°C (77°F).

Related Information

Nonsalicylate / Nonsteroidal Anti-inflammatory Agents *on page 1743*

♦ **Melpaque HP®** *see* Hydroquinone *on page 768*

Melphalan (MEL fa lan)

U.S. Brand Names Alkeran®

Synonyms L-PAM; L-Sarcolysin; Phenylalanine Mustard

Generic Available No

Pharmacologic Category Antineoplastic Agent, Alkylating Agent

Medication Safety Issues

Sound-alike/look-alike issues:
Melphalan may be confused with Mephyton®, Myleran®
Alkeran® may be confused with Alferon®, Leukeran®

Use Palliative treatment of multiple myeloma and nonresectable epithelial ovarian carcinoma; neuroblastoma, rhabdomyosarcoma, breast cancer

Mechanism of Action/Effect Alkylating agent which is a derivative of mechlorethamine that inhibits DNA and RNA synthesis via formation of carbonium ions; cross-links strands of DNA

Contraindications Hypersensitivity to melphalan or any component of the formulation; severe bone marrow suppression; patients whose disease was resistant to prior therapy; pregnancy

Warnings/Precautions The U.S. Food and Drug Administration (FDA) currently recommends that procedures for proper handling and disposal of antineoplastic agents be considered. Appropriate safety equipment is recommended for preparation, administration, and disposal of antineoplastics. If melphalan injection contacts the skin, wash and flush thoroughly with water. Melphalan is potentially mutagenic, carcinogenic, and teratogenic; produces amenorrhea. Reduce dosage or discontinue therapy if leukocyte count is <3000/mm^3 or platelet count is <100,000/mm^3; use with caution in patients with bone marrow suppression, impaired renal function, or who have received prior chemotherapy or irradiation; will cause amenorrhea. Toxicity to immunosuppressives is increased in the elderly. Start with lowest recommended adult doses. Signs of infection, such as fever and WBC rise, may not occur. Lethargy and confusion may be more prominent signs of infection.

Drug Interactions

Decreased Effect: Cimetidine and other H$_2$ antagonists: The reduction in gastric pH has been reported to decrease bioavailability of melphalan by 30%.

Increased Effect/Toxicity: Risk of nephrotoxicity of cyclosporine is increased by melphalan. Concomitant use of I.V. melphalan may cause serious GI toxicity.

Nutritional/Ethanol Interactions

Ethanol: Avoid ethanol (due to GI irritation).

Food: Food interferes with oral absorption.

Lab Interactions False-positive Coombs' test [direct]

Adverse Reactions

>10%: Hematologic: Myelosuppressive: Leukopenia and thrombocytopenia are the most common effects of melphalan; irreversible bone marrow failure has been reported

WBC: Moderate

(Continued)

Melphalan *(Continued)*

Platelets: Moderate
Onset: 7 days
Nadir: 8-10 days and 27-32 days
Recovery: 42-50 days
1% to 10%:
Cardiovascular: Vasculitis
Dermatologic: Vesiculation of skin, alopecia, pruritus, rash
Endocrine & metabolic: SIADH, sterility, amenorrhea
Gastrointestinal: Nausea and vomiting are mild; stomatitis and diarrhea are infrequent
Genitourinary: Hemorrhagic cystitis, bladder irritation
Hematologic: Anemia, agranulocytosis, hemolytic anemia
Hepatic: Transaminases increased (hepatitis, jaundice have been reported)
Respiratory: Pulmonary fibrosis, interstitial pneumonitis
Miscellaneous: Hypersensitivity, secondary malignancy

Overdosage/Toxicology Symptoms of overdose include hypocalcemia, pulmonary fibrosis, nausea and vomiting, and bone marrow suppression. Treatment is symptomatic and supportive.

Pharmacodynamics/Kinetics

Absorption: Oral: Variable and incomplete
Bioavailability: Unpredictable, decreasing from 85% to 58% with repeated doses
Time to Peak: Serum: ~2 hours
Half-Life Elimination: Terminal: 1.5 hours
Excretion: Oral: Feces (20% to 50%); urine (10% to 30% as unchanged drug)

Dosing

Adults & Elderly: Refer to individual protocols; dose should always be adjusted to patient response and weekly blood counts.

Multiple myeloma:
Oral: 6 mg/day initially adjusted as indicated **or** 0.15 mg/kg/day for 7 days **or** 0.25 mg/kg/day for 4 days; repeat at 4- to 6-week intervals.
I.V.: 16 mg/m^2 administered at 2-week intervals for 4 doses, then repeat monthly as per protocol for multiple myeloma.

Ovarian carcinoma: Oral: 0.2 mg/kg/day for 5 days, repeat every 4-5 weeks

High dose BMT: I.V.: 140-240 mg/m^2 as a single dose or divided into 2-5 daily doses. Infuse over 20-60 minutes.

Pediatrics: Oral (refer to individual protocols); dose should always be adjusted to patient response and weekly blood counts.

Various protocols: Oral: 4-20 mg/m^2/day for 1-21 days
Pediatric rhabdomyosarcoma: I.V.: 10-35 mg/m^2/dose every 21-28 days
High-dose melphalan with bone marrow transplantation for neuroblastoma: I.V.:
70-100 mg/m^2/day on day 7 and 6 before BMT **or**
140-220 mg/m^2 single dose before BMT **or**
50 mg/m^2/day for 4 days **or**
70 mg/m^2/day for 3 days

Renal Impairment:
Cl$_{cr}$ 10-50 mL/minute: Administer 75% of normal dose.
Cl$_{cr}$ <10 mL/minute: Administer 50% of normal dose.
  or
BUN >30 mg/dL: Reduce dose by 50%.
Serum creatinine >1.5 mg/dL: Reduce dose by 50%.
Hemodialysis effects: Unknown
CAPD effects: Unknown
CAVH effects: Unknown

Available Dosage Forms

Injection, powder for reconstitution: 50 mg [diluent contains ethanol and propylene glycol]]
Tablet: 2 mg

Monitoring and Teaching Issues

Physical Assessment: Use in presence of bone marrow suppression, impaired renal function, prior chemotherapy or irradiation (see Warnings/Precautions for specific use cautions). Assess potential for interactions with other pharmacological agent products patient may be taking (eg, cimetidine, cyclosporine; see Drug Interactions). For intravenous infusion see Administration and Reconstitution specifics. Assess results of laboratory tests and patient response regularly during therapy (oral or intravenous) (eg, myelosuppression [leukopenia], SIADH, diarrhea, bladder irritation [hematuria], interstitial pneumonitis; see Adverse Reactions). Teach patient proper use (oral), possible side effects/appropriate interventions, and adverse symptoms to report (see Patient Education).

Monitoring Laboratory Tests: CBC with differential, platelet count, serum electrolytes, serum uric acid

Patient Education: For intravenous infusion; report immediately any burning, swelling, pain, or redness at infusion or injection site. Take oral doses on an empty stomach, if possible, 1 hour before or 2 hours after meals. Avoid alcohol (may increase gastric irritation). Maintain adequate nutrition (small frequent meals may help) and adequate hydration (2-3 L/day of fluids) unless instructed to restrict fluid intake. You may be more susceptible to infection (avoid crowds and exposure to infection and do not have any vaccinations unless approved by prescriber). May cause hair loss (reversible); easy bleeding or bruising (use soft toothbrush or cotton swabs and frequent mouth care, use electric razor, avoid sharp knives or scissors); or nausea or vomiting (small frequent meals, frequent mouth care, chewing gum, or sucking lozenges may help). Report chest pain or palpitations; unusual fatigue; difficulty or pain on urination; unusual bruising/bleeding; respiratory difficulty; or pain or redness. **Pregnancy/breast-feeding precautions:** Inform prescriber if you are pregnant. Do not get pregnant during or for 1 month following therapy. Consult prescriber for instruction on appropriate barrier contraceptive measures. This drug may cause severe fetal defects. Breast-feeding is not recommended.

Dietary Considerations: Should be taken on an empty stomach (1 hour prior to or 2 hours after meals).

Geriatric Considerations: Toxicity to immunosuppressives is increased in the elderly. Start with lowest recommended adult doses. Signs of infection, such as fever and WBC rise, may not occur. Lethargy and confusion may be more prominent signs of infection.

Pregnancy Risk Factor: D

Lactation: Excretion in breast milk unknown/not recommended

Administration

Oral: Administer on an empty stomach.

I.V.: Due to limited stability, complete administration of I.V. dose should occur within 60 minutes of reconstitution

> I.V. infusion: I.V. dose is FDA-approved for administration as a single infusion over 15-20 minutes
>
> I.V. bolus: I.V. may be administered via central line and via peripheral vein as a rapid I.V. bolus; there have not been any unexpected or serious adverse events specifically related to rapid I.V. bolus administration; the most common adverse events were transient mild symptoms of hot flush and tingling sensation over the body
>
>> Central line: I.V. bolus doses of 17-200 mg/m² (reconstituted and not diluted) have been infused over 2-20 minutes
>>
>> Peripheral line: I.V. bolus doses of 2-23 mg/m² (reconstituted and not diluted) have been infused over 1-4 minutes

Reconstitution:

> Injection: Preparation: **The time between reconstitution/dilution and administration of parenteral melphalan must be kept to a minimum (<60 minutes) because reconstituted and diluted solutions are unstable.** Dissolve powder initially with 10 mL of diluent to a concentration of 5 mg/mL. **Immediately** dilute dose in NS to a concentration ≤0.45 mg/mL. If the solution is **highly unstable**, administration should occur within 1 hour of dissolution. Do not refrigerate solution; precipitation occurs.

Standard I.V. dilution:

> Dose/250-500 mL NS (concentration ≤0.45 mg/mL)
>
> **Must be prepared fresh;** solution is stable for 1 hour after dilution and must be administered within that time period.

Compatibility: Incompatible with D_5W, LR

Y-site administration: Incompatible with amphotericin B, chlorpromazine

Storage:

> Tablet: Store in refrigerator at 2°C to 8°C (36°F to 46°F); protect from light.
>
> Injection: Store at room temperature (15°C to 30°C). Protect from light.

♦ **Melquin-3®** *see* Hydroquinone *on page 768*

♦ **Melquin HP®** *see* Hydroquinone *on page 768*

Memantine (me MAN teen)

U.S. Brand Names Namenda™

Synonyms Memantine Hydrochloride

Generic Available No

Pharmacologic Category N-Methyl-D-Aspartate Receptor Antagonist

Use Treatment of moderate-to-severe dementia of the Alzheimer's type

Mechanism of Action/Effect Memantine reduces the decline in function in Alzheimer's disease; it has not been shown to prevent or slow neurodegeneration associated with this disease.

Contraindications Hypersensitivity to memantine or any component of the formulation

Warnings/Precautions Use caution with seizure disorders, hepatic impairment, or mild-to-moderate renal impairment. Use with severe renal impairment is not recommended. Clearance is significantly reduced by alkaline urine; use caution with medications, dietary changes, or patient conditions which may alter urine pH.

Drug Interactions

> **Increased Effect/Toxicity:** Clearance of memantine is decreased 80% at urinary pH 8; use caution with medications (carbonic anhydrase inhibitors, sodium bicarbonate) which may increase urinary pH.

Adverse Reactions

1% to 10%:

> Cardiovascular: Hypertension (4%), cardiac failure, syncope, cerebrovascular accident, transient ischemic attack
>
> Central nervous system: Dizziness (7%), confusion (6%), headache (6%), hallucinations (3%), pain (3%), somnolence (3%), fatigue (2%), aggressive reaction, ataxia, vertigo
>
> Dermatologic: Rash
>
> Gastrointestinal: Constipation (5%), vomiting (3%), weight loss
>
> Genitourinary: Micturition
>
> Hematologic: Anemia
>
> Hepatic: Alkaline phosphatase increased
>
> Neuromuscular & skeletal: Back pain (3%), hypokinesia
>
> Ocular: Cataract, conjunctivitis
>
> Respiratory: Cough (4%), dyspnea (2%), pneumonia

Overdosage/Toxicology Loss of consciousness, psychosis, restlessness, somnolence, stupor, and visual hallucinations were reported following ingestion of memantine 400 mg. In case of overdose, treatment should be symptomatic and supportive. Elimination may be increased by acidifying the urine.

(Continued)

Memantine (Continued)

Pharmacodynamics/Kinetics
Time to Peak: Serum: 3-7 hours
Protein Binding: 45%
Half-Life Elimination: Terminal: 60-80 hours
Metabolism: Forms three metabolites (minimal activity)
Excretion: Urine (57% to 82% unchanged); excretion affected by urine pH

Dosing
Adults & Elderly:
Alzheimer's disease: Oral: Initial: 5 mg/day; increase dose by 5 mg/day to a target dose of 20 mg/day; wait at least 1 week between dosage changes. Doses >5 mg/day should be given in 2 divided doses.
Suggested titration: 5 mg/day for ≥1 week; 5 mg twice daily for ≥1 week; 15 mg/day given in 5 mg and 10 mg separated doses for ≥1 week; then 10 mg twice daily.

Renal Impairment:
Moderate impairment: Consider dose reduction; specific recommendations are not available.
Severe impairment: Use is not recommended.

Available Dosage Forms
Tablet, as hydrochloride (Namenda™): 5 mg, 10 mg
Combination package (Namenda™) [titration pack contains 2 separate tablet formulations]: Memantine hydrochloride 5 mg (28s) and memantine hydrochloride 10 mg (21s)

Monitoring and Teaching Issues
Physical Assessment: Use caution in presence of seizure disorders, hepatic or renal impairment, and anything that causes alkaline urine (see Warnings/Precautions and Drug Interactions for use cautions). Assess therapeutic effectiveness and adverse reactions on a regular basis throughout therapy (eg, hypertension, CNS changes, rash, constipation; see Adverse Reactions). Teach patient possible side effects/appropriate interventions and adverse symptoms to report (see Patient Education).

Patient Education: Take as directed with or without food. May cause hypertension (monitor if recommended) or headache (consult prescriber for analgesic). Report increase in CNS changes (confusion, hallucinations, fatigue, aggressive reaction); chest pain or palpitations; dizziness or fainting; difficulty breathing or tightness in chest; rash; alteration in elimination patterns; or other persistent adverse reactions. **Breast-feeding precaution:** Consult prescriber if breast-feeding.

Dietary Considerations: May be taken with or without food.

Geriatric Considerations: In clinical trials, patients on memantine had less of a decline in cognitive function and activities of daily living (ADL) as compared to placebo. This was true for monotherapy with memantine, as well as combination therapy with donepezil, an acetylcholinesterase inhibitor.

Pregnancy Risk Factor: B
Lactation: Excretion in breast milk unknown/use caution

Administration
Storage: Store at controlled room temperature of 15°C to 30°C (59°F to 86°F).

- Memantine Hydrochloride *see* Memantine *on page* 947
- Menadol® [OTC] *see* Ibuprofen *on page* 777
- Menest® *see* Estrogens (Esterified) *on page* 569
- Meningococcal Polysaccharide Vaccine (Groups A, C, Y, and W-135) *see page* 1660
- Menomune®-A/C/Y/W-135 *see page* 1660
- Menopur® *see* Menotropins *on page* 948
- Menostar™ *see* Estradiol *on page* 552

Menotropins (men oh TROE pins)

U.S. Brand Names Menopur®; Pergonal® [DSC]; Repronex®
Generic Available No
Pharmacologic Category Gonadotropin; Ovulation Stimulator
Medication Safety Issues
Sound-alike/look-alike issues:
Repronex® may be confused with Regranex®

Use
Female:
In conjunction with hCG to induce ovulation and pregnancy in infertile females experiencing oligoanovulation or anovulation when the cause of anovulation is functional and not caused by primary ovarian failure (Pergonal®, Repronex®)
Stimulation of multiple follicle development in ovulatory patients as part of an assisted reproductive technology (ART) (Menopur®, Pergonal®, Repronex®)
Male: Stimulation of spermatogenesis in primary or secondary hypogonadotropic hypogonadism (Pergonal®)

Mechanism of Action/Effect Actions occur as a result of both follicle stimulating hormone (FSH) effects and luteinizing hormone (LH) effects; menotropins stimulate the development and maturation of the ovarian follicle (FSH), cause ovulation (LH), and stimulate the development of the corpus luteum (LH); in males it stimulates spermatogenesis (LH)

Contraindications Hypersensitivity to menotropins or any component of the formulation; primary ovarian failure as indicated by a high follicle-stimulating hormone (FSH) level; uncontrolled thyroid and adrenal dysfunction; abnormal bleeding of undetermined origin; intracranial lesion (ie, pituitary tumor); ovarian cyst or enlargement not due to polycystic ovary syndrome; infertility due to any cause other than anovulation (except candidates for *in vitro* fertilization); men with normal urinary gonadotropin concentrations, elevated gonadotropin levels indicating primary testicular failure; sex hormone-dependent tumors of the reproductive tract and accessory organs; pregnancy

Warnings/Precautions Advise patient of frequency and potential hazards of multiple pregnancy. To minimize the hazard of abnormal ovarian enlargement, use the lowest possible dose. Safety and efficacy have not been established in renal or hepatic impairment, or in pediatric and geriatric patients.

Adverse Reactions Adverse effects may vary according to specific product, route, and/or dosage.

Male:
>10%: Endocrine & metabolic: Gynecomastia
1% to 10%: Erythrocytosis (dyspnea, dizziness, anorexia, syncope, epistaxis)

Female:
>10%:
Central nervous system: Headache (up to 34%)
Gastrointestinal: Abdominal pain (up to 18%), nausea (up to 12%)
Genitourinary: OHSS (up to 13%, dose related)
Local: Injection site reaction (4% to 12%)

1% to 10%:
Cardiovascular: Flushing
Central nervous system: Dizziness, malaise, migraine
Endocrine & metabolic: Breast tenderness, hot flashes, menstrual irregularities
Gastrointestinal: Abdominal cramping, abdominal fullness, constipation, diarrhea, enlarged abdomen, vomiting
Genitourinary: Ectopic pregnancy, ovarian disease, vaginal hemorrhage
Local: Injection site edema/pain
Neuromuscular & skeletal: Back pain
Respiratory: Cough increased, respiratory disorder
Miscellaneous: Infection, flu-like syndrome

Frequency not defined:
Cardiovascular: Stroke, tachycardia, thrombosis (venous or arterial)
Central nervous system: Dizziness
Dermatologic: Angioedema, urticaria
Genitourinary: Adnexal torsion, hemoperitoneum, ovarian enlargement
Neuromuscular & skeletal: Limb necrosis
Respiratory: Acute respiratory distress syndrome, atelectasis, dyspnea, embolism, laryngeal edema pulmonary infarction tachypnea
Miscellaneous: Allergic reaction, anaphylaxis, rash

Overdosage/Toxicology Symptoms of overdose include ovarian hyperstimulation.

Pharmacodynamics/Kinetics
Excretion: Urine (~10% as unchanged drug)

Dosing
Adults:
Pergonal®: I.M.
Spermatogenesis (Male): Following pretreatment with hCG: 75 int. units 3 times/week and hCG 2000 units twice weekly until sperm is detected in the ejaculate (4-6 months); may then be increased to menotropins 150 int. units 3 times/week
Induction of ovulation (Female): 75 int. units for 7-12 days, followed by 10,000 units hCG one day after the last dose; repeated at least twice at same level before increasing dosage to 150 int. units

Repronex®: I.M., SubQ:
Induction of ovulation in patients with oligoanovulation (Female): Initial: 150 int. units daily for the first 5 days of treatment. Adjustments should not be made more frequently than once every 2 days and should not exceed 75-150 int. units per adjustment. Maximum daily dose should not exceed 450 int. units and dosing beyond 12 days is not recommended. If patient's response is appropriate, hCG 5000-10,000 units should be given one day following the last dose of Repronex®. Hold dose if serum estradiol is >2000 pg/mL, if the ovaries are abnormally enlarged, or if abdominal pain occurs; the patient should also be advised to refrain from intercourse. May repeat process if follicular development is inadequate or if pregnancy does not occur.
Assisted reproductive technologies (Female): Initial (in patients who have received GnRH agonist or antagonist pituitary suppression): 225 int. units; adjustments in dose should not be made more frequently than once every 2 days and should not exceed more than 75-150 int. units per adjustment. The maximum daily doses of Repronex® given should not exceed 450 int. units and dosing beyond 12 days is not recommended. Once adequate follicular development is evident, hCG (5000-10,000 units) should be administered to induce final follicular maturation in preparation for oocyte retrieval. Withhold treatment when ovaries are abnormally enlarged on last day of therapy (to reduce chance of developing OHSS).

Menopur®: SubQ:
Assisted reproductive technologies (ART): Initial (in patients who have received GnRH agonist for pituitary suppression): 225 int. units; adjustments in dose should not be made more frequently than once every 2 days and should not exceed more than 150 int. units per adjustment. The maximum daily dose given should not exceed 450 int. units and dosing beyond 20 days is not recommended. Once adequate follicular development is evident, hCG should be administered to induce final follicular maturation in preparation for oocyte retrieval. Withhold treatment when ovaries are abnormally enlarged on last day of therapy (to reduce chance of developing OHSS).

Available Dosage Forms [DSC] = Discontinued product
Injection, powder for reconstitution:
Menopur®: Follicle stimulating hormone activity 75 int. units and luteinizing hormone activity 75 int. units [packaged with diluent; contains lactose 21 mg]
Pergonal®: Follicle stimulating hormone activity 75 int. units and luteinizing hormone activity 75 int. units [packaged with diluent; contains lactose 10 mg] [DSC]
Repronex®: Follicle stimulating hormone activity 75 int. units and luteinizing hormone activity 75 int. units [packaged with diluent]
(Continued)

Menotropins *(Continued)*

Monitoring and Teaching Issues

Physical Assessment: Female: Assess knowledge/teach appropriate method for measuring basal body temperature to indicate ovulation. Stress importance of following prescriber's instructions for timing intercourse. If self-administered, assess/teach appropriate injection technique and needle disposal. **Pregnancy risk factor X:** Determine pregnancy status prior to beginning therapy.

Patient Education: Self injection: Follow prescriber's recommended schedule for injections. Multiple ovulations resulting in multiple pregnancies have been reported. Male infertility and/or breast enlargement may occur. You may experience headache, nausea, abdominal pain, flushing, dizziness, or menstrual irregularities. Report pain at injection site; enlarged breasts (male); respiratory difficulty; nosebleeds; acute abdominal discomfort; abdominal distention; fever; or warmth, swelling, weight gain, pain, or redness in calves.

Pregnancy Risk Factor: X

Pregnancy Issues: Ectopic pregnancy and congenital abnormalities have been reported. The incidence of congenital abnormality is similar during natural conception.

Lactation: Excretion in breast milk unknown/use caution

Administration

I.M.: Pergonal®, Repronex®: Administer deep in a large muscle.

Other: SubQ:

Menopur®: Administer to alternating sites of the abdomen. When administration to the lower abdomen is not possible, the injection may be given into the thigh.

Repronex®: Administer to alternating sites of the lower abdomen.

Reconstitution: After reconstitution inject immediately, discard any unused portion.

Storage: Lyophilized powder may be refrigerated or stored at room temperature.

Meperidine *(me PER i deen)*

U.S. Brand Names Demerol®; Meperitab®

Synonyms Isonipecaine Hydrochloride; Meperidine Hydrochloride; Pethidine Hydrochloride

Controlled Substance C-II

Generic Available Yes

Pharmacologic Category Analgesic, Narcotic

Medication Safety Issues

Sound-alike/look-alike issues:

Meperidine may be confused with meprobamate

Demerol® may be confused with Demulen®, Desyrel®, dicumarol, Dilaudid®, Dymelor®, Pamelor®

Use Management of moderate to severe pain; adjunct to anesthesia and preoperative sedation

Mechanism of Action/Effect Binds to opiate receptors in the CNS, causing inhibition of ascending pain pathways, altering the perception of and response to pain; produces generalized CNS depression

Contraindications Hypersensitivity to meperidine or any component of the formulation; patients receiving MAO inhibitors presently or in the past 14 days; pregnancy (prolonged use or high doses near term)

Warnings/Precautions An opioid-containing analgesic regimen should be tailored to each patient's needs and based upon the type of pain being treated (acute versus chronic), the route of administration, degree of tolerance for opioids (naive versus chronic user), age, weight, and medical condition. The optimal analgesic dose varies widely among patients. Doses should be titrated to pain relief/prevention. Use for chronic pain management not recommended. Oral meperidine not recommended for acute pain management.

Use with caution in patients with pulmonary, hepatic, renal disorders, or increased intracranial pressure; use with caution in patients with renal failure or seizure disorders or those receiving high-dose meperidine; normeperidine (an active metabolite and CNS stimulant) may accumulate and precipitate twitches, tremors, or seizures; some preparations contain sulfites which may cause allergic reaction; not recommended as a drug of first choice for the treatment of chronic pain in the elderly due to the accumulation of normeperidine; for acute pain, its use should be limited to 1-2 doses; tolerance or drug dependence may result from extended use. Use only with extreme caution **(if at all)** in patients with head injury or increased intracranial pressure (ICP); potential to elevate ICP may be greatly exaggerated in these patients.

Drug Interactions

Decreased Effect: Barbiturates may decrease the analgesic efficacy and increase the sedative effects of meperidine. Phenytoin may decrease the analgesic effects of meperidine.

Increased Effect/Toxicity: MAO inhibitors greatly potentiate the effects of meperidine; acute opioid overdosage symptoms can be seen, including severe toxic reactions. Concurrent use within 14 days of an MAO inhibitor is contraindicated. CNS depressants may potentiate the sedative effects of meperidine or increase respiratory depression. Phenothiazines may potentiate the sedative effects of meperidine and may increase the incidence of hypotension. Serotonin agonists, serotonin reuptake inhibitors, and tricyclic antidepressants may potentiate the effects of meperidine. In addition, concurrent therapy with these drugs potentially may increase the risk of serotonin syndrome. A number of drugs may increase meperidine metabolite concentrations (including acyclovir, cimetidine, and ritonavir).

Nutritional/Ethanol Interactions

Ethanol: Avoid or limit ethanol (may increase CNS depression). Watch for sedation.

Food: Glucose may cause hyperglycemia; monitor blood glucose concentrations.

Herb/Nutraceutical: Avoid valerian, St John's wort, kava kava, gotu kola (may increase CNS depression).

Lab Interactions Increased amylase (S), BSP retention, CPK (I.M. injections)

Adverse Reactions Frequency not defined.

Cardiovascular: Hypotension

Central nervous system: Fatigue, drowsiness, dizziness, nervousness, headache, restlessness, malaise, confusion, mental depression, hallucinations, paradoxical CNS stimulation, increased intracranial pressure, seizure (associated with metabolite accumulation)

Dermatologic: Rash, urticaria

Gastrointestinal: Nausea, vomiting, constipation, anorexia, stomach cramps, xerostomia, biliary spasm, paralytic ileus

Genitourinary: Ureteral spasms, decreased urination

Local: Pain at injection site

Neuromuscular & skeletal: Weakness

Respiratory: Dyspnea

Miscellaneous: Histamine release, physical and psychological dependence

Overdosage/Toxicology Symptoms of overdose include CNS depression, respiratory depression, mydriasis, bradycardia, pulmonary edema, chronic tremor, CNS excitability, and seizures. Treatment is symptomatic. Naloxone, 2 mg I.V. with repeat administration as necessary up to a total dose of 10 mg, can be used to reverse opiate effects. Naloxone should not be used to treat meperidine-induced seizures.

Pharmacodynamics/Kinetics
Onset of Action: Analgesic: Oral, SubQ, I.M.: 10-15 minutes; I.V.: ~5 minutes; Peak effect: Oral, SubQ, I.M.: ~1 hour

Duration of Action: Oral, SubQ, I.M.: 2-4 hours

Bioavailability: ~50% to 60%; increased with liver disease

Protein Binding: 65% to 75%

Half-Life Elimination:
Parent drug: Terminal phase: Neonates: 23 hours (range: 12-39 hours); Adults: 2.5-4 hours, Liver disease: 7-11 hours
Normeperidine (active metabolite): 15-30 hours; can accumulate with high doses or renal impairment

Metabolism: Hepatic; active metabolite (normeperidine)

Dosing
Adults: Note: Doses should be titrated to necessary analgesic effect. When changing route of administration, note that oral doses are about half as effective as parenteral dose. Oral route not recommended for chronic pain. These are guidelines and do not represent the maximum doses that may be required in all patients.

Pain (analgesic):
Oral: Initial: Opiate-naive: 50 mg every 3-4 hours as needed; usual dosage range: 50-150 mg every 2-4 hours as needed

I.M., SubQ: Initial: Opiate-naive: 50-75 mg every 3-4 hours as needed; patients with prior opiate exposure may require higher initial doses; usual dosage range: 50-150 mg every 2-4 hours as needed
Preoperatively: 50-100 mg given 30-90 minutes before the beginning of anesthesia

Slow I.V.: Initial: 5-10 mg every 5 minutes as needed

Patient-controlled analgesia (PCA): Usual concentration: 10 mg/mL
Initial dose: 10 mg
Demand dose: 1-5 mg (manufacturer recommendations); range 5-25 mg
Lockout interval: 5-10 minutes

Elderly: Note: Doses should be titrated to necessary analgesic effect. When changing route of administration, note that oral doses are about half as effective as parenteral dose. Oral route not recommended for chronic pain. These are guidelines and do not represent the maximum doses that may be required in all patients.

Oral: 50 mg every 4 hours
I.M.: 25 mg every 4 hours

Pediatrics:
Pain (analgesic): Oral, I.M., I.V., SubQ: Children: 1-1.5 mg/kg/dose every 3-4 hours as needed; 1-2 mg/kg as a single dose preoperative medication may be used; maximum 100 mg/dose. Oral therapy is discouraged.

Note: Doses should be titrated to necessary analgesic effect. When changing route of administration, note that oral doses are about half as effective as parenteral dose. Oral route not recommended for chronic pain. These are guidelines and do not represent the maximum doses that may be required in all patients.

Renal Impairment:
Cl_{cr} 10-50 mL/minute: Administer 75% of normal dose.
Cl_{cr} <10 mL/minute: Administer 50% of normal dose.
Note: Repeated use in renal impairment **should be avoided** due to potential accumulation of neuroexcitatory metabolite.

Hepatic Impairment: Increased narcotic effect in cirrhosis; reduction in dose is more important than for oral than I.V. route.

Available Dosage Forms
Injection, solution, as hydrochloride [ampul]: 25 mg/0.5 mL (0.5 mL); 25 mg/mL (1 mL); 50 mg/mL (1 mL, 1.5 mL, 2 mL); 75 mg/mL (1 mL); 100 mg/mL (1 mL)

Injection, solution, as hydrochloride [prefilled syringe]: 25 mg/mL (1 mL); 50 mg/mL (1 mL); 75 mg/mL (1 mL); 100 mg/mL (1 mL)

Injection, solution, as hydrochloride [for PCA pump]: 10 mg/mL (30 mL, 50 mL, 60 mL)

Injection, solution, as hydrochloride [vial]: 25 mg/mL (1 mL); 50 mg/mL (1 mL, 30 mL); 75 mg/mL (1 mL); 100 mg/mL (1 mL, 20 mL) [may contain sodium metabisulfite]

Syrup, as hydrochloride: 50 mg/5 mL (500 mL) [contains sodium benzoate]
Demerol®: 50 mg/5 mL (480 mL) [contains benzoic acid; banana flavor]

Tablet, as hydrochloride (Demerol®, Meperitab®): 50 mg, 100 mg

Monitoring and Teaching Issues
Physical Assessment: Assess other medications patient may be taking for additive or adverse interactions. Monitor therapeutic effectiveness and adverse reactions or overdose at beginning of therapy and at regular intervals with long-term use. Monitor frequently for need, may cause physical and/or psychological dependence. For inpatients, implement
(Continued)

Meperidine *(Continued)*

safety measures. Assess knowledge/teach patient appropriate use (if self-administered), adverse reactions to report, and appropriate interventions to reduce side effects. Discontinue slowly after prolonged use.

Patient Education: If self-administered, use exactly as directed; do not increase dose or frequency. Drug may cause physical and/or psychological dependence. While using this medication, do not use alcohol and other prescription or OTC medications (especially sedatives, tranquilizers, antihistamines, or pain medications) without consulting prescriber. Maintain adequate hydration (2-3 L/day of fluids) unless instructed to restrict fluid intake. May cause hypotension, dizziness, drowsiness, impaired coordination, or blurred vision (use caution when driving, climbing stairs, or changing position - rising from sitting or lying to standing, or when engaging in tasks requiring alertness until response to drug is known); loss of appetite, nausea, or vomiting (frequent mouth care, small frequent meals, chewing gum, or sucking lozenges may help); or constipation (increased exercise, fluids, fruit, or fiber may help; if unresolved, consult prescriber about use of stool softeners). Report chest pain, slow or rapid heartbeat, acute dizziness or persistent headache; changes in mental status; swelling of extremities or unusual weight gain; changes in urinary elimination; acute headache; back or flank pain or muscle spasms; blurred vision; skin rash; or shortness of breath. **Pregnancy/breast-feeding precautions:** Inform prescriber if you are or intend to become pregnant. Consult prescriber if breast-feeding.

Geriatric Considerations: Meperidine is not recommended as a drug of first choice for the treatment of chronic pain in the elderly due to the accumulation of its metabolite, normeperidine, which leads to serious CNS side effects (eg, tremor, seizures). For acute pain, its use should be limited to 1-2 doses.

Pregnancy Risk Factor: C/D (prolonged use or high doses at term)

Pregnancy Issues: Meperidine is known to cross the placenta, which may result in respiratory or CNS depression in the newborn.

Lactation: Enters breast milk/contraindicated (AAP rates "compatible")

Breast-Feeding Issues: Meperidine is excreted in breast milk and may cause CNS and/or respiratory depression in the nursing infant.

Administration

I.V.: Meperidine may be administered I.M. (preferably), SubQ, or I.V. IVP should be given slowly, use of a 10 mg/mL concentration has been recommended. For continuous I.V. infusions, a more dilute solution (eg, 1 mg/mL) should be used.

Compatibility: Stable in dextran 6% in dextrose, dextran 6% in NS, D₅LR, D₅¼NS, D₅½NS, D₅NS, D₅W, D₁₀W, LR, ½NS, NS

Y-site administration: Incompatible with allopurinol, amphotericin B cholesteryl sulfate complex, cefepime, cefoperazone, doxorubicin liposome, idarubicin, imipenem/cilastatin, minocycline

Compatibility in syringe: Incompatible with heparin, morphine, pentobarbital

Compatibility when admixed: Incompatible with aminophylline, amobarbital, floxacillin, furosemide, heparin, morphine, phenobarbital, phenytoin, thiopental

Storage: Meperidine injection should be stored at room temperature and protected from light and freezing. Protect oral dosage forms from light.

Related Information

Compatibility of Drugs *on page 1723*
Compatibility of Drugs in Syringe *on page 1725*
Narcotic / Opioid Analgesic Comparison *on page 1739*

♦ **Meperidine Hydrochloride** *see* Meperidine *on page 950*
♦ **Meperitab®** *see* Meperidine *on page 950*
♦ **Mephyton®** *see* Phytonadione *on page 1209*

Meprobamate *(me proe BA mate)*

U.S. Brand Names Miltown®

Synonyms Equanil

Controlled Substance C-IV

Generic Available Yes

Pharmacologic Category Antianxiety Agent, Miscellaneous

Medication Safety Issues

Sound-alike/look-alike issues:

Meprobamate may be confused with Mepergan, meperidine

Equanil may be confused with Elavil®

Use Management of anxiety disorders

Unlabeled/Investigational Use Demonstrated value for muscle contraction, headache, premenstrual tension, external sphincter spasticity, muscle rigidity, opisthotonos-associated with tetanus

Mechanism of Action/Effect Affects the thalamus and limbic system; also appears to inhibit multineuronal spinal reflexes

Contraindications Hypersensitivity to meprobamate, related compounds (including carisoprodol), or any component of the formulation; acute intermittent porphyria; pre-existing CNS depression; narrow-angle glaucoma; severe uncontrolled pain; pregnancy

Warnings/Precautions Physical and psychological dependence and abuse may occur; abrupt cessation may precipitate withdrawal. Use with caution in patients with depression or suicidal tendencies, or in patients with a history of drug abuse. May cause CNS depression, which may impair physical or mental abilities. Patients must be cautioned about performing tasks which require mental alertness (eg, operating machinery or driving). Effects with other sedative drugs or ethanol may be potentiated. Not recommended in children <6 years of age; allergic reaction may occur in patients with history of dermatological condition (usually by fourth dose). Use with caution in patients with renal or hepatic impairment, or with a history of seizures. Use caution in the elderly as it may cause confusion, cognitive impairment, or excessive sedation.

Drug Interactions

Increased Effect/Toxicity: CNS depressants (ethanol) may increase CNS depression.

Nutritional/Ethanol Interactions

Ethanol: Avoid ethanol (may increase CNS depression).

Herb/Nutraceutical: Avoid valerian, St John's wort, kava kava, gotu kola (may increase CNS depression).

Adverse Reactions Frequency not defined.

Cardiovascular: Syncope, peripheral edema, palpitation, tachycardia, arrhythmia

Central nervous system: Drowsiness, ataxia, dizziness, paradoxical excitement, confusion, slurred speech, headache, euphoria, chills, vertigo, paresthesia, overstimulation

Dermatologic: Rashes, purpura, dermatitis, Stevens-Johnson syndrome, petechiae, ecchymosis

Gastrointestinal: Diarrhea, vomiting, nausea

Hematologic: Leukopenia, eosinophilia, agranulocytosis, aplastic anemia

Neuromuscular & skeletal: Weakness

Ocular: Blurred vision, impairment of accommodation

Renal: Renal failure

Respiratory: Wheezing, dyspnea, bronchospasm, angioneurotic edema

Overdosage/Toxicology Symptoms of overdose include drowsiness, lethargy, ataxia, coma, hypotension, shock, and death. Treatment is supportive following attempts to enhance drug elimination.

Pharmacodynamics/Kinetics

Onset of Action: Sedation: ~1 hour

Half-Life Elimination: 10 hours

Metabolism: Hepatic

Excretion: Urine (8% to 20% as unchanged drug); feces (10% as metabolites)

Dosing

Adults: Oral: 400 mg 3-4 times/day, up to 2400 mg/day

Elderly: Oral (use lowest effective dose): Initial: 200 mg 2-3 times/day

Pediatrics: Oral: 6-12 years: 100-200 mg 2-3 times/day

Renal Impairment:

Cl_{cr} 10-50 mL/minute: Administer every 9-12 hours.

Cl_{cr} <10 mL/minute: Administer every 12-18 hours.

Moderately dialyzable (20% to 50%)

Hepatic Impairment: Probably necessary in patients with liver disease; no specific recommendations.

Available Dosage Forms Tablet: 200 mg, 400 mg

Monitoring and Teaching Issues

Physical Assessment: Assess other medications the patient may be taking for effectiveness and interactions. Assess for history of addiction; long-term use can result in dependence, abuse, or tolerance; periodically evaluate need for continued use. Monitor therapeutic effectiveness and adverse reactions or overdose at beginning of therapy and periodically with long-term use. Monitor for CNS depression. Taper dosage slowly when discontinuing. Assess knowledge/teach patient appropriate use, interventions to reduce side effects, and adverse symptoms to report.

Patient Education: Take exactly as directed; do not increase dose or frequency. Drug may cause physical and/or psychological dependence. Do not use alcohol or other prescription or OTC medications (especially pain medications, sedatives, antihistamines, or hypnotics) without consulting prescriber. Maintain adequate hydration (2-3 L/day of fluids) unless instructed to restrict fluid intake. You may experience drowsiness, lightheadedness, impaired coordination, dizziness, or blurred vision (use caution when driving or engaging in tasks requiring alertness until response to drug is known); nausea, vomiting, or dry mouth (small frequent meals, frequent mouth care, chewing gum, or sucking lozenges may help); or diarrhea (boiled milk, yogurt, or buttermilk may help). Report persistent CNS effects, skin rash or irritation, changes in urinary pattern, wheezing or respiratory difficulty, or worsening of condition. **Pregnancy/breast-feeding precautions:** Do not get pregnant while taking this medication; use appropriate contraceptive measures. Breast-feeding is not recommended.

Geriatric Considerations: Meprobamate is not considered a drug of choice in the elderly because of its potential to cause physical and psychological dependence. Interpretive guidelines from the Centers for Medicare and Medicaid Services (CMS) strongly discourage the use of meprobamate in residents of long-term care facilities.

Pregnancy Risk Factor: D

Lactation: Enters breast milk/not recommended

Breast-Feeding Issues: Breast milk concentrations are higher than plasma; effects are unknown.

Additional Information Withdrawal should be gradual over 1-2 weeks. Benzodiazepine and buspirone are better choices for treatment of anxiety disorders.

Related Information

Anxiolytic / Hypnotic Use in Long-Term Care Facilities *on page 1769*

Federal OBRA Regulations: Recommended Maximum Doses *on page 1773*

♦ **Meprobamate and Aspirin** *see Aspirin and Meprobamate* *on page 147*

♦ **Mepron®** *see Atovaquone* *on page 154*

Mequinol and Tretinoin (ME kwi nole & TRET i noyn)

U.S. Brand Names Solagé™

Synonyms Tretinoin and Mequinol

Generic Available No

Pharmacologic Category Retinoic Acid Derivative; Vitamin A Derivative; Vitamin, Topical

Use Treatment of solar lentigines; the efficacy of using Solagé™ daily for >24 weeks has not been established. The local cutaneous safety of Solagé™ in non-Caucasians has not been adequately established.

(Continued)

Mequinol and Tretinoin *(Continued)*

Dosing

Adults & Elderly: Solar lentigines: Topical: Apply twice daily to solar lentigines using the applicator tip while avoiding application to the surrounding skin. Separate application by at least 8 hours or as directed by physician.

Available Dosage Forms Liquid, topical: Mequinol 2% and tretinoin 0.01% (30 mL) [contains alcohol 78%; dispensed in applicator bottle]

Monitoring and Teaching Issues

Physical Assessment: Assess effectiveness and interactions of other medications. Monitor effectiveness of therapy and adverse effects at beginning of therapy and regularly with long-term use. Assess knowledge/teach patient appropriate use, possible side effects/interventions, and adverse symptoms to report. **Pregnancy risk factor X:** Determine that patient is not pregnant before beginning treatment and do not give to women of child-bearing age unless female is capable of complying with contraceptive measures 1 month prior to therapy, during therapy, and 1 month following therapy.

Patient Education: Use exactly as directed (use applicator tip, avoid application to surrounding skin, eyes, mouth, nose creases, or mucous membranes. Separate applications by at least 8 hours. Wait 30 minutes after application before applying make-up and do not bath or shower for 6 hours after application). Do not use more frequently than recommended. Do not use other vitamin A topical products; limit vitamin A intake. Avoid topical products with skin drying effects (eg, those containing alcohol, astringents, spices, lime, medicated soaps or shampoos, permanent wave solutions, depilatories or other hair removal products). You will be very sensitive to direct sunlight or sunlamps (use sunscreen, wear protective clothing and eyewear, and avoid direct exposure to sunlight or sunlamps). You may experience stinging, burning, or irritation after application. If skin reactions are severe or persistent, discontinue use and contact prescriber. **Pregnancy/breast-feeding precautions:** Inform prescriber if you are pregnant. Do not get pregnant 1 month before, during, or for 1 month following therapy. Consult prescriber for instruction on appropriate contraceptive measures. This drug may cause severe fetal defects. Do not donate blood during or for 1 month following therapy (same reason). Consult prescriber if breast-feeding.

Pregnancy Risk Factor: X

Lactation: Excretion in breast milk unknown/use caution

Related Information

Tretinoin (Oral) *on page 1514*
Tretinoin (Topical) *on page 1516*

Mercaptopurine *(mer kap toe PYOOR een)*

U.S. Brand Names Purinethol®

Synonyms 6-Mercaptopurine; 6-MP; NSC-755

Restrictions Note: I.V. formulation is not commercially available in the U.S.

Generic Available Yes

Pharmacologic Category Antineoplastic Agent, Antimetabolite

Medication Safety Issues

Sound-alike/look-alike issues:
Purinethol® may be confused with propylthiouracil

To avoid potentially serious dosage errors, the terms "6-mercaptopurine" or "6-MP" should be avoided; use of these terms has been associated with sixfold overdosages.

Use Treatment (maintenance and induction) of acute lymphoblastic leukemia (ALL)

Mechanism of Action/Effect Purine antagonist which inhibits DNA and RNA synthesis

Contraindications Hypersensitivity to mercaptopurine or any component of the formulation; patients whose disease showed prior resistance to mercaptopurine or thioguanine; severe liver disease, severe bone marrow suppression; pregnancy

Warnings/Precautions The U.S. Food and Drug Administration (FDA) currently recommends that procedures for proper handling and disposal of antineoplastic agents be considered. Mercaptopurine is potentially carcinogenic, and may be teratogenic; use with caution in patients with prior bone marrow suppression. Common signs of infection, such as fever and leukocytosis may not occur; lethargy and confusion may be more prominent signs of infection. Use caution with other hepatotoxic drugs or in dosages >2.5 mg/kg/day; hepatotoxicity may occur. Patients with genetic deficiency of thiopurine methyltransferase (TPMT) or concurrent therapy with drugs which may inhibit TPMT (eg, olsalazine) or xanthine oxidase (eg, allopurinol) may be sensitive to myelosuppressive effects.

To avoid potentially serious dosage errors, the terms "6-mercaptopurine" or "6-MP" should be avoided; use of these terms has been associated with sixfold overdosages.

Drug Interactions

Decreased Effect: Mercaptopurine inhibits the anticoagulation effect of warfarin by an unknown mechanism.

Increased Effect/Toxicity: Allopurinol can cause increased levels of mercaptopurine by inhibition of xanthine oxidase. Decrease dose of mercaptopurine by 75% when both drugs are used concomitantly. Seen only with oral mercaptopurine usage, not with I.V. May potentiate effect of bone marrow suppression (reduce mercaptopurine to 25% of dose). Synergistic liver toxicity between doxorubicin and mercaptopurine has been reported. Any agent which could potentially alter the metabolic function of the liver could produce higher drug levels and greater toxicities from either mercaptopurine or thioguanine (6-TG). Aminosalicylates (eg, olsalazine, mesalamine, sulfasalazine) may inhibit TPMT, increasing toxicity/myelosuppression of mercaptopurine.

Adverse Reactions

>10%:
Hematologic: Myelosuppression; leukopenia, thrombocytopenia, anemia
Onset: 7-10 days
Nadir: 14-16 days
Recovery: 21-28 days

Hepatic: Intrahepatic cholestasis and focal centralobular necrosis (40%), characterized by hyperbilirubinemia, increased alkaline phosphatase and AST, jaundice, ascites, encephalopathy; more common at doses >2.5 mg/kg/day. Usually occurs within 2 months of therapy but may occur within 1 week, or be delayed up to 8 years.

1% to 10%:

Central nervous system: Drug fever

Dermatologic: Hyperpigmentation, rash

Endocrine & metabolic: Hyperuricemia

Gastrointestinal: Nausea, vomiting, diarrhea, stomatitis, anorexia, stomach pain, mucositis

Renal: Renal toxicity

Overdosage/Toxicology Symptoms of overdose include nausea and vomiting (immediate); bone marrow suppression, hepatic necrosis, and gastroenteritis (delayed). Treatment is supportive. Efforts to minimize absorption (charcoal, gastric lavage) may be ineffective unless instituted within 60 minutes of ingestion.

Pharmacodynamics/Kinetics

Absorption: Variable and incomplete (16% to 50%)

Time to Peak: Serum: ~2 hours

Protein Binding: 19%

Half-Life Elimination: Age dependent: Children: 21 minutes; Adults: 47 minutes

Metabolism: Hepatic and via GI mucosa; hepatically via xanthine oxidase and methylation via TPMT to sulfate conjugates, 6-thiouric acid, and other inactive compounds; first-pass effect

Excretion: Urine; following high (1 g/m^2) I.V. doses, 20% to 40% as unchanged urine; at lower doses renal elimination minor

Dosing

Adults: Antineoplastic: Refer to individual protocols.

Induction: Oral: 2.5-5 mg/kg/day (100-200 mg)

Maintenance: Oral: 1.5-2.5 mg/kg/day **or** 80-100 mg/m^2/day given once daily

Note: In ALL, administration in the evening (vs morning administration) may lower the risk of relapse.

Dosage adjustment with concurrent allopurinol: Reduce mercaptopurine dosage to $\frac{1}{3}$ to $\frac{1}{2}$ the usual dose.

Dosage adjustment in TPMT-deficiency: Not established; substantial reductions are generally required only in homozygous deficiency.

Elderly: Due to renal decline with age, start with lower recommended doses for adults.

Pediatrics: Antineoplastic: Refer to individual protocols: Oral:

Induction: 2.5-5 mg/kg/day **or** 70-100 mg/m^2/day given once daily

Maintenance: 1.5-2.5 mg/kg/day **or** 50-75 mg/m^2/day given once daily

Note: In ALL, administration in the evening (vs morning administration) may lower the risk of relapse.

Renal Impairment: Dose should be reduced to avoid accumulation, but specific guidelines are not available.

Hemodialysis: Removed; supplemental dosing is usually required

Hepatic Impairment: Dose should be reduced to avoid accumulation, but specific guidelines are not available.

Available Dosage Forms Tablet [scored]: 50 mg

Monitoring and Teaching Issues

Physical Assessment: See Warnings/Precautions for specific use cautions (eg, do not use the terms "6-mercaptopurine" or "6-MP" when writing prescriptions; use of these terms has been associated with sixfold overdosage). Assess potential for interactions with other pharmacological agents patient may be taking (increased potential for liver toxicity or mercaptopurine toxicity; see Drug Interactions). Assess results of laboratory tests and adverse response on a regular basis and periodically following treatment (eg, hepatic function [jaundice, ascites, encephalopathy can occur some time following therapy], nutritional status [dehydration], myelosuppression [anemia, leukopenia], and renal status; see Adverse Reactions). Teach patient proper use, possible side effects/appropriate interventions (eg, importance of adequate hydration), and adverse symptoms to report (see Patient Education).

Monitoring Laboratory Tests: CBC with differential, platelet count, liver function, uric acid, renal function

Patient Education: Do not take any new medication during therapy unless approved by prescriber. Take daily oral dose at the same time each day. Preferable to take on an empty stomach, 1 hour before or 2 hours after meals. Maintain adequate hydration (2-3 L/day of fluids) unless instructed to restrict fluid intake. You may be more susceptible to infection (avoid crowds and exposure to infection and do not have any vaccinations without consulting prescriber). May cause nausea and vomiting, diarrhea, or loss of appetite (small frequent meals may help/request medication); weakness or lethargy (use caution when driving or engaging in tasks that require alertness until response to drug is known); mouth sores; or headache (consult prescriber for approved medications). Report signs of persistent fever; opportunistic infection (eg, fever, chills, sore throat, burning urination, fatigue); bleeding (eg, tarry stools, easy bruising); unresolved mouth sores; nausea or vomiting; swelling of extremities; respiratory difficulty; unusual weight gain; or changes in urinary pattern. **Pregnancy/breast-feeding precautions:** Inform prescriber if you are pregnant. Do not get pregnant while taking this medication. Consult prescriber for appropriate contraceptive measures. Do not breast-feed.

Dietary Considerations: Should not be administered with meals.

Geriatric Considerations: Toxicity to immunosuppressives is increased in the elderly. Start with lowest recommended adult doses. Signs of infection, such as fever and WBC rise, may not occur. Lethargy and confusion may be more prominent signs of infection.

(Continued)

Mercaptopurine *(Continued)*

Pregnancy Risk Factor: D
Lactation: Enters breast milk/contraindicated
Administration
I.V.: Administer by slow I.V. continuous infusion.
Reconstitution: Further dilute the 10 mg/mL reconstituted solution in normal saline or D_5W to a final concentration for administration of 1-2 mg/mL.
Storage: Store at room temperature.

♦ **6-Mercaptopurine** *see* Mercaptopurine *on page 954*
♦ **Mercapturic Acid** *see* Acetylcysteine *on page 45*
♦ **Meridia®** *see* Sibutramine *on page 1371*

Meropenem *(mer oh PEN em)*

U.S. Brand Names Merrem® I.V.
Generic Available No
Pharmacologic Category Antibiotic, Carbapenem
Use Intra-abdominal infections (complicated appendicitis and peritonitis) caused by viridans group streptococci, *E. coli*, *K. pneumoniae*, *P. aeruginosa*, *B. fragilis*, *B. thetaiotaomicron*, and *Peptostreptococcus* sp; also indicated for bacterial meningitis in pediatric patients >3 months of age caused by *S. pneumoniae*, *H. influenzae*, and *N. meningitidis*; meropenem has also been used to treat soft tissue infections, febrile neutropenia, and urinary tract infections
Mechanism of Action/Effect Inhibits cell wall synthesis in susceptible bacteria
Contraindications Hypersensitivity to meropenem, any component of the formulation, or other carbapenems (eg, imipenem); patients who have experienced anaphylactic reactions to other beta-lactams
Warnings/Precautions Pseudomembranous colitis and hypersensitivity reactions have occurred and often require immediate drug discontinuation. Thrombocytopenia has been reported in patients with significant renal dysfunction. Seizures have occurred in patients with underlying neurologic disorders (less frequent than with Primaxin®). Safety and efficacy have not been established for children <3 months of age. Superinfection possible with long courses of therapy.
Drug Interactions
Decreased Effect: Meropenem may decrease valproic acid serum concentrations to subtherapeutic levels.
Lab Interactions Increased SGPT, SGOT, alkaline phosphatase, LDH, bilirubin, platelets, eosinophils, BUN, creatinine; decreased platelets, hemoglobin/hematocrit, WBC; prolonged or shortened PT; prolonged PTT; positive direct or indirect Coombs' test; presence of urine red blood cells
Adverse Reactions 1% to 10%:
Central nervous system: Headache (2%)
Dermatologic: Rash (2% to 3%, includes diaper-area moniliasis in pediatrics), pruritus (1%)
Gastrointestinal: Diarrhea (4% to 5%), nausea/vomiting (1% to 4%), constipation (1%), oral moniliasis (up to 2% in pediatric patients), glossitis
Local: Inflammation at the injection site (2%), phlebitis/thrombophlebitis (1%), injection site reaction (1%)
Respiratory: Apnea (1%)
Miscellaneous: Sepsis (2%), septic shock (1%)
Overdosage/Toxicology No cases of acute overdose with resultant symptoms have been reported. Supportive therapy is recommended. Meropenem and metabolite are removable by dialysis.
Pharmacodynamics/Kinetics
Time to Peak: Tissue: 1 hour following infusion
Protein Binding: 2%
Half-Life Elimination:
Normal renal function: 1-1.5 hours
Cl_{cr} 30-80 mL/minute: 1.9-3.3 hours
Cl_{cr} 2-30 mL/minute: 3.82-5.7 hours
Metabolism: Hepatic; metabolized to open beta-lactam form (inactive)
Excretion: Urine (~25% as inactive metabolites)
Dosing
Adults & Elderly:
Susceptible infections: I.V.: 1 g every 8 hours
Pediatrics:
Intra-abdominal infections: I.V.:
Children >3 months (<50 kg): 20 mg/kg every 8 hours (maximum dose: 1 g every 8 hours)
Children >50 kg: 1 g every 8 hours
Meningitis: I.V.:
Children >3 months (<50 kg): 40 mg/kg every 8 hours (maximum dose: 2 g every 8 hours)
Children >50 kg: 2 g every 8 hours
Renal Impairment:
Cl_{cr} 26-50 mL/minute: Administer 1 g every 12 hours.
Cl_{cr} 10-25 mL/minute: Administer 500 mg every 12 hours.
Cl_{cr} <10 mL/minute: Administer 500 mg every 24 hours.
Meropenem and its metabolites are readily dialyzable.
Continuous arteriovenous hemofiltration: Dose as for Cl_{cr} 10-50 mL/minute.
Available Dosage Forms Injection, powder for reconstitution: 500 mg [contains sodium 45.1 mg as sodium carbonate (1.96 mEq)]; 1 g [contains sodium 90.2 mg as sodium carbonate (3.92 mEq)]

Monitoring and Teaching Issues

Physical Assessment: Assess results of culture and sensitivity tests and patient's allergy history prior to beginning treatment. Use caution in presence of renal impairment or neurologic disorder (see Warnings/Precautions for use cautions). See Administration for infusion specifics. Infusion site should be monitored closely to prevent phlebitis/thrombophlebitis. Assess renal and hepatic function and CBC, therapeutic effectiveness (resolution of infection), and adverse reactions (see Adverse Reactions). Teach patient proper use (according to formulation), possible side effects/appropriate interventions (eg, importance of adequate hydration), and adverse symptoms to report (refer to Patient Education).

Monitoring Laboratory Tests: Perform culture and sensitivity testing prior to initiating therapy. Monitor renal function, liver function, CBC.

Patient Education: This medication can only be given by infusion; report immediately any burning, pain, swelling, or redness at infusion site. Maintain adequate hydration (2-3 L/day of fluids) unless instructed to restrict fluid intake. May cause nausea or vomiting (small frequent meals, frequent mouth care, chewing gum, or sucking lozenges may help); diarrhea (boiled milk, buttermilk, or yogurt may help); or headache. Report persistent GI distress, diarrhea, mouth sores, respiratory difficulty, headache, or CNS changes (agitation, delirium). **Breast-feeding precaution:** Consult prescriber if breast-feeding.

Dietary Considerations: 1 g of meropenem contains 90.2 mg of sodium as sodium carbonate (3.92 mEq)

Geriatric Considerations: Adjust dose based on renal function.

Pregnancy Risk Factor: B

Lactation: Excretion in breast milk unknown/use caution

Breast-Feeding Issues: Although no teratogenic or infant harm has been found in studies, excretion in breast milk is not known and this drug should be used during lactation only if clearly indicated.

Administration

I.V.: Administer I.V. infusion over 15-30 minutes; I.V. bolus injection over 3-5 minutes.

Reconstitution: Meropenem infusion vials reconstituted with sodium chloride are stable for up to 2 hours at room temperature or for 18 hours refrigerated; reconstituted with dextrose 5% injections are stable for 1 hour at room temperature and 8 hours refrigerated. Mini bags with normal saline are stable for up to 24 hours refrigerated; with dextrose stable for 6 hours.

Compatibility:

Y-site administration: Incompatible with amphotericin B, diazepam, metronidazole

Compatibility when admixed: Incompatible with amphotericin B, metronidazole, multivitamins

Storage: Dry powder should be stored at controlled room temperature 20°C to 25°C (68°F to 77°F).

Related Information

Antimicrobial Drugs of Choice *on page 1792*
Community-Acquired Pneumonia in Adults *on page 1807*

♦ **Merrem® I.V.** *see* Meropenem *on page 956*

♦ **Meruvax® II** *see page 1660*

Mesalamine *(me SAL a meen)*

U.S. Brand Names Asacol®; Canasa™; Pentasa®; Rowasa®

Synonyms 5-Aminosalicylic Acid; Fisalamine; Mesalazine

Generic Available Yes: Rectal suspension

Pharmacologic Category 5-Aminosalicylic Acid Derivative

Medication Safety Issues

Sound-alike/look-alike issues:

Mesalamine may be confused with mecamylamine

Asacol® may be confused with Ansaid®, Os-Cal®

Use

Oral: Treatment and maintenance of remission of mildly to moderately active ulcerative colitis

Rectal: Treatment of active mild to moderate distal ulcerative colitis, proctosigmoiditis, or proctitis

Mechanism of Action/Effect Mesalamine (5-aminosalicylic acid) is the active component of sulfasalazine; the specific mechanism of action of mesalamine is unknown; however, it is thought that it modulates local chemical mediators of the inflammatory response, especially leukotrienes; action appears topical rather than systemic

Contraindications Hypersensitivity to mesalamine, sulfasalazine, salicylates, or any component of the formulation; Canasa™ suppositories contain saturated vegetable fatty acid esters (contraindicated in patients with allergy to these components)

Warnings/Precautions May cause an acute intolerance syndrome. Pericarditis should be considered in patients with chest pain; pancreatitis should be considered in patients with new abdominal complaints. Use with caution in patients with impaired hepatic or renal function. Postmarketing reports suggest an increased incidence of blood dyscrasias in patients >65 years of age. In addition, elderly may have difficulty administering and retaining rectal suppositories and decreased renal function; use with caution and monitor. Safety and efficacy in pediatric patients have not been established.

Rowasa® enema: Contains potassium metabisulfite; may cause anaphylactic reactions in patients with sulfite allergies.

Drug Interactions

Decreased Effect: Decreased digoxin bioavailability.

Increased Effect/Toxicity: Mesalamine may increase the risk of myelosuppression from azathioprine, mercaptopurine, and thioguanine.

Nutritional/Ethanol Interactions Food: Oral: Mesalamine serum levels may be decreased if taken with food.

(Continued)

Mesalamine *(Continued)*

Adverse Reactions Adverse effects vary depending upon dosage form. Effects as reported with tablets, unless otherwise noted:

>10%:

Central nervous system: Headache (suppository 14%), pain (14%)

Gastrointestinal: Abdominal pain (18%; enema 8%)

Genitourinary: Eructation (16%)

Respiratory: Pharyngitis (11%)

1% to 10%:

Cardiovascular: Chest pain (3%), peripheral edema (3%)

Central nervous system: Chills (3%), dizziness (suppository 3%), fever (enema 3%; suppository 1%), insomnia (2%), malaise (2%)

Dermatologic: Rash (6%; suppository 1%), pruritus (3%; enema 1%), acne (2%; suppository 1%)

Gastrointestinal: Abdominal pain (enema 8%; suppository 5%), colitis exacerbation (3%; suppository 1%), constipation (5%), diarrhea (suppository 3%), dyspepsia (6%), flatulence (enema 6%; suppository 5%), hemorrhoids (enema 1%), nausea (capsule/suppository 3%), nausea and vomiting (capsule 1%), rectal pain (enema 1%; suppository 2%), vomiting (5%)

Local: Pain on insertion of enema tip (enema 1%)

Neuromuscular & skeletal: Back pain (7%; enema 1%), arthralgia (5%), hypertonia (5%), myalgia (3%), arthritis (2%), leg/joint pain (enema 2%)

Ocular: Conjunctivitis (2%)

Respiratory: Flu-like syndrome (3%; enema 5%), cough increased (2%)

Miscellaneous: Diaphoresis (3%)

Overdosage/Toxicology Symptoms of overdose include decreased motor activity, diarrhea, vomiting, and renal function impairment. Treatment is supportive; emesis, gastric lavage, and follow with activated charcoal slurry.

Pharmacodynamics/Kinetics

Absorption: Rectal: Variable and dependent upon retention time, underlying GI disease, and colonic pH; Oral: Tablet: ~28%, Capsule: ~20% to 30%

Time to Peak: Serum: 4-7 hours

Half-Life Elimination: 5-ASA: 0.5-1.5 hours; acetyl-5-ASA: 5-10 hours

Metabolism: Hepatic and via GI tract to acetyl-5-aminosalicylic acid

Excretion: Urine (as metabolites); feces (<2%)

Dosing

Adults & Elderly:

Treatment of ulcerative colitis: Oral:

Capsule: 1 g 4 times/day

Tablet: 800 mg 3 times/day for 6 weeks

Maintenance of remission of ulcerative colitis: Oral:

Capsule: 1 g 4 times/day

Tablet: 1.6 g/day in divided doses

Distal ulcerative colitis, proctosigmoiditis, or proctitis: Rectal: Retention enema: 60 mL (4 g) at bedtime, retained overnight, approximately 8 hours

Active ulcerative proctitis: Rectal: Rectal suppository (Canasa™):

500 mg: Insert 1 suppository in rectum twice daily; may increase to 3 times/day if inadequate response is seen after 2 weeks

1000 mg: Insert 1 suppository in rectum daily at bedtime

Note: Suppositories should be retained for at least 1-3 hours to achieve maximum benefit.

Note: Some patients may require rectal and oral therapy concurrently.

Available Dosage Forms

Capsule, controlled release (Pentasa®): 250 mg

Suppository, rectal (Canasa™): 500 mg, 1000 mg [contains saturated vegetable fatty acid esters]

Suspension, rectal: 4 g/60 mL (7s) [contains potassium metabisulfite and sodium benzoate]

Rowasa®: 4 g/60 mL (7s, 28s) [contains potassium metabisulfite and sodium benzoate]

Tablet, delayed release [enteric coated] (Asacol®): 400 mg

Monitoring and Teaching Issues

Physical Assessment: Assess history of allergies prior to beginning treatment (eg, can cause anaphylactic reaction if patient is allergic to sulfites; see Contraindications). Use caution in presence of impaired hepatic or renal function (see Warnings/Precautions). Assess CBC and renal function regularly. Monitor therapeutic effectiveness (reduction of symptoms of colitis) and adverse reactions (eg, rash, edema, colitis exacerbation, decreased motor function; see Adverse Reactions). Teach patient proper use (according to formulation), possible side effects/appropriate interventions (eg, importance of adequate hydration), and adverse symptoms to report (see Patient Education).

Monitoring Laboratory Tests: CBC and renal function, particularly in elderly patients

Patient Education: Do not take any new medication during therapy unless approved by prescriber. Take as directed.

Oral: Do not chew or break tablets or capsules. Notify prescriber if whole or partial tablets are repeatedly found in stool.

Enemas: Shake well before using, retain for 8 hours or as long as possible. May cause staining of clothing and undergarments.

Suppository: Do not refrigerate. After removing foil wrapper, insert high in rectum without excessive handling (warmth will melt suppository). Retain suppositories for at least 1-3 hours to achieve maximum benefit. Report severe abdominal pain, unresolved diarrhea, jaundice, severe headache, any unusual pain (back, joint, muscle, swelling of extremities, or chest pain). May cause staining of clothing, undergarments; lubricating gel may be used if needed to assist insertion.

Enema and suppository: May cause staining of clothing, undergarments; lubricating gel may be used if needed to assist insertion.

Breast-feeding precaution: Consult prescriber if breast-feeding.

Dietary Considerations: Canasa™ rectal suppository contains saturated vegetable fatty acid esters.

Geriatric Considerations: Elderly may have difficulty administering and retaining rectal suppositories. Given renal function decline with aging, monitor serum creatinine often during therapy.

Pregnancy Risk Factor: B

Lactation: Excretion in breast milk unknown/use caution

Breast-Feeding Issues: Adverse effects (diarrhea) in a nursing infant have been reported while the mother received rectal administration of mesalamine within 12 hours after the first dose. The AAP recommends to monitor the infant stool for consistency and to use with caution.

Administration

Oral: Swallow capsules or tablets whole, do not chew or crush.

Other:

Rectal enema: Shake bottle well. Retain enemas for 8 hours or as long as practical.

Suppository: Remove foil wrapper; avoid excessive handling. Should be retained for at least 1-3 hours to achieve maximum benefit.

Storage:

Enema: Store at controlled room temperature. Use promptly once foil wrap is removed; contents may darken with time (do not use if dark brown)

Suppository: Store at controlled room temperature away from direct heat, light, and humidity; do not refrigerate

Tablet: Store at controlled room temperature

♦ **Mesalazine** *see* Mesalamine *on page 957*

Mesna (MES na)

U.S. Brand Names Mesnex®

Synonyms Sodium 2-Mercaptoethane Sulfonate

Generic Available Yes

Pharmacologic Category Antidote

Use Orphan drug: Prevention of hemorrhagic cystitis induced by ifosfamide

Unlabeled/Investigational Use Prevention of hemorrhagic cystitis induced by cyclophosphamide

Mechanism of Action/Effect Binds with and detoxifies urotoxic metabolites of ifosfamide and cyclophosphamide to prevent hemorrhagic cystitis induced by ifosfamide and cyclophosphamide

Contraindications Hypersensitivity to mesna or other thiol compounds, or any component of the formulation

Warnings/Precautions Examine morning urine specimen for hematuria prior to ifosfamide or cyclophosphamide treatment; if hematuria (>50 RBC/HPF) develops, reduce the ifosfamide/cyclophosphamide dose or discontinue the drug; will not prevent or alleviate other toxicities associated with ifosfamide or cyclophosphamide and will not prevent hemorrhagic cystitis in all patients. Allergic reactions have been reported; patients with autoimmune disorders may be at increased risk. Symptoms ranged from mild hypersensitivity to systemic anaphylactic reactions. I.V. formulation contains benzyl alcohol; do not use in neonates or infants.

Drug Interactions

Decreased Effect: Warfarin: Questionable alterations in coagulation control.

Lab Interactions False-positive urinary ketones with Multistix® or Labstix®

Adverse Reactions It is difficult to distinguish reactions from those caused by concomitant chemotherapy.

>10%: Gastrointestinal: Bad taste in mouth with oral administration (100%), vomiting (secondary to the bad taste after oral administration, or with high I.V. doses)

Pharmacodynamics/Kinetics

Bioavailability: Oral: 45% to 79%

Time to Peak: Plasma: 2-3 hours

Protein Binding: 69% to 75%

Half-Life Elimination: Parent drug: 24 minutes; Mesna disulfide: 72 minutes

Metabolism: Rapidly oxidized intravascularly to mesna disulfide; mesna disulfide is reduced in renal tubules back to mesna following glomerular filtration.

Excretion: Urine; as unchanged drug (18% to 26%) and metabolites

Dosing

Adults & Elderly: Prevention of toxicity: Refer to individual protocols.

I.V.: Recommended dose is 60% of the ifosfamide dose given in 3 divided doses (0, 4, and 8 hours after the start of ifosfamide)

Note: Alternative I.V. regimens include 80% of the ifosfamide dose given in 4 divided doses (0, 3, 6, and 9 hours after the start of ifosfamide) and continuous infusions

I.V./Oral: Recommended dose is 100% of the ifosfamide dose, given as 20% of the ifosfamide dose I.V. at hour 0, followed by 40% of the ifosfamide dose given orally 2 and 6 hours after start of ifosfamide

Pediatrics: Refer to adult dosing.

Available Dosage Forms

Injection, solution: 100 mg/mL (10 mL) [contains benzyl alcohol]

Tablet: 400 mg

Monitoring and Teaching Issues

Physical Assessment: Monitor laboratory results and assess frequently for hematuria/bladder hemorrhage.

Monitoring Laboratory Tests: Urinalysis

Patient Education: This drug is given to help prevent side effects of other chemotherapeutic agents you are taking. Report blood in urine. **Breast-feeding precaution:** Do not breast-feed.

(Continued)

Mesna *(Continued)*

Pregnancy Risk Factor: B

Lactation: Excretion in breast milk unknown/not recommended

Administration

Oral: Administer orally in tablet formulation or parenteral solution diluted in water, milk, juice, or carbonated beverages; patients who vomit within 2 hours of taking oral mesna should repeat the dose or receive I.V. mesna

I.V.: Administer by short (15-30 minutes) infusion or continuous (24 hour) infusion

Reconstitution: Dilute in 50-1000 mL NS, D_5W, or lactated Ringer's.

Compatibility: Stable in $D_5^1/_4NS$, $D_5^1/_3NS$, $D_5^1/_2NS$, D_5W, LR, NS

Y-site administration: Incompatible with amphotericin B cholesteryl sulfate complex

Compatibility in syringe: Incompatible with ifosfamide/epirubicin

Compatibility when admixed: Incompatible with carboplatin, cisplatin, ifosfamide/epirubicin

Storage: Store intact vials and tablets at controlled room temperature of 20°C to 25°C (68°F to 77°F). Opened multidose vials may be stored and used for use to 8 days after opening. Infusion solutions diluted in D_5W or lactated Ringer's are stable for at least 48 hours at room temperature. Solutions in NS are stable for at least 24 hours at room temperature. Solutions in plastic syringes are stable for 9 days under refrigeration, or at room or body temperature. Stability in syringes decreases if air is in the filled syringe. Solutions of mesna and ifosfamide in lactated Ringer's are stable for 7 days in a PVC ambulatory infusion pump reservoir. Mesna injection is stable for at least 7 days when diluted 1:2 or 1:5 with grape- and orange-flavored syrups or 11:1 to 1:100 in carbonated beverages for oral administration.

Additional Information A parenteral formulation without benzyl alcohol can be requested directly from the manufacturer.

♦ Mesnex® *see* Mesna *on page 959*

Mesoridazine *(mez oh RID a zeen)*

U.S. Brand Names Serentil® [DSC]

Synonyms Mesoridazine Besylate

Generic Available No

Pharmacologic Category Antipsychotic Agent, Typical, Phenothiazine

Medication Safety Issues

Sound-alike/look-alike issues:

Serentil® may be confused with selegiline, Serevent®, Seroquel®, sertraline, Serzone®, Sinequan®, Surgicel®

Use Management of schizophrenic patients who fail to respond adequately to treatment with other antipsychotic drugs, either because of insufficient effectiveness or the inability to achieve an effective dose due to intolerable adverse effects from these drugs

Unlabeled/Investigational Use Psychosis

Mechanism of Action/Effect Mesoridazine is a piperidine phenothiazine antipsychotic which blocks of postsynaptic CNS dopamine$_2$ receptors in the mesolimbic and mesocortical areas

Contraindications Hypersensitivity to mesoridazine or any component of the formulation (cross-reactivity between phenothiazines may occur); severe CNS depression and coma; prolonged QT interval (>450 msec), including prolongation due to congenital causes; history of arrhythmias; concurrent use of medications which prolong QT_c (including type Ia and type III antiarrhythmics, cyclic antidepressants, some fluoroquinolones, cisapride)

Warnings/Precautions Has been shown to prolong QT_c interval in a dose-dependent manner (associated with an increased risk of torsade de pointes). Patients should have a baseline ECG prior to initiation, and should not receive mesoridazine if baseline QT_c >450 msec. Mesoridazine should be discontinued in patients with a QT_c interval >500 msec. Potassium levels must be evaluated and normalized prior to and throughout treatment.

May cause hypotension, particularly with I.M. administration. Highly sedating, use with caution in disorders where CNS depression is a feature. Use with caution in Parkinson's disease. Caution in patients with hemodynamic instability; bone marrow suppression; predisposition to seizures; subcortical brain damage; severe cardiac, hepatic, renal, or respiratory disease. Esophageal dysmotility and aspiration have been associated with antipsychotic use; use with caution in patients at risk of pneumonia (ie, Alzheimer's disease). Caution in breast cancer or other prolactin-dependent tumors (may elevate prolactin levels). May alter temperature regulation or mask toxicity of other drugs due to antiemetic effects. May cause orthostatic hypotension - use with caution in patients at risk of this effect or those who would tolerate transient hypotensive episodes (cerebrovascular disease, cardiovascular disease, or other medications which may predispose).

Phenothiazines may cause anticholinergic effects (confusion, agitation, constipation, xerostomia, blurred vision, urinary retention). Therefore, they should be used with caution in patients with decreased gastrointestinal motility, urinary retention, BPH, xerostomia, or visual problems. Conditions which also may be exacerbated by cholinergic blockade include narrow-angle glaucoma (screening is recommended) and worsening of myasthenia gravis. Relative to other antipsychotics, mesoridazine has a high potency of cholinergic blockade.

May cause extrapyramidal symptoms, including pseudoparkinsonism, acute dystonic reactions, akathisia, and tardive dyskinesia (risk of these reactions is low relative to other neuroleptics). May be associated with neuroleptic malignant syndrome (NMS) or pigmentary retinopathy (particularly at doses >1 g/day).

Drug Interactions

Decreased Effect: Mesoridazine may inhibit the activity of bromocriptine and levodopa. Benztropine (and other anticholinergics) may inhibit the therapeutic response to mesoridazine and excess anticholinergic effects may occur. Mesoridazine and possibly other low potency antipsychotic may reverse the pressor effects of epinephrine.

Increased Effect/Toxicity: Use of mesoridazine with other agents known to prolong QT_c may increase the risk of malignant arrhythmias; concurrent use is contraindicated - includes type I and type III antiarrhythmics, TCAs, and some quinolone antibiotics (sparfloxacin, moxifloxacin, gatifloxacin). Mesoridazine may increase the effect and/or toxicity of antihypertensives, anticholinergics, lithium, CNS depressants (ethanol, narcotics), and trazodone. Metoclopramide may increase risk of extrapyramidal symptoms (EPS).

Nutritional/Ethanol Interactions

Ethanol: Avoid ethanol (may increase CNS depression).

Herb/Nutraceutical: Avoid valerian, St John's wort, kava kava, gotu kola (may increase CNS depression).

Lab Interactions Increased cholesterol (S), glucose; decreased uric acid (S)

Adverse Reactions Frequency not defined.

Cardiovascular: Hypotension, orthostatic hypotension, tachycardia, QT prolongation (dose dependent, up to 100% of patients at higher dosages), syncope, edema

Central nervous system: Pseudoparkinsonism, akathisia, dystonias, tardive dyskinesia, dizziness, drowsiness, restlessness, ataxia, slurred speech, neuroleptic malignant syndrome (NMS), impairment of temperature regulation, lowering of seizure threshold

Dermatologic: Increased sensitivity to sun, rash, itching, angioneurotic edema, dermatitis, discoloration of skin (blue-gray)

Endocrine & metabolic: Changes in menstrual cycle, libido (changes in), gynecomastia, lactation, galactorrhea

Gastrointestinal: Constipation, xerostomia, weight gain, nausea, vomiting, stomach pain

Genitourinary: Difficulty in urination, ejaculatory disturbances, impotence, enuresis, incontinence, priapism, urinary retention

Hematologic: Agranulocytosis, leukopenia, eosinophilia, thrombocytopenia, anemia, aplastic anemia

Hepatic: Cholestatic jaundice, hepatotoxicity

Neuromuscular & skeletal: Weakness, tremor, rigidity

Ocular: Pigmentary retinopathy, photophobia, blurred vision, cornea and lens changes

Respiratory: Nasal congestion

Miscellaneous: Diaphoresis (decreased), lupus-like syndrome

Overdosage/Toxicology Symptoms of overdose include deep sleep, coma, extrapyramidal symptoms, abnormal involuntary muscle movements, and hypotension. Monitor for cardiac arrhythmias and avoid use of drugs which prolong QT interval. Treatment is symptomatic and supportive.

Pharmacodynamics/Kinetics

Duration of Action: 4-6 hours

Absorption: Tablet: Erratic; Liquid: More dependable

Time to Peak: Serum: 2-4 hours; Steady-state serum: 4-7 days

Protein Binding: 91% to 99%

Half-Life Elimination: 24-48 hours

Excretion: Urine

Dosing

Adults:

Schizophrenia/psychoses:

Oral: 25-50 mg 3 times/day; maximum: 100-400 mg/day

Note: Concentrate may be diluted just prior to administration with distilled water, acidified tap water, orange or grape juice. Do not prepare and store bulk dilutions.

I.M.: Initial: 25 mg, repeat in 30-60 minutes as needed; optimal dosage range: 25-200 mg/day

Elderly: Behavioral symptoms associated with dementia:

Oral: Initial: 10 mg 1-2 times/day; if <10 mg/day is desired, consider administering 10 mg every other day. Increase dose at 4- to 7-day intervals by 10-25 mg/day; increase dose intervals (eg, twice daily, 3 times/day) as necessary to control response or side effects. Maximum daily dose: 250 mg. Gradual increases (titration) may prevent some side effects or decrease their severity.

I.M.: Initial: 25 mg; repeat doses in 30-60 minutes if necessary. Dose range: 25-200 mg/day. Elderly usually require less than maximal daily dose.

Renal Impairment: Not dialyzable (0% to 5%)

Available Dosage Forms [DSC] = Discontinued product

Injection, solution, as besylate [DSC]: 25 mg/mL (1 mL)

Liquid, oral, as besylate [DSC]: 25 mg/mL (118 mL) [contains alcohol 0.61%]

Tablet, as besylate [DSC]: 10 mg, 25 mg, 50 mg, 100 mg

Monitoring and Teaching Issues

Physical Assessment: Assess other medications patient is taking for effectiveness and interactions. Review ophthalmic screening and monitor laboratory results, therapeutic effectiveness, and adverse reactions at beginning of therapy and periodically with long-term use. Monitor CNS status. With I.M. or I.V. use, monitor closely for hypotension. **Note:** Avoid skin contact with oral or injection medication; may cause contact dermatitis (wash immediately with warm, soapy water). Initiate at lower doses and taper dosage slowly when discontinuing. Assess knowledge/teach patient appropriate use, interventions to reduce side effects, and adverse symptoms to report.

Monitoring Laboratory Tests: Baseline potassium, baseline liver and kidney function, lipid profile, CBC prior to and periodically during therapy, fasting blood glucose/Hgb A_{1c}, baseline (and periodic) serum potassium; BMI; monitor hepatic function (especially if fever with flu-like symptoms); baseline (and periodic) ECG; do not initiate if QT_c >450 msec (discontinue in QT_c 500 msec)

Patient Education: Use exactly as directed; do not increase dose or frequency. It may take 2-3 weeks to achieve desired results; do not discontinue without consulting prescriber. Dilute oral concentration with water, orange or grape juice. Do not take within 2 hours of any antacid. Avoid alcohol or caffeine and other prescription or OTC medications not approved by prescriber. Maintain adequate hydration (2-3 L/day of fluids) unless instructed to restrict fluid intake. Avoid skin contact with medication; may cause contact dermatitis (wash immediately with warm, soapy water). You may experience excess drowsiness,

(Continued)

Mesoridazine *(Continued)*

restlessness, dizziness, or blurred vision (use caution driving or when engaging in tasks requiring alertness until response to drug is known); dry mouth, nausea, vomiting (small frequent meals, frequent mouth care, chewing gum, or sucking lozenges may help); constipation (increased exercise, fluids, fruit, or fiber may help); postural hypotension (use caution climbing stairs or when changing position from lying or sitting to standing); urinary retention (void before taking medication); photosensitivity (use sunscreen, wear protective clothing and eyewear, and avoid direct sunlight); decreased perspiration (avoid strenuous exercise in hot environments); or changes in menstrual cycle, libido, ejaculation (will resolve when medication is discontinued). Report persistent CNS effects (eg, trembling fingers, altered gait or balance, excessive sedation, seizures, unusual movements, anxiety, abnormal thoughts, confusion, personality changes); chest pain, palpitations, rapid heartbeat, severe dizziness; unresolved urinary retention or changes in urinary pattern; menstrual pattern, change in libido, swelling or pain in breasts (male or female); vision changes; skin rash or yellowing of skin; respiratory difficulty; or worsening of condition.

Pregnancy/breast-feeding precautions: Inform prescriber if you are or intend to become pregnant. Do not breast-feed.

Geriatric Considerations: (See Warnings/Precautions, Adverse Reactions, and Overdose/Toxicology.) Elderly patients have an increased risk of adverse response to side effects or adverse reactions to antipsychotics.

Pregnancy Risk Factor: C

Lactation: Enters breast milk/contraindicated (AAP rates "of concern")

Administration

Oral: Dilute oral concentrate just prior to administration with distilled water, acidified tap water, orange or grape juice. Do not prepare and store bulk dilutions. Do not mix oral solutions of mesoridazine and lithium, these oral liquids are incompatible when mixed. **Note:** Avoid skin contact with oral medication; may cause contact dermatitis.

I.M.: Watch for hypotension when administering I.M.

I.V.: Watch for hypotension when administering I.V.

Reconstitution: Solutions may be diluted or mixed with fruit juices or other liquids but must be administered immediately after mixing; do not prepare bulk dilutions or store bulk dilutions.

Storage: Protect all dosage forms from light; clear or slightly yellow solutions may be used; should be dispensed in amber or opaque vials/bottles.

Related Information

Antipsychotic Agents *on page 1717*
Antipsychotic Medication Guidelines *on page 1766*
Federal OBRA Regulations: Recommended Maximum Doses *on page 1773*

♦ **Mesoridazine Besylate** *see* Mesoridazine *on page 960*

♦ **Mestinon®** *see* Pyridostigmine *on page 1287*

♦ **Mestinon® Timespan®** *see* Pyridostigmine *on page 1287*

Mestranol and Norethindrone *(MES tra nole & nor eth IN drone)*

U.S. Brand Names Necon® 1/50; Norinyl® 1+50; Ortho-Novum® 1/50

Synonyms Norethindrone and Mestranol; Ortho Novum 1/50

Generic Available Yes

Pharmacologic Category Contraceptive; Estrogen and Progestin Combination

Medication Safety Issues

Sound-alike/look-alike issues:

Norinyl® may be confused with Nardil®

Use Prevention of pregnancy

Unlabeled/Investigational Use Treatment of hypermenorrhea (menorrhagia); pain associated with endometriosis; dysmenorrhea; dysfunctional uterine bleeding

Mechanism of Action/Effect Combination hormonal contraceptives inhibit ovulation and also produce changes in the cervical mucus and endometrium creating an unfavorable environment for sperm penetration and nidation.

Contraindications Hypersensitivity to mestranol, norethindrone, or any component of the formulation; history of or current thrombophlebitis or venous thromboembolic disorders (including DVT, PE); active or recent (within 1 year) arterial thromboembolic disease (eg, stroke, MI); cerebral vascular disease, coronary artery disease, valvular heart disease with complications; severe hypertension; diabetes mellitus with vascular involvement; severe headache with focal neurological symptoms; known or suspected breast carcinoma, endometrial cancer, estrogen-dependent neoplasms, undiagnosed abnormal genital bleeding; hepatic dysfunction or tumor, cholestatic jaundice of pregnancy, jaundice with prior combination hormonal contraceptive use; major surgery with prolonged immobilization; heavy smoking (≥15 cigarettes/day) in patients >35 years of age; pregnancy

Warnings/Precautions Use with caution in patients with a history of thromboembolism, stroke, myocardial infarction, liver tumor, hypertension, cardiac, renal or hepatic insufficiency; use of any progestin during the first 4 months of pregnancy is not recommended; risk of cardiovascular side effects increases in those women who smoke cigarettes and in women >35 years of age. Use of oral contraceptives has been associated with a small increase in the frequency of breast cancer. Some studies suggest an increased risk of intraepithelial neoplasia may also be associated with oral contraceptive use. Not for use prior to menarche. Combination hormonal contraceptives do not protect against HIV infection or other sexually-transmitted diseases. The risk of cardiovascular side effects increases in women who smoke cigarettes, especially those who are >35 years of age; women who use combination hormonal contraceptives should be strongly advised not to smoke. Combination hormonal contraceptives may lead to increased risk of myocardial infarction, use with caution in patients with risk factors for coronary artery disease. May increase the risk of thromboembolism. Combination hormonal contraceptives may have a dose-related risk of vascular disease, hypertension, and gallbladder disease. Women with hypertension should be encouraged to use a nonhormonal form of contraception. The use of combination hormonal contraceptives has been associated with a slight increase in frequency of breast cancer, however, studies are not consistent. Combination hormonal contraceptives may cause glucose intolerance. Retinal thrombosis has been reported (rarely). Use with caution in patients with renal disease, conditions that may be aggravated by fluid retention, depression, or history of migraine. Not for use prior to menarche.

The minimum dosage combination of estrogen/progestin that will effectively treat the individual patient should be used. New patients should be started on products containing <50 mcg of estrogen per tablet.

Drug Interactions

Cytochrome P450 Effect:
Mestranol: **Substrate** of CYP2C19 (major); Based on active metabolite ethinyl estradiol: **Substrate** of CYP3A4 (major), 3A5-7 (minor); **Inhibits** CYP1A2 (weak), 2B6 (weak), 2C19 (weak), 3A4 (weak)

Norethindrone: **Substrate** of CYP3A4 (major); **Induces** CYP2C19 (weak)

Decreased Effect: CYP2C8/9 inhibitors may decrease the levels of ethinyl estradiol (active metabolite of mestranol); example inhibitors include delavirdine, fluconazole, gemfibrozil, ketoconazole, nicardipine, NSAIDs, pioglitazone, and sulfonamides. CYP3A4 inducers may decrease the levels of ethinyl estradiol (active metabolite of mestranol); example inducers include aminoglutethimide, carbamazepine, nafcillin, nevirapine, phenobarbital, phenytoin, and rifamycins. Combination hormonal contraceptives may decrease plasma levels of acetaminophen, clofibric acid, lorazepam, morphine, oxazepam, salicylic acid, temazepam. Contraceptive effect decreased by acitretin, aminoglutethimide, amprenavir, griseofulvin, lopinavir, nelfinavir, nevirapine, penicillins (effect not consistent), ritonavir, tetracyclines (effect not consistent) troglitazone. Combination hormonal contraceptives may decrease (or increase) the effects of coumarin derivatives.

Increased Effect/Toxicity: Acetaminophen and ascorbic acid may increase plasma levels of estrogen component. Atorvastatin and indinavir increase plasma levels of combination hormonal contraceptives. Combination hormonal contraceptives increase the plasma levels of alprazolam, chlordiazepoxide, cyclosporine, diazepam, prednisolone, selegiline, theophylline, tricyclic antidepressants. Combination hormonal contraceptives may increase (or decrease) the effects of coumarin derivatives.

Nutritional/Ethanol Interactions
Food: CNS effects of caffeine may be enhanced if oral contraceptives are used concurrently with caffeine. Grapefruit juice increases ethinyl estradiol concentrations and would be expected to increase progesterone serum levels as well; clinical implications are unclear.
Herb/Nutraceutical: St John's wort may decrease the effectiveness of combination hormonal contraceptives by inducing hepatic enzymes. Avoid dong quai and black cohosh (have estrogen activity). Avoid saw palmetto, red clover, ginseng.

Adverse Reactions Frequency not defined.
Cardiovascular: Arterial thromboembolism, cerebral hemorrhage, cerebral thrombosis, edema, hypertension, mesenteric thrombosis, MI

Central nervous system: Depression, dizziness, headache, migraine, nervousness, premenstrual syndrome, stroke

Dermatologic: Acne, erythema multiforme, erythema nodosum, hirsutism, loss of scalp hair, melasma (may persist), rash (allergic)

Endocrine & metabolic: Amenorrhea, breakthrough bleeding, breast enlargement, breast secretion, breast tenderness, carbohydrate intolerance, lactation decreased (postpartum), glucose tolerance decreased, libido changes, menstrual flow changes, sex hormone-binding globulins (SHBG) increased, spotting, temporary infertility (following discontinuation), thyroid-binding globulin increased, triglycerides increased

Gastrointestinal: Abdominal cramps, appetite changes, bloating, cholestasis, colitis, gallbladder disease, jaundice, nausea, vomiting, weight gain/loss

Genitourinary: Cervical erosion changes, cervical secretion changes, cystitis-like syndrome, vaginal candidiasis, vaginitis

Hematologic: Antithrombin III decreased, folate levels decreased, hemolytic uremic syndrome, norepinephrine induced platelet aggregability increased, porphyria, prothrombin increased; factors VII, VIII, IX, and X increased

Hepatic: Benign liver tumors, Budd-Chiari syndrome, cholestatic jaundice, hepatic adenomas

Local: Thrombophlebitis

Ocular: Cataracts, change in corneal curvature (steepening), contact lens intolerance, optic neuritis, retinal thrombosis

Renal: Impaired renal function

Respiratory: Pulmonary thromboembolism

Miscellaneous: Hemorrhagic eruption

Overdosage/Toxicology Toxicity is unlikely following single exposures of excessive doses. May cause withdrawal bleeding in females. Any treatment following emesis and charcoal administration should be supportive and symptomatic.

Pharmacodynamics/Kinetics
Metabolism:
Mestranol: Hepatic via demethylation to ethinyl estradiol

Pharmacokinetic Note: See Norethindrone monograph for additional information.

Dosing
Adults: Female: Contraception: Oral:
Schedule 1 (Sunday starter): Dose begins on first Sunday after onset of menstruation; if the menstrual period starts on Sunday, take first tablet that very same day. **With a Sunday start, an additional method of contraception should be used until after the first 7 days of consecutive administration.**

For 21-tablet package: Dosage is 1 tablet daily for 21 consecutive days, followed by 7 days off of the medication; a new course begins on the 8th day after the last tablet is taken.

For 28-tablet package: Dosage is 1 tablet daily without interruption.

(Continued)

Mestranol and Norethindrone *(Continued)*

Schedule 2 (Day 1 starter): Dose starts on first day of menstrual cycle taking 1 tablet daily.

For 21-tablet package: Dosage is 1 tablet daily for 21 consecutive days, followed by 7 days off of the medication; a new course begins on the 8th day after the last tablet is taken.

For 28-tablet package: Dosage is 1 tablet daily without interruption.

Note: If all doses have been taken on schedule and one menstrual period is missed, continue dosing cycle. If two consecutive menstrual periods are missed, pregnancy test is required before new dosing cycle is started.

Missed doses: Monophasic formulations (refer to package insert for complete information):

One dose missed: Take as soon as remembered or take 2 tablets next day

Two consecutive doses missed in the first 2 weeks: Take 2 tablets as soon as remembered or 2 tablets next 2 days. **An additional method of contraception should be used for 7 days after missed dose.**

Two consecutive doses missed in week 3 or three consecutive doses missed at any time: **An additional method of contraception must be used for 7 days after a missed dose:**

Schedule 1 (Sunday starter): Continue dose of 1 tablet daily until Sunday, then discard the rest of the pack, and a new pack should be started that same day.

Schedule 2 (Day 1 starter): Current pack should be discarded, and a new pack should be started that same day.

Pediatrics: Female: Contraception: Oral: See adult dosing; not to be used prior to menarche.

Renal Impairment: Specific guidelines not available; use with caution.

Hepatic Impairment: Contraindicated in patients with hepatic impairment.

Available Dosage Forms Tablet, monophasic formulations:

Necon® 1/50: Norethindrone 1 mg and mestranol 0.05 mg [21 light blue tablets and 7 white inactive tablets] (28s)

Norinyl® 1+50: Norethindrone 1 mg and mestranol 0.05 mg [21 white tablets and 7 orange inactive tablets] (28s)

Ortho-Novum® 1/50: Norethindrone 1 mg and mestranol 0.05 mg [21 yellow tablets and 7 green inactive tablets] (28s)

Monitoring and Teaching Issues

Physical Assessment: Monitor or teach patient to monitor blood pressure on a regular basis. Monitor or teach patient to monitor for occurrence of adverse effects and symptoms to report. Assess knowledge/teach importance of regular (monthly) blood pressure checks and annual physical assessment, Pap smear, and vision assessment. Teach importance of maintaining prescribed schedule of dosing. **Pregnancy risk factor X:** Do not use if patient is pregnant.

Patient Education: Oral contraceptives do not protect against HIV or other sexually-transmitted disease. Take exactly as directed by prescriber (also see package insert). Take at the same time each day. You are at risk of becoming pregnant if doses are missed. Detailed and complete information on dosing and missed doses can be found in the package insert. Be aware that some medications may reduce the effectiveness of oral contraceptives; an alternate form of contraception may be needed. Check all medicines (prescription and OTC), herbal, and alternative products with prescriber. It is important that you check your blood pressure monthly (on same day each month) and that you have an annual physical assessment, Pap smear, and vision assessment while taking this medication. Avoid smoking while taking this medication; smoking increases risk of adverse effects, including thromboembolic events and heart attacks. You may experience loss of appetite (small frequent meals will help); or constipation (increased exercise, fluids, fruit, fiber, or stool softeners may help). If you have diabetes, use accurate serum glucose testing to identify any changes in glucose tolerance; notify prescriber of significant changes so antidiabetic medication can be adjusted if necessary. Report immediately pain or muscle soreness; warmth, swelling, pain, or redness in calves; shortness of breath; sudden loss of vision; unresolved leg or foot swelling; change in menstrual pattern (unusual bleeding, amenorrhea, breakthrough spotting); breast tenderness that does not go away; acute abdominal cramping; signs of vaginal infection (drainage, pain, itching); CNS changes (blurred vision, confusion, acute anxiety, or unresolved depression); or significant weight gain (>5 lb/week). Notify prescriber of changes in contact lens tolerance. **Pregnancy/breast-feeding precautions:** This medication should not be used during pregnancy. If you suspect you may become pregnant, contact prescriber immediately. Consult prescriber if breast-feeding.

Dietary Considerations: Should be taken at same time each day.

Pregnancy Risk Factor: X

Pregnancy Issues: Pregnancy should be ruled out prior to treatment and discontinued if pregnancy occurs. In general, the use of combination hormonal contraceptives when inadvertently taken early in pregnancy have not been associated with teratogenic effects. Due to increased risk of thromboembolism postpartum, combination hormonal contraceptives should not be started earlier than 4-6 weeks following delivery. Hormonal contraceptives may be less effective in obese patients. An increase in oral contraceptive failure was noted in women with a BMI >27.3. Similar findings were noted in patients weighing ≥90 kg (198 lb) using the contraceptive patch.

Lactation: Enters breast milk/not recommended (AAP rates "compatible")

Breast-Feeding Issues: Jaundice and breast enlargement in the nursing infant have been reported following the use of combination hormonal contraceptives. May decrease the quality and quantity of breast milk; a nonhormonal form of contraception is recommended.

Administration

Oral: Administer at the same time each day. Administer at bedtime to minimize occurrence of adverse effects.

Storage: Store at controlled room temperature of 25°C (77°F).
Related Information
  Norethindrone *on page 1096*

- ◆ **Metacortandralone** *see* PrednisoLONE *on page 1245*
- ◆ **Metadate® CD** *see* Methylphenidate *on page 983*
- ◆ **Metadate™ ER** *see* Methylphenidate *on page 983*
- ◆ **Metaglip™** *see* Glipizide and Metformin *on page 717*
- ◆ **Metamucil® [OTC]** *see* Psyllium *on page 1284*
- ◆ **Metamucil® Smooth Texture [OTC]** *see* Psyllium *on page 1284*

Metformin *(met FOR min)*
U.S. Brand Names Fortamet™; Glucophage®; Glucophage® XR; Riomet™
Synonyms Metformin Hydrochloride
Generic Available Yes: Excludes solution
Pharmacologic Category Antidiabetic Agent, Biguanide
Medication Safety Issues
  Sound-alike/look-alike issues:
    Metformin may be confused with metronidazole
    Glucophage® may be confused with Glucotrol®, Glutofac®
Use Management of type 2 diabetes mellitus (noninsulin dependent, NIDDM) as monotherapy when hyperglycemia cannot be managed on diet alone. May be used concomitantly with a sulfonylurea or insulin to improve glycemic control.
Unlabeled/Investigational Use Treatment of HIV lipodystrophy syndrome
Mechanism of Action/Effect Decreases hepatic glucose production, decreasing intestinal absorption of glucose and improves insulin sensitivity (increases peripheral glucose uptake and utilization)
Contraindications Hypersensitivity to metformin or any component of the formulation; renal disease or renal dysfunction (serum creatinine ≥1.5 mg/dL in males or ≥1.4 mg/dL in females or abnormal creatinine clearance from any cause, including shock, acute myocardial infarction, or septicemia); congestive heart failure requiring pharmacological management; acute or chronic metabolic acidosis with or without coma (including diabetic ketoacidosis)

Note: Temporarily discontinue in patients undergoing radiologic studies in which intravascular iodinated contrast materials are utilized.
Warnings/Precautions Lactic acidosis is a rare, but potentially severe consequence of therapy with metformin. Lactic acidosis should be suspected in any diabetic patient receiving metformin who has evidence of acidosis when evidence of ketoacidosis is lacking. Discontinue metformin in clinical situations predisposing to hypoxemia, including conditions such as cardiovascular collapse, respiratory failure, acute myocardial infarction, acute congestive heart failure, and septicemia.

Metformin is substantially excreted by the kidney. The risk of accumulation and lactic acidosis increases with the degree of impairment of renal function. Patients with renal function below the limit of normal for their age should not receive metformin. In elderly patients, renal function should be monitored regularly; should not be used in any patient ≥80 years of age unless measurement of creatinine clearance verifies normal renal function. Use of concomitant medications that may affect renal function (ie, affect tubular secretion) may also affect metformin disposition. Metformin should be suspended in patients with dehydration and/or prerenal azotemia. Therapy should be suspended for any surgical procedures (resume only after normal intake resumed and normal renal function is verified). Metformin should also be temporarily discontinued for 48 hours in patients undergoing radiologic studies involving the intravascular administration of iodinated contrast materials (potential for acute alteration in renal function).

Avoid use in patients with impaired liver function. Patient must be instructed to avoid excessive acute or chronic ethanol use. Administration of oral antidiabetic drugs has been reported to be associated with increased cardiovascular mortality; metformin does not appear to share this risk. Safety and efficacy of metformin have been established for use in children ≥10 years of age; the extended release preparation is for use in patients ≥17 years of age.
Drug Interactions
  Decreased Effect: Drugs which tend to produce hyperglycemia (eg, diuretics, corticosteroids, phenothiazines, thyroid products, estrogens, oral contraceptives, phenytoin, nicotinic acid, sympathomimetics, calcium channel blocking drugs, isoniazid) may lead to a loss of glucose control.
  Increased Effect/Toxicity: Furosemide and cimetidine may increase metformin blood levels. Cationic drugs (eg, amiloride, digoxin, morphine, procainamide, quinidine, quinine, ranitidine, triamterene, trimethoprim, and vancomycin) which are eliminated by renal tubular secretion have the potential to increase metformin levels by competing for common renal tubular transport systems. Contrast agents may increase the risk of metformin-induced lactic acidosis; discontinue metformin prior to exposure and withhold for 48 hours.
Nutritional/Ethanol Interactions
  Ethanol: Avoid or limit ethanol (incidence of lactic acidosis may be increased; may cause hypoglycemia).
  Food: Food decreases the extent and slightly delays the absorption. May decrease absorption of vitamin B_{12} and/or folic acid.
  Herb/Nutraceutical: Caution with chromium, garlic, gymnema (may cause hypoglycemia).
Adverse Reactions
  >10%:
    Gastrointestinal: Nausea/vomiting (6% to 25%), diarrhea (10% to 53%), flatulence (12%)
    Neuromuscular & skeletal: Weakness (9%)
  1% to 10%:
    Cardiovascular: Chest discomfort, flushing, palpitation
    Central nervous system: Headache (6%), chills, dizziness, lightheadedness
(Continued)

Metformin *(Continued)*

Dermatologic: Rash

Endocrine & metabolic: Hypoglycemia

Gastrointestinal: Indigestion (7%), abdominal discomfort (6%), abdominal distention, abnormal stools, constipation, dyspepsia/ heartburn, taste disorder

Neuromuscular & skeletal: Myalgia

Respiratory: Dyspnea, upper respiratory tract infection

Miscellaneous: Decreased vitamin B_{12} levels (7%), increased diaphoresis, flu-like syndrome, nail disorder

Overdosage/Toxicology Hypoglycemia (10% of cases) or lactic acidosis (~32% of cases) may occur. Metformin is dialyzable with a clearance of up to 170 mL/minute. Hemodialysis may be useful for removal of accumulated drug from patients in whom metformin overdose is suspected. Treatment is supportive.

Pharmacodynamics/Kinetics

Onset of Action: Within days; maximum effects up to 2 weeks

Bioavailability: Absolute: Fasting: 50% to 60%

Protein Binding: Negligible

Half-Life Elimination: Plasma: 6.2 hours

Excretion: Urine (90% as unchanged drug)

Dosing

Adults: Note: Oral (allow 1-2 weeks between dose titrations): Generally, clinically significant responses are not seen at doses <1500 mg daily; however, a lower recommended starting dose and gradual increased dosage is recommended to minimize gastrointestinal symptoms

Management of type 2 diabetes mellitus: Oral:

Immediate release tablet or oral solution: Initial: 500 mg twice daily (give with the morning and evening meals) **or** 850 mg once daily; increase dosage incrementally.

Adjustment: Incremental dosing recommendations are based on dosage form:

500 mg tablet: One tablet/day at weekly intervals

850 mg tablet: One tablet/day every other week

Oral solution: 500 mg twice daily every other week

Note: Doses of up to 2000 mg/day may be given twice daily. If a dose >2000 mg/day is required, it may be better tolerated in three divided doses. Maximum recommended dose 2550 mg/day.

Extended release tablet: Initial: 500 mg once daily (with the evening meal); dosage may be increased by 500 mg weekly; maximum dose: 2000 mg once daily. If glycemic control is not achieved at maximum dose, may divide dose to 1000 mg twice daily. If doses >2000 mg/day are needed, switch to regular release tablets and titrate to maximum dose of 2550 mg/day.

Transfer from other antidiabetic agents: No transition period is generally necessary except when transferring from chlorpropamide. When transferring from chlorpropamide, care should be exercised during the first 2 weeks because of the prolonged retention of chlorpropamide in the body, leading to overlapping drug effects and possible hypoglycemia.

Concomitant metformin and oral sulfonylurea therapy: If patients have not responded to 4 weeks of the maximum dose of metformin monotherapy, consider a gradual addition of an oral sulfonylurea, even if prior primary or secondary failure to a sulfonylurea has occurred. Continue metformin at the maximum dose.

Failed sulfonylurea therapy: Patients with prior failure on glyburide may be treated by gradual addition of metformin. Initiate with glyburide 20 mg and metformin 500 mg daily. Metformin dosage may be increased by 500 mg/day at weekly intervals, up to a maximum of 2500 mg/day (dosage of glyburide maintained at 20 mg/day).

Concomitant metformin and insulin therapy:

Initial: 500 mg metformin once daily, continue current insulin dose; increase by 500 mg metformin weekly until adequate glycemic control is achieved

Maximum dose: 2500 mg metformin; 2000 mg metformin extended release

Note: Decrease insulin dose 10% to 25% when FPG <120 mg/dL; monitor and make further adjustments as needed

Elderly: The initial and maintenance dosing should be conservative, due to the potential for decreased renal function. Generally, elderly patients should **not** be titrated to the maximum dose of metformin. See Geriatric Considerations.

Pediatrics: Note: Allow 1-2 weeks between dose titrations: Generally, clinically significant responses are not seen at doses <1500 mg daily; however, a lower recommended starting dose and gradual increased dosage is recommended to minimize gastrointestinal symptoms

Management of type 2 diabetes mellitus: Children 10-16 years: Oral (500 mg tablet or oral solution): Initial: 500 mg twice daily (given with the morning and evening meals); increases in daily dosage should be made in increments of 500 mg at weekly intervals, given in divided doses, up to a maximum of 2000 mg/day

Renal Impairment: The plasma and blood half-life of metformin is prolonged and the renal clearance is decreased in proportion to the decrease in creatinine clearance. Per the manufacturer, metformin is contraindicated in the presence of renal dysfunction defined as a serum creatinine >1.5 mg/dL in males, or >1.4 mg/dL in females and in patients with abnormal clearance. Clinically, it has been recommended that metformin be avoided in patients with Cl_{cr} <60-70 mL/minute.

Hepatic Impairment: Avoid metformin; liver disease is a risk factor for the development of lactic acidosis during metformin therapy.

Available Dosage Forms

Solution, oral, as hydrochloride (Riomet™): 100 mg/mL (118 mL, 473 mL) [contains saccharin; cherry flavor]

Tablet, as hydrochloride (Glucophage®): 500 mg, 850 mg, 1000 mg

Tablet, extended release, as hydrochloride: 500 mg

Fortamet™: 500 mg, 1000 mg

Glucophage® XR: 500 mg, 750 mg

Monitoring and Teaching Issues

Physical Assessment: Assess potential for interactions with other prescriptions, OTC medications, or herbal products patient may be taking (eg, anything that may effect glucose levels). Assess results of laboratory tests, therapeutic effectiveness, and adverse response (eg, assess for signs and symptoms of vitamin B_{12} and/or folic acid deficiency; supplementation may be required). during therapy. Teach patient (or refer patient to diabetic educator for instruction) in appropriate use, possible side effects/appropriate interventions, and adverse symptoms to report.

Monitoring Laboratory Tests: Urine for glucose and ketones, fasting blood glucose, hemoglobin A_{1c}, and fructosamine. Initial and periodic monitoring of hematologic parameters (eg, hemoglobin/hematocrit and red blood cell indices) and renal function should be performed, at least annually. While megaloblastic anemia has been rarely seen with metformin, if suspected, vitamin B_{12} deficiency should be excluded.

Patient Education: Do not take any new medication during therapy unless approved by prescriber. Take as directed (may take with food to decrease GI upset). Do not chew or crush tablets. Parts of extended-release tablets may be excreted in the stool (normal). Do not change dosage or discontinue without consulting prescriber. Avoid overuse of alcohol (could cause severe reaction). It is important to follow dietary and lifestyle recommendations of prescriber. You will be instructed in signs of hypo- or hyperglycemia by prescriber or diabetic educator. May cause drowsiness or dizziness (use caution driving or engaging in potentially hazardous tasks until response to drug is known); nausea or vomiting (taking with meals, eating small frequent meals, frequent mouth care, or sucking lozenges may help); or abdominal distention, flatulence, diarrhea, constipation, or heartburn (if these persist consult prescriber for approved medication). Report immediately unusual weakness or fatigue; unusual muscle pain; persistent GI discomfort; dizziness or lightheadedness; sudden respiratory difficulty, chest discomfort, slow or irregular heartbeat; or other adverse reactions. **Breast-feeding precaution:** Breast-feeding is not recommended.

Dietary Considerations: Drug may cause GI upset; take with food (to decrease GI upset). Take at the same time each day. Dietary modification based on ADA recommendations is a part of therapy. Monitor for signs and symptoms of vitamin B_{12} and/or folic acid deficiency; supplementation may be required.

Geriatric Considerations: Limited data suggests that metformin's total body clearance may be decreased and AUC and half-life increased in older patients; presumably due to decreased renal clearance. Metformin has been well tolerated by the elderly but lower doses and frequent monitoring are recommended.

Pregnancy Risk Factor: B

Pregnancy Issues: Abnormal blood glucose levels are associated with a higher incidence of congenital abnormalities. Insulin is the drug of choice for the control of diabetes mellitus during pregnancy.

Lactation: Excretion in breast milk unknown/not recommended

Breast-Feeding Issues: It is not known if metformin is excreted in human breast milk (excretion occurs in animal models); insulin therapy should be considered in breast-feeding women.

Administration

Oral: Extended release dosage form should be swallowed whole; do not crush, break, or chew. Patients who are anorexic or NPO may need to have their dose held to avoid hypoglycemia.

Storage: Store tablets and oral solution at 20°C to 25°C (68°F to 77°F).

Related Information

Diabetes Mellitus Management *on page 1819*

- ♦ **Metformin and Glipizide** *see* Glipizide and Metformin *on page 717*
- ♦ **Metformin and Glyburide** *see* Glyburide and Metformin *on page 721*
- ♦ **Metformin and Rosiglitazone** *see* Rosiglitazone and Metformin *on page 1348*
- ♦ **Metformin Hydrochloride** *see* Metformin *on page 965*
- ♦ **Metformin Hydrochloride and Rosiglitazone Maleate** *see* Rosiglitazone and Metformin *on page 1348*
- ♦ **Methacholine** *see page 1625*

Methadone (METH a done)

U.S. Brand Names Dolophine®; Methadone Diskets®; Methadone Intensol™; Methadose®

Synonyms Methadone Hydrochloride

Controlled Substance C-II

Treatment of narcotic addiction: May only be dispensed by pharmacies or maintenance programs approved by the FDA and designated state authority. Prior approval must be obtained for doses >120 mg administered at a clinic or >100 mg to be taken at home.

Generic Available Yes

Pharmacologic Category Analgesic, Narcotic

Medication Safety Issues

Sound-alike/look-alike issues:

Methadone may be confused with Mephyton®, methylphenidate

Use Management of severe pain; detoxification and maintenance treatment of narcotic addiction (if used for detoxification and maintenance treatment of narcotic addiction, it must be part of an FDA-approved program)

Mechanism of Action/Effect Binds to opiate receptors in the CNS, causing inhibition of ascending pain pathways, altering the perception of and response to pain; produces generalized CNS depression

Contraindications Hypersensitivity to methadone or any component of the formulation; respiratory depression (in the absence of resuscitative equipment or in an unmonitored setting); acute bronchial asthma or hypercarbia; pregnancy (prolonged use or high doses near term)

Warnings/Precautions An opioid-containing analgesic regimen should be tailored to each patient's needs and based upon the type of pain being treated (acute versus chronic), the (Continued)

Methadone *(Continued)*

route of administration, degree of tolerance for opioids (naive versus chronic user), age, weight, and medical condition. The optimal analgesic dose varies widely among patients. Doses should be titrated to pain relief/prevention. Patients maintained on stable doses of methadone may need higher and/or more frequent doses in case of acute pain (eg, postoperative pain, physical trauma).

May prolong the QT interval; use caution in patients at risk for QT prolongation, with medications known to prolong the QT interval, or history of conduction abnormalities. QT interval prolongation and torsade de pointes may be associated with doses >200 mg/day, but have also been observed with lower doses. May cause severe hypotension; use caution with severe volume depletion or other conditions which may compromise maintenance of normal blood pressure. Use caution with cardiovascular disease or patients predisposed to dysrhythmias.

Methadone has a long half-life and risk of accumulation; because methadone's effects on respiration last much longer than its analgesic effects, the dose must be titrated slowly. May cause respiratory depression; use caution in patients with respiratory disease or pre-existing respiratory depression. Potential for drug dependency exists, abrupt cessation may precipitate withdrawal. Use caution in elderly, debilitated, or pediatric patients. Use with caution in patients with depression or suicidal tendencies, or in patients with a history of drug abuse. Tolerance or psychological and physical dependence may occur with prolonged use.

Use with caution in patients with hepatic, pulmonary, or renal function impairment. May cause CNS depression, which may impair physical or mental abilities. Patients must be cautioned about performing tasks which require mental alertness (eg, operating machinery or driving). Effects with other sedative drugs or ethanol may be potentiated. Elderly may be more sensitive to CNS depressant and constipating effects. Use with caution in patients with head injury or increased ICP, biliary tract dysfunction or pancreatitis; history of ileus or bowel obstruction, glaucoma, hyperthyroidism, hypothyroidism, adrenal insufficiency, prostatic hyperplasia or urinary stricture, CNS depression, toxic psychosis, alcoholism, delirium tremens, or kyphoscoliosis. Tablets contain excipients to deter use by injection.

Drug Interactions

Cytochrome P450 Effect: Substrate of CYP2C8/9 (minor), 2C19 (minor), 2D6 (minor), 3A4 (major); **Inhibits** CYP2D6 (moderate), 3A4 (weak)

Decreased Effect: Agonist/antagonist analgesics (buprenorphine, butorphanol, nalbuphine, pentazocine) may decrease analgesic effect of methadone and precipitate withdrawal symptoms; use is not recommended. Efavirenz and nevirapine may decrease levels of methadone (opioid withdrawal syndrome has been reported). Methadone may decrease bioavailability of didanosine and stavudine. Ritonavir (and combinations) may decrease levels of methadone; withdrawal symptoms have inconsistently been observed, monitor. CYP3A4 inducers may decrease the levels/effects of methadone (eg, aminoglutethimide, carbamazepine, nafcillin, nevirapine, phenobarbital, phenytoin, rifamycins). Monitor for methadone withdrawal. Larger doses of methadone may be required. Methadone may decrease the levels/effects of CYP2D6 prodrug substrates (eg, codeine, hydrocodone, oxycodone, tramadol).

Increased Effect/Toxicity: CYP3A4 inhibitors may increase the levels/effects of methadone (eg, azole antifungals, ciprofloxacin, clarithromycin, diclofenac, doxycycline, erythromycin, imatinib, isoniazid, nefazodone, nicardipine, propofol, protease inhibitors, quinidine, verapamil). Methadone may increase the levels/effects of CYP2D6 substrates (eg, amphetamines, selected beta-blockers, dextromethorphan, fluoxetine, lidocaine, mirtazapine, nefazodone, paroxetine, risperidone, ritonavir, thioridazine, tricyclic antidepressants, venlafaxine). Methadone may increase bioavailability and toxic effects of zidovudine. CNS depressants (including but not limited to opioid analgesics, general anesthetics, sedatives, hypnotics, ethanol) may cause respiratory depression, hypotension, profound sedation, or coma. Levels of desipramine may be increased by methadone. Effects/toxicity of QT_c interval-prolonging agents may be increased; use with caution (including but may not be limited to amitriptyline, astemizole, bepridil, disopyramide, erythromycin, haloperidol, imipramine, quinidine, pimozide, procainamide, sotalol, thioridazine).

Nutritional/Ethanol Interactions

Ethanol: Avoid ethanol (may increase CNS effects). Watch for sedation.

Herb/Nutraceutical: Avoid St John's wort (may decrease methadone levels; may increase CNS depression). Avoid valerian, kava kava, gotu kola (may increase CNS depression). Methadone is metabolized by CYP3A4 in the intestines; avoid concurrent use of grapefruit juice.

Lab Interactions
Increased thyroxine (S), aminotransferase [ALT (SGPT)/AST (SGOT)] (S)

Adverse Reactions
Frequency not defined. During prolonged administration, adverse effects may decrease over several weeks; however, constipation and sweating may persist.

Cardiovascular: Bradycardia, peripheral vasodilation, cardiac arrest, syncope, faintness, shock, hypotension, edema, arrhythmia, bigeminal rhythms, extrasystoles, tachycardia, torsade de pointes, ventricular fibrillation, ventricular tachycardia, ECG changes, QT interval prolonged, T-wave inversion, cardiomyopathy, flushing, heart failure, palpitation, phlebitis, orthostatic hypotension

Central nervous system: Euphoria, dysphoria, headache, insomnia, agitation, disorientation, drowsiness, dizziness, lightheadedness, sedation, confusion, seizure

Dermatologic: Pruritus, urticaria, rash, hemorrhagic urticaria

Endocrine & metabolic: Libido decreased, hypokalemia, hypomagnesemia, antidiuretic effect, amenorrhea

Gastrointestinal: Nausea, vomiting, constipation, anorexia, stomach cramps, xerostomia, biliary tract spasm, abdominal pain, glossitis, weight gain

Genitourinary: Urinary retention or hesitancy, impotence

Hematologic: Thrombocytopenia (reversible, reported in patients with chronic hepatitis)

Neuromuscular & skeletal: Weakness

Local: I.M./SubQ injection: Pain, erythema, swelling; I.V. injection: pruritus, urticaria, rash, hemorrhagic urticaria (rare)

Ocular: Miosis, visual disturbances

Respiratory: Respiratory depression, respiratory arrest, pulmonary edema

Miscellaneous: Physical and psychological dependence, death, diaphoresis

Overdosage/Toxicology Symptoms include respiratory depression, CNS depression, miosis, hypothermia, circulatory collapse, and convulsions. Treatment includes naloxone 2 mg I.V. (0.01 mg/kg for children), with repeat administration as necessary, up to a total of 10 mg, or as a continuous infusion. Nalmefene may also be used to reverse signs of intoxication.

Pharmacodynamics/Kinetics

Onset of Action: Oral: Analgesic: 0.5-1 hour; Parenteral: 10-20 minutes; Peak effect: Parenteral: 1-2 hours

Duration of Action: Oral: 6-8 hours, increases to 22-48 hours with repeated doses

Protein Binding: 85% to 90%

Half-Life Elimination: 8-59 hours; may be prolonged with alkaline pH, decreased during pregnancy

Metabolism: Hepatic; N-demethylation via CYP3A4 and 2D6 to inactive metabolites

Excretion: Urine (<10% as unchanged drug); increased with urine pH <6

Dosing

Adults: Note: These are guidelines and do not represent the maximum doses that may be required in all patients. Methadone accumulates with repeated doses and dosage may need reduction after 3-5 days to prevent CNS depressant effects. Some patients may benefit from every 8-12 hour dosing interval for chronic pain management. Doses should be titrated to appropriate effects.

Pain (analgesia):
Oral: Initial: 5-10 mg; dosing interval may range from 4-12 hours during initial therapy; decrease in dose or frequency may be required (~days 2-5) due to accumulation with repeated doses

Manufacturer's labeling: 2.5-10 mg every 3-4 hours as needed

I.V.: Manufacturers labeling: Initial: 2.5-10 mg every 8-12 hours in opioid-naive patients; titrate slowly to effect; may also be administered by SubQ or I.M. injection

Note: Conversion from oral to parenteral dose: Initial dose: Oral: parenteral: 2:1 ratio

Detoxification: Oral: 15-40 mg/day

Maintenance treatment of opiate dependence: Oral: 20-120 mg/day

Elderly: Oral, I.M.: 2.5 mg every 8-12 hours; refer to adult dosing.

Pediatrics: Note: These are guidelines and do not represent the maximum doses that may be required in all patients. Methadone accumulates with repeated doses and dosage may need reduction after 3-5 days to prevent CNS depressant effects. Some patients may benefit from every 8-12 hour dosing interval for chronic pain management. Doses should be titrated to appropriate effects.

Pain (analgesia):
Oral (unlabeled use): Initial: 0.1-0.2 mg/kg 4-8 hours initially for 2-3 doses, then every 6-12 hours as needed. Dosing interval may range from 4-12 hours during initial therapy; decrease in dose or frequency may be required (~ days 2-5) due to accumulation with repeated doses (maximum dose: 5-10 mg)

I.V. (unlabeled use): 0.1 mg/kg every 4-8 hours initially for 2-3 doses, then every 6-12 hours as needed. Dosing interval may range from 4-12 hours during initial therapy; decrease in dose or frequency may be required (~ days 2-5) due to accumulation with repeated doses (maximum dose: 5-8 mg)

Iatrogenic narcotic dependency (unlabeled): Oral: General guidelines: Initial: 0.05-0.1 mg/kg/dose every 6 hours; increase by 0.05 mg/kg/dose until withdrawal symptoms are controlled; after 24-48 hours, the dosing interval can be lengthened to every 12-24 hours; to taper dose, wean by 0.05 mg/kg/day; if withdrawal symptoms recur, taper at a slower rate

Renal Impairment: Cl$_{cr}$ <10 mL/minute: Administer 50% to 75% of normal dose.

Hepatic Impairment: Avoid in severe liver disease.

Available Dosage Forms

Injection, solution, as hydrochloride: 10 mg/mL (20 mL)

Solution, oral, as hydrochloride: 5 mg/5 mL (500 mL); 10 mg/5 mL (500 mL) [contains alcohol 8%; citrus flavor]

Solution, oral concentrate, as hydrochloride: 10 mg/mL (946 mL)

Methadone Intensol™: 10 mg/mL (30 mL)

Methadose®: 10 mg/mL (1000 mL) [cherry flavor or dye free, sugar free, unflavored]

Tablet, as hydrochloride (Dolophine®, Methadose®): 5 mg, 10 mg

Tablet, dispersible, as hydrochloride:

Methadose®: 40 mg

Methadone Diskets®: 40 mg [orange-pineapple flavor]

Monitoring and Teaching Issues

Physical Assessment: Assess other medications patient may be taking for additive or adverse interactions. Monitor therapeutic effectiveness and adverse reactions of overdose at beginning of therapy and at regular intervals with long-term use. May cause physical and/or psychological dependence. Monitor blood pressure, respiratory and CNS status (degree of sedation). For inpatients, implement safety measures. Assess knowledge/teach patient appropriate use (if self-administered) adverse reactions to report, and appropriate interventions to reduce side effects. Discontinue slowly after prolonged use.

Patient Education: If self-administered, use exactly as directed; do not increase dose or frequency. Drug may cause physical and/or psychological dependence. While using this medication, do not use alcohol and other prescription or OTC medications (especially sedatives, tranquilizers, antihistamines, or pain medications) without consulting prescriber. Maintain adequate hydration (2-3 L/day of fluids) unless instructed to restrict fluid intake. May cause hypotension, dizziness, drowsiness, impaired coordination, or blurred vision (use caution when driving, climbing stairs, or changing position - rising from sitting or lying to standing, or when engaging in tasks requiring alertness until response to drug is known); loss of appetite, nausea, or vomiting (frequent mouth care, small frequent meals, chewing gum, or sucking lozenges may help); or constipation (increased exercise, fluids, fruit, or (Continued)

Methadone *(Continued)*

fiber may help; if unresolved, consult prescriber about use of stool softeners). Report chest pain, slow or rapid heartbeat, acute dizziness or persistent headache; changes in mental status; swelling of extremities or unusual weight gain; changes in urinary elimination; acute headache; back or flank pain or muscle spasms; blurred vision; skin rash; or shortness of breath. **Pregnancy/breast-feeding precautions:** Inform prescriber if you are or intend to become pregnant. If you are breast-feeding, take medication immediately after breast-feeding or 3-4 hours prior to next feeding.

Geriatric Considerations: Because of its long half-life and risk of accumulation, methadone is not considered a drug of first choice in the elderly. The elderly may be particularly susceptible to the CNS depressant and constipating effects of narcotics. Adjust dose for renal function.

Pregnancy Risk Factor: C/D (prolonged use or high doses at term)

Pregnancy Issues: Teratogenic effects have been observed in some, but not all, animal studies. Data collected by the Teratogen Information System are complicated by maternal use of illicit drugs, nutrition, infection, and psychosocial circumstances. However, pregnant women in methadone treatment programs are reported to have improved fetal outcomes compared to pregnant women using illicit drugs. Methadone can be detected in the amniotic fluid, cord plasma, and newborn urine. Fetal growth, birth weight, length, and/or head circumference may be decreased in infants born to narcotic-addicted mothers treated with methadone during pregnancy. Growth deficits do not appear to persist; however, decreased performance on psychometric and behavioral tests has been found to continue into childhood. Abnormal fetal nonstress tests have also been reported. Withdrawal symptoms in the neonate may be observed up to 2-4 weeks after delivery. The manufacturer states that methadone should be used during pregnancy only if clearly needed. Because methadone clearance in pregnant women is increased and half-life is decreased during the 2nd and 3rd trimesters of pregnancy, withdrawal symptoms may be observed in the mother; dosage of methadone may need increased or dosing interval decreased during pregnancy.

Lactation: Enters breast milk/not recommended (AAP rates "compatible")

Breast-Feeding Issues: Peak methadone levels appear in breast milk 4-5 hours after an oral dose. Methadone has been detected in the plasma of some breast-fed infants whose mothers are taking methadone. Use during breast-feeding is not recommended, and the manufacturer recommends that women on high dose methadone maintenance who already are breast-feeding be instructed to wean breast-feeding gradually to avoid neonatal abstinence syndrome. Unless otherwise contraindicated (concurrent medical conditions, other medications of abuse), the AAP rates methadone "compatible" with breast-feeding.

Administration

Oral: Oral dose for detoxification and maintenance may be administered in fruit juice or water.

Compatibility: Stable in NS

Storage:

Injection: Store at controlled room temperature of 15°C to 30°C (59°F to 86°F). Protect from light.

Oral concentrate, oral solution, tablet: Store at controlled room temperature of 15°C to 30°C (59°F to 86°F).

Related Information

Narcotic / Opioid Analgesic Comparison *on page 1739*

♦ **Methadone Diskets®** *see Methadone on page 967*

♦ **Methadone Hydrochloride** *see Methadone on page 967*

♦ **Methadone Intensol™** *see Methadone on page 967*

♦ **Methadose®** *see Methadone on page 967*

♦ **Methaminodiazepoxide Hydrochloride** *see Chlordiazepoxide on page 308*

Methenamine *(meth EN a meen)*

U.S. Brand Names Hiprex®; Mandelamine®; Urex®

Synonyms Hexamethylenetetramine; Methenamine Hippurate; Methenamine Mandelate

Generic Available Yes

Pharmacologic Category Antibiotic, Miscellaneous

Medication Safety Issues

Sound-alike/look-alike issues:

Methenamine may be confused with methazolamide, methionine

Urex® may be confused with Eurax®, Serax®

Use Prophylaxis or suppression of recurrent urinary tract infections; urinary tract discomfort secondary to hypermotility

Mechanism of Action/Effect Methenamine is hydrolyzed to formaldehyde and ammonia in acidic urine; formaldehyde has nonspecific bactericidal action

Contraindications Hypersensitivity to methenamine or any component of the formulation; severe dehydration, renal insufficiency, hepatic insufficiency in patients receiving hippurate salt; concurrent treatment with sulfonamides

Warnings/Precautions Methenamine should not be used to treat infections outside of the lower urinary tract. Use with caution in patients with hepatic disease, gout, and the elderly; doses of 8 g/day for 3-4 weeks may cause bladder irritation. Use care to maintain an acid pH of the urine, especially when treating infections due to urea splitting organisms (eg, *Proteus* and strains of *Pseudomonas*); reversible increases in LFTs have occurred during therapy especially in patients with hepatic dysfunction. Hiprex® contains tartrazine dye.

Drug Interactions

Decreased Effect: Sodium bicarbonate and acetazolamide will decrease effect secondary to alkalinization of urine.

Increased Effect/Toxicity: Sulfonamides may precipitate in the urine; concurrent use is contraindicated.

Nutritional/Ethanol Interactions Food: Foods/diets which alkalinize urine pH >5.5 decrease therapeutic effect of methenamine.

Lab Interactions Increased catecholamines and VMA (U); decreased HIAA (U)

Adverse Reactions 1% to 10%:
Dermatologic: Rash (<4%)
Gastrointestinal: Nausea, dyspepsia (<4%)
Genitourinary: Dysuria (<4%)

Overdosage/Toxicology The drug is well tolerated. Treatment is supportive.

Pharmacodynamics/Kinetics
Absorption: Readily
Half-Life Elimination: 3-6 hours
Metabolism: Gastric juices: Hydrolyze 10% to 30% unless protected via enteric coating; Hepatic: ~10% to 25%
Excretion: Urine (~70% to 90% as unchanged drug) within 24 hours

Dosing
Adults & Elderly: Urinary tract infection: Oral:
Hippurate: 0.5-1 g twice daily
Mandelate: 1 g 4 times/day after meals and at bedtime
Pediatrics: Oral:
>2-6 years: *Mandelate:* 50-75 mg/kg/day in 3-4 doses or 0.25 g/30 lb 4 times/day
6-12 years:
Hippurate: 0.5-1 g twice daily
Mandelate: 50-75 mg/kg/day in 3-4 doses or 0.5 g 4 times/day
>12 years: Refer to adult dosing.
Renal Impairment: Cl_{cr} <50 mL/minute: Avoid use.

Available Dosage Forms
Tablet, as hippurate (Hiprex®, Urex®): 1 g [Hiprex® contains tartrazine dye]
Tablet, enteric coated, as mandelate (Mandelamine®): 500 mg, 1 g

Monitoring and Teaching Issues
Physical Assessment: See Warnings/Precautions for specific use cautions. Assess potential for interactions with other pharmacological agents patient may be taking (eg, anything that alkalizes urine or sulfonamides; see Drug Interactions). Assess therapeutic effectiveness (urinalysis; indicate resolution of infection) and adverse response (see Adverse Reactions). Teach patient proper use, possible side effects/appropriate interventions, and adverse symptoms to report (see Patient Education).
Monitoring Laboratory Tests: Urinalysis, periodic liver function
Patient Education: Take per recommended schedule, at regular intervals around-the-clock. Complete full course of therapy; do not skip doses. Maintain adequate hydration (2-3 L/day of fluids) unless instructed to restrict fluid intake. Avoid excessive citrus fruits, milk, or alkalizing medications. May cause nausea or vomiting or GI upset (small frequent meals, frequent mouth care, sucking lozenges, or chewing gum may help). Report pain on urination or blood in urine, skin rash, other persistent adverse effects, or if condition does not improve. **Pregnancy precaution:** Inform prescriber if you are or intend to become pregnant.
Dietary Considerations: Foods/diets which alkalinize urine pH >5.5 decrease activity of methenamine; cranberry juice can be used to acidify urine and increase activity of methenamine. Hiprex® contains tartrazine dye.
Geriatric Considerations: Methenamine has little, if any, role in the treatment or prevention of infections in patients with indwelling urinary (Foley) catheters. Furthermore, in noncatheterized patients, more effective antibiotics are available for the prevention or treatment of urinary tract infections. The influence of decreased renal function on the pharmacologic effects of methenamine results are unknown.
Pregnancy Risk Factor: C
Lactation: Enters breast milk/compatible
Breast-Feeding Issues: The concentration of methenamine hippurate in breast milk is approximately the same as that in the maternal plasma. The amount ingested by a breast-feeding infant is considered to be below a therapeutic dose.

Administration
Oral: Administer around-the-clock to promote less variation in effect. Foods/diets which alkalinize urine pH >5.5 decrease activity of methenamine.
Storage: Protect from excessive heat

Additional Information Should not be used to treat infections outside of the lower urinary tract. Methenamine has little, if any, role in the treatment or prevention of infections in patients with indwelling urinary (Foley) catheters. Furthermore, in noncatheterized patients, more effective antibiotics are available for the prevention or treatment of urinary tract infections. The influence of decreased renal function on the pharmacologic effects of methenamine results are unknown.

◆ **Methenamine Hippurate** *see* Methenamine *on page 970*
◆ **Methenamine Mandelate** *see* Methenamine *on page 970*
◆ **Methergine®** *see* Methylergonovine *on page 982*

Methimazole (meth IM a zole)
U.S. Brand Names Tapazole®
Synonyms Thiamazole
Generic Available Yes
Pharmacologic Category Antithyroid Agent
Medication Safety Issues
Sound-alike/look-alike issues:
Methimazole may be confused with metolazone
Use Palliative treatment of hyperthyroidism, return the hyperthyroid patient to a normal metabolic state prior to thyroidectomy, and to control thyrotoxic crisis that may accompany thyroidectomy. The use of antithyroid thioamides is as effective in elderly as they are in younger
(Continued)

Methimazole *(Continued)*

adults; however, the expense, potential adverse effects, and inconvenience (compliance, monitoring) make them undesirable. The use of radioiodine due to ease of administration and less concern for long-term side effects and reproduction problems (some older males) makes it a more appropriate therapy.

Mechanism of Action/Effect Inhibits the synthesis of thyroid hormones by blocking the oxidation of iodine in the thyroid gland, blocking iodine's ability to combine with tyrosine to form thyroxine and triiodothyronine (T_3), does not inactivate circulating T_4 and T_3

Contraindications Hypersensitivity to methimazole or any component of the formulation; nursing mothers (per manufacturer; however, expert analysis and the AAP state this drug may be used with caution in nursing mothers); pregnancy

Warnings/Precautions Use with extreme caution in patients receiving other drugs known to cause myelosuppression particularly agranulocytosis, patients >40 years of age. Avoid doses >40 mg/day (increased myelosuppression). May cause acneiform eruptions or worsen the condition of the thyroid.

Drug Interactions

Cytochrome P450 Effect: Inhibits CYP1A2 (weak), 2A6 (weak), 2B6 (weak), 2C8/9 (weak), 2C19 (weak), 2D6 (moderate), 2E1 (weak), 3A4 (weak)

Decreased Effect: Anticoagulant effect of warfarin may be decreased. Methimazole may decrease the levels/effects of CYP2D6 prodrug substrates (eg, codeine, hydrocodone, oxycodone, tramadol).

Increased Effect/Toxicity: Dosage of some drugs (including beta-blockers, digoxin, and theophylline) require adjustment during treatment of hyperthyroidism. Methimazole may increase the levels/effects of CYP2D6 substrates (eg, amphetamines, selected beta-blockers, dextromethorphan, fluoxetine, lidocaine, mirtazapine, nefazodone, paroxetine, risperidone, ritonavir, thioridazine, tricyclic antidepressants, venlafaxine).

Adverse Reactions Frequency not defined.

Cardiovascular: Edema

Central nervous system: Headache, vertigo, drowsiness, CNS stimulation, depression

Dermatologic: Skin rash, urticaria, pruritus, erythema nodosum, skin pigmentation, exfoliative dermatitis, alopecia

Endocrine & metabolic: Goiter

Gastrointestinal: Nausea, vomiting, stomach pain, abnormal taste, constipation, weight gain, salivary gland swelling

Hematologic: Leukopenia, agranulocytosis, granulocytopenia, thrombocytopenia, aplastic anemia, hypoprothrombinemia

Hepatic: Cholestatic jaundice, jaundice, hepatitis

Neuromuscular & skeletal: Arthralgia, paresthesia

Renal: Nephrotic syndrome

Miscellaneous: SLE-like syndrome

Overdosage/Toxicology Symptoms of overdose include nausea, vomiting, epigastric distress, headache, fever, arthralgia, pruritus, edema, pancytopenia, and signs of hypothyroidism. Management of overdose is supportive.

Pharmacodynamics/Kinetics

Onset of Action: Antithyroid: Oral: 12-18 hours

Duration of Action: 36-72 hours

Bioavailability: 80% to 95%

Protein Binding: Plasma: None

Half-Life Elimination: 4-13 hours

Metabolism: Hepatic

Excretion: Urine (80%)

Dosing

Adults & Elderly:

Hyperthyroidism: Oral: Administer in 3 equally divided doses at approximately 8-hour intervals

Initial: 15 mg/day for mild hyperthyroidism; 30-40 mg/day in moderately severe hyperthyroidism; 60 mg/day in severe hyperthyroidism; maintenance: 5-15 mg/day

Adjustment: Adjust dosage as required to achieve and maintain serum T_3, T_4, and TSH levels in the normal range. An elevated T_3 may be the sole indicator of inadequate treatment. An elevated TSH indicates excessive antithyroid treatment.

Pediatrics: Note: Administer in 3 equally divided doses at ~8-hour intervals.

Hyperthyroidism: Oral:

Initial: 0.4 mg/kg/day in 3 divided doses; maintenance: 0.2 mg/kg/day in 3 divided doses up to 30 mg/24 hours maximum

Alternatively: Initial: 0.5-0.7 mg/kg/day **or** 15-20 mg/m^2/day in 3 divided doses

Maintenance: $1/3$ to $2/3$ of the initial dose beginning when the patient is euthyroid

Maximum: 30 mg/24 hours

Available Dosage Forms

Tablet: 5 mg, 10 mg, 20 mg

Tapazole® 5 mg, 10 mg

Monitoring and Teaching Issues

Physical Assessment: Assess potential for interactions with other pharmacological agents patient may be taking (eg, extreme caution with anything that may cause myelosuppression, may increase or decrease levels/effects of other agents; see Warnings/Precautions and Drug Interactions). Assess results of laboratory tests at baseline and periodically. Monitor therapeutic effectiveness (clinical and laboratory indicators), and adverse reactions during therapy (eg, hyper-/hypothyroidism, rash, gastrointestinal upset, leukopenia, anemia, arthralgia; see Adverse Reactions). Teach patient proper use, possible side effects/appropriate interventions, and adverse symptoms to report (see Patient Education).

Monitoring Laboratory Tests: T_4, T_3, CBC with differential, liver function (baseline and as needed), serum thyroxine, free thyroxine index

Patient Education: Do not take any new medication during therapy unless approved by prescriber. Take as directed, at the same time each day, around-the-clock (eg, every 8 hours). Do not miss doses or make up missed doses. This drug will need to be taken for an extended period of time to achieve appropriate results. May cause nausea or vomiting (small frequent meals may help); or dizziness or drowsiness (use caution when driving or engaging in tasks that require alertness until response to drug is known). Report rash, fever, unusual bleeding or bruising, unresolved headache, yellowing of eyes or skin, changes in color of urine or feces, or unresolved malaise. **Pregnancy/breast-feeding precautions:** Inform prescriber if you are pregnant and do not get pregnant while taking this medicine. Consult prescriber for appropriate contraceptive measures. Consult prescriber if breast-feeding.

Dietary Considerations: Should be taken consistently in relation to meals every day.

Geriatric Considerations: The use of antithyroid thioamides is as effective in the elderly as in younger adults; however, the expense, potential adverse effects, and inconvenience (compliance, monitoring) make them undesirable.

Pregnancy Risk Factor: D

Pregnancy Issues: Hypothyroidism and congenital defects (rare) may occur.

Lactation: Enters breast milk/contraindicated (AAP rates "compatible")

Breast-Feeding Issues: Use with caution; consider monitoring thyroid function in the infant (weekly or biweekly)

Administration
Storage: Protect from light.

♦ Methitest™ *see* MethylTESTOSTERone *on page 988*

Methocarbamol (meth oh KAR ba mole)

U.S. Brand Names Robaxin®

Generic Available Yes: Tablet

Pharmacologic Category Skeletal Muscle Relaxant

Medication Safety Issues
Sound-alike/look-alike issues:
Methocarbamol may be confused with mephobarbital
Robaxin® may be confused with Rubex®

Use Treatment of muscle spasm associated with acute painful musculoskeletal conditions; supportive therapy in tetanus

Mechanism of Action/Effect Causes skeletal muscle relaxation by general CNS depression

Contraindications Hypersensitivity to methocarbamol or any component of the formulation; renal impairment (injection formulation)

Warnings/Precautions
Oral: Use caution with renal or hepatic impairment.
Injection: Rate of injection should not exceed 3 mL/minute; solution is hypertonic; avoid extravasation. Use with caution in patients with a history of seizures. Use caution with hepatic impairment.

Drug Interactions
Increased Effect/Toxicity: Increased effect/toxicity with CNS depressants.

Nutritional/Ethanol Interactions
Ethanol: Avoid ethanol (may increase CNS depression).
Herb/Nutraceutical: Avoid valerian, St John's wort, kava kava, gotu kola (may increase CNS depression).

Lab Interactions May cause color interference in certain screening tests for 5-HIAA using nitrosonaphthol reagent and in screening tests for urinary VMA using the Gitlow method.

Adverse Reactions Frequency not defined.
Cardiovascular: Flushing of face, bradycardia, hypotension, syncope
Central nervous system: Drowsiness, dizziness, lightheadedness, convulsion, vertigo, headache, fever, amnesia, confusion, insomnia, sedation, coordination impaired (mild)
Dermatologic: Allergic dermatitis, urticaria, pruritus, rash, angioneurotic edema
Gastrointestinal: Nausea, vomiting, metallic taste, dyspepsia
Hematologic: Leukopenia
Hepatic: Jaundice
Local: Pain at injection site, thrombophlebitis
Ocular: Nystagmus, blurred vision, diplopia, conjunctivitis
Renal: Renal impairment
Respiratory: Nasal congestion
Miscellaneous: Allergic manifestations, anaphylactic reaction

Overdosage/Toxicology Symptoms of overdose include cardiac arrhythmias, nausea, vomiting, drowsiness, and coma. Treatment is supportive.

Pharmacodynamics/Kinetics
Onset of Action: Muscle relaxation: Oral: ~30 minutes
Time to Peak: Serum: ~2 hours
Protein Binding: 46% to 50%
Half-Life Elimination: 1-2 hours
Metabolism: Hepatic via dealkylation and hydroxylation
Excretion: Urine (as metabolites)

Dosing
Adults:
Muscle spasm:
Oral: 1.5 g 4 times/day for 2-3 days (up to 8 g/day may be given in severe conditions), then decrease to 4-4.5 g/day in 3-6 divided doses
I.M., I.V.: 1 g every 8 hours if oral not possible; injection should not be used for more than 3 consecutive days. If condition persists, may repeat course of therapy after a drug-free interval of 48 hours.
Tetanus: I.V.: Initial dose: 1-3 g; may repeat dose every 6 hours until oral dosing is possible; injection should not be used for more than 3 consecutive days

(Continued)

Methocarbamol *(Continued)*

Elderly: Muscle spasm: Oral: Initial: 500 mg 4 times/day; titrate to response
Pediatrics:

Tetanus (recommended **only** for use in tetanus): I.V.: 15 mg/kg/dose or 500 mg/m²/dose, may repeat every 6 hours if needed; maximum dose: 1.8 g/m²/day for 3 days only

Muscle spasm: Children ≥16 years: Refer to adult dosing.

Renal Impairment: Do not administer parenteral formulation to patients with renal dysfunction.

Hepatic Impairment: Specific dosing guidelines are not available. Plasma protein binding and clearance are decreased; half-life is increased.

Available Dosage Forms

Injection, solution: 100 mg/mL (10 mL) [in polyethylene glycol; vial stopper contains latex]
Tablet: 500 mg, 750 mg

Monitoring and Teaching Issues

Physical Assessment: Assess other medications for excess CNS depression. Monitor effectiveness of therapy (according to rational for therapy) and adverse reactions at beginning and periodically during therapy. Monitor I.V. site closely to prevent extravasation. Assess knowledge/teach patient appropriate use, interventions to reduce side effects, and adverse symptoms to report.

Patient Education: Take exactly as directed. Do not increase dose or discontinue without consulting prescriber. Do not use alcohol, prescriptive or OTC antidepressants, sedatives, or pain medications without consulting prescriber. You may experience drowsiness, dizziness, lightheadedness (avoid driving or engaging in tasks requiring alertness until response to drug is known); or nausea or vomiting (small frequent meals, frequent mouth care, or sucking hard candy may help). Report excessive drowsiness or mental agitation, chest pain, skin rash, swelling of mouth/face, difficulty speaking, or vision changes. **Pregnancy/breast-feeding precautions:** Inform prescriber if you are or intend to become pregnant. Consult prescriber if breast-feeding.

Geriatric Considerations: There is no specific information on the use of skeletal muscle relaxants in the elderly. Methocarbamol has a short half-life, so it may be considered one of the safer agents in this class.

Pregnancy Risk Factor: C

Lactation: Excretion in breast milk unknown/use caution

Administration

Oral: Tablets may be crushed and mixed with food or liquid if needed. Avoid alcohol.

I.M.: A maximum of 5 mL can be administered into each gluteal region.

I.V.: Maximum rate: 3 mL/minute; injection should not be used for more than 3 consecutive days; may be administered undiluted

Reconstitution: Injection may be diluted to 4 mg/mL in sterile water, 5% dextrose, or 0.9% saline.

Storage:

Injection: Prior to dilution, store at controlled room temperature of 20°C to 25°C (68°F to 77°F). Injection when diluted to 4 mg/mL in sterile water, 5% dextrose, or 0.9% saline is stable for 6 days at room temperature; do **not** refrigerate after dilution
Tablet: Store at controlled room temperature of 20°C to 25°C (68°F to 77°F).

Methotrexate *(meth oh TREKS ate)*

U.S. Brand Names Rheumatrex®; Trexall™

Synonyms Amethopterin; Methotrexate Sodium; MTX; NSC-740

Generic Available Yes

Pharmacologic Category Antineoplastic Agent, Antimetabolite

Medication Safety Issues

Sound-alike/look-alike issues:

Methotrexate may be confused with metolazone, mitoxantrone

High alert medication: The Institute for Safe Medication Practices (ISMP) includes this medication among its list of drugs which have a heightened risk of causing significant patient harm when used in error.

Errors have occurred (resulting in death) when oral methotrexate was administered as "daily" dose instead of the recommended "weekly" dose.

Use Treatment of trophoblastic neoplasms; leukemias; psoriasis; rheumatoid arthritis (RA), including polyarticular-course juvenile rheumatoid arthritis (JRA); breast, head and neck, and lung carcinomas; osteosarcoma; soft-tissue sarcomas; carcinoma of gastrointestinal tract, esophagus, testes; lymphomas

Mechanism of Action/Effect Methotrexate is a folate antimetabolite that inhibits DNA synthesis. Methotrexate irreversibly binds to dihydrofolate reductase, inhibiting the formation of reduced folates, and thymidylate synthetase, resulting in inhibition of purine and thymidylic acid synthesis. Methotrexate is cell cycle specific for the S phase of the cycle.

The MOA in the treatment of rheumatoid arthritis is unknown, but may affect immune function. In psoriasis, methotrexate is thought to target rapidly proliferating epithelial cells in the skin.

Contraindications Hypersensitivity to methotrexate or any component of the formulation; severe renal or hepatic impairment; pre-existing profound bone marrow suppression in patients with psoriasis or rheumatoid arthritis, alcoholic liver disease, AIDS, pre-existing blood dyscrasias; pregnancy (in patients with psoriasis or rheumatoid arthritis); breast-feeding

Warnings/Precautions The U.S. Food and Drug Administration (FDA) currently recommends that procedures for proper handling and disposal of antineoplastic agents be considered.

May cause potentially life-threatening pneumonitis (may occur at any time during therapy and at any dosage); monitor closely for pulmonary symptoms, particularly dry, nonproductive cough. Methotrexate may cause photosensitivity and/or severe dermatologic reactions which are not dose-related. Methotrexate has been associated with acute and chronic hepatotoxicity, fibrosis, and cirrhosis. Risk is related to cumulative dose and prolonged exposure. Ethanol abuse, obesity, advanced age, and diabetes may increase the risk of hepatotoxic reactions.

Methotrexate may cause renal failure, gastrointestinal toxicity, or bone marrow depression. Use with caution in patients with renal impairment, peptic ulcer disease, ulcerative colitis, or pre-existing bone marrow suppression. Gastrointestinal toxicity may be severe: diarrhea and ulcerative stomatitis may require interruption of therapy; death from hemorrhagic enteritis or intestinal perforation has been reported. Methotrexate penetrates slowly into 3rd space fluids, such as pleural effusions or ascites, and exits slowly from these compartments (slower than from plasma). The potential for toxicity may be increased under these conditions. Dosage reduction may be necessary in patients with renal or hepatic impairment, ascites, and pleural effusion. Toxicity from methotrexate or any immunosuppressive is increased in the elderly.

Severe bone marrow suppression, aplastic anemia, and GI toxicity have occurred during concomitant administration with NSAIDs. Use caution when used with other hepatotoxic agents (azathioprine, retinoids, sulfasalazine). Methotrexate given concomitantly with radiotherapy may increase the risk of soft tissue necrosis and osteonecrosis. Immune suppression may lead to opportunistic infections.

For rheumatoid arthritis and psoriasis, immunosuppressive therapy should only be used when disease is active and less toxic; traditional therapy is ineffective. Discontinue therapy in RA or psoriasis if a significant decrease in hematologic components is noted. Methotrexate formulations and/or diluents containing preservatives should not be used for intrathecal or high-dose therapy. Methotrexate injection may contain benzyl alcohol and should not be used in neonates.

Drug Interactions

Decreased Effect: Cholestyramine may decrease levels of methotrexate. Corticosteroids may decrease uptake of methotrexate into leukemia cells. Administration of these drugs should be separated by 12 hours. Dexamethasone has been reported to not affect methotrexate influx into cells.

Increased Effect/Toxicity: Concurrent therapy with NSAIDs has resulted in severe bone marrow suppression, aplastic anemia, and GI toxicity. NSAIDs should not be used during moderate or high-dose methotrexate due to increased and prolonged methotrexate levels (may increase toxicity); NSAID use during treatment of rheumatoid arthritis has not been fully explored, but continuation of prior regimen has been allowed in some circumstances, with cautious monitoring. Salicylates may increase methotrexate levels, however salicylate doses used for prophylaxis of cardiovascular events are not likely to be of concern.

Penicillins, probenecid, sulfonamides, tetracyclines may increase methotrexate concentrations due to a reduction in renal tubular secretion; primarily a concern with high doses of methotrexate. Hepatotoxic agents (acitretin, azathioprine, retinoids, sulfasalazine) may increase the risk of hepatotoxic reactions with methotrexate.

Concomitant administration of cyclosporine with methotrexate may increase levels and toxicity of each. Methotrexate may increase mercaptopurine or theophylline levels. Methotrexate, when administered prior to cytarabine, may enhance the efficacy and toxicity of cytarabine; some combination treatment regimens (eg, hyper-CVAD) have been designed to take advantage of this interaction.

Concurrent use of live virus vaccines may result in infections.

Nutritional/Ethanol Interactions

Ethanol: Avoid ethanol (may be associated with increased liver injury).
Food: Methotrexate peak serum levels may be decreased if taken with food. Milk-rich foods may decrease methotrexate absorption. Folate may decrease drug response.
Herb/Nutraceutical: Avoid echinacea (has immunostimulant properties).

Adverse Reactions Note: Adverse reactions vary by route and dosage. Hematologic and/or gastrointestinal toxicities may be common at dosages used in chemotherapy; these reactions are much less frequent when used at typical dosages for rheumatic diseases.

>10%:
Central nervous system (with I.T. administration or very high-dose therapy):
Arachnoiditis: Acute reaction manifested as severe headache, nuchal rigidity, vomiting, and fever; may be alleviated by reducing the dose
Subacute toxicity: 10% of patients treated with 12-15 mg/m^2 of I.T. methotrexate may develop this in the second or third week of therapy; consists of motor paralysis of extremities, cranial nerve palsy, seizure, or coma. This has also been seen in pediatric cases receiving very high-dose I.V. methotrexate (when enough methotrexate can get across into the CSF).
Demyelinating encephalopathy: Seen months or years after receiving methotrexate; usually in association with cranial irradiation or other systemic chemotherapy
Dermatologic: Reddening of skin
Endocrine & metabolic: Hyperuricemia, defective oogenesis or spermatogenesis
Gastrointestinal: Ulcerative stomatitis, glossitis, gingivitis, nausea, vomiting, diarrhea, anorexia, intestinal perforation, mucositis (dose dependent; appears in 3-7 days after therapy, resolving within 2 weeks)
Emetic potential:
<100 mg: Moderately low (10% to 30%)
≥100 mg or <250 mg: Moderate (30% to 60%)
≥250 mg: Moderately high (60% to 90%)
Hematologic: Leukopenia, thrombocytopenia
Renal: Renal failure, azotemia, nephropathy
Respiratory: Pharyngitis

1% to 10%:
Cardiovascular: Vasculitis
Central nervous system: Dizziness, malaise, encephalopathy, seizure, fever, chills
Dermatologic: Alopecia, rash, photosensitivity, depigmentation or hyperpigmentation of skin
(Continued)

Methotrexate *(Continued)*

Endocrine & metabolic: Diabetes

Genitourinary: Cystitis

Hematologic: Hemorrhage

Myelosuppressive: This is the primary dose-limiting factor (along with mucositis) of methotrexate; occurs about 5-7 days after methotrexate therapy, and should resolve within 2 weeks

WBC: Mild

Platelets: Moderate

Onset: 7 days

Nadir: 10 days

Recovery: 21 days

Hepatic: Cirrhosis and portal fibrosis have been associated with chronic methotrexate therapy; acute elevation of liver enzymes are common after high-dose methotrexate, and usually resolve within 10 days.

Neuromuscular & skeletal: Arthralgia

Ocular: Blurred vision

Renal: Renal dysfunction: Manifested by an abrupt rise in serum creatinine and BUN and a fall in urine output; more common with high-dose methotrexate, and may be due to precipitation of the drug. The best treatment is prevention: Aggressively hydrate with 3 L/m^2/day starting 12 hours before therapy and continue for 24-36 hours; alkalinize the urine by adding 50 mEq of bicarbonate to each liter of fluid; keep urine flow over 100 mL/hour and urine pH >7.

Respiratory: Pneumonitis: Associated with fever, cough, and interstitial pulmonary infiltrates; treatment is to withhold methotrexate during the acute reaction; interstitial pneumonitis has been reported to occur with an incidence of 1% in patients with RA (dose 7.5-15 mg/week)

Overdosage/Toxicology Symptoms of overdose include nausea, vomiting, alopecia, melena, and renal failure.

Antidote: Leucovorin; administer as soon as toxicity is seen. Administer 10 mg/m^2 orally or parenterally. Follow with 10 mg/m^2 orally every 6 hours for 72 hours. After 24 hours following methotrexate administration, if the serum creatinine is ≥50% premethotrexate serum creatinine, increase leucovorin dose to 100 mg/m^2 every 3 hours until serum methotrexate level is <5 x 10^{-8} M. Hydration and alkalinization may be used to prevent precipitation of methotrexate or methotrexate metabolites in the renal tubules. Toxicity in low dose range is negligible, but may present mucositis and mild bone marrow suppression; severe bone marrow toxicity can result from overdose. Generally, neither peritoneal nor hemodialysis have been shown to increase elimination. However, effective clearance of methotrexate has been reported with acute, intermittent hemodialysis using a high-flux dialyzer. Leucovorin should be administered intravenously, never intrathecally, for overdoses of intrathecal methotrexate.

Pharmacodynamics/Kinetics

Onset of Action: Antirheumatic: 3-6 weeks; additional improvement may continue longer than 12 weeks

Absorption: Oral: Rapid; well absorbed at low doses (<30 mg/m^2), incomplete after large doses; I.M. injection: Complete

Time to Peak: Serum: Oral: 1-2 hours; I.M.: 30-60 minutes

Protein Binding: 50%

Half-Life Elimination: Low dose: 3-10 hours; High dose: 8-12 hours

Metabolism: <10%; degraded by intestinal flora to DAMPA by carboxypeptidase; hepatic aldehyde oxidase converts methotrexate to 7-OH methotrexate; polyglutamates are produced intracellularly and are just as potent as methotrexate; their production is dose- and duration-dependent and they are slowly eliminated by the cell once formed

Excretion: Urine (44% to 100%); feces (small amounts)

Dosing

Adults: Refer to individual protocols.

Note: Doses between 100 mg/m^2 to 500 mg/m^2 may require leucovorin rescue. Doses >500 mg/m^2 require leucovorin rescue.

Antineoplastic dosage range: I.V.: Range is wide from 30-40 mg/m^2/week to 100-12,000 mg/m^2 with leucovorin rescue

Trophoblastic neoplasms:

Oral, I.M.: 15-30 mg/day for 5 days; repeat in 7 days for 3-5 courses

I.V.: 11 mg/m^2 days 1 through 5 every 3 weeks

Head and neck cancer: Oral, I.M., I.V.: 25-50 mg/m^2 once weekly

Mycosis fungoides (cutaneous T-cell lymphoma): Oral, I.M.: Initial (early stages):

5-50 mg once weekly **or**

15-37.5 mg twice weekly

Bladder cancer: I.V.:

30 mg/m^2 day 1 and 8 every 3 weeks **or**

30 mg/m^2 day 1, 15, and 22 every 4 weeks

Breast cancer: I.V.: 30-60 mg/m^2 Day 1 and 8 every 3-4 weeks

Gastric cancer: I.V.:1500 mg/m^2 every 4 weeks

Lymphoma, non-Hodgkin's: I.V.:

30 mg/m^2 days 3 and 10 every 3 weeks **or**

120 mg/m^2 day 8 and 15 every 3-4 weeks **or**

200 mg/m^2 day 8 and 15 every 3 weeks **or**

400 mg/m^2 every 4 weeks for 3 cycles **or**

1 g/m^2 every 3 weeks **or**

1.5 g/m^2 every 4 weeks

Sarcoma: I.V.: 8-12 g/m^2 weekly for 2-4 weeks

Rheumatoid arthritis: Oral: 7.5 mg once weekly **or** 2.5 mg every 12 hours for 3 doses/week, not to exceed 20 mg/week

Psoriasis: Oral: 2.5-5 mg/dose every 12 hours for 3 doses given weekly **or** Oral, I.M.: 10-25 mg/dose given once weekly

Ectopic pregnancy: I.M., I.V.: 50 mg/m^2 single-dose

Elderly: Refer to individual protocols; adjust for renal impairment.

Rheumatoid arthritis/psoriasis: Oral: Initial: 5-7.5 mg/week, not to exceed 20 mg/week

Pediatrics: Refer to individual protocols.

Note: Doses between 100 mg/m^2 to 500 mg/m^2 may require leucovorin rescue. Doses >500 mg/m^2 require leucovorin rescue.

Dermatomyositis: Oral: 15-20 mg/m^2/week as a single dose once weekly **or** 0.3-1 mg/kg/dose once weekly

Juvenile rheumatoid arthritis: Oral, I.M.: 10 mg/m^2 once weekly, then 5-15 mg/m^2/week as a single dose **or** as 3 divided doses given 12 hours apart

Antineoplastic dosage range:

Oral, I.M.: 7.5-30 mg/m^2/week **or** every 2 weeks

I.V.: 10-18,000 mg/m^2 bolus dosing **or** continuous infusion over 6-42 hours

For dosing schedules, see table:

Methotrexate Dosing Schedules

Dose	Route	Frequency
Conventional		
15-20 mg/m^2	P.O.	Twice weekly
30-50 mg/m^2	P.O., I.V.	Weekly
15 mg/day for 5 days	P.O., I.M.	Every 2-3 weeks
Intermediate		
50-150 mg/m^2*	I.V. push	Every 2-3 weeks
240 mg/m^2*	I.V. infusion	Every 4-7 days
0.5-1 g/m^2**	I.V. infusion	Every 2-3 weeks
High		
1-25 g/m^2*	I.V. infusion	Every 1-3 weeks

*Doses between 100-500 mg/m^2 may require leucovorin rescue in some patients.

**Followed with leucovorin rescue - refer to Leucovorin monograph for details.

Pediatric solid tumors (high-dose): I.V.:

<12 years: 12-25 g/m^2

≥12 years: 8 g/m^2

Acute lymphocytic leukemia (intermediate-dose): I.V.: Loading: 100 mg/m^2 bolus dose, followed by 900 mg/m^2/day infusion over 23-41 hours.

Meningeal leukemia: I.T.: 10-15 mg/m^2 (maximum dose: 15 mg) **or** an age-based dosing regimen; one possible system is:

≤3 months: 3 mg/dose

4-11 months: 6 mg/dose

1 year: 8 mg/dose

2 years: 10 mg/dose

≥3 years: 12 mg/dose

Renal Impairment:

Cl$_{cr}$ 61-80 mL/minute: Reduce dose to 75%.

Cl$_{cr}$ 51-60 mL/minute: Reduce dose to 70%.

Cl$_{cr}$ 10-50 mL/minute: Reduce dose to 30% to 50%.

Cl$_{cr}$ <10 mL/minute: Avoid use.

Hemodialysis effects: Not dialyzable (0% to 5%)

Supplemental dose is not necessary.

Peritoneal dialysis effects: Supplemental dose is not necessary.

CAVH effects: Unknown

Hepatic Impairment:

Bilirubin 3.1-5 mg/dL or AST >180 units: Administer 75% of dose.

Bilirubin >5 mg/dL: Do not use.

Available Dosage Forms

Injection, powder for reconstitution [preservative free]: 20 mg, 1 g

Injection, solution, as sodium: 25 mg/mL (2 mL, 10 mL) [contains benzyl alcohol]

Injection, solution, as sodium [preservative free]: 25 mg/mL (2 mL, 4 mL, 8 mL, 10 mL)

Tablet, as sodium: 2.5 mg

Rheumatrex®: 2.5 mg

Trexall™: 5 mg, 7.5 mg, 10 mg, 15 mg

Tablet, as sodium [dose pack] (Rheumatrex® Dose Pack): 2.5 mg (4 cards with 2, 3, 4, 5, or 6 tablets each)

Monitoring and Teaching Issues

Physical Assessment: Use with caution in presence of renal impairment, peptic ulcer disease, ulcerative colitis, pre-existing bone marrow suppression (see Contraindications and Warnings/Precautions for specific use cautions and contraindications). Assess potential for interactions with other Pharmacological agents and herbal products patient may be using (eg, NSAIDs, salicylates, echinacea, or anything that may reduce renal tubular secretion,; see Drug Interactions). Assess results of baseline and frequent laboratory tests (see Monitoring Laboratory Tests). Monitor adverse reactions closely during therapy (eg, hyper- or hypothyroidism, pneumonitis [dry, nonproductive cough], ulcerative stomatitis [GI pain], renal failure [decreased urine output]; see Adverse Reactions). Teach patient proper use, possible side effects/appropriate interventions, and adverse symptoms to report (see Patient Education). **Pregnancy risk factor X:** Determine that patient is not pregnant before beginning treatment. Instruct patient of childbearing age (or males who may have intercourse with women of childbearing age) in appropriate use of contraceptive measures during therapy and for 3 months following treatment of males or 1 ovulatory cycle in female patients.

(Continued)

Methotrexate *(Continued)*

Monitoring Laboratory Tests: For prolonged use (especially rheumatoid arthritis, psoriasis) a baseline liver biopsy, repeated at each 1-1.5 g cumulative dose interval, should be performed; WBC and platelet counts every 4 weeks; CBC and creatinine, LFTs every 3-4 months; chest x-ray

Patient Education: Do not take any new medication during therapy unless approved by prescriber. **Infusion/injection:** Report immediately any redness, swelling, pain, or burning at infusion/injection site. It is very important to maintain adequate hydration (2-3 L/day of fluids) unless instructed to restrict fluid intake and nutrition (small frequent meals may help). Avoid alcohol to prevent serious side effects. You will be more susceptible to infection (avoid crowds and exposure to infection and do not have any vaccinations without consulting prescriber). May cause sensitivity to sunlight (use sunscreen, wear protective clothing, and eyewear); nausea or vomiting (small frequent meals, frequent mouth care, sucking lozenges, or chewing gum may help; if unresolved, contact prescriber); drowsiness, dizziness, numbness, or blurred vision (use caution when driving or engaging in tasks that require alertness until response to drug is known); loss of hair (may be reversible); color change of skin; permanent sterility; or mouth sores (frequent mouth care with soft toothbrush or cotton swabs and frequent rinses may help). Report immediately any rash, excessive or unusual fatigue, or respiratory difficulty. Report rapid heartbeat or palpitations, black or tarry stools, fever, chills, unusual bleeding or bruising, shortness of breath, persistent GI disturbances, diarrhea, constipation, pain on urination or change in urinary patterns, or any other persistent adverse effects. **Pregnancy/breast-feeding precautions:** Do not get pregnant while taking this medication. Consult prescriber for appropriate contraceptive measures. This drug may cause birth defects. Do not breast-feed.

Dietary Considerations:
Sodium content of 100 mg injection: 20 mg (0.86 mEq)
Sodium content of 100 mg (low sodium) injection: 15 mg (0.65 mEq)

Geriatric Considerations: Toxicity to methotrexate or any immunosuppressive is increased in the elderly. Must monitor carefully. For rheumatoid arthritis and psoriasis, immunosuppressive therapy should only be used when disease is active and less toxic, traditional therapy is ineffective. Recommended doses should be reduced when initiating therapy in the elderly due to possible decreased metabolism, reduced renal function, and presence of interacting diseases and drugs. Adjust dose as needed for renal function (Cl_{cr}).

Pregnancy Risk Factor: X (psoriasis, rheumatoid arthritis)

Lactation: Enters breast milk/contraindicated

Administration

I.M.: May be administered I.M.

I.V.: May be administered I.V.; I.V. administration may be as slow push, short bolus infusion, or 24- to 42-hour continuous infusion

Specific dosing schemes vary, but high dose should be followed by leucovorin calcium to prevent toxicity; refer to Leucovorin monograph *on page 875*

Other: May be administered I.T.

Reconstitution: Dilute powder with D_5W or NS to a concentration of ≤25 mg/mL (20 mg and 50 mg vials) and 50 mg/mL (1 g vial). Intrathecal solutions may be reconstituted to 2.5-5 mg/mL with NS, D_5W, lactated Ringer's, or Elliott's B solution. **Use preservative free preparations for intrathecal or high-dose administration.**

Compatibility: Stable in D_5NS, D_5W, NS

Y-site administration: Incompatible with chlorpromazine, gemcitabine, idarubicin, ifosfamide, midazolam, nalbuphine, promethazine, propofol

Compatibility when admixed: Incompatible with bleomycin

Storage: Store tablets and intact vials at room temperature (15°C to 25°C); protect from light. Solution diluted in D_5W or NS is stable for 24 hours at room temperature (21°C to 25°C). Reconstituted solutions with a preservative may be stored under refrigeration for up to 3 months, and up to 4 weeks at room temperature. Intrathecal dilutions are stable at room temperature for 7 days, but it is generally recommended that they be used within 4-8 hours.

Additional Information Latex-free products: 50 mg/2 mL, 100 mg/4 mL, and 250 mg/10 mL vials with and without preservatives by Immunex

Related Information
Maternal / Fetal Toxicology *on page 1762*

♦ **Methotrexate Sodium** *see* Methotrexate *on page 974*

Methoxsalen *(meth OKS a len)*

U.S. Brand Names 8-MOP®; Oxsoralen®; Oxsoralen-Ultra®; Uvadex®

Synonyms Methoxypsoralen; 8-Methoxypsoralen; 8-MOP

Generic Available No

Pharmacologic Category Psoralen

Use

Oral: Symptomatic control of severe, recalcitrant disabling psoriasis; repigmentation of idiopathic vitiligo; palliative treatment of skin manifestations of cutaneous T-cell lymphoma (CTCL)

Topical: Repigmentation of idiopathic vitiligo

Extracorporeal: Palliative treatment of skin manifestations of CTCL

Mechanism of Action/Effect Bonds covalently to pyrimidine bases in DNA, inhibits the synthesis of DNA, and suppresses cell division. The augmented sunburn reaction involves excitation of the methoxsalen molecule by radiation in the long-wave ultraviolet light (UVA), resulting in transference of energy to the methoxsalen molecule producing an excited state ("triplet electronic state"). The molecule, in this "triplet state", then reacts with cutaneous DNA.

Contraindications Hypersensitivity to methoxsalen (psoralens) or any component of the formulation; diseases associated with photosensitivity; cataract; invasive squamous cell cancer; aphakia; melanoma; pregnancy (Uvadex®)

Warnings/Precautions Serious burns may occur from ultraviolet radiation or sunlight even if exposed through glass if dose and/or exposure schedule is not maintained. Therapy may lead to increased risk of melanoma; this risk may be increased with fair skin or prior exposure to prolonged tar and UVB treatment, ionizing radiation, or arsenic. Methoxsalen concentrates in the lens; eyes should be shielded from light for 24 hours to prevent possible formation of cataracts. Soft-gelatin capsules and hard-gelatin capsule are not interchangeable. Use caution with basal cell carcinoma, hepatic, kidney, cardiac disease, or in the elderly. Use caution with other agents that may cause photosensitivity.

CTCL: For use only if inadequate response to other forms of therapy. Used in conjunction with long wave radiation of white blood cells using the UVAR® photopheresis system. Safety and efficacy in pediatric patients have not been established.

Psoriasis: For use only if inadequate response to other therapies when the diagnosis is biopsy proven. Administer only in conjunction with scheduled controlled doses of long wave ultraviolet (UVA) radiation (combination referred to as PUVA). Safety and efficacy in pediatric patients have not been established.

Vitiligo: Used in conjunction with controlled doses of long wave ultraviolet radiation or sunlight. Lotion should only be applied under direct supervision of prescriber and should not be dispensed to the patient. Safety and efficacy in children <12 years of age have not been established.

Drug Interactions

Cytochrome P450 Effect: Substrate of CYP2A6 (minor); **Inhibits** CYP1A2 (strong), 2A6 (strong), 2C8/9 (weak), 2C19 (weak), 2D6 (weak), 2E1 (weak), 3A4 (weak)

Increased Effect/Toxicity: Methoxsalen may increase the levels/effects of CYP1A2 substrates (eg, aminophylline, fluvoxamine, mexiletine, mirtazapine, ropinirole, theophylline, trifluoperazine) and CYP2A6 substrates (eg, dexmedetomidine, ifosfamide).

Nutritional/Ethanol Interactions Food: Methoxsalen serum concentrations may be increased if taken with food. Avoid furocoumarin-containing foods (limes, figs, parsley, celery, cloves, lemon, mustard, carrots).

Adverse Reactions Frequency not always defined.

Cardiovascular: Severe edema, hypotension

Central nervous system: Nervousness, vertigo, depression, dizziness, headache, malaise

Dermatologic: Painful blistering, burning, and peeling of skin; pruritus (10%), freckling, hypopigmentation, rash, cheilitis, erythema, itching, urticaria

Gastrointestinal: Nausea (10%)

Neuromuscular & skeletal: Loss of muscle coordination, leg cramps

Miscellaneous: Miliaria

Overdosage/Toxicology Symptoms of overdose include nausea and severe burns. Follow accepted treatment of severe burns. Keep room darkened until reaction subsides (8-24 hours or more).

Pharmacodynamics/Kinetics

Bioavailability: Bioavailability increased with soft-gelatin capsules compared to hard-gelatin capsules; exposure using UVAR® system is ~200 times less than with oral administration

Time to Peak: Time to peak, serum:

Hard-gelatin capsules: 1.5-6 hours (peak photosensitivity: ~4 hours)

Soft-gelatin capsules: 0.5-4 hours (peak photosensitivity: 1.5-2 hours)

Protein Binding: Reversibly bound to albumin

Half-Life Elimination: ~2 hours

Metabolism: Hepatic; forms metabolites

Excretion: Urine (~95% as metabolites)

Dosing

Adults & Elderly: Note: Refer to treatment protocols for UVA exposure guidelines.

Psoriasis: Oral: 10-70 mg 11/2-2 hours before exposure to UVA light; dose may be repeated 2-3 times per week, based on UVA exposure; doses must be given at least 48 hours apart; dosage is based upon patient's body weight and skin type:

<30 kg: 10 mg

30-50 kg: 20 mg

51-65 kg: 30 mg

66-80 kg: 40 mg

81-90 kg: 50 mg

91-115 kg: 60 mg

>115 kg: 70 mg

Vitiligo:

Oral (8-MOP®): 20 mg 2-4 hours before exposure to UVA light; dose may be repeated based on erythema and tenderness of skin; do not give on 2 consecutive days

Topical: Apply lotion 1-2 hours before exposure to UVA light, no more than once weekly

CTCL: Extracorporeal (Uvadex®): 200 mcg injected into the photoactivation bag during the collection cycle using the UVAR® photopheresis system (consult user's guide). Treatment schedule: Two consecutive days every 4 weeks for a minimum of 7 treatment cycles

Pediatrics: Vitiligo: Topical: Children >12 years: Refer to adult dosing.

Available Dosage Forms

Capsule:

8-MOP®: 10 mg [hard-gelatin capsule]

Oxsoralen-Ultra®: 10 mg [soft-gelatin capsule]

Lotion (Oxsoralen®): 1% (30 mL) [contains alcohol 71%]

Solution, for extracorporeal administration (Uvadex®): 20 mcg/mL (10 mL) **[not for injection]**

(Continued)

Methoxsalen (Continued)

Monitoring and Teaching Issues

Physical Assessment: Note: This drug is administered in conjunction with ultraviolet light or ultraviolet radiation therapy under supervision of provider. Assess potential for interactions with other pharmacological agents patient may be taking (eg, may increase or decrease levels/effects of other agents; see Warnings/Precautions). Patient should be monitored closely for adverse reactions (eg, hypotension, burns, hyperpigmentation, nausea). Teach patient proper use, side effects/appropriate interventions (eg, sunlight precautions), and adverse reactions to report (see Patient Education).

Patient Education: Do not take any new medication during therapy unless approved by prescriber. This medication is used in conjunction with specific ultraviolet treatment. Take as directed, with food or milk to reduce nausea. Consult prescriber for specific dietary instructions. Avoid use of any other skin treatments unless approved by prescriber. Control exposure to direct sunlight as per prescriber's instructions. If sunlight cannot be avoided, use sunblock (consult prescriber for specific SPF level); wear protective clothing and wraparound protective eyewear. Consult prescriber immediately if burning, blistering, or skin irritation occur. **Pregnancy/breast-feeding precautions:** Inform prescriber if you are or intend to become pregnant. Breast-feeding is not recommended.

Dietary Considerations: To reduce nausea, oral drug can be administered with food or milk or in 2 divided doses 30 minutes apart.

Pregnancy Risk Factor: C/D (Uvadex®)

Pregnancy Issues: Fetal toxicity has been observed in animal studies, however, there are no adequate and well-controlled studies in pregnant women. Use during pregnancy is not recommended. Women of childbearing potential should be advised to avoid pregnancy.

Lactation: Excretion in breast milk unknown/not recommended

Administration

Topical: Hands and fingers of person applying the lotion should be protected to prevent possible photosensitization and/or burns.

♦ **Methoxypsoralen** see Methoxsalen on page 978

♦ **8-Methoxypsoralen** see Methoxsalen on page 978

♦ **Methylacetoxyprogesterone** see MedroxyPROGESTERone on page 938

Methyldopa (meth il DOE pa)

Synonyms Aldomet; Methyldopate Hydrochloride

Generic Available Yes

Pharmacologic Category Alpha-Adrenergic Inhibitor

Medication Safety Issues

Sound-alike/look-alike issues:

Methyldopa may be confused with L-dopa, levodopa

Use Management of moderate to severe hypertension

Mechanism of Action/Effect Stimulation of central alpha-adrenergic receptors by a false transmitter that results in a decreased sympathetic outflow to the heart, kidneys, and peripheral vasculature

Contraindications Hypersensitivity to methyldopa or any component of the formulation; active hepatic disease; liver disorders previously associated with use of methyldopa; on MAO inhibitors; bisulfite allergy if using oral suspension or injectable

Warnings/Precautions May rarely produce hemolytic anemia and liver disorders; positive Coombs' test occurs in 10% to 20% of patients (perform periodic CBCs); sedation usually transient may occur during initial therapy or whenever the dose is increased. Use with caution in patients with previous liver disease or dysfunction, the active metabolites of methyldopa accumulate in uremia. Patients with impaired renal function may respond to smaller doses. Elderly patients may experience syncope (avoid by giving smaller doses). Tolerance may occur usually between the second and third month of therapy. Adding a diuretic or increasing the dosage of methyldopa frequently restores blood pressure control. Because of its CNS effects, methyldopa is not considered a drug of first choice in the elderly. Often considered the drug of choice for treatment of hypertension in pregnancy. Do not use injectable if bisulfite allergy.

Drug Interactions

Decreased Effect: Iron supplements can interact and cause a significant **increase** in blood pressure. Ferrous sulfate and ferrous gluconate decrease bioavailability. Barbiturates and TCAs may reduce response to methyldopa.

Increased Effect/Toxicity: Beta-blockers, MAO inhibitors, phenothiazines, and sympathomimetics (including epinephrine) may result in hypertension (sometimes severe) when combined with methyldopa. Methyldopa may increase lithium serum levels resulting in lithium toxicity. Levodopa may cause enhanced blood pressure lowering; methyldopa may also potentiate the effect of levodopa. Tolbutamide, haloperidol, and anesthetics effects/toxicity are increased with methyldopa.

Nutritional/Ethanol Interactions Herb/Nutraceutical: Avoid dong quai if using for hypertension (has estrogenic activity). Avoid ephedra, yohimbe, ginseng (may worsen hypertension). Avoid valerian, St John's wort, kava kava, gotu kola (may increase CNS depression). Avoid natural licorice (causes sodium and water retention and increases potassium loss). Avoid garlic (may have increased antihypertensive effect).

Lab Interactions Methyldopa interferes with the following laboratory tests: urinary uric acid, serum creatinine (alkaline picrate method), AST (colorimetric method), and urinary catecholamines (falsely high levels)

Adverse Reactions

>10%: Cardiovascular: Peripheral edema

1% to 10%:

Central nervous system: Drug fever, mental depression, anxiety, nightmares, drowsiness, headache

Gastrointestinal: Dry mouth

Overdosage/Toxicology Symptoms of overdose include hypotension, sedation, brady-cardia, dizziness, constipation or diarrhea, flatus, nausea, and vomiting. Treatment is supportive and symptomatic. Can be removed by hemodialysis.

Pharmacodynamics/Kinetics

Onset of Action: Peak effect: Hypotensive: Oral/parenteral: 3-6 hours

Duration of Action: 12-24 hours

Protein Binding: <15%

Half-Life Elimination: 75-80 minutes; End-stage renal disease: 6-16 hours

Metabolism: Intestinal and hepatic

Excretion: Urine (85% as metabolites) within 24 hours

Dosing

Adults: Hypertension:

Oral: Initial: 250 mg 2-3 times/day; increase every 2 days as needed (maximum dose: 3 g/day); usual dose range (JNC 7): 250-1000 mg/day in 2 divided doses

I.V.: 250-1000 mg every 6-8 hours; maximum: 1 g every 6 hours

Elderly: Oral: Initial: 125 mg 1-2 times/day; increase by 125 mg every 2-3 days as needed. Adjust for renal impairment. See Geriatric Considerations.

Pediatrics: Hypertension:

Oral: Initial: 10 mg/kg/day in 2-4 divided doses; increase every 2 days as needed to maximum dose of 65 mg/kg/day. Do not exceed 3 g/day.

I.V.: 5-10 mg/kg/dose every 6-8 hours up to a total dose of 65 mg/kg/24 hours or 3 g/24 hours

Renal Impairment:

Cl_{cr} >50 mL/minute: Administer every 8 hours.

Cl_{cr} 10-50 mL/minute: Administer every 8-12 hours.

Cl_{cr} <10 mL/minute: Administer every 12-24 hours.

Slightly dialyzable (5% to 20%)

Available Dosage Forms

Injection, solution, as methyldopate hydrochloride: 50 mg/mL (5 mL) [contains sodium bisulfite]

Tablet: 250 mg, 500 mg

Monitoring and Teaching Issues

Physical Assessment: See Warnings/Precautions for specific use cautions. Assess potential for interactions with other pharmacological agents or herbal products patient may be taking (eg, anything that affects blood pressure; see Drug Interactions). See Administration for infusion specifics. Assess CBC and liver enzymes regularly during therapy. Monitor therapeutic effectiveness (normotensive) and adverse reactions on a regular basis (eg, hypotension, bradycardia, CNS changes; see Adverse Reactions). Teach patient use, possible side effects/appropriate interventions, and adverse symptoms to report (see Patient Education).

Monitoring Laboratory Tests: CBC, liver enzymes, Coombs' test (direct)

Patient Education: Do not take any new medication during therapy unless approved by prescriber (especially any cough or cold remedies, diet pills, stay-awake medications). **Oral:** Take as directed. Do not skip dose or discontinue without consulting prescriber. Follow recommended diet and exercise program. This medication may cause altered color of urine (normal); drowsiness, dizziness, or impaired judgment (use caution when driving or engaging in tasks that require alertness until response to drug is known); postural hypotension (use caution when rising from sitting or lying position or when climbing stairs); or dry mouth or nausea (frequent mouth care or sucking lozenges may help). Report altered CNS status (eg, nightmares, depression, anxiety, increased nervousness); sudden weight gain (weigh yourself in the same clothes at the same time of day once a week); unusual or persistent swelling of ankles, feet, or extremities; palpitations or rapid heartbeat; persistent weakness, fatigue, or unusual bleeding; or other persistent side effects.

Dietary Considerations: Dietary requirements for vitamin B_{12} and folate may be increased with high doses of methyldopa.

Geriatric Considerations: Because of its CNS effects, methyldopa is not considered a drug of first choice in the elderly. Adjust dose for renal function.

Pregnancy Risk Factor: B

Pregnancy Issues: Crosses the placenta. Hypotension reported. A large amount of clinical experience with the use of these drugs for the management of hypertension during pregnancy is available. Available evidence suggests safe use during pregnancy.

Lactation: Enters breast milk/compatible

Breast-Feeding Issues: Crosses into breast milk at extremely low levels. AAP considers compatible with breast-feeding.

Administration

I.V.: Infuse over 30 minutes.

Compatibility: Stable in dextran 6% in NS, D_5NS, D_5W, sodium bicarbonate 5%, NS

Compatibility when admixed: Incompatible with amphotericin B, methohexital

Storage: Injectable dosage form is most stable at acid to neutral pH. Stability of parenteral admixture at room temperature (25°C) is 24 hours. Stability of parenteral admixture at refrigeration temperature (4°C) is 4 days.

Standard diluent: 250-500 mg/100 mL D_5W

Methyldopa and Hydrochlorothiazide

(meth il DOE pa & hye droe klor oh THYE a zide)

U.S. Brand Names Aldoril®

Synonyms Hydrochlorothiazide and Methyldopa

Generic Available Yes

Pharmacologic Category Antihypertensive Agent, Combination

Medication Safety Issues

Sound-alike/look-alike issues:

Aldoril® may be confused with Aldoclor®, Aldomet®, Elavil®

(Continued)

Methyldopa and Hydrochlorothiazide *(Continued)*

Use Management of moderate to severe hypertension

Dosing

Adults: Hypertension: Oral: 1 tablet 2-3 times/day for first 48 hours, then decrease or increase at intervals of not less than 2 days until an adequate response is achieved. Patients requiring higher doses may receive Aldoril® D30 once daily. Hydrochlorothiazide doses greater than 50 mg daily should be avoided.

Elderly: Refer to dosing in individual monographs.

Renal Impairment: Cl$_{cr}$ 30 mL/minute: Thiazides are recommended; loop diuretics are preferred.

Available Dosage Forms Tablet: Methyldopa 250 mg and hydrochlorothiazide 15 mg; methyldopa 250 mg and hydrochlorothiazide 25 mg

Aldoril® 25: Methyldopa 250 mg and hydrochlorothiazide 25 mg

Monitoring and Teaching Issues

Physical Assessment: See individual agents.

Patient Education: See individual agents. **Pregnancy precaution:** Inform prescriber if you are or intend to become pregnant.

Pregnancy Risk Factor: C

Lactation: Enters breast milk/compatible

Related Information

Hydrochlorothiazide *on page 751*
Methyldopa *on page 980*

- ◆ **Methyldopate Hydrochloride** *see Methyldopa on page 980*
- ◆ **Methylene Blue** *see page 1625*
- ◆ **Methylergometrine Maleate** *see Methylergonovine on page 982*

Methylergonovine (meth il er goe NOE veen)

U.S. Brand Names Methergine®

Synonyms Methylergometrine Maleate; Methylergonovine Maleate

Generic Available No

Pharmacologic Category Ergot Derivative

Medication Safety Issues

Sound-alike/look-alike issues:

Methylergonovine and terbutaline parenteral dosage forms look similar. Due to their contrasting indications, use care when administering these agents.

Use Prevention and treatment of postpartum and postabortion hemorrhage caused by uterine atony or subinvolution

Mechanism of Action/Effect Similar smooth muscle actions as seen with ergotamine; however, it affects primarily uterine smooth muscles producing sustained contractions and thereby shortens the third stage of labor

Contraindications Hypersensitivity to methylergonovine or any component of the formulation; ergot alkaloids are contraindicated with potent inhibitors of CYP3A4 (includes protease inhibitors, azole antifungals, and some macrolide antibiotics); hypertension; toxemia; pregnancy

Warnings/Precautions Use caution in patients with sepsis, obliterative vascular disease, hepatic, or renal involvement, or second stage of labor; administer with extreme caution if using intravenously. Pleural and peritoneal fibrosis have been reported with prolonged daily use. Cardiac valvular fibrosis has also been associated with ergot alkaloids.

Drug Interactions

Cytochrome P450 Effect: Substrate of CYP3A4 (major)

Decreased Effect: Effects of methylergonovine may be diminished by antipsychotics, metoclopramide/

Increased Effect/Toxicity: CYP3A4 inhibitors may increase the levels/effects of methylergonovine; example inhibitors include azole antifungals, ciprofloxacin, clarithromycin, diclofenac, doxycycline, erythromycin, imatinib, isoniazid, nefazodone, nicardipine, propofol, protease inhibitors, quinidine, and verapamil. Ergot alkaloids are contraindicated with potent CYP3A4 inhibitors. Methylergonovine may increase the effects of 5-HT$_1$ agonists (eg, sumatriptan), MAO inhibitors, sibutramine, and other serotonin agonists (serotonin syndrome). Severe vasoconstriction may occur when peripheral vasoconstrictors or beta-blockers are used in patients receiving ergot alkaloids; concurrent use is contraindicated.

Adverse Reactions Frequency not defined.

Cardiovascular: Acute MI, hypertension, temporary chest pain, palpitation

Central nervous system: Hallucinations, dizziness, seizure, headache

Endocrine & metabolic: Water intoxication

Gastrointestinal: Nausea, vomiting, diarrhea, foul taste

Local: Thrombophlebitis

Neuromuscular & skeletal: Leg cramps

Otic: Tinnitus

Renal: Hematuria

Respiratory: Dyspnea, nasal congestion

Miscellaneous: Diaphoresis

Overdosage/Toxicology Symptoms of overdose include prolonged gangrene, numbness in extremities, acute nausea, vomiting, abdominal pain, respiratory depression, hypotension, and seizures. Treatment is symptomatic and supportive.

Pharmacodynamics/Kinetics
Onset of Action: Oxytocic: Oral: 5-10 minutes; I.M.: 2-5 minutes; I.V.: Immediately
Duration of Action: Oral: ~3 hours; I.M.: ~3 hours; I.V.: 45 minutes
Absorption: Rapid
Bioavailability: Oral: 60%; I.M.: 78%
Time to Peak: Serum: Oral: 0.3-2 hours; I.M.: 0.2-0.6 hours
Half-Life Elimination: Biphasic: Initial: 1-5 minutes; Terminal: 0.5-2 hours
Metabolism: Hepatic
Excretion: Urine and feces

Dosing
Adults & Elderly: Prevention of hemorrhage:
Oral: 0.2 mg 3-4 times/day for 2-7 days
I.M., I.V.: 0.2 mg after delivery of anterior shoulder, after delivery of placenta, or during puerperium; may be repeated as required at intervals of 2-4 hours

Available Dosage Forms
Injection, solution, as maleate: 0.2 mg/mL (1 mL)
Tablet, as maleate: 0.2 mg

Monitoring and Teaching Issues
Physical Assessment: See Warning/Precautions for use cautions (eg, sepsis, obliterative vascular disease, hepatic, or renal involvement, hypertension). Assess potential for interactions with other pharmacological agents or herbal products patient may be taking (see Drug Interactions). Blood pressure, CNS status, and vaginal bleeding should be monitored on a regular basis, especially with infusion or injection (see Dosing for I.V. caution). Assess effectiveness (absence of hemorrhage) and adverse response (eg, ergotamine toxicity [headache, ringing in ears, nausea and vomiting, diarrhea, numbness or coldness of extremities, confusion, hallucinations, dyspnea, chest pain, convulsions]; see Adverse Reactions). Teach patient proper use (oral) and possible side effects/appropriate interventions (see Patient Education).
Patient Education: This drug will generally not be needed for more than a week. May cause nausea and vomiting (small frequent meals may help), dizziness, headache, or ringing in the ears (will reverse when drug is discontinued). Report any respiratory difficulty, acute headache, numb or cold extremities, or severe abdominal cramping. **Breast-feeding precaution:** Breast-feeding is not recommended.
Pregnancy Risk Factor: C
Pregnancy Issues: Prolonged constriction of the uterine vessels and/or increased myometrial tone may lead to reduced placental blood flow. This has contributed to fetal growth retardation in animals. Methylergonovine is intended for use after delivery of the infant.
Lactation: Enters breast milk/use caution

Administration
I.V.: Administer over ≥60 seconds. Should not be routinely administered I.V. because of possibility of inducing sudden hypertension and cerebrovascular accident.
Compatibility: Stable in NS
Storage:
Ampul: Store under refrigeration at 2°C to 8°C (36°F to 46°F). Protect from light.
Tablet: Store below 25°C (77°F).

- ♦ **Methylergonovine Maleate** *see* Methylergonovine *on page 982*
- ♦ **Methylin™** *see* Methylphenidate *on page 983*
- ♦ **Methylin™ ER** *see* Methylphenidate *on page 983*
- ♦ **Methylmorphine** *see* Codeine *on page 366*

Methylphenidate (meth il FEN i date)
U.S. Brand Names Concerta®; Metadate® CD; Metadate™ ER; Methylin™; Methylin™ ER; Ritalin®; Ritalin® LA; Ritalin-SR®
Synonyms Methylphenidate Hydrochloride
Controlled Substance C-II
Generic Available Yes: Tablet
Pharmacologic Category Central Nervous System Stimulant
Medication Safety Issues
Sound-alike/look-alike issues:
Methylphenidate may be confused with methadone
Ritalin® may be confused with Ismelin®, Rifadin®
Use Treatment of attention-deficit/hyperactivity disorder (ADHD); symptomatic management of narcolepsy
Unlabeled/Investigational Use Depression (especially elderly or medically ill)
Mechanism of Action/Effect Mild CNS stimulant; blocks the reuptake mechanism of dopaminergic neurons; appears to stimulate the cerebral cortex and subcortical structures similar to amphetamines
Contraindications Hypersensitivity to methylphenidate, any component of the formulation, or idiosyncrasy to sympathomimetic amines; marked anxiety, tension, and agitation; glaucoma; use during or within 14 days following MAO inhibitor therapy; Tourette's syndrome or tics
Warnings/Precautions Has demonstrated value as part of a comprehensive treatment program for ADHD. Safety and efficacy in children <6 years of age not established. Use with caution in patients with bipolar disorder, diabetes mellitus, cardiovascular disease, hyperthyroidism, seizure disorders, insomnia, porphyria, or hypertension. Use caution in patients with history of ethanol or drug abuse. May exacerbate symptoms of behavior and thought disorder in psychotic patients. Do not use to treat severe depression or fatigue states. Potential for drug dependency exists - avoid abrupt discontinuation in patients who have received for prolonged periods. Visual disturbances have been reported (rare). Stimulant use has been associated with growth suppression. Growth should be monitored during treatment. Stimulants may unmask tics in individuals with coexisting Tourette's syndrome. Concerta® should
(Continued)

Methylphenidate *(Continued)*

not be used in patients with esophageal motility disorders or pre-existing severe gastrointestinal narrowing (small bowel disease, short gut syndrome, history of peritonitis, cystic fibrosis, chronic intestinal pseudo-obstruction, Meckel's diverticulum).

Drug Interactions

Cytochrome P450 Effect: Substrate of CYP2D6 (major); **Inhibits** CYP2D6 (weak)

Decreased Effect: Effectiveness of antihypertensive agents may be decreased. Carbamazepine may decrease the effect of methylphenidate.

Increased Effect/Toxicity: Methylphenidate may cause hypertensive effects when used in combination with MAO inhibitors or drugs with MAO-inhibiting activity (linezolid). Risk may be less with selegiline (MAO type B selective at low doses); it is best to avoid this combination. CYP2D6 inhibitors may increase the levels/effects of methylphenidate; example inhibitors include chlorpromazine, delavirdine, fluoxetine, miconazole, paroxetine, pergolide, quinidine, quinine, ritonavir, and ropinirole. NMS has been reported in a patient receiving methylphenidate and venlafaxine. Methylphenidate may increase levels of phenytoin, phenobarbital, TCAs, and warfarin. Increased toxicity with clonidine and sibutramine.

Nutritional/Ethanol Interactions

Ethanol: Avoid ethanol (may cause CNS depression).

Food: Food may increase oral absorption; Concerta® formulation is not affected. Food delays early peak and high-fat meals increase C_{max} and AUC of Metadate® CD formulation.

Herb/Nutraceutical: Avoid ephedra (may cause hypertension or arrhythmias) and yohimbe (also has CNS stimulatory activity).

Adverse Reactions Frequency not defined.

Cardiovascular: Angina, cardiac arrhythmia, cerebral arteritis, cerebral occlusion, hyper-/hypotension, palpitation, pulse increase/decrease, tachycardia

Central nervous system: Depression, dizziness, drowsiness, fever, headache, insomnia, nervousness, neuroleptic malignant syndrome (NMS), Tourette's syndrome, toxic psychosis

Dermatologic: Erythema multiforme, exfoliative dermatitis, hair loss, rash, urticaria

Endocrine & metabolic: Growth retardation

Gastrointestinal: Abdominal pain, anorexia, diarrhea, nausea, vomiting, weight loss

Hematologic: Anemia, leukopenia, thrombocytopenic purpura

Hepatic: Liver function tests abnormal, hepatic coma, transaminases increased

Neuromuscular & skeletal: Arthralgia, dyskinesia

Ocular: Blurred vision

Renal: Necrotizing vasculitis

Respiratory: Cough increased, pharyngitis, sinusitis, upper respiratory tract infection

Miscellaneous: Accidental injury, hypersensitivity reactions

Overdosage/Toxicology Symptoms of overdose include vomiting, agitation, tremor, hyperpyrexia, muscle twitching, hallucinations, tachycardia, mydriasis, sweating, and palpitations. There is no specific antidote; treatment is supportive.

Pharmacodynamics/Kinetics

Onset of Action: Peak effect:

Immediate release tablet: Cerebral stimulation: ~2 hours

Extended release capsule (Metadate® CD): Biphasic; initial peak similar to immediate release product, followed by second rising portion (corresponding to extended release portion)

Sustained release tablet: 4-7 hours

Osmotic release tablet (Concerta®): Initial: 1-2 hours

Duration of Action: Immediate release tablet: 3-6 hours; Sustained release tablet: 8 hours

Absorption: Readily

Time to Peak: C_{max}: 6-8 hours

Half-Life Elimination: 2-4 hours

Metabolism: Hepatic via de-esterification to active metabolite

Excretion: Urine (90% as metabolites and unchanged drug)

Dosing

Adults & Elderly:

Narcolepsy: Oral: 10 mg 2-3 times/day, up to 60 mg/day

Depression: Oral: Initial: 2.5 mg every morning before 9 AM; dosage may be increased by 2.5-5 mg every 2-3 days as tolerated to a maximum of 20 mg/day. May be divided (eg, 7 AM and 12 noon), but should not be given after noon. Do not use sustained release product.

ADHD: Oral: Refer to pediatric dosing.

Note: Discontinue periodically to re-evaluate or if no improvement occurs within 1 month.

Pediatrics: Note: Oral: Discontinue periodically to re-evaluate or if no improvement occurs within 1 month.

ADHD: Oral: Children ≥6 years: Initial: 0.3 mg/kg/dose or 2.5-5 mg/dose given before breakfast and lunch; increase by 0.1 mg/kg/dose or by 5-10 mg/day at weekly intervals; usual dose: 0.5-1 mg/kg/day; maximum dose: 2 mg/kg/day or 90 mg/day

Extended release products:

Metadate™ ER, Methylin™ ER, Ritalin® SR: Duration of action is 8 hours. May be given in place of regular tablets, once the daily dose is titrated using the regular tablets and the titrated 8-hour dosage corresponds to sustained release tablet size.

Metadate® CD, Ritalin® LA: Initial: 20 mg once daily; may be adjusted in 10-20 mg increments at weekly intervals; maximum: 60 mg/day

Concerta®:

Initial dose:

Children not currently taking methylphenidate: 18 mg once daily in the morning

Children currently taking methylphenidate: **Note:** Dosing based on current regimen and clinical judgment; suggested dosing listed below:

Patients taking methylphenidate 5 mg 2-3 times/day or 20 mg/day sustained release formulation: 18 mg once every morning

Patients taking methylphenidate 10 mg 2-3 times/day or 40 mg/day sustained release formulation: 36 mg once every morning

Patients taking methylphenidate 15 mg 2-3 times/day or 60 mg/day sustained release formulation: 54 mg once every morning

Dose adjustment: May increase dose in increments of 18 mg; dose may be adjusted at weekly intervals. A dosage strength of 27 mg is available for situations in which a dosage between 18-36 mg is desired. Maximum dose should not exceed 2 mg/kg/day **or** 54 mg/day in children 6-12 years or 72 mg/day in children 13-17 years.

Available Dosage Forms

Capsule, extended release, as hydrochloride:
Metadate® CD: 10 mg, 20 mg, 30 mg
Ritalin® LA: 10 mg, 20 mg, 30 mg, 40 mg
Tablet, as hydrochloride (Methylin™, Ritalin®): 5 mg, 10 mg, 20 mg
Tablet, extended release, as hydrochloride: 20 mg
Concerta®: 18 mg, 27 mg, 36 mg, 54 mg [osmotic controlled release]
Metadate™ ER, Methylin™ ER: 10 mg, 20 mg
Tablet, sustained release, as hydrochloride (Ritalin-SR®): 20 mg

Monitoring and Teaching Issues

Physical Assessment: Assess effectiveness and interactions of other medications patient may be taking. Assess for history of addiction; long-term use can result in dependence, abuse, or tolerance. Evaluate periodically for need for continued use. After long-term use, taper dosage slowly when discontinuing. Assess results of laboratory tests, therapeutic effectiveness, and adverse reactions at beginning of therapy and periodically with long-term use. Assess knowledge/teach patient appropriate use, interventions to reduce side effects, and importance of reporting adverse symptoms promptly.

Patient Education: Take exactly as directed, 30-45 minutes before meals with a full glass of water. Do not change dosage or discontinue without consulting prescriber. Response may take some time. Do not crush or chew sustained release dosage forms. Tablets and sustained release tablets should be taken 30-45 minutes before meals. Concerta® may be taken with or without food, but must be taken with water, milk, or juice. Metadate® CD and Ritalin® LA capsules may be opened and the contents sprinkled onto a small amount (equal to 1 tablespoon) of applesauce. Swallow applesauce without chewing. Do not crush or chew capsule contents. Avoid alcohol, caffeine, or other stimulants. Maintain adequate hydration (2-3 L/day of fluids) unless instructed to restrict fluid intake. You may experience decreased appetite or weight loss (small frequent meals may help maintain adequate nutrition); or restlessness, impaired judgment, or dizziness, especially during early therapy (use caution when driving or engaging in tasks requiring alertness until response to drug is known). Report unresolved rapid heartbeat; excessive agitation, nervousness, insomnia, tremors, or dizziness; blackened stool; skin rash or irritation; or altered gait or movement. Concerta® tablet shell may appear intact in stool; this is normal. Pediatrics: Monitor growth. **Pregnancy/breast-feeding precautions:** Inform prescriber if you are or intend to become pregnant. Consult prescriber if breast-feeding.

Dietary Considerations: Should be taken 30-45 minutes before meals. Concerta® is not affected by food and should be taken with water, milk, or juice. Metadate® CD should be taken before breakfast. Metadate™ ER should be taken before breakfast and lunch.

Geriatric Considerations: Methylphenidate is often useful in treating elderly patients who are discouraged, withdrawn, apathetic, or disinterested in their activities. In particular, it is useful in patients who are starting a rehabilitation program but have resigned themselves to fail; these patients may not have a major depressive disorder; will not improve memory or cognitive function; use with caution in patients with dementia who may have increased agitation and confusion (see Dosing and Adverse Reactions).

Pregnancy Risk Factor: C

Lactation: Excretion in breast milk unknown/use caution

Administration

Oral: Do not crush or allow patient to chew sustained release dosage form. To effectively avoid insomnia, dosing should be completed by noon.

Concerta®: Administer dose once daily in the morning. May be taken with or without food, but must be taken with water, milk, or juice.

Metadate® CD, Ritalin® LA: Capsules may be opened and the contents sprinkled onto a small amount (equal to 1 tablespoon) of applesauce. Swallow applesauce without chewing. Do not crush or chew capsule contents.

Storage:

Immediate release tablet: Do not store above 30°C (86°F); protect from light
Extended release capsule: Store in dose pack provided at 25°C (77°F)
Sustained release tablet: Do not store above 30°C (86°F); protect from moisture
Osmotic controlled release tablet (Concerta®): Store at 25°C (77°F); protect from humidity

Additional Information Treatment with methylphenidate may include "drug holidays" or periodic discontinuation in order to assess the patient's requirements and to decrease tolerance and limit suppression of linear growth and weight. Specific patients may require 3 doses/day for treatment of ADHD (ie, additional dose at 4 PM).

Concerta® is an osmotic controlled release formulation (OROS®) of methylphenidate. The tablet has an immediate-release overcoat that provides an initial dose of methylphenidate within 1 hour. The overcoat covers a trilayer core. The trilayer core is composed of two layers containing the drug and excipients, and one layer of osmotic components. As water from the gastrointestinal tract enters the core, the osmotic components expand and methylphenidate is released.

Metadate® CD capsules contain a mixture of immediate release and extended release beads, designed to release 30% of the dose (6 mg) immediately and 70% (14 mg) over an extended period.

Ritalin® LA uses a combination of immediate release and enteric coated, delayed release beads.

♦ **Methylphenidate Hydrochloride** see Methylphenidate on page 983

♦ **Methylphenoxy-Benzene Propanamine** *see* Atomoxetine *on page 151*
♦ **Methylphytyl Napthoquinone** *see* Phytonadione *on page 1209*

MethylPREDNISolone (meth il pred NIS oh lone)

U.S. Brand Names Depo-Medrol®; Medrol®; Solu-Medrol®

Synonyms A-Methapred; 6-α-Methylprednisolone; Methylprednisolone Acetate; Methylprednisolone Sodium Succinate

Generic Available Yes: Sodium succinate injection, tablet

Pharmacologic Category Corticosteroid, Systemic

Medication Safety Issues
Sound-alike/look-alike issues:
MethylPREDNISolone may be confused with medroxyPROGESTERone, predniSONE
Depo-Medrol® may be confused with Solu-Medrol®
Medrol® may be confused with Mebaral®
Solu-Medrol® may be confused with Depo-Medrol®

Use Primarily as an anti-inflammatory or immunosuppressant agent in the treatment of a variety of diseases including those of hematologic, allergic, inflammatory, neoplastic, and autoimmune origin. Prevention and treatment of graft-versus-host disease following allogeneic bone marrow transplantation.

Unlabeled/Investigational Use Treatment of fibrosing-alveolitis phase of adult respiratory distress syndrome (ARDS)

Mechanism of Action/Effect In a tissue-specific manner, corticosteroids regulate gene expression subsequent to binding specific intracellular receptors and translocation into the nucleus. Corticosteroids exert a wide array of physiologic effects, including modulation of carbohydrate, protein, and lipid metabolism, and maintenance of fluid and electrolyte homeostasis. Moreover, cardiovascular, immunologic, musculoskeletal, endocrine, and neurologic physiology are influenced by corticosteroids.

Contraindications Hypersensitivity to methylprednisolone or any component of the formulation; viral, fungal, or tubercular skin lesions; administration of live virus vaccines; serious infections, except septic shock or tuberculous meningitis. Methylprednisolone formulations containing benzyl alcohol preservative are contraindicated in infants.

Warnings/Precautions Use with caution in patients with hyperthyroidism, cirrhosis, nonspecific ulcerative colitis, hypertension, osteoporosis, thromboembolic tendencies, CHF, convulsive disorders, myasthenia gravis, thrombophlebitis, peptic ulcer, diabetes, glaucoma, cataracts, or tuberculosis. Use caution in hepatic impairment. Acute adrenal insufficiency may occur with abrupt withdrawal after long-term therapy or with stress. Because of the risk of adverse effects, systemic corticosteroids should be used cautiously in the elderly, in the smallest possible dose, and for the shortest possible time.

Drug Interactions
Cytochrome P450 Effect: Substrate of CYP3A4 (minor); **Inhibits** CYP3A4 (weak)
Decreased Effect: Phenytoin, phenobarbital, rifampin increase clearance of methylprednisolone. Potassium-depleting diuretics enhance potassium depletion. Skin test antigens, immunizations decrease antibody response and increase potential infections.
Increased Effect/Toxicity: Methylprednisolone may increase circulating glucose levels; may need adjustments of insulin or oral hypoglycemics. Methylprednisolone increases cyclosporine and tacrolimus blood levels. Itraconazole increases corticosteroid levels.

Nutritional/Ethanol Interactions
Ethanol: Avoid ethanol (may increase gastric mucosal irritation).
Food: Methylprednisolone interferes with calcium absorption. Limit caffeine.
Herb/Nutraceutical: St John's wort may decrease methylprednisolone levels. Avoid cat's claw, echinacea (have immunostimulant properties).

Lab Interactions Interferes with skin tests

Adverse Reactions Frequency not defined.
Cardiovascular: Edema, hypertension, arrhythmia
Central nervous system: Insomnia, nervousness, vertigo, seizure, psychoses, pseudotumor cerebri, headache, mood swings, delirium, hallucinations, euphoria
Dermatologic: Hirsutism, acne, skin atrophy, bruising, hyperpigmentation
Endocrine & metabolic: Diabetes mellitus, adrenal suppression, hyperlipidemia, Cushing's syndrome, pituitary-adrenal axis suppression, growth suppression, glucose intolerance, hypokalemia, alkalosis, amenorrhea, sodium and water retention, hyperglycemia
Gastrointestinal: Increased appetite, indigestion, peptic ulcer, nausea, vomiting, abdominal distention, ulcerative esophagitis, pancreatitis
Hematologic: Transient leukocytosis
Neuromuscular & skeletal: Arthralgia, muscle weakness, osteoporosis, fractures
Ocular: Cataracts, glaucoma
Miscellaneous: Infections, hypersensitivity reactions, avascular necrosis, secondary malignancy, intractable hiccups

Overdosage/Toxicology When consumed in high doses for prolonged periods, systemic hypercorticism and adrenal suppression may occur. In these cases, discontinuation should be done judiciously. Arrhythmias and cardiovascular collapse are possible with rapid intravenous infusion of high-dose methylprednisolone. May mask signs and symptoms of infection.

Pharmacodynamics/Kinetics
Onset of Action: Peak effect (route dependent): Oral: 1-2 hours; I.M.: 4-8 days; Intra-articular: 1 week; methylprednisolone sodium succinate is highly soluble and has a rapid effect by I.M. and I.V. routes
Duration of Action: Route dependent: Oral: 30-36 hours; I.M.: 1-4 weeks; Intra-articular: 1-5 weeks; methylprednisolone acetate has a low solubility and has a sustained I.M. effect
Half-Life Elimination: 3-3.5 hours; reduced in obese
Excretion: Clearance: Reduced in obese
Dosing
Adults: Only sodium succinate may be given I.V.; methylprednisolone sodium succinate is highly soluble and has a rapid effect by I.M. and I.V. routes. Methylprednisolone acetate has a low solubility and has a sustained I.M. effect.

Anti-inflammatory or immunosuppressive:

Oral: 2-60 mg/day in 1-4 divided doses to start, followed by gradual reduction in dosage to the lowest possible level consistent with maintaining an adequate clinical response.

I.M. (sodium succinate): 10-80 mg/day once daily

I.M. (acetate): 10-80 mg every 1-2 weeks

I.V. (sodium succinate): 10-40 mg over a period of several minutes and repeated I.V. or I.M. at intervals depending on clinical response; when high dosages are needed, give 30 mg/kg over a period ≥30 minutes and may be repeated every 4-6 hours for 48 hours.

Status asthmaticus: I.V. (sodium succinate): Loading dose: 2 mg/kg/dose, then 0.5-1 mg/kg/dose every 6 hours for up to 5 days

Acute spinal cord injury: I.V. (sodium succinate): 30 mg/kg over 15 minutes, followed in 45 minutes by a continuous infusion of 5.4 mg/kg/hour for 23 hours

Lupus nephritis: High-dose "pulse" therapy: I.V. (sodium succinate): 1 g/day for 3 days

Aplastic anemia: I.V. (sodium succinate): 1 mg/kg/day or 40 mg/day (whichever dose is higher), for 4 days. After 4 days, change to oral and continue until day 10 or until symptoms of serum sickness resolve, then rapidly reduce over approximately 2 weeks.

Pneumonia in AIDS patients due to *Pneumocystis*: I.V.: 40-60 mg every 6 hours for 7-10 days

Arthritis: Intra-articular (acetate): Administer every 1-5 weeks.

Large joints: 20-80 mg

Small joints: 4-10 mg

Intralesional (acetate): 20-60 mg every 1-5 weeks

Elderly: Only sodium succinate salt may be given I.V. Use the lowest effective adult dose.

Pediatrics: Dosing should be based on the lesser of ideal body weight or actual body weight. **Only sodium succinate may be given I.V.;** methylprednisolone sodium succinate is highly soluble and has a rapid effect by I.M. and I.V. routes. Methylprednisolone acetate has a low solubility and has a sustained I.M. effect.

Anti-inflammatory or immunosuppressive: Oral, I.M., I.V. (sodium succinate): Children: 0.5-1.7 mg/kg/day **or** 5-25 mg/m²/day in divided doses every 6-12 hours; "Pulse" therapy: 15-30 mg/kg/dose over ≥30 minutes given once daily for 3 days

Status asthmaticus: Children: I.V. (sodium succinate): Loading dose: 2 mg/kg/dose, then 0.5-1 mg/kg/dose every 6 hours for up to 5 days

Acute spinal cord injury: I.V. (sodium succinate): 30 mg/kg over 15 minutes, followed in 45 minutes by a continuous infusion of 5.4 mg/kg/hour for 23 hours

Lupus nephritis: I.V. (sodium succinate): 30 mg/kg over ≥30 minutes every other day for 6 doses

Renal Impairment:

Hemodialysis effects: Slightly dialyzable (5% to 20%)

Administer dose posthemodialysis.

Available Dosage Forms

Injection, powder for reconstitution, as sodium succinate: 125 mg [strength expressed as base]

Solu-Medrol®: 40 mg, 125 mg, 500 mg, 1 g, 2 g [packaged with diluent; diluent contains benzyl alcohol; strength expressed as base]

Solu-Medrol®: 500 mg, 1 g

Injection, suspension, as acetate (Depo-Medrol®): 20 mg/mL (5 mL); 40 mg/mL (5 mL); 80 mg/mL (5 mL) [contains benzyl alcohol; strength expressed as base]

Injection, suspension, as acetate [single-dose vial] (Depo-Medrol®): 40 mg/mL (1 mL, 10 mL); 80 mg/mL (1 mL)

Tablet: 4 mg

Medrol®: 2 mg, 4 mg, 8 mg, 16 mg, 32 mg

Tablet, dose-pack: 4 mg (21s)

Medrol® Dosepack™: 4 mg (21s)

Monitoring and Teaching Issues

Physical Assessment: Assess effectiveness and interactions of other medications patient may be taking. Monitor for effectiveness of therapy and adverse reactions according to dose, route, and length of therapy (especially with systemic administration). Assess knowledge/teach patient appropriate use, possible side effects/interventions, and adverse symptoms to report (ie, opportunistic infection, adrenal suppression). Instruct patients with diabetes to monitor serum glucose levels closely; corticosteroids can alter glycemic response. Dose may need to be increased if patient is experiencing higher than normal levels of stress. When discontinuing, taper dose and frequency slowly.

Monitoring Laboratory Tests: Blood glucose, electrolytes

Patient Education: Maintain adequate nutritional intake; consult prescriber for possibility of special dietary instructions. If you have diabetes, monitor serum glucose closely and notify prescriber of any changes; this medication can alter glycemic response. Avoid alcohol. Inform prescriber if you are experiencing unusual stress; dosage may need to be adjusted. You will be susceptible to infection (avoid crowds and and exposure to infection). You may experience insomnia or nervousness; use caution when driving or engaging in tasks requiring alertness until response to drug is known. Report increased pain, swelling, or redness in area being treated; excessive or sudden weight gain; swelling of extremities; respiratory difficulty; muscle pain or weakness; change in menstrual pattern; vision changes; signs of hyperglycemia; signs of infection (eg, fever, chills, mouth sores, perianal itching, vaginal discharge); blackened stool; other persistent side effects; or worsening of condition. **Pregnancy/breast-feeding precautions:** Inform prescriber if you are or intend to become pregnant. Consult prescriber if breast-feeding.

Oral: Take as directed, with food or milk. Take once-a-day dose in the morning. Do not take more than prescribed or discontinue without consulting prescriber.

Intra-articular: Refrain from excessive use of joint following therapy, even if pain is gone.

Dietary Considerations: Should be taken after meals or with food or milk; need diet rich in pyridoxine, vitamin C, vitamin D, folate, calcium, phosphorus, and protein.

(Continued)

MethylPREDNISolone (Continued)

Sodium content of 1 g sodium succinate injection: 2.01 mEq; 53 mg of sodium succinate salt is equivalent to 40 mg of methylprednisolone base

Methylprednisolone acetate: Depo-Medrol®

Methylprednisolone sodium succinate: Solu-Medrol®

Geriatric Considerations: Because of the risk of adverse effects, systemic corticosteroids should be used cautiously in the elderly, in the smallest possible dose, and for the shortest possible time.

Pregnancy Risk Factor: C

Lactation: Excretion in breast milk unknown

Administration

Oral: Give oral formulation with meals to decrease GI upset. Give daily dose in the morning to mimic normal peak blood levels.

I.V.: Only sodium succinate formulation may be given I.V. Acetate salt should not be given I.V.

Parenteral: Methylprednisolone sodium succinate may be administered I.M. or I.V.; I.V. administration may be IVP over one to several minutes or IVPB or continuous I.V. infusion.

I.V.: Succinate:

Low dose: ≤1.8 mg/kg or ≤125 mg/dose: I.V. push over 3-15 minutes

Moderate dose: ≥2 mg/kg or 250 mg/dose: I.V. over 15-30 minutes

High dose: 15 mg/kg or ≥500 mg/dose: I.V. over ≥30 minutes

Doses >15 mg/kg or ≥1 g: Administer over 1 hour

Do **not** administer high-dose I.V. push; hypotension, cardiac arrhythmia, and sudden death have been reported in patients given high-dose methylprednisolone I.V. push over <20 minutes. Intermittent infusion over 15-60 minutes; maximum concentration: I.V. push 125 mg/mL.

Topical: For external use only. Apply sparingly.

Reconstitution: Reconstituted solutions of methylprednisolone sodium succinate should be stored at room temperature (15°C to 30°C) and used within 48 hours. Stability of parenteral admixture at room temperature (25°C) and at refrigeration temperature (4°C) is 48 hours.

Standard diluent (Solu-Medrol®): 40 mg/50 mL D₅W; 125 mg/50 mL D₅W

Minimum volume (Solu-Medrol®): 50 mL D₅W

Compatibility: Incompatible with D₅¹/₂NS

Y-site administration: Incompatible with allopurinol, amsacrine, ciprofloxacin, docetaxel, etoposide phosphate, filgrastim, gemcitabine, ondansetron, paclitaxel, propofol, sargramostim, vinorelbine

Compatibility in syringe: Incompatible with doxapram

Compatibility when admixed: Incompatible with calcium gluconate, glycopyrrolate, insulin (regular), metaraminol, nafcillin, penicillin G sodium

Storage: Intact vials of methylprednisolone sodium succinate should be stored at controlled room temperature.

Additional Information Sodium content of 1 g sodium succinate injection: 2.01 mEq; 53 mg of sodium succinate salt is equivalent to 40 mg of methylprednisolone base

Methylprednisolone acetate: Depo-Medrol®

Methylprednisolone sodium succinate: Solu-Medrol®

Related Information

Corticosteroids *on page 1731*

FDA Name Differentiation Project: The Use of Tall-Man Letters *on page 15*

♦ 6-α-**Methylprednisolone** *see* MethylPREDNISolone *on page 986*

♦ **Methylprednisolone Acetate** *see* MethylPREDNISolone *on page 986*

♦ **Methylprednisolone Sodium Succinate** *see* MethylPREDNISolone *on page 986*

MethylTESTOSTERone *(meth il tes TOS te rone)*

U.S. Brand Names Android®; Methitest™; Testred®; Virilon®

Controlled Substance C-III

Generic Available No

Pharmacologic Category Androgen

Medication Safety Issues

Sound-alike/look-alike issues:

MethylTESTOSTERone may be confused with medroxyPROGESTERone

Virilon® may be confused with Verelan®

Use

Male: Hypogonadism; delayed puberty; impotence and climacteric symptoms

Female: Palliative treatment of metastatic breast cancer

Mechanism of Action/Effect Male: Stimulates receptors in organs and tissues to promote growth and development of male sex organs and maintains secondary sex characteristics in androgen-deficient males.

Contraindications Hypersensitivity to methyltestosterone or any component of the formulation; in males, known or suspected carcinoma of the breast or the prostate; pregnancy

Warnings/Precautions Use with extreme caution in patients with liver or kidney disease or serious heart disease. May accelerate bone maturation without producing compensatory gain in linear growth.

Drug Interactions

Decreased Effect: Decreased oral anticoagulant effect

Increased Effect/Toxicity: Effects of oral anticoagulants and hypoglycemic agents may be increased. Toxicity may occur with cyclosporine; avoid concurrent use.

Adverse Reactions Frequency not defined.

Male: Virilism, priapism, prostatic hyperplasia, prostatic carcinoma, impotence, testicular atrophy, gynecomastia

Female: Virilism, menstrual problems (amenorrhea), breast soreness, hirsutism (increase in pubic hair growth) atrophy

Cardiovascular: Edema

Central nervous system: Headache, anxiety, depression

Dermatologic: Acne, "male pattern" baldness, seborrhea

Endocrine & metabolic: Hypercalcemia, hypercholesterolemia

Gastrointestinal: GI irritation, nausea, vomiting

Hematologic: Leukopenia, polycythemia

Hepatic: Hepatic dysfunction, hepatic necrosis, cholestatic hepatitis

Miscellaneous: Hypersensitivity reactions

Overdosage/Toxicology Abnormal liver function tests

Pharmacodynamics/Kinetics

Metabolism: Hepatic

Excretion: Urine

Dosing

Adults & Elderly: Note: Buccal absorption produces twice the androgenic activity of oral tablets.

Hypogonadism; delayed puberty; impotence and climacteric symptoms (males):
Oral: 10-40 mg/day
Buccal: 5-25 mg/day

Breast pain/engorgement (Female):
Oral: 80 mg/day for 3-5 days
Buccal: 40 mg/day for 3-5 days

Breast cancer (Female):
Oral: 50-200 mg/day
Buccal: 25-100 mg/day

Available Dosage Forms

Capsule (Android®, Testred®, Virilon®): 10 mg

Tablet (Methitest™): 10 mg

Monitoring and Teaching Issues

Physical Assessment: For use in children see pediatric reference. Use extreme caution in presence of liver, kidney, or heart disease (see Warnings/Precautions for use cautions). Assess potential for interactions with other pharmacological agents patient may be taking (eg, effects of hypoglycemic agents may be increased; see Drug Interactions). Assess therapeutic effects (according to purpose for use) and adverse response frequently during therapy (eg, virilism [male and female], edema, CNS changes [anxiety, depression], acne, baldness, GI irritation, leukopenia, hepatic dysfunction; see Adverse Reactions). Caution patients with diabetes; effects of hypoglycemic agents may be increased. Teach patient proper use, possible side effects/appropriate interventions, and adverse symptoms to report (see Patient Education). **Pregnancy risk factor X:** Determine that patient is not pregnant before beginning treatment. Instruct patients of childbearing age or males who may have intercourse with women of childbearing age on appropriate contraceptive measures.

Patient Education: Take as directed; do not discontinue without consulting prescriber. If you have diabetes, monitor serum glucose closely and notify prescriber of changes; this medication can alter hypoglycemic requirements. May cause acne, growth of body hair, loss of libido, impotence, menstrual irregularity (usually reversible); or nausea or vomiting (small frequent meals, frequent mouth care, sucking lozenges, or chewing gum may help). Report changes in menstrual pattern; deepening of voice or unusual growth of body hair; gynecomastia or breast soreness; priapism; fluid retention (swelling of ankles, feet, or hands, respiratory difficulty, or sudden weight gain); change in color of urine or stool; yellowing of eyes or skin; unusual bruising or bleeding; unusual fatigue or weakness; or other adverse reactions. **Pregnancy/breast-feeding precautions:** Inform prescriber if you are pregnant. Do not get pregnant or cause a pregnancy (males) during or for 1 month following therapy. Consult prescriber for instruction on appropriate contraceptive measures. This drug may cause severe fetal defects. Do not breast-feed.

Geriatric Considerations: Since elderly males have prostate changes with age, it would be best to obtain a PSA initially and periodically. Retention of sodium and water could be a problem in patients with CHF and hypertension.

Pregnancy Risk Factor: X

Lactation: Excretion in breast milk unknown/contraindicated

Related Information

FDA Name Differentiation Project: The Use of Tall-Man Letters *on page 15*

Metoclopramide (met oh kloe PRA mide)

U.S. Brand Names Reglan®

Generic Available Yes

Pharmacologic Category Antiemetic; Gastrointestinal Agent, Prokinetic

Medication Safety Issues

Sound-alike/look-alike issues:

Metoclopramide may be confused with metolazone

Reglan® may be confused with Megace®, Regonol®, Renagel®

Use Symptomatic treatment of diabetic gastric stasis; gastroesophageal reflux

Unlabeled/Investigational Use Postpyloric placement of enteral feeding tubes; prevention and/or treatment of nausea and vomiting associated with chemotherapy, radiation therapy, or postsurgery

Mechanism of Action/Effect Blocks dopamine receptors and (when given in higher doses) also blocks serotonin receptors in chemoreceptor trigger zone of the CNS; enhances the response to acetylcholine of tissue in upper GI tract causing enhanced motility and accelerated gastric emptying without stimulating gastric, biliary, or pancreatic secretions; increases lower esophageal sphincter tone

Contraindications Hypersensitivity to metoclopramide or any component of the formulation; GI obstruction, perforation or hemorrhage; pheochromocytoma; history of seizures

(Continued)

Metoclopramide *(Continued)*

Warnings/Precautions Use with caution in patients with Parkinson's disease and in patients with a history of mental illness; has been associated with extrapyramidal symptoms and depression. The frequency of EPS is higher in pediatric patients and adults <30 years of age; risk is increased at higher dosages. Extrapyramidal reactions typically occur within the initial 24-48 hours of treatment. Use caution with concurrent use of other drugs associated with EPS. Neuroleptic malignant syndrome (NMS) has been reported (rarely) with metoclopramide. Use lowest recommended doses initially; may cause transient increase in serum aldosterone; use caution in patients who are at risk of fluid overload (CHF, cirrhosis). Use caution in patients with hypertension or following surgical anastomosis/closure. Patients with NADH-cytochrome b5 reductase deficiency are at increased risk of methemoglobinemia and/or sulfhemoglobinemia. Use caution in patients with a history of seizures; risk of metoclopramide-associated seizures is increased. Abrupt discontinuation may (rarely) result in withdrawal symptoms (dizziness, headache, nervousness). Use caution and adjust dose in renal impairment.

Drug Interactions

Cytochrome P450 Effect: Substrate (minor) of CYP1A2, 2D6; **Inhibits** CYP2D6 (weak)

Decreased Effect: Anticholinergic agents antagonize metoclopramide's actions.

Increased Effect/Toxicity: Opiate analgesics may increase CNS depression. Metoclopramide may increase extrapyramidal symptoms (EPS) or risk when used concurrently with antipsychotic agents.

Nutritional/Ethanol Interactions Ethanol: Avoid ethanol (may increase CNS depression).

Lab Interactions Increased aminotransferase [ALT (SGPT)/AST (SGOT)] (S), amylase (S)

Adverse Reactions Adverse reactions are more common/severe at dosages used for prophylaxis of chemotherapy-induced emesis.

>10%:

Central nervous system: Restlessness, drowsiness, extrapyramidal symptoms (high-dose, up to 34%; 0.2% at doses of 30-40 mg/day)

Gastrointestinal: Diarrhea (may be dose-limiting)

Neuromuscular & skeletal: Weakness

1% to 10%:

Central nervous system: Insomnia, depression, confusion, headache

Dermatologic: Rash

Endocrine & metabolic: Breast tenderness, prolactin stimulation

Gastrointestinal: Nausea, xerostomia

Overdosage/Toxicology Symptoms of overdose include drowsiness, ataxia, extrapyramidal symptoms, seizures, methemoglobinemia (in infants). Disorientation, muscle hypertonia, irritability, and agitation are common. Metoclopramide often causes extrapyramidal symptoms (eg, dystonic reactions) requiring management with diphenhydramine 1-2 mg/kg (adults) up to a maximum of 50-100 mg I.M. or I.V. slow push followed by a maintenance dose (25-50 mg orally every 4-6 hours) for 48-72 hours. When these reactions are unresponsive to diphenhydramine, benztropine mesylate I.V. 1-2 mg (adults) may be effective. These agents are generally effective within 2-5 minutes. Methylene blue is not recommended in patients with G6PD deficiency who experience methemoglobinemia due to metoclopramide.

Pharmacodynamics/Kinetics

Onset of Action: Oral: 0.5-1 hour; I.V.: 1-3 minutes

Duration of Action: Therapeutic: 1-2 hours, regardless of route

Bioavailability: 80%

Time to Peak: Serum: Oral: 1-3 hours; I.M.: 2-3 hours; I.V.: Within 5 minutes; Rectal: 1-8 hours

Protein Binding: 30% to 40%, primarily to α_1-acid glycoprotein

Half-Life Elimination: May be dose dependent: Normal renal function: 4-7 hours

Excretion: Urine (70% to 85%, ~19% as unchanged drug); feces (2% to 3%)

Dosing

Adults:

Antiemetic (chemotherapy-induced emesis) (unlabeled): I.V.: 1-2 mg/kg 30 minutes before chemotherapy and every 2-4 hours, for a total of 5 doses (5-10 mg/kg)

Gastroesophageal reflux: Oral: 10-15 mg/dose up to 4 times/day 30 minutes before meals or food and at bedtime. Single doses of 20 mg are occasionally needed for provoking situations.

Gastrointestinal hypomotility (gastroparesis):

Oral: 10 mg 30 minutes before each meal and at bedtime for 2-8 weeks

I.V. (for severe symptoms): 10 mg over 1-2 minutes; 10 days of I.V. therapy may be necessary for best response.

Postoperative nausea and vomiting (unlabeled): I.M., I.V.: 10 mg near end of surgery; 20 mg doses may be used

Postpyloric feeding tube placement (unlabeled): I.M., I.V.: 10 mg

Elderly:

Antiemetic (chemotherapy-induced emesis) (unlabeled):

I.V.: 1-2 mg/kg/dose every 2-4 hours or (postsurgery); direct I.V. administration should be given slowly over 1-2 minutes.

I.M.: 10-20 mg (near end of surgery)

Diabetic gastroparesis:

Oral: Initial: 5 mg 30 minutes before meals and at bedtime for 2-8 weeks; increase if necessary to 10 mg doses.

I.V.: Initiate at 5 mg over 1-2 minutes; increase to 10 mg if necessary.

Gastroesophageal reflux: Oral: 5 mg 4 times/day, 30 minutes before meals and at bedtime; increase dose to 10 mg 4 times/day if no response at lower dose.

Postoperative nausea and vomiting (unlabeled): I.M.: 5 mg near end of surgery; may repeat dose if necessary.

Mykrox®: 0.5 mg once daily; may increase to 1 mg if response is inadequate; do not use more than 1 mg/day.

Pediatrics: Limited experience in pediatric patients. Doses used have generally ranged from 0.05 to 0.1 mg/kg administered once daily. Prolonged use is not recommended.

Renal Impairment: Not dialyzable (0% to 5%)

Available Dosage Forms Tablet, slow acting (Zaroxolyn®): 2.5 mg, 5 mg, 10 mg

Monitoring and Teaching Issues

Physical Assessment: Assess allergy history prior to beginning therapy (thiazides and sulfonamide derivatives). See Warnings/Precautions for use cautions (eg, severe hepatic dysfunction, diabetes, gout, renal impairment, high cholesterol, before or during surgery). Assess potential for interactions with other pharmacological agents and herbal products patient may be taking (eg, especially anything that will affect blood pressure; see Drug Interactions). Assess electrolytes and renal function, therapeutic effectiveness, and adverse reactions on a regular basis during therapy (eg, electrolyte imbalance, hypotension; see Adverse Reactions). Caution patients with diabetes (may see a change in glucose control). Teach patient proper use, possible side effects/appropriate interventions, and adverse symptoms to report (see Patient Education).

Monitoring Laboratory Tests: Serum electrolytes (potassium, sodium, chloride, bicarbonate), renal function

Patient Education: Do not take any new medication during therapy unless approved by prescriber (including any stimulants). Take exactly as directed, after breakfast. Include bananas or orange juice in daily diet but do not take potassium supplements without advice of prescriber. This medication does not replace other antihypertensive interventions; follow prescriber's instructions for diet and lifestyle changes. Weigh yourself weekly at the same time, in the same clothes. Report weight gain >5 lb/week. May cause dizziness or weakness (change position slowly when rising from sitting or lying, avoid driving or tasks requiring alertness until response to drug is known); nausea or loss of appetite (small frequent meals, frequent mouth care, chewing gum, or sucking lozenges may help); impotence (reversible); constipation (increased exercise, fluids, fruit, or fiber may help); or photosensitivity (use sunscreen, wear protective clothing and eyewear, and avoid direct sunlight). Report flu-like symptoms, headache, joint soreness or weakness, respiratory difficulty, skin rash, excessive fatigue, swelling of extremities, or respiratory difficulty. **Pregnancy/breast-feeding precautions:** Inform prescriber if you are pregnant. Consult prescriber if breast-feeding.

Dietary Considerations: Should be taken after breakfast; may require potassium supplementation

Geriatric Considerations: When metolazone is used in combination with other diuretics, there is an increased risk of azotemia and electrolyte depletion, particularly in the elderly, monitor closely. May be effective in patients with glomerular filtration rate <20 mL/minute. Metolazone is often used in combination with a loop diuretic in patients who are unresponsive to the loop diuretic alone.

Pregnancy Risk Factor: B (manufacturer); D (expert analysis)

Lactation: Enters breast milk/use caution

Administration

Oral: May be taken with food or milk. Take early in day to avoid nocturia. Take the last dose of multiple doses no later than 6 PM unless instructed otherwise.

Additional Information Metolazone 5 mg is approximately equivalent to hydrochlorothiazide 50 mg. When taken the day of surgery, it may cause hypovolemia and the hypertensive patient undergoing general anesthesia to have labile blood pressure; use with caution prior to surgery or perioperatively.

Related Information

Heart Failure *on page 1828*

Metoprolol (me toe PROE lole)

U.S. Brand Names Lopressor®; Toprol-XL®

Synonyms Metoprolol Succinate; Metoprolol Tartrate

Generic Available Yes: Injection, tablet (nonextended release)

Pharmacologic Category Beta Blocker, Beta₁ Selective

Medication Safety Issues

Sound-alike/look-alike issues:

Metoprolol may be confused with metaproterenol, metolazone, misoprostol

Toprol-XL® may be confused with Topamax®

Use Treatment of hypertension and angina pectoris; prevention of myocardial infarction, atrial fibrillation, flutter, symptomatic treatment of hypertrophic subaortic stenosis; to reduce mortality/hospitalization in patients with congestive heart failure (stable NYHA Class II or III) in patients already receiving ACE inhibitors, diuretics, and/or digoxin (sustained-release only)

Unlabeled/Investigational Use Treatment of ventricular arrhythmias, atrial ectopy, migraine prophylaxis, essential tremor, aggressive behavior

Mechanism of Action/Effect Selective inhibitor of beta₁-adrenergic receptors; competitively blocks beta₁-receptors, with little or no effect on beta₂-receptors at doses <100 mg; does not exhibit any membrane stabilizing or intrinsic sympathomimetic activity

Contraindications Hypersensitivity to metoprolol or any component of the formulation; sinus bradycardia; heart block greater than first degree (except in patients with a functioning artificial pacemaker); cardiogenic shock; uncompensated cardiac failure; pregnancy (2nd and 3rd trimesters)

Warnings/Precautions Use with caution in compensated heart failure; monitor closely for a worsening of the condition (efficacy has been demonstrated for metoprolol). Use caution in patients with PVD (can aggravate arterial insufficiency). Use caution with concurrent use of beta-blockers and either verapamil or diltiazem; bradycardia or heart block can occur. Avoid concurrent I.V. use of both agents. In general, beta-blockers should be avoided in patients with bronchospastic disease. Metoprolol, with B1 selectivity, should be used cautiously in bronchospastic disease with close monitoring. Beta-blockers may increase the risk of anaphylaxis (in predisposed patients) and blunt response to epinephrine. Use cautiously in *(Continued)*

Metoprolol *(Continued)*

patients with diabetes because it can mask prominent hypoglycemic symptoms. Can mask signs of thyrotoxicosis. Can cause fetal harm when administered in pregnancy. Use cautiously in the hepatically impaired. Use care with anesthetic agents which decrease myocardial function. Beta-blocker therapy should not be withdrawn abruptly (particularly in patients with CAD), but gradually tapered to avoid acute tachycardia, hypertension, and/or ischemia. Avoid use of extended release tablets (Toprol-XL®) in patients with known stricture/narrowing of the GI tract.

Drug Interactions

Cytochrome P450 Effect: Substrate of CYP2C19 (minor), 2D6 (major); **Inhibits** CYP2D6 (weak)

Decreased Effect: Decreased effect of beta-blockers with aluminum salts, barbiturates, calcium salts, cholestyramine, colestipol, NSAIDs, penicillins (ampicillin), rifampin, salicylates, and sulfinpyrazone due to decreased bioavailability and plasma levels. Beta-blockers may decrease the effect of sulfonylureas.

Increased Effect/Toxicity: CYP2D6 inhibitors may increase the levels/effects of metoprolol; example inhibitors include chlorpromazine, delavirdine, fluoxetine, miconazole, paroxetine, pergolide, quinidine, quinine, ritonavir, and ropinirole. Metoprolol may increase the effects of other drugs which slow AV conduction (digoxin, verapamil, diltiazem), alpha-blockers (prazosin, terazosin), and alpha-adrenergic stimulants (epinephrine, phenylephrine). Metoprolol may mask the tachycardia from hypoglycemia caused by insulin and oral hypoglycemics. In patients receiving concurrent therapy, the risk of hypertensive crisis is increased when either clonidine or the beta-blocker is withdrawn. Reserpine has been shown to enhance the effect of beta-blockers. Beta-blockers may increase the action or levels of ethanol, disopyramide, nondepolarizing muscle relaxants, and theophylline although the effects are difficult to predict.

Nutritional/Ethanol Interactions

Food: Food increases absorption. Metoprolol serum levels may be increased if taken with food.

Herb/Nutraceutical: Avoid dong quai if using for hypertension (has estrogenic activity). Avoid ephedra, yohimbe, ginseng (may worsen hypertension). Avoid garlic (may have increased antihypertensive effect).

Adverse Reactions

>10%:

Central nervous system: Drowsiness, insomnia

Endocrine & metabolic: Decreased sexual ability

1% to 10%:

Cardiovascular: Bradycardia, palpitation, edema, CHF, reduced peripheral circulation

Central nervous system: Mental depression

Gastrointestinal: Diarrhea or constipation, nausea, stomach discomfort

Respiratory: Bronchospasm

Miscellaneous: Cold extremities

Overdosage/Toxicology Symptoms of intoxication include cardiac disturbances, CNS toxicity, bronchospasm, hypoglycemia and hyperkalemia. The most common cardiac symptoms include hypotension and bradycardia. Atrioventricular block, intraventricular conduction disturbances, cardiogenic shock, and asystole may occur with severe overdose, especially with membrane-depressant drugs (eg, propranolol). CNS effects include convulsions, coma, and respiratory arrest. Treatment is symptom-directed and supportive.

Pharmacodynamics/Kinetics

Onset of Action: Peak effect: Antihypertensive: Oral: 1.5-4 hours

Duration of Action: 10-20 hours

Absorption: 95%

Bioavailability: Oral: 40% to 50%

Protein Binding: 8%

Half-Life Elimination: 3-4 hours; End-stage renal disease: 2.5-4.5 hours

Metabolism: Extensively hepatic; significant first-pass effect

Excretion: Urine (3% to 10% as unchanged drug)

Dosing

Adults:

Hypertension: Oral: 100-450 mg/day in 2-3 divided doses, begin with 50 mg twice daily and increase doses at weekly intervals to desired effect; usual dosage range (JNC 7): 50-100 mg/day

Extended release: Initial: 25-100 mg/day (maximum: 400 mg/day)

Angina, SVT, MI prophylaxis: Oral: 100-450 mg/day in 2-3 divided doses, begin with 50 mg twice daily and increase doses at weekly intervals to desired effect

Extended release: Initial: 100 mg/day (maximum: 400 mg/day)

Hypertension/ventricular rate control: I.V. (in patients having nonfunctioning GI tract): Initial: 1.25-5 mg every 6-12 hours; titrate initial dose to response. Initially, low doses may be appropriate to establish response; however, up to 15 mg every 3-6 hours has been employed.

Congestive heart failure: Oral (extended release): Initial: 25 mg once daily (reduce to 12.5 mg once daily in NYHA class higher than class II); may double dosage every 2 weeks as tolerated, up to 200 mg/day

Myocardial infarction (acute): I.V.: 5 mg every 2 minutes for 3 doses in early treatment of myocardial infarction; thereafter give 50 mg orally every 6 hours 15 minutes after last I.V. dose and continue for 48 hours; then administer a maintenance dose of 100 mg twice daily.

Elderly: Oral: Initial: 25 mg/day; usual dose range: 25-300 mg/day; increase at 1- to 2-week intervals.

Extended release: 25-50 mg/day initially as a single dose; increase at 1- to 2-week intervals.

Pediatrics:
Hypertension, arrhythmia: Oral: Children: 1-5 mg/kg/24 hours divided twice daily; allow 3 days between dose adjustments.
Renal Impairment: Hemodialysis: Administer dose posthemodialysis or administer 50 mg supplemental dose. Supplemental dose is not necessary following peritoneal dialysis.
Hepatic Impairment: Reduced dose is probably necessary.

Available Dosage Forms
Injection, solution, as tartrate (Lopressor®): 1 mg/mL (5 mL)
Tablet, as tartrate 25 mg, 50 mg, 100 mg
Lopressor®: 50 mg, 100 mg
Tablet, extended release, as succinate (Toprol-XL®): 25 mg, 50 mg, 100 mg, 200 mg [expressed as mg equivalent to tartrate]

Monitoring and Teaching Issues
Physical Assessment: Assess potential for interactions with other prescriptions, OTC medications, or herbal products patient may be taking. I.V.: See specifics above and monitor blood pressure and cardiac status. Assess therapeutic effectiveness and adverse reactions (eg, fluid balance, CHF, postural hypotension). Caution patients with diabetes to monitor serum glucose closely; may decrease the effect of sulfonylureas and can mask prominent hypoglycemic symptoms. Teach patient proper use (oral), possible side effects/appropriate interventions, and adverse symptoms to report.

Patient Education: I.V. use in emergency situations: Patient information is appropriate to patient condition.

Oral: Do not take any new medication during therapy unless approved by prescriber. Take exactly as directed. Do not change dosage or discontinue without consulting prescriber. Take pulse daily, prior to medication and follow prescriber's instruction about holding medication. Do not take with antacids. If you have diabetes, monitor serum sugar closely (drug may alter glucose tolerance or mask signs of hypoglycemia). May cause fatigue, dizziness, or postural hypotension (use caution when changing position from lying or sitting to standing, when driving, or when climbing stairs until response to medication is known); or alteration in sexual performance (reversible). Report unresolved swelling of extremities, respiratory difficulty or new cough, unresolved fatigue, unusual weight gain, unresolved constipation, or unusual muscle weakness. **Pregnancy/breast-feeding precautions:** Inform prescriber if you are or intend to become pregnant. Consult prescriber if breast-feeding.

Dietary Considerations: Regular tablets should be taken with food. Extended release tablets may be taken without regard to meals.

Geriatric Considerations: Due to alterations in the beta-adrenergic autonomic nervous system, beta-adrenergic blockade may result in less hemodynamic response than seen in younger adults.

Pregnancy Risk Factor: C (manufacturer); D (2nd and 3rd trimesters - expert analysis)

Pregnancy Issues: Metoprolol crosses the placenta. Beta-blockers have been associated with bradycardia, hypotension, and IUGR; IUGR is probably related to maternal hypertension. Available evidence suggests beta-blockers are generally safe during pregnancy (JNC 7). Cases of neonatal hypoglycemia have been reported following maternal use of beta-blockers at parturition or during breast-feeding. Monitor breast-fed infant for symptoms of beta-blockade.

Lactation: Enters breast milk/use caution (AAP rates "compatible")

Breast-Feeding Issues: Metoprolol is considered compatible by the AAP. However, monitor the infant for signs of beta-blockade (hypotension, bradycardia, etc) with long-term use.

Administration
Oral: Extended release tablets may be divided in half; do not crush or chew.
I.V.: When administered acutely for cardiac treatment, monitor ECG and blood pressure. May administer by rapid infusion (I.V. push) over 1 minute or by slow infusion (ie, 5-10 mg of metoprolol in 50 mL of fluid) over ~30 minutes. Necessary monitoring for surgical patients who are unable to take oral beta-blockers (prolonged ileus) has not been defined. Some institutions require monitoring of baseline and postinfusion heart rate and blood pressure when a patient's response to beta-blockade has not been characterized (ie, the patient's initial dose or following a change in dose). Consult individual institutional policies and procedures.

Compatibility: Stable in D_5W, NS
Y-site administration: Incompatible with amphotericin B cholesteryl sulfate complex
Storage:
Injection: Do not store above 30°C (86°F). Protect from light.
Tablet: Store between 15°C to 30°C (59°F to 86°F).

Related Information
Beta-Blockers on page 1720
Heart Failure on page 1828

◆ **Metoprolol Succinate** see Metoprolol on page 993
◆ **Metoprolol Tartrate** see Metoprolol on page 993
◆ **MetroCream®** see Metronidazole on page 995
◆ **MetroGel®** see Metronidazole on page 995
◆ **MetroGel-Vaginal®** see Metronidazole on page 995
◆ **MetroLotion®** see Metronidazole on page 995

Metronidazole (me troe NI da zole)
U.S. Brand Names Flagyl®; Flagyl ER®; Flagyl® I.V. RTU™; MetroCream®; MetroGel®; MetroGel-Vaginal®; MetroLotion®; Noritate®; Rozex™ [DSC]
Synonyms Metronidazole Hydrochloride
Generic Available Yes: Cream, infusion, tablet
Pharmacologic Category Amebicide; Antibiotic, Topical; Antibiotic, Miscellaneous; Antiprotozoal, Nitroimidazole
(Continued)

Metronidazole *(Continued)*

Medication Safety Issues

Sound-alike/look-alike issues:

Metronidazole may be confused with metformin.

Use Treatment of susceptible anaerobic bacterial and protozoal infections in the following conditions: Amebiasis, symptomatic and asymptomatic trichomoniasis; skin and skin structure infections; CNS infections; intra-abdominal infections (as part of combination regimen); systemic anaerobic infections; treatment of antibiotic-associated pseudomembranous colitis (AAPC), bacterial vaginosis; as part of a multidrug regimen for *H. pylori* eradication to reduce the risk of duodenal ulcer recurrence

Topical: Treatment of inflammatory lesions and erythema of rosacea

Unlabeled/Investigational Use Crohn's disease

Mechanism of Action/Effect Inhibits DNA synthesis in susceptible organisms

Contraindications Hypersensitivity to metronidazole, nitroimidazole derivatives, or any component of the formulation; pregnancy (1st trimester - found to be carcinogenic in rats)

Warnings/Precautions Use with caution in patients with liver impairment due to potential accumulation, blood dyscrasias; history of seizures, CHF, or other sodium retaining states; reduce dosage in patients with severe liver impairment, CNS disease, and severe renal failure (Cl$_{cr}$ <10 mL/minute); if *H. pylori* is not eradicated in patients being treated with metronidazole in a regimen, it should be assumed that metronidazole-resistance has occurred and it should not again be used; seizures and neuropathies have been reported especially with increased doses and chronic treatment; if this occurs, discontinue therapy

Drug Interactions

Cytochrome P450 Effect: Inhibits CYP2C8/9 (weak), 3A4 (moderate)

Decreased Effect: Phenytoin, phenobarbital (potentially other enzyme inducers) may decrease metronidazole half-life and effects.

Increased Effect/Toxicity: Ethanol may cause a disulfiram-like reaction. Warfarin and metronidazole may increase bleeding times (PT) which may result in bleeding. Cimetidine may increase metronidazole levels. Metronidazole may inhibit metabolism of cisapride, causing potential arrhythmias; avoid concurrent use. Metronidazole may increase lithium levels/toxicity. Metronidazole may increase the levels/effects of selected benzodiazepines, calcium channel blockers, cyclosporine, ergot derivatives, selected HMG-CoA reductase inhibitors, mirtazapine, nateglinide, nefazodone, sildenafil (and other PDE-5 inhibitors), tacrolimus, venlafaxine, and other CYP3A4 substrates.

Nutritional/Ethanol Interactions

Ethanol: The manufacturer recommends to avoid all ethanol or any ethanol-containing drugs (may cause disulfiram-like reaction characterized by flushing, headache, nausea, vomiting, sweating or tachycardia).

Food: Peak antibiotic serum concentration lowered and delayed, but total drug absorbed not affected.

Lab Interactions May cause falsely decreased AST and ALT levels.

Adverse Reactions

Systemic: Frequency not defined:

Cardiovascular: Flattening of the T-wave, flushing

Central nervous system: Ataxia, confusion, coordination impaired, dizziness, fever, headache, insomnia, irritability, seizure, vertigo

Dermatologic: Erythematous rash, urticaria

Endocrine & metabolic: Disulfiram-like reaction, dysmenorrhea, libido decreased

Gastrointestinal: Nausea (~12%), anorexia, abdominal cramping, constipation, diarrhea, furry tongue, glossitis, proctitis, stomatitis, unusual/metallic taste, vomiting, xerostomia

Genitourinary: Cystitis, darkened urine (rare), dysuria, incontinence, polyuria, vaginitis

Hematologic: Neutropenia (reversible), thrombocytopenia (reversible, rare)

Neuromuscular & skeletal: Peripheral neuropathy, weakness

Respiratory: Nasal congestion, rhinitis, sinusitis, pharyngitis

Miscellaneous: Flu-like syndrome, moniliasis

Topical: Frequency not defined:

Central nervous system: Headache

Dermatologic: Burning, contact dermatitis, dryness, erythema, irritation, pruritus, rash

Gastrointestinal: Unusual/metallic taste, nausea, constipation

Local: Local allergic reaction

Neuromuscular & skeletal: Tingling/numbness of extremities

Ocular: Eye irritation

Vaginal:

>10%: Genitourinary: Vaginal discharge (12%)

1% to 10%:

Central nervous system: Headache (5%), dizziness (2%)

Gastrointestinal: Gastrointestinal discomfort (7%), nausea and/or vomiting (4%), unusual/metallic taste (2%), diarrhea (1%)

Genitourinary: Vaginitis (10%), vulva/vaginal irritation (9%), pelvic discomfort (3%)

Hematologic: WBC increased (2%)

Overdosage/Toxicology Symptoms of overdose include nausea, vomiting, ataxia, seizures, and peripheral neuropathy. Treatment is symptomatic and supportive.

Pharmacodynamics/Kinetics

Absorption: Oral: Well absorbed; Topical: Concentrations achieved systemically after application of 1 g topically are 10 times less than those obtained after a 250 mg oral dose

Time to Peak: Serum: Oral: Immediate release: 1-2 hours

Protein Binding: <20%

Half-Life Elimination: Neonates: 25-75 hours; Others: 6-8 hours, prolonged with hepatic impairment; End-stage renal disease: 21 hours

Metabolism: Hepatic (30% to 60%)

Excretion: Urine (20% to 40% as unchanged drug); feces (6% to 15%)

Dosing

Adults:

Amebiasis: Oral: 500-750 mg every 8 hours for 5-10 days

Trichomoniasis: Oral: 250 mg every 8 hours for 7 days **or** 375 mg twice daily for 7 days **or** 2 g as a single dose

Anaerobic infections: Oral, I.V.: 500 mg every 6-8 hours, not to exceed 4 g/day

Antibiotic-associated pseudomembranous colitis: Oral: 250-500 mg 3-4 times/day for 10-14 days

Peptic ulcer disease: Eradication of *Helicobacter pylori*: Oral: 250-500 mg with meals and at bedtime for 14 days; requires combination therapy with at least one other antibiotic and an acid-suppressing agent (proton pump inhibitor or H_2 blocker)

Bacterial vaginosis:

Oral: 750 mg (extended release tablet) once daily for 7 days

Vaginal: One applicatorful (~37.5 mg metronidazole) once or twice daily for 5 days; apply once in morning and evening if using twice daily, if daily, use at bedtime

Acne rosacea: Topical:

0.75%: Apply and rub a thin film twice daily, morning and evening, to entire affected areas after washing. Significant therapeutic results should be noticed within 3 weeks. Clinical studies have demonstrated continuing improvement through 9 weeks of therapy.

1%: Apply thin film to affected area once daily.

Elderly: Use the lower end of the dosing recommendations for adults; do not administer as single dose as efficacy has not been established.

Pediatrics:

Anaerobic infections: Oral, I.V.:

Postnatal age >7 days:

1200-2000 g: 15 mg/kg/day in divided doses every 12 hours

>2000 g: 30 mg/kg/day in divided doses every 12 hours

Infants and Children:

Oral: 15-35 mg/kg/day in divided doses every 8 hours

I.V.: 30 mg/kg/day in divided doses every 6 hours

Colitis due to *Clostridium difficile*: Oral: 20 mg/kg/day divided every 6 hours. Maximum dose: 2 g/day

Amebiasis: Infants and Children: Oral: 35-50 mg/kg/day in divided doses every 8 hours for 10 days

Trichomoniasis: Infants and Children: Oral: 15-30 mg/kg/day in divided doses every 8 hours for 7 days

Renal Impairment:

Cl_{cr} <10 mL/minute: Administer 50% of dose or every 12 hours.

Hemodialysis effects: Extensively removed by hemodialysis and peritoneal dialysis (50% to 100%). Administer dose posthemodialysis. During peritoneal dialysis, dose as for Cl_{cr} <10 mL/minute.

Continuous arteriovenous or venovenous hemofiltration: Dose as for normal renal function

Hepatic Impairment: Unchanged in mild liver disease; reduce dosage in severe liver disease.

Available Dosage Forms [DSC] = Discontinued product

Capsule (Flagyl®): 375 mg

Cream, topical: 0.75% (45 g)

MetroCream®: 0.75% (45 g) [contains benzyl alcohol]

Noritate®: 1% (60 g)

Emulsion, topical (Rozex™): 0.75% (60 g) [contains benzyl alcohol] [DSC]

Gel, topical (MetroGel®): 0.75% (45 g)

Gel, vaginal (MetroGel-Vaginal®): 0.75% (70 g)

Infusion (Flagyl® I.V. RTU™) [premixed iso-osmotic sodium chloride solution]: 500 mg (100 mL) [contains sodium 14 mEq]

Lotion, topical (MetroLotion®): 0.75% (60 mL) [contains benzyl alcohol]

Tablet (Flagyl®): 250 mg, 500 mg

Tablet, extended release (Flagyl® ER): 750 mg

Monitoring and Teaching Issues

Physical Assessment: Assess effectiveness and interactions of other medications patient may be taking. Assess results of laboratory tests, therapeutic effectiveness, and adverse reactions according to dose, route of administration, and purpose of therapy. Assess knowledge/teach patient appropriate use, interventions to reduce side effects, and adverse symptoms to report.

Patient Education: Take exactly as directed. May take with or without food. Take with food if medication causes upset stomach. Avoid alcohol during and for 72 hours after last dose. With alcohol you may experience severe flushing, headache, nausea, vomiting, or chest and abdominal pain. May discolor urine (brown/black/dark) (normal). You may experience "metallic" taste disturbance or nausea or vomiting (small frequent meals, frequent mouth care, chewing gum, or sucking lozenges may help). Refrain from intercourse or use a contraceptive if being treated for trichomoniasis. Report unresolved or severe fatigue; weakness; fever or chills; mouth or vaginal sores; numbness, tingling, or swelling of extremities; respiratory difficulty; or lack of improvement or worsening of condition. **Pregnancy/breast-feeding precautions:** Inform prescriber if you are pregnant. Breast-feeding is not recommended.

Topical: Wash hands and area before applying. Apply medication thinly. Wash hands after applying. Avoid contact with eyes. Do not cover with occlusive dressing. Report severe skin irritation or if condition does not improve.

Dietary Considerations: Take on an empty stomach. Drug may cause GI upset; if GI upset occurs, take with food. Extended release tablets should be taken on an empty stomach (1 hour before or 2 hours after meals). Sodium content of 500 mg (I.V.): 322 mg

(Continued)

Metronidazole *(Continued)*

(14 mEq). The manufacturer recommends that ethanol be avoided during treatment and for 3 days after therapy is complete.

Geriatric Considerations: Adjust dose based on renal function.

Pregnancy Risk Factor: B (may be contraindicated in 1st trimester)

Pregnancy Issues: Crosses the placenta; contraindicated for the treatment of trichomoniasis during the first trimester of pregnancy, unless alternative treatment is inadequate. Until safety and efficacy for other indications have been established, use only during pregnancy when the benefit to the mother outweighs the potential risk to the fetus.

Lactation: Enters breast milk/not recommended (AAP rates "of concern")

Breast-Feeding Issues: It is suggested to stop breast-feeding for 12-24 hours following single dose therapy to allow excretion of dose.

Administration

Oral: May be taken with food to minimize stomach upset. Extended release tablets should be taken on an empty stomach (1 hour before or 2 hours after meals).

I.V.: Avoid contact between the drug and aluminum in the infusion set.

Topical: No disulfiram-like reactions have been reported after **topical** application, although metronidazole can be detected in the blood. Apply to clean, dry skin. Cosmetics may be used after application (wait at least 5 minutes after using lotion).

Reconstitution: Standard diluent: 500 mg/100 mL NS

Compatibility: Stable in D$_5$W, NS

Y-site administration: Incompatible with amphotericin B cholesteryl sulfate complex, aztreonam, filgrastim, meropenem, warfarin

Compatibility when admixed: Incompatible with aztreonam, dopamine, meropenem

Storage: Metronidazole injection should be stored at 15°C to 30°C and protected from light. Product may be refrigerated but crystals may form; crystals redissolve on warming to room temperature. Prolonged exposure to light will cause a darkening of the product. However, short-term exposure to normal room light does not adversely affect metronidazole stability. Direct sunlight should be avoided. Stability of parenteral admixture at room temperature (25°C): Out of overwrap stability: 30 days.

Related Information

Antimicrobial Drugs of Choice *on page 1792*
Helicobacter pylori Treatment *on page 1835*
I.V. to Oral Conversion *on page 1688*

* **Metronidazole, Bismuth Subsalicylate, and Tetracycline** *see* Bismuth Subsalicylate, Metronidazole, and Tetracycline *on page 199*

* **Metronidazole Hydrochloride** *see* Metronidazole *on page 995*

* **Metronidazole, Tetracycline, and Bismuth Subsalicylate** *see* Bismuth Subsalicylate, Metronidazole, and Tetracycline *on page 199*

* **Mevacor®** *see* Lovastatin *on page 925*

* **Mevinolin** *see* Lovastatin *on page 925*

Mexiletine *(MEKS i le teen)*

U.S. Brand Names Mexitil® [DSC]

Generic Available Yes

Pharmacologic Category Antiarrhythmic Agent, Class Ib

Use Management of serious ventricular arrhythmias; suppression of PVCs

Unlabeled/Investigational Use Diabetic neuropathy

Mechanism of Action/Effect Class IB antiarrhythmic, structurally related to lidocaine, which inhibits inward sodium current, decreases rate of rise of Phase 0, increases effective refractory period/action potential duration ratio

Contraindications Hypersensitivity to mexiletine or any component of the formulation; cardiogenic shock; second- or third-degree AV block (except in patients with a functioning artificial pacemaker)

Warnings/Precautions Can be proarrhythmic. May cause acute hepatic injury. Use cautiously in patients with first-degree block, pre-existing sinus node dysfunction, intraventricular conduction delays, significant hepatic dysfunction, hypotension, or severe CHF. Electrolytes disturbances alter response. Alterations in urinary pH may change urinary excretion. Rare hepatic toxicity may occur. Electrolyte abnormalities should be corrected before initiating therapy (can worsen CHF).

Drug Interactions

Cytochrome P450 Effect: Substrate (major) of CYP1A2, 2D6; **Inhibits** CYP1A2 (strong)

Decreased Effect: The levels/effects of mexiletine may be decreased by aminoglutethimide, carbamazepine, phenobarbital, rifampin, and other CYP1A2 inducers. Urinary acidifying agents may increase mexiletine levels.

Increased Effect/Toxicity: Mexiletine may increase the levels/effects of aminophylline, fluvoxamine, mirtazapine, ropinirole, trifluoperazine, or other CYP1A2 substrates. The levels/effects of mexiletine may be increased by inhibitors of CYP1A2 or 2D6; example inhibitors include amiodarone, chlorpromazine, ciprofloxacin, delavirdine, fluoxetine, fluvoxamine, ketoconazole, miconazole, norfloxacin, ofloxacin, paroxetine, pergolide, quinidine, quinine, ritonavir, rofecoxib, ropinirole, and other CYP1A2 or 2D6 inhibitors. Mexiletine may increase levels of theophylline and caffeine. Quinidine and urinary alkalinizers (antacids, sodium bicarbonate, acetazolamide) may increase mexiletine blood levels.

Nutritional/Ethanol Interactions Food: Food may decrease the rate, but not the extent of oral absorption; diets which affect urine pH can increase or decrease excretion of mexiletine. Avoid dietary changes that alter urine pH.

Lab Interactions Abnormal liver function test, positive ANA, thrombocytopenia

Adverse Reactions

>10%:

Central nervous system: Lightheadedness (11% to 25%), dizziness (20% to 25%), nervousness (5% to 10%), incoordination (10%)

Gastrointestinal: GI distress (41%), nausea/vomiting (40%)

Neuromuscular & skeletal: Trembling, unsteady gait, tremor (13%), ataxia (10% to 20%)

1% to 10%:

Cardiovascular: Chest pain (3% to 8%), premature ventricular contractions (1% to 2%), palpitation (4% to 8%), angina (2%), proarrhythmic (10% to 15% in patients with malignant arrhythmia)

Central nervous system: Confusion, headache, insomnia (5% to 7%), depression (2%)

Dermatologic: Rash (4%)

Gastrointestinal: Constipation or diarrhea (4% to 5%), xerostomia (3%), abdominal pain (1%)

Neuromuscular & skeletal: Weakness (5%), numbness of fingers or toes (2% to 4%), paresthesia (2%), arthralgia (1%)

Ocular: Blurred vision (5% to 7%), nystagmus (6%)

Otic: Tinnitus (2% to 3%)

Respiratory: Dyspnea (3%)

Overdosage/Toxicology Has a narrow therapeutic index and severe toxicity may occur slightly above the therapeutic range, especially with other antiarrhythmic drugs. Acute ingestion of twice the daily therapeutic dose is potentially life-threatening. Symptoms of overdose include sedation, confusion, coma, seizures, respiratory arrest and cardiac toxicity (sinus arrest, AV block, asystole, and hypotension). The QRS and QT intervals are usually normal, although they may be prolonged after massive overdose. Other effects include dizziness, paresthesia, tremor, ataxia, and GI disturbance. Treatment is symptomatic and supportive.

Pharmacodynamics/Kinetics

Absorption: Elderly have a slightly slower rate, but extent of absorption is the same as young adults

Time to Peak: 2-3 hours

Protein Binding: 50% to 70%

Half-Life Elimination: Adults: 10-14 hours (average: 14.4 hours elderly, 12 hours younger adults); prolonged with hepatic impairment or heart failure

Metabolism: Hepatic; low first-pass effect

Excretion: Urine (10% to 15% as unchanged drug); urinary acidification increases excretion, alkalinization decreases excretion

Dosing

Adults & Elderly: Arrhythmias: Oral: Initial: 200 mg every 8 hours (may load with 400 mg if necessary); adjust dose every 2-3 days; usual dose: 200-300 mg every 8 hours; maximum: 1.2 g/day (some patients respond to every 12-hour dosing). When switching from another antiarrhythmic, initiate a 200 mg dose 6-12 hours after stopping former agents, 3-6 hours after stopping procainamide.

Hepatic Impairment: Patients with hepatic impairment or CHF may require dose reduction; reduce dose to 25% to 30% of usual dose

Available Dosage Forms [DSC] = Discontinued product

Capsule, as hydrochloride: 150 mg, 200 mg, 250 mg

Mexitil®: 150 mg, 200 mg, 250 mg [DSC]

Monitoring and Teaching Issues

Physical Assessment: Assess other medications patient may be taking for effectiveness and interactions. Monitor cardiac status. Assess for CNS changes. Assess results of laboratory tests, therapeutic effectiveness, and adverse reactions at beginning of therapy, when titrating dosage, and on a regular basis with long-term therapy. **Note:** Mexiletine has a low toxic:therapeutic ratio and overdose may easily produce severe and life-threatening reactions. Assess knowledge/teach patient appropriate use, interventions to reduce side effects, and adverse symptoms to report.

Monitoring Laboratory Tests: Regular serum levels

Patient Education: Take exactly as directed with food or antacids, around-the-clock. Do not take additional doses or discontinue without consulting prescriber. Do not change diet without consulting prescriber. You will need regular cardiac checkups and blood tests while taking this medication. You may experience drowsiness or dizziness, numbness, or visual changes (use caution when driving or engaging in tasks requiring alertness until response to drug is known); nausea, vomiting, or heartburn (small frequent meals, frequent mouth care, chewing gum, or sucking lozenges may help); or headaches or sleep disturbances (usually temporary, if persistent consult prescriber). Report chest pain, palpitation, or erratic heartbeat; increased weight or swelling of hands or feet; chills, fever, or persistent sore throat; numbness, weakness, trembling, or unsteady gait; blurred vision or ringing in ears; or respiratory difficulty. **Pregnancy precaution:** Inform prescriber if you are or intend to become pregnant.

Pregnancy Risk Factor: C

Lactation: Enters breast milk/compatible

Administration

Oral: Administer with food. Administer around-the-clock to promote less variation in peak and trough serum levels.

Related Information

Antiarrhythmic Drugs *on page 1708*

- ◆ **Mexitil® [DSC]** *see* Mexiletine *on page 998*
- ◆ **Miacalcin®** *see* Calcitonin *on page 232*
- ◆ **Micaderm® [OTC]** *see* Miconazole *on page 999*
- ◆ **Micardis®** *see* Telmisartan *on page 1432*
- ◆ **Micardis® HCT** *see* Telmisartan and Hydrochlorothiazide *on page 1433*
- ◆ **Micatin® [OTC]** *see* Miconazole *on page 999*

Miconazole (mi KON a zole)

U.S. Brand Names Aloe Vesta® 2-n-1 Antifungal [OTC]; Baza® Antifungal [OTC]; Carrington Antifungal [OTC]; Femizol-M™ [OTC]; Fungoid® Tincture [OTC]; Lotrimin® AF Powder/Spray [OTC]; Micaderm® [OTC]; Micatin® [OTC]; Micro-Guard® [OTC]; Mitrazol™ [OTC]; Monistat® (Continued)

Miconazole *(Continued)*

1 Combination Pack [OTC]; Monistat® 3 [OTC]; Monistat® 7 [OTC]; Monistat-Derm®; Triple Care® Antifungal [OTC]; Zeasorb®-AF [OTC]

Synonyms Miconazole Nitrate

Generic Available Yes

Pharmacologic Category Antifungal Agent, Topical; Antifungal Agent, Vaginal

Medication Safety Issues

Sound-alike/look-alike issues:

Miconazole may be confused with Micronase®, Micronor®

Lotrimin® may be confused with Lotrisone®, Otrivin®

Micatin® may be confused with Miacalcin®

Use Treatment of vulvovaginal candidiasis and a variety of skin and mucous membrane fungal infections

Mechanism of Action/Effect Inhibits biosynthesis of ergosterol, damaging the fungal cell wall membrane, which increases permeability causing leaking of nutrients

Contraindications Hypersensitivity to miconazole or any component of the formulation

Warnings/Precautions For external use only; discontinue if sensitivity or irritation develop. Petrolatum-based vaginal products may damage rubber or latex condoms or diaphragms. Separate use by 3 days.

Drug Interactions

Cytochrome P450 Effect: Substrate of CYP3A4 (major); **Inhibits** CYP1A2 (moderate), 2A6 (strong), 2B6 (weak), 2C8/9 (strong), 2C19 (strong), 2D6 (strong), 2E1 (moderate), 3A4 (strong)

Decreased Effect: Amphotericin B may decrease antifungal effect of both agents. The levels/effects of miconazole may be decreased by aminoglutethimide, carbamazepine, nafcillin, nevirapine, phenobarbital, phenytoin, rifamycins or other CYP3A4 inducers. Miconazole may decrease the levels/effects of CYP2D6 prodrug substrates (eg, codeine, hydrocodone, oxycodone, tramadol).

Increased Effect/Toxicity: Note: The majority of reported drug interactions were observed following intravenous miconazole administration. Although systemic absorption following topical and/or vaginal administration is low, potential interactions due to CYP isoenzyme inhibition may occur (rarely). This may be particularly true in situations where topical absorption may be increased (ie, inflamed tissue).

Miconazole coadministered with warfarin has increased the anticoagulant effect of warfarin (including reports associated with vaginal miconazole therapy of as little as 3 days). Concurrent administration of cisapride is contraindicated due to an increased risk of cardiotoxicity. Miconazole may increase the serum levels/effects of amiodarone, amphetamines, benzodiazepines, beta-blockers, buspirone, busulfan, calcium channel blockers, citalopram, dexmedetomidine, dextromethorphan, diazepam, digoxin, docetaxel, fluoxetine, fluvoxamine, glimepiride, glipizide, ifosfamide, inhalational anesthetics, lidocaine, mesoridazine, methsuximide, mexiletine, mirtazapine, nateglinide, nefazodone, paroxetine, phenytoin, pioglitazone, propranolol, risperidone, ritonavir, ropinirole, rosiglitazone, sertraline, sirolimus, tacrolimus, theophylline, thioridazine, tricyclic antidepressants, trifluoperazine, trimetrexate, venlafaxine, vincristine, vinblastine, warfarin, zolpidem, and other substrates of CYP1A2, 2A6, 2C8/9, 2C19, 2D6, or 3A4. Selected benzodiazepines (midazolam and triazolam), cisapride, ergot alkaloids, selected HMG-CoA reductase inhibitors (lovastatin and simvastatin), and pimozide are generally contraindicated with strong CYP3A4 inhibitors. Mesoridazine and thioridazine are generally contraindicated with strong CYP2D6 inhibitors. When used with strong CYP3A4 inhibitors, dosage adjustment/limits are recommended for sildenafil and other PDE-5 inhibitors; consult individual monographs.

Nutritional/Ethanol Interactions Herb/Nutraceutical: St John's wort may decrease miconazole levels.

Lab Interactions Increased protein

Adverse Reactions Frequency not defined.

Topical: Allergic contact dermatitis, burning, maceration

Vaginal: Abdominal cramps, burning, irritation, itching

Pharmacodynamics/Kinetics

Absorption: Topical: Negligible

Protein Binding: 91% to 93%

Half-Life Elimination: Multiphasic: Initial: 40 minutes; Secondary: 126 minutes; Terminal: 24 hours

Metabolism: Hepatic

Excretion: Feces (~50%); urine (<1% as unchanged drug)

Dosing

Adults & Elderly:

Tinea pedis and tinea corporis: Topical: Apply twice daily for 4 weeks

Tinea cruris: Topical: Apply twice daily for 2 weeks

Vulvovaginal candidiasis: Vaginal:

Cream, 2%: Insert 1 applicatorful at bedtime for 7 days

Cream, 4%: Insert 1 applicatorful at bedtime for 3 days

Suppository, 100 mg: Insert 1 suppository at bedtime for 7 days

Suppository, 200 mg: Insert 1 suppository at bedtime for 3 days

Suppository, 1200 mg: Insert 1 suppository (a one-time dose); may be used at bedtime or during the day

Note: Many products are available as a combination pack, with a suppository for vaginal instillation and cream to relieve external symptoms. External cream may be used twice daily, as needed, for up to 7 days.

Pediatrics: Refer to adult dosing. **Note:** Not for OTC use in children <2 years.

Available Dosage Forms

Combination products: Miconazole nitrate vaginal suppository 200 mg (3s) and miconazole nitrate external cream 2%; Miconazole nitrate vaginal suppository 100 mg (7s) and miconazole nitrate external cream 2%

Monistat® 1 Combination Pack: Miconazole nitrate vaginal insert 1200 mg (1) and micona-zole external cream 2% (5 g) [Note: Do not confuse with 1-Day™ (formerly Monistat® 1) which contains tioconazole]

Monistat® 3 Combination Pack: Miconazole nitrate vaginal suppository 200 mg (3s) and miconazole nitrate external cream 2%

Monistat® 3 Cream Combination Pack: Miconazole nitrate vaginal cream 4% and micona-zole nitrate external cream 2%

Monistat® 7 Combination Pack:

Miconazole nitrate vaginal suppository 100 mg (7s) and miconazole nitrate external cream 2%

Miconazole nitrate vaginal cream 2% (7 prefilled applicators) and miconazole nitrate external cream 2%

Cream, topical, as nitrate: 2% (15 g, 30 g, 45 g)
Baza® Antifungal: 2% (4 g, 57 g, 142 g) [zinc oxide based formula]
Carrington Antifungal: 2% (150 g)
Micaderm®: 2% (30 g)
Micatin®: 2% (15 g)
Micro-Guard®, Mitrazol™: 2% (60 g)
Monistat-Derm®: 2% (15 g, 30 g, 85 g)
Triple Care® Antifungal: 2% (60 g, 98 g)

Cream, vaginal, as nitrate [prefilled or with single refillable applicator]: 2% (45 g)
Femizol-M™: 2% (47 g)
Monistat® 3: 4% (15 g, 25 g)
Monistat® 7: 2% (45 g)

Liquid, spray, as nitrate (Micatin®): 2% (90 mL, 105 mL)

Lotion, powder, as nitrate (Zeasorb®-AF): 2% (56 g) [contains alcohol 70%]

Ointment, topical, as nitrate: (Aloe Vesta® 2-n-1 Antifungal): 2% (60 g, 150 g)

Powder, topical, as nitrate:
Lotrimin® AF, Micatin®, Micro-Guard®: 2% (90 g)
Mitrazol™: 2% (30 g)
Zeasorb®-AF: 2% (70 g)

Powder spray, topical, as nitrate (Lotrimin® AF): 2% (100 g)

Suppository, vaginal, as nitrate: 100 mg (7s); 200 mg (3s)
Monistat® 3: 200 mg (3s)
Monistat® 7: 100 mg (7s)

Tincture, topical, as nitrate (Fungoid®): 2% (30 mL, 473 mL) [contains isopropyl alcohol 30%]

Monitoring and Teaching Issues

Physical Assessment: For topical use only. See Warnings/Precautions and Drug Interac-tions for use cautions. Caution patients with diabetes to test serum glucose regularly; may inhibit the metabolism of oral sulfonylureas. Teach patient proper use, possible side effects/appropriate interventions (eg, bleeding precautions), and adverse symptoms to report (see Patient Education).

Patient Education: Use full course of therapy as directed; do not discontinue without consulting prescriber. Some infections may require long periods of therapy. Practice good hygiene measures to prevent reinfection. If you have diabetes, you should test serum glucose regularly, this medication may inhibit the metabolism of oral sulfonylureas. Report persistent burning, itching, irritation, worsening of condition or lack of improvement to healthcare provider. **Pregnancy/breast-feeding precautions:** Inform prescriber if you are or intend to become pregnant. Consult prescriber if breast-feeding.

Topical: Wash and dry area before applying medication; apply thinly. Do not get in or near eyes. Not for use in children <2 years of age.

Vaginal: Consult with healthcare provider if using OTC product for a vaginal yeast infection for the first time. Insert high in vagina. Refrain from intercourse during treatment. Condoms and diaphragms may not be effective during therapy. Do not use tampons, douches, spermicides, or other vaginal products during treatment. Deodorant-free pads or panty shields may be used to protect clothing during use.

Geriatric Considerations: Assess patient's ability to self administer, may be difficult in patients with arthritis or limited range of motion.

Pregnancy Risk Factor: C

Lactation: Excretion in breast milk unknown/use caution

Midazolam (MID aye zoe lam)

Synonyms Midazolam Hydrochloride; Versed
Controlled Substance C-IV
Generic Available Yes
Pharmacologic Category Benzodiazepine
Medication Safety Issues
Sound-alike/look-alike issues:
Versed may be confused with VePesid®, Vistaril®
(Continued)

Midazolam *(Continued)*

Use Preoperative sedation and provides conscious sedation prior to diagnostic or radiographic procedures; ICU sedation (continuous infusion); intravenous anesthesia (induction); intravenous anesthesia (maintenance)

Unlabeled/Investigational Use Anxiety, status epilepticus

Mechanism of Action/Effect Binds to stereospecific benzodiazepine receptors on the postsynaptic GABA neuron at several sites within the central nervous system, including the limbic system, reticular formation. Enhancement of the inhibitory effect of GABA on neuronal excitability results by increased neuronal membrane permeability to chloride ions. This shift in chloride ions results in hyperpolarization (a less excitable state) and stabilization.

Contraindications Hypersensitivity to midazolam or any component of the formulation, including benzyl alcohol (cross-sensitivity with other benzodiazepines may exist); parenteral form is not for intrathecal or epidural injection; narrow-angle glaucoma; concurrent use of potent inhibitors of CYP3A4 (amprenavir, atazanavir, or ritonavir); pregnancy

Warnings/Precautions May cause severe respiratory depression, respiratory arrest, or apnea. Use with extreme caution, particularly in noncritical care settings. Appropriate resuscitative equipment and qualified personnel must be available for administration and monitoring. Initial dosing must be cautiously titrated and individualized, particularly in elderly or debilitated patients, hepatic impairment, or renal impairment, particularly if other CNS depressants (including opiates) are used concurrently. Initial doses in elderly or debilitated patients should not exceed 2.5 mg. Use with caution in patients with respiratory disease or impaired gag reflex. Use during upper airway procedures may increase risk of hypoventilation. Prolonged responses have been noted following extended administration by continuous infusion (possibly due to metabolite accumulation) or in the presence of drugs which inhibit midazolam metabolism.

May cause hypotension - hemodynamic events are more common in pediatric patients or patients with hemodynamic instability. Hypotension and/or respiratory depression may occur more frequently in patients who have received narcotic analgesics. Use with caution in obese patients, chronic renal failure, and CHF. Parenteral form contains benzyl alcohol - avoid rapid injection in neonates or prolonged infusions. Should not be used in shock, coma, or acute alcohol intoxication. Avoid intra-arterial administration or extravasation of parenteral formulation.

Causes CNS depression (dose-related) resulting in sedation, dizziness, confusion, or ataxia which may impair physical and mental capabilities. A minimum of 1 day should elapse after midazolam administration before attempting to drive or operate machinery. Use with caution in patients receiving other CNS depressants or psychoactive agents. Effects with other sedative drugs or ethanol may be potentiated. Benzodiazepines have been associated with falls and traumatic injury and should be used with extreme caution in patients who are at risk of these events (especially the elderly).

Midazolam causes anterograde amnesia. Paradoxical reactions, including hyperactive or aggressive behavior have been reported with benzodiazepines, particularly in adolescent/pediatric or psychiatric patients. Does not have analgesic, antidepressant, or antipsychotic properties.

Benzodiazepines have been associated with dependence and acute withdrawal symptoms on discontinuation or reduction in dose. Acute withdrawal, including seizures, may be precipitated after administration of flumazenil to patients receiving long-term benzodiazepine therapy.

Drug Interactions

Cytochrome P450 Effect: Substrate of CYP2B6 (minor), 3A4 (major); **Inhibits** CYP2C8/9 (weak), 3A4 (weak)

Decreased Effect: CYP3A4 inducers may decrease the levels/effects of midazolam; example inducers include aminoglutethimide, carbamazepine, nafcillin, nevirapine, phenobarbital, phenytoin, and rifamycins.

Increased Effect/Toxicity: CYP3A4 inhibitors may increase the levels/effects of midazolam; example inhibitors include azole antifungals, ciprofloxacin, clarithromycin, diclofenac, doxycycline, erythromycin, imatinib, isoniazid, nefazodone, nicardipine, propofol, protease inhibitors, quinidine, and verapamil. Use is contraindicated with amprenavir, atazanavir, and ritonavir. **If narcotics or other CNS depressants are administered concomitantly, the midazolam dose should be reduced by 30% if <65 years of age, or by at least 50% if >65 years of age.**

Nutritional/Ethanol Interactions

Ethanol: Avoid ethanol (may increase CNS depression).

Food: Grapefruit juice may increase serum concentrations of midazolam; avoid concurrent use with oral form.

Herb/Nutraceutical: Avoid concurrent use with St John's wort (may decrease midazolam levels, may increase CNS depression). Avoid concurrent use with valerian, kava kava, gotu kola (may increase CNS depression).

Adverse Reactions As reported in adults unless otherwise noted:

>10%: Respiratory: Decreased tidal volume and/or respiratory rate decrease, apnea (3% children)

1% to 10%:

Cardiovascular: Hypotension (3% children)

Central nervous system: Drowsiness (1%), oversedation, headache (1%), seizure-like activity (1% children)

Gastrointestinal: Nausea (3%), vomiting (3%)

Local: Pain and local reactions at injection site (4% I.M., 5% I.V.; severity less than diazepam)

Ocular: Nystagmus (1% children)

Respiratory: Cough (1%)

Miscellaneous: Physical and psychological dependence with prolonged use, hiccups (4%, 1% children), paradoxical reaction (2% children)

Overdosage/Toxicology Symptoms of overdose include respiratory depression, hypotension, coma, stupor, confusion, and apnea. Treatment for benzodiazepine overdose is supportive. Flumazenil has been shown to selectively block the binding of benzodiazepines to its receptor, resulting in reversal of CNS depression but not always respiratory depression.

Pharmacodynamics/Kinetics

Onset of Action: I.M.: Sedation: ~15 minutes; I.V.: 1-5 minutes; Peak effect: I.M.: 0.5-1 hour

Duration of Action: I.M.: Up to 6 hours; Mean: 2 hours

Absorption: Oral: Rapid

Bioavailability: Mean: 45%

Protein Binding: 95%

Half-Life Elimination: 1-4 hours; prolonged with cirrhosis, congestive heart failure, obesity, elderly

Metabolism: Extensively hepatic via CYP3A4

Excretion: Urine (as glucuronide conjugated metabolites); feces (~2% to 10%)

Dosing

Adults:

Note: The dose of midazolam needs to be individualized based on the patient's age, underlying diseases, and concurrent medications. Decrease dose (by ~30%) if narcotics or other CNS depressants are administered concomitantly. **Personnel and equipment needed for standard respiratory resuscitation should be immediately available during midazolam administration.**

Preoperative sedation:

I.M.: 0.07-0.08 mg/kg 30-60 minutes prior to surgery/procedure; usual dose: 5 mg; **Note:** Reduce dose in patients with COPD, high-risk patients, patients ≥60 years of age, and patients receiving other narcotics or CNS depressants

I.V.: 0.02-0.04 mg/kg; repeat every 5 minutes as needed to desired effect or up to 0.1-0.2 mg/kg

Intranasal (not an approved route): 0.2 mg/kg (up to 0.4 mg/kg in some studies); administer 30-45 minutes prior to surgery/procedure

Conscious sedation: I.V.: Initial: 0.5-2 mg slow I.V. over at least 2 minutes; slowly titrate to effect by repeating doses every 2-3 minutes if needed; usual total dose: 2.5-5 mg; use decreased doses in elderly.

Healthy Adults <60 years:

Initial: Some patients respond to doses as low as 1 mg; no more than 2.5 mg should be administered over a period of 2 minutes. Additional doses of midazolam may be administered after a 2-minute waiting period and evaluation of sedation after each dose increment. A total dose >5 mg is generally not needed. If narcotics or other CNS depressants are administered concomitantly, the midazolam dose should be reduced by 30%. *Refer to elderly dosing for patients ≥60 years, debilitated, or chronically ill.*

Maintenance: 25% of dose used to reach sedative effect

Anesthesia: I.V.:

Induction:

Unpremedicated patients: 0.3-0.35 mg/kg (up to 0.6 mg/kg in resistant cases)

Premedicated patients: 0.15-0.35 mg/kg

Maintenance: 0.05-0.3 mg/kg as needed, or continuous infusion 0.25-1.5 mcg/kg/minute

Sedation in mechanically-ventilated patients: I.V. continuous infusion: 100 mg in 250 mL D₅W or NS (if patient is fluid-restricted, may concentrate up to a maximum of 0.5 mg/mL); initial dose: 0.02-0.08 mg/kg (~1 mg to 5 mg in 70 kg adult) initially and either repeated at 5-15 minute intervals until adequate sedation is achieved or continuous infusion rates of 0.04-0.2 mg/kg/hour and titrate to reach desired level of sedation

Elderly: The dose of midazolam needs to be individualized based on the patient's age, underlying diseases, and concurrent medications. Decrease dose (by ~30%) if narcotics or other CNS depressants are administered concomitantly. **Personnel and equipment needed for standard respiratory resuscitation should be immediately available during midazolam administration.**

I.V.: Conscious sedation: Initial: 0.5 mg slow I.V.; give no more than 1.5 mg in a 2-minute period. If additional titration is needed, give no more than 1 mg over 2 minutes, waiting another 2 or more minutes to evaluate sedative effect. A total dose >3.5 mg is rarely necessary.

Pediatrics:

Notes: The dose of midazolam needs to be individualized based on the patient's age, underlying diseases, and concurrent medications. Decrease dose (by ~30%) if narcotics or other CNS depressants are administered concomitantly. **Personnel and equipment needed for standard respiratory resuscitation should be immediately available during midazolam administration.** Children <6 years may require higher doses and closer monitoring than older children; calculate dose on ideal body weight

Conscious sedation for procedures or preoperative sedation:

Oral: 0.25-0.5 mg/kg as a single dose preprocedure, up to a maximum of 20 mg; administer 30-40 minutes prior to procedure. Children <6 years, or less cooperative patients may require as much as 1 mg/kg as a single dose; 0.25 mg/kg may suffice for children 6-16 years of age.

Intranasal (not an approved route): 0.2 mg/kg (up to 0.4 mg/kg in some studies), administered 30-45 minutes prior to procedure

I.M.: 0.1-0.15 mg/kg 30-60 minutes before surgery or procedure; range 0.05-0.15 mg/kg; doses up to 0.5 mg/kg have been used in more anxious patients; maximum total dose: 10 mg

I.V.:

Infants <6 months: Limited information is available in nonintubated infants; dosing recommendations not clear; infants <6 months are at higher risk for airway obstruction and hypoventilation; titrate dose in small increments to desired effect; monitor carefully

(Continued)

Midazolam *(Continued)*

Infants 6 months to Children 5 years: Initial: 0.05-0.1 mg/kg; titrate dose carefully; total dose of 0.6 mg/kg may be required; usual maximum total dose: 6 mg

Children 6-12 years: Initial: 0.025-0.05 mg/kg; titrate dose carefully; total doses of 0.4 mg/kg may be required; usual maximum total dose: 10 mg

Children 12-16 years: Dose as adults; usual maximum total dose: 10 mg

Conscious sedation during mechanical ventilation: I.V.: Children: Loading dose: 0.05-0.2 mg/kg, followed by initial continuous infusion: 1-2 mcg/kg/minute; titrate to the desired effect; usual range: 0.4-6 mcg/kg/minute

Status epilepticus refractory to standard therapy: I.V.: Infants >2 months and Children: Loading dose: 0.15 mg/kg followed by a continuous infusion of 1 mcg/kg/minute; titrate dose upward every 5 minutes until clinical seizure activity is controlled; mean infusion rate required in 24 children was 2.3 mcg/kg/minute with a range of 1-18 mcg/kg/minute

Renal Impairment:

Hemodialysis: Supplemental dose is not necessary.

Peritoneal dialysis: Significant drug removal is unlikely based on physiochemical characteristics.

Available Dosage Forms

Injection, solution: 1 mg/mL (2 mL, 5 mL, 10 mL); 5 mg/mL (1 mL, 2 mL, 5 mL, 10 mL) [contains benzyl alcohol 1%]

Injection, solution [preservative free]: 1 mg/mL (2 mL, 5 mL); 5 mg/mL (1 mL, 2 mL)

Syrup: 2 mg/mL (118 mL) [contains sodium benzoate; cherry flavor]

Monitoring and Teaching Issues

Physical Assessment: Assess other medications the patient may be taking for effectiveness and interactions. For inpatient use, institute safety measures and monitor effectiveness and adverse reactions. For outpatients, monitor therapeutic effectiveness and adverse reactions at beginning of therapy and periodically with long-term use. **I.V.:** Monitor cardiac and respiratory status continuously. Monitor I.V. infusion site carefully for extravasation. **I.V./I.M.:** Monitor closely following administration. Bedrest and assistance with ambulation necessary for several hours. **Note:** Full recovery usually occurs within 2-3 hours, but may take 6 hours.

Patient Education: Avoid use of alcohol, prescription or OTC sedatives, or hypnotics for a minimum of 24 hours after administration. Avoid driving or engaging in any tasks that require alertness for 24 hours following administration. You may experience some loss of memory following administration. **Pregnancy/breast-feeding precautions:** Advise prescriber if you are pregnant; this medication is contraindicated for pregnant women. Breast-feeding is not recommended.

Dietary Considerations: Injection: Sodium content of 1 mL: 0.14 mEq

Geriatric Considerations: If concomitant CNS depressant medications are used in the elderly, the midazolam dose will be at least 50% less than doses used in healthy, young, unpremedicated patients (see Warnings/Precautions and Pharmacokinetics).

Pregnancy Risk Factor: D

Pregnancy Issues: Benzodiazepines cross the placenta. The association between benzodiazepine exposure and malformations remains controversial. A number of types of malformation have been reported (oral cleft, inguinal hernia, cardiac defects, spina bifida, dysmorphic facial features, skeletal defects); however, confounding factors make a clear association difficult. Overall, the risk to the fetus may be low. Nonteratogenic effects (including neonatal flaccidity, respiratory and feeding problems, and withdrawal symptoms) during the postnatal period have also been reported with benzodiazepine use.

Lactation: Enters breast milk/not recommended (AAP rates "of concern")

Administration

Oral: Do not mix with any liquid (such as grapefruit juice) prior to administration.

I.M.: Give deep I.M. into large muscle.

I.V.: Administer by slow I.V. injection over at least 2-5 minutes at a concentration of 1-5 mg/mL or by I.V. infusion. Continuous infusions should be administered via an infusion pump.

Other: Intranasal: Administer using a 1 mL needleless syringe into the nares over 15 seconds; use the 5 mg/mL injection; $^1/_2$ of the dose may be administered to each nare

Compatibility: Stable in D_5NS, D_5W, NS; **incompatible** with LR

Y-site administration: Incompatible with albumin, amphotericin B cholesteryl sulfate complex, ampicillin, bumetanide, butorphanol, ceftazidime, cefuroxime, clonidine, dexamethasone sodium succinate, floxacillin, foscarnet, fosphenytoin, furosemide, hydrocortisone sodium succinate, imipenem/cilastatin, methotrexate, nafcillin, omeprazole, sodium bicarbonate, thiopental, trimethoprim/sulfamethoxazole

Compatibility in syringe: Incompatible with dimenhydrinate, pentobarbital, perphenazine, prochlorperazine edisylate, ranitidine

Storage: Stable for 24 hours at room temperature/refrigeration; at a final concentration of 0.5 mg/mL, stable for up to 24 hours when diluted with D_5W or NS, or for up to 4 hours when diluted with lactated Ringer's; admixtures do not require protection from light for short-term storage

Additional Information Abrupt discontinuation after sustained use (generally >10 days) may cause withdrawal symptoms. For neonates, since both concentrations of the injection contain 1% benzyl alcohol, use the 5 mg/mL injection and dilute to 0.5 mg/mL with SWI without preservatives to decrease the amount of benzyl alcohol delivered to the neonate; with continuous infusion, midazolam may accumulate in peripheral tissues; use lowest effective infusion rate to reduce accumulation effects; midazolam is 3-4 times as potent as diazepam; paradoxical reactions associated with midazolam use in children (eg, agitation, restlessness, combativeness) have been successfully treated with flumazenil.

Related Information

Benzodiazepines *on page 1719*

Compatibility of Drugs in Syringe *on page 1725*

♦ **Midazolam Hydrochloride** *see* Midazolam *on page 1001*

Midodrine (MI doe dreen)

U.S. Brand Names Orvaten™; ProAmatine®

Synonyms Midodrine Hydrochloride

Generic Available Yes

Pharmacologic Category Alpha₁ Agonist

Medication Safety Issues

Sound-alike/look-alike issues:

ProAmatine® may be confused with protamine

Use Orphan drug: Treatment of symptomatic orthostatic hypotension

Unlabeled/Investigational Use Investigational: Management of urinary incontinence

Mechanism of Action/Effect Midodrine forms an active metabolite, desglymidodrine that is an alpha₁-agonist. This agent increases arteriolar and venous tone resulting in a rise in standing, sitting, and supine systolic and diastolic blood pressure in patient with orthostatic hypotension.

Contraindications Hypersensitivity to midodrine or any component of the formulation; severe organic heart disease; urinary retention; pheochromocytoma; thyrotoxicosis; persistent and significant supine hypertension

Warnings/Precautions Indicated for patients for whom orthostatic hypotension significantly impairs their daily life despite standard clinical care. Use is not recommended with supine hypertension. Caution should be exercised in patients with diabetes, visual problems (especially if receiving fludrocortisone), urinary retention (reduce initial dose), or hepatic dysfunction; monitor renal and hepatic function prior to and periodically during therapy; safety and efficacy has not been established in children; discontinue and re-evaluate therapy if signs of bradycardia occur.

Drug Interactions

Increased Effect/Toxicity: Concomitant fludrocortisone results in hypernatremia or an increase in intraocular pressure and glaucoma. Bradycardia may be accentuated with concomitant administration of cardiac glycosides, psychotherapeutics, and beta-blockers. Alpha agonists may increase the pressure effects and alpha antagonists may negate the effects of midodrine.

Adverse Reactions

>10%:

Cardiovascular: Supine hypertension (7% to 13%)

Dermatologic: Piloerection (13%), pruritus (12%)

Genitourinary: Urinary urgency, retention, or polyuria, dysuria (up to 13%)

Neuromuscular & skeletal: Paresthesia (18%)

1% to 10%:

Central nervous system: Chills (5%), pain (5%)

Dermatologic: Rash (2%)

Gastrointestinal: Abdominal pain

Overdosage/Toxicology

Symptoms of overdose include hypertension, piloerection, urinary retention

Treatment is symptomatic following gastric decontamination; alpha-sympatholytics and/or dialysis may be helpful

Pharmacodynamics/Kinetics

Onset of Action: ~1 hour

Duration of Action: 2-3 hours

Absorption: Rapid

Bioavailability: Desglymidodrine: 93%

Time to Peak: Desglymidodrine: 1-2 hours; Midodrine: 30 minutes

Protein Binding: Minimal

Half-Life Elimination: Desglymidodrine: ~3-4 hours; Midodrine: 25 minutes

Metabolism: Hepatic; midodrine is a prodrug which undergoes rapid deglycination to desglymidodrine (active metabolite); metabolism occurs in many tissues and plasma

Excretion: Urine (2% to 4%)

Clearance: Desglymidodrine: 385 mL/minute (predominantly by renal secretion)

Dosing

Adults & Elderly: Orthostatic hypotension: Oral: 10 mg 3 times/day during daytime hours (every 3-4 hours) when patient is upright (maximum: 40 mg/day)

Renal Impairment: 2.5 mg 3 times/day; gradually increase as tolerated.

Hemodialysis: Dialyzable

Available Dosage Forms Tablet, as hydrochloride: 2.5 mg, 5 mg, 10 mg

Monitoring and Teaching Issues

Physical Assessment: See Warnings/Precautions for use cautions (eg, diabetes, visual problems, urinary retention, hepatic dysfunction). Assess potential for interactions with other pharmacological agents and herbal products patient may be taking (eg, risk for increased bradycardia with cardiac glycosides, psychotherapeutics, beta blockers; see Drug Interactions). Assess therapeutic effectiveness (reduction of hypotension) and adverse reactions at beginning of therapy and periodically thereafter (eg, supine hypertension, urinary urgency/retention, rash; see Adverse Reactions). Note that standing blood pressure may be elevated 1 hour after administration and remain slightly elevated 3-4 hours. Teach patient possible side effects/appropriate interventions and adverse symptoms to report (see Patient Education).

Monitoring Laboratory Tests: Kidney and liver function tests

Patient Education: Do not take any new medication during therapy unless approved by prescriber (especially anything that may affect blood pressure; cough or cold medications, diet, weight reduction, stay-awake products). Take exactly as directed; take when sitting upright. Do not take within 4 hours of bedtime or when lying down for any length of time. Follow instructions for checking blood pressure and pulse routinely (same time of day; at least once per week). May cause urinary urgency or retention (void before taking or consult prescriber if difficulty persists); or dizziness, drowsiness, or headache (use caution when driving or engaging in tasks that require alertness until response to drug is known). Report

(Continued)

Midodrine *(Continued)*

skin rash, severe gastric upset or pain, muscle weakness or pain, or other persistent side effects. **Pregnancy/breast-feeding precautions:** Inform prescriber if you are or intend to become pregnant. Consult prescriber if breast-feeding.

Pregnancy Risk Factor: C

Lactation: Excretion in breast milk is unknown/use caution

Administration

Oral: Doses may be given in approximately 3- to 4-hour intervals (eg, shortly before or upon rising in the morning, at midday, in the late afternoon not later than 6 PM). Avoid dosing after the evening meal or within 4 hours of bedtime. Continue therapy only in patients who appear to attain symptomatic improvement during initial treatment. Standing systolic blood pressure may be elevated 15-30 mm Hg at 1 hour after a 10 mg dose. Some effect may persist for 2-3 hours.

♦ **Midodrine Hydrochloride** *see* Midodrine *on page 1005*

♦ **Midol® Maximum Strength Cramp Formula [OTC]** *see* Ibuprofen *on page 777*

♦ **Midrin®** *see* Acetaminophen, Isometheptene, and Dichloralphenazone *on page 42*

♦ **Mifeprex®** *see* Mifepristone *on page 1006*

Mifepristone *(mi FE pris tone)*

U.S. Brand Names Mifeprex®

Synonyms RU-486; RU-38486

Restrictions There are currently no clinical trials with mifepristone in oncology open in the U.S.; investigators wishing to obtain the agent for use in oncology patients must apply for a patient-specific IND from the FDA. Mifepristone will be supplied only to licensed physicians who sign and return a "Prescriber's Agreement." Distribution of mifepristone will be subject to specific requirements imposed by the distributor. Mifepristone will **not** be available to the public through licensed pharmacies. A patient medication guide is available and must be dispensed with the medication; the FDA-approved medication guide is available at www.fda.gov/cder/Offices/ODS/labeling.htm.

Generic Available No

Pharmacologic Category Abortifacient; Antineoplastic Agent, Hormone Antagonist; Antiprogestin

Medication Safety Issues

Sound-alike/look-alike issues:

Mifeprex® may be confused with Mirapex®

Use Medical termination of intrauterine pregnancy, through day 49 of pregnancy. Patients may need treatment with misoprostol and possibly surgery to complete therapy

Unlabeled/Investigational Use Treatment of unresectable meningioma; has been studied in the treatment of breast cancer, ovarian cancer, and adrenal cortical carcinoma

Mechanism of Action/Effect Mifepristone, a synthetic steroid, competitively binds to the intracellular progesterone receptor, blocking the effects of progesterone. When used for the termination of pregnancy, this leads to contraction-inducing activity in the myometrium. In the absence of progesterone, mifepristone acts as a partial progesterone agonist. Mifepristone also has weak antiglucocorticoid and antiandrogenic properties; it blocks the feedback effect of cortisol on corticotropin secretion.

Contraindications Hypersensitivity to mifepristone, misoprostol, other prostaglandins, or any component of the formulation; chronic adrenal failure; porphyrias; hemorrhagic disorder or concurrent anticoagulant therapy; pregnancy termination >49 days; intrauterine device (IUD) in place; ectopic pregnancy or undiagnosed adnexal mass; concurrent long-term corticosteroid therapy; inadequate or lack of access to emergency medical services; inability to understand effects and/or comply with treatment

Warnings/Precautions Patient must be instructed of the treatment procedure and expected effects. A signed agreement form must be kept in the patient's file. Physicians may obtain patient agreement forms, physician enrollment forms, and medical consultation directly from Danco Laboratories at 1-877-432-7596. Adverse effects (including blood transfusions, hospitalization, ongoing pregnancy, and other major complications) must be reported in writing to the medication distributor. To be administered only by physicians who can date pregnancy, diagnose ectopic pregnancies, provide access to surgical abortion (if needed), and can provide access to emergency care. Medication will be distributed directly to these physicians following signed agreement with the distributor. Must be administered under supervision by the qualified physician. Pregnancy is dated from day 1 of last menstrual period (presuming a 28-day cycle, ovulation occurring midcycle). Pregnancy duration can be determined using menstrual history and clinical examination. Ultrasound should be used if an ectopic pregnancy is suspected or if duration of pregnancy is uncertain. Ultrasonography may not identify all ectopic pregnancies, and healthcare providers should be alert for signs and symptoms which may be related to undiagnosed ectopic pregnancy in any patient who receives mifepristone.

Bleeding occurs and should be expected (average 9-16 days, may be ≥30 days). In some cases, bleeding may be prolonged and heavy, potentially leading to hypovolemic shock. Patients should be counseled to seek medical attention in cases of excessive bleeding; the manufacturer cites soaking through two thick sanitary pads per hour for two consecutive hours as an example of excessive bleeding. Bleeding may require blood transfusion (rare), curettage, saline infusions, and/or vasoconstrictors. Use caution in patients with severe anemia. Confirmation of pregnancy termination by clinical exam or ultrasound must be made 14 days following treatment. Manufacturer recommends surgical termination of pregnancy when medical termination fails or is not complete. Prescriber should determine in advance whether they will provide such care themselves or through other providers. Preventative measures to prevent rhesus immunization must be taken prior to surgical abortion. Prescriber should also give the patient clear instructions on whom to call and what to do in the event of an emergency following administration of mifepristone.

Bacterial infection have been reported following use of this product. In rare cases, these infections may be serious and/or fatal, with septic shock as a potential complication. A causal relationship has not been established. Sustained fever, abdominal pain, or pelvic tenderness should prompt evaluation; however, healthcare professionals are warned that atypical presentations of serious infection without these symptoms have also been noted.

Safety and efficacy have not been established for use in women with chronic cardiovascular, hypertensive, hepatic, respiratory, or renal disease, insulin-dependent diabetes mellitus, severe anemia, or heavy smokers. Women >35 years of age and smokers (>10 cigarettes/day) were excluded from clinical trials. Safety and efficacy in pediatric patients have not been established.

Drug Interactions

Cytochrome P450 Effect: **Substrate** of CYP3A4 (minor); **Inhibits** CYP2D6 (weak), 3A4 (weak)

Increased Effect/Toxicity: There are no reported interactions. It might be anticipated that the concurrent administration of mifepristone and a progestin would result in an attenuation of the effects of one or both agents.

Nutritional/Ethanol Interactions

Food: Do not take with grapefruit juice; grapefruit juice may inhibit mifepristone metabolism leading to increased levels.

Herb/Nutraceutical: Avoid St John's wort (may induce mifepristone metabolism, leading to decreased levels).

Lab Interactions hCG levels will not be useful to confirm pregnancy termination until at least 10 days following mifepristone treatment.

Adverse Reactions Vaginal bleeding and uterine cramping are expected to occur when this medication is used to terminate a pregnancy; 90% of women using this medication for this purpose also report adverse reactions. Bleeding or spotting occurs in most women for a period of 9-16 days. Up to 8% of women will experience some degree of bleeding or spotting for 30 days or more. In some cases, bleeding may be prolonged and heavy, potentially leading to hypovolemic shock.

>10%:
Central nervous system: Headache (2% to 31%), dizziness (1% to 12%)
Gastrointestinal: Abdominal pain (cramping) (96%), nausea (43% to 61%), vomiting (18% to 26%), diarrhea (12% to 20%)
Genitourinary: Uterine cramping (83%)
1% to 10%:
Cardiovascular: Syncope (1%)
Central nervous system: Fatigue (10%), fever (4%), insomnia (3%), anxiety (2%), fainting (2%)
Gastrointestinal: Dyspepsia (3%)
Genitourinary: Endometriosis/salpingitis/pelvic inflammatory disease (1%), pelvic pain (2%), uterine hemorrhage (5%), vaginitis (3%)
Hematologic: Decreased hemoglobin >2 g/dL (6%), anemia (2%), leukorrhea (2%)
Neuromuscular & skeletal: Back pain (9%), rigors (3%), leg pain (2%), weakness (2%)
Respiratory: Sinusitis (2%)
Miscellaneous: Viral infection (4%)

Overdosage/Toxicology In studies using 3 times the recommended dose for termination of pregnancy, no serious maternal adverse effects were reported. This medication is supplied in single-dose containers to be given under physician supervision, therefore, the risk of overdose should be low. In case of massive ingestion, treat symptomatically and monitor for signs of adrenal failure.

Pharmacodynamics/Kinetics

Time to Peak: 90 minutes

Protein Binding: 98% to albumin and α_1-acid glycoprotein

Half-Life Elimination: Terminal: 18 hours following a slower phase where 50% eliminated between 12-72 hours

Metabolism: Hepatic via CYP3A4 to three metabolites (may possess some antiprogestin and antiglucocorticoid activity)

Excretion: Feces (83%); urine (9%)

Dosing

Adults:

Termination of pregnancy: Oral: Treatment consists of three office visits by the patient; the patient must read medication guide and sign patient agreement prior to treatment:

Day 1: 600 mg (three 200 mg tablets) taken as a single dose under physician supervision

Day 3: Patient must return to the healthcare provider 2 days following administration of mifepristone; if termination of pregnancy cannot be confirmed using ultrasound or clinical examination: 400 mcg (two 200 mg tablets) of misoprostol; patient may need treatment for cramps or gastrointestinal symptoms at this time

Day 14: Patient must return to the healthcare provider ~14 days after administration of mifepristone; confirm complete termination of pregnancy by ultrasound or clinical exam. Surgical termination is recommended to manage treatment failures.

Dosing for unlabeled uses: Refer to individual protocols. The dose used in meningioma is usually 200 mg/day, continued based on toxicity and response.

Elderly: Safety and efficacy have not been established.

Renal Impairment: Safety and efficacy have not been established.

Hepatic Impairment: Safety and efficacy have not been established; use with caution due to CYP3A4 metabolism.

Available Dosage Forms Tablet: 200 mg

Monitoring and Teaching Issues

Physical Assessment: May only be administered under supervision of a qualified physician. Patient must be instructed in procedure and sign patient agreement forms. Assess results of laboratory tests and adverse reactions. Monitor for excessive bleeding. Monitor vital signs. Assess knowledge/teach patient interventions to reduce side effects, and

(Continued)

Mifepristone *(Continued)*

adverse reactions to report. **Pregnancy risk factor X:** This medication is used to terminate pregnancy.

Patient Education: This medication is used to terminate pregnancy under 7 weeks. It must be administered under direction of a qualified physician. You will need follow-up visits as directed by your prescriber (approximately 3 days and 14 days after treatment). Surgical termination of pregnancy may be required if medication fails; there is a risk of fetal malformation if treatment fails. You may experience vaginal bleeding and cramping that is heavier than a normal menstrual period; report immediately if severe or persistent. You may experience nausea, vomiting, and diarrhea. It is possible to get pregnant before your next period. Once the pregnancy has proved to be ended, contraception should be started before having sexual intercourse. Read carefully all information about this medication provided by your prescriber. **Pregnancy/breast-feeding precautions:** Your physician will give you a phone number to call for problems, questions, or emergencies; you should not use this medication if you do not have access to emergency care. You will be given a medication guide to help you understand this medication and its effects. It is important to review this carefully. Ask any questions you may have. You will also be required to sign a form saying that you understand the effects of this treatment and are able to return to the physician for follow-up appointments. Do not breast-feed. Discard breast milk for a few days following use of this medication.

Pregnancy Risk Factor: X

Pregnancy Issues: This medication is used to terminate pregnancy; there are no approved treatment indications for its use during pregnancy. Prostaglandins (including mifepristone and misoprostol) may have teratogenic effects when used during pregnancy.

Lactation: Excretion in breast milk unknown/contraindicated

Breast-Feeding Issues: Breast milk should be discarded for a few days following use of this medication.

Administration
Storage: Store at room temperature of 25°C (77°F).

Additional Information Medication will be distributed directly to qualified physicians following signed agreement with the distributor, Danco Laboratories. It will not be available through pharmacies.

Miglitol *(MIG li tol)*

U.S. Brand Names Glyset®

Generic Available No

Pharmacologic Category Antidiabetic Agent, Alpha-Glucosidase Inhibitor

Use Type 2 diabetes mellitus (noninsulin-dependent, NIDDM):

Monotherapy adjunct to diet to improve glycemic control in patients with type 2 diabetes mellitus (noninsulin-dependent, NIDDM) whose hyperglycemia cannot be managed with diet alone

Combination therapy with a sulfonylurea when diet plus either miglitol or a sulfonylurea alone do not result in adequate glycemic control. The effect of miglitol to enhance glycemic control is additive to that of sulfonylureas when used in combination.

Mechanism of Action/Effect In contrast to sulfonylureas, miglitol does not enhance insulin secretion. The antihyperglycemic action of miglitol results from a reversible inhibition of membrane-bound intestinal alpha-glucosidases which hydrolyze oligosaccharides and disaccharides to glucose and other monosaccharides in the brush border of the small intestine. In diabetic patients, this enzyme inhibition results in delayed glucose absorption and lowering of postprandial hyperglycemia.

Contraindications Hypersensitivity to miglitol or any of component of the formulation; diabetic ketoacidosis; inflammatory bowel disease; colonic ulceration; partial intestinal obstruction or predisposition to intestinal obstruction; chronic intestinal diseases associated with marked disorders of digestion or absorption or with conditions that may deteriorate as a result of increased gas formation in the intestine

Warnings/Precautions GI symptoms are the most common reactions. The incidence of abdominal pain and diarrhea tend to diminish considerably with continued treatment. Long-term clinical trials in diabetic patients with significant renal dysfunction (serum creatinine >2 mg/dL) have not been conducted. Treatment of these patients is not recommended. Because of its mechanism of action, miglitol administered alone should not cause hypoglycemia in the fasting of postprandial state. In combination with a sulfonylurea will cause a further lowering of blood glucose and may increase the hypoglycemic potential of the sulfonylurea.

Drug Interactions
Decreased Effect: Miglitol may decrease the absorption and bioavailability of digoxin, propranolol, and ranitidine. Digestive enzymes (amylase, pancreatin, charcoal) may reduce the effect of miglitol and should **not** be taken concomitantly.

Adverse Reactions
>10%: Gastrointestinal: Flatulence (42%), diarrhea (29%), abdominal pain (12%)
1% to 10%: Dermatologic: Rash

Overdosage/Toxicology An overdose of miglitol will not result in hypoglycemia. An overdose may result in transient increases in flatulence, diarrhea, and abdominal discomfort. No serious systemic reactions are expected in the event of an overdose.

Pharmacodynamics/Kinetics
Absorption: Saturable at high doses: 25 mg dose: Completely absorbed; 100 mg dose: 50% to 70% absorbed

Time to Peak: 2-3 hours
Protein Binding: <4%
Half-Life Elimination: ~2 hours
Metabolism: None
Excretion: Urine (as unchanged drug)

Dosing
Adults & Elderly: Type 2 diabetes (noninsulin dependent, NIDDM): Oral: 25 mg 3 times/day with the first bite of food at each meal; the dose may be increased to 50 mg 3 times/day after 4-8 weeks; maximum recommended dose: 100 mg 3 times/day
Renal Impairment: Miglitol is primarily excreted by the kidneys; there is little information of miglitol in patients with a Cl$_{cr}$ <25 mL/minute.
Hepatic Impairment: No adjustment necessary.
Available Dosage Forms Tablet: 25 mg, 50 mg, 100 mg

Monitoring and Teaching Issues
Physical Assessment: Assess results of laboratory tests, therapeutic effectiveness, and adverse response on a regular basis throughout therapy. Teach patient proper use (or refer patient to diabetic educator), possible side effects/appropriate interventions (eg, importance of adequate hydration), and adverse symptoms to report.
Monitoring Laboratory Tests: Blood glucose tests; measurement of glycosylated hemoglobin is recommended for the monitoring of long-term glycemic control.
Patient Education: Inform prescriber of all prescriptions, OTC medications, or herbal products you are taking, and any allergies you have. Do not take any new medication during therapy unless approved by prescriber. Take exactly as directed, with the first bite of each main meal. Do not change dosage or discontinue without first consulting prescriber. Do not take other medications with or within 2 hours of this medication unless advised by prescriber. Avoid alcohol. It is important to follow dietary and lifestyle recommendations of prescriber. You will be instructed in signs of hypo- or hyperglycemia by prescriber or diabetic educator. If combining this medication with other diabetic medication (eg, sulfonylureas, insulin), keep source of glucose (sugar) on hand in case hypoglycemia occurs. May cause mild side effects during first weeks of therapy (eg, bloating, flatulence, diarrhea, abdominal discomfort); these should diminish over time. Report severe or persistent side effects, fever, extended vomiting or flu, or change in color of urine or stool. **Breast-feeding precaution:** Breast-feeding is not recommended.
Pregnancy Risk Factor: B
Pregnancy Issues: Abnormal blood glucose levels are associated with a higher incidence of congenital abnormalities. Insulin is the drug of choice for the control of diabetes mellitus during pregnancy.
Lactation: Enters breast milk (small amounts)/not recommended

Administration
Oral: Should be taken orally at the start (with the first bite) of each main meal.

Related Information
Diabetes Mellitus Management *on page 1819*

Miglustat (MIG loo stat)

U.S. Brand Names Zavesca®
Synonyms OGT-918
Generic Available No
Pharmacologic Category Enzyme Inhibitor
Use Treatment of mild-to-moderate type 1 Gaucher disease when enzyme replacement therapy is not a therapeutic option
Mechanism of Action/Effect Miglustat inhibits the enzyme needed to produce glycosphingolipids and decreases the rate of glycosphingolipid glucosylceramide formation.
Contraindications Hypersensitivity to miglustat or any component of the formulation; pregnancy
Warnings/Precautions Peripheral neuropathy has been reported with use and neurologic monitoring is required. Tremor or exacerbations of existing tremor may occur; may resolve over time or respond to dosage reduction. Weigh risk versus benefit of therapy if patient develops numbness and tingling. Use caution in renal impairment. Safety and efficacy in severe type 1 Gaucher disease have not been established. Safety and efficacy in patients <18 or >65 years of age have not been established.

Drug Interactions
Decreased Effect: Miglustat increases the clearance of imiglucerase; combination therapy is not indicated.

Nutritional/Ethanol Interactions
Food: Food decreases the rate, but not the extent, of absorption.

Adverse Reactions Percentages reported from open-label, uncontrolled monotherapy trials.
>10%:
Central nervous system: Headache (21% to 22%), dizziness (up to 11%)
Gastrointestinal: Diarrhea (89%; up to 100% in other studies), weight loss (39% to 67%), abdominal pain (18% to 50%), flatulence (29% to 44%), nausea (14% to 22%), vomiting (4% to 11%), cramps (up to 11%)
Neuromuscular & skeletal: Tremor (11%; up to 30% in other studies), leg cramps (4% to 11%),
Ocular: visual disturbances (up to 17%)
1% to 10%:
Central nervous system: headache (up to 6%)
Endocrine & metabolic: Menstrual disorder (up to 6%)
Gastrointestinal: Anorexia (up to 7%), dyspepsia (up to 7%), epigastric pain (up to 6%)
Hematologic: Thrombocytopenia (6% to 7%)
Neuromuscular & skeletal: Paresthesia (up to 7%)
Overdosage/Toxicology Doses of up to 3000 mg/day were used in HIV-positive patients during clinical development. Dizziness, granulocytopenia, leukopenia, neutropenia, and paresthesia were observed.
(Continued)

Miglustat *(Continued)*

Pharmacodynamics/Kinetics
Bioavailability: 97%
Time to Peak: Plasma: 2-2.5 hours
Protein Binding: No binding to plasma proteins
Half-Life Elimination: 6-7 hours
Excretion: Urine (as unchanged drug)

Dosing
Adults: Type 1 Gaucher disease: Oral: 100 mg 3 times/day; dose may be reduced to 100 mg 1-2 times/day in patients with adverse effects (ie, tremor, GI distress)
Renal Impairment:
Cl_{cr} 50-75 mL/minute: 100 mg twice daily
Cl_{cr} 30-50 mL/minute: 100 mg once daily
Cl_{cr} <30 mL/minute: Not recommended

Available Dosage Forms Capsule: 100 mg

Monitoring and Teaching Issues
Physical Assessment: Use caution with renal impairment (see Warnings/Precautions for use cautions). Not to be used in combination with imiglucerase (see Drug Interactions). Assess results of neurological evaluations at beginning of therapy and every 6 months during therapy. Teach patient proper use, possible side effects/appropriate interventions, and adverse symptoms to report (see Patient Education). **Pregnancy risk factor X:** Determine that patient is not pregnant before beginning treatment. Do not give to women of childbearing age or males who may have intercourse with childbearing age females unless they are capable of complying with effective contraceptive measures during therapy. Men should continue contraceptive measures for 3 months following treatment.

Patient Education: Capsules should be swallowed whole and taken at the same time each day, with or without food. May cause headache and dizziness (use caution when driving or engaging in hazardous tasks until response to drug is known); nausea, vomiting, or loss of appetite (small frequent meals and good mouth care may help); or diarrhea (buttermilk, boiled milk, or yogurt may help). Notify prescriber at once of persistent diarrhea, numbness or tingling in extremities, change in vision, or other adverse effects. **Pregnancy/breast-feeding precautions:** Inform prescriber if you are pregnant. This drug can cause fetal abnormalities. Both females and males should use (consult prescriber) appropriate contraception during therapy. Males should continue contraceptive use for 3 months following therapy. Breast-feeding is not recommended.

Dietary Considerations: May be take, with or without food. Patients with diarrhea should avoid foods with high carbohydrate content.

Pregnancy Risk Factor: X

Pregnancy Issues: Decreased fetus weight, fetal loss, and difficult or delayed births were observed in animal studies. Women with reproduction potential should use effective contraception during therapy. In addition, adverse effects on spermatogenesis and reduced fertility were observed in male animal studies. The manufacturer recommends that male patients use reliable contraception during therapy and for 3 months following treatment.

Lactation: Excretion in breast milk unknown/not recommended

Administration
Oral: Capsules should be swallowed whole and taken at the same time each day. May be taken with or without food.

Storage: Store at 20°C to 25°C (68°F to 77°F).

- **Migranal®** *see* Dihydroergotamine *on page 457*
- **Migrin-A** *see* Acetaminophen, Isometheptene, and Dichloralphenazone *on page 42*
- **Milk of Magnesia** *see* Magnesium Hydroxide *on page 930*
- **Milliequivalent and Millimole Calculations and Conversions** *see page 1690*

Milrinone *(MIL ri none)*

U.S. Brand Names Primacor®
Synonyms Milrinone Lactate
Generic Available Yes
Pharmacologic Category Phosphodiesterase Enzyme Inhibitor
Medication Safety Issues
Sound-alike/look-alike issues:
Primacor® may be confused with Primaxin®
Use Short-term I.V. therapy of congestive heart failure; calcium antagonist intoxication
Mechanism of Action/Effect Phosphodiesterase inhibitor resulting in vasodilation
Contraindications Hypersensitivity to milrinone, inamrinone, or any component of the formulation; concurrent use of inamrinone
Warnings/Precautions Avoid in severe obstructive aortic or pulmonic valvular disease. Milrinone may aggravate outflow tract obstruction in hypertrophic subaortic stenosis. Supraventricular and ventricular arrhythmias have developed in high-risk patients. Ensure that ventricular rate controlled in atrial fibrillation/flutter prior to initiating milrinone. Not recommended for use in acute MI patients. Monitor and correct fluid and electrolyte problems. Adjust dose in renal dysfunction. Has not been demonstrated to be safe or effective for longer than 48 hours.

Adverse Reactions
>10%: Cardiovascular: Ventricular arrhythmia (ectopy 9%, NSVT 3%, sustained ventricular tachycardia 1%, ventricular fibrillation <1%); life-threatening arrhythmia are infrequent, often associated with underlying factors (eg, pre-existing arrhythmia, electrolyte disturbances, catheter insertion)
1% to 10%:
Cardiovascular: Supraventricular arrhythmia (4%), hypotension
Central nervous system: Headache
Overdosage/Toxicology Treatment is supportive and symptomatic.

Pharmacodynamics/Kinetics

Onset of Action: I.V.: 5-15 minutes

Serum level: I.V.: Following a 125 mcg/kg dose, peak plasma concentrations ~1000 ng/mL were observed at 2 minutes postinjection, decreasing to <100 ng/mL in 2 hours

Drug concentration levels:

Therapeutic:

Serum levels of 166 ng/mL, achieved during I.V. infusions of 0.25-1 mcg/kg/minute, were associated with sustained hemodynamic benefit in severe congestive heart failure patients over a 24-hour period

Maximum beneficial effects on cardiac output and pulmonary capillary wedge pressure following I.V. infusion have been associated with plasma milrinone concentrations of 150-250 ng/mL

Toxic: Serum concentrations >250-300 ng/mL have been associated with marked reductions in mean arterial pressure and tachycardia; however, more studies are required to determine the toxic serum levels for milrinone

Protein Binding: Plasma: ~70%

Half-Life Elimination: I.V.: 136 minutes in patients with congestive heart failure (CHF); patients with severe CHF have a more prolonged half-life, with values ranging from 1.7-2.7 hours. Patients with CHF have a reduction in the systemic clearance of milrinone, resulting in a prolonged elimination half-life. Alternatively, one study reported that 1 month of therapy with milrinone did not change the pharmacokinetic parameters for patients with CHF despite improvement in cardiac function.

Metabolism: Hepatic (12%)

Excretion: I.V.: Urine (85% as unchanged drug) within 24 hours; active tubular secretion is a major elimination pathway for milrinone

Clearance: I.V. bolus: 25.9 ± 5.7 L/hour (0.37 L/hour/kg); Severe congestive heart failure: 0.11-0.13 L/hour/kg. The reduction in clearance may be a result of reduced renal function. Creatinine clearance values were ½ those reported for healthy adults in patients with severe congestive heart failure (52 vs 119 mL/minute).

Dosing

Adults & Elderly: CHF/Hemodynamic support: I.V.: Loading dose: 50 mcg/kg administered over 10 minutes followed by a maintenance dose titrated according to the hemodynamic and clinical response, see table.

Maintenance Dosage	Dose Rate (mcg/kg/min)	Total Dose (mg/kg/24 h)
Minimum	0.375	0.59
Standard	0.500	0.77
Maximum	0.750	1.13

Renal Impairment:

Cl_{cr} 50 mL/minute/1.73 m^2: Administer 0.43 mcg/kg/minute.
Cl_{cr} 40 mL/minute/1.73 m^2: Administer 0.38 mcg/kg/minute.
Cl_{cr} 30 mL/minute/1.73 m^2: Administer 0.33 mcg/kg/minute.
Cl_{cr} 20 mL/minute/1.73 m^2: Administer 0.28 mcg/kg/minute.
Cl_{cr} 10 mL/minute/1.73 m^2: Administer 0.23 mcg/kg/minute.
Cl_{cr} 5 mL/minute/1.73 m^2: Administer 0.2 mcg/kg/minute.

Available Dosage Forms

Infusion [premixed in D_5W] (Primacor®): 200 mcg/mL (100 mL, 200 mL)
Injection, solution: 1 mg/mL (10 mL, 20 mL, 50 mL)
Primacor®: 1 mg/mL (10 mL, 20 mL, 50 mL)

Monitoring and Teaching Issues

Physical Assessment: Use infusion pump. Monitor cardiac/hemodynamic status continuously during therapy and serum potassium at regular intervals. Monitor for fluid retention.

Monitoring Laboratory Tests: Serum potassium

Patient Education: This drug can only be given intravenously. If you experience increased voiding call for assistance. Report pain at infusion site, numbness or tingling of extremities, or respiratory difficulty. **Pregnancy/breast-feeding precautions:** Inform prescriber if you are pregnant. Consult prescriber if breast-feeding.

Pregnancy Risk Factor: C

Lactation: Excretion in breast milk unknown

Administration

I.V.: Infuse via infusion pump.

Reconstitution: Stable at 0.2 mg/mL in 0.9% sodium chloride or D_5W for 72 hours at room temperature in normal light.

Standard dilution: For a final concentration of 0.2 mg/mL: Dilute Primacor® 1 mg/mL (20 mL) with 80 mL diluent (final volume: 100 mL); may also dilute 1 mg/mL (10 mL) with 40 mL diluent (final volume: 50 mL)

Compatibility: Stable in D_5W, LR, ½NS, NS
Y-site administration: Incompatible with furosemide, procainamide
Compatibility in syringe: Incompatible with furosemide
Compatibility when admixed: Incompatible with bumetanide, furosemide, procainamide

Storage: Colorless to pale yellow solution. Store at room temperature and protect from light.

Related Information

Inotropic and Vasoconstrictor Comparison *on page 1736*

♦ **Minocin®** *see Minocycline on page 1012*

Minocycline (mi noe SYE kleen)

U.S. Brand Names Dynacin®; Minocin®; myrac™

Synonyms Minocycline Hydrochloride

Generic Available Yes: Capsule, tablet

Pharmacologic Category Antibiotic, Tetracycline Derivative

Medication Safety Issues

Sound-alike/look-alike issues:

Dynacin® may be confused with Dyazide®, Dynabac®, DynaCirc®, Dynapen®

Minocin® may be confused with Indocin®, Lincocin®, Minizide®, Mithracin®, niacin

Use Treatment of susceptible bacterial infections of both gram-negative and gram-positive organisms; treatment of anthrax (inhalational, cutaneous, and gastrointestinal); acne; meningococcal carrier state; Rickettsial diseases (including Rocky Mountain spotted fever, Q fever); nongonococcal urethritis, gonorrhea; acute intestinal amebiasis

Mechanism of Action/Effect Inhibits bacterial protein synthesis by binding with the 30S and possibly the 50S ribosomal subunit(s) of susceptible bacteria; cell wall synthesis is not affected

Contraindications Hypersensitivity to minocycline, other tetracyclines, or any component of the formulation; pregnancy

Warnings/Precautions May cause permanent tooth discoloration; avoid use during tooth development (children ≤8 years of age) unless other drugs are not likely to be effective or are contraindicated. May be associated with increases in BUN secondary to antianabolic effects; use caution in patients with renal or hepatic insufficiency. CNS effects (lightheadedness, vertigo) may occur; patients must be cautioned about performing tasks which require mental alertness (eg, operating machinery or driving). Has been associated (rarely) with pseudotumor cerebri. May cause photosensitivity; discontinue if skin erythema occurs. May cause overgrowth of nonsusceptible organisms, including fungi; discontinue if superinfection occurs. Avoid use in children ≤8 years of age.

Drug Interactions

Decreased Effect: Although anecdotal reports suggest oral contraceptive efficacy could be reduced by tetracyclines, this has been refuted by more rigorous scientific and clinical data. Calcium-, magnesium-, or aluminum-containing antacids, bile acid sequestrants, bismuth, oral contraceptives, iron, zinc, sodium bicarbonate, penicillins, cimetidine, quinapril may decrease absorption of tetracyclines. Methoxyflurane anesthesia (when concurrent with tetracyclines) may cause fatal nephrotoxicity. Tetracyclines may reduce bactericidal efficacy of penicillins and cephalosporins.

Increased Effect/Toxicity: Minocycline may increase the effect of warfarin. Retinoic acid derivatives may increase risk of pseudotumor cerebri.

Nutritional/Ethanol Interactions

Food: Minocycline serum concentrations are not significantly altered if taken with food or dairy products.

Herb/Nutraceutical: Avoid dong quai, St John's wort (may also cause photosensitization).

Lab Interactions May cause interference with fluorescence test for urinary catecholamines (false elevations)

Adverse Reactions Frequency not defined.

Cardiovascular: Myocarditis, pericarditis, vasculitis

Central Nervous System: Bulging fontanels, convulsions, dizziness, fever, headache, hypoesthesia, paresthesia, pseudotumor cerebri, sedation, vertigo

Dermatologic: Alopecia, angioedema, epidermal necrolysis, erythema nodosum, erythematous rash, exfoliative dermatitis, hyperpigmentation of nails, maculopapular rash, photosensitivity, pigmentation of the skin and mucous membranes, pruritus, Stevens-Johnson syndrome, toxic erythema multiforme, urticaria

Endocrine & metabolic: Thyroid dysfunction

Gastrointestinal: Anorexia, diarrhea, dyspepsia, dysphagia, enamel hypoplasia, enterocolitis, esophageal ulcerations, esophagitis, glossitis, inflammatory lesions (oral/anogenital), moniliasis, nausea, oral cavity discoloration, pancreatitis, pseudomembranous colitis, stomatitis, tooth discoloration, vomiting

Genitourinary: Balanitis, vulvovaginitis

Hematologic: Agranulocytosis, eosinophilia, hemolytic anemia, leukopenia, neutropenia, pancytopenia, thrombocytopenia

Hepatic: Hepatic cholestasis, hepatic failure, hepatitis, hyperbilirubinemia, jaundice, liver enzyme increases

Neuromuscular & skeletal: Arthralgia, arthritis, bone discoloration, joint stiffness, joint swelling, myalgia

Otic: Hearing loss, tinnitus

Renal: Acute renal failure, BUN increased, interstitial nephritis

Respiratory: Asthma, bronchospasm, cough, dyspnea, pneumonitis, pulmonary infiltrate

Miscellaneous: Anaphylaxis, lupus erythematosus

Overdosage/Toxicology Symptoms of overdose include diabetes insipidus, nausea, anorexia, dizziness, vomiting, and diarrhea. Treatment is supportive. Not dialyzable (0% to 5%).

Pharmacodynamics/Kinetics

Absorption: Well absorbed

Protein Binding: 70% to 75%

Half-Life Elimination: 16 hours (range: 11-23 hours)

Excretion: Urine

Dosing

Adults & Elderly:

Susceptible infections: Oral, I.V.: 200 mg initially, followed by 100 mg every 12 hours, not to exceed 400 mg/24 hours

Acne: Oral: 50-100 mg daily

Chlamydial or *Ureaplasma urealyticum* infection, uncomplicated: Urethral, endocervical, or rectal: 100 mg every 12 hours for at least 7 days

Gonococcal infection, uncomplicated (males): Without urethritis or anorectal infection: 200 mg initially, followed by 100 mg every 12 hours for at least 4 days (cultures 2-3 days post-therapy)

Gonococcal infection, uncomplicated urethritis: 100 mg every 12 hours for 5 days

Meningococcal carrier state: 100 mg every 12 hours for 5 days

Mycobacterium marinum: 100 mg every 12 hours for 6-8 weeks (**Note:** Optimal doses have not been established)

Syphilis: 200 mg initially, followed by 100 mg every 12 hours for 10-15 days

Pediatrics: Children >8 years: Oral, I.V.: Initial: 4 mg/kg followed by 2 mg/kg/dose every 12 hours

Renal Impairment: Consider decreasing dose or increasing dosing interval; total daily dose should not exceed 200 mg.

Available Dosage Forms [DSC] = Discontinued product

Capsule (Dynacin®): 50 mg, 75 mg, 100 mg

Capsule, pellet-filled (Minocin®): 50 mg, 100 mg

Injection, powder for reconstitution (Minocin®): 100 mg [DSC]

Tablet (Dynacin®, myrac™): 50 mg, 75 mg, 100 mg

Monitoring and Teaching Issues

Physical Assessment: Assess results of culture and sensitivity tests and allergy history before beginning therapy. See Warnings/Precautions for use cautions (eg, renal insufficiency). Assess potential for interactions with other pharmacological agents or herbal products patient may be taking (eg, warfarin, antacids, hydantoins, carbamazepine; see Drug Interactions). **Infusion:** See Administration; infusion site must be closely monitored to prevent extravasation. Assess therapeutic effectiveness (resolution of infection) and adverse reactions on a regular basis during therapy (see Adverse Reactions). Teach patient proper use, possible side effects/appropriate interventions (eg, importance of adequate hydration), and adverse symptoms to report (see Patient Education).

Monitoring Laboratory Tests: Perform culture and sensitivity testing prior to initiating therapy.

Patient Education: Do not take any new medication during therapy unless approved by prescriber. Take at regular intervals around-the-clock; may be taken with food. Complete full course of therapy; do not discontinue even if condition is resolved. May cause photosensitivity reaction (avoid sun, use sunblock, or wear protective clothing); nausea (small frequent meals, frequent mouth care, chewing gum, or sucking lozenges may help); or diarrhea (boiled milk, buttermilk, or yogurt may help). Report rash or itching, unresolved nausea or diarrhea, change in urinary output (excess); or opportunistic infection (eg, fever, chills, sore throat, burning urination, fatigue). **Pregnancy/breast-feeding precautions:** Do not get pregnant while taking this medication. Consult prescriber for appropriate contraceptive measures. Consult prescriber if breast-feeding.

Dietary Considerations: May be taken with food or milk.

Geriatric Considerations: Minocycline has not been studied in the elderly but its CNS effects may limit its use (see Adverse Reactions). Dose reduction for renal function not necessary.

Pregnancy Risk Factor: D

Pregnancy Issues: May cause permanent discoloration (brown-gray) of teeth. Animal studies indicate possible tumorigenicity and impairment of fertility. Congenital anomalies have been reported postmarketing.

Lactation: Enters breast milk/not recommended (AAP rates "compatible")

Breast-Feeding Issues: Although tetracyclines are excreted in limited amounts, the potential for staining of unerupted teeth has led some experts to recommend against breast-feeding. The AAP identified tetracyclines as "compatible" with breast-feeding.

Administration

Oral: May be taken with food or milk. Administer with adequate fluid to decrease the risk of esophageal irritation and ulceration.

I.V.: Infuse I.V. minocycline slowly, usually over a 4- to 6-hour period.

Compatibility: Stable in D_5NS, D_5W, LR, NS

Y-site administration: Incompatible with allopurinol, amifostine, hydromorphone, meperidine, morphine, piperacillin/tazobactam, propofol, thiotepa

Compatibility in syringe: Incompatible with doxapram

Compatibility when admixed: Incompatible with rifampin

Related Information

Antimicrobial Drugs of Choice *on page 1792*

Mirtazapine (mir TAZ a peen)

U.S. Brand Names Remeron®; Remeron SolTab®

Restrictions A medication guide should be dispensed with each prescription. A template for the required MedGuides can be found on the FDA website at: http://www.fda.gov/cder/drug/antidepressants/labelTemplate.pdf

Generic Available Yes

Pharmacologic Category Antidepressant, Alpha-2 Antagonist

(Continued)

Mirtazapine (Continued)

Medication Safety Issues
Sound-alike/look-alike issues:
Remeron® may be confused with Premarin®, Zemuron®

Use Treatment of depression

Mechanism of Action/Effect
Mirtazapine is a tetracyclic antidepressant that works by its central presynaptic alpha$_2$-adrenergic antagonist effects, which results in increased release of norepinephrine and serotonin. It is also a potent antagonist of 5-HT$_2$ and 5-HT$_3$ serotonin receptors and H1 histamine receptors and a moderate peripheral alpha$_1$-adrenergic and muscarinic antagonist; it does not inhibit the reuptake of norepinephrine or serotonin.

Contraindications
Hypersensitivity to mirtazapine or any component of the formulation; use of MAO inhibitors within 14 days

Warnings/Precautions
Antidepressants increase the risk of suicidal thinking and behavior in children and adolescents with major depressive disorder (MDD) and other depressive disorders; consider risk prior to prescribing. All patients must be closely monitored for clinical worsening, suicidality, or unusual changes in behavior, especially during the initiation of therapy or following an increase or decrease in dosage. When used in children, the child's family or caregiver should be instructed to closely observe the patient and communicate condition with healthcare provider. A medication guide should be dispensed with each prescription. **Mirtazapine is not FDA approved for use in children.**

The possibility of a suicide attempt is inherent in major depression and may persist until remission occurs. Use caution in high-risk patients. Worsening depression and severe abrupt suicidality that are not part of the presenting symptoms may require discontinuation or modification of drug therapy. The patient's family or caregiver should be alerted to monitor patients for the emergence of suicidality and associated behaviors (such as agitation, irritability, hostility, impulsivity, and hypomania) and call healthcare provider.

May worsen psychosis in some patients or precipitate a shift to mania or hypomania in patients with bipolar disorder. Patients presenting with depressive symptoms should be screened for bipolar disorder. Monotherapy in patients with bipolar disorder should be avoided. **Mirtazapine is not FDA approved for the treatment of bipolar depression.**

Discontinue immediately if signs and symptoms of neutropenia/agranulocytosis occur. May cause sedation, resulting in impaired performance of tasks requiring alertness (eg, operating machinery or driving). Sedative effects may be additive with other CNS depressants and/or ethanol. The degree of sedation is moderate-high relative to other antidepressants. The risks of orthostatic hypotension or anticholinergic effects are low relative to other antidepressants. The incidence of sexual dysfunction with mirtazapine is generally lower than with SSRIs.

May increase appetite and stimulate weight gain. Weight gain of >7% of body weight reported in 7.5% of patients treated with mirtazapine compared to 0% for placebo; 8% of patients receiving mirtazapine discontinued treatment due to the weight gain. In an 8-week pediatric clinical trial, 49% of mirtazapine-treated patients had a weight gain of at least 7% (mean increase 4 kg) as compared to 5.7% of placebo-treated patients (mean increase 1 kg). May increase serum cholesterol and triglyceride levels.

Use caution in patients with a previous seizure disorder or condition predisposing to seizures such as brain damage, alcoholism, or concurrent therapy with other drugs which lower the seizure threshold. Use with caution in patients with hepatic or renal dysfunction and in elderly patients. SolTab® formulation contains phenylalanine.

Drug Interactions
Cytochrome P450 Effect: Substrate of CYP1A2 (major), 2C8/9 (minor), 2D6 (major), 3A4 (major); **Inhibits** CYP1A2 (weak), 3A4 (weak)

Decreased Effect: CYP1A2 inducers may decrease the levels/effects of mirtazapine; example inducers include aminoglutethimide, carbamazepine, phenobarbital, and rifampin. Decreased effect seen with clonidine. CYP3A4 inducers may decrease the levels/effects of mirtazapine; example inducers include aminoglutethimide, carbamazepine, nafcillin, nevirapine, phenobarbital, phenytoin, and rifamycins.

Increased Effect/Toxicity: Contraindicated with drugs which inhibit MAO (including linezolid, selegiline, sibutramine, and MAOIs); severe/fatal reactions may occur. CYP1A2 inhibitors may increase the levels/effects of mirtazapine; example inhibitors include amiodarone, ciprofloxacin, fluvoxamine, ketoconazole, norfloxacin, ofloxacin, and rofecoxib. CYP2D6 inhibitors may increase the levels/effects of mirtazapine; example inhibitors include chlorpromazine, delavirdine, fluoxetine, miconazole, paroxetine, pergolide, quinidine, quinine, ritonavir, and ropinirole. CYP3A4 inhibitors may increase the levels/effects of mirtazapine; example inhibitors include azole antifungals, ciprofloxacin, clarithromycin, diclofenac, doxycycline, erythromycin, imatinib, isoniazid, nefazodone, nicardipine, propofol, protease inhibitors, quinidine, and verapamil. Increased sedative effect seen with CNS depressants.

Nutritional/Ethanol Interactions
Ethanol: Avoid ethanol (may increase CNS depression).
Herb/Nutraceutical: Avoid St John's wort (may decrease mirtazapine levels). Avoid valerian, St John's wort, SAMe, kava kava (may increase CNS depression).

Adverse Reactions
>10%:
Central nervous system: Somnolence (54%)
Endocrine & metabolic: Increased cholesterol
Gastrointestinal: Constipation (13%), xerostomia (25%), increased appetite (17%), weight gain (12%; weight gain of >7% reported in 8% of adults, ≤49% of pediatric patients)
1% to 10%:
Cardiovascular: Hypertension, vasodilatation, peripheral edema (2%), edema (1%)
Central nervous system: Dizziness (7%), abnormal dreams (4%), abnormal thoughts (3%), confusion (2%), malaise
Endocrine & metabolic: Increased triglycerides
Gastrointestinal: Vomiting, anorexia, abdominal pain

Genitourinary: Urinary frequency (2%)

Neuromuscular & skeletal: Myalgia (2%), back pain (2%), arthralgia, trem[or], [weak]ness (8%)

Respiratory: Dyspnea (1%)

Miscellaneous: Flu-like symptoms (5%), thirst

Overdosage/Toxicology Experience with overdose is limited. Signs and symp[toms ha]ve included disorientation, drowsiness, impaired memory, and tachycardia. Treatmen[t sh]ould be symptomatic and supportive. Activated charcoal should be administered. Emesis is not recommended; however, gastric lavage with airway protection may be used in symptomatic patients or if performed soon after ingestion. Consider the possibility of multiple drug involvement.

Pharmacodynamics/Kinetics
Bioavailability: 50%

Time to Peak: Serum: 2 hours

Protein Binding: 85%

Half-Life Elimination: 20-40 hours; hampered with renal or hepatic impairment

Metabolism: Extensively hepatic via CYP1A2, 2C9, 2D6, 3A4 and via demethylation and hydroxylation

Excretion: Urine (75%) and feces (15%) as metabolites

Dosing
Adults: Depression: Oral: Initial: 15 mg nightly, titrate up to 15-45 mg/day with dose increases made no more frequently than every 1-2 weeks. There is an inverse relationship between dose and sedation.

Elderly: Initial: 7.5 mg/day as a single bedtime dose; increase by 7.5-15 mg/day every 1-2 weeks; usual dose: 15-30 mg/day; maximum dose: 45 mg/day

Renal Impairment:

Cl_{cr} 11-39 mL/minute: 30% decreased clearance

Cl_{cr} <10 mL/minute: 50% decreased clearance

Hepatic Impairment: Clearance is decreased by 30%.

Available Dosage Forms
Tablet (Remeron®): 15 mg, 30 mg, 45 mg

Tablet, orally-disintegrating: 15 mg, 30 mg

Remeron SolTab®:

15 mg [contains phenylalanine 2.6 mg/tablet; orange flavor]

30 mg [contains phenylalanine 5.2 mg/tablet; orange flavor]

45 mg [contains phenylalanine 7.8 mg/tablet; orange flavor]

Monitoring and Teaching Issues
Physical Assessment: Assess other medications patient may be taking for effectiveness and interactions. Has potential for psychological or physiological dependence, abuse, or tolerance. Monitor therapeutic effectiveness and adverse reactions at beginning of therapy and periodically with long-term use. Monitor for CNS depression/sedation. Monitor for clinical worsening and suicidal ideation. Taper dosage slowly when discontinuing. Assess knowledge/teach patient appropriate use, interventions to reduce side effects, and adverse symptoms to report.

Monitoring Laboratory Tests: CBC

Patient Education: Take exactly as directed; do not increase dose or frequency. It may take 2-3 weeks to achieve desired results. Take once-a-day dose at bedtime. Avoid alcohol, caffeine, and other prescription or OTC medications not approved by prescriber. Maintain adequate hydration (2-3 L/day of fluids) unless instructed to restrict fluid intake. You may experience drowsiness, dizziness, or lightheadedness (use caution when driving or engaging in tasks requiring alertness until response to drug is known); nausea, vomiting, anorexia, or dry mouth (small frequent meals, frequent mouth care, chewing gum, or sucking lozenges may help); or orthostatic hypotension (use caution when climbing stairs or changing position from lying or sitting to standing). Report persistent insomnia, agitation, or confusion; suicidal ideation; muscle cramping, tremors, weakness, or change in gait; breathlessness or respiratory difficulty; chest pain, palpitations, or rapid heartbeat; change in urinary pattern; vision changes or eye pain; yellowing of eyes or skin; pale stools/dark urine; or worsening of condition.

SolTab®: Open blister pack and place tablet on the tongue. Do not split tablet. Tablet is formulated to dissolve on the tongue without water.

Pregnancy/breast-feeding precautions: Inform prescriber if you are or intend to become pregnant. Breast-feeding is not recommended.

Dietary Considerations: Remeron SolTab® contains phenylalanine: 2.6 mg per 15 mg tablet; 5.2 mg per 30 mg tablet; 7.8 mg per 45 mg tablet

Pregnancy Risk Factor: C

Lactation: Excretion in breast milk unknown/not recommended

Administration
Storage: Store at controlled room temperature

SolTab®: Protect from light and moisture; use immediately upon opening tablet blister

Additional Information Note: At least 14 days should elapse between discontinuation of an MAO inhibitor and initiation of therapy with mirtazapine; at least 14 days should be allowed after discontinuing mirtazapine before starting an MAO inhibitor.

Related Information
Antidepressant Agents *on page 1713*

Antidepressant Medication Guidelines *on page 1765*

Misoprostol (mye soe PROST ole)
U.S. Brand Names Cytotec®

Generic Available Yes

Pharmacologic Category Prostaglandin

(Continued)

isoprostol *(Continued)*

Medication Safety Issues
Sound-alike/look-alike issues:
- Misoprostol may be confused with metoprolol
- Cytotec® may be confused with Cytoxan®, Sytobex®

Use Prevention of NSAID-induced gastric ulcers; medical termination of pregnancy of ≤49 days (in conjunction with mifepristone)

Unlabeled/Investigational Use Cervical ripening and labor induction; NSAID-induced nephropathy; fat malabsorption in cystic fibrosis

Mechanism of Action/Effect Misoprostol is a synthetic prostaglandin E_1 analog that replaces the protective prostaglandins consumed with prostaglandin-inhibiting therapies (eg, NSAIDs); has been shown to induce uterine contractions

Contraindications Hypersensitivity to misoprostol, prostaglandins, or any component of the formulation; pregnancy (when used to reduce NSAID-induced ulcers)

Warnings/Precautions Safety and efficacy have not been established in children <18 years of age. Use with caution in patients with renal impairment and the elderly. Not to be used in pregnant women or women of childbearing potential unless woman is capable of complying with effective contraceptive measures; therapy is normally begun on the second or third day of next normal menstrual period. Uterine perforation and/or rupture have been reported in association with intravaginal use to induce labor or with combined oral/intravaginal use to induce abortion. The manufacturer states that Cytotec® should not be used as a cervical-ripening agent for induction of labor. However, The American College of Obstetricians and Gynecologists (ACOG) continues to support this off-label use.

Drug Interactions
Increased Effect/Toxicity: Misoprostol may increase the effect of oxytocin; wait 6-12 hours after misoprostol administration before initiating oxytocin.

Nutritional/Ethanol Interactions Food: Misoprostol peak serum concentrations may be decreased if taken with food (not clinically significant).

Adverse Reactions
>10%: Gastrointestinal: Diarrhea, abdominal pain

1% to 10%:
- Central nervous system: Headache
- Gastrointestinal: Constipation, flatulence, nausea, dyspepsia, vomiting

Overdosage/Toxicology Symptoms of overdose include sedation, tremor, convulsions, dyspnea, abdominal pain, diarrhea, hypotension, and bradycardia. Treatment is symptom-directed and supportive.

Pharmacodynamics/Kinetics
Absorption: Rapid

Time to Peak: Serum: Active metabolite: Fasting: 15-30 minutes

Half-Life Elimination: Metabolite: 20-40 minutes

Metabolism: Hepatic; rapidly de-esterified to misoprostol acid (active)

Excretion: Urine (64% to 73%) and feces (15%) within 24 hours

Dosing
Adults:

Prevention of NSAID-induced ulcers: Oral: 200 mcg 4 times/day with food; if not tolerated, may decrease dose to 100 mcg 4 times/day with food or 200 mcg twice daily with food. Last dose of the day should be taken at bedtime.

Labor induction or cervical ripening (unlabeled use): Intravaginal: 25 mcg (¼ of 100 mcg tablet); may repeat at intervals no more frequent than every 3-6 hours. Do not use in patients with previous cesarean delivery or prior major uterine surgery.

Medical termination of pregnancy: Oral: Refer to Mifepristone monograph.

Elderly: Oral: 100-200 mcg 4 times/day with food; if 200 mcg 4 times/day not tolerated, reduce to 100 mcg 4 times/day or 200 mcg twice daily with food. **Note:** To avoid the diarrhea potential, doses can be initiated at 100 mcg/day and increased 100 mcg/day at 3-day intervals until desired dose is achieved; also, recommend administering with food to decrease diarrhea incidence.

Pediatrics: Children 8-16 years: Oral: Fat absorption in cystic fibrosis (unlabeled use): 100 mcg 4 times/day

Available Dosage Forms Tablet: 100 mcg, 200 mcg

Monitoring and Teaching Issues
Physical Assessment: Assess knowledge/teach appropriate antiulcer diet and lifestyle. Monitor renal function and fluid balance. **Pregnancy risk factor X:** Determine that patient is not pregnant before beginning treatment and do not give to women of childbearing age or to males who may have intercourse with women of childbearing age unless both male and female are capable of complying with contraceptive measures during therapy and for 1 month following therapy.

Patient Education: Take as directed; continue taking your NSAIDs while taking this medication. Take with meals or after meals to prevent nausea, diarrhea, and flatulence. Avoid using antacids. You may experience increased menstrual pain, or cramping; request analgesics. Report abnormal menstrual periods, spotting (may occur even in postmenstrual women), or severe menstrual bleeding. **Pregnancy/breast-feeding precautions:** When used to prevent NSAID-induced ulcers: Inform prescriber if you are pregnant. Do not get pregnant during or for 1 month following therapy. Male: Do not cause a female to become pregnant. Male/female: Consult prescriber for instruction on appropriate contraceptive measures. This drug may cause severe fetal defects, miscarriage, or abortion; do not share medication with others. Do not breast-feed.

Dietary Considerations: Should be taken with food; incidence of diarrhea may be lessened by having patient take dose right after meals.

Geriatric Considerations: Elderly, due to extensive use of NSAIDs and the high percentage of asymptomatic hemorrhage and perforation from NSAIDs, are at risk for NSAID-induced ulcers and may be candidates for misoprostol use. However, routine use for prophylaxis is not justified. Patients must be selected upon demonstration that they are at risk for NSAID-induced lesions. Misoprostol should not be used as a first-line therapy for gastric or duodenal ulcers.

Pregnancy Risk Factor: X

Pregnancy Issues: Misoprostol is an abortifacient. During pregnancy, use to prevent NSAID-induced ulcers is contraindicated. Reports of fetal death, congenital anomalies, uterine perforation, and abortion have been received after the use of misoprostol in pregnancy.

Lactation: Excretion in breast milk unknown/contraindicated

Breast-Feeding Issues: It is not known if misoprostol is excreted in human milk, however, because significant diarrhea may occur in a nursing infant, breast-feeding is contraindicated

Administration
  Oral: Incidence of diarrhea may be lessened by having patient take dose right after meals. Therapy is usually begun on the second or third day of the next normal menstrual period.

Storage: Store at or below 25°C (77°F).

♦ **Misoprostol and Diclofenac** *see Diclofenac and Misoprostol on page 444*

Mitomycin (mye toe MYE sin)

U.S. Brand Names Mutamycin®

Synonyms Mitomycin-C; Mitomycin-X; MTC; NSC-26980

Generic Available Yes

Pharmacologic Category Antineoplastic Agent, Antibiotic

Medication Safety Issues
  Sound-alike/look-alike issues:
    Mitomycin may be confused with mithramycin, mitotane, mitoxantrone, Mutamycin®
    Mutamycin® may be confused with mitomycin

Use Treatment of adenocarcinoma of stomach or pancreas, bladder cancer, breast cancer, or colorectal cancer

Unlabeled/Investigational Use Prevention of excess scarring in glaucoma filtration procedures in patients at high risk of bleb failure

Mechanism of Action/Effect Acts like an alkylating agent and produces DNA cross-linking (primarily with guanine and cytosine pairs); cell-cycle nonspecific; inhibits DNA and RNA synthesis; degrades preformed DNA, causes nuclear lysis and formation of giant cells. While not phase-specific *per se*, mitomycin has its maximum effect against cells in late G and early S phases.

Contraindications Hypersensitivity to mitomycin or any component of the formulation; platelet counts <75,000/mm³; leukocyte counts <3000/mm³ or serum creatinine >1.7 mg/dL; thrombocytopenia; coagulation disorders, increased bleeding tendency; pregnancy

Warnings/Precautions The U.S. Food and Drug Administration (FDA) currently recommends that procedures for proper handling and disposal of antineoplastic agents be considered. Use with caution in patients who have received radiation therapy or in the presence of hepatobiliary dysfunction; reduce dosage in patients who are receiving radiation therapy simultaneously. Hemolytic-uremic syndrome, potentially fatal, occurs in some patients receiving long-term therapy. It is correlated with total dose (single doses ≥60 mg or cumulative doses ≥50 mg/m²) and total duration of therapy (>5-11 months). **Mitomycin is a potent vesicant, may cause ulceration, necrosis, cellulitis, and tissue sloughing if infiltrated.**

Drug Interactions
  Increased Effect/Toxicity: *Vinca* alkaloids or doxorubicin may enhance cardiac toxicity when coadministered with mitomycin.

Nutritional/Ethanol Interactions Herb/Nutraceutical: Avoid black cohosh, dong quai in estrogen-dependent tumors.

Adverse Reactions
  >10%:
    Cardiovascular: CHF (3% to 15%) (doses >30 mg/m²)
    Central nervous system: Fever (14%)
    Dermatologic: Alopecia, nail banding/discoloration
    Gastrointestinal: Nausea, vomiting and anorexia (14%)
    Hematologic: Anemia (19% to 24%); myelosuppression, common, dose-limiting, delayed
      Onset: 3 weeks
      Nadir: 4-6 weeks
      Recovery: 6-8 weeks
  1% to 10%:
    Dermatologic: Rash
    Gastrointestinal: Stomatitis
    Neuromuscular: Paresthesias
    Renal: Creatinine increase (2%)
    Respiratory: Interstitial pneumonitis, infiltrates, dyspnea, cough (7%)

Overdosage/Toxicology Symptoms of overdose include bone marrow suppression, nausea, vomiting, and alopecia. Treatment is symptom-directed and supportive.

Pharmacodynamics/Kinetics
  Half-Life Elimination: 23-78 minutes; Terminal: 50 minutes
  Metabolism: Hepatic
  Excretion: Urine (<10% as unchanged drug), with elevated serum concentrations

Dosing
  Adults & Elderly: Refer to individual protocols:
    Single-agent therapy: I.V.: 20 mg/m² every 6-8 weeks
    Combination therapy: I.V.: 10 mg/m² every 6-8 weeks
    Bladder carcinoma: Intravesicular instillations (unapproved route): 20-40 mg/dose instilled into the bladder for 3 hours repeated up to 3 times/week for up to 20 procedures per course.
  (Continued)

Mitomycin (Continued)

Glaucoma surgery (unlabeled use): Dosages and techniques vary; 0.2-0.5 mg may be applied to a pledget (using a 0.2-0.5 mg/mL solution), and placed in contact with the surgical wound for 2-5 minutes; other protocols have been reported

Pediatrics: Refer to adult dosing.

Renal Impairment: Varying approaches to dosing adjustments have been published; one representative recommendation: Cl_{cr} <10 mL/minute: Administer 75% of normal dose

Note: The manufacturers state that products should not be given to patients with serum creatinine >1.7 mg/dL.

Hemodialysis: Unknown

CAPD effects: Unknown

CAVH effects: Unknown

Hepatic Impairment: Although some mitomycin may be excreted in the bile, no specific guidelines regarding dosage adjustment in hepatic impairment can be made.

Available Dosage Forms Injection, powder for reconstitution (Mutamycin®): 5 mg, 20 mg, 40 mg

Monitoring and Teaching Issues

Physical Assessment: Use caution in presence of hepatobiliary dysfunction (see Warnings/Precautions for specific use cautions). Assess potential for interactions with other pharmacological and herbal products patient may be taking (see Drug Interactions). See Administration for infusion specifics; infusion site must be closely monitored to prevent extravasation (eg, mitomycin is a potent vesicant, may cause ulceration, necrosis, cellulitis, and tissue sloughing if infiltrated). Assess results of laboratory tests and adverse reactions on a regular basis throughout therapy (eg, signs of CHF, hydration and nutritional status, and opportunistic infection; see Adverse Reactions). Teach patient possible side effects/appropriate interventions and adverse symptoms to report (see Patient Education).

Monitoring Laboratory Tests: Platelet count, CBC with differential, prothrombin time, renal and pulmonary function

Patient Education: Do not take any new medication during therapy unless approved by prescriber. This drug is administered intravenously; report immediately any redness, swelling, burning, or pain at infusion site. Maintain adequate hydration (2-3 L/day of fluids) unless instructed to restrict fluid intake and nutrition. You may be more susceptible to infection (avoid crowds and exposure to infection and do not have any vaccinations unless approved by prescriber). May cause nausea, vomiting, or anorexia (small frequent meals, frequent mouth care, chewing gum, or sucking lozenges may help); mouth sores (use soft toothbrush, waxed dental floss, and frequent mouth rinses); or loss of hair or discoloration of nails (may be reversible when therapy is discontinued). Report rash or itching, unresolved nausea or diarrhea; respiratory difficulty, swelling of extremities, sudden weight gain, or unusual cough; any numbness, tingling, or loss of sensation; or opportunistic infection (fever, chills, sore throat, burning urination, fatigue). **Pregnancy/breast-feeding precautions:** Do not get pregnant while taking this medication. Consult prescriber for appropriate contraceptive measures. Do not breast-feed.

Pregnancy Risk Factor: D

Pregnancy Issues: Mitomycin can cause fetal harm in humans. Animal studies show delayed fetal development, fetal external anomalies, and neonatal anomalies.

Lactation: Enters breast milk/contraindicated

Administration

I.V.: Vesicant. Administer slow I.V. push or by slow (15-30 minute) infusion via a freely-running dextrose or saline infusion. Consider using a central venous catheter.

Reconstitution: Dilute powder with SWFI or 0.9% sodium chloride to a concentration of 0.5-1 mg/mL.

Compatibility: Stable in LR

Y-site administration: Incompatible with aztreonam, cefepime, etoposide phosphate, filgrastim, gemcitabine, piperacillin/tazobactam, sargramostim, topotecan, vinorelbine

Compatibility when admixed: Incompatible with bleomycin

Storage: Store intact vials at controlled room temperature. Mitomycin solution is stable for 7 days at room temperature and 14 days when refrigerated if protected from light. Solution of 0.5 mg/mL in a syringe is stable for 7 days at room temperature and 14 days when refrigerated and protected from light.

Further dilution to 20-40 mcg/mL:

In normal saline: Stable for 12 hours at room temperature.

In sodium lactate: Stable for 24 hours at room temperature.

♦ **Mitomycin-C** see Mitomycin on page 1017

♦ **Mitomycin-X** see Mitomycin on page 1017

Mitotane (MYE toe tane)

U.S. Brand Names Lysodren®

Synonyms NSC-38721; o,p'-DDD

Generic Available No

Pharmacologic Category Antineoplastic Agent, Miscellaneous

Medication Safety Issues

Sound-alike/look-alike issues:

Mitotane may be confused with mitomycin

Use Treatment of adrenocortical carcinoma

Unlabeled/Investigational Use Treatment of Cushing's syndrome

Mechanism of Action/Effect Causes adrenal cortical atrophy; drug affects mitochondria in adrenal cortical cells and decreases production of cortisol; also alters the peripheral metabolism of steroids

Contraindications Hypersensitivity to mitotane or any component of the formulation

Warnings/Precautions The U.S. Food and Drug Administration (FDA) currently recommends that procedures for proper handling and disposal of antineoplastic agents be considered. Steroid replacement with glucocorticoid, and sometimes mineralocorticoid, is necessary. It has been recommended that replacement therapy be initiated at the start of therapy, rather than waiting for evidence of adrenal insufficiency. Because mitotane can increase the metabolism of hydrocortisone, higher than usual replacement doses of the latter may be required. Acute adrenal insufficiency may occur in the face of shock, trauma, or infection. Mitotane should be discontinued temporarily in this setting and appropriate steroid coverage should be administered.

Drug Interactions
    Decreased Effect: Mitotane may enhance the clearance of barbiturates and warfarin by induction of the hepatic microsomal enzyme system resulting in a decreased effect. Coadministration of spironolactone has resulted in negation of mitotane's effect. Mitotane may increase clearance of phenytoin by microsomal enzyme stimulation.
    Increased Effect/Toxicity: CNS depressants taken with mitotane may enhance CNS depression.

Nutritional/Ethanol Interactions Ethanol: Avoid ethanol (may increase CNS depression).

Adverse Reactions
  >10%:
    Central nervous system: CNS depression (32%), dizziness (15%)
    Dermatologic: Skin rash (12%)
    Gastrointestinal: Anorexia (24%), nausea (39%), vomiting (37%), diarrhea (13%)
    Neuromuscular & skeletal: Weakness (12%)
  1% to 10%:
    Central nervous system: Headache (5%), confusion (3%)
    Neuromuscular & skeletal: Muscle tremor (3%)

Overdosage/Toxicology Symptoms of overdose include diarrhea, vomiting, numbness of limbs, and weakness. Treatment is symptom-directed and supportive.

Pharmacodynamics/Kinetics
  Absorption: Oral: ~35% to 40%
  Time to Peak: Serum: 3-5 hours
  Half-Life Elimination: 18-159 days
  Metabolism: Hepatic and other tissues
  Excretion: Urine and feces (as metabolites)

Dosing
  Adults & Elderly: Adrenal carcinoma: Oral: Start at 1-6 g/day in divided doses, then increase incrementally to 8-10 g/day in 3-4 divided doses (maximum daily dose: 18 g)
  Pediatrics: Adrenal carcinoma: Oral: Children: 0.1-0.5 mg/kg or 1-2 g/day in divided doses increasing gradually to a maximum of 5-7 g/day
  Hepatic Impairment: Dose may need to be decreased in patients with liver disease.

Available Dosage Forms Tablet [scored]: 500 mg

Monitoring and Teaching Issues
  Physical Assessment: See Warnings/Precautions for use cautions (eg, steroid replacement information). Assess potential for interactions with other pharmacological agents or herbal products patient may be taking (eg, may increase or decrease levels/effects; see Drug Interactions). Assess therapeutic effectiveness and adverse response on a regular basis throughout therapy (eg, CNS depression, rash, nausea/vomiting, and muscle weakness; see Adverse Reactions). Teach patient proper use, possible side effects/appropriate interventions, and adverse symptoms to report (see Patient Education).
  Patient Education: Take as directed; do not alter dose or discontinue without consulting prescriber. Desired effects of this drug may not be seen for 2-3 months. Wear identification that alerts medical personnel that you are taking this drug in event of shock or trauma. Maintain adequate hydration (2-3 L/day of fluids) unless instructed to restrict fluid intake and nutrition. Avoid alcohol; may increase CNS depression. May cause dizziness, headache, confusion (avoid driving or performing tasks requiring alertness until response to drug is known); nausea, vomiting, or loss of appetite (small frequent meals, frequent mouth care, sucking lozenges, or chewing gum may help); or diarrhea (buttermilk, boiled milk, or yogurt may help). Report severe vomiting or diarrhea; muscular twitching, tremor, numbness, or weakness; or other persistent adverse effects. **Pregnancy/breast-feeding precautions:** Inform prescriber if you are or intend to become pregnant. Do not breast-feed.
  Pregnancy Risk Factor: C
  Lactation: Enters breast milk/contraindicated

Administration
  Storage: Protect from light. Store at room temperature.

Mitoxantrone (mye toe ZAN trone)

U.S. Brand Names Novantrone®
Synonyms DAD; DHAD; DHAQ; Dihydroxyanthracenedione Dihydrochloride; Mitoxantrone Hydrochloride CL-232315; Mitozantrone; NSC-301739
Generic Available No
Pharmacologic Category Antineoplastic Agent, Anthracenedione
Medication Safety Issues
  Sound-alike/look-alike issues:
    Mitoxantrone may be confused with methotrexate, mitomycin
Use Treatment of acute leukemias, lymphoma, breast cancer, pediatric sarcoma, progressive or relapsing-remitting multiple sclerosis, prostate cancer
Mechanism of Action/Effect Analogue of the anthracyclines, but different in mechanism of action, cardiac toxicity, and potential for tissue necrosis; inhibits DNA and RNA synthesis
Contraindications Hypersensitivity to mitoxantrone or any component of the formulation; multiple sclerosis with left ventricular ejection fraction (LVEF) <50% or clinically significant decrease in LVEF; pregnancy
Warnings/Precautions The FDA currently recommends that procedures for proper handling and disposal of antineoplastic agents be considered. Appropriate safety equipment is recommended for preparation, administration, and disposal of antineoplastics. If mitoxantrone contacts the skin, wash and flush thoroughly with water.
(Continued)

Mitoxantrone (Continued)

Dosage should be reduced in patients with impaired hepatobiliary function; not for treatment of multiple sclerosis in patients with concurrent hepatic impairment. Treatment may lead to severe myelosuppression; use with caution in patients with pre-existing myelosuppression. Do not use if baseline neutrophil count <1500 cells/mm³ (except for treatment of ANLL). May cause myocardial toxicity and potentially-fatal CHF; risk increases with cumulative dosing. Predisposing factors for mitoxantrone-induced cardiotoxicity include prior anthracycline therapy, prior cardiovascular disease, and mediastinal irradiation. Not for treatment of primary progressive multiple sclerosis. Has been associated with the development of secondary acute myelogenous leukemia and myelodysplasia when used in combination with other antineoplastic agents. For I.V. use only (not for intra-arterial or intrathecal injection). May cause urine, saliva, tears, and sweat to turn blue-green for 24 hours postinfusion. Whites of eyes may have blue-green tinge (this is normal).

Drug Interactions

Cytochrome P450 Effect: Inhibits CYP3A4 (weak)

Decreased Effect: Patients may experience impaired immune response to vaccines; possible infection after administration of live vaccines in patients receiving immunosuppressants.

Nutritional/Ethanol Interactions Herb/Nutraceutical: Avoid black cohosh, dong quai in estrogen-dependent tumors.

Adverse Reactions Reported with any indication; incidence varies based on treatment/dose

>10%:

Cardiovascular: Abnormal ECG, arrhythmia (3% to 18%), edema, nail bed changes

Central nervous system: Fatigue, fever, headache (6% to 13%)

Dermatologic: Alopecia (20% to 61%)

Endocrine & metabolic: Amenorrhea, menstrual disorder

Gastrointestinal: Abdominal pain, anorexia, nausea (29% to 76%), constipation, diarrhea (16% to 47%), GI bleeding, mucositis (10% to 29%), stomatitis, vomiting, weight gain/loss

Genitourinary: Abnormal urine, urinary tract infection

Hematologic: Decreased hemoglobin, leukopenia, lymphopenia, petechiae/bruising; myelosuppressive effects of chemotherapy:

WBC: Mild

Platelets: Mild

Onset: 7-10 days

Nadir: 14 days

Recovery: 21 days

Hepatic: Increased GGT

Neuromuscular & skeletal: Weakness (24%)

Respiratory: Cough, dyspnea, upper respiratory tract infection

Miscellaneous: Fungal infection, infection, sepsis

1% to 10%:

Cardiovascular: CHF (2% to 3%; risk is much lower with anthracyclines, some reports suggest cumulative doses >160 mg/mL cause CHF in ~10% of patients), ECG changes, hypotension, ischemia, LVEF decreased (≤5%)

Central nervous system: Chills, anxiety, depression, seizure

Dermatologic: Skin infection

Endocrine & metabolic: Hypocalcemia, hypokalemia, hyponatremia, hyperglycemia

Gastrointestinal: Dyspepsia, aphthosis

Genitourinary: Impotence, proteinuria, renal failure, sterility

Hematologic: Anemia, granulocytopenia, hemorrhage

Hepatic: Jaundice, increased SGOT, increased SGPT

Neuromuscular & skeletal: Back pain, myalgia, arthralgia

Ocular: Blurred vision, conjunctivitis

Renal: Hematuria

Respiratory: Pneumonia, rhinitis, sinusitis

Miscellaneous: Systemic infection, sweats, development of secondary leukemia

Overdosage/Toxicology Symptoms of overdose include leukopenia, tachycardia, and marrow hypoplasia. No known antidote. Treatment is symptom-directed and supportive.

Pharmacodynamics/Kinetics

Absorption: Oral: Poor

Protein Binding: >95%, 76% to albumin

Half-Life Elimination: Terminal: 23-215 hours; may be prolonged with hepatic impairment

Metabolism: Hepatic; pathway not determined

Excretion: Urine (6% to 11%) and feces as unchanged drug and metabolites

Dosing

Adults & Elderly: Refer to individual protocols. I.V. (may dilute in D₅W or NS):

Acute leukemias: I.V.: 8-12 mg/m²/day once daily for 4-5 days

Solid tumors: I.V.: 12-14 mg/m² every 3-4 weeks **or** 2-4 mg/m²/day for 5 days

Hormone-refractory prostate cancer: I.V.: 12-14 mg/m²

Multiple sclerosis: I.V.: 12 mg/m²

BMT high dose: I.V.: 24-48 mg/m² as a single dose; duration of infusion is 1-4 hours; generally combined with other high-dose chemotherapeutic drugs.

Pediatrics: Refer to individual protocols.

Acute leukemias: I.V. (may dilute in D₅W or NS):

Children ≤2 years: 0.4 mg/kg/day once daily for 3-5 days

Children >2 years: Refer to adult dosing.

Solid tumors: I.V.: Children: 18-20 mg/m² every 3-4 weeks **or** 5-8 mg/m² every week

Hepatic Impairment: Official dosage adjustment recommendations have not been established.

Moderate dysfunction (bilirubin 1.5-3 mg/dL): Some clinicians recommend a 50% dosage reduction.

Severe dysfunction (bilirubin >3.0 mg/dL) may require a dosage adjustment to 8 mg/m^2; some clinicians recommend a dosage reduction to 25% of dose.

Available Dosage Forms Injection, solution: 2 mg/mL (10 mL, 12.5 mL, 15 mL)

Monitoring and Teaching Issues

Physical Assessment: Use caution with hepatic impairment, cardiovascular disease, and mediastinal irradiation (see Warnings/Precautions for specific use cautions). See Administration for infusion specifics. Infusion site must be monitored closely to prevent extravasation. Assess results of laboratory tests, evidence of therapeutic effectiveness, and adverse response with each dose and throughout therapy (eg, arrhythmia, hypersensitivity reactions, myelosuppression [anemia], gastrointestinal upset [nutritional and hydration status], opportunistic infection, gout, CHF [rales, dyspnea, edema]; see Adverse Reactions). Teach patient possible side effects/appropriate interventions (eg, avoid crowds, maintain hydration) and adverse symptoms to report (see Patient Education).

Monitoring Laboratory Tests: CBC, serum uric acid, liver function, echocardiogram

Patient Education: Do not take any new medication during therapy unless approved by prescriber. This drug is only administered by infusion; report immediately any redness, swelling, burning, or pain at infusion site. Maintain adequate hydration (2-3 L/day of fluids) unless instructed to restrict fluid intake and nutrition. You will be more susceptible to infection (avoid crowds and exposure to infection and do not have any vaccinations without consulting prescriber). May cause urine, saliva, tears, sweat, and whites of eyes to turn blue-green for 24 hours postinfusion (this is normal). May cause nausea, vomiting, or GI upset (small frequent meals, frequent mouth care, chewing gum, or sucking lozenges may help); mouth sores (use soft toothbrush or cotton swabs, waxed dental floss, and frequent mouth rinses); headache, dizziness, or blurred vision (use caution when driving or engaging in tasks that are potentially hazardous until response to drug is known); or loss of hair (may be reversible). Report chest pain or palpitations; respiratory difficulty or constant cough; swelling of extremities or sudden weight gain; persistent fever or chills; or opportunistic infection (eg, fever, chills, sore throat, burning urination, fatigue); changed or decreased urine output. **Pregnancy/breast-feeding precautions:** Do not get pregnant while taking this medication. Consult prescriber for appropriate contraceptive measures. Do not breast-feed.

Pregnancy Risk Factor: D

Pregnancy Issues: May cause fetal harm if administered to a pregnant woman. Women with multiple sclerosis and who are biologically capable of becoming pregnant should have a pregnancy test prior to each dose. Mitoxantrone is excreted in human milk and significant concentrations (180 mg/mL) have been reported for 28 days after the last administration.

Lactation: Enters breast milk/contraindicated

Breast-Feeding Issues: Mitoxantrone is excreted in human milk and significant concentrations (180 mg/mL) have been reported for 28 days after the last administration. Because of the potential for serious adverse reactions in infants from mitoxantrone, breast-feeding should be discontinued before starting treatment.

Administration

I.V.: Irritant. Administered as a short (15-30 minutes) I.V. infusion; continuous 24-hour infusions are occasionally used. Although not generally recommended, mitoxantrone has been given as a rapid bolus over 1-3 minutes. High doses for bone marrow transplant are usually given as 1- to 4-hour infusions.

Reconstitution: Dilute in at least 50 mL of NS or D$_5$W.

Compatibility: Stable in in D$_5$NS, D$_5$W, NS

Y-site administration: Incompatible with amphotericin B cholesteryl sulfate complex, aztreonam, cefepime, doxorubicin liposome, paclitaxel, piperacillin/tazobactam, propofol

Compatibility when admixed: Incompatible with heparin

Storage: Store intact vials at 15°C to 25°C (59°F to 77°F); do not freeze. Opened vials may be stored at room temperature for 7 days or under refrigeration for up to 14 days. Solutions diluted for administration are stable for 7 days at room temperature or under refrigeration.

♦ **Mitoxantrone Hydrochloride CL-232315** see Mitoxantrone on page 1019

♦ **Mitozantrone** see Mitoxantrone on page 1019

♦ **Mitrazol™ [OTC]** see Miconazole on page 999

♦ **Mivacron®** see Mivacurium on page 1021

Mivacurium (mye va KYOO ree um)

U.S. Brand Names Mivacron®

Synonyms Mivacurium Chloride

Generic Available No

Pharmacologic Category Neuromuscular Blocker Agent, Nondepolarizing

Medication Safety Issues

Sound-alike/look-alike issues:

Mivacron® may be confused with Mevacor®

Use Adjunct to general anesthesia to facilitate endotracheal intubation and to relax skeletal muscles during surgery; to facilitate mechanical ventilation in ICU patients; does not relieve pain or produce sedation

Contraindications Hypersensitivity to mivacurium chloride, any component of the formulation, or other benzylisoquinolinium agents; use of multidose vials in patients with allergy to benzyl alcohol; pre-existing tachycardia

Warnings/Precautions Ventilation must be supported during neuromuscular blockade; does not counteract bradycardia produced by anesthetics/vagal stimulation; prolonged neuromuscular block may be seen in patients with reduced or atypical plasma cholinesterase activity (eg, pregnancy, liver or kidney disease, infections, peptic ulcer, anemia); patients homozygous for the atypical plasma cholinesterase gene are extremely sensitive to the neuromuscular blocking effect of mivacurium (use extreme caution if at all in those patients); duration prolonged in patients with renal and/or hepatic impairment; reduce initial dosage and inject

(Continued)

Mivacurium *(Continued)*

slowly (over 60 seconds) in patients in whom substantial histamine release would be potentially hazardous; certain clinical conditions may result in potentiation or antagonism of neuromuscular blockade (such as, potentiation by electrolyte abnormalities, neuromuscular diseases, or acidosis; antagonism with demyelinating lesions).

Increased sensitivity in patients with myasthenia gravis, Eaton-Lambert syndrome, resistance in burn patients (>30% of body) for period of 5-70 days postinjury; resistance in patients with muscle trauma, denervation, immobilization, infection. Cross-sensitivity with other neuromuscular-blocking agents may occur; use extreme caution in patients with previous anaphylactic reactions.

Drug Interactions

Decreased Effect: Effect of nondepolarizing neuromuscular blockers may be reduced by carbamazepine (chronic use), corticosteroids (also associated with myopathy - see increased effect), phenytoin (chronic use), sympathomimetics, and theophylline.

Increased Effect/Toxicity: Increased effects are possible with aminoglycosides, beta-blockers, clindamycin, calcium channel blockers, halogenated anesthetics, imipenem, ketamine, lidocaine, loop diuretics (furosemide), macrolides (case reports), magnesium sulfate, procainamide, quinidine, quinolones, tetracyclines, and vancomycin. May increase risk of myopathy when used with high-dose corticosteroids for extended periods. Drugs which inhibit acetylcholinesterase may prolong effect of mivacurium.

Adverse Reactions

>10%: Cardiovascular: Flushing of face

1% to 10%: Cardiovascular: Hypotension

Pharmacodynamics/Kinetics

Onset of Action: Neuromuscular blockade: I.V. (dose dependent): 1.5-3 minutes

Duration of Action: Short due to rapid hydrolysis by plasma cholinesterases; clinically effective block may last for 12-20 minutes; spontaneous recovery may be 95% complete in 25-30 minutes; duration shorter in children and may be slightly longer in elderly

Half-Life Elimination: 2 minutes (more active isomers only)

Metabolism: Via plasma cholinesterase, inactive metabolites

Excretion: Urine (<10%)

Dosing

Adults & Elderly: Note: Continuous infusion requires an infusion pump; dose should be based on ideal body weight

Neuromuscular blockade: Initial: I.V.: 0.15-0.25 mg/kg bolus followed by maintenance doses of 0.1 mg/kg at approximately 15-minute intervals; for prolonged neuromuscular block, initial infusion of 9-10 mcg/kg/minute is used upon evidence of spontaneous recovery from initial dose, usual infusion rate of 6-7 mcg/kg/minute (1-15 mcg/kg/minute) under balanced anesthesia; initial dose after succinylcholine for intubation (balanced anesthesia): Adults: 0.1 mg/kg

Pretreatment/priming: 10% of intubating dose given 3-5 minutes before initial dose

Pediatrics: Note: Continuous infusion requires an infusion pump; dose should be based on ideal body weight

Neuromuscular blockade: I.V.: Children 2-12 years (duration of action is shorter and dosage requirements are higher): 0.2 mg/kg followed by average infusion rate of 14 mcg/kg/minute (range: 5-31 mcg/kg/minute) upon evidence of spontaneous recovery from initial dose

Renal Impairment: 150 mcg/kg I.V. bolus; duration of action of blockade: 1.5 times longer in ESRD, may decrease infusion rates by as much as 50%, dependent on degree of renal impairment.

Hepatic Impairment: 150 mcg/kg I.V. bolus; duration of blockade: 3 times longer in ESLD, may decrease rate of infusion by as much as 50% in ESLD, dependent on the degree of impairment

Available Dosage Forms

Injection, solution [preservative free]: 2 mg/mL (5 mL, 10 mL)

Injection, solution: 2 mg/mL (20 mL, 50 mL) [with benzyl alcohol]

Monitoring and Teaching Issues

Physical Assessment: Only clinicians experienced in the use of neuromuscular blocking agents should administer and/or manage the use of mivacurium. Assess potential for interactions with other prescriptions, OTC medications, or herbal products patient may be taking (eg, other drugs that affect neuromuscular activity may increase/decrease neuromuscular block induced by mivacurium). Ventilatory support must be instituted and maintained until adequate respiratory muscle function and/or airway protection are assured. This drug does not cause anesthesia or analgesia; pain must be treated with appropriate agents. Continuous monitoring of vital signs, cardiac and respiratory status, and neuromuscular block (objective assessment with peripheral external nerve stimulator) are mandatory until full muscle tone has returned . Safety precautions must be maintained until full muscle tone has returned. **Note:** It may take longer for return of muscle tone in elderly persons or patients with myasthenia gravis, myopathy, other neuromuscular diseases, dehydration, electrolyte imbalance, or severe acid/base imbalance. Provide appropriate teaching/support prior to, during, and following administration.

Long-term use: Monitor vital signs and fluid levels regularly during treatment. Every 2- to 3-hour repositioning, and skin, mouth, and eye care is necessary while patient is sedated. Emotional and sensory support (auditory and environmental) should be provided.

Patient Education: Patient education should be appropriate for patient condition. Reassurance of constant monitoring and emotional support should precede and follow administration. Patients should be reminded as muscle tone returns not to attempt to change position or rise from bed without assistance and to report any skin rash, hives, pounding heartbeat, respiratory difficulty, or muscle tremors. **Pregnancy/breast-feeding precaution:** Inform prescriber if you are pregnant. Consult prescriber if breast-feeding.

Pregnancy Risk Factor: C
Lactation: Excretion in breast milk unknown/use caution

Administration

I.V.: Children require higher mivacurium infusion rates than adults; during opioid/nitrous oxide/oxygen anesthesia, the infusion rate required to maintain 89% to 99% neuromuscular block averages 14 mcg/kg/minute (range: 5-31). For adults and children, the amount of infusion solution required per hour depends upon the clinical requirements of the patient, the concentration of mivacurium in the infusion solution, and the patient's weight. The contribution of the infusion solution to the fluid requirements of the patient must be considered.

Compatibility: Stable in D_5LR, D_5NS, D_5W, LR, NS

Storage: Store at room temperature of 15°C to 25°C (59°F to 77°F); protect from direct ultraviolet light.

Additional Information Mivacurium is classified as a short-duration neuromuscular-blocking agent. Do not mix with barbiturates in the same syringe. Mivacurium does not appear to have a cumulative effect on the duration of blockade. It does not relieve pain or produce sedation.

Modafinil (moe DAF i nil)

U.S. Brand Names Provigil®
Controlled Substance C-IV
Generic Available No
Pharmacologic Category Stimulant

Use Improve wakefulness in patients with excessive daytime sleepiness associated with narcolepsy and shift work sleep disorder (SWSD); adjunctive therapy for obstructive sleep apnea/hypopnea syndrome (OSAHS)

Unlabeled/Investigational Use Attention-deficit/hyperactivity disorder (ADHD); treatment of fatigue in MS and other disorders

Mechanism of Action/Effect The exact mechanism of action is unclear, it does not appear to alter the release of dopamine or norepinephrine, it may exert its stimulant effects by decreasing GABA-mediated neurotransmission, although this theory has not yet been fully evaluated; several studies also suggest that an intact central alpha-adrenergic system is required for modafinil's activity; the drug increases high-frequency alpha waves while decreasing both delta and theta wave activity, and these effects are consistent with generalized increases in mental alertness

Contraindications Hypersensitivity to modafinil or any component of the formulation

Warnings/Precautions Use is not recommended with a history of angina, cardiac ischemia, recent history of myocardial infarction, left ventricular hypertrophy, or patients with mitral valve prolapse who have developed mitral valve prolapse syndrome with previous CNS stimulant use. Caution should be exercised when modafinil is given to patients with a history of psychosis; caution is warranted when operating machinery or driving, although functional impairment has not been demonstrated with modafinil, all CNS-active agents may alter judgment, thinking and/or motor skills. Stimulants may unmask tics in individuals with coexisting Tourette's syndrome. Use caution with renal or hepatic impairment. Safety and efficacy in children ≤16 years of age have not been established.

Drug Interactions

Cytochrome P450 Effect: Substrate of CYP3A4 (major); **Inhibits** CYP1A2 (weak), 2A6 (weak), 2C8/9 (weak), 2C19 (strong), 2E1 (weak), 3A4 (weak); **Induces** CYP1A2 (weak), 2B6 (weak), 3A4 (weak)

Decreased Effect: Modafinil may decrease serum concentrations of oral contraceptives, cyclosporine, and to a lesser degree, theophylline. The levels/effects of modafinil may be decreased by aminoglutethimide, carbamazepine, nafcillin, nevirapine, phenobarbital, phenytoin, rifamycins, and other CYP3A4 inducers. There is also evidence to suggest that modafinil may induce its own metabolism.

Increased Effect/Toxicity: Modafinil may increase the levels/effects of citalopram, diazepam, methsuximide, phenytoin, propranolol, sertraline, or other CYP2C19 substrates. Modafinil may increase levels of warfarin. In populations deficient in the CYP2D6 isoenzyme, where CYP2C19 acts as a secondary metabolic pathway, concentrations of tricyclic antidepressants and selective serotonin reuptake inhibitors may be increased during coadministration. The levels/effects of modafinil may be increased by azole antifungals, ciprofloxacin, clarithromycin, diclofenac, doxycycline, erythromycin, imatinib, isoniazid, nefazodone, nicardipine, propofol, protease inhibitors, quinidine, telithromycin, verapamil, or other CYP3A4 inhibitors.

Nutritional/Ethanol Interactions

Ethanol: Avoid or limit ethanol.
Food: Delays absorption, but does not affect bioavailability.

Adverse Reactions

>10%:
Central nervous system: Headache (34%, dose related)
Gastrointestinal: Nausea (11%)

1% to 10%:
Cardiovascular: Chest pain (3%), hypertension (3%), palpitation (2%), tachycardia (2%), vasodilation (2%), edema (1%)

(Continued)

Modafinil *(Continued)*

Central nervous system: Nervousness (7%), dizziness (5%), depression (2%), anxiety (5%, dose related), insomnia (5%), somnolence (2%), chills (1%), agitation (1%), confusion (1%), emotional lability (1%), vertigo (1%)

Gastrointestinal: Diarrhea (6%), dyspepsia (5%), xerostomia (4%), anorexia (4%), constipation (2%), flatulence (1%), mouth ulceration (1%), taste perversion (1%)

Genitourinary: Abnormal urine (1%), hematuria (1%), pyuria (1%)

Hematologic: Eosinophilia (1%)

Hepatic: Abnormal LFTs (2%)

Neuromuscular & skeletal: Back pain (6%), paresthesia (2%), dyskinesia (1%), hyperkinesia (1%), hypertonia (1%), neck rigidity (1%), tremor (1%)

Ocular: Amblyopia (1%), abnormal vision (1%), eye pain (1%)

Respiratory: Pharyngitis (4%), rhinitis (7%), lung disorder (2%), asthma (1%), epistaxis (1%)

Miscellaneous: Diaphoresis

Postmarketing and/or case reports: Agranulocytosis, mania, psychosis

Overdosage/Toxicology Symptoms of overdose include agitation, irritability, aggressiveness, confusion, nervousness, tremor, insomnia, palpitations, and elevations in hemodynamic parameters. Treatment is symptomatic and supportive. Cardiac monitoring is warranted.

Pharmacodynamics/Kinetics

Time to Peak: Serum: 2-4 hours

Protein Binding: 60%, primarily to albumin

Half-Life Elimination: Effective half-life: 15 hours; Steady-state: 2-4 days

Metabolism: Hepatic; multiple pathways including CYP3A4

Excretion: Urine (as metabolites, <10% as unchanged drug)

Pharmacokinetic Note: Modafinil is a racemic compound (10% *d*-isomer and 90% *l*-isomer at steady state), whose enantiomers have different pharmacokinetics.

Dosing

Adults:

ADHD (unlabeled use): Oral: 100-300 mg once daily

Narcolepsy, OSAHS: Oral: Initial: 200 mg as a single daily dose in the morning.

SWSD: Oral: Initial: 200 mg as a single dose taken ~1 hour prior to start of work shift.

Note: Doses of 400 mg/day, given as a single dose, have been well tolerated, but there is no consistent evidence that this dose confers additional benefit.

Elderly: Elimination of modafinil and its metabolites may be reduced as a consequence of aging and as a result, lower doses should be considered.

Pediatrics:

ADHD (unlabeled use): Oral: 50-100 mg once daily

Renal Impairment: Inadequate data to determine safety and efficacy in severe renal impairment.

Hepatic Impairment: Dose should be reduced to one-half of that recommended for patients with normal liver function.

Available Dosage Forms Tablet: 100 mg, 200 mg

Monitoring and Teaching Issues

Physical Assessment: Assess effectiveness and interactions of other medications, especially those that are metabolized by P450 enzymes. Note that modafinil has potential for abuse; caution patient about inappropriate or overuse. Assess knowledge/teach patient appropriate use, adverse symptoms to report. and interventions to reduce side effects.

Patient Education: Take exactly as prescribed; do not exceed recommended dosage without consulting prescriber. Avoid drinking alcohol. Do not share medication with anyone else. Void before taking medication. You may experience headache, nervousness, confusion, or dizziness (use caution when driving or engaging in tasks requiring alertness until response to drug is known); diarrhea (yogurt or buttermilk may help); or dry mouth or sore mouth, loss of appetite, or vomiting (small frequent meals, frequent mouth care, chewing gum, or sucking lozenges may help). If you have diabetes, monitor glucose levels closely. Report chest pain or palpitations; respiratory difficulty; excessive insomnia, CNS agitation, depression, or memory disturbances; vision changes; changes in urinary pattern or ejaculation disturbances; or persistent joint pain or stiffness. **Pregnancy/breast-feeding precautions:** Inform prescriber if you are or intend to become pregnant. Consult prescriber if breast-feeding.

Pregnancy Risk Factor: C

Pregnancy Issues: Embryotoxic effects have been observed in some, but not all animal studies. There are no adequate and well-controlled studies in pregnant women; use only when the potential risk of drug therapy is outweighed by the drug's benefits. Efficacy of steroidal contraceptives may be decreased; alternate means of contraception should be considered during therapy and for 1 month after modafinil is discontinued.

Lactation: Excretion in breast milk unknown/use caution

- ♦ **Modane® Bulk [OTC]** *see* Psyllium *on page 1284*
- ♦ **Modicon®** *see* Ethinyl Estradiol and Norethindrone *on page 589*
- ♦ **Modified Shohl's Solution** *see* Sodium Citrate and Citric Acid *on page 1382*
- ♦ **Moduretic® [DSC]** *see* Amiloride and Hydrochlorothiazide *on page 90*

Moexipril *(mo EKS i pril)*

U.S. Brand Names Univasc®

Synonyms Moexipril Hydrochloride

Generic Available No

Pharmacologic Category Angiotensin-Converting Enzyme (ACE) Inhibitor

Medication Safety Issues

Sound-alike/look-alike issues:

Moexipril may be confused with Monopril®

Use Treatment of hypertension, alone or in combination with thiazide diuretics; treatment of left ventricular dysfunction after myocardial infarction

Mechanism of Action/Effect Competitive inhibitor of angiotensin-converting enzyme (ACE); prevents conversion of angiotensin I to angiotensin II, a potent vasoconstrictor; results in lower levels of angiotensin II which causes an increase in plasma renin activity and a reduction in aldosterone secretion

Contraindications Hypersensitivity to moexipril, moexiprilat, or any component of the formulation; hypersensitivity or allergic reactions or angioedema related to previous treatment with an ACE inhibitor; pregnancy (2nd or 3rd trimester)

Warnings/Precautions Anaphylactic reactions can occur. Angioedema can occur at any time during treatment (especially following first dose). Angioedema may involve head and neck (potentially affecting the airway) or the intestine (presenting with abdominal pain). Careful blood pressure monitoring with first dose (hypotension can occur especially in volume depleted patients). Dosage adjustment needed in renal impairment. Use with caution in hypovolemia; collagen vascular diseases; valvular stenosis (particularly aortic stenosis); hyperkalemia; or before, during, or immediately after anesthesia. Avoid rapid dosage escalation which may lead to renal insufficiency. Rare toxicities associated with ACE inhibitors include cholestatic jaundice (which may progress to hepatic necrosis) and neutropenia/agranulocytosis with myeloid hyperplasia. Hypersensitivity reactions may be seen during hemodialysis with high-flux dialysis membranes (eg, AN69). Deterioration in renal function can occur with initiation. Use with caution in unilateral renal artery stenosis and pre-existing renal insufficiency.

Drug Interactions

Decreased Effect: Aspirin (high dose) may reduce the therapeutic effects of ACE inhibitors; at low dosages this does not appear to be significant. Rifampin may decrease the effect of ACE inhibitors. Antacids may decrease the bioavailability of ACE inhibitors (may be more likely to occur with captopril); separate administration times by 1-2 hours. NSAIDs, specifically indomethacin, may reduce the hypotensive effects of ACE inhibitors. More likely to occur in low renin or volume dependent hypertensive patients.

Increased Effect/Toxicity: Potassium supplements, co-trimoxazole (high dose), angiotensin II receptor antagonists (eg, candesartan, losartan, irbesartan), or potassium-sparing diuretics (amiloride, spironolactone, triamterene) may result in elevated serum potassium levels when combined with moexipril. ACE inhibitor effects may be increased by probenecid (increases levels of captopril). ACE inhibitors may increase serum concentrations/effects of digoxin, lithium, and sulfonylureas.

Diuretics have additive hypotensive effects with ACE inhibitors, and hypovolemia increases the potential for adverse renal effects of ACE inhibitors. In patients with compromised renal function, coadministration with NSAIDs may result in further deterioration of renal function. Allopurinol and ACE inhibitors may cause a higher risk of hypersensitivity reaction when taken concurrently.

Nutritional/Ethanol Interactions

Food: Food may delay and reduce peak serum levels.

Herb/Nutraceutical: Avoid dong quai if using for hypertension (has estrogenic activity). Avoid ephedra, yohimbe, ginseng (may worsen hypertension). Avoid garlic (may have increased antihypertensive effect).

Lab Interactions Increased BUN, creatinine, potassium, positive Coombs' [direct]; decreased cholesterol (S); may cause false-positive results in urine acetone determinations using sodium nitroprusside reagent

Adverse Reactions 1% to 10%:

Cardiovascular: Hypotension, peripheral edema

Central nervous system: Headache, dizziness, fatigue

Dermatologic: Rash, alopecia, flushing, rash

Endocrine & metabolic: Hyperkalemia, hyponatremia

Gastrointestinal: Diarrhea, nausea, heartburn

Genitourinary: Polyuria

Neuromuscular & skeletal: Myalgia

Renal: Reversible increases in creatinine or BUN

Respiratory: Cough, pharyngitis, upper respiratory infection, sinusitis

Overdosage/Toxicology Mild hypotension has been the primary toxic effect seen with acute overdose. Bradycardia may also occur. Hyperkalemia occurs even with therapeutic doses, especially in patients with renal insufficiency and those taking NSAIDs. Treatment is symptom-directed and supportive.

Pharmacodynamics/Kinetics

Onset of Action: Peak effect: 1-2 hours

Duration of Action: >24 hours

Bioavailability: Moexiprilat: 13%; reduced with food (AUC decreased by ~40%)

Time to Peak: 1.5 hours

Protein Binding: Plasma: Moexipril: 90%; Moexiprilat: 50% to 70%

Half-Life Elimination: Moexipril: 1 hour; Moexiprilat: 2-9 hours

Metabolism: Parent drug: Hepatic and via GI tract to moexiprilat, 1000 times more potent than parent

Excretion: Feces (50%)

Dosing

Adults: Hypertension, LV dysfunction (post MI): Oral: Initial: 7.5 mg once daily (in patients **not** receiving diuretics), 1 hour prior to a meal **or** 3.75 mg once daily (when combined with thiazide diuretics); maintenance dose: 7.5-30 mg/day in 1 or 2 divided doses 1 hour before meals

Elderly: Dose the same as adults; adjust for renal impairment. Tablet may be cut in half (3.75 mg) for starting therapy (see Renal Impairment and Additional Information).

Renal Impairment: $Cl_{cr} \leq 40$ mL/minute: Patients may be cautiously placed on 3.75 mg once daily, then upwardly titrated to a maximum of 15 mg/day.

Available Dosage Forms Tablet, as hydrochloride [film coated, scored]: 7.5 mg, 15 mg

(Continued)

Moexipril *(Continued)*

Monitoring and Teaching Issues

Physical Assessment: Use caution in presence of renal impairment; hypovolemia; collagen vascular diseases; valvular stenosis; hyperkalemia; or anesthesia (see Warnings/Precautions for specific use cautions). Assess potential for interactions with other pharmacological agents or herbal products patient may be taking (especially anything that may impact fluid balance or cardiac status; see Drug Interactions). Assess results of laboratory tests on a regular basis during therapy. Patient should be monitored closely for anaphylactic reaction or angioedema which can occur at any time during treatment and may involve head and neck. Assess therapeutic effectiveness (blood pressure) and adverse responses regularly (eg, hypotension, rash, diarrhea, myalgia, electrolyte imbalance; see Adverse Reactions). Teach patient proper use, possible side effects/appropriate interventions, and adverse symptoms to report (see Patient Education).

Monitoring Laboratory Tests: Electrolytes, CBC, renal function. If patient has renal impairment, a baseline WBC with differential and serum creatinine should be evaluated and monitored closely during the first 3 months of therapy.

Patient Education: Do not take any new medication during therapy unless approved by prescriber. Do not use potassium supplement or salt substitutes without consulting prescriber. Take exactly as directed; do not discontinue without consulting prescriber. Take first dose at bedtime. Take all doses on an empty stomach, 1 hour before or 2 hours after meals. This drug does not eliminate need for diet or exercise regimen as recommended by prescriber. May cause dizziness, fainting, or lightheadedness (use caution when driving or engaging in tasks that require alertness until response to drug is known); postural hypotension (use caution when rising from lying or sitting position or climbing stairs); or nausea, vomiting, abdominal pain, dry mouth, or transient loss of appetite (small frequent meals, frequent mouth care, sucking lozenges, or chewing gum may help). Report immediately unusual swelling of mouth, tongue, face, or throat. Report respiratory difficulty or unusual cough, rash, excessive urination, chest pain or palpitations; mouth sores; fever or chills; numbness, tingling, or pain in muscles; or other persistent adverse reactions. **Pregnancy/breast-feeding precautions:** Inform prescriber if you are or intend to become pregnant. This drug should not be used in the 2nd or 3rd trimester of pregnancy. Consult prescriber for appropriate contraceptive measures. Breast-feeding is not recommended.

Dietary Considerations: Administer on an empty stomach.

Geriatric Considerations: Due to frequent decreases in glomerular filtration (also creatinine clearance) with aging, elderly patients may have exaggerated responses to ACE inhibitors. Differences in clinical response due to hepatic changes are not observed.

Pregnancy Risk Factor: C/D (2nd and 3rd trimesters)

Pregnancy Issues: ACE inhibitors can cause fetal injury or death if taken during the 2nd or 3rd trimester. Discontinue ACE inhibitors as soon as pregnancy is detected.

Lactation: Excretion in breast milk unknown/use caution

Administration

Oral: Food may delay and reduce peak serum levels; take on an empty stomach, if possible.

Related Information

Angiotensin Agents *on page 1704*

Moexipril and Hydrochlorothiazide

(mo EKS i pril & hye droe klor oh THYE a zide)

U.S. Brand Names Uniretic®

Synonyms Hydrochlorothiazide and Moexipril

Generic Available No

Pharmacologic Category Antihypertensive Agent, Combination

Use Combination therapy for hypertension, however, not indicated for initial treatment of hypertension; replacement therapy in patients receiving separate dosage forms (for patient convenience); when monotherapy with one component fails to achieve desired antihypertensive effect, or when dose-limiting adverse effects limit upward titration of monotherapy

Dosing

Adults: Oral: 7.5-30 mg of moexipril, taken either in a single or divided dose one hour before meals; hydrochlorothiazide dose should be ≤50 mg/day

Elderly: Overall safety and efficacy are not different in elderly patients, although a higher moexipril AUC was observed in elderly patients. Greater sensitivity to effects may be observed in some older individuals. Refer to adult dosing.

Available Dosage Forms Tablet [film coated, scored]:

7.5/12.5: Moexipril hydrochloride 7.5 mg and hydrochlorothiazide 12.5 mg

15/12.5: Moexipril hydrochloride 15 mg and hydrochlorothiazide 12.5 mg

15/25: Moexipril hydrochloride 15 mg and hydrochlorothiazide 25 mg

Monitoring and Teaching Issues

Physical Assessment: See individual agents.

Patient Education: See individual agents. **Pregnancy/breast-feeding precautions:** Inform prescriber if you are or intend to become pregnant. Consult prescriber if breast-feeding.

Pregnancy Risk Factor: C/D (2nd and 3rd trimesters)

Lactation: Enters breast milk/use caution

Related Information

Hydrochlorothiazide *on page 751*

Moexipril *on page 1024*

♦ **Moexipril Hydrochloride** *see* Moexipril *on page 1024*

♦ **MOM** *see* Magnesium Hydroxide *on page 930*

Mometasone Furoate (moe MET a sone FYOOR oh ate)

U.S. Brand Names Elocon®; Nasonex®

Generic Available Yes: Ointment

Pharmacologic Category Corticosteroid, Nasal; Corticosteroid, Topical

Use Relief of the inflammatory and pruritic manifestations of corticosteroid-responsive dermatoses (medium potency topical corticosteroid); treatment of nasal symptoms of seasonal and perennial allergic rhinitis in adults and children ≥2 years of age; prevention of nasal symptoms associated with seasonal allergic rhinitis in children ≥12 years of age and adults; treatment of nasal polyps in adults

Mechanism of Action/Effect Corticosteroid with medium range potency. Reverses capillary permeability and release of inflammatory mediators (leukotrienes and prostaglandins); suppresses migration of polymorphonuclear leukocytes.

Contraindications Hypersensitivity to mometasone or any component of the formulation; fungal, viral, or tubercular skin lesions, herpes simplex or zoster

Warnings/Precautions

Nasal: Use caution if replacing systemic corticosteroid with nasal; may cause symptoms of withdrawal or acute adrenal insufficiency May cause suppression of hypothalamic-pituitary-adrenal (HPA) axis, particularly in younger children or in patients receiving high doses for prolonged periods. Controlled clinical studies have shown that intranasal corticosteroids may cause a reduction in growth velocity in pediatric patients; titrate to the lowest effective dose. May suppress the immune system, patients may be more susceptible to infection. Use with caution, if at all, in patients with systemic infections, active or quiescent tuberculosis infection, or ocular herpes simplex. Avoid exposure to chickenpox and measles.

Topical: May cause suppression of HPA axis, especially when used on large areas of the body, denuded areas, for prolonged periods of time or with an occlusive dressing. Pediatric patients may be more susceptible to systemic toxicity.

Drug Interactions

Cytochrome P450 Effect: Substrate of CYP3A4 (minor)

Adverse Reactions

Nasal:

>10%:

Central nervous system: Headache (17% to 26%)

Respiratory: Pharyngitis (10% to 12%), cough (7% to 13%), epistaxis (8% to 11%)

Miscellaneous: Viral infection (8% to 14%)

1% to 10%:

Cardiovascular: Chest pain

Endocrine & metabolic: Dysmenorrhea (1% to 5%)

Gastrointestinal: Vomiting (1% to 5%), diarrhea, dyspepsia, nausea

Neuromuscular & skeletal: Musculoskeletal pain (1% to 5%), arthralgia, myalgia

Ocular: Conjunctivitis

Otic: Earache, otitis media

Respiratory: Upper respiratory tract infection (5% to 6%), sinusitis (4% to 5%), asthma, bronchitis, nasal irritation, rhinitis, wheezing

Miscellaneous: Flu-like symptoms

Topical:

1% to 10%: Dermatologic: Bacterial skin infection, burning, furunculosis, pruritus, skin atrophy, tingling/stinging

Cataract formation, reduction in growth velocity, and HPA axis suppression have been reported with other corticosteroids

Pharmacodynamics/Kinetics

Absorption: Nasal: Mometasone furoate monohydrate: Undetectable in plasma; Ointment: 0.7%; increased by occlusive dressings

Protein Binding: Mometasone furoate: 98% to 99%

Half-Life Elimination: Elimination: I.V.: 5.8 hours

Metabolism: Mometasone furoate: Hepatic via CYP3A4; forms metabolite

Excretion: Bile, urine

Dosing

Adults & Elderly:

Treatment of seasonal and perennial allergic rhinitis: Nasal spray: 2 sprays (100 mcg) in each nostril daily

Prevention of seasonal and perennial allergic rhinitis: Nasal spray: 2 sprays (100 mcg) in each nostril daily beginning 2-4 weeks prior to pollen season

Treatment of corticosteroid-responsive dermatoses: Topical: Apply sparingly, do not use occlusive dressings. Therapy should be discontinued when control is achieved; if no improvement is seen in 2 weeks, reassessment of diagnosis may be necessary.

Cream, ointment: Apply a thin film to affected area once daily

Lotion: Apply a few drops to affected area once daily

Treatment of nasal polyps: Nasal spray: 2 sprays (100 mcg) in each nostril twice daily; 2 sprays (100 mcg) once daily may be effective in some patients

Pediatrics:

Treatment of seasonal and perennial allergic rhinitis treatment:

Nasal spray:

Children 2-11 years: 1 spray (50 mcg) in each nostril daily

Children ≥12 years: Refer to adult dosing.

Treatment of corticosteroid-responsive dermatoses: Topical:

Cream, ointment: Children ≥2 years: Refer to adult dosing. Do not use in pediatric patients for longer than 3 weeks.

Lotion: Children ≥12 years: Refer to adult dosing.

Available Dosage Forms

Cream, topical (Elocon®): 0.1% (15 g, 45 g)

Lotion, topical (Elocon®): 0.1% (30 mL, 60 mL) [contains isopropyl alcohol 40%]

Ointment, topical (Elocon®): 0.1% (15 g, 45 g)

Suspension, intranasal spray (Nasonex®): 50 mcg/spray (17 g) [delivers 120 sprays; contains benzalkonium chloride]

(Continued)

Mometasone Furoate *(Continued)*

Monitoring and Teaching Issues

Physical Assessment: Assess potential for interactions with other prescriptions, OTC medications, or herbal products patient may be taking. Assess patient response. Teach patient proper use (according to formulation), side effects/appropriate interventions, and symptoms to report.

Patient Education: For external use only. Do not take anything new during treatment without consulting prescriber. Use exactly as directed and for no longer than the period prescribed. **Pregnancy/breast-feeding precautions:** Inform prescriber if you are or intend to become pregnant. Consult prescriber if breast-feeding.

Nasal: Read complete instructions in package. Prime the pump as directed. Gently blow your nose to clear nostrils. Close one nostril. Tilt your head forward slightly and, keeping the bottle upright, carefully insert the nasal applicator into the other nostril. After the spray, breath gently inward through the nostril, then breath out through the mouth. Repeat in other nostril. You may experience headache, cough, or nosebleed. Report unusual chest pain, gastrointestinal upset, muscle pain, flu-like symptoms, other persistent adverse reactions, worsening of condition or failure to improve. Store at room temperature, away from light.

Topical: Do not use for eyes, mucous membranes, or open wounds. Use exactly as directed and for no longer than the period prescribed. Before using, wash and dry area gently. Apply in a thin layer (cream, ointment) or a few drops (lotion) and rub in lightly. Apply light dressing (if necessary) to area being treated. Do not use occlusive dressing unless so advised by prescriber. Avoid prolonged or excessive use around sensitive tissues, underarms, genital, or rectal areas. Avoid exposing treated area to direct sunlight (severe sunburn may occur). Inform prescriber if condition worsens (redness, swelling, irritation, signs of infection, or open sores) or fails to improve.

Pregnancy Risk Factor: C

Pregnancy Issues: There are no adequate and well-controlled studies using topical mometasone during pregnancy. However, intrauterine growth retardation has been reported with some topical steroids. Avoid use of large amounts for long periods of time during pregnancy.

Lactation: Excretion in breast milk unknown/use caution

Breast-Feeding Issues: Systemic corticosteroids are excreted in human milk. The extent of topical absorption is variable. Use with caution while breast-feeding; do not apply to nipples.

Administration

Inhalation: Nasal spray: Prior to first use, prime pump by actuating 10 times or until fine spray appears; may store for a maximum of 1 week without repriming. Spray should be administered once or twice daily, at a regular interval. Shake well prior to use.

Topical: Apply sparingly; avoid eyes, face, underarms, and groin. Do not wrap or bandage affected area.

Storage:

Cream: Store between 2°C to 25°C (36°F to 77°F).
Lotion: Store between 2°C to 30°C (36°F to 86°F).
Nasal spray: Store at room temperature of 15°C to 30°C (59°F to 86°F). Protect from light.
Ointment: Store at room temperature of 15°C to 30°C (59°F to 86°F).

Related Information

Corticosteroids *on page 1731*

- **Monacolin K** *see* Lovastatin *on page 925*
- **Monarc® M** *see* Antihemophilic Factor (Human) *on page 124*
- **Monistat® 1 Combination Pack [OTC]** *see* Miconazole *on page 999*
- **Monistat® 3 [OTC]** *see* Miconazole *on page 999*
- **Monistat® 7 [OTC]** *see* Miconazole *on page 999*
- **Monistat-Derm®** *see* Miconazole *on page 999*
- **Monoclate-P®** *see* Antihemophilic Factor (Human) *on page 124*
- **Monoclonal Antibody** *see* Muromonab-CD3 *on page 1038*
- **Monodox®** *see* Doxycycline *on page 496*
- **Mono-Gesic®** *see* Salsalate *on page 1354*
- **Monoket®** *see* Isosorbide Mononitrate *on page 841*
- **MonoNessa™** *see* Ethinyl Estradiol and Norgestimate *on page 593*
- **Monopril®** *see* Fosinopril *on page 681*

Montelukast *(mon te LOO kast)*

U.S. Brand Names Singulair®

Synonyms Montelukast Sodium

Generic Available No

Pharmacologic Category Leukotriene-Receptor Antagonist

Medication Safety Issues

Sound-alike/look-alike issues:

Singulair® may be confused with Sinequan®

Use Prophylaxis and chronic treatment of asthma in adults and children ≥1 year of age; relief of symptoms of seasonal allergic rhinitis in adults and children ≥2 years of age

Unlabeled/Investigational Use Acute asthma

Mechanism of Action/Effect Montelukast is a selective leukotriene receptor antagonist which inhibits cysteinyl leukotriene that is responsible for edema, smooth muscle contraction that is felt to be associated with the signs and symptoms of asthma.

Contraindications Hypersensitivity to montelukast or any component of the formulation

Warnings/Precautions Inform phenylketonuric patients that the chewable tablet contains phenylalanine. Montelukast is not FDA approved for use in the reversal of bronchospasm in acute asthma attacks; some clinicians, however, support its use. Should not be used as monotherapy for the treatment and management of exercise-induced bronchospasm. Has been associated with eosinophilic vasculitis (Churg-Strauss syndrome), usually following reduction or withdrawal of oral corticosteroids. Healthcare providers should be alert to eosinophilia, vasculitic rash, worsening pulmonary symptoms, cardiac complications, and/or neuropathy presenting in their patients. A casual association between montelukast and these underlying conditions has not been established. Safety and efficacy in children <1 year of age have not been established.

Drug Interactions

Cytochrome P450 Effect: Substrate (major) of CYP2C8/9, 3A4; **Inhibits** CYP2C8/9 (weak)

Decreased Effect: CYP2C8/9 inducers may decrease the levels/effects of montelukast; example inducers include carbamazepine, phenobarbital, phenytoin, rifampin, rifapentine, and secobarbital. CYP3A4 inducers may decrease the levels/effects of montelukast; example inducers include aminoglutethimide, carbamazepine, nafcillin, nevirapine, phenobarbital, phenytoin, and rifamycins.

Nutritional/Ethanol Interactions Herb/Nutraceutical: St John's wort may decrease montelukast levels.

Adverse Reactions (As reported in adults)

>10%: Central nervous system: Headache (18%)

1% to 10%:

Central nervous system: Dizziness (2%), fatigue (2%), fever (2%)

Dermatologic: Rash (2%)

Gastrointestinal: Dyspepsia (2%), dental pain (2%), gastroenteritis (2%), abdominal pain (3%)

Neuromuscular & skeletal: Weakness (2%)

Respiratory: Cough (3%), nasal congestion (2%), upper respiratory infection (2%)

Miscellaneous: Flu-like symptoms (4%), trauma (1%)

Overdosage/Toxicology No specific antidote

Remove unabsorbed material from the GI tract, employ clinical monitoring and institute supportive therapy if required

Pharmacodynamics/Kinetics

Duration of Action: >24 hours

Absorption: Rapid

Bioavailability: Tablet: 10 mg: Mean: 64%; 5 mg: 63% to 73%

Time to Peak: Serum: Tablet: 10 mg: 3-4 hours; 5 mg: 2-2.5 hours; 4 mg: 2 hours

Protein Binding: Plasma: >99%

Half-Life Elimination: Plasma: Mean: 2.7-5.5 hours

Metabolism: Extensively hepatic via CYP3A4 and 2C8/9

Excretion: Feces (86%); urine (<0.2%)

Dosing

Adults & Elderly:

Asthma or allergic seasonal rhinitis: Oral: One 10 mg tablet daily in the evening

Asthma, acute (unlabeled use): 10 mg as a single dose administered with first-line therapy

Pediatrics:

Asthma: Oral:

6-11 months (unlabeled use): 4 mg (oral granules) once daily, taken in the evening

12-23 months: 4 mg (oral granules) once daily, taken in the evening

Asthma or seasonal allergic rhinitis: Oral:

2-5 years: 4 mg (chewable tablet or oral granules) once daily, taken in the evening

6-14 years: Chew one 5 mg chewable tablet/day, taken in the evening

≥15 years: Refer to adult dosing.

Renal Impairment: No adjustment is necessary.

Hepatic Impairment: No adjustment necessary in mild-to-moderate hepatic disease. Patients with severe hepatic disease were **not** studied.

Available Dosage Forms

Granules: 4 mg/packet

Tablet: 10 mg

Tablet, chewable: 4 mg [contains phenylalanine 0.674 mg; cherry flavor]; 5 mg [contains phenylalanine 0.842 mg; cherry flavor]

Monitoring and Teaching Issues

Physical Assessment: Not for use in acute asthma attacks, including status asthmaticus. Assess effectiveness and interactions of other medications patient may be taking. Monitor effectiveness of therapy and adverse reactions at beginning of therapy and periodically with long-term use. Assess knowledge/teach patient appropriate use, interventions to reduce side effects, and adverse symptoms to report.

Patient Education: Do not stop other asthma medication unless advised by prescriber. Chewable tablet contains phenylalanine. Take every evening on a continuous basis; do not discontinue even if feeling better (this medication may help reduce incidence of acute attacks). Granules may be administered directly in the mouth or mixed with applesauce, carrots, rice, or ice cream (do not mix in liquids); administer within 15 minutes of opening packet. You may experience mild headache (mild analgesic may help); or fatigue or dizziness (use caution when driving). Report skin rash or itching, abdominal pain or persistent GI upset, unusual cough or congestion, feeling of numbness in arms or legs, flu-like illness, or worsening of asthmatic condition. **Breast-feeding precaution:** Consult prescriber if breast-feeding.

Dietary Considerations: Tablet, chewable: 4 mg strength contains phenylalanine 0.674 mg; 5 mg strength contains phenylalanine 0.842 mg

Pregnancy Risk Factor: B

Lactation: Excretion in breast milk unknown/use caution

Breast-Feeding Issues: Zafirlukast, another leukotriene receptor antagonist, is excreted in breast milk and use while breast-feeding is not recommended.

(Continued)

Montelukast *(Continued)*

Administration

Oral: Take dose in the evening. Granules may be administered directly in the mouth or mixed with applesauce, carrots, rice, or ice cream. Administer within 15 minutes of opening packet. Do not mix in liquids.

Storage: Store at room temperature of 15°C to 30°C (59°F to 86°F). Protect from moisture and light.

Granules: Use within 15 minutes of opening packet.

♦ **Montelukast Sodium** *see Montelukast on page 1028*

♦ **8-MOP®** *see Methoxsalen on page 978*

♦ **MoreDophilus® [OTC]** *see Lactobacillus on page 859*

Moricizine *(mor I siz een)*

U.S. Brand Names Ethmozine®

Synonyms Moricizine Hydrochloride

Generic Available No

Pharmacologic Category Antiarrhythmic Agent, Class I

Medication Safety Issues

Sound-alike/look-alike issues:

Ethmozine® may be confused with Erythrocin®, erythromycin

Use Treatment of ventricular tachycardia and life-threatening ventricular arrhythmias

Unlabeled/Investigational Use PVCs, complete and nonsustained ventricular tachycardia, atrial arrhythmias

Mechanism of Action/Effect Class I antiarrhythmic agent; reduces the fast inward current carried by sodium ions, shortens Phase I and Phase II repolarization, resulting in decreased action potential duration and effective refractory period

Contraindications Hypersensitivity to moricizine or any component of the formulation; pre-existing second- or third-degree AV block (except in patients with a functioning artificial pacemaker); right bundle branch block when associated with left hemiblock or bifascicular block (unless functional pacemaker in place); cardiogenic shock

Warnings/Precautions Can be proarrhythmic; watch for new rhythm disturbances or existing arrhythmias that worsen. Use cautiously in CAD, previous history of MI, CHF, and cardiomegaly. The CAST II trial demonstrated a decreased trend in survival for patients receiving moricizine. Dose-related increases in PR and QRS intervals occur. Use cautiously in patients with pre-existing conduction abnormalities, and significant hepatic impairment. Safety and efficacy have not been established in pediatric patients.

Drug Interactions

Cytochrome P450 Effect: Substrate of CYP3A4 (major); **Induces** CYP1A2 (weak), 3A4 (weak)

Decreased Effect: Moricizine may decrease levels of theophylline (50%) and diltiazem. CYP3A4 inducers may decrease the levels/effects of moricizine; example inducers include aminoglutethimide, carbamazepine, nafcillin, nevirapine, phenobarbital, phenytoin, and rifamycins.

Increased Effect/Toxicity: CYP3A4 inhibitors may increase the levels/effects of moricizine; example inhibitors include azole antifungals, ciprofloxacin, clarithromycin, diclofenac, doxycycline, erythromycin, imatinib, isoniazid, nefazodone, nicardipine, propofol, protease inhibitors, quinidine, and verapamil. Moricizine levels may be increased by cimetidine and diltiazem. Digoxin may result in additive prolongation of the PR interval when combined with moricizine (but not rate of second- and third-degree AV block). Drugs which may prolong QT interval (including cisapride, erythromycin, phenothiazines, cyclic antidepressants, and some quinolones) are contraindicated with type Ia antiarrhythmics. Moricizine has some type Ia activity, and caution should be used.

Nutritional/Ethanol Interactions Food: Moricizine peak serum concentrations may be decreased if taken with food.

Adverse Reactions

>10%: Central nervous system: Dizziness

1% to 10%:

Cardiovascular: Proarrhythmia, palpitation, cardiac death, ECG abnormalities, CHF

Central nervous system: Headache, fatigue, insomnia

Endocrine & metabolic: Decreased libido

Gastrointestinal: Nausea, diarrhea, ileus

Ocular: Blurred vision, periorbital edema

Respiratory: Dyspnea

Overdosage/Toxicology Has a narrow therapeutic index and severe toxicity may occur slightly above the therapeutic range, especially if combined with other antiarrhythmic drugs. Acute single ingestion of twice the daily therapeutic dose is life-threatening. Symptoms of overdose include increases in PR, QRS, QT intervals and amplitude of the T wave, AV block, bradycardia, hypotension, ventricular arrhythmias (monomorphic or polymorphic ventricular tachycardia), and asystole. Other symptoms include dizziness, blurred vision, headache, and GI upset.

Treatment is symptom-directed and supportive. **Note:** Type Ia antiarrhythmic agents should not be used to treat cardiotoxicity caused by type Ic drugs.

Pharmacodynamics/Kinetics
Bioavailability: 38%

Protein Binding: Plasma: 95%

Half-Life Elimination: Healthy volunteers: 3-4 hours; Cardiac disease: 6-13 hours

Metabolism: Significant first-pass effect; some enterohepatic recycling

Excretion: Feces (56%); urine (39%)

Dosing
Adults & Elderly: Ventricular arrhythmias: Oral: 200-300 mg every 8 hours, adjust dosage at 150 mg/day at 3-day intervals. See table for dosage recommendations of transferring from other antiarrhythmic agents to Ethmozine®. Hospitalization required to start therapy.

Moricizine

Transferred From	Start Ethmozine®
Encainide, propafenone, tocainide, or mexiletine	8-12 hours after last dose
Flecainide	12-24 hours after last dose
Procainamide	3-6 hours after last dose
Quinidine, disopyramide	6-12 hours after last dose

Renal Impairment: Start at 600 mg/day or less.

Hepatic Impairment: Start at 600 mg/day or less.

Available Dosage Forms Tablet, as hydrochloride: 200 mg, 250 mg, 300 mg

Monitoring and Teaching Issues
Physical Assessment: Assess other medications patient may be taking for effectiveness and interactions. Monitor cardiac status. Assess results of laboratory tests, therapeutic effectiveness, and adverse reactions at beginning of therapy, when titrating dosage, and on a regular basis with long-term therapy. **Note:** Moricizine has a low toxic:therapeutic ratio and overdose may easily produce severe and life-threatening reactions. Assess knowledge/teach patient appropriate use, interventions to reduce side effects, and adverse symptoms to report.

Monitoring Laboratory Tests: Electrolytes (correct any imbalance) prior to beginning therapy

Patient Education: Take exactly as directed; do not take additional doses or discontinue without consulting prescriber. You will need regular cardiac checkups and blood tests while taking this medication. You may experience dizziness or visual changes (use caution when driving or engaging in tasks requiring alertness until response to drug is known); nausea or vomiting (small frequent meals, frequent mouth care, chewing gum, or sucking lozenges may help); or headaches, sleep disturbances, or decreased libido (usually temporary, if persistent consult prescriber). Report chest pain, palpitation, or erratic heartbeat; increased weight or swelling of hands or feet; blurred vision or facial swelling; acute diarrhea; changes in bowel or bladder patterns; or respiratory difficulty. **Breast-feeding precaution:** Breast-feeding is not recommended.

Dietary Considerations: Best if taken on an empty stomach.

Geriatric Considerations: Due to moricizine binding to plasma albumin and alpha-glycoprotein, other highly bound drugs may displace moricizine. Since elderly may require multiple drugs, caution with highly bound drugs is necessary. Consider changes in renal and hepatic function with age and monitor closely since half-life may be prolonged.

Pregnancy Risk Factor: B

Lactation: Enters breast milk/not recommended

Related Information
Antiarrhythmic Drugs *on page 1708*

♦ **Moricizine Hydrochloride** *see Moricizine on page 1030*

Morphine Sulfate (MOR feen SUL fate)
U.S. Brand Names Astramorph/PF™; Avinza™; DepoDur™; Duramorph®; Infumorph®; Kadian®; MS Contin®; MSIR®; Oramorph SR®; RMS®; Roxanol™; Roxanol 100™; Roxanol™-T

Controlled Substance C-II

Generic Available Yes: Excludes capsule, controlled release tablet, sustained release tablet, extended release liposomal suspension for injection

Pharmacologic Category Analgesic, Narcotic

Medication Safety Issues
Sound-alike/look-alike issues:
Morphine may be confused with hydromorphone
Morphine sulfate may be confused with magnesium sulfate
Avinza™ may be confused with Evista®, Invanz®
Roxanol™ may be confused with Roxicet™

Avoid the MSO₄ abbreviation; errors have occurred with its use.

Use care when prescribing and/or administering morphine solutions. These products are available in different concentrations. Always prescribe dosage in mg; **not** by volume (mL).

Use Relief of moderate to severe acute and chronic pain; relief of pain of myocardial infarction; relief of dyspnea of acute left ventricular failure and pulmonary edema; preanesthetic medication

DepoDur™: Epidural (lumbar) single-dose management of surgical pain

Orphan drug: Infumorph®: Used in microinfusion devices for intraspinal administration in treatment of intractable chronic pain

Mechanism of Action/Effect Binds to opiate receptors in the CNS, causing inhibition of ascending pain pathways, altering the perception of and response to pain; produces generalized CNS depression

Contraindications Hypersensitivity to morphine sulfate or any component of the formulation; increased intracranial pressure; severe respiratory depression (in absence of resuscitative
(Continued)

Morphine Sulfate *(Continued)*

equipment or ventilatory support); acute or severe asthma; known or suspected paralytic ileus (sustained release products only); sustained release products are not recommended in acute/postoperative pain; pregnancy (prolonged use or high doses at term)

Warnings/Precautions An opioid-containing analgesic regimen should be tailored to each patient's needs and based upon the type of pain being treated (acute versus chronic), the route of administration, degree of tolerance for opioids (naive versus chronic user), age, weight, and medical condition. The optimal analgesic dose varies widely among patients. Doses should be titrated to pain relief/prevention. When used as an epidural injection, monitor for delayed sedation.

May cause respiratory depression; use with caution in patients with impaired respiratory function or severe hepatic dysfunction and in patients with hypersensitivity reactions to other phenanthrene derivative opioid agonists (codeine, hydrocodone, hydromorphone, levorphanol, oxycodone, oxymorphone). Infants <3 months of age are more susceptible to respiratory depression, use with caution and generally in reduced doses in this age group. May cause hypotension in patients with acute myocardial infarction. Tolerance or drug dependence may result from extended use. MS Contin® 200 mg tablets are for use only in opioid-tolerant patients requiring >400 mg/day. Infumorph® solutions are **for use in microinfusion devices only**; not for I.V., I.M., or SubQ administration.

Use caution in CNS depression, toxic psychosis, delirium tremens, or convulsive disorders. Sedation and psychomotor impairment are likely, and are additive with other CNS depressants or ethanol. Extended or sustained release dosage forms should not be crushed or chewed. Controlled-, extended-, or sustained-release products are not intended for "as needed (PRN)" use. Some preparations contain sulfites which may cause allergic reactions.

Use caution in renal impairment (metabolite accumulation); use caution in gastrointestinal motility disturbances (particularly with sustained release preparations), thyroid disorders (Addison's disease, myxedema, or hypothyroidism), prostatic hyperplasia, or urethral stricture.

Elderly and/or debilitated may be particularly susceptible to the CNS depressant and constipating effects of narcotics. May mask diagnosis or clinical course in patients with acute abdominal conditions.

Drug Interactions

Cytochrome P450 Effect: Substrate of CYP2D6 (minor)

Decreased Effect: Diuretic effects may be decreased (due to antidiuretic hormone release).

Increased Effect/Toxicity: CNS depressants (phenothiazines, tranquilizers, anxiolytics, sedatives, hypnotics, or alcohol), tricyclic antidepressants may potentiate the effects of morphine and other opiate agonists. Dextroamphetamine may enhance the analgesic effect of morphine and other opiate agonists. Concurrent use of MAO inhibitors and meperidine has been associated with significant adverse effects. Use caution with morphine. Some manufacturers recommend avoiding use within 14 days of MAO inhibitors.

Nutritional/Ethanol Interactions

Ethanol: Avoid ethanol (may increase CNS depression).

Food: Administration of oral morphine solution with food may increase bioavailability (ie, a report of 34% increase in morphine AUC when morphine oral solution followed a high-fat meal). The bioavailability of Oramorph SR® does not appear to be affected by food.

Herb/Nutraceutical: Avoid valerian, St John's wort, kava kava, gotu kola (may increase CNS depression).

Lab Interactions Increased aminotransferase [ALT (SGPT)/AST (SGOT)] (S)

Adverse Reactions Note: Percentages are based on a study in 19 chronic cancer pain patients (*J Pain Symptom Manage*, 1995, 10:416-22). Chronic use of various opioids in cancer pain is accompanied by similar adverse reactions; individual patient differences are unpredictable, and percentage may differ in acute pain (surgical) treatment.

Frequency not defined: Flushing, CNS depression, sedation, antidiuretic hormone release, physical and psychological dependence, diaphoresis

>10%:

Cardiovascular: Palpitations, hypotension, bradycardia

Central nervous system: Drowsiness (48%, tolerance usually develops to drowsiness with regular dosing for 1-2 weeks); dizziness (20%); confusion

Dermatologic: Pruritus (may be secondary to histamine release)

Gastrointestinal: Nausea (28%, tolerance usually develops to nausea and vomiting with chronic use); vomiting (9%); constipation (40%, tolerance develops very slowly if at all); xerostomia (78%)

Genitourinary: Urinary retention (16%)

Local: Pain at injection site

Neuromuscular & skeletal: Weakness

Miscellaneous: Histamine release

1% to 10%:

Central nervous system: Restlessness, headache, false feeling of well being

Gastrointestinal: Anorexia, GI irritation, paralytic ileus

Genitourinary: Decreased urination

Neuromuscular & skeletal: Trembling

Ocular: Vision problems

Respiratory: Respiratory depression, dyspnea

Overdosage/Toxicology Symptoms of overdose include respiratory depression, miosis, hypotension, bradycardia, apnea, and pulmonary edema. Treatment is symptomatic. Naloxone, 2 mg I.V. with repeat administration as necessary up to a total dose of 10 mg, can be used to reverse opiate effects.

Pharmacodynamics/Kinetics
Onset of Action: Oral: 1 hour; I.V.: 5-10 minutes
Duration of Action: Pain relief: Immediate release formulations: 4 hours; extended release epidural injection (DepoDur™): >48 hours
Absorption: Oral: Variable
Bioavailability: Oral: 17% to 33% (first-pass effect limits oral bioavailability; oral:parenteral effectiveness reportedly varies from 1:6 in opioid naive patients to 1:3 with chronic use)
Half-Life Elimination: Adults: 2-4 hours (immediate release forms)
Metabolism: Hepatic via conjugation with glucuronic acid to morphine-3-glucuronide (inactive), morphine-6-glucuronide (active), and in lesser amounts, morphine-3-6-diglucuronide; other minor metabolites include normorphine (active) and the 3-ethereal sulfate
Excretion: Urine (primarily as morphine-3-glucuronide, ~2% to 12% excreted unchanged); feces (~7% to 10%). It has been suggested that accumulation of morphine-6-glucuronide might cause toxicity with renal insufficiency. All of the metabolites (ie, morphine-3-glucuronide, morphine-6-glucuronide, and normorphine) have been suggested as possible causes of neurotoxicity (eg, myoclonus).

Dosing
Adults: Note: These are guidelines and do not represent the maximum doses that may be required in all patients. Doses should be titrated to pain relief/prevention.

Acute pain (moderate-to-severe):
Oral: Prompt release formulations: Opiate-naive: Initial: 10 mg every 3 to 4 hours as needed; patients with prior opiate exposure may require higher initial doses: usual dosage range: 10-30 mg every 3-4 hours as needed

Oral: Controlled-, extended-, or sustained-release formulations: **Note:** A patient's morphine requirement should be established using prompt-release formulations. Conversion to long-acting products may be considered when chronic, continuous treatment is required. Higher dosages should be reserved for use only in opioid-tolerant patients.

Capsules, extended release (Avinza™): Daily dose administered once daily (for best results, administer at same time each day)

Capsules, sustained release (Kadian®): Daily dose administered once daily or in 2 divided doses daily (every 12 hours)

Tablets, controlled release (MS Contin®), sustained release (Oramorph SR®), or extended release: Daily dose divided and administered every 8 or every 12 hours

I.V.: Initial: Opiate-naive: 2.5-5 mg every 3 to 4 hours; patients with prior opiate exposure may require higher initial doses. NOTE: Repeated doses (up to every 5 minutes if needed) in small increments (eg, 1-4 mg) may be preferred to larger and less frequent doses.

I.V., SubQ continuous infusion: 0.8-10 mg/hour; may increase depending on pain relief/adverse effects: usual range: up to 80 mg/hour although higher doses may be required Mechanically-ventilated patients (based on 70 kg patient): 0.7-10 mg every 1-2 hours as needed; infusion: 5-35 mg/hour

Patient-controlled analgesia (PCA): (Opiate-naive: Consider lower end of dosing range):
Usual concentration: 1 mg/mL
Demand dose: Usual: 1 mg; range: 0.5-2.5 mg
Lockout interval: 5-10 minutes

Epidural: **Note:** Administer with extreme caution and in reduced dosage to geriatric or debilitated patients.
Infusion:
Bolus dose: 1-6 mg
Infusion rate: 0.1-1 mg/hour
Maximum dose: 10 mg/24 hours
Single-dose (extended release, Depo-Dur™):
Cesarean section: 10 mg
Lower abdominal/pelvic surgery: 10-15 mg
Note: Some patients may benefit from a 20 mg dose, however, the incidence of adverse effects may be increased.

Intrathecal (I.T.): One-tenth of epidural dose; **Note:** Administer with extreme caution and in reduced dosage to geriatric or debilitated patients.
Opiate-naive: 0.2-1 mg/dose (may provide adequate relief for 24 hours); repeat doses **not** recommended except to establish initial IT dose.

I.M., SubQ: **Note:** Repeated SubQ administration causes local tissue irritation, pain, and induration.
Initial: Opiate-naive: 5-10 mg every 3-4 hours as needed; patients with prior opiate exposure may require higher initial doses; usual dosage range: 5-20 mg every 3-4 hours as needed

Rectal: 10-20 mg every 3-4 hours

Chronic pain: Patients taking opioids chronically may become tolerant and require doses higher than the usual dosage range to maintain the desired effect. Tolerance can be managed by appropriate dose titration. There is no optimal or maximal dose for morphine in chronic pain. The appropriate dose is one that relieves pain throughout its dosing interval without causing unmanageable side effects.

Elderly: Refer to adult dosing. Use with caution; may require reduced dosage in the elderly and debilitated patients.

Pediatrics: Note: These are guidelines and do not represent the maximum doses that may be required in all patients. Doses should be titrated to pain relief/prevention.

Acute pain (moderate-to-severe): Children >6 months and <50 kg:
Oral (prompt release): 0.15-0.3 mg/kg every 3-4 hours as needed
I.M.: 0.1 mg/kg every 3-4 hours as needed
I.V.: 0.05-0.1 mg/kg every 3-4 hours as needed
I.V. infusion: Range: 10-30 mcg/kg/hour

Sedation/analgesia for procedures: Adolescents >12 years: I.V.: 3-4 mg and repeat in 5 minutes if necessary

(Continued)

Morphine Sulfate (Continued)

Renal Impairment:
Cl_{cr} 10-50 mL/minute: Administer 75% of normal dose.
Cl_{cr} <10 mL/minute: Administer 50% of normal dose.

Hepatic Impairment: Unchanged in mild liver disease; substantial extrahepatic metabolism may occur. Excessive sedation may occur in cirrhosis.

Available Dosage Forms

Capsule (MSIR®): 15 mg, 30 mg

Capsule, extended release (Avinza™): 30 mg, 60 mg, 90 mg, 120 mg

Capsule, sustained release (Kadian®): 20 mg, 30 mg, 50 mg, 60 mg, 100 mg

Infusion [premixed in D_5W]: 0.2 mg/mL (250 mL, 500 mL); 1 mg/mL (100 mL, 250 mL, 500 mL)

Injection, extended release liposomal suspension [lumbar epidural injection, preservative free] (DepoDur™): 10 mg/mL (1 mL, 1.5 mL, 2 mL)

Injection, solution: 2 mg/mL (1 mL); 4 mg/mL (1 mL); 5 mg/mL (1 mL); 8 mg/mL (1 mL); 10 mg/mL (1 mL, 2 mL, 10 mL); 15 mg/mL (1 mL, 20 mL); 25 mg/mL (4 mL, 10 mL, 20 mL, 40 mL) [some preparations contain sodium metabisulfite]

Injection, solution [epidural, intrathecal, or I.V. infusion; preservative free]:
Astramorph/PF™: 0.5 mg/mL (2 mL, 10 mL); 1 mg/mL (2 mL, 10 mL)
Duramorph®: 0.5 mg/mL (10 mL); 1 mg/mL (10 mL)

Injection, solution [epidural or intrathecal infusion via microinfusion device; preservative free] (Infumorph®): 10 mg/mL (20 mL); 25 mg/mL (20 mL)

Injection, solution [I.V. infusion via PCA pump]: 1 mg/mL (50 mL); 5 mg/mL (50 mL)

Injection, solution [preservative free]: 0.5 mg/mL (10 mL); 1 mg/mL (10 mL, 30 mL); 10 mg/mL (10 mL); 15 mg/mL (20 mL); 25 mg/mL (4 mL, 10 mL, 20 mL); 50 mg/mL (10 mL, 20 mL, 50 mL)

Solution, oral: 10 mg/5 mL (5 mL, 10 mL, 100 mL, 500 mL); 20 mg/5 mL (100 mL, 500 mL); 20 mg/mL (30 mL, 120 mL, 240 mL)
MSIR®: 10 mg/5 mL (120 mL); 20 mg/5 mL (120 mL); 20 mg/mL (30 mL, 120 mL) [contains sodium benzoate] [DSC]
Roxanol™: 20 mg/mL (30 mL, 120 mL)
Roxanol 100™: 100 mg/5 mL (240 mL) [with calibrated spoon]
Roxanol™-T: 20 mg/mL (30 mL, 120 mL) [tinted, flavored]

Suppository, rectal (RMS®): 5 mg (12s), 10 mg (12s), 20 mg (12s), 30 mg (12s)

Tablet (MSIR®): 15 mg, 30 mg

Tablet, controlled release (MS Contin®): 15 mg, 30 mg, 60 mg, 100 mg, 200 mg

Tablet, extended release: 15 mg, 30 mg, 60 mg, 100 mg, 200 mg

Tablet, sustained release (Oramorph SR®): 15 mg, 30 mg, 60 mg, 100 mg

Monitoring and Teaching Issues

Physical Assessment: Assess other medications patient may be taking for additive or adverse interactions. Monitor vital signs, respiratory and CNS status, therapeutic effectiveness, and adverse reactions or overdose at regular intervals with long-term use. May cause physical and/or psychological dependence. For inpatients, implement safety measures. Assess knowledge/teach patient appropriate use (if self-administered), adverse reactions to report, and appropriate interventions to reduce side effects. Discontinue slowly after prolonged use.

Patient Education: If self-administered, use exactly as directed; do not increase dose or frequency. Do not crush or chew controlled release tablets. May cause physical and/or psychological dependence. While using this medication, do not use alcohol and other prescription or OTC medications (especially sedatives, tranquilizers, antihistamines, or pain medications) without consulting prescriber. Maintain adequate hydration (2-3 L/day of fluids) unless instructed to restrict fluid intake. May cause hypotension, dizziness, drowsiness, impaired coordination, or blurred vision (use caution when driving, climbing stairs, or changing position - rising from sitting or lying to standing, or when engaging in tasks requiring alertness until response to drug is known); loss of appetite, nausea, or vomiting (frequent mouth care, small frequent meals, chewing gum, or sucking lozenges may help); or constipation (increased exercise, fluids, fruit, or fiber may help; if unresolved, consult prescriber about use of stool softeners and/or laxatives). Report chest pain, slow or rapid heartbeat, acute dizziness, or persistent headache; changes in mental status; swelling of extremities or unusual weight gain; changes in urinary elimination or pain on urination; acute headache; back or flank pain; muscle spasms; blurred vision; skin rash; or shortness of breath. **Pregnancy/breast-feeding precautions:** Inform prescriber if you are or intend to become pregnant. If you are breast-feeding, take medication immediately after breast-feeding or 3-4 hours prior to next feeding.

Dietary Considerations: Morphine may cause GI upset; take with food if GI upset occurs. Be consistent when taking morphine with or without meals.

Geriatric Considerations: The elderly may be particularly susceptible to the CNS depressant and constipating effects of narcotics. For chronic administration of narcotic analgesics, morphine is preferable in the elderly due to its pharmacokinetics and side effect profile as compared to meperidine and methadone.

Pregnancy Risk Factor: C/D (prolonged use or high doses at term)

Pregnancy Issues: Morphine crosses the placenta. The frequency of congenital malformations has not been reported to be greater than expected in children from mothers treated with morphine during pregnancy. Reduced growth and behavioral abnormalities in offspring have been observed in animal studies. Neonates born to mothers receiving chronic opioids during pregnancy should be monitored for neonatal withdrawal syndrome.

DepoDur™ may be used in women undergoing cesarean section following clamping of the umbilical cord; not for use in vaginal labor and delivery.

Lactation: Enters breast milk/use caution (AAP rates "compatible")

Breast-Feeding Issues: Detectable serum levels of morphine can be found in infants following morphine administration to nursing mothers. Treatment of the mother with single doses of morphine is not expected to cause detrimental effects in nursing infants. Breast-feeding following chronic use or in neonates with hepatic or renal dysfunction may lead to higher levels of morphine in the infant and a risk of adverse effects. Some clinicians recommend administering morphine immediately after breast-feeding or 3-4 hours prior to the next feeding. Breast-feeding should be delayed for 48 hours after DepoDur™ administration.

Administration

Oral: Do not crush controlled release drug product, swallow whole. Kadian® can be opened and sprinkled on applesauce. Avinza™ can also be opened and sprinkled on applesauce; do not crush or chew the beads. Administration of oral morphine solution with food may increase bioavailability (not observed with Oramorph SR®).

I.V.: When giving morphine I.V. push, it is best to first dilute in 4-5 mL of sterile water, and then to administer slowly (eg, 15 mg over 3-5 minutes).

Other: Use preservative-free solutions for intrathecal or epidural use.

Epidural, extended release liposomal suspension (DepoDur™): May be administered undiluted or diluted up to 5 mL total volume in preservative-free NS. Do not use an in-line filter during administration. Not for I.V. or I.M. administration.

Resedation may occur following epidural administration; this may be delayed ≥48 hours in patients receiving extended-release (DepoDur™) injections.

Administration of an epidural test dose (lidocaine 1.5% and epinephrine 1:200,000) may affect the release of morphine from the liposomal preparation. Delaying the dose for an interval of at least 15 minutes following the test dose minimizes this pharmacokinetic interaction. Except for a test dose, other epidural local anesthetics should not be used before or after this product.

Reconstitution: Usual concentration for continuous I.V. infusion: 0.1-1 mg/mL in D_5W. DepoDur™ may be diluted in preservative-free NS to a volume of 5 mL.

Compatibility: Stable in dextran 6% in dextrose, dextran 6% in NS, D_5LR, $D_5^1/_4NS$, $D_5^1/_2NS$, D_5NS, D_5W, $D_{10}W$, LR, $^1/_2NS$, NS

Y-site administration: Incompatible with alatrofloxacin, amphotericin B cholesteryl sulfate complex, cefepime, doxorubicin liposome, minocycline, sargramostim

Compatibility in syringe: Incompatible with meperidine, thiopental

Compatibility when admixed: Incompatible with aminophylline, amobarbital, chlorothiazide, floxacillin, fluorouracil, heparin, meperidine, phenobarbital, phenytoin, sodium bicarbonate, thiopental

DepoDur™: Do not mix with other medications.

Storage:

Suppositories: Store at controlled room temperature 25°C (77°F). Protect from light.

Injection: Store at controlled room temperature. Protect from light. Degradation depends on pH and presence of oxygen; relatively stable in pH ≤4; darkening of solutions indicate degradation.

DepoDur™: Store under refrigeration, 2°C to 8°C (36°F to 46°F). Do not freeze. May store at room temperature for up to 7 days. Once vial is opened, use within 4 hours.

Related Information

Compatibility of Drugs *on page 1723*
Compatibility of Drugs in Syringe *on page 1725*
Narcotic / Opioid Analgesic Comparison *on page 1739*

♦ **Motofen®** *see* Difenoxin and Atropine *on page 450*
♦ **Motrin®** *see* Ibuprofen *on page 777*
♦ **Motrin® Children's [OTC]** *see* Ibuprofen *on page 777*
♦ **Motrin® IB [OTC]** *see* Ibuprofen *on page 777*
♦ **Motrin® Infants' [OTC]** *see* Ibuprofen *on page 777*
♦ **Motrin® Junior Strength [OTC]** *see* Ibuprofen *on page 777*
♦ **Motrin® Migraine Pain [OTC]** *see* Ibuprofen *on page 777*

Moxifloxacin (moxs i FLOKS a sin)

U.S. Brand Names Avelox®; Avelox® I.V.; Vigamox™
Synonyms Moxifloxacin Hydrochloride
Generic Available No
Pharmacologic Category Antibiotic, Ophthalmic; Antibiotic, Quinolone
Medication Safety Issues
Sound-alike/look-alike issues:
Avelox® may be confused with Avonex®

Use Treatment of mild-to-moderate community-acquired pneumonia, including multidrug-resistant *Streptococcus pneumoniae* (MDRSP); acute bacterial exacerbation of chronic bronchitis; acute bacterial sinusitis; uncomplicated skin infections; bacterial conjunctivitis (ophthalmic formulation)

Mechanism of Action/Effect Moxifloxacin is a quinolone antibiotic with bactericidal activity against susceptible gram negative and gram positive microorganisms.

Contraindications Hypersensitivity to moxifloxacin, other quinolone antibiotics, or any component of the formulation

Warnings/Precautions Use with caution in patients with significant bradycardia or acute myocardial ischemia. Moxifloxacin causes a concentration-dependent QT prolongation. Do not exceed recommended dose or infusion rate. Coadministration of moxifloxacin with other drugs that also prolong the QT interval or induce bradycardia should be avoided. Use with caution in individuals at risk of seizures (CNS disorders or concurrent therapy with medications which may lower seizure threshold). Discontinue in patients who experience significant CNS adverse effects (dizziness, hallucinations, suicidal ideation or actions). Not recommended in patients with moderate to severe hepatic insufficiency. Use with caution in diabetes; glucose regulation may be altered. Tendon inflammation and/or rupture have been reported with quinolone antibiotics. Risk may be increased with concurrent corticosteroids, particularly in the elderly. Discontinue at first signs or symptoms of tendon pain.

Severe hypersensitivity reactions, including anaphylaxis, have occurred with quinolone therapy. If an allergic reaction occurs (itching, urticaria, dyspnea or facial edema, loss of consciousness, tingling, cardiovascular collapse) discontinue drug immediately. Prolonged (Continued)

Moxifloxacin *(Continued)*

use may result in superinfection; pseudomembranous colitis may occur and should be considered in all patients who present with diarrhea. Quinolones may exacerbate myasthenia gravis, use with caution (rare, potentially life-threatening weakness of respiratory muscles may occur). Peripheral neuropathy may rarely occur.

Ophthalmic: Eye drops should not be injected subconjunctivally or introduced directly into the anterior chamber of the eye. Contact lenses should not be worn during therapy.

Drug Interactions
Decreased Effect: Concurrent administration of metal cations, including most antacids, oral electrolyte supplements, quinapril, sucralfate, and some didanosine formulations (chewable/buffered tablets and pediatric powder for oral suspension), may decrease quinolone levels; separate doses.

Increased Effect/Toxicity: Moxifloxacin may increase the effects/toxicity of glyburide and warfarin. Concomitant use with corticosteroids may increase the risk of tendon rupture. Concomitant use with other QT_c-prolonging agents (eg, Class Ia and Class III antiarrhythmics, erythromycin, cisapride, antipsychotics, and cyclic antidepressants) may result in arrhythmias, such as torsade de pointes.

Nutritional/Ethanol Interactions Food: Absorption is not affected by administration with a high-fat meal or yogurt.

Adverse Reactions
Systemic:

3% to 10%:
Central nervous system: Dizziness (3%)
Gastrointestinal: Nausea (7%), diarrhea (6%)

0.1% to 3%:
Cardiovascular: Chest pain, hypertension, palpitation, peripheral edema, QT prolongation, tachycardia
Central nervous system: Anxiety, chills, confusion, headache, insomnia, nervousness, pain, somnolence, tremor, vertigo
Dermatologic: Dry skin, pruritus, rash (maculopapular, purpuric, pustular)
Endocrine & metabolic: Serum chloride increased (≥2%), serum ionized calcium increased (≥2%), serum glucose decreased (≥2%)
Gastrointestinal: Abdominal pain, amylase increased, amylase decreased (≥2%), anorexia, constipation, dry mouth, dyspepsia, flatulence, glossitis, lactic dehydrogenase increased, stomatitis, taste perversion, vomiting
Hematologic: Eosinophilia, leukopenia, prothrombin time prolonged, increased INR, thrombocythemia, thrombocytopenia
Increased serum levels of the following (≥2%): MCH, neutrophils, WBC
Decreased serum levels of the following (≥2%): Basophils, eosinophils, hemoglobin, RBC, neutrophils
Hepatic: Bilirubin decreased (≥2%), cholestatic jaundice, GGTP increased, liver function test abnormal
Local: Injection site reaction
Neuromuscular & skeletal: Arthralgia, back pain, leg pain, myalgia, paresthesia, malaise, weakness
Renal: Serum albumin increased (≥2%)
Respiratory: Dyspnea, pharyngitis, pneumonia, rhinitis, sinusitis, PO_2 increased (≥2%)
Miscellaneous: Allergic reaction, infection, moniliasis, diaphoresis

Additional reactions with **ophthalmic** preparation: 1% to 6%: Conjunctivitis, dry eye, ocular discomfort, ocular hyperemia, ocular pain, ocular pruritus, subconjunctival hemorrhage, tearing, visual acuity decreased

Overdosage/Toxicology Potential symptoms of overdose may include CNS excitation, seizures, QT prolongation, and arrhythmias (including torsade de pointes). Patients should be monitored by continuous ECG in the event of an overdose. Management is supportive and symptomatic.

Pharmacodynamics/Kinetics
Absorption: Well absorbed; not affected by high fat meal or yogurt
Bioavailability: 90%
Protein Binding: 50%
Half-Life Elimination: Oral: 12 hours; I.V.: 15 hours
Metabolism: Hepatic (52% of dose) via glucuronide (14%) and sulfate (38%) conjugation
Excretion: Excretion: Approximately 45% of a dose is excreted in feces (25%) and urine (20%) as unchanged drug; Metabolites: Sulfate conjugates in feces, glucuronide conjugates in urine

Dosing
Adults & Elderly:
Acute bacterial sinusitis: Oral, I.V.: 400 mg every 24 hours for 10 days
Chronic bronchitis, acute bacterial exacerbation: Oral, I.V.: 400 mg every 24 hours for 5 days
Note: Avelox® ABC Pack™ (Avelox® Bronchitis Course) contains five tablets of 400 mg each.
Community-acquired pneumonia (including MDRSP): Oral, I.V.: 400 mg every 24 hours for 7-14 days
Uncomplicated skin infections: Oral, I.V.: 400 mg every 24 hours for 7 days
Bacterial conjunctivitis: Ophthalmic: Instill 1 drop into affected eye(s) 3 times/day for 7 days
Pediatrics: Bacterial conjunctivitis: Ophthalmic: Children ≥1 year: Refer to adult dosing.
Renal Impairment: No adjustment is necessary, including patients on hemodialysis or CAPD.
Hepatic Impairment: No dosage adjustment is required in mild to moderate hepatic insufficiency (Child-Pugh Classes A and B). Not recommended in patients with severe hepatic insufficiency.

Available Dosage Forms

Infusion [premixed in sodium chloride 0.8%] (Avelox® I.V.): 400 mg (250 mL)
Solution, ophthalmic (Vigamox™): 0.5% (3 mL)
Tablet [film coated]:
Avelox®: 400 mg
Avelox® ABC Pack [unit-dose pack]: 400 mg (5s)

Monitoring and Teaching Issues

Physical Assessment: Assess results of any culture and sensitivity tests and patient's allergy history before initiating therapy. Use caution with known CNS disorders, bradycardia, or hepatic impairment (see Warnings/Precautions for use cautions). Assess potential for interactions with other prescriptions, OTC medications, or herbal products patient may be taking (eg, increased risk of tendon rupture or arrhythmias; see Drug Interactions). See Administration for infusion specifics; if an allergic reaction occurs (itching, urticaria, dyspnea or facial edema, loss of consciousness, tingling, cardiovascular collapse), drug should be discontinued immediately and prescriber notified. Assess results of laboratory tests, therapeutic effectiveness (resolution of infection), and adverse effects (see Adverse Reactions). Teach patient proper use, possible side effects/appropriate interventions, and adverse symptoms to report (see Patient Education).

Monitoring Laboratory Tests: WBC

Patient Education: Do not take any new medication during therapy unless approved by prescriber. **Pregnancy/breast-feeding precautions:** Inform prescriber if you are or intend to become pregnant. Breast-feeding is not recommended.

I.V.: Report any redness, swelling, or pain at infusion site; any swelling of mouth, lips, tongue, or throat; chest pain or tightness; respiratory difficulty; back pain; itching; skin rash; tingling; tendon pain; dizziness; abnormal thinking; or anxiety.

Oral: Take exactly as directed with or without food. Do not take antacids 4 hours before or 8 hours after taking this medication. Do not miss a dose (take a missed dose as soon as possible, unless it is almost time for your next dose). Take entire prescription even if feeling better. Maintain adequate hydration (2-3 L/day of fluids) unless instructed to restrict fluid intake. May cause nausea, vomiting, taste perversion (small frequent meals, good mouth care, chewing gum, or sucking hard candy may help); headache, dizziness, insomnia, anxiety (use caution when driving or engaging in tasks requiring alertness until response to drug is known). Report immediately any swelling of mouth, lips, tongue or throat; chest pain or tightness; respiratory difficulty; back pain; itching; skin rash; tingling; tendon pain; confusion, dizziness, abnormal thinking, or anxiety; or insomnia. Report changes in voiding pattern; vaginal itching, burning, or discharge; vision changes or hearing; abnormal bruising or bleeding or blood in urine; or other adverse reactions.

Ophthalmic: Wash hands before instilling solution. Sit or lie down to instill. Open eye, look at ceiling, and instill prescribed amount of solution as directed. Close eye and roll eye in all directions, and apply gentle pressure to inner corner of eye. Do not touch tip of applicator or let tip of applicator touch eye (may cause eye infection, eye damage, or vision loss). Do not wear contact lenses during therapy. Temporary stinging, blurred vision, or dry eyes may occur. Report persistent pain, burning, excessive tearing, decreased visual acuity, swelling, itching, or worsening of condition.

Dietary Considerations: May be taken with or without food. Take 4 hours before or 8 hours after multiple vitamins, antacids, or other products containing magnesium, aluminum, iron, or zinc.

Pregnancy Risk Factor: C

Pregnancy Issues: Reports of arthropathy (observed in immature animals and reported rarely in humans) have limited the use of fluoroquinolones during pregnancy. Teratogenic effects were not observed with moxifloxacin in animal studies; however, delayed skeletal development and smaller fetuses were observed in some species. There are no adequate and well-controlled studies in pregnant women. Based on limited data, quinolones are not expected to be a major human teratogen. Although quinolone antibiotics should not be used as first-line agents during pregnancy, when considering treatment for life-threatening infection and/or prolonged duration of therapy, the potential risk to the fetus must be balanced against the severity of the potential illness.

Lactation: Excretion in breast milk unknown/not recommended

Breast-Feeding Issues: Other quinolones are known to be excreted in breast milk. The manufacturer recommends to discontinue nursing or to discontinue moxifloxacin.

Administration

I.V.: I.V.: Infuse over 60 minutes; do not infuse by rapid or bolus intravenous infusion
Compatibility: Stable in 0.9% NS, 1M sodium chloride, D_5W, $D_{10}W$, SWFI, LR
Do not add other medications to intravenous solution
Storage: Store at 25°C (77°F). I.V.: Do not refrigerate.

Related Information

Antimicrobial Drugs of Choice *on page 1792*
Community-Acquired Pneumonia in Adults *on page 1807*
Tuberculosis *on page 1864*

- ♦ Mucinex® [OTC] *see* Guaifenesin *on page 729*
- ♦ Mucinex®-D [OTC] *see* Guaifenesin and Pseudoephedrine *on page 733*
- ♦ Mucinex® DM [OTC] *see* Guaifenesin and Dextromethorphan *on page 731*
- ♦ Mucomyst® *see* Acetylcysteine *on page 45*
- ♦ Multitargeted Antifolate *see* Pemetrexed *on page 1169*
- ♦ Multitest CMI® *see page 1625*
- ♦ Mumps Skin Test Antigen *see page 1625*
- ♦ Mumpsvax® *see page 1660*
- ♦ Mumps Virus Vaccine (Live/Attenuated) *see page 1660*

Mupirocin (myoo PEER oh sin)

U.S. Brand Names Bactroban®; Bactroban® Nasal; Centany™
Synonyms Mupirocin Calcium; Pseudomonic Acid A
Generic Available Yes: Topical ointment
Pharmacologic Category Antibiotic, Topical
Medication Safety Issues
Sound-alike/look-alike issues:
Bactroban® may be confused with bacitracin, baclofen
Use
Intranasal: Eradication of nasal colonization with MRSA in adult patients and healthcare workers
Topical treatment of impetigo due to *Staphylococcus aureus*, beta-hemolytic *Streptococcus*, and *S. pyogenes*
Unlabeled/Investigational Use Intranasal: Surgical prophylaxis to prevent wound infections
Mechanism of Action/Effect Binds to bacterial isoleucyl transfer-RNA synthetase resulting in the inhibition of protein and RNA synthesis
Contraindications Hypersensitivity to mupirocin, polyethylene glycol, or any component of the formulation
Warnings/Precautions Potentially toxic amounts of polyethylene glycol contained in the vehicle may be absorbed percutaneously in patients with extensive burns or open wounds. Prolonged use may result in over growth of nonsusceptible organisms. For external use only. Not for treatment of pressure sores.
Adverse Reactions Frequency not defined.
Central nervous system: Dizziness, headache
Dermatologic: Pruritus, rash, erythema, dry skin, cellulitis, dermatitis
Gastrointestinal: Nausea, taste perversion
Local: Burning, stinging, tenderness, edema, pain
Respiratory: Rhinitis, upper respiratory tract infection, pharyngitis, cough
Pharmacodynamics/Kinetics
Absorption: Topical: Penetrates outer layers of skin; systemic absorption minimal through intact skin
Protein Binding: 95%
Half-Life Elimination: 17-36 minutes
Metabolism: Skin: 3% to monic acid
Excretion: Urine
Dosing
Adults & Elderly:
Impetigo: Topical: Apply small amount to affected area 2-5 times/day for 5-14 days.
Elimination of MRSA colonization: Nasal: Approximately one-half of the ointment from the single-use tube should be applied into one nostril and the other half into the other nostril twice daily for 5 days.
Pediatrics:
Topical: Children: Refer to adult dosing.
Nasal: ≥12 years: Refer to adult dosing.
Available Dosage Forms
Cream, topical, as calcium (Bactroban®): 2% (15 g, 30 g) [contains benzyl alcohol]
Ointment, intranasal, topical, as calcium (Bactroban® Nasal): 2% (1 g) [single-use tube]
Ointment, topical: 2% (22 g)
Bactroban®: 2% (22 g)
Centany™: 2% (15 g, 30 g)
Monitoring and Teaching Issues
Physical Assessment: See Warnings/Precautions for use cautions. Assess for effectiveness of therapy (resolution of infection). Teach patient appropriate application and use and adverse symptoms (see Adverse Reactions) to report.
Patient Education: For external use only. Wash hands before and after application. Apply thin film over affected areas exactly as directed. Avoid getting in eyes. Report rash, persistent burning, stinging, swelling, itching, or pain. Contact prescriber if no improvement is seen in 3-5 days. **Breast-feeding precaution:** Consult prescriber if breast-feeding.
Pregnancy Risk Factor: B
Lactation: Excretion in breast milk unknown/use caution
Administration
Topical: For external use only.
Compatibility: Do not mix with Aquaphor®, coal tar solution, or salicylic acid.
Additional Information Not for treatment of pressure sores; contains polyethylene glycol vehicle.

- ♦ Mupirocin Calcium *see* Mupirocin *on page 1038*

Muromonab-CD3 (myoo roe MOE nab see dee three)

U.S. Brand Names Orthoclone OKT® 3
Synonyms Monoclonal Antibody; OKT3
Generic Available No

Pharmacologic Category Immunosuppressant Agent

Use Treatment of acute allograft rejection in renal transplant patients; treatment of acute hepatic, kidney, and pancreas rejection episodes resistant to conventional treatment. Acute graft-versus-host disease following bone marrow transplantation resistant to conventional treatment.

Mechanism of Action/Effect Reverses graft rejection by binding to T cells and interfering with their function

Contraindications Hypersensitivity to OKT3 or any murine product; patients in fluid overload or those with >3% weight gain within 1 week prior to start of OKT3; mouse antibody titers >1:1000

Warnings/Precautions It is imperative, especially prior to the first few doses, that there be no clinical evidence of volume overload, uncontrolled hypertension, or uncompensated heart failure, including a clear chest x-ray and weight restriction of ≤3% above the patient's minimum weight during the week prior to injection.

May result in an increased susceptibility to infection; dosage of concomitant immunosuppressants should be reduced during OKT3 therapy; cyclosporine should be decreased to 50% usual maintenance dose and maintenance therapy resumed about 4 days before stopping OKT3.

Severe pulmonary edema has occurred in patients with fluid overload.

First dose effect (flu-like symptoms, anaphylactic-type reaction): may occur within 30 minutes to 6 hours up to 24 hours after the first dose and may be minimized by using the recommended regimens. See table.

Suggested Prevention/Treatment of Muromonab-CD3 First-Dose Effects

Adverse Reaction	Effective Prevention or Palliation	Supportive Treatment
Severe pulmonary edema	Clear chest x-ray within 24 hours preinjection; weight restriction to ≤3% gain over 7 days preinjection	Prompt intubation and oxygenation; 24 hours close observation
Fever, chills	15 mg/kg methylprednisolone sodium succinate 1 hour preinjection; fever reduction to <37.8°C (100°F) 1 hour preinjection; acetaminophen (1 g orally) and diphenhydramine (50 mg orally) 1 hour preinjection	Cooling blanket Acetaminophen prn
Respiratory effects	100 mg hydrocortisone sodium succinate 30 minutes postinjection	Additional 100 mg hydrocortisone sodium succinate prn for wheezing; if respiratory distress, give epinephrine 1:1000 (0.3 mL SubQ)

Cardiopulmonary resuscitation may be needed. If the patient's temperature is >37.8°C, reduce before administering OKT3

Drug Interactions

Decreased Effect: Decreased effect with immunosuppressive drugs.

Increased Effect/Toxicity: Recommend decreasing dose of prednisone to 0.5 mg/kg, azathioprine to 0.5 mg/kg (approximate 50% decrease in dose), and discontinuing cyclosporine while patient is receiving OKT3.

Adverse Reactions

>10%:

"First-dose" (cytokine release) effects: Onset: 1-3 hours after the dose; duration: 12-16 hours. Severity is mild to life-threatening. Signs and symptoms include fever, chilling, dyspnea, wheezing, chest pain, chest tightness, nausea, vomiting, and diarrhea. Hypervolemic pulmonary edema, nephrotoxicity, meningitis, and encephalopathy are possible. Reactions tend to decrease with repeated doses.

Cardiovascular: Tachycardia (including ventricular)

Central nervous system: Dizziness, faintness

Gastrointestinal: Diarrhea, nausea, vomiting

Hematologic: Transient lymphopenia

Neuromuscular & skeletal: Trembling

Respiratory: Dyspnea

1% to 10%:

Central nervous system: Headache

Neuromuscular & skeletal: Stiff neck

Ocular: Photophobia

Respiratory: Pulmonary edema

Pharmacodynamics/Kinetics

Duration of Action: 7 days after discontinuation

Time to Peak: Steady-state: Trough: 3-14 days

Dosing

Adults & Elderly: Treatment of acute allograft rejection or acute graft-versus-host disease: I.V. (refer to individual protocols): 5 mg/day once daily for 10-14 days

Pediatrics: Refer to individual protocols.

Treatment of acute allograft rejection or acute graft-versus-host disease: I.V.

Children <30 kg: 2.5 mg/day once daily for 7-14 days

Children >30 kg: 5 mg/day once daily for 7-14 days

or

Children <12 years: 0.1 mg/kg/day once daily for 10-14 days

Children ≥12 years: Refer to adult dosing.

(Continued)

Muromonab-CD3 (Continued)

Renal Impairment: Removal by dialysis: Molecular size of OKT3 is 150,000 daltons. Not dialyzed by most standard dialyzers; however, may be dialyzed by high flux dialysis. OKT3 will be removed by plasmapheresis. Administer following dialysis treatments.

Available Dosage Forms Injection, solution: 1 mg/mL (5 mL) [contains sodium 43 mg/5 mL]

Monitoring and Teaching Issues

Physical Assessment: Monitor pretreatment laboratory results prior to beginning therapy. Monitor closely for acute adverse pulmonary and cardiac effects, and anaphylactic-type effects during and for 24 hours following first infusion. Monitor vital signs, cardiac status, respiratory status, and adverse reactions on a regular basis. Assess knowledge/instruct patient about adverse reactions to report (eg, opportunistic infection) and appropriate interventions to reduce side effects.

Monitoring Laboratory Tests: Chest x-ray, CBC with differential, immunologic monitoring of T cells, serum levels of OKT3

Patient Education: There may be a severe reaction to the first infusion of this medication. You may experience high fever, chills, respiratory difficulty, or congestion. You will be closely monitored and comfort measures provided. Effects are substantially reduced with subsequent infusions. During the period of therapy and for some time after the regimen of infusions you will be susceptible to infection. People may wear masks and gloves while caring for you to protect you as much as possible from infection (avoid crowds and exposure to infection). You may experience dizziness, faintness, or trembling (use caution until response to medication is known); nausea or vomiting (small frequent meals, frequent mouth care); or sensitivity to direct sunlight (wear dark glasses, and protective clothing, use sunscreen, or avoid exposure to direct sunlight). Report chest pain or tightness; symptoms of respiratory infection, wheezing, or respiratory difficulty; vision change; or muscular trembling. **Pregnancy/breast-feeding precautions:** Inform prescriber if you are or intend to become pregnant. Do not breast-feed.

Dietary Considerations: Injection solution contains sodium 43 mg/5 mL.

Pregnancy Risk Factor: C

Lactation: Excretion in breast milk unknown/contraindicated

Administration

I.V.: Not for I.M. administration. Give I.V. push over <1 minute at a final concentration of 1 mg/mL. Methylprednisolone sodium succinate 1 mg/kg I.V. given prior to first muromonab-CD3 administration, and I.V. hydrocortisone sodium succinate 50-100 mg, given 30 minutes after administration are strongly recommended to decrease the incidence of reactions to the first dose.

Storage: Refrigerate; do not shake or freeze. Stable in Becton Dickinson syringe for 16 hours at room temperature or refrigeration.

♦ **Muse®** see Alprostadil on page 76

♦ **Mustargen®** see Mechlorethamine on page 935

♦ **Mustine** see Mechlorethamine on page 935

♦ **Mutamycin®** see Mitomycin on page 1017

♦ **Myambutol®** see Ethambutol on page 576

♦ **Mycelex®** see Clotrimazole on page 360

♦ **Mycelex®-7 [OTC]** see Clotrimazole on page 360

♦ **Mycelex® Twin Pack [OTC]** see Clotrimazole on page 360

♦ **Mycinettes® [OTC]** see Benzocaine on page 181

♦ **Mycobutin®** see Rifabutin on page 1322

♦ **Mycolog®-II [DSC]** see Nystatin and Triamcinolone on page 1104

Mycophenolate (mye koe FEN oh late)

U.S. Brand Names CellCept®; Myfortic®

Synonyms MMF; MPA; Mycophenolate Mofetil; Mycophenolate Sodium; Mycophenolic Acid

Generic Available No

Pharmacologic Category Immunosuppressant Agent

Use Prophylaxis of organ rejection concomitantly with cyclosporine and corticosteroids in patients receiving allogenic renal (CellCept®, Myfortic®), cardiac (CellCept®), or hepatic (CellCept®) transplants

Unlabeled/Investigational Use Treatment of rejection in liver transplant patients unable to tolerate tacrolimus or cyclosporine due to neurotoxicity; mild rejection in heart transplant patients; treatment of moderate-severe psoriasis; treatment of proliferative lupus nephritis

Mechanism of Action/Effect Inhibition of purine synthesis of human lymphocytes and proliferation of human lymphocytes

Contraindications Hypersensitivity to mycophenolate mofetil, mycophenolic acid, mycophenolate sodium, or any component of the formulation; intravenous formulation is contraindicated in patients who are allergic to polysorbate 80

Warnings/Precautions Risk for infection and development of lymphoproliferative disorders is increased. Patients should be monitored appropriately and given supportive treatment should these conditions occur. Toxicity may be increased in patients with renal impairment. Use caution with active peptic ulcer disease.

Mycophenolate mofetil is a potential teratogen; tablets should not be crushed, and capsules should not be opened or crushed. Avoid inhalation or direct contact with skin or mucous membranes of the powder contained in the capsules and the powder for oral suspension. Caution should be exercised in the handling and preparation of solutions of intravenous mycophenolate. Avoid skin contact with the intravenous solution and reconstituted suspension. If such contact occurs, wash thoroughly with soap and water, rinse eyes with plain water.

Theoretically, use should be avoided in patients with the rare hereditary deficiency of hypoxanthine-guanine phosphoribosyltransferase (such as Lesch-Nyhan or Kelley-Seegmiller syndrome). Intravenous solutions should be given over at least 2 hours; **never** administer intravenous solution by rapid or bolus injection.

CellCept® and Myfortic® dosage forms should not be used interchangeably due to differences in absorption.

Drug Interactions

Decreased Effect: Antacids decrease serum levels (C_{max} and AUC); **do not administer together.** Cholestyramine resin decreases serum levels; **do not administer together.** Avoid use of live vaccines; vaccinations may be less effective. Influenza vaccine may be of value. During concurrent use of oral contraceptives, progesterone levels are not significantly affected, however, effect on estrogen component varies; an additional form of contraception should be used.

Increased Effect/Toxicity: Acyclovir and ganciclovir levels may increase due to competition for tubular secretion of these drugs. Probenecid may increase mycophenolate levels due to inhibition of tubular secretion. High doses of salicylates may increase free fraction of mycophenolic acid. Azathioprine's bone marrow suppression may be potentiated; do not administer together.

Nutritional/Ethanol Interactions

Food: Decreases C_{max} of MPA by 40% following CellCept® administration and 33% following Myfortic® use; the extent of absorption is not changed

Herb/Nutraceutical: Avoid cat's claw, echinacea (have immunostimulant properties)

Adverse Reactions As reported in adults following oral dosing of CellCept® alone in renal, cardiac, and hepatic allograft rejection studies. In general, lower doses used in renal rejection patients had less adverse effects than higher doses. Rates of adverse effects were similar for each indication, except for those unique to the specific organ involved. The type of adverse effects observed in pediatric patients was similar to those seen in adults; abdominal pain, anemia, diarrhea, fever, hypertension, infection, pharyngitis, respiratory tract infection, sepsis, and vomiting were seen in higher proportion; lymphoproliferative disorder was the only type of malignancy observed. Percentages of adverse reactions were similar in studies comparing CellCept® to Myfortic® in patients following renal transplant.

>20%:

Cardiovascular: Hypertension (28% to 77%), peripheral edema (27% to 64%), edema (27% to 28%), tachycardia (20% to 22%)

Central nervous system: Pain (31% to 76%), headache (16% to 54%), insomnia (41% to 52%), fever (21% to 52%), anxiety (28%)

Dermatologic: Rash (22%)

Endocrine & metabolic: Hypercholesterolemia (41%), hypokalemia (32% to 37%)

Gastrointestinal: Abdominal pain (25% to 62%), nausea (20% to 54%), diarrhea (31% to 52%), constipation (18% to 41%), vomiting (33% to 34%), anorexia (25%), dyspepsia (22%)

Genitourinary: Urinary tract infection (37%)

Hematologic: Leukopenia (23% to 46%), leukocytosis (22% to 40%), hypochromic anemia (25%)

Hepatic: Liver function tests abnormal (25%), ascites (24%)

Neuromuscular & skeletal: Back pain (35% to 47%), weakness (35% to 43%), tremor (24% to 34%), paresthesia (21%)

Respiratory: Dyspnea (31% to 37%), respiratory tract infection (22% to 37%), cough (31%), lung disorder (22% to 30%)

Miscellaneous: Infection (18% to 27%), *Candida* (11% to 22%), herpes simplex (10% to 21%)

3% to <20%:

Cardiovascular: Angina, arrhythmia, arterial thrombosis, atrial fibrillation, atrial flutter, bradycardia, cardiac arrest, cardiac failure, CHF, extrasystole, facial edema, hypervolemia, hypotension, pallor, palpitation, pericardial effusion, peripheral vascular disorder, postural hypotension, supraventricular extrasystoles, supraventricular tachycardia, syncope, thrombosis, vasodilation, vasospasm, venous pressure increased, ventricular extrasystole, ventricular tachycardia

Central nervous system: Agitation, chills with fever, confusion, convulsion, delirium, depression, emotional lability, hallucinations, hypoesthesia, malaise, nervousness, psychosis, somnolence, thinking abnormal, vertigo

Dermatologic: Acne, alopecia, bruising, cellulitis, hirsutism, pruritus, skin carcinoma, skin hypertrophy

Endocrine & metabolic: Acidosis, Cushing's syndrome, dehydration, diabetes mellitus, gout, hypercalcemia, hyperlipemia, hyperphosphatemia, hyperuricemia, hypothyroidism, parathyroid disorder

Gastrointestinal: Abdomen enlarged, dry mouth, dysphagia, esophagitis, flatulence, gastritis, gastroenteritis, gastrointestinal hemorrhage, gastrointestinal moniliasis, gingivitis, gum hyperplasia, melena, mouth ulceration, oral moniliasis, stomach disorder, stomatitis

Genitourinary: Impotence, pelvic pain, prostatic disorder, urinary frequency, urinary incontinence, urinary retention, urinary tract disorder

Hematologic: Coagulation disorder, hemorrhage, pancytopenia, polycythemia, prothrombin time increased, thromboplastin increased

Hepatic: Alkaline phosphatase increased, alkalosis, bilirubinemia, cholangitis, cholestatic jaundice, GGT increased, hepatitis, jaundice, liver damage

Local: Abscess, ALT increased, AST increased

Neuromuscular & skeletal: Arthralgia, hypertonia, joint disorder, leg cramps, myalgia, myasthenia, neck pain, neuropathy, osteoporosis

Ocular: Amblyopia, cataract, conjunctivitis, eye hemorrhage, lacrimation disorder, vision abnormal

Otic: Deafness, ear disorder, ear pain, tinnitus

Renal: Albuminuria, creatinine increased, dysuria, hematuria, hydronephrosis, kidney failure, kidney tubular necrosis, oliguria

Respiratory: Apnea, asthma, atelectasis, bronchitis, epistaxis, hemoptysis, hiccup, hyperventilation, hypoxia, respiratory acidosis, lung edema, pharyngitis, pleural effusion,

(Continued)

Mycophenolate *(Continued)*

pneumonia, pneumothorax, pulmonary hypertension, respiratory moniliasis, rhinitis, sinusitis, sputum increased, voice alteration

Miscellaneous: CMV viremia/syndrome (12% to 14%), CMV tissue invasive disease (6% to 11%), herpes zoster cutaneous disease (4% to 10%), cyst, diaphoresis, flu-like syndrome, fungal dermatitis, healing abnormal, hernia, ileus infection, lactic dehydrogenase increased, peritonitis, pyelonephritis, scrotal edema, thirst

Overdosage/Toxicology There are no reported overdoses with mycophenolate. At plasma concentrations >100 mcg/mL, small amounts of the inactive metabolite MPAG are removed by hemodialysis. Excretion of the active metabolite, MPA, may be increased by using bile acid sequestrants (cholestyramine).

Pharmacodynamics/Kinetics

Onset of Action: Peak effect: Correlation of toxicity or efficacy is still being developed, however, one study indicated that 12-hour AUCs >40 mcg/mL/hour were correlated with efficacy and decreased episodes of rejection

T_{max}: Oral: MPA:
CellCept®: 1-1.5 hours
Myfortic®: 1.5-2.5 hours

Absorption: AUC values for MPA are lower in the early post-transplant period versus later (>3 months) post-transplant period. The extent of absorption in pediatrics is similar to that seen in adults, although there was wide variability reported.
Oral: Myfortic®: 93%

Bioavailability: Oral: CellCept®: 94%; Myfortic®: 72%

Protein Binding: MPA 97%, MPAG 82%

Half-Life Elimination:
CellCept®: MPA: Oral: 18 hours; I.V.: 17 hours
Myfortic®: MPA: Oral: 8-16 hours; MPAG: 13-17 hours

Metabolism: Hepatic and via GI tract; CellCept® is completely hydrolyzed in the liver to mycophenolic acid (MPA; active metabolite); enterohepatic recirculation of MPA may occur; MPA is glucuronidated to MPAG (inactive metabolite)

Excretion:
CellCept®: MPA: Urine (<1%), feces (6%); MPAG: Urine (87%)
Myfortic®: MPA: Urine (3%), feces; MPAG: Urine (>60%)

Dosing

Adults: The initial dose should be given as soon as possible following transplantation; intravenous solution may be given until the oral medication can be tolerated (up to 14 days)

Renal transplant:
CellCept®:
Oral: 1 g twice daily. Although a dose of 1.5 g twice daily was used in clinical trials and shown to be effective, no efficacy advantage was established. Patients receiving 2 g/day demonstrated an overall better safety profile than patients receiving 3 g/day. Doses >2 g/day are not recommended in these patients because of the possibility for enhanced immunosuppression as well as toxicities.
I.V.: 1 g twice daily
Myfortic®: Oral: 720 mg twice daily (1440 mg/day)

Cardiac transplantation:
Oral (CellCept®): 1.5 g twice daily
I.V. (CellCept®): 1.5 g twice daily

Hepatic transplantation:
Oral (CellCept®): 1.5 g twice daily
I.V. (CellCept®): 1 g twice daily

Dosing adjustment for toxicity (neutropenia): ANC <1.3 x 10^3/μL: Dosing should be interrupted or the dose reduced, appropriate diagnostic tests performed and patients managed appropriately

Elderly: Dosage is the same as younger patients, however, dosing should be cautious due to possibility of increased hepatic, renal, or cardiac dysfunction. Elderly patients may be at an increased risk of certain infections, gastrointestinal hemorrhage, and pulmonary edema, as compared to younger patients.

Pediatrics:

Renal transplant: Oral:
CellCept® suspension: 600 mg/m²/dose twice daily; maximum dose: 1 g twice daily
Alternatively, may use solid dosage forms according to BSA as follows:
BSA 1.25-1.5 m²: 750 mg capsule twice daily
BSA >1.5 m²: 1 g capsule or tablet twice daily
Myfortic®:
BSA <1.19 m²: Use of this formulation is not recommended
BSA 1.19-1.58 m²: 400 mg/m² twice daily (maximum: 1080 mg/day)
BSA >1.58 m²: 400 mg/m² twice daily (maximum: 1440 mg/day)

Renal Impairment:
Renal transplant: GFR <25 mL/minute in patients outside the immediate post-transplant period:
CellCept®: Doses of >1 g administered twice daily should be avoided; patients should also be carefully observed; no dose adjustments are needed in renal transplant patients experiencing delayed graft function postoperatively
Myfortic®: Cl_{cr} <25 mL/minute: Monitor carefully
Cardiac or liver transplant: No data available; mycophenolate may be used in cardiac or hepatic transplant patients with severe chronic renal impairment if the potential benefit outweighs the potential risk.
Hemodialysis: Not removed; supplemental dose is not necessary.
Peritoneal dialysis: Supplemental dose is not necessary.

Hepatic Impairment: No dosage adjustment is recommended for renal patients with severe hepatic parenchymal disease; however, it is not currently known whether dosage adjustments are necessary for hepatic disease with other etiologies.

Available Dosage Forms

Capsule, as mofetil (CellCept®): 250 mg

Injection, powder for reconstitution, as mofetil hydrochloride (CellCept®): 500 mg [contains polysorbate 80]

Powder for oral suspension, as mofetil (CellCept®): 200 mg/mL (225 mL) [provides 175 mL suspension following reconstitution; contains phenylalanine 0.56 mg/mL; mixed fruit flavor]

Tablet, as mofetil [film coated] (CellCept®): 500 mg [may contain ethyl alcohol]

Tablet, delayed release, as mycophenolic acid [film coated] (Myfortic®): 180 mg, 360 mg [formulated as a sodium salt]

Monitoring and Teaching Issues

Physical Assessment: Assess other medications patient may be taking for effectiveness and interactions. Assess results of laboratory tests, therapeutic effectiveness, and adverse reactions. Patients with diabetes should monitor glucose levels closely (this medication may alter glucose levels). Monitor/instruct patient on appropriate interventions to reduce side effects, to monitor for signs of opportunistic infection, and adverse reactions to report.

Monitoring Laboratory Tests: Renal and liver function, CBC

Patient Education: Take oral formulations as directed, preferably 1 hour before or 2 hours after meals. Do not take within 1 hour before or 2 hours after antacids or cholestyramine medications. Do not alter dose and do not discontinue without consulting prescriber. Maintain adequate hydration (2-3 L/day of fluids) during entire course of therapy unless instructed to restrict fluid intake. You will be susceptible to infection (avoid crowds and exposure to infection). May be at increased risk for skin cancer, wear protective clothing and use sunscreen with high protective factor to help limit exposure to sunlight and UV light. If you have diabetes, monitor glucose levels closely (drug may alter glucose levels). You may experience dizziness or trembling (use caution until response to medication is known); nausea or vomiting (small frequent meals, frequent mouth care may help); diarrhea (boiled milk, yogurt, or buttermilk may help); sores or white plaques in mouth (frequent rinsing of mouth and frequent mouth care may help); or muscle or back pain (mild analgesics may be recommended). Report chest pain; acute headache or dizziness; symptoms of respiratory infection, cough, or respiratory difficulty; unresolved GI effects; fatigue, chills, fever unhealed sores, white plaques in mouth; irritation in genital area or unusual discharge; unusual bruising or bleeding; or other unusual effects related to this medication. **Pregnancy/breast-feeding precautions:** Inform prescriber if you are or intend to become pregnant. Two reliable forms of contraception should be used prior to, during, and for 6 weeks after therapy. Breast-feeding is not recommended.

Dietary Considerations: Oral dosage formulations should be taken on an empty stomach to avoid variability in MPA absorption. However, in stable renal transplant patients, may be administered with food if necessary. Oral suspension contains 0.56 mg phenylalanine/mL; use caution if administered to patients with phenylketonuria.

Pregnancy Risk Factor: C (manufacturer)

Pregnancy Issues: There are no adequate and well-controlled studies using mycophenolate in pregnant women, however, it may cause fetal harm. Women of childbearing potential should have a negative pregnancy test prior to beginning therapy. Two reliable forms of contraception should be used prior to, during, and for 6 weeks after therapy.

Lactation: Excretion in breast milk unknown/not recommended

Breast-Feeding Issues: It is unknown if mycophenolate is excreted in human milk. Due to potentially serious adverse reactions, the decision to discontinue the drug or discontinue breast-feeding should be considered. Breast-feeding is not recommended during therapy or for 6 weeks after treatment is complete.

Administration

Oral: Oral dosage formulations (tablet, capsule, suspension) should be administered as soon as possible following transplantation. Oral dosage forms should be administered on an empty stomach to avoid variability in MPA absorption. The oral solution may be administered via a nasogastric tube (minimum 8 French, 1.7 mm interior diameter) and cannot be mixed with other medications. Delayed release tablets should not be crushed, cut, or chewed.

I.V.: Intravenous solutions should be given over at least 2 hours. Do not administer intravenous solution by rapid or bolus injection.

Reconstitution:

Oral suspension: Should be constituted by a pharmacist prior to dispensing to the patient and **not** mixed with any other medication. Closed bottle should be tapped to loosen the powder. Add 47 mL of water to the bottle and shake well for ~1 minute. Add another 47 mL of water to the bottle and shake well for an additional minute. Remove child-resistant cap and push bottle adapter into neck of the bottle; close bottle with child-resistant cap tightly to assure proper placement of adapter and status of child-resistant cap. Final concentration is 200 mg/mL of mycophenolate mofetil.

Injection: Does not contain an antibacterial preservative; therefore, reconstitution and dilution of the product must be done under aseptic conditions. Preparation of intravenous formulation should take place in a vertical laminar flow hood with the same precautions as antineoplastic agents.

I.V. preparation procedure Step 1:

a. Two vials of mycophenolate injection are used for preparing a 1 g dose, whereas 3 vials are needed for each 1.5 g dose. Reconstitute the contents of each vial by injecting 14 mL of 5% dextrose injection.

b. Gently shake the vial to dissolve the drug

c. Inspect the resulting slightly yellow solution for particulate matter and discoloration prior to further dilution. Discard the vial if particulate matter or discoloration is observed.

I.V. preparation procedure Step 2:

a. To prepare a 1 g dose, further dilute the contents of the two reconstituted vials into 140 mL of 5% dextrose in water. To prepare a 1.5 g dose, further dilute the contents of the three reconstituted vials into 210 mL of 5% dextrose in water. The final concentration of both solutions is 6 mg mycophenolate mofetil per mL.

(Continued)

Mycophenolate *(Continued)*

b. Inspect the infusion solution for particulate matter or discoloration. Discard the infusion solution if particulate matter or discoloration is observed.

Storage:

Capsules: Store at room temperature of 15°C to 39°C (59°F to 86°F).

Tablets: Store at room temperature of 15°C to 39°C (59°F to 86°F). Protect from light.

Oral suspension: Store powder for oral suspension at room temperature of 15°C to 39°C (59°F to 86°F). Once reconstituted, the oral solution may be stored at room temperature or under refrigeration. Do not freeze. The mixed suspension is stable for 60 days.

Injection: Store intact vials at room temperature 15°C to 30°C (59°F to 86°F). Stability of the infusion solution: 4 hours from reconstitution and dilution of the product. Store solutions at 15°C to 30°C (59°F to 86°F).

- ◆ **Mycophenolate Mofetil** *see* Mycophenolate *on page 1040*
- ◆ **Mycophenolate Sodium** *see* Mycophenolate *on page 1040*
- ◆ **Mycophenolic Acid** *see* Mycophenolate *on page 1040*
- ◆ **Mycostatin®** *see* Nystatin *on page 1103*
- ◆ **Mydfrin®** *see* Phenylephrine *on page 1200*
- ◆ **Mydriacyl®** *see page 1625*
- ◆ **Myfortic®** *see* Mycophenolate *on page 1040*
- ◆ **Mylanta® Children's [OTC]** *see* Calcium Carbonate *on page 235*
- ◆ **Myleran®** *see* Busulfan *on page 223*
- ◆ **Mylocel™** *see* Hydroxyurea *on page 771*
- ◆ **Mylotarg®** *see* Gemtuzumab Ozogamicin *on page 707*
- ◆ **myrac™** *see* Minocycline *on page 1012*
- ◆ **Mysoline®** *see* Primidone *on page 1251*
- ◆ **Mytelase®** *see* Ambenonium *on page 85*
- ◆ **Mytussin® AC** *see* Guaifenesin and Codeine *on page 731*
- ◆ **Mytussin® DAC** *see* Guaifenesin, Pseudoephedrine, and Codeine *on page 735*
- ◆ **Nabi-HB®** *see page 1660*
- ◆ **NAB-Paclitaxel** *see* Paclitaxel (Protein Bound) *on page 1146*

Nabumetone *(na BYOO me tone)*

U.S. Brand Names Relafen®

Generic Available Yes

Pharmacologic Category Nonsteroidal Anti-inflammatory Drug (NSAID), Oral

Use Management of osteoarthritis and rheumatoid arthritis

Unlabeled/Investigational Use Sunburn, mild to moderate pain

Mechanism of Action/Effect Nabumetone is a nonacidic NSAID that inhibits the production of inflammation and pain during arthritis. The active metabolite of nabumetone is felt to be the compound primarily responsible for therapeutic effect. Comparatively, the parent drug is a poor inhibitor of prostaglandin synthesis.

Contraindications Hypersensitivity to NSAIDs including aspirin, or any component of the formulation; should not be administered to patients with active peptic ulceration and those with severe hepatic impairment or in patients in whom nabumetone, aspirin, or other NSAIDs have induced asthma, urticaria, or other allergic-type reactions; fatal asthmatic reactions have occurred following NSAID administration; pregnancy (3rd trimester)

Warnings/Precautions Fatal asthmatic and anaphylactoid reactions have occurred in patients with "aspirin triad." Use with caution in patients with CHF, hypertension, dehydration, decreased renal or hepatic function, history of GI disease (bleeding, ulcers, or previous GI symptoms with NSAID use), or those receiving anticoagulants and/or corticosteroids. Use lowest effective dose for shortest period possible; bleeding risk has been correlated to dose and duration of therapy. Gastrointestinal bleeding may occur without prior symptoms of gastrointestinal irritation. Elderly are at a high risk for adverse effects from NSAIDs. As many as 60% of elderly can develop peptic ulceration and/or hemorrhage asymptomatically.

Use of NSAIDs can compromise existing renal function especially when Cl_{cr} <30 mL/minute. CNS adverse effects such as confusion, agitation, and hallucination are generally seen in overdose or high-dose situations; however, elderly may demonstrate these adverse effects at lower doses than younger adults. Withhold for at least 4-6 half-lives prior to surgical or dental procedures.

Drug Interactions

Decreased Effect: NSAIDs may decrease the effect of some antihypertensive agents, including ACE inhibitors, angiotensin receptor antagonists, and hydralazine. The efficacy of diuretics (loop and/or thiazide) may be decreased.

Increased Effect/Toxicity: NSAIDs may increase digoxin, methotrexate, and lithium serum concentrations. The renal adverse effects of ACE inhibitors may be potentiated by NSAIDs. Potential for bleeding may be increased with anticoagulants or antiplatelet agents. Concurrent use of corticosteroids may increase the risk of GI ulceration.

Nutritional/Ethanol Interactions

Ethanol: Avoid ethanol (may enhance gastric mucosal irritation).

Food: Nabumetone peak serum concentrations may be increased if taken with food or dairy products.

Herb/Nutraceutical: Avoid cat's claw, dong quai, evening primrose, feverfew, garlic, ginger, ginkgo, red clover, horse chestnut, green tea, ginseng (all have additional antiplatelet activity).

Adverse Reactions

>10%:

Central nervous system: Dizziness

Dermatologic: Rash

Gastrointestinal: Abdominal cramps, abdominal pain (12%), diarrhea (14%), dyspepsia (13%), heartburn, indigestion, nausea

1% to 10%:
    Central nervous system: Headache, nervousness
    Dermatologic: Itching
    Endocrine & metabolic: Fluid retention
    Gastrointestinal: Vomiting
    Otic: Tinnitus

Overdosage/Toxicology Symptoms of overdose include apnea, metabolic acidosis, coma, nystagmus, leukocytosis, and renal failure. Management of NSAID intoxication is supportive and symptomatic.

Pharmacodynamics/Kinetics
  Onset of Action: Several days
  Time to Peak: Serum: Metabolite: Oral: 3-6 hours; Synovial fluid: 4-12 hours
  Protein Binding: >99%
  Half-Life Elimination: Major metabolite: 24 hours
  Metabolism: Prodrug, rapidly metabolized to an active metabolite (6-methoxy-2-naphthylacetic acid); extensive first-pass effect
  Excretion: Urine (80%) and feces (10%) with little as unchanged drug

Dosing
  Adults: Osteoarthritis, rheumatoid arthritis: Oral: 1000 mg/day; an additional 500-1000 mg may be needed in some patients to obtain more symptomatic relief; may be administered once or twice daily.
  Elderly: Refer to adult dosing; do not exceed 2000 mg/day.

Available Dosage Forms Tablet: 500 mg, 750 mg

Monitoring and Teaching Issues
  Physical Assessment: Assess effectiveness and interactions of other medications patient may be taking. Assess results of laboratory tests, therapeutic effectiveness, and adverse reactions (eg, GI effects, hepatotoxicity, or ototoxicity) at beginning of therapy and periodically throughout therapy. Schedule ophthalmic evaluations for patients who develop eye complaints during long-term NSAID therapy. Assess knowledge/teach patient appropriate use, interventions to reduce side effects, and adverse symptoms to report.
  Monitoring Laboratory Tests: Patients with renal insufficiency: Baseline renal function followed by repeat test within weeks (to determine if renal function has deteriorated)
  Patient Education: Take this medication exactly as directed; do not increase dose without consulting prescriber. Do not crush tablets. Take with food or milk to reduce GI distress. Maintain adequate hydration (2-3 L/day of fluids) unless instructed to restrict fluid intake. Do not use alcohol, aspirin or aspirin-containing medication, or any other anti-inflammatory medications without consulting healthcare prescriber. You may experience drowsiness, dizziness, nervousness, or headache (use caution when driving or engaging in tasks requiring alertness until response to drug is known); anorexia, nausea, vomiting, or heartburn (small frequent meals, frequent oral care, sucking lozenges, or chewing gum may help); fluid retention (weigh yourself weekly and report unusual [3-5 lb/week] weight gain). GI bleeding, ulceration, or perforation can occur with or without pain; discontinue medication and contact prescriber if persistent abdominal pain or cramping, or blood in stool occurs. Report breathlessness, respiratory difficulty, or unusual cough; chest pain, rapid heartbeat, palpitations; unusual bruising/bleeding; blood in urine, stool, mouth, or vomitus; swollen extremities; skin rash or itching; acute fatigue; or hearing changes (ringing in ears).
  Pregnancy/breast-feeding precautions: Inform prescriber if you are pregnant. Breast-feeding is not recommended.
  Geriatric Considerations: In trials with nabumetone, no significant differences were noted between young and elderly in regards to efficacy and safety. However, elderly are at high risk for adverse effects from NSAIDs. As much as 60% of elderly can develop peptic ulceration and/or hemorrhage asymptomatically. The concomitant use of H_2 blockers, omeprazole, and sucralfate is not effective as prophylaxis with the exception of NSAID-induced duodenal ulcers which may be prevented by the use of ranitidine. Misoprostol is the only prophylactic agent proven effective. Also, concomitant disease and drug use contribute to the risk for GI adverse effects. Use lowest effective dose for shortest period possible. Consider renal function decline with age. Use of NSAIDs can compromise existing renal function especially when Cl_{cr} is ≤30 mL/minute. Tinnitus may be a difficult and unreliable indication of toxicity due to age-related hearing loss or eighth cranial nerve damage. CNS adverse effects such as confusion, agitation, and hallucination are generally seen in overdose or high-dose situations, but elderly may demonstrate these adverse effects at lower doses than younger adults.
  Pregnancy Risk Factor: C/D (3rd trimester)
  Lactation: Enters breast milk/not recommended

Related Information
  Nonsalicylate / Nonsteroidal Anti-inflammatory Agents *on page 1743*

- **NAC** *see* Acetylcysteine *on page 45*
- **N-Acetylcysteine** *see* Acetylcysteine *on page 45*
- **N-Acetyl-L-Cysteine** *see* Acetylcysteine *on page 45*
- **N-Acetyl-P-Aminophenol** *see* Acetaminophen *on page 38*

Nadolol (nay DOE lole)

U.S. Brand Names Corgard®
Generic Available Yes
Pharmacologic Category Beta-Adrenergic Blocker, Nonselective
Medication Safety Issues
  Sound-alike/look-alike issues:
    Nadolol may be confused with Mandol®
    Corgard® may be confused with Cognex®

Use Treatment of hypertension and angina pectoris; prophylaxis of migraine headaches
Mechanism of Action/Effect Competitively blocks response to beta$_1$- and beta$_2$-adrenergic stimulation; does not exhibit any membrane stabilizing or intrinsic sympathomimetic activity
(Continued)

Nadolol *(Continued)*

Contraindications Hypersensitivity to nadolol or any component of the formulation; bronchial asthma; sinus bradycardia; sinus node dysfunction; heart block greater than first degree (except in patients with a functioning artificial pacemaker); cardiogenic shock; uncompensated cardiac failure

Warnings/Precautions Administer only with extreme caution in patients with compensated heart failure, monitor for a worsening of the condition. Efficacy in heart failure has not been established for nadolol. Use caution with concurrent use of beta-blockers and either verapamil or diltiazem; bradycardia or heart block can occur. In general, patients with bronchospastic disease should not receive beta-blockers. Nadolol, if used at all, should be used cautiously in bronchospastic disease with close monitoring. Use cautiously in patients with diabetes because it can mask prominent hypoglycemic symptoms. Can mask signs of thyrotoxicosis. Can cause fetal harm when administered in pregnancy. Use cautiously in the renally impaired (dosage adjustments are required). Use care with anesthetic agents which decrease myocardial function. Beta-blocker therapy should not be withdrawn abruptly (particularly in patients with CAD), but gradually tapered to avoid acute tachycardia, hypertension, and/or ischemia.

Drug Interactions

Decreased Effect: Decreased effect of beta-blockers with aluminum salts, barbiturates, calcium salts, cholestyramine, colestipol, NSAIDs, penicillins (ampicillin), rifampin, salicylates, and sulfinpyrazone due to decreased bioavailability and plasma levels. Beta-blockers may decrease the effect of sulfonylureas (possibly hyperglycemia). Nonselective beta-blockers blunt the effect of beta-2 adrenergic agonists (albuterol).

Increased Effect/Toxicity: The heart rate lowering effects of nadolol are additive with other drugs which slow AV conduction (digoxin, verapamil, diltiazem). Concurrent use of alpha-blockers (prazosin, terazosin) with beta-blockers may increase risk of orthostasis. Nadolol may mask the tachycardia from hypoglycemia caused by insulin and oral hypoglycemics. In patients receiving concurrent therapy, the risk of hypertensive crisis is increased when either clonidine or the beta-blocker is withdrawn. Reserpine has been shown to enhance the effect of beta-blockers. Avoid using with alpha-adrenergic stimulants (phenylephrine, epinephrine, etc) which may have exaggerated hypertensive responses. Beta-blockers may affect the action or levels of ethanol, disopyramide, nondepolarizing muscle relaxants, and theophylline although the effects are difficult to predict. The vasoconstrictive effects of ergot alkaloids may be enhanced.

Nutritional/Ethanol Interactions Herb/Nutraceutical: Avoid dong quai if using for hypertension (has estrogenic activity). Avoid ephedra, garlic, yohimbe, ginseng (may worsen hypertension). Avoid natural licorice (causes sodium and water retention and increases potassium loss).

Adverse Reactions

>10%:

Central nervous system: Drowsiness, insomnia

Endocrine & metabolic: Decreased sexual ability

1% to 10%:

Cardiovascular: Bradycardia, palpitation, edema, CHF, reduced peripheral circulation

Central nervous system: Mental depression

Gastrointestinal: Diarrhea or constipation, nausea, vomiting, stomach discomfort

Respiratory: Bronchospasm

Miscellaneous: Cold extremities

Overdosage/Toxicology Symptoms of intoxication include cardiac disturbances, CNS toxicity, bronchospasm, hypoglycemia and hyperkalemia. The most common cardiac symptoms include hypotension and bradycardia. Atrioventricular block, intraventricular conduction disturbances, cardiogenic shock, and asystole may occur with severe overdose. CNS effects include convulsions, coma, and respiratory arrest. Treatment is symptom-directed and supportive. Glucagon has been used to reverse cardiac depression.

Pharmacodynamics/Kinetics

Duration of Action: 17-24 hours

Absorption: 30% to 40%

Time to Peak: Serum: 2-4 hours

Protein Binding: 28%

Half-Life Elimination: Adults: 10-24 hours, prolonged with renal impairment; End-stage renal disease: 45 hours

Excretion: Urine (as unchanged drug)

Dosing

Adults:

Hypertension, angina: Oral: Initial: 40-80 mg/day, increase dosage gradually by 40-80 mg increments at 3- to 7-day intervals until optimum clinical response is obtained with profound slowing of heart rate. Doses up to 160-240 mg/day in angina and 240-320 mg/day in hypertension may be necessary. Doses as high as 640 mg/day have been used. *Usual dosage range (JNC 7):* 40-120 mg once daily

Elderly: Oral: Initial: 20 mg/day; increase doses by 20 mg increments at 3- to 7-day intervals; usual dosage range: 20-240 mg/day. Adjust for renal impairment.

Renal Impairment:

Cl_{cr} 31-40 mL/minute: Administer every 24-36 hours or administer 50% of normal dose.

Cl_{cr} 10-30 mL/minute: Administer every 24-48 hours or administer 50% of normal dose.

Cl_{cr} <10 mL/minute: Administer every 40-60 hours or administer 25% of normal dose.

Hemodialysis effects: Moderately dialyzable (20% to 50%) via hemodialysis. Administer dose postdialysis or administer 40 mg supplemental dose. Supplemental dose is not necessary following peritoneal dialysis.

Hepatic Impairment: Reduced dose is probably necessary.

Available Dosage Forms Tablet: 20 mg, 40 mg, 80 mg, 120 mg, 160 mg

Monitoring and Teaching Issues

Physical Assessment: Assess other medications the patient may be taking for effectiveness and interactions. Assess blood pressure and heart rate prior to and following first dose, any change in dosage, and periodically thereafter. Monitor or advise patient to monitor weight and fluid balance, assess for signs of CHF, and assess therapeutic effectiveness. Monitor serum glucose levels of patients with diabetes since beta-blockers may alter glucose tolerance. Use/teach postural hypotension precautions.

Patient Education: Check pulse daily prior to taking medication. If pulse is <50, hold medication and consult prescriber. Take exactly as directed; do not adjust dosage or discontinue without consulting prescriber. May cause dizziness, fatigue, blurred vision; change position slowly (lying/sitting to standing) and use caution when driving or engaging in tasks that require alertness until response to drug is known. Exercise and increasing bulk or fiber in diet may help resolve constipation. If you have diabetes, monitor serum glucose closely (the drug may mask symptoms of hypoglycemia). Report swelling in feet or legs, respiratory difficulty or persistent cough, unresolved fatigue, unusual weight gain >5 lb/week, or unresolved constipation. **Pregnancy/breast-feeding precautions:** Inform prescriber if you are or intend to become pregnant. Consult prescriber if breast-feeding.

Dietary Considerations: May be taken without regard to meals.

Geriatric Considerations: Due to alterations in the beta-adrenergic autonomic nervous system, beta-adrenergic blockade may result in less hemodynamic response than seen in younger adults. Studies indicate that despite decreased sensitivity to the chronotropic effects of beta blockade with age, there appears to be an increased myocardial sensitivity to the negative inotropic effect during stress (eg, exercise). See Warnings/Precautions.

Pregnancy Risk Factor: C

Pregnancy Issues: No data available on crossing the placenta. Beta-blockers have been associated with bradycardia, hypotension, and IUGR; IUGR is probably related to maternal hypertension. Alternative beta-blockers are preferred for use during pregnancy due to limited data and prolonged half-life. Cases of neonatal hypoglycemia have been reported following maternal use of beta-blockers at parturition or during breast-feeding. Monitor breast-fed infant for symptoms of beta-blockade.

Lactation: Enters breast milk/use caution (AAP rates "compatible")

Breast-Feeding Issues: Considered compatible by the AAP. However, monitor the infant for signs of beta-blockade (hypotension, bradycardia, etc) with long-term use.

Related Information
Beta-Blockers *on page 1720*

Nafarelin (NAF a re lin)

U.S. Brand Names Synarel®

Synonyms Nafarelin Acetate

Generic Available No

Pharmacologic Category Gonadotropin Releasing Hormone Agonist

Medication Safety Issues
Sound-alike/look-alike issues:
Nafarelin may be confused with Anafranil®, enalapril

Use Treatment of endometriosis, including pain and reduction of lesions; treatment of central precocious puberty (gonadotropin-dependent precocious puberty) in children of both sexes

Mechanism of Action/Effect Potent synthetic decapeptide analogue of gonadotropin-releasing hormone (GnRH; LHRH) which is approximately 200 times more potent than GnRH in terms of pituitary release of luteinizing hormone (LH) and follicle-stimulating hormone (FSH)

Contraindications Hypersensitivity to GnRH, GnRH-agonist analogs, or any component of the formulation; undiagnosed abnormal vaginal bleeding; pregnancy

Warnings/Precautions Use with caution in patients with risk factors for decreased bone mineral content. Nafarelin therapy may pose an additional risk. Hypersensitivity reactions occur in 0.2% of the patients.

Adverse Reactions
>10%:
Central nervous system: Headache, emotional lability
Dermatologic: Acne
Endocrine & metabolic: Hot flashes, decreased libido, decreased breast size
Genitourinary: Vaginal dryness
Neuromuscular & skeletal: Myalgia
Respiratory: Nasal irritation
1% to 10%:
Cardiovascular: Edema, chest pain
Central nervous system: Insomnia
Dermatologic: Urticaria, rash, pruritus, seborrhea
Respiratory: Dyspnea

Pharmacodynamics/Kinetics
Time to Peak: Serum: 10-45 minutes
Protein Binding: Plasma: 80%

Dosing
Adults & Elderly: Endometriosis: Nasal: 1 spray (200 mcg) in 1 nostril each morning and the other nostril each evening starting on days 2-4 of menstrual cycle for 6 months
Pediatrics: Central precocious puberty: Nasal: 2 sprays (400 mcg) into each nostril in the morning 2 sprays (400 mcg) into each nostril in the evening. If inadequate suppression, may increase dose to 3 sprays (600 mcg) into alternating nostrils 3 times/day.

Available Dosage Forms Solution, intranasal spray, as acetate: 2 mg/mL (8 mL) [200 mcg/spray: 60 metered doses]

Monitoring and Teaching Issues
Physical Assessment: For treatment of precocious puberty, consult appropriate pediatric reference. Assess therapeutic effectiveness and adverse response. Teach patient (caregiver) proper use (correct timing and administration of nasal spray), possible side effects/appropriate interventions, and adverse symptoms to report. **Pregnancy risk factor X:** Determine that female patient is not pregnant before beginning therapy. Do not give to childbearing age female unless capable of complying with contraceptive use.

(Continued)

Nafarelin (Continued)

Patient Education: Endometriosis: You will begin this treatment between days 2-4 of your regular menstrual cycle. Use as directed, daily at the same time (arising and bedtime), and rotate nostrils. Maintain regular follow-up schedule. May cause hot flashes, flushing, or redness (cold clothes and cool environment may help); decreased or increased libido; emotional lability; weight gain; decreased breast size; or hirsutism. Report any breakthrough bleeding or continuing menstruation or musculoskeletal pain. Do not use a nasal decongestant within 30 minutes after nafarelin. **Pregnancy/breast-feeding precautions:** Inform prescriber if you are pregnant. Do not get pregnant while taking this medication. Consult prescriber for instruction on appropriate contraceptive measures. Do not breast-feed.

Pregnancy Risk Factor: X

Lactation: Enters breast milk/contraindicated

Administration

Inhalation: Nasal spray: Do not give to pregnant or breast-feeding patients. Do not use topical nasal decongestant for at least 30 minutes after nafarelin use.

Storage: Store at room temperature. Protect from light.

Additional Information Each spray delivers 200 mcg

♦ **Nafarelin Acetate** *see* Nafarelin *on page 1047*

Nafcillin (naf SIL in)

Synonyms Ethoxynaphthamido Penicillin Sodium; Nafcillin Sodium; Nallpen; Sodium Nafcillin

Generic Available Yes

Pharmacologic Category Antibiotic, Penicillin

Use Treatment of infections such as osteomyelitis, septicemia, endocarditis, and CNS infections caused by susceptible strains of staphylococci species

Mechanism of Action/Effect Interferes with bacterial cell wall synthesis during active multiplication, causing cell wall death and resultant bactericidal activity against susceptible bacteria

Contraindications Hypersensitivity to nafcillin, or any component of the formulation, or penicillins

Warnings/Precautions Extravasation of I.V. infusions should be avoided. Modification of dosage is necessary in patients with both severe renal and hepatic impairment. Elimination rate will be slow in neonates.

Drug Interactions

Cytochrome P450 Effect: Induces CYP3A4 (strong)

Decreased Effect: Chloramphenicol may decrease nafcillin efficacy. If taken concomitantly with warfarin, nafcillin may inhibit the anticoagulant response to warfarin. This effect may persist for up to 30 days after nafcillin has been discontinued. Subtherapeutic cyclosporine levels may result when taken concomitantly with nafcillin. Although anecdotal reports suggest oral contraceptive efficacy could be reduced by penicillins, this has been refuted by more rigorous scientific and clinical data. Nafcillin may decrease the levels/effects of benzodiazepines, calcium channel blockers, clarithromycin, cyclosporine, erythromycin, estrogens, mirtazapine, nateglinide, nefazodone, nevirapine, protease inhibitors, tacrolimus, venlafaxine, and other CYP3A4 substrates.

Increased Effect/Toxicity: Probenecid may cause an increase in nafcillin levels. Penicillins may increase the exposure to methotrexate during concurrent therapy; monitor.

Lab Interactions Positive Coombs' test (direct)

Adverse Reactions Frequency not defined.

Central nervous system: Pain, fever

Dermatologic: Rash

Gastrointestinal: Nausea, diarrhea

Hematologic: Agranulocytosis, bone marrow depression, neutropenia

Local: Pain, swelling, inflammation, phlebitis, skin sloughing, and thrombophlebitis at the injection site; oxacillin (less likely to cause phlebitis) is often preferred in pediatric patients

Renal: Interstitial nephritis (acute)

Miscellaneous: Hypersensitivity reactions

Overdosage/Toxicology Symptoms of penicillin overdose include neuromuscular hypersensitivity (eg, agitation, hallucinations, asterixis, encephalopathy, confusion, and seizures). Electrolyte imbalance may occur if the preparation contains potassium or sodium salts, especially in renal failure. Treatment is supportive or symptom-directed.

Pharmacodynamics/Kinetics

Time to Peak: Serum: I.M.: 30-60 minutes

Protein Binding: 70% to 90%

Half-Life Elimination:

Neonates: <3 weeks: 2.2-5.5 hours; 4-9 weeks: 1.2-2.3 hours

Children 3 months to 14 years: 0.75-1.9 hours

Adults: Normal renal/hepatic function: 30 minutes to 1.5 hours

Metabolism: Primarily hepatic; undergoes enterohepatic recirculation

Excretion: Primarily feces; urine (10% to 30% as unchanged drug)

Dosing

Adults & Elderly:

Susceptible infections:

I.M.: 500 mg every 4-6 hours

I.V.: 500-2000 mg every 4-6 hours

Pediatrics:

Susceptible infections: Children:

I.M.: 25 mg/kg twice daily

I.V.:

Mild to moderate infections: 50-100 mg/kg/day in divided doses every 6 hours

Severe infections: 100-200 mg/kg/day in divided doses every 4-6 hours

Maximum dose: 12 g/day

Renal Impairment: No adjustment is necessary.

Hemodialysis effects: Not dialyzable (0% to 5%) via hemodialysis. Supplemental dose is not necessary with hemo- or peritoneal dialysis or continuous arteriovenous or venovenous hemofiltration.

Hepatic Impairment: In patients with both hepatic and renal impairment, modification of dosage may be necessary; no data available.

Available Dosage Forms

Infusion [premixed iso-osmotic dextrose solution]: 1 g (50 mL); 2 g (100 mL)

Injection, powder for reconstitution, as sodium: 1 g, 2 g, 10 g

Monitoring and Teaching Issues

Physical Assessment: Assess results of culture and sensitivity tests and allergy history prior to starting therapy. See Warnings/Precautions for use cautions (eg, renal or hepatic impairment). Assess potential for interactions with other pharmacological agents patient may be taking (eg, Increased [toxic] or decreased [subtherapeutic] levels/effects; see Drug Interactions). Infusion/Injection site must be monitored closely to prevent extravasation (use ice packs). Assess for therapeutic effect (resolution of infection) and adverse reactions (eg, hypersensitivity, opportunistic infection [eg, fever, chills, unhealed sores, white plaques in mouth or vagina, purulent vaginal discharge, fatigue]; see Adverse Reactions). Teach patient possible side effects/appropriate interventions and adverse symptoms to report (see Patient Education).

Monitoring Laboratory Tests: Perform culture and sensitivity studies prior to initiating drug therapy. Monitor renal, hepatic, CBC with prolonged therapy.

Patient Education: Do not take any new medication during therapy unless approved by prescriber. This medication can only be administered by infusion or injection. Report immediately any redness, swelling, burning, or pain at injection/infusion site; difficulty breathing or swallowing; chest pain; or chills. May cause nausea (small frequent meals, frequent mouth care, chewing gum, or sucking lozenges may help); or opportunistic infection (eg, fever, chills, sore throat, burning urination, fatigue). Report persistent side effects or if condition does not respond to treatment. **Breast-feeding precaution:** Consult prescriber if breast-feeding.

Dietary Considerations: Sodium content of 1 g: 76.6 mg (3.33 mEq)

Geriatric Considerations: Nafcillin has not been studied exclusively in the elderly, however, given its route of elimination, dosage adjustments based upon age and renal function are not necessary. Consider sodium content in patients who may be sensitive to volume expansion (ie, CHF).

Pregnancy Risk Factor: B

Lactation: Enters breast milk/use caution

Administration

I.M.: Rotate injection sites.

I.V.: Vesicant. Administer around-the-clock to promote less variation in peak and trough serum levels. Infuse over 30-60 minutes.

Compatibility: Stable in dextran 40 10% in dextrose, D_5LR, $D_5\frac{1}{4}NS$, $D_5\frac{1}{2}NS$, D_5NS, D_5W, $D_{10}NS$, $D_{10}W$, LR, NS

Y-site administration: Incompatible with droperidol, fentanyl and droperidol, insulin (regular), labetalol, midazolam, nalbuphine, pentazocine, verapamil

Compatibility when admixed: Incompatible with ascorbic acid injection, aztreonam, bleomycin, cytarabine, gentamicin, hydrocortisone sodium succinate, methylprednisolone sodium succinate, promazine

Storage: Reconstituted parenteral solution is stable for 3 days at room temperature, 7 days when refrigerated, or 12 weeks when frozen. For I.V. infusion in NS or D_5W, solution is stable for 24 hours at room temperature and 96 hours when refrigerated.

♦ **Nafcillin Sodium** *see* Nafcillin *on page 1048*

♦ **NaHCO₃** *see* Sodium Bicarbonate *on page 1380*

Nalbuphine (NAL byoo feen)

U.S. Brand Names Nubain®

Synonyms Nalbuphine Hydrochloride

Generic Available Yes

Pharmacologic Category Analgesic, Narcotic

Medication Safety Issues

Sound-alike/look-alike issues:

Nubain® may be confused with Navane®, Nebcin®

Use Relief of moderate to severe pain; preoperative analgesia, postoperative and surgical anesthesia, and obstetrical analgesia during labor and delivery

Mechanism of Action/Effect Binds to opiate receptors in the CNS, causing inhibition of ascending pain pathways, altering the perception of and response to pain; produces generalized CNS depression

Contraindications Hypersensitivity to nalbuphine or any component, including sulfites; pregnancy (prolonged use or high dosages at term)

Warnings/Precautions Use with caution in patients with recent myocardial infarction, biliary tract surgery, or sulfite sensitivity; may produce respiratory depression; use with caution in women delivering premature infants; use with caution in patients with a history of drug dependence, head trauma or increased intracranial pressure, decreased hepatic or renal function, or pregnancy; tolerance or drug dependence may result from extended use

Drug Interactions

Increased Effect/Toxicity: Barbiturate anesthetics may increase CNS depression.

Nutritional/Ethanol Interactions

Ethanol: Avoid ethanol (may increase CNS depression).

Herb/Nutraceutical: Avoid valerian, St John's wort, kava kava, gotu kola (may increase CNS depression).

(Continued)

Nalbuphine *(Continued)*

Adverse Reactions

>10%:

Central nervous system: Fatigue, drowsiness

Miscellaneous: Histamine release

1% to 10%:

Cardiovascular: Hypotension

Central nervous system: Headache, nightmares, dizziness

Gastrointestinal: Anorexia, nausea, vomiting, dry mouth

Local: Pain at injection site

Neuromuscular & skeletal: Weakness

Overdosage/Toxicology Symptoms of overdose include CNS depression, respiratory depression, miosis, hypotension, and bradycardia. Treatment is symptomatic. Naloxone, 2 mg I.V. with repeat administration as necessary up to a total dose of 10 mg, can be used to reverse opiate effects.

Pharmacodynamics/Kinetics

Onset of Action: Peak effect: I.M.: 30 minutes; I.V.: 1-3 minutes

Half-Life Elimination: 3.5-5 hours

Metabolism: Hepatic

Excretion: Feces; urine ($\sim$7% as metabolites)

Dosing

Adults: Analgesic: I.M., I.V., SubQ: 10 mg/70 kg every 3-6 hours; maximum single dose: 20 mg; maximum daily dose: 160 mg

Elderly: Refer to adult dosing; use with caution.

Pediatrics: I.M., I.V., SubQ: Children 10 months to 14 years: Premedication: 0.2 mg/kg; maximum: 20 mg/dose

Renal Impairment: Use with caution and reduce dose.

Hepatic Impairment: Use with caution and reduce dose.

Available Dosage Forms

Injection, solution, as hydrochloride: 10 mg/mL (10 mL); 20 mg/mL (10 mL)

Injection, solution, as hydrochloride [preservative free]: 10 mg/mL (1 mL); 20 mg/mL (1 mL)

Monitoring and Teaching Issues

Physical Assessment: Assess effectiveness and interactions of other medications patient may be taking. Monitor therapeutic effectiveness (eg, pain relief) and adverse reactions at beginning of therapy and periodically throughout therapy. Monitor blood pressure, CNS and respiratory status, and degree of sedation at beginning of therapy and at regular intervals during use. For inpatients, implement safety measures. Generally used in conjunction with surgical anesthesia or during labor and delivery; however, if self-administered for relief of pain, assess knowledge/teach patient appropriate use, adverse reactions to report, and appropriate interventions to reduce side effects.

Patient Education: If self-administered, use exactly as directed; do not increase dose or frequency. Drug may cause physical and/or psychological dependence. While using this medication, do not use alcohol and other prescription or OTC medications (especially sedatives, tranquilizers, antihistamines, or pain medications) without consulting prescriber. Maintain adequate hydration (2-3 L/day of fluids) unless instructed to restrict fluid intake. May cause hypotension, dizziness, drowsiness, impaired coordination, or blurred vision (use caution when driving, climbing stairs, or changing position - rising from sitting or lying to standing, or when engaging in tasks requiring alertness until response to drug is known); loss of appetite, nausea, or vomiting (frequent mouth care, small frequent meals, chewing gum, or sucking lozenges may help); or constipation (increased exercise, fluids, fruit, or fiber may help; if unresolved, consult prescriber about use of stool softeners). Report chest pain, slow or rapid heartbeat, acute dizziness or persistent headache; changes in mental status; swelling of extremities or unusual weight gain; changes in urinary elimination or pain on urination; acute headache; back or flank pain or muscle spasms; blurred vision; skin rash; or shortness of breath. **Pregnancy/breast-feeding precautions:** Inform prescriber if you are or intend to become pregnant. If you are breast-feeding, take medication immediately after breast-feeding or 3-4 hours prior to next feeding.

Geriatric Considerations: The elderly may be particularly susceptible to CNS effects; monitor closely.

Pregnancy Risk Factor: B/D (prolonged use or high doses at term)

Pregnancy Issues: Severe fetal bradycardia has been reported following use in labor/delivery. Fetal bradycardia may occur when administered earlier in pregnancy (not documented). Use only if clearly needed, with monitoring to detect and manage possible adverse fetal effects. Naloxone has been reported to reverse bradycardia. Newborn should be monitored for respiratory depression or bradycardia following nalbuphine use in labor.

Lactation: Excretion in breast milk unknown/use caution

Administration

Compatibility: Stable in D_5NS, $D_{10}W$, LR, NS

Y-site administration: Incompatible with allopurinol, amphotericin B cholesteryl sulfate complex, cefepime, docetaxel, methotrexate, nafcillin, piperacillin/tazobactam, sargramostim, sodium bicarbonate

Compatibility in syringe: Incompatible with diazepam, ketorolac, pentobarbital

Related Information

Compatibility of Drugs in Syringe *on page 1725*

Narcotic / Opioid Analgesic Comparison *on page 1739*

- ◆ **Nalbuphine Hydrochloride** *see* Nalbuphine *on page 1049*
- ◆ **Naldecon Senior EX® [OTC]** *see* Guaifenesin *on page 729*
- ◆ **Nalfon®** *see* Fenoprofen *on page 616*
- ◆ **Nallpen** *see* Nafcillin *on page 1048*
- ◆ **N-Allylnoroxymorphine Hydrochloride** *see* Naloxone *on page 1052*

Nalmefene (NAL me feen)

U.S. Brand Names Revex®
Synonyms Nalmefene Hydrochloride
Generic Available No
Pharmacologic Category Antidote
Medication Safety Issues
Sound-alike/look-alike issues:
Revex® may be confused with Nimbex®, ReVia®

Use Complete or partial reversal of opioid drug effects, including respiratory depression induced by natural or synthetic opioids; reversal of postoperative opioid depression; management of known or suspected opioid overdose

Mechanism of Action/Effect Nalmefene acts as a competitive antagonist at opioid receptor sites, preventing or reversing the respiratory depression, sedation, and hypotension induced by opiates; no pharmacologic activity of its own (eg, opioid agonist activity) has been demonstrated

Contraindications Hypersensitivity to nalmefene, naltrexone, or any component of the formulation

Warnings/Precautions May induce symptoms of acute withdrawal in opioid-dependent patients; recurrence of respiratory depression is possible if the opioid involved is long-acting; observe patients until there is no reasonable risk of recurrent respiratory depression. Safety and efficacy have not been established in children. Avoid abrupt reversal of opioid effects in patients of high cardiovascular risk or who have received potentially cardiotoxic drugs. Pulmonary edema and cardiovascular instability have been reported in association with abrupt reversal with other narcotic antagonists. Animal studies indicate nalmefene may not completely reverse buprenorphine-induced respiratory depression.

Drug Interactions
Increased Effect/Toxicity: Potential increased risk of seizures may exist with use of flumazenil and nalmefene coadministration.

Adverse Reactions
>10%: Gastrointestinal: Nausea
1% to 10%:
Cardiovascular: Tachycardia, hyper-/hypotension, vasodilation
Central nervous system: Fever, dizziness, headache, chills
Gastrointestinal: Vomiting
Miscellaneous: Postoperative pain

Overdosage/Toxicology No reported symptoms with significant overdose. Large doses of opioids administered to overcome a full blockade of opioid antagonists, however, have resulted in adverse respiratory and circulatory reactions.

Pharmacodynamics/Kinetics
Onset of Action: I.M., SubQ: 5-15 minutes
Bioavailability: I.M., I.V., SubQ: 100%
Time to Peak: Serum: I.M.: 2.3 hours; I.V.: <2 minutes; SubQ: 1.5 hours
Protein Binding: 45%
Half-Life Elimination: 10.8 hours
Metabolism: Hepatic via glucuronide conjugation to metabolites with little or no activity
Excretion: Feces (17%); urine (<5% as unchanged drug)
Clearance: 0.8 L/hour/kg

Dosing
Adults & Elderly:
Reversal of postoperative opioid depression: I.V.: Blue labeled product (100 mcg/mL): Titrate to reverse the undesired effects of opioids; initial dose for nonopioid dependent patient: 0.25 mcg/kg followed by 0.25 mcg/kg incremental doses at 2- to 5-minute intervals. After a total dose >1 mcg/kg, further therapeutic response is unlikely.

Management of known/suspected opioid overdose: I.V.: Green labeled product (1000 mcg/mL): Initial: 0.5 mg/70 kg; may repeat with 1 mg/70 kg in 2-5 minutes. Further increase beyond a total dose of 1.5 mg/70 kg will not likely result in improved response and may result in cardiovascular stress and precipitated withdrawal syndrome. (If opioid dependency is suspected, administer a challenge dose of 0.1 mg/70 kg; if no withdrawal symptoms are observed in 2 minutes, the recommended doses can be administered).

Recurrence of respiratory depression: If noted, dose may again be titrated to clinical effect using incremental doses.

Loss of I.V. access: If I.V. access is lost or not readily obtainable, a single SubQ or I.M. dose of 1 mg may be effective in 5-15 minutes.

Renal Impairment: Not necessary with single uses, however, slow administration (over 60 seconds) of incremental doses is recommended to minimize hypertension and dizziness.

Hepatic Impairment: Not necessary with single uses, however, slow administration (over 60 seconds) of incremental doses is recommended to minimize hypertension and dizziness.

Available Dosage Forms Injection, solution: 100 mcg/mL (1 mL) [blue label]; 1000 mcg/mL (2 mL) [green label]

Monitoring and Teaching Issues
Physical Assessment: Assess patient for opioid dependency. Monitor vital signs, respiratory, and cardiac status carefully during infusion and for some time thereafter (effects may continue for several days, use nonopioid analgesics for pain).

Patient Education: This drug can only be administered I.V. You may experience drowsiness, dizziness, or blurred vision for several days; use caution when driving or engaging in tasks requiring alertness until response to drug is known. Small frequent meals and good mouth care may reduce any nausea or vomiting. Report yellowing of eyes or skin, unusual bleeding, dark or tarry stools, acute headache, or palpitations. **Breast-feeding precaution:** Wait 4 hours before breast-feeding.
(Continued)

Nalmefene (Continued)

Pregnancy Risk Factor: B
Pregnancy Issues: Limited information available
Lactation: Enters breast milk/use caution
Breast-Feeding Issues: Limited information available; do not use in lactating women if possible.

Administration
  I.M.: If I.V. access is lost or not readily obtainable, a single SubQ or I.M. dose of 1 mg may be effective in 5-15 minutes.
  I.V.: Slow administration (over 60 seconds) of incremental doses is recommended to minimize hypertension and dizziness.
  Compatibility: Stable in D_5LR, $D_5^{1}/_2NS$, D_5W, LR, sodium bicarbonate 5%, $^{1}/_2NS$, NS

Additional Information Proper steps should be used to prevent use of the incorrect dosage strength. The goal of treatment in the postoperative setting is to achieve reversal of excessive opioid effects without inducing a complete reversal and acute pain.

If opioid dependence is suspected, nalmefene should only be used in opioid overdose if the likelihood of overdose is high based on history or the clinical presentation of respiratory depression with concurrent pupillary constriction is present.

♦ **Nalmefene Hydrochloride** *see Nalmefene on page 1051*

Naloxone (nal OKS one)

U.S. Brand Names Narcan®
Synonyms N-Allylnoroxymorphine Hydrochloride; Naloxone Hydrochloride
Generic Available Yes
Pharmacologic Category Antidote
Medication Safety Issues
  Sound-alike/look-alike issues:
    Naloxone may be confused with naltrexone
    Narcan® may be confused with Marcaine®, Norcuron®

Use
  Complete or partial reversal of opioid depression, including respiratory depression, induced by natural and synthetic opioids, including propoxyphene, methadone, and certain mixed agonist-antagonist analgesics: nalbuphine, pentazocine, and butorphanol
  Diagnosis of suspected opioid tolerance or acute opioid overdose
  Adjunctive agent to increase blood pressure in the management of septic shock

Unlabeled/Investigational Use PCP and ethanol ingestion
Mechanism of Action/Effect Pure opioid antagonist that competes and displaces narcotics at opioid receptor sites
Contraindications Hypersensitivity to naloxone or any component of the formulation
Warnings/Precautions Due to an association between naloxone and acute pulmonary edema, use with caution in patients with cardiovascular disease or in patients receiving medications with potential adverse cardiovascular effects (eg, hypotension, pulmonary edema or arrhythmias). Excessive dosages should be avoided after use of opiates in surgery. Abrupt postoperative reversal may result in nausea, vomiting, sweating, tachycardia, hypertension, seizures, and other cardiovascular events (including pulmonary edema and arrhythmias). May precipitate withdrawal symptoms in patients addicted to opiates, including pain, hypertension, sweating, agitation, irritability; in neonates: shrill cry, failure to feed. Recurrence of respiratory depression is possible if the opioid involved is long-acting; observe patients until there is no reasonable risk of recurrent respiratory depression.

Drug Interactions
  Decreased Effect: Decreased effect of narcotic analgesics.
Adverse Reactions Frequency not defined.
  Cardiovascular: Hyper-/hypotension, tachycardia, ventricular arrhythmia, cardiac arrest
  Central nervous system: Irritability, anxiety, narcotic withdrawal, restlessness, seizure
  Gastrointestinal: Nausea, vomiting, diarrhea
  Neuromuscular & skeletal: Tremulousness
  Respiratory: Dyspnea, pulmonary edema, runny nose, sneezing
  Miscellaneous: Diaphoresis

Overdosage/Toxicology Naloxone is the drug of choice for respiratory depression that is known or suspected to be caused by overdose of an opiate or opioid. **Caution:** Naloxone's effects are due to its action on narcotic reversal, not due to any direct effect upon opiate receptors. Therefore, adverse events occur secondarily to reversal (withdrawal) of narcotic analgesia and sedation, which can cause severe reactions.

Pharmacodynamics/Kinetics
  Onset of Action: Endotracheal, I.M., SubQ: 2-5 minutes; I.V.: ~2 minutes
  Duration of Action: 20-60 minutes; since shorter than that of most opioids, repeated doses are usually needed
  Half-Life Elimination: Neonates: 1.2-3 hours; Adults: 1-1.5 hours
  Metabolism: Primarily hepatic via glucuronidation
  Excretion: Urine (as metabolites)

Dosing
  Adults & Elderly:
    Narcotic overdose:
      I.V. (preferred), I.M., intratracheal, SubQ: 0.4-2 mg every 2-3 minutes as needed; may need to repeat doses every 20-60 minutes. If no response is observed after 10 mg, question the diagnosis. **Note:** Use 0.1-0.2 mg increments in patients who are opioid dependent and in postoperative patients to avoid large cardiovascular changes.
      Continuous infusion: I.V.: If continuous infusion is required, calculate dosage/hour based on effective intermittent dose used and duration of adequate response seen; adult dose typically 0.25-6.25 mg/hour (short-term infusions as high as 2.4 mg/kg/hour have been tolerated in adults during treatment for septic shock); alternatively, continuous

infusion utilizes ⅔ of the initial naloxone bolus on an hourly basis; add 10 times this dose to each liter of D₅W and infuse at a rate of 100 mL/hour; ½ of the initial bolus dose should be readministered 15 minutes after initiation of the continuous infusion to prevent a drop in naloxone levels; increase infusion rate as needed to assure adequate ventilation

Pediatrics:
Postanesthesia narcotic reversal: I.M., I.V. (preferred), intratracheal, SubQ: Infants and Children: 0.01 mg/kg; may repeat every 2-3 minutes as needed based on response
Narcotic overdose:
I.M., I.V. (preferred), intratracheal, SubQ:
Birth (including premature infants) to 5 years or <20 kg: 0.1 mg/kg; repeat every 2-3 minutes if needed; may need to repeat doses every 20-60 minutes
>5 years or ≥20 kg: 2 mg/dose; if no response, repeat every 2-3 minutes; may need to repeat doses every 20-60 minutes
Continuous infusion: I.V.: Refer to adult dosing.

Available Dosage Forms
Injection, solution, as hydrochloride: 0.4 mg/mL (1 mL, 10 mL)
Narcan®: 0.4 mg/mL (1 mL)

Monitoring and Teaching Issues
Physical Assessment: Assess patient for opioid dependency. Monitor vital signs and cardiorespiratory status continuously during infusion, maintain patent airway.
Patient Education: If patient is responsive, instructions are individualized. This drug can only be administered I.V. Report respiratory difficulty, palpitations, or tremors. Breast-feeding precaution: Breast-feeding is not recommended.
Geriatric Considerations: In small trials, naloxone has shown temporary improvement in Alzheimer's disease; however, is not recommended for treatment.
Pregnancy Risk Factor: C
Pregnancy Issues: Consider benefit to the mother and the risk to the fetus before administering to a pregnant woman who is known or suspected to be opioid dependent. May precipitate withdrawal in both the mother and fetus.
Lactation: Excretion in breast milk unknown/not recommended
Breast-Feeding Issues: No data reported. Since naloxone is used for opiate reversal the concern should be on opiate drug levels in a breast-feeding mother and transfer to the infant rather than naloxone exposure. The safest approach would be **not** to breast-feed.

Administration
I.V.:
I.V. push: Administer over 30 seconds as undiluted preparation
I.V. continuous infusion: Dilute to 4 mcg/mL in D₅W or normal saline
Other: Intratracheal: Dilute to 1-2 mL with normal saline
Reconstitution: Stable in 0.9% sodium chloride and D₅W at 4 mcg/mL for 24 hours.
Compatibility: Stable in D₅W, NS
Y-site administration: Incompatible with amphotericin B cholesteryl sulfate complex
Storage: Store at 25°C (77°F). Protect from light.
Additional Information May contain methyl and propylparabens

♦ **Naloxone and Buprenorphine** *see* Buprenorphine and Naloxone *on page 218*
♦ **Naloxone Hydrochloride** *see* Naloxone *on page 1052*
♦ **Naloxone Hydrochloride and Pentazocine Hydrochloride** *see* Pentazocine *on page 1180*
♦ **Naloxone Hydrochloride Dihydrate and Buprenorphine Hydrochloride** *see* Buprenorphine and Naloxone *on page 218*

Naltrexone (nal TREKS one)

U.S. Brand Names Depade®; ReVia®
Synonyms Naltrexone Hydrochloride
Generic Available Yes
Pharmacologic Category Antidote
Medication Safety Issues
Sound-alike/look-alike issues:
Naltrexone may be confused with naloxone
ReVia® may be confused with Revex®
Use Treatment of ethanol dependence; blockade of the effects of exogenously administered opioids
Mechanism of Action/Effect Naltrexone (a pure opioid antagonist) is a cyclopropyl derivative of oxymorphone similar in structure to naloxone and nalorphine (a morphine derivative); it acts as a competitive antagonist at opioid receptor sites
Contraindications Hypersensitivity to naltrexone or any component of the formulation; narcotic dependence or current use of opioid analgesics; acute opioid withdrawal; failure to pass Narcan® challenge or positive urine screen for opioids; acute hepatitis; liver failure
Warnings/Precautions Dose-related hepatocellular injury is possible; the margin of separation between the apparent safe and hepatotoxic doses appear to be only fivefold or less. May precipitate withdrawal symptoms in patients addicted to opiates, including pain, hypertension, sweating, agitation, irritability; in neonates: shrill cry, failure to feed. Use with caution in patients with hepatic or renal impairment.

Patients who had been treated with naltrexone may respond to lower opioid doses than previously used. This could result in potentially life-threatening opioid intoxication. Patients should be aware that they may be more sensitive to lower doses of opioids after naltrexone treatment is discontinued. Use of naltrexone does not eliminate or diminish withdrawal symptoms.

Drug Interactions
Decreased Effect: Naltrexone decreases effects of opioid-containing products.
Increased Effect/Toxicity: Lethargy and somnolence have been reported with the combination of naltrexone and thioridazine.
(Continued)

Naltrexone *(Continued)*

Adverse Reactions

>10%:

Central nervous system: Insomnia, nervousness, headache, low energy

Gastrointestinal: Abdominal cramping, nausea, vomiting

Neuromuscular & skeletal: Arthralgia

1% to 10%:

Central nervous system: Increased energy, feeling down, irritability, dizziness, anxiety, somnolence

Dermatologic: Rash

Endocrine & metabolic: Polydipsia

Gastrointestinal: Diarrhea, constipation

Genitourinary: Delayed ejaculation, impotency

Overdosage/Toxicology Symptoms of overdose include clonic-tonic convulsions and respiratory failure. Patients receiving up to 800 mg/day for 1 week have shown no toxicity. Seizures and respiratory failure have been seen in animals.

Pharmacodynamics/Kinetics

Duration of Action: 50 mg: 24 hours; 100 mg: 48 hours; 150 mg: 72 hours

Absorption: Almost complete

Time to Peak: Serum: ~60 minutes

Protein Binding: 21%

Half-Life Elimination: 4 hours; 6-β-naltrexol: 13 hours

Metabolism: Extensive first-pass effect to 6-β-naltrexol

Excretion: Primarily urine (as metabolites and unchanged drug)

Dosing

Adults & Elderly: Opioid dependence or alcoholism (Do not give until patient is opioid-free for 7-10 days as required by urine analysis): Oral: 25 mg; if no withdrawal signs within 1 hour give another 25 mg; maintenance regimen is flexible, variable and individualized (50 mg/day to 100-150 mg 3 times/week).

Renal Impairment: Use caution.

Hepatic Impairment: Use caution. An increase in naltrexone AUC of approximately five- and 10-fold in patients with compensated or decompensated liver cirrhosis respectively, compared with normal liver function has been reported.

Available Dosage Forms

Tablet, as hydrochloride: 50 mg

Depade®: 25 mg, 50 mg, 100 mg

ReVia®: 25 mg

Monitoring and Teaching Issues

Physical Assessment: Do not use until patient has been opioid-free for 7-10 days. Assess carefully for several days following start of therapy for narcotic withdrawal symptoms or severe adverse reactions. Use non-narcotic analgesics for pain.

Monitoring Laboratory Tests: Periodic LFTs

Patient Education: This medication will help you achieve abstinence from opiates if taken as directed. Do not increase or change dose. Do not use opiates or any medications not approved by your prescriber during naltrexone therapy. You may experience drowsiness, dizziness, or blurred vision (use caution when driving or engaging in tasks requiring alertness until response to drug is known); abdominal cramping, nausea or vomiting (small frequent meals, frequent mouth care, chewing gum, or sucking lozenges may help); low energy; or decreased sexual function (reversible when drug is discontinued). Report yellowing of skin or eyes, change in color of stool or urine, increased perspiration or chills, acute headache, palpitations, or unusual joint pain. **Pregnancy/breast-feeding precautions:** Inform prescriber if you are or intend to become pregnant. Consult prescriber if breast-feeding.

Pregnancy Risk Factor: C

Lactation: Excretion in breast milk unknown

♦ **Naltrexone Hydrochloride** *see* Naltrexone *on page 1053*

♦ **Namenda™** *see* Memantine *on page 947*

Nandrolone *(NAN droe lone)*

Synonyms Nandrolone Decanoate; Nandrolone Phenpropionate

Controlled Substance C-III

Generic Available Yes

Pharmacologic Category Androgen

Use Control of metastatic breast cancer; management of anemia of renal insufficiency

Mechanism of Action/Effect Promotes tissue-building processes, increases production of erythropoietin, causes protein anabolism; increases hemoglobin and red blood cell volume

Contraindications Hypersensitivity to nandrolone or any component of the formulation; carcinoma of breast or prostate; nephrosis; pregnancy; not for use in infants

Warnings/Precautions Monitor diabetic patients carefully. Anabolic steroids may cause peliosis hepatis, liver cell tumors, and blood lipid changes with increased risk of arteriosclerosis. Use with caution in elderly patients, they may be at greater risk for prostatic hyperplasia. Use with caution in patients with cardiac, renal, or hepatic disease or epilepsy.

Drug Interactions

Increased Effect/Toxicity: Nandrolone may increase the effect of oral anticoagulants, insulin, oral hypoglycemic agents, adrenal steroids, or ACTH when taken together.

Lab Interactions Altered glucose tolerance tests

Adverse Reactions

Male:

Postpubertal:

>10%:

Dermatologic: Acne

Endocrine & metabolic: Gynecomastia
Genitourinary: Bladder irritability, priapism
1% to 10%:
Central nervous system: Insomnia, chills
Endocrine & metabolic: Decreased libido, hepatic dysfunction
Gastrointestinal: Nausea, diarrhea
Genitourinary: Prostatic hyperplasia (elderly)
Hematologic: Iron deficiency anemia, suppression of clotting factors
Prepubertal:
>10%:
Dermatologic: Acne
Endocrine & metabolic: Virilism
1% to 10%:
Central nervous system: Chills, insomnia
Dermatologic: Hyperpigmentation
Gastrointestinal: Diarrhea, nausea
Hematologic: Iron deficiency anemia, suppression of clotting
Female:
>10%: Endocrine & metabolic: Virilism
1% to 10%:
Central nervous system: Chills, insomnia
Endocrine & metabolic: Hypercalcemia
Gastrointestinal: Nausea, diarrhea
Hematologic: Iron deficiency anemia, suppression of clotting factors
Hepatic: Hepatic dysfunction

Pharmacodynamics/Kinetics
Onset of Action: 3-6 months
Duration of Action: Up to 30 days
Absorption: I.M.: 77%
Metabolism: Hepatic
Excretion: Urine

Dosing
Adults & Elderly:
Breast cancer, male/female (phenpropionate): I.M.: 50-100 mg/week
Anemia of renal insufficiency (decanoate): I.M.:
Male: 100-200 mg/week
Female: 50-100 mg/week
Note: Deep I.M. (into gluteal muscle):
Pediatrics: Deep I.M. (into gluteal muscle): Children 2-13 years (decanoate): 25-50 mg every 3-4 weeks

Available Dosage Forms Injection, solution, as decanoate [in sesame oil]: 100 mg/mL (2 mL); 200 mg/mL (1 mL) [contains benzyl alcohol]

Monitoring and Teaching Issues
Physical Assessment: Use caution is presence of cardiac, renal, or hepatic disease or epilepsy (see Warnings/precautions for use cautions). Assess potential for interactions with other pharmacological agents (see Drug Interactions). Assess results of LFTs, therapeutic effectiveness (according to purpose of use), and adverse response on a regular basis (adverse reactions may differ according to gender and age; see Adverse Reactions). Caution patients with diabetes to monitor serum glucose closely (may increase the effect of hypoglycemic agents). Teach patient possible side effects/appropriate interventions and adverse symptoms to report (see Patient Education). **Pregnancy risk factor X:** Determine that patient is not pregnant before starting therapy. Do not give to females of childbearing age unless patient is capable of complying with contraceptive use.

Monitoring Laboratory Tests: LFTs on a regular basis

Patient Education: Do not take any new medication during therapy unless approved by prescriber. This drug can only be given injection. Report immediately any redness, swelling, burning, or pain at injection site. If you have diabetes, monitor serum glucose closely and notify prescriber of significant changes (nandrolone may increase the effect of hypoglycemic agents). May cause nausea or vomiting (small frequent meals, frequent mouth care, sucking lozenges, or chewing gum may help); diarrhea (buttermilk, boiled milk, yogurt may help). **Male:** Acne, swelling of breasts, loss of libido, impotence. **Female:** Virilism, menstrual irregularity (usually reversible). Report changes in menstrual pattern; enlarged or painful breasts; deepening of voice or unusual growth of body hair; fluid retention (eg, swelling of ankles, feet, or hands, respiratory difficulty, or sudden weight gain); bladder irritability; unresolved CNS changes (eg, nervousness, chills, insomnia); change in color of urine or stool; yellowing of eyes or skin; unusual bruising or bleeding; or other adverse reactions. **Pregnancy/breast-feeding precautions:** Inform prescriber if you are pregnant. Do not get pregnant during or for 1 month following therapy. Consult prescriber for instruction on appropriate contraceptive measures. This drug may cause severe fetal defects. Do not breast-feed.

Pregnancy Risk Factor: X

Lactation: Excretion in breast milk unknown/contraindicated

Administration
I.M.: Inject deeply I.M., preferably into the gluteal muscle.

Additional Information Both phenpropionate and decanoate are injections in oil.

♦ **Nandrolone Decanoate** *see* Nandrolone *on page 1054*
♦ **Nandrolone Phenpropionate** *see* Nandrolone *on page 1054*
♦ **NapraPAC™** *see* Lansoprazole and Naproxen *on page 868*
♦ **Naprelan®** *see* Naproxen *on page 1056*
♦ **Naprosyn®** *see* Naproxen *on page 1056*

Naproxen (na PROKS en)

U.S. Brand Names Aleve® [OTC]; Anaprox®; Anaprox® DS; EC-Naprosyn®; Naprelan®; Naprosyn®; Pamprin® Maximum Strength All Day Relief [OTC]

Synonyms Naproxen Sodium

Generic Available Yes

Pharmacologic Category Nonsteroidal Anti-inflammatory Drug (NSAID), Oral

Medication Safety Issues

Sound-alike/look-alike issues:

Naproxen may be confused with Naprosyn®

Aleve® may be confused with Alesse®

Anaprox® may be confused with Anaspaz®, Avapro®

Naprelan® may be confused with Naprosyn®

Naprosyn® may be confused with Naprelan®, naproxen, Natacyn®, Nebcin®

Use Management of ankylosing spondylitis, osteoarthritis, and rheumatoid disorders (including juvenile rheumatoid arthritis); acute gout; mild to moderate pain; tendonitis, bursitis; dysmenorrhea; fever; migraine headache

Mechanism of Action/Effect Inhibits prostaglandin synthesis by decreasing the activity of the enzyme, cyclooxygenase, which results in decreased formation of prostaglandin precursors

Contraindications Hypersensitivity to naproxen, aspirin, other NSAIDs, or any component of the formulation; patients with "aspirin triad" (bronchial asthma, aspirin intolerance, rhinitis); pregnancy (3rd trimester)

Warnings/Precautions Fatal asthmatic and anaphylactoid reactions have occurred in patients with "aspirin triad." Use with caution in patients with CHF, hypertension, dehydration, decreased renal or hepatic function, history of GI disease (bleeding, ulcers, or previous GI symptoms with NSAID use), or those receiving anticoagulants and/or corticosteroids. Use lowest effective dose for shortest period possible; bleeding risk has been correlated to dose and duration of therapy. Gastrointestinal bleeding may occur without prior symptoms of gastrointestinal irritation. Elderly are at a high risk for adverse effects from NSAIDs. As many as 60% of elderly can develop peptic ulceration and/or hemorrhage asymptomatically.

Use of NSAIDs can compromise existing renal function especially when Cl_{cr} <30 mL/minute. CNS adverse effects such as confusion, agitation, and hallucination are generally seen in overdose or high-dose situations; however, elderly may demonstrate these adverse effects at lower doses than younger adults. Withhold for at least 4-6 half-lives prior to surgical or dental procedures.

OTC labeling: Recommended dosages should not be exceeded, due to an increased risk of GI bleeding. Consuming ≥3 alcoholic beverages/day may increase the risk of GI bleeding. When used for self-medication, patients should be instructed to contact healthcare provider if used for fever lasting >3 days or for pain lasting >10 days in adults or >3 days in children.

Drug Interactions

Cytochrome P450 Effect: Substrate (minor) of CYP1A2, 2C8/9

Decreased Effect: NSAIDs may decrease the effect of some antihypertensive agents, including ACE inhibitors, angiotensin receptor antagonists, and hydralazine. The efficacy of diuretics (loop and/or thiazide) may be decreased.

Increased Effect/Toxicity: Naproxen could displace other highly protein-bound drugs, increasing the effect of oral anticoagulants, hydantoins, salicylates, sulfonamides, and first-generation sulfonylureas. Naproxen and warfarin may cause a slight increase in free warfarin. Naproxen and probenecid may cause increased levels of naproxen. Naproxen and methotrexate may significantly increase and prolong blood methotrexate concentration, which may be severe or fatal. May increase lithium or cyclosporine levels. Corticosteroids may increase risk of GI ulceration.

Nutritional/Ethanol Interactions

Ethanol: Avoid or limit ethanol (may enhance gastric mucosal irritation).

Food: Naproxen absorption rate may be decreased if taken with food.

Herb/Nutraceutical: Avoid cat's claw, dong quai, evening primrose, feverfew, garlic, ginger, ginkgo, red clover, horse chestnut, green tea, ginseng (all have additional antiplatelet activity).

Lab Interactions Increased chloride (S), sodium (S), bleeding time

Adverse Reactions 1% to 10%:

Cardiovascular: Edema (3% to 9%), palpitations (<3%)

Central nervous system: Dizziness (3% to 9%), drowsiness (3% to 9%), headache (3% to 9%), lightheadedness (<3%), vertigo (<3%)

Dermatologic: Pruritus (3% to 9%), skin eruption (3% to 9%), rash, ecchymosis (3% to 9%), purpura (<3%)

Endocrine & metabolic: Fluid retention (3% to 9%)

Gastrointestinal: Abdominal pain (3% to 9%), constipation (3% to 9%), nausea (3% to 9%), heartburn (3% to 9%), diarrhea (<3%), dyspepsia (<3%), stomatitis (<3%), heartburn (<3%), flatulence, gross bleeding/perforation, indigestion, ulcers, vomiting

Genitourinary: Abnormal renal function

Hematologic: Hemolysis (3% to 9%), ecchymosis (3% to 9%), anemia, bleeding time increased

Hepatic: LFTS increased

Ocular: Visual disturbances (<3%)

Otic: Tinnitus (3% to 9%), hearing disturbances (<3%)

Respiratory: Dyspnea (3% to 9%)

Miscellaneous: Diaphoresis (<3%), thirst (<3%)

Overdosage/Toxicology Symptoms of overdose include drowsiness, heartburn, vomiting, CNS depression, leukocytosis, and renal failure. Management is supportive and symptomatic. Seizures tend to be very short-lived and often do not require drug treatment.

Pharmacodynamics/Kinetics

Onset of Action: Analgesic: 1 hour; Anti-inflammatory: ~2 weeks; Peak effect: Anti-inflammatory: 2-4 weeks

Duration of Action: Analgesic: ≤7 hours; Anti-inflammatory: ≤12 hours

Absorption: Almost 100%

Time to Peak: Serum: 1-4 hours

Protein Binding: >99%; increased free fraction in elderly

Half-Life Elimination: Normal renal function: 12-17 hours; End-stage renal disease: No change

Excretion: Urine (95%)

Dosing

Adults:

Acute gout: Oral: Initial: 750 mg, followed by 250 mg every 8 hours until attack subsides; **Note:** EC-Naprosyn® is not recommended

Rheumatoid arthritis, osteoarthritis, and ankylosing spondylitis: 500-1000 mg/day in 2 divided doses; may increase to 1.5 g/day of naproxen base for limited time period

Mild-to-moderate pain, dysmenorrhea, acute tendonitis, bursitis: Oral: Initial: 500 mg, then 250 mg every 6-8 hours; maximum: 1250 mg/day naproxen base

OTC labeling: Pain/fever:

Adults ≤65 years: 200 mg naproxen base every 8-12 hours; if needed, may take 400 mg naproxen base for the initial dose; maximum: 600 mg naproxen base/24 hours

Adults >65 years: Refer to elderly dosing.

Elderly: Refer to adult dosing and Geriatric Considerations.

OTC labeling: Pain/fever: Adults >65 years: 200 mg naproxen base every 12 hours

Pediatrics:

Fever: Oral: Children >2 years: 2.5-10 mg/kg/dose; maximum: 10 mg/kg/day

Juvenile arthritis: Oral: Children >2 years: 10 mg/kg/day in 2 divided doses

OTC labeling: Pain/fever: Oral: Children ≥12 years: Refer to adult dosing.

Renal Impairment: Cl$_{cr}$ <30 mL/minute: use is not recommended.

Available Dosage Forms

Caplet, as sodium (Aleve®, Pamprin® Maximum Strength All Day Relief): 220 mg [equivalent to naproxen 200 mg and sodium 20 mg]

Gelcap, as sodium (Aleve®): 220 mg [equivalent to naproxen 200 mg and sodium 20 mg]

Suspension, oral (Naprosyn®): 125 mg/5 mL (480 mL) [contains sodium 0.3 mEq/mL; orange-pineapple flavor]

Tablet (Naprosyn®): 250 mg, 375 mg, 500 mg

Tablet, as sodium: 220 mg [equivalent to naproxen 200 mg and sodium 20 mg]; 275 mg [equivalent to naproxen 250 mg and sodium 25 mg]; 550 mg [equivalent to naproxen 500 mg and sodium 50 mg]

Aleve®: 220 mg [equivalent to naproxen 200 mg and sodium 20 mg]

Anaprox®: 275 mg [equivalent to naproxen 250 mg and sodium 25 mg]

Anaprox® DS: 550 mg [equivalent to naproxen 500 mg and sodium 50 mg]

Tablet, controlled release, as sodium: 550 mg [equivalent to naproxen 500 mg and sodium 50 mg]

Naprelan®: 421.5 mg [equivalent to naproxen 375 mg and sodium 37.5 mg]; 550 mg [equivalent to naproxen 500 mg and sodium 50 mg]

Tablet, delayed release (EC-Naprosyn®): 375 mg, 500 mg

Monitoring and Teaching Issues

Physical Assessment: Assess effectiveness and interactions of other medications patient may be taking. Assess results of laboratory tests, therapeutic effectiveness, and adverse reactions (eg, GI effects, hepatotoxicity, or ototoxicity) at beginning of therapy and periodically throughout therapy. Schedule ophthalmic evaluations for patients who develop eye complaints during long-term NSAID therapy. Assess knowledge/teach patient appropriate use, interventions to reduce side effects, and adverse symptoms to report.

Monitoring Laboratory Tests: Periodic liver function, CBC, BUN, serum creatinine

Patient Education: Take this medication exactly as directed; do not increase dose without consulting prescriber. Do not crush tablets. Take with food or milk to reduce GI distress. Maintain adequate hydration (2-3 L/day of fluids) unless instructed to restrict fluid intake. Do not use alcohol, aspirin or aspirin-containing medication, or any other anti-inflammatory medications without consulting prescriber. You may experience drowsiness, dizziness, lightheadedness, or headache (use caution when driving or engaging in tasks requiring alertness until response to drug is known); anorexia, nausea, vomiting, or heartburn (small frequent meals, frequent mouth care, sucking lozenges, or chewing gum may help); or fluid retention (weigh yourself weekly and report unusual [3-5 lb/week] weight gain). GI bleeding, ulceration, or perforation can occur with or without pain; or discontinue medication and contact prescriber if persistent abdominal pain or cramping, or blood in stool occurs. Report breathlessness, respiratory difficulty, or unusual cough; chest pain, rapid heartbeat, palpitations; unusual bruising/bleeding; blood in urine, stool, mouth, or vomitus; swollen extremities; skin rash or itching; acute fatigue; or changes in eyesight (double vision, color changes, blurred vision), hearing, or ringing in ears. **Breast-feeding precautions:** Notify prescriber if you are or intend to become pregnant. Do not take this drug during last trimester of pregnancy.

Dietary Considerations: Drug may cause GI upset, bleeding, ulceration, perforation; take with food or milk to minimize GI upset.

Geriatric Considerations: Elderly are at high risk for adverse effects from NSAIDs. As much as 60% of elderly can develop peptic ulceration and/or hemorrhage asymptomatically. The concomitant use of H$_2$ blockers, omeprazole, and sucralfate is not effective as prophylaxis with the exception of NSAID-induced duodenal ulcers which may be prevented by the use of ranitidine. Misoprostol is the only prophylactic agent proven effective. Also, concomitant disease and drug use contribute to the risk for GI adverse effects. Use lowest effective dose for shortest period possible. Consider renal function decline with age. Use of NSAIDs can compromise existing renal function especially when Cl$_{cr}$ is ≤30 mL/minute. Tinnitus may be a difficult and unreliable indication of toxicity due to age-related hearing loss or eighth cranial nerve damage. CNS adverse effects such as confusion, agitation, and hallucination are generally seen in overdose or high-dose situations, but elderly may demonstrate these adverse effects at lower doses than younger adults.

(Continued)

Naproxen *(Continued)*

Pregnancy Risk Factor: C
Lactation: Enters breast milk/not recommended (AAP rates "compatible")

Administration
  Oral: Administer with food, milk, or antacids to decrease GI adverse effects
    Suspension: Shake suspension well before administration.
    Tablet, extended release: Swallow tablet whole; do not break, crush, or chew.
  Storage: Store oral suspension and tablet at 15°C to 30°C (59°F to 86°F).

Related Information
  Nonsalicylate / Nonsteroidal Anti-inflammatory Agents *on page 1743*

♦ **Naproxen and Lansoprazole** *see* Lansoprazole and Naproxen *on page 868*
♦ **Naproxen Sodium** *see* Naproxen *on page 1056*

Naratriptan *(NAR a trip tan)*

U.S. Brand Names Amerge®
Synonyms Naratriptan Hydrochloride
Generic Available No
Pharmacologic Category Serotonin 5-HT$_{1D}$ Receptor Agonist
Medication Safety Issues
  Sound-alike/look-alike issues:
    Amerge® may be confused with Altace®, Amaryl®
Use Treatment of acute migraine headache with or without aura
Mechanism of Action/Effect The therapeutic effect for migraine is due to serotonin agonist activity.
Contraindications Hypersensitivity to naratriptan or any component of the formulation; cerebrovascular, peripheral vascular disease (ischemic bowel disease), ischemic heart disease (angina pectoris, history of myocardial infarction, or proven silent ischemia); or in patients with symptoms consistent with ischemic heart disease, coronary artery vasospasm, or Prinzmetal's angina; uncontrolled hypertension or patients who have received within 24 hours another 5-HT agonist (sumatriptan, zolmitriptan) or ergotamine-containing product; patients with known risk factors associated with coronary artery disease; patients with severe hepatic or renal disease (Cl$_{cr}$ <15 mL/minute); do not administer naratriptan to patients with hemiplegic or basilar migraine
Warnings/Precautions Use only if there is a clear diagnosis of migraine. May cause vasospastic reactions resulting in colonic, peripheral, or coronary ischemia. Monitor closely, especially after the first dose. Patients who are at risk of CAD (based on risk factor evaluation) but have had a satisfactory cardiovascular evaluation may receive naratriptan, but extreme caution should be used; administration of the first dose in a setting with medical staff and equipment (ie, in a physician's office) is recommended, and ECG monitoring after the first dose should be considered. Periodically re-evaluate risk factors for CAD in patients receiving long-term intermittent treatment. Blood pressure may increase with the administration of naratriptan. If the patient does not respond to the first dose, re-evaluate the diagnosis of migraine before trying a second dose.

Drug Interactions
  Decreased Effect: Smoking increases the clearance of naratriptan.
  Increased Effect/Toxicity: Ergot-containing drugs (dihydroergotamine or methysergide) may cause vasospastic reactions when taken with naratriptan. Avoid concomitant use with ergots; separate dose of naratriptan and ergots by at least 24 hours. Oral contraceptives taken with naratriptan reduced the clearance of naratriptan ~30% which may contribute to adverse effects. Selective serotonin reuptake inhibitors (SSRIs) (eg, fluoxetine, fluvoxamine, paroxetine, sertraline) may cause lack of coordination, hyper-reflexia, or weakness and should be avoided when taking naratriptan.
Adverse Reactions 1% to 10%:
  Central nervous system: Dizziness, drowsiness, malaise/fatigue
  Gastrointestinal: Nausea, vomiting
  Neuromuscular & skeletal: Paresthesias
  Miscellaneous: Pain or pressure in throat or neck
Pharmacodynamics/Kinetics
  Onset of Action: 30 minutes
  Absorption: Well absorbed
  Bioavailability: 70%
  Time to Peak: 2-3 hours
  Protein Binding: Plasma: 28% to 31%
  Metabolism: Hepatic via CYP
  Excretion: Urine

Dosing
  Adults: Migraine: Oral: 1 mg to 2.5 mg at the onset of headache. It is recommended to use the lowest possible dose to minimize adverse effects. If headache returns or dose not fully resolve, the dose may be repeated after 4 hours. Do not exceed 5 mg in 24 hours.
  Elderly: Not recommended for use in the elderly.
  Renal Impairment:
    Cl$_{cr}$ 18-39 mL/minute: Initial: 1 mg; do not exceed 2.5 mg in 24 hours.
    Cl$_{cr}$ <15 mL/minute: Do not use.
  Hepatic Impairment: Contraindicated in patients with severe liver failure. The maximum dose is 2.5 mg in 24 hours for patients with mild or moderate liver failure. The recommended starting dose is 1 mg.
Available Dosage Forms Tablet: 1 mg, 2.5 mg
Monitoring and Teaching Issues
  Physical Assessment: See Contraindications and Warnings/Precautions for specific use cautions (eg, clear diagnosis of migraine). Assess potential for interactions with other pharmacological agents patient may be taking (eg, ergot containing drugs, SSRIs; see

Drug Interactions). Assess therapeutic effectiveness (relief of migraine) and adverse response (eg, drowsiness, nausea/vomiting, paresthesias; see Adverse Reactions), Teach patient proper use, possible side effects/appropriate interventions, and adverse symptoms to report (see Patient Education).

Patient Education: Do not take any new medication during therapy unless approved by prescriber (especially any other headache or pain medications). This drug is to be used to reduce your migraine, not to prevent or reduce the number of attacks. If headache returns or is not fully resolved, the dose may be repeated after 4 hours. If you have no relief with first dose, do not take a second dose without consulting prescriber. **Do not exceed 5 mg in 24 hours. Do not take within 24 hours of any other migraine medication without first consulting prescriber.** May cause dizziness, fatigue, or drowsiness (use caution when driving or engaging in tasks that require alertness until response to drug is known); or nausea or vomiting (small frequent meals, frequent mouth care, chewing gum, or sucking lozenges may help). Report immediately any chest pain, palpitations, or rapid heartbeat; tightness in throat or neck; or rash, itching, or hives. **Pregnancy/breast-feeding precautions:** Inform prescriber if you are or intend to become pregnant. Breast-feeding is not recommended.

Geriatric Considerations: Naratriptan was not studied in patients >65 years of age. Use in elderly patients is not recommended because of the presence of risk factors associated with adverse effects. These include the presence of coronary artery disease, decreased liver or renal function, and the risk of pronounced blood pressure increases.

Pregnancy Risk Factor: C

Lactation: Excretion in breast milk unknown/use caution

Administration

Oral: Do **not** crush or chew tablet; swallow whole with water.

Related Information

Antimigraine Drugs: 5-HT$_1$ Receptor Agonists *on page 1716*

♦ **Naratriptan Hydrochloride** *see Naratriptan on page 1058*

♦ **Narcan®** *see Naloxone on page 1052*

♦ **Narcotic / Opioid Analgesic Comparison** *see page 1739*

♦ **Nardil®** *see Phenelzine on page 1194*

♦ **Nasacort® [HFA]** *see Triamcinolone on page 1518*

♦ **Nasacort® AQ** *see Triamcinolone on page 1518*

♦ **NasalCrom® [OTC]** *see Cromolyn on page 374*

♦ **Nasarel®** *see Flunisolide on page 642*

♦ **Nasatab® LA** *see Guaifenesin and Pseudoephedrine on page 733*

♦ **Nascobal®** *see Cyanocobalamin on page 377*

♦ **Nasonex®** *see Mometasone Furoate on page 1026*

Natalizumab (na ta LIZ u mab)

U.S. Brand Names Tysabri®

Synonyms AN100226; Anti-4 Alpha Integrin; IgG4-Kappa Monoclonal Antibody

Generic Available No

Pharmacologic Category Monoclonal Antibody, Selective Adhesion-Molecule Inhibitor

Use Treatment of relapsing forms of multiple sclerosis

Unlabeled/Investigational Use Crohn's disease

Mechanism of Action/Effect Natalizumab inhibits the movement of white blood cells such as T-lymphocytes from the blood into areas of inflamed tissue. Treatment results in decreased frequency of relapse in multiple sclerosis.

Contraindications Hypersensitivity to natalizumab, murine proteins, or any component of the formulation; pregnancy

Warnings/Precautions During clinical studies, ~22% of patients experienced an infusion-related reaction; serious systemic hypersensitivity reactions occurred in <1% of patients. Severe reactions, including anaphylaxis, occur rarely; upon presentation, the infusion should be discontinued immediately. Retreatment is not recommended. Infusion-related reactions may occur more frequently in patients with antibody to natalizumab. Antibody formation (which occurs in about 10% of patients) is associated with a decrease in natalizumab levels and a decrease in the efficacy of natalizumab. Use caution in patients with a history of depression; closely monitor. Safety and efficacy have not been established in chronic progressive multiple sclerosis and in children (<18 years of age).

Drug Interactions

Increased Effect/Toxicity: Concomitant immunosuppressant therapy may increase the risk of infection. Interferon beta-1a may increase the levels of natalizumab (no dosage adjustment necessary).

Adverse Reactions

>10%:
Central nervous system: Headache (35%), fatigue (24%), depression (17%)
Genitourinary: Urinary tract infection (18%)
Neuromuscular & skeletal: Arthralgia (15%)
Respiratory: Lower respiratory infection (15%)
Miscellaneous: Infusion-related reaction (22%)

1% to 10%:
Cardiovascular: Chest discomfort (4%),
Central nervous system: Syncope (2%), suicidal ideation (1%)
Dermatologic: Rash (9%), dermatitis (5%), pruritus (4%), urticaria (2%)
Endocrine & metabolic: Menstrual irregularities (7%), amenorrhea (2%)
Gastrointestinal: Abdominal discomfort (10%), gastroenteritis (9%), cholelithiasis (1%)
Genitourinary: Urinary frequency (7%), vaginitis (8%)
Hepatic: Transaminase abnormal (5%)
Local: Bleeding at injection site (3%)
Neuromuscular & skeletal: Rigors (3%), tremor (3%)
Respiratory: Tonsillitis (5%), pneumonia (1%)

(Continued)

Natalizumab *(Continued)*

Miscellaneous: Allergic reaction (7%), infection (2%), anaphylaxis (1%)

Overdosage/Toxicology Safety of doses >300 mg has not been evaluated.

Pharmacodynamics/Kinetics
Half-Life Elimination: 7-15 days
Excretion: Clearance: 11-21 mL/hour

Dosing
Adults & Elderly:
Multiple sclerosis: I.V.: 300 mg infused over 1 hour every 4 weeks
Crohn's disease (unlabeled use): I.V.: 3-6 mg/kg, followed by a second infusion 4 weeks later

Renal Impairment: No adjustment recommended.
Hepatic Impairment: Not studied

Available Dosage Forms Injection, solution [preservative free]: 300 mg/15 mL (15 mL) [contains polysorbate-80]

Monitoring and Teaching Issues
Physical Assessment: Patient should be monitored closely for infusion-related reactions during and for 1 hour following infusion. If hypersensitivity reaction occurs, infusion should be promptly discontinued; retreatment is not recommended (see Warnings/Precautions). See Administration and Dosing specifics. Monitor effectiveness of treatment (reduction in relapses of MS) and adverse effects (opportunistic infection, excessive fatigue, depression; see Adverse Reactions). Teach patient/caregiver possible side effects, appropriate interventions, and adverse symptoms to report (see Patient Education).

Patient Education: This drug can only be administered by intravenous infusion. You will be monitored closely during and following infusion. Report immediately any skin rash, dizziness, nausea, flushing, difficulty breathing, chest pain, redness, or swelling at infusion site. Following infusion, you may experience headache or joint pain (consult prescriber for appropriate analgesic); unusual fatigue (adequate and frequent rest periods may help). Report any signs of urinary tract infection (itching, pain, discolored urine, or frequency of urination); lower respiratory infection (cough, difficulty breathing, chest tightness); chest discomfort or pain; unusual depression or suicidal ideation; or other persistent adverse effects. **Pregnancy/breast-feeding precautions:** Inform prescriber if you are or intend to be pregnant or breast-feed.

Pregnancy Risk Factor: C
Lactation: Excretion in breast milk unknown/not recommended
Breast-Feeding Issues: Immunoglobulin may be excreted in breast milk. Effects on infant are unknown. Manufacturer recommends that consideration be given to discontinuing breast-feeding during treatment.

Administration
I.V.: Solution may be warmed to room temperature prior to administration. Diluted solution should be infused over 1 hour; do not administer by I.V. bolus or push. Patients should be closely monitored for signs and symptoms of hypersensitivity during the infusion and for at least 1 hour after the infusion is complete. The infusion should be discontinued if a reaction occurs, and treatment of the reaction should be instituted. Following infusion, flush line with NS.

Reconstitution: Dilute natalizumab 300 mg in NS 100 mL. Gently invert to mix; do not shake.

Storage: Store concentrated solution under refrigeration between 2°C to 8°C (36°F to 46°F). Protect from light. Do not shake or freeze. Following dilution, may store refrigerated for use within up to 8 hours.

Nateglinide *(na te GLYE nide)*
U.S. Brand Names Starlix®
Generic Available No
Pharmacologic Category Antidiabetic Agent, Miscellaneous
Use Management of type 2 diabetes mellitus (noninsulin dependent, NIDDM) as monotherapy when hyperglycemia cannot be managed by diet and exercise alone; in combination with metformin or a thiazolidinedione to lower blood glucose in patients whose hyperglycemia cannot be controlled by exercise, diet, or a single agent alone

Mechanism of Action/Effect Increases insulin release from pancreatic beta cells; decreases postprandial hyperglycemia; not a sulfonylurea

Contraindications Hypersensitivity to nateglinide or any component of the formulation; diabetic ketoacidosis, with or without coma (treat with insulin); type 1 diabetes mellitus (insulin dependent, IDDM)

Warnings/Precautions Use with caution in patients with moderate-to-severe hepatic impairment. Use caution in severe renal dysfunction, elderly, malnourished, or patients with adrenal/pituitary dysfunction; may be more susceptible to glucose-lowering effects. All oral hypoglycemic agents are capable of producing hypoglycemia. Proper patient selection, dosage, and instructions to the patients are important to avoid hypoglycemic episodes. It may be necessary to discontinue nateglinide and administer insulin if the patient is exposed to stress (ie, fever, trauma, infection, surgery). Indicated for adjunctive therapy with metformin; not to be used as a substitute for metformin monotherapy. Combination treatment with sulfonylureas is not recommended (no additional benefit). Patients not adequately controlled on oral agents that stimulate insulin release (eg, glyburide) should not be switched to nateglinide or have nateglinide added to therapy. Safety and efficacy in pediatric patients have not been established.

Drug Interactions
Cytochrome P450 Effect: Substrate (major) of CYP2C8/9, 3A4; **Inhibits** CYP2C8/9 (weak)
Decreased Effect: CYP2C8/9 inducers may decrease the levels/effects of nateglinide; example inducers include carbamazepine, phenobarbital, phenytoin, rifampin, rifapentine, and secobarbital. CYP3A4 inducers may decrease the levels/effects of nateglinide;

example inducers include aminoglutethimide, carbamazepine, nafcillin, nevirapine, pheno-barbital, phenytoin, and rifamycins. Possible decreased hypoglycemic effect may be seen with thiazides, corticosteroids, thyroid products, and sympathomimetic drugs; monitor glucose closely when agents are initiated, modified, or discontinued.

Increased Effect/Toxicity: CYP2C8/9 inhibitors may increase the levels/effects of nateglinide; example inhibitors include delavirdine, fluconazole, gemfibrozil, ketoconazole, nicardipine, NSAIDs, pioglitazone, and sulfonamides. CYP3A4 inhibitors may increase the levels/effects of nateglinide; example inhibitors include azole antifungals, ciprofloxacin, clarithromycin, diclofenac, doxycycline, erythromycin, imatinib, isoniazid, nefazodone, nicardipine, propofol, protease inhibitors, quinidine, and verapamil. Possible increased hypoglycemic effect may be seen with salicylates, MAO inhibitors, and nonselective beta-adrenergic blocking agents; monitor glucose closely when agents are initiated, modified, or discontinued.

Nutritional/Ethanol Interactions

Ethanol: Avoid ethanol (increased risk of hypoglycemia).

Food: Rate of absorption is decreased and time to T_{max} is delayed when taken with food. Food does not affect AUC. Multiple peak plasma concentrations may be observed if fasting. Not affected by composition of meal.

Adverse Reactions As reported with nateglinide monotherapy:

1% to 10%:
Central nervous system: Dizziness (4%)
Endocrine & metabolic: Hypoglycemia (2%), increased uric acid
Gastrointestinal: Weight gain
Neuromuscular & skeletal: Arthropathy (3%)
Respiratory: Upper respiratory infection (10%)
Miscellaneous: Flu-like symptoms (4%)

Overdosage/Toxicology In case of overdose, hypoglycemic symptoms would be expected. Severe hypoglycemic reactions should be treated with intravenous glucose. Dialysis is not effective.

Pharmacodynamics/Kinetics

Onset of Action: Insulin secretion: ~20 minutes; Peak effect: 1 hour

Duration of Action: 4 hours

Absorption: Rapid

Bioavailability: 73%

Time to Peak: ≤1 hour

Protein Binding: 98%, primarily to albumin

Half-Life Elimination: 1.5 hours

Metabolism: Hepatic via hydroxylation followed by glucuronide conjugation via CYP2C9 (70%) and CYP3A4 (30%) to metabolites

Excretion: Urine (83%, 16% as unchanged drug); feces (10%)

Dosing

Adults & Elderly: Management of type 2 diabetes mellitus: Oral: Initial and maintenance dose: 120 mg 3 times/day, 1-30 minutes before meals; may be given alone or in combination with metformin or a thiazolidinedione; patients close to Hb A_{1c} goal may be started at 60 mg 3 times/day

Renal Impairment: No specific dosage adjustment is recommended for patients with mild-to-severe renal disease. Patients on dialysis showed reduced medication exposure and plasma protein binding. Patients with severe renal dysfunction are more susceptible to glucose-lowering effect; use with caution.

Hepatic Impairment: Increased serum levels are seen with mild hepatic insufficiency; no dosage adjustment is needed. Has not been studied in patients with moderate to severe liver disease; use with caution.

Available Dosage Forms Tablet: 60 mg, 120 mg

Monitoring and Teaching Issues

Physical Assessment: Assess potential for interactions with other prescriptions, OTC medications, or herbal products patient may be taking. Assess results of laboratory tests, therapeutic effectiveness, and adverse response on a regular basis throughout therapy. Teach patient proper use (or refer patient to diabetic educator), possible side effects/appropriate interventions (eg, importance of adequate hydration), and adverse symptoms to report.

Monitoring Laboratory Tests: Glucose and Hb A_{1c} levels, lipid profile

Patient Education: Do not take any new medication during therapy unless approved by prescriber. Take this medication exactly as directed, 1-30 minutes before a meal. If you skip a meal (or add an extra meal) skip (or add) a dose for that meal. Do not change dosage or discontinue without first consulting prescriber. Follow dietary and lifestyle recommendations of provider. You will be instructed in signs of hypo- or hyperglycemia by healthcare provide or diabetic educator; be alert for adverse hypoglycemia (tachycardia, profuse perspiration, tingling of lips and tongue, seizures, or change in sensorium) and follow prescriber's instructions for intervention. Note that unusual strenuous exercise, excessive alcohol intake, or acute reduction in caloric intake may increase risk of hypoglycemia. Persistent nausea or vomiting, or severely decreased dietary intake may increase risk of hyperglycemia. May cause mild side effects during first weeks of therapy (dizziness, weight gain, mild muscle aches or pain, or flu-like symptoms); if these do not diminish, notify prescriber. Report signs of respiratory infection or other persistent adverse effects. **Pregnancy/breast-feeding precautions:** Inform prescriber if you are or intend to become pregnant. Breast-feeding is not recommended.

Dietary Considerations: Nateglinide should be taken 1-30 minutes prior to meals. Scheduled dose should not be taken if meal is missed. Dietary modification based on ADA recommendations is a part of therapy. Decreases blood glucose concentration. Hypoglycemia may occur. Must be able to recognize symptoms of hypoglycemia (palpitations, sweaty palms, lightheadedness).

(Continued)

Nateglinide (Continued)

Pregnancy Risk Factor: C

Pregnancy Issues: Safety and efficacy in pregnant women have not been established. Do not use during pregnancy. Abnormal blood glucose levels are associated with a higher incidence of congenital abnormalities. Insulin is the drug of choice for the control of diabetes mellitus during pregnancy.

Lactation: Excretion in breast milk unknown/not recommended

Administration

Storage: Store at 25°C (77°F).

Additional Information An increase in weight was seen in nateglinide monotherapy, which was not seen when used in combination with metformin.

Related Information

Diabetes Mellitus Management *on page 1819*

♦ **Natrecor®** *see Nesiritide on page 1071*
♦ **Natriuretic Peptide** *see Nesiritide on page 1071*
♦ **Nature-Throid® NT** *see Thyroid on page 1469*
♦ **Navane®** *see Thiothixene on page 1467*
♦ **Navelbine®** *see Vinorelbine on page 1567*
♦ **Nebcin® [DSC]** *see Tobramycin on page 1489*
♦ **NebuPent®** *see Pentamidine on page 1178*
♦ **Necon® 0.5/35** *see Ethinyl Estradiol and Norethindrone on page 589*
♦ **Necon® 1/35** *see Ethinyl Estradiol and Norethindrone on page 589*
♦ **Necon® 1/50** *see Mestranol and Norethindrone on page 962*
♦ **Necon® 7/7/7** *see Ethinyl Estradiol and Norethindrone on page 589*
♦ **Necon® 10/11** *see Ethinyl Estradiol and Norethindrone on page 589*

Nedocromil (ne doe KROE mil)

U.S. Brand Names Alocril®; Tilade®

Synonyms Nedocromil Sodium

Generic Available No

Pharmacologic Category Mast Cell Stabilizer

Use

Aerosol: Maintenance therapy in patients with mild to moderate bronchial asthma

Ophthalmic: Treatment of itching associated with allergic conjunctivitis

Mechanism of Action/Effect Inhibits the activation of and mediator release from a variety of inflammatory cell types associated with asthma including eosinophils, neutrophils, macrophages, mast cells, monocytes, and platelets; it inhibits the release of histamine, leukotrienes, and slow-reacting substance of anaphylaxis; it inhibits the development of early and late bronchoconstriction responses to inhaled antigen

Contraindications Hypersensitivity to nedocromil or any component of the formulation

Warnings/Precautions

Aerosol: Safety and efficacy in children <6 years of age have not been established. If systemic or inhaled steroid therapy is at all reduced, monitor patients carefully. Nedocromil is **not** a bronchodilator and, therefore, should not be used for reversal of acute bronchospasm.

Ophthalmic solution: Users of contact lenses should not wear them during periods of symptomatic allergic conjunctivitis

Adverse Reactions

Inhalation aerosol:

>10%: Gastrointestinal: Unpleasant taste

1% to 10%:

Cardiovascular: Chest pain

Central nervous system: Dizziness, dysphonia, headache, fatigue

Dermatologic: Rash

Gastrointestinal: Nausea, vomiting, dyspepsia, diarrhea, abdominal pain, xerostomia, unpleasant taste

Hepatic: Increased ALT

Neuromuscular & skeletal: Arthritis, tremor

Respiratory: Cough, pharyngitis, rhinitis, bronchitis, upper respiratory infection, bronchospasm, increased sputum production

Ophthalmic solution:

>10%:

Central nervous system: Headache (40%)

Gastrointestinal: Unpleasant taste

Ocular: Burning, irritation, stinging

Respiratory: Nasal congestion

1% to 10%:

Ocular: Conjunctivitis, eye redness, photophobia

Respiratory: Asthma, rhinitis

Pharmacodynamics/Kinetics

Duration of Action: Therapeutic effect: 2 hours

Bioavailability: 7% to 9%

Protein Binding: Plasma: 89%

Half-Life Elimination: 1.5-2 hours

Excretion: Urine (as unchanged drug)

Dosing

Adults & Elderly:

Asthma: Inhalation: 2 inhalations 4 times/day; may reduce dosage to 2-3 times/day once desired clinical response to initial dose is observed. Drug has no known therapeutic systemic activity when delivered by inhalation.

Allergic conjunctivitis: Ophthalmic: 1-2 drops in each eye twice daily
Pediatrics: Children ≥6 years: Refer to adult dosing.

Available Dosage Forms
Aerosol for inhalation, as sodium (Tilade®): 1.75 mg/activation (16.2 g)
Solution, ophthalmic, as sodium (Alocril®): 2% (5 mL) [contains benzalkonium chloride]

Monitoring and Teaching Issues
Physical Assessment: Not for use during acute bronchospasm. Monitor effectiveness of therapy and adverse reactions at beginning of therapy and periodically with long-term use. Assess knowledge/teach patient appropriate use, interventions to reduce side effects, and adverse symptoms to report.

Patient Education: Aerosol: Do not use during acute bronchospasm. Use exactly as directed; do not use more often than instructed or discontinue without consulting prescriber. You may experience drowsiness, dizziness, fatigue, especially during early therapy (use caution when driving or engaging in tasks requiring alertness until response to drug is known); dry mouth, nausea, or vomiting (small frequent meals, frequent mouth care, chewing gum, or sucking lozenges may help). Report persistent runny nose, cough, cold symptoms; unresolved GI effects; skin rash; joint pain or tremor; or if breathing difficulty persists or worsens. **Breast-feeding precaution:** Consult prescriber if breast-feeding.

Inhaler: Review use with prescriber or follow package insert for directions. Prime with 3 activations prior to first use or if unused more than 7 days. Keep inhaler clean and unobstructed. Always rinse mouth and throat after use of inhaler to prevent advantageous infection. If you are also using a steroid bronchodilator, wait 10 minutes before using this aerosol.

Ophthalmic: Do not wear contact lenses with allergic conjunctivitis. For the eye only. Open eyes, look up, and pull lower lid down. Squeeze medicine into lower eyelid and close eye. Do not touch bottle tip to eye, eyelid, or other skin.

Geriatric Considerations: Elderly may have difficulty using inhaler delivery system, especially if they have physical or medical impairment (eg, Parkinson's disease, stroke). If this prophylactic modality is desired but patient cannot tolerate nedocromil inhalations, consider cromolyn sodium solution for nebulizer use.

Pregnancy Risk Factor: B
Lactation: Excretion in breast milk unknown/use caution

Administration
Storage: Store at 2°C to 30°C/36°F to 86°F. Do not freeze.

Additional Information Nedocromil has no known therapeutic systemic activity when delivered by inhalation.

Related Information
Inhalant Agents *on page 1734*

♦ **Nedocromil Sodium** *see* Nedocromil *on page 1062*

Nefazodone *(nef AY zoe done)*
U.S. Brand Names Serzone® [DSC]
Synonyms Nefazodone Hydrochloride
Restrictions A medication guide should be dispensed with each prescription. A template for the required MedGuides can be found on the FDA website at: http://www.fda.gov/cder/drug/antidepressants/labelTemplate.pdf
Generic Available Yes
Pharmacologic Category Antidepressant, Serotonin Reuptake Inhibitor/Antagonist
Medication Safety Issues
Sound-alike/look-alike issues:
Serzone® may be confused with selegiline, Serentil®, Seroquel®, sertraline
Use Treatment of depression
Unlabeled/Investigational Use Post-traumatic stress disorder
Mechanism of Action/Effect Inhibits neuronal reuptake of serotonin and norepinephrine; also blocks 5-HT$_2$ and 5-HT$_1$ receptors; has no significant affinity for alpha$_2$, beta-adrenergic, 5-HT$_{1A}$, cholinergic, dopaminergic, or benzodiazepine receptors
Contraindications Hypersensitivity to nefazodone, related compounds (phenylpiperazines), or any component of the formulation; liver injury due to previous nefazodone treatment, active liver disease, or elevated serum transaminases; concurrent use or use of MAO inhibitors within previous 14 days; use in a patient during the acute recovery phase of MI; concurrent use with carbamazepine, cisapride, or pimozide; concurrent therapy with triazolam or alprazolam is generally contraindicated (dosage must be reduced by 75% for triazolam and 50% for alprazolam; such reductions may not be possible with available dosage forms).
Warnings/Precautions Antidepressants increase the risk of suicidal thinking and behavior in children and adolescents with major depressive disorder (MDD) and other depressive disorders; consider risk prior to prescribing. All patients must be closely monitored for clinical worsening, suicidality, or unusual changes in behavior, especially during the initiation of therapy or following an increase or decrease in dosage. When used in children, the child's family or caregiver should be instructed to closely observe the patient and communicate condition with healthcare provider. A medication guide should be dispensed with each prescription. **Nefazodone is not FDA approved for use in children.**

The possibility of a suicide attempt is inherent in major depression and may persist until remission occurs. Use caution in high-risk patients. Worsening depression and severe abrupt suicidality that are not part of the presenting symptoms may require discontinuation or modification of drug therapy. The patient's family or caregiver should be alerted to monitor patients for the emergence of suicidality and associated behaviors (such as agitation, irritability, hostility, impulsivity, and hypomania) and call healthcare provider.

May worsen psychosis in some patients or precipitate a shift to mania or hypomania in patients with bipolar disorder. Patients presenting with depressive symptoms should be
(Continued)

Nefazodone *(Continued)*

screened for bipolar disorder. Monotherapy in patients with bipolar disorder should be avoided. **Nefazodone is not FDA approved for the treatment of bipolar depression.**

Cases of life-threatening hepatic failure have been reported (risk should be considered when choosing an agent for the treatment of depression); discontinue if clinical signs or symptoms suggest liver failure. May cause sedation, resulting in impaired performance of tasks requiring alertness (eg, operating machinery or driving). May increase the risks associated with electroconvulsive therapy. Consider discontinuing, when possible, prior to elective surgery. Therapy should not be abruptly discontinued in patients receiving high doses for prolonged periods. Rare reports of priapism have occurred. The incidence of sexual dysfunction with nefazodone is generally lower than with SSRIs.

The risk of sedation, conduction disturbances, orthostatic hypotension, or anticholinergic effects are very low relative to other antidepressants. Use with caution in patients with a history of cardiovascular disease (including previous MI, stroke, tachycardia, or conduction abnormalities). Use with caution in patients with urinary retention, benign prostatic hyperplasia, narrow-angle glaucoma, xerostomia, visual problems, constipation, or history of bowel obstruction (due to anticholinergic effects).

Use caution in patients with a previous seizure disorder or condition predisposing to seizures such as brain damage, alcoholism, or concurrent therapy with other drugs which lower the seizure threshold. Use with caution in patients with renal dysfunction and in elderly patients.

Drug Interactions

Cytochrome P450 Effect: Substrate (major) of CYP2D6, 3A4; **Inhibits** CYP1A2 (weak), 2B6 (weak), 2D6 (weak), 3A4 (strong)

Decreased Effect: Carbamazepine may reduce serum concentrations of nefazodone; concurrent administration should be avoided. The levels/effects of nefazodone may be decreased by aminoglutethimide, nafcillin, nevirapine, phenobarbital, phenytoin, and rifamycins and other CYP3A4 inducers.

Increased Effect/Toxicity: Concurrent use of carbamazepine, cisapride, or pimozide is contraindicated. Concurrent therapy with triazolam or alprazolam is generally contraindicated (dosage must be reduced by 75% for triazolam and 50% for alprazolam; such reductions may not be possible with available dosage forms). Concurrent use of ergot alkaloids and/or selected HMG-CoA reductase inhibitors (lovastatin and simvastatin) is generally contraindicated with strong CYP3A4 inhibitors.

Concurrent use of MAO inhibitors may lead to serotonin syndrome; avoid concurrent use or use within 14 days (includes phenelzine, isocarboxazid, and linezolid). Selegiline may increase the risk of serotonin syndrome, particularly at higher doses (>10 mg/day, where selectivity for MAO type B is decreased). Theoretically, concurrent use of buspirone, meperidine, serotonin agonists (sumatriptan and rizatriptan), SSRIs, and venlafaxine may result in serotonin syndrome.

Nefazodone may increase the serum levels/effects of antiarrhythmics (amiodarone, lidocaine, propafenone, quinidine), some antipsychotics (clozapine, haloperidol, mesoridazine, quetiapine, and risperidone), some benzodiazepines (triazolam is contraindicated; decrease alprazolam dose by 50%), buspirone (limit buspirone dose to <2.5 mg/day), Nefazodone may increase the levels/effects of calcium channel blockers, cyclosporine, mirtazapine, nateglinide, nefazodone, quinidine, sildenafil (and other PDE-5 inhibitors), tacrolimus, venlafaxine, and other CYP3A4 substrates. When used with strong CYP3A4 inhibitors, dosage adjustment/limits are recommended for sildenafil and other PDE-5 inhibitors; refer to individual monographs.

CYP3A4 inhibitors may increase The levels/effects of nefazodone may be increased by azole antifungals, chlorpromazine, ciprofloxacin, clarithromycin, delavirdine, diclofenac, doxycycline, erythromycin, fluoxetine, imatinib, isoniazid, miconazole, nicardipine, paroxetine, pergolide, propofol, protease inhibitors, quinidine, quinine, ritonavir, ropinirole, verapamil, and other CYP2D6 or 3A4 inhibitors.

Nutritional/Ethanol Interactions

Ethanol: Avoid ethanol (may increase CNS depression).

Food: Nefazodone absorption may be delayed and bioavailability may be decreased if taken with food.

Herb/Nutraceutical: Avoid valerian, St John's wort, SAMe, kava kava (may increase risk of serotonin syndrome and/or excessive sedation).

Adverse Reactions

>10%:
- Central nervous system: Headache, drowsiness, insomnia, agitation, dizziness
- Gastrointestinal: Xerostomia, nausea, constipation
- Neuromuscular & skeletal: Weakness

1% to 10%:
- Cardiovascular: Bradycardia, hypotension, peripheral edema, postural hypotension, vasodilation
- Central nervous system: Chills, fever, incoordination, lightheadedness, confusion, memory impairment, abnormal dreams, decreased concentration, ataxia, psychomotor retardation, tremor
- Dermatologic: Pruritus, rash
- Endocrine & metabolic: Breast pain, impotence, libido decreased
- Gastrointestinal: Gastroenteritis, vomiting, dyspepsia, diarrhea, increased appetite, thirst, taste perversion
- Genitourinary: Urinary frequency, urinary retention
- Hematologic: Hematocrit decreased
- Neuromuscular & skeletal: Arthralgia, hypertonia, paresthesia, neck rigidity, tremor
- Ocular: Blurred vision (9%), abnormal vision (7%), eye pain, visual field defect
- Otic: Tinnitus
- Respiratory: Bronchitis, cough, dyspnea, pharyngitis
- Miscellaneous: Flu syndrome, infection

Overdosage/Toxicology Symptoms of overdose include drowsiness, vomiting, hypotension, tachycardia, incontinence, and coma. Following initiation of essential overdose management, toxic symptoms should be treated.

Pharmacodynamics/Kinetics
Onset of Action: Therapeutic: Up to 6 weeks
Bioavailability: 20% (variable)
Time to Peak: Serum: 1 hour, prolonged in presence of food
Half-Life Elimination: Parent drug: 2-4 hours; active metabolites persist longer
Metabolism: Hepatic to three active metabolites: Triazoledione, hydroxynefazodone, and m-chlorophenylpiperazine (mCPP)
Excretion: Primarily urine (as metabolites); feces

Dosing
Adults: Depression: Oral: 200 mg/day, administered in two divided doses initially, with a range of 300-600 mg/day in two divided doses thereafter.
Elderly: Oral: Initial: 50 mg twice daily; increase dose to 100 mg twice daily in 2 weeks; usual maintenance dose: 200-400 mg/day
Pediatrics: Children and Adolescents: Depression (unlabeled use): Oral: Target dose: 300-400 mg/day (mean: 3.4 mg/kg)

Available Dosage Forms
Tablet, as hydrochloride: 50 mg, 100 mg, 150 mg, 200 mg, 250 mg
Serzone® [DSC]: 50 mg, 100 mg, 150 mg, 200 mg, 250 mg

Monitoring and Teaching Issues
Physical Assessment: Assess other medications patient may be taking for effectiveness and interactions. Monitor therapeutic effectiveness and adverse reactions at beginning of therapy and periodically with long-term use. Monitor for clinical worsening and suicidal ideation. Taper dosage slowly when discontinuing. Assess knowledge/teach patient appropriate use, interventions to reduce side effects, and adverse symptoms to report.
Monitoring Laboratory Tests: If AST/ALT increase >3 times ULN, the drug should be discontinued and not reintroduced.
Patient Education: Take exactly as directed; do not increase dose or frequency. It may take 2-3 weeks to achieve desired results. Avoid alcohol, caffeine, and other prescription or OTC medications not approved by prescriber. Maintain adequate hydration (2-3 L/day of fluids) unless instructed to restrict fluid intake. You may experience drowsiness, dizziness, or lightheadedness (use caution when driving or engaging in tasks requiring alertness until response to drug is known); nausea or vomiting (small frequent meals, frequent mouth care, chewing gum, or sucking lozenges may help); or orthostatic hypotension (use caution when climbing stairs or changing position from lying or sitting to standing). Report persistent insomnia or excessive daytime sedation; suicidal ideation; muscle cramping, tremors, weakness, tiredness, or change in gait; chest pain, palpitations, or rapid heartbeat; vision changes or eye pain; respiratory difficulty or breathlessness; malaise, loss of appetite, GI complaints, abdominal pain, or blood in stool; yellowing of skin or eyes (jaundice); or worsening of condition. **Pregnancy/breast-feeding precautions:** Inform prescriber if you are or intend to become pregnant. Breast-feeding is not recommended.
Geriatric Considerations: Data on nefazodone in the elderly is limited, specifically regarding efficacy. Clinical trials in adult patients have found it superior to placebo and similar to imipramine. Nefazodone's C_{max} and AUC have been reported to be increased twofold in the elderly and women after a single dose compared to younger patients, however, these differences were markedly reduced with multiple dosing.
Pregnancy Risk Factor: C
Lactation: Enters breast milk/not recommended
Breast-Feeding Issues: Drowsiness, lethargy, poor feeding, and failure to maintain body temperature have been reported in a nursing infant.

Administration
Oral: Dosing after meals may decrease lightheadedness and postural hypotension, but may also decrease absorption and therefore effectiveness.
Storage: Store at room temperature, below 40°C (104°F) in a tight container.

Additional Information May cause less sexual dysfunction than other antidepressants. Women and elderly receiving single doses attain significant higher peak concentrations than male volunteers.

Related Information
Antidepressant Agents on page 1713
Antidepressant Medication Guidelines on page 1765

♦ **Nefazodone Hydrochloride** see Nefazodone on page 1063

Nelfinavir (nel FIN a veer)
U.S. Brand Names Viracept®
Synonyms NFV
Generic Available No
Pharmacologic Category Antiretroviral Agent, Protease Inhibitor
Medication Safety Issues
Sound-alike/look-alike issues:
Nelfinavir may be confused with nevirapine
Viracept® may be confused with Viramune®
Use In combination with other antiretroviral therapy in the treatment of HIV infection
Mechanism of Action/Effect Inhibits HIV-1 protease enzyme; inhibition of the viral protease prevents cleavage of the gag-pol polyprotein resulting in the production of immature, noninfectious virions; cross-resistance with other protease inhibitors is possible, although, not known at this time
Contraindications Hypersensitivity to nelfinavir or any component of the formulation; concurrent therapy with amiodarone, ergot derivatives, midazolam, pimozide, quinidine, triazolam; additional medications which should not be coadministered (per manufacturer) include lovastatin and simvastatin
(Continued)

Nelfinavir *(Continued)*

Warnings/Precautions Nelfinavir is hepatically metabolized and has multiple drug interactions. A listing of medications that should not be used is available with each bottle and patients should be provided with this information. Use caution with hepatic impairment. Warn patients that redistribution of body fat can occur. New onset diabetes mellitus, exacerbation of diabetes, and hyperglycemia have been reported in HIV-infected patients receiving protease inhibitors. The oral powder contains phenylalanine; use caution in patients with phenylketonuria.

Drug Interactions

Cytochrome P450 Effect: Substrate of CYP2C8/9 (minor), 2C19 (major), 2D6 (minor), 3A4 (major); **Inhibits** CYP1A2 (weak), 2B6 (weak), 2C8/9 (weak), 2C19 (weak), 2D6 (weak), 3A4 (strong)

Decreased Effect: The levels/effects of nelfinavir may be decreased by aminoglutethimide, carbamazepine, nafcillin, nevirapine, phenobarbital, phenytoin, rifamycins, or other inducers of CYP2C19 or 3A4. Nelfinavir effects may be decreased by St John's wort. Nelfinavir may decrease the effects of delavirdine, methadone, and oral contraceptives

Increased Effect/Toxicity: Nelfinavir effects may be increased by azithromycin, delavirdine, and protease inhibitors. Nelfinavir may increase the levels/effects of selected benzodiazepines, calcium channel blockers, cyclosporine, mirtazapine, nateglinide, nefazodone, quinidine, sildenafil (and other PDE-5 inhibitors), tacrolimus, venlafaxine, and other CYP3A4 substrates. Selected benzodiazepines (midazolam, triazolam), cisapride, ergot alkaloids, selected HMG-CoA reductase inhibitors (lovastatin and simvastatin), and pimozide are generally contraindicated with strong CYP3A4 inhibitors. When used with strong CYP3A4 inhibitors, dosage adjustment/limits are recommended for sildenafil and other PDE-5 inhibitors; refer to individual monographs.

Nutritional/Ethanol Interactions

Food: Nelfinavir taken with food increases plasma concentration time curve (AUC) by two- to threefold. Do not administer with acidic food or juice (orange juice, apple juice, or applesauce) since the combination may have a bitter taste.

Herb/Nutraceutical: St John's wort may decrease nelfinavir serum concentrations; avoid concurrent use.

Adverse Reactions

>10%: Gastrointestinal: Diarrhea

2% to 10%:
Dermatologic: Rash
Gastrointestinal: Nausea, flatulence
Hematologic: Abnormal creatine kinase, hemoglobin, lymphocytes, neutrophils
Hepatic: Abnormal ALT, AST

Overdosage/Toxicology Limited data available; however, unabsorbed drug should be removed via gastric lavage and activated charcoal; significant symptoms beyond gastrointestinal disturbances are likely following acute overdose; hemodialysis will not be effective due to high protein binding of nelfinavir

Pharmacodynamics/Kinetics

Absorption: Food increases plasma concentration-time curve (AUC) by two- to threefold

Time to Peak: Serum: 2-4 hours

Protein Binding: 98%

Half-Life Elimination: 3.5-5 hours

Metabolism: Hepatic via CYP2C19 and 3A4; major metabolite has activity comparable to parent drug

Excretion: Feces (98% to 99%, 78% as metabolites, 22% as unchanged drug); urine (1% to 2%)

Dosing

Adults & Elderly: HIV infection: Oral: 1250 mg (5 tablets of 250 mg each) twice daily with food or 750 mg (3 tablets of 250 mg each) 3 times/day with food

Note: Dosage adjustments for nelfinavir when administered in combination with ritonavir: Nelfinavir 500-750 mg twice daily plus ritonavir 400 mg twice daily

Pediatrics: HIV infection: Oral: Children 2-13 years: 45-55 mg/kg twice daily **or** 25-35 mg/kg 3 times/day (maximum: 2500 mg/day); all doses should be taken with a meal. If tablets are unable to be taken, use oral powder in small amount of water, milk, formula, or dietary supplements; do not use acidic food/juice or store for >6 hours.

Renal Impairment: No adjustment is necessary.

Hepatic Impairment: Use caution.

Available Dosage Forms

Powder, oral: 50 mg/g (144 g) [contains phenylalanine 11.2 mg/g]
Tablet [film coated]: 250 mg, 625 mg

Monitoring and Teaching Issues

Physical Assessment: Use caution in presence of hepatic impairment (see Warnings/Precautions). Assess potential for interactions with other pharmacological agents and herbal products patient may be taking (nelfinavir has multiple drug interactions; a list of medications that should not be used is available with each bottle and patients should be provided with this information; see Drug Interactions). Assess therapeutic effectiveness and adverse response (see Adverse Reactions). Teach patient proper use, medication cautions, possible side effects/appropriate interventions, and adverse symptoms to report (refer to Patient Education).

Monitoring Laboratory Tests: Liver function tests, blood glucose levels, CBC with differential, CD4 cell count, plasma levels of HIV RNA

Patient Education: You will receive a list of medications that should not be taken with nelfinavir; however, do not take any new medication even if they are not on the list, unless approved by prescriber. This drug is not a cure for HIV and has not been shown to reduce the risk of transmitting HIV to others. Take exactly as directed with food. Mix powder with nonacid, noncitric fluids (orange juice, apple juice, or applesauce) and do not store reconstituted powder mixture for longer than 6 hours. If unable to swallow tablets whole, the tablet may be dissolved in water or crushed in food. Mixed or dissolved tablets must be consumed within 6 hours. If you miss a dose, take as soon as possible and return to your regular schedule (never take a double dose). Frequent blood tests may be required with prolonged therapy. May cause nausea or vomiting (small frequent meals, frequent mouth care, chewing gum, or sucking lozenges may help). Report rash; respiratory difficulty; CNS changes (migraine, confusion, suicidal ideation); muscular or skeletal pain, weakness, or tremors; or other adverse reactions. **Pregnancy/breast-feeding precautions:** Use appropriate barrier contraceptive measures (as alternative to oral contraceptives) to reduce risk of transmitting infection and potential pregnancy. Do not breast-feed.

Dietary Considerations: Should be taken as scheduled with food. Oral powder contains phenylalanine 11.2 mg/g.

Pregnancy Risk Factor: B

Pregnancy Issues: The Perinatal HIV Guidelines Working Group recommends nelfinavir as the preferred PI in combination regimens during pregnancy, especially with HAART for perinatal prophylaxis. A dose of 1250 mg twice daily has been shown to provide adequate plasma levels; 750 mg 3 times/day produced low and variable levels. Pregnancy and protease inhibitors are both associated with an increased risk of hyperglycemia. Glucose levels should be closely monitored. Health professionals are encouraged to contact the antiretroviral pregnancy registry to monitor outcomes of pregnant women exposed to antiretroviral medications (1-800-258-4263 or www.APRegistry.com).

Lactation: Enters breast milk/contraindicated

Breast-Feeding Issues: Nelfinavir is minimally excreted in breast milk. HIV-infected mothers are discouraged from breast-feeding to decrease potential transmission of HIV.

Administration

Oral: Mix powder or tablets in a small amount of water, milk, formula, soy milk, soy formula, or dietary supplement. Be sure entire contents is consumed to receive full dose. Do not use acidic food/juice to dilute due to bitter taste. One mixed, solution should be used immediately, but may be stored for up to 6 hours if refrigerated.

Storage: Store at room temperature. Oral powder (or dissolved tablets) diluted in nonacidic liquid is stable for 6 hours under refrigeration.

Related Information

Tuberculosis *on page 1864*

♦ Nembutal® *see* Pentobarbital *on page 1182*

♦ NeoDecadron® *see* Neomycin and Dexamethasone *on page 1068*

♦ Neo-Fradin™ *see* Neomycin *on page 1067*

Neomycin (nee oh MYE sin)

U.S. Brand Names Neo-Fradin™; Neo-Rx

Synonyms Neomycin Sulfate

Generic Available Yes

Pharmacologic Category Ammonium Detoxicant; Antibiotic, Aminoglycoside; Antibiotic, Topical

Medication Safety Issues

Sound-alike/look-alike issues:

Myciguent may be confused with Mycitracin®

Use Orally to prepare GI tract for surgery; topically to treat minor skin infections; treatment of diarrhea caused by *E. coli*; adjunct in the treatment of hepatic encephalopathy; bladder irrigation; ocular infections

Mechanism of Action/Effect Interferes with bacterial protein synthesis by binding to 30S ribosomal subunits

Contraindications Hypersensitivity to neomycin or any component of the formulation, or other aminoglycosides; intestinal obstruction

Warnings/Precautions Use with caution in patients with renal impairment, pre-existing hearing impairment (ototoxicity), neuromuscular disorders. Topical neomycin is a contact sensitizer with sensitivity occurring in 5% to 15% of patients treated with the drug. Symptoms include itching, reddening, edema, and failure to heal. Do not use as peritoneal lavage.

Drug Interactions

Decreased Effect: May decrease GI absorption of digoxin and methotrexate.

Increased Effect/Toxicity: Oral neomycin may potentiate the effects of oral anticoagulants. Neomycin may increase the adverse effects with other neurotoxic, ototoxic, or nephrotoxic drugs.

Adverse Reactions

Oral: >10%: Gastrointestinal: Nausea, diarrhea, vomiting, irritation or soreness of the mouth or rectal area

Topical: >10%: Dermatologic: Contact dermatitis

Overdosage/Toxicology Symptoms of overdose (rare due to poor oral bioavailability) include ototoxicity, nephrotoxicity, and neuromuscular toxicity. The treatment of choice following a single acute overdose appears to be maintenance of urine output of at least 3 mL/kg/hour during the acute treatment phase. Dialysis is of questionable value in enhancing aminoglycoside elimination. If required, hemodialysis is preferred over peritoneal dialysis in patients with normal renal function. Chelation with penicillin may be of benefit.

Pharmacodynamics/Kinetics

Absorption: Oral, percutaneous: Poor (3%)

Time to Peak: Serum: Oral: 1-4 hours

Half-Life Elimination: Age and renal function dependent: 3 hours

Metabolism: Slightly hepatic

Excretion: Feces (97% of oral dose as unchanged drug); urine (30% to 50% of absorbed drug as unchanged drug)

Dosing

Adults & Elderly:

Dermatologic infections: Topical: Topical solutions containing 0.1% to 1% neomycin have been used for irrigation

(Continued)

Neomycin *(Continued)*

Preoperative intestinal antisepsis: Oral: 1 g each hour for 4 doses then 1 g every 4 hours for 5 doses; or 1 g at 1 PM, 2 PM, and 11 PM on day preceding surgery as an adjunct to mechanical cleansing of the bowel and oral erythromycin; or 6 g/day divided every 4 hours for 2-3 days

Hepatic encephalopathy: Oral: 500-2000 mg every 6-8 hours or 4-12 g/day divided every 4-6 hours for 5-6 days

Chronic hepatic insufficiency: Oral: 4 g/day for an indefinite period

Pediatrics:

Preoperative intestinal antisepsis: Oral: Children: 90 mg/kg/day divided every 4 hours for 2 days; or 25 mg/kg at 1 PM, 2 PM, and 11 PM on the day preceding surgery as an adjunct to mechanical cleansing of the intestine and in combination with erythromycin base

Hepatic encephalopathy: Oral: Children: 50-100 mg/kg/day in divided doses every 6-8 hours or 2.5-7 g/m²/day divided every 4-6 days for 5-6 days not to exceed 12 g/day

Dermatologic infections: Topical: Children: Refer to adult dosing.

Available Dosage Forms

Powder, micronized, as sulfate [for prescription compounding] (Neo-Rx): (10 g, 100 g)

Solution, oral, as sulfate (Neo-Fradin™): 125 mg/5 mL (60 mL, 480 mL) [contains benzoic acid; cherry flavor]

Tablet, as sulfate: 500 mg

Monitoring and Teaching Issues

Physical Assessment: Assess effectiveness and interactions of other medications patient may be taking. Assess results of laboratory tests, therapeutic effectiveness, and adverse response (eg, ototoxicity, nephrotoxicity, neurotoxicity). Assess knowledge/teach patient appropriate use (application of cream/ointment), possible side effects/interventions, and adverse symptoms to report. Minimal absorption across GI mucosa or skin surfaces; however with ulceration, open or burned surfaces (especially large surfaces), absorption is possible.

Monitoring Laboratory Tests: Renal function; perform culture and sensitivity prior to initiating therapy.

Patient Education: Oral: Take as directed. Maintain adequate hydration (2-3 L/day of fluids) unless instructed to restrict fluid intake. You may experience nausea or vomiting (small frequent meals, frequent mouth care, sucking lozenges, or chewing gum may help); constipation (increased exercise, fluids, fruit, or fiber may help, or consult prescriber); or diarrhea (buttermilk, boiled milk, or yogurt may help). Report immediately any change in hearing; ringing or sense of fullness in ears; persistent diarrhea; changes in voiding patterns; or numbness, tingling, or pain in any extremity. **Pregnancy/breast-feeding precautions:** Inform prescriber if you are or intend to become pregnant. Consult prescriber if breast-feeding.

Pregnancy Risk Factor: C

Lactation: Excretion in breast milk unknown

Neomycin and Dexamethasone *(nee oh MYE sin & deks a METH a sone)*

U.S. Brand Names NeoDecadron®

Synonyms Dexamethasone and Neomycin

Generic Available No

Pharmacologic Category Antibiotic/Corticosteroid, Ophthalmic

Use Treatment of steroid responsive inflammatory conditions of the palpebral and bulbar conjunctiva, lid, cornea, and anterior segment of the globe

Dosing

Adults & Elderly: Inflammation/infection: Ophthalmic: Instill 1-2 drops in eye(s) every 3-4 hours

Available Dosage Forms Solution, ophthalmic: Neomycin sulfate 0.35% [3.5 mg/mL] and dexamethasone sodium phosphate 0.1% [1 mg/mL] (5 mL) [contains benzalkonium chloride and sodium bisulfite]

Monitoring and Teaching Issues

Physical Assessment: See individual agents.

Patient Education: See individual agents. **Pregnancy/breast-feeding precautions:** Inform prescriber if you are or intend to become pregnant. Consult prescriber if breast-feeding.

Pregnancy Risk Factor: C

Lactation: Excretion in breast milk unknown

Related Information

Dexamethasone *on page 424*

Neomycin *on page 1067*

Neomycin and Polymyxin B *(nee oh MYE sin & pol i MIKS in bee)*

U.S. Brand Names Neosporin® G.U. Irrigant

Synonyms Polymyxin B and Neomycin

Generic Available No

Pharmacologic Category Antibiotic, Topical

Use Short-term as a continuous irrigant or rinse in the urinary bladder to prevent bacteriuria and gram-negative rod septicemia associated with the use of indwelling catheters; to help prevent infection in minor cuts, scrapes, and burns

Dosing

Adults & Elderly: Bladder irrigation: **Not for I.V. injection;** add 1 mL irrigant to 1 liter isotonic saline solution and connect container to the inflow of lumen of 3-way catheter. Continuous irrigant or rinse in the urinary bladder for up to a maximum of 10 days with administration rate adjusted to patient's urine output; usually no more than 1 L of irrigant is used per day.

Pediatrics: Refer to adult dosing.

Available Dosage Forms Solution, irrigant: Neomycin 40 mg and polymyxin B sulfate 200,000 units per mL (1 mL, 20 mL)

Monitoring and Teaching Issues

Physical Assessment: See individual agents.

Patient Education: See individual agents. **Pregnancy/breast-feeding precautions:** Inform prescriber if you are or intend to become pregnant. Consult prescriber if breast-feeding.

Pregnancy Risk Factor: C/D (for G.U. irrigant)

Lactation: Excretion in breast milk unknown

Related Information

Neomycin *on page 1067*

Polymyxin B *on page 1228*

♦ **Neomycin, Bacitracin, and Polymyxin B** *see Bacitracin, Neomycin, and Polymyxin B on page 171*

♦ **Neomycin, Bacitracin, Polymyxin B, and Hydrocortisone** *see Bacitracin, Neomycin, Polymyxin B, and Hydrocortisone on page 172*

Neomycin, Colistin, Hydrocortisone, and Thonzonium

(neé oh MYE sin, koe LIS tin, hye droe KOR ti sone, & thon ZOE nee um)

U.S. Brand Names Coly-Mycin® S; Cortisporin®-TC

Synonyms Colistin, Neomycin, Hydrocortisone, and Thonzonium; Hydrocortisone, Neomycin, Colistin, and Thonzonium; Thonzonium, Neomycin, Colistin, and Hydrocortisone

Generic Available No

Pharmacologic Category Antibiotic/Corticosteroid, Otic

Use Treatment of superficial and susceptible bacterial infections of the external auditory canal; for treatment of susceptible bacterial infections of mastoidectomy and fenestration cavities

Dosing

Adults & Elderly: Ear inflammation/infection: Otic:

Calibrated dropper: 5 drops in affected ear 3-4 times/day

Dropper bottle: 4 drops in affected ear 3-4 times/day

Note: Alternatively, a cotton wick may be inserted in the ear canal and saturated with suspension every 4 hours; wick should be replaced at least every 24 hours

Pediatrics: Ear inflammation/infection: Otic:

Calibrated dropper: 4 drops in affected ear 3-4 times/day

Dropper bottle: 3 drops in affected ear 3-4 times/day

Note: Alternatively, a cotton wick may be inserted in the ear canal and saturated with suspension every 4 hours; wick should be replaced at least every 24 hours

Available Dosage Forms

Suspension, otic [drops]:

Coly-Mycin® S: Neomycin 0.33%, colistin 0.3%, hydrocortisone acetate 1%, and thonzonium bromide 0.05% (5 mL) [contains thimerosal; packaged with dropper]

Cortisporin®-TC: Neomycin 0.33%, colistin 0.3%, hydrocortisone acetate 1%, and thonzonium bromide 0.05% (10 mL) [contains thimerosal; packaged with dropper]

Monitoring and Teaching Issues

Physical Assessment: See individual agents.

Patient Education: Shake well before using.

Related Information

Hydrocortisone *on page 760*

Neomycin *on page 1067*

Neomycin, Polymyxin B, and Hydrocortisone

(neé oh MYE sin, pol i MIKS in bee, & hye droe KOR ti sone)

U.S. Brand Names AntibiOtic® Ear; Cortisporin® Cream; Cortisporin® Ophthalmic; Cortisporin® Otic; PediOtic®

Synonyms Hydrocortisone, Neomycin, and Polymyxin B; Polymyxin B, Neomycin, and Hydrocortisone

Generic Available Yes

Pharmacologic Category Antibiotic/Corticosteroid, Ophthalmic; Antibiotic/Corticosteroid, Otic; Topical Skin Product

Use Steroid-responsive inflammatory condition for which a corticosteroid is indicated and where bacterial infection or a risk of bacterial infection exists

Dosing

Adults & Elderly:

Note: Duration of use should be limited to 10 days unless otherwise directed by the physician. Otic solution is used **only** for swimmer's ear (infections of external auditory canal)

Auditory canal inflammation/infection: Otic: Instill 4 drops 3-4 times/day; otic suspension is the preferred otic preparation

Ocular inflammation/infection: Ophthalmic: Instill 1-2 drops 2-4 times/day, or more frequently as required for severe infections; in acute infections, instill 1-2 drops every 15-30 minutes gradually reducing the frequency of administration as the infection is controlled

Dermatologic inflammation/infection: Topical: Apply a thin layer 1-4 times/day. Therapy should be discontinued when control is achieved; if no improvement is seen, reassessment of diagnosis may be necessary.

Pediatrics:

Note: Duration of use should be limited to 10 days unless otherwise directed by the physician. Otic solution is used **only** for swimmer's ear (infections of external auditory canal).

Auditory canal inflammation/infection: Otic: Children: Instill 3 drops into affected ear 3-4 times/day.

(Continued)

Neomycin, Polymyxin B, and Hydrocortisone *(Continued)*

Ocular inflammation/infection: Children: Refer to adult dosing.
Dermatologic inflammation/infection: Children: Refer to adult dosing.

Available Dosage Forms
Cream, topical (Cortisporin®): Neomycin 3.5 mg, polymyxin B 10,000 units, and hydrocortisone 5 mg per g (7.5 g)

Solution, otic (AntibiOtic® Ear; Cortisporin®): Neomycin 3.5 mg, polymyxin B 10,000 units, and hydrocortisone 10 mg per mL (10 mL) [contains potassium metabisulfite]

Suspension, ophthalmic (Cortisporin®): Neomycin 3.5 mg, polymyxin B 10,000 units, and hydrocortisone 10 mg per mL (7.5 mL) [contains thimerosal]

Suspension, otic: Neomycin 3.5 mg, polymyxin B 10,000 units, and hydrocortisone 10 mg per mL (10 mL)

AntibiOtic® Ear, Cortisporin®: Neomycin 3.5 mg, polymyxin B 10,000 units, and hydrocortisone 10 mg per mL (10 mL) [contains thimerosal]

PediOtic®: Neomycin 3.5 mg, polymyxin B 10,000 units, and hydrocortisone 10 mg per mL (7.5 mL) [contains thimerosal]

Monitoring and Teaching Issues
Physical Assessment: See individual agents.
Patient Education:
Otic: Hold container in hand to warm; if drops are in suspension form, shake well for approximately 10 seconds, lie on your side with affected ear up; for adults hold the ear lobe up and back, for children hold the ear lobe down and back; instill drops in ear without inserting dropper into ear; maintain tilted ear for 2 minutes

Ophthalmic: May cause sensitivity to bright light; may cause temporary blurring of vision or stinging following administration, but discontinue product and see prescriber if problems persist or increase; to use, tilt head back and place medication in conjunctival sac and close eyes; apply light pressure on lacrimal sac for 1 minute

Cream: Discontinue product if irritation persists or increases

Pregnancy Risk Factor: C

Related Information
Hydrocortisone *on page 760*
Neomycin *on page 1067*
Polymyxin B *on page 1228*

♦ **Neomycin Sulfate** *see Neomycin on page 1067*
♦ **Neoral®** *see CycloSPORINE on page 383*
♦ **Neo-Rx** *see Neomycin on page 1067*
♦ **Neosporin® G.U. Irrigant** *see Neomycin and Polymyxin B on page 1068*
♦ **Neosporin® Neo To Go® [OTC]** *see Bacitracin, Neomycin, and Polymyxin B on page 171*
♦ **Neosporin® Ophthalmic Ointment** *see Bacitracin, Neomycin, and Polymyxin B on page 171*
♦ **Neosporin® Topical [OTC]** *see Bacitracin, Neomycin, and Polymyxin B on page 171*

Neostigmine *(nee oh STIG meen)*
U.S. Brand Names Prostigmin®
Synonyms Neostigmine Bromide; Neostigmine Methylsulfate
Generic Available Yes: Injection
Pharmacologic Category Acetylcholinesterase Inhibitor
Medication Safety Issues
Sound-alike/look-alike issues:
Prostigmin® may be confused with physostigmine

Use Diagnosis and treatment of myasthenia gravis; prevention and treatment of postoperative bladder distention and urinary retention; reversal of the effects of nondepolarizing neuromuscular-blocking agents after surgery
Mechanism of Action/Effect Inhibits destruction of acetylcholine by acetylcholinesterase which facilitates transmission of impulses across myoneural junction
Contraindications Hypersensitivity to neostigmine, bromides, or any component of the formulation; GI or GU obstruction
Warnings/Precautions Does **not** antagonize and may prolong the Phase I block of depolarizing muscle relaxants (eg, succinylcholine). Use with caution in patients with epilepsy, asthma, bradycardia, hyperthyroidism, cardiac arrhythmias, or peptic ulcer. Adequate facilities should be available for cardiopulmonary resuscitation when testing and adjusting dose for myasthenia gravis. Have atropine and epinephrine ready to treat hypersensitivity reactions. Overdosage may result in cholinergic crisis, this must be distinguished from myasthenic crisis. Anticholinesterase insensitivity can develop for brief or prolonged periods.
Drug Interactions
Decreased Effect: Antagonizes effects of nondepolarizing muscle relaxants (eg, pancuronium, tubocurarine). Atropine antagonizes the muscarinic effects of neostigmine.
Increased Effect/Toxicity: Neuromuscular blocking agent effects are increased when combined with neostigmine.
Lab Interactions Increased aminotransferase [ALT (SGPT)/AST (SGOT)] (S), amylase (S)
Adverse Reactions Frequency not defined.
Cardiovascular: Arrhythmias (especially bradycardia), hypotension, decreased carbon monoxide, tachycardia, AV block, nodal rhythm, nonspecific ECG changes, cardiac arrest, syncope, flushing
Central nervous system: Convulsions, dysarthria, dysphonia, dizziness, loss of consciousness, drowsiness, headache
Dermatologic: Skin rash, thrombophlebitis (I.V.), urticaria
Gastrointestinal: Hyperperistalsis, nausea, vomiting, salivation, diarrhea, stomach cramps, dysphagia, flatulence
Genitourinary: Urinary urgency
Neuromuscular & skeletal: Weakness, fasciculations, muscle cramps, spasms, arthralgia
Ocular: Small pupils, lacrimation

Respiratory: Increased bronchial secretions, laryngospasm, bronchiolar constriction, respiratory muscle paralysis, dyspnea, respiratory depression, respiratory arrest, bronchospasm

Miscellaneous: Diaphoresis (increased), anaphylaxis, allergic reactions

Overdosage/Toxicology Symptoms of overdose include muscle weakness, blurred vision, excessive sweating, tearing and salivation, nausea, vomiting, diarrhea, hypertension, bradycardia, muscle weakness, and paralysis. Atropine sulfate injection should be readily available as an antagonist for the effects of neostigmine.

Pharmacodynamics/Kinetics
Onset of Action: I.M.: 20-30 minutes; I.V.: 1-20 minutes

Duration of Action: I.M.: 2.5-4 hours; I.V.: 1-2 hours

Absorption: Oral: Poor, <2%

Half-Life Elimination: Normal renal function: 0.5-2.1 hours; End-stage renal disease: Prolonged

Metabolism: Hepatic

Excretion: Urine (50% as unchanged drug)

Dosing
Adults & Elderly:

Myasthenia gravis, diagnosis: I.M.: 0.02 mg/kg as a single dose

Myasthenia gravis, treatment:

Oral: 15 mg/dose every 3-4 hours up to 375 mg/day maximum

I.M., I.V., SubQ: 0.5-2.5 mg every 1-3 hours up to 10 mg/24 hours maximum

Reversal of nondepolarizing neuromuscular blockade after surgery in conjunction with atropine: I.V.: 0.5-2.5 mg; total dose not to exceed 5 mg; must administer atropine several minutes prior to neostigmine

Bladder atony: I.M., SubQ:

Prevention: 0.25 mg every 4-6 hours for 2-3 days

Treatment: 0.5-1 mg every 3 hours for 5 doses after bladder has emptied

Pediatrics:

Myasthenia gravis, diagnosis: I.M.: Children: 0.04 mg/kg as a single dose

Myasthenia gravis, treatment: Children:

Oral: 2 mg/kg/day divided every 3-4 hours

I.M., I.V., SubQ: 0.01-0.04 mg/kg every 2-4 hours

Reversal of nondepolarizing neuromuscular blockade after surgery in conjunction with atropine (must administer atropine several minutes prior to neostigmine): I.V.:

Infants: 0.025-0.1 mg/kg/dose

Children: 0.025-0.08 mg/kg/dose

Renal Impairment:

Cl_{cr} 10-50 mL/minute: Administer 50% of normal dose.

Cl_{cr} <10 mL/minute: Administer 25% of normal dose.

Available Dosage Forms
Injection, solution, as methylsulfate: 0.5 mg/mL (1 mL, 10 mL); 1 mg/mL (10 mL)

Tablet, as bromide: 15 mg

Monitoring and Teaching Issues
Physical Assessment: Used for MG diagnosis by physicians. For bladder atony, assess bladder adequacy prior to administering medication. Monitor therapeutic effectiveness and adverse effects (including cholinergic crisis). Teach patient symptoms to report.

Patient Education: Take this drug exactly as prescribed. You may experience visual difficulty (eg, blurring and dark adaptation, use caution at night) or urinary frequency. Promptly report any muscle weakness, respiratory difficulty, severe or unresolved diarrhea, persistent abdominal cramping or vomiting, sweating, or tearing. **Pregnancy/breast-feeding precautions:** Inform prescriber if you are pregnant. Breast-feeding is not recommended.

Geriatric Considerations: Many elderly will have diseases which may influence the use of neostigmine. Also, many elderly will need doses reduced 50% due to creatinine clearances in the 10-50 mL/minute range (common in the aged). Side effects or concomitant disease may warrant use of pyridostigmine.

Pregnancy Risk Factor: C

Lactation: Excretion in breast milk unknown/not recommended

Administration
I.M.: In the diagnosis of myasthenia gravis, all anticholinesterase medications should be discontinued for at least 8 hours before administering neostigmine.

Compatibility: Stable in NS

Additional Information In the diagnosis of myasthenia gravis, all anticholinesterase medications should be discontinued for at least 8 hours before administering neostigmine.

♦ **Neostigmine Bromide** *see Neostigmine on page 1070*

♦ **Neostigmine Methylsulfate** *see Neostigmine on page 1070*

♦ **NeoStrata AHA [OTC]** *see Hydroquinone on page 768*

♦ **Neo-Synephrine® Extra Strength [OTC]** *see Phenylephrine on page 1200*

♦ **Neo-Synephrine® Mild [OTC]** *see Phenylephrine on page 1200*

♦ **Neo-Synephrine® Ophthalmic** *see Phenylephrine on page 1200*

♦ **Neo-Synephrine® Regular Strength [OTC]** *see Phenylephrine on page 1200*

♦ **Nephro-Calci® [OTC]** *see Calcium Carbonate on page 235*

♦ **Nephro-Fer® [OTC]** *see Ferrous Fumarate on page 623*

Nesiritide (ni SIR i tide)
U.S. Brand Names Natrecor®

Synonyms B-Type Natriuretic Peptide (Human); hBNP; Natriuretic Peptide

Generic Available No

Pharmacologic Category Natriuretic Peptide, B-Type, Human; Vasodilator

(Continued)

Nesiritide *(Continued)*

Medication Safety Issues

High alert medication: The Institute for Safe Medication Practices (ISMP) includes this medication among its list of drugs which have a heightened risk of causing significant patient harm when used in error.

Use Treatment of acutely decompensated congestive heart failure (CHF) in patients with dyspnea at rest or with minimal activity

Mechanism of Action/Effect Binds to cell surface receptors in vasculature, resulting in smooth muscle cell relaxation. Has been shown to produce dose-dependent reductions in pulmonary capillary wedge pressure (PCWP) and systemic arterial pressure providing symptomatic improvements (dyspnea decreased) for several days.

Contraindications Hypersensitivity to natriuretic peptide or any component of the formulation; cardiogenic shock (when used as primary therapy); hypotension (systolic blood pressure <90 mm Hg)

Warnings/Precautions May cause hypotension; administer in clinical situations when blood pressure may be closely monitored. Use caution in patients systolic blood pressure <100 mm Hg (contraindicated if <90 mm Hg); more likely to experience hypotension. Effects may be additive with other agents capable of causing hypotension. Hypotensive effects may last for several hours.

Should not be used in patients with low filling pressures, or in patients with conditions which depend on venous return including significant valvular stenosis, restrictive or obstructive cardiomyopathy, constrictive pericarditis, and pericardial tamponade. May be associated with development of azotemia; use caution in patients with renal impairment or in patients where renal perfusion is dependent on renin-angiotensin-aldosterone system.

Monitor for allergic or anaphylactic reactions. Use caution with prolonged infusions; limited experience for infusions >48 hours. Safety and efficacy in pediatric patients have not been established.

Drug Interactions

Increased Effect/Toxicity: An increased frequency of symptomatic hypotension was observed with concurrent administration of ACE inhibitors. Other hypotensive agents are likely to have additive effects on hypotension. In patients receiving diuretic therapy leading to depletion of intravascular volume, the risk of hypotension and/or renal impairment may be increased. Nesiritide should be avoided in patients with low filling pressures.

Adverse Reactions Note: Frequencies cited below were recorded in VMAC trial at dosages similar to approved labeling. Higher frequencies have been observed in trials using higher dosages of nesiritide.

>10%:

Cardiovascular: Hypotension (total: 11%; symptomatic: 4% at recommended dose, up to 17% at higher doses)

Renal: Increased serum creatinine (28% with >0.5 mg/dL increase over baseline)

1% to 10%:

Cardiovascular: Ventricular tachycardia (3%)*, ventricular extrasystoles (3%)*, angina (2%)*, bradycardia (1%), tachycardia, atrial fibrillation, AV node conduction abnormalities

Central nervous system: Headache (8%)*, dizziness (3%)*, insomnia (2%), anxiety (3%), fever, confusion, paresthesia, somnolence, tremor

Dermatologic: Pruritus, rash

Gastrointestinal: Nausea (4%)*, abdominal pain (1%)*, vomiting (1%)*

Hematologic: Anemia

Local: Injection site reaction

Neuromuscular & skeletal: Back pain (4%), leg cramps

Ocular: Amblyopia

Respiratory: Cough (increased), hemoptysis, apnea

Miscellaneous: Increased diaphoresis

*Frequency less than or equal to placebo or other standard therapy

Overdosage/Toxicology No data. Symptoms of overdose would be expected to include excessive and/or prolonged hypotension. Treatment is symptomatic and supportive. Drug discontinuation and/or dosage reduction may be required.

Pharmacodynamics/Kinetics

Onset of Action: 15 minutes (60% of 3-hour effect achieved)

Duration of Action: >60 minutes (up to several hours) for systolic blood pressure; hemodynamic effects persist longer than serum half-life would predict

Time to Peak: 1 hour

Half-Life Elimination: Initial (distribution) 2 minutes; Terminal: 18 minutes

Metabolism: Proteolytic cleavage by vascular endopeptidases and proteolysis following receptor binding and cellular internalization

Excretion: Urine

Dosing

Adults & Elderly:

Congestive heart failure: I.V.: Initial: 2 mcg/kg (bolus); followed by continuous infusion at 0.01 mcg/kg/minute; **Note:** Should not be initiated at a dosage higher than initial recommended dose. At intervals of ≥3 hours, the dosage may be increased by 0.005 mcg/kg/minute (preceded by a bolus of 1 mcg/kg), up to a maximum of 0.03 mcg/kg/minute. Increases beyond the initial infusion rate should be limited to selected patients and accompanied by hemodynamic monitoring.

Patients experiencing hypotension during the infusion: Infusion should be interrupted. May attempt to restart at a lower dose (reduce initial infusion dose by 30% and omit bolus).

Renal Impairment: No adjustment required

Available Dosage Forms Injection, powder for reconstitution: 1.5 mg

Monitoring and Teaching Issues

Physical Assessment: Assess potential for interactions with other prescriptions, OTC medications, or herbal products patient may be taking (eg, other hypotensive agents or diuretics). Blood pressure and cardiac function should be monitored before and at frequent intervals during and for 24 hours following infusion (hemodynamic monitoring with larger doses). Assess results of laboratory tests and patient response on a regular basis throughout therapy (eg, hypersensitivity, hypotension). Teach patient possible side effects/appropriate interventions and adverse symptoms to report.

Patient Education: This medication can only be administered by infusion; you will be monitored closely during and following infusion. Report immediately any pain, burning, swelling at infusion site, or any signs of allergic reaction (eg, respiratory or swallowing difficulty, back pain, chest tightness, rash, hives, swelling of lips or mouth). Remain in bed until advised otherwise; call for assistance with turning or changing position. Report any chest pain, respiratory difficulty, confusion, nausea, leg cramps, or any other adverse effects. **Pregnancy/breast-feeding precautions:** Inform prescriber if you are or intend to become pregnant. Consult prescriber if breast-feeding.

Pregnancy Risk Factor: C

Lactation: Excretion in breast milk unknown/use caution

Administration

I.V.: Do not administer through a heparin-coated catheter (concurrent administration of heparin via a separate catheter is acceptable, per manufacturer).

Reconstitution: Reconstitute 1.5 mg vial with 5 mL of diluent removed from a premixed plastic I.V. bag (compatible with 5% dextrose, 0.9% sodium chloride, 5% dextrose and 0.45% sodium chloride, or 5% dextrose and 0.2% sodium chloride). Do not shake vial to dissolve (roll gently). Withdraw entire contents of vial and add to 250 mL I.V. bag. Resultant concentration of solution approximately 6 mcg/mL.

Compatibility: Incompatible with heparin, insulin, ethacrynate sodium, bumetanide, enalaprilat, hydralazine, and furosemide. Do not administer through the same catheter. Do not administer with any solution containing sodium metabisulfite. Catheter must be flushed between administration of nesiritide and physically incompatible drugs.

Storage: Vials may be stored at controlled room temperature of 20°C to 25°C (68°F to 77°F) or under refrigeration at 2°C to 8°C (36°F to 46°F). Following reconstitution, vials are stable under these conditions for up to 24 hours.

Additional Information The duration of symptomatic improvement with nesiritide following discontinuation of the infusion has been limited (generally lasting several days). Atrial natriuretic peptide, which is related to nesiritide, has been associated with increased vascular permeability. This has not been observed in clinical trials with nesiritide, but patients should be monitored for this effect.

Related Information

Heart Failure on page 1828

- **Neupogen®** see Filgrastim on page 627
- **Neurontin®** see Gabapentin on page 691
- **Neut®** see Sodium Bicarbonate on page 1380
- **Neutra-Phos® [OTC]** see Potassium Phosphate and Sodium Phosphate on page 1239
- **Neutra-Phos®-K [OTC]** see Potassium Phosphate on page 1238
- **NeuTrexin®** see Trimetrexate Glucuronate on page 1530

Nevirapine (ne VYE ra peen)

U.S. Brand Names Viramune®

Synonyms NVP

Restrictions An FDA-approved medication guide is available at www.fda.gov/cder/Offices/ODS/labeling.htm.

Generic Available No

Pharmacologic Category Antiretroviral Agent, Reverse Transcriptase Inhibitor (Non-nucleoside)

Medication Safety Issues

Sound-alike/look-alike issues:

Nevirapine may be confused with nelfinavir

Viramune® may be confused with Viracept®

Use In combination therapy with other antiretroviral agents for the treatment of HIV-1

Mechanism of Action/Effect Blocks the RNA-dependent DNA polymerase activity

Contraindications Hypersensitivity to nevirapine or any component of the formulation

Warnings/Precautions Severe hepatotoxic reactions may occur (fulminant and cholestatic hepatitis, hepatic necrosis) and, in some cases, have resulted in hepatic failure and death. Intensive monitoring is required during the initial 18 weeks of therapy to detect potentially life-threatening dermatologic, hypersensitivity, and hepatic reactions. The greatest risk of these reactions is within the initial 6 weeks of treatment. Patients with a history of chronic hepatitis (B or C) or increased baseline transaminase levels may be at increased risk of hepatotoxic reactions. Female gender and patients with increased CD4⁺-cell counts may be at substantially greater risk of hepatic events (often associated with rash). Therapy should not be started with elevated CD4⁺-cell counts unless the benefit of therapy outweighs the risk of serious hepatotoxicity (adult females: CD4⁺-cell counts >250 cells/mm³; adult males: CD4⁺-cell counts >400 cells/mm³).

Severe life-threatening skin reactions (eg, Stevens-Johnson syndrome, toxic epidermal necrolysis, hypersensitivity reactions with rash and organ dysfunction) have occurred. Nevirapine must be initiated with a 14-day lead-in dosing period to decrease the incidence of adverse effects.

If a severe dermatologic or hypersensitivity reaction occurs, or if signs and symptoms of hepatitis occur, nevirapine should be permanently discontinued. These may include a severe rash, or a rash associated with fever, blisters, oral lesions, conjunctivitis, facial edema, (Continued)

Nevirapine *(Continued)*

muscle or joint aches, general malaise, hepatitis, eosinophilia, granulocytopenia, lymphadenopathy, or renal dysfunction.

Consider alteration of antiretroviral therapies if disease progression occurs while patients are receiving nevirapine. Safety and efficacy have not been established in neonates.

Drug Interactions

Cytochrome P450 Effect: Substrate of CYP2B6 (minor), 2D6 (minor), 3A4 (major); **Inhibits** CYP1A2 (weak), 2D6 (weak), 3A4 (weak); **Induces** CYP2B6 (strong), 3A4 (strong)

Decreased Effect: The levels/effects of nevirapine may be decreased by aminoglutethimide, carbamazepine, nafcillin, nevirapine, phenobarbital, phenytoin, and rifamycins, and other CYP3A4 inducers; avoid concurrent use. Nevirapine may decrease the levels/effects of benzodiazepines, bupropion, calcium channel blockers, clarithromycin, cyclosporine, efavirenz, erythromycin, estrogens, mirtazapine, nateglinide, nefazodone, promethazine, selegiline, sertraline, tacrolimus, venlafaxine, and other CYP2B6 or 3A4 substrates. Nevirapine may decrease serum concentrations of some protease inhibitors (AUC of indinavir, lopinavir, nelfinavir, and saquinavir may be decreased, however, no effect noted with ritonavir); specific dosage adjustments have not been recommended; no adjustment recommended for ritonavir, unless combined with lopinavir (Kaletra™). Nevirapine may decrease the effectiveness of oral contraceptives; suggest alternate method or additional form of birth control. Nevirapine also decreases the effect of ketoconazole and methadone.

Increased Effect/Toxicity: Cimetidine, itraconazole, ketoconazole, and some macrolide antibiotics may increase nevirapine plasma concentrations. Concurrent administration of prednisone for the initial 14 days of nevirapine therapy was associated with an increased incidence and severity of rash. Rifabutin concentrations are increased by nevirapine.

Nutritional/Ethanol Interactions Herb/Nutraceutical: Nevirapine serum concentration may be decreased by St John's wort; avoid concurrent use.

Adverse Reactions Note: Potentially life-threatening nevirapine-associated adverse effects may present with the following symptoms: Abrupt onset of flu-like symptoms, abdominal pain, jaundice, or fever with or without rash; may progress to hepatic failure with encephalopathy. Skin rash is present in ~50% of cases.

Percentages of adverse effects vary by clinical trial:

>10%:

Dermatologic: Rash (grade 1/2: 13%; grade 3/4: 1.5%) is the most common toxicity; occurs most frequently within the first 6 weeks of therapy; women may be at higher risk than men

Hepatic: ALT >250 units/L (5% to 14%); symptomatic hepatic events (4%, range: up to 11%) are more common in women, women with CD4$^+$ cell counts >250 cells/mm^3, and men with CD4$^+$ cell counts >400 cells/mm^3

1% to 10%:

Central nervous system: Headache (1% to 4%), fatigue (up to 5%)

Gastrointestinal: Nausea (<1% to 9%), abdominal pain (<1% to 2%), diarrhea (up to 2%)

Hepatic: AST >250 units/L (4% to 8%); coinfection with hepatitis B or C and/or increased liver function tests at the beginning of therapy are associated with a greater risk of asymptomatic transaminase elevations (ALT or AST >5 times ULN: 6%, range: up to 9%) or symptomatic events occurring ≥6 weeks after beginning treatment

Overdosage/Toxicology Edema, erythema nodosum, fatigue, fever, headache, insomnia, nausea, pulmonary infiltrates, rash, vertigo, and weight loss have been reported following large doses.

Pharmacodynamics/Kinetics

Absorption: >90%

Time to Peak: Serum: 2-4 hours

Protein Binding: Plasma: 60%

Half-Life Elimination: Decreases over 2- to 4-week time with chronic dosing due to autoinduction (ie, half-life = 45 hours initially and decreases to 25-30 hours)

Metabolism: Extensively hepatic via CYP3A4 (hydroxylation to inactive compounds); may undergo enterohepatic recycling

Excretion: Urine (~81%, primarily as metabolites, <3% as unchanged drug); feces (~10%)

Dosing

Adults & Elderly: HIV infection: Oral: Initial: 200 mg once daily for 14 days; maintenance: 200 mg twice daily (in combination with an additional antiretroviral agents)

Note: If patient experiences a rash during the 14-day lead-in period, dose should not be increased until the rash has resolved. Discontinue if severe rash, or rash with constitutional symptoms, is noted. If a therapy is interrupted for >7 days, restart with initial dose for 14 days. Use of prednisone to prevent nevirapine-associated rash is not recommended. Permanently discontinue if symptomatic hepatic events occur.

Pediatrics:

HIV infection: Oral:

Children 2 months to <8 years: Initial: 4 mg/kg/dose once daily for 14 days; increase dose to 7 mg/kg/dose every 12 hours if no rash or other adverse effects occur; maximum dose: 200 mg/dose every 12 hours

Children ≥8 years: Initial: 4 mg/kg/dose once daily for 14 days; increase dose to 4 mg/kg/dose every 12 hours if no rash or other adverse effects occur; maximum dose: 200 mg/dose every 12 hours

Alternative pediatric dosing (unlabeled): 120-200 mg/m^2 every 12 hours; this dosing has been proposed due to the fact that dosing based on mg/kg may result in an abrupt decrease in dose at the 8th birthday, which may be inappropriate.

Note: If patient experiences a rash during the 14-day lead-in period, dose should not be increased until the rash has resolved. Discontinue if severe rash, or rash with constitutional symptoms, is noted. If therapy is interrupted for >7 days, restart with initial dose for 14 days. Use of prednisone to prevent nevirapine-associated rash is not recommended. Permanently discontinue if symptomatic hepatic events occur.

Renal Impairment:
Cl$_{cr}$ ≥20 mL/minute: No adjustment required
Hemodialysis: An additional 200 mg dose is recommended following dialysis.

Hepatic Impairment: Do not administer to patients with severe hepatic impairment. Discontinue (and do not reinitiate) if clinical hepatitis occurs.

Available Dosage Forms
Suspension, oral: 50 mg/5 mL (240 mL)
Tablet: 200 mg

Monitoring and Teaching Issues

Physical Assessment: Use caution in presence of hepatic impairment (for very specific use cautions/directions see Warnings/Precautions). See Dosing for 14 day lead-in dosing recommendations (to assess for hypersensitivity reactions prior to increasing to regular daily dose). Assess potential for interactions with extensive list of other pharmacological agents and herbal products (see Drug Interactions). Assess results of laboratory tests (especially LFTs at baseline and frequently during therapy; see Monitoring Laboratory Tests). Patient should be monitored very closely first weeks of therapy for symptoms of hypersensitivity/dermatologic reactions which may include (severe rash, rash with fever, blisters, oral lesions, conjunctivitis, facial edema, muscle or joint aches, general malaise, hepatitis, or renal dysfunction for first months of therapy; see Adverse Reactions). Teach patient proper use, possible side effects/appropriate interventions, and adverse symptoms to report (see Patient Education).

Monitoring Laboratory Tests: Monitor CBC and viral load. Liver function tests should be monitored at baseline, and intensively during the first 18 weeks of therapy (optimal frequency not established, some practitioners recommend more often than once a month, including prior to dose escalation, and at 2 weeks following dose escalation), then periodically throughout therapy; observe for CNS side effects. Assess/evaluate AST/ALT in any patients with a rash. Permanently discontinue if patient experiences severe rash, constitutional symptoms associated with rash, rash with elevated AST/ALT, or clinical hepatitis, Mild-to-moderate rash without AST/ALT elevation may continue treatment per discretion of prescriber. If mild-to-moderate urticarial rash, do not restart if treatment is interrupted.

Patient Education: Do not take any new medication during therapy unless approved by prescriber. This is not a cure for HIV and has not been shown to reduce the risk of transmitting HIV to others. The long-term effects of use are not known. Take as directed, with food. If unable to swallow tablets whole, the tablet may be dissolved in water or crushed in food. Shake suspension gently prior to use. Use oral syringe for volumes of 5 mL or less. When using dosing cups, rinse cup with water and drink. If you miss a dose, take as soon as possible and return to regular schedule (never take a double dose). Frequent blood tests may be required with prolonged therapy. If rash, blisters, or facial edema develops, stop medicine and contact prescriber immediately. May cause diarrhea (buttermilk, boiled milk, or yogurt may help); or headache (consult prescriber for approved analgesic). Report muscle or joint pain, general malaise, respiratory difficulty, persistent diarrhea or nausea, or pain or irritation in eyes. **Pregnancy/breast-feeding precautions:** Inform prescriber if you are or intend to become pregnant. Consult prescriber for appropriate contraceptives to reduce risk of transmitting infection and possible pregnancy. Do not breast-feed.

Pregnancy Risk Factor: C

Pregnancy Issues: Nevirapine crosses the placenta. Pharmacokinetics are not altered during pregnancy and dose adjustment is not needed. The Perinatal HIV Guidelines Working Group recommends nevirapine as the NNRTI for use during pregnancy. When used to prevent perinatal transmission in women who do not need therapy for their own health, use is not recommended if CD4$^+$ lymphocyte counts >250/mm^3 (monitor for liver toxicity during first 18 weeks of therapy). It may also be used in combination with zidovudine in HIV-infected women who are in labor, but have had no prior antiretroviral therapy, in order to reduce the maternal-fetal transmission of HIV. Health professionals are encouraged to contact the antiretroviral pregnancy registry to monitor outcomes of pregnant women exposed to antiretroviral medications (1-800-258-4263 or www.APRegistry.com).

Lactation: Enters breast milk/contraindicated

Breast-Feeding Issues: HIV-infected mothers are discouraged from breast-feeding to decrease potential transmission of HIV.

Administration
Oral: May be administered with or without food. May be administered with an antacid or didanosine. Shake suspension gently prior to administration.

Additional Information Potential compliance problems, frequency of administration, and adverse effects should be discussed with patients before initiating therapy to help prevent the emergence of resistance. Early virologic failure was observed with tenofovir and didanosine delayed release capsules, plus either efavirenz or nevirapine; use caution in treatment-naive patients with high baseline viral loads.

Related Information
Tuberculosis *on page 1864*

♦ **Nexium®** *see Esomeprazole on page 551*
♦ **NFV** *see Nelfinavir on page 1065*

Niacin (NYE a sin)

U.S. Brand Names Niacor®; Niaspan®; Slo-Niacin® [OTC]
Synonyms Nicotinic Acid; Vitamin B$_3$
Generic Available Yes
Pharmacologic Category Antilipemic Agent, Miscellaneous; Vitamin, Water Soluble
Medication Safety Issues
Sound-alike/look-alike issues:
Niacin may be confused with Minocin®, Niaspan®, Nispan®
Niaspan® may be confused with niacin
Nicobid® may be confused with Nitro-Bid®
(Continued)

Niacin *(Continued)*

Use Adjunctive treatment of dyslipidemias (alone or with lovastatin or bile acid sequestrant); peripheral vascular disease and circulatory disorders; treatment of pellagra; dietary supplement

Mechanism of Action/Effect Component of two coenzymes which is necessary for tissue respiration, lipid metabolism, and glycogenolysis; inhibits the synthesis of very low density lipoproteins

Contraindications Hypersensitivity to niacin, niacinamide, or any component of the formulation; hepatic disease; active peptic ulcer; severe hypotension; arterial hemorrhage

Warnings/Precautions Use caution in heavy ethanol users, unstable angina or MI, diabetes, renal disease, active gallbladder disease, gout, past history of hepatic disease, or allergies. Flushing is common; attenuated with a gradual dose increase. Monitor liver function tests.

Nutritional/Ethanol Interactions Ethanol: Avoid heavy use; avoid use around niacin dose.

Lab Interactions False elevations in some fluorometric determinations of urinary catecholamines; false-positive urine glucose (Benedict's reagent)

Adverse Reactions Frequency not defined.

Cardiovascular: Arrhythmias, atrial fibrillation, edema, flushing, hypotension, orthostasis, palpitation, syncope (rare), tachycardia

Central nervous system: Chills, dizziness, insomnia, migraine

Dermatologic: Acanthosis nigricans, dry skin, hyperpigmentation, maculopapular rash, pruritus, rash, urticaria

Endocrine & metabolic: Glucose tolerance decreased, gout, phosphorous levels decreased, uric acid level increased

Gastrointestinal: Abdominal pain, nausea, peptic ulcers, vomiting

Hepatic: Hepatic necrosis (rare), jaundice, liver enzymes elevated

Neuromuscular & skeletal: Myalgia, myopathy (with concurrent HMG-CoA reductase inhibitor), rhabdomyolysis (with concurrent HMG-CoA reductase inhibitor; rare), weakness

Ocular: Cystoid macular edema, toxic amblyopia

Respiratory: Dyspnea

Miscellaneous: Diaphoresis

Overdosage/Toxicology Symptoms of acute overdose include flushing, GI distress, and pruritus. Chronic excessive use has been associated with hepatitis. Antihistamines may relieve niacin-induced histamine release; otherwise treatment is symptomatic.

Pharmacodynamics/Kinetics

Absorption: Rapid and extensive

Time to Peak: Serum: Immediate release formulation: ~45 minutes; extended release formulation: 4-5 hours

Half-Life Elimination: 45 minutes

Metabolism: Extensive first-pass effects; converted to nicotinamide (dose dependent); niacinamide (30%) hepatically metabolized

Excretion: Urine (unchanged drug and metabolites); with larger doses, greater percentage as unchanged drug

Dosing

Adults & Elderly:

Recommended daily allowances:

Male: 25-50 years: 19 mg/day; >51 years: 15 mg/day

Female: 25-50 years: 15 mg/day; >51 years: 13 mg/day

Hyperlipidemia: Oral: Usual target dose: 1.5-6 g/day in 3 divided doses with or after meals using a dosage titration schedule; extended release: 375 mg to 2 g once daily at bedtime

Regular release formulation (Niacor®): Initial: 250 mg once daily (with evening meal); increase frequency and/or dose every 4-7 days to desired response or first-level therapeutic dose (1.5-2 g/day in 2-3 divided doses); after 2 months, may increase at 2- to 4-week intervals to 3 g/day in 3 divided doses

Extended release formulation (Niaspan®): 500 mg at bedtime for 4 weeks, then 1 g at bedtime for 4 weeks; adjust dose to response and tolerance; can increase to a maximum of 2 g/day, but only at 500 mg/day at 4-week intervals

Pellagra: Oral: 50-100 mg 3-4 times/day, maximum: 500 mg/day

Niacin deficiency: Oral: 10-20 mg/day, maximum: 100 mg/day

Pediatrics:

Pellagra: Oral: Children: 50-100 mg/dose 3 times/day

Recommended daily allowances:

0-0.5 years: 5 mg/day

0.5-1 year: 6 mg/day

1-3 years: 9 mg/day

4-6 years: 12 mg/day

7-10 years: 13 mg/day

RDA: Children and Adolescents:

Male:

11-14 years: 17 mg/day

15-18 years: 20 mg/day

19-24 years: 19 mg/day

Female: 11-24 years: 15 mg/day

Renal Impairment: Use with caution.

Hepatic Impairment: Not recommended for use in patients with significant or unexplained hepatic dysfunction.

Available Dosage Forms

Capsule, extended release: 125 mg, 250 mg, 400 mg, 500 mg

Capsule, timed release: 250 mg

Tablet: 50 mg, 100 mg, 250 mg, 500 mg

Niacor®: 500 mg

Tablet, controlled release (Slo-Niacin®): 250 mg, 500 mg, 750 mg

Tablet, extended release (Niaspan®): 500 mg, 750 mg, 1000 mg

Tablet, timed release: 250 mg, 500 mg, 750 mg, 1000 mg

Monitoring and Teaching Issues

Physical Assessment: Assess other medications patient may be taking for increased risk of drug/drug interactions. Teach patient appropriate use, interventions to reduce side effects, and adverse symptoms to report.

Monitoring Laboratory Tests: Blood glucose; liver function tests (dyslipidemia, high dose, prolonged therapy) pretreatment and every 6-12 weeks for first year then periodically; lipid profile; elevated uric acid levels have been reported

Patient Education: Take exactly as directed; do not exceed recommended dosage. Take with food to reduce incidence of GI upset. Do not crush sustained release capsules. You may experience flushing, sensation of heat, or headache; these reactions may be decreased by increasing dose slowly or by taking aspirin (consult prescriber) 30 minutes prior to taking niacin. You may experience dizziness, lightheadedness (use caution when driving or engaging in tasks requiring alertness until response to drug is known). Report persistent GI disturbance or changes in color of urine or stool. **Pregnancy/breast-feeding precautions:** Inform prescriber if you are pregnant. Consult prescriber if breast-feeding.

Dietary Considerations: Should be taken with meal; low-fat meal if treating hyperlipidemia. Avoid hot drinks around the time of niacin dose.

Pregnancy Risk Factor: A/C (dose exceeding RDA recommendation)

Lactation: Enters breast milk/consult prescriber

Administration

Oral: Administer with food. Niaspan® tablet strengths are not interchangeable. When switching from immediate release tablet, initiate Niaspan® at lower dose and titrate. Long-acting forms should not be crushed, broken, or chewed. Do not substitute long-acting forms for immediate release ones.

Related Information

Hyperlipidemia Management *on page 1836*
Lipid-Lowering Agents *on page 1738*

♦ **Niacor®** *see* Niacin *on page 1075*

♦ **Niaspan®** *see* Niacin *on page 1075*

NiCARdipine (nye KAR de peen)

U.S. Brand Names Cardene®; Cardene® I.V.; Cardene® SR

Synonyms Nicardipine Hydrochloride

Generic Available Yes: Capsule

Pharmacologic Category Calcium Channel Blocker

Medication Safety Issues

Sound-alike/look-alike issues:

NiCARdipine may be confused with niacinamide, NIFEdipine, nimodipine

Cardene® may be confused with Cardizem®, Cardura®, codeine

Use Chronic stable angina (immediate-release product only); management of essential hypertension (immediate and sustained release; parenteral only for short time that oral treatment is not feasible)

Unlabeled/Investigational Use Congestive heart failure

Mechanism of Action/Effect Inhibits calcium ion from entering the "slow channels" or select voltage-sensitive areas of vascular smooth muscle and myocardium during depolarization, producing a relaxation of coronary vascular smooth muscle and coronary vasodilation; increases myocardial oxygen delivery in patients with vasospastic angina

Contraindications Hypersensitivity to nicardipine or any component of the formulation; advanced aortic stenosis; severe hypotension; cardiogenic shock; ventricular tachycardia

Warnings/Precautions Blood pressure lowering should be done at a rate appropriate for the patient's condition. Rapid drops in blood pressure can lead to arterial insufficiency. Use with caution in CAD (can cause increase in angina), CHF (can worsen heart failure symptoms), and pheochromocytoma (limited clinical experience). Peripheral infusion sites (for I.V. therapy) should be changed ever 12 hours. Titrate I.V. dose cautiously in patients with CHF, renal, or hepatic dysfunction. Use the I.V. form cautiously in patients with portal hypertension (can cause increase in hepatic pressure gradient). Safety and efficacy have not been demonstrated in pediatric patients. Abrupt withdrawal may cause rebound angina in patients with CAD.

Drug Interactions

Cytochrome P450 Effect: Substrate of CYP1A2 (minor), 2C8/9 (minor), 2D6 (minor), 2E1 (minor), 3A4 (major); **Inhibits** CYP2C8/9 (strong), 2C19 (moderate), 2D6 (moderate), 3A4 (strong)

Decreased Effect: The levels/effects of nicardipine may be decreased by aminoglutethimide, carbamazepine, nafcillin, nevirapine, phenobarbital, phenytoin, rifamycins, and other CYP3A4 inducers. Nicardipine may decrease the levels/effects of CYP2D6 prodrug substrates (eg, codeine, hydrocodone, oxycodone, tramadol). Calcium may reduce the calcium channel blocker's effects, particularly hypotension.

Increased Effect/Toxicity: H_2 blockers (cimetidine) may increase the bioavailability of nicardipine. The levels/effects of nicardipine may be increased by azole antifungals, ciprofloxacin, clarithromycin, diclofenac, doxycycline, erythromycin, imatinib, isoniazid, nefazodone, propofol, protease inhibitors, quinidine, verapamil and other CYP3A4 inhibitors.

Nicardipine may increase the effect of vecuronium (reduce dose 25%). Nicardipine increase the levels/effects of amiodarone, amphetamines, selected benzodiazepines, selected beta-blockers, calcium channel blockers, cisapride, citalopram, cyclosporine, dextromethorphan, diazepam, ergot derivatives, fluoxetine, glimepiride, glipizide, HMG-CoA reductase inhibitors, lidocaine, methsuximide, mirtazapine, nateglinide, nefazodone, paroxetine, phenytoin, pioglitazone, propranolol, risperidone, ritonavir, rosiglitazone, sertraline, sildenafil (and other PDE-5 inhibitors), tacrolimus, thioridazine, tricyclic antidepressants, venlafaxine, warfarin, and other substrates of CYP2C8/9, 2C19, 2D6, or 3A4.

(Continued)

NiCARdipine *(Continued)*

Nutritional/Ethanol Interactions

Ethanol: Avoid ethanol (may increase CNS depression).

Food: Nicardipine average peak concentrations may be decreased if taken with food. Serum concentrations/toxicity of nicardipine may be increased by grapefruit juice; avoid concurrent use.

Herb/Nutraceutical: St John's wort may decrease levels. Avoid dong quai if using for hypertension (has estrogenic activity). Avoid ephedra, yohimbe, ginseng (may worsen hypertension). Avoid garlic (may have increased antihypertensive effect).

Adverse Reactions

1% to 10%:

Cardiovascular: Flushing (6% to 10%), palpitation (3% to 4%), tachycardia (1% to 4%), peripheral edema (dose related 7% to 8%), increased angina (dose related 6%), hypotension (I.V. 6%), orthostasis (I.V. 1%)

Central nervous system: Headache (6% to 15%), dizziness (4% to 7%), somnolence (4% to 6%), paresthesia (1%)

Dermatologic: Rash (1%)

Gastrointestinal: Nausea (2% to 5%), dry mouth (1%)

Genitourinary: Polyuria (1%)

Local: Injection site reaction (I.V. 1%)

Neuromuscular & skeletal: Weakness (4% to 6%), myalgia (1%)

Miscellaneous: Diaphoresis

Overdosage/Toxicology

The primary cardiac symptoms of calcium blocker overdose include hypotension and bradycardia. Noncardiac symptoms include confusion, stupor, nausea, vomiting, metabolic acidosis, and hyperglycemia. Following initial gastric decontamination, if possible, repeated calcium administration may promptly reverse the depressed cardiac contractility (but not sinus node depression or peripheral vasodilation). Glucagon and epinephrine may treat refractory hypotension. Glucagon and epinephrine also increase the heart rate (outside the U.S., 4-aminopyridine may be available as an antidote). Dialysis and hemoperfusion are not effective in enhancing elimination although repeat-dose activated charcoal may serve as an adjunct with sustained-release preparations.

Pharmacodynamics/Kinetics

Onset of Action: Oral: 1-2 hours; I.V.: 10 minutes; Hypotension: ~20 minutes

Duration of Action: 2-6 hours

Absorption: Oral: ~100%

Bioavailability: 35%

Time to Peak: Serum: 20-120 minutes

Protein Binding: 95%

Half-Life Elimination: 2-4 hours

Metabolism: Hepatic; extensive first-pass effect

Excretion: Urine (as metabolites)

Dosing

Adults & Elderly:

Angina: Immediate release: Oral: 20 mg 3 times/day; usual range: 60-120 mg/day; increase dose at 3-day intervals

Hypertension: Oral:

Immediate release: Initial: 20 mg 3 times/day; usual: 20-40 mg 3 times/day (allow 3 days between dose increases)

Sustained release: Initial: 30 mg twice daily, titrate up to 60 mg twice daily

Note: The total daily dose of immediate-release product may not automatically be equivalent to the daily sustained-release dose; use caution in converting.

Acute hypertension: I.V. (dilute to 0.1 mg/mL): Initial: 5 mg/hour increased by 2.5 mg/hour every 15 minutes to a maximum of 15 mg/hour; consider reduction to 3 mg/hour after response is achieved. Monitor and titrate to lowest dose necessary to maintain stable blood pressure.

Substitution for oral therapy (approximate equivalents):

20 mg every 8 hours oral, equivalent to 0.5 mg/hour I.V. infusion

30 mg every 8 hours oral, equivalent to 1.2 mg/hour I.V. infusion

40 mg every 8 hours oral, equivalent to 2.2 mg/hour I.V. infusion

Renal Impairment: Titrate dose beginning with 20 mg 3 times/day (immediate release) or 30 mg twice daily (sustained release). Specific guidelines for adjustment of I.V. nicardipine are not available, but careful monitoring/adjustment is warranted.

Hepatic Impairment: Starting dose: 20 mg twice daily (immediate release) with titration. Refer to "Note" in adult dosing. Specific guidelines for adjustment of I.V. nicardipine are not available, but careful monitoring/adjustment is warranted.

Available Dosage Forms

Capsule (Cardene®): 20 mg, 30 mg

Capsule, sustained release (Cardene® SR): 30 mg, 45 mg, 60 mg

Injection, solution (Cardene® IV): 2.5 mg/mL (10 mL)

Monitoring and Teaching Issues

Physical Assessment: Use caution with CAD and CHF (see Warnings/Precautions for use cautions). Assess potential for interactions with other pharmacological agents or herbal products patient may be taking (eg, increased risk for toxicity; see Drug Interactions). See Administration for infusion specifics; infusion site must be monitored closely to prevent extravasation; peripheral infusion sites should be changed ever 12 hours. Assess effectiveness (cardiac status and blood pressure) and adverse reactions when starting, adjusting dose, or discontinuing (eg, rash, hypotension, bradycardia, confusion, nausea; see Adverse Reactions). Teach patient proper use, possible side effects/appropriate interventions (eg, orthostatic precautions), and adverse symptoms to report (see Patient Education).

Patient Education: This medication may be administered by intravenous infusion; report immediately and swelling, redness, burning, or pain at infusion site. **Oral:** Take as directed; do not alter dose or decrease without consulting prescriber. Do not crush or chew sustained release forms; swallow whole. Take with nonfatty food. Avoid caffeine and alcohol. Consult prescriber before increasing exercise routine (decreased angina does not mean it is safe to increase exercise). May cause orthostatic hypotension (change position slowly from sitting or lying to standing, or when climbing stairs); sore mouth (inspect gums for swelling or redness; use soft toothbrush, waxed dental floss, and frequent mouth rinses); dizziness or fatigue (use caution when driving or engaging in tasks that require alertness until response to drug is known); or nausea and dry mouth (small frequent meals, frequent mouth care, chewing gum, or sucking lozenges may help). Report chest pain, palpitations, rapid heartbeat; swelling of extremities; muscle weakness or pain; respiratory difficulty; or nervousness. **Pregnancy/breast-feeding precautions:** Inform prescriber if you are or intend to become pregnant. Breast-feeding is not recommended.

Geriatric Considerations: Elderly may experience a greater hypotensive response. Constipation may be more of a problem in the elderly.

Pregnancy Risk Factor: C

Lactation: Enters breast milk/not recommended

Administration
Oral: Do not chew or crush the sustained release formulation, swallow whole. Do not open or cut capsules.

I.V.: Ampuls must be diluted before use. Administer as a slow continuous infusion.

Compatibility: Stable in D_5W with KCl 40 mEq, $D_5^1/_2NS$, D_5NS, D_5W, $^1/_2NS$, NS; **incompatible** with sodium bicarbonate 5%, LR

Y-site administration: Incompatible with furosemide, heparin, thiopental

Storage: I.V.: Store at room temperature. Protect from light. Freezing does not affect stability.

Related Information
Calcium Channel Blockers *on page 1722*
FDA Name Differentiation Project: The Use of Tall-Man Letters *on page 15*

♦ **Nicardipine Hydrochloride** *see NiCARdipine on page 1077*
♦ **NicoDerm® CQ® [OTC]** *see Nicotine on page 1079*
♦ **Nicorette® [OTC]** *see Nicotine on page 1079*

Nicotine (nik oh TEEN)
U.S. Brand Names Commit™ [OTC]; NicoDerm® CQ® [OTC]; Nicorette® [OTC]; Nicotrol® Inhaler; Nicotrol® NS; Nicotrol® Patch [OTC]

Synonyms Habitrol

Generic Available Yes: Transdermal patch and gum

Pharmacologic Category Smoking Cessation Aid

Medication Safety Issues
Sound-alike/look-alike issues:
NicoDerm® may be confused with Nitroderm
Nicorette® may be confused with Nordette®

Transdermal patch may contain conducting metal (eg, aluminum); remove patch prior to MRI.

Use Treatment to aid smoking cessation for the relief of nicotine withdrawal symptoms (including nicotine craving)

Unlabeled/Investigational Use Management of ulcerative colitis (transdermal)

Mechanism of Action/Effect Nicotine is one of two naturally-occurring alkaloids which exhibit their primary effects via autonomic ganglia stimulation. Nicotine is a potent ganglionic and central nervous system stimulant, the actions of which are mediated via nicotine-specific receptors. Stimulation of the central nervous system (CNS) is characterized by tremors and respiratory excitation. However, convulsions may occur with higher doses, along with respiratory failure secondary to both central paralysis and peripheral blockade to respiratory muscles.

Contraindications Hypersensitivity to nicotine or any component of the formulation; patients who are smoking during the postmyocardial infarction period; patients with life-threatening arrhythmias, or severe or worsening angina pectoris; active temporomandibular joint disease (gum); pregnancy; not for use in nonsmokers

Warnings/Precautions The risk versus the benefits must be weighed for each of these groups: patients with CAD, serious cardiac arrhythmias, vasospastic disease. Use caution in patients with hyperthyroidism, pheochromocytoma, or insulin-dependent diabetes. Use with caution in oropharyngeal inflammation and in patients with history of esophagitis, peptic ulcer, coronary artery disease, vasospastic disease, angina, hypertension, hyperthyroidism, pheochromocytoma, diabetes, severe renal dysfunction, and hepatic dysfunction. The inhaler should be used with caution in patients with bronchospastic disease (other forms of nicotine replacement may be preferred). Transdermal patch may contain conducting metal (eg, aluminum); remove patch prior to MRI. Cautious use of topical nicotine in patients with certain skin diseases. Hypersensitivity to the topical products can occur. Dental problems may be worsened by chewing the gum. Urge patients to stop smoking completely when initiating therapy. Safety and efficacy have not been established in pediatric patients.

Drug Interactions
Cytochrome P450 Effect: Substrate (minor) of CYP1A2, 2A6, 2B6, 2C8/9, 2C19, 2D6, 2E1, 3A4; **Inhibits** CYP2A6 (weak), 2E1 (weak)

Increased Effect/Toxicity: Nicotine increases the hemodynamic and AV blocking effects of adenosine; monitor. Cimetidine increases nicotine concentrations; therefore, may decrease amount of gum or patches needed. Monitor for treatment-emergent hypertension in patients treated with the combination of nicotine patch and bupropion.

Nutritional/Ethanol Interactions Food: Lozenge: Acidic foods/beverages decrease absorption of nicotine.

Adverse Reactions
Chewing gum/lozenge:
>10%:
Cardiovascular: Tachycardia
Central nervous system: Headache (mild)
(Continued)

Nicotine *(Continued)*

Gastrointestinal: Nausea, vomiting, indigestion, excessive salivation, belching, increased appetite

Miscellaneous: Mouth or throat soreness, jaw muscle ache, hiccups

1% to 10%:

Central nervous system: Insomnia, dizziness, nervousness

Endocrine & metabolic: Dysmenorrhea

Gastrointestinal: GI distress, eructation

Neuromuscular & skeletal: Muscle pain

Respiratory: Hoarseness

Miscellaneous: Hiccups

Transdermal systems:

>10%:

Central nervous system: Insomnia, abnormal dreams

Dermatologic: Pruritus, erythema

Local: Application site reaction

Respiratory: Rhinitis, cough, pharyngitis, sinusitis

1% to 10%:

Cardiovascular: Chest pain

Central nervous system: Dysphoria, anxiety, difficulty concentrating, dizziness, somnolence

Dermatologic: Rash

Gastrointestinal: Diarrhea, dyspepsia, nausea, xerostomia, constipation, anorexia, abdominal pain

Neuromuscular & skeletal: Arthralgia, myalgia

Overdosage/Toxicology Symptoms of overdose include nausea, vomiting, abdominal pain, mental confusion, diarrhea, salivation, tachycardia, respiratory and cardiovascular collapse. Treatment is symptomatic and supportive. Remove patch, rinse area with water, and dry. Do not use soap as this may increase absorption.

Pharmacodynamics/Kinetics

Onset of Action: Intranasal: More closely approximate the time course of plasma nicotine levels observed after cigarette smoking than other dosage forms

Duration of Action: Transdermal: 24 hours

Absorption: Transdermal: Slow

Time to Peak: Serum: Transdermal: 8-9 hours

Half-Life Elimination: 4 hours

Metabolism: Hepatic, primarily to cotinine ($\frac{1}{5}$ as active)

Excretion: Urine

Clearance: Renal: pH dependent

Dosing

Adults & Elderly:

Tobacco cessation (patients should be advised to completely stop smoking upon initiation of therapy):

Gum: Chew 1 piece of gum when urge to smoke, up to 30 pieces/day; most patients require 10-12 pieces of gum/day

Inhaler: Usually 6 to 16 cartridges per day; best effect was achieved by frequent continuous puffing (20 minutes); recommended duration of treatment is 3 months, after which patients may be weaned from the inhaler by gradual reduction of the daily dose over 6-12 weeks

Lozenge: Patients who smoke their first cigarette within 30 minutes of waking should use the 4 mg strength; otherwise the 2 mg strength is recommended.

Weeks 1-6: One lozenge every 1-2 hours

Weeks 7-9: One lozenge every 2-4 hours

Weeks 10-12: One lozenge every 4-8 hours

Note: Use at least 9 lozenges/day during first 6 weeks to improve chances of quitting; do not use more than one lozenge at a time (maximum: 5 lozenges every 6 hours, 20 lozenges/day)

Spray: 1-2 sprays/hour; do not exceed more than 5 doses (10 sprays) per hour; each dose (2 sprays) contains 1 mg of nicotine. **Warning:** A dose of 40 mg can cause fatalities

Transdermal patch: Apply new patch every 24 hours to nonhairy, clean, dry skin on the upper body or upper outer arm; each patch should be applied to a different site. **Note:** Adjustment may be required during initial treatment (move to higher dose if experiencing withdrawal symptoms; lower dose if side effects are experienced).

Habitrol®, NicoDerm CQ®:

Patients smoking ≥10 cigarettes/day: Begin with step 1 (21 mg/day) for 4-6 weeks, **followed by** step 2 (14 mg/day) for 2 weeks; **finish with** step 3 (7 mg/day) for 2 weeks

Patients smoking <10 cigarettes/day: Begin with step 2 (14 mg/day) for 6 weeks, **followed by** step 3 (7 mg/day) for 2 weeks

Note: Initial starting dose for patients <100 pounds, history of cardiovascular disease: 14 mg/day for 4-6 weeks, **followed by** 7 mg/day for 2-4 weeks

Note: Patients who are receiving >600 mg/day of cimetidine: Decrease to the next lower patch size

Nicotrol®: One patch daily for 6 weeks

Benefits of use of nicotine transdermal patches beyond 3 months have not been demonstrated

Ulcerative colitis (unlabeled use): Transdermal: Titrated to 22-25 mg/day

Available Dosage Forms

Gum, chewing, as polacrilex: 2 mg (48s, 108s); 4 mg (48s, 108s)

Nicorette®: 2 mg (48s, 50s, 108s, 110s, 168s, 170s, 192s, 200s, 216s); 4 mg (48s, 108s, 168s) [mint, fresh mint, orange, and original flavors]

Lozenge, as polacrilex (Commit™): 2 mg (48s, 72s) [contains phenylalanine 3.4 mg/lozenge; mint flavor]; 4 mg (48s, 72s) [contains phenylalanine 3.4 mg/lozenge; mint flavor]

Oral inhalation system (Nicotrol® Inhaler): 10 mg cartridge (delivering 4 mg nicotine) (168s) [each unit consists of 5 mouthpieces, 28 storage trays each containing 6 cartridges, and 1 storage case]

Patch, transdermal: 7 mg/24 (30s); 14 mg/24 hours (30s); 21 mg/24 hours (30s)

NicoDerm® CQ®: 7 mg/24 hours (14s); 14 mg/24 hours (14s); 21 mg/24 hours (14s) [available in tan or clear patch]

Nicotrol®: 15 mg/16 hours (7s, 14s) [step 1]; 10 mg/16 hours (14s) [step 2]; 5 mg/16 hours (14s) [step 3]

Solution, intranasal spray (Nicotrol® NS): 10 mg/mL (10 mL) [delivers 0.5 mg/spray; 200 sprays]

Monitoring and Teaching Issues

Physical Assessment: Monitor cardiac status and vital signs prior to, when beginning, and periodically during therapy. Monitor effectiveness of therapy (according to rational for therapy), and adverse reactions at beginning and periodically during therapy. Assess knowledge/teach patient appropriate use, interventions to reduce side effects, and adverse symptoms to report for prescribed form of drug. **Pregnancy risk factor D/X:** See Pregnancy Risk Factor for use cautions. Determine that patient is not pregnant before beginning treatment and do not give to women of childbearing age unless female is capable of complying with contraceptive measures.

Patient Education: Use exactly as directed; do not use more often than prescribed. Stop smoking completely during therapy. Do not smoke, chew tobacco, use snuff, nicotine gum, or any other form of nicotine. Nicotine overdose could occur.

Gum: Chew slowly for 30 minutes. Discard chewed gum away from access by children.

Lozenge: Allow to dissolve slowly in the mouth. Do not chew or swallow lozenge whole. Avoid food or drink 15 minutes prior to, during, or after lozenge.

Transdermal patch: Follow directions in package for dosing schedule and use. Do not cut patches or wear more than one patch at a time. Remove backing from patch and press immediately on skin. Hold for 10 seconds. Apply to clean, dry skin in different site each day. Do not touch eyes; wash hands after application. You may experience vivid dreams and sleep disturbances, dizziness or lightheadedness (use caution driving or when engaging in tasks requiring alertness until response to drug is known). For nausea, vomiting or GI upset, small frequent meals, chewing gum, and frequent oral care may help. Report persistent vomiting, diarrhea, chills, sweating, chest pain or palpitations, or burning or redness at application site.

Spray: Follow directions in package. Blow nose gently before use. Use 1-2 sprays/hour; do not exceed 5 doses (10 sprays) per hour. Excessive use can result in severe (even life-threatening) reactions. You may experience temporary stinging or burning after spray.

Pregnancy/breast-feeding precautions: Inform prescriber if you are pregnant. Do not get pregnant during or for 1 month following therapy. Consult prescriber for instruction on appropriate contraceptive measures. This drug may cause severe fetal defects. Do not breast-feed.

Dietary Considerations: Each lozenge contains phenylalanine 3.4 mg.

Geriatric Considerations: Must evaluate benefit in the elderly who may have chronic diseases mentioned (see Warnings/Precautions and Contraindications). The transdermal systems are as effective in the elderly as they are in younger adults; however, complaints of body aches, dizziness, and asthenia were reported more often in the elderly.

Pregnancy Risk Factor: D (transdermal); X (chewing gum)

Lactation: Excretion in breast milk unknown/contraindicated

Administration

Oral:

Gum: Should be chewed slowly to avoid jaw ache and to maximize benefit.

Lozenge: Should not be chewed or swallowed.

Topical: Do not cut patch; causes rapid evaporation, rendering the patch useless. Use of an aerosol corticosteroid may diminish local irritation under patches.

Other: Transdermal patch: Patches cannot be cut.

Storage: Store inhaler cartridge at room temperature not to exceed 30°C (86°F); protect cartridges from light

Additional Information A cigarette has 10-25 mg nicotine. Use of an aerosol corticosteroid may diminish local irritation under patches.

◆ **Nicotinic Acid** *see Niacin on page 1075*

◆ **Nicotrol® Inhaler** *see Nicotine on page 1079*

◆ **Nicotrol® NS** *see Nicotine on page 1079*

◆ **Nicotrol® Patch [OTC]** *see Nicotine on page 1079*

◆ **Nifediac™ CC** *see NIFEdipine on page 1081*

◆ **Nifedical™ XL** *see NIFEdipine on page 1081*

NIFEdipine (nye FED i peen)

U.S. Brand Names Adalat® CC; Afeditab™; Nifediac™ CC; Nifedical™ XL; Procardia®; Procardia XL®

Generic Available Yes

Pharmacologic Category Calcium Channel Blocker

Medication Safety Issues

Sound-alike/look-alike issues:

NIFEdipine may be confused with niCARdipine, nimodipine, nisoldipine

Procardia XL® may be confused with Cartia® XT

Use Angina and hypertension (sustained release only), pulmonary hypertension

Mechanism of Action/Effect Inhibits calcium ion from entering the "slow channels" or select voltage-sensitive areas of vascular smooth muscle and myocardium during depolarization, (Continued)

NIFEdipine *(Continued)*

producing a relaxation of coronary vascular smooth muscle and coronary vasodilation; increases myocardial oxygen delivery in patients with vasospastic angina

Contraindications Hypersensitivity to nifedipine or any component of the formulation; immediate release preparation for treatment of urgent or emergent hypertension; acute MI

Warnings/Precautions The use of sublingual short-acting nifedipine in hypertensive emergencies and pseudoemergencies is neither safe nor effective and SHOULD BE ABANDONED! Serious adverse events (cerebrovascular ischemia, syncope, heart block, stroke, sinus arrest, severe hypotension, acute myocardial infarction, ECG changes, and fetal distress) have been reported in relation to such use.

Blood pressure lowering should be done at a rate appropriate for the patient's condition. Rapid drops in blood pressure can lead to arterial insufficiency. Increased angina and/or MI has occurred with initiation or dosage titration of calcium channel blockers. Use caution in severe aortic stenosis. Use caution in patients with severe hepatic impairment (may need dosage adjustment). Abrupt withdrawal may cause rebound angina in patients with CAD. Use caution in CHF (may cause worsening of symptoms). Avoid use of extended release tablets (Procardia XL®) in patients with known stricture/narrowing of the GI tract. Avoid grapefruit juice during treatment with nifedipine.

Drug Interactions

Cytochrome P450 Effect: Substrate of CYP2D6 (minor), 3A4 (major); **Inhibits** CYP1A2 (moderate), 2C8/9 (weak), 2D6 (weak), 3A4 (weak)

Decreased Effect: Nifedipine may decrease quinidine serum levels. Calcium may reduce the hypotension from of calcium channel blockers. The levels/effects of nifedipine may be decreased by aminoglutethimide, carbamazepine, nafcillin, nevirapine, phenobarbital, phenytoin, rifamycins, and other CYP3A4 inducers.

Increased Effect/Toxicity: The levels/effects of nifedipine may be increased by azole antifungals, ciprofloxacin, clarithromycin, diclofenac, doxycycline, erythromycin, imatinib, isoniazid, nefazodone, nicardipine, propofol, protease inhibitors, quinidine, telithromycin, verapamil, and other CYP3A4 inhibitors. Cimetidine may also increase nifedipine levels. Nifedipine may increase the levels/effects of aminophylline, digoxin, fluvoxamine, mexiletine, mirtazapine, ropinirole, trifluoperazine, vincristine, and other CYP1A2 substrates. Digoxin, phenytoin, and vincristine levels may also be increased by nifedipine. Blood pressure-lowering effects may be additive with sildenafil, tadalafil, and vardenafil (use caution).

Nutritional/Ethanol Interactions

Ethanol: Avoid ethanol (may increase CNS depression).

Food: Nifedipine serum levels may be decreased if taken with food. Food may decrease the rate but not the extent of absorption of Procardia XL®. Increased therapeutic and vasodilator side effects, including severe hypotension and myocardial ischemia, may occur if nifedipine is taken by patients ingesting grapefruit.

Herb/Nutraceutical: St John's wort may decrease nifedipine levels. Avoid dong quai if using for hypertension (has estrogenic activity). Avoid ephedra, yohimbe, ginseng (may worsen hypertension). Avoid garlic (may have increased antihypertensive effect).

Adverse Reactions

>10%:

Cardiovascular: Flushing (10% to 25%), peripheral edema (dose related 7% to 10%; up to 50%)

Central nervous system: Dizziness/lightheadedness/giddiness (10% to 27%), headache (10% to 23%)

Gastrointestinal: Nausea/heartburn (10% to 11%)

Neuromuscular & skeletal: Weakness (10% to 12%)

≥1% to 10%:

Cardiovascular: Palpitations (≤2% to 7%), transient hypotension (dose related 5%), CHF (2%)

Central nervous system: Nervousness/mood changes (≤2% to 7%), shakiness (≤2%), jitteriness (≤2%), sleep disturbances (≤2%), difficulties in balance (≤2%), fever (≤2%), chills (≤2%)

Dermatologic: Dermatitis (≤2%), pruritus (≤2%), urticaria (≤2%)

Endocrine & metabolic: Sexual difficulties (≤2%)

Gastrointestinal: Diarrhea (≤2%), constipation (≤2%), cramps (≤2%), flatulence (≤2%), gingival hyperplasia (≤10%)

Neuromuscular & skeletal: Muscle cramps/tremor (≤2% to 8%), weakness (10%), inflammation (≤2%), joint stiffness (≤2%)

Ocular: Blurred vision (≤2%)

Respiratory: Dyspnea/cough/wheezing (6%), nasal congestion/sore throat (≤2% to 6%), chest congestion (≤2%), dyspnea (≤2%)

Miscellaneous: Diaphoresis (≤2%)

Overdosage/Toxicology Primary cardiac symptoms of calcium blocker overdose include hypotension and bradycardia. Noncardiac symptoms include confusion, stupor, nausea, vomiting, metabolic acidosis, and hyperglycemia. Following initial gastric decontamination, treat symptomatically.

Pharmacodynamics/Kinetics

Onset of Action: ~20 minutes

Bioavailability: Capsule: 45% to 75%; Sustained release: 65% to 86%

Protein Binding: Concentration dependent: 92% to 98%

Half-Life Elimination: Adults: Healthy: 2-5 hours, Cirrhosis: 7 hours; Elderly: 6.7 hours

Metabolism: Hepatic to inactive metabolites

Excretion: Urine

Dosing

Adults & Elderly:

Hypertension: Oral: Initial: 10 mg 3 times/day as capsules or 30 mg once daily as sustained release

Usual dose: 10-30 mg 3 times/day as capsules or 30-60 mg once daily as sustained release

Maximum: 120-180 mg/day

Note: Adjustment of sustained release formulations should be made at 7- to 14-day intervals

Pediatrics:

Hypertrophic cardiomyopathy (unlabeled use): Oral: Children: 0.6-0.9 mg/kg/24 hours in 3-4 divided doses

Hypertension: Oral: Adolescents: Refer to adult dosing.

Hepatic Impairment: Reduce oral dose by 50% to 60% in patients with cirrhosis.

Available Dosage Forms [DSC] = Discontinued product

Capsule, liquid-filled: 10 mg, 20 mg

Procardia®: 10 mg; 20 mg [DSC]

Tablet, extended release: 30 mg, 60 mg, 90 mg

Adalat® CC, Nifediac™ CC, Procardia XL®: 30 mg, 60 mg, 90 mg

Afeditab™, Nifedical™ XL: 30 mg, 60 mg

Monitoring and Teaching Issues

Physical Assessment: Use caution in severe aortic stenosis or severe hepatic impairment (see Warnings/Precautions for specific use cautions). Assess potential for interactions with other pharmacological agents or herbal products patient may be taking (eg, increased risk of hypotension, toxicities; see Drug Interactions). Assess therapeutic effectiveness (blood pressure and cardiac status) and adverse reactions when starting, adjusting dose, or discontinuing (see Adverse Reactions). Teach patient proper use, possible side effects/appropriate interventions (eg, orthostatic precautions), and adverse symptoms to report (see Patient Education).

Patient Education: Do not take any new medication during therapy unless approved by prescriber (especially anything that may act as a stimulant or depressant). Take as directed; do not alter dose or decrease without consulting prescriber. Do not crush or chew sustained release forms, swallow whole. Take with nonfatty food. Avoid caffeine, alcohol, and grapefruit juice. Consult prescriber before increasing exercise routine (decreased angina does not mean it is safe to increase exercise). May cause orthostatic hypotension (change position slowly from sitting or lying to standing, or when climbing stairs); sore mouth (inspect gums for swelling or redness; use soft toothbrush, waxed dental floss, and frequent mouth rinses); dizziness, difficulties in balance, or fatigue (use caution when driving or engaging in tasks that require alertness until response to drug is known); or nausea or heartburn (small frequent meals, frequent mouth care, chewing gum, or sucking lozenges may help). Report chest pain, palpitations, rapid heartbeat; swelling of extremities; muscle weakness or pain; respiratory difficulty; nervousness or mood change, rash; or vision changes. **Pregnancy precaution:** Inform prescriber if you are or intend to become pregnant.

Dietary Considerations: Capsule is rapidly absorbed orally if it is administered without food, but may result in vasodilator side effects; administration with low-fat meals may decrease flushing. Avoid grapefruit juice.

Geriatric Considerations: Elderly may experience a greater hypotensive response. Theoretically, constipation may be more of a problem in elderly patients. The half-life of nifedipine is extended in elderly patients (6.7 hours) as compared to younger subjects (3.8 hours).

Pregnancy Risk Factor: C

Pregnancy Issues: Hypotension, IUGR reported. IUGR probably related to maternal hypertension. May exhibit tocolytic effects.

Lactation: Enters breast milk/compatible

Breast-Feeding Issues: Crosses into breast milk. Available evidence suggests safe use during breast-feeding. AAP considers **compatible** with breast-feeding.

Administration

Oral: Extended release tablets should be swallowed whole; do not crush or chew.

Additional Information When measuring smaller doses from the liquid-filled capsules, consider the following concentrations (for Procardia®) 10 mg capsule = 10 mg/0.34 mL; 20 mg capsule = 20 mg/0.45 mL; may be used preoperative to treat hypertensive urgency.

Considerable attention has been directed to potential increases in mortality and morbidity when short-acting nifedipine is used in treating hypertension. The rapid reduction in blood pressure may precipitate adverse cardiovascular events. At this time, there is no indication for the use of short-acting calcium channel blocker therapy. Nifedipine also has potent negative inotropic effects and can worsen heart failure.

Related Information

Calcium Channel Blockers *on page 1722*

FDA Name Differentiation Project: The Use of Tall-Man Letters *on page 15*

♦ **Niftolid** *see* Flutamide *on page 658*

♦ **Nilandron®** *see* Nilutamide *on page 1083*

Nilutamide (ni LOO ta mide)

U.S. Brand Names Nilandron®

Synonyms RU-23908

Generic Available No

Pharmacologic Category Antiandrogen; Antineoplastic Agent, Antiandrogen

Use Treatment of metastatic prostate cancer

Mechanism of Action/Effect Nonsteroidal antiandrogen that inhibits androgen uptake or inhibits binding of androgen in target tissues

Contraindications Hypersensitivity to nilutamide or any component of the formulation; severe hepatic impairment; severe respiratory insufficiency

Warnings/Precautions May cause interstitial pneumonitis; the suggestive signs of pneumonitis most often occurred within the first 3 months of nilutamide treatment. Has been associated with severe hepatitis, which has resulted in fatality. In addition, foreign postmarketing

(Continued)

Nilutamide *(Continued)*

surveillance has revealed isolated cases of aplastic anemia (a causal relationship with nilutamide could not be ascertained).

May alter time for visual adaptation to darkness, ranging from seconds to a few minutes. This effect sometimes does not abate as drug treatment is continued. Caution patients who experience this effect about driving at night or through tunnels. This effect can be alleviated by wearing tinted glasses.

Drug Interactions

Cytochrome P450 Effect: Substrate of CYP2C19 (major); **Inhibits** CYP2C19 (weak)

Decreased Effect: CYP2C19 inducers may decrease the levels/effects of nilutamide; example inducers include aminoglutethimide, carbamazepine, phenytoin, and rifampin.

Increased Effect/Toxicity: CYP2C19 inhibitors may increase the levels/effects of nilutamide; example inhibitors include delavirdine, fluconazole, fluvoxamine, gemfibrozil, isoniazid, omeprazole, and ticlopidine.

Nutritional/Ethanol Interactions

Ethanol: Avoid ethanol. Up to 5% of patients may experience a systemic reaction (flushing, hypotension, malaise) when combined with nilutamide.

Herb/Nutraceutical: St John's wort may decrease nilutamide levels.

Adverse Reactions

>10%:

Central nervous system: Headache, insomnia

Endocrine & metabolic: Hot flashes (30% to 67%), gynecomastia (10%)

Gastrointestinal: Nausea (mild - 10% to 32%), abdominal pain (10%), constipation, anorexia

Genitourinary: Testicular atrophy (16%), libido decreased

Hepatic: Transaminases increased (8% to 13%; transient)

Ocular: Impaired dark adaptation (13% to 57%), usually reversible with dose reduction, may require discontinuation of the drug in 1% to 2% of patients

Respiratory: Dyspnea (11%)

1% to 10%:

Cardiovascular: Chest pain, edema, heart failure, hypertension, syncope

Central nervous system: Dizziness, drowsiness, malaise, hypoesthesia, depression

Dermatologic: Pruritus, alopecia, dry skin, rash

Endocrine & metabolic: Disulfiram-like reaction (hot flashes, rash) (5%); Flu-like syndrome, fever

Gastrointestinal: Vomiting, diarrhea, dyspepsia, GI hemorrhage, melena, weight loss, xerostomia

Genitourinary: Hematuria, nocturia

Hematologic: Anemia

Hepatic: Hepatitis (1%)

Neuromuscular & skeletal: Arthritis, paresthesia

Ocular: Chromatopsia (9%), abnormal vision (6% to 7%), cataracts, photophobia

Respiratory: Interstitial pneumonitis (2% - typically exertional dyspnea, cough, chest pain, and fever; most often occurring within the first 3 months of treatment); rhinitis

Miscellaneous: Diaphoresis

Overdosage/Toxicology
Symptoms of overdose may include nausea, vomiting, malaise, headache, dizziness, and elevated liver enzymes. Management is supportive. Dialysis is of no benefit.

Pharmacodynamics/Kinetics

Absorption: Rapid and complete

Protein Binding: 72% to 85%

Half-Life Elimination: Terminal: 23-87 hours; Metabolites: 35-137 hours

Metabolism: Hepatic, forms active metabolites

Excretion: Urine (up to 78% at 120 hours; <1% as unchanged drug); feces (1% to 7%)

Dosing

Adults & Elderly: Refer to individual protocols. Prostate cancer: Oral: 300 mg daily for 30 days starting the same day or day after surgical castration, then 150 mg/day

Available Dosage Forms Tablet: 150 mg

Monitoring and Teaching Issues

Physical Assessment: See Warnings/Precautions for use cautions. Assess potential for interactions with other pharmacological agents and herbal products patient may be taking (eg, agents that may increase or decrease levels/effects of nilutamide; see Drug Interactions). Assess results of chest x-rays and laboratory tests (see Monitoring Laboratory Tests) prior to and regularly during therapy. Assess effectiveness and adverse response (eg, signs of interstitial pneumonitis [dyspnea, chest pain, cough, fever], hepatitis, visual changes impaired dark adaptation; see Adverse Reactions). Teach patient proper use, possible side effects/appropriate interventions (eg, orthostatic precautions), and adverse symptoms to report (see Patient Education).

Monitoring Laboratory Tests: Chest x-rays prior to and regularly during treatment. Measure serum hepatic enzyme levels at baseline and at regular intervals (3 months). If transaminases increase over 2-3 times the upper limit of normal, discontinue treatment. Perform appropriate laboratory testing at the first symptom/sign of liver injury (eg, jaundice, dark urine, fatigue, abdominal pain, or unexplained GI symptoms).

Patient Education: Do not take any new medication during therapy unless approved by prescriber. Take as prescribed; do not change dosing schedule or stop taking without consulting prescriber. Avoid alcohol while taking this medication; may cause severe adverse reaction. Periodic laboratory tests are necessary while taking this medication. May cause loss of light accommodation (avoid night driving and use caution in poorly lighted or changing light situations such as tunnels); dizziness, confusion, or blurred vision (avoid driving or engaging in tasks that are potentially hazardous until response to drug is known); nausea or anorexia (small frequent meals, frequent mouth care, chewing gum, or sucking lozenges may help); or hot flashes, gynecomastia, decreased libido, impotence or sexual dysfunction (consult prescriber). Report any decreased respiratory function (eg, dyspnea, increased cough); unexplained fever; difficulty or painful voiding or blood in urine; or other persistent adverse effects.

Dietary Considerations: May be taken without regard to food.

Pregnancy Risk Factor: C

Lactation: Not indicated for use in women

Administration

   Storage: Store at room temperature of 15°C to 30°C (59°F to 86°F). Protect from light.

♦ **Nimbex®**   *see Cisatracurium on page 333*

Nimodipine   (nye MOE di peen)

U.S. Brand Names Nimotop®

Generic Available No

Pharmacologic Category Calcium Channel Blocker

Medication Safety Issues

   Sound-alike/look-alike issues:

   Nimodipine may be confused with niCARdipine, NIFEdipine

Use Spasm following subarachnoid hemorrhage from ruptured intracranial aneurysms regardless of the patients neurological condition postictus (Hunt and Hess grades I-V)

Mechanism of Action/Effect Nimodipine shares the pharmacology of other calcium channel blockers; animal studies indicate that nimodipine has a greater effect on cerebral arterials than other arterials; inhibits calcium ion from entering the "slow channels" or select voltage sensitive areas of vascular smooth muscle and myocardium during depolarization

Contraindications Hypersensitivity to nimodipine or any component of the formulation

Warnings/Precautions May cause reductions in blood pressure. Use caution in hepatic impairment. Intestinal pseudo-obstruction and ileus have been reported during the use of nimodipine. Use caution in patients with decreased GI motility or a history of bowel obstruction. Use caution when treating patients with increased intracranial pressure.

Drug Interactions

   Cytochrome P450 Effect: Substrate of CYP3A4 (major)

   Decreased Effect: CYP3A4 inducers may decrease the levels/effects of nimodipine; example inducers include aminoglutethimide, carbamazepine, nafcillin, nevirapine, phenobarbital, phenytoin, and rifamycins.

   Increased Effect/Toxicity: Calcium channel blockers and nimodipine may result in enhanced cardiovascular effects of other calcium channel blockers. Cimetidine, omeprazole, and valproic acid may increase serum nimodipine levels. The effects of antihypertensive agents may be increased by nimodipine. Blood pressure-lowering effects may be additive with sildenafil, tadalafil, and vardenafil (use caution). CYP3A4 inhibitors may increase the levels/effects of nimodipine; example inhibitors include azole antifungals, ciprofloxacin, clarithromycin, diclofenac, doxycycline, erythromycin, imatinib, isoniazid, nefazodone, nicardipine, propofol, protease inhibitors, quinidine, and verapamil.

Nutritional/Ethanol Interactions

   Food: Nimodipine has shown a 1.5-fold increase in bioavailability when taken with grapefruit juice; avoid concurrent use.

   Herb/Nutraceutical: St John's wort may decrease levels. Avoid dong quai if using for hypertension (has estrogenic activity). Avoid ephedra, yohimbe, ginseng (may worsen hypertension). Avoid garlic (may have increased antihypertensive effect).

Adverse Reactions 1% to 10%:

   Cardiovascular: Reductions in systemic blood pressure (1% to 8%)

   Central nervous system: Headache (1% to 4%)

   Dermatologic: Rash (1% to 2%)

   Gastrointestinal: Diarrhea (2% to 4%), abdominal discomfort (2%)

Overdosage/Toxicology Primary cardiac symptoms of calcium blocker overdose include hypotension and bradycardia. Noncardiac symptoms include confusion, stupor, nausea, vomiting, metabolic acidosis and hyperglycemia. Treat symptomatically.

Pharmacodynamics/Kinetics

   Bioavailability: 13%

   Time to Peak: Serum: ~1 hour

   Protein Binding: >95%

   Half-Life Elimination: 3 hours; prolonged with renal impairment

   Metabolism: Extensively hepatic

   Excretion: Urine (50%) and feces (32%) within 4 days

Dosing

   Adults & Elderly: Subarachnoid hemorrhage: Oral: 60 mg every 4 hours for 21 days, start therapy within 96 hours after subarachnoid hemorrhage.

   Renal Impairment: Not removed by hemo- or peritoneal dialysis; supplemental dose is not necessary.

   Hepatic Impairment: Reduce dosage to 30 mg every 4 hours in patients with liver failure.

Available Dosage Forms Capsule, liquid filled: 30 mg

Monitoring and Teaching Issues

   Physical Assessment: See Warnings/Precautions for use cautions (eg, hepatic impairment, history of bowel obstruction). Assess potential for interactions with other pharmacological agents and herbal products patient may be taking (eg, increased risk of hypotension with other antihypertensives; see Drug Interactions). Assess therapeutic effectiveness (blood pressure and cardiac status) and adverse response when starting or adjusting dose and periodically during long-term therapy (eg, rash, hypotension, diarrhea, confusion; see Adverse Reactions). Teach patient proper use, possible side effects/appropriate interventions, and adverse symptoms to report (see Patient Education).

   Patient Education: Do not take any new medication during therapy unless approved by prescriber. Take as directed; do not alter dose or decrease without consulting prescriber. Avoid grapefruit juice. May cause orthostatic hypotension (change position slowly from sitting or lying to standing, or when climbing stairs); headache (consult prescriber for (Continued)

Nimodipine *(Continued)*

approved analgesic); or diarrhea (buttermilk, boiled milk, or yogurt may help). Report chest pain, palpitations, slow heartbeat, respiratory difficulty, or other persistent adverse effects. **Pregnancy/breast-feeding precautions:** Inform prescriber if you are or intend to become pregnant. Breast-feeding is not recommended.

Geriatric Considerations: Elderly may experience a greater hypotensive response. Constipation may be more of a problem in the elderly.

Pregnancy Risk Factor: C

Lactation: Enters breast milk/not recommended

Administration

Oral: If the capsules cannot be swallowed, the liquid may be removed by making a hole in each end of the capsule with an 18-gauge needle and extracting the contents into a syringe. If given via NG tube, follow with a flush of 30 mL NS.

Related Information

Calcium Channel Blockers *on page 1722*

♦ **Nimotop®** *see* Nimodipine *on page 1085*

♦ **Nipent®** *see* Pentostatin *on page 1184*

Nisoldipine *(NYE sole di peen)*

U.S. Brand Names Sular®

Generic Available No

Pharmacologic Category Calcium Channel Blocker

Medication Safety Issues

Sound-alike/look-alike issues:

Nisoldipine may be confused with NIFEdipine

Use Management of hypertension, alone or in combination with other antihypertensive agents

Mechanism of Action/Effect As a dihydropyridine calcium channel blocker, structurally similar to nifedipine, nisoldipine impedes the movement of calcium ions into vascular smooth muscle and cardiac muscle. Dihydropyridines are potent vasodilators and are not as likely to suppress cardiac contractility and slow cardiac conduction as other calcium antagonists such as verapamil and diltiazem; nisoldipine is 5-10 times as potent a vasodilator as nifedipine.

Contraindications Hypersensitivity to nisoldipine, any component of the formulation, or other dihydropyridine calcium channel blockers

Warnings/Precautions May cause increased angina and/or myocardial infarction in patients with coronary artery disease (rare). Use with caution in patients with hypotension, CHF, and hepatic impairment. Blood pressure lowering must be done at a rate appropriate for the patient's condition.

Drug Interactions

Cytochrome P450 Effect: Substrate of CYP3A4 (major); **Inhibits** CYP1A2 (weak), 3A4 (weak)

Decreased Effect: CYP3A4 inducers may decrease the levels/effects of nisoldipine; example inducers include aminoglutethimide, carbamazepine, nafcillin, nevirapine, phenobarbital, phenytoin, and rifamycins. Calcium may decrease the hypotension from calcium channel blockers.

Increased Effect/Toxicity: CYP3A4 inhibitors may increase the levels/effects of nisoldipine; example inhibitors include azole antifungals, ciprofloxacin, clarithromycin, diclofenac, doxycycline, erythromycin, imatinib, isoniazid, nefazodone, nicardipine, propofol, protease inhibitors, quinidine, and verapamil. Calcium may reduce the calcium channel blocker's effects, particularly hypotension. Blood pressure-lowering effects may be additive with sildenafil, tadalafil, and vardenafil (use caution). Digoxin and nisoldipine may increase digoxin effect.

Nutritional/Ethanol Interactions

Food: Nisoldipine bioavailability may be increased if taken with high-lipid foods or with grapefruit juice. Avoid grapefruit products before and after dosing.

Herb/Nutraceutical: St John's wort may decrease nisoldipine levels. Avoid dong quai if using for hypertension (has estrogenic activity). Avoid ephedra, yohimbe, ginseng (may worsen hypertension). Avoid garlic (may have increased antihypertensive effect).

Adverse Reactions

>10%:

Cardiovascular: Peripheral edema (dose related 7% to 29%)

Central nervous system: Headache (22%)

1% to 10%:

Cardiovascular: Chest pain (2%), palpitation (3%), vasodilation (4%)

Central nervous system: Dizziness (3% to 10%)

Dermatologic: Rash (2%)

Gastrointestinal: Nausea (2%)

Respiratory: Pharyngitis (5%), sinusitis (3%), dyspnea (3%), cough (5%)

Overdosage/Toxicology Primary cardiac symptoms of calcium blocker overdose include hypotension and bradycardia. Noncardiac symptoms include confusion, stupor, nausea, vomiting, metabolic acidosis and hyperglycemia. Treat symptomatically.

Pharmacodynamics/Kinetics
Duration of Action: >24 hours

Absorption: Well absorbed

Bioavailability: 5%

Time to Peak: 6-12 hours

Half-Life Elimination: 7-12 hours

Metabolism: Extensively hepatic to inactive metabolites; first-pass effect

Excretion: Urine

Dosing
Adults:

Hypertension: Oral: Initial: 20 mg once daily, then increase by 10 mg/week (or longer intervals) to attain adequate control of blood pressure

Usual dose range (JNC 7): 10-40 mg once daily; doses >60 mg once daily are not recommended.

Elderly: Initial dose: 10 mg/day, increase by 10 mg/week (or longer intervals) to attain adequate blood pressure control. Those with hepatic disease should be started with 10 mg/day.

Hepatic Impairment: A starting dose not exceeding 10 mg/day is recommended for patients with hepatic impairment.

Available Dosage Forms Tablet, extended release: 10 mg, 20 mg, 30 mg, 40 mg

Monitoring and Teaching Issues
Physical Assessment: Use caution with hypotension, CHF, hepatic impairment (see Warnings/Precautions for use cautions). Assess potential for interactions with other pharmacological agents and herbal products patient may be taking (eg, increased potential for hypotension with other antihypertensives; see Drug Interactions). Assess therapeutic effectiveness (cardiac status and blood pressure) and adverse response when starting or adjusting dose and periodically during long-term therapy (eg, chest pain, dyspnea, cough, edema, rash, nausea, confusion; see Adverse Reactions and Overdose/Toxicology). Taper dose gradually (over 2 weeks) when discontinuing. Teach patient proper use, possible side effects/appropriate interventions, and adverse symptoms to report (see Patient Education).

Patient Education: Do not take any new medication during therapy unless approved by prescriber. Take exactly as directed; do not alter dose or decrease without consulting prescriber. Do not crush or chew capsules; swallow whole. Take with food, but avoid fatty food and grapefruit juice. This drug does not replace diet and other exercise recommendations of prescriber. May cause orthostatic hypotension (change position slowly when rising from sitting or lying, or when climbing stairs); headache (consult prescriber for approved analgesic); dizziness (use caution when driving or engaging in tasks that require alertness until response to drug is known); or nausea (small frequent meals, frequent mouth care, chewing gum, or sucking lozenges may help). Report chest pain, palpitations, irregular heartbeat; respiratory difficulty; unusual cough; rash; vision changes; anxiety, confusion, depression, or other CNS changes; or other persistent adverse reactions. **Pregnancy/breast-feeding precautions:** Inform prescriber if you are or intend to become pregnant. Consult prescriber if breast-feeding.

Geriatric Considerations: Elderly may experience a greater hypotensive response. Constipation may be more of a problem in the elderly. Calcium channel blockers are no more effective in the elderly than other therapies; however, they do not cause significant CNS effects which is an advantage over some antihypertensive agents.

Pregnancy Risk Factor: C

Lactation: Excretion in breast milk unknown

Administration
Oral: Administer at the same time each day to ensure minimal fluctuation of serum levels. Avoid high-fat diet.

Related Information
Calcium Channel Blockers *on page 1722*

♦ **Nitalapram** *see Citalopram on page 338*

Nitazoxanide (nye ta ZOX a nide)

U.S. Brand Names Alinia®

Synonyms NTZ

Generic Available No

Pharmacologic Category Antiprotozoal

Use Treatment of diarrhea caused by *Cryptosporidium parvum* or *Giardia lamblia*

Mechanism of Action/Effect Nitazoxanide is rapidly metabolized to the active metabolite tizoxanide *in vivo*. Nitazoxanide and its metabolite inhibit the growth of sporozoites and oocysts of *Cryptosporidium parvum* and trophozoites of *Giardia lamblia*.

Contraindications Hypersensitivity to nitazoxanide or any component of the formulation

Warnings/Precautions Use caution with renal or hepatic impairment. Safety and efficacy have not been established with HIV infection, immunodeficiency, or in children <1 year of age.

Nutritional/Ethanol Interactions Food: Food increases AUC.

Adverse Reactions Rates of adverse effects were similar to those reported with placebo.

1% to 10%:

Central nervous system: Headache (1% to 3%)

Gastrointestinal: Abdominal pain (7% to 8%), diarrhea (2% to 4%), nausea (3%), vomiting (1%)

Overdosage/Toxicology Treatment should be symptomatic and supportive.

(Continued)

Nitazoxanide (Continued)

Pharmacodynamics/Kinetics
Bioavailability: Relative bioavailability of suspension compared to tablet: 70%

Time to Peak: Plasma: Tizoxanide and tizoxanide glucuronide: 1-4 hours

Protein Binding: Tizoxanide: >99%

Metabolism: Hepatic, to an active metabolite, tizoxanide. Tizoxanide undergoes conjugation to form tizoxanide glucuronide. Nitazoxanide is not detectable in the serum following oral administration.

Excretion: Tizoxanide: Urine, bile, and feces; Tizoxanide glucuronide: Urine and bile

Dosing
Adults: Diarrhea caused by *Giardia lamblia*: Oral: 500 mg every 12 hours for 3 days

Pediatrics:

Diarrhea caused by *Cryptosporidium parvum*:
Children 12-47 months: 100 mg every 12 hours for 3 days
Children 4-11 years: 200 mg every 12 hours for 3 days

Diarrhea caused by *Giardia lamblia*:
Children 12-47 months: 100 mg every 12 hours for 3 days
Children 4-11 years: 200 mg every 12 hours for 3 days
Children ≥12 years: Refer to adult dosing.

Renal Impairment: Specific recommendations are not available; use with caution.

Hepatic Impairment: Specific recommendations are not available; use with caution.

Available Dosage Forms
Powder for oral suspension: 100 mg/5 mL (60 mL) [contains sucrose 1.48 g/5 mL, sodium benzoate; strawberry flavor]

Tablet: 500 mg

Alinia® 3-Day Therapy Packs™ [unit-dose pack]: 500 mg (6s)

Monitoring and Teaching Issues
Patient Education: Administer exactly as directed. Do not alter dose; administer with food. Shake suspension well before using. Store at room temperature and discard any unused portion of suspension after 7 days. May cause headache, abdominal pain, diarrhea, or vomiting. If severe or persistent, contact prescriber. **Breast-feeding precaution:** Consult prescriber if breast-feeding.

Dietary Considerations: Should be taken with food. Suspension contains sucrose 1.48 g/5 mL.

Pregnancy Risk Factor: B

Lactation: Excretion in breast milk unknown/use caution

Administration
Oral: Administer with food. Shake suspension well prior to administration.

Storage:

Suspension: Prior to and following reconstitution, store at room temperature of 15°C to 30°C (59°F to 86°F). Following reconstitution, discard unused portion of suspension after 7 days.

Tablet: Store at room temperature.

♦ Nitrek®   *see* Nitroglycerin *on page 1090*

♦ 4'-Nitro-3'-Trifluoromethylisobutyrantide   *see* Flutamide *on page 658*

♦ Nitro-Bid®   *see* Nitroglycerin *on page 1090*

♦ Nitro-Dur®   *see* Nitroglycerin *on page 1090*

Nitrofurantoin (nye troe fyoor AN toyn)

U.S. Brand Names Furadantin®; Macrobid®; Macrodantin®

Generic Available Yes: Excludes suspension

Pharmacologic Category Antibiotic, Miscellaneous

Use Prevention and treatment of urinary tract infections caused by susceptible gram-negative and some gram-positive organisms; *Pseudomonas*, *Serratia*, and most species of *Proteus* are generally resistant to nitrofurantoin

Mechanism of Action/Effect Inhibits several bacterial enzyme systems including acetyl coenzyme A interfering with metabolism and possibly cell wall synthesis

Contraindications Hypersensitivity to nitrofurantoin or any component of the formulation; renal impairment (anuria, oliguria, significantly elevated serum creatinine, or Cl_{cr}< 60 mL/minute); infants <1 month (due to the possibility of hemolytic anemia); pregnancy at term (38-42 weeks gestation), during labor and delivery, or when the onset of labor is imminent

Warnings/Precautions Use with caution in patients with G6PD deficiency or in patients with anemia. Therapeutic concentrations of nitrofurantoin are not attained in urine of patients with Cl_{cr}<60 mL/minute. Use with caution if prolonged therapy is anticipated due to possible pulmonary toxicity. Acute, subacute, or chronic (usually after 6 months of therapy) pulmonary reactions have been observed in patients treated with nitrofurantoin; if these occur, discontinue therapy immediately; monitor closely for malaise, dyspnea, cough, fever, radiologic evidence of diffuse interstitial pneumonitis or fibrosis. Rare, but severe hepatic reactions have been associated with nitrofurantoin (onset may be insidious); discontinue immediately if hepatitis occurs. Has been associated with peripheral neuropathy (rare); risk may be increased by renal impairment, diabetes, vitamin B deficiency, or electrolyte imbalance; use caution.

Drug Interactions
Decreased Effect: Antacids decrease absorption of nitrofurantoin.

Increased Effect/Toxicity: Probenecid decreases renal excretion of nitrofurantoin.

Nutritional/Ethanol Interactions
Ethanol: Avoid ethanol (may increase CNS depression).

Food: Nitrofurantoin serum concentrations may be increased if taken with food.

Lab Interactions False-positive urine glucose (Benedict's and Fehling's methods); no false positives with enzymatic tests

Adverse Reactions Frequency not defined.

Cardiovascular: Chest pain, cyanosis, ECG changes (associated with pulmonary toxicity)

Central nervous system: Chills, depression, dizziness, drowsiness, fatigue, fever, headache, pseudotumor cerebri, psychotic reaction

Dermatologic: Alopecia, erythema multiforme, exfoliative dermatitis, pruritus, rash, Stevens-Johnson syndrome

Gastrointestinal: Abdominal pain, *C. difficile*-colitis, constipation, diarrhea, dyspepsia, loss of appetite, nausea (most common), pancreatitis, sore throat, vomiting

Hematologic: Agranulocytosis, aplastic anemia, eosinophilia, hemolytic anemia, methemo-globinemia, thrombocytopenia

Hepatic: Cholestasis, hepatitis, hepatic necrosis, transaminases increased, jaundice (cholestatic)

Neuromuscular & skeletal: Arthralgia, numbness, paresthesia, peripheral neuropathy, weakness

Ocular: Amblyopia, nystagmus, optic neuritis (rare)

Respiratory: Cough, dyspnea, pneumonitis, pulmonary fibrosis

Miscellaneous: Hypersensitivity (including acute pulmonary hypersensitivity), lupus-like syndrome

Overdosage/Toxicology Symptoms of overdose include vomiting. Treatment is supportive.

Pharmacodynamics/Kinetics

Absorption: Well absorbed; macrocrystalline is absorbed more slowly due to slower dissolution (causes less GI distress)

Bioavailability: Increased with food

Protein Binding: 60% to 90%

Half-Life Elimination: 20-60 minutes; prolonged with renal impairment

Metabolism: Body tissues (except plasma) metabolize 60% of drug to inactive metabolites

Excretion:

Suspension: Urine (40%) and feces (small amounts) as metabolites and unchanged drug

Macrocrystals: Urine (20% to 25% as unchanged drug)

Dosing

Adults:

Treatment of UTI: Oral: 50-100 mg/dose every 6 hours (not to exceed 400 mg/24 hours)

Prophylaxis of UTI: Oral: 50-100 mg/dose at bedtime

Elderly: Refer to adult dosing (see Geriatric Considerations).

Pediatrics:

Treatment of UTI: Oral: Children >1 month: 5-7 mg/kg/day in divided doses every 6 hours; maximum: 400 mg/day

Chronic therapy: Oral: 1-2 mg/kg/day in divided doses every 12-24 hours; maximum: 100 mg/day

Renal Impairment:

Cl_{cr} <60 mL/minute: Contraindicated

Contraindicated in hemo- and peritoneal dialysis and continuous arteriovenous or venovenous hemofiltration.

Available Dosage Forms

Capsule, macrocrystal: 50 mg, 100 mg

Macrodantin®: 25 mg, 50 mg, 100 mg

Capsule, macrocrystal/monohydrate (Macrobid®): 100 mg

Suspension, oral (Furadantin®): 25 mg/5 mL (470 mL)

Monitoring and Teaching Issues

Physical Assessment: Assess results of culture and sensitivity test and assess patient's allergy history prior to beginning treatment. Use caution with G6PD deficiency, renal, hepatic, or respiratory impairment (see Warnings/Precautions for specific use cautions). Assess results periodic CBC and LFTs with long-term use. Monitor effectiveness (resolution of infection) and adverse response (eg, hypersensitivity, chest pain, pneumonitis [cough, dyspnea], rash, GI disturbance, anemia, jaundice; see Adverse Reactions). Advise patients with diabetes about use of Clinitest® (may cause false-positive urine glucose). Teach patient proper use, possible side effects/appropriate interventions, and adverse symptoms to report (see Patient Education).

Monitoring Laboratory Tests: CBC, periodic liver function. Perform culture and sensitivity prior to initiating therapy.

Patient Education: Do not take any new medication during therapy unless approved by prescriber. Take entire prescription, even if you are feeling better. Take with food. Suspension: Shake well before use. Maintain adequate hydration (2-3 L/day of fluids) unless instructed to restrict fluid intake. If you have diabetes, drug may cause false test results with Clinitest® urine glucose monitoring; use of another type of glucose monitoring is preferable. May cause nausea or vomiting (small frequent meals, frequent mouth care, sucking lozenges, or chewing gum may help); or diarrhea (buttermilk, boiled milk, or yogurt may help). Report immediately and rash; swelling of face, tongue, mouth, or throat; or chest tightness. Report if condition being treated worsens or does not improve by the time prescription is completed.

Geriatric Considerations: Because of nitrofurantoin's decreased efficacy in patients with a Cl_{cr} <60 mL/minute and its side effect profile, it is not an antibiotic of choice for acute or prophylactic treatment of urinary tract infections in the elderly. An increased rate of severe hepatic toxicity has been suggested by postmarketing reports.

Pregnancy Risk Factor: B (contraindicated at term)

Pregnancy Issues: Teratogenic effects have not been observed, however may cause hemolytic anemia in infants. Use of nitrofurantoin is contraindicated at term (38-42 weeks gestation), during labor and delivery, or when the onset of labor is imminent.

Lactation: Enters breast milk/not recommended (infants <1 month); AAP rates "compatible"

Breast-Feeding Issues: Excreted in trace amounts in breast milk; may cause hyperbilirubinemia or hemolytic anemia in infants (<1 month of age). AAP rates "compatible." Use caution in G6PD deficiency.

(Continued)

Nitrofurantoin (Continued)

Administration

Oral: Suspension: Shake well before use. Higher peak serum levels may cause increased GI upset. Give with meals to slow the rate of absorption and decrease adverse effects.

Storage: Store at room temperature 15°C to 30°C (59°F to 86°F).

♦ **Nitrogard®** see Nitroglycerin on page 1090

♦ **Nitrogen Mustard** see Mechlorethamine on page 935

Nitroglycerin (nye troe GLI ser in)

U.S. Brand Names Minitran™; Nitrek®; Nitro-Bid®; Nitro-Dur®; Nitrogard®; Nitrol® [DSC]; Nitrolingual®; NitroQuick®; Nitrostat®; Nitro-Tab®; NitroTime®

Synonyms Glyceryl Trinitrate; Nitroglycerol; NTG

Generic Available Yes: Capsule, injection, patch, tablet

Pharmacologic Category Vasodilator

Medication Safety Issues

Sound-alike/look-alike issues:

Nitroglycerin may be confused with nitroprusside

Nitro-Bid® may be confused with Nicobid®

Nitroderm may be confused with NicoDerm®

Nitrol® may be confused with Nizoral®

Nitrostat® may be confused with Hyperstat®, Nilstat®, nystatin

Nitroglycerin transdermal patches should be removed prior to defibrillation or MRI study.

Use Treatment of angina pectoris; I.V. for congestive heart failure (especially when associated with acute myocardial infarction); pulmonary hypertension; hypertensive emergencies occurring perioperatively (especially during cardiovascular surgery)

Unlabeled/Investigational Use Esophageal spastic disorders (sublingual)

Mechanism of Action/Effect Works by relaxation of smooth muscle, producing a vasodilator effect on the peripheral veins and arteries with more prominent effects on the veins. Primarily reduces cardiac oxygen demand by decreasing preload (left ventricular end-diastolic pressure); may modestly reduce afterload; dilates coronary arteries and improves collateral flow to ischemic regions

Contraindications Hypersensitivity to organic nitrates; hypersensitivity to isosorbide, nitroglycerin, or any component of the formulation; concurrent use with phosphodiesterase-5 (PDE-5) inhibitors (sildenafil, tadalafil, or vardenafil); angle-closure glaucoma (intraocular pressure may be increased); head trauma or cerebral hemorrhage (increase intracranial pressure); severe anemia; allergy to adhesive (transdermal product)

Additional contraindications for I.V. product: Hypotension; uncorrected hypovolemia; inadequate cerebral circulation; constrictive pericarditis; pericardial tamponade

Warnings/Precautions Severe hypotension can occur. Use with caution in volume depletion, hypotension, and right ventricular infarctions. Paradoxical bradycardia and increased angina pectoris can accompany hypotension. Orthostatic hypotension can also occur. Ethanol can accentuate this. Tolerance does develop to nitrates and appropriate dosing is needed to minimize this (drug-free interval). Safety and efficacy have not been established in pediatric patients. Avoid use of long-acting agents in acute MI or CHF; cannot easily reverse. Nitrate may aggravate angina caused by hypertrophic cardiomyopathy. Nitroglycerin transdermal patches should be removed prior to defibrillation or MRI study.

Drug Interactions

Decreased Effect: I.V. nitroglycerin may antagonize the anticoagulant effect of heparin (possibly only at high nitroglycerin dosages); monitor closely. May need to decrease heparin dosage when nitroglycerin is discontinued. Alteplase (tissue plasminogen activator) has a lesser effect when used with I.V. nitroglycerin; avoid concurrent use. Ergot alkaloids may cause an increase in blood pressure and decrease in antianginal effects; avoid concurrent use.

Increased Effect/Toxicity: Significant reduction of systolic and diastolic blood pressure with concurrent use of sildenafil, tadalafil, or vardenafil (contraindicated); do not administer sildenafil, tadalafil, or vardenafil within 24 hours of a nitrate preparation. Ethanol can cause hypotension when nitrates are taken 1 hour or more after ethanol ingestion.

Adverse Reactions

Spray or patch:

>10%: Central nervous system: Headache (patch 63%, spray 50%)

1% to 10%:

Cardiovascular: Hypotension (patch 4%), increased angina (patch 2%)

Central nervous system: Lightheadedness (patch 6%), syncope (patch 4%)

Topical, sublingual, intravenous: Frequency not defined:

Cardiovascular: Hypotension (infrequent), postural hypotension, crescendo angina (uncommon), rebound hypertension (uncommon), pallor, cardiovascular collapse, tachycardia, shock, flushing, peripheral edema

Central nervous system: Headache (most common), lightheadedness (related to blood pressure changes), syncope (uncommon), dizziness, restlessness

Gastrointestinal: Nausea, vomiting, bowel incontinence, xerostomia

Genitourinary: Urinary incontinence

Hematologic: Methemoglobinemia (rare, overdose)

Neuromuscular & skeletal: Weakness

Ocular: Blurred vision

Miscellaneous: Cold sweat

The incidence of hypotension and adverse cardiovascular events may be increased when used in combination with sildenafil (Viagra®).

Overdosage/Toxicology Symptoms of overdose include hypotension, throbbing headache, palpitations, bloody diarrhea, bradycardia, cyanosis, tissue hypoxia, metabolic acidosis, clonic convulsions, circulatory collapse, and methemoglobinemia with extremely large overdoses. Treatment is supportive and symptomatic. Methemoglobinemia should be treated with methylene blue (1-2 mg/kg over 5 minutes). Additional doses may be necessary (0.5-1 mg/kg) based on follow-up methemoglobin levels (obtained after 30 minutes).

Pharmacodynamics/Kinetics

Onset of Action: Sublingual tablet: 1-3 minutes; Translingual spray: 2 minutes; Buccal tablet: 2-5 minutes; Sustained release: 20-45 minutes; Topical: 15-60 minutes; Transdermal: 40-60 minutes; I.V. drip: Immediate

Peak effect: Sublingual tablet: 4-8 minutes; Translingual spray: 4-10 minutes; Buccal tablet: 4-10 minutes; Sustained release: 45-120 minutes; Topical: 30-120 minutes; Transdermal: 60-180 minutes; I.V. drip: Immediate

Duration of Action: Sublingual tablet: 30-60 minutes; Translingual spray: 30-60 minutes; Buccal tablet: 2 hours; Sustained release: 4-8 hours; Topical: 2-12 hours; Transdermal: 18-24 hours; I.V. drip: 3-5 minutes

Protein Binding: 60%

Half-Life Elimination: 1-4 minutes

Metabolism: Extensive first-pass effect

Excretion: Urine (as inactive metabolites)

Dosing

Adults & Elderly: Note: Hemodynamic and antianginal tolerance often develop within 24-48 hours of continuous nitrate administration. Nitrate-free interval (10-12 hours/day) is recommended to avoid tolerance development; gradually decrease dose in patients receiving NTG for prolonged period to avoid withdrawal reaction.

Angina/coronary artery disease:

Oral: 2.5-9 mg 2-4 times/day (up to 26 mg 4 times/day)

I.V.: 5 mcg/minute, increase by 5 mcg/minute every 3-5 minutes to 20 mcg/minute. If no response at 20 mcg/minute increase by 10 mcg/minute every 3-5 minutes, up to 200 mcg/minute.

Topical ointment: Include a nitrate free interval, ~10 to 12 hours; Apply 0.5" to 2" every 6 hours with a nitrate free interval.

Topical patch, transdermal: 0.2-0.4 mg/hour initially and titrate to doses of 0.4-0.8 mg/hour. Tolerance is minimized by using a patch-on period of 12-14 hours and patch-off period of 10-12 hours.

Buccal: Initial: 1 mg every 3-5 hours while awake (3 times/day); titrate dosage upward if angina occurs with tablet in place.

Sublingual: 0.2-0.6 mg every 5 minutes for maximum of 3 doses in 15 minutes; may also use prophylactically 5-10 minutes prior to activities which may provoke an attack.

Esophageal spastic disorders (unlabeled use): 0.3-0.4 mg 5 minutes before meals

Translingual: 1-2 sprays into mouth under tongue every 3-5 minutes for maximum of 3 doses in 15 minutes, may also be used 5-10 minutes prior to activities which may provoke an attack prophylactically.

Pediatrics:

Pulmonary hypertension: I.V. Continuous infusion: Children: Start 0.25-0.5 mcg/kg/minute and titrate by 1 mcg/kg/minute at 20- to 60-minute intervals to desired effect; usual dose: 1-3 mcg/kg/minute; maximum: 5 mcg/kg/minute

Note: Hemodynamic and antianginal tolerance often develop within 24-48 hours of continuous nitrate administration.

Available Dosage Forms [DSC] = Discontinued product

Aerosol, translingual spray (Nitrolingual®): 0.4 mg/metered spray (12 g) [contains alcohol 20%; 200 metered sprays]

Capsule, extended release (Nitro-Time®): 2.5 mg, 6.5 mg, 9 mg

Infusion [premixed in D₅W]: 0.1 mg/mL (250 mL, 500 mL); 0.2 mg/mL (250 mL); 0.4 mg/mL (250 mL, 500 mL)

Injection, solution: 5 mg/mL (5 mL, 10 mL) [contains alcohol and propylene glycol]

Ointment, topical:

Nitro-Bid®: 2% [20 mg/g] (30 g, 60 g)

Nitrol® [DSC]: 2% [20 mg/g] (3 g, 60 g)

Tablet, buccal, extended release (Nitrogard®): 2 mg, 3 mg

Tablet, sublingual (NitroQuick®, Nitrostat®, Nitro-Tab®): 0.3 mg, 0.4 mg, 0.6 mg

Transdermal system [once daily patch]: 0.1 mg/hour (30s); 0.2 mg/hour (30s); 0.4 mg/hour (30s); 0.6 mg/hour (30s)

Minitran™: 0.1 mg/hour (30s); 0.2 mg/hour (30s); 0.4 mg/hour (30s); 0.6 mg/hour (30s)

Nitrek®: 0.2 mg/hour (30s); 0.4 mg/hour (30s); 0.6 mg/hour (30s)

Nitro-Dur®: 0.1 mg/hour (30s); 0.2 mg/hour (30s); 0.3 mg/hour (30s); 0.4 mg/hour (30s); 0.6 mg/hour (30s); 0.8 mg/hour (30s)

Monitoring and Teaching Issues

Physical Assessment: See Warnings/Precautions for specific use cautions (eg, volume depletion, hypotension, and right ventricular infarctions). Assess potential for interactions with other pharmacological agents patient may be taking (eg, heparin, ergot alkaloids, sildenafil, tadalafil, or vardenafil; see Drug Interactions). See Administration specifics for different formulations. Assess therapeutic effectiveness (cardiac status) and adverse response (eg, hypotension, arrhythmias, CNS changes, GI disturbances; see Adverse Reactions). Dose should be reduced gradually when discontinuing after long-term therapy. Teach patient proper use (according to purpose and formulation), possible side effects/appropriate interventions (eg, drug-free intervals; remove transdermal patches for specific period of time), and adverse symptoms to report (see Patient Education).

Patient Education: Do not take any new medication during therapy unless approved by prescriber. Take as per directions (see below). Do not change brands without consulting prescriber. Do not discontinue abruptly. Keep medication in original container, tightly closed. If anginal chest pain is unresolved in 15 minutes, seek emergency medical help at once. Daily use may cause dizziness or lightheadedness (use caution when driving or engaging in hazardous activities until response to drug is known); headache (consult prescriber for approved analgesic); hypotension (use care when changing position from sitting or lying to standing, when climbing stairs, or when engaging in tasks that are potentially hazardous until response to drug is known); GI disturbances (small frequent (Continued)

Nitroglycerin *(Continued)*

meals, frequent mouth care, chewing gum, or sucking lozenges may help). Report acute headache, rapid heartbeat, unusual restlessness or dizziness, muscular weakness, or blurred vision or seeing abnormal colors. **Pregnancy/breast-feeding precautions:** Inform prescriber if you are or intend to become pregnant. Consult prescriber if breast-feeding.

Oral: Take as directed. Do not chew or swallow sublingual tablets; allow to dissolve under tongue. Sit down before using sublingual or buccal tablet. Do not chew or crush extended release capsules; swallow with 8 oz of water.

Spray: Spray directly on mucous membranes; do not inhale. Sit down before using spray form.

Topical: Spread prescribed amount thinly on applicator; rotate application sites.

Transdermal: Use as directed; place on hair-free area of skin, rotate sites (usually, patches will be removed for a period each day)

Geriatric Considerations: Caution should be used when using nitrate therapy in the elderly due to hypotension. Hypotension is enhanced in the elderly due to decreased baroreceptor response, decreased venous tone, and often hypovolemia (dehydration) or other hypotensive drugs. Elderly patients may be at greater risk of falling due to nitroglycerin-associated hypotension/orthostasis.

Pregnancy Risk Factor: C

Lactation: Excretion in breast milk unknown/use caution

Administration

Oral: Do not crush sublingual drug product.

I.V.: I.V. must be prepared in glass bottles and use special sets intended for nitroglycerin. glass I.V. bottles and administration sets provided by manufacturer.

Topical: Transdermal patches are labeled as mg/hour.

Reconstitution: Doses should be made in glass bottles, Excel® or PAB® containers; adsorption occurs to soft plastic (eg, PVC). Nitroglycerin diluted in D_5W or NS in glass containers is physically and chemically stable for 48 hours at room temperature and 7 days under refrigeration. In D_5W or NS in Excel®/PAB® containers is physically and chemically stable for 24 hours at room temperature and 14 days under refrigeration.

Standard diluent: 50 mg/250 mL D_5W; 50 mg/500 mL D_5W

Minimum volume: 100 mg/250 mL D_5W; concentration should not exceed 400 mcg/mL.

Compatibility: Stable in D_5LR, $D_5 \frac{1}{2}NS$, D_5NS, LR, $\frac{1}{2}NS$

Y-site administration: Incompatible with alteplase, levofloxacin

Compatibility when admixed: Dose is variable and may require titration, therefore it is not advisable to mix with other agents. **Incompatible** with hydralazine, phenytoin

Storage: Doses should be made in glass bottles, Excel® or PAB® containers. Adsorption occurs to soft plastic (eg, PVC). Premixed bottles are stable according to the manufacturer's expiration dating. Store sublingual tablets and ointment in tightly closed containers at 15°C to 30°C. Store spray at 25°C (excursions permitted to 15°C to 30°C (59°F to 86°F)).

Additional Information I.V. preparations contain alcohol and/or propylene glycol; may need to use nitrate-free interval (10-12 hours/day) to avoid tolerance development. Tolerance may possibly be reversed with acetylcysteine; gradually decrease dose in patients receiving NTG for prolonged period to avoid withdrawal reaction.

Concomitant use of sildenafil (Viagra®) or other phosphodiesterase-5 enzyme inhibitors (PDE-5) may precipitate acute hypotension, myocardial infarction, or death. Nitrates used in right ventricular infarction may induce acute hypotension. Nitrate use in severe pericardial effusion may reduce cardiac filling pressure and precipitate cardiac tamponade. In the management of heart failure, the combination of isosorbide dinitrate and hydralazine confers beneficial effects on disease progression and cardiac outcomes.

Related Information

Compatibility of Drugs *on page 1723*

- ◆ **Nitroglycerol** *see* Nitroglycerin *on page 1090*
- ◆ **Nitrol® [DSC]** *see* Nitroglycerin *on page 1090*
- ◆ **Nitrolingual®** *see* Nitroglycerin *on page 1090*
- ◆ **Nitropress®** *see* Nitroprusside *on page 1092*

Nitroprusside *(nye troe PRUS ide)*

U.S. Brand Names Nitropress®

Synonyms Nitroprusside Sodium; Sodium Nitroferricyanide; Sodium Nitroprusside

Generic Available Yes

Pharmacologic Category Vasodilator

Medication Safety Issues

Sound-alike/look-alike issues:

Nitroprusside may be confused with nitroglycerin

High alert medication: The Institute for Safe Medication Practices (ISMP) includes this medication among its list of drugs which have a heightened risk of causing significant patient harm when used in error.

Use Management of hypertensive crises; congestive heart failure; used for controlled hypotension to reduce bleeding during surgery

Mechanism of Action/Effect Causes peripheral vasodilation by direct action on venous and arteriolar smooth muscle, thus reducing peripheral resistance; will increase cardiac output by decreasing afterload; reduces aortal and left ventricular impedance

Contraindications Hypersensitivity to nitroprusside or any component of the formulation; treatment of compensatory hypertension (aortic coarctation, arteriovenous shunting); high output failure; congenital optic atrophy or tobacco amblyopia

Warnings/Precautions Except when used briefly or at low (<2 mcg/kg/minute) infusion rates, nitroprusside gives rise to large cyanide quantities. Do not use the maximum dose for more than 10 minutes. Use with extreme caution in patients with elevated intracranial pressure. Use extreme caution in patients with hepatic or renal dysfunction. Watch for cyanide toxicity in patients with impaired hepatic function. Use the lowest end of the dosage range with renal impairment. Thiocyanate toxicity occurs in patients with renal impairment or those on prolonged infusions. Continuous blood pressure monitoring is needed.

Adverse Reactions 1% to 10%:

Cardiovascular: Excessive hypotensive response, palpitation, substernal distress

Central nervous system: Disorientation, psychosis, headache, restlessness

Endocrine & metabolic: Thyroid suppression

Gastrointestinal: Nausea, vomiting

Neuromuscular & skeletal: Weakness, muscle spasm

Otic: Tinnitus

Respiratory: Hypoxia

Miscellaneous: Diaphoresis, thiocyanate toxicity

Overdosage/Toxicology Symptoms of overdose include hypotension, vomiting, hyperventilation, tachycardia, muscular twitching, hypothyroidism, cyanide or thiocyanate toxicity. Thiocyanate toxicity includes psychosis, hyper-reflexia, confusion, weakness, tinnitus, seizures, and coma; cyanide toxicity includes acidosis (decreased HCO_3, decreased pH, increased lactate), increase in mixed venous blood oxygen tension, tachycardia, altered consciousness, coma, convulsions, and almond smell on breath.

Nitroprusside has been shown to release cyanide in vivo with hemoglobin. Cyanide toxicity does not usually occur because of the rapid uptake of cyanide by erythrocytes and its eventual incorporation into thiocyanate in the liver. However, high doses, prolonged administration of nitroprusside, or reduced elimination can lead to cyanide poisoning or thiocyanate intoxication. Anemia and liver impairment pose a risk for cyanide accumulation, while renal impairment predisposes thiocyanate accumulation. If toxicity develops, airway support with oxygen therapy is appropriate, followed closely with antidotal therapy of amyl nitrate perles, sodium nitrate 300 mg I.V. for adults (range based on hemoglobin concentration: 6-12 mg/kg for children) and sodium thiosulfate 12.5 g I.V. for adults (range based on hemoglobin concentration: 0.95-1.95 mL/kg of the 25% solution for children); nitrates should not be administered to neonates and small children. Thiocyanate is dialyzable. May be mixed with sodium thiosulfate in I.V. to prevent cyanide toxicity.

Pharmacodynamics/Kinetics

Onset of Action: BP reduction <2 minutes

Duration of Action: 1-10 minutes

Half-Life Elimination: Parent drug: <10 minutes; Thiocyanate: 2.7-7 days

Metabolism: Nitroprusside is converted to cyanide ions in the bloodstream; decomposes to prussic acid which in the presence of sulfur donor is converted to thiocyanate (hepatic and renal rhodanase systems)

Excretion: Urine (as thiocyanate)

Dosing

Adults & Elderly:

Acute hypertension: I.V.: Initial: 0.3-0.5 mcg/kg/minute; increase in increments of 0.5 mcg/kg/minute, titrating to the desired hemodynamic effect or the appearance of headache or nausea; usual dose: 3 mcg/kg/minute; rarely need >4 mcg/kg/minute; maximum: 10 mcg/kg/minute. When >500 mcg/kg is administered by prolonged infusion of faster than 2 mcg/kg/minute, cyanide is generated faster than an unaided patient can handle.

Note: Administration requires the use of an infusion pump. Average dose: 5 mcg/kg/minute.

Pediatrics:

Pulmonary hypertension: I.V.: Children: Initial: 1 mcg/kg/minute by continuous I.V. infusion; increase in increments of 1 mcg/kg/minute at intervals of 20-60 minutes; titrating to the desired response; usual dose: 3 mcg/kg/minute, rarely need >4 mcg/kg/minute; maximum: 5 mcg/kg/minute.

Note: Administration requires the use of an infusion pump. Average dose: 5 mcg/kg/minute.

Renal Impairment: Limit use; accumulation of thiocyanate may occur.

Hepatic Impairment: Limit use; risk of cyanide toxicity.

Available Dosage Forms Injection, solution, as sodium: 25 mg/mL (2 mL)

Monitoring and Teaching Issues

Physical Assessment: See Warnings/Precautions for specific use cautions (eg, hepatic or renal impairment, elevated intracranial pressure). See Administration and Reconstitution for infusion specifics and warnings. Infusion site must be monitored closely to prevent extravasation. Continuous patient monitoring (including blood pressure) is needed. Assess adverse response (eg, acid/base balance, [metabolic acidosis is early sign of cyanide toxicity], disorientation, hypoxia, muscular twitching; see Adverse Reactions). Provide patient teaching according to patient condition (see Patient Education).

Patient Education: Patient condition should indicate extent of education and instruction needed. This drug can only be given I.V. You will be monitored at all times during infusion. Promptly report any chest pain or pain/burning at site of infusion, muscle twitching, disorientation. **Breast-feeding precaution:** Consult prescriber if breast-feeding.

Geriatric Considerations: Elderly patients may have an increased sensitivity to nitroprusside possibly due to a decreased baroreceptor reflex, altered sensitivity to vasodilating effects or a resistance of cardiac adrenergic receptors to stimulation by catecholamines.

Pregnancy Risk Factor: C

Lactation: Excretion in breast milk unknown

Administration

I.V.: I.V. infusion only, use only as an infusion with 5% dextrose in water. Infusion pump required. Not for direct injection.

Reconstitution: Brownish solution is usable, discard if bluish in color. Nitroprusside sodium should be reconstituted freshly by diluting 50 mg in 250-1000 mL of D_5W. Use only clear solutions; solutions of nitroprusside exhibit a color described as brownish, brown, brownish-pink, light orange, and straw. Solutions are highly sensitive to light. Exposure to (Continued)

Nitroprusside *(Continued)*

light causes decomposition, resulting in a highly colored solution of orange, dark brown or blue. **A blue color indicates almost complete degradation and breakdown to cyanide. Solutions should be wrapped with aluminum foil or other opaque material to protect from light (do as soon as possible).** Stability of parenteral admixture at room temperature (25°C) and at refrigeration temperature (4°C) is 24 hours.

Compatibility: Stable in LR

Y-site administration: Incompatible with levofloxacin

Compatibility when admixed: Incompatible with atracurium

Storage:

Use only clear solutions; solutions of nitroprusside exhibit a color described as brownish, brown, brownish-pink, light orange, and straw. Solutions are highly sensitive to light. Exposure to light causes decomposition, resulting in a highly colored solution of orange, dark brown or blue. **A blue color indicates almost complete degradation and breakdown to cyanide.**

Solutions should be wrapped with aluminum foil or other opaque material to protect from light (do as soon as possible)

Stability of parenteral admixture at room temperature (25°C) and at refrigeration temperature (4°C): 24 hours

- ♦ **Nitroprusside Sodium** *see* Nitroprusside *on page 1092*
- ♦ **NitroQuick®** *see* Nitroglycerin *on page 1090*
- ♦ **Nitrostat®** *see* Nitroglycerin *on page 1090*
- ♦ **Nitro-Tab®** *see* Nitroglycerin *on page 1090*
- ♦ **NitroTime®** *see* Nitroglycerin *on page 1090*
- ♦ **Nix® [OTC]** *see* Permethrin *on page 1190*

Nizatidine (ni ZA ti deen)

U.S. Brand Names Axid®; Axid® AR [OTC]

Generic Available Yes: Capsule

Pharmacologic Category Histamine H_2 Antagonist

Medication Safety Issues

Sound-alike/look-alike issues:

Axid® may be confused with Ansaid®

Use Treatment and maintenance of duodenal ulcer; treatment of benign gastric ulcer; treatment of gastroesophageal reflux disease (GERD); OTC tablet used for the prevention of meal-induced heartburn, acid indigestion, and sour stomach

Unlabeled/Investigational Use Part of a multidrug regimen for *H. pylori* eradication to reduce the risk of duodenal ulcer recurrence

Mechanism of Action/Effect Nizatidine is an H_2-receptor antagonist.

Contraindications Hypersensitivity to nizatidine or any component of the formulation; hypersensitivity to other H_2 antagonists (cross-sensitivity has been observed)

Warnings/Precautions Use with caution in children <12 years of age. Use with caution in patients with liver and renal impairment. Dosage modification required in patients with renal impairment.

Drug Interactions

Cytochrome P450 Effect: Inhibits 3A4 (weak)

Decreased Effect: May decrease the absorption of itraconazole or ketoconazole.

Nutritional/Ethanol Interactions Ethanol: Avoid ethanol (may cause gastric mucosal irritation).

Lab Interactions False-positive urine protein using Multistix®, gastric acid secretion test, skin tests allergen extracts, serum creatinine and serum transaminase concentrations, urine protein test

Adverse Reactions

>10%: Central nervous system: Headache (16%)

1% to 10%:

Central nervous system: Anxiety, dizziness, fever (reported in children), insomnia, irritability (reported in children), somnolence, nervousness

Dermatologic: Pruritus, rash

Gastrointestinal: Abdominal pain, anorexia, constipation, diarrhea, dry mouth, flatulence, heartburn, nausea, vomiting

Respiratory: Reported in children: Cough, nasal congestion, nasopharyngitis

Overdosage/Toxicology Symptoms of overdose include muscular tremor, vomiting, and rapid respiration. LD_{50} ~80 mg/kg. Treatment is symptomatic and supportive.

Pharmacodynamics/Kinetics

Absorption: >70%

Bioavailability: >70%

Time to Peak: Plasma: 0.5-3.0 hours

Protein Binding: 35% to α_1-acid glycoprotein

Half-Life Elimination: 1-2 hours; prolonged with renal impairment

Metabolism: Partially hepatic; forms metabolites

Excretion: Urine (90%; ~60% as unchanged drug); feces (<6%)

Dosing

Adults & Elderly:

Duodenal ulcer: Oral:

Treatment of active ulcer: 300 mg at bedtime or 150 mg twice daily

Maintenance of healed ulcer: 150 mg/day at bedtime

Gastric ulcer: Oral: 150 mg twice daily or 300 mg at bedtime

GERD: Oral: 150 mg twice daily

Meal-induced heartburn, acid indigestion, and sour stomach (OTC labeling): Oral: 75 mg tablet [OTC] twice daily, 30-60 minutes prior to consuming food or beverages

Eradication of *Helicobacter pylori* (unlabeled use): Oral: 150 mg twice daily; requires combination therapy

Pediatrics:
GERD (unlabeled use): Oral:
Children <12 years: 10 mg/kg/day in divided doses given twice daily; may not be as effective in children <12 years
Children ≥12 years: Refer to adult dosing.
Meal-induced heartburn, acid indigestion and sour stomach: Oral: Children ≥12 years: Refer to adult dosing.

Renal Impairment:
Active treatment:
Cl_{cr} 20-50 mL/minute: 150 mg/day
Cl_{cr} <20 mL/minute: 150 mg every other day
Maintenance treatment:
Cl_{cr} 20-50 mL/minute: 150 mg every other day
Cl_{cr} <20 mL/minute: 150 mg every 3 days

Available Dosage Forms
Capsule (Axid®): 150 mg, 300 mg
Solution, oral (Axid®): 15 mg/mL (480 mL) [bubble gum flavor]
Tablet (Axid® AR): 75 mg

Monitoring and Teaching Issues
Physical Assessment: Dose modification needed with renal impairment. Assess effectiveness (relief of clinical symptoms) and adverse response (eg, CNS changes [anxiety, irritability, nervousness], rash, GI disturbance; see Adverse Reactions). Teach patient proper use, possible side effects/appropriate interventions, and adverse symptoms to report (see Patient Education).

Patient Education: Do not take any new medication during therapy unless approved by prescriber. Take as directed; do not change dose or discontinue without consulting prescriber. Do not take within 1 hour of any antacids. Follow diet instructions of prescriber. May cause drowsiness (use caution when driving or engaging in tasks that require alertness until response to drug is known). Report rash, fever, sore throat, tarry stools, CNS changes (increased anxiety, irritability, nervousness), or muscle or joint pain. **Pregnancy precaution:** Inform prescriber if you are or intend to become pregnant.

Geriatric Considerations: H_2 blockers are the preferred drugs for treating peptic ulcer disorder (PUD) in the elderly due to cost and ease of administration. These agents are no less or more effective than any other therapy. The preferred agents (due to side effects and drug interaction profile and pharmacokinetics) are ranitidine, famotidine, and nizatidine. Treatment for PUD in the elderly is recommended for 12 weeks since their lesions are larger, and therefore, take longer to heal. Always adjust dose based upon creatinine clearance.

Pregnancy Risk Factor: B
Lactation: Enters breast milk/may be compatible
Breast-Feeding Issues: The amount of nizatidine excreted in breast milk is 0.1%.
Additional Information Giving dose at 6 PM (rather than 10 PM) may better suppress nocturnal acid secretion

- **Nizoral®** *see* Ketoconazole *on page 849*
- **Nizoral® A-D [OTC]** *see* Ketoconazole *on page 849*
- **N-Methylhydrazine** *see* Procarbazine *on page 1257*
- **No Doz® Maximum Strength [OTC]** *see* Caffeine *on page 229*
- **Nolvadex®** *see* Tamoxifen *on page 1424*
- **Nonsalicylate / Nonsteroidal Anti-inflammatory Agents** *see page 1743*
- **Nora-BE™** *see* Norethindrone *on page 1096*
- **Noradrenaline** *see* Norepinephrine *on page 1095*
- **Noradrenaline Acid Tartrate** *see* Norepinephrine *on page 1095*
- **Norco®** *see* Hydrocodone and Acetaminophen *on page 754*
- **Norcuron® [DSC]** *see* Vecuronium *on page 1555*
- **Nordeoxyguanosine** *see* Ganciclovir *on page 695*
- **Nordette®** *see* Ethinyl Estradiol and Levonorgestrel *on page 585*
- **Norditropin®** *see* Human Growth Hormone *on page 745*
- **Norditropin® NordiFlex®** *see* Human Growth Hormone *on page 745*

Norepinephrine (nor ep i NEF rin)
U.S. Brand Names Levophed®
Synonyms Levarterenol Bitartrate; Noradrenaline; Noradrenaline Acid Tartrate; Norepinephrine Bitartrate
Generic Available Yes
Pharmacologic Category Alpha/Beta Agonist
Use Treatment of shock which persists after adequate fluid volume replacement
Mechanism of Action/Effect Stimulates beta$_1$-adrenergic receptors and alpha-adrenergic receptors causing increased contractility and heart rate as well as vasoconstriction, thereby increasing systemic blood pressure and coronary blood flow; clinically alpha effects (vasoconstriction) are greater than beta effects (inotropic and chronotropic effects)
Contraindications Hypersensitivity to norepinephrine, bisulfites (contains metabisulfite), or any component of the formulation; hypotension from hypovolemia except as an emergency measure to maintain coronary and cerebral perfusion until volume could be replaced; mesenteric or peripheral vascular thrombosis unless it is a lifesaving procedure; during anesthesia with cyclopropane or halothane anesthesia (risk of ventricular arrhythmias)
Warnings/Precautions Assure adequate circulatory volume to minimize need for vasoconstrictors. Avoid hypertension; monitor blood pressure closely and adjust infusion rate. Infuse into a large vein if possible. Avoid infusion into leg veins. Watch I.V. site closely. Avoid extravasation. Never use leg veins for infusion sites.
(Continued)

Norepinephrine *(Continued)*

Drug Interactions

Decreased Effect: Alpha-blockers may blunt response to norepinephrine.

Increased Effect/Toxicity: The effects of norepinephrine may be increased by tricyclic antidepressants, MAO inhibitors, antihistamines (diphenhydramine, tripelennamine), beta-blockers (nonselective), guanethidine, ergot alkaloids, reserpine, and methyldopa. Atropine sulfate may block the reflex bradycardia caused by norepinephrine and enhances the vasopressor response.

Adverse Reactions Frequency not defined.

Cardiovascular: Bradycardia, arrhythmia, peripheral (digital) ischemia

Central nervous system: Headache (transient), anxiety

Local: Skin necrosis (with extravasation)

Respiratory: Dyspnea, respiratory difficulty

Overdosage/Toxicology

Symptoms of overdose include hypertension, sweating, cerebral hemorrhage, and convulsions. Infiltrate the area of extravasation with phentolamine 5-10 mg in 10-15 mL of saline solution; inject a small amount of this dilution into extravasated area; blanching should reverse immediately. Monitor site; if blanching should recur, additional injections of phentolamine may be needed.

Pharmacodynamics/Kinetics

Onset of Action: I.V.: Very rapid-acting

Duration of Action: Limited

Metabolism: Via catechol-o-methyltransferase (COMT) and monoamine oxidase (MAO)

Excretion: Urine (84% to 96% as inactive metabolites)

Dosing

Adults & Elderly: Note: Norepinephrine dosage is stated in terms of norepinephrine base and intravenous formulation is norepinephrine bitartrate.

Norepinephrine bitartrate 2 mg = norepinephrine base 1 mg

Hypotension/shock: Continuous I.V. infusion:

Adults: Initial: 0.5-1 mcg/minute and titrate to desired response; 8-30 mcg/minute is usual range; range used in clinical trials: 0.01-3 mcg/kg/minute;

ACLS dosing range: 0.5-30 mcg/minute

Rate of infusion: 4 mg in 500 mL D$_5$W

2 mcg/minute = 15 mL/hour

4 mcg/minute = 30 mL/hour

6 mcg/minute = 45 mL/hour

8 mcg/minute = 60 mL/hour

10 mcg/minute = 75 mL/hour

Pediatrics: Administration requires the use of an infusion pump

Note: Norepinephrine dosage is stated in terms of norepinephrine base and intravenous formulation is norepinephrine bitartrate.

Norepinephrine bitartrate 2 mg = Norepinephrine base 1 mg

Hypotension/shock: Continuous I.V. infusion: Children: Initial: 0.05-0.1 mcg/kg/minute; titrate to desired effect; maximum dose: 1-2 mcg/kg/minute

Available Dosage Forms Injection, solution, as bitartrate: 1 mg/mL (4 mL) [contains sodium metabisulfite]

Monitoring and Teaching Issues

Physical Assessment: Assess other medications patient may be taking. Monitor blood pressure and cardiac status, CNS status, skin temperature and color during and following infusion. Monitor fluid status. Assess infusion site frequently for extravasation. Blanching along vein pathway is a preliminary sign of extravasation.

Patient Education: This drug is used in emergency situations. Patient information is based on patient condition.

Pregnancy Risk Factor: C

Lactation: Excretion in breast milk unknown

Administration

I.V.: Administer into large vein to avoid the potential for extravasation; potent drug, must be diluted prior to use; do not administer NaHCO$_3$ through an I.V. line containing norepinephrine. Central line administration is required. Do not administer NaHCO$_3$ through an I.V. line containing norepinephrine.

Reconstitution: Dilute with D$_5$W or D$_5$NS, but not recommended to dilute in normal saline. Stability of parenteral admixture at room temperature (25°C) is 24 hours.

Compatibility: Stable in D$_5$NS, D$_5$W, LR; may dilute with D$_5$W or D$_5$NS, but not recommended to dilute in normal saline; not stable in alkaline solutions. Stability of parenteral admixture at room temperature (25°C) is 24 hours.

Y-site administration: Incompatible with insulin (regular), thiopental

Compatibility when admixed: Incompatible with aminophylline, amobarbital, chlorothiazide, chlorpheniramine, pentobarbital, phenobarbital, phenytoin, sodium bicarbonate, streptomycin, thiopental

Storage: Readily oxidized; protect from light. Do not use if brown coloration.

Related Information

Compatibility of Drugs *on page 1723*

Inotropic and Vasoconstrictor Comparison *on page 1736*

♦ **Norepinephrine Bitartrate** *see Norepinephrine on page 1095*

Norethindrone *(nor eth IN drone)*

U.S. Brand Names Aygestin®; Camila™; Errin™; Jolivette™; Micronor®; Nora-BE™; Nor-QD®

Synonyms Norethindrone Acetate; Norethisterone

Generic Available Yes

Pharmacologic Category Contraceptive; Progestin

Medication Safety Issues

Sound-alike/look-alike issues:

Micronor® may be confused with miconazole, Micronase®

Use Treatment of amenorrhea; abnormal uterine bleeding; endometriosis, oral contraceptive; **higher rate of failure with progestin only contraceptives**

Mechanism of Action/Effect Inhibits secretion of pituitary gonadotropin (LH) which prevents follicular maturation and ovulation; in the presence of adequate endogenous estrogen, transforms a proliferative endometrium to a secretory one

Contraindications Hypersensitivity to norethindrone or any component of the formulation; thromboembolic disorders; severe hepatic disease; breast cancer; undiagnosed vaginal bleeding; pregnancy

Warnings/Precautions Use of any progestin during the first 4 months of pregnancy is not recommended. Discontinue if sudden partial or complete loss of vision, proptosis, diplopia, or migraine occur. **There is a higher rate of failure with progestin only contraceptives.** Progestin-induced withdrawal bleeding occurs within 3-7 days after discontinuation of drug. Use with caution in patients with asthma, diabetes, seizure disorder, hyperlipidemias, migraine, cardiac or renal dysfunction, or psychic depression.

Drug Interactions

Cytochrome P450 Effect: Substrate of CYP3A4 (major); **Induces** CYP2C19 (weak)

Decreased Effect: Nelfinavir decreases the pharmacologic effect of norethindrone. CYP3A4 inducers may decrease the levels/effects of norethindrone; example inducers include aminoglutethimide, carbamazepine, nafcillin, nevirapine, phenobarbital, phenytoin, and rifamycins.

Nutritional/Ethanol Interactions

Food; Limit caffeine.

Herb/Nutraceutical: High-dose vitamin C (1 g/day) may increase adverse effects. Avoid St John's wort.

Lab Interactions Thyroid function test, metyrapone test, liver function tests, coagulation tests (prothrombin time, factors VII, VIII, IX, X)

Adverse Reactions

>10%:

Cardiovascular: Edema

Endocrine & metabolic: Breakthrough bleeding, spotting, changes in menstrual flow, amenorrhea

Gastrointestinal: Anorexia

Local: Pain at injection site

Neuromuscular & skeletal: Weakness

1% to 10%:

Cardiovascular: Edema

Central nervous system: Mental depression, fever, insomnia

Dermatologic: Melasma or chloasma, allergic rash with or without pruritus

Endocrine & metabolic: Increased breast tenderness

Gastrointestinal: Weight gain/loss

Genitourinary: Changes in cervical erosion and secretions

Hepatic: Cholestatic jaundice

Pharmacodynamics/Kinetics

Absorption: Oral, transdermal: Rapidly absorbed

Bioavailability: 64%

Time to Peak: 1-2 hours

Protein Binding: 61% to albumin, 36% to sex hormone-binding globulin (SHBG); SHBG capacity affected by plasma ethinyl estradiol levels

Half-Life Elimination: 5-14 hours

Metabolism: Oral: Hepatic via reduction and conjugation; first-pass effect

Excretion: Primarily urine (as metabolites)

Dosing

Adults:

Contraception (Females): Oral: Progesterone only: Norethindrone 0.35 mg every day of the year starting on first day of menstruation; if one dose is missed take as soon as remembered; then next tablet at regular time; if two doses are missed, take one of the missed doses, discard the other, and take daily dose at usual time; if three doses are missed, use another form of birth control until menses appear or pregnancy is ruled out

Amenorrhea and abnormal uterine bleeding: Oral:

Norethindrone: 5-20 mg/day on days 5-25 of menstrual cycle

Acetate salt (Aygestin®): 2.5-10 mg on days 5-25 of menstrual cycle

Endometriosis: Oral:

Norethindrone: 10 mg/day for 2 weeks; increase at increments of 5 mg/day every 2 weeks until 30 mg/day; continue for 6-9 months or until breakthrough bleeding demands temporary termination

Acetate salt (Aygestin®): 5 mg/day for 14 days; increase at increments of 2.5 mg/day every 2 weeks up to 15 mg/day; continue for 6-9 months or until breakthrough bleeding demands temporary termination

Pediatrics: Adolescents: Refer to adult dosing

Available Dosage Forms

Tablet (Camila™, Errin™, Jolivette™, Micronor®, Nora-BE™, Nor-QD®): 0.35 mg

Tablet, as acetate (Aygestin®): 5 mg

Monitoring and Teaching Issues

Physical Assessment: Assess patient knowledge/teach appropriate administration schedule and adverse signs to report. Teach appropriate breast self-exam and the need for regular breast self-exam and necessity of annual physical check-up with long-term use.

Pregnancy risk factor X: Determine that patient is not pregnant before beginning treatment.

(Continued)

Norethindrone *(Continued)*

Monitoring Laboratory Tests: Long-term therapy, annual Pap tests, mammogram

Patient Education: Take according to prescribed schedule. Follow instructions for regular self-breast exam. You may experience dizziness or lightheadedness; use caution when driving or engaging in tasks that require alertness until response to drug is known. Limit intake of caffeine. Avoid high-dose vitamin C. You may experience photosensitivity; use sunscreen, wear protective clothing and eyewear, and avoid direct sunlight. You may experience loss of hair (reversible), swelling of hands or feet, weight gain or loss. Report sudden severe headache or vomiting, disturbances of vision or speech, sudden blindness, numbness of weakness in an extremity, chest pain, calf pain, respiratory difficulty, weight gain >5 lb/week, depression or acute fatigue, unusual bleeding, spotting, or changes in menstrual flow. **Pregnancy/breast-feeding precautions:** Inform prescriber if you are pregnant. Consult prescriber if breast-feeding.

Dietary Considerations: Should be taken with food at same time each day.

Pregnancy Risk Factor: X

Lactation: Enters breast milk/use caution

Breast-Feeding Issues: Norethindrone can cause changes in milk production in the mother. Monitor infant growth. Use lowest possible dose of norethindrone for less effect on milk production.

Administration

Oral: Take with food.

♦ **Norethindrone Acetate** *see Norethindrone on page 1096*

♦ **Norethindrone Acetate and Ethinyl Estradiol** *see Ethinyl Estradiol and Norethindrone on page 589*

♦ **Norethindrone and Estradiol** *see Estradiol and Norethindrone on page 557*

♦ **Norethindrone and Mestranol** *see Mestranol and Norethindrone on page 962*

♦ **Norethisterone** *see Norethindrone on page 1096*

♦ **Norflex™** *see Orphenadrine on page 1124*

♦ **Norgesic™** *see Orphenadrine, Aspirin, and Caffeine on page 1125*

♦ **Norgesic™ Forte** *see Orphenadrine, Aspirin, and Caffeine on page 1125*

♦ **Norgestimate and Ethinyl Estradiol** *see Ethinyl Estradiol and Norgestimate on page 593*

Norgestrel *(nor JES trel)*

U.S. Brand Names Ovrette®

Generic Available No

Pharmacologic Category Contraceptive; Progestin

Use Prevention of pregnancy; **progestin only products have higher risk of failure in contraceptive use**

Mechanism of Action/Effect Inhibits secretion of pituitary gonadotropin (LH) which prevents follicular maturation and ovulation

Contraindications Hypersensitivity to norgestrel or any component of the formulation; hypersensitivity to tartrazine; thromboembolic disorders; severe hepatic disease; breast cancer; undiagnosed vaginal bleeding; pregnancy

Warnings/Precautions Discontinue if sudden loss of vision or if diplopia or proptosis occur. Use with caution in patients with a history of mental depression.

Drug Interactions

Cytochrome P450 Effect: Substrate of CYP3A4 (major)

Decreased Effect: CYP3A4 inducers may decrease the levels/effects of norgestrel; example inducers include aminoglutethimide, carbamazepine, nafcillin, nevirapine, phenobarbital, phenytoin, and rifamycins. Antibiotics (penicillins, tetracyclines, griseofulvin) were reported to decrease efficacy of oral contraceptives, but this has not been validated in more rigorous investigations.

Increased Effect/Toxicity: Oral contraceptives may increase toxicity of acetaminophen, anticoagulants, benzodiazepines, caffeine, corticosteroids, metoprolol, theophylline, and tricyclic antidepressants.

Nutritional/Ethanol Interactions

Food: CNS effects of caffeine may be enhanced if oral contraceptives are used concurrently with caffeine.

Herb/Nutraceutical: St John's wort may decrease levels. Avoid dong quai and black cohosh (have estrogen activity). Avoid saw palmetto, red clover, ginseng.

Lab Interactions Thyroid function tests, metyrapone test, liver function tests

Adverse Reactions Frequency not defined.

Cardiovascular: Embolism, cerebral thrombosis, edema

Central nervous system: Mental depression, fever, insomnia

Dermatologic: Melasma or chloasma, allergic rash with or without pruritus

Endocrine & metabolic: Breakthrough bleeding, spotting, changes in menstrual flow, amenorrhea, changes in cervical erosion and secretions, increased breast tenderness

Gastrointestinal: Weight gain/loss, anorexia

Hepatic: Cholestatic jaundice

Local: Thrombophlebitis

Neuromuscular & skeletal: Weakness

Overdosage/Toxicology

Toxicity is unlikely following single exposures of excessive doses.

Supportive treatment is adequate in most cases.

Pharmacodynamics/Kinetics

Absorption: Oral: Well absorbed

Protein Binding: >97% to sex hormone-binding globulin

Half-Life Elimination: ~20 hours

Metabolism: Primarily hepatic via reduction and conjugation

Excretion: Urine (as metabolites)

Dosing

Adults: Contraception: Oral: Administer daily, starting the first day of menstruation, take 1 tablet at the same time each day, every day of the year. If one dose is missed, take as soon as remembered, then next tablet at regular time; if two doses are missed, take 1 tablet as soon as it is remembered, followed by an additional dose that same day at the usual time. When one or two doses are missed, additional contraceptive measures should be used until 14 consecutive tablets have been taken. If three doses are missed, discontinue norgestrel and use an additional form of birth control until menses or pregnancy is ruled out.

Available Dosage Forms Tablet: 0.075 mg [contains tartrazine]

Monitoring and Teaching Issues

Physical Assessment: Monitor or teach patient to monitor blood pressure on a regular basis. Monitor or teach patient to monitor for occurrence of adverse effects and symptoms to report. Assess knowledge/teach importance of regular (monthly) blood pressure checks, annual physical assessment, Pap smear, and vision assessment. Teach importance of maintaining prescribed schedule of dosing (see Dosing for dosing and missed dose information). **Pregnancy risk factor X:** Do not use if patient is pregnant.

Patient Education: Take exactly as directed by prescriber (also see package insert). You are at risk of becoming pregnant if doses are missed. If you miss a dose, take as soon as possible or double the dose next day. If more than three doses are missed, contact prescriber for restarting directions. Use additional form of contraception during first week of taking this medication. Detailed and complete information on dosing and missed doses can be found in the package insert. Be aware that some medications may reduce the effectiveness of oral contraceptives; an alternate form of contraception may be needed. It is important that you check your blood pressure monthly (on same day each month) and that you have an annual physical assessment, Pap smear, and vision assessment while taking this medication. Avoid smoking while taking this medication; smoking increases risk of adverse effects, including thromboembolic events and heart attacks. You may experience loss of appetite (small frequent meals will help); or constipation (increased exercise, fluids, fruit, fiber, or stool softeners may help). If you have diabetes, use accurate serum glucose testing to identify any changes in glucose tolerance; notify prescriber of significant changes so antidiabetic medication can be adjusted if necessary. Report immediately pain or muscle soreness; warmth, swelling, or redness in calves; shortness of breath; sudden loss of vision; unresolved leg or foot swelling; change in menstrual pattern (unusual bleeding, amenorrhea, breakthrough spotting); breast tenderness that does not go away; acute abdominal cramping; signs of vaginal infection (drainage, pain, itching); CNS changes (blurred vision, confusion, acute anxiety, or unresolved depression); or significant weight gain (>5 lb/week). **Pregnancy/breast-feeding precautions:** This drug may cause severe fetal complication. If you suspect you may become pregnant, contact prescriber immediately. Consult prescriber if breast-feeding.

Dietary Considerations: Should be taken with food at same time each day.

Pregnancy Risk Factor: X

Lactation: Enters breast milk/use caution

♦ **Norinyl® 1+35** *see* Ethinyl Estradiol and Norethindrone *on page 589*

♦ **Norinyl® 1+50** *see* Mestranol and Norethindrone *on page 962*

♦ **Noritate®** *see* Metronidazole *on page 995*

♦ **Normal Human Serum Albumin** *see* Albumin *on page 58*

♦ **Normal Serum Albumin (Human)** *see* Albumin *on page 58*

♦ **Normodyne®** *see* Labetalol *on page 857*

♦ **Norpramin®** *see* Desipramine *on page 418*

♦ **Nor-QD®** *see* Norethindrone *on page 1096*

♦ **Nortrel™** *see* Ethinyl Estradiol and Norethindrone *on page 589*

♦ **Nortrel™ 7/7/7** *see* Ethinyl Estradiol and Norethindrone *on page 589*

Nortriptyline (nor TRIP ti leen)

U.S. Brand Names Pamelor®

Synonyms Nortriptyline Hydrochloride

Restrictions A medication guide should be dispensed with each prescription. A template for the required MedGuides can be found on the FDA website at: http://www.fda.gov/cder/drug/antidepressants/labelTemplate.pdf

Generic Available Yes: Excludes solution

Pharmacologic Category Antidepressant, Tricyclic (Secondary Amine)

Medication Safety Issues

Sound-alike/look-alike issues:

Nortriptyline may be confused with amitriptyline, desipramine, Norpramin®

Aventyl® HCl may be confused with Bentyl®

Pamelor® may be confused with Demerol®, Dymelor®

Use Treatment of symptoms of depression

Unlabeled/Investigational Use Chronic pain, anxiety disorders, enuresis, attention-deficit/hyperactivity disorder (ADHD); adjunctive therapy for smoking cessation

Mechanism of Action/Effect Traditionally believed to increase the synaptic concentration of serotonin and/or norepinephrine in the central nervous system by inhibition of their reuptake by the presynaptic neuronal membrane. However, additional receptor effects have been found including desensitization of adenyl cyclase, down regulation of beta-adrenergic receptors, and down regulation of serotonin receptors.

(Continued)

Nortriptyline *(Continued)*

Contraindications Hypersensitivity to nortriptyline and similar chemical class, or any component of the formulation; use of MAO inhibitors within 14 days; use in a patient during the acute recovery phase of MI; pregnancy

Warnings/Precautions Antidepressants increase the risk of suicidal thinking and behavior in children and adolescents with major depressive disorder (MDD) and other depressive disorders; consider risk prior to prescribing. All patients must be closely monitored for clinical worsening, suicidality, or unusual changes in behavior, especially during the initiation of therapy or following an increase or decrease in dosage. When used in children, the child's family or caregiver should be instructed to closely observe the patient and communicate condition with healthcare provider. A medication guide should be dispensed with each prescription. **Nortriptyline is not FDA approved for use in children.**

The possibility of a suicide attempt is inherent in major depression and may persist until remission occurs. Use caution in high-risk patients. Worsening depression and severe abrupt suicidality that are not part of the presenting symptoms may require discontinuation or modification of drug therapy. The patient's family or caregiver should be alerted to monitor patients for the emergence of suicidality and associated behaviors (such as agitation, irritability, hostility, impulsivity, and hypomania) and call healthcare provider.

May worsen psychosis in some patients or precipitate a shift to mania or hypomania in patients with bipolar disorder. Patients presenting with depressive symptoms should be screened for bipolar disorder. Monotherapy in patients with bipolar disorder should be avoided. **Nortriptyline is not FDA approved for the treatment of bipolar depression.**

The risk of sedation and orthostatic effects are low relative to other antidepressants. However, nortriptyline may result in impaired performance of tasks requiring alertness (eg, operating machinery or driving). Sedative effects may be additive with other CNS depressants and/or ethanol. The degree of anticholinergic blockade produced by this agent is moderate relative to other cyclic antidepressants, however, caution should still be used in patients with urinary retention, benign prostatic hyperplasia, narrow-angle glaucoma, xerostomia, visual problems, constipation, or history of bowel obstruction. May cause orthostatic hypotension (risk is low relative to other antidepressants) or conduction disturbances. Use with caution in patients with a history of cardiovascular disease (including previous MI, stroke, tachycardia, or conduction abnormalities). The risk conduction abnormalities with this agent is moderate relative to other antidepressants.

Consider discontinuing, when possible, prior to elective surgery. Therapy should not be abruptly discontinued in patients receiving high doses for prolonged periods. May alter glucose regulation - use caution in patients with diabetes. Use caution in patients with a previous seizure disorder or condition predisposing to seizures such as brain damage, alcoholism, or concurrent therapy with other drugs which lower the seizure threshold. May increase the risks associated with electroconvulsive therapy. Use with caution in hyperthyroid patients or those receiving thyroid supplementation. Use with caution in patients with hepatic or renal dysfunction and in elderly patients.

Drug Interactions

Cytochrome P450 Effect: Substrate of CYP1A2 (minor), 2C19 (minor), 2D6 (major), 3A4 (minor); **Inhibits** CYP2D6 (weak), 2E1 (weak)

Decreased Effect: Carbamazepine, phenobarbital, and rifampin may increase the metabolism of nortriptyline resulting in decreased effect of nortriptyline. Nortriptyline inhibits the antihypertensive response to bethanidine, clonidine, debrisoquin, guanadrel, guanethidine, guanabenz, or guanfacine. Cholestyramine and colestipol may bind TCAs and reduce their absorption; monitor for altered response.

Increased Effect/Toxicity: Nortriptyline increases the effects of amphetamines, anticholinergics, other CNS depressants (sedatives, hypnotics, ethanol), chlorpropamide, tolazamide, and warfarin. When used with MAO inhibitors, hyperpyrexia, hypertension, tachycardia, confusion, seizures, and **deaths have been reported** (serotonin syndrome). Serotonin syndrome has also been reported with ritonavir (rare). CYP2D6 inhibitors may increase the levels/effects of nortriptyline; example inhibitors include chlorpromazine, delavirdine, fluoxetine, miconazole, paroxetine, pergolide, quinidine, quinine, ritonavir, and ropinirole. Cimetidine, grapefruit juice, indinavir, methylphenidate, diltiazem, and verapamil may increase the serum concentrations of TCAs. Use of lithium with a TCA may increase the risk for neurotoxicity. Phenothiazines may increase concentration of some TCAs and TCAs may increase concentration of phenothiazines. Pressor response to I.V. epinephrine, norepinephrine, and phenylephrine may be enhanced in patients receiving TCAs (**Note:** Effect is unlikely with epinephrine or levonordefrin dosages typically administered as infiltration in combination with local anesthetics). Combined use of beta-agonists or drugs which prolong QT_c (including quinidine, procainamide, disopyramide, cisapride, sparfloxacin, gatifloxacin, moxifloxacin) with TCAs may predispose patients to cardiac arrhythmias. Use with altretamine may cause orthostatic hypotension.

Nutritional/Ethanol Interactions

Ethanol: Avoid ethanol (may increase CNS depression).

Food: Grapefruit juice may inhibit the metabolism of some TCAs and clinical toxicity may result.

Herb/Nutraceutical: Avoid valerian, St John's wort, SAMe, kava kava (may increase risk of serotonin syndrome and/or excessive sedation).

Lab Interactions Increased glucose

Adverse Reactions Frequency not defined.

Cardiovascular: Postural hypotension, arrhythmia, hypertension, heart block, tachycardia, palpitation, MI

Central nervous system: Confusion, delirium, hallucinations, restlessness, insomnia, disorientation, delusions, anxiety, agitation, panic, nightmares, hypomania, exacerbation of psychosis, incoordination, ataxia, extrapyramidal symptoms, seizure

Dermatologic: Alopecia, photosensitivity, rash, petechiae, urticaria, itching

Endocrine & metabolic: Sexual dysfunction, gynecomastia, breast enlargement, galactorrhea, increase or decrease in libido, increase in blood sugar, SIADH

Gastrointestinal: Xerostomia, constipation, vomiting, anorexia, diarrhea, abdominal cramps, black tongue, nausea, unpleasant taste, weight gain/loss

Genitourinary: Urinary retention, delayed micturition, impotence, testicular edema

Hematologic: Rarely agranulocytosis, eosinophilia, purpura, thrombocytopenia

Hepatic: Increased liver enzymes, cholestatic jaundice

Neuromuscular & skeletal: Tremor, numbness, tingling, paresthesia, peripheral neuropathy

Ocular: Blurred vision, eye pain, disturbances in accommodation, mydriasis

Otic: Tinnitus

Miscellaneous: Diaphoresis (excessive), allergic reactions

Overdosage/Toxicology Symptoms of overdose include agitation, confusion, hallucinations, urinary retention, hypothermia, hypotension, seizures, and ventricular tachycardia. Treatment is symptomatic and supportive. Alkalinization by sodium bicarbonate and/or hyperventilation may limit cardiac toxicity.

Pharmacodynamics/Kinetics

Onset of Action: Therapeutic: 1-3 weeks

Time to Peak: Serum: 7-8.5 hours

Protein Binding: 93% to 95%

Half-Life Elimination: 28-31 hours

Metabolism: Primarily hepatic; extensive first-pass effect

Excretion: Urine (as metabolites and small amounts of unchanged drug); feces (small amounts)

Dosing

Adults:

Depression: Oral: 25 mg 3-4 times/day up to 150 mg/day

Chronic urticaria, angioedema, nocturnal pruritus (unlabeled use): Oral: 75 mg/day

Smoking cessation (unlabeled use): Oral: 25-75 mg/day beginning 10-14 days before "quit" day; continue therapy for ≥12 weeks after "quit" day

Elderly: Note: Nortriptyline is one of the best tolerated TCAs in the elderly.

Initial: 10-25 mg at bedtime

Dosage can be increased by 25 mg every 3 days for inpatients and weekly for outpatients if tolerated.

Usual maintenance dose: 75 mg as a single bedtime dose or 2 divided doses; however, lower or higher doses may be required to stay within the therapeutic window.

Pediatrics:

Nocturnal enuresis (unlabeled use): Oral: 10-20 mg/day; titrate to a maximum of 40 mg/day

Depression (unlabeled use): Oral: 1-3 mg/kg/day

Hepatic Impairment: Lower doses and slower titration are recommended dependent on individualization of dosage.

Available Dosage Forms

Capsule, as hydrochloride: 10 mg, 25 mg, 50 mg, 75 mg

Pamelor®: 10 mg, 25 mg, 50 mg, 75 mg [may contain benzyl alcohol; 50 mg may also contain sodium bisulfite]

Solution, as hydrochloride (Pamelor®): 10 mg/5 mL (473 mL) [contains alcohol 4% and benzoic acid]

Monitoring and Teaching Issues

Physical Assessment: Assess potential for interactions with other prescriptions, OTC medications, or herbal products patient may be taking. Assess for suicidal tendencies before beginning therapy. May cause physiological or psychological dependence, tolerance, or abuse; periodically evaluate need for continued use. Assess therapeutic effectiveness (mental status, mood, affect) and adverse reactions (eg, suicidal ideation) at beginning of therapy and periodically with long-term use. Taper dosage slowly when discontinuing (allow 3-4 weeks between discontinuing this medication and starting another antidepressant). Caution patients with diabetes to monitor glucose levels closely; may increase or decrease serum glucose levels. Teach patient appropriate use, interventions to reduce side effects, and adverse symptoms to report.

Patient Education: Do not take any new medication during therapy unless approved by prescriber. Take exactly as directed; take once-a-day dose at bedtime. Do not increase dose or frequency; may take 2-3 weeks to achieve desired results. This drug may cause physical and/or psychological dependence. Avoid alcohol and grapefruit juice. Maintain adequate hydration (2-3 L/day of fluids) unless instructed to restrict fluid intake. May cause drowsiness, lightheadedness, impaired coordination, dizziness, or blurred vision (use caution when driving or engaging in tasks requiring alertness until response to drug is known); nausea, vomiting, loss of appetite, or disturbed taste (small frequent meals, good mouth care, chewing gum, or sucking lozenges may help); constipation (increased exercise, fluids, fruit, or fiber may help); urinary retention (void before taking medication); postural hypotension (use caution climbing stairs or when changing position from lying or sitting to standing); altered sexual drive or ability (reversible); or photosensitivity (use sunscreen, wear protective clothing and eyewear, and avoid direct sunlight). Report chest pain, palpitations, or rapid heartbeat; persistent adverse CNS effects (eg, suicidal ideation, nervousness, restlessness, insomnia, anxiety, excitation, headache, agitation, impaired coordination, changes in cognition); muscle cramping, weakness, tremors, or rigidity; blurred vision or eye pain; breast enlargement or swelling; yellowing of skin or eyes; or worsening of condition. **Pregnancy/breast-feeding precautions:** Inform prescriber if you pregnant. Do not get pregnant while taking this medication. Consult prescriber for appropriate contraceptive measures. Do not breast-feed.

Geriatric Considerations: Since nortriptyline is the least likely of the tricyclic antidepressants (TCAs) to cause orthostatic hypotension and one of the least anticholinergic and sedating TCAs, it is a preferred agent when a TCA is indicated. Data from a clinical trial comparing fluoxetine to tricyclics suggests that fluoxetine is significantly less effective than nortriptyline in hospitalized elderly patients with unipolar affective disorder, especially those with melancholia and concurrent cardiovascular disease.

(Continued)

Nortriptyline *(Continued)*

Pregnancy Risk Factor: D
Lactation: Enters breast milk/contraindicated (AAP rates "of concern")
Administration
Storage: Protect from light.
Related Information
Antidepressant Agents *on page 1713*
Antidepressant Medication Guidelines *on page 1765*
Federal OBRA Regulations: Recommended Maximum Doses *on page 1773*
Peak and Trough Guidelines *on page 1694*
Pharmacotherapy of Urinary Incontinence *on page 1858*

- Nortriptyline Hydrochloride *see* Nortriptyline *on page 1099*
- Norvasc® *see* Amlodipine *on page 99*
- Norvir® *see* Ritonavir *on page 1335*
- Nostril® [OTC] *see* Phenylephrine *on page 1200*
- Novantrone® *see* Mitoxantrone *on page 1019*
- Novarel™ *see* Chorionic Gonadotropin (Human) *on page 319*
- Novocain® *see* Procaine *on page 1256*
- Novolin® 70/30 *see* Insulin Preparations *on page 805*
- Novolin® L [DSC] *see* Insulin Preparations *on page 805*
- Novolin® N *see* Insulin Preparations *on page 805*
- Novolin® R *see* Insulin Preparations *on page 805*
- NovoLog® *see* Insulin Preparations *on page 805*
- NovoLog® Mix 70/30 *see* Insulin Preparations *on page 805*
- NovoSeven® *see* Factor VIIa (Recombinant) *on page 606*
- NPH Iletin® II *see* Insulin Preparations *on page 805*
- NPH, Insulin *see* Insulin Preparations *on page 805*
- NSC-740 *see* Methotrexate *on page 974*
- NSC-752 *see* Thioguanine *on page 1462*
- NSC-755 *see* Mercaptopurine *on page 954*
- NSC-762 *see* Mechlorethamine *on page 935*
- NSC-3053 *see* Dactinomycin *on page 397*
- NSC-3088 *see* Chlorambucil *on page 305*
- NSC-10363 *see* Megestrol *on page 942*
- NSC-13875 *see* Altretamine *on page 82*
- NSC-15200 *see* Gallium Nitrate *on page 694*
- NSC-26271 *see* Cyclophosphamide *on page 380*
- NSC-26980 *see* Mitomycin *on page 1017*
- NSC-27640 *see* Floxuridine *on page 632*
- NSC-38721 *see* Mitotane *on page 1018*
- NSC-49842 *see* VinBLAStine *on page 1563*
- NSC-63878 *see* Cytarabine *on page 389*
- NSC-67574 *see* VinCRIStine *on page 1564*
- NSC-77213 *see* Procarbazine *on page 1257*
- NSC-82151 *see* DAUNOrubicin Hydrochloride *on page 410*
- NSC-85998 *see* Streptozocin *on page 1399*
- NSC-89199' *see* Estramustine *on page 559*
- NSC-102816 *see* Azacitidine *on page 161*
- NSC-106977 (*Erwinia*) *see* Asparaginase *on page 141*
- NSC-109229 (*E. coli*) *see* Asparaginase *on page 141*
- NSC-109724 *see* Ifosfamide *on page 783*
- NSC-122758 *see* Tretinoin (Oral) *on page 1514*
- NSC-123127 *see* DOXOrubicin *on page 491*
- NSC-125066 *see* Bleomycin *on page 201*
- NSC-125973 *see* Paclitaxel *on page 1144*
- NSC-147834 *see* Flutamide *on page 658*
- NSC-180973 *see* Tamoxifen *on page 1424*
- NSC-218321 *see* Pentostatin *on page 1184*
- NSC-256439 *see* Idarubicin *on page 781*
- NSC-266046 *see* Oxaliplatin *on page 1127*
- NSC-301739 *see* Mitoxantrone *on page 1019*
- NSC-352122 *see* Trimetrexate Glucuronate *on page 1530*
- NSC-362856 *see* Temozolomide *on page 1436*
- NSC-373364 *see* Aldesleukin *on page 62*
- NSC-377526 *see* Leuprolide *on page 876*
- NSC-409962 *see* Carmustine *on page 260*
- NSC-606864 *see* Goserelin *on page 725*
- NSC-609699 *see* Topotecan *on page 1497*
- NSC-616348 *see* Irinotecan *on page 829*
- NSC-628503 *see* Docetaxel *on page 472*
- NSC-644954 *see* Pegaspargase *on page 1163*
- NSC-698037 *see* Pemetrexed *on page 1169*
- NSC-706363 *see* Arsenic Trioxide *on page 139*
- NSC-715055 *see* Gefitinib *on page 701*

- ♦ **NSC-718781** *see* Erlotinib *on page 540*
- ♦ **NTG** *see* Nitroglycerin *on page 1090*
- ♦ **N-Trifluoroacetyladriamycin-14-Valerate** *see* Valrubicin *on page 1546*
- ♦ **NTZ** *see* Nitazoxanide *on page 1087*
- ♦ **Nubain®** *see* Nalbuphine *on page 1049*
- ♦ **Nucofed® Expectorant** *see* Guaifenesin, Pseudoephedrine, and Codeine *on page 735*
- ♦ **Nucofed® Pediatric Expectorant** *see* Guaifenesin, Pseudoephedrine, and Codeine *on page 735*
- ♦ **Nucotuss® [DSC]** *see* Guaifenesin, Pseudoephedrine, and Codeine *on page 735*
- ♦ **NuLev™** *see* Hyoscyamine *on page 775*
- ♦ **NuLYTELY®** *see* Polyethylene Glycol-Electrolyte Solution *on page 1226*
- ♦ **Numorphan®** *see* Oxymorphone *on page 1141*
- ♦ **Nupercainal® Hydrocortisone Cream [OTC]** *see* Hydrocortisone *on page 760*
- ♦ **Nuquin HP®** *see* Hydroquinone *on page 768*
- ♦ **Nuromax®** *see* Doxacurium *on page 484*
- ♦ **Nutracort®** *see* Hydrocortisone *on page 760*
- ♦ **NutreStore™** *see* Glutamine *on page 719*
- ♦ **Nutropin®** *see* Human Growth Hormone *on page 745*
- ♦ **Nutropin AQ®** *see* Human Growth Hormone *on page 745*
- ♦ **Nutropin Depot® [DSC]** *see* Human Growth Hormone *on page 745*
- ♦ **NVB** *see* Vinorelbine *on page 1567*
- ♦ **NVP** *see* Nevirapine *on page 1073*
- ♦ **Nydrazid® [DSC]** *see* Isoniazid *on page 836*

Nystatin (nye STAT in)

U.S. Brand Names Bio-Statin®; Mycostatin®; Nystat-Rx®; Nystop®; Pedi-Dri®

Generic Available Yes: Cream, ointment, powder, suspension, tablet

Pharmacologic Category Antifungal Agent, Oral Nonabsorbed; Antifungal Agent, Topical; Antifungal Agent, Vaginal

Medication Safety Issues

Sound-alike/look-alike issues:

Nystatin may be confused with Nilstat®, Nitrostat®

Nilstat may be confused with Nitrostat®, nystatin

Use Treatment of susceptible cutaneous, mucocutaneous, and oral cavity fungal infections normally caused by the *Candida* species

Mechanism of Action/Effect Binds to sterols in fungal cell membrane, changing the cell wall permeability allowing for leakage of cellular contents and cell death

Contraindications Hypersensitivity to nystatin or any component of the formulation

Adverse Reactions

Frequency not defined: Dermatologic: Contact dermatitis, Stevens-Johnson syndrome

1% to 10%: Gastrointestinal: Nausea, vomiting, diarrhea, stomach pain

Overdosage/Toxicology Symptoms of overdose include nausea, vomiting, and diarrhea. Treatment is supportive.

Pharmacodynamics/Kinetics

Onset of Action: Symptomatic relief from candidiasis: 24-72 hours

Absorption: Topical: None through mucous membranes or intact skin; Oral: Poorly absorbed

Excretion: Feces (as unchanged drug)

Dosing

Adults & Elderly:

Oral candidiasis: Suspension (swish and swallow orally): 400,000-600,000 units 4 times/day; troche: 200,000-400,000 units 4-5 times/day

Mucocutaneous infections: Topical: Apply 2-3 times/day to affected areas; very moist topical lesions are treated best with powder.

Intestinal infections: Oral tablets: 500,000-1,000,000 units every 8 hours

Vaginal infections: Vaginal tablets: Insert 1 tablet/day at bedtime for 2 weeks. (May also be given orally.)

Note: Powder for compounding: $^1/_8$ teaspoon (500,000 units) to equal approximately $^1/_2$ cup of water; give 4 times/day

Pediatrics:

Oral candidiasis:

Suspension (swish and swallow orally):

Premature infants: 100,000 units 4 times/day

Infants: 200,000 units 4 times/day or 100,000 units to each side of mouth 4 times/day

Children: 400,000-600,000 units 4 times/day

Troche: Children: Refer to adult dosing.

Powder for compounding: Children: Refer to adult dosing.

Mucocutaneous infections: Children: Refer to adult dosing.

Available Dosage Forms [DSC] = Discontinued product

Capsule (Bio-Statin®): 500,000 units, 1 million units

Cream: 100,000 units/g (15 g, 30 g)

Mycostatin®: 100,000 units/g (30 g)

Lozenge (Mycostatin®): 200,000 units [DSC]

Ointment, topical: 100,000 units/g (15 g, 30 g)

Powder, for prescription compounding: 50 million units (10 g); 150 million units (30 g); 500 million units (100 g); 2 billion units (400 g)

Nystat-Rx®: 50 million units (10 g); 150 million units (30 g); 500 million units (100 g); 1 billion units (190 g); 2 billion units (350 g)

Powder, topical:

Mycostatin®: 100,000 units/g (15 g)

Nystop®: 100,000 units/g (15 g, 30 g, 60 g)

(Continued)

Nystatin *(Continued)*

Pedi-Dri®: 100,000 units/g (56.7 g)

Suspension, oral: 100,000 units/mL (5 mL, 60 mL, 480 mL)

Mycostatin® [DSC]: 100,000 units/mL (60 mL, 480 mL) [contains alcohol ≤1%; cherry-mint flavor]

Tablet: 500,000 units

Tablet, vaginal: 100,000 units (15s) [packaged with applicator]

Monitoring and Teaching Issues

Physical Assessment: Determine that cause of infection is fungal. Avoid skin contact when applying. Monitor therapeutic effectiveness, adverse reactions at beginning of therapy and periodically throughout therapy. Assess knowledge/teach patient appropriate use, interventions to reduce side effects, and adverse symptoms to report.

Patient Education: Take as directed. Maintain adequate hydration (2-3 L/day of fluids) unless instructed to restrict fluid intake. Do not allow medication to come in contact with eyes. Report persistent nausea, vomiting, or diarrhea; or if condition being treated worsens or does not improve. **Pregnancy precaution:** Inform prescriber if you are pregnant.

Oral tablets: Swallow whole; do not crush or chew.

Oral suspension: Shake well before using. Remove dentures, clean mouth (do not replace dentures until after using medications). Swish suspension in mouth for several minutes before swallowing.

Oral troches: Remove dentures, clean mouth (do not replace dentures until after using medication). Allow troche to dissolve in mouth; do not chew or swallow whole.

Topical: Wash and dry area before applying (do not reuse towels without washing, apply clean clothing after use). Report unresolved burning, redness, or swelling in treated areas.

Vaginal tablets: Wash hands before using. Lie down to insert high into vagina at bedtime.

Geriatric Considerations: For oral infections, patients who wear dentures must have them removed and cleaned in order to eliminate source of reinfection.

Pregnancy Risk Factor: B/C (oral)

Lactation: Does not enter breast milk/compatible (not absorbed orally)

Administration

Oral:

Suspension: Shake well before using. Should be swished about the mouth and retained in the mouth for as long as possible (several minutes) before swallowing.

Troches: Must be allowed to dissolve slowly and should not be chewed or swallowed whole.

Storage: Keep vaginal inserts in refrigerator. Protect from temperature extremes, moisture, and light.

Nystatin and Triamcinolone *(nye STAT in & trye am SIN oh lone)*

U.S. Brand Names Mycolog®-II [DSC]

Synonyms Triamcinolone and Nystatin

Generic Available Yes

Pharmacologic Category Antifungal Agent, Topical; Corticosteroid, Topical

Medication Safety Issues

Sound-alike/look-alike issues:

Mycolog®-II may be confused with Halog®

Use Treatment of cutaneous candidiasis

Dosing

Adults & Elderly: Cutaneous *Candida*: Topical: Apply sparingly 2-4 times/day,

Pediatrics: Refer to adult dosing.

Available Dosage Forms [DSC] = Discontinued product

Cream (Mycolog®-II [DSC]): Nystatin 100,000 units and triamcinolone acetonide 0.1% (15 g, 30 g, 60 g)

Ointment: Nystatin 100,000 units and triamcinolone acetonide 0.1% (15 g, 30 g, 60 g)

Mycolog®-II: Nystatin 100,000 units and triamcinolone acetonide 0.1% (15 g, 30 g, 60 g) [DSC]

Monitoring and Teaching Issues

Physical Assessment: See individual agents.

Patient Education: See individual agents. **Pregnancy/breast-feeding precautions:** Inform prescriber if you are or intend to become pregnant. Consult prescriber if breast-feeding.

Pregnancy Risk Factor: C

Lactation: Excretion in breast milk unknown

Related Information

Nystatin *on page 1103*

Triamcinolone *on page 1518*

- Nystat-Rx® *see* Nystatin *on page 1103*
- Nystop® *see* Nystatin *on page 1103*
- Nytol® Quick Caps [OTC] *see* DiphenhydrAMINE *on page 463*
- Nytol® Quick Gels [OTC] *see* DiphenhydrAMINE *on page 463*
- Obesity Treatment Guidelines for Adults *see page 1850*
- OCBZ *see* Oxcarbazepine *on page 1132*
- Octagam® *see* Immune Globulin (Intravenous) *on page 793*

Octreotide *(ok TREE oh tide)*

U.S. Brand Names Sandostatin®; Sandostatin LAR®

Synonyms Octreotide Acetate

Generic Available No

Pharmacologic Category Antidiarrheal; Somatostatin Analog

Medication Safety Issues

Sound-alike/look-alike issues:

Sandostatin® may be confused with Sandimmune®

Use Control of symptoms in patients with metastatic carcinoid and vasoactive intestinal peptide-secreting tumors (VIPomas); pancreatic tumors, gastrinoma, secretory diarrhea, acromegaly

Unlabeled/Investigational Use AIDS-associated secretory diarrhea, control of bleeding of esophageal varices, breast cancer, cryptosporidiosis, Cushing's syndrome, insulinomas, small bowel fistulas, postgastrectomy dumping syndrome, chemotherapy-induced diarrhea, graft-versus-host disease (GVHD) induced diarrhea, Zollinger-Ellison syndrome, congenital hyperinsulinism

Mechanism of Action/Effect Mimics natural somatostatin by inhibiting serotonin release, and the secretion of gastrin, VIP, insulin, glucagon, secretin, motilin, and pancreatic polypeptide. Decreases growth hormone and IGF-1 in acromegaly.

Contraindications Hypersensitivity to octreotide or any component of the formulation

Warnings/Precautions Dosage adjustment may be required to maintain symptomatic control; insulin requirements may be reduced as well as sulfonylurea requirements. Monitor patients for cholelithiasis. Use with caution in patients with renal impairment. Somatostatin analogs may affect glucose regulation; in type I diabetes, severe hypoglycemia may occur; in type II diabetes or nondiabetic patients, hyperglycemia may occur.

Drug Interactions

Decreased Effect: Octreotide may lower cyclosporine serum levels (case report of a transplant rejection due to reduction of serum cyclosporine levels). Codeine effect may be reduced.

Increased Effect/Toxicity: Octreotide may increase the effect of insulin or sulfonylurea agents which may result in hypoglycemia. Octreotide may increase serum levels of bromocriptine.

Adverse Reactions

>10%:

Cardiovascular: Sinus bradycardia (19% to 25%)

Endocrine & metabolic: Hyperglycemia (15% acromegaly, 27% carcinoid)

Gastrointestinal: Diarrhea (36% to 58% acromegaly), abdominal pain (30% to 44% acromegaly), flatulence (13% to 26% acromegaly), constipation (9% to 19% acromegaly), nausea (10% to 30%)

1% to 10%:

Cardiovascular: Flushing, edema, conduction abnormalities (9% to 10%), arrhythmia (3% to 9%)

Central nervous system: Fatigue, headache, dizziness, vertigo, anorexia, depression

Endocrine & metabolic: Hypoglycemia (2% acromegaly, 4% carcinoid), hyperglycemia (1%), hypothyroidism, galactorrhea

Gastrointestinal: Nausea, vomiting, diarrhea, constipation, abdominal pain, cramping, discomfort, fat malabsorption, loose stools, flatulence, tenesmus

Hepatic: Jaundice, hepatitis, increase LFTs, cholelithiasis has occurred, presumably by altering fat absorption and decreasing the motility of the gallbladder

Local: Pain at injection site (dose related)

Neuromuscular & skeletal: Weakness

Overdosage/Toxicology Symptoms of overdose include hypo- or hyperglycemia, blurred vision, dizziness, drowsiness, and loss of motor function. Well tolerated bolus doses up to 1000 mcg have failed to produce adverse effects.

Pharmacodynamics/Kinetics

Duration of Action: SubQ: 6-12 hours

Absorption: SubQ: Rapid

Bioavailability: SubQ: 100%

Protein Binding: 65% to lipoproteins

Half-Life Elimination: 60-110 minutes

Metabolism: Extensively hepatic

Excretion: Urine (32%)

Dosing

Adults & Elderly:

Carcinoid tumors:

SubQ, I.V.: Initial: 50 mcg 1-2 times/day; titrate dose based on response/tolerance. Range: 100-600 mcg/day in 2-4 divided doses

I.M. Depot injection: Patients must be stabilized on subcutaneous octreotide for at least 2 weeks before switching to the long-acting depot: Upon switch: 20 mg I.M. intragluteally every 4 weeks for 2-3 months, then the dose may be modified upon response

Dosage adjustment: See dosing for VIPomas.

VIPomas:

SubQ, I.V.: Initial 2 weeks: 200-300 mcg/day in 2-4 divided doses; titrate dose based on response/tolerance. Range: 150-750 mcg/day (doses >450 mcg/day are rarely required)

I.M. Depot injection: Patients must be stabilized on subcutaneous octreotide for at least 2 weeks before switching to the long-acting depot: Upon switch: 20 mg I.M. intragluteally every 4 weeks for 2-3 months, then the dose may be modified based upon response

Dosage adjustment for carcinoid tumors and VIPomas: After 2 months of depot injections the dosage may be continued or modified as follows:

Increase to 30 mg I.M. every 4 weeks if symptoms are inadequately controlled

Decrease to 10 mg I.M. every 4 weeks, for a trial period, if initially responsive to 20 mg dose

Dosage >30 mg is not recommended

Diarrhea: I.V.: Initial: 50-100 mcg every 8 hours; increase by 100 mcg/dose at 48-hour intervals; maximum dose: 500 mcg every 8 hours

Esophageal varices bleeding: I.V. bolus: 25-50 mcg followed by continuous I.V. infusion of 25-50 mcg/hour

(Continued)

Octreotide *(Continued)*

Acromegaly:

SubQ, I.V.: Initial: 50 mcg 3 times/day; titrate to achieve growth hormone levels <5 ng/mL or IGF-I (somatomedin C) levels <1.9 U/mL in males and <2.2 U/mL in females. Usual effective dose 100 mcg 3 times/day. Range 300-1500 mcg/day. **Note:** Should be withdrawn yearly for a 4 week interval in patients who have received irradiation. Resume if levels increase and signs/symptoms recur.

I.M. Depot injection: Patients must be stabilized on subcutaneous octreotide for at least 2 weeks before switching to the long-acting depot: Upon switch: 20 mg I.M. intragluteally every 4 weeks for 2-3 months, then the dose may be modified based upon response

Dosage adjustment for acromegaly: After 3 months of depot injections the dosage may be continued or modified as follows:

GH ≤1 ng/mL, IGF-1 is normal, symptoms controlled: Reduce octreotide LAR® to 10 mg I.M. every 4 weeks

GH ≤2.5 ng/mL, IGF-1 is normal, symptoms controlled: Maintain octreotide LAR® at 20 mg I.M. every 4 weeks

GH >2.5 ng/mL, IGF-1 is elevated, or symptoms uncontrolled: Increase octreotide LAR® to 30 mg I.M. every 4 weeks

Dosages >40 mg are not recommended

Pediatrics: Infants and Children:

Diarrhea: I.V., SubQ: Doses of 1-10 mcg/kg every 12 hours have been used in children beginning at the low end of the range and increasing by 0.3 mcg/kg/dose at 3-day intervals. Suppression of growth hormone (animal data) is of concern when used as long-term therapy.

Congenital hyperinsulinism (unlabeled use): SubQ: Doses of 3-40 mcg/kg/day have been used.

Renal Impairment: Half-life may be increased, requiring adjustment of maintenance dose.

Available Dosage Forms

Injection, microspheres for suspension, as acetate [depot formulation] (Sandostatin LAR®): 10 mg, 20 mg, 30 mg [with diluent and syringe]

Injection, solution, as acetate (Sandostatin®): 0.05 mg/mL (1 mL); 0.1 mg/mL (1 mL); 0.2 mg/mL (5 mL); 0.5 mg/mL (1 mL); 1 mg/mL (5 mL)

Monitoring and Teaching Issues

Physical Assessment: Use caution with diabetes, renal impairment (see Warnings/Precautions). Assess potential for interactions with other pharmacological agents patient may be taking (eg, may increase effect or insulin or sulfonylureas; see Drug Interactions). See Administration for I.V. and I.M. specifics. Assess results of laboratory tests with long-term therapy. Monitor therapeutic effectiveness according to purpose for use and adverse effects (eg, hypo- or hyperglycemia, bradycardia, diarrhea, GI disturbance, CNS changes, jaundice, blurred vision; see Adverse Reactions). Caution patients with diabetes to monitor serum glucose closely; may increase the effect of insulin or sulfonylureas, which may result in hypoglycemia. Teach patient proper use if self-administered (appropriate injection technique and syringe/needle disposal), possible side effects/appropriate interventions, and adverse symptoms to report (see Patient Education).

Monitoring Laboratory Tests: Vitamin B_{12} levels with chronic therapy

Patient Education: Do not take any new medication during therapy unless approved by prescriber (especially any other antidiarrheals or "stomach" medications). If self-administered, follow instructions for injection and syringe/needle disposal. Schedule injections between meals to decrease GI effects. Consult prescriber about appropriate diet. If you have diabetes, monitor serum glucose closely and notify prescriber of significant changes (this drug may increase the effects of insulin or sulfonylureas). May cause skin flushing; nausea or vomiting (small frequent meals, frequent mouth care, sucking lozenges, or chewing gum may help); or dizziness, fatigue, or drowsiness (use caution when driving or engaging in tasks that require alertness until response to drug is known). Report unusual weight gain, swelling of extremities, or respiratory difficulty; acute or persistent GI distress (eg, diarrhea, vomiting, constipation, abdominal pain); muscle weakness or tremors or loss of motor function; chest pain or palpitations; blurred vision; depression; or redness, swelling, burning, or pain at injection site. **Breast-feeding precaution:** Do not breast-feed.

Dietary Considerations: Schedule injections between meals to decrease GI effects.

Pregnancy Risk Factor: B

Lactation: Enters breast milk/contraindicated

Administration

I.M.: Depot formulation: Administer I.M. intragluteal; do not administer Sandostatin LAR® intravenously or subcutaneously; must be administered immediately after mixing

I.V.: Regular injection only (not suspension): IVP should be administered undiluted over 3 minutes. IVPB should be administered over 15-30 minutes. Continuous I.V. infusion rates have ranged from 25-50 mcg/hour for the treatment of esophageal variceal bleeding.

Other: Regular injection formulation (not depot) can be administered SubQ

Compatibility: Stable in D_5W, NS; **incompatible** with fat emulsion 10%.

The manufacturer states that octreotide solution is not compatible in TPN solutions due to the formation of a glycosyl octreotide conjugate which may have decreased activity; other sources give it limited compatibility.

Storage:

Solution: Octreotide is a clear solution and should be stored under refrigeration; may be stored at room temperature for up to 14 days when protected from light. Stability of parenteral admixture is stable in NS for 96 hours at room temperature (25°C) and in D_5W for 24 hours.

Suspension: Prior to dilution, store under refrigeration and protect from light; may be at room temperature for 30-60 minutes prior to use; use suspension immediately after preparation.

♦ **Octreotide Acetate** *see* Octreotide *on page 1104*

♦ **Ocufen®** *see* Flurbiprofen *on page 656*

♦ Ocuflox® *see* Ofloxacin *on page 1107*
♦ Ocusulf-10 *see* Sulfacetamide *on page 1403*

Ofloxacin (oh FLOKS a sin)

U.S. Brand Names Floxin®; Ocuflox®
Synonyms Floxin Otic Singles
Generic Available Yes: Tablet, ophthalmic solution
Pharmacologic Category Antibiotic, Quinolone
Medication Safety Issues
Sound-alike/look-alike issues:
Floxin® may be confused with Flexeril®
Ocuflox® may be confused with Ocufen®

Use Quinolone antibiotic for the treatment of acute exacerbations of chronic bronchitis, community-acquired pneumonia, skin and skin structure infections (uncomplicated), urethral and cervical gonorrhea (acute, uncomplicated), urethritis and cervicitis (nongonococcal), mixed infections of the urethra and cervix, pelvic inflammatory disease (acute), cystitis (uncomplicated), urinary tract infections (complicated), prostatitis
Ophthalmic: Treatment of superficial ocular infections involving the conjunctiva or cornea due to strains of susceptible organisms
Otic: Otitis externa, chronic suppurative otitis media, acute otitis media

Unlabeled/Investigational Use Epididymitis (gonorrhea)

Mechanism of Action/Effect Ofloxacin, a fluorinated quinolone, is a pyridine carboxylic acid derivative which exerts a broad spectrum bactericidal effect. It inhibits DNA gyrase inhibitor, an essential bacterial enzyme that maintains the superhelical structure of DNA. DNA gyrase is required for DNA replication and transcription, DNA repair, recombination, and transposition within the bacteria.

Contraindications Hypersensitivity to ofloxacin or other members of the quinolone group such as nalidixic acid, oxolinic acid, cinoxacin, norfloxacin, and ciprofloxacin; hypersensitivity to any component of the formulation

Warnings/Precautions Use with caution in patients with epilepsy or other CNS diseases which could predispose seizures. Use with caution in patients with renal or hepatic impairment. Has been associated with rare tendonitis or ruptured tendons (discontinue immediately with signs of inflammation or tendon pain). Risk may be increased with concurrent corticosteroids, particularly in the elderly. Discontinue at first sign of tendon inflammation or pain. Peripheral neuropathies have been linked to ofloxacin use; discontinue if numbness, tingling, or weakness develops.

Rare cases of torsade de pointes have been reported in patients receiving ofloxacin and other quinolones. Risk may be minimized by avoiding use in patients with known prolongation of the QT interval, bradycardia, hypokalemia, hypomagnesemia, cardiomyopathy, or in those receiving concurrent therapy with Class Ia or Class III antiarrhythmics.

Severe hypersensitivity reactions, including anaphylaxis, have occurred with quinolone therapy. Discontinue immediately if an allergic reaction occurs. Prolonged use may result in superinfection; pseudomembranous colitis may occur and should be considered in all patients who present with diarrhea. Quinolones may exacerbate myasthenia gravis.

Drug Interactions
Cytochrome P450 Effect: Inhibits CYP1A2 (strong)
Decreased Effect: Concurrent administration of metal cations, including most antacids, oral electrolyte supplements, quinapril, sucralfate, and some didanosine formulations (chewable/buffered tablets and pediatric powder for oral suspension), may decrease quinolone levels; separate doses.
Increased Effect/Toxicity: Ofloxacin may increase the effects/toxicity of CYP1A2 substrates (eg, aminophylline, fluvoxamine, mexiletine, mirtazapine, ropinirole, and trifluoperazine), glyburide, theophylline and warfarin. Concomitant use with corticosteroids may increase the risk of tendon rupture. Concomitant use with other QTc-prolonging agents (eg, Class Ia and Class III antiarrhythmics, erythromycin, cisapride, antipsychotics, and cyclic antidepressants) may result in arrhythmias such as torsade de pointes. Probenecid may increase ofloxacin levels.

Nutritional/Ethanol Interactions
Food: Ofloxacin average peak serum concentrations may be decreased by 20% if taken with food.
Herb/Nutraceutical: Avoid dong quai, St John's wort (may also cause photosensitization).

Adverse Reactions
Systemic:
1% to 10%:
Cardiovascular: Chest pain (1% to 3%)
Central nervous system: Headache (1% to 9%), insomnia (3% to 7%), dizziness (1% to 5%), fatigue (1% to 3%), somnolence (1% to 3%), sleep disorders (1% to 3%), nervousness (1% to 3%), pyrexia (1% to 3%)
Dermatologic: Rash/pruritus (1% to 3%)
Gastrointestinal: Diarrhea (1% to 4%), vomiting (1% to 4%), GI distress (1% to 3%), abdominal cramps (1% to 3%), flatulence (1% to 3%), abnormal taste (1% to 3%), xerostomia (1% to 3%), decreased appetite (1% to 3%), nausea (3% to 10%), constipation (1% to 3%)
Genitourinary: Vaginitis (1% to 5%), external genital pruritus in women (1% to 3%)
Ocular: Visual disturbances (1% to 3%)
Respiratory: Pharyngitis (1% to 3%)
Miscellaneous: Trunk pain

Ophthalmic: Frequency not defined:
Central nervous system: Dizziness
Gastrointestinal: Nausea
Ocular: Blurred vision, burning, chemical conjunctivitis/keratitis, discomfort, dryness, edema, eye pain, foreign body sensation, itching, photophobia, redness, stinging, tearing
(Continued)

Ofloxacin *(Continued)*

Otic:
>10%: Local: Application site reaction (<1% to 17%)
1% to 10%:
  Central nervous system: Dizziness (≤1%), vertigo (≤1%)
  Dermatologic: Pruritus (1% to 4%), rash (1%)
  Gastrointestinal: Taste perversion (7%)
  Neuromuscular & skeletal: Paresthesia (1%)

Overdosage/Toxicology Symptoms of overdose include acute renal failure, seizures, nausea, and vomiting. Treatment includes GI decontamination, if possible, and supportive care. Not removed by peritoneal or hemodialysis.

Pharmacodynamics/Kinetics

Absorption: Well absorbed; food causes only minor alterations
Bioavailability: Oral: 98%
Protein Binding: 20%
Half-Life Elimination: Biphasic: 5-7.5 hours and 20-25 hours (accounts for <5%); prolonged with renal impairment
Excretion: Primarily urine (as unchanged drug)

Dosing

Adults:

Chronic bronchitis (acute exacerbation), community-acquired pneumonia, skin and skin structure infections (uncomplicated): 400 mg every 12 hours for 10 days

Urethral and cervical gonorrhea (acute, uncomplicated): 400 mg as a single dose

Cervicitis/urethritis (nongonococcal) due to *C. trachomatis*, mixed infection of urethra and cervix due to *C. trachomatis* and *N. gonorrhoeae*: 300 mg every 12 hours for 7 days

Pelvic inflammatory disease (acute): 400 mg every 12 hours for 10-14 days

Cystitis (uncomplicated):
  Due to *E. coli* or *K. pneumoniae*: 200 mg every 12 hours for 3 days
  Due to other organisms: 200 mg every 12 hours for 7 days

UTI (complicated): 200 mg every 12 hours for 10 days

Prostatitis: 200 mg every 12 hours for 6 weeks

Epididymitis (gonorrhea; unlabeled use): 300 mg twice daily for 10 days

Conjunctivitis: Ophthalmic: Instill 1-2 drops in affected eye(s) every 2-4 hours for the first 2 days, then use 4 times/day for an additional 5 days.

Corneal ulcer: Ophthalmic: Instill 1-2 drops every 30 minutes while awake and every 4-6 hours after retiring for the first 2 days; beginning on day 3, instill 1-2 drops every hour while awake for 4-6 additional days; thereafter, 1-2 drops 4 times/day until clinical cure.

Chronic suppurative otitis media with perforated tympanic membranes: Otic: Instill 10 drops (or the contents of 2 single-dose containers) into affected ear twice daily for 14 days

Otitis externa: Otic: Instill 10 drops (or the contents of 2 single-dose containers) into affected ear(s) once daily for 7 days

Elderly: Oral: 200-400 mg every 12-24 hours (based on estimated renal function) for 7 days to 6 weeks depending on indication.

Pediatrics: Not for systemic use

Conjunctivitis: Ophthalmic: Children ≥1 year: Refer to adult dosing.

Corneal ulcer: Ophthalmic: Children ≥1 year: Refer to adult dosing.

Chronic suppurative otitis media with perforated tympanic membranes: Otic: Children >12 years: Refer to adult dosing.

Otitis externa: Otic:
  Children 6 months to 13 years: Instill 5 drops (or the contents to 1 single-dose container) into affected ear(s) once daily for 7 days
  Children ≥13 years: Refer to adult dosing.

Acute otitis media with tympanotomy tubes: Otic: Children 1-12 years: Instill 5 drops (or the contents of 1 single-dose container) into affected ear twice daily for 10 days.

Renal Impairment: Adults: Oral: After a normal initial dose, adjust as follows:
  Cl_{cr} 20-50 mL/minute: Administer usual dose every 24 hours
  Cl_{cr} <20 mL/minute: Administer half the usual dose every 24 hours
  Continuous arteriovenous or venovenous hemodiafiltration effects: Administer 300 mg every 24 hours

Hepatic Impairment: Severe impairment: Maximum dose: 400 mg/day

Available Dosage Forms

Solution, ophthalmic (Ocuflox®): 0.3% (5 mL, 10 mL) [contains benzalkonium chloride]
Solution, otic:
  Floxin®: 0.3% (5 mL, 10 mL) [contains benzalkonium chloride]
  Floxin® Otic Singles™: 0.3% (0.25 mL) [contains benzalkonium chloride; packaged as 2 single-dose containers per pouch, 10 pouches per carton, total net volume 5 mL]
Tablet (Floxin®): 200 mg, 300 mg, 400 mg

Monitoring and Teaching Issues

Physical Assessment: Assess results of culture and sensitivity tests and patient's allergy history before initiating therapy. Use caution with known CNS disorders, bradycardia, or hepatic impairment (see Warnings/Precautions for use cautions). Assess potential for interactions with other pharmacological agents and herbal products patient may be taking (eg, increased risk of tendon rupture or arrhythmias; see Drug Interactions). See administration specifics for different formulations (otic, ophthalmic, oral). Assess CBC, renal function and hepatic function with long-term therapy. Patient should be monitored for an allergic reaction occurs (itching, urticaria, dyspnea or facial edema, loss of consciousness, tingling, cardiovascular collapse); if allergic reactions occurs, drug should be discontinued. Monitor effectiveness (resolution of infection) and adverse effects (see Adverse Reactions). Teach patient appropriate use (according to formulation), possible side effects/appropriate interventions, and adverse symptoms to report (eg, allergic reaction, tendon pain; see Patient Education).

Monitoring Laboratory Tests: Perform culture and sensitivity studies before initiating therapy. Monitor CBC, renal and hepatic function periodically if therapy is prolonged.

Patient Education: Do not take any new medication during therapy unless approved by prescriber. Take as directed; on an empty stomach (1 hour before or 2 hours after meals, dairy products, antacids, or other medication). Complete full course of therapy, even if symptoms resolve. Maintain adequate hydration (2-3 L/day of fluids) unless instructed to restrict fluid intake. May cause dizziness, lightheadedness, or headache (use caution when driving or engaging in tasks that require alertness until response to drug is known); nausea, vomiting, or taste perversion (small frequent meals, frequent mouth care, sucking lozenges, or chewing gum may help). If inflammation or tendon pain occurs discontinue use immediately and report to prescriber. If sign of allergic reaction (eg, itching, urticaria, respiratory difficulty, facial edema or difficulty swallowing, loss of consciousness, tingling, chest pain, palpitations) occurs, discontinue use immediately and report to prescriber. Report GI disturbances; CNS changes (eg, excessive sleepiness, agitation, or tremors); skin rash; vision changes; respiratory difficulty; signs of opportunistic infection (eg, sore throat, chills, fever, burning, itching on urination, vaginal discharge, white plaques in mouth); or worsening of condition. **Pregnancy/breast-feeding precautions:** Inform prescriber if you are or intend to become pregnant. Breast-feeding is not recommended.

Ophthalmic: Wash hands before instilling solution. Sit or lie down to instill. Open eye, look at ceiling, and instill prescribed amount of solution as directed. Close eye and roll eye in all directions, and apply gentle pressure to inner corner of eye. Do not touch tip of applicator or let tip of applicator touch eye (may cause eye infection, eye damage, or vision loss). Do not wear contact lenses during therapy. Temporary stinging, blurred vision, dry eyes or a bad taste in your mouth may occur after installation. Report persistent pain, burning, excessive tearing, decreased visual acuity, swelling, itching, or worsening of condition.

Otic: Wash hands before and after applying drops. Lie with affected ear up and instill prescribed number of drops into ear. Remain on side with ear up for 5 minutes.

Geriatric Considerations: The risk of torsade de pointes and tendon inflammation and/or rupture associated with the concomitant use of corticosteroids and quinolones is increased in the elderly population. Dosage must be carefully adjusted to renal function. The half-life of ofloxacin may be prolonged, and serum concentrations are elevated in elderly patients even in the absence of overt renal impairment.

Pregnancy Risk Factor: C

Pregnancy Issues: Reports of arthropathy (observed in immature animals and reported rarely in humans) have limited the use of fluoroquinolones in pregnancy. Teratogenic effects were not observed with ofloxacin in animal studies; however, decreased fetal body weight and increased fetal mortality were observed in some species. Ofloxacin crosses the placenta. Although quinolone antibiotics should not be used as first-line agents during pregnancy, when considering treatment for life-threatening infection and/or prolonged duration of therapy, the potential risk to the fetus must be balanced against the severity of the potential illness.

Lactation: Enters breast milk/not recommended (AAP rates "compatible")

Breast-Feeding Issues: Following oral use, levels of ofloxacin in breast milk are similar to those in plasma. The manufacturer recommends to discontinue nursing or to discontinue ofloxacin.

Administration

Oral: Do not take within 2 hours of food or any antacids which contain zinc, magnesium, or aluminum.

Other:

Ophthalmic: For ophthalmic use only; avoid touching tip of applicator to eye or other surfaces.

Otic: Prior to use, warm solution by holding container in hands for 1-2 minutes. Patient should lie down with affected ear upward and medication instilled. Pump tragus 4 times to ensure penetration of medication. Patient should remain in this position for 5 minutes.

Related Information

I.V. to Oral Conversion *on page 1688*
Tuberculosis *on page 1864*

♦ **OGT-918** *see* Miglustat *on page 1009*

♦ **OKT3** *see* Muromonab-CD3 *on page 1038*

Olanzapine (oh LAN za peen)

U.S. Brand Names Zyprexa®; Zyprexa® Zydis®

Synonyms LY170053; Zyprexa Zydis

Generic Available No

Pharmacologic Category Antipsychotic Agent, Atypical

Medication Safety Issues

Sound-alike/look-alike issues:

Olanzapine may be confused with olsalazine

Zyprexa® may be confused with Celexa™, Zyrtec®

Use Treatment of the manifestations of schizophrenia; treatment of acute mania episodes associated with bipolar disorder (as monotherapy or in combination with lithium or valproate); maintenance treatment of bipolar disorder; acute agitation (patients with schizophrenia or bipolar mania)

Unlabeled/Investigational Use Treatment of psychotic symptoms; chronic pain

Mechanism of Action/Effect Olanzapine is a thienobenzodiazepine antipsychotic which is thought to work by antagonizing dopamine and serotonin activities. It is a selective monoaminergic antagonist with high affinity binding to serotonin 5-HT$_{2A}$ and 5-HT$_{2C}$, dopamine D$_{1-4}$, muscarinic M$_{1-5}$, histamine H$_1$ and alpha$_1$-adrenergic receptor sites. Olanzapine binds weakly to GABA-A, BZD, and beta-adrenergic receptors.

Contraindications Hypersensitivity to olanzapine or any component of the formulation
(Continued)

Olanzapine *(Continued)*

Warnings/Precautions Patients with dementia-related behavioral disorders treated with atypical antipsychotics are at an increased risk of death compared to placebo. Olanzapine is not approved for this indication.

Moderate to highly sedating, use with caution in disorders where CNS depression is a feature. Use with caution in Parkinson's disease; in patients with hemodynamic instability; bone marrow suppression; predisposition to seizures; subcortical brain damage; severe cardiac, hepatic, renal, or respiratory disease. Esophageal dysmotility and aspiration have been associated with antipsychotic use - use with caution in patients at risk of pneumonia (ie, Alzheimer's disease). Caution in breast cancer or other prolactin-dependent tumors (may elevate prolactin levels). May alter temperature regulation or mask toxicity of other drugs due to antiemetic effects. Life-threatening arrhythmias have occurred with therapeutic doses of some neuroleptics. An increased incidence of cerebrovascular adverse events (including fatalities) has been reported in elderly patients with dementia-related psychosis. Significant weight gain may occur.

May cause anticholinergic effects (constipation, xerostomia, blurred vision, urinary retention); therefore, they should be used with caution in patients with decreased gastrointestinal motility, urinary retention, BPH, xerostomia, or visual problems. Conditions which also may be exacerbated by cholinergic blockade include narrow-angle glaucoma (screening is recommended) and worsening of myasthenia gravis. Relative to other neuroleptics, olanzapine has a moderate potency of cholinergic blockade.

May cause extrapyramidal symptoms, including pseudoparkinsonism, acute dystonic reactions, akathisia, and tardive dyskinesia (risk of these reactions is very low relative to other neuroleptics). May be associated with neuroleptic malignant syndrome (NMS). May cause hyperglycemia; in some cases may be extreme and associated with ketoacidosis, hyperosmolar coma, or death. Use with caution in patients with diabetes or other disorders of glucose regulation; monitor for worsening of glucose control.

Drug Interactions

Cytochrome P450 Effect: Substrate (minor) of CYP1A2, 2D6; **Inhibits** CYP1A2 (weak), 2C8/9 (weak), 2C19 (weak), 2D6 (weak), 3A4 (weak)

Decreased Effect: Olanzapine levels may be decreased by cytochrome P450 enzyme inducers such as rifampin, omeprazole, and carbamazepine (also cigarette smoking). Olanzapine may antagonize the effects of levodopa and dopamine agonists.

Increased Effect/Toxicity: Olanzapine levels may be increased by CYP1A2 inhibitors such as cimetidine and fluvoxamine. Sedations from olanzapine is increased with ethanol or other CNS depressants. The risk of hypotension and orthostatic hypotension from olanzapine is increased by concurrent antihypertensives. Metoclopramide may increase risk of extrapyramidal symptoms (EPS).

Nutritional/Ethanol Interactions

Ethanol: Avoid ethanol (may increase CNS depression).

Herb/Nutraceutical: Avoid dong quai, St John's wort (may also cause photosensitization). Avoid kava kava, gotu kola, valerian, St John's wort (may increase CNS depression).

Adverse Reactions

>10%:

Central nervous system: Headache, somnolence, insomnia, agitation, nervousness, hostility, dizziness

Gastrointestinal: Dyspepsia, constipation, weight gain (clinically and long term)

Neuromuscular & skeletal: Weakness

1% to 10%:

Cardiovascular: Postural hypotension, tachycardia, hyper-/hypotension, peripheral edema, chest pain

Central nervous system: Dystonic reactions, parkinsonian events, amnesia, euphoria, stuttering, akathisia, anxiety, personality changes, fever, abnormal dreams, speech disorder

Dermatologic: Rash, bruising

Endocrine & metabolic: Prolactin increased, amenorrhea

Gastrointestinal: Xerostomia, abdominal pain, appetite increased, vomiting, salivation increased

Genitourinary: Premenstrual syndrome, incontinence

Hematologic: Leukopenia

Neuromuscular & skeletal: Arthralgia, neck rigidity, twitching, hypertonia, tremor, back pain, abnormal gait, akathisia, falling (particularly in older patients)

Ocular: Amblyopia

Respiratory: Rhinitis, cough, pharyngitis, dyspnea

Miscellaneous: Diaphoresis

Additional significant effects reported with I.M. administration: Articulation impairment, AV block, injection site pain, syncope

Overdosage/Toxicology Signs and symptoms of overdose include CNS depression (ranging from drowsiness to coma), extrapyramidal movements, fasciculations, hypotension (possible, though not described), miosis, respiratory depression, rhinitis (10%), slurred speech, tachycardia, trismus. Treatment is symptom-directed and supportive.

Pharmacodynamics/Kinetics

Absorption:

Oral: Well absorbed; not affected by food; tablets and orally-disintegrating tablets are bioequivalent

I.M.: Rapidly absorbed

Bioavailability: >57%

Time to Peak: Oral: ~6 hours; I.M.: 15-45 minutes

Maximum plasma concentrations after I.M. administration are 5 times higher than maximum plasma concentrations produced by an oral dose.

Protein Binding: Plasma: 93%, bound to albumin and alpha$_1$-glycoprotein

Half-Life Elimination: 21-54 hours; approximately 1.5 times greater in elderly

Metabolism: Highly metabolized via direct glucuronidation and cytochrome P450 mediated oxidation (CYP1A2, CYP2D6)

Excretion: Excretion: 40% removed via first pass metabolism; urine (57%, 7% as unchanged drug); feces (30%)

Clearance: 40% increase in olanzapine clearance in smokers

Pharmacokinetic Note: Tablets and orally-disintegrating tablets are bioequivalent.

Dosing

Adults:

Schizophrenia: Oral: Usual starting dose: 5-10 mg once daily; increase to 10 mg once daily within 5-7 days, thereafter adjust by 5 mg/day at 1-week intervals, up to a maximum of 20 mg/day. Doses as high as 30-50 mg per day have been used.

Acute mania associated with bipolar disorder: Oral:

Monotherapy: Usual starting dose: 10-15 mg once daily; increase by 5 mg/day at intervals of not less than 24 hours; maintenance: 5-20 mg/day; maximum dose: 20 mg/day

Combination therapy (with lithium or valproate): Initial: 10 mg once daily; dosing range: 5-20 mg/day

Agitation (acute, associated with bipolar disorder or schizophrenia): I.M.: Initial dose: 5-10 mg (a lower dose of 2.5 mg may be considered when clinical factors warrant); additional doses (2.5-10 mg) may be considered; however, 2-4 hours should be allowed between doses to evaluate response (maximum total daily dose: 30 mg, per manufacturer's recommendation)

Elderly:

Schizophrenia: Oral: Usual starting dose: 2.5 mg/day, increase as clinically indicated and monitor blood pressure; typical dosage range: 2.5-10 mg/day

Agitation: I.M.: Refer to adult dosing.

Pediatrics:

Schizophrenia/bipolar disorder: Oral: Initial: 2.5 mg/day; titrate as necessary to 20 mg/day (0.12-0.29 mg/kg/day)

Renal Impairment: Not removed by dialysis

Hepatic Impairment: Dosage adjustment may be necessary, however, there are no specific recommendations. Monitor closely.

Available Dosage Forms

Injection, powder for reconstitution (Zyprexa® IntraMuscular): 10 mg [contains lactose 50 mg]

Tablet (Zyprexa®): 2.5 mg, 5 mg, 7.5 mg, 10 mg, 15 mg, 20 mg

Tablet, orally-disintegrating (Zyprexa® Zydis®): 5 mg [contains phenylalanine 0.34 mg/tablet], 10 mg [contains phenylalanine 0.45 mg/tablet], 15 mg [contains phenylalanine 0.67 mg/tablet], 20 mg [contains phenylalanine 0.9 mg/tablet]

Monitoring and Teaching Issues

Physical Assessment: Assess potential for interactions with other prescriptions, OTC medications, or herbal products patient may be taking. Initiate at lower doses and taper dosage slowly when discontinuing. Instruct patients with diabetes to monitor blood glucose levels closely (may cause hyperglycemia). Monitor therapeutic effectiveness, and adverse reactions at beginning of therapy and periodically with long-term use. Monitor weight prior to initiating therapy and at least monthly. Consider titrating to a different antipsychotic agent for a weight gain greater than or equal to 5% of initial weight. Teach patient appropriate administration, interventions to reduce side effects, and adverse symptoms to report.

Monitoring Laboratory Tests: Fasting lipid profile and fasting blood glucose/Hgb A$_{1c}$ (prior to treatment, at 3 months, then annually); periodic assessment of hepatic transaminases (in patients with hepatic disease)

Patient Education: Do not take any new medication during therapy unless approved by prescriber. Use exactly as directed; do not increase dose or frequency. It may take 2-3 weeks to achieve desired results; do not discontinue without consulting prescriber. Avoid alcohol or caffeine and other prescription or OTC medications not approved by prescriber. For orally-disintegrating tablets, remove from foil blister by peeling back (do not push tablet through the foil). Place tablet in mouth immediately upon removal. Tablet dissolves rapidly in saliva and may be swallowed with or without liquid. Maintain adequate hydration (2-3 L/day of fluids) unless instructed to restrict fluid intake. If diabetic, you may experience increased blood sugars. Monitor blood sugars closely. If you have glaucoma periodic ophthalmic exams are recommended. You may experience excess drowsiness, restlessness, dizziness, or blurred vision (use caution driving or when engaging in tasks requiring alertness until response to drug is known); or constipation (increased exercise, fluids, fruit, or fiber may help). Report persistent CNS effects (eg, trembling fingers, altered gait or balance, excessive sedation, seizures, unusual movements, anxiety, abnormal thoughts, confusion, personality changes); unresolved constipation or GI effects; vision changes; respiratory difficulty; unusual cough or flu-like symptoms; or worsening of condition. **Pregnancy/breast-feeding precautions:** Inform prescriber if you are or intend to become pregnant. Breast-feeding is not recommended.

Dietary Considerations: Tablets may be taken with or without food/meals. Zyprexa® Zydis®: 5 mg tablet contains phenylalanine 0.34 mg; 10 mg tablet contains phenylalanine 0.45 mg; 15 mg tablet contains phenylalanine 0.67 mg; 20 mg tablet contains phenylalanine 0.9 mg

Geriatric Considerations: (See Warnings/Precautions and Adverse Reactions) Elderly patients have an increased risk of adverse response to side effects or adverse reactions to antipsychotics. A higher incidence of falls has been reported in elderly patients, particularly in debilitated patients. Olanzapine half-life that was 1.5 times that of younger (<65 years of age) adults; therefore, lower initial doses are recommended.

(Continued)

Olanzapine *(Continued)*

Pregnancy Risk Factor: C

Lactation: Enters breast milk/not recommended

Administration

Oral:

Tablet: May be administered with or without food/meals.

Orally-disintegrating tablet: Remove from foil blister by peeling back (do not push tablet through the foil). Place tablet in mouth immediately upon removal. Tablet dissolves rapidly in saliva and may be swallowed with or without liquid. May be administered with or without food/meals.

I.M.: Injection: For I.M. administration only; inject slowly, deep into muscle. If dizziness and/or drowsiness are noted, patient should remain recumbent until examination indicates postural hypotension and/or bradycardia are not a problem.

I.V.: Do not administer injection intravenously.

Reconstitution: Injection, powder for reconstitution: Reconstitute 10 mg vial with 2.1 mL SWFI; resulting solution is ~5 mg/mL. Use immediately (within 1 hour) following reconstitution. Discard any unused portion.

Storage:

Tablet and orally-disintegrating tablet: Store at room temperature of 20°C to 25°C (68°F to 77°F). Protect from light and moisture.

Injection, powder for reconstitution: Store at room temperature 20°C to 25°C (68°F to 77°F). Protect from light. Do not freeze.

Related Information

Antipsychotic Agents *on page 1717*

Antipsychotic Medication Guidelines *on page 1766*

Olanzapine and Fluoxetine *(oh LAN za peen & floo OKS e teen)*

U.S. Brand Names Symbyax™

Synonyms Fluoxetine and Olanzapine; Olanzapine and Fluoxetine Hydrochloride

Restrictions A medication guide should be dispensed with each prescription. A template for the required MedGuides can be found on the FDA website at: http://www.fda.gov/cder/drug/antidepressants/labelTemplate.pdf

Generic Available No

Pharmacologic Category Antidepressant, Selective Serotonin Reuptake Inhibitor; Antipsychotic Agent, Atypical

Use Treatment of depressive episodes associated with bipolar disorder

Dosing

Adults: Depression associated with bipolar disorder: Oral: Initial: Olanzapine 6 mg/fluoxetine 25 mg once daily in the evening. Dosing range: Olanzapine 6-12 mg/fluoxetine 25-50 mg. Use caution adjusting dose in patients predisposed to hypotension, in females, and in nonsmokers (metabolism may be decreased). Safety of daily doses of olanzapine >18 mg/fluoxetine >75 mg have not been evaluated.

Elderly: Oral: Initial: Olanzapine 6 mg/fluoxetine 25 mg once daily in the evening; use caution adjusting dose (metabolism may be decreased). Safety and efficacy have not been established in patients >65 years of age.

Hepatic Impairment: Initial: Olanzapine 6 mg/fluoxetine 25 mg once daily in the evening; use caution adjusting dose (metabolism may be decreased).

Available Dosage Forms

Capsule (Symbyax™):

6/25: Olanzapine 6 mg and fluoxetine 25 mg

6/50: Olanzapine 6 mg and fluoxetine 50 mg

12/25: Olanzapine 12 mg and fluoxetine 25 mg

12/50: Olanzapine 12 mg and fluoxetine 50 mg

Monitoring and Teaching Issues

Physical Assessment: See individual agents.

Patient Education: See individual agents. **Pregnancy/breast-feeding precautions:** Inform prescriber if you are pregnant. Breast-feeding is not recommended.

Pregnancy Risk Factor: C

Lactation: Enters breast milk/not recommended

Related Information

Fluoxetine *on page 649*

Olanzapine *on page 1109*

♦ **Olanzapine and Fluoxetine Hydrochloride** *see Olanzapine and Fluoxetine on page 1112*

Olmesartan *(ole me SAR tan)*

U.S. Brand Names Benicar™

Synonyms Olmesartan Medoxomil

Generic Available No

Pharmacologic Category Angiotensin II Receptor Blocker

Use Treatment of hypertension with or without concurrent use of other antihypertensive agents

Mechanism of Action/Effect As a selective and competitive, nonpeptide angiotensin II receptor antagonist, olmesartan blocks the vasoconstrictor and aldosterone-secreting effects of angiotensin II. Olmesartan increases urinary flow rate and in addition to being natriuretic and kaliuretic, increases excretion of chloride, magnesium, uric acid, calcium, and phosphate.

Contraindications Hypersensitivity to olmesartan or any component of the formulation; hypersensitivity to other A-II receptor antagonists; bilateral renal artery stenosis; pregnancy (2nd and 3rd trimesters)

Warnings/Precautions Avoid use or use a smaller dose in patients who are volume depleted; correct depletion first. Deterioration in renal function can occur with initiation. Use with caution in unilateral renal artery stenosis and pre-existing renal insufficiency; significant aortic/mitral stenosis. Safety and efficacy in pediatric patients have not been established.

Drug Interactions

Decreased Effect: NSAIDs may decrease the efficacy of olmesartan.

Increased Effect/Toxicity: The risk of hyperkalemia may be increased during concomitant use with potassium-sparing diuretics, potassium supplements, and trimethoprim; may increase risk of lithium toxicity.

Nutritional/Ethanol Interactions

Food: Does not affect olmesartan bioavailability.

Herb/Nutraceutical: Avoid ephedra, yohimbe, ginseng (may worsen hypertension). Avoid garlic (may have increased antihypertensive effect).

Adverse Reactions 1% to 10%:

Central nervous system: Dizziness (3%), headache

Endocrine & metabolic: Hyperglycemia, hypertriglyceridemia

Gastrointestinal: Diarrhea

Neuromuscular & skeletal: Back pain, CPK increased

Renal: Hematuria

Respiratory: Bronchitis, pharyngitis, rhinitis, sinusitis

Miscellaneous: Flu-like syndrome

Overdosage/Toxicology Hypotension and tachycardia may occur with significant overdose. Bradycardia is possible if vagal stimulation occurs. Treatment should be supportive.

Pharmacodynamics/Kinetics

Bioavailability: 26%

Time to Peak: 1-2 hours

Protein Binding: 99%

Half-Life Elimination: Terminal: 13 hours

Metabolism: Olmesartan medoxomil is hydrolyzed in the GI tract to active olmesartan. No further metabolism occurs.

Excretion: All as unchanged drug: Feces (50% to 65%); urine (35% to 50%)

Dosing

Adults: Antihypertensive: Oral: Initial: Usual starting dose is 20 mg once daily; if initial response is inadequate, may be increased to 40 mg once daily after 2 weeks. May administer with other antihypertensive agents if blood pressure inadequately controlled with olmesartan. Consider lower starting dose in patients with possible depletion of intravascular volume (eg, patients receiving diuretics).

Elderly: Initial: May start at 5-10 mg/day (due to concomitant disease or age changes).

Renal Impairment: No specific guidelines for dosage adjustment; patients undergoing hemodialysis have not been studied.

Hepatic Impairment: No adjustment necessary.

Available Dosage Forms Tablet [film coated], as medoxomil: 5 mg, 20 mg, 40 mg

Monitoring and Teaching Issues

Physical Assessment: Use caution in presence of volume depletion, renal insufficiency, aortic/mitral stenosis (see Warnings/Precautions for specific use cautions). Assess potential for interactions with other pharmacological agents and herbal products patient may be taking (see Drug Interactions). Assess effectiveness (blood pressure) and adverse response on a regular basis throughout therapy (eg, tachycardia, hypotension, diarrhea, bronchitis; see Adverse Reactions). Instruct patients with diabetes to monitor glucose levels closely (may cause hyperglycemia). Teach patient proper use, possible side effects/ appropriate interventions, and adverse symptoms to report (see Patient Education).

Patient Education: Do not take any new medication during therapy unless approved by prescriber. Do not use potassium supplement or salt substitutes without consulting prescriber. Take exactly as directed. Do not alter dose or discontinue without consulting prescriber. May be taken with or without food. This drug does not eliminate the need for diet or exercise regimen as recommended by prescriber. If you have diabetes, check glucose levels closely (drug may alter glucose levels). May cause headache or dizziness (use caution when driving or engaging in tasks that require alertness until response to drug is known); diarrhea (boiled milk, buttermilk, or yogurt may help); or back or joint pain (consult prescriber for approved analgesic). Report chest pain or palpitations; unrelieved headache; flu-like symptoms or upper respiratory infection; or other persistent adverse reactions. **Pregnancy/breast-feeding precautions:** Inform prescriber if you are or intend to become pregnant. This drug should not be used in the 2nd or 3rd trimester of pregnancy. Consult prescriber for appropriate contraceptive measures if necessary. Do not breast-feed.

Dietary Considerations: May be taken with or without food.

Pregnancy Risk Factor: C/D (2nd and 3rd trimesters)

Pregnancy Issues: The drug should be discontinued as soon as possible when pregnancy is detected. Drugs which act directly on renin-angiotensin can cause fetal and neonatal morbidity and death.

Lactation: Excretion in breast milk unknown/contraindicated

Administration

Oral: May be administered with or without food.

Storage: Store at 20°C to 25°C (68°F to 77°F).

Related Information

Angiotensin Agents *on page 1704*

Olmesartan and Hydrochlorothiazide

(ole me SAR tan & hye droe klor oh THYE a zide)

U.S. Brand Names Benicar HCT™

Synonyms Hydrochlorothiazide and Olmesartan Medoxomil; Olmesartan Medoxomil and Hydrochlorothiazide

Generic Available No

Pharmacologic Category Angiotensin II Receptor Blocker; Diuretic, Thiazide

(Continued)

Olmesartan and Hydrochlorothiazide (Continued)

Use Treatment of hypertension (not recommended for initial treatment)

Dosing

Adults & Elderly:

Hypertension: Oral: Dosage must be individualized; may be titrated at 2- to 4-week intervals.

Replacement therapy: May be substituted for titrated components.

Patients not controlled with single-agent therapy: Initiate by adding the lowest available dose of the alternative component (hydrochlorothiazide 12.5 mg or olmesartan 20 mg). Titrate to effect (maximum hydrochlorothiazide dose: 25 mg, maximum olmesartan dose: 40 mg).

Renal Impairment: Not recommended in patients with Cl_{cr} <30 mL/minute.

Available Dosage Forms

Tablet:

20/12.5: Olmesartan medoxomil 20 mg and hydrochlorothiazide 12.5 mg

40/12.5: Olmesartan medoxomil 40 mg and hydrochlorothiazide 12.5 mg

40/25: Olmesartan medoxomil 40 mg and hydrochlorothiazide 25 mg

Monitoring and Teaching Issues

Physical Assessment: See individual agents.

Patient Education: See individual agents. **Pregnancy/breast-feeding precautions:** Inform prescriber if you are or intend to become pregnant. Do not breast-feed.

Pregnancy Risk Factor: C/D (2nd and 3rd trimesters)

Lactation: Excretion in breast milk unknown/contraindicated

Related Information

Hydrochlorothiazide *on page 751*

Olmesartan *on page 1112*

- ◆ **Olmesartan Medoxomil** *see* Olmesartan *on page 1112*
- ◆ **Olmesartan Medoxomil and Hydrochlorothiazide** *see* Olmesartan and Hydrochlorothiazide *on page 1113*

Olopatadine (oh loe pa TA deen)

U.S. Brand Names Patanol®

Generic Available No

Pharmacologic Category Antihistamine; Ophthalmic Agent, Miscellaneous

Medication Safety Issues

Sound-alike/look-alike issues:

Patanol® may be confused with Platinol®

Use Treatment of the signs and symptoms of allergic conjunctivitis

Contraindications Hypersensitivity to olopatadine hydrochloride or any component of the formulation

Adverse Reactions

>5%: Central nervous system: Headache (7%)

<5%:

Central nervous system: Cold syndrome

Gastrointestinal: Taste perversion

Neuromuscular & skeletal: Weakness

Ocular: Burning, stinging, dry eyes, foreign body sensation, hyperemia, keratitis, eyelid edema, itching

Respiratory: Pharyngitis, rhinitis, sinusitis

Dosing

Adults & Elderly: Allergic conjunctivitis: Ophthalmic: 1 to 2 drops in affected eye(s) twice daily every 6 to 8 hours; results from an environmental study demonstrated that olopatadine was effective when dosed twice daily for up to 6 weeks

Available Dosage Forms Solution, ophthalmic: 0.1% (5 mL) [contains benzalkonium chloride]

Monitoring and Teaching Issues

Physical Assessment: Assess therapeutic response and adverse effects. Teach patient proper use, side effects/appropriate interventions, and symptoms to report.

Patient Education: For use in eyes only. Do not let tip of applicator touch eye; do not contaminate tip of applicator (may cause eye infection, eye damage, or vision loss). **Pregnancy precaution:** Inform prescriber if you are pregnant.

Pregnancy Risk Factor: C

Olsalazine (ole SAL a zeen)

U.S. Brand Names Dipentum®

Synonyms Olsalazine Sodium

Generic Available No

Pharmacologic Category 5-Aminosalicylic Acid Derivative

Medication Safety Issues

Sound-alike/look-alike issues:

Olsalazine may be confused with olanzapine

Dipentum® may be confused with Dilantin®

Use Maintenance of remission of ulcerative colitis in patients intolerant to sulfasalazine

Mechanism of Action/Effect The mechanism of action appears to be localized in the colon rather than systemic

Contraindications Hypersensitivity to olsalazine, salicylates, or any component of the formulation

Warnings/Precautions Diarrhea is a common adverse effect of olsalazine. Use with caution in patients with hypersensitivity to salicylates, sulfasalazine, or mesalamine.

Drug Interactions
    Increased Effect/Toxicity: Olsalazine has been reported to increase the prothrombin time in patients taking warfarin. Olsalazine may increase the risk of myelosuppression with azathioprine, mesalamine, or sulfasalazine.

Lab Interactions Increased ALT, AST (S)

Adverse Reactions
    >10%: Gastrointestinal: Diarrhea, cramps, abdominal pain
    1% to 10%:
        Central nervous system: Headache, fatigue, depression
        Dermatologic: Rash, itching
        Gastrointestinal: Nausea, heartburn, bloating, anorexia
        Neuromuscular & skeletal: Arthralgia

Overdosage/Toxicology Symptoms of overdose include decreased motor activity and diarrhea. Treatment is supportive.

Pharmacodynamics/Kinetics
    Absorption: <3%; very little intact olsalazine is systemically absorbed
    Time to Peak: ~1 hour
    Protein Binding: Plasma: >99%
    Half-Life Elimination: 56 minutes
    Metabolism: Primarily via colonic bacteria to active drug, 5-aminosalicylic acid
    Excretion: Primarily feces

Dosing
    Adults & Elderly: Ulcerative colitis: Oral: 1 g/day in 2 divided doses

Available Dosage Forms Capsule, as sodium: 250 mg

Monitoring and Teaching Issues
    Physical Assessment: Assess allergy history before initiating therapy (salicylates, sulfasalazine, or mesalamine). Assess effectiveness (reduction of clinical signs of ulcerative colitis) and adverse effects (eg, diarrhea; see Adverse Reactions). Teach patient proper use, possible side effects/appropriate interventions, and adverse symptoms to report (see Patient Education).

    Patient Education: Do not take any new medication during therapy unless approved by prescriber. Take as directed, with meals, in evenly divided doses. May cause flu-like symptoms or muscle pain (consult prescriber for approved analgesic); diarrhea (buttermilk, boiled milk, or yogurt may help); or nausea or loss of appetite (small frequent meals, frequent mouth care, sucking lozenges, or chewing gum may help). Report persistent diarrhea or abdominal cramping, skin rash or itching, or other adverse reactions. **Pregnancy/breast-feeding precautions:** Inform prescriber if you are or intend to become pregnant. Consult prescriber if breast-feeding.

    Dietary Considerations: Administer with food, increases residence of drug in body.

    Geriatric Considerations: No specific data is available on elderly to suggest the drug needs alterations in dose. Since so little is absorbed, dosing should not be changed for reasons of age. Diarrhea may pose a serious problem for elderly in that it may cause dehydration, electrolyte imbalance, hypotension, and confusion.

    Pregnancy Risk Factor: C

    Lactation: Enters breast milk/use caution (monitor for diarrhea)

Administration
    Oral: Take with food in evenly divided doses.

♦ **Olsalazine Sodium** *see* Olsalazine *on page 1114*

♦ **Omacor®** *see* Omega-3-Acid Ethyl Esters *on page 1117*

Omalizumab (oh mah lye ZOO mab)

U.S. Brand Names Xolair®

Synonyms rhuMAb-E25

Generic Available No

Pharmacologic Category Monoclonal Antibody, Anti-Asthmatic

Use Treatment of moderate-to-severe, persistent allergic asthma not adequately controlled with inhaled corticosteroids

Mechanism of Action/Effect Blocks the binding of IgE to mast cells and basophils, decreasing the allergic response, corticosteroid usage, and asthma exacerbations.

Contraindications Hypersensitivity to omalizumab or any component of the formulation; acute bronchospasm, status asthmaticus

Warnings/Precautions For use in patients with a documented reactivity to a perennial aeroallergen and with symptoms uncontrolled using inhaled corticosteroids; not used to control acute asthma symptoms. Dosing is based on pretreatment IgE serum levels and body weight. IgE levels remain elevated up to 1 year following treatment, therefore, levels taken during treatment can not be used as a dosage guide. Corticosteroid therapy should be tapered gradually, do not discontinue abruptly. Anaphylactic reactions have been reported within 2 hours of initial dose; appropriate medications for the treatment of hypersensitivity reactions should be available. Malignant neoplasm have been reported with use (<1%) in short-term studies; impact of long-term use is not known. Safety and efficacy in children <12 years of age have not been established.

Lab Interactions Total IgE levels are elevated for up to 1 year following treatment. Total serum IgE may be retested after interruption of therapy for 1 year or more.

Adverse Reactions
    >10%:
        Central nervous system: Headache (15%)
        Local: Injection site reaction (45%; placebo 43%), severe injection site reactions (12%; placebo 9%). Most reactions occurred within 1 hour, lasted <8 days, and decreased in frequency with additional dosing.
        Respiratory: Upper respiratory tract infection (23%), sinusitis (16%), pharyngitis (11%)
        Miscellaneous: Viral infection (23%)

(Continued)

Omalizumab *(Continued)*

1% to 10%:
Central nervous system: Pain (7%), fatigue (3%), dizziness (3%)
Dermatologic: Dermatitis (2%), pruritus (2%)
Neuromuscular & skeletal: Arthralgia (8%), leg pain (4%), arm pain (2%), fracture (2%)
Otic: Earache (2%)

Overdosage/Toxicology Limited data; single doses up to 4000 mg and cumulative doses up to 44,000 mg (over 20 weeks) have not been associated with toxicity.

Pharmacodynamics/Kinetics
Absorption: Slow following SubQ injection
Bioavailability: 62%
Time to Peak: 7-8 days
Half-Life Elimination: 26 days
Metabolism: Hepatic; IgG degradation by reticuloendothelial system and endothelial cells
Excretion: Primarily via hepatic degradation; intact IgG may be secreted in bile

Dosing
Adults & Elderly: Asthma: SubQ: Dose is based on pretreatment IgE serum levels and body weight. Dosing should not be adjusted based on IgE levels taken during treatment or <1 year following therapy; doses should be adjusted during treatment for significant changes in body weight

IgE ≥30-100 int. units/mL:
  30-90 kg: 150 mg every 4 weeks
  >90-150 kg: 300 mg every 4 weeks

IgE >100-200 int. units/mL:
  30-90 kg: 300 mg every 4 weeks
  >90-150 kg: 225 mg every 2 weeks

IgE >200-300 int. units/mL:
  30-60 kg: 300 mg every 4 weeks
  >60-90 kg: 225 mg every 2 weeks
  >90-150 kg: 300 mg every 2 weeks

IgE >300-400 int. units/mL:
  30-70 kg: 225 mg every 2 weeks
  >70-90 kg: 300 mg every 2 weeks
  >90 kg: Do not administer dose

IgE >400-500 int. units/mL:
  30-70 kg: 300 mg every 2 weeks
  >70-90 kg: 375 mg every 2 weeks
  >90 kg: Do not administer dose

IgE >500-600 int. units/mL:
  30-60 kg: 300 mg every 2 weeks
  >60-70 kg: 375 mg every 2 weeks
  >70 kg: Do not administer dose

IgE >600-700 int. units/mL:
  30-60 kg: 375 mg every 2 weeks
  >60 kg: Do not administer dose

Pediatrics: Asthma: Children ≥12 years: SubQ: Refer to adult dosing.

Available Dosage Forms Injection, powder for reconstitution [preservative free]: 150 mg [contains sucrose 145.5 g]

Monitoring and Teaching Issues
Physical Assessment: See Warnings/Precautions for use cautions (eg, appropriate use, anaphylactic reactions). For SubQ use only, see Storage and Reconstitution specifics. Assess patient response (relief of asthmatic symptoms) and adverse reactions (eg, hypersensitivity reaction, upper respiratory tract infection, viral infection, dermatitis, arthralgia; see Adverse Reactions) at beginning and periodically during therapy. Teach patient proper use if self-administered (storage, reconstitution, administration, needle/syringe disposal), possible side effects/interventions, and adverse symptoms to report (see Patient Education).

Monitoring Laboratory Tests: Baseline IgE; FEV_1, peak flow, and/or other pulmonary function tests

Patient Education: If self-administered, follow exact directions for storage, reconstitution, administration, and needle/syringe disposal. Report immediately any reaction at injection site (eg, redness, swelling, itching) or signs of allergic response (eg, chest pain, respiratory difficulty, skin rash). May cause headache or dizziness (use caution when driving or engaging in hazardous tasks until response to drug is known); or joint or bone pain, earache (consult prescriber for analgesic). Report unusual or increased respiratory difficulty, signs of infection, or skin rash. **Pregnancy/breast-feeding precautions:** Inform prescriber if you are or intend to become pregnant. Consult prescriber if you are breast-feeding.

Pregnancy Risk Factor: B
Lactation: Excretion in breast milk unknown/use caution
Breast-Feeding Issues: IgG is excreted in human milk and excretion of omalizumab is expected. Effects to nursing infant are not known; use with caution.

Administration
Other: For SubQ injection only; doses >150 mg should divided over more than one site. Injections may take 5-10 seconds to administer.

Reconstitution: Prepare using SWFI, USP only; add to upright vial and swirl gently for 5-10 seconds every 5 minutes until dissolved, may take >20 minutes to dissolve completely. Do not use if powder takes >40 minutes to dissolve.

Storage: Prior to reconstitution, store under refrigeration at 2°C to 8°C (36°F to 46°F); product may be shipped at room temperature. Following reconstitution, protect from direct sunlight. May be stored for up to 8 hours if refrigerated or 4 hours if stored at room temperature.

Omega-3-Acid Ethyl Esters (oh MEG a three AS id ETH il ES ters)

U.S. Brand Names Omacor®

Synonyms Ethyl Esters of Omega-3 Fatty Acids; Fish Oil

Pharmacologic Category Antilipemic Agent, Miscellaneous

Use Omacor®: Treatment of hypertriglyceridemia (≥500 mg/dL)

    Note: A number of OTC formulations containing omega-3 fatty acids are marketed as nutritional supplements; these do not have FDA-approved indications.

Unlabeled/Investigational Use Omacor®: Treatment of IgA nephropathy

Mechanism of Action/Effect Lowers serum triglycerides; possibly by increased metabolism or decreased synthesis of triglycerides

Contraindications Hypersensitivity to omega-3-acid ethyl esters or any component of the formulation

Warnings/Precautions Use with caution in patients with known allergy to fish. Should be used as an adjunct to diet and exercise only in those with very high triglyceride levels. Treatment of primary metabolic disorders (eg, diabetes, thyroid disease) and/or evaluation of the patient's medication regimen for possible etiologic agents should be completed prior to a decision to initiate therapy. If triglyceride levels do not adequately respond after 2 months of treatment with omega-3-acid ethyl esters, discontinue treatment. Prolongation of bleeding time has been observed in some clinical studies. Use caution in patients with coagulopathy or in those receiving therapeutic anticoagulation. Safety and efficacy have not been established in children (<18 years of age).

Drug Interactions

    Decreased Effect: Beta-blockers, estrogens, and thiazide diuretics may decrease the therapeutic effect of omega-3-acid ethyl esters.

    Increased Effect/Toxicity: Omega-3-acid ethyl esters may prolong bleeding time; effect of concurrent anticoagulant therapy or concurrent medications which may alter platelet function has not been evaluated. Thiazide diuretics may increase serum triglycerides. Omega-3-acid ethyl esters may augment the antihypertensive effect of beta blockers and thiazide diuretics.

Nutritional/Ethanol Interactions

    Ethanol: Monitor ethanol use (alcohol use may increase triglycerides).

Adverse Reactions

    Cardiovascular: Angina (1%)

    Central nervous system: Pain (2%)

    Dermatologic: Rash (2%)

    Gastrointestinal: Eructation (5%), dyspepsia (3%), taste perversion (3%)

    Neuromuscular and skeletal: Back pain (2%)

    Miscellaneous: Flu-like syndrome (4%), infection (4%)

Dosing

    Adults & Elderly:

        Hypertriglyceridemia: Oral: 4 g/day as a single daily dose or in 2 divided doses.

        Treatment of IgA nephropathy (unlabeled use): Oral: 4 g/day

    Renal Impairment: No dosage adjustment required.

Available Dosage Forms Capsule: 1 g [contains EPA ~465 mg and DHA ~375 mg]

Monitoring and Teaching Issues

    Physical Assessment: Do not use if allergic to fish. Encourage diet and exercise along with use of this medication.

    Monitoring Laboratory Tests: Triglycerides and other lipids (LDL-C) should be monitored at baseline and periodically. Hepatic transaminase levels, particularly ALT, should be monitored periodically.

    Patient Education: Do not use if allergic to fish. This medication should be used in addition to diet and exercise. Avoid alcohol use. You may experience flu-like syndrome, fever, burping, or an "upset stomach". Report any significant or continued problems to prescriber.

    Pregnancy/breast-feeding precautions: Inform prescriber if you are or intend to become pregnant. Consult prescriber before breast-feeding.

    Dietary Considerations: May be taken with meals. Dietary modification is important in the control of severe hypertriglyceridemia. Maintain dietary restrictions during therapy.

    Geriatric Considerations: Specific information about the safety and efficacy of omega-3-acid ethyl esters is limited. The manufacturer states there were no apparent differences between persons <60 and >60 years of age.

    Pregnancy Risk Factor: C

    Lactation: Excretion in breast milk unknown/use caution

Administration

    Oral: May be administered with meals.

    Storage: Store at 25°C (77°F); excursions permitted to 15°C to 30°C (59°F to 86°F). Do not freeze.

Omeprazole (oh ME pray zol)

U.S. Brand Names Prilosec®; Prilosec OTC™ [OTC]; Zegerid™

Generic Available Yes

Pharmacologic Category Proton Pump Inhibitor; Substituted Benzimidazole

Medication Safety Issues

    Sound-alike/look-alike issues:

        Prilosec® may be confused with Plendil®, Prevacid®, predniSONE, prilocaine, Prinivil®, Proventil®, Prozac®

Use Short-term (4-8 weeks) treatment of active duodenal ulcer disease or active benign gastric ulcer; treatment of heartburn and other symptoms associated with gastroesophageal reflux disease (GERD); short-term (4-8 weeks) treatment of endoscopically-diagnosed erosive esophagitis; maintenance healing of erosive esophagitis; long-term treatment of pathological hypersecretory conditions; as part of a multidrug regimen for *H. pylori* eradication to reduce the risk of duodenal ulcer recurrence; reduction of risk of upper gastrointestinal bleeding in critically-ill patients (Zegerid™)

(Continued)

Omeprazole *(Continued)*

OTC labeling: Short-term treatment of frequent, uncomplicated heartburn occurring ≥2 days/week

Unlabeled/Investigational Use Healing NSAID-induced ulcers; prevention of NSAID-induced ulcers

Mechanism of Action/Effect Suppresses gastric basal and stimulated acid secretion by inhibiting the parietal cell H+/K+ ATP pump

Contraindications Hypersensitivity to omeprazole, substituted benzimidazoles (ie, esomeprazole, lansoprazole, pantoprazole, rabeprazole), or any component of the formulation

Warnings/Precautions In long-term (2-year) studies in rats, omeprazole produced a dose-related increase in gastric carcinoid tumors. While available endoscopic evaluations and histologic examinations of biopsy specimens from human stomachs have not detected a risk from short-term exposure to omeprazole, further human data on the effect of sustained hypochlorhydria and hypergastrinemia is needed to rule out the possibility of an increased risk for the development of tumors in humans receiving long-term therapy. Bioavailability may be increased in the elderly, Asian population, and with hepatic dysfunction. Use Zegerid™ with caution in patients with Bartter's syndrome, hypokalemia, sodium-restricted diets, and respiratory alkalosis (contains sodium bicarbonate). Safety and efficacy have not been established in children <2 years of age. When used for self-medication (OTC), do not use for >14 days; treatment should not be repeated more often than every 4 months; OTC and oral suspension are not approved for use in children <18 years of age

Drug Interactions

Cytochrome P450 Effect: Substrate of CYP2A6 (minor), 2C8/9 (minor), 2C19 (major), 2D6 (minor), 3A4 (minor); **Inhibits** CYP1A2 (weak), 2C8/9 (moderate), 2C19 (strong), 2D6 (weak), 3A4 (weak); **Induces** CYP1A2 (weak)

Decreased Effect: Proton pump inhibitors may decrease the absorption of atazanavir, indinavir, itraconazole, and ketoconazole. The levels/effects of omeprazole may be decreased by aminoglutethimide, carbamazepine, phenytoin, rifampin, and other CYP2C19 inducers.

Increased Effect/Toxicity: Esomeprazole and omeprazole may increase the levels of benzodiazepines metabolized by oxidation (eg, diazepam, midazolam, triazolam) and carbamazepine. Elimination of phenytoin or warfarin may be prolonged when used concomitantly with omeprazole. Omeprazole may increase the levels/effects of amiodarone, citalopram, diazepam, fluoxetine, glimepiride, glipizide, methsuximide, nateglinide, phenytoin, pioglitazone, propranolol, rosiglitazone, sertraline, warfarin, and other CYP2C8/9 or 2C19 substrates.

Nutritional/Ethanol Interactions

Ethanol: Avoid ethanol (may cause gastric mucosal irritation).

Food: Food delays absorption. When Zegerid™ is given 1 hour after a meal, absorption is reduced.

Herb/Nutraceutical: St John's wort may decrease omeprazole levels.

Adverse Reactions

Zegerid™ oral powder for suspension:

>10%:

Central nervous system: Pyrexia (20%)

Endocrine & metabolic: Hypokalemia (12%), hyperglycemia (11%)

Respiratory: Nosocomial pneumonia (11%)

1% to 10%:

Cardiovascular: Hypotension (10%), hypertension (8%), atrial fibrillation (6%), ventricular tachycardia (5%), tachycardia (3%), supraventricular tachycardia (3%), edema (3%)

Central nervous system: Hyperpyrexia (5%), agitation (3%)

Dermatological: Rash (6%), decubitus ulcer (3%)

Endocrine & metabolic: Hypomagnesemia (10%), hypocalcemia (6%), hypophosphatemia (6%), fluid overload (5%), hypoglycemia (3%), hyponatremia (4%), hypernatremia (2%), hyperkalemia (2%)

Gastrointestinal: Constipation (5%), diarrhea (4%), hypomotility (2%)

Genitourinary: Urinary tract infection (2%)

Hematological: Thrombocytopenia (10%), anemia (8%), anemia increased (2%)

Hepatic: LFTs increased (2%)

Respiratory: ARDS (3%), respiratory failure (2%)

Miscellaneous: Sepsis (5%), oral candidiasis (4%), candidal infection (2%)

Capsule and tablet: 1% to 10%:

Central nervous system: Headache (3% to 7%), dizziness (2%)

Dermatologic: Rash (2%)

Gastrointestinal: Diarrhea (3% to 4%), abdominal pain (2% to 5 %), nausea (2% to 4%), vomiting (2% to 3%), flatulence (3%), acid regurgitation (2%), constipation (1% to 2%), taste perversion

Neuromuscular & skeletal: Weakness (1%), back pain (1%)

Respiratory: Upper respiratory infection (2%), cough (1%)

Overdosage/Toxicology Limited experience with overdose in humans. Symptoms include confusion, drowsiness, blurred vision, tachycardia, nausea, flushing, diaphoresis, headache, dry mouth. Treatment is symptom-directed and supportive.

Zegerid™: Also consider signs and symptoms of sodium bicarbonate overdose. Electrolytes (including sodium, potassium, calcium) may be altered; monitoring may be required.

Pharmacodynamics/Kinetics

Onset of Action: Antisecretory: ~1 hour; Peak effect: 2 hours

Duration of Action: 72 hours

Bioavailability: Oral: 30% to 40%; increased in Asian patients and patients with hepatic dysfunction

Protein Binding: 95%

Half-Life Elimination: Delayed release capsule: 0.5-1 hour; Oral suspension: 0.4-3.2 hours

Metabolism: Extensively hepatic to inactive metabolites
Excretion: Urine (77% as metabolites, very small amount as unchanged drug); feces
Dosing
Adults & Elderly:
Active duodenal ulcer: Oral: 20 mg/day for 4-8 weeks
Gastric ulcers: Oral: 40 mg/day for 4-8 weeks
Symptomatic GERD: Oral: 20 mg/day for up to 4 weeks
Erosive esophagitis: Oral: 20 mg/day for 4-8 weeks
Peptic ulcer disease: Eradication of *Helicobacter pylori*: Oral: Dose varies with regimen: 20 mg once daily **or** 40 mg/day as single dose or in 2 divided doses; requires combination therapy with antibiotics
Pathological hypersecretory conditions: Oral: Initial: 60 mg once daily; doses up to 120 mg 3 times/day have been administered; administer daily doses >80 mg in divided doses
Frequent heartburn (OTC labeling): Oral: 20 mg/day for 14 days; treatment may be repeated after 4 months if needed
Risk reduction of upper GI bleeding in critically-ill patients (Zegerid™):
Loading dose: Day 1: 40 mg every 6-8 hours for two doses
Maintenance dose: 40 mg/day for up to 14 days; therapy >14 days has not been evaluated
Pediatrics:
GERD or other acid-related disorders: Oral: Children ≥2 years:
<20 kg: 10 mg once daily
≥20 kg: 20 mg once daily
Renal Impairment: No adjustment is necessary.
Hepatic Impairment: Specific guidelines are not available; bioavailability is increased with chronic liver disease.
Available Dosage Forms
Capsule, delayed release: 10 mg, 20 mg
Prilosec®: 10 mg, 20 mg, 40 mg
Prilosec OTC™: 20 mg
Powder for oral suspension [packet] (Zegerid™): 20 mg (30s), 40 mg (30s) [both strengths contain sodium bicarbonate 1680 mg, equivalent to sodium 460 mg per packet]
Monitoring and Teaching Issues
Physical Assessment: Assess other medications patient may be taking for effectiveness and interactions (especially those dependent on cytochrome P450 metabolism or those dependent on a acid environment for absorption). Monitor effectiveness of therapeutic effectiveness and adverse reactions at beginning of therapy and periodically throughout therapy. Assess knowledge/teach appropriate use of this medication, interventions to reduce side effects, and adverse symptoms to report.
Patient Education: Take as directed, before eating. Do not crush or chew capsules. Capsule may be opened and contents added to applesauce. Avoid alcohol. You may experience anorexia; small frequent meals may help to maintain adequate nutrition. Report changes in urination or pain on urination, unresolved severe diarrhea, testicular pain, or changes in respiratory status. **Pregnancy/breast-feeding precautions:** Inform prescriber if you are or intend to become pregnant. Breast-feeding is not recommended.
Dietary Considerations:
Should be taken on an empty stomach; best if taken before breakfast.
Zegerid™: Take 1 hour before a meal; each 20 mg or 40 mg packet contains sodium bicarbonate 1680 mg (20 mEq), equivalent to sodium 460 mg (20 mEq) per dose
Geriatric Considerations: The incidence of side effects in the elderly is no different than that of younger adults (≤65 years) despite slight decrease in elimination and increase in bioavailability. Bioavailability may be increased in the elderly (≥65 years of age), however, dosage adjustments are not necessary.
Pregnancy Risk Factor: C
Pregnancy Issues: Crosses the placenta; congenital abnormalities have been reported sporadically following omeprazole use during pregnancy. Based on data collected by the Teratogen Information System (TERIS), it was concluded that therapeutic doses used during pregnancy would be unlikely to pose a substantial teratogenic risk (quantity/quality of data: fair). Because the possibility of harm still exists, the manufacturer recommends use during pregnancy only if the potential benefit to the mother outweighs the possible risk to the fetus. Zegerid™ contains sodium bicarbonate; chronic use may lead to systemic alkalosis, edema, and weight gain; metabolic alkalosis and fluid overload may occur in mother and fetus.
Lactation: Enters breast milk/not recommended
Administration
Oral:
Capsule: Should be swallowed whole; do not chew, crush, or open. Best if taken before breakfast. May be opened and contents added to applesauce. Administration via NG tube should be in an acidic juice.
Powder for oral suspension (Zegerid™): Administer 1 hour before a meal. Mix with 2 tablespoons of water; stir well and drink immediately. Rinse cup with water and drink.
Other: Nasogastric/orogastric tube: Powder for oral suspension (Zegerid™): Mix well with 20 mL of water and administer immediately; flush tube with an additional 20 mL of water. Suspend enteral feeding for 3 hours before and 1 hour after administering Zegerid™.
Storage: Store at 15°C to 30°C (59°F to 86°F).
Related Information
Helicobacter pylori Treatment *on page 1835*

♦ **Omnicef®** *see* Cefdinir *on page 270*
♦ **Oncaspar®** *see* Pegaspargase *on page 1163*

Ondansetron *(on DAN se tron)*
U.S. Brand Names Zofran®; Zofran® ODT
Synonyms GR38032R; Ondansetron Hydrochloride
(Continued)

Ondansetron (Continued)

Generic Available No
Pharmacologic Category Antiemetic; Selective 5-HT₃ Receptor Antagonist
Medication Safety Issues
Sound-alike/look-alike issues:
Zofran® may be confused with Zantac®, Zosyn®

Use Prevention of nausea and vomiting associated with moderately- to highly-emetogenic cancer chemotherapy; radiotherapy in patients receiving total body irradiation or fractions to the abdomen; prevention and treatment of postoperative nausea and vomiting

Generally **not** recommended for treatment of existing chemotherapy-induced emesis (CIE) or for prophylaxis of nausea from agents with a low emetogenic potential.

Unlabeled/Investigational Use Treatment of early-onset alcoholism
Mechanism of Action/Effect Selective 5-HT₃ receptor antagonist, blocking serotonin, both peripherally on vagal nerve terminals and centrally in the chemoreceptor trigger zone
Contraindications Hypersensitivity to ondansetron, other selective 5-HT₃ antagonists, or any component of the formulation
Warnings/Precautions Ondansetron should be used on a scheduled basis, not on an "as needed" (PRN) basis, since data support the use of this drug only in the prevention of nausea and vomiting (due to antineoplastic therapy) and not in the rescue of nausea and vomiting. Ondansetron should only be used in the first 24-48 hours of chemotherapy. Data do not support any increased efficacy of ondansetron in delayed nausea and vomiting. Does not stimulate gastric or intestinal peristalsis; may mask progressive ileus and/or gastric distension. Orally-disintegrating tablets contain phenylalanine.

Drug Interactions
Cytochrome P450 Effect: Substrate of CYP1A2 (minor), 2C8/9 (minor), 2D6 (minor), 2E1 (minor), 3A4 (major); **Inhibits** CYP1A2 (weak), 2C8/9 (weak), 2D6 (weak)
Decreased Effect: CYP3A4 inducers may decrease the levels/effects of ondansetron; example inducers include aminoglutethimide, carbamazepine, nafcillin, nevirapine, phenobarbital, phenytoin, and rifamycins. The manufacturer does not recommend dosage adjustment in patients receiving CYP3A4 inducers.

Nutritional/Ethanol Interactions
Food: Food increases the extent of absorption. The C_{max} and T_{max} do not change much.
Herb/Nutraceutical: St John's wort may decrease ondansetron levels.

Adverse Reactions
>10%:
Cardiovascular: Malaise/fatigue (9% to 13%)
Central nervous system: Headache (9% to 27%)
1% to 10%:
Central nervous system: Drowsiness (8%), fever (2% to 8%), dizziness (4% to 7%), anxiety (6%), cold sensation (2%)
Dermatologic: Pruritus (2% to 5%), rash (1%)
Gastrointestinal: Constipation (6% to 9%), diarrhea (3% to 7%)
Genitourinary: Gynecological disorder (7%), urinary retention (5%)
Hepatic: Increased ALT/AST (1% to 2%)
Local: Injection site reaction (4%)
Neuromuscular & skeletal: Paresthesia (2%)
Respiratory: Hypoxia (9%)

Overdosage/Toxicology Sudden transient blindness, severe constipation, hypotension, and vasovagal episode with transient secondary heart block have been reported in some cases of overdose. I.V. doses of up to 252 mg/day have been inadvertently given without adverse effects. There is no specific antidote. Treatment is symptom-directed and supportive.

Pharmacodynamics/Kinetics
Onset of Action: ~30 minutes
Bioavailability: Oral: 56% to 71%; Rectal: 58% to 74%
Time to Peak: Oral: ~2 hours
Protein Binding: Plasma: 70% to 76%
Half-Life Elimination: Children <15 years: 2-3 hours; Adults: 3-6 hours
Metabolism: Extensively hepatic via hydroxylation, followed by glucuronide or sulfate conjugation; CYP1A2, CYP2D6, and CYP3A4 substrate, some demethylation occurs
Excretion: Urine (44% to 60% as metabolites, 5% to 10% as unchanged drug); feces (~25%)

Dosing
Adults & Elderly:
Chemotherapy-induced emesis:
I.V.:
0.15 mg/kg 3 times/day beginning 30 minutes prior to chemotherapy **or**
0.45 mg/kg once daily **or**
8-10 mg 1-2 times/day **or**
24 mg or 32 mg once daily
Highly-emetogenic agents/single-day therapy: Oral: 24 mg given 30 minutes prior to the start of therapy
Moderately-emetogenic agents: Oral: 8 mg every 12 hours beginning 30 minutes before chemotherapy, continuously for 1-2 days after chemotherapy completed
Total body irradiation: Oral: 8 mg 1-2 hours before each daily fraction of radiotherapy
Single high-dose fraction radiotherapy to abdomen: Oral: 8 mg 1-2 hours before irradiation, then 8 mg every 8 hours after first dose for 1-2 days after completion of radiotherapy
Daily fractionated radiotherapy to abdomen: 8 mg 1-2 hours before irradiation, then 8 mg 8 hours after first dose for each day of radiotherapy
Postoperative nausea and vomiting (PONV):
Oral: 16 mg given one hour prior to induction of anesthesia

I.M., I.V.: 4 mg as a single dose immediately before induction of anesthesia, or shortly following procedure if vomiting occurs

Pediatrics:

Chemotherapy-induced emesis:

I.V.: Children 4-18 years: 0.15 mg/kg/dose administered 30 minutes prior to chemotherapy, 4 and 8 hours after the first dose **or** 0.45 mg/kg/day as a single dose

Oral:

4-11 years: 4 mg 30 minutes before chemotherapy; repeat 4 and 8 hours after initial dose, then 4 mg every 8 hours for 1-2 days after chemotherapy completed

≥12 years: Refer to adult dosing.

Postoperative nausea and vomiting (PONV): I.V.: Children 2-12 years:

≤40 kg: 0.1 mg/kg

>40 kg: 4 mg

Renal Impairment: No adjustment is necessary.

Hepatic Impairment: Maximum daily dose: 8 mg in patients with severe liver disease (Child-Pugh score ≥10)

Available Dosage Forms

Infusion, as hydrochloride [premixed in D_5W] (Zofran®): 32 mg (50 mL)

Injection, solution, as hydrochloride (Zofran®): 2 mg/mL (2 mL, 20 mL)

Solution, as hydrochloride (Zofran®): 4 mg/5 mL (50 mL) [contains sodium benzoate; strawberry flavor]

Tablet, as hydrochloride (Zofran®): 4 mg, 8 mg, 24 mg

Tablet, orally-disintegrating (Zofran® ODT): 4 mg, 8 mg [each strength contains phenylalanine <0.03 mg/tablet; strawberry flavor]

Monitoring and Teaching Issues

Physical Assessment: See Warnings/Precautions for use cautions. Assess potential for interactions with other pharmacological agents and herbal products patient may be taking (eg, may increase or decrease levels/effects of ondansetron; see Drug Interactions). See Administration for specifics according to formulation. Assess effectiveness (avoidance of nausea and vomiting) and adverse effects (dizziness, constipation, diarrhea, urinary retention, hypoxia; see Adverse Reactions). Teach patient appropriate use (according to formulation), possible side effects/appropriate interventions, and adverse symptoms to report (see Patient Education).

Patient Education: Do not take any other medication for nausea and vomiting with this medication unless approved by prescriber. If self-administered, take as directed. May cause drowsiness or dizziness (use caution when driving or engaging in tasks that require alertness until response to drug is known); or fatigue, diarrhea, constipation, or headache (request appropriate treatment from prescriber). Do not change position rapidly (rise slowly). Report persistent headache, excessive drowsiness; fever, numbness or tingling, or changes in elimination patterns (constipation or diarrhea); and chest pain or palpitations.

Orally-disintegrating tablets: Do not remove from blister until needed. Peel backing off the blister, do not push tablet through. Using dry hands, place tablet on tongue and allow to dissolve. Swallow with saliva.

Dietary Considerations: Take without regard to meals.

Potassium: Hypokalemia; monitor potassium serum concentration

Orally-disintegrating tablet contains <0.03 mg phenylalanine

Geriatric Considerations: Elderly have a slightly decreased hepatic clearance rate. This does not, however, require a dose adjustment.

Pregnancy Risk Factor: B

Lactation: Excretion in breast milk unknown/opportunity for use is minimal

Administration

Oral: Oral dosage forms should be given 30 minutes prior to chemotherapy; 1-2 hours before radiotherapy; 1 hour prior to the induction of anesthesia

Orally-disintegrating tablets: Do not remove from blister until needed. Peel backing off the blister, do not push tablet through. Using dry hands, place tablet on tongue and allow to dissolve. Swallow with saliva.

The I.V. preparation has been successful when administered orally.

I.M.: Should be given undiluted

I.V.: Give first dose 30 minutes prior to beginning chemotherapy; the I.V. preparation has been successful when administered orally

I.V. injection: Single doses for prevention of postoperative nausea and vomiting may be administered I.V. over 2-5 minutes as undiluted solution

IVPB: Dilute in 50-100 mL D_5W or NS (maximum concentration: 1 mg/mL). Infuse over 15-30 minutes; 24-hour continuous infusions have been reported, but are rarely used

Reconstitution: Prior to I.V. infusion, dilute in 50-100 mL D_5W or NS.

Compatibility: Stable in $D_5\frac{1}{2}$NS, D_5NS, D_5W, mannitol 10%, LR, NS, NS 3%; do not mix injection with alkaline solutions

Y-site administration: Incompatible with acyclovir, allopurinol, aminophylline, amphotericin B, amphotericin B cholesteryl sulfate complex, ampicillin, ampicillin/sulbactam, amsacrine, cefepime, cefoperazone, furosemide, ganciclovir, lorazepam, methylprednisolone sodium succinate, piperacillin, sargramostim, sodium bicarbonate

Storage:

Oral solution: Store between 15°C and 30°C (59°F and 86°F). Protect from light.

Tablet: Store between 2°C and 30°C (36°F and 86°F)

Vial: Store between 2°C and 30°C (36°F and 86°F). Protect from light. Stable when mixed in 5% dextrose or 0.9% sodium chloride for 48 hours at room temperature.

Related Information

Antiemetics for Chemotherapy-Induced Nausea and Vomiting *on page 1788*

♦ **Ondansetron Hydrochloride** *see* Ondansetron *on page 1119*

♦ **ONTAK®** *see* Denileukin Diftitox *on page 416*

♦ **Onxol™** *see* Paclitaxel *on page 1144*

♦ **OPC-13013** *see* Cilostazol *on page 323*

♦ **OPC-14597** *see* Aripiprazole *on page 137*
♦ **o,p'-DDD** *see* Mitotane *on page 1018*
♦ **Ophthetic®** *see page 1625*
♦ **Opium and Belladonna** *see* Belladonna and Opium *on page 177*

Opium Tincture (OH pee um TING chur)

Synonyms DTO; Opium Tincture, Deodorized
Controlled Substance C-II
Generic Available Yes
Pharmacologic Category Analgesic, Narcotic; Antidiarrheal
Medication Safety Issues
Sound-alike/look-alike issues:
Opium tincture may be confused with camphorated tincture of opium (paregoric)

Use care when prescribing opium tincture; each mL contains the equivalent of morphine 10 mg; paregoric contains the equivalent of morphine 0.4 mg/mL
Use Treatment of diarrhea or relief of pain
Mechanism of Action/Effect Contains many narcotic alkaloids including morphine; its mechanism for gastric motility inhibition is primarily due to this morphine content; it results in a decrease in digestive secretions, an increase in GI muscle tone, and therefore a reduction in GI propulsion
Contraindications Hypersensitivity to morphine sulfate or any component of the formulation; increased intracranial pressure; severe respiratory depression; severe hepatic or renal insufficiency; pregnancy (prolonged use or high dosages near term)
Warnings/Precautions Opium shares the toxic potential of opiate agonists, and usual precautions of opiate agonist therapy should be observed; some preparations contain sulfites which may cause allergic reactions; infants <3 months of age are more susceptible to respiratory depression, use with caution and generally in reduced doses in this age group; this is **not** paregoric, dose accordingly
Drug Interactions
Increased Effect/Toxicity: Opium tincture and CNS depressants, MAO inhibitors, tricyclic antidepressants may potentiate the effects of opiate agonists (eg, codeine, morphine). Dextroamphetamine may enhance the analgesic effect of opiate agonists.
Nutritional/Ethanol Interactions Ethanol: Avoid ethanol (may increase CNS depression).
Lab Interactions Increased aminotransferase [ALT (SGPT)/AST (SGOT)] (S)
Adverse Reactions Frequency not defined.
Cardiovascular: Palpitations, hypotension, bradycardia, peripheral vasodilation
Central nervous system: Drowsiness, dizziness, restlessness, headache, malaise, CNS depression, increased intracranial pressure, insomnia, mental depression
Gastrointestinal: Nausea, vomiting, constipation, anorexia, stomach cramps, biliary tract spasm
Genitourinary: Decreased urination, urinary tract spasm
Neuromuscular & skeletal: Weakness
Ocular: Miosis
Respiratory: Respiratory depression
Miscellaneous: Histamine release, physical and psychological dependence
Overdosage/Toxicology Primary attention should be directed to ensuring adequate respiratory exchange. Naloxone, 2 mg I.V. with repeat administration as necessary up to a total of 10 mg, can also be used to reverse toxic effects of the opiate.
Pharmacodynamics/Kinetics
Duration of Action: 4-5 hours
Absorption: Variable
Metabolism: Hepatic
Excretion: Urine
Dosing
Adults & Elderly:
Diarrhea: Oral: 0.3-1 mL/dose every 2-6 hours to maximum of 6 mL/24 hours
Analgesia: Oral: 0.6-1.5 mL/dose every 3-4 hours
Pediatrics:
Diarrhea: Oral: Children: 0.005-0.01 mL/kg/dose every 3-4 hours for a maximum of 6 doses/24 hours
Analgesia: Oral: Children: 0.01-0.02 mL/kg/dose every 3-4 hours
Available Dosage Forms Liquid: 10% (120 mL, 480 mL) [0.6 mL equivalent to morphine 6 mg; contains alcohol 19%]
Monitoring and Teaching Issues
Physical Assessment: Assess other medications patient may be taking for additive or adverse interactions. Monitor vital signs, effectiveness of pain relief, adverse reactions, and signs of overdose at beginning of therapy and at regular intervals with long-term use. May cause physical and/or psychological dependence. For inpatients, implement safety measures. Assess knowledge/teach patient appropriate use (if self-administered). Teach patient to monitor for adverse reactions, adverse reactions to report, and appropriate interventions to reduce side effects. Discontinue slowly after prolonged use.
Patient Education: If self-administered, use exactly as directed; do not increase dose or frequency. Drug may cause physical and/or psychological dependence. While using this medication, do not use alcohol and other prescription or OTC medications (especially sedatives, tranquilizers, antihistamines, or pain medications) without consulting prescriber. Maintain adequate hydration (2-3 L/day of fluids). May cause hypotension, dizziness, drowsiness, impaired coordination, or blurred vision (use caution when driving, climbing stairs, or changing position - rising from sitting or lying to standing, or when engaging in tasks requiring alertness until response to drug is known); or dry mouth (frequent mouth care, small frequent meals, chewing gum, or sucking lozenges may help). Report slow or rapid heartbeat, acute dizziness, or persistent headache; changes in mental status; swelling of extremities or unusual weight gain; changes in urinary elimination or pain on

urination; acute headache; trembling or muscle spasms; blurred vision; skin rash; or shortness of breath. **Pregnancy/breast-feeding precautions:** Inform prescriber if you are or intend to become pregnant. If you are breast-feeding, take medication immediately after breast-feeding or 3-4 hours prior to next feeding.

Pregnancy Risk Factor: B/D (prolonged use or high doses at term)

Lactation: Enters breast milk/use caution

Administration

Storage: Protect from light

- ♦ **Opium Tincture, Deodorized** *see* Opium Tincture *on page 1122*
- ♦ **Opticrom®** *see* Cromolyn *on page 374*
- ♦ **Opticyl®** *see page 1625*
- ♦ **Orabase®-B with Benzocaine [OTC]** *see* Benzocaine *on page 181*
- ♦ **Oracit®** *see* Sodium Citrate and Citric Acid *on page 1382*
- ♦ **Orajel® [OTC]** *see* Benzocaine *on page 181*
- ♦ **Orajel® Baby Teething [OTC]** *see* Benzocaine *on page 181*
- ♦ **Orajel® Baby Teething Nighttime [OTC]** *see* Benzocaine *on page 181*
- ♦ **Orajel® Denture Plus [OTC]** *see* Benzocaine *on page 181*
- ♦ **Orajel® Maximum Strength [OTC]** *see* Benzocaine *on page 181*
- ♦ **Orajel® Medicated Toothache [OTC]** *see* Benzocaine *on page 181*
- ♦ **Orajel® Mouth Sore [OTC]** *see* Benzocaine *on page 181*
- ♦ **Orajel® Multi-Action Cold Sore [OTC]** *see* Benzocaine *on page 181*
- ♦ **Orajel PM® [OTC]** *see* Benzocaine *on page 181*
- ♦ **Orajel® Ultra Mouth Sore [OTC]** *see* Benzocaine *on page 181*
- ♦ **Oramorph SR®** *see* Morphine Sulfate *on page 1031*
- ♦ **Oranyl [OTC]** *see* Pseudoephedrine *on page 1282*
- ♦ **Orap®** *see* Pimozide *on page 1213*
- ♦ **Orapred®** *see* PrednisoLONE *on page 1245*
- ♦ **ORG 946** *see* Rocuronium *on page 1343*
- ♦ **Organ-1 NR** *see* Guaifenesin *on page 729*
- ♦ **Organidin® NR** *see* Guaifenesin *on page 729*
- ♦ **ORG NC 45** *see* Vecuronium *on page 1555*

Orlistat (OR li stat)

U.S. Brand Names Xenical®

Generic Available No

Pharmacologic Category Lipase Inhibitor

Use Management of obesity, including weight loss and weight management when used in conjunction with a reduced-calorie diet; reduce the risk of weight regain after prior weight loss; indicated for obese patients with an initial body mass index (BMI) ≥30 kg/m² or ≥27 kg/m² in the presence of other risk factors

Mechanism of Action/Effect Inhibits gastric and pancreatic lipases, thus inhibiting the absorption of dietary fats (by 30% at doses of 120 mg 3 times/day)

Contraindications Hypersensitivity to orlistat or any component of the formulation; chronic malabsorption syndrome or cholestasis

Warnings/Precautions Patients should be advised to adhere to dietary guidelines; gastrointestinal adverse events may increase if taken with a diet high in fat (>30% total daily calories from fat). The daily intake of fat should be distributed over three main meals. If taken with any one meal very high in fat, the possibility of gastrointestinal effects increases. Patients should be counseled to take a multivitamin supplement that contains fat-soluble vitamins to ensure adequate nutrition because orlistat has been shown to reduce the absorption of some fat-soluble vitamins and beta-carotene. Some patients may develop increased levels of urinary oxalate following treatment; caution should be exercised when prescribing it to patients with a history of hyperoxaluria or calcium oxalate nephrolithiasis. As with any weight-loss agent, the potential exists for misuse in appropriate patient populations (eg, patients with anorexia nervosa or bulimia). Safety and efficacy have not been established in children <12 years of age. **Note:** Dispensing errors have been made between Xenical® (orlistat) and Xeloda® (capecitabine).

Drug Interactions

Decreased Effect: Orlistat may decrease amiodarone absorption (monitor). Coadministration with cyclosporine may decrease plasma levels of cyclosporine (administer cyclosporine 2 hours before or after orlistat and monitor). Orlistat does not alter the pharmacokinetics of warfarin, however, vitamin K absorption may be decreased during orlistat therapy (patients stabilized on warfarin should be monitored for changes in warfarin effects).

Nutritional/Ethanol Interactions

Fat-soluble vitamins: Absorption of vitamins A, D, E, and K may be decreased by orlistat. A multivitamin containing the fat-soluble vitamins (A, D, E, and K) should be administered once daily at least 2 hours before or after orlistat.

Adverse Reactions

>10%:

Central nervous system: Headache (31%)

Gastrointestinal: Oily spotting (27%), abdominal pain/discomfort (26%), flatus with discharge (24%), fatty/oily stool (20%), fecal urgency (22%), oily evacuation (12%), increased defecation (11%)

Neuromuscular & skeletal: Back pain (14%)

Respiratory: Upper respiratory infection (38%)

1% to 10%:

Central nervous system: Fatigue (7%), anxiety (5%), sleep disorder (4%)

Dermatologic: Dry skin (2%)

Endocrine & metabolic: Menstrual irregularities (10%)

(Continued)

Orlistat (Continued)

Gastrointestinal: Fecal incontinence (8%), nausea (8%), infectious diarrhea (5%), rectal pain/discomfort (5%), vomiting (4%)

Neuromuscular & skeletal: Arthritis (5%), myalgia (4%)

Otic: Otitis (4%)

Overdosage/Toxicology Single doses of 800 mg and multiple doses of up to 400 mg 3 times daily for 15 days have been studied in normal weight and obese patients without significant adverse findings. In case of significant overdose, it is recommended that the patient be observed for 24 hours.

Pharmacodynamics/Kinetics

Absorption: Minimal

Metabolism: Metabolized within the gastrointestinal wall; forms inactive metabolites

Excretion: Feces (83% as unchanged drug)

Dosing

Adults & Elderly: Obesity: Oral: 120 mg 3 times daily with each main meal containing fat (during or up to 1 hour after the meal); omit dose if meal is occasionally missed or contains no fat.

Pediatrics: Obesity: Children ≥12 years: Refer to adult dosing.

Available Dosage Forms Capsule: 120 mg

Monitoring and Teaching Issues

Physical Assessment: Assess effectiveness of other medications patient may be taking (especially anticoagulants). Monitor effectiveness of therapy, laboratory results, and adverse reactions at beginning of therapy and periodically during therapy. Assess knowledge/teach patient appropriate use, possible side effects/appropriate interventions, and adverse symptoms to report.

Patient Education: Take this medication exactly as ordered; do not alter prescribed dose without consulting prescriber. Maintain prescribed diet (high-fat meals may result in GI distress), exercise regimen, and vitamin supplements as prescribed. You may experience dizziness or lightheadedness (use caution when driving or engaging in tasks requiring alertness until response to drug is known) or increased flatus and fecal urgency (this may lessen with continued use). Report persistent back, muscle, or joint pain; signs of respiratory tract infection or flu-like symptoms; skin rash or irritation; or other reactions. **Breast-feeding precaution:** Breast-feeding is not recommended.

Dietary Considerations: Multivitamin supplements that contain fat-soluble vitamins should be taken once daily at least 2 hours before or after the administration of orlistat (ie, bedtime). Distribute the daily intake of fat over 3 main meals. Gastrointestinal effects of orlistat may increase if taken with any 1 meal very high in fat.

Pregnancy Risk Factor: B

Lactation: Excretion in breast milk unknown/not recommended

Related Information

Obesity Treatment Guidelines for Adults on page 1850

Orphenadrine (or FEN a dreen)

U.S. Brand Names Norflex™

Synonyms Orphenadrine Citrate

Generic Available Yes: Tablet

Pharmacologic Category Anti-Parkinson's Agent, Anticholinergic; Skeletal Muscle Relaxant

Medication Safety Issues

Sound-alike/look-alike issues:

Norflex™ may be confused with norfloxacin, Noroxin®

Use Treatment of muscle spasm associated with acute painful musculoskeletal conditions; supportive therapy in tetanus

Mechanism of Action/Effect Indirect skeletal muscle relaxant thought to work by central atropine-like effects; has some euphorogenic and analgesic properties

Contraindications Hypersensitivity to orphenadrine or any component of the formulation; glaucoma; GI obstruction; cardiospasm; myasthenia gravis

Warnings/Precautions Use with caution in patients with CHF or cardiac arrhythmias. Some products contain sulfites.

Drug Interactions

Cytochrome P450 Effect: Substrate (minor) of CYP1A2, 2B6, 2D6, 3A4; **Inhibits** CYP1A2 (weak), 2A6 (weak), 2B6 (weak), 2C8/9 (weak), 2C19 (weak), 2D6 (weak), 2E1 (weak), 3A4 (weak)

Increased Effect/Toxicity: Orphenadrine may increase potential for anticholinergic adverse effects of anticholinergic agents; includes drugs with high anticholinergic activity (diphenhydramine, TCAs, phenothiazines). Sedative effects of may be additive in concurrent use of orphenadrine and CNS depressants (monitor). Effects of levodopa may be decreased by orphenadrine. Monitor.

Nutritional/Ethanol Interactions

Ethanol: Avoid ethanol (may increase CNS depression).

Herb/Nutraceutical: St John's wort may decrease orphenadrine levels. Avoid valerian, St John's wort, kava kava, gotu kola (may increase CNS depression).

Adverse Reactions

>10%:

Central nervous system: Drowsiness, dizziness

Ocular: Blurred vision

1% to 10%:

Cardiovascular: Flushing of face, tachycardia, syncope

Dermatologic: Rash

Gastrointestinal: Nausea, vomiting, constipation

Genitourinary: Decreased urination

Neuromuscular & skeletal: Weakness

Ocular: Nystagmus, increased intraocular pressure
Respiratory: Nasal congestion

Overdosage/Toxicology Symptoms of overdose include blurred vision, tachycardia, confusion, seizures, respiratory arrest, and dysrhythmias. There is no specific treatment for antihistamine overdose. Clinical toxicity is due to blockade of cholinergic receptors. Lethal dose is 2-3 g; treatment is generally symptomatic. For anticholinergic overdose with severe life-threatening symptoms, physostigmine 1-2 mg I.V. slowly, may be given to reverse these effects.

Pharmacodynamics/Kinetics
Onset of Action: Peak effect: Oral: Within 2-4 hours
Duration of Action: 4-6 hours
Protein Binding: 20%
Half-Life Elimination: 14-16 hours
Metabolism: Extensively hepatic
Excretion: Primarily urine (8% as unchanged drug)

Dosing
Adults: Muscle spasms:
Oral: 100 mg twice daily
I.M., I.V.: 60 mg every 12 hours
Elderly: Not recommended for use in the elderly (see Geriatric Considerations).

Available Dosage Forms
Injection, solution, as citrate: 30 mg/mL (2 mL) [contains sodium bisulfite]
Tablet, extended release, as citrate: 100 mg

Monitoring and Teaching Issues
Physical Assessment: Monitor effectiveness of therapy (according to rational for therapy) and adverse reactions at beginning of therapy and periodically with long-term use. Do not discontinue abruptly; taper dosage slowly. Assess knowledge/teach patient appropriate use, interventions to reduce side effects, and adverse symptoms to report.
Patient Education: Take exactly as directed. Do not increase dose or discontinue without consulting prescriber. Do not chew or crush sustained release tablets. Do not use alcohol, prescriptive or OTC antidepressants, sedatives, or pain medications without consulting prescriber. You may experience drowsiness, dizziness, lightheadedness (avoid driving or engaging in tasks requiring alertness until response to drug is known); nausea or vomiting (small frequent meals, frequent mouth care, or sucking hard candy may help); constipation (increased exercise, fluids, fruit, or fibers may help); or decreased urination (void before taking medication). Report excessive drowsiness or mental agitation, chest pain, skin rash, swelling of mouth/face, difficulty speaking, or vision changes. **Pregnancy/breast-feeding precautions:** Inform prescriber if you are or intend to become pregnant. Consult prescriber if breast-feeding.
Geriatric Considerations: Because of its anticholinergic side effects, orphenadrine is not a drug of choice in the elderly.
Pregnancy Risk Factor: C
Lactation: Excretion in breast milk unknown

Administration
Oral: Do not crush sustained release drug product.

Orphenadrine, Aspirin, and Caffeine
(or FEN a dreen, AS pir in, & KAF een)

U.S. Brand Names Norgesic™; Norgesic™ Forte; Orphengesic; Orphengesic Forte
Synonyms Aspirin, Orphenadrine, and Caffeine; Caffeine, Orphenadrine, and Aspirin
Generic Available Yes
Pharmacologic Category Skeletal Muscle Relaxant
Medication Safety Issues
Sound-alike/look-alike issues:
Norgesic™ Forte may be confused with Norgesic 40®
Use Relief of discomfort associated with skeletal muscular conditions
Dosing
Adults: Muscular pain/spasms: Oral: 1-2 tablets 3-4 times/day
Elderly: Not recommended for use in the elderly; see individual agents
Available Dosage Forms
Tablet: Orphenadrine citrate 25 mg, aspirin 385 mg, and caffeine 30 mg; orphenadrine citrate 50 mg, aspirin 770 mg, and caffeine 60 mg
Norgesic™, Orphengesic: Orphenadrine citrate 25 mg, aspirin 385 mg, and caffeine 30 mg
Norgesic™ Forte, Orphengesic Forte: Orphenadrine citrate 50 mg, aspirin 770 mg, and caffeine 60 mg
Monitoring and Teaching Issues
Physical Assessment: Refer to Orphenadrine and Aspirin monographs (see Related Information).
Patient Education: Refer to Orphenadrine and Aspirin Monographs (see Related Information). **Pregnancy/breast-feeding precautions:** Inform prescriber if you are or intend to become pregnant. Consult prescriber if breast-feeding.
Pregnancy Risk Factor: D
Lactation: Enters breast milk/use caution due to aspirin content
Related Information
Aspirin on page 143
Orphenadrine on page 1124

- **Ortho-Cyclen®**   *see Ethinyl Estradiol and Norgestimate on page 593*
- **Ortho-Novum®**   *see Ethinyl Estradiol and Norethindrone on page 589*
- **Ortho-Novum® 1/50**   *see Mestranol and Norethindrone on page 962*
- **Ortho Tri-Cyclen®**   *see Ethinyl Estradiol and Norgestimate on page 593*
- **Ortho Tri-Cyclen® Lo**   *see Ethinyl Estradiol and Norgestimate on page 593*
- **Orudis® KT [OTC]**   *see Ketoprofen on page 851*
- **Oruvail®**   *see Ketoprofen on page 851*
- **Orvaten™**   *see Midodrine on page 1005*
- **Os-Cal® 500 [OTC]**   *see Calcium Carbonate on page 235*

Oseltamivir (oh sel TAM i vir)

U.S. Brand Names Tamiflu®

Generic Available No

Pharmacologic Category Antiviral Agent; Neuraminidase Inhibitor

Medication Safety Issues
Sound-alike/look-alike issues:
Tamiflu® may be confused with Thera-Flu®

Use Treatment of uncomplicated acute illness due to influenza (A or B) infection in adults and children >1 year of age who have been symptomatic for no more than 2 days; prophylaxis against influenza (A or B) infection in adults and adolescents ≥13 years of age

Mechanism of Action/Effect Thought to inhibit influenza virus by altering virus particle aggregation and release

Contraindications Hypersensitivity to oseltamivir or any component of the formulation

Warnings/Precautions Oseltamivir is not a substitute for the flu shot. Dosage adjustment is required for creatinine clearance between 10-30 mL/minute. Safety and efficacy in children (<18 years) have not been established for treatment regimens. Safety and efficacy have not been established for prophylactic use in patients <13 years of age. Also consider primary or concomitant bacterial infections. Safety and efficacy for treatment or prophylaxis in immuno-compromised patients have not been established.

Drug Interactions
Increased Effect/Toxicity: Cimetidine and amoxicillin have no effect on plasma concentrations. Probenecid increases oseltamivir carboxylate serum concentration by twofold. Dosage adjustments are not required.

Adverse Reactions
As seen with **treatment** doses: 1% to 10%:
Central nervous system: Insomnia (adults 1%), vertigo (adults 1%)
Gastrointestinal: Nausea (adults 10%), vomiting (adults 9%, children 15%), abdominal pain (children 5%)
Ocular: Conjunctivitis (children 1%)
Otic: Ear disorder (children 2%)
Respiratory: Epistaxis (children 3%)
Similar adverse effects were seen in **prophylactic** use, however, the incidence was generally less. The following reactions were seen more commonly with prophylactic use: Headache (20%), fatigue (8%), diarrhea (3%)

Overdosage/Toxicology Single doses of 1000 mg resulted in nausea and vomiting.

Pharmacodynamics/Kinetics
Absorption: Well absorbed
Bioavailability: 75% reaches systemic circulation in active form
Time to Peak: C_{max}: Oseltamivir: 65 ng/mL; Oseltamivir carboxylate: 348 ng/mL
Protein Binding: Plasma: Oseltamivir carboxylate: 3%; Oseltamivir: 42%
Half-Life Elimination: Oseltamivir carboxylate: 6-10 hours; similar in geriatrics (68-78 years)
Metabolism: Hepatic (90%) to oseltamivir carboxylate; neither the parent drug nor active metabolite has any effect on CYP.
Excretion: Urine (as carboxylate metabolite)

Dosing
Adults & Elderly:
Influenza prophylaxis: Oral: 75 mg once daily for at least 7 days; treatment should begin within 2 days of contact with an infected individual. During community outbreaks, dosing is 75 mg once daily. May be used for up to 6 weeks; duration of protection lasts for length of dosing period
Influenza treatment: Oral: 75 mg twice daily initiated within 2 days of onset of symptoms; duration of treatment: 5 days
Pediatrics:
Influenza prophylaxis: Adolescents ≥13 years: Oral: 75 mg once daily for at least 7 days; treatment should begin within 2 days of contact with an infected individual. During community outbreaks, dosing is 75 mg once daily. May be used for up to 6 weeks; duration of protection lasts for length of dosing period.
Influenza treatment: Oral:
Note: Initiate treatment within 2 days of onset of symptoms; duration of treatment: 5 days:
Children: 1-12 years:
≤15 kg: 30 mg twice daily
>15 kg - ≤23 kg: 45 mg twice daily
>23 kg - ≤40 kg: 60 mg twice daily
>40 kg: 75 mg twice daily
Adolescents ≥13 years: Refer to adult dosing.
Renal Impairment:
Cl_{cr} 10-30 mL/minute:
Treatment: Reduce dose to 75 mg once daily for 5 days.
Prophylaxis: Administer 75 mg every other day.
Cl_{cr} <10 mL/minute: Has not been studied.

Hepatic Impairment: Has not been evaluated

Available Dosage Forms

Capsule, as phosphate: 75 mg

Powder for oral suspension: 12 mg/mL (25 mL) [contains sodium benzoate; tutti-frutti flavor]

Monitoring and Teaching Issues

Physical Assessment: This is not a substitute for the influenza vaccine. Teach patient appropriate use, interventions to reduce side effects, and adverse reactions to report.

Patient Education: This is not a substitute for the flu shot. Must be taken within 2 days of onset of flu symptoms (eg, fever, cough, headache, fatigue, muscular weakness, and sore throat). Take as directed; do not increase dose or frequency, and do not miss a dose. You may experience nausea or vomiting (small frequent meals, good mouth care, chewing gum, or sucking hard candy may help). Report significant adverse effects to your prescriber. **Pregnancy/breast-feeding precautions:** Inform prescriber if you are or intend to become pregnant. Breast-feeding is not recommended.

Dietary Considerations: Take with or without food; take with food to improve tolerance.

Pregnancy Risk Factor: C

Lactation: Excretion in breast milk unknown/not recommended

Breast-Feeding Issues: Oseltamivir and its metabolite are excreted in the breast milk of lactating rats. It is unknown if they appear in human milk.

Administration

Reconstitution: Oral suspension: Reconstitute with 23 mL of water (to make 25 mL total suspension).

Storage:

Capsules: Store at 25°C (77°F).

Oral suspension: Store powder for suspension at 25°C (77°F). Once reconstituted, store suspension under refrigeration at 2°C to 8°C (36°F to 46°F); do not freeze. Use within 10 days of preparation.

♦ **OSI-774** *see* Erlotinib *on page 540*

♦ **Osmitrol®** *see* Mannitol *on page 932*

♦ **Osteoporosis Management** *see page 1853*

♦ **Oticaine** *see* Benzocaine *on page 181*

♦ **Otocaine™** *see* Benzocaine *on page 181*

♦ **Outgro® [OTC]** *see* Benzocaine *on page 181*

♦ **Ovace™** *see* Sulfacetamide *on page 1403*

♦ **Ovcon®** *see* Ethinyl Estradiol and Norethindrone *on page 589*

♦ **Overdose and Toxicology** *see page 1775*

♦ **Ovidrel®** *see* Chorionic Gonadotropin (Recombinant) *on page 320*

♦ **Ovrette®** *see* Norgestrel *on page 1098*

Oxaliplatin (ox AL i pla tin)

U.S. Brand Names Eloxatin™

Synonyms Diaminocyclohexane Oxalatoplatinum; L-OHP; NSC-266046

Generic Available No

Pharmacologic Category Antineoplastic Agent, Alkylating Agent

Medication Safety Issues

Sound-alike/look-alike issues:

Oxaliplatin may be confused with Aloxi™

Use Treatment of advanced colon cancer and advanced rectal carcinoma

Unlabeled/Investigational Use Head and neck cancer, nonsmall cell lung cancer, non-Hodgkin's lymphoma, ovarian cancer

Mechanism of Action/Effect Oxaliplatin is an alkylating agent. It binds to DNA, RNA, or proteins, disrupting DNA function. Cytotoxicity is cell-cycle nonspecific.

Contraindications Hypersensitivity to oxaliplatin, other platinum-containing compounds, or any component of the formulation; pregnancy

Warnings/Precautions The U.S. Food and Drug Administration (FDA) currently recommends that procedures for proper handling and disposal of antineoplastic agents be considered. Anaphylactic-like reaction may occur within minutes of oxaliplatin administration. Two different types of neuropathy may occur: First, acute (within first 2 days), reversible (resolves within 14 days), primarily peripheral symptoms that are often exacerbated by cold (may include pharyngolaryngeal dysesthesia); and secondly, a more persistent (>14 days) presentation that often interferes with daily activities (eg, writing, buttoning, swallowing), these symptoms may improve upon discontinuing treatment. May cause pulmonary fibrosis or hepatotoxicity. The presence of hepatic vascular disorders (including veno-occlusive disease) should be considered, especially in individuals developing portal hypertension or who present with increased liver function tests. Caution in renal dysfunction. Safety and efficacy in pediatric patients have not been established.

Drug Interactions

Increased Effect/Toxicity: Taxane derivatives may increase oxaliplatin toxicity if administered before the platin as a sequential infusion. Nephrotoxic agents may increase oxaliplatin toxicity. Prolonged prothrombin time and increased INR associated with hemorrhage have been reported in patients receiving oxaliplatin/fluorouracil/leucovorin concomitantly with oral anticoagulants.

Adverse Reactions Based on clinical trial data using oxaliplatin alone. Some adverse effects (eg, thrombocytopenia, hemorrhagic events, neutropenia) may be increased when therapy is combined with fluorouracil/leucovorin.

>10%:

Central nervous system: Fatigue (61%), fever (25%), pain (14%), headache (13%), insomnia (11%)

Gastrointestinal: Nausea (64%), diarrhea (46%), vomiting (37%), abdominal pain (31%), constipation (31%), anorexia (20%), stomatitis (14%)

Hematologic: Anemia (64%), thrombocytopenia (30%), leukopenia (13%)

(Continued)

Oxaliplatin *(Continued)*

Hepatic: SGOT increased (54%), SGPT increased (36%); total bilirubin increased (13%)

Neuromuscular & skeletal: Neuropathy (may be dose-limiting), peripheral (acute 56%, persistent 48%), back pain (11%)

Respiratory: Dyspnea (13%), cough (11%)

1% to 10%:

Cardiovascular: Edema (10%), chest pain (5%), flushing (3%), thrombosis (2% to 6%), thromboembolism (6% to 9%)

Central nervous system: Rigors (9%), dizziness (7%), hand-foot syndrome (1%)

Dermatologic: Rash (5%), alopecia (3%)

Endocrine & metabolic: Dehydration (5%), hypokalemia (3%)

Gastrointestinal: Dyspepsia (7%), taste perversion (5%), flatulence (3%), mucositis (2%), gastroesophageal reflux (1%), dysphagia (acute 1% to 2%)

Genitourinary: Dysuria (1%)

Hematologic: Neutropenia (7%)

Local: Injection site reaction (9%)

Neuromuscular & skeletal: Arthralgia (7%)

Ocular: Abnormal lacrimation (1%)

Renal: Serum creatinine increased (10%)

Respiratory: URI (7%), rhinitis (6%), epistaxis (2%), pharyngitis (2%), pharyngolaryngeal dysesthesia (1% to 2%)

Miscellaneous: Allergic reactions (3%), hiccup (2%)

Overdosage/Toxicology Overdose symptoms are extensions of known side effects (eg, thrombocytopenia, myelosuppression, nausea, vomiting, neurotoxicity, respiratory symptoms). Treatment should be supportive.

Pharmacodynamics/Kinetics

Protein Binding: >90% primarily albumin and gamma globulin (irreversible binding to platinum)

Half-Life Elimination: Distribution: Alpha phase: 0.4, Beta phase: 16.8 hours

Metabolism: Nonenzymatic (rapid and extensive), forms active and inactive derivatives

Excretion: Primarily urine

Dosing

Adults:

Colorectal cancer (labeled dosing): Refer to individual protocols. I.V.:

85 mg/m^2 every 2 weeks **or**

20-25 mg/m^2 days 1-5 every 3 weeks **or**

100-130 mg/m^2 every 2-3 weeks

Dosage adjustments for toxicity: Longer infusion times (over 6 hours instead of 2 hours) may mitigate acute toxicities. In patients experiencing persistent neurosensory events (grade 2) which do not resolve, a dose reduction may be considered. Grade 3 neurosensory events may prompt consideration to discontinue oxaliplatin (while fluorouracil/leucovorin are continued or decreased). After recovery from grade 3/4 gastrointestinal toxicity, grade 4 neutropenia, or grade 3/4 thrombocytopenia, a dosage reduction is recommended.

Elderly: No dosing adjustment recommended.

Renal Impairment: Use with caution; specific guidelines not established.

Available Dosage Forms

Injection, powder for reconstitution: 50 mg, 100 mg [contains lactose]

Injection, solution [preservative free]: 5 mg/mL (10 mL, 20 mL)

Monitoring and Teaching Issues

Physical Assessment: See Warnings/Precautions for use cautions (renal impairment). Assess potential for interactions with other pharmacological agents (eg, increased toxicity with taxane derivatives or nephrotoxic agents; see Drug Interactions). See Administration for infusion specifics. Patient must be observed closely for anaphylactic-like reactions (which can occur within minutes of administration; see Warnings/Precautions). Assess effectiveness and adverse reactions during and between each infusion (eg, pulmonary and hepatic toxicity, neuropathy, GI disturbance, anemia, chest pain, thromboembolism, abnormal lacrimation; see Adverse Reactions). Teach patient possible side effects/appropriate interventions and adverse symptoms to report (see Patient Education).

Patient Education: Do not take any new medication during therapy without consulting prescriber. This medication can only be administered by infusion; you will be monitored closely during and following infusion. Report immediately any pain, burning, swelling at infusion site, or any signs of allergic reaction (eg, respiratory or swallowing difficulty, back pain, chest tightness, rash, hives, swelling of lips or mouth). It is important that you maintain adequate nutrition (small frequent meals may help) and adequate hydration (2-3 L/day of fluids) unless instructed to restrict fluid intake. You will be susceptible to infection (avoid crowds and exposure to infection and do not have any vaccinations without consulting prescriber). May cause nausea, vomiting, loss of appetite, or taste perversion (small frequent meals, frequent mouth care, chewing gum, or sucking lozenges may help; if nausea/vomiting is unresolved, consult prescriber for approved antiemetic); mouth sores (use soft toothbrush or cotton swabs for mouth care); diarrhea (boiled milk, buttermilk, or yogurt may help); or loss of hair (reversible). Report any numbness, pain, tingling, or loss of sensation of extremities; chest pain or palpitations; swelling, pain, or hot areas in legs; unusual fatigue; unusual bruising or bleeding; respiratory difficulty; muscle cramps or twitching; change in hearing acuity; or other persistent adverse effects. **Pregnancy/ breast-feeding precautions:** Do not get pregnant while taking this medication; use appropriate barrier contraceptive measures. Breast-feeding is not recommended.

Pregnancy Risk Factor: D

Lactation: Excretion in breast milk unknown/not recommended

Administration

I.V.: Administer as I.V. infusion over 2-6 hours. Longer infusion times (eg, those approaching or equal to 6 hours) may mitigate signs/symptoms of acute reactions. Flush infusion line with D$_5$W prior to administration of any concomitant medication.

Reconstitution: Do not reconstitute using a chloride-containing solution (eg, NaCl). Further dilution with D$_5$W (250 or 500 mL) is required prior to administration. Reconstituted solution does not require protection from light.

Compatibility: Incompatible with alkaline solutions (eg, fluorouracil) and chloride-containing solutions. Flush infusion line with D$_5$W prior to, and following, administration of concomitant medications via same I.V. line.

Storage: Store in original outer carton at room temperature of 15°C to 30°C (59°F to 86°F); do not freeze. Protect from light. Diluted solution is stable up to 6 hours at room temperature of 20°C to 25°C (68°F to 77°F) or up to 24 hours under refrigeration at 2°C to 8°C (36°F to 46°F).

Oxaprozin (oks a PROE zin)

U.S. Brand Names Daypro®

Generic Available Yes

Pharmacologic Category Nonsteroidal Anti-inflammatory Drug (NSAID), Oral

Medication Safety Issues

Sound-alike/look-alike issues:

Daypro® may be confused with Diupres®

Oxaprozin may be confused with oxazepam

Use Acute and long-term use in the management of signs and symptoms of osteoarthritis and rheumatoid arthritis; juvenile rheumatoid arthritis

Mechanism of Action/Effect Inhibits prostaglandin synthesis by decreasing the activity of the enzyme, cyclooxygenase, which results in decreased formation of prostaglandin precursors

Contraindications Hypersensitivity to oxaprozin, aspirin, other NSAIDs, or any component of the formulation; advanced kidney disease; pregnancy (3rd trimester)

Warnings/Precautions Fatal asthmatic and anaphylactoid reactions have occurred in patients with "aspirin triad." Use with caution in patients with CHF, hypertension, dehydration, decreased renal or hepatic function, history of GI disease (bleeding, ulcers, or previous GI symptoms with NSAID use), or those receiving anticoagulants and/or corticosteroids. Use lowest effective dose for shortest period possible; bleeding risk has been correlated to dose and duration of therapy. Gastrointestinal bleeding may occur without prior symptoms of gastrointestinal irritation. Elderly are at a high risk for adverse effects from NSAIDs. As many as 60% of elderly can develop peptic ulceration and/or hemorrhage asymptomatically.

Use of NSAIDs can compromise existing renal function especially when Cl$_{cr}$ <30 mL/minute. CNS adverse effects such as confusion, agitation, and hallucination are generally seen in overdose or high-dose situations; however, elderly may demonstrate these adverse effects at lower doses than younger adults. Do not exceed 3200 mg/day. Withhold for at least 4-6 half-lives prior to surgical or dental procedures.

Rare cases of severe hepatic reactions (including necrosis, jaundice, fulminant hepatitis) have been reported. May cause mild photosensitivity reactions. Safety and efficacy have not been established in children <6 years of age.

Drug Interactions

Decreased Effect: Oxaprozin may decrease the effect of some antihypertensive agents (including ACE inhibitors and angiotensin antagonists) and diuretics.

Increased Effect/Toxicity: Oxaprozin may increase cyclosporine, digoxin, lithium, and methotrexate serum concentrations. The renal adverse effects of ACE inhibitors may be potentiated by NSAIDs. Corticosteroids may increase the risk of GI ulceration. The risk of bleeding with anticoagulants (warfarin, antiplatelet agents, low molecular weight heparins) may be increased.

Nutritional/Ethanol Interactions

Ethanol: Avoid ethanol (may enhance gastric mucosal irritation).

Herb/Nutraceutical: Avoid cat's claw, dong quai, evening primrose, feverfew, garlic, ginger, ginkgo, red clover, horse chestnut, green tea, ginseng (all have additional antiplatelet activity).

Lab Interactions False-positive urine immunoassay screening tests for benzodiazepines have been reported and may occur several days after discontinuing oxaprozin.

Adverse Reactions

1% to 10%:

Cardiovascular: Edema

Central nervous system: Confusion, depression, dizziness, headache, sedation, sleep disturbance, somnolence

Dermatologic: Pruritus, rash

Gastrointestinal: Abdominal distress, abdominal pain, anorexia, constipation, diarrhea, flatulence, gastrointestinal ulcer, gross bleeding with perforation, heartburn, nausea, vomiting

Hematologic: Anemia, bleeding time increased

Hepatic: Liver enzyme elevation

Otic: Tinnitus

Renal: Dysuria, renal function abnormal, urinary frequency

Overdosage/Toxicology Symptoms of overdose include acute renal failure, vomiting, drowsiness, and leukocytes. Management of NSAID intoxication is supportive and symptomatic. Since many NSAIDs undergo enterohepatic cycling, multiple doses of charcoal may be needed to reduce the potential for delayed toxicities.

(Continued)

Oxaprozin (Continued)

Pharmacodynamics/Kinetics

Onset of Action: Steady-state 4-7 days

Absorption: Almost complete

Time to Peak: 2-4 hours

Protein Binding: >99%

Half-Life Elimination: 40-50 hours

Metabolism: Hepatic via oxidation and glucuronidation; no active metabolites

Excretion: Urine (5% unchanged, 65% as metabolites); feces (35% as metabolites)

Dosing

Adults & Elderly:

Osteoarthritis: Oral: 600-1200 mg once daily; patients should be titrated to lowest dose possible; patients with low body weight should start with 600 mg daily

Rheumatoid arthritis: Oral: 1200 mg once daily; a one-time loading dose of up to 1800 mg/day or 26 mg/kg (whichever is lower) may be given

Note: Maximum: 1800 mg/day or 26 mg/kg (whichever is lower) in divided doses

Pediatrics:

Juvenile rheumatoid arthritis: Oral:

Note: Individualize to lowest effective dose.

Children 6-16 years:

22-31 kg: 600 mg once daily

32-54 kg: 900 mg once daily

≥55 kg: 1200 mg once daily

Renal Impairment: 600 mg once daily; dose may be increased to 1200 mg with close monitoring.

Hepatic Impairment: Use caution in patients with severe dysfunction.

Available Dosage Forms Tablet: 600 mg

Monitoring and Teaching Issues

Physical Assessment: Assess effectiveness and interactions of other medications patient may be taking. Assess results of laboratory tests, therapeutic effectiveness, and adverse reactions at beginning of therapy and periodically throughout therapy. Schedule ophthalmic evaluations for patients who develop eye complaints during long-term NSAID therapy. Assess knowledge/teach patient appropriate use, interventions to reduce side effects, and adverse symptoms to report.

Monitoring Laboratory Tests: CBC; hepatic, renal function

Patient Education: Take this medication exactly as directed; do not increase dose without consulting prescriber. Do not crush tablets. Take with food or milk to reduce GI distress. Maintain adequate hydration (2-3 L/day of fluids) unless instructed to restrict fluid intake. Do not use alcohol, aspirin or aspirin-containing medication, or any other anti-inflammatory medications without consulting prescriber. You may experience drowsiness, dizziness, or nervousness (use caution when driving or engaging in tasks requiring alertness until response to drug is known); anorexia, nausea, vomiting, or heartburn (small frequent meals, frequent mouth care, sucking lozenges, or chewing gum may help). GI bleeding, ulceration, or perforation can occur with or without pain. Discontinue medication and contact prescriber if persistent abdominal pain, cramping, or blood in stool occurs. Report vaginal bleeding; breathlessness, respiratory difficulty, or unusual cough; chest pain, rapid heartbeat, palpitations; unusual bruising or bleeding (blood in urine, mouth, or vomitus); swollen extremities; skin rash or itching; acute fatigue; or swelling of face, lips, tongue, or throat. **Pregnancy/breast-feeding precautions:** Inform prescriber if you are or intend to become pregnant. This drug should not be used in the 3rd trimester of pregnancy. Breast-feeding is not recommended.

Geriatric Considerations: Elderly are at high risk for adverse effects from NSAIDs. As much as 60% of elderly can develop peptic ulceration and/or hemorrhage asymptomatically. The concomitant use of H_2 blockers, omeprazole, and sucralfate is not generally effective as prophylaxis with the exception of NSAID-induced duodenal ulcers which may be prevented by the use of ranitidine. Misoprostol is the only prophylactic agent proven effective. Also, concomitant disease and drug use contribute to the risk for GI adverse effects. Use lowest effective dose for shortest period possible. Consider renal function decline with age. Use of NSAIDs can compromise existing renal function especially when Cl_{cr} is ≤30 mL/minute. Tinnitus may be a difficult and unreliable indication of toxicity due to age-related hearing loss or eighth cranial nerve damage. CNS adverse effects such as confusion, agitation, and hallucination are generally seen in overdose or high-dose situations, but elderly may demonstrate these adverse effects at lower doses than younger adults.

Pregnancy Risk Factor: C/D (3rd trimester)

Pregnancy Issues: Safety and efficacy in pregnant women have not been established. Exposure late in pregnancy may lead to premature closure of the ductus arteriosus and may inhibit uterine contractions.

Lactation: Excretion in breast milk unknown/not recommended

Administration

Storage: Store at 25°C (77°F). Protect from light. Keep bottle tightly closed.

Related Information

Nonsalicylate / Nonsteroidal Anti-inflammatory Agents *on page 1743*

Oxazepam (oks A ze pam)

U.S. Brand Names Serax®

Controlled Substance C-IV

Generic Available Yes: Capsule

Pharmacologic Category Benzodiazepine

Medication Safety Issues

Sound-alike/look-alike issues:

Oxazepam may be confused with oxaprozin, quazepam

Serax® may be confused with Eurax®, Urex®, Zyrtec®

Use Treatment of anxiety; management of ethanol withdrawal

Unlabeled/Investigational Use Anticonvulsant in management of simple partial seizures; hypnotic

Mechanism of Action/Effect Binds to stereospecific benzodiazepine receptors on the post-synaptic GABA neuron at several sites within the central nervous system, including the limbic system, reticular formation. Enhancement of the inhibitory effect of GABA on neuronal excitability results by increased neuronal membrane permeability to chloride ions. This shift in chloride ions results in hyperpolarization (a less excitable state) and stabilization.

Contraindications Hypersensitivity to oxazepam or any component of the formulation (cross-sensitivity with other benzodiazepines may exist); narrow-angle glaucoma (not in product labeling, however, benzodiazepines are contraindicated); not indicated for use in the treatment of psychosis; pregnancy

Warnings/Precautions May cause hypotension (rare) - use with caution in patients with cardiovascular or cerebrovascular disease, or in patients who would not tolerate transient decreases in blood pressure. Serax® 15 mg tablet contains tartrazine; use is not recommended in pediatric patients <6 years of age; dose has not been established between 6-12 years of age.

Use with caution in elderly or debilitated patients, patients with hepatic disease (including alcoholics), or renal impairment. Use with caution in patients with respiratory disease or impaired gag reflex. Avoid use in patients with sleep apnea.

Causes CNS depression (dose-related) resulting in sedation, dizziness, confusion, or ataxia which may impair physical and mental capabilities. Use with caution in patients receiving other CNS depressants or psychoactive agents. Benzodiazepines have been associated with falls and traumatic injury and should be used with extreme caution in patients who are at risk of these events (especially the elderly).

Use caution in patients with depression, particularly if suicidal risk may be present. Use with caution in patients with a history of drug dependence. Benzodiazepines have been associated with dependence and acute withdrawal symptoms on discontinuation or reduction in dose.

Benzodiazepines have been associated with anterograde amnesia. Paradoxical reactions, including hyperactive or aggressive behavior have been reported with benzodiazepines, particularly in adolescent/pediatric or psychiatric patients. Does not have analgesic, antidepressant, or antipsychotic properties.

Drug Interactions

Decreased Effect: Oral contraceptives may increase the clearance of oxazepam. Theophylline and other CNS stimulants may antagonize the sedative effects of oxazepam. Phenytoin may increase the clearance of oxazepam.

Increased Effect/Toxicity: Ethanol and other CNS depressants may increase the CNS effects of oxazepam. Oxazepam may decrease the antiparkinsonian efficacy of levodopa. Flumazenil may cause seizures if administered following long-term benzodiazepine treatment.

Nutritional/Ethanol Interactions

Ethanol: Avoid ethanol (may increase CNS depression).

Herb/Nutraceutical: Avoid valerian, St John's wort, kava kava, gotu kola (may increase CNS depression).

Adverse Reactions Frequency not defined.

Cardiovascular: Syncope (rare), edema

Central nervous system: Drowsiness, ataxia, dizziness, vertigo, memory impairment, headache, paradoxical reactions (excitement, stimulation of effect), lethargy, amnesia, euphoria

Dermatologic: Rash

Endocrine & metabolic: Decreased libido, menstrual irregularities

Genitourinary: Incontinence

Hematologic: Leukopenia, blood dyscrasias

Hepatic: Jaundice

Neuromuscular & skeletal: Dysarthria, tremor, reflex slowing

Ocular: Blurred vision, diplopia

Miscellaneous: Drug dependence

Overdosage/Toxicology Symptoms of overdose include somnolence, confusion, coma, hypoactive reflexes, dyspnea, hypotension, slurred speech, and impaired coordination. Treatment for benzodiazepine overdose is supportive. Flumazenil has been shown to selectively block the binding of benzodiazepines to CNS receptors, resulting in a reversal of benzodiazepine-induced CNS depression, but not respiratory depression due to toxicity.

Pharmacodynamics/Kinetics

Absorption: Almost complete

Time to Peak: Serum: 2-4 hours

Protein Binding: 86% to 99%

Half-Life Elimination: 2.8-5.7 hours

Metabolism: Hepatic to inactive compounds (primarily as glucuronides)

Excretion: Urine (as unchanged drug (50%) and metabolites)

Dosing

Adults:

Anxiety: Oral: 10-30 mg 3-4 times/day

Ethanol withdrawal: Oral: 15-30 mg 3-4 times/day

Hypnotic: Oral: 15-30 mg

Elderly: Oral: Anxiety: 10 mg 2-3 times/day; increase gradually as needed to a total of 30-45 mg/day. Dose titration should be slow to evaluate sensitivity.

Pediatrics:

Anxiety: Oral: Children: 1 mg/kg/day has been administered

(Continued)

Oxazepam *(Continued)*

Renal Impairment: Not dialyzable (0% to 5%)

Available Dosage Forms

Capsule: 10 mg, 15 mg, 30 mg

Tablet: 15 mg [contains tartrazine]

Monitoring and Teaching Issues

Physical Assessment: Assess other medications the patient may be taking for effectiveness and interactions. Assess for history of addiction; long-term use can result in dependence, abuse, or tolerance; periodically evaluate need for continued use. For inpatient use, institute safety measures and monitor effectiveness and adverse reactions. For outpatients, monitor therapeutic effectiveness and adverse reactions at beginning of therapy and periodically with long-term use. Can cause CNS depression (dose-related); monitor for sedation, dizziness, confusion, or ataxia which may impair physical and mental capabilities. Be alert to the possibility of suicide ideation. Taper dosage slowly when discontinuing. Assess knowledge/teach patient appropriate use, interventions to reduce side effects, and adverse symptoms to report.

Patient Education: Take exactly as directed; do not increase dose or frequency. It may take 2-3 weeks to achieve desired results. Drug may cause physical and/or psychological dependence. Do not use alcohol or other prescription or OTC medications (especially pain medications, sedatives, antihistamines, or hypnotics) without consulting prescriber. Maintain adequate hydration (2-3 L/day of fluids) unless instructed to restrict fluid intake. You may experience drowsiness, lightheadedness, impaired coordination, dizziness, or blurred vision (use caution when driving or engaging in tasks requiring alertness until response to drug is known); nausea, vomiting, or dry mouth (small frequent meals, frequent mouth care, chewing gum, or sucking lozenges may help); constipation (increased exercise, fluids, fruit, or fiber may help); altered sexual drive or ability (reversible); or photosensitivity (use sunscreen, wear protective clothing and eyewear, and avoid direct sunlight). Report persistent CNS effects (eg, confusion, depression, thoughts of suicide, increased sedation, excitation, headache, agitation, insomnia or nightmares, dizziness, fatigue, impaired coordination, changes in personality, or changes in cognition); changes in urinary pattern; muscle cramping, weakness, tremors, or rigidity; ringing in ears or visual disturbances; chest pain, palpitations, or rapid heartbeat; excessive perspiration, excessive GI symptoms (cramping, constipation, vomiting, anorexia); or worsening of condition. **Pregnancy/breast-feeding precautions:** Do not get pregnant while taking this medication; use appropriate contraceptive measures. Breast-feeding is not recommended.

Geriatric Considerations: Because of its relatively short half-life and its lack of active metabolites, oxazepam is recommended for use in the elderly when a benzodiazepine is indicated.

Pregnancy Risk Factor: D

Pregnancy Issues: Benzodiazepines cross the placenta. The association between benzodiazepine exposure and malformations remains controversial. A number of types of malformation have been reported (oral cleft, inguinal hernia, cardiac defects, spina bifida, dysmorphic facial features, skeletal defects); however, confounding factors make a clear association difficult. Overall, the risk to the fetus may be low. Nonteratogenic effects (including neonatal flaccidity, respiratory and feeding problems, and withdrawal symptoms) during the postnatal period have also been reported with benzodiazepine use.

Lactation: Enters breast milk/not recommended

Other Issues: Taper dosage gradually after long-term therapy, especially in epileptic patients. Abrupt withdrawal may cause tremors, nausea, vomiting, abdominal and/or muscle cramps.

Administration

Oral: Give orally in divided doses

Additional Information Not intended for management of anxieties and minor distresses associated with everyday life. Treatment longer than 4 months should be re-evaluated to determine the patient's need for the drug. Abrupt discontinuation after sustained use (generally >10 days) may cause withdrawal symptoms.

Related Information

Anxiolytic / Hypnotic Use in Long-Term Care Facilities *on page 1769*
Benzodiazepines *on page 1719*
Federal OBRA Regulations: Recommended Maximum Doses *on page 1773*

Oxcarbazepine *(ox car BAZ e peen)*

U.S. Brand Names Trileptal®

Synonyms GP 47680; OCBZ

Generic Available No

Pharmacologic Category Anticonvulsant, Miscellaneous

Use Monotherapy or adjunctive therapy in the treatment of partial seizures in adults and children (4-16 years of age) with epilepsy

Unlabeled/Investigational Use Bipolar disorder

Mechanism of Action/Effect Precise mechanism of action has not been determined. Believed to prevent the spread of seizures by decreasing propagation of synaptic impulses.

Contraindications Hypersensitivity to oxcarbazepine or any component of the formulation

Warnings/Precautions Clinically-significant hyponatremia (sodium <125 mmol/L) can develop during oxcarbazepine use; monitor serum sodium, particularly during the first 3 months of therapy or in patients at risk for hyponatremia. Potentially serious, sometimes fatal, dermatologic reactions (eg, Stevens-Johnson, toxic epidermal necrolysis) and multi-organ hypersensitivity reactions have been reported in adults and children; monitor for signs and symptoms of skin reactions and possible disparate manifestations associated with lymphatic, hepatic, renal and/or hematologic organ systems; gradual discontinuation and conversion to alternate therapy may be required. As with all antiepileptic drugs, oxcarbazepine should be withdrawn gradually to minimize the potential of increased seizure frequency. Use of oxcarbazepine has been associated with CNS related adverse events, most significant of these were cognitive symptoms including psychomotor slowing, difficulty with concentration, and speech or language problems, somnolence or fatigue, and coordination abnormalities, including ataxia and gait disturbances. Use caution in patients with previous hypersensitivity to carbamazepine (cross-sensitivity occurs in 25% to 30%). May reduce the efficacy of oral contraceptives (nonhormonal contraceptive measures are recommended).

Drug Interactions
Cytochrome P450 Effect: Inhibits CYP2C19 (weak); **Induces** CYP3A4 (strong)

Decreased Effect: Oxcarbazepine serum concentrations may be reduced by carbamazepine, phenytoin, phenobarbital, valproic acid and verapamil (decreases levels of active oxcarbazepine metabolite). Oxcarbazepine reduces the serum concentrations oral contraceptives; use alternative contraceptive measures. Oxcarbazepine may decrease the levels/effects of benzodiazepines, calcium channel blockers, clarithromycin, cyclosporine, erythromycin, estrogens, mirtazapine, nateglinide, nefazodone, nevirapine, protease inhibitors, tacrolimus, venlafaxine, and other CYP3A4 substrates.

Increased Effect/Toxicity: Serum concentrations of phenytoin and phenobarbital are increased by oxcarbazepine.

Nutritional/Ethanol Interactions
Ethanol: Avoid ethanol (may increase CNS depression).
Herb/Nutraceutical: St John's wort may decrease oxcarbazepine levels. Avoid evening primrose (seizure threshold decreased). Avoid valerian, St John's wort, kava kava, gotu kola.

Lab Interactions Thyroid function tests may depress serum T_4 without affecting T_3 levels or TSH.

Adverse Reactions As reported in adults with doses of up to 2400 mg/day (includes patients on monotherapy, adjunctive therapy, and those not previously on AEDs); incidence in children was similar.

>10%:
Central nervous system: Dizziness (22% to 49%), somnolence (20% to 36%), headache (13% to 32%, placebo 23%), ataxia (5% to 31%), fatigue (12% to 15%), vertigo (6% to 15%)
Gastrointestinal: Vomiting (7% to 36%), nausea (15% to 29%), abdominal pain (10% to 13%)
Neuromuscular & skeletal: Abnormal gait (5% to 17%), tremor (3% to 16%)
Ocular: Diplopia (14% to 40%), nystagmus (7% to 26%), abnormal vision (4% to 14%)
1% to 10%:
Cardiovascular: Hypotension (1% to 2%), leg edema (1% to 2%, placebo 1%)
Central nervous system: Nervousness (2% to 5%, placebo 1% to 2%), amnesia (4%), abnormal thinking (2% to 4%), insomnia (2% to 4%), speech disorder (1% to 3%), EEG abnormalities (2%), abnormal feelings (1% to 2%), agitation (1% to 2%, placebo 1%), confusion (1% to 2%, placebo 1%)
Dermatologic: Rash (4%), acne (1% to 2%)
Endocrine & metabolic: Hyponatremia (1% to 3%, placebo 1%)
Gastrointestinal: Diarrhea (5% to 7%), dyspepsia (5% to 6%), constipation (2% to 6%, placebo 0% to 4%), gastritis (1% to 2%, placebo 1%), weight gain (1% to 2%, placebo 1%)
Neuromuscular & skeletal: Weakness (3% to 6%, placebo 5%), back pain (4%), falling down (4%), abnormal coordination (1% to 4%, placebo 1% to 2%), dysmetria (1% to 3%), sprains/strains (2%), muscle weakness (1% to 2%)
Ocular: Abnormal accommodation (2%)
Respiratory: Upper respiratory tract infection (7%), rhinitis (2% to 5%, placebo 4%), chest infection (4%), epistaxis (4%), sinusitis (4%)

Overdosage/Toxicology Symptoms may include CNS depression (somnolence, ataxia). Treatment is symptomatic and supportive.

Pharmacodynamics/Kinetics
Absorption: Complete; food has no affect on rate or extent
Bioavailability: Decreased in children <8 years; increased in elderly >60 years
Time to Peak: Serum: 4.5 hours (3-13 hours)
Protein Binding: Serum: MHD: 40%
Half-Life Elimination: Parent drug: 2 hours; MHD: 9 hours; renal impairment (Cl_{cr} 30 mL/minute): 19 hours
Metabolism: Hepatic to 10-monohydroxy metabolite (MHD; active); MHD is further conjugated to DHD (inactive)
Excretion: Urine (95%, <1% as unchanged oxcarbazepine, 27% as unchanged MHD, 49% as MHD glucuronides); feces (<4%)

Dosing
Adults & Elderly:
Adjunctive therapy, partial seizures (epilepsy): Oral: Initial: 300 mg twice daily; dosage may be increased by 600 mg/day at approximate weekly intervals. Recommended daily dose is 1200 mg/day in 2 divided doses. Although daily doses >1200 mg/day demonstrated greater efficacy, most patients were unable to tolerate 2400 mg/day (due to CNS effects).

Conversion to monotherapy, partial seizures (epilepsy): Oral: Patients receiving concomitant antiepileptic drugs (AEDs): Initial: 300 mg twice daily while simultaneously reducing the dose of concomitant AEDs. Withdraw concomitant AEDs completely over 3-6 weeks, while increasing the oxcarbazine dose in increments of 600 mg/day at weekly intervals, reaching the maximum oxcarbazine dose (2400 mg/day) in about 2-4 weeks (lower doses have been effective in patients in whom monotherapy has been initiated).

Initiation of monotherapy, partial seizures (epilepsy): Oral: Patients not receiving prior AEDs: 300 mg twice daily (total dose 600 mg/day). Increase dose by 300 mg/day every third day to a dose of 1200 mg/day. Higher dosages (2400 mg/day) have been shown to be effective in patients converted to monotherapy from other AEDs.

Pediatrics:
Adjunctive treatment, partial seizures (epilepsy): Oral: Children 4-16 years:
Initial: 8-10 mg/kg/day (not to exceed 600 mg/day) given in a twice daily regimen.
(Continued)

Oxcarbazepine *(Continued)*

Maintenance: The target maintenance dose should be achieved over 2 weeks, and depends on weight of the child:

20-29 kg: 900 mg/day in 2 divided doses
29.1-39 kg: 1200 mg/day in 2 divided doses
>39 kg: 1800 mg/day in 2 divided doses

Conversion to monotherapy: Oxcarbazepine 8-10 mg/kg/day in twice daily divided doses, while simultaneously initiating the reduction of the dose of the concomitant antiepileptic drug; the concomitant drug should be withdrawn over 3-6 weeks. Oxcarbazepine dose may be increased by a maximum of 10 mg/kg/day at weekly intervals. See below for recommended total daily dose by weight.

Initiation of monotherapy: Oxcarbazepine should be initiated at 8-10 mg/kg/day in twice daily divided doses; doses may be titrated by 5 mg/kg/day every third day. See below for recommended total daily dose by weight.

Range of maintenance doses by weight during monotherapy:

20 kg: 600-900 mg/day
25-30 kg: 900-1200 mg/day
35-40 kg: 900-1500 mg/day
45 kg: 1200-1500 mg/day
50-55 kg: 1200-1800 mg/day
60-65 kg: 1200-2100 mg/day
70 kg: 1500-2100 mg/day

Renal Impairment: Cl_{cr} <30 mL/minute: Initial dose should be reduced by 50%, and the dosage increased slowly to achieve the desired clinical response.

Hepatic Impairment: No dosage adjustment recommended in mild to moderate hepatic impairment. Patients with severe hepatic impairment have not been evaluated.

Available Dosage Forms

Suspension, oral: 300 mg/5 mL (250 mL) [contains ethanol]
Tablet [film coated]: 150 mg, 300 mg, 600 mg

Monitoring and Teaching Issues

Physical Assessment: Assess complete allergy history (carbamazepine). Assess effectiveness and interactions of other medications. Monitor therapeutic effectiveness (seizure activity, frequency, duration, type), laboratory results, and adverse reactions (eg. sedation, CNS changes, visual changes). Dosage should be tapered when discontinuing to reduce risk of increased seizures. Assess knowledge/teach patient appropriate use, interventions to reduce side effects, and adverse reactions to report. **Note:** Oxcarbazepine may reduce the effectiveness of oral contraceptives, nonhormonal contraception is recommended.

Monitoring Laboratory Tests: Serum sodium (particularly during first 3 months of therapy); additional serum sodium monitoring is recommended during maintenance treatment in patients receiving other medications known to decrease sodium levels, in patients with signs/symptoms of hyponatremia, and in patients with an increase in seizure frequency or severity.

Patient Education: Take exactly as directed. Do not increase dose or frequency or discontinue without consulting prescriber. While using the medication do not use alcohol and other prescription or OTC medications (especially medications to relieve pain, induce sleep, reduce anxiety, treat or prevent cold, coughs, or allergies) unless approved by prescriber. Maintain adequate hydration (2-3 L/day of fluids) unless instructed to restrict fluid intake. You may experience drowsiness, dizziness, or blurred vision (use caution when driving or engaging in tasks requiring alertness until response to drug is known); nausea or vomiting (small frequent meals, good mouth care, chewing gum, or sucking hard candy may help, or contact prescriber). Report CNS changes, increase in seizure frequency or severity, mentation changes, changes in cognition or memory, acute fatigue or weakness, or insomnia; muscle cramping, weakness, or pain; rash or skin irritations; unusual bruising or bleeding (mouth, urine, stool); swelling of extremities; or other adverse response. **Pregnancy/breast-feeding precautions:** Inform prescriber if you are or intend to become pregnant. **Note:** Oxcarbazepine may reduce the effectiveness of oral contraceptives, nonhormonal contraception is recommended. Breast-feeding is not recommended.

Dietary Considerations: May be taken with or without food.

Geriatric Considerations: Studies in elderly volunteers (60-82 years of age) with both single dose (300 mg) and multiple doses (600 mg/day) reported in maximum plasma concentrations and AUC volumes becoming increased 30% to 60% higher than younger volunteers (18-32 years of age). These results were done to differences in creatinine clearance between the two groups. Since elderly may have Cl_{cr} <30 mL/minute, dose reductions may be needed. See dosing information.

Pregnancy Risk Factor: C

Pregnancy Issues: Although many epidemiological studies of congenital anomalies in infants born to women treated with various anticonvulsants during pregnancy have been reported, none of these investigations includes enough women treated with oxcarbazepine to assess possible teratogenic effects of this drug. Given that teratogenic effects have been observed in animal studies, and that oxcarbazepine is structurally related to carbamazepine (teratogenic in humans), use during pregnancy only if the benefit to the mother outweighs the potential risk to the fetus.

Lactation: Enters breast milk/not recommended

Breast-Feeding Issues: Oxcarbazepine and its active metabolite (MHD) are excreted in human breast milk. A milk-to-plasma concentration ratio of 0.5 was found for both. Because of the potential for serious adverse reactions to oxcarbazepine in nursing infants, a decision should be made whether to discontinue nursing or to discontinue the drug in nursing women.

Administration

Oral: Suspension: Prior to using for the first time, firmly insert the plastic adapter provided with the bottle. Cover adapter with child-resistant cap when not in use. Shake bottle for at least 10 seconds, remove child-resistant cap and insert the oral dosing syringe provided to withdraw appropriate dose. Dose may be taken directly from oral syringe or may be mixed in a small glass of water immediately prior to swallowing. Rinse syringe with warm water after use and allow to dry thoroughly. Discard any unused portion after 7 weeks of first opening bottle.

Storage: Store tablets and suspension at 25°C (77°F). Use suspension within 7 weeks of first opening container.

Related Information

Anticonvulsants By Seizure Type *on page 1712*

♦ **Oxpentifylline** *see* Pentoxifylline *on page 1185*

♦ **Oxsoralen®** *see* Methoxsalen *on page 978*

♦ **Oxsoralen-Ultra®** *see* Methoxsalen *on page 978*

Oxybutynin (oks i BYOO ti nin)

U.S. Brand Names Ditropan®; Ditropan® XL; Oxytrol™

Synonyms Oxybutynin Chloride

Generic Available Yes: Excludes extended release formulation or transdermal patch

Pharmacologic Category Antispasmodic Agent, Urinary

Medication Safety Issues

Sound-alike/look-alike issues:

Oxybutynin may be confused with OxyContin®

Ditropan® may be confused with Detrol®, diazepam, Diprivan®, dithranol

Transdermal patch may contain conducting metal (eg, aluminum); remove patch prior to MRI.

Use Antispasmodic for neurogenic bladder (urgency, frequency, urge incontinence) and uninhibited bladder

Mechanism of Action/Effect Direct antispasmodic effect on smooth muscle, also inhibits the action of acetylcholine on smooth muscle (exhibits $^1/_5$ the anticholinergic activity of atropine, but is 4-10 times the antispasmodic activity); does not block effects at skeletal muscle or at autonomic ganglia; increases bladder capacity, decreases uninhibited contractions, and delays desire to void; therefore, decreases urgency and frequency

Contraindications Hypersensitivity to oxybutynin or any component of the formulation; untreated glaucoma; partial or complete GI obstruction; GU obstruction; urinary retention; megacolon; toxic megacolon

Warnings/Precautions Use with caution in patients with urinary tract obstruction, angle-closure glaucoma (treated), hyperthyroidism, reflux esophagitis (including concurrent therapy with oral bisphosphonates or drugs which may increase the risk of esophagitis), heart disease, hepatic or renal disease, prostatic hyperplasia, autonomic neuropathy, ulcerative colitis (may cause ileus and toxic megacolon), hypertension, hiatal hernia, myasthenia gravis, ulcerative colitis, or intestinal atony. Transdermal patch may contain conducting metal (eg, aluminum); remove patch prior to MRI. Avoid use of extended release tablets (Ditropan® XL) in patients with known stricture/narrowing of the GI tract. Caution should be used in elderly due to anticholinergic activity (eg, confusion, constipation, blurred vision, and tachycardia). May increase the risk of heat prostration.

Drug Interactions

Cytochrome P450 Effect: Substrate of CYP3A4 (minor); **Inhibits** CYP2D6 (weak), 3A4 (weak)

Increased Effect/Toxicity: Additive sedation with CNS depressants and ethanol. Additive anticholinergic effects with antihistamines and anticholinergic agents.

Nutritional/Ethanol Interactions Ethanol: Use ethanol with caution (may increase CNS depression and toxicity). Watch for sedation.

Lab Interactions May suppress the wheal and flare reactions to skin test antigens.

Adverse Reactions

Oral:

>10%:

Central nervous system: Dizziness (6% to 16%), somnolence (12% to 13%)

Gastrointestinal: Xerostomia (61% to 71%), constipation (13%)

Genitourinary: Urination impaired (11%)

1% to 10%:

Cardiovascular: Palpitation (2% to <5%), peripheral edema (2% to <5%), hypertension (2% to <5%), vasodilation (2% to <5%)

Central nervous system: Headache (6% to 10%), pain (7%), confusion (2% to <5%), insomnia (2% to <5%), nervousness (2% to <5%)

Dermatologic: Dry skin (2% to <5%), skin rash (2% to <5%)

Gastrointestinal: Nausea (9% to 10%), dyspepsia (7%), abdominal pain (2% to 6%), diarrhea (5% to 9%), flatulence (2% to <5%), gastrointestinal reflux (2% to <5%), taste perversion (2% to <5%)

Genitourinary: Postvoid residuals increased (2% to 9%), urinary tract infection (5%)

Neuromuscular & skeletal: Weakness (2% to 7%)

Ocular: Blurred vision (8% to 9%), dry eyes (2% to 6%)

Respiratory: Rhinitis (6%), dry nasal and sinus membranes (2% to <5%)

Transdermal:

>10%: Local: Application site reaction (17%), pruritus (14%)

1% to 10%:

Gastrointestinal: Xerostomia (4% to 10%), diarrhea (3%), constipation (3%)

Genitourinary: Dysuria (2%)

Local: Erythema (6% to 8%), vesicles (3%), rash (3%)

Ocular: Vision changes (3%)

Overdosage/Toxicology Symptoms of overdose include hypotension, circulatory failure, psychotic behavior, flushing, respiratory failure, paralysis, tremor, irritability, seizures, delirium, hallucinations, and coma. Treatment is symptomatic and supportive. For anticholinergic overdose with severe life-threatening symptoms, physostigmine 1-2 mg I.V. slowly, may be given to reverse these effects.

(Continued)

Oxybutynin *(Continued)*

Pharmacodynamics/Kinetics
Onset of Action: Onset of action: Oral: 30-60 minutes; Peak effect: 3-6 hours
Duration of Action: 6-10 hours (up to 24 hours for extended release oral formulation)
Absorption: Oral: Rapid and well absorbed; Transdermal: High
Time to Peak: Serum: Oral: ~60 minutes; Transdermal: 24-48 hours
Half-Life Elimination: I.V.: ~2 hours (parent drug), 7-8 hours (metabolites)
Metabolism: Hepatic via CYP3A4; Oral: High first-pass metabolism; I.V.: Forms active and inactive metabolites
Excretion: Urine (<0.1%)

Dosing
Adults:
Bladder spasms:
Oral:
Regular release: 5 mg 2-3 times/day up to maximum of 5 mg 4 times/day
Extended release: Initial: 5-10 mg once daily, may increase in 5-10 mg increments; maximum: 30 mg daily
Transdermal: Apply one 3.9 mg/day patch twice weekly (every 3-4 days)
Note: Should be discontinued periodically to determine whether the patient can manage without the drug and to minimize resistance to the drug.

Elderly:
Oral: 2.5-5 mg 2-3 times/day
Transdermal: Refer to adult dosing. **Note:** Should be discontinued periodically to determine whether the patient can manage without the drug and to minimize resistance to the drug.

Pediatrics:
Bladder spasms: Oral: Children:
1-5 years (unlabeled use): 0.2 mg/kg/dose 2-4 times/day
>5 years: 5 mg twice daily, up to 5 mg 3 times/day maximum
>6 years: Extended release: 5 mg once daily; maximum dose: 20 mg/day

Available Dosage Forms
Syrup, as chloride (Ditropan®): 5 mg/5 mL (473 mL)
Tablet, as chloride (Ditropan®): 5 mg
Tablet, extended release, as chloride (Ditropan® XL): 5 mg, 10 mg, 15 mg
Transdermal system (Oxytrol™): 3.9 mg/day (8s, 24s) [39 cm²; total oxybutynin 36 mg]

Monitoring and Teaching Issues
Physical Assessment: Assess other prescriptions, OTC medications, or herbal products patient may be taking for interactions. Assess voiding pattern, incontinent episodes, frequency, urgency, distention, and urinary retention prior to beginning therapy and periodically with long-term use. Assess knowledge/teach patient appropriate use, possible side effects, and symptoms to report.

Patient Education: Take prescribed oral dose preferably on an empty stomach, 1 hour before or 2 hours after meals. Swallow extended-release tablets whole, do not chew or crush. You may experience dizziness, lightheadedness, or drowsiness (use caution when driving or engaging in tasks requiring alertness until response to drug is known); dry mouth or changes in appetite (small frequent meals, frequent mouth care, sucking lozenges, or chewing gum may help); constipation (increased exercise, fluids, fruit, fiber, or stool softener may help); decreased sexual ability (reversible with discontinuance of drug); or decreased sweating (use caution in hot weather, avoid extreme exercise or activity). Use alcohol with caution; may increase drowsiness. Report rapid heartbeat, palpitations, or chest pain; difficulty voiding; or vision changes.

Dietary Considerations: Food causes a slight delay in the absorption of the oral solution and bioavailability is deceased by ~25%. Absorption of the extended release tablet is not affected by food.

Geriatric Considerations: Caution should be used in the elderly due to anticholinergic activity (eg, confusion, constipation, blurred vision, and tachycardia). Start with lower doses. Transdermal dosage form may have less potential for these effects. Oxybutynin may cause memory problems in the elderly. A study of 12 healthy volunteers with an average age of 69 showed cognitive decline while taking the drug (*J Am Geriatr Soc*, 1998, L46:8-13).

Pregnancy Risk Factor: B
Lactation: Excretion in breast milk unknown/use caution
Breast-Feeding Issues: Suppression of lactation has been reported (rarely).

Administration
Oral: Immediate release tablets and solution should be administered on an empty stomach with water. Extended release tablets may be taken with or without food and must be swallowed whole; do not crush, divide, or chew.

Other: Transdermal: Apply to clean, dry skin on abdomen, hip, or buttock. Select a new site for each new system (avoid reapplication to same site within 7 days).

Storage: Store at controlled room temperature. Protect syrup from light. Keep transdermal patch in sealed pouch.

Related Information
Pharmacotherapy of Urinary Incontinence *on page 1858*

♦ **Oxybutynin Chloride** *see* Oxybutynin *on page 1135*

Oxycodone *(oks i KOE done)*
U.S. Brand Names OxyContin®; Oxydose™; OxyFast®; OxyIR®; Roxicodone™; Roxicodone™ Intensol™
Synonyms Dihydrohydroxycodeinone; Oxycodone Hydrochloride
Controlled Substance C-II
Generic Available Yes
Pharmacologic Category Analgesic, Narcotic

Medication Safety Issues

Sound-alike/look-alike issues:

Oxycodone may be confused with OxyContin®

OxyContin® may be confused with oxybutynin, oxycodone

Use Management of moderate to severe pain, normally used in combination with non-narcotic analgesics

OxyContin® is indicated for around-the-clock management of moderate to severe pain when an analgesic is needed for an extended period of time. **Note:** OxyContin® is not intended for use as an "as needed" analgesic or for immediately-postoperative pain management (should be used postoperatively only if the patient has received it prior to surgery or if severe, persistent pain is anticipated).

Mechanism of Action/Effect Binds to opiate receptors in the CNS, causing inhibition of ascending pain pathways, altering the perception of and response to pain; produces generalized CNS depression

Contraindications Hypersensitivity to oxycodone or any component of the formulation; significant respiratory depression; hypercarbia; acute or severe bronchial asthma; OxyContin® is also contraindicated in paralytic ileus (known or suspected); pregnancy (prolonged use or high doses at term)

Warnings/Precautions Use with caution in patients with hypersensitivity reactions to other phenanthrene derivative opioid agonists (morphine, hydrocodone, hydromorphone, levorphanol, oxycodone, oxymorphone), respiratory diseases including asthma, emphysema, or COPD. Use with caution in pancreatitis or biliary tract disease, acute alcoholism (including delirium tremens), adrenocortical insufficiency, CNS depression/coma, kyphoscoliosis (or other skeletal disorder which may alter respiratory function), hypothyroidism (including myxedema), prostatic hyperplasia, urethral stricture, and toxic psychosis.

Use with caution in the elderly, debilitated, severe hepatic or renal function. Hemodynamic effects (hypotension, orthostasis) may be exaggerated in patients with hypovolemia, concurrent vasodilating drugs, or in patients with head injury. Respiratory depressant effects and capacity to elevate CSF pressure may be exaggerated in presence of head injury, other intracranial lesion, or pre-existing intracranial pressure. Tolerance or drug dependence may result from extended use. Healthcare provider should be alert to problems of abuse, misuse, and diversion. Do **not** crush controlled-release tablets. Some preparations contain sulfites which may cause allergic reactions. OxyContin® 80 mg and 160 mg strengths are for use only in opioid-tolerant patients requiring high daily dosages >160 mg (80 mg formulation) or >320 mg (160 mg formulation).

Drug Interactions

Cytochrome P450 Effect: Substrate of CYP2D6 (major)

Increased Effect/Toxicity: MAO inhibitors may increase adverse symptoms. Cimetidine may increase narcotic analgesic serum levels resulting in toxicity. CNS depressants (barbiturates, ethanol) and TCAs may potentiate the sedative and respiratory depressive effects of morphine and other opiate agonists. Dextroamphetamine may enhance the analgesic effect of morphine and other opiate agonists.

Nutritional/Ethanol Interactions

Ethanol: Avoid ethanol (may increase CNS depression).

Food: When taken with a high-fat meal, peak concentration is 25% greater following a single OxyContin® 160 mg tablet as compared to two 80 mg tablets.

Herb/Nutraceutical: Avoid valerian, St John's wort, kava kava, gotu kola (may increase CNS depression).

Adverse Reactions

>10%:

Central nervous system: Fatigue, drowsiness, dizziness, somnolence

Dermatologic: Pruritus

Gastrointestinal: Nausea, vomiting, constipation

Neuromuscular & skeletal: Weakness

1% to 10%:

Cardiovascular: Postural hypotension

Central nervous system: Nervousness, headache, restlessness, malaise, confusion, anxiety, abnormal dreams, euphoria, thought abnormalities

Dermatologic: Rash

Gastrointestinal: Anorexia, stomach cramps, xerostomia, biliary spasm, abdominal pain, dyspepsia, gastritis

Genitourinary: Ureteral spasms, decreased urination

Local: Pain at injection site

Respiratory: Dyspnea, hiccups

Miscellaneous: Diaphoresis

Overdosage/Toxicology Symptoms of toxicity include CNS depression, respiratory depression, and miosis. Naloxone, 2 mg I.V. with repeat administration as necessary up to a total of 10 mg, can also be used to reverse toxic effects of the opiate.

Pharmacodynamics/Kinetics

Onset of Action: Pain relief: 10-15 minutes; Peak effect: 0.5-1 hour

Duration of Action: 3-6 hours; Controlled release: ≤12 hours

Half-Life Elimination: 2-3 hours

Metabolism: Hepatic

Excretion: Urine

Dosing

Adults & Elderly: Management of pain: Oral:

Regular or immediate release formulations: 2.5-5 mg every 6 hours as needed

Controlled release:

Opioid naive (not currently on opioid): 10 mg every 12 hours

Currently on opioid/ASA or acetaminophen or NSAID combination:

1-5 tablets: 10-20 mg every 12 hours

6-9 tablets: 20-30 mg every 12 hours

10-12 tablets: 30-40 mg every 12 hours

(Continued)

Oxycodone *(Continued)*

May continue the nonopioid as a separate drug.

Currently on opioids: Use standard conversion chart to convert daily dose to oxycodone equivalent. Divide daily dose in 2 (for every 12-hour dosing) and round down to nearest dosage form.

Note: 80 mg or 160 mg tablets are for use **only** in opioid-tolerant patients. Special safety considerations must be addressed when converting to OxyContin® doses ≥160 mg every 12 hours. Dietary caution must be taken when patients are initially titrated to 160 mg tablets.

Pediatrics: Oral: Regular or immediate release formulations:

6-12 years: 1.25 mg every 6 hours as needed

>12 years: 2.5 mg every 6 hours as needed

Hepatic Impairment: Reduce dosage in patients with severe liver disease.

Available Dosage Forms

Capsule, immediate release, as hydrochloride (OxyIR®): 5 mg

Solution, oral, as hydrochloride: 5 mg/5 mL (500 mL)

Roxicodone™: 5 mg/5 mL (5 mL, 500 mL) [contains alcohol]

Solution, oral concentrate, as hydrochloride: 20 mg/mL (30 mL)

Oxydose™: 20 mg/mL (30 mL) [contains sodium benzoate; berry flavor]

OxyFast®, Roxicodone™ Intensol™: 20 mg/mL (30 mL) [contains sodium benzoate]

Tablet, as hydrochloride: 5 mg

Roxicodone™: 5 mg, 15 mg, 30 mg

Tablet, controlled release, as hydrochloride (OxyContin®): 10 mg, 20 mg, 40 mg, 80 mg, 160 mg

Tablet, extended release, as hydrochloride: 80 mg

Monitoring and Teaching Issues

Physical Assessment: Assess other medications patient may be taking for additive or adverse interactions. Monitor for effectiveness of pain relief and monitor for signs of overdose. Monitor vital signs, CNS and respiratory status, and degree of sedation at beginning of therapy and at regular intervals with long-term use. May cause physical and/or psychological dependence. For inpatients, implement safety measures. Assess knowledge/teach patient appropriate use (if self-administered). Teach patient to monitor for adverse reactions, adverse reactions to report, and appropriate interventions to reduce side effects.

Patient Education: If self-administered, use exactly as directed; do not increase dose or frequency. Drug may cause physical or psychological dependence. Do not crush or chew controlled-release tablets. While using this medication, do not use alcohol and other prescription or OTC medications (especially sedatives, tranquilizers, antihistamines, or pain medications) without consulting prescriber. Maintain adequate hydration (2-3 L/day of fluids) unless instructed to restrict fluid intake. May cause hypotension, dizziness, drowsiness, impaired coordination, or blurred vision (use caution when driving, climbing stairs, or changing position - rising from sitting or lying to standing, or when engaging in tasks requiring alertness until response to drug is known); nausea, vomiting, or dry mouth (frequent mouth care, small frequent meals, chewing gum, or sucking lozenges may help); or constipation (increased exercise, fluids, fruit, or fiber may help; if unresolved, consult prescriber about use of stool softeners). Report persistent dizziness or headache; excessive fatigue or sedation; changes in mental status; changes in urinary elimination or pain on urination; weakness or trembling; blurred vision; or shortness of breath. **Pregnancy/breast-feeding precautions:** Inform prescriber if you are or intend to become pregnant. If you are breast-feeding, take medication immediately after breast-feeding or 3-4 hours prior to next feeding.

Dietary Considerations: Instruct patient to avoid high-fat meals when taking OxyContin® 160 mg tablets.

Geriatric Considerations: The elderly may be particularly susceptible to the CNS depressant and constipating effects of narcotics. Serum levels at a given dose may also be increased relative to concentrations in younger patients.

Pregnancy Risk Factor: B/D (prolonged use or high doses at term)

Pregnancy Issues: Use of narcotics during pregnancy may produce physical dependence in the neonate; respiratory depression may occur in the newborn if narcotics are used prior to delivery (especially high doses).

Lactation: Enters breast milk/use caution

Administration

Oral: Do not crush controlled-release tablets; 80 mg and 160 mg tablets are for use **only** in opioid-tolerant patients. Do not administer OxyContin® 160 mg tablet with a high-fat meal.

Storage: Tablets should be stored at room temperature.

Additional Information Prophylactic use of a laxative should be considered. OxyContin® 80 mg and 160 mg tablets are for use in opioid-tolerant patients only.

Related Information

Narcotic / Opioid Analgesic Comparison *on page 1739*

Oxycodone and Acetaminophen (oks i KOE done & a seet a MIN oh fen)

U.S. Brand Names Endocet®; Percocet®; Roxicet™; Roxicet™ 5/500; Tylox®

Synonyms Acetaminophen and Oxycodone

Controlled Substance C-II

Generic Available Yes

Pharmacologic Category Analgesic, Narcotic

Medication Safety Issues

Sound-alike/look-alike issues:

Percocet® may be confused with Percodan®

Roxicet™ may be confused with Roxanol™

Tylox® may be confused with Trimox®, Tylenol®, Wymox®, Xanax®

Use Management of moderate to severe pain

Dosing

Adults:

Note: Initial dose is based on the **oxycodone** content; however, the maximum daily dose is based on the **acetaminophen** content.

Management of pain: Doses should be given every 4-6 hours as needed and titrated to appropriate analgesic effects.

Maximum daily dose, based on acetaminophen content: Oral: 4 g/day.

Mild to moderate pain: Oral: Initial dose, **based on oxycodone content:** 5 mg

Severe pain: Oral: Initial dose, **based on oxycodone content:** 15-30 mg

Elderly: Doses should be titrated to appropriate analgesic effects: Oral: Initial dose, **based on oxycodone content:** 2.5-5 mg every 6 hours. Do not exceed 4 g/day of acetaminophen.

Pediatrics:

Note: Initial dose is based on the **oxycodone** content; however, the maximum daily dose is based on the **acetaminophen** content.

Management of pain: Doses should be given every 4-6 hours as needed and titrated to appropriate analgesic effects.

Mild to moderate pain: Oral: Initial dose, **based on oxycodone content:** 0.05-0.1 mg/kg/dose

Severe pain: Oral: Initial dose, **based on oxycodone content:** 0.3 mg/kg/dose

Maximum dose, based on acetaminophen content: Oral: Children <45 kg: 90 mg/kg/day; children >45 kg: 4 g/day

Hepatic Impairment: Dose should be reduced in patients with severe liver disease.

Available Dosage Forms

Caplet (Roxicet™ 5/500): Oxycodone hydrochloride 5 mg and acetaminophen 500 mg

Capsule: Oxycodone hydrochloride 5 mg and acetaminophen 500 mg

Tylox®: Oxycodone hydrochloride 5 mg and acetaminophen 500 mg [contains sodium benzoate and sodium metabisulfite]

Solution, oral (Roxicet™): Oxycodone hydrochloride 5 mg and acetaminophen 325 mg per 5 mL (5 mL, 500 mL) [contains alcohol <0.5%]

Tablet: Oxycodone hydrochloride 5 mg and acetaminophen 325 mg; oxycodone hydrochloride 7.5 mg and acetaminophen 325 mg; oxycodone hydrochloride 7.5 mg and acetaminophen 500 mg; oxycodone hydrochloride 10 mg and acetaminophen 325 mg; oxycodone hydrochloride 10 mg and acetaminophen 650 mg

Endocet® 5/325 [scored]: Oxycodone hydrochloride 5 mg and acetaminophen 325 mg

Endocet® 7.5/325: Oxycodone hydrochloride 7.5 mg and acetaminophen 325 mg

Endocet® 7.5/500: Oxycodone hydrochloride 7.5 mg and acetaminophen 500 mg

Endocet® 10/325: Oxycodone hydrochloride 10 mg and acetaminophen 325 mg

Endocet® 10/650: Oxycodone hydrochloride 10 mg and acetaminophen 650 mg

Percocet® 2.5/325: Oxycodone hydrochloride 2.5 mg and acetaminophen 325 mg

Percocet® 5/325 [scored]: Oxycodone hydrochloride 5 mg and acetaminophen 325 mg

Percocet® 7.5/325: Oxycodone hydrochloride 7.5 mg and acetaminophen 325 mg

Percocet® 7.5/500: Oxycodone hydrochloride 7.5 mg and acetaminophen 500 mg

Percocet® 10/325: Oxycodone hydrochloride 10 mg and acetaminophen 325 mg

Percocet® 10/650: Oxycodone hydrochloride 10 mg and acetaminophen 650 mg

Roxicet™ [scored]: Oxycodone hydrochloride 5 mg and acetaminophen 325 mg

Monitoring and Teaching Issues

Physical Assessment: See individual agents.

Patient Education: See individual agents. **Pregnancy/breast-feeding precautions:** Inform prescriber if you are or intend to become pregnant. Consult prescriber if breast-feeding.

Pregnancy Risk Factor: C/D (prolonged periods or high doses at term)

Lactation: Enters breast milk/use caution

Related Information

Acetaminophen *on page 38*

Oxycodone *on page 1136*

Oxycodone and Aspirin (oks i KOE done & AS pir in)

U.S. Brand Names Endodan®; Percodan®

Synonyms Aspirin and Oxycodone

Controlled Substance C-II

Generic Available Yes

Pharmacologic Category Analgesic, Narcotic

Medication Safety Issues

Sound-alike/look-alike issues:

Percodan® may be confused with Decadron®, Percocet®, Percogesic®, Periactin®

Use Management of moderate to severe pain

Dosing

Adults & Elderly: Analgesic: Oral (based on oxycodone combined salts): Percodan®: 1 tablet every 6 hours as needed for pain; maximum aspirin dose should not exceed 4 g/day.

Pediatrics: Analgesic: Oral (based on oxycodone combined salts): Maximum oxycodone: 5 mg/dose; maximum aspirin dose should not exceed 4 g/day. Doses should be given every 6 hours as needed.

Mild-to-moderate pain: Initial dose, **based on oxycodone content:** 0.05-0.1 mg/kg/dose

Severe pain: Initial dose, **based on oxycodone content:** 0.3 mg/kg/dose

Hepatic Impairment: Dose should be reduced in patients with severe liver disease.

Available Dosage Forms

Tablet: Oxycodone hydrochloride 4.5 mg, oxycodone terephthalate 0.38 mg, and aspirin 325 mg

Endodan®, Percodan®: Oxycodone hydrochloride 4.5 mg, oxycodone terephthalate 0.38 mg, and aspirin 325 mg

(Continued)

Oxycodone and Aspirin *(Continued)*

Monitoring and Teaching Issues
Physical Assessment: See individual agents.

Patient Education: See individual agents. **Pregnancy/breast-feeding precautions:** Inform prescriber if you are or intend to become pregnant. Consult prescriber if breast-feeding.

Pregnancy Risk Factor: D

Lactation: Enters breast milk/use caution

Related Information
Aspirin *on page 143*
Oxycodone *on page 1136*

Oxycodone and Ibuprofen *(oks i KOE done & eye byoo PROE fen)*

U.S. Brand Names Combunox™

Synonyms Ibuprofen and Oxycodone

Controlled Substance C-II

Generic Available No

Pharmacologic Category Analgesic, Narcotic; Nonsteroidal Anti-inflammatory Drug (NSAID), Oral

Use Short-term (≤7 days) management of acute, moderate-to-severe pain

Mechanism of Action/Effect
Based on **oxycodone** component: Binds to opiate receptors in the CNS, altering the perception of and response to pain; suppresses cough in medullary center; produces generalized CNS depression

Based on **ibuprofen** component: Inhibits prostaglandin synthesis by decreasing the activity of the enzyme, cyclooxygenase, which results in decreased formation of prostaglandin precursors

Contraindications Hypersensitivity to oxycodone, other opioids, ibuprofen, aspirin, other NSAIDs, or any component of the formulation; patients with suspected paralytic ileus; pregnancy (3rd trimester)

Warnings/Precautions Use with caution in elderly or debilitated patients, and those with severe hepatic or renal dysfunction, hypothyroidism, Addison's disease, prostatic hyperplasia, or urethral stricture. Respiratory depression is possible; use with caution in patients with underlying respiratory depression, acute or severe asthma, or hypercarbia. Patients with head injury, increased intracranial pressure, acute abdominal condition, active peptic ulcer disease, history of upper GI disease, impaired thyroid function, hypertension, edema, heart failure, and any bleeding disorder should use this agent cautiously. Patients are at risk for gastrointestinal ulceration and bleeding even during short-term therapy. Tolerance or drug dependence may result from extended use. Oxycodone suppresses the cough reflex; use caution postoperatively and in patients with pulmonary disease. Rare incidents of aseptic meningitis have been reported with ibuprofen's use. Safety and efficacy in pediatric patients have not been established.

Drug Interactions
Cytochrome P450 Effect:
Oxycodone: **Substrate** of CYP2D6
Ibuprofen: **Substrate** (minor) of CYP2C8/9, 2C19; **Inhibits** CYP2C8/9 (strong)

Decreased Effect: See individual agents.

Increased Effect/Toxicity: See individual agents.

Nutritional/Ethanol Interactions
Based on **oxycodone** component:
Ethanol: Avoid or limit ethanol (may increase CNS depression). Watch for sedation.
Based on **ibuprofen** component:
Ethanol: Avoid ethanol (may enhance gastric mucosal irritation).
Food: Food or milk are recommended to decrease gastric irritation.
Herb/Nutraceutical: Avoid cat's claw, dong quai, evening primrose, feverfew, garlic, ginger, ginkgo, red clover, horse chestnut, green tea, ginseng (all have antiplatelet activity).

Adverse Reactions
>10%:
Central nervous system: Dizziness (5% to 19%), somnolence (7% to 17%)
Gastrointestinal: Nausea (9% to 25%)
2% to 10%:
Cardiovascular: Vasodilation (<1% to 3%)
Central nervous system: Headache (10%), fever (3%)
Gastrointestinal: Constipation (<1% to 5%), vomiting (5%), diarrhea (2%), dyspepsia (<1% to 2%), flatulence (1%)
Neuromuscular & skeletal: Weakness (3%)
Miscellaneous: Diaphoresis (2%)

Overdosage/Toxicology Symptoms of toxicity may include respiratory depression, CNS depression, metabolic acidosis, seizures, hypotension, blood loss, coma, miosis, and renal failure. In cases of acute overdose, ipecac-induced emesis or gastric lavage may be used to empty the stomach. Emesis is most effective if within 30 minutes of ingestion, and is not recommended in patients who are not fully conscious or who have ingested >400 mg/kg of the ibuprofen component. Naloxone is the antidote for oxycodone. Repeat administration as necessary up to a total of 10 mg may be used to reverse toxic effects of the opiate. Treatment of NSAID overdose is supportive with symptomatic management as necessary; activated charcoal may be used to reduce the absorption and reabsorption of ibuprofen.

Pharmacodynamics/Kinetics
Absorption: Ibuprofen, oxycodone: rapidly absorbed
Bioavailability: Oxycodone: increased with food (25%)
Time to Peak: Ibuprofen: 1.6-3.1 hours; Oxycodone 1.3-2.1 hours
Protein Binding: Ibuprofen: 99%; Oxycodone: 45%
Half-Life Elimination: Ibuprofen: 1.8-2.6 hours; Oxycodone: 3.1-3.7 hours
Metabolism: Oxycodone: Hepatic to metabolites, noroxycodone (major), and oxymorphone (minor)
Excretion: Ibuprofen: Urine (<0.2% unchanged); Oxycodone: Urine (~4 % unchanged)
Pharmacokinetic Note: See individual agents.

Dosing
Adults: Pain: Oral: Take 1 tablet every 6 hours as needed (maximum: 4 tablets/24 hours); do not take for longer than 7 days

Available Dosage Forms Tablet [film-coated]: Oxycodone hydrochloride 5 mg and ibuprofen 400 mg

Monitoring and Teaching Issues
Physical Assessment: Assess other medications patient may be taking for additive or adverse interactions. Monitor for effectiveness of pain relief and monitor for signs of overdose. Monitor blood pressure, CNS and respiratory status, and degree of sedation at beginning of therapy and at regular intervals with long-term use. May cause physical and/or psychological dependence. For inpatients, implement safety measures (eg, side rails up, call light within reach, instructions to call for assistance). Assess knowledge/teach patient appropriate use (if self-administered). Teach patient to monitor for adverse reactions, adverse reactions to report, and appropriate interventions to reduce side effects.

Patient Education: If self-administered, use exactly as directed; do not increase dose or frequency. Drug may cause physical and/or psychological dependence. While using this medication, do not use alcohol and other prescription or OTC medications (especially sedatives, tranquilizers, antihistamines, or pain medications) without consulting prescriber. Maintain adequate hydration (2-3 L/day of fluids) unless instructed to restrict fluid intake. May cause hypotension, dizziness, drowsiness, impaired coordination, or blurred vision (use caution when driving, climbing stairs, or changing position - rising from sitting or lying to standing, or when engaging in tasks requiring alertness until response to drug is known); nausea, vomiting, (frequent mouth care, small frequent meals, chewing gum, or sucking lozenges may help); or constipation (increased exercise, fluids, fruit, or fiber may help; if unresolved, consult prescriber about use of stool softeners). Report persistent dizziness or headache; excessive fatigue or sedation; changes in mental status; gastrointestinal bleeding, unexplained weight gain, edema, blurred vision; or shortness of breath. **Pregnancy/breast-feeding precautions:** Inform prescriber if you are or intend to become pregnant. If you are breast-feeding, take medication immediately after breast-feeding or 3-4 hours prior to next feeding.

Dietary Considerations: Take with or without food.

Geriatric Considerations: Caution should be used when treating the elderly. May be more sensitive to the renal and gastrointestinal effects of ibuprofen and the respiratory effects of oxycodone.

Pregnancy Risk Factor: C/D (3rd trimester)

Lactation: Enters breast milk/contraindicated

Breast-Feeding Issues: Ibuprofen is not transferred to milk in significant quantities and is considered compatible with breast-feeding by AAP Oxycodone, however, is excreted in breast milk and withdrawal may occur in breast-fed infants when maternal opioid administration is discontinued. Discontinuation of either the opioid-containing medication (Combunox™) or breast-feeding is recommended.

Administration
Storage: Store between 15°C to 30°C (59°F to 86°F).

♦ **Oxycodone Hydrochloride** *see* Oxycodone *on page 1136*
♦ **OxyContin®** *see* Oxycodone *on page 1136*
♦ **Oxydose™** *see* Oxycodone *on page 1136*
♦ **OxyFast®** *see* Oxycodone *on page 1136*
♦ **OxyIR®** *see* Oxycodone *on page 1136*

Oxymorphone (oks i MOR fone)
U.S. Brand Names Numorphan®
Synonyms Oxymorphone Hydrochloride
Controlled Substance C-II
Generic Available No
Pharmacologic Category Analgesic, Narcotic
Medication Safety Issues
Sound-alike/look-alike issues:
Oxymorphone may be confused with oxymetholone

Use Management of moderate to severe pain and preoperatively as a sedative and a supplement to anesthesia

Mechanism of Action/Effect Oxymorphone hydrochloride (Numorphan®) is a potent narcotic analgesic with uses similar to those of morphine. The drug is a semisynthetic derivative of morphine (phenanthrene derivative) and is closely related to hydromorphone chemically (Dilaudid®).

Contraindications Hypersensitivity to oxymorphone or any component of the formulation; increased intracranial pressure; severe respiratory depression; pregnancy (prolonged use or high doses at term)

Warnings/Precautions Some preparations contain sulfites which may cause allergic reactions; infants <3 months of age are more susceptible to respiratory depression, use with caution and generally in reduced doses in this age group; use with caution in patients with impaired respiratory function or severe hepatic dysfunction and in patients with hypersensitivity reactions to other phenanthrene derivative opioid agonists (codeine, hydrocodone, (Continued)

Oxymorphone *(Continued)*

hydromorphone, levorphanol, oxycodone, oxymorphone); tolerance or drug dependence may result from extended use

Drug Interactions

Decreased Effect: Decreased effect with phenothiazines.

Increased Effect/Toxicity: Increased effect/toxicity with CNS depressants (phenothiazines, tranquilizers, anxiolytics, sedatives, hypnotics, alcohol), tricyclic antidepressants, and dextroamphetamine.

Nutritional/Ethanol Interactions

Ethanol: Avoid ethanol (may increase CNS depression).

Herb/Nutraceutical: Avoid valerian, St John's wort, kava kava, gotu kola (may increase CNS depression).

Adverse Reactions

>10%:

Cardiovascular: Hypotension

Central nervous system: Fatigue, drowsiness, dizziness

Gastrointestinal: Nausea, vomiting, constipation

Neuromuscular & skeletal: Weakness

Miscellaneous: Histamine release

1% to 10%:

Central nervous system: Nervousness, headache, restlessness, malaise, confusion

Gastrointestinal: Anorexia, stomach cramps, xerostomia, biliary spasm

Genitourinary: Decreased urination, ureteral spasms

Local: Pain at injection site

Respiratory: Dyspnea

Overdosage/Toxicology Symptoms of overdose include respiratory depression, miosis, hypotension, bradycardia, apnea, and pulmonary edema. Treatment of overdose includes maintaining patent airway and establishing an I.V. line. Naloxone, 2 mg I.V., with repeat administration as necessary up to a total of 10 mg, can also be used to reverse toxic effects of the opiate.

Pharmacodynamics/Kinetics

Onset of Action: Analgesic: I.V., I.M., SubQ: 5-10 minutes; Rectal: 15-30 minutes

Duration of Action: Analgesic: Parenteral, rectal: 3-4 hours

Metabolism: Hepatic via glucuronidation

Excretion: Urine

Dosing

Adults & Elderly: Analgesia: **Note:** More frequent dosing may be required.

I.M., SubQ: 0.5 mg initially, 1-1.5 mg every 4-6 hours as needed

I.V.: 0.5 mg initially

Rectal: 5 mg every 4-6 hours

Available Dosage Forms

Injection, solution, as hydrochloride: 1 mg (1 mL); 1.5 mg/mL (10 mL)

Suppository, rectal, as hydrochloride: 5 mg

Monitoring and Teaching Issues

Physical Assessment: Assess other medications patient may be taking for additive or adverse interactions. Monitor therapeutic effectiveness, adverse reactions, and signs of overdose at beginning of therapy and at regular intervals with long-term use. Monitor blood pressure, CNS and respiratory status, and degree of sedation. May cause physical and/or psychological dependence. For inpatients, implement safety measures. Assess knowledge/teach patient appropriate use (if self-administered). Teach patient to monitor for adverse reactions, adverse reactions to report, and appropriate interventions to reduce side effects.

Patient Education: If self-administered, use exactly as directed; do not increase dose or frequency or discontinue without consulting prescriber. Drug may cause physical and/or psychological dependence. While using this medication, do not use alcohol and other prescription or OTC medications (especially sedatives, tranquilizers, antihistamines, or pain medications) without consulting prescriber. Maintain adequate hydration (2-3 L/day of fluids) unless instructed to restrict fluid intake. May cause hypotension, dizziness, drowsiness, impaired coordination, or blurred vision (use caution when driving, climbing stairs, or changing position - rising from sitting or lying to standing, or when engaging in tasks requiring alertness until response to drug is known); nausea, vomiting or dry mouth (frequent mouth care, small frequent meals, chewing gum, or sucking lozenges may help); or constipation (increased exercise, fluids, fruit, or fiber may help; if unresolved, consult prescriber about use of stool softeners). Report persistent dizziness or headache; excessive fatigue or sedation; changes in mental status; changes in urinary elimination or pain on urination; weakness or trembling; blurred vision; or shortness of breath. **Pregnancy/breast-feeding precautions:** Inform prescriber if you are or intend to become pregnant. If you are breast-feeding, take medication immediately after breast-feeding or 3-4 hours prior to next feeding.

Geriatric Considerations: The elderly may be particularly susceptible to the CNS depressant and constipating effects of narcotics.

Pregnancy Risk Factor: B/D (prolonged use or high doses at term)

Lactation: Excretion in breast milk unknown/use caution

Administration

Storage: Refrigerate suppository.

Related Information

Narcotic / Opioid Analgesic Comparison *on page 1739*

♦ **Oxymorphone Hydrochloride** *see Oxymorphone on page 1141*

Oxytocin *(oks i TOE sin)*

U.S. Brand Names Pitocin®

Synonyms Pit

Generic Available Yes

Pharmacologic Category Oxytocic Agent

Medication Safety Issues

Sound-alike/look-alike issues:

Pitocin® may be confused with Pitressin®

Use Induction of labor at term; control of postpartum bleeding; adjunctive therapy in management of abortion

Mechanism of Action/Effect Produces rhythmic uterine contractions characteristic of delivery and stimulates breast milk flow during nursing

Contraindications Hypersensitivity to oxytocin or any component of the formulation; significant cephalopelvic disproportion; unfavorable fetal positions; fetal distress; hypertonic or hyperactive uterus; contraindicated vaginal delivery (invasive cervical cancer, active genital herpes, prolapse of the cord, cord presentation, total placenta previa, or vasa previa)

Warnings/Precautions To be used for medical rather than elective induction of labor. May produce antidiuretic effect (ie, water intoxication and excess uterine contractions). High doses or hypersensitivity to oxytocin may cause uterine hypertonicity, spasm, tetanic contraction, or rupture of the uterus. Severe water intoxication with convulsions, coma, and death has been associated with a slow oxytocin infusion over 24 hours.

Drug Interactions

Increased Effect/Toxicity: Dinoprostone and misoprostol may increase the effect of oxytocin; wait 6-12 hours after dinoprostone or misoprostol administration before initiating oxytocin.

Adverse Reactions Frequency not defined.

Fetus or neonate:

Cardiovascular: Arrhythmias (including premature ventricular contractions), bradycardia

Central nervous system: Brain or CNS damage (permanent), neonatal seizure

Hepatic: Neonatal jaundice

Ocular: Neonatal retinal hemorrhage

Miscellaneous: Fetal death, low Apgar score (5 minute)

Mother:

Cardiovascular: Arrhythmias, hypertensive episodes, premature ventricular contractions

Gastrointestinal: Nausea, vomiting

Genitourinary: Pelvic hematoma, postpartum hemorrhage, uterine hypertonicity, tetanic contraction of the uterus, uterine rupture, uterine spasm

Hematologic: Afibrinogenemia (fatal)

Miscellaneous: Anaphylactic reaction, subarachnoid hemorrhage

Overdosage/Toxicology Symptoms of overdose include tetanic uterine contractions, impaired uterine blood flow, amniotic fluid embolism, uterine rupture, SIADH, and seizures. Treatment is symptom-directed and supportive.

Pharmacodynamics/Kinetics

Onset of Action: Uterine contractions: I.M.: 3-5 minutes; I.V.: ~1 minute

Duration of Action: I.M.: 2-3 hour; I.V.: 1 hour

Half-Life Elimination: 1-5 minutes

Metabolism: Rapidly hepatic and via plasma (by oxytocinase) and to a smaller degree the mammary gland

Excretion: Urine

Dosing

Adults: Note: I.V. administration requires the use of an infusion pump.

Induction of labor: I.V.: 0.5-1 milliunits/minute; gradually increase dose in increments of 1-2 milliunits/minute until desired contraction pattern is established; dose may be decreased after desired frequency of contractions is reached and labor has progressed to 5-6 cm dilation. Infusion rates of 6 milliunits/minute provide oxytocin levels similar to those at spontaneous labor; rates of >9-10 milliunits/minute are rarely required.

Postpartum bleeding:

I.M.: Total dose of 10 units after delivery

I.V.: 10-40 units by I.V. infusion in 1000 mL of intravenous fluid at a rate sufficient to control uterine atony

Adjunctive treatment of abortion: I.V.: 10-20 milliunits/minute; maximum total dose: 30 units/12 hours

Available Dosage Forms

Injection, solution: 10 units/mL (1 mL, 10 mL)

Pitocin®: 10 units/mL (1 mL)

Monitoring and Teaching Issues

Physical Assessment: Monitor blood pressure, fluid intake and output, and labor closely if using oxytocin for induction; fetal monitoring is strongly recommended. **Pregnancy risk factor X.**

Patient Education: I.V./I.M.: Generally used in emergency situations. Drug teaching should be incorporated in other situational teaching. **Breast-feeding precaution:** Use caution.

Pregnancy Risk Factor: X

Pregnancy Issues: Reproduction studies have not been conducted. When used as indicated, teratogenic effects would not be expected. Nonteratogenic adverse reactions are reported in the neonate as well as the mother.

Lactation: Excretion in breast milk unknown/use caution

Breast-Feeding Issues: Endogenous levels of oxytocin naturally increase during breast-feeding.

Administration

I.V.: Refer to Reconstitution for dilution information. An infusion pump is required for administration.

Reconstitution: I.V.

Induction or stimulation of labor: Add oxytocin 10 units to NS or LR 1000 mL to yield a solution containing oxytocin 10 milliunits/mL; rotate solution to mix

(Continued)

Oxytocin *(Continued)*

Postpartum uterine bleeding: Add oxytocin 10-40 units to running I.V. infusion; maximum: 40 units/1000 mL

Adjunctive management of abortion: Add oxytocin 10 units to 500 mL of a physiologic saline solution or D$_5$W

Compatibility: Stable in dextran 6% in dextrose, dextran 6% in NS, D$_5$LR, D$_5$¼NS, D$_5$½NS, D$_5$NS, D$_5$W, D$_{10}$W, LR, ½NS, NS

Compatibility when admixed: Incompatible with fibrinolysin (human), norepinephrine, prochlorperazine edisylate, warfarin

Storage: Store oxytocin at 2°C to 8°C (36°F to 46°F); protect from freezing. Pitocin® may also be stored at 15°C to 25°C (59°F to 77°F) for up to 30 days.

◆ Oxytrol™ *see* Oxybutynin *on page 1135*

◆ Oysco 500 [OTC] *see* Calcium Carbonate *on page 235*

◆ Oyst-Cal 500 [OTC] *see* Calcium Carbonate *on page 235*

◆ P-071 *see* Cetirizine *on page 296*

◆ Pacerone® *see* Amiodarone *on page 93*

Paclitaxel *(PAK li taks el)*

U.S. Brand Names Onxol™; Taxol®

Synonyms NSC-125973

Generic Available Yes

Pharmacologic Category Antineoplastic Agent, Antimicrotubular; Antineoplastic Agent, Natural Source (Plant) Derivative

Medication Safety Issues

Sound-alike/look-alike issues:

Paclitaxel may be confused with paroxetine, Paxil®

Paclitaxel (conventional) may be confused with paclitaxel (protein-bound)

Taxol® may be confused with Abraxane™, Paxil®, Taxotere®

Use Treatment of breast, lung (small cell and nonsmall cell), and ovarian cancers

Mechanism of Action/Effect Paclitaxel promotes microtubule assembly by enhancing the action of tubulin dimers, stabilizing existing microtubules, and inhibiting their disassembly, interfering with the late G$_2$ mitotic phase, and inhibiting cell replication. In addition, the drug can distort mitotic spindles, resulting in the breakage of chromosomes. Paclitaxel may also suppress cell proliferation and modulate immune response.

Contraindications Hypersensitivity to paclitaxel, Cremophor® EL (polyoxyethylated castor oil), or any component of the formulation; pregnancy

Warnings/Precautions The FDA currently recommends that procedures for proper handling and disposal of antineoplastic agents be considered. All patients should be premedicated prior to Taxol® administration to prevent severe hypersensitivity reactions. Prolongation of the infusion (to ≥6 hours) plus premedication may minimize this effect.

Appropriate safety equipment is recommended for preparation, administration, and disposal of antineoplastics. If paclitaxel contacts the skin, wash and flush thoroughly with water.

When administered as sequential infusions, taxane derivatives (docetaxel, paclitaxel) should be administered before platinum derivatives (carboplatin, cisplatin) to limit myelosuppression. Elderly patients have an increased risk of toxicity (neutropenia, neuropathy).

Drug Interactions

Cytochrome P450 Effect: Substrate (major) of CYP2C8/9, 3A4; **Induces** CYP3A4 (weak)

Decreased Effect: CYP2C8/9 inducers may decrease the levels/effects of paclitaxel; example inducers include carbamazepine, phenobarbital, phenytoin, rifampin, rifapentine, and secobarbital. CYP3A4 inducers may decrease the levels/effects of paclitaxel; example inducers include aminoglutethimide, carbamazepine, nafcillin, nevirapine, phenobarbital, phenytoin, and rifamycins.

Increased Effect/Toxicity: CYP2C8/9 inhibitors may increase the levels/effects of paclitaxel; example inhibitors include delavirdine, fluconazole, gemfibrozil, ketoconazole, nicardipine, NSAIDs, pioglitazone, and sulfonamides. CYP3A4 inhibitors may increase the levels/effects of paclitaxel; example inhibitors include azole antifungals, ciprofloxacin, clarithromycin, diclofenac, doxycycline, erythromycin, imatinib, isoniazid, nefazodone, nicardipine, propofol, protease inhibitors, quinidine, and verapamil. In Phase I trials, myelosuppression was more profound when given after cisplatin than with alternative sequence. administered as sequential infusions, studies indicate a potential for increased toxicity when platinum derivatives (carboplatin, cisplatin) are administered before taxane derivatives (docetaxel, paclitaxel). Paclitaxel may increase doxorubicin levels/toxicity.

Nutritional/Ethanol Interactions Herb/Nutraceutical: Avoid black cohosh, dong quai in estrogen-dependent tumors. Avoid valerian, St John's wort, kava kava, gotu kola (may increase CNS depression).

Adverse Reactions

>10%:

Allergic: Appear to be primarily nonimmunologically mediated release of histamine and other vasoactive substances; almost always seen within the first hour of an infusion (~75% occur within 10 minutes of starting the infusion); incidence is significantly reduced by premedication

Cardiovascular: Bradycardia (transient, 25%)

Dermatologic: Alopecia (87%), venous erythema, tenderness, discomfort

Hematologic: Myelosuppression, leukopenia, neutropenia (6% to 21%), thrombocytopenia

Hepatic: Mild increases in liver enzymes

Onset: 8-11 days

Nadir: 15-21 days

Recovery: 21 days

Neurotoxicity: Sensory and/or autonomic neuropathy (numbness, tingling, burning pain), myopathy or myopathic effects (25% to 55%), and central nervous system toxicity. May be cumulative and dose-limiting. **Note:** Motor neuropathy is uncommon at doses <250 mg/m² ; sensory neuropathy is almost universal at doses >250 mg/m² ; myopathic effects are common with doses >250 mg/m² , generally occurring within 2-3 days of treatment, resolving over 5-6 days; pre-existing neuropathy may increase the risk of neuropathy.

Gastrointestinal: Severe, potentially dose-limiting mucositis, stomatitis (15%), most common at doses >390 mg/m²

Neuromuscular & skeletal: Arthralgia, myalgia

1% to 10%:

Cardiovascular: Myocardial infarction

Dermatologic: Phlebitis (2%)

Gastrointestinal: Mild nausea and vomiting (5% to 6%), diarrhea (5% to 6%)

Hematologic: Anemia

Pharmacodynamics/Kinetics

Protein Binding: 89% to 98%

Half-Life Elimination:

1- to 6-hour infusion: Mean (beta): 6.4 hours

3-hour infusion: Mean (terminal): 13.1-20.2 hours

24-hour infusion: Mean (terminal): 15.7-52.7 hours

Metabolism: Hepatic via CYP2C8/9 and 3A4; forms metabolites

Excretion: Feces (~70%, 5% as unchanged drug); urine (14%)

Clearance: Mean: Total body: After 1- and 6-hour infusions: 5.8-16.3 L/hour/m² ; After 24-hour infusions: 14.2-17.2 L/hour/m²

Dosing

Adults & Elderly: Note: Premedication with dexamethasone (20 mg orally or I.V. at 12 and 6 hours **or** 14 and 7 hours before the dose), diphenhydramine (50 mg I.V. 30-60 minutes prior to the dose), and cimetidine, famotidine or ranitidine (I.V. 30-60 minutes prior to the dose) is recommended

Ovarian carcinoma: I.V.: 135-175 mg/m² over 3 hours every 3 weeks **or** 50-80 mg/m² over 1-3 hours weekly **or** 1.4-4 mg/m²/day continuous infusion for 14 days every 4 weeks

Metastatic breast cancer: 175-250 mg/m² over 3 hours every 3 weeks **or** 50-80 mg/m² weekly **or** 1.4-4 mg/m²/day continuous infusion for 14 days every 4 weeks

Nonsmall cell lung carcinoma: 135 mg/m² over 24 hours every 3 weeks

AIDS-related Kaposi's sarcoma: 135 mg/m² over 3 hours every 3 weeks **or** 100 mg/m² over 3 hours every 2 weeks

Dosage modification for toxicity (solid tumors, including ovary, breast, and lung carcinoma): Courses of paclitaxel should not be repeated until the neutrophil count is ≥1500 cells/mm³ and the platelet count is ≥100,000 cells/mm³ ; reduce dosage by 20% for patients experiencing severe peripheral neuropathy or severe neutropenia (neutrophil <500 cells/mm³ for a week or longer)

Dosage modification for immunosuppression in advanced HIV disease: Paclitaxel should not be given to patients with HIV if the baseline or subsequent neutrophil count is <1000 cells/mm³ . Additional modifications include: Reduce dosage of dexamethasone in premedication to 10 mg orally; reduce dosage by 20% in patients experiencing severe peripheral neuropathy or severe neutropenia (neutrophil <500 cells/mm³ for a week or longer); initiate concurrent hematopoietic growth factor (G-CSF) as clinically indicated

Hepatic Impairment:

Note: These recommendations are based upon the patient's first course of therapy where the usual dose would be 135 mg/m² dose over 24 hours or the 175 mg/m² dose over 3 hours in patients with normal hepatic function. Dosage in subsequent courses should be based upon individual tolerance. Adjustments for other regimens are not available.

24-hour infusion:

If transaminase levels <2 times upper limit of normal (ULN) and bilirubin level ≤1.5 mg/dL: 135 mg/m²

If transaminase levels 2-<10 times ULN and bilirubin level ≤1.5 mg/dL: 100 mg/m²

If transaminase levels <10 times ULN and bilirubin level 1.6-7.5 mg/dL: 50 mg/m²

If transaminase levels ≥10 times ULN and bilirubin level >7.5 mg/dL: Avoid use

3-hour infusion:

If transaminase levels <10 times ULN and bilirubin level ≤1.25 times ULN: 175 mg/m²

If transaminase levels <10 times ULN and bilirubin level 1.26-2 times ULN: 135 mg/m²

If transaminase levels <10 times ULN and bilirubin level 2.01-5 times ULN: 90 mg/m²

If transaminase levels ≥10 times ULN and bilirubin level >5 times ULN: Avoid use

Available Dosage Forms Injection, solution: 6 mg/mL (5 mL, 16.7 mL, 50 mL) [contains alcohol and purified Cremophor® EL (polyoxyethylated castor oil)]

Onxol™: 6 mg/mL (5 mL, 25 mL, 50 mL) [contains alcohol] [contains alcohol and purified Cremophor® EL (polyoxyethylated castor oil)]

Taxol®: 6 mg/mL (5 mL, 16.7 mL, 50 mL) [contains alcohol and purified Cremophor® EL (polyoxyethylated castor oil)]

Monitoring and Teaching Issues

Physical Assessment: Note sequencing specifics; directions, taxane derivatives should be administered before platinum derivatives to limit myelosuppression (see Warnings/Precautions). Assess potential for interactions with other pharmacological agents and herbal products patient may be taking (eg, risk of increased or decreased levels/effects of paclitaxel; see Drug Interactions). See Administration for specific infusion directions. Premedication with dexamethasone, diphenhydramine and an H₂-blocker is recommended to reduce severe hypersensitivity reactions (see Dosing and Administration). Infusion site should be closely monitored to prevent extravasation. Assess results of laboratory tests prior to and regularly during therapy. Monitor adverse response prior to, during, and between each infusion (eg, hypersensitivity reactions, peripheral neuropathy [numbness, tingling, burning pain], myelosuppression [anemia, opportunistic infection], GI irritation [nausea, vomiting, mucositis, stomatitis]; see Adverse Reactions). Teach patient possible (Continued)

Paclitaxel *(Continued)*

side effects/appropriate interventions and adverse symptoms to report (see Patient Education).

Monitoring Laboratory Tests: CBC with differential and platelet count, liver and kidney function

Patient Education: Do not take any new medication during therapy unless approved by prescriber. This drug is given by infusion; report immediately any redness, swelling, burning, pain at infusion site or signs of allergic reaction (eg, respiratory or swallowing difficulty, chest tightness, rash, hives, swelling of lips or mouth). Maintain adequate hydration (2-3 L/day of fluids) unless instructed to restrict fluid intake and nutrition (frequent, small meals). You will be more susceptible to infection (avoid crowds and exposure to infection and do not have any vaccinations without consulting prescriber). May cause loss of hair (will grow back after therapy); nausea or vomiting (consult prescriber for approved antiemetic); weakness or lethargy (use caution when driving or engaging in tasks that require alertness until response to drug is known); or mouth sores (use good oral care, brush with soft toothbrush and use waxed dental floss). Report numbness or tingling in fingers or toes (use care to prevent injury); signs of opportunistic infection (fever, chills, sore throat, burning urination, fatigue); unusual bleeding (tarry stools, easy bruising, blood in stool, urine, or mouth); unresolved mouth sores; skin rash or itching; or other persistent adverse reactions. **Pregnancy/breast-feeding precautions:** Do not get pregnant while taking this medication. Consult prescriber for appropriate contraceptive measures. Do not breast-feed.

Geriatric Considerations: Elderly patients may have a higher incidence of severe neuropathy, severe myelosuppression, or cardiovascular events as compared to younger patients.

Pregnancy Risk Factor: D

Pregnancy Issues: Teratogenic effects have been observed in animal studies; women of childbearing potential should be advised to avoid becoming pregnant.

Lactation: Excretion in breast milk unknown/contraindicated

Breast-Feeding Issues: Antineoplastic agents are generally contraindicated.

Administration

I.V.: Irritant. Manufacturer recommends administration over 1-24 hours. Other routes are being studied. When administered as sequential infusions, taxane derivatives should be administered before platinum derivatives (cisplatin, carboplatin) to limit myelosuppression and to enhance efficacy.

Anaphylactoid-like reactions have been reported: Premedication with dexamethasone (20 mg orally or I.V. at 12 and 6 hours **or** 14 and 7 hours before the dose), diphenhydramine (50 mg I.V. 30-60 minutes prior to the dose), and cimetidine, famotidine or ranitidine (I.V. 30-60 minutes prior to the dose) is recommended.

Administer I.V. infusion over 1-24 hours; use of a 0.22 micron in-line filter and nonsorbing administration set is recommended during the infusion

Nonpolyvinyl (non-PVC) tubing (eg, polyethylene) should be used to minimize leaching. Formulated in a vehicle known as Cremophor® EL (polyoxyethylated castor oil). Cremophor® EL has been found to leach the plasticizer DEHP from polyvinyl chloride infusion bags or administration sets. Contact of the undiluted concentrate with plasticized polyvinyl chloride (PVC) equipment or devices is not recommended. Administer through I.V. tubing containing an in-line filter (NOT >0.22 μ) filter; administration through IVEX-2® filters (which incorporate short inlet and outlet polyvinyl chloride-coated tubing) has not resulted in significant leaching of DEHP.

Reconstitution: Dilute in D_5W, D_5LR, D_5NS, or NS to a concentration of of 0.3-1.2 mg/mL.

Compatibility: Stable in D_5W, D_5NS, D_5LR, NS

Y-site administration: Incompatible with amphotericin B, amphotericin B cholesteryl sulfate complex, chlorpromazine, doxorubicin liposome, hydroxyzine, methylprednisolone sodium succinate, mitoxantrone

Storage: Store intact vials at room temperature of 20°C to 25°C (68°F to 77°F). Protect from light. Per the manufacturer, reconstituted solution is stable for up to 27 hours at room temperature (25°C) and ambient light conditions. Other sources report that solutions in D_5W and NS are stable for up to 3 days at room temperature (25°C).

Paclitaxel should be dispensed in either glass or Excel™/PAB™ containers. Should also use **nonpolyvinyl** (non-PVC) tubing (eg, polyethylene) to minimize leaching. Formulated in a vehicle known as Cremophor® EL (polyoxyethylated castor oil). Cremophor® EL has been found to leach the plasticizer DEHP from polyvinyl chloride infusion bags or administration sets. Contact of the undiluted concentrate with plasticized polyvinyl chloride (PVC) equipment or devices is not recommended. Administer through I.V. tubing containing an in-line (NOT >0.22 μ) filter; administration through IVEX-2® filters (which incorporate short inlet and outlet polyvinyl chloride-coated tubing) has not resulted in significant leaching of DEHP.

Additional Information Sensory neuropathy is almost universal at doses >250 mg/m²; motor neuropathy is uncommon at doses <250 mg/m². Myopathic effects are common with doses >200 mg/m², generally occur within 2-3 days of treatment, and resolve over 5-6 days. Patients with pre-existing neuropathies from chemotherapy or coexisting conditions (eg, diabetes mellitus) may be at a higher risk.

Paclitaxel (Protein Bound) *(PAK li taks el PROE teen bownd)*

U.S. Brand Names Abraxane™

Synonyms BI-007; NAB-Paclitaxel; Protein-Bound Paclitaxel

Generic Available No

Pharmacologic Category Antineoplastic Agent, Antimicrotubular; Antineoplastic Agent, Natural Source (Plant) Derivative

Medication Safety Issues

Sound-alike/look-alike issues:

Paclitaxel (protein bound) may be confused with paclitaxel (conventional)

Abraxane™ may be confused with Paxil®, Taxol®, Taxotere®

Use Treatment of breast cancer (second-line)

Mechanism of Action/Effect Paclitaxel promotes microtubule assembly by enhancing the action of tubulin dimers, stabilizing existing microtubules, and inhibiting their disassembly, interfering with the late G_2 mitotic phase, and inhibiting cell replication. In addition, the drug can distort mitotic spindles, resulting in the breakage of chromosomes. Paclitaxel may also suppress cell proliferation and modulate immune response.

Contraindications Hypersensitivity to paclitaxel or any component of the formulation; baseline neutrophil count <1,500 cells/mm^3

Warnings/Precautions The U.S. Food and Drug Administration (FDA) currently recommends that procedures for proper handling and disposal of antineoplastic agents be considered.

Paclitaxel (protein-bound) is not interchangeable with Cremophor®-based paclitaxel. Use caution in neutropenia or thrombocytopenia; dosage adjustment recommended if severe drug-induced neutropenia lasts for ≥1 week; severe sensory neuropathy may occur; modified dosage recommended for subsequent courses of therapy. Use caution in hepatic and renal dysfunction. When administered as sequential infusions, taxane derivatives (docetaxel, paclitaxel) should be administered before platinum derivatives (carboplatin, cisplatin) to limit myelosuppression.

Drug Interactions

Cytochrome P450 Effect: Substrate (major) of CYP2C8/9, 3A4; **Induces** CYP3A4 (weak)

Decreased Effect: CYP2C8/9 inducers may decrease the levels/effects of paclitaxel; example inducers include carbamazepine, phenobarbital, phenytoin, rifampin, rifapentine, and secobarbital. CYP3A4 inducers may decrease the levels/effects of paclitaxel; example inducers include aminoglutethimide, carbamazepine, nafcillin, nevirapine, phenobarbital, phenytoin, and rifamycins.

Increased Effect/Toxicity: CYP2C8/9 inhibitors may increase the levels/effects of paclitaxel; example inhibitors include delavirdine, fluconazole, gemfibrozil, ketoconazole, nicardipine, NSAIDs, pioglitazone, and sulfonamides. CYP3A4 inhibitors may increase the levels/effects of paclitaxel; example inhibitors include azole antifungals, ciprofloxacin, clarithromycin, diclofenac, doxycycline, erythromycin, imatinib, isoniazid, nefazodone, nicardipine, propofol, protease inhibitors, quinidine, and verapamil. In Phase I trials, myelosuppression was more profound when given after cisplatin than with alternative sequence. administered as sequential infusions, studies indicate a potential for increased toxicity when platinum derivatives (carboplatin, cisplatin) are administered before taxane derivatives (docetaxel, paclitaxel). Paclitaxel may increase doxorubicin levels/toxicity.

Nutritional/Ethanol Interactions

Herb/Nutraceutical: Avoid black cohosh, dong quai in estrogen-dependent tumors. Avoid valerian, St John's wort, kava kava, gotu kola (may increase CNS depression).

Adverse Reactions

>10%:

Cardiovascular: EKG abnormal (60%)

Dermatologic: Alopecia (90%)

Gastrointestinal: Nausea (30%; severe 3%), diarrhea (26%; severe <1%), vomiting (18%; severe 4%)

Hematologic: Neutropenia (80%; grade 4 - 9%), anemia (33%; severe 1%)

Hepatic: AST increased (39%), alkaline phosphatase increased (36%)

Neuromuscular & skeletal: Sensory neuropathy (71%; severe 10%), asthenia (47%; severe 8%), myalgia/arthralgia (44%; severe 8%)

Ocular: Vision disturbance (13%; severe 1%)

Respiratory: Dyspnea (12%)

Miscellaneous: Infections (24%; primarily included oral candidiasis, respiratory tract infections, and pneumonia)

1% to 10%:

Cardiovascular: Edema (10%; severe 0%), hypotension (5%), Grade 3 cardiovascular events (3%; included chest pain, cardiac arrest, supraventricular tachycardia, edema, thrombosis, pulmonary thromboembolism, pulmonary emboli, and hypertension)

Central nervous system: Febrile neutropenia (2%)

Gastrointestinal: Mucositis (7%; severe < 1%)

Hematologic: Thrombocytopenia (2%), bleeding (2%)

Hepatic: Bilirubin increased (7%)

Local: Injection site reaction (1%)

Renal: Creatinine increased (11%; severe 1%)

Respiratory: Cough (6%)

Miscellaneous: Hypersensitivity reaction (4%)

Overdosage/Toxicology Overdose would likely result in severe bone marrow suppression, sensory neuropathy, and mucositis. Treatment should be supportive.

Pharmacodynamics/Kinetics

Protein Binding: 89% to 98%

Half-Life Elimination: Terminal: 27 hours

Metabolism: Hepatic via CYP3A4 and 2C8

Excretion: Urine (4% as unchanged drug, 1% as metabolites); feces (20%)

Clearance 15 L/hour/m^2

Dosing

Adults: Breast cancer: I.V.: 260 mg/m^2 every 3 weeks

Dosage adjustment for toxicity:

Severe neutropenia (<500 cells/mm^3) ≥1 week: Reduce dose to 220 mg/m^2 for subsequent courses

Recurrent severe neutropenia: Reduce dose to 180 mg/m^2

Severe sensory neuropathy: Reduce dose to 180 mg/m^2

Sensory neuropathy grade 3 or 4: Hold treatment until resolved to grade 1 or 2, then resume with reduced dose

(Continued)

Paclitaxel (Protein Bound) *(Continued)*

Renal Impairment: Safety not established for serum creatinine >2 mg/dL; use with caution.

Hepatic Impairment: Effects of hepatic dysfunction (serum bilirubin >1.5 mg/dL) unknown; dosage adjustment recommendations are not available.

Available Dosage Forms Injection, powder for reconstitution: 100 mg [contains human albumin 900 mg]

Monitoring and Teaching Issues

Physical Assessment: Assess other prescriptions, OTCs, or biologicals patient is taking (see Drug Interactions for discussion of potentially harmful interactions). Infusion site should be monitored to prevent extravasation. Vital signs (especially heart rate and blood pressure) and results of laboratory tests should be monitored during infusion. Assess for adverse reactions on a regular basis for duration of therapy (see Adverse Reactions). Teach patient/caregiver possible side effects, appropriate interventions, adverse symptoms to report, and pregnancy precautions (see Patient Education).

Monitoring Laboratory Tests: CBC, BP (during infusion)

Patient Education: Inform prescriber of all prescriptions, OTC medications, or herbal products you are taking, and any allergies you have. Do not take any new medication during therapy unless approved by prescriber. This drug can only be given by infusion. Report immediately any redness, swelling, burning, pain at infusion site or signs of allergic reaction (eg, respiratory or swallowing difficulty, chest tightness, rash, hives, swelling of lips or mouth). Maintain adequate hydration (2-3 L/day of fluids) unless instructed to restrict fluid intake and nutrition. You will be more susceptible to infection (avoid crowds and exposure to infection and do not have any vaccinations without consulting prescriber). May cause loss of hair (will grow back after therapy); experience nausea or vomiting (consult prescriber for approved antiemetic); feel weak or lethargic (use caution when driving or engaging in tasks that require alertness until response to drug is known); or mouth sores (use good oral care, bush with soft toothbrush and use waxed dental floss). Report numbness or tingling in fingers or toes (use care to prevent injury); signs of opportunistic infection (fever, chills, sore throat, burning urination, fatigue); unusual bleeding (tarry stools, easy bruising, or blood in stool, urine, or mouth); unresolved mouth sores; nausea or vomiting; or skin rash or itching. **Pregnancy/breast-feeding precautions:** Do not get pregnant while taking this medication. Consult prescriber for appropriate contraceptive measures. Do not breast-feed. Men should not father a child during therapy.

Pregnancy Risk Factor: D

Lactation: Excretion in breast milk unknown/not recommended

Breast-Feeding Issues: The manufacturer recommends that nursing be discontinued during paclitaxel (protein-bound) therapy.

Administration

I.V.: Administer over 30 minutes. Use of DEHP-free containers or administration sets is not necessary; do not use an in-line filter.

Reconstitution: Reconstitute vial with 20 mL NS (inject over 1 minute onto inside wall of vial, allow to sit for 5 minutes, then gently swirl until dissolved) to achieve 5 mg/mL solution. Inject dose for infusion into empty PVC bag. **Note:** Use of DEHP-free containers or administration sets is not necessary. Do not use an in-line filter.

Compatibility: Stable in NS. Formulation contains albumin; do not mix with other drugs.

Storage: Store intact vial at room temperature of 20°C to 25°C (68°F to 77°F) and protect from bright light. Reconstituted solution may be stored under refrigeration 2°C to 8°C (36°F to 46°F) for up to 8 hours. The solution for administration is stable for up to 8 hours at room temperature and ambient light.

- ♦ **Palgic®-D** *see* Carbinoxamine and Pseudoephedrine *on page 254*
- ♦ **Palgic®-DS** *see* Carbinoxamine and Pseudoephedrine *on page 254*
- ♦ **Palladone™** *see* Hydromorphone *on page 764*
- ♦ **Palmer's® Skin Success Eventone® Fade Cream [OTC]** *see* Hydroquinone *on page 768*

Palonosetron *(pal oh NOE se tron)*

U.S. Brand Names Aloxi™

Synonyms Palonosetron Hydrochloride; RS-25259; RS-25259-197

Generic Available No

Pharmacologic Category Antiemetic; Selective 5-HT$_3$ Receptor Antagonist

Medication Safety Issues

Sound-alike/look-alike issues:

Aloxi™ may be confused with oxaliplatin

Use Prevention of acute (within 24 hours) and delayed (2-5 days) chemotherapy-induced nausea and vomiting

Unlabeled/Investigational Use Prevention of postoperative vomiting

Mechanism of Action/Effect Selective 5-HT$_3$ receptor antagonist, blocking serotonin, both peripherally on vagal nerve terminals and centrally in the chemoreceptor trigger zone

Contraindications Hypersensitivity to palonosetron or any component of the formulation

Warnings/Precautions Use caution in patients allergic to other 5-HT$_3$ receptor antagonists; cross-reactivity is possible. Caution in patients with congenital QT syndrome or other risk factors for QT prolongation (eg, drugs, electrolyte abnormalities). Safety and efficacy in pediatric patients (<18 years of age) have not been established.

Drug Interactions

Cytochrome P450 Effect: Substrate (minor) of CYP1A2, 2D6, 3A4

Increased Effect/Toxicity: No drug interactions of concern have been identified.

Adverse Reactions

>10%: Dermatologic: Pruritus (8% to 22%)

1% to 10%:

Cardiovascular: Bradycardia (1%), hypotension (1%), tachycardia (nonsustained) (1%)

Central nervous system: Headache (6% to 9%), anxiety (1% to 5%), dizziness (1%)

Endocrine & metabolic: Hyperkalemia (1%)
Gastrointestinal: Constipation (5% to 10%), diarrhea (1%)
Neuromuscular & skeletal: Weakness (1%)

Overdosage/Toxicology Dose-ranging studies in humans using doses up to 25 times the recommended dose of 0.25 mg revealed no increase in the incidence of adverse effects compared to lower dose groups. Treatment is supportive.

Pharmacodynamics/Kinetics
Protein Binding: 62%
Half-Life Elimination: Terminal: 40 hours
Metabolism: ~50% metabolized via CYP enzymes (and likely other pathways) to relatively inactive metabolites; CYP1A2, 2D6, and 3A4 contribute to its metabolism
Excretion: Urine (80%, 40% as unchanged drug)

Dosing
Adults:
Chemotherapy-induced nausea and vomiting: I.V.: 0.25 mg 30 minutes prior to chemotherapy administration, day 1 of each cycle (doses should not be given more than once weekly)
Postoperative nausea and vomiting (unlabeled use): I.V.: 30 mcg/kg (used in hysterectomy, lower doses ineffective; no significant reduction in nausea at any dose)
Elderly: No dosage adjustment necessary.
Renal Impairment: No dosage adjustment necessary.
Hepatic Impairment: No dosage adjustment necessary.

Available Dosage Forms Injection, solution: 0.05 mg/mL (5 mL)

Monitoring and Teaching Issues
Physical Assessment: Assess allergy history (5-HT$_3$ receptor antagonists) prior to administering. See Warnings/Precautions for use cautions. See Administration for infusion specifics. Assess patient response and adverse reactions at beginning and periodically during therapy. Teach patient possible side effects/appropriate interventions, and adverse symptoms to report (see Patient Education).
Patient Education: This medication is only given by intravenous infusion. You will be monitored during infusion. Report immediately any chest pain, respiratory difficulty, pain or itching at infusion site. May cause dizziness, headache, or weakness (use caution when driving or engaging in hazardous tasks until response to drug is known). Report rash or any unusual or persistent adverse effects. **Pregnancy/breast-feeding precautions:** Breast-feeding is not recommended.
Pregnancy Risk Factor: B
Lactation: Excretion in breast milk unknown/not recommended
Breast-Feeding Issues: The extent to which palonosetron is excreted in breast milk, if at all, is unknown. Use in nursing women only if potential risks outweigh benefits.

Administration
I.V.: I.V.: Infuse over 30 seconds; flush I.V. line with NS prior to and following administration.
Compatibility: Stable in D$_5$W, NS, D$_5$1/2NS, and D$_5$LR
Y-site administration: Compatible: Doxorubicin, epirubicin
Storage: Store intact vials at controlled room temperature of 20°C to 25°C (68°F to 77°F); protect from freezing and light. Solutions of 5 mcg/mL and 30 mcg/mL in NS, D$_5$W, D$_5$1/2NS, and D$_5$LR injection are stable for 48 hours at room temperature and 14 days under refrigeration.

♦ **Palonosetron Hydrochloride** *see* Palonosetron *on page 1148*

♦ **Pamelor®** *see* Nortriptyline *on page 1099*

Pamidronate (pa mi DROE nate)

U.S. Brand Names Aredia®
Synonyms Pamidronate Disodium
Generic Available Yes
Pharmacologic Category Antidote; Bisphosphonate Derivative
Medication Safety Issues
Sound-alike/look-alike issues:
Aredia® may be confused with Adriamycin

Use Treatment of hypercalcemia associated with malignancy; treatment of osteolytic bone lesions associated with multiple myeloma or metastatic breast cancer; moderate to severe Paget's disease of bone

Mechanism of Action/Effect A bisphosphonate which inhibits bone resorption via actions on osteoclasts or on osteoclast precursors. Does not appear to produce any significant effects on renal tubular calcium handling and is poorly absorbed following oral administration (high oral doses have been reported effective); therefore, I.V. therapy is preferred.

Contraindications Hypersensitivity to pamidronate, other bisphosphonates, or any component of the formulation; pregnancy

Warnings/Precautions Osteonecrosis of the jaw has been reported in patients with cancer who were receiving chemotherapy, corticosteroids, and chronic bisphosphonate therapy; symptoms included nonhealing extraction socket or an exposed jawbone. Dental exams and preventative dentistry should be performed prior to placing patients with risk factors (eg, chemotherapy, corticosteroids, poor oral hygiene) on chronic bisphosphonate therapy. Invasive dental procedures should be avoided during treatment.

May cause deterioration in renal function. Use caution in patients with renal impairment and avoid in severe renal impairment. Assess serum creatinine prior to each dose; withhold dose in patients with bone metastases who experience deterioration in renal function. Leukemia has been observed with oral pamidronate and monitoring of white blood cell counts is suggested. Vein irritation and thrombophlebitis may occur with infusions. In elderly patients, monitor serum electrolytes periodically since elderly are often receiving diuretics which can result in decreases in serum calcium, potassium, and magnesium.
(Continued)

Pamidronate *(Continued)*

Drug Interactions

Increased Effect/Toxicity: Aminoglycosides may lower serum calcium levels with prolonged administration; concomitant use may have additive effect. Increased risk of hypocalcemia with concomitant loop diuretic use.

Adverse Reactions
As reported with hypercalcemia of malignancy; percentage of adverse effect varies upon dose and duration of infusion.

>10%:
    Central nervous system: Fever (18% to 26%), fatigue (12%)
    Endocrine & metabolic: Hypophosphatemia (9% to 18%), hypokalemia (4% to 18%), hypo-magnesemia (4% to 12%), hypocalcemia (1% to 12%)
    Gastrointestinal: Nausea (up to 18%), anorexia (1% to 12%)
    Local: Infusion site reaction (up to 18%)

1% to 10%:
    Cardiovascular: Atrial fibrillation (up to 6%), hypertension (up to 6%), syncope (up to 6%), tachycardia (up to 6%), atrial flutter (up to 1%), cardiac failure (up to 1%)
    Central nervous system: Somnolence (1% to 6%), psychosis (up to 4%), insomnia (up to 1%)
    Endocrine & metabolic: Hypothyroidism (6%)
    Gastrointestinal: Constipation (4% to 6%), stomatitis (up to 1%)
    Hematologic: Leukopenia (up to 4%), neutropenia (up to 1%), thrombocytopenia (up to 1%)
    Neuromuscular & skeletal: Myalgia (up to 1%)
    Renal: Uremia (up to 4%)
    Respiratory: Rales (up to 6%), rhinitis (up to 6%), upper respiratory tract infection (up to 3%)

Overdosage/Toxicology
Symptoms of overdose include hypocalcemia, ECG changes, seizures, bleeding, paresthesia, carpopedal spasm, and fever. Treat with I.V. calcium gluconate, and general supportive care; fever and hypotension can be treated with corticosteroids.

Pharmacodynamics/Kinetics

Onset of Action: 24-48 hours; Peak effect: Maximum: 5-7 days
Absorption: Poor; pharmacokinetic studies lacking
Half-Life Elimination: 21-35 hours
Metabolism: Not metabolized
Excretion: Biphasic; urine (~50% as unchanged drug) within 120 hours

Dosing

Adults & Elderly: Note: Drug must be diluted properly before administration and infused intravenously slowly. Due to risk of nephrotoxicity, doses should not exceed 90 mg.

    Hypercalcemia of malignancy: I.V.:
        Moderate cancer-related hypercalcemia (corrected serum calcium: 12-13.5 mg/dL): 60-90 mg, as a single dose, given as a slow infusion over 2-24 hours; dose should be diluted in 1000 mL 0.45% NaCl, 0.9% NaCl, or D_5W
        Severe cancer-related hypercalcemia (corrected serum calcium: >13.5 mg/dL): 90 mg, as a single dose, as a slow infusion over 2-24 hours; dose should be diluted in 1000 mL 0.45% NaCl, 0.9% NaCl, or D_5W
        Repeat dosing: A period of 7 days should elapse before the use of second course; repeat infusions every 2-3 weeks have been suggested, however, could be administered every 2-3 months according to the degree and of severity of hypercalcemia and/or the type of malignancy.
        Note: Some investigators have suggested a lack of a dose-response relationship. Courses of pamidronate for hypercalcemia may be repeated at varying intervals, depending on the duration of normocalcemia (median 2-3 weeks), but the manufacturer recommends a minimum interval between courses of 7 days. Oral etidronate at a dose of 20 mg/kg/day has been used to maintain the calcium lowering effect following I.V. bisphosphonates, although it is of limited effectiveness.

    Osteolytic bone lesions with multiple myeloma: I.V.: 90 mg in 500 mL D_5W, 0.45% NaCl or 0.9% NaCl administered over 4 hours on a monthly basis
    Osteolytic bone lesions with metastatic breast cancer: I.V.: 90 mg in 250 mL D_5W, 0.45% NaCl or 0.9% NaCl administered over 2 hours, repeated every 3-4 weeks
    Paget's disease: I.V.: 30 mg in 500 mL 0.45% NaCl, 0.9% NaCl or D_5W administered over 4 hours for 3 consecutive days

Renal Impairment: Not recommended in severe renal impairment (patients with bone metastases).

    Dosing adjustment in renal toxicity: In patients with bone metastases, treatment should be withheld in patients who experience deterioration in renal function (increase of serum creatinine ≥0.5 mg/dL in patients with normal baseline or ≥1.0 mg/dL in patients with abnormal baseline). Resumption of therapy may be considered when serum creatinine returns to within 10% of baseline.

Available Dosage Forms

Injection, powder for reconstitution, as disodium (Aredia®): 30 mg, 90 mg
Injection, solution: 3 mg/mL (10 mL); 6 mg/mL (10 mL); 9 mg/mL (10 mL)

Monitoring and Teaching Issues

Physical Assessment: Assess results of laboratory tests, therapeutic effectiveness, and adverse reactions. Teach patient lifestyle and dietary changes that will be beneficial, possible side effects, interventions to reduce side effects, and adverse reactions to report.

Monitoring Laboratory Tests: Serum electrolytes, monitor for hypocalcemia for at least 2 weeks after therapy; serum calcium, phosphate, magnesium, CBC with differential; monitor serum creatinine prior to each dose

Patient Education: Do not take any new medication during therapy unless approved by prescriber. This medication can only be administered intravenously; report immediately any difficulty breathing, chest tightness, difficulty swallowing, redness, swelling, or pain at infusion site. Avoid foods high in calcium or vitamins with mineral during infusion or for 2-3 hours after completion. You may experience nausea or vomiting (small frequent meals and good mouth care may help); recurrent bone pain (consult prescriber for analgesic);

increased fatigue (adequate rest is important); dizziness (use caution when driving or engaged in potentially dangerous tasks until response to drug is known). Report palpitations or rapid heart beat, unusual muscle twitching or spasms, persistent diarrhea/constipation, or acute bone pain, respiratory difficulty, or other persistent adverse effects. **Pregnancy/breast-feeding precautions:** Inform prescriber if you are pregnant. Do not get pregnant while taking this medication. Consult prescriber for appropriate contraceptive measures. Consult prescriber if breast-feeding.

Geriatric Considerations: Has not been studied exclusively in the elderly. Monitor serum electrolytes periodically since elderly are often receiving diuretics which can result in decreases in serum calcium, potassium, and magnesium.

Pregnancy Risk Factor: D

Pregnancy Issues: Pamidronate has been shown to cross the placenta and cause nonteratogenic embryo/fetal effects in animals. There are no adequate and well-controlled studies in pregnant women; manufacturer states pamidronate should not be used in pregnancy. Based on limited case reports, serum calcium levels in the newborn may be altered if pamidronate is administered during pregnancy. Bisphosphonates are incorporated into the bone matrix and gradually released over time. Theoretically, there may be a risk of fetal harm when pregnancy follows the completion of therapy.

Lactation: Excretion in breast milk unknown/use caution

Administration

I.V.: Drug must be properly diluted before administration and slowly infused intravenously (over at least 2 hours).

Reconstitution: Powder for injection: Reconstitute by adding 10 mL of sterile water for injection to each vial of lyophilized pamidronate disodium powder, the resulting solution will be 30 mg/10 mL or 90 mg/10 mL. The reconstituted solution is stable under refrigeration at 2°C to 8°C (36°F to 46°F) for 24 hours.

Pamidronate may be further diluted in 250-1000 mL of 0.45% or 0.9% sodium chloride or 5% dextrose; pamidronate should not be mixed with calcium-containing solutions (eg, Ringer's solution). Pamidronate solution for infusion is stable at room temperature for up to 24 hours.

Compatibility: Incompatible with calcium-containing infusion solutions such as lactated Ringer's

Storage: Do not store powder for reconstitution at temperatures above 30°C (86°F).

♦ **Pamidronate Disodium** see Pamidronate on page 1149
♦ **p-Aminoclonidine** see Apraclonidine on page 132
♦ **Pamprin® Maximum Strength All Day Relief [OTC]** see Naproxen on page 1056
♦ **Pan-B Antibody** see Rituximab on page 1338
♦ **Pancof®-EXP** see Dihydrocodeine, Pseudoephedrine, and Guaifenesin on page 457
♦ **Pancrease®** see Pancrelipase on page 1151
♦ **Pancrease® MT** see Pancrelipase on page 1151
♦ **Pancrecarb MS®** see Pancrelipase on page 1151

Pancrelipase (pan kre LI pase)

U.S. Brand Names Creon®; Ku-Zyme® HP; Lipram 4500; Lipram-CR; Lipram-PN; Lipram-UL; Pancrease®; Pancrease® MT; Pancrecarb MS®; Pangestyme™ CN; Pangestyme™ EC; Pangestyme™ MT; Pangestyme™ UL; Ultrase®; Ultrase® MT; Viokase®

Synonyms Lipancreatin

Generic Available Yes

Pharmacologic Category Enzyme

Use Replacement therapy in symptomatic treatment of malabsorption syndrome caused by pancreatic insufficiency

Unlabeled/Investigational Use Treatment of occluded feeding tubes

Mechanism of Action/Effect Replaces endogenous pancreatic enzymes to assist in digestion of protein, starch and fats

Contraindications Hypersensitivity to pork protein or any component of the formulation; acute pancreatitis or acute exacerbations of chronic pancreatic disease

Warnings/Precautions Pancrelipase is inactivated by acids. Use microencapsulated products whenever possible, since these products permit better dissolution of enzymes in the duodenum and protect the enzyme preparations from acid degradation in the stomach. Fibrotic strictures in the colon, some requiring surgery, have been reported with high doses; use caution, especially in children with cystic fibrosis. Use caution when adjusting doses or changing brands. Avoid inhalation of powder, may cause nasal and respiratory tract irritation.

Nutritional/Ethanol Interactions Food: Avoid placing contents of opened capsules on alkaline food (pH >5.5); pancrelipase may impair absorption of oral iron and folic acid.

Adverse Reactions Frequency not defined; occurrence of events may be dose related.

Central nervous system: Pain

Dermatologic: Rash

Endocrine & metabolic: Hyperuricemia

Gastrointestinal: Nausea, cramps, constipation, diarrhea, perianal irritation/inflammation (large doses), irritation of the mouth, abdominal pain, intestinal obstruction, vomiting, flatulence, melena, weight loss, fibrotic strictures, greasy stools

Ocular: Lacrimation

Renal: Hyperuricosuria

Respiratory: Sneezing, dyspnea, bronchospasm

Miscellaneous: Allergic reactions

Overdosage/Toxicology Symptoms of overdose include diarrhea, other transient intestinal upset, hyperuricosuria, and hyperuricemia. Treatment is supportive.

(Continued)

Pancrelipase *(Continued)*

Pharmacodynamics/Kinetics
Absorption: None; acts locally in GI tract
Excretion: Feces

Dosing
Adults & Elderly:
Malabsorption: Oral:
Powder: Actual dose depends on the condition being treated and the digestive requirements of the patient: 0.7 g ($^1/_4$ teaspoonful) with meals

Capsules/tablets: The following dosage recommendations are only an approximation for initial dosages. The actual dosage will depend on the condition being treated and the digestive requirements of the individual patient.

Note: Dosage adjustment: Adjust dose based on body weight and stool fat content. Total daily dose reflects ~3 meals/day and 2-3 snacks/day, with half the mealtime dose given with a snack. Older patients may need less units/kg due to increased weight, but decreased ingestion of fat/kg. Maximum dose: 2500 units of lipase/kg/meal (10,000 units of lipase/kg/day): 4000-48,000 units of lipase with meals and with snacks

Occluded feeding tubes (unlabeled use): One tablet of Viokase® crushed with one 325 mg tablet of sodium bicarbonate (to activate the Viokase®) in 5 mL of water can be instilled into the nasogastric tube and clamped for 5 minutes; then, flushed with 50 mL of tap water

Pediatrics:
Malabsorption: Oral:
Powder: Actual dose depends on the condition being treated and the digestive requirements of the patient: Children <1 year: Start with $^1/_8$ teaspoonful with feedings

Capsules/tablets: Children: Approximate initial dosages; actual dosage will depend on the condition being treated and the digestive requirements of the individual patient.
<1 year: 2000 units of lipase with meals
1-6 years: 4000-8000 units of lipase with meals and 4000 units with snacks
7-12 years: 4000-12,000 units of lipase with meals and snacks

Note: Dosage adjustment: Adjust dose based on body weight and stool fat content. Total daily dose reflects ~3 meals/day and 2-3 snacks/day, with half the mealtime dose given with a snack.

Available Dosage Forms
Capsule (Ku-Zyme® HP): Lipase 8000 units, protease 30,000 units, amylase 30,000 units
Capsule, delayed release:
Pangestyme™ CN-10: Lipase 10,000 units, protease 37,500 units, amylase 33,200 units
Pangestyme™ CN-20: Lipase 20,000 units, protease 75,000 units, amylase 66,400 units
Capsule, delayed release, enteric coated microspheres:
Creon® 5: Lipase 5000 units, protease 18,750 units, amylase 16,600 units
Creon® 10: Lipase 10,000 units, protease 37,500 units, amylase 33,200 units
Creon® 20: Lipase 20,000 units, protease 75,000 units, amylase 66,400 units
Lipram 4500: Lipase 4500 units, protease 25,000 units, amylase 20,000 units
Lipram-CR10: Lipase 10,000 units, protease 37,500 units, amylase 33,200 units
Lipram-CR20: Lipase 20,000 units, protease 75,000 units, amylase 66,400 units
Lipram-PN10: Lipase 10,000 units, protease 30,000 units, amylase 30,000 units
Lipram-PN16: Lipase 16,000 units, protease 48,000 units, amylase 48,000 units
Lipram-UL12: Lipase 12,000 units, protease 39,000 units, amylase 39,000 units
Lipram-UL18: Lipase 18,000 units, protease 58,500 units, amylase 58,500 units
Lipram-UL20: Lipase 20,000 units, protease 65,000 units, amylase 65,000 units
Pancrecarb MS-4®: Lipase 4000 units, protease 25,000 units, amylase 25,000 units [buffered]
Pancrecarb MS-8®: Lipase 8000 units, protease 45,000 units, amylase 40,000 units [buffered]
Capsule, enteric coated microspheres (Pancrease®, Pangestyme™ EC, Ultrase®): Lipase 4500 units, protease 25,000 units, amylase 20,000 units
Capsule, enteric coated microtablets:
Pancrease® MT 4: Lipase 4000 units, protease 12,000 units, amylase 12,000 units
Pancrease® MT 10: Lipase 10,000 units, protease 30,000 units, amylase 30,000 units
Pancrease® MT 16, Pangestyme™ MT 16: Lipase 16,000 units, protease 48,000 units, amylase 48,000 units
Pancrease® MT 20: Lipase 20,000 units, protease 44,000 units, amylase 56,000 units
Pangestyme™ UL 12: Lipase 12,000 units, protease 39,000 units, amylase 39,000 units
Pangestyme™ UL 18: Lipase 18,000 units, protease 58,500 units, amylase 58,500 units
Pangestyme™ UL 20: Lipase 20,000 units, protease 65,000 units, amylase 65,000 units
Capsule, enteric coated minitablets:
Ultrase® MT12: Lipase 12,000 units, protease 39,000 units, amylase 39,000 units
Ultrase® MT18: Lipase 18,000 units, protease 58,500 units, amylase 58,500 units
Ultrase® MT20: Lipase 20,000 units, protease 65,000 units, amylase 65,000 units
Powder (Viokase®): Lipase 16,800 units, protease 70,000 units, amylase 70,000 units per 0.7 g (227 g)
Tablet:
Viokase® 8: Lipase 8000 units, protease 30,000 units, amylase 30,000 units
Viokase® 16: Lipase 16,000 units, protease 60,000 units, amylase 60,000 units

Monitoring and Teaching Issues
Physical Assessment: See Warnings/Precautions for use cautions. Dosing and administration depends on purpose for use (see Dosing and Administration). Use caution preparing powder; if powder spills on skin, wash off immediately; do not inhale powder. Teach patient possible side effects/appropriate interventions and adverse symptoms to report (see Patient Education).

Patient Education: Do not take any new medication during therapy unless approved by prescriber. Take right before or with foods and swallow whole with a generous amount of liquid. Dairy products such as milk, custard, or ice cream may have a high pH and should be avoided. Do not crush or chew tablets or regular capsules. Delayed-release capsules containing enteric coated microspheres or microtablets may be opened and the contents sprinkled on soft food with a low pH such as applesauce, gelatin; apricot, banana, or sweet potato baby food; baby formula. **Powder:** If powder spills on skin, wash off immediately, do not inhale powder when preparing. You may experience some gastric discomfort. Report unusual rash, persistent GI upset; or respiratory difficulty. **Pregnancy/breast-feeding precautions:** Inform prescriber if you are or intend to become pregnant. Consult prescriber if breast-feeding.

Dietary Considerations: Should be used as part of a high-calorie diet, appropriate for age and clinical status. Administer with meals or snacks and swallow whole with a generous amount of liquid. Do not crush or chew. Delayed-release capsules containing enteric coated microspheres or microtablets may also be opened and the contents sprinkled on soft food with a low pH such as applesauce, gelatin; apricot, banana, or sweet potato baby food; baby formula. Dairy products such as milk, custard or ice cream may have a high pH and should be avoided.

Geriatric Considerations: No special considerations are necessary since drug is dosed to response; however, drug-induced diarrhea can result in unwanted side effects (confusion, hypotension, lethargy, fluid and electrolyte loss).

Pregnancy Risk Factor: B/C (product specific)

Lactation: Excretion in breast milk unknown/use caution

Breast-Feeding Issues: Systemic absorption and concentration in the breast milk is unlikely, but unknown.

Administration

Oral: Oral: Administer with meals or snacks and swallow whole with a generous amount of liquid. Do not crush or chew; retention in the mouth before swallowing may cause mucosal irritation and stomatitis. Delayed-release capsules containing enteric-coated microspheres or microtablets may also be opened and the contents sprinkled on soft food with a low pH that does not require chewing, such as applesauce, gelatin; apricot, banana, or sweet potato baby food; baby formula. Dairy products such as milk, custard, or ice cream may have a high pH and should be avoided. Avoid inhalation of powder, may cause nasal and respiratory tract irritation.

Storage: Store between 15°C to 25°C (59°F to 77°F). Keep in a dry place. Do not refrigerate.

Pancuronium (pan kyoo ROE nee um)

Synonyms Pancuronium Bromide; Pavulon [DSC]

Generic Available Yes

Pharmacologic Category Neuromuscular Blocker Agent, Nondepolarizing

Medication Safety Issues

Sound-alike/look-alike issues:

Pancuronium may be confused with pipecuronium

Use Adjunct to general anesthesia to facilitate endotracheal intubation and to relax skeletal muscles during surgery; to facilitate mechanical ventilation in ICU patients; does not relieve pain or produce sedation

Drug of choice for neuromuscular blockade except in patients with renal failure, hepatic failure, or cardiovascular instability or in situations not suited for pancuronium's long duration of action

Mechanism of Action/Effect Blocks neural transmission at the myoneural junction by binding with cholinergic receptor sites

Contraindications Hypersensitivity to pancuronium, bromide, or any component of the formulation

Warnings/Precautions Ventilation must be supported during neuromuscular blockade; use with caution in patients with renal and/or hepatic impairment (adjust dose appropriately); certain clinical conditions may result in potentiation or antagonism of neuromuscular blockade:

Potentiation: Electrolyte abnormalities, severe hyponatremia, severe hypocalcemia, severe hypokalemia, hypermagnesemia, neuromuscular diseases, acidosis, acute intermittent porphyria, renal failure, hepatic failure

Antagonism: Alkalosis, hypercalcemia, demyelinating lesions, peripheral neuropathies, diabetes mellitus

Increased sensitivity in patients with myasthenia gravis, Eaton-Lambert syndrome; resistance in burn patients (>30% of body) for period of 5-70 days postinjury; resistance in patients with muscle trauma, denervation, immobilization, infection. Cross-sensitivity with other neuromuscular-blocking agents may occur; use extreme caution in patients with previous anaphylactic reactions.

Drug Interactions

Decreased Effect: Effect of nondepolarizing neuromuscular blockers may be reduced by carbamazepine (chronic use), corticosteroids (also associated with myopathy - see increased effect), phenytoin (chronic use), sympathomimetics, and theophylline.

Increased Effect/Toxicity: Increased effects are possible with aminoglycosides, beta-blockers, clindamycin, calcium channel blockers, halogenated anesthetics, imipenem, ketamine, lidocaine, loop diuretics (furosemide), macrolides (case reports), magnesium sulfate, procainamide, quinidine, quinolones, tetracyclines, and vancomycin. May increase risk of myopathy when used with high-dose corticosteroids for extended periods.

Adverse Reactions Frequency not defined.

Cardiovascular: Elevation in pulse rate, elevated blood pressure and cardiac output, tachycardia, edema, skin flushing, circulatory collapse

Dermatologic: Rash, itching, erythema, burning sensation along the vein

Gastrointestinal: Excessive salivation

Neuromuscular & skeletal: Profound muscle weakness

Respiratory: Wheezing, bronchospasm

Miscellaneous: Hypersensitivity reaction

(Continued)

Pancuronium *(Continued)*

Causes of prolonged neuromuscular blockade: Excessive drug administration; cumulative drug effect, decreased metabolism/excretion (hepatic and/or renal impairment); accumulation of active metabolites; electrolyte imbalance (hypokalemia, hypocalcemia, hypermagnesemia, hypernatremia); hypothermia; drug interactions; increased sensitivity to muscle relaxants (eg, neuromuscular disorders such as myasthenia gravis or polymyositis)

Overdosage/Toxicology Symptoms of overdose include apnea, respiratory depression, and cardiovascular collapse. Pyridostigmine, neostigmine, or edrophonium in conjunction with atropine will usually antagonize the action of pancuronium.

Pharmacodynamics/Kinetics

Onset of Action: Peak effect: I.V.: 2-3 minutes

Duration of Action: Dose dependent: 60-100 minutes

Half-Life Elimination: 110 minutes

Metabolism: Hepatic (30% to 45%); active metabolite 3-hydroxypancuronium ($\frac{1}{3}$ to $\frac{1}{2}$ the activity of parent drug)

Excretion: Urine (55% to 70% as unchanged drug)

Dosing

Adults & Elderly: Administer I.V.; dose to effect; doses will vary due to interpatient variability; use ideal body weight for obese patients

Neuromuscular blockade: Initial: 0.06-0.1 mg/kg or 0.05 mg/kg after initial dose of succinylcholine for intubation; maintenance dose: 0.01 mg/kg 60-100 minutes after initial dose and then 0.01 mg/kg every 25-60 minutes

Pretreatment/priming: 10% of intubating dose given 3-5 minutes before initial dose

Neuromuscular blockade in the ICU: 0.05-0.1 mg/kg bolus followed by 0.8-1.7 mcg/kg/minute once initial recovery from bolus observed or 0.1-0.2 mg/kg every 1-3 hours

Pediatrics: Infants >1 month and Children: Refer to adult dosing.

Renal Impairment: Elimination half-life is doubled, plasma clearance is reduced, and rate of recovery is sometimes much slower.

Cl_{cr} 10-50 mL/minute: Administer 50% of normal dose.

Cl_{cr} <10 mL/minute: Do not use.

Hepatic Impairment: Elimination half-life is doubled, plasma clearance is doubled, recovery time is prolonged, volume of distribution is increased (50%) and results in a slower onset, higher total dosage, and prolongation of neuromuscular blockade. Patients with liver disease may develop slow resistance to nondepolarizing muscle relaxant. Large doses may be required and problems may arise in antagonism.

Available Dosage Forms Injection, solution, as bromide: 1 mg/mL (10 mL); 2 mg/mL (2 mL, 5 mL) [may contain benzyl alcohol]

Monitoring and Teaching Issues

Physical Assessment: Only clinicians experienced in the use of neuromuscular blocking drugs should administer and/or manage the use of pancuronium. Dosage and rate of administration should be individualized and titrated to the desired effect, according to relevant clinical factors, premedication, concomitant medications, age, and general condition of the patient. Ventilatory support must be instituted and maintained until adequate respiratory muscle function and/or airway protection are assured. Assess other medications for effectiveness and safety. Other drugs that affect neuromuscular activity may increase/decrease neuromuscular block induced by pancuronium. This drug does not cause anesthesia or analgesia; pain must be treated with appropriate analgesic agents. Continuous monitoring of vital signs, cardiac status, respiratory status, and degree of neuromuscular block (objective assessment with peripheral external nerve stimulator) is mandatory and until full muscle tone has returned. Muscle tone returns in a predictable pattern, starting with diaphragm, abdomen, chest, limbs, and finally muscles of the neck, face, and eyes. Safety precautions must be maintained until full muscle tone has returned. **Note:** It may take longer for return of muscle tone in obese or elderly patients or patients with renal or hepatic disease, myasthenia gravis, myopathy, other neuromuscular disease, dehydration, electrolyte imbalance, or severe acid/base imbalance. Provide appropriate patient teaching/support prior to and following administration.

Long-term use: Monitor fluid levels (intake and output) during and following infusion. Reposition patient and provide appropriate skin care, mouth care, and care of patient's eyes every 2-3 hours while sedated. Provide appropriate emotional and sensory support (auditory and environmental).

Pregnancy risk factor C. Breast-feeding is not recommended.

Patient Education: Patient will usually be unconscious prior to administration. Patient education should be appropriate to individual situation. Reassurance of constant monitoring and emotional support to reduce fear and anxiety should precede and follow administration. Following return of muscle tone, do not attempt to change position or rise from bed without assistance. Report immediately any skin rash or hives, pounding heartbeat, respiratory difficulty, or muscle tremors. **Pregnancy/breast-feeding precautions:** Inform prescriber if you are pregnant. Breast-feeding is not recommended.

Pregnancy Risk Factor: C

Lactation: Excretion in breast milk unknown/not recommended

Administration

I.V.: May be administered undiluted by rapid I.V. injection.

Compatibility: Stable in D_5NS, D_5W, LR, NS

Y-site administration: Incompatible with diazepam, thiopental

Storage: Refrigerate; however, is stable for up to 6 months at room temperature.

Additional Information Pancuronium is classified as a long-duration neuromuscular-blocking agent. Neuromuscular blockade will be prolonged in patients with decreased renal function. Pancuronium does not relieve pain or produce sedation. It may produce cumulative effect on duration of blockade. It produces tachycardia secondary to vagolytic activity and sympathetic stimulation.

♦ **Pancuronium Bromide** *see Pancuronium on page 1153*

- ◆ Pandel® *see* Hydrocortisone *on page 760*
- ◆ Pangestyme™ CN *see* Pancrelipase *on page 1151*
- ◆ Pangestyme™ EC *see* Pancrelipase *on page 1151*
- ◆ Pangestyme™ MT *see* Pancrelipase *on page 1151*
- ◆ Pangestyme™ UL *see* Pancrelipase *on page 1151*
- ◆ Panglobulin® *see* Immune Globulin (Intravenous) *on page 793*
- ◆ Panglobulin® NF *see* Immune Globulin (Intravenous) *on page 793*
- ◆ Panixine DisperDose™ *see* Cephalexin *on page 294*
- ◆ PanMist®-JR *see* Guaifenesin and Pseudoephedrine *on page 733*
- ◆ PanMist®-LA *see* Guaifenesin and Pseudoephedrine *on page 733*
- ◆ PanMist®-S *see* Guaifenesin and Pseudoephedrine *on page 733*
- ◆ Panretin® *see* Alitretinoin *on page 69*

Pantoprazole (pan TOE pra zole)

U.S. Brand Names Protonix®

Generic Available No

Pharmacologic Category Proton Pump Inhibitor; Substituted Benzimidazole

Medication Safety Issues

Sound-alike/look-alike issues:

Protonix® may be confused with Lotronex®, Lovenox®, protamine

Vials containing Protonix® I.V. for injection are not recommended for use with spiked I.V. system adaptors. Nurses and pharmacists have reported breakage of the glass vials during attempts to connect spiked I.V. system adaptors, which may potentially result in injury to healthcare professionals.

Use

Oral: Treatment and maintenance of healing of erosive esophagitis associated with GERD; reduction in relapse rates of daytime and nighttime heartburn symptoms in GERD; hypersecretory disorders associated with Zollinger-Ellison syndrome or other neoplastic disorders

I.V.: Short-term treatment (7-10 days) of patients with gastroesophageal reflux disease (GERD) and a history of erosive esophagitis; hypersecretory disorders associated with Zollinger-Ellison syndrome or other neoplastic disorders

Unlabeled/Investigational Use Peptic ulcer disease, active ulcer bleeding (parenteral formulation); adjunct treatment with antibiotics for *Helicobacter pylori* eradication

Mechanism of Action/Effect Suppresses gastric acid secretion by inhibiting the parietal cell H^+/K^+ ATP pump

Contraindications Hypersensitivity to pantoprazole, substituted benzamidazoles (ie, esomeprazole, lansoprazole, omeprazole, rabeprazole), or any component of the formulation

Warnings/Precautions Symptomatic response does not preclude gastric malignancy. Not indicated for maintenance therapy; safety and efficacy for use beyond 16 weeks have not been established. Prolonged treatment (typically >3 years) may lead to vitamin B_{12} malabsorption. Intravenous preparation contains edetate sodium (EDTA); use caution in patients who are risk for zinc deficiency if other EDTA-containing solutions are coadministered. Safety and efficacy in pediatric patients have not been established.

Drug Interactions

Cytochrome P450 Effect: Substrate of CYP2C19 (major), 3A4 (minor); **Inhibits** 2C8/9 (moderate); **Induces** CYP1A2 (weak), 3A4 (weak)

Decreased Effect: Proton pump inhibitors may decrease the absorption of atazanavir, indinavir, iron salts, itraconazole, and ketoconazole. The levels/effects of pantoprazole may be decreased by aminoglutethimide, carbamazepine, phenytoin, rifampin, and other CYP2C19 inducers.

Increased Effect/Toxicity: Pantoprazole may increase the levels/effects of amiodarone, fluoxetine, glimepiride, glipizide, nateglinide, phenytoin, pioglitazone, rosiglitazone, sertraline, warfarin, and other CYP2C8/9 substrates.

Nutritional/Ethanol Interactions

Ethanol: Avoid ethanol (may cause gastric mucosal irritation).

Herb/Nutraceutical: Prolonged treatment (typically >3 years) may lead to vitamin B_{12} malabsorption.

Lab Interactions False-positive urine screening tests for tetrahydrocannabinol (THC) have been reported in patients receiving proton pump inhibitors, including pantoprazole.

Adverse Reactions

1% to 10%:

Cardiovascular: Chest pain

Central nervous system: Pain, migraine, anxiety, dizziness

Endocrine & metabolic: Hyperglycemia (1%), hyperlipidemia

Gastrointestinal: Diarrhea (4%), constipation, dyspepsia, gastroenteritis, nausea, rectal disorder, vomiting

Genitourinary: Urinary frequency, urinary tract infection

Hepatic: Liver function test abnormality increased SGPT

Neuromuscular & skeletal: Weakness, back pain, neck pain, arthralgia, hypertonia

Respiratory: Bronchitis, increased cough, dyspnea, pharyngitis, rhinitis, sinusitis, upper respiratory tract infection

Miscellaneous: Flu syndrome, infection

Overdosage/Toxicology Treatment of an overdose would include appropriate supportive treatment. No adverse events were seen with ingestions of 400 and 600 mg doses. Pantoprazole is not removed by hemodialysis.

(Continued)

Pantoprazole *(Continued)*

Pharmacodynamics/Kinetics
Absorption: Well absorbed
Bioavailability: 77%
Time to Peak: Oral: 2.5 hours
Protein Binding: 98%, primarily to albumin
Half-Life Elimination: 1 hour
Metabolism: Extensively hepatic; CYP2C19 (demethylation), CYP3A4; no evidence that metabolites have pharmacologic activity
Excretion: Urine (71%); feces (18%)

Dosing
Adults & Elderly:
Erosive esophagitis associated with GERD:
Oral:
Treatment: 40 mg once daily for up to 8 weeks; an additional 8 weeks may be used in patients who have not healed after an 8-week course
Maintenance of healing: 40 mg once daily
Note: Lower doses (20 mg once daily) have been used successfully in mild GERD treatment and maintenance of healing
I.V.: 40 mg once daily for 7-10 days
Peptic ulcer disease: Eradication of *Helicobacter pylori* (unlabeled use): Oral: Doses up to 40 mg twice daily have been used as part of combination therapy
Hypersecretory disorders (including Zollinger-Ellison):
Oral: Initial: 40 mg twice daily; adjust dose based on patient needs; doses up to 240 mg/day have been administered
I.V.: 80 mg twice daily; adjust dose based on acid output measurements; 160-240 mg/day in divided doses has been used for a limited period (up to 7 days)
Prevention of rebleeding in peptic ulcer bleed (unlabeled use): I.V.: 80 mg, followed by 8 mg/hour infusion for 72 hours
Renal Impairment: No adjustment is required. Pantoprazole is not removed by hemodialysis.
Hepatic Impairment: No adjustment is required.
Available Dosage Forms [DSC] = Discontinued product; **Note:** Strength expressed as base:
Injection, powder for reconstitution, as sodium: 40 mg [original formulation] [DSC]
Injection, powder for reconstitution, as sodium: 40 mg [contains edetate sodium 1 mg]
Tablet, delayed release, as sodium: 20 mg, 40 mg

Monitoring and Teaching Issues
Physical Assessment: Assess other medications for effectiveness and interactions (cytochrome P450 enzyme substrate), especially those drugs where absorption is determined by an acidic gastric pH. Monitor therapeutic effectiveness and adverse effects at beginning of therapy and regularly with long-term use. Assess knowledge/teach patient appropriate use, possible side effects/interventions, and adverse symptoms to report.
Patient Education: Take as directed; do not alter dosage without consulting prescriber. Take at similar time each day. Swallow tablet whole (do not crush or chew). Avoid alcohol. You may experience dizziness, headache, or anxiety (use caution when driving or engaging in dangerous activities until response to medication is known); vomiting or loss of appetite (small frequent meals, frequent mouth care, sucking lozenges, or chewing gum may help); or diarrhea (boiled milk, yogurt, or buttermilk may help). Report persistent abdominal discomfort; chest pain or palpitations; acute headache; unresolved diarrhea; excessive fatigue; increased muscle, joint, or body pain; shortness of breath or wheezing; cold or flu symptoms; changes in urinary pattern; or other persistent adverse reactions.
Pregnancy/breast-feeding precautions: Inform prescriber if you are pregnant. Breast-feeding is not recommended.
Dietary Considerations:
Oral: May be taken with or without food; best if taken before breakfast.
I.V.: Due to EDTA in preparation, zinc supplementation may be needed in patients prone to zinc deficiency.
Pregnancy Risk Factor: B
Lactation: Enters breast milk/not recommended
Breast-Feeding Issues: Not recommended due to carcinogenicity in animal studies.

Administration
Oral: Tablets should be swallowed whole, do not crush or chew. Best if taken before breakfast.
I.V.: I.V.: Flush I.V. line before and after administration. Solutions prepared from original formulation must be infused through an inline filter. Solutions prepared from the EDTA-stabilized formulation do not require an in-line filter (per manufacturer).
2-minute infusion: The volume of reconstituted solution (4 mg/mL) to be injected may be administered intravenously over at least 2 minutes.
15-minute infusion: Infuse over 15 minutes at a rate not to exceed 3 mg/minute.
Reconstitution: Reconstitute with 10 mL NS (final concentration 4 mg/mL). Reconstituted solution may be given intravenously (over 2 minutes) or may be added to 100 mL D_5W, NS, or LR (for 15-minute infusion).
Compatibility: Y-site administration: Incompatible: Midazolam, zinc
Storage:
Oral: Store tablet at 15°C to 30°C (59°F to 77°F)
I.V.:
EDTA-stabilized formulation: Store at 20°C to 25°C (68°F to 77°F). Protect from light. When reconstituted with 10 mL NS (final concentration 4 mg/mL), solution is stable up to 2 hours at room temperature; protection from light not required. When diluted in 100 mL D_5W, LR, or NS, may be stored at room temperature for up to 22 hours.
Original formulation (discontinued): Store at 2°C to 8°C (36°F to 46°F). Protect from light. When reconstituted with 10 mL NS (final concentration 4 mg/mL), solution is stable up

to 2 hours at room temperature; protection from light not required. When diluted in 100 mL D₅W, LR, or NS, may be stored at room temperature for up to 12 hours.

Papaverine (pa PAV er een)

U.S. Brand Names Para-Time S.R.®

Synonyms Papaverine Hydrochloride; Pavabid [DSC]

Generic Available Yes

Pharmacologic Category Vasodilator

Use Oral: Relief of peripheral and cerebral ischemia associated with arterial spasm and myocardial ischemia complicated by arrhythmias

Unlabeled/Investigational Use Investigational: Parenteral: Various vascular spasms associated with muscle spasms as in myocardial infarction, angina, peripheral and pulmonary embolism, peripheral vascular disease, angiospastic states, and visceral spasm (ureteral, biliary, and GI colic); testing for impotence

Mechanism of Action/Effect Smooth muscle spasmolytic producing a generalized smooth muscle relaxation including: vasodilatation, GI sphincter relaxation, bronchiolar muscle relaxation, and potentially a depressed myocardium (with large doses); muscle relaxation may occur due to inhibition or cyclic nucleotide phosphodiesterase, increasing cyclic AMP; muscle relaxation is unrelated to nerve innervation; papaverine increases cerebral blood flow in normal subjects; oxygen uptake is unaltered

Contraindications Hypersensitivity to papaverine or any component of the formulation

Warnings/Precautions Use with caution in patients with glaucoma. Administer I.V. cautiously since apnea and arrhythmias may result. May, in large doses, depress cardiac conduction (eg, AV node) leading to arrhythmias. May interfere with levodopa therapy of Parkinson's disease. Hepatic hypersensitivity has been noted with jaundice, eosinophilia, and abnormal LFTs.

Drug Interactions

Decreased Effect: Papaverine decreases the effects of levodopa.

Nutritional/Ethanol Interactions Ethanol: Avoid ethanol (may increase CNS depression).

Adverse Reactions Frequency not defined.

Cardiovascular: Arrhythmias (with rapid I.V. use), flushing of the face, mild hypertension, tachycardia

Central nervous system: Drowsiness, headache, lethargy, sedation, vertigo

Gastrointestinal: Abdominal distress, anorexia, constipation, diarrhea, nausea

Hepatic: Chronic hepatitis, hepatic hypersensitivity

Respiratory: Apnea (with rapid I.V. use)

Overdosage/Toxicology Symptoms of overdose include nausea, vomiting, weakness, gastric distress, ataxia, hepatic dysfunction, drowsiness, nystagmus, hyperventilation, hypotension, and hypokalemia. Treatment is supportive.

Pharmacodynamics/Kinetics

Onset of Action: Oral: Rapid

Protein Binding: 90%

Half-Life Elimination: 0.5-1.5 hours

Metabolism: Rapidly hepatic

Excretion: Primarily urine (as metabolites)

Dosing

Adults & Elderly: Arterial spasm:

Oral, sustained release: 150-300 mg every 12 hours; in difficult cases: 150 mg every 8 hours

I.M., I.V.: 30-65 mg (rarely up to 120 mg); may repeat every 3 hours

Pediatrics: Arterial spasm: I.M., I.V.: 6 mg/kg/day in 4 divided doses

Available Dosage Forms

Capsule, sustained release, as hydrochloride (Para-Time SR®): 150 mg

Injection, solution, as hydrochloride: 30 mg/mL (2 mL, 10 mL)

Monitoring and Teaching Issues

Physical Assessment: See Warnings/Precautions for use cautions (eg, glaucoma, use of levodopa). I.V., I.M.: Blood pressure and heart rate should be monitored. Administer I.V. no faster than over 1-2 minutes. Oral: Blood pressure and heart rate should be monitored prior to therapy and at frequent intervals thereafter. Assess therapeutic effectiveness and adverse response (eg, arrhythmias, tachycardia, hypertension, or GI disturbance; see Adverse Reactions). Teach patient proper use, possible side effects/appropriate interventions, and adverse symptoms to report (see Patient Education).

Patient Education: Do not take any new medication during therapy (especially anything that will stimulate blood pressure) unless approved by prescriber. Take as directed; do not alter dose or discontinue without consulting prescriber. Swallow extended-release capsules whole; do not chew, crush, or dissolve. May cause dizziness, confusion, or blurred vision (avoid driving or engaging in tasks that require alertness until response to drug is known); or constipation (increased exercise, fluids, fruit, or fiber may help). Report rapid heartbeat or palpitations and CNS changes (eg, depression, persistent sedation or lethargy, or acute headache). **Pregnancy/breast-feeding precautions:** Inform prescriber if you are or intend to become pregnant. Breast-feeding is not recommended.

Dietary Considerations: May be taken with food.

Geriatric Considerations: Vasodilators have been used to treat dementia upon the premise that dementia is secondary to a cerebral blood flow insufficiency. The hypothesis is that if blood flow could be increased, cognitive function would be increased. This hypothesis is no longer valid. The use of vasodilators for cognitive dysfunction is not recommended or proven by appropriate scientific study.

Pregnancy Risk Factor: C

Lactation: Excretion in breast milk unknown/not recommended

Administration

I.V.: Rapid I.V. administration may result in arrhythmias and fatal apnea; administer no faster than over 1-2 minutes.

(Continued)

Papaverine *(Continued)*

Reconstitution: Solutions should be clear to pale yellow. Precipitates with lactated Ringer's.

Compatibility: Stable in dextran 6% in dextrose, dextran 6% in NS, D_5LR, $D_5{}^1/_4NS$, $D_5{}^1/_2NS$, D_5NS, D_5W, $D_{10}W$, $^1/_2NS$, NS; **incompatible** with LR

    Compatibility in syringe: Incompatible with diatrizoate meglumine 52%, diatrizoate sodium 8%

    Compatibility when admixed: Incompatible with aminophylline with trimecaine

Storage: Protect from heat or freezing. Refrigerate injection at 2°C to 8°C (35°F to 46°F).

- ♦ **Papaverine Hydrochloride** *see* Papaverine *on page 1157*
- ♦ **Para-Aminosalicylate Sodium** *see* Aminosalicylic Acid *on page 92*
- ♦ **Paracetamol** *see* Acetaminophen *on page 38*
- ♦ **Parafon Forte® DSC** *see* Chlorzoxazone *on page 315*
- ♦ **Paraplatin®** *see* Carboplatin *on page 255*
- ♦ **Parathyroid Hormone (1-34)** *see* Teriparatide *on page 1448*
- ♦ **Para-Time S.R.®** *see* Papaverine *on page 1157*
- ♦ **Parcopa™** *see* Levodopa and Carbidopa *on page 886*

Paregoric *(par e GOR ik)*

Synonyms Camphorated Tincture of Opium

Controlled Substance C-III

Generic Available Yes

Pharmacologic Category Analgesic, Narcotic

Medication Safety Issues

Sound-alike/look-alike issues:

Camphorated tincture of opium may be confused with opium tincture

Paregoric may be confused with Percogesic®

Use care when prescribing opium tincture; each mL contains the equivalent of morphine 10 mg; paregoric contains the equivalent of morphine 0.4 mg/mL

Use Treatment of diarrhea or relief of pain; neonatal opiate withdrawal

Mechanism of Action/Effect Increases smooth muscle tone in GI tract, decreases motility and peristalsis, diminishes digestive secretions

Contraindications Hypersensitivity to opium or any component of the formulation; diarrhea caused by poisoning until the toxic material has been removed; pregnancy (prolonged use or high doses)

Warnings/Precautions Use with caution in patients with respiratory, hepatic or renal dysfunction, severe prostatic hyperplasia, or history of narcotic abuse. Opium shares the toxic potential of opiate agonists, and usual precautions of opiate agonist therapy should be observed. Some preparations contain sulfites which may cause allergic reactions.

Drug Interactions

Increased Effect/Toxicity: Increased effect/toxicity with CNS depressants (eg, alcohol, narcotics, benzodiazepines, tricyclic antidepressants, MAO inhibitors, phenothiazine).

Nutritional/Ethanol Interactions Ethanol: Avoid ethanol (may increase CNS depression).

Lab Interactions Increased aminotransferase [ALT (SGPT)/AST (SGOT)] (S)

Adverse Reactions Frequency not defined.

Cardiovascular: Hypotension, peripheral vasodilation

Central nervous system: Drowsiness, dizziness, insomnia, CNS depression, mental depression, increased intracranial pressure, restlessness, headache, malaise

Gastrointestinal: Constipation, anorexia, stomach cramps, nausea, vomiting, biliary tract spasm

Genitourinary: Ureteral spasms, decreased urination, urinary tract spasm

Hepatic: Increased liver function tests

Neuromuscular & skeletal: Weakness

Ocular: Miosis

Respiratory: Respiratory depression

Miscellaneous: Physical and psychological dependence, histamine release

Overdosage/Toxicology Symptoms of overdose include hypotension, drowsiness, seizures, and respiratory depression. Naloxone, 2 mg I.V. with repeat administration as necessary up to a total of 10 mg, can be used to reverse opiate effects.

Pharmacodynamics/Kinetics

Metabolism: In terms of opium: Hepatic

Excretion: In terms of opium: Urine (primarily as morphine glucuronide conjugates and unchanged drug - morphine, codeine, papaverine, etc)

Dosing

Adults & Elderly: Diarrhea: Oral: 5-10 mL 1-4 times/day

Pediatrics:

Neonatal opiate withdrawal: Oral: 3-6 drops every 3-6 hours as needed, or initially 0.2 mL every 3 hours; increase dosage by approximately 0.05 mL every 3 hours until withdrawal symptoms are controlled; it is rare to exceed 0.7 mL/dose. Stabilize withdrawal symptoms for 3-5 days, then gradually decrease dosage over a 2- to 4-week period.

Diarrhea: Oral: Children: 0.25-0.5 mL/kg 1-4 times/day

Available Dosage Forms Liquid, oral: Morphine equivalent 2 mg/5 mL (473 mL) [equivalent to opium 20 mg powder; contains alcohol 45% and benzoic acid]

Monitoring and Teaching Issues

Physical Assessment: Monitor for excessive sedation, respiratory depression, or hypotension. Has potential for psychological or physiological dependence.

Patient Education: Take exactly as directed; do not increase dosage. May cause dependence with prolonged or excessive use. Avoid alcohol or any other prescription and OTC medications that may cause sedation (sleeping medications, some cough/cold remedies, antihistamines, etc). You may experience drowsiness, dizziness, or impaired judgment (use caution when driving or engaging in tasks that require alertness until response to drug is known) or postural hypotension (use caution when rising from sitting or lying position or when climbing stairs). You may experience nausea or loss of appetite (small frequent meals may help) or constipation (a laxative may be necessary). Report unresolved nausea, vomiting, respiratory difficulty (shortness of breath or decreased respirations), chest pain, or palpitations. **Pregnancy/breast-feeding precautions:** Inform prescriber if you are pregnant. If nursing, take immediately after feeding or 4-6 hour before next feeding.

Pregnancy Risk Factor: B/D (prolonged use or high doses)

Lactation: Enters breast milk/use caution

Breast-Feeding Issues: Information regarding use while breast-feeding is based on experience with morphine. Probably safe with low doses and by administering dose after breast-feeding to further minimize exposure to the drug. Monitor the infant for possible side effects related to opiates.

Administration

Storage: Store in light-resistant, tightly closed container

Additional Information Contains morphine 0.4 mg/mL and alcohol 45%. Do **not** confuse this product with opium tincture which is 25 times **more** potent; each 5 mL of paregoric contains 2 mg morphine equivalent, 0.02 mL anise oil, 20 mg benzoic acid, 20 mg camphor, 0.2 mL glycerin and alcohol; final alcohol content 45%; paregoric also contains papaverine and noscapine; because all of these additives may be harmful to neonates, **a 25-fold dilution of opium tincture** is often preferred for treatment of neonatal abstinence syndrome (opiate withdrawal).

♦ **Paremyd® Ophthalmic** *see page 1625*

Paricalcitol (pah ri KAL si tole)

U.S. Brand Names Zemplar®

Generic Available No

Pharmacologic Category Vitamin D Analog

Use Prevention and treatment of secondary hyperparathyroidism associated with chronic renal failure. Has been evaluated only in hemodialysis patients.

Mechanism of Action/Effect Synthetic vitamin D analog which has been shown to reduce PTH serum concentrations

Contraindications Hypersensitivity to paricalcitol or any component of the formulation; patients with evidence of vitamin D toxicity; hypercalcemia

Warnings/Precautions Chronic administration can place patients at risk of hypercalcemia, elevated calcium-phosphorus product, and metastatic calcification. It should not be used in patients with evidence of hypercalcemia or vitamin D toxicity.

Drug Interactions

Increased Effect/Toxicity: Phosphate or vitamin D-related compounds should not be taken concurrently. Digitalis toxicity is potentiated by hypercalcemia.

Adverse Reactions The three most frequently reported events in clinical studies were nausea, vomiting, and edema, which are commonly seen in hemodialysis patients.

>10%: Gastrointestinal: Nausea (13%)

1% to 10%:
  Cardiovascular: Palpitations, peripheral edema (7%)
  Central nervous system: Chills, malaise, fever, lightheadedness (5%)
  Gastrointestinal: Vomiting (8%), GI bleeding (5%), xerostomia (3%)
  Respiratory: Pneumonia (5%)
  Miscellaneous: Flu-like symptoms, sepsis

Overdosage/Toxicology Acute overdose may cause hypercalcemia. Monitor serum calcium and phosphorus closely during titration of paricalcitol. Dosage reduction/interruption may be required if hypercalcemia develops. Chronic use may predispose to metastatic calcification. Bone lesions may develop if parathyroid hormone is suppressed below normal.

Pharmacodynamics/Kinetics

Protein Binding: >99%

Excretion: Feces (74%) in healthy subjects; urine (16%); 51% to 59% as metabolites

Dosing

Adults & Elderly:

Hyperparathyroidism, secondary (prevention and treatment): I.V.: 0.04-0.1 mcg/kg (2.8-7 mcg) given as a bolus dose no more frequently than every other day at any time during dialysis; dose as high as 0.24 mcg/kg (16.8 mcg) have been administered safely. Usually start with 0.04 mcg/kg 3 times/week by I.V. bolus, increased by 0.04 mcg/kg every 2 weeks.

The dose of paricalcitol should be adjusted based on serum PTH levels, as follows:
  Same or increasing serum PTH level: Increase paricalcitol dose
  Serum PTH level decreased by <30%: Increase paricalcitol dose
  Serum PTH level decreased by >30% and <60%: Maintain paricalcitol dose
  Serum PTH level decrease by >60%: Decrease paricalcitol dose
  Serum PTH level 1.5-3 times upper limit of normal: Maintain paricalcitol dose

Pediatrics: Children >5 years: Refer to adult dosing.

Renal Impairment: Refer to adult dosing.

Hepatic Impairment: Kinetics have not been investigated in hepatically impaired patients.

Available Dosage Forms Injection, solution: 2 mcg/mL (1 mL); 5 mcg/mL (1 mL, 2 mL) [contains alcohol]

Monitoring and Teaching Issues

Physical Assessment: Assess results of laboratory tests. Monitor patient response and adverse effects. Monitor for signs and symptoms of vitamin D intoxication. Assess knowledge/instruct patient on safe and appropriate use of paricalcitol and dietary requirements.

Monitoring Laboratory Tests: Serum calcium and phosphorus should be monitored closely (eg, twice weekly) during dose titration. Monitor serum PTH. In trials, a mean PTH level reduction of 30% was achieved within 6 weeks.

(Continued)

Paricalcitol *(Continued)*

Patient Education: Take as directed; do not increase dosage without consulting prescriber. Adhere to diet as recommended (do not take any other phosphate or vitamin D related compounds while taking paricalcitol). You may experience nausea or vomiting (small frequent meals, frequent mouth care, chewing gums, or sucking lozenges may help); swelling of extremities (elevate feet when sitting); or lightheadedness or dizziness (use caution when driving or engaging in tasks requiring alertness until response to drug is known). Report persistent fever, gastric disturbances, abdominal pain or blood in stool, chest pain or palpitations, or signs of respiratory infection or flu. **Pregnancy/breast-feeding precautions:** Inform prescriber if you are or intend to become pregnant. Consult prescriber if breast-feeding.

Geriatric Considerations: Kinetics have not been investigated in geriatric patients.

Pregnancy Risk Factor: C

Lactation: Excretion in breast milk unknown/use caution

♦ **Pariprazole** *see* Rabeprazole *on page 1302*
♦ **Parlodel®** *see* Bromocriptine *on page 208*
♦ **Parnate®** *see* Tranylcypromine *on page 1508*

Paroxetine *(pa ROKS e teen)*

U.S. Brand Names Paxil®; Paxil CR™; Pexeva™

Synonyms Paroxetine Hydrochloride; Paroxetine Mesylate

Restrictions A medication guide should be dispensed with each prescription. A template for the required MedGuides can be found on the FDA website at: http://www.fda.gov/cder/drug/antidepressants/labelTemplate.pdf

Generic Available Yes: Tablet, as hydrochloride

Pharmacologic Category Antidepressant, Selective Serotonin Reuptake Inhibitor

Medication Safety Issues
Sound-alike/look-alike issues:
Paroxetine may be confused with paclitaxel, pyridoxine
Paxil® may be confused with Doxil®, paclitaxel, Plavix®, Taxol®

Use Treatment of depression in adults; treatment of panic disorder with or without agoraphobia; obsessive-compulsive disorder (OCD) in adults; social anxiety disorder (social phobia); generalized anxiety disorder (GAD); post-traumatic stress disorder (PTSD)

Paxil CR™: Treatment of depression; panic disorder; premenstrual dysphoric disorder (PMDD); social anxiety disorder (social phobia)

Unlabeled/Investigational Use May be useful in eating disorders, impulse control disorders, self-injurious behavior; premenstrual disorders, vasomotor symptoms of menopause; treatment of depression and obsessive-compulsive disorder (OCD) in children

Mechanism of Action/Effect Paroxetine is a selective serotonin reuptake inhibitor, chemically unrelated to tricyclic, tetracyclic, or other antidepressants; presumably, the inhibition of serotonin reuptake from brain synapse stimulated serotonin activity in the brain

Contraindications Hypersensitivity to paroxetine or any component of the formulation; use of MAO inhibitors or within 14 days; concurrent use with thioridazine or mesoridazine

Warnings/Precautions Antidepressants increase the risk of suicidal thinking and behavior in children and adolescents with major depressive disorder (MDD) and other depressive disorders; consider risk prior to prescribing. All patients must be closely monitored for clinical worsening, suicidality, or unusual changes in behavior, especially during the initiation of therapy or following an increase or decrease in dosage. When used in children, the child's family or caregiver should be instructed to closely observe the patient and communicate condition with healthcare provider. A medication guide should be dispensed with each prescription. **Paroxetine is not FDA approved for use in children.**

The possibility of a suicide attempt is inherent in major depression and may persist until remission occurs. Use caution in high-risk patients. Worsening depression and severe abrupt suicidality that are not part of the presenting symptoms may require discontinuation or modification of drug therapy. The patient's family or caregiver should be alerted to monitor patients for the emergence of suicidality and associated behaviors (such as agitation, irritability, hostility, impulsivity, and hypomania) and call healthcare provider.

May worsen psychosis in some patients or precipitate a shift to mania or hypomania in patients with bipolar disorder. Patients presenting with depressive symptoms should be screened for bipolar disorder. Monotherapy in patients with bipolar disorder should be avoided. **Paroxetine is not FDA approved for the treatment of bipolar depression.**

The potential for severe reaction exists when used with MAO inhibitors - serotonin syndrome (hyperthermia, muscular rigidity, mental status changes/agitation, autonomic instability) may occur. May increase the risks associated with electroconvulsive therapy. Has a low potential to impair cognitive or motor performance - caution operating hazardous machinery or driving. Low potential for sedation or anticholinergic effects relative to cyclic antidepressants.

Use caution in patients with a previous seizure disorder or condition predisposing to seizures such as brain damage, alcoholism, or concurrent therapy with other drugs which lower the seizure threshold. Use with caution in patients with hepatic or dysfunction and in elderly patients. May cause hyponatremia/SIADH. Use with caution in patients at risk of bleeding or receiving anticoagulant therapy - may cause impairment in platelet aggregation. Use with caution in patients with renal insufficiency or other concurrent illness (due to limited experience). May cause or exacerbate sexual dysfunction.

Upon discontinuation of paroxetine therapy, gradually taper dose and monitor for discontinuation symptoms (eg, dizziness, dysphoric mood, irritability, agitation, confusion, paresthesias). If intolerable symptoms occur following a decrease in dosage or upon discontinuation of therapy, then resuming the previous dose with a more gradual taper should be considered.

Drug Interactions
Cytochrome P450 Effect: Substrate of CYP2D6 (major); **Inhibits** CYP1A2 (weak), 2B6 (moderate), 2C8/9 (weak), 2C19 (weak), 2D6 (strong), 3A4 (weak)

Decreased Effect: Cyproheptadine, a serotonin antagonist, may inhibit the effects of serotonin reuptake inhibitors (paroxetine). Paroxetine may decrease the levels/effects of CYP2D6 prodrug substrates (eg, codeine, hydrocodone, oxycodone, tramadol).

Increased Effect/Toxicity: Paroxetine should not be used with nonselective MAO inhibitors (phenelzine, isocarboxazid) or other drugs with MAO inhibition (linezolid); fatal reactions have been reported. Wait 5 weeks after stopping fluoxetine before starting a nonselective MAO inhibitor and 2 weeks after stopping an MAO inhibitor before starting paroxetine. Concurrent selegiline has been associated with mania, hypertension, or serotonin syndrome (risk may be reduced relative to nonselective MAO inhibitors).

Paroxetine may inhibit the metabolism of thioridazine or mesoridazine, resulting in increased plasma levels and increasing the risk of QT_c interval prolongation. This may lead to serious ventricular arrhythmias, such as torsade de pointes-type arrhythmias and sudden death. Do not use together. Wait at least 5 weeks after discontinuing paroxetine prior to starting thioridazine.

The levels/effects of paroxetine may be increased by chlorpromazine, delavirdine, fluoxetine, miconazole, pergolide, quinidine, quinine, ritonavir, ropinirole, and other CYP2D6 inhibitors. Paroxetine may increase the levels/effects of amphetamines, selected beta-blockers, bupropion, dextromethorphan, fluoxetine, lidocaine, mirtazapine, nefazodone, promethazine, propofol, risperidone, ritonavir, sertraline, tricyclic antidepressants, venlafaxine, and other CYP2B6 or 2D6 substrates.

Concomitant use of paroxetine and NSAIDs, aspirin, or other drugs affecting coagulation has been associated with an increased risk of bleeding. Paroxetine may increase the hypoprothrombinemic response to warfarin. Paroxetine increases levels of procyclidine; this may result in increased anticholinergic effects; procyclidine dose reduction may be necessary.

Combined use of SSRIs and amphetamines, buspirone, meperidine, nefazodone, serotonin agonists (such as sumatriptan), sibutramine, other SSRIs, sympathomimetics, ritonavir, tramadol, and venlafaxine may increase the risk of serotonin syndrome. Combined use of sumatriptan (and other serotonin agonists) may result in toxicity; weakness, hyper-reflexia, and incoordination have been observed with sumatriptan and SSRIs. In addition, concurrent use may theoretically increase the risk of serotonin syndrome; includes sumatriptan, naratriptan, rizatriptan, and zolmitriptan. Concurrent lithium may increase risk of nephrotoxicity. Risk of hyponatremia may increase with concurrent use of loop diuretics (bumetanide, furosemide, torsemide).

Nutritional/Ethanol Interactions

Ethanol: Avoid ethanol.

Food: Peak concentration is increased, but bioavailability is not significantly altered by food.

Herb/Nutraceutical: Avoid valerian, St John's wort, SAMe, kava kava.

Lab Interactions Increased LFTs

Adverse Reactions

>10%:
  Central nervous system: Headache, somnolence, dizziness, insomnia
  Gastrointestinal: Nausea, xerostomia, constipation, diarrhea
  Genitourinary: Ejaculatory disturbances
  Neuromuscular & skeletal: Weakness
  Miscellaneous: Diaphoresis

1% to 10%:
  Cardiovascular: Palpitations, vasodilation, postural hypotension
  Central nervous system: Nervousness, anxiety, yawning, abnormal dreams, agitation
  Dermatologic: Rash
  Endocrine & metabolic: Libido decreased, delayed ejaculation
  Gastrointestinal: Anorexia, flatulence, vomiting, dyspepsia, taste perversion, weight gain
  Genitourinary: Urinary frequency, impotence
  Neuromuscular & skeletal: Tremor, paresthesia, myopathy, myalgia
  Ocular: Blurred vision
  Respiratory: Rhinitis

Overdosage/Toxicology Symptoms of overdose include somnolence, nausea, vomiting, hepatic dysfunction, drowsiness, sinus tachycardia, urinary retention, renal failure (acute), and dilated pupils. Convulsions, status epilepticus, and ventricular arrhythmias (including torsade de pointes) have been reported, as well as serotonin syndrome and manic reaction. There are no specific antidotes, following attempts at decontamination, treatment is supportive and symptomatic. Forced diuresis, dialysis, and hemoperfusion are unlikely to be beneficial.

Pharmacodynamics/Kinetics

Absorption: Completely absorbed following oral administration

Time to Peak: Immediate release: 5.2 hours; controlled release: 6-10 hours

Protein Binding: 93% to 95%

Half-Life Elimination: 21 hours (3-65 hours)

Metabolism: Extensively hepatic via CYP enzymes via oxidation and methylation; nonlinear pharmacokinetics may be seen with higher doses and longer duration of therapy. Saturation of CYP2D6 appears to account for the nonlinearity. C_{min} concentrations 70% to 80% greater in the elderly compared to nonelderly patients; clearance is also decreased.

Excretion: As metabolites in urine and bile; 2% as unchanged drug in urine

Dosing

Adults:

Depression: Oral:
  Paxil®, Pexeva™: Initial: 20 mg once daily, preferably in the morning; increase if needed by 10 mg/day increments at intervals of at least 1 week; maximum dose: 50 mg/day
  Paxil CR™: Initial: 25 mg once daily; increase if needed by 12.5 mg/day increments at intervals of at least 1 week; maximum dose: 62.5 mg/day

(Continued)

Paroxetine *(Continued)*

GAD (Paxil®): Oral: Initial: 20 mg once daily, preferably in the morning; doses of 20-50 mg/day were used in clinical trials, however, no greater benefit was seen with doses >20 mg. If dose is increased, adjust in increments of 10 mg/day at 1-week intervals.

OCD (Paxil®, Pexeva™): Oral: Initial: 20 mg once daily, preferably in the morning; increase if needed by 10 mg/day increments at intervals of at least 1 week; recommended dose: 40 mg/day; range: 20-60 mg/day; maximum dose: 60 mg/day

Panic disorder: Oral:

Paxil®, Pexeva™: Initial: 10 mg once daily, preferably in the morning; increase if needed by 10 mg/day increments at intervals of at least 1 week; recommended dose: 40 mg/day; range: 10-60 mg/day; maximum dose: 60 mg/day

Paxil CR™: Initial: 12.5 mg once daily; increase if needed by 12.5 mg/day at intervals of at least 1 week; maximum dose: 75 mg/day

PMDD (Paxil CR™): Oral: Initial: 12.5 mg once daily in the morning; may be increased to 25 mg/day; dosing changes should occur at intervals of at least 1 week. May be given daily throughout the menstrual cycle or limited to the luteal phase.

PTSD (Paxil®): Oral: Initial: 20 mg once daily, preferably in the morning; increase if needed by 10 mg/day increments at intervals of at least 1 week; range: 20-50 mg

Social anxiety disorder: Oral:

Paxil®: Initial: 20 mg once daily, preferably in the morning; recommended dose: 20 mg/day; range: 20-60 mg/day; doses >20 mg may not have additional benefit

Paxil CR™: Initial: 12.5 mg once daily, preferably in the morning; may be increased by 12.5 mg/day at intervals of at least 1 week; maximum dose: 37.5 mg/day

Menopause-associated vasomotor symptoms (unlabeled use, Paxil CR™): Oral: 12.5-25 mg/day

Elderly:

Depression, obsessive compulsive disorder, panic attack, social anxiety disorder:

Paxil®, Pexeva™: Oral: Initial: 10 mg/day; increase if needed by 10 mg/day increments at intervals of at least 1 week; maximum dose: 40 mg/day

Paxil CR™: Initial: 12.5 mg/day; increase if needed by 12.5 mg/day increments at intervals of at least 1 week; maximum dose: 50 mg/day

Pediatrics:

Depression (unlabeled use; not recommended by FDA): Oral: Initial: 10 mg/day and adjusted upward on an individual basis to 20 mg/day

OCD (unlabeled use): Oral: Initial: 10 mg/day and titrate up as necessary to 60 mg/day

Self-Injurious behavior (unlabeled use): Oral: 20 mg/day

Social phobia (unlabeled use): Oral: 2.5-15 mg/day

Renal Impairment:

Cl$_{cr}$ <30 mL/minute: Mean plasma concentrations ~4 times that seen in normal function.

Cl$_{cr}$ 30-60 mL/minute: Plasma concentrations 2 times that seen in normal function.

Paxil®, Pexeva™: Adults: Initial: 10 mg/day; increase if needed by 10 mg/day increments at intervals of at least 1 week; maximum dose: 40 mg/day

Paxil CR™: Initial: 12.5 mg/day; increase if needed by 12.5 mg/day increments at intervals of at least 1 week; maximum dose: 50 mg/day

Hepatic Impairment: In hepatic dysfunction, plasma concentration is 2 times that seen in normal function.

Paxil®, Pexeva™: Adults: Initial: 10 mg/day; increase if needed by 10 mg/day increments at intervals of at least 1 week; maximum dose: 40 mg/day

Paxil CR™: Initial: 12.5 mg/day; increase if needed by 12.5 mg/day increments at intervals of at least 1 week; maximum dose: 50 mg/day

Available Dosage Forms Note: Available as paroxetine hydrochloride or mesylate; mg strength refers to paroxetine

Suspension, oral, as hydrochloride (Paxil®): 10 mg/5 mL (250 mL) [orange flavor]

Tablet, as hydrochloride (Paxil®): 10 mg, 20 mg, 30 mg, 40 mg

Tablet, as mesylate (Pexeva™): 10 mg, 20 mg, 30 mg, 40 mg

Tablet, controlled release, as hydrochloride (Paxil CR™): 12.5 mg, 25 mg, 37.5 mg

Monitoring and Teaching Issues

Physical Assessment: Assess potential for interactions with other prescription or OTC medications or herbal products patient may be taking. Assess results of laboratory tests. Assess therapeutic effectiveness (according to rationale for prescribing), and adverse reactions at beginning of therapy and frequently with long-term use. Monitor for clinical worsening and suicidal ideation. Taper dosage slowly when discontinuing. Assess knowledge/teach patient appropriate use, interventions to reduce side effects, and adverse symptoms to report.

Monitoring Laboratory Tests: Hepatic and renal function

Patient Education: Take exactly as directed; do not increase dose or frequency or discontinue without consulting prescriber. It may take 2-3 weeks to achieve desired results. Take in the morning to reduce the incidence of insomnia (may be taken with or without food). Do not crush, break, or chew controlled release (Paxil CR™) tablets. Avoid alcohol, caffeine, and other prescription or OTC medications not approved by prescriber. Maintain adequate hydration (2-3 L/day of fluids) unless instructed to restrict fluid intake. You may experience drowsiness, dizziness, or lightheadedness (use caution when driving or engaging in tasks requiring alertness until response to drug is known); nausea, vomiting, anorexia, or dry mouth (small frequent meals, frequent mouth care, chewing gum, or sucking lozenges may help); or orthostatic hypotension (use caution when climbing stairs or changing position from lying or sitting to standing). Report persistent insomnia or excessive daytime sedation; muscle cramping, tremors, weakness, or change in gait; chest pain, palpitations, or rapid heartbeat; vision changes or eye pain; respiratory difficulty or breathlessness; abdominal pain or blood in stool; change in affect or thought processes, unusual agitation, or abnormal dreams; worsening of condition; or suicidal ideation. **Pregnancy/breast-feeding precautions:** Inform prescriber if you are or intend to become pregnant. Consult prescriber if breast-feeding.

Dietary Considerations: May be taken with or without food.

Geriatric Considerations: Paroxetine's favorable side effect profile make it a useful alternative to traditional tricyclic antidepressants. Paroxetine is the most sedating of the currently available selective serotonin reuptake inhibitors. Paroxetine's half-life is approximately 21 hours and it has no active metabolites.

Pregnancy Risk Factor: C

Pregnancy Issues: Teratogenic effects were not observed in animal studies. Nonteratogenic effects including respiratory distress, cyanosis, apnea, seizures, temperature instability, feeding difficulty, vomiting, hypoglycemia, hypo- or hypertonia, hyper-reflexia, jitteriness, irritability, constant crying, and tremor have been reported in the neonate immediately following delivery after exposure late in the third trimester. Adverse effects may be due to toxic effects of SSRI or drug discontinuation. There are no adequate and well-controlled studies in pregnant women. Use during pregnancy only if the potential benefit to the mother outweighs the possible risk to the fetus. If treatment during pregnancy is required, consider tapering therapy during the third trimester.

Lactation: Enters breast milk/use caution (AAP rates "of concern")

Administration

Oral: May be administered with or without food. Do not crush, break, or chew controlled release tablets.

Storage:

Suspension: Store at ≤25°C (≤77°F)

Tablet: Store at 15°C to 30°C (59°F to 86°F)

Additional Information Paxil CR™ incorporates a degradable polymeric matrix (Geomatrix™) to control dissolution rate over a period of 4-5 hours. An enteric coating delays the start of drug release until tablets have left the stomach.

Related Information

Antidepressant Agents *on page 1713*

Antidepressant Medication Guidelines *on page 1765*

- ♦ **Paroxetine Hydrochloride** *see* Paroxetine *on page 1160*
- ♦ **Paroxetine Mesylate** *see* Paroxetine *on page 1160*
- ♦ **PAS** *see* Aminosalicylic Acid *on page 92*
- ♦ **Paser**® *see* Aminosalicylic Acid *on page 92*
- ♦ **Patanol**® *see* Olopatadine *on page 1114*
- ♦ **Therapeutic Nursing Management of Side Effects** *see page 29*
- ♦ **Pavabid [DSC]** *see* Papaverine *on page 1157*
- ♦ **Pavulon [DSC]** *see* Pancuronium *on page 1153*
- ♦ **Paxil**® *see* Paroxetine *on page 1160*
- ♦ **Paxil CR™** *see* Paroxetine *on page 1160*
- ♦ **PCA** *see* Procainamide *on page 1254*
- ♦ **PCE**® *see* Erythromycin *on page 543*
- ♦ **Peak and Trough Guidelines** *see page 1694*
- ♦ **PediaCare**® **Decongestant Infants [OTC]** *see* Pseudoephedrine *on page 1282*
- ♦ **Pediapred**® *see* PrednisoLONE *on page 1245*
- ♦ **Pediarix™** *see page 1660*
- ♦ **Pediatex™-D** *see* Carbinoxamine and Pseudoephedrine *on page 254*
- ♦ **Pediatex™ HC** *see* Pseudoephedrine, Hydrocodone, and Chlorpheniramine *on page 1283*
- ♦ **Pediatric Dosage Estimations** *see page 1696*
- ♦ **Pediazole**® *see* Erythromycin and Sulfisoxazole *on page 546*
- ♦ **Pedi-Dri**® *see* Nystatin *on page 1103*
- ♦ **PediOtic**® *see* Neomycin, Polymyxin B, and Hydrocortisone *on page 1069*
- ♦ **PedvaxHIB**® *see page 1660*

Pegaspargase (peg AS par jase)

U.S. Brand Names Oncaspar®

Synonyms NSC-644954; PEG-L-Asparaginase

Generic Available No

Pharmacologic Category Antineoplastic Agent, Miscellaneous

Medication Safety Issues

Sound-alike/look-alike issues:

Pegaspargase may be confused with asparaginase

Use Treatment of acute lymphocytic leukemia, blast crisis of chronic lymphocytic leukemia (CLL), salvage therapy of non-Hodgkin's lymphoma; may be used in some patients who have had hypersensitivity reactions to *E. coli* asparaginase

Mechanism of Action/Effect Pegaspargase is a modified version of asparaginase. Leukemic cells, especially lymphoblasts, require exogenous asparagine; normal cells can synthesize asparagine. Pegaspargase contains L-asparaginase amidohydrolase type EC-2 which inhibits protein synthesis by deaminating asparagine to aspartic acid and ammonia in the plasma and extracellular fluid and therefore deprives tumor cells of the amino acid for protein synthesis. Asparaginase is cycle-specific for the G_1 phase of the cell cycle.

Contraindications Hypersensitivity to pegaspargase or any component of the formulation; pancreatitis or a history of pancreatitis; patients who have had significant hemorrhagic events associated with prior asparaginase therapy; previous serious allergic reactions, such as generalized urticaria, bronchospasm, laryngeal edema, hypotension, or other unacceptable adverse reactions to pegaspargase

Warnings/Precautions The U.S. Food and Drug Administration (FDA) currently recommends that procedures for proper handling and disposal of antineoplastic agents be considered.

Monitor for severe allergic reactions. Use cautiously in patients with an underlying coagulopathy or previous hematologic complications from asparaginase, hepatic dysfunction, hyperglycemia or diabetes, or pancreatitis. May be used cautiously in patients who have had *(Continued)*

Pegaspargase *(Continued)*

hypersensitivity reactions to *E. coli* asparaginase; however, up to 33% of patients who have an allergic reaction to *E. coli* asparaginase will also react to pegaspargase.

Drug Interactions

Decreased Effect: Asparaginase terminates methotrexate action by inhibition of protein synthesis and prevention of cell entry into the S Phase.

Increased Effect/Toxicity:

Aspirin, dipyridamole, heparin, warfarin, NSAIDs: Imbalances in coagulation factors have been noted with the use of pegaspargase - use with caution.

Vincristine and prednisone: An increased toxicity has been noticed when asparaginase is administered with VCR and prednisone.

Cyclophosphamide (decreased metabolism)

Mercaptopurine (increased hepatotoxicity)

Vincristine (increased neuropathy)

Prednisone (hyperglycemia)

Adverse Reactions In general, pegaspargase toxicities tend to be less frequent and appear somewhat later than comparable toxicities of asparaginase. Intramuscular rather than intravenous injection may decrease the incidence of coagulopathy, GI, hepatic, and renal toxicity.

>10%:

Cardiovascular: Edema

Central nervous system: Fatigue, disorientation (10%)

Gastrointestinal: Nausea, vomiting (50% to 60%), generally mild to moderate, but may be severe and protracted in some patients; anorexia (33%); abdominal pain (38%); diarrhea (28%); increased serum lipase and amylase

Hematologic: Hypofibrinogenemia and depression of clotting factors V and VII, variable decreases in factors VII and IX, severe protein C deficiency and decrease in antithrombin III - overt bleeding is uncommon, but may be dose-limiting, or fatal in some patients

Hypersensitivity: Acute allergic reactions, including fever, rash, urticaria, arthralgia, hypotension, angioedema, bronchospasm, anaphylaxis (10% to 30%) - dose-limiting in some patients

Neuromuscular & skeletal: Weakness (33%)

1% to 10%:

Cardiovascular: Hypotension, tachycardia, thrombosis

Dermatologic: Urticaria, erythema, lip edema

Endocrine & metabolic: Hyperglycemia (3%)

Gastrointestinal: Acute pancreatitis (1%)

Overdosage/Toxicology Symptoms of overdose include nausea and diarrhea.

Pharmacodynamics/Kinetics

Duration of Action: Asparaginase was measurable for at least 15 days following initial treatment with pegaspargase

Half-Life Elimination: 5.73 days; unaffected by age, renal or hepatic function

Metabolism: Systemically degraded

Excretion: Urine (trace amounts)

Dosing

Adults & Elderly: Refer to individual protocols.

Note: I.M. administration is preferred over I.V. administration. I.M. administration may decrease the incidence of hepatotoxicity, coagulopathy, and GI and renal disorders.

Acute lymphoblastic leukemia (ALL): I.M., I.V.: 2500 int. units/m^2 every 14 days

Pediatrics: Refer to individual protocols. I.M. administration is **preferred** over I.V. administration. I.M. administration may decrease the incidence of hepatotoxicity, coagulopathy, and GI and renal disorders.

Acute lymphoblastic leukemia: I.M., I.V.:

Body surface area <0.6 m^2: 82.5 int. units/kg every 14 days

Body surface area ≥0.6 m^2: 2500 int. units/m^2 every 14 days

Available Dosage Forms Injection, solution [preservative free]: 750 units/mL (5 mL)

Monitoring and Teaching Issues

Physical Assessment: Use caution with an underlying coagulopathy, hepatic dysfunction, hyperglycemia, diabetes, or pancreatitis (see Warnings/Precautions for specific use cautions). Assess potential for interactions with other pharmacological agents patient may be taking (eg, potential for toxicities; see Drug Interactions). I.V. See Administration for infusion specifics and anaphylactic precautions (have a freely-running I.V. in place and emergency medications on hand). Patient must be monitored closely during and for 1 hour following each infusion (anaphylactic reactions can occur with each dose; fever, rash, urticaria, arthralgia, hypotension, angioedema, bronchospasm, anaphylaxis). Assess laboratory tests and patient response with each dose (eg, GI disturbance [nausea, vomiting], depression of clotting factors, hypotension; see Adverse Reactions). **Note:** I.M. rather than I.V. administration may decrease the incidence of coagulopathy, GI, hepatic and renal toxicity. Teach patient possible side effects/appropriate interventions and adverse symptoms to report (see Patient Education).

Monitoring Laboratory Tests: Coagulation factors, amylase, liver enzymes, prothrombin time, renal function, blood glucose

Patient Education: This drug is given by infusion or injection; report immediately any redness, swelling, burning, or pain at infusion/injection site or any signs of allergic reaction (eg, respiratory or swallowing difficulty, chest tightness, rash, hives, swelling of lips or mouth). Maintain adequate hydration (2-3 L/day of fluids) unless instructed to restrict fluid intake and nutrition. You may be more susceptible to infection (avoid crowds and exposure to infection and do not have vaccinations without consulting prescriber). May cause nausea, vomiting, or loss of appetite (small frequent meals, frequent mouth care, chewing gum, or sucking lozenges may help); mouth sores (use soft toothbrush, waxed dental floss, and frequent mouth rinses); diarrhea (buttermilk, boiled milk, or yogurt may help); dizziness, drowsiness, syncope, or blurred vision (use caution when driving or engaging in tasks that require alertness until response to drug is known); increased sweating; decreased sexual drive; or cough. Report edema (eg, swelling of extremities or sudden weight gain); persistent nausea, vomiting, or diarrhea; unusual bleeding or bruising; black tarry stools; blood in urine or stool, pinpoint red spots on your skin; or weakness or fatigue. **Pregnancy/breast-feeding precautions:** Inform prescriber if you are or intend to become pregnant. Do not breast-feed.

Pregnancy Risk Factor: C

Pregnancy Issues: Based on limited reports in humans, the use of asparaginase does not seem to pose a major risk to the fetus when used in the 2nd and 3rd trimesters, or when exposure occurs prior to conception in either females or males. Because of the teratogenicity observed in animals and the lack of human data after 1st trimester exposure, asparaginase should be used cautiously, if at all, during this period.

Lactation: Enters breast milk/contraindicated

Administration

I.M.: Must only be given as a deep intramuscular injection into a large muscle.

I.V.:

Do not filter solution. May be given as a 1- to 2-hour I.V. infusion; **do not give I.V. push**. Some institutions recommend the following precautions for pegaspargase administration: Have parenteral epinephrine, diphenhydramine, and hydrocortisone available at the bedside; have a freely-running I.V. in place; have a physician readily accessible; monitor the patient closely for 30-60 minutes

Reconstitution: Avoid excessive agitation; do **not** shake.

Standard I.M. dilution: Do not exceed 2 mL volume per injection site

Standard I.V. dilution: Dose/100 mL NS or D_5W; stable for 48 hours at room temperature.

Storage: Refrigerate at 2°C to 8°C (36°F to 46°F). Do not use of cloudy or if precipitate is present. Do not use if stored at room temperature for >48 hours. Do **not** freeze. Do not use product if it is known to have been frozen. Single-use vial; discard unused portions.

Additional Information Obtain from Olsten Health Services 1-888-276-2217

♦ Pegasys® see Peginterferon Alfa-2a on page 1165

Peginterferon Alfa-2a (peg in ter FEER on AL fa too aye)

U.S. Brand Names Pegasys®

Synonyms Interferon Alfa-2a (PEG Conjugate); Pegylated Interferon Alfa-2a

Restrictions An FDA-approved medication guide is available at www.fda.gov/cder/Offices/ODS/labeling.htm; distribute to each patient to whom this medication is dispensed.

Generic Available No

Pharmacologic Category Interferon

Use Treatment of chronic hepatitis C (CHC), alone or in combination with ribavirin, in patients with compensated liver disease and histological evidence of cirrhosis (Child-Pugh class A) and patients with clinically-stable HIV disease

Mechanism of Action/Effect Alpha interferons are a family of proteins, produced by nucleated cells, that have antiviral, antiproliferative, and immune-regulating activity. There are 16 known subtypes of alpha interferons. Interferons interact with cells through high affinity cell surface receptors. Following activation, multiple effects can be detected including induction of gene transcription. Inhibits cellular growth, alters the state of cellular differentiation, interferes with oncogene expression, alters cell surface antigen expression, increases phagocytic activity of macrophages, and augments cytotoxicity of lymphocytes for target cells.

Contraindications Hypersensitivity to polyethylene glycol (PEG), interferon alfa, or any component of the formulation; autoimmune hepatitis; decompensated liver disease in cirrhotic CHC patients monoinfected (Child-Pugh score>6) or coinfected (Child-Pugh score ≥6, class B and C) with HIV; neonates and infants

Warnings/Precautions Severe acute hypersensitivity reactions have occurred rarely; prompt discontinuation is advised. Use caution with prior cardiovascular disease, endocrine disorders, autoimmune disorders, and pulmonary dysfunction. Discontinue treatment with worsening or persistently severe signs/symptoms of autoimmune, infectious, respiratory, or neuropsychiatric disorders (including depression and/or suicidal thoughts/behavior). Severe psychiatric adverse effects (including depression, suicidal ideation, and suicide attempt) may occur. Avoid use in severe psychiatric disorders; use caution in patients with a history of depression. Patients who experience dizziness, confusion, somnolence or fatigue should use caution when performing tasks which require mental alertness (eg, operating machinery or driving).

Hepatic decompensation and death have been associated with the use of alpha interferons including Pegasys®, in cirrhotic chronic hepatitis C patients; patients coinfected with HIV and receiving highly active antiretroviral therapy have shown an increased risk. Monitor hepatic function; discontinue if decompensation occurs (Child-Pugh score >6) in monoinfected patients and (Child-Pugh score ≥6, class B and C) in patients coinfected with HIV.

Use caution with renal dysfunction (Cl_{cr} <50 mL/minute). Patients with renal dysfunction should be monitored for signs/symptoms of toxicity (dosage adjustment required if toxicity occurs). Discontinue if new or worsening ophthalmologic disorders occur including retinal hemorrhages, cotton wool spots, and retinal artery or vein obstruction; visual exams are recommended in these instances, at the initiation of therapy, and periodically during therapy.

Use caution with baseline neutrophil count <1500/mm³, platelet count <90,000/mm³ or hemoglobin <10 g/dL. Discontinue therapy (at least temporarily) if ANC <500/mm³ or platelet count <25,000/mm³, colitis develops, or if known or suspected pancreatitis develops. Use caution in patients with an increased risk for severe anemia (eg, spherocytosis, history of GI bleeding).

Use caution in geriatric patients. Safety and efficacy have not been established in patients who have failed other alpha interferon therapy, received organ transplants, been infected with hepatitis B, been coinfected with HIV with a CD4⁺ cell count <100 cells/microL, or been treated for >48 weeks. Due to differences in dosage, patients should not change brands of interferon. Safety and efficacy have not been established in children.

(Continued)

Peginterferon Alfa-2a *(Continued)*

Drug Interactions

Cytochrome P450 Effect: Inhibits CYP1A2 (weak)

Decreased Effect: Prednisone may decrease the therapeutic effects of interferon alfa; interferon alfa may decrease the serum concentrations of melphalan

Increased Effect/Toxicity: Interferons may increase the risk of neutropenia when used with ACE inhibitors; fluorouracil concentrations doubled with interferon alfa-2b; interferon alfa may decrease the metabolism of theophylline and zidovudine; interferons may increase the anticoagulant effects of warfarin

Nutritional/Ethanol Interactions Ethanol: Avoid use in patients with hepatitis C virus.

Adverse Reactions Note: Percentages are reported for peginterferon alfa-2a in chronic hepatitis C (CHC) patients. Other percentages indicated as "with ribavirin" or "in HIV/CHC" are those which significantly exceed incidence reported for peginterferon monotherapy in CHC patients.

>10%:

Central nervous system: Headache (54%), fatigue (50%), pyrexia (37%; 41% with ribavirin), insomnia (19%; 30% with ribavirin), depression (18%), dizziness (16%), irritability/anxiety/nervousness (19%; 33% with ribavirin), pain (11%)

Dermatologic: Alopecia (23%; 28% with ribavirin), pruritus (12%; 19% with ribavirin), dermatitis (16% with ribavirin)

Gastrointestinal: Nausea/vomiting (24%), anorexia (17%; 24% with ribavirin), diarrhea (16%), weight loss (16% in HIV/CHC), abdominal pain (15%)

Hematologic: Neutropenia (21%; 27% with ribavirin; 40% in HIV/CHC), lymphopenia (14% with ribavirin), anemia (11% with ribavirin; 14% in HIV/CHC)

Local: Injection site reaction (22%)

Neuromuscular & skeletal: Weakness (56%; 65% with ribavirin), myalgia (37%), rigors (32%), arthralgia (28%)

Respiratory: Dyspnea (13% with ribavirin)

1% to 10%:

Central nervous system: Concentration impaired (8%), memory impaired (5%), mood alteration (3%; 9% in HIV/CHC)

Dermatologic: Dermatitis (8%), rash (5%), dry skin (4%; 10% with ribavirin), eczema (5% with ribavirin)

Endocrine & metabolic: Hypothyroidism (4%), hyperthyroidism (1%)

Gastrointestinal: Xerostomia (6%), dyspepsia (6% with ribavirin), weight loss (4%; 10% with ribavirin)

Hematologic: Thrombocytopenia (5%), platelets decreased <50,000/mm^3 (5%), lymphopenia (3%), anemia (2%)

Neuromuscular & skeletal: Back pain (9%)

Ocular: Blurred vision (4%)

Respiratory: Cough (4%; 10 % with ribavirin), dyspnea (4%), exertional dyspnea (4% with ribavirin)

Miscellaneous: Diaphoresis (6%), bacterial infection (3%; 5% in HIV/CHC)

Overdosage/Toxicology Experience with overdosage is limited and no serious reactions have been reported. Dose-limiting toxicities include fatigue, elevated liver enzymes, neutropenia and thrombocytopenia. In case of overdose, treatment should be symptom-directed and supportive. Hemodialysis and peritoneal dialysis are not effective.

Pharmacodynamics/Kinetics

Time to Peak: Serum: 72-96 hours

Half-Life Elimination: Terminal: 50-140 hours; increased with renal dysfunction

Dosing

Adults:

Chronic hepatitis C (monoinfection or coinfection with HIV): SubQ:

Monotherapy: 180 mcg once weekly for 48 weeks

Combination therapy with ribavirin: Recommended dosage: 180 mcg once/week with ribavirin (Copegus®)

Duration of therapy: Monoinfection (based on genotype):

Genotype 1,4: 48 weeks

Genotype 2,3: 24 weeks

Duration of therapy: Coinfection: 48 weeks

Dose modifications:

For moderate to severe adverse reactions: Initial: 135 mcg/week; may need decreased to 90 mcg/week in some cases

Based on hematologic parameters:

ANC <750/mm^3: 135 mcg/week

ANC <500/mm^3: Suspend therapy until >1000/mm^3, then restart at 90 mcg/week and monitor

Platelet count <50,000/mm^3: 90 mcg/week

Platelet count <25,000/mm^3: Discontinue therapy

Depression (severity based on DSM-IV criteria):

Mild depression: No dosage adjustment required; evaluate once weekly by visit/phone call. If depression remains stable, continue weekly visits. If depression improves, resume normal visit schedule

Moderate depression: Decrease interferon dose to 90-135 mcg once/week; evaluate once weekly with an office visit at least every other week. If depression remains stable, consider psychiatric evaluation and continue with reduced dosing. If symptoms improve and remain stable for 4 weeks, resume normal visit schedule; continue reduced dosing or return to normal dose.

Severe depression: Discontinue interferon permanently. Obtain immediate psychiatric consultation. Discontinue ribavirin if using concurrently.

Renal Impairment:

Cl$_{cr}$ <50 mL/minute: Use caution; monitor for toxicity

End-stage renal disease requiring hemodialysis: 135 mcg/week; monitor for toxicity

Hepatic Impairment: ALT progressively rising above baseline: Decrease dose to 135 mcg/week. If ALT continues to rise or is accompanied by increased bilirubin or hepatic decompensation, discontinue therapy immediately.

Available Dosage Forms
Injection, solution: 180 mcg/mL (1.2 mL) [contains benzyl alcohol]
Injection, solution [prefilled syringe]: 180 mcg/0.5 mL (0.5 mL) [contains benzyl alcohol; packaged with needles and alcohol swabs]

Monitoring and Teaching Issues
Physical Assessment: Assess potential for interactions with other prescriptions, OTC medications, or herbal products patient may be taking. Assess results of laboratory tests prior to and periodically during therapy. Evaluate for depression and other psychiatric symptoms before and during therapy; baseline eye examination and periodically in patients with baseline disorders; baseline echocardiogram in patients with cardiac disease; assess therapeutic effectiveness and adverse response at beginning of and at regular intervals during therapy. Teach patient proper use if self-administered (appropriate injection technique and syringe/needle disposal), possible side effects/appropriate interventions, and adverse symptoms to report.

Monitoring Laboratory Tests: Standard hematological tests should be performed prior to therapy, at week 2, and periodically. Standard biochemical tests should be performed prior to therapy, at week 4, and periodically. Baseline eye examination and periodically in patients with baseline disorders; baseline echocardiogram in patients with cardiac disease; serum HCV RNA levels after 12 weeks of treatment

Clinical studies tested as follows: CBC (including hemoglobin, WBC, and platelets) and chemistries (including liver function tests and uric acid) measured at weeks 1, 2, 4, 6, and 8, and then every 4 weeks; TSH measured every 12 weeks

In addition, the following baseline values were used as entrance criteria:
Platelet count ≥90,000/mm^3 (as low as 75,000/mm^3 in patients with cirrhosis or transition to cirrhosis)
ANC ≥1500/mm^3
Serum creatinine <1.5 times ULN
TSH and T$_4$ within normal limits or adequately controlled

Consider discontinuing treatment if virologic tests indicate no response by week 12.

Patient Education: Inform prescriber of all prescriptions, OTC medications, or herbal products you are taking, and any allergies you have. Do not take any new medication during therapy without consulting prescriber. This medication must be given by injection; if self-administered, follow exact instructions for injection and syringe/needle disposal. Avoid alcohol. You will need laboratory tests and ophthalmic exams prior to and during therapy. May cause headache, insomnia, dizziness (use caution when driving or engaging in potentially hazardous tasks until response to drug is known); loss of hair (will grow back after therapy); nausea or anorexia (small frequent meals or frequent mouth care may help); diarrhea (boiled milk, buttermilk, or yogurt may help); weakness; fatigue; muscle, skeletal, or joint pain; or increased perspiration. Report any severe or persistent adverse effects, including nausea, vomiting, or abdominal pain; severe depression, anxiety, or suicidal ideation; skin rash; pain, redness, or swelling at injection site; chest pain, palpitations, or respiratory difficulty. **Pregnancy/breast-feeding precautions:** Inform prescriber if you are or intend to become pregnant. Consult prescriber for appropriate contraceptive measures. Breast-feeding is not recommended.

Dietary Considerations: Avoid ethanol use in patients with hepatitis C virus.

Pregnancy Risk Factor: C; X when used with ribavirin

Pregnancy Issues: Animal teratogenicity studies have not been conducted; very high doses are abortifacient in Rhesus monkeys. Assumed to have abortifacient potential in humans. There are no adequate and well-controlled studies in pregnant women; use during pregnancy only if the potential benefit to the mother outweighs the possible risk to the fetus. Risk of maternal-infant transmission of hepatitis C is <5%. Reliable contraception should be used in women of childbearing potential.

Lactation: Excretion in breast milk unknown/not recommended

Administration
Other: SubQ: Administer in the abdomen or thigh. Rotate injection site. Do not use if solution contains particulate matter or is discolored. Discard unused solution. Administration should be done on the same day and at approximately the same time each week.

Storage: Store in refrigerator at 2°C to 8°C (36°F to 46°F). Do not freeze or shake; protect from light. Discard unused solution.

♦ **PEG-L-Asparaginase** see Pegaspargase on page 1163

Pegvisomant (peg VI soe mant)
U.S. Brand Names Somavert®
Synonyms B2036-PEG
Generic Available No
Pharmacologic Category Growth Hormone Receptor Antagonist
Use Treatment of acromegaly in patients resistant to or unable to tolerate other therapies
Mechanism of Action/Effect A recombinant human growth hormone (GH) antagonist that binds to GH receptors, leading to decreased serum concentrations of insulin-like growth factor-I (IGF-I) and other GH-responsive proteins.
Contraindications Hypersensitivity to polyethylene glycol or any component of the formulation
Warnings/Precautions Use caution with hepatic or renal disease, or in the elderly. Growth hormone (GH)-secreting tumor size and liver function should be carefully monitored. Interferes with commercially available GH assays; IGF-I levels not GH levels, should be used to adjust therapy. The manufacturer recommends the initial dose be administered under the supervision of prescribing health care provider. Safety and efficacy in pediatric patients have not been established.
(Continued)

Pegvisomant *(Continued)*

Drug Interactions
Decreased Effect: Pegvisomant may increase glucose tolerance; dose reduction of hypo-glycemic agents may be needed.

Increased Effect/Toxicity: Increased doses of pegvisomant may be needed when used with opioids.

Lab Interactions Interferes with measurement of serum GH concentrations by available GH assays.

Adverse Reactions
>10%:
Central nervous system: Pain (4% to 14%; placebo: 6%)
Gastrointestinal: Diarrhea (4% to 14%), nausea (8% to 14%)
Hepatic: Liver function tests abnormal (4% to 12%)
Local: Injection site reaction (4% to 11%)
Miscellaneous: Infection (23%), non-neutralizing anti-GH antibodies (17%; relevance unknown), flu-like syndrome (4% to 12%)

1% to 10%:
Cardiovascular: Hypertension (8%), chest pain (4% to 8%), peripheral edema (4% to 8%)
Central nervous system: Dizziness (4% to 8%; placebo: 6%)
Neuromuscular & skeletal: Back pain (4% to 8%), paresthesia (7%)
Respiratory: Sinusitis (4% to 8%)

Overdosage/Toxicology No specific experience with overdose. Fatigue reported at a dose of 80 mg/day for 7 days. In case of overdose, discontinue until IGF-I levels return to normal.

Pharmacodynamics/Kinetics
Absorption: 57%
Time to Peak: Serum: 33-77 hours
Half-Life Elimination: 6 days
Excretion: Urine (<1%)

Dosing
Adults & Elderly: Acromegaly: SubQ: Initial loading dose: 40 mg; maintenance dose: 10 mg once daily; doses may be adjusted by 5 mg in 4- to 6-week intervals based on IGF-I concentrations (maximum dose: 30 mg/day)

Hepatic Impairment:
Baseline liver function tests (LFT) >3 times ULN: Do not initiate treatment without compre-hensive work-up to determine cause; monitor closely if treatment is started.
LFT ≥3 times but <5 times ULN: Continue treatment, but monitor weekly if no signs or symptoms of hepatitis or liver injury; perform comprehensive hepatic work-up
LFT ≥5 times ULN or transaminase >3 times ULN associated with any increase in total bilirubin: Discontinue immediately and perform comprehensive hepatic work-up. If LFTs return to normal, may cautiously consider restarting therapy with frequent monitoring.
Signs or symptoms of hepatitis or hepatic injury: Evaluate liver function tests; discontinue if liver injury is confirmed

Available Dosage Forms Injection, powder for reconstitution [preservative free]: 10 mg, 15 mg, 20 mg [vial stopper contains latex; packaged with SWFI]

Monitoring and Teaching Issues
Physical Assessment: Assess potential for interactions with other prescriptions, OTC medications, and herbal products patient may be taking. Closely assess results of all laboratory tests at beginning and periodically during therapy. **Note:** First dose should be administered under supervision of prescriber. Assess therapeutic effectiveness and adverse reactions. Teach patient proper use (storage, reconstitution, injection technique, site rotation, and disposal of syringes/needles), possible side effects/appropriate interven-tions, and adverse symptoms to report. Instruct patients with diabetes on need to monitor glucose levels regularly; dose adjustment of hypoglycemic agent may be needed.

Monitoring Laboratory Tests: Serum glucose, serum IGF-I (every 4-6 weeks after initial dose and dosage change, every 6 months when normalized)
Liver function tests:
Normal at baseline: Monthly for first 6 months, quarterly for next 6 months, biannually for the next year
Elevated, but ≤3 times ULN: Monitor monthly for at least 1 year, then biannually the next year

Patient Education: Inform prescriber of all prescriptions, OTC medications, or herbal products you are taking, and any allergies you have. This medication may only be adminis-tered by injection. If instructed in self-injection, follow instructions exactly. Report immedi-ately any reaction at injection site (redness, swelling, itching). May cause diarrhea (buttermilk, boiled milk, or yogurt may help); nausea (frequent small meals and good mouth care may help); or signs of allergic response (chest pain, respiratory difficulty, skin rash). **Breast-feeding precaution:** Consult prescriber if breast-feeding.

Pregnancy Risk Factor: B
Lactation: Excretion in breast milk unknown/use caution

Administration
Other: For SubQ administration only; rotate injection site daily; may administer in upper arm, upper thigh, abdomen, or buttocks; do not rub injection site. The manufacturer recom-mends the initial dose be administered under the supervision of prescribing healthcare provider.

Reconstitution: Reconstitute with SWFI; gently roll, do not shake, in order to dissolve powder.

Storage: Store intact vials under refrigeration at 2°C to 8°C (36°F to 46°F); protect from freezing. Following reconstitution, use within 6 hours. Do not use solution if cloudy.

◆ Pegylated Interferon Alfa-2a *see* Peginterferon Alfa-2a *on page 1165*
◆ PemADD® [DSC] *see* Pemoline *on page 1170*
◆ PemADD® CT [DSC] *see* Pemoline *on page 1170*

Pemetrexed (pem e TREKS ed)

U.S. Brand Names Alimta®

Synonyms LY231514; MTA; Multitargeted Antifolate; NSC-698037; Pemetrexed Disodium

Pharmacologic Category Antineoplastic Agent, Antimetabolite; Antineoplastic Agent, Antimetabolite (Antifolate)

Use Treatment of malignant pleural mesothelioma in combination with cisplatin; treatment of nonsmall cell lung cancer

Unlabeled/Investigational Use Bladder, breast, cervical, colorectal, esophageal, gastric, head and neck, ovarian, pancreatic, and renal cell cancers

Mechanism of Action/Effect Disrupts folate-dependent metabolic processes essential for cell replication.

Contraindications Hypersensitivity to pemetrexed or any component of the formulation

Warnings/Precautions The U.S. Food and Drug Administration (FDA) currently recommends that procedures for proper handling and disposal of antineoplastic agents be considered. Prophylactic folic acid and vitamin B_{12} supplements are necessary to reduce hematologic and gastrointestinal toxicity. Folic acid and vitamin B_{12} should be started 1 week before the first dose of pemetrexed. Pretreatment with corticosteroids reduces the incidence and severity of cutaneous reactions. Use caution with hepatic dysfunction not due to metastases and in patients receiving concurrent nephrotoxins. Use caution when administering NSAIDs to patients with Cl_{cr} <80 mL/minutes. Patient should have an ANC ≥1500 cells/mm^3, platelets ≥100,000 cells/mm^3, and Cl_{cr} >45 mL/minutes before a dose is given. Use caution in patients with Cl_{cr} <45 mL/minute (use not recommended by manufacturer). Safety and efficacy have not been established in pediatric patients.

Drug Interactions

Increased Effect/Toxicity: NSAIDs may increase the toxicity of pemetrexed.

Nutritional/Ethanol Interactions Lower ANC nadirs occur in patients with elevated baseline cystathionine or homocysteine concentrations. Levels of these substances can be reduced by folic acid and vitamin B_{12} supplementation.

Adverse Reactions Note: Reported frequencies of adverse effects vary by indication/population and concurrent therapy.

>10%:

Cardiovascular: Chest pain (38% to 40%), edema (19%)

Central nervous system: Fatigue (80% to 87%), fever (17% to 26%), depression (11% to 14%)

Dermatologic: Rash (17% to 22%), alopecia (11%)

Gastrointestinal: Nausea (39% to 84%; grade 3/4 in 12%), vomiting (25% to 58%; grade 3/4 in 11%), constipation (30% to 44%), anorexia (35% to 62%), stomatitis/pharyngitis (20% to 28%), diarrhea (21% to 26%)

Hematologic: Neutropenia (11% to 58%), leukopenia (13% to 55%), anemia (33%), thrombocytopenia (9% to 27%)

Nadir: 8-10 days

Recovery: 12-17 days

Neuromuscular & skeletal: Neuropathy (17% to 29%), myalgia (13%)

Renal: Creatinine increased (3% to 16%)

Respiratory: Dyspnea (66%)

Miscellaneous: Infection (17% to 23%)

1% to 10%:

Cardiovascular: Thrombosis/embolism (4% to 7%), cardiac ischemia (3%)

Endocrine & metabolic: Dehydration (3% to 7%)

Gastrointestinal: Dysphagia/esophagitis/odynophagia (5% to 6%)

Renal: Renal failure (<1% to 2%)

Miscellaneous: Allergic reaction (2% to 8%)

Neuromuscular & skeletal: Arthralgia (8%)

Overdosage/Toxicology Toxicities include neutropenia, anemia, thrombocytopenia, mucositis, rash, infection, and diarrhea. Treatment is supportive and symptom-directed. Continuing leucovorin may help minimize additional hematologic toxicity. The intravenous leucovorin doses used in clinical trials were 100 mg/m^2 once, followed by 50 mg/m^2 every 6 hours for 8 days. It is unknown if pemetrexed is removed by hemodialysis.

Pharmacodynamics/Kinetics

Duration of Action: V_{dss}: 16.1 L

Protein Binding: ~81%

Half-Life Elimination: Normal renal function: 3.5 hours

Metabolism: Minimal

Excretion: Urine (70% to 90% as unchanged drug)

Dosing

Adults:

Nonsmall cell lung cancer: 500 mg/m^2 on day 1 of each 21-day cycle

Malignant pleural mesothelioma: I.V.: 500-600 mg/m^2 on day 1 of each 21-day cycle in combination with cisplatin.

Note: Start vitamin supplements 1 week before initial dose of pemetrexed. Folic acid 350-1000 mcg/day orally (continuing for 21 days after last dose of pemetrexed) and vitamin B_{12} 1000 mcg I.M. every 9 weeks. Dexamethasone 4 mg twice daily can be started the day before therapy, and continued the day of and the day after to minimize cutaneous reactions.

Dosage adjustments for toxicity:

General toxicity: Discontinue if patient has any grade 3 or 4 toxicity after two dose reductions (except grade 3 transaminase elevations) or immediately if grade 3 or 4 neurotoxicity develops

Hematologic toxicity: Upon recovery, reinitiate therapy

Nadir ANC <500/mm^3 and nadir platelets ≥50,000/mm^3: Reduce dose to 75% of previous dose of pemetrexed and cisplatin

Nadir platelets <50,000/mm^3: Reduce dose to 50% of previous dose of pemetrexed and cisplatin

(Continued)

Pemetrexed *(Continued)*

Nonhematologic toxicity (excluding neurotoxicity or ≥ grade 3 transaminase elevations):
Upon recovery, reinitiate therapy
Grade 3 or 4 toxicity (excluding mucositis or transaminase elevations): Reduce dose to 75% of previous dose of pemetrexed and cisplatin
Diarrhea requiring hospitalization: Reduce dose to 75% of previous dose of pemetrexed and cisplatin
Grade 3 or 4 mucositis: Reduce dose to 50% of previous dose of pemetrexed; continue cisplatin at 100% of previous dose

Neurotoxicity:
Common Toxicity Criteria (CTC) Grade 0-1: Continue at previous dose of pemetrexed and cisplatin.
CTC Grade 2: Continue at previous dose of pemetrexed; Reduce dose to 50% of previous dose of cisplatin.

Renal Impairment:
Cl_{cr} <45 mL/minute: No dosage adjustment guidelines are available; manufacturer recommends not using the drug.
Cl_{cr} ≥45 mL/minute: No dosage adjustment required.

Hepatic Impairment: No dosage adjustment required.

Available Dosage Forms Injection, powder for reconstitution: 500 mg

Monitoring and Teaching Issues

Physical Assessment: See Warnings/Precautions for use cautions (hepatic impairment) and premedication requirements (eg, start folic acid and vitamin B_{12} 1 week before first dose of pemetrexed; corticosteroids to reduce cutaneous reactions). Assess potential for interactions with other pharmacological agents (eg, NSAIDs and other agents with nephrotoxic potential; see Drug Interactions). Assess laboratory tests on regular schedule (see Monitoring Laboratory Tests). Monitor adverse response at frequent intervals during treatment (eg, chest pain, CNS changes, GI upset [nausea, vomiting, diarrhea, constipation], anemia, neuropathy, rash, infection; see Adverse Reactions). Teach patient appropriate interventions to reduce side effects and adverse symptoms to report (see Patient Education).

Monitoring Laboratory Tests: CBC (before each dose); serum creatinine, total bilirubin, ALT, AST (day 1 of each, or every other cycle)

Patient Education: This medication is only administered intravenously (with your cisplatin). Report immediately any burning, pain, itching, or redness at infusion site or any sudden feelings of anxiety, difficulty breathing, chest or back pain. It is important that you maintain adequate hydration (2-3 L/day of fluids) unless instructed to restrict fluid intake and adequate nutrition (frequent small meals may help). Maintain regularly scheduled dietary supplements (vitamin B_{12} and folic acid) as prescribed. May cause severe nausea, vomiting, constipation, or diarrhea (small frequent meals, and good mouth care are important; if persistent, consult prescriber for medication); mouth sores (use soft toothbrush or cotton swabs for mouth care). Report promptly any chest pain, skin rash, tingling or loss of sensation in extremities, difficulty breathing, fever, chills, unusual fatigue, or any other unusual symptoms. **Pregnancy/breast-feeding precautions:** Inform prescriber if you are pregnant. Do not get pregnant during therapy. Consult prescriber for instruction on appropriate contraceptive measures. This drug may cause severe fetal defects. Do not breast-feed.

Dietary Considerations: Initiate folic acid supplementation 1 week before first dose of pemetrexed, continue for full course of therapy, and for 21 days after last dose. Institute vitamin B_{12} 1 week before the first dose; administer every 9 weeks thereafter.

Pregnancy Risk Factor: D

Pregnancy Issues: In animal studies, was associated with fetotoxicity and teratogenicity when given on gestation days 6-15. Embryotoxicity also occurred. There are no adequate or well-controlled studies in pregnant women. Patients should avoid becoming pregnant while using this drug. If used during pregnancy or if patient becomes pregnant during therapy, patient should be educated about the potential hazards to the fetus.

Lactation: Excretion in breast milk unknown/not recommended

Administration

I.V.: Infuse over 10 minutes.

Reconstitution: Add 20 mL of 0.9% preservative free sodium chloride injection to make a 25 mg/mL solution. Gently swirl. Solution may be colorless to green-yellow. Further dilute in 50-200 mL of 0.9% sodium chloride for administration. Discard unused portion.

Compatibility: Physically **incompatible** with calcium-containing products.

Y-site administration: Incompatible: Amphotericin B, calcium gluconate, cefazolin sodium, cefotaxime sodium, cefotetan disodium, cefoxitin sodium, ceftazidime, chlorpromazine hydrochloride, ciprofloxacin, dobutamine hydrochloride, doxorubicin hydrochloride, doxycycline hyclate, droperidol, gemcitabine hydrochloride, gentamicin sulfate, irinotecan hydrochloride, metronidazole, minocycline hydrochloride, mitoxantrone hydrochloride, nalbuphine hydrochloride, ondansetron hydrochloride, prochlorperazine edisylate, tobramycin sulfate, topotecan hydrochloride

Storage: Store unopened vials at 25°C (77°F). Reconstituted and infusion solutions are stable for 24 hours when refrigerated or stored at room temperature.

♦ **Pemetrexed Disodium** *see Pemetrexed on page 1169*

Pemoline *(PEM oh leen)*

U.S. Brand Names Cylert®; PemADD® [DSC]; PemADD® CT [DSC]
Synonyms Phenylisohydantoin; PIO
Controlled Substance C-IV
Generic Available Yes
Pharmacologic Category Stimulant
Use Treatment of attention-deficit/hyperactivity disorder (ADHD) (not first-line)
Unlabeled/Investigational Use Narcolepsy

Mechanism of Action/Effect Blocks the reuptake mechanism of dopaminergic neurons, appears to act at the cerebral cortex and subcortical structures; CNS and respiratory stimulant with weak sympathomimetic effects; actions may be mediated via increase in CNS dopamine

Contraindications Hypersensitivity to pemoline or any component of the formulation; hepatic impairment (including abnormalities on baseline liver function tests); children <6 years of age; Tourette's syndrome; psychosis

Warnings/Precautions Not considered first-line therapy for ADHD due to association with hepatic failure. The manufacturer has recommended that signed informed consent following a discussion of risks and benefits must or should be obtained prior to the initiation of therapy. Therapy should be discontinued if a response is not evident after 3 weeks of therapy. Pemoline should not be started in patients with abnormalities in baseline liver function tests, and should be discontinued if clinically significant liver function test abnormalities are revealed at any time during therapy. Use with caution in patients with renal dysfunction or psychosis. In general, stimulant medications should be used with caution in patients with bipolar disorder, diabetes mellitus, cardiovascular disease, seizure disorders, insomnia, porphyria, or hypertension (although pemoline has been demonstrated to have a low potential to elevate blood pressure relative to other stimulants). May exacerbate symptoms of behavior and thought disorder in psychotic patients. Potential for drug dependency exists - avoid abrupt discontinuation in patients who have received for prolonged periods. Stimulant use has been associated with growth suppression, and careful monitoring is recommended.

Drug Interactions

Decreased Effect: Pemoline in combination with antiepileptic medications may decrease seizure threshold.

Increased Effect/Toxicity: Use caution when pemoline is used with other CNS-acting medications.

Nutritional/Ethanol Interactions Ethanol: Avoid ethanol (may increase CNS depression).

Adverse Reactions Frequency not defined.

Central nervous system: Insomnia, dizziness, drowsiness, mental depression, increased irritability, seizure, precipitation of Tourette's syndrome, hallucinations, headache, movement disorders

Dermatologic: Rash

Endocrine & metabolic: Suppression of growth in children

Gastrointestinal: Anorexia, weight loss, stomach pain, nausea

Hematologic: Aplastic anemia

Hepatic: Increased liver enzyme (usually reversible upon discontinuation), hepatitis, jaundice, hepatic failure

Overdosage/Toxicology Symptoms of overdose include tachycardia, hallucinations, and agitation. There is no specific antidote for intoxication and treatment is primarily supportive.

Pharmacodynamics/Kinetics

Onset of Action: Peak effect: 4 hours

Duration of Action: 8 hours

Time to Peak: Serum: 2-4 hours

Protein Binding: 50%

Half-Life Elimination: Children: 7-8.6 hours; Adults: 12 hours

Metabolism: Partially hepatic

Excretion: Urine; feces (negligible amounts)

Dosing

Adults & Elderly: ADHD: Oral: Initial: 37.5 mg given once daily in the morning, increase by 18.75 mg/day at weekly intervals; usual effective dose range: 56.25-75 mg/day; maximum: 112.5 mg/day; dosage range: 0.5-3 mg/kg/24 hours; significant benefit may not be evident until third or fourth week of administration.

Pediatrics: Children ≥6 years: Refer to adult dosing.

Renal Impairment: Cl_{cr} <50 mL/minute: Avoid use.

Available Dosage Forms [DSC] = Discontinued product

Tablet (Cylert®, PemADD® [DSC]): 18.75 mg, 37.5 mg, 75 mg

Tablet, chewable (Cylert®, PemADD® CT [DSC]): 37.5 mg

Monitoring and Teaching Issues

Physical Assessment: Assess effectiveness and interactions of other medications patient may be taking. After long-term use, taper dosage slowly when discontinuing. Monitor laboratory results, effectiveness of therapy, and adverse reactions at beginning of therapy and periodically with long-term use. Assess knowledge/teach patient appropriate use, interventions to reduce side effects, and adverse symptoms to report.

Monitoring Laboratory Tests: Liver enzymes (baseline and every 2 weeks)

Patient Education: Take exactly as directed; do not change dosage or discontinue without consulting prescriber. Response may take some time. Avoid alcohol, caffeine, or other stimulants. Maintain adequate hydration (2-3 L/day of fluids) unless instructed to restrict fluid intake. You may experience nausea, decreased appetite, or altered taste sensation (small frequent meals may help maintain adequate nutrition); or drowsiness, dizziness, or mental depression, especially during early therapy (use caution when driving or engaging in tasks requiring alertness until response to drug is known). Report unresolved rapid heartbeat; excessive agitation, nervousness, insomnia, tremors, dizziness, or seizures; skin rash or irritation; altered gait or movement; unusual mouth movements or vocalizations (Tourette's syndrome); yellowing of skin or eyes; or dark urine or pale stools.

Breast-feeding precaution: Breast-feeding is not recommended.

Pregnancy Risk Factor: B

Lactation: Excretion in breast milk unknown/not recommended

Administration

Oral: Administer medication in the morning.

Additional Information Treatment of ADHD should include "Drug Holidays" or periodic discontinuation of stimulant medication in order to assess the patient's requirements and to decrease tolerance and limit suppression of linear growth and weight. The labeling for Cylert® includes recommendations for liver function monitoring and a Patient Information Consent Form.

Penciclovir (pen SYE kloe veer)

U.S. Brand Names Denavir®

Generic Available No

Pharmacologic Category Antiviral Agent

Medication Safety Issues
Sound-alike/look-alike issues:
Denavir® may be confused with indinavir

Use Topical treatment of herpes simplex labialis (cold sores)

Mechanism of Action/Effect Phosphorylated in the virus-infected cells to penciclovir triphosphate, which competitively inhibits DNA polymerase in HSV-1 and HSV-2 strains. This prevents viral replication by inhibition of viral DNA synthesis. Some activity has been demonstrated against Epstein-Barr and varicella-zoster virus (VZV).

Contraindications Hypersensitivity to the penciclovir or any component of the formulation; previous and significant adverse reactions to famciclovir

Warnings/Precautions Apply only to herpes labialis on lips and face. Application to mucous membranes is not recommended. Effect has not been evaluated in immunocompromised patients.

Adverse Reactions
>10%: Dermatologic: Mild erythema (50%)
1% to 10%: Central nervous system: Headache (5.3%)

Overdosage/Toxicology Penciclovir is poorly absorbed if ingested orally. Adverse reactions related to oral ingestion are unlikely.

Pharmacodynamics/Kinetics
Absorption: Topical: None

Dosing
Adults & Elderly: Herpes simplex labialis (cold sores): Topical: Apply cream at the first sign or symptom of cold sore (eg, tingling, swelling); apply every 2 hours during waking hours for 4 days.
Pediatrics: Herpes simplex labialis (cold sores): Children ≥12 years: Refer to adult dosing.

Available Dosage Forms Cream: 1% (1.5 g)

Monitoring and Teaching Issues
Physical Assessment: Use for herpes labialis (cold sores) on lips and face; application to mucous membranes is not recommended. Teach patient appropriate application/use and adverse symptoms to report (see Patient Education).

Patient Education: This is not a cure for herpes (recurrences tend to appear within 3 months of original infection), nor will this medication reduce the risk of transmission to others when lesions are present. For external use only. Wash hands before and after application. Apply this film over affected areas at first sign of cold sore. Avoid use of other topical creams, lotions, or ointments unless approved by prescriber. You may experience headache, mild rash, or taste disturbances. Report lack of improvement or worsening of condition. **Breast-feeding precaution:** Consult prescriber if breast-feeding.

Pregnancy Risk Factor: B

Lactation: Excretion in breast milk unknown

Administration
Storage: Store at controlled room temperature of 20°C to 25°C (68°F to 77°F).

Additional Information Penciclovir is the active metabolite of the prodrug famciclovir. Penciclovir is an alternative to topical acyclovir for HSV-1 and HSV-2 infections. Neither drug will prevent recurring HSV attacks.

Penicillin G Benzathine (pen i SIL in jee BENZ a theen)

U.S. Brand Names Bicillin® L-A

Synonyms Benzathine Benzylpenicillin; Benzathine Penicillin G; Benzylpenicillin Benzathine

Generic Available No

Pharmacologic Category Antibiotic, Penicillin

Medication Safety Issues
Sound-alike/look-alike issues:
Penicillin may be confused with penicillamine
Bicillin® may be confused with Wycillin®
Bicillin® C-R (penicillin G benzathine and penicillin G procaine) may be confused with Bicillin® L-A (penicillin G benzathine). Penicillin G benzathine is the only product currently approved for the treatment of syphilis. Administration of penicillin G benzathine and penicillin G procaine combination instead of Bicillin® L-A may result in inadequate treatment response.

Penicillin G benzathine may only be administered by deep intramuscular injection; intravenous administration of penicillin G benzathine has been associated with cardiopulmonary arrest and death.

Use Active against some gram-positive organisms, few gram-negative organisms such as *Neisseria gonorrhoeae*, and some anaerobes and spirochetes; used in the treatment of syphilis; used only for the treatment of mild to moderately severe infections caused by organisms susceptible to low concentrations of penicillin G or for prophylaxis of infections caused by these organisms

Mechanism of Action/Effect Interferes with bacterial cell wall synthesis during active multiplication, causing cell wall death and resultant bactericidal activity against susceptible bacteria

Contraindications Hypersensitivity to penicillin or any component of the formulation

Warnings/Precautions Use with caution in patients with impaired renal function, seizure disorder. CDC and AAP do not currently recommend the use of penicillin G benzathine to treat congenital syphilis or neurosyphilis due to reported treatment failures and lack of published clinical data on its efficacy.

Drug Interactions

Decreased Effect: Tetracyclines may decrease penicillin effectiveness. Although anecdotal reports suggest oral contraceptive efficacy could be reduced by penicillins, this has been refuted by more rigorous scientific and clinical data.

Increased Effect/Toxicity: Probenecid increases penicillin levels. Aminoglycosides may lead to synergistic efficacy. Penicillins may increase the exposure to methotrexate during concurrent therapy; monitor.

Lab Interactions Positive Coombs' [direct], false-positive urinary and/or serum proteins; false-positive or negative urinary glucose using Clinitest®

Adverse Reactions Frequency not defined.

Central nervous system: Convulsions, confusion, drowsiness, myoclonus, fever

Dermatologic: Rash

Endocrine & metabolic: Electrolyte imbalance

Hematologic: Positive Coombs' reaction, hemolytic anemia

Local: Pain, thrombophlebitis

Renal: Acute interstitial nephritis

Miscellaneous: Anaphylaxis, hypersensitivity reactions, Jarisch-Herxheimer reaction

Overdosage/Toxicology Symptoms of penicillin overdose include neuromuscular hypersensitivity (eg, agitation, hallucinations, asterixis, encephalopathy, confusion, and seizures). Electrolyte imbalance may occur if the preparation contains potassium or sodium salts, especially in renal failure. Hemodialysis may be helpful to aid in removal of the drug from blood; otherwise, treatment is supportive or symptom-directed.

Pharmacodynamics/Kinetics

Duration of Action: Dose dependent: 1-4 weeks; larger doses result in more sustained levels

Absorption: I.M.: Slow

Time to Peak: Serum: 12-24 hours

Dosing

Adults & Elderly:

Group A streptococcal upper respiratory infection: I.M.: 1.2 million units as a single dose

Prophylaxis of recurrent rheumatic fever: I.M.: 1.2 million units every 3-4 weeks or 600,000 units twice monthly

Early syphilis: I.M.: 2.4 million units as a single dose in 2 injection sites

Syphilis of more than 1-year duration: I.M.: 2.4 million units in 2 injection sites once weekly for 3 doses

Note: Not indicated as single drug therapy for neurosyphilis, but may be given 1 time/week for 3 weeks following I.V. treatment (refer to Penicillin G monograph for dosing)

Pediatrics:

Asymptomatic congenital syphilis: I.M.: Neonates >1200g: 50,000 units/kg for 1 dose

Group A streptococcal upper respiratory infection: I.M.: Infants and Children: 25,000-50,000 units/kg as a single dose; maximum: 1.2 million units

Prophylaxis of recurrent rheumatic fever: I.M.: Infants and Children: 25,000-50,000 units/kg every 3-4 weeks; maximum: 1.2 million units/dose

Early syphilis: I.M.: Infants and Children: 50,000 units/kg as a single injection; maximum: 2.4 million units

Syphilis of more than 1-year duration: I.M.: Infants and Children: 50,000 units/kg every week for 3 doses; maximum: 2.4 million units/dose

Available Dosage Forms Injection, suspension [prefilled syringe] (Bicillin® L-A): 600,000 units/mL (1 mL, 2 mL, 4 mL)

Monitoring and Teaching Issues

Physical Assessment: Assess results of culture and sensitivity tests and patient's allergy history prior to starting therapy. Use with caution in presence of impaired renal function or history of seizures (see Warnings/Precautions). Assess potential for interactions with other pharmacological agents patient may be taking (eg, may increase or decrease levels/effects of penicillin; see Drug Interactions). Advise patients with diabetes about use of Clinitest®; may cause false readings. Assess for effectiveness (resolution of infection) and adverse reactions (eg, hypersensitivity reactions, opportunistic infection; see Adverse Reactions). Teach patient possible side effects/appropriate interventions and adverse symptoms to report (see Patient Education).

Monitoring Laboratory Tests: Perform culture and sensitivity before administering first dose.

Patient Education: This drug can only be given by injection. Report immediately any redness, swelling, burning, or pain at infusion site or any signs of allergic reaction (eg, respiratory or swallowing difficulty, chest tightness, rash, hives, swelling of lips or mouth). Maintain adequate hydration (2-3 L/day of fluids) unless instructed to restrict fluid intake. If being treated for sexually-transmitted disease, partner will also need to be treated. If you have diabetes, drug may cause false test results with Clinitest®; consult prescriber for alternative method of glucose monitoring. May cause confusion or drowsiness (use caution when driving or engaging in tasks that require alertness until response to drug is known). Report persistent adverse effects or signs of opportunistic infection (eg, fever, chills, unhealed sores, white plaques in mouth or vagina, purulent vaginal discharge, fatigue).

Pregnancy Risk Factor: B

Lactation: Enters breast milk/compatible

Administration

I.M.: Administer by deep I.M. injection in the upper outer quadrant of the buttock. Do **not** give I.V., intra-arterially, or SubQ. When doses are repeated, rotate the injection site.

Storage: Store in refrigerator.

Penicillin G (Parenteral/Aqueous)
(pen i SIL in jee, pa REN ter al, AYE kwee us)

U.S. Brand Names Pfizerpen®

Synonyms Benzylpenicillin Potassium; Benzylpenicillin Sodium; Crystalline Penicillin; Penicillin G Potassium; Penicillin G Sodium

Generic Available Yes

Pharmacologic Category Antibiotic, Penicillin

Medication Safety Issues
Sound-alike/look-alike issues:
Penicillin may be confused with penicillamine

Use Active against some gram-positive organisms, generally not *Staphylococcus aureus*; some gram-negative organisms such as *Neisseria gonorrhoeae*, and some anaerobes and spirochetes

Mechanism of Action/Effect Interferes with bacterial cell wall synthesis during active multiplication, causing cell wall death and resultant bactericidal activity against susceptible bacteria

Contraindications Hypersensitivity to penicillin or any component of the formulation

Warnings/Precautions Avoid intravascular or intra-arterial administration or injection into or near major peripheral nerves or blood vessels since such injections may cause severe and/or permanent neurovascular damage. Use with caution in patients with renal impairment (dosage reduction required), pre-existing seizure disorders.

Drug Interactions
Decreased Effect: Tetracyclines may decrease penicillin effectiveness. Although anecdotal reports suggest oral contraceptive efficacy could be reduced by penicillins, this has been refuted by more rigorous scientific and clinical data.

Increased Effect/Toxicity: Probenecid increases penicillin levels. Aminoglycosides may lead to synergistic efficacy. Penicillins may increase the exposure to methotrexate during concurrent therapy; monitor.

Lab Interactions False-positive or negative urinary glucose determination using Clinitest®; positive Coombs' [direct]; false-positive urinary and/or serum proteins

Adverse Reactions Frequency not defined.
Central nervous system: Convulsions, confusion, drowsiness, myoclonus, fever
Dermatologic: Rash
Endocrine & metabolic: Electrolyte imbalance
Hematologic: Positive Coombs' reaction, hemolytic anemia
Local: Thrombophlebitis
Renal: Acute interstitial nephritis
Miscellaneous: Anaphylaxis, hypersensitivity reactions, Jarisch-Herxheimer reaction

Overdosage/Toxicology Symptoms of penicillin overdose include neuromuscular hypersensitivity (eg, agitation, hallucinations, asterixis, encephalopathy, confusion, and seizures). Electrolyte imbalance may occur if the preparation contains potassium or sodium salts, especially in renal failure. Treatment is supportive or symptom-directed.

Pharmacodynamics/Kinetics
Time to Peak: Serum: I.M.: ~30 minutes; I.V. ~1 hour
Protein Binding: 65%
Half-Life Elimination:
Neonates: <6 days old: 3.2-3.4 hours; 7-13 days old: 1.2-2.2 hours; >14 days old: 0.9-1.9 hours
Children and Adults: Normal renal function: 20-50 minutes
End-stage renal disease: 3.3-5.1 hours
Metabolism: Hepatic (30%) to penicilloic acid
Excretion: Urine

Dosing
Adults & Elderly:
Susceptible infections: I.M., I.V.: 2-24 million units/day in divided doses every 4 hours depending on sensitivity of the organism and severity of the infection
Neurosyphilis: 18-24 million units/day in divided doses every 3-4 hours for 10-14 days
Pediatrics:
Susceptible infections: I.M., I.V.:
Infants:
<7 days, <2000 g: 50,000 units/kg/day in divided doses every 12 hours
<7 days, >2000 g: 50,000 units/kg/day in divided doses every 8 hours
>7 days, <2000 g: 75,000 units/kg/day in divided doses every 8 hours
>7 days, >2000 g: 100,000 units/kg/day in divided doses every 6 hours
Infants and Children (sodium salt is preferred in children): 100,000-250,000 units/kg/day in divided doses every 4 hours
Severe infections: Up to 400,000 units/kg/day in divided doses every 4 hours; maximum dose: 24 million units/day
Congenital syphilis:
Newborns: 50,000 units/kg/day I.V. every 8-12 hours for 10-14 days
Infants: 50,000 units/kg every 4-6 hours for 10-14 days
Disseminated gonococcal infections or gonococcus ophthalmia (if organism proven sensitive): 100,000 units/kg/day in 2 equal doses (4 equal doses/day for infants >1 week)
Gonococcal meningitis: 150,000 units/kg in 2 equal doses (4 doses/day for infants >1 week)
Renal Impairment: Dosage modification is required in patients with renal insufficiency.
Cl$_{cr}$ 30-50 mL/minute: Administer every 6 hours.
Cl$_{cr}$ 10-30 mL/minute: Administer every 8 hours.

Cl$_{cr}$ <10 mL/minute: Administer every 12 hours.

Moderately dialyzable (20% to 50%)

Continuous arteriovenous or venovenous hemofiltration: Dose as for Cl$_{cr}$ 10-50 mL/minute.

Available Dosage Forms

Infusion, as potassium [premixed iso-osmotic dextrose solution, frozen]: 1 million units (50 mL), 2 million units (50 mL), 3 million units (50 mL)

Injection, powder for reconstitution, as potassium (Pfizerpen®): 5 million units, 20 million units

Injection, powder for reconstitution, as sodium: 5 million units

Monitoring and Teaching Issues

Physical Assessment: Assess results of culture and sensitivity tests and patient's allergy history prior to starting therapy. Use with caution in presence of renal impairment or seizure disorder (see Warnings/Precautions). Assess potential for interactions with other pharmacological agents (eg, decreased or increased levels/effects of penicillin G; see Drug Interactions). See Administration for I.V. and I.M. specifics. Avoid intravascular or intra-arterial administration or injection into or near major peripheral nerves or blood vessels; may cause severe and/or permanent neurovascular damage. Advise patients with diabetes about use of Clinitest®; may cause false positive or negative. Assess effectiveness (resolution of infections) and adverse reactions (eg, hypersensitivity reactions, opportunistic infection [fever, chills, unhealed sores, white plaques in mouth or vagina, purulent vaginal discharge, fatigue], CNS changes, thrombophlebitis; see Adverse Reactions). Teach patient possible side effects/appropriate interventions and adverse symptoms to report (see Patient Education).

Monitoring Laboratory Tests: Perform culture and sensitivity before administering first dose.

Patient Education: This drug can only be given by injection or infusion. Report immediately any redness, swelling, burning, or pain at infusion site or any signs of allergic reaction (eg, respiratory or swallowing difficulty, chest tightness, rash, hives, swelling of lips or mouth). Maintain adequate hydration (2-3 L/day of fluids) unless instructed to restrict fluid intake. If being treated for sexually-transmitted disease, partner will also need to be treated. If you have diabetes, drug may cause false test results with Clinitest®, consult prescriber for alternative method of glucose monitoring. May cause confusion or drowsiness (use caution when driving or engaging in tasks that require alertness until response to drug is known). Report persistent adverse effects or signs of opportunistic infection (eg, fever, chills, unhealed sores, white plaques in mouth or vagina, purulent vaginal discharge, fatigue).

Geriatric Considerations: Despite a reported prolonged half-life, it is usually not necessary to adjust the dose of penicillin G or VK in the elderly to account for renal function changes with age, however, it is advised to calculate an estimated creatinine clearance and adjust dose accordingly. Consider sodium content in patients who may be sensitive to volume expansion (ie, CHF).

Pregnancy Risk Factor: B

Lactation: Enters breast milk/compatible

Administration

I.M.: Administer I.M. by deep injection in the upper outer quadrant of the buttock. Administer injection around-the-clock to promote less variation in peak and trough levels.

I.V.: While I.M. route is preferred route of administration, large doses should be administered by continuous I.V. infusion. Determine volume and rate of fluid administration required in a 24-hour period. Add appropriate daily dosage to this fluid. Rapid administration or excessive dosage can cause electrolyte imbalance, cardiac arrhythmias, and/or seizures.

Reconstitution: Reconstituted parenteral solution is stable for 7 days when refrigerated (2°C to 15°C). Penicillin G potassium for I.V. infusion in NS or D$_5$W, solution is stable for 24 hours at room temperature.

Compatibility: Inactivated in acidic or alkaline solutions

Penicillin G potassium: Stable in dextran 6% in dextrose, dextran 6% in NS, D$_5$LR, D$_5$¼NS, D$_5$½NS, D$_5$NS, D$_5$W, D$_{10}$W, LR, ½NS, NS, hetastarch 6%; **incompatible** with dextran 70 6% in dextrose, dextran 40 10% in dextrose

Compatibility in syringe: Incompatible with metoclopramide

Compatibility when admixed: Incompatible with aminoglycosides, aminophylline, amphotericin B, chlorpromazine, dopamine, floxacillin, hydroxyzine, metaraminol, pentobarbital, phenytoin, prochlorperazine mesylate, promazine, thiopental, vancomycin, vitamin B complex with C with oxytetracycline

Penicillin G sodium: Stable in dextran 40 10%; **incompatible** with fat emulsion 10%

Compatibility when admixed: Incompatible with amphotericin B, bleomycin, chlorpromazine, cytarabine, floxacillin, hydroxyzine, methylprednisolone sodium succinate, prochlorperazine mesylate, promethazine, vancomycin

Storage: Penicillin G potassium is stable at room temperature.

Additional Information 1 million units is approximately equal to 625 mg.

Penicillin G potassium injection:

Potassium content per million units: 65.6 mg (1.7 mEq)

Sodium content per million units: 23.5 mg (1.02 mEq)

Related Information

Antimicrobial Drugs of Choice *on page 1792*

♦ **Penicillin G Potassium** *see* Penicillin G (Parenteral/Aqueous) *on page 1174*

Penicillin G Procaine (pen i SIL in jee PROE kane)

Synonyms APPG; Aqueous Procaine Penicillin G; Procaine Benzylpenicillin; Procaine Penicillin G; Wycillin [DSC]

Generic Available Yes

Pharmacologic Category Antibiotic, Penicillin

Medication Safety Issues

Sound-alike/look-alike issues:

Penicillin G procaine may be confused with penicillin V potassium

Wycillin® may be confused with Bicillin®

(Continued)

Penicillin G Procaine *(Continued)*

Use Moderately severe infections due to *Treponema pallidum* and other penicillin G-sensitive microorganisms that are susceptible to low, but prolonged serum penicillin concentrations; anthrax due to *Bacillus anthracis* (postexposure) to reduce the incidence or progression of disease following exposure to aerolized *Bacillus anthracis*

Mechanism of Action/Effect Inhibits bacterial cell wall synthesis by binding to one or more of the penicillin binding proteins (PBPs); which in turn inhibits the final transpeptidation step of peptidoglycan synthesis in bacterial cell walls, thus inhibiting cell wall biosynthesis. Bacteria eventually lyse due to ongoing activity of cell wall autolytic enzymes (autolysins and murein hydrolases) while cell wall assembly is arrested.

Contraindications Hypersensitivity to penicillin, procaine, or any component of the formulation

Warnings/Precautions May need to modify dosage in patients with severe renal impairment, seizure disorders. Avoid I.V., intravascular, or intra-arterial administration of penicillin G procaine since severe and/or permanent neurovascular damage may occur. Use of penicillin for longer than 2 weeks may be associated with an increased risk for some adverse reactions (neutropenia, serum sickness).

Drug Interactions

Decreased Effect: Tetracyclines may decrease penicillin effectiveness. Although anecdotal reports suggest oral contraceptive efficacy could be reduced by penicillins, this has been refuted by more rigorous scientific and clinical data.

Increased Effect/Toxicity: Probenecid increases penicillin levels. Aminoglycosides may lead to synergistic efficacy. Penicillins may increase the exposure to methotrexate during concurrent therapy; monitor.

Lab Interactions Positive Coombs' [direct], false-positive urinary and/or serum proteins

Adverse Reactions Frequency not defined.

Cardiovascular: Myocardial depression, vasodilation, conduction disturbances

Central nervous system: Confusion, drowsiness, myoclonus, CNS stimulation, seizure

Hematologic: Positive Coombs' reaction, hemolytic anemia, neutropenia

Local: Pain at injection site, thrombophlebitis, sterile abscess at injection site

Renal: Interstitial nephritis

Miscellaneous: Pseudoanaphylactic reactions, hypersensitivity reactions, Jarisch-Herxheimer reaction, serum sickness

Overdosage/Toxicology Symptoms of penicillin overdose include neuromuscular hypersensitivity (eg, agitation, hallucinations, asterixis, encephalopathy, confusion, and seizures). Electrolyte imbalance may occur if the preparation contains potassium or sodium salts, especially in renal failure. Hemodialysis may be helpful to aid in removal of the drug from blood; otherwise, treatment is supportive or symptom-directed.

Pharmacodynamics/Kinetics

Duration of Action: Therapeutic: 15-24 hours

Absorption: I.M.: Slow

Time to Peak: Serum: 1-4 hours

Protein Binding: 65%

Metabolism: ~30% hepatically inactivated

Excretion: Urine (60% to 90% as unchanged drug)

Clearance: Renal: Delayed in neonates, young infants, and renal impairment

Dosing

Adults & Elderly:

Anthrax:

Inhalational (postexposure prophylaxis): I.M.: 1,200,000 units every 12 hours

Note: Overall treatment duration should be 60 days. Available safety data suggest continued administration of penicillin G procaine for longer than 2 weeks may incur additional risk of adverse reactions. Clinicians may consider switching to effective alternative treatment for completion of therapy beyond 2 weeks.

Cutaneous (treatment): I.M.: 600,000-1,200,000 units/day; alternative therapy is recommended in severe cutaneous or other forms of anthrax infection

Uncomplicated gonorrhea: I.M.: 1 g probenecid orally, then 4.8 million units procaine penicillin divided into 2 injection sites 30 minutes later

Endocarditis caused by susceptible viridans *Streptococcus* (when used in conjunction with an aminoglycoside): I.M.: 1.2 million units every 6 hours for 2-4 weeks

Neurosyphilis: I.M.: 2-4 million units/day with 500 mg probenecid by mouth 4 times/day for 10-14 days; **penicillin G aqueous I.V. is the preferred agent**

Pediatrics:

Susceptible infections: I.M.: Infants and Children: 25,000-50,000 units/kg/day in divided doses every 12-24 hours; not to exceed 4.8 million units/24 hours

Anthrax, inhalational (postexposure prophylaxis): I.M.: 25,000 units/kg every 12 hours (maximum: 1,200,000 units every 12 hours).

Note: Overall treatment duration should be 60 days. Available safety data suggest continued administration of penicillin G procaine for longer than 2 weeks may incur additional risk for adverse reactions. Clinicians may consider switching to effective alternative treatment for completion of therapy beyond 2 weeks.

Congenital syphilis: I.M.: 50,000 units/kg/day once daily for 10 days; if more than 1 day of therapy is missed, the entire course should be restarted

Renal Impairment:

Cl_{cr} 10-30 mL/minute: Administer every 8-12 hours.

Cl_{cr} <10 mL/minute: Administer every 12-18 hours.

Moderately dialyzable (20% to 50%)

Available Dosage Forms Injection, suspension: 600,000 units/mL (1 mL, 2 mL)

Monitoring and Teaching Issues

Physical Assessment: Assess results of culture and sensitivity tests and patient's allergy history prior to starting therapy. Use with caution in presence of renal impairment or seizure disorder (see Warnings/Precautions). Assess potential for interactions with other pharmacological agents (eg, decreased or increased levels/effects of penicillin G; see Drug Interactions). For deep I.M. injection only. Assess laboratory tests, effectiveness (resolution of infection), and adverse reactions (eg, hypersensitivity reactions, opportunistic infection [fever, chills, unhealed sores, white plaques in mouth or vagina, purulent vaginal discharge, fatigue]; see Adverse Reactions).Teach patient possible side effects/appropriate interventions and adverse symptoms to report (see Patient Education).

Monitoring Laboratory Tests: Periodic renal and hematologic function with prolonged therapy; WBC count; perform culture and sensitivity before administering first dose.

Patient Education: This drug is given by injection; report immediately any redness, swelling, burning, or pain at infusion site or any signs of allergic reaction (eg, respiratory or swallowing difficulty, chest tightness, rash, hives, swelling of lips or mouth). Maintain adequate hydration (2-3 L/day of fluids) unless instructed to restrict fluid intake. May cause confusion or drowsiness (use caution when driving or engaging in tasks that require alertness until response to drug is known). Report chest pain, palpitations, or irregular heartbeat; persistent adverse effects; or signs of opportunistic infection (eg, fever, chills, unhealed sores, white plaques in mouth or vagina, purulent vaginal discharge, fatigue).

Geriatric Considerations: Dosage does not usually need to be adjusted in the elderly, however, if multiple doses are to be given, adjust dose for renal function.

Pregnancy Risk Factor: B

Lactation: Enters breast milk/compatible

Administration

    I.M.: Procaine suspension is for deep I.M. injection only. Rotate the injection site. Do not inject in gluteal muscle in children <2 years of age.

    Storage: Store in refrigerator.

♦ **Penicillin G Sodium** *see* Penicillin G (Parenteral/Aqueous) *on page 1174*

Penicillin V Potassium (pen i SIL in vee poe TASS ee um)

U.S. Brand Names Veetids®

Synonyms Pen VK; Phenoxymethyl Penicillin

Generic Available Yes

Pharmacologic Category Antibiotic, Penicillin

Medication Safety Issues

    Sound-alike/look-alike issues:

        Penicillin V procaine may be confused with penicillin G potassium

Use Treatment of infections caused by susceptible organisms involving the respiratory tract, otitis media, sinusitis, skin, and urinary tract; prophylaxis in rheumatic fever

Mechanism of Action/Effect Inhibits bacterial cell wall synthesis by binding to one or more of the penicillin binding proteins (PBPs); which in turn inhibits the final transpeptidation step of peptidoglycan synthesis in bacterial cell walls, thus inhibiting cell wall biosynthesis. Bacteria eventually lyse due to ongoing activity of cell wall autolytic enzymes (autolysins and murein hydrolases) while cell wall assembly is arrested.

Contraindications Hypersensitivity to penicillin or any component of the formulation

Warnings/Precautions Use with caution in patients with severe renal impairment (modify dosage).

Drug Interactions

    Decreased Effect: Tetracyclines may decrease penicillin effectiveness. Although anecdotal reports suggest oral contraceptive efficacy could be reduced by penicillins, this has been refuted by more rigorous scientific and clinical data.

    Increased Effect/Toxicity: Probenecid increases penicillin levels. Aminoglycosides may cause synergistic efficacy. Penicillins may increase the exposure to methotrexate during concurrent therapy; monitor.

Nutritional/Ethanol Interactions Food: Decreases drug absorption rate; decreases drug serum concentration.

Lab Interactions False-positive or negative urinary glucose determination using Clinitest®; positive Coombs' [direct]; false-positive urinary and/or serum proteins

Adverse Reactions >10%: Gastrointestinal: Mild diarrhea, vomiting, nausea, oral candidiasis

Overdosage/Toxicology Symptoms of penicillin overdose include neuromuscular hypersensitivity (eg, agitation, hallucinations, asterixis, encephalopathy, confusion, and seizures). Electrolyte imbalance may occur if the preparation contains potassium or sodium salts, especially in renal failure. Hemodialysis may be helpful to aid in removal of the drug from blood; otherwise, treatment is supportive or symptom-directed.

Pharmacodynamics/Kinetics

    Absorption: 60% to 73%

    Time to Peak: Serum: 0.5-1 hour

    Protein Binding: Plasma: 80%

    Half-Life Elimination: 30 minutes; prolonged with renal impairment

    Excretion: Urine (as unchanged drug and metabolites)

Dosing

    Adults & Elderly:

        Systemic infections: Oral: 125-500 mg every 6-8 hours

        Prophylaxis of pneumococcal infections: Oral: 250 mg twice daily

        Prophylaxis of recurrent rheumatic fever: Oral: 250 mg twice daily

    Pediatrics:

        Systemic infections: Oral:

            <12 years: 25-50 mg/kg/day in divided doses every 6-8 hours; maximum dose: 3 g/day

            ≥12 years: 125-500 mg every 6-8 hours

        Prophylaxis of pneumococcal infections: Oral:

            <5 years: 125 mg twice daily

            ≥5 years: 250 mg twice daily

        Prophylaxis of recurrent rheumatic fever: Oral:

            <5 years: 125 mg twice daily

            ≥5 years: 250 mg twice daily

(Continued)

Penicillin V Potassium *(Continued)*

Renal Impairment:
Cl$_{cr}$ 10-50 mL/minute: Administer every 8-12 hours.
Cl$_{cr}$ <10 mL/minute: Administer every 12-16 hours.

Available Dosage Forms Note: 250 mg = 400,000 units
Powder for oral solution: 125 mg/5 mL (100 mL, 200 mL); 250 mg/5 mL (100 mL, 200 mL)
Tablet: 250 mg, 500 mg

Monitoring and Teaching Issues

Physical Assessment: Assess results of culture and sensitivity tests and patient's allergy history prior to starting therapy. Use with caution in presence of renal impairment (see Warnings/Precautions). Assess potential for interactions with other pharmacological agents (eg, decreased or increased levels/effects of penicillin V; see Drug Interactions). Assess results of laboratory tests, effectiveness (resolution of infection), and adverse reactions (eg, hypersensitivity reactions, opportunistic infection [fever, chills, unhealed sores, white plaques in mouth or vagina, purulent vaginal discharge, fatigue]; see Adverse Reactions). Advise patients with diabetes about use of Clinitest®; may cause false readings. Teach patient possible side effects/appropriate interventions and adverse symptoms to report (see Patient Education).

Monitoring Laboratory Tests: Periodic renal and hematologic function during prolonged therapy; perform culture and sensitivity before administering first dose

Patient Education: Take as directed at intervals around-the-clock, preferably on an empty stomach (1 hour before or 2 hours after a meal). Take entire prescription even if symptoms have resolved; do not skip doses or discontinue without consulting prescriber. Take a missed dose as soon as possible. If almost time for next dose, skip the missed dose and return to your regular schedule. Do not take a double dose. Maintain adequate hydration (2-3 L/day of fluids) unless instructed to restrict fluid intake. If you have diabetes, drug may cause false test results with Clinitest®, consult prescriber for alternative method of glucose monitoring. May cause nausea or vomiting (small frequent meals, frequent mouth care, chewing gum, or sucking lozenges may help); or diarrhea (buttermilk, boiled milk, or yogurt may help). Report persistent adverse effects; signs of opportunistic infection (eg, fever, chills, unhealed sores, white plaques in mouth or vagina, purulent vaginal discharge, fatigue); or signs of hypersensitivity reaction (rash; hives; itching; swelling of lips tongue, mouth, or throat).

Dietary Considerations: Take on an empty stomach 1 hour before or 2 hours after meals.

Pregnancy Risk Factor: B

Lactation: Enters breast milk (other penicillins are compatible with breast-feeding)

Breast-Feeding Issues: No data reported; however, other penicillins may be taken while breast-feeding.

Administration

Oral: Administer around-the-clock to promote less variation in peak and trough serum levels. Take on an empty stomach 1 hour before or 2 hours after meals, to enhance absorption, take until gone, do not skip doses.

Storage: Refrigerate suspension after reconstitution; discard after 14 days.

Additional Information 0.7 mEq of potassium per 250 mg penicillin V; 250 mg equals 400,000 units of penicillin

Related Information
Antimicrobial Drugs of Choice *on page 1792*

♦ **Pentam-300®** *see Pentamidine on page 1178*

Pentamidine *(pen TAM i deen)*

U.S. Brand Names NebuPent®; Pentam-300®

Synonyms Pentamidine Isethionate

Generic Available No

Pharmacologic Category Antibiotic, Miscellaneous

Use Treatment and prevention of pneumonia caused by *Pneumocystis carinii* (PCP)

Unlabeled/Investigational Use Treatment of trypanosomiasis and visceral leishmaniasis

Mechanism of Action/Effect Interferes with RNA/DNA synthesis and phospholipids leading to cell death in protozoa.

Contraindications Hypersensitivity to pentamidine isethionate or any component of the formulation (inhalation and injection)

Warnings/Precautions Use with caution in patients with diabetes mellitus, renal or hepatic dysfunction, hyper-/hypotension, leukopenia, thrombocytopenia, asthma, or hypo-/hyperglycemia.

Drug Interactions

Cytochrome P450 Effect: Substrate of CYP2C19 (major); **Inhibits** CYP2C8/9 (weak), 2C19 (weak), 2D6 (weak), 3A4 (weak)

Decreased Effect: CYP2C19 inducers may decrease the levels/effects of pentamidine; example inducers include aminoglutethimide, carbamazepine, phenytoin, and rifampin.

Increased Effect/Toxicity: CYP2C19 inhibitors may increase the levels/effects of pentamidine; example inhibitors include delavirdine, fluconazole, fluvoxamine, gemfibrozil, isoniazid, omeprazole, and ticlopidine. Pentamidine may potentiate the effect of other drugs which prolong QT interval (cisapride, sparfloxacin, gatifloxacin, moxifloxacin, pimozide, and type Ia and type III antiarrhythmics).

Nutritional/Ethanol Interactions Ethanol: Avoid ethanol (may increase CNS depression or aggravate hypoglycemia).

Adverse Reactions Injection (I); Aerosol (A)

>10%:
Cardiovascular: Chest pain (A - 10% to 23%)
Central nervous system: Fatigue (A - 50% to 70%); dizziness (A - 31% to 47%)
Dermatologic: Rash (31% to 47%)
Endocrine & metabolic: Hyperkalemia

Gastrointestinal: Anorexia (A - 50% to 70%), nausea (A - 10% to 23%)
Local: Local reactions at injection site
Renal: Increased creatinine (I - 23%)
Respiratory: Wheezing (A - 10% to 23%), dyspnea (A - 50% to 70%), cough (A - 31% to 47%), pharyngitis (10% to 23%)
1% to 10%:
Cardiovascular: Hypotension (I - 4%)
Central nervous system: Confusion/hallucinations (1% to 2%), headache (A - 1% to 5%)
Dermatologic: Rash (I - 3.3%)
Endocrine & metabolic: Hypoglycemia <25 mg/dL (I - 2.4%)
Gastrointestinal: Nausea/anorexia (I - 6%), diarrhea (A - 1% to 5%), vomiting
Hematologic: Severe leukopenia (I - 2.8%), thrombocytopenia <20,000/mm^3 (I - 1.7%), anemia (A - 1% to 5%)
Hepatic: Increased LFTs (I - 8.7%)

Overdosage/Toxicology Symptoms of overdose include hypotension, hypoglycemia, and cardiac arrhythmias. Treatment is supportive.

Pharmacodynamics/Kinetics
Absorption: I.M.: Well absorbed; Inhalation: Limited systemic absorption
Half-Life Elimination: Terminal: 6.4-9.4 hours; may be prolonged with severe renal impairment
Excretion: Urine (33% to 66% as unchanged drug)

Dosing
Adults & Elderly:
Treatment of PCP pneumonia: I.M., I.V. (I.V. preferred): 4 mg/kg/day once daily for 14 days
Prevention of PCP pneumonia: Inhalation: 300 mg every 4 weeks via Respirgard® II nebulizer
Pediatrics:
Treatment of PCP pneumonia: I.M., I.V. (I.V. preferred): Children: 4 mg/kg/day once daily for 10-14 days
Prevention of PCP pneumonia: Children:
I.M., I.V.: 4 mg/kg monthly or every 2 weeks
Inhalation (aerosolized pentamidine in children ≥5 years): 300 mg/dose given every 3-4 weeks via Respirgard® II inhaler (8 mg/kg dose has also been used in children <5 years)
Treatment of trypanosomiasis (unlabeled use): I.V.: 4 mg/kg/day once daily for 10 days
Renal Impairment:
Cl$_{cr}$ 10-50 mL/minute: Administer dose every 24-36 hours.
Cl$_{cr}$ <10 mL/minute: Administer dose every 48 hours.
Not removed by hemo- or peritoneal dialysis or continuous arteriovenous or venovenous hemofiltration. Supplemental dose is not necessary.

Available Dosage Forms
Injection, powder for reconstitution, as isethionate (Pentam-300®): 300 mg
Powder for nebulization, as isethionate (NebuPent®): 300 mg

Monitoring and Teaching Issues
Physical Assessment: Use with caution in presence of diabetes mellitus, renal or hepatic dysfunction, hyper- and hypotension, leukopenia, thrombocytopenia, asthma, or hypo- and hyperglycemia (see Warnings/Precautions). Assess potential for interactions with other pharmacological agents patient may be taking (eg, may increase or decrease levels/effects of pentamidine; see Drug Interactions). **I.V., I.M.:** Patients should be lying down. Blood pressure, cardiac status, and respiratory function should be monitored closely during I.V. administration or following I.M. injection. Assess results of laboratory tests, therapeutic response, and adverse reactions (eg, chest pain, hypotension, rash, confusion, hallucinations, hypoglycemia, dyspnea, cough; see Adverse Reactions). Teach patient proper use, possible side effects/appropriate interventions, and adverse symptoms to report (see Patient Education).
Monitoring Laboratory Tests: Liver and renal function, blood glucose, serum potassium and calcium, ECG, CBC with platelets
Patient Education: Do not take any new medication during therapy without consulting prescriber. I.V. or I.M. preparations must be given every day. Inhalant drug must be prepared and used with a nebulizer as directed once every 4 weeks. Frequent blood tests and blood pressure checks will be required while using this drug. PCP pneumonia may still occur despite pentamidine use. Maintain adequate hydration (2-3 L/day of fluids) unless instructed to restrict fluid intake. Avoid alcohol; may increase adverse symptoms. If diabetic, monitor glucose levels closely and frequently. May cause hypotension (use caution when rising from sitting or lying position or when climbing stairs); May cause metallic taste, nausea, vomiting, or anorexia (small frequent meals, frequent mouth care, chewing gum, or sucking lozenges may help). Report chest pain or irregular heartbeat; unusual confusion or hallucinations; rash; or unusual wheezing, coughing, or respiratory difficulty. **Pregnancy/breast-feeding precautions:** Inform prescriber if you are or intend to become pregnant. Do not breast-feed.
Geriatric Considerations: Ten percent of acquired immunodeficiency syndrome (AIDS) cases are in the elderly and this figure is expected to increase. Pentamidine has not as yet been studied exclusively in this population. Adjust dose for renal function.
Pregnancy Risk Factor: C
Lactation: Excretion in breast milk unknown/contraindicated

Administration
I.M.: Deep I.M.
I.V.: Do not use NS as a diluent. Infuse I.V. slowly over a period of at least 60 minutes or administer deep I.M.
Inhalation: Virtually undetectable amounts are transferred to healthcare personnel during aerosol administration.
(Continued)

Pentamidine *(Continued)*

Reconstitution: Powder for inhalation should be reconstituted with sterile water for injection. Powder for injection may be reconstituted with sterile water for injection or D_5W. **Do not use NS as a diluent.** Precipitation may occur if products are reconstituted with NS.

Compatibility: Solutions for injection (1-2.5 mg/mL) in D_5W are stable for at least 24 hours at room temperature. The manufacturer's labeling recommends D_5W, however, stability in NS has also been documented.

Y-site administration: Incompatible: Aldesleukin, cefazolin, cefoperazone, cefotaxime, cefoxitin, ceftazidime, ceftriaxone, fluconazole, foscarnet, linezolid

Storage: Store intact vials at controlled room temperature and protect from light. Do not refrigerate due to the possibility of crystallization. Reconstituted solutions (60-100 mg/mL) are stable for 48 hours at room temperature and do not require light protection. Diluted solutions for injection (1-2.5 mg/mL) in D_5W are stable for at least 24 hours at room temperature. The manufacturer recommends D_5W, however, stability in NS has also been documented; in addition, light protection is recommended by the manufacturer, but stability has been documented without protection from light.

Additional Information Virtually undetectable amounts are transferred to healthcare personnel during aerosol administration.

- ◆ **Pentamidine Isethionate** *see* Pentamidine *on page 1178*
- ◆ **Pentasa®** *see* Mesalamine *on page 957*

Pentazocine *(pen TAZ oh seen)*

U.S. Brand Names Talwin®; Talwin® NX

Synonyms Naloxone Hydrochloride and Pentazocine Hydrochloride; Pentazocine Hydrochloride; Pentazocine Hydrochloride and Naloxone Hydrochloride; Pentazocine Lactate

Controlled Substance C-IV

Generic Available Yes: Tablet

Pharmacologic Category Analgesic, Narcotic

Use Relief of moderate to severe pain; has also been used as a sedative prior to surgery and as a supplement to surgical anesthesia

Mechanism of Action/Effect Binds to opiate receptors in the CNS, causing inhibition of ascending pain pathways, altering the perception of and response to pain; produces generalized CNS depression; partial agonist-antagonist

Contraindications Hypersensitivity to pentazocine, naloxone, or any component of the formulation; increased intracranial pressure (unless the patient is mechanically ventilated); pregnancy (prolonged use or high doses at term)

Warnings/Precautions Use with caution in seizure-prone patients, acute myocardial infarction, patients undergoing biliary tract surgery, patients with renal and hepatic dysfunction, head trauma, increased intracranial pressure, and patients with a history of prior opioid dependence or abuse; pentazocine may precipitate opiate withdrawal symptoms in patients who have been receiving opiates regularly; injection contains sulfites which may cause allergic reaction; tolerance or drug dependence may result from extended use. Severe vascular complications have resulted from misuse (injection) of Talwin® tablet formulations.

Drug Interactions

Decreased Effect: May potentiate or reduce analgesic effect of opiate agonist (eg, morphine) depending on patients tolerance to opiates; can precipitate withdrawal in narcotic addicts.

Increased Effect/Toxicity: Increased effect/toxicity with tripelennamine (can be lethal), CNS depressants (eg, phenothiazines, tranquilizers, anxiolytics, sedatives, hypnotics, alcohol).

Nutritional/Ethanol Interactions Ethanol: Avoid ethanol (may increase CNS depression).

Adverse Reactions Frequency not defined.

Cardiovascular: Hypotension, circulatory depression, shock, tachycardia, syncope, flushing

Central nervous system: Malaise, headache, nightmares, insomnia, CNS depression, sedation, hallucinations, confusion, disorientation, dizziness, euphoria, drowsiness, lightheadedness, irritability, chills, excitement

Dermatologic: Rash, pruritus, dermatitis, urticaria, Stevens-Johnson syndrome, toxic epidermal necrolysis, erythema multiforme

Gastrointestinal: Nausea, vomiting, xerostomia, constipation, anorexia, diarrhea, abdominal distress

Genitourinary: Urinary retention

Hematologic: WBCs decreased, eosinophilia

Local: Tissue damage and irritation with I.M./SubQ use

Neuromuscular & skeletal: Weakness, tremor, paresthesia

Ocular: Blurred vision, miosis

Otic: Tinnitus

Respiratory: Dyspnea, respiratory depression (rare)

Miscellaneous: Physical and psychological dependence, facial edema, diaphoresis, anaphylaxis

Overdosage/Toxicology Symptoms of overdose include drowsiness, sedation, respiratory depression, and coma. Naloxone, 2 mg I.V., with repeat administration as necessary up to a total of 10 mg, can also be used to reverse toxic effects of the opiate.

Pharmacodynamics/Kinetics

Onset of Action: Oral, I.M., SubQ: 15-30 minutes; I.V.: 2-3 minutes

Duration of Action: Oral: 4-5 hours; Parenteral: 2-3 hours

Bioavailability: Oral: ~20%; increased to 60% to 70% with cirrhosis

Protein Binding: 60%

Half-Life Elimination: 2-3 hours; prolonged with hepatic impairment

Metabolism: Hepatic via oxidative and glucuronide conjugation pathways; extensive first-pass effect

Excretion: Urine (small amounts as unchanged drug)

Dosing

Adults: Analgesic:

Oral: 50 mg every 3-4 hours; may increase to 100 mg/dose if needed, but should not exceed 600 mg/day

I.M., SubQ: 30-60 mg every 3-4 hours; do **not** exceed 30 mg/dose (maximum: 360 mg/day)

I.V.: 30 mg every 3-4 hours; do **not** exceed 30 mg/dose (maximum: 360 mg/day)

Elderly: See Geriatric Considerations. Initial dose:

Oral: 50 mg every 4 hours

I.M.: 30 mg every 4 hours

Pediatrics:

Analgesia:

I.M.: Children:

5-8 years: 15 mg

8-14 years: 30 mg

Oral: Children >12 years: Refer to adult dosing.

Preoperative/preanesthetic: Children 1-16 years: 0.5 mg/kg

Renal Impairment:

Cl_{cr} 10-50 mL/minute: Administer 75% of normal dose.

Cl_{cr} <10 mL/minute: Administer 50% of normal dose.

Hepatic Impairment: Reduce dose or avoid use in patients with liver disease.

Available Dosage Forms

Injection, solution (Talwin®): 30 mg/mL (1 mL, 10 mL) [10 mL size contains sodium bisulfite]

Tablet (Talwin® NX): Pentazocine 50 mg and naloxone 0.5 mg

Monitoring and Teaching Issues

Physical Assessment: Assess other medications patient may be taking for additive or adverse interactions. Monitor therapeutic effectiveness, adverse reactions, and overdose at beginning of therapy and at regular intervals with long-term use. May cause physical and/or psychological dependence. For inpatients, implement safety measures. Assess knowledge/teach patient appropriate use (if self-administered), adverse reactions to report and appropriate interventions to reduce side effects.

Patient Education: If self-administered, use exactly as directed; do not increase dose or frequency. Drug may cause physical and/or psychological dependence. While using this medication, do not use alcohol and other prescription or OTC medications (especially sedatives, tranquilizers, antihistamines, or pain medications) without consulting prescriber. Maintain adequate hydration (2-3 L/day of fluids) unless instructed to restrict fluid intake. May cause hypotension, dizziness, drowsiness, impaired coordination, or blurred vision (use caution when driving, climbing stairs, or changing position - rising from sitting or lying to standing, or when engaging in tasks requiring alertness until response to drug is known); nausea, vomiting, loss of appetite, or dry mouth (frequent mouth care, small frequent meals, chewing gum, or sucking lozenges may help); or constipation (increased exercise, fluids, fruit, or fiber may help; if unresolved, consult prescriber about use of stool softeners). Report persistent dizziness or headache; excessive fatigue or sedation; changes in mental status; changes in urinary elimination or pain on urination; weakness or trembling; blurred vision; or shortness of breath. **Pregnancy/breast-feeding precautions:** Inform prescriber if you are or intend to become pregnant. Consult prescriber if breast-feeding.

Geriatric Considerations: Pentazocine is not recommended for use in the elderly because of its propensity to cause delirium and agitation. If pentazocine must be used, be sure to adjust dose for renal function.

Pregnancy Risk Factor: C/D (prolonged use or high doses at term)

Pregnancy Issues: Pentazocine was not found to be teratogenic in animal studies. Pentazocine and naloxone have been shown to cross the human placenta. Use should be avoided during labor and delivery of premature infants. Abstinence syndromes in the newborn have been reported after long-term use of pentazocine during pregnancy. Other adverse effects in the newborn have been reported following abuse of pentazocine during pregnancy; these effects may be due to pentazocine, other drugs abused, the mother's lifestyle, or a combination of all factors.

Lactation: Excretion in breast milk unknown/use caution

Breast-Feeding Issues: Excretion of pentazocine in breast milk is unknown; no data available for naloxone

Administration

I.M.: Rotate injection site; avoid intra-arterial injection

Other: Rotate injection site for SubQ use; avoid SubQ use unless absolutely necessary (may cause tissue damage); avoid intra-arterial injection

Compatibility:

Y-site administration: Incompatible with nafcillin

Compatibility in syringe: Incompatible with glycopyrrolate, heparin, pentobarbital

Compatibility when admixed: Incompatible with aminophylline, amobarbital, pentobarbital, phenobarbital, sodium bicarbonate

Storage: Injection: Store at room temperature, protect from heat and from freezing.

Additional Information Pentazocine hydrochloride: Talwin® NX tablet (with naloxone); naloxone is used to prevent abuse by dissolving tablets in water and using as injection.

Related Information

Compatibility of Drugs in Syringe *on page 1725*
Narcotic / Opioid Analgesic Comparison *on page 1739*

Pentazocine and Acetaminophen (pen TAZ oh seen & a seet a MIN oh fen)

U.S. Brand Names Talacen®

Synonyms Acetaminophen and Pentazocine; Pentazocine Hydrochloride and Acetaminophen

Controlled Substance C-IV

Generic Available Yes

Pharmacologic Category Analgesic Combination (Narcotic)

(Continued)

Pentazocine and Acetaminophen *(Continued)*

Medication Safety Issues
Sound-alike/look-alike issues:
Talacen® may be confused with Tegison®, Timoptic®, Tinactin®

Use Relief of mild to moderate pain

Dosing
Adults & Elderly: Analgesic: Oral: 1 caplet every 4 hours up to maximum of 6 caplets

Available Dosage Forms Caplet (Talacen®): Pentazocine 25 mg and acetaminophen 650 mg [contains sodium metabisulfite]

Monitoring and Teaching Issues
Physical Assessment: Assess patient for history of liver disease or ethanol abuse (acetaminophen and excessive ethanol may have adverse liver effects). Assess other medications patient may be taking for additive or adverse interactions (see Drug Interactions). Monitor therapeutic effectiveness, adverse reactions (see Adverse Reactions), and signs of overdose at beginning of therapy and at regular intervals with long-term use. May cause physical and/or psychological dependence. For inpatients, implement safety measures. Assess knowledge/teach patient appropriate use (if self-administered), adverse reactions to report, and appropriate interventions to reduce side effects (see Patient Education).

Patient Education: If self-administered, use exactly as directed; do not increase dose or frequency. Drug may cause physical and/or psychological dependence. Take with food or milk. While using this medication, do not use alcohol and other prescription or OTC medications (especially sedatives, tranquilizers, antihistamines, or pain medications) without consulting prescriber. Maintain adequate hydration (2-3 L/day of fluids) unless instructed to restrict fluid intake. May cause hypotension, dizziness, drowsiness, confusion, or nervousness (use caution when driving, climbing stairs, or changing position - rising from sitting or lying to standing, or when engaging in tasks requiring alertness until response to drug is known); nausea, dry mouth, decreased appetite, or gastric distress (frequent mouth care, frequent sips of fluids, chewing gum, or sucking lozenges may help); or constipation (increased exercise, fluids, fruit, or fiber may help; if unresolved, consult prescriber about use of stool softeners). Report chest pain, rapid heartbeat, or palpitations; persistent dizziness; change in mental status; shortness of breath or respiratory difficulty; unusual bleeding (stool, mouth, urine) or bruising; unusual fatigue and weakness; pain on urination; change in elimination patterns or change in color of urine or stool; or unresolved nausea or vomiting. **Pregnancy/breast-feeding precautions:** Inform prescriber if you are or intend to become pregnant. Consult prescriber if breast-feeding.

Pregnancy Risk Factor: C/D (prolonged use or high doses at term)

Lactation: Excretion in breast milk unknown/use caution

Related Information
Acetaminophen *on page 38*
Pentazocine *on page 1180*

♦ **Pentazocine Hydrochloride** *see* Pentazocine *on page 1180*
♦ **Pentazocine Hydrochloride and Acetaminophen** *see* Pentazocine and Acetaminophen *on page 1181*
♦ **Pentazocine Hydrochloride and Naloxone Hydrochloride** *see* Pentazocine *on page 1180*
♦ **Pentazocine Lactate** *see* Pentazocine *on page 1180*

Pentobarbital *(pen toe BAR bi tal)*
U.S. Brand Names Nembutal®
Synonyms Pentobarbital Sodium
Controlled Substance C-II
Generic Available No
Pharmacologic Category Anticonvulsant, Barbiturate; Barbiturate
Medication Safety Issues
Sound-alike/look-alike issues:
Pentobarbital may be confused with phenobarbital
Nembutal® may be confused with Myambutol®

Use Sedative/hypnotic; preanesthetic; high-dose barbiturate coma for treatment of increased intracranial pressure or status epilepticus unresponsive to other therapy

Mechanism of Action/Effect Short-acting barbiturate with sedative, hypnotic, and anticonvulsant properties. Barbiturates depress the sensory cortex, decrease motor activity, alter cerebellar function, and produce drowsiness, sedation, and hypnosis. In high doses, barbiturates exhibit anticonvulsant activity; barbiturates produce dose-dependent respiratory depression.

Contraindications Hypersensitivity to barbiturates or any component of the formulation; marked hepatic impairment; dyspnea or airway obstruction; porphyria; pregnancy

Warnings/Precautions Tolerance to hypnotic effect can occur; do not use for >2 weeks to treat insomnia. Potential for drug dependency exists, abrupt cessation may precipitate withdrawal, including status epilepticus in epileptic patients. Do not administer to patients in acute pain. Use caution in elderly, debilitated, renally impaired, hepatic dysfunction, or pediatric patients. May cause paradoxical responses, including agitation and hyperactivity, particularly in acute pain and pediatric patients. Use with caution in patients with depression or suicidal tendencies, or in patients with a history of drug abuse. Tolerance, psychological and physical dependence may occur with prolonged use.

May cause CNS depression, which may impair physical or mental abilities. Patients must be cautioned about performing tasks which require mental alertness (eg, operating machinery or driving). Effects with other sedative drugs or ethanol may be potentiated. Use of this agent as a hypnotic in the elderly is not recommended due to its long half-life and potential for physical and psychological dependence.

May cause respiratory depression or hypotension, particularly when administered intravenously. Use with caution in hemodynamically unstable patients or patients with respiratory disease. High doses (loading doses of 15-35 mg/kg given over 1-2 hours) have been utilized to induce pentobarbital coma, but these higher doses often cause hypotension requiring vasopressor therapy.

Drug Interactions

Cytochrome P450 Effect: Induces CYP2A6 (strong), 3A4 (strong)

Decreased Effect: Pentobarbital may decrease the levels/effects of benzodiazepines, calcium channel blockers, clarithromycin, cyclosporine, erythromycin, ifosfamide, mirtazapine, nateglinide, nefazodone, nevirapine, protease inhibitors, rifampin, tacrolimus, venlafaxine, and other CYP2A6 or 3A4 substrates. Barbiturates may increase the metabolism of estrogens and reduce the efficacy of oral contraceptives; an alternative method of contraception should be considered. Barbiturates inhibit the hypoprothrombinemic effects of oral anticoagulants via increased metabolism. Barbiturates may enhance the metabolism of methadone resulting in methadone withdrawal.

Increased Effect/Toxicity: When combined with other CNS depressants, ethanol, narcotic analgesics, antidepressants, or benzodiazepines, additive respiratory and CNS depression may occur. Barbiturates may enhance the hepatotoxic potential of acetaminophen overdoses. Chloramphenicol, MAO inhibitors, valproic acid, and felbamate may inhibit barbiturate metabolism. Barbiturates may impair the absorption of griseofulvin, and may enhance the nephrotoxic effects of methoxyflurane.

Nutritional/Ethanol Interactions Ethanol: Avoid ethanol (may increase CNS depression).

Lab Interactions Increased ammonia (B); decreased bilirubin (S)

Adverse Reactions Frequency not defined.

Cardiovascular: Bradycardia, hypotension, syncope

Central nervous system: Drowsiness, lethargy, CNS excitation or depression, impaired judgment, "hangover" effect, confusion, somnolence, agitation, hyperkinesia, ataxia, nervousness, headache, insomnia, nightmares, hallucinations, anxiety, dizziness

Dermatologic: Rash, exfoliative dermatitis, Stevens-Johnson syndrome

Gastrointestinal: Nausea, vomiting, constipation

Hematologic: Agranulocytosis, thrombocytopenia, megaloblastic anemia

Local: Pain at injection site, thrombophlebitis with I.V. use

Renal: Oliguria

Respiratory: Laryngospasm, respiratory depression, apnea (especially with rapid I.V. use), hypoventilation, apnea

Miscellaneous: Gangrene with inadvertent intra-arterial injection

Overdosage/Toxicology Symptoms of overdose include unsteady gait, slurred speech, confusion, jaundice, hypothermia, hypotension, respiratory depression, and coma. Treat symptomatically. Charcoal hemoperfusion may be beneficial in stage IV coma due to high serum concentration.

Pharmacodynamics/Kinetics

Onset of Action: I.M.: 10-15 minutes; I.V.: ~1 minute

Duration of Action: I.V.: 15 minutes

Protein Binding: 35% to 55%

Half-Life Elimination: Terminal: Children: 25 hours; Adults, healthy: 22 hours (range: 15-50 hours)

Metabolism: Extensively hepatic via hydroxylation and oxidation pathways

Excretion: Urine (<1% as unchanged drug)

Dosing

Adults:

Hypnotic:

I.M.: 150-200 mg

I.V.: Initial: 100 mg, may repeat every 1-3 minutes up to 200-500 mg total dose

Preoperative sedation: I.M.: 150-200 mg

Barbiturate coma in head injury patients or status epilepticus: I.V.: Loading dose: 5-10 mg/kg given slowly over 1-2 hours; monitor blood pressure and respiratory rate; maintenance infusion: initial: 1 mg/kg/hour; may increase to 2-3 mg/kg/hour; maintain burst suppression on EEG

Status epilepticus: I.V.: Loading dose: 2-15 mg/kg given slowly over 1-2 hours; maintenance infusion: 0.5-3 mg/kg/hour. **Note:** Intubation required; monitor hemodynamics

Elderly: Not recommended for use in the elderly (see Geriatric Considerations).

Pediatrics:

Hypnotic: I.M.: 2-6 mg/kg; maximum: 100 mg/dose

Preoperative/preprocedure sedation: ≥6 months:

Note: Limited information is available for infants <6 months of age.

I.M.: 2-6 mg/kg; maximum: 100 mg/dose

I.V.: 1-3 mg/kg to a maximum of 100 mg until asleep

Conscious sedation prior to a procedure: I.V.:

Children 5-12 years: I.V.: 2 mg/kg 5-10 minutes before procedures, may repeat one time

Adolescents: 100 mg prior to a procedure

Barbiturate coma in head injury patients: I.V.: Loading dose: 5-10 mg/kg given slowly over 1-2 hours; monitor blood pressure and respiratory rate; Maintenance infusion: Initial: 1 mg/kg/hour; may increase to 2-3 mg/kg/hour; maintain burst suppression on EEG

Status epilepticus: I.V.: **Note:** Intubation required; monitor hemodynamics: Loading dose: 5-15 mg/kg given slowly over 1-2 hours; maintenance infusion: 0.5-5 mg/kg/hour

Hepatic Impairment: Reduce dosage in patients with severe liver dysfunction.

Available Dosage Forms Injection, solution, as sodium: 50 mg/mL (20 mL, 50 mL) [contains alcohol 10% and propylene glycol 40%]

Monitoring and Teaching Issues

Physical Assessment: Assess effectiveness and interactions of other medications patient may be taking. Assess for history of addiction; long-term use can result in dependence, abuse, or tolerance. Periodically evaluate the need for continued use. **I.V.:** Keep patient under observation. Monitor cardio/respiratory status and institute patient safety precautions. Monitor effectiveness of therapy and adverse reactions.

(Continued)

Pentobarbital *(Continued)*

Patient Education: Patient instructions and information are determined by patient condition and therapeutic purpose. Drug may cause physical and/or psychological dependence. While using this medication, do not use alcohol and other prescription or OTC medications (especially pain medications, sedatives, antihistamines, or hypnotics) without consulting prescriber. Maintain adequate hydration (2-3 L/day of fluids) unless instructed to restrict fluid intake. You may experience drowsiness, dizziness, or blurred vision (use caution when driving or engaging in tasks requiring alertness until response to drug is known); nausea, vomiting, or loss of appetite (small frequent meals, frequent mouth care, chewing gum, or sucking lozenges may help); or constipation (increased exercise, fluids, fruit, or fiber may help). Report skin rash or irritation; CNS changes (confusion, depression, increased sedation, excitation, headache, insomnia, or nightmares); respiratory difficulty or shortness of breath; changes in urinary pattern or menstrual pattern; muscle weakness or tremors; or difficulty swallowing or feeling of tightness in throat. **Pregnancy/breast-feeding precautions:** Do not get pregnant; use appropriate contraceptive measures to prevent possible harm to the fetus. Do not breast-feed.

Geriatric Considerations: Use of this agent as a hypnotic in the elderly is not recommended due to its long half-life and addiction potential.

Pregnancy Risk Factor: D

Lactation: Enters breast milk/contraindicated

Administration

I.M.: Pentobarbital may be administered by deep I.M.: No more than 5 mL (250 mg) should be injected at any one site because of possible tissue irritation.

I.V.: Pentobarbital must be administered by slow I.V. injection. I.V. push doses can be given undiluted, but should be administered no faster than 50 mg/minute. Avoid intra-arterial injection. Has many incompatibilities when given I.V.

Compatibility: Stable in dextran 6% in dextrose, dextran 6% in NS, D_5LR, $D_5\frac{1}{4}NS$, $D_5\frac{1}{2}NS$, D_5NS, $D_{10}W$, LR, $\frac{1}{2}NS$

Y-site administration: Incompatible with amphotericin B cholesteryl sulfate complex

Compatibility in syringe: Incompatible with atropine with cimetidine, butorphanol, chlorpromazine, cimetidine, dimenhydrinate, diphenhydramine, droperidol, fentanyl, glycopyrrolate, hydroxyzine, meperidine, midazolam, nalbuphine, pentazocine, perphenazine, prochlorperazine edisylate, promazine, promethazine, ranitidine

Compatibility when admixed: Incompatible with cefazolin, chlorpheniramine, cimetidine, clindamycin, droperidol, ephedrine, fentanyl, hydrocortisone sodium succinate, hydroxyzine, insulin (regular), levorphanol, norepinephrine, pancuronium, penicillin G potassium, pentazocine, phenytoin, promazine, promethazine, streptomycin, triflupromazine, vancomycin

Storage: Protect from freezing. Aqueous solutions are not stable; a commercially available vehicle (containing propylene glycol) is more stable. When mixed with an acidic solution, precipitate may form. Use only clear solution.

Related Information

Anxiolytic / Hypnotic Use in Long-Term Care Facilities *on page 1769*
Compatibility of Drugs *on page 1723*
Compatibility of Drugs in Syringe *on page 1725*
Federal OBRA Regulations: Recommended Maximum Doses *on page 1773*

♦ **Pentobarbital Sodium** *see* Pentobarbital *on page 1182*

Pentostatin *(PEN toe stat in)*

U.S. Brand Names Nipent®

Synonyms CL-825; Co-Vidarabine; dCF; Deoxycoformycin; 2'-Deoxycoformycin; NSC-218321

Generic Available No

Pharmacologic Category Antineoplastic Agent, Antibiotic; Antineoplastic Agent, Antimetabolite

Medication Safety Issues

Sound-alike/look-alike issues:
Pentostatin may be confused with pentosan

Use Treatment of hairy cell leukemia; non-Hodgkin's lymphoma, cutaneous T-cell lymphoma

Mechanism of Action/Effect Results in cell death, probably through inhibiting DNA or RNA synthesis. Following a single dose, pentostatin has the ability to inhibit ADA for periods exceeding 1 week.

Contraindications Hypersensitivity to pentostatin or any component; pregnancy

Warnings/Precautions The FDA currently recommends that procedures for proper handling and disposal of antineoplastic agents be considered. Use extreme caution in the presence of renal insufficiency. Use with caution in patients with signs or symptoms of impaired hepatic function.

Preparation of pentostatin should be performed in a Class II laminar flow biologic safety cabinet. Appropriate safety equipment is recommended for preparation, administration, and disposal of antineoplastics. If pentostatin contacts the skin, wash and flush thoroughly with water.

Drug Interactions

Increased Effect/Toxicity: Increased toxicity with vidarabine and allopurinol; combined use with fludarabine may lead to severe, even fatal, pulmonary toxicity

Adverse Reactions

>10%:

Central nervous system: Fever, chills, headache
Dermatologic: Skin rash (25% to 30%), alopecia (10%)
Gastrointestinal: Mild to moderate nausea, vomiting (60%), stomatitis, diarrhea (13%), anorexia
Genitourinary: Acute renal failure (35%)

Hematologic: Thrombocytopenia (50%), dose-limiting in 25% of patients; anemia (40% to 45%), neutropenia, mild to moderate, not dose-limiting (11%)
Nadir: 7 days
Recovery: 10-14 days
Hepatic: Transaminases increased, mild-moderate, usually transient (30%); hepatitis (19%), usually reversible
Respiratory: Pulmonary edema (15%), may be exacerbated by fludarabine
Miscellaneous: Infection (57%; 35% severe, life-threatening)
1% to 10%:
Cardiovascular: Chest pain, arrhythmia, peripheral edema
Central nervous system: Opportunistic infection (8%); anxiety, confusion, depression, dizziness, insomnia, nervousness, somnolence, myalgia, malaise
Dermatologic: Dry skin, eczema, pruritus
Gastrointestinal: Constipation, flatulence, weight loss
Neuromuscular & skeletal: Paresthesia, weakness
Ocular: Moderate to severe keratoconjunctivitis, abnormal vision, eye pain
Otic: Ear pain
Respiratory: Dyspnea, pneumonia, bronchitis, pharyngitis, rhinitis, epistaxis, sinusitis (3% to 7%)

Overdosage/Toxicology Symptoms of overdose include severe renal, hepatic, pulmonary, and CNS toxicity. Treatment is supportive.

Pharmacodynamics/Kinetics
Half-Life Elimination: Distribution half-life: 30-85 minutes; Terminal: 5-15 hours
Excretion: Urine (~50% to 96%) within 24 hours (30% to 90% as unchanged drug)

Dosing
Adults & Elderly: Refer to individual protocols.
Refractory hairy cell leukemia:
4 mg/m^2 every other week **or**
4 mg/m^2 weekly for 3 weeks, then every 2 weeks **or**
5 mg/m^2 daily for 3 days every 3 weeks
Renal Impairment:
Cl$_{cr}$ <60 mL/minute: Use extreme caution.
Cl$_{cr}$ 50-60 mL/minute: Administer 2 mg/m^2/dose.
Hepatic Impairment:
Bilirubin 1.5-3 mg/dL or AST 60-180 units/L: Administer 75% of normal dose.
Bilirubin 3-5 mg/dL or AST >180 units/L: Administer 50% of normal dose.
Bilirubin >5 mg/dL: Do not administer.

Available Dosage Forms Injection, powder for reconstitution: 10 mg

Monitoring and Teaching Issues
Physical Assessment: Assess potential for adverse interactions with other pharmacological agents patient is taking (see Drug Interactions). See Administration for infusion specifics. Assess results of laboratory tests prior to and regularly during therapy. Monitor patient response closely (eg, nutritional status, renal function, myelosuppression [anemia], pulmonary edema, opportunistic infection; see Adverse Reactions). Teach patient possible side effects/appropriate interventions and adverse symptoms to report (see Patient Education).
Monitoring Laboratory Tests: CBC with differential, platelet count, liver function, serum uric acid, renal function
Patient Education: Do not take any new medications during therapy unless approved by prescriber. This drug can only be given by infusion on a specific schedule. Report immediately any redness, swelling, burning, or pain at infusion site; or signs of hypersensitivity (eg, respiratory or swallowing difficulty, chest tightness, rash, hives, swelling of lips or mouth). Maintain adequate hydration (2-3 L/day of fluids) unless instructed to restrict fluid intake. You may be more susceptible to infection (avoid crowds and exposure to infection and do not have any vaccinations without consulting prescriber). May cause nausea and vomiting, or loss of appetite (small frequent meals or frequent mouth care may help, or request medication from prescriber); headache (consult prescriber for approved analgesic); dizziness, confusion or lethargy (use caution when driving); or mouth sores (use frequent oral care with soft toothbrush or cotton swabs). Report signs of infection (eg, fever, chills, sore throat, mouth sores, burning urination, perianal itching, or vaginal discharge); unusual bruising or bleeding (eg, tarry stools, blood in urine, stool, or vomitus); vision changes or hearing; muscle tremors, weakness, or pain; CNS changes (eg, hallucinations, confusion, insomnia, seizures); or respiratory difficulty. **Pregnancy/breast-feeding precautions:** Do not get pregnant while taking this medication. Consult prescriber for appropriate contraceptive measures. Do not breast-feed.
Pregnancy Risk Factor: D
Lactation: Excretion in breast milk unknown/contraindicated

Administration
I.V.: Administer I.V. as a 15- to 30-minute infusion; continuous infusion regimens have been reported, but are not commonly used
I.V. bolus over ≥3-5 minutes in D$_5$W or NS at concentrations ≥2 mg/mL
Reconstitution: Reconstitute with SWFI to a concentration of 2 mg/mL. The injection may be further diluted with 25-50 mL NS or D$_5$W for infusion.
Compatibility: Stable in LR, NS
Storage: Vials are stable under refrigeration at 2°C to 8°C; reconstituted vials, or further dilutions, may be stored at room temperature exposed to ambient light; diluted solutions are stable for 24 hours in D$_5$W or 48 hours in NS or lactated Ringer's at room temperature; infusion with 5% dextrose injection USP or 0.9% sodium chloride injection USP does not interact with PVC-containing administration sets or containers

Pentoxifylline (pen toks I fi leen)
U.S. Brand Names Pentoxil®; Trental®
Synonyms Oxpentifylline
(Continued)

Pentoxifylline *(Continued)*

Generic Available Yes

Pharmacologic Category Blood Viscosity Reducer Agent

Medication Safety Issues

Sound-alike/look-alike issues:

Pentoxifylline may be confused with tamoxifen

Trental® may be confused with Bentyl®, Tegretol®, Trandate®

Use Treatment of intermittent claudication on the basis of chronic occlusive arterial disease of the limbs; may improve function and symptoms, but not intended to replace more definitive therapy

Unlabeled/Investigational Use AIDS patients with increased TNF, CVA, cerebrovascular diseases, diabetic atherosclerosis, diabetic neuropathy, gangrene, hemodialysis shunt thrombosis, vascular impotence, cerebral malaria, septic shock, sickle cell syndromes, and vasculitis

Mechanism of Action/Effect Mechanism of action remains unclear; is thought to reduce blood viscosity and improve blood flow by altering the rheology of red blood cells

Contraindications Hypersensitivity to pentoxifylline, xanthines, or any component of the formulation; recent cerebral and/or retinal hemorrhage

Warnings/Precautions Use with caution in patients with renal impairment or chronic occlusive arterial disease of the limbs.

Drug Interactions

Cytochrome P450 Effect: Inhibits CYP1A2 (weak)

Decreased Effect: Blood pressure changes (decreases) have been observed with the addition of pentoxifylline therapy in patients receiving antihypertensives.

Increased Effect/Toxicity: Pentoxifylline levels may be increased with cimetidine and other H_2 antagonists. May increase anticoagulation with warfarin. Pentoxifylline may increase the serum levels of theophylline.

Nutritional/Ethanol Interactions Food: Food may decrease rate but not extent of absorption. Pentoxifylline peak serum levels may be decreased if taken with food.

Lab Interactions Decreased calcium (S), magnesium (S); false-positive theophylline levels

Adverse Reactions 1% to 10%:

Central nervous system: Dizziness, headache

Gastrointestinal: Dyspepsia, nausea, vomiting

Overdosage/Toxicology Symptoms of overdose include hypotension, flushing, convulsions, deep sleep, agitation, bradycardia, and AV block. Treatment is supportive.

Pharmacodynamics/Kinetics

Absorption: Well absorbed

Time to Peak: Serum: 2-4 hours

Half-Life Elimination: Parent drug: 24-48 minutes; Metabolites: 60-96 minutes

Metabolism: Hepatic and via erythrocytes; extensive first-pass effect

Excretion: Primarily urine

Dosing

Adults & Elderly: Peripheral vascular disease: Oral: 400 mg 3 times/day with meals; may reduce to 400 mg twice daily if GI or CNS side effects occur

Available Dosage Forms

Tablet, controlled release (Trental®): 400 mg

Tablet, extended release (Pentoxil®): 400 mg

Monitoring and Teaching Issues

Physical Assessment: Assess potential for interactions with other prescriptions, OTC medications, or herbal products patient may be taking. Assess therapeutic effectiveness, and adverse reactions at regular intervals during therapy (eg, cardiac status and blood pressure). Teach patient proper use, possible side effects/appropriate interventions, and adverse symptoms to report.

Patient Education: Do not take any new medication during therapy unless approved by prescriber. This may relieve pain of claudication, but additional therapy may be recommended. Take as prescribed for full length of prescription. May cause dizziness (use caution when driving or engaging in tasks that are potentially hazardous until response to drug is known); or heartburn, nausea, or vomiting (small frequent meals, frequent mouth care, chewing gum, or sucking lozenges may help). Report chest pain; swelling of lips, mouth, or tongue; persistent headache; respiratory difficulty; rash; or unrelieved nausea or vomiting. Pregnancy/breast-feeding precautions: Inform prescriber if you are or intend to become pregnant. Consult prescriber if breast-feeding.

Dietary Considerations: May be taken with meals or food.

Geriatric Considerations: Pentoxifylline's value in the treatment of intermittent claudication is controversial. Walking distance improved statistically in some clinical trials, but the actual distance was minimal when applied to improving physical activity (see Dosing).

Pregnancy Risk Factor: C

Lactation: Enters breast milk/not recommended

Administration

Oral: Tablets should be swallowed whole; do not chew, break, or crush.

- **Pentoxil®** *see Pentoxifylline on page 1185*
- **Pen VK** *see Penicillin V Potassium on page 1177*
- **Pepcid®** *see Famotidine on page 608*
- **Pepcid® AC [OTC]** *see Famotidine on page 608*
- **Pepto-Bismol® [OTC]** *see Bismuth on page 197*
- **Pepto-Bismol® Maximum Strength [OTC]** *see Bismuth on page 197*
- **Percocet®** *see Oxycodone and Acetaminophen on page 1138*
- **Percodan®** *see Oxycodone and Aspirin on page 1139*
- **Perdiem® Fiber Therapy [OTC]** *see Psyllium on page 1284*

Pergolide (PER go lide)

U.S. Brand Names Permax®

Synonyms Pergolide Mesylate

Generic Available Yes

Pharmacologic Category Anti-Parkinson's Agent, Dopamine Agonist; Ergot Derivative

Medication Safety Issues

Sound-alike/look-alike issues:

Permax® may be confused with Bumex®, Pentrax®, Pernox®

Use Adjunctive treatment to levodopa/carbidopa in the management of Parkinson's disease

Unlabeled/Investigational Use Tourette's disorder, chronic motor or vocal tic disorder

Mechanism of Action/Effect Pergolide is a semisynthetic ergot alkaloid similar to bromocriptine but stated to be more potent (10-1000 times) and longer-acting; it is a centrally-active dopamine agonist stimulating both D_1 and D_2 receptors. Pergolide is believed to exert its therapeutic effect by directly stimulating postsynaptic dopamine receptors in the nigrostriatal system.

Contraindications Hypersensitivity to pergolide mesylate, other ergot derivatives, or any component of the formulation; ergot alkaloids are contraindicated with potent inhibitors of CYP3A4 (includes protease inhibitors, azole antifungals, and some macrolide antibiotics)

Warnings/Precautions Symptomatic hypotension occurs in 10% of patients. Use with caution in patients with a history of cardiac arrhythmias, hallucinations, or mental illness. Cardiac valvular, pleural, and peritoneal fibrosis have been reported with prolonged daily use. Avoid rapid dose reduction or abrupt discontinuation.

Pergolide has been associated with somnolence. Some patients have been reported to fall asleep during activities of daily living, including driving, while taking this medication. Not all patients exhibited somnolence prior to these events.

Drug Interactions

Cytochrome P450 Effect: Substrate of CYP3A4 (major); **Inhibits** CYP2D6 (strong), 3A4 (weak)

Decreased Effect: Effects of pergolide may be diminished by antipsychotics, metoclopramide. Pergolide may decrease the levels/effects of CYP2D6 prodrug substrates (eg, codeine, hydrocodone, oxycodone, tramadol).

Increased Effect/Toxicity: Effects of pergolide may be increased by levodopa (hallucinations) and MAO inhibitors. Pergolide may increase the levels/effects of amphetamines, selected beta-blockers, dextromethorphan, fluoxetine, lidocaine, mirtazapine, nefazodone, paroxetine, risperidone, ritonavir, thioridazine, tricyclic antidepressants, venlafaxine, and other CYP2D6 substrates. Pergolide may increase the levels/effects of sibutramine and other serotonin agonists (serotonin syndrome). The levels/effects of pergolide may be increased by azole antifungals, ciprofloxacin, clarithromycin, diclofenac, doxycycline, erythromycin, imatinib, isoniazid, nefazodone, nicardipine, propofol, protease inhibitors, quinidine, telithromycin, verapamil, and other CYP3A4 inhibitors.

Nutritional/Ethanol Interactions Ethanol: Avoid ethanol (may cause CNS depression).

Adverse Reactions

>10%:

Central nervous system: Dizziness (19%), hallucinations (14%), dystonia (12%), somnolence (10%), confusion (10%)

Gastrointestinal: Nausea (24%), constipation (11%)

Neuromuscular & skeletal: Dyskinesia (62%)

Respiratory: Rhinitis (12%)

1% to 10%:

Cardiovascular: Hypotension or postural hypotension (10%), peripheral edema (7%), chest pain (4%), vasodilation (3%), palpitation (2%), syncope (2%), arrhythmia (1%), hypertension (2%), MI (1%)

Central nervous system: Insomnia (8%), pain (7%), anxiety (6%), psychosis (2%), EPS (2%), incoordination (2%), chills (1%)

Dermatologic: Rash (3%)

Gastrointestinal: Diarrhea (6%), dyspepsia (6%), abdominal pain (6%), anorexia (5%), xerostomia (4%), vomiting (3%), dysphagia (1%), nausea (1%)

Hematologic: Anemia (1%)

Neuromuscular & skeletal: Myalgia (1%), neuralgia (1%)

Ocular: Abnormal vision (6%), diplopia (2%)

Respiratory: Dyspnea (5%), epistaxis (2%)

Miscellaneous: Flu syndrome (3%), hiccups (1%)

Overdosage/Toxicology Symptoms of overdose include vomiting, hypotension, agitation, hallucinations, ventricular extrasystoles, and possible seizures. Data on overdose is limited. Treatment is supportive.

Pharmacodynamics/Kinetics

Absorption: Well absorbed

Protein Binding: Plasma: 90%

Half-Life Elimination: 27 hours

Metabolism: Extensively hepatic

Excretion: Urine (~50%); feces (50%)

Dosing

Adults & Elderly:

Parkinson's disease: Oral: Start with 0.05 mg/day for 2 days, then increase dosage by 0.1 or 0.15 mg/day every 3 days over next 12 days, increase dose by 0.25 mg/day every 3 days until optimal therapeutic dose is achieved, up to 5 mg/day maximum; usual dosage range: 2-3 mg/day in 3 divided doses

Note: When adding pergolide to levodopa/carbidopa, the dose of the latter can usually and should be decreased. Patients no longer responsive to bromocriptine may benefit by being switched to pergolide.

Pediatrics: Children and Adolescents: Tourette's disorder, chronic motor or vocal disorder (unlabeled uses): Oral: Up to 300 mcg/day

(Continued)

Pergolide *(Continued)*

Available Dosage Forms Tablet: 0.05 mg, 0.25 mg, 1 mg

Monitoring and Teaching Issues

Physical Assessment: Assess effectiveness and interactions of other medications patient may be taking. Monitor blood pressure and level of sedation. Monitor therapeutic effectiveness and adverse reactions at beginning of therapy and periodically throughout therapy. Assess knowledge/teach patient appropriate use, interventions to reduce side effects, and adverse symptoms to report.

Patient Education: Take exactly as directed (may be prescribed in conjunction with levodopa/carbidopa); do not change dosage or discontinue without consulting prescriber. Therapeutic effects may take several weeks or months to achieve and you may need frequent monitoring during first weeks of therapy. Take with meals if GI upset occurs, before meals if dry mouth occurs, or after eating if drooling or if nausea occurs. Take at the same time each day. Maintain adequate hydration (2-3 L/day of fluids) unless instructed to restrict fluid intake; void before taking medication. Do not use alcohol and prescription or OTC sedatives or CNS depressants without consulting prescriber. You may experience drowsiness, dizziness, confusion, or vision changes (use caution when driving, climbing stairs, or engaging in tasks requiring alertness until response to drug is known); orthostatic hypotension (use caution when changing position - rising to standing from sitting or lying); constipation (increased exercise, fluids, fruit, or fiber may help); runny nose or flu-like symptoms (consult prescriber for appropriate relief); nausea, vomiting, loss of appetite, or stomach discomfort (small frequent meals, frequent mouth care, chewing gum, or sucking lozenges may help); or photosensitivity (use sunscreen, wear protective clothing and eyewear, and avoid direct sunlight). Report unresolved constipation or vomiting; chest pain, palpitations, irregular heartbeat; ringing in ears; CNS changes (hallucination, loss of memory, seizures, acute headache, nervousness, etc); painful or difficult urination; increased muscle spasticity, rigidity, or involuntary movements; skin rash; or significant worsening of condition. **Breast-feeding precaution:** Breast-feeding is not recommended.

Geriatric Considerations: High incidence of syncope and orthostatic hypotension upon initiation of therapy. Use with caution in patients prone to cardiac dysrhythmias and in patients with a history of confusion or hallucinations.

Pregnancy Risk Factor: B

Lactation: Excretion in breast milk unknown/not recommended

- ♦ **Pergolide Mesylate** *see* Pergolide *on page 1187*
- ♦ **Pergonal® [DSC]** *see* Menotropins *on page 948*
- ♦ **Periactin** *see* Cyproheptadine *on page 388*
- ♦ **Peri-Colace® *(reformulation)* [OTC]** *see* Docusate and Senna *on page 475*

Perindopril Erbumine *(per IN doe pril er BYOO meen)*

U.S. Brand Names Aceon®

Generic Available No

Pharmacologic Category Angiotensin-Converting Enzyme (ACE) Inhibitor

Use Treatment of stage I or II hypertension and congestive heart failure; treatment of left ventricular dysfunction after myocardial infarction

Mechanism of Action/Effect Competitive inhibitor of angiotensin-converting enzyme (ACE); prevents conversion of angiotensin I to angiotensin II, a potent vasoconstrictor; results in lower levels of angiotensin II which, in turn, causes an increase in plasma renin activity and a reduction in aldosterone secretion

Contraindications Hypersensitivity to perindopril or any component of the formulation; angioedema related to previous treatment with an ACE inhibitor; bilateral renal artery stenosis; pregnancy (2nd and 3rd trimesters)

Warnings/Precautions Angioedema can occur at any time during treatment (especially following first dose). Angioedema may involve head and neck (potentially affecting the airway) or the intestine (presenting with abdominal pain). Careful blood pressure monitoring with first dose (hypotension can occur especially in volume depleted patients). Dosage adjustment needed in renal impairment. Use with caution in hypovolemia; collagen vascular diseases; valvular stenosis (particularly aortic stenosis); hyperkalemia; or before, during, or immediately after anesthesia. Avoid rapid dosage escalation, which may lead to renal insufficiency. Rare toxicities associated with ACE inhibitors include cholestatic jaundice (which may progress to hepatic necrosis) and neutropenia/agranulocytosis with myeloid hyperplasia. Hypersensitivity reactions may be seen during hemodialysis with high-flux dialysis membranes (eg, AN69). Use with caution in unilateral renal artery stenosis and pre-existing renal insufficiency.

Drug Interactions

Decreased Effect: Aspirin (high dose) may reduce the therapeutic effects of ACE inhibitors; at low dosages this does not appear to be significant. Rifampin may decrease the effect of ACE inhibitors. Antacids may decrease the bioavailability of ACE inhibitors (may be more likely to occur with captopril); separate administration times by 1-2 hours. NSAIDs, specifically indomethacin, may reduce the hypotensive effects of ACE inhibitors. More likely to occur in low renin or volume dependent hypertensive patients.

Increased Effect/Toxicity: Potassium supplements, co-trimoxazole (high dose), angiotensin II receptor antagonists (eg, candesartan, losartan, irbesartan), or potassium-sparing diuretics (amiloride, spironolactone, triamterene) may result in elevated serum potassium levels when combined with perindopril. ACE inhibitor effects may be increased by phenothiazines or probenecid (increases levels of captopril). ACE inhibitors may increase serum concentrations/effects of digoxin, lithium, and sulfonlyureas.

Diuretics have additive hypotensive effects with ACE inhibitors, and hypovolemia increases the potential for adverse renal effects of ACE inhibitors. In patients with compromised renal function, coadministration with NSAIDs may result in further deterioration of renal function. Allopurinol and ACE inhibitors may cause a higher risk of hypersensitivity reaction when taken concurrently.

Nutritional/Ethanol Interactions

Food: Perindopril active metabolite concentrations may be lowered if taken with food.

Herb/Nutraceutical: Avoid dong quai if using for hypertension (has estrogenic activity). Avoid ephedra, yohimbe, ginseng (may worsen hypertension). Avoid garlic (may have increased antihypertensive effect).

Adverse Reactions

>10%: Central nervous system: Headache (23%)

1% to 10%:

Cardiovascular: edema (4%), chest pain (2%)

Central nervous system: Dizziness (8%), sleep disorders (3%), depression (2%), fever (2%), nervousness (1%)

Dermatologic: Rash (2%)

Endocrine & metabolic: Hyperkalemia (1%), increased triglycerides (1%)

Gastrointestinal: Nausea (2%), diarrhea (4%), vomiting (2%), dyspepsia (2%), abdominal pain (3%), flatulence (1%)

Genitourinary: Sexual dysfunction (male: 1%)

Hepatic: Increased ALT (2%)

Neuromuscular & skeletal: Back pain (6%), upper extremity pain (3%), lower extremity pain (5%), paresthesia (2%), joint pain (1%), myalgia (1%), arthritis (1%), weakness (8%)

Renal: Proteinuria (2%)

Respiratory: Cough (incidence is higher in women, 3:1) (12%), sinusitis (5%), rhinitis (5%), pharyngitis (3%)

Otic: Tinnitus (2%)

Miscellaneous: Viral infection (3%)

Note: Some reactions occurred at an incidence >1% but ≤ placebo.

Additional adverse effects associated with with **ACE inhibitors** include agranulocytosis (especially in patients with renal impairment or collagen vascular disease), neutropenia, decreases in creatinine clearance in some elderly hypertensive patients or those with chronic renal failure, and worsening of renal function in patients with bilateral renal artery stenosis or hypovolemic patients (diuretic therapy). In addition, a syndrome which may include fever, myalgia, arthralgia, interstitial nephritis, vasculitis, rash, eosinophilia and positive ANA, and elevated ESR has been reported with ACE inhibitors.

Overdosage/Toxicology Mild hypotension has been the primary toxic effect seen with acute overdose. Bradycardia may also occur. Hyperkalemia occurs even with therapeutic doses, especially in patients with renal insufficiency and those taking NSAIDs. Treatment is symptom-directed and supportive.

Pharmacodynamics/Kinetics

Onset of Action: Peak effect: 1-2 hours

Bioavailability: Perindopril: 65% to 95%

Time to Peak: Chronic therapy: Perindopril: 1 hour; Perindoprilat: 3-4 hours (maximum perindoprilat serum levels are 2-3 times higher and T_{max} is shorter following chronic therapy); CHF: Perindoprilat: 6 hours

Protein Binding: Perindopril: 60%; Perindoprilat: 10% to 20%

Half-Life Elimination: Parent drug: 1.5-3 hours; Metabolite: Effective: 3-10 hours, Terminal: 30-120 hours

Metabolism: Hydrolyzed hepatically to active metabolite, perindoprilat (~17% to 20% of a dose) and other inactive metabolites

Excretion: Urine (75%, 10% as unchanged drug)

Dosing

Adults:

Congestive heart failure: Oral: 4 mg once daily; increase at 1- to 2-week intervals; maximum: 16 mg/day

Hypertension: Oral: Initial: 4 mg/day but may be titrated to response; usual range: 4-8 mg/day; increase at 1- to 2-week intervals; maximum: 16 mg/day

Elderly: Due to greater bioavailability and lower renal clearance of the drug in elderly subjects, dose reduction of 50% is recommended.

Renal Impairment:

Cl_{cr} >60 mL/minute: Administer 4 mg/day.

Cl_{cr} 30-60 mL/minute: Administer 2 mg/day.

Cl_{cr} 15-29 mL/minute: Administer 2 mg every other day.

Cl_{cr} <15 mL/minute: Administer 2 mg on the day of dialysis.

Perindopril and its metabolites are dialyzable.

Available Dosage Forms Tablet: 2 mg, 4 mg, 8 mg

Monitoring and Teaching Issues

Physical Assessment: Use caution with renal impairment, hypovolemia; collagen vascular diseases; valvular stenosis, hyperkalemia; or anesthesia (see Warnings/Precautions for specific use cautions). Assess potential for interactions with other pharmacological agents and herbal products patient may be taking (other drugs may effect blood pressure or toxicities; see Drug Interactions). It is recommended that first dose is administered in prescriber's office with careful blood pressure monitoring (hypotension can occur especially with first dose and angioedema can occur at any time during treatment, especially following first dose). Assess results of laboratory tests and patient response at beginning of therapy, when adjusting dose, and periodically with long-term therapy (eg, BP [standing and sitting], cardiac status and fluid balance; see Adverse Reactions). Teach patient appropriate use, possible side effects/appropriate interventions, and adverse symptoms to report (see Patient Education).

Monitoring Laboratory Tests: Serum creatinine, electrolytes, and WBC with differential initially and repeated at 2-week intervals for at least 90 days (particularly important in patients with renal impairment at baseline).

Patient Education: Do not take any new medication during therapy without consulting prescriber. Take as directed; do not alter dose or discontinue without consulting prescriber. Take first dose at bedtime. Do not take potassium supplements or salt substitutes containing potassium without consulting prescriber. This drug does not eliminate need for

(Continued)

Perindopril Erbumine (Continued)

diet or exercise regimen as recommended by prescriber. May cause increased cough (if persistent or bothersome, contact prescriber); headache (consult prescriber for approved analgesic); postural hypotension (use caution when rising from lying or sitting position or climbing stairs); dizziness (use caution when driving or engaging in tasks that require alertness until response to drug is known); nausea or vomiting (small frequent meals, frequent mouth care, sucking lozenges, or chewing gum may help); or diarrhea (buttermilk, boiled milk, or yogurt may help). Report chest pain, respiratory difficulty or persistent cough, painful muscles or joints, rash, ringing in ears, or other persistent adverse reactions. **Pregnancy/breast-feeding precautions:** Inform prescriber if you are or intend to become pregnant. This drug should not be used in the 2nd or 3rd trimester of pregnancy. Consult prescriber for appropriate contraceptive measures if necessary. Consult prescriber if breast-feeding.

Pregnancy Risk Factor: D (especially 2nd and 3rd trimesters)

Pregnancy Issues: ACE inhibitors can cause fetal injury or death if taken during the 2nd or 3rd trimester. Discontinue ACE inhibitors as soon as pregnancy is detected.

Lactation: Enters breast milk (small amounts)/effect on infant unknown

Related Information

Angiotensin Agents *on page 1704*

♦ **Periostat®** *see* Doxycycline *on page 496*

♦ **Permax®** *see* Pergolide *on page 1187*

Permethrin *(per METH rin)*

U.S. Brand Names A200® Lice [OTC]; Acticin®; Elimite®; Nix® [OTC]; Rid® Spray [OTC]

Generic Available Yes: Excludes spray

Pharmacologic Category Antiparasitic Agent, Topical; Scabicidal Agent

Use Single-application treatment of infestation with *Pediculus humanus capitis* (head louse) and its nits or *Sarcoptes scabiei* (scabies); indicated for prophylactic use during epidemics of lice

Mechanism of Action/Effect Inhibits sodium ion influx through nerve cell membrane channels in parasites resulting in delayed repolarization and thus paralysis and death of the pest

Contraindications Hypersensitivity to pyrethroid, pyrethrin, chrysanthemums, or any component of the formulation; lotion is contraindicated for use in infants <2 months of age

Warnings/Precautions Treatment may temporarily exacerbate the symptoms of itching, redness, and swelling. For external use only.

Adverse Reactions 1% to 10%:

Dermatologic: Pruritus, erythema, rash of the scalp

Local: Burning, stinging, tingling, numbness or scalp discomfort, edema

Pharmacodynamics/Kinetics

Absorption: <2%

Metabolism: Hepatic via ester hydrolysis to inactive metabolites

Excretion: Urine

Dosing

Adults & Elderly:

Head lice: Topical: After hair has been washed with shampoo, rinsed with water and towel dried, apply a sufficient volume of creme rinse to saturate the hair and scalp; also apply behind the ears and at the base of the neck; leave on hair for 10 minutes before rinsing off with water; remove remaining nits. May repeat in 1 week if lice or nits still present; in areas of head lice resistance to 1% permethrin, 5% permethrin has been applied to clean, dry hair and left on overnight (8-14 hours) under a shower cap.

Scabies: Topical: Apply cream from head to toe; leave on for 8-14 hours before washing off with water; may reapply in 1 week if live mites appear. Time of application was limited to 6 hours before rinsing with soap and water.

Pediatrics:

Head lice: Topical: Children >2 months: Refer to adult dosing.

Scabies: Topical: Apply cream from head to toe; leave on for 8-14 hours before washing off with water; for infants, also apply on the hairline, neck, scalp, temple, and forehead; may reapply in 1 week if live mites appear. Permethrin 5% cream was shown to be safe and effective when applied to an infant <1 month of age with neonatal scabies; time of application was limited to 6 hours before rinsing with soap and water.

Available Dosage Forms

Cream, topical (Acticin®, Elimite®): 5% (60 g) [contains coconut oil]

Liquid, topical [creme rinse formulation] (Nix®): 1% (60 mL) [contains isopropyl alcohol 20%]

Lotion, topical: 1% (59 mL)

Solution, spray [for bedding and furniture]:

A200® Lice: 0.5% (180 mL)

Nix®: 0.25% (148 mL)

Rid®: 0.5% (150 mL)

Monitoring and Teaching Issues

Physical Assessment: Assess head, hair, and skin surfaces for presence of lice and nits. Assess knowledge/teach patient appropriate application and use and adverse symptoms to report.

Patient Education: For external use only. Do not apply to face and avoid contact with eyes or mucous membrane. Clothing and bedding must be washed in hot water or dry cleaned to kill nits. May need to treat all members of household and all sexual contacts concurrently. Wash all combs and brushes with permethrin and thoroughly rinse. **Breast-feeding precaution:** Consult prescriber if breast-feeding.

Cream rinse/lotion: Apply immediately after hair is shampooed, rinsed, and towel-dried. Apply enough to saturate hair and scalp (especially behind ears and on nape of neck). Leave on hair for 10 minutes before rinsing with water. Remove nits with fine-tooth comb. May repeat in 1 week if lice or nits are still present.

Cream: Apply from neck to toes. Bathe to remove drug after 8-14 hours. Repeat in 7 days if lice or nits are still present. Report if condition persists or infection occurs.

Geriatric Considerations: Because of its minimal absorption, permethrin is a drug of choice and is preferred over lindane.

Pregnancy Risk Factor: B

Lactation: Effect on infant unknown

Administration

Topical: Avoid contact with eyes and mucous membranes during application. Because scabies and lice are so contagious, use caution to avoid spreading or infecting oneself; wear gloves when applying

Cream rinse/lotion: Shake cream rinse well before using. Apply immediately after hair is shampooed, rinsed, and towel-dried. Apply enough to saturate hair and scalp (especially behind ears and on nape of neck). Leave on hair for 10 minutes before rinsing with water. Remove nits with fine-tooth comb. May repeat in 1 week if lice or nits are still present.

Cream: Apply from neck to toes. Bathe to remove drug after 8-14 hours. Repeat in 7 days if lice or nits are still present. Report if condition persists or infection occurs.

Perphenazine (per FEN a zeen)

Generic Available Yes

Pharmacologic Category Antipsychotic Agent, Typical, Phenothiazine

Medication Safety Issues

Sound-alike/look-alike issues:

Trilafon® may be confused with Tri-Levlen®

Use Treatment of schizophrenia; nausea and vomiting

Unlabeled/Investigational Use Ethanol withdrawal; dementia in elderly; Tourette's syndrome; Huntington's chorea; spasmodic torticollis; Reye's syndrome; psychosis

Mechanism of Action/Effect Perphenazine is a piperazine phenothiazine antipsychotic which blocks postsynaptic mesolimbic dopaminergic receptors in the brain; exhibits alpha-adrenergic blocking effect and depresses the release of hypothalamic and hypophyseal hormones

Contraindications Hypersensitivity to perphenazine or any component of the formulation (cross-reactivity between phenothiazines may occur); severe CNS depression; subcortical brain damage; bone marrow suppression; blood dyscrasias; coma

Warnings/Precautions May cause hypotension. May be sedating, use with caution in disorders where CNS depression is a feature. Use with caution in Parkinson's disease. Caution in patients with hemodynamic instability; predisposition to seizures; severe cardiac, hepatic, renal, or respiratory disease. Esophageal dysmotility and aspiration have been associated with antipsychotic use - use with caution in patients at risk of pneumonia (ie, Alzheimer's disease). Caution in breast cancer or other prolactin-dependent tumors (may elevate prolactin levels). May alter temperature regulation or mask toxicity of other drugs due to antiemetic effects. May alter cardiac conduction - life-threatening arrhythmias have occurred with therapeutic doses of phenothiazines. May cause orthostatic hypotension - use with caution in patients at risk of this effect or those who would tolerate transient hypotensive episodes (cerebrovascular disease, cardiovascular disease, or other medications which may predispose).

Due to anticholinergic effects, use with caution in patients with decreased gastrointestinal motility, urinary retention, BPH, xerostomia, visual problems, narrow-angle glaucoma (screening is recommended) and myasthenia gravis. Relative to other neuroleptics, perphenazine has a low potency of cholinergic blockade.

May cause extrapyramidal symptoms, including pseudoparkinsonism, acute dystonic reactions, akathisia, and tardive dyskinesia (risk of these reactions is moderate-high relative to other neuroleptics). May be associated with neuroleptic malignant syndrome (NMS) or pigmentary retinopathy.

Drug Interactions

Cytochrome P450 Effect: Substrate of CYP1A2 (minor), 2C8/9 (minor), 2C19 (minor), 2D6 (major), 3A4 (minor); **Inhibits** CYP1A2 (weak), 2D6 (weak)

Decreased Effect: Phenothiazines inhibit the ability of bromocriptine to lower serum prolactin concentrations. Benztropine (and other anticholinergics) may inhibit the therapeutic response to perphenazine and excess anticholinergic effects may occur. Cigarette smoking and barbiturates may enhance the hepatic metabolism of chlorpromazine. Antihypertensive effects of guanethidine and guanadrel may be inhibited by perphenazine. Perphenazine may inhibit the antiparkinsonian effect of levodopa. Perphenazine and possibly other low potency antipsychotics may reverse the pressor effects of epinephrine.

Increased Effect/Toxicity: CYP2D6 inhibitors may increase the levels/effects of perphenazine; example inhibitors include chlorpromazine, delavirdine, fluoxetine, miconazole, paroxetine, pergolide, quinidine, quinine, ritonavir, and ropinirole. Effects on CNS depression may be additive when perphenazine is combined with CNS depressants (narcotic analgesics, ethanol, barbiturates, cyclic antidepressants, antihistamines, or sedative-hypnotics). Perphenazine may increase the effects/toxicity of anticholinergics, antihypertensives, lithium (rare neurotoxicity), trazodone, or valproic acid. Concurrent use with TCA may produce increased toxicity or altered therapeutic response. Chloroquine and propranolol may increase perphenazine concentrations. Hypotension may occur when perphenazine is combined with epinephrine. May increase the risk of arrhythmia when combined with antiarrhythmics, cisapride, pimozide, sparfloxacin, or other drugs which prolong QT interval. Metoclopramide may increase risk of extrapyramidal symptoms (EPS).

Nutritional/Ethanol Interactions

Ethanol: Avoid ethanol (may increase CNS depression).

Herb/Nutraceutical: Avoid kava kava, gotu kola, valerian, St John's wort (may increase CNS depression).

Adverse Reactions Frequency not defined.

Cardiovascular: Hyper-/hypotension, orthostatic hypotension, tachycardia, bradycardia, dizziness, cardiac arrest

(Continued)

Perphenazine *(Continued)*

Central nervous system: Extrapyramidal symptoms (pseudoparkinsonism, akathisia, dystonias, tardive dyskinesia), dizziness, cerebral edema, seizure, headache, drowsiness, paradoxical excitement, restlessness, hyperactivity, insomnia, neuroleptic malignant syndrome (NMS), impairment of temperature regulation

Dermatologic: Rash, discoloration of skin (blue-gray), photosensitivity

Endocrine & metabolic: Hypoglycemia, hyperglycemia, galactorrhea, lactation, breast enlargement, gynecomastia, menstrual irregularity, amenorrhea, SIADH, libido (changes in)

Gastrointestinal: Constipation, weight gain, vomiting, stomach pain, nausea, xerostomia, salivation, diarrhea, anorexia, ileus

Genitourinary: Difficulty in urination, ejaculatory disturbances, incontinence, polyuria, ejaculating dysfunction, priapism

Hematologic: Agranulocytosis, leukopenia, eosinophilia, hemolytic anemia, thrombocytopenic purpura, pancytopenia

Hepatic: Cholestatic jaundice, hepatotoxicity

Neuromuscular & skeletal: Tremor

Ocular: Pigmentary retinopathy, blurred vision, cornea and lens changes

Respiratory: Nasal congestion

Miscellaneous: Diaphoresis

Overdosage/Toxicology Symptoms of overdose include deep sleep, dystonia, agitation, coma, abnormal involuntary muscle movements, hypotension, and arrhythmias (QT$_c$ prolongation, AV block, torsade de pointes, ventricular tachycardia/fibrillation). Children may have convulsive seizures.

Treatment is symptom-directed and supportive. Induction of emesis is not recommended. Peritoneal dialysis and hemodialysis are of no value. Gastric lavage and administration of activated charcoal together with a laxative should be considered. Cardiac function should be monitored for at least 5 days. Norepinephrine may be used to treat hypotension, but epinephrine should **not** be used.

Pharmacodynamics/Kinetics

Absorption: Oral: Well absorbed

Time to Peak: Serum: Perphenazine: 1-3 hours; 7-hydroxyperphenazine: 2-4 hours

Half-Life Elimination: Perphenazine: 9-12 hours; 7-hydroxyperphenazine: 11.3 hours

Metabolism: Extensively hepatic to metabolites via sulfoxidation, hydroxylation, dealkylation, and glucuronidation

Excretion: Urine and feces

Dosing

Adults:

Schizophrenia/psychoses: Oral: 4-16 mg 2-4 times/day not to exceed 64 mg/day

Nausea/vomiting: Oral: 8-16 mg/day in divided doses up to 24 mg/day

Elderly: Behavioral symptoms associated with dementia: Oral: Initial: 2-4 mg 1-2 times/day; increase at 4- to 7-day intervals by 2-4 mg/day. Increase dose intervals (bid, tid, etc) as necessary to control behavior response or side effects. Maximum daily dose: 32 mg; gradual increase (titration) and bedtime administration may prevent some side effects or decrease their severity.

Pediatrics:

Schizophrenia/psychoses: Oral:

1-6 years: 4-6 mg/day in divided doses

6-12 years: 6 mg/day in divided doses

>12 years: 4-16 mg 2-4 times/day

Renal Impairment: Not dialyzable (0% to 5%)

Hepatic Impairment: Dosage reductions should be considered in patients with liver disease although no specific guidelines are available.

Available Dosage Forms Tablet: 2 mg, 4 mg, 8 mg, 16 mg

Monitoring and Teaching Issues

Physical Assessment: Assess other medications patient is taking for effectiveness and interactions. Monitor ophthalmic screening, laboratory results, therapeutic effectiveness, and adverse reactions at beginning of therapy and periodically with long-term use. Monitor blood pressure; can cause orthostatic hypotension. Initiate at lower doses and taper dosage slowly when discontinuing. Assess knowledge/teach patient appropriate use, interventions to reduce side effects, and adverse symptoms to report.

Monitoring Laboratory Tests: Baseline liver and kidney function, CBC prior to and periodically during therapy, lipid profile, fasting blood glucose/Hgb A$_{1c}$; BMI

Patient Education: Use exactly as directed; do not increase dose or frequency. It may take 2-3 weeks to achieve desired results; do not discontinue without consulting prescriber. Do not take within 2 hours of any antacid. Avoid alcohol or caffeine and other prescription or OTC medications not approved by prescriber. Maintain adequate hydration (2-3 L/day of fluids) unless instructed to restrict fluid intake. Avoid skin contact with medication; may cause contact dermatitis (wash immediately with warm, soapy water). You may experience excess drowsiness, restlessness, dizziness, or blurred vision (use caution driving or when engaging in tasks requiring alertness until response to drug is known); dry mouth, nausea, vomiting (small frequent meals, frequent mouth care, chewing gum, or sucking lozenges may help); constipation (increased exercise, fluids, fruit, or fiber may help); postural hypotension (use caution climbing stairs or when changing position from lying or sitting to standing); urinary retention (void before taking medication); photosensitivity (use sunscreen, wear protective clothing and eyewear, and avoid direct sunlight); or decreased perspiration (avoid strenuous exercise in hot environments). Report persistent CNS effects (eg, trembling fingers, altered gait or balance, excessive sedation, seizures, unusual movements, anxiety, abnormal thoughts, confusion, personality changes); chest pain, palpitations, rapid heartbeat, severe dizziness; unresolved urinary retention or changes in urinary pattern; menstrual pattern, change in libido, or ejaculatory difficulty; vision changes; skin rash or yellowing of skin; respiratory difficulty; or worsening of condition. **Pregnancy/**

breast-feeding precautions: Inform prescriber if you are or intend to become pregnant. Breast-feeding is not recommended.

Geriatric Considerations: (See Warnings/Precautions, Adverse Reactions, and Over-dose/Toxicology.) Elderly patients have an increased risk of adverse response to side effects or adverse reactions to antipsychotics. Plasma levels at a given dose are increased in elderly patients. Older patients are also at higher risk of tardive dyskinesia, and prescribing should be approached in a manner which minimizes the development of this effect.

Pregnancy Risk Factor: C

Lactation: Enters breast milk/not recommended (AAP rates "of concern")

Administration

Storage: Store at 2°C to 25°C (36°F to 77°F). Protect from light.

Related Information

Antipsychotic Agents *on page 1717*
Antipsychotic Medication Guidelines *on page 1766*
Federal OBRA Regulations: Recommended Maximum Doses *on page 1773*

♦ **Persantine®** *see* Dipyridamole *on page 468*
♦ **Pethidine Hydrochloride** *see* Meperidine *on page 950*
♦ **Pexeva™** *see* Paroxetine *on page 1160*
♦ **PFA** *see* Foscarnet *on page 679*
♦ **Pfizerpen®** *see* Penicillin G (Parenteral/Aqueous) *on page 1174*
♦ **PGE₁** *see* Alprostadil *on page 76*
♦ **PGE₂** *see* Dinoprostone *on page 462*
♦ **PGI₂** *see* Epoprostenol *on page 534*
♦ **PGX** *see* Epoprostenol *on page 534*
♦ **Phanasin [OTC]** *see* Guaifenesin *on page 729*
♦ **Phanasin® Diabetic Choice [OTC]** *see* Guaifenesin *on page 729*
♦ **Pharmacotherapy of Urinary Incontinence** *see page 1858*
♦ **Phenadoz™** *see* Promethazine *on page 1265*

Phenazopyridine (fen az oh PEER i deen)

U.S. Brand Names Azo-Gesic® [OTC]; Azo-Standard® [OTC]; Prodium® [OTC]; Pyridium®; ReAzo [OTC]; Uristat® [OTC]; UTI Relief® [OTC]

Synonyms Phenazopyridine Hydrochloride; Phenylazo Diamino Pyridine Hydrochloride

Generic Available Yes

Pharmacologic Category Analgesic, Urinary

Medication Safety Issues

Sound-alike/look-alike issues:
Pyridium® may be confused with Dyrenium®, Perdiem®, pyridoxine, pyrithione

Use Symptomatic relief of urinary burning, itching, frequency and urgency in association with urinary tract infection or following urologic procedures

Mechanism of Action/Effect An azo dye which exerts local anesthetic or analgesic action on urinary tract mucosa through an unknown mechanism

Contraindications Hypersensitivity to phenazopyridine or any component of the formulation; kidney or liver disease; patients with a Cl_{cr} <50 mL/minute

Warnings/Precautions Does not treat infection, acts only as an analgesic; drug should be discontinued if skin or sclera develop a yellow color; use with caution in patients with renal impairment. Use of this agent in the elderly is limited since accumulation of phenazopyridine can occur in patients with renal insufficiency. Use is contraindicated in patients with a Cl_{cr} <50 mL/minute.

Lab Interactions Phenazopyridine may cause delayed reactions with glucose oxidase reagents (Clinistix®); cupric sulfate tests (Clinitest®) are not affected; interference may also occur with urine ketone tests (Acetest®, Ketostix®) and urinary protein tests; tests for urinary steroids and porphyrins may also occur

Adverse Reactions 1% to 10%:
Central nervous system: Headache, dizziness
Gastrointestinal: Stomach cramps

Overdosage/Toxicology Symptoms of overdose include methemoglobinemia, hemolytic anemia, skin pigmentation, and renal and hepatic impairment. For methemoglobinemia, the antidote is methylene blue 1-2 mg/kg I.V.

Pharmacodynamics/Kinetics

Metabolism: Hepatic and via other tissues

Excretion: Urine (65% as unchanged drug)

Dosing

Adults & Elderly: Urinary analgesic: Oral: 100-200 mg 3 times/day after meals for 2 days when used concomitantly with an antibacterial agent

Pediatrics: Urinary analgesic: Oral: Children: 12 mg/kg/day in 3 divided doses administered after meals for 2 days

Renal Impairment:
Cl_{cr} 50-80 mL/minute: Administer every 8-16 hours.
Cl_{cr} <50 mL/minute: Avoid use.

Available Dosage Forms Tablet, as hydrochloride: 100 mg, 200 mg
Azo-Gesic®, Azo-Standard®, Prodium®, Uristat®: 95 mg
ReAzo: 97 mg
Pyridium®: 100 mg, 200 mg [contains sodium benzoate]
UTI Relief®: 97.2 mg

Monitoring and Teaching Issues

Physical Assessment: Assess therapeutic effectiveness according to rational for use. Instruct patients with diabetes to use serum glucose monitoring (phenazopyridine may interfere with certain urine testing reagents). Teach patient appropriate use, side effects/appropriate interventions, and adverse symptoms to report.

(Continued)

Phenazopyridine *(Continued)*

Patient Education: Take exactly as directed. May discolor urine (orange/yellow); this is normal, but will also stain fabric. If you have diabetes, use serum glucose tests; this medication may interfere with accuracy of urine testing. Report persistent headache, dizziness, or stomach cramping. **Breast-feeding precaution:** Consult prescriber if breast-feeding.

Dietary Considerations: Should be taken after meals.

Geriatric Considerations: Use of this agent in the elderly is limited since accumulation of phenazopyridine can occur in patients with renal insufficiency. It should not be used in patients with a Cl_{cr} <50 mL/minute.

Pregnancy Risk Factor: B

Lactation: Excretion in breast milk unknown

♦ Phenazopyridine Hydrochloride *see Phenazopyridine on page 1193*

Phenelzine *(FEN el zeen)*

U.S. Brand Names Nardil®

Synonyms Phenelzine Sulfate

Restrictions A medication guide should be dispensed with each prescription. A template for the required MedGuides can be found on the FDA website at: http://www.fda.gov/cder/drug/antidepressants/labelTemplate.pdf

Generic Available No

Pharmacologic Category Antidepressant, Monoamine Oxidase Inhibitor

Medication Safety Issues

Sound-alike/look-alike issues:

Phenelzine may be confused with phenytoin

Nardil® may be confused with Norinyl®

Use Symptomatic treatment of atypical, nonendogenous, or neurotic depression

Unlabeled/Investigational Use Selective mutism

Mechanism of Action/Effect Thought to act by increasing endogenous concentrations of norepinephrine, dopamine, and serotonin through inhibition of the enzyme (monoamine oxidase) responsible for the breakdown of these neurotransmitters

Contraindications Hypersensitivity to phenelzine or any component of the formulation; uncontrolled hypertension; pheochromocytoma; hepatic disease; congestive heart failure; concurrent use of sympathomimetics (and related compounds), CNS depressants, ethanol, meperidine, bupropion, buspirone, guanethidine, serotonergic drugs (including SSRIs) - do not use within 5 weeks of fluoxetine discontinuation or 2 weeks of other antidepressant discontinuation; general anesthesia, local vasoconstrictors; spinal anesthesia (hypotension may be exaggerated); foods with a high content of tyramine, tryptophan, or dopamine, chocolate, or caffeine (may cause hypertensive crisis)

Warnings/Precautions Antidepressants increase the risk of suicidal thinking and behavior in children and adolescents with major depressive disorder (MDD) and other depressive disorders; consider risk prior to prescribing. All patients must be closely monitored for clinical worsening, suicidality, or unusual changes in behavior, especially during the initiation of therapy or following an increase or decrease in dosage. When used in children, the child's family or caregiver should be instructed to closely observe the patient and communicate condition with healthcare provider. A medication guide should be dispensed with each prescription. **Phenelzine is FDA approved for the treatment of depression in children ≥16 years of age.**

The possibility of a suicide attempt is inherent in major depression and may persist until remission occurs. Use caution in high-risk patients. Worsening depression and severe abrupt suicidality that are not part of the presenting symptoms may require discontinuation or modification of drug therapy. The patient's family or caregiver should be alerted to monitor patients for the emergence of suicidality and associated behaviors (such as agitation, irritability, hostility, impulsivity, and hypomania) and call healthcare provider.

May worsen psychosis in some patients or precipitate a shift to mania or hypomania in patients with bipolar disorder. Patients presenting with depressive symptoms should be screened for bipolar disorder. Monotherapy in patients with bipolar disorder should be avoided. **Phenelzine is not FDA approved for the treatment of bipolar depression.**

Use with caution in patients who are hyperactive, hyperexcitable, or who have glaucoma, hyperthyroidism, suicidal tendencies, or diabetes. Hypertensive crisis may occur with tyramine, tryptophan, or dopamine-containing foods. Should not be used in combination with other antidepressants. Hypotensive effects of antihypertensives (beta-blockers, thiazides) may be exaggerated. May cause orthostatic hypotension - use with caution in patients with hypotension or patients who would not tolerate transient hypotensive episodes (cardiovascular or cerebrovascular disease) - effects may be additive with other agents which cause orthostasis. Use with caution in patients at risk of seizures, or in patients receiving other drugs which may lower seizure threshold. Toxic reactions have occurred with dextromethorphan. Discontinue at least 48 hours prior to myelography. May increase the risks associated with electroconvulsive therapy. Consider discontinuing, when possible, prior to elective surgery.

Drug Interactions

Decreased Effect: Phenelzine (and other MAO inhibitors) inhibits the antihypertensive response to guanadrel or guanethidine; concurrent use is contraindicated.

Increased Effect/Toxicity: In general, the combined use of phenelzine with TCAs, venlafaxine, trazodone, dexfenfluramine, sibutramine, lithium, meperidine, fenfluramine, dextromethorphan, and SSRIs should be avoided due to the potential for severe adverse reactions (serotonin syndrome, death); avoid meperidine within 2 weeks of phenelzine use, allow 5 weeks between discontinuing fluoxetine and starting MAO inhibitors, allow at least 10 days after discontinuing MAO inhibitors and starting fluoxetine; concurrent use with dextromethorphan is contraindicated. MAO inhibitors (including phenelzine) may inhibit the metabolism of barbiturates and prolong their effect. Phenelzine in combination with amphetamines, other stimulants (methylphenidate), levodopa, metaraminol, reserpine, and decongestants (pseudoephedrine) may result in severe hypertensive reactions. Concurrent use with amphetamines, methylphenidate, metaraminol, and pseudoephedrine is contraindicated.

Foods (eg, cheese) and beverages (eg, ethanol) containing tyramine should be avoided; hypertensive crisis may result. Phenelzine may increase the pressor response of norepinephrine and may prolong neuromuscular blockade produced by succinylcholine. Tramadol may increase the risk of seizures and serotonin syndrome in patients receiving an MAO inhibitor. Phenelzine may produce additive hypoglycemic effect in patients receiving hypoglycemic agents and may produce delirium in patients receiving disulfiram. Concurrent use with bupropion is contraindicated; allow at least 14 days between discontinuing MAO inhibitors and starting bupropion. Concurrent use with buspirone may cause hypertension; wait at least 14 days between discontinuing one agent and starting the other.

Nutritional/Ethanol Interactions
Ethanol: Avoid ethanol (alcoholic beverages containing tyramine may induce a severe hypertensive response).
Food: Clinically-severe elevated blood pressure may occur if phenelzine is taken with tyramine-containing foods. Avoid foods containing tryptophan, dopamine, chocolate, or caffeine.

Lab Interactions Decreased glucose

Adverse Reactions Frequency not defined.
Cardiovascular: Orthostatic hypotension, edema
Central nervous system: Dizziness, headache, drowsiness, sleep disturbances, fatigue, hyper-reflexia, twitching, ataxia, mania
Dermatologic: Rash, pruritus
Endocrine & metabolic: Decreased sexual ability (anorgasmia, ejaculatory disturbances, impotence), hypernatremia, hypermetabolic syndrome
Gastrointestinal: Xerostomia, constipation, weight gain
Genitourinary: Urinary retention
Hematologic: Leukopenia
Hepatic: Hepatitis
Neuromuscular & skeletal: Weakness, tremor, myoclonus
Ocular: Blurred vision, glaucoma
Miscellaneous: Diaphoresis

Overdosage/Toxicology Symptoms of overdose include tachycardia, palpitations, muscle twitching, seizures, insomnia, restlessness, transient hypertension, hypotension, drowsiness, hyperpyrexia, and coma. Treatment is symptom-directed and supportive.

Pharmacodynamics/Kinetics
Onset of Action: Therapeutic: 2-4 weeks; geriatric patients receiving an average of 55 mg/day developed a mean platelet MAO activity inhibition of about 85%.
Duration of Action: May continue to have a therapeutic effect and interactions 2 weeks after discontinuing therapy
Absorption: Well absorbed
Half-Life Elimination: 11 hours
Metabolism: Oxidized via monoamine oxidase (primary pathway) and acetylation (minor pathway)
Excretion: Urine (primarily as metabolites and unchanged drug)

Dosing
Adults: Depression: Oral: 15 mg 3 times/day; may increase to 60-90 mg/day during early phase of treatment, then reduce dose for maintenance therapy slowly after maximum benefit is obtained. Takes 2-4 weeks for a significant response to occur.
Elderly: Oral: Initial: 7.5 mg/day; increase by 7.5-15 mg/day every 3-4 days as tolerated; usual therapeutic dose: 15-60 mg/day in 3-4 divided doses.
Pediatrics: Selective mutism (unlabeled use): Oral: 30-60 mg/day

Available Dosage Forms Tablet: 15 mg

Monitoring and Teaching Issues
Physical Assessment: Assess other medications patient may be taking for effectiveness and interactions. Monitor therapeutic effectiveness and adverse reactions at beginning of therapy and periodically with long-term use. Monitor blood pressure. Be alert to possibility of suicide ideation. Taper dosage slowly when discontinuing; allow 3-4 weeks between discontinuing phenelzine and starting another antidepressant. Advise patients with diabetes to monitor serum glucose closely (phenelzine may lower glucose level). Assess knowledge/teach patient appropriate use, interventions to reduce side effects (including tyramine-free diet; see Tyramine Content of Foods list *on page 1758*), and adverse symptoms to report.
Patient Education: Take exactly as directed; do not increase dose or frequency. It may take 2-3 weeks to achieve desired results. Avoid alcohol, caffeine, and other prescriptions or OTC medications not approved by prescriber. Avoid tyramine-containing foods (eg, pickles, aged cheese, wine). Maintain adequate hydration (2-3 L/day of fluids) unless instructed to restrict fluid intake. You may experience postural hypotension (use caution when climbing stairs or changing position from lying or sitting to standing); drowsiness, lightheadedness, dizziness (use caution when driving or engaging in tasks requiring alertness until response to drug is known); anorexia, dry mouth (small frequent meals, frequent mouth care, chewing gum, or sucking lozenges may help); constipation (increased exercise, fluids, fruit, or fiber may help); or diarrhea (buttermilk, yogurt, or boiled milk may help). If you have diabetes, monitor serum glucose closely (Nardil® may effect glucose levels). Report persistent insomnia; chest pain, palpitations, irregular or rapid heartbeat, or swelling of extremities; muscle cramping, tremors, or altered gait; blurred vision or eye pain; yellowing of eyes or skin; pale stools/dark urine; suicidal ideation; or worsening of condition. **Pregnancy/breast-feeding precautions:** Inform prescriber if you are or intend to become pregnant. Breast-feeding is not recommended.
Geriatric Considerations: MAO inhibitors are effective and generally well tolerated by older patients. Potential interactions with tyramine- or tryptophan-containing foods (see (Continued)

Phenelzine *(Continued)*

Warnings/Precautions) and other drugs, and adverse effects on blood pressure have limited the use of MAO inhibitors. They are usually reserved for patients who do not tolerate or respond to traditional "cyclic" or "second generation" antidepressants. Brain activity due to monoamine oxidase increases with age and even more so in patients with Alzheimer's disease. Therefore, MAO inhibitors may have an increased role in treating depressed patients with Alzheimer's disease. Phenelzine is less stimulating than tranylcypromine.

Pregnancy Risk Factor: C

Lactation: Excretion in breast milk unknown/not recommended

Administration

Storage: Protect from light

Additional Information Pyridoxine deficiency has occurred; symptoms include numbness and edema of hands; may respond to supplementation.

The MAO inhibitors are usually reserved for patients who do not tolerate or respond to other antidepressants. The brain activity of monoamine oxidase increases with age and even more so in patients with Alzheimer's disease. Therefore, the MAO inhibitors may have an increased role in patients with Alzheimer's disease who are depressed. Phenelzine is less stimulating than tranylcypromine.

Related Information

Antidepressant Agents *on page 1713*
Antidepressant Medication Guidelines *on page 1765*
Tyramine Content of Foods *on page 1758*

♦ **Phenelzine Sulfate** *see* Phenelzine *on page 1194*

♦ **Phenergan®** *see* Promethazine *on page 1265*

♦ **Phenergan® With Codeine** *see* Promethazine and Codeine *on page 1267*

Phenobarbital *(fee noe BAR bi tal)*

U.S. Brand Names Luminal® Sodium

Synonyms Phenobarbital Sodium; Phenobarbitone; Phenylethylmalonylurea

Controlled Substance C-IV

Generic Available Yes

Pharmacologic Category Anticonvulsant, Barbiturate; Barbiturate

Medication Safety Issues

Sound-alike/look-alike issues:
Phenobarbital may be confused with pentobarbital
Luminal® may be confused with Tuinal®

Use Management of generalized tonic-clonic (grand mal) and partial seizures; sedative

Unlabeled/Investigational Use Febrile seizures in children; may also be used for prevention and treatment of neonatal hyperbilirubinemia and lowering of bilirubin in chronic cholestasis; neonatal seizures; management of sedative/hypnotic withdrawal

Mechanism of Action/Effect Short-acting barbiturate with sedative, hypnotic, and anticonvulsant properties. Barbiturates depress the sensory cortex, decrease motor activity, alter cerebellar function, and produce drowsiness, sedation, and hypnosis. In high doses, barbiturates exhibit anticonvulsant activity; barbiturates produce dose-dependent respiratory depression.

Contraindications Hypersensitivity to barbiturates or any component of the formulation; marked hepatic impairment; dyspnea or airway obstruction; porphyria; pregnancy

Warnings/Precautions Potential for drug dependency exists, abrupt cessation may precipitate withdrawal, including status epilepticus in epileptic patients. Do not administer to patients in acute pain. Use caution in elderly, debilitated, renally or hepatic dysfunction, and pediatric patients. May cause paradoxical responses, including agitation and hyperactivity, particularly in acute pain and pediatric patients. Use with caution in patients with depression or suicidal tendencies, or in patients with a history of drug abuse. Tolerance, psychological and physical dependence may occur with prolonged use. May cause CNS depression, which may impair physical or mental abilities. Effects with other sedative drugs or ethanol may be potentiated. May cause respiratory depression or hypotension, particularly when administered intravenously. Use with caution in hemodynamically unstable patients (hypovolemic shock, CHF) or patients with respiratory disease. Due to its long half-life and risk of dependence, phenobarbital is not recommended as a sedative in the elderly. Use has been associated with cognitive deficits in children. Use with caution in patients with hypoadrenalism.

Drug Interactions

Cytochrome P450 Effect: Substrate of CYP2C8/9 (minor), 2C19 (major), 2E1 (minor); **Induces** CYP1A2 (strong), 2A6 (strong), 2B6 (strong), 2C8/9 (strong), 3A4 (strong)

Decreased Effect: Barbiturates may increase the metabolism of estrogens and reduce the efficacy of oral contraceptives; an alternative method of contraception should be considered. Barbiturates inhibit the hypoprothrombinemic effects of oral anticoagulants via increased metabolism. Barbiturates may enhance the metabolism of methadone resulting in methadone withdrawal. The levels/effects of phenobarbital may be decreased by aminoglutethimide, carbamazepine, phenytoin, rifampin, and other CYP2C19 inducers.

Phenobarbital may decrease the levels/effects of aminophylline, amiodarone, benzodiazepines, bupropion, calcium channel blockers, carbamazepine, citalopram, clarithromycin, cyclosporine, diazepam, efavirenz, erythromycin, estrogens, fluoxetine, fluvoxamine, glimepiride, glipizide, ifosfamide, losartan, methsuximide, mirtazapine, nateglinide, nefazodone, nevirapine, phenytoin, pioglitazone, promethazine, propranolol, protease inhibitors, proton pump inhibitors, rifampin, ropinirole, rosiglitazone, selegiline, sertraline, sulfonamides, tacrolimus, theophylline, venlafaxine, voriconazole, warfarin, zafirlukast, and other CYP1A2, 2A6, 2B6, 2C8/9, or 3A4 substrates.

Increased Effect/Toxicity: When combined with other CNS depressants, ethanol, narcotic analgesics, antidepressants, or benzodiazepines, additive respiratory and CNS depression may occur. Barbiturates may enhance the hepatotoxic potential of acetaminophen overdoses. Chloramphenicol, MAO inhibitors, valproic acid, and felbamate may inhibit barbiturate metabolism. Barbiturates may impair the absorption of griseofulvin, and may enhance the nephrotoxic effects of methoxyflurane. Concurrent use of phenobarbital with meperidine may result in increased CNS depression. Concurrent use of phenobarbital with primidone may result in elevated phenobarbital serum concentrations. The levels/ effects of phenobarbital may be increased by delavirdine, fluconazole, fluvoxamine, gemfibrozil, isoniazid, omeprazole, ticlopidine, and other CYP2C19 inhibitors.

Nutritional/Ethanol Interactions
Ethanol: Avoid ethanol (may increase CNS depression).
Food: May cause decrease in vitamin D and calcium.
Herb/Nutraceutical: Avoid evening primrose (seizure threshold decreased). Avoid valerian, St John's wort, kava kava, gotu kola (may increase CNS depression).

Lab Interactions Increased ammonia (B), LFTs, copper (serum); decreased bilirubin (S); assay interference of LDH

Adverse Reactions Frequency not defined.
Cardiovascular: Bradycardia, hypotension, syncope
Central nervous system: Drowsiness, lethargy, CNS excitation or depression, impaired judgment, "hangover" effect, confusion, somnolence, agitation, hyperkinesia, ataxia, nervousness, headache, insomnia, nightmares, hallucinations, anxiety, dizziness
Dermatologic: Rash, exfoliative dermatitis, Stevens-Johnson syndrome
Gastrointestinal: Nausea, vomiting, constipation
Hematologic: Agranulocytosis, thrombocytopenia, megaloblastic anemia
Local: Pain at injection site, thrombophlebitis with I.V. use
Renal: Oliguria
Respiratory: Laryngospasm, respiratory depression, apnea (especially with rapid I.V. use), hypoventilation
Miscellaneous: Gangrene with inadvertent intra-arterial injection

Overdosage/Toxicology Symptoms of overdose include unsteady gait, slurred speech, confusion, jaundice, hypothermia, hypotension, respiratory depression, and coma. In severe overdose, charcoal hemoperfusion may accelerate removal. Treatment is symptom-directed and supportive.

Pharmacodynamics/Kinetics
Onset of Action: Oral: Hypnosis: 20-60 minutes; I.V.: ~5 minutes; Peak effect: I.V.: ~30 minutes
Duration of Action: Oral: 6-10 hours; I.V.: 4-10 hours
Absorption: Oral: 70% to 90%
Time to Peak: Serum: Oral: 1-6 hours
Protein Binding: 20% to 45%; decreased in neonates
Half-Life Elimination: Neonates: 45-500 hours; Infants: 20-133 hours; Children: 37-73 hours; Adults: 53-140 hours
Metabolism: Hepatic via hydroxylation and glucuronide conjugation
Excretion: Urine (20% to 50% as unchanged drug)

Dosing
Adults:
Sedation: Oral, I.M.: 30-120 mg/day in 2-3 divided doses
Hypnotic: Oral, I.M., I.V., SubQ: 100-320 mg at bedtime
Preoperative sedation: I.M.: 100-200 mg 1-1.5 hours before procedure
Anticonvulsant/status epilepticus:
Loading dose: I.V.: 300-800 mg initially followed by 120-240 mg/dose at 20-minute intervals until seizures are controlled or a total dose of 1-2 g
Maintenance dose: Oral, I.V.: 1-3 mg/kg/day in divided doses or 50-100 mg 2-3 times/ day
Sedative/hypnotic withdrawal (unlabeled use): Initial daily requirement is determined by substituting phenobarbital 30 mg for every 100 mg pentobarbital used during tolerance testing; then daily requirement is decreased by 10% of initial dose.
Elderly: Geriatric patients should be started at the lowest recommended dose. Refer to adult dosing.
Pediatrics:
Sedation: Oral: Children: 2 mg/kg 3 times/day
Hypnotic: I.M., I.V., SubQ: Children: 3-5 mg/kg at bedtime
Preoperative sedation: Oral, I.M., I.V.: Children: 1-3 mg/kg 1-1.5 hours before procedure
Anticonvulsant/Status epilepticus (Loading dose): I.V.: Infants and Children: 10-20 mg/ kg in a single or divided dose; in select patients may administer additional 5 mg/kg/dose every 15-30 minutes until seizure is controlled or a total dose of 40 mg/kg is reached
Anticonvulsant maintenance dose: Oral, I.V.:
Infants: 5-8 mg/kg/day in 1-2 divided doses
Children:
1-5 years: 6-8 mg/kg/day in 1-2 divided doses
5-12 years: 4-6 mg/kg/day in 1-2 divided doses
>12 years: 1-3 mg/kg/day in divided doses or 50-100 mg 2-3 times/day
Renal Impairment:
Cl_{cr} <10 mL/minute: Administer every 12-16 hours.
Moderately dialyzable (20% to 50%)
Hepatic Impairment: Increased side effects may occur in severe liver disease. Monitor plasma levels and adjust dose accordingly.

Available Dosage Forms
Elixir: 20 mg/5 mL (5 mL, 7.5 mL, 15 mL, 473 mL, 946 mL, 4000 mL) [contains alcohol]
Injection, solution, as sodium: 60 mg/mL (1 mL); 130 mg/mL (1 mL) [contains alcohol]
Luminal® Sodium: 60 mg/mL (1 mL); 130 mg/mL (1 mL) [contains alcohol 10%]
Tablet: 15 mg, 30 mg, 32 mg, 60 mg, 65 mg, 100 mg
(Continued)

Phenobarbital *(Continued)*

Monitoring and Teaching Issues

Physical Assessment: Assess effectiveness and interactions of other medications patient may be taking. Assess for history of addiction; long-term use can result in dependence, abuse, or tolerance; periodically evaluate need for continued use. Monitor cardio/respiratory and CNS status; use safety precautions. Monitor effectiveness of therapy and adverse reactions. **Oral:** Monitor therapeutic effectiveness and adverse reactions at beginning of therapy and periodically with long-term use. Assess knowledge/teach patient appropriate use, possible side effects, and symptoms to report.

Monitoring Laboratory Tests: Phenobarbital serum concentrations, CBC, LFTs

Patient Education: I.M./I.V.: Patient instructions and information are determined by patient condition and therapeutic purpose. If self-administered, use exactly as directed; do not increase dose or frequency. Drug may cause physical and/or psychological dependence. While using this medication, do not use alcohol and other prescription or OTC medications (especially pain medications, sedatives, antihistamines, or hypnotics) without consulting prescriber. Maintain adequate hydration (2-3 L/day of fluids) unless instructed to restrict fluid intake. You may experience drowsiness, dizziness, or blurred vision (use caution when driving or engaging in tasks requiring alertness until response to drug is known); nausea, vomiting, or loss of appetite (small frequent meals, frequent mouth care, chewing gum, or sucking lozenges may help); or constipation (increased exercise, fluids, fruit, or fiber may help). Report skin rash or irritation; CNS changes (confusion, depression, increased sedation, excitation, headache, insomnia, or nightmares); respiratory difficulty or shortness of breath; changes in urinary pattern or menstrual pattern; muscle weakness or tremors; or difficulty swallowing or feeling of tightness in throat. **Pregnancy/ breast-feeding precautions:** Do not get pregnant while taking this medication; use appropriate contraceptive measures. Breast-feeding is not recommended.

Dietary Considerations: Vitamin D: Loss in vitamin D due to malabsorption; increase intake of foods rich in vitamin D. Supplementation of vitamin D and/or calcium may be necessary. Sodium content of injection (65 mg, 1 mL): 6 mg (0.3 mEq).

Geriatric Considerations: Due to its long half-life and risk of dependence, phenobarbital is not recommended as a sedative or hypnotic in the elderly. Interpretive guidelines from the Health Care Financing Administration discourage the use of this agent as a sedative/ hypnotic in long-term care residents.

Pregnancy Risk Factor: D

Pregnancy Issues: Crosses the placenta. Cardiac defect reported; hemorrhagic disease of newborn due to fetal vitamin K depletion may occur; may induce maternal folic acid deficiency; withdrawal symptoms observed in infant following delivery. Epilepsy itself, number of medications, genetic factors, or a combination of these probably influence the teratogenicity of anticonvulsant therapy. Benefit:risk ratio usually favors continued use during pregnancy.

Lactation: Enters breast milk/not recommended (AAP recommends use "with caution")

Breast-Feeding Issues: Sedation has been reported in nursing infants; infantile spasms may occur after weaning from breast milk. AAP recommends USE WITH CAUTION.

Administration

I.V.: Avoid rapid I.V. administration >50 mg/minute. Avoid intra-arterial injection.

Compatibility: Stable in dextran 6% in dextrose, dextran 6% in NS, D_5LR, $D_5\frac{1}{4}NS$, $D_5\frac{1}{2}NS$, D_5NS, D_5W, $D_{10}W$, LR, $\frac{1}{2}NS$, NS

Y-site administration: Incompatible with amphotericin B cholesteryl sulfate complex, hydromorphone

Compatibility in syringe: Incompatible with hydromorphone, pentazocine, ranitidine, sufentanil

Compatibility when admixed: Incompatible with chlorpromazine, cimetidine, clindamycin, dimenhydrinate, diphenhydramine, droperidol, ephedrine, hydralazine, hydrocortisone sodium succinate, hydroxyzine, insulin (regular), kanamycin, levorphanol, meperidine, morphine, norepinephrine, pancuronium, penicillin G, pentazocine, phenytoin, procaine, prochlorperazine edisylate, prochlorperazine mesylate, promazine, promethazine, streptomycin, succinylcholine, vancomycin

Storage: Protect elixir from light. Not stable in aqueous solutions. Use only clear solutions. Do not add to acidic solutions; precipitation may occur.

Additional Information Injectable solutions contain propylene glycol.

Related Information

Anticonvulsants By Seizure Type *on page 1712*
Compatibility of Drugs *on page 1723*
Peak and Trough Guidelines *on page 1694*

♦ **Phenobarbital, Hyoscyamine, Atropine, and Scopolamine** *see* Hyoscyamine, Atropine, Scopolamine, and Phenobarbital *on page 777*

♦ **Phenobarbital Sodium** *see* Phenobarbital *on page 1196*

♦ **Phenobarbitone** *see* Phenobarbital *on page 1196*

♦ **Phenoptic®** *see* Phenylephrine *on page 1200*

♦ **Phenoxymethyl Penicillin** *see* Penicillin V Potassium *on page 1177*

Phentolamine *(fen TOLE a meen)*

Synonyms Phentolamine Mesylate; Regitine [DSC]

Generic Available Yes

Pharmacologic Category Alpha$_1$ Blocker

Medication Safety Issues

Sound-alike/look-alike issues:

Phentolamine may be confused with phentermine, Ventolin®

Use Diagnosis of pheochromocytoma and treatment of hypertension associated with pheochromocytoma or other forms of hypertension caused by excess sympathomimetic amines; as treatment of dermal necrosis after extravasation of drugs with alpha-adrenergic effects (norepinephrine, dopamine, epinephrine)

Unlabeled/Investigational Use Treatment of pralidoxime-induced hypertension

Mechanism of Action/Effect Competitively blocks alpha-adrenergic receptors to produce brief antagonism of circulating epinephrine and norepinephrine to reduce hypertension caused by alpha effects of these catecholamines; also has a positive inotropic and chronotropic effect on the heart

Contraindications Hypersensitivity to phentolamine or any component of the formulation; renal impairment; coronary or cerebral arteriosclerosis; concurrent use with phosphodiesterase-5 (PDE-5) inhibitors including sildenafil (>25 mg), tadalafil, or vardenafil

Warnings/Precautions Myocardial infarction, cerebrovascular spasm and cerebrovascular occlusion have occurred following administration. Use with caution in patients with gastritis or peptic ulcer, tachycardia, or a history of cardiac arrhythmias.

Drug Interactions

Decreased Effect: Decreased effect of phentolamine with epinephrine and ephedrine.

Increased Effect/Toxicity: Phentolamine's toxicity is increased with ethanol (disulfiram reaction). Blood pressure-lowering effects are additive with sildenafil (use with extreme caution at a dose ≤25 mg), tadalafil (use is contraindicated by the manufacturer), and vardenafil (use is contraindicated by the manufacturer).

Lab Interactions Increased LFTs rarely

Adverse Reactions Frequency not defined.

Cardiovascular: Hypotension, tachycardia, arrhythmia, flushing, orthostatic hypotension

Central nervous system: Dizziness

Gastrointestinal: Nausea, vomiting, diarrhea

Neuromuscular & skeletal: Weakness

Respiratory: Nasal congestion

Case report: Pulmonary hypertension

Overdosage/Toxicology Symptoms of overdose include tachycardia, shock, vomiting, and dizziness. If fluid replacement is inadequate to treat hypotension, only alpha-adrenergic vasopressors such as norepinephrine should be used. Mixed agents such as epinephrine may cause more hypotension.

Pharmacodynamics/Kinetics

Onset of Action: I.M.: 15-20 minutes; I.V.: Immediate

Duration of Action: I.M.: 30-45 minutes; I.V.: 15-30 minutes

Half-Life Elimination: 19 minutes

Metabolism: Hepatic

Excretion: Urine (10% as unchanged drug)

Dosing

Adults & Elderly:

Treatment of alpha-adrenergic drug extravasation: SubQ:

Infiltrate area with a small amount (eg, 1 mL) of solution (made by diluting 5-10 mg in 10 mL of NS) within 12 hours of extravasation; do not exceed 0.1-0.2 mg/kg or 5 mg total

If dose is effective, normal skin color should return to the blanched area within 1 hour.

Diagnosis of pheochromocytoma: I.M., I.V.: 5 mg

Surgery for pheochromocytoma: Hypertension: I.M., I.V.: 5 mg given 1-2 hours before procedure and repeated as needed every 2-4 hours

Hypertensive crisis: I.V.: 5-20 mg

Treatment of pralidoxime-induced hypertension (unlabeled use): I.V.: 5 mg

Pediatrics:

Treatment of alpha-adrenergic drug extravasation: SubQ: Infiltrate area with a small amount (eg, 1 mL) of solution (made by diluting 5-10 mg in 10 mL of NS) within 12 hours of extravasation; do not exceed 0.1-0.2 mg/kg or 5 mg total

Diagnosis of pheochromocytoma: I.M., I.V.: 0.05-0.1 mg/kg/dose, maximum single dose: 5 mg

Surgery for pheochromocytoma: Hypertension: I.M., I.V.: 0.05-0.1 mg/kg/dose given 1-2 hours before procedure; repeat as needed every 2-4 hours until hypertension is controlled; maximum single dose: 5 mg.

Treatment of pralidoxime-induced hypertension (unlabeled use): I.V.: 1 mg

Available Dosage Forms Injection, powder for reconstitution, as mesylate: 5 mg

Monitoring and Teaching Issues

Physical Assessment: Use caution in presence of gastritis, peptic ulcer, tachycardia, or history of arrhythmias (see Warnings/Precautions). Assess potential for interactions with other pharmacological agents patient may be taking (eg, additive hypotensive effects and toxicity; see Drug Interactions). See Dosing and Administration for specifics and cautions according to purpose for use (eg, caution when used to treat extravasation). Assess patient response (eg, tachycardia, arrhythmias, hypo- and hypertension, nausea/vomiting; see Adverse Reactions). Teach patient adverse symptoms to report (see Patient Education).

Patient Education: This medication can only be administered by infusion or injection. Report immediately any pain at infusion/injection site. May cause orthostatic hypotension (use caution when changing position or call for assistance). Report dizziness, rapid heartbeat, feelings of weakness, or nausea/vomiting. **Pregnancy/breast-feeding precautions:** Inform prescriber if you are or intend to become pregnant. Consult prescriber if breast-feeding.

Pregnancy Risk Factor: C

Lactation: Excretion in breast milk unknown

Administration

I.V.:

Vasoconstrictor (alpha-adrenergic agonist) extravasation: Infiltrate the area of extravasation with multiple small injections using only 27- or 30-gauge needles and changing the needle between each skin entry. Be careful not to cause so much swelling of the extremity or digit that a compartment syndrome occurs. If infiltration is severe, may also need to consult vascular surgeon.

Pheochromocytoma: Inject each 5 mg over 1 minute.

Reconstitution: Reconstituted solution is stable for 48 hours at room temperature and 1 week when refrigerated.

Compatibility: Stable in NS

♦ **Phentolamine Mesylate**   *see* Phentolamine *on page 1198*
♦ **Phenylalanine Mustard**   *see* Melphalan *on page 945*
♦ **Phenylazo Diamino Pyridine Hydrochloride**   *see* Phenazopyridine *on page 1193*

Phenylephrine   (fen il EF rin)

U.S. Brand Names AK-Dilate®; AK-Nefrin®; Formulation R™ [OTC]; Medicone® [OTC]; Mydfrin®; Neo-Synephrine® Extra Strength [OTC]; Neo-Synephrine® Mild [OTC]; Neo-Synephrine® Ophthalmic; Neo-Synephrine® Regular Strength [OTC]; Nostril® [OTC]; Phenoptic®; Prefrin™ [DSC]; Relief® [OTC]; Vicks® Sinex® Nasal Spray [OTC]; Vicks® Sinex® UltraFine Mist [OTC]

Synonyms Phenylephrine Hydrochloride

Generic Available Yes: Excludes nasal drops and spray

Pharmacologic Category Alpha/Beta Agonist; Ophthalmic Agent, Antiglaucoma; Ophthalmic Agent, Mydriatic

Medication Safety Issues
Sound-alike/look-alike issues:
  Mydfrin® may be confused with Midrin®

Use Treatment of hypotension, vascular failure in shock; as a vasoconstrictor in regional analgesia; as a mydriatic in ophthalmic procedures and treatment of wide-angle glaucoma; supraventricular tachycardia

For OTC use as symptomatic relief of nasal and nasopharyngeal mucosal congestion, treatment of hemorrhoids, relief of redness of the eye due to irritation

Mechanism of Action/Effect Potent, direct-acting alpha-adrenergic stimulator with weak beta-adrenergic activity; causes vasoconstriction of the arterioles of the nasal mucosa and conjunctiva; activates the dilator muscle of the pupil to cause contraction; produces vasoconstriction of arterioles in the body; produces systemic arterial vasoconstriction

Contraindications Hypersensitivity to phenylephrine, bisulfite (some products contain metabisulfite), or any component of the formulation; hypertension; ventricular tachycardia

Warnings/Precautions Use with caution in the elderly, patients with hyperthyroidism, bradycardia, partial heart block, myocardial disease, or severe CAD. Not a substitute for volume replacement. Avoid hypertension; monitor blood pressure closely and adjust infusion rate. Infuse into a large vein if possible. Watch I.V. site closely. Avoid extravasation. With intranasal formulation use, rebound congestion can occur when the drug is discontinued after chronic use.

Drug Interactions
  Decreased Effect: Alpha- and beta-adrenergic blocking agents may have a decreased effect if taken with phenylephrine.

  Increased Effect/Toxicity: Phenylephrine, taken with sympathomimetics, may induce tachycardia or arrhythmias. If taken with MAO inhibitors or oxytocic agents, actions may be potentiated.

Nutritional/Ethanol Interactions Herb/Nutraceutical: Avoid ephedra, yohimbe (may cause CNS stimulation).

Adverse Reactions Frequency not defined.
  Cardiovascular: Reflex bradycardia, excitability, restlessness, arrhythmia (rare), precordial pain or discomfort, pallor, hypertension, severe peripheral and visceral vasoconstriction, decreased cardiac output
  Central nervous system: Headache, anxiety, dizziness, tremor, paresthesia, restlessness
  Endocrine & metabolic: Metabolic acidosis
  Local: I.V.: Extravasation which may lead to necrosis and sloughing of surrounding tissue, blanching of skin
  Neuromuscular & skeletal: Pilomotor response, weakness
  Renal: Decreased renal perfusion, reduced urine output, reduced urine output
  Respiratory: Respiratory distress

Overdosage/Toxicology Symptoms of overdose include vomiting, hypertension, palpitations, paresthesia, and ventricular extrasystoles. Treatment is supportive. In extreme cases, I.V. phentolamine may be used.

Pharmacodynamics/Kinetics
  Onset of Action: I.M., SubQ: 10-15 minutes; I.V.: Immediate
  Duration of Action: I.M.: 0.5-2 hours; I.V.: 15-30 minutes; SubQ: 1 hour
  Half-Life Elimination: 2.5 hours; prolonged after long-term infusion
  Metabolism: Hepatic, via intestinal monoamine oxidase to phenolic conjugates
  Excretion: Urine (90%)

Dosing
  Adults:
    Nasal congestion (therapy should not exceed 5 continuous days): Intranasal: Instill 1-2 sprays or instill 1-2 drops every 4 hours of 0.25% to 0.5% solution as needed; 1% solution may be used in adults in cases of extreme nasal congestion. Do not use nasal solutions more than 3 days.
    Hypotension/shock:
      I.V. bolus: 0.1-0.5 mg/dose every 10-15 minutes as needed (initial dose should not exceed 0.5 mg)
      I.V. infusion: 10 mg in 250 mL D₅W or NS (1:25,000 dilution) (40 mcg/mL); start at 100-180 mcg/minute (2-5 mL/minute; 50-90 drops/minute) initially; when blood pressure is stabilized, maintenance rate: 40-60 mcg/minute (20-30 drops/minute); rates up to 360 mcg/minute have been reported; dosing range: 0.4-9.1 mcg/kg/minute
      Note: Concentrations up to 100-500 mg in 250 mL have been used.
    Paroxysmal supraventricular tachycardia: I.V.: 0.25-0.5 mg/dose over 20-30 seconds
    Ocular procedures: Ophthalmic: Instill 1 drop of 2.5% or 10% solution, may repeat in 10-60 minutes as needed.

Reduction in ocular redness (OTC formulation): Ophthalmic: Instill 1-2 drops 0.12% solution into affected eye, up to 4 times/day; do not use for >72 hours

Hemorrhoids: Rectal:

Cream/ointment: Apply to clean dry area, up to 4 times/day; may be used externally or inserted rectally using applicator.

Suppository: Insert 1 suppository rectally, up to 4 times/day

Elderly:

Nasal decongestant: Administer 2-3 drops or 1-2 sprays every 4 hours of 0.125% to 0.25% solution as needed; do not use more than 3 days.

Ophthalmic preparations for pupil dilation: Instill 1 drop of 2.5% solution, may repeat in 1 hour if necessary.

Refer to adult dosing for other uses and Geriatric Considerations for cautions on I.V. use.

Pediatrics:

Ocular procedures: Ophthalmic:

Infants <1 year: Instill 1 drop of 2.5% 15-30 minutes before procedures

Children: Refer to adult dosing

Nasal congestion (therapy should not exceed 5 continuous days): Intranasal:

2-6 years: Instill 1 drop every 2-4 hours of 0.125% solution as needed

6-12 years: Instill 1-2 sprays or instill 1-2 drops every 4 hours of 0.25% solution as needed

>12 years: Refer to adult dosing.

Hypotension/shock: Children:

I.V. bolus: 5-20 mcg/kg/dose every 10-15 minutes as needed

I.V. infusion: 0.1-0.5 mcg/kg/minute

Paroxysmal supraventricular tachycardia: I.V.: Children: 5-10 mcg/kg/dose over 20-30 seconds

Hemorrhoids: Children >12 years: Refer to adult dosing.

Available Dosage Forms [DSC] = Discontinued product

Cream, rectal (Formulation R™): 0.25% (30 g, 60 g) [contains sodium benzoate]

Injection, solution, as hydrochloride: 1% [10 mg/mL] (1 mL) [may contain sodium metabisulfite]

Ointment, rectal (Formulation R™): 0.25% (30 g, 60 g) [contains benzoic acid]

Solution, intranasal drops, as hydrochloride:

Neo-Synephrine® Extra Strength: 1% (15 mL)

Neo-Synephrine® Regular Strength: 0.5% (15 mL)

Solution, intranasal spray, as hydrochloride:

Neo-Synephrine® Extra Strength: 1% (15 mL)

Neo-Synephrine® Mild: 0.25% (15 mL)

Neo-Synephrine® Regular Strength: 0.5% (15 mL)

Nostril®: 0.25% (15 mL); 0.5% (15 mL)

Vicks® Sinex®, Vicks® Sinex® UltraFine Mist: 0.5% (15 mL)

Solution, ophthalmic, as hydrochloride: 2.5% (2 mL, 3 mL, 5 mL, 15 mL) [may contain sodium bisulfite]

AK-Dilate®: 2.5% (2 mL, 15 mL); 10% (5 mL)

AK-Nefrin®: 0.12% (15 mL)

Mydfrin®: 2.5% (3 mL, 5 mL) [contains sodium bisulfite]

Neo-Synephrine®: 2.5% (15 mL); 10% (5 mL)

Neo-Synephrine® Viscous: 10% (5 mL)

Phenoptic®: 2.5% (15 mL)

Prefrin™ [DSC], Relief®: 0.12% (15 mL)

Suppository, rectal: 0.25% (12s)

Medicone®: 0.25% (18s, 24s)

Monitoring and Teaching Issues

Physical Assessment: Assess other medications patient may be taking for effectiveness and interactions. Monitor therapeutic effectiveness and adverse reactions according to use. **Parenteral:** Monitor arterial blood gases, vital signs, adverse reactions, and infusion site. **Nasal/ophthalmic:** Assess knowledge/teach patient appropriate use, interventions to reduce side effects, and adverse symptoms to report. Systemic absorption from ophthalmic instillation is minimal.

Monitoring Laboratory Tests: Parenteral use: Monitor arterial blood gases

Patient Education: Nasal decongestant: Do not use for more than 3 days in a row. Clear nose as much as possible before use. Tilt head back and instill recommended dose of drops or spray. Do not blow nose for 5-10 minutes. You may experience transient stinging or burning.

Ophthalmic: Do not let tip of applicator touch eye; do not contaminate tip of applicator (may cause eye infection, eye damage, or vision loss). Open eye, look at ceiling, and instill prescribed amount of solution. Close eye and roll eye in all directions, and apply gentle pressure to inner corner of eye for 1-2 minutes after instillation. Temporary stinging or blurred vision may occur. Report persistent pain, burning, double vision, severe headache, or if condition worsens.

Pregnancy/breast-feeding precautions: Inform prescriber if you are pregnant. Consult prescriber if breast-feeding.

Geriatric Considerations: Phenylephrine I.V. should be used with extreme caution in the elderly. The 10% ophthalmic solution has caused increased blood pressure in elderly patients and its use should, therefore, be avoided. Since topical decongestants can be obtained OTC, elderly patients should be counseled about their proper use and in what disease states they should be avoided (see Warnings/Precautions).

Pregnancy Risk Factor: C

Lactation: Enters breast milk/not recommended

Administration

I.V.: Concentration and rate of infusion can be calculated using the following formulas: Dilute 0.6 mg x weight (kg) to 100 mL; then the dose in mcg/kg/minute = 0.1 x the infusion rate in mL/hour.

(Continued)

Phenylephrine *(Continued)*

Reconstitution: Solution for injection:
I.V. infusion: May dilute 10 mg in 500 mL NS or D_5W.
I.V. injection: Dilute with SWFI to a concentration of 1 mg/mL.
Compatibility: Stable in dextran 6% in dextrose, dextran 6% in NS, D_5LR, $D_5^1/_4NS$, $D_5^1/_2NS$, D_5NS, D_5W, $D_{10}W$, LR, $^1/_2NS$, NS, sodium bicarbonate 5%
Y-site administration: Incompatible with thiopental

Storage:
Solution for injection: Store vials at controlled room temperature of 15°C to 30°C (59°F to 86°F). Protect from light. Do not use solution if brown or contains a precipitate.
Ophthalmic solution: Store at controlled room temperature. Protect from light and excessive heat.

Additional Information Phenylephrine allows for close titration of blood pressure and should be used in patients with hypotension or shock due to peripheral vasodilation. Phenylephrine should not constitute sole therapy in patients with hypotension due to aortic dysfunction or hypovolemia. An important benefit of this drug is the short half-life, allowing rapid changes in dosage with prompt appropriate blood pressure responses. When administered intravenously, it should be used in intensive care settings or under very close monitoring.

Related Information
Inotropic and Vasoconstrictor Comparison *on page 1736*

♦ **Phenylephrine and Promethazine** *see* Promethazine and Phenylephrine *on page 1268*

Phenylephrine and Pyrilamine *(fen il EF rin & peer IL a meen)*

U.S. Brand Names Pyrilafen Tannate; Viravan®
Synonyms Pyrilamine Tannate and Phenylephrine Tannate
Generic Available Yes: Suspension
Pharmacologic Category Antihistamine; Antihistamine/Decongestant Combination; Sympathomimetic
Use Symptomatic relief of nasal congestion and discharge associated with the common cold, sinusitis, allergic rhinitis, and other respiratory tract conditions

Dosing
Adults: Relief of cough, congestion (Viravan®): Oral: 5-10 mL of the suspension or 1-2 tablets every 12 hours
Pediatrics: Relief of cough, congestion (Viravan®): Oral:
Children 2-6 years: 2.5 mL of the suspension or $^1/_2$ tablet every 12 hours
Children 6-12 years: 5 mL of the suspension or $^1/_2$ to 1 tablet every 12 hours
Children >12 years: Refer to adult dosing.

Available Dosage Forms
Suspension:
Pyrilafen Tannate: Phenylephrine tannate 5 mg and pyrilamine tannate 30 mg per 5 mL (120 mL) [strawberry-black currant flavor]
Viravan®: Phenylephrine tannate 12.5 mg and pyrilamine tannate 30 mg per 5 mL (120 mL, 480 mL) [contains sodium benzoate; grape flavor]
Tablet, chewable (Viravan®): Phenylephrine tannate 25 mg and pyrilamine tannate 30 mg [dye free; grape flavor]

Monitoring and Teaching Issues
Pregnancy Risk Factor: C
Lactation: Excretion in breast milk unknown/contraindicated
Related Information
Phenylephrine *on page 1200*

♦ **Phenylephrine, Chlorpheniramine, and Carbetapentane** *see* Carbetapentane, Phenylephrine, and Chlorpheniramine *on page 253*
♦ **Phenylephrine, Diphenhydramine, and Hydrocodone** *see* Hydrocodone, Phenylephrine, and Diphenhydramine *on page 759*
♦ **Phenylephrine, Guaifenesin, and Hydrocodone** *see* Hydrocodone, Phenylephrine, and Guaifenesin *on page 760*
♦ **Phenylephrine Hydrochloride** *see* Phenylephrine *on page 1200*
♦ **Phenylephrine Hydrochloride, Hydrocodone Bitartrate, and Chlorpheniramine Maleate** *see* Phenylephrine, Hydrocodone, and Chlorpheniramine *on page 1202*

Phenylephrine, Hydrocodone, and Chlorpheniramine *(fen il EF rin, hye droe KOE done, & klor fen IR a meen)*

U.S. Brand Names Coughtuss; Cytuss HC; De-Chlor HC; De-Chlor HD; Endagen™-HD; Endal® HD Plus; H-C Tussive; Histinex® HC; Histussin® HC; Hydron CP; Hydro-PC II; Hydro PC II Plus; Maxi-Tuss HC®; Maxi-Tuss HCX; Mintuss HC; Mintuss HD; Mintuss MS; Relacon-HC; Rindal HD Plus; Uni-Tricof HC; Uni-Tuss HC; Vanex-HD®; Z-Cof HC
Synonyms Chlorpheniramine, Phenylephrine, and Hydrocodone; Dihydrocodeine Bitartrate, Phenylephrine Hydrochloride, and Chlorpheniramine Maleate; Hydrocodone, Phenylephrine, and Chlorpheniramine; Phenylephrine Hydrochloride, Hydrocodone Bitartrate, and Chlorpheniramine Maleate
Controlled Substance C-III
Generic Available Yes
Pharmacologic Category Antihistamine; Antihistamine/Decongestant/Antitussive; Antitussive; Decongestant
Use Symptomatic relief of cough and congestion associated with the common cold, sinusitis, or acute upper respiratory tract infections

Dosing
Adults: Cough and congestion: Oral:
Endagen™-HD, Vanex-HD®: 10 mL 3-4 times/day (maximum: 40 mL/24 hours)
Histinex® HC, Cytuss HC, Endal® HD Plus: 10 mL every 4 hours (maximum: 40 mL/24 hours)

Maxi-Tuss HC®, Maxi-Tuss HCX: 5 mL every 4 hours (maximum: 30 mL/24 hours)

Z-Cof HC: 5-10 mL every 4-6 hours (maximum: 40 mL/24 hours)

Pediatrics: Cough and congestion: Oral:

Children 2-6 years: *Z-Cof HC:* 1.25-2.5 mL every 4-6 hours (maximum: 10 mL/24 hours)

Children 6-12 years:

Endagen™-HD, Vanex-HD®: 5 mL 3-4 times/day (maximum: 20 mL/24 hours)

Histinex® HC, Cytuss HC, Endal® HD Plus: 5 mL every 4 hours (maximum: 20 mL/24 hours)

Maxi-Tuss HC®, Maxi-Tuss HCX: 2.5 mL every 4 hours (maximum: 15 mL/24 hours)

Z-Cof HC: 2.5-5 mL every 4-6 hours as needed (maximum: 20 mL/24 hours)

Available Dosage Forms

Liquid: Phenylephrine hydrochloride 5 mg, hydrocodone bitartrate 5 mg, and chlorpheniramine maleate 2 mg per 5 mL (480 mL); phenylephrine hydrochloride 10 mg, hydrocodone bitartrate 2.5 mg, and chlorpheniramine maleate 4 mg per 5 mL (480 mL); phenylephrine hydrochloride 10 mg, hydrocodone bitartrate 5 mg, and chlorpheniramine maleate 2 mg per 5 mL (480 mL)

Coughtuss: Phenylephrine hydrochloride 5 mg, hydrocodone bitartrate 5 mg, and chlorpheniramine maleate 2 mg per 5 mL (480 mL) [alcohol free, sugar free]

De-Chlor HC: Phenylephrine hydrochloride 10 mg, hydrocodone bitartrate 2.5 mg, and chlorpheniramine maleate 2 mg per 5 mL (480 mL) [cherry flavor]

De-Chlor HD: Phenylephrine hydrochloride 10 mg, hydrocodone bitartrate 2.5 mg, and chlorpheniramine maleate 4 mg per 5 mL (480 mL) [cherry flavor]

Endal® HD Plus: Phenylephrine hydrochloride 7.5 mg, hydrocodone bitartrate 3.5 mg, and chlorpheniramine maleate 2 mg per 5 mL (480 mL) [alcohol free, sugar free; black raspberry flavor]

Hydron CP: Phenylephrine hydrochloride 10 mg, hydrocodone bitartrate 5 mg, and chlorpheniramine maleate 2 mg per 5 mL (480 mL) [pineapple-orange flavor]

Hydro PC II Plus: Phenylephrine hydrochloride 7.5 mg, hydrocodone bitartrate 3.5 mg, and chlorpheniramine maleate 2 mg per 5 mL (480 mL) [strawberry flavor]

Maxi-Tuss HCX: Phenylephrine hydrochloride 12 mg, hydrocodone bitartrate 6 mg, and chlorpheniramine maleate 2 mg per 5 mL (480 mL) [alcohol free, sugar free; contains aspartame; vanilla bean flavor]

Relacon-HC: Phenylephrine hydrochloride 10 mg, hydrocodone bitartrate 3.5 mg, and chlorpheniramine maleate 2.5 mg per 5 mL (480 mL) [raspberry flavor]

Uni-Tricof HC: Phenylephrine hydrochloride 5 mg, hydrocodone bitartrate 1.67 mg, and chlorpheniramine maleate 2 mg per 5 mL (480 mL) [strawberry flavor]

Vanex-HD®: Phenylephrine hydrochloride 5 mg, hydrocodone bitartrate 1.7 mg, and chlorpheniramine maleate 2 mg per 5mL (480 mL) [dye free; cherry flavor]

Z-Cof HC: Phenylephrine hydrochloride 10 mg, hydrocodone bitartrate 3.5 mg, and chlorpheniramine maleate 2.5 mg per 5 mL (480 mL) [alcohol free, sugar free; raspberry flavor]

Syrup:

Cytuss HC: Phenylephrine hydrochloride 5 mg, hydrocodone bitartrate 2.5 mg, and chlorpheniramine maleate 2 mg per 5 mL (480 mL) [peach flavor]

Endagen™-HD: Phenylephrine hydrochloride 5 mg, hydrocodone bitartrate 1.7 mg, and chlorpheniramine maleate 2 mg per 5 mL (480 mL) [cherry flavor]

H-C Tussive: Phenylephrine hydrochloride 5 mg, hydrocodone bitartrate 2.5 mg, and chlorpheniramine maleate 2 mg per 5 mL (120 mL, 480 mL, 4000 mL) [orange-pineapple flavor]

Histinex® HC: Phenylephrine hydrochloride 5 mg, hydrocodone bitartrate 2.5 mg, and chlorpheniramine maleate 2 mg per 5 mL (480 mL, 960 mL) [alcohol free, sugar free; contains sodium benzoate]

Histussin® HC: Phenylephrine hydrochloride 5 mg, hydrocodone bitartrate 2.5 mg, and chlorpheniramine maleate 2 mg per 5 mL (480 mL) [alcohol free, sugar free; orange-pineapple flavor]

Hydro-PC II: Phenylephrine hydrochloride 7.5 mg, hydrocodone bitartrate 2 mg, and chlorpheniramine maleate 2 mg per 5 mL (480 mL) [strawberry flavor]

Maxi-Tuss HC®: Phenylephrine hydrochloride 10 mg, hydrocodone bitartrate 2.5 mg, and chlorpheniramine maleate 4 mg per 5 mL (480 mL) [orange flavor]

Mintuss HC: Phenylephrine hydrochloride 10 mg, hydrocodone bitartrate 2.5 mg, and chlorpheniramine maleate 2 mg per 5 mL (480 mL) [alcohol free; contains sodium benzoate; black cherry flavor]

Mintuss HD: Phenylephrine hydrochloride 10 mg, hydrocodone bitartrate 2.5 mg, and chlorpheniramine maleate 4 mg per 5 mL (480 mL) [alcohol free; contains sodium benzoate; cherry flavor]

Mintuss MS: Phenylephrine hydrochloride 10 mg, hydrocodone bitartrate 5 mg, and chlorpheniramine maleate 2 mg per 5 mL (480 mL) [alcohol free; contains sodium benzoate; orange flavor]

Rindal HD Plus: Phenylephrine hydrochloride 7.5 mg, hydrocodone bitartrate 3.5 mg, and chlorpheniramine maleate 2 mg per 5 mL (480 mL) [alcohol free, sugar free; contains sodium benzoate; black raspberry flavor]

Uni-Tuss HC: Phenylephrine hydrochloride 5 mg, hydrocodone bitartrate 1.67 mg, and chlorpheniramine maleate 2 mg per 5 mL (480 mL) [sugar free; orange flavor]

Monitoring and Teaching Issues

Pregnancy Risk Factor: C

Lactation: See individual agents.

Related Information

Phenylephrine *on page 1200*

◆ **Phenylephrine, Promethazine, and Codeine** *see* Promethazine, Phenylephrine, and Codeine *on page 1268*

Phenylephrine, Pyrilamine, and Dextromethorphan
(fen il EF rin, peer IL a meen, & deks troe meth OR fan)

U.S. Brand Names Codal-DM [OTC]; Codimal® DM [OTC]; Codituss DM [OTC]; Viravan®-DM

Synonyms Dextromethorphan Tannate, Pyrilamine Tannate, and Phenylephrine Tannate; Pyrilamine Maleate, Dextromethorphan Hydrobromide, and Phenylephrine Hydrochloride

Generic Available Yes

Pharmacologic Category Antihistamine; Antihistamine/Decongestant/Antitussive; Antitussive; Sympathomimetic

Use Symptomatic relief of cough, nasal congestion, and discharge associated with the common cold, sinusitis, allergic rhinitis, and other respiratory tract conditions

Dosing

Adults: Relief of cough, congestion: Oral:
  Codimal® DM: 10 mL every 4 hours; maximum: 60 mL/24 hours
  Viravan®-DM: 5-10 mL of the suspension or 1-2 tablets every 12 hours

Pediatrics: Relief of cough, congestion: Oral:
  Children 2-6 years (Viravan®-DM): 2.5 mL of the suspension or $^1/_2$ tablet every 12 hours
  Children 6-12 years:
    Codimal® DM: 5 mL every 4 hours; maximum: 30 mL/24 hours
    Viravan®-DM: 5 mL of the suspension or $^1/_2$ to 1 tablet every 12 hours
  Children >12 years: Refer to adult dosing.

Available Dosage Forms

Suspension (Viravan®-DM): Phenylephrine tannate 12.5 mg, pyrilamine tannate 30 mg, and dextromethorphan tannate 25 mg per 5 mL (480 mL) [contains sodium benzoate; grape flavor]

Syrup:
  Codal-DM: Phenylephrine hydrochloride 5 mg, pyrilamine maleate 8.33 mg, and dextromethorphan hydrobromide 10 mg (480 mL) [cherry flavor]
  Codimal® DM: Phenylephrine hydrochloride 5 mg, pyrilamine maleate 8.33 mg, and dextromethorphan hydrobromide 10 mg (120 mL, 480 mL) [alcohol free, dye free, sugar free; contains benzoic acid]
  Codituss DM: Phenylephrine hydrochloride 5 mg, pyrilamine maleate 8.33 mg, and dextromethorphan hydrobromide 10 mg (120 mL, 480 mL) [alcohol free, dye free, sugar free; cherry punch flavor]

Tablet, chewable (Viravan®-DM): Phenylephrine tannate 25 mg, pyrilamine tannate 30 mg, and dextromethorphan tannate 25 mg [dye free; grape flavor]

Monitoring and Teaching Issues

Pregnancy Risk Factor: C

Lactation: Excretion in breast milk unknown/contraindicated

Related Information

Phenylephrine *on page 1200*

◆ **Phenylethylmalonylurea** *see Phenobarbital on page 1196*

◆ **Phenylisohydantoin** *see Pemoline on page 1170*

◆ **Phenytek™** *see Phenytoin on page 1204*

Phenytoin (FEN i toyn)

U.S. Brand Names Dilantin®; Phenytek™

Synonyms Diphenylhydantoin; DPH; Phenytoin Sodium; Phenytoin Sodium, Extended; Phenytoin Sodium, Prompt

Generic Available Yes: Excludes chewable tablet, extended release capsule

Pharmacologic Category Antiarrhythmic Agent, Class Ib; Anticonvulsant, Hydantoin

Medication Safety Issues

Sound-alike/look-alike issues:
  Phenytoin may be confused with phenelzine, phentermine
  Dilantin® may be confused with Dilaudid®, diltiazem, Dipentum®

Use Management of generalized tonic-clonic (grand mal), complex partial seizures; prevention of seizures following head trauma/neurosurgery

Unlabeled/Investigational Use Ventricular arrhythmias, including those associated with digitalis intoxication, prolonged QT interval and surgical repair of congenital heart diseases in children; epidermolysis bullosa

Mechanism of Action/Effect Stabilizes neuronal membranes and decreases seizure activity by increasing efflux or decreasing influx of sodium ions across cell membranes in the motor cortex during generation of nerve impulses; prolongs effective refractory period and suppresses ventricular pacemaker automaticity, shortens action potential in the heart

Contraindications Hypersensitivity to phenytoin, other hydantoins, or any component of the formulation; pregnancy

Warnings/Precautions May increase frequency of petit mal seizures; I.V. form may cause hypotension, skin necrosis at I.V. site; avoid I.V. administration in small veins; use with caution in patients with porphyria; discontinue if rash or lymphadenopathy occurs; use with caution in patients with hepatic dysfunction, sinus bradycardia, SA block, or AV block; use with caution in elderly or debilitated patients, or in any condition associated with low serum albumin levels, which will increase the free fraction of phenytoin in the serum and, therefore, the pharmacologic response. Sedation, confusional states, or cerebellar dysfunction (loss of motor coordination) may occur at higher total serum concentrations, or at lower total serum concentrations when the free fraction of phenytoin is increased. Abrupt withdrawal may precipitate status epilepticus.

Drug Interactions

Cytochrome P450 Effect: Substrate of CYP2C8/9 (major), 2C19 (major), 3A4 (minor); **Induces** CYP2B6 (strong), 2C8/9 (strong), 2C19 (strong), 3A4 (strong)

Decreased Effect: Phenytoin may enhance the metabolism of estrogen and/or oral contraceptives, decreasing their clinical effect; an alternative method of contraception should be considered. Phenytoin may increase the metabolism of anticonvulsants including barbiturates, carbamazepine, ethosuximide, felbamate, lamotrigine, tiagabine, topiramate, and zonisamide. Valproic acid may increase, decrease, or have no effect on phenytoin serum concentrations. Phenytoin may also decrease the serum concentrations/effects of some antiarrhythmics (disopyramide, propafenone, quinidine, quetiapine) and tricyclic antidepressants may be reduced by phenytoin. Phenytoin may enhance the metabolism of doxycycline, decreasing its clinical effect; higher dosages may be required. Phenytoin may increase the metabolism of chloramphenicol or itraconazole.

Phenytoin may decrease the levels/effects of amiodarone, benzodiazepines, bupropion, calcium channel blockers, carbamazepine, citalopram, clarithromycin, clozapine, cyclosporine, efavirenz, erythromycin, estrogens, fluoxetine, glimepiride, glipizide, losartan, methsuximide, mirtazapine, nateglinide, nefazodone, nevirapine, phenytoin, pioglitazone, promethazine, propranolol, protease inhibitors, proton pump inhibitors, rosiglitazone, selegiline, sertraline, sulfonamides, tacrolimus, venlafaxine. voriconazole, warfarin, zafirlukast, and other CYP2B6, 2C8/9, 2C19, or 3A4 substrates.

The levels/effects of phenytoin may be decreased by aminoglutethimide, carbamazepine, phenobarbital, rifampin, rifapentine, secobarbital, and other CYP2C8/9 or 2C19 inducers. Clozapine and vigabatrin may reduce phenytoin serum concentrations. Ciprofloxacin may decrease serum phenytoin concentrations. Dexamethasone may decrease serum phenytoin concentrations. Replacement of folic acid has been reported to increase the metabolism of phenytoin, decreasing its serum concentrations and/or increasing seizures.

Initially, phenytoin increases the response to warfarin; this is followed by a decrease in response to warfarin. Phenytoin may inhibit the anti-Parkinson effect of levodopa. The duration of neuromuscular blockade from neuromuscular-blocking agents may be decreased by phenytoin. Phenytoin may enhance the metabolism of methadone resulting in methadone withdrawal. Phenytoin may decrease serum levels/effects of digitalis glycosides, theophylline, and thyroid hormones.

Several chemotherapeutic agents have been associated with a decrease in serum phenytoin levels; includes cisplatin, bleomycin, carmustine, methotrexate, and vinblastine. Enzyme-inducing anticonvulsant therapy may reduce the effectiveness of some chemotherapy regimens (specifically in ALL). Teniposide and methotrexate may be cleared more rapidly in these patients.

Increased Effect/Toxicity: The sedative effects of phenytoin may be additive with other CNS depressants including ethanol, barbiturates, sedatives, antidepressants, narcotic analgesics, and benzodiazepines. Selected anticonvulsants (felbamate, gabapentin, and topiramate) have been reported to increase phenytoin levels/effects. In addition, serum phenytoin concentrations may be increased by allopurinol, amiodarone, calcium channel blockers (including diltiazem and nifedipine), cimetidine, disulfiram, methylphenidate, metronidazole, omeprazole, selective serotonin reuptake inhibitors (SSRIs), ticlopidine, tricyclic antidepressants, trazodone, and trimethoprim.

The levels/effects of phenytoin may be increased by delavirdine, fluconazole, fluvoxamine, gemfibrozil, isoniazid, ketoconazole, nicardipine, NSAIDs, omeprazole, pioglitazone, sulfonamides, ticlopidine, and other CYP2C8/9 or 2C19 inhibitors.

Phenytoin enhances the conversion of primidone to phenobarbital resulting in elevated phenobarbital serum concentrations. Concurrent use of acetazolamide with phenytoin may result in an increased risk of osteomalacia. Concurrent use of phenytoin and lithium has resulted in lithium intoxication. Valproic acid (and sulfisoxazole) may displace phenytoin from binding sites; valproic acid may increase, decrease, or have no effect on phenytoin serum concentrations. Phenytoin transiently increased the response to warfarin initially; this is followed by an inhibition of the hypoprothrombinemic response. Phenytoin may enhance the hepatotoxic potential of acetaminophen overdoses. Concurrent use of dopamine and intravenous phenytoin may lead to an increased risk of hypotension.

Nutritional/Ethanol Interactions
Ethanol:
Acute use: Avoid or limit ethanol (inhibits metabolism of phenytoin). Watch for sedation.
Chronic use: Avoid or limit ethanol (stimulates metabolism of phenytoin).
Food: Phenytoin serum concentrations may be altered if taken with food. If taken with enteral nutrition, phenytoin serum concentrations may be decreased. Tube feedings decrease bioavailability; hold tube feedings 2 hours before and 2 hours after phenytoin administration. May decrease calcium, folic acid, and vitamin D levels.
Herb/Nutraceutical: Avoid evening primrose (seizure threshold decreased). Avoid valerian, St John's wort, kava kava, gotu kola (may increase CNS depression).

Lab Interactions Increased glucose, alkaline phosphatase (S); decreased thyroxine (S), calcium (S)

Adverse Reactions I.V. effects: Hypotension, bradycardia, cardiac arrhythmia, cardiovascular collapse (especially with rapid I.V. use), venous irritation and pain, thrombophlebitis

Effects not related to plasma phenytoin concentrations: Hypertrichosis, gingival hypertrophy, thickening of facial features, carbohydrate intolerance, folic acid deficiency, peripheral neuropathy, vitamin D deficiency, osteomalacia, systemic lupus erythematosus

Concentration-related effects: Nystagmus, blurred vision, diplopia, ataxia, slurred speech, dizziness, drowsiness, lethargy, coma, rash, fever, nausea, vomiting, gum tenderness, confusion, mood changes, folic acid depletion, osteomalacia, hyperglycemia

Related to elevated concentrations:
>20 mcg/mL: Far lateral nystagmus
>30 mcg/mL: 45° lateral gaze nystagmus and ataxia
>40 mcg/mL: Decreased mentation
>100 mcg/mL: Death

Cardiovascular: Hypotension, bradycardia, cardiac arrhythmia, cardiovascular collapse
Central nervous system: Psychiatric changes, slurred speech, dizziness, drowsiness, headache, insomnia
Dermatologic: Rash
Gastrointestinal: Constipation, nausea, vomiting, gingival hyperplasia, enlargement of lips
Hematologic: Leukopenia, thrombocytopenia, agranulocytosis
Hepatic: Hepatitis
(Continued)

Phenytoin *(Continued)*

Local: Thrombophlebitis

Neuromuscular & skeletal: Tremor, peripheral neuropathy, paresthesia

Ocular: Diplopia, nystagmus, blurred vision

Rarely seen effects: SLE-like syndrome, lymphadenopathy, hepatitis, Stevens-Johnson syndrome, blood dyscrasias, dyskinesias, pseudolymphoma, lymphoma, venous irritation and pain, coarsening of the facial features, hypertrichosis

Overdosage/Toxicology Symptoms of overdose include unsteady gait, slurred speech, confusion, nausea, hypothermia, fever, hypotension, respiratory depression, coma. Treatment is symptomatic.

Pharmacodynamics/Kinetics

Onset of Action: I.V.: ~0.5-1 hour

Absorption: Oral: Slow

Bioavailability: Form dependent

Time to Peak: Serum (form dependent): Oral: Extended-release capsule: 4-12 hours; Immediate release preparation: 2-3 hours

Protein Binding:

Neonates: ≥80% (≤20% free)

Infants: ≥85% (≤15% free)

Adults: 90% to 95%

Others: Decreased protein binding

Disease states resulting in a decrease in serum albumin concentration: Burns, hepatic cirrhosis, nephrotic syndrome, pregnancy, cystic fibrosis

Disease states resulting in an apparent decrease in affinity of phenytoin for serum albumin: Renal failure, jaundice (severe), other drugs (displacers), hyperbilirubinemia (total bilirubin >15 mg/dL), Cl_{cr} <25 mL/minute (unbound fraction is increased two- to threefold in uremia)

Half-Life Elimination: Oral: 22 hours (range: 7-42 hours)

Metabolism: Follows dose-dependent capacity-limited (Michaelis-Menten) pharmacokinetics with increased V_{max} in infants >6 months of age and children versus adults; major metabolite (via oxidation), HPPA, undergoes enterohepatic recirculation

Excretion: Urine (<5% as unchanged drug); as glucuronides

Clearance: Highly variable, dependent upon intrinsic hepatic function and dose administered; increased clearance and decreased serum concentrations with febrile illness

Dosing

Adults & Elderly:

Status epilepticus: I.V.: Loading dose: Manufacturer recommends 10-15 mg/kg, however, 15-25 mg/kg has been used clinically; maintenance dose: 300 mg/day or 5-6 mg/kg/day in 3 divided doses or 1-2 divided doses using extended release

Anticonvulsant: Oral: Loading dose: 15-20 mg/kg; based on phenytoin serum concentrations and recent dosing history; administer oral loading dose in 3 divided doses given every 2-4 hours to decrease GI adverse effects and to ensure complete oral absorption; maintenance dose: 300 mg/day or 5-6 mg/kg/day in 3 divided doses or 1-2 divided doses using extended release (range 200-1200 mg/day)

Pediatrics:

Status epilepticus: I.V.:

Infants and Children: Loading dose: 15-20 mg/kg in a single or divided dose; maintenance dose: Initial: 5 mg/kg/day in 2 divided doses, usual doses:

6 months to 3 years: 8-10 mg/kg/day

4-6 years: 7.5-9 mg/kg/day

7-9 years: 7-8 mg/kg/day

10-16 years: 6-7 mg/kg/day, some patients may require every 8 hours dosing

Anticonvulsant: Children: Oral: Refer to adult dosing.

Renal Impairment: Phenytoin level in serum may be difficult to interpret in renal failure. Monitoring of free (unbound) concentrations or adjustment to allow interpretation is recommended.

Hepatic Impairment: Safe in usual doses in mild liver disease; clearance may be substantially reduced in cirrhosis and plasma level monitoring with dose adjustment advisable. Free phenytoin levels should be monitored closely.

Available Dosage Forms

Capsule, extended release, as sodium:

Dilantin®: 30 mg [contains sodium benzoate], 100 mg

Phenytek™: 200 mg, 300 mg

Capsule, prompt release, as sodium: 100 mg

Injection, solution, as sodium: 50 mg/mL (2 mL, 5 mL) [contains alcohol]

Suspension, oral (Dilantin®): 125 mg/5 mL (240 mL) [contains alcohol <0.6%, sodium benzoate; orange-vanilla flavor]

Tablet, chewable (Dilantin®): 50 mg

Monitoring and Teaching Issues

Physical Assessment: Assess potential for numerous interactions with other prescriptions, OTC medications, or herbal products patient may be taking (see extensive list of Drug Interactions). Assess results of laboratory tests, therapeutic effectiveness, and adverse response when beginning therapy and at regular intervals during treatment. When discontinuing oral formulation, taper dose gradually; abrupt discontinuance can cause status epilepticus. I.V.: Monitor blood pressure. Infusion site should be monitored closely (vesicant). Patient should be monitored closely for adverse/toxic results. Teach patient proper use (oral), side effects/appropriate interventions, and adverse symptoms to report.

Monitoring Laboratory Tests: Plasma phenytoin level, CBC, liver function. **Note:** Serum phenytoin concentrations should be interpreted in terms of the unbound concentration. Adjustment should be made in patients with renal impairment and/or hypoalbuminemia.

Patient Education: Do not take any new medication during therapy without consulting prescriber. Take exactly as directed, preferably on an empty stomach. Do not alter dose or discontinue without consulting prescriber. Do not crush, break, or chew extended release

PHENYTOIN

capsules. Shake liquid suspension well before using. Follow recommended diet, avoid alcohol, and maintain adequate hydration (2-3 L/day of fluids) unless instructed to restrict fluid intake. May cause gum or mouth soreness (use good oral hygiene and have frequent dental exams); drowsiness, dizziness, nervousness, or headache (use caution when driving or engaging in tasks that require alertness until response to drug is known); or nausea or vomiting (small frequent meals, frequent mouth care, chewing gum, or sucking lozenges may help). Report chest pain, irregular heartbeat, or palpitations; slurred speech, unsteady gait, coordination difficulties, or change in mentation; skin rash; unresolved nausea, vomiting, or constipation; swollen glands; swollen, sore, or bleeding gums; unusual bruising or bleeding; acute persistent fatigue; vision changes; or other persistent adverse effects. **Pregnancy/breast-feeding precautions:** Do not get pregnant; use contraceptive measures to prevent possible harm to the fetus (effectiveness of oral contraceptives may be affected by phenytoin). Consult prescriber if breast-feeding.

Dietary Considerations:

Folic acid: Phenytoin may decrease mucosal uptake of folic acid; to avoid folic acid deficiency and megaloblastic anemia, some clinicians recommend giving patients on anticonvulsants prophylactic doses of folic acid and cyanocobalamin. However, folate supplementation may increase seizures in some patients (dose dependent). Discuss with healthcare provider prior to using any supplements.

Calcium: Hypocalcemia has been reported in patients taking prolonged high-dose therapy with an anticonvulsant. Some clinicians have given an additional 4000 units/week of vitamin D (especially in those receiving poor nutrition and getting no sun exposure) to prevent hypocalcemia.

Vitamin D: Phenytoin interferes with vitamin D metabolism and osteomalacia may result; may need to supplement with vitamin D

Tube feedings: Tube feedings decrease phenytoin absorption. To avoid decreased serum levels with continuous NG feeds, hold feedings for 2 hours prior to and 2 hours after phenytoin administration, if possible. There is a variety of opinions on how to administer phenytoin with enteral feedings. Be **consistent** throughout therapy.

Sodium content of 1 g injection: 88 mg (3.8 mEq)

Geriatric Considerations: Elderly may have low albumin which will increase free fraction and increase drug response. Monitor closely in those who are hypoalbuminemic. Free fraction measurements advised, also elderly may display a higher incidence of adverse effects (cardiovascular) when using the I.V. loading regimen; therefore, recommended to decrease loading I.V. dose to 25 mg/minute (see Warnings/Precautions).

Pregnancy Risk Factor: D

Pregnancy Issues: Phenytoin crosses the placenta. Congenital malformations (including a pattern of malformations termed the "fetal hydantoin syndrome" or "fetal anticonvulsant syndrome") have been reported in infants. Isolated cases of malignancies (including neuroblastoma) and coagulation defects in the neonate following delivery have also been reported. Epilepsy itself, the number of medications, genetic factors, or a combination of these probably influence the teratogenicity of anticonvulsant therapy.

Total plasma concentrations of phenytoin are decreased by 56% in the mother during pregnancy; unbound plasma (free) concentrations are decreased by 31%. Because protein binding is decreased, monitoring of unbound plasma concentrations is recommended. Concentrations should be monitored through the 8th week postpartum. The use of folic acid throughout pregnancy and vitamin K during the last month of pregnancy is recommended.

A pregnancy registry is available for women exposed to antiepileptic drug (including phenytoin) at the Genetics and Teratology Unit Massachusetts General Hospital, 1-888-233-2334.

Lactation: Enters breast milk/not recommended (AAP rates "compatible")

Breast-Feeding Issues: Phenytoin is excreted in breast milk; however, the amount to which the infant is exposed is considered small. The manufacturers of phenytoin do not recommend breast-feeding during therapy, however, the AAP considers it to be usually compatible. Women should be counseled of the possible risks and benefits associated with breast-feeding while on phenytoin.

Administration

Oral: Suspension: Shake well prior to use. Absorption is impaired when phenytoin suspension is given concurrently to patients who are receiving continuous nasogastric feedings. A method to resolve this interaction is to divide the daily dose of phenytoin and withhold the administration of nutritional supplements for 1-2 hours before and after each phenytoin dose.

I.M.: Although approved for I.M. use, I.M. administration is not recommended due to erratic absorption and pain on injection. Fosphenytoin may be considered.

I.V.: Vesicant. Fosphenytoin may be considered for loading in patients who are in status epilepticus, hemodynamically unstable or develop hypotension/bradycardia with I.V. administration of phenytoin. Phenytoin may be administered by IVP or IVPB administration. The maximum rate of I.V. administration is 50 mg/minute. Highly sensitive patients (eg, elderly, patients with pre-existing cardiovascular conditions) should receive phenytoin more slowly (eg, 20 mg/minute).

Other: SubQ administration is not recommended because of the possibility of local tissue damage.

Reconstitution: I.V.: Further dilution of the solution for I.V. infusion is controversial and no consensus exists as to the optimal concentration and length of stability. Stability is concentration and pH dependent. Based on limited clinical consensus, NS or LR are recommended diluents; dilutions of 1-10 mg/mL have been used and should be administered as soon as possible after preparation (some recommend to discard if not used within 4 hours). Do not refrigerate.

Compatibility: Incompatible with D$_5$NS, D$_5$W, fat emulsion 10%, LR, 1/2NS
  Compatibility in syringe: Incompatible with hydromorphone, sufentanil
  Compatibility when admixed: Incompatible with amikacin, aminophylline, bretylium, chloramphenicol, dimenhydrinate, diphenhydramine, dobutamine, hydroxyzine, insulin
(Continued)

1207

Phenytoin *(Continued)*

(regular), kanamycin, levorphanol, lidocaine, lincomycin, meperidine, metaraminol, morphine, nitroglycerin, norepinephrine, penicillin G potassium, pentobarbital, phenobarbital, phenylephrine, phytonadione, procainamide, procaine, prochlorperazine edisylate, promazine, promethazine, streptomycin, vancomycin, vitamin B complex with C

Storage:

Capsule, tablet: Store below 30°C (86°F); protect from light and moisture

Oral suspension: Store at room temperature of 20°C to 25°C (68°F to 77°F); protect from freezing and light.

Solution for injection: Store at room temperature of 15°C to 30°C (59°F to 86°F); use only clear solutions free of precipitate and haziness, slightly yellow solutions may be used. Precipitation may occur if solution is refrigerated and may dissolve at room temperature.

Related Information

Anticonvulsants By Seizure Type *on page 1712*
Maternal / Fetal Toxicology *on page 1762*
Peak and Trough Guidelines *on page 1694*

- ◆ **Phenytoin Sodium** *see* Phenytoin *on page 1204*
- ◆ **Phenytoin Sodium, Extended** *see* Phenytoin *on page 1204*
- ◆ **Phenytoin Sodium, Prompt** *see* Phenytoin *on page 1204*
- ◆ **Phillips'® Milk of Magnesia [OTC]** *see* Magnesium Hydroxide *on page 930*
- ◆ **Phillips'® Stool Softener Laxative [OTC]** *see* Docusate *on page 474*
- ◆ **PhosLo®** *see* Calcium Acetate *on page 235*
- ◆ **Phosphate, Potassium** *see* Potassium Phosphate *on page 1238*
- ◆ **Phosphonoformate** *see* Foscarnet *on page 679*
- ◆ **Phosphonoformic Acid** *see* Foscarnet *on page 679*
- ◆ **Photofrin®** *see* Porfimer *on page 1230*
- ◆ **Phrenilin® With Caffeine and Codeine** *see* Butalbital, Aspirin, Caffeine, and Codeine *on page 227*
- ◆ **p-Hydroxyampicillin** *see* Amoxicillin *on page 102*
- ◆ **Phylloquinone** *see* Phytonadione *on page 1209*

Physostigmine *(fye zoe STIG meen)*

Synonyms Eserine Salicylate; Physostigmine Salicylate; Physostigmine Sulfate

Generic Available Yes

Pharmacologic Category Acetylcholinesterase Inhibitor

Medication Safety Issues

Sound-alike/look-alike issues:

Physostigmine may be confused with Prostigmin®, pyridostigmine

Use Reverse toxic CNS effects caused by anticholinergic drugs

Mechanism of Action/Effect Inhibits destruction of acetylcholine by acetylcholinesterase which facilitates transmission of impulses across myoneural junction and prolongs the central and peripheral effects of acetylcholine

Contraindications Hypersensitivity to physostigmine or any component of the formulation; GI or GU obstruction; physostigmine therapy of drug intoxications should be used with extreme caution in patients with asthma, gangrene, severe cardiovascular disease, or mechanical obstruction of the GI tract or urogenital tract. In these patients, physostigmine should be used only to treat life-threatening conditions.

Warnings/Precautions Use with caution in patients with epilepsy, asthma, diabetes, gangrene, cardiovascular disease, bradycardia. Discontinue if excessive salivation or emesis, frequent urination or diarrhea occur. Reduce dosage if excessive sweating or nausea occurs. Administer I.V. slowly or at a controlled rate not faster than 1 mg/minute. Due to the possibility of hypersensitivity or overdose/cholinergic crisis, atropine should be readily available; not intended as a first-line agent for anticholinergic toxicity or Parkinson's disease.

Drug Interactions

Increased Effect/Toxicity: Increased toxicity with bethanechol, methacholine. Succinylcholine may increase neuromuscular blockade with systemic administration.

Lab Interactions Increased aminotransferase [ALT (SGPT)/AST (SGOT)] (S), amylase (S)

Adverse Reactions Frequency not defined.

Cardiovascular: Palpitations, bradycardia

Central nervous system: Restlessness, nervousness, hallucinations, seizure

Gastrointestinal: Nausea, salivation, diarrhea, stomach pain

Genitourinary: Frequent urge to urinate

Neuromuscular & skeletal: Muscle twitching

Ocular: Lacrimation, miosis

Respiratory: Dyspnea, bronchospasm, respiratory paralysis, pulmonary edema

Miscellaneous: Diaphoresis

Overdosage/Toxicology Symptoms of overdose include muscle weakness, blurred vision, excessive sweating, tearing and salivation, nausea, vomiting, bronchospasm, and seizures. If physostigmine is used in excess or in the absence of an anticholinergic overdose, patients may manifest signs of cholinergic toxicity. At this point, an anticholinergic agent (eg, atropine 0.015-0.05 mg/kg) may be necessary.

Pharmacodynamics/Kinetics
Onset of Action: ~5 minutes
Duration of Action: 0.5-5 hours
Absorption: I.M., SubQ: Readily absorbed
Half-Life Elimination: 15-40 minutes
Metabolism: Hepatic and via hydrolysis by cholinesterases

Dosing
Adults & Elderly:
Anticholinergic drug overdose:
I.M., I.V., SubQ: 0.5-2 mg to start; repeat every 20 minutes until response occurs or adverse effect occurs.
Repeat 1-4 mg every 30-60 minutes as life-threatening signs (arrhythmias, seizures, deep coma) recur; maximum I.V. rate: 1 mg/minute.
Pediatrics: Anticholinergic drug overdose (Reserve for life-threatening situations only): children: I.V.: 0.01-0.03 mg/kg/dose (maximum: 0.5 mg/minute). May repeat after 5-10 minutes to a maximum total dose of 2 mg or until response occurs or adverse cholinergic effects occur.

Available Dosage Forms Injection, solution, as salicylate: 1 mg/mL (2 mL) [contains benzyl alcohol and sodium metabisulfite]

Monitoring and Teaching Issues
Physical Assessment: When used to reverse neuromuscular block, patient must be monitored closely until full return of neuromuscular functioning. Assess bladder and sphincter adequacy prior to administering medication. Assess other medications patient may be taking for effectiveness and interactions. Monitor therapeutic effectiveness and adverse reactions (cholinergic crisis). Assess knowledge/teach patient appropriate use of ophthalmic forms, interventions to reduce side effects, and adverse symptoms to report.

Patient Education: Maintain adequate hydration (2-3 L/day of fluids) unless instructed to restrict fluid intake. May cause dizziness, drowsiness, or hypotension (rise slowly from sitting or lying position and use caution when driving or climbing stairs); vomiting or loss of appetite (small frequent meals, frequent mouth care, chewing gum, or sucking lozenges may help); or diarrhea (boiled milk, yogurt, or buttermilk may help). Report persistent abdominal discomfort; significantly increased salivation, sweating, tearing, or urination; flushed skin; chest pain or palpitations; acute headache; unresolved diarrhea; excessive fatigue, insomnia, dizziness, or depression; increased muscle, joint, or body pain; vision changes or blurred vision; or shortness of breath or wheezing. **Pregnancy/breast-feeding precautions:** Inform prescriber if you are or intend to become pregnant. Consult prescriber if breast-feeding.

Geriatric Considerations: Studies on the use of physostigmine in Alzheimer's disease have reported variable results. Doses generally were in the range of 2-4 mg 4 times/day. Limitations to the use of physostigmine include a short half-life requiring frequent dosing, variable absorption from the GI tract, and no commercially available oral product; therefore, not recommended for treatment of Alzheimer's disease.

Pregnancy Risk Factor: C
Lactation: Excretion in breast milk unknown

Administration
I.V.: Infuse slowly I.V. at a maximum rate of 0.5 mg/minute in children or 1 mg/minute in adults. Too rapid administration (I.V. rate not to exceed 1 mg/minute) can cause bradycardia, hypersalivation leading to respiratory difficulties and seizures.
Compatibility: Stable in dextran 6% in dextrose, dextran 6% in NS, D_5W, $D_{10}W$, D_5LR, $D_5\frac{1}{4}NS$, $D_5\frac{1}{2}NS$, D_5NS, fat emulsion 10%, LR, $\frac{1}{2}NS$, NS
Y-site administration: Incompatible with dobutamine
Compatibility when admixed: Incompatible with phenytoin, ranitidine
Storage: Do not use solution if cloudy or dark brown.

Related Information
Glaucoma Drug Therapy *on page 1827*

- Physostigmine Salicylate *see Physostigmine on page 1208*
- Physostigmine Sulfate *see Physostigmine on page 1208*
- Phytomenadione *see Phytonadione on page 1209*

Phytonadione (fye toe na DYE one)
U.S. Brand Names Mephyton®
Synonyms Methylphytyl Napthoquinone; Phylloquinone; Phytomenadione; Vitamin K_1
Generic Available Yes: Injection
Pharmacologic Category Vitamin, Fat Soluble
Medication Safety Issues
Sound-alike/look-alike issues:
Mephyton® may be confused with melphalan, methadone

Use Prevention and treatment of hypoprothrombinemia caused by drug-induced or anticoagulant-induced vitamin K deficiency, hemorrhagic disease of the newborn; phytonadione is more effective and is preferred to other vitamin K preparations in the presence of impending hemorrhage; oral absorption depends on the presence of bile salts

Mechanism of Action/Effect Promotes liver synthesis of clotting factors (II, VII, IX, X); however, the exact mechanism as to this stimulation is unknown. Menadiol is a water soluble form of vitamin K; phytonadione has a more rapid and prolonged effect than menadione; menadiol sodium diphosphate (K_4) is half as potent as menadione (K_3).

Contraindications Hypersensitivity to phytonadione or any component of the formulation

Warnings/Precautions Severe reactions resembling anaphylaxis or hypersensitivity have occurred rarely during or immediately after I.V. administration (even with proper dilution and rate of administration), as well as I.M. administration. Restrict I.V. administration for emergency use only. Allergic reactions have also occurred with I.M. and SubQ injection. Ineffective in hereditary hypoprothrombinemia, hypoprothrombinemia caused by severe liver
(Continued)

Phytonadione *(Continued)*

disease. Severe hemolytic anemia has been reported rarely in neonates following large doses (10-20 mg) of phytonadione.

Drug Interactions

Decreased Effect: The anticoagulant effects of warfarin, dicumarol, anisindione are reversed by phytonadione.

Pharmacodynamics/Kinetics

Onset of Action: Increased coagulation factors: Oral: 6-12 hours; Parenteral: 1-2 hours; prothrombin may become normal after 12-14 hours

Absorption: Oral: From intestines in presence of bile

Metabolism: Rapidly hepatic

Excretion: Urine and feces

Dosing

Adults & Elderly: SubQ is the preferred (per manufacturer) parenteral route; I.V. route should be restricted for emergency use only

Minimum daily requirement (not well established): 0.03 mcg/kg/day

Oral anticoagulant overdose: Oral, I.V., SubQ: 1-10 mg/dose depending on degree of INR elevation

Serious bleeding or major overdose: I.V. (slow infusion): 10 mg; may repeat every 12 hours (have required doses up to 25 mg)

Vitamin K deficiency (due to drugs, malabsorption or decreased synthesis of vitamin K):
Oral: 5-25 mg/24 hours
I.M., I.V., SubQ: 10 mg

Pediatrics: SubQ is the preferred (per manufacturer) parenteral route; I.V. route should be restricted for emergency use only.

Minimum daily requirement: Not well established
Infants: 1-5 mcg/kg/day

Hemorrhagic disease of the newborn:
Prophylaxis: I.M.: 0.5-1 mg within 1 hour of birth
Treatment: I.M., SubQ: 1-2 mg/dose/day

Oral anticoagulant overdose: Infants and Children:
No bleeding, rapid reversal needed, patient **will require** further oral anticoagulant therapy: SubQ, I.V.: 0.5-2 mg
No bleeding, rapid reversal needed, patient **will not require** further oral anticoagulant therapy: SubQ, I.V.: 2-5 mg
Significant bleeding, not life-threatening: SubQ, I.V.: 0.5-2 mg
Significant bleeding, life-threatening: I.V.: 5 mg over 10-20 minutes

Vitamin K deficiency (due to drugs, malabsorption or decreased synthesis of vitamin K): Infants and Children:
Oral: 2.5-5 mg/24 hours
I.M., I.V., SubQ: 1-2 mg/dose as a single dose

Available Dosage Forms

Injection, aqueous colloidal: 2 mg/mL (0.5 mL); 10 mg/mL (1 mL) [contains benzyl alcohol]
Tablet (Mephyton®): 5 mg

Monitoring and Teaching Issues

Physical Assessment: Note dosing specifics according to purpose for use. Assess results of laboratory tests and patient response (degree of bleeding). Teach patient proper use, possible side effects/appropriate interventions, and adverse symptoms to report.

Monitoring Laboratory Tests: PT

Patient Education: Do not take any new medication during therapy (especially any aspirin-containing products or NSAIDs) without consulting prescriber. Oral: Take only as directed; do not take more or more often than prescribed. Consult prescriber for recommended diet. Report bleeding gums; blood in urine, stool, or vomitus; unusual bruising or bleeding; or abdominal cramping. **Pregnancy precaution:** Inform prescriber if you are or intend to become pregnant.

Pregnancy Risk Factor: C

Lactation: Enters breast milk/compatible

Administration

I.V.: Dilute in normal saline, D₅W or D₅NS and infuse slowly; rate of infusion should not exceed 1 mg/minute. **This route should be used only if administration by another route is not feasible.** I.V. administration should not exceed 1 mg/minute; for I.V. infusion, dilute in PF (preservative free) D₅W or normal saline.

Storage: Protect injection from light at all times; may be autoclaved.

♦ **Pidorubicin** *see Epirubicin on page 527*
♦ **Pidorubicin Hydrochloride** *see Epirubicin on page 527*
♦ **Pilocar®** *see Pilocarpine on page 1210*

Pilocarpine *(pye loe KAR peen)*

U.S. Brand Names Isopto® Carpine; Pilocar®; Pilopine HS®; Salagen®

Synonyms Pilocarpine Hydrochloride

Generic Available Yes: Hydrochloride solution

Pharmacologic Category Cholinergic Agonist; Ophthalmic Agent, Antiglaucoma; Ophthalmic Agent, Miotic

Medication Safety Issues
Sound-alike/look-alike issues:
Isopto® Carpine may be confused with Isopto® Carbachol
Salagen® may be confused with Salacid®

Use

Ophthalmic: Management of chronic simple glaucoma, chronic and acute angle-closure glaucoma

Oral: Symptomatic treatment of xerostomia caused by salivary gland hypofunction resulting from radiotherapy for cancer of the head and neck or Sjögren's syndrome

Unlabeled/Investigational Use Counter effects of cycloplegics

Mechanism of Action/Effect Directly stimulates cholinergic receptors in the eye causing miosis (by contraction of the iris sphincter), loss of accommodation (by constriction of ciliary muscle), and lowering of intraocular pressure (with decreased resistance to aqueous humor outflow)

Contraindications Hypersensitivity to pilocarpine or any component of the formulation; acute inflammatory disease of the anterior chamber of the eye; in addition, tablets are also contraindicated in patients with uncontrolled asthma, angle-closure glaucoma, severe hepatic impairment

Warnings/Precautions Use caution with cardiovascular disease; patients may have difficulty compensating for transient changes in hemodynamics or rhythm induced by pilocarpine.

Ophthalmic products: May cause decreased visual acuity, especially at night or with reduced lighting.

Oral tablets: Use caution with controlled asthma, chronic bronchitis or COPD; may increase airway resistance, bronchial smooth muscle tone, and bronchial secretions. Use caution with cholelithiasis, biliary tract disease, nephrolithiasis; adjust dose with moderate hepatic impairment.

Drug Interactions

Cytochrome P450 Effect: Inhibits CYP2A6 (weak), 2E1 (weak), 3A4 (weak)

Decreased Effect: May decrease effects of anticholinergic drugs (atropine, ipratropium).

Increased Effect/Toxicity: Concurrent use with beta-blockers may cause conduction disturbances.

Nutritional/Ethanol Interactions Food: Avoid administering oral formulation with high-fat meal; fat decreases the rate of absorption, maximum concentration and increases the time it takes to reach maximum concentration.

Adverse Reactions

Ophthalmic: Frequency not defined:

Cardiovascular: Hypertension, tachycardia

Gastrointestinal: Diarrhea, nausea, salivation, vomiting

Ocular: Burning, ciliary spasm, conjunctival vascular congestion, corneal granularity (gel 10%), lacrimation, lens opacity, myopia, retinal detachment, supraorbital or temporal headache, visual acuity decreased

Respiratory: Bronchial spasm, pulmonary edema

Miscellaneous: Diaphoresis

Oral (frequency varies by indication and dose):

>10%:

Cardiovascular: Flushing (8% to 13%)

Central nervous system: Chills (3% to 15%), dizziness (5% to 12%), headache (11%)

Gastrointestinal: Nausea (6% to 15%)

Genitourinary: Urinary frequency (9% to 12%)

Neuromuscular & skeletal: Weakness (2% to 12%)

Respiratory: Rhinitis (5% to 14%)

Miscellaneous: Diaphoresis (29% to 68%)

1% to 10%:

Cardiovascular: Edema (<1% to 5%), facial edema, hypertension (3%), palpitation, tachycardia

Central nervous system: Pain (4%), fever, somnolence

Dermatologic: Pruritus, rash

Gastrointestinal: Diarrhea (4% to 7%), dyspepsia (7%), vomiting (3% to 4%), constipation, flatulence, glossitis, salivation increased, stomatitis, taste perversion

Genitourinary: Vaginitis, urinary incontinence

Neuromuscular & skeletal: Myalgias, tremor

Ocular: Lacrimation (6%), amblyopia (4%), abnormal vision, blurred vision, conjunctivitis

Otic: Tinnitus

Respiratory: Cough increased, dysphagia, epistaxis, sinusitis

Miscellaneous: Allergic reaction, voice alteration

Overdosage/Toxicology Symptoms of overdose include bronchospasm, bradycardia, involuntary urination, vomiting, hypotension, and tremor. Atropine is the treatment of choice for intoxications manifesting with significant muscarinic symptoms. Atropine I.V. 2-4 mg every 3-60 minutes should be repeated to control symptoms and then continued as needed for 1-2 days following acute ingestion. Epinephrine 0.1-1 mg SubQ may be useful for reversing severe cardiovascular or pulmonary sequelae.

Pharmacodynamics/Kinetics

Onset of Action:

Ophthalmic: Miosis: 10-30 minutes; Intraocular pressure reduction: 1 hour

Oral: 20 minutes

Duration of Action:

Ophthalmic: Miosis: 4-8 hours; Intraocular pressure reduction: 4-12 hours

Oral: 3-5 hours

Half-Life Elimination: Oral: 0.76-1.35 hours; increased with hepatic impairment

Excretion: Urine

Dosing

Adults & Elderly:

Glaucoma: Ophthalmic

Solution: Instill 1-2 drops up to 6 times/day; adjust the concentration and frequency as required to control elevated intraocular pressure.

Gel: Instill 0.5" ribbon into lower conjunctival sac once daily at bedtime.

To counteract the mydriatic effects of sympathomimetic agents (unlabeled use):

Ophthalmic solution: Instill 1 drop of a 1% solution in the affected eye.

(Continued)

Pilocarpine *(Continued)*

Xerostomia: Oral:
Following head and neck cancer: 5 mg 3 times/day, titration up to 10 mg 3 times/day may be considered for patients who have not responded adequately; do not exceed 2 tablets/dose
Sjögren's syndrome: 5 mg 4 times/day
Hepatic Impairment: Oral: Patients with moderate impairment: 5 mg 2 times/day regardless of indication; adjust dose based on response and tolerability. Do not use with severe impairment (Child-Pugh score 10-15)

Available Dosage Forms

Gel, ophthalmic, as hydrochloride (Pilopine HS®): 4% (3.5 g) [contains benzalkonium chloride]

Solution, ophthalmic, as hydrochloride: 1% (15 mL); 2% (15 mL); 4% (15 mL); 6% (15 mL) [may contain benzalkonium chloride]
Isopto® Carpine: 1% (15 mL); 2% (15 mL, 30 mL); 4% (15 mL, 30 mL); 6% (15 mL); 8% (15 mL) [contains benzalkonium chloride]
Pilocar®: 0.5% (15 mL); 1% (1 mL, 15 mL); 2% (1 mL, 15 mL); 3% (15 mL); 4% (1 mL, 15 mL); 6% (15 mL) [contains benzalkonium chloride]

Tablet, as hydrochloride (Salagen®): 5 mg, 7.5 mg

Monitoring and Teaching Issues

Physical Assessment: Monitor for adverse effects and response to treatment. Assess results of intraocular pressure testing, fundoscopic exam, and visual field testing on a periodic basis. Teach patient appropriate administration of ophthalmic solution.

Patient Education: Use as often as recommended. Avoid taking oral medication with a high fat meal.

Ophthalmic: Wash hands before using. Do not let tip of applicator touch eye; do not contaminate tip of applicator (may cause eye infection, eye damage, or vision loss). Sit or lie down. Open eye, look at ceiling, and instill prescribed amount of solution. Do not blink for 30 seconds, close eye and roll eye in all directions, and apply gentle pressure to inner corner of eye for 1-2 minutes. Temporary stinging or blurred vision may occur. You may experience altered dark adaptation; use caution when driving at night or in poorly lit environments. Report persistent pain, redness, burning, double vision, or severe headache. **Pregnancy/breast-feeding precautions:** Inform prescriber if you are pregnant. Breast-feeding is not recommended.

Geriatric Considerations: Assure the patient or a caregiver can adequately administer ophthalmic medication dosage form.

Pregnancy Risk Factor: C

Lactation: Excretion in breast milk unknown/not recommended

Administration

Oral: Avoid administering with high-fat meal. Fat decreases the rate of absorption, maximum concentration, and increases the time it takes to reach maximum concentration.

Other: Ophthalmic: If both solution and gel are used, the solution should be applied first, then the gel at least 5 minutes later. Following administration of the solution, finger pressure should be applied on the lacrimal sac for 1-2 minutes.

Storage:
Gel: Store at room temperature of 2°C to 27°C (36°F to 80°F). Do not freeze; avoid excessive heat.
Tablets: Store at controlled room temperature of 15°C to 30°C (59°F to 86°F).

Related Information

Glaucoma Drug Therapy *on page 1827*

◆ **Pilocarpine Hydrochloride** *see* Pilocarpine *on page 1210*
◆ **Pilopine HS®** *see* Pilocarpine *on page 1210*
◆ **Pima®** *see* Potassium Iodide *on page 1237*

Pimecrolimus *(pim e KROE li mus)*

U.S. Brand Names Elidel®

Generic Available No

Pharmacologic Category Immunosuppressant Agent; Topical Skin Product

Use Short-term and intermittent long-term treatment of mild to moderate atopic dermatitis in patients not responsive to conventional therapy or when conventional therapy is not appropriate

Mechanism of Action/Effect Inhibits T cell activation by blocking proinflammatory cytokine secretion.

Contraindications Hypersensitivity to pimecrolimus or any component of the formulation; Netherton's syndrome

Warnings/Precautions Topical calcineurin agents are considered second-line therapies in the treatment of atopic dermatitis/eczema, and should be limited to use in patients who have failed treatment with other therapies. They should be used for short-term and intermittent treatment using the minimum amount necessary for the control of symptoms should be used.

Do not apply to areas of active cutaneous viral infections; clinical infections at treatment sites should be cleared first. May be associated with increased risk of varicella zoster, herpes simplex viral infections, or eczema herpeticum. Consider discontinuation if lymphadenopathy or worsening of skin papillomas occur. Minimize or avoid natural/artificial sunlight exposure; can shorten time to skin tumor formation (animal study). Should not be used in immunocompromised patients. Use caution with CYP3A4 inhibitors in patients with widespread and/or erythrodermic disease. The use of Elidel® in children <2 years of age is not recommended, particularly since the effect on immune system development is unknown.

Drug Interactions

Cytochrome P450 Effect: Substrate of CYP3A4 (minor)

Increased Effect/Toxicity: CYP3A inhibitors may increase pimecrolimus levels in patients where increased absorption expected.

Adverse Reactions

>10%:

Central nervous system: Headache (7% to 25%), pyrexia (1% to 13%)

Local: Burning at application site (2% to 26%)

Respiratory: Nasopharyngitis (8% to 27%), cough (2% to 16%), upper respiratory tract infection (4% to 19%), bronchitis (0.4% to 11%)

Miscellaneous: Influenza (3% to 13%)

1% to 10%:

Dermatologic: Skin papilloma (warts) (up to 3%), molluscum contagiosum (0.7% to 2%), herpes simplex dermatitis (up to 2%)

Gastrointestinal: Diarrhea (0.6% to 8%), constipation (up to 4%)

Local: Irritation at application site (0.4% to 6%), erythema at application site (0.4% to 2%), pruritus at application site (0.6% to 6%)

Ocular: Eye infection (up to 1%)

Otic: Ear infection (0.6% to 6%)

Respiratory: Pharyngitis (0.7% to 8%), sinusitis (0.6% to 3%), nasal congestion (0.6% to 3%)

Miscellaneous: Viral infection (up to 7%), herpes simplex infection (0.4% to 4%), tonsillitis (0.4% to 6%)

Adverse events ≤ placebo: Abdominal pain, acne, arthralgia, asthma exacerbation, back pain, bacterial infection, conjunctivitis, dyspnea, dysmenorrhea, earache, epistaxis, folliculitis, hypersensitivity, impetigo, nausea, otitis media, pharyngitis (streptococcal), pneumonia, rhinorrhea, rhinitis, sinus congestion, skin infection, sore throat, Staphylococcal infection, toothache, urticaria, vomiting, wheezing

Overdosage/Toxicology No experience with overdose reported.

Pharmacodynamics/Kinetics

Absorption: Poor when applied to 13% to 62% body surface area for up to a year

Dosing

Adults & Elderly:

Mild to moderate atopic dermatitis: Topical: Apply thin layer to affected area twice daily; rub in gently and completely. **Note:** Continue as long as signs and symptoms persist; discontinue if resolution occurs; re-evaluate if symptoms persist >6 weeks.

Pediatrics: Children ≥2 years: Topical: Refer to adult dosing.

Available Dosage Forms Cream, topical: 1% (30 g, 60 g, 100 g)

Monitoring and Teaching Issues

Physical Assessment: See Administration directions. Assess knowledge/teach patient appropriate use, interventions to reduce side effects, and adverse symptoms to report.

Patient Education: This medication is for external use only. Do not use for any skin disorder except that for which it was prescribed. Avoid getting any medication in or close to eyes. Apply as often as directed by prescriber, in thin film to affected area. Do not cover with bandages or occlusive dressings. Wash and dry hands thoroughly before applying. Wash hands thoroughly after applying (if affected area is not on hands). Protect affected skin area from direct sunlight or UV light. Discontinue therapy after signs and symptoms have disappeared; restart treatment at first sign of recurrence. You may experience burning at sight of application, this will usually last less than 5 days, and go away as skin condition improves. You may experience headache, fever, cough, nasal or throat irritation, flu-like symptoms, diarrhea, or constipation; contact prescriber if these persist. Contact prescriber if skin condition worsens or if symptoms persist longer than 6 weeks. **Pregnancy/breast-feeding precautions:** Inform prescriber if you are or intend to become pregnant. Breast-feeding is not recommended.

Pregnancy Risk Factor: C

Lactation: Excretion in breast milk unknown/not recommended

Administration

Topical: Do not use with occlusive dressings. Burning at the application site is most common in first few days; improves as atopic dermatitis improves. Continue as long as signs and symptoms persist; discontinue if resolution occurs; re-evaluate if symptoms persist >6 weeks.

Storage: Store at 15°C to 30°C (59°F to 86°F). Do not freeze.

Pimozide (PI moe zide)

U.S. Brand Names Orap®

Generic Available No

Pharmacologic Category Antipsychotic Agent, Typical

Use Suppression of severe motor and phonic tics in patients with Tourette's disorder who have failed to respond satisfactorily to standard treatment

Unlabeled/Investigational Use Psychosis; reported use in individuals with delusions focused on physical symptoms (ie, preoccupation with parasitic infestation); Huntington's chorea

Mechanism of Action/Effect Pimozide, a diphenylbutylpiperidine antipsychotic, is a potent centrally-acting dopamine-receptor antagonist resulting in its characteristic neuroleptic effects

Contraindications Hypersensitivity to pimozide or any component of the formulation; severe CNS depression; coma; history of dysrhythmia; prolonged QT syndrome; concurrent use with QT$_c$-prolonging agents; hypokalemia or hypomagnesemia; concurrent use of drugs that are inhibitors of CYP3A4, including concurrent use of azole antifungals, fluvoxamine, macrolide antibiotics (such as clarithromycin or erythromycin), mesoridazine, nefazodone, protease inhibitors (ie, atazanavir, indinavir, nelfinavir, ritonavir, saquinavir), sertraline, thioridazine, zileuton, and ziprasidone; simple tics other than Tourette's

Warnings/Precautions May cause hypotension, use with caution in patients with autonomic instability. Moderately sedating, use with caution in disorders where CNS depression is a feature. Use with caution in Parkinson's disease. Caution in patients with hemodynamic instability; bone marrow suppression; predisposition to seizures; subcortical brain damage; severe cardiac, hepatic, renal, or respiratory disease. Esophageal dysmotility and aspiration (Continued)

Pimozide *(Continued)*

have been associated with antipsychotic use - use with caution in patients at risk of pneumonia (ie, Alzheimer's disease). Caution in breast cancer or other prolactin-dependent tumors (may elevate prolactin levels). May alter temperature regulation or mask toxicity of other drugs due to antiemetic effects. May alter cardiac conduction - life-threatening arrhythmias have occurred with high doses (>10 mg). May prolong QT interval predisposing patients to ventricular arrhythmias. Monitor ECG at baseline and periodically during dosage titration. May cause orthostatic hypotension - use with caution in patients at risk of this effect or those who would tolerate transient hypotensive episodes (cerebrovascular disease, cardiovascular disease, or other medications which may predispose).

May cause anticholinergic effects (confusion, agitation, constipation, xerostomia, blurred vision, urinary retention); therefore, they should be used with caution in patients with decreased gastrointestinal motility, urinary retention, BPH, xerostomia, or visual problems. Conditions which also may be exacerbated by cholinergic blockade include narrow-angle glaucoma (screening is recommended) and worsening of myasthenia gravis. Relative to neuroleptics, pimozide has a moderate potency of cholinergic blockade.

May cause extrapyramidal symptoms, including pseudoparkinsonism, acute dystonic reactions, akathisia, and tardive dyskinesia (risk of these reactions is high relative to other neuroleptics). May be associated with neuroleptic malignant syndrome (NMS) or pigmentary retinopathy.

Avoid grapefruit juice due to potential inhibition of pimozide metabolism.

Drug Interactions

Cytochrome P450 Effect: Substrate (major) of CYP1A2, 3A4; **Inhibits** CYP2C19 (weak), 2D6 (weak), 2E1 (weak), 3A4 (weak)

Decreased Effect: CYP1A2 inducers may decrease the levels/effects of pimozide; example inducers include aminoglutethimide, carbamazepine, phenobarbital, and rifampin. CYP3A4 inducers may decrease the levels/effects of pimozide; example inducers include aminoglutethimide, carbamazepine, nafcillin, nevirapine, phenobarbital, phenytoin, and rifamycins. Benztropine (and other anticholinergics) may inhibit the therapeutic response to pimozide. Antipsychotics such as pimozide inhibit the ability of bromocriptine to lower serum prolactin concentrations. The antihypertensive effects of guanethidine and guanadrel may be inhibited by pimozide. Pimozide may inhibit the antiparkinsonian effect of levodopa. Pimozide (and possibly other low potency antipsychotics) may reverse the pressor effects of epinephrine.

Increased Effect/Toxicity: Concurrent use with QT$_c$-prolonging agents is contraindicated including Class Ia and Class III antiarrhythmics, arsenic trioxide, chlorpromazine, dolasetron, droperidol, halofantrine, levomethadyl, mefloquine, pentamidine, probucol, tacrolimus, ziprasidone, mesoridazine, thioridazine, tricyclic antidepressants, and some quinolone antibiotics (sparfloxacin, moxifloxacin, and gatifloxacin).

CYP1A2 inhibitors may increase the levels/effects of pimozide; example inhibitors include amiodarone, ciprofloxacin, fluvoxamine, ketoconazole, norfloxacin, ofloxacin, and rofecoxib. Chloroquine, propranolol, and sulfadoxine-pyrimethamine also may increase pimozide concentrations. Concurrent use with TCA may produce increased toxicity or altered therapeutic response. Pimozide plus lithium may (rarely) produce neurotoxicity. Pimozide and CNS depressants (ethanol, narcotics) may produce additive CNS depressant effects. Pimozide with fluoxetine has been associated with the development of bradycardia (case report). Metoclopramide may increase risk of extrapyramidal symptoms (EPS).

CYP3A4 inhibitors may increase the levels/effects of pimozide; example inhibitors include azole antifungals, ciprofloxacin, clarithromycin, diclofenac, doxycycline, erythromycin, imatinib, isoniazid, nefazodone, nicardipine, propofol, protease inhibitors, quinidine, and verapamil. Concurrent use of strong CYP3A4 inhibitors with pimozide is contraindicated.

Nutritional/Ethanol Interactions

Ethanol: Avoid ethanol (may increase CNS depression).

Food: Pimozide serum concentration may be increased when taken with grapefruit juice; avoid concurrent use.

Herb/Nutraceutical: St John's wort may decrease pimozide levels. Avoid kava kava, gotu kola, valerian, St John's wort (may increase CNS depression).

Lab Interactions Increased prolactin (S)

Adverse Reactions

Frequencies >1% reported in adults (limited data) and/or children with Tourette's disorder:

Cardiovascular: Abnormal ECG (3%)

Central nervous system: Somnolence (up to 28% in children), sedation (14%), akathisia (8%), drowsiness (7%), hyperkinesias (6%), insomnia (2%), depression (2%), headache (1%), nervousness (1% to 8%)

Dermatologic: Rash (8%)

Gastrointestinal: Xerostomia (25%), constipation (20%), increased salivation (14%), diarrhea (5%), thirst (5%), appetite increased (5%), taste disturbance (5%), dysphagia (3%)

Genitourinary: Impotence (15%)

Neuromuscular & skeletal: Weakness (22%), muscle tightness (15%), rigidity (10%), myalgia (3%), torticollis (3%), tremor (3%)

Ocular: Visual disturbance (6% to 20%), accommodation decreased (20%)

Miscellaneous: Speech disorder (10%)

Frequency not established (reported in disorders other than Tourette's disorder):

Blood dyscrasias, breast edema, chest pain, dizziness, extrapyramidal symptoms (akathisia, akinesia, dystonia, pseudoparkinsonism, tardive dyskinesia); facial edema, gingival hyperplasia (case report), hyper-/hypotension, hyponatremia, jaundice, libido decreased, neuroleptic malignant syndrome, orthostatic hypotension, palpitation, periorbital edema, postural hypotension, QT$_c$ prolongation, seizure, tachycardia, ventricular arrhythmia, vomiting, weight gain/loss

Overdosage/Toxicology Symptoms of overdose include hypotension, respiratory depression, ECG abnormalities, extrapyramidal symptoms. Treatment is supportive and symptomatic. Epinephrine should not be used (consider norepinephrine or phenylephrine for hypotension).

Pharmacodynamics/Kinetics
  Absorption: 50%
  Time to Peak: Serum: 6-8 hours
  Protein Binding: 99%
  Half-Life Elimination: 50 hours
  Metabolism: Hepatic; significant first-pass effect
  Excretion: Urine

Dosing
  Adults:
    Tourette's disorder: Oral: Initial: 1-2 mg/day, then increase dosage as needed every other day; range is usually 7-16 mg/day; maximum: 10 mg/day or 0.2 mg/kg/day are not generally recommended.
    Note: Sudden unexpected deaths have occurred in patients taking doses >10 mg.
    Note: An ECG should be performed baseline and periodically thereafter, especially during dosage adjustment.
  Elderly: Recommend initial dose of 1 mg/day; periodically attempt gradual reduction of dose to determine if tic persists; follow up for 1-2 weeks before concluding the tic is a persistent disease phenomenon and not a manifestation of drug withdrawal. **Note:** An ECG should be performed baseline and periodically thereafter, especially during dosage adjustment.
  Pediatrics:
    Tourette's disorder: Oral:
      Children ≤12 years: Initial: 0.05 mg/kg preferably once at bedtime; may be increased every third day; usual range: 2-4 mg/day; do not exceed 10 mg/day (0.2 mg/kg/day)
      Children >12 years: Refer to adult dosing.
    Note: An ECG should be performed baseline and periodically thereafter, especially during dosage adjustment.
  Hepatic Impairment: Reduced dose is necessary.

Available Dosage Forms Tablet: 1 mg, 2 mg

Monitoring and Teaching Issues
  Physical Assessment: Assess other medications patient is taking for effectiveness and interactions. Assess patient/caregiver knowledge of rationale for therapy and risks involved. Assess results of ophthalmic exam and laboratory tests, blood pressure, therapeutic effectiveness, and adverse reactions at beginning of therapy and periodically with long-term use. Conduct baseline ECG and periodically during therapy (especially during dosage adjustment). Initiate at lower doses (see Dosing) and decrease dosage slowly when discontinuing. Assess knowledge/teach patient appropriate use, interventions to reduce side effects, and adverse symptoms to report.
  Monitoring Laboratory Tests: Lipid profile, fasting blood glucose/Hgb A_{1c}; BMI
  Patient Education: Use exactly as directed; do not increase dose or frequency. It may take 2-3 weeks to achieve desired results; do not discontinue without consulting prescriber. Avoid alcohol or caffeine and other prescription or OTC medications not approved by prescriber. Avoid grapefruit juice. Maintain adequate hydration (2-3 L/day of fluids) unless instructed to restrict fluid intake. You may experience excess drowsiness, restlessness, dizziness, or blurred vision (use caution driving or when engaging in tasks requiring alertness until response to drug is known); or constipation, dry mouth, anorexia (increased exercise, fluids, fruit, or fiber may help). Report persistent CNS effects (eg, trembling fingers, altered gait or balance, excessive sedation, seizures, unusual muscle or facial movements, anxiety, abnormal thoughts, confusion, personality changes); unresolved constipation or GI effects; breast swelling (male and female) or decreased sexual ability; vision changes; respiratory difficulty; unusual cough or flu-like symptoms; or worsening of condition. **Pregnancy/breast-feeding precautions:** Inform prescriber if you are or intend to become pregnant. Consult prescriber if breast-feeding.
  Geriatric Considerations: (See Warnings/Precautions, Adverse Reactions, and Overdose/Toxicology.) Elderly patients have an increased risk of adverse response to side effects or adverse reactions to antipsychotics.
  Pregnancy Risk Factor: C
  Lactation: Excretion in breast milk unknown

Additional Information Less sedation, but pimozide is more likely to cause acute extrapyramidal symptoms than chlorpromazine.

Related Information
  Antipsychotic Agents *on page 1717*
  Antipsychotic Medication Guidelines *on page 1766*

Pindolol *(PIN doe lole)*

Generic Available Yes

Pharmacologic Category Beta Blocker With Intrinsic Sympathomimetic Activity

Medication Safety Issues
  Sound-alike/look-alike issues:
    Pindolol may be confused with Parlodel®, Plendil®
    Visken® may be confused with Visine®

Use Management of hypertension

Unlabeled/Investigational Use Potential augmenting agent for antidepressants; ventricular arrhythmias/tachycardia, antipsychotic-induced akathisia, situational anxiety; aggressive behavior associated with dementia

Mechanism of Action/Effect Blocks both beta$_1$- and beta$_2$-receptors and has mild intrinsic sympathomimetic activity; pindolol has negative inotropic and chronotropic effects and can significantly slow AV nodal conduction. Augmentive action of antidepressants thought to be mediated via a serotonin 1A autoreceptor antagonism.

(Continued)

Pindolol *(Continued)*

Contraindications Hypersensitivity to pindolol, beta-blockers, or any component of the formulation; uncompensated congestive heart failure; cardiogenic shock; bradycardia, sinus node dysfunction, or heart block (2nd or 3rd degree) except in patients with a functioning artificial pacemaker; pulmonary edema; severe hyperactive airway disease (asthma or COPD); Raynaud's disease

Warnings/Precautions Administer very cautiously to patients with CHF, asthma, diabetes mellitus, hyperthyroidism. May mask signs and symptoms of thyrotoxicosis. Abrupt withdrawal of the drug should be avoided, drug should be discontinued over 1-2 weeks. Do not use in pregnant or nursing women. May potentiate hypoglycemia in a diabetic patient and mask signs and symptoms. Use with caution in patients with myasthenia gravis or peripheral vascular disease. May cause CNS depression; use caution in patients with a history of psychiatric illness. May potentiate anaphylactic reactions and/or blunt response to epinephrine treatment. Beta-blockers with intrinsic sympathomimetic activity (including pindolol) do not appear to be of benefit in CHF.

Drug Interactions

Cytochrome P450 Effect: Substrate of CYP2D6 (major); **Inhibits** CYP2D6 (weak)

Decreased Effect: Decreased levels/effect of pindolol with aluminum salts, barbiturates, calcium salts, cholestyramine, colestipol, NSAIDs, penicillins (ampicillin), rifampin, salicylates, and sulfinpyrazone due to decreased bioavailability and plasma levels. Beta-blockers may decrease the effect of sulfonylureas (possibly hyperglycemia). Nonselective beta-blockers blunt the effect of beta-2 adrenergic agonists (albuterol).

Increased Effect/Toxicity: CYP2D6 inhibitors may increase the levels/effects of pindolol; example inhibitors include chlorpromazine, delavirdine, fluoxetine, miconazole, paroxetine, pergolide, quinidine, quinine, ritonavir, and ropinirole. Pindolol may increase the effects of other drugs which slow AV conduction (digoxin, verapamil, diltiazem), alpha-blockers (prazosin, terazosin), and alpha-adrenergic stimulants (epinephrine, phenylephrine). Pindolol may mask the tachycardia from hypoglycemia caused by insulin and oral hypoglycemics. In patients receiving concurrent therapy, the risk of hypertensive crisis is increased when either clonidine or the beta-blocker is withdrawn. Reserpine has been shown to enhance the effect of beta-blockers. Beta-blockers may increase the action or levels of ethanol, disopyramide, nondepolarizing muscle relaxants, and theophylline although the effects are difficult to predict.

Nutritional/Ethanol Interactions Herb/Nutraceutical: Avoid dong quai if using for hypertension (has estrogenic activity). Avoid ephedra, yohimbe, ginseng (may worsen hypertension).

Adverse Reactions 1% to 10%:

Cardiovascular: Chest pain (3%), edema (6%)

Central nervous system: Nightmares/vivid dreams (5%), dizziness (9%), insomnia (10%), fatigue (8%), nervousness (7%), anxiety (<2%)

Dermatologic: Rash, itching (4%)

Gastrointestinal: Nausea (5%), abdominal discomfort (4%)

Neuromuscular & skeletal: Weakness (4%), paresthesia (3%), arthralgia (7%), muscle pain (10%)

Respiratory: Dyspnea (5%)

Overdosage/Toxicology Symptoms of intoxication include cardiac disturbances, CNS toxicity, bronchospasm, hypoglycemia, and hyperkalemia. The most common cardiac symptoms include hypotension and bradycardia. Atrioventricular block, intraventricular conduction disturbances, cardiogenic shock, and asystole may occur with severe overdose, especially with membrane-depressant drugs (eg, propranolol). CNS effects include convulsions, and coma. Respiratory arrest is commonly seen with propranolol and other membrane-depressant and lipid-soluble drugs. Treatment includes symptomatic treatment of seizures, hypotension, hyperkalemia, and hypoglycemia.

Pharmacodynamics/Kinetics

Absorption: Rapid, 50% to 95%

Time to Peak: Serum: 1-2 hours

Protein Binding: 50%

Half-Life Elimination: 2.5-4 hours; prolonged with renal impairment, age, and cirrhosis

Metabolism: Hepatic (60% to 65%) to conjugates

Excretion: Urine (35% to 50% as unchanged drug)

Dosing

Adults:

Hypertension: Oral: Initial: 5 mg twice daily, increase as necessary by 10 mg/day every 3-4 weeks (maximum daily dose: 60 mg); usual dose range (JNC 7): 10-40 mg twice daily.

Antidepressant augmentation (unlabeled use): Oral: 2.5 mg 3 times/day

Elderly: Oral: Initial: 5 mg once daily; increase as necessary by 5 mg/day every 3-4 weeks.

Renal Impairment: Reduction is necessary in severe impairment.

Hepatic Impairment: Reduce dose in severely impaired.

Available Dosage Forms Tablet: 5 mg, 10 mg

Monitoring and Teaching Issues

Physical Assessment: Assess potential for interactions with other prescriptions, OTC medications, or herbal products patient may be taking (eg, anything that affects blood pressure or cardiac status). Assess patient response at beginning of therapy, when adjusting dosage, and periodically with long-term therapy (eg, cardiac, respiratory, hemodynamic status). Caution patient to monitor serum glucose levels closely (may alter glucose tolerance, potentiate hypoglycemia, or mask symptoms of hypoglycemia). Teach patient appropriate use, possible side effects/appropriate interventions, and adverse symptoms to report.

Patient Education: Do not take any new medication during therapy unless approved by prescriber. Take exactly as directed. Do not alter dose or discontinue without consulting prescriber. If you have diabetes, monitor serum glucose closely (drug may alter glucose tolerance or mask signs of hypoglycemia). May cause nervousness, fatigue, dizziness, insomnia, or postural hypotension (use caution when changing position from lying or sitting to standing, when driving, or climbing stairs until response to medication is known); or nausea or abdominal discomfort (small frequent meals, frequent mouth care, chewing gum, or sucking lozenges may help). Report chest pain or swelling of extremities or unusual weight gain (>5 lb/week), unusual muscle weakness or pain; or other persistent adverse effects. **Breast-feeding precaution:** Consult prescriber if breast-feeding.

Dietary Considerations: May be taken without regard to meals.

Geriatric Considerations: Due to alterations in the beta-adrenergic autonomic nervous system, beta-adrenergic blockade may result in less hemodynamic response than seen in younger adults. Studies indicate that despite decreased sensitivity to the chronotropic effects of beta blockade with age, there appears to be an increased myocardial sensitivity to the negative inotropic effect during stress (eg, exercise). Controlled trials have shown the overall response rate for propranolol to be only 20% to 50% in elderly populations. Therefore, all beta-adrenergic blocking drugs may result in a decreased response as compared to younger adults (see Pharmacodynamics and Pharmacokinetics).

Pregnancy Risk Factor: B

Pregnancy Issues: Pindolol crosses the placenta. Beta-blockers have been associated with bradycardia, hypotension, and IUGR; IUGR is probably related to maternal hypertension. Available evidence suggests beta-blockers are generally safe during pregnancy (JNC 7). Cases of neonatal hypoglycemia have been reported following maternal use of beta-blockers at parturition or during breast-feeding. Monitor breast-fed infant for symptoms of beta-blockade.

Lactation: Enters breast milk/use caution

Breast-Feeding Issues: There is limited experience with pindolol; however, other beta-blockers like metoprolol are considered compatible by the AAP. Monitor the infant for signs of beta-blockade (hypotension, bradycardia, etc) with long-term use.

Related Information
Beta-Blockers *on page 1720*

♦ **Pink Bismuth** *see* Bismuth *on page 197*

♦ **PIO** *see* Pemoline *on page 1170*

Pioglitazone (pye oh GLI ta zone)

U.S. Brand Names Actos®

Generic Available No

Pharmacologic Category Antidiabetic Agent, Thiazolidinedione

Medication Safety Issues
Sound-alike/look-alike issues:
Actos® may be confused with Actidose®, Actonel®

Use

Type 2 diabetes mellitus (noninsulin dependent, NIDDM), monotherapy: Adjunct to diet and exercise, to improve glycemic control

Type 2 diabetes mellitus (noninsulin dependent, NIDDM), combination therapy with sulfonylurea, metformin, or insulin: When diet, exercise, and a single agent alone does not result in adequate glycemic control

Mechanism of Action/Effect Thiazolidinedione antidiabetic agent that lowers blood glucose by improving target cell response to insulin, without increasing pancreatic insulin secretion. It has a mechanism of action that is dependent on the presence of insulin for activity. Pioglitazone is a potent and selective agonist for peroxisome proliferator-activated receptor-gamma (PPARgamma). Activation of nuclear PPARgamma receptors influences the production of a number of gene products involved in glucose and lipid metabolism.

Contraindications Hypersensitivity to pioglitazone or any component of the formulation; active liver disease (transaminases >2.5 times the upper limit of normal at baseline); patients who have experienced jaundice during troglitazone therapy

Warnings/Precautions Should not be used in diabetic ketoacidosis. Mechanism requires the presence of insulin, therefore use in type 1 diabetes (insulin dependent, IDD) not recommended. May potentiate hypoglycemia when used in combination with sulfonylureas or insulin. Use with caution in premenopausal, anovulatory women - may result in a resumption of ovulation, increasing the risk of pregnancy. Use with caution in patients with anemia (may reduce hemoglobin and hematocrit). May increase plasma volume and/or increase cardiac hypertrophy. Use with caution in patients with edema. Monitor closely for signs and symptoms of heart failure (including weight gain, edema, or dyspnea). Not recommended for use in patients with NYHA Class III or IV heart failure, unless serum glucose control outweighs the risk of excessive fluid retention. Discontinue if heart failure develops. Use with caution in patients with minor elevations in transaminases (AST or ALT). Idiosyncratic hepatotoxicity has been reported with another thiazolidinedione agent (troglitazone) and postmarketing case reports of hepatitis (with rare hepatic failure) have been received for pioglitazone. Monitoring should include periodic determinations of liver function. Not for use in children <18 years of age.

Drug Interactions

Cytochrome P450 Effect: Substrate (major) of CYP2C8/9, 3A4; **Inhibits** CYP2C8/9 (strong), 2C19 (weak), 2D6 (moderate); **Induces** CYP3A4 (weak)

Decreased Effect: The levels/effects of pioglitazone may be decreased by aminoglutethimide, carbamazepine, nafcillin, nevirapine, phenobarbital, phenytoin, rifamycins, secobarbital, and other CYP2C8/9 or CYP3A4 inducers. Pioglitazone may decrease the levels/effects of CYP2D6 prodrug substrates (eg, codeine, hydrocodone, oxycodone, tramadol). Effects of oral contraceptives (hormonal) may be decreased, based on data from a related compound. This has not been specifically evaluated for pioglitazone. Bile acid sequestrants may decrease pioglitazone levels.

Increased Effect/Toxicity: Concomitant use with thioridazine is contraindicated, due to a risk of arrhythmias. The levels/effects of pioglitazone may be increased by azole antifungals, ciprofloxacin, clarithromycin, delavirdine, diclofenac, doxycycline, erythromycin, (Continued)

Pioglitazone *(Continued)*

fluconazole, gemfibrozil, imatinib, isoniazid, itraconazole, ketoconazole, nefazodone, nicardipine, NSAIDs, propofol, protease inhibitors, quinidine, sulfonamides, verapamil, and other CYP2C8/9 or 3A4 inhibitors.

Pioglitazone may increase the levels/effects of amiodarone, amphetamines, selected beta-blockers, dextromethorphan, fluoxetine, glimepiride, glipizide, lidocaine, mirtazapine, nateglinide, nefazodone, paroxetine, phenytoin, risperidone, ritonavir, rosiglitazone, sertraline, thioridazine, warfarin, and other CYP2D6 or 2C8/9 substrates.

Nutritional/Ethanol Interactions

Ethanol: Caution with ethanol (may cause hypoglycemia).

Food: Peak concentrations are delayed when administered with food, but the extent of absorption is not affected. Pioglitazone may be taken without regard to meals.

Herb/Nutraceutical: St John's wort may decrease levels. Caution with chromium, garlic, gymnema (may cause hypoglycemia).

Adverse Reactions

>10%:

Endocrine & metabolic: Serum triglycerides decreased, HDL-cholesterol increased

Gastrointestinal: Weight gain

Respiratory: Upper respiratory tract infection (13%)

1% to 10%:

Cardiovascular: Edema (5%) (in combination trials with sulfonylureas or insulin, the incidence of edema was as high as 15%)

Central nervous system: Headache (9%), fatigue (4%)

Endocrine & metabolic: Aggravation of diabetes mellitus (5%), hypoglycemia (range 2% to 15% when used in combination with sulfonylureas or insulin)

Hematologic: Anemia (1%)

Neuromuscular & skeletal: Myalgia (5%)

Respiratory: Sinusitis (6%), pharyngitis (5%)

Overdosage/Toxicology Experience in overdose is limited. Symptoms may include hypoglycemia. Treatment is supportive.

Pharmacodynamics/Kinetics

Onset of Action: Delayed; Peak effect: Glucose control: Several weeks

Time to Peak: ~2 hours

Protein Binding: 99.8%

Half-Life Elimination: Parent drug: 3-7 hours; Total: 16-24 hours

Metabolism: Hepatic (99%) via CYP2C8/9 and 3A4 to both active and inactive metabolites

Excretion: Urine (15% to 30%) and feces as metabolites

Dosing

Adults & Elderly: Type 2 diabetes: Oral:

Monotherapy: Initial: 15-30 mg once daily; if response is inadequate, the dosage may be increased in increments up to 45 mg once daily; maximum recommended dose: 45 mg once daily

Combination therapy:

Note: Maximum recommended dose: 45 mg/day

With sulfonylureas: Initial: 15-30 mg once daily; dose of sulfonylurea should be reduced if the patient reports hypoglycemia

With metformin: Initial: 15-30 mg once daily; it is unlikely that the dose of metformin will need to be reduced due to hypoglycemia

With insulin: Initial: 15-30 mg once daily; dose of insulin should be reduced by 10% to 25% if the patient reports hypoglycemia or if the plasma glucose falls to below 100 mg/dL.

Dosage adjustment in patients with CHF (NYHA Class II) in mono- or combination therapy: Oral: Initial: 15 mg once daily; may be increased after several months of treatment, with close attention to heart failure symptoms

Renal Impairment: No adjustment is necessary.

Hepatic Impairment: Clearance is significantly lower in hepatic impairment. Therapy should not be initiated if the patient exhibits active liver disease or increased transaminases (>2.5 times the upper limit of normal) at baseline.

Available Dosage Forms Tablet: 15 mg, 30 mg, 45 mg

Monitoring and Teaching Issues

Physical Assessment: Assess other medications patient may be taking. Assess results of laboratory tests. and response to therapy frequently until patient is stable. Monitor for adverse response. Assess knowledge/teach risks of hyper-/hypoglycemia, symptoms, and treatment. Refer patient to a diabetic educator, if available.

Monitoring Laboratory Tests: Hemoglobin A$_{1c}$; serum glucose; liver enzymes prior to initiation and periodically during treatment (per clinician judgment); if the ALT is increased to >2.5 times the upper limit of normal, liver function testing should be performed more frequently until the levels return to normal or pretreatment values. Patients with an elevation in ALT >3 times the upper limit of normal should be rechecked as soon as possible. If the ALT levels remain >3 times the upper limit of normal, therapy with pioglitazone should be discontinued.

Patient Education: Use exactly as directed; do not increase dose or frequency or discontinue without consulting prescriber. May be taken without regard to meals. Avoid or use caution with alcohol while taking this medication. If dose is missed, take as soon as possible. If dose is missed completely one day, do not double dose the next day. Follow dietary, exercise, and glucose monitoring instructions of prescriber (more frequent monitoring may be advised in periods of stress, trauma, surgery, increased exercise etc). Report respiratory infection, unusual weight gain, aggravation of hyper-/hypoglycemic condition, unusual swelling of extremities, shortness of breath, fatigue, yellowing of skin or eyes, dark urine, pale stool, nausea/vomiting, or muscle pain. **Pregnancy/breast-feeding precautions:** Inform prescriber if you are or intend to become pregnant. Use alternate means of contraception if using oral contraceptives. You may be at increased risk of pregnancy while taking this medication. Breast-feeding is not recommended.

Dietary Considerations: Management of type 2 diabetes mellitus (noninsulin dependent, NIDDM) should include diet control. May be taken without regard to meals.

Pregnancy Risk Factor: C

Pregnancy Issues: Treatment during mid-late gestation was associated with delayed parturition, embryotoxicity and postnatal growth retardation in animal models. Abnormal blood glucose levels are associated with a higher incidence of congenital abnormalities. Insulin is the drug of choice for the control of diabetes mellitus during pregnancy.

Lactation: Excretion in breast milk unknown/not recommended

Breast-Feeding Issues: In animal studies, pioglitazone has been found to be excreted in milk. It is not known whether pioglitazone is excreted in human milk. Should not be administered to a nursing woman.

Administration
  Oral: May be administered without regard to meals.

Related Information
  Diabetes Mellitus Management *on page 1819*

Piperacillin (pi PER a sil in)

Synonyms Piperacillin Sodium
Generic Available Yes
Pharmacologic Category Antibiotic, Penicillin
Use Treatment of susceptible infections such as septicemia, acute and chronic respiratory tract infections, skin and soft tissue infections, and urinary tract infections due to susceptible strains of *Pseudomonas*, *Proteus*, and *Escherichia coli* and *Enterobacter*; active against some streptococci and some anaerobic bacteria; febrile neutropenia (as part of combination regimen)

Mechanism of Action/Effect Inhibits bacterial cell wall synthesis by binding to one or more of the penicillin binding proteins (PBPs); which in turn inhibits the final transpeptidation step of peptidoglycan synthesis in bacterial cell walls, thus inhibiting cell wall biosynthesis. Bacteria eventually lyse due to ongoing activity of cell wall autolytic enzymes (autolysins and murein hydrolases) while cell wall assembly is arrested.

Contraindications Hypersensitivity to piperacillin, other penicillins, or any component of the formulation

Warnings/Precautions Dosage modification required in patients with impaired renal function; history of seizure activity; use with caution in patients with a history of beta-lactam allergy

Drug Interactions
  Decreased Effect: Tetracyclines may decrease penicillin effectiveness. High concentrations of piperacillin may cause physical inactivation of aminoglycosides and lead to potential toxicity in patients with mild-moderate renal dysfunction. Although anecdotal reports suggest oral contraceptive efficacy could be reduced by penicillins, this has been refuted by more rigorous scientific and clinical data.
  Increased Effect/Toxicity: Probenecid may increase penicillin levels. Neuromuscular blockers may increase duration of blockade. Penicillins may increase the exposure to methotrexate during concurrent therapy; monitor.

Lab Interactions May interfere with urinary glucose tests using cupric sulfate (Benedict's solution, Clinitest®); may inactivate aminoglycosides *in vitro*; false-positive urinary and serum proteins, positive Coombs' test [direct]

Adverse Reactions Frequency not defined.
  Central nervous system: Confusion, convulsions, drowsiness, fever, Jarisch-Herxheimer reaction
  Dermatologic: Rash
  Endocrine & metabolic: Electrolyte imbalance
  Hematologic: Abnormal platelet aggregation and prolonged PT (high doses), hemolytic anemia, Coombs' reaction (positive)
  Local: Thrombophlebitis
  Neuromuscular & skeletal: Myoclonus
  Renal: Acute interstitial nephritis
  Miscellaneous: Anaphylaxis, hypersensitivity reactions

Overdosage/Toxicology Symptoms of penicillin overdose include neuromuscular hypersensitivity (eg, agitation, hallucinations, asterixis, encephalopathy, confusion, and seizures). Electrolyte imbalance may occur if the preparation contains potassium or sodium salts, especially in renal failure. Hemodialysis may be helpful to aid in removal of the drug from blood; otherwise, treatment is supportive or symptom-directed.

Pharmacodynamics/Kinetics
  Absorption: I.M.: 70% to 80%
  Time to Peak: Serum: I.M.: 30-50 minutes
  Protein Binding: 22%
  Half-Life Elimination: Dose dependent; prolonged with moderately severe renal or hepatic impairment:

    Neonates: 1-5 days old: 3.6 hours; >6 days old: 2.1-2.7 hours
    Children: 1-6 months: 0.79 hour; 6 months to 12 years: 0.39-0.5 hour
    Adults: 36-80 minutes
  Excretion: Primarily urine; partially feces

Dosing
  Adults: Susceptible infections:
    I.M.: 2-3 g/dose every 6-12 hours; maximum: 24 g/24 hours
    I.V.: 3-4 g/dose every 4-6 hours; maximum: 24 g/24 hours
  Elderly: Adjust dose for renal impairment:
    I.M.: 1-2 g every 8-12 hours
    I.V.: 2-4 g every 6-8 hours
(Continued)

Piperacillin *(Continued)*

Pediatrics: Susceptible infections:

Infants and Children: I.M., I.V.: 200-300 mg/kg/day in divided doses every 4-6 hours

Note: In cystic fibrosis, dosages up to 350-500 mg/kg/day in divided doses every 4-6 hours have been used.

Renal Impairment:

Cl_{cr} 10-50 mL/minute: Administer every 6-8 hours.

Cl_{cr} <10 mL/minute: Administer every 8 hours.

Moderately dialyzable (20% to 50%)

Continuous arteriovenous or venovenous hemofiltration: Dose as for Cl_{cr} 10-50 mL/minute.

Available Dosage Forms Injection, powder for reconstitution: 2 g, 3 g, 4 g, 40 g

Monitoring and Teaching Issues

Physical Assessment: Assess results of culture and sensitivity tests and patient's allergy history prior to starting therapy. Use caution with impaired renal function and history of seizure activity (see Warnings/Precautions). Assess potential for interactions with other pharmacological agents patient may be taking (eg, may increase or decrease levels/effects of penicillin or increase risk of toxicity [aminoglycosides, neuromuscular blockers]; see Drug Interactions). Assess effectiveness (resolution of infection) and adverse reactions (eg, hypersensitivity reactions, opportunistic infection [fever, chills, unhealed sores, white plaques in mouth or vagina, purulent vaginal discharge, fatigue], confusion, convulsions, rash, thrombophlebitis; see Adverse Reactions). Advise patients with diabetes about use of Clinitest®. Teach patient possible side effects/appropriate interventions and adverse symptoms to report (see Patient Education).

Monitoring Laboratory Tests: Perform culture and sensitivity before administering first dose

Patient Education: Do not take any new medication during therapy unless approved by prescriber. This drug is given by injection or infusion; report immediately any redness, swelling, burning, or pain at infusion site or any signs of allergic reaction (eg, respiratory or swallowing difficulty, chest tightness, rash, hives, swelling of lips or mouth). Maintain adequate hydration (2-3 L/day of fluids) unless instructed to restrict fluid intake. If you have diabetes, drug may cause false test results with Clinitest®, consult prescriber for alternative method of glucose monitoring. May cause confusion or drowsiness (use caution when driving or engaging in tasks that require alertness until response to drug is known). Report chest pain, palpitations, or irregular heartbeat; persistent adverse effects.

Dietary Considerations: Sodium content of 1 g: 1.85 mEq

Geriatric Considerations: Antipseudomonal penicillins should not be used alone and are often combined with an aminoglycoside as empiric therapy for lower respiratory infection and sepsis in which gram-negative (including *Pseudomonas*) and/or anaerobes are of a high probability. Because of piperacillin's lower sodium content, it is preferred over ticarcillin in patients with a history of heart failure and/or renal or hepatic disease. Adjust dose for renal function.

Pregnancy Risk Factor: B

Lactation: Enters breast milk (small amounts - other penicillins are compatible with breast-feeding)

Administration

I.M.: Do not administer more than 2 g per injection site.

I.V.: Administer around-the-clock to promote less variation in peak and trough serum levels. Give at least 1 hour apart from aminoglycosides. Rapid administration can lead to seizures. Administer direct I.V. over 3-5 minutes. Intermittently infusion over 30 minutes.

Compatibility: Stable in dextran 6% in NS, D_5NS, D_5W, LR, NS, SWFI, bacteriostatic water

Y-site administration: Incompatible with amphotericin B cholesteryl sulfate complex, filgrastim, fluconazole, gatifloxacin, gemcitabine, ondansetron, sargramostim, vinorelbine

Compatibility when admixed: Incompatible with aminoglycosides

Storage: Reconstituted solution is stable (I.V. infusion) in NS or D_5W for 24 hours at room temperature, 7 days when refrigerated, or 4 weeks when frozen. After freezing, thawed solution is stable for 24 hours at room temperature or 48 hours when refrigerated. 40 g bulk vial should **not** be frozen after reconstitution.

Additional Information As of September 2002, piperacillin is not available from the manufacturer. This product is anticipated to return to the market in 2003.

Related Information

Antimicrobial Drugs of Choice *on page 1792*

Community-Acquired Pneumonia in Adults *on page 1807*

Piperacillin and Tazobactam Sodium

(pi PER a sil in & ta zoe BAK tam SOW dee um)

U.S. Brand Names Zosyn®

Synonyms Piperacillin Sodium and Tazobactam Sodium

Generic Available No

Pharmacologic Category Antibiotic, Penicillin

Medication Safety Issues

Sound-alike/look-alike issues:

Zosyn® may be confused with Zofran®, Zyvox™

Use Treatment of infections caused by susceptible organisms, including infections of the lower respiratory tract (community-acquired pneumonia, nosocomial pneumonia); urinary tract; skin and skin structures; gynecologic (endometritis, pelvic inflammatory disease); bone and joint infections; intra-abdominal infections (appendicitis with rupture/abscess, peritonitis); and septicemia. Tazobactam expands activity of piperacillin to include beta-lactamase producing strains of *S. aureus*, *H. influenzae*, *Bacteroides*, and other gram-negative bacteria.

Mechanism of Action/Effect Piperacillin interferes with bacterial cell wall synthesis during active multiplication, causing cell wall death and resultant bactericidal activity against susceptible bacteria; tazobactam prevents degradation of piperacillin by binding to the active side on beta-lactamase; tazobactam inhibits many beta-lactamases, including staphylococcal penicillinase and Richmond and Sykes Types II, III, IV, and V, including extended spectrum enzymes; it has only limited activity against Class I beta-lactamases other than Class 1C

Contraindications Hypersensitivity to penicillins, beta-lactamase inhibitors, or any component of the formulation

Warnings/Precautions Due to sodium load and to the adverse effects of high serum concentrations of penicillins, dosage modification is required in patients with impaired or underdeveloped renal function; use with caution in patients with seizures or in patients with history of beta-lactam allergy; safety and efficacy have not been established in children <12 years of age

Drug Interactions

Decreased Effect: Tetracyclines may decrease penicillin effectiveness. Aminoglycosides may cause physical inactivation of aminoglycosides in the presence of high concentrations of piperacillin and potential toxicity in patients with mild-moderate renal dysfunction. Although anecdotal reports suggest oral contraceptive efficacy could be reduced by penicillins, this has been refuted by more rigorous scientific and clinical data.

Increased Effect/Toxicity: Probenecid may increase penicillin levels. Neuromuscular blockers may increase duration of blockade. Penicillins may increase methotrexate exposure; clinical significance has not been established.

Lab Interactions Positive Coombs' [direct] test 3.8%, ALT, AST, bilirubin, and LDH

Adverse Reactions

>10%: Gastrointestinal: Diarrhea (11%)

1% to 10%:

Cardiovascular: Hypertension (2%)

Central nervous system: Insomnia (7%), headache (7% to 8%), agitation (2%), fever (2%), dizziness (1%)

Dermatologic: Rash (4%), pruritus (3%)

Gastrointestinal: Constipation (7% to 8%), nausea (7%), vomiting/dyspepsia (3%)

Hepatic: Transaminases increased

Respiratory: Rhinitis/dyspnea (~1%)

Miscellaneous: Serum sickness-like reaction

Several laboratory abnormalities have rarely been associated with piperacillin/tazobactam including reversible eosinophilia, and neutropenia (associated most often with prolonged therapy), positive direct Coombs' test, prolonged PT and aPTT, transient elevations of LFT, increases in creatinine

Overdosage/Toxicology Symptoms of penicillin overdose include neuromuscular hypersensitivity (eg, agitation, hallucinations, asterixis, encephalopathy, confusion, and seizures). Electrolyte imbalance may occur if the preparation contains potassium or sodium salts, especially in renal dysfunction. Hemodialysis may be helpful to aid in removal of the drug from blood; otherwise, treatment is supportive or symptom-directed.

Pharmacodynamics/Kinetics

Protein Binding: Piperacillin: ~26% to 33%; Tazobactam: 31% to 32%

Half-Life Elimination: Piperacillin: 1 hour; Metabolite: 1-1.5 hours; Tazobactam: 0.7-0.9 hour

Metabolism: Piperacillin: 6% to 9%; Tazobactam: ~26%

Excretion: Both piperacillin and tazobactam are directly proportional to renal function

Piperacillin: Urine (50% to 70%); feces (10% to 20%)

Tazobactam: Urine (26% as inactive metabolite) within 24 hours

Pharmacokinetic Note: Both AUC and peak concentrations are dose proportional. Hepatic impairment does not affect the kinetics of piperacillin or tazobactam significantly.

Dosing

Adults & Elderly:

Nosocomial pneumonia: I.V.: Piperacillin/tazobactam 4/0.5 g every 6 hours for 7-14 days (when used empirically, combination with an aminoglycoside is recommended; consider discontinuation of aminoglycoside if *P. aeruginosa* is not isolated)

Severe infections: I.V.: Piperacillin/tazobactam 4/0.5 g every 8 hours or 3/0.375 g every 6 hours for 7-10 days

Moderate infections: I.M.: Piperacillin/tazobactam 2/0.25 g every 6-8 hours; treatment should be continued for ≥7-10 days depending on severity of disease (**Note:** I.M. route not FDA-approved)

Pediatrics: Not FDA-approved for children <12 years of age.

Infants <6 months: I.V.: 150-300 mg of piperacillin component/kg/day in divided doses every 6-8 hours

Infants and Children ≥6 months: I.V.: 240 mg of piperacillin component/kg/day in divided doses every 8 hours; higher doses have been used for serious pseudomonal infections: 300-400 mg of piperacillin component/kg/day in divided doses every 6 hours.

Renal Impairment:

Cl_{cr} 20-40 mL/minute: Administer 2/0.25 g every 6 hours (3/0.375 g every 6 hours for nosocomial pneumonia)

Cl_{cr} <20 mL/minute: Administer 2/0.25 g every 8 hours (2/0.25 g every 6 hours for nosocomial pneumonia)

Hemodialysis: Administer 2/0.25 g every 12 hours (every 8 hours for nosocomial pneumonia) with an additional dose of 0.75 g after each dialysis

Continuous arteriovenous or venovenous hemodiafiltration effects: Dose as for Cl_{cr} 10-50 mL/minute

Hepatic Impairment: Hepatic impairment does not affect the kinetics of piperacillin or tazobactam significantly.

Available Dosage Forms Note: 8:1 ratio of piperacillin sodium/tazobactam sodium: Infusion [premixed iso-osmotic solution, frozen]:

2.25 g: Piperacillin 2 g and tazobactam 0.25 g (50 mL) [contains sodium 5.7 mEq (131 mg)]

3.375 g: Piperacillin 3 g and tazobactam 0.375 g (50 mL) [contains sodium 8.6 mEq (197 mg)]

4.5 g: Piperacillin 4 g and tazobactam 0.5 g (50 mL) [contains sodium 11.4 mEq (263 mg)]

(Continued)

Piperacillin and Tazobactam Sodium *(Continued)*

Injection, powder for reconstitution:
  2.25 g: Piperacillin 2 g and tazobactam 0.25 g [contains sodium 4.69 mEq (108 mg)]
  3.375 g: Piperacillin 3 g and tazobactam 0.375 g [contains sodium 7.04 mEq (162 mg)]
  4.5 g: Piperacillin 4 g and tazobactam 0.5 g [contains sodium 9.39 mEq (216 mg)]
  40.5 g: Piperacillin 36 g and tazobactam 4.5 g [contains sodium 84.5 mEq (1944 mg); bulk
  pharmacy vial]

Monitoring and Teaching Issues

Physical Assessment: Assess results of culture and sensitivity tests and patient's allergy history prior to starting therapy. Use caution with impaired renal function and history of seizure activity (see Warnings/Precautions). Assess potential for interactions with other pharmacological agents patient may be taking (eg, may increase or decrease levels/effects of penicillin or increase risk of toxicity [aminoglycosides, neuromuscular blockers]; see Drug Interactions). See Administration for infusion specifics. Assess effectiveness (resolution of infection) and adverse reactions (eg, hypersensitivity reactions, opportunistic infection [fever, chills, unhealed sores, white plaques in mouth or vagina, purulent vaginal discharge, fatigue], confusion, convulsions, rash, thrombophlebitis; see Adverse Reactions). Advise patients with diabetes about use of Clinitest®. Teach patient possible side effects/appropriate interventions and adverse symptoms to report (see Patient Education).

Monitoring Laboratory Tests: LFTs, creatinine, BUN, CBC with differential, serum electrolytes, urinalysis, PT, PTT; perform culture and sensitivity before administering first dose

Patient Education: This drug can only be given by injection or infusion; report immediately any redness, swelling, burning, or pain at infusion site or any signs of allergic reaction (eg, respiratory or swallowing difficulty, chest tightness, rash, hives, swelling of lips or mouth). Maintain adequate hydration (2-3 L/day of fluids) unless instructed to restrict fluid intake. If you have diabetes, drug may cause false test results with Clinitest®, consult prescriber for alternative method of glucose monitoring. May cause diarrhea (consult prescriber for approved medication); nausea or vomiting (small frequent meals, frequent mouth care, chewing gum, or sucking lozenges may help); or constipation (increased exercise, fluids, fruit, or fiber may help). Report acute or persistent headache; rash; CNS changes (eg, agitation, confusion, hallucinations, or seizures); persistent abdominal pain, cramping or diarrhea; unusual fever; or other persistent adverse effects. **Breast-feeding precaution:** Consult prescriber if breast-feeding.

Dietary Considerations:
  Infusion, premixed: 2.25 g contains sodium 5.7 mEq (131 mg); 3.375 g contains sodium 8.6 mEq (197 mg); 4.5 g contains sodium 11.4 mEq (263 mg)
  Injection, powder for reconstitution: 2.25 g contains sodium 4.69 mEq (108 mg); 3.375 g contains sodium 7.04 mEq (162 mg); 4.5 g contains sodium 9.39 mEq (216 mg); 40.5 g contains sodium 84.5 mEq (1944 mg, bulk pharmacy vial)

Geriatric Considerations: Has not been studied exclusively in the elderly.

Pregnancy Risk Factor: B

Lactation: Enters breast milk/use caution

Breast-Feeding Issues: Piperacillin is excreted in breast milk.

Administration

I.V.: Administer by I.V. infusion over 30 minutes. Discontinue primary infusion, if possible, during infusion and administer aminoglycosides separately from Zosyn®.

Reconstitution: Use single-dose vials immediately after reconstitution (discard unused portions after 24 hours at room temperature and 48 hours if refrigerated). Reconstitute with 5 mL of diluent per 1 g of piperacillin and then further dilute. Compatible diluents include NS, SW, dextran 6%, D_5W, D_5W with potassium chloride 40 mEq, bacteriostatic saline and water.

Compatibility: Stable in dextran 6% in NS, D_5W, NS, SWFI, bacteriostatic water; **incompatible** with LR

Y-site administration: Incompatible with acyclovir, alatrofloxacin, amphotericin B, amphotericin B cholesteryl sulfate complex, chlorpromazine, cisplatin, dacarbazine, daunorubicin, dobutamine, doxorubicin, doxorubicin liposome, doxycycline, droperidol, famotidine, ganciclovir, gatifloxacin, gemcitabine, haloperidol, hydroxyzine, idarubicin, minocycline, mitomycin, mitoxantrone, nalbuphine, prochlorperazine edisylate, promethazine, streptozocin

Storage: Store at controlled room temperature. After reconstitution, solution is stable in NS or D_5W for 24 hours at room temperature and 7 days when refrigerated.

Related Information

Piperacillin *on page 1219*

♦ **Piperacillin Sodium** *see* Piperacillin *on page 1219*

♦ **Piperacillin Sodium and Tazobactam Sodium** *see* Piperacillin and Tazobactam Sodium *on page 1220*

Pirbuterol *(peer BYOO ter ole)*

U.S. Brand Names Maxair™ Autohaler™

Synonyms Pirbuterol Acetate

Generic Available No

Pharmacologic Category Beta₂-Adrenergic Agonist

Use Prevention and treatment of reversible bronchospasm including asthma

Mechanism of Action/Effect Pirbuterol is a beta₂-adrenergic agonist with a similar structure to albuterol, specifically a pyridine ring has been substituted for the benzene ring in albuterol. The increased beta₂ selectivity of pirbuterol results from the substitution of a tertiary butyl group on the nitrogen of the side chain, which additionally imparts resistance of pirbuterol to degradation by monoamine oxidase and provides a lengthened duration of action in comparison to the less selective previous beta-agonist agents.

Contraindications Hypersensitivity to pirbuterol, albuterol, or any component of the formulation

Warnings/Precautions Optimize anti-inflammatory treatment before initiating maintenance treatment with pirbuterol. Do not use as a component of chronic therapy without an anti-inflammatory agent. Only the mildest form of asthma (Step 1 and/or exercise-induced) would not require concurrent use based upon asthma guidelines. Patient must be instructed to seek medical attention in cases where acute symptoms are not relieved or a previous level of response is diminished. The need to increase frequency of use may indicate deterioration of asthma, and treatment must not be delayed.

Use caution in patients with cardiovascular disease (arrhythmia or hypertension or CHF), convulsive disorders, diabetes, glaucoma, hyperthyroidism, or hypokalemia. Beta agonists may cause elevation in blood pressure, heart rate, and result in CNS stimulation/excitation. Beta$_2$ agonists may increase risk of arrhythmia, increase serum glucose, or decrease serum potassium.

Do not exceed recommended dose; serious adverse events including fatalities, have been associated with excessive use of inhaled sympathomimetics. Rarely, paradoxical broncho-spasm may occur with use of inhaled bronchodilating agents; this should be distinguished from inadequate response. All patients should utilize a spacer device when using a metered-dose inhaler. Safety and efficacy have not been established in children <12 years of age.

Drug Interactions

Decreased Effect: Decreased effect with beta-blockers.

Increased Effect/Toxicity: Increased toxicity with other beta agonists, MAO inhibitors, tricyclic antidepressants.

Adverse Reactions

>10%:

Central nervous system: Nervousness (7%)

Endocrine & metabolic: Serum glucose increased, serum potassium decreased

Neuromuscular & skeletal: Trembling (6%)

1% to 10%:

Cardiovascular: Palpitations (2%), tachycardia (1%)

Central nervous system: Headache (2%), dizziness (1%)

Gastrointestinal: Nausea (2%)

Respiratory: Cough (1%)

Overdosage/Toxicology Symptoms of overdose include tachycardia, tremor, hypertension, angina, and seizures. Hypokalemia also may occur. Cardiac arrest and death may be associated with abuse of beta-agonist bronchodilators. Treatment includes immediate discontinuation and symptomatic and supportive therapies. Cautious use of beta-adrenergic blocking agents may be considered in severe cases.

Pharmacodynamics/Kinetics

Onset of Action: Peak effect: Therapeutic: Oral: 2-3 hours with peak serum concentration of 6.2-9.8 mcg/L; Inhalation: 0.5-1 hour

Half-Life Elimination: 2-3 hours

Metabolism: Hepatic

Excretion: Urine (10% as unchanged drug)

Dosing

Adults & Elderly: Bronchospasm: Inhalation: 2 inhalations every 4-6 hours for prevention; 2 inhalations at an interval of at least 1-3 minutes, followed by a third inhalation in treatment of bronchospasm, not to exceed 12 inhalations/day

Pediatrics: Children ≥12 years: Refer to adult dosing.

Available Dosage Forms Aerosol for oral inhalation, as acetate:

Maxair™ Autohaler™: 14 g [400 inhalations; contains chlorofluorocarbons]

Monitoring and Teaching Issues

Physical Assessment: Assess effectiveness and interactions of other medications patient may be taking. Monitor effectiveness of therapy and adverse reactions at beginning of therapy and periodically with long-term use. For inpatient care, monitor vital signs and lung sounds prior to and periodically during therapy. Assess knowledge/teach patient appropriate use, interventions to reduce side effects, and adverse symptoms to report.

Monitoring Laboratory Tests: FEV$_1$, peak flow, and/or other pulmonary function tests; serum potassium, serum glucose (in selected patients)

Patient Education: Use exactly as directed. Do not use more often than recommended. Maintain adequate hydration (2-3 L/day of fluids) unless instructed to restrict fluid intake. You may experience nervousness, dizziness, or fatigue (use caution when driving or engaging in tasks requiring alertness until response to drug is known); or dry mouth or stomach upset (small frequent meals, frequent mouth care, chewing gum, or sucking hard candy may help). If you have diabetes, check blood sugar; blood glucose levels may be increased. Report unresolved GI upset; dizziness or fatigue; vision changes; chest pain, rapid heartbeat, or palpitations; nervousness or insomnia; muscle cramping or tremor; or unusual cough. **Pregnancy/breast-feeding precautions:** Inform prescriber if you are or intend to become pregnant. Consult prescriber if breast-feeding.

Aerosol: Store canister upside down; do not freeze. Shake canister before using. Sit when using medication. Close eyes when administering pirbuterol to avoid spray getting into eyes. Exhale slowly and completely through nose; inhale deeply through mouth while administering aerosol. Hold breath for 5-10 seconds after inhalation. Wait at least 1 full minute between inhalations. Wash mouthpiece between use. If more than one inhalation medication is used, use bronchodilator first and wait 5 minutes between medications.

Maxair™ Autohaler™: Hold upright. Raise lever so that it stays up and snaps into place. Shake well. Exhale. Seal lips tightly around mouthpiece, inhale deeply. A "click" will be heard and you will feel a soft puff when the medication has been triggered. Continue to take a full, deep breath. Remove inhaler from mouth, hold breath for 10 seconds, then exhale slowly. **Note:** A test-fire slide has been added to the bottom of the Autohaler™ actuator/mouthpiece. The inhaler should be primed prior to using for the first time or if it has not been used in 48 hours. To prime, remove mouthpiece; point mouthpiece away from yourself or others, and push the lever so that it stays up. Push the white test-fire slide

(Continued)

Pirbuterol (Continued)

located on the bottom of the mouthpiece to release the priming spray. In order to release a second priming spray, push lever to "down" position, then repeat steps. When two priming sprays have been done, return lever to "down" position.

Geriatric Considerations: Elderly patients may find it beneficial to utilize a spacer device when using a metered dose inhaler. Difficulty in using the inhaler often limits its effectiveness. The Maxair™ Autohaler™ may be easier for the elderly to use.

Pregnancy Risk Factor: C

Lactation: Excretion in breast milk unknown

Administration

Inhalation: Shake inhaler well before use.

Storage: Store between 15°C and 30°C (59°F and 86°F).

Related Information

Inhalant Agents *on page 1734*

♦ **Pirbuterol Acetate** *see* Pirbuterol *on page 1222*

Piroxicam *(peer OKS i kam)*

U.S. Brand Names Feldene®

Generic Available Yes

Pharmacologic Category Nonsteroidal Anti-inflammatory Drug (NSAID), Oral

Use Symptomatic treatment of acute and chronic rheumatoid arthritis and osteoarthritis

Unlabeled/Investigational Use Ankylosing spondylitis

Mechanism of Action/Effect Inhibits prostaglandin synthesis, acts on the hypothalamus heat-regulating center to reduce fever, blocks prostaglandin synthetase action which prevents formation of the platelet-aggregating substance thromboxane A_2; decreases pain receptor sensitivity. Other proposed mechanisms of action for salicylate anti-inflammatory action are lysosomal stabilization, kinin and leukotriene production, alteration of chemotactic factors, and inhibition of neutrophil activation. This latter mechanism may be the most significant pharmacologic action to reduce inflammation.

Contraindications Hypersensitivity to piroxicam, aspirin, other NSAIDs or any component of the formulation; active GI bleeding; pregnancy (3rd trimester or near term)

Warnings/Precautions Fatal asthmatic and anaphylactoid reactions have occurred in patients with "aspirin triad." Use with caution in patients with CHF, hypertension, dehydration, decreased renal or hepatic function, history of GI disease (bleeding, ulcers, or previous GI symptoms with NSAID use), or those receiving anticoagulants and/or corticosteroids. Use lowest effective dose for shortest period possible; bleeding risk has been correlated to dose and duration of therapy. Gastrointestinal bleeding may occur without prior symptoms of gastrointestinal irritation. Elderly are at a high risk for adverse effects from NSAIDs. As many as 60% of elderly can develop peptic ulceration and/or hemorrhage asymptomatically.

Use of NSAIDs can compromise existing renal function especially when Cl_{cr} <30 mL/minute. CNS adverse effects such as confusion, agitation, and hallucination are generally seen in overdose or high-dose situations; however, elderly may demonstrate these adverse effects at lower doses than younger adults. Withhold for at least 4-6 half-lives prior to surgical or dental procedures.

Drug Interactions

Cytochrome P450 Effect: Substrate of CYP2C8/9 (minor); **Inhibits** CYP2C8/9 (strong)

Decreased Effect: Decreased effect of diuretics, beta-blockers. Decreased effect with aspirin, antacids, and cholestyramine.

Increased Effect/Toxicity: Increased effect/toxicity of lithium and methotrexate (controversial). Piroxicam may increase the levels/effects of amiodarone, fluoxetine, glimepiride, glipizide, nateglinide, phenytoin, pioglitazone, rosiglitazone, sertraline, warfarin, and other CYP2C8/9 substrates.

Nutritional/Ethanol Interactions

Ethanol: Avoid ethanol (may enhance gastric mucosal irritation).

Food: Onset of effect may be delayed if piroxicam is taken with food.

Herb/Nutraceutical: Avoid cat's claw, dong quai, evening primrose, feverfew, garlic, red clover, horse chestnut, green tea, ginseng, ginkgo (all have additional antiplatelet activity).

Lab Interactions Increased chloride (S), sodium (S), bleeding time

Adverse Reactions

>10%:

Central nervous system: Dizziness

Dermatologic: Rash

Gastrointestinal: Abdominal cramps, heartburn, indigestion, nausea

1% to 10%:

Central nervous system: Headache, nervousness

Dermatologic: Itching

Endocrine & metabolic: Fluid retention

Gastrointestinal: Vomiting

Otic: Tinnitus

Overdosage/Toxicology Symptoms of overdose include nausea, epigastric distress, CNS depression, leukocytosis, and renal failure. Management of NSAID intoxication is supportive and symptomatic. Multiple doses of activated charcoal may interrupt enterohepatic recycling of some NSAIDs.

Pharmacodynamics/Kinetics

Onset of Action: Analgesic: ~1 hour; Peak effect: 3-5 hours

Protein Binding: 99%

Half-Life Elimination: 45-50 hours

Metabolism: Hepatic

Excretion: Primarily urine and feces (small amounts) as unchanged drug (5%) and metabolites

Dosing

Adults: Inflammation, rheumatoid arthritis: Oral: 10-20 mg/day once daily; although associated with increase in GI adverse effects, doses >20 mg/day have been used (ie, 30-40 mg/day); maximum dose: 20 mg/day

Elderly: Refer to adult dosing. **Note:** Some clinicians have used 10 mg every other day to initiate therapy in the elderly to help avoid side effects and produce therapeutic effect at minimal dose. Maximum dose: 20 mg/day

Pediatrics: Oral: Children: 0.2-0.3 mg/kg/day once daily; maximum dose: 15 mg/day

Hepatic Impairment: Reduced dose is necessary.

Available Dosage Forms Capsule: 10 mg, 20 mg

Monitoring and Teaching Issues

Physical Assessment: Assess effectiveness and interactions of other medications patient may be taking. Assess results of laboratory tests, therapeutic effectiveness, and adverse reactions (eg, GI effects, hepatotoxicity, ototoxicity) at beginning of therapy and periodically throughout therapy. Schedule ophthalmic evaluations for patients who develop eye complaints during long-term NSAID therapy. Advise patients with diabetes to use serum glucose testing. Assess knowledge/teach patient appropriate use, interventions to reduce side effects, and adverse symptoms to report.

Monitoring Laboratory Tests: Occult blood loss, hemoglobin, hematocrit, and periodic renal and hepatic function tests

Patient Education: Take this medication exactly as directed; do not increase dose without consulting prescriber. Do not break capsules. Take with food or milk to reduce GI distress. Maintain adequate hydration (2-3 L/day of fluids) unless instructed to restrict fluid intake. Do not use alcohol, aspirin or aspirin-containing medication, or any other anti-inflammatory medications without consulting prescriber. You may experience drowsiness, dizziness, or nervousness (use caution when driving or engaging in tasks requiring alertness until response to drug is known); anorexia, nausea, vomiting, flatulence, or heartburn (small frequent meals, frequent mouth care, sucking lozenges, or chewing gum may help); or fluid retention (weigh yourself weekly and report unusual weight gain [3-5 lb/week]). GI bleeding, ulceration, or perforation can occur with or without pain; discontinue medication and contact prescriber if persistent abdominal pain or cramping, or blood in stool occurs. Report unusual swelling of extremities or unusual weight gain; breathlessness, respiratory difficulty, or unusual cough; chest pain, rapid heartbeat, palpitations; unusual bruising/bleeding; blood in urine, stool, mouth, or vomitus; unusual fatigue; changes in urinary pattern (polyuria or anuria); skin rash or itching; or change in hearing or ringing in ears.

Pregnancy precaution: Inform prescriber if you are or intend to become pregnant. This drug should not be used in the 3rd trimester of pregnancy.

Dietary Considerations: May be taken with food to decrease GI adverse effect.

Geriatric Considerations: Elderly are at high risk for adverse effects from NSAIDs. As much as 60% of elderly can develop peptic ulceration and/or hemorrhage asymptomatically. The concomitant use of H_2 blockers, omeprazole, and sucralfate is not generally effective as prophylaxis with the exception of NSAID-induced duodenal ulcers which may be prevented by the use of ranitidine. Misoprostol is the only prophylactic agent proven effective. Also, concomitant disease and drug use contribute to the risk for GI adverse effects. Use lowest effective dose for shortest period possible. Consider renal function decline with age. Use of NSAIDs can compromise existing renal function especially when Cl_{cr} is ≤30 mL/minute. Tinnitus may be a difficult and unreliable indication of toxicity due to age-related hearing loss or eighth cranial nerve damage. CNS adverse effects such as confusion, agitation, and hallucination are generally seen in overdose or high-dose situations, but elderly may demonstrate these adverse effects at lower doses than younger adults.

Pregnancy Risk Factor: B/D (3rd trimester or near term)

Lactation: Enters breast milk (small amounts)/compatible

Related Information

Nonsalicylate / Nonsteroidal Anti-inflammatory Agents *on page 1743*

Podophyllum Resin (po DOF fil um REZ in)

U.S. Brand Names Podocon-25®

Synonyms Mandrake; May Apple; Podophyllin

Generic Available No

Pharmacologic Category Keratolytic Agent

Use Topical treatment of benign growths including external genital and perianal warts, papillomas, fibroids; compound benzoin tincture generally is used as the medium for topical application

Mechanism of Action/Effect Directly affects epithelial cell metabolism by arresting mitosis through binding to a protein subunit of spindle microtubules (tubulin)

Contraindications Not to be used on birthmarks, moles, or warts with hair growth; cervical, urethral, oral warts; not to be used by diabetic patient or patient with poor circulation; pregnancy

Warnings/Precautions Use of large amounts of drug should be avoided. Avoid contact with the eyes as it can cause severe corneal damage; do not apply to moles, birthmarks, or unusual warts. To be applied by prescriber only. For external use only; 25% solution should not be applied to or near mucous membranes.

Adverse Reactions 1% to 10%:

Dermatologic: Pruritus

Gastrointestinal: Nausea, vomiting, abdominal pain, diarrhea

Dosing

Adults & Elderly: Treatment of benign growths (warts, papillomas, fibroids): Topical: 10% to 25% solution in compound benzoin tincture; apply drug to dry surface, use 1 drop at a time allowing drying between drops until area is covered. Total volume should be limited to <0.5 mL per treatment session.

Condylomata acuminatum: 25% solution is applied daily. Use a 10% solution when applied to or near mucous membranes.

Verrucae: 25% solution is applied 3-5 times/day directly to the wart.

Pediatrics: Refer to adult dosing.

Available Dosage Forms Liquid, topical: 25% (15 mL) [in benzoin tincture]

Monitoring and Teaching Issues

Physical Assessment: Pregnancy risk factor X: Determine that patient is not pregnant before starting therapy. Do not give to sexually-active female patients unless capable of complying with contraceptive use. Breast-feeding is contraindicated.

Patient Education: Cover with occlusive dressing to prevent contact with unaffected skin. Wash off medication as instructed by professional who applied the treatment. **Pregnancy/breast-feeding precautions:** Inform prescriber if you are pregnant. Do not get pregnant during or for 1 month following therapy. Consult prescriber for instruction on appropriate contraceptive measures. This drug may cause severe fetal defects. Do not breast-feed.

Pregnancy Risk Factor: X

Lactation: Enters breast milk/contraindicated

Administration

Topical: Shake well before using. **Only to be applied by physician.** Solution should be washed off within 1-4 hours for genital and perianal warts and within 1-2 hours for accessible meatal warts. Use protective occlusive dressing around warts to prevent contact with unaffected skin. For external use only.

♦ **Poliovirus Vaccine (Inactivated)** see page 1660

♦ **Polycitra®-K** see Potassium Citrate and Citric Acid on page 1236

Polyethylene Glycol-Electrolyte Solution

(pol i ETH i leen GLY kol ee LEK troe lite soe LOO shun)

U.S. Brand Names Colyte®; GlycoLax™; GoLYTELY®; MiraLax™; NuLYTELY®; TriLyte™

Synonyms Electrolyte Lavage Solution

Generic Available Yes

Pharmacologic Category Cathartic; Laxative, Bowel Evacuant

Medication Safety Issues

Sound-alike/look-alike issues:

GoLYTELY® may be confused with NuLYTELY®

MiraLax™ may be confused with Mirapex®

NuLYTELY® may be confused with GoLYTELY®

Use Bowel cleansing prior to GI examination or following toxic ingestion (electrolyte containing solutions only); treatment of occasional constipation (MiraLax™)

Mechanism of Action/Effect Induces catharsis by strong electrolyte and osmotic effects

Contraindications Hypersensitivity to polyethylene glycol or any component of the formulation; gastrointestinal obstruction, gastric retention, bowel perforation, toxic colitis, megacolon

Warnings/Precautions Do not add flavorings as additional ingredients before use. Observe unconscious or semiconscious patients with impaired gag reflex or those who are otherwise prone to regurgitation or aspiration during administration. Use with caution in ulcerative colitis. Caution against the use of hot loop polypectomy. Do not use MiraLax™ for longer than 2 weeks.

Drug Interactions

Decreased Effect: Oral medications should not be administered within 1 hour of start of therapy.

Adverse Reactions Frequency not defined.

Dermatologic: Dermatitis, rash, urticaria

Gastrointestinal: Nausea, abdominal fullness, bloating, abdominal cramps, vomiting, anal irritation, diarrhea, flatulence

Pharmacodynamics/Kinetics
Onset of Action: Oral: Bowel cleansing: ~1-2 hours; Constipation: 48-96 hours

Dosing
Adults & Elderly:

Bowel cleansing prior to GI exam (solutions with electrolytes only):

Oral: 240 mL (8 oz) every 10 minutes, until 4 L are consumed or the rectal effluent is clear; rapid drinking of each portion is preferred to drinking small amounts continuously. Ideally, patients should fast for ~3-4 hours prior to administration; absolutely no solid food for at least 2 hours before the solution is given. The solution may be given via nasogastric tube to patients who are unwilling or unable to drink the solution.

Nasogastric tube: 20-30 mL/minute (1.2-1.8 L/hour); the first bowel movement should occur ~1 hour after the start of administration. Ideally, patients should fast for ~3-4 hours prior to administration; absolutely no solid food for at least 2 hours before the solution is given.

Occasional constipation (MiraLax™): Oral: 17 g of powder (~1 heaping tablespoon) dissolved in 8 oz of water; once daily; do not use for >2 weeks.

Pediatrics: Bowel cleansing (solutions with electrolytes only): Children ≥6 months: Ideally, patients should fast for ~3-4 hours prior to administration; absolutely no solid food for at least 2 hours before the solution is given.

Oral: 25-40 mL/kg/hour for 4-10 hours until rectal effluent is clear

Nasogastric tube: 25 mL/kg/hour until rectal effluent is clear

Available Dosage Forms
Powder, for oral solution: PEG 3350 240 g, sodium sulfate 22.72 g, sodium bicarbonate 6.72 g, sodium chloride 5.84 g, and potassium chloride 2.98 g (4000 mL)

Colyte®:

PEG 3350 240 g, sodium sulfate 22.72 g, sodium bicarbonate 6.72 g, sodium chloride 5.84 g, and potassium chloride 2.98 g (4000 mL) [available with citrus berry, lemon lime, cherry, and pineapple flavor packets]

PEG 3350 227.1 g, sodium sulfate 21.5 g, sodium bicarbonate 6.36 g, sodium chloride 5.53 g, and potassium chloride 2.82 g (4000 mL) [regular and pineapple flavor]

GlycoLax™: PEG 3350 17 g/packet (14s); PEG 3350 255 g (16 oz); PEG 3350 527 g (24 oz)

GoLYTELY®:

Disposable jug: PEG 3350 236 g, sodium sulfate 22.74 g, sodium bicarbonate 6.74 g, sodium chloride 5.86 g, and potassium chloride 2.97 g (4000 mL) [regular and pineapple flavor]

Packets: PEG 3350 227.1 g, sodium sulfate 21.5 g, sodium bicarbonate 6.36 g, sodium chloride 5.53 g, and potassium chloride 2.82 g (4000 mL) [regular flavor]

MiraLax™: PEG 3350 17 g/packet (12s); PEG 3350 255 g (14 oz); PEG 3350 527 g (26 oz)

NuLYTELY®: PEG 3350 420 g, sodium bicarbonate 5.72 g, sodium chloride 11.2 g, and potassium chloride 1.48 (4000 mL) [cherry, lemon-lime, and orange flavors]

TriLyte™: PEG 3350 420 g, sodium bicarbonate 5.72 g, sodium chloride 11.2 g, and potassium chloride 1.48 (4000 mL) [supplied with flavor packets]

Monitoring and Teaching Issues
Physical Assessment: See Contraindications, Warnings/Precautions, Drug Interactions, and Adverse Reactions for use cautions. Instruct patient in appropriate use (see above for specific instructions according to formulation and purpose).

Monitoring Laboratory Tests: Electrolytes, serum glucose, BUN, urine osmolality

Patient Education: Follow instructions exactly; directions will differ according to the formulation and the purpose for which this medication is taken. Do not eat any solid foods for at least 2-3 hours before taking and do not take any other oral medication for 1 hour before taking. For bowel cleansing prior to GI exam, take 240 mL (8 oz) every 10 minutes, until 4 L is consumed or the rectal effluent is clear. Rapid drinking of each portion is preferred to drinking small amounts continuously. The first bowel movement should occur approximately 1 hour after the start of administration. May cause abdominal bloating and distention before bowel starts to move. If severe discomfort or distention occurs, stop drinking temporarily or drink each portion at longer intervals until these symptoms disappear. Continue drinking until the watery stool is clear and free of solid matter. This usually requires at least 3 L. It is best to drink all of the solutions. Discard any unused portion. **Pregnancy/breast-feeding precautions:** Inform prescriber if you are or intend to become pregnant. Consult prescriber if breast-feeding.

Dietary Considerations: Bowel cleansing prior to GI exam: Ideally, the patient should fast for ~3-4 hours prior to administration, but in no case should solid food be given for at least 2 hours before the solution is given.

Pregnancy Risk Factor: C

Lactation: Excretion in breast milk unknown/use caution

Breast-Feeding Issues: Significant changes in the mother's fluid or electrolyte balance would not be expected.

Administration
Oral: Bowel cleansing prior to GI exam (solutions with electrolytes only): Oral: Rapid drinking of each portion is preferred to drinking small amounts continuously. Do not add flavorings as additional ingredients before use. Chilled solution often more palatable.

Reconstitution:
Powder for solution (with electrolytes): Use within 48 hours of preparation; refrigerate reconstituted solution; tap water may be used for preparation of the solution; shake container vigorously several times to ensure dissolution of powder. Do not add additional flavorings to solution.

MiraLax™: Dissolve powder in 8 ounces of water, juice, cola, or tea

Storage: Store at 15°C to 30°C (59°F to 86°F) before reconstitution.

Related Information
Laxatives, Classification and Properties *on page 1737*

Polyethylene Glycol-Electrolyte Solution and Bisacodyl
(pol i ETH i leen GLY kol ee LEK troe lite soe LOO shun & bis a KOE dil)

U.S. Brand Names HalfLytely® and Bisacodyl

Synonyms Electrolyte Lavage Solution

Generic Available No

Pharmacologic Category Laxative, Bowel Evacuant; Laxative, Stimulant

Use Bowel cleansing prior to GI examination

Dosing

  Adults & Elderly: Bowel cleansing: Oral:

    Bisacodyl: 4 tablets as a single dose. After bowel movement or 6 hours (whichever occurs first), initiate polyethylene glycol-electrolyte solution

    Polyethylene glycol-electrolyte solution: 8 ounces every 10 minutes until 2 L are consumed

Available Dosage Forms Kit (HalfLytely® and Bisacodyl) [each kit contains]:

  Powder for oral solution (HalfLytely®):PEG 3350 210 g, sodium bicarbonate 2.86 g, sodium chloride 5.6 g, potassium chloride 0.74 g (2000 mL) [sulfate-free, regular, cherry, lemon-lime, orange flavor]

  Tablet, delayed release: Bisacodyl: 5 mg (4s)

Monitoring and Teaching Issues

  Physical Assessment: Instruct patient in appropriate use and preparation.

  Patient Education: This preparation is intended to produce a watery stool which cleanses the bowel before examination. For best results, consume only clear liquids on the day of the examination unless otherwise directed by prescriber. Do not take antacids within 1 hour of taking the bisacodyl delayed-release tablets. Swallow all tablets (4) whole with water. Do not chew or crush. Expect the first bowel movement in approximately 1-6 hours after taking tablets. Wait for bowel movement (or maximum 6 hours), then drink the solution. Drink 8 ounces every 10 minutes. Drink all of the solution. Rapid drinking of each portion is better than drinking small amounts. A bowel movement should occur in approximately 1 hour after drinking the solution. You may experience bloating or abdominal distention before the bowels start to move. If severe discomfort or distention occurs, stop drinking the solution temporarily or drink each portion at longer intervals until symptoms disappear. **Pregnancy/ breast-feeding precaution:** Inform prescriber if you are or intend to become pregnant. Consult prescriber if breast-feeding.

  Pregnancy Risk Factor: C

  Lactation: Excretion in breast milk unknown/use caution

♦ **Polygam® S/D** *see* Immune Globulin (Intravenous) *on page 793*

Polymyxin B (pol i MIKS in bee)

U.S. Brand Names Poly-Rx

Synonyms Polymyxin B Sulfate

Generic Available Yes

Pharmacologic Category Antibiotic, Irrigation; Antibiotic, Miscellaneous

Use Treatment of acute infections caused by susceptible strains of *Pseudomonas aeruginosa*; used occasionally for gut decontamination; parenteral use of polymyxin B has mainly been replaced by less toxic antibiotics, reserved for life-threatening infections caused by organisms resistant to the preferred drugs (eg, pseudomonal meningitis - intrathecal administration)

Mechanism of Action/Effect Binds to phospholipids, alters permeability, and damages the bacterial cytoplasmic membrane permitting leakage of intracellular constituents

Contraindications Hypersensitivity to polymyxin B or any component of the formulation; concurrent use of neuromuscular blockers

Warnings/Precautions Use with caution in patients with impaired renal function (modify dosage) neurotoxic reactions are usually associated with high serum levels, found in patients with impaired renal function. Avoid concurrent or sequential use of other nephrotoxic and neurotoxic drugs, particularly bacitracin, colistin, and the aminoglycosides. The drug's neurotoxicity can result in respiratory paralysis from neuromuscular blockade, especially when the drug is given soon after anesthesia or muscle relaxants. Polymyxin B sulfate is toxic when given parenterally; avoid parenteral use whenever possible.

Drug Interactions

  Increased Effect/Toxicity: Increased/prolonged effect of neuromuscular blocking agents.

Adverse Reactions Frequency not defined.

  Cardiovascular: Facial flushing

  Central nervous system: Neurotoxicity (irritability, drowsiness, ataxia, perioral paresthesia, numbness of the extremities, and blurred vision); dizziness, drug fever, meningeal irritation with intrathecal administration

  Dermatologic: Urticarial rash

  Endocrine & metabolic: Hypocalcemia, hyponatremia, hypokalemia, hypochloremia

  Local: Pain at injection site

  Neuromuscular & skeletal: Neuromuscular blockade, weakness

  Renal: Nephrotoxicity

  Respiratory: Respiratory arrest

  Miscellaneous: Anaphylactoid reaction

Overdosage/Toxicology Symptoms of overdose include respiratory paralysis, ototoxicity, and nephrotoxicity. Supportive care is indicated as treatment.

Pharmacodynamics/Kinetics

  Absorption: Well absorbed from peritoneum; minimal from GI tract (except in neonates) from mucous membranes or intact skin

  Time to Peak: Serum: I.M.: ~2 hours

  Half-Life Elimination: 4.5-6 hours; prolonged with renal impairment

  Excretion: Urine (>60% primarily as unchanged drug)

Dosing

  Adults & Elderly:

    Ear canal infections (external): Otic (in combination with other drugs): Instill 1-2 drops, 3-4 times/day; should be used sparingly to avoid accumulation of excess debris.

Systemic infections:
  I.M.: 25,000-30,000 units/kg/day divided every 4-6 hours
  I.V.: 15,000-25,000 units/kg/day divided every 12 hours
  Intrathecal: 50,000 units/day for 3-4 days, then every other day for at least 2 weeks
  Note: Total daily dose should not exceed 2,000,000 units/day.
Bladder irrigation (in combination with 57 mg neomycin sulfate): Continuous irrigant or rinse in the urinary bladder for up to 10 days using 20 mg (equal to 200,000 units) added to 1 L of normal saline; usually no more than 1 L of irrigant is used per day unless urine flow rate is high; administration rate is adjusted to patient's urine output.
Topical irrigation or topical solution: 500,000 units/L of normal saline; topical irrigation should not exceed 2 million units/day in adults.
Ocular infections: Ophthalmic: A concentration of 0.1% to 0.25% is administered as 1-3 drops every hour, then increasing the interval as response indicates to 1-2 drops 4-6 times/day.

Pediatrics:
  Ear canal infections (external): Otic (in combination with other drugs): 1-2 drops, 3-4 times/day; should be used sparingly to avoid accumulation of excess debris
  Systemic infections: Infants <2 years:
    I.M.: Up to 40,000 units/kg/day divided every 6 hours (not routinely recommended due to pain at injection sites)
    I.V.: Up to 40,000 units/kg/day divided every 12 hours
    Intrathecal: 20,000 units/day for 3-4 days, then 25,000 units every other day for at least 2 weeks after CSF cultures are negative and CSF (glucose) has returned to within normal limits
    Children ≥2 years: Refer to adult dosing.

Renal Impairment:
  Cl_{cr} 20-50 mL/minute: Administer 75% to 100% of normal dose every 12 hours.
  Cl_{cr} 5-20 mL/minute: Administer 50% of normal dose every 12 hours.
  Cl_{cr} <5 mL/minute: Administer 15% of normal dose every 12 hours.

Available Dosage Forms
Injection, powder for reconstitution: 500,000 units
Powder [for prescription compounding] (Poly-Rx): 100 million units (13 g)

Monitoring and Teaching Issues
Physical Assessment: Assess results of culture and sensitivity tests and patient's allergy history prior to starting therapy. Use caution with impaired renal function (see Warnings/Precautions for use cautions). Assess potential for interactions with other pharmacological agents patient may be taking (eg, nephrotoxic and neurotoxic drugs, neuromuscular blocking agents; see Drug Interactions). See Administration for I.V. and I.M. specifics. Infusion site must be monitored closely to prevent extravasation; extravasation may cause serious injury with possible necrosis and tissue sloughing (rotate infusion site frequently). Assess effectiveness (resolution of infection) and adverse reactions (eg, renal function, neurotoxicity [irritability, drowsiness, ataxia, perioral paresthesia, numbness of the extremities, and blurring of vision]; neuromuscular blockade, rash, respiratory paralysis, ototoxicity; see Adverse Reactions). Teach patient possible side effects/appropriate interventions and adverse symptoms to report (see Patient Education).
Monitoring Laboratory Tests: Perform culture and sensitivity prior to beginning therapy. Establish baseline renal function prior to initiating therapy. Monitor renal function closely.
Patient Education: Used for wound irrigation/bladder irrigation/gut sterilization.

I.V.: Immediately report numbness or tingling of mouth, tongue, or extremities; constant blurring of vision; increased nervousness or irritability; excessive drowsiness; or respiratory difficulty. Immediately report swelling, redness, burning, or pain at infusion site.

Ophthalmic: Tilt head back, place medication into eyes (as frequently as prescribed), close eyes, apply light pressure over inside corner of the eye for 1 minute. Do not let tip of applicator touch eye; do not contaminate tip of applicator (may cause eye infection, eye damage, or vision loss). You may experience some stinging, burning, or temporary blurring of vision; use caution driving or when engaging in hazardous tasks until vision clears. Report any adverse effects including respiratory difficulty, unusual numbness, or tingling of mouth or tongue, increased nervousness or irritability, or excessive drowsiness.

Breast-feeding precaution: Consult prescriber if breast-feeding.
Pregnancy Risk Factor: B (per expert opinion)
Lactation: Excretion in breast milk unknown/use caution

Administration
I.M.: Administer into upper outer quadrant of gluteal muscle; however, I.M. route is not recommended due to severe pain at injection site.
I.V.: Infuse over 60-90 minutes.
Compatibility: Compatibility when admixed: Incompatible with amphotericin B, calcium chloride, calcium gluconate, cefazolin, chloramphenicol, chlorothiazide, heparin, magnesium sulfate
Storage: Prior to reconstitution, store at room temperature of 15°C to 30°C (59°F to 86°F) and protect from light. After reconstitution, store under refrigeration at 2°C to 8°C (36°F to 46°F). Discard any unused solution after 72 hours. **Incompatible** with strong acids/alkalies, calcium, magnesium, cephalothin, cefazolin, chloramphenicol, heparin, penicillins.

Additional Information 1 mg = 10,000 units

♦ **Poly-Rx** *see* Polymyxin B *on page 1228*
♦ **Polysporin® Ophthalmic** *see* Bacitracin and Polymyxin B *on page 171*
♦ **Polysporin® Topical [OTC]** *see* Bacitracin and Polymyxin B *on page 171*
♦ **Polythiazide and Prazosin** *see* Prazosin and Polythiazide *on page 1244*

Porfimer (POR fi mer)

U.S. Brand Names Photofrin®
Synonyms CL-184116; Dihematoporphyrin Ether; Porfimer Sodium
Generic Available No
Pharmacologic Category Antineoplastic Agent, Miscellaneous
Use Adjunct to laser light therapy for obstructing esophageal cancer, obstructing endobronchial nonsmall cell lung cancer (NSCLC), ablation of high-grade dysplasia in Barrett's esophagus
Unlabeled/Investigational Use Transitional cell carcinoma *in situ* of the urinary bladder; gastric and rectal cancers
Mechanism of Action/Effect Photosensitizing agent used in the photodynamic therapy (PDT) of tumors: cytotoxic and antitumor actions of porfimer are light and oxygen dependent. Cellular damage caused by porfimer PDT is a consequence of the propagation of radical reactions.
Contraindications Hypersensitivity to porfimer, porphyrins, or any component of the formulation; porphyria; tracheoesophageal or bronchoesophageal fistula; tumors eroding into a major blood vessel
Warnings/Precautions The U.S. Food and Drug Administration (FDA) currently recommends that procedures for proper handling and disposal of antineoplastic agents be considered. Photosensitivity reactions are common is patients are exposed to direct sunlight or bright indoor light (eg fluorescent lights, unshaded light bulbs, examination/operating lights). Photosensitivity may last 30-90 days. Ocular discomfort has been reported; for at least 30 days, when outdoors, patients should wear dark sunglasses which have an average white light transmittance of <4%. When treating endobronchial tumors, use caution if treatment-induced inflammation may obstruct airway.
Drug Interactions
  Decreased Effect: Compounds that quench active oxygen species or scavenge radicals (eg, dimethyl sulfoxide, beta-carotene, ethanol, mannitol) would be expected to decrease photodynamic therapy (PDT) activity. Allopurinol, calcium channel blockers, and some prostaglandin synthesis inhibitors could interfere with porfimer. Drugs that decrease clotting, vasoconstriction, or platelet aggregation could decrease the efficacy of PDT. Glucocorticoid hormones may decrease the efficacy of the treatment.
  Increased Effect/Toxicity: Concomitant administration of other photosensitizing agents (eg, tetracyclines, sulfonamides, phenothiazines, sulfonylureas, thiazide diuretics, griseofulvin) could increase the photosensitivity reaction.
Adverse Reactions
  >10%:
    Cardiovascular: Atrial fibrillation (10%), chest pain (5% to 22%)
    Central nervous system: Insomnia (14%), hyperthermia (31%)
    Dermatologic: Photosensitivity reaction (10% to 80%, minor reactions may occur in up to 100%)
    Gastrointestinal: Abdominal pain (20%), constipation (23%), dysphagia, nausea (24%), vomiting (17%)
    Genitourinary: Urinary tract irritation including frequency, urgency, nocturia, painful urination, or bladder spasm (~100% of bladder cancer patients)
    Hematologic: Anemia (26% of esophageal cancer patients)
    Neuromuscular & skeletal: Back pain
    Respiratory: Dyspnea (20%), pharyngitis (11%), pleural effusion (32% of esophageal cancer patients), pneumonia (18%), respiratory insufficiency
    Miscellaneous: Mild-moderate allergic-type reactions (34% of lung cancer patients)
  1% to 10%:
    Cardiovascular: Hyper-/hypotension (6% to 7%), edema, cardiac failure (6% to 7%), tachycardia (6%), chest pain (substernal)
    Central nervous system: Anxiety (7%), confusion (8%)
    Dermatologic: Increased hair growth, skin discoloration, skin wrinkles, skin nodules, increased skin fragility
    Endocrine & metabolic: Dehydration
    Gastrointestinal: Diarrhea (5%), dyspepsia (6%), eructation (5%), esophageal edema (8%), esophageal tumor bleeding, esophageal stricture, esophagitis, hematemesis, melena, weight loss, anorexia
    Genitourinary: Urinary tract infection
    Neuromuscular & skeletal: Weakness
    Respiratory: Coughing, tracheoesophageal fistula
    Miscellaneous: Moniliasis, surgical complication
Overdosage/Toxicology Laser treatment should not be given if an overdose of porfimer is administered. In the event of overdose, patients should protect their eyes and skin from direct sunlight or bright indoor lights for 30 days. Patients should be tested for residual photosensitivity. Porfimer is not dialyzable.
Pharmacodynamics/Kinetics
  Time to Peak: Serum: ~2 hours
  Protein Binding: Plasma: 90%
  Half-Life Elimination: Mean: 21.5 days (range: 11-28 days)
  Excretion: Feces
    Clearance: Plasma: Total: 0.051 mL/minute/kg
Dosing
  Adults & Elderly: Cancer photodynamic therapy: I.V.: 2 mg/kg, followed by exposure to the appropriate laser light
  Pediatrics: I.V. (refer to individual protocols): Children: Safety and efficacy have not been established.

Available Dosage Forms Injection, powder for reconstitution, as sodium: 75 mg

Monitoring and Teaching Issues

Physical Assessment: Assess potential for interactions with other pharmacological agents patient may be taking (eg, drugs that decrease the effect of PDT or porfimer or increase photosensitivity reaction; see Drug Interactions). See Administration specifics; infusion site must be monitored closely to prevent extravasation. Patients will be photosensitive and must be protected from direct sunlight or bright indoor light for 30-60 days after treatment. Ambient indoor light is, however, beneficial (should not stay in dark rooms). Assess patient response (eg, atrial fibrillation, hyper- and hypotension, hyperthermia, GI pain or upset, anemia, dyspnea, respiratory insufficiency, dehydration; see Adverse Reactions). Teach patient (caregiver) possible side effects/appropriate interventions and adverse symptoms to report (see Patient Education).

Patient Education: This drug is given by infusion, report immediately any redness, swelling, burning, or pain at infusion site. The infusion will be followed by laser light therapy. Maintain adequate hydration (2-3 L/day of fluids) unless instructed to restrict fluid intake. You will be highly sensitive to bright light. Avoid any exposure to sunlight or bright indoor light for at least 30-60 days following treatment (cover skin with protective clothing and wear dark sunglasses with light transmittance <4% when outdoors; severe blistering, burning, and skin/eye damage can result). Conventional sunscreens do not protect against photosensitization. After 30 days, test small area of skin (not face) for remaining sensitivity. Retest sensitivity if traveling to a different geographic area with greater sunshine. Exposure to indoor normal light is beneficial since it will help dissipate photosensitivity gradually. May cause nausea or vomiting (small frequent meals, frequent mouth care, sucking lozenges, or chewing gum may help); or constipation (increased exercise, fluids, fruit, or fiber may help). Report rapid heart rate, chest pain or palpitations, respiratory difficulty or air hunger, persistent fever or chills, foul-smelling urine or burning on urination, swelling of extremities, increased anxiety, confusion, or hallucination. **Pregnancy/breast-feeding precautions:** Inform prescriber if you are pregnant. Do not breast-feed.

Pregnancy Risk Factor: C

Pregnancy Issues: Animal studies have shown maternal and fetal toxicity, but no major malformations. Effective contraception is recommended for women of childbearing potential.

Lactation: Excretion in breast milk unknown/contraindicated

Administration

I.V.: Administer slow I.V. injection over 3-5 minutes.

Reconstitution: Reconstitute each vial of porfimer with 31.8 mL of either D_5W or NS injection resulting in a final concentration of 2.5 mg/mL. Shake well until dissolved. Do not mix porfimer with other drugs in the same solution. Protect the reconstituted product from bright light and use immediately.

Compatibility: Do not mix porfimer with other drugs in the same solution.

Storage: Store intact vials at controlled room temperature of 20°C to 25°C (68°F to 77°F). Reconstituted solutions are stable for 24 hours under refrigeration and protected from light.

♦ **Porfimer Sodium** *see* Porfimer *on page 1230*
♦ **Portia™** *see* Ethinyl Estradiol and Levonorgestrel *on page 585*
♦ **Post Peel Healing Balm [OTC]** *see* Hydrocortisone *on page 760*
♦ **Posture® [OTC]** *see* Calcium Phosphate (Tribasic) *on page 241*

Potassium Acetate (poe TASS ee um AS e tate)

Generic Available Yes

Pharmacologic Category Electrolyte Supplement, Parenteral

Medication Safety Issues

Consider special storage requirements for intravenous potassium salts; I.V. potassium salts have been administered IVP in error, leading to fatal outcomes.

Use Potassium deficiency; to avoid chloride when high concentration of potassium is needed, source of bicarbonate

Dosing

Adults & Elderly: I.V. doses should be incorporated into the patient's maintenance I.V. fluids, intermittent I.V. potassium administration should be reserved for severe depletion situations and requires ECG monitoring; doses listed as mEq of potassium

Treatment of hypokalemia: I.V.: 40-100 mEq/day
I.V. intermittent infusion (must be diluted prior to administration):
5-10 mEq/dose (maximum: 40 mEq/dose) to infuse over 2-3 hours (maximum: 40 mEq over 1 hour)
Note: Continuous cardiac monitor recommended for rates >0.5 mEq/hour
Potassium dosage/rate of infusion guidelines:
Serum potassium >2.5 mEq/L: Maximum infusion rate: 10 mEq/hour; maximum concentration: 40 mEq/L; maximum 24-hour dose: 200 mEq
Serum potassium <2.5 mEq/L: Maximum infusion rate: 40 mEq/hour; maximum concentration: 80 mEq/L; maximum 24-hour dose: 400 mEq

Pediatrics: I.V. doses should be incorporated into the patient's maintenance I.V. fluids, intermittent I.V. potassium administration should be reserved for severe depletion situations and requires ECG monitoring; doses listed as mEq of potassium.
Note: Use caution in premature neonates; potassium acetate for injection contains aluminum.

Treatment of hypokalemia: I.V.: 2-5 mEq/kg/day
I.V. intermittent infusion (must be diluted prior to administration): 0.5-1 mEq/kg/dose (maximum: 30 mEq/dose) to infuse at 0.3-0.5 mEq/kg/hour (maximum: 1 mEq/kg/hour)
Note: Continuous cardiac monitor recommended for rates >0.5 mEq/hour
Potassium dosage/rate of infusion guidelines:
Serum potassium >2.5 mEq/L: Maximum infusion rate: 10 mEq/hour; maximum concentration: 40 mEq/L; maximum 24-hour dose: 200 mEq

(Continued)

POTASSIUM ACETATE, POTASSIUM BICARBONATE, AND POTASSIUM CITRATE

Potassium Acetate *(Continued)*

Serum potassium <2.5 mEq/L: Maximum infusion rate: 40 mEq/hour; maximum concentration: 80 mEq/L; maximum 24-hour dose: 400 mEq

Renal Impairment: Use caution; potassium acetate injection contains aluminum.

Available Dosage Forms Injection, solution: 2 mEq/mL (20 mL, 50 mL, 100 mL); 4 mEq/mL (50 mL) [contains aluminum ≤200 mcg/mL]

Monitoring and Teaching Issues

Patient Education: This form of potassium may only be given I.V. Report immediately any burning or pain at infusion site, chest pain, palpitations, unusual weakness in muscles, tarry stools, or easy bruising.

Pregnancy Risk Factor: C

Potassium Acetate, Potassium Bicarbonate, and Potassium Citrate

(poe TASS ee um AS e tate, poe TASS ee um bye KAR bun ate, & poe TASS ee um SIT rate)

U.S. Brand Names Tri-K®

Synonyms Potassium Acetate, Potassium Citrate, and Potassium Bicarbonate; Potassium Bicarbonate, Potassium Acetate, and Potassium Citrate; Potassium Bicarbonate, Potassium Citrate, and Potassium Acetate; Potassium Citrate, Potassium Acetate, and Potassium Bicarbonate; Potassium Citrate, Potassium Bicarbonate, and Potassium Acetate

Generic Available No

Pharmacologic Category Electrolyte Supplement, Oral

Use Treatment or prevention of hypokalemia

Dosing

Adults & Elderly: Hypokalemia: Oral:
Prevention: 16-24 mEq/day in 2-4 divided doses
Treatment: 40-100 mEq/day in 2-4 divided doses

Pediatrics: Hypokalemia: Oral:
Children: 1-4 mEq/kg/24 hours in divided doses as required to maintain normal serum potassium

Available Dosage Forms Solution, oral: Potassium 45 mEq/15 mL (480 mL) [from potassium acetate 1500 mg, potassium bicarbonate 1500 mg, and potassium citrate 1500 mg per 15 mL]

Monitoring and Teaching Issues
Pregnancy Risk Factor: C

Related Information
Potassium Acetate *on page 1231*
Potassium Bicarbonate *on page 1232*
Potassium Citrate *on page 1235*

♦ **Potassium Acetate, Potassium Citrate, and Potassium Bicarbonate** *see* Potassium Acetate, Potassium Bicarbonate, and Potassium Citrate *on page 1232*

Potassium Acid Phosphate (poe TASS ee um AS id FOS fate)

U.S. Brand Names K-Phos® Original

Generic Available No

Pharmacologic Category Urinary Acidifying Agent

Use Acidifies urine and lowers urinary calcium concentration; reduces odor and rash caused by ammoniacal urine; increases the antibacterial activity of methenamine

Dosing

Adults & Elderly: Urine acidification: Oral: 1000 mg dissolved in 6-8 oz of water 4 times/day with meals and at bedtime; for best results, soak tablets in water for 2-5 minutes, then stir and swallow

Available Dosage Forms Tablet [scored]: 500 mg [phosphorus 114 mg and potassium 144 mg (3.7 mEq) per tablet; sodium free]

Monitoring and Teaching Issues

Patient Education: Dissolve tablets completely before drinking. Avoid taking magnesium, calcium, or aluminum antacids at the same time. Patients may pass old kidney stones when starting therapy. Notify physician if experiencing nausea, vomiting, or abdominal pain.

Pregnancy Risk Factor: C

Potassium Bicarbonate (poe TASS ee um bye KAR bun ate)

Generic Available Yes

Pharmacologic Category Electrolyte Supplement, Oral

Use Potassium deficiency, hypokalemia

Dosing

Adults & Elderly: Hypokalemia: Oral: 25 mEq 2-4 times/day
Pediatrics: Hypokalemia: Oral: Children: 1-4 mEq/kg/day

Available Dosage Forms Tablet for oral solution, effervescent: Potassium 25 mEq

Monitoring and Teaching Issues

Patient Education: Dissolve completely in 3-8 oz cold water, juice, or other suitable beverage and drink slowly.

Pregnancy Risk Factor: C

Potassium Bicarbonate and Potassium Chloride

(poe TASS ee um bye KAR bun ate & poe TASS ee um KLOR ide)

U.S. Brand Names K-Lyte/Cl®; K-Lyte/Cl® 50

Synonyms Potassium Bicarbonate and Potassium Chloride (Effervescent)

Generic Available No

Pharmacologic Category Electrolyte Supplement, Oral
Use Treatment or prevention of hypokalemia
Dosing
  Adults & Elderly: Hypokalemia: Oral:
    Prevention: 16-24 mEq/day in 2-4 divided doses
    Treatment: 40-100 mEq/day in 2-4 divided doses
Available Dosage Forms Tablet for oral solution, effervescent:
  K-Lyte/Cl®: Potassium chloride 25 mEq [potassium chloride 1.5 g and potassium bicarbonate 0.5 g; citrus or fruit punch flavor]
  K-Lyte/Cl® 50: Potassium chloride 50 mEq [potassium chloride 2.24 g and potassium bicarbonate 2 g; citrus flavor]
Monitoring and Teaching Issues
  Physical Assessment: Assess for adequate kidney function, use of ACE inhibitors, or potassium-sparing diuretics prior to starting therapy. Monitor cardiac status and serum potassium levels on a regular basis with long-term therapy. Instruct patient on appropriate diet and administration.
  Patient Education: Take as directed; do not take more than directed. Dissolve tablets in water or juice and stir before drinking. Do not take on an empty stomach; take with or after meals. Consult prescriber about increasing dietary potassium intake (eg, salt substitutes, orange juice, bananas). Report tingling of hands or feet, unresolved nausea or vomiting, chest pain, palpitations, persistent abdominal pain, muscle cramping or weakness, tarry stools, easy bruising, or unusual bleeding. **Pregnancy precaution:** Inform prescriber if you are pregnant.
  Pregnancy Risk Factor: C
  Lactation: Enters breast milk/compatible
Related Information
  Potassium Bicarbonate *on page 1232*
  Potassium Chloride *on page 1233*

♦ **Potassium Bicarbonate and Potassium Chloride (Effervescent)** *see* Potassium Bicarbonate and Potassium Chloride *on page 1232*

Potassium Bicarbonate and Potassium Citrate
(poe TASS ee um bye KAR bun ate & poe TASS ee um SIT rate)
U.S. Brand Names Effer-K™; Klor-Con®/EF; K-Lyte®; K-Lyte® DS
Synonyms Potassium Bicarbonate and Potassium Citrate (Effervescent)
Generic Available Yes
Pharmacologic Category Electrolyte Supplement, Oral
Medication Safety Issues
  Sound-alike/look-alike issues:
    Klor-Con® may be confused with Klaron®, K-Lor®
Use Treatment or prevention of hypokalemia
Dosing
  Adults & Elderly: Hypokalemia: Oral:
    Prevention: 16-24 mEq/day in 2-4 divided doses
    Treatment: 40-100 mEq/day in 2-4 divided doses
  Pediatrics: Hypokalemia: Oral: Children: 1-4 mEq/kg/24 hours in divided doses as required to maintain normal serum potassium
Available Dosage Forms Tablet, effervescent: Potassium 25 mEq
  Effer-K™: Potassium 25 mEq
  Klor-Con®/EF: Potassium 25 mEq [orange flavor]
  K-Lyte®: Potassium 25 mEq [lime or orange flavor]
  K-Lyte® DS: Potassium 50 mEq [lime or orange flavor]
Monitoring and Teaching Issues
  Patient Education: Dissolve completely in 3-8 oz cold water, juice, or other suitable beverage and drink slowly.
  Pregnancy Risk Factor: C
Related Information
  Potassium Bicarbonate *on page 1232*
  Potassium Citrate *on page 1235*

♦ **Potassium Bicarbonate and Potassium Citrate (Effervescent)** *see* Potassium Bicarbonate and Potassium Citrate *on page 1233*
♦ **Potassium Bicarbonate, Potassium Acetate, and Potassium Citrate** *see* Potassium Acetate, Potassium Bicarbonate, and Potassium Citrate *on page 1232*
♦ **Potassium Bicarbonate, Potassium Citrate, and Potassium Acetate** *see* Potassium Acetate, Potassium Bicarbonate, and Potassium Citrate *on page 1232*

Potassium Chloride (poe TASS ee um KLOR ide)
U.S. Brand Names K+8; K+10; Kaon-Cl-10®; Kaon-Cl® 20; Kay Ciel®; K+ Care®; K-Dur® 10; K-Dur® 20; K-Lor®; Klor-Con®; Klor-Con® 8; Klor-Con® 10; Klor-Con®/25; Klor-Con® M; Klotrix®; K-Tab®; microK®; microK® 10; Rum-K®
Synonyms KCl
Generic Available Yes
Pharmacologic Category Electrolyte Supplement, Oral; Electrolyte Supplement, Parenteral
Medication Safety Issues
  Sound-alike/look-alike issues:
    Kaon-Cl-10® may be confused with kaolin
    K-Dur® may be confused with Cardura®, Imdur®
    K-Lor® may be confused with Kaochlor®, Klor-Con®
    Klor-Con® may be confused with Klaron®, K-Lor®
    Klotrix® may be confused with liotrix
    microK® may be confused with Micronase®
(Continued)

Potassium Chloride *(Continued)*

High alert medication: The Institute for Safe Medication Practices (ISMP) includes this medication (I.V. formulation) among its list of drugs which have a heightened risk of causing significant patient harm when used in error.

Per JCAHO recommendations, concentrated electrolyte solutions should not be available in patient care areas.

Consider special storage requirements for intravenous potassium salts; I.V. potassium salts have been administered IVP in error, leading to fatal outcomes.

Use Treatment or prevention of hypokalemia

Contraindications Severe renal impairment, untreated Addison's disease, heat cramps, hyperkalemia, severe tissue trauma; solid oral dosage forms are contraindicated in patients in whom there is a structural, pathological, and/or pharmacologic cause for delay or arrest in passage through the GI tract; an oral liquid potassium preparation should be used in patients with esophageal compression or delayed gastric emptying time

Warnings/Precautions Use with caution in patients with cardiac disease, severe renal impairment, hyperkalemia.

Drug Interactions

Increased Effect/Toxicity: Potassium-sparing diuretics, salt substitutes, ACE inhibitors

Adverse Reactions

>10%: Gastrointestinal: Diarrhea, nausea, stomach pain, flatulence, vomiting (oral)

1% to 10%:

Cardiovascular: Bradycardia

Endocrine & metabolic: Hyperkalemia

Local: Local tissue necrosis with extravasation, pain at the site of injection

Neuromuscular & skeletal: Weakness

Respiratory: Dyspnea

Overdosage/Toxicology

Symptoms of overdose include muscle weakness, paralysis, peaked T waves, flattened P waves, prolongation of QRS complex, ventricular arrhythmias

Removal of potassium can be accomplished by various means; removal through the GI tract with Kayexalate® administration; by way of the kidney through diuresis, mineralocorticoid administration or increased sodium intake; by hemodialysis or peritoneal dialysis; or by shifting potassium back into the cells with insulin and glucose infusion or sodium bicarbonate; calcium chloride reverses cardiac effects.

Pharmacodynamics/Kinetics

Absorption: Well absorbed from upper GI tract

Excretion: Primarily urine; skin and feces (small amounts); most intestinal potassium reabsorbed

Dosing

Adults & Elderly: I.V. doses should be incorporated into the patient's maintenance I.V. fluids; intermittent I.V. potassium administration should be reserved for severe depletion situations in patients undergoing ECG monitoring.

Normal daily requirements: Oral, I.V.: 40-80 mEq/day

Prevention of hypokalemia during diuretic therapy: Oral: 20-40 mEq/day in 1-2 divided doses

Treatment of hypokalemia (guidelines):

Potassium >2.5 mEq/L:

Oral: 60-80 mEq/day plus additional amounts if needed

I.V.: 10 mEq over 1 hour with additional doses if needed

Potassium <2.5 mEq/L:

Oral: Up to 40-60 mEq initial dose, followed by further doses based on lab values

I.V.: Up to 40 mEq over 1 hour, with doses based on frequent lab monitoring; deficits at a plasma level of 2 mEq/L may be as high as 400-800 mEq of potassium

Acute hypokalemia:

I.V. intermittent infusion: 5-10 mEq/hour (continuous cardiac monitor recommended for rates >5 mEq/hour), not to exceed 40 mEq/hour; usual adult maximum per 24 hours: 400 mEq/day.

Potassium dosage/rate of infusion guidelines:

Serum potassium >2.5 mEq/L: Maximum infusion rate: 10 mEq/hour; maximum concentration: 40 mEq/L; maximum 24-hour dose: 200 mEq

Serum potassium <2.5 mEq/L: Maximum infusion rate: 40 mEq/hour; maximum concentration: 80 mEq/L; maximum 24-hour dose: 400 mEq

Pediatrics: I.V. doses should be incorporated into the patient's maintenance I.V. fluids; intermittent I.V. potassium administration should be reserved for severe depletion situations in patients undergoing ECG monitoring.

Normal daily requirements: Oral, I.V.:

Premature infants: 2-6 mEq/kg/24 hours

Term infants 0-24 hours: 0-2 mEq/kg/24 hours

Infants >24 hours: 1-2 mEq/kg/24 hours

Children: 2-3 mEq/kg/day

Prevention of hypokalemia during diuretic therapy: Oral: Children: 1-2 mEq/kg/day in 1-2 divided doses

Treatment of hypokalemia: Children:

Oral: 1-2 mEq/kg initially, then as needed based on frequently obtained lab values. If deficits are severe or ongoing losses are great, I.V. route should be considered.

I.V.: 1 mEq/kg over 1-2 hours initially, then repeated as needed based on frequently obtained lab values; severe depletion or ongoing losses may require >200% of normal limit needs

I.V. intermittent infusion: Dose should not exceed 1 mEq/kg/hour, or 40 mEq/hour; if it exceeds 0.5 mEq/kg/hour, physician should be at bedside and patient should have continuous ECG monitoring; usual pediatric maximum: 3 mEq/kg/day or 40 mEq/m²/ day

Available Dosage Forms

Capsule, extended release: 10 mEq [800 mg]
  microK® [microencapsulated]: 8 mEq [600 mg]
  microK 10 [microencapsulated]: 10 mEq [800 mg]
Infusion [premixed in D₅W]: 20 mEq (1000 mL); 30 mEq (1000 mL); 40 mEq (1000 mL)
Infusion [premixed in D₅W and LR]: 20 mEq (1000 mL); 30 mEq (1000 mL)
Infusion [premixed in D₅W and ¼NS]: 10 mEq (500 mL, 1000 mL); 20 mEq (1000 mL); 30 mEq (1000 mL); 40 mEq (1000 mL)
Infusion [premixed in D₅W and ½NS]: 20 mEq (1000 mL); 40 mEq (1000 mL)
Infusion [premixed in D₅ and NS]: 20 mEq (1000 mL); 40 mEq (1000 mL)
Infusion [premixed in D₅W and sodium chloride 0.3%]: 10 mEq (500 mL); 20 mEq (1000 mL)
Infusion [premixed in NS]: 20 mEq (1000 mL); 40 mEq (1000 mL)
Infusion [premixed in SWFI]: 10 mEq (50 mL, 100 mL); 20 mEq (50 mL, 100 mL); 30 mEq (100 mL); 40 mEq (100 mL)
Injection, solution [concentrate]: 2 mEq/mL (5 mL, 10 mL, 15 mL, 20 mL, 250 mL)
Powder, for oral solution: 20 mEq/packet (30s, 100s, 1000s)
  K+ Care®: 20 mEq/packet (30s) [fruit or orange flavor]
  K-Lor™: 20 mEq/packet (30s, 100s)
  Kay Ciel® 10%: 20 mEq/packet (30s, 100s) [sugar free]
  Klor-Con®: 20 mEq/packet (30s, 100s) [sugar free]
  Klor-Con®/25: 25 mEq/packet (30s, 100s) [sugar free]
Solution, oral: 20 mEq/15 mL (480 mL); 40 mEq/15 mL (480 mL)
  Kaon-Cl® 20: 40 mEq/15 mL (480 mL) [sugar free; contains alcohol; cherry flavor]
  Kay Ciel® 10%: 20 mEq/15 mL (120 mL, 480 mL) [sugar free; contains alcohol]
  Rum-K®: 20 mEq/10 mL (480 mL) [alcohol free, sugar free; butter/rum flavor]
Tablet, extended release: 8 mEq [600 mg]; 10 mEq [800 mg]; 20 mEq [1500 mg]
  K+8: 8 mEq [600 mg]
  K+10: 10 mEq [800 mg]
  K-Dur® 10 [microencapsulated]: 10 mEq [800 mg]
  K-Dur® 20 [microencapsulated]: 20 mEq [1500 mg; scored]
  K-Tab®: 10 mEq [800 mg]
  Kaon-Cl® 10 [film coated]: 10 mEq [800 mg]
  Klor-Con® 8: 8 mEq [600 mg; wax matrix]
  Klor-Con® 10: 10 mEq [800 mg; wax matrix]
  Klor-Con® M10 [microencapsulated]: 10 mEq [800 mg]
  Klor-Con® M15 [microencapsulated]: 15 mEq [1125 mg]
  Klor-Con® M20 [microencapsulated]: 20 mEq [1500 mg; scored]
Tablet, slow release [film coated] (Klotrix®): 10 mEq [800 mg; wax matrix]

Monitoring and Teaching Issues

Physical Assessment: Assess therapeutic response and adverse effects.
Monitoring Laboratory Tests: Serum potassium
Patient Education: Long-acting and wax matrix tablets should be swallowed whole; do not crush or chew. Powder must be dissolved in water before use. Take with food. Liquid can be diluted or dissolved in water or juice.
Dietary Considerations: Administer with plenty of fluid and/or food because of stomach irritation and discomfort.
Pregnancy Risk Factor: A

Administration

Oral: Wax matrix tablets must be swallowed and not allowed to dissolve in mouth.
I.V.: Potassium must be diluted prior to parenteral administration; maximum recommended concentration (peripheral line): 80 mEq/L; maximum recommended concentration (central line): 150 mEq/L or 15 mEq/100 mL; in severely fluid-restricted patients (with central lines): 200 mEq/L or 20 mEq/100 mL has been used; maximum rate of infusion, see Dosing, I.V. intermittent infusion
Compatibility: Stable in dextran 6% in dextrose, dextran 6% in NS, D₅LR, D₅¼NS, D₅½NS, D₅NS, D₅W, D₁₀W, D₂₀W, LR, ½NS, NS, sodium chloride 3%
  Y-site administration: Incompatible with amphotericin B cholesteryl sulfate complex, diazepam, ergotamine, phenytoin
  Compatibility when admixed: Incompatible with amphotericin B
Storage: Store at room temperature, protect from freezing; use only clear solutions; use admixtures within 24 hours

Related Information

Compatibility of Drugs *on page 1723*

Potassium Citrate (poe TASS ee um SIT rate)

U.S. Brand Names Urocit®-K
Generic Available No
Pharmacologic Category Alkalinizing Agent, Oral
Medication Safety Issues
  Sound-alike/look-alike issues:
    Urocit®-K may be confused with Urised®
Use Prevention of uric acid nephrolithiasis; prevention of calcium renal stones in patients with hypocitraturia; urinary alkalinizer when sodium citrate is contraindicated
Dosing
  Adults & Elderly: Alkalinizer, bicarbonate precursor: Oral: 10-20 mEq 3 times/day with meals up to 100 mEq/day
Available Dosage Forms Tablet: 540 mg [5 mEq]; 1080 mg [10 mEq]
Monitoring and Teaching Issues
  Physical Assessment: Assess effectiveness and interactions of other medications patient may be taking. Assess kidney function prior to starting therapy. Monitor cardiac status and serum potassium at beginning of therapy and at regular intervals with long-term therapy. Assess knowledge/teach patient appropriate use, recommended diet, and adverse symptoms to report.
(Continued)

Potassium Citrate *(Continued)*

Patient Education: Take as directed; do not take more than directed. Swallow tablet whole with full glass of water or juice and stir before sipping slowly, with or after meals (do not take on an empty stomach). Take any antacids 2 hours before or after potassium. Consult prescriber about advisability of increasing dietary potassium. Report tingling of hands or feet; unresolved nausea or vomiting; chest pain or palpitations; persistent abdominal pain; feelings of weakness, dizziness, listlessness, confusion; acute muscle weakness or cramping; blood in stool or tarry stools; or easy bruising or unusual bleeding.

Pregnancy Risk Factor: Not available

Lactation: Enters breast milk/compatible

Potassium Citrate and Citric Acid *(poe TASS ee um SIT rate & SI trik AS id)*

U.S. Brand Names Cytra-K; Polycitra®-K

Synonyms Citric Acid and Potassium Citrate

Generic Available Yes

Pharmacologic Category Alkalinizing Agent, Oral

Use Treatment of metabolic acidosis; alkalinizing agent in conditions where long-term maintenance of an alkaline urine is desirable

Dosing

Adults & Elderly: Urine alkalizing agent: Oral:

Powder: One packet dissolved in water after meals and at bedtime; adjust dose to urinary pH

Solution: 15-30 mL after meals and at bedtime; adjust dose based on urinary pH

Pediatrics: Urine alkalizing agent: Oral: Solution: 5-15 mL after meals and at bedtime; adjust dose based on urinary pH

Available Dosage Forms Note: Equivalent to potassium 2 mEq/mL and bicarbonate 2 mEq/mL

Powder:

Cytra-K: Potassium citrate 3300 mg and citric acid 1002 mg per packet (100s) [sugar free; fruit flavor]

Polycitra®-K: Potassium citrate 3300 mg and citric acid 1002 mg per packet (100s) [sugar free]

Solution:

Cytra-K: Potassium citrate 1100 mg and citric acid monohydrate 334 mg per 5 mL (480 mL) [alcohol free, sugar free; contains sodium benzoate; cherry flavor]

Polycitra®-K: Potassium citrate 1100 mg and citric acid monohydrate 334 mg per 5 mL (480 mL) [alcohol free, sugar free]

Monitoring and Teaching Issues

Physical Assessment: Assess kidney function prior to starting therapy. Monitor cardiac status and serum potassium at beginning of therapy and at regular intervals with long-term therapy. Assess knowledge/teach patient appropriate use, recommended diet, and adverse symptoms to report.

Patient Education: Take as directed; do not take more than directed. Dilute powder or solution in at least 6 oz of juice or water; stir and drink. May drink additional water or juice after dose. Take with or after meals (do not take on an empty stomach). Take any antacids 2 hours before or after potassium. Consult prescriber about advisability of increasing dietary potassium. Report tingling of hands or feet; unresolved nausea or vomiting; chest pain or palpitations; persistent abdominal pain; feelings of weakness, dizziness, listlessness, or confusion; acute muscle weakness or cramping; blood in stool or tarry stools; or easy bruising or unusual bleeding.

Pregnancy Risk Factor: A

Lactation: Excretion in breast milk unknown/compatible

Related Information

Potassium Citrate *on page 1235*

♦ **Potassium Citrate, Potassium Acetate, and Potassium Bicarbonate** *see* Potassium Acetate, Potassium Bicarbonate, and Potassium Citrate *on page 1232*

♦ **Potassium Citrate, Potassium Bicarbonate, and Potassium Acetate** *see* Potassium Acetate, Potassium Bicarbonate, and Potassium Citrate *on page 1232*

Potassium Gluconate *(poe TASS ee um GLOO coe nate)*

U.S. Brand Names Glu-K® [OTC]

Generic Available Yes

Pharmacologic Category Electrolyte Supplement, Oral

Use Treatment or prevention of hypokalemia

Dosing

Adults & Elderly: Note: Doses listed as mEq of potassium:

Normal daily requirement: Oral: 40-80 mEq/day

Prevention of hypokalemia during diuretic therapy: Oral: 16-24 mEq/day in 1-2 divided doses

Treatment of hypokalemia: Oral: 40-100 mEq/day in 2-4 divided doses

Pediatrics: Note: Doses listed as mEq of potassium:

Normal daily requirement: Oral: 2-3 mEq/kg/day

Prevention of hypokalemia during diuretic therapy: Oral: 1-2 mEq/kg/day in 1-2 divided doses

Treatment of hypokalemia: Oral: 2-5 mEq/kg/day in 2-4 divided doses

Available Dosage Forms

Tablet: 500 mg, 610 mg

Glu-K®: 486 mg

Tablet, timed release: 595 mg

Monitoring and Teaching Issues

Patient Education: Take with food, water, or fruit juice. Swallow tablets whole; do not crush or chew.

Pregnancy Risk Factor: A

Potassium Iodide (poe TASS ee um EYE oh dide)

U.S. Brand Names Iosat™ [OTC]; Pima®; SSKI®; ThyroSafe™ [OTC]; ThyroShield™ [OTC]

Synonyms KI; Lugol's Solution; Strong Iodine Solution

Generic Available Yes: Lugol's solution

Pharmacologic Category Antithyroid Agent; Expectorant

Use Expectorant for the symptomatic treatment of chronic pulmonary diseases complicated by mucous; reduce thyroid vascularity prior to thyroidectomy and management of thyrotoxic crisis; block thyroidal uptake of radioactive isotopes of iodine in a radiation emergency or other exposure to radioactive iodine

Unlabeled/Investigational Use Lymphocutaneous and cutaneous sporotrichosis

Dosing

Adults & Elderly:

RDA: 150 mcg (iodine)

Expectorant: Oral:

Pima®: 325-650 mg 3 times/day

SSKI®: 300-600 mg 3-4 times/day

Preoperative thyroidectomy: Oral: 50-250 mg (1-5 drops SSKI®) 3 times/day **or** 0.1-0.3 mL (3-5 drops) of strong iodine (Lugol's solution) 3 times/day; administer for 10 days before surgery

Radiation protectant to radioactive isotopes of iodine (Pima®): Oral: 195 mg once daily for 10 days; start 24 hours prior to exposure

To reduce risk of thyroid cancer following nuclear accident (Iosat™, ThyroSafe™, ThyroShield™): Oral: Children >68 kg and Adults (including pregnant/lactating women): Oral: 130 mg once daily. **Note:** Dosing should continue until risk of exposure has passed or other measures have are implemented.

Thyrotoxic crisis: Oral: 300-500 mg (6-10 drops SSKI®) 3 times/day or 1 mL strong iodine (Lugol's solution) 3 times/day

Sporotrichosis (cutaneous, lymphocutaneous; unlabeled use): Oral: Initial: 5 drops (SSKI®) 3 times/day; increase to 40-50 drops (SSKI®) 3 times/day as tolerated for 3-6 months

Pediatrics:

Expectorant: Oral (*Pima®*):

Children <3 years: 162 mg 3 times day

Children >3 years: 325 mg 3 times/day

Preoperative thyroidectomy: Refer to adult dosing.

Radiation protectant to radioactive isotopes of iodine (Pima®): Oral:

Infants up to 1 year: 65 mg once daily for 10 days; start 24 hours prior to exposure

Children >1 year: 130 mg once daily for 10 days; start 24 hours prior to exposure

To reduce risk of thyroid cancer following nuclear accident (Iosat™, ThyroSafe™, ThyroShield™): Oral:

Infants <1 month: 16.25 mg once daily

Children 1 month to 3 years: 32.5 mg once daily

Children 3-18 years: 65 mg once daily

Children >68 kg: Refer to adult dosing

Note: Dosing should continue until risk of exposure has passed or other measures are implemented.

Thyrotoxic crisis: Oral:

Infants <1 year: 150-250 mg (3-5 drops SSKI®) 3 times/day

Children: Refer to adult dosing.

Available Dosage Forms

Solution, oral:

SSKI®: 1 g/mL (30 mL, 240 mL) [contains sodium thiosulfate]

Lugol's solution, strong iodine: Potassium iodide 100 mg/mL and iodine 50 mg/mL (15 mL, 480 mL)

ThyroShield™: 65 mg/mL (30 mL) [black raspberry flavor]

Syrup (Pima®): 325 mg/5 mL (473 mL) [equivalent to iodide 249 mg/5 mL; black raspberry flavor]

Tablet:

Iosat™: 130 mg

ThyroSafe™: 65 mg [equivalent to iodine 50 mg]

Monitoring and Teaching Issues

Physical Assessment: See Contraindications, Warnings/Precautions, Drug Interactions, and Dosing for use cautions. Assess results of laboratory tests, therapeutic effectiveness (according to purpose for use), and adverse reactions (see Adverse Reactions and Overdose/Toxicology). Teach patient proper use, possible side effects/appropriate interventions, and adverse symptoms to report (see Patient Education).

Patient Education: Inform prescriber of all prescriptions, OTC medications, or herbal products you are taking, and any allergies you have. Do not take any new medication during therapy unless approved by prescriber. Take after meals. Dilute in 6 oz of water, fruit juice, milk, or broth. Do not exceed recommended dosage. May cause metallic taste, nausea, or vomiting (small frequent meals, frequent mouth care, chewing gum, or sucking lozenges may help); soreness of teeth or gums (use soft toothbrush and frequent mouth rinses); fever, headache, or sore joints (consult prescriber for approved medication); or acne or skin irritation. Discontinue and report any swelling of lips, mouth, or tongue; difficulty swallowing; chest pain or irregular heartbeat; unusual muscle weakness; or other persistent adverse effects. **Pregnancy/breast-feeding precautions:** Do not get pregnant while taking this medication. Consult prescriber for appropriate contraceptive measures. Consult prescriber if breast-feeding.

(Continued)

Potassium Iodide *(Continued)*

Pregnancy Risk Factor: D

Lactation: Enters breast milk/use caution (AAP rates "compatible")

Potassium Phosphate *(poe TASS ee um FOS fate)*

U.S. Brand Names Neutra-Phos®-K [OTC]

Synonyms Phosphate, Potassium

Generic Available Yes

Pharmacologic Category Electrolyte Supplement, Oral; Electrolyte Supplement, Parenteral

Medication Safety Issues

Sound-alike/look-alike issues:

Neutra-Phos®-K may be confused with K-Phos Neutral®

High alert medication: The Institute for Safe Medication Practices (ISMP) includes this medication (I.V. formulation) among its list of drugs which have a heightened risk of causing significant patient harm when used in error.

Per JCAHO recommendations, concentrated electrolyte solutions should not be available in patient care areas.

Consider special storage requirements for intravenous potassium salts; I.V. potassium salts have been administered IVP in error, leading to fatal outcomes.

Use Treatment and prevention of hypophosphatemia or hypokalemia

Contraindications Hyperphosphatemia, hyperkalemia, hypocalcemia, hypomagnesemia, renal failure

Warnings/Precautions Use with caution in patients with renal insufficiency, cardiac disease, metabolic alkalosis; admixture of phosphate and calcium in I.V. fluids can result in calcium phosphate precipitation.

Drug Interactions

Decreased Effect: Aluminum and magnesium-containing antacids or sucralfate can act as phosphate binders

Increased Effect/Toxicity: Potassium-sparing diuretics, salt substitutes, or ACE inhibitors; increased effect of digitalis

Nutritional/Ethanol Interactions Food: Avoid administering with oxalate (berries, nuts, chocolate, beans, celery, tomato) or phytate-containing foods (bran, whole wheat).

Lab Interactions Decreased ammonia (B)

Adverse Reactions

>10%: Gastrointestinal: Diarrhea, nausea, stomach pain, flatulence, vomiting

1% to 10%:

Cardiovascular: Bradycardia

Endocrine & metabolic: Hyperkalemia

Neuromuscular & skeletal: Weakness

Respiratory: Dyspnea

Overdosage/Toxicology

Symptoms of overdose include muscle weakness, paralysis, peaked T waves, flattened P waves, prolongation of QRS complex, ventricular arrhythmias, tetany, calcium-phosphate precipitation

Removal of potassium can be accomplished by various means; removal through the GI tract with Kayexalate® administration; by way of the kidney through diuresis, mineralocorticoid administration or increased sodium intake; by hemodialysis or peritoneal dialysis; or by shifting potassium back into the cells by insulin, glucose infusion, or sodium bicarbonate; calcium chloride reverses cardiac effects.

Dosing

Adults & Elderly: I.V. doses should be incorporated into the patient's maintenance I.V. fluids; intermittent I.V. infusion should be reserved for severe depletion situations in patients undergoing continuous ECG monitoring. It is difficult to determine total body phosphorus deficit; the following dosages are empiric guidelines:

Normal requirements elemental phosphorus: Oral:

Pregnancy lactation: Additional 400 mg/day

Adults: 800 mg

Treatment of hypophosphatemia: It is difficult to provide concrete guidelines for the treatment of severe hypophosphatemia because the extent of total body deficits and response to therapy are difficult to predict. Aggressive doses of phosphate may result in a transient serum elevation followed by redistribution into intracellular compartments or bone tissue. It is recommended that repletion of severe hypophosphatemia (<1 mg/dL in adults) be done I.V. because large doses of oral phosphate may cause diarrhea and intestinal absorption may be unreliable

Adult I.V. phosphate repletion:

Initial dose: 0.08 mmol/kg if recent uncomplicated hypophosphatemia

Initial dose: 0.16 mmol/kg if prolonged hypophosphatemia with presumed total body deficits; increase dose by 25% to 50% if patient symptomatic with severe hypophosphatemia

Do not exceed 0.24 mmol/kg/dose; administer over 6-12 hours by I.V. infusion. Some investigators have used more rapid infusions.

Note: With orders for I.V. phosphate, there is considerable confusion associated with the use of millimoles (mmol) versus milliequivalents (mEq) to express the phosphate requirement. Because inorganic phosphate exists as monobasic and dibasic anions, with the mixture of valences dependent on pH, ordering by mEq amounts is unreliable and may lead to large dosing errors. In addition, I.V. phosphate is available in the sodium and potassium salt; therefore, the content of these cations must be considered when ordering phosphate. The most reliable method of ordering I.V. phosphate is by millimoles, then specifying the potassium or sodium salt. For example, an order for 15 mmol of phosphate as potassium phosphate in one liter of normal saline. The dosing of phosphate should be 0.2-0.3 mmol/kg with a usual daily requirement of 30-60 mmol/day or 15 mmol of phosphate per liter of TPN or 15 mmol phosphate per 1000 calories of dextrose. Would also provide 22 mEq of potassium.

Maintenance:
I.V. solutions: 15-30 mmol/24 hours I.V. or 50-150 mmol/24 hours orally in divided doses
Oral: 1-2 capsules (250-500 mg phosphorus/8-16 mmol) 4 times/day; dilute as instructed

Pediatrics: I.V. doses should be incorporated into the patient's maintenance I.V. fluids; intermittent I.V. infusion should be reserved for severe depletion situations in patients undergoing continuous ECG monitoring. It is difficult to determine total body phosphorus deficit; the following are empiric guidelines

Note: Refer to notes under Adult dosing

Pediatric I.V. phosphate repletion:
Children: 0.25-0.5 mmol/kg **administer over 4-6 hours and repeat if symptomatic hypophosphatemia persists**; to assess the need for further phosphate administration, obtain serum inorganic phosphate after administration of the first dose and base further doses on serum levels and clinical status

Maintenance:
I.V. solutions: Children: 0.5-1.5 mmol/kg/24 hours I.V. or 2-3 mmol/kg/24 hours orally in divided doses
Oral:
Children <4 years: 1 capsule (250 mg phosphorus/8 mmol) 4 times/day; dilute as instructed
Children >4 years: Refer to adult dosing.

Available Dosage Forms
Injection, solution: Phosphate 3 mmol and potassium 4.4 mEq per mL (5 mL, 15 mL, 50 mL) [equivalent to phosphate 285 mg and potassium 170 mg per mL]
Powder for oral solution [packet] (Neutra-Phos®-K): Monobasic potassium phosphate and dibasic potassium phosphate/packet (100s) [equivalent to elemental phosphorus 250 mg and potassium 556 mg (14.2 mEq) per packet; sodium free]

Monitoring and Teaching Issues
Physical Assessment: Assess therapeutic response and adverse effects.
Monitoring Laboratory Tests: Serum potassium, phosphate
Patient Education: Empty contents of capsule into 3-4 oz of water; do not swallow the capsule. Take with food to reduce the risk of diarrhea.
Pregnancy Risk Factor: C

Administration
Compatibility: Stable in dextran 6% in dextrose, dextran 6% in NS, $D_{10}LR$, $D_5^1/_4NS$, $D_5^1/_2NS$, D_5NS, D_5W, $D_{10}W$, $^1/_2NS$, NS; **incompatible** with D_5LR, $D_{10}NS$, LR
Y-site administration: Incompatible with gatifloxacin
Compatibility when admixed: Incompatible with dobutamine

Potassium Phosphate and Sodium Phosphate
(poe TASS ee um FOS fate & SOW dee um FOS fate)

U.S. Brand Names K-Phos® MF; K-Phos® Neutral; K-Phos® No. 2; Neutra-Phos® [OTC]; Uro-KP-Neutral®
Synonyms Sodium Phosphate and Potassium Phosphate
Generic Available Yes
Pharmacologic Category Electrolyte Supplement, Oral
Medication Safety Issues
Sound-alike/look-alike issues:
K-Phos® Neutral may be confused with Neutra-Phos-K®
Use Treatment of conditions associated with excessive renal phosphate loss or inadequate GI absorption of phosphate; to acidify the urine to lower calcium concentrations; to increase the antibacterial activity of methenamine; reduce odor and rash caused by ammonia in urine
Dosing
Adults & Elderly: Note: All dosage forms to be mixed in 6-8 oz of water prior to administration
Phosphate supplement: Oral: Elemental phosphorus 250-500 mg 4 times/day after meals and at bedtime
Pediatrics: Note: All dosage forms to be mixed in 6-8 oz of water prior to administration
Phosphate supplement: Oral: Children ≥4 years: Elemental phosphorus 250 mg 4 times/day after meals and at bedtime
Available Dosage Forms
Powder, for oral suspension (Neutra-Phos®): Monobasic sodium, dibasic sodium, and potassium phosphate/packet (100s) [equivalent to elemental phosphorus 250 mg, sodium 164 mg (7.1 mEq), and potassium 278 mg (7.1 mEq) per packet]
Tablet:
K-Phos® MF: Potassium acid phosphate 155 mg and sodium acid phosphate 250 mg [equivalent to elemental phosphorus 125.6 mg, sodium 67 mg (2.9 mEq), and potassium 44.5 mg (1.1 mEq)]
K-Phos® Neutral: Dibasic sodium phosphate 852 mg, monobasic potassium phosphate 155 mg, and monobasic sodium phosphate 130 mg [equivalent to elemental phosphorus 250 mg, sodium 298 mg (13 mEq), and potassium 45 mg (1.1 mEq)]
K-Phos® No. 2: Potassium acid phosphate 305 mg and sodium acid phosphate 700 mg [equivalent to elemental phosphorus 250 mg, sodium 134 mg (5.8 mEq), and potassium 88 mg (2.3 mEq)]
Uro-KP-Neutral®: Sodium phosphate monobasic, dipotassium phosphate, and disodium phosphate [equivalent to elemental phosphorus 258 mg, phosphate 8 mmol, sodium 262.4 mg (10.8 mEq), and potassium 49.4 mg (1.3 mEq)]
Monitoring and Teaching Issues
Patient Education: Powder packets are to be mixed in 6-8 oz of water; following dilution, solution may be chilled to increase palatability. Tablets should be taken with a full glass of water.
(Continued)

Potassium Phosphate and Sodium Phosphate *(Continued)*

Pregnancy Risk Factor: C
Related Information
Potassium Phosphate *on page 1238*

♦ **Pounds / Kilograms Conversions** *see page 1697*
♦ **PPI-149** *see* Abarelix *on page 34*

Pramipexole *(pra mi PEKS ole)*
U.S. Brand Names Mirapex®
Generic Available No
Pharmacologic Category Anti-Parkinson's Agent, Dopamine Agonist
Medication Safety Issues
Sound-alike/look-alike issues:
Mirapex® may be confused with Mifeprex®, MiraLax™
Use Treatment of the signs and symptoms of idiopathic Parkinson's disease
Unlabeled/Investigational Use Treatment of depression
Mechanism of Action/Effect Pramipexole is a nonergot dopamine agonist with specificity for the D_2 subfamily dopamine receptor, and has also been shown to bind to D_3 and D_4 receptors. By binding to these receptors, it is thought that pramipexole can stimulate dopamine activity on the nerves of the striatum and substantia nigra.
Contraindications Hypersensitivity to pramipexole or any component of the formulation
Warnings/Precautions Caution should be taken in patients with renal insufficiency and in patients with pre-existing dyskinesias. May cause orthostatic hypotension; Parkinson's disease patients appear to have an impaired capacity to respond to a postural challenge. Use with caution in patients at risk of hypotension (such as those receiving antihypertensive drugs) or where transient hypotensive episodes would be poorly tolerated (cardiovascular disease or cerebrovascular disease). May cause hallucinations, particularly in older patients.

Although not reported for pramipexole, other dopaminergic agents have been associated with a syndrome resembling neuroleptic malignant syndrome on withdrawal or significant dosage reduction after long-term use. Dopaminergic agents from the ergot class have also been associated with fibrotic complications, such as retroperitoneum, lungs, and pleura.

Pramipexole has been associated with somnolence, particularly at higher dosages (>1.5 mg/day). In addition, patients have been reported to fall asleep during activities of daily living, including driving, while taking this medication. Patients should be advised of this issue, cautioned against driving or performing activities requiring alertness, and advised of factors which may increase risk (sleep disorders, other sedating medications, or concomitant medications which increase pramipexole concentrations). Patients should be instructed to report daytime somnolence or sleepiness to the prescriber.

Drug Interactions
Decreased Effect: Dopamine antagonists (antipsychotics, metoclopramide) may decrease the efficiency of pramipexole.
Increased Effect/Toxicity: Cimetidine in combination with pramipexole produced a 50% increase in AUC and a 40% increase in half-life. Drugs secreted by the cationic transport system (diltiazem, triamterene, verapamil, quinidine, quinine, ranitidine) decrease the clearance of pramipexole by ~20%.
Nutritional/Ethanol Interactions
Ethanol: Avoid ethanol (may increase CNS depression).
Food: Food intake does not affect the extent of drug absorption, although the time to maximal plasma concentration is delayed by 60 minutes when taken with a meal.
Herb/Nutraceutical: Avoid valerian, St John's wort, SAMe, kava kava (may increase risk of serotonin syndrome and/or excessive sedation).
Adverse Reactions
>10%:
Cardiovascular: Postural hypotension
Central nervous system: Asthenia, dizziness, somnolence, insomnia, hallucinations, abnormal dreams
Gastrointestinal: Nausea, constipation
Neuromuscular & skeletal: Weakness, dyskinesia, EPS
1% to 10%:
Cardiovascular: Edema, syncope, tachycardia, chest pain
Central nervous system: Malaise, confusion, amnesia, dystonias, akathisia, thinking abnormalities, myoclonus, hyperesthesia, paranoia, fever
Endocrine & metabolic: Decreased libido
Gastrointestinal: Anorexia, weight loss, xerostomia, dysphagia
Genitourinary: Urinary frequency, impotence, urinary incontinence
Neuromuscular & skeletal: Muscle twitching, leg cramps, arthritis, bursitis, myasthenia, gait abnormalities, hypertonia
Ocular: Vision abnormalities
Respiratory: Dyspnea, rhinitis
Pharmacodynamics/Kinetics
Bioavailability: 90%
Time to Peak: Serum: ~2 hours
Protein Binding: 15%
Half-Life Elimination: ~8 hours; Elderly: 12-14 hours
Excretion: Urine (90% as unchanged drug)
Dosing
Adults & Elderly: Parkinson's disease: Oral: Initial: 0.375 mg/day given in 3 divided doses; increase gradually by 0.125 mg/dose every 5-7 days; range: 1.5-4.5 mg/day.
Renal Impairment:
Cl_{cr} 35-59 mL/minute: Initial: 0.125 mg twice daily (maximum dose: 1.5 mg twice daily)
Cl_{cr} 15-34 mL/minute: Initial: 0.125 mg once daily (maximum dose: 1.5 mg once daily)

Cl_{cr} <15 mL/minute (or hemodialysis patients): Not adequately studied.

Available Dosage Forms Tablet, as dihydrochloride monohydrate: 0.125 mg, 0.25 mg, 0.5 mg, 1 mg, 1.5 mg

Monitoring and Teaching Issues

Physical Assessment: Assess potential for interactions with other prescriptions, OTC medications, or herbal products patient may be taking. Monitor blood pressure. Assess degree of somnolence. Assess for therapeutic effectiveness (improvement of symptoms) and adverse response. Teach patient appropriate use, interventions to reduce side effects, and adverse symptoms to report.

Patient Education: Do not take any new medication during therapy unless approved by prescriber. Take exactly as directed. Avoid alcohol. May cause drowsiness and extreme sedation or somnolence (use caution when driving or engaging in hazardous activities until response to drug is known); postural hypotension (use caution when changing position - rise slowly from sitting or lying position to standing and use caution when climbing stairs); constipation (increased exercise, fluids, fruit, or fiber may help); or urinary frequency. Consult prescriber about persistent adverse effects. **Pregnancy/breast-feeding precautions:** Inform prescriber if you are or intend to become pregnant. Breast-feeding is not recommended.

Dietary Considerations: May be taken with food to decrease nausea.

Pregnancy Risk Factor: C

Lactation: Excretion in breast milk unknown/not recommended

Breast-Feeding Issues: Prolactin secretion may be inhibited.

Administration

Oral: Doses should be titrated gradually in all patients to avoid the onset of intolerable side effects. The dosage should be increased to achieve a maximum therapeutic effect, balanced against the side effects of dyskinesia, hallucinations, somnolence, and dry mouth.

♦ **Prandin®** see Repaglinide on page 1311
♦ **Pravachol®** see Pravastatin on page 1241

Pravastatin (PRA va stat in)

U.S. Brand Names Pravachol®

Synonyms Pravastatin Sodium

Generic Available No

Pharmacologic Category Antilipemic Agent, HMG-CoA Reductase Inhibitor

Medication Safety Issues

Sound-alike/look-alike issues:

Pravachol® may be confused with Prevacid®, Prinivil®, propranolol

Use Use with dietary therapy for the following:

Primary prevention of coronary events: In hypercholesterolemic patients without established coronary heart disease to reduce cardiovascular morbidity (myocardial infarction, coronary revascularization procedures) and mortality.

Secondary prevention of cardiovascular events in patients with established coronary heart disease: To slow the progression of coronary atherosclerosis; to reduce cardiovascular morbidity (myocardial infarction, coronary vascular procedures) and to reduce mortality; to reduce the risk of stroke and transient ischemic attacks

Hyperlipidemias: Reduce elevations in total cholesterol, LDL-C, apolipoprotein B, and triglycerides (elevations of 1 or more components are present in Fredrickson type IIa, IIb, III, and IV hyperlipidemias)

Heterozygous familial hypercholesterolemia (HeFH): In pediatric patients, 8-18 years of age, with HeFH having LDL-C ≥190 mg/dL **or** LDL ≥160 mg/dL with positive family history of premature cardiovascular disease (CVD) or 2 or more CVD risk factors in the pediatric patient

Mechanism of Action/Effect Pravastatin is a competitive inhibitor of 3-hydroxy-3-methyl-glutaryl coenzyme A (HMG-CoA) reductase, which is the rate-limiting enzyme involved in de novo cholesterol synthesis.

Contraindications Hypersensitivity to pravastatin or any component of the formulation; active liver disease; unexplained persistent elevations of serum transaminases; pregnancy; breast-feeding

Warnings/Precautions Secondary causes of hyperlipidemia should be ruled out prior to therapy. Liver function must be monitored by periodic laboratory assessment. Rhabdomyolysis with acute renal failure has occurred. Risk may be increased with concurrent use of other drugs which may cause rhabdomyolysis (including gemfibrozil, fibric acid derivatives, or niacin at doses ≥1 g/day). Temporarily discontinue in any patient experiencing an acute or serious condition predisposing to renal failure secondary to rhabdomyolysis. Use caution in patients with previous liver disease or heavy ethanol use. Treatment in patients <8 years of age is not recommended.

Drug Interactions

Cytochrome P450 Effect: Substrate of CYP3A4 (minor); **Inhibits** CYP2C8/9 (weak), 2D6 (weak), 3A4 (weak)

Decreased Effect: Concurrent administration of cholestyramine or colestipol can decrease pravastatin absorption.

Increased Effect/Toxicity: Clofibrate, cyclosporine, fenofibrate, gemfibrozil, and niacin may increase the risk of myopathy and rhabdomyolysis. Imidazole antifungals (itraconazole, ketoconazole), P-glycoprotein inhibitors may increase pravastatin concentrations.

Nutritional/Ethanol Interactions

Ethanol: Consumption of large amounts of ethanol may increase the risk of liver damage with HMG-CoA reductase inhibitors.

Herb/Nutraceutical: St John's wort may decrease pravastatin levels.

Adverse Reactions As reported in short-term trials; safety and tolerability with long-term use were similar to placebo

(Continued)

Pravastatin *(Continued)*

1% to 10%:
    Cardiovascular: Chest pain (4%)
    Central nervous system: Headache (2% to 6%), fatigue (4%), dizziness (1% to 3%)
    Dermatologic: Rash (4%)
    Gastrointestinal: Nausea/vomiting (7%), diarrhea (6%), heartburn (3%)
    Hepatic: Transaminases increased (>3x normal on two occasions - 1%)
    Neuromuscular & skeletal: Myalgia (2%)
    Respiratory: Cough (3%)
    Miscellaneous: Influenza (2%)

Additional class-related events or case reports (not necessarily reported with pravastatin therapy): Angioedema, cataracts, depression, dyspnea, eosinophilia, erectile dysfunction, facial paresis, hypersensitivity reaction, impaired extraocular muscle movement, impotence, leukopenia, malaise, memory loss, ophthalmoplegia, paresthesia, peripheral neuropathy, photosensitivity, psychic disturbance, skin discoloration, thrombocytopenia, thyroid dysfunction, toxic epidermal necrolysis, transaminases increased, vomiting

Overdosage/Toxicology Treatment is symptomatic.

Pharmacodynamics/Kinetics
  Onset of Action: Several days; Peak effect: 4 weeks
  Absorption: Rapidly absorbed; average absorption 34%
  Bioavailability: 17%
  Time to Peak: Serum: 1-1.5 hours
  Protein Binding: 50%
  Half-Life Elimination: ~2-3 hours
  Metabolism: Hepatic to at least two metabolites
  Excretion: Feces (70%); urine (≤20%, 8% as unchanged drug)

Dosing
  Adults & Elderly:
    Hyperlipidemias, primary prevention of coronary events, secondary prevention of cardiovascular events: Oral: Initial: 40 mg once daily; titrate dosage to response (usual range: 10-80 mg) (maximum dose: 80 mg once daily)
    Dosage adjustment based on concomitant immunosuppressants (ie, cyclosporine): Oral: Initial: 10 mg/day, titrate with caution (maximum dose: 20 mg/day)
    Note: Doses should be individualized according to the baseline LDL-cholesterol levels, the recommended goal of therapy, and patient response; adjustments should be made at intervals of 4 weeks or more; doses may need adjusted based on concomitant medications

  Pediatrics:
    Heterozygous familial hypercholesterolemia (HeFH): Oral: Children:
      8-13 years: 20 mg/day
      14-18 years: 40 mg/day
    Dosage adjustment based on concomitant immunosuppressants (ie, cyclosporine): Refer to adult dosing.
    Note: Doses should be individualized according to the baseline LDL-cholesterol levels, the recommended goal of therapy, and patient response; adjustments should be made at intervals of 4 weeks or more; doses may need adjusted based on concomitant medications

  Renal Impairment: Initial: 10 mg/day
  Hepatic Impairment: Initial: 10 mg/day

Available Dosage Forms Tablet, as sodium: 10 mg, 20 mg, 40 mg, 80 mg

Monitoring and Teaching Issues
  Physical Assessment: See Warnings/Precautions for use cautions (eg, impaired liver function). Assess potential for interactions with other pharmacological agents or herbal products patient may be taking (eg, gemfibrozil, fibric acid derivatives, or niacin may increase risk of myopathy or rhabdomyolysis; see Drug Interactions). Assess LFTs prior to therapy and periodically (see Monitoring Laboratory Tests) and patient response on a regular basis throughout therapy (eg, rash, myalgia, blurred vision, abdominal pain, cough; see Adverse Reactions). Teach patient proper use (as adjunct to diet and exercise program), possible side effects/appropriate interventions, and adverse symptoms to report (see Patient Education). **Pregnancy risk factor X:** Determine that patient is not pregnant before starting therapy. Do not give to women of childbearing age unless they are capable of complying with effective contraceptive use. Instruct patient in appropriate contraceptive measures.

  Monitoring Laboratory Tests: Obtain baseline LFTs and total cholesterol profile; creatine phosphokinase due to possibility of myopathy. Repeat LFTs prior to elevation of dose. May be measured when clinically indicated and/or periodically thereafter.

  Patient Education: Take at same time each day with or without food. Follow cholesterol lowering diet and exercise regimen as prescribed. Avoid excess alcohol. You will have periodic blood tests to assess effectiveness. May cause mild nausea or vomiting (small frequent meals, frequent mouth care, chewing gum, or sucking lozenges may help); diarrhea (buttermilk, boiled milk, or yogurt may help); or headache (see prescriber for analgesic). Report chest pain; CNS changes (memory loss, depression, personality changes); numbness, weakness, tingling, pain, or cramping in extremities or muscles; vision changes; rash; or other persistent adverse reactions. **Pregnancy/breast-feeding precautions:** Inform prescriber if you are pregnant. Consult prescriber for appropriate contraceptive measures to use during and for 1 month following therapy. This drug may cause severe fetal defects. Do not donate blood during or for 1 month following therapy. Do not breast-feed.

  Dietary Considerations: May be taken without regard to meals. Before initiation of therapy, patients should be placed on a standard cholesterol-lowering diet for 6 weeks and the diet should be continued during drug therapy.

Geriatric Considerations: Effective and well tolerated in the elderly. No specific dosage recommendations. Clearance is reduced in older adults, resulting in an increase in AUC between 25% to 50%. However, substantial accumulation is not expected.

The definition of and, therefore, when to treat hyperlipidemia in older adults is a controversial issue. The National Cholesterol Education Program recommends that all adults maintain a plasma cholesterol <160 mg/dL. In elderly patients with one additional risk factor, goal LDL would decrease to <130 mg/dL. Pharmacologic treatment should be reserved for those who are unable to obtain a desirable plasma cholesterol concentration by diet alone and for whom the benefits of treatment are believed to outweigh the potential adverse effects, drug interactions, and cost of treatment.

Pregnancy Risk Factor: X

Pregnancy Issues: Safety and efficacy have not been established for use during pregnancy (treatment should be discontinued if pregnancy is recognized). Administer to women of childbearing potential only if conception is unlikely; females should be counseled on appropriate contraceptive methods.

Lactation: Enters breast milk/contraindicated

Administration

Oral: May be taken without regard to meals.

Storage: Store at 25°C (77°F); excursions permitted to 15°C to 30°C (59°F to 86°F). Protect from moisture and light.

Related Information

Hyperlipidemia Management *on page 1836*
Lipid-Lowering Agents *on page 1738*

♦ **Pravastatin and Aspirin** *see* Aspirin and Pravastatin *on page 148*

♦ **Pravastatin Sodium** *see* Pravastatin *on page 1241*

♦ **Pravigard™ PAC** *see* Aspirin and Pravastatin *on page 148*

Prazosin (PRA zoe sin)

U.S. Brand Names Minipress®

Synonyms Furazosin; Prazosin Hydrochloride

Generic Available Yes

Pharmacologic Category Alpha$_1$ Blocker

Medication Safety Issues

Sound-alike/look-alike issues:
Prazosin may be confused with prazepam, predniSONE

Use Treatment of hypertension

Unlabeled/Investigational Use Benign prostatic hyperplasia; Raynaud's syndrome

Mechanism of Action/Effect Competitively inhibits postsynaptic alpha-adrenergic receptors which results in vasodilation of veins and arterioles and a decrease in total peripheral resistance and blood pressure

Contraindications Hypersensitivity to quinazolines (doxazosin, prazosin, terazosin) or any component of the formulation; concurrent use with phosphodiesterase-5 (PDE-5) inhibitors including sildenafil (>25 mg), tadalafil, or vardenafil

Warnings/Precautions May cause significant orthostatic hypotension and syncope, especially with first dose. Risk is increased at doses >1 mg, hypovolemia, or in patients receiving concurrent beta-blocker therapy. Anticipate a similar effect if therapy is interrupted for a few days, if dosage is rapidly increased, or if another antihypertensive drug is introduced.

Drug Interactions

Decreased Effect: Decreased antihypertensive effect if taken with NSAIDs.

Increased Effect/Toxicity: Prazosin's hypotensive effect may be increased with beta-blockers, diuretics, ACE inhibitors, calcium channel blockers, other antihypertensive medications, sildenafil (use with extreme caution at a dose ≤25 mg), tadalafil (use is contraindicated by the manufacturer), and vardenafil (use is contraindicated by the manufacturer). Concurrent use with tricyclic antidepressants (TCAs) and low-potency antipsychotics may increase risk of orthostasis.

Nutritional/Ethanol Interactions

Ethanol: Avoid ethanol (may increase vasodilation).

Food: Food has variable effects on absorption.

Herb/Nutraceutical: Avoid dong quai if using for hypertension (has estrogenic activity). Avoid ephedra, yohimbe, ginseng (may worsen hypertension). Avoid saw palmetto (due to limited experience with this combination). Avoid garlic (may have increased antihypertensive effect).

Lab Interactions Increased urinary VMA 17%, norepinephrine metabolite 42%

Adverse Reactions

>10%: Central nervous system: Dizziness (10%)

1% to 10%:

Cardiovascular: Palpitations (5%), edema, orthostatic hypotension, syncope (1%)

Central nervous system: Headache (8%), drowsiness (8%), weakness (7%), vertigo, depression, nervousness

Dermatologic: Rash (1% to 4%)

Endocrine & metabolic: Decreased energy (7%)

Gastrointestinal: Nausea (5%), vomiting, diarrhea, constipation

Genitourinary: Urinary frequency (1% to 5%)

Ocular: Blurred vision, reddened sclera, xerostomia

Respiratory: Dyspnea, epistaxis, nasal congestion

Overdosage/Toxicology Symptoms of overdose include hypotension and drowsiness. Treatment is otherwise supportive and symptomatic.

(Continued)

Prazosin *(Continued)*

Pharmacodynamics/Kinetics
Onset of Action: BP reduction: ~2 hours; Maximum decrease: 2-4 hours
Duration of Action: 10-24 hours
Bioavailability: 43% to 82%
Protein Binding: 92% to 97%
Half-Life Elimination: 2-4 hours; prolonged with congestive heart failure
Metabolism: Extensively hepatic
Excretion: Urine (6% to 10% as unchanged drug)

Dosing
Adults:
Hypertension: Oral: Initial: 1 mg/dose 2-3 times/day; usual maintenance dose: 3-15 mg/day in divided doses 2-4 times/day; maximum daily dose: 20 mg
Hypertensive urgency: Oral: 10-20 mg once, may repeat in 30 minutes
Raynaud's (unlabeled use): Oral: 0.5-3 mg twice daily
Benign prostatic hyperplasia (unlabeled use): Oral: 2 mg twice daily
Elderly: Oral (first dose given at bedtime): Initial: 1 mg 1-2 times/day
Pediatrics: Oral: Children: Initial: 5 mcg/kg/dose (to assess hypotensive effects); usual dosing interval: every 6 hours; increase dosage gradually up to maximum of 25 mcg/kg/dose every 6 hours.

Available Dosage Forms Capsule, as hydrochloride: 1 mg, 2 mg, 5 mg

Monitoring and Teaching Issues
Physical Assessment: Assess potential for interactions with other pharmacological agents and herbal products patient may be taking (eg, anything that may increase hypotension [beta-blockers, diuretics, ACE inhibitors, calcium channel blockers, dong quai] and any PDE-5 inhibitors [sildenafil, tadalafil, vardenafil]; see Drug Interactions). Assess effectiveness (cardiac status and blood pressure) and adverse reactions at beginning of therapy and on a regular basis with long-term therapy (eg, orthostatic hypotension, rash, drowsiness, nausea, vomiting; see Adverse Reactions). When discontinuing, monitor blood pressure and taper dose slowly over 1 week or more. Teach patient proper use, possible side effects/appropriate interventions, and adverse symptoms to report (see Patient Education).
Patient Education: Do not take any new medication during therapy unless approved by prescriber. Take as directed with or without meals; do not skip dose or discontinue without consulting prescriber. Avoid alcohol. Follow recommended diet and exercise program. May cause drowsiness, dizziness, or impaired judgment (use caution when driving or engaging in tasks that require alertness until response to drug is known); postural hypotension (use caution when rising from sitting or lying position or when climbing stairs); or dry mouth or nausea (frequent mouth care or sucking lozenges may help). Report increased nervousness or depression; sudden weight gain (weigh yourself in the same clothes at the same time of day once a week); palpitations or rapid heartbeat; respiratory difficulty; muscle weakness, fatigue, or pain; vision changes or hearing; rash; changes in urinary pattern (void before taking medications); or other persistent side effects. **Pregnancy/breast-feeding precautions:** Inform prescriber if you are or intend to become pregnant. Consult prescriber if breast-feeding.
Geriatric Considerations: See Warnings/Precautions and Pharmacokinetics. Adverse effects such as dry mouth and urinary problems can be particularly bothersome in the elderly.
Pregnancy Risk Factor: C
Lactation: Excretion in breast milk unknown/use caution
Administration
Storage: Store in airtight container. Protect from light.

Prazosin and Polythiazide *(PRA zoe sin & pol i THYE a zide)*
U.S. Brand Names Minizide®
Synonyms Polythiazide and Prazosin
Generic Available No
Pharmacologic Category Antihypertensive Agent, Combination
Medication Safety Issues
Sound-alike/look-alike issues:
Minizide® may be confused with Minocin®
Use Management of mild to moderate hypertension
Dosing
Adults & Elderly: Hypertension: Oral: Initial: 1 capsule 2-3 times/day; maintenance: May be slowly increased to a total daily dose of 20 mg. Therapeutic dosages often used range from 6-15 mg in divided doses.
Available Dosage Forms Capsule:
Minizide® 1: Prazosin 1 mg and polythiazide 0.5 mg
Minizide® 2: Prazosin 2 mg and polythiazide 0.5 mg
Minizide® 5: Prazosin 5 mg and polythiazide 0.5 mg
Monitoring and Teaching Issues
Physical Assessment: See individual agents.
Patient Education: See individual agents. **Pregnancy/breast-feeding precautions:** Inform prescriber if you are or intend to become pregnant. Consult prescriber if breast-feeding.
Pregnancy Risk Factor: C
Lactation: Excretion in breast milk unknown
Related Information
Prazosin *on page 1243*

♦ Prazosin Hydrochloride *see Prazosin on page 1243*
♦ Precedex™ *see Dexmedetomidine on page 429*
♦ Precose® *see Acarbose on page 37*

♦ **Pred Forte®** *see* PrednisoLONE *on page 1245*
♦ **Pred Mild®** *see* PrednisoLONE *on page 1245*

PrednisoLONE (pred NISS oh lone)

U.S. Brand Names AK-Pred®; Bubbli-Pred™; Econopred® Plus; Orapred®; Pediapred®; Pred Forte®; Pred Mild®; Prelone®

Synonyms Deltahydrocortisone; Metacortandralone; Prednisolone Acetate; Prednisolone Acetate, Ophthalmic; Prednisolone Sodium Phosphate; Prednisolone Sodium Phosphate, Ophthalmic

Generic Available Yes

Pharmacologic Category Corticosteroid, Ophthalmic; Corticosteroid, Systemic

Medication Safety Issues
Sound-alike/look-alike issues:
PrednisoLONE may be confused with predniSONE
Pediapred® may be confused with Pediazole®

Use Treatment of palpebral and bulbar conjunctivitis; corneal injury from chemical, radiation, thermal burns, or foreign body penetration; endocrine disorders, rheumatic disorders, collagen diseases, dermatologic diseases, allergic states, ophthalmic diseases, respiratory diseases, hematologic disorders, neoplastic diseases, edematous states, and gastrointestinal diseases; resolution of acute exacerbations of multiple sclerosis

Mechanism of Action/Effect Decreases inflammation by suppression of migration of polymorphonuclear leukocytes and reversal of increased capillary permeability; suppresses the immune system by reducing activity and volume of the lymphatic system

Contraindications Hypersensitivity to prednisolone or any component of the formulation; acute superficial herpes simplex keratitis; live or attenuated virus vaccines; systemic fungal infections; varicella

Warnings/Precautions Use with caution in patients with hyperthyroidism, cirrhosis, nonspecific ulcerative colitis, hypertension, osteoporosis, thromboembolic tendencies, CHF, convulsive disorders, myasthenia gravis, thrombophlebitis, peptic ulcer, diabetes, or tuberculosis; acute adrenal insufficiency may occur with abrupt withdrawal after long-term therapy or with stress; young pediatric patients may be more susceptible to adrenal axis suppression from topical therapy.

Prolonged use of corticosteroids may result in glaucoma; damage to the optic nerve (not for treatment of optic neuritis), defects in visual acuity and fields of vision, and posterior subcapsular cataract formation may occur. Prolonged use may increase the incidence of secondary infection, mask acute infection (including fungal) or prolong or exacerbate viral infections. Avoid exposure to chickenpox. Corticosteroids should not treat ocular herpes simplex. Use following cataract surgery may delay healing or increase the incidence of bleb formation.

Corticosteroids should not be used for cerebral malaria. Use cautiously in the elderly.

Drug Interactions
Cytochrome P450 Effect: Substrate of CYP3A4 (minor); **Inhibits** CYP3A4 (weak)
Decreased Effect: Effects of prednisolone may be decreased by aminoglutethimide, antacids, barbiturates, CYP34 inducers, carbamazepine, nafcillin, nevirapine, phenobarbital, phenytoin, rifampin. Prednisolone may decrease the effects of isoniazid, skin tests, toxoids, warfarin, vaccines.
Increased Effect/Toxicity: Effects of prednisolone may be increased by azole antifungals, calcium channel blockers, cyclosporine, estrogens, ketoconazole, salicylates.

Nutritional/Ethanol Interactions
Ethanol: Avoid ethanol (may increase gastric mucosal irritation).
Food: Prednisolone interferes with calcium absorption. Limit caffeine.
Herb/Nutraceutical: St John's wort may decrease prednisolone levels. Avoid cat's claw, echinacea (have immunostimulant properties).

Lab Interactions Response to skin tests

Adverse Reactions Frequency not defined.
Ophthalmic formulation:
Endocrine & metabolic: Hypercorticoidism (rare)
Ocular: Conjunctival hyperemia, conjunctivitis, corneal ulcers, delayed wound healing, glaucoma, intraocular pressure increased, keratitis, loss of accommodation, optic nerve damage, mydriasis, posterior subcapsular cataract formation, ptosis, secondary ocular infection
Oral formulation:
Cardiovascular: CHF, edema, hypertension
Central nervous system: Convulsions, headache, insomnia, malaise, nervousness, psychic disorders, vertigo
Dermatologic: Bruising, diaphoresis increased, facial erythema, hirsutism, petechiae, skin test reaction suppression, thin fragile skin, urticaria
Endocrine & metabolic: Carbohydrate tolerance decreased, Cushing's syndrome, diabetes mellitus, growth suppression, hyperglycemia, hypokalemic alkalosis, menstrual irregularities, negative nitrogen balance, pituitary adrenal axis suppression, potassium loss
Gastrointestinal: Abdominal distention, increased appetite, indigestion, nausea, peptic ulcer, ulcerative esophagitis, weight gain
Hepatic: LFTs increased (usually reversible)
Neuromuscular & skeletal: Arthralgia, fractures, intracranial pressure with papilledema (usually after discontinuation), muscle mass decreased, muscle weakness, osteoporosis, steroid myopathy, tendon rupture, weakness
Ocular: Cataracts, exophthalmus, glaucoma, intraocular pressure increased
Respiratory: Epistaxis
Miscellaneous: Impaired wound healing

Overdosage/Toxicology When consumed in high doses for prolonged periods, systemic hypercorticism and adrenal suppression may occur, in those cases discontinuation of the corticosteroid should be done judiciously.
(Continued)

PrednisoLONE *(Continued)*

Pharmacodynamics/Kinetics
Duration of Action: 18-36 hours
Protein Binding: Concentration dependent: 65% to 91%; decreased in elderly
Half-Life Elimination: 3.6 hours; End-stage renal disease: 3-5 hours
Metabolism: Primarily hepatic, but also metabolized in most tissues, to inactive compounds
Excretion: Primarily urine (as glucuronides, sulfates, and unconjugated metabolites)

Dosing
Adults: Dose depends upon condition being treated and response of patient. Consider alternate day therapy for long-term therapy. Discontinuation of long-term therapy requires gradual withdrawal by tapering the dose. Patients undergoing unusual stress while receiving corticosteroids, should receive increased doses prior to, during, and after the stressful situation.

Usual dose (range): Oral: 5-60 mg/day
Rheumatoid arthritis: Oral: Initial: 5-7.5 mg/day, adjust dose as necessary
Multiple sclerosis: Oral: 200 mg/day for 1 week followed by 80 mg every other day for 1 month
Conjunctivitis: Ophthalmic (suspension/solution): Instill 1-2 drops into conjunctival sac every hour during day, every 2 hours at night until favorable response is obtained, then use 1 drop every 4 hours.
Dosing adjustment in hyperthyroidism: Prednisolone dose may need to be increased to achieve adequate therapeutic effects.

Elderly: Use lowest effective adult dose. Dose depends upon condition being treated and response of patient; alternate day dosing may be attempted in some disease states.

Pediatrics: Dose depends upon condition being treated and response of patient; dosage for infants and children should be based on severity of the disease and response of the patient rather than on strict adherence to dosage indicated by age, weight, or body surface area. Consider alternate day therapy for long-term therapy. Discontinuation of long-term therapy requires gradual withdrawal by tapering the dose. Patients undergoing unusual stress while receiving corticosteroids, should receive increased doses prior to, during, and after the stressful situation.

Acute asthma: Oral: 1-2 mg/kg/day in divided doses 1-2 times/day for 3-5 days
Anti-inflammatory or immunosuppressive dose: Oral: 0.1-2 mg/kg/day in divided doses 1-4 times/day
Nephrotic syndrome: Oral:
Initial (first 3 episodes): 2 mg/kg/day **or** 60 mg/m^2/day (maximum: 80 mg/day) in divided doses 3-4 times/day until urine is protein free for 3 consecutive days (maximum: 28 days); followed by 1-1.5 mg/kg/dose **or** 40 mg/m^2/dose given every other day for 4 weeks
Maintenance (for frequent relapses): 0.5-1 mg/kg/dose given every other day for 3-6 months
Conjunctivitis: Ophthalmic (suspension/solution): Children: Refer to adult dosing.
Dosing adjustment in hyperthyroidism: Refer to adult dosing.

Renal Impairment: Slightly dialyzable (5% to 20%)

Available Dosage Forms
Solution, ophthalmic, as sodium phosphate: 1% (5 mL, 10 mL, 15 mL) [contains benzalkonium chloride]
  AK-Pred®: 1% (5 mL, 15 mL) [contains benzalkonium chloride]
Solution, oral, as sodium phosphate: Prednisolone base 5 mg/5 mL (120 mL)
  Bubbli-Pred™: Prednisolone base 5 mg/5 mL (120 mL) [bubble gum flavor]
  Orapred®: 20 mg/5 mL (240 mL) [equivalent to prednisolone base 15 mg/5 mL; dye free; contains alcohol 2%, sodium benzoate; grape flavor]
  Pediapred®: 6.7 mg/5 mL (120 mL) [equivalent to prednisolone base 5 mg/5 mL; dye free; raspberry flavor]
Suspension, ophthalmic, as acetate: 1% (5 mL, 10 mL, 15 mL) [contains benzalkonium chloride]
  Econopred® Plus: 1% (5 mL, 10 mL) [contains benzalkonium chloride]
  Pred Forte®: 1% (1 mL, 5 mL, 10 mL, 15 mL) [contains benzalkonium chloride and sodium bisulfite]
  Pred Mild®: 0.12% (5 mL, 10 mL) [contains benzalkonium chloride and sodium bisulfite]
Syrup, as base: 5 mg/5 mL (120 mL); 15 mg/5 mL (240 mL, 480 mL)
  Prelone®: 15 mg/5 mL (240 mL, 480 mL) [contains alcohol 5%, benzoic acid; cherry flavor]
Tablet, as base: 5 mg

Monitoring and Teaching Issues
Physical Assessment: Assess other medications patient may be taking for effectiveness and interactions. Assess results of laboratory tests, therapeutic effectiveness, and adverse effects according to indications for therapy, dose, route, and duration of therapy. With systemic administration, patients with diabetes should monitor glucose levels closely. Assess knowledge/teach patient appropriate use, interventions to reduce side effects, and adverse symptoms to report. When used for long-term therapy (>10-14 days), do not discontinue abruptly; decrease dosage incrementally.

Monitoring Laboratory Tests: Blood glucose, electrolytes

Patient Education: Take exactly as directed; do not increase dose or discontinue abruptly without consulting prescriber. Avoid alcohol. Limit intake of caffeine or stimulants. Prescriber may recommend increased dietary vitamins, minerals, or iron. If you have diabetes, monitor glucose levels closely (antidiabetic medication may need to be adjusted). Inform prescriber if you are experiencing greater-than-normal levels of stress (medication may need adjustment). Some forms of this medication may cause GI upset (oral medication should be taken with meals to reduce GI upset; small frequent meals and frequent mouth care may reduce GI upset). You may be more susceptible to infection (avoid crowds and exposure to infection). Report promptly excessive nervousness or sleep disturbances; any signs of infection (sore throat, unhealed injuries); excessive growth of body hair or loss of skin color; vision changes; excessive or sudden weight gain (>3 lb/week); swelling of face or extremities; respiratory difficulty; muscle weakness; change in color of stools (black or tarry) or persistent abdominal pain; or worsening of condition or failure to improve.

Pregnancy precaution: Inform prescriber if you are or intend to become pregnant.

Ophthalmic: For ophthalmic use only. Wash hands before using. Tilt head back and look upward. Put drops of suspension inside lower eyelid. Close eye and roll eyeball in all directions. Do not blink for $^1\!/_2$ minute. Apply gentle pressure to inner corner of eye for 30 seconds. Do not use any other eye preparation for at least 10 minutes. Do not let tip of applicator touch eye; do not contaminate tip of applicator (may cause eye infection, eye damage, or vision loss). Do not share medication with anyone else. Wear sunglasses when in sunlight; you may be more sensitive to bright light. Inform prescriber if condition worsens or fails to improve or if you experience eye pain, disturbances of vision, or other adverse eye response.

Dietary Considerations: Should be taken after meals or with food or milk to decrease GI effects; increase dietary intake of pyridoxine, vitamin C, vitamin D, folate, calcium, and phosphorus.

Geriatric Considerations: Useful in patients with inability to activate prednisone (liver disease). Because of the risk of adverse effects, systemic corticosteroids should be used cautiously in the elderly, in the smallest possible dose, and for the shortest possible time.

Pregnancy Risk Factor: C

Lactation: Enters breast milk/use caution (AAP rates "compatible")

Administration

Oral: Give oral formulation with food or milk to decrease GI effects.

Related Information

Corticosteroids *on page 1731*

FDA Name Differentiation Project: The Use of Tall-Man Letters *on page 15*

♦ **Prednisolone Acetate** *see* PrednisoLONE *on page 1245*

♦ **Prednisolone Acetate, Ophthalmic** *see* PrednisoLONE *on page 1245*

♦ **Prednisolone and Sulfacetamide** *see* Sulfacetamide and Prednisolone *on page 1404*

♦ **Prednisolone Sodium Phosphate** *see* PrednisoLONE *on page 1245*

♦ **Prednisolone Sodium Phosphate, Ophthalmic** *see* PrednisoLONE *on page 1245*

PredniSONE (PRED ni sone)

U.S. Brand Names Prednisone Intensol™; Sterapred®; Sterapred® DS

Synonyms Deltacortisone; Deltadehydrocortisone

Generic Available Yes

Pharmacologic Category Corticosteroid, Systemic

Medication Safety Issues

Sound-alike/look-alike issues:

PredniSONE may be confused with methylPREDNISolone, Pramosone®, prazosin, predn-nisoLONE, Prilosec®, primidone, promethazine

Use Treatment of a variety of diseases including adrenocortical insufficiency, hypercalcemia, rheumatic, and collagen disorders; dermatologic, ocular, respiratory, gastrointestinal, and neoplastic diseases; organ transplantation and a variety of diseases including those of hematologic, allergic, inflammatory, and autoimmune in origin; not available in injectable form, prednisolone must be used

Unlabeled/Investigational Use Investigational: Prevention of postherpetic neuralgia and relief of acute pain in the early stages

Mechanism of Action/Effect Decreases inflammation by suppression of migration of poly-morphonuclear leukocytes and reversal of increased capillary permeability; suppresses the immune system by reducing activity and volume of the lymphatic system; suppresses adrenal function at high doses

Contraindications Hypersensitivity to prednisone or any component of the formulation; serious infections, except tuberculous meningitis; systemic fungal infections; varicella

Warnings/Precautions Use with caution in patients with hypothyroidism, cirrhosis, CHF, ulcerative colitis, thromboembolic disorders, and patients with an increased risk for peptic ulcer disease. Corticosteroids should be used with caution in patients with diabetes, hyper-tension, osteoporosis, glaucoma, cataracts, or tuberculosis. Use caution in hepatic impair-ment. May retard bone growth. Gradually taper dose to withdraw therapy. Because of the risk of adverse effects, systemic corticosteroids should be used cautiously in the elderly, in the smallest possible dose, and for the shortest possible time.

Drug Interactions

Cytochrome P450 Effect: Substrate of CYP3A4 (minor); **Induces** CYP2C19 (weak), 3A4 (weak)

Decreased Effect: Decreased effect with barbiturates, phenytoin, rifampin; decreased effect of salicylates, vaccines, and toxoids.

Increased Effect/Toxicity: Concurrent use with NSAIDs may increase the risk of GI ulceration.

Nutritional/Ethanol Interactions

Ethanol: Avoid ethanol (may increase gastric mucosal irritation)

Food: Prednisone interferes with calcium absorption, Limit caffeine.

Herb/Nutraceutical: St John's wort may decrease prednisone levels. Avoid cat's claw, echi-nacea (have immunostimulant properties).

Lab Interactions Response to skin tests

Adverse Reactions

>10%:

Central nervous system: Insomnia, nervousness

Gastrointestinal: Increased appetite, indigestion

1% to 10%:

Dermatologic: Hirsutism

Endocrine & metabolic: Diabetes mellitus, glucose intolerance, hyperglycemia

Neuromuscular & skeletal: Arthralgia

Ocular: Cataracts, glaucoma

Respiratory: Epistaxis

(Continued)

PredniSONE *(Continued)*

Overdosage/Toxicology When consumed in high doses for prolonged periods, systemic hypercorticism and adrenal suppression may occur. In those cases, discontinuation of the corticosteroid should be done judiciously.

Pharmacodynamics/Kinetics
Protein Binding: Concentration dependent: 65% to 91%

Half-Life Elimination: Normal renal function: 2.5-3.5 hours

Metabolism: Hepatically converted from prednisone (inactive) to prednisolone (active); may be impaired with hepatic dysfunction

Pharmacokinetic Note: See Prednisolone monograph for complete information.

Dosing
Adults: Dose depends upon condition being treated and response of patient; consider alternate day therapy for long-term therapy. Discontinuation of long-term therapy requires gradual withdrawal by tapering the dose.

Physiologic replacement: Oral: 4-5 mg/m²/day

Immunosuppression/chemotherapy adjunct: Oral: Range: 5-60 mg/day in divided doses 1-4 times/day

Allergic reaction (contact dermatitis): Oral:
Day 1: 30 mg divided as 10 mg before breakfast, 5 mg at lunch, 5 mg at dinner, 10 mg at bedtime
Day 2: 5 mg at breakfast, 5 mg at lunch, 5 mg at dinner, 10 mg at bedtime
Day 3: 5 mg 4 times/day (with meals and at bedtime)
Day 4: 5 mg 3 times/day (breakfast, lunch, bedtime)
Day 5: 5 mg 2 times/day (breakfast, bedtime)
Day 6: 5 mg before breakfast

Acute asthma: 1-2 mg/kg/day in divided doses 1-2 times/day for 3-5 days

Asthma maintenance:
Moderate persistent: Inhaled corticosteroid (medium dose) or inhaled corticosteroid (low-medium dose) with a long-acting bronchodilator
Severe persistent: Inhaled corticosteroid (high dose) and corticosteroid tablets or syrup long term: 2 mg/kg/day, generally not to exceed 60 mg/day

Pneumonia due to *Pneumocystis carinii*: Oral:
40 mg twice daily for 5 days **followed by**
40 mg once daily for 5 days **followed by**
20 mg once daily for 11 days or until antimicrobial regimen is completed

Thyrotoxicosis: Oral: 60 mg/day
Note: Dosing adjustment in hyperthyroidism: Prednisone dose may need to be increased to achieve adequate therapeutic effects

Chemotherapy (refer to individual protocols): Oral: Range: 20 mg/day to 100 mg/m²/day

Rheumatoid arthritis: Oral: Use lowest possible daily dose (often ≤7.5 mg/day)

Idiopathic thrombocytopenia purpura (ITP): Oral: 60 mg daily for 4-6 weeks, gradually tapered over several weeks

Systemic lupus erythematosus (SLE): Oral:
Acute: 1-2 mg/kg/day in 2-3 divided doses
Maintenance: Reduce to lowest possible dose, usually <1 mg/kg/day as single dose (morning)

Elderly: Refer to adult dosing; use the lowest effective dose. Oral dose depends upon condition being treated and response of patient. Alternate day dosing may be attempted.

Pediatrics: Note: Dose depends upon condition being treated and response of patient; dosage for infants and children should be based on severity of the disease and response of the patient rather than on strict adherence to dosage indicated by age, weight, or body surface area. Consider alternate day therapy for long-term therapy. Discontinuation of long-term therapy requires gradual withdrawal by tapering the dose.

Physiologic replacement: Oral: Children: 4-5 mg/m²/day

Anti-inflammatory or immunosuppressive dose: Oral: 0.05-2 mg/kg/day divided 1-4 times/day

Acute asthma: Oral: 1-2 mg/kg/day in divided doses 1-2 times/day for 3-5 days
Alternatively (for 3- to 5-day "burst"):
<1 year: 10 mg every 12 hours
1-4 years: 20 mg every 12 hours
5-13 years: 30 mg every 12 hours
>13 years: 40 mg every 12 hours

Asthma long-term therapy (alternative dosing by age): Oral:
<1 year: 10 mg every other day
1-4 years: 20 mg every other day
5-13 years: 30 mg every other day
>13 years: 40 mg every other day

Asthma maintenance: Children ≥5 years: Refer to adult dosing.

Nephrotic syndrome: Oral:
Initial (first 3 episodes): 2 mg/kg/day **or** 60 mg/m²/day (maximum: 80 mg/day) in divided doses 3-4 times/day until urine is protein free for 3 consecutive days (maximum: 28 days); followed by 1-1.5 mg/kg/dose **or** 40 mg/m²/dose given every other day for 4 weeks
Maintenance dose (for frequent relapses): 0.5-1 mg/kg/dose given every other day for 3-6 months

Renal Impairment: Hemodialysis effects: Supplemental dose is not necessary.

Available Dosage Forms
Solution, oral: 1 mg/mL (5 mL, 120 mL, 500 mL) [contains alcohol 5%, sodium benzoate; vanilla flavor]
Solution, oral concentrate (Prednisone Intensol™): 5 mg/mL (30 mL) [contains alcohol 30%]

Tablet: 1 mg, 2.5 mg, 5 mg, 10 mg, 20 mg, 50 mg
  Sterapred®: 5 mg [supplied as 21 tablet 6-day unit-dose package or 48 tablet 12-day unit-dose package]
  Sterapred® DS: 10 mg [supplied as 21 tablet 6-day unit-dose package or 48 tablet 12-day unit-dose package]

Monitoring and Teaching Issues

Physical Assessment: Assess effectiveness and interactions of other medications patient may be taking. Monitor for effectiveness of therapy and adverse reactions according to dose and length of therapy. Assess knowledge/teach patient appropriate use, possible side effects/interventions, and adverse symptoms to report (ie, opportunistic infection, adrenal suppression). Instruct patients with diabetes to monitor serum glucose levels closely; corticosteroids can alter glucose tolerance. Dose may need to be increased if patient is experiencing higher than normal levels of stress. When discontinuing, taper dose and frequency slowly.

Monitoring Laboratory Tests: Blood glucose, electrolytes

Patient Education: Take exactly as directed. Do not take more than prescribed dose and do not discontinue abruptly; consult prescriber. Take with or after meals. Take once-a-day dose with food in the morning. Avoid alcohol. Limit intake of caffeine or stimulants. Maintain adequate nutrition; consult prescriber for possibility of special dietary recommendations. If you have diabetes, monitor serum glucose closely and notify prescriber of changes; this medication can alter hypoglycemic requirements. Notify prescriber if you are experiencing higher than normal levels of stress; medication may need adjustment. Periodic ophthalmic examinations will be necessary with long-term use. You will be susceptible to infection (avoid crowds and exposure to infection). You may experience insomnia or nervousness; use caution when driving or engaging in tasks requiring alertness until response to drug is known. Report weakness, change in menstrual pattern, vision changes, signs of hyperglycemia, signs of infection (eg, fever, chills, mouth sores, perianal itching, vaginal discharge), other persistent side effects, or worsening of condition.

Dietary Considerations: Should be taken after meals or with food or milk; increase dietary intake of pyridoxine, vitamin C, vitamin D, folate, calcium, and phosphorus.

Geriatric Considerations: Because of the risk of adverse effects, systemic corticosteroids should be used cautiously in the elderly, in the smallest possible dose, and for the shortest possible time.

Pregnancy Risk Factor: B

Pregnancy Issues: Crosses the placenta. Immunosuppression reported in 1 infant exposed to high-dose prednisone plus azathioprine throughout gestation. One report of congenital cataracts. Available evidence suggests safe use during pregnancy.

Lactation: Enters breast milk/compatible

Breast-Feeding Issues: Crosses into breast milk. No data on clinical effects on the infant. AAP considers **compatible** with breast-feeding.

Administration

Oral: Take with food to decrease GI upset.

Additional Information Tapering of corticosteroids after a short course of therapy (<7-10 days) is generally not required unless the disease/inflammatory process is slow to respond. Tapering after prolonged exposure is dependent upon the individual patient, duration of corticosteroid treatments, and size of steroid dose. Recovery of the HPA axis may require several months. Subtle but important HPA axis suppression may be present for as long as several months after a course of as few as 10-14 days duration. Testing of HPA axis (cosyntropin) may be required, and signs/symptoms of adrenal insufficiency should be monitored in patients with a history of use.

Related Information

Corticosteroids *on page 1731*
FDA Name Differentiation Project: The Use of Tall-Man Letters *on page 15*

Primaquine (PRIM a kween)

Synonyms Primaquine Phosphate; Prymaccone

Generic Available Yes

Pharmacologic Category Aminoquinoline (Antimalarial)

Use Treatment of malaria

Unlabeled/Investigational Use Prevention of malaria; treatment *Pneumocystis carinii* pneumonia

Mechanism of Action/Effect Eliminates the primary tissue exoerythrocytic forms of *P. falciparum*; disrupts mitochondria and binds to DNA

Contraindications Hypersensitivity to primaquine, similar alkaloids, or any component of the formulation; acutely ill patients who have a tendency to develop granulocytopenia (rheumatoid arthritis, SLE); patients receiving other drugs capable of depressing the bone marrow (eg, quinacrine and primaquine)

Warnings/Precautions Use with caution in patients with G6PD deficiency, NADH methemoglobin reductase deficiency. Do not exceed recommended dosage.

Drug Interactions

Cytochrome P450 Effect: Substrate of CYP3A4 (major); **Inhibits** CYP1A2 (strong), 2D6 (weak), 3A4 (weak); **Induces** CYP1A2 (weak)

Decreased Effect: The levels/effects of primaquine may be decreased by aminoglutethimide, carbamazepine, nafcillin, nevirapine, phenobarbital, phenytoin, rifamycins, and other CYP3A4 inducers.

Increased Effect/Toxicity: Increased toxicity/levels with quinacrine. Primaquine may increase the levels/effects of aminophylline, fluvoxamine, mexiletine, mirtazapine, ropinirole, theophylline, trifluoperazine, and other CYP1A2 substrates.

Nutritional/Ethanol Interactions Ethanol: Avoid ethanol (due to GI irritation).

Adverse Reactions Frequency not defined.

Cardiovascular: Arrhythmias

Central nervous system: Headache

Dermatologic: Pruritus

Gastrointestinal: Abdominal pain, nausea, vomiting

Hematologic: Agranulocytosis, hemolytic anemia in G6PD deficiency, leukopenia, leukocytosis, methemoglobinemia in NADH-methemoglobin reductase-deficient individuals

Ocular: Interference with visual accommodation

Overdosage/Toxicology Symptoms of acute overdose include abdominal cramps, vomiting, cyanosis, methemoglobinemia (possibly severe), leukopenia, acute hemolytic anemia (often significant), and granulocytopenia. With chronic overdose, symptoms include ototoxicity and retinopathy. Treatment is supportive.

Pharmacodynamics/Kinetics

Absorption: Well absorbed

Time to Peak: Serum: 1-2 hours

Half-Life Elimination: 3.7-9.6 hours

Metabolism: Hepatic to carboxyprimaquine (active)

Excretion: Urine (small amounts as unchanged drug)

Dosing

Adults & Elderly: Dosage expressed as mg of base (15 mg base = 26.3 mg primaquine phosphate)

Treatment of malaria: To decrease risk of delayed primary attacks and prevent relapse: Oral: 15 mg/day (base) once daily for 14 days or 45 mg base once weekly for 8 weeks

CDC treatment recommendations: Begin therapy during last 2 weeks of, or following a course of, suppression with chloroquine or a comparable drug

Note: A second course (30 mg/day) for 14 days may be required in patients with relapse. Higher initial doses (30 mg/day) have also been used following exposure in S.E. Asia or Somalia.

Prevention of malaria (unlabeled use): Initiate prior to travel and continue for 7 days after departure from malaria-endemic area: Oral: 30 mg once daily

Pneumonia due to *Pneumocystis carinii* (unlabeled use): Oral: 30 mg once daily for 21 days (in conjunction with clindamycin)

Pediatrics: Dosage expressed as mg of base (15 mg base = 26.3 mg primaquine phosphate)

Treatment of malaria: To Decrease risk of delayed primary attacks and prevent relapse: Oral: 0.3 mg base/kg/day once daily for 14 days (not to exceed 15 mg/day) or 0.9 mg base/kg once weekly for 8 weeks not to exceed 45 mg base/week

CDC treatment recommendations: Begin therapy during last 2 weeks of, or following a course of, suppression with chloroquine or a comparable drug

Note: A second course (30 mg/day) for 14 days may be required in patients with relapse. Higher initial doses (30 mg/day) have also been used following exposure in S.E. Asia or Somalia.

Prevention of malaria (unlabeled use): Oral: Initiate prior to travel and continue for 7 days after departure from malaria-endemic area: 0.5 mg/kg once daily

Available Dosage Forms Tablet, as phosphate: 26.3 mg [15 mg base]

Monitoring and Teaching Issues

Physical Assessment: See Warnings/Precautions for use cautions. Assess potential for interactions with other pharmacological agents patient may be taking (eg, may increase or decrease levels/effects of primaquine; see Drug Interactions). Assess results of laboratory tests, effectiveness according to purpose for use, and adverse reactions periodically during therapy (eg, arrhythmias, rash, GI disturbance, cyanosis, anemia, visual changes; see Adverse Reactions). Teach patient appropriate use, possible side effects/interventions, and adverse symptoms to report (see Patient Education).

Monitoring Laboratory Tests: Periodic CBC, visual color check of urine, glucose, electrolytes; if hemolysis suspected, check: CBC, haptoglobin, peripheral smear, urinalysis dipstick for occult blood

Patient Education: Do not take any new medication during therapy unless approved by prescriber. It is important to complete full course of therapy for full effect. May be taken with meals to decrease GI upset and bitter aftertaste. Avoid alcohol. You should have regular ophthalmic exams (every 4-6 months) if using this medication over extended periods. May cause nausea, vomiting, or loss of appetite (small frequent meals, frequent mouth care, sucking lozenges, or chewing gum may help). Report persistent GI disturbance, chest pain or palpitation, unusual fatigue, easy bruising or bleeding, visual or hearing disturbances, changes in urine (darkening, tinged with red, decreased volume), or any other persistent adverse reactions. **Pregnancy/breast-feeding precautions:** Inform prescriber if you are or intend to become pregnant. Consult prescriber if breast-feeding.

Pregnancy Risk Factor: C

Lactation: Excretion in breast milk unknown

Administration

    Oral: Take with meals to decrease adverse GI effects. Drug has a bitter taste.

♦ **Primaquine Phosphate** *see Primaquine on page 1250*

♦ **Primatene® Mist [OTC]** *see Epinephrine on page 525*

♦ **Primaxin®** *see Imipenem and Cilastatin on page 787*

Primidone (PRI mi done)

U.S. Brand Names Mysoline®

Synonyms Desoxyphenobarbital; Primaclone

Generic Available Yes

Pharmacologic Category Anticonvulsant, Miscellaneous; Barbiturate

Medication Safety Issues

    Sound-alike/look-alike issues:

        Primidone may be confused with predniSONE

Use Management of grand mal, psychomotor, and focal seizures

Unlabeled/Investigational Use Benign familial tremor (essential tremor)

Mechanism of Action/Effect Decreases neuron excitability, raises seizure threshold similar to phenobarbital; primidone has two active metabolites, phenobarbital and phenylethylmalonamide (PEMA); PEMA may enhance the activity of phenobarbital

Contraindications Hypersensitivity to primidone, phenobarbital, or any component of the formulation; porphyria; pregnancy

Warnings/Precautions Use with caution in patients with renal or hepatic impairment, pulmonary insufficiency; abrupt withdrawal may precipitate status epilepticus. Potential for drug dependency exists. Do not administer to patients in acute pain. Use caution in elderly, debilitated, or pediatric patients - may cause paradoxical responses. May cause CNS depression, which may impair physical or mental abilities. Patients must cautioned about performing tasks which require mental alertness (eg, operating machinery or driving). Effects with other sedative drugs or ethanol may be potentiated. Use with caution in patients with depression or suicidal tendencies, or in patients with a history of drug abuse. Tolerance or psychological and physical dependence may occur with prolonged use. Primidone's metabolite, phenobarbital, has been associated with cognitive deficits in children. Use with caution in patients with hypoadrenalism.

Drug Interactions

    Cytochrome P450 Effect: Metabolized to phenobarbital; **Induces** CYP1A2 (strong), 2B6 (strong), 2C8/9 (strong), 3A4 (strong)

    Decreased Effect: Barbiturates may increase the metabolism of estrogens and reduce the efficacy of oral contraceptives; an alternative method of contraception should be considered. Barbiturates inhibit the hypoprothrombinemic effects of oral anticoagulants via increased metabolism. Barbiturates may enhance the metabolism of methadone resulting in methadone withdrawal. The levels/effects of primidone may be decreased by aminoglutethimide, carbamazepine, phenytoin, rifampin, and other CYP2C19 inducers.

    Primidone may decrease the levels/effects of aminophylline, amiodarone, benzodiazepines, bupropion, calcium channel blockers, carbamazepine, citalopram, clarithromycin, cyclosporine, diazepam, efavirenz, erythromycin, estrogens, fluoxetine, fluvoxamine, glimepiride, glipizide, ifosfamide, losartan, methsuximide, mirtazapine, nateglinide, nefazodone, nevirapine, phenytoin, pioglitazone, promethazine, propranolol, protease inhibitors, proton pump inhibitors, rifampin, ropinirole, rosiglitazone, selegiline, sertraline, sulfonamides, tacrolimus, theophylline, venlafaxine. voriconazole, warfarin, zafirlukast, and other CYP1A2, 2A6, 2B6, 2C8/9, or 3A4 substrates.

    Increased Effect/Toxicity: When combined with other CNS depressants, ethanol, narcotic analgesics, antidepressants, or benzodiazepines, additive respiratory and CNS depression may occur. Barbiturates may enhance the hepatotoxic potential of acetaminophen overdoses. Chloramphenicol, MAO inhibitors, valproic acid, and felbamate may inhibit barbiturate metabolism. Barbiturates may impair the absorption of griseofulvin, and may enhance the nephrotoxic effects of methoxyflurane. Concurrent use of phenobarbital with meperidine may result in increased CNS depression. Concurrent use of phenobarbital with primidone may result in elevated phenobarbital serum concentrations. CYP2C19 inhibitors may increase the levels/effects of primidone; example inhibitors include delavirdine, fluconazole, fluvoxamine, gemfibrozil, isoniazid, omeprazole, and ticlopidine.

Nutritional/Ethanol Interactions

    Ethanol: Avoid ethanol (may increase CNS depression).

    Food: Protein-deficient diets increase duration of action of primidone.

    Herb/Nutraceutical: Avoid valerian, St John's wort, kava kava, gotu kola (may increase CNS depression).

Lab Interactions Increased alkaline phosphatase (S); decreased calcium (S)

Adverse Reactions Frequency not defined.

    Central nervous system: Drowsiness, vertigo, ataxia, lethargy, behavior change, fatigue, hyperirritability

    Dermatologic: Rash

    Gastrointestinal: Nausea, vomiting, anorexia

(Continued)

Primidone *(Continued)*

Genitourinary: Impotence

Hematologic: Agranulocytopenia, agranulocytosis, anemia

Ocular: Diplopia, nystagmus

Overdosage/Toxicology Symptoms of overdose include unsteady gait, slurred speech, confusion, jaundice, hypothermia, fever, hypotension, coma, and respiratory arrest. Assure adequate hydration and renal function. Urinary alkalinization with I.V. sodium bicarbonate also helps to enhance elimination. Repeat oral doses of activated charcoal significantly reduce the half-life of primidone through nonrenal elimination. Hemodialysis or hemoperfusion is of uncertain value. Patients in stage IV coma due to high serum drug levels may require charcoal hemoperfusion.

Pharmacodynamics/Kinetics

Bioavailability: 60% to 80%

Time to Peak: Serum: ~4 hours

Protein Binding: 99%

Half-Life Elimination: Age dependent: Primidone: 10-12 hours; PEMA: 16 hours; Phenobarbital: 52-118 hours

Metabolism: Hepatic to phenobarbital (active) and phenylethylmalonamide (PEMA)

Excretion: Urine (15% to 25% as unchanged drug and active metabolites)

Dosing

Adults & Elderly:

Essential tremor (unlabeled use): 750 mg early in divided doses

Seizure disorders (grand mal, psychomotor, and focal): Oral: Initial: 125-250 mg/day at bedtime; increase by 125-250 mg/day every 3-7 days; usual dose: 750-1500 mg/day in divided doses 3-4 times/day with maximum dosage of 2 g/day.

Pediatrics: Seizure disorders (grand mal, psychomotor, and focal): Oral:

Children <8 years: Initial: 50-125 mg/day given at bedtime; increase by 50-125 mg/day increments every 3-7 days; usual dose: 10-25 mg/kg/day in divided doses 3-4 times/day.

Children ≥8 years: Refer to adult dosing.

Renal Impairment:

Cl_{cr} 50-80 mL/minute: Administer every 8 hours.

Cl_{cr} 10-50 mL/minute: Administer every 8-12 hours.

Cl_{cr} <10 mL/minute: Administer every 12-24 hours.

Moderately dialyzable (20% to 50%)

Administer dose postdialysis or administer supplemental 30% dose.

Hepatic Impairment: Increased side effects may occur in severe liver disease. Monitor plasma levels and adjust dose accordingly.

Available Dosage Forms Tablet: 50 mg, 250 mg [generic tablet may contain sodium benzoate]

Monitoring and Teaching Issues

Physical Assessment: Assess effectiveness and interactions of other medications patient may be taking. Monitor therapeutic effectiveness, laboratory values, and adverse reactions at beginning of therapy and periodically with long-term use. Taper dosage slowly when discontinuing. Assess knowledge/teach patient appropriate use and seizure precautions, interventions to reduce side effects, and adverse symptoms to report.

Monitoring Laboratory Tests: Serum primidone and phenobarbital concentration, CBC. Monitor CBC at 6-month intervals to compare with baseline obtained at start of therapy. Since elderly patients metabolize phenobarbital at a slower rate than younger adults, it is suggested to measure both primidone and phenobarbital levels together.

Patient Education: Take exactly as directed; do not increase dose or frequency or discontinue without consulting prescriber. Drug may cause physical and/or psychological dependence. While using this medication, do not use alcohol and other prescription or OTC medications (especially pain medications, sedatives, antihistamines, or hypnotics) without consulting prescriber. Maintain adequate hydration (2-3 L/day of fluids) unless instructed to restrict fluid intake. You may experience drowsiness, dizziness, or blurred vision (use caution when driving or engaging in tasks requiring alertness until response to drug is known); nausea, vomiting, or loss of appetite (small frequent meals, frequent mouth care, chewing gum, or sucking lozenges may help); or impotence (reversible). Wear identification of epileptic status and medications. Report behavioral or CNS changes (confusion, depression, increased sedation, excitation, headache, insomnia, or lethargy); muscle weakness, or tremors; unusual bruising or bleeding (mouth, urine, stool); or worsening of seizure activity or loss of seizure control. **Pregnancy/breast-feeding precautions:** Do not get pregnant while taking this drug; use appropriate contraceptive measures. Consult prescriber if breast-feeding.

Dietary Considerations: Folic acid: Low erythrocyte and CSF folate concentrations. Megaloblastic anemia has been reported. To avoid folic acid deficiency and megaloblastic anemia, some clinicians recommend giving patients on anticonvulsants prophylactic doses of folic acid and cyanocobalamin.

Geriatric Considerations: Due to CNS effects, monitor closely when initiating drug in the elderly. Since elderly metabolize phenobarbital at a slower rate than younger adults, it is suggested to measure both primidone and phenobarbital levels together. Adjust dose for renal function in the elderly when initiating or changing dose.

Pregnancy Risk Factor: D

Pregnancy Issues: Crosses the placenta. Dysmorphic facial features; hemorrhagic disease of newborn due to fetal vitamin K depletion, maternal folic acid deficiency may occur. Epilepsy itself, number of medications, genetic factors, or a combination of these probably influence the teratogenicity of anticonvulsant therapy. Benefit:risk ratio usually favors continued use during pregnancy.

Lactation: Enters breast milk/not recommended (AAP recommends use "with caution")

Breast-Feeding Issues: Sedation and feeding problems may occur in nursing infants. AAP recommends USE WITH CAUTION.

Administration
  Storage: Protect from light.
Related Information
  Anticonvulsants By Seizure Type *on page 1712*
  Peak and Trough Guidelines *on page 1694*

- **Primsol**® *see* Trimethoprim *on page 1528*
- **Principen**® *see* Ampicillin *on page 115*
- **Prinivil**® *see* Lisinopril *on page 906*
- **Prinzide**® *see* Lisinopril and Hydrochlorothiazide *on page 908*
- **Pristinamycin** *see* Quinupristin and Dalfopristin *on page 1300*
- **ProAmatine**® *see* Midodrine *on page 1005*

Probenecid (proe BEN e sid)

Synonyms Benemid [DSC]
Generic Available Yes
Pharmacologic Category Uricosuric Agent
Medication Safety Issues
  Sound-alike/look-alike issues:
    Probenecid may be confused with Procanbid®
Use Prevention of gouty arthritis; hyperuricemia; prolongation of beta-lactam effect (ie, serum levels)
Mechanism of Action/Effect Competitively inhibits the reabsorption of uric acid at the proximal convoluted tubule, thereby promoting its excretion and reducing serum uric acid levels; increases plasma levels of weak organic acids (penicillins, cephalosporins, or other beta-lactam antibiotics) by competitively inhibiting their renal tubular secretion
Contraindications Hypersensitivity to probenecid or any component of the formulation; high-dose aspirin therapy; moderate to severe renal impairment; children <2 years of age
Warnings/Precautions Use with caution in patients with peptic ulcer. Use extreme caution in the use of probenecid with penicillin in patients with renal insufficiency. Probenecid may not be effective in patients with a creatinine clearance <30-50 mL/minute. May cause exacerbation of acute gouty attack.
Drug Interactions
  Cytochrome P450 Effect: Inhibits CYP2C19 (weak)
  Decreased Effect: Salicylates (high-dose) may decrease uricosuria. Decreased urinary levels of nitrofurantoin may decrease efficacy.
  Increased Effect/Toxicity: Increases methotrexate toxic potential. Probenecid increases the serum concentrations of quinolones and beta-lactams such as penicillins and cephalosporins. Also increases levels/toxicity of acyclovir, diflunisal, ketorolac, thiopental, benzodiazepines, dapsone, fluoroquinolones, methotrexate, NSAIDs, sulfonylureas, zidovudine.
Lab Interactions False-positive glucosuria with Clinitest®
Adverse Reactions Frequency not defined.
  Cardiovascular: Flushing of face
  Central nervous system: Headache, dizziness
  Dermatologic: Rash, itching
  Gastrointestinal: Anorexia, nausea, vomiting, sore gums
  Genitourinary: Painful urination
  Hematologic: Aplastic anemia, hemolytic anemia, leukopenia
  Hepatic: Hepatic necrosis
  Neuromuscular & skeletal: Gouty arthritis (acute)
  Renal: Renal calculi, nephrotic syndrome, urate nephropathy
  Miscellaneous: Anaphylaxis
Overdosage/Toxicology Symptoms of overdose include nausea, vomiting, tonic-clonic seizures, and coma. Activated charcoal is especially effective at binding probenecid, for GI decontamination.
Pharmacodynamics/Kinetics
  Onset of Action: Effect on penicillin levels: 2 hours
  Absorption: Rapid and complete
  Time to Peak: Serum: 2-4 hours
  Half-Life Elimination: Dose dependent: Normal renal function: 6-12 hours
  Metabolism: Hepatic
  Excretion: Urine
Dosing
  Adults & Elderly:
    Hyperuricemia with gout: Oral: 250 mg twice daily for 1 week; increase to 250-500 mg/day; may increase by 500 mg/month, if needed, to maximum of 2-3 g/day (dosages may be increased by 500 mg every 6 months if serum urate concentrations are controlled)
    Prolong penicillin serum levels: Oral: 500 mg 4 times/day
    Gonorrhea: Oral: 1 g 30 minutes before penicillin, ampicillin, or amoxicillin
    Neurosyphilis: Oral: Aqueous procaine penicillin 2.4 million units/day I.M. plus probenecid 500 mg 4 times/day for 10-14 days
  Pediatrics:
    Note: Note recommended in children <2 years of age.
    Prolong penicillin serum levels: Oral: Children 2-14 years: 25 mg/kg starting dose, then 40 mg/kg/day given 4 times/day
    Treatment of gonorrhea: Oral: Children <45 kg: 25 mg/kg x 1 (maximum: 1 g/dose) 30 minutes before penicillin, ampicillin, or amoxicillin
  Renal Impairment: Cl_{cr} <50 mL/minute: Avoid use.
Available Dosage Forms Tablet: 500 mg
Monitoring and Teaching Issues
  Physical Assessment: Assess effectiveness and interactions of other medications patient may be taking. Monitor therapeutic effectiveness, laboratory values, and adverse reactions
(Continued)

Probenecid *(Continued)*

at beginning of therapy and periodically with long-term use. Assess knowledge/teach patient appropriate use, interventions to reduce side effects, and adverse symptoms to report.

Monitoring Laboratory Tests: Uric acid, renal function, CBC

Patient Education: Take as directed; do not discontinue without consulting prescriber. May take 6-12 months to reduce gouty attacks (attacks may increase in frequency and severity for first few months of therapy). Take with food or antacids or alkaline ash foods (milk, nuts, beets, spinach, turnip greens). Maintain adequate hydration (2-3 L/day of fluids) unless instructed to restrict fluid intake. Avoid aspirin or aspirin-containing substances. If you have diabetes, use serum glucose monitoring. If you experience severe headache, contact prescriber for medication. You may experience dizziness or lightheadedness (use caution when driving, changing position, or engaging in tasks requiring alertness until response to drug is known); or nausea, vomiting, indigestion, or loss of appetite (small frequent meals, frequent mouth care, chewing gum, or sucking lozenges may help). Report skin rash or itching, persistent headache, blood in urine or painful urination, excessive tiredness or easy bruising or bleeding, or sore gums. **Breast-feeding precaution:** Consult prescriber if breast-feeding.

Dietary Considerations: Drug may cause GI upset; take with food if GI upset. Drink plenty of fluids.

Geriatric Considerations: Since probenecid loses its effectiveness when the Cl_{cr} is <30 mL/minute, its usefulness in the elderly is limited.

Pregnancy Risk Factor: B

Lactation: Excretion in breast milk unknown

Additional Information Avoid fluctuation in uric acid (increase or decrease); may precipitate gout attack. Use of sodium bicarbonate or potassium citrate is suggested until serum uric acid normalizes and tophaceous deposits disappear.

♦ **Probenecid and Colchicine** *see Colchicine and Probenecid on page 370*

♦ **Probiotica® [OTC]** *see Lactobacillus on page 859*

Procainamide *(proe kane A mide)*

U.S. Brand Names Procanbid®

Synonyms PCA; Procainamide Hydrochloride; Procaine Amide Hydrochloride

Generic Available Yes

Pharmacologic Category Antiarrhythmic Agent, Class Ia

Medication Safety Issues

Sound-alike/look-alike issues:

"PCA" abbreviation should not be used when writing orders for this medication; has been misread as "patient controlled analgesia"

Procanbid® may be confused with probenecid

Pronestyl® may be confused with Ponstel®

Use Treatment of ventricular tachycardia (VT), premature ventricular contractions, paroxysmal atrial tachycardia (PSVT), and atrial fibrillation (AF); prevent recurrence of ventricular tachycardia, paroxysmal supraventricular tachycardia, atrial fibrillation or flutter

Unlabeled/Investigational Use ACLS guidelines:

Intermittent/recurrent VF or pulseless VT not responsive to earlier interventions

Monomorphic VT (EF >40%, no CHF)

Polymorphic VT with normal baseline QT interval

Wide complex tachycardia of unknown type (EF >40%, no CHF, patient stable)

Refractory paroxysmal SVT

Atrial fibrillation or flutter (EF >40%, no CHF) including pre-excitation syndrome

Mechanism of Action/Effect Decreases myocardial excitability and conduction velocity and may depress myocardial contractility, by increasing the electrical stimulation threshold of ventricle, His-Purkinje system and through direct cardiac effects

Contraindications Hypersensitivity to procaine, other ester-type local anesthetics, or any component of the formulation; complete heart block (except in patients with a functioning artificial pacemaker); second-degree AV block (without a functional pacemaker); various types of hemiblock (without a functional pacemaker); SLE; torsade de pointes; concurrent cisapride use; QT prolongation

Warnings/Precautions Monitor and adjust dose to prevent QT_c prolongation. Watch for proarrhythmic effects. May precipitate or exacerbate CHF. Reduce dosage in renal impairment. May increase ventricular response rate in patients with atrial fibrillation or flutter; control AV conduction before initiating. Correct hypokalemia before initiating therapy; hypokalemia may worsen toxicity. Use caution in digoxin-induced toxicity (can further depress AV conduction). Reduce dose if first-degree heart block occurs. Use caution with concurrent use of other antiarrhythmics. Avoid use in myasthenia gravis (may worsen condition). Hypersensitivity reactions can occur.

Potentially fatal blood dyscrasias have occurred with therapeutic doses; close monitoring is recommended during the first 3 months of therapy.

Long-term administration leads to the development of a positive antinuclear antibody (ANA) test in 50% of patients which may result in a drug-induced lupus erythematosus-like syndrome (in 20% to 30% of patients); discontinue procainamide with SLE symptoms and choose an alternative agent

Drug Interactions

Cytochrome P450 Effect: Substrate of CYP2D6 (major)

Increased Effect/Toxicity: Amiodarone, cimetidine, ofloxacin (and potentially other renally eliminated quinolones), ranitidine, and trimethoprim increase procainamide and NAPA blood levels; consider reducing procainamide dosage by 25% with concurrent use. Cisapride and procainamide may increase the risk of malignant arrhythmia; concurrent use is contraindicated. Procainamide may potentiate neuromuscular blockade of neuromuscular-blocking agents. CYP2D6 inhibitors may increase the levels/effects of procainamide;

example inhibitors include chlorpromazine, delavirdine, fluoxetine, miconazole, paroxetine, pergolide, quinidine, quinine, ritonavir, and ropinirole.

Drugs which may prolong the QT interval include amiodarone, amitriptyline, bepridil, cisapride, disopyramide, erythromycin, haloperidol, imipramine, pimozide, quinidine, sotalol, mesoridazine, thioridazine, and some quinolone antibiotics (sparfloxacin, gatifloxacin, moxifloxacin); concurrent use may result in additional prolongation of the QT interval.

Nutritional/Ethanol Interactions
Ethanol: Avoid ethanol (acute ethanol administration reduces procainamide serum concentrations).

Herb/Nutraceutical: Avoid ephedra (may worsen arrhythmia).

Adverse Reactions >1%:
Cardiovascular: Hypotension (I.V., up to 5%)

Dermatologic: Rash

Gastrointestinal: Diarrhea (3% to 4%), nausea, vomiting, taste disorder, GI complaints (3% to 4%)

Overdosage/Toxicology
Procainamide has a low toxic:therapeutic ratio and may easily produce fatal intoxication (acute toxic dose: 5 g in adults). Symptoms of overdose include sinus bradycardia, sinus node arrest or asystole, P-R, QRS, or QT interval prolongation, torsade de pointes (polymorphous ventricular tachycardia), and depressed myocardial contractility, which along with alpha-adrenergic or ganglionic blockade, may result in hypotension and pulmonary edema. Other effects are seizures, coma, and respiratory arrest. Treatment is symptomatic and effects usually respond to conventional therapies. **Note:** Do not use other Type 1A or 1C antiarrhythmic agents to treat ventricular tachycardia. Sodium bicarbonate may treat wide QRS intervals or hypotension. Markedly impaired conduction or high degree AV block, unresponsive to bicarbonate, indicates consideration of a pacemaker.

Pharmacodynamics/Kinetics
Onset of Action: I.M. 10-30 minutes

Bioavailability: Oral: 75% to 95%

Time to Peak: Serum: Capsule: 45 minutes to 2.5 hours; I.M.: 15-60 minutes

Protein Binding: 15% to 20%

Half-Life Elimination:
Procainamide (hepatic acetylator, phenotype, cardiac and renal function dependent):
Children: 1.7 hours; Adults: 2.5-4.7 hours; Anephric: 11 hours

NAPA (renal function dependent):
Children: 6 hours; Adults: 6-8 hours; Anephric: 42 hours

Metabolism: Hepatic via acetylation to produce N-acetyl procainamide (NAPA) (active metabolite)

Excretion: Urine (25% as NAPA)

Dosing
Adults & Elderly: Dose must be titrated to patient's response.

Antiarrhythmic:
Oral: 250-500 mg/dose every 3-6 hours or 500 mg to 1 g every 6 hours extended release; usual dose: 50 mg/kg/24 hours; maximum: 4 g/24 hours

I.M.: 0.5-1 g every 4-8 hours until oral therapy is possible

I.V. (infusion requires use of an infusion pump):
Loading dose: 15-18 mg/kg administered as slow infusion over 25-30 minutes or 100-200 mg/dose repeated every 5 minutes as needed to a total dose of 1 g
Maintenance dose: 1-4 mg/minute by continuous infusion.

Infusion rate: 2 g/250 mL (I.V. infusion requires use of an infusion pump):
1 mg/minute: 7.5 mL/hour
2 mg/minute: 15 mL/hour
3 mg/minute: 22.5 mL/hour
4 mg/minute: 30 mL/hour
5 mg/minute: 37.5 mL/hour
6 mg/minute: 45 mL/hour

Intermittent/recurrent VF or pulseless VT:
Initial: 20-30 mg/minute (maximum: 50 mg/minute if necessary), up to a total of 17 mg/kg.

ACLS guidelines: I.V.: Infuse 20 mg/minute until arrhythmia is controlled, hypotension occurs, QRS complex widens by 50% of its original width, or total of 17 mg/kg is given.

Note: Reduce to 12 mg/kg in setting of cardiac or renal dysfunction

I.V. maintenance infusion: 1-4 mg/minute; monitor levels and do not exceed 3 mg/minute for >24 hours in adults with renal failure.

Pediatrics: Must be titrated to patient's response:

Arrhythmias:
Oral: 15-50 mg/kg/24 hours divided every 3-6 hours

I.M.: 50 mg/kg/24 hours divided into doses of $1/8$ to $1/4$ every 3-6 hours in divided doses until oral therapy is possible

I.V. (infusion requires use of an infusion pump):
Load: 3-6 mg/kg/dose over 5 minutes not to exceed 100 mg/dose; may repeat every 5-10 minutes to maximum of 15 mg/kg/load
Maintenance as continuous I.V. infusion: 20-80 mcg/kg/minute; maximum: 2 g/24 hours

Renal Impairment:
Cl_{cr} 10-50 mL/minute: Administer every 6-12 hours.

Cl_{cr} <10 mL/minute: Administer every 8-24 hours.

Dialysis:
Procainamide: Moderately hemodialyzable (20% to 50%): 200 mg supplemental dose posthemodialysis is recommended.

N-acetylprocainamide: Not dialyzable (0% to 5%)

Procainamide/N-acetylprocainamide: Peritoneal dialysis: Not dialyzable (0% to 5%)

(Continued)

Procainamide *(Continued)*

Procainamide/N-acetylprocainamide: Replace by blood level during continuous arterio-venous or venovenous hemofiltration.

Hepatic Impairment: Reduce dose by 50%.

Available Dosage Forms

Capsule, as hydrochloride: 250 mg, 500 mg

Injection, solution, as hydrochloride: 100 mg/mL (10 mL); 500 mg/mL (2 mL) [contains sodium metabisulfite]

Tablet, extended release, as hydrochloride: 500 mg, 750 mg, 1000 mg

Procanbid®: 500 mg, 1000 mg

Monitoring and Teaching Issues

Physical Assessment: Assess other medications patient may be taking for effectiveness and interactions. I.V. requires use of infusion pump and continuous cardiac and hemody-namic monitoring. Assess results of laboratory tests, therapeutic effectiveness, and adverse reactions at beginning of therapy, when titrating dosage, and on a regular basis with long-term therapy. **Note:** Procainamide has a low TI and overdose may easily produce severe and life-threatening reactions. Assess knowledge/teach patient appropriate use, interventions to reduce side effects, and adverse symptoms to report.

Monitoring Laboratory Tests: CBC with differential, platelet count

Patient Education: Oral: Take exactly as directed; do not take additional doses or discon-tinue without consulting prescriber. Avoid alcohol. You will need regular cardiac checkups and blood tests while taking this medication. You may experience dizziness, lightheaded-ness, or visual changes (use caution when driving or engaging in tasks requiring alertness until response to drug is known); loss of appetite (small frequent meals, frequent mouth care, chewing gum, or sucking lozenges may help); headaches (prescriber may recom-mend mild analgesic); or diarrhea (yogurt or boiled milk may help; if persistent consult prescriber). Report chest pain, palpitation, or erratic heartbeat; increased weight or swelling of hands or feet; acute diarrhea; or unusual fatigue and tiredness. **Pregnancy/breast-feeding precautions:** Inform prescriber if you are or intend to become pregnant. Consult prescriber if breast-feeding.

Dietary Considerations: Should be taken with water on an empty stomach.

Geriatric Considerations: Monitor closely since clearance is reduced in those >60 years of age. If clinically possible, start doses at lowest recommended dose. Also, elderly frequently have drug therapy which may interfere with the use of procainamide. Adjust dose for renal function in the elderly.

Pregnancy Risk Factor: C

Lactation: Enters breast milk/use caution (AAP rates "compatible")

Breast-Feeding Issues: Considered compatible by the AAP. However, the AAP stated concern regarding long-term effects and potential for infant toxicity. Use caution and monitor closely if continuing to breast-feed while taking procainamide.

Administration

Oral: Do **not** crush or chew extended release drug products.

I.V.: Must dilute prior to I.V. administration; maximum rate: 50 mg/minute; give around-the-clock to promote less variation in peak and trough serum levels.

Reconstitution: Minimum volume: 1 g/250 mL NS/D$_5$W

Stability of admixture at room temperature in D$_5$W or NS is 24 hours. Some information indicates that procainamide may be subject to greater decomposition in D$_5$W unless the admixture is refrigerated or the pH is adjusted. Procainamide is believed to form an association complex with dextrose - the bioavailability of procainamide in this complex is not known and the complex formation is reversible.

Compatibility: Stable in ½NS, NS, SWFI

Y-site administration: Incompatible with milrinone

Compatibility when admixed: Incompatible with esmolol, ethacrynate, milrinone, phen-ytoin

Storage: Procainamide may be stored at room temperature up to 27°C; however, refrigera-tion retards oxidation, which causes color formation. The solution is initially colorless but may turn slightly yellow on standing. Injection of air into the vial causes the solution to darken. Solutions darker than a light amber should be discarded.

Related Information

Antiarrhythmic Drugs *on page 1708*

Peak and Trough Guidelines *on page 1694*

♦ **Procainamide Hydrochloride** *see* Procainamide *on page 1254*

Procaine *(PROE kane)*

U.S. Brand Names Novocain®

Synonyms Procaine Hydrochloride

Generic Available Yes

Pharmacologic Category Local Anesthetic

Use Produces spinal anesthesia and epidural and peripheral nerve block by injection and infiltration methods

Mechanism of Action/Effect Blocks both the initiation and conduction of nerve impulses by decreasing the neuronal membrane's permeability to sodium ions, which results in inhibition of depolarization with resultant blockade of conduction

Contraindications Hypersensitivity to procaine, PABA, parabens, other ester local anes-thetics, or any component of the formulation

Warnings/Precautions Patients with cardiac diseases, hyperthyroidism, or other endocrine diseases may be more susceptible to toxic effects of local anesthetics. Some preparations contain metabisulfite.

Drug Interactions

Decreased Effect: Decreased effect of sulfonamides with the PABA metabolite of procaine, chloroprocaine, and tetracaine. Decreased/increased effect of vasopressors, ergot alkaloids, and MAO inhibitors on blood pressure when using anesthetic solutions with a vasoconstrictor.

Adverse Reactions 1% to 10%: Local: Burning sensation at site of injection, tissue irritation, pain at injection site

Overdosage/Toxicology Treatment is symptomatic and supportive. Termination of anesthesia by pneumatic tourniquet inflation should be attempted when procaine is administered by infiltration or regional injection.

Pharmacodynamics/Kinetics
Onset of Action: 2-5 minutes
Duration of Action: Patient, type of block, concentration, and method of anesthesia dependent: 0.5-1.5 hours
Half-Life Elimination: 7.7 minutes
Metabolism: Rapidly hydrolyzed by plasma enzymes to para-aminobenzoic acid and diethylaminoethanol (80% conjugated before elimination)
Excretion: Urine (as metabolites and some unchanged drug)

Dosing
Adults & Elderly: Spinal anesthesia, epidural and peripheral nerve block: Injection and infiltration methods: Dose varies with procedure, desired depth, and duration of anesthesia, desired muscle relaxation, vascularity of tissues, physical condition, and age of patient.
Pediatrics: Dose varies with procedure, desired depth, and duration of anesthesia, desired muscle relaxation, vascularity of tissues, physical condition, and age of patient.

Available Dosage Forms Injection, solution, as hydrochloride: 1% (30 mL); 2% (30 mL)
Novocain®: 1% [10 mg/mL] (2 mL, 6 mL, 30 mL); 2% [20 mg/mL] (30 mL); 10% (2 mL)

Monitoring and Teaching Issues
Physical Assessment: Monitor response, degree of pain sensation, and injection site.
Epidural: Monitor CNS status.
Patient Education: The purpose of this medication is to reduce pain sensation. Report local burning or pain at injection site. **Pregnancy/breast-feeding precautions:** Inform prescriber if you are or intend to become pregnant. Consult prescriber if breast-feeding.
Pregnancy Risk Factor: C
Lactation: Excretion in breast milk unknown

Administration
Other: Prior to instillation of anesthetic agent, withdraw plunger to ensure needle is not in artery or vein; resuscitative equipment should be available when local anesthetics are administered
Compatibility: Stable in dextran 6% in dextrose, dextran 6% in NS, D_5LR, $D_5^1/_4NS$, $D_5^1/_2NS$, D_5NS, D_5W, $D_{10}W$, LR, $^1/_2NS$, NS
Compatibility when admixed: Incompatible with amobarbital, amphotericin B, chlorothiazide, magnesium sulfate, phenobarbital, phenytoin, sodium bicarbonate

♦ **Procaine Amide Hydrochloride** see Procainamide on page 1254
♦ **Procaine Benzylpenicillin** see Penicillin G Procaine on page 1175
♦ **Procaine Hydrochloride** see Procaine on page 1256
♦ **Procaine Penicillin G** see Penicillin G Procaine on page 1175
♦ **Procanbid®** see Procainamide on page 1254

Procarbazine (proe KAR ba zeen)

U.S. Brand Names Matulane®
Synonyms Benzmethyzin; N-Methylhydrazine; NSC-77213; Procarbazine Hydrochloride
Generic Available No
Pharmacologic Category Antineoplastic Agent, Alkylating Agent
Medication Safety Issues
Sound-alike/look-alike issues:
Procarbazine may be confused with dacarbazine
Matulane® may be confused with Modane®

Use Treatment of Hodgkin's disease
Unlabeled/Investigational Use Treatment of non-Hodgkin's lymphoma, brain tumors, melanoma, lung cancer, multiple myeloma
Mechanism of Action/Effect Mechanism of action is not clear, methylating of nucleic acids; inhibits DNA, RNA, and protein synthesis; may damage DNA directly and suppresses mitosis; metabolic activation required by host
Contraindications Hypersensitivity to procarbazine or any component of the formulation; pre-existing bone marrow aplasia; ethanol ingestion; pregnancy
Warnings/Precautions The U.S. Food and Drug Administration (FDA) currently recommends that procedures for proper handling and disposal of antineoplastic agents be considered. Use with caution in patients with pre-existing renal or hepatic impairment. Procarbazine possesses MAO inhibitor activity. Procarbazine is a carcinogen which may cause acute leukemia. Procarbazine may cause infertility.

Drug Interactions
Increased Effect/Toxicity: Procarbazine exhibits weak MAO inhibitor activity. Foods containing high amounts of tyramine should, therefore, be avoided. When an MAO inhibitor is given with food high in tyramine, hypertensive crisis, intracranial bleeding, and headache have been reported.

Sympathomimetic amines (epinephrine and amphetamines) and antidepressants (tricyclics) should be used cautiously with procarbazine. Barbiturates, narcotics, phenothiazines, and other CNS depressants can cause somnolence, ataxia, and other symptoms of CNS depression. Ethanol has caused a disulfiram-like reaction with procarbazine. May result in headache, respiratory difficulties, nausea, vomiting, sweating, thirst, hypotension, and flushing.

Nutritional/Ethanol Interactions
Ethanol: Use ethanol and ethanol-containing products cautiously.
(Continued)

Procarbazine *(Continued)*

Food: Clinically severe and possibly life-threatening elevations in blood pressure may occur if procarbazine is taken with tyramine-containing foods.

Adverse Reactions Frequency not defined.

Central nervous system: Reports of neurotoxicity with procarbazine generally originate from early usage with single agent oral (continuous) or I.V. dosing; CNS depression is commonly reported to be additive with other CNS depressants

Hematologic: Myelosuppression, hemolysis in patients with G6PD deficiency

Gastrointestinal: Nausea and vomiting (60% to 90%); increasing the dose in a stepwise fashion over several days may minimize this

Genitourinary: Reproductive dysfunction >10% (in animals, hormone treatment has prevented azoospermia)

Respiratory: Pulmonary toxicity (<1%); the most commonly reported pulmonary toxicity is a hypersensitivity pneumonitis which responds to steroids and discontinuation of the drug. At least one report of persistent pulmonary fibrosis has been reported, however, a higher incidence (18%) of pulmonary toxicity (fibrosis) was reported when procarbazine was given prior to BCNU (BCNU alone does cause pulmonary fibrosis).

Miscellaneous: Second malignancies (cumulative incidence 2% to 15% reported with MOPP combination therapy)

Overdosage/Toxicology Symptoms of overdose include arthralgia, alopecia, paresthesia, bone marrow suppression, hallucinations, nausea, vomiting, diarrhea, seizures, and coma. Treatment is supportive. Adverse effects such as marrow toxicity may begin as late as 2 weeks after exposure.

Pharmacodynamics/Kinetics

Absorption: Rapid and complete

Half-Life Elimination: 1 hour

Metabolism: Hepatic and renal

Excretion: Urine and respiratory tract (<5% as unchanged drug, 70% as metabolites)

Dosing

Adults: Refer to individual protocols.

Chemotherapy: Oral: Initial: 2-4 mg/kg/day in single or divided doses for 7 days then increase dose to 4-6 mg/kg/day until response is obtained or leukocyte count decreased <4000/mm^3 or the platelet count decreased <100,000/mm^3; maintenance: 1-2 mg/kg/day

Elderly: Refer to adult dosing; use with caution. Adjust for renal impairment.

Pediatrics: Refer to individual protocols. Dose based on patient's ideal weight if the patient is obese or has abnormal fluid retention. Oral (may be given as a single daily dose or in 2-3 divided doses): Children:

BMT aplastic anemia conditioning regimen: 12.5 mg/kg/dose every other day for 4 doses

Hodgkin's disease: MOPP/IC-MOPP regimens: 100 mg/m^2/day for 14 days and repeated every 4 weeks

Neuroblastoma and medulloblastoma: Doses as high as 100-200 mg/m^2/day once daily have been used.

Renal Impairment: Use with caution, may result in increased toxicity; decrease dose if serum creatinine >2 mg/dL

Hepatic Impairment: Use with caution; may result in increased toxicity; decrease dose if total bilirubin >3 mg/dL

Available Dosage Forms Capsule, as hydrochloride: 50 mg

Monitoring and Teaching Issues

Physical Assessment: Assess potential for interactions with other pharmacological agents patient may be taking (eg, CNS depressants increase risk of adverse reactions; see Drug Interactions). Emetic potential is high; antiemetic is generally required. Assess results of laboratory tests and patient response frequently (eg, neurotoxicity, nausea, vomiting, pneumonitis, arthralgia, or paresthesia; see Adverse Reactions). Instruct patient about dietary and alcohol cautions (procarbazine has some MAO inhibitory effects, can result in life-threatening hypertension with tyramine [see Tyramine Content of Foods list *on page 1758*]; alcohol may cause disulfiram-like reaction). Teach patient proper use, possible side effects/appropriate interventions, and adverse symptoms to report (see Patient Education).

Monitoring Laboratory Tests: CBC with differential, platelet and reticulocyte count, urinalysis, liver and renal function

Patient Education: Do not take any new medication during therapy unless approved by prescriber. Take as directed. Avoid alcohol; may cause acute disulfiram reaction (headache, respiratory difficulties, nausea, vomiting, sweating, thirst, hypotension, and flushing). Avoid tyramine-containing foods (eg, aged cheese, chocolate, pickles, aged meat, wine, etc), could cause serious hypertensive effects. Maintain adequate hydration (2-3 L/day of fluids) unless instructed to restrict fluid intake. You will be more sensitive to infection (avoid crowds and exposure to infection and do not have any vaccinations without consulting prescriber). May cause considerable nausea or vomiting (consult prescriber for approved antiemetic); mental depression, nervousness, insomnia, nightmares, dizziness, confusion, or lethargy (use caution when driving or engaging in tasks that require alertness until response to drug is known); rash, hair loss, or hyperpigmentation (reversible), loss of libido, sterility, or amenorrhea. Report persistent fever, chills, sore throat; unusual bleeding; blood in urine, stool (black stool), or vomitus; unresolved depression; mania; hallucinations; nightmares; disorientation; seizures; chest pain or palpitations; respiratory difficulty; or vision changes. **Pregnancy/breast-feeding precautions:** Inform prescriber if you are pregnant. Do not get pregnant during or for 1 month following therapy. Males: Do not cause a female to become pregnant. Males/females: Consult prescriber for instruction on appropriate barrier contraceptive measures. This drug may cause severe fetal defects. Breast-feeding is not recommended.

Pregnancy Risk Factor: D
Lactation: Excretion in breast milk unknown/not recommended
Administration
　Storage: Protect from light
Related Information
　Tyramine Content of Foods *on page 1758*

♦ **Procarbazine Hydrochloride** *see* Procarbazine *on page 1257*

♦ **Procardia®** *see* NIFEdipine *on page 1081*

♦ **Procardia XL®** *see* NIFEdipine *on page 1081*

♦ **Procetofene** *see* Fenofibrate *on page 615*

♦ **Prochieve™** *see* Progesterone *on page 1262*

Prochlorperazine (proe klor PER a zeen)

U.S. Brand Names Compazine® [DSC]; Compro™
Synonyms Chlormeprazine; Prochlorperazine Edisylate; Prochlorperazine Maleate
Generic Available Yes: Injection, tablet, suppository
Pharmacologic Category Antiemetic; Antipsychotic Agent, Typical, Phenothiazine
Medication Safety Issues
　Sound-alike/look-alike issues:
　　Prochlorperazine may be confused with chlorproMAZINE
　　Compazine® may be confused with Copaxone®, Coumadin®
Use Management of nausea and vomiting; psychosis; anxiety
Unlabeled/Investigational Use Behavioral syndromes in dementia
Mechanism of Action/Effect Prochlorperazine is a piperazine phenothiazine antipsychotic which blocks postsynaptic mesolimbic dopaminergic D_1 and D_2 receptors in the brain, including the medullary chemoreceptor trigger zone; exhibits a strong alpha-adrenergic and anticholinergic blocking effect and depresses the release of hypothalamic and hypophyseal hormones; believed to depress the reticular activating system, thus affecting basal metabolism, body temperature, wakefulness, vasomotor tone and emesis
Contraindications Hypersensitivity to prochlorperazine or any component of the formulation (cross-reactivity between phenothiazines may occur); severe CNS depression; coma; should not be used in children <2 years of age or <10 kg
Warnings/Precautions May be sedating; use with caution in disorders where CNS depression is a feature. May impair physical or mental abilities; patients must be cautioned about performing tasks which require mental alertness (eg, operating machinery or driving). Effects with other sedative drugs or ethanol may be potentiated. Avoid use in Reye's syndrome. Use with caution in Parkinson's disease; hemodynamic instability; bone marrow suppression; predisposition to seizures; subcortical brain damage; and in severe cardiac, hepatic, renal or respiratory disease. Caution in breast cancer or other prolactin-dependent tumors (may elevate prolactin levels). May alter temperature regulation or mask toxicity of other drugs due to antiemetic effects. May alter cardiac conduction - life threatening arrhythmias have occurred with therapeutic doses of phenothiazines. May cause orthostatic hypotension; use with caution in patients at risk of hypotension or where transient hypotensive episodes would be poorly tolerated (cardiovascular disease or cerebrovascular disease). Hypotension may occur following administration, particularly when parenteral form is used or in high dosages.

Due to anticholinergic effects, use with caution in patients with decreased gastrointestinal motility, urinary retention, BPH, xerostomia, visual problems, narrow-angle glaucoma (screening is recommended) and myasthenia gravis. May cause extrapyramidal symptoms, including pseudoparkinsonism, acute dystonic reactions, akathisia and tardive dyskinesia. May be associated with neuroleptic malignant syndrome (NMS).

Drug Interactions
　Decreased Effect: Barbiturates and carbamazepine may increase the metabolism of prochlorperazine, lowering its serum levels. Benztropine (and other anticholinergics) may inhibit the therapeutic response to prochlorperazine. Antipsychotics such as prochlorperazine inhibit the ability of bromocriptine to lower serum prolactin concentrations. The antihypertensive effects of guanethidine and guanadrel may be inhibited by prochlorperazine. Prochlorperazine may inhibit the antiparkinsonian effect of levodopa. Prochlorperazine (and possibly other low potency antipsychotics) may reverse the pressor effects of epinephrine.
　Increased Effect/Toxicity: Chloroquine, propranolol, and sulfadoxine-pyrimethamine may increase prochlorperazine concentrations. Concurrent use with TCA may produce increased toxicity or altered therapeutic response. Prochlorperazine plus lithium may rarely produce neurotoxicity. Prochlorperazine may produce additive CNS depressant effects with CNS depressants (ethanol, narcotics). Metoclopramide may increase risk of extrapyramidal symptoms (EPS).
Nutritional/Ethanol Interactions
　Ethanol: Avoid ethanol (may increase CNS depression).
　Food: Limit caffeine.
　Herb/Nutraceutical: Avoid dong quai, St John's wort (may also cause photosensitization). Avoid kava kava, gotu kola, valerian, St John's wort (may increase CNS depression).
Lab Interactions False-positives for phenylketonuria, urinary amylase, uroporphyrins, urobilinogen
Adverse Reactions Frequency not defined.
　Cardiovascular: Hyper-/hypotension, orthostatic hypotension, tachycardia, bradycardia, dizziness, cardiac arrest
　Central nervous system: Extrapyramidal signs (pseudoparkinsonism, akathisia, dystonias, tardive dyskinesia), dizziness, cerebral edema, seizure, headache, drowsiness, paradoxical excitement, restlessness, hyperactivity, insomnia, neuroleptic malignant syndrome (NMS), impairment of temperature regulation
　Dermatologic: Rash, discoloration of skin (blue-gray), photosensitivity
(Continued)

1259

Prochlorperazine *(Continued)*

Endocrine & metabolic: Hypoglycemia, hyperglycemia, galactorrhea, lactation, breast enlargement, gynecomastia, menstrual irregularity, amenorrhea, SIADH, libido (changes in)

Gastrointestinal: Constipation, weight gain, vomiting, stomach pain, nausea, xerostomia, salivation, diarrhea, anorexia, ileus

Genitourinary: Difficulty in urination, ejaculatory disturbances, incontinence, polyuria, ejaculating dysfunction, priapism

Hematologic: Agranulocytosis, leukopenia, eosinophilia, hemolytic anemia, thrombocytopenic purpura, pancytopenia

Hepatic: Cholestatic jaundice, hepatotoxicity

Neuromuscular & skeletal: Tremor

Ocular: Pigmentary retinopathy, blurred vision, cornea and lens changes

Respiratory: Nasal congestion

Miscellaneous: Diaphoresis

Overdosage/Toxicology Symptoms of overdose include deep sleep, coma, extrapyramidal symptoms, abnormal involuntary muscle movements, and hypotension. Treatment is symptom-directed and supportive.

Pharmacodynamics/Kinetics

Onset of Action: Oral: 30-40 minutes; I.M.: 10-20 minutes; Rectal: ~60 minutes

Duration of Action: I.M., oral extended-release: 12 hours; Rectal, immediate release: 3-4 hours

Bioavailability: Oral: 12.5%

Half-Life Elimination: Oral: 3-5 hours; I.V.: ~7 hours

Metabolism: Primarily hepatic; N-desmethyl prochlorperazine (major active metabolite)

Dosing

Adults:

Antiemetic:

Oral: 5-10 mg 3-4 times/day; usual maximum: 40 mg/day

I.M.: 5-10 mg every 3-4 hours; usual maximum: 40 mg/day

I.V.: 2.5-10 mg; maximum 10 mg/dose or 40 mg/day; may repeat dose every 3-4 hours as needed

Rectal: 25 mg twice daily

Surgical nausea/vomiting: Adults:

I.M.: 5-10 mg 1-2 hours before induction; may repeat once if necessary

I.V.: 5-10 mg 15-30 minutes before induction; may repeat once if necessary

Antipsychotic:

Oral: 5-10 mg 3-4 times/day; doses up to 150 mg/day may be required in some patients for treatment of severe disturbances.

I.M.: 10-20 mg every 4-6 hours may be required in some patients for treatment of severe disturbances; change to oral as soon as possible.

Nonpsychotic anxiety: Oral: Usual dose: 15-20 mg/day in divided doses; do not give doses >20 mg/day or for longer than 12 weeks

Elderly: Dementia behavior (nonpsychotic, unlabeled use): Initial: 2.5-5 mg 1-2 times/day; increase dose at 4- to 7-day intervals by 2.5-5 mg/day. Increase dosing intervals (twice daily, 3 times/day, etc) as necessary to control response or side effects. Maximum daily dose should probably not exceed 75 mg in the elderly. Gradual increases (titration) may prevent some side effects or decrease their severity. See Geriatric Considerations.

Pediatrics: Not recommended in children <10 kg or <2 years.

Antiemetic:

Oral, rectal:

>10 kg: 0.4 mg/kg/24 hours in 3-4 divided doses; **or**

9-14 kg: 2.5 mg every 12-24 hours as needed; maximum: 7.5 mg/day

14-18 kg: 2.5 mg every 8-12 hours as needed; maximum: 10 mg/day

18-39 kg: 2.5 mg every 8 hours or 5 mg every 12 hours as needed; maximum: 15 mg/day

I.M.: 0.1-0.15 mg/kg/dose; usual: 0.13 mg/kg/dose; change to oral as soon as possible.

Antipsychotic: Children 2-12 years:

Oral, rectal: 2.5 mg 2-3 times/day; increase dosage as needed to maximum daily dose of 20 mg for 2-5 years and 25 mg for 6-12 years.

I.M.: 0.13 mg/kg/dose; change to oral as soon as possible.

Renal Impairment: Not dialyzable (0% to 5%)

Available Dosage Forms [DSC] = Discontinued product

Injection, solution, as edisylate: 5 mg/mL (2 mL, 10 mL) [contains benzyl alcohol]

Suppository, rectal: 2.5 mg (12s), 5 mg (12s), 25 mg (12s) [may contain coconut and palm oil]

Compazine®: 2.5 mg (12s), 5 mg (12s), 25 mg (12s) [contains coconut and palm oils] [DSC]

Compro™: 25 mg (12s) [contains coconut and palm oils]

Tablet, as maleate: 5 mg, 10 mg

Monitoring and Teaching Issues

Physical Assessment: Assess all other medications patient may be taking. For I.V., continuously monitor blood pressure and heart rate during administration. Monitor blood pressure and heart rate, fluid balance, and dehydration. Monitor for seizures, especially with known seizure disorder. Monitor for excessive sedation, neuromuscular malignant syndrome, autonomic instability (eg, anticholinergic effects), and extrapyramidal symptoms.

Monitoring Laboratory Tests: Baseline liver and kidney function, CBC prior to and periodically during therapy, lipid profile, fasting blood glucose/Hgb A_{1c}; BMI

Patient Education: Take exact amount as prescribed. Do not change brand names. Do not crush or chew tablets or capsules. Do not discontinue without consulting prescriber. Avoid alcohol or other sedatives or sleep-inducing drugs. Avoid skin contact with drug; wash immediately with warm soapy water. You may experience appetite changes; small frequent meals may help. Maintain adequate hydration (2-3 L/day of fluids) unless instructed to restrict fluid intake. May cause dizziness, tremors, or visual disturbance (especially during early therapy); use caution when driving or engaging in tasks that require alertness until response to drug is known. Do not change position rapidly (rise slowly). May cause photosensitivity reaction; use sunscreen, wear protective clothing and eyewear, and avoid direct sunlight. Report immediately any changes in gait or muscular tremors. Report unresolved changes in voiding or elimination (constipation or diarrhea), acute dizziness or unresolved sedation, vision changes, palpitations, yellowing of skin or eyes, or changes in color of urine or stool (pink or red brown urine is expected). **Pregnancy/breast-feeding precautions:** Inform prescriber if you are or intend to become pregnant. Breast-feeding is not recommended.

Dietary Considerations: Increase dietary intake of riboflavin; should be administered with food or water. Rectal suppositories may contain coconut and palm oil.

Geriatric Considerations: Due to side effect profile (dystonias, EPS) this is not a preferred drug in the elderly for antiemetic therapy.

Pregnancy Risk Factor: C

Pregnancy Issues: Crosses the placenta. Isolated reports of congenital anomalies, however, some included exposures to other drugs. Available evidence with use of occasional low doses suggests safe use during pregnancy.

Lactation: Enters breast milk/not recommended

Administration

I.V.: I.V. doses should be given as a short (~30 minute) infusion or by slow (5-10 minutes) IVP to avoid orthostatic hypotension.

Compatibility: Stable in dextran 6% in dextrose, dextran 6% in NS, D_5W, $D_{10}W$, D_5LR, $D_5\frac{1}{4}NS$, $D_5\frac{1}{2}NS$, D_5NS, LR, $\frac{1}{2}NS$, NS

Y-site administration: Incompatible with aldesleukin, allopurinol, amifostine, amphotericin B cholesteryl sulfate complex, aztreonam, cefepime, etoposide phosphate, fludarabine, foscarnet, filgrastim, gemcitabine, piperacillin/tazobactam

Compatibility in syringe: Incompatible with dimenhydrinate, ketorolac, midazolam, morphine tartrate, pentobarbital, thiopental

Compatibility when admixed: Incompatible with aminophylline, amphotericin B, ampicillin, calcium salts, cephalothin, foscarnet, chloramphenicol, chlorothiazide, floxacillin, furosemide, heparin, hydrocortisone sodium succinate, methohexital, midazolam, penicillin G sodium, phenobarbital, phenytoin, thiopental

Storage:

Injection: Intact vials/ampuls for injection are stable at room temperature. Protect from light. Clear or slightly yellow solutions may be used.

I.V. infusion: Injection may be diluted in 50-100 mL NS or D_5W.

Suppository: May require refrigeration.

Tablet: Stable at room temperature.

Additional Information Not recommended as an antipsychotic due to inferior efficacy compared to other phenothiazines.

Related Information

Antiemetics for Chemotherapy-Induced Nausea and Vomiting *on page 1788*

Antipsychotic Medication Guidelines *on page 1766*

Compatibility of Drugs in Syringe *on page 1725*

- ♦ **Prochlorperazine Edisylate** *see* Prochlorperazine *on page 1259*
- ♦ **Prochlorperazine Maleate** *see* Prochlorperazine *on page 1259*
- ♦ **Procrit®** *see* Epoetin Alfa *on page 531*
- ♦ **Proctocort®** *see* Hydrocortisone *on page 760*
- ♦ **ProctoCream® HC** *see* Hydrocortisone *on page 760*
- ♦ **Proctofene** *see* Fenofibrate *on page 615*
- ♦ **Procto-Kit™** *see* Hydrocortisone *on page 760*
- ♦ **Procto-Pak™** *see* Hydrocortisone *on page 760*
- ♦ **Proctosert** *see* Hydrocortisone *on page 760*
- ♦ **Proctosol-HC®** *see* Hydrocortisone *on page 760*
- ♦ **Proctozone-HC™** *see* Hydrocortisone *on page 760*

Procyclidine (proe SYE kli deen)

U.S. Brand Names Kemadrin®

Synonyms Procyclidine Hydrochloride

Generic Available No

Pharmacologic Category Anticholinergic Agent; Anti-Parkinson's Agent, Anticholinergic

Medication Safety Issues

Sound-alike/look-alike issues:

Kemadrin® may be confused with Coumadin®

Use Relieves symptoms of parkinsonian syndrome and drug-induced extrapyramidal symptoms

Mechanism of Action/Effect Thought to act by blocking excess acetylcholine at cerebral synapses; many of its effects are due to its pharmacologic similarities with atropine; it exerts an antispasmodic effect on smooth muscle, is a potent mydriatic; inhibits salivation

Contraindications Hypersensitivity to procyclidine or any component of the formulation; angle-closure glaucoma; myasthenia gravis; safe use in children not established

Warnings/Precautions Use with caution in hot weather or during exercise. Elderly patients frequently develop increased sensitivity and require strict dosage regulation - side effects may be more severe in elderly patients with atherosclerotic changes. Use with caution in patients with tachycardia, cardiac arrhythmias, hypertension, hypotension, prostatic hyperplasia (especially in the elderly) or any tendency toward urinary retention, liver or kidney disorders and obstructive disease of the GI or GU tract. When given in large doses or to susceptible patients, may cause weakness and inability to move particular muscle groups.

Drug Interactions

Decreased Effect: May increase gastric degradation of levodopa and decrease the amount of levodopa absorbed by delaying gastric emptying; the opposite may be true for digoxin. (Continued)

Procyclidine *(Continued)*

Therapeutic effects of cholinergic agents (tacrine, donepezil) and neuroleptics may be antagonized.

Increased Effect/Toxicity: Central and/or peripheral anticholinergic syndrome can occur when administered with amantadine, rimantadine, narcotic analgesics, phenothiazines and other antipsychotics (especially with high anticholinergic activity), tricyclic antidepressants, quinidine and some other antiarrhythmics, and antihistamines.

Nutritional/Ethanol Interactions Ethanol: Avoid ethanol.

Adverse Reactions Frequency not defined.

Cardiovascular: Tachycardia, palpitation

Central nervous system: Confusion, drowsiness, headache, loss of memory, fatigue, ataxia, giddiness, lightheadedness

Dermatologic: Dry skin, increased sensitivity to light, rash

Gastrointestinal: Constipation, xerostomia, dry throat, nausea, vomiting, epigastric distress

Genitourinary: Difficult urination

Neuromuscular & skeletal: Weakness

Ocular: Increased intraocular pain, blurred vision, mydriasis

Respiratory: Dry nose

Miscellaneous: Diaphoresis (decreased)

Overdosage/Toxicology Symptoms of overdose include disorientation, hallucinations, delusions, blurred vision, dysphagia, absent bowel sounds, hyperthermia, hypertension, and urinary retention. For anticholinergic overdose with severe life-threatening symptoms, physostigmine 1-2 mg SubQ or I.V. slowly, may be given to reverse these effects.

Pharmacodynamics/Kinetics

Onset of Action: 30-40 minutes

Duration of Action: 4-6 hours

Dosing

Adults: Parkinson's disease or treatment of EPS: Oral: 2.5 mg 3 times/day after meals; if tolerated, gradually increase dose, to a maximum of 20 mg/day if necessary.

Elderly: Oral: Initial: 2.5 mg once or twice daily, gradually increasing as necessary. Avoid use if possible (see Geriatric Considerations).

Hepatic Impairment: Decrease dose to a twice daily dosing regimen.

Available Dosage Forms Tablet, as hydrochloride [scored]: 5 mg

Monitoring and Teaching Issues

Physical Assessment: Assess effectiveness and interactions of other medications patient may be taking. Monitor therapeutic effectiveness, renal function, and adverse reactions (eg, anticholinergic syndrome) at beginning of therapy and periodically throughout therapy. Assess knowledge/teach patient appropriate use, interventions to reduce side effects, and adverse symptoms to report.

Patient Education: Take exactly as directed (after meals); do not increase, decrease, or discontinue without consulting prescriber. Take at the same time each day. Do not use alcohol, prescription or OTC sedatives, or CNS depressants without consulting prescriber. You may experience drowsiness, dizziness, confusion, and blurred vision (use caution when driving, climbing stairs, or engaging in tasks requiring alertness until response to drug is known); increased susceptibility to heat stroke, decreased perspiration (use caution in hot weather, maintain adequate fluids and reduce exercise activity); constipation (increased exercise, fluids, fruit, or fiber may help); or dry skin or nasal passages (consult prescriber for appropriate relief). Report unresolved constipation, chest pain or palpitations, respiratory difficulty, CNS changes (hallucination, loss of memory, nervousness, etc), painful or difficult urination, increased muscle spasticity or rigidity, skin rash, or significant worsening of condition. **Pregnancy/breast-feeding precautions:** Inform prescriber if you are or intend to become pregnant. Breast-feeding is not recommended.

Dietary Considerations: Should be taken after meals to minimize stomach upset.

Geriatric Considerations: Anticholinergic agents are generally not well tolerated in the elderly and their use should be avoided when possible (see Warnings/Precautions, Adverse Reactions). In the elderly, anticholinergic agents should not be used as prophylaxis against extrapyramidal symptoms. Elderly patients frequently develop increased sensitivity and require strict dosage regulation - side effects may be more severe in elderly patients with atherosclerotic changes.

Pregnancy Risk Factor: C

Lactation: Excretion in breast milk unknown/not recommended

Administration

Oral: Should be administered after meals to minimize stomach upset.

♦ **Procyclidine Hydrochloride** *see* Procyclidine *on page 1261*

♦ **Prodium® [OTC]** *see* Phenazopyridine *on page 1193*

♦ **Profen Forte®** *see* Guaifenesin and Pseudoephedrine *on page 733*

♦ **Profen II®** *see* Guaifenesin and Pseudoephedrine *on page 733*

Progesterone *(proe JES ter one)*

U.S. Brand Names Crinone®; Prochieve™; Prometrium®

Synonyms Pregnenedione; Progestin

Generic Available Yes: Injection

Pharmacologic Category Progestin

Use

Oral: Prevention of endometrial hyperplasia in nonhysterectomized, postmenopausal women who are receiving conjugated estrogen tablets; secondary amenorrhea

I.M.: Amenorrhea; abnormal uterine bleeding due to hormonal imbalance

Intravaginal gel: Part of assisted reproductive technology (ART) for infertile women with progesterone deficiency; secondary amenorrhea

Mechanism of Action/Effect Natural steroid hormone that induces secretory changes in the endometrium, promotes mammary gland development, relaxes uterine smooth muscle, blocks follicular maturation and ovulation, and maintains pregnancy

Contraindications Hypersensitivity to progesterone or any component of the formulation; undiagnosed abnormal vaginal bleeding; history of or current thrombophlebitis or venous thromboembolic disorders (including DVT, PE); active or recent (within 1 year) arterial thromboembolic disease (eg, stroke, MI); carcinoma of the breast or genital organs; hepatic dysfunction or disease; missed abortion; diagnostic test for pregnancy; pregnancy (see Pregnancy Implications)

The following are also contraindicated in patients with allergies to their inactive ingredient:
Crinone® and Prochieve™ vaginal gels contain palm oil
Prometrium® capsules contain peanut oil
Oil for injection contains sesame oil

Warnings/Precautions Use caution with cardiovascular disease or dysfunction. Progestins used in combination with estrogen may increase the risks of hypertension, myocardial infarction (MI), stroke, pulmonary emboli (PE), and deep vein thrombosis; incidence of these effects was shown to be significantly increased in postmenopausal women using conjugated equine estrogens (CEE) in combination with medroxyprogesterone acetate (MPA). Similar risk should be assumed with other progestins. Progestins in combination with estrogens should not be used to prevent coronary heart disease.

The risk of dementia may be increased in postmenopausal women; increased incidence was observed in women ≥65 years of age taking CEE in combination with MPA. An increased risk of invasive breast cancer was observed in postmenopausal women using CEE in combination with MPA. An increase in abnormal mammograms has also been reported with estrogen and progestin therapy.

Discontinue pending examination in cases of sudden partial or complete vision loss, sudden onset of proptosis, diplopia, or migraine; discontinue permanently if papilledema or retinal vascular lesions are observed on examination. Use with caution in patients with diseases that may be exacerbated by fluid retention, including asthma, epilepsy, migraine, diabetes or renal dysfunction. Use caution with history of depression. Patients should be warned that progesterone might cause transient dizziness or drowsiness during initial therapy. Whenever possible, progestins in combination with estrogens should be discontinued at least 4-6 weeks prior to surgeries associated with an increased risk of thromboembolism or during periods of prolonged immobilization. Progestins used in combination with estrogen should be used for shortest duration possible consistent with treatment goals. Conduct periodic risk:benefit assessments.

Drug Interactions

Cytochrome P450 Effect: Substrate of CYP1A2 (minor), 2A6 (minor), 2C8/9 (minor), 2C19 (major), 2D6 (minor), 3A4 (major); **Inhibits** CYP2C8/9 (weak), 2C19 (weak), 3A4 (weak)

Decreased Effect: CYP2C19 inducers may decrease the levels/effects of progesterone; example inducers include aminoglutethimide, carbamazepine, phenytoin, and rifampin. CYP3A4 inducers may decrease the levels/effects of progesterone; example inducers include aminoglutethimide, carbamazepine, nafcillin, nevirapine, phenobarbital, phenytoin, and rifamycins.

Increased Effect/Toxicity: Ketoconazole may increase the bioavailability of progesterone. Progesterone may increase concentrations of estrogenic compounds during concurrent therapy with conjugated estrogens.

Nutritional/Ethanol Interactions

Food: Food increases oral bioavailability.
Herb/Nutraceutical: St John's wort may decrease progesterone levels.

Lab Interactions Thyroid function, metyrapone, liver function, coagulation tests, endocrine function tests

Adverse Reactions

Injection (I.M.):
Cardiovascular: Edema
Central nervous system: Depression, fever, insomnia, somnolence
Dermatologic: Acne, allergic rash (rare), alopecia, hirsutism, pruritus, rash, urticaria
Endocrine & metabolic: Amenorrhea, breakthrough bleeding, breast tenderness, galactorrhea, menstrual flow changes, spotting
Gastrointestinal: Nausea, weight gain, weight loss
Genitourinary: Cervical erosion changes, cervical secretion changes
Hepatic: Cholestatic jaundice
Local: Pain at the injection site
Miscellaneous: Anaphylactoid reactions

Oral capsule (percentages reported when used in combination with or cycled with conjugated estrogens):
>10%:
Central nervous system: Headache (10% to 31%), dizziness (15% to 24%), depression (19%)
Endocrine & metabolic: Breast tenderness (27%), breast pain (6% to 16%)
Gastrointestinal: Abdominal pain (6% to 12%), abdominal bloating (10% to 20%)
Genitourinary: Urinary problems (11%)
Neuromuscular & skeletal: Joint pain (20%), musculoskeletal pain (6% to 12%)
Miscellaneous: Viral infection (7% to 12%)
5% to 10%:
Cardiovascular: Chest pain (7%)
Central nervous system: Fatigue (8% to 9%), emotional lability (6%), irritability (5% to 8%), worry (8%)
Gastrointestinal: Nausea/vomiting (8%), diarrhea (8%)
Respiratory: Upper respiratory tract infection (5%), cough (8%)
Miscellaneous: Night sweats (7%)
(Continued)

Progesterone *(Continued)*

Vaginal gel (percentages reported with ART); also refer to oral capsule reactions listing for additional effects noted with progesterone:

>10%:

Central nervous system: Somnolence (27%), headache (13% to 17%), nervousness (16%), depression (11%)

Endocrine & metabolic: Breast enlargement (40%), breast pain (13%), libido decreased (11%)

Gastrointestinal: Constipation (27%), nausea (7% to 22%), cramps (15%), abdominal pain (12%)

Genitourinary: Perineal pain (17%), nocturia (13%)

5% to 10%:

Central nervous system: Pain (8%), dizziness (5%)

Gastrointestinal: Diarrhea (8%), bloating (7%), vomiting (5%)

Genitourinary: Vaginal discharge (7%), dyspareunia (6%), genital moniliasis (5%), genital pruritus (5%)

Neuromuscular & skeletal: Arthralgia (8%)

Overdosage/Toxicology Toxicity is unlikely following single exposure of excessive doses. Supportive treatment is adequate in most cases.

Pharmacodynamics/Kinetics

Absorption: Vaginal gel: Prolonged; Absorption half-life: 25-50 hours

Time to Peak: Oral: Within 3 hours

Protein Binding: 96% to 99%

Half-Life Elimination: Vaginal gel: 5-20 minutes

Metabolism: Hepatic

Excretion: Urine, bile, feces

Dosing

Adults & Elderly: Female:

Amenorrhea: I.M.: 5-10 mg/day for 6-8 consecutive days

Amenorrhea, secondary:

Intravaginal gel: 45 mg (4% gel) every other day for 6 doses; if response is inadequate, may increase to 90 mg (8% gel) at same schedule

Oral: 400 mg every evening for 10 days

ART in patients who require progesterone supplementation:

Intravaginal gel: 90 mg (8% gel) once daily. If pregnancy occurs, may continue treatment for 10-12 weeks.

ART in patients with partial or complete ovarian failure:

Intravaginal gel: 90 mg (8% gel) twice daily. If pregnancy occurs, continue treatment for 10-12 weeks.

Endometrial hyperplasia prevention (in postmenopausal women with a uterus who are receiving daily conjugated estrogen tablets): Oral: 200 mg as a single daily dose every evening for 12 days sequentially per 28-day cycle

Functional uterine bleeding: I.M.: 5-10 mg/day for 6 doses

Available Dosage Forms

Capsule (Prometrium®): 100 mg, 200 mg [contains peanut oil]

Gel, vaginal (Crinone®, Prochieve™): 4% (45 mg); 8% (90 mg) [contains palm oil; prefilled applicators]

Injection, oil: 50 mg/mL (10 mL) [contains benzyl alcohol 10%, sesame oil]

Monitoring and Teaching Issues

Physical Assessment: Assess potential for interactions with other prescriptions, OTC medications, or herbal products patient may be taking. Assess therapeutic effectiveness and patient response (eg, blood pressure, mammogram, and results of Pap smears and pregnancy tests before beginning treatment and at least annually with vaginal insert). Teach patient proper use according to formulation, possible side effects/appropriate interventions (eg, annual physicals, Pap smears, and vision assessment), and adverse symptoms to report.

Patient Education: Do not take any new medication during therapy unless approved by prescriber. Use exactly as directed. It is important that you have an annual physical assessment, Pap smear, and vision assessment while taking this medication. May cause temporary dizziness or drowsiness (use caution when driving or engaging in tasks that are potentially hazardous until response to drug is known). Report immediately muscle pain or soreness; warmth, swelling, or redness in calves; shortness of breath; sudden loss or change in vision; change in menstrual pattern (unusual bleeding, amenorrhea, breakthrough spotting); breast tenderness that does not go away; acute abdominal cramping; signs of vaginal infection (drainage, pain, itching); or CNS changes (eg, blurred vision, confusion, acute anxiety, or unresolved depression).

Vaginal gel: A small amount of gel will remain in the applicator following insertion. Administer into the vagina directly from sealed applicator. Remove applicator from wrapper; holding applicator by thickest end, shake down to move contents to thin end; while holding applicator by flat section of thick end, twist off tab; gently insert into vagina and squeeze thick end of applicator.

Geriatric Considerations: Not a progestin of choice in the elderly for hormonal cycling.

Pregnancy Risk Factor: B (Prometrium®, per manufacturer); none established for vaginal gel or injection (contraindicated)

Pregnancy Issues: There is an increased risk of minor birth defects in children whose mothers take progesterones during the first 4 months of pregnancy. Hypospadias has been reported in male and mild masculinization of the external genitalia has been reported in female babies exposed during the first trimester. Cleft lip, cleft palate, congenital heart disease, patent ductus arteriosus, ventricular septal defect, intrauterine death, and spontaneous abortion have been noted in case reports following use of oral progesterone during pregnancy. High doses of progesterone would be expected to impair fertility. According to the American College of Obstetricians and Gynecologists, additional studies are needed to evaluate the use of progesterone to reduce the risk of preterm birth. If needed, use should be restricted to women with history of previous spontaneous abortion at <37 weeks. The vaginal gel is indicated for use in ART.

Lactation: Enters breast milk/use caution (AAP rates "compatible")

Administration

I.M.: Administer deep I.M. only

Other: Vaginal gel: (A small amount of gel will remain in the applicator following insertion): Administer into the vagina directly from sealed applicator. Remove applicator from wrapper; holding applicator by thickest end, shake down to move contents to thin end; while holding applicator by flat section of thick end, twist off tab; gently insert into vagina and squeeze thick end of applicator.

For use at altitudes above 2500 feet: Remove applicator from wrapper; hold applicator on both sides of bubble in the thick end; using a lancet, make a single puncture in the bubble to relieve air pressure; holding applicator by thickest end, shake down to move contents to thin end; while holding applicator by flat section of thick end, twist off tab; gently insert into vagina and squeeze thick end of applicator.

Storage: Store at controlled room temperature.

Promethazine (proe METH a zeen)

U.S. Brand Names Phenadoz™; Phenergan®; Promethegan™

Synonyms Promethazine Hydrochloride

Generic Available Yes

Pharmacologic Category Antiemetic; Antihistamine; Phenothiazine Derivative; Sedative

Medication Safety Issues

Sound-alike/look-alike issues:

Promethazine may be confused with chlorproMAZINE, predniSONE, promazine

Phenergan® may be confused with Phenaphen®, Phrenilin®, Theragran®

Use Symptomatic treatment of various allergic conditions; antiemetic; motion sickness; sedative; postoperative pain (adjunctive therapy); anesthetic (adjunctive therapy); anaphylactic reactions (adjunctive therapy)

Mechanism of Action/Effect Blocks postsynaptic mesolimbic dopaminergic receptors in the brain; exhibits a strong alpha-adrenergic blocking effect and depresses the release of hypothalamic and hypophyseal hormones; competes with histamine for the H_1-receptor; reduces stimuli to the brainstem reticular system

Contraindications Hypersensitivity to promethazine or any component of the formulation (cross-reactivity between phenothiazines may occur); coma; treatment of lower respiratory tract symptoms, including asthma; children <2 years of age

Warnings/Precautions Do not give SubQ or intra-arterially, necrotic lesions may occur. Injection may contain sulfites which may cause allergic reactions in some patients. Rapid I.V. administration may produce a transient fall in blood pressure; rate of administration should not exceed 25 mg/minute. Slow I.V. administration may produce a slightly elevated blood pressure. Not considered an antihistamine of choice in the elderly.

May be sedating and may impair physical or mental abilities. Effects with other sedative drugs or ethanol may be potentiated. Use with caution in Parkinson's disease, hemodynamic instability, bone marrow suppression, subcortical brain damage, and in severe cardiac, hepatic, renal, or respiratory disease. Avoid use in Reye's syndrome. Respiratory fatalities have been reported in children <2 years of age. In children ≥2 years, use the lowest possible dose; other drugs with respiratory depressant effects should be avoided. May lower seizure threshold; use caution in persons with seizure disorders or in persons using narcotics or local anesthetics which may also affect seizure threshold. Caution in breast cancer or other prolactin-dependent tumors (may elevate prolactin levels). May alter temperature regulation or mask toxicity of other drugs due to antiemetic effects. May alter cardiac conduction (life-threatening arrhythmias have occurred with therapeutic doses of phenothiazines). May cause orthostatic hypotension. Use caution in cardiovascular or cerebrovascular disease.

Due to anticholinergic effects, use caution in patients with decreased gastrointestinal motility, urinary retention, BPH, xerostomia, visual problems, narrow-angle glaucoma, and myasthenia gravis. May cause extrapyramidal symptoms, including pseudoparkinsonism, acute dystonic reactions, akathisia, and tardive dyskinesia. May be associated with neuroleptic malignant syndrome (NMS). Ampuls contain sodium metabisulfite.

Drug Interactions

Cytochrome P450 Effect: Substrate (major) of CYP2B6, 2D6; **Inhibits** CYP2D6 (weak)

Decreased Effect: CYP2B6 inducers may decrease the levels/effects of promethazine; example inducers include carbamazepine, nevirapine, phenobarbital, phenytoin, and rifampin. Benztropine (and other anticholinergics) may inhibit the therapeutic response to promethazine. Promethazine may inhibit the ability of bromocriptine to lower serum prolactin concentrations. The antihypertensive effects of guanethidine and guanadrel may be inhibited by promethazine. Promethazine may inhibit the antiparkinsonian effect of levodopa. Promethazine (and possibly other low potency antipsychotics) may reverse the pressor effects of epinephrine.

Increased Effect/Toxicity: CYP2B6 inhibitors may increase the levels/effects of promethazine; example inhibitors include desipramine, paroxetine, and sertraline. CYP2D6 inhibitors may increase the levels/effects of promethazine; example inhibitors include chlorpromazine, delavirdine, fluoxetine, miconazole, paroxetine, pergolide, quinidine, quinine, ritonavir, and ropinirole. Chloroquine, propranolol, and sulfadoxine-pyrimethamine also may increase promethazine concentrations. Concurrent use with TCA may produce (Continued)

Promethazine *(Continued)*

increased toxicity or altered therapeutic response. Promethazine plus lithium may rarely produce neurotoxicity. Concurrent use of promethazine and CNS depressants (ethanol, narcotics) may produce additive depressant effects.

Nutritional/Ethanol Interactions

Ethanol: Avoid ethanol (may increase CNS depression).

Herb/Nutraceutical: Avoid valerian, St John's wort, kava kava, gotu kola (may increase CNS depression).

Lab Interactions Alters the flare response in intradermal allergen tests

Adverse Reactions

Cardiovascular: Bradycardia, hypertension, nonspecific QT changes, postural hypotension, tachycardia

Central nervous system: Akathisia, catatonic states, confusion, delirium, disorientation, dizziness, drowsiness, dystonias, euphoria, excitation, extrapyramidal symptoms, fatigue, hallucinations, hysteria, insomnia, lassitude, nervousness, neuroleptic malignant syndrome, nightmares, pseudoparkinsonism, sedation, seizure, somnolence, tardive dyskinesia

Dermatologic: Angioneurotic edema, dermatitis, photosensitivity, skin pigmentation (slate gray), urticaria

Endocrine & metabolic: Amenorrhea, breast engorgement, gynecomastia, hyper-/hypoglycemia, lactation

Gastrointestinal: Constipation, nausea, vomiting, xerostomia

Genitourinary: Ejaculatory disorder, impotence, urinary retention

Hematologic: Agranulocytosis, aplastic anemia, eosinophilia, hemolytic anemia, leukopenia, thrombocytopenia, thrombocytopenic purpura

Hepatic: Jaundice

Neuromuscular & skeletal: Incoordination, tremor

Ocular: Blurred vision, corneal and lenticular changes, diplopia, epithelial keratopathy, pigmentary retinopathy

Otic: Tinnitus

Respiratory: Apnea, asthma, nasal congestion, respiratory depression

Overdosage/Toxicology Symptoms of overdose include CNS depression, respiratory depression, possible CNS stimulation, dry mouth, fixed and dilated pupils, and hypotension. Treatment is symptom-directed and supportive. Epinephrine should not be used. Hemodialysis: Not dialyzable (0% to 5%)

Pharmacodynamics/Kinetics

Onset of Action: I.M.: ~20 minutes; I.V.: 3-5 minutes

Peak effect: C_{max}: 9.04 ng/mL (suppository); 19.3 ng/mL (syrup)

Duration of Action: 2-6 hours

Absorption:

I.M.: Bioavailability may be greater than with oral or rectal administration

Oral: Rapid and complete; large first pass effect limits systemic bioavailability

Time to Peak: Maximum serum concentration: 4.4 hours (syrup); 6.7-8.6 hours (suppositories)

Protein Binding: 93%

Half-Life Elimination: 9-16 hours

Metabolism: Hepatic; primarily oxidation; forms metabolites

Excretion: Primarily urine and feces (as inactive metabolites)

Dosing

Adults & Elderly:

Allergic conditions (including allergic reactions to blood or plasma):

Oral, rectal: 25 mg at bedtime **or** 12.5 mg before meals and at bedtime (range: 6.25-12.5 mg 3 times/day)

I.M., I.V.: 25 mg, may repeat in 2 hours when necessary; switch to oral route as soon as feasible

Antiemetic: Oral, I.M., I.V., rectal: 12.5-25 mg every 4-6 hours as needed

Motion sickness: Oral, rectal: 25 mg 30-60 minutes before departure, then every 12 hours as needed

Sedation: Oral, I.M., I.V., rectal: 12.5-50 mg/dose

Pediatrics:

Allergic conditions: Children ≥2 years: Oral, rectal: 0.1 mg/kg/dose (maximum: 12.5 mg) every 6 hours during the day and 0.5 mg/kg/dose (maximum: 25 mg) at bedtime as needed

Antiemetic: Children ≥2 years: Oral, I.M., I.V., rectal: 0.25-1 mg/kg 4-6 times/day as needed (maximum: 25 mg/dose)

Motion sickness: Children ≥2 years: Oral, rectal: 0.5 mg/kg/dose 30 minutes to 1 hour before departure, then every 12 hours as needed (maximum dose: 25 mg twice daily)

Sedation: Children ≥2 years: Oral, I.M., I.V., rectal: 0.5-1 mg/kg/dose every 6 hours as needed (maximum: 50 mg/dose)

Available Dosage Forms [DSC] = Discontinued product

Injection, solution, as hydrochloride: 25 mg/mL (1 mL); 50 mg/mL (1 mL)

Phenergan®: 25 mg/mL (1 mL); 50 mg/mL (1 mL) [contains sodium metabisulfite]

Suppository, rectal, as hydrochloride: 12.5 mg, 25 mg, 50 mg

Phenadoz™: 12.5 mg, 25 mg

Phenergan®, Promethegan™: 12.5 mg, 25 mg, 50 mg

Syrup, as hydrochloride: 6.25 mg/5 mL (120 mL, 480 mL) [contains alcohol]

Tablet, as hydrochloride: 12.5 mg, 25 mg, 50 mg

Phenergan®: 12.5 mg [DSC], 25 mg, 50 mg [DSC]

Monitoring and Teaching Issues

Physical Assessment: Use caution in presence of Parkinson's disease, cardiovascular or cerebrovascular disease, hemodynamic instability, bone marrow suppression, and history of seizures (see Warnings/Precautions for multiple use cautions). Assess potential for interactions with other pharmacological agents and herbal products patient may be taking (see Drug Interactions). See Administration specifics for I.V. and I.M. use (do not give

SubQ or intra-arterially; necrotic lesions may occur). Assess for effectiveness (according to purpose for use) and adverse response (eg, sedation, bradycardia, akathisia, delirium, extrapyramidal symptoms, dermatitis, gastrointestinal upset, urinary retention, blurred vision, or respiratory depression; see Adverse Reactions). May be sedating and impair physical or mental abilities; use and teach sedation safety measures (eg, side rails up, call light within reach). Teach patient appropriate use (oral), interventions to reduce side effects, and adverse symptoms to report (see Patient Education).

Patient Education: Do not take any new medication during therapy unless approved by prescriber (especially anything that may cause CNS depression). Take this drug as prescribed; do not increase dosage. Avoid alcohol; may increase CNS depression. May cause dizziness, drowsiness, or blurred vision (use caution when driving or engaging in tasks requiring alertness until response to drug is known); or nausea, dry mouth, appetite disturbances (small frequent meals, frequent mouth care, chewing gum, or sucking lozenges may help). Report unusual weight gain, unresolved nausea or diarrhea, chest pain or palpitations, excess sedation or stimulation, or sore throat or respiratory difficulty. **Pregnancy/breast-feeding precautions:** Inform prescriber if you are or intend to become pregnant. Breast-feeding is not recommended.

Dietary Considerations: Increase dietary intake of riboflavin.

Geriatric Considerations: Because promethazine is a phenothiazine (and can, therefore, cause side effects such as extrapyramidal symptoms), it is not considered an antihistamine of choice in the elderly.

Pregnancy Risk Factor: C

Pregnancy Issues: Crosses the placenta. Possible respiratory depression if drug is administered near time of delivery; behavioral changes, EEG alterations, impaired platelet aggregation reported with use during labor. Available evidence with use of occasional low doses suggests safe use during pregnancy.

Lactation: Excretion in breast milk unknown/not recommended

Administration

I.M.: Preferred route of administration; administer into deep muscle

I.V.: Due to the possibility of orthostatic hypotension, I.V. administration is not the preferred route. Solution for injection may be diluted in 25-100 mL NS or D_5W (maximum concentration of 25 mg/mL) and infused over 15-30 minutes at a rate ≤25 mg/minute.

Other: Not for SubQ or intra-arterial administration.

Compatibility: Stable in dextran 6% in dextrose, dextran 6% in NS, D_5W, $D_{10}W$, D_5LR, $D_5^{1}/_4NS$, $D_5^{1}/_2NS$, D_5NS, LR, $^{1}/_2NS$, NS

Y-site administration: Incompatible with aldesleukin, allopurinol, amphotericin B cholesteryl sulfate complex, cefazolin, cefepime, cefoperazone, cefotetan, doxorubicin liposome, foscarnet, methotrexate, piperacillin/tazobactam

Compatibility in syringe: Incompatible with cefotetan, chloroquine, diatrizoate sodium 75%, diatrizoate meglumine 52% with diatrizoate sodium 8%, diatrizoate meglumine 34.3% with diatrizoate sodium 35%, dimenhydrinate, heparin, iodipamide meglumine 52%, iothalamate meglumine 60%, iothalamate sodium 80%, ketorolac, pentobarbital, thiopental

Compatibility when admixed: Incompatible with aminophylline, chloramphenicol, chlorothiazide, dimenhydrinate, floxacillin, furosemide, heparin, hydrocortisone sodium succinate, methohexital, penicillin G sodium, pentobarbital, phenobarbital, phenytoin, thiopental

Storage:

Injection: Prior to dilution, store at room temperature; protect from light. Solutions in NS or D_5W are stable for 24 hours at room temperature.

Suppositories: Store refrigerated at 2°C to 8°C (36°F to 46°F).

Tablets: Store at room temperature. Protect from light.

Related Information

Compatibility of Drugs in Syringe *on page 1725*

Promethazine and Codeine (proe METH a zeen & KOE deen)

U.S. Brand Names Phenergan® With Codeine

Synonyms Codeine and Promethazine

Controlled Substance C-V

Generic Available Yes

Pharmacologic Category Antihistamine/Antitussive

Medication Safety Issues

Sound-alike/look-alike issues:

Phenergan® may be confused with Phenaphen®, Phrenilin®, Theragran®

Use Temporary relief of coughs and upper respiratory symptoms associated with allergy or the common cold

Dosing

Adults: Upper respiratory symptoms: Oral: 10-20 mg/dose every 4-6 hours as needed; maximum: 120 mg codeine/day; or 5-10 mL every 4-6 hours as needed

Elderly: Refer to dosing in individual monographs.

Pediatrics: Upper respiratory symptoms: Oral (in terms of codeine):

Children: 1-1.5 mg/kg/day every 4 hours as needed; maximum: 30 mg/day **or**

2-6 years: 1.25-2.5 mL every 4-6 hours or 2.5-5 mg/dose every 4-6 hours as needed; maximum: 30 mg codeine/day

6-12 years: 2.5-5 mL every 4-6 hours as needed or 5-10 mg/dose every 4-6 hours as needed; maximum: 60 mg codeine/day

Available Dosage Forms Syrup: Promethazine hydrochloride 6.25 mg and codeine phosphate 10 mg per 5 mL (120 mL, 473 mL, 3840 mL) [contains alcohol]

Phenergan® with Codeine: Promethazine hydrochloride 6.25 mg and codeine phosphate 10 mg per 5 mL (120 mL) [contains alcohol 7% and sodium benzoate]

(Continued)

Promethazine and Codeine *(Continued)*

Monitoring and Teaching Issues
Physical Assessment: See individual agents.

Patient Education: See individual agents. **Pregnancy/breast-feeding precautions:** Inform prescriber if you are or intend to become pregnant. Breast-feeding is not recommended.

Pregnancy Risk Factor: C

Lactation: Enters breast milk (codeine)/not recommended

Related Information
Codeine *on page 366*
Promethazine *on page 1265*

Promethazine and Dextromethorphan
(proe METH a zeen & deks troe meth OR fan)

Synonyms Dextromethorphan and Promethazine

Generic Available Yes

Pharmacologic Category Antihistamine/Antitussive

Use Temporary relief of coughs and upper respiratory symptoms associated with allergy or the common cold

Dosing
Adults: Cough and upper respiratory symptoms: Oral: 5 mL every 4-6 hours, up to 30 mL in 24 hours

Elderly: Refer to dosing in individual monographs.

Pediatrics: Cough and upper respiratory symptoms: Oral: Children:
2-6 years: 1.25-2.5 mL every 4-6 hours up to 10 mL in 24 hours
6-12 years: 2.5-5 mL every 4-6 hours up to 20 mL in 24 hours

Available Dosage Forms Syrup: Promethazine hydrochloride 6.25 mg and dextromethorphan hydrobromide 15 mg per 5 mL (120 mL, 480 mL, 4000 mL) [contains alcohol 7%]

Monitoring and Teaching Issues
Physical Assessment: See individual agents.

Patient Education: See individual agents. **Pregnancy/breast-feeding precautions:** Inform prescriber if you are or intend to become pregnant. Breast-feeding is not recommended.

Pregnancy Risk Factor: C

Lactation: Excretion in breast milk unknown/not recommended

Related Information
Promethazine *on page 1265*

Promethazine and Phenylephrine (proe METH a zeen & fen il EF rin)

Synonyms Phenylephrine and Promethazine

Generic Available Yes

Pharmacologic Category Antihistamine/Decongestant Combination

Use Temporary relief of upper respiratory symptoms associated with allergy or the common cold

Dosing
Adults: Upper respiratory symptoms: Oral: 5 mL every 4-6 hours, not to exceed 30 mL in 24 hours

Elderly: Refer to dosing in individual monographs.

Pediatrics: Upper respiratory symptoms: Oral: Children:
2-6 years: 1.25 mL every 4-6 hours, not to exceed 7.5 mL in 24 hours
6-12 years: 2.5 mL every 4-6 hours, not to exceed 15 mL in 24 hours
>12 years: Refer to adult dosing.

Available Dosage Forms Syrup: Promethazine hydrochloride 6.25 mg and phenylephrine hydrochloride 5 mg per 5 mL (120 mL, 473 mL) [contains alcohol]

Monitoring and Teaching Issues
Physical Assessment: See individual agents.

Patient Education: See individual agents. **Pregnancy/breast-feeding precautions:** Inform prescriber if you are or intend to become pregnant. Breast-feeding is not recommended.

Pregnancy Risk Factor: C

Lactation: Excretion in breast milk unknown/not recommended

Related Information
Phenylephrine *on page 1200*
Promethazine *on page 1265*

♦ **Promethazine Hydrochloride** *see* Promethazine *on page 1265*

Promethazine, Phenylephrine, and Codeine
(proe METH a zeen, fen il EF rin, & KOE deen)

Synonyms Codeine, Promethazine, and Phenylephrine; Phenylephrine, Promethazine, and Codeine

Controlled Substance C-V

Generic Available Yes

Pharmacologic Category Antihistamine/Decongestant/Antitussive

Use Temporary relief of coughs and upper respiratory symptoms including nasal congestion

Dosing
Adults: Cough and upper respiratory symptoms: Oral: 5 mL every 4-6 hours, not to exceed 30 mL/24 hours

Elderly: Refer to dosing in individual monographs.

Pediatrics: Cough and upper respiratory symptoms: Oral:
Children (expressed in terms of codeine dosage): 1-1.5 mg/kg/day every 4 hours, maximum: 30 mg/day **or**

<2 years: Not recommended

2-6 years:
  Weight 25 lb: 1.25-2.5 mL every 4-6 hours, not >6 mL/24 hours
  Weight 30 lb: 1.25-2.5 mL every 4-6 hours, not >7 mL/24 hours
  Weight 35 lb: 1.25-2.5 mL every 4-6 hours, not >8 mL/24 hours
  Weight 40 lb: 1.25-2.5 mL every 4-6 hours, not >9 mL/24 hours

6 to <12 years: 2.5-5 mL every 4-6 hours, not >15 mL/24 hours

Available Dosage Forms Syrup: Promethazine hydrochloride 6.25 mg, phenylephrine hydrochloride 5 mg, and codeine phosphate 10 mg per 5 mL with alcohol 7% (120 mL, 480 mL) [contains alcohol]

Monitoring and Teaching Issues
  Physical Assessment: See individual agents.
  Patient Education: See individual agents. **Pregnancy/breast-feeding precautions:** Inform prescriber if you are or intend to become pregnant. Breast-feeding is not recommended.
  Pregnancy Risk Factor: C
  Lactation: Enters breast milk/not recommended

Related Information
  Codeine *on page 366*
  Phenylephrine *on page 1200*
  Promethazine *on page 1265*

♦ **Promethegan™** *see* Promethazine *on page 1265*

♦ **Prometrium®** *see* Progesterone *on page 1262*

♦ **Promit®** *see* Dextran 1 *on page 434*

♦ **Pronap-100®** *see* Propoxyphene and Acetaminophen *on page 1272*

Propafenone (proe pa FEEN one)

U.S. Brand Names Rythmol®; Rythmol® SR
Synonyms Propafenone Hydrochloride
Generic Available Yes
Pharmacologic Category Antiarrhythmic Agent, Class Ic
Use Treatment of life-threatening ventricular arrhythmias
  Rythmol® SR: Maintenance of normal sinus rhythm in patients with symptomatic atrial fibrillation
Unlabeled/Investigational Use Supraventricular tachycardias, including those patients with Wolff-Parkinson-White syndrome
Mechanism of Action/Effect Propafenone is a class 1c antiarrhythmic agent which possesses local anesthetic properties, blocks the fast inward sodium current, and slows the rate of increase of the action potential. Prolongs conduction and refractoriness in all areas of the myocardium, with a slightly more pronounced effect on intraventricular conduction; it prolongs effective refractory period, reduces spontaneous automaticity and exhibits some beta-blockade activity.
Contraindications Hypersensitivity to propafenone or any component of the formulation; sinoatrial, AV, and intraventricular disorders of impulse generation and/or conduction (except in patients with a functioning artificial pacemaker); sinus bradycardia; cardiogenic shock; uncompensated cardiac failure; hypotension; bronchospastic disorders; uncorrected electrolyte abnormalities; concurrent use of ritonavir (see Drug Interactions)
Warnings/Precautions Patients with bronchospastic disease should generally not receive this drug. May worsen CHF in some patients. May cause or unmask a variety of conduction disturbances, or lead to the development of new arrhythmias (proarrhythmic events). May alter pacing and sensing thresholds of artificial pacemakers. May prolong QT_c interval; use caution with other QT_c-prolonging drugs. Administer cautiously in significant hepatic dysfunction.
Drug Interactions
  Cytochrome P450 Effect: Substrate of CYP1A2 (minor), 2D6 (major), 3A4 (minor); **Inhibits** CYP1A2 (weak), 2C8/9 (weak), 2D6 (weak)
  Decreased Effect: Enzyme inducers (phenobarbital, phenytoin, rifabutin, rifampin) may decrease propafenone blood levels.
  Increased Effect/Toxicity: Cimetidine and quinidine may increase propafenone levels. Ritonavir may increase propafenone levels; concurrent use is contraindicated. CYP2D6 inhibitors may increase the levels/effects of propafenone; example inhibitors include chlorpromazine, delavirdine, fluoxetine, miconazole, paroxetine, pergolide, quinine, and ropinirole. Digoxin (reduce dose by 25%), metoprolol, propranolol, theophylline, and warfarin blood levels are increased by propafenone. Use caution with Class Ia and Class III antiarrhythmics, erythromycin, cisapride, antipsychotics, and cyclic antidepressants; QT_c-prolonging effects may be additive with propafenone.
Nutritional/Ethanol Interactions
  Food: Propafenone serum concentrations may be increased if taken with food.
  Herb/Nutraceutical: St John's wort may decrease propafenone levels. Avoid ephedra (may worsen arrhythmia).
Adverse Reactions 1% to 10%:
  Cardiovascular: New or worsened arrhythmia (proarrhythmic effect) (2% to 10%), angina (2% to 5%), CHF (1% to 4%), ventricular tachycardia (1% to 3%), palpitation (1% to 3%), AV block (first-degree) (1% to 3%), syncope (1% to 2%), increased QRS interval (1% to 2%), chest pain (1% to 2%), PVCs (1% to 2%), bradycardia (1% to 2%), edema (0% to 1%), bundle branch block (0% to 1%), atrial fibrillation (1%), hypotension (0% to 1%), intraventricular conduction delay (0% to 1%)
  Central nervous system: Dizziness (4% to 15%), fatigue (2% to 6%), headache (2% to 5%), ataxia (0% to 2%), insomnia (0% to 2%), anxiety (1% to 2%), drowsiness (1%)
  Dermatologic: Rash (1% to 3%)
(Continued)

Propafenone *(Continued)*

Gastrointestinal: Nausea/vomiting (2% to 11%), unusual taste (3% to 23%), constipation (2% to 7%), dyspepsia (1% to 3%), diarrhea (1% to 3%), xerostomia (1% to 2%), anorexia (1% to 2%), abdominal pain (1% to 2%), flatulence (0% to 1%)

Neuromuscular & skeletal: Tremor (0% to 1%), arthralgia (0% to 1%), weakness (1% to 2%)

Ocular: Blurred vision (1% to 6%)

Respiratory: Dyspnea (2% to 5%)

Miscellaneous: Diaphoresis (1%)

Overdosage/Toxicology Propafenone has a narrow therapeutic index and severe toxicity may occur slightly above the therapeutic range, especially if combined with other antiarrhythmic drugs. Acute single ingestion of twice the daily therapeutic dose is life-threatening. Symptoms of overdose include increased P-R, QRS, or QT intervals and amplitude of the T wave, AV block, bradycardia, hypotension, ventricular arrhythmias (monomorphic or polymorphic ventricular tachycardia), and asystole. Other symptoms include dizziness, blurred vision, headache, and GI upset. Treatment is supportive. **Note:** Class 1A antiarrhythmic agents should not be used to treat cardiotoxicity caused by Class 1C drugs. Sodium bicarbonate may reverse QRS prolongation, bradycardia, and hypotension. Ventricular pacing may be needed.

Pharmacodynamics/Kinetics

Absorption: Well absorbed

Bioavailability: 150 mg: 3.4%; 300 mg: 10.6%

Time to Peak: 150 mg dose: 2 hours; 300 mg dose: 3 hours

Half-Life Elimination: Single dose (100-300 mg): 2-8 hours; Chronic dosing: 10-32 hours

Metabolism: Hepatic; two genetically determined metabolism groups exist: fast or slow metabolizers; 10% of Caucasians are slow metabolizers; exhibits nonlinear pharmacokinetics; when dose is increased from 300-900 mg/day, serum concentrations increase tenfold; this nonlinearity is thought to be due to saturable first-pass effect

Dosing

Adults & Elderly: Note: Patients who exhibit significant widening of QRS complex or second- or third-degree AV block may need dose reduction.

Ventricular arrhythmias: Oral:

Immediate release tablet: Initial: 150 mg every 8 hours, increase at 3- to 4-day intervals up to 300 mg every 8 hours.

Extended release capsule: Initial: 225 mg every 12 hours; dosage increase may be made at a minimum of 5-day intervals; may increase to 325 mg every 12 hours; if further increase is necessary, may increase to 425 mg every 12 hours

Hepatic Impairment: Reduction is necessary; however, specific guidelines are not available.

Available Dosage Forms

Capsule, extended release, as hydrochloride: 225 mg, 325 mg, 425 mg

Tablet, as hydrochloride: 150 mg, 225 mg, 300 mg

Monitoring and Teaching Issues

Physical Assessment: Assess other medications patient may be taking for effectiveness and interactions. Assess therapeutic effectiveness, and adverse reactions at beginning of therapy, when titrating dosage, and on a regular basis with long-term therapy. Monitor cardiac status closely. **Note:** Propafenone has a low TI and overdose may easily produce severe and life-threatening reactions. Assess knowledge/teach patient appropriate use, interventions to reduce side effects, and adverse symptoms to report.

Patient Education: Take exactly as directed; do not take additional doses or discontinue without consulting prescriber. You will need regular cardiac checkups. You may experience dizziness, drowsiness, or visual changes (use caution when driving or engaging in tasks requiring alertness until response to drug is known); abnormal taste, nausea or vomiting, or loss of appetite (small frequent meals, frequent mouth care, chewing gum, or sucking lozenges may help); headaches (prescriber may recommend mild analgesic); or diarrhea (yogurt or boiled milk may help; if persistent consult prescriber). Report chest pain, palpitation, or erratic heartbeat; respiratory difficulty, increased weight or swelling of hands or feet; acute persistent diarrhea or constipation; or vision changes.

Dietary Considerations:

Capsule: May be taken without regard to food.

Tablet: Should be taken at the same time in relation to meals each day, either always with meals or always between meals.

Geriatric Considerations: Elderly may have age-related decreases in hepatic Phase I metabolism. Propafenone is dependent upon liver metabolism, therefore, monitor closely in the elderly and adjust dose more gradually during initial treatment (see Warnings/Precautions). No differences in clearance noted with impaired renal function and, therefore, no adjustment for renal function in the elderly is necessary.

Pregnancy Risk Factor: C

Lactation: Enters breast milk/use caution

Administration

Oral: Capsules should be swallowed whole; do not crush or chew.

Storage: Store at 25°C (77°F). Excursions permitted to 15°C to 30°C (59°F to 86°F).

Related Information

Antiarrhythmic Drugs *on page 1708*

♦ **Propafenone Hydrochloride** *see* Propafenone *on page 1269*

♦ **Proparacaine** *see page 1625*

♦ **Proparacaine and Fluorescein** *see page 1625*

♦ **Propecia®** *see* Finasteride *on page 629*

♦ **Prophylaxis for Exposure to Communicable Diseases** *see page 1859*

Propoxyphene (proe POKS i feen)

U.S. Brand Names Darvon®; Darvon-N®

Synonyms Dextropropoxyphene; Propoxyphene Hydrochloride; Propoxyphene Napsylate

Controlled Substance C-IV

Generic Available Yes: Capsule

Pharmacologic Category Analgesic, Narcotic

Medication Safety Issues
Sound-alike/look-alike issues:
Propoxyphene may be confused with proparacaine
Darvon® may be confused with Devrom®, Diovan®
Darvon-N® may be confused with Darvocet-N®

Use Management of mild to moderate pain

Mechanism of Action/Effect Binds to opiate receptors in the CNS, causing inhibition of ascending pain pathways, altering the perception of and response to pain; produces generalized CNS depression

Contraindications Hypersensitivity to propoxyphene or any component of the formulation

Warnings/Precautions When given in excessive doses, either alone or in combination with other CNS depressants, propoxyphene is a major cause of drug-related deaths; do not exceed recommended dosage; give with caution in patients dependent on opiates, substitution may result in acute opiate withdrawal symptoms. Avoid use in severely depressed or suicidal patients. Tolerance or drug dependence may result from extended use. Propoxyphene should be used with caution in patients with renal or hepatic dysfunction or in the elderly; consider dosing adjustment.

Drug Interactions

Cytochrome P450 Effect: Inhibits CYP2C8/9 (weak), 2D6 (weak), 3A4 (weak)

Decreased Effect: Decreased effect with cigarette smoking.

Increased Effect/Toxicity: CNS depressants (phenothiazines, tranquilizers, anxiolytics, sedatives, hypnotics, or alcohol) may potentiate pharmacologic effects. Propoxyphene may inhibit the metabolism and increase the serum concentrations of carbamazepine, phenobarbital, MAO inhibitors, tricyclic antidepressants, and warfarin.

Nutritional/Ethanol Interactions
Ethanol: Avoid or limit ethanol (may increase CNS depression). Watch for sedation.
Food: May decrease rate of absorption, but may slightly increase bioavailability.

Lab Interactions False-positive methadone test; increased LFTs; decreased glucose (S), 17-OHCS (U)

Adverse Reactions Frequency not defined.
Cardiovascular: Hypotension, bundle branch block
Central nervous system: Dizziness, lightheadedness, sedation, paradoxical excitement and insomnia, fatigue, drowsiness, mental depression, hallucinations, paradoxical CNS stimulation, increased intracranial pressure, nervousness, headache, restlessness, malaise, confusion, dysphoria, vertigo
Dermatologic: Rash, urticaria
Endocrine & metabolic: Hypoglycemia, urinary 17-OHCS decreased
Gastrointestinal: Anorexia, stomach cramps, xerostomia, biliary spasm, nausea, vomiting, constipation, paralytic ileus, abdominal pain
Genitourinary: Urination decreased, ureteral spasms
Hepatic: LFTs increased, jaundice
Neuromuscular & skeletal: Weakness
Ocular: Visual disturbances
Respiratory: Dyspnea
Miscellaneous: Psychologic and physical dependence with prolonged use, histamine release, hypersensitivity reaction

Overdosage/Toxicology Symptoms of overdose include CNS disturbances, respiratory depression, hypotension, pulmonary edema, and seizures. Naloxone, 2 mg I.V. with repeat administration as necessary up to a total of 10 mg, can also be used to reverse toxic effects of the opiate. Charcoal is very effective (>95%) at binding propoxyphene.

Pharmacodynamics/Kinetics

Onset of Action: 0.5-1 hour

Duration of Action: 4-6 hours

Half-Life Elimination: Adults: Parent drug: 6-12 hours; Norpropoxyphene: 30-36 hours

Metabolism: Hepatic to active metabolite (norpropoxyphene) and inactive metabolites; first-pass effect

Excretion: Urine (primarily as metabolites)

Dosing

Adults: Pain management: Oral:
Hydrochloride: 65 mg every 3-4 hours as needed for pain; maximum: 390 mg/day
Napsylate: 100 mg every 4 hours as needed for pain; maximum: 600 mg/day

Elderly: Pain management: Oral:
Hydrochloride: 65 mg every 4-6 hours as needed for pain
Napsylate: 100 mg every 4-6 hours as needed for pain

Pediatrics: Pain management: Oral: Children: Doses for children are not well established; doses of the hydrochloride of 2-3 mg/kg/d divided every 6 hours have been used.

Renal Impairment: Serum concentrations of propoxyphene may be increased or elimination may be delayed. Avoid use in Cl_{cr} <10 mL/minute. Specific dosing recommendations not available for less severe impairment.
Not dialyzable (0% to 5%)

Hepatic Impairment: Serum concentrations of propoxyphene may be increased or elimination may be delayed. Specific dosing recommendations not available.

Available Dosage Forms
Capsule, as hydrochloride (Darvon®): 65 mg
Tablet, as napsylate (Darvon-N®): 100 mg
(Continued)

Propoxyphene *(Continued)*

Monitoring and Teaching Issues

Physical Assessment: Assess other medications patient may be taking for effectiveness and interactions. Monitor therapeutic effectiveness, cardio/respiratory and CNS status, adverse reactions and signs of overdose at beginning of therapy and periodically with long-term use. Assess knowledge/teach patient appropriate use, interventions to reduce side effects, and adverse symptoms to report.

Patient Education: Take as directed; do not take a larger dose or more often than prescribed. Do not use alcohol, other prescription or OTC sedatives, tranquilizers, antihistamines, or pain medications without consulting prescriber. May cause dizziness, drowsiness, or impaired judgment; avoid driving or engaging in tasks requiring alertness until response to drug is known. If you experience vomiting or loss of appetite, frequent mouth care, small frequent meals, chewing gum, or sucking lozenges may help. Increased fluid intake, exercise, fiber in diet may help with constipation (if unresolved consult prescriber). Report unresolved nausea or vomiting, respiratory difficulty or shortness of breath, or unusual weakness. **Pregnancy/breast-feeding precautions:** Inform prescriber if you are or intend to become pregnant.

Dietary Considerations: May administer with food if gastrointestinal distress occurs.

Geriatric Considerations: The elderly may be particularly susceptible to the CNS depressant effects of narcotics.

Pregnancy Risk Factor: C/D (prolonged use)

Pregnancy Issues: Withdrawal symptoms have been reported in the neonate following propoxyphene use during pregnancy. Teratogenic effects have also been noted in case reports. Opioid analgesics are considered pregnancy risk factor D if used for prolonged periods or in large doses near term.

Lactation: Enters breast milk/use caution (AAP rates "compatible")

Breast-Feeding Issues: Propoxyphene and norpropoxyphene are excreted in breast milk.

Administration

Oral: Should be administered with glass of water on an empty stomach. Food may decrease rate of absorption, but may slightly increase bioavailability.

Storage: Store at controlled room temperature of 15°C to 30°C (59°F to 86°F).

Additional Information 100 mg of napsylate = 65 mg of hydrochloride

Propoxyphene hydrochloride: Darvon®

Propoxyphene napsylate: Darvon-N®

Related Information

Narcotic / Opioid Analgesic Comparison *on page 1739*

Propoxyphene and Acetaminophen

(proe POKS i feen & a seet a MIN oh fen)

U.S. Brand Names Darvocet A500™; Darvocet-N® 50; Darvocet-N® 100; Pronap-100®

Synonyms Propoxyphene Hydrochloride and Acetaminophen; Propoxyphene Napsylate and Acetaminophen

Controlled Substance C-IV

Generic Available Yes

Pharmacologic Category Analgesic Combination (Narcotic)

Medication Safety Issues

Sound-alike/look-alike issues:

Darvocet-N® may be confused with Darvon-N®

Use Management of mild to moderate pain

Dosing

Adults & Elderly:

Pain management: Oral:

Darvocet A500™, Darvocet-N® 100: 1 tablet every 4 hours as needed; maximum: 600 mg propoxyphene napsylate/day

Darvocet-N® 50: 1-2 tablets every 4 hours as needed; maximum: 600 mg propoxyphene napsylate/day

Note: Formulations contain significant amounts of acetaminophen; intake should be limited to <4 g acetaminophen/day (less in patients with hepatic impairment/ethanol abuse)

Renal Impairment: Serum concentrations of propoxyphene may be increased or elimination may be delayed; specific dosing recommendations not available.

Hepatic Impairment: Serum concentrations of propoxyphene may be increased or elimination may be delayed; specific dosing recommendations not available.

Available Dosage Forms Tablet: Propoxyphene hydrochloride 65 mg and acetaminophen 650 mg, propoxyphene napsylate 100 mg, and acetaminophen 650 mg

Darvocet A500™: Propoxyphene napsylate 100 mg and acetaminophen 500 mg [contains lactose]

Darvocet-N® 50: Propoxyphene napsylate 50 mg and acetaminophen 325 mg

Darvocet-N® 100, Pronap-100®: Propoxyphene napsylate 100 mg and acetaminophen 650 mg

Monitoring and Teaching Issues

Physical Assessment: See individual agents.

Patient Education: See individual agents. **Pregnancy precaution:** Inform prescriber if you are or intend to become pregnant.

Pregnancy Risk Factor: C

Lactation: Enters breast milk/compatible

Related Information

Acetaminophen *on page 38*
Propoxyphene *on page 1271*

Propoxyphene, Aspirin, and Caffeine
(proe POKS i feen, AS pir in, & KAF een)

U.S. Brand Names Darvon® Compound

Synonyms Aspirin, Caffeine, and Propoxyphene; Caffeine, Propoxyphene, and Aspirin; Propoxyphene Hydrochloride, Aspirin, and Caffeine

Controlled Substance C-IV

Generic Available No

Pharmacologic Category Analgesic Combination (Narcotic)

Medication Safety Issues
Sound-alike/look-alike issues:
Darvon® may be confused with Devrom®, Diovan®

Use Treatment of mild-to-moderate pain

Dosing
Adults: Pain: Oral: One capsule (providing propoxyphene 65 mg) every 4 hours as needed; maximum propoxyphene 390 mg/day. This will also provide aspirin 389 mg and caffeine 32.4 mg per capsule.

Elderly: Refer to adult dosing. Consider increasing dosing interval.

Renal Impairment: Serum concentrations of propoxyphene may be increased or elimination may be delayed; specific dosing recommendations not available. Avoid use with Cl_{cr} <10 mL/minute.

Hepatic Impairment: Serum concentrations or propoxyphene may be increased or elimination may be delayed; specific dosing recommendations not available.

Available Dosage Forms Capsule (Darvon® Compound 65): Propoxyphene hydrochloride 65 mg, aspirin 389 mg, and caffeine 32.4 mg

Monitoring and Teaching Issues
Physical Assessment: See individual agents.

Pregnancy Risk Factor: C

Lactation: Enters breast milk/use caution

Related Information
Aspirin *on page 143*
Propoxyphene *on page 1271*

Propranolol (proe PRAN oh lole)

U.S. Brand Names Inderal®; Inderal® LA; InnoPran XL™; Propranolol Intensol™

Synonyms Propranolol Hydrochloride

Generic Available Yes: Excludes capsule

Pharmacologic Category Antiarrhythmic Agent, Class II; Beta-Adrenergic Blocker, Nonselective

Medication Safety Issues
Sound-alike/look-alike issues:
Propranolol may be confused with Pravachol®, Propulsid®
Inderal® may be confused with Adderall®, Enduron®, Enduronyl®, Imdur®, Imuran®, Inderide®, Isordil®, Toradol®
Inderal® 40 may be confused with Enduronyl® Forte

Use Management of hypertension; angina pectoris; pheochromocytoma; essential tremor; tetralogy of Fallot cyanotic spells; arrhythmias (such as atrial fibrillation and flutter, AV nodal re-entrant tachycardias, and catecholamine-induced arrhythmias); prevention of myocardial infarction; migraine headache; symptomatic treatment of hypertrophic subaortic stenosis

Unlabeled/Investigational Use Tremor due to Parkinson's disease; ethanol withdrawal; aggressive behavior; antipsychotic-induced akathisia; prevention of bleeding esophageal varices; anxiety; schizophrenia; acute panic; gastric bleeding in portal hypertension; thyrotoxicosis

Mechanism of Action/Effect Nonselective beta-adrenergic blocker (class II antiarrhythmic); competitively blocks response to beta$_1$- and beta$_2$-adrenergic stimulation which results in decreases in heart rate, myocardial contractility, blood pressure, and myocardial oxygen demand

Contraindications Hypersensitivity to propranolol, beta-blockers, or any component of the formulation; uncompensated congestive heart failure (unless the failure is due to tachyarrhythmias being treated with propranolol); cardiogenic shock, bradycardia or heart block (2nd or 3rd degree); pulmonary edema, severe hyperactive airway disease (asthma or COPD), Raynaud's disease; pregnancy (2nd and 3rd trimesters)

Warnings/Precautions Administer cautiously in compensated heart failure and monitor for a worsening of the condition (efficacy of propranolol in CHF has not been demonstrated). Beta-blocker therapy should not be withdrawn abruptly (particularly in patients with CAD), but gradually tapered (over 2 weeks) to avoid acute tachycardia, hypertension, and/or ischemia. Use caution in patient with peripheral vascular disease. Use caution with concurrent use of beta-blockers and either verapamil or diltiazem; bradycardia or heart block can occur. Avoid concurrent I.V. use of both agents. Use cautiously in patients with diabetes; may mask prominent hypoglycemic symptoms. May mask signs of thyrotoxicosis. Can cause fetal harm when administered in pregnancy. Use cautiously in hepatic dysfunction (dosage adjustment required). Use care with anesthetic agents which decrease myocardial function. Not indicated for hypertensive emergencies.

(Continued)

Propranolol (Continued)

Drug Interactions

Cytochrome P450 Effect: Substrate of CYP1A2 (major), 2C19 (minor), 2D6 (major), 3A4 (minor); **Inhibits** CYP1A2 (weak), 2D6 (weak)

Decreased Effect: CYP1A2 inducers may decrease the levels/effects of propranolol; example inducers include aminoglutethimide, carbamazepine, phenobarbital, and rifampin. Aluminum salts, calcium salts, cholestyramine, colestipol, NSAIDs, penicillins (ampicillin), salicylates, and sulfinpyrazone decrease effect of beta-blockers due to decreased bioavailability and plasma levels. Beta-blockers may decrease the effect of sulfonylureas. Ascorbic acid decreases propranolol Cp_{max} and AUC and increases the T_{max} significantly resulting in a greater decrease in the reduction of heart rate, possibly due to decreased absorption and first pass metabolism (n=5). Nefazodone decreased peak plasma levels and AUC of propranolol and increases time to reach steady-state; monitoring of clinical response is recommended. Nonselective beta-blockers blunt the response to beta-2 adrenergic agonists (albuterol).

Increased Effect/Toxicity: CYP1A2 inhibitors may increase the levels/effects of propranolol; example inhibitors include amiodarone, ciprofloxacin, fluvoxamine, ketoconazole, norfloxacin, ofloxacin, and rofecoxib. CYP2D6 inhibitors may increase the levels/effects of propranolol; example inhibitors include chlorpromazine, delavirdine, fluoxetine, miconazole, paroxetine, pergolide, quinidine, quinine, ritonavir, and ropinirole. The heart rate-lowering effects of propranolol are additive with other drugs which slow AV conduction (digoxin, verapamil, diltiazem). Reserpine increases the effects of propranolol. Concurrent use of propranolol may increase the effects of alpha-blockers (prazosin, terazosin), alpha-adrenergic stimulants (epinephrine, phenylephrine), and the vasoconstrictive effects of ergot alkaloids. Propranolol may mask the tachycardia from hypoglycemia caused by insulin and oral hypoglycemics. In patients receiving concurrent therapy, the risk of hypertensive crisis is increased when either clonidine or the beta-blocker is withdrawn. Beta-blockers may increase the action or levels of ethanol, disopyramide, nondepolarizing muscle relaxants, and theophylline although the effects are difficult to predict. Propranolol may increase the bioavailability of serotonin 5-HT_{1D} receptor agonists. Propranolol may decrease the metabolism of lidocaine.

Beta-blocker effects may be enhanced by oral contraceptives, flecainide, haloperidol (hypotensive effects), cimetidine, hydralazine, phenothiazines, propafenone, thyroid hormones (when hypothyroid patient is converted to euthyroid state). Beta-blockers may increase the effect/toxicity of flecainide, haloperidol (hypotensive effects), hydralazine, phenothiazines, acetaminophen, anticoagulants (warfarin), and benzodiazepines.

Nutritional/Ethanol Interactions

Ethanol: Ethanol may decrease plasma levels of propranolol by increasing metabolism.

Food: Propranolol serum levels may be increased if taken with food. Protein-rich foods may increase bioavailability; a change in diet from high carbohydrate/low protein to low carbohydrate/high protein may result in increased oral clearance.

Cigarette: Smoking may decrease plasma levels of propranolol by increasing metabolism.

Herb/Nutraceutical: Avoid dong quai if using for hypertension (has estrogenic activity). Avoid ephedra, yohimbe, ginseng (may worsen hypertension or arrhythmia). Avoid natural licorice (causes sodium and water retention and increases potassium loss). Avoid garlic (may have increased antihypertensive effect).

Lab Interactions Increased thyroxine (S)

Adverse Reactions Frequency not defined.

Cardiovascular: Bradycardia, CHF, reduced peripheral circulation, chest pain, hypotension, impaired myocardial contractility, worsening of AV conduction disturbance, cardiogenic shock, Raynaud's syndrome, mesenteric thrombosis (rare)

Central nervous system: Mental depression, lightheadedness, amnesia, emotional lability, confusion, hallucinations, dizziness, insomnia, fatigue, vivid dreams, lethargy, cold extremities, vertigo, syncope, cognitive dysfunction, psychosis, hypersomnolence

Dermatologic: Alopecia, contact dermatitis, eczematous eruptions, erythema multiforme, exfoliative dermatitis, hyperkeratosis, nail changes, pruritus, psoriasiform eruptions, rash, ulcerative lichenoid, urticaria, Stevens-Johnson syndrome, toxic epidermal necrolysis

Endocrine & metabolic: Hypoglycemia, hyperglycemia, hyperlipidemia, hyperkalemia

Gastrointestinal: Diarrhea, nausea, vomiting, stomach discomfort, constipation, anorexia

Genitourinary: Impotence, proteinuria (rare), oliguria (rare), interstitial nephritis (rare), Peyronie's disease

Hematologic: Agranulocytosis, thrombocytopenia, thrombocytopenic purpura

Neuromuscular & skeletal: Weakness, carpal tunnel syndrome (rare), paresthesia, myotonus, polyarthritis, arthropathy

Ocular: Hyperemia of the conjunctiva, decreased tear production, decreased visual acuity, mydriasis

Respiratory: Wheezing, pharyngitis, bronchospasm, pulmonary edema, respiratory distress, laryngospasm

Miscellaneous: Lupus-like syndrome (rare), anaphylactic/anaphylactoid allergic reaction

Overdosage/Toxicology Symptoms of intoxication include cardiac disturbances, CNS toxicity, bronchospasm, hypoglycemia, and hyperkalemia. The most common cardiac symptoms include hypotension and bradycardia. Atrioventricular block, intraventricular conduction disturbances, cardiogenic shock, and asystole may occur with severe overdose, especially with membrane-depressant drugs (eg, propranolol). CNS effects include convulsions and coma. Respiratory arrest is commonly seen with propranolol and other membrane-depressant and lipid-soluble drugs. Treatment is symptom-directed and supportive.

Pharmacodynamics/Kinetics

Onset of Action: Beta-blockade: Oral: 1-2 hours

Duration of Action: ~6 hours

Bioavailability: 30% to 40%; may be increased with Down syndrome

Protein Binding: Newborns: 68%; Adults: 93%

Half-Life Elimination: Neonates and Infants: Possible increased half-life; Children: 3.9-6.4 hours; Adults: 4-6 hours

Metabolism: Hepatic to active and inactive compounds; extensive first-pass effect

Excretion: Urine (96% to 99%)

Dosing

Adults:

Akathisia: Oral: 30-120 mg/day in 2-3 divided doses

Angina: Oral: 80-320 mg/day in doses divided 2-4 times/day

Long-acting formulation: Initial: 80 mg once daily; maximum dose: 320 mg once daily

Essential tremor: Oral: 20-40 mg twice daily initially; maintenance doses: usually 120-320 mg/day

Hypertension: Initial: 40 mg twice daily; increase dosage every 3-7 days; usual dose: ≤320 mg divided in 2-3 doses/day; maximum daily dose: 640 mg; usual dosage range (JNC 7): 40-160 mg/day in 2 divided doses

Long-acting formulation: Initial: 80 mg once daily; usual maintenance: 120-160 mg once daily; maximum daily dose: 640 mg; usual dosage range (JNC 7): 60-180 mg/day once daily

Hypertrophic subaortic stenosis: Oral: 20-40 mg 3-4 times/day

Long-acting formulation: 80-160 mg once daily

Migraine headache prophylaxis: Oral: Initial: 80 mg/day divided every 6-8 hours; increase by 20-40 mg/dose every 3-4 weeks to a maximum of 160-240 mg/day given in divided doses every 6-8 hours; if satisfactory response not achieved within 6 weeks of starting therapy, drug should be withdrawn gradually over several weeks

Long-acting formulation: Initial: 80 mg once daily; effective dose range: 160-240 mg once daily

Myocardial infarction prophylaxis: Oral: 180-240 mg/day in 3-4 divided doses

Pheochromocytoma: Oral: 30-60 mg/day in divided doses

Tachyarrhythmias:

Oral: 10-30 mg/dose every 6-8 hours

I.V. (in patients having nonfunctional GI tract): 1 mg/dose slow IVP; repeat every 5 minutes up to a total of 5 mg; titrate initial dose to desired response

Thyrotoxicosis:

Oral: 10-40 mg/dose every 6 hours

I.V.: 1-3 mg/dose slow IVP as a single dose

Elderly: Tachyarrhythmias: Initial: 10 mg twice daily; increase dosage every 3-7 days; usual dose range: 10-320 mg given 1-2 times/day. Refer to adult dosing for additional uses.

Pediatrics:

Hypertension:

Oral: Initial: 0.5-1 mg/kg/day in divided doses every 6-12 hours; increase gradually every 5-7 days; maximum: 16 mg/kg/24 hours

I.V.: 0.01-0.05 mg/kg over 1 hour; maximum dose: 10 mg

Migraine headache prophylaxis: Oral: Initial: 2-4 mg/kg/day **or**

≤35 kg: 10-20 mg 3 times/day

>35 kg: 20-40 mg 3 times/day

Tachyarrhythmias:

Oral: Initial: 0.5-1 mg/kg/day in divided doses every 6-8 hours; titrate dosage upward every 3-7 days; usual dose: 2-6 mg/kg/day; higher doses may be needed; do not exceed 16 mg/kg/day or 60 mg/day

I.V.: 0.01-0.1 mg/kg/dose slow IVP over 10 minutes; maximum dose: 1 mg for infants; 3 mg for children

Tetralogy spells:

Oral: Palliation: Initial: 1 mg/kg/day every 6 hours; if ineffective, may increase dose after 1 week by 1 mg/kg/day to a maximum of 5 mg/kg/day, if patient becomes refractory, may increase slowly to a maximum of 10-15 mg/kg/day. Allow 24 hours between dosing changes.

I.V.: 0.01-0.2 mg/kg/dose infused over 10 minutes; maximum initial dose: 1 mg

Thyrotoxicosis: Oral:

2 mg/kg/day, divided every 6-8 hours, titrate to effective dose

Adolescents: Refer to adult dosing.

Renal Impairment:

Not dialyzable (0% to 5%); supplemental dose is not necessary.

Peritoneal dialysis effects: Supplemental dose is not necessary.

Hepatic Impairment: Marked slowing of heart rate may occur in cirrhosis with conventional doses; low initial dose and regular heart rate monitoring.

Available Dosage Forms

Capsule, extended release, as hydrochloride (InnoPran XL™): 80 mg, 120 mg

Capsule, sustained release, as hydrochloride (Inderal® LA): 60 mg, 80 mg, 120 mg, 160 mg

Injection, solution, as hydrochloride (Inderal®): 1 mg/mL (1 mL)

Solution, oral, as hydrochloride: 4 mg/mL (5 mL, 500 mL); 8 mg/mL (500 mL) [strawberry-mint flavor; contains alcohol 0.6%]

Solution, oral concentrate, as hydrochloride (Propranolol Intensol™): 80 mg/mL (30 mL)

Tablet, as hydrochloride (Inderal®): 10 mg, 20 mg, 40 mg, 60 mg, 80 mg

Monitoring and Teaching Issues

Physical Assessment: Assess effectiveness and interactions of other medications patient may be taking. Monitor therapeutic effectiveness and adverse reactions when starting or adjusting dosage. I.V. infusion requires hemodynamic monitoring. Monitor serum glucose closely in patients with diabetes. Beta-blockers may alter serum glucose levels. Assess knowledge/teach patient appropriate use, orthostatic precautions, interventions to reduce side effects, and adverse symptoms to report.

(Continued)

Propranolol *(Continued)*

Patient Education: Take exactly as directed; do not increase, decrease, or discontinue without consulting prescriber. Tablets may be crushed and taken with liquids. Do not chew or crush long-acting forms; take whole. Take at the same time each day. Do not alter dietary intake of protein or carbohydrates without consulting prescriber. You may experience orthostatic hypotension, dizziness, drowsiness, or blurred vision (use caution when driving, climbing stairs, or changing position - rising from sitting or lying to standing; or engaging in tasks requiring alertness until response to drug is known); nausea, vomiting, or stomach discomfort (small frequent meals, frequent mouth care, chewing gum, or sucking lozenges may help); or decreased sexual ability (reversible). If you have diabetes, monitor serum glucose closely. Report unusual swelling of extremities, respiratory difficulty, unresolved cough, unusual weight gain, cold extremities, persistent diarrhea, confusion, hallucinations, headache, nervousness, lack of improvement, or worsening of condition.
Pregnancy/breast-feeding precautions: Inform prescriber if you are or intend to become pregnant. Consult prescriber if breast-feeding.

Dietary Considerations: Tablets should be taken on an empty stomach; capsules may be taken with or without food, but should always be taken consistently (with food or on an empty stomach)

Geriatric Considerations: Since bioavailability increased in the elderly, about twofold geriatric patients may require lower maintenance doses, therefore, as serum and tissue concentrations increase beta$_1$ selectivity diminishes; due to alterations in the beta-adrenergic autonomic nervous system, beta-adrenergic blockade may result in less hemodynamic response than seen in younger adults.

Pregnancy Risk Factor: C (manufacturer); D (2nd and 3rd trimesters - expert analysis)

Pregnancy Issues: Propranolol crosses the placenta. Beta-blockers have been associated with bradycardia, hypotension, and IUGR. IUGR is probably related to maternal hypertension. Available evidence suggests beta-blockers are generally safe during pregnancy (JNC 7). Cases of neonatal hypoglycemia have been reported following maternal use of beta-blockers at parturition or during breast-feeding. Monitor breast-fed infant for symptoms of beta-blockade.

Lactation: Enters breast milk/use caution (AAP rates "compatible")

Breast-Feeding Issues: Propranolol is excreted in breast milk and is considered compatible by the AAP. It is recommended that the infant be monitored for signs or symptoms of beta-blockade (hypotension, bradycardia, etc) with long-term use.

Administration

Oral: Do not crush long-acting forms.

I.V.: I.V. dose is much smaller than oral dose. When administered acutely for cardiac treatment, monitor ECG and blood pressure. May administer by rapid infusion (I.V. push) at a rate of 1 mg/minute or by slow infusion over ~30 minutes. Necessary monitoring for surgical patients who are unable to take oral beta-blockers (prolonged ileus) has not been defined. Some institutions require monitoring of baseline and postinfusion heart rate and blood pressure when a patient's response to beta-blockade has not been characterized (ie, the patient's initial dose or following a change in dose). Consult individual institutional policies and procedures.

Compatibility: Stable in $D_5^{1}/_2NS$, D_5NS, D_5W, LR, $^1/_2NS$, NS

Y-site administration: Incompatible with amphotericin B cholesteryl sulfate complex, diazoxide
Compatibility in syringe: Incompatible with HCO_3
Compatibility when admixed: Incompatible with HCO_3

Storage: Protect injection from light. Solutions have maximum stability at pH of 3 and decompose rapidly in alkaline pH. Propranolol is stable for 24 hours at room temperature in D_5W or NS.

Related Information
Antiarrhythmic Drugs *on page 1708*
Beta-Blockers *on page 1720*

Propranolol and Hydrochlorothiazide

(proe PRAN oh lole & hye droe klor oh THYE a zide)

U.S. Brand Names Inderide®

Synonyms Hydrochlorothiazide and Propranolol

Generic Available Yes

Pharmacologic Category Antihypertensive Agent, Combination

Medication Safety Issues
Sound-alike/look-alike issues:
Inderide® may be confused with Inderal®

Use Management of hypertension

Dosing
Adults & Elderly:
Hypertension: Oral: Dose is individualized; typical dosages of **hydrochlorothiazide**: 12.5-50 mg/day; initial dose of **propranolol** 80 mg/day
Note: Daily dose of tablet form should be divided into 2 daily doses; may be used to maximum dosage of up to 160 mg of propranolol; higher dosages would result in higher than optimal thiazide dosages.

Available Dosage Forms Tablet (Inderide®):
40/25: Propranolol hydrochloride 40 mg and hydrochlorothiazide 25 mg
80/25: Propranolol hydrochloride 80 mg and hydrochlorothiazide 25 mg

Monitoring and Teaching Issues
Physical Assessment: See individual agents.
Patient Education: See individual agents. **Pregnancy precaution:** Inform prescriber if you are or intend to become pregnant.

Pregnancy Risk Factor: C
Lactation: Enters breast milk/compatible
Related Information
Hydrochlorothiazide *on page 751*
Propranolol *on page 1273*

♦ **Propranolol Hydrochloride** *see* Propranolol *on page 1273*
♦ **Propranolol Intensol™** *see* Propranolol *on page 1273*
♦ **Proprinal [OTC]** *see* Ibuprofen *on page 777*
♦ **Propulsid®** *see* Cisapride *on page 332*
♦ **Propylene Glycol Diacetate, Acetic Acid, and Hydrocortisone** *see* Acetic Acid, Propylene Glycol Diacetate, and Hydrocortisone *on page 44*
♦ **Propylene Glycol Diacetate, Hydrocortisone, and Acetic Acid** *see* Acetic Acid, Propylene Glycol Diacetate, and Hydrocortisone *on page 44*
♦ **2-Propylpentanoic Acid** *see* Valproic Acid and Derivatives *on page 1543*

Propylthiouracil (proe pil thye oh YOOR a sil)

Synonyms PTU
Generic Available Yes
Pharmacologic Category Antithyroid Agent
Medication Safety Issues
Sound-alike/look-alike issues:
Propylthiouracil may be confused with Purinethol®
"PTU" abbreviation should not be used when writing orders for this medication; has been misread as "6-MP" (mercaptopurine)
Use Palliative treatment of hyperthyroidism as an adjunct to ameliorate hyperthyroidism in preparation for surgical treatment or radioactive iodine therapy; management of thyrotoxic crisis
Mechanism of Action/Effect Inhibits the synthesis of thyroid hormones by blocking the oxidation of iodine in the thyroid gland; blocks synthesis of thyroxine and triiodothyronine
Contraindications Hypersensitivity to propylthiouracil or any component of the formulation; pregnancy
Warnings/Precautions Use with caution in patients >40 years of age because PTU may cause hypoprothrombinemia and bleeding. Use with extreme caution in patients receiving other drugs known to cause agranulocytosis; may cause agranulocytosis, thyroid hyperplasia, thyroid carcinoma (usage >1 year). Discontinue in the presence of agranulocytosis, aplastic anemia, ANCA-positive vasculitis, hepatitis, unexplained fever, or exfoliative dermatitis. Safety and efficacy have not been established in children <6 years of age.
Drug Interactions
Decreased Effect: Oral anticoagulant activity is increased only until metabolic effect stabilizes. Anticoagulants may be potentiated by antivitamin K effect of propylthiouracil. Correction of hyperthyroidism may alter disposition of beta-blockers, digoxin, and theophylline, necessitating a dose reduction of these agents.
Increased Effect/Toxicity: Propylthiouracil may increase the anticoagulant activity of warfarin.
Nutritional/Ethanol Interactions Food: Propylthiouracil serum levels may be altered if taken with food.
Adverse Reactions Frequency not defined.
Cardiovascular: Edema, cutaneous vasculitis, leukocytoclastic vasculitis, ANCA-positive vasculitis
Central nervous system: Fever, drowsiness, vertigo, headache, drug fever, dizziness, neuritis
Dermatologic: Skin rash, urticaria, pruritus, exfoliative dermatitis, alopecia, erythema nodosum
Endocrine & metabolic: Goiter, weight gain, swollen salivary glands
Gastrointestinal: Nausea, vomiting, loss of taste perception, stomach pain, constipation
Hematologic: Leukopenia, agranulocytosis, thrombocytopenia, bleeding, aplastic anemia
Hepatic: Cholestatic jaundice, hepatitis
Neuromuscular & skeletal: Arthralgia, paresthesia
Renal: Nephritis, glomerulonephritis, acute renal failure
Respiratory: Interstitial pneumonitis, alveolar hemorrhage
Miscellaneous: SLE-like syndrome
Overdosage/Toxicology Symptoms of overdose include nausea, vomiting, epigastric pain, headache, fever, arthralgia, pruritus, edema, pancytopenia, epigastric distress, headache, fever, CNS stimulation, or depression. Treatment is supportive. Monitor bone marrow response. Forced diuresis, dialysis, and charcoal hemoperfusion have been used to enhance elimination.
Pharmacodynamics/Kinetics
Onset of Action: Therapeutic: 24-36 hours; Peak effect: Remission: 4 months of continued therapy
Duration of Action: 2-3 hours
Bioavailability: 80% to 95%
Time to Peak: Serum: ~1 hour
Protein Binding: 75% to 80%
Half-Life Elimination: 1.5-5 hours; End-stage renal disease: 8.5 hours
Metabolism: Hepatic
Excretion: Urine (35%)
Dosing
Adults:
Hyperthyroidism: Oral: Initial: 300-450 mg/day in divided doses every 8 hours (severe hyperthyroidism may require 600-1200 mg/day); maintenance: 100-150 mg/day in divided doses every 8-12 hours
Note: Administer in 3 equally divided doses at approximately 8-hour intervals. Adjust dosage to maintain T_3, T_4, and TSH levels in normal range; elevated T_3 may be sole
(Continued)

Propylthiouracil (Continued)

indicator of inadequate treatment. Elevated TSH indicates excessive antithyroid treatment.

Elderly: Use lower dose recommendations; adjust for renal impairment.
Initial: 150-300 mg/day in divided doses every 8 hours
Maintenance: 100-150 mg/day in divided doses every 8-12 hours

Pediatrics:
Hyperthyroidism: Oral: Children: Initial: 5-7 mg/kg/day **or** 150-200 mg/m^2/day in divided doses every 8 hours **or**
6-10 years: 50-150 mg/day
>10 years: 150-300 mg/day
Maintenance: Determined by patient response **or** $^1/_3$ to $^2/_3$ of the initial dose in divided doses every 8-12 hours. This usually begins after 2 months on an effective initial dose.

Note: Administer in 3 equally divided doses at approximately 8-hour intervals. Adjust dosage to maintain T_3, T_4, and TSH levels in normal range; elevated T_3 may be sole indicator of inadequate treatment. Elevated TSH indicates excessive antithyroid treatment.

Renal Impairment:
Cl$_{cr}$ 10-50 mL/minute: Administer 75% of normal dose.
Cl$_{cr}$ <10 mL/minute: Administer 50% of normal dose.

Available Dosage Forms Tablet: 50 mg

Monitoring and Teaching Issues

Physical Assessment: See Warnings/Precautions for use cautions. Assess potential for interactions with other medications/herbal agents and herbal products patient may be taking (eg, increased anticoagulant activity; see Drug Interactions). Assess results of laboratory tests, effectiveness according to use, and adverse response (eg, rash, goiter, nausea, vomiting, leukopenia, agranulocytosis, anemia, jaundice, arthralgia, CNS stimulation, or depression; see Adverse Reactions). Teach patient proper use, possible side effects/appropriate interventions, and adverse symptoms to report (see Patient Education).

Monitoring Laboratory Tests: CBC with differential, prothrombin time, liver and thyroid function (T_4, T_3, TSH); periodic blood counts are recommended for chronic therapy

Patient Education: Take as directed at the same time each day at around-the-clock intervals and in relation to meals, either always with meals or always between meals. Do not miss doses or make up missed doses. This drug may need to be taken for an extended period of time to achieve appropriate results and you may need periodic blood tests to assess effectiveness of therapy. May cause nausea or vomiting (small frequent meals may help); constipation (increased exercise, fluids, fruit, or fiber may help); or dizziness or drowsiness (use caution when driving or engaging in tasks that require alertness until response to drug is known). Report rash, skin eruptions, or loss of hair; fever; unusual bleeding or bruising; unusual weight gain (>5 lb/week); unresolved headache or fever; yellowing of eyes or skin; changes in color of urine or feces; or joint or muscle pain or weakness. **Pregnancy/breast-feeding precautions:** Inform prescriber if you are pregnant. Do not get pregnant while taking this medication. Consult prescriber for appropriate contraceptive measures. Consult prescriber if breast-feeding.

Dietary Considerations: Administer at the same time in relation to meals each day, either always with meals or always between meals.

Geriatric Considerations: The use of antithyroid thioamides is as effective in the elderly as they are in younger adults; however, the expense, potential adverse effects, and inconvenience (compliance, monitoring) make them undesirable. The use of radioiodine, due to ease of administration and less concern for long-term side effects and reproduction problems, makes it a more appropriate therapy.

Pregnancy Risk Factor: D

Pregnancy Issues: Crosses the placenta and may induce goiter and hypothyroidism in the developing fetus (cretinism). May need to monitor infant's thyroid function periodically.

Lactation: Enters breast milk/use caution (AAP rates "compatible")

Additional Information Preferred over methimazole in thyroid storm due to inhibition of peripheral conversion as well as synthesis of thyroid hormone.

- ♦ **2-Propylvaleric Acid** *see* Valproic Acid and Derivatives *on page 1543*
- ♦ **Proscar®** *see* Finasteride *on page 629*
- ♦ **Prostacyclin** *see* Epoprostenol *on page 534*
- ♦ **Prostaglandin E$_1$** *see* Alprostadil *on page 76*
- ♦ **Prostaglandin E$_2$** *see* Dinoprostone *on page 462*
- ♦ **Prostigmin®** *see* Neostigmine *on page 1070*
- ♦ **Prostin E$_2$®** *see* Dinoprostone *on page 462*
- ♦ **Prostin F$_2$ Alpha®** *see page 1625*
- ♦ **Prostin VR Pediatric®** *see* Alprostadil *on page 76*

Protamine Sulfate (PROE ta meen SUL fate)

Generic Available Yes

Pharmacologic Category Antidote

Medication Safety Issues
Sound-alike/look-alike issues:
Protamine may be confused with ProAmatine®, protamine, Protopam®, Protropin®

Use Treatment of heparin overdosage; neutralize heparin during surgery or dialysis procedures

Unlabeled/Investigational Use Treatment of low molecular weight heparin (LMWH) overdose

Mechanism of Action/Effect Combines with strongly acidic heparin to form a stable complex (salt) neutralizing the anticoagulant activity of both drugs

Contraindications Hypersensitivity to protamine or any component of the formulation

Warnings/Precautions For I.V. use only. May not be totally effective in some patients following cardiac surgery despite adequate doses. May cause hypersensitivity reaction in patients with a history of allergy to fish (have epinephrine 1:1000 available) and in patients sensitized to protamine (via protamine zinc insulin). Rapid administration can cause severe hypotensive and anaphylactoid-like reactions. Heparin rebound associated with anticoagulation and bleeding has been reported to occur occasionally. Symptoms typically occur 8-9 hours after protamine administration, but may occur as long as 18 hours later.

Adverse Reactions Frequency not defined.

Cardiovascular: Sudden fall in blood pressure, bradycardia, flushing, hypotension

Central nervous system: Lassitude

Gastrointestinal: Nausea, vomiting

Hematologic: Hemorrhage

Respiratory: Dyspnea, pulmonary hypertension

Miscellaneous: Hypersensitivity reactions

Overdosage/Toxicology Symptoms of overdose include hypertension. May cause hemorrhage. Doses exceeding 100 mg may cause paradoxical anticoagulation.

Pharmacodynamics/Kinetics

Duration of Action: Onset of action: I.V.: Heparin neutralization: ~5 minutes

Dosing

Adults & Elderly:

Heparin neutralization: I.V.: Protamine dosage is determined by the dosage of heparin; 1 mg of protamine neutralizes 90 USP units of heparin (lung) and 115 USP units of heparin (intestinal); maximum dose: 50 mg

Heparin overdosage, following intravenous administration: I.V.: Since blood heparin concentrations decrease rapidly **after** administration, adjust the protamine dosage depending upon the duration of time since heparin administration as follows: See table.

Time Elapsed	Dose of Protamine (mg) to Neutralize 100 units of Heparin
Immediate	1-1.5
30-60 min	0.5-0.75
>2 h	0.25-0.375

Heparin overdosage, following SubQ injection: I.V.: 1-1.5 mg protamine per 100 units heparin; this may be done by a portion of the dose (eg, 25-50 mg) given slowly I.V. followed by the remaining portion as a continuous infusion over 8-16 hours (the expected absorption time of the SubQ heparin dose)

LMWH overdose (unlabeled use):

Enoxaparin: 1 mg protamine for each mg of enoxaparin; if PTT prolonged 2-4 hours after first dose, consider additional dose of 0.5 mg for each mg of enoxaparin.

Dalteparin or tinzaparin: 1 mg protamine for each 100 anti-Xa int. units of dalteparin or tinzaparin; if PTT prolonged 2-4 hours after first dose, consider additional dose of 0.5 mg for each 100 anti-Xa int. units of dalteparin or tinzaparin.

Note: Antifactor Xa activity never completely neutralized (maximum: ~60% to 75%). Excessive protamine doses may worsen bleeding potential.

Pediatrics: Refer to adult dosing.

Available Dosage Forms Injection, solution, as sulfate [preservative free]: 10 mg/mL (5 mL, 25 mL)

Monitoring and Teaching Issues

Physical Assessment: Assess results of laboratory tests and therapeutic effectiveness frequently during therapy. Monitor closely for adverse response. Assess knowledge/teach patient possible side effects and adverse symptoms to report.

Monitoring Laboratory Tests: Coagulation test, aPTT or ACT

Patient Education: Report any respiratory difficulty, rash or flushing, feeling of warmth, tingling or numbness, dizziness, or disorientation. **Pregnancy/breast-feeding precautions:** Inform prescriber if you are pregnant. Consult prescriber if breast-feeding.

Pregnancy Risk Factor: C

Lactation: Excretion in breast milk unknown

Administration

I.V.: For I.V. use only. Administer slow IVP (50 mg over 10 minutes). Rapid I.V. infusion causes hypotension. Reconstitute vial with 5 mL sterile water. Resulting solution equals 10 mg/mL. Inject without further dilution over 1-3 minutes; maximum of 50 mg in any 10-minute period.

Reconstitution: Reconstitute vial with 5 mL sterile water; if using protamine in neonates, reconstitute with preservative-free sterile water for injection; resulting solution equals 10 mg/mL.

Compatibility: Stable in D_5W, NS

Compatibility in syringe: Incompatible with diatrizoate meglumine 52%, diatrizoate sodium 8%, diatrizoate sodium 60%, ioxaglate meglumine 39.3%, ioxaglate sodium 19.6%

Compatibility when admixed: Incompatible with cephalosporins, penicillins

Storage: Refrigerate; avoid freezing. Remains stable for at least 2 weeks at room temperature; preservative-free formulation does not require refrigeration.

♦ **Protein-Bound Paclitaxel** see Paclitaxel (Protein Bound) on page 1146
♦ **Protein C (Activated), Human, Recombinant** see Drotrecogin Alfa on page 501
♦ **Protirelin** see page 1625
♦ **Protonix®** see Pantoprazole on page 1155
♦ **Protopic®** see Tacrolimus on page 1419

Protriptyline (proe TRIP ti leen)

U.S. Brand Names Vivactil®

Synonyms Protriptyline Hydrochloride

(Continued)

Protriptyline *(Continued)*

Restrictions A medication guide should be dispensed with each prescription. A template for the required MedGuides can be found on the FDA website at: http://www.fda.gov/cder/drug/antidepressants/labelTemplate.pdf

Generic Available No

Pharmacologic Category Antidepressant, Tricyclic (Secondary Amine)

Use Treatment of depression

Mechanism of Action/Effect Increases the synaptic concentration of serotonin and/or norepinephrine in the central nervous system by inhibition of their reuptake by the presynaptic neuronal membrane

Contraindications Hypersensitivity to protriptyline (cross-reactivity to other cyclic antidepressants may occur) or any component of the formulation; use of MAO inhibitors within 14 days; use of cisapride; use in a patient during the acute recovery phase of MI

Warnings/Precautions Antidepressants increase the risk of suicidal thinking and behavior in children and adolescents with major depressive disorder (MDD) and other depressive disorders; consider risk prior to prescribing. All patients must be closely monitored for clinical worsening, suicidality, or unusual changes in behavior, especially during the initiation of therapy or following an increase or decrease in dosage. When used in children, the child's family or caregiver should be instructed to closely observe the patient and communicate condition with healthcare provider. A medication guide should be dispensed with each prescription. **Protriptyline is FDA approved for the treatment of depression in adolescents.**

The possibility of a suicide attempt is inherent in major depression and may persist until remission occurs. Use caution in high-risk patients. Worsening depression and severe abrupt suicidality that are not part of the presenting symptoms may require discontinuation or modification of drug therapy. The patient's family or caregiver should be alerted to monitor patients for the emergence of suicidality and associated behaviors (such as agitation, irritability, hostility, impulsivity, and hypomania) and call healthcare provider.

May worsen psychosis in some patients or precipitate a shift to mania or hypomania in patients with bipolar disorder. Patients presenting with depressive symptoms should be screened for bipolar disorder. Monotherapy in patients with bipolar disorder should be avoided. **Protriptyline is not FDA approved for the treatment of bipolar depression.**

Although the degree of sedation is low relative to other antidepressant agents, protriptyline may cause sedation, resulting in impaired performance of tasks requiring alertness (eg, operating machinery or driving). Sedative effects may be additive with other CNS depressants and/or ethanol. Protriptyline may aggravate aggressive behavior. Consider discontinuing, when possible, prior to elective surgery. Therapy should not be abruptly discontinued in patients receiving high doses for prolonged periods. May alter glucose regulation - use with caution in patients with diabetes.

May cause orthostatic hypotension or conduction abnormalities (risks are moderate relative to other antidepressants). Use with caution in patients with a history of cardiovascular disease (including previous MI, stroke, tachycardia, or conduction abnormalities). The degree of anticholinergic blockade produced by this agent is moderate relative to other cyclic antidepressants, however, caution should still be used in patients with urinary retention, benign prostatic hyperplasia, narrow-angle glaucoma, xerostomia, visual problems, constipation, or history of bowel obstruction.

Use caution in patients with a previous seizure disorder or condition predisposing to seizures such as brain damage, alcoholism, or concurrent therapy with other drugs which lower the seizure threshold. May increase the risks associated with electroconvulsive therapy. Use with caution in hyperthyroid patients or those receiving thyroid supplementation. Use with caution in patients with hepatic or renal dysfunction and in elderly patients.

Drug Interactions

Cytochrome P450 Effect: Substrate of CYP2D6 (major)

Decreased Effect: Carbamazepine, phenobarbital, and rifampin may increase the metabolism of protriptyline, decreasing its effects. Protriptyline inhibits the antihypertensive response to bethanidine, clonidine, debrisoquin, guanadrel, guanethidine, guanabenz, guanfacine. Cimetidine and methylphenidate may decrease the metabolism of protriptyline. Cholestyramine and colestipol may bind TCAs and reduce their absorption.

Increased Effect/Toxicity: Protriptyline increases the effects of amphetamines, anticholinergics, other CNS depressants (sedatives, hypnotics, or ethanol), chlorpropamide, tolazamide, and warfarin. When used with MAO inhibitors, hyperpyrexia, hypertension, tachycardia, confusion, seizures, and **deaths have been reported** (serotonin syndrome). The SSRIs (to varying degrees), cimetidine, grapefruit juice, indinavir, methylphenidate, ritonavir, quinidine, diltiazem, and verapamil inhibit the metabolism of TCAs. Levels/effects of protriptyline may be increased by chlorpromazine, delavirdine, fluoxetine, miconazole, paroxetine, pergolide, quinidine, quinine, ritonavir, ropinirole, and other CYP2D6 inhibitors. Use of lithium with a TCA may increase the risk for neurotoxicity. Phenothiazines may increase concentration of some TCAs and TCAs may increase concentration of phenothiazines. Pressor response to I.V. epinephrine, norepinephrine, and phenylephrine may be enhanced in patients receiving TCAs (**Note:** Effect is unlikely with epinephrine or levonordefrin dosages typically administered as infiltration in combination with local anesthetics). Combined use of beta-agonists or drugs which prolong QT_c (including quinidine, procainamide, disopyramide, cisapride, sparfloxacin, gatifloxacin, moxifloxacin) with TCAs may predispose patients to cardiac arrhythmias.

Nutritional/Ethanol Interactions

Ethanol: Avoid ethanol (may increase CNS depression).

Food: Grapefruit juice may inhibit the metabolism of some TCAs and clinical toxicity may result.

Herb/Nutraceutical: Avoid valerian, St John's wort, SAMe, kava kava (may increase risk of serotonin syndrome and/or excessive sedation).

Lab Interactions Increased glucose

Adverse Reactions Frequency not defined.

Cardiovascular: Arrhythmias, hyper-/hypotension, MI, stroke, heart block, tachycardia, palpitation

Central nervous system: Dizziness, drowsiness, headache, confusion, delirium, hallucinations, restlessness, insomnia, nightmares, fatigue, delusions, anxiety, agitation, hypomania, exacerbation of psychosis, panic, seizure, incoordination, ataxia, EPS

Dermatologic: Alopecia, photosensitivity, rash, petechiae, urticaria, itching

Endocrine & metabolic: Breast enlargement, galactorrhea, SIADH, gynecomastia, increased or decreased libido

Gastrointestinal: Xerostomia, constipation, unpleasant taste, weight gain/loss, increased appetite, nausea, diarrhea, heartburn, vomiting, anorexia, trouble with gums, decreased lower esophageal sphincter tone may cause GE reflux

Genitourinary: Difficult urination, impotence, testicular edema

Hematologic: Agranulocytosis, leukopenia, eosinophilia, thrombocytopenia, purpura

Hepatic: Cholestatic jaundice, increased liver enzymes

Neuromuscular & skeletal: Fine muscle tremor, weakness, tremor, numbness, tingling

Ocular: Blurred vision, eye pain, increased intraocular pressure

Otic: Tinnitus

Miscellaneous: Diaphoresis (excessive), allergic reactions

Overdosage/Toxicology Symptoms of overdose include confusion, hallucinations, urinary retention, hypotension, tachycardia, seizures, and hyperthermia. Following initiation of essential overdose management, toxic symptoms should be treated. Ventricular arrhythmias often respond to systemic alkalinization (sodium bicarbonate 0.5-2 mEq/kg I.V.) Physostigmine (1-2 mg I.V. slowly for adults) may be indicated for reversing life-threatening cardiac arrhythmias.

Pharmacodynamics/Kinetics
Time to Peak: Serum: 24-30 hours
Protein Binding: 92%
Half-Life Elimination: 54-92 hours (average: 74 hours)
Metabolism: Extensively hepatic via N-oxidation, hydroxylation, and glucuronidation; first-pass effect (10% to 25%)
Excretion: Urine

Dosing
Adults: Depression: Oral: 15-60 mg in 3-4 divided doses
Elderly: Oral: Initial: 5-10 mg/day; increase every 3-7 days by 5-10 mg; usual dose: 15-20 mg/day
Pediatrics: Depression: Oral: Adolescents: 15-20 mg/day

Available Dosage Forms Tablet, as hydrochloride [film coated]: 5 mg, 10 mg

Monitoring and Teaching Issues
Physical Assessment: Assess potential for interactions with other prescriptions, OTC medications, or herbal products patient may be taking (see extensive list of Drug Interactions). Assess for suicidal tendencies before beginning therapy. May cause physiological or psychological dependence, tolerance, or abuse; periodically evaluate need for continued use. Assess therapeutic effectiveness (mental status, mood, affect) and adverse reactions (eg, suicidal ideation) at beginning of therapy and periodically with long-term use. Taper dosage slowly when discontinuing (allow 3-4 weeks between discontinuing this medication and starting another antidepressant). Caution patients with diabetes to monitor glucose levels closely; may increase or decrease serum glucose levels. Teach patient appropriate use, interventions to reduce side effects, and adverse symptoms to report.

Patient Education: Do not take any new medication during therapy unless approved by prescriber. Take exactly as directed; take once-a-day dose at bedtime. Do not increase dose or frequency; may take 2-3 weeks to achieve desired results. This drug may cause physical and/or psychological dependence. Avoid alcohol and grapefruit juice. Maintain adequate hydration (2-3 L/day of fluids) unless instructed to restrict fluid intake. May cause drowsiness, lightheadedness, impaired coordination, dizziness, or blurred vision (use caution when driving or engaging in tasks requiring alertness until response to drug is known); nausea, vomiting, loss of appetite, or disturbed taste (small frequent meals, good mouth care, chewing gum, or sucking lozenges may help); constipation (increased exercise, fluids, fruit, or fiber may help); urinary retention (void before taking medication); postural hypotension (use caution climbing stairs or when changing position from lying or sitting to standing); altered sexual drive or ability (reversible); or photosensitivity (use sunscreen, wear protective clothing and eyewear, and avoid direct sunlight). Report chest pain, palpitations, or rapid heartbeat; persistent adverse CNS effects (eg, suicidal ideation, nervousness, restlessness, insomnia, anxiety, excitation, headache, agitation, impaired coordination, changes in cognition); muscle cramping, weakness, tremors, or rigidity; blurred vision or eye pain; breast enlargement or swelling; yellowing of skin or eyes; or worsening of condition. **Pregnancy/breast-feeding precautions:** Inform prescriber if you are or intend to become pregnant. Breast-feeding is not recommended.

Dietary Considerations: May be taken with food to decrease GI distress.

Geriatric Considerations: Little data on use in the elderly. Strong anticholinergic properties which may limit protriptyline's use; more often stimulating rather than sedating effects.

Pregnancy Risk Factor: C

Lactation: Excretion in breast milk unknown/not recommended

Related Information
Antidepressant Agents *on page 1713*
Antidepressant Medication Guidelines *on page 1765*
Federal OBRA Regulations: Recommended Maximum Doses *on page 1773*

♦ **Protriptyline Hydrochloride** *see* Protriptyline *on page 1279*

♦ **Protropin® [DSC]** *see* Human Growth Hormone *on page 745*

♦ **Proventil®** *see* Albuterol *on page 59*

♦ **Proventil® HFA** *see* Albuterol *on page 59*

♦ **Proventil® Repetabs®** *see* Albuterol *on page 59*

- ♦ **Provera®** see MedroxyPROGESTERone on page 938
- ♦ **Provigil®** see Modafinil on page 1023
- ♦ **Provocholine®** see page 1625
- ♦ **Prozac®** see Fluoxetine on page 649
- ♦ **Prozac® Weekly™** see Fluoxetine on page 649
- ♦ **Prudoxin™** see Doxepin on page 487
- ♦ **Prymaccone** see Primaquine on page 1250
- ♦ **PS-341** see Bortezomib on page 203

Pseudoephedrine (soo doe e FED rin)

U.S. Brand Names Biofed [OTC]; Contact® Cold [OTC]; Dimetapp® 12-Hour Non-Drowsy Extentabs® [OTC]; ElixSure® Congestion [OTC]; Genaphed® [OTC]; Kidkare Decongestant [OTC]; Kodet SE [OTC]; Oranyl [OTC]; PediaCare® Decongestant Infants [OTC]; Silfedrine Children's [OTC]; Simply Stuffy™ [OTC]; Sudafed® [OTC]; Sudafed® 12 Hour [OTC]; Sudafed® 24 Hour [OTC]; Sudafed® Children's [OTC]; Sudodrin [OTC]; SudoGest [OTC]; Sudo-Tab® [OTC]

Synonyms d-Isoephedrine Hydrochloride; Pseudoephedrine Hydrochloride; Pseudoephedrine Sulfate

Generic Available Yes: Liquid, syrup, tablet

Pharmacologic Category Alpha/Beta Agonist

Medication Safety Issues

Sound-alike/look-alike issues:

Dimetapp® may be confused with Dermatop®, Dimetabs®, Dimetane®

Sudafed® may be confused with Sufenta®

Use Temporary symptomatic relief of nasal congestion due to common cold, upper respiratory allergies, and sinusitis; also promotes nasal or sinus drainage

Mechanism of Action/Effect Directly stimulates alpha-adrenergic receptors of respiratory mucosa causing vasoconstriction; directly stimulates beta-adrenergic receptors causing bronchial relaxation, increased heart rate and contractility

Contraindications Hypersensitivity to pseudoephedrine or any component of the formulation; with or within 14 days of MAO inhibitor therapy

Warnings/Precautions Use with caution in patients >60 years of age. Administer with caution to patients with hypertension, hyperthyroidism, diabetes mellitus, cardiovascular disease, ischemic heart disease, increased intraocular pressure, or prostatic hyperplasia. Elderly patients are more likely to experience adverse reactions to sympathomimetics. Overdosage may cause hallucinations, seizures, CNS depression, and death. When used for self-medication (OTC), notify prescriber if symptoms do not improve within 7 days or are accompanied by fever.

Drug Interactions

Decreased Effect: Decreased effect of methyldopa, reserpine.

Increased Effect/Toxicity: MAO inhibitors may increase blood pressure effects of pseudoephedrine. Sympathomimetic agents may increase toxicity.

Nutritional/Ethanol Interactions

Food: Onset of effect may be delayed if pseudoephedrine is taken with food.

Herb/Nutraceutical: Avoid ephedra, yohimbe (may cause hypertension).

Lab Interactions Interferes with urine detection of amphetamine (false-positive)

Adverse Reactions Frequency not defined.

Cardiovascular: Tachycardia, palpitation, arrhythmia

Central nervous system: Nervousness, transient stimulation, insomnia, excitability, dizziness, drowsiness, convulsions, hallucinations, headache

Gastrointestinal: Nausea, vomiting

Genitourinary: Dysuria

Neuromuscular & skeletal: Weakness, tremor

Respiratory: Dyspnea

Miscellaneous: Diaphoresis

Overdosage/Toxicology Symptoms of overdose include seizures, nausea, vomiting, cardiac arrhythmias, hypertension, agitation, hallucinations, and death. There is no specific antidote for pseudoephedrine intoxication. Treatment is primarily supportive.

Pharmacodynamics/Kinetics

Onset of Action: Decongestant: Oral: 15-30 minutes

Duration of Action: Immediate release tablet: 4-6 hours; Extended release: ≤12 hours

Absorption: Rapid

Half-Life Elimination: 9-16 hours

Metabolism: Partially hepatic

Excretion: Urine (70% to 90% as unchanged drug, 1% to 6% as active norpseudoephedrine); dependent on urine pH and flow rate; alkaline urine decreases renal elimination of pseudoephedrine

Dosing

Adults: Nasal congestion: Oral: 30-60 mg every 4-6 hours, sustained release: 120 mg every 12 hours; maximum: 240 mg/24 hours

Elderly: Nasal congestion: 30-60 mg every 6 hours as needed

Pediatrics: Nasal congestion: Oral: General dosing guidelines:

<2 years: 4 mg/kg/day in divided doses every 6 hours

2-5 years: 15 mg every 4-6 hours; maximum: 60 mg/24 hours

6-12 years: 30 mg every 4-6 hours; maximum: 120 mg/24 hours

Renal Impairment: Reduce dose.

Available Dosage Forms

Caplet, extended release, as hydrochloride (Contact® Cold, Sudafed® 12 Hour): 120 mg

Liquid, as hydrochloride: 30 mg/5 mL (120 mL, 480 mL)

Silfedrine Children's: 15 mg/5 mL (120 mL, 480 mL) [alcohol and sugar free; grape flavor]

Simply Stuffy™: 15 mg/5 mL (120 mL) [alcohol free; contains sodium benzoate; cherry berry flavor]

      Sudafed® Children's: 15 mg/5 mL (120 mL) [alcohol and sugar free; contains sodium benzoate; grape flavor]

Liquid, oral drops, as hydrochloride:

    Dimetapp® Decongestant Infant Drops: 7.5 mg/0.8 mL (15 mL) [alcohol free; contains sodium benzoate; grape flavor]

    Kidkare Decongestant: 7.5 mg/0.8 mL (30 mL) [alcohol free; contains benzoic acid and sodium benzoate; cherry flavor]

    PediaCare® Decongestant: 7.5 mg/0.8 mL (15 mL) [alcohol free, dye free; contains benzoic acid, sodium benzoate; fruit flavor]

Syrup, as hydrochloride:

    Biofed: 30 mg/5 mL (120 mL, 240 mL, 480 mL, 3840 mL) [alcohol free; contains sodium benzoate]

    ElixSure® Congestion: 15 mg/5 mL (120 mL) [grape bubble gum flavor]

Tablet, as hydrochloride: 30 mg, 60 mg

    Genaphed®, Kodet SE, Oranyl, Sudafed®, Sudodrin, Sudo-Tab®: 30 mg

    SudoGest: 30 mg, 60 mg

Tablet, chewable, as hydrochloride (Sudafed® Children's): 15 mg [sugar free; contains phenylalanine 0.78 mg/tablet; orange flavor]

Tablet, extended release, as hydrochloride:

    Dimetapp® 12-Hour Non-Drowsy Extentabs®: 120 mg

    Sudafed® 24 Hour: 240 mg

Monitoring and Teaching Issues

Physical Assessment: Assess effectiveness and interactions of other medications patient may be taking. Monitor effectiveness of therapy and adverse reactions at beginning of therapy and periodically with long-term use. Assess knowledge/teach patient appropriate use, interventions to reduce side effects, and adverse symptoms to report.

Patient Education: Take only as prescribed; do not exceed prescribed dose or frequency. Do not chew or crush timed release forms. Maintain adequate hydration (2-3 L/day of fluids) unless instructed to restrict fluid intake. You may experience nervousness, insomnia, dizziness, or drowsiness (use caution when driving or engaging in tasks requiring alertness until response to drug is known). Report persistent CNS changes (dizziness, tremor, agitation, or convulsions); respiratory difficulty; chest pain, palpitations, or rapid heartbeat; muscle tremor; or lack of improvement or worsening of condition. **Pregnancy/breast-feeding precautions:** Inform prescriber if you are or intend to become pregnant. Consult prescriber if breast-feeding.

Dietary Considerations: Should be taken with water or milk to decrease GI distress.

Geriatric Considerations: Elderly patients should be counseled about the proper use of over-the-counter cough and cold preparations. Elderly are more predisposed to adverse effects of sympathomimetics since they frequently have cardiovascular diseases and diabetes mellitus as well as multiple drug therapies. It may be advisable to treat with a short-acting/immediate-release formulation before initiating sustained-release/long-acting formulations.

Pregnancy Risk Factor: C

Lactation: Enters breast milk/use caution (AAP rates "compatible")

Administration

Oral: Do not crush extended release drug product, swallow whole.

Related Information

    Pharmacotherapy of Urinary Incontinence *on page 1858*

♦ **Pseudoephedrine and Acrivastine** *see Acrivastine and Pseudoephedrine on page 47*

♦ **Pseudoephedrine and Carbinoxamine** *see Carbinoxamine and Pseudoephedrine on page 254*

♦ **Pseudoephedrine and Fexofenadine** *see Fexofenadine and Pseudoephedrine on page 627*

♦ **Pseudoephedrine and Guaifenesin** *see Guaifenesin and Pseudoephedrine on page 733*

♦ **Pseudoephedrine and Loratadine** *see Loratadine and Pseudoephedrine on page 919*

♦ **Pseudoephedrine, Guaifenesin, and Codeine** *see Guaifenesin, Pseudoephedrine, and Codeine on page 735*

♦ **Pseudoephedrine Hydrochloride** *see Pseudoephedrine on page 1282*

♦ **Pseudoephedrine Hydrochloride, Guaifenesin, and Dihydrocodeine Bitartrate** *see Dihydrocodeine, Pseudoephedrine, and Guaifenesin on page 457*

♦ **Pseudoephedrine Hydrochloride, Hydrocodone Bitartrate, and Chlorpheniramine Maleate** *see Pseudoephedrine, Hydrocodone, and Chlorpheniramine on page 1283*

♦ **Pseudoephedrine, Hydrocodone, and Carbinoxamine** *see Hydrocodone, Carbinoxamine, and Pseudoephedrine on page 759*

Pseudoephedrine, Hydrocodone, and Chlorpheniramine

(soo doe e FED rin, hye droe KOE done, & klor fen IR a meen)

U.S. Brand Names Coldcough HC; Cordron-HC; Detuss; Histinex® PV; Hydron PSC; Hydro-Tussin™ HC; Hyphed; Pediatex™ HC; P-V-Tussin® Syrup; Q-V Tussin; Tussend® Syrup; Tussend® Tablet

Synonyms Chlorpheniramine, Pseudoephedrine, and Hydrocodone; Hydrocodone, Chlorpheniramine, and Pseudoephedrine; Pseudoephedrine Hydrochloride, Hydrocodone Bitartrate, and Chlorpheniramine Maleate

Controlled Substance C-III

Generic Available Yes: Excludes tablet

Pharmacologic Category Antihistamine; Antihistamine/Decongestant/Antitussive; Antitussive; Decongestant

Use Temporary relief of cough, congestion, and sneezing due to colds, respiratory infections, or hay fever

(Continued)

Pseudoephedrine, Hydrocodone, and Chlorpheniramine
(Continued)

Dosing
Adults: Cough and congestion: Oral:

Histinex® PV, Pediatex™ HC, P-V-Tussin®, Tussend®: 10 mL or 1 tablet every 4-6 hours; do not exceed 4 doses in 24 hours

Hydro-Tussin™ HC: 5-10 mL or 1 tablet every 4-6 hours; do not exceed 4 doses in 24 hours

Pediatrics: Cough and congestion: Oral: Children:

2-6 years:

Hydro-Tussin™ HC: 1.25-2.5 mL every 4-6 hours; do not exceed 4 doses in 24 hours

Histinex® PV, Pediatex™ HC, P-V-Tussin®: 2.5 mL every 4-6 hours; do not exceed 4 doses in 24 hours

6-12 years:

Histinex® PV, Pediatex™ HC, P-V-Tussin®, Tussend®: 5 mL or ¹/₂ tablet every 4-6 hours; do not exceed 4 doses in 24 hours

Hydro-Tussin™ HC: 2.5-5 mL or ¹/₂ tablet every 4-6 hours; do not exceed 4 doses in 24 hours

>12 years: Refer to adult dosing.

Available Dosage Forms
Liquid:

Cordron-HC: Pseudoephedrine hydrochloride 20 mg, hydrocodone bitartrate 1.67 mg, and chlorpheniramine maleate 2.5 mg per 5 mL (480 mL) [vanilla mint flavor]

Detuss: Pseudoephedrine hydrochloride 30 mg, hydrocodone bitartrate 5 mg, and chlorpheniramine maleate 2 mg per 5 mL (480 mL) [alcohol free; vanilla flavor]

Hydron PSC: Pseudoephedrine hydrochloride 30 mg, hydrocodone bitartrate 5 mg, and chlorpheniramine maleate 2 mg per 5 mL (480 mL) [vanilla flavor]

Pediatex™ HC: Pseudoephedrine hydrochloride 20 mg, hydrocodone bitartrate 1.67 mg, and chlorpheniramine maleate 2.5 mg per 5 mL (480 mL) [alcohol free, sugar free; vanilla mint flavor]

Syrup:

Coldcough HC: Pseudoephedrine hydrochloride 15 mg, hydrocodone bitartrate 3 mg, and chlorpheniramine maleate 2 mg per 5 mL (480 mL) [alcohol free, dye free, sugar free; grape flavor]

Histinex® PV: Pseudoephedrine hydrochloride 30 mg, hydrocodone bitartrate 2.5 mg, and chlorpheniramine maleate 2 mg per 5 mL (480 mL) [alcohol free, sugar free; apricot flavor]

Hydro-Tussin™ HC; Pseudoephedrine hydrochloride 15 mg, hydrocodone bitartrate 3 mg, and chlorpheniramine maleate 2 mg per 5 mL (480 mL) [alcohol free, dye free, sugar free]

Hyphed: Pseudoephedrine hydrochloride 30 mg, hydrocodone bitartrate 2.5 mg, and chlorpheniramine maleate 2 mg per 5 mL (480 mL) [contains alcohol 5%; raspberry flavor]

P-V-Tussin®, Q-V Tussin, Tussend®: Pseudoephedrine hydrochloride 30 mg, hydrocodone bitartrate 2.5 mg, and chlorpheniramine maleate 2 mg per 5 mL (480 mL) [contains alcohol 5%; banana flavor]

Tablet [scored] (Tussend®): Pseudoephedrine hydrochloride 60 mg, hydrocodone bitartrate 5 mg, and chlorpheniramine maleate 4 mg

Monitoring and Teaching Issues
Physical Assessment: See individual agents.

Pregnancy Risk Factor: C

Lactation: Enters breast milk/contraindicated

Related Information
Pseudoephedrine *on page 1282*

Psyllium (SIL i yum)

U.S. Brand Names Fiberall®; Genfiber® [OTC]; Hydrocil® [OTC]; Konsyl® [OTC]; Konsyl-D® [OTC]; Konsyl® Easy Mix [OTC]; Konsyl® Orange [OTC]; Metamucil® [OTC]; Metamucil® Smooth Texture [OTC]; Modane® Bulk [OTC]; Perdiem® Fiber Therapy [OTC]; Reguloid® [OTC]; Serutan® [OTC]

Synonyms Plantago Seed; Plantain Seed; Psyllium Hydrophilic Mucilloid

Generic Available Yes: Powder

Pharmacologic Category Antidiarrheal; Laxative, Bulk-Producing

Medication Safety Issues

Sound-alike/look-alike issues:

Fiberall® may be confused with Feverall®

Hydrocil® may be confused with Hydrocet®

Modane® may be confused with Matulane®, Moban®

Perdiem® may be confused with Pyridium®

Use Treatment of chronic atonic or spastic constipation and in constipation associated with rectal disorders; management of irritable bowel syndrome; labeled for OTC use as fiber supplement, treatment of constipation

Mechanism of Action/Effect Adsorbs water in the intestine to form a viscous liquid which promotes peristalsis and reduces transit time

Contraindications Hypersensitivity to psyllium or any component of the formulation; fecal impaction; GI obstruction

Warnings/Precautions Products must be taken with adequate fluid. Use with caution in patients with esophageal strictures, ulcers, stenosis, or intestinal adhesions. Elderly may have insufficient fluid intake which may predispose them to fecal impaction and bowel obstruction.

Drug Interactions

Decreased Effect: Decreased effect of warfarin, digitalis, potassium-sparing diuretics, salicylates, tetracyclines, nitrofurantoin when taken together. Separate administration times to reduce potential for drug-drug interaction.

Adverse Reactions Frequency not defined.

Gastrointestinal: Esophageal or bowel obstruction, diarrhea, constipation, abdominal cramps

Respiratory: Bronchospasm

Miscellaneous: Anaphylaxis upon inhalation in susceptible individuals, rhinoconjunctivitis

Overdosage/Toxicology Symptoms of overdose include abdominal pain, diarrhea, and constipation.

Pharmacodynamics/Kinetics

Onset of Action: 12-24 hours; Peak effect: 2-3 days

Absorption: None; small amounts of grain extracts present in the preparation have been reportedly absorbed following colonic hydrolysis

Dosing

Adults & Elderly:

Constipation, IBS: Oral (administer at least 2 hours before or after other drugs): Take 1 dose up to 3 times/day; all doses should be followed with 8 oz of water or liquid

Capsule: 4 capsules/dose (range: 2-6); swallow capsules one at a time

Powder: 1 rounded tablespoonful/dose (1 teaspoonful/dose for many sugar free or select concentrated products) mixed in 8 oz liquid

Tablet: 1 tablet/dose

Wafer: 2 wafers/dose

Pediatrics:

Constipation: Oral (administer at least 2 hours before or after other drugs):

Children 6-11 years: Approximately ½ adult dosage

Children ≥12 years: Refer to adult dosing.

Available Dosage Forms

Capsule (Metamucil®): 0.52 g [provides 3 g dietary fiber per 6 capsules]

Granules:

Perdiem® Fiber Therapy: 4 g/teaspoon (250 g)

Serutan®: 2.5 g/teaspoon (510 g) [contains sodium benzoate]

Powder: 3.4 g/dose (unit-dose packets, 397 g)

Fiberall®: 3.5 g/dose (454 g) [sugar free; contains phenylalanine; orange flavor]

Genfiber®: 3.4 g/dose (397 g, 595 g) [regular and orange flavors]

Hydrocil® Instant: 3.5 g/dose (300 g)

Konsyl®: 6 g/dose (6 g unit-dose packets, 300 g, 450 g) [sodium and sugar free; regular and orange flavors]

Konsyl-D®: 3.4 g/dose (6.5 g unit-dose packets, 325 g, 500 g) [contains dextrose]

Konsyl® Easy Mix: 6 g/dose (6 g unit-dose packets, 250 g) [sodium and sugar free]

Konsyl® Orange: 3.4 g/dose (12 g unit-dose packets, 425 g, 538 g) [contains sucrose]

Metamucil®: 3.4 g/dose (390 g, 570 g, 870 g, 1254 g) [regular or orange flavor]

Metamucil® Smooth Texture: 3.4 g/dose (unit-dose packets, 609 g, 912 g, 1368 g) [orange flavor]

Metamucil® Smooth Texture: 3.4 g/dose (12 g unit-dose packets, 300 g, 450 g, 660 g, 699 g) [sugar free; contains phenylalanine 25 mg/teaspoon; regular or orange flavor]

Modane® Bulk: 3.4 g/dose (390 g)

Reguloid®: 3.4 g/dose (300 g, 390 g, 450 g, 570 g) [regular and orange flavor; also available sugar free]

Wafers (Metamucil®): 3.4 g/dose (24s) [apple crisp and cinnamon spice flavors]

Monitoring and Teaching Issues

Physical Assessment: Use caution with esophageal strictures, ulcers, stenosis, or intestinal adhesions (see Warnings/Precautions). Teach patient proper use (according to formulation), possible side effects/appropriate interventions (adequate fluid intake), and adverse symptoms to report (see Patient Education).

Patient Education: Take as directed. Granules/powder: Mix in large glass of water or juice (8 oz or more) and drink immediately. Mix carefully; do not inhale powder. Separate this medication from other medications by at least 1 hour. Results may begin in 12 hours; full results may take 2-3 days. Do not increase dose. It is very important to maintain adequate hydration (2-3 L/day of fluids) unless instructed to restrict fluid intake. Report persistent constipation; watery diarrhea; difficulty, pain, or choking with swallowing; respiratory difficulty; or unusual coughing.

Dietary Considerations: Products should be taken with large amount of fluids. Some products contain aspartame, dextrose, or sucrose, as well as additional ingredients. Check individual product information for caloric and nutritional value.

Fiberall® (sugar free formulation) contains phenylalanine.

Metamucil® Smooth Texture (sugar free formulation) contains phenylalanine 25 mg per teaspoonful.

Geriatric Considerations: Elderly may have insufficient fluid intake which may predispose them to fecal impaction and bowel obstruction. Patients should have a 1 month trial, with at least 14 g/day, before effects in bowel function are determined. Bloating and flatulence are mostly a problem in first 4 weeks of therapy.

(Continued)

Psyllium (Continued)

Pregnancy Risk Factor: B
Lactation: Excretion in breast milk unknown/compatible
Administration
    Oral: Inhalation of psyllium dust may cause sensitivity to psyllium (eg, runny nose, watery eyes, wheezing). Drink a full glass of liquid with each dose. Powder must be mixed in a glass of water or juice. Separate dose from other drug therapies.
Related Information
    Laxatives, Classification and Properties *on page 1737*

- **Psyllium Hydrophilic Mucilloid** *see* Psyllium *on page 1284*
- **Pteroylglutamic Acid** *see* Folic Acid *on page 669*
- **PTU** *see* Propylthiouracil *on page 1277*
- **Pulmicort Respules®** *see* Budesonide *on page 210*
- **Pulmicort Turbuhaler®** *see* Budesonide *on page 210*
- **Pulmozyme®** *see* Dornase Alfa *on page 482*
- **Purinethol®** *see* Mercaptopurine *on page 954*
- **P-V-Tussin® Syrup** *see* Pseudoephedrine, Hydrocodone, and Chlorpheniramine *on page 1283*

Pyrazinamide (peer a ZIN a mide)

Synonyms Pyrazinoic Acid Amide
Generic Available Yes
Pharmacologic Category Antitubercular Agent
Use Adjunctive treatment of tuberculosis in combination with other antituberculosis agents
Mechanism of Action/Effect Converted to pyrazinoic acid in susceptible strains of *Mycobacterium* which lowers the pH of the environment; bacteriostatic or bactericidal depending on the drug's concentration at the site of infection
Contraindications Hypersensitivity to pyrazinamide or any component of the formulation; acute gout; severe hepatic damage
Warnings/Precautions Administer with at least one other effective agent for tuberculosis; use with caution in patients with renal failure, chronic gout, diabetes mellitus, or porphyria. Use with caution in patients receiving concurrent medications associated with hepatotoxicity (particularly with rifampin), or in patients with a history of alcoholism (even if ethanol consumption is discontinued during therapy).
Drug Interactions
    Increased Effect/Toxicity: Combination therapy with rifampin and pyrazinamide has been associated with severe and fatal hepatotoxic reactions.
Lab Interactions Reacts with Acetest® and Ketostix® to produce pinkish-brown color.
Adverse Reactions 1% to 10%:
    Central nervous system: Malaise
    Gastrointestinal: Nausea, vomiting, anorexia
    Neuromuscular & skeletal: Arthralgia, myalgia
Overdosage/Toxicology Symptoms of overdose include gout, gastric upset, and hepatic damage (mild). Treatment is supportive.
Pharmacodynamics/Kinetics
    Absorption: Well absorbed
    Time to Peak: Serum: Within 2 hours
    Protein Binding: 50%
    Half-Life Elimination: 9-10 hours
    Metabolism: Hepatic
    Excretion: Urine (4% as unchanged drug)
    Pharmacokinetic Note: Bacteriostatic or bactericidal depending on drug's concentration at infection site.
Dosing
    Adults:
        Tuberculosis treatment: Oral (dosing is based on lean body weight):
            Daily therapy: 15-30 mg/kg/day
                40-55 kg: 1000 mg
                56-75 kg: 1500 mg
                76-90 kg: 2000 mg (maximum dose regardless of weight)
            Twice weekly directly observed therapy (DOT): 50 mg/kg
                40-55 kg: 2000 mg
                56-75 kg: 3000 mg
                76-90 kg: 4000 mg (maximum dose regardless of weight)
            Three times/week DOT: 25-30 mg/kg (maximum: 2.5 g)
                40-55 kg: 1500 mg
                56-75 kg: 2500 mg
                76-90 kg: 3000 mg (maximum dose regardless of weight)
        Note: Used as part of a multidrug regimen. Treatment regimens consist of an initial 2-month phase, followed by a continuation phase of 4 or 7 additional months; frequency of dosing may differ depending on phase of therapy.
    Elderly: Start with a lower daily dose (15 mg/kg) and increase as tolerated.
    Pediatrics:
        Tuberculosis treatment: Oral:
            Daily therapy: 15-30 mg/kg/day (maximum: 2 g/day)
            Twice weekly directly observed therapy (DOT): 50 mg/kg/dose (maximum: 4 g/dose)
        See "Note" in adult dosing.
    Renal Impairment:
        Cl$_{cr}$ <50 mL/minute: Avoid use or reduce dose to 12-20 mg/kg/day.
        Avoid use in hemo- and peritoneal dialysis as well as continuous arteriovenous or venovenous hemofiltration.

Hepatic Impairment: Reduce dose.

Available Dosage Forms Tablet: 500 mg

Monitoring and Teaching Issues

Physical Assessment: Use caution in presence of renal failure, chronic gout, diabetes mellitus, porphyria, or history of alcoholism (see Warnings/Precautions). Avoid combination with other pharmacological agents associated with hepatotoxicity, especially concurrent use with rifampin (see Drug Interactions). Schedule and assess results of laboratory tests and chest x-ray regularly. Teach patient proper use and necessity of scheduled laboratory tests, possible side effects/appropriate interventions, and adverse symptoms to report (see Patient Education).

Monitoring Laboratory Tests: Periodic liver function, serum uric acid, sputum culture, chest x-ray 2-3 months into treatment and at completion

Patient Education: Take as directed, with food. It is imperative to take for full length of therapy; do not miss doses and do not discontinue without consulting prescriber. You will need regular medical follow-up and laboratory tests while taking this medication. May cause nausea or loss of appetite (small frequent meals, frequent mouth care, sucking lozenges, or chewing gum may help). Report change in color of urine, pale stools, easy bruising or bleeding, blood in urine or difficulty urinating, yellowing of skin or eyes, extreme joint pain, unusual fever, or unresolved nausea or vomiting, **Pregnancy precaution:** Inform prescriber if you are or intend to become pregnant.

Geriatric Considerations: Pyrazinamide is used in the 2-month intensive treatment phase of a 6-month treatment plan. Most elderly acquired their *Mycobacterium tuberculosis* infection before effective chemotherapy was available; however, older persons with new infections (not reactivation), or who are from areas where drug-resistant *M. tuberculosis* is endemic, or who are HIV-infected should receive 3-4 drug therapies including pyrazinamide.

Pregnancy Risk Factor: C

Lactation: Enters breast milk

Related Information

Tuberculosis *on page 1864*

♦ **Pyrazinamide, Rifampin, and Isoniazid** *see* Rifampin, Isoniazid, and Pyrazinamide *on page 1326*

♦ **Pyrazinoic Acid Amide** *see* Pyrazinamide *on page 1286*

♦ **Pyridium®** *see* Phenazopyridine *on page 1193*

Pyridostigmine (peer id oh STIG meen)

U.S. Brand Names Mestinon®; Mestinon® Timespan®; Regonol®

Synonyms Pyridostigmine Bromide

Generic Available Yes: Tablet

Pharmacologic Category Acetylcholinesterase Inhibitor

Medication Safety Issues

Sound-alike/look-alike issues:

Pyridostigmine may be confused with physostigmine

Mestinon® may be confused with Metatensin®

Regonol® may be confused with Reglan®, Renagel®

Use Symptomatic treatment of myasthenia gravis; antidote for nondepolarizing neuromuscular blockers

Military use: Pretreatment for Soman nerve gas exposure

Mechanism of Action/Effect Inhibits destruction of acetylcholine by acetylcholinesterase which facilitates transmission of impulses across myoneural junction

Contraindications Hypersensitivity to pyridostigmine, bromides, or any component of the formulation; GI or GU obstruction

Warnings/Precautions Use with caution in patients with epilepsy, asthma, bradycardia, hyperthyroidism, cardiac arrhythmias, or peptic ulcer. Use with caution in renal impairment (lower dosages may be required). Adequate facilities should be available for cardiopulmonary resuscitation when testing and adjusting dose for myasthenia gravis. Have atropine and epinephrine ready to treat hypersensitivity reactions. Overdosage may result in cholinergic crisis, this must be distinguished from myasthenic crisis. Anticholinesterase insensitivity can develop for brief or prolonged periods. Safety and efficacy in pediatric patients have not been established. Regonol® injection contains 1% benzyl alcohol as the preservative (not intended for use in newborns).

Drug Interactions

Decreased Effect: Neuromuscular blockade reversal effect of pyridostigmine may be decreased by aminoglycosides, quinolones, tetracyclines, bacitracin, colistin, polymyxin B, sodium colistimethate, quinidine, elevated serum magnesium concentrations.

Increased Effect/Toxicity: Increased effect of depolarizing neuromuscular blockers (succinylcholine). Increased toxicity with edrophonium. Increased bradycardia/hypotension with beta-blockers.

Lab Interactions Increased aminotransferase [ALT (SGPT)/AST (SGOT)] (S), amylase (S)

Adverse Reactions Frequency not defined.

Cardiovascular: Arrhythmias (especially bradycardia), hypotension, decreased carbon monoxide, tachycardia, AV block, nodal rhythm, nonspecific ECG changes, cardiac arrest, syncope, flushing

Central nervous system: Convulsions, dysarthria, dysphonia, dizziness, loss of consciousness, drowsiness, headache

Dermatologic: Skin rash, thrombophlebitis (I.V.), urticaria

Gastrointestinal: Hyperperistalsis, nausea, vomiting, salivation, diarrhea, stomach cramps, dysphagia, flatulence, abdominal pain

Genitourinary: Urinary urgency

Neuromuscular & skeletal: Weakness, fasciculations, muscle cramps, spasms, arthralgia, myalgia

Ocular: Small pupils, lacrimation, amblyopia

(Continued)

Pyridostigmine *(Continued)*

Respiratory: Increased bronchial secretions, laryngospasm, bronchiolar constriction, respiratory muscle paralysis, dyspnea, respiratory depression, respiratory arrest, bronchospasm

Miscellaneous: Diaphoresis (increased), anaphylaxis, allergic reactions

Overdosage/Toxicology Symptoms of overdose include muscle weakness, blurred vision, excessive sweating, tearing and salivation, nausea, vomiting, diarrhea, hypertension, bradycardia, and paralysis. Atropine is the treatment of choice for intoxications manifesting significant muscarinic symptoms. Atropine I.V. 2-4 mg every 3-60 minutes should be repeated to control symptoms and then continued as needed for 1-2 days following acute ingestion. Monitor cardiac function and support ventilation.

Pharmacodynamics/Kinetics

Onset of Action: Oral, I.M.: 15-30 minutes; I.V. injection: 2-5 minutes

Duration of Action: Oral: Up to 6-8 hours (due to slow absorption); I.V.: 2-3 hours

Absorption: Oral: Very poor (10% to 20%)

Bioavailability: 10% to 20%

Half-Life Elimination: 1-2 hours; Renal failure: ≤6 hours

Metabolism: Hepatic

Excretion: Urine (80% to 90% as unchanged drug)

Dosing

Adults & Elderly:

Myasthenia gravis:

Oral: Highly individualized dosing ranges: 60-1500 mg/day, usually 600 mg/day divided into 5-6 doses, spaced to provide maximum relief

Sustained release formulation: Highly individualized dosing ranges: 180-540 mg once or twice daily (doses separated by at least 6 hours); **Note:** Most clinicians reserve sustained release dosage form for bedtime dose only.

I.M. or slow I.V. Push: To supplement oral dosage pre- and postoperatively during labor and postpartum, during myasthenic crisis, or when oral therapy is impractical): ~1/30th of oral dose; observe patient closely for cholinergic reactions

I.V. infusion: To supplement oral dosage pre- and postoperatively, during labor and postpartum, during myasthenic crisis, or when oral therapy is impractical): Initial: 2 mg/hour with gradual titration in increments of 0.5-1 mg/hour, up to a maximum rate of 4 mg/hour

Pretreatment for Soman nerve gas exposure (military use): Oral: 30 mg every 8 hours beginning several hours prior to exposure; discontinue at first sign of nerve agent exposure, then begin atropine and pralidoxime

Reversal of nondepolarizing muscle relaxants: I.V.: 0.1-0.25 mg/kg/dose; 10-20 mg is usually sufficient* (Full recovery usually occurs ≤15 minutes, but ≥30 minutes may be required).

Note: Atropine sulfate (0.6-1.2 mg) I.V. immediately prior to pyridostigmine to minimize side effects:

Pediatrics:

Myasthenia gravis:

Oral: Children: 7 mg/kg/24 hours divided into 5-6 doses. Most clinicians reserve sustained release dosage form for bedtime dose only.

I.M., slow I.V. push: Children: 0.05-0.15 mg/kg/dose

Reversal of nondepolarizing muscle relaxants: I.V.: Children: Dosing range: 0.1-0.25 mg/kg/dose*

Note: Atropine sulfate (0.6-1.2 mg) I.V. immediately prior to pyridostigmine to minimize side effects:

Renal Impairment: Lower dosages may be required due to prolonged elimination; no specific recommendations have been published.

Available Dosage Forms

Injection, solution, as bromide:

Mestinon®: 5 mg/mL (2 mL)

Regonol®: 5 mg/mL (2 mL) [contains benzyl alcohol]

Syrup, as bromide (Mestinon®): 60 mg/5 mL (480 mL) [raspberry flavor; contains alcohol 5%, sodium benzoate]

Tablet, as bromide (Mestinon®): 60 mg

Tablet, sustained release, as bromide (Mestinon® Timespan®): 180 mg

Monitoring and Teaching Issues

Physical Assessment: When used to reverse neuromuscular block (anesthesia or excessive acetylcholine), monitor patient safety until full return of neuromuscular functioning. Assess bladder and sphincter adequacy prior to administering medication. Monitor therapeutic effectiveness and adverse reactions (eg, cholinergic crisis). Assess knowledge/teach patient appropriate use (self-injections, oral), interventions to reduce side effects, and adverse symptoms to report.

Patient Education: This drug will not cure myasthenia gravis, but may help reduce symptoms. Use as directed; do not increase dose or discontinue without consulting prescriber. Take extended release tablets at bedtime; do not chew or crush extended release tablets. Maintain adequate hydration (2-3 L/day of fluids) unless instructed to restrict fluid intake. May cause dizziness, drowsiness, or hypotension (rise slowly from sitting or lying position and use caution when driving or climbing stairs); vomiting or loss of appetite (small frequent meals, frequent mouth care, chewing gum, or sucking lozenges may help); or diarrhea (boiled milk, yogurt, or buttermilk may help). Report persistent abdominal discomfort; significantly increased salivation, sweating, tearing, or urination; flushed skin; chest pain or palpitations; acute headache; unresolved diarrhea; excessive fatigue, insomnia, dizziness, or depression; increased muscle, joint, or body pain; vision changes or blurred vision; or shortness of breath or wheezing.

Geriatric Considerations: See Warnings/Precautions and Adverse Reactions.

Pregnancy Risk Factor: B

Pregnancy Issues: Safety has not been established for use during pregnancy. The potential benefit to the mother should outweigh the potential risk to the fetus. When pyridostigmine is needed in myasthenic mothers, giving dose parenterally 1 hour before completion of the second stage of labor may facilitate delivery and protect the neonate during the immediate postnatal state.

Lactation: Enters breast milk/compatible

Breast-Feeding Issues: Neonates of myasthenia gravis mothers may have difficulty in sucking and swallowing (as well as breathing). Neonatal pyridostigmine may be indicated by symptoms (confirmed by edrophonium test).

Administration

Oral: Do **not** crush sustained release tablet.

Storage:

Injection: Protect from light.

Tablet:

30 mg: Store under refrigeration at 2°C to 8°C (36°F to 46°F) and protect from light. Stable at room temperature for up to 3 months.

Mestinon®: Store at 25°C (77°F). Protect from moisture.

♦ Pyridostigmine Bromide see Pyridostigmine on page 1287

Pyridoxine (peer i DOKS een)

U.S. Brand Names Aminoxin® [OTC]

Synonyms Pyridoxine Hydrochloride; Vitamin B₆

Generic Available Yes

Pharmacologic Category Vitamin, Water Soluble

Medication Safety Issues

Sound-alike/look-alike issues:

Pyridoxine may be confused with paroxetine, pralidoxime, Pyridium®

Use Prevention and treatment of vitamin B_6 deficiency, pyridoxine-dependent seizures in infants; adjunct to treatment of acute toxicity from isoniazid, cycloserine, or hydralazine overdose

Mechanism of Action/Effect Precursor to pyridoxal, which functions in the metabolism of proteins, carbohydrates, and fats; pyridoxal also aids in the release of liver and muscle-stored glycogen and in the synthesis of GABA (within the central nervous system) and heme

Contraindications Hypersensitivity to pyridoxine or any component of the formulation

Warnings/Precautions Dependence and withdrawal may occur with doses >200 mg/day.

Drug Interactions

Decreased Effect: Pyridoxine may decrease serum levels of levodopa, phenobarbital, and phenytoin (patients taking levodopa without carbidopa should avoid supplemental vitamin B_6 >5 mg per day, which includes multivitamin preparations).

Lab Interactions Urobilinogen

Adverse Reactions Frequency not defined.

Central nervous system: Headache, seizure (following very large I.V. doses), sensory neuropathy

Endocrine & metabolic: Decreased serum folic acid secretions

Gastrointestinal: Nausea

Hepatic: Increased AST

Neuromuscular & skeletal: Paresthesia

Miscellaneous: Allergic reactions

Overdosage/Toxicology Symptoms of overdose include ataxia and sensory neuropathy with doses of 50 mg to 2 g daily over prolonged periods.

Pharmacodynamics/Kinetics

Absorption: Enteral, parenteral: Well absorbed

Half-Life Elimination: 15-20 days

Metabolism: Via 4-pyridoxic acid (active form) and other metabolites

Excretion: Urine

Dosing

Adults & Elderly:

Recommended daily allowance (RDA):

Male: 1.7-2.0 mg

Female: 1.4-1.6 mg

Dietary deficiency: Oral: 10-20 mg/day for 3 weeks

Drug-induced neuritis (eg, isoniazid, hydralazine, penicillamine, cycloserine): Oral:

Treatment: 100-200 mg/24 hours

Prophylaxis: 25-100 mg/24 hours

Treatment of seizures and/or coma from acute isoniazid toxicity: A dose of pyridoxine hydrochloride equal to the amount of INH ingested can be given I.M./I.V. in divided doses together with other anticonvulsants; if the amount INH ingested is not known, administer 5 g I.V. pyridoxine.

Treatment of acute hydralazine toxicity: A pyridoxine dose of 25 mg/kg in divided doses I.M./I.V. has been used.

Pediatrics:

Recommended daily allowance (RDA):

1-3 years: 0.9 mg

4-6 years: 1.3 mg

7-10 years: 1.6 mg

Pyridoxine-dependent Infants:

Oral: 2-100 mg/day

I.M., I.V., SubQ: 10-100 mg

Dietary deficiency: Oral: Children: 5-25 mg/24 hours for 3 weeks, then 1.5-2.5 mg/day in multiple vitamin product

(Continued)

Pyridoxine *(Continued)*

Drug-induced neuritis (eg, isoniazid, hydralazine, penicillamine, cycloserine): Oral: Children:
Treatment: 10-50 mg/24 hours
Prophylaxis: 1-2 mg/kg/24 hours

Treatment of seizures and/or coma from acute isoniazid toxicity: A dose of pyridoxine hydrochloride equal to the amount of INH ingested can be given I.M./I.V. in divided doses together with other anticonvulsants. If the amount INH ingested is not known, administer 5 g I.V. pyridoxine.

Treatment of acute hydralazine toxicity; A pyridoxine dose of 25 mg/kg in divided doses I.M./I.V. has been used.

Available Dosage Forms
Capsule, as hydrochloride: 250 mg
Injection, solution, as hydrochloride: 100 mg/mL (1 mL)
Tablet, as hydrochloride: 25 mg, 50 mg, 100 mg, 250 mg, 500 mg
Tablet, enteric coated, as hydrochloride (Aminoxin®): 20 mg

Monitoring and Teaching Issues
Physical Assessment: Assess effectiveness and interactions of other medications patient may be taking. Monitor effectiveness of therapy and adverse effects at beginning of therapy and regularly with long-term use. Assess knowledge/teach patient appropriate use, dietary instructions, interventions to reduce side effects, and adverse symptoms to report.

Patient Education: Take exactly as directed. Do not take more than recommended. Do not exceed recommended intake of dietary B₆ (eg, red meat, bananas, potatoes, yeast, lima beans, and whole grain cereals). You may experience burning or pain at injection site; notify prescriber if this persists. **Pregnancy precaution:** Inform prescriber if you are pregnant.

Geriatric Considerations: Use with caution in patients with Parkinson's disease treated with levodopa.

Pregnancy Risk Factor: A/C (dose exceeding RDA recommendation)

Lactation: Enters breast milk/compatible

Breast-Feeding Issues: Crosses into breast milk; possible inhibition of lactation at doses >600 mg/day. AAP considers **compatible** with breast-feeding.

Administration
I.M.: Burning may occur at the injection site after I.M. or SubQ administration.
I.V.: Seizures have occurred following I.V. administration of very large doses.
Compatibility: Stable in fat emulsion 10%
Storage: Protect from light.

Related Information
Anticonvulsants By Seizure Type *on page 1712*

♦ **Pyridoxine Hydrochloride** *see* Pyridoxine *on page 1289*
♦ **Pyrilafen Tannate** *see* Phenylephrine and Pyrilamine *on page 1202*
♦ **Pyrilamine Maleate, Dextromethorphan Hydrobromide, and Phenylephrine Hydrochloride** *see* Phenylephrine, Pyrilamine, and Dextromethorphan *on page 1204*
♦ **Pyrilamine Tannate and Phenylephrine Tannate** *see* Phenylephrine and Pyrilamine *on page 1202*

Pyrimethamine *(peer i METH a meen)*

U.S. Brand Names Daraprim®

Generic Available No

Pharmacologic Category Antimalarial Agent

Medication Safety Issues
Sound-alike/look-alike issues:
Daraprim® may be confused with Dantrium®, Daranide®

Use Prophylaxis of malaria due to susceptible strains of plasmodia; used in conjunction with quinine and sulfadiazine for the treatment of uncomplicated attacks of chloroquine-resistant *P. falciparum* malaria; used in conjunction with fast-acting schizonticide to initiate transmission control and suppression cure; synergistic combination with sulfonamide in treatment of toxoplasmosis

Mechanism of Action/Effect Inhibits parasitic dihydrofolate reductase, resulting in inhibition of vital tetrahydrofolic acid synthesis

Contraindications Hypersensitivity to pyrimethamine or any component of the formulation; chloroguanide; resistant malaria; megaloblastic anemia secondary to folate deficiency

Warnings/Precautions When used for more than 3-4 days, it may be advisable to give leucovorin to prevent hematologic complications. Use with caution in patients with impaired renal or hepatic function or with possible G6PD. Use caution in patients with seizure disorders or possible folate deficiency (eg, malabsorption syndrome, pregnancy, alcoholism).

Drug Interactions
Cytochrome P450 Effect: Inhibits CYP2C8/9 (moderate), 2D6 (moderate)
Decreased Effect: Pyrimethamine may decrease the levels/effects of CYP2D6 prodrug substrates (eg, codeine, hydrocodone, oxycodone, tramadol).
Increased Effect/Toxicity: Serum levels of antipsychotic agents may be increased by pyrimethamine. Sulfonamides (synergy), methotrexate, TMP/SMZ, and zidovudine may increase the risk of bone marrow suppression. Pyrimethamine may increase the levels/effects of amiodarone, amphetamines, selected beta-blockers, dextromethorphan, fluoxetine, glimepiride, glipizide, lidocaine, mirtazapine, nateglinide, nefazodone, paroxetine, phenytoin, pioglitazone, risperidone, ritonavir, rosiglitazone, sertraline, thioridazine, tricyclic antidepressants, venlafaxine, warfarin, and other CYP2C8/9 or 2D6 substrates.

Adverse Reactions Frequency not defined.
Cardiovascular: Arrhythmias (large doses)
Central nervous system: Depression, fever, insomnia, lightheadedness, malaise, seizure

Dermatologic: Abnormal skin pigmentation, dermatitis, erythema multiforme, rash, Stevens-Johnson syndrome, toxic epidermal necrolysis

Gastrointestinal: Anorexia, abdominal cramps, vomiting, diarrhea, xerostomia, atrophic glossitis

Genitourinary: Hematuria

Hematologic: Megaloblastic anemia, leukopenia, pancytopenia, thrombocytopenia, pulmonary eosinophilia

Miscellaneous: Anaphylaxis

Overdosage/Toxicology Symptoms of overdose include megaloblastic anemia, leukopenia, thrombocytopenia, anorexia, CNS stimulation, seizures, nausea, vomiting, and hematemesis. Following GI decontamination, leucovorin should be administered in an I.M. or I.V. dosage of 5-15 mg/day or orally for 5-7 days, or as required to reverse symptoms of folic acid deficiency. Provide other supportive treatment as required.

Pharmacodynamics/Kinetics

Onset of Action: ~1 hour

Absorption: Well absorbed

Time to Peak: Serum: 1.5-8 hours

Protein Binding: 80% to 87%

Half-Life Elimination: 80-95 hours

Metabolism: Hepatic

Excretion: Urine (20% to 30% as unchanged drug)

Dosing

Adults & Elderly:

Malaria chemoprophylaxis (for areas of chloroquine-resistant *P. falciparum*): Oral: Begin prophylaxis 2 weeks before entering endemic area: 25 mg once weekly. Dosage should be continued for all age groups for at least 6-10 weeks after leaving endemic areas

Chloroquine-resistant *P. falciparum* malaria (when used in conjunction with quinine and sulfadiazine): Oral: 25 mg twice daily for 3 days

Toxoplasmosis: Oral: 50-75 mg/day together with 1-4 g of a sulfonamide for 1-3 weeks depending on patient's tolerance and response, then reduce dose by 50% and continue for 4-5 weeks **or** 25-50 mg/day for 3-4 weeks

Prophylaxis for first episode of *Toxoplasma gondii*: Oral: 50 mg once weekly with dapsone, plus oral folinic acid 25 mg once weekly

Prophylaxis to prevent recurrence of *Toxoplasma gondii*: Oral: 25-50 mg once daily in combination with sulfadiazine or clindamycin, plus oral folinic acid 10-25 mg daily. Atovaquone plus oral folinic acid 10 mg daily has also been used in combination with pyrimethamine.

Pediatrics:

Malaria chemoprophylaxis (for areas with chloroquine-resistant *P. falciparum*): Oral: Begin prophylaxis 2 weeks before entering endemic area:

Children: 0.5 mg/kg once weekly, not to exceed 25 mg/dose

or

<4 years: 6.25 mg once weekly

4-10 years: 12.5 mg once weekly

Children >10 years: Refer to adult dosing

Note: Dosage should be continued for all age groups for at least 6-10 weeks after leaving endemic areas.

Chloroquine-resistant *P. falciparum* malaria (when used in conjunction with quinine and sulfadiazine): Oral:

Children:

<10 kg: 6.25 mg/day once daily for 3 days

10-20 kg: 12.5 mg/day once daily for 3 days

20-40 kg: 25 mg/day once daily for 3 days

Toxoplasmosis:

Infants (congenital toxoplasmosis): Oral: 1 mg/kg once daily for 6 months with sulfadiazine then every other month with sulfa, alternating with spiramycin.

Children: Loading dose: 2 mg/kg/day divided into 2 equal daily doses for 1-3 days (maximum: 100 mg/day) followed by 1 mg/kg/day divided into 2 doses for 4 weeks; maximum: 25 mg/day

With sulfadiazine or trisulfapyrimidines: 2 mg/kg/day divided every 12 hours for 3 days, followed by 1 mg/kg/day once daily or divided twice daily for 4 weeks given with trisulfapyrimidines or sulfadiazine

Prophylaxis for first episode of *Toxoplasma gondii*: Oral:

Children ≥1 month of age: 1 mg/kg/day once daily with dapsone, plus oral folinic acid 5 mg every 3 days

Adolescents: Refer to adult dosing.

Prophylaxis to prevent recurrence of *Toxoplasma gondii*: Oral:

Children ≥1 month of age: 1 mg/kg/day once daily given with sulfadiazine or clindamycin, plus oral folinic acid 5 mg every 3 days

Adolescents: Refer to adult dosing.

Available Dosage Forms Tablet: 25 mg

Monitoring and Teaching Issues

Physical Assessment: See Warnings/Precautions for specific use cautions (eg, concurrent use of leucovorin to prevent hematologic complications). Assess potential for interactions with other pharmacological agents patient may be taking (eg, increased potential for toxicities; see Drug Interactions). Assess results of laboratory tests, effectiveness according to purpose for use, and adverse reactions periodically during therapy (eg, arrhythmias, rash, GI disturbance, hematuria, megaloblastic anemia; see Adverse Reactions). Teach patient appropriate use, possible side effects/interventions, and adverse symptoms to report (see Patient Education).

Monitoring Laboratory Tests: CBC, including platelet counts twice weekly; liver and renal function

(Continued)

Pyrimethamine *(Continued)*

Patient Education: Do not take any new medication during therapy unless approved by prescriber. Take with meals. Tablets may be crushed to prepare oral suspensions of the drug in water, cherry syrup, or sucrose-containing solutions at a concentration of 1 mg/mL of liquid. It is important to complete full course of therapy for full effect. Regular blood tests will be necessary during therapy. If used for prophylaxis, consult with prescriber in order to begin 2 weeks before traveling to endemic areas, continue during travel period, and for 6-10 weeks following return. May cause GI distress or loss of appetite (small frequent meals, frequent mouth care, sucking lozenges, or chewing gum may help); dizziness, lightheadedness, insomnia, or changes in mentation (use caution when driving or with tasks that require alertness until response to drug is known); or changes in skin pigmentation or rash. Report persistent GI disturbance (nausea, vomiting, diarrhea, cramping); chest pain or palpitation; unusual fatigue, easy bruising, bleeding, or bloody emesis; or other adverse reactions. **Pregnancy/breast-feeding precautions:** Inform prescriber if you are or intend to become pregnant. Consult prescriber if breast-feeding.

Pregnancy Risk Factor: C

Pregnancy Issues: There are no adequate or well-controlled studies in pregnant women. If administered during pregnancy (ie, for toxoplasmosis), supplementation of folate (or folinic acid) is strongly recommended (5 mg/day). Pregnancy should be avoided during therapy.

Lactation: Enters breast milk/not recommended (AAP rates "compatible")

Breast-Feeding Issues: Pyrimethamine enters breast milk and may result in significant systemic concentrations in breast-fed infants. AAP rates as "compatible" (although the manufacturer does not recommend its use during breast-feeding). The effect of concurrent therapy with sulfonamide or dapsone (frequently used with pyrimethamine as combination treatment) must be considered.

Administration

Oral: Administer with meals to minimize GI distress.

Storage: Store at 15°C to 25°C (59°F to 77°F). Protect from light.

Additional Information Leucovorin may be administered in a dosage of 3-9 mg/day for 3 days or 5 mg every 3 days or as required to reverse symptoms of or to prevent hematologic problems due to folic acid deficiency

♦ Q-Tussin [OTC] *see* Guaifenesin *on page 729*

♦ Quelicin® *see* Succinylcholine *on page 1400*

♦ Quelicin® Injection *see page 1625*

♦ Questran® *see* Cholestyramine Resin *on page 316*

♦ Questran® Light *see* Cholestyramine Resin *on page 316*

Quetiapine *(kwe TYE a peen)*

U.S. Brand Names Seroquel®

Synonyms Quetiapine Fumarate

Generic Available No

Pharmacologic Category Antipsychotic Agent, Atypical

Medication Safety Issues

Sound-alike/look-alike issues:

Seroquel® may be confused with Serentil®, Serzone®, Sinequan®

Use Treatment of schizophrenia; treatment of acute manic episodes associated with bipolar disorder (as monotherapy or in combination with lithium or valproate)

Unlabeled/Investigational Use Autism, psychosis (children)

Mechanism of Action/Effect Mechanism of action of quetiapine (dibenzothiazepine antipsychotic), as with other antipsychotic drugs, is unknown. However, it has been proposed that this drug's antipsychotic activity is mediated through a combination of dopamine type 2 and serotonin type 2 antagonism.

Antagonism at receptors other than dopamine and 5-HT$_2$ with similar receptor affinities may explain some of the other effects of quetiapine. The drug's antagonism of histamine H$_1$-receptors may explain the somnolence observed with it. The drug's antagonism of adrenergic alpha$_1$-receptors may explain the orthostatic hypotension observed with it.

Contraindications Hypersensitivity to quetiapine or any component of the formulation; severe CNS depression; bone marrow suppression; blood dyscrasias; severe hepatic disease, coma

Warnings/Precautions Patients with dementia-related behavioral disorders treated with atypical antipsychotics are at an increased risk of death compared to placebo. Quetiapine is not approved for this indication.

May be sedating, use with caution in disorders where CNS depression is a feature. Use with caution in Parkinson's disease. May cause orthostatic hypotension; use caution in patients predisposed to hypotension or with hemodynamic instability; prior myocardial infarction, cerebrovascular disease or ischemic heart disease. Caution in patients with hypercholesterolemia; thyroid disease; predisposition to seizures; subcortical brain damage; hepatic impairment; or severe cardiac, renal, or respiratory disease. May alter temperature regulation or mask toxicity of other drugs due to antiemetic effects. May alter cardiac conduction - life-threatening arrhythmias have occurred with therapeutic doses of neuroleptics.

Due to anticholinergic effects, use with caution in patients with decreased gastrointestinal motility, urinary retention, BPH, xerostomia, visual problems, narrow-angle glaucoma (screening is recommended), and myasthenia gravis. Relative to other antipsychotics, quetiapine has a moderate potency of cholinergic blockade. Risk of neuroleptic malignant syndrome, extrapyramidal symptoms or tardive dyskinesias appears to be very low relative to other antipsychotics. May cause hyperglycemia; in some cases may be extreme and associated with ketoacidosis, hyperosmolar coma, or death. Use with caution in patients with diabetes or other disorders of glucose regulation; monitor for worsening of glucose control.

Has been noted to cause cataracts in animals, lens examination on initiation of therapy and every 6 months is recommended.

The possibility of a suicide attempt is inherent in psychotic illness or bipolar disorder; use caution in high-risk patients during initiation of therapy. Prescriptions should be written for the smallest quantity consistent with good patient care.

Drug Interactions

Cytochrome P450 Effect: Substrate of CYP2D6 (minor), 3A4 (major)

Decreased Effect: Thioridazine increases quetiapine's clearance (by 65%), decreasing serum levels. CYP3A4 inducers may decrease the levels/effects of quetiapine. Example inducers include aminoglutethimide, carbamazepine, nafcillin, nevirapine, phenobarbital, phenytoin, and rifamycins.

Increased Effect/Toxicity: Quetiapine increases levels of lorazepam. The effects of other centrally-acting drugs, sedatives, or ethanol may be potentiated by quetiapine. Quetiapine may enhance the effects of antihypertensive agents. CYP3A4 inhibitors may increase the levels/effects of quetiapine; example inhibitors include azole antifungals, ciprofloxacin, clarithromycin, diclofenac, doxycycline, erythromycin, imatinib, isoniazid, nefazodone, nicardipine, propofol, protease inhibitors, quinidine, and verapamil; ketoconazole increased serum concentrations of quetiapine by 335%. Concomitant use of quetiapine and divalproex increased the mean maximum plasma concentration of quetiapine at by 17% at steady state (the mean oral clearance of valproic acid was increased by 11%). Cimetidine increases blood levels of quetiapine (quetiapine's clearance is reduced by 20%). Metoclopramide may increase risk of extrapyramidal symptoms (EPS).

Nutritional/Ethanol Interactions

Ethanol: Avoid ethanol (may cause excessive impairment in cognition/motor function).

Food: In healthy volunteers, administration of quetiapine with food resulted in an increase in the peak serum concentration and AUC (each by ~15%) compared to the fasting state.

Herb/Nutraceutical: St John's wort may decrease quetiapine levels. Avoid valerian, St John's wort, kava kava, gotu kola (may increase CNS depression).

Adverse Reactions

>10%:
Central nervous system: Agitation, dizziness, headache, somnolence
Endocrine & metabolic: Cholesterol increased (11%), triglycerides increased (17%)
Gastrointestinal: Weight gain (≥7% body weight, dose related), xerostomia

1% to 10%:
Cardiovascular: Postural hypotension, tachycardia, palpitation, peripheral edema
Central nervous system: Anxiety, fever, pain
Dermatologic: Rash
Gastrointestinal: Abdominal pain (dose related), constipation, dyspepsia (dose related), anorexia, vomiting, gastroenteritis
Hematologic: Leukopenia
Hepatic: AST increased, ALT increased, GGT increased
Neuromuscular & skeletal: Dysarthria, back pain, weakness, tremor, hypertonia, dysarthria
Ocular: Amblyopia
Respiratory: Rhinitis, pharyngitis, cough, dyspnea
Miscellaneous: Diaphoresis, flu-like syndrome

Pharmacodynamics/Kinetics

Absorption: Rapidly absorbed following oral administration
Bioavailability: 9% ± 4%; tablet is 100% bioavailable relative to solution
Time to Peak: Plasma: 1.5 hours
Protein Binding: Plasma: 83%
Half-Life Elimination: Mean: Terminal: ~6 hours
Metabolism: Primarily hepatic; via CYP3A4; forms two inactive metabolites
Excretion: Urine (73% as metabolites, <1% as unchanged drug); feces (20%)

Dosing

Adults:

Schizophrenia/psychosis: Oral: 25-100 mg 2-3 times/day; usual starting dose 25 mg twice daily, increased in increments of 25-50 mg 2-3 times/day on the second or third day. By the fourth day, the dose should be in the range of 300-400 mg/day in 2-3 divided doses. Further adjustments may be made, as needed, at intervals of at least 2 days in adjustments of 25-50 mg twice daily. Usual maintenance range: 150-750 mg/day.

Mania: Oral: Initial: 50 mg twice daily on day 1, increase dose in increments of 100 mg/day to 200 mg twice daily on day 4; may increase to a target dose of 800 mg/day by day 6 at increments of ≤200 mg/day. Usual dosage range: 400-800 mg/day

Note: Dose reductions should be attempted periodically to establish lowest effective dose in patients with psychosis or to establish need to continue treating agitated symptoms in demented older adults. Patients being restarted after 1 week of no drug need to be titrated as above.

Elderly: Lower clearance in elderly patients (40%), resulting in higher concentrations. Dosage adjustment may be required.

Pediatrics: Children and Adolescents:

Autism (unlabeled use): Oral: 100-350 mg/day (1.6-5.2 mg/kg/day)

Psychosis and mania (unlabeled use): Oral: Initial: 25 mg twice daily; titrate as necessary to 450 mg/day

Renal Impairment: No dosage adjustment required: 25% lower mean oral clearance of quetiapine than normal subjects; however, plasma concentrations similar to normal subjects receiving the same dose.

Hepatic Impairment: Lower clearance in hepatic impairment (30%), may result in higher concentrations. Dosage adjustment may be required.
Oral: Initial: 25 mg/day, increase dose by 25-50 mg/day to effective dose, based on clinical response and tolerability to patient

Available Dosage Forms Tablet, as fumarate: 25 mg, 100 mg, 200 mg, 300 mg [contains lactose]

Monitoring and Teaching Issues

Physical Assessment: Assess other medications patient is taking for effectiveness and interactions (especially drugs affected by P450 enzymes). Assess results of laboratory (Continued)

Quetiapine *(Continued)*

tests, therapeutic effectiveness, and adverse reactions at beginning of therapy and periodically with long-term use. Evaluate for cataracts before initiating treatment and every 6 months during chronic treatment. Monitor weight prior to initiating therapy and at least monthly. Consider titrating to a different antipsychotic agent for weight gain greater than or equal to 5% of initial weight. Initiate at lower doses and taper dosage slowly when discontinuing. Assess knowledge/teach patient appropriate use, interventions to reduce side effects, and adverse symptoms to report.

Monitoring Laboratory Tests: Fasting lipid profile and fasting blood glucose/Hgb A_{1c} (prior to treatment, at 3 months, then annually)

Patient Education: Use exactly as directed; do not increase dose or frequency. It may take 2-3 weeks to achieve desired results; do not discontinue without consulting prescriber. Avoid alcohol or caffeine and other prescriptions or OTC medications not approved by prescriber. Maintain adequate hydration (2-3 L/day of fluids) unless instructed to restrict fluid intake. If diabetic, you may experience increased blood sugars. Monitor blood closely. You may experience excess drowsiness, restlessness, dizziness, or blurred vision (use caution driving or when engaging in tasks requiring alertness until response to drug is known); mouth sores or GI upset (small frequent meals, frequent mouth care, chewing gum, or sucking lozenges may help); constipation (increased exercise, fluids, fruit, or fiber may help); or postural hypotension (use caution climbing stairs or when changing position from lying or sitting to standing). Report persistent CNS effects (eg, somnolence, agitation, insomnia); severe dizziness; vision changes; respiratory difficulty; or worsening of condition. **Pregnancy/breast-feeding precautions:** Inform prescriber if you are or intend to become pregnant. Breast-feeding is not recommended.

Dietary Considerations: May be taken with or without food.

Geriatric Considerations: (See Warnings/Precautions, Adverse Reactions, and Overdose/Toxicology.) Elderly patients have an increased risk of adverse response to side effects or adverse reactions to antipsychotics.

Pregnancy Risk Factor: C

Lactation: Excretion in breast milk unknown/not recommended

Related Information
Antipsychotic Agents *on page 1717*
Antipsychotic Medication Guidelines *on page 1766*
Federal OBRA Regulations: Recommended Maximum Doses *on page 1773*

♦ **Quetiapine Fumarate** *see* Quetiapine *on page 1292*

♦ **Quibron®-T** *see* Theophylline *on page 1457*

♦ **Quibron®-T/SR** *see* Theophylline *on page 1457*

♦ **Quinaglute® Dura-Tabs® [DSC]** *see* Quinidine *on page 1296*

♦ **Quinalbarbitone Sodium** *see* Secobarbital *on page 1362*

Quinapril *(KWIN a pril)*

U.S. Brand Names Accupril®

Synonyms Quinapril Hydrochloride

Generic Available Yes

Pharmacologic Category Angiotensin-Converting Enzyme (ACE) Inhibitor

Medication Safety Issues
Sound-alike/look-alike issues:
  Accupril® may be confused with Accolate®, Accutane®, AcipHex®, Monopril®

Use Management of hypertension; treatment of congestive heart failure

Unlabeled/Investigational Use Treatment of left ventricular dysfunction after myocardial infarction

Mechanism of Action/Effect Competitive inhibitor of angiotensin-converting enzyme (ACE); prevents conversion of angiotensin I to angiotensin II, a potent vasoconstrictor; results in lower levels of angiotensin II which causes an increase in plasma renin activity and a reduction in aldosterone secretion

Contraindications Hypersensitivity to quinapril or any component of the formulation; angioedema related to previous treatment with an ACE inhibitor; bilateral renal artery stenosis; patients with idiopathic or hereditary angioedema; pregnancy (2nd and 3rd trimesters)

Warnings/Precautions Anaphylactic reactions can occur. Angioedema can occur at any time during treatment (especially following first dose). Angioedema may involve head and neck (potentially affecting the airway) or the intestine (presenting with abdominal pain). Careful blood pressure monitoring with first dose (hypotension can occur especially in volume depleted patients). Dosage adjustment needed in renal impairment. Use with caution in hypovolemia; collagen vascular diseases; valvular stenosis (particularly aortic stenosis); hyperkalemia; or before, during, or immediately after anesthesia. Avoid rapid dosage escalation, which may lead to renal insufficiency. Rare toxicities associated with ACE inhibitors include cholestatic jaundice (which may progress to hepatic necrosis) and neutropenia/agranulocytosis with myeloid hyperplasia. Hypersensitivity reactions may be seen during hemodialysis with high-flux dialysis membranes (eg, AN69). Use with caution in unilateral renal artery stenosis and pre-existing renal insufficiency. Deterioration in renal function can occur with initiation. Due to rare hepatotoxic reactions, discontinue if jaundice or marked elevation of transaminases occurs.

Drug Interactions

Decreased Effect: Quinapril may reduce the absorption of quinolones and tetracycline antibiotics. Aspirin (high dose) may reduce the therapeutic effects of ACE inhibitors; at low dosages this does not appear to be significant. Rifampin may decrease the effect of ACE inhibitors. Antacids may decrease the bioavailability of ACE inhibitors (may be more likely to occur with captopril); separate administration times by 1-2 hours. NSAIDs, specifically indomethacin, may reduce the hypotensive effects of ACE inhibitors.

Increased Effect/Toxicity: Potassium supplements, co-trimoxazole (high dose), angiotensin II receptor antagonists (eg, candesartan, losartan, irbesartan), or potassium-sparing diuretics (amiloride, spironolactone, triamterene) may result in elevated serum potassium levels when combined with quinapril. ACE inhibitor effects may be increased by phenothi- azines or probenecid (increases levels of captopril). ACE inhibitors may increase serum concentrations/effects of digoxin, lithium, and sulfonylureas.

Diuretics have additive hypotensive effects with ACE inhibitors, and hypovolemia increases the potential for adverse renal effects of ACE inhibitors. In patients with compromised renal function, coadministration with NSAIDs may result in further deterioration of renal function. Allopurinol and ACE inhibitors may cause a higher risk of hypersensitivity reaction when taken concurrently.

Nutritional/Ethanol Interactions Herb/Nutraceutical: Avoid dong quai if using for hyperten- sion (has estrogenic activity). Avoid ephedra, yohimbe, ginseng (may worsen hypertension). Avoid garlic (may have increased antihypertensive effect).

Adverse Reactions Note: Frequency ranges include data from hypertension and heart failure trials. Higher rates of adverse reactions have generally been noted in patients with CHF. However, the frequency of adverse effects associated with placebo is also increased in this population.

1% to 10%:

Cardiovascular: Hypotension (3%), chest pain (2%), first-dose hypotension (up to 3%)
Central nervous system: Dizziness (4% to 8%), headache (2% to 6%), fatigue (3%)
Dermatologic: Rash (1%)
Endocrine & metabolic: Hyperkalemia (2%)
Gastrointestinal: Vomiting/nausea (1% to 2%), diarrhea (2%)
Neuromuscular & skeletal: Myalgias (2% to 5%), back pain (1%)
Renal: Increased BUN/serum creatinine (2%, transient elevations may occur with a higher frequency), worsening of renal function (in patients with bilateral renal artery stenosis or hypovolemia)
Respiratory: Upper respiratory symptoms, cough (2% to 4%; up to 13% in some studies), dyspnea (2%)

Overdosage/Toxicology Mild hypotension has been the primary toxic effect seen with acute overdose. Bradycardia may also occur. Hyperkalemia occurs even with therapeutic doses, especially in patients with renal insufficiency and those taking NSAIDs. Treatment is symptom-directed and supportive.

Pharmacodynamics/Kinetics

Onset of Action: 1 hour

Duration of Action: 24 hours

Absorption: Quinapril: ≥60%

Time to Peak: Serum: Quinapril: 1 hour; Quinaprilat: ~2 hours

Protein Binding: Quinapril: 97%; Quinaprilat: 97%

Half-Life Elimination: Quinapril: 0.8 hours; Quinaprilat: 3 hours; increases as Cl_{cr} decreases

Metabolism: Rapidly hydrolyzed to quinaprilat, the active metabolite

Excretion: Urine (50% to 60% primarily as quinaprilat)

Dosing

Adults:

Hypertension: Oral: Initial: 10-20 mg once daily, adjust according to blood pressure response at peak and trough blood levels; initial dose may be reduced to 5 mg in patients receiving diuretic therapy if the diuretic is continued.
Usual dose range (JNC 7): 10-40 mg once daily

Congestive heart failure or post-MI: Oral: Initial: 5 mg once daily, titrated at weekly intervals to 20-40 mg daily in 2 divided doses

Elderly: Oral: Initial: 2.5-5 mg/day; increase dosage at increments of 2.5-5 mg at 1- to 2-week intervals; adjust for renal impairment.

Renal Impairment: Lower initial doses should be used; after initial dose (if tolerated), administer initial dose twice daily; may be increased at weekly intervals to optimal response:

Hypertension: Oral: Initial:
Cl_{cr} >60 mL/minute: Administer 10 mg/day
Cl_{cr} 30-60 mL/minute: Administer 5 mg/day
Cl_{cr} 10-30 mL/minute: Administer 2.5 mg/day

Congestive heart failure: Oral: Initial:
Cl_{cr} >30 mL/minute: Administer 5 mg/day
Cl_{cr} 10-30 mL/minute: Administer 2.5 mg/day

Hepatic Impairment: In patients with alcoholic cirrhosis, hydrolysis of quinapril to quinaprilat is impaired; however, the subsequent elimination of quinaprilat is unaltered.

Available Dosage Forms Tablet, as hydrochloride: 5 mg, 10 mg, 20 mg, 40 mg

Monitoring and Teaching Issues

Physical Assessment: Use caution in presence of renal impairment; hypovolemia; collagen vascular diseases; valvular stenosis; hyperkalemia; or before, during, or immedi- ately after anesthesia (see Warnings/Precautions for specific use cautions). Assess poten- tial for interactions with other pharmacological agents or herbal products patient may be taking (especially anything that may impact fluid balance or cardiac status; see Drug Interactions). May be advisable to administer first dose in prescriber's office with careful blood pressure monitoring (hypotension or angioedema can occur at any time during treatment, especially following first dose). Assess results of laboratory tests, effectiveness (blood pressure and cardiac status), and adverse response on a regular basis during therapy (eg, hypovolemia, angioedema, postural hypotension; see Adverse Reactions). Teach patient proper use, possible side effects/appropriate interventions, and adverse symptoms to report (see Patient Education).

Monitoring Laboratory Tests: CBC, renal function tests, electrolytes; if patient has renal impairment, a baseline WBC with differential and serum creatinine should be evaluated and monitored closely during the first 3 months of therapy

Patient Education: Do not take any new medication during therapy unless approved by prescriber. Take as directed; do not alter dose or discontinue without consulting prescriber.
(Continued)

Quinapril *(Continued)*

Take first dose at bedtime or when sitting down (hypotension may occur). This drug does not eliminate need for diet or exercise regimen as recommended by prescriber. May cause increased cough (if persistent or bothersome, contact prescriber); postural hypotension (use caution when rising from lying or sitting position or climbing stairs); headache (consult prescriber for approved analgesic); dizziness (use caution when driving or engaging in tasks that require alertness until response to drug is known); nausea or vomiting (small frequent meals, frequent mouth care, sucking lozenges, or chewing gum may help); or muscle or back pain (consult prescriber for approved analgesic). Report immediately any swelling of face, mouth, lips, tongue, or throat; chest pain or respiratory difficulty. Report persistent cough; persistent pain in muscles, joints, or back; skin rash; or other persistent adverse reactions. **Pregnancy/breast-feeding precautions:** Inform prescriber if you are or intend to become pregnant. This drug should not be used in the 2nd or 3rd trimester of pregnancy. Consult prescriber for appropriate contraceptive measures if necessary. Consult prescriber if breast-feeding.

Geriatric Considerations: Due to frequent decreases in glomerular filtration (also creatinine clearance) with aging, elderly patients may have exaggerated responses to ACE inhibitors. Differences in clinical response due to hepatic changes are not observed.

Pregnancy Risk Factor: C/D (2nd and 3rd trimesters)

Pregnancy Issues: ACE inhibitors can cause fetal injury or death if taken during the 2nd or 3rd trimester. Discontinue ACE inhibitors as soon as pregnancy is detected.

Lactation: Excretion in breast milk unknown

Administration

Reconstitution: Unstable in aqueous solutions. To prepare solution for oral administration, mix prior to administration and use within 10 minutes.

Storage: Store at room temperature.

Related Information

Angiotensin Agents *on page 1704*
Heart Failure *on page 1828*

Quinapril and Hydrochlorothiazide

(KWIN a pril & hye droe klor oh THYE a zide)

U.S. Brand Names Accuretic®; Quinaretic

Synonyms Hydrochlorothiazide and Quinapril

Generic Available Yes

Pharmacologic Category Angiotensin-Converting Enzyme (ACE) Inhibitor; Antihypertensive; Diuretic, Thiazide

Use Treatment of hypertension (not for initial therapy)

Dosing

Adults:

Hypertension: Oral:

Patients with inadequate response to quinapril monotherapy: Quinapril 10 mg/ hydrochlorothiazide 12.5 mg **or** quinapril 20 mg/hydrochlorothiazide 12.5 mg once daily

Patients with adequate blood pressure control on hydrochlorothiazide 25 mg/day, but significant potassium loss: Quinapril 10 mg/hydrochlorothiazide 12.5 mg **or** quinapril 20 mg/hydrochlorothiazide 12.5 mg once daily

Note: Clinical trials of quinapril/hydrochlorothiazide combinations used quinapril doses of 2.5-40 mg/day and hydrochlorothiazide doses of 6.25-25 mg/day.

Elderly: If previous response to individual components is unknown, initial dose selection should be cautious, at the low end of adult dosage range; titration should occur at 1- to 2-week intervals.

Pediatrics: Safety and efficacy have not been established.

Renal Impairment: Cl$_{cr}$ <30 mL/minute/1.73 m^2 or serum creatinine ≤3 mg/dL: Use is not recommended.

Available Dosage Forms Tablet:

10/12.5: Quinapril 10 mg and hydrochlorothiazide 12.5 mg
20/12.5: Quinapril 20 mg and hydrochlorothiazide 12.5 mg
20/25: Quinapril 20 mg and hydrochlorothiazide 25 mg

Monitoring and Teaching Issues

Physical Assessment: See individual agents.

Patient Education: See individual agents. **Pregnancy/breast-feeding precautions:** Do not get pregnant while taking this medication. Consult prescriber for appropriate contraceptive measures. Consult prescriber if breast-feeding.

Pregnancy Risk Factor: C (1st trimester); D (2nd and 3rd trimesters)

Lactation: Enters breast milk/use caution

Related Information

Hydrochlorothiazide *on page 751*
Quinapril *on page 1294*

♦ **Quinapril Hydrochloride** *see Quinapril on page 1294*

♦ **Quinaretic** *see Quinapril and Hydrochlorothiazide on page 1296*

Quinidine *(KWIN i deen)*

U.S. Brand Names Quinaglute® Dura-Tabs® [DSC]

Synonyms Quinidine Gluconate; Quinidine Polygalacturonate; Quinidine Sulfate

Generic Available Yes

Pharmacologic Category Antiarrhythmic Agent, Class Ia

Medication Safety Issues

Sound-alike/look-alike issues:
Quinidine may be confused with clonidine, quinine, Quinora®

Use Prophylaxis after cardioversion of atrial fibrillation and/or flutter to maintain normal sinus rhythm; prevent recurrence of paroxysmal supraventricular tachycardia, paroxysmal AV junctional rhythm, paroxysmal ventricular tachycardia, paroxysmal atrial fibrillation, and atrial or ventricular premature contractions; has activity against *Plasmodium falciparum* malaria

Mechanism of Action/Effect Class 1a antiarrhythmic agent; depresses phase O of the action potential; decreases myocardial excitability and conduction velocity, and myocardial contractility by decreasing sodium influx during depolarization and potassium efflux in repolarization; also reduces calcium transport across cell membrane

Contraindications Hypersensitivity to quinidine or any component of the formulation; thrombocytopenia; thrombocytopenic purpura; myasthenia gravis; heart block greater than first degree; idioventricular conduction delays (except in patients with a functioning artificial pacemaker); those adversely affected by anticholinergic activity; concurrent use of quinolone antibiotics which prolong QT interval, cisapride, amprenavir, or ritonavir

Warnings/Precautions Monitor and adjust dose to prevent excessive QT_c prolongation. May cause new or worsened arrhythmia (proarrhythmic effect). May precipitate or exacerbate CHF. Reduce dosage in hepatic impairment. In patients with atrial fibrillation or flutter, block the AV node before initiating. Correct hypokalemia before initiating therapy; hypokalemia may worsen toxicity. Use may cause digoxin-induced toxicity (adjust digoxin's dose). Use caution with concurrent use of other antiarrhythmics. Hypersensitivity reactions can occur. Can unmask sick sinus syndrome (causes bradycardia). Has been associated with severe hepatotoxic reactions, including granulomatous hepatitis. Hemolysis may occur in patients with G6PD (glucose-6-phosphate dehydrogenase) deficiency.

Drug Interactions

Cytochrome P450 Effect: Substrate of CYP2C8/9 (minor), 2E1 (minor), 3A4 (major); **Inhibits** CYP2C8/9 (weak), 2D6 (strong), 3A4 (strong)

Decreased Effect: The levels/effects of quinidine may be decreased by aminoglutethimide, carbamazepine, nafcillin, nevirapine, phenobarbital, phenytoin, rifamycins, and other CYP3A4 inducers. Quinidine may decrease the levels/effects of CYP2D6 prodrug substrates (eg, codeine, hydrocodone, oxycodone, tramadol).

Increased Effect/Toxicity: Effects may be additive with drugs which prolong the QT interval, including amiodarone, amitriptyline, bepridil, cisapride (use is contraindicated), disopyramide, erythromycin, haloperidol, imipramine, pimozide, procainamide, sotalol, thioridazine, and some quinolones (sparfloxacin, gatifloxacin, moxifloxacin - concurrent use is contraindicated). Concurrent use of amprenavir, or ritonavir is contraindicated. Quinidine increases digoxin serum concentrations; digoxin dosage may need to be reduced (by 50%) when quinidine is initiated; new steady-state digoxin plasma concentrations occur in 5-7 days.

Quinidine may increase the levels/effects of amphetamines, selected beta-blockers, selected benzodiazepines, calcium channel blockers, cisapride, cyclosporine, dextromethorphan, ergot alkaloids, fluoxetine, selected HMG-CoA reductase inhibitors, lidocaine, mesoridazine, mirtazapine, nateglinide, nefazodone, paroxetine, risperidone, ritonavir, sildenafil (and other PDE-5 inhibitors), tacrolimus, thioridazine, tricyclic antidepressants, venlafaxine, and other substrates of CYP2D6 or 3A4. Selected benzodiazepines (midazolam and triazolam), cisapride, ergot alkaloids, selected HMG-CoA reductase inhibitors (lovastatin and simvastatin), mesoridazine, pimozide, and thioridazine are generally contraindicated with strong CYP3A4 inhibitors. When used with strong CYP3A4 inhibitors, dosage adjustment/limits are recommended for sildenafil and other PDE-5 inhibitors; refer to individual monographs.

The levels/effects of quinidine may be increased by azole antifungals, ciprofloxacin, clarithromycin, diclofenac, doxycycline, erythromycin, imatinib, isoniazid, nefazodone, nicardipine, propofol, protease inhibitors (amprenavir and ritonavir are contraindicated), verapamil, and other CYP3A4 inhibitors. Quinidine potentiates nondepolarizing and depolarizing muscle relaxants. When combined with quinidine, amiloride may cause prolonged ventricular conduction leading to arrhythmias. Urinary alkalinizers (antacids, sodium bicarbonate, acetazolamide) increase quinidine blood levels. Warfarin effects may be increased by quinidine.

Nutritional/Ethanol Interactions

Food: Dietary salt intake may alter the rate and extent of quinidine absorption. A decrease in dietary salt may lead to an increase in quinidine serum concentrations. Avoid changes in dietary salt intake. Quinidine serum levels may be increased if taken with food. Food has a variable effect on absorption of sustained release formulation. The rate of absorption of quinidine may be decreased following the ingestion of grapefruit juice. In addition, CYP3A4 metabolism of quinidine may be reduced by grapefruit juice. Grapefruit juice should be avoided. Excessive intake of fruit juices or vitamin C may decrease urine pH and result in increased clearance of quinidine with decreased serum concentration. Alkaline foods may result in increased quinidine serum concentrations.

Herb/Nutraceutical: St John's wort may decrease quinidine levels. Avoid ephedra (may worsen arrhythmia).

Adverse Reactions

Frequency not defined: Hypotension, syncope

>10%:

Cardiovascular: QT_c prolongation (modest prolongation is common, however, excessive prolongation is rare and indicates toxicity)

Central nervous system: Lightheadedness (15%)

Gastrointestinal: Diarrhea (35%), upper GI distress, bitter taste, diarrhea, anorexia, nausea, vomiting, stomach cramping (22%)

1% to 10%:

Cardiovascular: Angina (6%), palpitation (7%), new or worsened arrhythmia (proarrhythmic effect)

Central nervous system: Syncope (1% to 8%), headache (7%), fatigue (7%), sleep disturbance (3%), tremor (2%), nervousness (2%), incoordination (1%)

Dermatologic: Rash (5%)

Neuromuscular & skeletal: Weakness (5%)

(Continued)

Quinidine *(Continued)*

Ocular: Blurred vision
Otic: Tinnitus
Respiratory: Wheezing

Note: Cinchonism, a syndrome which may include tinnitus, high-frequency hearing loss, deafness, vertigo, blurred vision, diplopia, photophobia, headache, confusion, and delirium has been associated with quinidine use. Usually associated with chronic toxicity, this syndrome has also been described after brief exposure to a moderate dose in sensitive patients. Vomiting and diarrhea may also occur as isolated reactions to therapeutic quinidine levels.

Overdosage/Toxicology Has a low toxic:therapeutic ratio and may easily produce fatal intoxication (acute toxic dose: 1 g in adults). Symptoms of overdose include sinus bradycardia, sinus node arrest or asystole, P-R, QRS, or QT interval prolongation, torsade de pointes (polymorphous ventricular tachycardia), and depressed myocardial contractility, which along with alpha-adrenergic or ganglionic blockade, may result in hypotension and pulmonary edema. Other effects are anticholinergic (dry mouth, dilated pupils, and delirium) as well as seizures, coma, and respiratory arrest. Treatment is symptomatic and effects usually respond to conventional therapies. **Note:** Do not use other Class 1A or 1C antiarrhythmic agents to treat ventricular tachycardia. Sodium bicarbonate may treat wide QRS intervals or hypotension. Markedly impaired conduction or high degree AV block, unresponsive to bicarbonate, indicates consideration of a pacemaker.

Pharmacodynamics/Kinetics

Bioavailability: Sulfate: 80%; Gluconate: 70%
Protein Binding:
Newborns: 60% to 70%; decreased protein binding with cyanotic congenital heart disease, cirrhosis, or acute myocardial infarction
Adults: 80% to 90%
Half-Life Elimination: Plasma: Children: 2.5-6.7 hours; Adults: 6-8 hours; prolonged with elderly, cirrhosis, and congestive heart failure
Metabolism: Extensively hepatic (50% to 90%) to inactive compounds
Excretion: Urine (15% to 25% as unchanged drug)

Dosing

Adults & Elderly:
Note: Dosage expressed in terms of the salt: 267 mg of quinidine gluconate = 275 mg of quinidine polygalacturonate = 200 mg of quinidine sulfate.

Test dose for idiosyncratic reaction: Oral, I.M.: 200 mg administered several hours before full dosage (to determine possibility of idiosyncratic reaction)
Antiarrhythmic:
Oral:
Sulfate: 100-600 mg/dose every 4-6 hours; begin at 200 mg/dose and titrate to desired effect (maximum daily dose: 3-4 g)
Gluconate: 324-972 mg every 8-12 hours
I.M.: 400 mg/dose every 4-6 hours
I.V.: 200-400 mg/dose diluted and given at a rate ≤10 mg/minute

Pediatrics:
Note: Dosage expressed in terms of the salt: 267 mg of quinidine gluconate = 200 mg of quinidine sulfate.

Test dose for idiosyncratic reaction (sulfate, oral or gluconate, I.M.): Children: 2 mg/kg or 60 mg/m^2
Antiarrhythmic: Oral (quinidine sulfate): Children: 15-60 mg/kg/day in 4-5 divided doses or 6 mg/kg every 4-6 hours; usual 30 mg/kg/day or 900 mg/m^2/day given in 5 daily doses
I.V. **not** recommended (quinidine gluconate): Children: 2-10 mg/kg/dose given at a rate ≤10 mg/minute every 3-6 hours as needed

Renal Impairment:
Cl$_{cr}$ <10 mL/minute: Administer 75% of normal dose.
Hemodialysis effects: Slightly hemodialyzable (5% to 20%); 200 mg supplemental dose posthemodialysis is recommended; not dialyzable (0% to 5%) by peritoneal dialysis.

Hepatic Impairment: Larger loading dose may be indicated; reduce maintenance doses by 50% and monitor serum levels closely.

Available Dosage Forms [DSC] = Discontinued product
Injection, solution, as gluconate: 80 mg/mL (10 mL) [equivalent to quinidine base 50 mg]
Tablet, as sulfate: 200 mg, 300 mg
Tablet, extended release, as gluconate: 324 mg [equivalent to quinidine base 202 mg]
Quinaglute® Dura-Tabs®: 324 mg [equivalent to quinidine base 202 mg] [DSC]
Tablet, extended release, as sulfate: 300 mg [equivalent to quinidine base 249 mg]

Monitoring and Teaching Issues

Physical Assessment: Assess other medications patient may be taking for effectiveness and interactions. I.V. requires use of infusion pump and continuous cardiac and hemodynamic monitoring. Assess results of laboratory tests, therapeutic effectiveness (monitor cardiac functioning closely), and adverse reactions at beginning of therapy, when titrating dosage, and on a regular basis with long-term therapy. **Note:** Quinidine has a low TI and overdose may easily produce severe and life-threatening reactions. Assess knowledge/teach patient appropriate use, interventions to reduce side effects, and adverse symptoms to report.

Monitoring Laboratory Tests: Routine CBC, liver and renal function during long-term administration

Patient Education: Take exactly as directed, around-the-clock; do not take additional doses or discontinue without consulting prescriber. Do not crush, chew, or break sustained release dosage forms. Do not take with grapefruit juice. You will need regular cardiac checkups and blood tests while taking this medication. You may experience dizziness, drowsiness, or visual changes (use caution when driving or engaging in tasks requiring alertness until response to drug is known); abnormal taste, nausea or vomiting, or loss of appetite (small frequent meals, frequent mouth care, chewing gum, or sucking lozenges may help); headaches (prescriber may recommend mild analgesic); or diarrhea (yogurt or boiled milk may help; if persistent consult prescriber). Report chest pain, palpitation, or erratic heartbeat; respiratory difficulty or wheezing; CNS changes (confusion, delirium, fever, consistent dizziness); skin rash; sense of fullness or ringing in ears; or vision changes. **Pregnancy precaution:** Inform prescriber if you are or intend to become pregnant.

Dietary Considerations: Administer with food or milk to decrease gastrointestinal irritation. Avoid changes in dietary salt intake.

Geriatric Considerations: Clearance may be decreased with a resultant increased half-life. Must individualize dose. Bioavailability and half-life are increased in the elderly due to decreases in both renal and hepatic function with age.

Pregnancy Risk Factor: C

Lactation: Enters breast milk/compatible

Administration

Oral: Do not crush, chew, or break sustained release dosage forms. Give around-the-clock to promote less variation in peak and trough serum levels.

I.V.: Give around-the-clock to promote less variation in peak and trough serum levels. Maximum I.V. infusion rate: 10 mg/minute. Minimize use of PVC tubing to enhance bioavailability.

Compatibility: Stable in D_5W, NS

Y-site administration: Incompatible with furosemide

Compatibility when admixed: Incompatible with atracurium

Storage: Do not use discolored parenteral solution.

Related Information

Antiarrhythmic Drugs *on page 1708*

Peak and Trough Guidelines *on page 1694*

♦ **Quinidine Gluconate** *see* Quinidine *on page 1296*

♦ **Quinidine Polygalacturonate** *see* Quinidine *on page 1296*

♦ **Quinidine Sulfate** *see* Quinidine *on page 1296*

Quinine (KWYE nine)

Synonyms Quinine Sulfate

Generic Available Yes

Pharmacologic Category Antimalarial Agent

Medication Safety Issues

Sound-alike/look-alike issues:

Quinine may be confused with quinidine

Use In conjunction with other antimalarial agents, suppression or treatment of chloroquine-resistant *P. falciparum* malaria; treatment of *Babesia microti* infection in conjunction with clindamycin

Unlabeled/Investigational Use Prevention and treatment of nocturnal recumbency leg muscle cramps

Mechanism of Action/Effect Depresses oxygen uptake and carbohydrate metabolism; intercalates into DNA, disrupting the parasite's replication and transcription; affects calcium distribution within muscle fibers and decreases the excitability of the motor end-plate region; cardiovascular effects similar to quinidine

Contraindications Hypersensitivity to quinine or any component of the formulation; tinnitus, optic neuritis, G6PD deficiency; history of black water fever; thrombocytopenia with quinine or quinidine; pregnancy

Warnings/Precautions Use with caution in patients with cardiac arrhythmias (quinine has quinidine-like activity) and in patients with myasthenia gravis.

Drug Interactions

Cytochrome P450 Effect: Substrate (minor) of CYP1A2, 2C19, 3A4; **Inhibits** CYP2C8/9 (moderate), 2D6 (strong), 3A4 (weak)

Decreased Effect: Phenobarbital, phenytoin, and rifampin may decrease quinine serum concentrations. Quinine may decrease the levels/effects of CYP2D6 prodrug substrates (eg, codeine, hydrocodone, oxycodone, tramadol).

Increased Effect/Toxicity: Quinine may increase the levels/effects of CYP2D6 substrates (eg, amphetamines, selected beta-blockers, dextromethorphan, fluoxetine, lidocaine, mirtazapine, nefazodone, paroxetine, risperidone, ritonavir, thioridazine, tricyclic antidepressants, venlafaxine). Beta-blockers with quinine may increase bradycardia. Quinine may enhance warfarin anticoagulant effect. Quinine potentiates nondepolarizing and depolarizing muscle relaxants. Quinine may increase plasma concentration of digoxin. Closely monitor digoxin concentrations. Digoxin dosage may need to be reduced (by one-half) when quinine is initiated. New steady-state digoxin plasma concentrations occur in 5-7 days. Verapamil, amiodarone, alkalinizing agents, and cimetidine may increase quinine serum concentrations.

Nutritional/Ethanol Interactions Herb/Nutraceutical: St John's wort may decrease quinine levels.

Lab Interactions Positive Coombs' [direct]

Adverse Reactions Frequency not defined.

Central nervous system: Severe headache

Gastrointestinal: Nausea, vomiting, diarrhea

Ocular: Blurred vision

Otic: Tinnitus

Miscellaneous: Cinchonism (risk of cinchonism is directly related to dose and duration of therapy)

Overdosage/Toxicology Symptoms of mild toxicity include nausea, vomiting, and cinchonism. Severe intoxication may cause ataxia, obtundation, convulsions, coma, and respiratory arrest. With massive intoxication quinidine-like cardiotoxicity (hypotension, QRS and QT interval prolongation, AV block, and ventricular arrhythmias) may be fatal. Retinal toxicity (Continued)

Quinine *(Continued)*

occurs 9-10 hours after ingestion (blurred vision, impaired color perception, constriction of visual fields and blindness). Other toxic effects include hypokalemia, hypoglycemia, hemolysis, and congenital malformations when taken during pregnancy. Treatment includes symptomatic therapy with conventional agents. **Note:** Avoid Type 1A and 1C antiarrhythmic drugs. Treat cardiotoxicity with sodium bicarbonate. Dialysis and hemoperfusion procedures are ineffective in enhancing elimination.

Pharmacodynamics/Kinetics
Absorption: Readily, mainly from upper small intestine
Time to Peak: Serum: 1-3 hours
Protein Binding: 70% to 95%
Half-Life Elimination: Children: 6-12 hours; Adults: 8-14 hours
Metabolism: Primarily hepatic
Excretion: Feces and saliva; urine (<5% as unchanged drug)

Dosing
Adults & Elderly:
Treatment of chloroquine-resistant malaria: Oral: 650 mg every 8 hours for 3-7 days with tetracycline
Suppression of malaria: Oral: 325 mg twice daily and continued for 6 weeks after exposure
Babesiosis: Oral: 650 mg every 6-8 hours for 7 days
Leg cramps: Oral: 200-300 mg at bedtime

Pediatrics:
Treatment of chloroquine-resistant malaria: Oral: Children: 25-30 mg/kg/day in divided doses every 8 hours for 3-7 days with tetracycline (consider risk versus benefit in children <8 years of age)
Babesiosis: Oral: Children: 25 mg/kg/day divided every 8 hours for 7 days

Renal Impairment:
Cl_{cr} 10-50 mL/minute: Administer every 8-12 hours or 75% of normal dose.
Cl_{cr} <10 mL/minute: Administer every 24 hours or 30% to 50% of normal dose.
Not removed by hemo- or peritoneal dialysis; dose for Cl_{cr} <10 mL/minute.
Continuous arteriovenous or venovenous hemofiltration: Dose as for Cl_{cr} 10-50 mL/minute.

Available Dosage Forms
Capsule, as sulfate: 200 mg, 325 mg
Tablet, as sulfate: 260 mg

Monitoring and Teaching Issues
Physical Assessment: Assess allergy history prior to beginning therapy. Use caution in presence of cardiac arrhythmias (quinine has quinidine-like activity) and myasthenia gravis (see Warnings/Precautions). Assess potential for interactions with other pharmacological agents patient may be taking (eg, may increase or decrease levels/effects and toxicity [eg, digoxin, beta blockers, warfarin, oxycodone, lidocaine]; see Drug Interactions). Assess effectiveness (according to purpose for therapy) and adverse reactions (see Adverse Reactions). Teach patient appropriate use, possible side effects/interventions, and adverse symptoms to report (see Patient Education). **Pregnancy risk factor X:** Determine that patient is not pregnant before starting therapy. Do not give to females of childbearing age unless patient is capable of complying with contraceptive use during and for 2 months following therapy.

Monitoring Laboratory Tests: Monitor CBC with platelet count, liver function tests, blood glucose, ophthalmologic examination

Patient Education: Do not take any new medication during therapy unless approved by prescriber (avoid use of any aluminum-containing antacids). Take on schedule as directed, with full 8 oz glass of water. Take with or without food. Do not open, crush, or chew sustained release preparations. Do not increase dose without consulting prescriber; overdose can cause severe systemic effects. You will need to return for follow-up blood tests. May cause severe headache (consult prescriber for approved analgesic); nausea or vomiting (small frequent meals, frequent mouth care, chewing gum, or sucking lozenges may help); or diarrhea (buttermilk, boiled milk, or yogurt may help). Report any vision changes (eg, blurring, night-blindness, double vision); ringing in ears; or other persistent side effects. Seek emergency help for chest pain, respiratory difficulty, or seizures. **Pregnancy precautions:** Inform prescriber if you are pregnant. Consult prescriber for appropriate contraceptive measures to use during and for 2 months following therapy. This drug may cause fetal defects. Do not donate blood during or for 1 month following therapy.

Dietary Considerations: May be taken with food.

Geriatric Considerations: Efficacy in nocturnal leg cramps is not well supported in the medical and pharmacy literature, however, some patients do respond. Nonresponders should be evaluated for other possible etiologies.

Pregnancy Risk Factor: X
Lactation: Enters breast milk/compatible

Administration
Oral: Do not crush sustained release preparations. Avoid use of aluminum-containing antacids because of drug absorption problems. Swallow dose whole to avoid bitter taste. May be administered with food.
Storage: Protect from light.

♦ **Quinine Sulfate** *see Quinine on page 1299*
♦ **Quinol** *see Hydroquinone on page 768*
♦ **Quintex HC** *see Hydrocodone, Phenylephrine, and Guaifenesin on page 760*

Quinupristin and Dalfopristin *(kwi NYOO pris tin & dal FOE pris tin)*
U.S. Brand Names Synercid®
Synonyms Pristinamycin; RP-59500
Generic Available No
Pharmacologic Category Antibiotic, Streptogramin

Use Treatment of serious or life-threatening infections associated with vancomycin-resistant *Enterococcus faecium* bacteremia; treatment of complicated skin and skin structure infections caused by methicillin-susceptible *Staphylococcus aureus* or *Streptococcus pyogenes*

Has been studied in the treatment of a variety of infections caused by *Enterococcus faecium* (not *E. fecalis*) including vancomycin-resistant strains. May also be effective in the treatment of serious infections caused by *Staphylococcus* species including those resistant to methicillin.

Mechanism of Action/Effect Quinupristin/dalfopristin inhibits bacterial protein synthesis by binding to different sites on the 50S bacterial ribosomal subunit thereby inhibiting protein synthesis.

Contraindications Hypersensitivity to quinupristin, dalfopristin, pristinamycin, or virginiamycin, or any component of the formulation

Warnings/Precautions Use with caution in patients with hepatic or renal dysfunction. May cause pain and phlebitis when infused through a peripheral line (not relieved by hydrocortisone or diphenhydramine). May inhibit the metabolism of many drugs metabolized by CYP3A4. Concurrent therapy with cisapride (which may prolong QT_c interval and lead to arrhythmias) should be avoided. Superinfection may occur. As with many antibiotics, antibiotic-associated colitis and pseudomembranous colitis may occur. May cause arthralgias, myalgias, and hyperbilirubinemia.

Drug Interactions

Cytochrome P450 Effect: Quinupristin: **Inhibits** CYP3A4 (weak)

Increased Effect/Toxicity: The manufacturer states that quinupristin/dalfopristin may increase cisapride concentrations and cause QT_c prolongation, and recommends to avoid concurrent use with cisapride. Quinupristin/dalfopristin may increase cyclosporine concentrations; monitor.

Adverse Reactions

>10%:

Hepatic: Hyperbilirubinemia (3% to 35%)

Local: Inflammation at infusion site (38% to 42%), local pain (40% to 44%), local edema (17% to 18%), infusion site reaction (12% to 13%)

Neuromuscular & skeletal: Arthralgia (up to 47%), myalgia (up to 47%)

1% to 10%:

Central nervous system: Pain (2% to 3%), headache (2%)

Dermatologic: Pruritus (2%), rash (2%)

Endocrine & metabolic: Hyperglycemia (1%)

Gastrointestinal: Nausea (3% to 5%), diarrhea (3%), vomiting (3% to 4%)

Hematologic: Anemia (3%)

Hepatic: GGT increased (2%), LDH increased (3%)

Local: Thrombophlebitis (2%)

Neuromuscular & skeletal: CPK increased (2%)

Overdosage/Toxicology Symptoms may include dyspnea, emesis, tremors and ataxia. Treatment is supportive. Not removed by hemodialysis or peritoneal dialysis.

Pharmacodynamics/Kinetics

Protein Binding: Moderate

Half-Life Elimination: Quinupristin: 0.85 hour; Dalfopristin: 0.7 hour (mean elimination half-lives, including metabolites: 3 and 1 hours, respectively)

Metabolism: To active metabolites via nonenzymatic reactions

Excretion: Feces (75% to 77% as unchanged drug and metabolites); urine (15% to 19%)

Dosing

Adults & Elderly:

Vancomycin-resistant *Enterococcus faecium*: I.V.: 7.5 mg/kg every 8 hours

Complicated skin and skin structure infection: I.V.: 7.5 mg/kg every 12 hours

Pediatrics: Limited information: Dosages similar to adult dosing have been used in the treatment of complicated skin/soft tissue infections and infections caused by vancomycin-resistant *Enterococcus faecium*

CNS shunt infection due to vancomycin-resistant *Enterococcus faecium*: I.V.: 7.5 mg/kg/dose every 8 hours. Concurrent intrathecal doses of 1-2 mg/day have been administered for up to 68 days.

Renal Impairment: No adjustment is necessary in renal failure, hemodialysis, or peritoneal dialysis.

Hepatic Impairment: Pharmacokinetic data suggest dosage adjustment may be necessary; however, specific recommendations have not been proposed.

Available Dosage Forms

Injection, powder for reconstitution:

500 mg: Quinupristin 150 mg and dalfopristin 350 mg

600 mg: Quinupristin 180 mg and dalfopristin 420 mg

Monitoring and Teaching Issues

Physical Assessment: Assess allergy history prior to starting treatment. Use caution in presence of hepatic or renal impairment (see Warnings/Precautions). Assess effectiveness and interactions of other pharmacological agents (see Drug Interactions). See Administration (prior to starting infusion) for exact infusion protocols to prevent severe venous irritation. Infusion site must be closely monitored. Assess effectiveness (reduction of infection) and adverse reactions (eg, arthralgia, headache, rash, hyperglycemia, opportunistic infection [fever, chills, sore throat, burning urination, fatigue], pseudomembranous, hyperbilirubinemia, dyspnea, ataxia; see Adverse Reactions). Teach patient possible side effects/interventions, and adverse symptoms to report (see Patient Education).

Monitoring Laboratory Tests: Culture and sensitivity

Patient Education: This drug is only administered by infusion; report immediately any pain, irritation, redness, burning, or swelling at infusion site. You may experience other side effects. Report headache, rash, nausea, vomiting, diarrhea, pain, heat, or swelling in muscle areas, especially in lower extremities; respiratory difficulty, tremors, or difficulty speaking. **Breast-feeding precaution:** Consult prescriber if breast-feeding.

(Continued)

Quinupristin and Dalfopristin *(Continued)*

Pregnancy Risk Factor: B

Lactation: Excretion in breast milk unknown/use caution

Administration
I.V.: Line should be flushed with 5% dextrose in water prior to and following administration. Incompatible with saline. Infusion should be completed over 60 minutes (toxicity may be increased with shorter infusion). Compatible (Y-site injection) with aztreonam, ciprofloxacin, haloperidol, metoclopramide or potassium chloride when admixed in 5% dextrose in water. Also compatible (Y-site injection) with fluconazole (used as undiluted solution). If severe venous irritation occurs following peripheral administration of quinupristin/dalfopristin diluted in 250 mL 5% dextrose in water, consideration should be given to increasing the infusion volume to 500 mL or 750 mL, changing the infusion site, or infusing by a peripherally inserted central catheter (PICC) or a central venous catheter.

Reconstitution: Reconstitute single dose vial with 5 mL of 5% dextrose in water or sterile water for injection. Swirl gentle to dissolve - do not shake (to limit foam formation). The reconstituted solution should be diluted within 30 minutes. Stability of the diluted solution prior to the infusion is established as 5 hours at room temperature or 54 hours if refrigerated at 2°C to 8°C. Reconstituted solution should be added to at least 250 mL of 5% dextrose in water for peripheral administration (increase to 500 mL or 750 mL if necessary to limit venous irritation). An infusion volume of 100 mL may be used for central line infusions. Do not freeze solution.

Storage: Store unopened vials under refrigeration (2°C to 8°C/36°F to 46°F).

Related Information
Antimicrobial Drugs of Choice *on page 1792*

- ♦ Quixin™ *see* Levofloxacin *on page 888*
- ♦ QVAR® *see* Beclomethasone *on page 175*
- ♦ Q-V Tussin *see* Pseudoephedrine, Hydrocodone, and Chlorpheniramine *on page 1283*
- ♦ R 14-15 *see* Erlotinib *on page 540*
- ♦ R-3827 *see* Abarelix *on page 34*
- ♦ RabAvert® *see page 1660*

Rabeprazole *(ra BE pray zole)*

U.S. Brand Names AcipHex®

Synonyms Pariprazole

Generic Available No

Pharmacologic Category Proton Pump Inhibitor; Substituted Benzimidazole

Medication Safety Issues

Sound-alike/look-alike issues:

AcipHex® may be confused with Acephen®, Accupril®, Aricept®

Rabeprazole may be confused with aripiprazole

Use Short-term (4-8 weeks) treatment and maintenance of erosive or ulcerative gastroesophageal reflux disease (GERD); symptomatic GERD; short-term (up to 4 weeks) treatment of duodenal ulcers; long-term treatment of pathological hypersecretory conditions, including Zollinger-Ellison syndrome; *H. pylori* eradication (in combination with amoxicillin and clarithromycin)

Unlabeled/Investigational Use Maintenance of duodenal ulcer

Mechanism of Action/Effect Suppresses gastric acid secretion by inhibiting the parietal cell H^+/K^+ ATP pump

Contraindications Hypersensitivity to rabeprazole, substituted benzimidazoles (ie, esomeprazole, lansoprazole, omeprazole, pantoprazole), or any component of the formulation

Warnings/Precautions Use caution in severe hepatic impairment. Relief of symptoms with rabeprazole does not preclude the presence of a gastric malignancy

Drug Interactions
Cytochrome P450 Effect: Substrate (major) of CYP2C19, 3A4; **Inhibits** CYP2C19 (moderate), 2DC (weak), 3A4 (weak)

Decreased Effect: Proton pump inhibitors may decrease the absorption of atazanavir, indinavir, itraconazole, and ketoconazole. The levels/effects of rabeprazole may be decreased by aminoglutethimide, carbamazepine, nafcillin, nevirapine, phenobarbital, phenytoin, rifampin, and other CYP2C19 or 3A4 inducers.

Increased Effect/Toxicity: Rabeprazole may increase the levels/effects of citalopram, diazepam, methsuximide, phenytoin, propranolol, sertraline, or other CYP2C19 substrates.

Nutritional/Ethanol Interactions

Ethanol: Avoid ethanol (may cause gastric mucosal irritation).

Food: High-fat meals may delay absorption, but C_{max} and AUC are not altered.

Adverse Reactions 1% to 10%: Central nervous system: Headache

Overdosage/Toxicology No experience with large overdose; rabeprazole is not dialyzable. Treatment of overdosage should be symptomatic and supportive.

Pharmacodynamics/Kinetics
Onset of Action: 1 hour
Duration of Action: 24 hours
Absorption: Oral: Well absorbed within 1 hour
Bioavailability: Oral: 52%
Time to Peak: Plasma: 2-5 hours
Protein Binding: Serum: 94.8% to 97.5%
Half-Life Elimination: Dose dependent: 0.85-2 hours
Metabolism: Hepatic via CYP3A and 2C19 to inactive metabolites
Excretion: Urine (90% primarily as thioether carboxylic acid); remainder in feces

Dosing
Adults & Elderly:
GERD: Oral: 20 mg once daily for 4-8 weeks; maintenance: 20 mg once daily
Duodenal ulcer: Oral: 20 mg/day before breakfast for 4 weeks
Eradication of *H. pylori*: Oral: 20 mg twice daily for 7 days; to be administered with amoxicillin 1000 mg and clarithromycin 500 mg, also given twice daily for 7 days.
Hypersecretory conditions: Oral: 60 mg once daily; dose may need to be adjusted as necessary. Doses as high as 100 mg once daily and 60 mg twice daily have been used.
Renal Impairment: No dosage adjustment required.
Hepatic Impairment:
Mild to moderate: Elimination decreased; no dosage adjustment required.
Severe: Use caution.

Available Dosage Forms Tablet, delayed release, enteric coated, as sodium: 20 mg

Monitoring and Teaching Issues
Physical Assessment: Assess other medications, especially those dependent on cytochrome P450 metabolism (eg, digoxin) and those requiring acid environment for absorption (eg, ketoconazole, ampicillin). Monitor therapeutic effectiveness (reduction in symptoms) and adverse reactions and toxicity. Assess knowledge/teach patient appropriate use, interventions to reduce side effects, and adverse reactions to report.
Patient Education: Take as directed. Swallow whole, do not crush, split, or chew. Follow recommended diet and activity instructions. Avoid alcohol. You may experience headache (use of mild analgesic may help) or other side effects. Report these to prescriber if they persist. **Breast-feeding precaution:** Breast-feeding is not recommended.
Dietary Considerations: May be taken with or without food; best if taken before breakfast.
Geriatric Considerations: No difference in efficacy or safety was noted in elderly subjects as compared to younger subjects. No dosage adjustment is necessary in the elderly.
Pregnancy Risk Factor: B
Lactation: Excretion in breast milk unknown/not recommended

Administration
Oral: May be administered with or without food; best if taken before breakfast. Do not crush, split, or chew tablet. May be administered with an antacid.
Storage: Rapidly degraded in acid conditions.

Related Information
Helicobacter pylori Treatment *on page 1835*

♦ **Rabies Immune Globulin (Human)** *see page 1660*
♦ **Rabies Virus Vaccine** *see page 1660*
♦ **rAHF** *see* Antihemophilic Factor (Recombinant) *on page 127*
♦ **R-Albuterol** *see* Levalbuterol *on page 879*

Raloxifene (ral OKS i feen)

U.S. Brand Names Evista®
Synonyms Keoxifene Hydrochloride; Raloxifene Hydrochloride
Generic Available No
Pharmacologic Category Selective Estrogen Receptor Modulator (SERM)
Medication Safety Issues
Sound-alike/look-alike issues:
Evista® may be confused with Avinza™
Use Prevention and treatment of osteoporosis in postmenopausal women
Mechanism of Action/Effect A selective estrogen receptor modulator, meaning that it affects some of the same receptors that estrogen does, but not all, and in some instances, it antagonizes or blocks estrogen; it acts like estrogen to prevent bone loss and improve lipid profiles (decreases total and LDL-cholesterol but does not raise triglycerides), but it has the potential to block some estrogen effects such as those that lead to breast cancer and uterine cancer
Contraindications Hypersensitivity to raloxifene or any component of the formulation; active thromboembolic disorder; pregnancy (not intended for use in premenopausal women)
Warnings/Precautions Use caution in patients with history of or at high risk for venous thromboembolism/pulmonary embolism; patients with cardiovascular disease; history of cervical/uterine carcinoma; renal/hepatic insufficiency (however, pharmacokinetic data are lacking); concurrent use of estrogens; women with a history of elevated triglycerides in response to treatment with oral estrogens (or estrogen/progestin). Discontinue at least 72 hours prior to and during prolonged immobilization (postoperative recovery or prolonged bedrest).
Drug Interactions
Decreased Effect: Ampicillin and cholestyramine reduce raloxifene absorption/blood levels.
Increased Effect/Toxicity: Raloxifene has the potential to interact with highly protein-bound drugs (increase effects of either agent). Use caution with highly protein-bound drugs, warfarin, clofibrate, indomethacin, naproxen, ibuprofen, diazepam, phenytoin, or tamoxifen.
(Continued)

Raloxifene *(Continued)*

Nutritional/Ethanol Interactions Ethanol: Avoid ethanol (may increase risk of osteoporosis).

Adverse Reactions Note: Has been associated with increased risk of thromboembolism (DVT, PE) and superficial thrombophlebitis; risk is similar to reported risk of HRT

≥2%:

Cardiovascular: Chest pain

Central nervous system: Migraine, depression, insomnia, fever

Dermatologic: Rash

Endocrine & metabolic: Hot flashes

Gastrointestinal: Nausea, dyspepsia, vomiting, flatulence, gastroenteritis, weight gain

Genitourinary: Vaginitis, urinary tract infection, cystitis, leukorrhea

Neuromuscular & skeletal: Leg cramps, arthralgia, myalgia, arthritis

Respiratory: Sinusitis, pharyngitis, cough, pneumonia, laryngitis

Miscellaneous: Infection, flu syndrome, diaphoresis

Overdosage/Toxicology Incidence of overdose in humans has not been reported. In an 8-week study of postmenopausal women, a dose of raloxifene 600 mg/day was safely tolerated. No mortality was seen after a single oral dose in rats or mice at 810 times the human dose for rats and 405 times the human dose for mice. There is no specific antidote for raloxifene.

Pharmacodynamics/Kinetics

Onset of Action: 8 weeks

Absorption: ~60%

Bioavailability: ~2%

Protein Binding: >95% to albumin and α-glycoprotein

Half-Life Elimination: 27.7-32.5 hours

Metabolism: Extensive first-pass effect

Excretion: Primarily feces; urine (0.2%)

Dosing

Adults & Elderly: Osteoporosis prevention or treatment (postmenopausal women): Oral: 1 tablet (60 mg) daily; may be administered any time of the day without regard to meals.

Hepatic Impairment: Avoid use; safety has not been established.

Available Dosage Forms Tablet, as hydrochloride: 60 mg

Monitoring and Teaching Issues

Physical Assessment: Use caution with history or risk of venous thromboembolism/ pulmonary embolism, cardiovascular disease, cervical/uterine carcinoma, or concurrent use of estrogens (see Warnings/Precautions for specific use cautions). Assess potential for interactions with other pharmacological agents (eg, highly protein-bound drugs, warfarin, clofibrate, indomethacin, naproxen, ibuprofen, diazepam, phenytoin, or tamoxifen; see Drug Interactions). Assess results of laboratory work, effectiveness (repeat BMI is best measure of osteoporosis treatment) and adverse response (eg, DVT, PE, chest pain, migraine, rash, hot flashes, vaginitis, UTI, myalgia, cough; see Adverse Reactions). Teach patient appropriate use, possible side effects/appropriate interventions, and adverse symptoms to report (eg, thromboembolism; see Patient Education). **Pregnancy risk factor X:** Determine that patient is not pregnant before starting therapy. For use in postmenopausal women only.

Monitoring Laboratory Tests: Monitor lipid profile, bone mineral density

Patient Education: Do not take any new medication during therapy unless approved by prescriber. Avoid alcohol (ethanol may increase risk of osteoporosis). May be taken at any time of day without regard to meals. This medication is given to reduce incidence of osteoporosis; it will not reduce menopausal hot flashes or flushing (cool environment may reduce hot flashes). May cause flu-like symptoms at beginning of therapy (these will resolve with use); GI disturbances (eg, nausea, vomiting, dyspepsia; small frequent meals, frequent mouth care, chewing gum, or sucking lozenges may help); or joint pain (consult prescriber for approved analgesic). Report immediately any pain, redness, warmth, or cramping in leg muscles; sudden chest pain; or respiratory difficulty. Report fever, acute migraine, insomnia or emotional depression, unusual weight gain (>5 lb/week), unresolved gastric distress, urinary infection or vaginal burning or itching, or unusual cough. **Pregnancy/breast-feeding precautions:** Inform prescriber if you are pregnant. For use in postmenopausal women only. Do not breast-feed.

Geriatric Considerations: No need to cycle with progesterone.

Pregnancy Risk Factor: X

Pregnancy Issues: Raloxifene should not be used by pregnant women or by women planning to become pregnant in the immediate future.

Lactation: Contraindicated

Administration

Oral: Raloxifene should be stopped 72 hours prior to or during prolonged immobilization due to risk of thromboembolic events.

Additional Information The decrease in estrogen-related adverse effects with the selective estrogen-receptor modulators in general and raloxifene in particular should improve compliance and decrease the incidence of cardiovascular events and fractures while not increasing breast cancer.

♦ **Raloxifene Hydrochloride** *see Raloxifene on page 1303*

Ramipril *(ra MI pril)*

U.S. Brand Names Altace®

Generic Available No

Pharmacologic Category Angiotensin-Converting Enzyme (ACE) Inhibitor

Medication Safety Issues

Sound-alike/look-alike issues:

Ramipril may be confused with enalapril, Monopril®

Altace® may be confused with alteplase, Amaryl®, Amerge®, Artane®

Use Treatment of hypertension, alone or in combination with thiazide diuretics; treatment of congestive heart failure; treatment of left ventricular dysfunction after myocardial infarction; to reduce risk of heart attack, stroke, and death in patients at increased risk for these problems

Mechanism of Action/Effect Ramipril is an ACE inhibitor which prevents the formation of angiotensin II from angiotensin I and exhibits pharmacologic effects that are similar to captopril. Ramipril must undergo conversion in the liver to its biologically active metabolite, ramiprilat. The pharmacodynamic effects of ramipril result from the high-affinity, competitive, reversible binding of ramiprilat to angiotensin-converting enzyme thus preventing the formation of the potent vasoconstrictor angiotensin II.

Contraindications Hypersensitivity to ramipril or any component of the formulation; prior hypersensitivity (including angioedema) to ACE inhibitors; bilateral renal artery stenosis; pregnancy (2nd and 3rd trimesters)

Warnings/Precautions Angioedema can occur at any time during treatment (especially following first dose). Angioedema may involve head and neck (potentially affecting the airway) or the intestine (presenting with abdominal pain). Careful blood pressure monitoring with first dose (hypotension can occur especially in volume depleted patients). Dosage adjustment needed in renal impairment. Use with caution in hypovolemia; collagen vascular diseases; valvular stenosis (particularly aortic stenosis); hyperkalemia; or before, during, or immediately after anesthesia. Avoid rapid dosage escalation, which may lead to renal insufficiency. Rare toxicities associated with ACE inhibitors include cholestatic jaundice (which may progress to hepatic necrosis) and neutropenia/agranulocytosis with myeloid hyperplasia. Hypersensitivity reactions may be seen during hemodialysis with high-flux dialysis membranes (eg, AN69). Use with caution in unilateral renal artery stenosis and pre-existing renal insufficiency.

Drug Interactions

Decreased Effect: Aspirin (high dose) may reduce the therapeutic effects of ACE inhibitors; at low dosages this does not appear to be significant. Rifampin may decrease the effect of ACE inhibitors. Antacids may decrease the bioavailability of ACE inhibitors (may be more likely to occur with captopril); separate administration times by 1-2 hours. NSAIDs, specifically indomethacin, may reduce the hypotensive effects of ACE inhibitors. More likely to occur in low renin or volume dependent hypertensive patients.

Increased Effect/Toxicity: Potassium supplements, co-trimoxazole (high dose), angiotensin II receptor antagonists (eg, candesartan, losartan, irbesartan), or potassium-sparing diuretics (amiloride, spironolactone, triamterene) may result in elevated serum potassium levels when combined with ramipril. ACE inhibitor effects may be increased by phenothiazines or probenecid (increases levels of captopril). ACE inhibitors may increase serum concentrations/effects of digoxin, lithium, and sulfonylureas.

Diuretics have additive hypotensive effects with ACE inhibitors, and hypovolemia increases the potential for adverse renal effects of ACE inhibitors. In patients with compromised renal function, coadministration with NSAIDs may result in further deterioration of renal function. Allopurinol and ACE inhibitors may cause a higher risk of hypersensitivity reaction when taken concurrently.

Nutritional/Ethanol Interactions Herb/Nutraceutical: Avoid dong quai if using for hypertension (has estrogenic activity). Avoid ephedra, yohimbe, ginseng (may worsen hypertension). Avoid garlic (may have increased antihypertensive effect).

Lab Interactions Increases BUN, creatinine, potassium, positive Coombs' [direct]; decreases cholesterol (S); may cause false-positive results in urine acetone determinations using sodium nitroprusside reagent

Adverse Reactions Note: Frequency ranges include data from hypertension and heart failure trials. Higher rates of adverse reactions have generally been noted in patients with CHF. However, the frequency of adverse effects associated with placebo is also increased in this population.

>10%: Respiratory: Cough (increased) (7% to 12%)

1% to 10%:
  Cardiovascular: Hypotension (11%), angina (3%), postural hypotension (2%), syncope (2%)
  Central nervous system: Headache (1% to 5%), dizziness (2% to 4%), fatigue (2%), vertigo (2%)
  Endocrine & metabolic: Hyperkalemia (1% to 10%)
  Gastrointestinal: Nausea/vomiting (1% to 2%)
  Neuromuscular & skeletal: Chest pain (noncardiac) (1%)
  Renal: Renal dysfunction (1%), elevation in serum creatinine (1% to 2%), increased BUN (<1% to 3%); transient elevations of creatinine and/or BUN may occur more frequently
  Respiratory: Cough (estimated 1% to 10%)

Worsening of renal function may occur in patients with bilateral renal artery stenosis or in hypovolemia. In addition, a syndrome which may include fever, myalgia, arthralgia, interstitial nephritis, vasculitis, rash, eosinophilia and positive ANA, and elevated ESR has been reported with ACE inhibitors. Risk of pancreatitis and agranulocytosis may be increased in patients with collagen vascular disease or renal impairment.

Overdosage/Toxicology Mild hypotension has been the primary toxic effect seen with acute overdose. Bradycardia may also occur. Hyperkalemia occurs even with therapeutic doses, especially in patients with renal insufficiency and those taking NSAIDs. Treatment is symptom-directed and supportive.
(Continued)

Ramipril *(Continued)*

Pharmacodynamics/Kinetics

Onset of Action: 1-2 hours

Duration of Action: 24 hours

Absorption: Well absorbed (50% to 60%)

Time to Peak: Serum: ~1 hour

Half-Life Elimination: Ramiprilat: Effective: 13-17 hours; Terminal: >50 hours

Metabolism: Hepatic to the active form, ramiprilat

Excretion: Urine (60%) and feces (40%) as parent drug and metabolites

Dosing

Adults:

Hypertension: Oral: 2.5-5 mg once daily, maximum: 20 mg/day

To reduce the risk of MI, stroke, and death from cardiovascular causes: Oral: Initial: 2.5 mg once daily for 1 week, then 5 mg once daily for the next 3 weeks, then increase as tolerated to 10 mg once daily (may be given as divided dose)

Left ventricular dysfunction postmyocardial infarction: Oral: Initial: 2.5 mg twice daily titrated upward, if possible, to 5 mg twice daily.

Note: The dose of any concomitant diuretic should be reduced. If the diuretic cannot be discontinued, initiate therapy with 1.25 mg. After the initial dose, the patient should be monitored carefully until blood pressure has stabilized.

Elderly: Refer to adult dosing (see Geriatric Considerations). Adjust for renal function for elderly since glomerular filtration rates are decreased; may see exaggerated hypotensive effects if renal clearance is not considered.

Renal Impairment:

Cl_{cr} <40 mL/minute: Administer 25% of normal dose.

Renal failure and hypertension: Administer 1.25 mg once daily, titrated upward as possible.

Renal failure and heart failure: Administer 1.25 mg once daily, increasing to 1.25 mg twice daily up to 2.5 mg twice daily as tolerated.

Available Dosage Forms Capsule: 1.25 mg, 2.5 mg, 5 mg, 10 mg

Monitoring and Teaching Issues

Physical Assessment: Use caution in presence of renal impairment; hypovolemia; collagen vascular diseases; valvular stenosis; hyperkalemia; or before, during, or immediately after anesthesia (see Warnings/Precautions for specific use cautions). Assess potential for interactions with other pharmacological agents or herbal products patient may be taking (especially anything that may impact fluid balance or cardiac status; see Drug Interactions). May be advisable to administer first dose in prescriber's office with careful blood pressure monitoring (hypotension or angioedema can occur at any time during treatment, especially following first dose). Assess results of laboratory tests, effectiveness (blood pressure and cardiac status), and adverse response on a regular basis during therapy (eg, cough, renal dysfunction, nausea/vomiting, hypovolemia, angioedema, postural hypotension; see Adverse Reactions). Teach patient proper use, possible side effects/appropriate interventions, and adverse symptoms to report (see Patient Education).

Monitoring Laboratory Tests: CBC, renal function tests, electrolytes; if patient has renal impairment, a baseline WBC with differential and serum creatinine should be evaluated and monitored closely during the first 3 months of therapy

Patient Education: Do not take any new medication during therapy unless approved by prescriber. Take as directed; do not alter dose or discontinue without consulting prescriber. Take first dose at bedtime or when sitting down (hypotension may occur). This drug does not eliminate need for diet or exercise regimen as recommended by prescriber. May cause increased cough (if persistent or bothersome, contact prescriber); postural hypotension (use caution when rising from lying or sitting position or climbing stairs); headache (consult prescriber for approved analgesic); dizziness (use caution when driving or engaging in tasks that require alertness until response to drug is known); nausea or vomiting (small frequent meals, frequent mouth care, sucking lozenges, or chewing gum may help); or muscle or back pain (consult prescriber for approved analgesic). Report immediately any swelling of face, mouth, lips, tongue, or throat; chest pain or respiratory difficulty. Report persistent cough; persistent pain in muscles, joints, or back; skin rash; or other persistent adverse reactions. **Pregnancy/breast-feeding precautions:** Inform prescriber if you are or intend to become pregnant. This drug should not be used in the 2nd or 3rd trimester of pregnancy. Consult prescriber for appropriate contraceptive measures if necessary. Consult prescriber if breast-feeding.

Geriatric Considerations: Due to frequent decreases in glomerular filtration (also creatinine clearance) with aging, elderly patients may have exaggerated responses to ACE inhibitors. Differences in clinical response due to hepatic changes are not observed.

Pregnancy Risk Factor: C/D (2nd and 3rd trimesters)

Pregnancy Issues: ACE inhibitors can cause fetal injury or death if taken during the 2nd or 3rd trimester. Discontinue ACE inhibitors as soon as pregnancy is detected.

Lactation: Enters breast milk/not recommended

Breast-Feeding Issues: The manufacturer states that after single dose studies, ramipril was not excreted in breast milk; however, since the amount excreted with daily dosing is unknown, nursing while taking ramipril is not recommended.

Administration

Oral: Capsule is usually swallowed whole, but may be may be mixed in water, apple juice, or applesauce.

Storage: Store at controlled room temperature.

Related Information

Angiotensin Agents *on page 1704*
Heart Failure *on page 1828*

♦ **Raniclor™** *see* Cefaclor *on page 266*

Ranitidine (ra NI ti deen)

U.S. Brand Names Zantac®; Zantac® 75 [OTC]; Zantac® EFFERdose®

Synonyms Ranitidine Hydrochloride

Generic Available Yes; Excludes effervescent tablet, injection

Pharmacologic Category Histamine H_2 Antagonist

Medication Safety Issues

Sound-alike/look-alike issues:

Ranitidine may be confused with amantadine, rimantadine

Zantac® may be confused with Xanax®, Zarontin®, Zofran®, Zyrtec®

Use

Zantac®: Short-term and maintenance therapy of duodenal ulcer, gastric ulcer, gastroesophageal reflux, active benign ulcer, erosive esophagitis, and pathological hypersecretory conditions; as part of a multidrug regimen for *H. pylori* eradication to reduce the risk of duodenal ulcer recurrence

Zantac® 75 [OTC]: Relief of heartburn, acid indigestion, and sour stomach

Unlabeled/Investigational Use Recurrent postoperative ulcer, upper GI bleeding, prevention of acid-aspiration pneumonitis during surgery, and prevention of stress-induced ulcers

Mechanism of Action/Effect Competitive inhibition of histamine at H_2-receptors, gastric acid secretion, gastric volume and hydrogen ion concentration are reduced

Contraindications Hypersensitivity to ranitidine or any component of the formulation

Warnings/Precautions Use with caution in patients with hepatic impairment; dosage modification required in patients with renal impairment; long-term therapy may be associated with vitamin B_{12} deficiency

Drug Interactions

Cytochrome P450 Effect: Substrate (minor) of CYP1A2, 2C19, 2D6; **Inhibits** CYP1A2 (weak), 2D6 (weak)

Decreased Effect:

Decreased effect: Variable effects on warfarin; antacids may decrease absorption of ranitidine; ketoconazole and itraconazole absorptions are decreased; may produce altered serum levels of procainamide and ferrous sulfate; decreased effect of nondepolarizing muscle relaxants, cefpodoxime, cyanocobalamin (decreased absorption), diazepam, oxaprozin

Decreased toxicity of atropine

Increased Effect/Toxicity: Increased the effect/toxicity of cyclosporine (increased serum creatinine), gentamicin (neuromuscular blockade), glipizide, glyburide, midazolam (increased concentrations), metoprolol, pentoxifylline, phenytoin, quinidine, and triazolam.

Nutritional/Ethanol Interactions

Ethanol: Avoid ethanol (may cause gastric mucosal irritation).

Food: Does not interfere with absorption of ranitidine.

Lab Interactions False-positive urine protein using Multistix®, gastric acid secretion test, skin test allergen extracts, serum creatinine and serum transaminase concentrations, urine protein test

Adverse Reactions Frequency not defined.

Cardiovascular: Atrioventricular block, bradycardia, premature ventricular beats, tachycardia, vasculitis

Central nervous system: Agitation, dizziness, depression, hallucinations, headache, insomnia, malaise, mental confusion, somnolence, vertigo

Dermatologic: Alopecia, erythema multiforme, rash

Endocrine & metabolic: Gynecomastia, impotence, increased prolactin levels, loss of libido

Gastrointestinal: Abdominal discomfort/pain, constipation, diarrhea, nausea, pancreatitis, vomiting

Hematologic: Acquired hemolytic anemia, agranulocytosis, aplastic anemia, granulocytopenia, leukopenia, pancytopenia, thrombocytopenia

Hepatic: Hepatic failure, hepatitis

Local: Transient pain, burning or itching at the injection site

Neuromuscular & skeletal: Arthralgia, involuntary motor disturbance, myalgia

Ocular: Blurred vision

Renal: Increased serum creatinine

Miscellaneous: Anaphylaxis, angioneurotic edema, hypersensitivity reactions

Overdosage/Toxicology Symptoms of overdose include abnormal gait, hypotension, and adverse effects seen with normal use. Treatment is primarily symptomatic and supportive.

Pharmacodynamics/Kinetics

Absorption: Oral: 50%

Bioavailability: Oral: 48%

Time to Peak: Serum: Oral: 2-3 hours; I.M.: ≤15 minutes

Protein Binding: 15%

Half-Life Elimination:

Oral: Normal renal function: 2.5-3 hours; Cl_{cr} 25-35 mL/minute: 4.8 hours

I.V.: Normal renal function: 2-2.5 hours

Metabolism: Hepatic to N-oxide, S-oxide, and N-desmethyl metabolites

Excretion: Urine: Oral: 30%, I.V.: 70% (as unchanged drug); feces (as metabolites)

Dosing

Adults & Elderly:

Duodenal ulcer: Oral: Treatment: 150 mg twice daily, or 300 mg once daily after the evening meal or at bedtime; maintenance: 150 mg once daily at bedtime

Eradication of *Helicobacter pylori*: Oral: 150 mg twice daily; requires combination therapy

Pathological hypersecretory conditions:

Oral: 150 mg twice daily; adjust dose or frequency as clinically indicated; doses of up to 6 g/day have been used

(Continued)

Ranitidine *(Continued)*

I.V.: Continuous infusion for Zollinger-Ellison: 1 mg/kg/hour; measure gastric acid output at 4 hours, if >10 mEq or if patient is symptomatic, increase dose in increments of 0.5 mg/kg/hour; doses of up to 2.5 mg/kg/hour have been used

Gastric ulcer, benign: Oral: 150 mg twice daily; maintenance: 150 mg once daily at bedtime

Erosive esophagitis: Oral: Treatment: 150 mg 4 times/day; maintenance: 150 mg twice daily

Prevention of heartburn: Oral: Zantac®75 [OTC]: 75 mg 30-60 minutes before eating food or drinking beverages which cause heartburn; maximum: 150 mg in 24 hours; do not use for more than 14 days

Patients not able to take oral medication:

I.M.: 50 mg every 6-8 hours

I.V.: Intermittent bolus or infusion: 50 mg every 6-8 hours

Continuous I.V. infusion: 6.25 mg/hour

Pediatrics:

Duodenal and gastric ulcer:

Oral: Children 1 month to 16 years:

Treatment: 2-4 mg/kg/day divided twice daily; maximum treatment dose: 300 mg/day

Maintenance: 2-4 mg/kg once daily; maximum maintenance dose: 150 mg/day

I.V.: 2-4 mg/kg/day divided every 6-8 hours; maximum: 150 mg/day

GERD and erosive esophagitis: Children 1 month to 16 years:

Oral: 5-10 mg/kg/day divided twice daily; maximum: GERD: 300 mg/day, erosive esophagitis: 600 mg/day

I.V.: 2-4 mg/kg/day divided every 6-8 hours; maximum: 150 mg/day **or as an alternative**

Continuous infusion: Initial: 1 mg/kg/dose for one dose followed by infusion of 0.08-0.17 mg/kg/hour or 2-4 mg/kg/day

Prevention of heartburn: Oral: Children ≥12 years: Zantac® 75 [OTC]: 75 mg 30-60 minutes before eating food or drinking beverages which cause heartburn; maximum: 150 mg/24 hours; do not use for more than 14 days

Renal Impairment: Adults: Cl_{cr} <50 mL/minute:

Oral: 150 mg every 24 hours; adjust dose cautiously if needed

I.V.: 50 mg every 18-24 hours; adjust dose cautiously if needed

Hemodialysis: Adjust dosing schedule so that dose coincides with the end of hemodialysis.

Hepatic Impairment: Patients with hepatic impairment may have minor changes in ranitidine half-life, distribution, clearance, and bioavailability; dosing adjustments are not necessary; monitor patient.

Available Dosage Forms

Capsule, as hydrochloride: 150 mg, 300 mg

Infusion, as hydrochloride [premixed in NaCl 0.45%; preservative free] (Zantac®): 50 mg (50 mL)

Injection, solution, as hydrochloride (Zantac®): 25 mg/mL (2 mL, 6 mL, 40 mL) [contains phenol 0.5% as preservative]

Syrup, as hydrochloride: 15 mg/mL (10 mL) [contains alcohol 7.5%; peppermint flavor]

Zantac®: 15 mg/mL (473 mL) [contains alcohol 7.5%; peppermint flavor]

Tablet, as hydrochloride: 75 mg [OTC], 150 mg, 300 mg

Zantac®: 150 mg, 300 mg

Zantac® 75: 75 mg

Tablet, effervescent, as hydrochloride (Zantac® EFFERdose®): 25 mg [contains sodium 1.33 mEq/tablet, phenylalanine 2.81 mg/tablet, and sodium benzoate]; 150 mg [contains sodium 7.96 mEq/tablet, phenylalanine 16.84 mg/tablet, and sodium benzoate]

Monitoring and Teaching Issues

Physical Assessment: See Contraindications, Warnings/Precautions (eg, use caution with renal or hepatic impairment). Assess potential for interactions with other pharmacological agents patient may be taking (eg, may increase or decrease levels/effects and toxicity; see Drug Interactions). Assess results of laboratory tests, effectiveness, and adverse reactions (eg, bradycardia, PVCs, tachycardia, CNS changes [depression, hallucinations, confusion, malaise], rash, gynecomastia, GI disturbance, hepatic failure, etc; see Adverse Reactions). Teach patient appropriate use, possible side effects/appropriate interventions, and adverse symptoms to report (see Patient Education).

Monitoring Laboratory Tests: AST, ALT, serum creatinine; when used to prevent stress-related GI bleeding, measure the intragastric pH and try to maintain pH >4; occult blood with GI bleeding; monitor renal function and adjust dosage as indicated

Patient Education: Do not take any new medication during therapy without consulting prescriber. Take exactly as directed; do not increase dose, may take several days before you notice relief. Allow 1 hour between any other antacids (if approved by prescriber) and ranitidine. Avoid alcohol. Follow diet as prescriber recommends. May cause drowsiness, dizziness, or fatigue (use caution when driving or engaging in tasks requiring alertness until response to drug is known). Report chest pain or irregular heartbeat; skin rash; CNS changes (mental confusion, hallucinations, somnolence); unusual persistent weakness or lethargy; yellowing of skin or eyes; or change in color of urine or stool. **Breast-feeding precaution:** Consult prescriber if breast-feeding.

Dietary Considerations: Oral dosage forms may be taken with or without food.

Zantac® EFFERdose®:

Effervescent tablet 25 mg contains sodium 1.33 mEq/tablet and phenylalanine 2.81 mg/tablet

Effervescent tablet 150 mg contains sodium 7.96 mEq/tablet and phenylalanine 16.84 mg/tablet

Geriatric Considerations: H_2 blockers are the preferred drugs for treating PUD in elderly due to cost and ease of administration. These agents are no less or more effective than any other therapy. The preferred agents, due to side effects and drug interaction profile and pharmacokinetics are ranitidine, famotidine, and nizatidine. Treatment for PUD in elderly is recommended for 12 weeks since their lesions are larger; therefore, take longer to heal. Always adjust dose based upon creatinine clearance. Serum half-life is increased to 3-4 hours in elderly patients.

Pregnancy Risk Factor: B

Pregnancy Issues: Ranitidine crosses the placenta, teratogenic effects to the fetus have not been reported. Use with caution during pregnancy.

Lactation: Enters breast milk/use caution

Administration

Oral: EFFERdose®:

25 mg tablet: Dissolve in at least 5 mL (1 teaspoonful) of water; wait until completely dissolved before administering

150 mg tablet: Dissolve each dose in 6-8 ounces of water before drinking

I.M.: No dilution is needed

I.V.:

Intermittent bolus: Dilute vials to 2.5 mg/mL; infuse at 4 mL/minute (5 minutes)

Intermittent infusion: Dilute vials to 0.5 mg/mL; infuse at 5-7 mL/minute (15-20 minutes)

Continuous I.V. infusion: Administer at 6.25 mg/hour and titrate dosage based on gastric pH by continuous infusion over 24 hours

Reconstitution: Vials can be mixed with NS or D_5W; solutions are stable for 48 hours at room temperature

Intermittent bolus injection: Dilute to maximum of 2.5 mg/mL

Intermittent infusion: Dilute to maximum of 0.5 mg/mL

Compatibility: Injection: Do not add other medications to premixed bag. Stable in $D_5^{1}/_2NS$, D_5W, $D_{10}W$, fat emulsion 10%, LR, NS, sodium bicarbonate 5%

Y-site administration: Incompatible with amphotericin B cholesteryl sulfate complex, hetastarch, insulin (regular)

Compatibility in syringe: Incompatible with hydroxyzine, methotrimeprazine, midazolam, pentobarbital, phenobarbital

Compatibility when admixed: Incompatible with amphotericin B, atracurium, cefamandole, cefazolin, cefoxitin, ceftazidime, cefuroxime, ethacrynate, metaraminol, phytonadione

Storage:

Injection: Vials; Store between 4°C to 30°C (39°F to 86°F); protect from light. Solution is a clear, colorless to yellow solution; slight darkening does not affect potency.

Premixed bag: Store between 2°C to 25°C (36°F to 77°F); protect from light.

EFFERdose® formulations: Store between 2°C to 30°C (36°F to 86°F).

Syrup; Store between 4°C to 25°C (39°F to 77°F); protect from light.

Tablets; Store in dry place, between 15°C to 30°C (59°F to 86°F); protect from light.

Related Information

Compatibility of Drugs in Syringe *on page 1725*

♦ **Ranitidine Hydrochloride** *see* Ranitidine *on page 1307*

♦ **Rapamune®** *see* Sirolimus *on page 1377*

♦ **Raptiva™** *see* Efalizumab *on page 508*

Rasburicase (ras BYOOR i kayse)

U.S. Brand Names Elitek™

Generic Available No

Pharmacologic Category Enzyme; Enzyme, Urate-Oxidase (Recombinant)

Use Initial management of uric acid levels in pediatric patients with leukemia, lymphoma, and solid tumor malignancies receiving anticancer therapy expected to result in tumor lysis and elevation of plasma uric acid

Mechanism of Action/Effect Converts uric acid to allantoin (an inactive and soluble metabolite of uric acid); it does not inhibit the formation of uric acid.

Contraindications Hypersensitivity, hemolytic or methemoglobinemia reactions to rasburicase or any component of the formulation; glucose-6-phosphatase dehydrogenase (G6PD) deficiency

Warnings/Precautions Hypersensitivity reactions (including anaphylaxis), methemoglobinemia, and severe hemolysis have been reported; reactions may occur at any time during treatment (including the initial dose); discontinue **immediately and permanently** in patients developing any of these reactions. Hemolysis may be associated with G6PD deficiency; patients at higher risk for G6PD deficiency should be screened prior to therapy. Enzymatic degradation of uric acid in blood samples will occur if left at room temperature; specific guidelines for the collection of plasma uric acid samples must be followed. Rasburicase is immunogenic and can elicit an antibody response; studies in healthy volunteers detected neutralizing antibodies from 1-6 weeks after exposure and lasted for up to 494 days. Safety and efficacy have been established for a single treatment course; administration of more than one course is not recommended. Administer concurrently with standard intravenous hydration therapy. Efficacy in adults has not been established.

Lab Interactions Specific handling procedures must be followed to prevent the degradation of uric acid in plasma samples. Blood must be collected in prechilled tubes containing heparin anticoagulant. Samples must then be **immediately** immersed in an ice water bath. Prepare samples by centrifugation in a precooled centrifuge (4°C). Samples must be kept in ice water bath and analyzed within 4 hours of collection.

Adverse Reactions As reported in patients receiving rasburicase with antitumor therapy versus active-control:

>10%:

Central nervous system: Fever (5% to 46%), headache (26%)

Dermatologic: Rash (13%)

Gastrointestinal: Vomiting (50%), nausea (27%), abdominal pain (20%), constipation (20%), mucositis (2% to 15%), diarrhea (≤1% to 20%)

1% to 10%:

Hematologic: Neutropenia with fever (4%), neutropenia (2%)

Respiratory: Respiratory distress (3%)

Miscellaneous: Sepsis (3%)

(Continued)

Rasburicase *(Continued)*

Overdosage/Toxicology No cases of overdose have been reported; low or undetectable serum levels of uric acid would be expected. Treatment should be symptom-directed and supportive.

Pharmacodynamics/Kinetics

Half-Life Elimination: Elimination: Pediatric patients: 18 hours

Dosing

Adults: Refer to pediatric dosing. Insufficient data collected in adult patients to determine response to treatment.

Elderly: Refer to pediatric dosing. Insufficient data collected in geriatric patients to determine response to treatment.

Pediatrics:

Management of uric acid levels: I.V.: Children: 0.15 mg/kg or 0.2 mg/kg once daily for 5 days (manufacturer-recommended duration); begin chemotherapy 4-24 hours after the first dose

Note: Limited data suggest that a single prechemotherapy dose (versus multiple-day administration) may be sufficiently efficacious. Monitoring electrolytes, hydration status, and uric acid concentrations are necessary to identify the need for additional doses. Other clinical manifestations of tumor lysis syndrome (eg, hyperphosphatemia, hypocalcemia, and hyperkalemia) may occur.

Available Dosage Forms Injection, powder for reconstitution: 1.5 mg [packaged with three 1 mL ampuls of diluent]

Monitoring and Teaching Issues

Physical Assessment: See Warnings/Precautions (eg, severe hypersensitivity reactions) use cautions. See Administration for infusion specifics. Patient must be observed closely for hypersensitivity reaction (which can occur within minutes of administration). Assess effectiveness and adverse reactions prior to initiating therapy and on a regular basis throughout therapy (see Adverse Reactions). Teach patient (caregiver) possible side effects/appropriate interventions and adverse symptoms to report (see Patient Education).

Patient Education: This medication is only administered by infusion; you will be monitored closely during and following infusion. Report immediately any pain, burning, swelling at infusion site, or any signs of allergic reaction (eg, respiratory or swallowing difficulty, back pain, chest tightness, rash, hives, swelling of lips or mouth, chills). Report headache, nausea, vomiting, constipation, or fever.

Pregnancy Risk Factor: C

Lactation: Excretion in breast milk unknown/not recommended

Administration

I.V.: To be given as an I.V. infusion over 30 minutes; do **not** administer as a bolus infusion. Do **not** filter during infusion. If not possible to administer through a separate line, I.V. line should be flushed with at least 15 mL saline prior to and following rasburicase infusion.

Reconstitution: Reconstitute each vial with 1 mL of the provided diluent. Mix by gently swirling; do **not** shake or vortex. Discard if discolored or containing particulate matter. Total dose should be further diluted in NS to a final volume of 50 mL. Both the reconstituted and final solution may be stored up to 24 hours at 2°C to 8°C (36°F to 46°F). Discard unused product.

Storage: Prior to reconstitution, store with diluent at 2°C to 8°C (36°F to 46°F). Do not freeze; protect from light.

- ReAzo [OTC] *see* Phenazopyridine *on page 1193*
- Rebetol® *see* Ribavirin *on page 1318*
- Rebetron® *see* Interferon Alfa-2b and Ribavirin *on page 814*
- Rebif® *see* Interferon Beta-1a *on page 819*
- Recombinant Hirudin *see* Lepirudin *on page 872*
- Recombinant Human Deoxyribonuclease *see* Dornase Alfa *on page 482*
- Recombinant Human Follicle Stimulating Hormone *see* Follitropins *on page 670*
- Recombinant Human Luteinizing Hormone *see* Lutropin Alfa *on page 928*
- Recombinant Human Parathyroid Hormone (1-34) *see* Teriparatide *on page 1448*
- Recombinant Plasminogen Activator *see* Reteplase *on page 1314*
- Recombinate™ *see* Antihemophilic Factor (Recombinant) *on page 127*
- Recombivax HB® *see page 1660*
- Red Cross™ Canker Sore [OTC] *see* Benzocaine *on page 181*
- Redutemp® [OTC] *see* Acetaminophen *on page 38*
- ReFacto® *see* Antihemophilic Factor (Recombinant) *on page 127*
- Refenesen Plus [OTC] *see* Guaifenesin and Pseudoephedrine *on page 733*
- Refludan® *see* Lepirudin *on page 872*
- Regitine [DSC] *see* Phentolamine *on page 1198*
- Reglan® *see* Metoclopramide *on page 989*
- Regonol® *see* Pyridostigmine *on page 1287*
- Regular Iletin® II *see* Insulin Preparations *on page 805*
- Regular, Insulin *see* Insulin Preparations *on page 805*
- Reguloid® [OTC] *see* Psyllium *on page 1284*
- Relacon-HC *see* Phenylephrine, Hydrocodone, and Chlorpheniramine *on page 1202*
- Relafen® *see* Nabumetone *on page 1044*
- Relefact® TRH Injection *see page 1625*
- Relenza® *see* Zanamivir *on page 1582*
- Relief® [OTC] *see* Phenylephrine *on page 1200*
- Relpax® *see* Eletriptan *on page 512*
- Remeron® *see* Mirtazapine *on page 1013*
- Remeron SolTab® *see* Mirtazapine *on page 1013*

♦ **Remicade®** *see* Infliximab *on page 803*
♦ **Reminyl®** *see* Galantamine *on page 693*
♦ **Renagel®** *see* Sevelamer *on page 1370*
♦ **Renova®** *see* Tretinoin (Topical) *on page 1516*

Repaglinide (re pa GLI nide)

U.S. Brand Names Prandin®
Generic Available No
Pharmacologic Category Antidiabetic Agent, Miscellaneous
Medication Safety Issues
Sound-alike/look-alike issues:
Prandin® may be confused with Avandia®

Use Management of type 2 diabetes mellitus (noninsulin dependent, NIDDM); may be used in combination with metformin or thiazolidinediones

Mechanism of Action/Effect Nonsulfonylurea hypoglycemic agent which blocks ATP-dependent potassium channels, depolarizing the membrane and facilitating calcium entry through calcium channels. Increased intracellular calcium stimulates insulin release from the pancreatic beta cells.

Contraindications Hypersensitivity to repaglinide or any component of the formulation; diabetic ketoacidosis, with or without coma (treat with insulin); type 1 diabetes (insulin dependent, IDDM)

Warnings/Precautions Use with caution in patients with hepatic or renal impairment. All oral hypoglycemic agents are capable of producing hypoglycemia. Proper patient selection, dosage, and instructions to the patients are important to avoid hypoglycemic episodes. It may be necessary to discontinue repaglinide and administer insulin if the patient is exposed to stress (fever, trauma, infection, surgery). Safety and efficacy have not been established in pediatric patients. Not indicated for use in combination with NPH insulin.

Drug Interactions
Cytochrome P450 Effect: Substrate of CYP2C8/9 (major), 3A4 (major)
Decreased Effect: CYP2C8/9 inducers may decrease the levels/effects of repaglinide; example inducers include carbamazepine, phenobarbital, phenytoin, rifampin, rifapentine, and secobarbital. CYP3A4 inducers may decrease the levels/effects of repaglinide; example inducers include aminoglutethimide, carbamazepine, nafcillin, nevirapine, phenobarbital, phenytoin, and rifamycins.
Increased Effect/Toxicity: Concurrent use of other hypoglycemic agents may increase risk of hypoglycemia. Gemfibrozil may increase the serum concentration of repaglinide (resulting in severe, prolonged hypoglycemia), and the addition of itraconazole may augment the effects of gemfibrozil on repaglinide. CYP2C8/9 inhibitors may increase the levels/effects of repaglinide; example inhibitors include delavirdine, fluconazole, gemfibrozil, ketoconazole, nicardipine, NSAIDs, pioglitazone, and sulfonamides. CYP3A4 inhibitors may increase the levels/effects of repaglinide; example inhibitors include azole antifungals, ciprofloxacin, clarithromycin, diclofenac, doxycycline, erythromycin, imatinib, isoniazid, nefazodone, nicardipine, propofol, protease inhibitors, quinidine, and verapamil.

Nutritional/Ethanol Interactions
Ethanol: Avoid ethanol (may cause hypoglycemia).
Food: When given with food, the AUC of repaglinide is decreased.
Herb/Nutraceutical: St John's wort may decrease repaglinide levels. Avoid gymnema, garlic (may cause hypoglycemia).

Adverse Reactions
>10%:
Central nervous system: Headache (9% to 11%)
Endocrine & metabolic: Hypoglycemia (16% to 31%)
Respiratory: Upper respiratory tract infection (10% to 16%)
1% to 10%:
Cardiovascular: Chest pain (2% to 3%), ischemia (4%)
Gastrointestinal: Nausea (3% to 5%), heartburn (2% to 4%), vomiting (2% to 3%) constipation (2% to 3%), diarrhea (4% to 5%), tooth disorder (<1% to 2%)
Genitourinary: Urinary tract infection (2% to 3%)
Neuromuscular & skeletal: Arthralgia (3% to 6%), back pain (5% to 6%), paresthesia (2% to 3%)
Respiratory: Sinusitis (3% to 6%), rhinitis (3% to 7%), bronchitis (2% to 6%)
Miscellaneous: Allergy (1% to 2%)

Overdosage/Toxicology Symptoms of severe hypoglycemia include seizures, cerebral damage, tingling of lips and tongue, nausea, yawning, confusion, agitation, tachycardia, sweating, convulsions, stupor, and coma. Management includes glucose administration (oral for milder hypoglycemia or by injection in more severe forms) and symptomatic treatment.

Pharmacodynamics/Kinetics
Onset of Action: Single dose: Increased insulin levels: ~15-60 minutes
Duration of Action: 4-6 hours
Absorption: Rapid and complete
Bioavailability: Mean absolute: ~56%
Time to Peak: Plasma: ~1 hour
Protein Binding: Plasma: >98%
Half-Life Elimination: 1 hour
Metabolism: Hepatic via CYP3A4 isoenzyme and glucuronidation to inactive metabolites
Excretion: Within 96 hours: Feces (~90%, <2% as parent drug); Urine (~8%)

Dosing
Adults & Elderly:
Type 2 diabetes: Oral:
Note: Doses should be taken within 15 minutes of the meal, but time may vary from immediately preceding the meal to as long as 30 minutes before the meal
Patients not previously treated or whose Hb A₁c is <8%: Initial: 0.5 mg before each meal
(Continued)

Repaglinide *(Continued)*

Patients previously treated with blood glucose-lowering agents whose Hb A$_{1c}$ is ≥8%: Initial: 1 or 2 mg before each meal.

Dose adjustment: Determine dosing adjustments by blood glucose response, usually fasting blood glucose. Double the preprandial dose up to 4 mg until satisfactory blood glucose response is achieved. At least 1 week should elapse to assess response after each dose adjustment.

Dose range: 0.5-4 mg taken with meals. Repaglinide may be dosed prandial 2, 3 or 4 times/day in response to changes in the patient's meal pattern. Maximum recommended daily dose: 16 mg.

Patients receiving other oral hypoglycemic agents: When repaglinide is used to replace therapy with other oral hypoglycemic agents, it may be started the day after the final dose is given. Observe patients carefully for hypoglycemia because of potential overlapping of drug effects. When transferred from longer half-life sulfonylureas (eg, chlorpropamide), close monitoring may be indicated for up to ≥1 week.

Note: Combination therapy: If repaglinide monotherapy does not result in adequate glycemic control, metformin or a thiazolidinedione may be added. Or, if metformin or thiazolidinedione therapy does not provide adequate control, repaglinide may be added. The starting dose and dose adjustments for combination therapy are the same as repaglinide monotherapy. Carefully adjust the dose of each drug to determine the minimal dose required to achieve the desired pharmacologic effect. Failure to do so could result in an increase in the incidence of hypoglycemic episodes. Use appropriate monitoring of FPG and Hb A$_{1c}$ measurements to ensure that the patient is not subjected to excessive drug exposure or increased probability of secondary drug failure. If glucose is not achieved after a suitable trial of combination therapy, consider discontinuing these drugs and using insulin.

Renal Impairment:

Cl$_{cr}$ 40-80 mL/minute (mild to moderate renal dysfunction): Initial dosage adjustment does not appear to be necessary.

Cl$_{cr}$ 20-40 mL/minute: Initiate 0.5 mg with meals; titrate carefully.

Hepatic Impairment: Use conservative initial and maintenance doses. Use longer intervals between dosage adjustments.

Available Dosage Forms Tablet: 0.5 mg, 1 mg, 2 mg

Monitoring and Teaching Issues

Physical Assessment: Assess potential for interactions with other prescriptions, OTC medications, or herbal products patient may be taking (especially anything that is metabolized via the cytochrome P450 isoenzyme 3A4 route). Assess results of laboratory tests and patient response on a regular basis throughout therapy. Teach patient proper use (or refer patient to diabetic educator), possible side effects/appropriate interventions, and adverse symptoms to report (eg, signs of hypoglycemia).

Monitoring Laboratory Tests: Fasting blood glucose and glycosylated hemoglobin (Hb A$_{1c}$) levels

Patient Education: Do not take any new medication during therapy without consulting prescriber. Take this medication exactly as directed (3-4 times a day) 15-30 minutes prior to a meal. If you skip a meal (or add an extra meal) skip (or add) a dose for that meal. Do not change dosage or discontinue without consulting prescriber. Follow dietary and lifestyle directions of prescriber or diabetic educator. Avoid alcohol. You will be instructed in signs of hypo- or hyperglycemia by prescriber or diabetic educator; be alert for adverse hypoglycemia (lightheadedness, tachycardia or palpitations, sweaty palms or profuse perspiration, yawning, tingling of lips and tongue, seizures, or change in sensorium) and follow prescriber's instructions for intervention. May cause headache or mild GI effects during first weeks of therapy (nausea, vomiting, diarrhea, constipation, heartburn), if these do not diminish, consult prescriber for approved medication. Report chest pain; respiratory difficulty or symptoms of upper respiratory infection; urinary tract infection (burning or itching on urination); muscle pain or back pain; or other adverse effects. **Pregnancy/breast-feeding precautions:** Inform prescriber if you are or intend to become pregnant. Breast-feeding is not recommended.

Dietary Considerations: Administer repaglinide 15-30 minutes before meals. Dietary modification based on ADA recommendations is a part of therapy. May cause hypoglycemia. Must be able to recognize symptoms of hypoglycemia (palpitations, tachycardia, sweaty palms, diaphoresis, lightheadedness).

Geriatric Considerations: Repaglinide has not been studied exclusively in the elderly; information from the manufacturer states that no differences in its effectiveness or adverse effects had been identified between persons younger than and older than 65 years of age. How "tightly" a geriatric patient's blood glucose should be controlled is controversial; however, a fasting blood glucose <150 mg/dL is now an acceptable endpoint. Such a decision should be based on the patient's functional status, how well he/she recognizes hypoglycemic or hyperglycemic symptoms, and how to respond to them and their other disease states.

Pregnancy Risk Factor: C

Pregnancy Issues: Safety in pregnant women has not been established. Use during pregnancy only if clearly needed. Abnormal blood glucose levels are associated with a higher incidence of congenital abnormalities. Insulin is the drug of choice for the control of diabetes mellitus during pregnancy.

Lactation: Excretion in breast milk unknown/not recommended

Breast-Feeding Issues: It is not known whether repaglinide is excreted in breast milk. Because the potential for hypoglycemia in nursing infants may exist, decide whether to discontinue repaglinide or discontinue breast-feeding. If repaglinide is discontinued and if diet alone is inadequate for controlling blood glucose, consider insulin therapy.

Administration

Oral: Administer repaglinide 15-30 minutes before meals. Patients who are anorexic or NPO, may need to have their dose held to avoid hypoglycemia.

Storage: Do not store above 25°C (77°F). Protect from moisture.

Related Information

Diabetes Mellitus Management *on page 1819*

♦ **Repan®** *see* Butalbital, Acetaminophen, and Caffeine *on page 225*

♦ **Repronex®** *see* Menotropins *on page 948*

♦ **Requip®** *see* Ropinirole *on page 1345*

♦ **Rescriptor®** *see* Delavirdine *on page 413*

♦ **Resectisol®** *see* Mannitol *on page 932*

Reserpine (re SER peen)

Generic Available Yes

Pharmacologic Category Rauwolfia Alkaloid

Medication Safety Issues

Sound-alike/look-alike issues:

Reserpine may be confused with Risperdal®, risperidone

Use Management of mild to moderate hypertension

Unlabeled/Investigational Use Management of tardive dyskinesia, schizophrenia

Mechanism of Action/Effect Reduces blood pressure via depletion of sympathetic biogenic amines (norepinephrine and dopamine); this also commonly results in sedative effects

Contraindications Hypersensitivity to reserpine or any component of the formulation; active peptic ulcer disease; ulcerative colitis; history of mental depression (especially with suicidal tendencies); MAO inhibitors

Warnings/Precautions Use extreme caution in treating patients with a history of depression; watch for signs and symptoms of depression. Discontinue at the first sign of depression. Use cautiously in patients with a history of PUD (increases GI motility and secretion) or gallstones (biliary colic may be precipitated). Preoperative withdrawal does not ensure circulatory stability. Make anesthesiologist aware of medical regimen. Avoid in severe renal impairment. Avoid use with MAO inhibitors.

Drug Interactions

Decreased Effect: Tricyclic antidepressants may increase antihypertensive effect.

Increased Effect/Toxicity: Reserpine may cause hypertensive reactions in patients receiving an MAO inhibitor; use an alternative antihypertensive. Reserpine may increase the effect of beta-blockers. May increase effects of CNS depressants and/or ethanol. May increase the effects/toxicity of levodopa, quinidine, procainamide, and digitalis glycosides.

Nutritional/Ethanol Interactions

Ethanol: Avoid ethanol (may increase CNS depression).

Herb/Nutraceutical: Avoid dong quai if using for hypertension (has estrogenic activity). Avoid ephedra, yohimbe (may worsen hypertension). Avoid valerian, St John's wort, kava kava, gotu kola (may increase CNS depression). Avoid garlic (may have increased antihypertensive effect).

Lab Interactions Decreased catecholamines (U)

Adverse Reactions Frequency not defined.

Cardiovascular: Peripheral edema, arrhythmia, bradycardia, chest pain, PVC, hypotension

Central nervous system: Dizziness, headache, nightmares, nervousness, drowsiness, fatigue, mental depression, parkinsonism, dull sensorium, syncope, paradoxical anxiety

Dermatologic: Rash, pruritus, flushing of skin

Gastrointestinal: Anorexia, diarrhea, dry mouth, nausea, vomiting, increased salivation, weight gain, increased gastric acid secretion

Genitourinary: Impotence, decreased libido

Hematologic: Thrombocytopenia purpura

Ocular: Blurred vision

Respiratory: Nasal congestion, dyspnea, epistaxis

Overdosage/Toxicology Symptoms of overdose include hypotension, bradycardia, CNS depression, sedation, coma, hypothermia, miosis, tremor, diarrhea, and vomiting. Treatment is symptom-directed and supportive. Anticholinergic agents may be useful in reducing parkinsonian effects and bradycardia.

Pharmacodynamics/Kinetics

Onset of Action: Antihypertensive: 3-6 days

Duration of Action: 2-6 weeks

Absorption: ~40%

Protein Binding: 96%

Half-Life Elimination: 50-100 hours

Metabolism: Extensively hepatic (>90%)

Excretion: Feces (30% to 60%); urine (10%)

Dosing

Adults:

Hypertension: Oral: Initial: 0.5 mg/day for 1-2 weeks; 0.1 mg may be given every other day to achieve a dose of 0.05 mg once daily (full antihypertensive effects may take as long as 3 weeks).

Usual dose range (JNC 7): 0.05-0.25 mg once daily

Tardive dyskinesia/schizophrenia (unlabeled use): Oral: Initial: 0.5 mg/day; usual range: 0.1-1 mg

Elderly: Oral: Initial: 0.05 mg once daily increasing by 0.05 mg every week as necessary (full antihypertensive effects may take as long as 3 weeks).

Pediatrics: Children: Hypertension: 0.01-0.02 mg/kg/24 hours divided every 12 hours; maximum dose: 0.25 mg/day (not recommended in children)

Renal Impairment:

Cl$_{cr}$ <10 mL/minute: Avoid use.

Not removed by hemo- or peritoneal dialysis; supplemental dose is not necessary.

Available Dosage Forms Tablet: 0.1 mg, 0.25 mg

(Continued)

Reserpine *(Continued)*

Monitoring and Teaching Issues

Physical Assessment: Use caution with history of depression, history of PUD, or gall-stones (see Warnings/Precautions for specific use cautions). Assess potential for interactions with other pharmacological agents and herbal products patient may be taking (eg, increased hypotensive effect [TCAs], hypertensive reaction [MAOIs, ephedra, yohimbe], increased effects of toxicity [CNS depressants]; see Drug Interactions). Assess blood pressure and cardiac status prior to starting therapy, during first doses, when changing dose, and regularly thereafter (eg, arrhythmia, hypotension, CNS changes [nervousness, depression], Parkinsonism, rash, diarrhea, nausea, vomiting; see Adverse Reactions) Teach patient proper use, possible side effects/appropriate interventions, and adverse symptoms to report (see Patient Education).

Patient Education: Do not take any new medication during therapy without consulting prescriber (especially any sleep remedies or stimulants). Take as directed; do not alter dose or discontinue without consulting prescriber. May take up to 2 weeks to see effects of therapy. Avoid alcohol and maintain recommended diet. May cause mild nervousness, dizziness, or fatigue (use caution when driving or engaging in hazardous activities until response to drug is known); orthostatic hypotension (use caution when rising from sitting or lying position or when climbing stairs until response to therapy is known): nausea or loss of appetite (small frequent meals or sucking lozenges may help); constipation (increased exercise, fluids, fruit, or fiber may help); nasal stuffiness (avoid OTC medications and consult prescriber for approved medication); or impotence (will resolve when medication is discontinued). Report chest pain, rapid heartbeat, or palpitations; respiratory difficulty; sudden increase in weight; swelling in ankles or hands; black tarry stools; or unusual feelings of depression, alteration in gait or balance, or other adverse reactions. **Pregnancy/breast-feeding precautions:** Inform prescriber if you are or intend to become pregnant. Consult prescriber if breast-feeding.

Geriatric Considerations: Some studies advocate the use of reserpine because of its low cost, long half-life, and efficacy, but it is generally not considered a first-line drug. If it is to be used, doses should not exceed 0.25 mg and the patient should be monitored for depressed mood.

Pregnancy Risk Factor: C

Lactation: Enters breast milk/use caution

Administration

Storage: Protect oral dosage forms from light.

Additional Information Adverse effects are usually dose related, mild, and infrequent when administered for the management of hypertension.

- ♦ **Resource® GlutaSolve® [OTC]** *see* Glutamine *on page 719*
- ♦ **Respa-DM®** *see* Guaifenesin and Dextromethorphan *on page 731*
- ♦ **Respaire®-60 SR** *see* Guaifenesin and Pseudoephedrine *on page 733*
- ♦ **Respaire®-120 SR** *see* Guaifenesin and Pseudoephedrine *on page 733*
- ♦ **Restasis™** *see* CycloSPORINE *on page 383*
- ♦ **Restoril®** *see* Temazepam *on page 1434*
- ♦ **Retavase®** *see* Reteplase *on page 1314*

Reteplase *(RE ta plase)*

U.S. Brand Names Retavase®

Synonyms Recombinant Plasminogen Activator; r-PA

Generic Available No

Pharmacologic Category Thrombolytic Agent

Use Management of acute myocardial infarction (AMI); improvement of ventricular function; reduction of the incidence of CHF and the reduction of mortality following AMI

Mechanism of Action/Effect Reteplase initiates local fibrinolysis by binding to fibrin in a thrombus (clot) and converting entrapped plasminogen to plasmin. Dissolution of thrombus occluding a coronary artery restores perfusion to ischemic myocardium. Reteplase is manufactured by recombinant DNA technology using *E. coli.*

Contraindications Hypersensitivity to reteplase or any component of the formulation; active internal bleeding; history of cerebrovascular accident; recent intracranial or intraspinal surgery or trauma; intracranial neoplasm, arteriovenous malformations, or aneurysm; known bleeding diathesis; severe uncontrolled hypertension

Warnings/Precautions Concurrent heparin anticoagulation can contribute to bleeding; careful attention to all potential bleeding sites. I.M. injections and nonessential handling of the patient should be avoided. Venipunctures should be performed carefully and only when necessary. If arterial puncture is necessary, use an upper extremity vessel that can be manually compressed. If serious bleeding occurs then the infusion of anistreplase and heparin should be stopped.

For the following conditions the risk of bleeding is higher with use of reteplase and should be weighed against the benefits of therapy: recent major surgery (eg, CABG, obstetrical delivery, organ biopsy, previous puncture of noncompressible vessels), cerebrovascular disease, recent gastrointestinal or genitourinary bleeding, recent trauma including CPR, hypertension (systolic BP >180 mm Hg and/or diastolic BP >110 mm Hg), high likelihood of left heart thrombus (eg, mitral stenosis with atrial fibrillation), acute pericarditis, subacute bacterial endocarditis, hemostatic defects including ones caused by severe renal or hepatic dysfunction, significant hepatic dysfunction, pregnancy, diabetic hemorrhagic retinopathy or other hemorrhagic ophthalmic conditions, septic thrombophlebitis or occluded AV cannula at seriously infected site, advanced age (eg, >75 years), patients receiving oral anticoagulants, any other condition in which bleeding constitutes a significant hazard or would be particularly difficult to manage because of location.

Coronary thrombolysis may result in reperfusion arrhythmias. Follow standard MI management. Rare anaphylactic reactions can occur. Safety and efficacy in pediatric patients have not been established.

Drug Interactions

Decreased Effect: Aminocaproic acid (antifibrinolytic agent) may decrease effectiveness of thrombolytic agents.

Increased Effect/Toxicity: The risk of bleeding associated with reteplase may be increased by oral anticoagulants (warfarin), heparin, low molecular weight heparins, and drugs which affect platelet function (eg, NSAIDs, dipyridamole, ticlopidine, clopidogrel, IIb/IIIa antagonists). Concurrent use with aspirin and heparin may increase the risk of bleeding; however, aspirin and heparin were used concomitantly with reteplase in the majority of patients in clinical studies.

Adverse Reactions Bleeding is the most frequent adverse effect associated with reteplase. Heparin and aspirin have been administered concurrently with reteplase in clinical trials. The incidence of adverse events is a reflection of these combined therapies, and are comparable with comparison thrombolytics.

>10%: Local: Injection site bleeding (4.6% to 48.6%)

1% to 10%:

Gastrointestinal: Bleeding (1.8% to 9.0%)

Genitourinary: Bleeding (0.9% to 9.5%)

Hematologic: Anemia (0.9% to 2.6%)

Other adverse effects noted are frequently associated with MI (and therefore may or may not be attributable to Retavase®) and include arrhythmia, hypotension, cardiogenic shock, pulmonary edema, cardiac arrest, reinfarction, pericarditis, tamponade, thrombosis, and embolism.

Overdosage/Toxicology Symptoms of overdose include increased incidence of intracranial bleeding. Treatment is supportive.

Pharmacodynamics/Kinetics

Onset of Action: Thrombolysis: 30-90 minutes

Half-Life Elimination: 13-16 minutes

Excretion: Feces and urine

Clearance: Plasma: 250-450 mL/minute

Dosing

Adults & Elderly:

Acute MI (thrombolysis): I.V.: 10 units I.V. over 2 minutes, followed by a second dose 30 minutes later of 10 units I.V. over 2 minutes; withhold second dose if serious bleeding or anaphylaxis occurs.

Pediatrics: Not recommended

Available Dosage Forms Injection, powder for reconstitution [preservative free]: 10.4 units [equivalent to reteplase 18.1 mg; packaged with sterile water for injection]

Monitoring and Teaching Issues

Physical Assessment: Use caution when there is significant risk of bleeding (see Warnings/Precautions for specific use cautions). Assess potential risk interactions with other pharmacological and herbal products patient may be taking (especially those medications that may affect coagulation or platelet function; see Drug Interactions). See Administration for infusion specifics. Patient should be closely monitored for bleeding during and following treatment; infusion site, neurological status (eg, intracranial hemorrhage), vital signs, and ECG (see Adverse Reactions). Bleeding precautions should be maintained; avoid I.M. injections, venipunctures (unless absolutely necessary), and nonessential handling of the patient. If arterial puncture is necessary, use an upper extremity vessel that can be manually compressed. Patient instructions determined by patient condition (see Patient Education).

Monitoring Laboratory Tests: CBC, PTT, signs and symptoms of bleeding, ECG monitoring

Patient Education: Inform prescriber of all medication or herbal products you are taking. This medication is only administered by infusion; you will be monitored closely during and after treatment. You will have a tendency to bleed easily; use caution to prevent injury (use electric razor, and soft toothbrush). Also use caution when handling knives, needles, or anything sharp. Follow instructions for strict bedrest to reduce the risk of injury. If bleeding occurs, report immediately and apply pressure to bleeding spot until bleeding stops completely. Report unusual pain (acute headache, joint pain, chest pain); unusual bruising or bleeding; blood in urine, stool, or vomitus; bleeding gums; vision changes; or respiratory difficulty. **Pregnancy/breast-feeding precautions:** Inform prescriber if you are or intend to become pregnant. Consult prescriber if breast-feeding.

Pregnancy Risk Factor: C

Lactation: Excretion in breast milk unknown/use caution

Administration

I.V.: Infuse over 2 minutes.

Reconstitution: Reteplase should be reconstituted using the diluent, syringe, needle, and dispensing pin provided with each kit.

Storage: Dosage kits should be stored at 2°C to 25°C (36°F to 77°F) and remain sealed until use in order to protect from light.

* **r-hCG** *see Chorionic Gonadotropin (Recombinant) on page 320*
* **Rheumatrex®** *see Methotrexate on page 974*
* **rhFSH-alpha** *see Follitropins on page 670*
* **rhFSH-beta** *see Follitropins on page 670*
* **RhIG** *see Rh₀(D) Immune Globulin on page 1316*
* **Rhinocort® Aqua®** *see Budesonide on page 210*
* **r-hLH** *see Lutropin Alfa on page 928*

Rh₀(D) Immune Globulin (ar aych oh (dee) i MYUN GLOB yoo lin)

U.S. Brand Names BayRho-D® Full-Dose; BayRho-D® Mini-Dose; MICRhoGAM®; RhoGAM®; Rhophylac®; WinRho SDF®

Synonyms RhIG; Rho(D) Immune Globulin (Human); RhoIGIV; RhoIVIM

Generic Available No

Pharmacologic Category Immune Globulin

Use

Suppression of Rh isoimmunization: Use in the following situations when an Rh₀(D)-negative individual is exposed to Rh₀(D)-positive blood: During delivery of an Rh₀(D)-positive infant; abortion; amniocentesis; chorionic villus sampling; ruptured tubal pregnancy; abdominal trauma; transplacental hemorrhage. Used when the mother is Rh₀(D) negative, the father of the child is either Rh₀(D) positive or Rh₀(D) unknown, the baby is either Rh₀(D) positive or Rh₀(D) unknown.

Transfusion: Suppression of Rh isoimmunization in Rh₀(D)-negative female children and female adults in their childbearing years transfused with Rh₀(D) antigen-positive RBCs or blood components containing Rh₀(D) antigen-positive RBCs

Treatment of idiopathic thrombocytopenic purpura (ITP): Used in the following nonsplenectomized Rh₀(D) positive individuals: Children with acute or chronic ITP, adults with chronic ITP, children and adults with ITP secondary to HIV infection

Mechanism of Action/Effect

Rh suppression: Suppresses the immune response and antibody formation of Rh₀(D) negative individuals to Rh₀(D) positive red blood cells.

ITP: Coats the patients Rh₀(D) positive red blood cells with antibody, so that as they are cleared by the spleen, the spleens ability to clear antibody-coated cells is saturated, sparing the platelets.

Contraindications Hypersensitivity to immune globulins or any component of the formulation; prior sensitization to Rh₀(D)

Warnings/Precautions As a product of human plasma, may potentially transmit disease; screening of donors, as well as testing and/or inactivation of certain viruses reduces this risk. Not for replacement therapy in immune globulin deficiency syndromes. Use caution with IgA deficiency, may contain trace amounts of IgA; patients who are IgA deficient may have the potential for developing IgA antibodies, anaphylactic reactions may occur. Administer I.M. injections with caution in patients with thrombocytopenia or coagulation disorders.

ITP: Do not administer I.M. or SubQ; administer dose I.V. only. Safety and efficacy not established in Rh₀(D) negative or splenectomized patients. Decrease dose with hemoglobin <10 g/dL; use with extreme caution if hemoglobin <8 g/dL

Rh₀(D) suppression: For use in the mother; do not administer to the neonate.

Drug Interactions

Decreased Effect: Rh₀(D) immune globulin may interfere with the response of live vaccines; vaccines should not be administered within 3 months after Rh₀(D)

Lab Interactions Some infants born to women given Rh₀(D) antepartum have a weakly positive Coombs' test at birth. Fetal-maternal hemorrhage may cause false blood-typing result in the mother; when there is any doubt to the patients' Rh type, Rh₀(D) immune globulin should be administered

Adverse Reactions Frequency not defined.

Cardiovascular: Hypotension, pallor, tachycardia, vasodilation

Central nervous system: Chills, dizziness, fever, headache, malaise, somnolence

Dermatologic: Pruritus, rash

Gastrointestinal: Abdominal pain, diarrhea, nausea, vomiting

Hematologic: Hemoglobin decreased (patients with ITP), intravascular hemolysis (patients with ITP)

Hepatic: LDH increased

Local: Injection site reaction: Discomfort, induration, mild pain, redness, swelling

Neuromuscular & skeletal: Back pain, hyperkinesia, myalgia, weakness

Miscellaneous: Anaphylaxis, diaphoresis

Overdosage/Toxicology No symptoms are likely, however, high doses have been associated with a mild, transient hemolytic anemia. Treatment is supportive.

Pharmacodynamics/Kinetics

Onset of Action: Onset of platelet increase: ITP: 1-3 days

Duration of Action: Suppression of Rh isoimmunization: ~12 weeks; Treatment of ITP: 3-4 weeks

Time to Peak: Plasma: I.M.: 5-10 days

Half-Life Elimination: 21-30 days

Dosing

Adults:

ITP: WinRho SDF®: I.V.:

Initial: 50 mcg/kg as a single injection, or can be given as a divided dose on separate days. If hemoglobin is <10 g/dL: Dose should be reduced to 25-40 mcg/kg

Subsequent dosing: 25-60 mcg/kg can be used if required to elevate platelet count

Maintenance dosing if patient **did respond** to initial dosing: 25-60 mcg/kg based on platelet and hemoglobin levels:

Maintenance dosing if patient **did not respond** to initial dosing:

Hemoglobin 8-10 g/dL: Redose between 25-40 mcg/kg

Hemoglobin >10 g/dL: Redose between 50-60 mcg/kg

Hemoglobin <8 g/dL: Use with caution

Rh_o(D) suppression: Note: One "full dose" (300 mcg) provides enough antibody to prevent Rh sensitization if the volume of RBC entering the circulation is ≤15 mL. When >15 mL is suspected, a fetal red cell count should be performed to determine the appropriate dose.

Pregnancy:

Antepartum prophylaxis: In general, dose is given at 28 weeks. If given early in pregnancy, administer every 12 weeks to ensure adequate levels of passively acquired anti-Rh

BayRho-D® Full Dose, RhoGAM®: I.M.: 300 mcg

Rhophylac®, WinRho SDF®: I.M., I.V.: 300 mcg

Postpartum prophylaxis: In general, dose is administered as soon as possible after delivery, preferably within 72 hours. Can be given up to 28 days following delivery

BayRho-D® Full Dose, RhoGAM®: I.M.: 300 mcg

Rhophylac®: I.M., I.V.: 300 mcg

WinRho SDF®: I.M., I.V.: 120 mcg

Threatened abortion, any time during pregnancy (with continuation of pregnancy):

BayRho-D® Full Dose, RhoGAM®: I.M.: 300 mcg; administer as soon as possible

Rhophylac®, WinRho SDF®: I.M./I.V.: 300 mcg; administer as soon as possible

Abortion, miscarriage, termination of ectopic pregnancy:

BayRho-D®, RhoGAM®: I.M.: ≥13 weeks gestation: 300 mcg.

BayRho-D® Mini Dose, MICRhoGAM®: <13 weeks gestation: I.M.: 50 mcg

Rhophylac®: I.M., I.V.: 300 mcg

WinRho SDF®: I.M., I.V.: After 34 weeks gestation: 120 mcg; administer immediately or within 72 hours

Amniocentesis, chorionic villus sampling:

BayRho-D®, RhoGAM®: I.M.: At 15-18 weeks gestation or during the 3rd trimester: 300 mcg. If dose is given between 13-18 weeks, repeat at 26-28 weeks and within 72 hours of delivery.

Rhophylac®: I.M., I.V.: 300 mcg

WinRho SDF®: I.M., I.V.:

Before 34 weeks gestation: 300 mcg; administer immediately, repeat dose every 12 weeks during pregnancy

After 34 weeks gestation: 120 mcg, administered immediately or within 72 hours

Abdominal trauma, manipulation:

BayRho-D®, RhoGAM®: I.M.: 2nd or 3rd trimester: 300 mcg. If dose is given between 13-18 weeks, repeat at 26-28 weeks and within 72 hours of delivery.

Rhophylac®: I.M., I.V.: 300 mcg

WinRho SDF®: I.M., I.V.: After 34 weeks gestation: 120 mcg; administer immediately or within 72 hours

Transfusion:

BayRho-D®, RhoGAM®: I.M.: Multiply the volume of Rh positive whole blood administered by the hematocrit of the donor unit to equal the volume of RBCs transfused. The volume of RBCs is then divided by 15 mL, providing the number of 300 mcg doses (vials/syringes) to administer. If the dose calculated results in a fraction, round up to the next higher whole 300 mcg dose (vial/syringe).

WinRho SDF®: Administer within 72 hours after exposure of incompatible blood transfusions or massive fetal hemorrhage.

I.V.: Calculate dose as follows; administer 600 mcg every 8 hours until the total dose is administered:

Exposure to Rh_o(D) positive whole blood: 9 mcg/mL blood

Exposure to Rh_o(D) positive red blood cells: 18 mcg/mL cells

I.M.: Calculate dose as follows; administer 1200 mcg every 12 hours until the total dose is administered:

Exposure to Rh_o(D) positive whole blood: 12 mcg/mL blood

Exposure to Rh_o(D) positive red blood cells: 24 mcg/mL cells

Rhophylac®: I.M., I.V.:20 mcg per 2 mL transfused blood or 1 mL erythrocyte concentrate

Pediatrics: ITP, transfusion: WinRho SDF®: Refer to adult dosing.

Available Dosage Forms

Injection, solution [preservative free]:

BayRho-D® Full-Dose, RhoGAM®: 300 mcg [for I.M. use only]

BayRho-D® Mini-Dose, MICRhoGAM®: 50 mcg [for I.M. use only]

Rhophylac®: 300 mcg/2 mL (2 mL) [1500 int. units; for I.M. or I.V. use]

Injection, powder for reconstitution [preservative free] (WinRho SDF®): 120 mcg [600 int. units], 300 mcg [1500 int. units], 1000 mcg [5000 int. units] [for I.M. or I.V. use]

Monitoring and Teaching Issues

Physical Assessment: Assess results of laboratory tests, therapeutic effectiveness, and adverse reactions. Teach patient possible side effects, interventions to reduce side effects, and adverse reactions to report.

Monitoring Laboratory Tests: CBC, renal function

Patient Education: Do not have live virus vaccinations within 3 months of receiving this medication. This medication can only be administered by injection or infusion; report immediately any difficulty breathing, chills, rapid heart beat, back rash, pain, or redness, swelling, or pain at injection site. You may experience headache or mild headache (consult prescriber for appropriate analgesic). Report any acute or persistent adverse effects.

Pregnancy precautions: Inform prescriber if you are pregnant or plan to become pregnant.

Pregnancy Risk Factor: C

Pregnancy Issues: Animal studies have not been conducted. Available evidence suggests that Rh_o(D) immune globulin administration during pregnancy does not harm the fetus or affect future pregnancies.

(Continued)

Rh₀(D) Immune Globulin *(Continued)*

Lactation: Does not enter breast milk

Administration

I.M.: Administer into the deltoid muscle of the upper arm or anterolateral aspect of the upper thigh. Avoid gluteal region due to risk of sciatic nerve injury. If large doses (>5 mL) are needed, administration in divided doses at different sites is recommended.

I.V.: WinRho SDF®: Infuse over 3-5 minutes. Do not administer with other medications.

Reconstitution: WinRho SDF®: Dilute with provided NS only. Inject diluent slowly into vial and gently swirl until dissolved; do not shake. Following reconstitution, may store at room temperature for up to 12 hours. Discard unused portion.

Storage: Store at 2°C to 8°C (35°F to 46°F). Do not freeze.

Rhophylac®: Stored at this temperature, Rhophylac® has a shelf life of 36 months. Protect from light.

Additional Information A "full dose" of Rh₀(D) immune globulin has previously been referred to as a 300 mcg dose. It is not the actual anti-D content. Although dosing has traditionally been expressed in mcg, potency is listed in int. units.

Ribavirin *(rye ba VYE rin)*

U.S. Brand Names Copegus®; Rebetol®; Ribasphere™; Virazole®

Synonyms RTCA; Tribavirin

Restrictions An FDA-approved medication guide is available at www.fda.gov/cder/Offices/ODS/labeling.htm; distribute to each patient to whom this medication is dispensed for the treatment of hepatitis C.

Generic Available Yes: Capsule

Pharmacologic Category Antiviral Agent

Medication Safety Issues

Sound-alike/look-alike issues:

Ribavirin may be confused with riboflavin

Use

Inhalation: Treatment of patients with respiratory syncytial virus (RSV) infections; specially indicated for treatment of severe lower respiratory tract RSV infections in patients with an underlying compromising condition (prematurity, bronchopulmonary dysplasia and other chronic lung conditions, congenital heart disease, immunodeficiency, immunosuppression), and recent transplant recipients

Oral capsule:

In combination with interferon alfa-2b (Intron® A) injection for the treatment of chronic hepatitis C in patients with compensated liver disease who have relapsed after alpha interferon therapy or were previously untreated with alpha interferons

In combination with peginterferon alfa-2b (PEG-Intron®) injection for the treatment of chronic hepatitis C in patients with compensated liver disease who were previously untreated with alpha interferons

Oral solution: In combination with interferon alfa 2b (Intron® A) injection for the treatment of chronic hepatitis C in patients ≥3 years of age with compensated liver disease who were previously untreated with alpha interferons or patients ≥18 years of age who have relapsed after alpha interferon therapy

Oral tablet: In combination with peginterferon alfa-2a (Pegasys®) injection for the treatment of chronic hepatitis C in patients with compensated liver disease who were previously untreated with alpha interferons (includes patients with histological evidence of cirrhosis [Child-Pugh class A] and patients with clinically-stable HIV disease)

Unlabeled/Investigational Use Used in other viral infections including influenza A and B and adenovirus

Mechanism of Action/Effect Inhibits viral protein synthesis

Contraindications Hypersensitivity to ribavirin or any component of the formulation; women of childbearing age who will not use contraception reliably; pregnancy

Additional contraindications for oral formulation: Male partners of pregnant women; Cl_cr < 50 mL/minute; hemoglobinopathies (eg, thalassemia major, sickle cell anemia); as monotherapy for treatment of chronic hepatitis C; patients with autoimmune hepatitis, anemia, severe heart disease

Refer to individual monographs for Interferon Alfa-2b (Intron® A) and Peginterferon Alfa-2a (Pegasys®) for additional contraindication information.

Warnings/Precautions Negative pregnancy test is required before initiation and monthly thereafter. Avoid pregnancy in female patients and female partners of male patients, during therapy, and for at least 6 months after treatment; two forms of contraception should be used. Elderly patients are more susceptible to adverse effects; use caution. Safety and efficacy have not been established in patients who have failed other alpha interferon therapy, received organ transplants, or been coinfected with hepatitis B or HIV (Copegus® may be used in HIV coinfected patients unless CD4+ cell count is <100 cells/microL). Safety and efficacy have not been established in patients <3 years of age.

Inhalation: Use with caution in patients requiring assisted ventilation because precipitation of the drug in the respiratory equipment may interfere with safe and effective patient ventilation;

monitor carefully in patients with COPD and asthma for deterioration of respiratory function. Ribavirin is potentially mutagenic, tumor-promoting, and gonadotoxic. Although anemia has not been reported with inhalation therapy, consider monitoring for anemia 1-2 weeks post-treatment. Pregnant healthcare workers may consider unnecessary occupational exposure; ribavirin has been detected in healthcare workers' urine. Healthcare professionals or family members who are pregnant (or may become pregnant) should be counseled about potential risks of exposure and counseled about risk reduction strategies.

Oral: Severe psychiatric events have occurred including depression and suicidal behavior during combination therapy. Avoid use in patients with a psychiatric history; discontinue if severe psychiatric symptoms occur. Hemolytic anemia is a significant toxicity; usually occurring within 1-2 weeks. Assess cardiac disease before initiation. Anemia may worsen underlying cardiac disease; use caution. If any deterioration in cardiovascular status occurs, discontinue therapy. Use caution in pulmonary disease; pulmonary symptoms have been associated with administration. Discontinue therapy in suspected/confirmed pancreatitis or if hepatic decompensation occurs. Use caution in patients with sarcoidosis (exacerbation reported).

Drug Interactions

Decreased Effect: Decreased effect of lamivudine, stavudine, and zidovudine (*in vitro*).

Increased Effect/Toxicity: Concomitant use of ribavirin and nucleoside analogues may increase the risk of developing lactic acidosis (includes adefovir, didanosine, lamivudine, stavudine, zalcitabine, zidovudine). Concurrent therapy of zidovudine with ribavirin/interferon alfa-2a may cause increased risk of severe anemia and/or severe neutropenia. Concurrent use with didanosine has been noted to increase the risk of pancreatitis and/or peripheral neuropathy in addition to lactic acidosis. Suspend therapy if signs/symptoms of toxicity are present.

Nutritional/Ethanol Interactions Food: Oral: High-fat meal increases the AUC and C_{max}.

Adverse Reactions

Inhalation:

1% to 10%:

Central nervous system: Fatigue, headache, insomnia

Gastrointestinal: Nausea, anorexia

Hematologic: Anemia

Note: Incidence of adverse effects (approximate) in healthcare workers: Headache (51%); conjunctivitis (32%); rhinitis, nausea, rash, dizziness, pharyngitis, and lacrimation (10% to 20%)

Oral (all adverse reactions are documented while receiving combination therapy with interferon alpha-2b or interferon alpha-2a; percentages as reported in adults):

>10%:

Central nervous system: Fatigue (60% to 70%)*, headache (43% to 66%)*, fever (32% to 46%)*, insomnia (26% to 41%), depression (20% to 36%)*, irritability (23% to 32%), dizziness (14% to 26%), impaired concentration (10% to 14%)*, emotional lability (7% to 12%)*

Dermatologic: Alopecia (27% to 36%), pruritus (13% to 29%), dry skin (13% to 24%), rash (5% to 28%), dermatitis (up to 16%)

Gastrointestinal: Nausea (33% to 47%), anorexia (21% to 32%), weight decrease (10% to 29%), diarrhea (10% to 22%), dyspepsia (8% to 16%), vomiting (9% to 14%)*, abdominal pain (8% to 13%), xerostomia (up to 12%), RUQ pain (up to 12%)

Hematologic: Neutropenia (8% to 27%; 40% with HIV coinfection), hemoglobin decreased (25% to 36%), hyperbilirubinemia (24% to 34%), anorexia (24% to 26%), anemia (11% to 17%), lymphopenia (12% to 14%), absolute neutrophil count <0.5 x 10^9/L (5% to 11%), thrombocytopenia (<1% to 14%), hemolytic anemia (10% to 13%), WBC decreased

Neuromuscular & skeletal: Myalgia (40% to 64%)*, rigors (40% to 48%), arthralgia (22% to 34%)*, musculoskeletal pain (19% to 28%)

Respiratory: Dyspnea (13% to 26%), cough (7% to 23%), pharyngitis (up to 13%), sinusitis (up to 12%)*, nasal congestion

Miscellaneous: Flu-like syndrome (13% to 18%)*, viral infection (up to 12%), diaphoresis increased (up to 11%)

*Similar to interferon alone

1% to 10%:

Cardiovascular: Chest pain (5% to 9%)*, flushing (up to 4 %)

Central nervous system: Mood alteration (up to 6%; 9% with HIV coinfection), memory impairment (up to 6%), malaise (up to 6%), nervousness (~5%)*

Dermatologic: Eczema (4% to 5%)

Endocrine & metabolic: Hypothyroidism (up to 5%)

Gastrointestinal: Taste perversion (4% to 9%), constipation (up to 5%)

Genitourinary: Menstrual disorder (up to 7%)

Hematologic: Hepatomegaly (up to 4%)

Neuromuscular & skeletal: Weakness (9% to 10%), back pain (5%)

Optic: Conjunctivitis (up to 6%), blurred vision (up to 5%)

Respiratory: Rhinitis (up to 8%), exertional dyspnea (up to 7%)

Miscellaneous: Fungal infection (up to 6%)

*Similar to interferon alone

Incidence of anorexia, headache, fever, suicidal ideation, and vomiting are higher in children.

Overdosage/Toxicology Treatment is symptom-directed and supportive. Not effectively removed by hemodialysis.

Pharmacodynamics/Kinetics

Absorption: Inhalation: Systemic; dependent upon respiratory factors and method of drug delivery; maximal absorption occurs with the use of aerosol generator via endotracheal tube; highest concentrations in respiratory tract and erythrocytes

Bioavailability: Oral: 64%

Time to Peak: Serum: Inhalation: At end of inhalation period; Oral capsule: Multiple doses: 3 hours

(Continued)

Ribavirin *(Continued)*

Protein Binding: Oral: None
Half-Life Elimination: Plasma:
  Children: Inhalation: 6.5-11 hours
  Adults: Oral:
    Capsule, single dose (Rebetol®, Ribasphere™): 24 hours in healthy adults, 44 hours with chronic hepatitis C infection (increases to ~298 hours at steady state)
    Tablet, single dose (Copegus®): 120-170 hours
Metabolism: Hepatically and intracellularly (forms active metabolites); may be necessary for drug action
Excretion: Inhalation: Urine (40% as unchanged drug and metabolites); Oral capsule: Urine (61%), feces (12%)

Dosing
Adults & Elderly:
Chronic hepatitis C (in combination with peginterferon alfa-2a): Oral tablet (Copegus®):
  Monoinfection, genotype 1,4:
    <75 kg: 1000 mg/day, in 2 divided doses for 48 weeks
    ≥75 kg: 1200 mg/day, in 2 divided doses for 48 weeks
  Monoinfection, genotype 2,3: 800 mg/day, in 2 divided doses, for 24 weeks
  Coinfection with HIV: 800 mg/day in 2 divided doses for 48 weeks
  Note: Also refer to Peginterferon Alfa-2a monograph
Chronic hepatitis C (in combination with interferon alfa-2b): Oral capsule (Rebetol®, Ribasphere™):
  Note: Also refer to Interferon Alfa-2b/Ribavirin combination pack monograph
  ≤75 kg: 400 mg in the morning, then 600 mg in the evening
  >75 kg: 600 mg in the morning, then 600 mg in the evening
  Note: If HCV-RNA is undetectable at 24 weeks, duration of therapy is 48 weeks. In patients who relapse following interferon therapy, duration of dual therapy is 24 weeks.
Chronic hepatitis C (in combination with peginterferon alfa-2b): Oral capsule (Rebetol®, Ribasphere™): 400 mg twice daily; duration of therapy is 1 year; after 24 weeks of treatment, if serum HCV-RNA is not below the limit of detection of the assay, consider discontinuation.
Dosage adjustment for toxicity: Oral (capsule, solution, tablet):
  Patient without cardiac history:
    Hemoglobin <10 g/dL: Decrease dose to 600 mg/day
    Hemoglobin <8.5 g/dL: Permanently discontinue treatment
  Patient with cardiac history:
    Hemoglobin has decreased ≥2 g/dL during any 4-week period of treatment: Decrease dose to 600 mg/day
    Hemoglobin <12 g/dL after 4 weeks of reduced dose: Permanently discontinue treatment
Pediatrics:
RSV infection: Infants and Children:
  Aerosol inhalation: Use with Viratek® small particle aerosol generator (SPAG-2): A concentration of 20 mg/mL (6 g reconstituted with 300 mL of sterile water without preservatives)
  Aerosol only: 12-18 hours/day for 3 days, up to 7 days in length
Chronic hepatitis C (in combination with interferon alfa-2b): Oral solution should be used in children 3-5 years of age, children ≤25 kg, or those unable to swallow capsules.
  Capsule/oral solution: Children ≥3 years: 15 mg/kg/day in 2 divided doses.
  Capsule dosing recommendations:
    25-36 kg: 400 mg/day (200 mg morning and evening)
    37-49 kg: 600 mg/day (200 mg in the morning and two 200 mg capsules in the evening)
    50-61 kg: 800 mg/day (two 200 mg capsules morning and evening)
    >61 kg: Refer to adult dosing.
  Note: Duration of therapy is 48 weeks in pediatric patients with genotype 1 and 24 weeks in patients with genotype 2,3. Discontinue treatment in any patient if HCV-RNA is not below the limit of detection of the assay after 24 weeks of therapy.
  Note: Also refer to Interferon Alfa-2b/Ribavirin combination pack monograph.
Dosage adjustment for toxicity: Oral (capsule, solution, tablet):
  Patient without cardiac history:
    Hemoglobin <10 g/dL: 7.5 mg/kg/day
    Hemoglobin <8.5 g/dL: Refer to adult dosing.
  Patient with cardiac history:
    Hemoglobin has decreased ≥2 g/dL during any 4-week period of treatment: 7.5 mg/kg/day
    Hemoglobin <12 g/dL after 4 weeks of reduced dose: Refer to adult dosing.
Renal Impairment: Cl$_{cr}$ <50 mL/minute: Oral is route contraindicated.

Available Dosage Forms
Capsule (Rebetol®, Ribasphere™): 200 mg
Powder for aerosol (Virazole®): 6 g
Solution, oral (Rebetol®): 40 mg/mL (100 mL) [contains sodium benzoate; bubble gum flavor]
Tablet (Copegus®): 200 mg

Monitoring and Teaching Issues
Physical Assessment: See Warnings/Precautions for use cautions (eg, mechanical ventilation, cardiac disease, liver disease, psychiatric history). See specific cautions for healthcare professionals' exposure risks with inhalation formulation. Assess results of laboratory tests, effectiveness (respiratory status), and adverse reactions (see Adverse Reactions). Teach patient proper use (according to formulation), possible side effects/appropriate interventions, and adverse symptoms to report (eg, CNS effects [headache, fatigue, irritability, impaired concentration], GI disturbance [nausea, vomiting, anorexia], hematologic [anemia], myalgia, rigors, dyspnea; see Patient Education). **Pregnancy risk factor X:** Determine that patient is not pregnant before beginning treatment. Do not give to women of

childbearing age or males who may have intercourse with childbearing women unless both male and female are capable of complying with using two effective forms of contraception during therapy and 6 months following therapy.

Monitoring Laboratory Tests:
Inhalation: Respiratory function, CBC
Oral: CBC with differential (pretreatment, 2- and 4 weeks after initiation); pretreatment and monthly pregnancy test for women of childbearing age; LFTs, TSH, HCV-RNA after 24 weeks of therapy; ECG in patients with pre-existing cardiac disease

Patient Education: For oral administration, take as directed. Follow directions for aerosol device. Do not allow pregnant women or women of childbearing age to handle medication. Maintain adequate hydration (2-3 L/day of fluids) unless instructed to restrict fluid intake. You will need regular blood tests while taking this drug. You may experience increased susceptibility to infection (avoid crowds and exposure to infection and do not have any vaccinations without consulting prescriber). May cause confusion, impaired concentration, or headache (use cautions when driving or engaging in potentially hazardous tasks until response to drug is known); nausea, vomiting, or anorexia (small frequent meals, frequent mouth care, chewing gum, or sucking lozenges may help); diarrhea (buttermilk, boiled milk, or yogurt may relieve diarrhea); or loss of hair (reversible). Report rash, infection (fever, chills, unusual bleeding or bruising, or unhealed sores or white plaques in mouth); tingling, weakness, or pain in extremities; or other persistent adverse effects. **Pregnancy/breast-feeding precautions:** Inform prescriber if you are pregnant. Both males and females should use appropriate contraceptive measures during and for 60-90 days following end of therapy. Do not allow family members or friends who are pregnant (or may become pregnant) to handle inhalation powder. This drug may cause serious fetal defects. Consult prescriber for appropriate contraceptive measures. Do not donate blood during or for 6 months following therapy. Breast-feeding is not recommended.

Dietary Considerations: When used in combination with interferon alfa-2b, capsules and solution may be taken with or without food, but always in a consistent manner in regard to food intake (ie, always take with food or always take on an empty stomach). When used in combination with peginterferon alfa 2b, capsules should be taken with food. Tablets should be taken with food.

Pregnancy Risk Factor: X

Pregnancy Issues: Produced significant embryocidal and/or teratogenic effects in all animal studies at ~0.01 times the maximum recommended daily human dose. Use is contraindicated in pregnancy. Negative pregnancy test is required before initiation and monthly thereafter. Avoid pregnancy in female patients and female partners of male patients during therapy by using two effective forms of contraception; continue contraceptive measures for at least 6 months after completion of therapy. If patient or female partner becomes pregnant during treatment, she should be counseled about potential risks of exposure. If pregnancy occurs during use or within 6 months after treatment, report to company (800-593-2214).

Lactation: Excretion in breast milk unknown/not recommended

Administration
Oral: Administer concurrently with interferon alfa injection. Capsule should not be opened, crushed, chewed, or broken. Capsules are not for use in children <5 years of age. Use oral solution for children 3-5 years, those ≤25 kg, or those who cannot swallow capsules.
Capsule, in combination with interferon alfa-2b: May be administered with or without food, but always in a consistent manner in regard to food intake.
Capsule, in combination with peginterferon alfa 2b: Administer with food.
Solution, in combination with interferon alfa-2b: May be administered with or without food, but always in a consistent manner in regard to food intake.
Tablet: Should be administered with food.

Inhalation: Ribavirin should be administered in well-ventilated rooms (at least 6 air changes/hour). In mechanically-ventilated patients, ribavirin can potentially be deposited in the ventilator delivery system depending on temperature, humidity, and electrostatic forces; this deposition can lead to malfunction or obstruction of the expiratory valve, resulting in inadvertently high positive end-expiratory pressures. The use of one-way valves in the inspiratory lines, a breathing circuit filter in the expiratory line, and frequent monitoring and filter replacement have been effective in preventing these problems. Solutions in SPAG-2 unit should be discarded at least every 24 hours and when the liquid level is low before adding newly reconstituted solution. Should not be mixed with other aerosolized medication.

Reconstitution: Inhalation: Do not use any water containing an antimicrobial agent to reconstitute drug. Reconstituted solution is stable for 24 hours at room temperature.

Compatibility: Inhalation: Should not be mixed with other aerosolized medication

Storage:
Inhalation: Store vials in a dry place at 15°C to 25°C (59°F to 78°F).
Oral: Store at 15°C to 30°C (59°F to 86°F). Solution may also be refrigerated at 2°C to 8°C (36°F to 46°F).

♦ **Ribavirin and Interferon Alfa-2b Combination Pack** *see* Interferon Alfa-2b and Ribavirin *on page 814*

♦ **Ribo-100** *see* Riboflavin *on page 1321*

Riboflavin (RYE boe flay vin)

U.S. Brand Names Ribo-100
Synonyms Lactoflavin; Vitamin B_2; Vitamin G
Generic Available Yes
Pharmacologic Category Vitamin, Water Soluble
Medication Safety Issues
Sound-alike/look-alike issues:
Riboflavin may be confused with ribavirin
Use Prevention of riboflavin deficiency and treatment of ariboflavinosis
(Continued)

Riboflavin *(Continued)*

Mechanism of Action/Effect Component of flavoprotein enzymes that work together, which are necessary for normal tissue respiration; also needed for activation of pyridoxine and conversion of tryptophan to niacin

Warnings/Precautions Riboflavin deficiency often occurs in the presence of other B vitamin deficiencies.

Drug Interactions

Decreased Effect: Decreased absorption with probenecid.

Lab Interactions Large doses may interfere with urinalysis based on spectrometry. May cause false elevations in fluorometric determinations of catecholamines and urobilinogen.

Adverse Reactions Frequency not defined: Genitourinary: Discoloration of urine (yellow-orange)

Pharmacodynamics/Kinetics

Absorption: Readily via GI tract, however, food increases extent; decreased with hepatitis, cirrhosis, or biliary obstruction

Half-Life Elimination: Biologic: 66-84 minutes

Metabolism: None

Excretion: Urine (9%) as unchanged drug

Dosing

Adults & Elderly:

Riboflavin deficiency: Oral: 5-30 mg/day in divided doses

Recommended daily allowance: Oral: 1.2-1.7 mg

Pediatrics:

Riboflavin deficiency: Oral: Children: 2.5-10 mg/day in divided doses

Recommended daily allowance: Oral: Children: 0.4-1.8 mg

Available Dosage Forms

Tablet: 25 mg, 50 mg, 100 mg

Ribo-100: 100 mg

Monitoring and Teaching Issues

Physical Assessment: Assess knowledge/teach patient appropriate use, dietary instruction, possible side effects, and adverse symptoms to report.

Patient Education: Take with food. Large doses may cause bright yellow or orange urine.

Pregnancy Risk Factor: A/C (dose exceeding RDA recommendation)

Lactation: Enters breast milk/compatible

Additional Information Dietary sources of riboflavin include liver, kidney, dairy products, green vegetables, eggs, whole grain cereals, yeast, and mushroom.

♦ **Rid-A-Pain Dental Drops [OTC]** *see* Benzocaine *on page 181*

♦ **Rid® Spray [OTC]** *see* Permethrin *on page 1190*

Rifabutin *(rif a BYOO tin)*

U.S. Brand Names Mycobutin®

Synonyms Ansamycin

Generic Available No

Pharmacologic Category Antibiotic, Miscellaneous; Antitubercular Agent

Medication Safety Issues

Sound-alike/look-alike issues:

Rifabutin may be confused with rifampin

Use Prevention of disseminated *Mycobacterium avium* complex (MAC) in patients with advanced HIV infection

Unlabeled/Investigational Use Utilized in multidrug regimens for treatment of MAC

Mechanism of Action/Effect Inhibits DNA-dependent RNA polymerase at the beta subunit which prevents chain initiation

Contraindications Hypersensitivity to rifabutin, any other rifamycins, or any component of the formulation; rifabutin is contraindicated in patients with a WBC <1000/mm³ or a platelet count <50,000/mm³

Warnings/Precautions Rifabutin as a single agent must not be administered to patients with active tuberculosis since its use may lead to the development of tuberculosis that is resistant to both rifabutin and rifampin. Rifabutin should be discontinued in patients with AST >500 units/L or if total bilirubin is >3 mg/dL. Use with caution in patients with liver impairment. Modification of dosage should be considered in patients with renal impairment.

Drug Interactions

Cytochrome P450 Effect: Substrate (major) of CYP1A2, 3A4; **Induces** CYP3A4 (strong)

Decreased Effect: Rifabutin may decrease the levels/effects of alfentanil, amiodarone, angiotensin II receptor blockers (irbesartan, losartan), CYP3A4 substrates (eg, clarithromycin, erythromycin, mirtazapine, nefazodone, venlafaxine), 5-HT₃ antagonists, imidazole antifungals, aprepitant, barbiturates, benzodiazepines (metabolized by oxidation), beta blockers, buspirone, calcium channel blockers, chloramphenicol, corticosteroids, cyclosporine, dapsone, disopyramide, estrogen and progestin contraceptives, fluconazole, gefitinib, HMG-CoA reductase inhibitors, methadone, morphine, phenytoin, propafenone, protease inhibitors, quinidine, repaglinide, reverse transcriptase inhibitors (non-nucleoside), tacrolimus, tamoxifen, terbinafine, tocainide, tricyclic antidepressants, warfarin, zaleplon, zolpidem. The effects of rifabutin may be decreased by CYP3A4 inducers (eg, aminoglutethimide, carbamazepine, nafcillin, nevirapine, phenobarbital, phenytoin).

Increased Effect/Toxicity: Rifabutin may increase the therapeutic effect of clopidogrel; concurrent use with isoniazid may increase risk of hepatotoxicity; the levels/toxicity of rifabutin may be increased by imidazole antifungals, macrolide antibiotics, and protease inhibitors

Nutritional/Ethanol Interactions Food: High-fat meal may decrease the rate but not the extent of absorption.

Adverse Reactions

>10%:
Dermatologic: Rash (11%)
Genitourinary: Discoloration of urine (30%)
Hematologic: Neutropenia (25%), leukopenia (17%)
1% to 10%:
Central nervous system: Headache (3%)
Gastrointestinal: Vomiting/nausea (3%), abdominal pain (4%), diarrhea (3%), anorexia (2%), flatulence (2%), eructation (3%)
Hematologic: Anemia, thrombocytopenia (5%)
Hepatic: Increased AST/ALT (7% to 9%)
Neuromuscular & skeletal: Myalgia

Overdosage/Toxicology Symptoms of overdose include nausea, vomiting, hepatotoxicity, lethargy, CNS disturbances, and depression. Treatment is supportive. Hemodialysis will remove rifabutin; however, its effect on outcome is unknown.

Pharmacodynamics/Kinetics

Absorption: Readily, 53%
Bioavailability: Absolute: HIV: 20%
Time to Peak: Serum: 2-4 hours
Protein Binding: 85%
Half-Life Elimination: Terminal: 45 hours (range: 16-69 hours)
Metabolism: To active and inactive metabolites
Excretion: Urine (10% as unchanged drug, 53% as metabolites); feces (10% as unchanged drug, 30% as metabolites)

Dosing

Adults & Elderly:
Disseminated MAC in advanced HIV infection:
Prophylaxis: Oral: 300 mg once daily (alone or in combination with azithromycin)
Treatment (unlabeled use): Oral:
Patients not receiving NNRTIs or protease inhibitors:
Initial phase: 5 mg/kg daily (maximum: 300 mg)
Second phase: 5 mg/kg daily or twice weekly
Patients receiving nelfinavir, amprenavir, indinavir: Reduce dose to 150 mg/day; no change in dose if administered twice weekly

Pediatrics:
Disseminated MAC in advanced HIV infection: Children >1 year:
Prophylaxis: Oral: 5 mg/kg daily; higher dosages have been used in limited trials
Treatment (unlabeled use): Oral: Patients not receiving NNRTIs or protease inhibitors:
Initial phase (2 weeks to 2 months): 10-20 mg/kg daily (maximum: 300 mg).
Second phase: 10-20 mg/kg daily (maximum: 300 mg) or twice weekly

Renal Impairment: Cl_{cr} <30 mL/minute: Reduce dose by 50%

Available Dosage Forms Capsule: 150 mg

Monitoring and Teaching Issues

Physical Assessment: Not to be used as single agent. Use caution with renal or hepatic impairment (see Warnings/Precautions for specific use cautions). Assess potential for interactions with other pharmacological agents patient may be taking (eg, increased levels/effects and increased risk of toxicity [risk of hepatotoxicity increases with isoniazid] and decreased levels/effects [eg, oral contraceptives, oral anticoagulants, some oral hypoglycemics, beta blockers, 4-HT$_3$ antagonists]; see Drug Interactions for extensive list). Assess results of laboratory tests, effectiveness (prevention of MAC in patient with HIV), and adverse response (eg, anemia, neutropenia, or GI disturbance; see Adverse Reactions and Overdose/Toxicology). Teach patient proper use, possible side effects/appropriate interventions, and adverse symptoms to report (see Patient Education).

Monitoring Laboratory Tests: Periodic liver function, CBC with differential, platelet count

Patient Education: Do not take any new medication during therapy without consulting prescriber. Take as directed, with or without food. Complete full course of therapy; do not skip doses. Will discolor urine, stool, saliva, tears, sweat, and other body fluid a red-brown color. Stains on clothing or contact lenses are permanent. Report skin rash; persistent vomiting or diarrhea; fever, chills, or flu-like symptoms; dark urine or pale stools; unusual bleeding or bruising; or confusion, depression, or fatigue. Effectiveness of oral/systemic contraceptives may be impaired; consult prescriber for appropriate contraceptives. **Breast-feeding precaution:** Consult prescriber if breast-feeding.

Dietary Considerations: May be taken with meals or without food or mix with applesauce.

Pregnancy Risk Factor: B

Lactation: Excretion in breast milk unknown

Administration

Oral: Rifabutin is best taken on an empty stomach but may be taken with meals to minimize nausea or vomiting.

♦ **Rifadin®** *see Rifampin on page 1323*
♦ **Rifamate®** *see Rifampin and Isoniazid on page 1326*
♦ **Rifampicin** *see Rifampin on page 1323*

Rifampin (RIF am pin)

U.S. Brand Names Rifadin®
Synonyms Rifampicin
Generic Available Yes
Pharmacologic Category Antibiotic, Miscellaneous; Antitubercular Agent
Medication Safety Issues
Sound-alike/look-alike issues:
Rifampin may be confused with rifabutin, Rifamate®, rifapentine
Rifadin® may be confused with Ritalin®
Rimactane® may be confused with rimantadine
(Continued)

Rifampin *(Continued)*

Use Management of active tuberculosis in combination with other agents; elimination of menin-gococci from the nasopharynx in asymptomatic carriers

Unlabeled/Investigational Use Prophylaxis of *Haemophilus influenzae* type b infection; *Legionella* pneumonia; used in combination with other anti-infectives in the treatment of staphylococcal infections; treatment of *M. leprae* infections

Mechanism of Action/Effect Inhibits bacterial RNA synthesis by binding to the beta subunit of DNA-dependent RNA polymerase, blocking RNA transcription

Contraindications Hypersensitivity to rifampin, any rifamycins, or any component of the formulation; concurrent use of amprenavir, saquinavir/ritonavir (possibly other protease inhibitors)

Warnings/Precautions Use with caution and modify dosage in patients with liver impairment. Discontinue therapy if clinical symptoms or any signs of significant hepatocellular damage develop. Use with caution in patients with porphyria. Not for use in meningococcal disease, only for short-term treatment of asymptomatic carrier states. Use with caution in patients receiving concurrent medications associated with hepatotoxicity (particularly with pyrazina-mide), or in patients with a history of alcoholism (even if ethanol consumption is discontinued during therapy).

Monitor for compliance and effects including hypersensitivity, thrombocytopenia in patients on intermittent therapy. May discolor urine, feces, saliva, sweat, tears, and CSF (red/orange); remove soft contact lenses during therapy. Regimens of 600 mg once or twice weekly have been associated with a high incidence of adverse reactions including a flu-like syndrome. I.V. formulation is not intended for I.M. or SubQ administration.

Drug Interactions

  Cytochrome P450 Effect: Substrate (major) of CYP2A6, 2C8/9, 3A4; **Induces** CYP1A2 (strong), 2A6 (strong), 2B6 (strong), 2C8/9 (strong), 2C19 (strong), 3A4 (strong)

  Decreased Effect: Rifampin may decrease the levels/effects of the following drugs: Aceta-minophen, alfentanil, amiodarone, angiotensin II receptor blockers (irbesartan and losartan), 5-HT$_3$ antagonists, imidazole antifungals, aprepitant, barbiturates, benzodiaze-pines (metabolized by oxidation), beta blockers, buspirone, calcium channel blockers, chloramphenicol, corticosteroids, cyclosporine; CYP1A2, 2A6, 2B6, 2C8/9, 2C19, and 3A4 substrates (eg, aminophylline, amiodarone, bupropion, fluoxetine, fluvoxamine, ifosfamide, methsuximide, mirtazapine, nateglinide, pioglitazone, promethazine, proton pump inhibi-tors, ropinirole, rosiglitazone, selegiline, sertraline, theophylline, venlafaxine, and zafirlukast); dapsone, disopyramide, estrogen and progestin contraceptives, fexofenadine, fluconazole, fusidic acid, gefitinib, HMG-CoA reductase inhibitors, methadone, morphine, phenytoin, propafenone, protease inhibitors, quinidine, repaglinide, reverse transcriptase inhibitors (non-nucleoside), sulfonylureas, tacrolimus, tamoxifen, terbinafine, tocainide, tricyclic antidepressants, warfarin, zaleplon, zidovudine, zolpidem. The effects of rifampin may be decreased by CYP2A6, 2C8/9, and 3A4 inducers (eg, aminoglutethimide, barbitu-rates, carbamazepine, nafcillin, nevirapine, and phenytoin).

  Increased Effect/Toxicity: Rifampin may increase the therapeutic effect of clopidogrel; concurrent use with isoniazid, pyrazinamide, or protease inhibitors (amprenavir, saquinavir/ritonavir) may increase risk of hepatotoxicity; macrolide antibiotics may increase levels/toxicity of rifampin

Nutritional/Ethanol Interactions

  Ethanol: Avoid ethanol (may increase risk of hepatotoxicity).

  Food: Food decreases the extent of absorption; rifampin concentrations may be decreased if taken with food.

  Herb/Nutraceutical: St John's wort may decrease rifampin levels.

Lab Interactions Positive Coombs' reaction [direct], inhibit standard assay's ability to measure serum folate and B$_{12}$

Adverse Reactions

  Frequency not defined:

    Cardiovascular: Edema, flushing

    Central nervous system: Ataxia, behavioral changes, concentration impaired, confusion, dizziness, drowsiness, fatigue, fever, headache, numbness, psychosis

    Dermatologic: Pemphigoid reaction, pruritus, urticaria

    Endocrine & metabolic: Adrenal insufficiency, menstrual disorders

    Hematologic: Agranulocytosis, DIC, eosinophilia, hemoglobin decreased, hemolysis, hemolytic anemia, leukopenia, thrombocytopenia (especially with high-dose therapy)

    Hepatic: Hepatitis (rare), jaundice

    Neuromuscular & skeletal: Myalgia, osteomalacia, weakness

    Ocular: Exudative conjunctivitis, visual changes

  1% to 10%:

    Dermatologic: Rash (1% to 5%)

    Gastrointestinal (1% to 2%): Anorexia, cramps, diarrhea, epigastric distress, flatulence, heartburn, nausea, pseudomembranous colitis, pancreatitis vomiting

    Hepatic: LFTs increased (up to 14%)

Overdosage/Toxicology Symptoms of overdose include nausea, vomiting, hepatotoxicity, lethargy, and CNS depression. Treatment is supportive. Plasma rifampin concentrations are not significantly affected by hemodialysis or peritoneal dialysis.

Pharmacodynamics/Kinetics

  Duration of Action: ≤24 hours

  Absorption: Oral: Well absorbed; food may delay or slightly reduce peak

  Time to Peak: Serum: Oral: 2-4 hours

  Protein Binding: 80%

  Half-Life Elimination: 3-4 hours, prolonged with hepatic impairment; End-stage renal disease: 1.8-11 hours

Metabolism: Hepatic; undergoes enterohepatic recirculation

Excretion: Feces (60% to 65%) and urine (~30%) as unchanged drug

Dosing

Adults & Elderly:

Tuberculosis therapy (drug susceptible): Oral, I.V.: **Note:** A four-drug regimen (isoniazid, rifampin, pyrazinamide, and ethambutol) is preferred for the initial, empiric treatment of TB. When the drug susceptibility results are available, the regimen should be altered as appropriate.

Daily therapy: 10 mg/kg/day (maximum: 600 mg/day)

Twice weekly directly observed therapy (DOT): 10 mg/kg (maximum: 600 mg); 3 times/week: 10 mg/kg (maximum: 600 mg)

Latent tuberculosis infection (LTBI): As an alternative to isoniazid: Oral, I.V.: 10 mg/kg/day (maximum: 600 mg/day) **Note:** Combination with pyrazinamide should not generally be offered (*MMWR*, Aug 8, 2003).

***H. influenzae* prophylaxis (unlabeled use):** Oral, I.V.: 600 mg every 24 hours for 4 days

Leprosy (unlabeled use): Oral, I.V.:

Multibacillary: 600 mg once monthly for 24 months in combination with ofloxacin and minocycline

Paucibacillary: 600 mg once monthly for 6 months in combination with dapsone

Single lesion: 600 mg as a single dose in combination with ofloxacin 400 mg and minocycline 100 mg

Meningococcal meningitis prophylaxis: Oral, I.V.: 600 mg every 12 hours for 2 days

Nasal carriers of *Staphylococcus aureus* (unlabeled use): Oral, I.V.: 600 mg/day for 5-10 days in combination with other antibiotics

Synergy for *Staphylococcus aureus* infections (unlabeled use): Oral, I.V.: 300-600 mg twice daily with other antibiotics

Pediatrics:

Tuberculosis therapy (drug susceptible): Oral, I.V.:

Infants and Children <12 years:

Daily therapy: 10-20 mg/kg/day usually as a single dose (maximum: 600 mg/day)

Twice weekly directly observed therapy (DOT): 10-20 mg/kg (maximum: 600 mg)

See "Note" in adult dosing.

Latent tuberculosis infection (LTBI): As an alternative to isoniazid: Children: 10-20 mg/kg/day (maximum: 600 mg/day) for 6 months

***H. influenzae* prophylaxis (unlabeled use):** Oral, I.V.: Infants and Children: 20 mg/kg/day every 24 hours for 4 days, not to exceed 600 mg/dose

Meningococcal prophylaxis: Oral:

<1 month: 10 mg/kg/day in divided doses every 12 hours for 2 days

Infants and Children: 20 mg/kg/day in divided doses every 12 hours for 2 days (maximum: 600 mg/dose)

Nasal carriers of *Staphylococcus aureus* (unlabeled use): Oral, I.V.: 15 mg/kg/day divided every 12 hours for 5-10 days in combination with other antibiotics

Renal Impairment: Plasma rifampin concentrations are not significantly affected by hemodialysis or peritoneal dialysis.

Hepatic Impairment: Dose reductions are necessary to reduce hepatotoxicity.

Available Dosage Forms

Capsule (Rifadin®): 150 mg, 300 mg

Injection, powder for reconstitution (Rifadin®): 600 mg

Monitoring and Teaching Issues

Physical Assessment: Use caution in presence of liver disease, porphyria, alcoholism (see Warnings/Precautions for use cautions). Assess potential for interactions with other pharmacological agents patient may be taking (eg, increased levels/effects with increased risk of toxicity [risk of hepatotoxicity increases with isoniazid or pyrazinamide] and decreased levels/effects [eg, oral contraceptives, oral anticoagulants, some oral hypoglycemics, beta blockers, 4-HT$_3$ antagonists]; see Drug Interactions for extensive list). See Administration for infusion specifics; infusion site must be monitored to prevent extravasation. Assess results of periodic laboratory tests and patient response (eg, rash, CNS changes [confusion, numbness, ataxia], leukopenia, anemia, myalgia, visual changes, gastrointestinal disturbance [anorexia, nausea, vomiting, diarrhea]; see Adverse Reactions). Teach patient proper use (importance of compliance), possible side effects/appropriate interventions, and adverse symptoms to report (see Patient Education).

Monitoring Laboratory Tests: Periodic monitoring of liver function (AST, ALT), CBC; sputum culture, chest x-ray 2-3 months into treatment

Patient Education: Do not take any new medication during therapy without consulting prescriber. Take as prescribed, on an empty stomach, 1 hour before or 2 hours after meals. Complete full course of therapy; do not skip doses. Will discolor urine, stool, saliva, tears, sweat, and other body fluid a red-brown color. Stains on contact lenses and clothing are permanent. Report persistent vomiting or diarrhea; rash; fever, chills, or flu-like symptoms; unusual bruising or bleeding; or other persistent adverse effects. **Pregnancy precaution:** Inform prescriber if you are or intend to become pregnant. This drug may interfere with effectiveness of oral/systemic contraceptives; consult prescriber for alternative contraceptive measures.

Dietary Considerations: Rifampin should be taken on an empty stomach.

Geriatric Considerations: Rifampin, in combination with isoniazid, is the foundation of tuberculosis treatment. Since most older patients acquired their *Mycobacterium tuberculosis* infection before effective chemotherapy was available, either a 9-month regimen of isoniazid and rifampin or a 6-month regimen of isoniazid and rifampin with pyrazinamide (the first 2 months) should be effective.

Pregnancy Risk Factor: C

Lactation: Enters breast milk/not recommended (AAP rates "compatible")

Administration

Oral: Administer on an empty stomach with a glass of water (ie, 1 hour prior to, or 2 hours after meals or antacids) to increase total absorption (food may delay and reduce the (Continued)

Rifampin *(Continued)*

amount of rifampin absorbed). The compounded oral suspension must be shaken well before using. May mix contents of capsule with applesauce or jelly.

I.M.: Do not administer I.M. or SubQ

I.V.: Administer I.V. preparation once daily by slow I.V. infusion over 30 minutes to 3 hours at a final concentration not to exceed 6 mg/mL.

Reconstitution: Reconstitute powder for injection with SWFI; prior to injection, dilute in appropriate volume of compatible diluent (eg, 100 mL D$_5$W).

Compatibility:

Y-site administration: Incompatible with diltiazem

Compatibility when admixed: Incompatible with minocycline

Storage: Rifampin powder is reddish brown. Intact vials should be stored at room temperature and protected from excessive heat and light. Reconstituted vials are stable for 24 hours at room temperature

Stability of parenteral admixture at room temperature (25°C) is 4 hours for D$_5$W and 24 hours for NS

Related Information

Antimicrobial Drugs of Choice *on page 1792*
Prophylaxis for Exposure to Communicable Diseases *on page 1859*
Tuberculosis *on page 1864*

Rifampin and Isoniazid *(RIF am pin & eye soe NYE a zid)*

U.S. Brand Names Rifamate®

Synonyms Isoniazid and Rifampin

Generic Available No

Pharmacologic Category Antibiotic, Miscellaneous

Medication Safety Issues

Sound-alike/look-alike issues:

Rifamate® may be confused with rifampin

Use Management of active tuberculosis; see individual agents for additional information

Dosing

Adults: Tuberculosis: Oral: 2 capsules/day

Elderly: Refer to dosing in individual monographs.

Available Dosage Forms Capsule: Rifampin 300 mg and isoniazid 150 mg

Monitoring and Teaching Issues

Physical Assessment: See individual agents.

Patient Education: See individual agents. **Pregnancy precaution:** Inform prescriber if you are or intend to become pregnant.

Pregnancy Risk Factor: C

Lactation: Enters breast milk/compatible

Related Information

Isoniazid *on page 836*
Rifampin *on page 1323*

Rifampin, Isoniazid, and Pyrazinamide

(RIF am pin, eye soe NYE a zid, & peer a ZIN a mide)

U.S. Brand Names Rifater®

Synonyms Isoniazid, Rifampin, and Pyrazinamide; Pyrazinamide, Rifampin, and Isoniazid

Generic Available No

Pharmacologic Category Antibiotic, Miscellaneous

Use Management of active tuberculosis; see individual agents for additional information

Dosing

Adults: Tuberculosis: Oral: Patients weighing:

≤44 kg: 4 tablets

45-54 kg: 5 tablets

≥55 kg: 6 tablets

Doses should be administered in a single daily dose.

Elderly: Refer to dosing in individual monographs.

Available Dosage Forms Tablet: Rifampin 120 mg, isoniazid 50 mg, and pyrazinamide 300 mg

Monitoring and Teaching Issues

Physical Assessment: See individual agents.

Patient Education: See individual agents. **Pregnancy/breast-feeding precautions:** Inform prescriber if you are or intend to become pregnant. Consult prescriber if breast-feeding.

Pregnancy Risk Factor: C

Lactation: Excretion in breast milk unknown

Related Information

Isoniazid *on page 836*
Pyrazinamide *on page 1286*
Rifampin *on page 1323*

Rifapentine *(RIF a pen teen)*

U.S. Brand Names Priftin®

Generic Available No

Pharmacologic Category Antitubercular Agent

Medication Safety Issues

Sound-alike/look-alike issues:

Rifapentine may be confused with rifampin

Use Treatment of pulmonary tuberculosis; rifapentine must always be used in conjunction with at least one other antituberculosis drug to which the isolate is susceptible; it may also be necessary to add a third agent (either streptomycin or ethambutol) until susceptibility is known.

Mechanism of Action/Effect Inhibits DNA-dependent RNA polymerase in susceptible strains of *Mycobacterium tuberculosis* (but not in mammalian cells). Rifapentine is bactericidal against both intracellular and extracellular MTB organisms. Strains which are resistant to other rifamycins including rifampin are likely to be resistant to rifapentine. Cross-resistance does not appear between rifapentine and other nonrifamycin antimycobacterial agents.

Contraindications Hypersensitivity to rifapentine, rifampin, rifabutin, any rifamycin analog, or any component of the formulation

Warnings/Precautions Compliance with dosing regimen is absolutely necessary for successful drug therapy. Patients with abnormal liver tests and/or liver disease should only be given rifapentine when absolutely necessary and under strict medical supervision. Monitoring of liver function tests should be carried out prior to therapy and then every 2-4 weeks during therapy if signs of liver disease occur or worsen, rifapentine should be discontinued. Pseudomembranous colitis has been reported to occur with various antibiotics including other rifamycins. If this is suspected, rifapentine should be stopped and the patient treated with specific and supportive treatment. Experience in treating TB in HIV-infected patients is limited.

Rifapentine may produce a red-orange discoloration of body tissues/fluids including skin, teeth, tongue, urine, feces, saliva, sputum, tears, sweat, and cerebral spinal fluid. Contact lenses may become permanently stained.

Drug Interactions

Cytochrome P450 Effect: Induces CYP2C8/9 (strong), 3A4 (strong)

Decreased Effect: Rifapentine may decrease the levels/effects of the following drugs: alfentanil, amiodarone, angiotensin II receptor blockers (irbesartan, losartan), 5-HT$_3$ antagonists, imidazole antifungals, aprepitant, barbiturates, benzodiazepines (metabolized by oxidation), beta blockers, buspirone, calcium channel blockers, corticosteroids, cyclosporine; CYP2C8/9 and 3A4 substrates (eg, amiodarone, clarithromycin, erythromycin, fluoxetine, mirtazapine, nateglinide, nefazodone, nevirapine, pioglitazone, rosiglitazone, sertraline, venlafaxine, and zafirlukast); dapsone, disopyramide, estrogen and progestin contraceptives, fluconazole, gefitinib, HMG-CoA reductase inhibitors, methadone, morphine, phenytoin, propafenone, protease inhibitors, quinidine, repaglinide, reverse transcriptase inhibitors (non-nucleoside), tacrolimus, tamoxifen, terbinafine, tocainide, tricyclic antidepressants, warfarin, zaleplon, zidovudine, and zolpidem.

Increased Effect/Toxicity: Rifapentine may increase the therapeutic effect of clopidogrel; concurrent use with isoniazid may increase risk of hepatotoxicity

Nutritional/Ethanol Interactions Food: Food increases AUC and maximum serum concentration by 43% and 44% respectively as compared to fasting conditions.

Lab Interactions Rifampin has been shown to inhibit standard microbiological assays for serum folate and vitamin B$_{12}$. This should be considered for rifapentine; therefore, alternative assay methods should be considered.

Adverse Reactions

>10%: Endocrine & metabolic: Hyperuricemia (most likely due to pyrazinamide from initiation phase combination therapy)

1% to 10%:

Cardiovascular: Hypertension

Central nervous system: Headache, dizziness

Dermatologic: Rash, pruritus, acne

Gastrointestinal: Anorexia, nausea, vomiting, dyspepsia, diarrhea

Hematologic: Neutropenia, lymphopenia, anemia, leukopenia, thrombocytosis

Hepatic: Increased ALT/AST

Neuromuscular & skeletal: Arthralgia, pain

Renal: Pyuria, proteinuria, hematuria, urinary casts

Respiratory: Hemoptysis

Overdosage/Toxicology There is no experience with treatment of acute overdose with rifapentine; experience with other rifamycins suggests that gastric lavage to help adsorb any remaining drug from the GI tract. Hemodialysis or forced diuresis is not expected to enhance elimination of unchanged rifapentine in an overdose.

Pharmacodynamics/Kinetics

Absorption: Food increases AUC and C$_{max}$ by 43% and 44% respectively.

Bioavailability: ~70%

Time to Peak: Serum: 5-6 hours

Protein Binding: Rifapentine and 25-desacetyl metabolite: 97.7% and 93.2%, primarily to albumin

Half-Life Elimination: Rifapentine: 14-17 hours; 25-desacetyl rifapentine: 13 hours

Metabolism: Hepatic; hydrolyzed by an esterase and esterase enzyme to form the active metabolite 25-desacetyl rifapentine

Excretion: Urine (17% primarily as metabolites)

Dosing

Adults & Elderly: Note: Rifapentine should not be used alone; initial phase should include a 3- to 4-drug regimen.

Tuberculosis, intensive phase (initial 2 months) of short-term therapy: 600 mg (four 150 mg tablets) given twice weekly (with an interval of not less than 72 hours between doses); following the intensive phase, treatment should continue with rifapentine 600 mg once weekly for 4 months in combination with INH or appropriate agent for susceptible organisms.

Available Dosage Forms Tablet [film coated]: 150 mg

Monitoring and Teaching Issues

Physical Assessment: For use in combination with other antitubercular medications. Use caution in presence of liver disease (see Warnings/Precautions for use cautions). Assess potential for interactions with other pharmacological agents patient may be taking (eg, increased levels/effects with increased risk of toxicity [risk of hepatotoxicity increases with (Continued)

Rifapentine *(Continued)*

isoniazid] and decreased levels/effects [eg, oral contraceptives, oral anticoagulants, some oral hypoglycemics, beta blockers, 4-HT$_3$ antagonists]; see Drug Interactions for extensive list). Assess results of periodic laboratory tests and patient response (eg, hypertension, rash, leukopenia, anemia, myalgia, GI disturbance [anorexia, nausea, vomiting, diarrhea], hemoptysis; see Adverse Reactions). Teach patient proper use (importance of compliance), possible side effects/appropriate interventions, and adverse symptoms to report (see Patient Education).

Monitoring Laboratory Tests: Perform baseline liver function tests at beginning of therapy. Patients with pre-existing hepatic problems should have liver function tests monitored every 2-4 weeks during therapy. Perform CBC monthly.

Patient Education: Inform prescriber of all prescriptions, OTC medications, or herbal products you are taking, and any allergies you have. Do not take any new medication during therapy without consulting prescriber. Take as prescribed, preferably on an empty stomach, 1 hour before or 2 hours after meals. Complete full course of therapy; do not skip doses. Will discolor urine, stool, saliva, tears, sweat, and other body fluid a red-brown color. Stains on contact lenses or clothing are permanent. Report changes in urinary pattern or pain on urination; vomiting; fever, chills, or flu-like symptoms; muscle weakness or unusual fatigue; dark urine, pale stools, or unusual bleeding or bruising; yellowing skin or eyes; skin rash; swelling of extremities; chest pain or palpitations; or persistent GI upset. **Pregnancy/breast-feeding precautions:** Inform prescriber if you are or intend to become pregnant. This drug may interfere with effectiveness of oral contraceptives; consult prescriber for alternative contraceptive measures. Do not breast-feed.

Pregnancy Risk Factor: C

Lactation: Excretion in breast milk unknown/contraindicated

Breast-Feeding Issues: May discolor breast milk

Administration

Storage: Store at room temperature (15°C to 30°C; 59°F to 86°F). Protect from excessive heat and humidity.

Additional Information Rifapentine has only been studied in patients with tuberculosis receiving a 6-month short-course intensive regimen approval. Outcomes have been based on 6-month follow-up treatment observed in clinical trial 008 as a surrogate for the 2-year follow-up generally accepted as evidence for efficacy in the treatment of pulmonary tuberculosis.

Related Information

Tuberculosis *on page 1864*

♦ **Rifater®** *see* Rifampin, Isoniazid, and Pyrazinamide *on page 1326*
♦ **rIFN-A** *see* Interferon Alfa-2a *on page 809*
♦ **rIFN beta-1a** *see* Interferon Beta-1a *on page 819*
♦ **rIFN beta-1b** *see* Interferon Beta-1b *on page 821*
♦ **Rilutek®** *see* Riluzole *on page 1328*

Riluzole *(RIL yoo zole)*

U.S. Brand Names Rilutek®

Synonyms 2-Amino-6-Trifluoromethoxy-Benzothiazole; RP-54274

Generic Available No

Pharmacologic Category Glutamate Inhibitor

Use Treatment of amyotrophic lateral sclerosis (ALS); riluzole can extend survival or time to tracheostomy

Mechanism of Action/Effect Mechanism of action is not known. Pharmacologic properties include inhibitory effect on glutamate release, inactivation of voltage-dependent sodium channels; and ability to interfere with intracellular events that follow transmitter binding at excitatory amino acid receptors

Contraindications Severe hypersensitivity reactions to riluzole or any component of the formulation

Warnings/Precautions Among 4000 patients given riluzole for ALS, there were 3 cases of marked neutropenia (ANC <500/mm³), all seen within the first 2 months of treatment. Use with caution in patients with concomitant renal insufficiency. Use with caution in patients with current evidence or history of abnormal liver function; do not administer if baseline liver function tests are elevated. The elderly, female, or Japanese patients may have decreased clearance of riluzole; use with caution. May cause dizziness or somnolence; caution should be used performing tasks which require alertness (operating machinery or driving).

Drug Interactions

Cytochrome P450 Effect: Substrate of CYP1A2 (major)

Decreased Effect: CYP1A2 inducers may decrease the levels/effects of riluzole; example inducers include aminoglutethimide, carbamazepine, phenobarbital, and rifampin.

Increased Effect/Toxicity: CYP1A2 inhibitors may increase the levels/effects of riluzole; example inhibitors include amiodarone, ciprofloxacin, fluvoxamine, ketoconazole, norfloxacin, ofloxacin, and rofecoxib.

Nutritional/Ethanol Interactions

Ethanol: Avoid ethanol (due to CNS depression and possible risk of liver toxicity).

Food: A high-fat meal decreases absorption of riluzole (decreasing AUC by 20% and peak blood levels by 45%). Charbroiled food may increase riluzole elimination.

Adverse Reactions

>10%:

Gastrointestinal: Nausea (12% to 21%)

Neuromuscular & skeletal: Weakness (15% to 20%)

Respiratory: Lung function decreased (10% to 16%)

1% to 10%:

Cardiovascular: Edema, hypertension, tachycardia

Central nervous system: Agitation, circumoral paresthesia, depression, dizziness, headache, insomnia, malaise, somnolence, tremor, vertigo

Dermatologic: Alopecia, eczema, pruritus

Gastrointestinal: Abdominal pain, anorexia, diarrhea, dyspepsia, flatulence, oral moniliasis, stomatitis, vomiting

Hepatic: Liver function tests increased

Neuromuscular & skeletal: Arthralgia, back pain

Respiratory: Cough increased, rhinitis, sinusitis

Miscellaneous: Aggravation reaction

Overdosage/Toxicology Methemoglobinemia has been reported with overdose. No specific antidote or treatment information is available. Treatment should be supportive and directed toward alleviating symptoms.

Pharmacodynamics/Kinetics

Absorption: 90%; high-fat meal decreases AUC by 20% and peak blood levels by 45%

Bioavailability: Oral: Absolute: 60%

Protein Binding: Plasma: 96%, primarily to albumin and lipoproteins

Half-Life Elimination: 12 hours

Metabolism: Extensively hepatic to six major and a number of minor metabolites via CYP1A2 dependent hydroxylation and glucuronidation

Excretion: Urine (90%; 85% as metabolites, 2% as unchanged drug) and feces (5%) within 7 days

Dosing

Adults & Elderly:

ALS treatment: Oral: 50 mg every 12 hours; no increased benefit can be expected from higher daily doses, but adverse events are increased.

Dosage adjustment in smoking: Cigarette smoking is known to induce CYP1A2; patients who smoke cigarettes would be expected to eliminate riluzole faster. There is no information, however, on the effect of, or need for, dosage adjustment in these patients.

Dosage adjustment in special populations: Females and Japanese patients may possess a lower metabolic capacity to eliminate riluzole compared with male and Caucasian subjects, respectively.

Renal Impairment: Use with caution in patients with concomitant renal insufficiency.

Hepatic Impairment: Use with caution in patients with current evidence or history of abnormal liver function indicated by significant abnormalities in serum transaminase, bilirubin or GGT levels. Baseline elevations of several LFTs (especially elevated bilirubin) should preclude use of riluzole.

Available Dosage Forms Tablet: 50 mg [film coated]

Monitoring and Teaching Issues

Physical Assessment: Assess effectiveness and interactions of other medications patient may be taking. Assess results of laboratory tests, therapeutic effectiveness, and adverse reactions (decreased liver function) at beginning of therapy and periodically throughout therapy. Assess knowledge/teach patient appropriate use, interventions to reduce side effects, and adverse symptoms to report.

Monitoring Laboratory Tests: Monitor serum aminotransferases including ALT levels before and during therapy. Evaluate serum ALT levels every month during the first 3 months of therapy, every 3 months during the remainder of the first year and periodically thereafter. Evaluate ALT levels more frequently in patients who develop elevations. Maximum increases in serum ALT usually occurred within 3 months after the start of therapy and were usually transient when <5 times ULN.

In trials, if ALT levels were <5 times ULN, treatment continued and ALT levels usually returned to below 2 times ULN within 2-6 months. Treatment in studies was discontinued, however, if ALT levels exceed 5 times ULN, so that there is no experience with continued treatment of ALS patients once ALT values exceed 5 times ULN.

If a decision is made to continue treatment in patients when the ALT exceeds 5 times ULN, frequent monitoring (at least weekly) of complete liver function is recommended. Discontinue treatment if ALT exceeds 10 times ULN or if clinical jaundice develops.

Patient Education: This drug will not cure or stop disease but it may slow progression. Take as directed, at the same time each day, preferably on an empty stomach, 1 hour before or 2 hours after meals. Avoid alcohol. You may experience increased spasticity, dizziness or sleepiness; use caution when driving or engaging in tasks requiring alertness until response to drug is known. Small frequent meals, frequent mouth care, chewing gum, or sucking lozenges may reduce nausea, vomiting, or anorexia. Report fever; severe vomiting, diarrhea, or constipation; change in color of urine or stool; yellowing of skin or eyes; acute back pain or muscle pain; or worsening of condition. **Pregnancy/breast-feeding precautions:** Inform prescriber if you are or intend to become pregnant. Consult prescriber if breast-feeding.

Dietary Considerations: Take at least 1 hour before, or 2 hours after, a meal.

Geriatric Considerations: In clinical trials, no difference was demonstrated between elderly and younger adults. However, renal and hepatic changes with age can be expected to result in higher serum concentrations of the parent drug and its metabolites.

Pregnancy Risk Factor: C

Lactation: Excretion in breast milk unknown/not recommended

Administration

Oral: Administer at the same time each day, 1 hour before or 2 hours after a meal.

Storage: Store at 20°C to 25°C (68°F to 77°F). Protect from bright light.

Rimantadine (ri MAN ta deen)

U.S. Brand Names Flumadine®

Synonyms Rimantadine Hydrochloride

Generic Available Yes: Tablet

Pharmacologic Category Antiviral Agent

Medication Safety Issues

Sound-alike/look-alike issues:

Rimantadine may be confused with amantadine, ranitidine, Rimactane®

(Continued)

Rimantadine *(Continued)*

Flumadine® may be confused with fludarabine, flunisolide, flutamide

Use Prophylaxis (adults and children >1 year of age) and treatment (adults) of influenza A viral infection

Mechanism of Action/Effect Exerts its inhibitory effect on three antigenic subtypes of influenza A virus (H1N1, H2N2, H3N2) early in the viral replicative cycle, possibly inhibiting the uncoating process; it has no activity against influenza B virus and is two- to eightfold more active than amantadine

Contraindications Hypersensitivity to drugs of the adamantine class, including rimantadine and amantadine, or any component of the formulation

Warnings/Precautions Use with caution in patients with renal and hepatic dysfunction. Avoid use, if possible, in patients with recurrent and eczematoid dermatitis, uncontrolled psychosis, or severe psychoneurosis. An increase in seizure incidence may occur in patients with seizure disorders. Discontinue drug if seizures occur. Consider the development of resistance during rimantadine treatment of the index case as likely if failure of rimantadine prophylaxis among family contact occurs and if index case is a child. Viruses exhibit cross-resistance between amantadine and rimantadine.

Drug Interactions

Decreased Effect: Acetaminophen may cause a small reduction in AUC and peak concentration of rimantadine. Peak plasma and AUC concentrations of rimantadine are slightly reduced by aspirin.

Increased Effect/Toxicity: Cimetidine increases blood levels/toxicity of rimantadine.

Nutritional/Ethanol Interactions Food: Food does not affect rate or extent of absorption

Adverse Reactions 1% to 10%:

Cardiovascular: Orthostatic hypotension, edema

Central nervous system: Dizziness (2%), confusion, headache (1%), insomnia (2%), difficulty in concentrating, anxiety (1%), restlessness, irritability, hallucinations; incidence of CNS side effects may be less than that associated with amantadine

Gastrointestinal: Nausea (3%), vomiting (2%), xerostomia (2%), abdominal pain (1%), anorexia (2%)

Genitourinary: Urinary retention

Overdosage/Toxicology Agitation, hallucinations, ventricular cardiac arrhythmias (torsade de pointes and PVCs), slurred speech, anticholinergic effects (dry mouth, urinary retention and mydriasis), ataxia, tremor, myoclonus, seizures, and death have been reported with amantadine, a related drug. Treatment is symptomatic (do not use physostigmine). Tachyarrhythmias may be treated with beta-blockers such as propranolol. Dialysis is not recommended except possibly in renal failure.

Pharmacodynamics/Kinetics

Onset of Action: Antiviral activity: No data exist establishing a correlation between plasma concentration and antiviral effect

Absorption: Tablets and syrup formulations are equally absorbed

Time to Peak: 6 hours

Half-Life Elimination: 25.4 hours; prolonged with elderly

Metabolism: Extensively hepatic

Excretion: Urine (<25% as unchanged drug)

Clearance: Hemodialysis does not contribute to clearance

Dosing

Adults:

Prophylaxis of influenza A: Oral: 100 mg twice daily

Treatment of influenza A: Oral: 100 mg twice daily

Elderly: Prophylaxis and treatment: Oral: Decrease to 100 mg/day in elderly patients (see Geriatric Considerations).

Pediatrics:

Prophylaxis of influenza A: Oral:

Children <10 years: 5 mg/kg once daily; maximum: 150 mg

Children >10 years: Refer to adult dosing.

Renal Impairment: Cl_{cr} ≤10 mL/minute: Administer 50% of normal dose.

Hepatic Impairment: Administer 50% normal dose with severe hepatic impairment.

Available Dosage Forms

Syrup, as hydrochloride: 50 mg/5 mL (240 mL) [raspberry flavor]

Tablet, as hydrochloride: 100 mg

Monitoring and Teaching Issues

Physical Assessment: Use caution with hepatic or renal impairment, seizure disorders (see Warnings/Precautions for use cautions). Assess effectiveness (resolution of infection) and adverse reactions (eg, hypotension, CNS changes [confusion, anxiety, agitation], GI upset, anticholinergic effects [dry mouth, urinary retention, mydriases]; see Adverse Reactions). Teach patient appropriate use, possible side effects/interventions (eg, postural hypotension), and adverse symptoms to report (see Patient Education).

Patient Education: Do not take any new medication during therapy unless approved by prescriber. Take as directed. Complete full course of therapy even if feeling better. Take a missed dose as soon as possible. If almost time for next dose, skip the missed dose and return to your regular schedule. Do not take a double dose. May cause orthostatic hypotension (use caution when changing position [rising from sitting or lying] or climbing stairs until response is known). Report CNS changes (eg, confusion, insomnia, anxiety, restlessness, irritability, hallucinations); difficulty urinating; or severe nausea or vomiting. **Pregnancy/breast-feeding precautions:** Inform prescriber if you are or intend to become pregnant. Do not breast-feed.

Geriatric Considerations: Adverse CNS and GI effects occur frequently if dosage is not adjusted. Monitor GI effects in the elderly or patients with renal or hepatic impairment. Dosing must be individualized (100 mg 1-2 times/day). It is recommended that nursing home patients receive 100 mg/day (see Pharmacodynamics/Kinetics).

Pregnancy Risk Factor: C

Lactation: Enters breast milk/contraindicated

Breast-Feeding Issues: Use in nursing mothers due to potential adverse effect in infants; rimantadine is concentrated in milk.

Administration

Oral: Initiation of rimantadine within 48 hours of the onset of influenza A illness halves the duration of illness and significantly reduces the duration of viral shedding and increased peripheral airways resistance. Continue therapy for 5-7 days after symptoms begin.

♦ **Rimantadine Hydrochloride** *see* Rimantadine *on page 1329*

♦ **Rimso®-50** *see* Dimethyl Sulfoxide *on page 462*

♦ **Rindal HD Plus** *see* Phenylephrine, Hydrocodone, and Chlorpheniramine *on page 1202*

♦ **Riomet™** *see* Metformin *on page 965*

♦ **Riopan Plus® [OTC] [DSC]** *see* Magaldrate and Simethicone *on page 929*

♦ **Riopan Plus® Double Strength [OTC] [DSC]** *see* Magaldrate and Simethicone *on page 929*

Risedronate (ris ED roe nate)

U.S. Brand Names Actonel®

Synonyms Risedronate Sodium

Generic Available No

Pharmacologic Category Bisphosphonate Derivative

Use Paget's disease of the bone; treatment and prevention of glucocorticoid-induced osteoporosis; treatment and prevention of osteoporosis in postmenopausal women

Mechanism of Action/Effect A bisphosphonate which inhibits bone resorption via actions on osteoclasts or on osteoclast precursors; decreases the rate of bone resorption, leading to an indirect increase in bone mineral density. In Paget's disease, characterized by disordered resorption and formation of bone, inhibition of resorption leads to an indirect decrease in bone formation; but the newly-formed bone has a more normal architecture.

Contraindications Hypersensitivity to risedronate, bisphosphonates, or any component of the formulation; hypocalcemia; abnormalities of the esophagus which delay esophageal emptying such as stricture or achalasia; inability to stand or sit upright for at least 30 minutes; severe renal impairment (Cl$_{cr}$ <30 mL/minute)

Warnings/Precautions Bisphosphonates may cause upper gastrointestinal disorders such as dysphagia, esophageal ulcer, and gastric ulcer. Use caution in patients with renal impairment; hypocalcemia must be corrected before therapy initiation with alendronate; ensure adequate calcium and vitamin D intake, especially for patients with Paget's disease in whom the pretreatment rate of bone turnover may be greatly elevated.

Drug Interactions

Decreased Effect: Calcium supplements and antacids interfere with absorption of risedronate (take at a different time of the day than risedronate).

Nutritional/Ethanol Interactions

Ethanol: Avoid ethanol (may increase risk of osteoporosis).

Food: Food may reduce absorption (similar to other bisphosphonates); mean oral bioavailability is decreased when given with food.

Adverse Reactions

Seen in patients taking 30 mg/day for Paget's disease:

>10%:

Central nervous system: Headache (18%)

Dermatologic: Rash (11%)

Gastrointestinal: Diarrhea (20%), abdominal pain (11%)

Neuromuscular & skeletal: Arthralgia (33%)

Miscellaneous: Flu-like syndrome (10%)

1% to 10%:

Cardiovascular: Peripheral edema (8%)

Central nervous system: Chest pain (7%), dizziness (7%)

Gastrointestinal: Nausea (10%), constipation (7%), belching (3%), colitis (3%, placebo 3%)

Neuromuscular & skeletal: Weakness (5%), bone pain (5%, placebo 5%), leg cramps (3%, placebo 3%), myasthenia (3%)

Ocular: Amblyopia (3%, placebo 3%), dry eye (3%)

Otic: Tinnitus (3%, placebo 3%)

Respiratory: Sinusitis (5%), bronchitis (3%, placebo 5%)

Miscellaneous: Neoplasm (3%)

Seen in patient taking 5 mg/day for osteoporosis (events similar to those seen with placebo)

>10%:

Central nervous system: Pain (14%)

Gastrointestinal: Abdominal pain (12%), diarrhea (11%), nausea (11%)

Genitourinary: Urinary tract infection (11%)

Neuromuscular & skeletal: Back pain (26%), arthralgia (24%)

1% to 10%:

Cardiovascular: Hypertension (10%), chest pain (5%), cardiovascular disorder (2%), angina (2%)

Central nervous system: Depression (7%), dizziness (6%), insomnia (5%), anxiety (4%), vertigo (3%)

Dermatologic: Rash (8%), bruising (4%), pruritus (3%), skin carcinoma (2%)

Gastrointestinal: Flatulence (5), gastritis (2%), gastrointestinal disorder (2%), rectal disorder (2%), tooth disorder (2%)

Genitourinary: Cystitis (4%)

Hematologic: Anemia (2%)

Neuromuscular & skeletal: Joint disorder (7%), myalgia (7%), neck pain (5%), asthenia (5%), bone pain (5%), bone disorder (4%), neuralgia (4%), leg cramps (4%), bursitis (3%), tendon disorder (3%), hypertonia (2%), paresthesia (2%)

(Continued)

Risedronate *(Continued)*

Ocular: Cataract (6%), conjunctivitis (3%)
Otic: Otitis media (2%)
Respiratory: Pharyngitis (6%), rhinitis (6%), dyspnea (4%), pneumonia (3%)
Miscellaneous: Neoplasm (3%), hernia (3%)

Overdosage/Toxicology Symptoms of overdose include hypocalcemia, hypophosphatemia, and upper GI adverse events (upset stomach, heartburn, esophagitis, gastritis, or ulcer). Gastric lavage may remove unabsorbed drug. Treat with milk or antacids to bind risedronate; dialysis would not be beneficial.

Pharmacodynamics/Kinetics
Onset of Action: May require weeks
Absorption: Rapid
Bioavailability: Poor, ~0.54% to 0.75%
Protein Binding: ~24%
Half-Life Elimination: Terminal: 480 hours
Metabolism: None
Excretion: Urine (up to 80%); feces (as unabsorbed drug)

Dosing
Adults:
Paget's disease of bone: Oral: 30 mg once daily for 2 months
Note: Retreatment may be considered (following post-treatment observation of at least 2 months) if relapse occurs, or if treatment fails to normalize serum alkaline phosphatase. For retreatment, the dose and duration of therapy are the same as for initial treatment. No data are available on more than one course of retreatment.
Osteoporosis (postmenopausal) prevention and treatment: Oral: 5 mg once daily; efficacy for use longer than 1 year has not been established; **alternatively,** a dose of 35 mg once weekly has been demonstrated to be effective
Osteoporosis (glucocorticoid-induced) prevention and treatment: Oral: 5 mg once daily
Note: Risedronate should be taken at least 30 minutes before the first food or drink of the day other than water. Patients should receive supplemental calcium and vitamin D if dietary intake is inadequate.
Elderly: Dosage adjustment is not necessary in patients with Cl_{cr} ≥30 mL/minute.
Renal Impairment: Cl_{cr} <30 mL/minute: Not recommended

Available Dosage Forms Tablet, as sodium: 5 mg, 30 mg, 35 mg

Monitoring and Teaching Issues
Physical Assessment: Ascertain that patient is capable of complying with administration directions before starting treatment and able to remain in standing or sitting position for 30 minutes. Use caution with renal impairment and correct any hypocalcemia before treatment (see Warnings/Precautions for use cautions). Assess results of laboratory tests, therapeutic effectiveness according to purpose for use, and adverse reactions (eg, rash, diarrhea, arthralgia, peripheral edema, gastrointestinal disturbance [nausea, vomiting, diarrhea], visual changes, hypocalcemia, hypophosphatemia; see Adverse Reactions). Teach patient appropriate use and administration of medication (see Administration), lifestyle, and dietary changes that will have a beneficial impact on Paget's disease or osteoporosis, possible side effects, interventions to reduce side effects, and adverse reactions to report (see Patient Education).

Monitoring Laboratory Tests: Alkaline phosphatase should be periodically measured; serum calcium, phosphorus, and possibly potassium due to its drug class. Use of absorptiometry may assist in noting benefit in osteoporosis.

Patient Education: In order to be effective, this medication must be taken exactly as directed with a full glass of water first thing in the morning, at least 30 minutes before the first food or beverage of the day. Wait at least 30 minutes after taking this medication before taking anything else. Stay in sitting or standing position for 30 minutes following administration and until after the first food of the day to reduce potential for esophageal irritation. Consult prescriber to determine necessity of lifestyle changes (eg, decreased smoking, decreased alcohol intake, dietary supplements of calcium, or increased dietary vitamin D). Avoid alcohol (ethanol may increase risk of osteoporosis). You may experience GI upset (eg, flatulence, bloating, nausea, acid regurgitation; small frequent meals may help). Report unresolved muscle twitching or bone pain or leg cramps; acute abdominal pain; chest pain, palpitations, or swollen extremities; disturbed vision or excessively dry eyes; ringing in the ears; or persistent flu-like symptoms. Also notify prescriber at once if experiencing difficulty swallowing, pain when swallowing, or severe or persistent heartburn. **Pregnancy/breast-feeding precautions:** Inform prescriber if you are or intend to become pregnant or if you are breast-feeding.

Dietary Considerations: Take ≥30 minutes before the first food or drink of the day other than water.

Pregnancy Risk Factor: C

Pregnancy Issues: Teratogenic and nonteratogenic embryo/fetal effects have been reported in animal studies. There are no adequate and well-controlled studies in pregnant women. Bisphosphonates are incorporated into the bone matrix and gradually released over time. Theoretically, there may be a risk of fetal harm when pregnancy follows the completion of therapy. Based on limited case reports with pamidronate, serum calcium levels in the newborn may be altered if administered during pregnancy.

Lactation: Excretion in breast milk unknown/not recommended

Breast-Feeding Issues: The manufacturer recommends discontinuing nursing or discontinuing risedronate.

Administration
Oral: Risedronate should be administered 30 or more minutes before the first food or drink of the day other than water. Risedronate should be taken in an upright position with a full glass (6-8 oz) of plain water and the patient should avoid lying down for 30 minutes to minimize the possibility of GI side effects.

Storage: Store at room temperature of 20°C to 25°C (68°F to 77°F).

RISPERIDONE

♦ **Risedronate Sodium** *see* Risedronate *on page 1331*

♦ **Risperdal®** *see* Risperidone *on page 1333*

♦ **Risperdal® Consta™** *see* Risperidone *on page 1333*

♦ **Risperdal® M-Tabs™** *see* Risperidone *on page 1333*

Risperidone (ris PER i done)

U.S. Brand Names Risperdal®; Risperdal® Consta™; Risperdal® M-Tabs™
Synonyms Risperdal M-Tabs™
Generic Available No
Pharmacologic Category Antipsychotic Agent, Atypical
Medication Safety Issues
Sound-alike/look-alike issues:
Risperidone may be confused with reserpine
Risperdal® may be confused with lisinopril, reserpine

Use Treatment of schizophrenia; treatment of acute mania or mixed episodes associated with bipolar I disorder (as monotherapy or in combination with lithium or valproate)

Unlabeled/Investigational Use Behavioral symptoms associated with dementia in elderly; treatment of Tourette's disorder; treatment of pervasive developmental disorder and autism in children and adolescents

Mechanism of Action/Effect Risperidone is a benzisoxazole antipsychotic, mixed serotonin-dopamine antagonist that binds to 5-HT$_2$-receptors in the CNS and in the periphery with a very high affinity; binds to dopamine-D$_2$ receptors with less affinity. The binding affinity to the dopamine-D$_2$ receptor is 20 times lower than the 5-HT$_2$ affinity. The addition of serotonin antagonism to dopamine antagonism (classic neuroleptic mechanism) is thought to improve negative symptoms of psychoses and reduce the incidence of extrapyramidal side effects. Alpha$_1$, alpha$_2$ adrenergic, and histaminergic receptors are also antagonized with high affinity. Risperidone has low to moderate affinity for 5-HT$_{1C}$, 5-HT$_{1D}$, and 5-HT$_{1A}$ receptors, weak affinity for D$_1$ and no affinity for muscarinics or beta$_1$ and beta$_2$ receptors

Contraindications Hypersensitivity to risperidone or any component of the formulation

Warnings/Precautions Patients with dementia-related behavioral disorders treated with atypical antipsychotics are at an increased risk of death compared to placebo. Risperidone is not approved for this indication.

Low to moderately sedating, use with caution in disorders where CNS depression is a feature. Use with caution in Parkinson's disease; in patients with hemodynamic instability; bone marrow suppression; predisposition to seizures; subcortical brain damage; or severe cardiac, hepatic, renal, or respiratory disease. Neuroleptics may cause swallowing difficulties, caution in patients predisposed to aspiration. Use with caution in breast cancer or other prolactin-dependent tumors (may elevate prolactin levels).

May cause orthostasis; an increased incidence of cerebrovascular events has been associated with risperidone use in elderly demented patients. Use with caution in patients with cardiovascular diseases (eg, heart failure, history of myocardial infarction or ischemia, cerebrovascular disease, conduction abnormalities). Use caution in patients receiving medications for hypertension (orthostatic effects may be exacerbated) or in patients with hypovolemia or dehydration. May alter cardiac conduction (low risk relative to other neuroleptics); life-threatening arrhythmias have occurred with therapeutic doses of neuroleptics.

Risperidone has a low potential for anticholinergic effects, but should be used with caution in patients with decreased gastrointestinal motility, urinary retention, BPH, xerostomia, visual problems, narrow-angle glaucoma (screening is recommended), and myasthenia gravis.

May cause extrapyramidal symptoms including pseudoparkinsonism, acute dystonic reactions, akathisia, and tardive dyskinesia (risk of these reactions is dose dependent and low relative to other neuroleptics). May be associated with neuroleptic malignant syndrome (NMS). May cause hyperglycemia; in some cases may be extreme and associated with ketoacidosis, hyperosmolar coma, or death. Use with caution in patients with diabetes or other disorders of glucose regulation; monitor for worsening of glucose control.

The possibility of a suicide attempt is inherent in psychotic illness or bipolar disorder; use caution in high-risk patients during initiation of therapy. Prescriptions should be written for the smallest quantity consistent with good patient care.

Drug Interactions
Cytochrome P450 Effect: Substrate of CYP2D6 (major), 3A4 (minor); **Inhibits** CYP2D6 (weak), 3A4 (weak)
Decreased Effect: Risperidone may antagonize effects of levodopa. Carbamazepine decreases risperidone serum concentrations.
Increased Effect/Toxicity: CYP2D6 inhibitors may increase the levels/effects of risperidone; example inhibitors include chlorpromazine, delavirdine, fluoxetine, miconazole, paroxetine, pergolide, quinidine, quinine, ritonavir, and ropinirole. Risperidone may enhance the hypotensive effects of antihypertensive agents. Clozapine decreases clearance of risperidone. Metoclopramide may increase risk of extrapyramidal symptoms (EPS).

Nutritional/Ethanol Interactions
Ethanol: Avoid ethanol (may increase CNS depression).
Herb/Nutraceutical: Avoid kava kava, gotu kola, valerian, St John's wort (may increase CNS depression).

Adverse Reactions
Frequency not defined: Gastrointestinal: Dysphagia, esophageal dysmotility
>10%:
Central nervous system: Insomnia, agitation, anxiety, headache, extrapyramidal symptoms (dose dependent), dizziness (I.M. injection)
Gastrointestinal: Weight gain
Respiratory: Rhinitis (I.M. injection)
1% to 10%:
Cardiovascular: Hypotension (especially orthostatic), tachycardia
(Continued)

Risperidone *(Continued)*

Central nervous system: Sedation, dizziness (oral formulation), restlessness, dystonic reactions, pseudoparkinsonism, tardive dyskinesia, neuroleptic malignant syndrome, altered central temperature regulation, nervousness, fatigue, somnolence, hallucination, tremor, hypoesthesia, akathisia

Dermatologic: Photosensitivity (rare), rash, dry skin, seborrhea, acne

Endocrine & metabolic: Amenorrhea, galactorrhea, gynecomastia, sexual dysfunction

Gastrointestinal: Constipation, GI upset, xerostomia, dyspepsia, vomiting, abdominal pain, nausea, anorexia, diarrhea, weight changes

Genitourinary: Polyuria

Neuromuscular & skeletal: Myalgia

Ocular: Abnormal vision

Respiratory: Rhinitis (oral formulation), cough, sinusitis, pharyngitis, dyspnea

Pharmacodynamics/Kinetics

Absorption:

Oral: Rapid and well absorbed; food does not affect rate or extent

Injection: <1% absorbed initially; main release occurs at ~3 weeks and is maintained from 4-6 weeks

Bioavailability: Solution: 70%; Tablet: 66%; orally-disintegrating tablets are bioequivalent to tablets

Time to Peak: Plasma: Oral: Risperidone: Within 1 hour; 9-hydroxyrisperidone: Extensive metabolizers: 3 hours; Poor metabolizers: 17 hours

Protein Binding: Plasma: Risperidone 90%; 9-hydroxyrisperidone: 77%

Half-Life Elimination: Active moiety (risperidone and its active metabolite 9-hydroxyrisperidone)

Oral: 20 hours (mean)

Extensive metabolizers: Risperidone: 3 hours; 9-hydroxyrisperidone: 21 hours

Poor metabolizers: Risperidone: 20 hours; 9-hydroxyrisperidone: 30 hours

Injection: 3-6 days; related to microsphere erosion and subsequent absorption of risperidone

Metabolism: Extensively hepatic via CYP2D6 to 9-hydroxyrisperidone (similar pharmacological activity as risperidone); *N*-dealkylation is a second minor pathway

Excretion: Urine (70%); feces (15%)

Dosing

Adults:

Bipolar mania: Oral: Recommended starting dose: 2-3 mg once daily; if needed, adjust dose by 1 mg/day in intervals ≥24 hours; dosing range: 1-6 mg/day.

Schizophrenia:

Oral: Recommended starting dose: 0.5-1 mg twice daily; slowly increase to the optimum range of 3-6 mg/day; may be given as a single daily dose once maintenance dose is achieved; daily dosages >10 mg does not appear to confer any additional benefit, and the incidence of extrapyramidal symptoms is higher than with lower doses.

I.M. (Risperdal® Consta™): 25 mg every 2 weeks; some patients may benefit from larger doses; maximum dose not to exceed 50 mg every 2 weeks. Dosage adjustments should not be made more frequently than every 4 weeks.

Note: Oral risperidone (or other antipsychotic) should be administered with the initial injection of Risperdal® Consta™ and continued for 3 weeks (then discontinued) to maintain adequate therapeutic plasma concentrations prior to main release phase of risperidone from injection site.

Tourette's disorder (unlabeled use): Oral: Initial: 0.5 mg; titrate to 2-4 mg/day

Elderly: In elderly patients, a starting dose of 0.25-0.5 mg once or twice daily is recommended, and titration should progress slowly. Increase dose by 0.5 mg twice daily at weekly intervals if possible; if rapid escalation is needed, increase by 1 mg twice daily every 3 days to achieve a target dose of 3 mg twice daily. Target dose in dementia: 0.75-1.25 mg/day. Additional monitoring of renal function and orthostatic blood pressure may be warranted. If once-a-day dosing in the elderly or debilitated patient is considered, a twice daily regimen should be used to titrate to the target dose, and this dose should be maintained for 2-3 days prior to attempts to switch to a once-daily regimen.

Pediatrics: Children and Adolescents:

Autism (unlabeled use): Oral: Initial: 0.25 mg at bedtime; titrate to 1 mg/day (0.1 mg/kg/day)

Bipolar disorder (unlabeled use): Oral: Initial: 0.5 mg; titrate to 0.5-3 mg/day

Pervasive developmental disorder (unlabeled use): Oral: Initial: 0.25 mg twice daily; titrate up 0.25 mg/day every 5-7 days; optimal dose range: 0.75-3 mg/day

Schizophrenia (unlabeled use): Oral: Initial: 0.5 mg once or twice daily; titrate as necessary up to 2-6 mg/day

Tourette's disorder (unlabeled use): Refer to adult dosing.

Renal Impairment: Oral: Starting dose of 0.25-0.5 mg twice daily; clearance of the active moiety is decreased by 60% in patients with moderate to severe renal disease compared to healthy subjects.

Hepatic Impairment: Oral: Starting dose of 0.25-0.5 mg twice daily; the mean free fraction of risperidone in plasma was increased by 35% compared to healthy subjects.

Available Dosage Forms

Injection, microspheres for reconstitution, extended release (Risperdal® Consta™): 25 mg, 37.5 mg, 50 mg [supplied in a dose-pack containing vial with active ingredient in microsphere formulation, prefilled syringe with diluent, needle-free vial access device, and safety needle]

Solution, oral: 1 mg/mL (30 mL) [contains benzoic acid]

Tablet: 0.25 mg, 0.5 mg, 1 mg, 2 mg, 3 mg, 4 mg

Tablet, orally disintegrating (Risperdal® M-Tabs™): 0.5 mg [contains phenylalanine 0.14 mg]; 1 mg [contains phenylalanine 0.28 mg]; 2 mg [contains phenylalanine 0.56 mg]

Monitoring and Teaching Issues

Physical Assessment: Assess potential for interactions with other prescriptions, OTC medications, or herbal products patient may be taking. Monitor results of periodic ophthalmic exams. Assess therapeutic effectiveness and adverse reactions at beginning of therapy and periodically with long-term use. Monitor weight prior to initiating therapy and at least monthly. Initiate at lower doses and taper dosage slowly when discontinuing. Teach patient appropriate use, possible side effects, interventions to reduce side effects, and adverse symptoms to report.

Monitoring Laboratory Tests: Fasting lipid profile and fasting blood glucose/Hgb A_{1c} (prior to treatment, at 3 months, then annually)

Patient Education: Do not take any new medication during therapy unless approved by prescriber. Use exactly as directed; do not increase dose or frequency. It may take several weeks to achieve desired results; do not discontinue without consulting prescriber. Dilute solution with water, milk, or orange juice; do not dilute with beverages containing tannin or pectinate (eg, colas, tea). Avoid alcohol or caffeine unless approved by prescriber. Maintain adequate hydration (2-3 L/day of fluids) unless instructed to restrict fluid intake. If diabetic, you may experience increased blood sugars. Monitor blood sugars closely. You may experience excess sedation, drowsiness, restlessness, dizziness, or blurred vision (use caution driving or when engaging in tasks requiring alertness until response to drug is known); dry mouth, nausea, or GI upset (small frequent meals, frequent mouth care, chewing gum, or sucking lozenges may help); postural hypotension (use caution climbing stairs or when changing position from lying or sitting to standing); or urinary retention (void before taking medication). Report persistent CNS effects (eg, trembling fingers, altered gait or balance, excessive sedation, seizures, unusual muscle or skeletal movements, anxiety, abnormal thoughts, confusion, personality changes); chest pain, palpitations, rapid heartbeat, severe dizziness; swelling or pain in breasts (male and female), altered menstrual pattern, sexual dysfunction; pain or difficulty on urination; vision changes; skin rash or yellowing of skin; respiratory difficulty; or worsening of condition. **Pregnancy/breast-feeding precautions:** Inform prescriber if you are or intend to become pregnant. Do not breast-feed.

Dietary Considerations: May be taken with or without food. Risperdal® M-Tabs™ contain phenylalanine.

Geriatric Considerations: (See Warnings/Precautions, Adverse Reactions, Elderly Dosing, and Overdose/Toxicology.) Elderly patients have an increased risk of adverse response to side effects or adverse reactions to antipsychotics.

Pregnancy Risk Factor: C

Lactation: Enters breast milk/contraindicated

Breast-Feeding Issues: Risperidone and its metabolite are excreted in breast milk; it is recommended that women not breast feed during therapy or for 12 weeks after the last injection if using Risperdal® Consta™.

Administration

Oral: Oral solution can be mixed with water, coffee, orange juice, or low-fat milk, but is **not compatible** with cola or tea. May be administered with or without food.

Risperdal® M-Tabs™ should not be removed from blister pack until administered. Using dry hands, place immediately on tongue. Tablet will dissolve within seconds, and may be swallowed with or without liquid. Do not split or chew.

I.M.: Risperdal® Consta™ should be administered I.M. into the upper outer quadrant of the gluteal area. Injection should alternate between the two buttocks. Do not combine two different dosage strengths into one single administration. Do not substitute any components of the dose-pack; administer with needle provided.

Reconstitution: Risperdal® Consta™: Bring to room temperature prior to reconstitution. Reconstitute with provided diluent only. Shake vigorously to mix; will form thick, milky suspension. Following reconstitution, store at room temperature and use within 6 hours. If suspension settles prior to use, shake vigorously to resuspend.

Storage: Risperdal® Consta™: Store in refrigerator at 2°C to 8°C (36°F to 46°F) and protect from light. May be stored at room temperature of 25°C (77°F) for up to 7 days prior to administration.

Additional Information Risperdal® Consta™ is an injectable formulation of risperidone using the extended release Medisorb® drug-delivery system; small polymeric microspheres degrade slowly, releasing the medication at a controlled rate.

Related Information

Antipsychotic Agents *on page 1717*
Antipsychotic Medication Guidelines *on page 1766*
Federal OBRA Regulations: Recommended Maximum Doses *on page 1773*

♦ **Ritalin®** *see* Methylphenidate *on page 983*
♦ **Ritalin® LA** *see* Methylphenidate *on page 983*
♦ **Ritalin-SR®** *see* Methylphenidate *on page 983*

Ritonavir (ri TOE na veer)

U.S. Brand Names Norvir®
Generic Available No
Pharmacologic Category Antiretroviral Agent, Protease Inhibitor
Medication Safety Issues
Sound-alike/look-alike issues:
Ritonavir may be confused with Retrovir®
Norvir® may be confused with Norvasc®

Use Treatment of HIV infection; should always be used as part of a multidrug regimen (at least three antiretroviral agents)

Mechanism of Action/Effect Ritonavir prevents cleavage of protein precursors essential for HIV infection of new cells and viral replication. Saquinavir- and zidovudine-resistant HIV isolates are generally susceptible to ritonavir. Used in combination therapy, resistance to ritonavir develops slowly; strains resistant to ritonavir are cross-resistant to indinavir and saquinavir.
(Continued)

Ritonavir *(Continued)*

Contraindications Hypersensitivity to ritonavir or any component of the formulation; concurrent amiodarone, bepridil, cisapride, dihydroergotamine, ergonovine, ergotamine, flecainide, lovastatin, methylergonovine, midazolam, pimozide, propafenone, quinidine, simvastatin, St John's wort, triazolam, and voriconazole

Warnings/Precautions Use caution in patients with hepatic insufficiency. Safety and efficacy have not been established in children <2 years of age. Use caution with benzodiazepines, rifabutin, sildenafil, and certain analgesics (meperidine, piroxicam, propoxyphene). Selected HMG-CoA reductase inhibitors are contraindicated (see Contraindications); atorvastatin should be used at the lowest possible dose, while fluvastatin or pravastatin may be safer alternatives. Avoid concurrent use of St John's wort. Warn patients that redistribution of fat may occur.

Drug Interactions

    Cytochrome P450 Effect: Substrate of CYP1A2 (minor), 2B6 (minor), 2D6 (minor), 3A4 (major); **Inhibits** CYP2C8/9 (weak), 2C19 (weak), 2D6 (strong), 2E1 (weak), 3A4 (strong); **Induces** CYP1A2 (weak), 2C8/9 (weak), 3A4 (weak)

    Decreased Effect: The administration of didanosine (buffered formulation) should be separated from ritonavir by 2.5 hours to limit interaction with ritonavir. Concurrent use of rifampin, rifabutin, dexamethasone, and many anticonvulsants may lower serum concentration of ritonavir. Ritonavir may reduce the concentration of ethinyl estradiol which may result in loss of contraception (including combination products). Theophylline concentrations may be reduced in concurrent therapy. Levels of didanosine and zidovudine may be decreased by ritonavir, however, no dosage adjustment is necessary. Voriconazole serum levels are reduced by ritonavir (concurrent use is contraindicated). In addition, ritonavir may decrease the serum concentrations of the following drugs: Atovaquone, divalproex, lamotrigine, methadone, phenytoin, warfarin. The levels/effects of ritonavir may be decreased by aminoglutethimide, carbamazepine, nafcillin, nevirapine, phenobarbital, phenytoin, rifamycins, and other CYP3A4 inducers. Ritonavir may decrease the levels/effects of CYP2D6 prodrug substrates (eg, codeine, hydrocodone, oxycodone, tramadol).

    Increased Effect/Toxicity: Concurrent use of amiodarone, bepridil, cisapride, ergot alkaloids (dihydroergotamine, ergonovine, methylergonovine), flecainide, lovastatin, midazolam, pimozide, propafenone, quinidine, simvastatin, and triazolam is contraindicated.

    Saquinavir's serum concentrations are increased by ritonavir; the dosage of both agents should be reduced to 400 mg twice daily. Concurrent therapy with amprenavir may result in increased serum concentrations: dosage adjustment is recommended. Metronidazole or disulfiram may cause disulfiram reaction (oral solution contains 43% ethanol). Serum levels/effects of corticosteroids (eg, dexamethasone, fluticasone, prednisone) and immunosuppressants (cyclosporine, sirolimus, tacrolimus; monitor) may be increased by ritonavir. Serum concentrations of meperidine's neuroexcitatory metabolite (normeperidine) are increased by ritonavir, which may increase the risk of CNS toxicity/seizures. Rifabutin and rifabutin metabolite serum concentrations may be increased by ritonavir; reduce rifabutin dose to 150 mg every other day.

    Ritonavir may increase the levels/effects of amphetamines, selected beta-blockers, selected benzodiazepines (midazolam and triazolam contraindicated), calcium channel blockers (bepridil contraindicated), cisapride (contraindicated), dextromethorphan, ergot alkaloids (contraindicated), fluoxetine, lidocaine, HMG-CoA reductase inhibitors (lovastatin and simvastatin are contraindicated), mesoridazine, mirtazapine, nateglinide, nefazodone, paroxetine, pimozide (contraindicated), propafenone (contraindicated), risperidone, sildenafil (and other PDE-5 inhibitors), thioridazine, tricyclic antidepressants, venlafaxine, and other substrates of CYP2D6 or 3A4. Mesoridazine and thioridazine are generally contraindicated with strong CYP2D6 inhibitors. When used with strong CYP3A4 inhibitors, dosage adjustment/limits are recommended for sildenafil and other PDE-5 inhibitors; refer to individual monographs.

Nutritional/Ethanol Interactions

    Food: Food enhances absorption.

    Herb/Nutraceutical: St John's wort may decrease ritonavir serum levels. Avoid use.

Adverse Reactions Protease inhibitors cause dyslipidemia which includes elevated cholesterol and triglycerides and a redistribution of body fat centrally to cause increased abdominal girth, buffalo hump, facial atrophy, and breast enlargement. These agents also cause hyperglycemia.

    >10%:

        Endocrine & metabolic: Triglycerides increased

        Gastrointestinal: Diarrhea, nausea, vomiting, taste perversion

        Hematologic: Anemia, WBCs decreased

        Hepatic: GGT increased

        Neuromuscular & skeletal: Weakness

    1% to 10%:

        Cardiovascular: Vasodilation

        Central nervous system: Fever, headache, malaise, dizziness, insomnia, somnolence, thinking abnormally

        Dermatologic: Rash

        Endocrine & metabolic: Hyperlipidemia, uric acid increased, glucose increased

        Gastrointestinal: Abdominal pain, anorexia, constipation, dyspepsia, flatulence, local throat irritation

        Hematologic: Neutropenia, eosinophilia, neutrophilia, prolonged PT, leukocytosis

        Hepatic: LFTs increased

        Neuromuscular & skeletal: CPK increased, myalgia, paresthesia

        Respiratory: Pharyngitis

        Miscellaneous: Diaphoresis, potassium increased, calcium increased

Overdosage/Toxicology Human experience is limited; there is no specific antidote for overdose with ritonavir. Oral solution contains 43% ethanol by volume, potentially causing significant ethanol-related toxicity in younger patients. Dialysis is unlikely to be beneficial in significant removal of the drug. Charcoal or gastric lavage may be useful to remove unabsorbed drug.

Pharmacodynamics/Kinetics

Absorption: Variable, with or without food

Protein Binding: 98% to 99%

Half-Life Elimination: 3-5 hours

Metabolism: Hepatic; five metabolites, low concentration of an active metabolite achieved in plasma (oxidative); see Drug Interactions

Excretion: Urine (negligible amounts)

Dosing

Adults & Elderly:

HIV infection: Oral: 600 mg twice daily; dose escalation tends to avoid nausea that many patients experience upon initiation of full dosing. Escalate the dose as follows: 300 mg twice daily for 1 day, 400 mg twice daily for 2 days, 500 mg twice daily for 1 day, then 600 mg twice daily. Ritonavir may be better tolerated when used in combination with other antiretrovirals by initiating the drug alone and subsequently adding the second agent within 2 weeks.

Dosage adjustments for ritonavir when administered in combination therapy:

Amprenavir: Adjustments necessary for each agent:

    Amprenavir 1200 mg with ritonavir 200 mg once daily **or**

    Amprenavir 600 mg with ritonavir 100 mg twice daily

Amprenavir plus efavirenz (3-drug regimen): Amprenavir 1200 mg twice daily plus ritonavir 200 mg twice daily plus efavirenz at standard dose

Indinavir: Adjustments necessary for agent:

    Indinavir 800 mg twice daily plus ritonavir 100-200 mg twice daily **or**

    Indinavir 400 mg twice daily plus ritonavir 400 mg twice daily

Nelfinavir or saquinavir: Ritonavir 400 mg twice daily

Rifabutin: Decrease rifabutin dose to 150 mg every other day

Pediatrics:

HIV infection: Oral: Children ≥2 years: 250 mg/m^2 twice daily; titrate dose upward to 400 mg/m^2 twice daily (maximum: 600 mg twice daily)

Hepatic Impairment: No adjustment required in mild or moderate impairment; however, careful monitoring is required in moderate hepatic impairment (levels may be decreased); caution advised with severe impairment (no data available).

Available Dosage Forms

Capsule: 100 mg [contains ethanol and polyoxyl 35 castor oil]

Solution: 80 mg/mL (240 mL) [contains ethanol and polyoxyl 35 castor oil; peppermint and caramel flavor]

Monitoring and Teaching Issues

Physical Assessment: Use caution with hepatic impairment (see Warnings/Precautions). Assess potential for interactions with other pharmacological agents and herbal products patient may be taking (multiple liver enzyme interactions that increase or decrease levels/effects of multiple other drugs [increased potential for severe toxicity or loss of effectiveness]; see Drug Interactions for extensive list and cautions). Assess result of laboratory tests, patient response (CD4 count and viral load), and adverse reactions at regular intervals during therapy (eg, gastrointestinal disturbance [nausea, vomiting, diarrhea], anemia, hyperlipidemia and redistribution of body fat, rash, CNS effects [malaise, insomnia, abnormal thinking], electrolyte imbalance; see Adverse Reactions). Teach patient proper use, possible side effects/appropriate interventions (eg, glucose testing; protease inhibitors may cause hyperglycemia [exacerbation or new-onset diabetes]), use of appropriate contraceptives (protease inhibitors may decrease effectiveness of oral contraceptives), and adverse symptoms to report (see Patient Education).

Monitoring Laboratory Tests: Triglycerides, cholesterol, LFTs, CBC, CPK, uric acid, viral load, CD4 count, glucose

Patient Education: Do not take any new medication during therapy unless approved by prescriber. Ritonavir is not a cure for HIV, nor has it been shown to reduce transmission of HIV. Take as directed with meals. Mix liquid formulation with chocolate milk or liquid nutritional supplement. Capsules may be stored in refrigerator (do not freeze or expose to excessive heat) or stored at room temperature if used within 30 days. Protect from light. Solution should be stored at room temperature. Do not refrigerate. Maintain adequate hydration (2-3 L/day of fluids) unless instructed to restrict fluid intake. Ritonavir may be prescribed with a combination of other medications; time these medications as directed by prescriber. You may be advised to check your glucose levels (this drug can cause exacerbation or new-onset diabetes). May cause body changes due to redistribution of body fat, facial atrophy, or breast enlargement (normal effects of drug); dizziness, insomnia, abnormal thinking (use caution when driving or engaging in potentially hazardous tasks until response to drug is known); nausea, vomiting, or taste perversion (small frequent meals, frequent mouth care, chewing gum, or sucking lozenges may help); muscle weakness (consult prescriber for approved analgesic); or headache or insomnia (consult prescriber for medication). Report any persistent adverse effect. **Pregnancy/breast-feeding precautions:** May reduce effectiveness of some oral/systemic contraceptives. Consult prescriber for appropriate contraceptive measures. Do not breast-feed.

Dietary Considerations: Should be taken with food. Oral solution contains 43% ethanol by volume.

Pregnancy Risk Factor: B

Pregnancy Issues: Early studies have shown lower plasma levels during pregnancy compared to postpartum. If needed during pregnancy, use in combination with another PI to boost levels of second PI. Pregnancy and protease inhibitors are both associated with an increased risk of hyperglycemia. Glucose levels should be closely monitored. The Perinatal HIV Guidelines Working Group considers ritonavir to be an alternative PI for use during pregnancy. Healthcare professionals are encouraged to contact the antiretroviral pregnancy registry to monitor outcomes of pregnant women exposed to antiretroviral medications (1-800-258-4263 or www.APRegistry.com).

(Continued)

Ritonavir *(Continued)*

Lactation: Enters breast milk/contraindicated

Breast-Feeding Issues: Ritonavir is minimally excreted in breast milk. HIV-infected mothers are discouraged from breast-feeding to decrease potential transmission of HIV.

Administration

Oral: Administer with food. Liquid formulations usually have an unpleasant taste. Consider mixing it with chocolate milk or a liquid nutritional supplement.

Storage:

Capsule: Store under refrigeration at 2°C to 8°C (36°F to 46°F); may be left out at room temperature of <25°C (<77°F) if used within 30 days. Protect from light. Avoid exposure to excessive heat.

Solution: Store at room temperature at 20°C to 25°C (68°F to 77°F). Do not refrigerate.

Additional Information Potential compliance problems, frequency of administration and adverse effects should be discussed with patients before initiating therapy to help prevent the emergence of resistance.

Related Information

Tuberculosis *on page 1864*

♦ **Ritonavir and Lopinavir** *see Lopinavir and Ritonavir on page 916*

♦ **Rituxan®** *see Rituximab on page 1338*

Rituximab *(ri TUK si mab)*

U.S. Brand Names Rituxan®

Synonyms Anti-CD20 Monoclonal Antibody; C2B8; C2B8 Monoclonal Antibody; IDEC-C2B8; Pan-B Antibody

Generic Available No

Pharmacologic Category Antineoplastic Agent, Monoclonal Antibody

Medication Safety Issues

Sound-alike/look-alike issues:

Rituxan® may be confused with Remicade®

Use Treatment of relapsed or refractory CD20 positive, B-cell non-Hodgkin's lymphoma

Mechanism of Action/Effect Binds to the CD20 antigen on B-lymphocytes and recruits immune effector functions to mediate B-cell lysis *in vitro*. The antibody induces cell death in the DHL-4 human B-cell lymphoma line.

Contraindications Type I hypersensitivity or anaphylactic reactions to murine proteins or any component of the formulation

Warnings/Precautions Severe infusion related reactions have been reported (77% following the first dose). Hypotension, bronchospasm, and angioedema have occurred as part of an infusion-related symptom complex; hypoxia, pulmonary infiltrates, acute respiratory distress syndrome, myocardial infarction, ventricular fibrillation, or cardiogenic shock may occur in the most severe cases. Risk factors associated with fatal outcomes include chronic lymphocytic leukemia, female gender, mantle cell lymphoma, or pulmonary infiltrates. Treatment of these reactions is symptomatic (antihistamines, bronchodilators, saline infusion); pretreatment with diphenhydramine and acetaminophen is recommended. In most cases, patients who have experienced nonlife-threatening reactions have been able to complete the full course of therapy. Rituximab is associated with hypersensitivity reactions which may respond to adjustments in the infusion rate. Medications for the treatment of hypersensitivity reactions (eg, epinephrine, antihistamines, corticosteroids) should be available for immediate use. Discontinue infusions in the event of serious or life-threatening cardiac arrhythmias. Reactivation of Hepatitis B has been reported in association with rituximab (rare); consider screening in high-risk patients.

Tumor lysis syndrome leading to acute renal failure requiring dialysis may occur 12-24 hours following the first dose. Consider prophylaxis in patients at high risk. Severe and sometimes fatal mucocutaneous reactions have been reported, occurring from 1-13 weeks following exposure. Use caution with cardiac or pulmonary disease, prior cardiopulmonary events and with high numbers of circulating malignant cells (≥25000/mm³). Safety and efficacy in pediatric patients have not been established.

Adverse Reactions Note: Abdominal pain, anemia, dyspnea, hypotension, and neutropenia are more common in patients with bulky disease.

>10%:

Central nervous system: Fever (53%), chills (33%), headache (19%), pain (12%)

Dermatologic: Rash (15%), pruritus (14%), angioedema (11%)

Gastrointestinal: Nausea (23%), abdominal pain (14%)

Hematologic: Lymphopenia (48%; Grade 3/4: 40%; mean duration 14 days), leukopenia (14%; Grade 3/4: 4%), neutropenia (14%; Grade 3/4: 6%; mean duration 13 days), thrombocytopenia (12%; Grade 3/4: 2%)

Neuromuscular & skeletal: Weakness (26%)

Respiratory: Cough (13%), rhinitis (12%)

Miscellaneous: Infection (31%), night sweats (15%)

Infusion-related reactions: Chills, fever, rigors, dizziness, hypertension, myalgia, nausea, pruritus, rash and vomiting (first dose 77%; fourth dose 30%; eighth dose 14%)

1% to 10%:

Cardiovascular: Dizziness (10%), hypotension (10%), peripheral edema (8%), hypertension (6%), anxiety (5%), flushing (5%)

Central nervous system: Agitation (<5%), depression (<5%), edema (<5%), insomnia (<5%), malaise (<5%), nervousness (<5%), somnolence (<5%), vertigo (<5%)

Dermatologic: Urticaria (8%)

Endocrine & metabolic: Hyperglycemia (9%), hypoglycemia (<5%)

Gastrointestinal: Diarrhea (10%), vomiting (10%), anorexia (<5%), weight loss (<5%)

Hematologic: Anemia (8%; Grade 3/4: 3%)

Local: Pain at the injection site (<5%)

Neuromuscular & skeletal: Arthralgia (10%), back pain (10%), myalgia (10%), arthritis (<5%), hyperkinesia (<5%), hypertonia (<5%), hypoesthesia (<5%), neuritis (<5%), neuropathy (<5%), paresthesia (<5%)

Ocular: Conjunctivitis (<5%), lacrimation disorder (<5%)

Respiratory: Throat irritation (9%), bronchospasm (8%), dyspnea (7%), sinusitis (6%), dyspepsia (<5%)

Miscellaneous: LDH increased (7%)

Overdosage/Toxicology There has been no experience with overdosage in human clinical trials; single doses higher than 500 mg/m^2 have not been tested

Pharmacodynamics/Kinetics

Duration of Action: Detectable in serum 3-6 months after completion of treatment; B-cell recovery begins ~6 months following completion of treatment; median B-cell levels return to normal by 12 months following completion of treatment

Absorption: I.V.: Immediate and results in a rapid and sustained depletion of circulating and tissue-based B cells

Half-Life Elimination:
>100 mg/m^2: 4.4 days (range 1.6-10.5 days)
375 mg/m^2: 50 hours (following first dose) to 174 hours (following fourth dose)

Excretion: Uncertain; may undergo phagocytosis and catabolism in the reticuloendothelial system (RES)

Dosing

Adults & Elderly: Non-Hodgkin's lymphoma: I.V. infusion (refer to individual protocols):
Manufacturer's labeling: 375 mg/m^2 once weekly for 4-8 weeks
or
100 mg/m^2 I.V. day 1, then 375 mg/m^2 3 times/week for 11 doses has also been reported (cycles may be repeated in patients with refractory or relapsed disease)

Retreatment following disease progression: 375 mg/m^2 once weekly for 4 doses

Combination therapy with ibritumomab: 250 mg/m^2 I.V. day 1; repeat in 7-9 days with ibritumomab (also see Ibritumomab monograph):

Rituximab dose in combination with ibritumomab:

Step 1: 250 mg/m^2 at an initial rate of 50 mg/hour. If hypersensitivity or infusion-related events do not occur, increase infusion in increments of 50 mg/hour every 30 minutes, to a maximum of 400 mg/hour. Infusions should be temporarily slowed or interrupted if hypersensitivity or infusion related events occur. The infusion may be resumed at $^1/_2$ the previous rate upon improvement of symptoms.

Step 2: 250 mg/m^2 at an initial rate of 100 mg/hour (50 mg/hour if infusion-related events occurred with the first infusion). If hypersensitivity or infusion-related events do not occur, increase infusion in increments of 100 mg/hour every 30 minutes, to a maximum of 400 mg/hour, as tolerated.

Available Dosage Forms Injection, solution [preservative free]: 10 mg/mL (10 mL, 50 mL)

Monitoring and Teaching Issues

Physical Assessment: Assess patient history to mouse antibodies prior to therapy. See Warning/Precautions for specifics about severe infusion related reactions and use cautions (cardiac or pulmonary disease and prior cardiopulmonary events). See Administration for infusion specifics. Patient must be monitored closely during and following each infusion; severe infusion related reactions can include chills, fever, rigors, dizziness, hypo- or hypertension, angioedema, respiratory distress, myalgia, nausea, pruritus, rash, and vomiting; acute tumor lysis syndrome leading to acute renal failure 12-24 hours after first dose and severe mucocutaneous reactions can occur from 1-13 weeks following treatment. Preinfusion treatment with diphenhydramine and acetaminophen is recommended and epinephrine, antihistamines, corticosteroids should be immediately available in event of infusion reaction. Assess results of laboratory tests prior to, during, and following therapy (see Monitoring Laboratory Tests). Teach patient possible side effects of treatment/appropriate interventions and adverse reactions to report (see Patient Education).

Monitoring Laboratory Tests: CBC with differential, peripheral CD20+ cells. Patients with elevated HAMA/HACA titers may have an allergic reaction when treated with rituximab or other antibodies from a mouse genetic source.

Patient Education: This medication is only administered by infusion. You may experience a reaction during the infusion of this medication including high fever, chills, respiratory difficulty, or congestion. You will be closely monitored and comfort measures provided. Maintain adequate hydration (2-3 L/day of fluids during entire course of therapy) unless instructed to restrict fluid intake. You will be susceptible to infection and people may wear masks and gloves while caring for you to protect you as much as possible (avoid crowds and exposure to infection and do not have any vaccinations without consulting prescriber). May cause dizziness or trembling (use caution until response to medication is known); nausea, vomiting, or loss of appetite (small frequent meals, frequent mouth care may help); diarrhea (increase dietary fiber, buttermilk, or yogurt); bone or muscle pain (ask prescriber for appropriate analgesic). Report persistent dizziness, swelling of extremities, unusual weight gain, chest pain or tightness; symptoms of respiratory infection (wheezing, bronchospasms, or difficulty breathing); unresolved GI disturbance (nausea, vomiting); skin rash or redness; opportunistic infection (sore or irritated throat; unusual and persistent fatigue, chills, fever, unhealed sores, white plaques in mouth or genital area; unusual bruising or bleeding); or other unusual effects related to this medication. **Pregnancy/breast-feeding precautions:** Inform prescriber if you are or intend to become pregnant. Do not breast-feed.

Pregnancy Risk Factor: C

Lactation: Excretion in breast milk unknown/contraindicated

Breast-Feeding Issues: The manufacturer recommends discontinuing breast-feeding until circulating levels of rituximab are no longer detectable.

Administration

I.V.: Do **not** administer as an I.V. push or short bolus. Rituximab is associated with hypersensitivity reactions which may respond to adjustments in the infusion rate.

Initial infusion: Start rate of 50 mg/hour; if there is no reaction, increase the rate 50 mg/hour every 30 minutes, to a maximum of 400 mg/hour.

(Continued)

Rituximab *(Continued)*

Subsequent infusions: Start at 100 mg/hour; if there is no reaction, increase the rate 100 mg/hour every 30 minutes, to a maximum of 400 mg/hour.

Note: If a reaction occurs, slow or stop the infusion. If the reaction abates, restart infusion at 50% of the previous dose.

Reconstitution: Withdraw necessary amount of rituximab and dilute to a final concentration of 1-4 mg/mL into an infusion bag containing either 0.9% sodium chloride or 5% dextrose in water.

Storage: Store under refrigeration; protect vials from direct sunlight. Solutions for infusion are stable at 2°C to 8°C/36°F to 46°F for 24 hours and at room temperature for an additional 12 hours.

Rivastigmine (ri va STIG meen)

U.S. Brand Names Exelon®

Synonyms ENA 713; Rivastigmine Tartrate; SDZ ENA 713

Generic Available No

Pharmacologic Category Acetylcholinesterase Inhibitor (Central)

Use Mild to moderate dementia from Alzheimer's disease

Mechanism of Action/Effect A deficiency of cortical acetylcholine is thought to account for some of the symptoms of Alzheimer's disease; rivastigmine increases acetylcholine in the central nervous system through reversible inhibition of its hydrolysis by cholinesterase

Contraindications Hypersensitivity to rivastigmine, other carbamate derivatives, or any component of the formulation

Warnings/Precautions Significant nausea, vomiting, anorexia, and weight loss are associated with use, occurring more frequently in women and during the titration phase. Use caution in patients with a history of peptic ulcer disease or concurrent NSAID use. Caution in patients undergoing anesthesia who will receive succinylcholine-type muscle relaxation, patients with sick sinus syndrome, bradycardia or supraventricular conduction conditions, urinary obstruction, seizure disorders, or pulmonary conditions such as asthma or COPD. There are no trials evaluating the safety and efficacy in children.

Drug Interactions

Decreased Effect: Anticholinergic agents effects may be reduced with rivastigmine.

Increased Effect/Toxicity:

Beta-blockers without ISA activity may increase risk of bradycardia.

Calcium channel blockers (diltiazem or verapamil) may increase risk of bradycardia.

Cholinergic agonists effects may be increased with rivastigmine.

Cigarette use increases the clearance of rivastigmine by 23%.

Depolarizing neuromuscular blocking agents effects may be increased with rivastigmine.

Digoxin may increase risk of bradycardia.

Nutritional/Ethanol Interactions

Cigarette use: Increases the clearance of rivastigmine by 23%.

Ethanol: Avoid ethanol (due to risk of sedation; may increase GI irritation).

Food: Food delays absorption by 90 minutes, lowers C_{max} by 30% and increases AUC by 30%.

Adverse Reactions

>10%:

Central nervous system: Dizziness (21%), headache (17%)

Gastrointestinal: Nausea (47%), vomiting (31%), diarrhea (19%), anorexia (17%), abdominal pain (13%)

2% to 10%:

Cardiovascular: Syncope (3%), hypertension (3%)

Central nervous system: Fatigue (9%), insomnia (9%), confusion (8%), depression (6%), anxiety (5%), malaise (5%), somnolence (5%), hallucinations (4%), aggressiveness (3%)

Gastrointestinal: Dyspepsia (9%), constipation (5%), flatulence (4%), weight loss (3%), eructation (2%)

Genitourinary: Urinary tract infection (7%)

Neuromuscular & skeletal: Weakness (6%), tremor (4%)

Respiratory: Rhinitis (4%)

Miscellaneous: Increased diaphoresis (4%), flu-like syndrome (3%)

>2% (but frequency equal to placebo): Chest pain, peripheral edema, vertigo, back pain, arthralgia, pain, bone fracture, agitation, nervousness, delusion, paranoid reaction, upper respiratory tract infection, infection, cough, pharyngitis, bronchitis, rash, urinary incontinence.

<2% (Limited to important or life-threatening symptoms; reactions may be at a similar frequency to placebo): Fever, edema, allergy, periorbital or facial edema, hypothermia, hypotension, postural hypotension, cardiac failure, ataxia, convulsions, apraxia, aphasia, dysphonia, hyperkinesia, hypertonia, hypokinesia, migraine, neuralgia, peripheral neuropathy, hypothyroidism, peptic ulcer, gastroesophageal reflux, GI hemorrhage, intestinal obstruction, pancreatitis, colitis, atrial fibrillation, bradycardia, AV block, bundle branch block, sick sinus syndrome, cardiac arrest, supraventricular tachycardia, tachycardia, abnormal hepatic function, cholecystitis, dehydration, arthritis, angina pectoris, MI, epistaxis, hematoma, thrombocytopenia, purpura, delirium, emotional lability, psychosis, anemia, bronchospasm, apnea, rash (maculopapular, eczema, bullous, exfoliative, psoriaform, erythematous), urticaria, acute renal failure, peripheral ischemia, pulmonary embolism, thrombosis, thrombophlebitis, intracranial hemorrhage, conjunctival hemorrhage, diplopia, glaucoma, lymphadenopathy, leukocytosis.

Overdosage/Toxicology In cases of asymptomatic overdoses, rivastigmine should be held for 24 hours. Cholinergic crisis, caused by significant acetylcholinesterase inhibition, is characterized by severe nausea, vomiting, salivation, sweating, bradycardia, hypotension, respiratory depression, collapse, and convulsions. Treatment is supportive and symptomatic. Dialysis would not be helpful.

Pharmacodynamics/Kinetics

Absorption: Fasting: Rapid and complete within 1 hour

Bioavailability: 40%

Time to Peak: 1 hour

Protein Binding: 40%

Half-Life Elimination: 1.5 hours

Metabolism: Extensively via cholinesterase-mediated hydrolysis in the brain; metabolite undergoes N-demethylation and/or sulfate conjugation hepatically; minimal CYP involvement; linear kinetics at 3 mg twice daily, but nonlinear at higher doses

Excretion: Urine (97% as metabolites); feces (0.4%)

Dosing

Adults & Elderly: Alzheimer's dementia: Oral: Initial: 1.5 mg twice daily for 2 weeks; if tolerated, may be increased to 3 mg twice daily; further increases may be attempted no more frequently than every 2 weeks, to 4.5 mg twice daily and then to 6 mg twice daily; maximum dose: 6 mg twice daily. If gastrointestinal adverse events occur, the patient should be instructed to discontinue treatment for several doses then restart at the same or next lower dosage level; antiemetics have been used to control GI symptoms. If treatment is interrupted for longer than several days, restart the treatment at the lowest dose and titrate as previously described.

Renal Impairment: Dosage adjustments are not recommended, however, titrate the dose to the individual's tolerance.

Hepatic Impairment: Clearance is significantly reduced in mild to moderately impaired patients. Although dosage adjustments are not recommended, use lowest possible dose and titrate according to individual's tolerance. May consider waiting >2 weeks between dosage adjustments.

Available Dosage Forms

Capsule: 1.5 mg, 3 mg, 4.5 mg, 6 mg

Solution, oral: 2 mg/mL (120 mL) [contains sodium benzoate]

Monitoring and Teaching Issues

Physical Assessment: Assess bladder and sphincter adequacy prior to administering medication. Assess other medications for effectiveness and interactions. Monitor therapeutic effectiveness and adverse reactions at beginning of therapy and regularly with long-term use. Assess cognitive function at periodic intervals. Assess knowledge/teach patient appropriate use, possible side effects/appropriate interventions, and adverse symptoms to report.

Patient Education: This drug is not a cure for Alzheimer's disease, but it may reduce the symptoms. Use as directed; do not increase dose or discontinue without consulting prescriber. Swallow capsule whole with meals (do not crush or chew). Liquid can be swallowed directly from syringe or mixed with water, milk, or juice; stir well and drink within 4 hours of mixing. Maintain adequate hydration (2-3 L/day of fluids) unless instructed to restrict fluid intake. Avoid alcohol. May cause dizziness, drowsiness, or postural hypotension (rise slowly from sitting or lying position and use caution when driving or climbing stairs); vomiting or loss of appetite (small frequent meals, frequent mouth care, sucking lozenges, or chewing gum may help); diarrhea (buttermilk, boiled milk, or yogurt may help); or constipation (increased exercise, fluids, fruit, or fiber may help); or urinary frequency. Report persistent abdominal discomfort, diarrhea, or constipation; significantly increased salivation, sweating, tearing, or urination; chest pain, palpitations, acute headache; CNS changes (eg, excessive fatigue, agitation, insomnia, dizziness, confusion, aggressiveness, depression); increased muscle, joint, or body pain; vision changes or blurred vision; shortness of breath, coughing, or wheezing; skin rash; or other persistent adverse reactions. **Breast-feeding precaution:** Consult prescriber if breast-feeding.

Dietary Considerations: Should be taken with meals.

Pregnancy Risk Factor: B

Lactation: Excretion in breast milk unknown/use caution

Administration

Oral: Should be administered with meals (breakfast or dinner). Capsule should be swallowed whole. Liquid form is available for patients who cannot swallow capsules (can be swallowed directly from syringe or mixed with water, milk, or juice). Stir well and drink within 4 hours of mixing.

Storage: Store below 77°F (25°C). Store solution in an upright position and protect from freezing.

♦ **Rivastigmine Tartrate** see Rivastigmine on page 1340

Rizatriptan (rye za TRIP tan)

U.S. Brand Names Maxalt®; Maxalt-MLT®

Synonyms MK462

Generic Available No

Pharmacologic Category Serotonin 5-HT₁D Receptor Agonist

Use Acute treatment of migraine with or without aura

Mechanism of Action/Effect Selective agonist for serotonin (5-HT-₁D receptor) in cranial arteries to cause vasoconstriction and reduce sterile inflammation associated with antidromic neuronal transmission correlating with relief of migraine

Contraindications Hypersensitivity to rizatriptan or any component of the formulation; documented ischemic heart disease or Prinzmetal's angina; uncontrolled hypertension; basilar or hemiplegic migraine; during or within 2 weeks of MAO inhibitors; during or within 24 hours of treatment with another 5-HT₁ agonist, or an ergot-containing or ergot-type medication (eg, methysergide, dihydroergotamine)

Warnings/Precautions Use only in patients with a clear diagnosis of migraine. May cause vasospastic reactions resulting in colonic, peripheral, or coronary ischemia. Use with caution in elderly or patients with hepatic or renal impairment (including dialysis patients), history of hypersensitivity to sumatriptan or adverse effects from sumatriptan, and in patients at risk of coronary artery disease. (as predicted by presence of risk factors); establish absence of (Continued)

Rizatriptan *(Continued)*

cardiovascular disease and administer initial dose in appropriately staffed setting (physician's office). Do not use with ergotamines. May increase blood pressure transiently; may cause coronary vasospasm (less than sumatriptan); avoid in patients with signs/symptoms suggestive of reduced arterial flow (ischemic bowel, Raynaud's) which could be exacerbated by vasospasm.

Patients who experience sensations of chest pain/pressure/tightness or symptoms suggestive of angina following dosing should be evaluated for coronary artery disease or Prinzmetal's angina before receiving additional doses.

Reconsider diagnosis of migraine if no response to initial dose. Long-term effects on vision have not been evaluated.

Drug Interactions

Increased Effect/Toxicity: Use within 24 hours of another selective 5-HT$_1$ antagonist or ergot-containing drug should be avoided due to possible additive vasoconstriction. Use with propranolol increased plasma concentration of rizatriptan by 70%. Rarely, concurrent use with SSRIs results in weakness and incoordination; monitor closely. MAO inhibitors and nonselective MAO inhibitors increase concentration of rizatriptan.

Nutritional/Ethanol Interactions Food: Food delays absorption.

Adverse Reactions 1% to 10%:

Cardiovascular: Systolic/diastolic blood pressure increases (5-10 mm Hg), chest pain (5%), palpitation

Central nervous system: Dizziness, drowsiness, fatigue (13% to 30%, dose related)

Dermatologic: Skin flushing

Endocrine & metabolic: Mild increase in growth hormone, hot flashes

Gastrointestinal: Nausea, abdominal pain, dry mouth (<5%)

Respiratory: Dyspnea

Pharmacodynamics/Kinetics

Onset of Action: ~30 minutes

Duration of Action: 14-16 hours

Bioavailability: 40% to 50%

Time to Peak: 1-1.5 hours

Protein Binding: 14%

Half-Life Elimination: 2-3 hours

Metabolism: Via monoamine oxidase-A; first-pass effect

Excretion: Urine (82%, 8% to 16% as unchanged drug); feces (12%)

Dosing

Adults & Elderly: Note: In patients with risk factors for coronary artery disease, following adequate evaluation to establish the absence of coronary artery disease, the initial dose should be administered in a setting where response may be evaluated (physician's office or similarly staffed setting). ECG monitoring may be considered.

Migraine: Oral: 5-10 mg, repeat after 2 hours if significant relief is not attained; maximum: 30 mg in a 24-hour period (use 5 mg dose in patients receiving propranolol with a maximum of 15 mg in 24 hours)

Note: For orally-disintegrating tablets (Maxalt-MLT®): Patient should be instructed to place tablet on tongue and allow to dissolve. Dissolved tablet will be swallowed with saliva.

Available Dosage Forms

Tablet, as benzoate (Maxalt®): 5 mg, 10 mg

Tablet, orally-disintegrating, as benzoate (Maxalt-MLT®): 5 mg [contains phenylalanine 1.05 mg/tablet; peppermint flavor]; 10 mg [contains phenylalanine 2.1 mg/tablet; peppermint flavor]

Monitoring and Teaching Issues

Physical Assessment: For use only with clear diagnosis of migraine. Assess potential for interactions with other pharmacological agents patient may be taking (eg, ergot containing drugs, SSRIs; see Drug Interactions). Assess effectiveness (relief of migraine) and adverse response (eg, drowsiness, nausea/vomiting, chest pain, palpitations; see Adverse Reactions). Teach patient proper use, possible side effects/appropriate interventions, and adverse symptoms to report (see Patient Education).

Monitoring Laboratory Tests: Consider monitoring vital signs and ECG with first dose in patients with unrecognized coronary disease, such as patients with significant hypertension, hypercholesterolemia, obese patients, patients with diabetes, smokers with other risk factors, or strong family history of coronary artery disease

Patient Education: Do not take any new medication during therapy unless approved by prescriber (especially any other headache or pain medicine). This drug is to be used to reduce your migraine, not to prevent or reduce the number of attacks. Follow exact instructions for use. For orally-disintegrating tablets (Maxalt-MLT®), do not open blister pack before using. Open with dry hands, place on tongue, and allow to dissolve (dissolved tablet will be swallowed with saliva). Do not crush, break, or chew. Do not take within 24 hours of any other migraine medication without first consulting prescriber. If first dose brings relief, second dose may be taken anytime after 2 hours if migraine returns. Do not take more than two doses without consulting prescriber. May cause dizziness or drowsiness (use caution when driving or engaging in tasks requiring alertness until response to drug is known); dry mouth (frequent mouth care and sucking on lozenges may help); skin flushing or hot flashes (cool clothes or a cool environment may help); or mild abdominal discomfort or nausea or vomiting. Report immediately any chest pain, palpitations, or irregular heartbeat; severe dizziness, acute headache, stiff or painful neck or facial swelling; muscle weakness or pain; changes in mental acuity; blurred vision or eye pain; or excessive perspiration or urination. **Pregnancy/breast-feeding precautions:** Inform prescriber if you are or intend to become pregnant. Breast-feeding is not recommended.

Dietary Considerations: Orally-disintegrating tablet contains phenylalanine (1.05 mg per 5 mg tablet, 2.10 mg per 10 mg tablet).

Pregnancy Risk Factor: C
Lactation: Excretion in breast milk unknown/use caution
Administration
    Storage: Store in blister pack until administration.
Related Information
    Antimigraine Drugs: 5-HT$_1$ Receptor Agonists *on page 1716*

Rocuronium (roe kyoor OH nee um)

U.S. Brand Names Zemuron®
Synonyms ORG 946; Rocuronium Bromide
Generic Available No
Pharmacologic Category Neuromuscular Blocker Agent, Nondepolarizing
Medication Safety Issues
    Sound-alike/look-alike issues:
        Zemuron® may be confused with Remeron®
Use Adjunct to general anesthesia to facilitate both rapid sequence and routine endotracheal intubation and to relax skeletal muscles during surgery; to facilitate mechanical ventilation in ICU patients; does not relieve pain or produce sedation
Contraindications Hypersensitivity to rocuronium or any component of the formulation
Warnings/Precautions Use with caution in patients with valvular heart disease, pulmonary disease, hepatic impairment; ventilation must be supported during neuromuscular blockade; certain clinical conditions may result in potentiation or antagonism of neuromuscular blockade:

    Potentiation: Electrolyte abnormalities, severe hyponatremia, severe hypocalcemia, severe hypokalemia, hypermagnesemia, neuromuscular diseases, acidosis, acute intermittent porphyria, renal failure, hepatic failure
    Antagonism: Alkalosis, hypercalcemia, demyelinating lesions, peripheral neuropathies, diabetes mellitus

Increased sensitivity in patients with myasthenia gravis, Eaton-Lambert syndrome; resistance in burn patients (>30% of body) for period of 5-70 days postinjury; resistance in patients with muscle trauma, denervation, immobilization, infection. Cross-sensitivity with other neuromuscular-blocking agents may occur; use extreme caution in patients with previous anaphylactic reactions.
Drug Interactions
    Decreased Effect: Effect of nondepolarizing neuromuscular blockers may be reduced by carbamazepine (chronic use), corticosteroids (also associated with myopathy - see increased effect), phenytoin (chronic use), sympathomimetics, and theophylline.
    Increased Effect/Toxicity: Increased effects are possible with aminoglycosides, beta-blockers, clindamycin, calcium channel blockers, halogenated anesthetics, imipenem, ketamine, lidocaine, loop diuretics (furosemide), macrolides (case reports), magnesium sulfate, procainamide, quinidine, quinolones, tetracyclines, and vancomycin. May increase risk of myopathy when used with high- dose corticosteroids for extended periods.
Adverse Reactions >1%: Cardiovascular: Transient hypotension and hypertension
Overdosage/Toxicology
    Symptoms of overdose include prolonged skeletal muscle block, muscle weakness and apnea
    Treatment is maintenance of a patent airway and controlled ventilation until recovery of normal neuromuscular block is observed, further recovery may be facilitated by administering an anticholinesterase agent (eg, neostigmine, edrophonium, or pyridostigmine) with atropine, to antagonize the skeletal muscle relaxation; support of the cardiovascular system with fluids and pressors may be necessary
Pharmacodynamics/Kinetics
    Onset of Action: Good intubation conditions in 1-2 minutes; maximum neuromuscular blockade within 4 minutes
    Duration of Action: ~30 minutes (with standard doses, increases with higher doses)
    Half-Life Elimination: 60-70 minutes
    Metabolism: Minimally hepatic; 17-desacetylrocuronium (5% to 10% activity of parent drug)
    Excretion: Feces (50%); urine (30%)
Dosing
    Adults & Elderly: Administer I.V.; dose to effect; doses will vary due to interpatient variability; use ideal body weight for obese patients
    (Continued)

Rocuronium *(Continued)*

Tracheal intubation: I.V.:

Initial: 0.6 mg/kg is expected to provide approximately 31 minutes of clinical relaxation under opioid/nitrous oxide/oxygen anesthesia with neuromuscular block sufficient for intubation attained in 1-2 minutes; lower doses (0.45 mg/kg) may be used to provide 22 minutes of clinical relaxation with median time to neuromuscular block of 1-3 minutes; maximum blockade is achieved in <4 minutes

Maximum: 0.9-1.2 mg/kg may be given during surgery under opioid/nitrous oxide/oxygen anesthesia without adverse cardiovascular effects and is expected to provide 58-67 minutes of clinical relaxation; neuromuscular blockade sufficient for intubation is achieved in <2 minutes with maximum blockade in <3 minutes

Maintenance: 0.1, 0.15, and 0.2 mg/kg administered at 25% recovery of control T_1 (defined as 3 twitches of train-of-four) provides a median of 12, 17, and 24 minutes of clinical duration under anesthesia

Rapid sequence intubation: 0.6-1.2 mg/kg in appropriately premedicated and anesthetized patients with excellent or good intubating conditions within 2 minutes

Continuous infusion: Initial: 0.01-0.012 mg/kg/minute only after early evidence of spontaneous recovery of neuromuscular function is evident; infusion rates have ranged from 0.004-0.016 mg/kg/minute.

ICU neuromuscular blockade: 10 mcg/kg/minute; adjust dose to maintain appropriate degree of neuromuscular blockade (eg, 1 or 2 twitches on train-of-four)

Pediatrics: Administer I.V.; dose to effect; doses will vary due to interpatient variability; use ideal body weight for obese patients

Tracheal intubation: I.V.: Children:

Initial: 0.6 mg/kg under halothane anesthesia produce excellent to good intubating conditions within 1 minute and will provide a median time of 41 minutes of clinical relaxation in children 3 months to 1 year of age, and 27 minutes in children <3 years

Maintenance: 0.075-0.125 mg/kg administered upon return of T_1 to 25% of control provides clinical relaxation for 7-10 minutes

Available Dosage Forms Injection, solution, as bromide: 10 mg/mL (5 mL, 10 mL)

Monitoring and Teaching Issues

Physical Assessment: Only clinicians experienced in the use of neuromuscular blocking agents should administer and/or manage the use of mivacurium. Assess potential for interactions with other prescription or OTC medications or herbal products patient may be taking (eg, other drugs that affect neuromuscular activity may increase/decrease neuromuscular block induced by rocuronium). Dosage and rate of administration should be individualized and titrated to the desired effect, according to relevant clinical factors, premedication, concomitant medication, age, and general condition of the patient. Ventilatory support must be instituted and maintained until adequate respiratory muscle function and/or airway protection are assured. This drug does not cause anesthesia or analgesia; pain must be treated with appropriate agents. Continuous monitoring of vital signs, cardiac and respiratory status, and neuromuscular block (objective assessment with peripheral external nerve stimulator) are mandatory until full muscle tone has returned. Safety precautions must be maintained until full muscle tone has returned. Muscle tone returns in a predictable pattern; starting with diaphragm, abdomen, chest, limbs, and finally muscles of the neck, face, and eyes. **Note:** It may take longer for return of muscle tone in obese or elderly persons or patients with renal or hepatic disease, myasthenia gravis, myopathy, other neuromuscular diseases, dehydration, electrolyte imbalance, or severe acid/base imbalance. Provide appropriate teaching/support prior to, during, and following administration.

Long-term use: Vital signs and fluid levels should be monitored regularly during treatment. Every 2- to 3-hour repositioning, and skin, mouth, and eye care is necessary while patient is sedated. Emotional and sensory support (auditory and environmental) should be provided.

Patient Education: Patient education should be appropriate for patient condition. Reassurance of constant monitoring and emotional support should precede and follow administration. Patients should be reminded as muscle tone returns not to attempt to change position or rise from bed without assistance and to report and skin rash, hives, pounding heartbeat, respiratory difficulty, or muscle tremors. **Pregnancy/breast-feeding precautions:** Inform prescriber if you are pregnant. Consult prescriber if breast-feeding.

Pregnancy Risk Factor: C

Lactation: Excretion in breast milk unknown/use caution

Administration

I.V.: Administer I.V. only; may be given undiluted as a bolus injection or via a continuous infusion using an infusion pump

Storage: Store under refrigeration (2°C to 8°C), do not freeze; when stored at room temperature, it is stable for 30 days; unlike vecuronium, it is stable in 0.9% sodium chloride and 5% dextrose in water, this mixture should be used within 24 hours of preparation

Additional Information Rocuronium is classified as an intermediate-duration neuromuscular-blocking agent. Do not mix in the same syringe with barbiturates. Rocuronium does not relieve pain or produce sedation.

Ropinirole (roe PIN i role)

U.S. Brand Names Requip®

Synonyms Ropinirole Hydrochloride

Generic Available No

Pharmacologic Category Anti-Parkinson's Agent, Dopamine Agonist

Medication Safety Issues

Sound-alike/look-alike issues:

Ropinirole may be confused with ropivacaine

Use Treatment of idiopathic Parkinson's disease; in patients with early Parkinson's disease who were not receiving concomitant levodopa therapy as well as in patients with advanced disease on concomitant levodopa

Contraindications Hypersensitivity to ropinirole or any component of the formulation

Warnings/Precautions Syncope, sometimes associated with bradycardia, was observed in association with ropinirole in both early Parkinson's disease (without levodopa) patients and advanced Parkinson's disease (with levodopa) patients. Use with caution in patients at risk of hypotension (ie, those receiving antihypertensive drugs) or where transient hypotensive episodes would be poorly tolerated (cardiovascular disease or cerebrovascular disease). Parkinson's patients being treated with dopaminergic agonists ordinarily require careful monitoring for signs and symptoms of postural hypotension, especially during dose escalation, and should be informed of this risk. May cause hallucinations. Use with caution in patients with pre-existing dyskinesia, severe hepatic or renal dysfunction.

Patients treated with ropinirole have reported falling asleep while engaging in activities of daily living. Discontinue if significant daytime sleepiness or episodes of falling asleep occur. The significance of data concerning retinal changes observed in animal studies remains uncertain.

Other dopaminergic agents have been associated with a syndrome resembling neuroleptic malignant syndrome on withdrawal or significant dosage reduction after long-term use.

Drug Interactions

Cytochrome P450 Effect: Substrate of CYP1A2 (major), 3A4 (minor); **Inhibits** CYP1A2 (weak), 2D6 (strong)

Decreased Effect: The levels/effects of ropinirole may be decreased by aminoglutethimide, carbamazepine, phenobarbital, rifampin, and other CYP1A2 inducers. Antipsychotics, cigarette smoking, and metoclopramide may reduce the effect or serum concentrations of ropinirole. Ropinirole may decrease the levels/effects of CYP2D6 prodrug substrates (eg, codeine, hydrocodone, oxycodone, tramadol).

Increased Effect/Toxicity: The levels/effects of ropinirole may be increased by amiodarone, ciprofloxacin, fluvoxamine, ketoconazole, norfloxacin, ofloxacin, rofecoxib, and other CYP1A2 inhibitors. Estrogens may also reduce the metabolism of ropinirole; dosage adjustments may be needed. Ropinirole may increase the levels/effects of amphetamines, selected beta-blockers, dextromethorphan, fluoxetine, lidocaine, mirtazapine, nefazodone, paroxetine, risperidone, ritonavir, thioridazine, tricyclic antidepressants, venlafaxine, and other CYP2D6 substrates.

Nutritional/Ethanol Interactions

Ethanol: Avoid ethanol (may increase CNS depression).

Herb/Nutraceutical: Avoid kava kava, gotu kola, valerian, St John's wort (may increase CNS depression).

Adverse Reactions

Early Parkinson's disease (without levodopa):

>10%:

Cardiovascular: Syncope (12%)

Central nervous system: Dizziness (40%), somnolence (40%), fatigue (11%)

Gastrointestinal: Nausea (60%), vomiting (12%)

Miscellaneous: Viral infection (11%)

1% to 10%:

Cardiovascular: Dependent/leg edema (6% to 7%), orthostasis (6%), hypertension (5%), chest pain (4%), flushing (3%), palpitation (3%), peripheral ischemia (3%), hypotension (2%), tachycardia (2%)

Central nervous system: Pain (8%), confusion (5%), hallucinations (5%, dose related), hypoesthesia (4%), amnesia (3%), malaise (3%), vertigo (2%), yawning (3%)

Gastrointestinal: Constipation (>5%), dyspepsia (10%), abdominal pain (6%), xerostomia (5%), anorexia (4%), flatulence (3%)

Genitourinary: Urinary tract infection (5%), impotence (3%)

Hepatic: Elevated alkaline phosphatase (3%)

Neuromuscular & skeletal: Weakness (6%)

Ocular: Abnormal vision (6%), xerophthalmia (2%)

Respiratory: Pharyngitis (6%), rhinitis (4%), sinusitis (4%), dyspnea (3%)

Miscellaneous: Diaphoresis (increased) (6%)

Advanced Parkinson's disease (with levodopa):

>10%:

Central nervous system: Dizziness (26%), somnolence (20%), headache (17%)

Gastrointestinal: Nausea (30%)

Neuromuscular & skeletal: Dyskinesias (34%)

1% to 10%:

Cardiovascular: Syncope (3%), hypotension (2%)

Central nervous system: Hallucinations (10%, dose related), aggravated parkinsonism, confusion (9%), pain (5%), paresis (3%), amnesia (5%), anxiety (6%), abnormal dreaming (3%), insomnia

Gastrointestinal: Abdominal pain (9%), vomiting (7%), constipation (6%), diarrhea (5%), dysphagia (2%), flatulence (2%), increased salivation (2%), xerostomia, weight loss (2%)

Genitourinary: Urinary tract infection

Hematologic: Anemia (2%)

(Continued)

Ropinirole *(Continued)*

Neuromuscular & skeletal: Falls (10%), arthralgia (7%), tremor (6%), hypokinesia (5%), paresthesia (5%), arthritis (3%)

Respiratory: Upper respiratory tract infection (9%), dyspnea (3%)

Miscellaneous: Injury, increased diaphoresis (7%), viral infection, increased drug level (7%)

Other adverse effects (all phase 2/3 trials):

1% to 10%:

Central nervous system: Neuralgia (>1%)

Renal: Elevated BUN (>1%)

Overdosage/Toxicology No reports of intentional overdose; symptoms reported with accidental overdosage were agitation, increased dyskinesia, sedation, orthostatic hypotension, chest pain, confusion, nausea, and vomiting. It is anticipated that the symptoms of overdose will be related to its dopaminergic activity. General supportive measures are recommended. Vital signs should be maintained, if necessary. Removal of any unabsorbed material (eg, by gastric lavage) should be considered. Removal by hemodialysis is unlikely.

Pharmacodynamics/Kinetics

Absorption: Not affected by food

Bioavailability: Absolute: 55%

Time to Peak: ~1-2 hours; T_{max} increased by 2.5 hours when taken with food

Half-Life Elimination: ~6 hours

Metabolism: Extensively hepatic via CYP1A2 to inactive metabolites; first-pass effect

Excretion: Clearance: Reduced by 30% in patients >65 years of age

Dosing

Adults & Elderly:

Parkinson's disease: Oral:

Initial: Recommended starting dose is 0.25 mg 3 times/day;

Adjustment:

Note: The dosage should be increased to achieve a maximum therapeutic effect, balanced against the principal side effects of nausea, dizziness, somnolence and dyskinesia. Based on individual patient response, the dosage should be titrated with weekly increments as described below:

- Week 1: 0.25 mg 3 times/day; total daily dose: 0.75 mg
- Week 2: 0.5 mg 3 times/day; total daily dose: 1.5 mg
- Week 3: 0.75 mg 3 times/day; total daily dose: 2.25 mg
- Week 4: 1 mg 3 times/day; total daily dose: 3 mg

After week 4, if necessary, daily dosage may be increased by 1.5 mg per day on a weekly basis up to a dose of 9 mg/day, and then by up to 3 mg/day weekly to a total of 24 mg/day

Renal Impairment: Removal by hemodialysis is unlikely.

Available Dosage Forms Tablet, as hydrochloride: 0.25 mg, 0.5 mg, 1 mg, 2 mg, 3 mg, 4 mg, 5 mg

Monitoring and Teaching Issues

Physical Assessment: Assess potential for interactions with other prescriptions, OTC medications, or herbal products patient may be taking. Assess therapeutic effectiveness and adverse responses on a regular basis during therapy. Monitor for CNS depression/somnolence. Teach patient proper use, side effects/appropriate interventions, and adverse reactions to report.

Patient Education: Take exactly as directed, without regard to food. May cause dizziness, sudden, overwhelming sleepiness (use caution when driving or engaging in tasks that require alertness until response to drug is known); postural hypotension (use caution and avoid quick moves when rising from sitting or lying position, when climbing stairs, or engaging in activities that require quick movements); or nausea, vomiting, lack of appetite, or mouth sores (small frequent meals, frequent mouth care, chewing gum, or sucking lozenges may help). Report unusual and persistent sleepiness; chest pain or palpitations; CNS changes (confusion, hallucinations, amnesia, abnormal dreaming, insomnia); skeletal weakness or increased random tremors or movements, gait changes, or difficulty walking; signs of urinary tract or respiratory infection (pain or burning on urination, pus or blood in urine, or unusual cough and chest tightness); or unusual persistent adverse reactions. **Pregnancy/breast-feeding precautions:** Inform prescriber if you are or intend to become pregnant. Breast-feeding is not recommended.

Dietary Considerations: May be taken with or without food.

Pregnancy Risk Factor: C

Lactation: Excretion in breast milk unknown/not recommended

Additional Information If therapy with a drug known to be a potent inhibitor of CYP1A2 is stopped or started during treatment with ropinirole, adjustment of ropinirole dose may be required. Ropinirole binds to melanin-containing tissues (ie, eyes, skin) in pigmented rats. After a single dose, long-term retention of drug was demonstrated, with a half-life in the eye of 20 days; not known if ropinirole accumulates in these tissues over time.

- ♦ **Ropinirole Hydrochloride** *see* Ropinirole *on page 1345*

Rosiglitazone *(roh si GLI ta zone)*

U.S. Brand Names Avandia®

Generic Available No

Pharmacologic Category Antidiabetic Agent, Thiazolidinedione

Medication Safety Issues

Sound-alike/look-alike issues:

Avandia® may be confused with Avalide®, Coumadin®, Prandin®

Use Type 2 diabetes mellitus (noninsulin dependent, NIDDM):

Monotherapy: Improve glycemic control as an adjunct to diet and exercise

Combination therapy: In combination with a sulfonylurea, metformin, or insulin, or sulfonylurea plus metformin when diet, exercise, and a single agent do not result in adequate
glycemic control

Mechanism of Action/Effect Thiazolidinedione antidiabetic agent that lowers blood glucose
by improving target cell response to insulin, without increasing pancreatic insulin secretion. It
has a mechanism of action that is dependent on the presence of insulin for activity.

Contraindications Hypersensitivity to rosiglitazone or any component of the formulation;
active liver disease (transaminases >2.5 times the upper limit of normal at baseline); contraindicated in patients who previously experienced jaundice during troglitazone therapy

Warnings/Precautions Should not be used in diabetic ketoacidosis. Mechanism requires the
presence of insulin, therefore use in type 1 diabetes (insulin dependent, IDDM) is not recommended. Use with caution in premenopausal, anovulatory women; may result in resumption
of ovulation, increasing the risk of pregnancy. May result in hormonal imbalance; development of menstrual irregularities should prompt reconsideration of therapy. Use with caution in
patients with anemia or depressed leukocyte counts (may reduce hemoglobin, hematocrit,
and/or WBC). May increase plasma volume and/or increase cardiac hypertrophy. Assess for
fluid accumulation in patients with unusually rapid weight gain. Use with caution in patients
with edema. Monitor closely for signs and symptoms of heart failure, , unless serum glucose
control outweighs the risk of excessive fluid retention. Not recommended for use in patients
with NYHA Class III or IV heart failure, unless serum glucose control outweighs the risk of
excessive fluid retention. Discontinue if heart failure develops. Use with caution in patients
with elevated transaminases (AST or ALT). Idiosyncratic hepatotoxicity has been reported
with another thiazolidinedione agent (troglitazone) and (rarely) with rosiglitazone; discontinue
if jaundice occurs. Monitoring should include periodic determinations of liver function. Safety
and efficacy in pediatric patients have not been established.

Drug Interactions
Cytochrome P450 Effect: Substrate of CYP2C8/9 (major); **Inhibits** CYP2C8/9
(moderate), 2C19 (weak), 2D6 (weak)
Decreased Effect: The levels/effects of rosiglitazone may be decreased by carbamazepine, phenobarbital, phenytoin, rifampin, rifapentine, and secobarbital, and other CYP2C8/
9 inducers. Bile acid sequestrants may decrease rosiglitazone levels.
Increased Effect/Toxicity: The levels/effects of rosiglitazone may be increased by
delavirdine, fluconazole, gemfibrozil, ketoconazole, nicardipine, NSAIDs, pioglitazone,
sulfonamides, and other CYP2C8/9 inhibitors. Gemfibrozil may increase rosiglitazone
levels; severe hypoglycemic episodes have been reported. Rosiglitazone may increase the
levels/effects of amiodarone, fluoxetine, glimepiride, glipizide, nateglinide, phenytoin, pioglitazone, sertraline, warfarin, and other CYP2C8/9 substrates.

Nutritional/Ethanol Interactions
Ethanol: Avoid ethanol (may cause hypoglycemia).
Food: Peak concentrations are lower by 28% and delayed when administered with food, but
these effects are not believed to be clinically significant.
Herb/Nutraceutical: Avoid garlic, gymnema (may cause hypoglycemia).

Adverse Reactions Rare cases of hepatocellular injury have been reported in men in their
60s within 2-3 weeks after initiation of rosiglitazone therapy. LFTs in these patients revealed
severe hepatocellular injury which responded with rapid improvement of liver function and
resolution of symptoms upon discontinuation of rosiglitazone. Patients were also receiving
other potentially hepatotoxic medications (*Ann Intern Med*, 2000, 132:121-4; 132:164-6). The
rate of certain adverse reactions (eg, anemia, edema, hypoglycemia) may be higher with
some combination therapies.

>10%: Endocrine & metabolic: Weight gain, increase in total cholesterol, increased
LDL-cholesterol, increased HDL-cholesterol
1% to 10%:
Cardiovascular: Edema (5%)
Central nervous system: Headache (6%), fatigue (4%)
Endocrine & metabolic: Hyperglycemia (4%), hypoglycemia (1%; increased with insulin to
12% to 14%)
Gastrointestinal: Diarrhea (2%)
Hematologic: Anemia (2%)
Neuromuscular & skeletal: Back pain (4%)
Respiratory: Upper respiratory tract infection (10%), sinusitis (3%)
Miscellaneous: Injury (8%)

Overdosage/Toxicology Experience in overdose is limited. Symptoms may include hypoglycemia. Treatment is supportive.

Pharmacodynamics/Kinetics
Onset of Action: Delayed; Maximum effect: Up to 12 weeks
Bioavailability: 99%
Time to Peak: 1 hour; delayed with food
Protein Binding: 99.8%
Half-Life Elimination: 3-4 hours
Metabolism: Hepatic (99%) via CYP2C8; minor metabolism via CYP2C9
Excretion: Urine (64%) and feces (23%) as metabolites

Dosing
Adults & Elderly: Type 2 diabetes: Oral:
Monotherapy: Initial: 4 mg daily as a single daily dose or in divided doses twice daily. If
response is inadequate after 8-12 weeks of treatment, the dosage may be increased to 8
mg daily as a single daily dose or in divided doses twice daily. In clinical trials, the 4 mg
twice-daily regimen resulted in the greatest reduction in fasting plasma glucose and Hb
A$_{1c}$.
Combination therapy: When adding rosiglitazone to existing therapy, continue current
dose(s) of previous agents:
With sulfonylureas or metformin (or sulfonylurea plus metformin): Initial: 4 mg daily as a
single daily dose or in divided doses twice daily. If response is inadequate after 8-12
weeks of treatment, the dosage may be increased to 8 mg daily as a single daily dose
(Continued)

Rosiglitazone *(Continued)*

or in divided doses twice daily. Reduce dose of sulfonylurea if hypoglycemia occurs. It is unlikely that the dose of metformin will need to be reduced to hypoglycemia.

With insulin: Initial: 4 mg daily as a single daily dose or in divided doses twice daily. Dose of insulin should be reduced by 10% to 25% if the patient reports hypoglycemia or if the plasma glucose falls to <100 mg/dL. Doses of rosiglitazone >4 mg/day are not indicated in combination with insulin.

Renal Impairment: No adjustment is necessary.

Hepatic Impairment: Clearance is significantly lower in hepatic impairment. Therapy should not be initiated if the patient exhibits active liver disease of increased transaminases (>2.5 times the upper limit of normal) at baseline.

Available Dosage Forms Tablet: 2 mg, 4 mg, 8 mg

Monitoring and Teaching Issues

Physical Assessment: Monitor laboratory results closely. Assess other prescriptions, OTC medications, or herbal products patient may be taking. Assess for signs of fluid retention and congestive heart failure. Monitor weight. Monitor response to therapy closely until response is stable. Advise women using oral contraceptives about need for alternative method of contraception. Assess knowledge/teach risks of hyper-/hypoglycemia, its symptoms, treatment, and predisposing conditions. Refer patient to a diabetic educator, if possible. Teach appropriate use of medication, interventions to reduce side effects, and adverse reactions to report.

Monitoring Laboratory Tests: Hemoglobin A_{1c}, serum glucose; liver enzymes (prior to initiation of therapy, then periodically thereafter). Patients with an elevation in ALT >3 times the upper limit of normal should be rechecked as soon as possible. If the ALT levels remain >3 times the upper limit of normal, therapy with rosiglitazone should be discontinued.

Patient Education: May be taken without regard to meals. Follow directions of prescriber. If dose is missed at the usual meal, take it with next meal. Do not double dose if daily dose is missed completely. Monitor urine or serum glucose as recommended by prescriber. More frequent monitoring is required during periods of stress, trauma, surgery, pregnancy, increased activity or exercise. Avoid alcohol. Report chest pain, rapid heartbeat or palpitations, abdominal pain, fever, rash, hypoglycemia reactions, yellowing of skin or eyes, dark urine or light stool, or unusual fatigue or nausea/vomiting. Report unusually rapid weight gain; swelling of ankles, legs, or abdomen; or weakness or shortness of breath. **Pregnancy/breast-feeding precautions:** In anovulatory, premenopausal women, ovulation may occur, increasing the risk of pregnancy. Adequate contraception is recommended. Use alternate means of contraception if using oral contraceptives. Breast-feeding is not recommended.

Dietary Considerations: Management of type 2 diabetes mellitus (noninsulin dependent, NIDDM) should include diet control. May be taken without regard to meals.

Pregnancy Risk Factor: C

Pregnancy Issues: Treatment during mid to late gestation was associated with fetal death and growth retardation in animal models. Abnormal blood glucose levels are associated with a higher incidence of congenital abnormalities. Insulin is the drug of choice for the control of diabetes mellitus during pregnancy. In anovulatory, premenopausal women, ovulation may occur, increasing the risk of pregnancy; adequate contraception is recommended.

Lactation: Excretion in breast milk unknown/not recommended

Breast-Feeding Issues: In animal studies, rosiglitazone has been found to be excreted in milk. It is not known whether rosiglitazone is excreted in human milk. Should not be administered to a nursing woman.

Administration

Storage: Store at 25°C (77°F); excursions permitted to 15°C to 30°C (59°F to 86°F). Protect from light.

Related Information

Diabetes Mellitus Management *on page 1819*

Rosiglitazone and Metformin *(roh si GLI ta zone & met FOR min)*

U.S. Brand Names Avandamet™

Synonyms Metformin and Rosiglitazone; Metformin Hydrochloride and Rosiglitazone Maleate; Rosiglitazone Maleate and Metformin Hydrochloride

Generic Available No

Pharmacologic Category Antidiabetic Agent, Biguanide; Antidiabetic Agent, Thiazolidinedione

Use Management of type 2 diabetes mellitus (noninsulin dependent, NIDDM) in patients who are already treated with the combination of rosiglitazone and metformin, or who are not adequately controlled on metformin alone. Used as an adjunct to diet and exercise to lower the blood glucose when hyperglycemia cannot be controlled satisfactorily by diet and exercise alone

Dosing

Adults: Type 2 diabetes mellitus: Oral: Initial dose should be based on current dose of rosiglitazone and/or metformin; daily doses should be divided and given with meals

Patients inadequately controlled on metformin alone: Initial dose: Rosiglitazone 4 mg/day plus current dose of metformin

Patients inadequately controlled on rosiglitazone alone: Initial dose: Metformin 1000 mg/day plus current dose of rosiglitazone

Note: When switching from combination rosiglitazone and metformin as separate tablets: Use current dose

Dose adjustment: Doses may be increased as increments of rosiglitazone 4 mg and/or metformin 500 mg, up to the maximum dose; doses should be titrated gradually.

After a change in the metformin dosage, titration can be done after 1-2 weeks

After a change in the rosiglitazone dosage, titration can be done after 8-12 weeks

Maximum dose: Rosiglitazone 8 mg/metformin 2000 mg daily

Elderly: The initial and maintenance dosing should be conservative, due to the potential for decreased renal function (monitor). Generally, elderly patients should not be titrated to the maximum. Do not use in patients ≥80 years unless normal renal function has been established.

Renal Impairment: Do not use with renal disease or renal dysfunction (serum creatinine ≥1.5 mg/dL in males or ≥1.4 mg/dL in females or abnormal clearance).

Hepatic Impairment: Do not use with active liver disease or ALT >2.5 times the upper limit of normal.

Available Dosage Forms Tablet [film coated]:

1/500: Rosiglitazone 1 mg and metformin 500 mg

2/500: Rosiglitazone 2 mg and metformin 500 mg

4/500: Rosiglitazone 4 mg and metformin 500 mg

2/1000: Rosiglitazone 2 mg and metformin 1000 mg

4/1000: Rosiglitazone 4 mg and metformin 1000 mg

Monitoring and Teaching Issues

Physical Assessment: Assess allergy history prior to beginning therapy. See Contraindications, Warnings/Precautions, and Dosing for use cautions. Assess potential for interactions with other prescriptions, OTC medications, or herbal products patient may be taking (eg, anything that may affect glucose levels; see Drug Interactions). Assess results of laboratory tests (see Monitoring Laboratory Tests), therapeutic effectiveness, and adverse response (eg, hypoglycemia, vitamin B_{12} and/or folic acid deficiency; see Adverse Reactions and Overdose/Toxicology) at regular intervals during therapy. Teach patient proper use or refer patient to diabetic educator for instruction, possible side effects/appropriate interventions, and adverse symptoms to report (see Patient Education).

Patient Education: Inform prescriber of all prescriptions, OTC medications, or herbal products you are taking, and any allergies you have. Do not take any new medication during therapy without consulting prescriber. This medication is used to control diabetes; it is not a cure. Take exactly as directed with a meal at the same time(s) each day. Avoid alcohol; may cause severe reaction. Monitor glucose as recommended by prescriber. Maintain regular prescribed dietary intake and exercise routine (consult prescriber or diabetic educator) and always carry a quick source of sugar with you. Contact prescriber immediately if you experience a hypoglycemic reaction. May cause headache, nausea, or diarrhea during first weeks of therapy; consult prescriber if these persist. Report chest pain, rapid heartbeat, or palpitations; hypo- or hyperglycemic reactions; persistent, unusual fatigue; muscle pain or weakness; nausea or vomiting; rapid weight gain; swelling of extremities; or respiratory difficulty. **Pregnancy/breast-feeding precautions:** Inform prescriber if you are or intend to become pregnant. Use alternate means of contraception if using oral contraceptives. Breast-feeding is not recommended.

Pregnancy Risk Factor: C

Lactation: Excretion in breast milk unknown/not recommended

Related Information

Metformin *on page 965*

Rosiglitazone *on page 1346*

♦ **Rosiglitazone Maleate and Metformin Hydrochloride** *see* Rosiglitazone and Metformin *on page 1348*

Rosuvastatin (roe SOO va sta tin)

U.S. Brand Names Crestor®

Synonyms Rosuvastatin Calcium

Generic Available No

Pharmacologic Category Antilipemic Agent, HMG-CoA Reductase Inhibitor

Use Used with dietary therapy for hyperlipidemias to reduce elevations in total cholesterol (TC), LDL-C, apolipoprotein B, and triglycerides (TG) in patients with primary hypercholesterolemia (elevations of 1 or more components are present in Fredrickson type IIa, IIb, and IV hyperlipidemias); treatment of homozygous familial hypercholesterolemia (FH)

Mechanism of Action/Effect Inhibitor of 3-hydroxy-3-methylglutaryl coenzyme A (HMG-CoA) reductase, the rate limiting enzyme in cholesterol synthesis (reduces the production of mevalonic acid from HMG-CoA); lowers TC, LDL-C, TG and improves HDL:LDL ratio

Contraindications Hypersensitivity to rosuvastatin or any component of the formulation; active liver disease; unexplained persistent elevations of serum transaminases (>3 times ULN); pregnancy; breast-feeding

Warnings/Precautions Secondary causes of hyperlipidemia should be ruled out prior to therapy. Liver function must be monitored by periodic laboratory assessment. Use with caution in patients who consume large amounts of ethanol or have a history of liver disease. Rhabdomyolysis with acute renal failure has occurred. Discontinue in any patient in which CPK levels are markedly elevated (>10 times ULN) or if myopathy is suspected/diagnosed. An increased incidence of rosuvastatin-associated myopathy has been reported during concomitant therapy with fibric acid derivatives, niacin, cyclosporine, and in certain subgroups of the Asian population. Risk is also elevated at higher dosages of rosuvastatin. Patients should be instructed to report unexplained muscle pain, tenderness, or weakness, particularly if associated with fever and/or malaise. Use caution in patients predisposed to myopathy (eg, renal failure, advanced age, inadequately treated hypothyroidism). Temporarily withhold in patients experiencing an acute or serious condition predisposing to renal failure secondary to rhabdomyolysis (sepsis, hypotension, major surgery, trauma, severe metabolic or endocrine or electrolyte disorders, uncontrolled seizures). Safety and efficacy have not been established in children (limited experience with homozygous FH in patients >8 years of age).
(Continued)

Rosuvastatin *(Continued)*

Drug Interactions
Cytochrome P450 Effect: Substrate (minor) of CYP2C9, 3A4

Decreased Effect: Plasma concentrations of rosuvastatin may be decreased when given with magnesium/aluminum hydroxide-containing antacids; antacids should be administered at least 2 hours after rosuvastatin. Cholestyramine and colestipol (bile acid sequestrants) may reduce absorption of several HMG-CoA reductase inhibitors; separate administration times by at least 4 hours; cholesterol-lowering effects are additive.

Increased Effect/Toxicity: Cyclosporine may increase serum concentrations of rosuvastatin (up to 10-fold); limit dose to 5 mg/day. Serum concentrations of rosuvastatin may be increased (doubled) during concurrent administration of gemfibrozil; combination should be avoided; limit dose to 10 mg/day. Clofibrate, fenofibrate, or niacin may increase the risk of myopathy and rhabdomyolysis with HMG-CoA reductase inhibitors; the effects on lipids may be additive. The anticoagulant effects of warfarin may be increased by rosuvastatin (monitor). Rosuvastatin increases serum concentrations of hormonal contraceptives (ethinyl estradiol and norgestrel).

Nutritional/Ethanol Interactions Ethanol: Avoid excessive ethanol consumption (due to potential hepatic effects).

Adverse Reactions
1% to 10%:

Cardiovascular: Chest pain, hypertension, peripheral edema, palpitation

Central nervous system: Headache (6%), depression, dizziness, insomnia, pain, anxiety, neuralgia, vertigo

Dermatologic: Rash

Gastrointestinal: Pharyngitis (9%), diarrhea, dyspepsia, nausea, abdominal pain, constipation, gastroenteritis, vomiting

Hematologic: Anemia, bruising

Neuromuscular & skeletal: Myalgia (3%), weakness, back pain, arthritis, arthralgia, hypertonia, paresthesia

Respiratory: Bronchitis, rhinitis, sinusitis, cough

Miscellaneous: Flu-like syndrome

Adverse reactions reported with other HMG-CoA reductase inhibitors include a hypersensitivity syndrome (symptoms may include anaphylaxis, angioedema, arthralgia, erythema multiforme, eosinophilia, hemolytic anemia, lupus syndrome, photosensitivity, polymyalgia rheumatica, positive ANA, purpura, Stevens-Johnson syndrome, toxic epidermal necrolysis, urticaria, vasculitis)

Overdosage/Toxicology No specific experience in overdose. Treatment is supportive. Rosuvastatin is not removed by hemodialysis. CNS vascular lesions and corneal opacities have been reported following high-dose, long-term exposure to HMG-CoA reductase inhibitors in animal studies. The relationship to human exposures has not been established.

Pharmacodynamics/Kinetics
Onset of Action: Within 1 week; maximal at 4 weeks

Bioavailability: 20% (high first-pass extraction by liver)

Time to Peak: Plasma: 3-5 hours

Protein Binding: 90%

Half-Life Elimination: 19 hours

Metabolism: Hepatic (10%), via CYP2C9 (1 active metabolite identified)

Excretion: Feces (90%), primarily as unchanged drug

Pharmacokinetic Note: Asian patients have been noted to have increased bioavailability.

Dosing
Adults & Elderly:

Heterozygous familial and nonfamilial hypercholesterolemia; mixed dyslipidemia: Oral:

Initial dose:

General dosing: 10 mg once daily (20 mg in patients with severe hypercholesterolemia)

Conservative dosing: Patients requiring less aggressive treatment or predisposed to myopathy (including patients of Asian descent): 5 mg once daily

Titration: After 2 weeks, may be increased by 5-10 mg once daily; dosing range: 5-40 mg/day (maximum dose: 40 mg once daily)

Note: The 40 mg dose should be reserved for patients who have not achieved goal cholesterol levels on a dose of 20 mg/day, including patients switched from another HMG-CoA reductase inhibitor.

Homozygous familial hypercholesterolemia (HFH): Oral: Initial: 20 mg once daily (maximum dose: 40 mg/day)

Dosage adjustment with concomitant medications: Oral:

Cyclosporine: Rosuvastatin dose should not exceed 5 mg/day

Gemfibrozil: Rosuvastatin dose should not exceed 10 mg/day

Dosage adjustment for persistent, unexplained proteinuria while on 40 mg/day: Reduce dose and evaluate causes.

Renal Impairment:

Mild to moderate impairment: No dosage adjustment required.

Cl_{cr} <30 mL/minute/1.73 m^2: Initial: 5 mg/day; do not exceed 10 mg once daily

Available Dosage Forms Tablet, as calcium: 5 mg, 10 mg, 20 mg, 40 mg

Monitoring and Teaching Issues
Physical Assessment: See Warnings/Precautions for use cautions (eg, impaired liver function). Assess potential for interactions with other pharmacological agents or herbal products patient may be taking (eg, gemfibrozil, fibric acid derivatives, or niacin may increase risk of myopathy or rhabdomyolysis; see Drug Interactions). Assess LFTs prior to therapy and periodically (see Monitoring Laboratory Tests) and patient response on a regular basis throughout therapy (eg, rash, myalgia, blurred vision, abdominal pain, cough; see Adverse Reactions). Teach patient proper use (as adjunct to diet and exercise program), possible side effects/appropriate interventions, and adverse symptoms to report

(see Patient Education). **Pregnancy risk factor X:** Determine that patient is not pregnant before starting therapy. Do not give to women of childbearing age unless they are capable of complying with effective contraceptive use. Instruct patient in appropriate contraceptive measures.

Monitoring Laboratory Tests: Total cholesterol, LDL, and HDL cholesterol; liver function tests should be determined at baseline (prior to initiation), 3 months following initiation, and 3 months after any increase in dose; baseline CPK (recheck CPK in any patient with symptoms suggestive of myopathy)

Patient Education: Take at same time each day with or without food. Follow cholesterol lowering diet and exercise regimen as prescribed. Avoid excess alcohol. You will have periodic blood tests to assess effectiveness. You may experience constipation (increased exercise, fluids, fiber, and fruit may help); headache, dressing, dizziness, insomnia (use caution when driving or engaged in potentially hazardous tasks until response to drug in known). Report unusual chest pain, swelling of extremities, weight gain of >5 lb/week, or persistent cough. Contact prescriber immediately with persistent muscle or skeletal pain, joint pain, or numbness, or any sign of allergic reactions (skin rash, difficulty breathing, tightness in throat, choking sensation, swelling of mouth or face). **Pregnancy/breast-feeding precautions:** Inform prescriber if you are pregnant. Do not get pregnant during and for 1 month following therapy. Consult prescriber for appropriate contraceptive measures. This drug may cause severe fetal defects. Do not donate blood during or for 1 month following therapy. Do not breast feed.

Dietary Considerations: May be taken with or without food.

Pregnancy Risk Factor: X

Pregnancy Issues: Use in women of childbearing potential only if they are highly unlikely to conceive; discontinue if pregnancy occurs.

Lactation: Excretion in breast milk unknown/contraindicated

Administration

Oral: May be administered with or without food.

Storage: Store between 20°C and 25°C (68°F to 77°F). Protect from moisture.

Related Information

Hyperlipidemia Management *on page 1836*

Lipid-Lowering Agents *on page 1738*

- ♦ **Rosuvastatin Calcium** *see Rosuvastatin on page 1349*
- ♦ **Rowasa®** *see Mesalamine on page 957*
- ♦ **Roxanol™** *see Morphine Sulfate on page 1031*
- ♦ **Roxanol 100™** *see Morphine Sulfate on page 1031*
- ♦ **Roxanol™-T** *see Morphine Sulfate on page 1031*
- ♦ **Roxicet™** *see Oxycodone and Acetaminophen on page 1138*
- ♦ **Roxicet™ 5/500** *see Oxycodone and Acetaminophen on page 1138*
- ♦ **Roxicodone™** *see Oxycodone on page 1136*
- ♦ **Roxicodone™ Intensol™** *see Oxycodone on page 1136*
- ♦ **Rozex™ [DSC]** *see Metronidazole on page 995*
- ♦ **RP-6976** *see Docetaxel on page 472*
- ♦ **RP-54274** *see Riluzole on page 1328*
- ♦ **RP-59500** *see Quinupristin and Dalfopristin on page 1300*
- ♦ **r-PA** *see Reteplase on page 1314*
- ♦ **RS-25259** *see Palonosetron on page 1148*
- ♦ **RS-25259-197** *see Palonosetron on page 1148*
- ♦ **RTCA** *see Ribavirin on page 1318*
- ♦ **RU-486** *see Mifepristone on page 1006*
- ♦ **RU-23908** *see Nilutamide on page 1083*
- ♦ **RU-38486** *see Mifepristone on page 1006*
- ♦ **Rubella Virus Vaccine (Live)** *see page 1660*
- ♦ **Rubex®** *see DOXOrubicin on page 491*
- ♦ **Rubidomycin Hydrochloride** *see DAUNOrubicin Hydrochloride on page 410*
- ♦ **Rum-K®** *see Potassium Chloride on page 1233*
- ♦ **Rythmol®** *see Propafenone on page 1269*
- ♦ **Rythmol® SR** *see Propafenone on page 1269*

Sacrosidase (sak ROE si dase)

U.S. Brand Names Sucraid®

Generic Available No

Pharmacologic Category Enzyme, Gastrointestinal

Use Orphan drug: Oral replacement therapy in sucrase deficiency, as seen in congenital sucrase-isomaltase deficiency (CSID)

Mechanism of Action/Effect Sacrosidase is a naturally-occurring gastrointestinal enzyme which breaks down the disaccharide sucrose to its monosaccharide components. Hydrolysis is necessary to allow absorption of these nutrients.

Contraindications Hypersensitivity to yeast, yeast products, or glycerin

Warnings/Precautions Hypersensitivity reactions to sacrosidase, including bronchospasm, have been reported. Administer initial doses in a setting where acute hypersensitivity reactions may be treated within a few minutes. Skin testing for hypersensitivity may be performed prior to administration to identify patients at risk.

Drug Interactions

Increased Effect/Toxicity: Drug-drug interactions have not been evaluated.

Nutritional/Ethanol Interactions Food: May be inactivated or denatured if administered with fruit juice, warm or hot food or liquids. Since isomaltase deficiency is not addressed by supplementation of sacrosidase, adherence to a low-starch diet may be required.

(Continued)

Sacrosidase *(Continued)*

Adverse Reactions 1% to 10%: Gastrointestinal: Abdominal pain, vomiting, nausea, diarrhea, constipation

Overdosage/Toxicology Symptoms may include epigastric pain, drowsiness, lethargy, nausea, and vomiting. Gastrointestinal bleeding may occur. Rare manifestations include hypertension, respiratory depression, coma, and acute renal failure. Treatment is symptomatic and supportive. Forced diuresis, hemodialysis and/or urinary alkalinization are not likely to be useful.

Pharmacodynamics/Kinetics

Absorption: Amino acids

Metabolism: GI tract to individual amino acids

Dosing

Adults & Elderly: Sucrase deficiency: Oral: 17,000 int. units (2 mL) per meal or snack. Doses should be diluted with 2-4 ounces of water, milk or formula with each meal or snack. Approximately one-half of the dose may be taken before, and the remainder of a dose taken at the completion of each meal or snack.

Pediatrics: Children >15 kg: Refer to adult dosing.

Available Dosage Forms Solution, oral: 8500 int. units per mL (118 mL)

Monitoring and Teaching Issues

Physical Assessment: See Warnings/Precautions for use cautions (eg, hypersensitivity testing). Monitor effectiveness of therapy and adverse reactions at beginning of therapy and periodically with long-term use (see Adverse Reactions). Assess knowledge/teach patient appropriate use, interventions to reduce side effects, and adverse symptoms to report (see Patient Education).

Patient Education: Use exactly as directed. Dilute dose in 2-4 oz of water, milk, or formula; do not dilute with fruit juice or warm or cold liquids. Take half the dose at beginning of meal and half the dose at end of meal. Maintain adequate hydration (2-3 L/day of fluids unless instructed to restrict fluid intake). Follow prescriber's recommended diet exactly. You may experience headache or nervousness (use caution when driving or engaging in tasks requiring alertness until response to drug is known); or nausea, vomiting, or GI disturbance (frequent mouth care, chewing gum, or sucking hard candy may help). Report immediately skin rash or respiratory difficulty; persistent vomiting, abdominal pain, or blood in stools; change in CNS status (depression, agitation, lethargy); or other adverse response. **Pregnancy precaution:** Inform prescriber if you are or intend to become pregnant.

Pregnancy Risk Factor: C

Lactation: Enters breast milk/compatible

Administration

Storage: Store under refrigeration at 4°C to 8°C (36°F to 46°F). Protect from heat or light.

Additional Information Oral solution contains 50% glycerol.

- ♦ **Safe Prescription Writing** *see page 17*
- ♦ **Safe Tussin® 30 [OTC]** *see* Guaifenesin and Dextromethorphan *on page 731*
- ♦ **Saizen®** *see* Human Growth Hormone *on page 745*
- ♦ **Salagen®** *see* Pilocarpine *on page 1210*
- ♦ **Salbutamol** *see* Albuterol *on page 59*
- ♦ **Salflex®** *see* Salsalate *on page 1354*
- ♦ **Salicylazosulfapyridine** *see* Sulfasalazine *on page 1409*
- ♦ **Salicylsalicylic Acid** *see* Salsalate *on page 1354*

Salmeterol *(sal ME te role)*

U.S. Brand Names Serevent® Diskus®

Synonyms Salmeterol Xinafoate

Generic Available No

Pharmacologic Category Beta$_2$-Adrenergic Agonist

Medication Safety Issues

Sound-alike/look-alike issues:

Salmeterol may be confused with Salbutamol

Serevent® may be confused with Serentil®

Use Maintenance treatment of asthma and in prevention of bronchospasm with reversible obstructive airway disease, including patients with symptoms of nocturnal asthma, who require regular treatment with inhaled, short-acting beta$_2$ agonists; prevention of exercise-induced bronchospasm; maintenance treatment of bronchospasm associated with COPD

Mechanism of Action/Effect Relaxes bronchial smooth muscle by selective action on beta$_2$-receptors with little effect on heart rate; because salmeterol acts locally in the lung, therapeutic effect is not predicted by plasma levels

Contraindications Hypersensitivity to salmeterol, adrenergic amines, or any component of the formulation; need for acute bronchodilation

Warnings/Precautions Salmeterol is not meant to relieve acute asthmatic symptoms. Acute episodes should be treated with short-acting beta$_2$ agonist. Optimize anti-inflammatory treatment before initiating maintenance treatment with salmeterol. Do not use as a component of chronic therapy without an anti-inflammatory agent. Patient must be instructed to seek medical attention in cases where acute symptoms are not relieved by short-acting beta-agonist (**not** salmeterol) or a previous level of response is diminished. Treatment must not be delayed.

Use caution in patients with cardiovascular disease (arrhythmia or hypertension or CHF), convulsive disorders, diabetes, glaucoma, hyperthyroidism, hepatic impairment, or hypokalemia. Beta agonists may cause elevation in blood pressure, heart rate, and result in CNS stimulation/excitation. Beta$_2$ agonists may increase risk of arrhythmia, increase serum glucose, or decrease serum potassium.

In a large, randomized clinical trial (SMART), salmeterol was associated with a small, but statistically significant increase in asthma-related deaths (when added to usual asthma therapy); risk may be greater in African-American patients versus Caucasians.

Do not exceed recommended dose; serious adverse events including fatalities, have been associated with excessive use of inhaled sympathomimetics. Rarely, paradoxical broncho-spasm may occur with use of inhaled bronchodilating agents; this should be distinguished from inadequate response. Safety and efficacy have not been established in children <4 years of age.

Drug Interactions

Cytochrome P450 Effect: Substrate of CYP3A4 (major)

Decreased Effect: Beta-adrenergic blockers (eg, propranolol)

Increased Effect/Toxicity: MAO inhibitors and TCAs may increase toxicity of salmeterol (wait 2 weeks after discontinuing MAO inhibitors or TCA before initiating salmeterol therapy).

Adverse Reactions

>10%:

Central nervous system: Headache

Endocrine & metabolic: Serum glucose increased, serum potassium decreased

Respiratory: Pharyngitis

1% to 10%:

Cardiovascular: Tachycardia, palpitation, elevation or depression of blood pressure, cardiac arrhythmia

Central nervous system: Nervousness, CNS stimulation, hyperactivity, insomnia, malaise, dizziness

Gastrointestinal: GI upset, diarrhea, nausea

Neuromuscular & skeletal: Tremors (may be more common in the elderly), myalgia, back pain, arthralgia

Respiratory: Upper respiratory infection, cough, bronchitis

Overdosage/Toxicology Symptoms of overdose include tachycardia, tremor, hypertension, angina, and seizures. Hypokalemia also may occur. Cardiac arrest and death may be associated with abuse of beta-agonist bronchodilators. Treatment includes immediate discontinuation and symptomatic and supportive therapies. Cautious use of beta-adrenergic blocking agents may be considered in severe cases.

Pharmacodynamics/Kinetics

Onset of Action: Asthma: 30-48 minutes, COPD: 2 hours; Peak effect: 2-4 hours, COPD: 3.27-4.75 hours

Duration of Action: 12 hours

Protein Binding: 96%

Half-Life Elimination: 5.5 hours

Metabolism: Hepatically hydroxylated

Excretion: Feces (60%), urine (25%)

Dosing

Adults & Elderly:

Asthma, maintenance and prevention: Inhalation, powder (Serevent® Diskus®): One inhalation (50 mcg) twice daily (~12 hours apart)

Exercise-induced asthma, prevention: One inhalation (50 mcg) at least 30 minutes prior to exercise; additional doses should not be used for 12 hours; should not be used in individuals already receiving salmeterol twice daily

COPD (maintenance treatment of associated bronchospasm): One inhalation (50 mcg) twice daily (~12 hours apart)

Pediatrics: Asthma (maintenance/prevention) and exercise-induced asthma (prevention): Inhalation, powder (Serevent® Diskus®): Children ≥4 years: Refer to adult dosing.

Available Dosage Forms Powder for oral inhalation (Serevent® Diskus®): 50 mcg (28s, 60s) [delivers 46 mcg/inhalation; contains lactose]

Monitoring and Teaching Issues

Physical Assessment: Not for use to relieve acute asthmatic attacks. Assess effectiveness and interactions of other medications patient may be taking. Monitor effectiveness of therapy and adverse reactions at beginning of therapy and periodically with long-term use. Monitor for increased use of short-acting beta₂-agonist inhalers; may be marker of a deteriorating asthma condition. For inpatient care, monitor vital signs and lung sounds prior to and periodically during therapy. Assess knowledge/teach patient appropriate use, interventions to reduce side effects, and adverse symptoms to report

Monitoring Laboratory Tests: FEV₁, peak flow, and/or other pulmonary function tests

Patient Education: Use exactly as directed (see Administration below). Do not use more often than recommended (excessive use may result in tolerance, overdose may result in serious adverse effects) and do not discontinue without consulting prescriber. Do not use for acute attacks. Maintain adequate hydration (2-3 L/day of fluids) unless instructed to restrict fluid intake. You may experience nervousness, dizziness, or fatigue (use caution when driving or engaging in tasks requiring alertness until response to drug is known); or dry mouth, stomach upset (small frequent meals, frequent mouth care, chewing gum, or sucking hard candy may help). If you have diabetes, check blood sugar; blood glucose level may be increased. Report unresolved GI upset; dizziness or fatigue; vision changes; chest pain, rapid heartbeat, or palpitations; insomnia; nervousness or hyperactivity; muscle cramping, tremors, or pain; unusual cough; or skin rash. **Pregnancy/breast-feeding precautions:** Inform prescriber if you are or intend to become pregnant. Consult prescriber if breast-feeding.

Geriatric Considerations: Geriatric patients were included in four clinical studies of salmeterol; no apparent differences in efficacy and safety were noted in geriatric patients compared to younger adults. Because salmeterol is only to be used for prevention of bronchospasm, patients also need a short-acting beta-agonist to treat acute attacks. Elderly patients should be carefully counseled about which inhaler to use and the proper scheduling of doses; a spacer device may be utilized to maximize effectiveness.

(Continued)

Salmeterol *(Continued)*

Pregnancy Risk Factor: C

Lactation: Enters breast milk/use caution

Administration

Inhalation: Not to be used for the relief of acute attacks. Not for use with a spacer device. Administer with Diskus® in a level, horizontal position. Do not wash mouthpiece; Diskus® should be kept dry.

Storage: Inhalation powder (Serevent® Diskus®): Store at controlled room temperature 20°C to 25°C (68°F to 77°F) in a dry place away from direct heat or sunlight. Stable for 6 weeks after removal from foil pouch.

Related Information

Inhalant Agents *on page 1734*

♦ **Salmeterol and Fluticasone** *see* Fluticasone and Salmeterol *on page 664*

♦ **Salmeterol Xinafoate** *see* Salmeterol *on page 1352*

Salsalate *(SAL sa late)*

U.S. Brand Names Amigesic®; Disalcid® [DSC]; Mono-Gesic®; Salflex®

Synonyms Disalicylic Acid; Salicylsalicylic Acid

Generic Available Yes

Pharmacologic Category Salicylate

Medication Safety Issues

Sound-alike/look-alike issues:

Salsalate may be confused with sucralfate, sulfasalazine

Use Treatment of minor pain or fever; arthritis

Mechanism of Action/Effect Inhibits prostaglandin synthesis, acts on the hypothalamus heat-regulating center to reduce fever, blocks prostaglandin synthetase action which prevents formation of the platelet-aggregating substance thromboxane A_2

Contraindications Hypersensitivity to salsalate or any component of the formulation; GI ulcer or bleeding; pregnancy (3rd trimester)

Warnings/Precautions Use with caution in patients with platelet and bleeding disorders, renal dysfunction, erosive gastritis, or peptic ulcer disease, dehydration, previous nonreaction does not guarantee future safe taking of medication.

Drug Interactions

Decreased Effect: Decreased effect with urinary alkalinizers, antacids, and corticosteroids. Decreased effect of uricosurics and spironolactone.

Increased Effect/Toxicity: Increased effect/toxicity of oral anticoagulants, hypoglycemics, and methotrexate.

Nutritional/Ethanol Interactions

Ethanol: Avoid ethanol (may enhance gastric mucosal irritation).

Food: Salsalate peak serum levels may be delayed if taken with food.

Herb/Nutraceutical: Avoid cat's claw, dong quai, evening primrose, feverfew, garlic, ginger, ginkgo, red clover, horse chestnut, green tea, ginseng (all have additional antiplatelet activity).

Lab Interactions False-negative results for glucose oxidase urinary glucose tests (Clinistix®); false-positives using the cupric sulfate method (Clinitest®); also, interferes with Gerhardt test, VMA determination; 5-HIAA, xylose tolerance test and T_3 and T_4

Adverse Reactions

>10%: Gastrointestinal: Nausea, heartburn, stomach pain, dyspepsia

1% to 10%:

Central nervous system: Fatigue

Dermatologic: Rash

Gastrointestinal: Gastrointestinal ulceration

Hematologic: Hemolytic anemia

Neuromuscular & skeletal: Weakness

Respiratory: Dyspnea

Miscellaneous: Anaphylactic shock

Overdosage/Toxicology Symptoms of overdose include respiratory alkalosis, hyperpnea, tachypnea, tinnitus, headache, hyperpyrexia, metabolic acidosis, hypoglycemia, and coma. Nomograms, such as the "Done" nomogram, can be very helpful for estimating the severity of aspirin poisoning and for directing treatment using serum salicylate levels. Treatment can also be based upon symptomatology.

Pharmacodynamics/Kinetics

Onset of Action: Therapeutic: 3-4 days of continuous dosing

Absorption: Complete, from small intestine

Half-Life Elimination: 7-8 hours

Metabolism: Hepatically hydrolyzed to two moles of salicylic acid (active)

Excretion: Primarily urine

Dosing

Adults & Elderly: Pain, inflammation (arthritis): Oral: 3 g/day in 2-3 divided doses

Renal Impairment: Patients with end-stage renal disease undergoing hemodialysis: Administer 750 mg twice daily with an additional 500 mg after dialysis.

Available Dosage Forms [DSC] = Discontinued product

Tablet: 500 mg, 750 mg

Amigesic®, Disalcid® [DSC]: 500 mg, 750 mg

Mono-Gesic®, Salflex®: 750 mg

Monitoring and Teaching Issues

Physical Assessment: Assess effectiveness and interactions of other medications patient may be taking. Assess results of laboratory tests, therapeutic effectiveness, and adverse reactions (eg, GI effects, unusual bleeding, hepatotoxicity) at beginning of therapy and periodically throughout therapy. Schedule ophthalmic evaluations for patients who are on long-term NSAID therapy. Assess knowledge/teach patient appropriate use, interventions to reduce side effects, and adverse symptoms to report.

Patient Education: Take this medication exactly as directed; do not increase dose without consulting prescriber. Do not crush tablets. Take with food or milk to reduce GI distress. Maintain adequate hydration (2-3 L/day of fluids) unless instructed to restrict fluid intake. Do not use alcohol, aspirin or aspirin-containing medication, or any other anti-inflammatory medications without consulting prescriber. You may experience drowsiness (use caution when driving or engaging in tasks requiring alertness until response to drug is known); or nausea or heartburn (small frequent meals, frequent mouth care, sucking lozenges, or chewing gum may help). GI bleeding, ulceration, or perforation can occur with or without pain; discontinue medication and contact prescriber if persistent abdominal pain or cramping, or blood in stool occurs. Report breathlessness or respiratory difficulty; unusual bruising or bleeding; blood in urine, stool, mouth, or vomitus; unusual fatigue; skin rash or itching; change in urinary pattern; or change in hearing or ringing in ears. **Pregnancy/breast-feeding precautions:** Inform prescriber if you are or intend to become pregnant. This drug should not be used in the 3rd trimester of pregnancy. Do not breast-feed.

Dietary Considerations: May be taken with food to decrease GI distress.

Geriatric Considerations: Elderly are at high risk for adverse effects from NSAIDs. As much as 60% of elderly can develop peptic ulceration and/or hemorrhage asymptomatically. The concomitant use of H_2 blockers, omeprazole, and sucralfate is not effective as prophylaxis with the exception of NSAID-induced duodenal ulcers which may be prevented by the use of ranitidine. Misoprostol is the only prophylactic agent proven effective. Also, concomitant disease and drug use contribute to the risk for GI adverse effects. Use lowest effective dose for shortest period possible. Consider renal function decline with age. Use of NSAIDs can compromise existing renal function especially when Cl_{cr} is ≤ 30 mL/minute. Tinnitus may be a difficult and unreliable indication of toxicity due to age-related hearing loss or eighth cranial nerve damage. CNS adverse effects such as confusion, agitation, and hallucinations are generally seen in overdose or high-dose situations, but elderly may demonstrate these adverse effects at lower doses than younger adults.

Pregnancy Risk Factor: C/D (3rd trimester)

Lactation: Enters breast milk/contraindicated

Breast-Feeding Issues: Salsalate is metabolized to salicylate which is contraindicated while breast-feeding.

Additional Information Does not appear to inhibit platelet aggregation

Related Information

Nonsalicylate / Nonsteroidal Anti-inflammatory Agents *on page 1743*

♦ **Salt Poor Albumin** *see* Albumin *on page 58*

♦ **Sal-Tropine**™ *see* Atropine *on page 158*

♦ **Sandimmune**® *see* CycloSPORINE *on page 383*

♦ **Sandostatin**® *see* Octreotide *on page 1104*

♦ **Sandostatin LAR**® *see* Octreotide *on page 1104*

♦ **Santyl**® *see* Collagenase *on page 372*

Saquinavir (sa KWIN a veer)

U.S. Brand Names Fortovase®; Invirase®

Synonyms Saquinavir Mesylate

Generic Available No

Pharmacologic Category Antiretroviral Agent, Protease Inhibitor

Medication Safety Issues

Sound-alike/look-alike issues:

Saquinavir may be confused with Sinequan®

Fortovase® may be confused with Invirase®

Invirase® may be confused with Fortovase®

Use Treatment of HIV infection; used in combination with at least two other antiretroviral agents

Mechanism of Action/Effect As an inhibitor of HIV protease, saquinavir prevents the cleavage of viral polyprotein precursors which are needed to generate functional proteins in and maturation of HIV-infected cells

Contraindications Hypersensitivity to saquinavir or any component of the formulation; exposure to direct sunlight without sunscreen or protective clothing; severe hepatic impairment; coadministration with amiodarone, bepridil, cisapride, flecainide, midazolam, pimozide, propafenone, quinidine, rifampin, triazolam, or ergot derivatives

Warnings/Precautions Use caution in patients with hepatic insufficiency. May exacerbate pre-existing hepatic dysfunction; use with caution in patients with hepatitis B or C and in cirrhosis. May be associated with fat redistribution (buffalo hump, increased abdominal girth, breast engorgement, facial atrophy). Use caution in hemophilia. May increase cholesterol and/or triglycerides; hypertriglyceridemia may increase risk of pancreatitis.

Saquinavir interacts with multiple medications (including herbal products) when given concurrently; refer to Drug Interactions. Fortovase® and Invirase® are not bioequivalent and should not be used interchangeably; only Fortovase® should be used to initiate therapy. Fortovase® is recommended when saquinavir will be given as the sole protease inhibitor; Invirase® may be used only if combined with ritonavir. Safety and efficacy have not been established in children <16 years of age.

Drug Interactions

Cytochrome P450 Effect: Substrate of CYP2D6 (minor), 3A4 (major); **Inhibits** CYP2C8/9 (weak), 2C19 (weak), 2D6 (weak), 3A4 (moderate)

Decreased Effect: The levels/effects of saquinavir may be reduced by aminoglutethimide, carbamazepine, nafcillin, nevirapine, phenobarbital, phenytoin, rifamycins, and other CYP3A4 inducers. Loss of efficacy and potential resistance may occur. Concurrent use with rifampin is contraindicated.

(Continued)

Saquinavir (Continued)

Serum concentrations of methadone may be decreased; an increased dose may be needed when administered with saquinavir. Serum levels of the hormones in oral contraceptives may decrease significantly with administration of saquinavir. Patients should use alternative methods of contraceptives during saquinavir therapy.

Serum levels of saquinavir and efavirenz may be decreased with concurrent use; saquinavir should not be used as the sole protease inhibitor with efavirenz or nevirapine.

Dexamethasone may decrease serum concentrations of saquinavir; use with caution. Serum concentrations of saquinavir are decreased and levels of rifabutin are increased when used together. Saquinavir should not be used as the sole protease inhibitor when given with rifabutin.

Increased Effect/Toxicity: Concurrent use of amiodarone, bepridil, cisapride, flecainide, midazolam, pimozide, propafenone, quinidine, rifampin, triazolam, or ergot derivatives is contraindicated.

Saquinavir may increase the levels/effects of selected benzodiazepines, calcium channel blockers, cisapride, cyclosporine, ergot alkaloids, selected HMG-CoA reductase inhibitors, mirtazapine, nateglinide, nefazodone, pimozide, quinidine, sildenafil (and other PDE-5 inhibitors), tacrolimus, venlafaxine, and other CYP3A4 substrates. The effects of warfarin may also be increased.

Serum concentrations of saquinavir may be increased by azole antifungals (itraconazole, ketoconazole); dose adjustment was not needed at the study dose when used for a limited time (ketoconazole 400 mg once daily and Fortovase® 1200 mg 3 times/day). Saquinavir serum concentrations may be increased by delavirdine. Indinavir and ritonavir may increase serum levels of saquinavir. Serum levels of saquinavir and nelfinavir may be increased with concurrent use. Lopinavir/ritonavir (combination product) may increase serum levels of saquinavir. Refer to Dosing.

Serum concentrations of saquinavir and clarithromycin may both be increased. Dose adjustment not was not needed at the study dose when used for 7 days (clarithromycin 500 mg twice daily and Fortovase® 1200 mg 3 times/day); dosage adjustment of clarithromycin is recommended in patients with renal impairment.

Serum concentrations of saquinavir are decreased and levels of rifabutin are increased when used together. Saquinavir should not be used as the sole protease inhibitor when given with rifabutin.

Nutritional/Ethanol Interactions

Food: A high-fat meal maximizes bioavailability. Saquinavir levels may increase if taken with grapefruit juice.

Herb/Nutraceutical: Saquinavir serum concentrations may be decreased by St John's wort; avoid concurrent use. Garlic capsules may decrease saquinavir serum concentrations; avoid use if saquinavir is the only protease inhibitor.

Adverse Reactions Protease inhibitors cause dyslipidemia which includes elevated cholesterol and triglycerides and a redistribution of body fat centrally to cause increased abdominal girth, buffalo hump, facial atrophy, and breast enlargement. These agents also cause hyperglycemia.

10%: Gastrointestinal: Diarrhea, nausea

1% to 10%:

Cardiovascular: Chest pain

Central nervous system: Anxiety, depression, fatigue, headache, insomnia, pain

Dermatologic: Rash, verruca

Endocrine & metabolic: Hyperglycemia, hypoglycemia, hyperkalemia, libido disorder, serum amylase increased

Gastrointestinal: Abdominal discomfort, abdominal pain, appetite decreased, buccal mucosa ulceration, constipation, dyspepsia, flatulence, taste alteration, vomiting

Hepatic: AST increased, ALT increased, bilirubin increased

Neuromuscular & skeletal: Paresthesia, weakness, CPK increased

Renal: Creatinine kinase increased

Pharmacodynamics/Kinetics

Absorption: Poor; increased with high fat meal; Fortovase® has improved absorption over Invirase®

Bioavailability: Invirase®: ~4%; Fortovase®: 12% to 15%

Protein Binding: Plasma: ~98%

Metabolism: Extensively hepatic via CYP3A4; extensive first-pass effect

Excretion: Feces (81% to 88%), urine (1% to 3%) within 5 days

Dosing

Adults:

HIV infection: Oral: **Note:** Fortovase® and Invirase® are not bioequivalent and should not be used interchangeably; only Fortovase® should be used to initiate therapy:

Fortovase®: 1200 mg (six 200 mg capsules) 3 times/day within 2 hours after a meal in combination with a nucleoside analog or 1000 mg (five 200 mg capsules) twice daily in combination with ritonavir 100 mg twice daily

Invirase®: 1000 mg (five 200 mg capsules or two 500 mg tablets) twice daily given in combination with ritonavir 100 mg twice daily. This combination should be given together and within 2 hours after a full meal in combination with a nucleoside analog.

Note: Dosage adjustments of Fortovase® when administered in combination therapy:

Delavirdine: Fortovase® 800 mg 3 times/day

Lopinavir and ritonavir (Kaletra™): Fortovase® 800 mg twice daily

Nelfinavir: Fortovase® 800 mg twice daily

Elderly: Clinical studies did not include sufficient numbers of patients ≥65 years of age. Use caution due to increased frequency of organ dysfunction.

Pediatrics:

HIV infection: Oral:

Children and Adolescents <16 years: Safety and efficacy have not been established; dosages of 50 mg/kg/dose 3 times/day are under study.

Children ≥16 years: Refer to adult dosing.

Available Dosage Forms Note: Strength expressed as base.

Capsule, as mesylate (Invirase®): 200 mg [contains lactose 63.3 mg/capsule]

Capsule, soft gelatin, as base (Fortovase®): 200 mg

Tablet, as base (Invirase®): 500 mg

Monitoring and Teaching Issues

Physical Assessment: Use caution with hepatic impairment (may increase hepatic dysfunction caused by hepatitis), diabetes (may exacerbate hyperglycemia); see Warnings/Precautions for specific use cautions. Assess potential for interactions with other pharmacological agents and herbal products patient may be taking (impacts multiple liver enzymes that can increase or decrease levels/effects [eg, increase potential for severe toxicity or loss of effectiveness] when used concurrently with multiple other drugs; see Drug Interactions for extensive list and cautions). Assess result of laboratory tests, patient response (CD4 count and viral load), and adverse reactions at regular intervals during therapy (eg, gastrointestinal disturbance [nausea, vomiting, diarrhea], anemia, hyperlipidemia and redistribution of body fat, rash, CNS effects [malaise, insomnia, abnormal thinking], electrolyte imbalance, opportunistic infection; see Adverse Reactions). Teach patient proper use, possible side effects/appropriate interventions (eg, glucose testing; protease inhibitors may cause hyperglycemia [exacerbation or new-onset diabetes]), use of barrier contraceptives (protease inhibitors may decrease effectiveness of oral contraceptives), and adverse symptoms to report (see Patient Education).

Monitoring Laboratory Tests: CBC, renal and liver function, electrolytes, triglycerides, cholesterol, glucose, CD4 cell count, plasma levels of HIV RNA

Patient Education: Do not take any new medication during therapy unless approved by prescriber. This medication is not a cure for HIV, nor has it been found to reduce transmission of HIV. Take as directed, within 2 hours after a meal. Avoid grapefruit juice. Maintain adequate hydration (2-3 L/day of fluids unless instructed to restrict fluid intake). Saquinavir may be prescribed with a combination of other medications; time these medications as directed by prescriber. This drug can cause exacerbation of diabetes or new onset diabetes (if you have diabetes, check your glucose levels frequently); if you experience increased thirst or hunger, increased urination, weight lose, or dry, itchy skin contact prescriber. Avoid exposure to direct sunlight (wear protective clothing and use sunblock). May cause body changes due to redistribution of body fat, facial atrophy, or breast enlargement (normal effects of drug); dizziness, insomnia, abnormal thinking (use caution when driving or engaging in potentially hazardous tasks until response to drug is known); nausea, vomiting, or taste perversion (small frequent meals, frequent mouth care, chewing gum, or sucking lozenges may help); mouth sores (frequent oral care is necessary); muscle weakness (consult prescriber for approved analgesic); headache; or insomnia (consult prescriber for medication). Report any persistent adverse effects. **Pregnancy/breast-feeding precautions:** May reduce effectiveness of some oral systemic contraceptives. Consult prescriber for appropriate contraceptive measures. Do not breast-feed. Do not breast-feed.

Dietary Considerations: Administer within 2 hours of a meal. Invirase® capsules contain lactose 63.3 mg/capsule (not expected to induce symptoms of intolerance).

Pregnancy Risk Factor: B

Pregnancy Issues: Saquinavir soft gelatin capsules (Fortovase®) provide adequate levels when used in normal doses during pregnancy; pharmacokinetic data not available for Invirase®. The Perinatal HIV Guidelines Working Group considers Fortovase® and ritonavir to be a preferred combination for use during pregnancy. Pregnancy and protease inhibitors are both associated with an increased risk of hyperglycemia. Glucose levels should be closely monitored. Health professionals are encouraged to contact the antiretroviral pregnancy registry to monitor outcomes of pregnant women exposed to antiretroviral medications (1-800-258-4263 or www.APRegistry.com).

Lactation: Enters breast milk/contraindicated

Breast-Feeding Issues: Saquinavir is minimally excreted in breast milk. HIV-infected mothers are discouraged from breast-feeding to decrease postnatal transmission of HIV.

Administration

Oral: Take saquinavir within 2 hours after a full meal. Avoid direct sunlight when taking saquinavir. When used with ritonavir, saquinavir and ritonavir should be administered at the same time.

Storage:

Fortovase®: Store in refrigerator. Stable for 3 months when stored at room temperature.

Invirase®: Store at room temperature.

Additional Information The indication for saquinavir for the treatment of HIV infection is based on changes in surrogate markers. At present, there are no results from controlled clinical trials evaluating the effect of regimens containing saquinavir on patient survival or the clinical progression of HIV infection, such as the occurrence of opportunistic infections or malignancies; in cell culture, saquinavir is additive to synergistic with AZT, ddC, and DDI without enhanced toxicity. According to the manufacturer, Invirase® will be phased out over time and completely replaced by Fortovase®. Potential compliance problems, frequency of administration and adverse effects should be discussed with patients before initiating therapy to help prevent the emergence of resistance.

Related Information

Tuberculosis on page 1864

♦ **Saquinavir Mesylate** see Saquinavir on page 1355

♦ **Sarafem™** see Fluoxetine on page 649

Sargramostim (sar GRAM oh stim)

U.S. Brand Names Leukine®

Synonyms GM-CSF; Granulocyte-Macrophage Colony Stimulating Factor; rGM-CSF

Generic Available No

Pharmacologic Category Colony Stimulating Factor

Medication Safety Issues

Sound-alike/look-alike issues:

Leukine® may be confused with Leukeran®

Use

Myeloid reconstitution after autologous bone marrow transplantation: Non-Hodgkin's lymphoma (NHL), acute lymphoblastic leukemia (ALL), Hodgkin's lymphoma, metastatic breast cancer

Myeloid reconstitution after allogeneic bone marrow transplantation

Peripheral stem cell transplantation: Metastatic breast cancer, non-Hodgkin's lymphoma, Hodgkin's lymphoma, multiple myeloma

Orphan drug:

Acute myelogenous leukemia (AML) following induction chemotherapy in older adults to shorten time to neutrophil recovery and to reduce the incidence of severe and life-threatening infections and infections resulting in death

Bone marrow transplant (allogeneic or autologous) failure or engraftment delay

Safety and efficacy of GM-CSF given simultaneously with cytotoxic chemotherapy have not been established. Concurrent treatment may increase myelosuppression.

Mechanism of Action/Effect Stimulates proliferation, differentiation and functional activity of neutrophils, eosinophils, monocytes, and macrophages; see table.

Comparative Effects — G-CSF vs GM-CSF

Proliferation/Differentiation	G-CSF (Filgrastim)	GM-CSF (Sargramostim)
Neutrophils	Yes	Yes
Eosinophils	No	Yes
Macrophages	No	Yes
Neutrophil migration	Enhanced	Inhibited

Contraindications Hypersensitivity to sargramostim, yeast-derived products, or any component of the formulation; concurrent myelosuppressive chemotherapy or radiation therapy. The solution for injection contains benzyl alcohol and should not be used in neonates.

Warnings/Precautions Simultaneous administration, or administration 24 hours preceding/following cytotoxic chemotherapy or radiotherapy is not recommended. Use with caution in patients with pre-existing cardiac problems, hypoxia, fluid retention, pulmonary infiltrates or CHF, renal or hepatic impairment. rapid increase in peripheral blood counts. If ANC is >20,000/mm³, or platelets >500,000/mm³ decrease dose by 50% or discontinue drug (counts will fall to normal within 3-7 days after discontinuing drug). Growth factor potential: caution with myeloid malignancies. Precaution should be exercised in the usage of GM-CSF in any malignancy with myeloid characteristics. GM-CSF can potentially act as a growth factor for any tumor type, particularly myeloid malignancies. Tumors of nonhematopoietic origin may have surface receptors for GM-CSF.

Drug Interactions

Increased Effect/Toxicity: Lithium, corticosteroids may potentiate myeloproliferative effects.

Adverse Reactions

>10%:

Cardiovascular: Hypotension, tachycardia, flushing, and syncope may occur with the first dose of a cycle ("first-dose effect"); peripheral edema (11%)

Central nervous system: Headache (26%)

Dermatologic: Rash, alopecia

Endocrine & metabolic: Polydypsia

Gastrointestinal: Diarrhea (52% to 89%), stomatitis, mucositis

Local: Local reactions at the injection site (~50%)

Neuromuscular & skeletal: Myalgia (18%), arthralgia (21%), bone pain

Renal: Increased serum creatinine (14%)

Respiratory: Dyspnea (28%)

1% to 10%:

Cardiovascular: Transient supraventricular arrhythmia; chest pain; capillary leak syndrome; pericardial effusion (4%)

Central nervous system: Headache

Gastrointestinal: Nausea, vomiting

Hematologic: Leukocytosis, thrombocytopenia

Neuromuscular & skeletal: Weakness

Respiratory: Cough; pleural effusion (1%)

Overdosage/Toxicology Symptoms of overdose include dyspnea, malaise, nausea, fever, headache, and chills. Discontinue drug and wait for levels to fall. Treatment is supportive. Monitor CBC, respiratory symptoms, and fluid status. Discontinue drug and wait for levels to fall, monitor for pulmonary edema. Toxicity of GM-CSF is dose dependent. Severe reactions such as capillary leak syndrome are seen at higher doses (>15 mcg/kg/day).

Pharmacodynamics/Kinetics

Onset of Action: Increase in WBC: 7-14 days

Duration of Action: WBCs return to baseline within 1 week of discontinuing drug

Time to Peak: Serum: SubQ: 1-2 hours

Half-Life Elimination: 2 hours

Dosing

Adults & Elderly:

Existing clinical data suggest that starting GM-CSF between 24 and 72 hours subsequent to chemotherapy may provide optimal neutrophil recover. Continue therapy until the occurrence of an absolute neutrophil count of 10,000/µL after the neutrophil nadir.

The available data suggest that rounding the dose to the nearest vial size may enhance patient convenience and reduce costs without clinical detrement.

Myeloid reconstitution after peripheral stem cell, allogeneic or autologous bone marrow transplant: I.V.: 250 mcg/m^2/day for 21 days to begin 2-4 hours after the marrow infusion on day 0 of autologous bone marrow transplant or ≥24 hours after chemotherapy or 12 hours after last dose of radiotherapy.

If a severe adverse reaction occurs, reduce or temporarily discontinue the dose until the reaction abates.

If blast cells appear or progression of the underlying disease occurs, disrupt treatment.

Interrupt or reduce the dose by half if ANC is >20,000 cells/mm^3

Patients should not receive sargramostim until the postmarrow infusion ANC is <500 cells/mm^3.

Neutrophil recovery following chemotherapy in AML: I.V.: 250 mcg/m^2/day over a 4-hour period starting approximately day 11 or 4 days following the completion of induction chemotherapy, if day 10 bone marrow is hypoblastic with <5% blasts.

If a second cycle of chemotherapy is necessary, administer ~4 days after the completion of chemotherapy if the bone marrow is hypoblastic with <5% blasts.

Continue sargramostim until ANC is >1500 cells/mm^3 for consecutive days or a maximum of 42 days.

Discontinue sargramostim immediately if leukemic regrowth occurs.

If a severe adverse reaction occurs, reduce the dose by 50% or temporarily discontinue the dose until the reaction abates.

Mobilization of peripheral blood progenitor cells: I.V.: 250 mcg/m^2/day over 24 hours or SubQ once daily.

Continue the same dose through the period of PBPC collection.

The optimal schedule for PBPC collection has not been established (usually begun by day 5 and performed daily until protocol specified targets are achieved).

If WBC >50,000 cells/mm^3, reduce the dose by 50%.

If adequate numbers of progenitor cells are not collected, consider other mobilization therapy.

Postperipheral blood progenitor cell transplantation: I.V.: 250 mcg/m^2/day over 24 hours or SubQ once daily beginning immediately following infusion of progenitor cells and continuing until ANC is >1500 for 3 consecutive days is attained.

BMT failure or engraftment delay: I.V.: 250 mcg/m^2/day for 14 days as a 2-hour infusion.

The dose can be repeated after 7 days off therapy if engraftment has not occurred.

If engraftment still has not occurred, a third course of 500 mcg/m^2/day for 14 days may be tried after another 7 days off therapy; if there is still no improvement, it is unlikely that further dose escalation will be beneficial.

If a severe adverse reaction occurs, reduce or temporarily discontinue the dose until the reaction abates.

If blast cells appear or disease progression occurs, discontinue treatment.

Note: Doses may be given via I.V. infusion over ≥2 hours or SubQ

Pediatrics: Refer to adult dosing.

Available Dosage Forms

Injection, powder for reconstitution: 250 mcg

Injection, solution: 500 mcg/mL (1 mL) [contains benzyl alcohol]

Monitoring and Teaching Issues

Physical Assessment: Use caution with pre-existing cardiac problems, hypoxia, fluid retention, pulmonary infiltrates, CHF, renal or hepatic impairment (see Warnings/Precautions for specific use cautions). See Administration and Reconstitution for specific infusion directions. Patient must be monitored closely for "first dose effect" (hypotension, tachycardia, flushing, syncope) with the first dose of a cycle. Assess results of laboratory tests closely (see Monitoring Laboratory Tests). Assess patient response and adverse reactions frequently during therapy (eg, fluid balance [I & O], rash, hypotension, tachycardia, GI disturbance [diarrhea, stomatitis, mucositis], myalgia, bone pain; see Adverse Reactions). Teach patient use if self-administered SubQ (eg, appropriate injection technique and syringe/needle disposal), possible side effects/appropriate interventions, and adverse symptoms to report (see Patient Education).

Monitoring Laboratory Tests: To avoid potential complications of excessive leukocytosis (WBC >50,000 cells/mm^3, ANC >20,000 cells/mm^3), a CBC with differential is recommended twice per week during therapy. Sargramostim therapy should be interrupted or the dose reduced by half if the ANC is >20,000 cells/mm^3. Monitoring of renal and hepatic function in patients displaying renal or hepatic dysfunction prior to initiation of treatment is recommended and at least biweekly during sargramostim administration.

Patient Education: Do not take any new medication during therapy without consulting prescriber. If administered by infusion; report any redness, swelling, pain, or burning at infusion site. **SubQ** (self injection): Follow exact direction for injection and disposal of syringe/needle; report redness, pain, or signs of infections at injection site. You will require frequent blood tests during treatment. May cause bone, joint, or muscle pain (request analgesic); nausea and vomiting (small frequent meals may help); or hair loss (reversible); diarrhea (buttermilk, boiled milk, or yogurt may help). Report chest pain or palpitations, signs or symptoms of edema (eg, swollen extremities, difficulty breathing, rapid weight gain); onset of severe headache; acute back or chest pain; muscular tremors or seizure

(Continued)

Sargramostim *(Continued)*

activity; or other persistent adverse effects. **Pregnancy/breast-feeding precautions:** Inform prescriber if you are or intend to become pregnant. Consult prescriber if breast-feeding.

Pregnancy Risk Factor: C

Lactation: Excretion in breast milk unknown

Administration

I.V.: Can premedicate with analgesics and antipyretics; control bone pain with non-narcotic analgesics. I.V. infusion should be over at least 2 hours; incompatible with dextrose-containing solutions. An in-line membrane filter should not be used for intravenous injection.

Other: Administer by SubQ (undiluted). Do not shake solution. When administering GM-CSF subcutaneously, rotate injection sites.

Reconstitution:

Solution for injection: May be stored for up to 20 days at 2°C to 8°C (36°F to 46°F) once the vial has been entered. Discard remaining solution after 20 days.

Powder for injection: May be reconstituted with preservative free SWFI or bacteriostatic water for injection (with benzyl alcohol 0.9%). Preparations made with SWFI should be administered as soon as possible, and discarded within 6 hours of reconstitution. Preparations made with bacteriostatic water maybe stored for up to 20 days at 2°C to 8°C (36°F to 46°F). Gently swirl to reconstitute; do not shake.

Sargramostim may also be further diluted in 0.9% sodium chloride to a concentration of ≥10 mcg/mL for I.V. infusion administration; this diluted solution is stable for 48 hours at room temperature and refrigeration.

If the final concentration of sargramostim is <10 mcg/mL, human albumin should be added to the saline prior to the addition of sargramostim to prevent absorption of the components to the delivery system. It is recommended that 1 mg of human albumin/1 mL of 0.9% sodium chloride (eg, 1 mL of 5% human albumin/50 mL of 0.9% sodium chloride) be added.

Standard diluent: Dose ≥250 mcg/25 mL NS

Compatibility: Stable in NS, SWFI, bacteriostatic water; **incompatible** with dextrose-containing solutions

Y-site administration: Incompatible with acyclovir, ampicillin, ampicillin/sulbactam, cefoperazone, chlorpromazine, ganciclovir, haloperidol, hydrocortisone sodium phosphate, hydrocortisone sodium succinate, hydromorphone, hydroxyzine, imipenem/cilastatin, lorazepam, methylprednisolone sodium succinate, mitomycin, morphine, nalbuphine, ondansetron, piperacillin, sodium bicarbonate, tobramycin

Storage: Sargramostim should be stored at 2°C to 8°C (36°F to 46°F). Vials should not be frozen or shaken.

Additional Information Reimbursement Hotline (Leukine®): 1-800-321-4669

♦ **Sarnol®-HC [OTC]** *see* Hydrocortisone *on page 760*

♦ **SB-265805** *see* Gemifloxacin *on page 706*

♦ **SC 33428** *see* Idarubicin *on page 781*

♦ **SCH 13521** *see* Flutamide *on page 658*

♦ **S-Citalopram** *see* Escitalopram *on page 547*

♦ **Scopace™** *see* Scopolamine Derivatives *on page 1360*

♦ **Scopolamine Butylbromide** *see* Scopolamine Derivatives *on page 1360*

Scopolamine Derivatives *(skoe POL a meen dah RIV ah tives)*

U.S. Brand Names Isopto® Hyoscine; Scopace™; Transderm Scōp®

Synonyms Hyoscine Butylbromide; Hyoscine Hydrobromide; Scopolamine Butylbromide; Scopolamine Hydrobromide

Generic Available Yes

Pharmacologic Category Anticholinergic Agent

Medication Safety Issues

Transdermal patch may contain conducting metal (eg, aluminum); remove patch prior to MRI.

Use

Scopolamine hydrobromide:

Injection: Preoperative medication to produce amnesia, sedation, and decrease salivary and respiratory secretions

Ophthalmic: Produce cycloplegia and mydriasis; treatment of iridocyclitis

Oral: Symptomatic treatment of postencephalitic parkinsonism and paralysis agitans; inhibits excessive motility and hypertonus of the genitourinary or gastrointestinal tract in such conditions as the irritable colon syndrome, mild dysentery, diverticulitis, pylorospasm, and cardiospasm

Transdermal: Prevention of nausea/vomiting associated with anesthesia or opiate analgesia; prevention of motion sickness

Scopolamine butylbromide:

Oral/injection: Treatment of smooth muscle spasm of the genitourinary or gastrointestinal tract; injection may also be used to prior to radiological/diagnostic procedures to prevent spasm

Mechanism of Action/Effect Blocks the action of acetylcholine at parasympathetic sites in smooth muscle, secretory glands and the CNS; increases cardiac output, dries secretions, antagonizes histamine and serotonin

Contraindications Hypersensitivity to scopolamine or any component of the formulation; narrow-angle glaucoma; acute hemorrhage; paralytic ileus, GI or GU obstruction; thyrotoxicosis; tachycardia secondary to cardiac insufficiency; myasthenia gravis

Warnings/Precautions Use with caution with hepatic or renal impairment since adverse CNS effects occur more often in these patients; use with caution in infants and children since they may be more susceptible to adverse effects of scopolamine; use with caution in patients with GI obstruction, prostatic hyperplasia (nonobstructive), or urinary retention. Discontinue if patient reports unusual visual disturbances or pain within the eye. Use caution in hiatal hernia, reflux esophagitis, and ulcerative colitis. Scopolamine (hyoscine) hydrobromide should not be interchanged with scopolamine butylbromide formulations; dosages are not equivalent. Transdermal patch may contain conducting metal (eg, aluminum); remove patch prior to MRI.

Drug Interactions

Decreased Effect: Decreased effect of acetaminophen, levodopa, ketoconazole, digoxin, riboflavin, and potassium chloride in wax matrix preparations.

Increased Effect/Toxicity: Adverse anticholinergic effects may be additive with other anticholinergic agents (includes tricyclic antidepressants, antihistamines, and phenothiazines). Sedative effects of other CNS depressants may be additive with scopolamine.

Nutritional/Ethanol Interactions Ethanol: Avoid ethanol (may increase CNS depression).

Adverse Reactions Frequency not defined.

Ophthalmic: Note: Systemic adverse effects have been reported following ophthalmic administration.

Cardiovascular: Vascular congestion, edema

Central nervous system: Drowsiness

Dermatologic: Eczematoid dermatitis

Ocular: Blurred vision, photophobia, local irritation, increased intraocular pressure, follicular conjunctivitis, exudate

Respiratory: Congestion

Systemic:

Cardiovascular: Orthostatic hypotension, ventricular fibrillation, tachycardia, palpitation

Central nervous system: Confusion, drowsiness, headache, loss of memory, ataxia, fatigue

Dermatologic: Dry skin, increased sensitivity to light, rash

Endocrine & metabolic: Decreased flow of breast milk

Gastrointestinal: Constipation, xerostomia, dry throat, dysphagia, bloated feeling, nausea, vomiting

Genitourinary: Dysuria

Local: Irritation at injection site

Neuromuscular & skeletal: Weakness

Ocular: Increased intraocular pain, blurred vision

Respiratory: Dry nose

Miscellaneous: Diaphoresis (decreased)

Overdosage/Toxicology Symptoms of overdose include dilated pupils, flushed skin, tachycardia, hypertension, and ECG abnormalities. CNS manifestations resemble acute psychosis. CNS depression, circulatory collapse, respiratory failure, and death can occur. For a scopolamine overdose with severe life-threatening symptoms, physostigmine 1-2 mg SubQ or I.V. slowly should be given to reverse toxic effects.

Pharmacodynamics/Kinetics

Onset of Action: Oral, I.M.: 0.5-1 hour; I.V.: 10 minutes

Peak effect: 20-60 minutes; may take 3-7 days for full recovery; transdermal: 24 hours

Duration of Action: Oral, I.M.: 4-6 hours; I.V.: 2 hours

Absorption: Tertiary salts (hydrobromide) are well absorbed; quaternary salts (butylbromide) are poorly absorbed (local concentrations in the GI tract following oral dosing may be high)

Half-Life Elimination: 4.8 hours

Metabolism: Hepatic

Excretion: Urine (as metabolites)

Dosing

Adults & Elderly: Note: Scopolamine (hyoscine) hydrobromide should not be interchanged with scopolamine butylbromide formulations. Dosages are not equivalent.

Scopolamine hydrobromide:

Preoperative:

I.M., I.V., SubQ: 0.3-0.65 mg; may be repeated every 4-6 hours

Transdermal patch: Apply 2.5 cm^2 patch to hairless area behind ear the night before surgery or 1 hour prior to cesarean section (the patch should be applied no sooner than 1 hour before surgery for best results and removed 24 hours after surgery)

Motion sickness: Transdermal: Apply 1 disc behind the ear at least 4 hours prior to exposure and every 3 days as needed; effective if applied as soon as 2-3 hours before anticipated need, best if 12 hours before

Refraction: Ophthalmic: Instill 1-2 drops of 0.25% to eye(s) 1 hour before procedure

Iridocyclitis: Ophthalmic: Instill 1-2 drops of 0.25% to eye(s) up to 4 times/day

Parkinsonism, spasticity, motion sickness: Oral: 0.4-0.8 mg as a range; the dosage may be cautiously increased in parkinsonism and spastic states.

Scopolamine butylbromide:

Gastrointestinal/genitourinary spasm (Buscopan® [CAN]; not available in the U.S.):

Oral: 10-20 mg daily (1-2 tablets); maximum: 6 tablets/day

I.M., I.V., SubQ: 10-20 mg; maximum: 100 mg/day. Intramuscular injections should be administered 10-15 minutes prior to radiological/diagnostic procedures

Pediatrics:

Scopolamine hydrobromide:

Preoperative: I.M., SubQ: 6 mcg/kg/dose (maximum: 0.3 mg/dose) every 6-8 hours

Refraction: Ophthalmic: Instill 1 drop of 0.25% to eye(s) twice daily for 2 days before procedure

Iridocyclitis: Ophthalmic: Instill 1 drop of 0.25% to eye(s) up to 3 times/day

Available Dosage Forms [CAN] = Canadian brand name

Injection, solution, as hydrobromide: 0.4 mg/mL (1 mL)

Injection, solution, as hyoscine-N-butylbromide (Buscopan® [CAN]): 20 mg/mL [not available in U.S.]

Solution, ophthalmic, as hydrobromide (Isopto® Hyoscine): 0.25% (5 mL, 15 mL) [contains benzalkonium chloride]

Tablet, as hyoscine-N-butylbromide (Buscopan® [CAN]): 10 mg [not available in U.S.]

(Continued)

Scopolamine Derivatives *(Continued)*

Tablet, soluble, as hydrobromide (Scopace™): 0.4 mg

Transdermal system (Transderm Scōp®): 1.5 mg (4s) [releases ~1 mg over 72 hours]

Monitoring and Teaching Issues

Physical Assessment: Assess potential for interactions with other prescriptions, OTC medications, or herbal products patient may be taking (eg, ergot-containing drugs). When used preoperatively, safety precautions should be observed and patient should be advised about blurred vision. For all uses, assess therapeutic effectiveness and adverse reactions. Teach patient appropriate use (according to formulation and purpose), interventions to reduce side effects, and adverse symptoms to report. Systemic effects have been reported following ophthalmic administration.

Patient Education: Use as directed. May cause drowsiness, confusion, impaired judgment, or vision changes (use caution when driving or engaging in tasks requiring alertness until response to drug is known); dry mouth, nausea, or vomiting (small frequent meals, frequent mouth care, chewing gum, or sucking lozenges may help); orthostatic hypotension (use caution when climbing stairs and when rising from lying or sitting position); constipation (increased exercise, fluids, fruit, or fiber may help; if not effective consult prescriber); increased sensitivity to heat and decreased perspiration (avoid extremes of heat, reduce exercise in hot weather); or decreased milk if breast-feeding. Report hot, dry, flushed skin; blurred vision or vision changes; difficulty swallowing; chest pain, palpitations, or rapid heartbeat; painful or difficult urination; increased confusion, depression, or loss of memory; rapid or difficult respirations; muscle weakness or tremors; or eye pain.

Pregnancy precaution: Inform prescriber if you are or intend to become pregnant.

Transdermal: Apply patch behind ear the day before traveling. Wash hands before and after applying, and avoid contact with the eyes. Do not remove for 3 days.

Ophthalmic: Instill as often as recommended. Wash hands before using. Do not let tip of applicator touch eye; do not contaminate tip of applicator (may cause eye infection, eye damage, or vision loss). Sit or lie down, open eye, look at ceiling, and instill prescribed amount of solution. Do not blink for 30 seconds, close eye and roll eye in all directions, and apply gentle pressure to inner corner of eye for 1-2 minutes. Temporary stinging or blurred vision may occur.

Geriatric Considerations: Because of its long duration of action as a mydriatic agent, it should be avoided in elderly patients. Anticholinergic agents are not well tolerated in the elderly and their use should be avoided when possible.

Pregnancy Risk Factor: C

Lactation: Enters breast milk/use caution (AAP rates "compatible")

Administration

I.V.:

Hydrobromide: Inject over 2-3 minutes

Butylbromide: Inject at a rate of 1 mL/minute

Topical: Topical disc is programmed to deliver *in vivo* 1 mg over 3 days. Once applied, do not remove the patch for 3 full days. Apply to hairless area of skin behind the ear. Wash hands before and after applying the disc to avoid drug contact with eyes.

Storage: Store tablets and/or injection at room temperature of 15°C to 30°C. Protect injection from light.

Hydrobromide injection: Avoid acid solutions, hydrolysis occurs at pH <3

Butylbromide injection: Stable in D_5W, NS, $D_{10}W$, and LR for up to 8 hours

- **Scopolamine Hydrobromide** *see* Scopolamine Derivatives *on page 1360*
- **Scopolamine, Hyoscyamine, Atropine, and Phenobarbital** *see* Hyoscyamine, Atropine, Scopolamine, and Phenobarbital *on page 777*
- **Scot-Tussin® Expectorant [OTC]** *see* Guaifenesin *on page 729*
- **Scot-Tussin® Senior [OTC]** *see* Guaifenesin and Dextromethorphan *on page 731*
- **SDZ ENA 713** *see* Rivastigmine *on page 1340*
- **Seasonale®** *see* Ethinyl Estradiol and Levonorgestrel *on page 585*

Secobarbital *(see koe BAR bi tal)*

U.S. Brand Names Seconal®

Synonyms Quinalbarbitone Sodium; Secobarbital Sodium

Controlled Substance C-II

Generic Available No

Pharmacologic Category Barbiturate

Medication Safety Issues

Sound-alike/look-alike issues:

Seconal® may be confused with Sectral®

Use Preanesthetic agent; short-term treatment of insomnia

Mechanism of Action/Effect Interferes with transmission of impulses from the thalamus to the cortex of the brain resulting in an imbalance in central inhibitory and facilitatory mechanisms

Contraindications Hypersensitivity to barbiturates or a component of the formulation; marked hepatic impairment; dyspnea or airway obstruction; porphyria; pregnancy

Warnings/Precautions Should be used only after evaluation of potential causes of sleep disturbance. Failure of sleep disturbance to resolve after 7-10 days may indicate psychiatric or medical illness. Do not administer to patients in acute pain. Use caution in elderly patients, debilitated patients, hepatic impairment, renally impairment, or pediatric patients. May cause paradoxical responses, including agitation and hyperactivity, particularly in acute pain and pediatric patients. Use with caution in patients with depression or suicidal tendencies, or in patients with a history of drug abuse. Tolerance, psychological and physical dependence may occur with prolonged use. May cause CNS depression, which may impair physical or mental abilities. Effects with other sedative drugs or ethanol may be potentiated. May cause respiratory depression or hypotension, Use with caution in hemodynamically unstable patients or patients with respiratory disease.

Drug Interactions

Cytochrome P450 Effect: Induces CYP2A6 (strong), 2C8/9 (strong)

Decreased Effect: Barbiturates, such as secobarbital, are hepatic enzyme inducers, and may increase the metabolism of antipsychotics, some beta-blockers (unlikely with atenolol and nadolol), calcium channel blockers, chloramphenicol, cimetidine, corticosteroids, cyclosporine, disopyramide, doxycycline, ethosuximide, felbamate, furosemide, griseofulvin, lamotrigine, phenytoin, propafenone, quinidine, tacrolimus, TCAs, and theophylline. Barbiturates may increase the metabolism of estrogens and reduce the efficacy of oral contraceptives; an alternative method of contraception should be considered. Barbiturates inhibit the hypoprothrombinemic effects of oral anticoagulants via increased metabolism. Barbiturates may enhance the metabolism of methadone resulting in methadone withdrawal.

Increased Effect/Toxicity: Increased toxicity when combined with other CNS depressants, antidepressants, benzodiazepines, chloramphenicol, or valproic acid; respiratory and CNS depression may be additive. MAO inhibitors may prolong the effect of secobarbital. Barbiturates may enhance the hepatotoxic potential of acetaminophen (due to an increased formation of toxic metabolites). Chloramphenicol may inhibit the metabolism of barbiturates.

Nutritional/Ethanol Interactions

Ethanol: Avoid ethanol (may increase CNS depression).

Herb/Nutraceutical: Avoid valerian, St John's wort, kava kava, gotu kola (may increase CNS depression).

Adverse Reactions Frequency not defined.

Cardiovascular: Hypotension

Central nervous system: Dizziness, lightheadedness, "hangover" effect, drowsiness, CNS depression, fever, confusion, mental depression, unusual excitement, nervousness, faint feeling, headache, insomnia, nightmares, hallucinations

Dermatologic: Exfoliative dermatitis, rash, Stevens-Johnson syndrome

Gastrointestinal: Nausea, vomiting, constipation

Hematologic: Agranulocytosis, megaloblastic anemia, thrombocytopenia, thrombophlebitis, urticaria apnea

Local: Pain at injection site

Respiratory: Respiratory depression, laryngospasm

Overdosage/Toxicology Symptoms of overdose include unsteady gait, slurred speech, confusion, jaundice, hypothermia, fever, hypotension, respiratory depression, and coma. Charcoal hemoperfusion or hemodialysis may be useful, especially in the presence of very high serum barbiturate levels when the patient is in shock, coma, or renal failure. Forced alkaline diuresis is of no value in the treatment of intoxications with short-acting barbiturates.

Pharmacodynamics/Kinetics

Onset of Action: Onset of hypnosis: 15-30 minutes

Duration of Action: 3-4 hours with 100 mg dose

Time to Peak: Serum: Within 2-4 hours

Protein Binding: 45% to 60%

Half-Life Elimination: 15-40 hours, mean: 28 hours

Metabolism: Hepatic, by microsomal enzyme system

Excretion: Urine (as inactive metabolites, small amounts as unchanged drug)

Dosing

Adults: Insomnia (hypnotic): Oral: 100 mg/dose at bedtime; range: 100-200 mg/dose

Elderly: Not recommended for use in the elderly (see Geriatric Considerations).

Pediatrics:

Preoperative sedation: Oral: Children: 2-6 mg/kg (maximum dose: 100 mg/dose) 1-2 hours before procedure

Sedation: Oral: Children: 6 mg/kg/day divided every 8 hours

Renal Impairment: Slightly dialyzable (5% to 20%)

Available Dosage Forms Capsule, as sodium: 100 mg

Monitoring and Teaching Issues

Physical Assessment: Assess effectiveness and interactions of other medications patient may be taking. Assess patient for history of addiction; long-term use can result in dependence, abuse, or tolerance and evaluate periodically for need for continued use. Assess for CNS depression. Monitor vital signs and respiratory status. After long-term use, taper dosage slowly when discontinuing. **I.V.:** Monitor infusion site frequently; patient should be carefully monitored and safety/seizure precautions observed. **Oral:** For inpatient use, institute safety measures. For outpatient use, monitor effectiveness and adverse reactions at beginning of therapy and periodically with long-term use. Assess knowledge/teach patient appropriate use, interventions to reduce side effects, and adverse symptoms to report.

Patient Education: Use exactly as directed; do not increase dose or frequency or discontinue without consulting prescriber. Drug may cause physical and/or psychological dependence. While using this medication, do not use alcohol or other prescription or OTC medications (especially, pain medications, sedatives, antihistamines, or hypnotics) without consulting prescriber. Maintain adequate hydration (2-3 L/day of fluids) unless instructed to restrict fluid intake. You may experience drowsiness, dizziness, or blurred vision (use caution when driving or engaging in tasks requiring alertness until response to drug is known); nausea or vomiting (small frequent meals, frequent mouth care, chewing gum, or sucking lozenges may help); or constipation (increased exercise, fluids, fruit, or fiber may help). Report skin rash or irritation; CNS changes (confusion, depression, increased sedation, excitation, headache, insomnia, or nightmares); respiratory difficulty or shortness of breath; difficulty swallowing or feeling of tightness in throat; unusual weakness or unusual bleeding in mouth, urine, or stool; or other unanticipated adverse effects. **Pregnancy/breast-feeding precautions:** Do not get pregnant while taking this medication. Use appropriate contraceptive measures. Consult prescriber if breast-feeding.

(Continued)

Secobarbital *(Continued)*

Geriatric Considerations: Use of this agent in the elderly is not recommended due to its long half-life and addiction potential.

Pregnancy Risk Factor: D

Lactation: Enters breast milk/use caution (AAP rates "compatible")

Administration

I.V.: Maximum infusion rate: 50 mg/15 seconds; avoid intra-arterial injection.

Reconstitution: Do not shake vial during reconstitution, rotate ampul. Aqueous solutions are not stable, reconstitute with aqueous polyethylene glycol. Aqueous (sterile water) solutions should be used within 30 minutes. Do not use bacteriostatic water for injection or lactated Ringer's.

Compatibility: I.V. formulation: **Incompatible** with benzquinamide (in syringe), cimetidine (same syringe), codeine, erythromycin, glycopyrrolate (same syringe), hydrocortisone, insulin, levorphanol, methadone, norepinephrine, pentazocine, phenytoin, sodium bicarbonate, tetracycline, and vancomycin

Related Information

Anxiolytic / Hypnotic Use in Long-Term Care Facilities *on page 1769*
Compatibility of Drugs in Syringe *on page 1725*
Federal OBRA Regulations: Recommended Maximum Doses *on page 1773*

♦ **Secobarbital Sodium** *see Secobarbital on page 1362*

♦ **Seconal®** *see Secobarbital on page 1362*

♦ **Secretin** *see page 1625*

♦ **Secretin Ferring Powder** *see page 1625*

♦ **Selected Adverse Effects** *see page 1673*

Selegiline *(se LE ji leen)*

U.S. Brand Names Eldepryl®

Synonyms Deprenyl; L-Deprenyl; Selegiline Hydrochloride

Generic Available Yes

Pharmacologic Category Antidepressant, Monoamine Oxidase Inhibitor; Anti-Parkinson's Agent, MAO Type B Inhibitor

Medication Safety Issues

Sound-alike/look-alike issues:

Selegiline may be confused with Serentil®, sertraline, Serzone®, Stelazine®

Eldepryl® may be confused with Elavil®, enalapril

Use Adjunct in the management of parkinsonian patients in which levodopa/carbidopa therapy is deteriorating

Unlabeled/Investigational Use Early Parkinson's disease; attention-deficit/hyperactivity disorder (ADHD); negative symptoms of schizophrenia; extrapyramidal symptoms; depression; Alzheimer's disease (studies have shown some improvement in behavioral and cognitive performance)

Mechanism of Action/Effect Potent monoamine oxidase (MAO) type B inhibitor; MAO type B plays a major role in the metabolism of dopamine; selegiline may also increase dopaminergic activity by interfering with dopamine reuptake at the synapse

Contraindications Hypersensitivity to selegiline or any component of the formulation; concomitant use of meperidine

Warnings/Precautions Increased risk of nonselective MAO inhibition occurs with doses >10 mg/day. A MAO inhibitor type "B", there should **not** be a problem with tyramine-containing products as long as the typical doses are employed, however, rare reactions have been reported. The possibility of a suicide attempt is inherent in major depression and may persist until remission occurs. Use caution in high-risk patients during initiation of therapy. Prescriptions should be written for the smallest quantity consistent with good patient care.

Drug Interactions

Cytochrome P450 Effect: Substrate of CYP1A2 (minor), 2A6 (minor), 2B6 (major), 2C8/9 (major), 2D6 (minor), 3A4 (minor); **Inhibits** CYP1A2 (weak), 2A6 (weak), 2C8/9 (weak), 2C19 (weak), 2D6 (weak), 2E1 (weak), 3A4 (weak)

Decreased Effect: CYP2B6 inducers may decrease the levels/effects of selegiline; example inducers include carbamazepine, nevirapine, phenobarbital, phenytoin, and rifampin. CYP2C8/9 inducers may decrease the levels/effects of selegiline; example inducers include carbamazepine, phenobarbital, phenytoin, rifampin, rifapentine, and secobarbital.

Increased Effect/Toxicity: CYP2B6 inhibitors may increase the levels/effects of selegiline; example inhibitors include desipramine, paroxetine, and sertraline. CYP2C8/9 inhibitors may increase the levels/effects of selegiline; example inhibitors include delavirdine, fluconazole, gemfibrozil, ketoconazole, nicardipine, NSAIDs, and sulfonamides. Concurrent use of selegiline (high dose) in combination with amphetamines, methylphenidate, dextromethorphan, fenfluramine, meperidine, nefazodone, sibutramine, tramadol, trazodone, tricyclic antidepressants, and venlafaxine may result in serotonin syndrome; these combinations are best avoided. Concurrent use of selegiline with an SSRI may result in mania or hypertension; it is generally best to avoid these combinations. Selegiline (>10 mg/day) in combination with tyramine (cheese, ethanol) may increase the pressor response; avoid high tyramine-containing foods in patients receiving >10 mg/day of selegiline. The toxicity of levodopa (hypertension), lithium (hyperpyrexia), and reserpine may be increased by MAO inhibitors.

Nutritional/Ethanol Interactions

Ethanol: Avoid ethanol. Avoid beverages containing tyramine (wine [Chianti and hearty red] and beer).

Food: Selegiline may cause sudden and severe high blood pressure when taken with food high in tyramine (cheeses, sour cream, yogurt, pickled herring, chicken liver, canned figs, raisins, bananas, avocados, soy sauce, broad bean pods, yeast extracts, meats prepared with tenderizers, and many foods aged to improve flavor). Small amounts of caffeine may produce irregular heartbeat or high blood pressure and can interact with this medication for up to 2 weeks after stopping its use.

Herb/Nutraceutical: Avoid valerian, St John's wort, SAMe, kava kava (may increase risk of serotonin syndrome and/or excessive sedation).

Adverse Reactions Frequency not defined.

Cardiovascular: Orthostatic hypotension, hypertension, arrhythmia, palpitation, angina, tachycardia, peripheral edema, bradycardia, syncope

Central nervous system: Hallucinations, dizziness, confusion, anxiety, depression, drowsiness, behavior/mood changes, dreams/nightmares, fatigue, delusions

Dermatologic: Rash, photosensitivity

Gastrointestinal: Xerostomia, nausea, vomiting, constipation, weight loss, anorexia, diarrhea, heartburn

Genitourinary: Nocturia, prostatic hyperplasia, urinary retention, sexual dysfunction

Neuromuscular & skeletal: Tremor, chorea, loss of balance, restlessness, bradykinesia

Ocular: Blepharospasm, blurred vision

Miscellaneous: Diaphoresis (increased)

Overdosage/Toxicology Symptoms of overdose include tachycardia, palpitations, muscle twitching, and seizures. Both hypertension or hypotension can occur with intoxication. While treating hypertension, care is warranted to avoid sudden drops in blood pressure, since this may worsen MAO inhibitor toxicity. Cardiac arrhythmias are best treated with phenytoin or procainamide. Treatment is generally symptom-directed and supportive.

Pharmacodynamics/Kinetics

Onset of Action: Therapeutic: Within 1 hour

Duration of Action: 24-72 hours

Half-Life Elimination: Steady state: 10 hours

Metabolism: Hepatic to amphetamine and methamphetamine

Dosing

Adults: Parkinson's disease: Oral: 5 mg twice daily with breakfast and lunch or 10 mg in the morning

Elderly: Oral: Initial: 5 mg in the morning; may increase to a total of 10 mg/day.

Pediatrics: Children and Adolescents: ADHD (unlabeled use): Oral: 5-15 mg/day

Available Dosage Forms

Capsule, as hydrochloride (Eldepryl®): 5 mg

Tablet, as hydrochloride: 5 mg

Monitoring and Teaching Issues

Physical Assessment: Assess effectiveness and interactions of other medications patient may be taking. Monitor therapeutic effectiveness according to rationale for therapy and adverse reactions at beginning of therapy and periodically throughout therapy. Monitor blood pressure. Be alert to thoughts of suicide. Patient should be cautioned against eating foods high in tyramine (see Tyramine Content of Foods list *on page 1758*). Assess knowledge/teach patient appropriate use, interventions to reduce side effects, and adverse symptoms to report.

Patient Education: Take exactly as directed (may be prescribed in conjunction with levodopa/carbidopa); do not change dosage or discontinue without consulting prescriber. Therapeutic effects may take several weeks or months to achieve and you may need frequent monitoring during first weeks of therapy. Take with meals if GI upset occurs, before meals if dry mouth occurs, or after eating if drooling or if nausea occurs. Take at the same time each day. Avoid tyramine-containing foods (low potential for reaction). Maintain adequate hydration (2-3 L/day of fluids) unless instructed to restrict fluid intake; void before taking medication. Do not use alcohol and prescription or OTC sedatives or CNS depressants without consulting prescriber. You may experience drowsiness, dizziness, confusion, or vision changes (use caution when driving, climbing stairs, or engaging in tasks requiring alertness until response to drug is known); orthostatic hypotension (use caution when changing position - rising to standing from sitting or lying); constipation (increased exercise, fluids, fruit, or fiber may help); runny nose or flu-like symptoms (consult prescriber for appropriate relief); or nausea, vomiting, loss of appetite, or stomach discomfort (small frequent meals, frequent mouth care, chewing gum, or sucking lozenges may help). Report unresolved constipation or vomiting; chest pain, palpitations, irregular heartbeat; CNS changes (hallucination, loss of memory, seizures, acute headache, nervousness, thoughts of suicide, etc); painful or difficult urination; increased muscle spasticity, rigidity, or involuntary movements; skin rash; or significant worsening of condition. **Pregnancy/breast-feeding precautions:** Inform prescriber if you are or intend to become pregnant. Consult prescriber if breast-feeding.

Geriatric Considerations: Selegiline is also being studied in Alzheimer's disease, but further studies are needed to assess its usefulness. Do not use at daily doses exceeding 10 mg/day because of the risks associated with nonselective inhibition of MAO.

Pregnancy Risk Factor: C

Lactation: Excretion in breast milk unknown

Additional Information When adding selegiline to levodopa/carbidopa, the dose of the latter can usually be decreased. Studies are investigating the use of selegiline in early Parkinson's disease to slow the progression of the disease.

Related Information

Tyramine Content of Foods *on page 1758*

♦ Selegiline Hydrochloride *see* Selegiline *on page 1364*

♦ Semprex®-D *see* Acrivastine and Pseudoephedrine *on page 47*

♦ Senexon® [OTC] *see* Senna *on page 1365*

Senna (SEN na)

U.S. Brand Names Agoral® Maximum Strength Laxative [OTC]; Evac-U-Gen [OTC]; ex-lax® [OTC]; ex-lax® Maximum Strength [OTC]; Fletcher's® Castoria® [OTC]; Senexon® [OTC]; Senna-Gen® [OTC]; Sennatural™ [OTC]; Senokot® [OTC]; Senokot® Children's [OTC]; SenokotXTRA® [OTC]; X-Prep® [OTC]

Generic Available Yes: Tablet

(Continued)

Senna *(Continued)*

Pharmacologic Category Laxative, Stimulant

Medication Safety Issues
Sound-alike/look-alike issues:
Senexon® may be confused with Cenestin®
Senokot® may be confused with Depakote®

Use Short-term treatment of constipation; evacuate the colon for bowel or rectal examinations

Contraindications Per Commission E: Intestinal obstruction, acute intestinal inflammation (eg, Crohn's disease), colitis ulcerosa, appendicitis, abdominal pain of unknown origin; pregnancy

Warnings/Precautions Not recommended for over-the-counter (OTC) use in patients experiencing stomach pain, nausea, vomiting, or a sudden change in bowel movements which lasts >2 weeks. Not recommended for OTC use in children <2 years of age.

Adverse Reactions Frequency not defined: Gastrointestinal: Nausea, vomiting, diarrhea, abdominal cramps

Dosing
Adults & Elderly:
Bowel evacuation: Oral: OTC labeling: Usual dose: Sennosides 130 mg (X-Prep® 75 mL) between 2-4 PM the afternoon of the day prior to procedure
Constipation: Oral: OTC ranges: Sennosides 15 mg once daily (maximum: 70-100 mg/day, divided twice daily)

Pediatrics:
Bowel evacuation: OTC labeling: Children ≥12 years: Refer to adult dosing.
Constipation: OTC ranges: Children:
2-6 years:
Sennosides: Initial: 3.75 mg once daily (maximum: 15 mg/day, divided twice daily)
Senna concentrate: 33.3 mg/mL: 5-10 mL up to twice daily
6-12 years:
Sennosides: Initial: 8.6 mg once daily (maximum: 50 mg/day, divided twice daily)
Senna concentrate: 33.3 mg/mL: 10-30 mL up to twice daily
≥12 years: Refer to adult dosing.

Available Dosage Forms
Granules (Senokot®): Sennosides 15 mg/teaspoon (60 g, 180 g, 360 g) [cocoa flavor]
Liquid:
Agoral® Maximum Strength Laxative: Sennosides 25 mg/15 mL (480 mL) [contains sodium 19.6 mg/15 mL; marshmallow and raspberry flavors]
X-Prep®: Sennosides 8.8 mg/5 mL (75 mL) [alcohol free; contains sugar 50 g/75 mL; available individually or in a kit]
Liquid concentrate:
Fletcher's® Castoria®: Senna concentrate 33.3 mg/mL (75 mL) [alcohol free; contains sodium benzoate; root beer flavor]
Syrup:
Senokot®: Sennosides 8.8 mg/5 mL (240 mL) [alcohol free; cocoa flavor]
Senokot® Children's: Sennosides 8.8 mg/5 mL (74 mL) [alcohol free; chocolate flavor]
Tablet: Sennosides 8.6 mg
ex-lax®: Sennosides USP 15 mg [contains sodium benzoate]
ex-lax® Maximum Strength: Sennosides USP 25 mg [contains sodium benzoate]
Sennatural™, Senokot®, Senexon®, Senna-Gen®: Sennosides 8.6 mg
SenokotXTRA®: Sennosides 17 mg
Tablet, chewable:
ex-lax®: Sennosides USP 15 mg [chocolate flavor]
Evac-U-Gen: Sennosides 10 mg

Monitoring and Teaching Issues
Patient Education: May discolor urine or feces (yellow, brown, pink, red, or violet); may cause dependence with prolonged or excessive use. Bowel movements usually occur within 6-12 hours after a dose. Notify prescriber for failure to have a bowel movement after the first dose or for rectal bleeding. OTC labeling does not recommend for use longer than 1 week, use in children <2 years, or in women who are pregnant or breast-feeding.
Dietary Considerations: Liquid may be administered with fruit juice or milk to mask taste. X-Prep® liquid contains sugar 50 g/75 mL.

Administration
Oral: Once daily doses should be taken at bedtime. Granules may be eaten plain, sprinkled on food, or mixed in liquids
Additional Information Some products that may have previously been labeled as standardized senna concentrate are now labeled as sennosides. For example, Senokot® tablets, previously labeled as standardized senna concentrate 187 mg, are now labeled as sennosides 8.6 mg. The actual content of senna in this product did not change. Individual product labeling should be consulted prior to dosing.

Related Information
Laxatives, Classification and Properties *on page 1737*

♦ **Senna and Docusate** *see* Docusate and Senna *on page 475*
♦ **Senna-Gen® [OTC]** *see* Senna *on page 1365*
♦ **Senna-S** *see* Docusate and Senna *on page 475*
♦ **Sennatural™ [OTC]** *see* Senna *on page 1365*
♦ **Senokot® [OTC]** *see* Senna *on page 1365*
♦ **Senokot® Children's [OTC]** *see* Senna *on page 1365*
♦ **Senokot-S® [OTC]** *see* Docusate and Senna *on page 475*
♦ **SenokotXTRA® [OTC]** *see* Senna *on page 1365*
♦ **Sensipar™** *see* Cinacalcet *on page 326*
♦ **Sensorcaine®** *see* Bupivacaine *on page 214*
♦ **Sensorcaine®-MPF** *see* Bupivacaine *on page 214*

- **Septra®** *see* Sulfamethoxazole and Trimethoprim *on page 1407*
- **Septra® DS** *see* Sulfamethoxazole and Trimethoprim *on page 1407*
- **Serax®** *see* Oxazepam *on page 1130*
- **Serentil® [DSC]** *see* Mesoridazine *on page 960*
- **Serevent® Diskus®** *see* Salmeterol *on page 1352*
- **Sermorelin Acetate** *see page 1625*
- **Seromycin®** *see* CycloSERINE *on page 382*
- **Serophene®** *see* ClomiPHENE *on page 349*
- **Seroquel®** *see* Quetiapine *on page 1292*
- **Serostim®** *see* Human Growth Hormone *on page 745*
- **Serotonin Syndrome** *see page 1680*

Sertaconazole (ser ta KOE na zole)

U.S. Brand Names Ertaczo™
Synonyms Sertaconazole Nitrate
Generic Available No
Pharmacologic Category Antifungal Agent, Topical
Use Topical treatment of tinea pedis (athlete's foot)
Mechanism of Action/Effect Alters fungal cell wall membrane permeability
Contraindications Hypersensitivity to sertaconazole, other imidazoles (manufacturer-based contraindication), or any component of the formulation
Warnings/Precautions Discontinue drug if sensitivity or chemical irritation occurs. For external use only; not for ophthalmic or intravaginal use. Hypersensitivity to one imidazole antifungal may result in cross-reactivity with another. Safety and efficacy have not been established in pediatric patients <12 years of age.
Adverse Reactions 1% to 10%: Dermatologic: Burning, contact dermatitis, dry skin, tenderness
Pharmacodynamics/Kinetics
 Absorption: Topical: Minimal
Dosing
 Adults & Elderly: Tinea pedis: Topical: Apply between toes and to surrounding healthy skin twice daily for 4 weeks
 Pediatrics: Tinea pedis: Topical: Children ≥12 years: Refer to adult dosing.
Available Dosage Forms Cream, topical, as nitrate: 2% (15 g, 30 g)
Monitoring and Teaching Issues
 Physical Assessment: For external use only; not for ophthalmic or intravaginal use. Teach patient proper use, appropriate interventions to reduce side effects, and adverse symptoms to report (see Patient Education).
 Patient Education: This medication is for topical use only. Avoid contact with eyes, nose, mouth, and other mucous membranes. Use exactly as directed. Wash feet and dry thoroughly. Apply to affected area between toes and to surrounding healthy skin. Avoid use of occlusive dressing. Wash hands thoroughly after application; infection can be spread to other parts of your body or to other persons. Wear socks that keep your feet dry and change them frequently if you perspire heavily. Do not share foot wear with others. May cause dry skin, mild tenderness, or slight discomfort (burning) after application. Stop using and contact prescriber if burning or tenderness persists or if other adverse skin reactions occur. **Pregnancy/breast-feeding precautions:** Inform prescriber if you are or intend to become pregnant or breast-feed.
 Pregnancy Risk Factor: C
 Lactation: Excretion in breast milk unknown/use caution
Administration
 Topical: For external use only. Apply to affected area between toes and to surrounding healthy skin. Make sure skin is dry before applying. Avoid use of occlusive dressing. Avoid contact with eyes, nose, mouth, and other mucous membranes.
 Storage: Store at 25°C (77°F).

- **Sertaconazole Nitrate** *see* Sertaconazole *on page 1367*

Sertraline (SER tra leen)

U.S. Brand Names Zoloft®
Synonyms Sertraline Hydrochloride
Restrictions A medication guide should be dispensed with each prescription. A template for the required MedGuides can be found on the FDA website at: http://www.fda.gov/cder/drug/antidepressants/labelTemplate.pdf
Generic Available No
Pharmacologic Category Antidepressant, Selective Serotonin Reuptake Inhibitor
Medication Safety Issues
 Sound-alike/look-alike issues:
  Sertraline may be confused with selegiline, Serentil®
  Zoloft® may be confused with Zocor®
Use Treatment of major depression; obsessive-compulsive disorder (OCD); panic disorder; post-traumatic stress disorder (PTSD); premenstrual dysphoric disorder (PMDD); social anxiety disorder
Unlabeled/Investigational Use Eating disorders; generalized anxiety disorder (GAD); impulse control disorders
Mechanism of Action/Effect Antidepressant with selective inhibitory effects on presynaptic serotonin (5-HT) reuptake and only very weak effects on norepinephrine and dopamine neuronal uptake
Contraindications Hypersensitivity to sertraline or any component of the formulation; use of MAO inhibitors within 14 days; concurrent use of pimozide; concurrent use of sertraline oral concentrate with disulfiram
(Continued)

Sertraline *(Continued)*

Warnings/Precautions Antidepressants increase the risk of suicidal thinking and behavior in children and adolescents with major depressive disorder (MDD) and other depressive disorders; consider risk prior to prescribing. All patients must be closely monitored for clinical worsening, suicidality, or unusual changes in behavior, especially during the initiation of therapy or following an increase or decrease in dosage. When used in children, the child's family or caregiver should be instructed to closely observe the patient and communicate condition with healthcare provider. A medication guide should be dispensed with each prescription. **Sertraline is FDA approved for the treatment of OCD in children ≥6 years of age.**

The possibility of a suicide attempt is inherent in major depression and may persist until remission occurs. Use caution in high-risk patients. Worsening depression and severe abrupt suicidality that are not part of the presenting symptoms may require discontinuation or modification of drug therapy. The patient's family or caregiver should be alerted to monitor patients for the emergence of suicidality and associated behaviors (such as agitation, irritability, hostility, impulsivity, and hypomania) and call healthcare provider.

May worsen psychosis in some patients or precipitate a shift to mania or hypomania in patients with bipolar disorder. Patients presenting with depressive symptoms should be screened for bipolar disorder. Monotherapy in patients with bipolar disorder should be avoided. **Sertraline is not FDA approved for the treatment of bipolar depression.**

The potential for severe reaction exists when used with MAO inhibitors - serotonin syndrome (hyperthermia, muscular rigidity, mental status changes/agitation, autonomic instability) may occur. Has a very low potential to impair cognitive or motor performance. However, caution patients regarding activities requiring alertness until response to sertraline is known. Does not appear to potentiate the effects of alcohol, however, ethanol use is not advised.

Use caution in patients with a previous seizure disorder or condition predisposing to seizures such as brain damage, alcoholism, or concurrent therapy with other drugs which lower the seizure threshold. May increase the risks associated with electroconvulsive therapy. Use with caution in patients with hepatic or renal dysfunction and in elderly patients. May cause hyponatremia/SIADH. Use with caution in patients with renal insufficiency or other concurrent illness (due to limited experience). Sertraline acts as a mild uricosuric; use with caution in patients at risk of uric acid nephropathy. Use with caution in patients at risk of bleeding or receiving anticoagulant therapy; may cause impairment in platelet aggregation. Use with caution in patients where weight loss is undesirable. May cause or exacerbate sexual dysfunction.

Use oral concentrate formulation with caution in patients with latex sensitivity; dropper dispenser contains dry natural rubber. Monitor growth in pediatric patients. Discontinuation symptoms (eg, dysphoric mood, irritability, agitation, confusion, anxiety, insomnia, hypomania) may occur upon abrupt discontinuation. Taper dose when discontinuing therapy.

Drug Interactions

Cytochrome P450 Effect: Substrate of CYP2B6 (minor), 2C8/9 (minor), 2C19 (major), 2D6 (major), 3A4 (minor); **Inhibits** CYP1A2 (weak), 2B6(moderate), 2C8/9 (weak), 2C19 (moderate), 2D6 (moderate), 3A4 (moderate)

Decreased Effect: The levels/effects of sertraline may be decreased by aminoglutethimide, carbamazepine, phenytoin, rifampin, and other CYP2C19 inducers. Sertraline may decrease the metabolism of tolbutamide; monitor for changes in glucose control. Sertraline may decrease the levels/effects of CYP2D6 prodrug substrates (eg, codeine, hydrocodone, oxycodone, tramadol).

Increased Effect/Toxicity: Sertraline should not be used with nonselective MAO inhibitors (phenelzine, isocarboxazid) or other drugs with MAO inhibition (linezolid); fatal reactions have been reported. Wait 5 weeks after stopping sertraline before starting a nonselective MAO inhibitor and 2 weeks after stopping an MAO inhibitor before starting sertraline. Concurrent selegiline has been associated with mania, hypertension, or serotonin syndrome (risk may be reduced relative to nonselective MAO inhibitors). Sertraline may increase serum concentrations of pimozide; concurrent use is contraindicated. Avoid use of oral concentrate with disulfiram.

Sertraline may inhibit the metabolism of thioridazine or mesoridazine, resulting in increased plasma levels and increasing the risk of QT$_c$ interval prolongation. This may lead to serious ventricular arrhythmias, such as torsade de pointes-type arrhythmias and sudden death. Do not use together. Wait at least 5 weeks after discontinuing sertraline prior to starting thioridazine.

Sertraline may increase the levels/effects of levels/effects of amphetamines, selected beta-blockers, bupropion, selected benzodiazepines, calcium channel blockers, cisapride, cyclosporine, dextromethorphan, ergot alkaloids, fluoxetine, selected HMG-CoA reductase inhibitors, lidocaine, mesoridazine, mirtazapine, nateglinide, nefazodone, paroxetine,promethazine, propofol, risperidone, ritonavir, selegiline, sildenafil (and other PDE-5 inhibitors), tacrolimus, thioridazine, tricyclic antidepressants, venlafaxine, and other substrates of CYP2B6, 2D6 or 3A4. Sertraline may increase the hypoprothrombinemic response to warfarin.

The levels/effects of sertraline may be increased by chlorpromazine, delavirdine, fluconazole, fluoxetine, fluvoxamine, gemfibrozil, isoniazid, miconazole, omeprazole, paroxetine, pergolide, quinidine, quinine, ritonavir, ropinirole, ticlopidine, and other CYP2C19 or 2D6 inhibitors.

Combined use of SSRIs and amphetamines, buspirone, meperidine, nefazodone, serotonin agonists (such as sumatriptan), sibutramine, other SSRIs, sympathomimetics, ritonavir, tramadol, and venlafaxine may increase the risk of serotonin syndrome. Combined use of sumatriptan (and other serotonin agonists) may result in toxicity; weakness, hyper-reflexia, and incoordination have been observed with sumatriptan and SSRIs. In addition, concurrent use may theoretically increase the risk of serotonin syndrome; includes sumatriptan, naratriptan, rizatriptan, and zolmitriptan.

Concurrent lithium may increase risk of nephrotoxicity. Risk of hyponatremia may increase with concurrent use of loop diuretics (bumetanide, furosemide, torsemide). Concomitant use of sertraline and NSAIDs, aspirin, or other drugs affecting coagulation has been associated with an increased risk of bleeding; monitor.

Nutritional/Ethanol Interactions
Ethanol: Avoid ethanol (may increase CNS depression).
Food: Sertraline average peak serum levels may be increased if taken with food.
Herb/Nutraceutical: Avoid valerian, St John's wort, kava kava, gotu kola (may increase CNS depression).

Lab Interactions Increased (minor) triglycerides (S), LFTs; decreased uric acid (S)

Adverse Reactions
>10%:
  Central nervous system: Insomnia, somnolence, dizziness, headache, fatigue
  Gastrointestinal: Xerostomia, diarrhea, nausea
  Genitourinary: Ejaculatory disturbances
1% to 10%:
  Cardiovascular: Palpitations
  Central nervous system: Agitation, anxiety, nervousness
  Dermatologic: Rash
  Endocrine & metabolic: Decreased libido
  Gastrointestinal: Constipation, anorexia, dyspepsia, flatulence, vomiting, weight gain
  Genitourinary: Micturition disorders
  Neuromuscular & skeletal: Tremors, paresthesia
  Ocular: Visual difficulty, abnormal vision
  Otic: Tinnitus
  Miscellaneous: Diaphoresis (increased)

Additional adverse reactions reported in pediatric patients (frequency >2%): Aggressiveness, epistaxis, hyperkinesia, purpura, sinusitis, urinary incontinence

Overdosage/Toxicology Among 634 patients who overdosed on sertraline alone, 8 resulted in a fatal outcome. Symptoms of overdose include somnolence, vomiting, tachycardia, nausea, dizziness, agitation, and tremor. Treatment is symptomatic and supportive.

Pharmacodynamics/Kinetics
Absorption: Slow
Bioavailability: 88%
Time to Peak: Plasma: 4.5-8.4 hours
Protein Binding: 98%
Half-Life Elimination: Parent drug: 26 hours; Metabolite N-desmethylsertraline: 66 hours (range: 62-104 hours)
Metabolism: Hepatic; extensive first-pass metabolism
Excretion: Urine and feces

Dosing
Adults:
Depression/OCD: Oral: Initial: 50 mg/day
  Note: May increase daily dose, at intervals of not less than 1 week, to a maximum of 200 mg/day. If somnolence is noted, give at bedtime.
Panic disorder, PTSD, social anxiety disorder: Oral: Initial: 25 mg once daily; increased after 1 week to 50 mg once daily (see "Note" above)
Premenstrual dysphoric disorder (PMDD): 50 mg/day either daily throughout menstrual cycle **or** limited to the luteal phase of menstrual cycle, depending on physician assessment. Patients not responding to 50 mg/day may benefit from dose increases (50 mg increments per menstrual cycle) up to 150 mg/day when dosing throughout menstrual cycle **or** up to 100 mg day when dosing during luteal phase only. If a 100 mg/day dose has been established with luteal phase dosing, a 50 mg/day titration step for 3 days should be utilized at the beginning of each luteal phase dosing period.
Elderly: Oral: Initial: 25 mg/day in the morning; increase by 25 mg/day increments every 2-3 days if tolerated to 50-100 mg/day; additional increases may be necessary; maximum: 200 mg/day.
Pediatrics:
OCD: Oral: Children:
  6-12 years: Initial: 25 mg once daily
  13-17 years: Initial: 50 mg once daily
  May increase daily dose, at intervals of not less than 1 week, to a maximum: 200 mg/day. If somnolence is noted, give at bedtime.
Renal Impairment: Multiple-dose pharmacokinetics are unaffected by renal impairment. Hemodialysis effect: Not removed by hemodialysis
Hepatic Impairment: Sertraline is extensively metabolized by the liver. Caution should be used in patients with hepatic impairment. A lower dose or less frequent dosing should be used.

Available Dosage Forms Note: Available as sertraline hydrochloride; mg strength refers to sertraline
Solution, oral concentrate: 20 mg/mL (60 mL) [contains alcohol 12%]
Tablet: 25 mg, 50 mg, 100 mg

Monitoring and Teaching Issues
Physical Assessment: Assess other medications patient may be taking for effectiveness and interactions. Assess mental status for worsening of depression, suicidal ideation, anxiety, social functioning, mania, or panic attack (especially during initiation of therapy and when dosage is changed). Taper dosage slowly when discontinuing. Assess knowledge/teach patient appropriate use, interventions to reduce side effects, and adverse symptoms to report. Pediatric patients: Monitor growth pattern.
Patient Education: Take exactly as directed; do not increase dose or frequency; or discontinue use abruptly. It may take 2-3 weeks to achieve desired results. Take in the morning to reduce the incidence of insomnia. Avoid alcohol, caffeine, and other prescription or OTC medications not approved by prescriber. Maintain adequate hydration (2-3 L/
(Continued)

Sertraline *(Continued)*

day of fluids) unless instructed to restrict fluid intake. You may experience drowsiness, dizziness, or lightheadedness (use caution when driving or engaging in tasks requiring alertness until response to drug is known); nausea, vomiting, anorexia, or dry mouth (small frequent meals, frequent mouth care, chewing gum, or sucking lozenges may help); postural hypotension (use caution when climbing stairs or changing position from sitting or lying to standing); urinary pattern changes (void before taking medication); or male sexual dysfunction (reversible). Report persistent insomnia or daytime sedation, agitation, nervousness, fatigue; muscle cramping, tremors, weakness, or change in gait; chest pain, palpitations, or swelling of extremities; vision changes or eye pain; hearing changes (ringing in ears); respiratory difficulty or breathlessness; skin rash or irritation; suicidal ideation; or worsening of condition. **Pregnancy/breast-feeding precautions:** Inform prescriber if you are or intend to become pregnant. Breast-feeding is not recommended.

Geriatric Considerations: Sertraline's favorable side effect profile makes it a useful alternative to the traditional tricyclic antidepressants. Its potential stimulation effect and anorexia may be bothersome.

Pregnancy Risk Factor: C

Pregnancy Issues: Nonteratogenic effects including respiratory distress, cyanosis, apnea, seizures, temperature instability, feeding difficulty, vomiting, hypoglycemia, hypo- or hypertonia, hyper-reflexia, jitteriness, irritability, constant crying, and tremor have been reported in the neonate immediately following delivery after exposure of other SSRIs late in the third trimester. Adverse effects may be due to toxic effects of SSRI or drug discontinuation. In some cases, may present clinically as serotonin syndrome. There are no adequate and well-controlled studies in pregnant women. Use during pregnancy only if the potential benefit to the mother outweighs the possible risk to the fetus. If treatment during pregnancy is required, consider tapering therapy during the third trimester.

Lactation: Enters breast milk/not recommended (AAP rates "of concern")

Administration

Oral: Oral concentrate: Must be diluted before use. Immediately before administration, use the dropper provided to measure the required amount of concentrate; mix with 4 ounces ($^1/_2$ cup) of water, ginger ale, lemon/lime soda, lemonade, or orange juice **only**. Do not mix with any other liquids than these. The dose should be taken immediately after mixing; do not mix in advance. A slight haze may appear after mixing; this is normal. **Note:** Use with caution in patients with latex sensitivity; dropper dispenser contains dry natural rubber.

Storage: Tablets and oral solution should be stored at controlled room temperature of 15°C to 30°C (59°F to 86°F).

Additional Information Buspirone (15-60 mg/day) may be useful in treatment of sexual dysfunction during treatment with a selective serotonin reuptake inhibitor. May exacerbate tics in Tourette's syndrome.

Related Information

Antidepressant Agents *on page 1713*
Antidepressant Medication Guidelines *on page 1765*

♦ **Sertraline Hydrochloride** *see Sertraline on page 1367*

♦ **Serutan® [OTC]** *see Psyllium on page 1284*

♦ **Serzone® [DSC]** *see Nefazodone on page 1063*

Sevelamer *(se VEL a mer)*

U.S. Brand Names Renagel®

Synonyms Sevelamer Hydrochloride

Generic Available No

Pharmacologic Category Phosphate Binder

Medication Safety Issues

Sound-alike/look-alike issues:
Renagel® may be confused with Reglan®, Regonol®

Use Reduction of serum phosphorous in patients with end-stage renal disease

Mechanism of Action/Effect Sevelamer (a polymeric compound) binds phosphate within the intestinal lumen, limiting absorption and decreasing serum phosphate concentrations without altering calcium, aluminum, or bicarbonate concentrations.

Contraindications Hypersensitivity to sevelamer or any component of the formulation; hypophosphatemia; bowel obstruction

Warnings/Precautions Use with caution in patients with gastrointestinal disorders including dysphagia, swallowing disorders, severe gastrointestinal motility disorders, or major gastrointestinal surgery. May cause reductions in vitamin D, E, K, and folic acid absorption. Long-term studies of carcinogenic potential have not been completed. Capsules should not be taken apart or chewed.

Drug Interactions

Decreased Effect: Sevelamer may bind to some drugs in the gastrointestinal tract and decrease their absorption. When changes in absorption of oral medications may have significant clinical consequences (such as antiarrhythmic and antiseizure medications), these medications should be taken at least 1 hour before or 3 hours after a dose of sevelamer.

Adverse Reactions

>10%:
Cardiovascular: Hypotension (11%), thrombosis (10%)
Central nervous system: Headache (10%)
Endocrine & metabolic: Decreased absorption of vitamins D, E, K and folic acid
Gastrointestinal: Diarrhea (16%), dyspepsia (5% to 11%), vomiting (12%)
Neuromuscular & skeletal: Pain (13%)
Miscellaneous: Infection (15%)
1% to 10%:
Cardiovascular: Hypertension (9%)
Gastrointestinal: Nausea (7%), flatulence (4%), diarrhea (4%), constipation (2%)

Respiratory: Cough (4%)

Overdosage/Toxicology Sevelamer is not absorbed systemically. There are no reports of overdosage in patients.

Pharmacodynamics/Kinetics
Absorption: None
Excretion: Feces

Dosing
Adults & Elderly: Reduction of serum phosphorous (ESRD): Oral:
Patients not taking a phosphate binder: 800-1600 mg 3 times/day with meals; the initial dose may be based on serum phosphorous.
Phosphorous: Initial:
>6.0 mg/dL and <7.5 mg/dL: 800 mg 3 times/day
≥7.5 mg/dL and <9.0 mg/dL: 1200-1600 mg 3 times/day
≥9.0 mg/dL: 1600 mg 3 times/day
Adjustment: Dosage should be adjusted based on serum phosphorous concentration, with a goal of lowering to <6.0 mg/dL; maximum daily dose studied was equivalent to 30 capsules/day.

Available Dosage Forms
Capsule, as hydrochloride: 403 mg
Tablet, as hydrochloride: 400 mg, 800 mg

Monitoring and Teaching Issues
Physical Assessment: Assess knowledge/teach patient appropriate use, possible side effects/interventions, and adverse symptoms to report. Monitor blood pressure.
Monitoring Laboratory Tests: Serum phosphorus
Patient Education: Take as directed, with meals. Do not break or chew capsules or tablets (contents will expand in water). You may experience headache or dizziness (use caution when driving or engaging in tasks requiring alertness until response to drug is known); nausea or vomiting (small frequent meals, frequent mouth care, or sucking hard candy may help); diarrhea (yogurt or buttermilk may help); hypotension (use caution when rising from sitting or lying position or when climbing stairs or bending over); or mild neuromuscular pain or stiffness (mild analgesic may help). Report persistent adverse reactions. **Pregnancy/breast-feeding precautions:** Inform prescriber if you are or intend to become pregnant. Consult prescriber if breast-feeding.
Pregnancy Risk Factor: C
Pregnancy Issues: Because sevelamer may cause a reduction in the absorption of some vitamins, it should be used with caution in pregnant women.
Lactation: Excretion in breast milk unknown/use caution (not absorbed systemically but may alter maternal nutrition)
Breast-Feeding Issues: It is not known whether sevelamer is excreted in human milk. Because sevelamer may cause a reduction in the absorption of some vitamins, it should be used with caution in nursing women.

Administration
Storage: Store at controlled room temperature.
Additional Information Switching patients from calcium acetate to sevelamer: 667 mg of calcium acetate is equivalent to 800 mg sevelamer

♦ **Sevelamer Hydrochloride** *see Sevelamer on page 1370*

Sibutramine (si BYOO tra meen)

U.S. Brand Names Meridia®
Synonyms Sibutramine Hydrochloride Monohydrate
Controlled Substance C-IV; recommended only for obese patients with a body mass index ≥30 kg/m^2 or ≥27 kg/m^2 in the presence of other risk factors such as hypertension, diabetes, and/or dyslipidemia
Generic Available No
Pharmacologic Category Anorexiant
Use Management of obesity, including weight loss and maintenance of weight loss; should be used in conjunction with a reduced-calorie diet
Mechanism of Action/Effect Sibutramine blocks the neuronal uptake of norepinephrine, serotonin, and (to a lesser extent) dopamine
Contraindications Hypersensitivity to sibutramine or any component of the formulation; during or within 2 weeks of MAO inhibitors (eg, phenelzine, selegiline) or concomitant centrally-acting appetite suppressants; anorexia nervosa; bulimia nervosa; uncontrolled or poorly-controlled hypertension; congestive heart failure; coronary heart disease; conduction disorders (arrhythmias); stroke; concurrent use of serotonergic agents (eg, SSRIs sumatriptan, dihydroergotamine, dextromethorphan, meperidine, pentazocine, fentanyl, lithium)
Warnings/Precautions Use with caution in renal impairment or hepatic dysfunction, seizure disorder, hypertension, gallstones, narrow-angle glaucoma, nursing mothers, and elderly patients. Primary pulmonary hypertension (PPH), a rare and frequently fatal pulmonary disease, has been reported to occur in patients receiving other agents with serotonergic activity which have been used as anorexiants. Although not reported in clinical trials, it is possible that sibutramine may share this potential, and patients should be monitored closely. Rare cases of bleeding have been reported; use caution in patients with bleeding disorders. Stimulants may unmask tics in individuals with coexisting Tourette's syndrome. Sibutramine may have the potential to potentiate or impair judgment or motor skills.

Serious, potentially life-threatening toxicities may occur when thyroid hormones (at dosages above usual daily hormonal requirements) are used in combination with sympathomimetic amines to induce weight loss.

Safety and efficacy have not been established with severe renal or hepatic dysfunction or in children <16 years of age.
(Continued)

Sibutramine *(Continued)*

Drug Interactions
Cytochrome P450 Effect: Substrate of CYP3A4 (major)

Decreased Effect: Inducers of CYP3A4 (including phenytoin, phenobarbital, carbamazepine, and rifampin) theoretically may reduce sibutramine serum concentrations.

Increased Effect/Toxicity: Serotonergic agents such as buspirone, selective serotonin reuptake inhibitors (eg, citalopram, fluoxetine, fluvoxamine, paroxetine, sertraline), sumatriptan (and similar serotonin agonists), dihydroergotamine, lithium, tryptophan, some opioid/analgesics (eg, meperidine, tramadol), and venlafaxine, when combined with sibutramine may result in serotonin syndrome. Dextromethorphan, MAO inhibitors and other drugs that can raise the blood pressure (eg decongestants, centrally-acting weight loss products, amphetamines, and amphetamine-like compounds) can increase the possibility of sibutramine-associated cardiovascular complications. Sibutramine may increase serum levels of tricyclic antidepressants. CYP3A4 inhibitors may increase the levels/effects of sibutramine; example inhibitors include azole antifungals, ciprofloxacin, clarithromycin, diclofenac, doxycycline, erythromycin, imatinib, isoniazid, nefazodone, nicardipine, propofol, protease inhibitors, quinidine, and verapamil.

Nutritional/Ethanol Interactions
Ethanol: Avoid excess ethanol ingestion.

Herb/Nutraceutical: St John's wort may decrease sibutramine levels.

Adverse Reactions
Frequency not defined.

Central nervous system: Thinking abnormal, agitation, fever

Dermatologic: Pruritus

Endocrine & metabolic: Menstrual disorders/irregularities

Gastrointestinal: Diarrhea, flatulence, gastroenteritis, tooth disorder

Neuromuscular & Skeletal: Arthritis, hypertonia, leg cramps

Ocular: Amblyopia

Respiratory: Bronchitis, dyspnea

>10%

Central nervous system: Headache, insomnia

Gastrointestinal: Anorexia, xerostomia, constipation

Respiratory: Rhinitis

1% to 10%

Cardiovascular: Tachycardia, vasodilation, hypertension, palpitation, chest pain, edema

Central nervous system: Migraine, dizziness, nervousness, anxiety, depression, somnolence, CNS stimulation, emotional liability

Dermatologic: Acne, herpes simplex, rash

Endocrine & metabolic: Dysmenorrhea

Gastrointestinal: Appetite increased, nausea, dyspepsia, gastritis, vomiting, taste perversion, abdominal pain, rectal disorder

Genitourinary: Urinary tract infection, vaginal *Monilia*

Hepatic: Abnormal LFTs

Neuromuscular & skeletal: Weakness, arthralgia, back pain, neck pain, myalgia

Otic: Ear disorder, ear pain

Respiratory: Pharyngitis, sinusitis, cough, laryngitis

Miscellaneous: Diaphoresis, flu-like syndrome, allergic reactions, thirst

Overdosage/Toxicology
Symptoms of overdose include hypertension, tachycardia, headache, and palpitations. Treatment is supportive.

Pharmacodynamics/Kinetics
Absorption: Rapid

Time to Peak: Within 3-4 hours

Protein Binding: Plasma: 94% to 97%

Metabolism: Hepatic; undergoes first-pass metabolism via CYP3A4; forms metabolites (active)

Excretion: Primarily urine (77%); feces

Dosing
Adults: Obesity: Oral: Initial: 10 mg once daily; after 4 weeks may titrate up to 15 mg once daily as needed and tolerated (may be used for up to 2 years, per manufacturer labeling).

Elderly: Use with caution; adjust dose based on renal or hepatic function.

Hepatic Impairment: No adjustment necessary for mild to moderate liver failure. Sibutramine is contraindicated in patients with severe liver failure.

Available Dosage Forms
Capsule, as hydrochloride: 5 mg, 10 mg, 15 mg

Monitoring and Teaching Issues
Physical Assessment: Assess effectiveness and interactions of other medications patient may be taking. Monitor vital signs, weight, and adverse reactions at start of therapy, when changing dosage, and at regular intervals during therapy. Assess knowledge/teach patient appropriate use, possible side effects, and symptoms to report.

Patient Education: Take exactly as directed; do not increase dose or frequency without consulting prescriber. May be taken with meals (do not take at bedtime). Avoid alcohol, caffeine, or OTC medications that act as stimulants. You may experience restlessness, dizziness, sleepiness (use caution when driving or engaging in tasks requiring alertness until response to drug is known); insomnia (taking medication early in morning may help, warm milk, and quiet environment at bedtime may help); increased appetite, nausea or vomiting (small frequent meals, frequent mouth care may help); constipation (increased exercise, fluids, fruit, or fiber may help); diarrhea (buttermilk, boiled milk, or yogurt may help); or altered menstrual periods (reversible when drug is discontinued). Report chest pain, palpitations, or irregular heartbeat; excessive nervousness, excitation, or sleepiness; back pain, muscle weakness, or tremors; CNS changes (acute headache, aggressiveness, restlessness, excitation, sleep disturbances); menstrual pattern changes; rash; blurred vision; runny nose, sinusitis, cough, or respiratory difficulty. **Pregnancy/breast-feeding precautions:** Inform prescriber if you are or intend to become pregnant. Breast-feeding is not recommended.

Dietary Considerations: Sibutramine, as an appetite suppressant, is the most effective when combined with a low calorie diet and behavior modification counseling.

Pregnancy Risk Factor: C

Lactation: Excretion in breast milk unknown/not recommended

Administration

Oral: May take with or without food.

Storage: Store at room temperature of 15°C to 30°C (59°F to 86°F).

Additional Information Physicians should carefully evaluate patients for history of drug abuse and follow such patients closely, observing them for signs of misuse or abuse (eg, development of tolerance, excessive increases of doses, drug seeking behavior).

Unlike dexfenfluramine and fenfluramine, the medication does not cause the release of serotonin from neurons. Tests done on humans show no evidence of valvular heart disease and experiments done on animals show no evidence of the neurotoxicity which was found in similar testing using animals treated with fenfluramine and dexfenfluramine; has minimal potential for abuse.

Related Information

Obesity Treatment Guidelines for Adults *on page 1850*

- ♦ **Sibutramine Hydrochloride Monohydrate** *see* Sibutramine *on page 1371*
- ♦ **Silace [OTC]** *see* Docusate *on page 474*
- ♦ **Siladryl® Allergy [OTC]** *see* DiphenhydrAMINE *on page 463*
- ♦ **Siladryl® DAS [OTC]** *see* DiphenhydrAMINE *on page 463*
- ♦ **Silapap® Children's [OTC]** *see* Acetaminophen *on page 38*
- ♦ **Silapap® Infants [OTC]** *see* Acetaminophen *on page 38*
- ♦ **Sildec** *see* Carbinoxamine and Pseudoephedrine *on page 254*

Sildenafil (sil DEN a fil)

U.S. Brand Names Viagra®

Synonyms UK92480

Generic Available No

Pharmacologic Category Phosphodiesterase-5 Enzyme Inhibitor

Medication Safety Issues

Sound-alike/look-alike issues:

Viagra® may be confused with Allegra®, Vaniqa™

Use Treatment of erectile dysfunction

Unlabeled/Investigational Use Psychotropic-induced sexual dysfunction; primary pulmonary hypertension

Mechanism of Action/Effect Sildenafil enhances the effect of nitric oxide by inhibiting phosphodiesterase type 5 (PDE-5), resulting in smooth muscle relaxation and inflow of blood into the corpus cavernosum with sexual stimulation.

Contraindications Hypersensitivity to sildenafil or any component of the formulation; concurrent use of organic nitrates (nitroglycerin) in any form (potentiates the hypotensive effects)

Warnings/Precautions A thorough medical history and physical examination to diagnose erectile dysfunction should be undertaken to determine potential underlying causes and appropriate treatment. There is a potential cardiac risk associated with sexual activity which may need to be considered in patients with cardiovascular disease before starting sildenafil therapy. Use with caution in patients predisposed to priapism (ie, sickle cell anemia, multiple myeloma or leukemia). Use with caution in patients with anatomical deformation of the penis (ie, angulation, cavernosal fibrosis, or Peyronie's disease). Use of sildenafil with other approaches to treat erectile dysfunction is **not** recommended. May cause hypotension; use caution in patients with MI, stroke, or life-threatening arrhythmia (within last 6 months); resting hypotension or hypertension; history of unstable angina or cardiac failure; and retinitis pigmentosa.

Drug Interactions

Cytochrome P450 Effect: Substrate of CYP2C8/9 (minor), 3A4 (major); **Inhibits** CYP1A2 (weak), 2C8/9 (weak), 2C19 (weak), 2D6 (weak), 2E1 (weak), 3A4 (weak)

Decreased Effect: Enzyme inducers (including phenytoin, carbamazepine, phenobarbital, rifampin) may decrease the serum concentration and efficacy of sildenafil.

Increased Effect/Toxicity: Sildenafil potentiates the hypotensive effects of nitrates (amyl nitrate, isosorbide dinitrate, isosorbide mononitrate, nitroglycerin); severe reactions have occurred and concurrent use is contraindicated. Concomitant use of alpha-blockers (doxazosin) may lead to symptomatic hypotension in some patients (sildenafil in doses >25 mg should not be given within 4 hours of administering an alpha-blocker).

CYP3A4 inhibitors may increase the levels/effects of sildenafil; example inhibitors include azole antifungals, ciprofloxacin, clarithromycin, diclofenac, doxycycline, erythromycin, imatinib, isoniazid, nefazodone, nicardipine, propofol, protease inhibitors, quinidine, and verapamil. Sildenafil may potentiate the effect of other antihypertensives. Sildenafil may potentiate bleeding in patients receiving heparin. Reduce sildenafil dose to 25 mg/24 hours in patients receiving azole antifungals or protease inhibitors.

Nutritional/Ethanol Interactions

Food: Amount and rate of absorption of sildenafil is reduced when taken with a high-fat meal. Serum concentrations/toxicity may be increased with grapefruit juice; avoid concurrent use.

Herb/Nutraceutical: St John's wort may decrease sildenafil levels.

Adverse Reactions

>10%: Central nervous system: Headache

Note: Dyspepsia and abnormal vision (color changes, blurred or increased sensitivity to light) occurred at an incidence of >10% with doses of 100 mg.

1% to 10%:

Cardiovascular: Flushing

Central nervous system: Dizziness

Dermatologic: Rash

Genitourinary: Urinary tract infection

(Continued)

Sildenafil *(Continued)*

Ophthalmic: Abnormal vision (color changes, blurred or increased sensitivity to light)

Respiratory: Nasal congestion

<2% (Limited to important of life-threatening): Allergic reaction, angina pectoris anorgasmia, asthma, AV block, cardiac arrest, cardiomyopathy, cataract, cerebral thrombosis, colitis, dyspnea, edema, exfoliative dermatitis, eye hemorrhage, gout, heart failure, hyperglycemia, hypotension, migraine, myocardial ischemia, neuralgia, photosensitivity, postural hypotension, priapism, rectal hemorrhage, seizure, shock, syncope, vertigo

Overdosage/Toxicology In studies with healthy volunteers of single doses up to 800 mg, adverse events were similar to those seen at lower doses but incidence rates were increased

Pharmacodynamics/Kinetics
Onset of Action: ~60 minutes
Duration of Action: 2-4 hours
Absorption: Rapid
Bioavailability: 40%
Time to Peak: 30-120 minutes
Protein Binding: Plasma: ~96%
Half-Life Elimination: 4 hours
Metabolism: Hepatic via CYP3A4 (major) and CYP2C9 (minor route)
Excretion: Feces (80%); urine (13%)

Dosing
Adults:
Erectile dysfunction: Oral: 50 mg tablet, approximately 1 hour before sexual activity (30 minutes - 4 hours). An initial and maximum dose of 25 mg is recommended in patients with factors which may increase sildenafil levels (age >65, hepatic impairment, severe renal impairment, and concomitant use of inhibitors of CYP3A4 such as erythromycin, ketoconazole, and itraconazole). Adjust dose in other patients based on effectiveness or tolerance, decrease to 25 mg or increase to the maximum daily dose of 100 mg. Do not take more than once daily.

Primary pulmonary hypertension (unlabeled use): Oral: 25 mg twice daily, titrated based on response. Dosages up to 100 mg 5 times/day have been used (limited data).

Elderly: Initial: 25 mg, 1 hour before sexual activity. Age >65 years was associated with increased serum sildenafil concentrations which may increase side effects and efficacy.

Renal Impairment: Cl_{cr} <30 mL/minute: Initial: 25 mg, 1 hour before sexual activity.

Hepatic Impairment: Hepatic impairment; cirrhosis: Initial: 25 mg, 1 hour before sexual activity.

Available Dosage Forms Tablet, as citrate: 25 mg, 50 mg, 100 mg

Monitoring and Teaching Issues
Physical Assessment: Monitor other medications patient may be taking for effectiveness and interactions. Instruct patient on appropriate use and cautions, possible side effects, and symptoms to report.

Patient Education: Inform prescriber of all other medications you are taking; serious side effects can result when sildenafil is used with nitrates and some other medications. Do not combine sildenafil with other approaches to treating erectile dysfunction without consulting prescriber. **Note:** Sildenafil provides no protection against sexually-transmitted diseases, including HIV. You may experience headache, flushing, or abnormal vision (color changes, blurred or increased sensitivity to light); use caution when driving at night or in poorly lit environments. Report immediately acute allergic reactions; chest pain or palpitations; persistent dizziness; sign of urinary tract infection; skin rash; respiratory difficulty; genital swelling; or other adverse reactions. If erection lasts longer than 4 hours, contact prescriber immediately; permanent damage to the penis can occur.

Pregnancy Risk Factor: B
Pregnancy Issues: Sildenafil is not indicated for use in women.
Breast-Feeding Issues: Sildenafil is not indicated for use in women.

Administration
Oral: Administer orally ~1 hour before sexual activity (may be used anytime from 4 hours to 30 minutes before).

Storage: Store tablets at controlled room temperature of 15°C to 30°C (59°F to 86°F).

Additional Information Sildenafil is ~10 times more selective for PDE-5 as compared to PDE6. This enzyme is found in the retina and is involved in phototransduction. At higher plasma levels, interference with PDE6 is believed to be the basis for changes in color vision noted in some patients.

♦ **Silexin® [OTC]** *see* Guaifenesin and Dextromethorphan *on page 731*
♦ **Silfedrine Children's [OTC]** *see* Pseudoephedrine *on page 1282*
♦ **Silphen® [OTC]** *see* DiphenhydrAMINE *on page 463*
♦ **Siltussin DAS [OTC]** *see* Guaifenesin *on page 729*
♦ **Siltussin DM [OTC]** *see* Guaifenesin and Dextromethorphan *on page 731*
♦ **Siltussin DM DAS [OTC]** *see* Guaifenesin and Dextromethorphan *on page 731*
♦ **Siltussin SA [OTC]** *see* Guaifenesin *on page 729*
♦ **Silvadene®** *see* Silver Sulfadiazine *on page 1374*

Silver Sulfadiazine *(SIL ver sul fa DYE a zeen)*

U.S. Brand Names Silvadene®; SSD®; SSD® AF; Thermazene®
Generic Available Yes
Pharmacologic Category Antibiotic, Topical
Use Prevention and treatment of infection in second and third degree burns
Mechanism of Action/Effect Acts upon the bacterial cell wall and cell membrane. Bactericidal for many gram-negative and gram-positive bacteria and is effective against yeast. Active against *Pseudomonas aeruginosa, Pseudomonas maltophilia, Enterobacter* species, *Klebsiella* species, *Serratia* species, *Escherichia coli, Proteus mirabilis, Morganella morganii,*

Providencia rettgeri, *Proteus vulgaris*, *Providencia* species, *Citrobacter* species, *Acinetobacter calcoaceticus*, *Staphylococcus aureus*, *Staphylococcus epidermidis*, *Enterococcus* species, *Candida albicans*, *Corynebacterium diphtheriae*, and *Clostridium perfringens*

Contraindications Hypersensitivity to silver sulfadiazine or any component of the formulation; premature infants or neonates <2 months of age (sulfonamides may displace bilirubin and cause kernicterus); pregnancy (approaching or at term)

Warnings/Precautions Use with caution in patients with G6PD deficiency, renal impairment, or history of allergy to other sulfonamides. Sulfadiazine may accumulate in patients with impaired hepatic or renal function. Use of analgesic might be needed before application. Systemic absorption is significant and adverse reactions may be due to sulfa component.

Drug Interactions
Decreased Effect: Topical proteolytic enzymes are inactivated by silver sulfadiazine.

Adverse Reactions Frequency not defined.
Dermatologic: Itching, rash, erythema multiforme, discoloration of skin, photosensitivity
Hematologic: Hemolytic anemia, leukopenia, agranulocytosis, aplastic anemia
Hepatic: Hepatitis
Renal: Interstitial nephritis
Miscellaneous: Allergic reactions may be related to sulfa component

Pharmacodynamics/Kinetics
Absorption: Significant percutaneous absorption of silver sulfadiazine can occur especially when applied to extensive burns
Time to Peak: Serum: 3-11 days of continuous therapy
Half-Life Elimination: 10 hours; prolonged with renal impairment
Excretion: Urine (~50% as unchanged drug)

Dosing
Adults & Elderly: Antiseptic, burns: Topical: Apply once or twice daily
Pediatrics: Refer to adult dosing.

Available Dosage Forms
Cream, topical: 1% [10 mg/g] (25 g, 85 g, 400 g)
Silvadene®, Thermazene®: 1% (20 g, 50 g, 85 g, 400 g, 1000 g)
SSD®: 1% (25 g, 50 g, 85 g, 400 g)
SSD® AF: 1% (50 g, 400 g)

Monitoring and Teaching Issues
Physical Assessment: Assess allergy history before treatment (sulfonamides). Use caution in patients with G6PD deficiency or renal impairment (see Warnings/Precautions). Assess results of laboratory tests, therapeutic effectiveness (development of granulation), adverse response (eg, rash, irritation, burning, itching of unburned area, hepatic or hematological response with long-term use or use over large areas; see Adverse Reactions).
Monitoring Laboratory Tests: Serum electrolytes, urinalysis, renal function, CBC in patients with extensive burns on long-term treatment
Patient Education: Usually applied by professional in burn care setting. Patient instruction should be appropriate to extent of burn and patient understanding.
Pregnancy Risk Factor: B
Lactation: For external use

Administration
Topical: Apply with a sterile-gloved hand. Apply to a thickness $^1/_{16}$". Burned area should be covered with cream at all times.
Storage: Discard if cream is darkened (reacts with heavy metals resulting in release of silver).

Additional Information Contains methylparaben and propylene glycol

♦ **Simethicone and Magaldrate** *see* Magaldrate and Simethicone *on page 929*
♦ **Simply Sleep® [OTC]** *see* DiphenhydrAMINE *on page 463*
♦ **Simply Stuffy™ [OTC]** *see* Pseudoephedrine *on page 1282*
♦ **Simulect®** *see* Basiliximab *on page 174*

Simvastatin (SIM va stat in)

U.S. Brand Names Zocor®
Generic Available No
Pharmacologic Category Antilipemic Agent, HMG-CoA Reductase Inhibitor
Medication Safety Issues
Sound-alike/look-alike issues:
Zocor® may be confused with Cozaar®, Yocon®, Zoloft®

Use Used with dietary therapy for the following:
Secondary prevention of cardiovascular events in hypercholesterolemic patients with established coronary heart disease (CHD) or at high risk for CHD: To reduce cardiovascular morbidity (myocardial infarction, coronary revascularization procedures) and mortality; to reduce the risk of stroke and transient ischemic attacks
Hyperlipidemias: To reduce elevations in total cholesterol, LDL-C, apolipoprotein B, and triglycerides in patients with primary hypercholesterolemia (elevations of 1 or more components are present in Fredrickson type IIa, IIb, III, and IV hyperlipidemias); treatment of homozygous familial hypercholesterolemia
Heterozygous familial hypercholesterolemia (HeFH): In adolescent patients (10-17 years of age, females >1 year postmenarche) with HeFH having LDL-C ≥190 mg/dL **or** LDL ≥160 mg/dL with positive family history of premature cardiovascular disease (CVD), or 2 or more CVD risk factors in the adolescent patient

Mechanism of Action/Effect Simvastatin is a derivative of lovastatin that acts by competitively inhibiting 3-hydroxy-3-methylglutaryl-coenzyme A (HMG-CoA) reductase, the enzyme that catalyzes the rate-limiting step in cholesterol biosynthesis; lowers total and LDL-cholesterol with increase in HDL

Contraindications Hypersensitivity to simvastatin or any component of the formulation; acute liver disease; unexplained persistent elevations of serum transaminases; pregnancy; breast-feeding
(Continued)

Simvastatin (Continued)

Warnings/Precautions Secondary causes of hyperlipidemia should be ruled out prior to therapy. Liver function must be monitored by laboratory assessment. Rhabdomyolysis with acute renal failure has occurred. Risk is dose-related and is increased with concurrent use of lipid-lowering agents which may cause rhabdomyolysis (gemfibrozil, fibric acid derivatives, or niacin at doses ≥1 g/day) or during concurrent use with potent CYP3A4 inhibitors (including amiodarone, clarithromycin, cyclosporine, erythromycin, itraconazole, ketoconazole, nefazodone, grapefruit juice in large quantities, verapamil, or protease inhibitors such as indinavir, nelfinavir, or ritonavir). Weigh the risk versus benefit when combining any of these drugs with simvastatin. Temporarily discontinue in any patient experiencing an acute or serious condition predisposing to renal failure secondary to rhabdomyolysis. Use with caution in patients who consume large amounts of ethanol or have a history of liver disease. Safety and efficacy have not been established in patients <10 years or in premenarcheal girls.

Drug Interactions

Cytochrome P450 Effect: Substrate of CYP3A4 (major); **Inhibits** CYP2C8/9 (weak), 2D6 (weak)

Decreased Effect: When taken within 1 before or up to 2 hours after cholestyramine, a decrease in absorption of simvastatin can occur.

Increased Effect/Toxicity: Risk of myopathy/rhabdomyolysis may be increased by concurrent use of lipid-lowering agents which may cause rhabdomyolysis (gemfibrozil, fibric acid derivatives, or niacin at doses ≥1 g/day), or during concurrent use of strong CYP3A4 inhibitors.

CYP3A4 inhibitors may increase the levels/effects of simvastatin; example inhibitors include azole antifungals, ciprofloxacin, clarithromycin, diclofenac, doxycycline, erythromycin, imatinib, isoniazid, nefazodone, nicardipine, propofol, protease inhibitors, quinidine, and verapamil. In large quantities (ie, >1 quart/day), grapefruit juice may also increase simvastatin serum concentrations, increasing the risk of rhabdomyolysis. In general, concurrent use with CYP3A4 inhibitors is not recommended; manufacturer recommends limiting simvastatin dose to 20 mg/day when used with amiodarone or verapamil, and 10 mg/day when used with cyclosporine, gemfibrozil, or fibric acid derivatives.

The anticoagulant effect of warfarin may be increased by simvastatin. Cholesterol-lowering effects are additive with bile-acid sequestrants (colestipol and cholestyramine).

Nutritional/Ethanol Interactions

Ethanol: Avoid excessive ethanol consumption (due to potential hepatic effects).

Food: Simvastatin serum concentration may be increased when taken with grapefruit juice; avoid concurrent intake of large quantities (>1 quart/day).

Herb/Nutraceutical: St John's wort may decrease simvastatin levels.

Adverse Reactions 1% to 10%:

Gastrointestinal: Constipation (2%), dyspepsia (1%), flatulence (2%)

Neuromuscular & skeletal: CPK elevation (>3x normal on one or more occasions - 5%)

Respiratory: Upper respiratory infection (2%)

Additional class-related events or case reports (not necessarily reported with simvastatin therapy): Alopecia, alteration in taste, anaphylaxis, angioedema, anorexia, anxiety, arthritis, cataracts, chills, cholestatic jaundice, cirrhosis, decreased libido, depression, dermatomyositis, dryness of skin/mucous membranes, dyspnea, elevated transaminases, eosinophilia, erectile dysfunction/impotence, erythema multiforme, facial paresis, fatty liver, fever, flushing, fulminant hepatic necrosis, gynecomastia, hemolytic anemia, hepatitis, hepatoma, hyperbilirubinemia, hypersensitivity reaction, impaired extraocular muscle movement, increased alkaline phosphatase, increased CPK (>10x normal), increased ESR, increased GGT, leukopenia, malaise, memory loss, myopathy, nail changes, nodules, ophthalmoplegia, pancreatitis, paresthesia, peripheral nerve palsy, peripheral neuropathy, photosensitivity, polymyalgia rheumatica, positive ANA, pruritus, psychic disturbance, purpura, rash, renal failure (secondary to rhabdomyolysis), rhabdomyolysis, skin discoloration, Stevens-Johnson syndrome, systemic lupus erythematosus-like syndrome, thrombocytopenia, thyroid dysfunction, toxic epidermal necrolysis, tremor, urticaria, vasculitis, vertigo, vomiting

Overdosage/Toxicology Very few adverse events. Treatment is symptomatic.

Pharmacodynamics/Kinetics

Onset of Action: >3 days; Peak effect: 2 weeks

Absorption: 85%

Bioavailability: <5%

Time to Peak: 1.3-2.4 hours

Protein Binding: ~95%

Half-Life Elimination: Unknown

Metabolism: Hepatic via CYP3A4; extensive first-pass effect

Excretion: Feces (60%); urine (13%)

Dosing

Adults: Note: Doses should be individualized according to the baseline LDL-cholesterol levels, the recommended goal of therapy, and the patient's response; adjustments should be made at intervals of 4 weeks or more; doses may need adjusted based on concomitant medications

Homozygous familial hypercholesterolemia: Oral: 40 mg once daily in the evening **or** 80 mg/day (given as 20 mg, 20 mg, and 40 mg evening dose)

Prevention of cardiovascular events, hyperlipidemias: Oral: 20-40 mg once daily in the evening; range: 5-80 mg/day

Patients requiring only moderate reduction of LDL-cholesterol: May be started at 10 mg once daily

Patients requiring reduction of >45% in low-density lipoprotein (LDL) cholesterol: May be started at 40 mg once daily in the evening

Patients with CHD or at high risk for CHD: Dosing should be started at 40 mg once daily in the evening; simvastatin may be started simultaneously with diet

Dosage adjustment for simvastatin with concomitant medications:

Cyclosporine: Initial: 5 mg, should **not** exceed 10 mg/day

Fibrates or niacin: Dose should **not** exceed 10 mg/day

Amiodarone or verapamil: Dose should **not** exceed 20 mg/day

Elderly: Oral: Initial: Maximum reductions in LDL-cholesterol may be achieved with daily dose ≤20 mg.

Pediatrics: HeFH: Oral: Children 10-17 years (females >1 year postmenarche): 10 mg once daily in the evening; range: 10-40 mg/day (maximum: 40 mg/day)

Dosage adjustment with concomitant medications: With concomitant cyclosporine, fibrates, niacin, amiodarone, or verapamil: Refer to adult dosing.

Note: Doses should be individualized according to the baseline LDL-cholesterol levels, the recommended goal of therapy, and the patient's response; adjustments should be made at intervals of 4 weeks or more; doses may need adjusted based on concomitant medications

Renal Impairment: Because simvastatin does not undergo significant renal excretion, modification of dose should not be necessary in patients with mild to moderate renal insufficiency.

Severe renal impairment: Cl_{cr} <10 mL/minute: Initial: 5 mg/day with close monitoring.

Available Dosage Forms Tablet: 5 mg, 10 mg, 20 mg, 40 mg, 80 mg

Monitoring and Teaching Issues

Physical Assessment: See Warnings/Precautions for use cautions (eg, impaired liver function). Assess potential for interactions with other pharmacological agents or herbal products patient may be taking (eg, gemfibrozil, fibric acid derivatives, niacin may increase risk of myopathy or rhabdomyolysis; see Drug Interactions). Assess LFTs prior to therapy and periodically (see Monitoring Laboratory Tests) and patient response on a regular basis throughout therapy (eg, rash, myalgia, blurred vision, abdominal pain, cough; see Adverse Reactions). Teach patient proper use (as adjunct to diet and exercise program), possible side effects/appropriate interventions, and adverse symptoms to report (see Patient Education). **Pregnancy risk factor X:** Determine that patient is not pregnant before starting therapy. Do not give to women of childbearing age unless they are capable of complying with effective contraceptive use. Instruct patient in appropriate contraceptive measures.

Monitoring Laboratory Tests: Creatine phosphokinase levels due to possibility of myopathy; serum cholesterol (total and fractionated)

Obtain liver function tests prior to initiation dose and thereafter when clinically indicated. Patients titrated to the 80 mg dose should be tested prior to initiation and 3 months after initiating the 80 mg dose. Thereafter, periodic monitoring (ie, semiannually) is recommended for the first year of treatment. Patients with elevated transaminase levels should have a second (confirmatory) test and frequent monitoring until values normalize. Discontinue if increase in ALT/AST is persistently >3 times ULN.

Patient Education: Do not take any new medication during therapy without consulting prescriber. Take at same time each day with or without food. Follow cholesterol-lowering diet and exercise regimen as prescribed. Avoid grapefruit juice and excessive alcohol while taking this medication You will have periodic blood tests to assess effectiveness. May cause mild GI upset (should diminish with use); constipation (increased exercise, fluids, fiber, and fruit may help); headache, dizziness, insomnia (use caution when driving or engaged in potentially hazardous tasks until response to drug is known). Report unusual chest pain, swelling of extremities, weight gain of >5 lb/week, persistent cough; CNS changes (dizziness, memory loss, depression, or vision changes). Contact prescriber immediately with persistent muscle or skeletal pain, joint pain, or numbness, or any sign of allergic reactions (skin rash, difficulty breathing, tightness in throat, choking sensation, swelling of mouth or face). **Pregnancy/breast-feeding precautions:** Inform prescriber if you are pregnant. Do not get pregnant during and for 1 month following therapy. Consult prescriber for appropriate contraceptive measures. This drug may cause severe fetal defects. Do not donate blood during or for 1 month following therapy. Do not breast feed.

Geriatric Considerations: Effective and well tolerated in the elderly. The definition of and, therefore, when to treat hyperlipidemia in the elderly is a controversial issue. The National Cholesterol Education Program recommends that all adults maintain a plasma cholesterol <160 mg/dL. In elderly patients with one additional risk factor, goal LDL would decrease to <130 mg/dL. Pharmacologic treatment should be reserved for those who are unable to obtain a desirable plasma cholesterol concentration by diet alone and for whom the benefits of treatment are believed to outweigh the potential adverse effects, drug interactions, and cost of treatment.

Pregnancy Risk Factor: X

Lactation: Excretion in breast milk unknown/contraindicated

Breast-Feeding Issues: Excretion in breast milk is unknown, but would be expected; other medications in this class are excreted in human milk. Breast-feeding is contraindicated.

Administration

Oral: May be taken without regard to meals.

Storage: Tablets should be stored in tightly-closed containers at temperatures between 5°C to 30°C (41°F to 86°F).

Related Information

Hyperlipidemia Management *on page 1836*

Lipid-Lowering Agents *on page 1738*

♦ **Sincalide** *see page 1625*

♦ **Sinemet**® *see* Levodopa and Carbidopa *on page 886*

♦ **Sinemet® CR** *see* Levodopa and Carbidopa *on page 886*

♦ **Sinequan**® *see* Doxepin *on page 487*

♦ **Singulair**® *see* Montelukast *on page 1028*

♦ **Sirdalud**® *see* Tizanidine *on page 1487*

Sirolimus (sir OH li mus)

U.S. Brand Names Rapamune®

Generic Available No

(Continued)

Sirolimus *(Continued)*

Pharmacologic Category Immunosuppressant Agent

Use Prophylaxis of organ rejection in patients receiving renal transplants, in combination with corticosteroids and cyclosporine (cyclosporine may be withdrawn in low-to-moderate immunological risk patients after 2-4 months, in conjunction with an increase in sirolimus dosage)

Unlabeled/Investigational Use Investigational: Immunosuppression in other forms of solid organ transplantation

Mechanism of Action/Effect Sirolimus inhibits T-lymphocyte activation and proliferation in response to antigenic and cytokine stimulation. Its mechanism differs from other immunosuppressants. It inhibits acute rejection of allografts and prolongs graft survival.

Contraindications Hypersensitivity to sirolimus or any component of the formulation

Warnings/Precautions Immunosuppressive agents, including sirolimus, increase the risk of infection and may be associated with the development of lymphoma. Only physicians experienced in the management of organ transplant patients should prescribe sirolimus. May increase serum lipids (cholesterol and triglycerides). Use with caution in patients with hyperlipidemia. May decrease GFR and increase serum creatinine. Use caution in patients with renal impairment, or when used concurrently with medications which may alter renal function. Monitor renal function closely when combined with cyclosporine; consider dosage adjustment or discontinue in patients with increasing serum creatinine. Has been associated with an increased risk of lymphocele. Cases of interstitial lung disease (eg, pneumonitis, bronchiolitis obliterans organizing pneumonia, pulmonary fibrosis) have been observed; risk may be increased with higher trough levels. Avoid concurrent use of strong CYP3A4 inhibitors or strong inducers of either CYP3A4 or P-glycoprotein. Anaphylactic reactions have been reported. May increase sensitivity to UV light; use appropriate sun protection.

Sirolimus is neither approved nor recommended for use in liver transplant patients; studies indicate an association with an increase risk of hepatic artery thrombosis and graft failure in these patients. Cases of bronchial anastomotic dehiscence have been reported in lung transplant patients when sirolimus was used as part of an immunosuppressive regimen; most of these reactions were fatal. Use in patients with lung transplants is not recommended. Safety and efficacy of cyclosporine withdrawal in high-risk patients is not currently recommended. Safety and efficacy in children <13 years of age, or in adolescent patients <18 years of age considered at high immunological risk, have not been established.

Drug Interactions

Cytochrome P450 Effect: Substrate of CYP3A4 (major); **Inhibits** CYP3A4 (weak)

Decreased Effect: CYP3A4 inducers may decrease the levels/effects of sirolimus; example inducers include aminoglutethimide, carbamazepine, nafcillin, nevirapine, phenobarbital, phenytoin, and rifamycins.

Increased Effect/Toxicity: Cyclosporine increases sirolimus concentrations during concurrent therapy, and cyclosporine levels may be increased; sirolimus should be taken 4 hours after cyclosporine oral solution (modified) and/or cyclosporine capsules (modified). CYP3A4 inhibitors may increase the levels/effects of sirolimus; example inhibitors include azole antifungals, ciprofloxacin, clarithromycin, diclofenac, diltiazem, doxycycline, erythromycin, imatinib, isoniazid, nefazodone, nicardipine, propofol, protease inhibitors, quinidine, and verapamil; avoid concurrent use. Vaccination may be less effective and use of live vaccines should be avoided during sirolimus therapy.

Nutritional/Ethanol Interactions

Food: Do not administer with grapefruit juice; may decrease clearance of sirolimus. Ingestion with high-fat meals decreases peak concentrations but increases AUC by 35%. Sirolimus should be taken consistently either with or without food to minimize variability.

Herb/Nutraceutical: St John's wort may decrease sirolimus levels; avoid concurrent use. Avoid cat's claw, echinacea (have immunostimulant properties).

Adverse Reactions Incidence of many adverse effects is dose related

>20%:

Cardiovascular: Hypertension (39% to 49%), peripheral edema (54% to 64%), edema (16% to 24%), chest pain (16% to 24%)

Central nervous system: Fever (23% to 34%), headache (23% to 34%), pain (24% to 33%), insomnia (13% to 22%)

Dermatologic: Acne (20% to 31%)

Endocrine & metabolic: Hypercholesterolemia (38% to 46%), hypophosphatemia (15% to 23%), hyperlipidemia (38% to 57%), hypokalemia (11% to 21%)

Gastrointestinal: Abdominal pain (28% to 36%), nausea (25% to 36%), vomiting (19% to 25%), diarrhea (25% to 42%), constipation (28% to 38%), dyspepsia (17% to 25%), weight gain (8% to 21%)

Genitourinary: Urinary tract infection (20% to 33%)

Hematologic: Anemia (23% to 37%), thrombocytopenia (13% to 40%)

Neuromuscular & skeletal: Arthralgia (25% to 31%), weakness (22% to 40%), back pain (16% to 26%), tremor (21% to 31%)

Renal: Increased serum creatinine (35% to 40%)

Respiratory: Dyspnea (22% to 30%), upper respiratory infection (20% to 26%), pharyngitis (16% to 21%)

3% to 20%:

Cardiovascular: Atrial fibrillation, CHF, hypervolemia, hypotension, palpitation, peripheral vascular disorder, postural hypotension, syncope, tachycardia, thrombosis, vasodilation, venous thromboembolism

Central nervous system: Chills, malaise, anxiety, confusion, depression, dizziness, emotional lability, hypoesthesia, hypotonia, insomnia, neuropathy, somnolence

Dermatologic: Dermatitis (fungal), hirsutism, pruritus, skin hypertrophy, dermal ulcer, ecchymosis, cellulitis, rash (10% to 20%)

Endocrine & metabolic: Cushing's syndrome, diabetes mellitus, glycosuria, acidosis, dehydration, hypercalcemia, hyperglycemia, hyperphosphatemia, hypocalcemia, hypoglycemia, hypomagnesemia, hyponatremia, hyperkalemia (12% to 17%)

Gastrointestinal: Enlarged abdomen, anorexia, dysphagia, eructation, esophagitis, flatulence, gastritis, gastroenteritis, gingivitis, gingival hyperplasia, ileus, mouth ulceration, oral moniliasis, stomatitis, weight loss

Genitourinary: Pelvic pain, scrotal edema, testis disorder, impotence

Hematologic: Leukocytosis, polycythemia, TTP, hemolytic-uremic syndrome, hemorrhage, leukopenia (9% to 15%)

Hepatic: Abnormal liver function tests, alkaline phosphatase increased, ascites, LDH increased, transaminases increased

Local: Thrombophlebitis

Neuromuscular & skeletal: Increased CPK, arthrosis, bone necrosis, leg cramps, myalgia, osteoporosis, tetany, hypertonia, paresthesia

Ocular: Abnormal vision, cataract, conjunctivitis

Otic: Ear pain, deafness, otitis media, tinnitus

Renal: Increased BUN, albuminuria, bladder pain, dysuria, hematuria, hydronephrosis, kidney pain, tubular necrosis, nocturia, oliguria, pyuria, nephropathy (toxic), urinary frequency, urinary incontinence, urinary retention

Respiratory: Asthma, atelectasis, bronchitis, cough, epistaxis, hypoxia, lung edema, pleural effusion, pneumonia, rhinitis, sinusitis

Miscellaneous: Abscess, diaphoresis, facial edema, flu-like syndrome, hernia, infection, lymphadenopathy, lymphocele, peritonitis, sepsis

Overdosage/Toxicology Experience with overdosage has been limited. Dose-limiting toxicities include immune suppression. Reported symptoms of overdose include atrial fibrillation. Treatment is supportive, dialysis is not likely to facilitate removal.

Pharmacodynamics/Kinetics
Absorption: Rapid
Bioavailability: Oral solution: 14%; Oral tablet: 18%
Time to Peak: 1-2 hours
Protein Binding: 92%, primarily to albumin
Half-Life Elimination: Mean: 62 hours
Metabolism: Extensively hepatic via CYP3A; P-glycoprotein-mediated efflux into gut lumen
Excretion: Feces (91%); urine (2%)

Dosing
Adults & Elderly:
Immunosuppression: Oral:
<40 kg: Loading dose: 3 mg/m^2 (day 1); followed by a maintenance of 1 mg/m^2/day.
≥40 kg: Loading dose: For *de novo* transplant recipients, a loading dose of 3 times the daily maintenance dose should be administered on day 1 of dosing. Maintenance dose: 2 mg/day. Doses should be taken 4 hours after cyclosporine, and should be taken consistently either with or without food.
Maintenance therapy after withdrawal of cyclosporine:
Following 2-4 months of combined therapy, withdrawal of cyclosporine may be considered in low-to-moderate risk patients. Cyclosporine withdrawal in not recommended in high immunological risk patients. Cyclosporine should be discontinued over 4-8 weeks, and a necessary increase in the dosage of sirolimus (up to fourfold) should be anticipated due to removal of metabolic inhibition by cyclosporine and to maintain adequate immunosuppressive effects.
Sirolimus dosages should be adjusted to maintain trough concentrations of 12-24 ng/mL. Dosage should be adjusted at intervals of 7-14 days to account for the long half-life of sirolimus. Considerable increases in dosage may require an additional loading dose, calculated as the difference between the target concentration and the current concentration, multiplied by a factor of 3. Loading doses >40 mg may be administered over two days. Serum concentrations should not be used as the sole basis for dosage adjustment (monitor clinical signs/symptoms, tissue biopsy, and laboratory parameters).
Pediatrics:
Immunosuppression: Oral: Children ≥13 years: Loading dose: 3 mg/m^2 (day 1); followed by a maintenance of 1 mg/m^2/day.
Renal Impairment: No adjustment is necessary.
Hepatic Impairment: Reduce maintenance dose by approximately 33% in hepatic impairment. Loading dose is unchanged.

Available Dosage Forms
Solution, oral [bottle]: 1 mg/mL (60 mL, 150 mL) [contains ethanol 1.5% to 2.5%; packaged with 1 mL, 2 mL, or 5 mL oral syringes]
Solution, oral [unit-dose pouch]: 1 mg/mL (1 mL, 2 mL, 5 mL) [contains ethanol 1.5% to 2.5%; packaged in cartons of 30]
Tablet: 1 mg, 2 mg, 5 mg

Monitoring and Teaching Issues
Physical Assessment: Assess effectiveness and interactions of other medications. Assess results of laboratory tests at beginning and periodically during therapy, therapeutic effectiveness, and adverse reactions and toxicity. Monitor blood pressure and renal function. Assess knowledge/teach patient appropriate use, interventions to reduce side effects, and adverse reactions to report.
Monitoring Laboratory Tests: Monitor sirolimus levels in pediatric patients, patients ≥13 years of age weighing <40 kg, patients with hepatic impairment, or on concurrent potent inhibitors or inducers of CYP3A4, and/or if cyclosporine dosing is markedly reduced or discontinued. Also monitor serum cholesterol and triglycerides and serum creatinine. Routine therapeutic drug level monitoring is not required in most patients. Serum concentrations should not be used as the sole basis for dosage adjustment, especially during withdrawal of cyclosporine (monitor clinical signs/symptoms, tissue biopsy, and laboratory parameters).
Patient Education: Take as directed; do not alter dose or discontinue without consulting prescriber. Do not ever mix sirolimus solution with anything other than water or orange juice (avoid taking with grapefruit juice). May be taken with or without food, but should be taken consistently with regard to food (always on an empty stomach or always with food). (Continued)

Sirolimus *(Continued)*

Consult prescriber about timing of any other prescribed or OTC medications. Maintain adequate hydration (2-3 L/day of fluids) unless instructed to restrict fluid intake. You will be susceptible to infection (avoid crowds and exposure to infection). If you have diabetes, monitor glucose levels closely (drug may alter glucose levels). Limit exposure to sunlight by wearing protective clothing or sunscreen. You may experience nausea, vomiting, loss of appetite (small frequent meals, good mouth care, chewing gum, or sucking hard candy may help); constipation (increase exercise, fluids, fruit, or fiber may help); or diarrhea (yogurt or buttermilk); or muscle or back pain (mild analgesic). Inform prescriber of any adverse effects including, but not limited to, unresolved GI problems; respiratory difficulty, cough, infection; skin rash or irritation; headache, insomnia, anxiety, confusion, emotional lability; changes in voiding pattern, burning, itching, or pain on urination; persistent bone, joint, or muscle cramping, pain or weakness; chest pain, palpitations, swelling of extremities; weight gain of 3-5 pounds per week; vision changes or hearing; or any other adverse reactions. **Pregnancy/breast-feeding precautions:** Inform prescriber if you are or intend to become pregnant. Breast-feeding is not recommended.

Dietary Considerations: Take consistently, with or without food, to minimize variability of absorption.

Pregnancy Risk Factor: C

Pregnancy Issues: Embryotoxicity and fetotoxicity may occur, as evidenced by increased mortality, reduced fetal weights and delayed ossification. Effective contraception must be initiated before therapy with sirolimus and continued for 12 weeks after discontinuation.

Lactation: Excretion in breast milk unknown/not recommended

Administration

Oral: Amber oral dose syringe should be used to withdraw solution from the bottle. Syringe should then be emptied, or, if a pouch is used, the entire contents should be squeezed out into a glass or plastic cup. The solution in the cup should be mixed with at least 2 ounces of water or orange juice. No other liquids should be used for dilution. Patient should drink diluted solution immediately. The cup should then be refilled with an additional 4 ounces of water or orange juice, stirred vigorously, and the patient should drink the contents at once.

Storage:

Oral solution: Protect from light and store under refrigeration, 2°C to 8°C (36°F to 46°F). A slight haze may develop in refrigerated solutions, but the quality of the product is not affected. After opening, solution should be used in 1 month. If necessary, may be stored at temperatures up to 25°C (77°F) for several days after opening (up to 24 hours for pouches and not >15 days for bottles). Product may be stored in amber syringe for a maximum of 24 hours (at room temperature or refrigerated). Discard syringe after use. Solution should be used immediately following dilution.

Tablet: Store at room temperature of 20°C to 25°C (68°F to 77°F). Protect from light.

Additional Information Sirolimus tablets and oral solution are not bioequivalent, due to differences in absorption. Clinical equivalence was seen using 2 mg tablet and 2 mg solution. It is not known if higher doses are also clinically equivalent.

- ◆ **SK** *see Streptokinase on page 1395*
- ◆ **SK and F 104864** *see Topotecan on page 1497*
- ◆ **Skeeter Stik [OTC]** *see Benzocaine on page 181*
- ◆ **Skelid®** *see Tiludronate on page 1477*
- ◆ **SKF 104864** *see Topotecan on page 1497*
- ◆ **SKF 104864-A** *see Topotecan on page 1497*
- ◆ **Skin Test Antigens, Multiple** *see page 1625*
- ◆ **Sleepinal® [OTC]** *see DiphenhydrAMINE on page 463*
- ◆ **Slo-Niacin® [OTC]** *see Niacin on page 1075*
- ◆ **Slow FE® [OTC]** *see Ferrous Sulfate on page 624*
- ◆ **Slow-Mag® [OTC]** *see Magnesium Chloride on page 929*
- ◆ **Smallpox Vaccine** *see page 1660*
- ◆ **SMZ-TMP** *see Sulfamethoxazole and Trimethoprim on page 1407*
- ◆ **(+)-(S)-N-Methyl-γ-(1-Naphthyloxy)-2-Thiophenepropylamine Hydrochloride** *see Duloxetine on page 503*
- ◆ **Sodium 2-Mercaptoethane Sulfonate** *see Mesna on page 959*
- ◆ **Sodium Acid Carbonate** *see Sodium Bicarbonate on page 1380*
- ◆ **Sodium Benzoate and Caffeine** *see Caffeine on page 229*

Sodium Bicarbonate *(SOW dee um bye KAR bun ate)*

U.S. Brand Names Brioschi® [OTC]; Neut®

Synonyms Baking Soda; NaHCO$_3$; Sodium Acid Carbonate; Sodium Hydrogen Carbonate

Generic Available Yes

Pharmacologic Category Alkalinizing Agent; Antacid; Electrolyte Supplement, Oral; Electrolyte Supplement, Parenteral

Use Management of metabolic acidosis; gastric hyperacidity; as an alkalinization agent for the urine; treatment of hyperkalemia; management of overdose of certain drugs, including tricyclic antidepressants and aspirin

Mechanism of Action/Effect Dissociates to provide bicarbonate ion which neutralizes hydrogen ion concentration and raises blood and urinary pH

Contraindications Alkalosis, hypernatremia, severe pulmonary edema, hypocalcemia, unknown abdominal pain

Warnings/Precautions Use of I.V. NaHCO$_3$ should be reserved for documented metabolic acidosis and for hyperkalemia-induced cardiac arrest. Routine use in cardiac arrest is not recommended. Avoid extravasation, tissue necrosis can occur due to the hypertonicity of NaHCO$_3$. May cause sodium retention especially if renal function is impaired; not to be used in treatment of peptic ulcer; use with caution in patients with CHF, edema, cirrhosis, or renal failure. Not the antacid of choice for the elderly because of sodium content and potential for systemic alkalosis.

Drug Interactions

Decreased Effect: Decreased effect/levels of lithium, chlorpropamide, and salicylates due to urinary alkalinization.

Increased Effect/Toxicity: Increased toxicity/levels of amphetamines, ephedrine, pseudo-ephedrine, flecainide, quinidine, and quinine due to urinary alkalinization.

Nutritional/Ethanol Interactions Herb/Nutraceutical: Concurrent doses with iron may decrease iron absorption.

Adverse Reactions Frequency not defined.

Cardiovascular: Cerebral hemorrhage, CHF (aggravated), edema

Central nervous system: Tetany

Gastrointestinal: Belching, flatulence (with oral), gastric distension

Endocrine & metabolic: Hypernatremia, hyperosmolality, hypocalcemia, hypokalemia, increased affinity of hemoglobin for oxygen-reduced pH in myocardial tissue necrosis when extravasated, intracranial acidosis, metabolic alkalosis, milk-alkali syndrome (especially with renal dysfunction)

Respiratory: Pulmonary edema

Overdosage/Toxicology Symptoms of overdose include hypocalcemia, hypokalemia, hypernatremia, and seizures. Treatment is symptom-directed and supportive.

Pharmacodynamics/Kinetics

Onset of Action: Oral: Rapid; I.V.: 15 minutes

Duration of Action: Oral: 8-10 minutes; I.V.: 1-2 hours

Absorption: Oral: Well absorbed

Excretion: Urine (<1%)

Dosing

Adults & Elderly:

Cardiac arrest: Initial: 1 mEq/kg/dose one time; maintenance: 0.5 mEq/kg/dose every 10 minutes or as indicated by arterial blood gases

Note: Routine use of $NaHCO_3$ is not recommended and should be given only after adequate alveolar ventilation has been established and effective cardiac compressions are provided

Metabolic acidosis: I.V.: Dosage should be based on the following formula if blood gases and pH measurements are available:

HCO_3^-(mEq) = 0.2 x weight (kg) x base deficit (mEq/L)

Administer $1/2$ dose initially, then remaining $1/2$ dose over the next 24 hours; monitor pH, serum HCO_3^-, and clinical status

Note: If acid-base status is not available: 2-5 mEq/kg I.V. infusion over 4-8 hours; subsequent doses should be based on patient's acid-base status

Hyperkalemia: I.V.: 1 mEq/kg over 5 minutes

Chronic renal failure: Oral: Initiate when plasma HCO_3^- <15 mEq/L Start with 20-36 mEq/day in divided doses, titrate to bicarbonate level of 18-20 mEq/L

Renal tubular acidosis: Oral:

Distal: 0.5-2 mEq/kg/day in 4-5 divided doses

Proximal: Initial: 5-10 mEq/kg/day; maintenance: Increase as required to maintain serum bicarbonate in the normal range

Urine alkalinization: Oral: Initial: 48 mEq (4 g), then 12-24 mEq (1-2 g) every 4 hours; dose should be titrated to desired urinary pH; doses up to 16 g/day (200 mEq) in patients <60 years and 8 g (100 mEq) in patients >60 years

Antacid: Oral: 325 mg to 2 g 1-4 times/day

Pediatrics:

Cardiac arrest: I.V.: Infants and Children: I.V.: 0.5-1 mEq/kg/dose repeated every 10 minutes or as indicated by arterial blood gases; rate of infusion should not exceed 10 mEq/minute; neonates and children <2 years of age should receive 4.2% (0.5 mEq/mL) solution.

Note: Routine use of $NaHCO_3$ is not recommended and should be given only after adequate alveolar ventilation has been established and effective cardiac compressions are provided

Metabolic acidosis: I.V.; Infants and Children: Dosage should be based on the following formula if blood gases and pH measurements are available:

HCO_3^-(mEq) = 0.3 x weight (kg) x base deficit (mEq/L)

Administer $1/2$ dose initially, then remaining $1/2$ dose over the next 24 hours; monitor pH, serum HCO_3^-, and clinical status

Note: If acid-base status is not available: Dose for older Children: 2-5 mEq/kg I.V. infusion over 4-8 hours; subsequent doses should be based on patient's acid-base status.

Chronic renal failure: Oral: Children: Initiate when plasma HCO_3^- <15 mEq/L: 1-3 mEq/kg/day

Renal tubular acidosis, distal: Oral: Children: 2-3 mEq/kg/day

Renal tubular acidosis, proximal: Children: Initial: 5-10 mEq/kg/day; maintenance: Increase as required to maintain serum bicarbonate in the normal range

Urine alkalinization: Oral: Children: 1-10 mEq (84-840 mg)/kg/day in divided doses every 4-6 hours; dose should be titrated to desired urinary pH.

Available Dosage Forms

Granules, effervescent (Brioschi®): 6 g, 120 g, 240 g [lemon flavor]

Infusion [premixed in sterile water]: 5% (500 mL)

Injection, solution:

4.2% [42 mg/mL = 5 mEq/10 mL] (10 mL)

5% [50 mg/mL = 5.95 mEq/10 mL] (500 mL)

7.5% [75 mg/mL = 8.92 mEq/10 mL] (50 mL)

8.4% [84 mg/mL = 10 mEq/10 mL] (10 mL, 50 mL)

Neut®: 4% [40 mg/mL = 2.4 mEq/5 mL] (5 mL)

Powder: 120 g, 480 g

Tablet: 325 mg [3.8 mEq]; 650 mg [7.6 mEq]

(Continued)

Sodium Bicarbonate *(Continued)*

Monitoring and Teaching Issues

Physical Assessment: Assess other medications patient may be taking for effectiveness and interactions. **I.V.:** Monitor therapeutic effectiveness, adverse reactions, and infusion site (if extravasation occurs, elevate extravasation site and apply warm compresses). Monitor for signs of fluid retention. Teach patient adverse symptoms to report. **Oral:** Monitor effectiveness of treatment and adverse response. Assess knowledge/teach patient appropriate use, interventions to reduce side effects, and adverse symptoms to report.

Patient Education: Do not use for chronic gastric acidity. Take as directed. Chew tablets thoroughly and follow with a full glass of water, preferably on an empty stomach (2 hours before or after food). Take at least 2 hours before or after any other medications. Report CNS effects (eg, irritability, confusion); muscle rigidity or tremors; swelling of feet or ankles; respiratory difficulty; chest pain or palpitations; respiratory changes; or tarry stools. **Pregnancy precaution:** Inform prescriber if you are or intend to become pregnant.

Dietary Considerations: Oral product should be administered 1-3 hours after meals. Sodium content of injection 50 mL, 8.4% = 1150 mg = 50 mEq; each 6 mg of $NaHCO_3$ contains 12 mEq sodium; 1 mEq $NaHCO_3$ = 84 mg

Geriatric Considerations: Not the antacid of choice for the elderly because of sodium content and potential for systemic alkalosis (see maximum daily dose under Dosage).

Pregnancy Risk Factor: C

Lactation: Enters breast milk/compatible

Administration

I.V.: Vesicant.

Compatibility: Stable in dextran 6% in dextrose, dextran 6% in NS, $D_5{}^1\!/_4NS$, $D_5{}^1\!/_2NS$, D_5NS, D_5W, $D_{10}W$, $^1\!/_2NS$, NS; incompatible with acids, acidic salts, alkaloid salts, calcium salts, catecholamines, and atropine

Y-site administration: Incompatible with allopurinol, amiodarone, amphotericin B cholesteryl sulfate complex, calcium chloride, doxorubicin liposome, idarubicin, imipenem/cilastatin inamrinone, leucovorin, midazolam, nalbuphine, ondansetron, oxacillin, sargramostim, verapamil, vincristine, vindesine, vinorelbine

Compatibility in syringe: Incompatible with etidocaine, glycopyrrolate, mepivacaine, metoclopramide, thiopental

Compatibility when admixed: Incompatible with amiodarone, ascorbic acid injection, carboplatin, carmustine, cefotaxime, ciprofloxacin, cisplatin, dobutamine, dopamine, epinephrine, hydromorphone, imipenem/cilastatin, isoproterenol, labetalol, levorphanol, magnesium sulfate, meropenem, morphine, norepinephrine, pentazocine, procaine, streptomycin, succinylcholine, ticarcillin/clavulanate potassium, vitamin B complex with C

Storage: Store injection at room temperature. Protect from heat and from freezing. Use only clear solutions.

Related Information

Compatibility of Drugs *on page 1723*

Sodium Citrate and Citric Acid *(SOW dee um SIT rate & SI trik AS id)*

U.S. Brand Names Bicitra®; Cytra-2; Oracit®

Synonyms Modified Shohl's Solution

Generic Available Yes

Pharmacologic Category Alkalinizing Agent, Oral

Use Treatment of metabolic acidosis; alkalinizing agent in conditions where long-term maintenance of an alkaline urine is desirable

Dosing

Adults & Elderly: Systemic alkalization: Oral: 10-30 mL with water after meals and at bedtime

Pediatrics: Systemic alkalization: Oral: Infants and Children: 2-3 mEq/kg/day in divided doses 3-4 times/day **or** 5-15 mL with water after meals and at bedtime

Available Dosage Forms Note: Equivalent to sodium 1 mEq/mL and bicarbonate 1 mEq/mL

Solution, oral: Sodium citrate 500 mg and citric acid 334 mg per 5 mL (480 mL)

Bicitra®: Sodium citrate 500 mg and citric acid 334 mg per 5 mL (480 mL) [sugar free; grape flavor]

Cytra-2: Sodium citrate 500 mg and citric acid 334 mg per 5 mL (480 mL) [alcohol free, dye free, sugar free; grape flavor]

Oracit®: Sodium citrate 490 mg and citric acid 640 mg per 5 mL (15 mL, 30 mL, 480 mL, 3840 mL)

Monitoring and Teaching Issues

Physical Assessment: Assess kidney function prior to starting therapy. Monitor cardiac status and serum potassium at beginning of therapy and at regular intervals with long-term therapy. Assess knowledge/teach patient appropriate use, possible side effects, and adverse symptoms to report.

Patient Education: Take as often as directed, after meals, and at least 2 hours before or after any other medications. Dilute with 1-3 oz of water and follow with additional water; chilling solution prior to taking will help to improve taste. You may experience diarrhea or nausea and vomiting; if severe, contact prescriber. Report CNS changes status (eg, irritability, tremors, confusion); swelling of feet or ankles; respiratory difficulty or palpitations; abdominal pain or tarry stools.

Pregnancy Risk Factor: Not established

Lactation: Excretion in breast milk unknown/compatible

♦ **Sodium Ferric Gluconate** *see* Ferric Gluconate *on page 622*

♦ **Sodium Hyaluronate** *see page 1625*

♦ **Sodium Hydrogen Carbonate** *see* Sodium Bicarbonate *on page 1380*

♦ **Sodium Nafcillin** *see* Nafcillin *on page 1048*

♦ **Sodium Nitroferricyanide** *see* Nitroprusside *on page 1092*

♦ **Sodium Nitroprusside** *see* Nitroprusside *on page 1092*

♦ **Sodium PAS** *see* Aminosalicylic Acid *on page 92*

♦ **Sodium Phosphate and Potassium Phosphate** *see* Potassium Phosphate and Sodium Phosphate *on page 1239*

Sodium Polystyrene Sulfonate (SOW dee um pol ee STYE reen SUL fon ate)

U.S. Brand Names Kayexalate®; Kionex™; SPS®

Generic Available Yes

Pharmacologic Category Antidote

Medication Safety Issues

Sound-alike/look-alike issues:

Kayexalate® may be confused with Kaopectate®

Always prescribe either one-time doses or as a specific number of doses (eg, 15 g q6h x 2 doses). Scheduled doses with no dosage limit could be given for days leading to dangerous hypokalemia.

Use Treatment of hyperkalemia

Mechanism of Action/Effect Removes potassium by exchanging sodium ions for potassium ions in the intestine before the resin is passed from the body; exchange capacity is 1 mEq/g *in vivo*, and *in vitro* capacity is 3.1 mEq/g, therefore, a wide range of exchange capacity exists such that close monitoring of serum electrolytes is necessary

Contraindications Hypersensitivity to sodium polystyrene sulfonate or any component of the formulation; hypernatremia, hypokalemia, obstructive bowel disease

Warnings/Precautions Use with caution in patients with severe CHF, hypertension, edema, or renal failure. Large oral doses may cause fecal impaction (especially in the elderly). Enema will reduce the serum potassium faster than oral administration, but the oral route will result in a greater reduction over several hours.

Drug Interactions

Increased Effect/Toxicity: Systemic alkalosis and seizure has occurred after cation-exchange resins were administered with nonabsorbable cation-donating antacids and laxatives (eg, magnesium hydroxide, aluminum carbonate). Digitalis toxicity may occur with hypokalemia.

Adverse Reactions Frequency not defined.

Endocrine & metabolic: Hypernatremia, hypokalemia, hypocalcemia, hypomagnesemia

Gastrointestinal: Anorexia, colonic necrosis (rare), constipation, fecal impaction, intestinal obstruction (due to concretions in association with aluminum hydroxide), nausea, vomiting

Overdosage/Toxicology Symptoms of overdose include hyperkalemia including cardiac dysrhythmias, confusion, irritability, ECG changes, muscle weakness, and GI effects. Treatment is supportive, limited to management of fluid and electrolytes.

Pharmacodynamics/Kinetics

Onset of Action: 2-24 hours

Absorption: None

Excretion: Completely feces (primarily as potassium polystyrene sulfonate)

Dosing

Adults & Elderly: Hyperkalemia:

Oral: 15 g (60 mL) 1-4 times/day

Rectal: 30-50 g every 6 hours

Pediatrics: Hyperkalemia:

Oral: Children: 1 g/kg/dose every 6 hours

Rectal: Children: 1 g/kg/dose every 2-6 hours (in small children and infants, employ lower doses by using the practical exchange ratio of 1 mEq K$^+$/g of resin as the basis for calculation)

Available Dosage Forms

Powder for suspension, oral/rectal:

Kayexalate®: 480 g

Kionex™: 454 g

Suspension, oral/rectal: 15 g/60 mL (60 mL, 120 mL, 200 mL, 500 mL) [with sorbitol and alcohol]

SPS®: 15 g/60 mL (60 mL, 120 mL, 480 mL) [contains alcohol 0.3% and sorbitol; cherry flavor]

Monitoring and Teaching Issues

Physical Assessment: Assess results of laboratory tests. Monitor ECG until potassium levels are normal. Monitor for adverse reactions and teach patient interventions and importance of reporting adverse symptoms promptly.

Monitoring Laboratory Tests: Serum electrolytes, calcium, magnesium

Patient Education: Emergency instructions depend on patient's condition. You will be monitored for effects of this medication and frequent blood tests may be necessary. Oral: Take as directed. Mix well with a full glass of liquid (not orange juice). You may experience nausea or vomiting (small frequent meals, frequent mouth care, chewing gum, or sucking lozenges may help); or constipation or fecal impaction (increased dietary fluids and exercise may help). Report persistent constipation or GI distress; chest pain or rapid heartbeat; or mental confusion or muscle weakness. **Pregnancy/breast-feeding precautions:** Inform prescriber if you are pregnant. Consult prescriber if breast-feeding.

Dietary Considerations: Do **not** mix in orange juice. Sodium content of 1 g: 31 mg (1.3 mEq).

Geriatric Considerations: Large doses in the elderly may cause fecal impaction and intestinal obstruction. Best to administer using sorbitol 70% as vehicle.

Pregnancy Risk Factor: C

Lactation: Excretion in breast milk unknown/use caution

Administration

Oral: Administer oral (or NG) as ~25% sorbitol solution; never mix in orange juice. Chilling the oral mixture will increase palatability.

(Continued)

Sodium Polystyrene Sulfonate *(Continued)*

Other: Rectal: Enema route is less effective than oral administration. Administer cleansing enema first. Retain enema in colon for at least 30-60 minutes and for several hours, if possible. Enema should be followed by irrigation with normal saline to prevent necrosis.

Storage: Store prepared suspensions at 15°C to 30°C (59°F to 86°F); store repackaged product in refrigerator and use within 14 days; freshly prepared suspensions should be used within 24 hours; do not heat resin suspension

Additional Information 1 g of resin binds approximately 1 mEq of potassium

♦ **Sodium Sulfacetamide** *see* Sulfacetamide *on page 1403*

♦ **Solagé™** *see* Mequinol and Tretinoin *on page 953*

♦ **Solaquin® [OTC]** *see* Hydroquinone *on page 768*

♦ **Solaquin Forte®** *see* Hydroquinone *on page 768*

♦ **Solaraze™** *see* Diclofenac *on page 442*

♦ **Solarcaine® [OTC]** *see* Benzocaine *on page 181*

♦ **Solarcaine® Aloe Extra Burn Relief [OTC]** *see* Lidocaine *on page 898*

♦ **Solia™** *see* Ethinyl Estradiol and Desogestrel *on page 578*

Solifenacin *(sol i FEN a sin)*

U.S. Brand Names VESIcare®

Synonyms Solifenacin Succinate

Generic Available No

Pharmacologic Category Anticholinergic Agent

Use Treatment of overactive bladder with symptoms of urinary frequency, urgency, or urge incontinence

Mechanism of Action/Effect Inhibits muscarinic receptors resulting in decreased urinary bladder contraction, increased residual urine volume, and decreased detrusor muscle pressure.

Contraindications Hypersensitivity to solifenacin or any component of the formulation; urinary retention; gastric retention; uncontrolled narrow-angle glaucoma.

Warnings/Precautions Use with caution in patients with bladder outflow obstruction, gastrointestinal obstructive disorders, and decreased gastrointestinal motility. Use with caution in patients with controlled (treated) narrow-angle glaucoma. Dosage adjustment is required for patients with renal or hepatic impairment. Patients on potent CYP3A4 inhibitors require lower dose. Safety and efficacy in pediatric patients have not been established.

Drug Interactions

Cytochrome P450 Effect: Substrate of CYP3A4 (major)

Decreased Effect: CYP3A4 inducers may decrease the levels/effects of solifenacin; example inducers include aminoglutethimide, carbamazepine, nafcillin, nevirapine, phenobarbital, and phenytoin.

Increased Effect/Toxicity: CYP3A4 inhibitors may increase the levels/effects of solifenacin; example inhibitors include azole antifungals, ciprofloxacin, clarithromycin, diclofenac, doxycycline, erythromycin, ketoconazole, imatinib, isoniazid, nefazodone, nicardipine, propofol, protease inhibitors, quinidine and verapamil; solifenacin dose should not exceed 5 mg/day.

Nutritional/Ethanol Interactions

Food: Grapefruit juice may increase the serum level effects of solifenacin.

Herb/Nutraceutical: St John's wort (*Hypericum*) may decrease the levels/effects of solifenacin.

Adverse Reactions Adverse reactions are dose related.

>10%: Gastrointestinal: Xerostomia (11% to 28%), constipation (5% to 13%)

1% to 10%:

Cardiovascular: Edema (up to 1%), hypertension (up to 1%)

Central nervous system: Dizziness (2%), fatigue (1% to 2%), depression (up to 1%)

Gastrointestinal: Nausea (2% to 3%), dyspepsia (1% to 4%), upper abdominal pain (1% to 2%), vomiting (up to 1%)

Genitourinary: Urinary tract infection (3% to 5%), urinary retention (up to 1%)

Ocular: Blurred vision (4% to 5%), dry eyes (up to 2%)

Respiratory: Cough (up to 1%), pharyngitis (up to 1%)

Miscellaneous: Influenza (1% to 2%)

Overdosage/Toxicology Overdosage can potentially result in severe central anticholinergic effects. Treatment should include gastric lavage and supportive measures.

Pharmacodynamics/Kinetics

Bioavailability: 90%

Time to Peak: Plasma: 3-8 hours

Protein Binding: 98% bound to alpha$_1$-acid glycoprotein

Half-Life Elimination: 45-68 hours following chronic dosing

Metabolism: Extensively hepatic; via N-oxidation and 4 R-hydroxylation, forms one active and three inactive metabolites; primary pathway for elimination is via CYP3A4 route

Excretion: Urine 69% (<15% as unchanged drug); feces 23%

Dosing

Adults: Overactive bladder: Oral: 5 mg/day; if tolerated, may increase to 10 mg/day.

Elderly: Base dosing on renal/hepatic function.

Renal Impairment: Use with caution in reduced renal function; Cl$_{cr}$ <30 mL/minute: 5 mg/day

Hepatic Impairment: Use with caution in reduced hepatic function: Moderate: 5 mg/day; Severe: Not recommended

Available Dosage Forms Tablet: 5 mg, 10 mg

Monitoring and Teaching Issues

Physical Assessment: Assess other prescriptions and OTC medications the patient may be taking to avoid duplications and interactions. Assess knowledge/teach patient appropriate use, side effects, and symptoms to report. Monitor therapeutic response to medication; urination pattern.

Patient Education: Maintain adequate hydration (2-3 L/day) unless instructed to restrict fluid intake by prescriber. This medication may cause dry mouth (sucking on lozenges or hard candy may help). You may be more susceptible to heat prostration due to decreased ability to sweat. Use caution in hot weather (maintain adequate fluids, reduce exercise activity, rest frequently). You may experience constipation (increased exercise, fluids, fruit/fiber may help), nausea, vomiting, blurred vision and dry eyes. Report difficulty, pain, or burning on urination. **Pregnancy/breast-feeding precautions:** Inform prescriber if you are or intend to become pregnant. Consult prescriber before breast-feeding.

Geriatric Considerations: In patients with Cl_{cr} <30 mL/minute, doses >5 mg/day are not recommended.

Pregnancy Risk Factor: C

Lactation: Excretion in breast milk unknown/not recommended

Administration

Oral: Swallow tablet whole; may take with liquids, without regard to food.

Storage: Store at room temperature between 15°C to 30°C (59°F to 86°F).

Sorbitol (SOR bi tole)

Generic Available Yes

Pharmacologic Category Genitourinary Irrigant; Laxative, Miscellaneous

Use Genitourinary irrigant in transurethral prostatic resection or other transurethral resection or other transurethral surgical procedures; diuretic; humectant; sweetening agent; hyperosmotic laxative; facilitate the passage of sodium polystyrene sulfonate through the intestinal tract

Mechanism of Action/Effect A polyalcoholic sugar with osmotic cathartic actions

Contraindications Anuria

Warnings/Precautions Use with caution in patients with severe cardiopulmonary or renal impairment and in patients unable to metabolize sorbitol; large volumes may result in fluid overload and/or electrolyte changes.

Adverse Reactions Frequency not defined.

Cardiovascular: Edema

Endocrine & metabolic: Fluid and electrolyte losses, hyperglycemia, lactic acidosis

Gastrointestinal: Diarrhea, nausea, vomiting, abdominal discomfort, xerostomia

Overdosage/Toxicology Symptoms of overdose include nausea, diarrhea, fluid and electrolyte loss. Treatment is supportive to ensure fluid and electrolyte balance.

Pharmacodynamics/Kinetics

Onset of Action: 0.25-1 hour

Absorption: Oral, rectal: Poor

Metabolism: Primarily hepatic to fructose

Dosing

Adults & Elderly:

Hyperosmotic laxative (as single dose, at infrequent intervals):

Oral: 30-150 mL (as 70% solution)

Rectal enema: 120 mL as 25% to 30% solution

Adjunct to sodium polystyrene sulfonate: 15 mL as 70% solution orally until diarrhea occurs (10-20 mL/2 hours) or 20-100 mL as an oral vehicle for the sodium polystyrene sulfonate resin

When administered with charcoal:

Oral: 4.3 mL/kg of 70% sorbitol with 1 g/kg of activated charcoal every 4 hours until first stool containing charcoal is passed

Transurethral surgical procedures: Irrigation: Topical: 3% to 3.3% as transurethral surgical procedure irrigation

Pediatrics:

Hyperosmotic laxative (as single dose, at infrequent intervals):

Children 2-11 years:

Oral: 2 mL/kg (as 70% solution)

Rectal enema: 30-60 mL as 25% to 30% solution

Children >12 years: Oral, Rectal enema: Refer to adult dosing.

When administered with charcoal: Oral: Children: 4.3 mL/kg of 35% sorbitol with 1 g/kg of activated charcoal

Available Dosage Forms

Solution, genitourinary irrigation: 3% (1500 mL, 3000 mL); 3.3% (2000 mL, 4000 mL)

Solution, oral: 70% (480 mL, 3840 mL)

(Continued)

Sorbitol *(Continued)*

Monitoring and Teaching Issues

Physical Assessment: When used as cathartic, determine cause of constipation before use. Assess knowledge/teach patient about use of nonpharmacological interventions to prevent constipation.

Monitoring Laboratory Tests: Electrolytes

Patient Education: Cathartic: Use of cathartics on a regular basis will have adverse effects. Increased exercise, increased fluid intake, or increased dietary fruit and fiber may be effective in preventing and resolving constipation. **Breast-feeding precaution:** Consult prescriber if breast-feeding.

Geriatric Considerations: Causes for constipation must be evaluated prior to initiating treatment. Nonpharmacological dietary treatment should be initiated before laxative use. Sorbitol is as effective as lactulose but is much less expensive.

Pregnancy Risk Factor: C

Lactation: Excretion in breast milk unknown

Administration

Storage: Protect from freezing. Avoid storage in temperatures >150°F.

Related Information

Laxatives, Classification and Properties *on page 1737*

♦ **Sorine®** *see Sotalol on page 1386*

Sotalol *(SOE ta lole)*

U.S. Brand Names Betapace®; Betapace AF®; Sorine®

Synonyms Sotalol Hydrochloride

Generic Available Yes

Pharmacologic Category Antiarrhythmic Agent, Class II; Antiarrhythmic Agent, Class III; Beta-Adrenergic Blocker, Nonselective

Medication Safety Issues

Sound-alike/look-alike issues:
Sotalol may be confused with Stadol®
Betapace® may be confused with Betapace AF®
Betapace AF® may be confused with Betapace®

Use Treatment of documented ventricular arrhythmias (ie, sustained ventricular tachycardia), that in the judgment of the physician are life-threatening; maintenance of normal sinus rhythm in patients with symptomatic atrial fibrillation and atrial flutter who are currently in sinus rhythm. Manufacturer states substitutions should not be made for Betapace AF® since Betapace AF® is distributed with a patient package insert specific for atrial fibrillation/flutter.

Mechanism of Action/Effect

Beta-blocker which contains both beta-adrenoreceptor-blocking (Vaughan Williams Class II) and cardiac action potential duration prolongation (Vaughan Williams Class III) properties

Class II effects: Increased sinus cycle length, slowed heart rate, decreased AV nodal conduction, and increased AV nodal refractoriness

Class III effects: Prolongation of the atrial and ventricular monophasic action potentials, and effective refractory prolongation of atrial muscle, ventricular muscle, and atrioventricular accessory pathways in both the antegrade and retrograde directions

Sotalol is a racemic mixture of *d*- and *l*-sotalol; both isomers have similar Class III antiarrhythmic effects while the *l*-isomer is responsible for virtually all of the beta-blocking activity

Sotalol has both beta$_1$- and beta$_2$-receptor blocking activity

The beta-blocking effect of sotalol is a noncardioselective [half maximal at about 80 mg/day and maximal at doses of 320-640 mg/day]. Significant beta blockade occurs at oral doses as low as 25 mg/day.

Significant Class III effects are seen only at oral doses ≥160 mg/day.

Contraindications Hypersensitivity to sotalol or any component of the formulation; bronchial asthma; sinus bradycardia; second- and third-degree AV block (unless a functioning pacemaker is present); congenital or acquired long QT syndromes; cardiogenic shock; uncontrolled congestive heart failure. Betapace AF® is contraindicated in patients with significantly reduced renal filtration (Cl$_{cr}$ <40 mL/minute).

Warnings/Precautions Must be initiated (or reinitiated) in a setting with continuous monitoring and staff familiar with the recognition and treatment of life-threatening arrhythmias. Patients must be monitored with continuous ECG for a minimum of 3 days (on their maintenance dose). Use cautiously in the renally-impaired (dosage adjustment required). Creatinine clearance must be calculated prior to dosing.

Monitor and adjust dose to prevent QT$_c$ prolongation. Concurrent use with other QT$_c$-prolonging drugs (including Class I and Class III antiarrhythmics) is generally not recommended; withhold for 3 half-lives. Watch for proarrhythmic effects. Correct electrolyte imbalances before initiating (especially hypokalemia and hyperkalemia). Consider pre-existing conditions such as sick sinus syndrome before initiating. Conduction abnormalities can occur particularly sinus bradycardia. Use cautiously within the first 2 weeks post-MI (experience limited), in compensated heart failure, diabetes, or in patients with PVD. Beta-blocker therapy should not be withdrawn abruptly (particularly in patients with CAD), but gradually tapered to avoid acute tachycardia, hypertension, and/or ischemia. Use caution with concurrent use of beta-blockers and either verapamil or diltiazem; bradycardia or heart block can occur. Can mask signs of thyrotoxicosis. Use care with anesthetic agents which decrease myocardial function.

Drug Interactions

Decreased Effect: Decreased effect of sotalol may occur with aluminum-magnesium antacids (if taken within 2 hours), aluminum salts, barbiturates, calcium salts, cholestyramine, colestipol, NSAIDs, penicillins (ampicillin), rifampin, salicylates, and sulfinpyrazone due to decreased bioavailability and plasma levels. Beta-blockers may decrease the effect of sulfonylureas. Beta-agonists such as albuterol, terbutaline may have less of a therapeutic effect when administered concomitantly.

Increased Effect/Toxicity: Increased effect/toxicity of beta-blockers with calcium blockers since there may be additive effects on AV conduction or ventricular function. Other agents which prolong QT interval, including Class I antiarrhythmic agents, bepridil, cisapride, erythromycin, haloperidol, pimozide, phenothiazines, tricyclic antidepressants, and specific quinolones (including sparfloxacin, gatifloxacin, moxifloxacin) may increase the effect of sotalol on the prolongation of QT interval. Amiodarone may cause additive effects on QT_c prolongation as well as decreased heart rate, and has been associated with cardiac arrest in patients receiving some beta-blockers. When used concurrently with clonidine, sotalol may increase the risk of rebound hypertension after or during withdrawal of either agent. Beta-blocker and catecholamine depleting agents (reserpine or guanethidine) may result in additive hypotension or bradycardia. Beta-blockers may increase the action or levels of ethanol, nondepolarizing muscle relaxants, and theophylline although the effects are difficult to predict.

Nutritional/Ethanol Interactions
Food: Sotalol peak serum concentrations may be decreased if taken with food.
Herb/Nutraceutical: Avoid ephedra (may worsen arrhythmia).

Adverse Reactions
>10%:
  Cardiovascular: Bradycardia (16%), chest pain (16%), palpitation (14%)
  Central nervous system: Fatigue (20%), dizziness (20%), lightheadedness (12%)
  Neuromuscular & skeletal: Weakness (13%)
  Respiratory: Dyspnea (21%)
1% to 10%:
  Cardiovascular: CHF (5%), peripheral vascular disorders (3%), edema (8%), abnormal ECG (7%), hypotension (6%), proarrhythmia (5%), syncope (5%)
  Central nervous system: Mental confusion (6%), anxiety (4%), headache (8%), sleep problems (8%), depression (4%)
  Dermatologic: Itching/rash (5%)
  Endocrine & metabolic: Sexual ability decreased (3%)
  Gastrointestinal: Diarrhea (7%), nausea/vomiting (10%), stomach discomfort (3% to 6%), flatulence (2%)
  Genitourinary: Impotence (2%)
  Hematologic: Bleeding (2%)
  Neuromuscular & skeletal: Paresthesia (4%), extremity pain (7%), back pain (3%)
  Ocular: Visual problems (5%)
  Respiratory: Upper respiratory problems (5% to 8%), asthma (2%)

Overdosage/Toxicology Symptoms of intoxication include cardiac disturbances, CNS toxicity, bronchospasm, hypoglycemia and hyperkalemia. The most common cardiac symptoms include hypotension and bradycardia; atrioventricular block, intraventricular conduction disturbances, cardiogenic shock, and asystole may occur with severe overdose, especially with membrane-depressant drugs (eg, propranolol); CNS effects include convulsions, coma, and respiratory arrest is commonly seen with propranolol and other membrane-depressant and lipid-soluble drugs.

Treatment includes symptomatic treatment of seizures, hypotension, hyperkalemia and hypoglycemia. Bradycardia and hypotension resistant to atropine, isoproterenol or pacing may respond to glucagon. Wide QRS defects caused by the membrane-depressant poisoning may respond to hypertonic sodium bicarbonate. Repeat-dose charcoal, hemoperfusion, or hemodialysis may be helpful in removal of only those beta-blockers with a small V_d, long half-life, or low intrinsic clearance (acebutolol, atenolol, nadolol, sotalol).

Pharmacodynamics/Kinetics
Onset of Action: Rapid, 1-2 hours; Peak effect: 2.5-4 hours
Duration of Action: 8-16 hours
Absorption: Decreased 20% to 30% by meals compared to fasting
Bioavailability: 90% to 100%
Protein Binding: None
Half-Life Elimination: 12 hours; Children: 9.5 hours; terminal half-life decreases with age <2 years (may by ≥1 week in neonates)
Metabolism: None
Excretion: Urine (as unchanged drug)

Dosing
Adults & Elderly: Sotalol should be initiated and doses increased in a hospital with facilities for cardiac rhythm monitoring and assessment. Proarrhythmic events can occur after initiation of therapy and with each upward dosage adjustment.

  Ventricular arrhythmias (Betapace®, Sorine®): Oral:
    Initial: 80 mg twice daily; dose may be increased gradually to 240-320 mg/day; allow 3 days between dosing increments (to attain steady-state plasma concentrations and to allow monitoring of QT intervals).
    Usual range: Most patients respond to 160-320 mg/day in 2-3 divided doses.
    Maximum: Some patients, with life-threatening refractory ventricular arrhythmias, may require doses as high as 480-640 mg/day; prescribed ONLY when the potential benefit outweighs the increased of adverse events.
  Atrial fibrillation or atrial flutter (Betapace AF®): Oral: Initial: 80 mg twice daily
    Note: If the initial dose does not reduce the frequency of relapses of atrial fibrillation/flutter and is tolerated without excessive QT prolongation (not >520 msec) after 3 days, the dose may be increased to 120 mg twice daily. This may be further increased to 160 mg twice daily if response is inadequate and QT prolongation is not excessive.
Pediatrics: Sotalol should be initiated and doses increased in a hospital with facilities for cardiac rhythm monitoring and assessment. Proarrhythmic events can occur after initiation of therapy and with each upward dosage adjustment.

  Note: The safety and efficacy of sotalol in children have not been established
  Supraventricular arrhythmias: Oral: **Note:** Dosing per manufacturer, based on pediatric pharmacokinetic data; wait at least 36 hours between dosage adjustments to allow monitoring of QT intervals

(Continued)

Sotalol *(Continued)*

Children ≤2 years: Dosage should be adjusted (decreased) by plotting of the child's age on a logarithmic scale; see graph or refer to manufacturer's package labeling.

Sotalol Age Factor Nomogram for Patients ≤2 Years of Age

Adapted from U.S. Food and Drug Administration.
http://www.fda.gov/cder/foi/label/2001/2115s3lbl.PDF

Children >2 years: Initial: 90 mg/m²/day in 3 divided doses; may be incrementally increased to a maximum of 180 mg/m²/day

Renal Impairment: Adults: Impaired renal function can increase the terminal half-life, resulting in increased drug accumulation. Sotalol (Betapace AF®) is contraindicated per the manufacturer for treatment of atrial fibrillation/flutter in patients with a Cl_{cr} <40 mL/minute.

Ventricular arrhythmias (Betapace®, Sorine®):
Cl_{cr} >60 mL/minute: Administer every 12 hours.
Cl_{cr} 30-60 mL/minute: Administer every 24 hours.
Cl_{cr} 10-30 mL/minute: Administer every 36-48 hours.
Cl_{cr} <10 mL/minute: Individualize dose.

Atrial fibrillation/flutter (Betapace AF®):
Cl_{cr} >60 mL/minute: Administer every 12 hours.
Cl_{cr} 40-60 mL/minute: Administer every 24 hours.
Cl_{cr} <40 mL/minute: Use is contraindicated.

Dialysis: Hemodialysis would be expected to reduce sotalol plasma concentrations because sotalol is not bound to plasma proteins and does not undergo extensive metabolism. Administer dose postdialysis or administer supplemental 80 mg dose. Peritoneal dialysis does not remove sotalol; supplemental dose is not necessary.

Available Dosage Forms Tablet, as hydrochloride: 80 mg, 80 mg [AF], 120 mg, 120 mg [AF], 160 mg, 160 mg [AF], 240 mg
Betapace® [light blue]: 80 mg, 120 mg, 160 mg, 240 mg
Betapace AF® [white]: 80 mg, 120 mg, 160 mg
Sorine® [white]: 80 mg, 120 mg, 160 mg, 240 mg

Monitoring and Teaching Issues

Physical Assessment: Assess potential for interactions with other prescriptions, OTC medications, or herbal products patient may be taking. Assess blood pressure and heart rate prior to and following first dose and with any change in dosage. Assess results of laboratory tests, therapeutic effectiveness, and adverse effects (eg, cardiac and pulmonary status). Advise patients with diabetes to monitor glucose levels closely (beta-blockers may alter glucose tolerance). Do not discontinue abruptly; dose should be tapered gradually. Teach patient appropriate use, possible side effects/interventions (hypotension precautions), and adverse symptoms to report.

Monitoring Laboratory Tests: Serum magnesium, potassium

Patient Education: Do not take any new medications without consulting prescriber. Take exactly as directed; do not adjust dosage or discontinue without consulting prescriber. Take pulse daily (prior to medication) and follow prescriber's instruction about holding of medication. If you have diabetes, monitor serum sugar closely (drug may alter glucose tolerance or mask signs of hypoglycemia). May cause fatigue, dizziness, lightheadedness, or postural hypotension (use caution when changing position from lying or sitting to standing, when driving, or climbing stairs until response to medication is known); alteration in sexual performance (reversible); nausea or vomiting (small frequent meals, frequent mouth care, sucking lozenges, or chewing gum may help); or diarrhea (boiled milk, buttermilk, or yogurt may help). Report immediately any chest pain, palpitations, irregular heartbeat; swelling of extremities, respiratory difficulty, new cough, or unusual fatigue; persistent nausea, vomiting, or diarrhea; or unusual muscle weakness. **Breast-feeding precaution:** Consult prescriber if breast-feeding.

Dietary Considerations: Administer on an empty stomach.

Geriatric Considerations: Since elderly frequently have Cl_{cr} <60 mL/minute, attention to dose, creatinine clearance, and monitoring is important. Make dosage adjustments at 3-day intervals or after 5-6 doses at any dosage.

Pregnancy Risk Factor: B

Pregnancy Issues: There are no adequate and well-controlled studies in pregnant women. Beta-blockers have been associated with bradycardia, hypotension, and IUGR; IUGR is probably related to maternal hypertension. Sotalol has been shown to cross the placenta, and is found in amniotic fluid; therefore, sotalol should be used during pregnancy only if the potential benefit outweighs the potential risk. Cases of neonatal hypoglycemia have been reported following maternal use of beta-blockers at parturition or during breast-feeding. Monitor breast-fed infant for symptoms of beta-blockade.

Lactation: Enters breast milk/use caution (AAP rates "compatible")

Breast-Feeding Issues: Sotalol is considered compatible by the AAP. It is recommended that the infant be monitored for signs or symptoms of beta-blockade (hypotension, brady-cardia, etc) with long-term use.

Administration

Storage: Store at 25°C (77°F). Excursions permitted to 15°C to 30°C (59°F to 86°F).

Additional Information Pharmacokinetics in children are more relevant for BSA than age.

Related Information

Antiarrhythmic Drugs *on page 1708*

Beta-Blockers *on page 1720*

♦ **Sotalol Hydrochloride** *see Sotalol on page 1386*

♦ **Sotret®** *see Isotretinoin on page 842*

♦ **SPA** *see Albumin on page 58*

♦ **Spacol [DSC]** *see Hyoscyamine on page 775*

♦ **Spacol T/S [DSC]** *see Hyoscyamine on page 775*

Sparfloxacin *(spar FLOKS a sin)*

U.S. Brand Names Zagam®

Generic Available No

Pharmacologic Category Antibiotic, Quinolone

Medication Safety Issues

Sound-alike/look-alike issues:

Zagam® may be confused with Zyban®

Use Treatment of adults with community-acquired pneumonia caused by *C. pneumoniae, H. influenzae, H. parainfluenzae, M. catarrhalis, M. pneumoniae* or *S. pneumoniae*; treatment of acute bacterial exacerbations of chronic bronchitis caused by *C. pneumoniae, E. cloacae, H. influenzae, H. parainfluenzae, K. pneumoniae, M. catarrhalis, S. aureus* or *S. pneumoniae*

Mechanism of Action/Effect Inhibits DNA-gyrase in susceptible organisms; inhibits relaxation of supercoiled DNA and promotes breakage of double-stranded DNA

Contraindications Hypersensitivity to sparfloxacin, any component of the formulation, or other quinolones; a concurrent administration with drugs which increase the QT interval including amiodarone, bepridil, bretylium, cisapride, disopyramide, furosemide, procaina-mide, quinidine, sotalol, albuterol, chloroquine, halofantrine, phenothiazines, prednisone, and tricyclic antidepressants

Warnings/Precautions Not recommended in children <18 years of age, other quinolones have caused transient arthropathy in children; CNS stimulation may occur (tremor, restless-ness, confusion, and very rarely hallucinations or seizures); use with caution in patients with known or suspected CNS disorder or renal dysfunction; prolonged use may result in superin-fection. Moderate to severe photosensitivity reactions may occur in patients exposed to direct or indirect sunlight, or to artificial ultraviolet light. Patients should avoid unnecessary sunlight exposure during treatment and for 5 days following therapy. Pseudomembranous colitis may occur and should be considered in patients who present with diarrhea. Tendon inflammation and/or rupture have been reported with other quinolone antibiotics. Risk may be increased with concurrent corticosteroids, particularly in the elderly. Discontinue at first sign of tendon inflammation or pain.

Severe hypersensitivity reactions, including anaphylaxis, have occurred with quinolone therapy. If an allergic reaction occurs (itching, urticaria, dyspnea, facial edema, loss of consciousness, tingling, cardiovascular collapse), discontinue drug immediately. Although quinolones may exacerbate myasthenia gravis, sparfloxacin appears to be an exception; caution is still warranted.

Drug Interactions

Decreased Effect: Concurrent administration of metal cations, including most antacids, oral electrolyte supplements, quinapril, sucralfate, and some didanosine formulations (chewable/buffered tablets and pediatric powder for oral suspension), may decrease quinolone levels; separate doses.

Increased Effect/Toxicity: Sparfloxacin may increase the effects/toxicity of glyburide and warfarin. Concomitant use with corticosteroids may increase the risk of tendon rupture. Concomitant use with other QT_c-prolonging agents (eg, Class Ia and Class III antiar-rhythmics, erythromycin, cisapride, antipsychotics, and cyclic antidepressants) may result in arrhythmias such as torsade de pointes. Probenecid may increase sparfloxacin levels.

Nutritional/Ethanol Interactions Herb/Nutraceutical: Avoid dong quai, St John's wort (may also cause photosensitization).

Adverse Reactions 1% to 10%:

Cardiovascular: QT_c interval prolongation (1%), vasodilation (1%)

Central nervous system: Insomnia (2%), dizziness (2%), headache (4%)

Dermatologic: Photosensitivity reaction (8%; severe <1%), pruritus (2%)

Gastrointestinal: Diarrhea (5%), dyspepsia (2%), nausea (4%), abdominal pain (2%), vomiting (1%), flatulence (1%), taste perversion (2%)

Hepatic: Increased LFTs

(Continued)

Sparfloxacin *(Continued)*

Overdosage/Toxicology Symptoms include acute renal failure and seizures. Treatment consists of GI decontamination and supportive care; it is not known if sparfloxacin is dialyzable.

Pharmacodynamics/Kinetics

Absorption: Unaffected by food or milk; reduced ~50% by concurrent administration of aluminum- and magnesium-containing antacids

Time to Peak: 3-5 hours

Protein Binding: 45%

Half-Life Elimination: Mean terminal: 20 hours (range: 16-30 hours)

Metabolism: Hepatic, primarily by phase II glucuronidation

Excretion: Excretion: Urine (50%; ~10% as unchanged drug); feces (50%)

Dosing

Adults & Elderly: Susceptible infections: Oral: Loading dose: 400 mg on day 1; maintenance dose: 200 mg/day for 10 days total therapy

Renal Impairment: Cl_{cr} <50 mL/minute: Administer 400 mg on day 1 as a loading dose, then 200 mg every 48 hours for a total of 8 additional days of therapy (total 6 tablets).

Available Dosage Forms Tablet [film coated]: 200 mg

Monitoring and Teaching Issues

Physical Assessment: Perform culture and sensitivity tests and assess patient's allergy history before initiating therapy. Use caution with known CNS disorders, bradycardia, or renal impairment (see Warnings/Precautions for use cautions). Assess potential for interactions with other pharmacological agents and herbal products patient may be taking (eg, increased risk of arrhythmias; see Drug Interactions). If severe allergic reactions occurs (itching, urticaria, dyspnea or facial edema, loss of consciousness, tingling, cardiovascular collapse), drug should be discontinued immediately. Assess results of laboratory tests, therapeutic effectiveness (resolution of infection), and adverse effects (photosensitivity, rash, gastrointestinal disturbance [diarrhea, nausea, vomiting, pain]; see Adverse Reactions). Teach patient proper use, possible side effects/appropriate interventions (eg, photosensitivity), and adverse symptoms to report (eg, opportunistic infection). See Patient Education.

Monitoring Laboratory Tests: Perform culture and sensitivity prior to beginning therapy. Monitor CBC, renal and hepatic function periodically if therapy is prolonged.

Patient Education: Do not take any new medication during therapy without consulting prescriber. Take as directed, at the same time each day. Antacids containing aluminum or magnesium or products containing iron, zinc, or calcium (vitamins) should be taken more that 4 hours after sparfloxacin. Take entire prescription even if feeling better. If dose is missed take as soon as possible, do not double doses. Maintain adequate hydration (2-3 L/day of fluids) unless instructed to restrict fluid intake. May cause photosensitivity (use sunscreen, wear protective clothing and eyewear, and avoid direct sunlight during and for several days following therapy); dizziness, lightheadedness, or anxiety (use caution when driving or engaging in tasks that require alertness until response to drug is known); nausea, vomiting, or dry mouth (small frequent meals, frequent mouth care, sucking lozenges, or chewing gum may help). If inflammation or tendon pain occurs, discontinue use immediately and report to prescriber. If allergic reaction occurs (itching urticaria, respiratory difficulty, facial edema or difficulty swallowing, loss of consciousness, tingling, chest pain, palpitations), discontinue immediately and report to prescriber. Report palpitations or chest pain; persistent diarrhea or constipation; or signs of superinfection (unusual fever or chills; vaginal itching or foul-smelling vaginal discharge; easy bruising or bleeding). **Pregnancy/breast-feeding precautions:** Inform prescriber if you are or intend to become pregnant. Do not breast-feed.

Dietary Considerations: May be taken without regard to meals; should be taken at the same time each day.

Geriatric Considerations: Elderly patients may be more susceptible to the cardiac adverse effects of sparfloxacin. Adjust dose based on renal function; evaluate patient's drug regimen prior to initiating therapy to avoid or make allowances for possible drug interactions since elderly frequently have diseases requiring medications that can interact with quinolones.

Pregnancy Risk Factor: C

Pregnancy Issues: Reports of arthropathy (observed in immature animals and reported rarely in humans) have limited the use of fluoroquinolones in pregnancy. Teratogenic effects were not reported with sparfloxacin in animal studies. Based on limited data, quinolones are not expected to be a major human teratogen. Although quinolone antibiotics should not be used as first-line agents during pregnancy, when considering treatment for life-threatening infection and/or prolonged duration of therapy, the potential risk to the fetus must be balanced against the severity of the potential illness.

Lactation: Enters breast milk/not recommended

Breast-Feeding Issues: The manufacturer recommends to discontinue nursing or to discontinue sparfloxacin.

Administration

Oral: May be taken without regard to meals, however, should be administered at the same time each day. Antacids containing aluminum or magnesium; products containing iron, zinc, or calcium; and sucralfate and didanosine should all be given >4 hours after sparfloxacin.

♦ SPD417 *see* Carbamazepine *on page 249*

Spectinomycin *(spek ti noe MYE sin)*

U.S. Brand Names Trobicin®

Synonyms Spectinomycin Hydrochloride

Generic Available No

Pharmacologic Category Antibiotic, Miscellaneous

Medication Safety Issues
Sound-alike/look-alike issues:
Trobicin® may be confused with tobramycin

Use Treatment of uncomplicated gonorrhea

Mechanism of Action/Effect A bacteriostatic antibiotic that selectively binds to the 30s subunits of ribosomes, and thereby inhibiting bacterial protein synthesis

Contraindications Hypersensitivity to spectinomycin or any component of the formulation

Warnings/Precautions Since spectinomycin is ineffective in the treatment of syphilis and may mask symptoms, all patients should be tested for syphilis at the time of diagnosis and 3 months later.

Overdosage/Toxicology Symptoms of overdose include paresthesia, dizziness, blurring of vision, ototoxicity, renal damage, nausea, sleeplessness, decrease in hemoglobin

Pharmacodynamics/Kinetics
Duration of Action: Up to 8 hours
Absorption: I.M.: Rapid and almost complete
Time to Peak: ~1 hour
Half-Life Elimination: 1.7 hours
Excretion: Urine (70% to 100% as unchanged drug)

Dosing
Adults & Elderly:
Uncomplicated gonorrhea (urethral, cervical, pharyngeal, or rectal): I.M.: 2 g deep I.M. or 4 g where antibiotic resistance is prevalent 1 time; 4 g (10 mL) dose should be given as two 5 mL injections, followed by adequate chlamydial treatment (doxycycline 100 mg twice daily for 7 days)
Disseminated gonococcal infection: I.M.: 2 g every 12 hours
Pediatrics: Gonorrhea: I.M.: Children:
<45 kg: 40 mg/kg/dose 1 time (ceftriaxone preferred)
≥45 kg: Refer to adult dosing.
Children >8 years who are allergic to PCNS/cephalosporins may be treated with oral tetracycline.
Renal Impairment: Hemodialysis effects: 50% removed by hemodialysis

Available Dosage Forms Injection, powder for reconstitution, as hydrochloride: 2 g [diluent contains benzyl alcohol]

Monitoring and Teaching Issues
Physical Assessment: Assess knowledge/teach patient sexually transmitted disease precautions. Monitor effectiveness and evaluate laboratory results.
Monitoring Laboratory Tests: Test for syphilis before treatment and 3 months later (see Warnings/Precautions).
Patient Education: This medication can only be administered I.M. You will need to return for follow-up blood tests. Report redness, irritation, pain, swelling or sign of infection at injection site. Report dizziness, blurring of vision, ototoxicity, nausea or sleeplessness.
Breast-feeding precaution: Consult prescriber if breast-feeding.
Pregnancy Risk Factor: B
Lactation: Enters breast milk/effect on infant unknown

Administration
I.M.: For I.M. use only.
Reconstitution: Use reconstituted solutions within 24 hours; reconstitute with supplied diluent only.

♦ **Spectinomycin Hydrochloride** see Spectinomycin on page 1390
♦ **Spectracef™** see Cefditoren on page 271
♦ **Spiriva®** see Tiotropium on page 1485

Spironolactone (speer on oh LAK tone)
U.S. Brand Names Aldactone®
Generic Available Yes
Pharmacologic Category Diuretic, Potassium-Sparing; Selective Aldosterone Blocker
Medication Safety Issues
Sound-alike/look-alike issues:
Aldactone® may be confused with Aldactazide®

Use Management of edema associated with excessive aldosterone excretion; hypertension; primary hyperaldosteronism; hypokalemia; treatment of hirsutism; cirrhosis of liver accompanied by edema or ascites

Unlabeled/Investigational Use Female acne (adjunctive therapy); hirsutism; hypertension (pediatric); diuretic (pediatric)

Mechanism of Action/Effect Competes with aldosterone for receptor sites in the distal renal tubules, increasing sodium chloride and water excretion while conserving potassium and hydrogen ions; may block the effect of aldosterone on arteriolar smooth muscle as well

Contraindications Hypersensitivity to spironolactone or any component of the formulation; anuria; acute renal insufficiency; significant impairment of renal excretory function; hyperkalemia; pregnancy (pregnancy-induced hypertension - per expert analysis)

Warnings/Precautions Avoid potassium supplements, potassium-containing salt substitutes, a diet rich in potassium, or other drugs that can cause hyperkalemia. Monitor for fluid and electrolyte imbalances. Gynecomastia is related to dose and duration of therapy. Diuretic therapy should be carefully used in severe hepatic dysfunction; electrolyte and fluid shifts can cause or exacerbate encephalopathy. Discontinue use prior to adrenal vein catheterization.

Drug Interactions
Decreased Effect: The effects of digoxin (loss of positive inotropic effect) and mitotane may be reduced by spironolactone. Salicylates and NSAIDs (indomethacin) may decrease the natriuretic effect of spironolactone.
Increased Effect/Toxicity: Concurrent use of spironolactone with other potassium-sparing diuretics, potassium supplements, angiotensin receptor antagonists, co-trimoxazole (high dose), and ACE inhibitors can increase the risk of hyperkalemia, especially in patients with (Continued)

Spironolactone *(Continued)*

renal impairment. Cholestyramine can cause hyperchloremic acidosis in cirrhotic patients; avoid concurrent use.

Nutritional/Ethanol Interactions
Food: Food increases absorption.
Herb/Nutraceutical: Avoid natural licorice (due to mineralocorticoid activity)

Lab Interactions May cause false elevation in serum digoxin concentrations measured by RIA.

Adverse Reactions Incidence of adverse events is not always reported. (Mean daily dose: 26 mg)

Cardiovascular: Edema (2%, placebo 2%)
Central nervous system: Disorders (23%, placebo 21%) which may include drowsiness, lethargy, headache, mental confusion, drug fever, ataxia, fatigue
Dermatologic: Maculopapular, erythematous cutaneous eruptions, urticaria, hirsutism, eosinophilia
Endocrine & metabolic: Gynecomastia (men 9%; placebo 1%), breast pain (men 2%; placebo 0.1%), serious hyperkalemia (2%, placebo 1%), hyponatremia, dehydration, hyperchloremic metabolic acidosis in decompensated hepatic cirrhosis, inability to achieve or maintain an erection, irregular menses, amenorrhea, postmenopausal bleeding
Gastrointestinal: Disorders (29%, placebo 29%) which may include anorexia, nausea, cramping, diarrhea, gastric bleeding, ulceration, gastritis, vomiting
Genitourinary: Disorders (12%, placebo 11%)
Hematologic: Agranulocytosis
Hepatic: Cholestatic/hepatocellular toxicity
Renal: Increased BUN concentration
Respiratory: Disorders (32%, placebo 34%)
Miscellaneous: Deepening of the voice, anaphylactic reaction, breast cancer

Overdosage/Toxicology Symptoms of overdose include drowsiness, confusion, clinical signs of dehydration and electrolyte imbalance, and hyperkalemia. Ingestion of large amounts of potassium-sparing diuretics may result in life-threatening hyperkalemia. This can be treated with I.V. glucose, with concurrent regular insulin. Sodium bicarbonate may also be used as a temporary measure. If needed, Kayexalate® oral or rectal solutions in sorbitol may also be used.

Pharmacodynamics/Kinetics
Time to Peak: Serum: 1-3 hours (primarily as the active metabolite)
Protein Binding: 91% to 98%
Half-Life Elimination: 78-84 minutes
Metabolism: Hepatic to multiple metabolites, including canrenone (active)
Excretion: Urine and feces

Dosing
Adults: To reduce delay in onset of effect, a loading dose of 2 or 3 times the daily dose may be administered on the first day of therapy. Oral:

Edema, hypokalemia: 25-200 mg/day in 1-2 divided doses
Hypertension (JNC 7): 25-50 mg/day in 1-2 divided doses
Diagnosis of primary aldosteronism: 100-400 mg/day in 1-2 divided doses
Acne in women (unlabeled use): 25-200 mg once daily
Hirsutism in women (unlabeled use): 50-200 mg/day in 1-2 divided doses
CHF, severe (with ACE inhibitor and a loop diuretic ± digoxin): 25 mg/day, increased or reduced depending on individual response and evidence of hyperkalemia
Elderly: Oral: Initial: 25-50 mg/day in 1-2 divided doses; increase by 25-50 mg every 5 days as needed. Adjust for renal impairment.
Pediatrics: Administration with food increases absorption. To reduce delay in onset of effect, a loading dose of 2 or 3 times the daily dose may be administered on the first day of therapy.

Edema, hypertension (unlabeled use): Oral: Children 1-17 years: Initial: 1 mg/kg/day divided every 12-24 hours (maximum dose: 3.3 mg/kg/day, up to 100 mg/day)
Diagnosis of primary aldosteronism (unlabeled use): Oral: 125-375 mg/m²/day in divided doses

Renal Impairment:
Cl_{cr} 10-50 mL/minute: Administer every 12-24 hours.
Cl_{cr} <10 mL/minute: Avoid use.

Available Dosage Forms Tablet: 25 mg, 50 mg, 100 mg

Monitoring and Teaching Issues
Physical Assessment: See Warnings/Precautions for use cautions. Diuretic effect may be delayed 2-3 days and antihypertensive effect may be delayed 2-3 weeks (see Dosing for loading dose recommendations). Assess potential for interactions with other pharmacological agents patient may be taking (eg, anything that will increase risk of hyperkalemia; see Drug Interactions). Assess serum electrolytes and hepatic function on a regular basis during therapy. Monitor effectiveness (fluid status) and adverse reactions periodically (eg, CNS changes [drowsiness, headache, confusion], rash, gynecomastia, dehydration, hyperkalemia, jaundice; see Adverse Reactions). Teach patient appropriate use, possible side effects/appropriate interventions, and symptoms to report (see Patient Education).
Monitoring Laboratory Tests: Serum electrolytes (potassium, sodium), renal function
Patient Education: Take as directed, with meals. Avoid any potassium supplements (vitamin/mineral products), potassium-containing salt substitutes, natural licorice, or extra dietary intake of potassium. Weigh yourself weekly at the same time, in the same clothes, and report weight loss >5 lb/week. May cause dizziness, drowsiness, confusion, or headache (use caution when driving or engaging in tasks requiring alertness until response to drug is known); nausea, vomiting, or dry mouth (small frequent meals, frequent mouth care, sucking lozenges, or chewing gum may help); or decreased sexual ability, gynecomastia, impotence, menstrual irregularities (reversible with discontinuing of medication).

Report mental confusion; clumsiness; persistent fatigue, chills, numbness, or muscle weakness in hands, feet, or face; acute persistent diarrhea; chest pain, rapid heartbeat, or palpitations; excessive thirst; respiratory difficulty; breast tenderness or increased body hair in females; or breast enlargement or inability to achieve erection in males. **Pregnancy precaution:** Do not get pregnant while taking this medication. Consult prescriber for appropriate contraceptive measures.

Dietary Considerations: Should be taken with food to decrease gastrointestinal irritation and to increase absorption. Excessive potassium intake (eg, salt substitutes, low-salt foods, bananas, nuts) should be avoided.

Geriatric Considerations: See Warnings/Precautions. When used in combination with ACE inhibitors, monitor patient for hyperkalemia.

Pregnancy Risk Factor: C/D in pregnancy-induced hypertension (per expert analysis)

Pregnancy Issues: Teratogenic effects were not observed in animal studies; however, doses used were less than or equal to equivalent doses in humans. The antiandrogen effects of spironolactone have been shown to cause feminization of the male fetus in animal studies. Two case reports did not demonstrate this effect in humans however, the authors caution that adequate data is lacking. Diuretics are generally avoided in pregnancy due to the theoretical risk that decreased plasma volume may cause placental insufficiency. Diuretics should not be used during pregnancy in the presence of reduced placental perfusion (eg, pre-eclampsia, intrauterine growth restriction).

Lactation: Enters breast milk/not recommended (AAP rates "compatible")

Breast-Feeding Issues: The active metabolite of spironolactone has been found in breast milk. Effects to humans are not known; however, this metabolite was found to be carcinogenic in rats. The manufacturer recommends discontinuing spironolactone or using an alternative method of feeding.

Administration

Storage: Protect from light.

Additional Information Maximum diuretic effect may be delayed 2-3 days and maximum hypertensive effects may be delayed 2-3 weeks.

Related Information

Heart Failure *on page 1828*

- **Spironolactone and Hydrochlorothiazide** *see* Hydrochlorothiazide and Spironolactone *on page 753*
- **Sporanox®** *see* Itraconazole *on page 846*
- **Sprintec™** *see* Ethinyl Estradiol and Norgestimate *on page 593*
- **SPS®** *see* Sodium Polystyrene Sulfonate *on page 1383*
- **SSD®** *see* Silver Sulfadiazine *on page 1374*
- **SSD® AF** *see* Silver Sulfadiazine *on page 1374*
- **SSKI®** *see* Potassium Iodide *on page 1237*
- **Stadol®** *see* Butorphanol *on page 227*
- **Stadol® NS [DSC]** *see* Butorphanol *on page 227*
- **Stagesic®** *see* Hydrocodone and Acetaminophen *on page 754*
- **Stalevo™** *see* Levodopa, Carbidopa, and Entacapone *on page 888*
- **Starlix®** *see* Nateglinide *on page 1060*
- **Staticin® [DSC]** *see* Erythromycin *on page 543*

Stavudine (STAV yoo deen)

U.S. Brand Names Zerit®

Synonyms d4T

Generic Available No

Pharmacologic Category Antiretroviral Agent, Reverse Transcriptase Inhibitor (Nucleoside)

Medication Safety Issues

Sound-alike/look-alike issues:

Zerit® may be confused with Ziac®

Use Treatment of HIV infection in combination with other antiretroviral agents

Mechanism of Action/Effect Inhibits reverse transcriptase of the human immunodeficiency virus (HIV)

Contraindications Hypersensitivity to stavudine or any component of the formulation

Warnings/Precautions Use with caution in patients who demonstrate previous hypersensitivity to zidovudine, didanosine, zalcitabine, pre-existing bone marrow suppression, renal insufficiency, or peripheral neuropathy. Peripheral neuropathy may be the dose-limiting side effect. Zidovudine should not be used in combination with stavudine. Lactic acidosis and severe hepatomegaly with steatosis have been reported with stavudine use, including fatal cases. Risk may be increased in obesity, prolonged nucleoside exposure, or in female patients. Suspend therapy in patients with suspected lactic acidosis; consider discontinuation of stavudine if lactic acidosis is confirmed. Pregnant women may be at increased risk of lactic acidosis and liver damage. Severe motor weakness (resembling Guillain-Barré syndrome) has also been reported (including fatal cases, usually in association with lactic acidosis); manufacturer recommends discontinuation if motor weakness develops (with or without lactic acidosis). Pancreatitis (including some fatal cases) has occurred during combination therapy (didanosine with or without hydroxyurea). Risk increased when used in combination regimen with didanosine and hydroxyurea. Suspend therapy with agents toxic to the pancreas (including stavudine, didanosine, or hydroxyurea) in patients with suspected pancreatitis.

Drug Interactions

Decreased Effect: Zidovudine inhibits intracellular phosphorylation of stavudine; concurrent use not recommended. Doxorubicin may inhibit intracellular phosphorylation of stavudine; use with caution. Ribavirin may inhibit intracellular phosphorylation of stavudine; use with caution.

Increased Effect/Toxicity: Risk of pancreatitis may be increased with concurrent didanosine use; cases of fatal lactic acidosis have been reported with this combination when used during pregnancy (use only if clearly needed). Risk of hepatotoxicity or pancreatitis

(Continued)

Stavudine *(Continued)*

may be increased with concurrent hydroxyurea use. Zalcitabine may increase risk of peripheral neuropathy; concurrent use not recommended.

Adverse Reactions All adverse reactions reported below were similar to comparative agent, zidovudine, except for peripheral neuropathy, which was greater for stavudine. Selected adverse events reported as monotherapy or in combination therapy include:

>10%:
Central nervous system: Headache
Dermatologic: Rash
Gastrointestinal: Nausea, vomiting, diarrhea
Hepatic: Hepatic transaminases increased
Neuromuscular & skeletal: Peripheral neuropathy
Miscellaneous: Amylase increased
1% to 10%: Hepatic: Bilirubin increased

Overdosage/Toxicology Acute toxicity was not reported following administration of 12-24 times the recommended dose in adults. Peripheral neuropathy and hepatic toxicity have been reported following chronic overdose. Stavudine may be removed by hemodialysis.

Pharmacodynamics/Kinetics
Bioavailability: 86.4%
Time to Peak: Serum: 1 hour
Half-Life Elimination: 1-1.6 hours
Metabolism: Undergoes intracellular phosphorylation to an active metabolite
Excretion: Urine (40% as unchanged drug)

Dosing
Adults: HIV infection (in combination with other antiretrovirals): Oral:
≥60 kg: 40 mg every 12 hours
<60 kg: 30 mg every 12 hours
Dosing adjustment for toxicity: If symptoms of peripheral neuropathy occur, discontinue until symptoms resolve. Treatment may then be resumed at 50% the recommended dose. If symptoms recur at lower dose, permanent discontinuation should be considered.
Elderly: Older patients should be closely monitored for signs and symptoms of peripheral neuropathy. Dosage should be carefully adjusted to renal function.
Pediatrics: HIV infection: Oral:
Newborns (Birth to 13 days): 0.5 mg/kg every 12 hours
Children:
>14 days and <30 kg: 1 mg/kg every 12 hours
≥30 kg: 30 mg every 12 hours
Renal Impairment:
Children: Specific recommendations not available. Reduction in dose or increase in dosing interval should be considered.
Adults:
Cl_{cr} >50 mL/minute:
≥60 kg: 40 mg every 12 hours
<60 kg: 30 mg every 12 hours
Cl_{cr} 26-50 mL/minute:
≥60 kg: 20 mg every 12 hours
<60 kg: 15 mg every 12 hours
Cl_{cr} 10-25 mL/minute, hemodialysis (administer dose after hemodialysis on day of dialysis):
≥60 kg: 20 mg every 24 hours
<60 kg: 15 mg every 24 hours

Available Dosage Forms
Capsule: 15 mg, 20 mg, 30 mg, 40 mg
Powder, for oral solution: 1 mg/mL (200 mL) [dye-free; fruit flavor]

Monitoring and Teaching Issues
Physical Assessment: Use caution in presence of impaired hepatic or renal function (see Warnings/Precautions for specific use cautions). Assess potential for interactions with other pharmacological agents patient may be taking (eg, increased risk of toxicity; see Drug Interactions). Assess results of laboratory tests, therapeutic effectiveness, and adverse reactions on a regular basis throughout therapy (eg, nausea/vomiting [dehydration], rash, peripheral neuropathy, opportunistic infection; see Adverse Reactions). Monitor patients closely for several months following discontinuation of therapy for chronic hepatitis B and clinical exacerbations. Teach patient proper use (importance of adhering to full treatment regimen), possible side effects/appropriate interventions, and adverse symptoms to report (see Patient Education).
Monitoring Laboratory Tests: Liver function, viral load
Patient Education: Do not take any new medication during therapy unless approved by prescriber. Stavudine is not a cure for HIV or hepatitis B, nor has it been found to reduce transmission. You will need frequent blood tests to adjust dosage for maximum therapeutic effect. Take as directed for full course of therapy; do not discontinue (even if feeling better). Take with or without food. Shake solution before using. This may be prescribed as part of a multidrug regiment; it is vital that you maintain that regimen and time medications as instructed. May cause loss of appetite or change in taste (sucking on lozenges, chewing gum, or small frequent meals may help); dizziness or numbness (use caution when driving or engaging in tasks that require alertness until response to drug is known); or headache, fever, or muscle pain (an analgesic may be recommended). Report persistent lethargy or unusual fatigue; yellowing of eyes, pale stool and dark urine; acute headache, severe nausea or vomiting, respiratory difficulty, loss of sensation, rash; signs of opportunistic infection (burning on urination, perineal itching, white plaques in mouth, unhealed sores, persistent sore throat or cough); or other persistent adverse effects. **Pregnancy/breast-feeding precautions:** Inform prescriber if you are or intend to become pregnant. Do not breast-feed.

Dietary Considerations: May be taken without regard to meals.

Pregnancy Risk Factor: C

Pregnancy Issues: Cases of fatal and nonfatal lactic acidosis, with or without pancreatitis, have been reported in pregnant women. It is not known if pregnancy itself potentiates this known side effect; however, pregnant women may be at increased risk of lactic acidosis and liver damage. Hepatic enzymes and electrolytes should be monitored frequently during the 3rd trimester of pregnancy. Pharmacokinetics of stavudine are not significantly altered during pregnancy; dose adjustments are not needed. The Perinatal HIV Guidelines Working Group considers stavudine to be an alternative NRTI in dual nucleoside combination regimens; use with didanosine only if no alternatives are available, do not use with zidovudine. Health professionals are encouraged to contact the antiretroviral pregnancy registry to monitor outcomes of pregnant women exposed to antiretroviral medications (1-800-258-4263 or www.APRegistry.com).

Lactation: Excretion in breast milk unknown/contraindicated

Breast-Feeding Issues: HIV-infected mothers are discouraged from breast-feeding to decrease potential transmission of HIV.

Administration

Oral: May be administered without regard to meals. Oral solution should be shaken vigorously prior to use.

Storage: Capsules and powder for reconstitution may be stored at room temperature. Reconstituted oral solution should be refrigerated and is stable for 30 days.

Additional Information Potential compliance problems, frequency of administration and adverse effects should be discussed with patients before initiating therapy to help prevent the emergence of resistance.

♦ **Stelazine®** [DSC] *see* Trifluoperazine *on page 1523*

♦ **Sterapred®** *see* PredniSONE *on page 1247*

♦ **Sterapred® DS** *see* PredniSONE *on page 1247*

♦ **STI571** *see* Imatinib *on page 785*

♦ **Stimate™** *see* Desmopressin *on page 422*

♦ **Sting-Kill** [OTC] *see* Benzocaine *on page 181*

♦ **St. Joseph® Adult Aspirin** [OTC] *see* Aspirin *on page 143*

♦ **Strattera™** *see* Atomoxetine *on page 151*

♦ **Streptase®** *see* Streptokinase *on page 1395*

Streptokinase (strep toe KYE nase)

U.S. Brand Names Streptase®

Synonyms SK

Generic Available No

Pharmacologic Category Thrombolytic Agent

Use Thrombolytic agent used in treatment of recent severe or massive deep vein thrombosis, pulmonary emboli, myocardial infarction, and occluded arteriovenous cannulas

Mechanism of Action/Effect Activates the conversion of plasminogen to plasmin by forming a complex, exposing plasminogen-activating site, and cleaving a peptide bond that converts plasminogen to plasmin; plasmin degrades fibrin, fibrinogen and other procoagulant proteins into soluble fragments; effective both outside and within the formed thrombus/embolus

Contraindications Hypersensitivity to anistreplase, streptokinase, or any component of the formulation; active internal bleeding; history of CVA; recent (within 2 months) intracranial or intraspinal surgery or trauma; intracranial neoplasm, arteriovenous malformation, or aneurysm; known bleeding diathesis; severe uncontrolled hypertension

Warnings/Precautions Concurrent heparin anticoagulation can contribute to bleeding; careful attention to all potential bleeding sites. I.M. injections and nonessential handling of the patient should be avoided. Venipunctures should be performed carefully and only when necessary. If arterial puncture is necessary, use an upper extremity vessel that can be manually compressed. If serious bleeding occurs then the infusion of streptokinase and heparin should be stopped.

For the following conditions the risk of bleeding is higher with use of thrombolytics and should be weighed against the benefits of therapy: recent (within 10 days) major surgery (eg, CABG, obstetrical delivery, organ biopsy, previous puncture of noncompressible vessels), cerebrovascular disease, recent (within 10 days) gastrointestinal or genitourinary bleeding, recent trauma (within 10 days) including CPR, hypertension (systolic BP >180 mm Hg and/or diastolic BP >110 mm Hg), high likelihood of left heart thrombus (eg, mitral stenosis with atrial fibrillation), acute pericarditis, subacute bacterial endocarditis, hemostatic defects including ones caused by severe renal or hepatic dysfunction, significant hepatic dysfunction, pregnancy, diabetic hemorrhagic retinopathy or other hemorrhagic ophthalmic conditions, septic thrombophlebitis or occluded AV cannula at seriously infected site, advanced age (eg, >75 years), patients receiving oral anticoagulants, any other condition in which bleeding constitutes a significant hazard or would be particularly difficult to manage because of location.

Coronary thrombolysis may result in reperfusion arrhythmias. Hypotension, occasionally severe, can occur (not from bleeding or anaphylaxis). Follow standard MI management. Rare anaphylactic reactions can occur. Cautious repeat administration in patients who have received anistreplase or streptokinase within 1 year (streptokinase antibody may decrease effectiveness or risk of allergic reactions). Safety and efficacy in pediatric patients have not been established.

Streptokinase is not indicated for restoration of patency of intravenous catheters. Serious adverse events relating to the use of streptokinase in the restoration of patency of occluded intravenous catheters have involved the use of high doses of streptokinase in small volumes (250,000 international units in 2 mL). Uses of lower doses of streptokinase in infusions over several hours, generally into partially occluded catheters, or local instillation into the catheter lumen and subsequent aspiration, have been described in the medical *(Continued)*

Streptokinase *(Continued)*

literature. Healthcare providers should consider the risk for potentially life-threatening reactions (hypersensitivity, apnea, bleeding) associated with the use of streptokinase in the management of occluded intravenous catheters.

Drug Interactions

Decreased Effect: Antifibrinolytic agents (aminocaproic acid) may decrease effectiveness to thrombolytic agents.

Increased Effect/Toxicity: The risk of bleeding with streptokinase is increased by oral anticoagulants (warfarin), heparin, low molecular weight heparins, and drugs which affect platelet function (eg, NSAIDs, dipyridamole, ticlopidine, clopidogrel, IIb/IIIa antagonists). Although concurrent use with aspirin and heparin may increase the risk of bleeding. Aspirin and heparin were used concomitantly with streptokinase in the majority of patients in clinical studies of MI.

Nutritional/Ethanol Interactions Herb/Nutraceutical: Avoid cat's claw, dong quai, evening primrose, feverfew, red clover, horse chestnut, garlic, green tea, ginseng, ginkgo (all have additional antiplatelet activity).

Adverse Reactions As with all drugs which may affect hemostasis, bleeding is the major adverse effect associated with streptokinase. Hemorrhage may occur at virtually any site. Risk is dependent on multiple variables, including the dosage administered, concurrent use of multiple agents which alter hemostasis, and patient predisposition (including hypertension). Rapid lysis of coronary artery thrombi by thrombolytic agents may be associated with reperfusion-related atrial and/or ventricular arrhythmia.

>10%:
   Cardiovascular: Hypotension
   Local: Injection site bleeding
1% to 10%:
   Central nervous system: Fever (1% to 4%)
   Dermatologic: Bruising, rash, pruritus
   Gastrointestinal: Gastrointestinal hemorrhage, nausea, vomiting
   Genitourinary: Genitourinary hemorrhage
   Hematologic: Anemia
   Neuromuscular & skeletal: Muscle pain
   Ocular: Eye hemorrhage, periorbital edema
   Respiratory: Bronchospasm, epistaxis
   Miscellaneous: Diaphoresis hemorrhage, gingival hemorrhage

Additional cardiovascular events associated with use in MI: Asystole, AV block, cardiac arrest, cardiac tamponade, cardiogenic shock, electromechanical dissociation, heart failure, mitral regurgitation, myocardial rupture, pericardial effusion, pericarditis, pulmonary edema, recurrent ischemia/infarction, thromboembolism, ventricular tachycardia

Overdosage/Toxicology Symptoms of overdose include epistaxis, bleeding gums, hematoma, spontaneous ecchymoses, and oozing at the catheter site. If uncontrollable bleeding occurs, discontinue infusion. Whole blood or blood products may be used to reverse bleeding.

Pharmacodynamics/Kinetics

Onset of Action: Activation of plasminogen occurs almost immediately

Duration of Action: Fibrinolytic effect: Several hours; Anticoagulant effect: 12-24 hours

Half-Life Elimination: 83 minutes

Excretion: By circulating antibodies and the reticuloendothelial system

Dosing

Adults & Elderly: I.V.:

   Note: Antibodies to streptokinase remain for at least 3-6 months after initial dose: See Warnings/Precautions. An intradermal skin test of 100 units has been suggested to predict allergic response to streptokinase. If a positive reaction is not seen after 15-20 minutes, a therapeutic dose may be administered.

   Guidelines for acute myocardial infarction (AMI): I.V.: 1.5 million units over 60 minutes
      Administration:
      Dilute two 750,000 unit vials of streptokinase with 5 mL dextrose 5% in water (D$_5$W) each, gently swirl to dissolve.
      Add this dose of the 1.5 million units to 150 mL D$_5$W.
      This should be infused over 60 minutes; an in-line filter ≥0.45 micron should be used.
      Monitor for the first few hours for signs of anaphylaxis or allergic reaction. **Infusion should be slowed if lowering of 25 mm Hg in blood pressure or terminated if asthmatic symptoms appear.**
      Note: If heparin is administered, start when aPTT is less than 2 times the upper limit of control; do not use a bolus, but initiate infusion adjusted to a target a PTT of 1.5-2 times the upper limit of control. If heparin is not administered by infusion, initiate 7500-12,500 units SubQ every 12 hours.

   Guidelines for acute pulmonary embolism (APE): I.V.: 3 million unit dose over 24 hours
      Administration:
      Dilute four 750,000 unit vials of streptokinase with 5 mL dextrose 5% in water (D$_5$W) each, gently swirl to dissolve.
      Add this dose of 3 million units to 250 mL D$_5$W, an in-line filter ≥0.45 micron should be used.
      Administer 250,000 units (23 mL) over 30 minutes followed by 100,000 units/hour (9 mL/hour) for 24 hours.
      Monitor for the first few hours for signs of anaphylaxis or allergic reaction. **Infusion should be slowed if blood pressure is lowered by 25 mm Hg or if asthmatic symptoms appear.**
      Begin heparin 1000 units/hour about 3-4 hours after completion of streptokinase infusion or when PTT is <100 seconds.

   Guidelines for thromboses: I.V.: Administer 250,000 units to start, then 100,000 units/hour for 24-72 hours depending on location.

Cannula occlusion: 250,000 units into cannula, clamp for 2 hours, then aspirate contents and flush with normal saline; **Not recommended; see Warnings/Precautions**

Pediatrics: Children: Safety and efficacy not established; limited studies have used the following doses.

Thromboses: I.V.: Initial (loading dose): 2000 units/kg followed by 2000 units/kg/hour for 6-12 hours **or** initial (loading dose): 3500-4000 units/kg over 30 minutes followed by I.V. continuous infusion: 1000-1500 units/kg/hour; doseshould be individualized based on response.

Clotted catheter: I.V.: **Note:** Not recommended due to possibility of allergic reactions with repeated doses: 10,000-25,000 units diluted in NS to a final volume equivalent to catheter volume; instill into catheter and leave in place for 1 hour, then aspirate contents out of catheter and flush catheter with normal saline.

Available Dosage Forms Injection, powder for reconstitution: 250,000 units, 750,000 units, 1,500,000 units

Monitoring and Teaching Issues

Physical Assessment: Weigh benefits against risks when bleeding/hemorrhage constitutes a significant hazard (see Warnings/Precautions). **Note:** Streptokinase is not indicated for restoration of patency of intravenous catheters; life-threatening reactions are associated with this use. Assess potential for interactions with other pharmacological agents and herbal products patient may be taking (especially those medications that may affect coagulation [warfarin] or platelet function [NSAIDs, dipyridamole, ticlopidine, clopidogrel]; see Drug Interactions). Assess results of laboratory results. See Administration for infusion specifics (infusion pump is required). Patient should be closely monitored for bleeding during and following treatment; infusion site, neurological status (eg, intracranial hemorrhage), vital signs, ECG (reperfusion arrhythmias); see Adverse Reactions. Bedrest and bleeding precautions should be maintained; avoid I.M. injections, venipuncture (unless absolutely necessary), and nonessential handling of the patient. If arterial puncture is necessary, use an upper extremity vessel that can be manually compressed. Patient instructions determined by patient condition (see Patient Education).

Monitoring Laboratory Tests: PT, aPTT, platelet count, hematocrit, fibrinogen concentration

Patient Education: Inform prescriber of all medications and herbal products you are taking. This medication is only administered by infusion; you will be monitored closely during and after treatment. Immediately report burning, pain, redness, swelling, or oozing at infusion site, sudden acute headache, joint pain, chest pain, or altered vision. Following infusion, you will have a tendency to bleed easily; use caution to prevent injury (use electric razor, soft toothbrush, and caution with knives, needles, or anything sharp) and follow instructions for strict bedrest to reduce the risk of injury. If bleeding does occur, report immediately and apply pressure to bleeding spot until bleeding stops completely. Report unusual pain (acute headache, joint pain, chest pain); unusual bruising or bleeding; blood in urine, stool, or vomitus; bleeding gums; vision changes; or respiratory difficulty. **Pregnancy/breast-feeding precautions:** Inform prescriber if you are or intend to become pregnant. Consult prescriber if breast-feeding.

Geriatric Considerations: Investigators applied analysis to data for patients ≥75 years of age from two large trials studying the impact of streptokinase on patient outcome after acute myocardial infarction. Their conclusion was that age alone is not a contraindication to the use of streptokinase and that thrombolytic therapy is cost-effective and is beneficial toward the survival of elderly patients. Additional studies are needed to determine if a weight-adjusted dose will maintain efficacy but decrease adverse events such as stroke.

Pregnancy Risk Factor: C

Lactation: Excretion in breast milk unknown

Administration

I.M.: Do **not** administer by intramuscular injection.

I.V.: For I.V. or intracoronary use only. Infusion pump is required. Use in-line filter >0.8 micron.

Reconstitution: Reconstituted solutions should be refrigerated and are stable for 24 hours.

Compatibility: Stable in D_5W, NS; **incompatible** with dextrans

Storage: Streptokinase, a white lyophilized powder, may have a slight yellow color in solution due to the presence of albumin. Intact vials should be stored at room temperature. Stability of parenteral admixture at room temperature (25°C) is 8 hours and at refrigeration (4°C) is 24 hours.

Streptomycin (strep toe MYE sin)

Synonyms Streptomycin Sulfate

Generic Available Yes

Pharmacologic Category Antibiotic, Aminoglycoside; Antitubercular Agent

Medication Safety Issues

Sound-alike/look-alike issues:

Streptomycin may be confused with streptozocin

Use Part of combination therapy of active tuberculosis; used in combination with other agents for treatment of streptococcal or enterococcal endocarditis, mycobacterial infections, plague, tularemia, and brucellosis

Mechanism of Action/Effect Inhibits bacterial protein synthesis by binding directly to the 30S ribosomal subunits causing faulty peptide sequence to form in the protein chain

Contraindications Hypersensitivity to streptomycin or any component of the formulation; pregnancy

Warnings/Precautions Use with caution in patients with pre-existing vertigo, tinnitus, hearing loss, neuromuscular disorders, or renal impairment. Modify dosage in patients with renal impairment. Aminoglycosides are associated with nephrotoxicity or ototoxicity. The ototoxicity may be proportional to the amount of drug given and the duration of treatment. Tinnitus or vertigo are indications of vestibular injury and impending hearing damage. Renal damage is usually reversible.

(Continued)

Streptomycin *(Continued)*

Drug Interactions

Increased Effect/Toxicity: Increased/prolonged effect with depolarizing and nondepolarizing neuromuscular blocking agents. Concurrent use with amphotericin or loop diuretics may increase nephrotoxicity.

Lab Interactions False-positive urine glucose with Benedict's solution

Adverse Reactions Frequency not defined.

Cardiovascular: Hypotension

Central nervous system: Neurotoxicity, drowsiness, headache, drug fever, paresthesia

Dermatologic: Skin rash

Gastrointestinal: Nausea, vomiting

Hematologic: Eosinophilia, anemia

Neuromuscular & skeletal: Arthralgia, weakness, tremor

Otic: Ototoxicity (auditory), ototoxicity (vestibular)

Renal: Nephrotoxicity

Respiratory: Difficulty in breathing

Overdosage/Toxicology Symptoms of overdose include ototoxicity, nephrotoxicity, and neuromuscular toxicity. The treatment of choice following a single acute overdose appears to be maintenance of urine output of at least 3 mL/kg/hour during the acute treatment phase. Dialysis is of questionable value in enhancing aminoglycoside elimination. If required, hemodialysis is preferred over peritoneal dialysis in patients with normal renal function. Chelation with penicillins is experimental.

Pharmacodynamics/Kinetics

Absorption: I.M.: Well absorbed

Time to Peak: I.M.: Within 1 hour

Protein Binding: 34%

Half-Life Elimination: Newborns: 4-10 hours; Adults: 2-4.7 hours, prolonged with renal impairment

Excretion: Urine (90% as unchanged drug); feces, saliva, sweat, and tears (<1%)

Dosing

Adults:

Tuberculosis: I.M.:

Daily therapy: I.M.: 15 mg/kg/day (maximum: 1 g)

Directly observed therapy (DOT), twice weekly: I.M.: 25-30 mg/kg (maximum: 1.5 g)

Directly observed therapy (DOT), 3 times/week: I.M.: 25-30 mg/kg (maximum: 1 g)

Enterococcal endocarditis: I.M.: 1 g every 12 hours for 2 weeks, 500 mg every 12 hours for 4 weeks in combination with penicillin

Streptococcal endocarditis: I.M., I.V.: 1 g every 12 hours for 1 week, 500 mg every 12 hours for 1 week

Tularemia: I.M., I.V.: 1-2 g/day in divided doses for 7-10 days or until patient is afebrile for 5-7 days

Plague: I.M., I.V.: 2-4 g/day in divided doses until the patient is afebrile for at least 3 days

Elderly: Intramuscular: 10 mg/kg/day, not to exceed 750 mg/day; dosing interval should be adjusted for renal function. Some authors suggest not to give more than 5 days/week or give as 20-25 mg/kg/dose twice weekly.

Pediatrics:

Tuberculosis: I.M., I.V.: Children:

Daily therapy: 20-40 mg/kg/day (maximum: 1 g/day)

Directly observed therapy (DOT), twice weekly: 20-40 mg/kg (maximum: 1 g)

Directly observed therapy DOT, 3 times/week: 25-30 mg/kg (maximum: 1 g)

Renal Impairment:

Cl$_{cr}$ 10-50 mL/minute: Administer every 24-72 hours.

Cl$_{cr}$ <10 mL/minute: Administer every 72-96 hours.

Removed by hemo- and peritoneal dialysis: Administer dose postdialysis.

Available Dosage Forms Injection, powder for reconstitution, as sulfate: 1 g

Monitoring and Teaching Issues

Physical Assessment: Assess for allergy history prior to starting therapy. See Warnings/Precautions for use cautions. Assess potential for interactions with other pharmacological agents patient may be taking (eg, increased risk of toxicity with other nephrotoxic or ototoxic drugs; see Drug Interactions). Assess results of laboratory tests, effectiveness (resolution of infection), and adverse effects on a regular basis during therapy (eg, ototoxicity [auditory or vestibular], neurotoxicity [drowsiness, paresthesia], nephrotoxicity [I & O, hematuria, edema]; see Adverse Reactions). Teach patient possible side effects/appropriate interventions and adverse symptoms to report (see Patient Education).

Monitoring Laboratory Tests: Hearing (audiogram), BUN, creatinine; serum concentration of the drug should be monitored. Perform culture and sensitivity prior to initiating therapy.

Patient Education: Do not take any new medication during therapy without consulting prescriber. This medication can only be given by I.M. injection. Therapy for TB may last several months. Do not discontinue even if you are feeling better. Maintain adequate hydration (2-3 L/day of fluids unless instructed to restrict fluid intake). May cause headache or dizziness (use caution when driving or engaging in tasks requiring alertness until response to drug is known); or nausea, vomiting, or loss of appetite (small frequent meals, frequent mouth care, sucking lozenges, or chewing gum may help). Report immediately change in hearing or sense of fullness in ears; pain, weakness, tremors, or numbness in muscles; unusual clumsiness or change in strength or altered gait; change in urinary pattern or back pain; or respiratory difficulty or chest pain. **Pregnancy precaution:** Do not get pregnant while taking this medication. Consult prescriber for appropriate contraceptive measures.

Geriatric Considerations: Streptomycin is indicated for persons from endemic areas of drug-resistant *Mycobacterium tuberculosis* or who are HIV infected. Since most older patients acquired the *M. tuberculosis* infection prior to the availability of effective chemo-therapy, isoniazid and rifampin are usually effective unless resistant organisms are suspected or the patient is HIV infected. Adjust dose interval for renal function.

Pregnancy Risk Factor: D

Lactation: Enters breast milk/compatible

Administration

I.M.: Inject deep I.M. into large muscle mass.

I.V.: I.V. administration is not recommended. Has been administered intravenously over 30-60 minutes.

Compatibility:

Compatibility in syringe: Incompatible with heparin

Compatibility when admixed: Incompatible with amobarbital, amphotericin B, chlorothi-azide, heparin, methohexital, norepinephrine, pentobarbital, phenobarbital, phenytoin, sodium bicarbonate

Storage: Depending upon manufacturer, reconstituted solution remains stable for 2-4 weeks when refrigerated and 24 hours at room temperature. Exposure to light causes darkening of solution without apparent loss of potency.

Related Information

Antimicrobial Drugs of Choice *on page 1792*

Tuberculosis *on page 1864*

♦ **Streptomycin Sulfate** *see* Streptomycin *on page 1397*

Streptozocin (strep toe ZOE sin)

U.S. Brand Names Zanosar®

Synonyms NSC-85998

Generic Available No

Pharmacologic Category Antineoplastic Agent, Alkylating Agent

Medication Safety Issues

Sound-alike/look-alike issues:

Streptozocin may be confused with streptomycin

Use Treatment of metastatic islet cell carcinoma of the pancreas, carcinoid tumor and syndrome, Hodgkin's disease, palliative treatment of colorectal cancer

Mechanism of Action/Effect Interferes with the normal function of DNA by alkylation and cross-linking the strands of DNA, and by possible protein modification

Contraindications Pregnancy

Warnings/Precautions The U.S. Food and Drug Administration (FDA) currently recom-mends that procedures for proper handling and disposal of antineoplastic agents be consid-ered. Renal toxicity is dose-related and cumulative and may be severe or fatal.

Drug Interactions

Decreased Effect: Phenytoin results in negation of streptozocin cytotoxicity.

Increased Effect/Toxicity: Doxorubicin toxicity may be increased with concurrent use of streptozocin. Manufacturer recommends doxorubicin dosage adjustment be considered.

Adverse Reactions

>10%:

Gastrointestinal: Nausea and vomiting (100%)

Hepatic: Increased LFTs

Miscellaneous: Hypoalbuminemia

Renal: BUN increased, Cl_{cr} decreased, hypophosphatemia, nephrotoxicity (25% to 75%), proteinuria, renal dysfunction (65%), renal tubular acidosis

1% to 10%:

Endocrine & metabolic: Hypoglycemia (6%)

Gastrointestinal: Diarrhea (10%)

Local: Pain at injection site

Overdosage/Toxicology Symptoms of overdose include bone marrow suppression, nausea, and vomiting. Treatment of bone marrow suppression is supportive.

Pharmacodynamics/Kinetics

Duration of Action: Disappears from serum in 4 hours

Half-Life Elimination: 35-40 minutes

Metabolism: Rapidly hepatic

Excretion: Urine (60% to 70% as metabolites); exhaled gases (5%); feces (1%)

Dosing

Adults & Elderly: Antineoplastic: Refer to individual protocols.

Single agent therapy: I.V.: 1-1.5 g/m² weekly for 6 weeks followed by a 4-week rest period

Combination therapy: I.V.: 0.5-1 g/m² for 5 consecutive days followed by a 4- to 6-week rest period

Pediatrics: Refer to adult dosing.

Renal Impairment:

Cl_{cr} 10-50 mL/minute: Administer 75% of dose.

Cl_{cr} <10 mL/minute: Administer 50% of dose.

Hepatic Impairment: Dose should be reduced in patients with severe liver disease.

Available Dosage Forms Injection, powder for reconstitution: 1 g

Monitoring and Teaching Issues

Physical Assessment: Antiemetic should be administered prior to therapy (emetic poten-tial 100%). Assess potential for interactions with other pharmacological agents (see Drug Interactions). See Administration for infusion specifics. Infusion site should be monitored closely to prevent extravasation. Assess results of laboratory tests and patient response regularly during therapy (see Adverse Reactions; eg, nephrotoxicity/renal dysfunction [I & O, hematuria, edema, BUN], hepatotoxicity [jaundice, fatigue, LFTs], hypoglycemia, diar-rhea [dehydration]). Patients with diabetes should monitor glucose levels closely (may precipitate hypoglycemia). Teach patient (or caregiver) possible side effects/appropriate interventions and adverse symptoms to report (see Patient Education).

(Continued)

Streptozocin *(Continued)*

Monitoring Laboratory Tests: Liver function tests, CBC, renal function tests (BUN, serum creatinine) at baseline and weekly during therapy

Patient Education: Do not take any new medication during therapy without consulting prescriber. This drug is only given by intravenous infusion; report immediately any redness, swelling, pain, or burning at infusion site. Maintain adequate hydration (2-3 L/day of fluids) unless instructed to restrict fluid intake. You will be more sensitive to infection (avoid crowds and exposure to infection and do not have any vaccinations without consulting prescriber). If you have diabetes, monitor glucose levels closely; may cause hypoglycemia. May cause nausea and vomiting (consult prescriber for antiemetic); nervousness, dizziness, confusion, or lethargy (use caution when driving or engaging in tasks requiring alertness until response to drug is known); or loss of body hair (reversible when treatment is finished). Report unusual back pain, change in urinary pattern; persistent fever, chills, or sore throat; unusual bleeding; blood in urine, vomitus, or stool; chest pain, palpitations, or respiratory difficulty; or swelling of feet or lower legs. **Pregnancy/breast-feeding precautions:** Inform prescriber if you are pregnant. Do not get pregnant during or for 1 month following therapy. Males: Do not cause a female to become pregnant. Males/females: Consult prescriber for instruction on appropriate barrier contraceptive measures. This drug may cause severe fetal damage. Do not breast-feed.

Pregnancy Risk Factor: D

Lactation: Enters breast milk/contraindicated

Administration

I.V.: Administer as short (30-60 minutes) or 6-hour infusion; may be given by rapid I.V. push

Reconstitution: Dilute powder with 9.5 mL SWFI or NS to a concentration of 100 mg/mL.

Compatibility: Stable in D_5W, NS

Y-site administration: Incompatible with allopurinol, aztreonam, cefepime, piperacillin/tazobactam

Storage: Store intact vials under refrigeration; vials are stable for one year at room temperature. Solution reconstituted with 9.5 mL SWFI or NS to a concentration of 100 mg/mL is stable for 48 hours at room temperature and 96 hours under refrigeration. Further dilution in D_5W or NS is stable for 48 hours at room temperature and 96 hours under refrigeration when protected from light.

♦ **Striant**™ *see* Testosterone *on page 1450*

♦ **Strong Iodine Solution** *see* Potassium Iodide *on page 1237*

♦ **Sublimaze®** *see* Fentanyl *on page 618*

♦ **Suboxone®** *see* Buprenorphine and Naloxone *on page 218*

♦ **Subutex®** *see* Buprenorphine *on page 216*

Succinylcholine *(suks in il KOE leen)*

U.S. Brand Names Anectine® [DSC]; Quelicin®

Synonyms Succinylcholine Chloride; Suxamethonium Chloride

Generic Available Yes

Pharmacologic Category Neuromuscular Blocker Agent, Depolarizing

Use Adjunct to general anesthesia to facilitate both rapid sequence and routine endotracheal intubation and to relax skeletal muscles during surgery; to reduce the intensity of muscle contractions of pharmacologically- or electrically-induced convulsions; does not relieve pain or produce sedation

Mechanism of Action/Effect Acts similar to acetylcholine, produces depolarization of the motor endplate at the myoneural junction which causes sustained flaccid skeletal muscle paralysis produced by state of accommodation that developes in adjacent excitable muscle membranes

Contraindications Hypersensitivity to succinylcholine or any component of the formulation; personal or familial history of malignant hyperthermia; myopathies associated with elevated serum creatine phosphokinase (CPK) values; narrow-angle glaucoma, penetrating eye injuries; disorders of plasma pseudocholinesterase

Warnings/Precautions Use with caution in pediatrics and adolescents secondary to undiagnosed skeletal muscle myopathy and potential for ventricular dysrhythmias and cardiac arrest resulting from hyperkalemia; use with caution in patients with pre-existing hyperkalemia, paraplegia, extensive or severe burns, extensive denervation of skeletal muscle because of disease or injury to the CNS or with degenerative or dystrophic neuromuscular disease; may increase vagal tone

Drug Interactions

Increased Effect/Toxicity:

Increased toxicity: Anticholinesterase drugs (neostigmine, physostigmine, or pyridostigmine) in combination with succinylcholine can cause cardiorespiratory collapse; cyclophosphamide, oral contraceptives, lidocaine, thiotepa, pancuronium, lithium, magnesium salts, aprotinin, chloroquine, metoclopramide, terbutaline, and procaine enhance and prolong the effects of succinylcholine

Prolonged neuromuscular blockade: Inhaled anesthetics, local anesthetics, calcium channel blockers, antiarrhythmics (eg, quinidine or procainamide), antibiotics (eg, aminoglycosides, tetracyclines, vancomycin, clindamycin), immunosuppressants (eg, cyclosporine)

Lab Interactions Increased potassium (S)

Adverse Reactions

>10%:

Ocular: Increased intraocular pressure

Miscellaneous: Postoperative stiffness

1% to 10%:

Cardiovascular: Bradycardia, hypotension, cardiac arrhythmia, tachycardia

Gastrointestinal: Intragastric pressure, salivation

Causes of prolonged neuromuscular blockade: Excessive drug administration; cumulative drug effect, decreased metabolism/excretion (hepatic and/or renal impairment); accumulation of active metabolites; electrolyte imbalance (hypokalemia, hypocalcemia, hypermagnesemia, hypernatremia); hypothermia; drug interactions; increased sensitivity to muscle relaxants (eg, neuromuscular disorders such as myasthenia gravis or polymyositis)

Overdosage/Toxicology

Symptoms of overdose include respiratory paralysis and cardiac arrest.

Bradyarrhythmias can often be treated with atropine 0.1 mg (infants). Do not treat with anticholinesterase drugs (eg, neostigmine, physostigmine) since this may worsen its toxicity by interfering with its metabolism.

Pharmacodynamics/Kinetics

Onset of Action: I.M.: 2-3 minutes; I.V.: Complete muscular relaxation: 30-60 seconds

Duration of Action: I.M.: 10-30 minutes; I.V.: 4-6 minutes with single administration

Metabolism: Rapidly hydrolyzed by plasma pseudocholinesterase

Dosing

Adults & Elderly: Neuromuscular blockade: Dose to effect; doses will vary due to interpatient variability; use ideal body weight for obese patients

I.M.: 2.5-4 mg/kg, total dose should not exceed 150 mg

I.V.: 1-1.5 mg/kg, up to 150 mg total dose

Maintenance: 0.04-0.07 mg/kg every 5-10 minutes as needed

Continuous infusion: 10-100 mcg/kg/minute (or 0.5-10 mg/minute); dilute to concentration of 1-2 mg/mL in D_5W or NS

Note: Initial dose of succinylcholine must be increased when nondepolarizing agent pretreatment used because of the antagonism between succinylcholine and nondepolarizing neuromuscular blocking agents

Pediatrics: Neuromuscular blockade: I.V.:

Note: Because of the risk of malignant hyperthermia, use of continuous infusions is not recommended in infants and children:

Small Children: Intermittent: Initial: 2 mg/kg/dose one time; maintenance: 0.3-0.6 mg/kg/dose at intervals of 5-10 minutes as necessary

Older Children and Adolescents: Intermittent: Initial: 1 mg/kg/dose one time; maintenance: 0.3-0.6 mg/kg every 5-10 minutes as needed

Hepatic Impairment: Dose should be reduced in patients with severe liver disease.

Available Dosage Forms [DSC] = Discontinued product

Injection, solution, as chloride: 20 mg/mL (10 mL) [may contain benzyl alcohol]

Anectine® [DSC]: 20 mg/mL (10 mL)

Quelicin®: 20 mg/mL (5 mL, 10 mL); 50 mg/mL (10 mL); 100 mg/mL (10 mL)

Monitoring and Teaching Issues

Physical Assessment: Only clinicians experienced in the use of neuromuscular-blocking drugs should administer and/or manage the use of succinylcholine. Dosage and rate of administration should be individualized and titrated to the desired effect, according to relevant clinical factors, premedication, concomitant medications, age, and general condition of patient. Ventilatory support must be instituted and maintained until adequate respiratory muscle function and/or airway protection are assured. Assess other medications for effectiveness and safety. Other drugs that affect neuromuscular activity may increase/decrease neuromuscular block induced by succinylcholine. This drug does not cause anesthesia or analgesia; pain must be treated with appropriate analgesic agents. Continuous monitoring of vital signs, cardiac status, respiratory status, and degree of neuromuscular block (objective assessment with external nerve stimulator) is mandatory during infusion and until full muscle tone has returned. Muscle tone returns in a predictable pattern, starting with limbs, abdomen, chest diaphragm, intercostals, and finally muscles of the neck, face, and eyes. Safety precautions must be maintained until full muscle tone has returned. Provide appropriate patient teaching/support prior to and following administration.

Monitoring Laboratory Tests: Serum potassium and calcium

Patient Education: Patient will usually be unconscious prior to administration. Education should be appropriate to individual situation. Reassurance of constant monitoring and emotional support to reduce fear and anxiety should precede and follow administration. Following return of muscle tone, do not attempt to change position or rise from bed without assistance. Report immediately any skin rash or hives, pounding heartbeat, respiratory difficulty, or muscle tremors. **Pregnancy/breast-feeding precautions:** Inform prescriber if you are pregnant. Consult prescriber if breast-feeding.

Pregnancy Risk Factor: C

Lactation: Excretion in breast milk unknown/use caution

Administration

I.M.: I.M. injections should be made deeply, preferably high into deltoid muscle.

I.V.: May be given by rapid I.V. injection without further dilution.

Compatibility:

Stable in dextran 6% in dextrose, dextran 6% in NS, D_5LR, $D_5^1/_4NS$, $D_5^1/_2NS$, D_5NS, D_5W, $D_{10}W$, LR, $^1/_2NS$, NS

Y-site administration: Incompatible with thiopental

Compatibility when admixed: Incompatible with methohexital, nafcillin, sodium bicarbonate, thiopental

Storage: Refrigerate at 2°C to 8°C (36°F to 46°F); however, remains stable for ≤3 months unrefrigerated; powder form does not require refrigeration. Stability of parenteral admixture at refrigeration temperature (4°C) is 24 hours in D_5W or NS.

Related Information

Diagnostics and Surgical Aids *on page 1625*

♦ **Succinylcholine Chloride** *see* Succinylcholine *on page 1400*

♦ **Sucraid®** *see* Sacrosidase *on page 1351*

Sucralfate (soo KRAL fate)

U.S. Brand Names Carafate®

Synonyms Aluminum Sucrose Sulfate, Basic

Generic Available Yes

Pharmacologic Category Gastrointestinal Agent, Miscellaneous

Medication Safety Issues

Sound-alike/look-alike issues:

Sucralfate may be confused with salsalate

Carafate® may be confused with Cafergot®

Use Short-term management of duodenal ulcers; maintenance of duodenal ulcers

Unlabeled/Investigational Use Gastric ulcers; suspension may be used topically for treatment of stomatitis due to cancer chemotherapy and other causes of esophageal and gastric erosions; GERD, esophagitis; treatment of NSAID mucosal damage; prevention of stress ulcers; postsclerotherapy for esophageal variceal bleeding

Mechanism of Action/Effect Forms a complex by binding with positively charged proteins in exudates, forming a viscous paste-like, adhesive substance, when combined with gastric acid adheres to the damaged mucosal area. This selectively forms a protective coating that protects the lining against peptic acid, pepsin, and bile salts.

Contraindications Hypersensitivity to sucralfate or any component of the formulation

Warnings/Precautions Successful therapy with sucralfate should not be expected to alter the posthealing frequency of recurrence or the severity of duodenal ulceration. Use with caution in patients with chronic renal failure who have an impaired excretion of absorbed aluminum. Because of the potential for sucralfate to alter the absorption of some drugs, take other medications 2 hours before sucralfate when alterations in bioavailability are believed to be critical. Do not give antacids within 30 minutes of administration.

Drug Interactions

Decreased Effect: Sucralfate may alter the absorption of digoxin, phenytoin (hydantoins), warfarin, ketoconazole, quinidine, quinolones, tetracycline, theophylline. Because of the potential for sucralfate to alter the absorption of some drugs; separate administration (take other medications at least 2 hours before sucralfate). The potential for decreased absorption should be considered when alterations in bioavailability are believed to be critical.

Nutritional/Ethanol Interactions Food: Sucralfate may interfere with absorption of vitamin A, vitamin D, vitamin E, and vitamin K.

Adverse Reactions 1% to 10%: Gastrointestinal: Constipation

Overdosage/Toxicology Toxicity is minimal, may cause constipation

Pharmacodynamics/Kinetics

Onset of Action: Paste formation and ulcer adhesion: 1-2 hours

Duration of Action: Up to 6 hours

Absorption: Oral: <5%

Metabolism: None

Excretion: Urine (small amounts as unchanged compounds)

Dosing

Adults & Elderly:

Stress ulcer prophylaxis: Oral: 1 g 4 times/day

Stress ulcer treatment: Oral: 1 g every 4 hours

Treatment of duodenal ulcer: Oral:

Initial treatment: 1 g 4 times/day, 1 hour before meals or food and at bedtime for 4-8 weeks, or alternatively 2 g twice daily; treatment is recommended for 4-8 weeks in adults, the elderly will require 12 weeks.

Maintenance/prophylaxis of duodenal ulcer: 1 g twice daily

Stomatitis (unlabeled use): Oral: 1 g/10 mL suspension; swish and spit or swish and swallow 4 times/day.

Pediatrics: Dose not established, doses of 40-80 mg/kg/day divided every 6 hours have been used

Stomatitis (unlabeled use): Oral: Children: 2.5-5 mL (1 g/10 mL suspension), swish and spit or swish and swallow 4 times/day

Renal Impairment: Aluminum salt is minimally absorbed (<5%), however, may accumulate in renal failure.

Available Dosage Forms

Suspension, oral: 1 g/10 mL (10 mL)

Carafate®: 1 g/10 mL (420 mL)

Tablet (Carafate®): 1 g

Monitoring and Teaching Issues

Physical Assessment: Use caution in presence of renal failure (see Warnings/Precautions for use cautions). Assess potential for interactions with other pharmacological agents patient may be taking (eg, will affect absorption of concurrently administered drugs; see Drug Interactions). Assess effectiveness (reduction in clinical symptoms) and adverse reactions (see Adverse Reactions). Teach patient proper use (eg, timing of other medications), possible side effects (eg, constipation) and interventions, and adverse symptoms to report (see Patient Education).

Patient Education: Take recommended dose with water on an empty stomach, 1 hour before or 2 hours after meals. Take any other medications (including vitamin supplements) at least 2 hours before taking sucralfate. Do not take antacids (if prescribed) within 30 minutes of taking sucralfate. May cause constipation (increased exercise, fluids, fruit, or fiber may help). If constipation persists, consult prescriber for approved stool softener.

Dietary Considerations: Administer with water on an empty stomach.

Geriatric Considerations: Caution should be used in the elderly due to reduced renal function. Patients with Cl$_{cr}$ <30 mL/minute may be at risk for aluminum intoxication. Due to low side effect profile, this may be an agent of choice in the elderly with PUD.

Pregnancy Risk Factor: B
Lactation: Enters breast milk/compatible
Administration
   Oral: Tablet may be broken or dissolved in water before ingestion. Administer with water on an empty stomach.
   Storage: Suspension: Shake well. Refrigeration is **not** necessary; do **not** freeze.

♦ Sucrets® [OTC] *see* Dyclonine *on page 505*
♦ Sudafed® [OTC] *see* Pseudoephedrine *on page 1282*
♦ Sudafed® 12 Hour [OTC] *see* Pseudoephedrine *on page 1282*
♦ Sudafed® 24 Hour [OTC] *see* Pseudoephedrine *on page 1282*
♦ Sudafed® Children's [OTC] *see* Pseudoephedrine *on page 1282*
♦ Sudafed® Non-Drying Sinus [OTC] *see* Guaifenesin and Pseudoephedrine *on page 733*
♦ Sudodrin [OTC] *see* Pseudoephedrine *on page 1282*
♦ SudoGest [OTC] *see* Pseudoephedrine *on page 1282*
♦ Sudo-Tab® [OTC] *see* Pseudoephedrine *on page 1282*
♦ Sular® *see* Nisoldipine *on page 1086*
♦ Sulbactam and Ampicillin *see* Ampicillin and Sulbactam *on page 118*
♦ Sulf-10® *see* Sulfacetamide *on page 1403*

Sulfacetamide (sul fa SEE ta mide)

U.S. Brand Names AK-Sulf®; Bleph®-10; Carmol® Scalp; Klaron®; Ocusulf-10; Ovace™; Sulf-10®
Synonyms Sodium Sulfacetamide; Sulfacetamide Sodium
Generic Available Yes: Ointment, solution
Pharmacologic Category Antibiotic, Ophthalmic; Antibiotic, Sulfonamide Derivative
Medication Safety Issues
   Sound-alike/look-alike issues:
      Bleph®-10 may be confused with Blephamide®
      Klaron® may be confused with Klor-Con®
Use
   Ophthalmic: Treatment and prophylaxis of conjunctivitis due to susceptible organisms; corneal ulcers; adjunctive treatment with systemic sulfonamides for therapy of trachoma
   Dermatologic: Scaling dermatosis (seborrheic); bacterial infections of the skin; acne vulgaris
Mechanism of Action/Effect Interferes with bacterial growth by inhibiting bacterial folic acid synthesis through competitive antagonism of PABA
Contraindications Hypersensitivity to sulfacetamide, sulfonamides, or any component of the formulation
Warnings/Precautions Severe reactions to sulfonamides have been reported, regardless of route of administration; reactions may include Stevens-Johnson syndrome, toxic epidermal necrolysis, fulminant hepatic necrosis, or blood dyscrasias. Chemical similarities are present among sulfonamides, sulfonylureas, carbonic anhydrase inhibitors, thiazides, and loop diuretics (except ethacrynic acid). Use in patients with sulfonamide allergy is specifically contraindicated in product labeling; however, a risk of cross-reaction exists in patients with allergy to any of these compounds; avoid use when previous reaction has been severe.

Ophthalmic: Inactivated by purulent exudates containing PABA; use with caution in severe dry eye; ointment may retard corneal epithelial healing. For topical application to the eye only; not for injection. Safety and efficacy have not been established in children <2 months of age.

Dermatologic: Use caution if applied to denuded or abraded skin. Some products contain sodium metabisulfite which may cause allergic reactions in certain individuals. For external use only; avoid contact with eyes. Safety and efficacy have not been established in children <12 years of age.
Drug Interactions
   Decreased Effect: Silver containing products are incompatible with sulfacetamide solutions.
Adverse Reactions Frequency not defined.
   Cardiovascular: Edema
   Dermatologic: Burning, erythema, irritation, itching, stinging, Stevens-Johnson syndrome
   Ocular (following ophthalmic application): Burning, conjunctivitis, conjunctival hyperemia, corneal ulcers, stinging
   Miscellaneous: Allergic reactions, systemic lupus erythematosus
Pharmacodynamics/Kinetics
   Half-Life Elimination: 7-13 hours
   Excretion: When absorbed, primarily urine (as unchanged drug)
Dosing
   Adults & Elderly:
      Conjunctivitis: Ophthalmic:
         Ointment: Apply to lower conjunctival sac 1-4 times/day and at bedtime
         Solution: Instill 1-2 drops several times daily up to every 2-3 hours in lower conjunctival sac during waking hours and less frequently at night; increase dosing interval as condition responds. Usual duration of treatment: 7-10 days
           Trachoma: Instill 2 drops into the conjunctival sac every 2 hours; must be used in conjunction with systemic therapy
      Acne: Topical: Apply thin film to affected area twice daily
      Seborrheic dermatitis: Topical: Apply at bedtime and allow to remain overnight; in severe cases, may apply twice daily. Duration of therapy is usually 8-10 applications; dosing interval may be increased as eruption subsides. Applications once or twice weekly, or every other week may be used to prevent eruptions.
      Secondary cutaneous bacterial infections: Topical: Apply 2-4 times/day until infection clears
(Continued)

Sulfacetamide *(Continued)*

Pediatrics:
Conjunctivitis: Ophthalmic: Children >2 months: Refer to adult dosing.
Dermatologic: Topical: Children >12 years: Refer to adult dosing.

Available Dosage Forms
Lotion, as sodium:
Carmol® Scalp: 10% (85 g) [contains urea 10%]
Klaron®: 10% (120 mL) [contains sodium metabisulfite]
Ovace™: 10% (180 mL, 360 mL)
Ointment, ophthalmic, as sodium (AK-Sulf®): 10% (3.5 g)
Solution, ophthalmic, as sodium: 10% (15 mL)
Bleph®-10: 10% (5 mL, 15 mL) [contains benzalkonium chloride]
Ocusulf-10: 10% (15 mL)
Sulf-10®: 10% (1 mL)

Monitoring and Teaching Issues
Physical Assessment: Assess for previous sulfonamide allergy (see Warnings/Precautions). Assess effectiveness (resolution of infection). Teach patient appropriate use (ophthalmic/topical), interventions to reduce side effects, and adverse symptoms to report (see Patient Education).
Patient Education: Do not take any new medication during therapy without consulting prescriber. Use as directed. Complete full course of therapy even if condition appears improved. **Pregnancy/breast-feeding precautions:** Inform prescriber if you are pregnant. Consult prescriber if breast-feeding.

Ophthalmic: Store at room temperature. Shake solution before using. Apply prescribed amount as often as directed. Wash hands before using. Do not let tip of applicator touch eye; do not contaminate tip of applicator (may cause eye infection, eye damage, or vision loss). When using solution, tilt head back and look upward. Gently pull down lower lid and put drop(s) in inner corner of eye. When using ointment, place medicine inside the lower lid, close eye, and roll eyeball in all directions. Do not blink for 30 seconds. Apply gentle pressure to inner corner of eye for 30 seconds. Wipe away excess from skin around eye. Do not use any other eye preparation for at least 10 minutes. Do not share medication with anyone else. May cause sensitivity to bright light (dark glasses may help); temporary stinging or blurred vision may occur. Inform prescriber if you experience eye pain, redness, burning, watering, dryness, double vision, puffiness around eye, vision changes, or other adverse eye response; worsening of condition or lack of improvement within 3-4 days.

Topical: For external use only. Apply a thin film of lotion to affected area as often as directed. Do not cover with occlusive dressing. Report increased skin redness, irritation, or development of open sores; or if condition worsens or does not improve.
Geriatric Considerations: Assess whether patient can adequately instill drops or ointment.
Pregnancy Risk Factor: C
Pregnancy Issues: Use of systemic sulfonamides during pregnancy may cause kernicterus in the newborn; the amount of systemic absorption following topical administration is not known. Use during pregnancy only if clearly needed.
Lactation: Excretion in breast milk unknown/use caution
Breast-Feeding Issues: The amount of systemic absorption following topical administration is not known. When used orally, small amounts of sulfonamides are excreted in breast milk.

Administration
Topical:
Scalp lotion: Shampoo hair with a nonirritating shampoo prior to application. Part hair in sections and apply small quantities of lotion to scalp; rub in gently. Brush hair for 2-3 minutes. May discolor white fabric.
Acne lotion: Shake well before using.
Compatibility: Incompatible with silver and zinc sulfate. Sulfacetamide is inactivated by blood or purulent exudates.
Storage: Store at controlled room temperature.
Ophthalmic solution: Solution may be used if yellow; do not use if darkened.
Carmol® Scalp treatment: Do not freeze; may be used if slightly discolored.

Sulfacetamide and Prednisolone *(sul fa SEE ta mide & pred NIS oh lone)*
U.S. Brand Names Blephamide®; Vasocidin®
Synonyms Prednisolone and Sulfacetamide
Generic Available Yes: Suspension
Pharmacologic Category Antibiotic/Corticosteroid, Ophthalmic
Medication Safety Issues
Sound-alike/look-alike issues:
Blephamide® may be confused with Bleph®-10
Vasocidin® may be confused with Vasodilan®
Use Steroid-responsive inflammatory ocular conditions where infection is present or there is a risk of infection; ophthalmic suspension may be used as an otic preparation
Dosing
Adults & Elderly: Conjunctivitis: Ophthalmic:
Ointment: Apply to lower conjunctival sac 1-4 times/day
Solution: Instill 1-3 drops every 2-3 hours while awake
Pediatrics: Conjunctivitis: Ophthalmic: Children >2 months: Refer to adult dosing.
Available Dosage Forms
Ointment, ophthalmic:
Blephamide®: Sulfacetamide sodium 10% and prednisolone acetate 0.2% (3.5 g)
Vasocidin®: Sulfacetamide sodium 10% and prednisolone acetate 0.5% (3.5 g)
Suspension, ophthalmic: Sulfacetamide sodium 10% and prednisolone sodium phosphate 0.25% (5 mL, 10 mL)

Blephamide®: Sulfacetamide sodium 10% and prednisolone acetate 0.2% (5 mL, 10 mL) [contains benzalkonium chloride]

Vasocidin®: Sulfacetamide sodium 10% and prednisolone sodium phosphate: 0.25% (5 mL, 10 mL)

Monitoring and Teaching Issues

Physical Assessment: See individual components listed under Related Information.

Patient Education: Eye drops will burn upon instillation. Ointment will cause blurred vision. Do not touch container to eye. Wait at least 10 minutes before using another eye preparation. May cause sensitivity to sunlight. Notify physician if condition does not improve in 3-4 days. **Pregnancy precaution:** Notify prescriber if you are or intend to become pregnant.

Pregnancy Risk Factor: C

Related Information

PrednisoLONE on page 1245
Sulfacetamide on page 1403

♦ **Sulfacetamide Sodium** see Sulfacetamide on page 1403

Sulfacetamide Sodium and Fluorometholone
(sul fa SEE ta mide SOW dee um & flure oh METH oh lone)

U.S. Brand Names FML-S®

Synonyms Fluorometholone and Sulfacetamide

Generic Available No

Pharmacologic Category Antibiotic/Corticosteroid, Ophthalmic

Use Steroid-responsive inflammatory ocular conditions where infection is present or there is a risk of infection

Dosing

Adults & Elderly: Conjunctivitis: Ophthalmic: Instill 1 drop into affected eye(s) 4 times/day

Note: Dose may be decreased, but should not be discontinued prematurely; re-evaluation should occur if improvement is not seen within 2 days. In chronic conditions, dosing frequency should be gradually decreased prior to discontinuing treatment.

Pediatrics: Conjunctivitis: Ophthalmic: Children >2 years: Refer to adult dosing.

Available Dosage Forms Suspension, ophthalmic: Sulfacetamide sodium 10% and fluorometholone 0.1% (5 mL, 10 mL) [contains benzalkonium chloride]

Monitoring and Teaching Issues

Physical Assessment: See individual agents.

Patient Education: Pregnancy precaution: Notify prescriber if you are or intend to become pregnant.

Pregnancy Risk Factor: C

Lactation: Enters breast milk/not recommended

Related Information

Fluorometholone on page 646
Sulfacetamide on page 1403

SulfaDIAZINE (sul fa DYE a zeen)

Generic Available Yes

Pharmacologic Category Antibiotic, Sulfonamide Derivative

Medication Safety Issues

Sound-alike/look-alike issues:

SulfaDIAZINE may be confused with sulfasalazine, sulfiSOXAZOLE

Use Treatment of urinary tract infections and nocardiosis; adjunctive treatment in toxoplasmosis; uncomplicated attack of malaria

Unlabeled/Investigational Use Rheumatic fever prophylaxis

Mechanism of Action/Effect Interferes with bacterial growth by inhibiting bacterial folic acid synthesis through competitive antagonism of PABA

Contraindications Hypersensitivity to any sulfa drug or any component of the formulation; porphyria; children <2 months of age unless indicated for the treatment of congenital toxoplasmosis; sunscreens containing PABA; pregnancy (at term)

Warnings/Precautions Use with caution in patients with impaired hepatic function or impaired renal function, G6PD deficiency; dosage modification required in patients with renal impairment; fluid intake should be maintained ≥1500 mL/day, or administer sodium bicarbonate to keep urine alkaline; more likely to cause crystalluria because it is less soluble than other sulfonamides. Chemical similarities are present among sulfonamides, sulfonylureas, carbonic anhydrase inhibitors, thiazides, and loop diuretics (except ethacrynic acid). Use in patients with sulfonamide allergy is specifically contraindicated in product labeling, however, a risk of cross-reaction exists in patients with allergy to any of these compounds; avoid use when previous reaction has been severe.

Drug Interactions

Cytochrome P450 Effect: Substrate of CYP2C8/9 (major), 2E1 (minor), 3A4 (minor); **Inhibits** CYP2C8/9 (strong)

Decreased Effect: The levels/effects of sulfadiazine may be decreased by carbamazepine, phenobarbital, phenytoin, rifampin, rifapentine, secobarbital, and other CYP2C8/9 inducers. Decreased effect with PABA or PABA metabolites of drugs (eg, procaine, proparacaine, tetracaine, sunblock).

Increased Effect/Toxicity: Increased effect of oral anticoagulants and oral hypoglycemic agents. Sulfadiazine may increase the levels/effects of amiodarone, fluoxetine, glimepiride, glipizide, nateglinide, phenytoin, pioglitazone, rosiglitazone, sertraline, warfarin, and other CYP2C8/9 substrates.

Nutritional/Ethanol Interactions

Food: Avoid large quantities of vitamin C or acidifying agents (cranberry juice) to prevent crystalluria.

Herb/Nutraceutical: Avoid dong quai, St John's wort (may also cause photosensitization).

Adverse Reactions Frequency not defined.

Central nervous system: Fever, dizziness, headache

(Continued)

SulfaDIAZINE *(Continued)*

Dermatologic: Lyell's syndrome, Stevens-Johnson syndrome, itching, rash, photosensitivity

Endocrine & metabolic: Thyroid function disturbance

Gastrointestinal: Anorexia, nausea, vomiting, diarrhea

Genitourinary: Crystalluria

Hematologic: Granulocytopenia, leukopenia, thrombocytopenia, aplastic anemia, hemolytic anemia

Hepatic: Hepatitis, jaundice

Renal: Hematuria, acute nephropathy, interstitial nephritis

Miscellaneous: Serum sickness-like reactions

Overdosage/Toxicology Symptoms of overdose include drowsiness, dizziness, anorexia, abdominal pain, nausea, vomiting, hemolytic anemia, acidosis, jaundice, fever, and agranulocytosis. Doses as little as 2-5 g/day may produce toxicity. The aniline radical is responsible for hematologic toxicity. High volume diuresis may aid in elimination and prevention of renal failure. Leucovorin 5-15 mg/day has been used to speed recovery of bone marrow.

Pharmacodynamics/Kinetics

Absorption: Well absorbed

Time to Peak: Within 3-6 hours

Half-Life Elimination: 10 hours

Metabolism: Via N-acetylation

Excretion: Urine (43% to 60% as unchanged drug, 15% to 40% as metabolites)

Dosing

Adults & Elderly:

Toxoplasmosis: Oral: 2-6 g/day divided every 6 hours in conjunction with pyrimethamine 50-75 mg/day and with supplemental folinic acid

Asymptomatic meningococcal carriers: 1 g twice daily for 2 days

Nocardiosis: 4-8 g/day for a minimum of 6 weeks

Prevention of recurrent attacks of rheumatic fever (unlabeled use): 1 g/day

Pediatrics:

Asymptomatic meningococcal carriers: Oral:

Infants 1-12 months: 500 mg once daily for 2 days

Children 1-12 years: 500 mg twice daily for 2 days

Congenital toxoplasmosis: Oral:

Newborns and Children <2 months: 100 mg/kg/day divided every 6 hours in conjunction with pyrimethamine 1 mg/kg/day once daily and supplemental folinic acid 5 mg every 3 days for 6 months

Children >2 months: 25-50 mg/kg/dose 4 times/day

Toxoplasmosis: Oral:

Children >2 months: Loading dose: 75 mg/kg; maintenance dose: 120-150 mg/kg/day, maximum dose: 6 g/day; divided every 4-6 hours in conjunction with pyrimethamine 2 mg/kg/day divided every 12 hours for 3 days followed by 1 mg/kg/day once daily with supplemental folinic acid

Prevention of recurrent attacks of rheumatic fever (unlabeled use): Oral: >30 kg: 1 g/day; <30 kg: 0.5 g/day

Available Dosage Forms Tablet: 500 mg

Monitoring and Teaching Issues

Physical Assessment: Assess for allergy history prior to starting therapy (sulfonamides). Use caution with impaired hepatic function or G6PD deficiency (see Warnings/Precautions for use cautions). Assess potential for interactions with other pharmacological agents and herbal products patient may be taking (eg, may increase or decrease levels/effects of concurrently administered drugs; see Drug Interactions). Assess effectiveness (reduced clinical symptoms) and patient response (see Adverse Reactions; eg, rash, photosensitivity, GI disturbance [nausea, vomiting, anorexia], anemia, jaundice, hematuria). Teach patient proper use, possible side effects/appropriate interventions, and adverse symptoms to report (see Patient Education).

Monitoring Laboratory Tests: Perform culture and sensitivity prior to initiating therapy.

Patient Education: Inform prescriber of any allergies you have. Do not take any new medication during therapy without consulting prescriber. Take as directed, at regular intervals around-the-clock. Take on an empty stomach, 1 hour before or 2 hours after meals with full glass of water. Complete full course of therapy even if you are feeling better. Take a missed dose as soon as possible. If almost time for next dose, skip the missed dose and return to your regular schedule. Do not take a double dose. Avoid large quantities of vitamin C. Maintain adequate hydration to prevent kidney damage (2-3 L/day of fluids) unless instructed to restrict fluid intake. May cause dizziness or headache (use caution when driving or engaging in tasks requiring alertness until response to drug is known); photosensitivity (use sunblock, wear protective clothing and eyewear, and avoid direct sunlight); nausea, vomiting, or loss of appetite (small frequent meals, frequent mouth care, sucking lozenges, or chewing gum may help). Report skin rash, persistent nausea, vomiting, or diarrhea; opportunistic infection (sore throat, fever, vaginal itching or discharge, unusual bruising or bleeding, fatigue); blood in urine or change in urinary pattern; persistent headache; abdominal pain; or respiratory difficulty. **Pregnancy/breast-feeding precautions:** Inform prescriber if you are or intend to become pregnant. Do not breast-feed.

Dietary Considerations: Supplemental folinic acid should be administered to reverse symptoms or prevent problems due to folic acid deficiency.

Pregnancy Risk Factor: B/D (at term)

Lactation: Enters breast milk/contraindicated

Administration

Oral: Tablets may be crushed to prepare oral suspension of the drug in water or with a sucrose-containing solution. Aqueous suspension with concentrations of 100 mg/mL should be stored in the refrigerator and used within 7 days. Administer around-the-clock to promote less variation in peak and trough serum levels.

Related Information FDA Name Differentiation Project: The Use of Tall-Man Letters *on page 15*

Sulfamethoxazole and Trimethoprim
(sul fa meth OKS a zole & trye METH oh prim)

U.S. Brand Names Bactrim™; Bactrim™ DS; Septra®; Septra® DS

Synonyms Co-Trimoxazole; SMZ-TMP; Sulfatrim; TMP-SMZ; Trimethoprim and Sulfamethoxazole

Generic Available Yes

Pharmacologic Category Antibiotic, Sulfonamide Derivative; Antibiotic, Miscellaneous

Medication Safety Issues
Sound-alike/look-alike issues:
Bactrim™ may be confused with bacitracin, Bactine®
Co-trimoxazole may be confused with clotrimazole
Septra® may be confused with Ceptaz®, Sectral®, Septa®

Use
Oral treatment of urinary tract infections due to *E. coli*, *Klebsiella* and *Enterobacter* sp, *M. morganii*, *P. mirabilis* and *P. vulgaris*; acute otitis media in children and acute exacerbations of chronic bronchitis in adults due to susceptible strains of *H. influenzae* or *S. pneumoniae*; treatment and prophylaxis of *Pneumocystis carinii* pneumonitis (PCP), traveler's diarrhea due to enterotoxigenic *E. coli*; treatment of enteritis caused by *Shigella flexneri* or *Shigella sonnei*

I.V. treatment or severe or complicated infections when oral therapy is not feasible, for documented PCP, empiric treatment of PCP in immune compromised patients; treatment of documented or suspected shigellosis, typhoid fever, *Nocardia asteroides* infection, or other infections caused by susceptible bacteria

Unlabeled/Investigational Use Cholera and *Salmonella*-type infections and nocardiosis; chronic prostatitis; as prophylaxis in neutropenic patients with *P. carinii* infections, in leukemics, and in patients following renal transplantation, to decrease incidence of PCP; treatment of *Cyclospora* infection, typhoid fever, *Nocardia asteroides* infection

Mechanism of Action/Effect Sulfamethoxazole interferes with bacterial folic acid synthesis; trimethoprim inhibits enzymes of the folic acid pathway

Contraindications Hypersensitivity to any sulfa drug, trimethoprim, or any component of the formulation; porphyria; megaloblastic anemia due to folate deficiency; infants <2 months of age; marked hepatic damage; severe renal disease; pregnancy (at term)

Warnings/Precautions Use with caution in patients with G6PD deficiency, impaired renal or hepatic function. Adjust dosage in patients with renal impairment. Injection vehicle contains benzyl alcohol and sodium metabisulfite. Fatalities associated with severe reactions including Stevens-Johnson syndrome, toxic epidermal necrolysis, hepatic necrosis, agranulocytosis, aplastic anemia, and other blood dyscrasias. Discontinue use at first sign of rash. Elderly patients and patients with HIV appear at greater risk for more severe adverse reactions. May cause hypoglycemia (particularly in malnourished, renal, or hepatic impairment). Use caution in patients with porphyria or thyroid dysfunction. May cause hyperkalemia. Slow acetylators may be more prone to adverse reactions.

Chemical similarities are present among sulfonamides, sulfonylureas, carbonic anhydrase inhibitors, thiazides, and loop diuretics (except ethacrynic acid). Use in patients with sulfonamide allergy is specifically contraindicated in product labeling, however, a risk of cross-reaction exists in patients with allergy to any of these compounds; avoid use when previous reaction has been severe.

Drug Interactions
Cytochrome P450 Effect:
Sulfamethoxazole: **Substrate** of CYP2C8/9 (major), 3A4 (minor); **Inhibits** CYP2C8/9 (moderate)
Trimethoprim: **Substrate** (major) of CYP2C8/9, 3A4; **Inhibits** CYP2C8/9 (moderate)

Decreased Effect: The levels/effects of sulfamethoxazole may be decreased by carbamazepine, phenobarbital, phenytoin, rifampin, rifapentine, secobarbital, and other CYP2C8/9 inducers. Although occasionally recommended to limit or reverse hematologic toxicity of high-dose sulfamethoxazole/trimethoprim, concurrent use has been associated with a decreased effectiveness in treating *Pneumocystis carinii*.

Increased Effect/Toxicity: Sulfamethoxazole/trimethoprim may increase toxicity of methotrexate. Sulfamethoxazole/trimethoprim may increase the serum levels of procainamide. Concurrent therapy with pyrimethamine (in doses >25 mg/week) may increase the risk of megaloblastic anemia. Sulfamethoxazole/trimethoprim may increase the levels/effects of amiodarone, fluoxetine, glimepiride, glipizide, nateglinide, phenytoin, pioglitazone, rosiglitazone, sertraline, warfarin, and other CYP2C8/9 substrates.

ACE Inhibitors, angiotensin receptor antagonists, or potassium-sparing diuretics may increase the risk of hyperkalemia. Concurrent use with cyclosporine may result in an increased risk of nephrotoxicity when used with sulfamethoxazole/trimethoprim. Trimethoprim may increase the serum concentration of dapsone.

Nutritional/Ethanol Interactions Herb/Nutraceutical: Avoid dong quai, St John's wort (may also cause photosensitization).

Lab Interactions Increased creatinine (Jaffé alkaline picrate reaction); increased serum methotrexate by dihydrofolate reductase method; does not interfere with RAI method

Adverse Reactions The most common adverse reactions include gastrointestinal upset (nausea, vomiting, anorexia) and dermatologic reactions (rash or urticaria). Rare, life-threatening reactions have been associated with co-trimoxazole, including severe dermatologic reactions and hepatotoxic reactions. Most other reactions listed are rare, however, frequency cannot be accurately estimated.

Cardiovascular: Allergic myocarditis
Central nervous system: Confusion, depression, hallucinations, seizure, aseptic meningitis, peripheral neuritis, fever, ataxia, kernicterus in neonates
(Continued)

Sulfamethoxazole and Trimethoprim *(Continued)*

Dermatologic: Rashes, pruritus, urticaria, photosensitivity; rare reactions include erythema multiforme, Stevens-Johnson syndrome, toxic epidermal necrolysis, exfoliative dermatitis, and Henoch-Schönlein purpura

Endocrine & metabolic: Hyperkalemia (generally at high dosages), hypoglycemia

Gastrointestinal: Nausea, vomiting, anorexia, stomatitis, diarrhea, pseudomembranous colitis, pancreatitis

Hematologic: Thrombocytopenia, megaloblastic anemia, granulocytopenia, eosinophilia, pancytopenia, aplastic anemia, methemoglobinemia, hemolysis (with G6PD deficiency), agranulocytosis

Hepatic: Hepatotoxicity (including hepatitis, cholestasis, and hepatic necrosis), hyperbilirubinemia, transaminases increased

Neuromuscular & skeletal: Arthralgia, myalgia, rhabdomyolysis

Renal: Interstitial nephritis, crystalluria, renal failure, nephrotoxicity (in association with cyclosporine), diuresis

Respiratory: Cough, dyspnea, pulmonary infiltrates

Miscellaneous: Serum sickness, angioedema, periarteritis nodosa (rare), systemic lupus erythematosus (rare)

Overdosage/Toxicology Symptoms of overdose include nausea, vomiting, GI distress, hematuria, and crystalluria. Bone marrow suppression may occur. Treatment is supportive. Adequate fluid intake is essential. Peritoneal dialysis is not effective and hemodialysis is only moderately effective in removing co-trimoxazole. Leucovorin 5-15 mg/day may accelerate hematologic recovery.

Pharmacodynamics/Kinetics

Absorption: Oral: Almost completely, 90% to 100%

Time to Peak: Serum: Within 1-4 hours

Protein Binding: SMX: 68%, TMP: 45%

Half-Life Elimination: SMX: 9 hours, TMP: 6-17 hours; both are prolonged in renal failure

Metabolism: SMX: N-acetylated and glucuronidated; TMP: metabolized to oxide and hydroxylated metabolites

Excretion: Both are excreted in urine as metabolites and unchanged drug

Pharmacokinetic Note: Effects of aging on the pharmacokinetics of both agents has been variable; increase in half-life and decreases in clearance have been associated with reduced creatinine clearance

Dosing

Adults & Elderly: Dosage recommendations are based on the trimethoprim component. Double-strength tablets are equivalent to sulfamethoxazole 800 mg and trimethoprim 160 mg.

Urinary tract infection:
Oral: One double-strength tablet every 12 hours for 10-14 days
I.V.: 8-10 mg TMP/kg/day in divided doses every 6, 8, or 12 hours for up to 14 days with severe infections

Chronic bronchitis: Oral: One double-strength tablet every 12 hours for 10-14 days

Shigellosis:
Oral: One double strength tablet every 12 hours for 5 days
I.V.: 8-10 mg TMP/kg/day in divided doses every 6, 8, or 12 hours for up to 5 days

Travelers' diarrhea: Oral: One double strength tablet every 12 hours for 5 days

Sepsis: I.V.: 20 TMP/kg/day divided every 6 hours

***Pneumocystis carinii*:**
Prophylaxis: Oral: 1 double strength tablet daily or 3 times/week
Treatment: Oral, I.V.: 15-20 mg TMP/kg/day in 3-4 divided doses

Cyclospora (unlabeled use): Oral, I.V.: 160 mg TMP twice daily for 7-10 days

Nocardia (unlabeled use): Oral, I.V.: 640 mg TMP/day in divided doses for several months (duration is controversial; an average of 7 months has been reported)

Pediatrics: Recommendations are based on the trimethoprim component.

General dosing guidelines: Children >2 months:
Mild-to-moderate infections: Oral: 8-12 mg TMP/kg/day in divided doses every 12 hours

Serious infection:
Oral: 20 mg TMP/kg/day in divided doses every 6 hours
I.V.: 8-12 mg TMP/kg/day in divided doses every 6 hours

Acute otitis media: Oral: 8 mg TMP/kg/day in divided doses every 12 hours for 10 days

Urinary tract infection:
Treatment:
Oral: 6-12 mg TMP/kg/day in divided doses every 12 hours
I.V.: 8-10 mg TMP/kg/day in divided doses every 6, 8, or 12 hours for up to 4 days with serious infections
Prophylaxis: Oral: 2 mg TMP/kg/dose daily or 5 mg TMP/kg/dose twice weekly

***Pneumocystis*:**
Treatment: Oral, I.V.: 15-20 mg TMP/kg/day in divided doses every 6-8 hours
Prophylaxis: Oral, 150 mg TMP/m^2/day in divided doses every 12 hours for 3 days/ week; dose should not exceed trimethoprim 320 mg and sulfamethoxazole 1600 mg daily
Alternative prophylaxis dosing schedules include:
150 mg TMP/m^2/day as a single daily dose 3 times/week on consecutive days
or
150 mg TMP/m^2/day in divided doses every 12 hours administered 7 days/week
or
150 mg TMP/m^2/day in divided doses every 12 hours administered 3 times/week on alternate days

Shigellosis:
Oral: 8 mg TMP/kg/day in divided doses every 12 hours for 5 days
I.V.: 8-10 mg TMP/kg/day in divided doses every 6, 8, or 12 hours for up to 5 days

Cyclospora (unlabeled use): Oral, I.V.: 5 mg TMP/kg twice daily for 7-10 days

Renal Impairment:
Cl$_{cr}$ 15-30 mL/minute: Administer 50% of recommended dose.
Cl$_{cr}$ <15 mL/minute: Not recommended

Available Dosage Forms Note: The 5:1 ratio (SMX:TMP) remains constant in all dosage forms.

Injection, solution: Sulfamethoxazole 80 mg and trimethoprim 16 mg per mL (5 mL, 10 mL, 30 mL, 50 mL) [contains propylene glycol ~400 mg/mL, alcohol, benzyl alcohol, and sodium metabisulfite]

Suspension, oral: Sulfamethoxazole 200 mg and trimethoprim 40 mg per 5 mL (20 mL, 480 mL) [contains alcohol]

Septra®: Sulfamethoxazole 200 mg and trimethoprim 40 mg per 5 mL (100 mL, 480 mL) [contains alcohol 0.26% and sodium benzoate; cherry and grape flavors]

Tablet: Sulfamethoxazole 400 mg and trimethoprim 80 mg
Bactrim™: Sulfamethoxazole 400 mg and trimethoprim 80 mg [contains sodium benzoate]
Septra®: Sulfamethoxazole 400 mg and trimethoprim 80 mg

Tablet, double strength: Sulfamethoxazole 800 mg and trimethoprim 160 mg
Bactrim™ DS: Sulfamethoxazole 800 mg and trimethoprim 160 mg [contains sodium benzoate]
Septra® DS: Sulfamethoxazole 800 mg and trimethoprim 160 mg

Monitoring and Teaching Issues

Physical Assessment: Assess results of culture and sensitivity tests and patient's allergy history prior to therapy. Use caution in presence of G6PD deficiency, impaired renal or hepatic function, thyroid dysfunction (see Warnings/Precautions). Assess potential for interactions with other pharmacological agents or herbal products patient may be taking (see Drug Interactions). See I.V. Administration for infusion specifics. Assess therapeutic response (according to purpose for use) and adverse effects (reactions are usually rare; however, severe dermatologic and hepatotoxic reactions have been reported; see Adverse Reactions). Advise patients with diabetes to monitor glucose levels closely; may cause hypoglycemia. Teach patient possible side effects/appropriate interventions and adverse symptoms to report (eg, rash, persistent gastrointestinal upset; refer to Patient Education).

Monitoring Laboratory Tests: Perform culture and sensitivity testing prior to initiating therapy; serum potassium, creatinine, BUN

Patient Education: Do not take any new medication during therapy unless approved by prescriber. Take oral medication with 8 oz of water on an empty stomach, 1 hour before or 2 hours after meals, for best absorption. Finish all medication; do not skip doses. If you have diabetes you should monitor your glucose levels closely; may cause hypoglycemia. May cause increased sensitivity to sunlight (use sunblock, wear protective clothing and dark glasses, and avoid direct exposure to sunlight); or nausea or vomiting (small frequent meals, frequent mouth care, sucking lozenges, or chewing gum may help). Report immediately rash; palpitations or chest pain; CNS changes (eg, hallucinations, abnormal anxiety, seizures); sore throat, unusual coughing, or shortness of breath; blackened stool; unusual bruising or bleeding; edema; or blood in urine or changes in urinary pattern. **Pregnancy/breast-feeding precautions:** Inform prescriber if you are or intend to become pregnant or breast-feed.

Dietary Considerations: Should be taken with 8 oz of water on empty stomach.

Geriatric Considerations: Elderly patients appear at greater risk for more severe adverse reactions. Adjust dose based on renal function.

Pregnancy Risk Factor: C/D (at term - expert analysis)

Pregnancy Issues: Do not use at term to avoid kernicterus in the newborn and use during pregnancy only if risks outweigh the benefits since folic acid metabolism may be affected.

Lactation: Enters breast milk/contraindicated (AAP rates "compatible with restrictions")

Breast-Feeding Issues: Sulfonamides are excreted in low concentrations in breast milk. Use during breast feeding in infants <2 months of age is contraindicated according to the manufacturer. The AAP considers use during breast-feeding "compatible" in full term neonates; however, breast-feeding is not recommended if the infant is ill, stressed, or premature **or** if the infant has glucose-6-phosphate dehydrogenase deficiency or hyperbilirubinemia.

Administration

I.V.: Infuse over 60-90 minutes, must dilute well before giving.

Reconstitution: Injection: Less soluble in more alkaline pH. Solution must be diluted prior to administration. The manufacturer recommends dilution as follows:
Stability of parenteral admixture at room temperature (25°C):
5 mL/125 mL D$_5$W; stable for 6 hours
5 mL/100 mL D$_5$W; stable for 4 hours
5 mL/75 mL D$_5$W; stable for 2 hours
Studies have also confirmed limited stability in NS; detailed references should be consulted.

Compatibility: Stable in D$_5$½NS, LR, ½NS
Y-site administration: Incompatible with fluconazole, midazolam, vinorelbine
Compatibility when admixed: Incompatible with fluconazole, verapamil

Storage:
Injection: Store at room temperature; do not refrigerate. Less soluble in more alkaline pH. Protect from light. Following dilution, store at room temperature; do not refrigerate.
Suspension, tablet: Store at room temperature. Protect from light.

Related Information

Antimicrobial Drugs of Choice *on page 1792*
I.V. to Oral Conversion *on page 1688*
Trimethoprim *on page 1528*

Sulfasalazine (sul fa SAL a zeen)

U.S. Brand Names Azulfidine®; Azulfidine® EN-tabs®
Synonyms Salicylazosulfapyridine
(Continued)

Sulfasalazine *(Continued)*

Generic Available Yes: Tablet; excludes delayed release

Pharmacologic Category 5-Aminosalicylic Acid Derivative

Medication Safety Issues
Sound-alike/look-alike issues:
Sulfasalazine may be confused with salsalate, sulfaDIAZINE, sulfiSOXAZOLE
Azulfidine® may be confused with Augmentin®, azathioprine

Use Management of ulcerative colitis; enteric coated tablets are also used for rheumatoid arthritis (including juvenile rheumatoid arthritis) in patients who inadequately respond to analgesics and NSAIDs

Unlabeled/Investigational Use Ankylosing spondylitis, collagenous colitis, Crohn's disease, psoriasis, psoriatic arthritis, juvenile chronic arthritis

Mechanism of Action/Effect Acts locally in the colon to decrease the inflammatory response and systemically interferes with secretion by inhibiting prostaglandin synthesis

Contraindications Hypersensitivity to sulfasalazine, sulfa drugs, salicylates, or any component of the formulation; porphyria; GI or GU obstruction; pregnancy (at term)

Warnings/Precautions Use with caution in patients with renal impairment; impaired hepatic function or urinary obstruction, blood dyscrasias, severe allergies or asthma, or G6PD deficiency; may cause folate deficiency (consider providing 1 mg/day folate supplement). Chemical similarities are present among sulfonamides, sulfonylureas, carbonic anhydrase inhibitors, thiazides, and loop diuretics (except ethacrynic acid). Use in patients with sulfonamide allergy is specifically contraindicated in product labeling, however, a risk of cross-reaction exists in patients with allergy to any of these compounds; avoid use when previous reaction has been severe. Safety and efficacy have not been established in children <2 years of age.

Drug Interactions
Decreased Effect: Decreased effect with iron, digoxin and PABA or PABA metabolites of drugs (eg, procaine, proparacaine, tetracaine).

Increased Effect/Toxicity: Sulfasalazine may increase hydantoin levels. Effects of thiopental, oral hypoglycemics, and oral anticoagulants may be increased. Sulfasalazine may increase the risk of myelosuppression with azathioprine, mercaptopurine, or thioguanine (due to TPMT inhibition); may also increase the toxicity of methotrexate. Risk of thrombocytopenia may be increased with thiazide diuretics. Concurrent methenamine may increase risk of crystalluria.

Nutritional/Ethanol Interactions
Food: May impair folate absorption.
Herb/Nutraceutical: Avoid dong quai, St John's wort (may also cause photosensitization)

Adverse Reactions
>10%:
Central nervous system: Headache (33%)
Dermatologic: Photosensitivity
Gastrointestinal: Anorexia, nausea, vomiting, diarrhea (33%), gastric distress
Genitourinary: Reversible oligospermia (33%)
<3%:
Dermatologic: Urticaria/pruritus (<3%)
Hematologic: Hemolytic anemia (<3%), Heinz body anemia (<3%)
Additional events reported with sulfonamides and/or 5-ASA derivatives: Cholestatic jaundice, eosinophilia pneumonitis, erythema multiforme, fibrosing alveolitis, hepatic necrosis, Kawasaki-like syndrome, SLE-like syndrome, pericarditis, seizure, transverse myelitis

Overdosage/Toxicology Symptoms of overdose include drowsiness, dizziness, anorexia, abdominal pain, nausea, vomiting, hemolytic anemia, acidosis, jaundice, fever, and agranulocytosis. The aniline radical is responsible for hematologic toxicity. High volume diuresis may aid in elimination and prevention of renal failure. Leucovorin 5-15 mg/day has been used to speed recovery of bone marrow.

Pharmacodynamics/Kinetics
Absorption: 10% to 15% as unchanged drug from small intestine
Half-Life Elimination: 5.7-10 hours
Metabolism: Via colonic intestinal flora to sulfapyridine and 5-aminosalicylic acid (5-ASA); following absorption, sulfapyridine undergoes N-acetylation and ring hydroxylation while 5-ASA undergoes N-acetylation
Excretion: Primarily urine (as unchanged drug, components, and acetylated metabolites)

Dosing
Adults & Elderly:
Ulcerative colitis: Oral: Initial: 1 g 3-4 times/day, 2 g/day maintenance in divided doses; may initiate therapy with 0.5-1 g/day
Rheumatoid arthritis: Oral (enteric coated tablet): Initial: 0.5-1 g/day; increase weekly to maintenance dose of 2 g/day in 2 divided doses; maximum: 3 g/day (if response to 2 g/day is inadequate after 12 weeks of treatment)

Pediatrics:
Ulcerative colitis: Oral: Children ≥2 years: Initial: 40-60 mg/kg/day in 3-6 divided doses; maintenance dose: 20-30 mg/kg/day in 4 divided doses
Juvenile rheumatoid arthritis: Oral (enteric coated tablet): Children ≥6 years: 30-50 mg/kg/day in 2 divided doses; Initial: Begin with 1/4 to 1/3 of expected maintenance dose; increase weekly; maximum: 2 g/day typically

Renal Impairment:
Cl_{cr} 10-30 mL/minute: Administer twice daily.
Cl_{cr} <10 mL/minute: Administer once daily.

Hepatic Impairment: Avoid use.

Available Dosage Forms
Tablet (Azulfidine®): 500 mg
Tablet, delayed release, enteric coated (Azulfidine® EN-tabs®): 500 mg

Monitoring and Teaching Issues

Physical Assessment: Assess for allergy history prior to starting therapy (sulfa drugs, salicylates). Use caution with renal impairment, urinary obstruction, blood dyscrasias, G6PD deficiency (see Warnings/Precautions for use cautions). Assess potential for interactions with other pharmacological agents patient may be taking (eg, may increase or decrease levels/effects of concurrently administered drugs; see Drug Interactions). Assess effectiveness (reduced clinical symptoms) and patient response (see Adverse Reactions; eg, photosensitivity, GI disturbance [nausea, vomiting, anorexia], anemia, jaundice, hematuria). Caution patients with diabetes to monitor glucose levels closely (may cause altered effect of oral hypoglycemic agents). Teach patient proper use, possible side effects/appropriate interventions, and adverse symptoms to report (see Patient Education).

Patient Education: Inform prescriber of any allergies you have. Do not take any new medication during therapy without consulting prescriber. Take as directed, at regular intervals around-the-clock with food. Do not crush, chew, or dissolve coated tablets. Complete full course of therapy even if you are feeling better. Take a missed dose as soon as possible. If almost time for next dose, skip the missed dose and return to your regular schedule. Do not take a double dose. Maintain adequate hydration to prevent kidney damage (2-3 L/day of fluids) unless instructed to restrict fluid intake. If you have diabetes, monitor glucose levels closely (may cause decreased effect of oral hypoglycemic agents). May cause dizziness or headache (use caution when driving or engaging in tasks requiring alertness until response to drug is known); photosensitivity (use sunblock, wear protective clothing and eyewear, and avoid direct sunlight); or nausea, vomiting, or loss of appetite (small frequent meals, frequent mouth care, sucking lozenges, or chewing gum may help). Report rash; persistent nausea, vomiting, or diarrhea; opportunistic infection (sore throat, fever, vaginal itching or discharge, unusual bruising or bleeding, fatigue); blood in urine or change in urinary pattern; swelling of face, lips, or tongue, tightness in chest, bad cough, blue skin color, or other persistent adverse effects. **Pregnancy/breast-feeding precautions:** Inform prescriber if you are or intend to become pregnant. Consult prescriber if breast-feeding.

Dietary Considerations: Since sulfasalazine impairs folate absorption, consider providing 1 mg/day folate supplement.

Geriatric Considerations: Adjust dose for renal function (see Additional Information).

Pregnancy Risk Factor: B/D (at term)

Lactation: Enters breast milk/use caution (AAP recommends use "with caution")

Breast-Feeding Issues: Sulfonamides are excreted in human breast milk and may cause kernicterus in the newborn. Although sulfapyridine has poor bilirubin-displacing ability, use with caution in women who are breast-feeding. The AAP classifies this agent to be used with caution since adverse effects have been reported in nursing infants.

Administration

Oral: GI intolerance is common during the first few days of therapy (give with meals).

Storage: Protect from light.

◆ **Sulfatrim** *see* Sulfamethoxazole and Trimethoprim *on page 1407*

Sulfinpyrazone (sul fin PEER a zone)

Synonyms Anturane

Generic Available Yes

Pharmacologic Category Uricosuric Agent

Use Treatment of chronic gouty arthritis and intermittent gouty arthritis

Unlabeled/Investigational Use To decrease the incidence of sudden death postmyocardial infarction

Mechanism of Action/Effect Acts by increasing the urinary excretion of uric acid, thereby decreasing blood urate levels; this effect is therapeutically useful in treating patients with acute intermittent gout, chronic tophaceous gout, and acts to promote resorption of tophi; also has antithrombic and platelet inhibitory effects

Contraindications Hypersensitivity to sulfinpyrazone, phenylbutazone, other pyrazoles, or any component of the formulation; active peptic ulcer; GI inflammation; blood dyscrasias; pregnancy (near term)

Warnings/Precautions Safety and efficacy are not established in children <18 years of age. Use with caution in patients with impaired renal function and urolithiasis.

Drug Interactions

Cytochrome P450 Effect: Substrate of CYP2C8/9 (major), 3A4 (minor); **Inhibits** CYP2C8/9 (moderate); **Induces** CYP3A4 (weak)

Decreased Effect: CYP2C8/9 inducers may decrease the levels/effects of sulfinpyrazone; example inducers include carbamazepine, phenobarbital, phenytoin, rifampin, rifapentine, and secobarbital. Decreased effect/levels of theophylline, verapamil. Decreased uricosuric activity with salicylates, niacins.

Increased Effect/Toxicity: Risk of acetaminophen hepatotoxicity is increased, while therapeutic effects may be reduced. Sulfinpyrazone may increase the levels/effects of CYP2C8/9 substrates (eg, amiodarone, fluoxetine, glimepiride, glipizide, nateglinide, phenytoin, pioglitazone, rosiglitazone, sertraline, warfarin).

Nutritional/Ethanol Interactions Herb/Nutraceutical: Avoid dong quai, St John's wort (may also cause photosensitization).

Lab Interactions Decreased uric acid (S)

Adverse Reactions Frequency not defined.

Cardiovascular: Flushing

Central nervous system: Dizziness, headache

Dermatologic: Dermatitis, rash

Gastrointestinal (most frequent adverse effects): Nausea, vomiting, stomach pain

Genitourinary: Polyuria

Hematologic: Anemia, leukopenia, increased bleeding time (decreased platelet aggregation)

Hepatic: Hepatic necrosis

Renal: Nephrotic syndrome, uric acid stones

(Continued)

Sulfinpyrazone *(Continued)*

Overdosage/Toxicology Symptoms of overdose include drowsiness, dizziness, anorexia, abdominal pain, nausea, vomiting, hemolytic anemia, acidosis, jaundice, fever, and agranulocytosis. The aniline radical is responsible for hematologic toxicity. High volume diuresis may aid in elimination and prevention of renal failure. Leucovorin 5-15 mg/day has been used to speed recovery of bone marrow.

Pharmacodynamics/Kinetics
Absorption: Rapid and complete
Time to Peak: Serum: 1.6 hours
Half-Life Elimination: 2.7-6 hours
Metabolism: Hepatic to two active metabolites
Excretion: Urine (22% to 50% as unchanged drug)

Dosing
Adults & Elderly: Gouty arthritis: Oral: 100-200 mg twice daily increasing to 400 mg twice daily, monitoring uric acid concentrations; decrease to 200 mg/day as a maintenance dose; maximum daily dose: 800 mg
Renal Impairment: Cl_{cr} <50 mL/minute: Avoid use.

Available Dosage Forms Tablet: 100 mg

Monitoring and Teaching Issues
Physical Assessment: Assess effectiveness and interactions of other medications patient may be taking. Monitor therapeutic effectiveness (eg, frequency and severity of gouty attacks), laboratory values, and adverse reactions at beginning of therapy and periodically with long-term use. Assess knowledge/teach patient appropriate use, interventions to reduce side effects, and adverse symptoms to report.
Monitoring Laboratory Tests: Serum and urinary uric acid, CBC
Patient Education: Take as directed, with meals or antacids and a full glass of water. Avoid aspirin, aspirin-containing medications, or acetaminophen products and avoid large quantities of vitamin C. It is very important to maintain adequate hydration (2-3 L/day of fluids) to prevent kidney damage unless instructed to restrict fluid intake. You may experience nausea or vomiting (small frequent meals, frequent mouth care, chewing gum, or sucking lozenges may help). Report skin rash, persistent stomach pain, painful urination or bloody urine, unusual bruising or bleeding, fatigue, or yellowing of eyes or skin. **Pregnancy/breast-feeding precautions:** Inform prescriber if you are or intend to become pregnant. Consult prescriber if breast-feeding.
Dietary Considerations: Should be taken with food or milk.
Geriatric Considerations: Since sulfinpyrazone loses its effectiveness when the Cl_{cr} is <50 mL/minute, its usefulness in the elderly is limited.
Pregnancy Risk Factor: C/D (near term - expert analysis)
Lactation: Excretion in breast milk unknown

SulfiSOXAZOLE *(sul fi SOKS a zole)*

U.S. Brand Names Gantrisin®
Synonyms Sulfisoxazole Acetyl; Sulphafurazole
Generic Available Yes: Tablet
Pharmacologic Category Antibiotic, Sulfonamide Derivative
Medication Safety Issues
Sound-alike/look-alike issues:
SulfiSOXAZOLE may be confused with sulfaDIAZINE, sulfamethoxazole, sulfasalazine
Gantrisin® may be confused with Gastrosed™
Use Treatment of urinary tract infections, otitis media, *Chlamydia*; nocardiosis
Mechanism of Action/Effect Interferes with bacterial growth by inhibiting bacterial folic acid synthesis through competitive antagonism of PABA
Contraindications Hypersensitivity to sulfisoxazole, any sulfa drug, or any component of the formulation; porphyria; infants <2 months of age (sulfas compete with bilirubin for protein binding sites); patients with urinary obstruction; sunscreens containing PABA; pregnancy (at term)
Warnings/Precautions Use with caution in patients with G6PD deficiency (hemolysis may occur), hepatic or renal impairment; dosage modification required in patients with renal impairment; risk of crystalluria should be considered in patients with impaired renal function. Chemical similarities are present among sulfonamides, sulfonylureas, carbonic anhydrase inhibitors, thiazides, and loop diuretics (except ethacrynic acid). Use in patients with sulfonamide allergy is specifically contraindicated in product labeling, however, a risk of cross-reaction exists in patients with allergy to any of these compounds; avoid use when previous reaction has been severe.
Drug Interactions
Cytochrome P450 Effect: Substrate of CYP2C8/9 (major); **Inhibits** CYP2C8/9 (strong)
Decreased Effect: Decreased effect with PABA or PABA metabolites of drugs (eg, procaine, proparacaine, tetracaine), thiopental. May decrease cyclosporine levels.
Increased Effect/Toxicity: Sulfisoxazole may increase the levels/effects of amiodarone, fluoxetine, glimepiride, glipizide, nateglinide, phenytoin, pioglitazone, rosiglitazone, sertraline, warfarin, and other CYP2C8/9 substrates. May increase the effect of methotrexate. Risk of adverse reactions (thrombocytopenia purpura) may be increased by thiazide diuretics.
Nutritional/Ethanol Interactions
Food: Interferes with folate absorption.
Herb/Nutraceutical: Avoid dong quai, St John's wort (may also cause photosensitization).
Lab Interactions False-positive protein in urine; false-positive urine glucose with Clinitest®
Adverse Reactions Frequency not defined.
Cardiovascular: Vasculitis
Central nervous system: Fever, dizziness, headache
Dermatologic: Itching, rash, photosensitivity, Lyell's syndrome, Stevens-Johnson syndrome
Endocrine & metabolic: Thyroid function disturbance

Gastrointestinal: Anorexia, nausea, vomiting, diarrhea

Genitourinary: Crystalluria, hematuria,

Hematologic: Granulocytopenia, leukopenia, thrombocytopenia, aplastic anemia, hemolytic anemia

Hepatic: Jaundice, hepatitis

Renal: Interstitial nephritis

Miscellaneous: Serum sickness-like reactions

Overdosage/Toxicology Symptoms of overdose include drowsiness, dizziness, anorexia, abdominal pain, nausea, vomiting, hemolytic anemia, acidosis, jaundice, fever, and agranulocytosis. Doses as little as 2-5 g/day may produce toxicity. The aniline radical is responsible for hematologic toxicity. High volume diuresis may aid in elimination and prevention of renal failure. Leucovorin 5-15 mg/day has been used to speed recovery of bone marrow.

Pharmacodynamics/Kinetics

Absorption: Sulfisoxazole acetyl is hydrolyzed in GI tract to sulfisoxazole which is readily absorbed

Time to Peak: Serum: 2-3 hours

Protein Binding: 85% to 88%

Half-Life Elimination: 4-7 hours; prolonged with renal impairment

Metabolism: Hepatic via acetylation and glucuronide conjugation to inactive compounds

Excretion: Urine (95%, 40% to 60% as unchanged drug) within 24 hours

Dosing

Adults & Elderly: Susceptible infections: Oral: 2-4 g stat, 4-8 g/day in divided doses every 4-6 hours

Pediatrics: Not for use in patients <2 months of age:

Children >2 months: Oral: Initial: 75 mg/kg, followed by 120-150 mg/kg/day in divided doses every 4-6 hours; not to exceed 6 g/day

Renal Impairment:

Cl_{cr} 10-50 mL/minutes: Administer every 8-12 hours.

Cl_{cr} <10 mL/minute: Administer every 12-24 hours.

Hemodialysis effects: >50% is removed by hemodialysis.

Available Dosage Forms

Suspension, oral, pediatric, as acetyl (Gantrisin®): 500 mg/5 mL (480 mL) [contains alcohol 0.3%; raspberry flavor]

Tablet: 500 mg

Monitoring and Teaching Issues

Physical Assessment: Assess for allergy history prior to starting therapy (sulfa drugs). Use caution with hepatic or renal impairment, G6PD deficiency (see Warnings/Precautions for use cautions). Assess potential for interactions with other pharmacological agents patient may be taking (eg, may increase or decrease levels/effects of concurrently administered drugs; see Drug Interactions). Assess effectiveness (reduced clinical symptoms) and patient response (see Adverse Reactions; eg, photosensitivity, GI disturbance [nausea, vomiting, anorexia], anemia, jaundice, hematuria). Caution patients with diabetes to monitor glucose levels closely (may cause altered response to oral hypoglycemics and may cause false-positive urine glucose with Clinitest®). Teach patient proper use, possible side effects/appropriate interventions, and adverse symptoms to report (see Patient Education).

Monitoring Laboratory Tests: CBC, urinalysis, renal function. Obtain specimen for culture prior to first dose.

Patient Education: Inform prescriber of any allergies you have. Do not take any new medication during therapy without consulting prescriber. Take as directed with a full glass of water, at regular intervals around-the-clock. Complete full course of therapy even if you are feeling better. Take a missed dose as soon as possible. If almost time for next dose, skip the missed dose and return to your regular schedule. Do not take a double dose. Maintain adequate hydration to prevent kidney damage (2-3 L/day of fluids) unless instructed to restrict fluid intake. If you have diabetes, this medication may cause increased effect of oral hypoglycemics; monitor glucose levels closely; may alter Clinitest® response; use of alternative method of glucose monitoring is preferable. May cause dizziness or headache (use caution when driving or engaging in tasks requiring alertness until response to drug is known); photosensitivity (use sunblock, wear protective clothing and eyewear, and avoid direct sunlight); or nausea, vomiting, or loss of appetite (small frequent meals, frequent mouth care, sucking lozenges, or chewing gum may help). Report persistent nausea, vomiting, or diarrhea; opportunistic infection (sore throat, fever, vaginal itching or discharge, unusual bruising or bleeding, fatigue); blood in urine or change in urinary pattern; swelling of face, lips, or tongue; tightness in chest; bad cough; or other persistent adverse effects. **Pregnancy precaution:** Inform prescriber if you are or intend to become pregnant.

Dietary Considerations: Should be taken with a glass of water on an empty stomach.

Geriatric Considerations: Sulfisoxazole is an effective anti-infective agent. Most prescribers prefer the combination of sulfamethoxazole and trimethoprim for its dual mechanism of action. Trimethoprim penetrates the prostate. Adjust dose for renal function.

Pregnancy Risk Factor: B/D (near term)

Lactation: Enters breast milk/compatible

Administration

Oral: Administer around-the-clock to promote less variation in peak and trough serum levels.

Storage: Protect from light.

Related Information

FDA Name Differentiation Project: The Use of Tall-Man Letters *on page 15*

♦ **Sulfisoxazole Acetyl** *see* SulfiSOXAZOLE *on page 1412*

♦ **Sulfisoxazole and Erythromycin** *see* Erythromycin and Sulfisoxazole *on page 546*

Sulindac (sul IN dak)

U.S. Brand Names Clinoril®

Generic Available Yes

Pharmacologic Category Nonsteroidal Anti-inflammatory Drug (NSAID), Oral

Medication Safety Issues

Sound-alike/look-alike issues:

Clinoril® may be confused with Cleocin®, Clozaril®, Oruvail®

Use Management of inflammatory disease, rheumatoid disorders, acute gouty arthritis, ankylosing spondylitis, bursitis, tendonitis

Mechanism of Action/Effect Inhibits prostaglandin synthesis by decreasing the activity of the enzyme, cyclooxygenase, which results in decreased formation of prostaglandin precursors

Contraindications Hypersensitivity to sulindac, any component of the formulation, aspirin or other NSAIDs; pregnancy (3rd trimester)

Warnings/Precautions Fatal asthmatic and anaphylactoid reactions have occurred in patients with "aspirin triad." Use with caution in patients with CHF, hypertension, dehydration, decreased renal or hepatic function, history of GI disease (bleeding, ulcers, or previous GI symptoms with NSAID use), or those receiving anticoagulants and/or corticosteroids. Use lowest effective dose for shortest period possible; bleeding risk has been correlated to dose and duration of therapy. Gastrointestinal bleeding may occur without prior symptoms of gastrointestinal irritation. Elderly are at a high risk for adverse effects from NSAIDs. As many as 60% of elderly can develop peptic ulceration and/or hemorrhage asymptomatically.

Use of NSAIDs can compromise existing renal function especially when Cl_{cr} <30 mL/minute. CNS adverse effects such as confusion, agitation, and hallucination are generally seen in overdose or high-dose situations; however, elderly may demonstrate these adverse effects at lower doses than younger adults. Withhold for at least 4-6 half-lives prior to surgical or dental procedures.

Drug Interactions

Decreased Effect: Decreased effect of diuretics, beta-blockers, hydralazine, and captopril.

Increased Effect/Toxicity: Increased toxicity with probenecid, NSAIDs. Increased toxicity of digoxin, anticoagulants, methotrexate, lithium, aminoglycosides antibiotics (reported in neonates), cyclosporine (increased nephrotoxicity), and potassium-sparing diuretics (hyperkalemia).

Nutritional/Ethanol Interactions

Ethanol: Avoid ethanol (may enhance gastric mucosal irritation).

Food: Food may decrease the rate but not the extent of oral absorption. The therapeutic effect of sulindac may be decreased if taken with food.

Herb/Nutraceutical: Avoid cat's claw, dong quai, evening primrose, feverfew, garlic, ginger, ginkgo, red clover, horse chestnut, green tea, ginseng (all have additional antiplatelet activity).

Lab Interactions Increased chloride (S), sodium (S), bleeding time

Adverse Reactions 1% to 10%:

Cardiovascular: Edema

Central nervous system: Dizziness, headache, nervousness

Dermatologic: Pruritus, rash

Gastrointestinal: GI pain, heartburn, nausea, vomiting, diarrhea, constipation, flatulence, anorexia, abdominal cramps

Otic: Tinnitus

Overdosage/Toxicology Symptoms of overdose include dizziness, vomiting, nausea, abdominal pain, hypotension, coma, stupor, metabolic acidosis, leukocytosis, and renal failure. Management of NSAID intoxication is supportive and symptomatic. Seizures tend to be short-lived and often do not require drug treatment.

Pharmacodynamics/Kinetics

Onset of Action: Analgesic: ~1 hour

Duration of Action: 12-24 hours

Absorption: 90%

Half-Life Elimination: Parent drug: 7 hours; Active metabolite: 18 hours

Metabolism: Hepatic; prodrug requiring metabolic activation to sulfide metabolite (active) for therapeutic effects and to sulfone metabolites (inactive)

Excretion: Urine (50%); feces (25%)

Dosing

Adults & Elderly: Note: Maximum therapeutic response may not be realized for up to 3 weeks.

Pain, inflammation: Oral: 150-200 mg twice daily or 300-400 mg once daily; not to exceed 400 mg/day.

Pediatrics: Dose not established

Hepatic Impairment: Dose reduction is necessary.

Available Dosage Forms [DSC] = Discontinued product

Tablet: 150 mg, 200 mg

Clinoril®: 150 mg [DSC]; 200 mg

Monitoring and Teaching Issues

Physical Assessment: Assess effectiveness and interactions of other medications patient may be taking. Assess results of laboratory tests, therapeutic effectiveness according to purpose for therapy, and adverse reactions (eg, GI bleeding, hepatotoxicity, ototoxicity) at beginning of therapy and periodically throughout therapy. Schedule ophthalmic evaluations for patients who are taking NSAIDs for long periods of time. Assess knowledge/teach patient appropriate use, interventions to reduce side effects, and adverse symptoms to report.

Monitoring Laboratory Tests: Liver enzymes, BUN, serum creatinine, CBC, platelets

Patient Education: Take this medication exactly as directed; do not increase dose without consulting prescriber. Take with food or milk to reduce GI distress. Maintain adequate hydration (2-3 L/day of fluids) unless instructed to restrict fluid intake. Do not use alcohol, aspirin or aspirin-containing medication, or any other anti-inflammatory medications without consulting prescriber. Regularly scheduled ophthalmic exams are advised with long-term use of NSAIDs. You may experience dizziness, nervousness, or headache (use caution when driving or engaging in tasks requiring alertness until response to drug is known); nausea, vomiting, or heartburn (small frequent meals, frequent mouth care, sucking lozenges, or chewing gum may help); or constipation (increased exercise, fluids, fruit, or fiber may help). GI bleeding, ulceration, or perforation can occur with or without pain; discontinue medication and contact prescriber if persistent abdominal pain, cramping, or blood in stool occurs. Report breathlessness or respiratory difficulty; unusual bruising or bleeding; blood in urine, stool, mouth, or vomitus; unusual fatigue; skin rash or itching; change in urinary pattern; or change in hearing or ringing in ears. **Pregnancy/breast-feeding precautions:** Inform prescriber if you are or intend to become pregnant. This drug should not be used in the 3rd trimester of pregnancy. Consult prescriber if breast-feeding.

Dietary Considerations: Drug may cause GI upset, bleeding, ulceration, perforation; take with food or milk to minimize GI upset.

Geriatric Considerations: Elderly are at high risk for adverse effects from NSAIDs. As much as 60% of elderly who develop NSAID complications can develop peptic ulceration and/or hemorrhage asymptomatically. The concomitant use of H_2 blockers, omeprazole, and sucralfate is not effective as prophylaxis with the exception of NSAID-induced duodenal ulcers which may be prevented by the use of ranitidine. Misoprostol is the only prophylactic agent proven effective. Also, concomitant disease and drug use contribute to the risk for GI adverse effects. Use lowest effective dose for shortest period possible. Consider renal function decline with age. Use of NSAIDs can compromise existing renal function especially when Cl_{cr} is ≤30 mL/minute. Tinnitus may be a difficult and unreliable indication of toxicity due to age-related hearing loss or eighth cranial nerve damage. CNS adverse effects such as confusion, agitation, and hallucination are generally seen in overdose or high-dose situations, but elderly may demonstrate these adverse effects at lower doses than younger adults.

Pregnancy Risk Factor: B/D (3rd trimester)

Lactation: Excretion in breast milk unknown

Administration

Oral: Should be administered with food or milk.

Related Information

Nonsalicylate / Nonsteroidal Anti-inflammatory Agents *on page 1743*

♦ **Sulphafurazole** *see* SulfiSOXAZOLE *on page 1412*

Sumatriptan (soo ma TRIP tan SUKS i nate)

U.S. Brand Names Imitrex®

Synonyms Sumatriptan Succinate

Generic Available No

Pharmacologic Category Serotonin 5-HT$_{1D}$ Receptor Agonist

Medication Safety Issues

Sound-alike/look-alike issues:

Sumatriptan may be confused with somatropin, zolmitriptan

Use

Oral, SubQ: Acute treatment of migraine with or without aura

SubQ: Acute treatment of cluster headache episodes

Mechanism of Action/Effect Selective agonist for serotonin (5-HT$_{1D}$ receptor) in cranial arteries to cause vasoconstriction and reduces sterile inflammation associated with antidromic neuronal transmission correlating with relief of migraine

Contraindications Hypersensitivity to sumatriptan or any component of the formulation; patients with ischemic heart disease or signs or symptoms of ischemic heart disease (including Prinzmetal's angina, angina pectoris, myocardial infarction, silent myocardial ischemia); cerebrovascular syndromes (including strokes, transient ischemic attacks); peripheral vascular syndromes (including ischemic bowel disease); uncontrolled hypertension; use within 24 hours of ergotamine derivatives; use within 24 hours of another 5-HT$_1$ agonist; concurrent administration or within 2 weeks of discontinuing an MAO inhibitor, specifically MAO type A inhibitors; management of hemiplegic or basilar migraine; prophylactic treatment of migraine; severe hepatic impairment; not for I.V. administration

Warnings/Precautions Sumatriptan is indicated only in patients ≥18 years of age with a clear diagnosis of migraine or cluster headache. Cardiac events, cerebral/subarachnoid hemorrhage, and stroke have been reported with 5-HT$_1$ agonist administration. Do not give to patients with risk factors for CAD until a cardiovascular evaluation has been performed. If the evaluation is satisfactory, the healthcare provider should administer the first dose and cardiovascular status should be periodically evaluated.

Significant elevation in blood pressure, including hypertensive crisis, has also been reported on rare occasions in patients with and without a history of hypertension. Vasospasm-related reactions have been reported other than coronary artery vasospasm. Peripheral vascular ischemia and colonic ischemia with abdominal pain and bloody diarrhea have occurred.

Use with caution in patients with history of seizure disorder or in patients with a lowered seizure threshold. Safety and efficacy in pediatric patients have not been established.

Drug Interactions

Increased Effect/Toxicity: Increased toxicity with ergot-containing drugs, avoid use, wait 24 hours from last ergot containing drug (dihydroergotamine, or methysergide) before administering sumatriptan. MAO inhibitors decrease clearance of sumatriptan increasing the risk of systemic sumatriptan toxic effects. Sumatriptan may enhance CNS toxic effects when taken with selective serotonin reuptake inhibitors (SSRIs) like fluoxetine, fluvoxamine, paroxetine, or sertraline. **Note:** Use cautiously in patients receiving concomitant medications that can lower the seizure threshold.

(Continued)

Sumatriptan *(Continued)*

Adverse Reactions

Injection:

>10%:

Central nervous system: Dizziness (12%), warm/hot sensation (11%)

Local: Pain at injection site (59%)

Neuromuscular & skeletal: Tingling (13%)

1% to 10%:

Cardiovascular: Chest pain/tightness/heaviness/pressure (2% to 3%), hyper-/hypotension (1%)

Central nervous system: Burning (7%), feeling of heaviness (7%), flushing (7%), pressure sensation (7%), feeling of tightness (5%), drowsiness (3%), malaise/fatigue (1%), feeling strange (2%), headache (2%), tight feeling in head (2%), cold sensation (1%), anxiety (1%)

Gastrointestinal: Abdominal discomfort (1%), dysphagia (1%)

Neuromuscular & skeletal: Neck, throat, and jaw pain/tightness/pressure (2% to 5%), mouth/tongue discomfort (5%), weakness (5%), myalgia (2%); muscle cramps (1%), numbness (5%)

Ocular: Vision alterations (1%)

Respiratory: Nasal disorder/discomfort (2%), throat discomfort (3%)

Miscellaneous: Diaphoresis (2%)

Nasal spray:

>10%: Gastrointestinal: Bad taste (13% to 24%), nausea (11% to 13%), vomiting (11% to 13%)

1% to 10%:

Central nervous system: Dizziness (1% to 2%)

Respiratory: Nasal disorder/discomfort (2% to 4%), throat discomfort (1% to 2%)

Tablet:

1% to 10%:

Cardiovascular: Chest pain/tightness/heaviness/pressure (1% to 2%), hyper-/hypotension (1%), palpitation (1%), syncope (1%)

Central nervous system: Burning (1%), dizziness (>1%), drowsiness (>1%), malaise/fatigue (2% to 3%), headache (>1%), nonspecified pain (1% to 2%, placebo 1%), vertigo (<1% to 2%), migraine (>1%), sleepiness (>1%)

Gastrointestinal: Diarrhea (1%), nausea (>1%), vomiting (>1%), hyposalivation (>1%)

Genitourinary: Hematuria (1%)

Hematologic: Hemolytic anemia (1%)

Neuromuscular & skeletal: Neck, throat, and jaw pain/tightness/pressure (2% to 3%), paresthesia (3% to 5%), myalgia (1%), numbness (1%)

Otic: Ear hemorrhage (1%), hearing loss (1%), sensitivity to noise (1%), tinnitus (1%)

Respiratory: Allergic rhinitis (1%), dyspnea (1%), nasal inflammation (1%), nose/throat hemorrhage (1%), sinusitis (1%), upper respiratory inflammation (1%)

Miscellaneous: Hypersensitivity reactions (1%), nonspecified pressure/tightness/heaviness (1% to 3%, placebo 2%); warm/cold sensation (2% to 3%, placebo 2%)

Overdosage/Toxicology Single oral doses ≤400 mg, injectable doses ≤16 mg, and nasal doses of 40 mg have been reported without adverse effects. Treatment of overdose should be supportive and symptomatic. Monitor for at least 12 hours or until signs and symptoms subside. It is not known if hemodialysis or peritoneal dialysis is effective.

Pharmacodynamics/Kinetics

Onset of Action: ~30 minutes

Bioavailability: SubQ: 97% ± 16% of that following I.V. injection; Oral: 15%

Time to Peak: Serum: 5-20 minutes

Protein Binding: 14% to 21%

Half-Life Elimination: Injection, tablet: 2.5 hours; Nasal spray: 2 hours

Metabolism: Hepatic, primarily via MAO-A isoenzyme

Excretion:

Injection: Urine (38% as indole acetic acid metabolite, 22% as unchanged drug)

Nasal spray: Urine (42% as indole acetic acid metabolite, 3% as unchanged drug)

Tablet: Urine (60% as indole acetic acid metabolite, 3% as unchanged drug); feces (40%)

Dosing

Adults:

Migraine:

Oral: A single dose of 25 mg, 50 mg, or 100 mg (taken with fluids). If a satisfactory response has not been obtained at 2 hours, a second dose may be administered. Results from clinical trials show that initial doses of 50 mg and 100 mg are more effective than doses of 25 mg, and that 100 mg doses do not provide a greater effect than 50 mg and may have increased incidence of side effects. Although doses of up to 300 mg/day have been studied, the total daily dose should not exceed 200 mg. The safety of treating an average of >4 headaches in a 30-day period have not been established.

Intranasal: Single dose of 5, 10, or 20 mg administered in one nostril; a 10 mg dose may be achieved by administration of a single 5 mg dose in each nostril; if headache returns, the dose may be repeated once after 2 hours, not to exceed a total daily dose of 40 mg. The safety of treating an average of >4 headaches in a 30-day period has not been established.

SubQ: 6 mg; a second injection may be administered at least 1 hour after the initial dose, but not more than two injections in a 24-hour period. If side effects are dose-limiting, lower doses may be used.

Cluster headache: Refer to dosing under "Migraine, SubQ"

Renal Impairment: Dosage adjustment is not necessary.

Hepatic Impairment: Bioavailability of oral sumatriptan is increased with liver disease. If treatment is needed, do not exceed single doses of 50 mg. The nasal spray has not been studied in patients with hepatic impairment, however, because the spray does not undergo first-pass metabolism, levels would not be expected to alter. Use of all dosage forms is contraindicated with severe hepatic impairment.

Available Dosage Forms Note: Expressed as sumatriptan base

Injection, solution, as succinate: 12 mg/mL (0.5 mL)

Solution, intranasal spray: 5 mg (100 µL unit dose spray device); 20 mg (100 µL unit dose spray device)

Tablet, as succinate: 25 mg, 50 mg, 100 mg

Monitoring and Teaching Issues

Physical Assessment: For use only with a clear diagnosis of migraine or cluster headaches. Use caution with for CAD or history of seizure disorder (see Warnings/Precautions for use cautions). Assess potential for interactions with other pharmacological agents patient may be taking (eg, ergot-containing drugs, MAO inhibitors, SSRIs; see Drug Interactions). See Administration for specifics of SubQ, intranasal, oral formulation use. Assess therapeutic effectiveness (relief of headaches) and adverse response (eg, dizziness, tingling, drowsiness, myalgia, vision alternation, nausea, vomiting; reactions differ according to formulation; see Adverse Reactions). Teach patient proper use according to formulation (eg, with SubQ, appropriate injection technique and syringe/needle disposal), possible side effects/appropriate interventions, and adverse symptoms to report (see Patient Education).

Patient Education: Take at first sign of migraine attack. This drug is to be used to reduce your migraine, not to prevent or reduce the number of attacks. Follow exact instructions for use. Do not take any form of this drug within 24 hours of any other migraine medication without consulting prescriber. May cause dizziness, fatigue, or drowsiness (use caution when driving or engaging in tasks that require alertness until response to drug is known); or nausea or vomiting (small frequent meals, frequent mouth care, chewing gum, or sucking on lozenges may help). Report chest tightness or pain; excessive drowsiness; acute abdominal pain; skin rash or burning sensation; muscle weakness, soreness, or numbness; respiratory difficulty; or any other persistent adverse reactions. **Pregnancy/breast-feeding precautions:** Inform prescriber if you are or intend to become pregnant. Consult prescriber if breast-feeding.

Nasal spray: Administer dose into one nostril. If headache returns or is not fully resolved after the first dose, the dose may be repeated after 2 hours. Do not exceed 40 mg in 24 hours.

Oral: If headache returns or is not fully resolved after first dose, the dose may be repeated after 2 hours. Do not exceed 200 mg in 24 hours. Take whole with fluids.

SubQ: If headache returns or is not fully resolved after first dose, the dose may be repeated after 1 hour. Do not exceed two injections in 24 hours.

Geriatric Considerations: Use cautiously in the elderly, particularly since many elderly have cardiovascular disease which would put them at risk for cardiovascular adverse effects. Safety and efficacy in the elderly (>65 years) have not been established. Pharmacokinetic disposition is, however, similar to that in young adults.

Pregnancy Risk Factor: C

Lactation: Enters breast milk/use caution (AAP rates "compatible")

Breast-Feeding Issues: The amount of sumatriptan an infant would be exposed to following breast-feeding is considered to be small (although the mean milk-to-plasma ratio is ~4.9, weight adjusted doses estimates suggest breast-fed infants receive 3.5% of a maternal dose). Expressing and discarding the milk for 8 hours after a single dose is suggested to reduce the amount present even further. The half-life of sumatriptan in breast milk is 2.22 hours.

Administration

Oral: Oral: Should be taken with fluids as soon as symptoms appear.

I.V.: Do **not** administer I.V.; may cause coronary vasospasm.

Other: Administer injection formulation subcutaneously.

Storage: Store at 2°C to 20°C (36°F to 86°F). Protect from light.

Related Information

Antimigraine Drugs: 5-HT₁ Receptor Agonists on page 1716

+ **Synthroid®** *see* Levothyroxine *on page 895*
+ **Syrup of Ipecac** *see* Ipecac Syrup *on page 824*
+ **T₄** *see* Levothyroxine *on page 895*
+ **T-20** *see* Enfuvirtide *on page 519*
+ **Tabloid®** *see* Thioguanine *on page 1462*

Tacrine (TAK reen)

U.S. Brand Names Cognex®
Synonyms Tacrine Hydrochloride; Tetrahydroaminoacrine; THA
Generic Available No
Pharmacologic Category Acetylcholinesterase Inhibitor (Central)
Medication Safety Issues
  Sound-alike/look-alike issues:
    Cognex® may be confused with Corgard®
Use Treatment of mild to moderate dementia of the Alzheimer's type
Mechanism of Action/Effect Centrally-acting cholinesterase inhibitor. It elevates acetylcholine in cerebral cortex by slowing the degradation of acetylcholine.
Contraindications Hypersensitivity to tacrine, acridine derivatives, or any component of the formulation; patients previously treated with tacrine who developed jaundice
Warnings/Precautions The use of tacrine has been associated with elevations in serum transaminases; serum transaminases (specifically ALT) must be monitored throughout therapy; use extreme caution in patients with current evidence of a history of abnormal liver function tests; use caution in patients with urinary tract obstruction (bladder outlet obstruction or prostatic hyperplasia), asthma, and sick-sinus syndrome, bradycardia, or conduction abnormalities (tacrine may cause bradycardia and/or heart block). Also, patients with cardiovascular disease, asthma, or peptic ulcer should use cautiously. Adverse cardiovascular events may also occur in patients without known cardiac disease. Use with caution in patients with a history of seizures. May cause nausea, vomiting, or loose stools. Abrupt discontinuation or dosage decrease may worsen cognitive function. May be associated with neutropenia.
Drug Interactions
  Cytochrome P450 Effect: Substrate of CYP1A2 (major); **Inhibits** CYP1A2 (weak)
  Decreased Effect: CYP1A2 inducers may decrease the levels/effects of tacrine; example inducers include aminoglutethimide, carbamazepine, phenobarbital, rifampin, and cigarette smoking. Tacrine may worsen Parkinson's disease and inhibit the effects of levodopa. Tacrine may antagonize the therapeutic effect of anticholinergic agents (benztropine, trihexyphenidyl).
  Increased Effect/Toxicity: CYP1A2 inhibitors may increase the levels/effects of tacrine; example inhibitors include amiodarone, ciprofloxacin, fluvoxamine, ketoconazole, norfloxacin, ofloxacin, and rofecoxib. Tacrine in combination with other cholinergic agents (eg, ambenonium, edrophonium, neostigmine, pyridostigmine, bethanechol), will likely produce additive cholinergic effects. Tacrine in combination with beta-blockers may produce additive bradycardia. Tacrine may increase the levels/effect of succinylcholine and theophylline. in elevated plasma levels. Fluvoxamine, enoxacin, and cimetidine increase tacrine concentrations via enzyme inhibition (CYP1A2).
Nutritional/Ethanol Interactions Food: Food decreases bioavailability.
Adverse Reactions
  >10%:
    Central nervous system: Headache, dizziness
    Gastrointestinal: Nausea, vomiting, diarrhea
    Miscellaneous: Transaminases increased
  1% to 10%:
    Cardiovascular: Flushing
    Central nervous system: Confusion, ataxia, insomnia, somnolence, depression, anxiety, fatigue
    Dermatologic: Rash
    Gastrointestinal: Dyspepsia, anorexia, abdominal pain, flatulence, constipation, weight loss
    Neuromuscular & skeletal: Myalgia, tremor
    Respiratory: Rhinitis
Overdosage/Toxicology Provide general supportive measures. Can cause cholinergic crisis characterized by severe nausea, vomiting, salivation, sweating, bradycardia, hypotension, collapse, and convulsions. Increased muscle weakness is a possibility and may result in death if respiratory muscles are involved.

Tertiary anticholinergics, such as atropine, may be used as an antidote for overdose. I.V. atropine sulfate titrated to effect is recommended at an initial dose of 1-2 mg I.V. with subsequent doses based upon clinical response. Atypical increases in blood pressure and heart rate have been reported with other cholinomimetics when coadministered with quaternary anticholinergics such as glycopyrrolate.
Pharmacodynamics/Kinetics
  Absorption: Oral: Rapid
  Bioavailability: Absolute: 17%
  Time to Peak: Plasma: 1-2 hours
  Protein Binding: Plasma: 55%
  Half-Life Elimination: Serum: 2-4 hours; Steady-state: 24-36 hours
  Metabolism: Extensively by CYP450 to multiple metabolites; first pass effect
Dosing
  Adults & Elderly:
    Alzheimer's disease: Oral: Initial: 10 mg 4 times/day; may increase by 40 mg/day adjusted every 6 weeks; maximum: 160 mg/day; best administered separate from meal times.

    Dose adjustment based upon transaminase elevations:
      ALT ≤3 times ULN*: Continue titration

ALT >3 to ≤5 times ULN*: Decrease dose by 40 mg/day, resume when ALT returns to normal

ALT >5 times ULN*: Stop treatment, may rechallenge upon return of ALT to normal

*ULN = upper limit of normal

Note: Patients with clinical jaundice confirmed by elevated total bilirubin (>3 mg/dL) should not be rechallenged with tacrine

Hepatic Impairment: Patients with clinical jaundice confirmed by elevated total bilirubin (>3 mg/dL) should not be rechallenged with tacrine.

Available Dosage Forms Capsule, as hydrochloride: 10 mg, 20 mg, 30 mg, 40 mg

Monitoring and Teaching Issues

Physical Assessment: Assess bladder and sphincter adequacy prior to administering medication. Assess other medications patient may be taking for effectiveness and interactions. Assess results of laboratory tests throughout therapy, therapeutic effectiveness, and adverse reactions (eg, cholinergic crisis). Assess knowledge/teach patient appropriate use, interventions to reduce side effects, and adverse symptoms to report.

Monitoring Laboratory Tests: ALT (SGPT) levels and other liver enzymes at least every other week from weeks 4-16 weeks, then monitor once every 3 months

Patient Education: This medication will not cure the disease, but may help reduce symptoms. Use as directed; do not increase dose or discontinue without consulting prescriber. Maintain adequate hydration (2-3 L/day of fluids) unless instructed to restrict fluid intake. May cause dizziness, sedation, or hypotension (rise slowly from sitting or lying position and use caution when driving or climbing stairs); vomiting or loss of appetite (small frequent meals, frequent mouth care, or chewing gum, or sucking lozenges may help); or diarrhea (boiled milk, yogurt, or buttermilk may help). Report persistent abdominal discomfort; significantly increased salivation, sweating, tearing, or urination; flushed skin; chest pain or palpitations; acute headache; unresolved diarrhea; excessive fatigue, insomnia, dizziness, or depression; increased muscle, joint, or body pain; vision changes or blurred vision; shortness of breath or wheezing; or signs of jaundice (yellowing of eyes or skin, dark colored urine or light colored stool, abdominal pain, or easy fatigue). **Pregnancy/breast-feeding precautions:** Inform prescriber if you are or intend to become pregnant. Breast-feeding is not recommended.

Dietary Considerations: Give with food if GI side effects are intolerable.

Geriatric Considerations: Tacrine is currently FDA-approved for the treatment of Alzheimer's disease, it is clearly not a cure. At least 25% of patients may not tolerate the drug and only 50% of patients demonstrate some improvement in symptoms or a slowing of deterioration. While worth a trial in mild to moderate dementia of the Alzheimer's type, patients and their families must be counseled about the limitations of the drug and the importance of regular monitoring of liver function tests. No specific dosage adjustments are necessary due to age.

Pregnancy Risk Factor: C

Lactation: Excretion in breast milk unknown/not recommended

♦ **Tacrine Hydrochloride** *see* Tacrine *on page 1418*

Tacrolimus (ta KROE li mus)

U.S. Brand Names Prograf®; Protopic®

Synonyms FK506

Generic Available No

Pharmacologic Category Immunosuppressant Agent; Topical Skin Product

Medication Safety Issues

Sound-alike/look-alike issues:

Prograf® may be confused with Gengraf®

Use

Oral/injection: Potent immunosuppressive drug used in liver or kidney transplant recipients

Topical: Moderate to severe atopic dermatitis in patients not responsive to conventional therapy or when conventional therapy is not appropriate

Unlabeled/Investigational Use Potent immunosuppressive drug used in heart, lung, small bowel transplant recipients; immunosuppressive drug for peripheral stem cell/bone marrow transplantation

Mechanism of Action/Effect Suppresses cellular immunity (inhibits T-lymphocyte activation)

Contraindications Hypersensitivity to tacrolimus or any component of the formulation

Warnings/Precautions

Oral/injection: Insulin-dependent post-transplant diabetes mellitus (PTDM) has been reported (1% to 20%); risk increases in African-American and Hispanic kidney transplant patients. Increased susceptibility to infection and the possible development of lymphoma may occur after administration of tacrolimus. Nephrotoxicity and neurotoxicity have been reported, especially with higher doses; to avoid excess nephrotoxicity do not administer simultaneously with cyclosporine; monitoring of serum concentrations (trough for oral therapy) is essential to prevent organ rejection and reduce drug-related toxicity; tonic clonic seizures may have been triggered by tacrolimus. A period of 24 hours should elapse between discontinuation of cyclosporine and the initiation of tacrolimus. Use caution in renal or hepatic dysfunction, dosing adjustments may be required. Delay initiation if postoperative oliguria occurs. Use may be associated with the development of hypertension (common). Myocardial hypertrophy has been reported (rare). Each mL of injection contains polyoxyl 60 hydrogenated castor oil (HCO-60) (200 mg) and dehydrated alcohol USP 80% v/v. Anaphylaxis has been reported with the injection, use should be reserved for those patients not able to take oral medications.

Topical: Topical calcineurin agents are considered second-line therapies in the treatment of atopic dermatitis/eczema, and should be limited to use in patients who have failed treatment with other therapies. They should be used for short-term and intermittent treatment using the minimum amount necessary for the control of symptoms should be used.

Infections at the treatment site should be cleared prior to therapy. Patients with atopic dermatitis are predisposed to skin infections, including eczema herpeticum, varicella zoster, (Continued)

Tacrolimus *(Continued)*

and herpes simplex. Discontinue use in patients with unknown cause of lymphadenopathy or acute infectious mononucleosis. Not recommended for use in patients with Netherton's syndrome. Safety not established in patients with generalized erythroderma. The use of Protopic® in children <2 years of age is not recommended, particularly since the effect on immune system development is unknown.

Drug Interactions

Cytochrome P450 Effect: Substrate of CYP3A4 (major); **Inhibits** CYP3A4 (weak)

Decreased Effect: Antacids impair tacrolimus absorption (separate administration by at least 2 hours). St John's wort may reduce tacrolimus serum concentrations (avoid concurrent use). CYP3A4 inducers may decrease the levels/effects of tacrolimus; example inducers include aminoglutethimide, carbamazepine, nafcillin, nevirapine, phenobarbital, phenytoin, and rifamycins. Caspofungin and sirolimus may decrease the serum concentrations of tacrolimus.

Increased Effect/Toxicity: Amphotericin B and other nephrotoxic antibiotics have the potential to increase tacrolimus-associated nephrotoxicity. Cisapride and metoclopramide may increase tacrolimus levels. Synergistic immunosuppression results from concurrent use of cyclosporine. Voriconazole may increase tacrolimus serum concentrations; decrease tacrolimus dosage by 66% when initiating voriconazole. CYP3A4 inhibitors may increase the levels/effects of tacrolimus; example inhibitors include azole antifungals, ciprofloxacin, clarithromycin, diclofenac, doxycycline, erythromycin, imatinib, isoniazid, nefazodone, nicardipine, propofol, protease inhibitors, quinidine, and verapamil. Calcium channel blockers (dihydropyridine) may increase tacrolimus serum concentrations (monitor).

Nutritional/Ethanol Interactions

Ethanol: Localized flushing (redness, warm sensation) may occur at application site of topical tacrolimus following ethanol consumption.

Food: Decreases rate and extent of absorption. High-fat meals have most pronounced effect (35% decrease in AUC, 77% decrease in C_{max}). Grapefruit juice, CYP3A4 inhibitor, may increase serum level and/or toxicity of tacrolimus; avoid concurrent use.

Herb/Nutraceutical: St John's wort: May reduce tacrolimus serum concentrations (avoid concurrent use).

Adverse Reactions

Oral, I.V.:

≥15%:

Cardiovascular: Chest pain, hypertension

Central nervous system: Dizziness, headache, insomnia, tremor (headache and tremor are associated with high whole blood concentrations and may respond to decreased dosage)

Dermatologic: Pruritus, rash

Endocrine & metabolic: Diabetes mellitus, hyperglycemia, hyperkalemia, hyperlipemia, hypomagnesemia, hypophosphatemia

Gastrointestinal: Abdominal pain, constipation, diarrhea, dyspepsia, nausea, vomiting

Genitourinary: Urinary tract infection

Hematologic: Anemia, leukocytosis, thrombocytopenia

Hepatic: Ascites

Neuromuscular & skeletal: Arthralgia, back pain, weakness, paresthesia

Renal: Abnormal kidney function, increased creatinine, oliguria, urinary tract infection, increased BUN

Respiratory: Atelectasis, dyspnea, increased cough

3% to 15% (Limited to important or life-threatening symptoms):

Cardiovascular: Abnormal ECG, angina pectoris, deep thrombophlebitis, hemorrhage, hypotension, postural hypotension, thrombosis

Central nervous system: Agitation, amnesia, anxiety, confusion, depression, encephalopathy, hallucinations, psychosis, somnolence

Dermatologic: Acne, alopecia, exfoliative dermatitis, hirsutism, photosensitivity reaction, skin discoloration

Endocrine & metabolic: Cushing's syndrome, decreased bicarbonate, decreased serum iron, diabetes mellitus, hypercalcemia, hypercholesterolemia, hyperphosphatemia

Gastrointestinal: Dysphagia, esophagitis, GI perforation/hemorrhage, ileus

Hematologic: Coagulation disorder, decreased prothrombin, leukopenia

Hepatic: Cholangitis, jaundice, hepatitis

Neuromuscular & skeletal: Incoordination, myasthenia, neuropathy, osteoporosis

Respiratory: Asthma, pneumothorax, pulmonary edema

Miscellaneous: Abscess, allergic reaction, flu-like syndrome, peritonitis, sepsis

Topical (as reported in children and adults, unless otherwise noted):

>10%:

Central nervous system: Headache (5% to 20%), fever (1% to 21%)

Dermatologic: Skin burning (43% to 58%), pruritus (41% to 46%), erythema (12% to 28%)

Respiratory: Increased cough (18% children)

Miscellaneous: Flu-like syndrome (23% to 28%), allergic reaction (4% to 12%)

1% to 10%:

Cardiovascular: Peripheral edema (3% to 4% adults)

Central nervous system: Hyperesthesia (3% to 7% adults), pain (1% to 2%)

Dermatologic: Skin tingling (2% to 8%), acne (4% to 7% adults), localized flushing (following ethanol consumption 3% to 7% adults), folliculitis (2% to 6%), urticaria (1% to 6%), rash (2% to 5%), pustular rash (2% to 4%), vesiculobullous rash (4% children), contact dermatitis (3% to 4%), cyst (1% to 3% adults), eczema herpeticum (1% to 2%), fungal dermatitis (1% to 2% adults), sunburn (1% to 2% adults), dry skin (1% children)

Endocrine & metabolic: Dysmenorrhea (4% women)

Gastrointestinal: Diarrhea (3% to 5%), dyspepsia (1% to 4% adults), abdominal pain (3% children), vomiting (1% adults), gastroenteritis (adults 2%), nausea (1% children)

Neuromuscular & skeletal: Myalgia (2% to 3% adults), weakness (2% to 3% adults), back pain (2% adults)

Ocular: Conjunctivitis (2% adults)

Otic: Otitis media (12% children)

Respiratory: Rhinitis (6% children), sinusitis (2% to 4% adults), bronchitis (2% adults), pneumonia (1% adults)

Miscellaneous: Varicella/herpes zoster (1% to 5%), lymphadenopathy (3% children)

Overdosage/Toxicology Symptoms are extensions of immunosuppressive activity and adverse effects. Symptomatic and supportive treatment is required. Hemodialysis is not effective.

Pharmacodynamics/Kinetics

Absorption: Better in resected patients with a closed stoma; unlike cyclosporine, clamping of the T-tube in liver transplant patients does not alter trough concentrations or AUC

Oral: Incomplete and variable; food within 15 minutes of administration decreases absorption (27%)

Topical: Serum concentrations range from undetectable to 20 ng/mL (<5 ng/mL in majority of adult patients studied)

Bioavailability: Oral: Adults: 7% to 28%, Children: 10% to 52%; Topical: <0.5%; Absolute: Unknown

Time to Peak: 0.5-4 hours

Protein Binding: 99%

Half-Life Elimination: Variable, 21-61 hours in healthy volunteers

Metabolism: Extensively hepatic via CYP3A4 to eight possible metabolites (major metabolite, 31-demethyl tacrolimus, shows same activity as tacrolimus *in vitro*)

Excretion: Feces (~92%); feces/urine (<1% as unchanged drug)

Dosing

Adults & Elderly:

Kidney transplant:

Oral: Initial dose: 0.2 mg/kg/day in 2 divided doses, given every 12 hours; initial dose may be given within 24 hours of transplant, but should be delayed until renal function has recovered; African-American patients may require larger doses to maintain trough concentration

Typical whole blood trough concentrations: Months 1-3: 7- 20 ng/mL; months 4-12: 5-15 ng/mL

I.V.: **Note:** I.V. route should only be used in patients not able to take oral medications, anaphylaxis has been reported. Initial dose: 0.03-0.05 mg/kg/day as a continuous infusion; begin no sooner than 6 hours post-transplant, starting at lower end of the dosage range; adjunctive therapy with corticosteroids is recommended; continue only until oral medication can be tolerated

Liver transplant:

Oral: Initial dose: 0.1-0.15 mg/kg/day in 2 divided doses, given every 12 hours; begin oral dose no sooner than 6 hours post-transplant; adjunctive therapy with corticosteroids is recommended; if switching from I.V. to oral, the oral dose should be started 8-12 hours after stopping the infusion

Typical whole blood trough concentrations: Months 1-12: 5-20 ng/mL

I.V.: **Note:** I.V. route should only be used in patients not able to take oral medications, anaphylaxis has been reported. Initial dose: 0.03-0.05 mg/kg/day as a continuous infusion; begin no sooner than 6 hours post-transplant starting at lower end of the dosage range; adjunctive therapy with corticosteroids is recommended; continue only until oral medication can be tolerated

Prevention of graft-vs-host disease: I.V.: 0.03 mg/kg/day as continuous infusion

Atopic dermatitis (moderate to severe): Topical: Apply 0.03% or 0.1% ointment to affected area twice daily; rub in gently and completely; continue applications for 1 week after symptoms have cleared

Pediatrics:

Liver transplant:

Note: Patients without pre-existing renal or hepatic dysfunction have required and tolerated higher doses than adults to achieve similar blood concentrations. It is recommended that therapy be initiated at high end of the recommended adult I.V. and oral dosing ranges; dosage adjustments may be required.

Oral: Initial dose: 0.15-0.20 mg/kg/day in 2 divided doses, given every 12 hours; begin oral dose no sooner than 6 hours post-transplant; adjunctive therapy with corticosteroids is recommended; if switching from I.V. to oral, the oral dose should be started 8-12 hours after stopping the infusion

Typical whole blood trough concentrations: Months 1-12: 5-20 ng/mL

I.V.: **Note:** I.V. route should only be used in patients not able to take oral medications, anaphylaxis has been reported. Initial dose: 0.03-0.05 mg/kg/day as a continuous infusion; begin no sooner than 6 hours post-transplant; adjunctive therapy with corticosteroids is recommended; continue only until oral medication can be tolerated

Moderate to severe atopic dermatitis: Topical: Children ≥2 years: Apply 0.03% ointment to affected area twice daily; rub in gently and completely; continue applications for 1 week after symptoms have cleared

Renal Impairment: Evidence suggests that lower doses should be used. Patients should receive doses at the lowest value of the recommended I.V. and oral dosing ranges. Further reductions in dose below these ranges may be required. Tacrolimus therapy should usually be delayed up to 48 hours or longer in patients with postoperative oliguria.

Hemodialysis: Not removed by hemodialysis; supplemental dose is not necessary.

Peritoneal dialysis: Significant drug removal is unlikely based on physiochemical characteristics.

Hepatic Impairment: Use of tacrolimus in liver transplant recipients experiencing post-transplant hepatic impairment may be associated with increased risk of developing renal insufficiency related to high whole blood levels of tacrolimus. The presence of moderate-to-severe hepatic dysfunction (serum bilirubin >2 mg/dL) appears to affect the metabolism of FK506. The half-life of the drug was prolonged and the clearance reduced

(Continued)

Tacrolimus *(Continued)*

after I.V. administration. The bioavailability of FK506 was also increased after oral administration. The higher plasma concentrations as determined by ELISA, in patients with severe hepatic dysfunction are probably due to the accumulation of FK506 metabolites of lower activity. These patients should be monitored closely and dosage adjustments should be considered. Some evidence indicates that lower doses could be used in these patients.

Available Dosage Forms

Capsule (Prograf®): 0.5 mg, 1 mg, 5 mg

Injection, solution (Prograf®): 5 mg/mL (1 mL) [contains dehydrated alcohol 80% and polyoxyl 60 hydrogenated castor oil]

Ointment, topical (Protopic®): 0.03% (30 g, 60 g, 100 g); 0.1% (30 g, 60 g, 100 g)

Monitoring and Teaching Issues

Physical Assessment: Assess other medications patient may be taking for effectiveness and interactions. Monitor blood pressure frequently. Assess results of laboratory tests prior to, during, and following therapy. Monitor response to therapy and adverse reactions. Patients with diabetes should be advised to monitor glucose levels closely (this medication may alter glucose levels). Monitor/instruct patient on appropriate use, interventions to reduce side effects, to monitor for signs of opportunistic infection, and adverse reactions to report.

Monitoring Laboratory Tests: Renal function, hepatic function, serum electrolytes, glucose. Since pharmacokinetics show great inter- and intrapatient variability over time, monitoring of serum concentrations (trough for oral therapy) has proven helpful to prevent organ rejection and reduce drug-related toxicity. Measure 3 times/week for first few weeks, then gradually decrease frequency as patient stabilizes.

Patient Education: Take as directed, on an empty stomach. Be consistent with timing and consistency of meals if GI intolerance occurs (per manufacturer). Do not take within 2 hours before or after antacids. Do not alter dose and do not discontinue without consulting prescriber. Maintain adequate hydration (2-3 L/day of fluids) during entire course of therapy unless instructed to restrict fluid intake. You will be susceptible to infection (avoid crowds and exposure to infection). If you have diabetes, monitor glucose levels closely (drug may alter glucose levels). You may experience nausea, vomiting, loss of appetite (small frequent meals, frequent mouth care may help); diarrhea (boiled milk, yogurt, or buttermilk may help); constipation (increased exercise, fluids, fruit, fluid, or fiber may help; if unresolved, consult prescriber); or muscle or back pain (mild analgesics may be recommended). Report chest pain; acute headache or dizziness; symptoms of respiratory infection, cough, or respiratory difficulty; unresolved GI effects; fatigue, chills, fever, unhealed sores, white plaques in mouth, irritation in genital area; unusual bruising or bleeding; pain or irritation on urination or change in urinary patterns; rash or skin irritation; or other unusual effects.

Topical: Before applying, wash area gently and thoroughly. Apply in thin film to affected area. Do not cover skin with bandages. Wash hands only if not treating skin on the hands. Protect skin from sunlight or exposure to UV light. Consult prescriber if breast-feeding.

Pregnancy/breast-feeding precautions: Inform prescriber if you are or intend to become pregnant. Do not breast-feed.

Dietary Considerations: Capsule: Take on an empty stomach; be consistent with timing and composition of meals if GI intolerance occurs (per manufacturer).

Pregnancy Risk Factor: C

Pregnancy Issues: Tacrolimus crosses the placenta and reaches concentrations four times greater than maternal plasma concentrations. Neonatal hyperkalemia and renal dysfunction have been reported.

Lactation: Enters breast milk/contraindicated

Breast-Feeding Issues: Concentrations in breast milk are equivalent to plasma concentrations; breast-feeding is not advised.

Administration

I.V.: Administer by I.V. continuous infusion only (use infusion pump). Tacrolimus is dispensed in a 50 mL glass container with no overfill. It is intended to be infused over 24 hours. Polyolefin administration sets should be used. Dilute with 0.9% sodium chloride or D_5W to a concentration of 0.004-0.02 mg/mL prior to administration.

Storage:

Injection: Prior to dilution, store at 5°C to 25°C (41°F to 77°F). Polyvinyl-containing sets (eg, Venoset®, Accuset®) adsorb significant amounts of the drug, and their use may lead to a lower dose being delivered to the patient. FK506 admixtures prepared in 5% dextrose injection or 0.9% sodium chloride injection should be stored in polyolefin containers or glass bottles. Infusion of FK506 through PVC tubings did not result in decreased concentration of the drug, however, loss by absorption may be more important when lower concentrations of FK506 are used. Stable for 24 hours in D_5W or NS in glass or polyolefin containers.

Capsules and ointment: Store at room temperature 25°C (77°F).

Additional Information Additional dosing considerations:

Switch from I.V. to oral therapy: Threefold increase in dose

Pediatric patients: About 2 times higher dose compared to adults

Liver dysfunction: Decrease I.V. dose; decrease oral dose

Renal dysfunction: Does not affect kinetics; decrease dose to decrease levels if renal dysfunction is related to the drug

Tadalafil *(tah DA la fil)*

U.S. Brand Names Cialis®

Synonyms GF196960

Generic Available No

Pharmacologic Category Phosphodiesterase-5 Enzyme Inhibitor

Use Treatment of erectile dysfunction

Mechanism of Action/Effect Tadalafil enhances the effect of nitric oxide (NO) by inhibiting phosphodiesterase type 5 (PDE-5), which is responsible for degradation of cGMP in the corpus cavernosum; when sexual stimulation causes local release of NO, inhibition of PDE-5 by tadalafil causes increased levels of cGMP in the corpus cavernosum, resulting in smooth muscle relaxation and inflow of blood to the corpus cavernosum. At recommended doses, it has no effect in the absence of sexual stimulation.

Contraindications Hypersensitivity to tadalafil or any component of the formulation; concurrent use of organic nitrates (nitroglycerin) in any form; concurrent use of alpha-adrenergic antagonists (except tamsulosin 0.4 mg/day)

Warnings/Precautions There is a degree of cardiac risk associated with sexual activity; therefore, physicians may wish to consider the cardiovascular status of their patients prior to initiating any treatment for erectile dysfunction. Use caution in patients with left ventricular outflow obstruction (aortic stenosis or IHSS); may be more sensitive to hypotensive actions. Use caution in patients receiving strong CYP3A4 inhibitors, the elderly, or those with hepatic impairment or renal impairment; dosage adjustment/limitation is needed. Use caution in patients with peptic ulcer disease.

Agents for the treatment of erectile dysfunction should be used with caution in patients with anatomical deformation of the penis (angulation, cavernosal fibrosis, or Peyronie's disease), or in patients who have conditions which may predispose them to priapism (sickle cell anemia, multiple myeloma, leukemia). All patients should be instructed to seek medical attention if erection persists >4 hours. The safety and efficacy of tadalafil with other treatments for erectile dysfunction have not been studied and are, therefore, not recommended as combination therapy.

Safety and efficacy have not been studied in patients with the following conditions, therefore, use in these patients is not recommended: Arrhythmias, hypotension, uncontrolled hypertension, unstable angina or angina during intercourse, cardiac failure (NYHA Class II or greater), recent myocardial infarction, or stroke within the last 6 months. A minority of patients with retinitis pigmentosa have genetic disorders of retinal phosphodiesterases. There is no safety information on the administration of tadalafil to these patients; administer with caution.

Drug Interactions
Cytochrome P450 Effect: Substrate of CYP3A4 (major)

Nutritional/Ethanol Interactions
Ethanol: Substantial consumption of ethanol may increase the risk of hypotension and orthostasis. Lower ethanol consumption has not been associated with significant changes in blood pressure or increase in orthostatic symptoms.
Food: Rate and extent of absorption are not affected by food. Grapefruit juice may increase serum levels/toxicity of tadalafil. Do not give more than a single 10 mg dose of tadalafil more frequently than every 72 hours in patients who regularly consume grapefruit juice.

Adverse Reactions
>10%:
Central nervous system: Headache (11% to 15%)
Gastrointestinal: Dyspepsia (4% to 10%)
2% to 10%:
Cardiovascular: Flushing (2% to 3%)
Neuromuscular & skeletal: CPK increased (2%), back pain (3% to 6%), myalgia (1% to 3%)
Respiratory: Nasal congestion (2% to 3%)
Miscellaneous: Limb pain (1% to 3%)

Overdosage/Toxicology Symptoms similar to those seen at lower doses (headache, back pain, myalgias). Treatment is symptomatic and supportive.

Pharmacodynamics/Kinetics
Onset of Action: Within 1 hour
Duration of Action: Up to 36 hours
Time to Peak: Plasma: 2 hours
Protein Binding: 94%
Half-Life Elimination: 17.5 hours
Metabolism: Hepatic, via CYP3A4 to metabolites (inactive)
Excretion: Feces (61%, as metabolites); urine (36%, as metabolites)

Dosing
Adults:
Erectile dysfunction: Oral: 10 mg prior to anticipated sexual activity (dosing range: 5-20 mg); to be given as one single dose and not given more than once daily. **Note:** Erectile function may be improved for up to 36 hours following a single dose; adjust dose.
Dosing adjustment with concomitant medications: CYP3A4 inhibitors: Dose reduction of tadalafil is recommended with strong CYP3A4 inhibitors. The dose of tadalafil should not exceed 10 mg, and tadalafil should not be taken more frequently than once every 72 hours. Examples of such inhibitors include azole antifungals, clarithromycin, diclofenac, doxycycline, erythromycin, imatinib, isoniazid, nefazodone, nicardipine, propofol, protease inhibitors, quinidine, and verapamil.
Elderly: Dosage is based on renal function; refer to dosing in renal impairment.
Renal Impairment:
Cl_{cr} 31-50 mL/minute: Initial dose 5 mg once daily; maximum dose 10 mg not to be given more frequently than every 48 hours.
Cl_{cr} <30 mL/minute or hemodialysis: Maximum dose 5 mg.
Hepatic Impairment:
Mild-to-moderate hepatic impairment (Child-Pugh class A or B): Dose should not exceed 10 mg once daily.
Severe hepatic impairment: Use is not recommended.

Available Dosage Forms Tablet: 5 mg, 10 mg, 20 mg

Monitoring and Teaching Issues
Physical Assessment: Assess potential for interactions with other prescription, OTC medications, or herbal products patient may be using. Assess for therapeutic effectiveness
(Continued)

Tadalafil *(Continued)*

and adverse reactions. Instruct patient on appropriate use and cautions, possible side effects, and symptoms to report.

Patient Education: Inform prescriber of all other prescriptions, OTC medications, or herbal products you are taking and any allergies you have; serious side effects can result when tadalafil is used with some other medications. Do not combine tadalafil with other approaches to treating erectile dysfunction without consulting prescriber. **Note:** This drug provides no protection against sexually-transmitted diseases, including HIV. Take exactly as directed; do not take more often than prescribed. You may experience headache, fatigue, dizziness, or blurred vision (use caution when driving or engaging in hazardous tasks until response to drug is known); back or limb pain (consult prescriber for appropriate analgesic). Report immediately chest pain, palpitations; respiratory difficulty; unusual dizziness; sign of urinary tract infection; skin rash; genital swelling or priapism, erection lasting >4 hours, or other persistent adverse reactions.

Dietary Considerations: May be taken with or without food.

Geriatric Considerations: No significant differences in pharmacokinetics were seen in elderly men versus younger men. Dosing should be adjusted for renal function. Since older adults often have concomitant diseases, many of which may be contraindicated with the use of tadalafil, prescriber should complete a thorough review of diseases and medications prior to prescribing tadalafil.

Pregnancy Risk Factor: B

Administration

Oral: May be administered with or without food, prior to anticipated sexual activity.

Storage: Store at controlled room temperature of 15°C to 30°C (59°F to 86°F).

- ♦ **Tagamet®** *see* Cimetidine *on page 324*
- ♦ **Tagamet® HB 200 [OTC]** *see* Cimetidine *on page 324*
- ♦ **Talacen®** *see* Pentazocine and Acetaminophen *on page 1181*
- ♦ **Talwin®** *see* Pentazocine *on page 1180*
- ♦ **Talwin® NX** *see* Pentazocine *on page 1180*
- ♦ **TAM** *see* Tamoxifen *on page 1424*
- ♦ **Tambocor™** *see* Flecainide *on page 631*
- ♦ **Tamiflu®** *see* Oseltamivir *on page 1126*

Tamoxifen *(ta MOKS i fen)*

U.S. Brand Names Nolvadex®

Synonyms ICI-46474; NSC-180973; TAM; Tamoxifen Citrate

Restrictions An FDA-approved medication guide is available at www.AstraZeneca-us.com/pi/Nolvadex.pdf. Distribute to each female patient who is using tamoxifen to decrease risk of developing breast cancer or who has ductal carcinoma *in situ.*

Generic Available Yes

Pharmacologic Category Antineoplastic Agent, Estrogen Receptor Antagonist

Medication Safety Issues

Sound-alike/look-alike issues:

Tamoxifen may be confused with pentoxifylline, Tambocor™

Use Palliative or adjunctive treatment of advanced breast cancer; reduce the incidence of breast cancer in women at high risk; reduce risk of invasive breast cancer in women with ductal carcinoma *in situ* (DCIS); metastatic female and male breast cancer; treatment of melanoma, desmoid tumors

Unlabeled/Investigational Use Treatment of mastalgia, gynecomastia, pancreatic carcinoma; induction of ovulation; treatment of precocious puberty in females, secondary to McCune-Albright syndrome

Mechanism of Action/Effect Competitively binds to estrogen receptors on tumors and other tissue targets, producing a nuclear complex that decreases DNA synthesis and inhibits estrogen effects; nonsteroidal agent with potent antiestrogenic properties which compete with estrogen for binding sites in breast and other tissues; cells accumulate in the G_0 and G_1 phases; therefore, tamoxifen is cytostatic rather than cytocidal.

Contraindications Hypersensitivity to tamoxifen or any component of the formulation; concurrent warfarin therapy (when used for cancer risk reduction); pregnancy

Warnings/Precautions Serious and life-threatening events (including stroke, pulmonary emboli, and uterine malignancy) have occurred at an incidence greater than placebo during use for cancer risk reduction; these events are rare, but require consideration in risk:benefit evaluation. An increased incidence of thromboembolic events has been associated with use for breast cancer; risk may increase with chemotherapy addition; use caution in individuals with a history of thromboembolic events. Use with caution in patients with leukopenia, thrombocytopenia, or hyperlipidemias. Decreased visual acuity, retinopathy, corneal changes, and increased incidence of cataracts have been reported. Hypercalcemia has occurred in patients with bone metastasis. Significant bone loss of the lumbar spine and hip was associated with use in premenopausal women. Liver abnormalities such as cholestasis, hepatitis, and hepatic necrosis have occurred; hepatocellular carcinomas have been reported in some studies, relationship to treatment is unclear. Endometrial hyperplasia and polyps have occurred. Increased risk of uterine or endometrial cancer; monitor.

Drug Interactions

Cytochrome P450 Effect: Substrate of CYP2A6 (minor), 2B6 (minor), 2C8/9 (major), 2D6 (major), 2E1 (minor), 3A4 (major); **Inhibits** CYP2B6 (weak), 2C8/9 (weak), 3A4 (weak)

Decreased Effect: CYP2C8/9 inducers may decrease the levels/effects of tamoxifen; example inducers include carbamazepine, phenobarbital, phenytoin, rifampin, rifapentine, and secobarbital. CYP3A4 inducers may decrease the levels/effects of tamoxifen; example inducers include aminoglutethimide, carbamazepine, nafcillin, nevirapine, phenobarbital, phenytoin, and rifamycins. Letrozole serum levels may be reduced by tamoxifen.

Increased Effect/Toxicity: Allopurinol and tamoxifen results in exacerbation of allopurinol-induced hepatotoxicity. Cyclosporine serum levels may be increased when taken with tamoxifen. Concomitant use of warfarin is contraindicated when used for risk reduction; results in significant enhancement of the anticoagulant effects of warfarin. CYP2C8/9 inhibitors may increase the levels/effects of tamoxifen; example inhibitors include delavirdine, fluconazole, gemfibrozil, ketoconazole, nicardipine, NSAIDs, pioglitazone, and sulfonamides. CYP2D6 inhibitors may increase the levels/effects of tamoxifen; example inhibitors include chlorpromazine, delavirdine, fluoxetine, miconazole, paroxetine, pergolide, quinidine, quinine, ritonavir, and ropinirole. CYP3A4 inhibitors may increase the levels/effects of tamoxifen; example inhibitors include azole antifungals, ciprofloxacin, clarithromycin, diclofenac, doxycycline, erythromycin, imatinib, isoniazid, nefazodone, nicardipine, propofol, protease inhibitors, quinidine, and verapamil.

Nutritional/Ethanol Interactions Herb/Nutraceutical: Avoid black cohosh, dong quai in estrogen-dependent tumors.

Lab Interactions T$_4$ elevations (which may be explained by increases in thyroid-binding globulin) have been reported; not accompanied by clinical hyperthyroidism

Adverse Reactions Note: Differences in the frequency of some adverse events may be related to use for a specific indication.

>10%:
- Cardiovascular: Flushing (33%)
- Central nervous system: Mood changes (up to 12%)
- Dermatologic: Skin changes (19%)
- Endocrine & metabolic: Hot flashes (3% to 80%), fluid retention (32%), altered menses (13% to 25%), amenorrhea (16%)
- Gastrointestinal: Nausea (5% to 26%), weight loss (23%)
- Genitourinary: Vaginal bleeding (up to 23%), vaginal discharge (30% to 55%)

1% to 10%:
- Cardiovascular: Edema (4%)
- Central nervous system: Fatigue (4%), depression (2%)
- Dermatologic: Alopecia (<1% to 5%)
- Endocrine & metabolic: Oligomenorrhea (9%), menstrual disorder (6%)
- Gastrointestinal: Constipation (up to 4%), abdominal cramps (1%), anorexia (1%)
- Genitourinary: Ovarian cyst (3%)
- Hematologic: Thrombocytopenia (<1% to 10%)
- Hepatic: SGOT increased (5%), serum bilirubin increased (2%)
- Neuromuscular & skeletal: Bone pain (6%), musculoskeletal pain (3%), pain (3%)
- Renal: Serum creatinine increased (up to 2%)
- Respiratory: Cough (4%)
- Miscellaneous: Infection/sepsis (up to 6%), allergic reaction (up to 3%)

Overdosage/Toxicology Symptoms of overdose include hypercalcemia and edema. Provide general supportive care.

Pharmacodynamics/Kinetics
- **Absorption:** Well absorbed
- **Time to Peak:** Serum: 5 hours
- **Protein Binding:** 99%
- **Half-Life Elimination:** Distribution: 7-14 hours; Elimination: 5-7 days; Metabolites: 14 days
- **Metabolism:** Hepatic (via CYP3A4) to major metabolites, N-desmethyl tamoxifen (major) and 4-hydroxytamoxifen (minor), and a tamoxifen derivative (minor); undergoes enterohepatic recirculation
- **Excretion:** Feces (26% to 51%); urine (9% to 13%)

Dosing
Adults & Elderly: Refer to individual protocols.
Breast cancer treatment:
  Metastatic (males and females) or adjuvant therapy (females): Oral: 20-40 mg/day; daily doses >20 mg should be given in 2 divided doses (morning and evening)
  DCIS (females): Oral: 20 mg once daily for 5 years
Breast cancer prevention (high-risk females): Oral: 20 mg/day for 5 years
Note: Higher dosages (up to 700 mg/day) have been investigated for use in modulation of multidrug resistance (MDR), but are not routinely used in clinical practice.
Induction of ovulation (unlabeled use): Oral: 5-40 mg twice daily for 4 days
Pediatrics: Female: Precocious puberty and McCune-Albright syndrome (unlabeled use): Oral: A dose of 20 mg/day has been reported in patients 2-10 years of age; safety and efficacy have not been established for treatment of longer than 1 year duration

Available Dosage Forms Tablet, as citrate: 10 mg, 20 mg

Monitoring and Teaching Issues
Physical Assessment: Use caution in presence of leukopenia, thrombocytopenia, or hyperlipidemia (see Warnings/Precautions for specific use cautions). Assess potential for interactions with other pharmacological agents and herbal products patient may be taking (may increase or decrease levels/effects of tamoxifen or other drugs administered concurrently [eg, concomitant use of warfarin significantly increases anticoagulant effects of warfarin; see Drug Interactions). Assess results of CBC and platelet counts, therapeutic effectiveness (eg, complaints of bone pain is usually an indication of a good therapeutic effectiveness and will usually subside as treatment continues), and adverse reactions (see Adverse Reactions; eg, edema, fluid retention, hot flashes, vaginal bleeding, constipation, rash). Teach patient proper use, possible side effects/appropriate interventions (eg, periodic ophthalmic evaluations with long-term use), and adverse symptoms to report (see Patient Education).

Monitoring Laboratory Tests: WBC and platelet counts

Patient Education: Do not take any new medication during therapy without consulting prescriber. Take exactly as directed. It is important to maintain adequate hydration (2-3 L/day of fluids) unless instructed to restrict fluid intake and adequate nutrition (small frequent meals may help). You should schedule an annual ophthalmic examination as this medication is used long-term. You may experience hot flashes, hair loss, loss of libido (these will subside when treatment is completed). Bone pain may indicate a good therapeutic responses (consult prescriber for mild analgesics). May cause nausea or vomiting (small frequent meals, frequent mouth care, sucking lozenges, or chewing gum may help); or (Continued)

Tamoxifen *(Continued)*

photosensitivity (use sunscreen, wear protective clothing and eyewear, and avoid direct sunlight). Notify prescriber if menstrual irregularities or vaginal bleeding occur. Report unusual bleeding or bruising, severe weakness, sedation, mental changes, swelling or pain in calves, respiratory difficulty, or any vision changes. **Pregnancy/breast-feeding precautions:** Do not get pregnant while taking this medication. Consult prescriber for appropriate contraceptive measures. Do not breast-feed.

Geriatric Considerations: Studies have shown tamoxifen to be effective in the treatment of primary breast cancer in elderly women. Comparative studies with other antineoplastic agents in elderly women with breast cancer had more favorable survival rates with tamoxifen. Initiation of hormone therapy rather than chemotherapy is justified for elderly patients with metastatic breast cancer who are responsive.

Pregnancy Risk Factor: D

Pregnancy Issues: There are no adequate and well-controlled studies in pregnant women. For sexually-active women of childbearing age, initiate during menstruation (negative β-hCG immediately prior to initiation in women with irregular cycles). Tamoxifen may induce ovulation. Barrier or nonhormonal contraceptives are recommended. Pregnancy should be avoided for 2 months after treatment has been discontinued.

Lactation: Excretion in breast milk unknown/contraindicated

Breast-Feeding Issues: Tamoxifen has been shown to inhibit lactation.

Administration

Storage: Store at room temperature of 20°C to 25°C (68°F to 77°F).

Additional Information Oral clonidine is being studied for the treatment of tamoxifen-induced "hot flashes." The tumor flare reaction may indicate a good therapeutic response, and is often considered a good prognostic factor.

♦ **Tamoxifen Citrate** *see Tamoxifen on page 1424*

Tamsulosin *(tam SOO loe sin)*

U.S. Brand Names Flomax®

Synonyms Tamsulosin Hydrochloride

Generic Available No

Pharmacologic Category Alpha₁ Blocker

Medication Safety Issues
Sound-alike/look-alike issues:
Flomax® may be confused with Fosamax®, Volmax®

Use Treatment of signs and symptoms of benign prostatic hyperplasia (BPH)

Mechanism of Action/Effect Antagonizes alpha₁ₐ adrenoreceptors in the prostate which mediate the dynamic component of urine flow obstruction by regulating smooth muscle tone of the bladder neck and prostate. When given to patients with BPH, blockade of alpha receptors leads to relaxation of these muscles, resulting in an improvement in urine flow rate and symptoms. Alpha blockade does not influence the static component of urinary obstruction, which is related to tissue proliferation.

Contraindications Hypersensitivity to tamsulosin or any component of the formulation; concurrent use with phosphodiesterase-5 (PDE-5) inhibitors including sildenafil (>25 mg), tadalafil (if tamsulosin dose >0.4 mg/day), or vardenafil

Warnings/Precautions Not intended for use as an antihypertensive drug. May cause orthostasis, syncope or dizziness. Patients should avoid situations where injury may occur as a result of syncope. Rule out prostatic carcinoma before beginning therapy with tamsulosin.

Drug Interactions

Cytochrome P450 Effect: Substrate (major) of CYP2D6, 3A4

Decreased Effect: CYP3A4 inducers may decrease the levels/effects of tamsulosin; example inducers include aminoglutethimide, carbamazepine, nafcillin, nevirapine, phenobarbital, phenytoin, and rifamycins.

Increased Effect/Toxicity: Alpha-adrenergic blockers and calcium channel blockers may increase risk of hypotension. Risk of first-dose orthostatic hypotension may increase with beta-blockers. Cimetidine may decrease tamsulosin clearance. Blood pressure-lowering effects are additive with sildenafil (use with extreme caution), tadalafil (may be used when tamsulosin dose is ≤0.4 mg/day), and vardenafil (use is contraindicated by the manufacturer).

CYP2D6 inhibitors may increase the levels/effects of tamsulosin; example inhibitors include chlorpromazine, delavirdine, fluoxetine, miconazole, paroxetine, pergolide, quinidine, quinine, ritonavir, and ropinirole. CYP3A4 inhibitors may increase the levels/effects of tamsulosin; example inhibitors include azole antifungals, ciprofloxacin, clarithromycin, diclofenac, doxycycline, erythromycin, imatinib, isoniazid, nefazodone, nicardipine, propofol, protease inhibitors, quinidine, and verapamil.

Nutritional/Ethanol Interactions
Food: Fasting increases bioavailability by 30% and peak concentration 40% to 70%.
Herb/Nutraceutical: Avoid saw palmetto (due to limited experience with this combination).

Adverse Reactions
>10%:
Cardiovascular: Studies specific for orthostatic hypotension: Overall, at least one positive test was observed in 16% of patients receiving 0.4 mg and 19% of patients receiving the 0.8 mg dose. "First-dose" orthostatic hypotension following a 0.4 mg dose was reported as 7% at 4 hours postdose and 6% at 8 hours postdose.
Central nervous system: Headache (19% to 21%), dizziness (15% to 17%)
Genitourinary: Abnormal ejaculation (8% to 18%)
Respiratory: Rhinitis (13% to 18%)
1% to 10%:
Cardiovascular: Chest pain (~4%)
Central nervous system: Somnolence (3% to 4%), insomnia (1% to 2%), vertigo (0.6% to 1%)
Endocrine & metabolic: Libido decreased (1% to 2%)

Gastrointestinal: Diarrhea (4% to 6%), nausea (3% to 4%), stomach discomfort (2% to 3%), bitter taste (2% to 3%)

Neuromuscular & skeletal: Weakness (8% to 9%), back pain (7% to 8%)

Ocular: Amblyopia (0.2% to 2%)

Respiratory: Pharyngitis (5% to 6%), cough (3% to 5%), sinusitis (2% to 4%)

Miscellaneous: Infection (9% to 11%), tooth disorder (1% to 2%)

Overdosage/Toxicology Symptoms of overdose include headache and hypotension. Treatment is supportive.

Pharmacodynamics/Kinetics

Absorption: >90%

Bioavailability: Fasting: 30% increase

Time to Peak: Fasting: 4-5 hours; With food: 6-7 hours

Steady-state: By the fifth day of once daily dosing

Protein Binding: 94% to 99%, primarily to alpha$_1$ acid glycoprotein (AAG)

Half-Life Elimination: Healthy volunteers: 9-13 hours; Target population: 14-15 hours

Metabolism: Hepatic via CYP; metabolites undergo extensive conjugation to glucuronide or sulfate

Excretion: Urine (76%, <10% as unchanged drug); feces (21%)

Dosing

Adults & Elderly: Benign prostatic hyperplasia (BPH): Oral: 0.4 mg once daily ~30 minutes after the same meal each day; dose may be increased after 2-4 weeks to 0.8 mg once daily in patients who fail to respond. If therapy is interrupted for several days, restart with 0.4 mg once daily.

Renal Impairment:

Cl_{cr} ≥10 mL/minute: No adjustment needed.

Cl_{cr} <10 mL/minute: Not studied.

Available Dosage Forms Capsule, as hydrochloride: 0.4 mg

Monitoring and Teaching Issues

Physical Assessment: Not for use as an antihypertensive (see Warnings/Precautions for use cautions). Assess potential for interactions with other pharmacological agents patient may be taking (eg, increased risk of hypotension; see Drug Interactions). Assess results of periodic lipid panels, therapeutic effectiveness (improved urine flow), and adverse reactions at beginning of therapy and on a regular basis with long-term therapy (eg, "first dose" orthostatic hypotension, headache, GI disturbance [nausea, vomiting], cough; see Adverse Reactions). When discontinuing, dose should be tapered and blood pressure monitored closely. Teach patient proper use, possible side effects/appropriate interventions, and adverse symptoms to report (see Patient Education).

Monitoring Laboratory Tests: Periodic lipid panels

Patient Education: Do not take any new medication during therapy without consulting prescriber. Take as directed; do not skip dose or discontinue without consulting prescriber. May cause drowsiness, dizziness, or impaired judgment with first doses (use caution when driving or engaging in tasks that require alertness until response to drug is known); postural hypotension (use caution when rising from sitting or lying position or when climbing stairs); nausea (frequent mouth care or sucking lozenges may help); urinary incontinence (void before taking medication); ejaculatory disturbance (reversible, may resolve with continued use of drug); diarrhea (buttermilk, boiled milk, or yogurt may help); palpitations or rapid heartbeat; respiratory difficulty, unusual cough, or sore throat; or other persistent side effects. Report palpitations or rapid heartbeat; respiratory difficulty; muscle weakness, fatigue, or pain; vision or hearing changes; rash; changes in urinary pattern (void before taking medications); or other persistent side effects.

Dietary Considerations: Take once daily, 30 minutes after the same meal each day.

Geriatric Considerations: Metabolism of tamsulosin may be slower, and older patients may be more sensitive to the orthostatic hypotension caused by this medication. A 40% higher exposure (AUC) is anticipated in patients between 55 and 75 years of age as compared to younger subjects (20-32 years).

Pregnancy Risk Factor: B

Lactation: Not indicated for use in women

Administration

Oral: Capsules should be swallowed whole; do not crush, chew, or open.

Tazarotene (taz AR oh teen)

U.S. Brand Names Avage™; Tazorac®

Generic Available No

Pharmacologic Category Keratolytic Agent

(Continued)

Tazarotene *(Continued)*

Use Topical treatment of facial acne vulgaris; topical treatment of stable plaque psoriasis of up to 20% body surface area involvement; mitigation (palliation) of facial skin wrinkling, facial mottled hyper/hypopigmentation, and benign facial lentigines

Contraindications Hypersensitivity to tazarotene, other retinoids or vitamin A derivatives (isotretinoin, tretinoin, etretinate), or any component of the formulation; use in women of childbearing potential who are unable to comply with birth control requirements; pregnancy (negative pregnancy test required)

Warnings/Precautions Women of childbearing potential must use adequate contraceptive measures because of potential teratogenicity. May cause photosensitivity; exposure to sunlight should be avoided unless deemed medically necessary, and in such cases, exposure should be minimized (including use of sunscreens/protective clothing) during use of tazarotene. Risk may be increased by concurrent therapy with known photosensitizers (thiazides, tetracyclines, fluoroquinolones, phenothiazines, sulfonamides). For external use only; avoid contact with eyes, eyelids, and mouth. Not for use on eczematous, broken, or sunburned skin; not for treatment of lentigo maligna. Avoid application over extensive areas; specifically, safety and efficacy of gel applied over >20% of BSA have not been established. Safety and efficacy in children <12 years of age have not been established.

Drug Interactions

Increased Effect/Toxicity: Increased toxicity may occur with sulfur, benzoyl peroxide, salicylic acid, resorcinol, or any product with strong drying effects (including alcohol-containing compounds) due to increased drying actions. May augment phototoxicity of sensitizing medications (thiazides, tetracyclines, fluoroquinolones, phenothiazines, sulfonamides).

Adverse Reactions Percentage of incidence varies with formulation and/or strength:

>10%: Dermatologic: Burning/stinging, desquamation, dry skin, erythema, pruritus, skin pain, worsening of psoriasis

1% to 10%: Dermatologic: Contact dermatitis, discoloration, fissuring, hypertriglyceridemia, inflammation, irritation, localized bleeding, rash

Frequency not defined:
Dermatologic: Photosensitization
Neuromuscular & skeletal: Peripheral neuropathy

Overdosage/Toxicology

Excessive topical use may lead to marked redness, peeling, or discomfort. Oral ingestion may lead to the same adverse effects as those associated with excessive oral intake of Vitamin A (hypervitaminosis A) or other retinoids.

Treatment: If oral ingestion occurs, monitor the patient and administer appropriate supportive measures as necessary

Pharmacodynamics/Kinetics

Duration of Action: Therapeutic: Psoriasis: Effects have been observed for up to 3 months after a 3-month course of topical treatment

Absorption: Minimal following cutaneous application (≤6% of dose)

Protein Binding: >99%

Half-Life Elimination: 18 hours

Metabolism: Prodrug, rapidly metabolized via esterases to an active metabolite (tazarotenic acid) following topical application and systemic absorption; tazarotenic acid undergoes further hepatic metabolism

Excretion: Urine and feces (as metabolites)

Dosing

Adults & Elderly: Note: In patients experiencing excessive pruritus, burning, skin redness, or peeling, discontinue until integrity of the skin is restored, or reduce dosing to an interval the patient is able to tolerate.

Acne: Topical: Tazorac® cream/gel 0.1%: Cleanse the face gently. After the skin is dry, apply a thin film of tazarotene (2 mg/cm^2) once daily, in the evening, to the skin where the acne lesions appear; use enough to cover the entire affected area

Palliation of fine facial wrinkles, facial mottled hyper/hypopigmentation, benign facial lentigines: Topical: Avage™: Apply a pea-sized amount once daily to clean dry face at bedtime; lightly cover entire face including eyelids if desired. Emollients or moisturizers may be applied before or after; if applied before tazarotene, ensure cream or lotion has absorbed into the skin and has dried completely.

Psoriasis: Topical:

Tazorac® cream/gel 0.05% or 0.1%: Apply once daily, in the evening, to psoriatic lesions using enough (2 mg/cm^2) to cover only the lesion with a thin film to no more than 20% of body surface area. If a bath or shower is taken prior to application, dry the skin before applying. Unaffected skin may be more susceptible to irritation, avoid application to these areas. **Note:** In patients experiencing excessive pruritus, burning, skin redness, or peeling, discontinue until integrity of the skin is restored, or reduce dosing to an interval the patient is able to tolerate.

Pediatrics: Note: In patients experiencing excessive pruritus, burning, skin redness, or peeling, discontinue until integrity of the skin is restored, or reduce dosing to an interval the patient is able to tolerate.

Acne: Children ≥12 years: Topical: Tazorac® cream/gel 0.1%: Cleanse the face gently. After the skin is dry, apply a thin film of tazarotene (2 mg/cm^2) once daily, in the evening, to the skin where the acne lesions appear; use enough to cover the entire affected area

Psoriasis: Children ≥12 years: Topical: Tazorac® gel 0.05% or 0.1%: Apply once daily, in the evening, to psoriatic lesions using enough (2 mg/cm^2) to cover only the lesion with a thin film to no more than 20% of body surface area. If a bath or shower is taken prior to application, dry the skin before applying. Unaffected skin may be more susceptible to irritation, avoid application to these areas.

Palliation of fine facial wrinkles, facial mottled hyper/hypopigmentation, benign facial lentigines: Children ≥17 years: Topical: Avage™: Refer to adult dosing.

Available Dosage Forms
Cream:

Avage™: 0.1% (15 g, 30 g) [contains benzyl alcohol]

Tazorac®: 0.05% (15 g, 30 g, 60 g); 0.1% (15 g, 30 g, 60 g) [contains benzyl alcohol]

Gel (Tazorac®): 0.05% (30 g, 100 g); 0.1% (30 g, 100 g) [contains benzyl alcohol]

Monitoring and Teaching Issues
Physical Assessment: Assess potential for interactions with other prescriptions, OTC medications, or herbal products patient may be taking (eg, accumulated photosensitivity). Assess therapeutic effectiveness and adverse response on a regular basis during therapy. Teach patient proper use, side effects/appropriate interventions, and adverse reactions to report. **Pregnancy risk factor X:** Determine that patient is not pregnant before beginning treatment. Do not give to women of childbearing age unless they are capable of complying with contraceptive use. Instruct patients of childbearing age about appropriate contraceptive measures.

Patient Education: This medication is for external use only; avoid using near eyes or mouth. Use exactly as directed; do not use more than recommended (severe skin reactions may occur). Avoid any other skin products (including cosmetics or personal products that may contain medications, spices, alcohols, or irritants) that are not approved by your prescriber. May cause photosensitivity, which will cause severe rash or burning (use sunblock SPF 15 or higher, wear protective clothing and eyewear, and avoid direct sunlight, sunlamps, or tanning beds). Report redness or discoloration, irritation, open sores, bleeding, burning, stinging, excessive dryness, or swelling of skin; or worsening of condition. **Pregnancy/breast-feeding precautions:** Inform prescriber if you are pregnant. Do not get pregnant during treatment. Consult prescriber for instruction on appropriate contraceptive measures. This drug may cause severe fetal defects. Do not allow anyone who may be or become pregnant to touch this medication. Consult prescriber if breast-feeding.

Application: Wash affected area gently and completely dry before applying medication. Apply a thin layer to cover affected area. Wash off any medication that gets on unaffected skin areas and wash hands thoroughly after application.

Geriatric Considerations: No differences in safety or efficacy were seen when the cream formulation was administered to patients >65 years of age; may experience increased sensitivity. Increased incidence of adverse effects and lower treatment success rates were observed with the gel formulation in the treatment of psoriasis.

Pregnancy Risk Factor: X

Pregnancy Issues: May cause fetal harm if administered to a pregnant woman. A negative pregnancy test should be obtained 2 weeks prior to treatment; treatment should begin during a normal menstrual period.

Lactation: Excretion in breast milk unknown/use caution

Administration
Topical: Do not apply to eczematous or sunburned skin; apply thin film to affected areas; avoid eyes and mouth

Storage: Store at room temperature of 25°C (77°F), away from heat and direct light; do not freeze.

♦ **Tazicef®** *see* Ceftazidime *on page 283*

♦ **Tazorac®** *see* Tazarotene *on page 1427*

♦ **Taztia XT™** *see* Diltiazem *on page 459*

♦ **3TC** *see* Lamivudine *on page 861*

♦ **3TC, Abacavir, and Zidovudine** *see* Abacavir, Lamivudine, and Zidovudine *on page 34*

♦ **T-Cell Growth Factor** *see* Aldesleukin *on page 62*

♦ **TCGF** *see* Aldesleukin *on page 62*

♦ **TCN** *see* Tetracycline *on page 1452*

♦ **TDF** *see* Tenofovir *on page 1441*

Tegaserod (teg a SER od)
U.S. Brand Names Zelnorm®

Synonyms HTF919; Tegaserod Maleate

Generic Available No

Pharmacologic Category Serotonin 5-HT$_4$ Receptor Agonist

Use Short-term treatment of constipation-predominate irritable bowel syndrome (IBS) in women; treatment of chronic idiopathic constipation

Mechanism of Action/Effect Normalizes impaired motility by stimulating peristalsis and decreasing transit time in the gastrointestinal tract.

Contraindications Hypersensitivity to tegaserod or any component of the formulation; severe renal impairment; moderate or severe hepatic impairment; history of bowel obstruction, symptomatic gallbladder disease, suspected sphincter of Oddi dysfunction, or abdominal adhesions. Treatment should **not** be started in patients with diarrhea or in those who experience diarrhea frequently.

Warnings/Precautions Has been associated with rare intestinal ischemic events. Discontinue immediately with new or sudden worsening abdominal pain or rectal bleeding. Diarrhea may occur after the start of treatment, most cases reported as a single episode within the first week of therapy, and may resolve with continued dosing. However, serious consequences of diarrhea (hypovolemia, syncope) have been reported. Patients should be warned to contact healthcare provider immediately if they develop severe diarrhea, or diarrhea with severe cramping, abdominal pain, or dizziness. Use caution with mild hepatic impairment. Safety and efficacy have not been established in males or patients <18 years of age.

Nutritional/Ethanol Interactions Food: Bioavailability is decreased by 40% to 65% and C$_{max}$ is decreased by 20% to 40% when taken with food. T$_{max}$ is prolonged from 1 hour up to 2 hours when taken following a meal, but decreased to 0.7 hours when taken 30 minutes before a meal.

(Continued)

Tegaserod *(Continued)*

Adverse Reactions
>10%:
  Central nervous system: Headache (15%)
  Gastrointestinal: Abdominal pain (12%)
1% to 10%:
  Central nervous system: Dizziness (4%), migraine (2%)
  Gastrointestinal: Diarrhea (9%; severe <1%), nausea (8%), flatulence (6%)
  Neuromuscular & skeletal: Back pain (5%), arthropathy (2%), leg pain (1%)

Overdosage/Toxicology Treatment should be symptom-directed and supportive. Diarrhea, headache, abdominal pain, orthostatic hypotension, flatulence, nausea, and vomiting were reported in healthy volunteers with doses of 90-180 mg. Unlikely to be removed by dialysis.

Pharmacodynamics/Kinetics
Bioavailability: Fasting: 10%
Time to Peak: 1 hour
Protein Binding: 98% primarily to α_1-acid glycoprotein
Half-Life Elimination: I.V.: 11 ± 5 hours
Metabolism: GI: Hydrolysis in the stomach; Hepatic: oxidation, conjugation, and glucuronidation; metabolite (negligible activity); significant first-pass effect
Excretion: Feces (~66% as unchanged drug); urine (~33% as metabolites)

Dosing
Adults & Elderly:
  IBS with constipation: Female: Oral: 6 mg twice daily, before meals, for 4-6 weeks; may consider continuing treatment for an additional 4-6 weeks in patients who respond initially.
  Chronic idiopathic constipation: Oral: 6 mg twice daily, before meals; the need for continued therapy should be reassessed periodically

Renal Impairment: C_{max} and AUC of the inactive metabolite are increased with renal impairment.
Mild to moderate impairment: No dosage adjustment recommended
Severe impairment: Use is contraindicated

Hepatic Impairment: C_{max} and AUC of tegaserod are increased with hepatic impairment.
Mild impairment: No dosage adjustment recommended; however, user caution
Moderate to severe impairment: Use is contraindicated

Available Dosage Forms Tablet: 2 mg, 6 mg

Monitoring and Teaching Issues
Physical Assessment: Use caution with hepatic impairment (see Warnings/Precautions for use cautions). Assess therapeutic effectiveness (improved bowel function) and adverse response when beginning therapy and at regular intervals during treatment (eg, clinically-significant diarrhea [hypovolemia, hypotension, syncope] or ischemic colitis [including rectal bleeding, bloody diarrhea, abdominal pain]; see Adverse Reactions). Teach patient appropriate use, side effects/appropriate interventions, and adverse symptoms to report (see Patient Education).

Patient Education: Do not take any new medication during therapy without consulting prescriber. Take exactly as directed, on an empty stomach, at least 30 minutes before meals. If you miss a dose, skip that dose and continue with regular schedule; do not double doses. May cause headache or dizziness (use caution when driving or engaging in tasks requiring alertness until response to drug is known); nausea or vomiting (small frequent meals, frequent mouth care, chewing gum, or sucking lozenges may help); or diarrhea (should resolve within a week). Report immediately if you experience severe diarrhea, bloody diarrhea, rectal bleeding, abdominal cramping or pain, or dizziness. **Breast-feeding precaution:** Breast-feeding is not recommended.

Dietary Considerations: Take on an empty stomach, 30 minutes before meals.

Pregnancy Risk Factor: B

Lactation: Excretion in breast milk unknown/not recommended

Administration
Oral: Administer 30 minutes before meals.
Storage: Store at controlled room temperature of 15°C to 30°C (59°F to 86°F). Protect from moisture.

Additional Information In clinical trials, constipation was defined as <3 bowel movements per week, hard or lumpy stools, or straining with a bowel movement.

- **Tegaserod Maleate** *see* Tegaserod *on page 1429*
- **Tegretol®** *see* Carbamazepine *on page 249*
- **Tegretol®-XR** *see* Carbamazepine *on page 249*

Telithromycin *(tel ith roe MYE sin)*
U.S. Brand Names Ketek®
Synonyms HMR 3647
Generic Available No
Pharmacologic Category Antibiotic, Ketolide
Use Treatment of community-acquired pneumonia (mild-to-moderate) caused by susceptible strains of *Streptococcus pneumoniae* (including multidrug-resistant isolates), *Haemophilus influenzae*, *Chlamydia pneumoniae*, *Moraxella catarrhalis*, and *Mycoplasma pneumoniae*; treatment of bacterial exacerbation of chronic bronchitis caused by susceptible strains of *S. pneumoniae*, *H. influenzae* and *Moraxella catarrhalis*; treatment of acute bacterial sinusitis caused by *Streptococcus pneumoniae*, *Haemophilus influenzae*, *Moraxella catarrhalis*, and *Staphylococcus aureus*
Unlabeled/Investigational Use Approved in Canada for use in the treatment of tonsillitis/pharyngitis due to *S. pyogenes* (as an alternative to beta-lactam antibiotics when necessary/appropriate)

Mechanism of Action/Effect Inhibits bacterial protein synthesis by binding to two sites on the 50S ribosomal subunit.

Contraindications Hypersensitivity to telithromycin, macrolide antibiotics, or any component of the formulation; concurrent use of cisapride or pimozide

Warnings/Precautions May prolong QT_c interval, leading to a risk of ventricular arrhythmias; closely-related antibiotics have been associated with malignant ventricular arrhythmias and torsade de pointes. Avoid in patients with prolongation of QT_c interval due to congenital causes, history of long QT syndrome, uncorrected electrolyte disturbances (hypokalemia or hypomagnesemia), significant bradycardia (<50 bpm), or concurrent therapy with QT_c-prolonging drugs (eg, class Ia and class III antiarrhythmics). Avoid use in patients with a prior history of confirmed cardiogenic syncope or ventricular arrhythmias while receiving macrolide antibiotics or other QT_c-prolonging drugs. Use caution in renal impairment (dosage adjustment required). Use caution in patients with myasthenia gravis (use only if suitable alternatives are not available). Inform patients of potential for blurred vision, which may interfere with ability to operate machinery or drive; use caution until effects are known. Safety and efficacy not established in pediatric patients <13 years of age per Canadian approved labeling and <18 years of age per U.S. approved labeling. Pseudomembranous colitis has been reported.

Drug Interactions

Cytochrome P450 Effect: Substrate of CYP1A2 (minor), 3A4 (major); **Inhibits** CYP2D6 (weak), 3A4 (strong)

Decreased Effect: The levels/effects of telithromycin may be decreased by aminoglutethimide, carbamazepine, nafcillin, nevirapine, phenobarbital, phenytoin, rifamycins, and other CYP3A4 inducers; avoid concurrent use.

Increased Effect/Toxicity: Concurrent use of cisapride or pimozide is contraindicated. Concurrent use with antiarrhythmics (eg, class Ia and class III) or other drugs which prolong QT_c (eg, gatifloxacin, mesoridazine, moxifloxacin, pimozide, sparfloxacin, thioridazine) may be additive; serious arrhythmias may occur. Neuromuscular-blocking agents may be potentiated by telithromycin.

Telithromycin may increase the levels/effects of selected benzodiazepines, calcium channel blockers, cyclosporine, ergot alkaloids, selected HMG-CoA reductase inhibitors, mirtazapine, nateglinide, nefazodone, pimozide, quinidine, sildenafil (and other PDE-5 inhibitors), tacrolimus, venlafaxine, and other CYP3A4 substrates. Selected benzodiazepines (midazolam, triazolam), and selected HMG-CoA reductase inhibitors (atorvastatin, lovastatin and simvastatin) are generally contraindicated with strong CYP3A4 inhibitors. When used with strong CYP3A4 inhibitors, dosage adjustment/limits are recommended for sildenafil and other PDE-5 inhibitors; refer to individual monographs.

The levels/effects of telithromycin may be increased by azole antifungals, ciprofloxacin, clarithromycin, diclofenac, doxycycline, erythromycin, imatinib, isoniazid, nefazodone, nicardipine, propofol, protease inhibitors, quinidine, verapamil, and other CYP3A4 inhibitors.

Adverse Reactions

2% to 10%:

Central nervous system: Headache (2% to 6%), dizziness (3% to 4%)

Gastrointestinal: Diarrhea (10%), nausea (7% to 8%), vomiting (2% to 3%), loose stools (2%), dysgeusia (2%)

≥0.2% to <2%:

Central nervous system: Vertigo, fatigue, somnolence, insomnia

Dermatologic: Rash

Gastrointestinal: Abdominal distension, abdominal pain, anorexia, constipation, dyspepsia, flatulence, gastritis, gastroenteritis, GI upset, glossitis, stomatitis, watery stools, xerostomia

Genitourinary: Vaginal candidiasis

Hematologic: Platelets increased

Hepatic: Transaminases increased, hepatitis

Ocular: Blurred vision, accommodation delayed, diplopia

Miscellaneous: Candidiasis, diaphoresis increased, exacerbation of myasthenia gravis (rare)

Additional effects also reported with telithromycin:

Cardiovascular: Bundle branch block, palpitation, QT_c prolongation, vasculitis

Central nervous system: Abnormal dreams, nervousness, tremor

Endocrine & metabolic: Appetite decreased, hypokalemia, hyperkalemia

Gastrointestinal: Esophagitis, pharyngolaryngeal pain, pseudomembranous colitis, reflux esophagitis, tooth discoloration

Genitourinary: Vaginal irritation, urine discoloration, polyuria

Hematologic: Anemia, coagulation disorder, leukopenia, neutropenia, thrombocytopenia, lymphopenia

Hepatic: Cholestasis

Neuromuscular & skeletal: Weakness

Renal: Serum creatinine increased

Miscellaneous: Hypersensitivity

Overdosage/Toxicology Treatment should be symptomatic and supportive. ECG and electrolytes should be monitored.

(Continued)

Telithromycin *(Continued)*

Pharmacodynamics/Kinetics

Absorption: Rapid

Bioavailability: 57% (significant first-pass metabolism)

Time to Peak: Plasma: 1 hour

Protein Binding: 60% to 70%

Half-Life Elimination: 10 hours

Metabolism: Hepatic, via CYP3A4 (50%) and non-CYP-mediated pathways

Excretion: Urine (13% unchanged drug, remainder as metabolites); feces (7%)

Dosing

Adults & Elderly:

Tonsillitis/pharyngitis (unlabeled U.S. indication): Oral: 800 mg once daily for 5 days

Acute exacerbation of chronic bronchitis, acute bacterial sinusitis: Oral: 800 mg once daily for 5 days

Community-acquired pneumonia: Oral: 800 mg once daily for 7-10 days

Pediatrics: Tonsillitis/pharyngitis (unlabeled U.S. indication): Children ≥13 years: Oral: Refer to adult dosing.

Renal Impairment:

Cl$_{cr}$ <30 mL/minute:

U.S. product labeling: 600 mg once daily; when renal impairment is accompanied by hepatic impairment, reduce dosage to 400 mg once daily

Canadian product labeling: Reduce dose to 400 mg once daily

Hemodialysis: Administer following dialysis

Hepatic Impairment: No adjustment recommended, unless concurrent severe renal impairment is present.

Available Dosage Forms

Tablet [film coated]: 300 mg [not available in Canada], 400 mg

Ketek Pak™ [blister pack]: 400 mg (10s) [packaged as 10 tablets/card; 2 tablets/blister]

Monitoring and Teaching Issues

Physical Assessment: Assess for previous allergy history prior to therapy. Use caution in renal impairment, prolonged QT or ventricular disease, or myasthenia gravis (see Warning/Precautions for cautious use). Assess for potential interactions with other pharmacological agents patient may be using (eg, potential for increased risk of arrhythmias, decreased of levels/effects of telithromycin; see Drug Interactions). Assess therapeutic effectiveness (resolution of infection) and adverse reactions (eg, gastrointestinal disturbance [nausea, vomiting, diarrhea], CNS [vertigo, insomnia], rash, opportunistic infection, QT$_c$ prolongation; see Adverse Reactions). Teach patient proper use, possible side effects/appropriate interventions, and adverse symptoms to report (see Patient Education).

Monitoring Laboratory Tests: Culture and sensitivity

Patient Education: Take as directed, with or without food. Do not chew or crush tablets. Take complete prescription even if you are feeling better. May cause dizziness or blurred vision (use caution when driving or engaging in tasks that require alertness until response to drug is known); nausea, vomiting, abdominal pain (frequent small meals and frequent mouth care may help), constipation (increased dietary fluid and fibers may help), diarrhea (consult prescriber if persistent). Report chest pain, palpitations, irregular heart beat, flushing or facial swelling; CNS disturbance (dizziness, headache, anxiety, abnormal dreams, tremor); unusual muscle weakness or cramping; rash; or other persistent adverse effects.

Dietary Considerations: May be taken with or without food.

Geriatric Considerations: Bioavailability (57%) equivalent in persons ≥65 years compared to younger adults; although a 1.4- to 2-fold increase in AUC found in older adults. No dosage adjustment required. See dosing information.

Pregnancy Risk Factor: C

Lactation: Excretion in breast milk unknown/use caution

Administration

Oral: May be administered with or without food.

Storage: Store at room temperature between 15°C and 30°C.

Telmisartan *(tel mi SAR tan)*

U.S. Brand Names Micardis®

Generic Available No

Pharmacologic Category Angiotensin II Receptor Blocker

Use Treatment of hypertension; may be used alone or in combination with other antihypertensive agents

Mechanism of Action/Effect Telmisartan is a nonpeptide angiotensin receptor antagonist. Angiotensin II acts as a vasoconstrictor. In addition to causing direct vasoconstriction, angiotensin II also stimulates the release of aldosterone. Once aldosterone is released, sodium as well as water are reabsorbed. The end result is an elevation in blood pressure. Telmisartan binds to the AT1 angiotensin II receptor. This binding prevents angiotensin II from binding to the receptor thereby blocking the vasoconstriction and the aldosterone secreting effects of angiotensin II.

Contraindications Hypersensitivity to telmisartan or any component of the formulation; hypersensitivity to other A-II receptor antagonists; bilateral renal artery stenosis; pregnancy (2nd and 3rd trimesters)

Warnings/Precautions Avoid use or use a smaller dose in patients who are volume depleted; correct depletion first. Deterioration in renal function can occur with initiation. Use with caution in unilateral renal artery stenosis and pre-existing renal insufficiency; significant aortic/mitral stenosis. Use with caution in patients who have biliary obstructive disorders or hepatic dysfunction.

Drug Interactions

Cytochrome P450 Effect: Inhibits CYP2C19 (weak)

Decreased Effect: Telmisartan decreased the trough concentrations of warfarin during concurrent therapy, however, INR was not affected.

Increased Effect/Toxicity: Telmisartan may increase serum digoxin concentrations. Potassium salts/supplements, co-trimoxazole (high dose), ACE inhibitors, and potassium-sparing diuretics (amiloride, spironolactone, triamterene) may increase the risk of hyperkalemia with telmisartan.

Nutritional/Ethanol Interactions Herb/Nutraceutical: Avoid dong quai if using for hypertension (has estrogenic activity). Avoid ephedra, yohimbe, ginseng (may worsen hypertension). Avoid garlic (may have increased antihypertensive effect).

Adverse Reactions May be associated with worsening of renal function in patients dependent on renin-angiotensin-aldosterone system.

1% to 10%:
Cardiovascular: Hypertension (1%), chest pain (1%), peripheral edema (1%)
Central nervous system: Headache (1%), dizziness (1%), pain (1%), fatigue (1%)
Gastrointestinal: Diarrhea (3%), dyspepsia (1%), nausea (1%), abdominal pain (1%)
Genitourinary: Urinary tract infection (1%)
Neuromuscular & skeletal: Back pain (3%), myalgia (1%)
Respiratory: Upper respiratory infection (7%), sinusitis (3%), pharyngitis (1%), cough (2%)
Miscellaneous: Flu-like syndrome (1%)

Overdosage/Toxicology Symptoms of overdose may include hypotension, dizziness, and tachycardia. Vagal stimulation may result in bradycardia. Treatment is supportive.

Pharmacodynamics/Kinetics

Onset of Action: 1-2 hours; Peak effect: 0.5-1 hours

Duration of Action: Up to 24 hours

Bioavailability: Dose dependent: 42% to 58%

Protein Binding: >99.5%

Half-Life Elimination: Terminal: 24 hours

Metabolism: Hepatic via conjugation to inactive metabolites; not metabolized via CYP

Excretion: Feces (97%)
Clearance: Total body: 800 mL/minute

Pharmacokinetic Note: Orally active, not a prodrug.

Dosing

Adults: Hypertension: Oral: Initial: 40 mg once daily; usual maintenance dose range: 20-80 mg/day. Patients with volume depletion should be initiated on the lower dosage with close supervision.

Elderly: Initial: 20 mg/day; usual maintenance dose range: 20-80 mg/day

Hepatic Impairment: Supervise patients closely.

Available Dosage Forms Tablet: 20 mg, 40 mg, 80 mg

Monitoring and Teaching Issues

Physical Assessment: Use caution in presence of renal or hepatic impairment or aortic/mitral stenosis (see Warnings/Precautions for specific use cautions). Assess potential for interactions with other pharmacological agents and herbal products patient may be taking (eg, increased risk of hypercalcemia or increased hypotensive effects; see Drug Interactions). Assess results of laboratory tests, therapeutic effectiveness (reduced hypertension), and adverse response on a regular basis during therapy (eg, hypotension, diarrhea, URI, cough; see Adverse Reactions). Teach patient proper use, need for regular blood pressure monitoring, possible side effects/appropriate interventions, and adverse symptoms to report (see Patient Education).

Monitoring Laboratory Tests: Monitor electrolytes, serum creatinine, BUN, urinalysis, symptomatic hypotension, and tachycardia

Patient Education: Do not take any new medication during therapy without consulting prescriber. Take exactly as directed and do not alter dose or discontinue without consulting prescriber. Monitor blood pressure on a regular basis at same time of day; as advised by prescriber. This drug does not eliminate need for diet or exercise regimen as recommended by prescriber. May cause dizziness, fainting, or lightheadedness (use caution when driving or engaging in tasks that require alertness until response to drug is known); or postural hypotension (use caution when rising from lying or sitting position or climbing stairs). Report unusual weight gain and swelling of ankles, hands, face, lips, throat, or tongue; persistent fatigue; dry cough or respiratory difficulty; palpitations or chest pain; CNS changes; GI disturbances; muscle or bone pain, cramping, or tremors; change in urinary pattern; changes in hearing or vision; or other adverse response. **Pregnancy/breast-feeding precautions:** Inform prescriber if you are or intend to become pregnant. This drug should not be used in the 2nd or 3rd trimester of pregnancy. Consult prescriber for appropriate contraceptive measures if necessary. Breast-feeding is not recommended.

Dietary Considerations: May be taken without regard to food.

Pregnancy Risk Factor: C (1st trimester); D (2nd and 3rd trimesters)

Pregnancy Issues: The drug should be discontinued as soon as possible when pregnancy is detected. Drugs which act directly on renin-angiotensin can cause fetal and neonatal morbidity and death.

Lactation: Enters breast milk/not recommended

Related Information

Angiotensin Agents *on page 1704*

♦ **Telmisartan and HCTZ** *see* Telmisartan and Hydrochlorothiazide *on page 1433*

Telmisartan and Hydrochlorothiazide
(tel mi SAR tan & hye droe klor oh THYE a zide)

U.S. Brand Names Micardis® HCT

Synonyms HCTZ and Telmisartan; Hydrochlorothiazide and Telmisartan; Telmisartan and HCTZ

Generic Available No

(Continued)

Telmisartan and Hydrochlorothiazide *(Continued)*

Pharmacologic Category Angiotensin II Receptor Blocker Combination; Antihypertensive Agent, Combination; Diuretic, Thiazide

Use Treatment of hypertension; combination product should not be used for initial therapy

Dosing

Adults: Hypertension: Oral: Replacement therapy: Combination product can be substituted for individual titrated agents. Initiation of combination therapy when monotherapy has failed to achieve desired effects:

Patients currently on telmisartan: Initial dose if blood pressure is not currently controlled on monotherapy of 80 mg telmisartan: Telmisartan 80 mg/hydrochlorothiazide 12.5 mg once daily; may titrate up to telmisartan 160 mg/hydrochlorothiazide 25 mg if needed.

Patients currently on HCTZ: Initial dose if blood pressure is not currently controlled on monotherapy of 25 mg once daily: Telmisartan 80 mg/hydrochlorothiazide 12.5 mg once daily or telmisartan 80 mg/hydrochlorothiazide 25 mg once daily; may titrate up to telmisartan 160 mg/hydrochlorothiazide 25 mg if blood pressure remains uncontrolled after 2-4 weeks of therapy. Patients who develop hypokalemia may be switched to telmisartan 80 mg/hydrochlorothiazide 12.5 mg.

Elderly: Refer to adult dosing. Monitor renal function.

Renal Impairment:
Cl_{cr} >30 mL/minute: Usual recommended dose
Cl_{cr} ≤30 mL/minute: Not recommended

Hepatic Impairment: Dosing should be started at telmisartan 40 mg/hydrochlorothiazide 12.5 mg. Do **not** use in patients with severe hepatic impairment.

Available Dosage Forms Tablet:
40/12.5: Telmisartan 40 mg and hydrochlorothiazide 12.5 mg
80/12.5: Telmisartan 80 mg and hydrochlorothiazide 12.5 mg
80/25: Telmisartan 80 mg and hydrochlorothiazide 25 mg

Monitoring and Teaching Issues

Physical Assessment: See individual agents.

Patient Education: See individual agents. **Pregnancy/breast-feeding precautions:** Use appropriate contraceptive measures; do not get pregnant while taking this drug. Inform prescriber if you are or intend to become pregnant. Breast-feeding is not recommended.

Pregnancy Risk Factor: C (1st trimester); D (2nd and 3rd trimesters)

Lactation: Enters breast milk/not recommended

Related Information
Hydrochlorothiazide *on page 751*
Telmisartan *on page 1432*

Temazepam *(te MAZ e pam)*

U.S. Brand Names Restoril®

Controlled Substance C-IV

Generic Available Yes

Pharmacologic Category Benzodiazepine

Medication Safety Issues
Sound-alike/look-alike issues:
Temazepam may be confused with flurazepam, lorazepam
Restoril® may be confused with Vistaril®, Zestril®

Use Short-term treatment of insomnia

Unlabeled/Investigational Use Treatment of anxiety; adjunct in the treatment of depression; management of panic attacks

Mechanism of Action/Effect Binds to stereospecific benzodiazepine receptors on the postsynaptic GABA neuron at several sites within the central nervous system, including the limbic system, reticular formation. Enhancement of the inhibitory effect of GABA on neuronal excitability results by increased neuronal membrane permeability to chloride ions. This shift in chloride ions results in hyperpolarization (a less excitable state) and stabilization.

Contraindications Hypersensitivity to temazepam or any component of the formulation (cross-sensitivity with other benzodiazepines may exist); narrow-angle glaucoma (not in product labeling, however, benzodiazepines are contraindicated); pregnancy

Warnings/Precautions As a hypnotic, should be used only after evaluation of potential causes of sleep disturbance. Failure of sleep disturbance to resolve after 7-10 days may indicate psychiatric or medical illness. Use is not recommended in patients with depressive disorders or psychoses. Avoid use in patients with sleep apnea. Use with caution in patients receiving concurrent CYP3A4 inhibitors, particularly when these agents are added to therapy. Use with caution in elderly or debilitated patients, patients with hepatic disease (including alcoholics), renal impairment, respiratory disease, impaired gag reflex, or obese patients.

Causes CNS depression (dose-related) which may impair physical and mental capabilities. Use with caution in patients receiving other CNS depressants or psychoactive agents. Benzodiazepines have been associated with falls and traumatic injury and should be used with extreme caution in patients who are at risk of these events (especially the elderly). May cause physical or psychological dependence - use with caution in patients with a history of drug dependence.

Benzodiazepines have been associated with anterograde amnesia. Paradoxical reactions, including hyperactive or aggressive behavior, have been reported with benzodiazepines, particularly in adolescent/pediatric or psychiatric patients. Does not have analgesic, antidepressant, or antipsychotic properties.

Drug Interactions

Cytochrome P450 Effect: Substrate (minor) of CYP2B6, 2C8/9, 2C19, 3A4

Decreased Effect: Oral contraceptives may increase the clearance of temazepam. Temazepam may decrease the antiparkinsonian efficacy of levodopa. Theophylline and other CNS stimulants may antagonize the sedative effects of temazepam. Carbamazepine, rifampin, rifabutin may enhance the metabolism of temazepam and decrease its therapeutic effect.

Increased Effect/Toxicity: Temazepam potentiates the CNS depressant effects of narcotic analgesics, barbiturates, phenothiazines, ethanol, antihistamines, MAO inhibitors, sedative-hypnotics, and cyclic antidepressants. Serum levels of temazepam may be increased by inhibitors of CYP3A4, including cimetidine, ciprofloxacin, clarithromycin, clozapine, diltiazem, disulfiram, digoxin, erythromycin, ethanol, fluconazole, fluoxetine, fluvoxamine, grapefruit juice, isoniazid, itraconazole, ketoconazole, labetalol, levodopa, loxapine, metoprolol, metronidazole, miconazole, nefazodone, omeprazole, phenytoin, rifabutin, rifampin, troleandomycin, valproic acid, and verapamil.

Nutritional/Ethanol Interactions
Ethanol: Avoid ethanol (may increase CNS depression).
Food: Serum levels may be increased by grapefruit juice.
Herb/Nutraceutical: St John's wort may decrease temazepam levels. Avoid valerian, St John's wort, kava kava, gotu kola (may increase CNS depression).

Adverse Reactions
1% to 10%:
Central nervous system: Confusion, dizziness, drowsiness, fatigue, anxiety, headache, lethargy, hangover, euphoria, vertigo
Dermatologic: Rash
Endocrine & metabolic: Decreased libido
Gastrointestinal: Diarrhea
Neuromuscular & skeletal: Dysarthria, weakness
Ocular: Blurred vision
Miscellaneous: Diaphoresis

Overdosage/Toxicology Symptoms of overdose include somnolence, confusion, coma, hypoactive reflexes, dyspnea, hypotension, slurred speech, and impaired coordination. Treatment for benzodiazepine overdose is supportive. Flumazenil has been shown to selectively block the binding of benzodiazepines to CNS receptors, resulting in a reversal of benzodiazepine-induced CNS depression but not always respiratory depression due to toxicity.

Pharmacodynamics/Kinetics
Time to Peak: Serum: 2-3 hours
Protein Binding: 96%
Half-Life Elimination: 9.5-12.4 hours
Metabolism: Hepatic
Excretion: Urine (80% to 90% as inactive metabolites)

Dosing
Adults: Insomnia: Oral: 15-30 mg at bedtime
Elderly: 15 mg in elderly or debilitated patients
Available Dosage Forms Capsule: 15 mg, 30 mg
Restoril®: 7.5 mg, 15 mg, 30 mg

Monitoring and Teaching Issues
Physical Assessment: For short-term use. Assess effectiveness and interactions of other medications patient may be taking. Assess for history of addiction (long-term use can result in dependence, abuse, or tolerance) and periodically evaluate need for continued use. After long-term use, taper dosage slowly when discontinuing. For inpatient use, institute safety measures and monitor effectiveness and adverse reactions. For outpatients, monitor therapeutic effectiveness and adverse reactions (eg, CNS depression) at beginning of therapy and periodically with long-term use. Assess knowledge/teach patient appropriate use, interventions to reduce side effects, and adverse symptoms to report. **Pregnancy risk factor X:** Determine that patient is not pregnant before starting therapy. Do not give to sexually-active female patients unless capable of complying with contraceptive use.

Patient Education: Use exactly as directed; do not increase dose or frequency or discontinue without consulting prescriber. Drug may cause physical and/or psychological dependence. May take with food to decrease GI upset. While using this medication, do not use alcohol or other prescription or OTC medications (especially, pain medications, sedatives, antihistamines, or hypnotics) without consulting prescriber. Maintain adequate hydration (2-3 L/day of fluids) unless instructed to restrict fluid intake. You may experience drowsiness, dizziness, lightheadedness, or blurred vision (use caution when driving or engaging in tasks requiring alertness until response to drug is known); or dry mouth or GI discomfort (small frequent meals, frequent mouth care, chewing gum, or sucking lozenges may help). Report CNS changes (confusion, depression, increased sedation, excitation, headache, abnormal thinking, insomnia, or nightmares, memory impairment, impaired coordination); muscle pain or weakness; respiratory difficulty; persistent dizziness, chest pain, or palpitations; alterations in normal gait; vision changes; or ineffectiveness of medication. **Pregnancy/breast-feeding precautions:** Inform prescriber if you are pregnant. Do not get pregnant during or for 1 month following therapy. Consult prescriber for instruction on appropriate contraceptive measures. This drug may cause severe fetal defects. Breast-feeding is not recommended.

Geriatric Considerations: Because of its lack of active metabolites, temazepam is recommended in the elderly when a benzodiazepine hypnotic is indicated. Hypnotic use should be limited to 10-14 days. If insomnia persists, the patient should be evaluated for etiology.

Pregnancy Risk Factor: X

Pregnancy Issues: Benzodiazepines cross the placenta. The association between benzodiazepine exposure and malformations remains controversial. A number of types of malformation have been reported (oral cleft, inguinal hernia, cardiac defects, spina bifida, dysmorphic facial features, skeletal defects); however, confounding factors make a clear association difficult. Overall, the risk to the fetus may be low. Nonteratogenic effects (including neonatal flaccidity, respiratory and feeding problems, and withdrawal symptoms) during the postnatal period have also been reported with benzodiazepine use.

Lactation: Enters breast milk/not recommended (AAP rates "of concern")

Other Issues: Taper dosage gradually after long-term therapy. Abrupt withdrawal may cause tremors, nausea, vomiting, abdominal and/or muscle cramps.
(Continued)

Temazepam (Continued)

Additional Information Abrupt discontinuation after sustained use (generally >10 days) may cause withdrawal symptoms.

Related Information

Anxiolytic / Hypnotic Use in Long-Term Care Facilities *on page 1769*
Benzodiazepines *on page 1719*
Federal OBRA Regulations: Recommended Maximum Doses *on page 1773*

♦ **Temodar®** *see* Temozolomide *on page 1436*

Temozolomide (te moe ZOE loe mide)

U.S. Brand Names Temodar®
Synonyms NSC-362856; TMZ
Generic Available No
Pharmacologic Category Antineoplastic Agent, Alkylating Agent
Use Treatment of adult patients with refractory (first relapse) anaplastic astrocytoma who have experienced disease progression on nitrosourea and procarbazine; newly-diagnosed glioblastoma multiforme
Unlabeled/Investigational Use Glioma, melanoma
Mechanism of Action/Effect Prodrug, hydrolyzed to MTIC [(methyl-triazene-1-yl)-imidazole-4-carboxamide] (active form). The cytotoxic effects of MTIC are manifested through alkylation of DNA (O^6, N^7 of guanine).
Contraindications Hypersensitivity to temozolomide or any component of the formulation; hypersensitivity to dacarbazine (since both drugs are metabolized to MTIC); pregnancy
Warnings/Precautions The U.S. Food and Drug Administration (FDA) currently recommends that procedures for proper handling and disposal of antineoplastic agents be considered. *Pneumocystis carinii* pneumonia (PCP) may occur; risk is increased in those receiving steroids or longer dosing regimens; PCP prophylaxis is required with radiotherapy for the 42-day regimen. Myelosuppression may occur; an increased incidence has been reported in geriatric and female patients; prior to dosing, absolute neutrophil count (ANC) should be ≥1.5 X 10^9/L and platelet count ≥100 X 10^9/L. Use caution in patients with severe hepatic or renal impairment. Safety and efficacy in pediatric patients have not been established.
Nutritional/Ethanol Interactions Food: Food reduces rate and extent of absorption.
Adverse Reactions Adverse reactions are listed as the combined incidence in studies for treatment of newly-diagnosed glioblastoma multiforme during the maintenance phase (after radiotherapy) and refractory anaplastic astrocytoma in adults.

>10%:
Cardiovascular: Peripheral edema (up to 11%)
Central nervous system: Fatigue (34% to 61%), headache (23% to 41%), fatigue (34% to 61%), convulsions (11% to 23%), hemiparesis (18%), dizziness (5% to 12%), fever (up to 13%), coordination abnormality (up to 11%). In the case of CNS malignancies, it is difficult to distinguish the relative contributions of temozolomide and progressive disease to CNS symptoms.
Dermatologic: Alopecia (55% - maintenance phase after radiotherapy), rash (8% to 13%)
Gastrointestinal: Nausea (49% to 53%), vomiting (29% to 42%), constipation (22% to 33%), anorexia (9% to 27%), diarrhea (10% to 16%)
Hematologic: Lymphopenia (grade 3/4 in 55%), thrombocytopenia (grade 3/4 in 4% to 19%), neutropenia (grade 3/4 in 8% to 14%), leukopenia (grade 3/4 in 11%)
Neuromuscular & skeletal: Weakness (7% to 13%)
Miscellaneous: Viral infection (up to 11%)

1% to 10%:
Central nervous system: Ataxia (8%), memory impairment (up to 7%), confusion (5%), anxiety (7%), depression (up to 6%), amnesia (up to 10%), paresis (up to 8%), somnolence (up to 9%), insomnia (4% to 10%)
Dermatologic: Rash (8% to 13%), pruritus (5% to 8%), dry skin (up to 5%), radiation injury (2% - maintenance phase after radiotherapy), erythema (1%)
Endocrine & metabolic: Hypercorticism (8%), breast pain (up to 6%)
Gastrointestinal: Dysphagia (up to 7%), abdominal pain (5% to 9%), stomatitis (up to 9%), weight gain (up to 5%)
Genitourinary: Micturition frequency increased (up to 6%), incontinence (up to 8%), urinary tract infection (up to 8%)
Hematologic: Anemia (8%; grade 3/4 in up to 4%)
Neuromuscular & skeletal: Paresthesia (up to 9%), back pain (up to 8%), arthralgia (up to 6%), abnormal gait (up to 6%), myalgia (up to 5%),
Ocular: Diplopia (5%); vision abnormality (blurred vision, visual deficit, vision changes) (5% to 8%)
Respiratory: Pharyngitis (up to 8%), sinusitis (up to 6%), cough (5% to 8%), upper respiratory tract infection (up to 8%), dyspnea (5%)
Miscellaneous: Taste perversion (up to 5%), allergic reaction (up to 3%)

Overdosage/Toxicology Dose-limiting toxicity is hematological. In the event of an overdose, hematological evaluation is necessary. Treatment is supportive.

Pharmacodynamics/Kinetics
Bioavailability: 100%
Time to Peak: Empty stomach: 1 hour
Protein Binding: 15%
Half-Life Elimination: Mean: Parent drug: 1.8 hours
Metabolism: Prodrug, hydrolyzed to the active form, MTIC; MTIC is eventually eliminated as CO_2 and 5-aminoimidazole-4-carboxamide (AIC), a natural constituent in urine
Excretion: Urine (~38%); parent drug 6%); feces 0.8%

Dosing
Adults: Oral (refer to individual protocols):
Anaplastic astrocytoma (refractory): Initial dose: 150 mg/m²/day for 5 days; repeat every 28 days. Subsequent doses of 100-200 mg/m²/day; based upon hematologic

tolerance. This monthly-cycle regimen may be preceded by a 6- to 7-week regimen of 75 mg/m^2/day.

ANC <1000/mm^3 or platelets <50,000/mm^3 on day 22 or day 29 (day 1 of next cycle): Postpone therapy until ANC >1500/mm^3 and platelets >100,000/mm^3; reduce dose by 50 mg/m^2/day for subsequent cycle

ANC 1000-1500/mm^3 or platelets 50,000-100,000/mm^3 on day 22 or day 29 (day 1 of next cycle): Postpone therapy until ANC >1500/mm^3 and platelets >100,000/mm^3; maintain initial dose

ANC >1500/mm^3 and platelets >100,000/mm^3 on day 22 or day 29 (day 1 of next cycle): Increase dose to or maintain dose at 200 mg/m^2/day for 5 days for subsequent cycle

Glioblastoma multiforme (high-grade glioma):
Concomitant phase: 75 mg/m^2/day for 42 days with radiotherapy (60Gy administered in 30 fractions). **Note:** PCP prophylaxis is required during concomitant phase and should continue in patients who develop lymphocytopenia until recovery (common toxicity criteria [CTC] ≤1). Obtain weekly CBC.

ANC ≥1500/mm^3, platelet count ≥100,000/mm^3, and nonhematologic CTC ≤grade 1 (excludes alopecia, nausea/vomiting): Temodar® 75 mg/m^2/day may be continued throughout the 42-day concomitant period up to 49 days

Dosage modification:
ANC ≥500/mm^3 but <1500/mm^3 **or** platelet count ≥10,000/mm^3 but <100,000/mm^3 **or** nonhematologic CTC grade 2 (excludes alopecia, nausea/vomiting): Interrupt therapy

ANC <500/mm^3 **or** platelet count <10,000/mm^3 **or** nonhematologic CTC grade 3/4 (excludes alopecia, nausea/vomiting): Discontinue therapy

Maintenance phase (consists of 6 treatment cycles): Begin 4 weeks after concomitant phase completion. **Note:** Each subsequent cycle is 28 days (consisting of 5 days of drug treatment followed by 23 days without treatment). Draw CBC within 48 hours of day 22; hold next cycle and do weekly CBC until ANC >1500/mm^3 and platelet count >100,000/mm^3; dosing modification should be based on lowest blood counts and worst nonhematologic toxicity during the previous cycle.

Cycle 1: 150 mg/m^2/day for 5 days

Dosage modification for next cycle:
ANC <1000/mm^3, platelet count <50,000/mm^3, or nonhematologic CTC grade 3 (excludes for alopecia, nausea/vomiting) during previous cycle: Decrease dose by 50 mg/m^2/day for 5 days, unless dose has already been lowered to 100 mg/m^2/day, then discontinue therapy.

If dose reduction <100 mg/m^2/day is required or nonhematologic CTC grade 4 (excludes for alopecia, nausea/vomiting), or if the same grade 3 nonhematologic toxicity occurs after dose reduction: Discontinue therapy

Cycle 2: 200 mg/m^2/day for 5 days unless prior toxicity, then refer to Dosage Modifications under "Cycle 1" and give adjusted dose for 5 days

Cycles 3-6: Continue with previous cycle's dose for 5 days unless toxicity has occurred then, refer to Dosage Modifications under "Cycle 1" and give adjusted dose for 5 days

Elderly: Patients ≥70 years of age had a higher incidence of grade 4 neutropenia and thrombocytopenia in the first cycle of therapy than patients <70 years of age.

Renal Impairment: Caution should be used when administered to patients with severe renal impairment (Cl$_{cr}$ <39 mL/minute).

Hepatic Impairment: Caution should be used when administering to patients with severe hepatic impairment.

Available Dosage Forms Capsule: 5 mg, 20 mg, 100 mg, 250 mg

Monitoring and Teaching Issues
Physical Assessment: Use caution in presence of severe hepatic or renal impairment (see Warnings/Precautions for use cautions). Assess results of CBC, effectiveness (reduction in symptoms), and adverse effects (eg, CNS [convulsions, fatigue, impaired coordination, ataxia], gastrointestinal disturbance [nausea, vomiting, constipation], myelosuppression, rash, opportunistic infection, vision disturbance, cough; see Adverse Reactions). Teach patient proper use, possible side effects, and appropriate interventions (see Patient Education).

Monitoring Laboratory Tests: CBC

Patient Education: Do not take any new medication during therapy without consulting prescriber. Take exactly as directed. Take on an empty stomach (1 hour before or 2 hours after meals or at bedtime) to reduce GI upset. Do not open, crush, or chew capsules; swallow whole with full 8 oz glass of water. May cause blurred visions, diplopia, headache, dizziness, confusion, fatigue, anxiety, insomnia, or impaired coordination (use caution when driving or engaging in tasks requiring alertness until response to medication is known); or nausea, vomiting, or loss of appetite (small frequent meals, good mouth care, chewing gum, or sucking hard candy may help). Report chest pain, palpitations, acute headache, persistent visual disturbances; unresolved GI problems; itching or burning on urination or vaginal discharge; acute joint, back, bone, or muscle pain; respiratory difficulty, unusual cough, or respiratory infection; or other adverse reactions. **Pregnancy/breast-feeding precautions:** Inform prescriber if you pregnant. Do not get pregnant while taking this medication. Consult prescriber for appropriate barrier contraceptive measures. Breast-feeding is not recommended.

Dietary Considerations: The incidence of nausea/vomiting is decreased when the drug is taken on an empty stomach.

Pregnancy Risk Factor: D

Pregnancy Issues: May cause fetal harm when administered to pregnant women. Male and female patients should avoid pregnancy while receiving drug.

Lactation: Excretion in breast milk unknown/not recommended

Administration
Oral: Capsules should not be opened or chewed but swallowed whole with a glass of water. May be administered on an empty stomach to reduce nausea and vomiting. Bedtime administration may be advised.

Storage: Store at controlled room temperature (15°C to 10°C/59°F to 86°F).

Tenecteplase (ten EK te plase)

U.S. Brand Names TNKase™

Generic Available No

Pharmacologic Category Thrombolytic Agent

Medication Safety Issues

Sound-alike/look-alike issues:

TNKase™ may be confused with t-PA

Use Thrombolytic agent used in the management of acute myocardial infarction for the lysis of thrombi in the coronary vasculature to restore perfusion and reduce mortality.

Mechanism of Action/Effect Initiates fibrinolysis by binding to fibrin and converting plasminogen to plasmin.

Contraindications Hypersensitivity to tenecteplase or any component of the formulation; active internal bleeding; history of stroke; intracranial/intraspinal surgery or trauma within 2 months; intracranial neoplasm; arteriovenous malformation or aneurysm; bleeding diathesis; severe uncontrolled hypertension

Warnings/Precautions Stop antiplatelet agents and heparin if serious bleeding occurs. Avoid I.M. injections and nonessential handling of the patient for a few hours after administration. Monitor for bleeding complications. Venipunctures should be performed carefully and only when necessary. If arterial puncture is necessary then use an upper extremity that can be compressed manually. For the following conditions the risk of bleeding is higher with use of tenecteplase and should be weighed against the benefits: recent major surgery, cerebrovascular disease, recent GI or GU bleed, recent trauma, uncontrolled HTN (systolic BP ≥180 mm Hg and/or diastolic BP ≥110 mm Hg), suspected left heart thrombus, acute pericarditis, subacute bacterial endocarditis, hemostatic defects, severe hepatic dysfunction, pregnancy, hemorrhagic diabetic retinopathy or other hemorrhagic ophthalmic conditions, septic thrombophlebitis or occluded AV cannula at seriously infected site, advanced age (>75 years of age), anticoagulants, recent administration of GP IIb/IIIa inhibitors. Coronary thrombolysis may result in reperfusion arrhythmias. Caution should be used with readministration of tenecteplase. Safety and efficacy has not been established in pediatric patients. Cholesterol embolism has rarely been reported.

Drug Interactions

Decreased Effect: Aminocaproic acid (antifibrinolytic agent) may decrease effectiveness.

Increased Effect/Toxicity: Drugs which affect platelet function (eg, NSAIDs, dipyridamole, ticlopidine, clopidogrel, IIb/IIIa antagonists) may potentiate the risk of hemorrhage; use with caution.

Heparin and aspirin: Use with aspirin and heparin may increase bleeding. However, aspirin and heparin were used concomitantly with tenecteplase in the majority of patients in clinical studies.

Warfarin or oral anticoagulants: Risk of bleeding may be increased during concurrent therapy.

Adverse Reactions As with all drugs which may affect hemostasis, bleeding is the major adverse effect associated with tenecteplase. Hemorrhage may occur at virtually any site. Risk is dependent on multiple variables, including the dosage administered, concurrent use of multiple agents which alter hemostasis, and patient predisposition. Rapid lysis of coronary artery thrombi by thrombolytic agents may be associated with reperfusion-related arterial and/or ventricular arrhythmia. The incidence of stroke and bleeding increase in patients >65 years.

>10%:

Hematologic: Bleeding (22% minor: ASSENT-2 trial)

Local: Hematoma (12% minor)

1% to 10%:

Central nervous system: Stroke (2%)

Gastrointestinal: GI hemorrhage (1% major, 2% minor), epistaxis (2% minor)

Genitourinary: GU bleeding (4% minor)

Hematologic: Bleeding (5% major: ASSENT-2 trial)

Local: Bleeding at catheter puncture site (4% minor), hematoma (2% major)

Respiratory: Pharyngeal bleeding (3% minor)

Additional cardiovascular events associated with use in MI: Cardiogenic shock, arrhythmia, AV block, pulmonary edema, heart failure, cardiac arrest, recurrent myocardial ischemia, myocardial reinfarction, myocardial rupture, cardiac tamponade, pericarditis, pericardial effusion, mitral regurgitation, thrombosis, embolism, electromechanical dissociation, hypotension, fever, nausea, vomiting

Overdosage/Toxicology Increased incidence of bleeding

Pharmacodynamics/Kinetics

Half-Life Elimination: 90-130 minutes

Metabolism: Primarily hepatic

Excretion: Clearance: Plasma: 99-119 mL/minute

Dosing

Adults:

Coronary thrombosis/AMI: I.V.: The recommended total dose should not exceed 50 mg and is based on weight. Administer as a bolus over 5 seconds:

<60 kg: 30 mg dose

≥60 to <70 kg: 35 mg

≥70 to <80 kg: 40 mg

≥80 to <90 kg: 45 mg

≥90 kg: 50 mg

Note: All patients received 150-325 mg of aspirin as soon as possible and then daily. Intravenous heparin was initiated as soon as possible and PTT was maintained between 50-70 seconds.

Elderly: Refer to adult dosing. Although dosage adjustments are not recommended, the elderly have a higher incidence of morbidity and mortality with the use of tenecteplase. The 30-day mortality in the ASSENT-2 trial was 2.5% for patients younger than 65 years, 8.5% for patients between 65 and 74 years, and 16.2% for patients 75 years and older. The intracranial hemorrhage rate was 0.4% for patient younger than 65 years, 1.6% for patients between 65 and 74 years, and 1.7% for patients 75 years and older. The risks and benefits of use should be weighted carefully in the elderly.

Renal Impairment: No adjustment is necessary.

Hepatic Impairment: Severe hepatic failure is a relative contraindication. Recommendations were not made for mild or moderate hepatic impairment.

Available Dosage Forms Injection, powder for reconstitution, recombinant: 50 mg [packaged with diluent and syringe]

Monitoring and Teaching Issues

Physical Assessment: Weigh benefits against risks of use in conditions where bleeding constitutes a significant hazard or would be particularly difficult to manage because of location (see Warnings/Precautions). Assess potential for interactions with other pharmacological agents and herbal products patient may be taking (especially those medications that may affect coagulation [warfarin] or platelet function [NSAIDs, dipyridamole, ticlopidine, clopidogrel]; see Drug Interactions). See Administration for infusion specifics. Patient should be closely monitored for bleeding during and following treatment; infusion site, neurological status (eg, intracranial hemorrhage), vital signs, ECG (reperfusion arrhythmias); see Adverse Reactions. Arrhythmias may occur; antiarrhythmic drugs should be immediately available. Bedrest and bleeding precautions should be maintained; avoid I.M. injections, venipuncture (unless absolutely necessary) and nonessential handling of the patient. If arterial puncture is necessary, use an upper extremity vessel that can be manually compressed. Patient instructions determined by patient condition (see Patient Education).

Monitoring Laboratory Tests: CBC, PTT, signs and symptoms of bleeding, ECG monitoring

Patient Education: Inform prescriber of all medication or herbal products you are taking. This medication is only administered by infusion; you will be monitored closely during and after treatment. Immediately report burning, pain, redness, swelling, or oozing at infusion site, sudden acute headache, joint pain, chest pain, or altered vision. Following infusion you will have a tendency to bleed easily; use caution to prevent injury (use electric razor, soft toothbrush, and caution with knives, needles, or anything sharp) and follow instructions for strict bedrest to reduce the risk of injury. If bleeding does occur, report immediately and apply pressure to bleeding spot until bleeding stops completely. Report unusual pain (acute headache, joint pain, chest pain); unusual bruising or bleeding; blood in urine, stool, or vomitus; bleeding gums; vision changes; or respiratory difficulty. **Pregnancy/breast-feeding precautions:** Inform prescriber if you are or intend to become pregnant or breast-feed.

Pregnancy Risk Factor: C

Lactation: Use caution

Administration

I.V.: Tenecteplase should be reconstituted using the supplied 10 mL syringe with TwinPak™ Dual Cannula Device and 10 mL SWFI. Do not shake when reconstituting. Slight foaming is normal; will dissipate if left standing for several minutes. Any unused solution should be discarded. The reconstituted solution is 5 mg/mL. Dextrose-containing lines must be flushed with a saline solution before and after administration. Check frequently for signs of bleeding. Avoid I.M. injections and nonessential handling of patient.

Reconstitution: Tenecteplase should be reconstituted using the supplied 10 mL syringe with TwinPak™ Dual Cannula Device and 10 mL sterile water for injection. Tenecteplase is incompatible with dextrose solutions. Dextrose-containing lines must be flushed with a saline solution before and after administration. Administer as a single I.V. bolus over 5 seconds. If reconstituted and not used immediately, store in refrigerator and use within 8 hours.

Storage: Store at room temperature not to exceed 30°C (86°F) or under refrigeration 2°C to 8°C (36°F to 46°F).

Teniposide (ten i POE side)

U.S. Brand Names Vumon

Synonyms EPT; VM-26

Generic Available No

Pharmacologic Category Antineoplastic Agent, Miscellaneous

Use Treatment of acute lymphocytic leukemia, small cell lung cancer

Mechanism of Action/Effect Inhibits mitotic activity; inhibits cells from entering mitosis

Contraindications Hypersensitivity to teniposide, Cremophor® EL (polyoxyethylated castor oil), or any component of the formulation; pregnancy

Warnings/Precautions The U.S. Food and Drug Administration (FDA) currently recommends that procedures for proper handling and disposal of antineoplastic agents be considered. Teniposide injection contains benzyl alcohol and should be avoided in neonates. The injection contains about 43% alcohol; the possible CNS depressant effect, especially with higher doses of teniposide, should be considered.

Drug Interactions

Cytochrome P450 Effect: Substrate of CYP3A4 (major); **Inhibits** CYP2C8/9 (weak), 3A4 (weak)

Decreased Effect: CYP3A4 inducers may decrease the levels/effects of teniposide; example inducers include aminoglutethimide, carbamazepine, nafcillin, nevirapine, phenobarbital, phenytoin, and rifamycins.

Increased Effect/Toxicity: May increase toxicity of methotrexate. Sodium salicylate, sulfamethizole, and tolbutamide displace teniposide from protein-binding sites which could cause substantial increases in free drug levels, resulting in potentiation of toxicity. Concurrent use of vincristine may increase the incidence of peripheral neuropathy. CYP3A4 (Continued)

Teniposide (Continued)

inhibitors may increase the levels/effects of teniposide; example inhibitors include azole antifungals, ciprofloxacin, clarithromycin, diclofenac, doxycycline, erythromycin, imatinib, isoniazid, nefazodone, nicardipine, propofol, protease inhibitors, quinidine, and verapamil.

Nutritional/Ethanol Interactions Herb/Nutraceutical: St John's wort may decrease teniposide levels.

Adverse Reactions

>10%:

Gastrointestinal: Mucositis (75%); diarrhea, nausea, vomiting (20% to 30%); anorexia

Hematologic: Myelosuppression, leukopenia, neutropenia (95%), thrombocytopenia (65% to 80%), anemia

Onset: 5-7 days

Nadir: 7-10 days

Recovery: 21-28 days

1% to 10%:

Cardiovascular: Hypotension (2%), associated with rapid (<30 minutes) infusions

Dermatologic: Alopecia (9%), rash (3%)

Miscellaneous: Anaphylactoid reactions (5%) (fever, rash, hyper-/hypotension, dyspnea, bronchospasm), usually seen with rapid (<30 minutes) infusions

Overdosage/Toxicology Symptoms of overdose include bone marrow suppression, leukopenia, thrombocytopenia, nausea, and vomiting. Treatment is supportive.

Pharmacodynamics/Kinetics

Protein Binding: 99.4%

Half-Life Elimination: 5 hours

Metabolism: Extensively hepatic

Excretion: Urine (44%, 21% as unchanged drug); feces (≤10%)

Dosing

Adults & Elderly:

Antineoplastic: I.V. (refer to individual protocols): 50-180 mg/m^2 once or twice weekly for 4-6 weeks or 20-60 mg/m^2/day for 5 days

Small cell lung cancer: I.V.: 80-90 mg/m^2/day for 5 days every 4-6 weeks

Dosage adjustment in Down syndrome patient: Reduce initial dosing give the first course at half the usual dose. Patients with both Down syndrome and leukemia may be especially sensitive to myelosuppressive chemotherapy.

Pediatrics:

Antineoplastic: I.V. (refer to individual protocols): 130 mg/m^2/week, increasing to 150 mg/m^2 after 3 weeks and up to 180 mg/m^2 after 6 weeks

Acute lymphoblastic leukemia (ALL): I.V.: 165 mg/m^2 twice weekly for 8-9 doses **or** 250 mg/m^2 weekly for 4-8 weeks

Renal Impairment: Data is insufficient, but dose adjustments may be necessary in patient with significant renal impairment.

Hepatic Impairment: Data is insufficient, but dose adjustments may be necessary in patient with significant hepatic impairment.

Available Dosage Forms Injection, solution: 10 mg/mL (5 mL) [contains benzyl alcohol, dehydrated alcohol, and polyoxyethylated castor oil]

Monitoring and Teaching Issues

Physical Assessment: Assess potential for interactions with other pharmacological agents or herbal products patient may be taking (eg, potential for increased or decreased levels/effects and risk of toxicity; see Drug Interactions). Premedication with antiemetic may be beneficial. See Administration for infusion specifics. Infusion site should be closely monitored to prevent extravasation. Patient should be monitored closely during infusion for possible hypotension (may require discontinuing infusion and administering supportive therapy) or hypersensitivity reactions (chills, fever, tachycardia, dyspnea, hypotension). Assess results of laboratory tests, therapeutic effectiveness, and adverse reactions prior to each infusion and throughout therapy (eg, mucositis, diarrhea, myelosuppression, leukopenia; see Adverse Reactions). Teach patient possible side effects/appropriate interventions and adverse symptoms to report (see Patient Education).

Monitoring Laboratory Tests: CBC, platelet count

Patient Education: Do not take any new medication during therapy without consulting prescriber. This medication is only administered by infusion; report immediately any swelling, pain, burning, or redness at infusion site and hypersensitivity reactions (chills, fever, chest pain, difficulty breathing or swallowing). It is important to maintain adequate hydration (2-3 L/day of fluids) unless instructed to restrict fluid intake and adequate nutrition (small frequent meals may help). You will be more susceptible to infection (avoid crowds and exposure to infection and do not have any vaccinations without consulting prescriber). May cause nausea or vomiting (small frequent meals, frequent mouth care, sucking lozenges, or chewing gum may help); diarrhea (buttermilk, boiled milk, or yogurt may help); or loss of hair (reversible). Report unusual bleeding or bruising, persistent fever or chills, sore throat, sores in mouth or vagina, or respiratory difficulty. **Pregnancy/breast-feeding precautions:** Do not get pregnant while taking this medication. Consult prescriber for appropriate contraceptive measures. Breast-feeding is not recommended.

Pregnancy Risk Factor: D

Lactation: Not recommended

Administration

I.V.: Irritant. Slow I.V. infusion over ≥30 minutes.

Reconstitution: Reconstituted solutions are stable at room temperature for up to 24 hours after preparation. Teniposide must be diluted with either D$_5$W or 0.9% sodium chloride solutions to a final concentration of 0.1, 0.2, 0.4, or 1 mg/mL. In order to prevent extraction of the plasticizer DEHP, **solutions should be prepared in non-DEHP-containing containers such as glass or polyolefin containers.** The use of polyvinyl chloride (PVC) containers is not recommended. Administer 1 mg/mL solutions within 4 hours of preparation to reduce the potential for precipitation. Precipitation may occur at any concentration.

Compatibility: Stable in D$_5$W, LR, NS
Y-site administration: Incompatible with Idarubicin, heparin
Storage: Store ampuls in refrigerator at 2°C to 8°C (36°F to 46°F).

Tenofovir (te NOE fo veer)

U.S. Brand Names Viread®
Synonyms PMPA; TDF; Tenofovir Disoproxil Fumarate
Generic Available No
Pharmacologic Category Antiretroviral Agent, Reverse Transcriptase Inhibitor (Nucleotide)
Use Management of HIV infections in combination with at least two other antiretroviral agents
Mechanism of Action/Effect Tenofovir blocks replication of HIV virus by inhibiting the reverse transcriptase enzyme. It is chemically similar to adenosine 5'-monophosphate (a nucleotide), which is required to form DNA.
Contraindications Hypersensitivity to tenofovir or any component of the formulation
Warnings/Precautions Lactic acidosis and severe hepatomegaly with steatosis have been reported with nucleoside analogues, including fatal cases; use with caution in patients with risk factors for liver disease (risk may be increased in obese patients or prolonged exposure) and suspend treatment in any patient who develops clinical or laboratory findings suggestive of lactic acidosis (transaminase elevation may/may not accompany hepatomegaly and steatosis).

Use caution in renal impairment (Cl$_{cr}$ <50 mL/minute; dosage adjustment required. May cause osteomalacia and/or renal toxicity; monitor renal function and possible bone abnormalities during therapy. Use caution in hepatic impairment. All patients with HIV should be tested for HBV prior to initiation of treatment. Safety and efficacy of tenofovir during coinfection of HIV and HBV have not been established; acute, severe exacerbations of HBV have been reported following tenofovir discontinuation. In HBV coinfected patients, monitor hepatic function closely for several months following discontinuation. Safety and efficacy have not been established in pediatric patients.

Drug Interactions
Cytochrome P450 Effect: Inhibits CYP1A2 (weak)
Decreased Effect: Serum levels of lopinavir and/or ritonavir may be decreased by tenofovir. Tenofovir may decrease serum concentrations of atazanavir, resulting in a loss of virologic response (specific atazanavir dosing recommendations provided by manufacturer).
Increased Effect/Toxicity: Concurrent use has been noted to increase serum concentrations/exposure to didanosine and its metabolites, potentially increasing the risk of didanosine toxicity (pancreatitis, peripheral neuropathy, or lactic acidosis); use caution and monitor closely; suspend therapy if signs/symptoms of toxicity are present. Drugs which may compete for renal tubule secretion (including acyclovir, cidofovir, ganciclovir, valacyclovir, valganciclovir) may increase the serum concentrations of tenofovir. Drugs causing nephrotoxicity may reduce elimination of tenofovir. Lopinavir/ritonavir may increase serum concentrations of tenofovir.
Nutritional/Ethanol Interactions Food: Fatty meals may increase the bioavailability of tenofovir. Tenofovir may be taken with or without food.
Adverse Reactions Clinical trials involved addition to prior antiretroviral therapy. Frequencies listed are treatment-emergent adverse effects noted at higher frequency than in the placebo group.
>10%: Gastrointestinal: Nausea (8% to 11%), diarrhea (11% to 16%)
1% to 10%:
  Central nervous system: Headache (5% to 8%), depression (5% to 8%), dizziness (1% to 3%), insomnia (1% to 4%)
  Endocrine & metabolic: Glycosuria (3%, frequency equal to placebo); other metabolic effects (hyperglycemia, hypertriglyceridemia) noted at frequencies less than placebo
  Gastrointestinal: Vomiting (4% to 7%), flatulence (3% to 4%), abdominal pain (4% to 7%), anorexia (3% to 4%)
  Hematologic: Neutropenia (1% to 2%)
  Hepatic: Transaminases increased (2% to 4%)
  Neuromuscular & skeletal: Weakness (7% to 11%), back pain (3% to 4%), myalgia (3% to 4%), neuropathy (1% to 3%)

Note: Uncommon, but significant adverse reactions reported with other reverse transcriptase inhibitors include pancreatitis, peripheral neuropathy, and myopathy.
Overdosage/Toxicology Limited experience with overdose. Treatment is supportive.
Pharmacodynamics/Kinetics
Bioavailability: Fasting: 25%; increases ~40% with high-fat meal
Time to Peak: Serum: Fasting: 1 hour; With food: 2 hours
Protein Binding: 7% to serum proteins
Metabolism: Tenofovir disoproxil fumarate (TDF) is converted intracellularly by hydrolysis (by non-CYP enzymes) to tenofovir, then phosphorylated to the active tenofovir diphosphate
Excretion: Urine (70% to 80%) via filtration and active secretion, primarily as unchanged tenofovir
Dosing
Adults: HIV infection: Oral: 300 mg once daily
Renal Impairment:
  Cl$_{cr}$ 30-49 mL/minute: 300 mg every 48 hours
  Cl$_{cr}$ 10-29 mL/minute: 300 mg twice weekly
    Cl$_{cr}$ <10 mL/minute without dialysis: No recommendation available.
  Hemodialysis: 300 mg every 7 days or after ~12 hours of dialysis
Available Dosage Forms Tablet, as disoproxil fumarate: 300 mg [equivalent to 245 mg tenofovir disoproxil]
(Continued)

Tenofovir (Continued)

Monitoring and Teaching Issues

Physical Assessment: Use caution in renal or hepatic impairment (see Warnings/Precautions for specific use cautions). Assess potential for interactions with other pharmacological agents patient may be taking (concurrent use with other antiretroviral nephrotoxic or hepatotoxic drugs may increase potential for severe toxicities; see Drug Interactions). Assess results of laboratory tests, therapeutic response (CD4 count and viral load), and adverse reactions on a regular basis throughout therapy (eg, lactic acidosis [elevated transaminases], GI disturbance [nausea, vomiting, diarrhea], neutropenia, myalgia, peripheral neuropathy; see Adverse Reactions). Teach patient proper use, possible side effects/appropriate interventions, and adverse symptoms to report (see Patient Education).

Monitoring Laboratory Tests: CBC with differential, reticulocyte count, serum creatine kinase, CD4 cell count, HIV RNA plasma levels, renal and hepatic function tests, bone density (long-term), serum phosphorus; testing for HBV is recommended prior to the initiation of antiretroviral therapy

Patients with HIV and HVB coinfection should be monitored for several months following tenofovir discontinuation.

Patient Education: Do not take any new medication during therapy without consulting prescriber. Take exactly as directed with food (space other medications as instructed). This drug will not cure HIV, nor will it prevent transmission; use appropriate precautions to prevent spread to other persons. Maintain adequate hydration (2-3 L/day of fluids unless instructed to restrict fluid intake). You may be susceptible to infection (avoid crowds and exposure to infection and do not have any vaccinations without consulting prescriber). May cause nausea, vomiting, loss of appetite (small frequent meals, frequent mouth care, chewing gum, or sucking lozenges may help); or diarrhea (boiled milk, yogurt, or buttermilk may help). Report immediately any loss of sensation, numbness, or tingling in fingers, toes, or feet; persistent unresolved abdominal distress (nausea, vomiting, diarrhea); signs of opportunistic infection (burning on urination, perineal itching, white plaques in mouth, unhealed sores, persistent sore throat or cough); changes in urine color or output; swelling of extremities, or other persistent adverse effects. **Pregnancy/breast-feeding precautions:** Inform prescriber if you are pregnant and do not get pregnant while taking this medicine. Do not breast-feed.

Dietary Considerations: May be taken with or without food. Consider calcium and vitamin D supplementation in patients with history of bone fracture or osteopenia.

Pregnancy Risk Factor: B

Pregnancy Issues: There are no adequate and well-controlled studies in pregnant women. Animal studies have shown decreased fetal growth and reduced fetal bone porosity. Clinical studies in children have shown bone demineralization with chronic use. Use in pregnancy only if clearly needed. Cases of lactic acidosis/hepatic steatosis syndrome have been reported in pregnant women receiving nucleoside analogues. It is not known if pregnancy itself potentiates this known side effect; however, pregnant women may be at increased risk of lactic acidosis and liver damage. Hepatic enzymes and electrolytes should be monitored frequently during the 3rd trimester of pregnancy in women receiving nucleoside analogues. Health professionals are encouraged to contact the Antiretroviral Pregnancy Registry to monitor outcomes of pregnant women exposed to antiretroviral medications (1-800-258-4263 or www.APRegistry.com).

Lactation: Excretion in breast milk unknown/contraindicated

Breast-Feeding Issues: HIV-infected mothers are discouraged from breast-feeding to decrease potential transmission of HIV.

Administration

Oral: May be administered with or without food.

Storage: Store at 25°C (77°F); excursions permitted to 15°C to 30°C (59°F to 86°F).

Additional Information Approval was based on two clinical trials involving patients who were previously treated with antiretrovirals with continued evidence of HIV replication despite therapy. The risk:benefit ratio for untreated patients has not been established (studies currently ongoing), however, patients who received tenofovir showed significant decreases in HIV replication as compared to continuation of standard therapy.

A high rate of early virologic nonresponse was observed when abacavir, lamivudine, and tenofovir were used as the initial regimen in treatment-naive patients. A high rate of early virologic nonresponse was also observed when didanosine, lamivudine, and tenofovir were used as the initial regimen in treatment-naive patients. Use of either of these combinations is not recommended; patients currently on either of these regimens should be closely monitored for modification of therapy. Early virologic failure was also observed with tenofovir and didanosine delayed release capsules, plus either efavirenz or nevirapine; use caution in treatment-naive patients with high baseline viral loads.

♦ **Tenofovir and Emtricitabine** *see* Emtricitabine and Tenofovir *on page 515*

♦ **Tenofovir Disoproxil Fumarate** *see* Tenofovir *on page 1441*

♦ **Tenoretic®** *see* Atenolol and Chlorthalidone *on page 151*

♦ **Tenormin®** *see* Atenolol *on page 149*

♦ **Tenuate®** *see* Diethylpropion *on page 449*

♦ **Tenuate® Dospan®** *see* Diethylpropion *on page 449*

♦ **Tequin®** *see* Gatifloxacin *on page 698*

♦ **Terazol® 3** *see* Terconazole *on page 1447*

♦ **Terazol® 7** *see* Terconazole *on page 1447*

Terazosin (ter AY zoe sin)

U.S. Brand Names Hytrin®

Generic Available Yes

Pharmacologic Category Alpha₁ Blocker

Use Management of mild to moderate hypertension; alone or in combination with other agents such as diuretics or beta-blockers; benign prostate hyperplasia (BPH)

Mechanism of Action/Effect Alpha$_1$-specific blocking agent with minimal alpha$_2$ effects; this allows peripheral postsynaptic blockade, with the resultant decrease in arterial tone, while preserving the negative feedback loop which is mediated by the peripheral presynaptic alpha$_2$-receptors; terazosin relaxes the smooth muscle of the bladder neck, thus reducing bladder outlet obstruction

Contraindications Hypersensitivity to quinazolines (doxazosin, prazosin, terazosin) or any component of the formulation; concurrent use with phosphodiesterase-5 (PDE-5) inhibitors including sildenafil (>25 mg), tadalafil, or vardenafil

Warnings/Precautions Can cause significant orthostatic hypotension and syncope, especially with first dose. Prostate cancer should be ruled out before starting for BPH. Anticipate a similar effect if therapy is interrupted for a few days, if dosage is rapidly increased, or if another antihypertensive drug is introduced.

Drug Interactions

  Decreased Effect: Decreased antihypertensive response with NSAIDs. Alpha-blockers reduce the response to pressor agents (norepinephrine).

  Increased Effect/Toxicity: Terazosin's hypotensive effect is increased with beta-blockers, diuretics, ACE inhibitors, calcium channel blockers, other antihypertensive medications, sildenafil (use with extreme caution at a dose ≤25 mg), tadalafil (use is contraindicated by the manufacturer), and vardenafil (use is contraindicated by the manufacturer).

Nutritional/Ethanol Interactions Herb/Nutraceutical: Avoid dong quai if using for hypertension (has estrogenic activity). Avoid ephedra, yohimbe, ginseng (may worsen hypertension). Avoid saw palmetto. Avoid garlic (may have increased antihypertensive effect).

Adverse Reactions Asthenia, postural hypotension, dizziness, somnolence, nasal congestion/rhinitis, and impotence were the only events noted in clinical trials to occur at a frequency significantly greater than placebo (p <0.05).

  >10%:
    Central nervous system: Dizziness, headache
    Neuromuscular & skeletal: Muscle weakness
  1% to 10%:
    Cardiovascular: Edema, palpitation, chest pain, peripheral edema (3%), orthostatic hypotension (3% to 4%), tachycardia
    Central nervous system: Fatigue, nervousness, drowsiness
    Gastrointestinal: Dry mouth
    Genitourinary: Urinary incontinence
    Ocular: Blurred vision
    Respiratory: Dyspnea, nasal congestion

Overdosage/Toxicology Symptoms of overdose include hypotension, drowsiness, and shock. Treatment is supportive and symptomatic.

Pharmacodynamics/Kinetics
  Onset of Action: 1-2 hours
  Absorption: Rapid
  Time to Peak: Serum: ~1 hour
  Protein Binding: 90% to 95%
  Half-Life Elimination: 9.2-12 hours
  Metabolism: Extensively hepatic
  Excretion: Feces (60%); urine (40%)

Dosing
  Adults & Elderly:
    Hypertension: Oral: Initial: 1 mg at bedtime; slowly increase dose to achieve desired blood pressure, up to 20 mg/day; usual dose range (JNC 7): 1-20 mg once daily
    Benign prostatic hyperplasia: Oral: Initial: 1 mg at bedtime, increasing as needed; most patients require 10 mg day. If no response after 4-6 weeks of 10 mg/day, may increase to 20 mg/day.

Available Dosage Forms
  Capsule (Hytrin®): 1 mg, 2 mg, 5 mg, 10 mg
  Tablet: 1 mg, 2 mg, 5 mg, 10 mg

Monitoring and Teaching Issues

  Physical Assessment: See Warnings/Precautions for use cautions. Assess potential for interactions with other pharmacological agents and herbal products patient may be taking (especially anything that may decrease antihypertensive response [NSAIDs, ephedra, yohimbe, ginseng] or increase hypotensive effect [beta-blockers, diuretics, ACE inhibitors]; see Drug Interactions). Assess therapeutic effectiveness (blood pressure) and adverse reactions at beginning of therapy and on a regular basis with long-term therapy (see Adverse Reactions; eg, hypotension, dizziness, somnolence, impotence). When discontinuing, dose should be tapered and blood pressure monitored closely. Teach patient proper use, possible side effects/appropriate interventions, and adverse symptoms to report (see Patient Education).

  Patient Education: Do not take any new medication during therapy unless approved by prescriber (especially anything that can impact blood pressure; cough medicines, stay-awake products, sleep remedies, stimulants). Take as directed; at bedtime. Do not skip dose or discontinue without consulting prescriber. Follow recommended diet and exercise program. May cause drowsiness, dizziness, or impaired judgment (use caution when driving or engaging in tasks that require alertness until response to drug is known); postural hypotension (use caution when rising from sitting or lying position or when climbing stairs); dry mouth or nausea (frequent mouth care or sucking lozenges may help); urinary incontinence (void before taking medication); or sexual dysfunction (reversible, may resolve with continued use). Report altered CNS status (eg, fatigue, lethargy, confusion, nervousness); sudden weight gain (weigh yourself in the same clothes at the same time of day once a week); unusual or persistent swelling of ankles, feet, or extremities; palpitations or rapid heartbeat; respiratory difficulty; muscle weakness; or other persistent side effects. **Pregnancy/breast-feeding precautions:** Inform prescriber if you are or intend to become pregnant. Consult prescriber if breast-feeding.

(Continued)

Terazosin *(Continued)*

Dietary Considerations: May be taken without regard to meals at the same time each day.

Geriatric Considerations: Adverse reactions such as dry mouth and urinary problems can be particularly bothersome in the elderly.

Pregnancy Risk Factor: C

Lactation: Excretion in breast milk unknown

Related Information

Pharmacotherapy of Urinary Incontinence *on page 1858*

Terbinafine *(TER bin a feen)*

U.S. Brand Names Lamisil®; Lamisil® AT™ [OTC]

Synonyms Terbinafine Hydrochloride

Generic Available No

Pharmacologic Category Antifungal Agent, Oral; Antifungal Agent, Topical

Medication Safety Issues

Sound-alike/look-alike issues:

Terbinafine may be confused with terbutaline

Lamisil® may be confused with Lamictal®, Lomotil®

Use Active against most strains of *Trichophyton mentagrophytes, Trichophyton rubrum*; may be effective for infections of *Microsporum gypseum* and *M. nanum, Trichophyton verrucosum, Epidermophyton floccosum, Candida albicans,* and *Scopulariopsis brevicaulis*

Oral: Onychomycosis of the toenail or fingernail due to susceptible dermatophytes

Topical: Antifungal for the treatment of tinea pedis (athlete's foot), tinea cruris (jock itch), and tinea corporis (ringworm) [OTC/prescription formulations]; tinea versicolor [prescription formulations]

Contraindications Hypersensitivity to terbinafine, naftifine, or any component of the formulation

Warnings/Precautions While rare, the following complications have been reported and may require discontinuation of therapy: Changes in the ocular lens and retina, pancytopenia, neutropenia, Stevens-Johnson syndrome, toxic epidermal necrolysis. Rare cases of hepatic failure, including fatal cases, have been reported following oral treatment of onychomycosis. Not recommended for use in patients with active or chronic liver disease. Discontinue if symptoms or signs of hepatobiliary dysfunction or cholestatic hepatitis develop. If irritation/sensitivity develop with topical use, discontinue therapy. Oral products are not recommended for use with pre-existing liver or renal disease (≤50 mL/minute GFR). **Use caution in writing and/or filling prescription/orders. Confusion between Lamictal® (lamotrigine) and Lamisil® (terbinafine) has occurred.**

Drug Interactions

Cytochrome P450 Effect: Substrate (minor) of 1A2, 2C8/9, 2C19, 3A4; **Inhibits** CYP2D6 (strong); **Induces** CYP3A4 (weak)

Decreased Effect: Terbinafine may decrease the levels/effects of CYP2D6 prodrug substrates (eg, codeine, hydrocodone, oxycodone, tramadol).

Increased Effect/Toxicity: Terbinafine may increase the levels/effects of amphetamines, beta-blockers, dextromethorphan, fluoxetine, lidocaine, mirtazapine, nefazodone, paroxetine, risperidone, ritonavir, thioridazine, tricyclic antidepressants, venlafaxine, and other CYP2D6 substrates. The effects of warfarin may be increased.

Adverse Reactions

Oral:

1% to 10%:

Central nervous system: Headache, dizziness, vertigo

Dermatologic: Rash, pruritus, urticaria

Gastrointestinal: Diarrhea, dyspepsia, abdominal pain, appetite decrease, taste disturbance

Hematologic: Lymphocytopenia

Hepatic: Liver enzymes increased

Ocular: Visual disturbance

Topical: 1% to 10%:

Dermatologic: Pruritus, contact dermatitis, irritation, burning, dryness

Local: Irritation, stinging

Pharmacodynamics/Kinetics

Absorption: Topical: Limited (<5%); Oral: >70%

Bioavailability: Oral: 40%

Time to Peak: Plasma: 1-2 hours

Protein Binding: Plasma: >99%

Half-Life Elimination: Topical: 22-26 hours; Oral: Terminal half-life: 200-400 hours; very slow release of drug from skin and adipose tissues occurs; effective half-life: ~36 hours

Metabolism: Hepatic; no active metabolites; first-pass effect (40%); little effect on CYP

Excretion: Urine (70% to 75%)

Dosing

Adults & Elderly:

Superficial mycoses (onychomycosis): Oral:

Fingernail: 250 mg/day for up to 6 weeks; may be given in two divided doses

Toenail: 250 mg/day for 12 weeks; may be given in two divided doses

Systemic mycosis: Oral: 250-500 mg/day for up to 16 months

Athlete's foot (tinea pedis): Topical:

Cream: Apply to affected area twice daily for at least 1 week, not to exceed 4 weeks [OTC/prescription formulations]

Solution: Apply to affected area twice daily for 7 days [OTC/prescription formulations]:

Ringworm and jock itch (tinea corporis, tinea cruris): Topical:

Cream: Apply to affected area once or twice daily for at least 1 week, not to exceed 4 weeks [OTC formulations]

Solution: Apply to affected area once daily for 7 days in tinea corporis and tinea cruris [OTC formulations]; apply to affected area twice daily for 7 days in tinea versicolor [prescription formulation]

Pediatrics:
Athlete's foot (tinea pedis), ringworm (tinea corporis), jock itch (tinea cruris): Children ≥12 years: Topical cream, solution: Refer to adult dosing.
Oral (unlabeled use in children):
10-20 kg: 62.5 mg/day
20-40 kg: 125 mg/day
>40 kg: 250 mg/day
Treatment duration:
Tinea pedis: 2 weeks
Tinea capitis: 2-4 weeks
Onychomycosis: Fingernails: 6 weeks; Toenails: 12 weeks

Renal Impairment: GFR <50 mL/minute: Oral administration is not recommended.

Hepatic Impairment: Clearance is decreased by ~50% with hepatic cirrhosis; use is not recommended.

Available Dosage Forms
Cream, as hydrochloride (Lamisil® AT™): 1% (15 g, 30 g)
Solution, as hydrochloride [topical spray] (Lamisil®, Lamisil® AT™): 1% (30 mL)
Tablet (Lamisil®): 250 mg

Monitoring and Teaching Issues
Physical Assessment: Use oral formulation with caution in presence of liver or renal impairment (see Warnings/Precautions for use cautions). Due to potential toxicity, the manufacturer recommends confirmation of diagnosis testing of nail specimens prior to treatment of onychomycosis. Assess potential for interactions with other pharmacological agents patient may be taking (may increase levels/effects of amphetamines, beta-blockers, ritonavir, risperidone, TCAs and other CYP2D6 substrates; see Drug Interactions). Assess results of laboratory tests, therapeutic effectiveness (according to purpose for use) and adverse reactions at beginning of therapy and on a regular basis with long-term therapy (will differ according to formulation and purpose for use; see Adverse Reactions). If irritation develops with topical use, discontinue therapy. If signs of hepatic dysfunction occur with oral formulation, discontinue use. Teach patient proper use, possible side effects/appropriate interventions, and adverse symptoms to report (see Patient Education).

Patient Education: Do not take any new medication during therapy without consulting prescriber. Use exactly as directed. Take tablets at same time of day, with or without regard to meals. Take full prescription even if symptoms appear resolved; may take several months for full treatment (inadequate treatment may result in reinfection). May cause altered taste (normal). Report unusual fatigue; persistent loss of appetite, nausea or vomiting; dark urine/pale stool; or other persistent adverse response. **Breast-feeding precaution:** Breast-feeding is not recommended.

Topical: (cream or spray) for topical use only. Wash and dry nails thoroughly before applying. Avoid contact with eyes, nose, or mouth. Do not use occlusive dressings. Report irritation, itching, burning or skin around nail. Full clinical effect may require several months due to the time required for a new nail to grow.

Pregnancy Risk Factor: B
Pregnancy Issues: Avoid use in pregnancy since treatment of onychomycosis is postponable.
Lactation: Enters breast milk/not recommended
Breast-Feeding Issues: Although minimal concentrations of terbinafine cross into breast milk after topical use, oral or topical treatment during lactation should be avoided.

Administration
Storage:
Cream: Store at 5°C to 30°C (41°F to 86°F).
Solution: Store at 5°C to 25°C (41°F to 77°F). Do not refrigerate.
Tablet: Store below 25°C (77°F). Protect from light.

Additional Information Due to potential toxicity, the manufacturer recommends confirmation of diagnosis testing of nail specimens prior to treatment of onychomycosis. Patients should not be considered therapeutic failures until they have been symptom-free for 2-4 weeks off following a course of treatment; GI complaints usually subside with continued administration.

A meta-analysis of efficacy studies for toenail infections revealed that weighted average mycological cure rates for continuous therapy were 36.7% (griseofulvin), 54.7% (itraconazole), and 77% (terbinafine). Cure rate for 4-month pulse therapy for itraconazole and terbinafine were 73.3% and 80%. Additionally, the final outcome measure of final costs per cured infections for continuous therapy was significantly lower for terbinafine.

♦ **Terbinafine Hydrochloride** *see Terbinafine on page 1444*

Terbutaline (ter BYOO ta leen)
U.S. Brand Names Brethine®
Synonyms Brethaire [DSC]; Bricanyl [DSC]
Generic Available Yes
Pharmacologic Category Beta₂-Adrenergic Agonist
Medication Safety Issues
Sound-alike/look-alike issues:
Terbutaline may be confused with terbinafine, TOLBUTamide
Use Bronchodilator in reversible airway obstruction and bronchial asthma; tocolytic agent
Unlabeled/Investigational Use Tocolytic agent (management of preterm labor)
Mechanism of Action/Effect Relaxes bronchial smooth muscle by action on beta₂-receptors with less effect on heart rate
Contraindications Hypersensitivity to terbutaline or any component of the formulation; cardiac arrhythmias associated with tachycardia; tachycardia caused by digitalis intoxication (Continued)

Terbutaline *(Continued)*

Warnings/Precautions When used for tocolysis, there is some risk of maternal pulmonary edema, which has been associated with the following risk factors, excessive hydration, multiple gestation, occult sepsis and underlying cardiac disease. To reduce risk, limit fluid intake to 2.5-3 L/day, limit sodium intake, maintain maternal pulse to <130 beats/minute.

Use caution in patients with cardiovascular disease (arrhythmia or hypertension or CHF), convulsive disorders, diabetes, glaucoma, hyperthyroidism, or hypokalemia. Beta agonists may cause elevation in blood pressure, heart rate, and result in CNS stimulation/excitation. Beta$_2$ agonists may increase risk of arrhythmia, increase serum glucose, or decrease serum potassium.

When used as a bronchodilator, optimize anti-inflammatory treatment before initiating maintenance treatment with terbutaline. Do not use as a component of chronic therapy without an anti-inflammatory agent. Only the mildest form of asthma (Step 1 and/or exercise-induced) would not require concurrent use based upon asthma guidelines. Patient must be instructed to seek medical attention in cases where acute symptoms are not relieved or a previous level of response is diminished. The need to increase frequency of use may indicate deterioration of asthma, and treatment must not be delayed.

Do not exceed recommended dose; serious adverse events including fatalities, have been associated with excessive use of inhaled sympathomimetics. Rarely, paradoxical bronchospasm may occur with use of inhaled bronchodilating agents; this should be distinguished from inadequate response.

Drug Interactions

Decreased Effect: Decreased effect with beta-blockers.

Increased Effect/Toxicity: Increased toxicity with MAO inhibitors, tricyclic antidepressants.

Nutritional/Ethanol Interactions Herb/Nutraceutical: Avoid ephedra, yohimbe (may cause CNS stimulation).

Adverse Reactions

>10%:
  Central nervous system: Nervousness, restlessness
  Endocrine & metabolic: Serum glucose increased, serum potassium decreased
  Neuromuscular & skeletal: Trembling
1% to 10%:
  Cardiovascular: Tachycardia, hypertension
  Central nervous system: Dizziness, drowsiness, headache, insomnia
  Gastrointestinal: Xerostomia, nausea, vomiting, bad taste in mouth
  Neuromuscular & skeletal: Muscle cramps, weakness
  Miscellaneous: Diaphoresis

Overdosage/Toxicology Symptoms of overdose include tachycardia, tremor, hypertension, angina, and seizures. Hypokalemia also may occur. Cardiac arrest and death may be associated with abuse of beta-agonist bronchodilators. Treatment includes immediate discontinuation and symptomatic and supportive therapies. Cautious use of beta-adrenergic blocking agents may be considered in severe cases.

Pharmacodynamics/Kinetics

Onset of Action: Oral: 30-45 minutes; SubQ: 6-15 minutes
Bioavailability: SubQ doses are more bioavailable than oral
Protein Binding: 25%
Half-Life Elimination: 11-16 hours
Metabolism: Hepatic to inactive sulfate conjugates
Excretion: Urine

Dosing

Adults & Elderly:
  Asthma or bronchoconstriction:
    Oral: 5 mg/dose every 6 hours 3 times/day; if side effects occur, reduce dose to 2.5 mg every 6 hours; not to exceed 15 mg in 24 hours.
    SubQ: 0.25 mg/dose repeated in 15-30 minutes for one time only; a total dose of 0.5 mg should not be exceeded within a 4-hour period.
  Premature labor (tocolysis):
    Acute: I.V. 2.5-10 mcg/minute; increased gradually every 10-20 minutes. Effective maximum dosages from 17.5-30 mcg/minute have been use with caution. Duration of infusion is at least 12 hours.
    Maintenance: Oral: 2.5-10 mg every 4-6 hours for as long as necessary to prolong pregnancy depending on patient tolerance

Pediatrics:
  Asthma or bronchoconstriction:
    Oral: Children:
      <12 years: Initial: 0.05 mg/kg/dose 3 times/day, increased gradually as required; maximum: 0.15 mg/kg/dose 3-4 times/day or a total of 5 mg/24 hours
      12-15 years: 2.5 mg every 6 hours 3 times/day; not to exceed 7.5 mg in 24 hours
      >15 years: 5 mg/dose every 6 hours 3 times/day; if side effects occur, reduce dose to 2.5 mg every 6 hours; not to exceed 15 mg in 24 hours
    SubQ: Children:
      <12 years: 0.005-0.01 mg/kg/dose to a maximum of 0.3 mg/dose every 15-20 minutes for 3 doses
      ≥12 years: Refer to adult dosing.

Renal Impairment:
  Cl$_{cr}$ 10-50 mL/minute: Administer 50% of normal dose.
  Cl$_{cr}$ <10 mL/minute: Avoid use.

Available Dosage Forms

Injection, solution, as sulfate: 1 mg/mL (1 mL)
Tablet, as sulfate: 2.5 mg, 5 mg

Monitoring and Teaching Issues

Physical Assessment: Respiratory use: Assess effectiveness and interactions of other medications patient may be taking. Monitor therapeutic effectiveness and adverse reactions at beginning of therapy and periodically with long-term use. For inpatient care, monitor vital signs and lung sounds prior to and periodically during therapy. Assess knowledge/teach patient appropriate use, interventions to reduce side effects, and adverse symptoms to report. **Preterm labor use: Inpatient:** Monitor maternal vital signs; respiratory, cardiac, and electrolyte status; frequency, duration, and intensity of contractions; and fetal heart rate. **Outpatients:** Assess knowledge/teach patient appropriate use, interventions to reduce side effects, and adverse symptoms to report.

Monitoring Laboratory Tests: FEV$_1$, peak flow, and/or other pulmonary function tests; serum potassium, serum glucose (in selected patients)

Tocolysis: If patient receives therapy for more than 1 week, monitor serum glucose.

Patient Education: Use exactly as directed. Do not use more often than recommended (excessive use may result in tolerance, overdose may result in serious adverse effects) and do not discontinue without consulting prescriber. Maintain adequate hydration (2-3 L/day of fluids) unless instructed to restrict fluid intake. If you have diabetes, monitor blood sugar closely. Serum glucose may be elevated. You may experience nervousness, dizziness, or fatigue (use caution when driving or engaging in tasks requiring alertness until response to drug is known); or dry mouth, stomach upset (small frequent meals, frequent mouth care, chewing gum, or sucking hard candy may help). Report unresolved GI upset; dizziness or fatigue; vision changes; chest pain, rapid heartbeat, or palpitations; insomnia, nervousness, or hyperactivity; muscle cramping, tremors, or pain; unusual cough; or rash (hypersensitivity).

Preterm labor: Notify prescriber immediately if labor resumes or adverse side effects are noted.

Pregnancy Risk Factor: B

Lactation: Enters breast milk/compatible

Administration

Oral: Administer around-the-clock to promote less variation in peak and trough serum levels.

I.V.: Use infusion pump.

Compatibility: Stable in D$_5$W, $^1/_2$NS, NS

    Compatibility when admixed: Incompatible with bleomycin

Storage: Store injection at room temperature. Protect from heat, light, and from freezing. Use only clear solutions.

Related Information

Inhalant Agents *on page 1734*

Terconazole (ter KONE a zole)

U.S. Brand Names Terazol® 3; Terazol® 7

Synonyms Triaconazole

Generic Available No

Pharmacologic Category Antifungal Agent, Vaginal

Medication Safety Issues

Sound-alike/look-alike issues:

Terconazole may be confused with tioconazole

Use Local treatment of vulvovaginal candidiasis

Mechanism of Action/Effect Triazole ketal antifungal agent; involves inhibition of fungal cytochrome P450

Contraindications Hypersensitivity to terconazole or any component of the formulation

Warnings/Precautions Should be discontinued if sensitization or irritation occurs. Microbiological studies (KOH smear and/or cultures) should be repeated in patients not responding to terconazole in order to confirm the diagnosis and rule out other pathogens.

Adverse Reactions 1% to 10%:

Central nervous system; Fever, chills

Gastrointestinal: Abdominal pain

Genitourinary: Vulvar/vaginal burning, dysmenorrhea

Pharmacodynamics/Kinetics

Absorption: Extent of systemic absorption after vaginal administration may be dependent on presence of a uterus; 5% to 8% in women who had a hysterectomy versus 12% to 16% in nonhysterectomy women

Dosing

Adults & Elderly: Vulvovaginal candidiasis: Intravaginal:

Terazol® 3 vaginal cream: Insert 1 applicatorful intravaginally at bedtime for 3 consecutive days.

Terazol® 7 vaginal cream: Insert 1 applicatorful intravaginally at bedtime for 7 consecutive days.

Terazol® 3 vaginal suppository: Insert 1 suppository intravaginally at bedtime for 3 consecutive days.

Available Dosage Forms

Cream, vaginal:

Terazol® 7: 0.4% (45 g) [packaged with measured-dose applicator]

Terazol® 3: 0.8% (20 g) [packaged with measured-dose applicator]

Suppository, vaginal (Terazol® 3): 80 mg (3s) [may contain coconut and/or palm kernel oil]

Monitoring and Teaching Issues

Physical Assessment: Assess knowledge/teach patient appropriate administration, possible side effects/interventions, and adverse symptoms to report.

Patient Education: Complete full course of therapy as directed. Insert vaginally as directed by prescriber or see package insert. Sexual partner may experience irritation of penis; best to refrain from intercourse during period of treatment. Suppositories may cause breakdown of rubber/latex products such as diaphragms; avoid concurrent use. Report persistent vaginal burning, itching, irritation, or discharge. **Pregnancy/breast-feeding precautions:** Inform prescriber if you are or intend to become pregnant. Consult prescriber if breast-feeding.

(Continued)

Terconazole *(Continued)*

Geriatric Considerations: Assess patient's ability to self-administer; may be difficult in patients with arthritis or limited range of motion.

Pregnancy Risk Factor: C

Lactation: Excretion in breast milk unknown/not recommended

Administration

Storage: Store at room temperature of 13°C to 30°C (59°F to 86°F).

Additional Information Watch for local irritation; assist patient in administration, if necessary; assess patient's ability to self-administer, may be difficult in patients with arthritis or limited range of motion

Teriparatide *(ter i PAR a tide)*

U.S. Brand Names Forteo™

Synonyms Parathyroid Hormone (1-34); Recombinant Human Parathyroid Hormone (1-34); rhPTH(1-34)

Restrictions An FDA-approved medication guide is available at www.fda.gov/cder/Offices/ODS/labeling.htm; distribute to each patient to whom this medication is dispensed.

Generic Available No

Pharmacologic Category Parathyroid Hormone Analog

Use Treatment of osteoporosis in postmenopausal women at high risk of fracture; treatment of primary or hypogonadal osteoporosis in men at high risk of fracture

Mechanism of Action/Effect An analog of parathyroid hormone, teriparatide stimulates osteoblast function, increases gastrointestinal calcium absorption, and increases renal tubular reabsorption of calcium. Treatment with teriparatide increases bone mineral density, bone mass, and strength. In postmenopausal women, it has been shown to decrease osteoporosis-related fractures.

Contraindications Hypersensitivity to teriparatide or any component of the formulation

Warnings/Precautions In animal studies, teriparatide has been associated with an increase in osteosarcoma; risk was dependent on both dose and duration. Use of teriparatide for longer than 2 years is not recommended. Avoid use in patients with an increased risk of osteosarcoma (including Paget's disease, prior radiation, unexplained elevation of alkaline phosphatase, or in patients with open epiphyses). Do not use in patients with a history of skeletal metastases, hyperparathyroidism, or pre-existing hypercalcemia. Exclude metabolic bone disease other than osteoporosis prior to initiating therapy. Use caution in patients with active or recent urolithiasis. Use caution in patients at risk of orthostasis (including concurrent antihypertensive therapy), or in patients who may not tolerate transient hypotension (cardiovascular or cerebrovascular disease). Use caution in patients with renal or hepatic impairment (limited data available concerning safety and efficacy). Not approved for use in pediatric patients.

Drug Interactions

Increased Effect/Toxicity: Digitalis serum concentrations are not affected, however, transient hypercalcemia may increase risk of digitalis toxicity (case reports).

Nutritional/Ethanol Interactions

Ethanol: Excessive intake may increase risk of osteoporosis.

Herb/Nutraceutical: Ensure adequate calcium and vitamin D intake.

Adverse Reactions 1% to 10%:

Cardiovascular: Chest pain (3%), syncope (3%)

Central nervous system: Dizziness (8%), depression (4%), vertigo (4%)

Dermatologic: Rash (5%)

Endocrine & metabolic: Hypercalcemia (transient increases noted 4-6 hours postdose in 11% of women and 6% of men)

Gastrointestinal: Nausea (9%), dyspepsia (5%), vomiting (3%), tooth disorder (2%)

Genitourinary: Hyperuricemia (3%)

Neuromuscular & skeletal: Arthralgia (10%), weakness (9%), leg cramps (3%)

Respiratory: Rhinitis (10%), pharyngitis (6%), dyspnea (4%), pneumonia (4%)

Miscellaneous: Antibodies to teriparatide (3% of women in long-term treatment; hypersensitivity reactions or decreased efficacy were not associated in preclinical trials)

Overdosage/Toxicology No specific experience in overdose. Symptoms may include hypercalcemia, hypotension, headache, nausea, vomiting, and hypotension. Treatment is supportive (monitor serum calcium and phosphorus).

Pharmacodynamics/Kinetics

Bioavailability: 95%

Half-Life Elimination: Serum: I.V.: 5 minutes; SubQ: 1 hour

Metabolism: Hepatic (nonspecific proteolysis)

Excretion: Urine (as metabolites)

Dosing

Adults: Osteoporosis: SubQ: 20 mcg once daily; **Note:** Initial administration should occur under circumstances in which the patient may sit or lie down, in the event of orthostasis.

Renal Impairment: No dosage adjustment required. Bioavailability and half-life increase with Cl$_{cr}$ <30 mL/minute.

Available Dosage Forms Injection, solution: 250 mcg/mL (3 mL) [prefilled syringe, delivers teriparatide 20 mcg/dose]

Monitoring and Teaching Issues

Physical Assessment: Use caution with existing cardiovascular or cerebrovascular disease and renal or hepatic impairments (see Warnings/Precautions for use cautions). Initial administration should occur where patient may sit or lie down, in the event of orthostasis. Assess results of laboratory tests prior to and periodically during therapy (see Monitoring Laboratory Tests). Assess therapeutic effectiveness and adverse response at beginning of and regular intervals during therapy (eg, chest pain, hypotension, nausea, vomiting, arthralgia, leg cramps, dyspnea, see Adverse Reactions). Teach patient proper use (administration with injector "pen" and disposal), possible side effects/appropriate interventions (diet with adequate calcium and vitamin D), and adverse symptoms to report (see Patient Education).

Monitoring Laboratory Tests: Serum calcium, serum phosphorus

Patient Education: Do not take any new medication during therapy without consulting prescriber. Use injector pen and dispose of pen exactly as instructed; (refer to Forteo™ user manual dispensed with the medication); rotate injection sites in thigh or abdominal wall. Sit when administering to reduce possibility of falling or injury. Avoid excess alcohol (may increase risk of osteoporosis) and follow dietary instructions of prescriber. May cause dizziness (use caution when driving or engaged in potentially hazardous tasks until response to drug is known); nausea, vomiting, or upset stomach (small frequent meals or frequent mouth care may help); muscle or skeletal pain, weakness, or cramping (consult prescriber for approved analgesic). Report chest pain or palpitations; respiratory difficulty; or other persistent adverse effects. **Pregnancy/breast-feeding precautions:** Inform prescriber if you are or intend to become pregnant. Breast-feeding is not recommended.

Geriatric Considerations: No age-related differences in pharmacokinetics have been seen. In studies, no significant difference was seen in either efficacy or adverse effects between older patients and younger patients. Teriparatide should be considered as a last resort in patents who cannot tolerate or have not responded to other treatments for osteoporosis.

Pregnancy Risk Factor: C

Lactation: Excretion in breast milk unknown/not recommended

Breast-Feeding Issues: Indicated for use in postmenopausal women. No studies have been conducted to determine excretion in breast milk. Not recommended for use in breast-feeding women.

Administration

Other: Administer by subcutaneous injection into the thigh or abdominal wall. Initial administration should occur under circumstances in which the patient may sit or lie down, in the event of orthostasis.

Storage: Store at 2°C to 8°C (36°F to 46°F). Protect from light. Do not freeze. Discard pen 28 days after first injection.

Additional Information Teriparatide was formerly marketed as a diagnostic agent (Perithar™); that agent was withdrawn from the market in 1997. Teriparatide (Forteo™) is manufactured through recombinant DNA technology using a strain of *E. coli*.

♦ **Teslac**® *see* Testolactone *on page 1449*
♦ **TESPA** *see* Thiotepa *on page 1466*
♦ **Tessalon**® *see* Benzonatate *on page 183*
♦ **Testim**™ *see* Testosterone *on page 1450*

Testolactone (tes toe LAK tone)

U.S. Brand Names Teslac®

Controlled Substance C-III

Generic Available No

Pharmacologic Category Androgen

Medication Safety Issues
Sound-alike/look-alike issues:
Testolactone may be confused with testosterone

Use Palliative treatment of advanced or disseminated breast carcinoma

Mechanism of Action/Effect Testolactone is a synthetic testosterone derivative without significant androgen activity. The drug inhibits steroid aromatase activity, thereby blocking the production of estradiol and estrone from androgen precursors such as testosterone and androstenedione. Unfortunately, the enzymatic block provided by testolactone is transient and is usually limited to a period of 3 months.

Contraindications Hypersensitivity to testolactone or any component of the formulation; treatment of breast cancer in men

Warnings/Precautions Use with caution in hepatic, renal, or cardiac disease; prolonged use may cause drug-induced hepatic disease; history of porphyria. For use in postmenopausal women or in premenopausal women without ovarian function only. Safety and efficacy in pediatric patients have not been established.

Drug Interactions
Increased Effect/Toxicity: Increased effects of oral anticoagulants.

Lab Interactions Plasma estradiol concentrations by RIA

Adverse Reactions Frequency not defined.
Cardiovascular: Edema, blood pressure increased
Central nervous system: Malaise
Dermatologic: Maculopapular rash, alopecia (rare)
Endocrine & metabolic: Hypercalcemia
Gastrointestinal: Anorexia, diarrhea, nausea, edema of the tongue
Neuromuscular & skeletal: Paresthesias, peripheral neuropathies
Miscellaneous: Nail growth disturbance (rare)

Pharmacodynamics/Kinetics
Absorption: Well absorbed
Metabolism: Hepatic (forms metabolites)
Excretion: Urine

Dosing
Adults & Elderly: Breast carcinoma (palliative): Female: Oral: 250 mg 4 times/day for at least 3 months; desired response may take as long as 3 months.

Available Dosage Forms Tablet: 50 mg

Monitoring and Teaching Issues
Physical Assessment: Use caution in hepatic, renal, or cardiac disease (see Warnings/Precautions for use cautions). May increase effects of oral anticoagulants (see Drug Interactions). Monitor effectiveness of therapy, laboratory tests, and adverse response (Continued)

Testolactone *(Continued)*

(see Adverse Reactions). Assess knowledge/teach patient appropriate use, possible side effects/appropriate interventions, and adverse symptoms to report (see Patient Education).

Monitoring Laboratory Tests: Plasma calcium levels

Patient Education: Take as directed; do not discontinue without consulting prescriber. Effectiveness of therapy may take several months. Maintain adequate hydration (2-3 L/day of fluids) unless instructed to restrict fluid intake and diet and exercise program recommended by prescriber. You may experience nausea or vomiting (small frequent meals, frequent mouth care, sucking lozenges, or chewing gum may help). Report fluid retention (swelling of ankles, feet, or hands; respiratory difficulty or sudden weight gain); numbness, tingling, or swelling of fingers, toes, or face; skin rash, redness, or irritation; or other adverse reactions. **Pregnancy precaution:** Breast-feeding is not recommended.

Pregnancy Risk Factor: C

Lactation: Excretion in breast milk unknown/not recommended

♦ **Testopel®** *see* Testosterone *on page 1450*

Testosterone *(tes TOS ter one)*

U.S. Brand Names Androderm®; AndroGel®; Delatestryl®; Depo®-Testosterone; Striant™; Testim™; Testopel®

Synonyms Testosterone Cypionate; Testosterone Enanthate

Controlled Substance C-III

Generic Available No

Pharmacologic Category Androgen

Medication Safety Issues

Sound-alike/look-alike issues:

Testosterone may be confused with testolactone

Testoderm® may be confused with Estraderm®

Transdermal patch may contain conducting metal (eg, aluminum); remove patch prior to MRI.

Use

Injection: Androgen replacement therapy in the treatment of delayed male puberty; male hypogonadism (primary or hypogonadotropic); inoperable female breast cancer (enanthate only)

Pellet: Androgen replacement therapy in the treatment of delayed male puberty; male hypogonadism (primary or hypogonadotropic)

Buccal, topical: Male hypogonadism (primary or hypogonadotropic)

Mechanism of Action/Effect Principal endogenous androgen responsible for promoting the growth and development of the male sex organs and maintaining secondary sex characteristics in androgen-deficient males

Contraindications Hypersensitivity to testosterone or any component of the formulation (including soy); severe renal or cardiac disease; benign prostatic hyperplasia with obstruction; undiagnosed genital bleeding; males with carcinoma of the breast or prostate; pregnancy

Warnings/Precautions When used to treat delayed male puberty, perform radiographic examination of the hand and wrist every 6 months to determine the rate of bone maturation. May accelerate bone maturation without producing compensating gain in linear growth. Has both androgenic and anabolic activity; the anabolic action may enhance hypoglycemia. Use caution in elderly patients or patients with other demographic factors which may increase the risk of prostatic carcinoma; careful monitoring is required. May cause fluid retention; use caution in patients with cardiovascular disease or other edematous conditions. Prolonged use has been associated with serious hepatic effects (hepatitis, hepatic neoplasms, cholestatic hepatitis, jaundice). May potentiate sleep apnea in some male patients (obesity or chronic lung disease). Transdermal patch may contain conducting metal (eg, aluminum); remove patch prior to MRI. Gels and buccal system have not been evaluated in males <18 years of age; safety and efficacy of injection have not been established in males <12 years of age.

Drug Interactions

Cytochrome P450 Effect: Substrate (minor) of CYP2B6, 2C8/9, 2C19, 3A4; **Inhibits** CYP3A4 (weak)

Increased Effect/Toxicity: Warfarin and testosterone: Effects of oral anticoagulants may be enhanced. Testosterone may increase levels of oxyphenbutazone. May enhance fluid retention from corticosteroids.

Nutritional/Ethanol Interactions Herb/Nutraceutical: St John's wort may decrease testosterone levels.

Lab Interactions May cause a decrease in creatinine and creatine excretion and an increase in the excretion of 17-ketosteroids, thyroid function tests.

Adverse Reactions Frequency not defined.

Cardiovascular: Flushing, edema

Central nervous system: Excitation, aggressive behavior, sleeplessness, anxiety, mental depression, headache

Dermatologic: Hirsutism (increase in pubic hair growth), acne

Endocrine & metabolic: Menstrual problems (amenorrhea), virilism, breast soreness, gynecomastia, hypercalcemia, hypoglycemia

Gastrointestinal: Nausea, vomiting, GI irritation

Following buccal administration: Bitter taste, gum edema, gum or mouth irritation, gum tenderness, taste perversion

Genitourinary: Prostatic hyperplasia, prostatic carcinoma, impotence, testicular atrophy, epididymitis, priapism, bladder irritability

Hepatic: Hepatic dysfunction, cholestatic hepatitis, hepatic necrosis

Hematologic: Leukopenia, polycythemia, suppression of clotting factors

Miscellaneous: Hypersensitivity reactions

Pharmacodynamics/Kinetics

Duration of Action: Route and ester dependent; I.M.: Cypionate and enanthate esters have longest duration, ≤2-4 weeks

Absorption: Transdermal gel: ~10% of dose
Protein Binding: 98% bound to sex hormone-binding globulin (40%) and albumin
Half-Life Elimination: 10-100 minutes
Metabolism: Hepatic; forms metabolites
Excretion: Urine (90%); feces (6%)

Dosing

Adults & Elderly:

Inoperable breast cancer (females): I.M.: Testosterone enanthate: 200-400 mg every 2-4 weeks

Male hypogonadism or hypogonadotropic hypogonadism:
Oral (buccal): 30 mg twice daily (every 12 hours) applied to the gum region above the incisor tooth
Pellet (for subcutaneous implantation): Hypogonadism, delayed puberty: 150-450 mg every 3-6 months
Transdermal:
Androderm®: Initial: Apply 5 mg/day once nightly to clean, dry area on the back, abdomen, upper arms, or thighs (do **not** apply to scrotum); dosing range: 2.5-7.5 mg/day; in nonvirilized patients, dose may be initiated at 2.5 mg/day
AndroGel®, Testim™: 5 g (to deliver 50 mg of testosterone with 5 mg systemically absorbed) applied once daily (preferably in the morning) to clean, dry, intact skin of the shoulder and upper arms. AndroGel® may also be applied to the abdomen. Dosage may be increased to a maximum of 10 g (100 mg). **(Do not apply testosterone gel to the genitals.)**

Delayed puberty in males: I.M. (cypionate or enanthate ester) : 50-200 mg every 2-4 weeks for a limited duration

Male hypogonadism: I.M. (cypionate or enanthate ester) 50-400 mg every 2-4 weeks

Pediatrics: Adolescents:

Male hypogonadism:
I.M.:
Initiation of pubertal growth: 40-50 mg/m^2/dose (cypionate or enanthate ester) monthly until the growth rate falls to prepubertal levels
Terminal growth phase: 100 mg/m^2/dose (cypionate or enanthate ester) monthly until growth ceases
Maintenance virilizing dose: 100 mg/m^2/dose (cypionate or enanthate ester) twice monthly
SubQ: Pellet (for subcutaneous implantation): Refer to adult dosing.

Delayed puberty (male):
I.M.: 40-50 mg/m^2/dose monthly (cypionate or enanthate ester) for 6 months
SubQ: Pellet (for subcutaneous implantation): Refer to adult dosing.

Hepatic Impairment: Reduce dose.

Available Dosage Forms

Gel, topical:
AndroGel®:
25 mg/2.5 g (30s); 50 mg/5 g (30s) [1% unit-dose packet]
1.25 g/dose (75 g) [1% metered-dose pump; provides 60 doses]
Testim™: 50 mg/5 g (30s) [1% unit-dose tube]
Injection, in oil, as cypionate (Depo® Testosterone): 100 mg/mL (10 mL); 200 mg/mL (1 mL, 10 mL) [contains benzyl alcohol, benzyl benzoate, and cottonseed oil]
Injection, in oil, as enanthate (Delatestryl®): 200 mg/mL (1 mL [prefilled syringe; contains sesame oil]; 5 mL [multidose vial; contains sesame oil])
Mucoadhesive, for buccal application [buccal system] (Striant™): 30 mg
Pellet, for subcutaneous implantation (Testopel®): 75 mg (1 pellet/vial)
Transdermal system (Androderm®): 2.5 mg/day (60s); 5 mg/day (30s)

Monitoring and Teaching Issues

Physical Assessment: (For use in children see pediatric reference). See Warnings/Precautions for use cautions. Assess potential for interactions with other pharmacological agents and herbal products patient may be taking (eg, effects of warfarin may be enhanced; may increase fluid retention with corticosteroids; see Drug Interactions). Assess results of laboratory tests (see Monitoring Laboratory Tests), therapeutic effectiveness (according to purpose for use), and adverse reactions regularly during therapy (see Adverse Reactions). Caution patients with diabetes, may cause hypoglycemic reaction. Teach patient proper use (according to formulation), possible side effects/appropriate interventions, and adverse symptoms to report (see Patient Education). **Pregnancy risk factor X:** Determine that patient is not pregnant before beginning treatment. Instruct patients of childbearing age or males who may have intercourse with women of child-bearing age on appropriate contraceptive measures.

Monitoring Laboratory Tests: Periodic liver function tests, PSA, cholesterol, hemoglobin and hematocrit; radiologic examination of wrist and hand every 6 months (when using in prepubertal children)
Androderm®: Morning serum testosterone levels following application the previous evening
Gel: Morning serum testosterone levels 14 days after start of therapy

Patient Education: Use exactly as directed according to formulation. For topical application (patch or gel) or buccal application, follow directions that accompany package. If using self-administered injections, follow prescriber's directions for injection procedure and disposal of syringes/needles. If you have diabetes, monitor serum glucose closely and notify prescriber of changes; this medication may alter hypoglycemic requirements. You may experience acne, growth of body hair, loss of libido, impotence, or menstrual irregularity (usually reversible); or nausea or vomiting (small frequent meals, frequent mouth care, sucking lozenges, or chewing gum may help). Report changes in menstrual pattern; enlarged or painful breasts; deepening of voice or unusual growth of body hair; persistent penile erection; fluid retention (swelling of ankles, feet, or hands, respiratory difficulty or sudden weight gain); unresolved changes in CNS (nervousness, chills, insomnia, depression, aggressiveness); altered urinary patterns; change in color of urine or stool; yellowing of eyes or skin; unusual bruising or bleeding; or other persistent adverse reactions.
(Continued)

Testosterone *(Continued)*

Dietary Considerations: Testosterone USP may be synthesized from soy. Food and beverages have not been found to interfere with buccal system; ensure system is in place following eating, drinking, or brushing teeth.

Geriatric Considerations: Geriatric patients may have an increased risk of prostatic hyperplasia or prostatic carcinoma.

Pregnancy Risk Factor: X

Pregnancy Issues: Testosterone may cause adverse effects, including masculinization of the female fetus, if used during pregnancy. Females who are or may become pregnant should also avoid skin-to-skin contact to areas where testosterone has been applied topically on another person.

Lactation: Enters breast milk/contraindicated

Administration

Oral: Striant™: One mucoadhesive for buccal application (buccal system) should be applied to a comfortable area above the incisor tooth. Apply flat side of system to gum. Rotate to alternate sides of mouth with each application. Hold buccal system firmly in place for 30 seconds to ensure adhesion. The buccal system should adhere to gum for 12 hours. If the buccal system falls out, replace with a new system. If the system falls out within 4 hours of next dose, the new buccal system should remain in place until the time of the following scheduled dose. System will soften and mold to shape of gum as it absorbs moisture from mouth. Do not chew or swallow the buccal system. The buccal system will not dissolve; gently remove by sliding downwards from gum; avoid scratching gum.

I.M.: Warm injection to room temperature and shaking vial will help redissolve crystals that have formed after storage. Administer by deep I.M. injection into the upper outer quadrant of the gluteus maximus.

Topical:

Transdermal:

Androderm®: Apply patch to clean, dry area of skin on the arm, back, or upper buttocks. Following patch removal, mild skin irritation may be treated with OTC hydrocortisone cream. A small amount of triamcinolone acetonide 0.1% cream may be applied under the system to decrease irritation; do not use ointment. Patch should be applied nightly. Rotate administration sites, allowing 7 days between applying to the same site.

Gel: AndroGel®, Testim™: Apply gel (preferably in the morning) to clean, dry, intact skin of the shoulder and upper arms (AndroGel® may also be applied to the abdomen). Upon opening the packet(s), the entire contents should be squeezed into the palm of the hand and immediately applied to the application site(s). Alternatively, a portion may be squeezed onto palm of hand and applied, repeating the process until entire packet has been applied. Application sites should be allowed to dry for a few minutes prior to dressing. Hands should be washed with soap and water after application. **Do not apply testosterone gel to the genitals.**

Storage:

Androderm®: Store at room temperature. Do not store outside of pouch. Excessive heat may cause system to burst.

AndroGel®, Delatestryl®, Striant™, Testim™: Store at room temperature.

Depo® Testosterone: Store at room temperature. Protect from light.

Testopel®: Store in a cool location.

♦ **Testosterone Cypionate** *see* Testosterone *on page 1450*

♦ **Testosterone Enanthate** *see* Testosterone *on page 1450*

♦ **Testred®** *see* MethylTESTOSTERone *on page 988*

♦ **Tetanus Antitoxin** *see page 1660*

♦ **Tetanus Immune Globulin (Human)** *see page 1660*

♦ **Tetanus Toxoid (Adsorbed)** *see page 1660*

♦ **Tetanus Toxoid (Fluid)** *see page 1660*

Tetracycline *(tet ra SYE kleen)*

U.S. Brand Names Sumycin®

Synonyms Achromycin; TCN; Tetracycline Hydrochloride

Generic Available Yes: Capsule

Pharmacologic Category Antibiotic, Tetracycline Derivative

Medication Safety Issues

Sound-alike/look-alike issues:

Tetracycline may be confused with tetradecyl sulfate

Achromycin may be confused with actinomycin, Adriamycin PFS®

Use Treatment of susceptible bacterial infections of both gram-positive and gram-negative organisms; also infections due to *Mycoplasma*, *Chlamydia*, and *Rickettsia*; indicated for acne, exacerbations of chronic bronchitis, and treatment of gonorrhea and syphilis in patients that are allergic to penicillin; as part of a multidrug regimen for *H. pylori* eradication to reduce the risk of duodenal ulcer recurrence

Mechanism of Action/Effect Inhibits protein synthesis of susceptible bacteria; bacteriostatic - causes call death.

Contraindications Hypersensitivity to tetracycline or any component of the formulation; do not administer to children ≤8 years of age; pregnancy

Warnings/Precautions Use of tetracyclines during tooth development may cause permanent discoloration of the teeth and enamel, hypoplasia and retardation of skeletal development and bone growth with risk being the greatest for children <4 years and those receiving high doses; use with caution in patients with renal or hepatic impairment (eg, elderly); dosage modification required in patients with renal impairment since it may increase BUN as an antianabolic agent; pseudotumor cerebri has been reported with tetracycline use (usually resolves with discontinuation); outdated drug can cause nephropathy; superinfection possible; use protective measure to avoid photosensitivity

Drug Interactions

Cytochrome P450 Effect: Substrate of CYP3A4 (major); **Inhibits** CYP3A4 (moderate)

Decreased Effect: Calcium, magnesium- or aluminum-containing antacids, iron, zinc, sodium bicarbonate, sucralfate, didanosine, or quinapril may decrease tetracycline absorption. Therapeutic effect of penicillins may be reduced with coadministration of tetracycline. Although anecdotal reports suggest oral contraceptive efficacy could be reduced by tetracyclines, this has been refuted by more rigorous scientific and clinical data. The levels/effects of tetracycline may be decreased by aminoglutethimide, carbamazepine, nafcillin, nevirapine, phenobarbital, phenytoin, rifamycins, and other CYP3A4 inducers.

Increased Effect/Toxicity: Methoxyflurane anesthesia when concurrent with tetracycline may cause fatal nephrotoxicity. Warfarin with tetracyclines may cause increased anticoagulation. Tetracycline may increase the levels/effects of selected benzodiazepines, calcium channel blockers, cisapride, cyclosporine, ergot alkaloids, selected HMG-CoA reductase inhibitors, mirtazapine, nateglinide, nefazodone, pimozide, quinidine, sildenafil (and other PDE-5 inhibitors), tacrolimus, venlafaxine, and other CYP3A4 substrates.

Nutritional/Ethanol Interactions

Food: Tetracycline serum concentrations may be decreased if taken with dairy products.

Herb/Nutraceutical: Avoid dong quai, St John's wort (may also cause photosensitization)

Lab Interactions

False-negative urine glucose with Clinistix®

Adverse Reactions

Frequency not defined.

Cardiovascular: Pericarditis

Central nervous system: Intracranial pressure increased, bulging fontanels in infants, pseudotumor cerebri, paresthesia

Dermatologic: Photosensitivity, pruritus, pigmentation of nails, exfoliative dermatitis

Endocrine & metabolic: Diabetes insipidus syndrome

Gastrointestinal: Discoloration of teeth and enamel hypoplasia (young children), nausea, diarrhea, vomiting, esophagitis, anorexia, abdominal cramps, antibiotic-associated pseudomembranous colitis, staphylococcal enterocolitis, pancreatitis

Hematologic: Thrombophlebitis

Hepatic: Hepatotoxicity

Renal: Acute renal failure, azotemia, renal damage

Miscellaneous: Superinfection, anaphylaxis, hypersensitivity reactions, candidal superinfection

Overdosage/Toxicology

Symptoms of overdose include nausea, anorexia, and diarrhea. Treatment is supportive.

Pharmacodynamics/Kinetics

Absorption: Oral: 75%

Time to Peak: Serum: Oral: 2-4 hours

Protein Binding: ~65%

Half-Life Elimination: Normal renal function: 8-11 hours; End-stage renal disease: 57-108 hours

Excretion: Urine (60% as unchanged drug); feces (as active form)

Dosing

Adults & Elderly: Antibacterial: Oral:

Systemic infection: Oral: 250-500 mg/dose every 6 hours

Peptic ulcer disease: Eradication of *Helicobacter pylori*: 500 mg 2-4 times/day depending on regimen; requires combination therapy with at least one other antibiotic and an acid-suppressing agent (proton pump inhibitor or H_2 blocker)

Periodontitis: 250 mg every 6 hours until improvement (usually 10 days)

Pediatrics: Antibacterial, systemic: Children >8 years: Oral: 25-50 mg/kg/day in divided doses every 6 hours

Renal Impairment:

Cl_{cr} 50-80 mL/minute: Administer every 8-12 hours.

Cl_{cr} 10-50 mL/minute: Administer every 12-24 hours.

Cl_{cr} <10 mL/minute: Administer every 24 hours.

Slightly dialyzable (5% to 20%) via hemo- and peritoneal dialysis or via continuous arteriovenous or venovenous hemofiltration; supplemental dose is not necessary.

Hepatic Impairment: Avoid use or maximum dose is 1 g/day.

Available Dosage Forms

Capsule, as hydrochloride: 250 mg, 500 mg

Suspension, oral, as hydrochloride (Sumycin®): 125 mg/5 mL (480 mL) [contains sodium benzoate and sodium metabisulfite; fruit flavor]

Tablet, as hydrochloride (Sumycin®): 250 mg, 500 mg

Monitoring and Teaching Issues

Physical Assessment: Assess results of culture and sensitivity tests and patient's allergy history prior to beginning therapy. Use caution with renal or hepatic impairment (see Warnings/Precautions for use cautions). Assess potential interactions with other pharmacological agents and herbal products patient may be using (eg, may decrease levels/effects of penicillins and CYP3A4 inducers, increase levels/effects of warfarin and CYP3A4 substrates; see Drug Interactions). Assess results of laboratory tests, therapeutic effectiveness (resolution of infection), and adverse reactions at beginning of and periodically throughout therapy (see Adverse Reactions; eg, nausea, diarrhea, pericarditis, photosensitivity, rash, opportunistic infection, hypersensitivity). Caution patients with diabetes to monitor glucose levels closely (may cause false-positive urine glucose with Clinitest®). Assess knowledge/teach patient appropriate use, interventions to reduce side effects, and adverse symptoms to report (see Patient Education).

Monitoring Laboratory Tests: Renal, hepatic, and hematologic function; WBC. Perform culture and sensitivity studies prior to initiating therapy to determine the causative organism and its susceptibility to tetracycline.

Patient Education: Do not take any new medication during therapy without consulting prescriber. Take this medication exactly as directed. Preferable to take on an empty stomach, 1 hour before or 2 hours after meals. Take at regularly scheduled times, (Continued)

Tetracycline *(Continued)*

around-the-clock. Avoid antacids, iron, or dairy products within 2 hours of taking tetracycline. Take all of the prescription even if you see an improvement in your condition. You may experience photosensitivity (use sunscreen, wear protective clothing and eyewear, and avoid direct sunlight); dizziness or lightheadedness (use caution when driving or engaging in tasks requiring alertness until response to drug is known); or nausea/vomiting (small frequent meals, frequent mouth care, chewing gum, or sucking lozenges may help). Report rash or intense itching, yellowing of skin or eyes, fever or chills, blackened stool, vaginal itching or discharge, foul-smelling stools, excessive thirst or urination, acute headache, unresolved diarrhea, respiratory difficulty, condition does not improve, or worsening of condition. **Pregnancy/breast-feeding precautions:** Do not get pregnant while taking this medication. Use appropriate contraceptive measures. Breast-feeding is not recommended.

Geriatric Considerations: The role of tetracycline has decreased because of the emergence of resistant organisms. Doxycycline is the tetracycline of choice when one is indicated because of its better GI absorption, less interactions with divalent cations, longer half-life, and the fact that the majority is cleared by nonrenal mechanisms.

Pregnancy Risk Factor: D

Pregnancy Issues: Tetracyclines cross the placenta and enter fetal circulation; may cause permanent discoloration of teeth if used during the last half of pregnancy.

Lactation: Enters breast milk/not recommended (AAP rates "compatible")

Breast-Feeding Issues: Negligible absorption by infant; potential to stain infants' unerupted teeth

Administration

Oral: Oral should be given on an empty stomach (ie, 1 hour prior to, or 2 hours after meals) to increase total absorption. Administer at least 1-2 hours prior to, or 4 hours after antacid because aluminum and magnesium cations may chelate with tetracycline and reduce its total absorption. Administer around-the-clock to promote less variation in peak and trough serum levels.

Storage: Outdated tetracyclines have caused a Fanconi-like syndrome (nausea, vomiting, acidosis, proteinuria, glycosuria, aminoaciduria, polydipsia, polyuria, hypokalemia). Protect oral dosage forms from light.

Related Information

Antimicrobial Drugs of Choice *on page 1792*
Compatibility of Drugs *on page 1723*
Helicobacter pylori Treatment *on page 1835*
Maternal / Fetal Toxicology *on page 1762*

♦ **Tetracycline, Bismuth Subsalicylate, and Metronidazole** *see* Bismuth Subsalicylate, Metronidazole, and Tetracycline *on page 199*

♦ **Tetracycline Hydrochloride** *see* Tetracycline *on page 1452*

♦ **Tetracycline, Metronidazole, and Bismuth Subsalicylate** *see* Bismuth Subsalicylate, Metronidazole, and Tetracycline *on page 199*

♦ **Tetrahydroaminoacrine** *see* Tacrine *on page 1418*

♦ **Tetrahydrocannabinol** *see* Dronabinol *on page 499*

♦ **Teveten®** *see* Eprosartan *on page 536*

♦ **Teveten® HCT** *see* Eprosartan and Hydrochlorothiazide *on page 537*

♦ **Tev-Tropin™** *see* Human Growth Hormone *on page 745*

♦ **Texacort®** *see* Hydrocortisone *on page 760*

♦ **TG** *see* Thioguanine *on page 1462*

♦ **6-TG** *see* Thioguanine *on page 1462*

♦ **THA** *see* Tacrine *on page 1418*

Thalidomide *(tha LI doe mide)*

U.S. Brand Names Thalomid®

Restrictions Thalidomide is approved for marketing only under a special distribution program. This program, called the "System for Thalidomide Education and Prescribing Safety" (STEPS), has been approved by the FDA. Prescribing and dispensing of thalidomide is restricted to prescribers and pharmacists registered with the program. Prior to dispensing, an authorization number must be obtained (1-888-423-5436) from Celgene (write authorization number on prescription). No more than a 4-week supply should be dispensed. Blister packs should be dispensed intact (do not repackage capsules). Prescriptions must be filled within 7 days.

Generic Available No

Pharmacologic Category Immunosuppressant Agent; Tumor Necrosis Factor (TNF) Blocking Agent

Medication Safety Issues
Sound-alike/look-alike issues:
Thalidomide may be confused with flutamide

Use Treatment and maintenance of cutaneous manifestations of erythema nodosum leprosum

Unlabeled/Investigational Use Treatment of Crohn's disease; treatment or prevention of graft-versus-host reactions after bone marrow transplantation; AIDS-related aphthous stomatitis; Behçet's syndrome; Waldenström's macroglobulinemia; Langerhans cell histiocytosis; may be effective in rheumatoid arthritis, discoid lupus erythematosus, and erythema multiforme

Mechanism of Action/Effect A derivative of glutethimide; mode of action for immunosuppression is unclear; inhibition of neutrophil chemotaxis and decreased monocyte phagocytosis may occur; may cause 50% to 80% reduction of tumor necrosis factor - alpha.

Contraindications Hypersensitivity to thalidomide or any component of the formulation; neuropathy (peripheral); pregnancy or women in childbearing years unless alternative therapies are inappropriate and adequate precautions are taken to avoid pregnancy; patient unable to comply with STEPS™ program.

Warnings/Precautions Effective contraception must be used for at least 4 weeks before initiating therapy, during therapy, and for 4 weeks following discontinuation of thalidomide. Males (even those vasectomized) must use a latex condom during any sexual contact with women of childbearing age. May cause sedation; patients must be warned to use caution when performing tasks which require alertness. Use caution in patients with renal or hepatic impairment, neurological disorders, cardiovascular disease, or constipation.

Thalidomide has been associated with the development of peripheral neuropathy, which may be irreversible. Consider immediate discontinuation, if clinically appropriate, in patients who develop neuropathy. Use caution in patients with a history of seizures, concurrent therapy with drugs which alter seizure threshold, or conditions which predispose to seizures. May cause neutropenia; discontinue therapy if absolute neutrophil count decrease to <750/mm^3. Use caution in patients with HIV infection; has been associated with increased viral loads.

May cause orthostasis and/or bradycardia; use with caution in patients with cardiovascular disease or in patients who would not tolerate transient hypotensive episodes. Thrombotic events have been reported in patients receiving thalidomide, generally in patients with other risk factors for thrombosis (neoplastic disease, inflammatory disease, or concurrent therapy with other drugs which may cause thrombosis). Safety and efficacy have not been established in children <12 years of age.

Drug Interactions

Increased Effect/Toxicity: Thalidomide may enhance the sedative activity of other drugs such as ethanol, barbiturates, reserpine, and chlorpromazine. Drugs which may cause peripheral neuropathy should be used with caution in patients receiving thalidomide. Women using any drug which may decrease the serum concentrations and/or efficacy of hormonal contraceptives must use 2 other methods of contraception or abstain from heterosexual contact. Thalidomide may be associated with increased risk of serious infection when used in combination with anakinra.

Nutritional/Ethanol Interactions

Ethanol: Avoid ethanol (may increase sedation).

Herb/Nutraceutical: Avoid cat's claw (has immunostimulant properties).

Adverse Reactions

Controlled clinical trials: ENL:

>10%:

Central nervous system: Somnolence (37.5%), headache (12.5%)

Dermatologic: Rash (20.8%)

1% to 10%:

Cardiovascular: Peripheral edema

Central nervous system: Dizziness (4.2%), vertigo (8.3%), chills, malaise (8.3%),

Dermatologic: Dermatitis (fungal) (4.2%), nail disorder (4.2%), pruritus (8.3%), rash (maculopapular) (4.2%)

Gastrointestinal (4.2%): Constipation, diarrhea, nausea, moniliasis, tooth pain, abdominal pain

Genitourinary: Impotence (8.2%)

Neuromuscular & skeletal: Asthenia (8.3%), pain (8.3%), back pain (4.2%), neck pain (4.2%), neck rigidity (4.2%), tremor (4.2%)

Respiratory (4.2%): Pharyngitis, rhinitis, sinusitis

HIV-seropositive:

General: An increased viral load has been noted in patients treated with thalidomide. This is of uncertain clinical significance

>10%:

Central nervous system: Somnolence (36% to 37%), dizziness (18.7% to 19.4%), fever (19.4% to 21.9%), headache (16.7% to 18.7%)

Dermatologic: Rash (25%), maculopapular rash (16.7% to 18.7%), acne (3.1% to 11.1%)

Gastrointestinal: AST increase (2.8% to 12.5%), diarrhea (11.1% to 18.7%), nausea (≤12.5%), oral moniliasis (6.3% to 11.1%)

Hematologic: Leukopenia (16.7% to 25%), anemia (5.6% to 12.5%)

Neuromuscular & skeletal: Paresthesia (5.6% to 15.6%), weakness (5.6% to 21.9%)

Miscellaneous: Diaphoresis (≤12.5%), lymphadenopathy (5.6% to 12.5%)

1% to 10%:

Cardiovascular: Peripheral edema (3.1% to 8.3%)

Central nervous system: Nervousness (2.8% to 9.4%), insomnia (≤9.4%), agitation (≤9.4%), chills (≤9.4%), neuropathy (up to 8% in HIV-seropositive patients)

Dermatologic: Dermatitis (fungal) (5.6% to 9.4%), nail disorder (≤3.1%), pruritus (2.8% to 6.3%)

Gastrointestinal: Anorexia (2.8% to 9.4%), constipation (2.8% to 9.4%), dry mouth (8.3% to 9.4%), flatulence (8.3% to 9.4%), multiple abnormalities LFTs (≤9.4%), abdominal pain (2.8% to 3.1%)

Neuromuscular & skeletal: Back pain (≤5%), pain (≤3.1%)

Respiratory: Pharyngitis (6.3% to 8.3%), sinusitis (3.1% to 8.3%)

Miscellaneous: Accidental injury (≤5.6%), infection (6.3% to 8.3%)

Pharmacodynamics/Kinetics

Time to Peak: Plasma: 2-6 hours

Protein Binding: 55% to 66%

Half-Life Elimination: 5-7 hours

Metabolism: Nonenzymatic hydrolysis in plasma; forms multiple metabolites

Excretion: Urine (<1%)

Dosing

Adults & Elderly:

Cutaneous ENL: Oral:

Initial dose: 100-300 mg/day taken once daily at bedtime with water (at least 1 hour after evening meal)

Adjustments to initial dose:

Patients weighing <50 kg: Initiate at lower end of the dosing range

(Continued)

Thalidomide *(Continued)*

Severe cutaneous reaction or previously requiring high dose: May be initiated at 400 mg/day; doses may be divided, but taken 1 hour after meals

Duration and tapering/maintenance:

Dosing should continue until active reaction subsides (usually at least 2 weeks), then tapered in 50 mg decrements every 2-4 weeks

Note: Patients who flare during tapering or with a history or requiring prolonged maintenance should be maintained on the minimum dosage necessary to control the reaction. Efforts to taper should be repeated every 3-6 months, in increments of 50 mg every 2-4 weeks.

Behçet's syndrome (unlabeled use): Oral: 100-400 mg/day

Graft-vs-host reactions (unlabeled use): Oral: 100-1600 mg/day; usual initial dose: 200 mg 4 times/day for use up to 700 days

AIDS-related aphthous stomatitis (unlabeled use): Oral: 200 mg twice daily for 5 days, then 200 mg/day for up to 8 weeks

Discoid lupus erythematosus (unlabeled use): Oral: 100-400 mg/day; maintenance dose: 25-50 mg

Pediatrics: Graft-vs-host reactions (unlabeled use): Oral: Children: 3 mg/kg 4 times/day

Available Dosage Forms Capsule: 50 mg, 100 mg, 200 mg

Monitoring and Teaching Issues

Physical Assessment: Patient must be capable of complying with STEPS™ program (see Use). Instruct patient on risks of pregnancy, appropriate contraceptive measures (see Patient Education), and necessity for frequent pregnancy testing (schedule pregnancy testing at time of dispensing and give patient schedule in writing). Assess other medications patient may be taking for possible interactions (see Drug Interactions). Monitor closely for signs of neuropathy, neutropenia, and CNS depression. Instruct patient on signs and symptoms to report (see Patient Education), and appropriate interventions for adverse reactions.

Pregnancy risk factor X: Pregnancy test is required within 24 hours prior to beginning therapy, weekly during first month of therapy, and monthly thereafter for all women of childbearing age. Effective contraception with at least two reliable forms of contraception must be used for 1 month prior to beginning therapy, during therapy, and for 1 month following discontinuance of therapy. Women who have undergone a hysterectomy or have been postmenopausal for at least 24 consecutive months are the only exception. Do not prescribe, administer, or dispense to women of childbearing age or males who may have intercourse with women of childbearing age unless both female and male are capable of complying with contraceptive measures. Even males who have undergone vasectomy must acknowledge these risks in writing, and must use a latex condom during any sexual contact with women of childbearing age. Oral and written warnings concerning contraception and the hazards of thalidomide must be conveyed to females and males and they must acknowledge their understanding in writing. Parents or guardians must consent and sign acknowledgment for patients between 12 and 18 years of age following therapy. Breast-feeding is contraindicated.

Monitoring Laboratory Tests: Pregnancy testing is required within 24 hours of initiation of therapy, weekly during the first 4 weeks, then every 4 weeks in women with regular menstrual cycles or every 2 weeks in women with irregular menstrual cycles. In HIV-seropositive patients: monitor viral load after 1 and 3 months, then every 3 months. CBS initially and periodically during therapy. Consider monitoring of sensory nerve application potential amplitudes at baseline and every 6 months to detect asymptomatic neuropathy.

Patient Education: You will be given oral and written instructions about the necessity of using two methods of contraception and and the necessity of keeping return visits for pregnancy testing. Do not donate blood while taking this medicine. Male patients should not donate sperm. Avoid extensive handling of capsules; capsules should remain in blister pack until ingestion. If exposed to the powder content from broken capsules or body fluids from patients receiving thalidomide, the exposed area should be washed with soap and water. You may experience postural hypotension (use caution when rising from lying or sitting position); sleepiness; dizziness; headaches; lack of concentration (use caution when driving, climbing stairs, or engaging in tasks requiring alertness until response to drug is known); nausea or vomiting or loss of appetite (small frequent meals, frequent mouth care, chewing gum, or sucking lozenges may help); constipation or diarrhea; oral thrush (frequent mouth care is necessary); or sexual dysfunction (reversible). Report any of the above if persistent or severe. Report chest pain or palpitations or swelling of extremities; back, neck, or muscle pain or stiffness; numbness or pain in extremities; skin rash or eruptions; increased nervousness, anxiety, or insomnia; or any other symptom of adverse reactions. **Pregnancy/breast-feeding precautions:** Do not get pregnant (females) or cause pregnancy (males) during treatment. The use of two forms of contraception are required for 1 month prior to therapy, during therapy, and for 1 month following discontinuation of therapy. Pregnancy tests will be routinely conducted during therapy. Do not breast-feed while taking this medication or for 1 month following discontinuation.

Dietary Considerations: Should be taken at least 1 hour after the evening meal.

Pregnancy Risk Factor: X

Pregnancy Issues: Embryotoxic with limb defects noted from the 27th to 40th gestational day of exposure; all cases of phocomelia occur from the 27th to 42nd gestational day; fetal cardiac, gastrointestinal, and genitourinary tract abnormalities have also been described. Effective contraception must be used for at least 4 weeks before initiating therapy, during therapy, and for 4 weeks following discontinuation of thalidomide. Males (even those vasectomized) must use a latex condom during any sexual contact with women of childbearing age. Risk to the fetus from semen of male patients is unknown.

Lactation: Excretion in breast milk unknown/not recommended

Breast-Feeding Issues: Due to the potential for serious adverse reactions in the infant, a decision should be made to discontinue nursing or discontinue treatment with thalidomide.

Administration
Oral: Avoid extensive handling of capsules; capsules should remain in blister pack until ingestion. If exposed to the powder content from broken capsules or body fluids from patients receiving thalidomide, the exposed area should be washed with soap and water.
Storage: Store at 15°C to 30°C (50°F to 86°F). Protect from light. Keep in original package.
Related Information
Maternal / Fetal Toxicology *on page 1762*

♦ **Thalitone**® *see* Chlorthalidone *on page 314*
♦ **Thalomid**® *see* Thalidomide *on page 1454*
♦ **THC** *see* Dronabinol *on page 499*
♦ **Theo-24**® *see* Theophylline *on page 1457*
♦ **Theochron**® *see* Theophylline *on page 1457*
♦ **Theolair**™ *see* Theophylline *on page 1457*
♦ **Theolair-SR**® **[DSC]** *see* Theophylline *on page 1457*

Theophylline (thee OFF i lin)

U.S. Brand Names Elixophyllin®; Quibron®-T; Quibron®-T/SR; Theo-24®; Theochron®; Theolair™; Theolair-SR® [DSC]; T-Phyl®; Uniphyl®
Synonyms Theophylline Anhydrous
Generic Available Yes: Elixir, extended release tablet, infusion, oral solution
Pharmacologic Category Theophylline Derivative
Medication Safety Issues
Sound-alike/look-alike issues:
Theolair™ may be confused with Thiola®, Thyrolar®
Use Treatment of symptoms and reversible airway obstruction due to chronic asthma, chronic bronchitis, or COPD
Mechanism of Action/Effect Causes bronchodilatation, diuresis, CNS and cardiac stimulation, and gastric acid secretion by blocking phosphodiesterase which increases tissue concentrations of cyclic adenine monophosphate (cAMP) which in turn promotes catecholamine stimulation of lipolysis, glycogenolysis, and gluconeogenesis and induces release of epinephrine from adrenal medulla cells.
Contraindications Hypersensitivity to theophylline or any component of the formulation; premixed injection may contain corn-derived dextrose and its use is contraindicated in patients with allergy to corn-related products
Warnings/Precautions If a patient develops signs and symptoms of theophylline toxicity (eg, persistent, repetitive vomiting), a serum theophylline level should be measured and subsequent doses held. Due to potential saturation of theophylline clearance at serum levels in or (in some patients) less than the therapeutic range, dosage adjustment should be made in small increments (maximum: 25%). Due to wider interpatient variability, theophylline serum level measurements must be used to optimize therapy and prevent serious toxicity. Use with caution in patients with peptic ulcer, hyperthyroidism, seizure disorders, hypertension, and patients with cardiac arrhythmias (excluding bradyarrhythmias).
Drug Interactions
Cytochrome P450 Effect: Substrate of CYP1A2 (major), 2C8/9 (minor), 2D6 (minor), 2E1 (major), 3A4 (major); **Inhibits** CYP1A2 (weak)
Decreased Effect: CYP1A2 inducers may decrease the levels/effects of theophylline; example inducers include aminoglutethimide, carbamazepine, phenobarbital, and rifampin. CYP3A4 inducers may decrease the levels/effects of theophylline; example inducers include aminoglutethimide, carbamazepine, nafcillin, nevirapine, phenobarbital, phenytoin, and rifamycins.
Increased Effect/Toxicity: CYP1A2 inhibitors may increase the levels/effects of theophylline; example inhibitors include amiodarone, ciprofloxacin, fluvoxamine, ketoconazole, norfloxacin, ofloxacin, and rofecoxib. CYP2E1 inhibitors may increase the levels/effects of theophylline; example inhibitors include disulfiram, isoniazid, and miconazole. Changes in diet may affect the elimination of theophylline. CYP3A4 inhibitors may increase the levels/effects of theophylline; example inhibitors include azole antifungals, ciprofloxacin, clarithromycin, diclofenac, doxycycline, erythromycin, imatinib, isoniazid, nefazodone, nicardipine, propofol, protease inhibitors, quinidine, and verapamil.
Nutritional/Ethanol Interactions Food: Food does not appreciably affect the absorption of liquid, fast-release products, and most sustained release products; however, food may induce a sudden release (dose-dumping) of once-daily sustained release products resulting in an increase in serum drug levels and potential toxicity. Avoid excessive amounts of caffeine. Avoid extremes of dietary protein and carbohydrate intake. Changes in diet may affect the elimination of theophylline; charbroiled foods may increase elimination, reducing half-life by 50%.
Adverse Reactions
Adverse reactions/theophylline serum level: (Adverse effects do not necessarily occur according to serum levels. Arrhythmia and seizure can occur without seeing the other adverse effects.)
15-25 mcg/mL: GI upset, diarrhea, nausea/vomiting, abdominal pain, nervousness, headache, insomnia, agitation, dizziness, muscle cramp, tremor
25-35 mcg/mL: Tachycardia, occasional PVC
>35 mcg/mL: Ventricular tachycardia, frequent PVC, seizure
Uncommon at serum theophylline concentrations ≤20 mcg/mL
1% to 10%:
Cardiovascular: Tachycardia
Central nervous system: Nervousness, restlessness
Gastrointestinal: Nausea, vomiting
Overdosage/Toxicology Symptoms of overdose include nausea, vomiting, insomnia, irritability, tachycardia, seizures, tonic-clonic seizures, insomnia, and circulatory failure. If seizures have not occurred, induce vomiting; ipecac syrup is preferred. Do not induce emesis in the presence of impaired consciousness. Repeated doses of charcoal have been shown to be
(Continued)

Theophylline *(Continued)*

effective in enhancing the total body clearance of theophylline. Do not repeat charcoal doses if an ileus is present. Charcoal hemoperfusion may be considered if serum theophylline levels exceed 40 mcg/mL, the patient is unable to tolerate repeat oral charcoal administrations, or if severe toxic symptoms are present. Clearance with hemoperfusion is better than clearance from hemodialysis. Administer a cathartic, especially if sustained release agents were used. Phenobarbital administered prophylactically may prevent seizures.

Pharmacodynamics/Kinetics

Onset of Action: I.V.: <30 minutes

Absorption: Oral (formulation dependent): ≤100%

Protein Binding: 40%, primarily to albumin

Half-Life Elimination: Highly variable and age, liver and cardiac function, lung disease, and smoking history dependent

Metabolism: Children >1 year and Adults: Hepatic; involves CYP1A2, 2E1 and 3A4; forms active metabolites (caffeine and 3-methylxanthine)

Excretion: Urine: Neonates: 50% unchanged; Children >3 months and Adults: 10% unchanged

Dosing

Adults: Bronchodilation/respiratory stimulant:

Initial dosage recommendation: Loading dose (to achieve a serum concentration of about 10 mcg/mL; loading doses should be given using a rapidly absorbed oral product **not** a sustained release product):

If no theophylline has been administered in the previous 24 hours: 4-6 mg/kg theophylline

If theophylline has been administered in the previous 24 hours: Administer 1/2 loading dose; 2-3 mg/kg theophylline can be given in emergencies when serum concentrations are not available

On the average, for every 1 mg/kg theophylline given, blood concentrations will rise 2 mcg/mL

Maintenance dose: See table.

Maintenance Dose for Acute Symptoms

Population Group	Oral Theophylline (mg/kg/day)	I.V. Aminophylline
Otherwise healthy nonsmoking adults (including elderly patients)	10 (not to exceed 900 mg/day)	0.5 mg/kg/h
Cardiac decompensation, cor pulmonale, and/or liver dysfunction	5 (not to exceed 400 mg/day)	0.25 mg/kg/h

Note: For continuous I.V. infusion, divide total daily dose by 24 = mg/kg/h.

Bronchodilation: Oral:

Nonsustained release: 16-20 mg/kg/day divided into 4 doses/day

Sustained release: 9-13 mg/kg/day divided into 2-3 doses/day

Note: These recommendations, based on mean clearance rates for age or risk factors, were calculated to achieve a serum concentration of 10 mcg/mL. In healthy adults, a slow-release product can be used (9-13 mg/kg in divided dose). The total daily dose can be divided every 8-12 hours.

Dosage in obese patients: Use ideal body weight for obese patients. Dose should be adjusted further based on serum concentrations. Guidelines for obtaining theophylline serum concentrations are shown in the table under Monitoring Laboratory Tests.

Elderly: Elderly patients should be started with a 25% reduction in the adult dose.

Pediatrics:

Loading dose:

Apnea of prematurity: Neonates: Oral: 4 mg/kg/dose

Maintenance Dose for Acute Symptoms

Population Group	Oral Theophylline (mg/kg/day)
Premature infant or newborn to 6 wk (for apnea/bradycardia)[1]	4
6 wk to 6 mo[1]	10
Infants 6 mo to 1 y[1]	12-18
Children 1-9 y	20-24
Children 9-12 y, adolescent daily smokers of cigarettes or marijuana, and otherwise healthy adult smokers <50 y	16
Adolescents 12-16 y (nonsmokers)	13
Otherwise healthy nonsmoking adults (including elderly patients)	10 (not to exceed 900 mg/day)
Cardiac decompensation, cor pulmonale, and/or liver dysfunction	5 (not to exceed 400 mg/day)

[1]**Alternative dosing regimen for full-term infants <1 year of age:**

Total daily dose (mg) = [(0.2 x age in weeks) + 5] x weight (kg)

Postnatal age <26 weeks: Total daily dose divided every 8 hours

Postnatal age >26 weeks: Total daily dose divided every 6 hours

Treatment of acute bronchospasm: Infants and Children: Oral (to achieve a serum level of about 10 mcg/mL; loading doses should be given using a rapidly absorbed oral product **not** a sustained release product):

If no theophylline has been administered in the previous 24 hours: 5 mg/kg theophylline

If theophylline has been administered in the previous 24 hours: 2.5 mg/kg theophylline may be given in emergencies when serum levels are not available

Note: A modified loading dose (mg/kg) may be calculated (when the serum level is known) by: [Blood level desired - blood level measured] divided by 2 (for every 1 mg/kg theophylline given, the blood level will rise by approximately 2 mcg/mL)

Maintenance dose: See table on previous page.

Note: These recommendations, based on mean clearance rates for age or risk factors, were calculated to achieve a serum level of 10 mcg/mL (5 mcg/mL for newborns with apnea/bradycardia). In newborns and infants, a fast-release oral product can be used. The total daily dose can be divided every 12 hours in newborns and every 6-8 hours in infants. In children and healthy adults, a slow-release product can be used. The total daily dose can be divided every 8-12 hours.

Note: Use ideal body weight for obese patients

Adjustment of dose: Dose should be further adjusted based on serum levels. Guidelines for drawing theophylline serum levels are shown in the table.

Guidelines for Drawing Theophylline Serum Levels

Dosage Form	Time to Draw Level
I.V. bolus	30 min after end of 30-min infusion
I.V. continuous infusion	12-24 h after initiation of infusion
P.O. liquid, fast-release tab	Peak: 1 h postdose after at least 1 day of therapy Trough: Just before a dose after at least 1 day of therapy
P.O. slow-release product	Peak: 4 h postdose after at least 1 day of therapy Trough: Just before a dose after at least 1 day of therapy

Available Dosage Forms [DSC] = Discontinued product

Capsule, extended release (Theo-24®): 100 mg, 200 mg, 300 mg, 400 mg [24 hours]

Elixir (Elixophyllin®): 80 mg/15 mL (480 mL) [contains alcohol 20%; fruit flavor]

Infusion [premixed in D₅W]: 0.8 mg/mL (500 mL, 1000 mL); 1.6 mg/mL (250 mL, 500 mL); 2 mg/mL (100 mL); 3.2 mg/mL (250 mL); 4 mg/mL (50 mL, 100 mL)

Solution, oral: 80 mg/15 mL (15 mL, 18.75 mL, 500 mL) [dye free, sugar free; contains alcohol 0.4% and benzoic acid; orange flavor]

Tablet, controlled release:

T-Phyl®: 200 mg [12 hours; contains cetostearyl alcohol]

Uniphyl®: 400 mg, 600 mg [24 hours; contains cetostearyl alcohol]

Tablet, extended release: 100 mg, 200 mg, 300 mg, 450 mg

Theochron®: 100 mg, 200 mg, 300 mg [12-24 hours]

Tablet, immediate release:

Quibron®-T: 300 mg

Theolair™: 125 mg, 250 mg

Tablet, sustained release (Quibron®-T/SR): 300 mg [8-12 hours]

Tablet, timed release (Theolair™-SR [DSC]): 300 mg, 500 mg

Monitoring and Teaching Issues

Physical Assessment: Assess effectiveness and interactions of other medications patient may be taking. Monitor effectiveness of therapy (respiratory rate, lung sounds, characteristics of cough and sputum) and adverse reactions at beginning of therapy and periodically with long-term use. For inpatient care, monitor vital signs and lung sounds prior to and periodically during therapy. Assess knowledge/teach patient appropriate use, interventions to reduce side effects, and adverse symptoms to report.

Monitoring Laboratory Tests: Therapeutic levels:

Asthma: 10-15 mg/mL (peak level)

Toxic concentration: >20 mg/mL

Patient Education: Take exactly as directed; do not exceed recommended dosage. Avoid smoking (smoking may interfere with drug absorption as well as exacerbate condition for which medication is prescribed). If you are smoking when dosage is prescribed; inform prescriber if you stop smoking (dosage may need to be adjusted to prevent toxicity). Preferable to take on empty stomach, 1 hour before or 2 hours after meals, with a full glass of water. Do not chew or crush sustained release forms; capsules may be opened and contents sprinkled on soft food (do not chew beads). Avoid dietary stimulants (eg, caffeine, tea, colas, or chocolate; may increase adverse side effects). Maintain adequate hydration (2-3 L/day of fluids) unless instructed to restrict fluid intake. You may experience nausea, vomiting, or lose of appetite (small frequent meals, frequent mouth care, chewing gum, or sucking lozenges may help). Report acute insomnia or restlessness, chest pain or rapid heartbeat, emotional lability or agitation, muscle tremors or cramping, acute headache, abdominal pain and cramping, blackened stool, or worsening of respiratory condition. **Pregnancy precaution:** Inform prescriber if you are or intend to become pregnant.

Dietary Considerations: Should be taken with water 1 hour before or 2 hours after meals. Premixed injection may contain corn-derived dextrose and its use is contraindicated in patients with allergy to corn-related products.

Geriatric Considerations: Although there is a great intersubject variability for half-lives of methylxanthines (2-10 hours), elderly as a group have slower hepatic clearance. Therefore, use lower initial doses and monitor closely for response and adverse reactions. Additionally, elderly are at greater risk for toxicity due to concomitant disease (eg, CHF, arrhythmias), and drug use (eg, cimetidine, ciprofloxacin); see Warnings/Precautions and Drug Interactions.

Pregnancy Risk Factor: C

Pregnancy Issues: Theophylline crosses the placenta; adverse effects may be seen in the newborn. Theophylline metabolism may change during pregnancy; monitor serum levels. (Continued)

Theophylline *(Continued)*

Lactation: Enters breast milk/compatible (AAP rates "compatible")

Breast-Feeding Issues: Irritability may be observed in the nursing infant.

Administration

Oral: Long-acting preparations should be taken with a full glass of water, swallowed whole, or cut in half if scored. Do **not** crush. Extended release capsule forms may be opened and the contents sprinkled on soft foods; do **not** chew beads.

Compatibility: Stable in D_5W

Y-site administration: Incompatible with hetastarch, phenytoin

Compatibility when admixed: Incompatible with ascorbic acid injection, ceftriaxone, cimetidine

Additional Information Theophylline salt / theophylline content (percent)

Theophylline anhydrous (eg, most oral solids): 100% theophylline

Theophylline monohydrate (eg, oral solutions): 91% theophylline

Aminophylline (theophylline) (eg, injection): 80% (79% to 86%) theophylline

Oxtriphylline (choline theophylline) (eg, Choledyl®): 64% theophylline

Related Information

Peak and Trough Guidelines *on page 1694*

♦ **Theophylline Anhydrous** *see Theophylline on page 1457*

♦ **TheraCys®** *see page 1660*

♦ **Theramycin Z®** *see Erythromycin on page 543*

♦ **Thermazene®** *see Silver Sulfadiazine on page 1374*

Thiabendazole *(thye a BEN da zole)*

U.S. Brand Names Mintezol®

Synonyms Tiabendazole

Generic Available No

Pharmacologic Category Anthelmintic

Use Treatment of strongyloidiasis, cutaneous larva migrans, visceral larva migrans, dracunculiasis, trichinosis, and mixed helminthic infections

Unlabeled/Investigational Use Cutaneous larva migrans (topical application)

Mechanism of Action/Effect Inhibits helminth-specific mitochondrial fumarate reductase

Contraindications Hypersensitivity to thiabendazole or any component of the formulation; not for use as prophylactic treatment of enterobiasis (pinworm) infestation

Warnings/Precautions Use with caution in patients with renal or hepatic impairment, malnutrition or anemia, or dehydration. Causes sedation; caution must be used in performing tasks which require alertness. Not suitable treatment for mixed infections with *Ascaris*. Ophthalmic changes may occur and persist >1 year. Safety and efficacy are limited in children <14 kg (30 lb).

Drug Interactions

Cytochrome P450 Effect: Substrate of CYP1A2 (minor); **Inhibits** CYP1A2 (strong)

Increased Effect/Toxicity: Thiabendazole may increase the levels/effects of aminophylline, fluvoxamine, mexiletine, mirtazapine, ropinirole, theophylline, trifluoperazine, and other CYP1A2 substrates.

Lab Interactions Increased glucose

Adverse Reactions Frequency not defined.

Central nervous system: Seizures, hallucinations, delirium, dizziness, drowsiness, headache, chills

Dermatologic: Rash, Stevens-Johnson syndrome, pruritus, angioedema

Endocrine & metabolic: Hyperglycemia

Gastrointestinal: Anorexia, diarrhea, nausea, vomiting, drying of mucous membranes, abdominal pain

Genitourinary: Malodor of urine, hematuria, crystalluria, enuresis

Hematologic: Leukopenia

Hepatic: Jaundice, cholestasis, hepatic failure, hepatotoxicity

Neuromuscular & skeletal: Numbness, incoordination

Ocular: Abnormal sensation in eyes, blurred vision, dry eyes, Sicca syndrome, vision decreased, xanthopsia

Otic: Tinnitus

Renal: Nephrotoxicity

Miscellaneous: Anaphylaxis, hypersensitivity reactions, lymphadenopathy

Overdosage/Toxicology Symptoms of overdose include altered mental status and visual problems. Treatment is supportive.

Pharmacodynamics/Kinetics

Absorption: Rapid and well absorbed

Time to Peak: Oral suspension: Within 1-2 hours

Half-Life Elimination: 1.2 hours

Metabolism: Rapidly hepatic; metabolized to 5-hydroxy form

Excretion: Urine (90%) and feces (5%) primarily as conjugated metabolites

Dosing

Adults & Elderly: Note: Purgation is not required prior to use; drinking of fruit juice aids in expulsion of worms by removing the mucous to which the intestinal tapeworms attach themselves.

Parasitic infections: Oral: 50 mg/kg/day divided every 12 hours; maximum: 3 g/day

Treatment duration:

Strongyloidiasis: For 2 consecutive days

Cutaneous larva migrans: For 2 consecutive days; if active lesions are still present 2 days after completion, a second course of treatment is recommended.

Visceral larva migrans: For 7 consecutive days

Trichinosis: For 2-4 consecutive days; optimal dosage not established.

Dracunculosis: 50-75 mg/kg/day divided every 12 hours for 3 days

Cutaneous larva migrans: Topical (unlabeled): Apply directly to larval tracks 2-3 times/day for up to 2 weeks; application frequencies may range from 2-6 times/day. **Note:** Not available as a topical formulation; oral suspension (10% to 15%) has been used topically, as well as a number of extemporaneous formulations.

Pediatrics: Parasitic infections: Children: Refer to adult dosing.

Renal Impairment: Use with caution.

Hepatic Impairment: Use with caution.

Available Dosage Forms
Suspension, oral: 500 mg/5 mL (120 mL)
Tablet, chewable: 500 mg [orange flavor]

Monitoring and Teaching Issues

Physical Assessment: See Warnings/Precautions and Drug Interactions for use cautions. Worm infestations are easily transmitted, all close family members should be treated. Instruct patient/caregiver on appropriate use, transmission prevention, possible side effects/appropriate interventions, and adverse symptoms to report (see Patient Education).

Patient Education: Take exactly as directed for full course of medication. Tablets may be chewed, swallowed whole, or crushed and mixed with food. Increase dietary intake of fruit juices. All family members and close friends should also be treated. To reduce possibility of reinfection, wash hands and scrub nails carefully with soap and hot water before handling food, before eating, and before and after toileting. Keep hands out of mouth. Disinfect toilet daily and launder bed lines, undergarments, and nightclothes daily with hot water and soap. Do not go barefoot and do not sit directly on grass or ground. May cause dizziness, fainting, or lightheadedness (use caution when driving or engaging in tasks requiring alertness until response to drug is known); or abdominal pain, nausea, dry mouth, or vomiting (small frequent meals, frequent mouth care, sucking lozenges, or chewing gum may help). Report skin rash or itching, unresolved diarrhea or vomiting, CNS changes (hallucinations, delirium, and acute headache), change in color of urine or stool, or easy bruising or unusual bleeding. **Pregnancy/breast-feeding precautions:** Inform prescriber if you are pregnant. Breast-feeding is not recommended.

Pregnancy Risk Factor: C

Lactation: Excretion in breast milk unknown/not recommended

♦ **Thiamazole** see Methimazole on page 971

♦ **Thiamilate® [OTC]** see Thiamine on page 1461

Thiamine (THYE a min)

U.S. Brand Names Thiamilate® [OTC]

Synonyms Aneurine Hydrochloride; Thiamine Hydrochloride; Thiaminium Chloride Hydrochloride; Vitamin B_1

Generic Available Yes

Pharmacologic Category Vitamin, Water Soluble

Medication Safety Issues
Sound-alike/look-alike issues:
Thiamine may be confused with Tenormin®, Thorazine®

Use Treatment of thiamine deficiency including beriberi, Wernicke's encephalopathy syndrome, and peripheral neuritis associated with pellagra, alcoholic patients with altered sensorium; various genetic metabolic disorders

Mechanism of Action/Effect An essential coenzyme in carbohydrate metabolism by combining with adenosine triphosphate to form thiamine pyrophosphate

Contraindications Hypersensitivity to thiamine or any component of the formulation

Warnings/Precautions Use with caution with parenteral route (especially I.V.) of administration.

Nutritional/Ethanol Interactions Food: High carbohydrate diets may increase thiamine requirement.

Lab Interactions False-positive for uric acid using the phosphotungstate method and for urobilinogen using the Ehrlich's reagent; large doses may interfere with the spectrophotometric determination of serum theophylline concentration

Pharmacodynamics/Kinetics
Absorption: Oral: Adequate; I.M.: Rapid and complete
Excretion: Urine (as unchanged drug and as pyrimidine after body storage sites become saturated)

Dosing
Adults & Elderly:
Recommended daily allowance: >14 years: 1-1.5 mg
Thiamine deficiency (beriberi): I.M. or I.V. 5-30 mg/dose 3 times/day (if critically ill); then orally 5-30 mg/day in single or divided doses 3 times/day for 1 month
Wernicke's encephalopathy: I.V., I.M.: Initial: 100 mg I.V., then 50-100 mg/day I.M. or I.V. until consuming a regular, balanced diet
Dietary supplement (depends on caloric or carbohydrate content of the diet): Oral: 1-2 mg/day
Note: The above doses can be found in multivitamin preparations.
Metabolic disorders: Oral: 10-20 mg/day (dosages up to 4 g/day in divided doses have been used)

Pediatrics:
Recommended daily allowance:
<6 months: 0.3 mg
6 months to 1 year: 0.4 mg
1-3 years: 0.7 mg
4-6 years: 0.9 mg
7-10 years: 1 mg
11-14 years: 1.1-1.3 mg
>14 years: 1-1.5 mg

(Continued)

Thiamine *(Continued)*

Thiamine deficiency (beriberi):
Children: I.M., I.V.: 10-25 mg/dose daily (if critically ill), or 10-50 mg/dose orally every day for 2 weeks, then 5-10 mg/dose orally daily for 1 month

Dietary supplement (depends on caloric or carbohydrate content of the diet): Oral:
Infants: 0.3-0.5 mg/day

Children: 0.5-1 mg/day

Note: The above doses can be found in multivitamin preparations

Available Dosage Forms
Injection, solution, as hydrochloride: 100 mg/mL (2 mL)

Tablet, as hydrochloride: 50 mg, 100 mg, 250 mg, 500 mg

Tablet, enteric coated, as hydrochloride (Thiamilate®): 20 mg

Monitoring and Teaching Issues
Physical Assessment: Assess knowledge/teach patient appropriate administration (injection technique and needle disposal if I.M. self-administered) and dietary instruction.

Patient Education: Take exactly as directed; do not discontinue without consulting prescriber (deficiency state can occur in as little as 3 weeks). Follow dietary instructions (dietary sources include legumes, pork, beef, whole grains, yeast, fresh vegetables). **Pregnancy precaution:** Inform prescriber if you are or intend to become pregnant.

Dietary Considerations: Dietary sources include legumes, pork, beef, whole grains, yeast, and fresh vegetables. A deficiency state can occur in as little as 3 weeks following total dietary absence.

Pregnancy Risk Factor: A/C (dose exceeding RDA recommendation)

Lactation: Enters breast milk/compatible

Administration
I.M.: Parenteral form may be administered by I.M. or slow I.V. injection.

I.V.: Doses are usually administered over 1-2 minutes.

Compatibility: Stable in dextran 6% in dextrose, dextran 6% in NS, D$_5$LR, D$_5$1/4NS, D$_5$1/2NS, D$_5$NS, D$_5$W, D$_{10}$W, fat emulsion 10%, LR, 1/2NS, NS

Storage: Protect oral dosage forms from light.

Additional Information Single vitamin deficiency is rare; evaluate for other deficiencies

♦ **Thiamine Hydrochloride** *see* Thiamine *on page 1461*

♦ **Thiaminium Chloride Hydrochloride** *see* Thiamine *on page 1461*

Thioguanine *(thye oh GWAH neen)*

U.S. Brand Names Tabloid®

Synonyms 2-Amino-6-Mercaptopurine; NSC-752; TG; 6-TG; 6-Thioguanine; Tioguanine

Generic Available No

Pharmacologic Category Antineoplastic Agent, Antimetabolite (Purine Antagonist)

Use Treatment of acute myelogenous (nonlymphocytic) leukemia; treatment of chronic myelogenous leukemia and granulocytic leukemia

Mechanism of Action/Effect Purine analog that is incorporated into DNA and RNA resulting in the blockage of synthesis and metabolism of purine nucleotides

Contraindications Hypersensitivity to thioguanine or any component of the formulation; pregnancy

Warnings/Precautions The U.S. Food and Drug Administration (FDA) currently recommends that procedures for proper handling and disposal of antineoplastic agents be considered. Use with caution and reduce dose of thioguanine in patients with renal or hepatic impairment. Not recommended for long-term continuous therapy due to potential for hepatotoxicity (hepatic veno-occlusive disease). Discontinue in patients with evidence of hepatotoxicity, including signs associated with portal hypertension. Caution with history of previous therapy resistance with either thioguanine or mercaptopurine (there is usually complete cross resistance between these two). Thioguanine is potentially carcinogenic and teratogenic. Patients with genetic deficiency of thiopurine methyltransferase (TPMT) or who are receiving drugs which inhibit this enzyme (mesalazine, olsalazine, sulfasalazine) may be highly sensitive to myelosuppressive effects.

Drug Interactions
Increased Effect/Toxicity: Allopurinol can be used in full doses with thioguanine unlike mercaptopurine. Use with busulfan may cause hepatotoxicity and esophageal varices. Aminosalicylates (olsalazine, mesalamine, sulfasalazine) may inhibit TPMT, increasing toxicity/myelosuppression of thioguanine.

Nutritional/Ethanol Interactions Food: Enhanced absorption if administered between meals.

Adverse Reactions
>10%: Hematologic: Myelosuppressive:
WBC: Moderate

Platelets: Moderate

Onset (days): 7-10

Nadir (days): 14

Recovery (days): 21

1% to 10%:
Dermatologic: Skin rash

Endocrine & metabolic: Hyperuricemia

Gastrointestinal: Mild nausea or vomiting, anorexia, stomatitis, diarrhea

Neuromuscular & skeletal: Unsteady gait

Overdosage/Toxicology Symptoms of overdose include bone marrow suppression, nausea, vomiting, malaise, hypertension, and sweating. Treatment is supportive. Dialysis is not useful.

Pharmacodynamics/Kinetics
Absorption: 30% (highly variable)
Time to Peak: Serum: Within 8 hours
Half-Life Elimination: Terminal: 11 hours
Metabolism: Hepatic; rapidly and extensively via TPMT to 2-amino-6-methylthioguanine (active) and inactive compounds
Excretion: Urine

Dosing
Adults & Elderly: Total daily dose can be given at one time; is sometimes ordered as 6-thioguanine, with 6 being part of the drug name and not some kind of unit or strength.

Antineoplastic: Oral: Refer to individual protocols: 2-3 mg/kg/day calculated to nearest 20 mg or 75-200 mg/m²/day in 1-2 divided doses for 5-7 days or until remission is attained

Pediatrics: Total daily dose can be given at one time; is sometimes ordered as 6-thioguanine, with 6 being part of the drug name and not a unit or strength.

Antineoplastic: Oral (refer to individual protocols):
Infants and Children <3 years: Combination drug therapy for acute nonlymphocytic leukemia: 3.3 mg/kg/day in divided doses twice daily for 4 days
Children >3 years: Refer to adult dosing.

Renal Impairment: Reduce dose.
Hepatic Impairment: Reduce dose.

Available Dosage Forms
Injection, powder for reconstitution: 75 mg [investigational in U.S.]
Tablet [scored]: 40 mg

Monitoring and Teaching Issues
Physical Assessment: Use caution with renal or hepatic impairment (see Warnings/Precautions for specific use cautions). Assess potential for interactions with other pharmacological agents patient may be taking (see Drug Interactions). Assess results of laboratory tests (Monitoring Laboratory Tests) and patient response weekly when beginning therapy, then monthly (eg, myelosuppression, nausea, vomiting, malaise, rash, diarrhea; see Adverse Reactions). Teach patient appropriate use, possible side effects/appropriate interventions (eg, importance of adequate hydration), and adverse symptoms to report (see Patient Education).

Monitoring Laboratory Tests: CBC with differential and platelet count; liver function tests (weekly when beginning therapy then monthly, more frequently in patients with liver disease or concurrent hepatotoxic drugs); serum uric acid, renal function; some laboratories offer testing for TPMT deficiency

Patient Education: Do not take any new medication during therapy unless approved by prescriber. Take exactly as directed. Maintain adequate hydration (2-3 L/day of fluids) unless instructed to restrict fluid intake. May cause nausea and vomiting, diarrhea, or loss of appetite (small frequent meals may help/request medication); weakness or lethargy (use caution when driving or engaging in tasks requiring alertness until response to drug is known); mouth sores (use good oral care); or headache (request medication). You will be susceptible to infection (avoid crowds and exposure to infection). Report signs or symptoms of infection (eg, fever, chills, sore throat, burning urination, fatigue); bleeding (eg, tarry stools, easy bruising); vision changes; unresolved mouth sores, nausea, or vomiting; CNS changes (hallucinations); or respiratory difficulty. **Pregnancy/breast-feeding precautions:** Do not get pregnant. Consult prescriber for appropriate contraceptive measures. The drug may cause permanent sterility and may cause birth defects. Consult prescriber if breast-feeding.

Pregnancy Risk Factor: D
Lactation: Excretion in breast milk unknown

Administration
Reconstitution: Reconstitute parenteral preparation with 5 mL SWFI, NS, or D₅W to yield a 15 mg/mL solution.
Storage:
Tablet: Store at room temperature.
Injection (investigational in U.S.): Store intact vials under refrigeration (2°C to 8°C). The reconstituted solution is stable for at least 24 hours under refrigeration. Further dilutions for infusion are stable for 24 hours at room temperature or under refrigeration.

♦ **6-Thioguanine** *see* Thioguanine *on page 1462*
♦ **Thiophosphoramide** *see* Thiotepa *on page 1466*

Thioridazine (thye oh RID a zeen)
U.S. Brand Names Mellaril® [DSC]; Thioridazine Intensol™
Synonyms Thioridazine Hydrochloride
Generic Available Yes
Pharmacologic Category Antipsychotic Agent, Typical, Phenothiazine
Medication Safety Issues
Sound-alike/look-alike issues:
Thioridazine may be confused with thiothixene, Thorazine®
Mellaril® may be confused with Elavil®, Mebaral®

Use Management of schizophrenic patients who fail to respond adequately to treatment with other antipsychotic drugs, either because of insufficient effectiveness or the inability to achieve an effective dose due to intolerable adverse effects from those medications
Unlabeled/Investigational Use Psychosis
Mechanism of Action/Effect Thioridazine is a piperidine phenothiazine which blocks postsynaptic mesolimbic dopaminergic receptors in the brain; exhibits a strong alpha-adrenergic blocking effect and depresses the release of hypothalamic and hypophyseal hormones
Contraindications Hypersensitivity to thioridazine or any component of the formulation (cross-reactivity between phenothiazines may occur); severe CNS depression; circulatory
(Continued)

Thioridazine *(Continued)*

collapse; severe hypotension; bone marrow suppression; blood dyscrasias; coma; in combination with other drugs that are known to prolong the QT$_c$ interval; in patients with congenital long QT syndrome or a history of cardiac arrhythmias; concurrent use with medications that inhibit the metabolism of thioridazine (fluoxetine, paroxetine, fluvoxamine, propranolol, pindolol); patients known to have genetic defect leading to reduced levels of activity of CYP2D6

Warnings/Precautions Thioridazine has dose-related effects on ventricular repolarization leading to QT$_c$ prolongation, a potentially life-threatening effect. Therefore, it should be reserved for patients with schizophrenia who have failed to respond to adequate levels of other antipsychotic drugs. May cause orthostatic hypotension - use with caution in patients at risk of this effect or those who would tolerate transient hypotensive episodes (cerebrovascular disease, cardiovascular disease, or other medications which may predispose).

Highly sedating, use with caution in disorders where CNS depression is a feature. Use with caution in Parkinson's disease. Caution in patients with hemodynamic instability; bone marrow suppression; predisposition to seizures; subcortical brain damage; severe cardiac, hepatic, renal, or respiratory disease. Esophageal dysmotility and aspiration have been associated with antipsychotic use - use with caution in patients at risk of pneumonia (ie, Alzheimer's disease). Caution in breast cancer or other prolactin-dependent tumors (may elevate prolactin levels). May alter temperature regulation or mask toxicity of other drugs due to antiemetic effects.

Due to anticholinergic effects, use caution in patients with decreased gastrointestinal motility, urinary retention, BPH, xerostomia, visual problems, narrow-angle glaucoma (screening is recommended) and myasthenia gravis. Relative to other neuroleptics, thioridazine has a high potency of cholinergic blockade.

May cause extrapyramidal symptoms, including pseudoparkinsonism, acute dystonic reactions, akathisia, and tardive dyskinesia (risk of these reactions is low relative to other neuroleptics). May be associated with neuroleptic malignant syndrome (NMS). Doses exceeding recommended doses may cause pigmentary retinopathy.

Drug Interactions

Cytochrome P450 Effect: Substrate of CYP2C19 (minor), 2D6 (major); **Inhibits** CYP1A2 (weak), 2C8/9 (weak), 2D6 (moderate), 2E1 (weak)

Decreased Effect: Aluminum salts may decrease the absorption of phenothiazines. The efficacy of amphetamines may be diminished by antipsychotics; in addition, amphetamines may increase psychotic symptoms; avoid concurrent use. Anticholinergics may inhibit the therapeutic response to phenothiazines and excess anticholinergic effects may occur (includes benztropine, trihexyphenidyl, biperiden, and drugs with significant anticholinergic activity). Chlorpromazine (and possibly other low potency antipsychotics) may diminish the pressor effects of epinephrine. The antihypertensive effects of guanethidine or guanadrel may be inhibited by phenothiazines. Phenothiazines may inhibit the antiparkinsonian effect of levodopa. Enzyme inducers may enhance the hepatic metabolism of phenothiazines; larger doses may be required; includes rifampin, rifabutin, barbiturates, phenytoin, and cigarette smoking. Thioridazine may decrease the levels/effects of CYP2D6 prodrug substrates (eg, codeine, hydrocodone, oxycodone, tramadol).

Increased Effect/Toxicity: Concurrent use fluvoxamine, propranolol, and pindolol. The levels/effects of thioridazine may be increased by chlorpromazine, delavirdine, fluoxetine, miconazole, paroxetine, pergolide, quinidine, quinine, ritonavir, ropinirole, and other CYP2D6 inhibitors. **Thioridazine is contraindicated with strong inhibitors of this enzyme.**

Drugs which alter the QT$_c$ interval may be additive with thioridazine, increasing the risk of malignant arrhythmias; includes type Ia antiarrhythmics, TCAs, and some quinolone antibiotics (sparfloxacin, moxifloxacin and gatifloxacin). **These agents are contraindicated with thioridazine.** Potassium depleting agents may increase the risk of serious arrhythmias with thioridazine (includes many diuretics, aminoglycosides, and amphotericin).

Phenothiazines inhibit the ability of bromocriptine to lower serum prolactin concentrations. The sedative effects of CNS depressants or ethanol may be additive with phenothiazines. Phenothiazines and trazodone may produce additive hypotensive effects. Metoclopramide may increase risk of extrapyramidal symptoms (EPS). Concurrent use of antihypertensives may result in additive hypotensive effects (particularly orthostasis).

Thioridazine may increase the levels/effects of amphetamines, beta-blockers, dextromethorphan, fluoxetine, lidocaine, mirtazapine, nefazodone, paroxetine, risperidone, ritonavir, tricyclic antidepressants, venlafaxine, and other CYP2D6 substrates. **Concurrent use with fluvoxamine is contraindicated.**

Phenothiazines may produce neurotoxicity with lithium; this is a rare effect. Rare cases of respiratory paralysis have been reported with concurrent use of phenothiazines and polypeptide antibiotics. Naltrexone in combination with thioridazine has been reported to cause lethargy and somnolence. Phenylpropanolamine has been reported to result in cardiac arrhythmias when combined with thioridazine.

Nutritional/Ethanol Interactions

Ethanol: Avoid ethanol (may increase CNS depression).

Herb/Nutraceutical: Avoid kava kava, valerian, St John's wort, gotu kola (may increase CNS depression). Avoid dong quai, St John's wort (may also cause photosensitization).

Lab Interactions False-positives for phenylketonuria, urinary amylase, uroporphyrins, urobilinogen

Adverse Reactions Frequency not defined.

Cardiovascular: Hypotension, orthostatic hypotension, peripheral edema, ECG changes

Central nervous system: EPS (pseudoparkinsonism, akathisia, dystonias, tardive dyskinesia), dizziness, drowsiness, neuroleptic malignant syndrome (NMS), impairment of temperature regulation, lowering of seizure threshold, seizure

Dermatologic: Increased sensitivity to sun, rash, discoloration of skin (blue-gray)

Endocrine & metabolic: Changes in menstrual cycle, libido (changes in), breast pain, galactorrhea, amenorrhea

Gastrointestinal: Constipation, weight gain, nausea, vomiting, stomach pain, xerostomia, nausea, vomiting, diarrhea

Genitourinary: Difficulty in urination, ejaculatory disturbances, urinary retention, priapism

Hematologic: Agranulocytosis, leukopenia

Hepatic: Cholestatic jaundice, hepatotoxicity

Neuromuscular & skeletal: Tremor

Ocular: Pigmentary retinopathy, blurred vision, cornea and lens changes

Respiratory: Nasal congestion

Overdosage/Toxicology Symptoms of overdose include deep sleep, coma, extrapyramidal symptoms, abnormal involuntary muscle movements, hypotension, and arrhythmias.

Immediate cardiac monitoring, including continuous electrocardiographic monitoring, to detect arrhythmias. Avoid use of medications that also prolong the QT_c interval, such as disopyramide, procainamide, and quinidine. Following initiation of essential overdose management, toxic symptom treatment and supportive treatment should be initiated. Hypotension usually responds to I.V. fluids or Trendelenburg positioning. If unresponsive to these measures, the use of a parenteral inotrope may be required (eg, norepinephrine 0.1-0.2 mcg/kg/minute titrated to response); do not use epinephrine or dopamine. Seizures commonly respond to diazepam (I.V. 5-10 mg bolus in adults every 15 minutes if needed up to a total of 30 mg; I.V. 0.25-0.4 mg/kg/dose up to a total of 10 mg in children) or to phenytoin. Avoid barbiturates (may potentiate respiratory depression). Neuroleptics often cause extrapyramidal symptoms (eg, dystonic reactions) requiring management with diphenhydramine 1-2 mg/kg (adults) up to a maximum of 50 mg I.M. or I.V. slow push followed by a maintenance dose for 48-72 hours. When these reactions are unresponsive to diphenhydramine, benztropine mesylate I.V. 1-2 mg (adults) may be effective. These agents are generally effective within 2-5 minutes.

Pharmacodynamics/Kinetics

Duration of Action: 4-5 days

Time to Peak: Serum: ~1 hour

Half-Life Elimination: 21-25 hours

Dosing

Adults:

Schizophrenia/psychosis: Oral: Initial: 50-100 mg 3 times/day with gradual increments as needed and tolerated; maximum: 800 mg/day in 2-4 divided doses

Depressive disorders, dementia: Oral: Initial: 25 mg 3 times/day; maintenance dose: 20-200 mg/day

Elderly: Behavioral symptoms associated with dementia: Oral: Initial: 10-25 mg 1-2 times/day; increase at 4- to 7-day intervals by 10-25 mg/day; increase dose intervals (once daily, twice daily, etc) as necessary to control response or side effects. Maximum daily dose: 400 mg; gradual increases (titration) may prevent some side effects or decrease their severity.

Pediatrics:

Schizophrenia/psychosis: Oral:

Children >2-12 years: Range: 0.5-3 mg/kg/day in 2-3 divided doses; usual: 1 mg/kg/day; maximum: 3 mg/kg/day

Children >12 years: Refer to adult dosing.

Behavior problems: Oral:

Children >2-12 years: Initial: 10 mg 2-3 times/day, increase gradually.

Children >12 years: Refer to adult dosing.

Severe psychoses: Oral:

Children >2-12 years: Initial: 25 mg 2-3 times/day, increase gradually.

Children >12 years: Refer to adult dosing.

Renal Impairment: Not dialyzable (0% to 5%)

Available Dosage Forms

Solution, oral concentrate, as hydrochloride (Thioridazine Intensol™): 30 mg/mL (120 mL); 100 mg/mL (120 mL) [contains alcohol <0.5%; fruit-mint flavor]

Tablet, as hydrochloride: 10 mg, 15 mg, 25 mg, 50 mg, 100 mg, 150 mg, 200 mg

Monitoring and Teaching Issues

Physical Assessment: Assess other medications patient is taking for effectiveness and interactions. Review ophthalmic exam and monitor laboratory results, therapeutic effectiveness (mental status, mood, affect, gait), and adverse reactions at beginning of therapy and periodically with long-term use. Monitor for CNS depression/level of sedation. Avoid skin contact with liquid medication; may cause contact dermatitis (wash immediately with warm, soapy water). Initiate at lower doses and taper dosage slowly when discontinuing. Assess knowledge/teach patient appropriate use, interventions to reduce side effects, and adverse symptoms to report.

Monitoring Laboratory Tests: Baseline ECG; serum potassium, lipid profile, fasting blood glucose and Hgb A_{1c}; BMI; do not initiate if QT_c >450 msec

Patient Education: Use exactly as directed; do not increase dose or frequency. Do not discontinue without consulting prescriber. Tablets/capsules may be taken with food. Mix oral solution with 2-4 oz of liquid (eg, juice, milk, water, pudding). Do not take within 2 hours of any antacid. Store away from light. Avoid alcohol or caffeine and other prescription or OTC medications not approved by prescriber. Maintain adequate hydration (2-3 L/day of fluids) unless instructed to restrict fluid intake. Avoid skin contact with liquid medication; may cause contact dermatitis (wash immediately with warm, soapy water). May turn urine red-brown (normal). You may experience excess drowsiness, lightheadedness, dizziness, or blurred vision (use caution driving or when engaging in tasks requiring alertness until response to drug is known); nausea, vomiting, or dry mouth (small frequent meals, frequent mouth care, chewing gum, or sucking lozenges may help); constipation (increased exercise, fluids, fruit, or fiber may help); postural hypotension (use caution climbing stairs or when changing position from lying or sitting to standing); urinary retention (void before taking medication); ejaculatory dysfunction (reversible); decreased perspiration (avoid

(Continued)

Thioridazine (Continued)

strenuous exercise in hot environments); or photosensitivity (use sunscreen, wear protective clothing and eyewear, and avoid direct sunlight). Report persistent CNS effects (eg, trembling fingers, altered gait or balance, excessive sedation, seizures, unusual movements, anxiety, abnormal thoughts, confusion, personality changes); chest pain, palpitations, rapid heartbeat, severe dizziness; unresolved urinary retention or changes in urinary pattern; altered menstrual pattern, change in libido, swelling or pain in breasts (male or female); vision changes; skin rash, irritation, or changes in color of skin (gray-blue); or worsening of condition. **Pregnancy/breast-feeding precautions:** Inform prescriber if you are or intend to become pregnant. Breast-feeding is not recommended.

Geriatric Considerations: (See Warnings/Precautions, Adverse Reactions, and Overdose/Toxicology.) Elderly patients have an increased risk of adverse response to side effects or adverse reactions to antipsychotics.

Pregnancy Risk Factor: C

Lactation: Excretion in breast milk unknown/not recommended

Administration

Oral: Oral concentrate must be diluted in 2-4 oz of liquid (eg, water, fruit juice, carbonated drinks, milk, or pudding) before administration. Do not take antacid within 2 hours of taking drug. Thioridazine concentrate is not compatible with carbamazepine suspension; schedule dosing at least 1-2 hours apart from each other. **Note:** Avoid skin contact with oral suspension or solution; may cause contact dermatitis.

Storage: Protect all dosage forms from light.

Related Information

Antipsychotic Agents *on page 1717*
Antipsychotic Medication Guidelines *on page 1766*
Federal OBRA Regulations: Recommended Maximum Doses *on page 1773*

- ◆ **Thioridazine Hydrochloride** *see* Thioridazine *on page 1463*
- ◆ **Thioridazine Intensol™** *see* Thioridazine *on page 1463*

Thiotepa (thye oh TEP a)

Synonyms TESPA; Thiophosphoramide; Triethylenethiophosphoramide; TSPA

Generic Available Yes

Pharmacologic Category Antineoplastic Agent, Alkylating Agent

Use Treatment of superficial tumors of the bladder; palliative treatment of adenocarcinoma of breast or ovary; lymphomas and sarcomas; controlling intracavitary effusions caused by metastatic tumors; I.T. use: CNS leukemia/lymphoma, CNS metastases

Mechanism of Action/Effect Alkylating agent that reacts with DNA phosphate groups to produce cross-linking of DNA strands leading to inhibition of DNA, RNA, and protein synthesis; mechanism of action has not been explored as thoroughly as the other alkylating agents, it is presumed that the aziridine rings open and react as nitrogen mustard; reactivity is enhanced at a lower pH

Contraindications Hypersensitivity to thiotepa or any component of the formulation; severe myelosuppression with leukocyte count <3000/mm^3 or platelet count <150,000 mm^3, except in stem cell transplant; pregnancy

Warnings/Precautions The U.S. Food and Drug Administration (FDA) currently recommends that procedures for proper handling and disposal of antineoplastic agents be considered. Appropriate safety equipment is recommended for preparation, administration, and disposal of antineoplastics. If thiotepa contacts the skin, wash and flush thoroughly with water. Potentially mutagenic, carcinogenic, and teratogenic. Reduce dosage in patients with hepatic, renal, or bone marrow damage.

Drug Interactions

Cytochrome P450 Effect: Inhibits CYP2B6 (weak)

Increased Effect/Toxicity: Other alkylating agents or irradiation used concomitantly with thiotepa intensifies toxicity rather than enhancing therapeutic response. Prolonged muscular paralysis and respiratory depression may occur when neuromuscular blocking agents are administered. Succinylcholine and other neuromuscular blocking agents' action can be prolonged due to thiotepa inhibiting plasma pseudocholinesterase.

Nutritional/Ethanol Interactions

Ethanol: Avoid ethanol (due to GI irritation).

Herb/Nutraceutical: Avoid black cohosh, dong quai in estrogen-dependent tumors.

Adverse Reactions

>10%:

Hematopoietic: Dose-limiting toxicity which is dose related and cumulative; moderate to severe leukopenia and severe thrombocytopenia have occurred. Anemia and pancytopenia may become fatal, so careful hematologic monitoring is required; intravesical administration may cause bone marrow suppression as well.

Hematologic: Myelosuppressive:
WBC: Moderate
Platelets: Severe
Onset: 7-10 days
Nadir: 14 days
Recovery: 28 days

Local: Pain at injection site

1% to 10%:

Central nervous system: Dizziness, fever, headache

Dermatologic: Alopecia, rash, pruritus, hyperpigmentation with high-dose therapy

Endocrine & metabolic: Hyperuricemia

Gastrointestinal: Anorexia, nausea and vomiting rarely occur
Emetic potential: Low (<10%)

Genitourinary: Hemorrhagic cystitis

Renal: Hematuria

Miscellaneous: Tightness of the throat, allergic reactions

Overdosage/Toxicology Symptoms of overdose include nausea, vomiting, precipitation of uric acid in kidney tubules, bone marrow suppression, and bleeding. Therapy is supportive only. Thiotepa is dialyzable. Transfusions of whole blood or platelets have been proven beneficial.

Pharmacodynamics/Kinetics
Absorption: Intracavitary instillation: Unreliable (10% to 100%) through bladder mucosa; I.M.: variable
Half-Life Elimination: Terminal: Dose-dependent clearance: 109 minutes
Metabolism: Extensively hepatic
Excretion: Urine (as metabolites and unchanged drug)

Dosing
Adults & Elderly: Refer to individual protocols. Dosing must be based on the clinical and hematologic response of the patient.

Usual dose (range):
I.M., I.V., SubQ: 30-60 mg/m^2 once weekly
I.V.: 0.3-0.4 mg/kg by rapid I.V. administration every 1-4 weeks, **or** 0.2 mg/kg or 6-8 mg/m^2/day for 4-5 days every 2-4 weeks
I.M.: 15-30 mg in various schedules have been given
Intracavitary: 0.6-0.8 mg/kg or 30-60 mg weekly
Intrapericardial: 15-30 mg
Intrathecal: 10-15 mg or 5-11.5 mg/m^2

Pediatrics: Refer to individual protocols; dosing must be based on the clinical and hematologic response of the patient. Children: Sarcomas: I.V.: 25-65 mg/m^2 as a single dose every 21 days.

Renal Impairment: Use with extreme caution, reduced dose may be warranted.

Available Dosage Forms Injection, powder for reconstitution: 15 mg, 30 mg

Monitoring and Teaching Issues
Physical Assessment: Assess potential for interactions with other pharmacological agents patient may be taking (eg, other alkylating agents or irradiation used concomitantly with thiotepa intensifies toxicity; prolonged muscular paralysis and respiratory depression may occur when neuromuscular blocking agents are administered; see Drug Interactions). See Administration for infusion specifics. Monitor results of laboratory tests closely (eg, anemia and pancytopenia can become fatal). Assess adverse response on a regular basis (eg, myelosuppression, leukopenia, hematuria; see Adverse Reactions). Teach patient possible side effects/appropriate interventions (eg, importance of adequate hydration) and adverse symptoms to report (see Patient Education).

Monitoring Laboratory Tests: CBC with differential, platelet count, uric acid, urinalysis

Patient Education: Do not take any new medication during therapy unless approved by prescriber (especially aspirin or aspirin-containing products). If administered by infusion: report immediately any redness, pain, swelling, or burning at infusion site. You will require regular blood tests to assess response to therapy. Maintain adequate hydration to prevent kidney damage (2-3 L/day of fluids) unless instructed to restrict fluid intake. You may have increased sensitivity to infection (avoid crowds and exposure to infection and do not have any vaccinations unless approved by prescriber). May cause nausea, vomiting, or loss of appetite (small frequent meals, chewing gum, or sucking lozenges may help); rash; or hair loss. Report unusual bleeding or bruising; persistent fever or chills; sore throat; sores in mouth or vagina; blackened stool; or respiratory difficulty. **Pregnancy/breast-feeding precautions:** Inform prescriber if you are pregnant. Do not get pregnant (females) or cause a pregnancy (males) during therapy and for 1 month following completion of therapy. Consult prescriber for instruction on appropriate barrier contraceptive measures. This drug may cause severe fetal defects. Breast-feeding is not recommended.

Pregnancy Risk Factor: D
Lactation: Enters breast milk/not recommended

Administration
I.V.: Administer either as a short (10-60 minute) infusion or 1-2 minute push; a 1 mg/mL solution is considered isotonic; not a vesicant
Other: Intravesical lavage: Instill directly into the bladder and retain for at least 2 hours; patient should be repositioned every 15-30 minutes for maximal exposure
Reconstitution: Reconstitute each vial with SWFI to make a 10 mg/mL solution. Solutions for infusion should be diluted to a concentration ≥5 mg/mL in 5% dextrose or 1, 3, or 5 mg/mL in 0.9% sodium chloride injection. Solutions for intravesicular administration should be diluted in 30-60 mL SWFI or NS. Solutions for intrathecal administration should be diluted in 1-5 mL NS or Elliott's B Solution.
Compatibility:
Y-site administration: Incompatible with cisplatin, filgrastim, minocycline, vinorelbine
Compatibility when admixed: Incompatible with cisplatin
Storage: Store intact vials under refrigeration (2°C to 8°C) and protect from light. Reconstituted solutions (10 mg/mL in SWFI) are stable for up to 28 days under refrigeration (4°C to 8°C) or 7 days at room temperature (25°C).
Solutions for infusion in D$_5$W (≥5 mg/mL) are stable for 14 days under refrigeration (4°C) or 3 days at room temperature (23°C).
Solutions for infusion in NS (1, 3, or 5 mg/mL) are stable for 48 hours under refrigeration (4°C to 8°C) or 24 hours at room temperature (25°C). Solutions in NS at a concentration of ≤0.5 mg/mL are stable for <1 hour.

Additional Information A 1 mg/mL solution is considered isotonic.

Thiothixene (thye oh THIKS een)
U.S. Brand Names Navane®
Synonyms Tiotixene
Generic Available Yes
Pharmacologic Category Antipsychotic Agent, Typical
(Continued)

Thiothixene *(Continued)*

Medication Safety Issues
Sound-alike/look-alike issues:
Thiothixene may be confused with thioridazine
Navane® may be confused with Norvasc®, Nubain®

Use Management of schizophrenia

Unlabeled/Investigational Use Psychotic disorders

Mechanism of Action/Effect Thiothixene is a thioxanthene antipsychotic which elicits anti-psychotic activity by postsynaptic blockade of CNS dopamine receptors resulting in inhibition of dopamine-mediated effects; also has alpha-adrenergic blocking activity

Contraindications Hypersensitivity to thiothixene or any component of the formulation; severe CNS depression; circulatory collapse; blood dyscrasias; coma

Warnings/Precautions May be sedating, use with caution in disorders where CNS depression is a feature. Use with caution in Parkinson's disease. Caution in patients with hemodynamic instability; predisposition to seizures; subcortical brain damage; bone marrow suppression; severe cardiac, hepatic, renal, or respiratory disease. Esophageal dysmotility and aspiration have been associated with antipsychotic use - use with caution in patients at risk of pneumonia (ie, Alzheimer's disease). Caution in breast cancer or other prolactin-dependent tumors (may elevate prolactin levels). May alter temperature regulation or mask toxicity of other drugs due to antiemetic effects. May alter cardiac conduction - life-threatening arrhythmias have occurred with therapeutic doses of neuroleptics. May cause orthostatic hypotension - use with caution in patients at risk of this effect or those who would tolerate transient hypotensive episodes (cerebrovascular disease, cardiovascular disease, or other medications which may predispose). Safety and efficacy in children <12 years of age have not been established.

May cause anticholinergic effects, use caution in patients with decreased gastrointestinal motility, urinary retention, BPH, xerostomia, visual problems, narrow-angle glaucoma (screening is recommended), and myasthenia gravis. Relative to other neuroleptics, thiothixene has a low potency of cholinergic blockade.

May cause extrapyramidal symptoms, including pseudoparkinsonism, acute dystonic reactions, akathisia, and tardive dyskinesia (risk of these reactions is high relative to other neuroleptics). May be associated with neuroleptic malignant syndrome (NMS) or pigmentary retinopathy.

Drug Interactions

Cytochrome P450 Effect: Substrate of CYP1A2 (major); **Inhibits** CYP2D6 (weak)

Decreased Effect: CYP1A2 inducers may decrease the levels/effects of thiothixene; example inducers include aminoglutethimide, carbamazepine, phenobarbital, and rifampin. Thiothixene inhibits the activity of guanadrel, guanethidine, levodopa, and bromocriptine. Benztropine (and other anticholinergics) may inhibit the therapeutic response to thiothixene. Thiothixene and low potency antipsychotics may reverse the pressor effects of epinephrine.

Increased Effect/Toxicity: CYP1A2 inhibitors may increase the levels/effects of thiothixene; example inhibitors include amiodarone, ciprofloxacin, fluvoxamine, ketoconazole, norfloxacin, ofloxacin, and rofecoxib. Thiothixene and CNS depressants (ethanol, narcotics) may produce additive CNS depressant effects. Thiothixene may increase the effect/toxicity of antihypertensives, benztropine (and other anticholinergic agents), lithium, trazodone, and TCAs. Thiothixene's concentrations may be increased by chloroquine, sulfadoxine-pyrimethamine, and propranolol. Metoclopramide may increase risk of extrapyramidal symptoms (EPS).

Nutritional/Ethanol Interactions
Ethanol: Avoid ethanol (may increase CNS depression).
Herb/Nutraceutical: Avoid kava kava, valerian, St John's wort, gotu kola (may increase CNS depression).

Lab Interactions Increased cholesterol (S), glucose; decreased uric acid (S); may cause false-positive pregnancy test

Adverse Reactions Frequency not defined.
Cardiovascular: Hypotension, tachycardia, syncope, nonspecific ECG changes
Central nervous system: Extrapyramidal signs (pseudoparkinsonism, akathisia, dystonias, lightheadedness, tardive dyskinesia), dizziness, drowsiness, restlessness, agitation, insomnia
Dermatologic: Discoloration of skin (blue-gray), rash, pruritus, urticaria, photosensitivity
Endocrine & metabolic: Changes in menstrual cycle, libido (changes in), breast pain, galactorrhea, lactation, amenorrhea, gynecomastia, hyperglycemia, hypoglycemia
Gastrointestinal: Weight gain, nausea, vomiting, stomach pain, constipation, xerostomia, increased salivation
Genitourinary: Difficulty in urination, ejaculatory disturbances, impotence
Hematologic: Leukopenia, leukocytes
Neuromuscular & skeletal: Tremors
Ocular: Pigmentary retinopathy, blurred vision
Respiratory: Nasal congestion
Miscellaneous: Diaphoresis

Overdosage/Toxicology Symptoms of overdose include muscle twitching, drowsiness, dizziness, rigidity, tremor, hypotension, and cardiac arrhythmias. Treatment is symptom-directed and supportive.

Pharmacodynamics/Kinetics
Half-Life Elimination: >24 hours with chronic use
Metabolism: Extensively hepatic

Dosing
Adults:
Mild to moderate psychosis: Oral: 2 mg 3 times/day, up to 20-30 mg/day; more severe psychosis: Initial: 5 mg 2 times/day, may increase gradually, if necessary; maximum: 60 mg/day

Rapid tranquilization of the agitated patient (administered every 30-60 minutes):
Oral: 5-10 mg; average total dose for tranquilization: 15-30 mg

Elderly: Nonpsychotic patients, dementia behavior: Initial: 1-2 mg 1-2 times/day; increase dose at 4- to 7-day intervals by 1-2 mg/day. Increase dosing intervals (bid, tid, etc) as necessary to control response or side effects; maximum daily dose: 30 mg. Gradual increases in dose may prevent some side effects or decrease their severity.

Pediatrics:
Children <12 years (unlabeled use): Oral: 0.25 mg/kg/24 hours in divided doses (dose not well established; use not recommended)

Children >12 years: Mild to moderate psychosis: Refer to adult dosing.

Renal Impairment: Not dialyzable (0% to 5%)

Available Dosage Forms [DSC] = Discontinued product

Capsule: 1 mg, 2 mg, 5 mg, 10 mg
   Navane®: 1 mg, 2 mg, 5 mg, 10 mg, 20 mg

Solution, oral concentrate, as hydrochloride [DSC]: 5 mg/mL (120 mL) [fruit flavor]

Monitoring and Teaching Issues

Physical Assessment: Assess other medications patient is taking for effectiveness and interactions. Review ophthalmic exam and monitor laboratory results, therapeutic effectiveness, and adverse reactions at beginning of therapy and periodically with long-term use. Avoid skin contact with liquid medication; may cause contact dermatitis (wash immediately with warm, soapy water). Initiate at lower doses and taper dosage slowly when discontinuing. Assess knowledge/teach patient appropriate use, interventions to reduce side effects, and adverse symptoms to report.

Monitoring Laboratory Tests: Lipid profile, fasting blood glucose, Hgb A_{1c}; BMI

Patient Education: Use exactly as directed; do not increase dose or frequency. Do not discontinue without consulting prescriber. Capsules may be taken with food. Mix oral solution with 2-4 oz of liquid (eg, juice, milk, water, pudding). Do not take within 2 hours of any antacid. Avoid alcohol or caffeine and other prescription or OTC medications not approved by prescriber. Maintain adequate hydration (2-3 L/day of fluids) unless instructed to restrict fluid intake. May turn urine red-brown (normal). You may experience excess drowsiness, lightheadedness, dizziness, or blurred vision (use caution driving or when engaging in tasks requiring alertness until response to drug is known); nausea or vomiting (small frequent meals, frequent mouth care, chewing gum, or sucking lozenges may help); constipation (increased exercise, fluids, fruit, or fiber may help); postural hypotension (use caution climbing stairs or when changing position from lying or sitting to standing); urinary retention (void before taking medication); ejaculatory dysfunction (reversible); decreased perspiration (avoid strenuous exercise in hot environments); or photosensitivity (use sunscreen, wear protective clothing and eyewear, and avoid direct sunlight). Report persistent CNS effects (eg, trembling fingers, altered gait or balance, excessive sedation, seizures, unusual movements, anxiety, abnormal thoughts, confusion, personality changes); chest pain, palpitations, rapid heartbeat, severe dizziness; unresolved urinary retention or changes in urinary pattern; altered menstrual pattern, change in libido, swelling or pain in breasts (male or female); vision changes; skin rash, irritation, or changes in color of skin (gray-blue); or worsening of condition. **Pregnancy/breast-feeding precautions:** Inform prescriber if you are or intend to become pregnant. Breast-feeding is not recommended.

Geriatric Considerations: (See Warnings/Precautions, Adverse Reactions, and Overdose/Toxicology.) Elderly patients have an increased risk of adverse response to side effects or adverse reactions to antipsychotics.

Pregnancy Risk Factor: C

Lactation: Excretion in breast milk unknown/not recommended

Administration

Oral: Oral (concentrate) solution: Dilute immediately before administration with water, fruit juice, milk, etc. **Note:** Avoid skin contact with oral medication; may cause contact dermatitis.

Related Information

Antipsychotic Agents *on page 1717*
Federal OBRA Regulations: Recommended Maximum Doses *on page 1773*

♦ **Thonzonium, Neomycin, Colistin, and Hydrocortisone** *see* Neomycin, Colistin, Hydrocortisone, and Thonzonium *on page 1069*

♦ **Thorazine® [DSC]** *see* ChlorproMAZINE *on page 312*

♦ **Thorets [OTC]** *see* Benzocaine *on page 181*

♦ **Thrombinar®** *see page 1625*

♦ **Thrombin, Topical** *see page 1625*

♦ **Thrombogen®** *see page 1625*

♦ **Thrombostat®** *see page 1625*

♦ **Thymocyte-Stimulating Factor** *see* Aldesleukin *on page 62*

♦ **Thypinone® Injection** *see page 1625*

♦ **Thyrogen®** *see page 1625*

Thyroid (THYE roid)

U.S. Brand Names Armour® Thyroid; Nature-Throid® NT; Westhroid®

Synonyms Desiccated Thyroid; Thyroid Extract; Thyroid USP

Generic Available Yes

Pharmacologic Category Thyroid Product

Use Replacement or supplemental therapy in hypothyroidism; pituitary TSH suppressants (thyroid nodules, thyroiditis, multinodular goiter, thyroid cancer), thyrotoxicosis, diagnostic suppression tests

Mechanism of Action/Effect The primary active compound is T_3 (triiodothyronine), which may be converted from T_4 (thyroxine) and then circulates throughout the body to influence growth and maturation of various tissues
(Continued)

Thyroid *(Continued)*

Contraindications Hypersensitivity to beef or pork or any component of the formulation; recent myocardial infarction; thyrotoxicosis uncomplicated by hypothyroidism; uncorrected adrenal insufficiency

Warnings/Precautions Ineffective for weight reduction. High doses may produce serious or even life-threatening toxic effects particularly when used with some anorectic drugs. Use cautiously in patients with pre-existing cardiovascular disease (angina, CHD), elderly since they may be more likely to have compromised cardiovascular function. Chronic hypothyroidism predisposes patients to coronary artery disease. Desiccated thyroid contains variable amounts of T_3, T_4, and other triiodothyronine compounds which are more likely to cause cardiac signs or symptoms due to fluctuating levels. Should avoid use in the elderly for this reason. Many clinicians consider levothyroxine to be the drug of choice for thyroid replacement.

Drug Interactions

Decreased Effect: Thyroid hormones increase the therapeutic need for oral hypoglycemics or insulin. Cholestyramine can bind thyroid and reduce its absorption. Phenytoin may decrease thyroxine serum levels. Thyroid hormone may decrease effect of oral sulfonylureas.

Increased Effect/Toxicity: Thyroid may potentiate the hypoprothrombinemic effect of oral anticoagulants. Tricyclic antidepressants (TAD) coadministered with thyroid hormone may increase potential for toxicity of both drugs.

Lab Interactions Many drugs may have effects on thyroid function tests: para-aminosalicylic acid, aminoglutethimide, amiodarone, barbiturates, carbamazepine, chloral hydrate, clofibrate, colestipol, corticosteroids, danazol, diazepam, estrogens, ethionamide, fluorouracil, I.V. heparin, insulin, lithium, methadone, methimazole, mitotane, nitroprusside, oxyphenbutazone, phenylbutazone, PTU, perphenazine, phenytoin, propranolol, salicylates, sulfonylureas, and thiazides.

Overdosage/Toxicology Chronic excessive use results in signs and symptoms of hyperthyroidism, weight loss, nervousness, sweating, tachycardia, insomnia, heat intolerance, palpitations, vomiting, psychosis, fever, seizures, angina, arrhythmias, and CHF in those predisposed.

Reduce dose or temporarily discontinue therapy. Hypothalamic-pituitary-thyroid axis will return to normal in 6-8 weeks. Serum T_4 levels do not correlate well with toxicity. In massive acute ingestion, reduce GI absorption and give general supportive care.

Pharmacodynamics/Kinetics

Absorption: T_4: 48% to 79%; T_3: 95%; desiccated thyroid contains thyroxine, liothyronine, and iodine (primarily bound)

Half-Life Elimination: Serum: Liothyronine: 1-2 days; Thyroxine: 6-7 days

Metabolism: Thyroxine: Largely converted to liothyronine

Dosing

Adults: Hypothyroidism: Oral: Initial: 15-30 mg; increase with 15 mg increments every 2-4 weeks; use 15 mg in patients with cardiovascular disease or myxedema. Maintenance dose: Usually 60-120 mg/day; monitor TSH and clinical symptoms.

Note: Thyroid cancer requires larger amounts than replacement therapy.

Elderly: Not recommended for use in the elderly (see Geriatric Considerations).

Pediatrics: Hypothyroidism: Oral: See table.

Recommended Pediatric Dosage for Congenital Hypothyroidism

Age	Daily Dose (mg)	Daily Dose/kg (mg)
0-6 mo	15-30	4.8-6
6-12 mo	30-45	3.6-4.8
1-5 y	45-60	3-3.6
6-12 y	60-90	2.4-3
>12 y	>90	1.2-1.8

Available Dosage Forms

Capsule: 15 mg, 30 mg, 60 mg, 90 mg, 120 mg, 180 mg, 240 mg

Tablet: 30 mg, 32.5 mg, 60 mg, 65 mg, 120 mg, 130 mg, 180 mg

Armour® Thyroid: 15 mg, 30 mg, 60 mg, 90 mg, 120 mg, 180 mg, 240 mg, 300 mg

Nature-Throid® NT, Westhroid®: 32.4 mg, 64.8 mg, 129.6 mg, 194.4 mg

Monitoring and Teaching Issues

Physical Assessment: Use caution with cardiovascular disease and advanced age; ineffective for weight reduction (see Warnings/Precautions for use cautions). Assess potential for interactions with other pharmacological agents and herbal products patient may be taking (eg, may decrease level/effect of oral hypoglycemics, increase risk of toxicity with TCAs and some anorexiants; see Drug Interactions). Assess results of laboratory tests at baseline and regularly during therapy. **Note:** Many drugs may effect thyroid function tests when assessing results of thyroid function tests. Monitor for hyperthyroidism (weight loss, nervousness, sweating, tachycardia, insomnia, heat intolerance, palpitations, vomiting, psychosis, fever, seizures, angina, arrhythmias; see Adverse Reactions). Caution patients with diabetes to monitor glucose levels closely (may increase need for oral hypoglycemics or insulin). Teach patient appropriate use, possible side effects/appropriate interventions, and adverse symptoms to report (see Patient Education).

Monitoring Laboratory Tests: Monitor T_4 and TSH. TSH is the most reliable guide for evaluating adequacy of thyroid replacement dosage. TSH may be elevated during the first few months of thyroid replacement despite patients being clinically euthyroid. In cases where T_4 remains low and TSH is within normal limits, an evaluation of "free" (unbound) T_4 is needed to evaluate further increase in dosage.

Patient Education: Do not take any new medication during therapy unless approved by prescriber. Thyroid replacement therapy is generally for life. Take as directed, in the morning before breakfast. Do not take antacids or iron preparations within 8 hours of thyroid medication. Do not change brands and do not discontinue without consulting prescriber. Consult prescriber if drastically increasing or decreasing intake of goitrogenic food (eg, asparagus, cabbage, peas, turnip greens, broccoli, spinach, Brussels sprouts, lettuce, soybeans). If you have diabetes, monitor glucose levels closely (may increase need for oral hypoglycemics or insulin). Report chest pain, rapid heart rate, palpitations, heat intolerance, excessive sweating, increased nervousness, agitation, or lethargy.

Dietary Considerations: Should be taken on an empty stomach.

Geriatric Considerations: Desiccated thyroid contains variable amounts of T_3, T_4, and other triiodothyronine compounds which are more likely to cause cardiac signs or symptoms due to fluctuating levels. Should avoid use in the elderly for this reason. Many clinicians consider levothyroxine to be the drug of choice.

Pregnancy Risk Factor: A

Lactation: Enters breast milk/compatible

- ◆ **Thyroid Extract** *see* Thyroid *on page 1469*
- ◆ **Thyroid USP** *see* Thyroid *on page 1469*
- ◆ **ThyroSafe™ [OTC]** *see* Potassium Iodide *on page 1237*
- ◆ **ThyroShield™ [OTC]** *see* Potassium Iodide *on page 1237*
- ◆ **Thyrotropin Alpha** *see page 1625*
- ◆ **Tiabendazole** *see* Thiabendazole *on page 1460*

Tiagabine (tye AG a been)

U.S. Brand Names Gabitril®

Synonyms Tiagabine Hydrochloride

Generic Available No

Pharmacologic Category Anticonvulsant, Miscellaneous

Medication Safety Issues
Sound-alike/look-alike issues:
Tiagabine may be confused with tizanidine

Use Adjunctive therapy in adults and children ≥12 years of age in the treatment of partial seizures

Mechanism of Action/Effect The exact mechanism by which tiagabine exerts antiseizure activity is not definitively known; however, *in vitro* experiments demonstrate that it enhances the activity of gamma aminobutyric acid (GABA), the major neuroinhibitory transmitter in the nervous system; it is thought that binding to the GABA uptake carrier inhibits the uptake of GABA into presynaptic neurons, allowing an increased amount of GABA to be available to postsynaptic neurons; based on *in vitro* studies, tiagabine does not inhibit the uptake of dopamine, norepinephrine, serotonin, glutamate, or choline

Contraindications Hypersensitivity to tiagabine or any component of the formulation

Warnings/Precautions New-onset seizures and status epilepticus have been associated with tiagabine use when taken for unlabeled indications. Often these seizures have occurred shortly after the initiation of treatment or shortly after a dosage increase. Seizures have also occurred with very low doses or after several months of therapy. In most cases, patients were using concomitant medications (eg, antidepressants, antipsychotics, stimulants, narcotics). In these instances, the discontinuation of tiagabine, followed by an evaluation for an underlying seizure disorder, is suggested. Use for unapproved indications, however, has not been proven to be safe or effective and is not recommended. When tiagabine is used as an adjunct in partial seizures (an FDA-approved indication), it should not be abruptly discontinued because of the possibility of increasing seizure frequency, unless safety concerns require a more rapid withdrawal. Rarely, nonconvulsive status epilepticus has been reported following abrupt discontinuation or dosage reduction.

Use with caution in patients with hepatic impairment. Experience in patients not receiving enzyme-inducing drugs has been limited; caution should be used in treating any patient who is not receiving one of these medications (decreased dose and slower titration may be required). Weakness, sedation, and confusion may occur with tiagabine use. Patients must be cautioned about performing tasks which require mental alertness (eg, operating machinery or driving). Effects with other sedative drugs or ethanol may be potentiated. Animal studies suggest that tiagabine may bind to retina and uvea; however, no treatment-related ophthalmoscopic changes were seen long-term; periodic monitoring may be considered. May cause serious rash, including Stevens-Johnson syndrome. Safety and efficacy have not been established in children <12 years of age.

Drug Interactions

Cytochrome P450 Effect: Substrate of 3A4 (major)

Decreased Effect: CYP3A4 inducers may decrease the levels/effects of tiagabine; example inducers include aminoglutethimide, carbamazepine, nafcillin, nevirapine, phenobarbital, phenytoin, and rifamycins.

Increased Effect/Toxicity: CYP3A4 inhibitors may increase the levels/effects of tiagabine; example inhibitors include azole antifungals, ciprofloxacin, clarithromycin, diclofenac, doxycycline, erythromycin, imatinib, isoniazid, nefazodone, nicardipine, propofol, protease inhibitors, quinidine, and verapamil. Valproate increased free tiagabine concentrations (*in vitro*) by 40%.

Nutritional/Ethanol Interactions

Ethanol: Avoid ethanol (may increase CNS depression).

Food: Food reduces the rate but not the extent of absorption.

Herb/Nutraceutical: St John's wort may decrease tiagabine levels. Avoid valerian, St John's wort, kava kava, gotu kola (may increase CNS depression).

Adverse Reactions

>10%:

Central nervous system: Concentration decreased, dizziness, nervousness, somnolence

Gastrointestinal: Nausea

(Continued)

Tiagabine (Continued)

Neuromuscular & skeletal: Weakness, tremor

1% to 10%:

Cardiovascular: Chest pain, edema, hypertension, palpitation, peripheral edema, syncope, tachycardia, vasodilation

Central nervous system: Agitation, ataxia, chills, confusion, difficulty with memory, confusion, depersonalization, depression, euphoria, hallucination, hostility, insomnia, malaise, migraine, paranoid reaction, personality disorder, speech disorder

Dermatologic: Alopecia, bruising, dry skin, pruritus, rash

Gastrointestinal: Abdominal pain, diarrhea, gingivitis, increased appetite, mouth ulceration, stomatitis, vomiting, weight gain/loss

Neuromuscular & skeletal: Abnormal gait, arthralgia, dysarthria, hyper-/hypokinesia, hyper-/hypotonia, myasthenia, myalgia, myoclonus, neck pain, paresthesia, reflexes decreased, stupor, twitching, vertigo

Ocular: Abnormal vision, amblyopia, nystagmus

Otic: Ear pain, hearing impairment, otitis media, tinnitus

Respiratory: Bronchitis, cough, dyspnea, epistaxis, pneumonia

Miscellaneous: Allergic reaction, cyst, diaphoresis, flu-like syndrome, lymphadenopathy

Overdosage/Toxicology Somnolence, impaired consciousness, agitation, confusion, speech difficulty, hostility, depression, weakness, myoclonus, and seizures may occur. Treatment is supportive.

Pharmacodynamics/Kinetics

Absorption: Rapid (45 minutes); prolonged with food

Bioavailability: Oral: Absolute: 90%

Time to Peak: Plasma: 45 minutes

Protein Binding: 96%, primarily to albumin and α_1-acid glycoprotein

Half-Life Elimination: 2-5 hours when administered with enzyme inducers; 7-9 hours when administered without enzyme inducers

Metabolism: Hepatic via CYP (primarily 3A4)

Excretion: Feces (63%); urine (25%); 2% as unchanged drug; primarily as metabolites

Dosing

Adults & Elderly: Partial seizures (adjunct): Oral:

Patients receiving enzyme-inducing AED regimens: 4 mg once daily for 1 week; may increase by 4-8 mg weekly to response or up to 56 mg daily in 2-4 divided doses

Patients **not** receiving enzyme-inducing AED regimens: The estimated plasma concentrations of tiagabine in patients not taking enzyme-inducing medications is twice that of patients receiving enzyme-inducing AEDs. Lower doses are required; slower titration may be necessary.

Pediatrics: Partial seizures: Oral:

Patients receiving enzyme-inducing AED regimens: Children 12-18 years: 4 mg once daily for 1 week; may increase to 8 mg daily in 2 divided doses for 1 week; then may increase by 4-8 mg weekly to response or up to 32 mg daily in 2-4 divided doses

Patients **not** receiving enzyme-inducing AED regimens: Refer to adult dosing.

Available Dosage Forms Tablet, as hydrochloride: 2 mg, 4 mg, 12 mg, 16 mg

Monitoring and Teaching Issues

Physical Assessment: Assess effectiveness and interactions of other medications patient may be taking. Monitor therapeutic effectiveness (seizure activity, force, type, duration), laboratory values, and adverse reactions at beginning of therapy and periodically with long-term use. Taper dosage slowly when discontinuing. Assess knowledge/teach patient appropriate use, seizure safety precautions, interventions to reduce side effects, and adverse symptoms to report.

Monitoring Laboratory Tests: A therapeutic range for tiagabine has not been established. Monitor complete blood counts, renal function tests, liver function tests, and routine blood chemistry.

Patient Education: Take exactly as directed; do not increase dose or frequency or discontinue without consulting prescriber. While using this medication, do not use alcohol and other prescription or OTC medications (especially pain medications, sedatives, antihistamines, or hypnotics) without consulting prescriber. Maintain adequate hydration (2-3 L/day of fluids) unless instructed to restrict fluid intake. You may experience drowsiness, dizziness, disturbed concentration, or blurred vision (use caution when driving or engaging in tasks requiring alertness until response to drug is known); or nausea, vomiting, or loss of appetite (small frequent meals, frequent mouth care, chewing gum, or sucking lozenges may help). Wear identification of epileptic status and medications. Report behavioral or CNS changes; skin rash; muscle cramping, weakness, tremors, changes in gait; vision difficulties; persistent GI distress (cramping, pain, vomiting); chest pain, irregular heartbeat, or palpitations; cough or respiratory difficulty; or worsening of seizure activity or loss of seizure control. **Pregnancy/breast-feeding precautions:** Inform prescriber if you are or intend to become pregnant. Breast-feeding is not recommended.

Dietary Considerations: Take with food.

Geriatric Considerations: There has been limited clinical experience with geriatric patients during clinical evaluation - use with caution.

Pregnancy Risk Factor: C

Lactation: Enters breast milk/not recommended

Related Information

Anticonvulsants By Seizure Type on page 1712

♦ **Tiagabine Hydrochloride** see Tiagabine on page 1471

♦ **Tiazac®** see Diltiazem on page 459

♦ **Ticar®** see Ticarcillin on page 1472

Ticarcillin (tye kar SIL in)

U.S. Brand Names Ticar®

Synonyms Ticarcillin Disodium

Generic Available No

Pharmacologic Category Antibiotic, Penicillin

Medication Safety Issues

Sound-alike/look-alike issues:

Ticar® may be confused with Tigan®

Use Treatment of susceptible infections such as septicemia, acute and chronic respiratory tract infections, skin and soft tissue infections, and urinary tract infections due to susceptible strains of *Pseudomonas*, and other gram-negative bacteria

Mechanism of Action/Effect Interferes with bacterial cell wall synthesis during active multiplication, causing cell wall death and resultant bactericidal activity against susceptible bacteria

Contraindications Hypersensitivity to ticarcillin, any component of the formulation, or penicillins

Warnings/Precautions Due to sodium load and adverse effects (anemia, neuropsychological changes), use with caution and modify dosage in patients with renal impairment. Serious and occasionally severe or fatal hypersensitivity (anaphylactoid) reactions have been reported in patients on penicillin therapy (especially with a history of beta-lactam hypersensitivity and/or a history of sensitivity to multiple allergens). Use with caution in patients with seizures.

Drug Interactions

Decreased Effect: Tetracyclines may decrease penicillin effectiveness. Aminoglycosides may cause physical inactivation of aminoglycosides in the presence of high concentrations of ticarcillin and potential toxicity in patients with mild-moderate renal dysfunction. Although anecdotal reports suggest oral contraceptive efficacy could be reduced by penicillins, this has been refuted by more rigorous scientific and clinical data.

Increased Effect/Toxicity: Probenecid may increase penicillin levels. Neuromuscular blockers may have an increased duration of action (neuromuscular blockade). Penicillins may increase the exposure to methotrexate during concurrent therapy; monitor.

Lab Interactions False-positive urinary or serum protein, positive Coombs' test

Adverse Reactions Frequency not defined.

Central nervous system: Confusion, convulsions, drowsiness, fever, Jarisch-Herxheimer reaction

Dermatologic: Rash

Endocrine & metabolic: Electrolyte imbalance

Gastrointestinal: *Clostridium difficile* colitis

Hematologic: Bleeding, eosinophilia, hemolytic anemia, leukopenia, neutropenia, positive Coombs' reaction, thrombocytopenia

Hepatic: Hepatotoxicity, jaundice

Local: Thrombophlebitis

Neuromuscular & skeletal: Myoclonus

Renal: Interstitial nephritis (acute)

Miscellaneous: Anaphylaxis, hypersensitivity reactions

Overdosage/Toxicology Symptoms of penicillin overdose include neuromuscular hypersensitivity (eg, agitation, hallucinations, asterixis, encephalopathy, confusion, and seizures). Electrolyte imbalance may occur if the preparation contains potassium or sodium salts, especially in renal failure. Hemodialysis may be helpful to aid in removal of the drug from blood; otherwise, treatment is supportive or symptom-directed.

Pharmacodynamics/Kinetics

Absorption: I.M.: 86%

Time to Peak: Serum: I.M.: 30-75 minutes

Protein Binding: 45% to 65%

Half-Life Elimination:

Neonates: <1 week old: 3.5-5.6 hours; 1-8 weeks old: 1.3-2.2 hours

Children 5-13 years: 0.9 hour

Adults: 66-72 minutes; prolonged with renal and/or hepatic impairment

Excretion: Almost entirely urine (as unchanged drug and metabolites); feces (3.5%)

Dosing

Adults:

Susceptible infections: I.M., I.V.: 1-4 g every 4-6 hours, usual dose: 3 g I.V. every 4-6 hours

Note: Ticarcillin is generally given I.V., I.M. injection is only for the treatment of uncomplicated urinary tract infections and dose should not exceed 2 g/injection when administered I.M.

Elderly: I.V.: 3 g every 4-6 hours; adjust dosing interval for renal impairment

Pediatrics:

Susceptible infections: I.M., I.V.: Infants and Children:

Systemic infections: I.V.: 200-300 mg/kg/day in divided doses every 4-6 hours

Urinary tract infections: I.M., I.V.: 50-100 mg/kg/day in divided doses every 6-8 hours

Maximum dose: 24 g/day

Note: Ticarcillin is generally given I.V., I.M. injection is only for the treatment of uncomplicated urinary tract infections and dose should not exceed 2 g/injection when administered I.M.

Renal Impairment:

Cl_{cr} 30-60 mL/minute: 2 g every 4 hours or 3 g every 8 hours

Cl_{cr} 10-30 mL/minute: 2 g every 8 hours or 3 g every 12 hours

Cl_{cr} <10 mL/minute: 2 g every 12 hours

Moderately dialyzable (20% to 50%)

Continuous arteriovenous or venovenous hemodiafiltration effects: Dose as for Cl_{cr} 10-50 mL/minute

Available Dosage Forms Injection, powder for reconstitution, as disodium: 3 g, 20 g

(Continued)

Ticarcillin *(Continued)*

Monitoring and Teaching Issues

Physical Assessment: Perform culture and sensitivity test and assess patient's allergy history prior to starting therapy. Use caution with seizure history (see Warnings/Precautions). Assess potential for interactions with other pharmacological agents patient may be taking (see Drug Interactions). See Administration for infusion/injection specifics. Assess results of laboratory tests, therapeutic effectiveness, and adverse reactions (eg, hypersensitivity reactions, opportunistic infection; see Adverse Reactions). Advise patients with diabetes about use of Clinitest®; may cause false reading. Teach patient possible side effects/appropriate interventions and adverse symptoms to report (see Patient Education).

Monitoring Laboratory Tests: Serum electrolytes, bleeding time, and periodic tests of renal, hepatic, and hematologic function; perform culture and sensitivity before administering first dose.

Patient Education: Do not take any new medication during therapy unless approved by prescriber. This drug is only given by injection or infusion; report immediately any redness, swelling, burning, or pain at infusion site or any signs of allergic reaction (eg, respiratory or swallowing difficulty, chest tightness, rash, hives, swelling of lips or mouth). Maintain adequate hydration (2-3 L/day of fluids) unless instructed to restrict fluid intake. If you have diabetes, drug may cause false test results with Clinitest®, consult prescriber for alternative method of glucose monitoring. May cause confusion or drowsiness (use caution when driving or engaging in tasks that require alertness until response to drug is known). Report persistent diarrhea or abdominal pain (do not use antidiarrheal medication without consulting prescriber); bloody urine or stool; muscle pain; mouth sores; respiratory difficulty; skin rash; or signs of opportunistic infection (eg, fever, chills, unhealed sores, white plaques in mouth or vagina, purulent vaginal discharge, fatigue).

Dietary Considerations: Sodium content of 1 g: 119.6-149.5 mg (5.2-6.5 mEq)

Geriatric Considerations: When used as empiric therapy or for documented pseudomonal pneumonia, it is best to combine with an aminoglycoside such as gentamicin or tobramycin. High sodium may limit use in patients with congestive heart failure. Adjust dose for renal function.

Pregnancy Risk Factor: B

Lactation: Enters breast milk/compatible

Administration

I.M.: Do not give more than 2 g per injection.

I.V.: Administer around-the-clock. Administer 1 hour apart from aminoglycosides. Intermittently infusion over 30 minutes to 2 hours.

Compatibility: Stable in D_5W, LR, NS, SWFI

> **Y-site administration: Incompatible** with amphotericin B cholesteryl sulfate complex, fluconazole
>
> **Compatibility in syringe: Incompatible** with doxapram
>
> **Compatibility when admixed: Incompatible** with gentamicin, aminoglycosides

Storage: Reconstituted solution is stable for 72 hours at room temperature and 14 days when refrigerated or 30 days when frozen. For I.V. infusion in NS or D_5W.

Related Information

Antimicrobial Drugs of Choice *on page 1792*

Ticarcillin and Clavulanate Potassium

(tye kar SIL in & klav yoo LAN ate poe TASS ee um)

U.S. Brand Names Timentin®

Synonyms Ticarcillin and Clavulanic Acid

Generic Available No

Pharmacologic Category Antibiotic, Penicillin

Use Treatment of infections of lower respiratory tract, urinary tract, skin and skin structures, bone and joint, and septicemia caused by susceptible organisms. Clavulanate expands activity of ticarcillin to include beta-lactamase producing strains of *S. aureus, H. influenzae, Bacteroides* species, and some other gram-negative bacilli

Mechanism of Action/Effect Ticarcillin interferes with bacterial cell wall synthesis during active multiplication, causing cell wall death and resultant bactericidal activity against susceptible bacteria; clavulanic acid prevents degradation of ticarcillin by binding to the active site on beta-lactamase

Contraindications Hypersensitivity to ticarcillin, clavulanate, any penicillin, or any component of the formulation

Warnings/Precautions Use with caution and modify dosage in patients with renal impairment. Serious and occasionally fatal hypersensitivity (anaphylactoid) reactions have been reported in patients on penicillin therapy. These reactions are more likely to occur in individuals with a history of cephalosporin hypersensitivity and/or a history of sensitivity to multiple allergens.

Drug Interactions

Decreased Effect: Tetracyclines may decrease penicillin effectiveness. Aminoglycosides may cause physical inactivation of aminoglycosides in the presence of high concentrations of ticarcillin and potential toxicity in patients with mild-moderate renal dysfunction. Although anecdotal reports suggest oral contraceptive efficacy could be reduced by penicillins, this has been refuted by more rigorous scientific and clinical data.

Increased Effect/Toxicity: Probenecid may increase penicillin levels. Neuromuscular blockers may have an increased duration of action (neuromuscular blockade). Penicillins may increase the exposure to methotrexate during concurrent therapy; monitor.

Lab Interactions Positive Coombs' test, false-positive urinary proteins

Adverse Reactions Frequency not defined.

Central nervous system: Confusion, convulsions, drowsiness, fever, Jarisch-Herxheimer reaction

Dermatologic: Rash, erythema multiforme, toxic epidermal necrolysis, Stevens-Johnson syndrome

Endocrine & metabolic: Electrolyte imbalance

Gastrointestinal: *Clostridium difficile* colitis

Hematologic: Bleeding, hemolytic anemia, leukopenia, neutropenia, positive Coombs' reaction, thrombocytopenia

Hepatic: Hepatotoxicity, jaundice

Local: Thrombophlebitis

Neuromuscular & skeletal: Myoclonus

Renal: Interstitial nephritis (acute)

Miscellaneous: Anaphylaxis, hypersensitivity reactions

Overdosage/Toxicology Symptoms of overdose include neuromuscular hypersensitivity and seizures. Hemodialysis may be helpful to aid in removal of the drug from blood; otherwise, treatment is supportive or symptom-directed.

Pharmacodynamics/Kinetics

Protein Binding:

Clavulanic acid: 9% to 30%

Half-Life Elimination:

Clavulanic acid: 66-90 minutes

Metabolism:

Clavulanic acid: Hepatic

Excretion:

Clavulanic acid: Urine (45% as unchanged drug)

Clearance: Does not affect clearance of ticarcillin

Pharmacokinetic Note: See Ticarcillin monograph.

Dosing

Adults:

Systemic infections: I.V.: 3.1 g (ticarcillin 3 g plus clavulanic acid 0.1 g) every 4-6 hours; maximum: 18-24 g/day

Urinary tract infections: I.V.: 3.1 g every 6-8 hours

Elderly: I.V.: 3.1 g every 4-6 hours; adjust for renal function.

Pediatrics:

Systemic infections:

Children <60 kg: 200-300 mg of ticarcillin component/kg/day in divided doses every 4-6 hours

Children >60 kg: 3.1 g (ticarcillin 3 g plus clavulanic acid 0.1 g) every 4-6 hours; maximum: 24 g/day

Renal Impairment:

Cl_{cr} 30-60 mL/minute: Administer 2 g every 4 hours or 3.1 g every 8 hours.

Cl_{cr} 10-30 mL/minute: Administer 2 g every 8 hours or 3.1 g every 12 hours.

Cl_{cr} <10 mL/minute: Administer 2 g every 12 hours.

Cl_{cr} <10 mL/minute with hepatic dysfunction: 2 g every 24 hours.

Moderately dialyzable (20% to 50%)

Continuous arteriovenous or venovenous hemodiafiltration effects: Dose as for Cl_{cr} 10-50 mL/minute.

Peritoneal dialysis: Administer 3.1 g every 12 hours.

Hemodialysis: Administer 2 g every 12 hours; supplemented with 3.1 g after each dialysis.

Hepatic Impairment: Cl_{cr} <10 mL/minute with hepatic dysfunction: Administer 2 g every 24 hours.

Available Dosage Forms

Infusion [premixed, frozen]: Ticarcillin 3 g and clavulanate acid 0.1 g (100 mL) [contains sodium 4.51 mEq and potassium 0.15 mEq per g]

Injection, powder for reconstitution: Ticarcillin 3 g and clavulanate acid 0.1 g (3.1 g, 31 g) [contains sodium 4.51 mEq and potassium 0.15 mEq per g]

Monitoring and Teaching Issues

Physical Assessment: Assess for allergy history prior to starting therapy. See Contraindications and Warnings/Precautions for use cautions. Assess potential for interactions with other prescriptions, OTC medications, or herbal products patient may be taking (see Drug Interactions). Advise patients with diabetes about use of Clinitest®. Assess results of laboratory tests, therapeutic effectiveness, and adverse reactions (eg, hypersensitivity reactions, opportunistic infection; see Adverse Reactions and Overdose/Toxicology). Teach patient possible side effects/appropriate interventions and adverse symptoms to report (see Patient Education).

Monitoring Laboratory Tests: Serum electrolytes, bleeding time, and periodic tests of renal, hepatic, and hematologic function; perform culture and sensitivity before administering first dose.

Patient Education: Inform prescriber of all prescriptions, OTC medications, or herbal products you are taking, and any allergies you have. Do not take any new medication during therapy unless approved by prescriber. This drug can only be given by injection or infusion. Report immediately any redness, swelling, burning, or pain at infusion site or any signs of allergic reaction (eg, respiratory or swallowing difficulty, chest tightness, rash, hives, swelling of lips or mouth). Maintain adequate hydration (2-3 L/day of fluids) unless instructed to restrict fluid intake. If you have diabetes, drug may cause false test results with Clinitest®, consult prescriber for alternative method of glucose monitoring. May cause confusion or drowsiness (use caution when driving or engaging in tasks that require alertness until response to drug is known). Report persistent diarrhea or abdominal pain (do not use antidiarrheal medication without consulting prescriber); fever, chills, unhealed sores, bloody urine or stool, muscle pain, mouth sores, respiratory difficulty, or skin rash; or signs of opportunistic infection (eg, fever, chills, unhealed sores, white plaques in mouth or vagina, purulent vaginal discharge, fatigue).

Dietary Considerations: Sodium content of 1 g: 4.51 mEq; potassium content of 1 g: 0.15 mEq

Geriatric Considerations: When used as empiric therapy or for a documented pseudomonal pneumonia, it is best to combine with an aminoglycoside such as gentamicin

(Continued)

Ticarcillin and Clavulanate Potassium *(Continued)*

or tobramycin. High sodium content may limit use in patients with congestive heart failure. Adjust dose for renal function.

Pregnancy Risk Factor: B

Lactation: Enters breast milk (other penicillins are compatible with breast-feeding)

Administration

I.V.: Infuse over 30 minutes. Administer 1 hour apart from aminoglycosides. Give around-the-clock.

Compatibility: Stable in D_5W, LR, NS, SWFI

Y-site administration: Incompatible with alatrofloxacin, amphotericin B cholesteryl sulfate complex

Compatibility when admixed: Incompatible with sodium bicarbonate, aminoglycosides

Storage: Reconstituted solution is stable for 6 hours at room temperature and 72 hours when refrigerated. I.V. infusion in NS is stable for 24 hours at room temperature, 7 days when refrigerated, or 30 days when frozen. Darkening of solution indicates loss of potency of clavulanate potassium.

Related Information

Ticarcillin *on page 1472*

Ticlopidine *(tye KLOE pi deen)*

U.S. Brand Names Ticlid®

Synonyms Ticlopidine Hydrochloride

Generic Available Yes

Pharmacologic Category Antiplatelet Agent

Use Platelet aggregation inhibitor that reduces the risk of thrombotic stroke in patients who have had a stroke or stroke precursors. **Note:** Due to its association with life-threatening hematologic disorders, ticlopidine should be reserved for patients who are intolerant to aspirin, or who have failed aspirin therapy. Adjunctive therapy (with aspirin) following successful coronary stent implantation to reduce the incidence of subacute stent thrombosis.

Unlabeled/Investigational Use Protection of aortocoronary bypass grafts, diabetic microangiopathy, ischemic heart disease, prevention of postoperative DVT, reduction of graft loss following renal transplant

Mechanism of Action/Effect Ticlopidine is an inhibitor of platelet function with a mechanism which is different from other antiplatelet drugs. The drug significantly increases bleeding time. This effect may not be solely related to ticlopidine's effect on platelets. The prolongation of the bleeding time caused by ticlopidine is further increased by the addition of aspirin in *ex vivo* experiments. Although many metabolites of ticlopidine have been found, none have been shown to account for *in vivo* activity.

Contraindications Hypersensitivity to ticlopidine or any component of the formulation; active pathological bleeding such as PUD or intracranial hemorrhage; severe liver dysfunction; hematopoietic disorders (neutropenia, thrombocytopenia, a past history of TTP)

Warnings/Precautions Use with caution in patients who may have an increased risk of bleeding (such as, ulcers). Consider discontinuing 10-14 days before elective surgery. Use caution in mixing with other antiplatelet drugs. Use with caution in patients with severe liver disease or severe renal impairment (experience is limited). May cause life-threatening hematologic reactions, including neutropenia, agranulocytosis, thrombotic thrombocytopenia purpura (TTP), and aplastic anemia. Routine monitoring is required. Monitor for signs and symptoms of neutropenia including WBC count. Discontinue if the absolute neutrophil count falls to <1200/mm^3 or if the platelet count falls to <80,000/mm^3.

Drug Interactions

Cytochrome P450 Effect: Substrate of CYP3A4 (major); **Inhibits** CYP1A2 (weak), 2C8/9 (weak), 2C19 (strong), 2D6 (moderate), 2E1 (weak), 3A4 (weak)

Decreased Effect: Decreased effect of ticlopidine with antacids (decreased absorption). Ticlopidine may decrease the effect of digoxin or cyclosporine. The levels/effects of ticlopidine may be decreased by aminoglutethimide, carbamazepine, nafcillin, nevirapine, phenobarbital, phenytoin, rifamycins, and other CYP3A4 inducers. Ticlopidine may decrease the levels/effects of CYP2D6 prodrug substrates (eg, codeine, hydrocodone, oxycodone, tramadol).

Increased Effect/Toxicity: Ticlopidine may increase effect/toxicity of aspirin, anticoagulants, theophylline, and NSAIDs. Cimetidine may increase ticlopidine blood levels. Ticlopidine may increase the levels/effects of amphetamines, selected beta-blockers, citalopram, dextromethorphan, diazepam, fluoxetine, lidocaine, methsuximide, mirtazapine, nefazodone, paroxetine, phenytoin, sertraline, risperidone, ritonavir, thioridazine, tricyclic antidepressants, venlafaxine, and other CYP2C19 or 2D6 substrates.

Nutritional/Ethanol Interactions

Food: Ticlopidine bioavailability may be increased (20%) if taken with food. High-fat meals increase absorption, antacids decrease absorption.

Herb/Nutraceutical: Avoid cat's claw, dong quai, evening primrose, feverfew, garlic, ginkgo, ginger, red clover, horse chestnut, green tea, ginseng (all have additional antiplatelet activity).

Lab Interactions Increased cholesterol (S), alkaline phosphatase, transaminases (S)

Adverse Reactions As with all drugs which may affect hemostasis, bleeding is associated with ticlopidine. Hemorrhage may occur at virtually any site. Risk is dependent on multiple variables, including the use of multiple agents which alter hemostasis and patient susceptibility.

>10%:
   Endocrine & metabolic: Increased total cholesterol (increases of ~8% to 10% within 1 month of therapy)
   Gastrointestinal: Diarrhea (13%)
1% to 10%:
   Central nervous system: Dizziness (1%)
   Dermatologic: Rash (5%), purpura (2%), pruritus (1%)
   Gastrointestinal: Nausea (7%), dyspepsia (7%), gastrointestinal pain (4%), vomiting (2%), flatulence (2%), anorexia (1%)
   Hematologic: Neutropenia (2%)
   Hepatic: Abnormal liver function test (1%)

Overdosage/Toxicology Symptoms of overdose include ataxia, seizures, vomiting, abdominal pain, and hematologic abnormalities. Specific treatments are lacking. Treatment is symptomatic and supportive.

Pharmacodynamics/Kinetics
   Onset of Action: ~6 hours; Peak effect: 3-5 days; serum levels do not correlate with clinical antiplatelet activity
   Half-Life Elimination: 24 hours
   Metabolism: Extensively hepatic; has at least one active metabolite

Dosing
   Adults:
      Stroke prevention: Oral: 250 mg twice daily with food
      Coronary artery stenting (initiate after successful implantation): Oral: 250 mg twice daily with food (in combination with antiplatelet doses of aspirin) for up to 30 days
   Elderly: 250 mg twice daily with food; dosage in older patients has not been determined; however, in two large clinical trials, the average age of subjects was 63 and 66 years. A dosage decrease may be necessary if bleeding develops.

Available Dosage Forms Tablet, as hydrochloride: 250 mg

Monitoring and Teaching Issues
   Physical Assessment: Monitor effectiveness of therapy (laboratory results) frequently at beginning of treatment and regularly thereafter. Monitor and teach patient bleeding precautions, possible side effects, and adverse symptoms to report.
   Monitoring Laboratory Tests: CBC with differential and platelet counts every 2 weeks starting the second week through the third month of treatment; more frequent monitoring is recommended for patients whose absolute neutrophil counts have been consistently declining or are 30% less than baseline values. Liver function tests (alkaline phosphatase and transaminases) should be performed in the first 4 months of therapy if liver dysfunction is suspected.
   Patient Education: Take exact dosage prescribed, with food. Do not use aspirin or aspirin-containing medications and OTC medications without consulting prescriber. You may experience easy bleeding or bruising (use soft toothbrush or cotton swabs and frequent mouth care, use electric razor, avoid sharp knives or scissors). Report unusual bleeding or bruising, persistent fever, sore throat, weakness, paleness, changes in neurological status; blood in urine, stool, or vomitus; delayed healing of any wounds; skin rash; yellowing of skin or eyes; changes in color of urine or stool; pain or burning on urination; respiratory difficulty; or skin rash. **Breast-feeding precaution:** Consult prescriber if breast-feeding.
   Dietary Considerations: Should be taken with food to reduce stomach upset.
   Geriatric Considerations: Because of the risk of neutropenia and its relative expense as compared with aspirin, ticlopidine should only be used in patients with a documented intolerance to aspirin.
   Pregnancy Risk Factor: B
   Lactation: Excretion in breast milk unknown

Administration
   Oral: Administer with food.

♦ **Ticlopidine Hydrochloride** *see* Ticlopidine *on page 1476*
♦ **Tigan®** *see* Trimethobenzamide *on page 1527*
♦ **Tikosyn™** *see* Dofetilide *on page 476*
♦ **Tilade®** *see* Nedocromil *on page 1062*

Tiludronate (tye LOO droe nate)

U.S. Brand Names Skelid®
Synonyms Tiludronate Disodium
Generic Available No
Pharmacologic Category Bisphosphonate Derivative
Use Treatment of Paget's disease of the bone in patients who have a level of serum alkaline phosphatase (SAP) at least twice the upper limit of normal, or who are symptomatic, or who are at risk for future complications of their disease
Mechanism of Action/Effect A bisphosphonate which inhibits osteoclast activity, reducing enzymatic and transport processes that lead to resorption of bone. At least two possible mechanisms may be involved: detachment of osteoclasts from the bone surface (due to inhibition of protein-tyrosine-phosphatase) and inhibition of the osteoclastic proton pump, required to alter local pH to solubilize ions and bone matrix during resorption.
Contraindications Hypersensitivity to bisphosphonates or any component of the formulation
Warnings/Precautions Not recommended in severe renal impairment (Cl_{cr} <30 mL/minute). May cause upper gastrointestinal problems (eg, dysphagia, esophageal diseases, gastritis, duodenitis, ulcers).
Drug Interactions
   Decreased Effect: Concurrent administration of calcium salts, aluminum- or magnesium-containing antacids, and aspirin markedly decrease absorption/bioavailability (by 50% to 60%) of tiludronate if given within 2 hours of a dose.
(Continued)

Tiludronate *(Continued)*

Increased Effect/Toxicity: Administration of indomethacin increases bioavailability of tiludronate two- to fourfold.

Nutritional/Ethanol Interactions Food: In single-dose studies, the bioavailability of tiludronate was reduced by 90% when an oral dose was administered with, or 2 hours after, a standard breakfast compared to the same dose administered after an overnight fast and 4 hours before a standard breakfast.

Adverse Reactions The following events occurred >2% and at a frequency greater than placebo:

1% to 10%:
Cardiovascular: Chest pain (3%), edema (3%)
Central nervous system: Dizziness (4%), paresthesia (4%)
Dermatologic: Rash (3%), skin disorder (3%)
Gastrointestinal: Nausea (9%), diarrhea (9%), heartburn (5%), vomiting (4%), flatulence (3%)
Neuromuscular & skeletal: Arthrosis (3%)
Ocular: cataract (3%), conjunctivitis (3%), glaucoma (3%)
Respiratory: Rhinitis (5%), sinusitis (5%), cough (3%), pharyngitis (3%)

Overdosage/Toxicology Hypocalcemia is a potential consequence of overdose. Treatment is supportive.

Pharmacodynamics/Kinetics
Onset of Action: Delayed, may require several weeks
Absorption: Rapid
Bioavailability: 6%; reduced by food
Time to Peak: Plasma: ~2 hours
Protein Binding: 90%, primarily to albumin
Half-Life Elimination: Healthy volunteers: 50 hours; Pagetic patients: 150 hours
Metabolism: Little, if any
Excretion: Urine (60% as unchanged drug) within 13 days

Dosing
Adults & Elderly: Paget's disease: Oral: 400 mg (2 tablets of tiludronic acid) daily for a period of 3 months
Renal Impairment: Tiludronate is excreted renally. It is not recommended for use in patients with severe renal impairment (Cl_{cr} <30 mL/minute) and is not removed by dialysis.

Available Dosage Forms Tablet, tiludronic acid: 200 mg [equivalent to 240 mg tiludronate disodium]

Monitoring and Teaching Issues
Physical Assessment: Ascertain that patient is capable of complying with administration directions before starting treatment (eg, able to remain in standing or sitting position for 30 minutes). Use caution with renal impairment. Assess results of laboratory tests, therapeutic effectiveness, and adverse reactions (eg, rash, diarrhea, arthralgia, peripheral edema, GI disturbance [nausea, vomiting, diarrhea], visual changes, hypocalcemia, hypophosphatemia; see Adverse Reactions). Teach patient appropriate use and administration of medication, lifestyle and dietary changes that will have a beneficial impact on Paget's disease, possible side effects, interventions to reduce side effects, and adverse reactions to report (see Patient Education).
Monitoring Laboratory Tests: Serum calcium, alkaline phosphatase
Patient Education: Do not take any new medication during therapy unless approved by prescriber. In order to be effective, this medication must be taken exactly as directed, with a full glass of water; do not take within 2 hours of food. Remain standing or sitting for at least 30 minutes after taking this medication before eating. Do not remove medication from foil strip until ready to be used. Do not take aspirin, antacids or vitamin supplements containing calcium, magnesium, or aluminum within 2 hours. Consult prescriber to determine recommended lifestyle changes (eg, decreased smoking, decreased alcohol intake, dietary supplements of calcium, or increased dietary vitamin D). Notify prescriber at once if experiencing difficulty swallowing, pain when swallowing, or severe or persistent heartburn. May cause mild/temporary skin rash; or abdominal pain, diarrhea, or constipation (report if persistent). Report persistent muscle or bone pain or leg cramps; chest pain, palpitations, or swollen extremities; disturbed vision; ringing in the ears; unusual weakness or significantly increased perspiration. **Pregnancy/breast-feeding precautions:** Inform prescriber if you are or intend to become pregnant. Consult prescriber if breast-feeding.
Dietary Considerations: Do not take within 2 hours of food.
Pregnancy Risk Factor: C
Pregnancy Issues: Teratogenic and nonteratogenic embryo/fetal effects have been reported in animal studies. There are no adequate and well-controlled studies in pregnant women. Bisphosphonates are incorporated into the bone matrix and gradually released over time. Theoretically, there may be a risk of fetal harm when pregnancy follows the completion of therapy. Based on limited case reports with pamidronate, serum calcium levels in the newborn may be altered if administered during pregnancy.
Lactation: Excretion in breast milk unknown/use caution
Administration
Oral: Take with 6-8 oz of plain water. Do not take within 2 hours of food, aspirin, indomethacin, or calcium-, magnesium-, or aluminum-containing medications.
Storage: Do not remove tablet from foil strips until they are to be used.

♦ Tiludronate Disodium *see* Tiludronate *on page 1477*
♦ Timentin® *see* Ticarcillin and Clavulanate Potassium *on page 1474*

Timolol *(TYE moe lole)*

U.S. Brand Names Betimol®; Blocadren®; Istalol™; Timoptic®; Timoptic® OcuDose®; Timoptic-XE®
Synonyms Timolol Hemihydrate; Timolol Maleate

Generic Available Yes; Excludes hemihydrate ophthalmic solutions

Pharmacologic Category Beta-Adrenergic Blocker, Nonselective; Ophthalmic Agent, Antiglaucoma

Medication Safety Issues

Sound-alike/look-alike issues:

Timolol may be confused with atenolol, Tylenol®

Timoptic® may be confused with Talacen®, Viroptic®

Use Ophthalmic dosage form used in treatment of elevated intraocular pressure such as glaucoma or ocular hypertension; oral dosage form used for treatment of hypertension and angina, to reduce mortality following myocardial infarction, and for prophylaxis of migraine

Mechanism of Action/Effect Blocks both beta$_1$- and beta$_2$-adrenergic receptors, reduces intraocular pressure by reducing aqueous humor production or possibly outflow; reduces blood pressure by blocking adrenergic receptors and decreasing sympathetic outflow, produces a negative chronotropic and inotropic activity through an unknown mechanism

Contraindications Hypersensitivity to timolol or any component of the formulation; sinus bradycardia; sinus node dysfunction; heart block greater than first degree (except in patients with a functioning artificial pacemaker); cardiogenic shock; uncompensated cardiac failure; bronchospastic disease; pregnancy (2nd and 3rd trimesters)

Warnings/Precautions Administer cautiously in compensated heart failure and monitor for a worsening of the condition. Beta-blocker therapy should not be withdrawn abruptly (particularly in patients with CAD), but gradually tapered to avoid acute tachycardia, hypertension, and/or ischemia. Use caution with concurrent use of beta-blockers and either verapamil or diltiazem; bradycardia or heart block can occur. Beta-blockers can aggravate symptoms in patients with peripheral vascular disease. Patients with bronchospastic disease should generally not receive beta-blockers - monitor closely if used in patients at risk of bronchospasm. Use cautiously in patients with diabetes; may mask prominent hypoglycemic symptoms. May mask signs of thyrotoxicosis. Use cautiously in severe renal impairment: marked hypotension can occur in patients maintained on hemodialysis. Use care with anesthetic agents which decrease myocardial function. Can worsen myasthenia gravis. Similar reactions found with systemic administration may occur with topical (ophthalmic) administration.

Drug Interactions

Cytochrome P450 Effect: Substrate of CYP2D6 (major); **Inhibits** CYP2D6 (weak)

Decreased Effect: Decreased effect of timolol with aluminum salts, barbiturates, calcium salts, cholestyramine, colestipol, NSAIDs, penicillins (ampicillin), rifampin, salicylates, and sulfinpyrazone due to decreased bioavailability and plasma levels. Beta-blockers may decrease the effect of sulfonylureas. Beta-blockers may affect the action or levels of ethanol, disopyramide, nondepolarizing muscle relaxants, and theophylline, although the effects are difficult to predict.

Increased Effect/Toxicity: CYP2D6 inhibitors may increase the levels/effects of timolol; example inhibitors include chlorpromazine, delavirdine, fluoxetine, miconazole, paroxetine, pergolide, quinidine, quinine, ritonavir, and ropinirole. The heart rate-lowering effects of timolol are additive with other drugs which slow AV conduction (digoxin, verapamil, diltiazem). Reserpine increases the effects of timolol. Concurrent use of timolol may increase the effects of alpha-blockers (prazosin, terazosin), alpha-adrenergic stimulants (epinephrine, phenylephrine), and the vasoconstrictive effects of ergot alkaloids. Timolol may mask the tachycardia from hypoglycemia caused by insulin and oral hypoglycemics. In patients receiving concurrent therapy, the risk of hypertensive crisis is increased when either clonidine or the beta-blocker is withdrawn. Beta-blockers may increase the action or levels of ethanol, disopyramide, nondepolarizing muscle relaxants, and theophylline although the effects are difficult to predict.

Adverse Reactions

Ophthalmic:

>10%: Ocular: Burning, stinging

1% to 10%:

Cardiovascular: Hypertension

Central nervous system: Headache

Ocular: Blurred vision, cataract, conjunctival injection, itching, visual acuity decreased

Miscellaneous: Infection

Systemic:

1% to 10%:

Cardiovascular: Bradycardia

Central nervous system: Fatigue, dizziness

Respiratory: Dyspnea

Frequency not defined (reported with any dosage form):

Cardiovascular: Angina pectoris, arrhythmia, bradycardia, cardiac failure, cardiac arrest, cerebral vascular accident, cerebral ischemia, edema, hypotension, heart block, palpitation, Raynaud's phenomenon

Central nervous system: Anxiety, confusion, depression, disorientation, dizziness, hallucinations, insomnia, memory loss, nervousness, nightmares, somnolence

Dermatologic: Alopecia, angioedema, pseudopemphigoid, psoriasiform rash, psoriasis exacerbation, rash, urticaria

Endocrine & metabolic: Hypoglycemia masked, libido decreased

Gastrointestinal: Anorexia, diarrhea, dyspepsia, nausea, xerostomia

Genitourinary: Impotence, retoperitoneal fibrosis

Hematologic: Claudication

Neuromuscular & skeletal: Myasthenia gravis exacerbation, paresthesia

Ocular: Blepharitis, conjunctivitis, corneal sensitivity decreased, cystoid macular edema, diplopia, dry eyes, foreign body sensation, keratitis, ocular discharge, ocular pain, ptosis, refractive changes, tearing, visual disturbances

Otic: Tinnitus

Respiratory: Bronchospasm, cough, dyspnea, nasal congestion, pulmonary edema, respiratory failure

Miscellaneous: Allergic reactions, cold hands/feet, Peyronie's disease, systemic lupus erythematosus

(Continued)

Timolol *(Continued)*

Overdosage/Toxicology Symptoms of intoxication include cardiac disturbances, CNS toxicity, bronchospasm, hypoglycemia and hyperkalemia. The most common cardiac symptoms include hypotension and bradycardia. Atrioventricular block, intraventricular conduction disturbances, cardiogenic shock, and asystole may occur with severe overdose, especially with membrane-depressant drugs (eg, propranolol). CNS effects including convulsions, coma, and respiratory arrest are commonly seen with propranolol and other membrane-depressant and lipid-soluble drugs. Treatment is symptom-directed and supportive. Timolol is not readily dialyzable.

Pharmacodynamics/Kinetics

Onset of Action:
Hypotensive: Oral: 15-45 minutes; Peak effect: 0.5-2.5 hours
Intraocular pressure reduction: Ophthalmic: 30 minutes; Peak effect: 1-2 hours

Duration of Action: ~4 hours; Ophthalmic: Intraocular: 24 hours

Protein Binding: 60%

Half-Life Elimination: 2-2.7 hours; prolonged with renal impairment

Metabolism: Extensively hepatic; extensive first-pass effect

Excretion: Urine (15% to 20% as unchanged drug)

Dosing

Adults & Elderly:

Glaucoma: Ophthalmic:
Solution: Initial: 0.25% solution, instill 1 drop twice daily; increase to 0.5% solution if response not adequate; decrease to 1 drop/day if controlled; do not exceed 1 drop twice daily of 0.5% solution.
Istalol™: Instill 1 drop (0.5% solution) once daily in the morning.
Gel-forming solution (Timoptic-XE):* Instill 1 drop (either 0.25% or 0.5%) once daily

Hypertension: Oral: Initial: 10 mg twice daily, increase gradually every 7 days, usual dosage: 20-40 mg/day in 2 divided doses; maximum: 60 mg/day.

Prevention of myocardial infarction: Oral: 10 mg twice daily initiated within 1-4 weeks after infarction.

Migraine prophylaxis: Oral: Initial: 10 mg twice daily, increase to maximum of 30 mg/day.

Pediatrics: Children: Ophthalmic: Refer to adult dosing.

Available Dosage Forms [DSC] = Discontinued product;

Note: Strength expressed as base.

Gel-forming solution, ophthalmic, as maleate: 0.25% (5 mL); 0.5% (2.5 mL, 5 mL)
Timoptic-XE®: 0.25% (2.5 mL [DSC], 5 mL); 0.5% (2.5 mL [DSC], 5 mL)

Solution, ophthalmic, as hemihydrate (Betimol®): 0.25% (5 mL, 10 mL, 15 mL); 0.5% (5 mL, 10 mL, 15 mL) [contains benzalkonium chloride]

Solution, ophthalmic, as maleate: 0.25% (5 mL, 10 mL, 15 mL); 0.5% (5 mL, 10 mL, 15 mL) [contains benzalkonium chloride]

Istalol™: 0.5% (10 mL) [contains benzalkonium chloride and potassium sorbate]
Timoptic®: 0.25% (5 mL, 10 mL); 0.5% (5 mL, 10 mL) [contains benzalkonium chloride]

Solution, ophthalmic, as maleate [preservative free] (Timoptic® OcuDose®): 0.25% (0.2 mL); 0.5% (0.2 mL) [single use]

Tablet, as maleate (Blocadren®): 5 mg, 10 mg, 20 mg

Monitoring and Teaching Issues

Physical Assessment: Assess other medications patient may be taking for effectiveness and interactions. Monitor therapeutic effectiveness (according to purpose of therapy) and adverse reactions at beginning of therapy and regularly with long-term therapy. Monitor blood pressure periodically. Assess knowledge/teach patient appropriate use, interventions to reduce side effects, and adverse symptoms to report.

Patient Education: Oral: Take exact dose prescribed; do not increase, decrease, or discontinue dosage without consulting prescriber. Take at the same time each day. If you have diabetes, monitor serum glucose closely. May cause postural hypotension (use caution when rising from sitting or lying position or climbing stairs); dizziness, drowsiness, or blurred vision (use caution when driving or engaging in tasks requiring alertness until response to drug is known); decreased sexual ability (reversible); or nausea or vomiting (small frequent meals or frequent mouth care may help). Report swelling of extremities, respiratory difficulty, or new cough; weight gain (>3 lb/week); unresolved diarrhea or vomiting; or cold blue extremities. **Pregnancy/breast-feeding precautions:** Inform prescriber if you are or intend to become pregnant. Consult prescriber if breast-feeding.

Ophthalmic: For ophthalmic use only. Apply prescribed amount as often as directed. Wash hands before using. Do not let tip of applicator touch eye; do not contaminate tip of applicator (may cause eye infection, eye damage, or vision loss). Tilt head back and look upward. Gently pull down lower lid and put drop(s) inside lower eyelid at inner corner. Close eye and roll eyeball in all directions. Do not blink for 1/2 minute. Apply gentle pressure to inner corner of eye for 30 seconds. Wipe away excess from skin around eye. Do not use any other eye preparation for at least 10 minutes. Do not share medication with anyone else. Temporary stinging or blurred vision may occur. If using Istalol™, remove contact lenses prior to administration. Lenses may be reinserted 15 minutes following administration. Immediately report any adverse cardiac or CNS effects (usually signifies overdose). Report persistent eye pain, redness, burning, watering, dryness, double vision, puffiness around eye, vision changes, other adverse eye response, worsening of condition or lack of improvement.

Dietary Considerations: Oral product should be administered with food at the same time each day.

Geriatric Considerations: Due to alterations in the beta-adrenergic autonomic nervous system, beta-adrenergic blockade may result in less hemodynamic response than seen in younger adults.

Pregnancy Risk Factor: C (manufacturer); D (2nd and 3rd trimesters - expert analysis)

Pregnancy Issues: Timolol was shown to cross the placenta in an *in vitro* perfusion study. Beta-blockers have been associated with bradycardia, hypotension, hypoglycemia, and intrauterine growth rate (IUGR); IUGR is probably related to maternal hypertension. Available evidence suggests beta-blockers are generally safe during pregnancy (JNC 7). Cases of neonatal hypoglycemia have been reported following maternal use of beta-blockers at parturition or during breast-feeding. Bradycardia and arrhythmia have been reported in an infant following ophthalmic administration of timolol during pregnancy.

Lactation: Enters breast milk/use caution (AAP rates "compatible")

Breast-Feeding Issues: Timolol is excreted in breast milk following oral and ophthalmic administration, and is considered compatible by the AAP. It is recommended that the infant be monitored for signs or symptoms of beta-blockade (hypotension, bradycardia, etc) with long-term use.

Administration

Other: Administer other topically-applied ophthalmic medications at least 10 minutes before Timoptic-XE®; wash hands before use; invert closed bottle and shake once before use; remove cap carefully so that tip does not touch anything; hold bottle between thumb and index finger; use index finger of other hand to pull down the lower eyelid to form a pocket for the eye drop and tilt head back; place the dispenser tip close to the eye and gently squeeze the bottle to administer 1 drop; remove pressure after a single drop has been released; **do not allow the dispenser tip to touch the eye**; replace cap and store bottle in an upright position in a clean area; do **not** enlarge hole of dispenser; do **not** wash tip with water, soap, or any other cleaner. Some ophthalmic solutions contain benzalkonium chloride; wait at least 10 minutes after instilling solution before inserting soft contact lenses.

Storage: Ophthalmic drops: Store at room temperature. Protect from light and freezing.
Timoptic Occudose®: Store in the protective foil wrap and use within 1 month after opening foil package.

Related Information
Beta-Blockers *on page 1720*
Glaucoma Drug Therapy *on page 1827*

Tinidazole (tye NI da zole)

U.S. Brand Names Tindamax™

Generic Available No

Pharmacologic Category Amebicide; Antibiotic, Miscellaneous; Antiprotozoal, Nitroimidazole

Use Treatment of trichomoniasis caused by *T. vaginalis*; treatment of giardiasis caused by *G. duodenalis* (*G. lamblia*); treatment of intestinal amebiasis and amebic liver abscess caused by *E. histolytica*

Mechanism of Action/Effect After diffusing into the organism, it is proposed that tinidazole causes cytotoxicity by damaging DNA and preventing further DNA synthesis.

Contraindications Hypersensitivity to tinidazole, nitroimidazole derivatives (including metronidazole), or any component of the formulation; pregnancy (1st trimester); breast-feeding

Warnings/Precautions Use caution with CNS diseases; seizures and peripheral neuropathy have been reported with tinidazole and other nitroimidazole derivatives. Use caution with current or history of blood dyscrasias or hepatic impairment. When used for amebiasis, not indicated for the treatment of asymptomatic cyst passage. Safety and efficacy have not been established in children ≤3 years of age.

Drug Interactions

Cytochrome P450 Effect: Substrate of CYP3A4 (minor)

Decreased Effect: Specific interaction studies have not been conducted. Refer to Metronidazole monograph *on page 995.*

Increased Effect/Toxicity: Specific interaction studies have not been conducted. Refer to Metronidazole monograph *on page 995.*

Nutritional/Ethanol Interactions

Ethanol: The manufacturer recommends to avoid all ethanol or any ethanol-containing drugs (may cause disulfiram-like reaction characterized by flushing, headache, nausea, vomiting, sweating or tachycardia).

Food: Peak antibiotic serum concentration lowered and delayed, but total drug absorbed not affected.

Lab Interactions May interfere with AST, ALT, triglycerides, glucose, and LDH testing

Adverse Reactions

1% to 10%:

Central nervous system: Fatigue/malaise (1% to 2%), dizziness (≤1%), headache (≤1%)

Gastrointestinal: Metallic/bitter taste (4% to 6%), nausea (3% to 5%), anorexia (2% to 3%), dyspepsia/cramps/epigastric discomfort (1% to 2%), vomiting (1% to 2%), constipation (≤1%)

Neuromuscular & skeletal: Weakness (1% to 2%)

Frequency not defined.

Cardiovascular: Flushing, palpitation

Central nervous system: Ataxia, coma, confusion, convulsions, depression, drowsiness, fever, giddiness, insomnia, vertigo

Dermatologic: Angioedema, pruritus, rash, urticaria

Gastrointestinal: Diarrhea, furry tongue, oral candidiasis, salivation, stomatitis, thirst, tongue discoloration, xerostomia

Genitourinary: Urine darkened, vaginal discharge increased

Hematologic: Leukopenia (transient), neutropenia (transient), thrombocytopenia (reversible)

Hepatic: Transaminases increased

(Continued)

Tinidazole *(Continued)*

Neuromuscular & skeletal: Arthralgia, arthritis, myalgia, peripheral neuropathy (transient, includes numbness and paresthesia)

Respiratory: Bronchospasm, dyspnea, pharyngitis

Miscellaneous: Burning sensation, *Candida* overgrowth, diaphoresis

Overdosage/Toxicology Treatment should be symptomatic and supportive. Hemodialysis may be considered (43% removed during a 6-hour session).

Pharmacodynamics/Kinetics

Absorption: Rapid and complete

Protein Binding: 12%

Half-Life Elimination: 13 hours

Metabolism: Hepatic via CYP3A4 (primarily); undergoes oxidation, hydroxylation and conjugation; forms a metabolite

Excretion: Urine (20% to 25%); feces (12%)

Dosing

Adults:

Amebiasis, intestinal: Oral: 2 g/day for 3 days

Amebiasis, liver abscess: Oral: 2 g/day for 3-5 days

Giardiasis: Oral: 2 g as a single dose

Trichomoniasis: Oral: 2 g as a single dose; sexual partners should be treated at the same time

Pediatrics:

Amebiasis, intestinal: Oral: Children >3 years: 50 mg/kg/day for 3 days (maximum dose: 2 g/day)

Amebiasis, liver abscess: Oral: Children >3 years: 50 mg/kg/day for 3-5 days (maximum dose: 2 g/day)

Giardiasis: Oral: Children >3 years: 50 mg/kg as a single dose (maximum dose: 2 g)

Renal Impairment: Adjustment not necessary. An additional dose equal to 1/2 the usual dose, should be administered at the end of hemodialysis if tinidazole is administered on a day hemodialysis occurs.

Hepatic Impairment: Specific recommendations are not available; use with caution.

Available Dosage Forms Tablet, scored: 250 mg, 500 mg

Monitoring and Teaching Issues

Physical Assessment: Assess potential for interactions with other prescriptions, OTC medications, or herbal products patient may be taking. Assess therapeutic effectiveness (symptoms and laboratory tests) and adverse response. Teach patient appropriate use, interventions to reduce side effects, and adverse symptoms to report.

Patient Education: Do not take any new medications during therapy without consulting prescriber. Take exactly as directed. Avoid all alcohol while taking this medication; may cause unpleasant reaction (flushing, nausea, vomiting, sweating, headache, rapid heart beat). Refrain from sexual intercourse or use contraceptive if being treated for trichomoniasis. May cause headache, drowsiness or dizziness (use caution when climbing stairs, driving, or engaged in potentially hazardous tasks until response to drug is known); mild gastrointestinal disturbance (nausea, vomiting, constipation, diarrhea, metallic/bitter taste, abdominal discomfort) small frequent meals, frequent mouth care, chewing gum or sucking lozenges may help. Report severe fatigue or weakness; chest pain or palpitations; swelling of lips or mouth, other persistent adverse reactions, lack of improvement or worsening of condition. **Pregnancy/breast-feeding precautions:** Inform prescriber if you are or intend to become pregnant. Breast-feeding is contraindicated.

Dietary Considerations: Take with food. The manufacturer recommends that ethanol be avoided during treatment and for 3 days after therapy is complete.

Pregnancy Risk Factor: C

Pregnancy Issues: Tinidazole crosses the placenta and enters the fetal circulation. Use during the first trimester is contraindicated.

Lactation: Enters breast milk/not recommended

Breast-Feeding Issues: Breast-feeding should be discontinued during therapy and for 3 days after the last dose.

Administration

Oral: Administer with food.

Storage: Store at controlled room temperature of 20°C to 25°C (68°F to 77°F). Protect from light.

Tinzaparin *(tin ZA pa rin)*

U.S. Brand Names Innohep®

Synonyms Tinzaparin Sodium

Generic Available No

Pharmacologic Category Low Molecular Weight Heparin

Use Treatment of acute symptomatic deep vein thrombosis, with or without pulmonary embolism, in conjunction with warfarin sodium

Mechanism of Action/Effect Standard heparin consists of components with molecular weights ranging from 4000-30,000 daltons with a mean of 16,000 daltons. Heparin acts as an anticoagulant by enhancing the inhibition rate of clotting proteases by antithrombin III, impairing normal hemostasis and inhibition of factor Xa. Low molecular weight heparins have a small effect on the activated partial thromboplastin time and strongly inhibit factor Xa. The primary inhibitory activity of tinzaparin is through antithrombin. Tinzaparin is derived from porcine heparin that undergoes controlled enzymatic depolymerization. The average molecular weight of tinzaparin ranges between 5500 and 7500 daltons which is distributed as (<10%) 2000 daltons (60% to 72%) 2000-8000 daltons, and (22% to 36%) >8000 daltons. The antifactor Xa activity is approximately 100 int. units/mg.

Contraindications Hypersensitivity to tinzaparin sodium, heparin, sulfites, benzyl alcohol, pork products, or any component of the formulation; active major bleeding; heparin-induced thrombocytopenia (current or history of)

Warnings/Precautions Patients with recent or anticipated neuraxial anesthesia (epidural or spinal anesthesia) are at risk of spinal or epidural hematoma and subsequent paralysis. Consider risk versus benefit prior to neuraxial anesthesia; risk is increased by concomitant agents which may alter hemostasis, as well as traumatic or repeated epidural or spinal puncture, and indwelling epidural catheters. Patient should be observed closely for signs and symptoms of neurological impairment. Not to be used interchangeably (unit for unit) with heparin or any other low molecular weight heparins.

Monitor patient closely for signs or symptoms of bleeding. Certain patients are at increased risk of bleeding. Risk factors include bacterial endocarditis; congenital or acquired bleeding disorders; active ulcerative or angiodysplastic GI diseases; severe uncontrolled hypertension; hemorrhagic stroke; use shortly after brain, spinal, or ophthalmologic surgery; patients treated concomitantly with platelet inhibitors; recent GI bleeding; thrombocytopenia or platelet defects; severe liver disease; hypertensive or diabetic retinopathy; or in patients undergoing invasive procedures. Monitor platelet count closely. Rare cases of thrombocytopenia have occurred. Manufacturer recommends discontinuation of therapy if platelets are <100,000/mm^3.

Safety and efficacy in pediatric patients has not been established. Use with caution in the elderly (delayed elimination may occur). Heparin can cause hyperkalemia by affecting aldosterone; similar reactions could occur with LMWHs. Monitor for hyperkalemia. For subcutaneous injection only, do not mix with other injections or infusions. Clinical experience is limited in patients with BMI >40 kg.

Drug Interactions

Increased Effect/Toxicity: Drugs which affect platelet function (eg, aspirin, NSAIDs, dipyridamole, ticlopidine, clopidogrel, sulfinpyrazone, dextran) may potentiate the risk of hemorrhage. Thrombolytic agents increase the risk of hemorrhage.

Warfarin: Risk of bleeding may be increased during concurrent therapy. Tinzaparin is commonly continued during the initiation of warfarin therapy to assure anticoagulation and to protect against possible transient hypercoagulability

Lab Interactions Asymptomatic increases in AST (SGOT) (8.8%) and ALT (SGPT) (13%) have been reported. Elevations were >3 times the upper limit of normal and were reversible and rarely associated with increases in bilirubin.

Adverse Reactions As with all anticoagulants, bleeding is the major adverse effect of tinzaparin. Hemorrhage may occur at virtually any site. Risk is dependent on multiple variables.

>10%:
  Hepatic: Increased ALT (13%)
  Local: Injection site hematoma (16%)
1% to 10%:
  Cardiovascular: Angina pectoris, chest pain (2%), hyper-/hypotension, tachycardia
  Central nervous system: Confusion, dizziness, fever (2%), headache (2%), insomnia, pain (2%)
  Dermatologic: Bullous eruption, pruritus, rash (1%), skin disorder
  Gastrointestinal: Constipation (1%), dyspepsia, flatulence, nausea (1%), nonspecified gastrointestinal disorder, vomiting (1%)
  Genitourinary: Dysuria, urinary retention, urinary tract infection (4%)
  Hematologic: Anemia, hematoma, hemorrhage (2%), thrombocytopenia (1%)
  Hepatic: Increased AST (9%)
  Local: Deep vein thrombosis, injection site hematoma
  Neuromuscular & skeletal: Back pain (2%)
  Renal: Hematuria (1%)
  Respiratory: Dyspnea (1%), epistaxis (2%), pneumonia, pulmonary embolism (2%), respiratory disorder
  Miscellaneous: Impaired healing, infection, unclassified reactions

Overdosage/Toxicology Overdose may lead to bleeding; bleeding may occur at any site. In case of overdose, discontinue medication, apply pressure to bleeding site if possible, and replace volume and hemostatic blood elements as required. If these measures are ineffective, or if bleeding is severe, protamine sulfate may be administered at 1 mg per every 100 anti-Xa int. units of tinzaparin.

Pharmacodynamics/Kinetics

Onset of Action: 2-3 hours
Bioavailability: 87%
Time to Peak: 4-5 hours
Half-Life Elimination: 3-4 hours
Metabolism: Partially metabolized by desulphation and depolymerization
Excretion: Urine

Dosing

Adults & Elderly: Treatment of DVT: SubQ: 175 anti-Xa int. units/kg of body weight once daily. Warfarin sodium should be started when appropriate. Administer tinzaparin for at least 6 days and until patient is adequately anticoagulated with warfarin.
  Note: To calculate the volume of solution to administer per dose: Volume to be administered (mL) = patient weight (kg) x 0.00875 mL/kg (may be rounded off to the nearest 0.05 mL)

Renal Impairment: Patients with severe renal impairment had a 24% decrease in clearance, use with caution.

Hepatic Impairment: No adjustment necessary.

Available Dosage Forms Injection, solution: 20,000 anti-Xa int. units/mL (2 mL) [contains benzyl alcohol and sodium metabisulfite]

Monitoring and Teaching Issues

Physical Assessment: Use caution in the presence of increased risk of bleeding (see Warnings/Precautions for specific use cautions). Assess potential for interactions with other pharmacological agents and herbal products patient may be taking (especially anything that will impact coagulation or platelet aggregation; see Drug Interactions). Assess results of laboratory tests on a regular basis. Monitor therapeutic effectiveness, (Continued)

Tinzaparin *(Continued)*

and adverse response (eg, bleeding at any source, rash, angina, confusion, urinary retention, dyspnea; see Adverse Reactions). Observe and teach bleeding precautions. Teach
patient use if self-administered (appropriate injection technique and syringe/needle
disposal), possible side effects/appropriate interventions (eg, bleeding precautions), and
adverse symptoms to report (see Patient Education).

Monitoring Laboratory Tests: CBC including platelet count and hematocrit or hemoglobin, and stool for occult blood; the monitoring of PT and/or PTT is not necessary.
Patients receiving both warfarin and tinzaparin should have their INR drawn just prior to the
next scheduled dose of tinzaparin.

Patient Education: Do not take any new medication during therapy unless approved by
prescriber. This drug can only be administered by injection. If self-administered, use
exactly as directed and follow instructions for syringe disposal. Do not alter dosage or
discontinue without consulting prescriber. You may have a tendency to bleed easily while
taking this drug (brush teeth with soft brush, use waxed dental floss, use electric razor,
avoid scissors or sharp knives, and avoid potentially harmful activities). Report immediately
any unusual bleeding or bruising (eg, mouth, nose, blood in urine or stool); chest pain or
palpitations; confusion, dizziness, or headache; skin rash or itching; persistent GI upset
(eg, nausea, vomiting, abdominal pain, acute constipation); warmth, swelling, pain, or
redness in calves or other areas; back or muscle pain; respiratory difficulties; or other
persistent adverse reactions. **Pregnancy/breast-feeding precautions:** Inform prescriber
if you are pregnant or intend to become pregnant or breast-feed.

Pregnancy Risk Factor: B

Pregnancy Issues: There are no adequate and well-controlled studies in pregnant women.
Cases of teratogenic effects and/or fetal death have been reported (relationship to
tinzaparin not established). Use during pregnancy only if clearly needed. Pregnant women,
or those who become pregnant while receiving tinzaparin, should be informed of the
potential risks to the fetus.

Lactation: Excretion in breast milk unknown/use caution

Administration

I.V.: Patient should be lying down or sitting. Administer by deep SubQ injection, alternating
between the left and right anterolateral and left and right posterolateral abdominal wall.
Vary site daily. The entire needle should be introduced into the skin fold formed by the
thumb and forefinger. Hold the skin fold until injection is complete. To minimize bruising, do
not rub the injection site.

Storage: Store at 25°C (77°F). Excursions permitted to 15°C to 30°C (59°F to 86°F).

Additional Information Contains sodium metabisulfite and benzyl alcohol, 10 mg/mL

Related Information

Anticoagulants, Injectable *on page 1711*

♦ **Tinzaparin Sodium** *see* Tinzaparin *on page 1482*

Tioconazole *(tye oh KONE a zole)*

U.S. Brand Names 1-Day™ [OTC]; Vagistat®-1 [OTC]

Generic Available No

Pharmacologic Category Antifungal Agent, Vaginal

Medication Safety Issues

Sound-alike/look-alike issues:
Tioconazole may be confused with terconazole

Use Local treatment of vulvovaginal candidiasis

Mechanism of Action/Effect A 1-substituted imidazole derivative with a broad antifungal
spectrum against a wide variety of dermatophytes and yeasts

Contraindications Hypersensitivity to tioconazole or any component of the formulation

Warnings/Precautions For vaginal use only. Petrolatum-based vaginal products may
damage rubber or latex condoms or diaphragms. Separate use by 3 days.

Drug Interactions

Cytochrome P450 Effect: Inhibits CYP1A2 (weak), 2A6 (weak), 2C8/9 (weak), 2C19
(weak), 2D6 (weak), 2E1 (weak)

Adverse Reactions Frequency not defined.

Central nervous system: Headache

Gastrointestinal: Abdominal pain

Dermatologic: Burning, desquamation

Genitourinary: Discharge, dyspareunia, dysuria, irritation, itching, nocturia, vaginal pain, vaginitis, vulvar swelling

Pharmacodynamics/Kinetics

Onset of Action: Some improvement: Within 24 hours; Complete relief: Within 7 days

Absorption: Intravaginal: Systemic (small amounts)

Excretion: Urine and feces

Dosing

Adults & Elderly: Vulvovaginal candidiasis: Vaginal: Insert 1 applicatorful in vagina, just
prior to bedtime, as a single dose

Available Dosage Forms Ointment, vaginal: 6.5% (4.6 g) [with applicator]

Monitoring and Teaching Issues

Physical Assessment: Assess knowledge/teach patient appropriate administration,
possible side effects/interventions, and adverse symptoms to report.

Patient Education: Consult with healthcare provider if treating a vaginal yeast infection for
the first time. Insert high into the vagina. Refrain from intercourse during treatment. May
interact with condoms and vaginal contraceptive diaphragms (ie, weaken latex); do not rely
on these products for 3 days following treatment. Do not use tampons, douches, spermicides, or other vaginal products during treatment. Although product is used for a single day,
relief from symptoms usually takes longer than 1 day. Report persistent (>3 days) vaginal
burning, irritation, or discharge. **Breast-feeding precaution:** Breast-feeding is not recommended.

Pregnancy Risk Factor: C
Lactation: Excretion in breast milk unknown/not recommended
Administration
 Storage: Store at room temperature.

♦ **Tioguanine** *see Thioguanine on page 1462*
♦ **Tiotixene** *see Thiothixene on page 1467*

Tiotropium (ty oh TRO pee um)

U.S. Brand Names Spiriva®
Synonyms Tiotropium Bromide Monohydrate
Pharmacologic Category Anticholinergic Agent
Medication Safety Issues
 Sound-alike/look-alike issues:
  Spiriva® may be confused with Inspra™
Use Maintenance treatment of bronchospasm associated with COPD (bronchitis and emphysema)
Mechanism of Action/Effect Blocks the action of acetylcholine at parasympathetic sites in bronchial smooth muscle causing bronchodilation
Contraindications Hypersensitivity to tiotropium, its derivatives, or any component of the formulation (contains lactose); not for use as an acute ("rescue") bronchodilator
Warnings/Precautions Not indicated for the initial treatment of acute episodes of bronchospasm; use with caution in patients with myasthenia gravis, narrow-angle glaucoma, prostatic hyperplasia, or bladder neck obstruction; avoid inadvertent instillation of powder into the eyes. Immediate hypersensitivity reactions may occur. Use caution in renal impairment. Safety and efficacy have not been established in pediatric patients.
Drug Interactions
 Cytochrome P450 Effect: Substrate (minor) of CYP2D6, 3A4
 Increased Effect/Toxicity: Increased toxicity with anticholinergics or drugs with anticholinergic properties.
Adverse Reactions
 >10%:
  Gastrointestinal: Xerostomia (16%)
  Respiratory: Upper respiratory tract infection (41% vs 37% with placebo), sinusitis (11% vs 9% with placebo), pharyngeal irritation (frequency not specified)
 1% to 10%:
  Cardiovascular: Angina, edema (dependent, 5%)
  Central nervous system: Paresthesia, depression
  Dermatologic: Rash (4%)
  Endocrine & metabolic: Hypercholesterolemia, hyperglycemia
  Gastrointestinal: Dyspepsia (6%), abdominal pain (5%), constipation (4%), vomiting (4%), reflux, ulcerative stomatitis
  Genitourinary: Urinary tract infection (7%)
  Neuromuscular & skeletal: Myalgia (4%), leg pain, skeletal pain
  Ocular: Cataract
  Respiratory: Pharyngitis (9%), rhinitis (6%), epistaxis (4%), dysphonia, laryngitis
  Miscellaneous: Infection (4%), moniliasis (4%), allergic reaction, herpes zoster
Overdosage/Toxicology Conjunctivitis and xerostomia have been observed with doses up to 141 micrograms. Other symptoms of overdose include drying of respiratory secretions, cough, nausea, GI distress, blurred vision or impaired visual accommodation, headache, and nervousness. Acute overdose with tiotropium by inhalation is unlikely since it is so poorly absorbed. However, if poisoning occurs, it can be treated like any other anticholinergic toxicity. An anticholinergic overdose with severe life-threatening symptoms may be treated with physostigmine 1-2 mg SubQ or I.V. slowly.
Pharmacodynamics/Kinetics
 Absorption: Poorly absorbed from GI tract, systemic absorption may occur from lung.
 Bioavailability: Following inhalation: 19.5%; oral solution: 2% to 3%
 Time to Peak: Plasma: 5 minutes (following inhalation)
 Protein Binding: 72%
 Half-Life Elimination: 5-6 days
 Metabolism: Hepatic (minimal), via CYP2D6 and CYP3A4
 Excretion: Urine (74% as unchanged drug)
Dosing
 Adults & Elderly: COPD: Oral inhalation: Contents of 1 capsule (18 mcg) inhaled once daily using HandiHaler® device
 Renal Impairment: Plasma concentrations increase in renal impairment. Use caution; no specific dosage adjustment recommended.
Available Dosage Forms Powder for oral inhalation [capsule]: 18 mcg/capsule [contains lactose; packaged in 6s or 30s with HandiHaler® device]
Monitoring and Teaching Issues
 Physical Assessment: Assess potential for interactions with other prescription or OTC medications or herbal products patient may be taking. Assess results of pulmonary tests prior to and periodically during therapy. Assess therapeutic effectiveness and adverse response at beginning of therapy and at regular intervals during therapy. Teach patient proper use, appropriate interventions to reduce side effects, and adverse symptoms to report.
 Monitoring Laboratory Tests: FEV_1, peak flow (or other pulmonary function studies)
 Patient Education: Use inhaler and medication as instructed - once daily, at same time each day. Do not use more often than prescribed. Do not use as an acute "rescue" bronchodilator. May cause nausea or vomiting (small frequent meals and frequent mouth care may help);hyperglycemia (if diabetic, monitor serum glucose closely); muscle or skeletal pain (consult prescriber for appropriate analgesic). Report swelling of face, mouth, or tongue; skin rash; chest pain or palpitations; persistent gastrointestinal effects; muscle
(Continued)

Tiotropium *(Continued)*

or skeletal pain or weakness; change in vision; respiratory changes, sore throat, or flu-like symptoms. **Pregnancy/breast-feeding precautions:** Inform prescriber if you are or intent to be pregnant. Breast-feeding is not recommended.

Administration of HandiHaler® Inhaler: Remove capsule from blister pack immediately before using. Place capsule in capsule-chamber in the base of inhaler. Close mouthpiece until a click is heard, leaving dustcap open. Exhale fully (do not exhale into inhaler). Place mouthpiece gently between teeth, closing lips around inhaled, tilt head back slightly, and inhale once rapidly, steadily and deeply. (the capsule may vibration may be heard within the inhaler, but you will not sense the medication as it is inhaled.) Hold breath as long as possible. Remove inhaler from mouth before exhaling. If any powder remains in capsule, repeat inhalation again. Throw away empty capsule. After using inhaler, rinse mouth with water and spit out rinse water. Do not store capsule in inhaler and always keep inhaler and capsules dry.

Geriatric Considerations: Assess patient's ability to use the HandiHaler®. In elderly patients, renal clearance of tiotropium was decreased and plasma concentrations were increased, due to decreased renal function. No significant difference in adverse effects were seen in young vs older patients. No dosage adjustments are recommended due to age or renal function. However, the manufacturer recommends monitoring patients with moderate-to-severe renal impairment.

Pregnancy Risk Factor: C

Lactation: Excretion in breast milk unknown/use caution

Administration

Oral: For inhalation, not to be swallowed

Inhalation: Administer once daily at the same time each day. Remove capsule from foil blister immediately before use. Place capsule in the capsule-chamber in the base of the HandiHaler® Inhaler. Must only use the HandiHaler® Inhaler. Close mouthpiece until a click is heard, leaving dustcap open. Exhale fully. Do not exhale into inhaler. Tilt head slightly back and inhale (rapidly, steadily and deeply); the capsule vibration may be heard within the device. Hold breath as long as possible. If any powder remains in capsule, exhale and inhale again. Repeat until capsule is empty. Throw away empty capsule; do not leave in inhaler. Do not use a spacer with the HandiHaler® Inhaler. Always keep capsules and inhaler dry.

Delivery of dose: Instruct patient to place mouthpiece gently between teeth, closing lips around inhaler. Instruct patient to inhale deeply and hold breath held for 5-10 seconds. The amount of drug delivered is small, and the individual will not sense the medication as it is inhaled. Remove mouthpiece prior to exhalation. Patient should not breathe out through the mouthpiece. After use of the inhaler, patient should rinse mouth/oropharynx with water and spit out rinse solution.

Storage: Store between 15°C and 25°C. Do not store capsules in HandiHaler® device. Capsules should be stored in the blister pack and only removed immediately before use. After first capsule in the strip is used, the 2 remaining capsules should be used over the next 2 days.

♦ **Tiotropium Bromide Monohydrate** *see* Tiotropium *on page 1485*

Tirofiban *(tye roe FYE ban)*

U.S. Brand Names Aggrastat®

Synonyms MK383; Tirofiban Hydrochloride

Generic Available No

Pharmacologic Category Antiplatelet Agent, Glycoprotein IIb/IIIa Inhibitor

Medication Safety Issues

Sound-alike/look-alike issues:

Aggrastat® may be confused with Aggrenox®, argatroban

Use In combination with heparin, is indicated for the treatment of acute coronary syndrome, including patients who are to be managed medically and those undergoing PTCA or atherectomy. In this setting, it has been shown to decrease the rate of a combined endpoint of death, new myocardial infarction or refractory ischemia/repeat cardiac procedure.

Mechanism of Action/Effect A reversible antagonist of fibrinogen binding to the GP IIb/IIIa receptor, the major platelet surface receptor involved in platelet aggregation. Platelet aggregation inhibition is reversible following cessation of the infusion.

Contraindications Hypersensitivity to tirofiban or any component of the formulation; active internal bleeding or a history of bleeding diathesis within the previous 30 days; history of intracranial hemorrhage, intracranial neoplasm, arteriovenous malformation, or aneurysm; history of thrombocytopenia following prior exposure; history of CVA within 30 days or any history of hemorrhagic stroke; major surgical procedure or severe physical trauma within the previous month; history, symptoms, or findings suggestive of aortic dissection; severe hypertension (systolic BP >180 mm Hg and/or diastolic BP >110 mm Hg); concomitant use of another parenteral GP IIb/IIIa inhibitor; acute pericarditis

Warnings/Precautions Bleeding is the most common complication. Watch closely for bleeding, especially the arterial access site for the cardiac catheterization. Prior to pulling the sheath, heparin should be discontinued for 3-4 hours and ACT <180 seconds or aPTT <45 seconds. Use standard compression techniques after sheath removal. Watch the site closely afterwards for further bleeding. Use with extreme caution in patients with platelet counts <150,000/mm³, patients with hemorrhagic retinopathy, and chronic dialysis patients. Use caution with administration of other drugs affecting hemostasis. Adjust the dose with severe renal dysfunction (Cl_cr <30 mL/minute). The use of tirofiban, aspirin and heparin together causes more bleeding than aspirin and heparin alone.

Drug Interactions

Decreased Effect: Levothyroxine and omeprazole decrease tirofiban levels; however, the clinical significance of this interaction remains to be demonstrated.

Increased Effect/Toxicity: Use of tirofiban with aspirin and heparin is associated with an increase in bleeding over aspirin and heparin alone; however, efficacy of tirofiban is improved. Risk of bleeding is increased when used with thrombolytics, oral anticoagulants, NSAIDs, dipyridamole, ticlopidine, and clopidogrel. Avoid concomitant use of other IIb/IIIa antagonists. Cephalosporins which contain the MTT side chain may theoretically increase the risk of hemorrhage.

Adverse Reactions Bleeding is the major drug-related adverse effect. Patients received background treatment with aspirin and heparin. Major bleeding was reported in 1.4% to 2.2%; minor bleeding in 10.5% to 12%; transfusion was required in 4% to 4.3%.

>1% (nonbleeding adverse events):
Cardiovascular: Bradycardia (4%), coronary artery dissection (5%), edema (2%)
Central nervous system: Dizziness (3%), fever (>1%), headache (>1%), vasovagal reaction (2%)
Gastrointestinal: Nausea (>1%)
Genitourinary: Pelvic pain (6%)
Hematologic: Thrombocytopenia: <90,000/mm^3 (1.5%), <50,000/mm^3 (0.3%)
Neuromuscular & skeletal: Leg pain (3%)
Miscellaneous: Diaphoresis (2%)

Overdosage/Toxicology The most frequent manifestation of overdose is bleeding. Treatment is cessation of therapy and assessment of transfusion. Tirofiban is dialyzable.

Pharmacodynamics/Kinetics
Half-Life Elimination: 2 hours
Metabolism: Minimally hepatic
Excretion: Urine (65%) and feces (25%) primarily as unchanged drug
Clearance: Elderly: Reduced by 19% to 26%

Dosing
Adults & Elderly: Acute coronary syndromes: I.V.: Initial rate of 0.4 mcg/kg/minute for 30 minutes and then continued at 0.1 mcg/kg/minute. Dosing should be continued through angiography and for 12-24 hours after angioplasty or atherectomy.
Renal Impairment: Cl$_{cr}$ <30 mL/minute: Reduce dose to 50% of normal rate.

Available Dosage Forms
Infusion, as hydrochloride [premixed in sodium chloride]: 50 mcg/mL (100 mL, 250 mL)
Injection, solution, as hydrochloride: 250 mcg/mL (50 mL)

Monitoring and Teaching Issues
Physical Assessment: Monitor vital signs and laboratory results prior to, during, and after therapy. Assess infusion insertion site during and after therapy. Monitor closely for bleeding and teach bleeding precautions.
Monitoring Laboratory Tests: Platelet count, persistent reductions <90,000/mm^3 may require interruption or discontinuation of infusion. Hemoglobin and hematocrit should be monitored prior to treatment, within 6 hours following loading infusion, and at least daily thereafter during therapy. Platelet count may need to be monitored earlier in patients who received prior glycoprotein IIb/IIa antagonists. Because tirofiban requires concurrent heparin therapy, aPTT levels should also be followed.
Patient Education: Emergency use may dictate depth of patient education. This medication can only be administered I.V. You will have a tendency to bleed easily following this medication. Use caution to prevent injury (use electric razor, use soft toothbrush, use caution with sharps). If bleeding occurs, apply pressure to bleeding spot until bleeding stops completely. Report unusual bruising or bleeding (eg, blood in urine, stool, or vomitus; bleeding gums, vaginal bleeding, nosebleeds); unusual and persistent fever; dizziness or vision changes; back, leg, or pelvic pain; or persistent nausea or vomiting. **Breast-feeding precaution:** Do not breast-feed.
Pregnancy Risk Factor: B
Lactation: Excretion in breast milk unknown/contraindicated

Administration
I.V.: Infuse over 30 minutes. Tirofiban injection must be diluted to a concentration of 50 mcg/mL (premixed solution does not require dilution). Unused solution should be discarded. Do not administer via the same IV line as diazepam.
Compatibility: Stable in D$_5$¹/₂NS, D$_5$W, NS
Y-site administration: Incompatible with diazepam
Storage: Store at 25°C (77°F); do not freeze. Protect from light during storage.

♦ **Tirofiban Hydrochloride** *see* Tirofiban *on page 1486*
♦ **Titralac™ [OTC]** *see* Calcium Carbonate *on page 235*
♦ **Titralac™ Extra Strength [OTC]** *see* Calcium Carbonate *on page 235*

Tizanidine (tye ZAN i deen)

U.S. Brand Names Zanaflex®
Synonyms Sirdalud®
Generic Available Yes
Pharmacologic Category Alpha$_2$-Adrenergic Agonist
Medication Safety Issues
Sound-alike/look-alike issues:
Tizanidine may be confused with tiagabine
Use Skeletal muscle relaxant used for treatment of muscle spasticity
Unlabeled/Investigational Use Tension headaches, low back pain, and trigeminal neuralgia
Contraindications Hypersensitivity to tizanidine or any component of the formulation; concomitant therapy with fluvoxamine
Warnings/Precautions Reduce dose in patients with liver or renal disease. May cause significant orthostatic hypotension or bradycardia; use with caution in patients with hypotension or cardiac disease. Tizanidine clearance is reduced by more than 50% in elderly patients with renal insufficiency (Cl$_{cr}$ <25 mL/minute) compared to healthy elderly subjects; this may lead to a longer duration of effects and, therefore, should be used with caution in renally-impaired patients. Take consistently with or without food.
(Continued)

Tizanidine *(Continued)*

Drug Interactions

Cytochrome P450 Effect: Substrate of CYP1A2 (major)

Increased Effect/Toxicity: Oral contraceptives may decrease the clearance of tizanidine. Additive hypotensive effects may be seen with diuretics, other alpha adrenergic agonists, or antihypertensives; CNS depression with baclofen or other CNS depressants. CYP1A2 inhibitors may increase the levels/effects of tizanidine; example inhibitors include amiodarone, ciprofloxacin, fluvoxamine, ketoconazole, norfloxacin, ofloxacin, and rofecoxib. Fluvoxamine may increase levels/effects (eg, hypotension) of tizanidine.

Nutritional/Ethanol Interactions

Ethanol: Avoid ethanol (may increase CNS depression).

Food: The tablet and capsule dosage forms are not bioequivalent when administered with food. Food increases both the time to peak concentration and the extent of absorption for both the tablet and capsule. However, maximal concentrations of tizanidine achieved when administered with food were increased by 30% for the tablet, but decreased by 20% for the capsule. Under fed conditions, the capsule is ~80% bioavailable relative to the tablet.

Herb/Nutraceutical: Avoid valerian, St John's wort, kava kava, gotu kola (may increase CNS depression). Avoid black cohosh, California poppy, coleus, golden seal, hawthorn, mistletoe, periwinkle, quinine, shepherd's purse (may increase hypotensive effects).

Adverse Reactions

>10%:
Cardiovascular: Hypotension (16% to 33%)
Central nervous system: Somnolence (48%), dizziness (16%)
Gastrointestinal: Xerostomia (49%)
Neuromuscular & skeletal: Weakness (41%)

1% to 10%:
Cardiovascular: Bradycardia (2% to 10%)
Central nervous system:, Nervousness (3%), speech disorder (3%)
Gastrointestinal: Constipation (4%), vomiting (3%), pharyngitis (3%)
Genitourinary: UTI (10%), urinary frequency (3%)
Hepatic: Liver enzymes increased (3%)
Neuromuscular & skeletal: Dyskinesia (3%)
Ocular: Blurred vision (3%)
Respiratory: Rhinitis (3%)
Miscellaneous: Infection (6%), flu (3%)

Overdosage/Toxicology

Symptoms of overdose include dry mouth, bradycardia, hypotension

Treatment: Lavage (within 2 hours of ingestion) with activated charcoal; benzodiazepines for seizure control; atropine can be given for treatment of bradycardia; flumazenil has been used to reverse coma successfully; forced diuresis is not helpful; multiple dosing of activated charcoal may be helpful. Following attempts to enhance drug elimination, hypotension should be treated with I.V. fluids and/or Trendelenburg positioning.

Pharmacodynamics/Kinetics

Duration of Action: 3-6 hours

Bioavailability: 40%

Time to Peak:
Fasting state: Capsule, tablet: 1 hour
Fed state: Capsule: 3-4 hours, Tablet: 1.5 hours

Protein Binding: 30%

Half-Life Elimination: 2 hours

Metabolism: Extensively hepatic

Excretion: Urine (60%); feces (20%)

Dosing

Adults & Elderly:
Spasticity: Usual initial dose: 4 mg, may increase by 2-4 mg as needed for satisfactory reduction of muscle tone every 6-8 hours to a maximum of three doses in any 24 hour period
Range: 2-4 mg 3 times/day
Maximum dose: 36 mg/day

Renal Impairment: May require dose reductions or less frequent dosing

Hepatic Impairment: May require dose reductions or less frequent dosing.

Available Dosage Forms

Capsule: 2 mg, 4 mg, 6 mg
Tablet: 2 mg, 4 mg

Monitoring and Teaching Issues

Physical Assessment: Assess potential for interactions with other prescriptions, OTC medications, or herbal products patient may be taking. Assess results of laboratory tests, therapeutic effectiveness, and adverse reactions on a regular basis throughout therapy. Teach patient proper use, possible side effects/appropriate interventions, and adverse symptoms to report.

Patient Education: Take exactly as directed; do not change dosage or discontinue without consulting prescriber. If you miss a dose, take the missed dose as soon as possible if it is within an hour or so of the regular time. If not within an hour or so, skip the missed dose and go back to your regular dosing schedule. Do not double doses. Avoid alcohol. May cause dizziness, nervousness, insomnia, or daytime drowsiness (use caution when driving or engaging in tasks that require alertness until response to drug is known); postural hypotension (use caution and avoid quick moves when rising from sitting or lying position, climbing stairs, or engaging in activities that require quick movements); or nausea, vomiting, dry mouth, mouth sores, or upset stomach (small frequent meals, frequent mouth care, chewing gum, or sucking lozenges may help). Report persistent dizziness or GI symptoms; chest pain or palpitations; CNS disturbances (delusions, confusion); muscle weakness or tremors; rash; respiratory difficulty; or other persistent adverse effects. **Pregnancy/breast-feeding precautions:** Inform prescriber if you are or intend to become pregnant. Breast-feeding is not recommended.

Dietary Considerations: Food affects the absorption of tizanidine. Take consistently with or without food.

Pregnancy Risk Factor: C

Lactation: Excretion in breast milk unknown/not recommended

Administration

Oral: Capsules may be opened and contents sprinkled on food; however, extent of absorption is increased up to 20% relative to administration of the capsule under fasted conditions.

- ◆ **TMP** *see* Trimethoprim *on page 1528*
- ◆ **TMP-SMZ** *see* Sulfamethoxazole and Trimethoprim *on page 1407*
- ◆ **TMZ** *see* Temozolomide *on page 1436*
- ◆ **TNKase™** *see* Tenecteplase *on page 1438*
- ◆ **TOBI®** *see* Tobramycin *on page 1489*
- ◆ **TobraDex®** *see* Tobramycin and Dexamethasone *on page 1492*

Tobramycin (toe bra MYE sin)
U.S. Brand Names AKTob®; Nebcin® [DSC]; TOBI®; Tobrex®
Synonyms Tobramycin Sulfate
Generic Available Yes; Excludes ophthalmic ointment, solution for nebulization
Pharmacologic Category Antibiotic, Aminoglycoside; Antibiotic, Ophthalmic
Medication Safety Issues
Sound-alike/look-alike issues:
Tobramycin may be confused with Trobicin®
AKTob® may be confused with AK-Trol®
Nebcin® may be confused with Inapsine®, Naprosyn®, Nubain®
Tobrex® may be confused with TobraDex®
Use Treatment of documented or suspected infections caused by susceptible gram-negative bacilli including *Pseudomonas aeruginosa*; topically used to treat superficial ophthalmic infections caused by susceptible bacteria. Tobramycin solution for inhalation is indicated for the management of cystic fibrosis patients (>6 years of age) with *Pseudomonas aeruginosa*.
Mechanism of Action/Effect Interferes with bacterial protein synthesis by binding to 30S and 50S ribosomal subunits resulting in a defective bacterial cell membrane
Contraindications Hypersensitivity to tobramycin, other aminoglycosides, or any component of the formulation; pregnancy (injection/inhalation)
Warnings/Precautions Use with caution in patients with renal impairment, pre-existing auditory or vestibular impairment, and in patients with neuromuscular disorders. Dosage modification required in patients with impaired renal function (I.M. & I.V.). Aminoglycosides are associated with significant nephrotoxicity or ototoxicity; the ototoxicity is directly proportional to the amount of drug given and the duration of treatment. Tinnitus or vertigo are indications of vestibular injury. Ototoxicity is often irreversible, while renal damage is usually reversible.
Drug Interactions
Increased Effect/Toxicity: Increased antimicrobial effect of tobramycin with extended spectrum penicillins (synergistic). Neuromuscular blockers may have an increased duration of action (neuromuscular blockade). Amphotericin B, cephalosporins, and loop diuretics may increase the risk of nephrotoxicity.
Lab Interactions Increased protein, BUN, aminotransferase [AST (SGOT)/ALT (SGPT)] (S), alkaline phosphatase, creatinine; decreased magnesium, potassium, sodium, calcium (S)
Adverse Reactions
Injection: Frequency not defined:
Central nervous system: Confusion, disorientation, dizziness, fever, headache, lethargy, vertigo
Dermatologic: Exfoliative dermatitis, itching, rash, urticaria
Endocrine & metabolic: Serum calcium, magnesium, potassium, and/or sodium decreased
Gastrointestinal: Diarrhea, nausea, vomiting
Hematologic: Anemia, eosinophilia, granulocytopenia, leukocytosis, leukopenia, thrombocytopenia
Hepatic: ALT, AST, bilirubin, and/or LDH increased
Local: Pain at the injection site
Otic: Hearing loss, tinnitus, ototoxicity (auditory), ototoxicity (vestibular), roaring in the ears
Renal: BUN increased, cylindruria, serum creatinine increased, oliguria, proteinuria

Inhalation:
>10%:
Gastrointestinal: Sputum discoloration (21%)
Respiratory: Voice alteration (13%)
1% to 10%:
Central nervous system: Malaise (6%)
Otic: Tinnitus (3%)
Overdosage/Toxicology Symptoms of overdose include ototoxicity, nephrotoxicity, and neuromuscular toxicity. Treatment of choice following a single acute overdose appears to be maintenance of urine output of at least 3 mL/kg/hour during the acute treatment phase. Dialysis is of questionable value in enhancing aminoglycoside elimination. If required, hemodialysis is preferred over peritoneal dialysis in patients with normal renal function. Chelation with penicillins is investigational.
Pharmacodynamics/Kinetics
Absorption: I.M.: Rapid and complete
Time to Peak: Serum: I.M.: 30-60 minutes; I.V.: ~30 minutes
Protein Binding: <30%
Half-Life Elimination:
Neonates: ≤1200 g: 11 hours; >1200 g: 2-9 hours
(Continued)

Tobramycin *(Continued)*

Adults: 2-3 hours; directly dependent upon glomerular filtration rate

Adults with impaired renal function: 5-70 hours

Excretion: Normal renal function: Urine (~90% to 95%) within 24 hours

Dosing

Adults: Individualization is **critical** because of the low therapeutic index.

Use of ideal body weight (IBW) for determining the mg/kg/dose appears to be more accurate than dosing on the basis of total body weight (TBW). In morbid obesity, dosage requirement may best be estimated using a dosing weight of IBW + 0.4 (TBW - IBW).

Initial and periodic plasma drug levels (eg, peak and trough with conventional dosing) should be determined, particularly in critically-ill patients with serious infections or in disease states known to significantly alter aminoglycoside pharmacokinetics (eg, cystic fibrosis, burns, or major surgery).

I.M., I.V.:

Severe life-threatening infections:

Conventional dosing: 2-2.5 mg/kg/dose every 8-12 hours; to ensure adequate peak concentrations early in therapy, higher initial dosages may be considered in selected patients (eg, edema, septic shock, postsurgery, and/or trauma).

Once-daily dosing: Some clinicians suggest a daily dose of 4-7 mg/kg for all patients with normal renal function; this dose is at least as efficacious with similar, if not less, toxicity than conventional dosing.

Urinary tract infection: 1.5 mg/kg/dose

Synergy (for gram-positive infections): 1 mg/kg/dose

Ocular infections: Ophthalmic:

Ointment: Apply 2-3 times/day; for severe infections, apply every 3-4 hours

Solution: Instill 1-2 drops every 4 hours; for severe infections, instill 2 drops every 30-60 minutes initially, then reduce to less frequent intervals

Pulmonary infections: Inhalation:

Standard aerosolized tobramycin: 60-80 mg 3 times/day

High-dose regimen: 300 mg every 12 hours (do not administer doses >6 hours apart); administer in repeated cycles of 28 days on drug followed by 28 days off drug

Elderly: Dosage should be based on an estimate of ideal body weight.

I.M., I.V.: 1.5-5 mg/kg/day in 1-2 divided doses

I.V.: Once daily or extended interval: 5-7 mg/kg/dose given every 24, 36, or 48 hours based on Cl_{cr} (see Renal Impairment and Geriatric Considerations).

Pediatrics: Individualization is **critical** because of the low therapeutic index

Use of ideal body weight (IBW) for determining the mg/kg/dose appears to be more accurate than dosing on the basis of total body weight (TBW). In morbid obesity, dosage requirement may best be estimated using a dosing weight of IBW + 0.4 (TBW - IBW).

Susceptible systemic infections: I.M., I.V.:

Infants and Children <5 years: 2.5 mg/kg/dose every 8 hours

Children >5 years: 2-2.5 g/kg/dose every 8 hours

Ocular infection: Ophthalmic: Children ≥2 months: See adult dosing.

Cystic fibrosis:

I.M., I.V.: 2.5-3.3 mg/kg every 6-8 hours

Inhalation:

Standard aerosolized tobramycin: 40-80 mg 2-3 times/day

High-dose regimen (TOBI®): Children ≥6 years: See adult dosing.

Note: Some patients may require larger or more frequent doses if serum levels document the need (eg, cystic fibrosis or febrile granulocytopenic patients). Also see drug level monitoring information in adult dosing.

Renal Impairment: I.M., I.V.:

Conventional dosing:

Cl_{cr} ≥60 mL/minute: Administer every 8 hours.

Cl_{cr} 40-60 mL/minute: Administer every 12 hours.

Cl_{cr} 20-40 mL/minute: Administer every 24 hours.

Cl_{cr} 10-20 mL/minute: Administer every 48 hours.

Cl_{cr} <10 mL/minute: Administer every 72 hours.

High-dose therapy: Interval may be extended (eg, every 48 hours) in patients with moderate renal impairment (Cl_{cr} 30-59 mL/minute) and/or adjusted based on serum level determinations.

Dialyzable; 30% removal of aminoglycosides occurs during 4 hours of HD - administer dose after dialysis and follow levels.

Continuous arteriovenous or venovenous hemofiltration: Dose as for Cl_{cr} of 10-40 mL/minute and follow levels.

Administration via CAPD fluid:

Gram-negative infection: 4-8 mg/L (4-8 mcg/mL) of CAPD fluid

Gram-positive infection (ie, synergy): 3-4 mg/L (3-4 mcg/mL) of CAPD fluid

Administration IVPB/I.M.: Dose as for Cl_{cr} <10 mL/minute and follow levels.

Hepatic Impairment: Monitor plasma concentrations.

Available Dosage Forms [DSC] = Discontinued product

Injection, powder for reconstitution (Nebcin® [DSC]): 1.2 g

Injection, solution, as sulfate: 10 mg/mL (2 mL, 8 mL); 40 mg/mL (2 mL, 30 mL, 50 mL) [may contain sodium metabisulfite]

Nebcin®: 40 mg/mL (2 mL) [contains sodium bisulfite] [DSC]

Ointment, ophthalmic (Tobrex®): 0.3% (3.5 g)

Solution for nebulization [preservative free] (TOBI®): 60 mg/mL (5 mL)

Solution, ophthalmic (AKTob®, Tobrex®): 0.3% (5 mL) [contains benzalkonium chloride]

Monitoring and Teaching Issues

Physical Assessment: Assess effectiveness and interactions of other medications patient may be taking. Assess patient's hearing level before, during, and following therapy. Monitor therapeutic effectiveness, laboratory values, and adverse reactions (eg, ototoxicity and nephrotoxicity) at beginning of therapy and periodically throughout therapy. Assess knowledge/teach patient appropriate use, interventions to reduce side effects, and adverse symptoms to report.

Monitoring Laboratory Tests: Urinalysis, BUN, serum creatinine, plasma tobramycin levels (as appropriate to dosing method). Peak levels are drawn 30 minutes after the end of a 30-minute infusion or 1 hour after initiation of infusion or I.M. injection. The trough is drawn just before the next dose. Levels are typically obtained after the third dose in conventional dosing. Perform culture and sensitivity studies prior to initiating therapy to determine the causative organism and its susceptibility to tobramycin.

Patient Education: Systemic: Maintain adequate hydration (2-3 L/day of fluids) unless instructed to restrict fluid intake. Report decreased urine output, swelling of extremities, respiratory difficulty, vaginal itching or discharge, rash, diarrhea, oral thrush, unhealed wounds, dizziness, change in hearing acuity or ringing in ears, or worsening of condition. **Pregnancy/breast-feeding precautions:** Inform prescriber if you are pregnant. Breast-feeding is not recommended.

Ophthalmic: Use as frequently as recommended; do not overuse. Do not let tip of applicator touch eye; do not contaminate tip of applicator (may cause eye infection, eye damage, or vision loss). Sit down, tilt head back, instill solution or drops inside lower eyelid, and roll eyeball in all directions. Close eye and apply gentle pressure to inner corner of eye for 30 seconds. May experience temporary stinging or blurred vision. Do not use any other eye preparation for 10 minutes. Inform prescriber if condition worsens or does not improve in 3-4 days.

Dietary Considerations: May require supplementation of calcium, magnesium, potassium.

Geriatric Considerations: Aminoglycosides are important therapeutic interventions for susceptible organisms and as empiric therapy in seriously ill patients. Their use is not without risk of toxicity; however, these risks can be minimized if initial dosing is adjusted for estimated renal function and appropriate monitoring is performed. High-dose, once-daily aminoglycosides have been advocated as an alternative to traditional dosing regimens. To date, there is little information on the safety and efficacy of these regimens in persons with a creatinine clearance <60 mL/minute/70 kg. A dosing nomogram based upon creatinine clearance has been proposed. Additional studies comparing high-dose, once-daily aminoglycosides to traditional dosing regimens in the elderly are needed before once-daily aminoglycoside dosing can be routinely adopted to this patient population.

Pregnancy Risk Factor: D (injection, inhalation); B (ophthalmic)

Pregnancy Issues: Aminoglycosides, including tobramycin, cross the placenta. The manufacturers of Nebcin® and TOBI® have a labeled pregnancy category of D based on reports of bilateral congenital deafness in children whose mothers used streptomycin during pregnancy. The risk of teratogenic effects and deafness following *in utero* exposure to tobramycin is considered to be small and some resources consider the pregnancy risk factor to be C. The manufacturer of Tobrex® states that animal studies have not shown harm to the fetus; however, no adequate and well-controlled studies have been conducted in pregnant women.

Lactation: Enters breast milk/not recommended

Breast-Feeding Issues: Tobramycin is excreted into breast milk. The actual amount following inhalation or topical therapy is not known. The AAP considers a related antibiotic, gentamicin, usually compatible with breast-feeding.

Administration

I.V.: Infuse over 30-60 minutes. Give penicillins or cephalosporins at least 1 hour apart from tobramycin.

Inhalation: TOBI®: To be inhaled over ~15 minutes using a handheld nebulizer.

Topical: Ophthalmic solution: Allow 5 minutes between application of "multiple-drop" therapy.

Other: Ophthalmic: Contact lenses should not be worn during treatment of ophthalmic infections.

Ointment: Do not touch tip of tube to eye. Instill ointment into pocket between eyeball and lower lid; patient should look downward before closing eye.

Solution: contact lenses should not be worn during treatment of ophthalmic infections. Allow 5 minutes between application of "multiple-drop" therapy.

Suspension: Shake well before using; Tilt head back, instill suspension in conjunctival sac and close eye(s). Do not touch dropper to eye. Apply light finger pressure on lacrimal sac for 1 minute following instillation.

Reconstitution: Stability of parenteral admixture at room temperature (25°C) and at refrigeration temperature (4°C) is 48 hours. Standard diluent: Dose/100 mL NS; minimum volume: 50 mL NS

Compatibility: Stable in dextran 40 10% in dextrose, D₅NS, D₅W, D₁₀W, mannitol 20%, LR, NS

Y-site administration: Incompatible with allopurinol, amphotericin B cholesteryl sulfate complex, cefoperazone, heparin, hetastarch, indomethacin, propofol, sargramostim

Compatibility in syringe: Incompatible with cefamandole, clindamycin, heparin

Compatibility when admixed: Incompatible with cefamandole, cefepime, cefotaxime, cefotetan, floxacillin, heparin, penicillins

Storage:

Injection: Stable at room temperature both as the clear, colorless solution and as the dry powder. Reconstituted solutions remain stable for 24 hours at room temperature and 96 hours when refrigerated.

Ophthalmic solution: Store at 8°C to 27°C (46°F to 80°F).

Solution, for inhalation (TOBI®): Store under refrigeration at 2°C to 8°C (36°F to 46°F); may be stored in foil pouch at room temperature of 25°C (77°F) for up to 28 days. Avoid intense light. Solution may darken over time; however, do not use if cloudy or contains particles.

(Continued)

Tobramycin (Continued)

Additional Information Once-daily dosing: Higher peak serum drug concentration to MIC ratios, demonstrated aminoglycoside postantibiotic effect, decreased renal cortex drug uptake, and improved cost-time efficiency are supportive reasons for the use of once daily dosing regimens for aminoglycosides. Current research indicates these regimens to be as effective for nonlife-threatening infections, with no higher incidence of nephrotoxicity, than those requiring multiple daily doses. Doses are determined by calculating the entire day's dose via usual multiple dose calculation techniques and administering this quantity as a single dose. Doses are then adjusted to maintain mean serum concentrations above the MIC(s) of the causative organism(s). (Example: 2.5-5 mg/kg as a single dose; expected Cp_{max}: 10-20 mcg/mL and Cp_{min}: <1 mcg/mL). Further research is needed for universal recommendation in all patient populations and gram-negative disease; exceptions may include those with known high clearance (eg, children, patients with cystic fibrosis, or burns who may require shorter dosage intervals) and patients with renal function impairment for whom longer than conventional dosage intervals are usually required.

Related Information

Antimicrobial Drugs of Choice *on page 1792*
Peak and Trough Guidelines *on page 1694*

Tobramycin and Dexamethasone (toe bra MYE sin & deks a METH a sone)

U.S. Brand Names TobraDex®

Synonyms Dexamethasone and Tobramycin

Generic Available No

Pharmacologic Category Antibiotic/Corticosteroid, Ophthalmic

Medication Safety Issues

Sound-alike/look-alike issues:
  TobraDex® may be confused with Tobrex®

Use Treatment of external ocular infection caused by susceptible gram-negative bacteria and steroid responsive inflammatory conditions of the palpebral and bulbar conjunctiva, lid, cornea, and anterior segment of the globe

Dosing

Adults & Elderly: Ocular infection/inflammation: Ophthalmic: Instill 1-2 drops of solution every 4 hours; apply ointment 2-3 times/day; for severe infections apply ointment every 3-4 hours, or solution 2 drops every 30-60 minutes initially, then reduce to less frequent intervals

Pediatrics: Ocular infection/inflammation: Children: Refer to adult dosing.

Available Dosage Forms

Ointment, ophthalmic: Tobramycin 0.3% and dexamethasone 0.1% (3.5 g)
Suspension, ophthalmic: Tobramycin 0.3% and dexamethasone 0.1% (2.5 mL, 5 mL, 10 mL) [contains benzalkonium chloride]

Monitoring and Teaching Issues

Physical Assessment: See individual agents.

Patient Education: Shake suspension well before using. Do not touch dropper to eye. Apply light finger pressure on lacrimal sac for one minute following instillation. Notify physician if condition fails to improve or worsens.

Pregnancy Risk Factor: C

Lactation: Excretion in breast milk unknown/use caution

Related Information

Dexamethasone *on page 424*
Tobramycin *on page 1489*

♦ **Tobramycin and Loteprednol Etabonate** *see Loteprednol and Tobramycin on page 925*

♦ **Tobramycin Sulfate** *see Tobramycin on page 1489*

♦ **Tobrex®** *see Tobramycin on page 1489*

♦ **Tofranil®** *see Imipramine on page 789*

♦ **Tofranil-PM®** *see Imipramine on page 789*

Tolcapone (TOLE ka pone)

U.S. Brand Names Tasmar®

Generic Available No

Pharmacologic Category Anti-Parkinson's Agent, COMT Inhibitor

Use Adjunct to levodopa and carbidopa for the treatment of signs and symptoms of idiopathic Parkinson's disease

Mechanism of Action/Effect Tolcapone is a selective and reversible inhibitor of cate-chol-o-methyltransferase (COMT)

Contraindications Hypersensitivity to tolcapone or any component of the formulation

Warnings/Precautions Due to reports of fatal liver injury, reserve for use only in patients who do not have severe movement abnormalities and who do not respond to or who are not appropriate candidates for other available treatments. Use with caution in patients with pre-existing dyskinesias, hepatic impairment, or severe renal impairment. May cause/exacerbate orthostatic hypotension (common in Parkinson's disease) use caution in patients at risk or where transient hypotensive episodes would be poorly tolerated. Monitor carefully for signs and symptoms of postural hypotension, especially during dose escalation, and inform patient of this risk. May cause hallucinations, which may improve with reduction in levodopa therapy. Use with caution in patients with lower gastrointestinal disease or an increased risk of dehydration - tolcapone has been associated with delayed development of diarrhea (onset after 2-12 weeks).

It is not recommended that patients receive tolcapone concomitantly with nonselective MAO inhibitors (see Drug Interactions). Selegiline is a selective MAO type B inhibitor and can be taken with tolcapone.

Although not reported for tolcapone, other dopaminergic agents have been associated with a syndrome resembling neuroleptic malignant syndrome on withdrawal or significant dosage reduction after long-term use. Dopaminergic agents from the ergot class have also been associated with fibrotic complications, such as retroperitoneum, lungs, and pleura.

Drug Interactions

Cytochrome P450 Effect: Inhibits CYP2C8/9 (weak)

Increased Effect/Toxicity: Tolcapone may decrease the metabolism and increase the side effects of COMT substrates (eg, apomorphine, bitolterol, dobutamine, dopamine, epinephrine, norepinephrine, isoproterenol, isoetharine, and methyldopa). Effects on mental status may be additive with other CNS depressants; includes barbiturates, benzodiazepines, TCAs, antipsychotics, ethanol, narcotic analgesics, and other sedative-hypnotics. Concurrent use of nonselective MAO inhibitors with tolcapone may increase the risk of cardiovascular side effects; selective MAO inhibitors (eg, selegiline) appear to pose limited risk.

Nutritional/Ethanol Interactions

Ethanol: Avoid ethanol (may increase CNS depression).

Food: Tolcapone, taken with food within 1 hour before or 2 hours after the dose, decreases bioavailability by 10% to 20%.

Avoid valerian, St John's wort, kava kava, gotu kola (may increase CNS depression).

Adverse Reactions

>10%:

Cardiovascular: Orthostatic hypotension

Central nervous system: Sleep disorder, excessive dreaming, somnolence, headache

Gastrointestinal: Nausea, diarrhea, anorexia

Neuromuscular & skeletal: Dyskinesia, dystonia, muscle cramps

1% to 10%:

Central nervous system: Hallucinations, fatigue, loss of balance, hyperkinesia

Gastrointestinal: Vomiting, constipation, xerostomia, abdominal pain, flatulence, dyspepsia

Genitourinary: Urine discoloration

Neuromuscular & skeletal: Paresthesia, stiffness

Miscellaneous: Diaphoresis (increased)

Pharmacodynamics/Kinetics

Absorption: Rapid

Bioavailability: 65%

Time to Peak: ~2 hours

Protein Binding: >99.0%

Half-Life Elimination: 2-3 hours

Metabolism: Glucuronidation

Excretion: Urine and feces (40%)

Dosing

Adults & Elderly: Parkinson's disease: Oral: Initial: 100-200 mg 3 times/day; levodopa therapy may need to be decreased upon initiation of tolcapone.

Available Dosage Forms Tablet: 100 mg, 200 mg

Monitoring and Teaching Issues

Physical Assessment: Assess effectiveness and interactions of other medications patient may be taking. Monitor therapeutic effectiveness (eg, mental status, involuntary movements) and adverse reactions at beginning of therapy and periodically throughout therapy. Monitor for CNS depression. Monitor blood pressure. Assess knowledge/teach patient appropriate use, interventions to reduce side effects, and adverse symptoms to report.

Patient Education: Take exactly as directed (may be prescribed in conjunction with levodopa/carbidopa); do not change dosage or discontinue without consulting prescriber. Therapeutic effects may take several weeks or months to achieve and you may need frequent monitoring during first weeks of therapy. Best to take 2 hours before or after a meal; however, may be taken with meals if GI upset occurs. Take at the same time each day. Maintain adequate hydration (2-3 L/day of fluids) unless instructed to restrict fluid intake. Do not use alcohol and prescription or OTC sedatives or CNS depressants without consulting prescriber. Urine or perspiration may appear darker. You may experience drowsiness, dizziness, confusion, or vision changes (use caution when driving, climbing stairs, or engaging in tasks requiring alertness until response to drug is known); orthostatic hypotension (use caution when changing position - rising to standing from sitting or lying); increased susceptibility to heat stroke, decreased perspiration (use caution in hot weather; maintain adequate fluids and reduce exercise activity); constipation (increased exercise, fluids, or fruit, or fiber may help); dry skin or nasal passages (consult prescriber for appropriate relief); or nausea, vomiting, loss of appetite, or stomach discomfort (small frequent meals, frequent mouth care, chewing gum, or sucking lozenges may help). Report unresolved constipation or vomiting; chest pain or irregular heartbeat; respiratory difficulty; acute headache or dizziness; CNS changes (hallucination, loss of memory, nervousness, etc); painful or difficult urination; abdominal pain or blood in stool; increased muscle spasticity, rigidity, or involuntary movements; skin rash; or significant worsening of condition. **Pregnancy/breast-feeding precautions:** Inform prescriber if you are or intend to become pregnant. Do not breast-feed.

Pregnancy Risk Factor: C

Lactation: Excretion in breast milk unknown/contraindicated

Tolterodine (tole TER oh deen)

U.S. Brand Names Detrol®; Detrol® LA

Synonyms Tolterodine Tartrate

Generic Available No

Pharmacologic Category Anticholinergic Agent

Medication Safety Issues

Sound-alike/look-alike issues:

Detrol® may be confused with Ditropan®

Use Treatment of patients with an overactive bladder with symptoms of urinary frequency, urgency, or urge incontinence

(Continued)

Tolterodine *(Continued)*

Mechanism of Action/Effect Tolterodine is a competitive antagonist of muscarinic receptors. In animal models, tolterodine demonstrates selectivity for urinary bladder receptors over salivary receptors. Urinary bladder contraction is mediated by muscarinic receptors. Tolterodine increases residual urine volume and decreases detrusor muscle pressure.

Contraindications Hypersensitivity to tolterodine or any component of the formulation; urinary retention; gastric retention; uncontrolled narrow-angle glaucoma; myasthenia gravis

Warnings/Precautions Use with caution in patients with bladder flow obstruction, may increase the risk of urinary retention. Use with caution in patients with gastrointestinal obstructive disorders (ie pyloric stenosis), may increase the risk of gastric retention. Use with caution in patients with controlled (treated) narrow-angle glaucoma; metabolized in the liver and excreted in the urine and feces, dosage adjustment is required for patients with renal or hepatic impairment. Patients on CYP3A4 inhibitors require lower dose. Safety and efficacy in pediatric patients have not been established.

Drug Interactions

Cytochrome P450 Effect: Substrate of CYP2C8/9 (minor), 2C19 (minor), 2D6 (major), 3A4 (major)

Decreased Effect: CYP3A4 inducers may decrease the levels/effects of tolterodine; example inducers include aminoglutethimide, carbamazepine, nafcillin, nevirapine, phenobarbital, phenytoin, and rifamycins.

Increased Effect/Toxicity: CYP2D6 inhibitors may increase the levels/effects of tolterodine; example inhibitors include chlorpromazine, delavirdine, fluoxetine, miconazole, paroxetine, pergolide, quinidine, quinine, ritonavir, and ropinirole. No dosage adjustment was needed in patients coadministered tolterodine and fluoxetine. CYP3A4 inhibitors may increase the levels/effects of tolterodine; example inhibitors include azole antifungals, ciprofloxacin, clarithromycin, diclofenac, doxycycline, erythromycin, imatinib, isoniazid, nefazodone, nicardipine, propofol, protease inhibitors, quinidine, and verapamil.

Nutritional/Ethanol Interactions

Food: Increases bioavailability (~53% increase) of tolterodine tablets, but does not affect the pharmacokinetics of tolterodine extended release capsules; adjustment of dose is not needed. As a CYP3A4 inhibitor, grapefruit juice may increase the serum level and/or toxicity of tolterodine, but unlikely secondary to high oral bioavailability.

Herb/Nutraceutical: St John's wort (*Hypericum*) appears to induce CYP3A enzymes.

Adverse Reactions As reported with immediate release tablet, unless otherwise specified

>10%: Gastrointestinal: Dry mouth (35%; extended release capsules 23%)

1% to 10%:

Cardiovascular: Chest pain (2%)

Central nervous system: Headache (7%; extended release capsules 6%), somnolence (3%; extended release capsules 3%), fatigue (4%; extended release capsules 2%), dizziness (5%; extended release capsules 2%), anxiety (extended release capsules 1%)

Dermatologic: Dry skin (1%)

Gastrointestinal: Abdominal pain (5%; extended release capsules 4%), constipation (7%; extended release capsules 6%), dyspepsia (4%; extended release capsules 3%), diarrhea (4%), weight gain (1%)

Genitourinary: Dysuria (2%; extended release capsules 1%)

Neuromuscular & skeletal: Arthralgia (2%)

Ocular: Abnormal vision (2%; extended release capsules 1%), dry eyes (3%; extended release capsules 3%)

Respiratory: Bronchitis (2%), sinusitis (extended release capsules 2%)

Overdosage/Toxicology Overdosage with tolterodine can potentially result in severe central anticholinergic effects and should be treated accordingly. ECG monitoring is recommended in the event of overdosage.

Pharmacodynamics/Kinetics

Absorption: Immediate release tablet: Rapid

Bioavailability: Immediate release tablet: 77%; increased with food

Time to Peak: Immediate release tablet: 1-2 hours; Extended release tablet: 2-6 hours

Protein Binding: Highly bound to alpha$_1$-acid glycoprotein

Half-Life Elimination:

Immediate release tablet: Extensive metabolizers: ~2 hours; Poor metabolizers: ~10 hours

Extended release capsule: Extensive metabolizers: ~7 hours; Poor metabolizers: ~18 hours

Metabolism: Extensively hepatic, primarily via CYP2D6 (some metabolites share activity) and 3A4 (minor pathway). In patients with a genetic deficiency of CYP2D6, metabolism via 3A4 predominates. Forms three active metabolites.

Excretion: Urine (77% as unchanged drug, 5% to 14% as metabolites, <1% as metabolites in poor metabolizers); feces (17%, <1% as unchanged drug, <2.5% in poor metabolizers)

Dosing

Adults & Elderly: Treatment of overactive bladder: Oral:

Immediate release tablet: 2 mg twice daily; the dose may be lowered to 1 mg twice daily based on individual response and tolerability

Dosing adjustment in patients concurrently taking CYP3A4 inhibitors: 1 mg twice daily

Extended release capsule: 4 mg once a day; dose may be lowered to 2 mg daily based on individual response and tolerability

Dosing adjustment in patients concurrently taking CYP3A4 inhibitors: 2 mg daily

Pediatrics: Safety and efficacy in pediatric patients have not been established

Renal Impairment: Use with caution (studies conducted in patients with Cl$_{cr}$ 10-30 mL/minute):

Immediate release tablet: 1 mg twice daily

Extended release capsule: 2 mg daily

Hepatic Impairment:

Immediate release tablet: 1 mg twice daily

Extended release capsule: 2 mg daily

Available Dosage Forms
Capsule, extended release, as tartrate (Detrol® LA): 2 mg, 4 mg
Tablet, as tartrate (Detrol®): 1 mg, 2 mg

Monitoring and Teaching Issues
Physical Assessment: Assess potential for interactions with other prescriptions, OTC medications, or herbal products patient may be taking (eg, ergot-containing drugs). Assess therapeutic effectiveness and adverse reactions. Teach patient appropriate use (according to formulation and purpose), interventions to reduce side effects, and adverse symptoms to report.

Patient Education: Take as directed, preferably with food. Do not break, crush, or chew extended release medication. May cause headache (consult prescriber for a mild analgesic); dizziness, nervousness, or sleepiness (use caution when driving, climbing stairs, or engaging in tasks requiring alertness until response to drug is known); or abdominal discomfort, diarrhea, constipation, nausea, or vomiting (small frequent meals, increased exercise, adequate hydration may help). Report back pain, muscle spasms, alteration in gait, or numbness of extremities; unresolved or persistent constipation, diarrhea, or vomiting; or symptoms of upper respiratory infection or flu. Report immediately any chest pain or palpitations, difficulty urinating, or pain on urination. **Pregnancy/breast-feeding precautions:** Inform prescriber if you are or intend to become pregnant. Breast-feeding is not recommended.

Pregnancy Risk Factor: C

Lactation: Excretion in breast milk unknown/not recommended

Administration
Storage: Store at room temperature, protect from light

Related Information
Pharmacotherapy of Urinary Incontinence *on page 1858*

◆ **Tolterodine Tartrate** *see* Tolterodine *on page 1493*

◆ **Tomoxetine** *see* Atomoxetine *on page 151*

◆ **Topamax®** *see* Topiramate *on page 1495*

◆ **Topicaine® [OTC]** *see* Lidocaine *on page 898*

Topiramate (toe PYRE a mate)
U.S. Brand Names Topamax®

Generic Available No

Pharmacologic Category Anticonvulsant, Miscellaneous

Medication Safety Issues
Sound-alike/look-alike issues:
Topamax® may be confused with Toprol-XL®

Use In adults and pediatric patients, adjunctive therapy for partial onset seizures and adjunctive therapy of primary generalized tonic-clonic seizures; treatment of seizures associated with Lennox-Gastaut syndrome; prophylaxis of migraine headache

Unlabeled/Investigational Use Infantile spasms, neuropathic pain, cluster headache

Mechanism of Action/Effect Blocks sodium channels in neurons and enhances GABA activity

Contraindications Hypersensitivity to topiramate or any component of the formulation

Warnings/Precautions Use with caution in patients with hepatic, respiratory, or renal impairment. Topiramate may decrease serum bicarbonate concentrations (up to 67% of patients); treatment-emergent metabolic acidosis is less common. Risk may be increased in patients with a predisposing condition (organ dysfunction, ketogenic diet, or concurrent treatment with other drugs which may cause acidosis). Monitor serum bicarbonate as well as potential complications of chronic acidosis (nephrolithiasis, osteomalacia, and reduced growth rates in children). The risk of kidney stones is about 2-4 times that of the untreated population, the risk of this event may be reduced by increasing fluid intake.

Sedation, psychomotor slowing, confusion, paresthesias, and mood disturbances may occur with topiramate use. Topiramate has been associated with secondary angle-closure glaucoma in adults and children, typically within 1 month of initiation; discontinue in patients with acute onset of decreased visual acuity or ocular pain. Hyperammonemia with or without encephalopathy may occur; use with caution in patients with inborn errors of metabolism or decreased hepatic mitochondrial activity. Topiramate may be associated (rarely) with severe oligohydrosis and hyperthermia, most frequently in children; use caution and monitor closely during strenuous exercise, during exposure to high environmental temperature, or in patients receiving drugs with anticholinergic activity.

Avoid abrupt withdrawal of topiramate therapy, it should be withdrawn/tapered slowly to minimize the potential of increased seizure frequency. Safety and efficacy have not been established in children <2 years of age.

Drug Interactions
Cytochrome P450 Effect: Inhibits CYP2C19 (weak); **Induces** CYP3A4 (weak)

Decreased Effect: Phenytoin can decrease topiramate levels by as much as 48%, carbamazepine reduces it by 40%. Digoxin levels and ethinyl estradiol blood levels are decreased when coadministered with topiramate. Hyperammonemia (with or without encephalopathy) has been reported in patients who tolerated valproic acid or topiramate alone; these drugs may modestly decrease the serum concentrations of the other drug.

Increased Effect/Toxicity: Concomitant administration with other CNS depressants will increase its sedative effects. Coadministration with other carbonic anhydrase inhibitors may increase the chance of nephrolithiasis and/or hyperthermia (includes acetazolamide). Topiramate may increase phenytoin concentration by 25%. Concurrent administration with anticholinergic drugs may increase the risk of oligohydrosis and/or hyperthermia (includes drugs with high anticholinergic activity such as antihistamines, cyclic antidepressants, and antipsychotics); use caution.

Nutritional/Ethanol Interactions
Ethanol: Avoid ethanol (may increase CNS depression).
Food: Ketogenic diet may increase the possibility of acidosis.
(Continued)

Topiramate *(Continued)*

Herb/Nutraceutical: Avoid evening primrose (seizure threshold decreased).

Adverse Reactions

>10%:

Central nervous system: Dizziness, ataxia, somnolence, psychomotor slowing, nervousness, memory difficulties, speech problems, fatigue

Endocrine & metabolic: Serum bicarbonate decreased (up to 67%; marked reductions to <17 mEq/L have been reported in up to 11% of patients)

Gastrointestinal: Nausea

Neuromuscular & skeletal: Paresthesia, tremor

Ocular: Nystagmus, diplopia, abnormal vision

Respiratory: Upper respiratory infection

1% to 10%:

Cardiovascular: Chest pain, edema

Central nervous system: Language problems, abnormal coordination, confusion, depression, difficulty concentrating, hypoesthesia, hallucination, psychosis, suicide attempt

Endocrine & metabolic: Hot flashes; metabolic acidosis (hyperchloremia, nonanion gap); dehydration

Gastrointestinal: Dyspepsia, abdominal pain, anorexia, constipation, xerostomia, gingivitis, weight loss, diarrhea, vomiting

Genitourinary: Impotence, dysuria

Neuromuscular & skeletal: Myalgia, weakness, back pain, leg pain, rigors, hypertonia, arthralgia

Ocular: Conjunctivitis

Otic: Hearing decreased

Renal: Nephrolithiasis, renal calculus

Respiratory: Pharyngitis, sinusitis, epistaxis

Miscellaneous: Flu-like symptoms

Overdosage/Toxicology Signs and symptoms of overdose include convulsions, drowsiness, speech disturbance, blurred vision, diplopia, impaired mentation, lethargy, and metabolic acidosis. Activated charcoal has not been shown to adsorb topiramate and is therefore not recommended. Hemodialysis can remove the drug; however, most cases do not require removal and instead are best treated with supportive measures.

Pharmacodynamics/Kinetics

Absorption: Good; unaffected by food

Bioavailability: 80%

Time to Peak: Serum: ~2-4 hours

Protein Binding: 15% to 41%

Half-Life Elimination: Mean: Adults: Normal renal function: 21 hours; shorter in pediatric patients; clearance is 50% higher in pediatric patients

Metabolism: Hepatic via P450

Excretion: Urine (~70% to 80% as unchanged drug)

Dialyzable: ~30%

Dosing

Adults:

Partial onset seizures (adjunctive therapy), primary generalized tonic-clonic seizures (adjunctive therapy): Oral: Initial: 25-50 mg/day; titrate in increments of 25-50 mg per week until an effective daily dose is reached; the daily dose may be increased by 25 mg at weekly intervals for the first 4 weeks; thereafter, the daily dose may be increased by 25-50 mg weekly to an effective daily dose (usually at least 400 mg); usual maximum dose: 1600 mg/day

Note: A more rapid titration schedule has been previously recommended (ie, 50 mg/week), and may be attempted in some clinical situations; however, this may reduce the patient's ability to tolerate topiramate.

Migraine prophylaxis: Oral: Initial: 25 mg/day, titrated at weekly intervals in 25 mg increments, up to the recommended total daily dose of 100 mg/day given in 2 divided doses

Cluster headache (unlabeled uses): Oral: Initial: 25 mg/day, titrated at weekly intervals in 25 mg increments, up to 200 mg/day

Elderly: Most older adults have creatinine clearances <70 mL/min; obtain a serum creatinine and calculate creatinine clearance prior to initiation of therapy. An initial dose of 25 mg/day may be recommended, followed by incremental increases of 25 mg at weekly intervals until an effective dose is reached; refer to adult dosing for titration schedule.

Pediatrics: Children 2-16 years: Partial onset seizures (adjunctive therapy), primary generalized tonic-clonic seizures (adjunctive therapy), and seizures associated with Lennox-Gastaut syndrome: Oral: Initial dose titration should begin at 25 mg (or less, based on a range of 1-3 mg/kg/day) nightly for the first week. Dosage may be increased in increments of 1-3 mg/kg/day (administered in two divided doses) at 1- or 2-week intervals to a total daily dose of 5-9 mg/kg/day.

Renal Impairment: Cl_{cr} <70 mL/minute: Administer 50% dose and titrate more slowly.

Hemodialysis: Supplemental dose may be needed during hemodialysis

Dialyzable: ~30%

Hepatic Impairment: Clearance may be reduced.

Available Dosage Forms

Capsule, sprinkle: 15 mg, 25 mg

Tablet: 25 mg, 50 mg, 100 mg, 200 mg

Monitoring and Teaching Issues

Physical Assessment: Assess effectiveness and interactions of other medications patient may be taking. Monitor therapeutic effectiveness (seizure activity, force, type, duration), laboratory values, and adverse reactions at beginning of therapy and periodically with long-term use. Taper dosage slowly when discontinuing. Assess knowledge/teach patient appropriate use, seizure safety precautions, interventions to reduce side effects, and adverse symptoms to report.

Monitoring Laboratory Tests: Recommended monitoring includes serum bicarbonate at baseline and periodically during treatment. Ammonia level in patients with unexplained lethargy, vomiting, or mental status changes.

Patient Education: Take exactly as directed; do not increase dose or frequency or discontinue without consulting prescriber. While using this medication, do not use alcohol and other prescription or OTC medications (especially pain medications, sedatives, antihistamines, or hypnotics) without consulting prescriber. Maintain adequate hydration (2-3 L/day of fluids) unless instructed to restrict fluid intake; possibly to prevent the inflammation of kidney stones and dehydration. You may be at risk for decreased sweating and increased body temperature, especially in hot weather. You may experience drowsiness, dizziness, disturbed concentration, memory changes, or blurred vision (use caution when driving or engaging in tasks requiring alertness until response to drug is known); or mouth sores, nausea, vomiting, or loss of appetite (small frequent meals, frequent mouth care, chewing gum, or sucking lozenges may help). Wear identification of epileptic status and medications. Report behavioral or CNS changes; skin rash; muscle cramping, weakness, tremors, changes in gait; chest pain, irregular heartbeat, or palpitations; hearing loss; cough or respiratory difficulty; or worsening of seizure activity or loss of seizure control. Seek immediate medical evaluation if you experience sudden vision changes and/or periorbital pain. **Pregnancy/breast-feeding precautions:** Inform prescriber if you are pregnant or intend to become pregnant. Breast-feeding is not recommended.

Geriatric Considerations: Since drug is renally excreted and most elderly will have creatinine clearance <70 mL/minute, doses must be reduced 50% and titrated more slowly. Obtain a serum creatinine and calculate creatinine clearance prior to starting therapy. Follow the recommended titration schedule and adjust time intervals to meet patient's needs.

Pregnancy Risk Factor: C

Pregnancy Issues: No studies in pregnant women; use only if benefit to the mother outweighs the risk to the fetus. Postmarketing experience includes reports of hypospadias following *in vitro* exposure to topiramate.

Lactation: Enters breast milk/not recommended

Breast-Feeding Issues: Based on limited data, topiramate was found in breast milk; low concentrations were detected in nursing infants.

Administration

Oral: May be administered without regard to meals

Capsule sprinkles: May be swallowed whole or opened to sprinkle the contents on soft food (drug/food mixture should not be chewed).

Tablet: Because of bitter taste, tablets should not be broken.

Storage: Store at room temperature; protect capsules from moisture.

Additional Information May be associated with weight loss in some patients

Related Information

Anticonvulsants By Seizure Type *on page 1712*

♦ **TOPO** *see* Topotecan *on page 1497*

♦ **Toposar®** *see* Etoposide *on page 599*

Topotecan (toe poe TEE kan)

U.S. Brand Names Hycamtin®

Synonyms Hycamptamine; NSC-609699; SK and F 104864; SKF 104864; SKF 104864-A; TOPO; Topotecan Hydrochloride; TPT

Generic Available No

Pharmacologic Category Antineoplastic Agent, Natural Source (Plant) Derivative

Medication Safety Issues

Sound-alike/look-alike issues:

Hycamtin® may be confused with Hycomine®

Use Treatment of ovarian cancer, small cell lung cancer

Unlabeled/Investigational Use Investigational: Treatment of nonsmall cell lung cancer, sarcoma (pediatrics)

Mechanism of Action/Effect Binds to topoisomerase I and stabilizes the cleavable complex so that religation of the cleaved DNA strand cannot occur. This results in the accumulation of cleavable complexes and single-strand DNA breaks. Topotecan acts in S phase.

Contraindications Hypersensitivity to topotecan or any component of the formulation; severe bone marrow depression; pregnancy; breast-feeding

Warnings/Precautions The U.S. Food and Drug Administration (FDA) currently recommends that procedures for proper handling and disposal of antineoplastic agents be considered. Appropriate safety equipment is recommended for preparation, administration, and disposal of antineoplastics. Monitor bone marrow function. Should only administer to patients with adequate bone marrow reserves, baseline neutrophils at least 1500 cells/mm³ and platelet counts at least 100,000/mm³. Use caution in renal impairment.

Drug Interactions

Increased Effect/Toxicity: Concurrent administration of TPT and G-CSF in clinical trials results in severe myelosuppression. If G-CSF is to be used, manufacturer recommends that it should not be initiated until 24 hours after the completion of treatment with topotecan. Concurrent *in vitro* exposure to TPT and the topoisomerase II inhibitor etoposide results in no altered effect; sequential exposure results in potentiation. Concurrent exposure to TPT and 5-azacytidine results in potentiation both *in vitro* and *in vivo*. Myelosuppression was more severe when given in combination with cisplatin.

Nutritional/Ethanol Interactions Ethanol: Avoid ethanol (due to GI irritation).

Lab Interactions None known

Adverse Reactions

>10%:

Central nervous system: Headache, fatigue, fever, pain

Dermatologic: Alopecia (reversible), rash

(Continued)

Topotecan (Continued)

Gastrointestinal: Nausea, vomiting, diarrhea, constipation, abdominal pain, stomatitis, anorexia

Hematologic: Myelosuppressive: Principle dose-limiting toxicity; white blood cell count nadir is 8-11 days and is more frequent than thrombocytopenia (at lower doses); recover is usually within 21 days and cumulative toxicity has not been noted.

Neuromuscular & skeletal: Weakness

Respiratory: Dyspnea (22%), cough

1% to 10%:

Hepatic: Transient increases in liver enzymes

Neuromuscular & skeletal: Paresthesia

Pharmacodynamics/Kinetics

Absorption: Oral: ~30%

Protein Binding: 35%

Half-Life Elimination: 2-3 hours

Metabolism: Undergoes a rapid, pH-dependent opening of the lactone ring to yield a relatively inactive hydroxy acid in plasma

Excretion: Urine (30%) within 24 hours

Dosing

Adults & Elderly: Refer to individual protocols.

Metastatic ovarian cancer and small cell lung cancer:

IVPB: 1.5 mg/m^2/day for 5 days; repeated every 21 days (neutrophil count should be >1500/mm^3 and platelet count should be >100,000/mm^3)

I.V. continuous infusion: 0.2-0.7 mg/m^2/day for 7-21 days

Dosage adjustment for hematological effects: If neutrophil count <1500/mm^3, reduce dose by 0.25 mg/m^2/day for 5 days for next cycle

Renal Impairment:

Cl$_{cr}$ 20-39 mL/minute: Administer 50% of normal dose.

Cl$_{cr}$ <20 mL/minute: Do not use, insufficient data available.

Hemodialysis: Supplemental dose is not necessary.

CAPD effects: Unknown

CAVH effects: Unknown

Hepatic Impairment: Bilirubin 1.5-10 mg/dL: No adjustment necessary.

Available Dosage Forms Injection, powder for reconstitution, as hydrochloride: 4 mg [base]

Monitoring and Teaching Issues

Physical Assessment: Use caution in renal impairment (see Warnings/Precautions for use cautions). Note cautions and recommendation in Drug Interactions. Assess results of laboratory tests and adverse reactions prior to each infusion and throughout therapy (eg, signs of myelosuppression, renal function [I & O, edema]; GI disturbance [nausea, vomiting, diarrhea, pain]; dyspnea; see Adverse Reactions). Teach patient possible side effects/appropriate interventions and adverse symptoms to report (see Patient Education).

Monitoring Laboratory Tests: CBC with differential and platelet count, renal function tests

Patient Education: Do not take any new medication during therapy unless approved by prescriber. This drug is administered by intravenous infusion: report immediately any burning, pain, redness, swelling at infusion site or sudden chest pain, difficulty breathing or swallowing, or chills. Maintain adequate hydration (3-4 L/day of fluids) unless instructed to restrict fluid intake during therapy. Maintain good oral hygiene (use soft toothbrush or cotton applicators several times a day and rinse mouth frequently). You will be more susceptible to infection (avoid crowds and exposure to infection and do not have any vaccinations without consulting prescriber). May cause nausea or vomiting (small frequent meals, frequent mouth care, sucking lozenges, or chewing gum may help); hair loss (will regrow after treatment is completed). Report unresolved nausea, or vomiting; alterations in urinary pattern (increased or decreased); opportunistic infection (fever, chills, unusual bruising or bleeding, fatigue, purulent vaginal discharge, unhealed mouth sores); chest pain, respiratory difficulty, unexplained weakness or fatigue; or other persistent effects. **Pregnancy/breast-feeding precautions:** Inform prescriber if you are pregnant. Do not get pregnant or cause a pregnancy (males) while taking this medication. Consult prescriber for appropriate contraceptive measures (may cause severe fetal defects). Do not breast-feed.

Pregnancy Risk Factor: D

Pregnancy Issues: May cause fetal harm in pregnant women.

Lactation: Excretion in breast milk unknown/contraindicated

Administration

I.V.: Administer IVPB over 30 minutes or by 24-hour continuous infusion.

Reconstitution: Reconstitute vials with 4 mL SWFI, D$_5$, or NS; may be further diluted in 50-100 mL D$_5$W or NS for infusion.

Compatibility: Stable in D$_5$W, NS

Y-site administration: Incompatible with dexamethasone sodium phosphate, fluorouracil, mitomycin

Storage: Store intact vials of lyophilized powder for injection at room temperature and protected from light. Reconstituted solution is stable for 24 hours at room temperature or up to 7 days under refrigeration. Diluted in 50-100 mL D$_5$W or NS is stable for 24 hours at room temperature or up to 7 days under refrigeration.

♦ **Topotecan Hydrochloride** *see* Topotecan *on page 1497*

♦ **Toprol-XL®** *see* Metoprolol *on page 993*

♦ **Toradol®** *see* Ketorolac *on page 853*

Toremifene (TORE em i feen)

U.S. Brand Names Fareston®

Synonyms FC1157a; Toremifene Citrate

Generic Available No

Pharmacologic Category Antineoplastic Agent, Estrogen Receptor Antagonist

Use Treatment of advanced breast cancer; management of desmoid tumors and endometrial carcinoma

Mechanism of Action/Effect Nonsteroidal agent that competitively binds to estrogen receptors on tumors and other tissue targets (including breast and other tissues), producing a nuclear complex that decreases DNA synthesis and inhibits estrogen effects. Cells accumulate in the G_0 and G_1 phases; therefore, toremifene is cytostatic rather than cytocidal.

Contraindications Hypersensitivity to toremifene or any component of the formulation; pregnancy

Warnings/Precautions Hypercalcemia and tumor flare have been reported in some breast cancer patients with bone metastases during the first weeks of treatment. Tumor flare is a syndrome of diffuse musculoskeletal pain and erythema with increased size of tumor lesions that later regress. It is often accompanied by hypercalcemia. Tumor flare does not imply treatment failure or represent tumor progression. Institute appropriate measures if hypercalcemia occurs, and if severe, discontinue treatment. Drugs that decrease renal calcium excretion (eg, thiazide diuretics) may increase the risk of hypercalcemia in patients receiving toremifene. Leukopenia and thrombocytopenia have been reported rarely. Use cautiously in patients with anemia, hepatic failure, or thromboembolic disease.

Drug Interactions

Cytochrome P450 Effect: Substrate of CYP1A2 (minor), 3A4 (major)

Decreased Effect: CYP3A4 inducers may decrease the levels/effects of toremifene; example inducers include aminoglutethimide, carbamazepine, nafcillin, nevirapine, phenobarbital, phenytoin, and rifamycins.

Increased Effect/Toxicity: Concurrent therapy with warfarin results in significant enhancement of anticoagulant effects; has been speculated that a decrease in antitumor effect of tamoxifen may also occur due to alterations in the percentage of active tamoxifen metabolites.

Adverse Reactions

>10%:
Endocrine & metabolic: Vaginal discharge, hot flashes
Gastrointestinal: Nausea, vomiting
Miscellaneous: Diaphoresis

1% to 10%:
Cardiovascular: Thromboembolism: Tamoxifen has been associated with the occurrence of venous thrombosis and pulmonary embolism; arterial thrombosis has also been described in a few case reports; cardiac failure, MI, edema
Central nervous system: Dizziness
Endocrine & metabolic: Hypercalcemia may occur in patients with bone metastases; galactorrhea and vitamin deficiency, menstrual irregularities
Genitourinary: Vaginal bleeding or discharge, endometriosis, priapism, possible endometrial cancer
Ocular: Ophthalmologic effects (visual acuity changes, cataracts, or retinopathy), corneal opacities, dry eyes

Overdosage/Toxicology Theoretically, overdose may manifest as an increase of antiestrogenic effects such as hot flashes; estrogenic effects such as vaginal bleeding; or nervous system disorders such as vertigo, dizziness, ataxia, and nausea. No specific antidote exists and treatment is symptomatic.

Pharmacodynamics/Kinetics

Absorption: Well absorbed

Time to Peak: Serum: ~3 hours

Protein Binding: Plasma: >99.5%, primarily to albumin

Half-Life Elimination: ~5 days

Metabolism: Extensively hepatic, principally by CYP3A4 to N-demethyltoremifene, which is also antiestrogenic but with weak *in vivo* antitumor potency

Excretion: Primarily feces; urine (10%) during a 1-week period

Dosing

Adults & Elderly: Refer to individual protocols.
Metastatic breast carcinoma: Oral: 60 mg once daily, generally continued until disease progression is observed

Renal Impairment: No adjustment is necessary.

Hepatic Impairment: Toremifene is extensively metabolized in the liver and dosage adjustments may be indicated in patients with liver disease; however, no specific guidelines have been developed.

Available Dosage Forms Tablet: 60 mg

Monitoring and Teaching Issues

Physical Assessment: Use caution with anemia, hepatic failure, or thromboembolic disease (see Warnings/Precautions for specific use cautions). Assess potential for interactions with other pharmacological agents patient may be taking (drugs that decrease renal calcium excretion [eg, thiazide diuretics] may increase the risk of hypercalcemia, use with warfarin increases anticoagulant effect, CYP3A4 inducers [eg, carbamazepine, nafcillin, phenobarbital, phenytoin] may decrease the levels/effects of toremifene; see Drug Interactions). Monitor laboratory tests on a regular basis throughout therapy. Monitor adverse reactions regularly (eg, thromboembolism, MI, edema, hypercalcemia, endometriosis, nausea, vomiting, vision changes; see Adverse Reactions). Teach patient proper use, possible side effects/appropriate interventions and adverse symptoms to report (see Patient Education).

Monitoring Laboratory Tests: Obtain periodic complete blood counts, calcium levels, and liver function tests. Closely monitor patients with bone metastases for hypercalcemia during the first few weeks of treatment. Leukopenia and thrombocytopenia have been reported rarely; monitor leukocyte and platelet counts during treatment.

Patient Education: Do not take any new medication during therapy unless approved by prescriber. Take as directed, without regard to food. You may experience an initial "flare" of this disease (eg, increased bone pain and hot flashes), which will subside with continued use. May cause nausea, vomiting, or loss of appetite (frequent mouth care, small frequent
(Continued)

Toremifene *(Continued)*

meals, chewing gum, or sucking lozenges may help); dizziness (use caution when driving, climbing stairs, or engaging in tasks requiring alertness until response to drug is known); or loss of hair (reversible). Report vomiting that occurs immediately after taking medication; chest pain, palpitations, or swollen extremities; vaginal bleeding, hot flashes, or excessive perspiration; unusual coughing, or respiratory difficulty; or any vision changes or dry eyes.
Pregnancy/breast-feeding precautions: Do not get pregnant while taking this medication. Consult prescriber for appropriate contraceptive measures. Do not breast-feed.

Pregnancy Risk Factor: D

Lactation: Excretion in breast milk unknown/contraindicated

Administration
   Storage: Store at 25°C (77°F); excursions permitted to 15°C to 30°C (59°F to 86°F). Protect from heat and light.

Additional Information Increase of bone pain usually indicates a good therapeutic response

♦ **Toremifene Citrate** *see* Toremifene *on page 1498*

Torsemide *(TORE se mide)*

U.S. Brand Names Demadex®

Generic Available Yes: Tablet

Pharmacologic Category Diuretic, Loop

Medication Safety Issues
   Sound-alike/look-alike issues:
      Torsemide may be confused with furosemide
      Demadex® may be confused with Denorex®

Use Management of edema associated with congestive heart failure and hepatic or renal disease; used alone or in combination with antihypertensives in treatment of hypertension; I.V. form is indicated when rapid onset is desired

Mechanism of Action/Effect Inhibits reabsorption of sodium and chloride in the ascending loop of Henle and distal renal tubule, interfering with the chloride-binding cotransport system, thus causing increased excretion of water, sodium, chloride, magnesium, and calcium; does not alter GFR, renal plasma flow, or acid-base balance

Contraindications Hypersensitivity to torsemide, any component of the formulation, or any sulfonylureas; anuria

Warnings/Precautions Ototoxicity has been associated with loop diuretics and has been seen with oral torsemide. Do not administer intravenously in less than 2 minutes; single doses should not exceed 200 mg. Avoid electrolyte imbalances in cirrhosis that might lead to hepatic encephalopathy. Monitor fluid status and renal function in an attempt to prevent dehydration, oliguria, azotemia, and reversible increases in BUN and creatinine. Monitor closely for electrolyte imbalances particularly hypokalemia and correct when necessary. Coadministration with antihypertensives may increase the risk of hypotension.

Chemical similarities are present among sulfonamides, sulfonylureas, carbonic anhydrase inhibitors, thiazides, and loop diuretics (except ethacrynic acid). Use in patients with sulfonylurea allergy is specifically contraindicated in product labeling, however, a risk of cross-reaction exists in patients with allergy to any of these compounds; avoid use when previous reaction has been severe.

Drug Interactions
   Cytochrome P450 Effect: Substrate of CYP2C8/9 (major); **Inhibits** CYP2C19 (weak)
   Decreased Effect: Torsemide action may be reduced with probenecid. Diuretic action may be impaired in patients with cirrhosis and ascites if used with salicylates. Glucose tolerance may be decreased when used with sulfonylureas. CYP2C8/9 inducers may decrease the levels/effects of torsemide; example inducers include carbamazepine, phenobarbital, phenytoin, rifampin, rifapentine, and secobarbital. Torsemide efficacy may be decreased with NSAIDs.
   Increased Effect/Toxicity: Torsemide-induced hypokalemia may predispose to digoxin toxicity and may increase the risk of arrhythmia with drugs which may prolong QT interval, including type Ia and type III antiarrhythmic agents, cisapride, and some quinolones (sparfloxacin, gatifloxacin, and moxifloxacin). The risk of toxicity from lithium and salicylates (high dose) may be increased by loop diuretics. Hypotensive effects and/or adverse renal effects of ACE inhibitors and NSAIDs are potentiated by bumetanide-induced hypovolemia. The effects of peripheral adrenergic-blocking drugs or ganglionic blockers may be increased by bumetanide.

Torsemide may increase the risk of ototoxicity with other ototoxic agents (aminoglycosides, cis-platinum), especially in patients with renal dysfunction. Synergistic diuretic effects occur with thiazide-type diuretics. Diuretics tend to be synergistic with other antihypertensive agents, and hypotension may occur.

Nutritional/Ethanol Interactions Herb/Nutraceutical: Avoid dong quai if using for hypertension (has estrogenic activity). Avoid ephedra, yohimbe, ginseng (may worsen hypertension). Avoid garlic (may have increased antihypertensive effect).

Adverse Reactions 1% to 10%:
   Cardiovascular: Edema (1.1%), ECG abnormality (2%), chest pain (1.2%)
   Central nervous system: Headache (7.3%), dizziness (3.2%), insomnia (1.2%), nervousness (1%)
   Endocrine & metabolic: Hyperglycemia, hyperuricemia, hypokalemia
   Gastrointestinal: Diarrhea (2%), constipation (1.8%), nausea (1.8%), dyspepsia (1.6%), sore throat (1.6%)
   Genitourinary: Excessive urination (6.7%)
   Neuromuscular & skeletal: Weakness (2%), arthralgia (1.8%), myalgia (1.6%)
   Respiratory: Rhinitis (2.8%), cough increase (2%)

Overdosage/Toxicology Symptoms include electrolyte depletion, volume depletion, hypotension, dehydration, and circulatory collapse. Electrolyte depletion may manifest as weakness, dizziness, mental confusion, anorexia, lethargy, vomiting, and cramps. Treatment is supportive.

Pharmacodynamics/Kinetics
Onset of Action: Diuresis: 30-60 minutes; Peak effect: 1-4 hours

Duration of Action: ~6 hours

Absorption: Oral: Rapid

Bioavailability: 80% to 90%

Protein Binding: Plasma: ~97% to 99%

Half-Life Elimination: 2-4; Cirrhosis: 7-8 hours

Metabolism: Hepatic (80%) via CYP

Excretion: Urine (20% as unchanged drug)

Dosing
Adults:

Note: The oral form may be given regardless of meal times. Patients may be switched from the I.V. form to the oral and vice-versa with no change in dose.

Congestive heart failure: Oral, I.V.: 10-20 mg once daily; may increase gradually for chronic treatment by doubling dose until the diuretic response is apparent (for acute treatment. I.V. dose may be repeated every 2 hours with double the dose as needed).

Chronic renal failure: Oral, I.V.: 20 mg once daily; increase as above.

Hepatic cirrhosis: Oral, I.V.: 5-10 mg once daily with an aldosterone antagonist or a potassium-sparing diuretic; increase as above.

Hypertension: Oral, I.V.: 2.5-5 mg once daily; increase to 10 mg after 4-6 weeks if an adequate hypotensive response is not apparent. If still not effective, an additional antihypertensive agent may be added.

Elderly: Usual starting dose should be 5 mg; refer to adult dosing.

Available Dosage Forms
Injection, solution: 10 mg/mL (2 mL, 5 mL)

Tablet: 5 mg, 10 mg, 20 mg, 100 mg

Monitoring and Teaching Issues
Physical Assessment: Assess for allergy to sulfonylurea before beginning therapy. See Warnings/Precautions for use cautions. Assess potential for interactions with other pharmacological agents or herbal products the patient may be taking (especially anything that may impact fluid balance or increase potential for ototoxicity or hypotension; see Drug Interactions). For intravenous use see Administration specifics. Assess results of laboratory tests (electrolytes), therapeutic effectiveness, and adverse response on a regular basis during therapy (eg, dehydration, electrolyte imbalance, postural hypotension; see Adverse Reactions). Caution patients with diabetes about closely monitoring glucose levels (glucose tolerance may be decreased). Teach patient appropriate use, possible side effects/appropriate interventions, and adverse symptoms to report (see Patient Education).

Monitoring Laboratory Tests: Renal function, electrolytes

Patient Education: Do not take any new medication during therapy unless approved by prescriber. Take as directed, with food or milk (to reduce GI distress), early in the day, or if twice daily, take last dose in afternoon in order to avoid sleep disturbance and achieve maximum therapeutic effect. Include orange juice or bananas (or other potassium-rich foods) in daily diet. Do not take potassium supplements without consulting prescriber. Weigh yourself each day, at the same time, in the same clothes when beginning therapy, and weekly on long-term therapy; report unusual or unanticipated weight gain or loss. May cause postural hypotension (change position slowly when rising from sitting or lying); transient drowsiness, blurred vision, or dizziness (avoid driving or engaging in tasks that require alertness until response to drug is known); reduced tolerance to heat (avoid strenuous activity in hot weather or excessively hot showers); or constipation (increased exercise and increased dietary fiber, fruit, or fluids may help). Report unusual weight gain or loss (>5 lb/week), swelling of ankles and hands; persistent fatigue; unresolved constipation or diarrhea; weakness, fatigue, or dizziness; vomiting; cramps; change in hearing; or chest pain or palpitations. **Breast-feeding precaution:** Consult prescriber if breast-feeding.

Pregnancy Risk Factor: B

Pregnancy Issues: A decrease in fetal weight, an increase in fetal resorption, and delayed fetal ossification has occurred in animal studies.

Lactation: Excretion in breast milk unknown/use caution

Administration
I.V.: I.V. injections should be given over ≥2 minutes.

Compatibility: Stable in D$_5$W, NS, ½NS

Additional Information 10-20 mg torsemide is approximately equivalent to furosemide 40 mg or bumetanide 1 mg.

Related Information
Heart Failure on page 1828

Tositumomab and Iodine I 131 Tositumomab
(toe si TYOO mo mab & EYE oh dyne eye one THUR tee one toe si TYOO mo mab)

U.S. Brand Names Bexxar®

Synonyms Anti-CD20-Murine Monoclonal Antibody I-131; B1; B1 Antibody; 131 I Anti-B1 Antibody; 131 I-Anti-B1 Monoclonal Antibody; Iodine I 131 Tositumomab and Tositumomab; Tositumomab I-131

Generic Available No

Pharmacologic Category Antineoplastic Agent, Monoclonal Antibody; Radiopharmaceutical

Use Treatment of relapsed or refractory CD20 positive, low-grade, follicular, or transformed non-Hodgkin's lymphoma

(Continued)

Tositumomab and Iodine I 131 Tositumomab *(Continued)*

Mechanism of Action/Effect Tositumomab is a murine IgG2a lambda monoclonal antibody which binds to the CD20 antigen, expressed on B-lymphocytes and on >90% of B-cell non-Hodgkin's lymphomas. Iodine I 131 tositumomab is a radio-iodinated derivative of tositumomab covalently linked to iodine 131. The possible actions of the regimen include apoptosis, complement-dependent cytotoxicity, antibody-dependent cellular cytotoxicity, and cell death. Administration results in depletion of CD20 positive cells.

Contraindications Hypersensitivity to murine proteins or any component of the formulation; pregnancy; breast-feeding

Warnings/Precautions Hypersensitivity reactions (including anaphylaxis) have been reported. Patients should be screened for human antimouse antibodies (HAMA); may be at increased risk of allergic or serious hypersensitivity reactions. Hematologic toxicity was reported to be the most common adverse effect with 27% patients requiring supportive care. Severe or life-threatening cytopenias (NCI CTC grade 3 or 4) have been reported in a large number of patients; may be prolonged and severe. Secondary malignancies have been reported following use.

Treatment involves radioactive isotopes; appropriate precautions in handling and administration must be followed. Patients must be instructed in measures to minimize exposure of others. Women of childbearing potential should be advised of potential fetal risk; effective contraceptive measures should be used for 12 months following treatment (males and females). Treatment may lead to hypothyroidism; patients should receive thyroid-blocking medications prior to the start of therapy. Patients should be premedicated to prevent infusion related reactions. For a single course of therapy only; multiple courses or use in combination with other chemotherapy or irradiation have not been studied.

Safety has not been established in patients with >25% lymphoma marrow involvement, platelet count <100,000 cells/mm^3 or neutrophil count <1500 cells/mm^3. Use caution with cardiovascular disease, renal, or hepatic impairment. Safety and efficacy have not been established with impaired renal function or in pediatric patients.

Drug Interactions

Decreased Effect: No formal drug interaction studies have been conducted. The ability of patients receiving tositumomab to generate humoral response (primary or anamnestic) to vaccination is unknown; safety of live vaccines has not been established.

Increased Effect/Toxicity: No formal drug interaction studies have been conducted.

Lab Interactions May interfere with tests using murine antibody technology.

Adverse Reactions

>10%:

Central nervous system: Fever (37%), pain (19%), chills (18%), headache (16%)

Dermatologic: Rash (17%)

Endocrine & metabolic: Hypothyroidism (7% to 19%)

Gastrointestinal: Nausea (36%), abdominal pain (15%), vomiting (15%), anorexia (14%), diarrhea (12%)

Hematologic:

Neutropenia (grade 3 or 4, 63%); thrombocytopenia (grade 3 or 4, 53%)

Time to nadir: 4-7 weeks

Duration: 30 days (>90 days in 5% to 7% of patients)

Neuromuscular & skeletal: Weakness (46%), myalgia (13%)

Respiratory: Cough (21%), pharyngitis (12%), dyspnea (11%)

Miscellaneous: Infusion-related reactions (26%, occurred within 14 days of infusion, included bronchospasm, chills, dyspnea, fever, hypotension, nausea, rigors, diaphoresis), infection (21%), HAMA-positive seroconversion (11%; up to 21% at 1 year)

1% to 10%:

Cardiovascular: Hypotension (7% to 10%), peripheral edema (9%), chest pain (7%), vasodilation (5%)

Central nervous system: Dizziness (5%), somnolence (5%)

Dermatologic: Pruritus (10%)

Gastrointestinal: Constipation (6%), dyspepsia (6%), weight loss (6%)

Local: Injection site hypersensitivity

Neuromuscular & skeletal: Arthralgia (10%), back pain (8%), neck pain (6%)

Respiratory: Rhinitis (10%), pneumonia (6%), laryngismus

Miscellaneous: Diaphoresis (8%), hypersensitivity reaction (6%), secondary leukemia/myelodysplastic syndrome (3%; up to 6% at 5 years), anaphylactoid reaction, secondary malignancies, serum sickness

Overdosage/Toxicology Grade 4 hematologic toxicity lasting 18 days was reported in one patient accidentally receiving a total body dose of 88 cGy. Monitor for cytopenias and radiation-related toxicity.

Pharmacodynamics/Kinetics

Half-Life Elimination: Tositumomab:

Elimination: 36-48 hours

Terminal half-life decreased with high tumor burden, splenomegaly, or bone marrow involvement

Clearance: Blood: 68.2 mg/hour

Excretion: Iodine-131: Urine (98%) and decay

Dosing

Adults: I.V.: Dosing consists of four components administered in 2 steps. Thyroid protective agents (SSKI, Lugol's solution or potassium iodide), acetaminophen and diphenhydramine should be given prior to or with treatment. Refer to Additional Information.

Step 1: Dosimetric step (Day 0):

Tositumomab 450 mg in NS 50 mL administered over 60 minutes

Iodine I 131 tositumomab (containing I-131 5.0 mCi and tositumomab 35mg) in NS 30 mL administered over 20 minutes

Note: Whole body dosimetry and biodistribution should be determined on Day 0; days 2, 3, or 4; and day 6 or 7 prior to administration of Step 2. If biodistribution is not acceptable, do not administer the therapeutic step. On day 6 or 7, calculate the patient specific activity of iodine I 131 tositumomab to deliver 75 cGy TBD or 65 cGy TBD (in mCi).

Step 2: Therapeutic step (Day 7):
Tositumomab 450 mg in NS 50 mL administered over 60 minutes
Iodine I 131 tositumomab:
Platelets ≥150,000/mm³: Iodine I 131 calculated to deliver 75 cGy total body irradiation and tositumomab 35 mg over 20 minutes
Platelets ≥100,000/mm³ and <150,000/mm³: Iodine I 131 calculated to deliver 65 cGy total body irradiation and tositumomab 35 mg over 20 minutes

Available Dosage Forms Note: Not all components are shipped from the same facility. When ordering, ensure that all will arrive on the same day.
Kit [dosimetric package] (Bexxar®): Tositumomab 225 mg/16.1 mL [2 vials], tositumomab 35 mg/2.5 mL [1 vial], and iodine I 131 tositumomab 0.1 mg/mL and 0.61mCi/mL (20 mL) [1 vial]
Kit [therapeutic package] (Bexxar®): Tositumomab 225 mg/16.1 mL [2 vials], tositumomab 35 mg/2.5 mL [1 vial], and iodine I 131 tositumomab 1.1 mg/mL and 5.6 mCi/mL (20 mL) [1 or 2 vials]

Monitoring and Teaching Issues

Physical Assessment: Use caution with cardiovascular disease, renal, or hepatic impairment (see Warnings/Precautions for specific use cautious). This is a one time, step-wise treatment that requires specific timing of several steps; see Dosing, Administration, and Additional Information for detailed directions. Assess results of laboratory tests prior to and immediately after therapy, and regularly thereafter. Patient must be monitored closely for infusion related reactions can occur up to 14 days of infusion (bronchospasm, chills, dyspnea, fever, hypotension, nausea, rigors, diaphoresis). Assess for signs of any adverse response (eg, GI disturbance [nausea, vomiting, pain, diarrhea], hematologic toxicity [neutropenia, thrombocytopenia], myalgia, cough, dyspnea, hypothyroidism; see Adverse Reactions). Teach patient possible side effects/appropriate interventions and adverse symptoms to report (see Patient Education). **Pregnancy risk factor X:** Determine that patient is not pregnant before starting therapy. Do not give to females of childbearing age or males having intercourse with females of childbearing age unless capable of complying with contraceptive use during therapy and for 12 months following therapy.

Monitoring Laboratory Tests: CBC with differential (prior to therapy and at least weekly); TSH (prior to therapy and yearly); serum creatinine (immediately prior to administration)
Following infusion of the iodine I 131 tositumomab dosimetric dose, the total body gamma camera counts and whole body images should be taken within 1 hour of the infusion and prior to urination, and 2-4 days after the infusion and following urination, and 6-7 days after the infusion and following urination.

Patient Education: Do not take any new medications during therapy without consulting prescriber. This treatment is only administered by intravenous infusion. You will be closely monitored prior to, during, and following all infusions; report immediately any immediate chills, nausea, diaphoresis; difficulty swallowing or breathing; or tightness in chest or chest pain. You will need frequent laboratory tests following therapy to assess effectiveness and response. Other medication may be prescribed related to this therapy. Take as directed; do not stop or alter dosage without consulting prescriber. You may experience nausea, vomiting, abdominal pain (if persistent, contact prescriber for medication); or loss of appetite (small frequent meals and frequent mouth care may help). Report immediately any chills, persistent or acute headache, fever, rash, swelling of extremities, chest pain, muscle or back pain, upper respiratory symptoms (sore throat, runny nose, persistent cough, pneumonia), signs of infection, or other adverse reactions. **Pregnancy/breast-feeding precautions:** Inform prescriber if you are pregnant. Do not get pregnant (females) or cause a pregnancy (males) during therapy or for 12 months following therapy. Consult prescriber for appropriate contraceptives. This medication will cause severe fetal defects. Do not give blood during therapy of for 12 months following therapy. Do not breast-feed.

Pregnancy Risk Factor: X

Lactation: Enters breast milk/contraindicated

Breast-Feeding Issues: Radioiodine and immunoglobulins are excreted in breast milk. Quantity of radioiodine may be greater than maternal serum concentrations. Women should be advised to discontinue nursing prior to therapy.

Administration

I.V.: Reduce the rate of infusion by 50% for mild-to-moderate infusion-related toxicities; interrupt for severe toxicity. Once severe toxicity has resolved, infusion may be restarted at half the previous rate. The same IV tubing set with an in-line 0.22 micron filter should be used for the entire dosimetric or therapeutic step. Changing filters may result in loss of drug. Prior to infusion, patients should be premedicated and a thyroid-protective agent should be started.

Reconstitution:
Tositumomab: Withdraw and discard 32 mL of saline from a 50 mL bag of NS. Add contents of both 225 mg vials of tositumomab (total 32 mL) to remaining NS to make a final volume of 50 mL. Gently mix by inverting bag, do not shake.
Iodine I 131 tositumomab: Calculate volume required for an iodine I 131 tositumomab activity of 5 mCi (specification sheet provided with product). If the amount of tositumomab contained in the iodine I 131 tositumomab solution contains <35 mg of tositumomab, use the 35 mg vial of tositumomab to prepare a final concentration of tositumomab 35 mg. Using NS, the final volume should equal 30 mL.

Storage:
Tositumomab: Store under refrigeration at 2°C to 8°C (36°F to 46°F); protect from strong light; do not freeze. Following dilution, tositumomab is stable for 24 hour when refrigerated or 8 hours at room temperature.
Iodine I 131 tositumomab: Store frozen at less than or equal to -20°C in the original lead pots. Allow 60 minutes for thawing at ambient temperature. Solutions for infusion are stable for up to 8 hours at 2°C to 8°C (36°F to 46°F) or room temperature.

(Continued)

Tositumomab and Iodine I 131 Tositumomab *(Continued)*

Additional Information Thyroid protective agent: One of the following agents should be used starting at least 24 hours prior to the dosimetric dose and continued for 2 weeks after the therapeutic dose. Therapy should not begin without using one of the following agents:
SSKI: 4 drops 3 times/day
Lugol's solution: 20 drops 3 times/day
Potassium iodide: 130 mg once daily

♦ **Tositumomab I-131** *see* Tositumomab and Iodine I 131 Tositumomab *on page 1501*

♦ **Touro® DM** *see* Guaifenesin and Dextromethorphan *on page 731*

♦ **Touro LA®** *see* Guaifenesin and Pseudoephedrine *on page 733*

♦ **tPA** *see* Alteplase *on page 79*

♦ **T-Phyl®** *see* Theophylline *on page 1457*

♦ **TPT** *see* Topotecan *on page 1497*

♦ **tRA** *see* Tretinoin (Oral) *on page 1514*

♦ **Tracrium®** *see* Atracurium *on page 157*

Tramadol *(TRA ma dole)*

U.S. Brand Names Ultram®

Synonyms Tramadol Hydrochloride

Generic Available Yes

Pharmacologic Category Analgesic, Non-narcotic

Medication Safety Issues
Sound-alike/look-alike issues:
Tramadol may be confused with Toradol®, Trandate®, Voltaren®
Ultram® may be confused with Ultane®, Voltaren®

Use Relief of moderate to moderately-severe pain

Mechanism of Action/Effect Binds to μ-opiate receptors in the CNS causing inhibition of ascending pain pathways, altering the perception of and response to pain; also inhibits the reuptake of norepinephrine and serotonin, which also modifies the ascending pain pathway

Contraindications Hypersensitivity to tramadol, opioids, or any component of the formulation; opioid-dependent patients; acute intoxication with alcohol, hypnotics, centrally-acting analgesics, opioids, or psychotropic drugs

Warnings/Precautions Should be used only with extreme caution in patients receiving MAO inhibitors. May cause CNS depression and/or respiratory depression, particularly when combined with other CNS depressants. Use with caution and reduce dosage when administered to patients receiving other CNS depressants. An increased risk of seizures may occur in patients receiving serotonin reuptake inhibitors (SSRIs or anorectics), tricyclic antidepressants, other cyclic compounds (including cyclobenzaprine, promethazine), neuroleptics, MAO inhibitors, or drugs which may lower seizure threshold. Patients with a history of seizures, or with a risk of seizures (head trauma, metabolic disorders, CNS infection, or malignancy, or during ethanol/drug withdrawal) are also at increased risk.

Elderly patients and patients with chronic respiratory disorders may be at greater risk of adverse events. Use with caution in patients with increased intracranial pressure or head injury. Use tramadol with caution and reduce dosage in patients with liver disease or renal dysfunction and in patients with myxedema, hypothyroidism, or hypoadrenalism. Not recommended during pregnancy or in nursing mothers. Tolerance or drug dependence may result from extended use (withdrawal symptoms have been reported); abrupt discontinuation should be avoided. Tapering of dose at the time of discontinuation limits the risk of withdrawal symptoms. Safety and efficacy in pediatric patients have not been established.

Drug Interactions

Cytochrome P450 Effect: Substrate of CYP2D6 (major), 3A4 (minor)

Decreased Effect: CYP2D6 inhibitors may decrease the effects of tramadol; example inhibitors include chlorpromazine, delavirdine, fluoxetine, miconazole, paroxetine, pergolide, quinidine, quinine, ritonavir, and ropinirole. Carbamazepine may decrease analgesic efficacy of tramadol (half-life decreases 33% to 50%) and may increase the risk of seizures in patients requiring anticonvulsants.

Increased Effect/Toxicity: Amphetamines may increase the risk of seizures with tramadol. Cimetidine increases the half-life of tramadol by 20% to 25%. SSRIs may increase the risk of seizures with tramadol. Tricyclic antidepressants may increase the risk of seizures. Linezolid may be associated with increased risk of seizures (due to MAO inhibition). MAO inhibitors may increases the risk of seizures. It is not clear if drugs with selective MAO type B inhibition are safer than nonselective agents. Avoid drugs with MAO activity (ie, linezolid). Naloxone may increase the risk of seizures in tramadol overdose. Neuroleptic agents may increase the risk of tramadol-associated seizures and may have additive CNS depressant effects. Opioids may increase the risk of seizures, and may have additive CNS depressant effects. Quinidine (and other inhibitors of CYP2D6) may increase the tramadol serum concentrations.

Nutritional/Ethanol Interactions
Ethanol: Avoid ethanol (may increase CNS depression).
Food: Does not affect the rate or extent of absorption.
Herb/Nutraceutical: Avoid valerian, St John's wort, kava kava, gotu kola (may increase CNS depression).

Adverse Reactions Incidence of some adverse effects may increase over time
>10%:
Central nervous system: Dizziness, headache, somnolence, vertigo
Gastrointestinal: Constipation, nausea
1% to 10%:
Cardiovascular: Vasodilation
Central nervous system: Agitation, anxiety, confusion, coordination impaired, emotional lability, euphoria, hallucinations, malaise, nervousness, sleep disorder, tremor
Dermatologic: Pruritus, rash

Endocrine & metabolic: Menopausal symptoms

Gastrointestinal: Abdominal pain, anorexia, diarrhea, dry mouth, dyspepsia, flatulence, vomiting

Genitourinary: Urinary frequency, urinary retention

Neuromuscular & skeletal: Hypertonia, spasticity, weakness

Ocular: Miosis, visual disturbance

Miscellaneous: Diaphoresis

Overdosage/Toxicology Symptoms of overdose include CNS and respiratory depression, lethargy, coma, seizure, cardiac arrest, and death. Treatment may include naloxone 2 mg I.V. (0.01 mg/kg children) with repeat administration as needed up to 18 mg. Naloxone may increase the risk of seizures in tramadol overdose.

Pharmacodynamics/Kinetics

Onset of Action: ~1 hour

Duration of Action: 9 hours

Absorption: Rapid and complete

Bioavailability: 75%

Time to Peak: 2 hours

Protein Binding: Plasma: 20%

Half-Life Elimination: Tramadol: ~6 hours; Active metabolite: 7 hours; prolonged in elderly, hepatic or renal impairment

Metabolism: Extensively hepatic via demethylation, glucuronidation, and sulfation; has pharmacologically active metabolite formed by CYP2D6

Excretion: Urine (as metabolites)

Dosing

Adults:

Moderate to severe chronic pain: Oral: 50-100 mg every 4-6 hours, not to exceed 400 mg/day

Note: For patients not requiring rapid onset of effect, tolerability may be improved by starting dose at 25 mg/day and titrating dose by 25 mg every 3 days, until reaching 25 mg 4 times/day. Dose may then be increased by 50 mg every 3 days as tolerated, to reach dose of 50 mg 4 times/day.

Elderly: Oral: >75 years: 50-100 mg every 4-6 hours not to exceed 300 mg/day; see renal or hepatic dosing.

Renal Impairment: Cl$_{cr}$ <30 mL/minute: Administer 50-100 mg dose every 12 hours; maximum: 200 mg/day.

Hepatic Impairment: Cirrhosis: Recommended dose is 50 mg every 12 hours.

Available Dosage Forms Tablet, as hydrochloride: 50 mg

Monitoring and Teaching Issues

Physical Assessment: Assess other medications patient may be taking for additive or adverse interactions. Monitor therapeutic effectiveness and adverse reactions or overdose at beginning of therapy and periodically during therapy. May cause physical and/or psychological dependence. Taper dose when discontinuing to avoid withdrawal symptoms. Assess knowledge/teach patient appropriate use, interventions to reduce side effects, and adverse symptoms to report.

Patient Education: If self-administered, use exactly as directed; do not increase dose or frequency. Drug may cause physical and/or psychological dependence. While using this medication, do not use alcohol and other prescription or OTC medications (especially pain medications, sedatives, antihistamines, or cough preparations) without consulting prescriber. Maintain adequate hydration (2-3 L/day of fluids) unless instructed to restrict fluid intake. You may experience drowsiness, dizziness, or blurred vision (use caution when driving or engaging in tasks requiring alertness until response to drug is known); nausea, vomiting, or loss of appetite (small frequent meals, frequent mouth care, chewing gum, or sucking lozenges may help); or constipation (increased exercise, fluids, fruit, or fiber may help). Report severe unresolved constipation, respiratory difficulty or shortness of breath, excessive sedation or increased insomnia and restlessness, changes in urinary pattern or menstrual pattern, seizures, muscle weakness or tremors, or chest pain or palpitations. **Pregnancy/breast-feeding precautions:** Inform prescriber if you are or intend to become pregnant. Do not breast-feed.

Dietary Considerations: May be taken with or without food.

Geriatric Considerations: One study in the elderly found that tramadol 50 mg was similar in efficacy as acetaminophen 300 mg with codeine 30 mg.

Pregnancy Risk Factor: C

Pregnancy Issues: Tramadol has been shown to cross the placenta. Postmarketing reports following tramadol use during pregnancy include neonatal seizures, withdrawal syndrome, fetal death and stillbirth. Not recommended for use during labor and delivery.

Lactation: Enters breast milk/contraindicated

Breast-Feeding Issues: Not recommended for postdelivery analgesia in nursing mothers.

Administration

Storage: Store at controlled room temperature of 25°C (77°F).

♦ **Tramadol Hydrochloride** *see* Tramadol *on page 1504*

♦ **Trandate®** *see* Labetalol *on page 857*

Trandolapril (tran DOE la pril)

U.S. Brand Names Mavik®

Generic Available No

Pharmacologic Category Angiotensin-Converting Enzyme (ACE) Inhibitor

Use Management of hypertension alone or in combination with other antihypertensive agents; treatment of left ventricular dysfunction after myocardial infarction

Unlabeled/Investigational Use As a class, ACE inhibitors are recommended in the treatment of systolic congestive heart failure

Mechanism of Action/Effect Competitive inhibitor of angiotensin-converting enzyme (ACE); prevents conversion of angiotensin I to angiotensin II, a potent vasoconstrictor; results in (Continued)

Trandolapril *(Continued)*

lower levels of angiotensin II which causes an increase in plasma renin activity and a reduction in aldosterone secretion

Contraindications Hypersensitivity to trandolapril or any component of the formulation; history of angioedema-related to previous treatment with an ACE inhibitor; bilateral renal artery stenosis; pregnancy (2nd and 3rd trimesters)

Warnings/Precautions Angioedema can occur at any time during treatment (especially following first dose). Angioedema may involve head and neck (potentially affecting the airway) or the intestine (presenting with abdominal pain). Careful blood pressure monitoring with first dose (hypotension can occur especially in volume depleted patients). Dosage adjustment needed in severe renal dysfunction (Cl$_{cr}$ <30 mL/minute) or in hepatic cirrhosis. Use with caution in hypovolemia; collagen vascular diseases; valvular stenosis (particularly aortic stenosis); hyperkalemia; or before, during, or immediately after anesthesia. Avoid rapid dosage escalation, which may lead to renal insufficiency. Rare toxicities associated with ACE inhibitors include cholestatic jaundice (which may progress to hepatic necrosis) and neutropenia/agranulocytosis with myeloid hyperplasia. Use with caution in unilateral renal artery stenosis and pre-existing renal insufficiency.

Drug Interactions

Decreased Effect: Aspirin (high dose) may reduce the therapeutic effects of ACE inhibitors; at low dosages this does not appear to be significant. Rifampin may decrease the effect of ACE inhibitors. Antacids may decrease the bioavailability of ACE inhibitors (may be more likely to occur with captopril); separate administration times by 1-2 hours. NSAIDs, specifically indomethacin, may reduce the hypotensive effects of ACE inhibitors. More likely to occur in low renin or volume dependent hypertensive patients.

Increased Effect/Toxicity: Potassium supplements, co-trimoxazole (high dose), angiotensin II receptor antagonists (eg, candesartan, losartan, irbesartan), or potassium-sparing diuretics (amiloride, spironolactone, triamterene) may result in elevated serum potassium levels when combined with trandolapril. ACE inhibitor effects may be increased by phenothiazines or probenecid (increases levels of captopril). ACE inhibitors may increase serum concentrations/effects of digoxin, lithium, and sulfonlyureas.

Diuretics have additive hypotensive effects with ACE inhibitors, and hypovolemia increases the potential for adverse renal effects of ACE inhibitors. In patients with compromised renal function, coadministration with NSAIDs may result in further deterioration of renal function. Allopurinol and ACE inhibitors may cause a higher risk of hypersensitivity reaction when taken concurrently.

Nutritional/Ethanol Interactions Herb/Nutraceutical: Avoid dong quai if using for hypertension (has estrogenic activity). Avoid ephedra, yohimbe, ginseng (may worsen hypertension). Avoid garlic (may have increased antihypertensive effect).

Adverse Reactions Note: Frequency ranges include data from hypertension and heart failure trials. Higher rates of adverse reactions have generally been noted in patients with CHF. However, the frequency of adverse effects associated with placebo is also increased in this population.

>1%:
Cardiovascular: Hypotension (<1% to 11%), bradycardia (<1% to 4.7%), intermittent claudication (3.8%), stroke (3.3%)
Central nervous system: Dizziness (1.3% to 23%), syncope (5.9%), asthenia (3.3%)
Endocrine & metabolic: Elevated uric acid (15%), hyperkalemia (5.3%), hypocalcemia (4.7%)
Gastrointestinal: Dyspepsia (6.4%), gastritis (4.2%)
Neuromuscular & skeletal: Myalgia (4.7%)
Renal: Elevated BUN (9%), elevated serum creatinine (1.1% to 4.7%) Respiratory: Cough (1.9% to 35%)

Overdosage/Toxicology Mild hypotension has been the primary toxic effect seen with acute overdose. Bradycardia may also occur. Hyperkalemia occurs even with therapeutic doses, especially in patients with renal insufficiency and those taking NSAIDs. Treatment is symptom-directed and supportive.

Pharmacodynamics/Kinetics

Onset of Action: 1-2 hours; Peak effect: Reduction in blood pressure: 6 hours

Duration of Action: Prolonged; 72 hours after single dose

Absorption: Rapid

Time to Peak: Parent: 1 hour; Active metabolite trandolaprilat: 4-10 hours

Protein Binding: 80%

Half-Life Elimination:
Trandolapril: 6 hours; Trandolaprilat: Effective: 10 hours, Terminal: 24 hours

Metabolism: Hepatically hydrolyzed to active metabolite, trandolaprilat

Excretion: Urine (as metabolites)
Clearance: Reduce dose in renal failure; creatinine clearances ≤30 mL/minute result in accumulation of active metabolite

Dosing

Adults & Elderly:

Hypertension: Oral; Initial dose in patients not receiving a diuretic: 1 mg/day (2 mg/day in black patients). Adjust dosage according to the blood pressure response. Make dosage adjustments at intervals of ≥1 week. Most patients have required dosages of 2-4 mg/day. There is a little experience with doses >8 mg/day. Patients inadequately treated with once daily dosing at 4 mg may be treated with twice daily dosing. If blood pressure is not adequately controlled with trandolapril monotherapy, a diuretic may be added.
Usual dose range (JNC 7): 1-4 mg once daily

Heart failure postmyocardial infarction or left ventricular dysfunction postmyocardial infarction: Oral: Initial: 1 mg/day; titrate patients (as tolerated) towards the target dose of 4 mg/day. If a 4 mg dose is not tolerated, patients can continue therapy with the greatest tolerated dose.

Renal Impairment: Cl$_{cr}$ ≤30 mL/minute: Administer lowest doses, starting at 0.5 mg/day.

Hepatic Impairment: Patients with hepatic cirrhosis: Start dose at 0.5 mg.

Available Dosage Forms Tablet: 1 mg, 2 mg, 4 mg

Monitoring and Teaching Issues

Physical Assessment: Use caution in presence of renal impairment; hypovolemia; collagen vascular diseases; valvular stenosis; hyperkalemia; or before, during, or immediately after anesthesia (see Warnings/Precautions for specific use cautions). Assess potential for interactions with other pharmacological agents or herbal products patient may be taking (especially anything that may impact fluid balance or cardiac status; see Drug Interactions). Assess results of laboratory tests, therapeutic effectiveness, and adverse response with first doses and on a regular basis during therapy (eg, hypovolemia, angioedema, postural hypotension; see Adverse Reactions). Teach patient proper use, possible side effects/appropriate interventions, and adverse symptoms to report (see Patient Education).

Monitoring Laboratory Tests: CBC, electrolytes, renal function; if patient has renal impairment, a baseline WBC with differential and serum creatinine should be evaluated and monitored closely during the first 3 months of therapy.

Patient Education: Do not take any new medication during therapy unless approved by prescriber. Take exactly as directed; do not discontinue without consulting prescriber. Do not take antacids within 2 hours of this medication. Take first dose at bedtime. This drug does not eliminate need for diet or exercise regimen as recommended by prescriber. May cause dizziness, fainting, or lightheadedness (use caution when driving or engaging in tasks that require alertness until response to drug is known); postural hypotension (use caution when rising from lying or sitting position or climbing stairs); or diarrhea (buttermilk, boiled milk, yogurt may help). Report immediately any swelling of face, mouth, lips, tongue or throat. Report chest pain or palpitations; swelling of extremities, mouth, or tongue; skin rash; respiratory difficulty or unusual cough; or other persistent adverse reactions. **Pregnancy/breast-feeding precautions:** Inform prescriber if you are or intend to become pregnant. This drug should not be used in the 2nd or 3rd trimester of pregnancy. Consult prescriber for appropriate contraceptive measures if necessary. Do not breast-feed.

Geriatric Considerations: Due to frequent decreases in glomerular filtration (also creatinine clearance) with aging, elderly patients may have exaggerated responses to ACE inhibitors. Differences in clinical response due to hepatic changes are not observed.

Pregnancy Risk Factor: C/D (2nd and 3rd trimesters)

Pregnancy Issues: ACE inhibitors can cause fetal injury or death if taken during the 2nd or 3rd trimester. Discontinue ACE inhibitors as soon as pregnancy is detected.

Lactation: Enters breast milk/contraindicated

Related Information

Angiotensin Agents *on page 1704*

Heart Failure *on page 1828*

Trandolapril and Verapamil (tran DOE la pril & ver AP a mil)

U.S. Brand Names Tarka®

Synonyms Verapamil and Trandolapril

Generic Available No

Pharmacologic Category Antihypertensive Agent, Combination

Use Combination drug for the treatment of hypertension, however, not indicated for initial treatment of hypertension; replacement therapy in patients receiving separate dosage forms (for patient convenience); when monotherapy with one component fails to achieve desired antihypertensive effect, or when dose-limiting adverse effects limit upward titration of monotherapy

Dosing

Adults: Hypertension: Oral: Individualize dose. Patients receiving trandolapril (up to 8 mg) and verapamil (up to 240 mg) in separate tablets may wish to receive Tarka® at equivalent dosages once daily.

Elderly: Refer to dosing in individual monographs.

Renal Impairment: Usual regimen need not be adjusted unless patient's creatinine clearance is <30 mL/minute. Titration of individual components must be done prior to switching to combination product

Hepatic Impairment: Has not been evaluated in hepatic impairment. Verapamil is hepatically metabolized, adjustment of dosage in hepatic impairment is recommended.

Available Dosage Forms

Tablet, combination [trandolapril component is immediate release, verapamil component is sustained release]:

Trandolapril 1 mg and verapamil hydrochloride 240 mg

Trandolapril 2 mg and verapamil hydrochloride 180 mg

Trandolapril 2 mg and verapamil hydrochloride 240 mg

Trandolapril 4 mg and verapamil hydrochloride 240 mg

Monitoring and Teaching Issues

Physical Assessment: See individual agents.

Patient Education: See individual agents. **Pregnancy/breast-feeding precautions:** Inform prescriber if you are or intend to become pregnant. Do not breast-feed.

Pregnancy Risk Factor: C/D (2nd and 3rd trimesters)

Lactation: Enters breast milk/contraindicated

Related Information

Trandolapril *on page 1505*

Verapamil *on page 1560*

♦ **Transamine Sulphate** *see* Tranylcypromine *on page 1508*

♦ **Transderm Scōp®** *see* Scopolamine Derivatives *on page 1360*

♦ *trans*-Retinoic Acid *see* Tretinoin (Oral) *on page 1514*

♦ *trans*-Retinoic Acid *see* Tretinoin (Topical) *on page 1516*

♦ **Tranxene®** *see* Clorazepate *on page 359*

♦ **Tranxene® SD™**   *see* Clorazepate *on page 359*

♦ **Tranxene® SD™-Half Strength**   *see* Clorazepate *on page 359*

♦ **Tranxene T-Tab®**   *see* Clorazepate *on page 359*

Tranylcypromine (tran il SIP roe meen)

U.S. Brand Names Parnate®
Synonyms Transamine Sulphate; Tranylcypromine Sulfate
Restrictions A medication guide should be dispensed with each prescription. A template for the required MedGuides can be found on the FDA website at: http://www.fda.gov/cder/drug/antidepressants/labelTemplate.pdf
Generic Available No
Pharmacologic Category Antidepressant, Monoamine Oxidase Inhibitor
Use Treatment of major depressive episode without melancholia
Unlabeled/Investigational Use Post-traumatic stress disorder
Mechanism of Action/Effect Thought to act by increasing endogenous concentrations of epinephrine, norepinephrine, dopamine, and serotonin through inhibition of the enzyme (monoamine oxidase) responsible for the breakdown of these neurotransmitters
Contraindications Hypersensitivity to tranylcypromine or any component of the formulation; uncontrolled hypertension; pheochromocytoma; hepatic or renal disease; cerebrovascular defect; cardiovascular disease (CHF); concurrent use of sympathomimetics (and related compounds), CNS depressants, ethanol, meperidine, bupropion, buspirone, dexfenfluramine, dextromethorphan, guanethidine, and serotonergic drugs (including SSRIs) - do not use within 5 weeks of fluoxetine discontinuation or 2 weeks of other antidepressant discontinuation; general anesthesia (discontinue 10 days prior to elective surgery); local vasoconstrictors; spinal anesthesia (hypotension may be exaggerated); foods which are high in tyramine, tryptophan, or dopamine, chocolate, or caffeine.
Warnings/Precautions Antidepressants increase the risk of suicidal thinking and behavior in children and adolescents with major depressive disorder (MDD) and other depressive disorders; consider risk prior to prescribing. All patients must be closely monitored for clinical worsening, suicidality, or unusual changes in behavior, especially during the initiation of therapy or following an increase or decrease in dosage. When used in children, the child's family or caregiver should be instructed to closely observe the patient and communicate condition with healthcare provider. A medication guide should be dispensed with each prescription. **Tranylcypromine is FDA approved for the treatment of depression in children ≥16 years of age.**

The possibility of a suicide attempt is inherent in major depression and may persist until remission occurs. Use caution in high-risk patients. Worsening depression and severe abrupt suicidality that are not part of the presenting symptoms may require discontinuation or modification of drug therapy. The patient's family or caregiver should be alerted to monitor patients for the emergence of suicidality and associated behaviors (such as agitation, irritability, hostility, impulsivity, and hypomania) and call healthcare provider.

May worsen psychosis in some patients or precipitate a shift to mania or hypomania in patients with bipolar disorder. Patients presenting with depressive symptoms should be screened for bipolar disorder. Monotherapy in patients with bipolar disorder should be avoided. **Tranylcypromine is not FDA approved for the treatment of bipolar depression.**

Use with caution in patients who are hyperactive, hyperexcitable, or who have glaucoma, hyperthyroidism, or diabetes; avoid use of meperidine within 2 weeks of tranylcypromine use. Toxic reactions have occurred with dextromethorphan. Hypertensive crisis may occur with tyramine, tryptophan, or dopamine-containing foods. Should not be used in combination with other antidepressants.

Hypotensive effects of antihypertensives (beta-blockers, thiazides) may be exaggerated. May cause orthostatic hypotension (especially at dosages >30 mg/day) - use with caution in patients with hypotension or patients who would not tolerate transient hypotensive episodes - effects may be additive when used with other agents known to cause orthostasis (phenothiazines).

Use with caution in patients at risk of seizures, or in patients receiving other drugs which may lower seizure threshold. Discontinue at least 48 hours prior to myelography. May increase the risks associated with electroconvulsive therapy. Consider discontinuing, when possible, prior to elective surgery. Use with caution in patients receiving disulfiram. Use with caution in patients with renal impairment.

Drug Interactions
Cytochrome P450 Effect: Inhibits CYP1A2 (moderate), 2A6 (strong), 2C8/9 (weak), 2C19 (moderate), 2D6 (moderate), 2E1 (weak), 3A4 (weak)
Decreased Effect: Tranylcypromine inhibits the antihypertensive response to guanadrel or guanethidine. Tranylcypromine may decrease the levels/effects of CYP2D6 prodrug substrates (eg, codeine, hydrocodone, oxycodone, tramadol).
Increased Effect/Toxicity: In general, the combined use of tranylcypromine with TCAs, venlafaxine, trazodone, dexfenfluramine, sibutramine, lithium, meperidine, fenfluramine, dextromethorphan, and SSRIs should be avoided due to the potential for severe adverse reactions (serotonin syndrome, death). Tranylcypromine in combination with amphetamines, other stimulants (methylphenidate), levodopa, metaraminol, buspirone, bupropion, reserpine, and decongestants (pseudoephedrine) may result in severe hypertensive reactions. MAO inhibitors (including tranylcypromine) may inhibit the metabolism of barbiturates and prolong their effect. Foods (eg, cheese) and beverages (eg, ethanol) containing tyramine should be avoided; hypertensive crisis may result.

Tranylcypromine may increase the levels/effects of aminophylline, amphetamines, selected beta-blockers, citalopram, dexmedetomidine, dextromethorphan, diazepam, fluvoxamine, ifosfamide, lidocaine, mesoridazine, mexiletine, methsuximide, mirtazapine, nefazodone, paroxetine, phenytoin, propranolol, risperidone, ritonavir, ropinirole, sertraline, theophylline, thioridazine, tricyclic antidepressants, trifluoperazine, venlafaxine, and other substrates of CYP1A2, 2A6, 2C19, or 2D6.

Tranylcypromine may increase the pressor response of norepinephrine and may prolong neuromuscular blockade produced by succinylcholine. Tramadol may increase the risk of seizures and serotonin syndrome in patients receiving an MAO inhibitor. Tranylcypromine may produce additive hypoglycemic effect in patients receiving hypoglycemic agents and may produce delirium in patients receiving disulfiram. Tryptophan combined use with an MAO inhibitor has been reported to cause disorientation, confusion, anxiety, delirium, agitation, hypomanic signs, ataxia, and myoclonus; concurrent use is contraindicated.

Nutritional/Ethanol Interactions

Ethanol: Avoid ethanol (many contain tyramine).

Food: Clinically-severe elevated blood pressure may occur if tranylcypromine is taken with tyramine-containing food. Avoid foods containing tryptophan or dopamine, chocolate or caffeine.

Herb/Nutraceutical: Avoid valerian, St John's wort, SAMe, ginseng. Avoid ginkgo (may lead to MAO inhibitor toxicity). Avoid ephedra, yohimbe (can cause hypertension).

Lab Interactions Decreased glucose

Adverse Reactions Frequency not defined.

Cardiovascular: Orthostatic hypotension, edema

Central nervous system: Dizziness, headache, drowsiness, sleep disturbances, fatigue, hyper-reflexia, twitching, ataxia, mania, akinesia, confusion, disorientation, memory loss

Dermatologic: Rash, pruritus, urticaria, localized scleroderma, cystic acne (flare), alopecia

Endocrine & metabolic: Sexual dysfunction (anorgasmia, ejaculatory disturbances, impotence), hypernatremia, hypermetabolic syndrome, SIADH

Gastrointestinal: Xerostomia, constipation, weight gain

Genitourinary: Urinary retention, incontinence

Hematologic: Leukopenia, agranulocytosis

Hepatic: Hepatitis

Neuromuscular & skeletal: Weakness, tremor, myoclonus

Ocular: Blurred vision, glaucoma

Miscellaneous: Diaphoresis

Overdosage/Toxicology Symptoms of overdose include tachycardia, palpitations, muscle twitching, seizures, insomnia, transient hypotension, hypertension, hyperpyrexia, and coma. Treatment is symptom-directed and supportive.

Pharmacodynamics/Kinetics

Onset of Action: Therapeutic: 2-3 weeks continued dosing

Time to Peak: Serum: ~2 hours

Half-Life Elimination: 90-190 minutes

Excretion: Urine

Dosing

Adults & Elderly: Depression: Oral: 10 mg twice daily for 2 weeks, increase by 10 mg increments at 1- to 3-week intervals; maximum: 60 mg/day

Hepatic Impairment: Use with care and monitor plasma levels and patient response closely.

Available Dosage Forms Tablet, as sulfate: 10 mg

Monitoring and Teaching Issues

Physical Assessment: Assess other medications patient may be taking for effectiveness and interactions. Evaluate need for continued therapy on a regular basis. Assess results of laboratory tests, therapeutic effectiveness according to rationale for therapy, and adverse reactions at beginning of therapy and periodically with long-term use. Monitor blood pressure. Monitor for CNS depression. Taper dosage slowly when discontinuing. Assess knowledge/teach patient appropriate use, interventions to reduce side effects, and adverse symptoms to report.

Monitoring Laboratory Tests: Blood glucose

Patient Education: Take exactly as directed; do not increase dose or frequency. It may take 2-3 weeks to achieve desired results. Take in the morning to reduce the incidence of insomnia. Avoid alcohol, caffeine, and other prescription or OTC medications not approved by prescriber. Avoid tyramine-containing foods (eg, pickles, aged cheese, wine); see prescriber for complete list of foods to be avoided. Maintain adequate hydration (2-3 L/day of fluids) unless instructed to restrict fluid intake. You may experience drowsiness, dizziness, or blurred vision (use caution when driving or engaging in tasks requiring alertness until response to drug is known); anorexia or dry mouth (small frequent meals, frequent mouth care, chewing gum, or sucking lozenges may help); constipation (increased exercise, fluids, fruit, or fiber may help); diarrhea (buttermilk, yogurt, or boiled milk may help); or orthostatic hypotension (use caution when climbing stairs or changing position from lying or sitting to standing); or altered sexual ability (reversible). Report persistent excessive sedation; muscle cramping, tremors, weakness, or change in gait; chest pain, palpitations, rapid heartbeat, or swelling of extremities; vision changes; suicidal ideation; or worsening of condition. **Pregnancy/breast-feeding precautions:** Inform prescriber if you are or intend to become pregnant. Breast-feeding is not recommended.

Dietary Considerations: Avoid food which contains high amounts of tyramine. Avoid foods containing tryptophan or dopamine, including chocolate and caffeine.

Geriatric Considerations: MAO inhibitors are effective and generally well tolerated by older patients. Potential interactions with tyramine- or tryptophan-containing foods (see Warnings/Precautions), other drugs, and adverse effects on blood pressure have limited use of MAO inhibitors. They are usually reserved for patients who do not tolerate or respond to traditional "cyclic" or "second generation" antidepressants. Tranylcypromine is the preferred MAO inhibitor because its enzymatic-blocking effects are more rapidly reversed. The brain activity of monoamine oxidase increases with age and even more so in patients with Alzheimer's disease. Therefore, MAO inhibitors may have an increased role in treating depressed patients with Alzheimer's disease.

Pregnancy Risk Factor: C

Lactation: Excretion in breast milk unknown/not recommended

Additional Information Tranylcypromine has a more rapid onset of therapeutic effect than other MAO inhibitors, but causes more severe hypertensive reactions.

(Continued)

Tranylcypromine *(Continued)*

Related Information
Antidepressant Agents *on page 1713*
Antidepressant Medication Guidelines *on page 1765*
Tyramine Content of Foods *on page 1758*

♦ **Tranylcypromine Sulfate** *see* Tranylcypromine *on page 1508*

Trastuzumab *(tras TU zoo mab)*

U.S. Brand Names Herceptin®

Generic Available No

Pharmacologic Category Monoclonal Antibody

Use

Single agent for the treatment of patients with metastatic breast cancer whose tumors overexpress the HER-2/*neu* protein and who have received one or more chemotherapy regimens for their metastatic disease

Combination therapy with paclitaxel for the treatment of patients with metastatic breast cancer whose tumors overexpress the HER-2/*neu* protein and who have not received chemotherapy for their metastatic disease

Unlabeled/Investigational Use Treatment of ovarian, gastric, colorectal, endometrial, lung, bladder, prostate, and salivary gland tumors

Mechanism of Action/Effect Trastuzumab is a monoclonal antibody which binds to the extracellular domain of the human epidermal growth factor receptor 2 protein (HER-2). It mediates antibody-dependent cellular cytotoxicity against cells which overproduce HER-2.

Contraindications Hypersensitivity to trastuzumab, Chinese hamster ovary cell proteins, or any component of the formulation. No specific contraindications noted in product labeling. However, patients experiencing severe hypersensitivity reactions have been reported to have repeat episodes despite pretreatment with antihistamines and corticosteroids.

Warnings/Precautions Congestive heart failure associated with trastuzumab may be severe and has been associated with disabling cardiac failure, death, mural thrombus, and stroke. Left ventricular function should be evaluated in all patients prior to and during treatment with trastuzumab. Discontinuation should be strongly considered in patients who develop a clinically significant decrease in ejection fraction during therapy. Combination therapy which includes anthracyclines and cyclophosphamide increases the incidence and severity of cardiac dysfunction. Extreme caution should be used when treating patients with pre-existing cardiac disease or dysfunction, and in patients with previous exposure to anthracyclines. Advanced age may also predispose to cardiac toxicity. Use with caution in patients with known hypersensitivity to trastuzumab, Chinese hamster ovary cell preparations or any component of this product.

Serious adverse events, including hypersensitivity reaction (anaphylaxis), infusion reactions (including fatalities), and pulmonary events (including adult respiratory distress syndrome) have been associated with trastuzumab. Most of these events occur within 24 hours of infusion, however, delayed reactions have occurred. Use with caution in pre-existing pulmonary disease. Discontinuation of trastuzumab should be strongly considered in any patient who develops anaphylaxis, angioedema, or acute respiratory distress syndrome. Retreatment of patients who experienced severe hypersensitivity reactions has been attempted (with premedication). Some patients tolerated retreatment, while others experienced a second severe reaction. When used in combination with myelosuppressive chemotherapy, trastuzumab may increase the incidence of neutropenia (moderate-to-severe) and febrile neutropenia.

Drug Interactions

Increased Effect/Toxicity: Paclitaxel may result in a decrease in clearance of trastuzumab, increasing serum concentrations. Combined use with anthracyclines or cyclophosphamide may increase the incidence/severity of cardiac dysfunction. Trastuzumab may increase the incidence of neutropenia and/or febrile neutropenia when used in combination with myelosuppressive chemotherapy.

Adverse Reactions Note: The most common adverse effects are infusion-related, occurring in up to 40% of patients, consisting of fever and chills (mild to moderate, often with other systemic symptoms). Treatment with acetaminophen, diphenhydramine, and/or meperidine is usually effective.

>10%:

Central nervous system: Pain (47%), fever (36%), chills (32%), headache (26%)

Dermatologic: Rash (18%)

Gastrointestinal: Nausea (33%), diarrhea (25%), vomiting (23%), abdominal pain (22%), anorexia (14%)

Neuromuscular & skeletal: Weakness (42%), back pain (22%)

Respiratory: Cough (26%), dyspnea (22%), rhinitis (14%), pharyngitis (12%)

Miscellaneous: Infection (20%); infusion reaction (40%, chills and fever most common)

1% to 10%:

Cardiovascular: Peripheral edema (10%), CHF (7%), tachycardia (5%)

Central nervous system: Insomnia (14%), dizziness (13%), paresthesia (9%), depression (6%), peripheral neuritis (2%), neuropathy (1%)

Dermatologic: Herpes simplex (2%), acne (2%)

Genitourinary: Urinary tract infection (5%)

Hematologic: Anemia (4%), leukopenia (3%)

Neuromuscular & skeletal: Bone pain (7%), arthralgia (6%)

Respiratory: Sinusitis (9%)

Miscellaneous: Flu syndrome (10%), accidental injury (6%), allergic reaction (3%)

Overdosage/Toxicology There is no experience with overdose in human clinical trials. Treatment is supportive.

Pharmacodynamics/Kinetics
Half-Life Elimination: Mean: 5.8 days (range: 1-32 days)
Dosing
Adults & Elderly:
Metastatic breast carcinoma: I.V.:
Loading dose: 4 mg/kg over 90 minutes; do not administer as an I.V. bolus or I.V. push.
Maintenance dose: 2 mg/kg once weekly (may be infused over 30 minutes if prior infusions are well tolerated).
Renal Impairment: No adjustment is necessary.
Hepatic Impairment: No adjustment necessary.
Available Dosage Forms Injection, powder for reconstitution: 440 mg [packaged with bacteriostatic water for injection; diluent contains benzyl alcohol]
Monitoring and Teaching Issues
Physical Assessment: Monitor therapeutic effectiveness and adverse reactions. Monitor vital signs during infusion. Assess knowledge/teach patient interventions to reduce side effects and adverse symptoms to report.
Patient Education: This medication can only be administered by infusion. Report immediately any adverse reactions during infusion (eg, respiratory difficulty, chills, fever, headache, backache, or nausea/vomiting) so appropriate medication can be administered. You will be susceptible to infection (avoid crowds and exposure to infection). You may experience dizziness or weakness (use caution when driving or engaging in tasks requiring alertness until response to drug is known); nausea or vomiting (small frequent meals, frequent mouth care, chewing gum, or sucking lozenges may help); diarrhea (boiled milk, yogurt, or buttermilk may help); or headache, back or joint pain (mild analgesics may offer relief). Report persistent GI effects; sore throat, runny nose, or respiratory difficulty; chest pain, irregular heartbeat, palpitations, swelling of extremities, or unusual weight gain; muscle or joint weakness, numbness, or pain; skin rash or irritation; itching or pain on urination; unhealed sores, white plaques in mouth or genital area, unusual bruising or bleeding; or other unusual adverse effects. **Breast-feeding precaution:** Breast-feeding is not recommended.
Pregnancy Risk Factor: B
Lactation: Excretion in breast milk unknown/not recommended
Breast-Feeding Issues: It is not known whether trastuzumab is secreted in human milk. Because many immunoglobulins are secreted in milk, and the potential for serious adverse reactions exists, patients should discontinue nursing during treatment and for 6 months after the last dose.
Administration
I.V.: Administered by I.V. infusion; loading doses are infused over 90 minutes; maintenance doses may be infused over 30 minutes if tolerated.
Reconstitution: Reconstitute each vial with 20 mL of bacteriostatic sterile water for injection. Do not shake. If patient has a known hypersensitivity to benzyl alcohol, it may be reconstituted with sterile water for injection.
Storage: Store intact vials under refrigeration (2°C to 8°C/36°F to 46°F) prior to reconstitution. Stable for 28 days after reconstitution if refrigerated; do not freeze. If sterile water for injection without preservative is used for reconstitution, it must be used immediately. After dilution in 0.9% sodium chloride for injection in polyethylene bags, solution is stable for 24 hours.

♦ **Travatan**® *see Travoprost on page 1511*

Travoprost (TRA voe prost)
U.S. Brand Names Travatan®
Generic Available No
Pharmacologic Category Prostaglandin, Ophthalmic
Medication Safety Issues
Sound-alike/look-alike issues:
Travatan® may be confused with Xalatan®
Use Reduction of elevated intraocular pressure in patients with open-angle glaucoma or ocular hypertension who are intolerant of the other IOP-lowering medications or insufficiently responsive (failed to achieve target IOP determined after multiple measurements over time) to another IOP-lowering medication
Contraindications Hypersensitivity to travoprost or any component of the formulation; pregnancy
Warnings/Precautions May permanently change/increase brown pigmentation of the iris, the eyelid skin, and eyelashes. In addition, may increase the length and/or number of eyelashes (may vary between eyes); changes occur slowly and may not be noticeable for months or years. Bacterial keratitis may be caused by inadvertent contamination of multiple-dose ophthalmic solutions. Use caution in patients with intraocular inflammation, aphakic patients, pseudophakic patients with a torn posterior lens capsule, or patients with risk factors for macular edema. Contains benzalkonium chloride; remove contacts prior to administration and wait 15 minutes before reinserting. Contact with contents of vial should be avoided in women who are pregnant or attempting to become pregnant; in case of accidental exposure to the skin, wash the exposed area with soap and water immediately. Safety and efficacy have not been determined for use in patients with renal or hepatic impairment, angle-closure-, inflammatory-, or neovascular glaucoma. Safety and efficacy in pediatric patients have not been established.
Adverse Reactions
>10%: Ocular: Hyperemia (35% to 50%)
5% to 10%: Ocular: Decreased visual acuity, eye discomfort, foreign body sensation, pain, pruritus
1% to 5%:
Cardiovascular: Angina pectoris, bradycardia, hyper-/hypotension
Central nervous system: Depression, pain, anxiety, headache
Endocrine & metabolic: Hypercholesterolemia
(Continued)

Travoprost *(Continued)*

Gastrointestinal: Dyspepsia

Genitourinary: Prostate disorder, urinary incontinence

Neuromuscular & skeletal: Arthritis, back pain, chest pain

Ocular (1% to 4%): Abnormal vision, blepharitis, blurred vision, conjunctivitis, dry eye, iris discoloration, keratitis, lid margin crusting, photophobia, subconjunctival hemorrhage, cataract, tearing, periorbital skin discoloration (darkening), eyelash darkening, eyelash growth increased

Respiratory: Bronchitis, sinusitis

Pharmacodynamics/Kinetics

Onset of Action: ~2 hours; Peak effect: 12 hours

Duration of Action: Plasma levels decrease to <10 pg/mL within 1 hour

Absorption: Via cornea

Metabolism: Hydrolyzed by esterases in the cornea to active free acid; systemically; the free acid is metabolized to inactive metabolites

Dosing

Adults & Elderly: Glaucoma (open angle) or ocular hypertension: Ophthalmic: Instill 1 drop into affected eye(s) once daily in the evening; do not exceed once-daily dosing (may decrease IOP-lowering effect). If used with other topical ophthalmic agents, separate administration by at least 5 minutes.

Available Dosage Forms Solution, ophthalmic: 0.004% (2.5 mL, 5 mL) [contains benzalkonium chloride]

Monitoring and Teaching Issues

Physical Assessment: Assess potential for interactions with other prescriptions, OTC medications, or herbal products patient may be taking. Monitor patient response and adverse effects. Teach patient proper use, side effects/appropriate interventions, and symptoms to report.

Patient Education: For use in eyes only. Wash hands before instilling. Sit or lie down to instill. Open eye, look at ceiling, and instill prescribed amount of solution. Apply gentle pressure to inner corner of eye. Do not let tip of applicator touch eye; do not contaminate tip of applicator (may cause eye infection, eye damage, or vision loss). Contact prescriber concerning continued use of drops if eye infection develops, trauma occurs to the eye, and prior to eye surgery. This product contains benzalkonium chloride which may be adsorbed by contact lenses; remove contacts prior to administration and wait 15 minutes before reinserting. May cause permanent changes in eye color (increases the amount of brown pigment in the iris), eyelid, and eyelashes. May also increase the length and/or number of eyelashes. Changes may occur slowly (months to years). May be used with other eye drops to lower intraocular pressure. If using more than one eye drop medicine, wait at least 5 minutes in between application of each medication. Notify prescriber if conjunctivitis or eyelid reactions occur with use of this product. **Pregnancy precautions:** Do not use if you are pregnant or attempting to become pregnant. In case of accidental contact with the solution, wash skin with soap and water immediately. Consult prescriber if breast-feeding.

Pregnancy Risk Factor: C

Pregnancy Issues: May interfere with the maintenance of pregnancy. Do not use during pregnancy or in women attempting to become pregnant. Teratogenic effects in humans are not known.

Lactation: Excretion in breast milk unknown/use caution

Administration

Other: May be used with other eye drops to lower intraocular pressure. If using more than one ophthalmic product, wait at least 5 minutes in between application of each medication. Remove contact lenses prior to administration and wait 15 minutes before reinserting.

Storage: Store between 2°C to 25°C (36°F to 77°F); discard within 6 weeks of removing from sealed pouch

Additional Information The IOP-lowering effect was shown to be 7-8 mm Hg in clinical studies. The mean IOP reduction in African-American patients was up to 1.8 mm Hg greater than in non-African-American patients. The reason for this effect is unknown.

Related Information

Glaucoma Drug Therapy *on page 1827*

Trazodone *(TRAZ oh done)*

U.S. Brand Names Desyrel®

Synonyms Trazodone Hydrochloride

Restrictions A medication guide should be dispensed with each prescription. A template for the required MedGuides can be found on the FDA website at: http://www.fda.gov/cder/drug/antidepressants/labelTemplate.pdf

Generic Available Yes

Pharmacologic Category Antidepressant, Serotonin Reuptake Inhibitor/Antagonist

Medication Safety Issues

Sound-alike/look-alike issues:

Desyrel® may be confused with Demerol®, Delsym®, Zestril®

Use Treatment of depression

Unlabeled/Investigational Use Potential augmenting agent for antidepressants, hypnotic

Mechanism of Action/Effect Inhibits reuptake of serotonin, causes adrenoreceptor subsensitivity, and induces significant changes in 5HT presynaptic receptor adrenoreceptors. Trazodone also significantly blocks histamine (H1) and alpha₁ adrenergic receptors.

Contraindications Hypersensitivity to trazodone or any component of the formulation

Warnings/Precautions Antidepressants increase the risk of suicidal thinking and behavior in children and adolescents with major depressive disorder (MDD) and other depressive disorders; consider risk prior to prescribing. All patients must be closely monitored for clinical worsening, suicidality, or unusual changes in behavior, especially during the initiation of therapy or following an increase or decrease in dosage. When used in children, the child's family or caregiver should be instructed to closely observe the patient and communicate condition with healthcare provider. A medication guide should be dispensed with each prescription. **Trazodone is not FDA approved for use in children.**

The possibility of a suicide attempt is inherent in major depression and may persist until remission occurs. Use caution in high-risk patients. Worsening depression and severe abrupt suicidality that are not part of the presenting symptoms may require discontinuation or modification of drug therapy. The patient's family or caregiver should be alerted to monitor patients for the emergence of suicidality and associated behaviors (such as agitation, irritability, hostility, impulsivity, and hypomania) and call healthcare provider.

May worsen psychosis in some patients or precipitate a shift to mania or hypomania in patients with bipolar disorder. Patients presenting with depressive symptoms should be screened for bipolar disorder. Monotherapy in patients with bipolar disorder should be avoided. **Trazodone is not FDA approved for the treatment of bipolar depression.**

Priapism, including cases resulting in permanent dysfunction, has occurred with the use of trazodone. Not recommended for use in a patient during the acute recovery phase of MI. Trazodone should be initiated with caution in patients who are receiving concurrent or recent therapy with a MAO inhibitor.

The risks of sedation and/or postural hypotension are high relative to other antidepressants. Trazodone frequently causes sedation, which may result in impaired performance of tasks requiring alertness (eg, operating machinery or driving). Sedative effects may be additive with other CNS depressants and ethanol. Use with caution in patients with a history of cardiovascular disease (including previous MI, stroke, tachycardia, or conduction abnormalities). The risk of conduction abnormalities with this agent is low relative to other antidepressants.

Consider discontinuing, when possible, prior to elective surgery. Therapy should not be abruptly discontinued in patients receiving high doses for prolonged periods. Use caution in patients with a previous seizure disorder or condition predisposing to seizures such as brain damage, alcoholism, or concurrent therapy with other drugs which lower the seizure threshold. Use with caution in patients with hepatic or renal dysfunction and in elderly patients.

Drug Interactions
Cytochrome P450 Effect: Substrate of CYP2D6 (minor), 3A4 (major); **Inhibits** CYP2D6 (moderate), 3A4 (weak)

Decreased Effect: Trazodone inhibits the hypotensive response to clonidine. The levels/effects of trazodone may be decreased by aminoglutethimide, carbamazepine, nafcillin, nevirapine, phenobarbital, phenytoin, rifamycins, and other CYP3A4 inducers. Trazodone may decrease the levels/effects of CYP2D6 prodrug substrates (eg, codeine, hydrocodone, oxycodone, tramadol).

Increased Effect/Toxicity: Trazodone, in combination with other serotonergic agents (buspirone, MAO inhibitors), may produce additive serotonergic effects, including serotonin syndrome. Trazodone, in combination with other psychotropics (low potency antipsychotics), may result in additional hypotension. Fluoxetine may inhibit the metabolism of trazodone resulting in elevated plasma levels.

Trazodone may increase the levels/effects of amphetamines, beta-blockers, dextromethorphan, fluoxetine, lidocaine, mirtazapine, nefazodone, paroxetine, risperidone, ritonavir, thioridazine, tricyclic antidepressants, venlafaxine, and other CYP2D6 substrates. The levels/effects of trazodone may be increased by azole antifungals, ciprofloxacin, clarithromycin, diclofenac, doxycycline, erythromycin, imatinib, isoniazid, nefazodone, nicardipine, propofol, protease inhibitors, quinidine, telithromycin, verapamil, and other CYP3A4 inhibitors.

Nutritional/Ethanol Interactions
Ethanol: Avoid ethanol (may increase CNS depression).
Food: Time to peak serum levels may be increased if trazodone is taken with food.
Herb/Nutraceutical: Avoid valerian, St John's wort, SAMe, kava kava (may increase risk of serotonin syndrome and/or excessive sedation).

Adverse Reactions
>10%:
Central nervous system: Dizziness, headache, sedation
Gastrointestinal: Nausea, xerostomia
Ocular: Blurred vision
1% to 10%:
Cardiovascular: Syncope, hyper-/hypotension, edema
Central nervous system: Confusion, decreased concentration, fatigue, incoordination
Gastrointestinal: Diarrhea, constipation, weight gain/loss
Neuromuscular & skeletal: Tremor, myalgia
Respiratory: Nasal congestion

Overdosage/Toxicology Symptoms of overdose include drowsiness, vomiting, hypotension, tachycardia, incontinence, coma, and priapism. Treatment is symptom-directed and supportive.

Pharmacodynamics/Kinetics
Onset of Action: Therapeutic (antidepressant): 1-3 weeks; sleep aid: 1-3 hours
Time to Peak: Serum: 30-100 minutes; delayed with food (up to 2.5 hours)
Protein Binding: 85% to 95%
Half-Life Elimination: 7-8 hours, two compartment kinetics
Metabolism: Hepatic via CYP3A4 to an active metabolite (mCPP)
Excretion: Primarily urine; secondarily feces

Dosing
Adults:
Depression: Oral: Initial: 150 mg/day in 3 divided doses (may increase by 50 mg/day every 3-7 days); maximum: 600 mg/day
Note: Therapeutic effects may take up to 6 weeks. Therapy is normally maintained for 6-12 months after optimum response is reached to prevent recurrence of depression.

(Continued)

Trazodone *(Continued)*

Sedation/hypnotic (unlabeled use): Oral: 25-50 mg at bedtime (often in combination with daytime SSRIs). May increase up to 200 mg at bedtime.

Elderly: Oral: 25-50 mg at bedtime with 25-50 mg/day dose increase every 3 days for inpatients and weekly for outpatients, if tolerated; usual dose: 75-150 mg/day

Pediatrics:

Depression (unlabeled use):

Children 6-12 years: Initial: 1.5-2 mg/kg/day in divided doses; increase gradually every 3-4 days as needed; maximum: 6 mg/kg/day in 3 divided doses

Adolescents: Initial: 25-50 mg/day; increase to 100-150 mg/day in divided doses

Available Dosage Forms Tablet, as hydrochloride: 50 mg, 100 mg, 150 mg, 300 mg

Monitoring and Teaching Issues

Physical Assessment: Assess potential and monitor closely for interactions with other prescriptions, OTC medications, or herbal products patient may be taking. Assess results of laboratory tests, therapeutic effectiveness according to rationale for therapy, and adverse reactions at beginning of therapy and periodically with long-term use. Initiate at lower doses and taper dosage slowly when discontinuing (allow 3-4 weeks between discontinuing Desyrel® and starting another antidepressant). Teach patient appropriate use, side effects/appropriate interventions, and adverse symptoms to report.

Monitoring Laboratory Tests: Baseline liver function prior to and periodically during therapy

Patient Education: Do not take any new medication during therapy unless approved by prescriber. Take exactly as directed; do not increase dose or frequency. It may take 2-4 weeks to achieve desired results. Take after meals. Avoid excessive alcohol and caffeine. Maintain adequate hydration (2-3 L/day of fluids) unless instructed to restrict fluid intake. You may experience drowsiness, lightheadedness, dizziness (use caution when driving or engaging in tasks requiring alertness until response to drug is known); postural hypotension (use caution when climbing stairs or changing position from lying or sitting to standing); nausea, dry mouth (small frequent meals, frequent mouth care, chewing gum, or sucking lozenges may help); constipation (increased exercise, fluids, fruit, or fiber may help); or diarrhea (buttermilk, yogurt, or boiled milk may help). Report persistent dizziness or headache; muscle cramping, tremors, or altered gait; blurred vision or eye pain; chest pain or irregular heartbeat; suicidal ideation; or worsening of condition. Report prolonged or inappropriate erections. **Pregnancy/breast-feeding precautions:** Inform prescriber if you are or intend to become pregnant. Do not breast-feed.

Geriatric Considerations: Very sedating, but little anticholinergic effects.

Pregnancy Risk Factor: C

Lactation: Enters breast milk/use caution (AAP rates "of concern")

Administration

Oral: Dosing after meals may decrease lightheadedness and postural hypotension.

Related Information

Antidepressant Agents *on page 1713*

Antidepressant Medication Guidelines *on page 1765*

Federal OBRA Regulations: Recommended Maximum Doses *on page 1773*

♦ **Trazodone Hydrochloride** *see* Trazodone *on page 1512*

♦ **Treatment of Sexually-Transmitted Infections** *see page 1861*

♦ **Trelstar™ Depot** *see* Triptorelin *on page 1533*

♦ Trelstar™ LA *see* Triptorelin *on page 1533*

♦ **Trental®** *see* Pentoxifylline *on page 1185*

♦ **Tretinoin and Mequinol** *see* Mequinol and Tretinoin *on page 953*

♦ **Tretinoin, Fluocinolone Acetonide, and Hydroquinone** *see* Fluocinolone, Hydroquinone, and Tretinoin *on page 644*

Tretinoin (Oral) (TRET i noyn, oral)

U.S. Brand Names Vesanoid®

Synonyms All-*trans*-Retinoic Acid; ATRA; NSC-122758; Ro 5488; tRA; *trans*-Retinoic Acid

Generic Available No

Pharmacologic Category Antineoplastic Agent, Miscellaneous

Medication Safety Issues

Sound-alike/look-alike issues:

Tretinoin may be confused with trientine

Use Induction of remission in patients with acute promyelocytic leukemia (APL), French American British (FAB) classification M3 (including the M3 variant)

Mechanism of Action/Effect Tretinoin appears to bind one or more nuclear receptors and inhibits clonal proliferation and/or granulocyte differentiation

Contraindications Sensitivity to parabens, vitamin A, other retinoids, or any component of the formulation; pregnancy

Warnings/Precautions Patients with acute promyelocytic leukemia (APL) are at high risk and can have severe adverse reactions to tretinoin. Administer under the supervision of a physician who is experienced in the management of patients with acute leukemia and in a facility with laboratory and supportive services sufficient to monitor drug tolerance and to protect and maintain a patient compromised by drug toxicity, including respiratory compromise.

May cause retinoic acid-APL (RA-APL) syndrome (fever, dyspnea, pulmonary infiltrates, pleural/pericardial effusions, cardiac dysfunction). May be treated with high-dose steroids. The majority of patients do not require termination of tretinoin therapy. During treatment, rapidly evolving leukocytosis is associated with a higher risk of life-threatening complications.

Not to be used in women of childbearing potential unless the woman is capable of complying with effective contraceptive measures; therapy is normally begun on the second or third day of next normal menstrual period; two reliable methods of effective contraception must be used during therapy and for 1 month after discontinuation of therapy, unless abstinence is the chosen method. Within one week prior to the institution of tretinoin therapy, the patient should have blood or urine collected for a serum or urine pregnancy test with a sensitivity of at least 50 mIU/L. When possible, delay tretinoin therapy until a negative result from this test is obtained. When a delay is not possible, place the patient on two reliable forms of contraception. Repeat pregnancy testing and contraception counseling monthly throughout the period of treatment.

Initiation of therapy with tretinoin may be based on the morphological diagnosis of APL. Confirm the diagnosis of APL by detection of the t(15;17) genetic marker by cytogenetic studies. If these are negative, PML/RARα fusion should be sought using molecular diagnostic techniques. The response rate of other AML subtypes to tretinoin has not been demonstrated. Retinoids have been associated with pseudotumor cerebri (benign intracranial hypertension), especially in children. Concurrent use of other drugs associated with this effect (eg, tetracyclines) may increase risk. Up to 60% of patients experienced reversible hypercholesterolemia or hypertriglyceridemia. Monitor liver function during treatment.

Drug Interactions
Cytochrome P450 Effect: Substrate (minor) of CYP2A6, 2B6, 2C8/9; **Inhibits** CYP2C8/9 (weak); **Induces** CYP2E1 (weak)

Increased Effect/Toxicity: Ketoconazole increases the mean plasma AUC of tretinoin. Concurrent use with antifibrinolytic agents (eg, aminocaproic acid, aprotinin, tranexamic acid) may increase risk of thrombosis. Concurrent use with tetracyclines may increase risk of pseudotumor cerebri.

Nutritional/Ethanol Interactions
Ethanol: Avoid ethanol (may increase CNS depression).

Food: Absorption of retinoids has been shown to be enhanced when taken with food.

Herb/Nutraceutical: St John's wort may decrease tretinoin levels. Avoid dong quai, St John's wort (may also cause photosensitization). Avoid additional vitamin A supplementation. May lead to vitamin A toxicity.

Adverse Reactions
Virtually all patients experience some drug-related toxicity, especially headache, fever, weakness and fatigue. These adverse effects are seldom permanent or irreversible nor do they usually require therapy interruption.

>10%:
Cardiovascular: Peripheral edema (52%), chest discomfort (32%), edema (29%), arrhythmias (23%), flushing (23%), hypotension (14%), hypertension (11%)

Central nervous system: Headache (86%), fever (83%), malaise (66%), pain (37%), dizziness (20%), anxiety (17%), insomnia (14%), depression (14%), confusion (11%)

Dermatologic: Skin/mucous membrane dryness (77%), pruritus (20%), rash (54%), alopecia (14%)

Endocrine & metabolic: Hypercholesterolemia and/or hypertriglyceridemia (60%)

Gastrointestinal: Nausea/vomiting (57%), liver function tests increased (50% to 60%), GI hemorrhage (34%), abdominal pain (31%), mucositis (26%), diarrhea (23%), constipation (17%), dyspepsia (14%), abdominal distention (11%), weight gain (23%), weight loss (17%), xerostomia, anorexia (17%)

Hematologic: Hemorrhage (60%), leukocytosis (40%), disseminated intravascular coagulation (26%)

Local: Phlebitis (11%), injection site reactions (17%)

Neuromuscular & skeletal: Bone pain (77%), myalgia (14%), paresthesia (17%)

Ocular: Visual disturbances (17%)

Otic: Earache/ear fullness (23%)

Renal: Renal insufficiency (11%)

Respiratory: Upper respiratory tract disorders (63%), dyspnea (60%), respiratory insufficiency (26%), pleural effusion (20%), pneumonia (14%), rales (14%), expiratory wheezing (14%), dry nose

Miscellaneous: Infection (58%), shivering (63%), retinoic acid-acute promyelocytic leukemia syndrome (25%), diaphoresis increased (20%)

1% to 10%:
Cardiovascular: Cerebral hemorrhage (9%), pallor (6%), cardiac failure (6%), cardiac arrest (3%), MI (3%), enlarged heart (3%), heart murmur (3%), ischemia, stroke (3%), myocarditis (3%), pericarditis (3%), pulmonary hypertension (3%), secondary cardiomyopathy (3%)

Central nervous system: Intracranial hypertension (9%), agitation (9%), hallucination (6%), agnosia (3%), aphasia (3%), cerebellar edema (3%), cerebral hemorrhage (9%), seizures(3%), coma (3%), CNS depression (3%), dysarthria (3%), encephalopathy (3%), hypotaxia (3%), light reflex absent (3%), spinal cord disorder (3%), unconsciousness (3%), dementia (3%), forgetfulness (3%), somnolence (3%), slow speech (3%), hypothermia (3%)

Dermatologic: Cellulitis (8%), photosensitivity

Endocrine & metabolic: Acidosis (3%)

Gastrointestinal: Hepatosplenomegaly (9%), hepatitis (3%), ulcer (3%)

Genitourinary: Dysuria (9%), acute renal failure (3%), micturition frequency (3%), renal tubular necrosis (3%), enlarged prostate (3%)

Hepatic: Ascites (3%), hepatitis

Neuromuscular & skeletal: Tremor (3%), leg weakness (3%), hyporeflexia, dysarthria, facial paralysis, hemiplegia, flank pain, asterixis, abnormal gait (3%), bone inflammation (3%)

Ocular: Dry eyes, visual acuity change (6%), visual field deficit (3%)

Otic: Hearing loss

Renal: Acute renal failure, renal tubular necrosis

Respiratory: Lower respiratory tract disorders (9%), pulmonary infiltration (6%), bronchial asthma (3%), pulmonary/larynx edema

Miscellaneous: Face edema

Overdosage/Toxicology
Symptoms of overdose include transient headache, facial flushing, cheilosis, abdominal pain, dizziness, and ataxia. All signs or symptoms have been transient and have resolved without apparent residual effects.

(Continued)

Tretinoin (Oral) *(Continued)*

Pharmacodynamics/Kinetics
Time to Peak: Serum: 1-2 hours
Protein Binding: >95%
Half-Life Elimination: Terminal: Parent drug: 0.5-2 hours
Metabolism: Hepatic via CYP; primary metabolite: 4-oxo-all-*trans*-retinoic acid
Excretion: Urine (63%); feces (30%)

Dosing
Adults & Elderly:
Acute promyelocytic leukemia (APL): Oral:
Remission induction: 45 mg/m²/day in 2-3 divided doses for up to 30 days after complete remission (maximum duration of treatment: 90 days)
Remission maintenance: 45-200 mg/m²/day in 2-3 divided doses for up to 12 months.
Note: Optimal consolidation or maintenance regimens have not been determined. All patients should therefore receive a standard consolidation or maintenance chemotherapy regimen for APL after induction therapy with tretinoin unless otherwise contraindicated.
Pediatrics: APL induction of remission, remission maintenance: Oral: Refer to adult dosing.
Available Dosage Forms Capsule: 10 mg [contains soybean oil and parabens]

Monitoring and Teaching Issues
Physical Assessment: To be administered under the supervision of a physician who is experienced in the management of patients with acute leukemia. See extensive and specific Warnings/Precautions for use cautions. Assess potential for interactions with other pharmacological agents and herbal products patient may be taking (see Drug Interactions). Assess results of laboratory tests closely. Patient will require close monitoring (eg, cardiac, CNS, and respiratory status) on a frequent basis during therapy; see Adverse Reactions. Teach patient appropriate use, possible side effects/ interventions, and adverse symptoms to report (see Patient Education).
Monitoring Laboratory Tests: Monitor the patient's hematologic profile, coagulation profile, liver function results and triglyceride and cholesterol levels frequently. Consider temporary discontinuation if LFTs are >5 times the upper limit of normal.
Patient Education: Do not take any new medication during therapy unless approved by prescriber. Take with food. Do not crush, chew, or dissolve capsules. Maintain adequate hydration (2-3 L/day of fluids) unless instructed to restrict fluid intake. Avoid alcohol, foods containing vitamin A, and foods with high fat content. May cause lethargy, dizziness, visual changes, confusion, anxiety (avoid driving or engaging in tasks requiring alertness until response to drug is known); nausea, vomiting, loss of appetite, or dry mouth (small frequent meals, chewing gum, or sucking lozenges may help); photosensitivity (use sunscreen, wear protective clothing and eyewear, and avoid direct sunlight); dry, itchy skin; or dry or irritated eyes (avoid contact lenses). Report persistent vomiting or diarrhea, respiratory difficulty, unusual bleeding or bruising, acute GI pain, bone pain, swelling of extremities, unusual weight gain, or vision changes immediately. **Pregnancy/breast-feeding precautions:** Do not get pregnant (females) or cause a pregnancy (males) while taking this medication and for 1 month following completion of therapy. Consult prescriber for appropriate contraceptive measures. Breast-feeding is not recommended.
Dietary Considerations: To enhance absorption, some clinicians recommend giving with a fatty meal. Capsule contains soybean oil.
Pregnancy Risk Factor: D
Pregnancy Issues: Oral tretinoin is teratogenic and fetotoxic in rats at doses 1000 and 500 times the topical human dose, respectively.
Lactation: Enters breast milk/not recommended

Administration
Oral: Administer with meals; do not crush capsules
Storage: Store capsule at 15°C to 30°C (59°F to 86°F). Protect from light.

Tretinoin (Topical) (TRET i noyn, TOP i kal)
U.S. Brand Names Altinac™; Avita®; Renova®; Retin-A®; Retin-A® Micro
Synonyms Retinoic Acid; *trans*-Retinoic Acid; Vitamin A Acid
Generic Available Yes: Cream, gel
Pharmacologic Category Retinoic Acid Derivative
Medication Safety Issues
Sound-alike/look-alike issues:
Tretinoin may be confused with trientine
Use Treatment of acne vulgaris; photodamaged skin; palliation of fine wrinkles, mottled hyperpigmentation, and tactile roughness of facial skin as part of a comprehensive skin care and sun avoidance program
Unlabeled/Investigational Use Some skin cancers
Mechanism of Action/Effect Keratinocytes in the sebaceous follicle become less adherent which allows for easy removal; decreases microcomedone formation
Contraindications Hypersensitivity to tretinoin or any component of the formulation; sunburn
Warnings/Precautions Use with caution in patients with eczema; avoid excessive exposure to sunlight and sunlamps; avoid contact with abraded skin, mucous membranes, eyes, mouth, angles of the nose. Palliation of fine wrinkles, mottled hyperpigmentation, and tactile roughness of facial skin: Do not use the 0.05% cream for longer than 48 weeks or the 0.02% cream for longer than 52 weeks. Not for use on moderate- to heavily-pigmented skin. Gel is flammable; do not expose to high temperatures or flame.
Drug Interactions
Cytochrome P450 Effect: Substrate (minor) of CYP2A6, 2B6, 2C8/9; **Inhibits** CYP2C8/9 (weak); **Induces** CYP2E1 (weak)
Increased Effect/Toxicity: Topical application of sulfur, benzoyl peroxide, salicylic acid, resorcinol, or any product with strong drying effects potentiates adverse reactions with tretinoin.

Photosensitizing medications (thiazides, tetracyclines, fluoroquinolones, phenothiazines, sulfonamides) augment phototoxicity and should not be used when treating palliation of fine wrinkles, mottled hyperpigmentation, and tactile roughness of facial skin.

Nutritional/Ethanol Interactions

Food: Avoid excessive intake of vitamin A (cod liver oil, halibut fish oil).

Herb/Nutraceutical: Avoid dong quai, St John's wort (may also cause photosensitization). Avoid excessive amounts of vitamin A supplements.

Adverse Reactions

>10%: Dermatologic: Excessive dryness, erythema, scaling of the skin, pruritus

1% to 10%:

Dermatologic: Hyperpigmentation or hypopigmentation, photosensitivity, initial acne flare-up

Local: Edema, blistering, stinging

Overdosage/Toxicology Excessive application may lead to marked redness, peeling or discomfort. Oral ingestion of the topical product may lead to the same adverse reactions seen with excessive vitamin A intake (increased intracranial pressure, jaundice, ascites, cutaneous desquamation; symptoms of acute overdose [12,000 units/kg] include nausea, vomiting, and diarrhea); toxic signs of an overdose commonly respond to drug discontinuation, and generally return to normal spontaneously within a few days to weeks. Toxic signs of a topical overdose commonly respond to drug discontinuation, and generally resolve spontaneously within a few days to weeks.

When confronted with signs of increased intracranial pressure, treatment with mannitol (0.25 g/kg I.V. up to 1 g/kg/dose repeated every 5 minutes as needed), dexamethasone (1.5 mg/kg I.V. load followed with 0.375 mg/kg every 6 hours for 5 days), and/or hyperventilation should be employed.

Pharmacodynamics/Kinetics

Absorption: Minimal

Metabolism: Hepatic for the small amount absorbed

Excretion: Urine and feces

Dosing

Adults:

Acne vulgaris: Topical: Begin therapy with a weaker formulation of tretinoin (0.025% cream, 0.04% microsphere gel, or 0.01% gel) and increase the concentration as tolerated; apply once daily to acne lesions before retiring or on alternate days; if stinging or irritation develop, decrease frequency of application

Palliation of fine wrinkles, mottled hyperpigmentation, and tactile roughness of facial skin: Topical: Pea-sized amount of the 0.02% or 0.05% cream applied to entire face once daily in the evening

Elderly: Use of the 0.02% cream in patients 65-71 years of age showed similar improvement in fine wrinkles as seen in patients <65 years. Safety and efficacy of the 0.02% cream have not been established in patients >71 years of age. Safety and efficacy of the 0.05% cream have not been established in patients >50 years of age.

Pediatrics: Children >12 years: Acne vulgaris: Topical: Refer to adult dosing.

Available Dosage Forms

Cream, topical: 0.025% (20 g, 45 g); 0.05% (20 g, 45 g); 0.1% (20 g, 45 g)

Altinac™: 0.025% (20 g, 45 g); 0.05% (20 g, 45 g); 0.1% (20 g, 45 g)

Avita®: 0.025% (20 g, 45 g)

Renova®: 0.02% (40 g); 0.05% (40 g, 60 g)

Retin-A®: 0.025% (20 g, 45 g); 0.05% (20 g, 45 g); 0.1% (20 g, 45 g)

Gel, topical: 0.025% (15 g, 45 g)

Avita®: 0.025% (15 g, 45 g)

Retin-A®: 0.01% (15 g, 45 g); 0.025% (15 g, 45 g)

Retin-A® Micro [microsphere gel]: 0.04% (20 g, 45 g); 0.1% (20 g, 45 g)

Liquid, topical (Retin-A®): 0.05% (28 mL)

Monitoring and Teaching Issues

Physical Assessment: Assess knowledge/instruct patient on appropriate application, possible adverse effects, and symptoms to report.

Patient Education: For once-daily use, do not overuse. Avoid increased intake of vitamin A. Thoroughly wash hands before applying. Wash area to be treated at least 30 minutes before applying. Do not wash face more frequently than 2-3 times a day. Do not apply to areas near your mouth, eyes, corners of your nose, or open sores. Avoid using topical preparations that contain alcohol or harsh chemicals during treatment. It may take several weeks before the full benefit of the medication is seen. You may experience increased sensitivity to sunlight; protect skin with sunblock (minimum SPF 15), wear protective clothing, and avoid direct sunlight. Stop treatment and inform prescriber if rash, skin irritation, redness, scaling, or excessive dryness occurs. When used for hyperpigmentation and tactile redness of facial skin, wrinkles will not be eliminated. Must be used in combination with a comprehensive skin care program. **Pregnancy precaution:** Inform prescriber if you are pregnant.

Gel: Flammable; do not expose to flame and do not smoke during use.

Pregnancy Risk Factor: C

Pregnancy Issues: High doses may be teratogenic and fetotoxic. Tretinoin does not appear to be teratogenic when used topically since it is rapidly metabolized by the skin; however, there are rare reports of fetal defects. Use for acne only if benefit to mother outweighs potential risk to fetus. During pregnancy, do not use for palliation of fine wrinkles, mottled hyperpigmentation, and tactile roughness of facial skin.

Lactation: Enters breast milk/compatible

Administration

Topical: Palliation of fine wrinkles, mottled hyperpigmentation, and tactile roughness of facial skin: Cream: Prior to application, gently wash face with a mild soap. Pat dry. Wait 20-30 minutes to apply cream. Avoid eyes, ears, nostrils, and mouth.

Storage: Store at 25°C (77°F); gel is flammable, keep away from heat and flame

♦ **Trexall™** *see Methotrexate on page 974*

♦ **Triaconazole** *see Terconazole on page 1447*

Triamcinolone (trye am SIN oh lone)

U.S. Brand Names Aristocort®; Aristocort® A; Aristocort® Forte; Aristospan®; Azmacort®; Kenalog®; Kenalog-10®; Kenalog-40®; Kenalog® in Orabase®; Nasacort® [HFA]; Nasacort® AQ; Triderm®; Tri-Nasal®

Synonyms Triamcinolone Acetonide, Aerosol; Triamcinolone Acetonide, Parenteral; Triamcinolone Diacetate, Oral; Triamcinolone Diacetate, Parenteral; Triamcinolone Hexacetonide; Triamcinolone, Oral

Generic Available Yes: Cream, lotion, ointment, paste

Pharmacologic Category Corticosteroid, Adrenal; Corticosteroid, Inhalant (Oral); Corticosteroid, Nasal; Corticosteroid, Systemic; Corticosteroid, Topical

Medication Safety Issues
Sound-alike/look-alike issues:
Kenalog® may be confused with Ketalar®
Nasacort® may be confused with NasalCrom®

Use
Nasal inhalation: Management of seasonal and perennial allergic rhinitis in patients ≥6 years of age
Oral inhalation: Control of bronchial asthma and related bronchospastic conditions
Oral topical: Adjunctive treatment and temporary relief of symptoms associated with oral inflammatory lesions and ulcerative lesions resulting from trauma
Systemic: Adrenocortical insufficiency, rheumatic disorders, allergic states, respiratory diseases, systemic lupus erythematosus (SLE), and other diseases requiring anti-inflammatory or immunosuppressive effects
Topical: Inflammatory dermatoses responsive to steroids

Mechanism of Action/Effect Decreases inflammation by suppression of migration of polymorphonuclear leukocytes and reversal of increased capillary permeability; suppresses the immune system by reducing activity and volume of the lymphatic system; suppresses adrenal function at high doses

Contraindications Hypersensitivity to triamcinolone or any component of the formulation; systemic fungal infections; serious infections (except septic shock or tuberculous meningitis); primary treatment of status asthmaticus; fungal, viral, or bacterial infections of the mouth or throat (oral topical formulation)

Warnings/Precautions Not to be used in status asthmaticus or for the relief of acute bronchospasm. May cause suppression of hypothalamic-pituitary-adrenal (HPA) axis, particularly in younger children or in patients receiving high doses for prolonged periods. Fatalities have occurred due to adrenal insufficiency in asthmatic patients during and after transfer from systemic corticosteroids to aerosol steroids; aerosol steroids do **not** provide the systemic steroid needed to treat patients having trauma, surgery, or infections. Withdrawal and discontinuation of the corticosteroid should be done slowly and carefully

Orally-inhaled and intranasal corticosteroids may cause a reduction in growth velocity in pediatric patients, which appears to be related to dose and duration of exposure.

May suppress the immune system, patients may be more susceptible to infection. Use with caution in patients with systemic infections or ocular herpes simplex. Avoid exposure to chickenpox and measles. Corticosteroids should be used with caution in patients with diabetes, hypertension, osteoporosis, peptic ulcer, glaucoma, cataracts, or tuberculosis. Use caution in hepatic impairment.

Oral topical: Discontinue if local irritation or sensitization should develop. If significant regeneration or repair of oral tissues has not occurred in seven days, re-evaluation of the etiology of the oral lesion is advised.

Drug Interactions
Decreased Effect: Decreased effect with barbiturates and phenytoin. Rifampin increased metabolism of triamcinolone. Vaccine and toxoid effects may be reduced.

Increased Effect/Toxicity: Salicylates or NSAIDs coadministered oral corticosteroids may increase risk of GI ulceration.

Nutritional/Ethanol Interactions
Ethanol: Avoid ethanol (may enhance gastric mucosal irritation).
Food: Triamcinolone interferes with calcium absorption.
Herb/Nutraceutical: Avoid cat's claw, echinacea (have immunostimulant properties).

Adverse Reactions
Systemic: Frequency not defined:
Cardiovascular: CHF, hypertension
Central nervous system: Convulsions, fever, headache, intracranial pressure increased, vertigo
Dermatologic: Bruising, facial erythema, petechiae, photosensitivity, rash, thin/fragile skin, wound healing impaired
Endocrine & metabolic: Adrenocortical/pituitary unresponsiveness (particularly during stress), carbohydrate tolerance decreased, cushingoid state, diabetes mellitus (manifestations of latent disease), fluid retention, growth suppression (children), hypokalemic alkalosis, menstrual irregularities, negative nitrogen balance, potassium loss, sodium retention
Gastrointestinal: Abdominal distention, diarrhea, dyspepsia, nausea, oral *Monilia* (oral inhaler), pancreatitis, peptic ulcer, ulcerative esophagitis, weight gain
Local: Skin atrophy (at the injection site)
Neuromuscular & skeletal: Femoral/humeral head aseptic necrosis, muscle mass decreased, muscle weakness, osteoporosis, pathologic fracture of long bones, steroid myopathy, vertebral compression fractures

Ocular: Cataracts, intraocular pressure increased, exophthalmos, glaucoma

Respiratory: Cough increased (nasal spray), epistaxis (nasal inhaler/spray), pharyngitis (nasal spray/oral inhaler), sinusitis (oral inhaler), voice alteration (oral inhaler)

Miscellaneous: Anaphylaxis, diaphoresis increased, suppression to skin tests

Topical: Frequency not defined:

Dermatologic: Itching, allergic contact dermatitis, dryness, folliculitis, skin infection (secondary), itching, hypertrichosis, acneiform eruptions, hypopigmentation, skin maceration, skin atrophy, striae, miliaria, perioral dermatitis, atrophy of oral mucosa

Local: Burning, irritation

Overdosage/Toxicology When consumed in high doses for prolonged periods, systemic hypercorticism and adrenal suppression may occur. In those cases, discontinuation of the corticosteroid should be done judiciously.

Pharmacodynamics/Kinetics

Duration of Action: Oral: 8-12 hours

Absorption: Topical: Systemic

Time to Peak: I.M.: 8-10 hours

Half-Life Elimination: Biologic: 18-36 hours

Dosing

Adults & Elderly: The lowest possible dose should be used to control the condition; when dose reduction is possible, the dose should be reduced gradually. Parenteral dose is usually 1/3 to 1/2 the oral dose given every 12 hours. In life-threatening situations, parenteral doses larger than the oral dose may be needed.

Adrenocortical insufficiency: Oral: Range: 4-12 mg/day

Allergic rhinitis (perennial or seasonal):

Nasal spray: 220 mcg/day as 2 sprays in each nostril once daily

Nasal inhaler: Initial: 220 mcg/day as 2 sprays in each nostril once daily; may increase dose to 440 mcg/day (given once daily or divided and given 2 or 4 times/day)

Oral (acute treatment only): Range: 8-12 mg/day

Asthma:

Oral: 8-16 mg/day

Oral inhalation: 200 mcg 3-4 times/day **or** 400 mcg twice daily; maximum dose: 1600 mcg/day

Carditis (acute rheumatic): Oral: Initial: 20-60 mg/day; reduce dose during maintenance therapy

Dermatoses (steroid-responsive, including contact/atopic dermatitis):

Oral: Initial: 8-16 mg/day

Injection:

Acetonide: Intradermal: Initial: 1 mg

Diacetate: Intralesional, sublesional: Range: 5-48 mg, dependent upon size of lesion; maximum 12.5 mg/injection site, 25 mg/lesion, 75 mg/week; usual treatment course: 2-3 injections at 1- to 2-week intervals

Hexacetonide: Intralesional, sublesional: up to 0.5 mg/square inch of affected skin

Topical:

Cream, ointment: Apply thin film to affected areas 2-4 times/day

Spray: Apply to affected area 3-4 times/day

Ophthalmic disorders: Oral: 12-40 mg/day

Oral inflammatory lesions/ulcers: Oral topical: Press a small dab (about 1/4 inch) to the lesion until a thin film develops; a larger quantity may be required for coverage of some lesions. For optimal results, use only enough to coat the lesion with a thin film; do not rub in.

Rheumatic or arthritic disorders:

Oral: Range: 8-16 mg/day

Lupus (SLE): Initial: 20-32 mg/day, some patients may need initial doses ≥48 mg; reduce dose during maintenance therapy

Intra-articular (or similar injection as designated):

Acetonide: Intra-articular, intrabursal, tendon sheaths: Initial: Smaller joints: 2.5-5 mg, larger joints: 5-15 mg

Triamcinolone Dosing

	Acetonide	Diacetate	Hexacetonide
Intrasynovial	2.5-40 mg	5-40 mg	
Intralesional	1-30 mg (usually 1 mg per injection site); 10 mg/mL suspension usually used	5-48 mg (not >25 mg per lesion)	Up to 0.5 mg/sq inch affected area
Sublesional	1-30 mg		
Systemic I.M.	2.5-60 mg/dose (usual adult dose: 60 mg; may repeat with 20-100 mg dose when symptoms recur)	~40 mg/wk	
Intra-articular	2.5-40 mg	2-40 mg	2-20 mg average
large joints	5-15 mg		10-20 mg
small joints	2.5-5 mg		2-6 mg
Tendon sheaths	2.5-10 mg		
Intradermal	1 mg/site		

(Continued)

Triamcinolone *(Continued)*

Diacetate: Intra-articular, Intrasynovial: Range: 5-40 mg; duration of effect varies from 1 week to 2 months, although more frequent dosing may be needed in acutely inflamed joints.

Average dose: Knee: 25 mg, finger: 2-5 mg

Hexacetonide: Intra-articular: Initial range: 2-20 mg/day

I.M.:

Acetonide: Range: 2.5-60 mg/day; Initial: 60 mg

Diacetate: Initial range: 3-48 mg/day; average dose: 40 mg/week

See table on previous page.

Pediatrics:

Allergic rhinitis (perennial or seasonal):

Nasal spray:

Children 6-11 years: 110 mcg/day as 1 spray in each nostril once daily.

Children ≥12 years: Refer to adult dosing.

Nasal inhaler:

Children 6-11 years: Initial: 220 mcg/day as 2 sprays in each nostril once daily

Children ≥12 years: Refer to adult dosing.

Asthma:

Oral: 8-16 mg/day

Oral inhalation:

Children 6-12 years: 100-200 mcg 3-4 times/day **or** 200-400 mcg twice daily; maximum dose: 1200 mcg

Children >12 years: Refer to adult dosing.

Rheumatic conditions: I.M. (acetonide): Range: 2.5-60 mg/day

Children 6-12 years: Initial: 40 mg

Children ≥12 years: Refer to adult dosing.

Available Dosage Forms

Aerosol for nasal inhalation, as acetonide [CFC free] (Nasacort® [HFA]): 55 mcg/inhalation (9.3 g) [100 doses]

Aerosol for nasal inhalation, as acetonide [spray]:

Nasacort® AQ: 55 mcg/inhalation (16.5 g) [120 doses]

Tri-Nasal®: 50 mcg/inhalation (15 mL) [120 doses]

Aerosol for oral inhalation, as acetonide (Azmacort®): 100 mcg per actuation (20 g) [240 actuations]

Aerosol, topical, as acetonide (Kenalog®): 0.2 mg/2-second spray (63 g)

Cream, as acetonide: 0.025% (15 g, 80 g); 0.1% (15 g, 80 g, 454 g, 2270 g); 0.5% (15 g)

Aristocort® A: 0.025% (15 g, 60 g); 0.1% (15 g, 60 g); 0.5% (15 g) [contains benzyl alcohol]

Kenalog®: 0.1% (15 g, 60 g, 80 g); 0.5% (20 g)

Triderm®: 0.1% (30 g, 85 g)

Injection, suspension, as acetonide:

Kenalog-10®: 10 mg/mL (5 mL) [contains benzyl alcohol; not for I.V. or I.M. use]

Kenalog-40®: 40 mg/mL (1 mL, 5 mL, 10 mL) [contains benzyl alcohol; not for I.V. or intradermal use]

Injection, suspension, as diacetate:

Aristocort®: 25 mg/mL (5 mL) [contains benzyl alcohol; not for I.V. use]

Aristocort® Forte: 40 mg/mL (1 mL, 5mL) [contains benzyl alcohol; not for I.V. use]

Injection, suspension, as hexacetonide (Aristospan®): 5 mg/mL (5 mL); 20 mg/mL (1 mL, 5 mL) [contains benzyl alcohol; not for I.V. use]

Lotion, as acetonide (Kenalog®): 0.025% (60 mL); 0.1% (60 mL)

Ointment, topical, as acetonide: 0.025% (80 g); 0.1% (15 g, 80 g, 454 g)

Aristocort® A, Kenalog®: 0.1% (15 g, 60 g)

Paste, oral, topical, as acetonide (Kenalog® in Orabase®): 0.1% (5 g)

Tablet (Aristocort®): 4 mg [contains lactose and sodium benzoate]

Monitoring and Teaching Issues

Physical Assessment: Assess other medications patient may be taking for effectiveness and interactions. Assess results of laboratory tests, therapeutic effectiveness, and adverse effects according to indications for therapy, dose, route (systemic or topical), and duration of therapy. With systemic administration, patients with diabetes should monitor glucose levels closely (corticosteroids may alter glucose levels). Assess knowledge/teach patient appropriate use, interventions to reduce side effects, and adverse symptoms to report. When used for long-term therapy (>10-14 days) do not discontinue abruptly; decrease dosage incrementally.

Patient Education: Take exactly as directed; do not increase dose or discontinue abruptly without consulting prescriber. Take oral medication with or after meals. Avoid alcohol. Limit intake of caffeine or stimulants. Prescriber may recommend increased dietary vitamins, minerals, or iron. If you have diabetes, monitor glucose levels closely (antidiabetic medication may need to be adjusted). Inform prescriber if you are experiencing greater than normal levels of stress (medication may need adjustment). Some forms of this medication may cause GI upset (oral medication may be taken with meals to reduce GI upset; or small frequent meals and frequent mouth care may reduce GI upset). You may be more susceptible to infection (avoid crowds and exposure to infection). Report promptly excessive nervousness or sleep disturbances; any signs of infection (sore throat, unhealed injuries); excessive growth of body hair or loss of skin color; vision changes; excessive or sudden weight gain (>3 lb/week); swelling of face or extremities; respiratory difficulty; muscle weakness; change in color of stools (black or tarry) or persistent abdominal pain; or worsening of condition or failure to improve. **Pregnancy/breast-feeding precautions:** Inform prescriber if you are or intend to become pregnant. Consult prescriber if breast-feeding.

Aerosol: Shake gently before use. Use at regular intervals, no more frequently than directed. Not for use during acute asthmatic attack. Follow directions that accompany product. Rinse mouth and throat after use to prevent candidiasis. Do not use intranasal product if you have a nasal infection, nasal injury, or recent nasal surgery. If using two products, consult prescriber in which order to use the two products. Report unusual cough or spasm; persistent nasal bleeding, burning, or irritation; or worsening of condition.

Inhalation: Sit when using. Take deep breaths for 3-5 minutes, and clear nasal passages before administration (use decongestant as needed). Hold breath for 5-10 seconds after use, and wait 1-3 minutes between inhalations. Follow package insert instructions for use. Do not exceed maximum dosage. If also using inhaled bronchodilator, use before triamcinolone. Rinse mouth and throat after use to reduce aftertaste and prevent candidiasis.

Topical: For external use only. Not for eyes or mucous membranes or open wounds. Apply in very thin layer to occlusive dressing. Apply dressing to area being treated. Avoid prolonged or excessive use around sensitive tissues, genital, or rectal areas. Inform prescriber if condition worsens (swelling, redness, irritation, pain, open sores) or fails to improve.

Dietary Considerations: May be taken with food to decrease GI distress.

Geriatric Considerations: Because of the risk of adverse effects, systemic corticosteroids should be used cautiously in the elderly, in the smallest possible dose, and for the shortest possible time. Azmacort® (metered dose inhaler) comes with its own spacer device attached and may be easier to use in older patients.

Pregnancy Risk Factor: C

Pregnancy Issues: There are no adequate and well-controlled studies in pregnant women, however, triamcinolone is teratogenic in animals; use during pregnancy with caution. Increased incidence of cleft palate, neonatal adrenal suppression, low birth weight, and cataracts in the infant has been reported following corticosteroid use during pregnancy. In general, the use of large amounts, or prolonged use, of topical corticosteroids during pregnancy should be avoided. In the mother, corticosteroids may increase calcium and potassium excretion, elevate blood pressure, and cause salt and water retention.

Lactation: Excretion in breast milk unknown/use caution

Breast-Feeding Issues: It is not known if triamcinolone is excreted in breast milk, however, other corticosteroids are excreted. Prednisone and prednisolone are excreted in breast milk; the AAP considers them to be "usually compatible" with breast-feeding. Hypertension was reported in a nursing infant when a topical corticosteroid was applied to the nipples of the mother.

Administration

Oral: Tablet: Once-daily doses should be given in the morning.

I.M.: Inject I.M. dose deep in large muscle mass, avoid deltoid.

Inhalation:

Intranasal: Spray/inhaler: Shake well prior to use. Gently blow nose to clear nostrils.

Oral: Shake well prior to use. Rinse mouth and throat after using inhaler to prevent candidiasis. Use spacer device provided with Azmacort®.

Topical:

Oral topical: Apply small dab to lesion until a thin film develops; do not rub in. Apply at bedtime or after meals if applications are needed throughout the day.

Topical: Apply a thin film sparingly and avoid topical application on the face. Do not use on open skin or wounds. Do not occlude area unless directed.

Other: Avoid subcutaneous administration.

Reconstitution: Injection, suspension:

Diacetate suspension: May dilute prior to use using NS or equal parts of NS and procaine 1%. Diluted suspension stable ~1 week. Avoid diluents containing parabens or preservatives (may cause flocculation). Suspensions for intralesional use may be diluted to 1:1 or 1:10 concentration.

Hexacetonide suspension: Avoid diluents containing parabens or preservatives (may cause flocculation). Diluted suspension stable ~1 week. Suspension for intralesional use, may be diluted with D_5NS, $D_{10}NS$ or SWFI to a 1:1, 1:2, or 1:4 concentration. Solutions for intra-articular use, may be diluted with lidocaine 1% or 2%.

Storage: Store at room temperature. Avoid freezing.

Injection, suspension: Shake well prior to use.

Topical spray: Avoid excessive heat.

Additional Information 16 mg triamcinolone is equivalent to 100 mg cortisone (no mineralocorticoid activity).

Effects of inhaled/intranasal steroids on growth have been observed in the absence of laboratory evidence of HPA axis suppression, suggesting that growth velocity is a more sensitive indicator of systemic corticosteroid exposure in pediatric patients than some commonly used tests of HPA axis function. The long-term effects of this reduction in growth velocity associated with orally-inhaled and intranasal corticosteroids, including the impact on final adult height, are unknown. The potential for "catch up" growth following discontinuation of treatment with inhaled corticosteroids has not been adequately studied.

Related Information

Asthma *on page 1799*

Corticosteroids *on page 1731*

Inhalant Agents *on page 1734*

♦ **Triamcinolone Acetonide, Aerosol** *see Triamcinolone on page 1518*

♦ **Triamcinolone Acetonide, Parenteral** *see Triamcinolone on page 1518*

♦ **Triamcinolone and Nystatin** *see Nystatin and Triamcinolone on page 1104*

♦ **Triamcinolone Diacetate, Oral** *see Triamcinolone on page 1518*

♦ **Triamcinolone Diacetate, Parenteral** *see Triamcinolone on page 1518*

♦ **Triamcinolone Hexacetonide** *see Triamcinolone on page 1518*

♦ **Triamcinolone, Oral** *see Triamcinolone on page 1518*

♦ **Triaminic® Thin Strips™ Cough and Runny Nose [OTC]** *see DiphenhydrAMINE on page 463*

♦ **Triamterene and Hydrochlorothiazide** *see Hydrochlorothiazide and Triamterene on page 754*

Triazolam (trye AY zoe lam)

U.S. Brand Names Halcion®

Controlled Substance C-IV

Generic Available Yes

Pharmacologic Category Benzodiazepine

Medication Safety Issues

Sound-alike/look-alike issues:

Triazolam may be confused with alprazolam

Halcion® may be confused with halcinonide, Haldol®

Use Short-term treatment of insomnia

Mechanism of Action/Effect Binds to stereospecific benzodiazepine receptors on the postsynaptic GABA neuron at several sites within the central nervous system, including the limbic system, reticular formation. Enhancement of the inhibitory effect of GABA on neuronal excitability results by increased neuronal membrane permeability to chloride ions. This shift in chloride ions results in hyperpolarization (a less excitable state) and stabilization.

Contraindications Hypersensitivity to triazolam or any component of the formulation (cross-sensitivity with other benzodiazepines may exist); concurrent therapy with atazanavir, ketoconazole, itraconazole, nefazodone, and ritonavir; pregnancy

Warnings/Precautions As a hypnotic, should be used only after evaluation of potential causes of sleep disturbance. Failure of sleep disturbance to resolve after 7-10 days may indicate psychiatric or medical illness. Prescription should be written for a maximum of 7-10 days and should not be prescribed in quantities exceeding a 1-month supply. Abrupt discontinuation after sustained use (generally >10 days) may cause withdrawal symptoms. Use is not recommended in patients with depressive disorders or psychoses. Avoid use in patients with sleep apnea. Use with caution in elderly or debilitated patients, patients with hepatic disease (including alcoholics), renal impairment, respiratory disease, impaired gag reflex, or obese patients. Use caution with potent CYP3A4 inhibitors, as they may significantly decreased the clearance of triazolam.

Causes CNS depression (dose-related) which may impair physical and mental capabilities. Use with caution in patients receiving other CNS depressants or psychoactive agents. Benzodiazepines have been associated with falls and traumatic injury and should be used with extreme caution in patients who are at risk of these events (especially the elderly). May cause physical or psychological dependence - use with caution in patients with a history of drug dependence.

Benzodiazepines have been associated with anterograde amnesia. Paradoxical reactions, including hyperactive or aggressive behavior, have been reported with benzodiazepines, particularly in adolescent/pediatric or psychiatric patients. Does not have analgesic, antidepressant, or antipsychotic properties.

Drug Interactions

Cytochrome P450 Effect: Substrate of CYP3A4 (major); **Inhibits** CYP2C8/9 (weak)

Decreased Effect: CYP3A4 inducers may decrease the levels/effects of triazolam; example inducers include aminoglutethimide, carbamazepine, nafcillin, nevirapine, phenobarbital, phenytoin, and rifamycins.

Increased Effect/Toxicity: Sedative and/or respiratory depressive effects may be additive with other CNS depressants. CYP3A4 inhibitors may increase the levels/effects of triazolam; example inhibitors include azole antifungals, ciprofloxacin, clarithromycin, diclofenac, doxycycline, erythromycin, imatinib, isoniazid, nefazodone, nicardipine, propofol, protease inhibitors, quinidine, and verapamil. Concurrent use of some strong CYP3A4 inhibitors (including azole antifungals, nefazodone, and protease inhibitors) has been contraindicated by the manufacturers. Oral contraceptives may decrease the clearance and increase the half-life of triazolam (monitor for increased triazolam effect).

Nutritional/Ethanol Interactions

Ethanol: Avoid ethanol (may increase CNS depression).

Food: Food may decrease the rate of absorption. Triazolam serum concentration may be increased by grapefruit juice; avoid concurrent use.

Herb/Nutraceutical: St John's wort may decrease levels. Avoid valerian, St John's wort, kava kava, gotu kola (may increase CNS depression).

Adverse Reactions

>10%: Central nervous system: Drowsiness, anteriograde amnesia

1% to 10%:

Central nervous system: Headache, dizziness, nervousness, lightheadedness, ataxia

Gastrointestinal: Nausea, vomiting

Overdosage/Toxicology Symptoms of overdose include somnolence, confusion, coma, diminished reflexes, dyspnea, and hypotension. Treatment for benzodiazepine overdose is supportive. Flumazenil has been shown to selectively block the binding of benzodiazepines to CNS receptors, resulting in reversal of benzodiazepine-induced CNS depression but not always respiratory depression.

Pharmacodynamics/Kinetics

Onset of Action: Hypnotic: 15-30 minutes

Duration of Action: 6-7 hours

Protein Binding: 89%

Half-Life Elimination: 1.7-5 hours

Metabolism: Extensively hepatic

Excretion: Urine (as unchanged drug and metabolites)

Dosing

Adults: Note: Onset of action is rapid, patient should be in bed when taking medication.

Insomnia (short-term): Oral: 0.125-0.25 mg at bedtime (maximum dose: 0.5 mg/day)

Dental (preprocedure): Oral: 0.25 mg taken the evening before oral surgery; or 0.25 mg 1 hour before procedure

Elderly: Oral: Insomnia (short-term use): 0.0625-0.125 mg at bedtime; maximum dose: 0.25 mg/day (see Geriatric Considerations)

Hepatic Impairment: Reduce dose or avoid use in cirrhosis.

Available Dosage Forms Tablet: 0.125 mg, 0.25 mg [contains sodium benzoate]

Monitoring and Teaching Issues

Physical Assessment: Assess other medications patient may be taking for effectiveness and interactions. Assess for history of addiction; long-term use can result in dependence, abuse, or tolerance; periodically evaluate need for continued use. For inpatient use, institute safety measures and monitor effectiveness and adverse reactions. For outpatients, monitor therapeutic effectiveness and adverse reactions at beginning of therapy and periodically with long-term use. Monitor for CNS depression. Taper dosage slowly when discontinuing. Assess knowledge/teach patient appropriate use, interventions to reduce side effects, and adverse symptoms to report. **Pregnancy risk factor X:** Determine that patient is not pregnant before starting therapy. Do not give to sexually-active female patients unless capable of complying with contraceptive use.

Patient Education: Take exactly as directed; do not increase dose or frequency. Drug may cause physical and/or psychological dependence. Do not use alcohol or other prescription or OTC medications (especially pain medications, sedatives, antihistamines, or hypnotics) without consulting prescriber. Maintain adequate hydration (2-3 L/day of fluids) unless instructed to restrict fluid intake. You may experience drowsiness, lightheadedness, impaired coordination, dizziness, or blurred vision (use caution when driving or engaging in tasks requiring alertness until response to drug is known); nausea, vomiting, or dry mouth (small frequent meals, frequent mouth care, chewing gum, or sucking lozenges may help); constipation (increased exercise, fluids, fruit, or fiber may help); altered sexual drive or ability (reversible); or photosensitivity (use sunscreen, wear protective clothing and eyewear, and avoid direct sunlight). Report persistent CNS effects (eg, memory impairment, confusion, depression, increased sedation, excitation, headache, agitation, insomnia or nightmares, dizziness, fatigue, impaired coordination, changes in personality, or changes in cognition); changes in urinary pattern; muscle cramping, weakness, tremors, or rigidity; ringing in ears or visual disturbances; chest pain, palpitations, or rapid heartbeat; excessive perspiration; excessive GI symptoms (cramping, constipation, vomiting, anorexia); or worsening of condition. **Pregnancy/breast-feeding precautions:** Inform prescriber if you are pregnant. Do not get pregnant during or for 1 month following therapy. Consult prescriber for instruction on appropriate contraceptive measures. This drug may cause severe fetal defects. Breast-feeding is not recommended.

Geriatric Considerations: Due to the higher incidence of CNS adverse reactions and its short half-life, this benzodiazepine is not a drug of first choice. For short-term only.

Pregnancy Risk Factor: X

Pregnancy Issues: Benzodiazepines cross the placenta. The association between benzodiazepine exposure and malformations remains controversial. A number of types of malformation have been reported (oral cleft, inguinal hernia, cardiac defects, spina bifida, dysmorphic facial features, skeletal defects); however, confounding factors make a clear association difficult. Overall, the risk to the fetus may be low. Nonteratogenic effects (including neonatal flaccidity, respiratory and feeding problems, and withdrawal symptoms) during the postnatal period have also been reported with benzodiazepine use.

Lactation: Excretion in breast milk unknown/not recommended

Breast-Feeding Issues: It is not known if triazolam is excreted in breast milk; however, other benzodiazepines are known to be excreted in breast milk. The AAP rates use of related agents as "of concern" and breast-feeding is not recommended.

Administration

Oral: May take with food. Tablet may be crushed or swallowed whole. Onset of action is rapid, patient should be in bed when taking medication.

Related Information

Anxiolytic / Hypnotic Use in Long-Term Care Facilities *on page 1769*

Benzodiazepines *on page 1719*

Federal OBRA Regulations: Recommended Maximum Doses *on page 1773*

♦ **Tribavirin** *see* Ribavirin *on page 1318*

♦ **Tricalcium Phosphate** *see* Calcium Phosphate (Tribasic) *on page 241*

♦ **Trichloroacetaldehyde Monohydrate** *see* Chloral Hydrate *on page 303*

♦ **Trichophyton Skin Test** *see page 1625*

♦ **TriCor®** *see* Fenofibrate *on page 615*

♦ **Tricosal** *see* Choline Magnesium Trisalicylate *on page 317*

♦ **Triderm®** *see* Triamcinolone *on page 1518*

♦ **Triethylenethiophosphoramide** *see* Thiotepa *on page 1466*

Trifluoperazine (trye floo oh PER a zeen)

U.S. Brand Names Stelazine® [DSC]

Synonyms Trifluoperazine Hydrochloride

Generic Available Yes: Tablet

Pharmacologic Category Antipsychotic Agent, Typical, Phenothiazine

Medication Safety Issues

Sound-alike/look-alike issues:

Trifluoperazine may be confused with triflupromazine, trihexyphenidyl

Stelazine® may be confused with selegiline

Use Treatment of schizophrenia

Unlabeled/Investigational Use Management of psychotic disorders

Mechanism of Action/Effect Trifluoperazine is a piperazine phenothiazine antipsychotic which blocks postsynaptic mesolimbic dopaminergic receptors in the brain; exhibits alpha-adrenergic blocking effect and depresses the release of hypothalamic and hypophyseal hormones

Contraindications Hypersensitivity to trifluoperazine or any component of the formulation (cross-reactivity between phenothiazines may occur); severe CNS depression; bone marrow suppression; blood dyscrasias; severe hepatic disease; coma

(Continued)

Trifluoperazine *(Continued)*

Warnings/Precautions May result in hypotension, particularly after I.M. administration. May be sedating, use with caution in disorders where CNS depression is a feature. Use with caution in Parkinson's disease. Caution in patients with hemodynamic instability; predisposition to seizures; subcortical brain damage; hepatic impairment; severe cardiac, renal, or respiratory disease. Esophageal dysmotility and aspiration have been associated with antipsychotic use - use with caution in patients at risk of pneumonia (ie, Alzheimer's disease). Caution in breast cancer or other prolactin-dependent tumors (may elevate prolactin levels). May alter temperature regulation or mask toxicity of other drugs due to antiemetic effects. May alter cardiac conduction - life-threatening arrhythmias have occurred with therapeutic doses of phenothiazines. May cause orthostatic hypotension - use with caution in patients at risk of this effect or those who would tolerate transient hypotensive episodes (cerebrovascular disease, cardiovascular disease or other medications which may predispose). Safety in children <6 months of age has not been established.

Due to anticholinergic effects, should be used with caution in patients with decreased gastrointestinal motility, urinary retention, BPH, xerostomia, visual problems, narrow-angle glaucoma (screening is recommended) and myasthenia gravis. Relative to other antipsychotics, trifluoperazine has a low potency of cholinergic blockade.

May cause extrapyramidal symptoms, including pseudoparkinsonism, acute dystonic reactions, akathisia, and tardive dyskinesia (risk of these reactions is high relative to other neuroleptics). May be associated with neuroleptic malignant syndrome (NMS) or pigmentary retinopathy.

Drug Interactions

Cytochrome P450 Effect: Substrate of CYP1A2 (major)

Decreased Effect: CYP1A2 inducers may decrease the levels/effects of trifluoperazine; example inducers include aminoglutethimide, carbamazepine, phenobarbital, and rifampin. Phenothiazines inhibit the effects of levodopa, guanadrel, guanethidine, and bromocriptine. Benztropine (and other anticholinergics) may inhibit the therapeutic response to trifluoperazine and excess anticholinergic effects may occur. Cigarette smoking may enhance the hepatic metabolism of trifluoperazine. Trifluoperazine and possibly other low potency antipsychotics may reverse the pressor effects of epinephrine.

Increased Effect/Toxicity: CYP1A2 inhibitors may increase the levels/effects of trifluoperazine; example inhibitors include amiodarone, ciprofloxacin, fluvoxamine, ketoconazole, norfloxacin, ofloxacin, and rofecoxib. Trifluoperazine's effects on CNS depression may be additive when trifluoperazine is combined with CNS depressants (narcotic analgesics, ethanol, barbiturates, cyclic antidepressants, antihistamines, or sedative-hypnotics). Trifluoperazine may increase the effects/toxicity of anticholinergics, antihypertensives, lithium (rare neurotoxicity), trazodone, or valproic acid. Concurrent use with TCA may produce increased toxicity or altered therapeutic response. Chloroquine and propranolol may increase trifluoperazine concentrations. Hypotension may occur when trifluoperazine is combined with epinephrine. May increase the risk of arrhythmia when combined with antiarrhythmics, cisapride, pimozide, sparfloxacin, or other drugs which prolong QT interval. Metoclopramide may increase risk of extrapyramidal symptoms (EPS).

Nutritional/Ethanol Interactions

Ethanol: Avoid ethanol (may increase CNS depression).

Herb/Nutraceutical: Avoid kava kava, gotu kola, valerian, St John's wort (may increase CNS depression). Avoid dong quai, St John's wort (may also cause photosensitization).

Lab Interactions False-positive for phenylketonuria; increased cholesterol (S), glucose; decreased uric acid (S)

Adverse Reactions Frequency not defined.

Cardiovascular: Hypotension, orthostatic hypotension, cardiac arrest

Central nervous system: Extrapyramidal signs (pseudoparkinsonism, akathisia, dystonias, tardive dyskinesia), dizziness, headache, neuroleptic malignant syndrome (NMS), impairment of temperature regulation, lowering of seizure threshold

Dermatologic: Increased sensitivity to sun, rash, discoloration of skin (blue-gray), photosensitivity

Endocrine & metabolic: Changes in menstrual cycle, libido (changes in), breast pain, hyperglycemia, hypoglycemia, gynecomastia, lactation, galactorrhea

Gastrointestinal: Constipation, weight gain, nausea, vomiting, stomach pain, xerostomia

Genitourinary: Difficulty in urination, ejaculatory disturbances, urinary retention, priapism

Hematologic: Agranulocytosis, leukopenia, pancytopenia, thrombocytopenic purpura, eosinophilia, hemolytic anemia, aplastic anemia

Hepatic: Cholestatic jaundice, hepatotoxicity

Neuromuscular & skeletal: Tremor

Ocular: Pigmentary retinopathy, cornea and lens changes

Respiratory: Nasal congestion

Overdosage/Toxicology Symptoms of overdose include deep sleep, coma, extrapyramidal symptoms, abnormal involuntary muscle movements, hypo- or hypertension, and cardiac arrhythmias. Treatment is symptom-directed and supportive.

Pharmacodynamics/Kinetics

Half-Life Elimination: >24 hours with chronic use

Metabolism: Extensively hepatic

Dosing

Adults:

Schizophrenia/psychoses:

Oral:

Outpatients: 1-2 mg twice daily

Hospitalized or well supervised patient: Initial: 2-5 mg twice daily with optimum response in the 15-20 mg/day range; do not exceed 40 mg/day.

I.M.: 1-2 mg every 4-6 hours as needed up to 10 mg/24 hours maximum

Nonpsychotic anxiety: Oral: 1-2 mg twice daily; maximum: 6 mg/day; therapy for anxiety should not exceed 12 weeks; do not exceed 6 mg/day for longer than 12 weeks when treating anxiety; agitation, jitteriness, or insomnia may be confused with original neurotic or psychotic symptoms.

Elderly:

Schizophrenia/psychoses:

Oral: Refer to adult dosing. Dose selection should start at the low end of the dosage range and titration must be gradual.

I.M.: Initial: 1 mg every 4-6 hours; increase at 1 mg increments; do not exceed 6 mg/day

Behavioral symptoms associated with dementia behavior: Oral: Initial: 0.5-1 mg 1-2 times/day; increase dose at 4- to 7-day intervals by 0.5-1 mg/day; increase dosing intervals (bid, tid, etc) as necessary to control response or side effects. Maximum daily dose: 40 mg. Gradual increases (titration) may prevent some side effects or decrease their severity.

Pediatrics: Children 6-12 years: Schizophrenia/psychoses:

Oral: Hospitalized or well supervised patients: Initial: 1 mg 1-2 times/day, gradually increase until symptoms are controlled or adverse effects become troublesome; maximum: 15 mg/day.

I.M.: 1 mg twice daily

Renal Impairment: Not dialyzable (0% to 5%)

Available Dosage Forms [DSC] = Discontinued product

Injection, solution, as hydrochloride (Stelazine®): 2 mg/mL (10 mL) [contains benzyl alcohol] [DSC]

Tablet, as hydrochloride: 1 mg, 2 mg, 5 mg, 10 mg

Stelazine®: 5 mg [DSC]

Monitoring and Teaching Issues

Physical Assessment: Assess other medications patient is taking for effectiveness and interactions. Review ophthalmic exam and monitor laboratory results, therapeutic effectiveness according to rationale for therapy, and adverse reactions at beginning of therapy and periodically with long-term use. With I.M. use, monitor closely for hypotension. **Note:** Avoid skin contact with liquid medication; may cause contact dermatitis (wash immediately with warm, soapy water). Initiate at lower doses and taper dosage slowly when discontinuing. Assess knowledge/teach patient appropriate use, interventions to reduce side effects, and adverse symptoms to report.

Monitoring Laboratory Tests: Lipid profile, fasting blood glucose, Hgb A_{1c}; BMI

Patient Education: Use exactly as directed; do not increase dose or frequency. Do not discontinue without consulting prescriber. Tablets/capsules may be taken with food. Do not take within 2 hours of any antacid. Avoid alcohol or caffeine and other prescription or OTC medications not approved by prescriber. Maintain adequate hydration (2-3 L/day of fluids) unless instructed to restrict fluid intake. You may experience excess drowsiness, lightheadedness, dizziness, or blurred vision (use caution driving or when engaging in tasks requiring alertness until response to drug is known); nausea or vomiting (small frequent meals, frequent mouth care, chewing gum, or sucking lozenges may help); constipation (increased exercise, fluids, fruit, or fiber may help); postural hypotension (use caution climbing stairs or when changing position from lying or sitting to standing); urinary retention (void before taking medication); ejaculatory dysfunction (reversible); decreased perspiration (avoid strenuous exercise in hot environments); or photosensitivity (use sunscreen, wear protective clothing and eyewear, and avoid direct sunlight). Report persistent CNS effects (eg, trembling fingers, altered gait or balance, excessive sedation, seizures, unusual movements, anxiety, abnormal thoughts, confusion, personality changes); chest pain, palpitations, rapid heartbeat, severe dizziness; unresolved urinary retention or changes in urinary pattern; altered menstrual pattern, changes in libido, swelling or pain in breasts (male or female); vision changes; skin rash, irritation, or changes in color of skin (gray-blue); or worsening of condition. **Pregnancy/breast-feeding precautions:** Inform prescriber if you are or intend to become pregnant. Breast-feeding is not recommended.

Dietary Considerations: May be taken with food to decrease GI distress.

Geriatric Considerations: (See Warnings/Precautions, Adverse Reactions, and Overdose/Toxicology.) Elderly patients have an increased risk of adverse response to side effects or adverse reactions to antipsychotics.

Pregnancy Risk Factor: C

Lactation: Enters breast milk/not recommended (AAP rates "of concern")

Administration

I.M.: Give I.M. injection deep in upper outer quadrant of buttock.

Storage: Store injection at room temperature. Protect from heat and from freezing. Use only clear or slightly yellow solutions.

Additional Information Do not exceed 6 mg/day for longer than 12 weeks when treating anxiety. Agitation, jitteriness, or insomnia may be confused with original neurotic or psychotic symptoms.

Related Information

Antipsychotic Agents on page 1717
Antipsychotic Medication Guidelines on page 1766

♦ **Trifluoperazine Hydrochloride** see Trifluoperazine on page 1523
♦ **Trifluorothymidine** see Trifluridine on page 1525

Trifluridine (trye FLURE i deen)

U.S. Brand Names Viroptic®

Synonyms F_3T; Trifluorothymidine

Generic Available Yes

Pharmacologic Category Antiviral Agent, Ophthalmic

Medication Safety Issues

Sound-alike/look-alike issues:

Viroptic® may be confused with Timoptic®

Use Treatment of primary keratoconjunctivitis and recurrent epithelial keratitis caused by herpes simplex virus types I and II

(Continued)

Trifluridine *(Continued)*

Mechanism of Action/Effect Interferes with viral replication by incorporating into viral DNA in place of thymidine, inhibiting thymidylate synthetase resulting in the formation of defective proteins

Contraindications Hypersensitivity to trifluridine or any component of the formulation

Warnings/Precautions Mild local irritation of conjunctiva and cornea may occur when instilled but usually is a transient effect.

Adverse Reactions 1% to 10%: Local: Burning, stinging

Pharmacodynamics/Kinetics

Absorption: Ophthalmic: Systemic absorption negligible, corneal penetration adequate

Dosing

Adults & Elderly: Herpes keratoconjunctivitis, keratitis: Ophthalmic: Instill 1 drop into affected eye every 2 hours while awake, to a maximum of 9 drops/day, until re-epithelialization of corneal ulcer occurs. Then use 1 drop every 4 hours for another 7 days. Do **not** exceed 21 days of treatment. If improvement has not taken place in 7-14 days, consider another form of therapy.

Available Dosage Forms Solution, ophthalmic: 1% (7.5 mL)

Monitoring and Teaching Issues

Physical Assessment: Monitor effectiveness of therapy, not for long-term use (see Dosing). Teach patient appropriate use, interventions to reduce side effects, and adverse symptoms to report (see Patient Education).

Patient Education: For ophthalmic use only. Store in refrigerator; do not use discolored solution. Apply prescribed amount as often as directed. Wash hands before using. Do not let tip of applicator touch eye; do not contaminate tip of applicator (may cause eye infection, eye damage, or vision loss). Tilt head back and look upward. Gently pull down lower lid and put drop(s) in inner corner of eye. Close eye and roll eyeball in all directions. Do not blink for 1/2 minute. Apply gentle pressure to inner corner of eye for 30 seconds. Wipe away excess from skin around eye. Do not use any other eye preparation for at least 10 minutes. Do not touch tip of applicator to eye or contaminate tip of applicator. Do not share medication with anyone else. May cause sensitivity to bright light (dark glasses may help); or temporary stinging or blurred vision may occur. Inform prescriber if you experience eye pain, redness, burning, watering, dryness, double vision, puffiness around eye, vision changes, or other adverse eye response; or worsening of condition or lack of improvement within 7-14 days. **Pregnancy/breast-feeding precautions:** Inform prescriber if you are pregnant. Consult prescriber if breast-feeding.

Geriatric Considerations: Assess ability to self-administer.

Pregnancy Risk Factor: C

Lactation: Excretion in breast milk unknown

Administration

Storage: Refrigerate at 2°C to 8°C (36°F to 46°F). Storage at room temperature may result in a solution altered pH which could result in ocular discomfort upon administration and/or decreased potency.

Trihexyphenidyl *(trye heks ee FEN i dil)*

Synonyms Artane; Benzhexol Hydrochloride; Trihexyphenidyl Hydrochloride

Generic Available Yes

Pharmacologic Category Anticholinergic Agent; Anti-Parkinson's Agent, Anticholinergic

Medication Safety Issues

Sound-alike/look-alike issues:

Trihexyphenidyl may be confused with trifluoperazine

Artane may be confused with Altace®, Anturane®, Aramine®

Use Adjunctive treatment of Parkinson's disease; treatment of drug-induced extrapyramidal symptoms

Mechanism of Action/Effect Exerts a direct inhibitory effect on the parasympathetic nervous system. It also has a relaxing effect on smooth musculature; exerted both directly on the muscle itself and indirectly through parasympathetic nervous system (inhibitory effect)

Contraindications Hypersensitivity to trihexyphenidyl or any component of the formulation; narrow-angle glaucoma; pyloric or duodenal obstruction; stenosing peptic ulcers; bladder neck obstructions; achalasia; myasthenia gravis

Warnings/Precautions Use with caution in hot weather or during exercise, especially when administered concomitantly with other atropine-like drugs to chronically-ill patients, alcoholics, patients with CNS disease, or persons doing manual labor in a hot environment. Elderly patients require strict dosage regulation. Use with caution in patients with tachycardia, cardiac arrhythmias, hypertension, hypotension, prostatic hyperplasia or any tendency toward urinary retention, liver or kidney disorders, and obstructive disease of the GI or GU tract. May exacerbate mental symptoms when used to treat extrapyramidal symptoms. When given in large doses or to susceptible patients, may cause weakness. Does not improve symptoms of tardive dyskinesias.

Drug Interactions

Decreased Effect: May increase gastric degradation of levodopa and decrease the amount of levodopa absorbed by delaying gastric emptying; the opposite may be true for digoxin. Therapeutic effects of cholinergic agents (tacrine, donepezil, rivastigmine, galantamine) and neuroleptics may be antagonized.

Increased Effect/Toxicity: Central and/or peripheral anticholinergic syndrome can occur when administered with amantadine, rimantadine, narcotic analgesics, phenothiazines and other antipsychotics (especially with high anticholinergic activity), tricyclic antidepressants, MAO inhibitors, quinidine and some other antiarrhythmics, and antihistamines. CNS depressants (cannabinoids, ethanol, barbiturates, and narcotic analgesics) may have additive effects with trihexyphenidyl; an abuse potential exits.

Nutritional/Ethanol Interactions Ethanol: Avoid ethanol (may increase CNS depression).

Adverse Reactions Frequency not defined.

Cardiovascular: Tachycardia

Central nervous system: Confusion, agitation, euphoria, drowsiness, headache, dizziness, nervousness, delusions, hallucinations, paranoia

Dermatologic: Dry skin, increased sensitivity to light, rash

Gastrointestinal: Constipation, xerostomia, dry throat, ileus, nausea, vomiting, parotitis

Genitourinary: Urinary retention

Neuromuscular & skeletal: Weakness

Ocular: Blurred vision, mydriasis, increase in intraocular pressure, glaucoma, blindness (long-term use in narrow-angle glaucoma)

Respiratory: Dry nose

Miscellaneous: Diaphoresis (decreased)

Overdosage/Toxicology Symptoms of overdose include blurred vision, urinary retention, and tachycardia. For anticholinergic overdose with severe life-threatening symptoms, physostigmine 1-2 mg SubQ or I.V. slowly, may be given to reverse these effects.

Pharmacodynamics/Kinetics
Onset of Action: Peak effect: Within 1 hour
Time to Peak: Serum: 1-1.5 hours
Half-Life Elimination: 3.3-4.1 hours
Excretion: Primarily urine

Dosing
Adults: Parkinson's disease or drug-induced EPS: Oral: Initial: 1-2 mg/day, increase by 2 mg increments at intervals of 3-5 days; usual dose: 5-15 mg/day in 3-4 divided doses

Elderly: Parkinsonism: Oral: 1 mg on first day, increase by 2 mg every 3-5 days as needed until a total of 6-10 mg/day (in 3-4 divided doses) is reached. If the patient is on concomitant levodopa therapy, the daily dose is reduced to 1-2 mg 3 times/day. Avoid use if possible (see Geriatric Considerations).

Available Dosage Forms
Elixir, as hydrochloride: 2 mg/5 mL (480 mL)
Tablet, as hydrochloride: 2 mg, 5 mg

Monitoring and Teaching Issues
Physical Assessment: Assess effectiveness and interactions of other medications patient may be taking. Monitor renal function, therapeutic effectiveness, and adverse reactions (eg, anticholinergic syndrome) at beginning of therapy and periodically throughout therapy. Intraocular pressure monitoring and gonioscopic evaluations should be performed periodically. Assess knowledge/teach patient appropriate use, interventions to reduce side effects, and adverse symptoms to report.

Patient Education: Take exactly as directed; with meals if GI upset occurs, before meals if dry mouth occurs, after eating if drooling or if nausea occurs. Take at the same time each day. Maintain adequate hydration (2-3 L/day of fluids) unless instructed to restrict fluid intake; void before taking medication. Do not use alcohol and all prescription or OTC sedatives or CNS depressants without consulting prescriber. You may experience drowsiness, confusion, or vision changes (use caution when driving, climbing stairs, or engaging in tasks requiring alertness until response to drug is known); increased susceptibility to heat stroke, decreased perspiration (use caution in hot weather; maintain adequate fluids and reduce exercise activity); constipation (increased exercise, fluids, fruit, or fiber may help); or dry skin or nasal passages (consult prescriber for appropriate relief). Report unresolved constipation; chest pain or palpitations; respiratory difficulty; CNS changes (hallucination, loss of memory, nervousness, etc); painful or difficult urination; increased muscle spasticity or rigidity; skin rash; or significant worsening of condition. **Pregnancy/breast-feeding precautions:** Inform prescriber if you are or intend to become pregnant. Consult prescriber if breast-feeding.

Geriatric Considerations: Anticholinergic agents are generally not well tolerated in the elderly and their use should be avoided when possible. Elderly patients require strict dosage regulation. In the elderly, anticholinergic agents should not be used as prophylaxis against extrapyramidal symptoms.

Pregnancy Risk Factor: C
Lactation: Excretion in breast milk unknown/use caution
Breast-Feeding Issues: Anticholinergic agents may suppress lactation.

Administration
Oral: Tolerated best if given in 3 daily doses and with food. High doses may be divided into 4 doses, at meal times and at bedtime. Patients may be switched to sustained-action capsules when stabilized on conventional dosage forms.

Additional Information Incidence and severity of side effects are dose related. Patients may be switched to sustained-action capsules when stabilized on conventional dosage forms.

♦ **Trihexyphenidyl Hydrochloride** see Trihexyphenidyl on page 1526
♦ **TriHIBit®** see page 1660
♦ **Tri-K®** see Potassium Acetate, Potassium Bicarbonate, and Potassium Citrate on page 1232
♦ **Trileptal®** see Oxcarbazepine on page 1132
♦ **Tri-Levlen®** see Ethinyl Estradiol and Levonorgestrel on page 585
♦ **Trilisate® [DSC]** see Choline Magnesium Trisalicylate on page 317
♦ **Tri-Luma™** see Fluocinolone, Hydroquinone, and Tretinoin on page 644
♦ **TriLyte™** see Polyethylene Glycol-Electrolyte Solution on page 1226

Trimethobenzamide (trye meth oh BEN za mide)

U.S. Brand Names Tigan®
Synonyms Trimethobenzamide Hydrochloride
Generic Available Yes: Injection
Pharmacologic Category Anticholinergic Agent; Antiemetic
Medication Safety Issues
Sound-alike/look-alike issues:
Tigan® may be confused with Tiazac®, Ticar®
Use Treatment of nausea and vomiting
(Continued)

Trimethobenzamide *(Continued)*

Mechanism of Action/Effect Acts centrally to inhibit the medullary chemoreceptor trigger zone

Contraindications Hypersensitivity to trimethobenzamide, benzocaine (or similar local anesthetics), or any component of the formulation; injection contraindicated in children; suppositories contraindicated in premature infants or neonates

Warnings/Precautions May mask emesis due to Reye's syndrome or mimic CNS effects of Reye's syndrome in patients with emesis of other etiologies. Use in patients with acute vomiting should be avoided. May cause drowsiness; patient should avoid tasks requiring alertness (eg, driving, operating machinery). May cause extrapyramidal symptoms (EPS) which may be confused with CNS symptoms of primary disease responsible for emesis.

Nutritional/Ethanol Interactions Ethanol: Concomitant use should be avoided.

Adverse Reactions Frequency not defined.
Cardiovascular: Hypotension
Central nervous system: Coma, depression, disorientation, dizziness, drowsiness, EPS, headache, opisthotonos, Parkinson-like syndrome, seizure
Hematologic: Blood dyscrasias
Hepatic: Jaundice
Neuromuscular & skeletal: Muscle cramps
Ocular: Blurred vision
Miscellaneous: Hypersensitivity reactions

Overdosage/Toxicology Symptoms of overdose include hypotension, seizures, CNS depression, cardiac arrhythmias, disorientation, and confusion. Treatment is symptom-directed and supportive.

Pharmacodynamics/Kinetics
Onset of Action: Antiemetic: Oral: 10-40 minutes; I.M.: 15-35 minutes
Duration of Action: 3-4 hours
Absorption: Rectal: ~60%
Bioavailability: Oral: 100%
Time to Peak: Oral: 45 minutes; I.M.: 30 minutes
Half-Life Elimination: 7-9 hours
Excretion: Urine (30% to 50%)

Dosing
Adults & Elderly: Nausea, vomiting:
Oral: 250-300 mg 3-4 times/day
I.M., rectal: 200 mg 3-4 times/day
Pediatrics: *Note:* Rectal use is contraindicated in neonates and premature infants.
Nausea, vomiting: Oral, rectal: Children:
<14 kg: 100 mg 3-4 times/day
14-40 kg: 100-200 mg 3-4 times/day

Available Dosage Forms [DSC] = Discontinued product
Capsule, as hydrochloride: 300 mg
Tigan®: 300 mg
Injection, solution, as hydrochloride: 100 mg/mL (2 mL)
Tigan®: 100 mg/mL (2 mL, 20 mL)
Suppository, rectal, as hydrochloride (Tigan®): 100 mg [DSC], 200 mg [contains benzocaine]

Monitoring and Teaching Issues
Physical Assessment: See Warnings/Precautions, (eg, GI or GU obstruction) for use cautions. Assess therapeutic effectiveness, and adverse reactions with first dose and on a regular basis during therapy (eg, hypovolemia, angioedema, postural hypotension; see Adverse Reactions). Teach patient appropriate use (if self-administered injection teach injection technique and syringe disposal), possible side effects/interventions, and adverse symptoms to report (see Patient Education).

Patient Education: Do not take any new medication during therapy unless approved by prescriber. Take capsule as directed before meals; do not increase dose and do not discontinue without consulting prescriber. If using injection formulation; follow directions for injection and disposal of syringe. May cause drowsiness, blurred vision (use caution when driving or engaging in tasks that require alertness until response to drug is known), or diarrhea (buttermilk or yogurt may help). Report chest pain or palpitations, persistent dizziness or blurred vision, or CNS changes (disorientation, depression, confusion). **Pregnancy/breast-feeding precautions:** Inform prescriber if you are or intend to become pregnant. Consult prescriber if breast-feeding.

Pregnancy Risk Factor: C
Lactation: Excretion in breast milk unknown

Administration
I.M.: Administer I.M. only. Inject deep into upper outer quadrant of gluteal muscle.
Storage: Store capsules, injection solution, and suppositories at room temperature.

♦ **Trimethobenzamide Hydrochloride** *see Trimethobenzamide on page 1527*

Trimethoprim *(trye METH oh prim)*

U.S. Brand Names Primsol®; Proloprim®
Synonyms TMP
Generic Available Yes: Tablet
Pharmacologic Category Antibiotic, Miscellaneous
Medication Safety Issues
Sound-alike/look-alike issues:
Trimethoprim may be confused with trimethaphan
Proloprim® may be confused with Prolixin®, Protropin®

Use Treatment of urinary tract infections due to susceptible strains of *E. coli, P. mirabilis, K. pneumoniae, Enterobacter* sp and coagulase-negative *Staphylococcus* including *S. saprophyticus*; acute otitis media in children; acute exacerbations of chronic bronchitis in adults; in combination with other agents for treatment of toxoplasmosis, *Pneumocystis carinii*; treatment of superficial ocular infections involving the conjunctiva and cornea

Mechanism of Action/Effect Inhibits folic acid reduction to tetrahydrofolate, and thereby inhibits microbial growth

Contraindications Hypersensitivity to trimethoprim or any component of the formulation; megaloblastic anemia due to folate deficiency

Warnings/Precautions Use with caution in patients with impaired renal or hepatic function or with possible folate deficiency

Drug Interactions

Cytochrome P450 Effect: Substrate (major) of CYP2C8/9, 3A4; **Inhibits** CYP2C8/9 (moderate)

Decreased Effect: The levels/effects of trimethoprim may be decreased by aminoglutethimide, carbamazepine, nafcillin, nevirapine, phenobarbital, phenytoin, rifampin, rifapentine, secobarbital, and other CYP2C8/9 or 3A4 inducers.

Increased Effect/Toxicity: Increased effect/toxicity/levels of phenytoin. Concurrent use with ACE inhibitors increases risk of hyperkalemia. Increased myelosuppression with methotrexate. May increase levels of digoxin. Concurrent use with dapsone may increase levels of dapsone and trimethoprim. Concurrent use with procainamide may increase levels of procainamide and trimethoprim. Trimethoprim may increase the levels/effects of amiodarone, fluoxetine, glimepiride, glipizide, nateglinide, phenytoin, pioglitazone, rosiglitazone, sertraline, warfarin, and other CYP2C8/9 substrates.

Adverse Reactions Frequency not defined.

Central nervous system: Aseptic meningitis (rare), fever

Dermatologic: Maculopapular rash (3% to 7% at 200 mg/day; incidence higher with larger daily doses), erythema multiforme (rare), exfoliative dermatitis (rare), pruritus (common), phototoxic skin eruptions, Stevens-Johnson syndrome (rare), toxic epidermal necrolysis (rare)

Endocrine & metabolic: Hyperkalemia, hyponatremia

Gastrointestinal: Epigastric distress, glossitis, nausea, vomiting

Hematologic: Leukopenia, megaloblastic anemia, methemoglobinemia, neutropenia, thrombocytopenia

Hepatic: Liver enzyme elevation, cholestatic jaundice (rare)

Renal: BUN and creatinine increased

Miscellaneous: Anaphylaxis, hypersensitivity reactions

Overdosage/Toxicology Symptoms of acute toxicity include nausea, vomiting, confusion, and dizziness. Chronic overdose results in bone marrow suppression. Treatment of acute overdose is supportive following GI decontamination. Use oral leucovorin 5-15 mg/day for treatment of chronic overdose. Hemodialysis is only moderately effective in eliminating drug.

Pharmacodynamics/Kinetics

Absorption: Readily and extensive

Time to Peak: Serum: 1-4 hours

Protein Binding: 42% to 46%

Half-Life Elimination: 8-14 hours; prolonged with renal impairment

Metabolism: Partially hepatic

Excretion: Urine (60% to 80%) as unchanged drug

Dosing

Adults & Elderly: Susceptible infections: Oral: 100 mg every 12 hours or 200 mg every 24 hours for 10 days; longer treatment periods may be necessary for prostatitis (ie, 4-16 weeks)

Pediatrics: Oral: Children (>2 months or age): 4 mg/kg/day in divided doses every 12 hours

Renal Impairment:

Cl$_{cr}$ 15-30 mL/minute: Administer 100 mg every 18 hours or 50 mg every 12 hours.

Cl$_{cr}$ <15 mL/minute: Administer 100 mg every 24 hours or avoid use.

Moderately dialyzable (20% to 50%)

Available Dosage Forms

Solution, oral (Primsol®): 50 mg (base)/5 mL (480 mL) [contains sodium benzoate; bubble gum flavor]

Tablet: 100 mg

Proloprim®: 100 mg, 200 mg

Monitoring and Teaching Issues

Physical Assessment: Perform culture and sensitivity prior to initiating therapy. See Warnings/Precautions for use cautions. Assess potential for interactions with other pharmacological agents patient may be taking (eg, risk of increased or decreased levels/effects with other medications; see Drug Interactions). Assess results of laboratory tests with long-term therapy. Monitor effectiveness (resolution of infection) and adverse reactions (eg, rash, electrolyte imbalance [K, NA], anemia, neutropenia, elevated LFTs, nausea, vomiting, confusion; see Adverse Reactions). Teach patient possible side effects/appropriate interventions and adverse symptoms to report (see Patient Education).

Monitoring Laboratory Tests: Periodic CBC and serum potassium during long-term therapy. Perform culture and sensitivity prior to initiating therapy.

Patient Education: Do not take any new medication during therapy unless approved by prescriber. Take exactly as recommended. Complete full course of therapy even if feeling better; do not skip doses. Maintain adequate hydration (2-3 L/day of fluids) unless instructed to restrict fluid intake. May cause nausea, vomiting, or GI upset (small frequent meals, frequent mouth care, sucking lozenges, or chewing gum may help). Report skin rash, redness, or irritation; feelings of acute fatigue or weakness; unusual bleeding or bruising; or other persistent adverse effects. **Pregnancy precaution:** Inform prescriber if you are or intend to become pregnant. Consult prescriber if breast-feeding.

Dietary Considerations: May cause folic acid deficiency, supplements may be needed. Should be taken with milk or food.

Geriatric Considerations: Trimethoprim is often used in combination with sulfamethoxazole; it can be used alone in patients who are allergic to sulfonamides; adjust dose for renal function (see Pharmacokinetics and Dosing).

(Continued)

Trimethoprim *(Continued)*

Pregnancy Risk Factor: C
Pregnancy Issues: Because trimethoprim may interfere with folic acid metabolism, consider using only if the potential benefit to the mother outweighs the possible risk to the fetus.
Lactation: Enters breast milk/use caution (AAP rates "compatible")
Administration
Oral: Administer with milk or food.
Storage: Protect the 200 mg tablet from light.

♦ **Trimethoprim and Sulfamethoxazole** *see* Sulfamethoxazole and Trimethoprim *on page 1407*

Trimetrexate Glucuronate *(tri me TREKS ate gloo KYOOR oh nate)*

U.S. Brand Names NeuTrexin®
Synonyms NSC-352122
Generic Available No
Pharmacologic Category Antineoplastic Agent, Miscellaneous
Use Alternative therapy for the treatment of moderate-to-severe *Pneumocystis carinii* pneumonia (PCP) in immunocompromised patients, including patients with acquired immunodeficiency syndrome (AIDS), who are intolerant of, or are refractory to, co-trimoxazole therapy or for whom co-trimoxazole and pentamidine are contraindicated. **Concurrent folinic acid (leucovorin) must always be administered.**
Unlabeled/Investigational Use Treatment of nonsmall cell lung cancer, metastatic colorectal cancer, metastatic head and neck cancer, pancreatic adenocarcinoma
Mechanism of Action/Effect Exerts effects through potent inhibition of the enzyme dihydrofolate reductase (DHFR)
Contraindications Hypersensitivity to trimetrexate, methotrexate, leucovorin, or any component of the formulation; severe existing myelosuppression; pregnancy
Warnings/Precautions The U.S. Food and Drug Administration (FDA) currently recommends that procedures for proper handling and disposal of antineoplastic agents be considered. Appropriate safety equipment is recommended for preparation, administration, and disposal of antineoplastics. If trimetrexate contacts the skin, immediately wash with soap and water. **Must be administered with concurrent leucovorin to avoid potentially serious or life-threatening toxicities.** Leucovorin therapy must extend for 72 hours past the last dose of trimetrexate. Hypersensitivity/allergic-type reactions have been reported, primarily when given as a bolus infusion, at higher than recommended doses for PCP, or in combination with fluorouracil or leucovorin. Use with caution in patients with mild myelosuppression, severe hepatic or renal dysfunction, hypoproteinemia, hypoalbuminemia, or previous extensive myelosuppressive therapies.
Drug Interactions
Increased Effect/Toxicity: Cimetidine, clotrimazole, and ketoconazole may decrease trimetrexate metabolism, resulting in increased serum levels. Trimetrexate may increase toxicity (infections) of live virus vaccines.
Adverse Reactions
>10%:
Hematologic: Neutropenia
Hepatic: LFTs increased
1% to 10%:
Central nervous system: Seizures, fever
Dermatologic: Rash
Gastrointestinal: Stomatitis, nausea, vomiting
Hematologic: Thrombocytopenia, anemia
Neuromuscular & skeletal: Peripheral neuropathy
Renal: Increased serum creatinine
Miscellaneous: Flu-like illness, hypersensitivity reactions, anaphylactoid reactions
Pharmacodynamics/Kinetics
Half-Life Elimination: 15-17 hours
Metabolism: Extensively hepatic
Dosing
Adults & Elderly: Note: Concurrent leucovorin 20 mg/m^2 every 6 hours must be administered daily (oral or I.V.) during treatment and for 72 hours past the last dose of trimetrexate glucuronate.
Pneumonia caused by *Pneumocystis carinii*: I.V.: 45 mg/m^2 once daily for 21 days; alternative dosing based on weight:
<50 kg: Trimetrexate glucuronate 1.5 mg/kg/day; leucovorin 0.6 mg/kg 4 times/day
50-80 kg: Trimetrexate glucuronate 1.2 mg/kg/day; leucovorin 0.5 mg/kg/4 times/day
>80 kg: Trimetrexate glucuronate 1 mg/kg/day; leucovorin 0.5 mg/kg/4 times/day
Note: Oral doses of leucovorin should be rounded up to the next higher 25 mg increment.
Antineoplastic (unlabeled use): I.V.: 6-16 mg/m^2 once daily for 5 days every 21-28 days **or** 150-200 mg/m^2 every 2 weeks
Hepatic Impairment: Although it may be necessary to reduce the dose in patients with liver dysfunction, no specific recommendations exist.
Available Dosage Forms Injection, powder for reconstitution: 25 mg, 200 mg
Monitoring and Teaching Issues
Physical Assessment: Use caution with myelosuppression, hepatic or renal dysfunction, low protein or albumin (see Warnings/Precautions for specific use cautions). Must be administered with concurrent leucovorin to avoid potentially serious or life-threatening toxicities. Leucovorin therapy must extend for 72 hours past the last dose of trimetrexate. Assess potential for interactions with other pharmacological agents patient may be taking (see Drug Interactions). Assess results of laboratory tests at baseline and periodically during therapy. Monitor therapeutic effectiveness, and adverse reactions (eg, rash,

nausea, vomiting, anemia, peripheral neuropathy, increased LFTs; see Adverse Reactions). Teach patient possible side effects/appropriate interventions and adverse symptoms to report (see Patient Education).

Monitoring Laboratory Tests: Absolute neutrophil counts (ANC), platelet count, renal function tests (serum creatinine, BUN), hepatic function (ALT, AST, alkaline phosphatase)

Patient Education: Do not take any new medication during therapy unless approved by prescriber (especially aspirin or aspirin-containing products.). This medication is only administered by intravenous infusion; report immediately any redness, swelling, or pain at infusion site. Maintain adequate hydration (2-3 L/day of fluids) unless instructed to restrict fluid intake. You may be more susceptible to infection (avoid crowds and exposure to infection and do not have any vaccinations unless approved by prescriber). Report persistent fever, chills, or joint pain; numbness or tingling of extremities; vomiting, nausea, or acute abdominal pain; mouth sores; increased bruising or bleeding; blood in urine or stool; changes in sensorium (eg, confusion, hallucinations, seizures); increased respiratory difficulty; or acute persistent malaise or weakness. **Pregnancy/breast-feeding precautions:** Inform prescriber if you are pregnant. Do not get pregnant while taking this medication or for 1 month after completing therapy. Consult prescriber for appropriate contraceptive measures. Do not breast-feed.

Geriatric Considerations: No specific recommendations are available for the elderly. Use with caution in patients with liver dysfunction (see Dosing).

Pregnancy Risk Factor: D

Lactation: Excretion in breast milk unknown/contraindicated

Administration

I.V.: Infuse over 60 minutes.

Reconstitution: Reconstitute with D_5W or SWFI to a concentration of 12.5 mg/mL. Do not use if cloudy or if precipitate forms. Following reconstitution, the solution should be used immediately, but is stable for 6 hours at room temperature or 24 hours under refrigeration. Prior to administration, solution should be further diluted with D_5W to a concentration of 0.25 mg/mL to 2 mg/mL. This final diluted solution is stable under refrigeration or at room temperature for 24 hours.

Compatibility: Stable in D_5W, SWFI

Precipitate occurs with leucovorin or any solution containing chloride ion.

Y-site administration: Incompatible with foscarnet, indomethacin

Compatibility when admixed: Incompatible with chloride-containing solutions, leucovorin

Storage: Prior to reconstitution, vials should stored at controlled room temperature of 20°C to 25°C (68°F to 77°F). Protect from light.

Additional Information Not a vesicant; methotrexate derivative

Trimipramine (trye MI pra meen)

U.S. Brand Names Surmontil®

Synonyms Trimipramine Maleate

Restrictions A medication guide should be dispensed with each prescription. A template for the required MedGuides can be found on the FDA website at: http://www.fda.gov.cder/drug/antidepressants/labelTemplate.pdf

Generic Available No

Pharmacologic Category Antidepressant, Tricyclic (Tertiary Amine)

Medication Safety Issues

Sound-alike/look-alike issues:

Trimipramine may be confused with triamterene, trimeprazine

Use Treatment of depression

Mechanism of Action/Effect Increases the synaptic concentration of serotonin and/or norepinephrine in the central nervous system by inhibition of their reuptake by the presynaptic neuronal membrane

Contraindications Hypersensitivity to trimipramine, any component of the formulation, or other dibenzodiazepines; use of MAO inhibitors within 14 days; use in a patient during the acute recovery phase of MI

Warnings/Precautions Antidepressants increase the risk of suicidal thinking and behavior in children and adolescents with major depressive disorder (MDD) and other depressive disorders; consider risk prior to prescribing. All patients must be closely monitored for clinical worsening, suicidality, or unusual changes in behavior, especially during the initiation of therapy or following an increase or decrease in dosage. When used in children, the child's family or caregiver should be instructed to closely observe the patient and communicate condition with healthcare provider. A medication guide should be dispensed with each prescription. **Trimipramine is not FDA approved for use in children.**

The possibility of a suicide attempt is inherent in major depression and may persist until remission occurs. Use caution in high-risk patients. Worsening depression and severe abrupt suicidality that are not part of the presenting symptoms may require discontinuation or modification of drug therapy. The patient's family or caregiver should be alerted to monitor patients for the emergence of suicidality and associated behaviors (such as agitation, irritability, hostility, impulsivity, and hypomania) and call healthcare provider.

May worsen psychosis in some patients or precipitate a shift to mania or hypomania in patients with bipolar disorder. Patients presenting with depressive symptoms should be screened for bipolar disorder. Monotherapy in patients with bipolar disorder should be avoided. **Trimipramine is not FDA approved for the treatment of bipolar depression.**

The degree of sedation, anticholinergic effects, orthostasis, and conduction abnormalities are high relative to other antidepressants. Trimipramine often causes drowsiness/sedation, resulting in impaired performance of tasks requiring alertness (eg, operating machinery or driving). Sedative effects may be additive with other CNS depressants and/or ethanol. Use with caution in patients with a history of cardiovascular disease (including previous MI, stroke, tachycardia, or conduction abnormalities). Use with caution in patients with urinary retention, (Continued)

Trimipramine *(Continued)*

benign prostatic hyperplasia, narrow-angle glaucoma, xerostomia, visual problems, constipation, or a history of bowel obstruction.

May alter glucose control - use with caution in patients with diabetes. Consider discontinuing, when possible, prior to elective surgery. Therapy should not be abruptly discontinued in patients receiving high doses for prolonged periods. May lower seizure threshold - use caution in patients with a previous seizure disorder or condition predisposing to seizures such as brain damage, alcoholism, or concurrent therapy with other drugs which lower the seizure threshold. May increase the risks associated with electroconvulsive therapy. Use with caution in hyperthyroid patients or those receiving thyroid supplementation. Use with caution in patients with hepatic or renal dysfunction and in elderly patients.

Drug Interactions

Cytochrome P450 Effect: Substrate (major) of CYP2C19, 2D6, 3A4

Decreased Effect: CYP2C19 inducers may decrease the levels/effects of trimipramine; example inducers include aminoglutethimide, carbamazepine, phenytoin, and rifampin. Trimipramine inhibits the antihypertensive response to bethanidine, clonidine, debrisoquin, guanadrel, guanethidine, guanabenz, and guanfacine. Cholestyramine and colestipol may bind TCAs and reduce their absorption; monitor for altered response. CYP3A4 inducers may decrease the levels/effects of trimipramine; example inducers include aminoglutethimide, carbamazepine, nafcillin, nevirapine, phenobarbital, phenytoin, and rifamycins.

Increased Effect/Toxicity: Pressor response to I.V. epinephrine, norepinephrine, and phenylephrine may be enhanced in patients receiving TCAs (**Note:** Effect is unlikely with epinephrine or levonordefrin dosages typically administered as infiltration in combination with local anesthetics). Trimipramine increases the effects of amphetamines, anticholinergics, other CNS depressants (sedatives, hypnotics, or ethanol), chlorpropamide, tolazamide, and warfarin. When used with MAO inhibitors, hyperpyrexia, hypertension, tachycardia, confusion, seizures, and **deaths have been reported** (serotonin syndrome). Serotonin syndrome has also been reported with ritonavir (rare).

CYP2C19 inhibitors may increase the levels/effects of trimipramine; example inhibitors include delavirdine, fluconazole, fluvoxamine, gemfibrozil, isoniazid, omeprazole, and ticlopidine. CYP2D6 inhibitors may increase the levels/effects of trimipramine; example inhibitors include chlorpromazine, delavirdine, fluoxetine, miconazole, paroxetine, pergolide, quinidine, quinine, ritonavir, and ropinirole. CYP3A4 inhibitors may increase the levels/effects of trimipramine; example inhibitors include azole antifungals, ciprofloxacin, clarithromycin, diclofenac, doxycycline, erythromycin, imatinib, isoniazid, nefazodone, nicardipine, propofol, protease inhibitors, quinidine, and verapamil. Use of lithium with a TCA may increase the risk for neurotoxicity. Phenothiazines may increase concentration of some TCAs and TCAs may increase concentration of phenothiazines. Combined use of beta-agonists or drugs which prolong QT$_c$ (including quinidine, procainamide, disopyramide, cisapride, sparfloxacin, gatifloxacin, moxifloxacin) with TCAs may predispose patients to cardiac arrhythmias.

Nutritional/Ethanol Interactions

Ethanol: Avoid ethanol (may increase CNS depression).

Food: Grapefruit juice may inhibit the metabolism of some TCAs and clinical toxicity may result.

Herb/Nutraceutical: Avoid valerian, St John's wort, SAMe, kava kava (may increase risk of serotonin syndrome and/or excessive sedation).

Lab Interactions Increased glucose

Adverse Reactions Frequency not defined.

Cardiovascular: Arrhythmias, hyper-/hypotension, tachycardia, palpitation, heart block, stroke, MI

Central nervous system: Headache, exacerbation of psychosis, confusion, delirium, hallucinations, nervousness, restlessness, delusions, agitation, insomnia, nightmares, anxiety, seizure, drowsiness

Dermatologic: Photosensitivity, rash, petechiae, itching

Endocrine & metabolic: Sexual dysfunction, breast enlargement, galactorrhea, SIADH

Gastrointestinal: Xerostomia, constipation, increased appetite, nausea, unpleasant taste, weight gain, diarrhea, heartburn, vomiting, anorexia, trouble with gums, decreased lower esophageal sphincter tone may cause GE reflux

Genitourinary: Difficult urination, urinary retention, testicular edema

Hematologic: Agranulocytosis, eosinophilia, purpura, thrombocytopenia

Hepatic: Cholestatic jaundice, increased liver enzymes

Neuromuscular & skeletal: Tremors, numbness, tingling, paresthesia, incoordination, ataxia, peripheral neuropathy, extrapyramidal symptoms

Ocular: Blurred vision, eye pain, disturbances in accommodation, mydriasis, increased intraocular pressure

Otic: Tinnitus

Miscellaneous: Allergic reactions

Overdosage/Toxicology Symptoms of overdose include agitation, confusion, hallucinations, urinary retention, hypothermia, hypotension, tachycardia, and cardiac arrhythmias. Following initiation of essential overdose management, toxic symptoms should be treated.

Ventricular arrhythmias and ECG changes (QRS widening) often respond to systemic alkalinization (sodium bicarbonate 0.5-2 mEq/kg I.V.). Physostigmine (1-2 mg I.V. slowly for adults) may be indicated for reversing life-threatening cardiac arrhythmias. Treatment is symptomatic and supportive.

Pharmacodynamics/Kinetics
Bioavailability: 18% to 63%
Protein Binding: 95%; free drug: 3% to 7%
Half-Life Elimination: 16-40 hours
Metabolism: Hepatic; significant first-pass effect
Excretion: Urine

Dosing
Adults: Depression: Oral: 50-150 mg/day as a single bedtime dose up to a maximum of 200 mg/day for outpatients and 300 mg/day for inpatients
Elderly: Oral: Initial: 25 mg at bedtime; increase by 25 mg/day every 3 days for inpatients and weekly for outpatients, as tolerated, to a maximum of 100 mg/day (see Geriatric Considerations).

Available Dosage Forms Capsule, as maleate: 25 mg, 50 mg, 100 mg

Monitoring and Teaching Issues
Physical Assessment: Assess other medications patient may be taking for effectiveness and interactions. Monitor therapeutic effectiveness according to rationale for therapy, and adverse reactions at beginning of therapy and periodically with long-term use. Monitor for CNS depression, thoughts of suicide. Taper dosage slowly when discontinuing (allow 3-4 weeks between discontinuing Surmontil® and starting another antidepressant). Assess knowledge/teach patient appropriate use, interventions to reduce side effects, and adverse symptoms to report.

Patient Education: Take exactly as directed; do not increase dose or frequency. It may take 2-3 weeks to achieve desired results. Take at bedtime. Avoid alcohol, caffeine, and other prescription or OTC medications not approved by prescriber. Maintain adequate hydration (2-3 L/day of fluids) unless instructed to restrict fluid intake. You may experience drowsiness, lightheadedness, dizziness, or blurred vision (use caution when driving or engaging in tasks requiring alertness until response to drug is known); nausea, altered taste, dry mouth (small frequent meals, frequent mouth care, chewing gum, or sucking lozenges may help); constipation (increased exercise, fluids, fruit, or fiber may help); diarrhea (buttermilk, yogurt, or boiled milk may help); increased appetite (monitor dietary intake to avoid excess weight gain); postural hypotension (use caution when climbing stairs or changing position from lying or sitting to standing); urinary retention (void before taking medication); or sexual dysfunction (reversible). Report persistent CNS effects (eg, insomnia, restlessness, fatigue, anxiety, impaired cognitive function, seizures, suicide ideation); muscle cramping or tremors; chest pain, palpitations, rapid heartbeat, swelling of extremities, or severe dizziness; unresolved urinary retention; vision changes or eye pain; yellowing of eyes or skin; pale stools/dark urine; suicidal ideation; or worsening of condition. **Pregnancy/breast-feeding precautions:** Inform prescriber if you are or intend to become pregnant. Do not breast-feed.

Geriatric Considerations: Similar to doxepin in its side effect profile. Has not been well studied in the elderly. Very anticholinergic and, therefore, not considered a drug of first choice in the elderly when selecting an antidepressant.

Pregnancy Risk Factor: C
Lactation: Enters breast milk/contraindicated

Administration
Storage: Solutions stable at a pH of 4-5; turns yellowish or reddish on exposure to light. Slight discoloration does not affect potency; marked discoloration is associated with loss of potency. Capsules stable for 3 years following date of manufacture.

Additional Information May cause alterations in bleeding time.

Related Information
Antidepressant Agents *on page 1713*
Antidepressant Medication Guidelines *on page 1765*
Federal OBRA Regulations: Recommended Maximum Doses *on page 1773*

- ◆ **Trimipramine Maleate** *see Trimipramine on page 1531*
- ◆ **Trimox®** *see Amoxicillin on page 102*
- ◆ **Tri-Nasal®** *see Triamcinolone on page 1518*
- ◆ **TriNessa™** *see Ethinyl Estradiol and Norgestimate on page 593*
- ◆ **Tri-Norinyl®** *see Ethinyl Estradiol and Norethindrone on page 589*
- ◆ **Tripedia®** *see page 1660*
- ◆ **Triphasil®** *see Ethinyl Estradiol and Levonorgestrel on page 585*
- ◆ **Triple Antibiotic** *see Bacitracin, Neomycin, and Polymyxin B on page 171*
- ◆ **Triple Care® Antifungal [OTC]** *see Miconazole on page 999*
- ◆ **Tri-Previfem™** *see Ethinyl Estradiol and Norgestimate on page 593*
- ◆ **Triptoraline** *see Triptorelin on page 1533*

Triptorelin (trip toe REL in)

U.S. Brand Names Trelstar™ Depot; Trelstar™ LA
Synonyms AY-25650; CL-118,532; D-Trp(6)-LHRH; Triptoraline; Triptorelin Pamoate; Tryptoreline
Generic Available No
Pharmacologic Category Gonadotropin Releasing Hormone Agonist
Use Palliative treatment of advanced prostate cancer as an alternative to orchiectomy or estrogen administration
Unlabeled/Investigational Use Treatment of endometriosis, growth hormone deficiency, hyperandrogenism, *in vitro* fertilization, ovarian carcinoma, pancreatic carcinoma, precocious puberty, uterine leiomyomata
Mechanism of Action/Effect Causes suppression of ovarian and testicular steroidogenesis due to decreased levels of LH and FSH with subsequent decrease in testosterone (male) and estrogen (female) levels. After chronic and continuous administration, usually 2-4 weeks after initiation, a sustained decrease in LH and FSH secretion occurs.
(Continued)

Triptorelin *(Continued)*

Contraindications Hypersensitivity to triptorelin or any component of the formulation, other LHRH agonists or LHRH; pregnancy

Warnings/Precautions Transient increases in testosterone can lead to worsening symptoms (bone pain, hematuria, bladder outlet obstruction) of prostate cancer during the first few weeks of therapy. Cases of spinal cord compression have been reported with LHRH agonists. Hypersensitivity reactions including angioedema and anaphylaxis have rarely occurred. Safety and efficacy has not established in pediatric population.

Drug Interactions

Decreased Effect: Not studied. Hyperprolactinemic drugs (dopamine antagonists such as antipsychotics, and metoclopramide) are contraindicated.

Increased Effect/Toxicity: Not studied. Hyperprolactinemic drugs (dopamine antagonists such as antipsychotics, and metoclopramide) are contraindicated.

Lab Interactions Pituitary-gonadal function may be suppressed with chronic administration and for up to 8 weeks after triptorelin therapy has been discontinued.

Adverse Reactions As reported with Trelstar™ Depot and Trelstar™ LA; frequency of effect may vary by product:

>10%:

Central nervous system: Headache (30% to 60%)

Endocrine & metabolic: Hot flashes (95% to 100%), glucose increased, hemoglobin decreased, RBC count decreased

Hepatic: Alkaline phosphatase increased, ALT increased, AST increased

Neuromuscular & skeletal: Skeletal pain (12% to 13%)

Renal: BUN increased

1% to 10%:

Cardiovascular: Leg edema (6%), hypertension (4%), chest pain (2%), peripheral edema (1%)

Central nervous system: Dizziness (1% to 3%), pain (2% to 3%), emotional lability (1%), fatigue (2%), insomnia (2%)

Dermatologic: Rash (2%), pruritus (1%)

Endocrine & metabolic: Alkaline phosphatase increased (2%), breast pain (2%), gynecomastia (2%), libido decreased (2%), tumor flare (8%)

Gastrointestinal: Nausea (3%), anorexia (2%), constipation (2%), dyspepsia (2%), vomiting (2%), abdominal pain (1%), diarrhea (1%)

Genitourinary: Dysuria (5%), impotence (2% to 7%), urinary retention (1%), urinary tract infection (1%)

Hematologic: Anemia (1%)

Local: Injection site pain (4%)

Neuromuscular & skeletal: Leg pain (2% to 5%), back pain (3%), arthralgia (2%), leg cramps (2%), myalgia (1%), weakness (1%)

Ocular: Conjunctivitis (1%), eye pain (1%)

Respiratory: Cough (2%), dyspnea (1%), pharyngitis (1%)

Postmarketing and/or case reports: Anaphylaxis, angioedema, hypersensitivity reactions, spinal cord compression, renal dysfunction

Overdosage/Toxicology Accidental or intentional overdose unlikely. If it were to occur, supportive and symptomatic treatment would be indicated.

Pharmacodynamics/Kinetics

Absorption: Oral: Not active

Time to Peak: 1-3 hours

Protein Binding: None

Half-Life Elimination: 2.8 ± 1.2 hours

Moderate to severe renal impairment: 6.5-7.7 hours

Hepatic impairment: 7.6 hours

Metabolism: Unknown; unlikely to involve CYP; no known metabolites

Excretion: Urine (42% as intact peptide); hepatic

Dosing

Adults & Elderly: Advanced prostate carcinoma: I.M.: 3.75 mg once monthly

Renal Impairment: Specific guidelines are not available.

Hepatic Impairment: Specific guidelines are not available.

Available Dosage Forms Injection, powder for reconstitution, as pamoate [also available packaged with Debioclip™ (prefilled syringe containing sterile water)]:

Trelstar™ Depot: 3.75 mg

Trelstar™ LA: 11.25 mg

Monitoring and Teaching Issues

Physical Assessment: Assess results of laboratory tests, therapeutic effectiveness, and adverse response. Teach patient possible side effects/appropriate interventions and adverse symptoms to report. **Pregnancy risk factor X:** Used to treat advanced prostate cancer.

Monitoring Laboratory Tests: Serum testosterone levels, prostate-specific antigen

Patient Education: This medication can only be administered by injection. Report swelling, pain, or burning at injection site. May cause disease flare (increased bone pain), blood in urine, or urinary retention during early treatment (usually resolves within 1 week); impotence; or hot flashes (cool cloth on forehead, cool environment, and light clothing may help; contact prescriber if these become intolerable). Report any persistent adverse GI upset; chest pain, rapid heartbeat, or palpations; numbness in extremities; acute headache; alterations in urinary pattern; or other persistent adverse effects. **Pregnancy/breast-feeding precautions:** This drug will cause severe fetal defects. Do not breast-feed.

Pregnancy Risk Factor: X
Pregnancy Issues: Contraindicated in women who are or may become pregnant.
Lactation: Excretion in breast milk unknown/contraindicated
Administration
  I.M.: Must be administered under the supervision of a physician. Administer by I.M. injection into the buttock; alternate injection sites.
  Debioclip™: Follow manufacturer's instructions for mixing prior to use.
  Reconstitution: Reconstitute with 2 mL sterile water for injection. Shake well to obtain a uniform suspension. Withdraw the entire contents into the syringe and inject immediately.
  Storage:
    Trelstar™ Depot: Store at 15°C to 30°C (59°F to 86°F)
    Trelstar™ LA: Store at 20°C to 25°C (68°F to 77°F)

- ◆ **Triptorelin Pamoate** *see* Triptorelin *on page 1533*
- ◆ **Trisenox**™ *see* Arsenic Trioxide *on page 139*
- ◆ **Tri-Sprintec**™ *see* Ethinyl Estradiol and Norgestimate *on page 593*
- ◆ **Tri-Vent**™ **HC** *see* Hydrocodone, Carbinoxamine, and Pseudoephedrine *on page 759*
- ◆ **Trivora**® *see* Ethinyl Estradiol and Levonorgestrel *on page 585*
- ◆ **Trizivir**® *see* Abacavir, Lamivudine, and Zidovudine *on page 34*
- ◆ **Trobicin**® *see* Spectinomycin *on page 1390*
- ◆ **Trocaine**® **[OTC]** *see* Benzocaine *on page 181*
- ◆ **Tropicacyl**® *see page 1625*
- ◆ **Tropicamide** *see page 1625*
- ◆ **Trusopt**® *see* Dorzolamide *on page 483*
- ◆ **Truvada**™ *see* Emtricitabine and Tenofovir *on page 515*
- ◆ **Tryptoreline** *see* Triptorelin *on page 1533*
- ◆ **TSPA** *see* Thiotepa *on page 1466*
- ◆ **T-Stat**® **[DSC]** *see* Erythromycin *on page 543*
- ◆ **T-Tab**® *see* Clorazepate *on page 359*
- ◆ **Tuberculosis** *see page 1864*
- ◆ **Tums**® **[OTC]** *see* Calcium Carbonate *on page 235*
- ◆ **Tums**® **500 [OTC]** *see* Calcium Carbonate *on page 235*
- ◆ **Tums**® **E-X [OTC]** *see* Calcium Carbonate *on page 235*
- ◆ **Tums**® **Extra Strength Sugar Free [OTC]** *see* Calcium Carbonate *on page 235*
- ◆ **Tums**® **Smooth Dissolve [OTC]** *see* Calcium Carbonate *on page 235*
- ◆ **Tums**® **Ultra [OTC]** *see* Calcium Carbonate *on page 235*
- ◆ **Tussafed**® **HC** *see* Hydrocodone, Phenylephrine, and Guaifenesin *on page 760*
- ◆ **Tussend**® **Syrup** *see* Pseudoephedrine, Hydrocodone, and Chlorpheniramine *on page 1283*
- ◆ **Tussend**® **Tablet** *see* Pseudoephedrine, Hydrocodone, and Chlorpheniramine *on page 1283*
- ◆ **Tussi-12**® *see* Carbetapentane and Chlorpheniramine *on page 253*
- ◆ **Tussi-12 S**™ *see* Carbetapentane and Chlorpheniramine *on page 253*
- ◆ **Tussin [OTC]** *see* Guaifenesin *on page 729*
- ◆ **TussiNate**™ *see* Hydrocodone, Phenylephrine, and Diphenhydramine *on page 759*
- ◆ **Tussi-Organidin**® **DM NR [DSC]** *see* Guaifenesin and Dextromethorphan *on page 731*
- ◆ **Tussi-Organidin**® **NR** *see* Guaifenesin and Codeine *on page 731*
- ◆ **Tussi-Organidin**® **S-NR** *see* Guaifenesin and Codeine *on page 731*
- ◆ **Tussizone-12 RF**™ *see* Carbetapentane and Chlorpheniramine *on page 253*
- ◆ **Twelve Resin-K** *see* Cyanocobalamin *on page 377*
- ◆ **Twilite**® **[OTC]** *see* DiphenhydrAMINE *on page 463*
- ◆ **Twinrix**® *see page 1660*
- ◆ **Tylenol**® **[OTC]** *see* Acetaminophen *on page 38*
- ◆ **Tylenol**® **8 Hour [OTC]** *see* Acetaminophen *on page 38*
- ◆ **Tylenol**® **Arthritis Pain [OTC]** *see* Acetaminophen *on page 38*
- ◆ **Tylenol**® **Children's [OTC]** *see* Acetaminophen *on page 38*
- ◆ **Tylenol**® **Extra Strength [OTC]** *see* Acetaminophen *on page 38*
- ◆ **Tylenol**® **Infants [OTC]** *see* Acetaminophen *on page 38*
- ◆ **Tylenol**® **Junior Strength [OTC]** *see* Acetaminophen *on page 38*
- ◆ **Tylenol**® **Sore Throat [OTC]** *see* Acetaminophen *on page 38*
- ◆ **Tylenol**® **With Codeine** *see* Acetaminophen and Codeine *on page 41*
- ◆ **Tylox**® *see* Oxycodone and Acetaminophen *on page 1138*
- ◆ **Typhim Vi**® *see page 1660*
- ◆ **Typhoid Vaccine** *see page 1660*
- ◆ **Tyramine Content of Foods** *see page 1758*
- ◆ **Tysabri**® *see* Natalizumab *on page 1059*
- ◆ **U-90152S** *see* Delavirdine *on page 413*
- ◆ **UCB-P071** *see* Cetirizine *on page 296*
- ◆ **UK** *see* Urokinase *on page 1536*
- ◆ **UK-88,525** *see* Darifenacin *on page 407*
- ◆ **UK92480** *see* Sildenafil *on page 1373*
- ◆ **UK109496** *see* Voriconazole *on page 1570*
- ◆ **Ultram**® *see* Tramadol *on page 1504*
- ◆ **Ultraprin [OTC]** *see* Ibuprofen *on page 777*
- ◆ **Ultrase**® *see* Pancrelipase *on page 1151*
- ◆ **Ultrase**® **MT** *see* Pancrelipase *on page 1151*
- ◆ **Unasyn**® *see* Ampicillin and Sulbactam *on page 118*
- ◆ **Uniphyl**® *see* Theophylline *on page 1457*

♦ **Uniretic®** *see* Moexipril and Hydrochlorothiazide *on page 1026*

♦ **Unisom® Maximum Strength SleepGels® [OTC]** *see* DiphenhydrAMINE *on page 463*

♦ **Unithroid®** *see* Levothyroxine *on page 895*

♦ **Uni-Tricof HC** *see* Phenylephrine, Hydrocodone, and Chlorpheniramine *on page 1202*

♦ **Uni-Tuss HC** *see* Phenylephrine, Hydrocodone, and Chlorpheniramine *on page 1202*

♦ **Univasc®** *see* Moexipril *on page 1024*

♦ **Urecholine®** *see* Bethanechol *on page 190*

♦ **Urex®** *see* Methenamine *on page 970*

♦ **Uristat® [OTC]** *see* Phenazopyridine *on page 1193*

♦ **Urocit®-K** *see* Potassium Citrate *on page 1235*

♦ **Urofollitropin** *see* Follitropins *on page 670*

Urokinase (yoor oh KIN ase)

U.S. Brand Names Abbokinase® [DSC]

Synonyms UK

Generic Available No

Pharmacologic Category Thrombolytic Agent

Use Thrombolytic agent for the lysis of acute massive pulmonary emboli or pulmonary emboli with unstable hemodynamics

Unlabeled/Investigational Use Thrombolytic agent used in treatment of recent severe or massive deep vein thrombosis, myocardial infarction, and occluded I.V. or dialysis cannulas

Mechanism of Action/Effect Promotes thrombolysis by directly activating plasminogen to plasmin, which degrades fibrin, fibrinogen, and other procoagulant plasma proteins

Contraindications Hypersensitivity to urokinase or any component of the formulation; active internal bleeding; history of CVA; recent (within 2 months) intracranial or intraspinal surgery or trauma; intracranial neoplasm, arteriovenous malformation, or aneurysm; known bleeding diathesis; severe uncontrolled hypertension

Warnings/Precautions Concurrent heparin anticoagulation can contribute to bleeding; careful attention to all potential bleeding sites. I.M. injections and nonessential handling of the patient should be avoided. Venipunctures should be performed carefully and only when necessary. If arterial puncture is necessary, use an upper extremity vessel that can be manually compressed. If serious bleeding occurs, then the infusion of urokinase and heparin should be stopped.

For the following conditions the risk of bleeding is higher with use of anistreplase and should be weighed against the benefits of therapy: recent (within 10 days) major surgery (eg, CABG, obstetrical delivery, organ biopsy, previous puncture of noncompressible vessels), cerebrovascular disease, recent (within 10 days) gastrointestinal or genitourinary bleeding, recent trauma (within 10 days) including CPR, hypertension (systolic BP >180 mm Hg and/or diastolic BP >110 mm Hg), high likelihood of left heart thrombus (eg, mitral stenosis with atrial fibrillation), acute pericarditis, subacute bacterial endocarditis, hemostatic defects including ones caused by severe renal or hepatic dysfunction, significant hepatic dysfunction, pregnancy, diabetic hemorrhagic retinopathy or other hemorrhagic ophthalmic conditions, septic thrombophlebitis or occluded AV cannula at seriously infected site, advanced age (eg, >75 years), patients receiving oral anticoagulants, any other condition in which bleeding constitutes a significant hazard or would be particularly difficult to manage because of location.

Coronary thrombolysis may result in reperfusion arrhythmias. Follow standard MI management. Rare anaphylactoid reactions can occur. Safety and efficacy in pediatric patients have not been established.

Drug Interactions

Decreased Effect: Aminocaproic acid (an antifibrinolytic agent) may decrease the effectiveness of thrombolytic therapy.

Increased Effect/Toxicity: Oral anticoagulants (warfarin), heparin, low molecular weight heparins, and drugs which affect platelet function (eg, NSAIDs, dipyridamole, ticlopidine, clopidogrel, IIb/IIIa antagonists) may potentiate the risk of hemorrhage.

Adverse Reactions As with all drugs which may affect hemostasis, bleeding is the major adverse effect associated with urokinase. Hemorrhage may occur at virtually any site. Risk is dependent on multiple variables, including the dosage administered, concurrent use of multiple agents which alter hemostasis, and patient predisposition.

>10%: Local: Injection site: Bleeding (5% decrease in hematocrit reported in 37% patients; most bleeding occurring at external incisions or injection sites, but also reported in other areas)

Overdosage/Toxicology Symptoms of overdose include epistaxis, bleeding gums, hematoma, spontaneous ecchymoses, and oozing at the catheter site. In the event of overdose, stop the infusion and reverse bleeding with blood products that contain clotting factors.

Pharmacodynamics/Kinetics

Onset of Action: I.V.: Fibrinolysis occurs rapidly

Duration of Action: ≥4 hours

Half-Life Elimination: 6.4-18.8 minutes

Excretion: Urine and feces (small amounts)

Dosing

Adults & Elderly:

Acute pulmonary embolism: I.V.: Loading: 4400 int. units/kg over 10 minutes; maintenance: 4400 int. units/kg/hour for 12 hours. Following infusion, anticoagulation treatment is recommended to prevent recurrent thrombosis. Do not start anticoagulation until aPTT has decreased to less than twice the normal control value. If heparin is used, do not administer loading dose. Treatment should be followed with oral anticoagulants.

Deep vein thrombosis (unlabeled use): I.V.: Loading: 4400 units/kg over 10 minutes, then 4400 units/kg/hour for 12 hours

Myocardial infarction (unlabeled use): Intracoronary: 750,000 units over 2 hours (6000 units/minute over up to 2 hours)

Occluded I.V. catheters (unlabeled use):

5000 units in each lumen over 1-2 minutes, leave in lumen for 1-4 hours, then aspirate. May repeat with 10,000 units in each lumen if 5000 units fails to clear the catheter. **Do not infuse into the patient.** Volume to instill into catheter is equal to the volume of the catheter. Will not dissolve drug precipitate or anything other than blood products.

I.V. infusion: 200 units/kg/hour in each lumen for 12-48 hours at a rate of at least 20 mL/ hour

Dialysis patient: 5000 units is administered in each lumen over 1-2 minutes; leave urokinase in lumen for 1-2 days, then aspirate.

Pediatrics: Children: Deep vein thrombosis, pulmonary embolus, or occluded catheter: I.V.: Refer to adult dosing.

Available Dosage Forms [DSC] = Discontinued product

Injection, powder for reconstitution: 250,000 int. units [contains human albumin 250 mg and mannitol 25 mg] [DSC]

Monitoring and Teaching Issues

Physical Assessment: Weigh benefits against risks when bleeding/hemorrhage constitute a significant hazard (see Warnings/Precautions). Assess potential for interactions with other pharmacological agents and herbal products patient may be taking (especially those medications that may affect coagulation [warfarin] or platelet function [NSAIDs, dipyridamole, ticlopidine, clopidogrel]; see Drug Interactions). See Administration for infusion specifics (infusion pump is required). Assess results of laboratory results. Patient should be closely monitored for bleeding during and following treatment; infusion site, neurological status (eg, intracranial hemorrhage), vital signs, ECG (reperfusion arrhythmias); see Adverse Reactions. Bedrest and bleeding precautions should be maintained; avoid I.M. injections, venipuncture (unless absolutely necessary) and nonessential handling of the patient. If arterial puncture is necessary, use an upper extremity vessel that can be manually compressed. Patient instructions determined by patient condition (see Patient Education).

Monitoring Laboratory Tests: CBC, platelet count, aPTT, urinalysis

Patient Education: Inform prescriber of all medications or herbal products you are taking. This medication is only administered by infusion; you will be monitored closely during and after treatment. Immediately report burning, pain, redness, swelling, or oozing at infusion site, sudden acute headache, joint pain, chest pain, or altered vision. Following infusion you will have a tendency to bleed easily; use caution to prevent injury (use electric razor, soft toothbrush, and caution with knives, needles, or anything sharp) and follow instructions for strict bedrest to reduce the risk of injury. If bleeding does occur, report immediately and apply pressure to bleeding spot until bleeding stops completely. Report unusual pain (acute headache, joint pain, chest pain); unusual bruising or bleeding; blood in urine, stool, or vomitus; bleeding gums; vision changes; or respiratory difficulty. **Pregnancy/ breast-feeding precautions:** Inform prescriber if you are or intend to become pregnant. Consult prescriber if breast-feeding.

Pregnancy Risk Factor: B

Lactation: Excretion in breast milk unknown/use caution

Administration

I.V.: Solution may be filtered using a 0.22 or 0.45 micron filter during I.V. therapy. Administer using a pump which can deliver a total volume of 195 mL. The loading dose should be administered at 90 mL/hour over 10 minutes. The maintenance dose should be administered at 15 mL/hour over 12 hours. I.V. tubing should be flushed with NS or D_5W to ensure total dose is administered.

Reconstitution: Reconstitute vial with 5 mL sterile water for injection (preservative free) by gently rolling and tilting; do not shake. Contains no preservatives; should not be reconstituted until immediately before using; discard unused portion. Solution will look pale and straw colored. May filter through ≤0.45 micron filter.

Compatibility: Stable in NS

Storage: Prior to reconstitution, store in refrigerator at 2°C to 8°C (36°F to 46°F). Prior to infusion, solution should be further diluted in D_5W or NS.

♦ **Uro-KP-Neutral®** *see* Potassium Phosphate and Sodium Phosphate *on page 1239*

♦ **Urolene Blue®** *see page 1625*

♦ **Uro-Mag® [OTC]** *see* Magnesium Oxide *on page 931*

♦ **Uroxatral™** *see* Alfuzosin *on page 68*

♦ **Urso 250™** *see* Ursodiol *on page 1537*

♦ **Ursodeoxycholic Acid** *see* Ursodiol *on page 1537*

Ursodiol (ER soe dye ole)

U.S. Brand Names Actigall®; Urso 250™; Urso Forte™

Synonyms Ursodeoxycholic Acid

Generic Available Yes: Capsule

Pharmacologic Category Gallstone Dissolution Agent

Use Actigall®: Gallbladder stone dissolution; prevention of gallstones in obese patients experiencing rapid weight loss; Urso®: Primary biliary cirrhosis

Unlabeled/Investigational Use Liver transplantation

Mechanism of Action/Effect Decreases the cholesterol content of bile and bile stones by reducing the secretion of cholesterol from the liver and the fractional reabsorption of cholesterol by the intestines. Mechanism of action in primary biliary cirrhosis is not clearly defined.

Contraindications Hypersensitivity to ursodiol, bile acids, or any component of the formulation; not to be used with cholesterol, radiopaque, bile pigment stones, or stones >20 mm in diameter; allergy to bile acids

Warnings/Precautions Gallbladder stone dissolution may take several months of therapy. Complete dissolution may not occur and recurrence of stones within 5 years has been observed in 50% of patients. Use with caution in patients with a nonvisualizing gallbladder and those with chronic liver disease.

(Continued)

Ursodiol *(Continued)*

Drug Interactions
Decreased Effect: Decreased effect with aluminum-containing antacids, cholestyramine, colestipol, clofibrate, and oral contraceptives (estrogens).

Adverse Reactions
>10%:
Central nervous system: Headache (up to 25%), dizziness (up to 17%)
Gastrointestinal: In treatment of primary biliary cirrhosis: Constipation (up to 26%)
1% to 10%:
Dermatologic: Rash (<1% to 3%), alopecia (<1% to 5%)
Gastrointestinal:
In gallstone dissolution: Most GI events (diarrhea, nausea, vomiting) are similar to placebo and attributable to gallstone disease.
In treatment of primary biliary cirrhosis: Diarrhea (1%)
Hematologic: Leukopenia (3%)
Miscellaneous: Allergy (5%)

Overdosage/Toxicology Symptoms of overdose include diarrhea. No specific therapy for diarrhea or overdose.

Pharmacodynamics/Kinetics
Half-Life Elimination: 100 hours
Metabolism: Undergoes extensive enterohepatic recycling; following hepatic conjugation and biliary secretion, the drug is hydrolyzed to active ursodiol, where it is recycled or transformed to lithocholic acid by colonic microbial flora
Excretion: Feces

Dosing
Adults & Elderly:
Gallstone dissolution: Oral: 8-10 mg/kg/day in 2-3 divided doses; use beyond 24 months is not established; obtain ultrasound images at 6-month intervals for the first year of therapy; 30% of patients have stone recurrence after dissolution
Gallstone prevention: Oral: 300 mg twice daily
Primary biliary cirrhosis: Oral: 13-15 mg/kg/day in 2-4 divided doses (with food)

Available Dosage Forms
Capsule (Actigall®): 300 mg
Tablet:
Urso 250™: 250 mg
Urso Forte™: 500 mg

Monitoring and Teaching Issues
Physical Assessment: Use caution with a nonvisualizing gallbladder and chronic liver disease (see Warnings/Precautions for use cautions). Assess results of laboratory tests, therapeutic effectiveness, and adverse reactions (see Adverse Reactions). Teach patient proper use and possible side effects signs to report (see Patient Education).

Monitoring Laboratory Tests:
Gallstone disease: ALT, AST, ALP; sonogram may be required
Hepatic disease: Monitor hepatic function tests frequently

Patient Education: Take medication as directed with food. Do not take aluminum containing antacids within 2 hours of taking ursodiol. Drug will need to be taken for 1-3 months after stone is dissolved and stones may recur. Report any persistent nausea, vomiting, abdominal pain, or yellowing of skin or eyes. **Breast-feeding precaution:** Consult prescriber if breast-feeding.

Dietary Considerations: Urso® should be taken with food.

Geriatric Considerations: No specific clinical studies in the elderly. Would recommend starting at lowest recommended dose with scheduled monitoring.

Pregnancy Risk Factor: B

Lactation: Excretion in breast milk unknown

Administration
Oral: Do not administer with aluminum-based antacids. If aluminum based antacids are needed, administer 2 hours after ursodiol. Urso® should be taken with food.

Storage: Do not store above 30°C (86°F)

- **Urso Forte™** *see Ursodiol on page 1537*
- **UTI Relief® [OTC]** *see Phenazopyridine on page 1193*
- **Uvadex®** *see Methoxsalen on page 978*
- **Vagifem®** *see Estradiol on page 552*
- **Vagistat®-1 [OTC]** *see Tioconazole on page 1484*

Valacyclovir *(val ay SYE kloe veer)*

U.S. Brand Names Valtrex®
Synonyms Valacyclovir Hydrochloride
Generic Available No
Pharmacologic Category Antiviral Agent, Oral
Medication Safety Issues
Sound-alike/look-alike issues:
Valtrex® may be confused with Valcyte™
Valacyclovir may be confused with valganciclovir

Use Treatment of herpes zoster (shingles) in immunocompetent patients; treatment of first-episode genital herpes; episodic treatment of recurrent genital herpes; suppression of recurrent genital herpes and reduction of heterosexual transmission of genital herpes in immunocompetent patients; suppression of genital herpes in HIV-infected individuals; treatment of herpes labialis (cold sores)

Mechanism of Action/Effect Valacyclovir is rapidly converted to acyclovir before it exerts its antiviral activity against HSV-1, HSV-2, or VZV. Inhibits viral DNA synthesis and replication.

Contraindications Hypersensitivity to valacyclovir, acyclovir, or any component of the formulation

Warnings/Precautions Thrombotic thrombocytopenic purpura/hemolytic uremic syndrome has occurred in immunocompromised patients (at doses of 8 g/day); use caution and adjust the dose in elderly patients or those with renal insufficiency and in patients receiving concurrent nephrotoxic agents. For genital herpes, treatment should begin as soon as possible after the first signs and symptoms (within 72 hours of onset of first diagnosis or within 24 hours of onset of recurrent episodes). For herpes zoster, treatment should begin within 72 hours of onset of rash. For cold sores, treatment should begin at with earliest symptom (tingling, itching, burning). Safety and efficacy in prepubertal patients have not been established.

Drug Interactions
  Decreased Effect: Cimetidine and/or probenecid has decreased the rate but not the extent of valacyclovir conversion to acyclovir leading to decreased effectiveness of valacyclovir.
  Increased Effect/Toxicity: Valacyclovir and acyclovir have increased CNS side effects with zidovudine and probenecid.

Adverse Reactions
  >10%: Central nervous system: Headache (14% to 35%)
  1% to 10%:
    Central nervous system: Dizziness (2% to 4%), depression (0% to 7%)
    Endocrine: Dysmenorrhea (≤1% to 8%)
    Gastrointestinal: Abdominal pain (2% to 11%), vomiting (<1% to 6%), nausea (6% to 15%)
    Hematologic: Leukopenia (≤1%), thrombocytopenia (≤1%)
    Hepatic: AST increased (1% to 4%)
    Neuromuscular & skeletal: Arthralgia (≤1 to 6%)

Overdosage/Toxicology Precipitation in renal tubules may occur. Treatment is symptomatic and includes hemodialysis, especially if compromised renal function develops.

Pharmacodynamics/Kinetics
  Absorption: Rapid
  Bioavailability: ~55% once converted to acyclovir
  Protein Binding: 13.5% to 17.9%
  Half-Life Elimination: Normal renal function: Adults: 2.5-3.3 hours (acyclovir), ~30 minutes (valacyclovir); End-stage renal disease: 14-20 hours (acyclovir)
  Metabolism: Hepatic; valacyclovir is rapidly and nearly completely converted to acyclovir and L-valine by first-pass effect; acyclovir is hepatically metabolized to a very small extent by aldehyde oxidase and by alcohol and aldehyde dehydrogenase (inactive metabolites)
  Excretion: Urine, primarily as acyclovir (88%). **Note:** Following oral administration of radio-labeled valacyclovir, 46% of the label is eliminated in the feces (corresponding to nonabsorbed drug), while 47% of the radiolabel is eliminated in the urine.

Dosing
  Adults & Elderly:
    Herpes labialis (cold sores): Oral: 2 g twice daily for 1 day (separate doses by ~12 hours)
    Herpes zoster (shingles): Oral: 1 g 3 times/day for 7 days
    Genital herpes: Oral:
      Initial episode: 1 g twice daily for 10 days
      Recurrent episode: 500 mg twice daily for 3 days
      Reduction of transmission: 500 mg once daily (source partner)
      Suppressive therapy:
        Immunocompetent patients: 1000 mg once daily (500 mg once daily in patients with <9 recurrences per year)
        HIV-infected patients (CD4 ≥100 cells/mm³): 500 mg twice daily
  Pediatrics: Herpes labialis (cold sores): Adolescents: Refer to adult dosing.
  Renal Impairment:
    Herpes zoster: Adults:
      Cl_cr 30-49 mL/minute: 1 g every 12 hours
      Cl_cr 10-29 mL/minute: 1 g every 24 hours
      Cl_cr <10 mL/minute: 500 mg every 24 hours
    Genital herpes: Adults:
      Initial episode:
        Cl_cr 10-29 mL/minute: 1 g every 24 hours
        Cl_cr <10 mL/minute: 500 mg every 24 hours
      Recurrent episode: Cl_cr <10-29 mL/minute: 500 mg every 24 hours
      Suppressive therapy: Cl_cr <10-29 mL/minute:
        For usual dose of 1 g every 24 hours, decrease dose to 500 mg every 24 hours
        For usual dose of 500 mg every 24 hours, decrease dose to 500 mg every 48 hours
        HIV-infected patients: 500 mg every 24 hours
    Herpes labialis: Adolescents and Adults:
      Cl_cr 30-49 mL/minute: 1 g every 12 hours for 2 doses
      Cl_cr 10-29 mL/minute: 500 mg every 12 hours for 2 doses
      Cl_cr <10 mL/minute: 500 mg as a single dose
    Hemodialysis: Dialyzable (~33% removed during 4-hour session); administer dose postdialysis
    Chronic ambulatory peritoneal dialysis/continuous arteriovenous hemofiltration dialysis: Pharmacokinetic parameters are similar to those in patients with ESRD; supplemental dose not needed following dialysis

Available Dosage Forms Caplet: 500 mg, 1000 mg

Monitoring and Teaching Issues
  Physical Assessment: Use caution with renal insufficiency and with concurrent nephrotoxic agents (see Warnings/Precautions and Drug Interactions). Assess therapeutic effectiveness (resolution of clinical symptoms) and adverse responses (eg, CNS changes [dizziness, depression], nausea, vomiting, dysmenorrhea, arthralgia; see Adverse Reactions). Teach patient appropriate use, possible side effects/appropriate interventions, and adverse symptoms to report (See Patient Education).

(Continued)

Valacyclovir *(Continued)*

Monitoring Laboratory Tests: Urinalysis, BUN, serum creatinine, liver enzymes, CBC

Patient Education: This medication is not a cure for genital herpes; it is not known if it will prevent transmission to others. Take as directed, with or without food. Begin use at first sign of herpes. Maintain adequate hydration (2-3 L/day of fluids) unless instructed to restrict fluid intake. May cause headache, dizziness (use caution when driving or engaging in potentially hazardous tasks until response to drug is known); or nausea, vomiting, abdominal pain (small frequent meals, frequent mouth care, chewing gum, or sucking lozenges may help). Immediately report difficulty swallowing or breathing, rash, hives, or changes in menses. **Breast-feeding precaution:** Consult prescriber if breast-feeding.

Dietary Considerations: May be taken with or without food.

Geriatric Considerations: More convenient dosing and increased bioavailability, without increasing side effects, make valacyclovir a favorable choice compared to acyclovir. Has been shown to accelerate resolution of postherpetic pain. Adjust dose for renal impairment.

Pregnancy Risk Factor: B

Pregnancy Issues: Teratogenicity registry has shown no increased rate of birth defects than that of the general population; however, the registry is small and use during pregnancy is only warranted if the potential benefit to the mother justifies the risk of the fetus.

Lactation: Enters breast milk/use caution

Breast-Feeding Issues: Peak concentrations in breast milk range from 0.5-2.3 times the corresponding maternal acyclovir serum concentration. This is expected to provide a nursing infant with a dose of acyclovir equivalent to ~0.6 mg/kg/day following ingestion of valacyclovir 500 mg twice daily by the mother. Use with caution while breast-feeding.

Administration

Oral: If GI upset occurs, administer with meals.

Storage: Store at 15°C to 25°C (59°F to 77°F).

♦ **Valacyclovir Hydrochloride** *see Valacyclovir on page 1538*
♦ **Valcyte™** *see Valganciclovir on page 1541*

Valdecoxib *(val de KOKS ib)*

U.S. Brand Names Bextra®

Generic Available No

Pharmacologic Category Nonsteroidal Anti-inflammatory Drug (NSAID), COX-2 Selective

Use Relief of signs and symptoms of osteoarthritis and adult rheumatoid arthritis; treatment of primary dysmenorrhea

Mechanism of Action/Effect Inhibits cyclooxygenase-2 (COX-2) and as a result, prostaglandin synthesis resulting in decreased pain.

Contraindications Hypersensitivity to valdecoxib, sulfonamides, or any component of the formulation; patients who have experienced asthma, urticaria, or allergic-type reactions to aspirin or NSAIDs; acute pain following CABG; pregnancy (3rd trimester)

Warnings/Precautions Gastrointestinal irritation, ulceration, bleeding, and perforation may occur with NSAIDs. Use with caution in patients with a history of GI bleeding, ulcers, or risk factor for GI bleeding. Anaphylactic/anaphylactoid reactions may occur, even with no prior exposure to valdecoxib. Serious dermatologic reactions (including life-threatening Stevens-Johnson syndrome and erythema multiforme) have been reported; discontinue in any patients who develop rash or any signs of hypersensitivity. Use with caution in patients with decreased renal function, hepatic disease, CHF, hypertension, fluid retention, dehydration, or asthma. Carefully evaluate individual cardiovascular risk profiles prior to prescribing COX-2 inhibitors. COX-2 inhibitors may not be appropriate in patients with cardiovascular disease or in patients with significant risk factors for cardiovascular disease. Use caution in patients with known or suspected deficiency of cytochrome P450 isoenzyme 2C9. Use in patients with severe hepatic impairment (Child-Pugh Class C) is not recommended. Use in patients following CABG has been associated with an increase in thromboembolic events, including MI, stroke, DVT, and PE. Safety and efficacy have not been established for patients <18 years of age.

Drug Interactions

Cytochrome P450 Effect: Substrate (minor) of CYP2C8/9, 3A4; **Inhibits** CYP2C8/9 (weak), 2C19 (weak)

Decreased Effect: ACE inhibitors, angiotensin II antagonists, hydralazine, loop and thiazide diuretics effects reduced.

Increased Effect/Toxicity: Anticoagulants and antiplatelet drugs may increase risk of bleeding. Warfarin efficacy may increase. Corticosteroids may increase risk of GI ulceration. Cyclosporine, dextromethorphan, lithium levels increased. Serum concentrations/toxicity of methotrexate may be increased. Azole antifungals may increase valdecoxib concentrations.

Nutritional/Ethanol Interactions

Ethanol: Avoid ethanol (may enhance gastric mucosal irritation).

Food: Time to peak level is delayed by 1-2 hours when taken with high-fat meal, but other parameters are unaffected.

Herb/Nutraceutical: Avoid cat's claw, dong quai, evening primrose, feverfew, garlic, ginger, ginkgo, red clover, horse chestnut, green tea, ginseng (may cause increased risk of bleeding).

Adverse Reactions 2% to 10%:

Cardiovascular: Peripheral edema (2% to 3%), hypertension (2%)

Central nervous system: Headache (5% to 9%), dizziness (3%)

Dermatologic: Rash (1% to 2%)

Gastrointestinal: Dyspepsia (8% to 9%), abdominal pain (7% to 8%), nausea (6% to 7%), diarrhea (5% to 6%), flatulence (3% to 4%), abdominal fullness (2%)

Neuromuscular & skeletal: Back pain (2% to 3%), myalgia (2%)

Otic: Earache, tinnitus

Respiratory: Upper respiratory tract infection (6% to 7%), sinusitis (2% to 3%)

Miscellaneous: Influenza-like symptoms (2%)

Overdosage/Toxicology Symptoms of overdose may include epigastric pain, drowsiness, lethargy, nausea, and vomiting; gastrointestinal bleeding may occur. Rare manifestations include hypertension, respiratory depression, coma, and acute renal failure. Treatment is symptomatic and supportive. Forced diuresis, hemodialysis, hemoperfusion, and/or urinary alkalinization may not be useful.

Pharmacodynamics/Kinetics
Onset of Action: Dysmenorrhea: 60 minutes
Bioavailability: 83%
Time to Peak: 2.25-3 hours
Protein Binding: 98%
Half-Life Elimination: 8-11 hours
Metabolism: Extensively hepatic via CYP3A4 and 2C9; glucuronidation; forms metabolite (active)
Excretion: Primarily urine (as metabolites)

Dosing
Adults & Elderly:
Osteoarthritis and rheumatoid arthritis: Oral: 10 mg once daily; **Note:** No additional benefits seen with 20 mg/day
Primary dysmenorrhea: Oral: 20 mg twice daily as needed
Pediatrics: Not indicated for pediatric patients.
Renal Impairment: Not recommended for use in advanced disease.
Hepatic Impairment: Not recommended for use in advanced liver dysfunction (Child-Pugh Class C).

Available Dosage Forms Tablet: 10 mg, 20 mg

Monitoring and Teaching Issues
Physical Assessment: Assess effectiveness and interactions of other prescription, OTC, or herbal medication patient may be taking. Assess allergy history (salicylates, NSAIDs). Monitor for effectiveness of therapy and adverse reactions. Assess knowledge/teach patient appropriate use, interventions to reduce possible side effects, and adverse symptoms to report.
Patient Education: Use exactly as directed. May be taken with food to reduce GI upset. Do not take with antacids. Avoid alcohol, aspirin, or other medication unless approved by prescriber. Maintain adequate hydration (2-3 L/day of fluids) unless instructed to restrict fluid intake. GI bleeding, ulceration, or perforation can occur with or without pain. Stop taking medication and report immediately abdominal tenderness, stomach pain or cramping; unusual bleeding or bruising; or blood in vomitus, stool, or urine. You may experience dizziness, confusion, or blurred vision (avoid driving or engaging in tasks requiring alertness until response to drug is known); or anorexia, nausea, vomiting (small frequent meals, frequent mouth care, chewing gum or sucking lozenges may help). Report any skin rash, muscle aches, unusual fatigue, lethargy, yellowing of skin or eyes, flu-like symptoms, easy bruising or bleeding, sudden weight gain, changes in urinary pattern, respiratory difficulty, or signs of upper respiratory infection. **Pregnancy/breast-feeding precautions:** Inform prescriber if you are or intend to become pregnant. This drug should not be used in the 3rd trimester of pregnancy. Breast-feeding is not recommended.
Dietary Considerations: May be taken with or without food.
Pregnancy Risk Factor: C/D (3rd trimester)
Pregnancy Issues: Use should be avoided in late pregnancy because it may cause premature closure of the ductus arteriosus.
Lactation: Excretion in breast milk unknown/not recommended

Administration
Oral: Avoid dehydration. Encourage patient to drink plenty of fluids.
Storage: Store at 15°C to 30°C (59°F to 86°F).

Related Information
Nonsalicylate / Nonsteroidal Anti-inflammatory Agents *on page 1743*

Valganciclovir (val gan SYE kloh veer)

U.S. Brand Names Valcyte™
Synonyms Valganciclovir Hydrochloride
Generic Available No
Pharmacologic Category Antiviral Agent
Medication Safety Issues
Sound-alike/look-alike issues:
Valcyte™ may be confused with Valium®, Valtrex®
Valganciclovir may be confused with valacyclovir

Use Treatment of cytomegalovirus (CMV) retinitis in patients with acquired immunodeficiency syndrome (AIDS); prevention of CMV disease in high-risk patients (donor CMV positive/ recipient CMV negative) undergoing kidney, heart, or kidney/pancreas transplantation

Mechanism of Action/Effect Valganciclovir is a prodrug of ganciclovir, and is rapidly metabolized in the body to form ganciclovir. Ganciclovir inhibits the formation of viral DNA within infected cells, blocking reproduction of the virus.

Contraindications Hypersensitivity to valganciclovir, ganciclovir, acyclovir, or any component of the formulation; absolute neutrophil count <500/mm³; platelet count <25,000/mm³; hemoglobin <8 g/dL

Warnings/Precautions Dosage adjustment or interruption of valganciclovir therapy may be necessary in patients with neutropenia and/or thrombocytopenia and patients with impaired renal function. Not approved for use in children. Due to differences in bioavailability, valganciclovir tablets cannot be substituted for ganciclovir capsules on a one-to-one basis. Not indicated for use in liver transplant patients (higher incidence of tissue-invasive CMV relative to oral ganciclovir was observed in trials). Safety and efficacy not established in pediatric patients.
(Continued)

Valganciclovir *(Continued)*

Drug Interactions

Decreased Effect: Reported for ganciclovir: A decrease in blood levels of ganciclovir AUC may occur when used with didanosine.

Increased Effect/Toxicity: Reported for ganciclovir: Immunosuppressive agents may increase hematologic toxicity of ganciclovir. Imipenem/cilastatin may increase seizure potential. Oral ganciclovir increases blood levels of zidovudine, although zidovudine decreases steady-state levels of ganciclovir. Since both drugs have the potential to cause neutropenia and anemia, some patients may not tolerate concomitant therapy with these drugs at full dosage. Didanosine levels are increased with concurrent ganciclovir. Other nephrotoxic drugs (eg, amphotericin and cyclosporine) may have additive nephrotoxicity with ganciclovir.

Nutritional/Ethanol Interactions Food: Coadministration with a high-fat meal increased AUC by 30%.

Adverse Reactions

>10%:
Central nervous system: Fever (31%), headache (9% to 22%), insomnia (16%)
Gastrointestinal: Diarrhea (16% to 41%), nausea (8% to 30%), vomiting (21%), abdominal pain (15%)
Hematologic: Granulocytopenia (11% to 27%), anemia (8% to 26%)
Ocular: Retinal detachment (15%)

1% to 10%:
Central nervous system: Peripheral neuropathy (9%), paresthesia (8%), seizure (<5%), psychosis, hallucinations (<5%), confusion (<5%), agitation (<5%)
Hematologic: Thrombocytopenia (8%), pancytopenia (<5%), bone marrow depression (<5%), aplastic anemia (<5%), bleeding (potentially life-threatening due to thrombocytopenia <5%)
Renal: Decreased renal function (<5%)
Miscellaneous: Local and systemic infection, including sepsis (<5%); allergic reaction (<5%)

Overdosage/Toxicology
Symptoms of overdose with ganciclovir include neutropenia, vomiting, hypersalivation, bloody diarrhea, cytopenia, and testicular atrophy. Treatment is supportive. Hemodialysis removes 50% of the drug. Hydration may be of some benefit.

Pharmacodynamics/Kinetics

Absorption: Well absorbed; high-fat meal increases AUC by 30%
Bioavailability: With food: 60%
Protein Binding: 1% to 2%
Half-Life Elimination: Ganciclovir: 4.08 hours, prolonged with renal impairment; Severe renal impairment: Up to 68 hours
Metabolism: Converted to ganciclovir by intestinal mucosal cells and hepatocytes
Excretion: Urine (primarily as ganciclovir)

Dosing

Adults & Elderly:
CMV retinitis: Oral:
Induction (active retinitis): 900 mg twice daily for 21 days (with food)
Maintenance: Following induction treatment, or for patients with inactive CMV retinitis who require maintenance therapy: Recommended dose: 900 mg once daily (with food)
Prevention of CMV disease following transplantation: Oral: 900 mg once daily (with food) beginning within 10 days of transplantation; continue therapy until 100 days post-transplantation.

Renal Impairment:
Induction dose:
Cl_{cr} 40-59 mL/minute: 450 mg twice daily
Cl_{cr} 25-39 mL/minute: 450 mg once daily
Cl_{cr} 10-24 mL/minute: 450 mg every 2 days
Maintenance dose:
Cl_{cr} 40-59 mL/minute: 450 mg once daily
Cl_{cr} 25-39 mL/minute: 450 mg every 2 days
Cl_{cr} 10-24 mL/minute: 450 mg twice weekly
Note: Valganciclovir is not recommended in patients receiving hemodialysis. For patients on hemodialysis (Cl_{cr} <10 mL/minute), it is recommended that ganciclovir be used (dose adjusted as specified for ganciclovir).

Available Dosage Forms Tablet, as hydrochloride: 450 mg [valganciclovir hydrochloride 496.3 mg equivalent to valganciclovir 450 mg]

Monitoring and Teaching Issues

Physical Assessment: Use caution with renal impairment (see Warnings/Precautions for use cautions). Assess potential for interactions with other pharmacological agents patient may be taking (eg, increased risk of nephrotoxicity and hematologic toxicity; see Drug Interactions). Assess results of laboratory tests (see Monitoring Laboratory Tests), therapeutic effectiveness (reduction in clinical symptoms), and adverse response on a regular basis during therapy (eg, peripheral neuropathy, neutropenia, anemia, nephrotoxicity, retinal detachment, vomiting, bloody diarrhea; see Adverse Reactions). Teach proper use, possible side effects/appropriate interventions, and adverse symptoms to report (See Patient Education).

Monitoring Laboratory Tests: Retinal exam (at least every 4-6 weeks), CBC, platelet counts, serum creatinine

Patient Education: Do not take any new medication (especially any eye medication) during therapy unless approved by prescriber. This medication is not a cure for CMV retinitis. Take exactly as directed; do not alter dosage or discontinue without consulting prescriber. You will need frequent and regular laboratory tests and ophthalmic exams while taking this medication. Maintain adequate hydration (2-3 L/day of fluids) unless instructed to restrict fluid intake. You may be more susceptible to infection (avoid crowds or exposure to infection and do not have any vaccinations unless approved by prescriber). May cause headache or insomnia (use caution when driving or engaging in hazardous tasks until response to drug is known); nausea or vomiting (small frequent meals, good mouth care, sucking lozenges, or chewing gum may help); diarrhea (boiled milk, yogurt, or buttermilk may help); or photosensitivity (use sunscreen, wear protective clothing and eyewear, and avoid direct sunlight). Report any worsening of eye condition; infection (fever; chills; unusual bleeding or bruising, white plaques in mouth or vaginal discharge); CNS disturbances (eg, hallucinations, confusion, nightmares); or weakness or loss of feeling in nerves or muscles. **Pregnancy/breast-feeding precautions:** Inform prescriber if you are pregnant. Males and females should use appropriate contraceptive measures during and for 90 days following end of therapy. Do not breast-feed.

Dietary Considerations: Should be taken with meals.

Pregnancy Risk Factor: C

Pregnancy Issues: Valganciclovir is converted to ganciclovir and shares its reproductive toxicity. Ganciclovir may adversely affect spermatogenesis and fertility; due to its mutagenic potential, contraceptive precautions for female and male patients need to be followed during and for at least 90 days after therapy with this drug.

Lactation: Excretion in breast milk unknown/contraindicated

Breast-Feeding Issues: HIV-infected mothers are discouraged from breast-feeding to decrease the potential transmission of HIV.

Administration

Oral: Avoid direct contact with broken or crushed tablets. Consideration should be given to handling and disposal according to guidelines issued for antineoplastic drugs. However, there is no consensus on the need for these precautions.

Storage: Store at 25°C (77°F), excursions permitted to 15°C to 30°C (59°F to 86°F).

- ◆ **Valganciclovir Hydrochloride** *see* Valganciclovir *on page 1541*
- ◆ **Valium**® *see* Diazepam *on page 439*
- ◆ **Valorin [OTC]** *see* Acetaminophen *on page 38*
- ◆ **Valorin Extra [OTC]** *see* Acetaminophen *on page 38*
- ◆ **Valproate Semisodium** *see* Valproic Acid and Derivatives *on page 1543*
- ◆ **Valproate Sodium** *see* Valproic Acid and Derivatives *on page 1543*
- ◆ **Valproic Acid** *see* Valproic Acid and Derivatives *on page 1543*

Valproic Acid and Derivatives (val PROE ik AS id & dah RIV ah tives)

U.S. Brand Names Depacon®; Depakene®; Depakote® Delayed Release; Depakote® ER; Depakote® Sprinkle®

Synonyms Dipropylacetic Acid; Divalproex Sodium; DPA; 2-Propylpentanoic Acid; 2-Propylvaleric Acid; Valproate Semisodium; Valproate Sodium; Valproic Acid

Generic Available Yes: Valproic acid, valproate sodium

Pharmacologic Category Anticonvulsant, Miscellaneous

Medication Safety Issues

Sound-alike/look-alike issues:

Depakene® may be confused with Depakote®

Depakote® may be confused with Depakene®, Depakote® ER, Senokot®

Use Monotherapy and adjunctive therapy in the treatment of patients with complex partial seizures; monotherapy and adjunctive therapy of simple and complex absence seizures; adjunctive therapy patients with multiple seizure types that include absence seizures

Mania associated with bipolar disorder (Depakote®)

Migraine prophylaxis (Depakote®, Depakote® ER)

Unlabeled/Investigational Use Behavior disorders in Alzheimer's disease; status epilepticus

Mechanism of Action/Effect Causes increased availability of gamma-aminobutyric acid (GABA), an inhibitory neurotransmitter, to brain neurons or may enhance the action of GABA or mimic its action at postsynaptic receptor sites

Contraindications Hypersensitivity to valproic acid, derivatives, or any component of the formulation; hepatic dysfunction; urea cycle disorders; pregnancy

Warnings/Precautions Hepatic failure resulting in fatalities has occurred in patients; children <2 years of age are at considerable risk; other risk factors include organic brain disease, mental retardation with severe seizure disorders, congenital metabolic disorders, and patients on multiple anticonvulsants. Hepatotoxicity has been reported after 3 days to 6 months of therapy. Monitor patients closely for appearance of malaise, weakness, facial edema, anorexia, jaundice, and vomiting; may cause severe thrombocytopenia, inhibition of platelet aggregation and bleeding; tremors may indicate overdosage; use with caution in patients receiving other anticonvulsants.

Cases of life-threatening pancreatitis, occurring at the start of therapy or following years of use, have been reported in adults and children. Some cases have been hemorrhagic with rapid progression of initial symptoms to death.

May cause teratogenic effects such as neural tube defects (eg, spina bifida). Use in women of childbearing potential requires that benefits of use in mother be weighed against the potential risk to fetus, especially when used for conditions not associated with permanent injury or risk of death (eg, migraine).

Hyperammonemic encephalopathy, sometimes fatal, has been reported following the initiation of valproate therapy in patients with known or suspected urea cycle disorders (UCD), particularly those with ornithine transcarbamylase deficiency. Although a rare genetic disorder, UCD evaluation should be considered for the following patients, prior to the start of therapy: History of unexplained encephalopathy or coma; encephalopathy associated with protein load; pregnancy or postpartum encephalopathy; unexplained mental retardation; history of elevated plasma ammonia or glutamine; history of cyclical vomiting and lethargy; episodic extreme irritability, ataxia; low BUN or protein avoidance; family history of UCD or unexplained infant deaths (particularly male); signs or symptoms of UCD (hyperammonemia, encephalopathy, respiratory alkalosis). Patients who develop symptoms of hyperammonemic (Continued)

Valproic Acid and Derivatives *(Continued)*

encephalopathy during therapy with valproate should receive prompt evaluation for UCD and valproate should be discontinued.

Hyperammonemia may occur with therapy and may be present with normal liver function tests. Ammonia levels should be measured in patients who develop unexplained lethargy and vomiting, or changes in mental status. Discontinue therapy if ammonia levels are increased and evaluate for possible UCD.

In vitro studies have suggested valproate stimulates the replication of HIV and CMV viruses under experimental conditions. The clinical consequence of this is unknown, but should be considered when monitoring affected patients.

Anticonvulsants should not be discontinued abruptly because of the possibility of increasing seizure frequency; valproate should be withdrawn gradually to minimize the potential of increased seizure frequency, unless safety concerns require a more rapid withdrawal. Concomitant use with clonazepam may induce absence status.

CNS depression may occur with valproate use. Patients must be cautioned about performing tasks which require mental alertness (operating machinery or driving). Effects with other sedative drugs or ethanol may be potentiated.

Drug Interactions

Cytochrome P450 Effect: For valproic acid: **Substrate** (minor) of CYP2A6, 2B6, 2C8/9, 2C19, 2E1; **Inhibits** CYP2C8/9 (weak), 2C19 (weak), 2D6 (weak), 3A4 (weak); **Induces** CYP2A6 (weak)

Decreased Effect: Valproic acid may displace clozapine from protein binding site resulting in decreased clozapine serum concentrations. Cholestyramine (and possibly colestipol) may bind valproic acid in GI tract, decreasing absorption. Acyclovir may reduce valproic acid levels. Mefloquine may decrease serum concentration of valproic acid. Carbapenem antibiotics (ertapenem, imipenem, meropenem) may decrease valproic acid concentrations to subtherapeutic levels; monitor.

Increased Effect/Toxicity: Absence seizures have been reported in patients receiving VPA and clonazepam. Valproic acid may increase, decrease, or have no effect on carbamazepine and phenytoin levels. Valproic acid may increase serum concentrations of carbamazepine - epoxide (active metabolite). Valproic acid may increase serum concentrations of diazepam, lamotrigine, nimodipine, and phenobarbital, and tricyclic antidepressants. Chlorpromazine (and possibly other phenothiazines), macrolide antibiotics (clarithromycin, erythromycin, troleandomycin), felbamate, and isoniazid may inhibit the metabolism of valproic acid. Aspirin or other salicylates may displace valproic acid from protein-binding sites, leading to acute toxicity.

Nutritional/Ethanol Interactions

Ethanol: Avoid ethanol (may increase CNS depression).

Food: Food may delay but does not affect the extent of absorption. Valproic acid serum concentrations may be decreased if taken with food. Milk has no effect on absorption.

Herb/Nutraceutical: Avoid evening primrose (seizure threshold decreased)

Lab Interactions
Valproic acid may cause abnormalities in liver function tests; false-positive result for urine ketones; accuracy of thyroid function tests

Adverse Reactions

Adverse reactions reported when used as monotherapy for complex partial seizure:

>10%:
Central nervous system: Somnolence (18% to 30%), dizziness (13% to 18%), insomnia (9% to 15%), nervousness (7% to 11%)

Dermatologic: Alopecia (13% to 24%)

Gastrointestinal: Nausea (26% to 34%), diarrhea (19% to 23%), vomiting (15% to 23%), abdominal pain (9% to 12%), dyspepsia (10% to 11%), anorexia (4% to 11%)

Hematologic: Thrombocytopenia (1% to 24%)

Neuromuscular & skeletal: Tremor (19% to 57%), weakness (10% to 21%)

Respiratory: Respiratory tract infection (13% to 20%), pharyngitis (2% to 8%), dyspnea (1% to 5%)

1% to 10%:
Cardiovascular: Hypertension, palpitation, peripheral edema (3% to 8%), tachycardia, chest pain

Central nervous system: Amnesia (4% to 7%), abnormal dreams, anxiety, confusion, depression (4% to 5%), malaise, personality disorder

Dermatologic: Bruising (4% to 5%), dry skin, petechia, pruritus, rash

Endocrine & metabolic: Amenorrhea, dysmenorrhea

Gastrointestinal: Eructation, flatulence, hematemesis, increased appetite, pancreatitis, periodontal abscess, taste perversion, weight gain (4% to 9%)

Genitourinary: Urinary frequency, urinary incontinence, vaginitis

Hepatic: AST and ALT increased

Neuromuscular & skeletal: Abnormal gait, arthralgia, back pain, hypertonia, incoordination, leg cramps, myalgia, myasthenia, paresthesia, twitching

Ocular: Amblyopia/blurred vision (4% to 8%), abnormal vision, nystagmus (1% to 7%)

Otic: Deafness, otitis media, tinnitus (1% to 7%)

Respiratory: Epistaxis, increased cough, pneumonia, sinusitis

Additional adverse effects: Frequency not defined:
Cardiovascular: Bradycardia

Central nervous system: Aggression, ataxia, behavioral deterioration, cerebral atrophy (reversible), dementia, emotional upset, encephalopathy (rare), fever, hallucinations, headache, hostility, hyperactivity, hypoesthesia, incoordination, Parkinsonism, psychosis, vertigo

Dermatologic: Cutaneous vasculitis, erythema multiforme, photosensitivity, Stevens-Johnson syndrome, toxic epidermal necrolysis (rare)

Endocrine & metabolic: Breast enlargement, galactorrhea, hyperammonemia, hyponatremia, inappropriate ADH secretion, irregular menses, parotid gland swelling, polycystic ovary disease (rare), abnormal thyroid function tests

Genitourinary: Enuresis, urinary tract infection

Hematologic: Anemia, aplastic anemia, bone marrow suppression, eosinophilia, hematoma formation, hemorrhage, hypofibrinogenemia, intermittent porphyria, leukopenia, lymphocytosis, macrocytosis, pancytopenia

Hepatic: Bilirubin increased, hyperammonemic encephalopathy (in patients with UCD)

Neuromuscular & skeletal: Asterixis, bone pain, dysarthria

Ocular: Diplopia, "spots before the eyes"

Renal: Fanconi-like syndrome (rare, in children)

Miscellaneous: Anaphylaxis, decreased carnitine, hyperglycinemia, lupus

Overdosage/Toxicology Symptoms of overdose include coma, deep sleep, motor restlessness, and visual hallucinations. Supportive treatment is necessary. Naloxone has been used to reverse CNS depressant effects, but may block the action of other anticonvulsants.

Pharmacodynamics/Kinetics

Bioavailability: Extended release: 90% of I.V. dose and 81% to 90% of delayed release dose

Time to Peak: Serum: 1-4 hours; Divalproex (enteric coated): 3-5 hours

Protein Binding: Dose dependent: 80% to 90%

Half-Life Elimination: Increased in neonates and with liver disease; Children: 4-14 hours; Adults: 9-16 hours

Metabolism: Extensively hepatic via glucuronide conjugation and mitochondrial beta-oxidation. The relationship between dose and total valproate concentration is nonlinear; concentration does not increase proportionally with the dose, but increases to a lesser extent due to saturable plasma protein binding. The kinetics of unbound drug are linear.

Excretion: Urine (30% to 50% as glucuronide conjugate, 3% as unchanged drug)

Dosing

Adults & Elderly:

Seizures:

Oral: Initial: 10-15 mg/kg/day in 1-3 divided doses; increase by 5-10 mg/kg/day at weekly intervals until therapeutic levels are achieved; maintenance: 30-60 mg/kg/day. Adult usual dose: 1000-2500 mg/day. **Note:** Regular release and delayed release formulations are usually given in 2-4 divided doses/day, extended release formulation (Depakote® ER) is usually given once daily. Conversion to Depakote® ER from a stable dose of Depakote® may require an increase in the total daily dose between 8% and 20% to maintain similar serum concentrations.

I.V.: Administer as a 60-minute infusion (≤20 mg/minute) with the same frequency as oral products; switch patient to oral products as soon as possible. Alternatively, rapid infusions have been given: ≤15 mg/kg over 5-10 minutes (1.5-3 mg/minute).

Rectal (unlabeled): Dilute syrup 1:1 with water for use as a retention enema; loading dose: 17-20 mg/kg one time; maintenance: 10-15 mg/kg/dose every 8 hours

Status epilepticus (unlabeled use):

Loading dose: I.V.: 15-25 mg/kg administered at 3 mg/kg/minute

Maintenance dose: I.V. infusion: 1-4 mg/kg/hour; titrate dose as needed based upon patient response and evaluation of drug-drug interactions

Mania:

Oral: 750-1500 mg/day in divided doses; dose should be adjusted as rapidly as possible to desired clinical effect; a loading dose of 20 mg/kg may be used; maximum recommended dosage: 60 mg/kg/day

Migraine prophylaxis: Oral:

Extended release tablets: 500 mg once daily for 7 days, then increase to 1000 mg once daily; adjust dose based on patient response; usual dosage range 500-1000 mg/day

Delayed release tablets: 250 mg twice daily; adjust dose based on patient response, up to 1000 mg/day

Pediatrics: Seizures: Oral, I.V., Rectal: Children >10 years: Refer to adult dosing.

Renal Impairment: A 27% reduction in clearance of unbound valproate is seen in patients with Cl_{cr} <10 mL/minute. Hemodialysis reduces valproate concentrations by 20%, therefore no dose adjustment is needed in patients with renal failure. Protein binding is reduced, monitoring only total valproate concentrations may be misleading.

Hepatic Impairment: Dosage reduction is required. Clearance is decreased with liver impairment. Hepatic disease is also associated with decreased albumin concentrations and 2- to 2.6-fold increase in the unbound fraction. Free concentrations of valproate may be elevated while total concentrations appear normal.

Available Dosage Forms

Capsule, as valproic acid (Depakene®): 250 mg

Capsule, sprinkles, as divalproex sodium (Depakote® Sprinkle®): 125 mg

Injection, solution, as valproate sodium (Depacon®): 100 mg/mL (5 mL)

Syrup, as valproic acid: 250 mg/5 mL (5 mL, 480 mL)

Depakene®: 250 mg/5 mL (480 mL)

Tablet, delayed release, as divalproex sodium (Depakote®): 125 mg, 250 mg, 500 mg

Tablet, extended release, as divalproex sodium (Depakote® ER): 250 mg, 500 mg

Monitoring and Teaching Issues

Physical Assessment: Assess effectiveness and interactions of other medications patient may be taking. **I.V.:** Keep patient under observation, observe safety/seizure precautions, and monitor therapeutic effectiveness (type of seizure activity, force, and duration). Monitor vital signs; neurological, cardiac, and respiratory status. For outpatients, monitor therapeutic effect, laboratory values, and adverse reactions at beginning of therapy and periodically with long-term use. Taper dosage slowly when discontinuing. Assess knowledge/teach patient seizure safety precautions, appropriate use, interventions to reduce side effects, and adverse symptoms to report. **Note:** Valproic acid will alter results of urine ketones (use serum glucose testing) and reduce effectiveness of oral contraceptives (use alternative form of contraception to prevent pregnancy). Some adverse reactions including hepatic failure and thrombocytopenia can occur 3 days to 6 months after beginning therapy.

(Continued)

Valproic Acid and Derivatives *(Continued)*

Monitoring Laboratory Tests: Liver enzymes, CBC with platelets, ammonium levels

Patient Education: When used to treat generalized seizures, patient instructions are determined by patient's condition and ability to understand. Oral: Take as directed; do not alter dose or timing of medication. Do not increase dose or take more than recommended. Do not crush or chew capsule or enteric-coated pill. While using this medication, do not use alcohol and other prescription or OTC medications (especially pain medications, sedatives, antihistamines, or hypnotics) without consulting prescriber. Maintain adequate hydration (2-3 L/day of fluids) unless instructed to restrict fluid intake. If you have diabetes, monitor serum glucose closely (valproic acid will alter results of urine ketones). Report alterations in menstrual cycle; abdominal cramps, unresolved diarrhea, vomiting, or constipation; skin rash; unusual bruising or bleeding; blood in urine, stool, or vomitus; malaise; weakness; facial swelling; yellowing of skin or eyes; persistent abdominal pain; excessive sedation; or restlessness. **Pregnancy/breast-feeding precautions:** Do not get pregnant while taking this medication; use appropriate contraceptive measures. Consult prescriber if breast-feeding.

Dietary Considerations: Valproic acid may cause GI upset; take with large amount of water or food to decrease GI upset. May need to split doses to avoid GI upset.

Coated particles of divalproex sodium may be mixed with semisolid food (eg, applesauce or pudding) in patients having difficulty swallowing; particles should be swallowed and not chewed

Valproate sodium oral solution will generate valproic acid in carbonated beverages and may cause mouth and throat irritation; do not mix valproate sodium oral solution with carbonated beverages; sodium content of valproate sodium syrup (5 mL): 23 mg (1 mEq)

Pregnancy Risk Factor: D

Pregnancy Issues: Crosses the placenta. Neural tube, cardiac, facial (characteristic pattern of dysmorphic facial features), skeletal, multiple other defects reported. Epilepsy itself, number of medications, genetic factors, or a combination of these probably influence the teratogenicity of anticonvulsant therapy. Risk of neural tube defects with use during first 30 days of pregnancy warrants discontinuation prior to pregnancy and through this period of possible. Use in women of childbearing potential requires that benefits of use in mother be weighed against the potential risk to fetus, especially when used for conditions not associated with permanent injury or risk of death (eg, migraine).

Lactation: Enters breast milk/use caution (AAP considers "compatible")

Breast-Feeding Issues: Crosses into breast milk. AAP considers **compatible** with breast-feeding.

Administration

Oral: Do not crush delayed release or extended release drug product or capsules.

I.V.: Depacon®: Following dilution to final concentration, administer over 60 minutes at a rate of ≤20 mg/minute. Alternatively, single doses up to 15 mg/kg have been administered as a rapid infusion over 5-10 minutes (1.5-3 mg/kg/minute).

Reconstitution: Injection should be diluted in 50 mL of a compatible diluent; is physically compatible and chemically stable in D₅W, NS, and LR for at least 24 hours when stored in glass or PVC.

Storage: Store vials at room temperature 15°C to 30°C (59°F to 86°F).

Additional Information Extended release tablets have 10% to 20% less fluctuation in serum concentration than delayed release tablets. Extended release tablets are not bioequivalent to delayed release tablets.

Related Information

Anticonvulsants By Seizure Type *on page 1712*
Maternal / Fetal Toxicology *on page 1762*
Peak and Trough Guidelines *on page 1694*

Valrubicin *(val ROO bi sin)*

U.S. Brand Names Valstar® [DSC]

Synonyms AD3L; *N*-Trifluoroacetyladriamycin-14-Valerate

Generic Available No

Pharmacologic Category Antineoplastic Agent, Anthracycline

Medication Safety Issues

Sound-alike/look-alike issues:

Valstar® may be confused with valsartan

Use Intravesical therapy of BCG-refractory carcinoma *in situ* of the urinary bladder

Mechanism of Action/Effect Blocks function of DNA topoisomerase II; inhibits DNA synthesis, causes extensive chromosomal damage, and arrests cell development; unlike other anthracyclines, does not appear to intercalate DNA

Contraindications Hypersensitivity to anthracyclines, Cremophor® EL, or any component of the formulation; concurrent urinary tract infection or small bladder capacity (unable to tolerate a 75 mL instillation)

Warnings/Precautions The U.S. Food and Drug Administration (FDA) currently recommends that procedures for proper handling and disposal of antineoplastic agents be considered. Appropriate safety equipment is recommended for preparation, administration, and disposal of antineoplastics. If valrubicin contacts the skin, wash and flush thoroughly with water. Do not administer if mucosal integrity of bladder has been compromised or bladder perforation is present. Irritable bladder symptoms may occur during instillation and retention. Caution in patients with severe irritable bladder symptoms. Valrubicin should be used cautiously (if at all) in patients having a history of hypersensitivity reactions to other medications prepared with Cremophor® EL, although not reported with valrubicin.

Drug Interactions

Decreased Effect: No specific drug interactions studies have been performed. Systemic exposure to valrubicin is negligible, and interactions are unlikely.

Increased Effect/Toxicity: No specific drug interactions studies have been performed. Systemic exposure to valrubicin is negligible, and interactions are unlikely.

Adverse Reactions

>10%: Genitourinary: Frequency (61%), dysuria (56%), urgency (57%), bladder spasm (31%), hematuria (29%), bladder pain (28%), urinary incontinence (22%), cystitis (15%), urinary tract infection (15%)

1% to 10%:

Cardiovascular: Chest pain (2%), vasodilation (2%), peripheral edema (1%)

Central nervous system: Headache (4%), malaise (4%), dizziness (3%), fever (2%)

Dermatologic: Rash (3%)

Endocrine & metabolic: Hyperglycemia (1%)

Gastrointestinal: Abdominal pain (5%), nausea (5%), diarrhea (3%), vomiting (2%), flatulence (1%)

Genitourinary: Nocturia (7%), burning symptoms (5%), urinary retention (4%), urethral pain (3%), pelvic pain (1%), hematuria (microscopic) (3%)

Hematologic: Anemia (2%)

Neuromuscular & skeletal: Weakness (4%), back pain (3%), myalgia (1%)

Respiratory: Pneumonia (1%)

Overdosage/Toxicology Inadvertent paravenous extravasation has not been associated with skin ulceration or necrosis. Myelosuppression is possible following inadvertent systemic administration, or following significant systemic absorption from intravesical instillation.

Pharmacodynamics/Kinetics

Absorption: Well absorbed into bladder tissue, negligible systemic absorption. Trauma to mucosa may increase absorption, and perforation greatly increases absorption with significant systemic myelotoxicity.

Metabolism: Negligible after intravesical instillation and 2 hour retention

Excretion: Urine when expelled from urinary bladder (98.6% as intact drug; 0.4% as N-trifluoroacetyladriamycin)

Dosing

Adults & Elderly: Urinary carcinoma in situ: Intravesical: 800 mg once weekly for 6 weeks

Renal Impairment: No adjustment is necessary.

Hepatic Impairment: No adjustment necessary.

Available Dosage Forms [DSC] = Discontinued product

Injection, solution [DSC]: 40 mg/mL (5 mL) [contains Cremophor® EL 50% (polyoxyethyleneglycol triricinoleate) and dehydrated alcohol 50%]

Monitoring and Teaching Issues

Physical Assessment: This medication is administered by a physician through a urinary bladder catheter, using aseptic technique. **Note:** Caution must be used to prevent exposure to this mediation (see Warnings/Precautions). Assess patient response during and following instillation (genitourinary [frequency, urgency, incontinence or dysuria, bladder spasm or pain, hematuria, urinary tract infection], rash, nausea, vomiting, myalgia, hyperglycemia; see Adverse Reactions). Instruct patient on appropriate interventions to reduce side effects and adverse symptoms to report (See Patient Education).

Monitoring Laboratory Tests: Cystoscopy, biopsy, and urine cytology every 3 months for recurrence or progression

Patient Education: This medication will be instilled into your bladder through a catheter to be retained for as long as possible. Your urine will be red tinged for the next 24 hours; report promptly if this continues for a longer period. May cause altered urination patterns (frequency, dysuria, or incontinence), some bladder pain, pain on urination, or pelvic pain; report if these persist. If you have diabetes, monitor glucose levels closely (may cause hyperglycemia). It is important that you maintain adequate hydration (2-3 L/day of fluids) unless instructed to restrict fluid intake. May cause dizziness or fatigue (use caution when driving or engaging in tasks requiring alertness until response to drug is known); or nausea, vomiting, or taste disturbance (small frequent meals, frequent mouth care, chewing gum, or sucking lozenges may help). Report chest pain or palpitations; persistent dizziness; swelling of extremities; persistent nausea, vomiting, diarrhea, or abdominal pain; muscle weakness, pain, or tremors; unusual cough or respiratory difficulty; or other adverse effects. **Pregnancy/breast-feeding precautions:** Inform prescriber if you are pregnant. Do not get pregnant while taking this medication and for 1 month following therapy; consult prescriber for appropriate contraceptives. Breast-feeding is not recommended.

Pregnancy Risk Factor: C

Lactation: Excretion in breast milk unknown/not recommended

Breast-Feeding Issues: It is not known whether valrubicin is secreted in human milk. Because many immunoglobulins are secreted in milk, and the potential for serious adverse reactions exists, a decision should be made whether to discontinue nursing or discontinue the drug, taking into account the importance of the drug to the mother.

Administration

I.V.: Valrubicin is administered as an intravesicular bladder lavage, usually in 75 mL of 0.9% sodium chloride injection. The drug is retained in the bladder for 2 hours, then voided. Due to the Cremophor® EL diluent, valrubicin should be administered through non-PVC tubing.

Reconstitution: Allow vial to warm to room temperature without heating. Dilute 800 mg (20 mL) with 55 mL NS.

Storage: Store unopened vials under refrigeration at 2°C to 8°C (36°F to 48°F). Stable for 12 hours when diluted in 0.9% sodium chloride.

Valsartan (val SAR tan)

U.S. Brand Names Diovan®

Generic Available No

Pharmacologic Category Angiotensin II Receptor Blocker

Medication Safety Issues

Sound-alike/look-alike issues:

Valsartan may be confused with losartan, Valstar™

Diovan® may be confused with Darvon®, Dioval®, Zyban®

(Continued)

Valsartan *(Continued)*

Use Alone or in combination with other antihypertensive agents in treating essential hypertension; treatment of heart failure (NYHA Class II-IV) in patients intolerant to angiotensin converting enzyme (ACE) inhibitors

Mechanism of Action/Effect Valsartan produces direct antagonism of the angiotensin II (AT2) receptors. Valsartan blocks the vasoconstrictor and aldosterone-secreting effects of angiotensin II. It displaces angiotensin II from the AT1 receptor and produces its blood pressure lowering effects by antagonizing AT1-induced vasoconstriction, aldosterone release, catecholamine release, arginine vasopressin release, water intake, and hypertrophic responses. This action results in more efficient blockade of the cardiovascular effects of angiotensin II and fewer side effects than the ACE inhibitors.

Contraindications Hypersensitivity to valsartan or any component of the formulation; hypersensitivity to other A-II receptor antagonists; bilateral renal artery stenosis; pregnancy (2nd and 3rd trimesters)

Warnings/Precautions Avoid use or use a smaller dose in patients who are volume depleted; correct depletion first. Deterioration in renal function can occur with initiation. Use with caution in unilateral renal artery stenosis and pre-existing renal insufficiency; significant aortic/mitral stenosis. Use caution in patients with severe renal impairment or significant hepatic dysfunction.

Heart failure: Concomitant use of valsartan, an ACE inhibitor, and a beta-blocker is not recommended; this combination has been associated with unfavorable outcomes in clinical trials. Monitor renal function closely in patients with severe heart failure; changes in renal function should be anticipated and dosage adjustments of valsartan or concomitant medications may be needed.

Drug Interactions

Cytochrome P450 Effect: Inhibits CYP2C8/9 (weak)

Decreased Effect: Phenobarbital, ketoconazole, troleandomycin, sulfaphenazole

Increased Effect/Toxicity: Valsartan blood levels may be increased by cimetidine and monoxidine; clinical effect is unknown. Concurrent use of potassium salts/supplements, co-trimoxazole (high dose), ACE inhibitors, and potassium-sparing diuretics (amiloride, spironolactone, triamterene) may increase the risk of hyperkalemia.

Nutritional/Ethanol Interactions

Food: Decreases rate and extent of absorption by 50% and 40%, respectively.

Herb/Nutraceutical: Avoid dong quai if using for hypertension (has estrogenic activity). Avoid ephedra, yohimbe, ginseng (may worsen hypertension). Avoid garlic (may have increased antihypertensive effect).

Adverse Reactions

Hypertension: Similar incidence to placebo; independent of race, age, and gender.

>1%:

Central nervous system: Dizziness (2% to 8%), fatigue (2%)

Endocrine & metabolic: Serum potassium increased (4.4%)

Gastrointestinal: Abdominal pain (2%)

Hematologic: Neutropenia (1.9%)

Respiratory: Cough (2.6% versus 1.5% in placebo)

Miscellaneous: Viral infection (3%)

>1% but frequency ≤ placebo: Headache, upper respiratory infection, cough, diarrhea, rhinitis, sinusitis, nausea, pharyngitis, edema, arthralgia

Heart failure:

>10%: Central nervous system: Dizziness (17%)

1% to 10%:

Cardiovascular: Hypotension (7%), postural hypotension (2%)

Central nervous system: Fatigue (3%)

Endocrine & metabolic: Hyperkalemia (2%)

Gastrointestinal: Diarrhea (5%)

Neuromuscular & skeletal: Arthralgia (3%), back pain (3%)

Renal: Creatinine increased >50% (4%)

Overdosage/Toxicology Only mild toxicity (hypotension, bradycardia, hyperkalemia) has been reported with large overdoses (up to 5 g of captopril and 300 mg of enalapril). No fatalities have been reported. Treatment is symptomatic. Not removed by hemodialysis.

Pharmacodynamics/Kinetics

Onset of Action: Peak antihypertensive effect: 2-4 weeks

Bioavailability: 25% (range 10% to 35%)

Time to Peak: 2-4 hours

Protein Binding: 95%, primarily albumin

Half-Life Elimination: 6 hours

Metabolism: To inactive metabolite

Excretion: Feces (83%) and urine (13%) as unchanged drug

Dosing

Adults & Elderly:

Hypertension: Oral: Initial: 80 mg or 160 mg once daily (in patients who are not volume depleted); majority of effect within 2 weeks, maximal effects in 4-6 weeks; dose may be increased to achieve desired effect; maximum recommended dose: 320 mg/day

Heart failure: Oral: Initial: 40 mg twice daily; titrate dose to 80-160 mg twice daily, as tolerated; maximum daily dose: 320 mg. **Note:** Do not use with ACE inhibitors and beta blockers.

Renal Impairment:

Cl_{cr} >10 mL/minute: No dosage adjustment necessary.

Dialysis: Not significantly removed.

Hepatic Impairment: Mild to moderate liver disease: ≤80 mg/day

Available Dosage Forms Tablet: 40 mg, 80 mg, 160 mg, 320 mg

Monitoring and Teaching Issues

Physical Assessment: Use caution with volume depletion, impaired renal or hepatic function, aortic/mitral stenosis (see Warnings/Precautions for use cautions). Assess effectiveness and interactions of other pharmacological agents and herbal products patients may be taking (eg, concurrent use of potassium supplements, ACE inhibitors, potassium-sparing diuretics may increase risk of hyperkalemia; see Drug Interactions). Assess results of laboratory tests at baseline and periodically. Monitor therapeutic effectiveness (reduced hypertension) and adverse response on a regular basis during therapy (eg, dizziness, bradycardia, cough, headache, nausea, hypotension, hyperkalemia; see Adverse Reactions). Teach patient appropriate use according to drug form and purpose of therapy, possible side effects/appropriate interventions, and adverse symptoms to report (see Patient Education).

Monitoring Laboratory Tests: Baseline and periodic electrolyte panels, renal and liver function, urinalysis

Patient Education: Do not take any new medication during therapy unless approved by prescriber (especially sleep remedies or antisleep, cough or cold remedies, or weight loss products). Take exactly as directed and do not discontinue without consulting prescriber. This drug does not eliminate need for diet or exercise regimen as recommended by prescriber. May cause dizziness, fainting, or lightheadedness (use caution when driving or engaging in tasks that require alertness until response to drug is known); postural hypotension (use caution when rising from lying or sitting position or climbing stairs); diarrhea (boiled milk, buttermilk, or yogurt may help); or decreased libido (will resolve). Report chest pain or palpitations; unrelenting headache; swelling of extremities, face, or tongue; muscle weakness or pain; respiratory difficulty or unusual cough; flu-like symptoms; or other persistent adverse reactions. **Pregnancy/breast-feeding precautions:** Inform prescriber if you are or intend to become pregnant. This drug should not be used in the 2nd or 3rd trimester of pregnancy. Consult prescriber for appropriate contraceptive measures if necessary. Do not breast-feed.

Dietary Considerations: Avoid salt substitutes which contain potassium. May be taken with or without food.

Pregnancy Risk Factor: C/D (2nd and 3rd trimesters)

Pregnancy Issues: Medications which act on the renin-angiotensin system are reported to have the following fetal/neonatal effects: Hypotension, neonatal skull hypoplasia, anuria, renal failure, and death; oligohydramnios is also reported. These effects are reported to occur with exposure during the 2nd and 3rd trimesters. Valsartan should be discontinued as soon as possible after pregnancy is detected.

Lactation: Excretion in breast milk unknown/contraindicated

Administration

Oral: Administer with or without food.

Storage: Store at controlled room temperature of 15°C to 30°C (59°F to 86°F). Protect from moisture.

Additional Information Valsartan may have an advantage over losartan due to minimal metabolism requirements and consequent use in mild to moderate hepatic impairment.

Related Information

Angiotensin Agents *on page 1704*

Valsartan and Hydrochlorothiazide

(val SAR tan & hye droe klor oh THYE a zide)

U.S. Brand Names Diovan HCT®

Synonyms Hydrochlorothiazide and Valsartan

Generic Available No

Pharmacologic Category Angiotensin II Receptor Blocker Combination; Antihypertensive Agent, Combination; Diuretic, Thiazide

Medication Safety Issues

Sound-alike/look-alike issues:

Diovan® may be confused with Darvon®, Dioval®, Zyban®

Use Treatment of hypertension (not indicated for initial therapy)

Dosing

Adults & Elderly: Hypertension: Oral: Dose is individualized (combination substituted for individual components); dose may be titrated after 3-4 weeks of therapy.

Usual recommended starting dose of valsartan: 80 mg or 160 mg once daily when used as monotherapy in patients who are not volume depleted

Renal Impairment: Cl$_{cr}$ ≤30 mL/minute: Use of combination not recommended. Contraindicated in patients with anuria.

Hepatic Impairment: Use with caution.

Available Dosage Forms Tablet:

80 mg/12.5 mg: Valsartan 80 mg and hydrochlorothiazide 12.5 mg
160 mg/12.5 mg: Valsartan 160 mg and hydrochlorothiazide 12.5 mg
160 mg/25 mg: Valsartan 160 mg and hydrochlorothiazide 25 mg

Monitoring and Teaching Issues

Physical Assessment: See individual agents.

Patient Education: See individual agents. **Pregnancy/breast-feeding precautions:** Inform prescriber if you are or intend to become pregnant. Breast-feeding is not recommended.

Pregnancy Risk Factor: C/D (2nd and 3rd trimester)

Lactation: Excretion in breast milk unknown/not recommended

Related Information

Hydrochlorothiazide *on page 751*
Valsartan *on page 1547*

♦ **Valstar® [DSC]** *see* Valrubicin *on page 1546*

♦ **Valtrex®** *see* Valacyclovir *on page 1538*

♦ **Vancocin®** *see* Vancomycin *on page 1550*

Vancomycin (van koe MYE sin)

U.S. Brand Names Vancocin®

Synonyms Vancomycin Hydrochloride

Generic Available Yes: Injection

Pharmacologic Category Antibiotic, Miscellaneous

Medication Safety Issues

Sound-alike/look-alike issues:

I.V. vancomycin may be confused with Invanz®

Vancomycin may be confused with vecuronium

Use Treatment of patients with infections caused by staphylococcal species and streptococcal species; used orally for staphylococcal enterocolitis or for antibiotic-associated pseudomembranous colitis produced by *C. difficile*

Mechanism of Action/Effect Inhibits bacterial cell wall synthesis

Contraindications Hypersensitivity to vancomycin or any component of the formulation; avoid in patients with previous severe hearing loss

Warnings/Precautions Use with caution in patients with renal impairment or those receiving other nephrotoxic or ototoxic drugs. Dosage modification is required in patients with impaired renal function (especially elderly).

Drug Interactions

Increased Effect/Toxicity: Increased toxicity with other ototoxic or nephrotoxic drugs. Increased neuromuscular blockade with most neuromuscular blocking agents.

Adverse Reactions

Oral:

>10%: Gastrointestinal: Bitter taste, nausea, vomiting

1% to 10%:

Central nervous system: Chills, drug fever

Hematologic: Eosinophilia

Parenteral:

>10%:

Cardiovascular: Hypotension accompanied by flushing

Dermatologic: Erythematous rash on face and upper body (red neck or red man syndrome - infusion rate related)

1% to 10%:

Central nervous system: Chills, drug fever

Dermatologic: Rash

Hematologic: Eosinophilia, reversible neutropenia

Overdosage/Toxicology Symptoms of overdose include ototoxicity and nephrotoxicity. There is no specific therapy for overdose with vancomycin. Care is symptomatic and supportive. Peritoneal filtration and hemofiltration (not dialysis) have been shown to reduce the serum concentration of vancomycin. High flux dialysis may remove up to 25% of the drug.

Pharmacodynamics/Kinetics

Absorption: Oral: Poor; I.M.: Erratic; Intraperitoneal: ~38%

Time to Peak: Serum: I.V.: 45-65 minutes

Protein Binding: 10% to 50%

Half-Life Elimination: Biphasic: Terminal:

Newborns: 6-10 hours

Infants and Children 3 months to 4 years: 4 hours

Children >3 years: 2.2-3 hours

Adults: 5-11 hours; significantly prolonged with renal impairment

End-stage renal disease: 200-250 hours

Excretion: I.V.: Urine (80% to 90% as unchanged drug); Oral: Primarily feces

Dosing

Adults:

Systemic infections: I.V.: Initial dosage recommendation: Normal renal function: 1 g every 12 hours **or** select individualized dosage based on weight (10-15 mg/kg)

Note: Select interval based on estimated Cl_{cr} >60 mL/minute every 12 hours, 40-60 mL/minute every 24 hours, <40 mL/minute every 24 hours; monitor levels.

Prophylaxis for bacterial endocarditis: I.V.:

Dental, oral, or upper respiratory tract surgery: 1 g 1 hour before surgery

GI/GU procedure: 1 g plus 1.5 mg/kg gentamicin 1 hour prior to surgery

CNS infections:

Intrathecal: **Note:** Vancomycin is available as a powder for injection and may be diluted to 1-5 mg/mL concentration in preservative-free 0.9% sodium chloride for administration into the CSF. Dose: Up to 20 mg/day

Antibiotic lock technique (for catheter infections): 2 mg/mL in SWI/NS or D_5W; instill 3-5 mL into catheter port as a flush solution instead of heparin lock. (**Note:** Do not mix with any other solutions.)

Intrathecal: 20 mg/day; vancomycin is available as a powder for injection and may be diluted to 1-5 mg/mL concentration in preservative free 0.9% sodium chloride for administration into the CSF.

Pseudomembranous colitis produced by *C. difficile*: Oral: 125 mg 4 times/day for 10 days. **Note:** Due to the emergence of resistant enterococci, the use of vancomycin is limited in most settings

Elderly: Elderly patients may require greater dosage reduction than expected. Best to individualize therapy; dose (mg/kg/24 hours) = $(0.227 \times Cl_{cr})$ + 5.67. Refer to adult dosing.

Pediatrics:

Systemic infections: Initial dosage recommendation: I.V.:

Neonates:

Postnatal age ≤7 days:

<1200 g: 15 mg/kg/dose every 24 hours

≥1200 g: 10 mg/kg/dose divided every 8 hours

>2000 g: 15 mg/kg/dose every 12 hours

Postnatal age >7 days:

<1200 g: 15 mg/kg/dose every 24 hours

≥1200 g: 10 mg/kg/dose divided every 8 hours

Infants >1 month and Children: 40 mg/kg/day in divided doses every 6 hours

Prophylaxis for bacterial endocarditis: I.V.:

Dental, oral, or upper respiratory tract surgery: 20 mg/kg 1 hour prior to the procedure

GI/GU procedure: 20 mg/kg plus gentamicin 2 mg/kg 1 hour prior to surgery

CNS infections:

Intrathecal: **Note:** Vancomycin is available as a powder for injection and may be diluted to 1-5 mg/mL concentration in preservative-free 0.9% sodium chloride for administration into the CSF

Neonates: 5-10 mg/day

Children: 5-20 mg/day

I.V.: Infants >1 month and Children with staphylococcal central nervous system infection: 60 mg/kg/day in divided doses every 6 hours

Antibiotic lock technique (for catheter infections): 2 mg/mL in SWI/NS or D_5W; instill 3-5 mL into catheter port as a flush solution instead of heparin lock (**Note:** Do not mix with any other solutions)

Pseudomembranous colitis produced by *C. difficile:* **Oral:**

Neonates: 10 mg/kg/day in divided doses

Children: 40 mg/kg/day in divided doses, added to fluids

Note: Use is restricted in most settings

Renal Impairment: Vancomycin levels should be monitored in patients with any renal impairment.

Cl_{cr} >60 mL/minute: Start with 1 g or 10-15 mg/kg/dose every 12 hours.

Cl_{cr} 40-60 mL/minute: Start with 1 g or 10-15 mg/kg/dose every 24 hours.

Cl_{cr} <40 mL/minute: Will need longer intervals; determine by serum concentration monitoring.

Hemodialysis: Not dialyzable (0% to 5%); generally not removed; exception minimal-moderate removal by some of the newer high-flux filters. Dose may need to be administered more frequently. Monitor serum concentrations.

Continuous ambulatory peritoneal dialysis (CAPD): Not significantly removed; administration via CAPD fluid: 15-30 mg/L (15-30 mcg/mL) of CAPD fluid.

Continuous arteriovenous hemofiltration: Dose as for Cl_{cr} 10-40 mL/minute.

Antibiotic lock technique (for catheter infections): 2 mg/mL in SWI/NS or D_5W; instill 3-5 mL into catheter port as a flush solution instead of heparin lock (**Note:** Do not mix with any other solutions).

Hepatic Impairment: Reduce dose by 60%.

Available Dosage Forms

Capsule (Vancocin®): 125 mg, 250 mg

Infusion [premixed in iso-osmotic dextrose] (Vancocin®): 500 mg (100 mL); 1 g (200 mL)

Injection, powder for reconstitution: 500 mg, 1 g, 5 g, 10 g

Monitoring and Teaching Issues

Physical Assessment: Assess results of culture and sensitivity tests and patient's allergy history prior to first dose. Use caution with renal impairment (see Warnings/Precautions). Assess potential for interactions with other pharmacological agents patient may be taking (eg, concurrent use with anything that is ototoxic or nephrotoxic increases risk of toxicity; see Drug Interactions). See Administration for infusion specifics (premedication with antihistamines may prevent or minimize "Red man" reaction). Infusion site must be monitored closely to prevent extravasation. Assess results of laboratory tests, therapeutic effectiveness (resolution of infection), and adverse response on a regular basis during therapy (eg, hypotension, rash, neutropenia, nausea, vomiting, auditory changes; see Adverse Reactions). Teach patient appropriate use (oral), possible side effects/appropriate interventions, and adverse symptoms to report (See Patient Education).

Monitoring Laboratory Tests: Perform culture and sensitivity studies prior to first dose. Periodic renal function, urinalysis, serum vancomycin concentrations, WBC, audiogram with prolonged use. Obtain drug levels after the third dose unless otherwise directed. Peaks are drawn 1 hour after the completion of a 1- to 2-hour infusion. Troughs are obtained just before the next dose.

Patient Education: Do not take any new medication during therapy unless approved by prescriber. With I.V. use, report immediately any chills; pain, swelling, or redness at infusion site; or respiratory difficulty. **Pregnancy/breast-feeding precautions:** Inform prescriber if you are or intend to become pregnant. Consult prescriber if breast-feeding.

Oral: Take as directed with food, for as long as prescribed. Maintain adequate hydration (2-3 L/day of fluids) unless instructed to restrict fluid intake.

Oral/I.V.: May cause nausea, vomiting, or GI upset (small frequent meals, frequent mouth care, sucking lozenges, or chewing gum may help). Report rash or hives; chills or fever; persistent GI disturbances; opportunistic infection (sore throat, chills, fever, burning, itching on urination, vaginal discharge, white plaques in mouth); respiratory difficulty; decreased urine output; chest pain or palpitations; changes in hearing or fullness in ears; or worsening of condition.

Dietary Considerations: May be taken with food.

Geriatric Considerations: As a result of age-related changes in renal function and volume of distribution, accumulation and toxicity are a risk in the elderly. Careful monitoring and dosing adjustment is necessary.

Pregnancy Risk Factor: C

Lactation: Enters breast milk/use caution

Breast-Feeding Issues: Vancomycin is excreted in breast milk but is poorly absorbed from the gastrointestinal tract. Therefore, systemic absorption would not be expected. Theoretically, vancomycin in the GI tract may affect the normal bowel flora in the infant, resulting in diarrhea.

(Continued)

Vancomycin *(Continued)*

Administration

Oral: May be administered with food.

I.M.: Do not administer I.M.

I.V.: Administer vancomycin by I.V. intermittent infusion over at least 60 minutes at a final concentration not to exceed 5 mg/mL. If a maculopapular rash appears on the face, neck, trunk, and/or upper extremities (Red man syndrome), slow the infusion rate to over 1$^1/_2$ to 2 hours and increase the dilution volume. Hypotension, shock, and cardiac arrest (rare) have also been reported with too rapid of infusion. Reactions are often treated with antihistamines and possibly steroids.

Extravasation treatment: Monitor I.V. site closely; extravasation will cause serious injury with possible necrosis and tissue sloughing. Rotate infusion site frequently.

Reconstitution: Vancomycin reconstituted intravenous solutions are stable for 14 days at room temperature or refrigeration. Stability of parenteral admixture at room temperature (25°C) or refrigeration temperature (4°C) is 7 days.

Standard diluent: 500 mg/150 mL D_5W; 750 mg/250 mL D_5W; 1 g/250 mL D_5W

Minimum volume: Maximum concentration is 5 mg/mL to minimize thrombophlebitis.

Compatibility: Stable in dextran 6% in NS, D_5LR, D_5NS, D_5W, $D_{10}W$, LR, NS

Y-site administration: Incompatible with albumin, amphotericin B cholesteryl sulfate complex, cefepime, gatifloxacin, heparin, idarubicin, omeprazole

Compatibility in syringe: Incompatible with heparin

Compatibility when admixed: Incompatible with amobarbital, chloramphenicol, chlorothiazide, dexamethasone sodium phosphate, penicillin G potassium, pentobarbital, phenobarbital, phenytoin

Additional Information Because of its long half-life, vancomycin should be dosed on an every 12 hour basis; monitoring of peak and trough serum levels is advisable. The "red man syndrome" characterized by skin rash and hypotension is not an allergic reaction but rather is associated with too rapid infusion of the drug. To alleviate or prevent the reaction, infuse vancomycin at a rate of ≥30 minutes for each 500 mg of drug being administered (eg, 1 g over ≥60 minutes); 1.5 g over ≥90 minutes.

Related Information

Antimicrobial Drugs of Choice *on page 1792*
Compatibility of Drugs *on page 1723*
Peak and Trough Guidelines *on page 1694*

- **Vancomycin Hydrochloride** *see* Vancomycin *on page 1550*
- **Vanex-HD**® *see* Phenylephrine, Hydrocodone, and Chlorpheniramine *on page 1202*
- **Vaniqa**™ *see* Eflornithine *on page 511*
- **Vanos**™ *see* Fluocinonide *on page 645*
- **Vanoxide-HC**® *see* Benzoyl Peroxide and Hydrocortisone *on page 183*
- **Vantin**® *see* Cefpodoxime *on page 280*
- **VAQTA**® *see page 1660*

Vardenafil *(var DEN a fil)*

U.S. Brand Names Levitra®

Synonyms Vardenafil Hydrochloride

Generic Available No

Pharmacologic Category Phosphodiesterase-5 Enzyme Inhibitor

Medication Safety Issues

Sound-alike/look-alike issues:

Levitra® may be confused with Lexiva™

Use Treatment of erectile dysfunction

Mechanism of Action/Effect Vardenafil enhances the effect of nitric oxide by inhibiting phosphodiesterase type 5 (PDE-5), resulting in smooth muscle relaxation and inflow of blood into the corpus cavernosum with sexual stimulation.

Contraindications Hypersensitivity to vardenafil or any component of the formulation; concurrent use of organic nitrates (nitroglycerin; scheduled dosing or as needed); concomitant use of alpha blockers

Warnings/Precautions There is a degree of cardiac risk associated with sexual activity; therefore, physicians may wish to consider the patient's cardiovascular status prior to initiating any treatment for erectile dysfunction. Use caution in patients with anatomical deformation of the penis (angulation, cavernosal fibrosis, or Peyronie's disease) and in patients who have conditions which may predispose them to priapism (sickle cell anemia, multiple myeloma, leukemia). Patients should be instructed to seek medical attention if erection persists >4 hours.

Not recommended for use in patients with congenital QT prolongation or those taking Class Ia or III antiarrhythmics. Use caution with effective CYP3A4 inhibitors, the elderly, or those with hepatic impairment (Child-Pugh class B); dosage adjustment is needed.

Safety and efficacy have not been studied in patients with the following conditions, therefore, use in these patients is not recommended at this time: Hypotension, uncontrolled hypertension, unstable angina, severe cardiac failure; a life-threatening arrhythmia, myocardial infarction,or stroke within the last 6 months; severe hepatic impairment (Child-Pugh class C); end-stage renal disease requiring dialysis; retinitis pigmentosa or other degenerative retinal disorders. The safety and efficacy of vardenafil with other treatments for erectile dysfunction have not been studied and are not recommended as combination therapy.

Drug Interactions

Cytochrome P450 Effect: Substrate of CYP2C (minor), 3A5 (minor), 3A4 (major)

Increased Effect/Toxicity: CYP3A4 inhibitors may increase the levels/effects of vardenafil; example inhibitors include azole antifungals, ciprofloxacin, clarithromycin, diclofenac, doxycycline, erythromycin, imatinib, isoniazid, nefazodone, nicardipine, propofol, protease inhibitors, quinidine, and verapamil. Alpha blockers and nitroglycerin may lead to excessive hypotension; concomitant use is contraindicated.

Nutritional/Ethanol Interactions

Food: High-fat meals decrease maximum serum concentration 18% to 50%. Serum concentrations/toxicity may be increased with grapefruit juice; avoid concurrent use.

Adverse Reactions

>10%:
Cardiovascular: Flushing (11%)
Central nervous system: Headache (15%)

2% to 10%:
Central nervous system: Dizziness (2%)
Gastrointestinal: Dyspepsia (4%), nausea (2%)
Neuromuscular & skeletal: CPK increased (2%)
Respiratory: Rhinitis (9%), sinusitis (3%)
Miscellaneous: Flu-like syndrome (3%)

Overdosage/Toxicology Doses of up to 120 mg caused back pain, myalgia, and/or abnormal vision in healthy volunteers. Treatment should be symptomatic and supportive.

Pharmacodynamics/Kinetics

Absorption: Rapid

Bioavailability: 15%; Elderly (≥65 years): 52%; Hepatic impairment (Child-Pugh class B): 160%

Time to Peak: Plasma: 0.5-2 hours

Half-Life Elimination: Terminal: Vardenafil and metabolite: 4-5 hours

Metabolism: Hepatic via CYP3A4 (major), CYP2C and 3A5 (minor); forms metabolite (active)

Excretion: Feces (91% to 95% as metabolites); urine (2% to 6%)
Clearance: 56 L/hour

Dosing

Adults:

Erectile dysfunction: Oral: 10 mg 60 minutes prior to sexual activity; dosing range: 5-20 mg; to be given as one single dose and not given more than once daily

Dosing adjustment with concomitant medications:
Erythromycin: Maximum vardenafil dose: 5 mg/24 hours
Indinavir: Maximum vardenafil dose: 2.5 mg/24 hours
Itraconazole:
200 mg/day: Maximum vardenafil dose: 5 mg/24 hours
400 mg/day: Maximum vardenafil dose: 2.5 mg/24 hours
Ketoconazole:
200 mg/day: Maximum vardenafil dose: 5 mg/24 hours
400 mg/day: Maximum vardenafil dose: 2.5 mg/24 hours
Ritonavir: Maximum vardenafil dose: 2.5 mg/72 hours

Elderly: Erectile dysfunction: Elderly ≥65 years: Oral: Initial: 5 mg 60 minutes prior to sexual activity; to be given as one single dose and not given more than once daily.

Renal Impairment: Dose adjustment not needed for mild, moderate, or severe impairment; use has not been studied in patients on renal dialysis.

Hepatic Impairment: Child-Pugh class B: Initial: 5 mg 60 minutes prior to sexual activity (maximum dose: 10 mg); to be given as one single dose and not given more than once daily.

Available Dosage Forms Tablet, as hydrochloride [film-coated]: 2.5 mg, 5 mg, 10 mg, 20 mg

Monitoring and Teaching Issues

Physical Assessment: Assess potential for interactions with other prescriptions, OTC medications, and herbal products patient may be taking. Teach patient proper use, possible side effects/appropriate interventions, and adverse symptoms to report.

Patient Education: Do not take any new medication during therapy without consulting prescriber. Use exactly as directed 60 minutes prior to sexual activity without regard to meals; avoid taking with high-fat meals or grapefruit juice. Do not combine with other approaches to treating erectile dysfunction without consulting prescriber. **Note:** This medication does not provide protection against sexually-transmitted diseases, including HIV. You may experience headache, flushing, or blurred vision (use caution when driving at night or in poorly lit environments until response is known). Report immediately chest pain; acute head pain; respiratory difficulty; allergic response (chills, fever, respiratory difficulty, rash); genital swelling; erection lasting >4 hours; or other adverse reactions.

Dietary Considerations: May take with or without food

Geriatric Considerations: In adults ≥65 years of age, vardenafil plasma concentrations were higher than younger males (mean C_{max} was 34% higher), therefore, initial dose should be lower than the usual adult dose. See Pharmacokinetics and Dosing. Since older adults often have concomitant diseases, many of which may be contraindicated with the use of vardenafil, the prescriber should complete a thorough review of diseases and medications prior to prescribing vardenafil.

Pregnancy Risk Factor: B

Lactation: Vardenafil is not indicated for use in women.

Administration

Oral: May be administered with or without food, 60 minutes prior to sexual activity.

Storage: Store at controlled room temperature of 15°C to 30°C (59°F to 86°F).

Vasopressin (vay soe PRES in)

U.S. Brand Names Pitressin®

Synonyms ADH; Antidiuretic Hormone; 8-Arginine Vasopressin

Generic Available No

Pharmacologic Category Antidiuretic Hormone Analog; Hormone, Posterior Pituitary

Medication Safety Issues

Sound-alike/look-alike issues:

Pitressin® may be confused with Pitocin®

Use Treatment of diabetes insipidus; prevention and treatment of postoperative abdominal distention; differential diagnosis of diabetes insipidus

Unlabeled/Investigational Use Adjunct in the treatment of GI hemorrhage and esophageal varices; pulseless ventricular tachycardia (VT)/ventricular fibrillation (VF); vasodilatory shock (septic shock); out-of-hospital asystole

Mechanism of Action/Effect Increases cyclic adenosine monophosphate (cAMP) which increases water permeability at the renal tubule resulting in decreased urine volume and increased osmolality. Causes peristalsis by directly stimulating the smooth muscle in the GI tract.

Contraindications Hypersensitivity to vasopressin or any component of the formulation

Warnings/Precautions Use with caution in patients with seizure disorders, migraine, asthma, vascular disease, renal disease, cardiac disease, chronic nephritis with nitrogen retention, goiter with cardiac complications, arteriosclerosis. I.V. infiltration may lead to severe vasoconstriction and localized tissue necrosis, gangrene of extremities or tongue, and ischemic colitis.

Drug Interactions

Decreased Effect: Lithium, epinephrine, demeclocycline, heparin, and ethanol block antidiuretic activity to varying degrees.

Increased Effect/Toxicity: Chlorpropamide, urea, clofibrate, carbamazepine, and fludrocortisone potentiate antidiuretic response.

Nutritional/Ethanol Interactions Ethanol: Avoid ethanol (due to effects on ADH).

Adverse Reactions Frequency not defined.

Cardiovascular: Increased blood pressure, arrhythmia, venous thrombosis, vasoconstriction (with higher doses), angina, MI

Central nervous system: Pounding in the head, fever, vertigo

Dermatologic: Urticaria, circumoral pallor

Gastrointestinal: Flatulence, abdominal cramps, nausea, vomiting

Genitourinary: Uterine contraction

Neuromuscular & skeletal: Tremor

Respiratory: Bronchial constriction

Miscellaneous: Diaphoresis

Overdosage/Toxicology Symptoms of overdose include drowsiness, weight gain, confusion, listlessness, and water intoxication. Water intoxication requires withdrawal of the drug. Severe intoxication may require osmotic diuresis and loop diuretics.

Pharmacodynamics/Kinetics

Onset of Action: Nasal: 1 hour

Duration of Action: Nasal: 3-8 hours; I.M., SubQ: 2-8 hours

Half-Life Elimination: Nasal: 15 minutes; Parenteral: 10-20 minutes

Metabolism: Nasal/Parenteral: Hepatic, renal

Excretion: Nasal: Urine; Parenteral: SubQ: Urine (5% as unchanged drug) after 4 hours

Dosing

Adults & Elderly:

Diabetes insipidus:

Note: Dosage is highly variable; titrated based on serum and urine sodium and osmolality in addition to fluid balance and urine output

I.M., SubQ: 5-10 units 2-4 times/day as needed (dosage range 5-60 units/day)

Continuous I.V. infusion: 0.5 milliunit/kg/hour (0.0005 unit/kg/hour); double dosage as needed every 30 minutes to a maximum of 0.01 unit/kg/hour

Intranasal: Administer on cotton pledget, as nasal spray, or by dropper

Abdominal distention: I.M.: 5 units stat, 10 units every 3-4 hours

GI hemorrhage (unlabeled use):

Continuous I.V. infusion: 0.5 milliunits/kg/hour (0.0005 unit/kg/hour); double dosage as needed every 30 minutes to a maximum of 10 milliunits/kg/hour

I.V.: Initial: 0.2-0.4 unit/minute, then titrate dose as needed; if bleeding stops, continue at same dose for 12 hours, taper off over 24-48 hours.

Out-of-hospital asystole (unlabeled use): Adults: I.V.: 40 units; if spontaneous circulation is not restored in 3 minutes, then repeat dose

Pulseless VT/VF (ACLS protocol): I.V.: 40 units (as a single dose only); if no I.V. access, administer 40 units diluted with NS (to a total volume of 10 mL) endotracheally

Vasodilatory shock/septic shock (unlabeled use): I.V.: Vasopressin has been used in doses of 0.01-0.1 units/minute for the treatment of septic shock. Doses >0.05 units/minute may have more cardiovascular side effects. Most case reports have used 0.04 units/minute continuous infusion as a fixed dose.

Pediatrics:

Diabetes insipidus:

Note: Dosage is highly variable; titrated based on serum and urine sodium and osmolality in addition to fluid balance and urine output

I.M., SubQ:

Children: 2.5-10 units 2-4 times/day as needed

Continuous I.V. infusion: Children: 0.5 milliunit/kg/hour (0.0005 unit/kg/hour); double dosage as needed every 30 minutes to a maximum of 0.01 unit/kg/hour

Intranasal: Administer on cotton pledget, as nasal spray, or by dropper

GI hemorrhage (unlabeled use): I.V. infusion: Dilute in NS or D_5W to 0.1-1 unit/mL

Children: Initial: 0.002-0.005 units/kg/minute; titrate dose as needed; maximum: 0.01 unit/kg/minute; continue at same dosage (if bleeding stops) for 12 hours, then taper off over 24-48 hours

Hepatic Impairment: Some patients respond to much lower doses with cirrhosis.

Available Dosage Forms Injection, solution: 20 units/mL (0.5 mL, 1 mL, 10 mL)

Pitressin®: 20 units/mL (1 mL)

Monitoring and Teaching Issues

Physical Assessment: See Warnings/Precautions for specific use cautions (eg, seizures, migraine, vascular, renal, cardiac disease, atherosclerosis). Assess potential for interactions with other pharmacological agents patient may be taking (eg, concurrent use that will block or enhance antidiuretic response; see Drug Interactions). See Administration for intravenous or intranasal use. I.V. requires use of infusion pump and close monitoring to prevent extravasation (may cause severe necrosis and gangrene). Assess results of laboratory tests, therapeutic effectiveness, and adverse response on a regular basis during therapy (eg, cardiac status, blood pressure, CNS status, fluid balance, signs or symptoms of water intoxication, or intranasal irritation; see Adverse Reactions). Teach patient possible side effects/appropriate interventions and adverse symptoms to report (see Patient Education).

Monitoring Laboratory Tests: Serum and urine sodium, urine specific gravity, urine and serum osmolality

Patient Education: Do not take any new medication during therapy unless approved by prescriber. Avoid alcohol. This drug will usually be administered by infusion or injection; report immediately any redness, swelling, pain, or burning at infusion/injection site. When self-administered, follow directions exactly. May cause dizziness, drowsiness (use caution when driving or engaging in potentially hazardous tasks until response to drug is known); nausea, vomiting, cramping (small frequent meals, frequent mouth care, chewing gum, or sucking lozenges may help). Report persistent nausea, vomiting, abdominal cramps; tremor, acute headache, or dizziness; chest pain or irregular heartbeat; respiratory difficulty or excess perspiration; CNS changes (confusion, drowsiness); or runny nose or painful nasal membranes (intranasal application).

Geriatric Considerations: Elderly patients should be cautioned not to increase their fluid intake beyond that sufficient to satisfy their thirst in order to avoid water intoxication and hyponatremia. Under experimental conditions, the elderly have shown to have a decreased responsiveness to vasopressin with respect to its effects on water homeostasis.

Pregnancy Risk Factor: C

Pregnancy Issues: Animal reproduction studies have not been conducted. Vasopressin and desmopressin have been used safely during pregnancy based on case reports.

Lactation: Enters breast milk/use caution

Breast-Feeding Issues: Based on case reports, vasopressin and desmopressin have been used safely during nursing.

Administration

I.V.:

GI hemorrhage: Administration requires the use of an infusion pump and should be administered in a peripheral line.

Vasodilatory shock: Administration through a central catheter is recommended.

Infusion rates:

100 units in 500 mL D_5W rate
- 0.1 unit/minute: 30 mL/hour
- 0.2 units/minute: 60 mL/hour
- 0.3 units/minute: 90 mL/hour
- 0.4 units/minute: 120 mL/hour
- 0.5 units/minute: 150 mL/hour
- 0.6 units/minute: 180 mL/hour

Topical: Topical administration on nasal mucosa: Administer injectable vasopressin on cotton plugs, as nasal spray, or by dropper. Should not be inhaled.

Compatibility: Stable in D_5W, NS

Storage: Store injection at room temperature. Protect from heat and from freezing. Use only clear solutions.

Additional Information Vasopressin increases factor VIII levels and may be useful in hemophiliacs.

◆ **Vasotec®** see Enalapril on page 515

◆ **VCR** see VinCRIStine on page 1564

Vecuronium (ve KYOO roe ni um)

U.S. Brand Names Norcuron® [DSC]

Synonyms ORG NC 45

Generic Available Yes

Pharmacologic Category Neuromuscular Blocker Agent, Nondepolarizing

Medication Safety Issues

Sound-alike/look-alike issues:

Vecuronium may be confused with vancomycin

Norcuron® may be confused with Narcan®

Use Adjunct to general anesthesia to facilitate endotracheal intubation and to relax skeletal muscles during surgery; to facilitate mechanical ventilation in ICU patients; does not relieve pain or produce sedation

Mechanism of Action/Effect Blocks acetylcholine from binding to receptors on motor endplate inhibiting depolarization

Contraindications Hypersensitivity to vecuronium or any component of the formulation

Warnings/Precautions Ventilation must be supported during neuromuscular blockade; certain clinical conditions may result in potentiation or antagonism of neuromuscular blockade:

(Continued)

Vecuronium *(Continued)*

Potentiation: Electrolyte abnormalities, severe hyponatremia, severe hypocalcemia, severe hypokalemia, hypermagnesemia, neuromuscular diseases, acidosis, acute intermittent porphyria, renal failure, hepatic failure

Antagonism: Alkalosis, hypercalcemia, demyelinating lesions, peripheral neuropathies, diabetes mellitus

Increased sensitivity in patients with myasthenia gravis, Eaton-Lambert syndrome; resistance in burn patients (>30% of body) for period of 5-70 days postinjury; resistance in patients with muscle trauma, denervation, immobilization, infection; use with caution in patients with hepatic or renal impairment; does not counteract bradycardia produced by anesthetics/vagal stimulation. Cross-sensitivity with other neuromuscular-blocking agents may occur; use extreme caution in patients with previous anaphylactic reactions.

Drug Interactions

Increased Effect/Toxicity: Increased effects are possible with aminoglycosides, beta-blockers, clindamycin, calcium channel blockers, halogenated anesthetics, imipenem, ketamine, lidocaine, loop diuretics (furosemide), macrolides (case reports), magnesium sulfate, procainamide, quinidine, quinolones, tetracyclines, and vancomycin. May increase risk of myopathy when used with high- dose corticosteroids for extended periods.

Overdosage/Toxicology

Symptoms of overdose include prolonged skeletal muscle weakness and apnea cardiovascular collapse.

Use neostigmine, edrophonium, or pyridostigmine with atropine to antagonize skeletal muscle relaxation; support of ventilation and the cardiovascular system through mechanical means, fluids, and pressors may be necessary.

Pharmacodynamics/Kinetics

Onset of Action: Good intubation conditions: Within 2.5-3 minutes; Maximum neuromuscular blockade: Within 3-5 minutes

Duration of Action: 20-40 minutes

Half-Life Elimination: 51-80 minutes

Metabolism: Active metabolite: 3-desacetyl vecuronium ($1/2$ the activity of parent drug)

Excretion: Primarily feces (40% to 75%); urine (30% as unchanged drug and metabolites)

Dosing

Adults & Elderly:

Neuromuscular blockade: I.V. (do not administer I.M.):

Initial: 0.08-0.1 mg/kg or 0.04-0.06 mg/kg after initial dose of succinylcholine for intubation

Maintenance: 0.01-0.015 mg/kg 25-40 minutes after initial dose, then 0.01-0.015 mg/kg every 12-15 minutes (higher doses will allow less frequent maintenance doses); may be administered as a continuous infusion at 0.8-2 mcg/kg/minute

Pretreatment/priming: Adults: 10% of intubating dose given 3-5 minutes before initial dose

Neuromuscular blockade in ICU patients: Adults: 0.05-0.1 mg/kg bolus followed by 0.8-1.7 mcg/kg/minute once initial recovery from bolus observed or 0.1-0.2 mg/kg/dose every 1 hour

Pediatrics:

Neuromuscular blockade: I.V. (do not administer I.M.):

Infants >7 weeks to 1 year: Initial: 0.08-0.1 mg/kg/dose; maintenance: 0.05-0.1 mg/kg/ every 60 minutes as needed

Children >1 year: Refer to adult dosing.

Hepatic Impairment: Dose reductions are necessary in patients with liver disease.

Available Dosage Forms Injection, powder for reconstitution, as bromide: 10 mg, 20 mg [may be supplied with diluent containing benzyl alcohol]

Monitoring and Teaching Issues

Physical Assessment: Only clinicians experienced in the use of neuromuscular blocking drugs should administer and/or manage the use of vecuronium. Dosage and rate of administration should be individualized and titrated to the desired effect, according to relevant clinical factors, premedication, concomitant medications, age, and general condition of patient. Ventilatory support must be instituted and maintained until adequate respiratory muscle function and/or airway protection are assured. Assess other medications for effectiveness and safety. Other drugs that affect neuromuscular activity may increase/decrease neuromuscular block induced by vecuronium; monitor and adjust dosage as necessary. This drug does not cause anesthesia or analgesia; pain must be treated with appropriate analgesic agents. Continuous monitoring of vital signs, cardiac status, respiratory status, and degree of neuromuscular block (objective assessment with peripheral external nerve stimulator) is mandatory during infusion and until full muscle tone has returned. Muscle tone returns in a predictable pattern, starting with diaphragm, abdomen, chest, limbs, and finally muscles of the neck, face, and eyes. Safety precautions must be maintained until full muscle tone has returned. **Note:** It may take longer for return of muscle tone in obese or elderly patients or patients with renal or hepatic disease, myasthenia gravis, myopathy, other neuromuscular disease, dehydration, electrolyte imbalance, or severe acid/base imbalance. Provide appropriate patient teaching /support prior to and following administration.

Long-term use: Monitor fluid levels (intake and output) during and following infusion. Reposition patient and provide appropriate skin care, mouth care, and care of patient's eyes every 2-3 hours while sedated. Provide appropriate emotional and sensory support (auditory and environmental).

Patient Education: Patient will usually be unconscious prior to administration. Patient education should be appropriate to individual situation. Reassurance of constant monitoring and emotional support to reduce fear and anxiety should precede and follow administration. Following return of muscle tone, do not attempt to change position or rise from bed without assistance. Report immediately any skin rash or hives, pounding heartbeat, respiratory difficulty, or muscle tremors. **Pregnancy/breast-feeding precautions:** Inform prescriber if you are or intend to become pregnant. Consult prescriber if breast-feeding.

Pregnancy Risk Factor: C

Pregnancy Issues: Use in cesarean section has been reported. Umbilical venous concentrations were 11% of maternal.

Lactation: Excretion in breast milk unknown/use caution

Administration

I.V.: Concentration of 1 mg/mL may be administered by rapid I.V. injection. May further dilute reconstituted vial to 0.1-0.2 mg/mL in a compatible solution for I.V. infusion. Concentration of 1 mg/mL may be used for I.V. infusion in fluid-restricted patients.

Reconstitution: Reconstitute with compatible solution for injection to final concentration of 1 mg/mL.

Compatibility:

Incompatible with alkaline solutions/medications.

Y-Site administration: Incompatible with thiopental

Compatibility in syringe: Incompatible with thiopental

Storage: Store intact vials of powder for injection at room temperature 15°C to 30°C (59°F to 86°F). Vials reconstituted with bacteriostatic water for injection (BWFI) may be stored for 5 days under refrigeration or at room temperature. Vials reconstituted with other compatible diluents (nonbacteriostatic) should be stored under refrigeration and used within 24 hours.

Additional Information Vecuronium is classified as an intermediate-duration neuromuscular-blocking agent. It produces minimal, if any, histamine release; does not relieve pain or produce sedation. It may produce cumulative effect on duration of blockade.

♦ **Veetids®** *see* Penicillin V Potassium *on page 1177*

♦ **Velcade™** *see* Bortezomib *on page 203*

♦ **Velivet™** *see* Ethinyl Estradiol and Desogestrel *on page 578*

♦ **Velosef®** *see* Cephradine *on page 295*

♦ **Velosulin® BR (Buffered) [DSC]** *see* Insulin Preparations *on page 805*

Venlafaxine (VEN la faks een)

U.S. Brand Names Effexor®; Effexor® XR

Restrictions A medication guide should be dispensed with each prescription. A template for the required MedGuides can be found on the FDA website at: http://www.fda.gov/cder drug/antidepressants/labelTemplate.pdf

Generic Available No

Pharmacologic Category Antidepressant, Serotonin/Norepinephrine Reuptake Inhibitor

Use Treatment of major depressive disorder; generalized anxiety disorder (GAD), social anxiety disorder (social phobia)

Unlabeled/Investigational Use Obsessive-compulsive disorder (OCD), chronic fatigue syndrome; hot flashes; neuropathic pain; attention-deficit/hyperactivity disorder (ADHD) and autism in children

Mechanism of Action/Effect Venlafaxine and its active metabolite o-desmethylvenlafaxine (ODV) are potent inhibitors of neuronal serotonin and norepinephrine reuptake and weak inhibitors of dopamine reuptake. Venlafaxine and ODV have no significant activity for muscarinic cholinergic, H_1-histaminergic, or $alpha_2$-adrenergic receptors. Venlafaxine and ODV do not possess MAO-inhibitory activity.

Contraindications Hypersensitivity to venlafaxine or any component of the formulation; use of MAO inhibitors within 14 days; should not initiate MAO inhibitor within 7 days of discontinuing venlafaxine

Warnings/Precautions Antidepressants increase the risk of suicidal thinking and behavior in children and adolescents with major depressive disorder (MDD) and other depressive disorders; consider risk prior to prescribing. All patients must be closely monitored for clinical worsening, suicidality, or unusual changes in behavior, especially during the initiation of therapy or following an increase or decrease in dosage. When used in children, the child's family or caregiver should be instructed to closely observe the patient and communicate condition with healthcare provider. A medication guide should be dispensed with each prescription. **Venlafaxine is not FDA approved for use in children.**

The possibility of a suicide attempt is inherent in major depression and may persist until remission occurs. Use caution in high-risk patients. Worsening depression and severe abrupt suicidality that are not part of the presenting symptoms may require discontinuation or modification of drug therapy. The patient's family or caregiver should be alerted to monitor patients for the emergence of suicidality and associated behaviors (such as agitation, irritability, hostility, impulsivity, and hypomania) and call healthcare provider.

May worsen psychosis in some patients or precipitate a shift to mania or hypomania in patients with bipolar disorder. Patients presenting with depressive symptoms should be screened for bipolar disorder. Monotherapy in patients with bipolar disorder should be avoided. **Venlafaxine is not FDA approved for the treatment of bipolar depression.**

The potential for severe reactions exists when used with MAO inhibitors (myoclonus, diaphoresis, hyperthermia, NMS features, seizures, and death). May cause sustained increase in blood pressure or tachycardia, use caution in patients with recent history of MI, unstable heart disease, or hyperthyroidism; may cause increase in anxiety, nervousness, insomnia; may cause weight loss (use with caution in patients where weight loss is undesirable); may cause increases in serum cholesterol. Use caution with hepatic or renal impairment. Venlafaxine has been associated with the development of SIADH and hyponatremia.

May increase the risks associated with electroconvulsive therapy. Use cautiously in patients with a history of seizures. The risks of cognitive or motor impairment, as well as the potential for anticholinergic effects are very low. May cause or exacerbate sexual dysfunction. May impair platelet aggregation, resulting in bleeding.

Abrupt discontinuation or dosage reduction after extended (≥6 weeks) therapy may lead to agitation, dysphoria, nervousness, anxiety, and other symptoms. When discontinuing (Continued)

Venlafaxine *(Continued)*

therapy, dosage should be tapered gradually over at least a 2-week period. If intolerable symptoms occur following a decrease in dosage or upon discontinuation of therapy, then resuming the previous dose with a more gradual taper should be considered. Use caution in patients with increased intraocular pressure or at risk of acute narrow-angle glaucoma.

Drug Interactions

Cytochrome P450 Effect: Substrate of CYP2C8/9 (minor), 2C19 (minor), 2D6 (major), 3A4 (major); **Inhibits** CYP2B6 (weak), 2D6 (weak), 3A4 (weak)

Decreased Effect: Serum levels of indinavir may be reduced be venlafaxine (AUC reduced by 28%); clinical significance not determined. CYP3A4 inducers may decrease the levels/ effects of venlafaxine; example inducers include aminoglutethimide, carbamazepine, nafcillin, nevirapine, phenobarbital, phenytoin, and rifamycins.

Increased Effect/Toxicity: Concurrent use of MAO inhibitors (phenelzine, isocarboxazid), or drugs with MAO inhibitor activity (linezolid) may result in serotonin syndrome; should not be used within 2 weeks of each other. Selegiline may have a lower risk of this effect, particularly at low dosages, due to selectivity for MAO type B. In addition, concurrent use of buspirone, lithium, meperidine, nefazodone, selegiline, serotonin agonists (sumatriptan, naratriptan), sibutramine, SSRIs, trazodone, or tricyclic antidepressants may increase the risk of serotonin syndrome. Serum levels of haloperidol may be increased by venlafaxine. CYP2D6 inhibitors may increase the levels/effects of venlafaxine; example inhibitors include chlorpromazine, delavirdine, fluoxetine, miconazole, paroxetine, pergolide, quinidine, quinine, ritonavir, and ropinirole. CYP3A4 inhibitors may increase the levels/effects of venlafaxine; example inhibitors include azole antifungals, ciprofloxacin, clarithromycin, diclofenac, doxycycline, erythromycin, imatinib, isoniazid, nefazodone, nicardipine, propofol, protease inhibitors, quinidine, and verapamil.

Nutritional/Ethanol Interactions

Ethanol: Avoid ethanol (may increase CNS effects).

Herb/Nutraceutical: Avoid valerian, St John's wort, SAMe, kava kava, tryptophan (may increase risk of serotonin syndrome and/or excessive sedation).

Lab Interactions Increased thyroid, uric acid, glucose, potassium, AST, cholesterol (S)

Adverse Reactions

≥10%:

Central nervous system: Headache (25%), somnolence (23%), dizziness (19%), insomnia (18%), nervousness (13%)

Gastrointestinal: Nausea (37%), xerostomia (22%), constipation (15%), anorexia (11%)

Genitourinary: Abnormal ejaculation/orgasm (12%)

Neuromuscular & skeletal: Weakness (12%)

Miscellaneous: Diaphoresis (12%)

1% to 10%:

Cardiovascular: Vasodilation (4%), hypertension (dose related; 3% in patients receiving <100 mg/day, up to 13% in patients receiving >300 mg/day), tachycardia (2%), chest pain (2%), postural hypotension (1%)

Central nervous system: Anxiety (6%), abnormal dreams (4%), yawning (3%), agitation (2%), confusion (2%), abnormal thinking (2%), depersonalization (1%), depression (1%)

Dermatologic: Rash (3%), pruritus (1%)

Endocrine & metabolic: Decreased libido

Gastrointestinal: Diarrhea (8%), vomiting (6%), dyspepsia (5%), flatulence (3%), taste perversion (2%), weight loss (1%)

Genitourinary: Impotence (6%), urinary frequency (3%), impaired urination (2%), orgasm disturbance (2%), urinary retention (1%)

Neuromuscular & skeletal: Tremor (5%), hypertonia (3%), paresthesia (3%), twitching (1%)

Ocular: Blurred vision (6%), mydriasis (2%)

Otic: Tinnitus (2%)

Miscellaneous: Infection (6%), chills (3%), trauma (2%)

Overdosage/Toxicology Symptoms of overdose include somnolence and occasionally tachycardia. Most overdoses resolve with only supportive treatment. Use of activated charcoal, inductions of emesis, or gastric lavage should be considered for acute ingestion. Forced diuresis, dialysis, and hemoperfusion not effective due to large volume of distribution.

Pharmacodynamics/Kinetics

Absorption: Oral: 92% to 100%; food has no significant effect on absorption of venlafaxine or formation of the active metabolite O-desmethylvenlafaxine (ODV)

Bioavailability: Absolute: ~45%

Time to Peak:

Immediate release: Venlafaxine: 2 hours, ODV: 3 hours

Extended release: Venlafaxine: 5.5 hours, ODV: 9 hours

Protein Binding: Bound to human plasma protein: Venlafaxine 27%, ODV 30%

Half-Life Elimination: Venlafaxine: 3-7 hours; ODV: 9-13 hours; Steady-state plasma: Venlafaxine/ODV: Within 3 days of multiple dose therapy

Prolonged with cirrhosis and dialysis:

Adults: Cirrhosis: Venlafaxine: ~30%, ODV: ~60%

Adults: Dialysis: Venlafaxine: ~180%, ODV: ~142%

Metabolism: Hepatic via CYP2D6 to active metabolite, O-desmethylvenlafaxine (ODV); other metabolites include N-desmethylvenlafaxine and N,O-didesmethylvenlafaxine

Excretion: Urine (~87%, 5% as unchanged drug, 29% as unconjugated ODV, 26% as conjugated ODV, 27% as minor metabolites) within 48 hours

Clearance at steady state: Venlafaxine: 1.3 ± 0.6 L/hour/kg, ODV: 0.4 ± 0.2 L/hour/kg

Clearance decreased with:

Cirrhosis: Adults: Venlafaxine: ~50%, ODV: ~30%

Severe cirrhosis: Adults: Venlafaxine: ~90%

Renal impairment (Cl_{cr} 10-70 mL/minute): Adults: Venlafaxine: ~24%

Dialysis: Adults: Venlafaxine: ~57%, ODV: ~56%; due to large volume of distribution, a significant amount of drug is not likely to be removed.

Dosing
Adults:
Depression:

Immediate-release tablets: 75 mg/day, administered in 2 or 3 divided doses, taken with food; dose may be increased in 75 mg/day increments at intervals of at least 4 days, up to 225-375 mg/day

Extended-release capsules: 75 mg once daily taken with food; for some new patients, it may be desirable to start at 37.5 mg/day for 4-7 days before increasing to 75 mg once daily; dose may be increased by up to 75 mg/day increments every 4 days as tolerated, up to a maximum of 225 mg/day

GAD, social anxiety disorder: *Extended-release capsules:* 75 mg once daily taken with food; for some new patients, it may be desirable to start at 37.5 mg/day for 4-7 days before increasing to 75 mg once daily; dose may be increased by up to 75 mg/day increments every 4 days as tolerated, up to a maximum of 225 mg/day

Note: When discontinuing this medication after more than 1 week of treatment, it is generally recommended that the dose be tapered. If venlafaxine is used for 6 weeks or longer, the dose should be tapered over 2 weeks when discontinuing its use.

Elderly: No specific recommendations for elderly, but may be best to start lower at 25-50 mg twice daily and increase as tolerated by 25 mg/dose. Extended-release formulation: 37.5 mg once daily, increase by 37.5 mg every 4-7 days as tolerated

Pediatrics: Children and Adolescents:

ADHD (unlabeled use): Initial: 12.5 mg/day

Children <40 kg: Increase by 12.5 mg/week to maximum of 50 mg/day in 2 divided doses

Children ≥40 kg: Increase by 25 mg/week to maximum of 75 mg/day in 3 divided doses.

Mean dose: 60 mg or 1.4 mg/kg administered in 2-3 divided doses

Autism (unlabeled use): Oral: Initial: 12.5 mg/day; adjust to 6.25-50 mg/day

Renal Impairment:

Cl$_{cr}$ 10-70 mL/minute: Decrease dose by 25%.

Hemodialysis: Decrease total daily dose by 50% given after completion of dialysis.

Hepatic Impairment: Reduce total dosage by 50%.

Available Dosage Forms

Capsule, extended release, as hydrochloride (Effexor® XR): 37.5 mg, 75 mg, 150 mg

Tablet, as hydrochloride (Effexor®): 25 mg, 37.5 mg, 50 mg, 75 mg, 100 mg

Monitoring and Teaching Issues

Physical Assessment: Assess other medications patient may be taking for effectiveness and interactions. Monitor for worsening of depression or suicidality, especially during initiation of therapy or with dose increases or decreases. Monitor therapeutic effectiveness according to rationale for therapy and adverse reactions at beginning of therapy and periodically with long-term use. Taper dosage slowly when discontinuing. Assess knowledge/teach patient appropriate use, interventions to reduce side effects, and adverse symptoms to report.

Monitoring Laboratory Tests: Cholesterol

Patient Education: Take exactly as directed; do not increase dose or frequency. It may take 2-3 weeks to achieve desired results. Take with food. Extended release capsules should be swallowed whole; do not crush or chew. Alternatively, contents may be emptied onto a spoonful of applesauce and swallowed without chewing. Avoid alcohol, caffeine, and other prescription or OTC medications not approved by prescriber. Maintain adequate hydration (2-3 L/day of fluids) unless instructed to restrict fluid intake. You may experience excess drowsiness or insomnia, lightheadedness, dizziness, or blurred vision (use caution when driving or engaging in tasks requiring alertness until response to drug is known); headache, nausea, vomiting, anorexia, altered taste, dry mouth (small frequent meals, frequent mouth care, chewing gum, or sucking lozenges may help); constipation (increased exercise, fluids, fruit, or fiber may help); diarrhea (buttermilk, yogurt, or boiled milk may help); postural hypotension (use caution when climbing stairs or changing position from lying or sitting to standing); urinary retention (void before taking medication); or sexual dysfunction (reversible). Report persistent CNS effects (eg, insomnia, restlessness, fatigue, anxiety, abnormal thoughts, suicidal ideation, confusion, personality changes, impaired cognitive function); muscle cramping or tremors; chest pain, palpitations, rapid heartbeat, swelling of extremities, or severe dizziness; unresolved urinary retention; vision changes or eye pain; hearing changes or ringing in ears; skin rash or irritation; or worsening of condition. **Pregnancy/breast-feeding precautions:** Inform prescriber if you are or intend to become pregnant. Do not breast-feed.

Dietary Considerations: Should be taken with food.

Geriatric Considerations: Has not been studied exclusively in the elderly, however, its low anticholinergic activity, minimal sedation, and hypotension makes this a potentially valuable antidepressant in treating elderly with depression. No dose adjustment is necessary for age alone, additional studies are necessary; adjust dose for renal function in the elderly.

Pregnancy Risk Factor: C

Pregnancy Issues: Teratogenic effects were not observed in animal studies. Nonteratogenic effects including respiratory distress, cyanosis, apnea, seizures, temperature instability, feeding difficulty, vomiting, hypoglycemia, hypo- or hypertonia, hyper-reflexia, jitteriness, irritability, constant crying, and tremor have been reported in the neonate immediately following delivery after exposure late in the third trimester. Adverse effects may be due to toxic effects of SNRI or drug discontinuation. There are no adequate and well-controlled studies in pregnant women. Use during pregnancy only if the potential benefit to the mother outweighs the possible risk to the fetus. If treatment during pregnancy is required, consider tapering therapy during the third trimester.

Lactation: Enters breast milk/not recommended

Breast-Feeding Issues: The manufacturer recommends discontinuing nursing or discontinuing venlafaxine, depending upon the importance of the drug to the mother.

(Continued)

Venlafaxine (Continued)

Administration

Oral: Administer with food.

Extended release capsule: Swallow capsule whole; do not crush or chew. Alternatively, contents may be sprinkled on a spoonful of applesauce and swallowed immediately without chewing; followed with a glass of water to ensure complete swallowing of the pellets.

Related Information

Antidepressant Agents *on page 1713*
Antidepressant Medication Guidelines *on page 1765*

♦ **Venofer**® *see Iron Sucrose on page 834*
♦ **Venoglobulin**®-Š [DSC] *see Immune Globulin (Intravenous) on page 793*
♦ **Ventolin**® HFA *see Albuterol on page 59*
♦ **VePesid**® *see Etoposide on page 599*

Verapamil (ver AP a mil)

U.S. Brand Names Calan®; Calan® SR; Covera-HS®; Isoptin® SR; Verelan®; Verelan® PM

Synonyms Iproveratril Hydrochloride; Verapamil Hydrochloride

Generic Available Yes

Pharmacologic Category Antiarrhythmic Agent, Class IV; Calcium Channel Blocker

Medication Safety Issues

Sound-alike/look-alike issues:

Verapamil may be confused with Verelan®
Calan® may be confused with Colace®
Covera-HS® may be confused with Provera®
Isoptin® may be confused with Isopto® Tears
Verelan® may be confused with verapamil, Virilon®, Voltaren®

Use Orally for treatment of angina pectoris (vasospastic, chronic stable, unstable) and hypertension; I.V. for supraventricular tachyarrhythmias (PSVT, atrial fibrillation, atrial flutter)

Unlabeled/Investigational Use Migraine; hypertrophic cardiomyopathy; bipolar disorder (manic manifestations)

Mechanism of Action/Effect Inhibits calcium ion from entering the "slow channels" or select voltage-sensitive areas of vascular smooth muscle and myocardium during depolarization. Produces a relaxation of coronary vascular smooth muscle and coronary vasodilation. Increases myocardial oxygen delivery in patients with vasospastic (Prinzmetal's) angina. Slows automaticity and conduction of AV node.

Contraindications Hypersensitivity to verapamil or any component of the formulation; severe left ventricular dysfunction; hypotension (systolic pressure <90 mm Hg) or cardiogenic shock; sick sinus syndrome (except in patients with a functioning artificial pacemaker); second- or third-degree AV block (except in patients with a functioning artificial pacemaker); atrial flutter or fibrillation and an accessory bypass tract (WPW, Lown-Ganong-Levine syndrome)

Warnings/Precautions Avoid use in heart failure; can exacerbate condition. Can cause hypotension. Rare increases in liver function tests can be observed. Can cause first-degree AV block or sinus bradycardia. Other conduction abnormalities are rare. Use caution when using verapamil together with a beta-blocker. Avoid use of I.V. verapamil with an I.V. beta-blocker; can result in asystole. Use caution in patients with hypertrophic cardiomyopathy (IHSS). Use with caution in patients with attenuated neuromuscular transmission (Duchenne's muscular dystrophy, myasthenia gravis). Adjust the dose in severe renal dysfunction and hepatic dysfunction. Verapamil significantly increases digoxin serum concentrations (adjust digoxin's dose). May prolong recovery from nondepolarizing neuromuscular-blocking agents.

Drug Interactions

Cytochrome P450 Effect: Substrate of CYP1A2 (minor), 2B6 (minor), 2C8/9 (minor), 2C18 (minor), 2E1 (minor), 3A4 (major); **Inhibits** CYP1A2 (weak), 2C8/9 (weak), 2D6 (weak), 3A4 (moderate)

Decreased Effect: The levels/effects of verapamil may be decreased by aminoglutethimide, carbamazepine, nafcillin, nevirapine, phenobarbital, phenytoin, rifamycins, and other CYP3A4 inducers. Lithium levels may be decreased by verapamil. Nafcillin decreases plasma concentration of verapamil.

Increased Effect/Toxicity: Use of verapamil with amiodarone, beta-blockers, or flecainide may lead to bradycardia and decreased cardiac output. Aspirin and concurrent verapamil use may increase bleeding times. Lithium neurotoxicity may result when verapamil is added. Effect of nondepolarizing neuromuscular blocker is prolonged by verapamil. Grapefruit juice may increase verapamil serum concentrations. Blood pressure-lowering effects may be additive with sildenafil, tadalafil, and vardenafil (use caution).

Cisapride levels may be increased by verapamil, potentially resulting in life-threatening arrhythmias; avoid concurrent use. Verapamil may increase the levels/effects of selected benzodiazepines, other calcium channel blockers, cyclosporine, ergot alkaloids, selected HMG-CoA reductase inhibitors, mirtazapine, nateglinide, nefazodone, pimozide, quinidine, sildenafil (and other PDE-5 inhibitors), tacrolimus, venlafaxine, and other CYP3A4 substrates. In addition, serum concentrations of the following drugs may be increased by verapamil: Alfentanil, digoxin, doxorubicin, ethanol, prazosin, and theophylline.

The levels/effects of verapamil may be increased by azole antifungals, ciprofloxacin, clarithromycin, diclofenac, doxycycline, erythromycin, imatinib, isoniazid, nefazodone, nicardipine, propofol, protease inhibitors, quinidine, and other CYP3A4 inhibitors.

Nutritional/Ethanol Interactions

Ethanol: Avoid or limit ethanol (may increase ethanol levels).
Food: Grapefruit juice may increase the serum concentration of verapamil; avoid concurrent use.

Herb/Nutraceutical: St John's wort may decrease levels. Avoid dong quai if using for hypertension (has estrogenic activity). Avoid ephedra, yohimbe, ginseng (may worsen arrhythmia or hypertension). Avoid garlic (may have increased antihypertensive effect).

Lab Interactions Increased alkaline phosphatase, CPK, LDH, aminotransferase [AST (SGOT)/ALT (SGPT)] (S)

Adverse Reactions
>10%: Gastrointestinal: Gingival hyperplasia (19%)
1% to 10%:
Cardiovascular: Bradycardia (1.4% oral, 1.2% I.V.); first-, second-, or third-degree AV block (1.2% oral, unknown I.V.); CHF (1.8% oral); hypotension (2.5% oral, 3% I.V.); peripheral edema (1.9% oral), symptomatic hypotension (1.5% I.V.); severe tachycardia (1% I.V.)
Central nervous system: Dizziness (3.3% oral, 1.2% I.V.), fatigue (1.7% oral), headache (2.2% oral, 1.2% I.V.)
Dermatologic: Rash (1.2% oral)
Gastrointestinal: Constipation (12% up to 42% in clinical trials), nausea (2.7% oral, 0.9% I.V.)
Respiratory: Dyspnea (1.4% oral)

Overdosage/Toxicology Primary cardiac symptoms of calcium blocker overdose include hypotension and bradycardia (second- or third-degree atrioventricular block, or sinus arrest with junctional rhythm). Intraventricular conduction is usually not affected so QRS duration is normal (verapamil does prolong the PR interval).

Noncardiac symptoms include confusion, stupor, nausea, vomiting, metabolic acidosis and hyperglycemia. Following initial gastric decontamination, if possible, repeated calcium administration may promptly reverse depressed cardiac contractility (but not sinus node depression or peripheral vasodilation). Large doses of calcium chloride (up to 1 g/hour for 24 hours) have been used in refractory cases. Glucagon, epinephrine, and amrinone may treat refractory hypotension. Glucagon and epinephrine also increase heart rate (outside the U.S., 4-aminopyridine may be available as an antidote). Dialysis and hemoperfusion are not effective in enhancing elimination although repeat-dose activated charcoal may serve as an adjunct with sustained-release preparations.

Pharmacodynamics/Kinetics
Onset of Action: Oral (immediate release tablets): Peak effect: 2 hours; I.V.: Peak effect: 1-5 minutes
Duration of Action: Oral: Immediate release tablets: 6-8 hours; I.V.: 10-20 minutes
Bioavailability: Oral: 20% to 30%
Protein Binding: 90%
Half-Life Elimination: Infants: 4.4-6.9 hours; Adults: Single dose: 2-8 hours, Multiple doses: Up to 12 hours; prolonged with hepatic cirrhosis
Metabolism: Hepatic via multiple CYP isoenzymes; extensive first-pass effect
Excretion: Urine (70%, 3% to 4% as unchanged drug); feces (16%)

Dosing
Adults:
Angina: Oral: Initial: 80-120 mg twice daily (elderly or small stature: 40 mg twice daily); range: 240-480 mg/day in 3-4 divided doses
Hypertension: Oral:
Immediate release: 80 mg 3 times/day; usual dose range (JNC 7): 80-320 mg/day in 2 divided doses
Sustained release: 240 mg/day; usual dose range (JNC 7): 120-360 mg/day in 1-2 divided doses; 120 mg/day in the elderly or small patients (no evidence of additional benefit in doses >360 mg/day)
Extended release:
Covera-HS®: Usual dose range (JNC 7): 120-360 mg once daily (once-daily dosing is recommended at bedtime)
Verelan® PM: Usual dose range: 200-400 mg once daily at bedtime
Arrhythmia (SVT): I.V.: 2.5-5 mg (over 2 minutes); second dose of 5-10 mg (~0.15 mg/kg) may be given 15-30 minutes after the initial dose if patient tolerates, but does not respond to initial dose; maximum total dose: 20 mg

Elderly:
Oral: 120-480 mg/24 hours divided 3-4 times/day
Sustained release: 120 mg/day; adjust dose after 24 hours by increases of 120 mg/day. When switching from immediate release forms, total daily dose may remain the same. Controlled onset: initiate therapy with 180 mg in the evening; titrate upward as needed to obtain desired response and avoiding adverse effects.

Pediatrics: Children: SVT:
I.V.:
<1 year: 0.1-0.2 mg/kg over 2 minutes; repeat every 30 minutes as needed
1-15 years: 0.1-0.3 mg/kg over 2 minutes; maximum: 5 mg/dose, may repeat dose in 15 minutes if adequate response not achieved; maximum for second dose: 10 mg/dose
Oral (dose not well established):
1-5 years: 4-8 mg/kg/day in 3 divided doses **or** 40-80 mg every 8 hours
>5 years: 80 mg every 6-8 hours

Renal Impairment: Cl_{cr} <10 mL/minute: Administer 50% to 75% of normal dose.
Hepatic Impairment: In cirrhosis, reduce dose to 20% to 50% of normal and monitor ECG.

Available Dosage Forms
Caplet, sustained release (Calan® SR): 120 mg, 180 mg, 240 mg
Capsule, extended release: 120 mg, 180 mg, 240 mg
Verelan® PM: 100 mg, 200 mg, 300 mg
Capsule, sustained release, as hydrochloride (Verelan®): 120 mg, 180 mg, 240 mg, 360 mg
Injection, solution, as hydrochloride: 2.5 mg/mL (2 mL, 4 mL)
Tablet, as hydrochloride (Calan®): 40 mg, 80 mg, 120 mg
Tablet, extended release: 120 mg, 180 mg, 240 mg
Covera-HS®: 180 mg, 240 mg
Tablet, sustained release, as hydrochloride (Isoptin® SR): 120 mg, 180 mg, 240 mg
(Continued)

Verapamil *(Continued)*

Monitoring and Teaching Issues

Physical Assessment: Assess other medications patient may be taking for effectiveness and interactions. I.V. requires use of infusion pump and continuous cardiac and hemodynamic monitoring. Assess results of laboratory tests, therapeutic effectiveness, and adverse reactions when beginning therapy, when titrating dosage, and periodically during long-term oral therapy. Assess knowledge/teach patient appropriate use (oral), interventions to reduce side effects, and adverse symptoms to report.

Patient Education: Oral: Take as directed. Do not alter dosage or discontinue therapy without consulting prescriber. Do not crush or chew sustained or extended release forms. Avoid grapefruit juice; avoid (or limit) alcohol and caffeine. You may experience dizziness or lightheadedness (use caution when driving or engaging in tasks requiring alertness until response to drug is known); nausea or vomiting (small frequent meals, frequent mouth care, chewing gum, or sucking lozenges may help); constipation (increased exercise, fluids, fruit, or fiber may help); or diarrhea (buttermilk, boiled milk, or yogurt may help). Report chest pain, palpitations, or irregular heartbeat; unusual cough, respiratory difficulty, or swelling of extremities (feet/ankles); muscle tremors or weakness; confusion or acute lethargy; or skin irritation or rash. **Pregnancy precaution:** Inform prescriber if you are or intend to become pregnant.

Dietary Considerations: Calan® SR and Isoptin® SR products may be taken with food or milk, other formulations may be administered without regard to meals; sprinkling contents of Verelan® or Verelan® PM capsule onto applesauce does not affect oral absorption.

Geriatric Considerations: Elderly may experience a greater hypotensive response. Theoretically, constipation may be more of a problem in the elderly. Calcium channel blockers are no more effective in the elderly than other therapies, however, they do not cause significant CNS effects, which is an advantage over some antihypertensive agents. Generic verapamil products which are bioequivalent in young adults may not be bioequivalent in the elderly. Use generics cautiously.

Pregnancy Risk Factor: C

Pregnancy Issues: Crosses the placenta. One report of suspected heart block when used to control fetal supraventricular tachycardia. May exhibit tocolytic effects.

Lactation: Enters breast milk (small amounts)/not recommended

Breast-Feeding Issues: Crosses into breast milk; manufacturer recommends to discontinue breast-feeding while taking verapamil. AAP considers **compatible** with breast-feeding.

Administration

Oral: Do not crush or chew sustained or extended release products.

Calan® SR, Isoptin® SR: Administer with food.

Verelan®, Verelan® PM: Capsules may be opened and the contents sprinkled on 1 tablespoonful of applesauce, then swallowed without chewing.

I.V.: Rate of infusion: Over 2 minutes

Compatibility: Stable in dextran 40 10% in NS, dextran 75 6% in NS, D$_5$LR, D$_5$¹/$_2$NS, D$_5$NS, D$_5$W, LR, ¹/$_2$NS, NS

Y-site administration: Incompatible with albumin, amphotericin B cholesteryl sulfate complex, ampicillin, nafcillin, oxacillin, propofol, sodium bicarbonate

Compatibility when admixed: Incompatible with albumin, amphotericin B, floxacillin, hydralazine, trimethoprim/sulfamethoxazole

Storage: Store injection at room temperature. Protect from heat and from freezing. Use only clear solutions. Protect I.V. solution from light.

Related Information

Antiarrhythmic Drugs *on page 1708*

Calcium Channel Blockers *on page 1722*

Compatibility of Drugs *on page 1723*

VinBLAStine (vin BLAS teen)

Synonyms NSC-49842; Vinblastine Sulfate; VLB

Generic Available Yes

Pharmacologic Category Antineoplastic Agent, Natural Source (Plant) Derivative; Antineoplastic Agent, Vinca Alkaloid

Medication Safety Issues

Sound-alike/look-alike issues:

VinBLAStine may be confused with vinCRIStine, vinorelbine

Use Treatment of Hodgkin's and non-Hodgkin's lymphoma, testicular, lung, head and neck, breast, and renal carcinomas, Mycosis fungoides, Kaposi's sarcoma, histiocytosis, choriocarcinoma, and idiopathic thrombocytopenic purpura

Mechanism of Action/Effect Vinblastine arrests cell cycle growth in metaphase. Also inhibits RNA synthesis and amino acid metabolism resulting in inhibition of metabolic pathways and cell growth.

Contraindications For I.V. use only; **I.T. use may result in death**; hypersensitivity to vinblastine or any component of the formulation; severe bone marrow suppression or presence of bacterial infection not under control prior to initiation of therapy; pregnancy

Warnings/Precautions The U.S. Food and Drug Administration (FDA) currently recommends that procedures for proper handling and disposal of antineoplastic agents be considered. Vinblastine is a moderate vesicant; avoid extravasation; extravasation may cause tissue damage and pain. Discontinue immediately if extravasation occurs (remaining portion of dose to be infused through another vein). Dosage modification required in patients with impaired liver function and neurotoxicity. Using small amounts of drug daily for long periods may cause neurotoxicity and is therefore not advised. For I.V. use only. **Intrathecal administration results in death.** Use with caution in patients with cachexia or ulcerated skin. Monitor closely for shortness of breath or bronchospasm in patients receiving mitomycin C.

Drug Interactions

Cytochrome P450 Effect: Substrate of CYP2D6 (minor), 3A4 (major); **Inhibits** CYP2D6 (weak), 3A4 (weak)

Decreased Effect: CYP3A4 inducers may decrease the levels/effects of vinblastine; example inducers include aminoglutethimide, carbamazepine, nafcillin, nevirapine, phenobarbital, phenytoin (may reduce vinblastine serum concentrations), and rifamycins.

Increased Effect/Toxicity: CYP3A4 inhibitors may increase the levels/effects of vinblastine; example inhibitors include azole antifungals, ciprofloxacin, clarithromycin, diclofenac, doxycycline, erythromycin, imatinib, isoniazid, nefazodone, nicardipine, propofol, protease inhibitors, quinidine, and verapamil.

Previous or simultaneous use with mitomycin-C has resulted in acute shortness of breath and severe bronchospasm within minutes or several hours after *Vinca* alkaloid injection and may occur up to 2 weeks after the dose of mitomycin. Mitomycin-C in combination with administration of VLB may cause acute shortness of breath and severe bronchospasm, onset may be within minutes or several hours after VLB injection.

Nutritional/Ethanol Interactions Herb/Nutraceutical: St John's wort may decrease vinblastine levels. Avoid black cohosh, dong quai in estrogen-dependent tumors.

Adverse Reactions

>10%:

Dermatologic: Alopecia

Endocrine & metabolic: SIADH

Gastrointestinal: Diarrhea (less common), stomatitis, anorexia, metallic taste

Hematologic: May cause severe bone marrow suppression and is the dose-limiting toxicity of VLB (unlike vincristine); severe granulocytopenia and thrombocytopenia may occur following the administration of VLB and nadir 5-10 days after treatment

Myelosuppression (primarily leukopenia, may be dose limiting)

Onset: 4-7 days

Nadir: 5-10 days

Recovery: 4-21 days

1% to 10%:

Cardiovascular: Hypertension, Raynaud's phenomenon

Central nervous system: Depression, malaise, headache, seizure

Dermatologic: Rash, photosensitivity, dermatitis

Endocrine & metabolic: Hyperuricemia

Gastrointestinal: Constipation, abdominal pain, nausea (mild), vomiting (mild), paralytic ileus, stomatitis

Genitourinary: Urinary retention

Neuromuscular & skeletal: Jaw pain, myalgia, paresthesia

Respiratory: Bronchospasm

Overdosage/Toxicology Symptoms of overdose include bone marrow suppression, mental depression, paresthesia, loss of deep tendon reflexes, and neurotoxicity. There are no antidotes for vinblastine. Treatment is supportive and symptomatic, including fluid restriction or hypertonic saline (3% sodium chloride) for drug-induced secretion of inappropriate antidiuretic hormone (SIADH).

Pharmacodynamics/Kinetics

Protein Binding: 99%

Half-Life Elimination: Biphasic: Initial: 0.164 hours; Terminal: 25 hours

Metabolism: Hepatic to active metabolite

Excretion: Feces (95%); urine (<1% as unchanged drug)

Dosing

Adults & Elderly: Refer to individual protocols.

Antineoplastic (typical dosages): I.V.: 4-20 mg/m² (0.1-0.5 mg/kg) every 7-10 days **or** 5-day continuous infusion of 1.5-2 mg/m²/day **or** 0.1-0.5 mg/kg/week

(Continued)

VinBLAStine *(Continued)*

Pediatrics: Refer to adult dosing.

Renal Impairment: Not removed by hemodialysis

Hepatic Impairment:

Serum bilirubin 1.5-3.0 mg/dL or AST 60-180 units: Administer 50% of normal dose.
Serum bilirubin 3.0-5.0 mg/dL: Administer 25% of dose.
Serum bilirubin >5.0 mg/dL or AST >180 units: Omit dose.

Available Dosage Forms

Injection, powder for reconstitution, as sulfate: 10 mg

Injection, solution, as sulfate: 1 mg/mL (10 mL) [contains benzyl alcohol]

Monitoring and Teaching Issues

Physical Assessment: Use caution with impaired liver function (see Warnings/Precautions for specific for use cautions). Assess potential for interactions with other pharmacological agents and herbal products patient may be taking (eg, previous or concurrent use mitomycin-C can cause severe reaction; see Drug Interactions). Premedication with antiemetic is advisable. Infusion site must be monitored closely to prevent extravasation (vesicant will cause tissue damage and necrosis). Assess results of laboratory tests and renal function, and adverse reactions prior to each infusion and throughout therapy (eg, SIADH, bone marrow suppression, leukopenia, hypertension, gastrointestinal disturbance, myalgia, depression, paresthesia; see Adverse Reactions). Teach patient possible side effects/appropriate interventions and adverse symptoms to report (See Patient Education).

Monitoring Laboratory Tests: CBC with differential and platelet count, serum uric acid, hepatic function

Patient Education: Do not take any new medication during therapy unless approved by prescriber. This medication is only administered by infusion; report immediately any redness, swelling, burning, or pain at infusion site; sudden difficulty breathing or swelling, chest pain, chills. Maintain adequate hydration (2-3 L/day of fluids) unless instructed to restrict fluid intake and nutrition (small frequent meals will help). You will be more susceptible to infection (avoid crowds and exposure to infection and do not have any vaccinations unless approved by prescriber). May cause hair loss (will grow back after therapy); nausea or vomiting (request antiemetic); photosensitivity (use sunscreen, wear protective clothing and eyewear, and avoid direct sunlight); feelings of extreme weakness or lethargy (use caution when driving or engaging in tasks requiring alertness until response to drug is known); or mouth sores (use soft toothbrush, waxed dental floss, and frequent oral care). Report persistent constipation, abdominal pain; numbness or tingling in fingers or toes (use care to prevent injury); weakness or pain in muscles or jaw; signs of infection (eg, fever, chills, sore throat, burning urination, fatigue); unusual bleeding (eg, tarry stools, easy bruising, blood in stool, urine, or mouth); unresolved mouth sores; skin rash or itching; or respiratory difficulty. **Pregnancy/breast-feeding precautions:** Do not get pregnant (females) or cause a pregnancy (males) during this therapy. Consult prescriber for appropriate contraceptive measures. Breast-feeding is not recommended.

Pregnancy Risk Factor: D

Lactation: Enters breast milk/not recommended

Administration

I.V.: Vesicant. Drug is for I.V. administration only. **Fatal if given intrathecally.** Administer vinblastine I.V., usually as a slow (2-3 minutes) push, or a bolus (5- to 15-minute) infusion. It is occasionally given as a 24-hour continuous infusion.

Reconstitution: Reconstitute to a concentration of 1 mg/mL with bacteriostatic water, bacteriostatic NS, SWFI, NS, or D_5W; for infusion, may be diluted with 50-1000 mL Ns or D_5W.

Compatibility: Stable in D_5W, LR, NS, bacteriostatic water

Y-site administration: Incompatible with cefepime, furosemide

Compatibility in syringe: Incompatible with furosemide

Storage: Store intact vials under refrigeration (2°C to 8°C) and protect from light. Solutions reconstituted in bacteriostatic water or bacteriostatic NS are stable for 21 days at room temperature or under refrigeration.

Note: Must be dispensed in overwrap which bears the statement "Do not remove covering until the moment of injection. Fatal if given intrathecally. For I.V. use only." Syringes should be labeled: "Fatal if given intrathecally. For I.V. use only."

Additional Information Allopurinol may be given to prevent uric acid nephropathy.

Related Information

FDA Name Differentiation Project: The Use of Tall-Man Letters *on page 15*

♦ **Vinblastine Sulfate** *see* VinBLAStine *on page 1563*

♦ **Vincasar PFS®** *see* VinCRIStine *on page 1564*

VinCRIStine *(vin KRIS teen)*

U.S. Brand Names Vincasar PFS®

Synonyms LCR; Leurocristine Sulfate; NSC-67574; VCR; Vincristine Sulfate

Generic Available Yes

Pharmacologic Category Antineoplastic Agent, Natural Source (Plant) Derivative; Antineoplastic Agent, Vinca Alkaloid

Medication Safety Issues

Sound-alike/look-alike issues:

VinCRIStine may be confused with vinBLAStine

Oncovin® may be confused with Ancobon®

To prevent fatal inadvertent intrathecal injection, it is recommended that all doses be dispensed in a small minibag; do not dispense in a syringe.

Use Treatment of leukemias, Hodgkin's disease, non-Hodgkin's lymphomas, Wilms' tumor, neuroblastoma, rhabdomyosarcoma

Mechanism of Action/Effect Binds to microtubular protein of the mitotic spindle causing metaphase arrest; cell-cycle phase specific in the M and S phases

Contraindications Hypersensitivity to vincristine or any component of the formulation; **for I.V. use only, fatal if given intrathecally**; patients with demyelinating form of Charcot-Marie-Tooth syndrome; pregnancy

Warnings/Precautions For I.V. use only. The U.S. Food and Drug Administration (FDA) currently recommends that procedures for proper handling and disposal of antineoplastic agents be considered. Appropriate safety equipment is recommended for preparation, administration, and disposal of antineoplastics. If vincristine contacts the skin, wash and flush thoroughly with water.

Dosage modification required in patients with impaired hepatic function or who have pre-existing neuromuscular disease. Drug is a vesicant. Avoid extravasation. Use with caution in the elderly. Avoid eye contamination. Observe closely for shortness of breath, bronchospasm, especially in patients treated with mitomycin C. Alterations in mental status such as depression, confusion, or insomnia; constipation, paralytic ileus, and urinary tract disturbances may occur. All patients should be on a prophylactic bowel management regimen. Administer allopurinol to prevent uric acid nephropathy.

Intrathecal administration of VCR has uniformly caused death; VCR should never be administered by this route. Neurologic effects of VCR may be additive with those of other neurotoxic agents and spinal cord irradiation.

Drug Interactions

Cytochrome P450 Effect: Substrate of CYP3A4 (major); **Inhibits** CYP3A4 (weak)

Decreased Effect: Digoxin levels may decrease with combination chemotherapy. CYP3A4 inducers may decrease the levels/effects of vincristine; example inducers include aminoglutethimide, carbamazepine, nafcillin, nevirapine, phenobarbital, phenytoin, and rifamycins.

Increased Effect/Toxicity: Vincristine should be given 12-24 hours before asparaginase to minimize toxicity (may decrease the hepatic clearance of vincristine). Acute pulmonary reactions may occur with mitomycin-C. Previous or simultaneous use with mitomycin-C has resulted in acute shortness of breath and severe bronchospasm within minutes or several hours after *Vinca* alkaloid injection and may occur up to 2 weeks after the dose of mitomycin.

CYP3A4 inhibitors may increase the levels/effects of vincristine. Example inhibitors include azole antifungals, ciprofloxacin, clarithromycin, diclofenac, doxycycline, erythromycin, imatinib, isoniazid, nefazodone, nicardipine, propofol, protease inhibitors, quinidine, and verapamil. Digoxin plasma levels and renal excretion may decrease with combination chemotherapy including vincristine.

Nutritional/Ethanol Interactions Herb/Nutraceutical: St John's wort may decrease vincristine levels.

Adverse Reactions

>10%:

Dermatologic: Alopecia occurs in 20% to 70% of patients

Extravasation: VCR is a vesicant and can cause tissue irritation and necrosis if infiltrated; if extravasation occurs, follow institutional policy, which may include hyaluronidase and hot compresses

Vesicant chemotherapy

1% to 10%:

Cardiovascular: Orthostatic hypotension or hypertension, hyper-/hypotension

Central nervous system: Motor difficulties, seizure, headache, CNS depression, cranial nerve paralysis, fever

Dermatologic: Rash

Endocrine & metabolic: Hyperuricemia

SIADH: Rarely occurs, but may be related to the neurologic toxicity; may cause symptomatic hyponatremia with seizure; the increase in serum ADH concentration usually subsides within 2-3 days after onset

Gastrointestinal: Constipation and possible paralytic ileus secondary to neurologic toxicity; oral ulceration, abdominal cramps, anorexia, metallic taste, bloating, nausea (mild), vomiting, weight loss, diarrhea

Local: Phlebitis

Neurologic: Alterations in mental status such as depression, confusion, or insomnia; constipation, paralytic ileus, and urinary tract disturbances may occur. All patients should be on a prophylactic bowel management regimen. Cranial nerve palsies, headaches, jaw pain, optic atrophy with blindness have been reported. Intrathecal administration of VCR has uniformly caused death; VCR should **never** be administered by this route. Neurologic effects of VCR may be additive with those of other neurotoxic agents and spinal cord irradiation.

Neuromuscular & skeletal: Jaw pain, leg pain, myalgia, cramping, numbness, weakness

Peripheral neuropathy: Frequently the dose-limiting toxicity of VCR. Most frequent in patients >40 years of age; occurs usually after an average of 3 weekly doses, but may occur after just one dose. Manifested as loss of the deep tendon reflexes in the lower extremities, numbness, tingling, pain, paresthesia of the fingers and toes (stocking glove sensation), and "foot drop" or "wrist drop"

Ocular: Photophobia

Overdosage/Toxicology Symptoms of overdose include bone marrow suppression, mental depression, paresthesia, loss of deep tendon reflexes, alopecia, and nausea. Severe symptoms may occur with 3-4 mg/m^2.

There are no antidotes for vincristine. Treatment is supportive and symptomatic, including fluid restriction or hypertonic saline (3% sodium chloride) for drug-induced secretion of inappropriate antidiuretic hormone (SIADH). Case reports suggest that folinic acid may be helpful in treating vincristine overdose. It is suggested that 100 mg folinic acid be given I.V. every 3 hours for 24 hours, then every 6 hours for 48 hours. This is in addition to supportive care. The use of pyridoxine, leucovorin factor, cyanocobalamin, or thiamine has been used with little success for drug-induced peripheral neuropathy.

(Continued)

VinCRIStine *(Continued)*

Pharmacodynamics/Kinetics
Absorption: Oral: Poor

Protein Binding: 75%

Half-Life Elimination: Terminal: 24 hours

Metabolism: Extensively hepatic

Excretion: Feces (~80%); urine (<1% as unchanged drug)

Dosing
Adults & Elderly: Note: Doses are often capped at 2 mg; however, this may reduce the efficacy of the therapy and may not be advisable. Refer to individual protocols; orders for single doses >2.5 mg or >5 mg/treatment cycle should be verified with the specific treatment regimen and/or an experienced oncologist prior to dispensing.

Antineoplastic (typical dosages): I.V.: 0.4-1.4 mg/m^2, may repeat every week **or**
0.4-0.5 mg/day continuous infusion for 4 days every 4 weeks **or**
0.25-0.5 mg/m^2/day continuous infusion for 5 days every 4 weeks

Pediatrics: Refer to individual protocols. **Note:** Doses are often capped at 2 mg; however, this may reduce the efficacy of the therapy and may not be advisable. Orders for single doses >2.5 mg or >5 mg/treatment cycle should be verified with the specific treatment regimen and/or an experienced oncologist prior to dispensing.

Antineoplastic (typical dosages): I.V.:
Children ≤10 kg or BSA <1 m^2: Initial therapy: 0.05 mg/kg once weekly then titrate dose; maximum single dose: 2 mg
Children >10 kg or BSA ≥1 m^2: 1-2 mg/m^2, may repeat once weekly for 3-6 weeks; maximum single dose: 2 mg

Neuroblastoma: I.V. continuous infusion with doxorubicin: 1 mg/m^2/day for 72 hours

Hepatic Impairment:
Serum bilirubin 1.5-3.0 mg/dL or AST 60-180 units: Administer 50% of normal dose.
Serum bilirubin 3.0-5.0 mg/dL: Administer 25% of dose.
Serum bilirubin >5.0 mg/dL or AST >180 units: Omit dose.

Available Dosage Forms Injection, solution, as sulfate: 1 mg/mL (1 mL, 2 mL)

Monitoring and Teaching Issues
Physical Assessment: Use caution with impaired liver function (see Warnings/Precautions for specific for use cautions). Assess potential for interactions with other pharmacological agents and herbal products patient may be taking (eg, previous or concurrent use with mitomycin-C can cause severe reaction; see Drug Interactions). Premedication with antiemetic is advisable. Infusion site must be monitored closely to prevent extravasation (vesicant will cause tissue damage and necrosis). May cause severe constipation, paralytic ileus, intestinal obstruction, necrosis, and/or perforation; prophylactic bowel management regimen may be advisable. Assess results of laboratory tests, hepatic function, and adverse reactions prior to each infusion and throughout therapy (eg, CNS [motor difficulties, seizure, depression], neuromuscular [myalgia, cramping], peripheral neuropathy, photophobia; see Adverse Reactions). Teach patient possible side effects/appropriate interventions and adverse symptoms to report (see Patient Education).

Monitoring Laboratory Tests: Serum electrolytes (sodium), hepatic function, CBC, serum uric acid

Patient Education: Do not take any new medication during therapy unless approved by prescriber. This medication can only be administered by infusion; report immediately any redness, swelling, burning, or pain at infusion site. Maintain adequate hydration (2-3 L/day of fluids) unless instructed to restrict fluid intake and nutrition (small frequent meals will help). You will be more susceptible to infection (avoid crowds and exposure to infection and do not have any vaccinations unless approved by prescriber). May cause hair loss (will grow back after therapy); nausea or vomiting (request antiemetic); photosensitivity (use sunscreen, wear protective clothing and eyewear, and avoid direct sunlight); feelings of extreme weakness or lethargy (use caution when driving or engaging in tasks requiring alertness until response to drug is known); or mouth sores (use soft toothbrush, waxed dental floss, and frequent oral care). Report persistent constipation, abdominal pain; numbness or tingling in fingers or toes (use care to prevent injury); weakness, numbness, or pain in muscles or extremities; signs of infection (eg, fever, chills, sore throat, burning urination, fatigue); unusual bleeding (eg, tarry stools, easy bruising, blood in stool, urine, or mouth); unresolved mouth sores; skin rash or itching; or respiratory difficulty. **Pregnancy/breast-feeding precautions:** Do not get pregnant (females) or cause a pregnancy (males) during this therapy. Consult prescriber for appropriate contraceptive measures. Breast-feeding is not recommended.

Pregnancy Risk Factor: D

Lactation: Enters breast milk/not recommended

Administration
I.V.: Vesicant. For I.V. use only. **Fatal if given intrathecally.** Usually administered as slow (1-2 minutes) push or short (10-15 minutes) infusion; 24-hour continuous infusions are occasionally used

Other: Intralesional injection has been reported for Kaposi's sarcoma

Reconstitution: Solutions for I.V. infusion may be mixed in NS or D$_5$W.

Compatibility: Stable in D$_5$W, LR, NS
Y-site administration: Incompatible with cefepime, furosemide, idarubicin, sodium bicarbonate
Compatibility in syringe: Incompatible with furosemide

Storage: Store intact vials at refrigeration (2°C to 8°C). Protect from light. Solutions reconstituted in NS or D$_5$W are stable for 21 days at room temperature or under refrigeration.

Related Information
FDA Name Differentiation Project: The Use of Tall-Man Letters *on page 15*

◆ **Vincristine Sulfate** *see* VinCRIStine *on page 1564*

Vinorelbine (vi NOR el been)

U.S. Brand Names Navelbine®

Synonyms Dihydroxydeoxynorvinkaleukoblastine; NVB; Vinorelbine Tartrate

Generic Available Yes

Pharmacologic Category Antineoplastic Agent, Natural Source (Plant) Derivative; Antineoplastic Agent, Vinca Alkaloid

Medication Safety Issues
Sound-alike/look-alike issues:
Vinorelbine may be confused with vinBLAStine

Use Treatment of nonsmall cell lung cancer

Unlabeled/Investigational Use Treatment of breast cancer, ovarian carcinoma, Hodgkin's disease, non-Hodgkin's lymphoma

Mechanism of Action/Effect Mitotic inhibition that causes metaphase arrest in neoplastic cells

Contraindications For I.V. use only; **I.T. use may result in death**; hypersensitivity to vinorelbine or any component of the formulation; severe bone marrow suppression (granulocyte counts <1000 cells/mm³); pregnancy

Warnings/Precautions The U.S. Food and Drug Administration (FDA) currently recommends that procedures for proper handling and disposal of antineoplastic agents be considered. Avoid extravasation; dosage modification required in patients with impaired liver function and neurotoxicity. Frequently monitor patients for myelosuppression both during and after therapy. Granulocytopenia is dose-limiting. **Intrathecal administration may result in death.** Use with caution in patients with cachexia or ulcerated skin.

Acute shortness of breath and severe bronchospasm have been reported, most commonly when administered with mitomycin. Fatal cases of interstitial pulmonary changes and ARDS have also been reported. May cause severe constipation (grade 3-4), paralytic ileus, intestinal obstruction, necrosis, and/or perforation.

Drug Interactions
Cytochrome P450 Effect: Substrate of CYP2D6 (minor), 3A4 (major); **Inhibits** CYP2D6 (weak), 3A4 (weak)

Decreased Effect: CYP3A4 inducers may decrease the levels/effects of vinorelbine; example inducers include aminoglutethimide, carbamazepine, nafcillin, nevirapine, phenobarbital, phenytoin, and rifamycins.

Increased Effect/Toxicity: Previous or simultaneous use with mitomycin-C has resulted in acute shortness of breath and severe bronchospasm within minutes or several hours after *Vinca* alkaloid injection and may occur up to 2 weeks after the dose of mitomycin. CYP3A4 inhibitors may increase the levels/effects of vinorelbine; example inhibitors include azole antifungals, ciprofloxacin, clarithromycin, diclofenac, doxycycline, erythromycin, imatinib, isoniazid, nefazodone, nicardipine, propofol, protease inhibitors, quinidine, and verapamil. Incidence of granulocytopenia is significantly higher in cisplatin/vinorelbine combination therapy than with single-agent vinorelbine.

Nutritional/Ethanol Interactions Herb/Nutraceutical: St John's wort may decrease vinorelbine levels.

Adverse Reactions
>10%:
Central nervous system: Fatigue (27%)
Dermatologic: Alopecia (12%)
Gastrointestinal: Nausea (44%, severe <2%) and vomiting (20%) are most common and are easily controlled with standard antiemetics; constipation (35%), diarrhea (17%)
Emetic potential: Moderate (30% to 60%)
Hematologic: May cause severe bone marrow suppression and is the dose-limiting toxicity of vinorelbine; severe granulocytopenia (90%) may occur following the administration of vinorelbine; leukopenia (92%), anemia (83%)
Myelosuppressive:
WBC: Moderate - severe
Onset: 4-7 days
Nadir: 7-10 days
Recovery: 14-21 days
Hepatic: Elevated SGOT (67%), elevated total bilirubin (13%)
Local: Injection site reaction (28%), injection site pain (16%)
Neuromuscular & skeletal: Weakness (36%), peripheral neuropathy (20% to 25%)
1% to 10%:
Cardiovascular: Chest pain (5%)
Gastrointestinal: Paralytic ileus (1%)
Hematologic: Thrombocytopenia (5%)
Local: Extravasation: Vesicant and can cause tissue irritation and necrosis if infiltrated; if extravasation occurs, follow institutional policy, which may include hyaluronidase and hot compresses; phlebitis (7%)
Vesicant chemotherapy
Neuromuscular & skeletal: Mild to moderate peripheral neuropathy manifested by paresthesia and hyperesthesia, loss of deep tendon reflexes (<5%); myalgia (<5%), arthralgia (<5%), jaw pain (<5%)
Respiratory: Dyspnea (3% to 7%)

Overdosage/Toxicology Symptoms of overdose include bone marrow suppression, mental depression, paresthesia, loss of deep tendon reflexes, and neurotoxicity. There are no antidotes for vinorelbine. Treatment is supportive and symptomatic, including fluid restriction or hypertonic saline (3% sodium chloride) for drug-induced secretion of inappropriate antidiuretic hormone (SIADH).
(Continued)

Vinorelbine (Continued)

Pharmacodynamics/Kinetics

Absorption: Unreliable; must be given I.V.

Bioavailability: Oral: 26% to 45%

Protein Binding: 80% to 90%

Half-Life Elimination: Triphasic: Terminal: 27.7-43.6 hours

Metabolism: Extensively hepatic to two metabolites, deacetylvinorelbine (active) and vinorelbine N-oxide

Excretion: Feces (46%); urine (18%, 10% to 12% as unchanged drug)

Clearance: Plasma: Mean: 0.97-1.26 L/hour/kg

Dosing

Adults & Elderly: Refer to individual protocols.

Nonsmall cell lung cancer: I.V.:

Single-agent therapy: 30 mg/m^2 every 7 days

Combination therapy with cisplatin: 25 mg/m^2 every 7 days (with cisplatin 100 mg/m^2 every 4 weeks); **Alternatively:** 30 mg/m^2 in combination with cisplatin 120 mg/m^2 on days 1 and 29, then every 6 weeks.

Dosage adjustment in hematological toxicity (based on granulocyte counts):

Granulocytes ≥1500 cells/mm^3 on day of treatment: Administer 100% of starting dose.

Granulocytes 1000-1499 cells/mm^3 on day of treatment: Administer 50% of starting dose.

Granulocytes <1000 cells/mm^3 on day of treatment: Do not administer. Repeat granulocyte count in 1 week. If 3 consecutive doses are held because granulocyte count is <1000 cells/mm^3, discontinue vinorelbine.

Adjustment: For patients who, during treatment, have experienced fever or sepsis while granulocytopenic or had 2 consecutive weekly doses held due to granulocytopenia, subsequent doses of vinorelbine should be:

75% of starting dose for granulocytes ≥1500 cells/mm^3

37.5% of starting dose for granulocytes 1000-1499 cells/mm^3

Renal Impairment: No dose adjustments are required for renal insufficiency.

Hepatic Impairment:

Serum bilirubin ≤2 mg/dL: Administer 100% of starting dose.

Serum bilirubin 2.1-3 mg/dL: Administer 50% of starting dose.

Serum bilirubin >3 mg/dL: Administer 25% of starting dose.

In patients with concurrent hematologic toxicity and hepatic impairment, administer the lower doses determined from the above recommendations under Adult Dosing.

Available Dosage Forms Injection, solution, as tartrate [preservative free]: 10 mg/mL (1 mL, 5 mL)

Monitoring and Teaching Issues

Physical Assessment: See Warnings/Precautions for specific use cautions. Assess potential for interactions with other pharmacological agents and herbal products patient may be taking (eg, CYP3A4 inducers [eg, carbamazepine, nafcillin, phenobarbital] may decrease levels/effects of vinorelbine; CYP3A4 inhibitors [eg, azole antifungals, clarithromycin, erythromycin, protease inhibitors] may increase levels effects of vinorelbine; see Drug Interactions). Premedication with antiemetic is advisable. May cause severe constipation, paralytic ileus, intestinal obstruction, necrosis, and/or perforation; prophylactic bowel management regimen may be advisable. See Administration for infusion specifics. Infusion site must be monitored closely to prevent extravasation (may cause tissue damage and necrosis). Assess results of laboratory tests and monitor for adverse reactions prior to each infusion and throughout therapy (see Adverse Reactions). Teach patient possible side effects/appropriate interventions and adverse symptoms to report (see Patient Education).

Monitoring Laboratory Tests: CBC with differential and platelet count, hepatic function

Patient Education: Do not take any new medication during therapy unless approved by prescriber. This medication can only be administered by infusion; report immediately any redness, swelling, burning, or pain at infusion site. Maintain adequate hydration (2-3 L/day of fluids) unless instructed to restrict fluid intake and nutrition (small frequent meals will help). You will be more susceptible to infection (avoid crowds and exposure to infection and do not have any vaccinations unless approved by prescriber). May cause hair loss (will grow back after therapy); nausea or vomiting (request antiemetic); photosensitivity (use sunscreen, wear protective clothing and eyewear, and avoid direct sunlight); feelings of weakness or lethargy (use caution when driving or engaging in tasks requiring alertness until response to drug is known); or mouth sores (use soft toothbrush, waxed dental floss and frequent oral care). Report persistent constipation or abdominal pain; numbness or tingling in fingers or toes (use care to prevent injury); weakness, numbness, or pain in muscles or extremities; signs of infection (eg, fever, chills, sore throat, burning urination, fatigue); unusual bleeding (eg, tarry stools, easy bruising, blood in stool, urine, or mouth); unresolved mouth sores; skin rash or itching; or respiratory difficulty. **Pregnancy/breast-feeding precautions:** Do not get pregnant (females) or cause a pregnancy (males) during this therapy. Consult prescriber for appropriate contraceptive measures. Do not breast-feed.

Pregnancy Risk Factor: D

Lactation: Excretion in breast milk unknown/contraindicated

Administration

I.V.: FATAL IF GIVEN INTRATHECALLY. Administer as a direct intravenous push or rapid bolus, over 6-10 minutes (up to 30 minutes). Longer infusions may increase the risk of pain and phlebitis. Intravenous doses should be followed by 150-250 mL of saline or dextrose to reduce the incidence of phlebitis and inflammation. **CENTRAL LINE ONLY** for IVPB administration.

Reconstitution: Dilute in 10-50 mL D$_5$W or NS.

Compatibility: Stable in D$_5$¹/₂NS, D$_5$W, LR, NS, ¹/₂NS

Y-site administration: Incompatible with acyclovir, allopurinol, aminophylline, amphotericin B, amphotericin B cholesteryl sulfate complex, ampicillin, cefazolin, cefoperazone, cefotetan, ceftriaxone, cefuroxime, co-trimoxazole, fluorouracil, furosemide, ganciclovir, methylprednisolone sodium succinate, mitomycin, piperacillin, sodium bicarbonate, thiotepa

Storage: Store intact vials under refrigeration (2°C to 8°C) and protect from light; vials are stable at room temperature for up to 72 hours. Dilutions in D_5W or NS are stable for 24 hours at room temperature.

- ◆ **Vinorelbine Tartrate** *see* Vinorelbine *on page 1567*
- ◆ **Viokase®** *see* Pancrelipase *on page 1151*
- ◆ **Viosterol** *see* Ergocalciferol *on page 538*
- ◆ **Viracept®** *see* Nelfinavir *on page 1065*
- ◆ **Viramune®** *see* Nevirapine *on page 1073*
- ◆ **Viravan®** *see* Phenylephrine and Pyrilamine *on page 1202*
- ◆ **Viravan®-DM** *see* Phenylephrine, Pyrilamine, and Dextromethorphan *on page 1204*
- ◆ **Virazole®** *see* Ribavirin *on page 1318*
- ◆ **Viread®** *see* Tenofovir *on page 1441*
- ◆ **Virilon®** *see* MethylTESTOSTERone *on page 988*
- ◆ **Viroptic®** *see* Trifluridine *on page 1525*
- ◆ **Viscoat®** *see page 1625*
- ◆ **Vistaril®** *see* HydrOXYzine *on page 773*
- ◆ **Vistide®** *see* Cidofovir *on page 321*
- ◆ **Vitamin A Acid** *see* Tretinoin (Topical) *on page 1516*
- ◆ **Vitamin B₁** *see* Thiamine *on page 1461*
- ◆ **Vitamin B₂** *see* Riboflavin *on page 1321*
- ◆ **Vitamin B₃** *see* Niacin *on page 1075*
- ◆ **Vitamin B₆** *see* Pyridoxine *on page 1289*
- ◆ **Vitamin B₁₂** *see* Cyanocobalamin *on page 377*
- ◆ **Vitamin B₁₂** *see* Hydroxocobalamin *on page 769*
- ◆ **Vitamin D₂** *see* Ergocalciferol *on page 538*

Vitamin E (VYE ta min ee)

U.S. Brand Names Aqua Gem E® [OTC]; Aquasol E® [OTC]; E-Gems® [OTC]; Key-E® [OTC]; Key-E® Kaps [OTC]

Synonyms *d*-Alpha Tocopherol; *dl*-Alpha Tocopherol

Generic Available Yes

Pharmacologic Category Vitamin, Fat Soluble

Medication Safety Issues

Sound-alike/look-alike issues:

Aquasol E® may be confused with Anusol®

Use Prevention and treatment hemolytic anemia secondary to vitamin E deficiency, dietary supplement

Unlabeled/Investigational Use To reduce the risk of bronchopulmonary dysplasia or retrolental fibroplasia in infants exposed to high concentrations of oxygen; prevention and treatment of tardive dyskinesia and Alzheimer's disease

Mechanism of Action/Effect Prevents oxidation of vitamin A and C; protects polyunsaturated fatty acids in membranes from attack by free radicals and protects red blood cells against hemolysis

Contraindications Hypersensitivity to vitamin E or any component of the formulation; I.V. route

Warnings/Precautions May induce vitamin K deficiency. Necrotizing enterocolitis has been associated with oral administration of large dosages (eg, >200 units/day) of a hyperosmolar vitamin E preparation in low birth weight infants.

Drug Interactions

Decreased Effect: Vitamin E may impair the hematologic response to iron in children with iron-deficiency anemia; monitor.

Increased Effect/Toxicity: Vitamin E may alter the effect of vitamin K actions on clotting factors resulting in an increase hypoprothrombinemic response to warfarin; monitor.

Pharmacodynamics/Kinetics

Absorption: Oral: Depends on presence of bile; reduced in conditions of malabsorption, in low birth weight premature infants, and as dosage increases; water miscible preparations are better absorbed than oil preparations

Metabolism: Hepatic to glucuronides

Excretion: Feces

Dosing

Adults & Elderly: One unit of vitamin E = 1 mg *dl*-alpha-tocopherol acetate. Oral:

Recommended daily allowance (RDA): 15 mg (22.5 units); upper limit of intake should not exceed 1000 mg/day

Pregnant female:

≤18 years: 15 mg (22.5 units); upper level of intake should not exceed 800 mg/day

19-50 years: 15 mg (22.5 units); upper level of intake should not exceed 1000 mg/day

Lactating female:

≤18 years: 19 mg (28.5 units); upper level of intake should not exceed 800 mg/day

19-50 years: 19 mg (28.5 units); upper level of intake should not exceed 1000 mg/day

Vitamin E deficiency: 60-75 units/day

Prevention of vitamin E deficiency: Oral: 30 units/day

Cystic fibrosis: Oral: 100-400 units/day

Beta-thalassemia: Oral: 750 units/day

Sickle cell disease: Oral: 450 units/day

Alzheimer's disease: Oral: 1000 units twice daily

Tardive dyskinesia: Oral: 1600 units/day

Superficial dermatologic irritation: Topical: Apply a thin layer over affected area.

(Continued)

Vitamin E *(Continued)*

Pediatrics: One unit of vitamin E = 1 mg *dl*-alpha-tocopherol acetate. Oral:

Recommended daily allowance (RDA):
Premature infants ≤3 months: 17 mg (25 units)
Infants:
  ≤6 months: 3 mg (4.5 units)
  7-12 months: 4 mg (6 units)
Children:
  1-3 years: 6 mg (9 units); upper limit of intake should not exceed 200 mg/day
  4-8 years: 7 mg (10.5 units); upper limit of intake should not exceed 300 mg/day
  9-13 years: 11 mg (16.5 units); upper limit of intake should not exceed 600 mg/day
  14-18 years: 15 mg (22.5 units); upper limit of intake should not exceed 800 mg/day

Vitamin E deficiency:
Children (with malabsorption syndrome): 1 unit/kg/day of water miscible vitamin E (to raise plasma tocopherol concentrations to the normal range within 2 months and to maintain normal plasma concentrations)

Prevention of retinopathy of prematurity or BPD secondary to O₂ therapy (AAP considers this use investigational and routine use is not recommended):
Retinopathy prophylaxis: 15-30 units/kg/day to maintain plasma levels between 1.5-2 mcg/mL (may need as high as 100 units/kg/day)

Cystic fibrosis, beta-thalassemia may require higher daily maintenance doses:
Cystic fibrosis: Oral: 100-400 units/day
Beta-thalassemia: Oral: 750 units/day

Available Dosage Forms
Capsule: 100 units, 200 units, 400 units, 500 units, 600 units, 1000 units
  Aqua Gem E®: 200 units, 400 units
  E-Gems®: 30 units, 100 units, 600 units, 800 units, 1000 units, 1200 units
  Key-E® Kaps: 200 units, 400 units
Cream: 100 units/g (60 g)
  Key-E®: 30 units/g (60 g, 120 g, 480 g)
Oil: 100 units/0.25 mL (60 mL); 1150 units/0.25 mL (30 mL, 60 mL, 120 mL)
  E-Gems®: 100 units/10 drops (15 mL, 60 mL)
Ointment, topical (Key-E®): 30 units/g (60 g, 120 g, 480 g)
Powder (Key-E®): 700 units/dose (15 g, 75 g, 1000 g)
Solution, oral drops (Aquasol E®): 15 units/0.3 mL (12 mL, 30 mL)
Spray (Key-E®): 30 units/3 seconds (105 g)
Suppository (Key-E®): 30 units (12s, 24s)
Tablet: 100 units, 200 units, 400 units, 500 units, 800 units
  Key-E®: 100 units, 200 units, 400 units

Monitoring and Teaching Issues
Physical Assessment: Assess effectiveness and interactions of other medications patient may be taking. Assess knowledge/teach patient appropriate use (according to formulation prescribed) and adverse symptoms to report.
Monitoring Laboratory Tests: Monitor plasma tocopherol concentrations (normal range: 6-14 mcg/mL)
Patient Education: Take exactly as directed; do not take more than the recommended dose. Do not use mineral oil or other vitamin E supplements without consulting prescriber. Report persistent nausea, vomiting, or cramping; or gonadal dysfunction. **Pregnancy precaution:** Inform prescriber if you are pregnant.
Pregnancy Risk Factor: A/C (dose exceeding RDA recommendation)
Lactation: Excretion in breast milk unknown/compatible

Administration
Oral: Swallow capsules whole, do not crush or chew.
Storage: Protect from light.
Additional Information 1 mg *dl*-alpha tocopheryl acetate = 1 int. unit

- **Vitamin G** *see* Riboflavin *on page 1321*
- **Vitamin K₁** *see* Phytonadione *on page 1209*
- **Vitrasert®** *see* Ganciclovir *on page 695*
- **Vivactil®** *see* Protriptyline *on page 1279*
- **Vivarin® [OTC]** *see* Caffeine *on page 229*
- **Vivelle®** *see* Estradiol *on page 552*
- **Vivelle-Dot®** *see* Estradiol *on page 552*
- **Vivotif Berna®** *see page 1660*
- **VLB** *see* VinBLAStine *on page 1563*
- **VM-26** *see* Teniposide *on page 1439*
- **Volmax® [DSC]** *see* Albuterol *on page 59*
- **Voltaren®** *see* Diclofenac *on page 442*
- **Voltaren Ophthalmic®** *see* Diclofenac *on page 442*
- **Voltaren®-XR** *see* Diclofenac *on page 442*

Voriconazole *(vor i KOE na zole)*
U.S. Brand Names VFEND®
Synonyms UK109496
Generic Available No
Pharmacologic Category Antifungal Agent, Oral; Antifungal Agent, Parenteral
Use Treatment of invasive aspergillosis; treatment of esophageal candidiasis; treatment of candidemia (in non-neutropenic patients); treatment of *Candida* deep tissue infections; treatment of serious fungal infections caused by *Scedosporium apiospermum* and *Fusarium* spp (including *Fusarium solani*) in patients intolerant of, or refractory to, other therapy

Mechanism of Action/Effect Interferes with fungal cytochrome P450 activity, decreasing ergosterol synthesis (principal sterol in fungal cell membrane) and inhibiting fungal cell membrane formation.

Contraindications Hypersensitivity to voriconazole or any component of the formulation (cross-reaction with other azole antifungal agents may occur but has not been established, use caution); coadministration of CYP3A4 substrates which may lead to QT_c prolongation (cisapride, pimozide, or quinidine); coadministration with barbiturates (long acting), carbamazepine, efavirenz, ergot alkaloids, rifampin, rifabutin, ritonavir, and sirolimus; pregnancy (unless risk:benefit justifies use)

Warnings/Precautions Visual changes are commonly associated with treatment. Patients should be warned to avoid tasks which depend on vision, including operating machinery or driving. Changes are reversible on discontinuation following brief exposure/treatment regimens (≤28 days).

Serious hepatic reactions (including hepatitis, cholestasis, and fulminant hepatic failure) have occurred during treatment, primarily in patients with serious concomitant medical conditions. However, hepatotoxicity has occurred in patients with no identifiable risk factors. Use caution in patients with pre-existing hepatic impairment (dose adjustment required).

Voriconazole tablets contain lactose; avoid administration in hereditary galactose intolerance, Lapp lactase deficiency, or glucose-galactose malabsorption. Suspension contains sucrose; use caution with fructose intolerance, sucrose-isomaltase deficiency, or glucose-galactose malabsorption. Avoid/limit use of intravenous formulation in patients with renal impairment; intravenous formulation contains excipient sulfobutyl ether beta-cyclodextrin (SBECD), which may accumulate in renal insufficiency. Infusion-related reactions may occur with intravenous dosing. Consider discontinuation of infusion if reaction is severe.

Use caution in patients with an increased risk of arrhythmia (concurrent QT_c-prolonging drugs, hypokalemia, cardiomyopathy, or prior cardiotoxic therapy). Use caution in patients receiving concurrent non-nucleoside reverse transcriptase inhibitors (efavirenz is contraindicated).

Avoid use in pregnancy, unless an evaluation of the potential benefit justifies possible risk to the fetus. Safety and efficacy have not been established in children <12 years of age.

Drug Interactions

Cytochrome P450 Effect: Substrate of CYP2C8/9 (major), 2C19 (major), 3A4 (minor); **Inhibits** CYP2C8/9 (weak), 2C19 (weak), 3A4 (moderate)

Decreased Effect: The levels/effects of voriconazole may be decreased by aminoglutethimide, carbamazepine, efavirenz, nevirapine, phenytoin, phenobarbital, secobarbital, rifampin, ritonavir, and other CYP2C8/9 or 2C19 inducers. Rifampin decreases voriconazole's serum concentration to levels which are no longer effective; avoid concurrent use. When used with phenytoin, prospective adjustment of voriconazole dosage is recommended. Serum levels of voriconazole may be decreased by efavirenz or nevirapine.

Increased Effect/Toxicity: Voriconazole may increase the serum concentrations of cisapride, pimozide leading to malignant arrhythmias; use is contraindicated. Concurrent use of QT_c-prolonging agents (including class Ia and III antiarrhythmics) may increase risk of arrhythmias. Serum levels of ergot alkaloids may be increased by voriconazole, leading to ergot toxicity; concurrent use is contraindicated. Rifabutin serum levels are increased by voriconazole; concurrent use is contraindicated. Serum concentrations of busulfan, docetaxel, and dofetilide may be increased; avoid concurrent use.

Serum concentrations of immunosuppressants (cyclosporine, sirolimus, and tacrolimus) may be increased; concurrent use of sirolimus is contraindicated. Decrease cyclosporine dosage by 50% when initiating voriconazole, decreased tacrolimus dosage by 66% when initiating voriconazole.

Serum levels of voriconazole may be increased by delavirdine. Indinavir did not appear to alter voriconazole serum concentrations during concurrent treatment; other protease inhibitors may result in increased voriconazole concentrations.

Voriconazole may increase the serum concentrations of buspirone, methylprednisolone, quinidine, sulfonylureas, trimetrexate, vinca alkaloids, or zolpidem. Voriconazole may increase the levels/effects of benzodiazepines, calcium channel blockers, selected HMG-CoA reductase inhibitors mirtazapine, nateglinide, nefazodone, sildenafil (and other PDE-5 inhibitors), tacrolimus, venlafaxine, and other CYP3A4 substrates. In addition, the anticoagulant effect of warfarin may be increased.

Changes in gastric acidity (due to H_2 antagonists or proton pump inhibitors) do not appear to significantly affect voriconazole absorption. However, voriconazole may significantly increase serum levels of omeprazole. For omeprazole dosages >40 mg/day, reduce omeprazole dosage by 50%. Serum levels of other proton pump inhibitors may also be increased.

Nutritional/Ethanol Interactions

Food: May decrease voriconazole absorption. Voriconazole should be taken 1 hour before or 1 hour after a meal. Avoid grapefruit juice (may increase voriconazole serum levels).

Herb/Nutraceutical: St John's wort may decrease voriconazole levels.

Adverse Reactions Note: Includes adverse reactions reported from all trials, including trials conducted in immunocompromised patients; cause:effect relationship not established for many reactions

>10%: Ocular: Visual changes (photophobia, color changes, increased or decreased visual acuity, or blurred vision occur in ~30%)

1% to 10%:

Cardiovascular: Tachycardia (3%), hyper-/hypotension (2%), vasodilation (2%), peripheral edema (1%)

Central nervous system: Fever (6%), chills (4%), headache (3%), hallucinations (3%), dizziness (1%)

Dermatologic: Rash (6%), pruritus (1%)

Endocrine & metabolic: Hypokalemia (2%), hypomagnesemia (1%)

(Continued)

Voriconazole *(Continued)*

Gastrointestinal: Nausea (6%), vomiting (5%), abdominal pain (2%), diarrhea (1%), xerostomia (1%)

Hematologic: Thrombocytopenia (1%)

Hepatic: Alkaline phosphatase increased (4%), transaminases increased (2%), AST increased (2%), ALT increased (2%), cholestatic jaundice (1%)

Renal: Acute renal failure (1%)

Overdosage/Toxicology Limited experience in overdose. Symptoms may include changes in vision, cholinergic symptoms (salivation, mydriasis), and CNS depression. Following intravenous overdose, toxicity from the vehicle, SBECD, may also occur. Both voriconazole and the intravenous vehicle may be eliminated via hemodialysis.

Pharmacodynamics/Kinetics

Absorption: Well absorbed after oral administration

Bioavailability: 96%

Time to Peak: 1-2 hours

Protein Binding: 58%

Half-Life Elimination: Variable, dose dependent

Metabolism: Hepatic, nonlinear (via CYP isoenzymes)

Excretion: Urine (as inactive metabolites)

Dosing

Adults & Elderly:

Invasive aspergillosis and other serious fungal infections: I.V.: Initial: Loading dose: 6 mg/kg every 12 hours for 2 doses; followed by maintenance dose of 4 mg/kg every 12 hours

Candidemia and other deep tissue *Candida* infections: I.V.: Initial: Loading dose 6 mg/kg every 12 hours for 2 doses; followed by maintenance dose of 3-4 mg/kg every 12 hours

Note: *Conversion to oral dosing:*

Patients <40 kg: 100 mg every 12 hours; increase to 150 mg every 12 hours in patients who fail to respond adequately

Patients ≥40 kg: 200 mg every 12 hours; increase to 300 mg every 12 hours in patients who fail to respond adequately

Esophageal candidiasis: Oral:

Patients <40 kg: 100 mg every 12 hours

Patients ≥40 kg: 200 mg every 12 hours

Note: Treatment should continue for a minimum of 14 days, and for at least 7 days following resolution of symptoms.

Dosage adjustment in patients unable to tolerate treatment:

I.V.: Dose may be reduced to 3 mg/kg every 12 hours

Oral: Dose may be reduced in 50 mg increments to a minimum dosage of 200 mg every 12 hours in patients weighing ≥40 kg (100 mg every 12 hours in patients <40 kg)

Dosage adjustment in patients receiving concomitant phenytoin:

I.V.: Increase maintenance dosage to 5 mg/kg every 12 hours

Oral: Increase dose from 200 mg to 400 mg every 12 hours in patients ≥40 kg (100 mg to 200 mg every 12 hours in patients <40 kg)

Pediatrics:

Children <12 years: No data available

Children ≥12 years: Refer to adult dosing.

Renal Impairment: In patients with Cl_{cr} <50 mL/minute, accumulation of the intravenous vehicle (SBECD) occurs. After initial loading dose, oral voriconazole should be administered to these patients, unless an assessment of the benefit:risk to the patient justifies the use of I.V. voriconazole. Monitor serum creatinine and change to oral voriconazole therapy when possible.

Hepatic Impairment:

Mild to moderate hepatic dysfunction (Child-Pugh class A and B): Following standard loading dose, reduce maintenance dosage by 50%

Severe hepatic impairment: Should only be used if benefit outweighs risk; monitor closely for toxicity

Available Dosage Forms

Injection, powder for reconstitution: 200 mg [contains SBECD 3200 mg]

Powder for oral suspension: 200 mg/5 mL (70 mL) [contains sodium benzoate and sucrose; orange flavor]

Tablet: 50 mg, 200 mg [contains lactose]

Monitoring and Teaching Issues

Physical Assessment: Assess allergy history prior to beginning therapy. Use caution with hepatic impairment, increased risk of arrhythmia (see Warnings/Precautions for specific use cautions). Assess potential for interactions with pharmacological agents and herbal products patient may be taking (eg, risk for increased or decreased levels/effects of voriconazole; see Drug Interactions for detailed list). Assess results of laboratory tests (see Monitoring Laboratory Tests), therapeutic effectiveness (resolution of fungal infection), and adverse response on a regular basis, (eg, vision changes [photophobia, changed visual acuity, blurred vision], hepatic toxicity [increased liver enzymes, jaundice], tachycardia; see Adverse Reactions). Teach patient use, possible side effects (eg, vision changes) and interventions, and adverse symptoms to report (see Patient Education).

Patient Education: Do not take any new medication during therapy unless approved by prescriber. Take full course of medication as ordered. Preferable to take on empty stomach (1 hour before or 2 hours after a meal). Avoid grapefruit juice while taking this medication. Maintain adequate hydration (2-3 L/day of fluids) unless instructed to restrict fluid intake. You may experience headache, dizziness, blurred vision, photophobia, or changes in visual acuity (use caution when driving or engaging in tasks that require alertness until response to drug is known; vision changes are reversible on discontinuation following brief treatment); or nausea or vomiting (small frequent meals, frequent mouth care, sucking lozenges, or chewing gum may help). Report immediately any change in vision. Report skin rash; chest pain, palpitations, or rapid heartbeat; fever, chills, or hallucinations; persistent GI upset; urinary pattern changes; yellowing of skin or eyes; changes in color of stool or urine; or any other persistent side effects. **Pregnancy/breast-feeding precautions:** Inform prescriber if you are pregnant. Do not get pregnant while taking this drug. Fetal harm can occur. Consult prescriber for appropriate contraceptive measures. Breast-feeding is not recommended.

Dietary Considerations: Oral: Should be taken 1 hour before or 1 hour after a meal. Voriconazole tablets contain lactose; avoid administration in hereditary galactose intolerance, Lapp lactase deficiency, or glucose-galactose malabsorption. Suspension contains sucrose; use caution with fructose intolerance, sucrose-isomaltase deficiency, or glucose-galactose malabsorption.

Pregnancy Risk Factor: D

Pregnancy Issues: Voriconazole can cause fetal harm when administered to a pregnant woman. Should be used in pregnant woman only if benefit to mother justifies potential risk to the fetus.

Lactation: Excretion in breast milk unknown/not recommended

Breast-Feeding Issues: Excretion in breast milk has not been investigated; avoid breast-feeding until additional data are available.

Administration

Oral: Administer 1 hour before or 1 hour after a meal.

I.V.: Infuse over 1-2 hours (rate not to exceed 3 mg/kg/hour)

Reconstitution:

Powder for injection: Reconstitute 200 mg vial with 19 mL of sterile water for injection (use of automated syringe is not recommended). Resultant solution (20 mL) has a concentration of 10 mg/mL. Must dilute to 0.5-5 mg/mL prior to infusion.

Powder for oral suspension: Add 46 mL of water to the bottle to make 40 mg/mL suspension. Discard unused portion after 14 days.

Compatibility: Stable in LR, $\frac{1}{2}$NS, NS, D_5W, D_5LR, D_5NS, $D_5\frac{1}{2}NS$; **incompatible** with alkaline solutions, bicarbonate, aminofusin 10%, electrolyte solutions.

Storage:

Powder for injection: Store at 15°C to 30°C (59°F to 86°F). Reconstituted solutions are stable for up to 24 hours under refrigeration at 2°C to 8°C (36°F to 46°F).

Powder for oral suspension: Store at 2°C to 8°C (36°F to 46°F). Reconstituted oral suspension may be stored at 15°C to 30°C (59°F to 86°F).

Tablets: Store at 15°C to 30°C (59°F to 86°F).

◆ **VoSol® HC**   see Acetic Acid, Propylene Glycol Diacetate, and Hydrocortisone on page 44

◆ **VoSpire ER™**   see Albuterol on page 59

◆ **VP-16**   see Etoposide on page 599

◆ **VP-16-213**   see Etoposide on page 599

◆ **Vumon**   see Teniposide on page 1439

◆ **Vytorin™**   see Ezetimibe and Simvastatin on page 606

Warfarin (WAR far in)

U.S. Brand Names Coumadin®; Jantoven™

Synonyms Warfarin Sodium

Generic Available Yes: Tablet

Pharmacologic Category Anticoagulant, Coumarin Derivative

Medication Safety Issues

Sound-alike/look-alike issues:

Coumadin® may be confused with Avandia®, Cardura®, Compazine®, Kemadrin®

High alert medication: The Institute for Safe Medication Practices (ISMP) includes this medication among its list of drugs which have a heightened risk of causing significant patient harm when used in error.

Use Prophylaxis and treatment of venous thrombosis, pulmonary embolism and thromboembolic disorders; atrial fibrillation with risk of embolism and as an adjunct in the prophylaxis of systemic embolism after myocardial infarction

Unlabeled/Investigational Use Prevention of recurrent transient ischemic attacks and to reduce risk of recurrent myocardial infarction

Mechanism of Action/Effect Interferes with hepatic synthesis of vitamin K-dependent coagulation factors (II, VII, IX, X)

Contraindications Hypersensitivity to warfarin or any component of the formulation; hemorrhagic tendencies; hemophilia; thrombocytopenia purpura; leukemia; recent or potential surgery of the eye or CNS; major regional lumbar block anesthesia or surgery resulting in large, open surfaces; patients bleeding from the GI, respiratory, or GU tract; threatened abortion; aneurysm; ascorbic acid deficiency; history of bleeding diathesis; prostatectomy; continuous tube drainage of the small intestine; polyarthritis; diverticulitis; emaciation; malnutrition; cerebrovascular hemorrhage; eclampsia/pre-eclampsia; blood dyscrasias; severe uncontrolled or malignant hypertension; severe hepatic disease; pericarditis or pericardial effusion; subacute bacterial endocarditis; visceral carcinoma; following spinal puncture and other diagnostic or therapeutic procedures with potential for significant bleeding; history of warfarin-induced necrosis; an unreliable, noncompliant patient; alcoholism; patient who has a history of falls or is a significant fall risk; pregnancy

Warnings/Precautions Use care in the selection of patients appropriate for this treatment. Ensure patient cooperation especially from the alcoholic, illicit drug user, demented, or psychotic patient. Use with caution in trauma, acute infection (antibiotics and fever may alter affects), renal insufficiency, prolonged dietary insufficiencies (vitamin K deficiency), moderate-severe hypertension, polycythemia vera, vasculitis, open wound, active TB, history of PUD, anaphylactic disorders, indwelling catheters, severe diabetes, thyroid disease, severe renal disease, and menstruating and postpartum women. Use with caution in protein C deficiency.

(Continued)

Warfarin (Continued)

Hemorrhage is the most serious risk of therapy. Patient must be instructed to report bleeding, accidents, or falls. Patient must also report any new or discontinued medications, herbal or alternative products used, significant changes in smoking or dietary habits. Necrosis or gangrene of the skin and other tissues can occur (rarely) due to early hypercoagulability. "Purple toes syndrome," due to cholesterol microembolization, may rarely occur (often after several weeks of therapy). Women may be at risk of developing ovarian hemorrhage at the time of ovulation. The elderly may be more sensitive to anticoagulant therapy.

Drug Interactions

Cytochrome P450 Effect: Substrate of CYP1A2 (minor), 2C8/9 (major), 2C19 (minor), 3A4 (minor); **Inhibits** CYP2C8/9 (moderate), 2C19 (weak)

Decreased Effect: CYP2C8/9 inducers may decrease the levels/effects of warfarin; example inducers include carbamazepine, phenobarbital, phenytoin, rifampin, rifapentine, and secobarbital. Also see table.

Decreased Anticoagulant Effects

Induction of Enzymes		Increased Procoagulant Factors	Decreased Drug Absorption	Other
Antithyroid drugs	Nafcillin	Estrogens	Aluminum hydroxide	Ethchlorvynol
Barbiturates	Phenytoin	Oral contraceptives	Cholestyramine[1]	Griseofulvin
Bosentan	Rifampin	Vitamin K (including	Colestipol[1]	Spironolactone[2]
Carbamazepine		nutritional supplements)		Sucralfate
Glutethimide				
Griseofulvin				

Decreased anticoagulant effect may occur when these drugs are administered with oral anticoagulants.

[1]Cholestyramine and colestipol may increase the anticoagulant effect by binding vitamin K in the gut; yet, the decreased drug absorption appears to be of more concern.

[2]Diuretic-induced hemoconcentration with subsequent concentration of clotting factors has been reported to decrease the effects of oral anticoagulants.

Increased Effect/Toxicity: CYP2C8/9 inhibitors may increase the levels/effects of warfarin (eg, delavirdine, fluconazole, gemfibrozil, ketoconazole, nicardipine, NSAIDs, sulfonamides). Warfarin may increase the levels/effects of CYP2C8/9 substrates (eg, amiodarone, fluoxetine, glimepiride, glipizide, nateglinide, phenytoin, pioglitazone, rosiglitazone, sertraline).

Also see tables.

Increased Bleeding Tendency

Inhibit Platelet Aggregation	Inhibit Procoagulant Factors	Ulcerogenic Drugs
Cephalosporins	Antimetabolites	Adrenal corticosteroids
Clopidogrel	Quinidine	Indomethacin
Dipyridamole	Quinine	Potassium products
Indomethacin	Salicylates	Salicylates
Penicillin, parenteral		
Salicylates		
Sulfinpyrazone		
Ticlopidine		

Use of these agents with oral anticoagulants may increase the chances of hemorrhage.

Enhanced Anticoagulant Effects

Decrease Vitamin K	Displace Anticoagulant	Inhibit Metabolism	Other
Oral antibiotics:	Chloral hydrate	Allopurinol	Acetaminophen
Can ↑/↓ INR.	Clofibrate	Amiodarone	Anabolic steroids
Check INR 3 days	Diazoxide	Azole antifungals	Capecitabine
after a patient	Ethacrynic acid	Capecitabine	Celecoxib
begins antibiotics to	Miconazole (including	Chloramphenicol	Clarithromycin
see the INR value	intravaginal use)	Chlorpropamide	Clofibrate
and adjust the	Nalidixic acid	Cimetidine	Danazol
warfarin dose	Salicylates	Ciprofloxacin	Erythromycin
accordingly	Sulfonamides	Co-trimoxazole	Fenofibrate
	Sulfonylureas	Disulfiram	Gemfibrozil
		Ethanol	Glucagon
		(acute ingestion)[1]	Influenza vaccine
		Flutamide	Propranolol
		Isoniazid	Propylthiouracil
		Metronidazole	Ranitidine
		Norfloxacin	Rofecoxib
		Ofloxacin	SSRIs
		Omeprazole	Sulindac
		Phenytoin	Tetracycline
		Propafenone	Thyroid drugs
		Propoxyphene	Vitamin E
		Quinidine	(≥400 int. units)
		"Statins"[2]	
		Sulfinpyrazone	
		Sulfonamides	
		Tamoxifen	
		Tolbutamide	
		Zafirlukast	
		Zileuton	

[1]The hypoprothrombinemic effect of oral anticoagulants has been reported to be both increased and decreased during chronic and excessive alcohol ingestion. Data are insufficient to predict the direction of this interaction in alcoholic patients.

[2]Particularly lovastatin and fluvastatin; others (atorvastatin, pravastatin) rarely associated with increased PT.

Nutritional/Ethanol Interactions

Ethanol: Avoid ethanol. Acute ethanol ingestion (binge drinking) decreases the metabolism of warfarin and increases PT/INR. Chronic daily ethanol use increases the metabolism of warfarin and decreases PT/INR.

Food: The anticoagulant effects of warfarin may be decreased if taken with foods rich in vitamin K. Vitamin E may increase warfarin effect. Cranberry juice may increase warfarin effect.

Herb/Nutraceutical: St John's wort may decrease warfarin levels. Alfalfa contains large amounts of vitamin K as do many enteral products. Coenzyme Q_{10} may decrease response to warfarin. Avoid cat's claw, dong quai, bromelains, evening primrose, feverfew, red clover, horse chestnut, garlic, green tea, ginseng, ginkgo (all have additional antiplatelet activity).

Lab Interactions Increased aPTT

Adverse Reactions As with all anticoagulants, bleeding is the major adverse effect of warfarin. Hemorrhage may occur at virtually any site. Risk is dependent on multiple variables, including the intensity of anticoagulation and patient susceptibility.

Additional adverse effects are often related to idiosyncratic reactions, and the frequency cannot be accurately estimated.

Cardiovascular: Vasculitis, edema, hemorrhagic shock

Central nervous system: Fever, lethargy, malaise, asthenia, pain, headache, dizziness, stroke

Dermatologic: Rash, dermatitis, bullous eruptions, urticaria, pruritus, alopecia

Gastrointestinal: Anorexia, nausea, vomiting, stomach cramps, abdominal pain, diarrhea, flatulence, gastrointestinal bleeding, taste disturbance, mouth ulcers

Genitourinary: Priapism, hematuria

Hematologic: Hemorrhage, leukopenia, unrecognized bleeding sites (eg, colon cancer) may be uncovered by anticoagulation, retroperitoneal hematoma, agranulocytosis

Hepatic: Hepatic injury, jaundice, transaminases increased

Neuromuscular & skeletal: Paresthesia, osteoporosis

Respiratory: Hemoptysis, epistaxis, pulmonary hemorrhage, tracheobronchial calcification

Miscellaneous: Hypersensitivity/allergic reactions

Skin necrosis/gangrene, due to paradoxical local thrombosis, is a known but rare risk of warfarin therapy. Its onset is usually within the first few days of therapy and is frequently localized to the limbs, breast or penis. The risk of this effect is increased in patients with protein C or S deficiency.

"Purple toes syndrome," caused by cholesterol microembolization, also occurs rarely. Typically, this occurs after several weeks of therapy, and may present as a dark, purplish, mottled discoloration of the plantar and lateral surfaces. Other manifestations of cholesterol microembolization may include rash; livedo reticularis; gangrene; abrupt and intense pain in lower extremities; abdominal, flank, or back pain; hematuria, renal insufficiency; hypertension; cerebral ischemia; spinal cord infarction; or other symptom of vascular compromise.

Overdosage/Toxicology Symptoms of overdose include internal or external hemorrhage and hematuria. Avoid emesis and lavage to avoid possible trauma and incidental bleeding. When an overdose occurs, the drug should be immediately discontinued and vitamin K_1 (phytonadione) may be administered, up to 25 mg I.V. for adults. When hemorrhage occurs, fresh frozen plasma transfusions can help control bleeding by replacing clotting factors. In urgent bleeding, prothrombin complex concentrates may be needed.

Management of elevated INR: See table.

Management of Elevated INR

INR	Patient Situation	Action
>3 and <5	No bleeding or need for rapid reversal (ie, no need for surgery)	Omit next few warfarin dose and/or restart at lower dose when INR approaches desired range. If only minimally above range, then no dosage reduction may be required.
>5 and <9.0	No bleeding or need for rapid reversal	Omit next 1-2 doses, monitor INR more frequently, and restart at lower dose when INR approaches target range **or** omit dose and give 1-2.5 mg vitamin K_1 orally (use this if patient has risk factors for bleeding).
	No bleeding but reversal needed for surgery or dental extraction within 24 hours	2-4 mg vitamin K_1 orally (expected reversal within 24 hours); give additional 1-2 mg if INR remains high at 24 hours.
>9.0 and <20.0	No bleeding	Stop warfarin, give 3-5 mg vitamin K_1 orally; follow INR closely; repeat vitamin K_1 if needed. Reassess need and dose of warfarin when INR approaches desirable range.
Rapid reversal required (ie, INR >20)	Serious bleeding or major warfarin overdose	Stop warfarin, give 10 mg vitamin K_1 by slow I.V. infusion. May repeat vitamin K_1 every 12 hours and give fresh plasma transfusion or prothrombin complex concentrate as needed. When appropriate, heparin can be given until the patient becomes responsive to warfarin.

Pharmacodynamics/Kinetics

Onset of Action: Anticoagulation: Oral: 36-72 hours; Peak effect: Full therapeutic effect: 5-7 days; INR may increase in 36-72 hours

(Continued)

Warfarin *(Continued)*

Duration of Action: 2-5 days

Absorption: Oral: Rapid

Half-Life Elimination: 20-60 hours; Mean: 40 hours; highly variable among individuals

Metabolism: Hepatic

Dosing

Adults:

Prevention/treatment of thrombosis/embolism:

I.V. (administer as a slow bolus injection): 2-5 mg/day

Oral: Initial dosing must be individualized. Consider the patient (hepatic function, cardiac function, age, nutritional status, concurrent therapy, risk of bleeding) in addition to prior dose response (if available) and the clinical situation. Start 5-10 mg daily for 2 days. Adjust dose according to INR results; usual maintenance dose ranges from 2-10 mg daily (individual patients may require loading and maintenance doses outside these general guidelines).

Note: Lower starting doses may be required for patients with hepatic impairment, poor nutrition, CHF, elderly, or a high risk of bleeding. Higher initial doses may be reasonable in selected patients (ie, receiving enzyme-inducing agents and with low risk of bleeding).

Elderly: Oral: Initial dose ≤5 mg. Usual maintenance dose: 2-5 mg/day. The elderly tend to require lower dosages to produce a therapeutic level of anticoagulation (due to changes in the pattern of warfarin metabolism).

Pediatrics:

Prevention/treatment of thrombosis: Oral: Infants and Children: 0.05-0.34 mg/kg/day; infants <12 months of age may require doses at or near the high end of this range; consistent anticoagulation may be difficult to maintain in children <5 years of age.

Hepatic Impairment: Monitor effect at usual doses. The response to oral anticoagulants may be markedly enhanced in obstructive jaundice, hepatitis, and cirrhosis. Prothrombin index should be closely monitored.

Available Dosage Forms

Injection, powder for reconstitution, as sodium (Coumadin®): 5 mg

Tablet, as sodium (Coumadin®, Jantoven™): 1 mg, 2 mg, 2.5 mg, 3 mg, 4 mg, 5 mg, 6 mg, 7.5 mg, 10 mg

Monitoring and Teaching Issues

Physical Assessment: Use caution with any condition that increases risk of bleeding (eg, dietary vitamin K or C deficiency, hypertension, open wounds, TB, PUD, diabetes, thyroid or renal disease, recent surgery; see Contraindications and Warnings/Precautions for specific detailed use cautions). Assess potential for interactions with other pharmacological agents and herbal products patient may be taking (especially those medications that may affect coagulation or platelet aggregation; see Drug Interaction). Assess results of laboratory tests closely. Patient should be monitored frequently for adverse reactions (eg, bleeding from any site, rash, urticaria, gastrointestinal upset, abdominal pain, diarrhea, hypersensitivity reaction; see Adverse Reactions). Teach patient possible side effects/ appropriate interventions (eg, safety precautions) and adverse symptoms to report (see Patient Education). **Pregnancy risk factor X:** Determine that patient is not pregnant before beginning treatment. Teach patients of childbearing age appropriate use of contraceptives.

Monitoring Laboratory Tests: Prothrombin time (desirable range usually 1.5-2 times the control), hematocrit, INR (desirable range usually 2.0-3.0 with standard therapy, 2.5-3.5 with high-dose therapy)

Patient Education: It is imperative that you inform prescriber of all prescriptions, OTC medications, or herbal products you are taking. Do not take any new medication during therapy unless approved by prescriber. Take exactly as directed; if dose is missed, take as soon as possible. Do not double dose. Follow diet and activity as recommended by prescriber; check with prescriber before changing diet. Avoid alcohol. Do not make major changes in your dietary intake of vitamin K (green vegetables). You will have a tendency to bleed easily while taking this drug (use soft toothbrush, waxed dental floss, electric razor, and avoid scissors or sharp knives and potentially harmful activities). May cause nausea, vomiting, disturbed taste (small frequent meals, frequent mouth care, sucking lozenges, or chewing gum may help). Report any unusual bleeding or bruising (eg, bleeding gums, nosebleed, blood in urine, dark stool, bloody emesis, heavier than usual menses, or menstrual irregularities); skin rash or irritation; unusual fever; persistent nausea or GI upset; pain in joints or back; swelling or pain at injection site, unhealed wounds. **Pregnancy precautions:** Do not get pregnant while taking this medication. Consult prescriber for appropriate contraceptive measures.

Dietary Considerations: Foods high in vitamin K (eg, beef liver, pork liver, green tea and leafy green vegetables) inhibit anticoagulant effect. Do not change dietary habits once stabilized on warfarin therapy; a balanced diet with a consistent intake of vitamin K is essential; avoid large amounts of alfalfa, asparagus, broccoli, Brussels sprouts, cabbage, cauliflower, green teas, kale, lettuce, spinach, turnip greens, watercress decrease efficacy of warfarin. It is recommended that the diet contain a CONSISTENT vitamin K content of 70-140 mcg/day. Check with healthcare provider before changing diet.

Geriatric Considerations: Before committing an elderly patient to long-term anticoagulation therapy, their risk for bleeding complications secondary to falls, drug interactions, living situation, and cognitive status should be considered. A risk of bleeding complications has been associated with increased age.

Pregnancy Risk Factor: X

Pregnancy Issues: Oral anticoagulants cross the placenta and produce fetal abnormalities. Warfarin should not be used during pregnancy because of significant risks. Adjusted-dose heparin can be given safely throughout pregnancy in patients with venous thromboembolism.

Lactation: Does not enter breast milk, only metabolites are excreted (AAP rates "compatible")

Breast-Feeding Issues: Warfarin does not pass into breast milk and can be given to nursing mothers (AAP rates "compatible"). However, limited data suggests prolonged PT may occur in some infants. Women who are breast-feeding should be carefully monitored to avoid excessive anticoagulation. Evaluation of coagulation tests and vitamin K status of breast-feeding infant is considered prudent.

Administration

Oral: Do not take with food. Take at the same time each day.

I.V.: Administer as a slow bolus injection over 1-2 minutes. Avoid all I.M. injections.

Reconstitution: Injection is stable for 4 hours at room temperature after reconstitution with 2.7 mL of sterile water (yields 2 mg/mL solution).

Compatibility: Stable in D_5LR, $D_5^{1}/_2NS$, D_5NS, D_5W, $D_{10}W$

Y-site administration: Incompatible with aminophylline, bretylium, ceftazidime, cimetidine, ciprofloxacin, dobutamine, esmolol, gentamicin, labetalol, metronidazole, promazine, lactated Ringer's

Compatibility in syringe: Incompatible with heparin

Storage: Protect from light.

Related Information
Anticoagulants, Injectable *on page 1711*
Anticoagulant Therapy Guidelines *on page 1784*
Maternal / Fetal Toxicology *on page 1762*
Overdose and Toxicology *on page 1775*
Peak and Trough Guidelines *on page 1694*

♦ **Warfarin Sodium** *see* Warfarin *on page 1573*
♦ **WelChol®** *see* Colesevelam *on page 370*
♦ **Wellbutrin®** *see* BuPROPion *on page 219*
♦ **Wellbutrin SR®** *see* BuPROPion *on page 219*
♦ **Wellbutrin XL™** *see* BuPROPion *on page 219*
♦ **Westcort®** *see* Hydrocortisone *on page 760*
♦ **Westhroid®** *see* Thyroid *on page 1469*
♦ **WinRho SDF®** *see* $Rh_o(D)$ Immune Globulin *on page 1316*
♦ **WR-2721** *see* Amifostine *on page 86*
♦ **WR-139007** *see* Dacarbazine *on page 394*
♦ **WR-139013** *see* Chlorambucil *on page 305*
♦ **WR-139021** *see* Carmustine *on page 260*
♦ **Wycillin [DSC]** *see* Penicillin G Procaine *on page 1175*
♦ **Xalatan®** *see* Latanoprost *on page 869*
♦ **Xanax®** *see* Alprazolam *on page 74*
♦ **Xanax XR®** *see* Alprazolam *on page 74*
♦ **Xeloda®** *see* Capecitabine *on page 244*
♦ **Xenical®** *see* Orlistat *on page 1123*
♦ **Xigris®** *see* Drotrecogin Alfa *on page 501*
♦ **XiraTuss** *see* Carbetapentane, Phenylephrine, and Chlorpheniramine *on page 253*
♦ **Xolair®** *see* Omalizumab *on page 1115*
♦ **Xopenex®** *see* Levalbuterol *on page 879*
♦ **Xopenex HFA™** *see* Levalbuterol *on page 879*
♦ **X-Prep® [OTC]** *see* Senna *on page 1365*
♦ **Xylocaine®** *see* Lidocaine *on page 898*
♦ **Xylocaine® MPF** *see* Lidocaine *on page 898*
♦ **Xylocaine® MPF With Epinephrine** *see* Lidocaine and Epinephrine *on page 901*
♦ **Xylocaine® Viscous** *see* Lidocaine *on page 898*
♦ **Xylocaine® With Epinephrine** *see* Lidocaine and Epinephrine *on page 901*
♦ **Yasmin®** *see* Ethinyl Estradiol and Drospirenone *on page 581*
♦ **YM-08310** *see* Amifostine *on page 86*
♦ **Yodoxin®** *see* Iodoquinol *on page 824*
♦ **Z4942** *see* Ifosfamide *on page 783*
♦ **Zaditor™** *see* Ketotifen *on page 855*

Zafirlukast (za FIR loo kast)

U.S. Brand Names Accolate®
Synonyms ICI-204,219
Generic Available No
Pharmacologic Category Leukotriene-Receptor Antagonist
Medication Safety Issues
Sound-alike/look-alike issues:
Accolate® may be confused with Accupril®, Accutane®, Aclovate®
Use Prophylaxis and chronic treatment of asthma in adults and children ≥5 years of age
Mechanism of Action/Effect Leukotrienes are inflammatory mediators of asthma. Zafirlukast blocks leukotriene receptors and is able to reduce bronchoconstriction and inflammatory cell infiltration.
Contraindications Hypersensitivity to zafirlukast or any component of the formulation
Warnings/Precautions The clearance of zafirlukast is reduced in patients with stable alcoholic cirrhosis such that the C_{max} and AUC are approximately 50% to 60% greater than those of normal adults.

Zafirlukast is not indicated for use in the reversal of bronchospasm in acute asthma attacks, including status asthmaticus. Therapy with zafirlukast can be continued during acute exacerbations of asthma.
(Continued)

Zafirlukast *(Continued)*

An increased proportion of zafirlukast patients >55 years of age reported infections as compared to placebo-treated patients. These infections were mostly mild or moderate in intensity and predominantly affected the respiratory tract. Infections occurred equally in both sexes, were dose-proportional to total milligrams of zafirlukast exposure and were associated with coadministration of inhaled corticosteroids.

Hepatic adverse events (including hepatitis, hyperbilirubinemia, and hepatic failure) have been reported. Female patients may be at greater risk. Discontinue **immediately** if liver dysfunction is suspected. Periodic testing of liver function may be considered (early detection is generally believed to improve the likelihood of recovery). If hepatic dysfunction is suspected (due to clinical signs/symptoms) liver function tests should be measured immediately. Do not resume or restart if hepatic function tests are consistent with dysfunction.

Rare cases of eosinophilic vasculitis (Churg-Strauss) have been reported in patients receiving zafirlukast (usually, but not always, associated with reduction in concurrent steroid dosage). No causal relationship established.

Drug Interactions

Cytochrome P450 Effect: Substrate of CYP2C8/9 (major); **Inhibits** CYP1A2 (weak), 2C8/9 (moderate), 2C19 (weak), 2D6 (weak), 3A4 (weak)

Decreased Effect: The levels/effects of zafirlukast may be decreased by carbamazepine, phenobarbital, phenytoin, rifampin, rifapentine, secobarbital, and other CYP2C8/9 inducers. Zafirlukast concentrations may be reduced by erythromycin.

Increased Effect/Toxicity: Zafirlukast concentrations are increased by aspirin. Zafirlukast may increase theophylline levels. Zafirlukast may increase the levels/effects of amiodarone, fluoxetine, glimepiride, glipizide, nateglinide, phenytoin, pioglitazone, rosiglitazone, sertraline, warfarin, and other CYP2C8/9 substrates.

Nutritional/Ethanol Interactions Food: Decreases bioavailability of zafirlukast by 40%.

Adverse Reactions

>10%: Central nervous system: Headache (12.9%)

1% to 10%:
Central nervous system: Dizziness, pain, fever
Gastrointestinal: Nausea, diarrhea, abdominal pain, vomiting, dyspepsia
Hepatic: SGPT elevation
Neuromuscular & skeletal: Back pain, myalgia, weakness

Overdosage/Toxicology There is no experience with overdose in humans to date. Treatment is supportive.

Pharmacodynamics/Kinetics

Bioavailability: Reduced 40% with food

Time to Peak: Serum: 3 hours

Protein Binding: >99%, primarily to albumin

Half-Life Elimination: 10 hours

Metabolism: Extensively hepatic via CYP2C9

Excretion: Urine (10%); feces

Dosing

Adults & Elderly: Asthma: Oral: 20 mg twice daily

Pediatrics: Asthma: Oral:
Children 5-11 years: 10 mg twice daily. Safety and effectiveness have not been established in children <5 years of age.
Children ≥12 years: Refer to adult dosing.

Hepatic Impairment: Clearance of zafirlukast is reduced with a greater C_{max} and AUC of 50% to 60% in patients with alcoholic cirrhosis.

Available Dosage Forms Tablet: 10 mg, 20 mg

Monitoring and Teaching Issues

Physical Assessment: Not for use in acute asthma attack. Assess effectiveness and interactions of other medications patient may be taking. Monitor effectiveness of therapy and adverse reactions at beginning of therapy and periodically with long-term use. Monitor for liver dysfunction. Assess knowledge/teach patient appropriate use, interventions to reduce side effects, and adverse symptoms to report.

Monitoring Laboratory Tests: Monitor for improvements in air flow; periodic monitoring of LFTs may be considered (not proved to prevent serious injury, but early detection may enhance recovery)

Patient Education: Do not use during acute bronchospasm. Take regularly as prescribed, even during symptom-free periods. This medication should be taken on an empty stomach, 1 hour before or 2 hours after meals. Do not take more than recommended or discontinue use without consulting prescriber. Do not stop taking other antiasthmatic medications unless instructed by prescriber. Avoid aspirin or aspirin-containing medications unless approved by prescriber. You may experience headache, drowsiness, dizziness, or blurred vision (use caution when driving or engaging in tasks requiring alertness until response to drug is known); or gastric upset, nausea, or vomiting (small frequent meals, frequent mouth care, chewing gum, or sucking lozenges may help). Report persistent CNS or GI symptoms; muscle or back pain; weakness, fever, chills; yellowing of skin or eyes; dark urine or pale stool; or skin rash. Contact prescriber immediately if experiencing right upper abdominal pain, nausea, fatigue, itching, flu-like symptoms; swelling of the eyes, face, neck, or throat; anorexia; or worsening of condition. **Breast-feeding precaution:** Do not breast-feed.

Dietary Considerations: Should be taken on an empty stomach (1 hour before or 2 hours after meals).

Geriatric Considerations: The mean dose (mg/kg) normalized AUC and C_{max} increase and plasma clearance decreases with increasing age. In patients >65 years of age, there is a two- to threefold greater C_{max} and AUC compared to younger adults. Some studies have demonstrated slightly higher adverse effect reports in elderly compared to younger adults: Headache (4.7%), diarrhea and nausea (1.8%), and pharyngitis (1.3%). No changes in dose recommended for elderly.

Pregnancy Risk Factor: B
Lactation: Enters breast milk/contraindicated
Administration
  Oral: Administer 1 hour before or 2 hours after meals.
  Storage: Store tablets at controlled room temperature (20°C to 25°C; 68°F to 77°F); protect from light and moisture; dispense in original airtight container

♦ **Zagam®** *see* Sparfloxacin *on page 1389*

Zalcitabine (zal SITE a been)

U.S. Brand Names Hivid®
Synonyms ddC; Dideoxycytidine
Generic Available No
Pharmacologic Category Antiretroviral Agent, Reverse Transcriptase Inhibitor (Nucleoside)
Use In combination with at least two other antiretrovirals in the treatment of patients with HIV infection; it is not recommended that zalcitabine be given in combination with didanosine, stavudine, or lamivudine due to overlapping toxicities, virologic interactions, or lack of clinical data
Mechanism of Action/Effect Inhibits cell protein synthesis leading to cell death with viral replication.
Contraindications Hypersensitivity to zalcitabine or any component of the formulation
Warnings/Precautions Careful monitoring of pancreatic enzymes and liver function tests in patients with a history of pancreatitis, increased amylase, those on parenteral nutrition or with a history of ethanol abuse; discontinue use immediately if pancreatitis is suspected; lactic acidosis and severe hepatomegaly and failure have rarely occurred with zalcitabine resulting in fatality (stop treatment if lactic acidosis or hepatotoxicity occur); some cases may possibly be related to underlying hepatitis B; use with caution in patients on digitalis, or with CHF, renal failure, or hyperphosphatemia; zalcitabine can cause severe peripheral neuropathy; avoid use, if possible, in patients with pre-existing neuropathy or at risk of developing neuropathy. Risk factors include CD4 counts <50 cells/mm^3, diabetes mellitus, weight loss, other drugs known to cause peripheral neuropathy.
Drug Interactions
  Decreased Effect: It is not recommended that zalcitabine be given in combination with didanosine, stavudine, or lamivudine due to overlapping toxicities, virologic interactions, or lack of clinical data. Doxorubicin and lamivudine have been shown *in vitro* to decrease zalcitabine phosphorylation. Magnesium/aluminum-containing antacids and metoclopramide may decrease the absorption of zalcitabine.
  Increased Effect/Toxicity: Amphotericin, foscarnet, and aminoglycosides may potentiate the risk of developing peripheral neuropathy or other toxicities associated with zalcitabine by interfering with the renal elimination of zalcitabine. Other drugs associated with peripheral neuropathy include chloramphenicol, cisplatin, dapsone, disulfiram, ethionamide, glutethimide, gold, hydralazine, iodoquinol, isoniazid, metronidazole, nitrofurantoin, phenytoin, ribavirin, and vincristine. Concomitant use with zalcitabine may increase risk of peripheral neuropathy. Concomitant use of zalcitabine with didanosine is not recommended. Concomitant use of ribavirin and nucleoside analogues may increase the risk of developing lactic acidosis (includes adefovir, didanosine, lamivudine, stavudine, zalcitabine, zidovudine).
Nutritional/Ethanol Interactions Food: Food decreases peak plasma concentrations by 39%. Extent and rate of absorption may be decreased with food.
Lab Interactions May cause abnormalities in CBC, WBC, hemoglobin, platelet count, AST, ALT, or alkaline phosphatase.
Adverse Reactions
  >10%:
    Central nervous system: Fever (5% to 17%), malaise (2% to 13%)
    Neuromuscular & skeletal: Peripheral neuropathy (28%)
  1% to 10%:
    Central nervous system: Headache (2%), dizziness (1%), fatigue (4%), seizure (1.3%)
    Dermatologic: Rash (2% to 11%), pruritus (3% to 5%)
    Endocrine & metabolic: Hypoglycemia (2% to 6%), hyponatremia (4%), hyperglycemia (1% to 6%)
    Gastrointestinal: Nausea (3%), dysphagia (1% to 4%), anorexia (4%), abdominal pain (3% to 8%), vomiting (1% to 3%), diarrhea (<1% to 10%), weight loss, oral ulcers (3% to 7%), increased amylase (3% to 8%)
    Hematologic: Anemia (occurs as early as 2-4 weeks), granulocytopenia (usually after 6-8 weeks)
    Hepatic: Abnormal hepatic function (9%), hyperbilirubinemia (2% to 5%)
    Neuromuscular & skeletal: Myalgia (1% to 6%), foot pain
    Respiratory: Pharyngitis (2%), cough (6%), nasal discharge (4%)
Overdosage/Toxicology Symptoms of overdose include delayed peripheral neurotoxicity. Treatment is supportive.
Pharmacodynamics/Kinetics
  Absorption: Well, but variable; decreased 39% with food
  Bioavailability: >80%
  Protein Binding: <4%
  Half-Life Elimination: 2.9 hours; Renal impairment: ≤8.5 hours
  Metabolism: Intracellularly to active triphosphorylated agent
  Excretion: Urine (>70% as unchanged drug)
Dosing
  Adults & Elderly: HIV infection (component of combination therapy): Oral: Daily dose: 0.75 mg every 8 hours
  Pediatrics: HIV infection: Oral:
    Children <13 years: Safety and efficacy have not been established.
    Adolescents: Refer to adult dosing.
(Continued)

Zalcitabine (Continued)

Renal Impairment:
Cl$_{cr}$ 10-40 mL/minute: Administer 0.75 mg every 12 hours.
Cl$_{cr}$ <10 mL/minute: Administer 0.75 mg every 24 hours.
Moderately dialyzable (20% to 50%)

Available Dosage Forms Tablet: 0.375 mg, 0.75 mg

Monitoring and Teaching Issues

Physical Assessment: See Warnings/Precautions for use cautions. Assess potential for interactions with other pharmacological agents or herbal products patient may be taking (eg, especially those that increase risk of peripheral neuropathy; see Drug Interactions). Assess results of laboratory tests, therapeutic effectiveness (CD4 counts, viral load), and adverse reactions (see Adverse Reactions) on a regular basis throughout therapy. Teach patient proper use (see Administration and Storage), possible side effects/appropriate interventions, and adverse symptoms to report (see Patient Education).

Monitoring Laboratory Tests: CBC and serum chemistry (prior to initiation and appropriate intervals), renal function, CD4 counts, serum amylase, triglyceride, calcium, viral load

Patient Education: Do not take any new medication during therapy unless approved by prescriber. This is not a cure for HIV nor has it been found to reduce transmission of HIV. Take as directed, around-the-clock, preferably on an empty stomach, 1 hour before or 2 hours after meals. Do not take antacids or other medication within 1 hour of taking this medication. Maintain adequate hydration (2-3 L/day of fluids) unless instructed to restrict fluid intake. May cause headache, dizziness, fatigue (use caution when driving or engaging in potentially hazardous tasks until response to drug is known); nausea, vomiting, lack of appetite, mouth sores (small frequent meals, frequent mouth care, chewing gum, or sucking lozenges may help). Report muscle weakness or pain; tingling, numbness, or pain in toes or fingers; weakness of extremities; chest pain, palpitations, or rapid heartbeat; swelling of extremities; weight gain or loss >5 lb/week; signs of infection (eg, fever, chills, sore throat, burning urination, fatigue); unusual bleeding (eg, tarry stools, easy bruising, or blood in stool, urine, or mouth); skin rash or irritation. **Pregnancy/breast-feeding precautions:** Inform prescriber if you are or intend to become pregnant. Do not breast-feed.

Pregnancy Risk Factor: C

Pregnancy Issues: It is not known if zalcitabine crosses the human placenta. Animal studies have shown zalcitabine to be teratogenic, developmental toxicities were also observed. Cases of lactic acidosis/hepatic steatosis syndrome have been reported in pregnant women receiving nucleoside analogue drugs. It is not known if pregnancy itself potentiates this known side effect; however, pregnant women may be at increased risk of lactic acidosis and liver damage. Hepatic enzymes and electrolytes should be monitored frequently during the 3rd trimester of pregnancy in women receiving nucleoside analogues. Health professionals are encouraged to contact the antiretroviral pregnancy registry to monitor outcomes of pregnant women exposed to antiretroviral medications (1-800-258-4263 or www.APRegistry.com).

Lactation: Excretion in breast milk unknown/contraindicated

Breast-Feeding Issues: HIV-infected mothers are discouraged from breast-feeding to decrease potential transmission of HIV.

Administration

Oral: Food decreases absorption; take on an empty stomach. Administer around-the-clock. Do not take at the same time with dapsone.

Storage: Tablets should be stored in tightly closed bottles at room temperature (59°F to 86°F)

Additional Information Potential compliance problems, frequency of administration and adverse effects should be discussed with patients before initiating therapy to help prevent the emergence of resistance.

Zaleplon (ZAL e plon)

U.S. Brand Names Sonata®

Controlled Substance C-IV

Generic Available No

Pharmacologic Category Hypnotic, Nonbenzodiazepine

Use Short-term (7-10 days) treatment of insomnia (has been demonstrated to be effective for up to 5 weeks in controlled trial)

Mechanism of Action/Effect Zaleplon is unrelated to benzodiazepines, barbiturates, or other hypnotics. However, it interacts with the benzodiazepine GABA receptor complex. Nonclinical studies have shown that it binds selectively to the brain omega-1 receptor situated on the alpha subunit of the GABA-A receptor complex.

Contraindications Hypersensitivity to zaleplon or any component of the formulation

Warnings/Precautions Failure of sleep disturbance to resolve after 7-10 days may indicate psychiatric and/or medical illness. Use with caution in patients with depression, particularly if suicidal risk may be present. Use with caution in patients with a history of drug dependence. Abrupt discontinuance may lead to withdrawal symptoms. May impair physical and mental capabilities; caution in patients receiving other CNS depressants or psychoactive medications. Effects with other sedative drugs or ethanol may be potentiated. Use with caution in the elderly, those with compromised respiratory function, or renal and hepatic impairment. Because of the rapid onset of action, zaleplon should be administered immediately prior to bedtime or after the patient has gone to bed and is having difficulty falling asleep. Capsules contain tartrazine (FDC yellow #5); avoid in patients with sensitivity (caution in patients with asthma).

Drug Interactions

Cytochrome P450 Effect: Substrate of CYP3A4 (minor)

Increased Effect/Toxicity: Zaleplon potentiates the CNS effects of CNS depressants, including ethanol, anticonvulsants, antipsychotics, barbiturates, benzodiazepines, narcotic agonists, and other sedative agents. Cimetidine increases concentrations of zaleplon. Avoid concurrent use or use 5 mg zaleplon as starting dose in patient receiving cimetidine.

Nutritional/Ethanol Interactions

Ethanol: Avoid ethanol (may increase CNS depression).

Food: High fat meal prolonged absorption; delayed t_{max} by 2 hours, and reduced C_{max} by 35%.

Herb/Nutraceutical: St John's wort may decrease zaleplon levels. Avoid valerian, St John's wort, kava kava, gotu kola (may increase CNS depression).

Adverse Reactions

1% to 10%:

Cardiovascular: Peripheral edema, chest pain

Central nervous system: Amnesia, anxiety, depersonalization, dizziness, hallucinations, hypoesthesia, somnolence, vertigo, malaise, depression, lightheadedness, impaired coordination, fever, migraine

Dermatologic: Photosensitivity reaction, rash, pruritus

Gastrointestinal: Abdominal pain, anorexia, colitis, dyspepsia, nausea, constipation, xerostomia

Genitourinary: Dysmenorrhea

Neuromuscular & skeletal: Paresthesia, tremor, myalgia, weakness, back pain, arthralgia

Ocular: Abnormal vision, eye pain

Otic: Hyperacusis

Miscellaneous: Parosmia

Overdosage/Toxicology Symptoms include CNS depression, ranging from drowsiness to coma. Mild overdose is associated with drowsiness, confusion, and lethargy. Serious case may result in ataxia, respiratory depression, hypotension, hypotonia, coma, and rarely death. Treatment is supportive.

Pharmacodynamics/Kinetics

Onset of Action: Rapid; Peak effect: ~1 hour

Duration of Action: 6-8 hours

Absorption: Rapid and almost complete

Bioavailability: 30%

Time to Peak: Serum: 1 hour

Protein Binding: 60% ± 15%

Half-Life Elimination: 1 hour

Metabolism: Extensive, primarily via aldehyde oxidase to form 5-oxo-zaleplon and to a lesser extent by CYP3A4 to desethylzaleplon; all metabolites are pharmacologically inactive

Excretion: Urine (primarily metabolites, <1% as unchanged drug)

Clearance: Plasma: Oral: 3 L/hour/kg

Dosing

Adults: Insomnia (short-term use): Oral: 10 mg at bedtime (range: 5-20 mg)

Elderly: Reduce dose to 5 mg at bedtime

Renal Impairment: No adjustment for mild to moderate renal impairment; use in severe renal impairment has not been adequately studied.

Hepatic Impairment: Mild to moderate impairment: 5 mg; not recommended for use in patients with severe hepatic impairment.

Available Dosage Forms Capsule: 5 mg, 10 mg [contains tartrazine]

Monitoring and Teaching Issues

Physical Assessment: Evaluate etiology of insomnia; failure of sleep disturbance after 7-10 days may indicate psychiatric and/or medical illness. Assess effectiveness and interactions of other medications. Evaluate risk for suicide and assess for history of addiction (long-term use may result in dependence, abuse, or tolerance). Prescription quantities should not exceed a 1 month supply; periodically evaluate need for continued use. For inpatient use, institute safety measures and monitor effectiveness and adverse reactions. For outpatients, monitor therapeutic effectiveness and adverse reactions at beginning of therapy and periodically with long-term use. Assess knowledge/teach patient appropriate use, interventions to reduce side effects, and adverse reactions to report.

Patient Education: Take exactly as directed; immediately before bedtime, or when you cannot fall asleep. Do not alter dosage or frequency, may be habit forming. Avoid alcohol and other prescription or OTC medications (especially medications to relieve pain, induce sleep, reduce anxiety, treat or prevent cold, coughs, or allergies) unless approved by prescriber. You may experience drowsiness, dizziness, somnolence, vertigo, lightheadedness, blurred vision (avoid driving or engaging in activities that require alertness until response to drug is known); photosensitivity (avoid exposure to direct sunlight, wear protective clothing, and sunscreen); nausea or GI discomfort (small frequent meals, good mouth care, chewing gum, or sucking hard candy may help); constipation (increase exercise, fluids, fruit, or fiber may help); or menstrual disturbances (reversible when drug is discontinued). Discontinue drug and report any severe CNS disturbances (hallucinations, acute nervousness or anxiety, persistent sleepiness or lethargy, impaired coordination, amnesia, or impaired thought processes); skin rash or irritation; eye pain or major vision changes; respiratory difficulty; chest pain; ear pain; or muscle weakness or pain. **Pregnancy/breast-feeding precautions:** Inform prescriber if you are or intend to become pregnant. Breast-feeding is not recommended.

Pregnancy Risk Factor: C

Pregnancy Issues: Benzodiazepines cross the placenta. The association between benzodiazepine exposure and malformations remains controversial. A number of types of malformation have been reported (oral cleft, inguinal hernia, cardiac defects, spina bifida, dysmorphic facial features, skeletal defects); however, confounding factors make a clear association difficult. Overall, the risk to the fetus may be low. Nonteratogenic effects (including neonatal flaccidity, respiratory and feeding problems, and withdrawal symptoms) during the postnatal period have also been reported with benzodiazepine use.

(Continued)

Zaleplon (Continued)

Lactation: Enters breast milk/not recommended

Administration

Oral: Administer immediately before bedtime or when the patient is in bed and cannot fall asleep.

Storage: Store at controlled room temperature of 20°C to 25°C (68°F to 77°F); protect from light

Additional Information Prescription quantities should not exceed a 1-month supply.

Related Information

Anxiolytic / Hypnotic Use in Long-Term Care Facilities *on page 1769*

♦ **Zanaflex®** *see* Tizanidine *on page 1487*

Zanamivir (za NA mi veer)

U.S. Brand Names Relenza®

Generic Available No

Pharmacologic Category Antiviral Agent; Neuraminidase Inhibitor

Use Treatment of uncomplicated acute illness due to influenza virus in adults and children ≥7 years of age; should not be used in patients with underlying airway disease. Treatment should only be initiated in patients who have been symptomatic for no more than 2 days.

Unlabeled/Investigational Use Investigational: Prophylaxis against influenza A/B infections

Mechanism of Action/Effect Zanamivir inhibits influenza virus neuraminidase enzymes, potentially altering virus particle aggregation and release.

Contraindications Hypersensitivity to zanamivir or any component of the formulation

Warnings/Precautions Patients must be instructed in the use of the delivery system. No data are available to support the use of this drug in patients who begin treatment after 48 hours of symptoms, as a prophylactic treatment for influenza, or in patients with significant underlying medical conditions. Bronchospasm, decreased lung function, and other serious adverse reactions, including those with fatal outcomes, have been reported. Not recommended for use in patients with underlying chronic airway disease, such as asthma or COPD, due to lack of efficacy and risk of serious adverse effects. For a patient with an underlying airway disease where a medical decision has been made to use zanamivir, a fast-acting bronchodilator should be made available, and used prior to each dose. Discontinue if bronchospasm occur or if there is a decline in respiratory function. Consider primary or concomitant bacterial infections. Not a substitute for influenza vaccine. Powder for oral inhalation contains lactose.

Drug Interactions

Decreased Effect: No clinically significant pharmacokinetic interactions are predicted.

Increased Effect/Toxicity: No clinically significant pharmacokinetic interactions are predicted.

Adverse Reactions Most adverse reactions occurred at a frequency which was equal to the control (lactose vehicle).

>1.5%:

Central nervous system: Headache (2%), dizziness (2%)

Gastrointestinal: Nausea (3%), diarrhea (3% adults, 2% children), vomiting (1% adults, 2% children)

Respiratory: Sinusitis (3%), bronchitis (2%), cough (2%), other nasal signs and symptoms (2%), infection (ear, nose, and throat; 2% adults, 5% children)

Overdosage/Toxicology Information is limited, and symptoms appear similar to reported adverse events from clinical studies.

Pharmacodynamics/Kinetics

Absorption: Inhalation: 4% to 17%

Protein Binding: Plasma: <10%

Half-Life Elimination: Serum: 2.5-5.1 hours

Metabolism: None

Excretion: Urine (as unchanged drug); feces (unabsorbed drug)

Dosing

Adults & Elderly:

Treatment of influenza: Inhalation: 2 inhalations (10 mg total) twice daily for 5 days. Two doses should be taken on the first day of dosing, regardless of interval, while doses should be spaced by approximately 12 hours on subsequent days.

Prophylaxis of influenza (investigational use): Inhalation: 2 inhalations (10 mg) once daily for duration of exposure period (6 weeks has been used in clinical trial)

Pediatrics: Influenza treatment: Children ≥7 years: Refer to adult dosing.

Available Dosage Forms Powder for oral inhalation: 5 mg/blister (20s) [4 blisters per Rotadisk® foil pack, 5 Rotadisk® per package; packaged with Diskhaler® inhalation device; contains lactose]

Monitoring and Teaching Issues

Physical Assessment: This is **not** a substitute for the influenza vaccine. Therapy must be started within 48 hours of first influenza symptoms. Teach patient appropriate use (inhalation device), interventions to reduce side effects, and adverse reactions to report.

Patient Education: Use delivery device exactly as directed; complete full 5-day regimen, even if symptoms improve sooner. If you have asthma or COPD you may be at risk for bronchospasm; see prescriber for appropriate bronchodilator before using zanamivir. Stop using this medication and contact your physician if you experience shortness of breath, increased wheezing, or other signs of bronchospasm. You may experience dizziness or headache (use caution when driving or engaging in hazardous tasks until response to drug is known). Report unresolved diarrhea, vomiting, or nausea; acute fever or muscle pain; or other acute and persistent adverse effects. **Pregnancy/breast-feeding precautions:** Inform prescriber if you are or intend to become pregnant. Consult prescriber if breast-feeding.

Pregnancy Risk Factor: C

Lactation: Excretion in breast milk unknown/use caution

Breast-Feeding Issues: Zanamivir has been shown to be excreted in the milk of animals, but its excretion in human milk is unknown. Caution should be used when zanamivir is administered to a nursing mother.

Administration

Inhalation: Must be used with Diskhaler® delivery device. Patients who are scheduled to use an inhaled bronchodilator should use their bronchodilator prior to zanamivir.

Storage: Store at room temperature (25°C) 77°F. Do not puncture blister until taking a dose using the Diskhaler®.

Additional Information Majority of patients included in clinical trials were infected with influenza A, however, a number of patients with influenza B infections were also enrolled. Patients with lower temperature or less severe symptoms appeared to derive less benefit from therapy. No consistent treatment benefit was demonstrated in patients with chronic underlying medical conditions.

Ziconotide (zi KOE no tide)

U.S. Brand Names Prialt®

Generic Available No

Pharmacologic Category Analgesic, Non-narcotic; Calcium Channel Blocker, N-Type

Use Management of severe chronic pain in patients requiring intrathecal (I.T.) therapy and are intolerant or refractory to other therapies

Mechanism of Action/Effect Ziconotide selectively binds to N-type voltage sensitive calcium channels located on the afferent nerves of the dorsal horn in the spinal cord. This binding is thought to block N-type calcium channels, leading to a blockade of excitatory neurotransmitter release and reducing sensitivity to painful stimuli.

Contraindications Hypersensitivity to ziconotide or any component of the formulation; history of psychosis; I.V. administration

I.T. administration is contraindicated in patients with infection at the injection site, uncontrolled bleeding, or spinal canal obstruction that impairs CSF circulation

Warnings/Precautions Severe psychiatric symptoms and neurological impairment have been reported; interrupt or discontinue therapy if cognitive impairment, hallucinations, mood changes, or changes in consciousness occur. Cognitive impairment may appear gradually during treatment and is generally reversible after discontinuation. Use caution in the elderly; may experience confusion. Patients should be instructed to use caution in performing tasks which require alertness (eg, operating machinery or driving). May have additive effects with opiates or other CNS-depressant medications. Does not potentiate opiate-induced respiratory depression. Will not prevent or relieve symptoms associated with opiate withdrawal and opiates should not be abruptly discontinued. Unlike opioids, ziconotide therapy can be interrupted abruptly or discontinued without evidence of withdrawal. Meningitis may occur with use of I.T. pumps and treatment may require removal of system and discontinuation of therapy. Safety and efficacy have not been established with renal or hepatic dysfunction, or in pediatric patients.

Drug Interactions

Increased Effect/Toxicity: May enhance the adverse/toxic effects of other CNS depressants

Adverse Reactions Percentages reported when using the slow (21-day) titration schedule; frequencies may be higher with faster titration.

(Continued)

Ziconotide *(Continued)*

>10%:

Central nervous system: Dizziness (47%), somnolence (22%), confusion (18%), ataxia (16%), headache (15%), memory impairment (12%), pain (11%)

Gastrointestinal: Nausea (41%), diarrhea (19%), vomiting (15%)

Neuromuscular & skeletal: Weakness (22%), gait disturbances (15%), hypertonia (11%)

2% to 10%:

Cardiovascular: Chest pain, edema, hyper or hypotension, postural hypotension, tachycardia, vasodilation

Central nervous system: Anxiety (9%), speech disorder (9%), aphasia (8%), dysesthesia (7%), fever (7%), hallucinations (7%), nervousness (7%), vertigo (7%), agitation, chills, depression, dreams abnormal, emotional lability, hostility, hyperesthesia, insomnia, malaise, neuralgia, paranoid reaction, stupor

Dermatologic: Bruising, cellulitis, diaphoresis, dry skin, pruritus, rash

Endocrine & metabolic: Hypokalemia

Gastrointestinal: Anorexia (10%), abdominal pain, constipation, dehydration, dyspepsia, taste perversion, weight loss, xerostomia

Genitourinary: Urinary retention (9%), dysuria, urinary incontinence, urinary tract infection, urination impaired

Hematologic: Anemia

Local: Catheter complication, catheter site pain, pump site complication, pump site mass, pump site pain

Neuromuscular & skeletal: Paresthesia (7%), arthralgia, arthritis, back pain, incoordination, leg cramps, myalgia, myasthenia, neck pain, neck rigidity, reflexes decreased, tremor

Ocular: Vision abnormal (10%), nystagmus (8%), diplopia, photophobia,

Otic: Tinnitus

Renal: CPK increased (<2%)

Respiratory: Bronchitis, cough, dyspnea, pharyngitis, pneumonia, rhinitis, sinusitis

Miscellaneous: Flu-like syndrome, infection, CSF abnormalities, meningitis

Overdosage/Toxicology Exaggerated pharmacological effects, including ataxia, confusion, dizziness, garbled speech, hypotension, nausea, nystagmus, sedation, spinal myoclonus, stupor, unresponsiveness, vomiting and word-finding difficulty, are reported at doses >19.2 mcg/day. Respiratory depression was not observed. In case of overdose, ziconotide can be discontinued temporarily or withdrawn; additional treatment should be symptom directed and supportive. Opioid antagonists are not effective. Most patients recover within 24 hours of discontinuing ziconotide therapy.

Pharmacodynamics/Kinetics

Protein Binding: 50%

Half-Life Elimination: I.V.: 1-1.6 hours (plasma); I.T.: 2.9-6.5 hours (CSF)

Metabolism: Metabolized via endopeptidases and exopeptidases present on multiple organs including kidney, liver, lung; degraded to peptide fragments and free amino acids

Excretion: I.V.: Urine (<1%)

Dosing

Adults: Chronic pain: I.T.: Initial dose: 2.4 mcg/day (0.1 mcg/hour)

Dose may be titrated by ≤2.4 mcg/day (0.1 mcg/hour) at intervals ≥2-3 times/week to a maximum dose of 19.2 mcg/day (0.8 mcg/hour) by day 21; average dose at day 21: 6.9 mcg/day (0.29 mcg/hour). A faster titration should be used only if the urgent need for analgesia outweighs the possible risk to patient safety.

Dosage adjustment for toxicity: Cognitive impairment: Reduce dose or discontinue. Effects are generally reversible within 2 weeks of discontinuation.

Elderly: Refer to adult dosing. Use with caution.

Available Dosage Forms Injection, solution, as acetate [preservative free]: 100 mcg/mL (1 mL, 2 mL, 5 mL); 25 mcg/mL (20 mL)

Monitoring and Teaching Issues

Physical Assessment: Assess other medications patient may be taking for effectiveness and interactions. This medication is given intrathecally via an implanted pump. Monitor for therapeutic response. Monitor for changes in behavior, cognitive impairment, hallucinations, or changes in mood or consciousness. Assess knowledge/teach patient appropriate use, interventions to reduce side effects, and adverse symptoms to report.

Patient Education: You may experience dizziness, sleepiness, or lightheadedness (use caution when driving or engaging in tasks requiring alertness until response to drug is known); nausea or vomiting (small frequent meals, frequent mouth care, chewing gum, or sucking lozenges may help); constipation (increased exercise, fluids, fruit, or fiber may help); or diarrhea (buttermilk, boiled milk, or yogurt may help), loss of appetite. Report chest pain, swelling of extremities (feet/ankles); muscle weakness and poor coordination; hallucinations, confusion, or extreme weakness. **Pregnancy/breast-feeding precaution:** Inform prescriber if you are or intend to become pregnant. Consult prescriber if breast-feeding.

Geriatric Considerations: See Warnings/Precautions, Adverse Reactions, and Dosing. Manufacturer reports that in all trials there was a higher incidence of confusion in the elderly compared to younger adults.

Pregnancy Risk Factor: C

Lactation: Excretion in breast milk unknown/not recommended

Breast-Feeding Issues: The manufacturer recommends discontinuing breast-feeding or discontinuing ziconotide.

Administration

I.V.: Not for I.V. administration

Other: Not for I.V. administration. **For I.T. administration only** using a Medtronic SynchroMed® EL, SynchroMed® II Infusion System or Simms Deltec Cadd Micro® External Microinfusion Device and Catheter.

Medtronic SynchroMed® EL or SynchroMed® II Infusion Systems:

Naive pump priming (first time use with ziconotide): Use 2mL of undiluted ziconotide 25 mcg/mL solution to rinse the internal surfaces of the pump; repeat twice for a total of 3 rinses

Initial pump fill: Use only undiluted 25 mcg/mL solution and fill pump after priming. Following the initial fill only, adsorption on internal device surfaces will occur, requiring the use of the undiluted solution and refill within 14 days.

Pump refills: Contents should be emptied prior to refill. Subsequent pump refills should occur at least every 40 days if using diluted solution or every 60 days if using undiluted solution

Simms Deltec Cadd Micro® External Microinfusion Device and Catheter: Refer to manufacturers' manual for initial fill and refill instructions

Reconstitution: Preservative free NS should be used when dilution is needed.

Simms Deltec Cadd Micro® External Microinfusion Device and Catheter: Initial fill: Dilute to final concentration of 5 mcg/mL

Storage: Prior to use, store vials at 2°C to 8°C (36°F to 46°F); once diluted, may be stored at 2°C to 8°C (36°F to 46°F) for 24 hours. Do not freeze. Protect from light.

When using the Medtronic SynchroMed® EL or SynchroMed® II Infusion System, solutions expire as follows:

25 mcg/mL: Undiluted:
 Initial fill: Use within 14 days
 Refill: use within 60 days
100 mcg/mL
 Undiluted: Refill: Use within 60 days
 Diluted: Refill: Use within 40 days

Zidovudine (zye DOE vyoo deen)

U.S. Brand Names Retrovir®
Synonyms Azidothymidine; AZT; Compound S; ZDV
Generic Available No
Pharmacologic Category Antiretroviral Agent, Reverse Transcriptase Inhibitor (Nucleoside)
Medication Safety Issues
Sound-alike/look-alike issues:
Azidothymidine may be confused with azathioprine, aztreonam
Retrovir® may be confused with ritonavir
Use Management of patients with HIV infections in combination with at least two other antiretroviral agents; for prevention of maternal/fetal HIV transmission as monotherapy
Unlabeled/Investigational Use Postexposure prophylaxis for HIV exposure as part of a multidrug regimen
Mechanism of Action/Effect Zidovudine is a thymidine analog which interferes with the HIV virus that results in inhibition of viral replication.
Contraindications Life-threatening hypersensitivity to zidovudine or any component of the formulation
Warnings/Precautions Often associated with hematologic toxicity including granulocytopenia, severe anemia requiring transfusions, or (rarely) pancytopenia. Use with caution in patients with bone marrow compromise (granulocytes <1000 cells/mm^3 or hemoglobin <9.5 mg/dL); dosage adjustment may be required in patients who develop anemia or neutropenia. Lactic acidosis and severe hepatomegaly with steatosis have been reported, including fatal cases; use with caution in patients with risk factors for liver disease (risk may be increased in obese patients or prolonged exposure) and suspend treatment with zidovudine in any patient who develops clinical or laboratory findings suggestive of lactic acidosis (transaminase elevation may/may not accompany hepatomegaly and steatosis). Prolonged use has been associated with symptomatic myopathy. Reduce dose in patients with renal impairment.
Drug Interactions
Cytochrome P450 Effect: Substrate (minor) of CYP2A6, 2C8/9, 2C19, 3A4
Decreased Effect: *In vitro* evidence suggests zidovudine's antiretroviral activity may be antagonized by doxorubicin and ribavirin; avoid concurrent use. Zidovudine may decrease the antiviral activity of stavudine (based on *in vitro* data); avoid concurrent use.
Increased Effect/Toxicity: Coadministration of zidovudine with drugs that are nephrotoxic (amphotericin B), cytotoxic (flucytosine, vincristine, vinblastine, doxorubicin, interferon), inhibit glucuronidation or excretion (acetaminophen, cimetidine, indomethacin, lorazepam, probenecid, aspirin), or interfere with RBC/WBC number or function (acyclovir, ganciclovir, pentamidine, dapsone). Clarithromycin may increase blood levels of zidovudine (although total body exposure was unaffected, peak plasma concentrations were increased). Valproic acid significantly increases zidovudine's blood levels (believed due to inhibition first pass metabolism). Concomitant use of ribavirin and nucleoside analogues may increase the risk of developing lactic acidosis (includes adefovir, didanosine, lamivudine, stavudine, zalcitabine, zidovudine).
Adverse Reactions
>10%:
Central nervous system: Severe headache (42%), fever (16%)
Dermatologic: Rash (17%)
Gastrointestinal: Nausea (46% to 61%), anorexia (11%), diarrhea (17%), pain (20%), vomiting (6% to 25%)
Hematologic: Anemia (23% in children), leukopenia, granulocytopenia (39% in children)
Neuromuscular & skeletal: Weakness (19%)
1% to 10%:
Central nervous system: Malaise (8%), dizziness (6%), insomnia (5%), somnolence (8%)
Dermatologic: Hyperpigmentation of nails (bluish-brown)
Gastrointestinal: Dyspepsia (5%)
Hematologic: Changes in platelet count
Neuromuscular & skeletal: Paresthesia (6%)
Overdosage/Toxicology Symptoms of overdose include nausea, vomiting, ataxia, and granulocytopenia. Erythropoietin, thymidine, and cyanocobalamin have been used experimentally
(Continued)

Zidovudine *(Continued)*

to treat zidovudine-induced hematopoietic toxicity, yet none are presently specified as the agent of choice. Treatment is supportive.

Pharmacodynamics/Kinetics

Absorption: Oral: 66% to 70%

Time to Peak: Serum: 30-90 minutes

Protein Binding: 25% to 38%

Half-Life Elimination: Terminal: 60 minutes

Metabolism: Hepatic via glucuronidation to inactive metabolites; extensive first-pass effect

Excretion:
Oral: Urine (72% to 74% as metabolites, 14% to 18% as unchanged drug)
I.V.: Urine (45% to 60% as metabolites, 18% to 29% as unchanged drug)

Dosing

Adults & Elderly:

Prevention of maternal-fetal HIV transmission: Maternal (per AIDSinfo guidelines): 100 mg 5 times/day **or** 200 mg 3 times/day **or** 300 mg twice daily. Begin at 14-34 weeks gestation and continue until start of labor.

During labor and delivery, administer zidovudine I.V. at 2 mg/kg over 1 hour followed by a continuous I.V. infusion of 1 mg/kg/hour until the umbilical cord is clamped

HIV infection:
Oral: 300 mg twice daily or 200 mg 3 times/day
I.V.: 1-2 mg/kg/dose (infused over 1 hour) administered every 4 hours around-the-clock (6 doses/day)

Prevention of HIV following needlesticks (unlabeled use): Oral: 200 mg 3 times/day plus lamivudine 150 mg twice daily; a protease inhibitor (eg, indinavir) may be added for high risk exposures; begin therapy within 2 hours of exposure if possible

Note: Patients should receive I.V. therapy only until oral therapy can be administered

Pediatrics:

Prevention of maternal-fetal HIV transmission (in neonates):
Note: Dosing should begin 8-12 hours after birth and continue for the first 6 weeks of life.
Oral:
Full-term infants: 2 mg/kg/dose every 6 hours
Infants ≥30 weeks and <35 weeks gestation at birth: 2 mg/kg/dose every 12 hours; at 2 weeks of age, advance to 2 mg/kg/dose every 8 hours
Infants <30 weeks gestation at birth: 2 mg/kg/dose every 12 hours; at 4 weeks of age, advance to 2 mg/kg/dose every 8 hours
I.V. (infants unable to receive oral dosing):
Full term: 1.5 mg/kg/dose every 6 hours
Infants ≥30 weeks and <35 weeks gestation at birth: 1.5 mg/kg/dose every 12 hours; at 2 weeks of age, advance to 1.5 mg/kg/dose every 8 hours
Infants <30 weeks gestation at birth: 1.5 mg/kg/dose every 12 hours; at 4 weeks of age, advance to 1.5 mg/kg/dose every 8 hours
During labor and delivery, administer zidovudine I.V. at 2 mg/kg over 1 hour followed by a continuous I.V. infusion of 1 mg/kg/hour until the umbilical cord is clamped

Treatment of HIV infection:
Oral: Children 3 months to 12 years:
160 mg/m^2/dose every 8 hours; dosage range: 90 mg/m^2/dose to 180 mg/m^2/dose every 6-8 hours; some Working Group members use a dose of 180 mg/m^2 every 12 hours when using in drug combinations with other antiretroviral compounds, but data on this dosing in children is limited
I.V. continuous infusion: 20 mg/m^2/hour
I.V. intermittent infusion: 120 mg/m^2/dose every 6 hours

Renal Impairment: Cl$_{cr}$ <10 mL/minute: May require minor dose adjustment.
Hemodialysis: At least partially removed by hemo- and peritoneal dialysis. Administer dose after hemodialysis or administer 100 mg supplemental dose. During CAPD, dose as for Cl$_{cr}$ <10 mL/minute.
Continuous arteriovenous or venovenous hemodiafiltration effects: Administer 100 mg every 8 hours.

Hepatic Impairment: Reduce dose by 50% or double dosing interval in patients with cirrhosis.

Available Dosage Forms

Capsule: 100 mg
Injection, solution [preservative free]: 10 mg/mL (20 mL)
Syrup: 50 mg/5 mL (240 mL) [contains sodium benzoate; strawberry flavor]
Tablet: 300 mg

Monitoring and Teaching Issues

Physical Assessment: See Warnings/Precautions for specific use cautions (eg, hepatic or renal impairment). Assess potential for interactions with other pharmacological agents and herbal products patient may be taking (eg, increased risk of nephrotoxicity, hepatotoxicity, lactic acidosis; see Drug Interactions). Assess results of laboratory tests and patient response (eg, CNS changes, hematological changes, and gastrointestinal disturbances; see Adverse Reaction) on a regular basis throughout therapy. Teach patient proper use, possible side effects/appropriate interventions, and adverse symptoms to report (see Patient Education).

Monitoring Laboratory Tests: Monitor CBC and platelet count at least every 2 weeks, MCV, serum creatinine kinase, CD4 cell count, viral load

Patient Education: Do not take any new medication during therapy unless approved by prescriber. This drug will not cure HIV; use appropriate precautions to prevent spread of HIV to other persons. Take as directed; may be taken without regard to food. Take around-the-clock. Maintain adequate hydration (2-3 L/day of fluids) unless instructed to restrict fluid intake. You may be more susceptible to infection (avoid crowds and exposure to infection and do not have any vaccinations unless approved by prescriber). May cause headache or insomnia; if these persist notify prescriber. Report unresolved nausea or vomiting; signs of infection (eg, fever, chills, sore throat, burning urination, flu-like symptoms, fatigue); unusual bleeding (eg, tarry stools, easy bruising, or blood in stool, urine, or mouth); pain, tingling, or numbness of toes or fingers; skin rash or irritation; or muscle weakness or tremors. **Pregnancy/breast-feeding precautions:** Inform prescriber if you are or intend to become pregnant. Breast-feeding is not recommended.

Dietary Considerations: May be taken without regard to food.

Pregnancy Risk Factor: C

Pregnancy Issues: Zidovudine crosses the placenta. The use of zidovudine reduces the maternal-fetal transmission of HIV by ~70% and should be considered for antenatal and intrapartum therapy whenever possible. The Perinatal HIV Guidelines Working Group considers zidovudine the preferred NRTI for use in combination regimens during pregnancy. In HIV infected mothers not previously on antiretroviral therapy, treatment may be delayed until after 10-12 weeks gestation. Cases of lactic acidosis/hepatic steatosis syndrome have been reported in pregnant women receiving nucleoside analogues. It is not known if pregnancy itself potentiates this known side effect; however, pregnant women may be at increased risk of lactic acidosis and liver damage. Hepatic enzymes and electrolytes should be monitored frequently during the 3rd trimester of pregnancy in women receiving nucleoside analogues. Health professionals are encouraged to contact the antiretroviral pregnancy registry to monitor outcomes of pregnant women exposed to antiretroviral medications (1-800-258-4263 or www.APRegistry.com).

Lactation: Enters breast milk/not recommended

Breast-Feeding Issues: HIV-infected mothers are discouraged from breast-feeding to decrease potential transmission of HIV.

Other Issues: Anemia occurs usually after 4-6 weeks of therapy. Dose adjustments and/or transfusions may be required.

Administration

Oral: Administer around-the-clock to promote less variation in peak and trough serum levels. Oral zidovudine may be administered without regard to food.

I.M.: Do not give I.M.

I.V.: Avoid rapid infusion or bolus injection

Neonates: Infuse over 30 minutes

Adults: Infuse over 1 hour

Reconstitution: Solution for injection should be diluted with D₅W to a concentration of ≤4 mg/mL; the solution is physically and chemically stable for 24 hours at room temperature and 48 hours if refrigerated. Attempt to administer diluted solution within 8 hours, if stored at room temperature or 24 hours if refrigerated to minimize potential for microbially contaminated solutions.

Compatibility: Stable in D₅W, NS; incompatible with blood products and protein solutions

Storage: Store undiluted vials at room temperature and protect from light.

Additional Information Potential compliance problems, frequency of administration and adverse effects should be discussed with patients before initiating therapy to help prevent the emergence of resistance.

♦ **Zidovudine, Abacavir, and Lamivudine** *see* Abacavir, Lamivudine, and Zidovudine *on page 34*

Zidovudine and Lamivudine (zye DOE vyoo deen & la MI vyoo deen)

U.S. Brand Names Combivir®

Synonyms AZT + 3TC; Lamivudine and Zidovudine

Generic Available No

Pharmacologic Category Antiretroviral Agent, Reverse Transcriptase Inhibitor (Nucleoside)

Medication Safety Issues

Sound-alike/look-alike issues:

Combivir® may be confused with Combivent®, Epivir®

Use Treatment of HIV infection when therapy is warranted based on clinical and/or immunological evidence of disease progression. Combivir® given twice daily, provides an alternative regimen to lamivudine 150 mg twice daily plus zidovudine 600 mg/day in divided doses; this drug form reduces capsule/tablet intake for these two drugs to 2 per day instead of up to 8.

Dosing

Adults: Treatment of HIV infection: Oral: 1 tablet twice daily. Because this is a fixed-dose combination product, avoid use in patients requiring dosage reduction including children <12 years of age, renally impaired patients with a creatinine clearance ≤50 mL/minute, patients with low body weight (<50 kg or 110 pounds), or those experiencing dose-limiting adverse effects.

Elderly: See Geriatric Considerations.

Pediatrics: Children >12 years: Refer to adult dosing.

Available Dosage Forms Tablet: Zidovudine 300 mg and lamivudine 150 mg

Monitoring and Teaching Issues

Physical Assessment: See individual agents.

Patient Education: Combivir® is not a cure for HIV and you may continue to experience HIV-associated illness. Major toxicities are neutropenia and/or anemia; have blood counts checked regularly while on therapy. **Pregnancy/breast-feeding precautions:** Inform prescriber if you are or intend to become pregnant. Do not breast-feed.

Pregnancy Risk Factor: C

Lactation: See individual agents.

Related Information

Lamivudine *on page 861*

Zidovudine *on page 1585*

♦ **Zilactin®-B [OTC]** *see* Benzocaine *on page 181*

♦ **Zilactin® Baby [OTC]** *see* Benzocaine *on page 181*

♦ **Zilactin-L® [OTC]** *see* Lidocaine *on page 898*

Zileuton (zye LOO ton)

U.S. Brand Names Zyflo™ [DSC]

Generic Available No

Pharmacologic Category 5-Lipoxygenase Inhibitor

Use Prophylaxis and chronic treatment of asthma in children ≥12 years of age and adults

Mechanism of Action/Effect Specific inhibitor of 5-lipoxygenase and thus inhibits leukotriene (LTB4, LTC4, LTD4 and LTE4) formation. Leukotrienes are substances that induce numerous biological effects including augmentation of neutrophil and eosinophil migration, neutrophil and monocyte aggregation, leukocyte adhesion, increased capillary permeability and smooth muscle contraction.

Contraindications Hypersensitivity to zileuton or any component of the formulation; active liver disease or transaminase elevations greater than or equal to three times the upper limit of normal (≥3 times ULN)

Warnings/Precautions Elevations of one or more liver function tests may occur during therapy. These laboratory abnormalities may progress, remain unchanged or resolve with continued therapy. Use with caution in patients who consume substantial quantities of ethanol or have a past history of liver disease. Zileuton is not indicated for use in the reversal of bronchospasm in acute asthma attacks, including status asthmaticus. Zileuton can be continued during acute exacerbations of asthma.

Drug Interactions

Cytochrome P450 Effect: Substrate (minor) of CYP1A2, 2C8/9, 3A4; **Inhibits** CYP1A2 (weak)

Increased Effect/Toxicity: Zileuton increases concentrations/effects of of beta-blockers (propranolol), theophylline, and warfarin. Potentially, it may increase levels of many drugs, including cisapride, due to inhibition of CYP3A4.

Nutritional/Ethanol Interactions

Ethanol: Avoid ethanol (may increase CNS depression).

Herb/Nutraceutical: St John's wort may decrease zileuton levels.

Adverse Reactions

>10%:

Central nervous system: Headache (24.6%)

Hepatic: ALT elevation (12%)

1% to 10%:

Cardiovascular: Chest pain

Central nervous system: Pain, dizziness, fever, insomnia, malaise, nervousness, somnolence

Gastrointestinal: Dyspepsia, nausea, abdominal pain, constipation, flatulence

Hematologic: Low white blood cell count

Neuromuscular & skeletal: Myalgia, arthralgia, weakness

Ocular: Conjunctivitis

Overdosage/Toxicology Symptoms of overdose: Human experience is limited. Oral minimum lethal doses in mice and rats were 500-1000 mg/kg and 300-1000 mg/kg, respectively (providing >3 and 9 times the systemic exposure achieved at the maximum recommended human daily oral dose, respectively). No deaths occurred, but nephritis was reported in dogs at an oral dose of 1000 mg/kg. Treat symptomatically; institute supportive measures as required.

Pharmacodynamics/Kinetics

Absorption: Rapid

Bioavailability: Unknown

Time to Peak: Serum: 1.7 hours

Protein Binding: 93%

Half-Life Elimination: 2.5 hours

Metabolism: Several metabolites in plasma and urine; metabolized via CYP1A2, 2C9, and 3A4

Excretion: Urine (~95% primarily as metabolites); feces (~2%)

Dosing

Adults & Elderly:

Asthma: Oral: 600 mg 4 times/day with meals and at bedtime

Pediatrics: Asthma: Oral: Children ≥12 years: Refer to adult dosing.

Renal Impairment: Dosing adjustment is **not** necessary in renal impairment or renal failure (even during dialysis).

Hepatic Impairment: Contraindicated in patients with active liver disease.

Available Dosage Forms Tablet: 600 mg

Monitoring and Teaching Issues

Physical Assessment: Not for use to relieve acute asthmatic attacks. Assess effectiveness and interactions of other medications patient may be taking. Monitor results of laboratory tests, therapeutic effectiveness, and adverse reactions at beginning of therapy and periodically with long-term use. For inpatient care, monitor vital signs and lung sounds prior to and periodically during therapy. Assess knowledge/teach patient appropriate use, interventions to reduce side effects, and adverse symptoms to report.

Monitoring Laboratory Tests: Liver function tests

Patient Education: This medication is not for an acute asthmatic attack; in acute attack, follow instructions of prescriber. Do not stop other asthma medication unless advised by prescriber. Take with meals and at bedtime on a continuous bases; do not discontinue even if feeling better (this medication may help reduce incidence of acute attacks). Avoid alcohol and other medications unless approved by your prescriber. You may experience mild headache (mild analgesic may help); fatigue or dizziness (use caution when driving); or nausea or heartburn (small frequent meals, frequent mouth care, sucking lozenges, or chewing gum may help). Report persistent headache, chest pain, rapid heartbeat, or palpitations; skin rash or itching; unusual bleeding (eg, tarry stools, easy bruising, or blood in stool, urine, or mouth); skin rash or irritation; muscle weakness or tremors; redness, irritation, or infections of the eye; or worsening of asthmatic condition. **Pregnancy/**

breast-feeding precautions: Inform prescriber if you are or intend to become pregnant. Consult prescriber if breast-feeding.

Geriatric Considerations: No differences in the pharmacokinetics found between younger adults and elderly; no dosage adjustments necessary. However, monitor liver effects closely as with any patient regardless of age.

Pregnancy Risk Factor: C

Lactation: Excretion in breast milk unknown

Breast-Feeding Issues: Zileuton and its metabolites are excreted in rat milk; it is not known if zileuton is excreted in breast milk.

Administration

Oral: Can be administered without regard to meals (ie, with or without food).

♦ Zinacef® *see* Cefuroxime *on page 290*

♦ Zinecard® *see* Dexrazoxane *on page 432*

Ziprasidone (zi PRAY si done)

U.S. Brand Names Geodon®

Synonyms Zeldox; Ziprasidone Hydrochloride; Ziprasidone Mesylate

Generic Available No

Pharmacologic Category Antipsychotic Agent, Atypical

Use Treatment of schizophrenia; treatment of acute manic or mixed episodes associated with bipolar disorder with or without psychosis; acute agitation in patients with schizophrenia

Unlabeled/Investigational Use Tourette's syndrome

Mechanism of Action/Effect Ziprasidone is a benzylisothiazolylpiperazine antipsychotic which blocks a number of CNS receptors, including dopamine, serotonin, alpha$_1$ adrenergic, and histamine receptors. Also inhibits reuptake of serotonin and epinephrine. Results in improvement in positive and negative symptoms of schizophrenia.

Contraindications Hypersensitivity to ziprasidone or any component of the formulation; history (or current) prolonged QT; congenital long QT syndrome; recent myocardial infarction; history of arrhythmias; uncompensated heart failure; concurrent use of other QT$_c$-prolonging agents including amiodarone, arsenic trioxide, bretylium, chlorpromazine, cisapride, class Ia antiarrhythmics (quinidine, procainamide), dofetilide, dolasetron, droperidol, halofantrine, ibutilide, levomethadyl, mefloquine, mesoridazine, pentamidine, pimozide, probucol, some quinolone antibiotics (moxifloxacin, sparfloxacin, gatifloxacin), sotalol, tacrolimus, and thioridazine

Warnings/Precautions May result in QT$_c$ prolongation (dose-related), which has been associated with the development of malignant ventricular arrhythmias (torsade de pointes) and sudden death. Observed prolongation was greater than with other atypical antipsychotic agents (risperidone, olanzapine, quetiapine), but less than with thioridazine. Avoid hypokalemia, hypomagnesemia. Use caution in patients with bradycardia. Discontinue in patients found to have persistent QT$_c$ intervals >500 msec. Patients with symptoms of dizziness, palpitations, or syncope should receive further cardiac evaluation.

May cause extrapyramidal symptoms. Antipsychotic use may also be associated with neuroleptic malignant syndrome (NMS). Use with caution in patients at risk of seizures.

May cause orthostatic hypotension. Atypical antipsychotics have been associated with development of hyperglycemia. There is limited documentation with ziprasidone and specific risk associated with this agent is not known. Use caution in patients with diabetes or other disorders of glucose regulation; monitor for worsening of glucose control.

Cognitive and/or motor impairment (sedation) is common with ziprasidone. Use with caution in disorders where CNS depression is a feature. Use with caution in Parkinson's disease. Use with caution in patients at risk of aspiration pneumonia (ie, Alzheimer's disease). Caution in breast cancer or other prolactin-dependent tumors. Use caution in renal or hepatic impairment. Ziprasidone has been associated with a fairly high incidence of rash (5%). Safety and efficacy have not been established in pediatric patients.

The possibility of a suicide attempt is inherent in psychotic illness or bipolar disorder; use caution in high-risk patients during initiation of therapy. Prescriptions should be written for the smallest quantity consistent with good patient care.

Drug Interactions

Cytochrome P450 Effect: Substrate (minor) of CYP1A2, 3A4; **Inhibits** CYP2D6 (weak), 3A4 (weak)

Decreased Effect: Carbamazepine may decrease serum concentrations of ziprasidone. Other enzyme-inducing agents may share this potential. Amphetamines may decrease the efficacy of ziprasidone. Ziprasidone may inhibit the efficacy of levodopa.

Increased Effect/Toxicity:

Ketoconazole may increase serum concentrations of ziprasidone. Other CYP3A4 inhibitors may share this potential.

Concurrent use with QT$_c$-prolonging agents may result in additive effects on cardiac conduction, potentially resulting in malignant or lethal arrhythmias. Concurrent use is contraindicated; includes amiodarone, arsenic trioxide, bretylium, chlorpromazine, cisapride; class Ia antiarrhythmics (quinidine, procainamide); dofetilide, dolasetron, droperidol, halofantrine, ibutilide, levomethadyl, mefloquine, mesoridazine, pentamidine, pimozide, probucol; some quinolone antibiotics (moxifloxacin, sparfloxacin, gatifloxacin); sotalol, tacrolimus, and thioridazine. Potassium- or magnesium-depleting agents (diuretics, aminoglycosides, cyclosporine, and amphotericin B) may increase the risk of QT$_c$ prolongation. Antihypertensive agents may increase the risk of orthostatic hypotension. CNS depressants may increase the degree of sedation caused by ziprasidone. Metoclopramide may increase risk of extrapyramidal symptoms (EPS).

Nutritional/Ethanol Interactions

Ethanol: Avoid ethanol (may increase CNS depression).

Food: Administration with food increases serum levels twofold. Grapefruit juice may increase serum concentration of ziprasidone.

(Continued)

Ziprasidone *(Continued)*

Herb/Nutraceutical: St John's wort may decrease serum levels of ziprasidone, due to a potential effect on CYP3A4. This has not been specifically studied. Avoid kava kava, chamomile (may increase CNS depression).

Lab Interactions Increased cholesterol, triglycerides, eosinophils

Adverse Reactions Note: Although minor QT_c prolongation (mean 10 msec at 160 mg/day) may occur more frequently (incidence not specified), clinically-relevant prolongation (>500 msec) was rare (0.06%) and less than placebo (0.23%).

>10%:
  Central nervous system: Extrapyramidal symptoms (2% to 31%), somnolence (8% to 31%), headache (3% to 18%), dizziness (3% to 16%)
  Gastrointestinal: Nausea (4% to 12%) 1% to 10%:
  Cardiovascular: Chest pain (5%), postural hypotension (5%), hypertension (2% to 3%), bradycardia (2%), tachycardia (2%), vasodilation (1%), chills, confusion, delirium, facial edema, hostility, hypertension, orthostatic hypotension, vertigo
  Central nervous system: Akathisia (2% to 10%), anxiety (2% to 5%) insomnia (3%), agitation (2%), speech disorder (2%), personality disorder (2%), psychosis (1%), akinesia, amnesia, ataxia, coordination abnormal, dystonia, fever, hypothermia, oculogyric crisis
  Dermatologic: Rash (4%), fungal dermatitis (2%)
  Endocrine & metabolic: Dysmenorrhea (2%)
  Gastrointestinal: Weight gain (10%), constipation (2% to 9%), dyspepsia (1% to 8%), diarrhea (3% to 5%), vomiting (3% to 5%), salivation increased (4%), xerostomia (1% to 5%), tongue edema (3%), abdominal pain (2%), anorexia (2%), dysphagia (2%), rectal hemorrhage (2%), tooth disorder (1%), buccoglossal syndrome
  Genitourinary: Priapism (1%)
  Local: Injection site pain (7% to 9%)
  Neuromuscular & skeletal: Weakness (2% to 6%), hypoesthesia (2%), myalgia (2%), paresthesia (2%), back pain (1%), cogwheel rigidity (1%), hypertonia (1%), abnormal gait, choreoathetosis, dysarthria, dyskinesia, hyperkinesia, hypokinesia, hypotonia, neuropathy, tremor, twitching
  Ocular: Vision abnormal (3% to 6%), diplopia
  Respiratory: Infection (8%), rhinitis (1% to 4%), cough (3%), pharyngitis (3%), dyspnea (2%)
  Miscellaneous: Diaphoresis (2%), furunculosis (2%), flu syndrome (1%), photosensitivity reaction, withdrawal syndrome

Overdosage/Toxicology Reported symptoms include somnolence, slurring of speech, and hypertension. Acute extrapyramidal symptoms may also occur. Treatment is symptom-directed and supportive. Not removed by dialysis.

Pharmacodynamics/Kinetics
Absorption: Well absorbed
Bioavailability: Oral (with food): 60% (up to twofold increase with food); I.M.: 100%
Time to Peak: Oral: 6-8 hours; I.M.: ≤60 minutes
Protein Binding: 99%, primarily to albumin and alpha$_1$-acid glycoprotein
Half-Life Elimination: Oral: 7 hours; I.M.: 2-5 hours
Metabolism: Extensively hepatic, primarily via aldehyde oxidase; less than $^1/_3$ of total metabolism via CYP3A4 and CYP1A2 (minor)
Excretion: Feces (66%) and urine (20%) as metabolites; little as unchanged drug (1% urine, 4% feces)
  Clearance: 7.5 mL/minute/kg

Dosing
Adults:
  Bipolar mania: Oral: Initial: 40 mg twice daily (with food)
    Adjustment: May increase to 60 or 80 mg twice daily on second day of treatment; average dose 40-80 mg twice daily.
  Schizophrenia: Oral: Initial: 20 mg twice daily (with food)
    Adjustment: Increases (if indicated) should be made no more frequently than every 2 days; ordinarily patients should be observed for improvement over several weeks before adjusting the dose.
    Maintenance: Range 20-100 mg twice daily; however, dosages >80 mg twice daily are generally not recommended.
  Acute agitation (schizophrenia): I.M.: 10 mg every 2 hours **or** 20 mg every 4 hours (maximum: 40 mg/day). Oral therapy should replace I.M. administration as soon as possible.
Elderly: No dosage adjustment is recommended; consider initiating at a low end of the dosage range, with slower titration.
Pediatrics:
  Tourette's syndrome (unlabeled use): Children and adolescents: Oral: 5-40 mg/day
Renal Impairment:
  Oral: No dosage adjustment is recommended
  I.M.: Cyclodextrin, an excipient in the I.M. formulation, is cleared by renal filtration; use with caution.
  Ziprasidone is not removed by hemodialysis.
Hepatic Impairment: No adjustment necessary.

Available Dosage Forms
Capsule, as hydrochloride: 20 mg, 40 mg, 60 mg, 80 mg
Injection, powder for reconstitution, as mesylate: 20 mg

Monitoring and Teaching Issues
Physical Assessment: Assess seizure risk (seizure history, ethanol use, head trauma, brain damage, or current therapy with medications that reduce seizure threshold) and cardiac status (bradycardia, QT prolongation) before starting therapy. Assess other medications patient may be taking for effectiveness and interactions (especially those

dependent on cytochrome P450 metabolism). Monitor closely for therapeutic effectiveness and adverse reactions at beginning and at regular periods throughout therapy. Monitor weight prior to initiating therapy and at least monthly. Consider titrating to a different antipsychotic agent for a weight gain ≥5% of initial weight. Assess knowledge/teach appropriate use of this medication, interventions to reduce side effects, and adverse symptoms to report.

Monitoring Laboratory Tests: Serum potassium and magnesium; fasting lipid profile and fasting blood glucose, Hgb A_{1c} (prior to treatment, at 3 months, then annually).

Patient Education: Use this mediation exactly as directed; do not alter dosage or discontinue without consulting prescriber; may take 2-3 weeks to achieve desired results. Do not share this medication with anyone else. Avoid alcohol, caffeine, other prescription or OTC medication unless approved by prescriber. Maintain adequate hydration (2-3 L/day of fluids) unless instructed to restrict fluid intake. If diabetic, you may experience increased blood sugars. Monitor blood sugars closely. You may experience drowsiness, lightheadedness, impaired coordination, dizziness, or blurred vision (use caution when driving or engaging in tasks hazardous tasks until response to drug is known); dry mouth, nausea, or GI upset (small frequent meals, good mouth care, sucking lozenges or chewing gum may help); postural hypotension (rise slowly when changing position from lying or sitting to standing or when climbing stairs); urinary retention (void before taking medication); or constipation (increased exercise, fluids, fruit, or fiber may help). Report immediately persistent CNS effects (eg, trembling, altered gait or balance, excessive sedation, seizures, unusual muscle or skeletal movements, excessive anxiety, hallucinations, nightmares, suicidal thoughts, or confusion); swelling or pain in breasts (male or female); altered menstrual pattern; sexual dysfunction; alteration in urinary pattern; vision changes; rash; respiratory difficulty; or chest pain or palpitations. **Pregnancy/breast-feeding precautions:** Inform prescriber if you are or intend to become pregnant. Breast-feeding is not recommended.

Pregnancy Risk Factor: C

Pregnancy Issues: Developmental toxicity demonstrated in animals. There are no adequate and well-controlled studies in pregnant women. Use only if potential benefit justifies risk to the fetus.

Lactation: Excretion in breast milk unknown/not recommended

Administration

Oral: Administer with food.

I.M.: Injection: For I.M. administration only.

Reconstitution: Each vial should be reconstituted with 1.2 mL SWI; shake vigorously; will form a pale, pink solution containing 20 mg/mL ziprasidone.

Storage:

Capsule: Store at controlled room temperature of 15°C to 30°C (59°F to 86°F).

Vials for injection: Prior to reconstitution, store at controlled room temperature of 15°C to 30°C (59°F to 86°F); protect from light. Following reconstitution, injection may be stored at room temperature up to 24 hours, or up to 7 days if refrigerated; protect from light.

Additional Information The increased potential to prolong QT_c, as compared to other available antipsychotic agents, should be considered in the evaluation of available alternatives.

Related Information

Antipsychotic Agents *on page 1717*

Zoledronic Acid (ZOE le dron ik AS id)

U.S. Brand Names Zometa®

Synonyms CGP-42446; Zoledronate

Generic Available No

Pharmacologic Category Adjuvant Analgesic, Bisphosphonate

Use Treatment of hypercalcemia of malignancy and bone metastases of solid tumors

Unlabeled/Investigational Use Investigational: Prevention of bone metastases from breast or prostate cancer; treatment of metabolic bone diseases

Mechanism of Action/Effect A bisphosphonate which inhibits bone resorption via actions on osteoclasts or on osteoclast precursors; inhibits osteoclastic activity and skeletal calcium release induced by tumors. Decreases serum calcium and phosphorus, and increases their elimination.

Contraindications Hypersensitivity to zoledronic acid, other bisphosphonates, or any component of the formulation; pregnancy

Warnings/Precautions Osteonecrosis of the jaw has been reported in patients with cancer who were receiving chemotherapy, corticosteroids, and chronic bisphosphonate therapy; symptoms included nonhealing extraction socket or an exposed jawbone. Dental exams and preventative dentistry should be performed prior to placing patients with risk factors (eg, chemotherapy, corticosteroids, poor oral hygiene) on chronic bisphosphonate therapy. Invasive dental procedures should be avoided during treatment.

Use caution in renal dysfunction; dosage adjustment required. Renal toxicity has been reported with doses >4 mg or infusions administered over 15 minutes. Risk factors for renal (Continued)

Zoledronic Acid *(Continued)*

deterioration include pre-existing renal insufficiency and repeated doses of zoledronic acid and other bisphosphonates. Dehydration and the use of other nephrotoxic drugs which may contribute to renal deterioration should be identified and managed. Use is not recommended in patients with severe renal impairment (serum creatinine >3 mg/dL) and bone metastases (limited data); use in patients with hypercalcemia of malignancy and severe renal impairment should only be done if the benefits outweigh the risks. Renal function should be assessed prior to treatment; if decreased after treatment, additional treatments should be withheld until renal function returns to within 10% of baseline. Adequate hydration is required during treatment (urine output ~2 L/day); avoid overhydration, especially in patients with heart failure; diuretics should not be used before correcting hypovolemia. Renal deterioration, resulting in renal failure and dialysis has occurred in patients treated with zoledronic acid after single and multiple infusions at recommended doses of 4 mg over 15 minutes.

Use caution in patients with aspirin-sensitive asthma (may cause bronchoconstriction), hepatic dysfunction, and the elderly. Women of childbearing age should be advised against becoming pregnant. Safety and efficacy in pediatric patients have not been established.

Drug Interactions
Increased Effect/Toxicity: Aminoglycosides may also lower serum calcium levels; loop diuretics increase risk of hypocalcemia; thalidomide increases renal toxicity

Adverse Reactions
>10%:
Cardiovascular: Leg edema (up to 19%)
Central nervous system: Fatigue (36%), fever (30% to 44%), headache (up to 18%), insomnia (15%), anxiety (9% to 14%), dizziness (14%), agitation (13%), depression (12%)
Dermatologic: Alopecia (11%)
Endocrine & metabolic: Hypophosphatemia (13%), hypokalemia (12%), dehydration (up to 12%)
Gastrointestinal: Nausea (29% to 45%), constipation (27% to 28%), vomiting (14% to 30%), diarrhea (17% to 22%), abdominal pain (12% to 16%)
Genitourinary: Urinary tract infection (11% to 14%)
Hematologic: Anemia (22% to 29%), neutropenia (11%)
Neuromuscular & skeletal: Myalgia (21%), paresthesia (18%), arthralgia (up to 18%) skeletal pain (12%)
Respiratory: Dyspnea (22% to 24%), cough (12% to 19%)
Miscellaneous Moniliasis (12%)
1% to 10%:
Cardiovascular: Hypotension (10%), chest pain
Central nervous system: Hypoesthesia (10%)
Dermatologic: Dermatitis (10%)
Endocrine & metabolic: Hypomagnesemia (up to 10%), hypocalcemia, hypophosphatemia (9%), hypermagnesemia (Grade 3: 2%)
Gastrointestinal: Anorexia (9%), mucositis, dysphagia
Genitourinary: Urinary tract infection (14%)
Hematologic: Thrombocytopenia, pancytopenia, granulocytopenia
Neuromuscular & skeletal: Rigors (10%), weakness
Renal: Serum creatinine increased
Respiratory: Pleural effusion, upper respiratory tract infection (8%)
Symptoms of hypercalcemia include polyuria, nephrolithiasis, anorexia, nausea, vomiting, constipation, weakness, fatigue, confusion, stupor, and coma. These may not be drug-related adverse events, but related to the underlying metabolic condition.

Overdosage/Toxicology Clinically significant hypocalcemia, hypophosphatemia, and hypomagnesemia may occur.

Pharmacodynamics/Kinetics
Onset of Action: Maximum effect may not been seen for 7 days.
Protein Binding: ~22%
Half-Life Elimination: Triphasic; Terminal: 146 hours
Excretion: Urine (39% ± 16% as unchanged drug) within 24 hours; feces (<3%)

Dosing
Adults & Elderly:
Hypercalcemia of malignancy (albumin-corrected serum calcium ≥12 mg/dL): I.V.: 4 mg (maximum) given as a single dose infused over **no less than 15 minutes**; patients should be adequately hydrated prior to treatment (restoring urine output to ~2 L/day). Monitor serum calcium and wait at least 7 days before considering retreatment. Dosage adjustment may be needed in patients with decreased renal function following treatment.
Multiple myeloma or metastatic bone lesions from solid tumors: I.V.: 4 mg given over 15 minutes every 3-4 weeks
Note: Patients should receive a daily calcium supplement and multivitamin containing vitamin D

Renal Impairment:
Renal impairment:
Cl_{cr} >60 mL/minute: 4 mg
Cl_{cr} 50-60 mL/minute: 3.5 mg
Cl_{cr} 40-49 mL/minute: 3.3 mg
Cl_{cr} 30-39 mL/minute: 3 mg

Renal toxicity:
Hypercalcemia of malignancy: Evidence of renal deterioration: Evaluate risk versus benefit.
Bone metastases: Evidence of renal deterioration: Discontinue further dosing until renal function returns to within 10% of baseline: renal deterioration defined as follows:
Normal baseline creatinine: Increase of 0.5 mg/dL
Abnormal baseline creatinine: Increase of 1 mg/dL

Reinitiate dose at the same dose administered prior to treatment interruption.

Hepatic Impairment: Specific guidelines are not available.

Available Dosage Forms Injection, solution: 4 mg/5 mL (5 mL) [as monohydrate 4.264 mg]

Monitoring and Teaching Issues

Physical Assessment: Use caution with aspirin-sensitive asthma, hepatic dysfunction, advanced age (see Warnings/Precautions for specific cautions). Assess potential for interactions with other pharmacological agents and herbal products patient may be taking (see Drug Interactions). Note recommendations for daily calcium and vitamin D supplements. Assess results of laboratory tests and patient response to therapy (see Adverse Reactions). Teach patient possible side effects/appropriate interventions (eg, need for adequate hydration) and adverse symptoms to report (See Patient Education).

Monitoring Laboratory Tests: Monitor serum creatinine prior to each dose. Serum electrolytes, phosphate, magnesium, and hemoglobin/hematocrit should be evaluated regularly. Monitor serum calcium to assess response and avoid over treatment.

Patient Education: This medication is only administered intravenously. Avoid vitamins during infusion or for 2-3 hours after completion. Maintain adequate hydration (2-3 L/day of fluids) unless instructed to restrict fluid intake. You may experience some nausea or vomiting (small frequent meals, good mouth care, sucking lozenges, or chewing gum may help) or recurrent bone pain (consult prescriber for analgesic). Report unusual muscle twitching or spasms, severe diarrhea/constipation, acute bone pain, or other persistent adverse effects. **Pregnancy/breast-feeding precautions:** Inform prescriber if you are or intend to become pregnant. Do not get pregnant during therapy. Consult prescriber for instructions on appropriate contraceptive measures. This drug may cause fetal defects. Breast-feeding is not recommended.

Dietary Considerations: Multiple myeloma or metastatic bone lesions from solid tumors: Take daily calcium supplement (500 mg) and daily multivitamin (with 400 int. units vitamin D).

Pregnancy Risk Factor: D

Pregnancy Issues: Animal studies resulted in embryotoxicity and losses. May cause fetal harm when administered to a pregnant woman. Use only if the benefit to the mother outweighs the potential risk to the fetus.

Lactation: Excretion in breast milk unknown/not recommended

Administration

I.V.: In order to prevent renal toxicity, infuse solution over at least 15 minutes.

Reconstitution: Dilute solution for injection in 100 mL NS or D_5W prior to administration. Infusion of solution must be completed within 24 hours

Compatibility: Incompatible with calcium-containing solutions (eg, LR)

Storage: Store intact vials at 25°C (77°F).

Zolmitriptan (zohl mi TRIP tan)

U.S. Brand Names Zomig®; Zomig-ZMT™

Synonyms 311C90

Generic Available No

Pharmacologic Category Serotonin 5-HT$_{1D}$ Receptor Agonist

Medication Safety Issues

Sound-alike/look-alike issues:

Zolmitriptan may be confused with sumatriptan

Use Acute treatment of migraine with or without aura

Mechanism of Action/Effect Zolmitriptan is a selective 5-HT$_{1B/1D}$ agonist

Contraindications Hypersensitivity to zolmitriptan or any component of the formulation; ischemic heart disease or Prinzmetal's angina; signs or symptoms of ischemic heart disease; uncontrolled hypertension; symptomatic Wolff-Parkinson-White syndrome or arrhythmias associated with other cardiac accessory conduction pathway disorders; use with ergotamine derivatives (within 24 hours of); use within 24 hours of another 5-HT$_1$ agonist; concurrent administration or within 2 weeks of discontinuing an MAO inhibitor; management of hemiplegic or basilar migraine

Warnings/Precautions Zolmitriptan is indicated only in patient populations with a clear diagnosis of migraine. Not for prophylactic treatment of migraine headaches. Cardiac events (including myocardial infarction, ventricular arrhythmia, cardiac arrest, and death) have been reported with 5-HT$_1$ agonist administration. Should not be given to patients who have risk factors for CAD without adequate cardiac evaluation. Patients with suspected CAD should have cardiovascular evaluation to rule out CAD before considering zolmitriptan's use; if cardiovascular evaluation negative, first dose would be safest if given in the healthcare provider's office. Periodic evaluation of those without cardiovascular disease, but with continued risk factors should be done. Significant elevation in blood pressure, including hypertensive crisis, has also been reported. Vasospasm-related reactions have been reported other than coronary artery vasospasm. Peripheral vascular ischemia and colonic ischemia with abdominal pain and bloody diarrhea have occurred. Use with caution in patients with hepatic impairment. Zomig-ZMT™ tablets contain phenylalanine. Safety and efficacy not established in patients <18 years of age.

Drug Interactions

Cytochrome P450 Effect: Substrate of CYP1A2 (minor)

Increased Effect/Toxicity: Ergot-containing drugs may lead to vasospasm; cimetidine, MAO inhibitors, oral contraceptives, propranolol increase levels of zolmitriptan; concurrent use with SSRIs and sibutramine may lead to serotonin syndrome.

Nutritional/Ethanol Interactions Ethanol: Limit use (may have additive CNS toxicity).

Lab Interactions No interferences have been identified

Adverse Reactions Percentages noted from oral preparations.

1% to 10%:

Cardiovascular: Chest pain (2% to 4%), palpitation (up to 2%)

Central nervous system: Dizziness (6% to 10%), somnolence (5% to 8%), pain (2% to 3%), vertigo (≤2%)

(Continued)

Zolmitriptan *(Continued)*

Gastrointestinal: Nausea (4% to 9%), xerostomia (3% to 5%), dyspepsia (1% to 3%), dysphagia (≤2%)

Neuromuscular & skeletal: Paresthesia (5% to 9%), weakness (3% to 9%), warm/cold sensation (5% to 7%), hypoesthesia (1% to 2%), myalgia (1% to 2%), myasthenia (up to 2%)

Miscellaneous: Neck/throat/jaw pain (4% to 10%), diaphoresis (up to 3%), allergic reaction (up to 1%)

Overdosage/Toxicology Treatment is symptom-directed and supportive. It is not known if hemodialysis or peritoneal dialysis is effective.

Pharmacodynamics/Kinetics

Onset of Action: 0.5-1 hour

Absorption: Well absorbed

Bioavailability: 40%

Time to Peak: Serum: Tablet: 1.5 hours; Orally-disintegrating tablet and nasal spray: 3 hours

Protein Binding: 25%

Half-Life Elimination: 2.8-3.7 hours

Metabolism: Converted to an active N-desmethyl metabolite (2-6 times more potent than zolmitriptan)

Excretion: Urine (~60% to 65% total dose); feces (30% to 40%)

Dosing

Adults:

Migraine headache:

Oral:

Tablet: Initial: ≤2.5 mg at the onset of migraine headache; may break 2.5 mg tablet in half

Orally-disintegrating tablet: Initial: 2.5 mg at the onset of migraine headache

Nasal spray: Initial: 1 spray (5 mg) at the onset of migraine headache

Note: Use the lowest possible dose to minimize adverse events. If the headache returns, the dose may be repeated after 2 hours; do not exceed 10 mg within a 24-hour period. Controlled trials have not established the effectiveness of a second dose if the initial one was ineffective

Elderly: No dosage adjustment needed, but elderly patients are more likely to have underlying cardiovascular disease and should have careful evaluation of cardiovascular system before prescribing.

Renal Impairment: No dosage adjustment recommended. There is a 25% reduction in zolmitriptan's clearance in patients with severe renal impairment (Cl$_{cr}$ 5-25 mL/minute)

Hepatic Impairment: Administer with caution in patients with liver disease, generally using doses <2.5 mg. Patients with moderate-to-severe hepatic impairment may have decreased clearance of zolmitriptan, and significant elevation in blood pressure was observed in some patients.

Available Dosage Forms

Solution, nasal spray [single dose] (Zomig®): 5 mg/0.1 mL (0.1 mL)

Tablet (Zomig®): 2.5 mg, 5 mg

Tablet, orally-disintegrating (Zomig-ZMT™): 2.5 mg [contains phenylalanine 2.81 mg/tablet; orange flavor]; 5 mg [contains phenylalanine 5.62 mg/tablet; orange flavor]

Monitoring and Teaching Issues

Physical Assessment: For use only with a clear diagnosis of migraine headaches. Use caution in presence of cardiovascular risk factors and hepatic impairment (see Warnings/Precautions for use cautions). Assess potential for interactions with other pharmacological agents and herbal products patient may be taking (eg, ergot-containing drugs; see Drug Interactions). Assess effectiveness and adverse response (eg, chest pain, nausea, dizziness, paresthesia, myalgia, pain; see Adverse Reactions). Teach patient proper use (according to formulation), possible side effects/appropriate interventions, and adverse symptoms to report (see Patient Education).

Patient Education: This drug is to be used to reduce your migraine, not to prevent or reduce the number of attacks. Follow exact instructions for use. Remove orally-disintegrating tablet from blister package just before using, place on tongue, and allow to dissolve. Do not crush, break, or chew. Regular tablet may be broken in half for use. Follow package directions for nasal spray. Do not take within 24 hours of any other migraine medication without first consulting prescriber. If first dose brings relief, second dose may be taken anytime after 2 hours if migraine returns. If you have no relief with first dose, do not take a second dose without consulting prescriber. Do not exceed 10 mg in 24 hours. May cause dizziness or drowsiness (use caution when driving or engaging in tasks requiring alertness until response to drug is known); or dry mouth (frequent mouth care and sucking on lozenges may help). Report immediately any chest pain, heart throbbing, or tightness in throat; swelling of eyelids, face, or lips; skin rash or hives; easy bruising; blood in urine, stool, or vomitus; pain or itching with urination; or pain, warmth, or numbness in extremities. **Pregnancy/breast-feeding precautions:** Inform prescriber if you are or intend to become pregnant. Consult prescriber if breast-feeding.

Geriatric Considerations: Zolmitriptan use in the elderly patient has not been studied.

Pregnancy Risk Factor: C

Pregnancy Issues: In pregnant animals, zolmitriptan caused embryolethality and fetal abnormalities at doses ≥11 times the equivalent human dose.

Lactation: Excretion in breast milk unknown/use caution

Administration

Oral: Administer as soon as migraine headache starts. Tablets may be broken. Orally-disintegrating tablets: Must be taken whole; do not break, crush or chew; place on tongue and allow to dissolve; administration with liquid is not required

Other: Nasal spray: Administer as soon as migraine headache starts. Blow nose gently prior to use. After removing protective cap, instill device into nostril. Block opposite nostril;

breathe in gently through nose while pressing plunger of spray device. One dose (5 mg) is equal to 1 spray in 1 nostril.

Storage: Store at 20°C to 25°C (68°F to 77°F); protect from light and moisture

Additional Information Not recommended if the patient has risk factors for heart disease (high blood pressure, high cholesterol, obesity, diabetes, smoking, strong family history of heart disease, postmenopausal woman, or a male >40 years of age).

This agent is intended to relieve migraine, but not to prevent or reduce the number of attacks. Use only to treat an actual migraine attack.

Related Information

Antimigraine Drugs: 5-HT$_1$ Receptor Agonists *on page 1716*

♦ **Zoloft**® *see* Sertraline *on page 1367*

Zolpidem (zole PI dem)

U.S. Brand Names Ambien®

Synonyms Zolpidem Tartrate

Controlled Substance C-IV

Generic Available No

Pharmacologic Category Hypnotic, Nonbenzodiazepine

Medication Safety Issues

Sound-alike/look-alike issues:

Ambien® may be confused with Ambi 10®

Use Short-term treatment of insomnia

Mechanism of Action/Effect Structurally dissimilar to benzodiazepine, however, has much or all of its actions explained by its effects on benzodiazepine (BZD) receptors, especially the omega-1 receptor; retains hypnotic and much of the anxiolytic properties of the BZD, but has reduced effects on skeletal muscle and seizure threshold.

Contraindications Hypersensitivity to zolpidem or any component of the formulation

Warnings/Precautions Should be used only after evaluation of potential causes of sleep disturbance. Failure of sleep disturbance to resolve after 7-10 days may indicate psychiatric or medical illness. Use with caution in patients with decreased respiratory function or or depression. Behavioral changes have been associated with sedative-hypnotics. Causes CNS depression, which may impair physical and mental capabilities. Effects with other sedative drugs or ethanol may be potentiated. Closely monitor elderly or debilitated patients for impaired cognitive or motor performance; not recommended for use in children <18 years of age. Avoid use in patients with sleep apnea or a history of sedative-hypnotic abuse.

Drug Interactions

Cytochrome P450 Effect: Substrate of CYP1A2 (minor), 2C8/9 (minor), 2C19 (minor), 2D6 (minor), 3A4 (major)

Decreased Effect: CYP3A4 inducers may decrease the levels/effects of zolpidem; example inducers include aminoglutethimide, carbamazepine, nafcillin, nevirapine, phenobarbital, phenytoin, and rifamycins.

Increased Effect/Toxicity: Use of zolpidem in combination with other centrally-acting drugs may produce additive CNS depression. CYP3A4 inhibitors may increase the levels/effects of zolpidem; example inhibitors include azole antifungals, ciprofloxacin, clarithromycin, diclofenac, doxycycline, erythromycin, imatinib, isoniazid, nefazodone, nicardipine, propofol, protease inhibitors, quinidine, and verapamil.

Nutritional/Ethanol Interactions

Ethanol: Avoid ethanol (may increase CNS depression).

Herb/Nutraceutical: St John's wort may decrease zolpidem levels. Avoid valerian, St John's wort, kava kava, gotu kola (may increase CNS depression).

Lab Interactions Increased aminotransferase [ALT (SGPT)/AST (SGOT)], bilirubin (S); decreased RAI uptake

Adverse Reactions 1% to 10%:

Cardiovascular: Palpitations

Central nervous system: Headache, drowsiness, dizziness, lethargy, lightheadedness, depression, abnormal dreams, amnesia

Dermatologic: Rash

Gastrointestinal: Nausea, diarrhea, xerostomia, constipation

Respiratory: Sinusitis, pharyngitis

Overdosage/Toxicology Symptoms of overdose include coma and hypotension. Treatment for overdose is supportive. Rarely is mechanical ventilation required. Flumazenil has been shown to selectively block binding to CNS receptors, resulting in a reversal of CNS depression, but not always respiratory depression.

Pharmacodynamics/Kinetics

Onset of Action: 30 minutes

Duration of Action: 6-8 hours

Absorption: Rapid

Protein Binding: 92%

Half-Life Elimination: 2-2.6 hours; Cirrhosis: Up to 9.9 hours

Metabolism: Hepatic to inactive metabolites

Dosing

Adults:

Insomnia: Oral: 10 mg immediately before bedtime; maximum: 10 mg (duration of therapy should be limited to 7-10 days)

Elderly: 5 mg immediately before bedtime

Renal Impairment: Not dialyzable

Hepatic Impairment: Decrease dose to 5 mg.

Available Dosage Forms

Tablet, as tartrate: 5 mg, 10 mg

Ambien® PAK™ [dose pack]: 5 mg (30s), 10 mg (30s)

(Continued)

Zolpidem *(Continued)*

Monitoring and Teaching Issues

Physical Assessment: For short-term use. Assess effectiveness and interactions of other medications patient may be taking. Assess for history of addiction; long-term use can result in dependence, abuse, or tolerance; periodically evaluate need for continued use. After long-term use, taper dosage slowly when discontinuing. Monitor for CNS depression. For inpatient use, institute safety measures and monitor effectiveness and adverse reactions. For outpatients, monitor for effectiveness of therapy and adverse reactions at beginning of therapy and periodically with long-term use. Assess knowledge/teach patient appropriate use, interventions to reduce side effects, and adverse symptoms to report.

Patient Education: Use exactly as directed; do not increase dose or frequency or discontinue without consulting prescriber. Drug may cause physical and/or psychological dependence. While using this medication, do not use alcohol or other prescription or OTC medications (especially, pain medications, sedatives, antihistamines, or hypnotics) without consulting prescriber. Maintain adequate hydration (2-3 L/day of fluids) unless instructed to restrict fluid intake. You may experience drowsiness, dizziness, or blurred vision (use caution when driving or engaging in tasks requiring alertness until response to drug is known); nausea (small frequent meals, frequent mouth care, chewing gum, or sucking lozenges may help); or diarrhea (buttermilk, boiled milk, yogurt may help). Report CNS changes (confusion, depression, increased sedation, excitation, headache, abnormal thinking, insomnia, or nightmares); muscle pain or weakness; respiratory difficulty; chest pain or palpitations; or ineffectiveness of medication. **Breast-feeding precaution:** Consult prescriber if breast-feeding.

Geriatric Considerations: In doses >5 mg, there was subjective evidence of impaired sleep on the first post-treatment night. There have been few reports of increased hypotension and/or falls in the elderly with this drug. Can be considered a drug of choice in the elderly when a hypnotic is indicated.

Pregnancy Risk Factor: B

Pregnancy Issues: Benzodiazepines cross the placenta. The association between benzodiazepine exposure and malformations remains controversial. A number of types of malformation have been reported (oral cleft, inguinal hernia, cardiac defects, spina bifida, dysmorphic facial features, skeletal defects); however, confounding factors make a clear association difficult. Overall, the risk to the fetus may be low. Nonteratogenic effects (including neonatal flaccidity, respiratory and feeding problems, and withdrawal symptoms) during the postnatal period have also been reported with benzodiazepine use.

Lactation: Enters breast milk/use caution (AAP rates "compatible")

Additional Information Causes less disturbances in sleep stages as compared to benzodiazepines. Time spent in sleep stages 3 and 4 are maintained; decreases sleep latency. Should not be prescribed in quantities exceeding a 1-month supply.

Related Information

Anxiolytic / Hypnotic Use in Long-Term Care Facilities *on page 1769*

- **Zolpidem Tartrate** *see Zolpidem on page 1595*
- **Zometa®** *see Zoledronic Acid on page 1591*
- **Zomig®** *see Zolmitriptan on page 1593*
- **Zomig-ZMT™** *see Zolmitriptan on page 1593*
- **Zonalon®** *see Doxepin on page 487*
- **Zonegran®** *see Zonisamide on page 1596*

Zonisamide *(zoe NIS a mide)*

U.S. Brand Names Zonegran®

Generic Available No

Pharmacologic Category Anticonvulsant, Miscellaneous

Use Adjunct treatment of partial seizures in children >16 years of age and adults with epilepsy

Unlabeled/Investigational Use Bipolar disorder

Mechanism of Action/Effect The exact mechanism of action is not known. May stabilize neuronal membranes and suppress neuronal hypersynchronization through action at sodium and calcium channels. Does not affect GABA activity.

Contraindications Hypersensitivity to zonisamide, sulfonamides, or any component of the formulation

Warnings/Precautions Rare, but potentially fatal sulfonamide reactions have occurred following the use of zonisamide. These reactions include Stevens-Johnson syndrome and toxic epidermal necrolysis, usually appearing within 2-16 weeks of drug initiation. Discontinue zonisamide if rash develops. Chemical similarities are present among sulfonamides, sulfonylureas, carbonic anhydrase inhibitors, thiazides, and loop diuretics (except ethacrynic acid). Use in patients with sulfonamide allergy is specifically contraindicated in product labeling, however, a risk of cross-reaction exists in patients with allergy to any of these compounds; avoid use when previous reaction has been severe.

Decreased sweating (oligohydrosis) and hyperthermia requiring hospitalization have been reported in children. Discontinue zonisamide in patients who develop acute renal failure or a significant sustained increase in creatinine/BUN concentration. Kidney stones have been reported. Use cautiously in patients with renal or hepatic dysfunction. Significant CNS effects include psychiatric symptoms, psychomotor slowing, and fatigue or somnolence. Fatigue and somnolence occur within the first month of treatment, most commonly at doses of 300-500 mg/day. Abrupt withdrawal may precipitate seizures; discontinue or reduce doses gradually. Safety and efficacy in children <16 years of age has not been established.

Drug Interactions

Cytochrome P450 Effect: Substrate of CYP2C19 (minor), 3A4 (major)

Decreased Effect: CYP3A4 inducers may decrease the levels/effects of zonisamide; example inducers include aminoglutethimide, carbamazepine, nafcillin, nevirapine, phenobarbital, phenytoin, and rifamycins.

Increased Effect/Toxicity: Sedative effects may be additive with other CNS depressants; monitor for increased effect (includes barbiturates, benzodiazepines, narcotic analgesics, ethanol, and other sedative agents). CYP3A4 inhibitors may increase the levels/effects of zonisamide; example inhibitors include azole antifungals, ciprofloxacin, clarithromycin, diclofenac, doxycycline, erythromycin, imatinib, isoniazid, nefazodone, nicardipine, propofol, protease inhibitors, quinidine, and verapamil.

Nutritional/Ethanol Interactions

Ethanol: Avoid ethanol (may increase CNS depression).

Food: Food delays time to maximum concentration, but does not affect bioavailability.

Adverse Reactions Adjunctive Therapy: Frequencies noted in patients receiving other anticonvulsants:

>10%:

Central nervous system: Somnolence (17%), dizziness (13%)

Gastrointestinal: Anorexia (13%)

1% to 10%:

Central nervous system: Headache (10%), agitation/irritability (9%), fatigue (8%), tiredness (7%), ataxia (6%), confusion (6%), decreased concentration (6%), memory impairment (6%), depression (6%), insomnia (6%), speech disorders (5%), mental slowing (4%), anxiety (3%), nervousness (2%), schizophrenic/schizophreniform behavior (2%), difficulty in verbal expression (2%), status epilepticus (1%), tremor (1%), convulsion (1%), hyperesthesia (1%), incoordination (1%)

Dermatologic: Rash (3%), bruising (2%), pruritus (1%)

Gastrointestinal: Nausea (9%), abdominal pain (6%), diarrhea (5%), dyspepsia (3%), weight loss (3%), constipation (2%), dry mouth (2%), taste perversion (2%), vomiting (1%)

Neuromuscular & skeletal: Paresthesia (4%), weakness (1%), abnormal gait (1%)

Ocular: Diplopia (6%), nystagmus (4%), amblyopia (1%)

Otic: Tinnitus (1%)

Respiratory: Rhinitis (2%), pharyngitis (1%), increased cough (1%)

Miscellaneous: Flu-like syndrome (4%) accidental injury (1%)

Overdosage/Toxicology No specific antidotes are available; experience with doses >800 mg/day is limited. Emesis or gastric lavage, with airway protection, should be done following a recent overdose. General supportive care and close observation are indicated. Renal dialysis may not be effective due to low protein binding (40%).

Pharmacodynamics/Kinetics

Time to Peak: 2-6 hours

Protein Binding: 40%

Half-Life Elimination: 63 hours

Metabolism: Hepatic via CYP3A4; forms N-acetyl zonisamide and 2-sulfamoylacetyl phenol (SMAP)

Excretion: Urine (62%, 35% as unchanged drug, 65% as metabolites); feces (3%)

Dosing

Adults:

Adjunctive treatment of partial seizures: Oral: Initial: 100 mg/day. Dose may be increased to 200 mg/day after 2 weeks. Further dosage increases to 300 mg and 400 mg/day can then be made with a minimum of 2 weeks between adjustments, in order to reach steady state at each dosage level. Doses of up to 600 mg/day have been studied, however, there is no evidence of increased response with doses >400 mg/day.

Mania (unlabeled use): Oral: Initial: 100-200 mg/day; maximum: 600 mg/day

Elderly: Data from clinical trials is insufficient for patients older than 65. Begin dosing at the low end of the dosing range.

Pediatrics: Children >16 years: Refer to adult dosing.

Renal Impairment: Slower titration and frequent monitoring are indicated in patients with renal or hepatic disease. There is insufficient experience regarding dosing/toxicity in patients with estimated GFR <50 mL/minute. Marked renal impairment (Cl_{cr} <20 mL/minute) was associated with a 35% increase in AUC.

Hepatic Impairment: Slower titration and frequent monitoring are indicated.

Available Dosage Forms Capsule: 25 mg, 50 mg, 100 mg

Monitoring and Teaching Issues

Physical Assessment: Assess other medications patient may be taking for increased risk of drug/drug interactions. Monitor therapeutic effectiveness, laboratory results, and adverse reactions at beginning of therapy and periodically with long-term use. Observe and teach seizure precautions. Assess knowledge/teach patient appropriate use, interventions to reduce side effects, and adverse symptoms to report.

Patient Education: Take exactly as directed, as the same time each day, with or without food. Do not increase frequency, alter dose, or discontinue without consulting prescriber. If you miss a dose, take as soon as possible. If it is almost time for your next dose, skip the missed dose. Do not chew, crush, or open capsules; swallow whole. Maintain adequate hydration (2-3 L/day of fluids) unless instructed to restrict fluid intake. Avoid grapefruit juice while on this medication. While using this medication, avoid alcohol, herbal remedies, OTC or prescriptions drugs (especially pain medication, antihistamines, psychiatric medications, sedatives, or hypnotics) unless approved by your prescriber. Wear/carry identification of epileptic status and medications. You may experience drowsiness, dizziness, or blurred vision (use caution when driving or engaging in tasks requiring alertness until response to drug is known); or nausea, vomiting, constipation, dry mouth, or loss of appetite (small frequent meals, frequent mouth care, chewing gum, or sucking hard candy may help). Report CNS changes (changes in speech patterns, mentation changes, changes in cognition or memory, unusual thought patterns, coordination difficulties, or excessive drowsiness); respiratory difficulty or tightening of the throat; swelling of mouth, lips, or tongue; muscle cramping, weakness, or pain; rash or skin irritations; unusual bruising or bleeding (mouth, urine, stool); fever, sore throat, sores in your mouth; swelling of extremities; sudden back pain, pain on urination, or dark/bloody urine (signs of kidney stones); or other

(Continued)

Zonisamide *(Continued)*

adverse response including change in seizure type or frequency. **Pregnancy/ breast-feeding precautions:** Inform prescriber if you are or intend to become pregnant. Do not breast-feed.

Dietary Considerations: May be taken with or without food.

Pregnancy Risk Factor: C

Pregnancy Issues: Fetal abnormalities and death have been reported in animals, however, there are no studies in pregnant women.

Lactation: Excretion in breast milk unknown/contraindicated

Breast-Feeding Issues: Based on limited case reports, it appears zonisamide is excreted in breast milk. Use during lactation only if the potential benefits outweigh the potential risks.

Administration
Storage: Store at controlled room temperature 25°C (77°F). Protect from moisture and light.

Related Information
Anticonvulsants By Seizure Type *on page 1712*

CONTROLLED SUBSTANCE INDEX

CONTROLLED SUBSTANCE INDEX

PHARMACOLOGIC CATEGORY INDEX

Antitussive/Decongestant/Expectorant

Antiviral Agent

Antiviral Agent, Ophthalmic

Antiviral Agent, Oral

Appetite Stimulant

Aromatase Inhibitor

Barbiturate

Benzodiazepine

Beta-Adrenergic Blocker, Nonselective

Beta Blocker, Beta$_1$ Selective

Beta Blocker With Alpha-Blocking Activity

Beta Blocker With Intrinsic Sympathomimetic Activity

Beta$_1$- & Beta$_2$-Adrenergic Agonist Agent

Beta$_2$-Adrenergic Agonist

APPENDIX

TABLE OF CONTENTS

APPENDIX *(Continued)*

DIAGNOSTICS AND SURGICAL AIDS

Agent	Use
Apraclonidine (Iopidine®)	Prevention and treatment of postsurgical intraocular pressure elevation
Benzylpenicilloyl-Polylysine (Pre-Pen®)	Adjunct in assessing the risk of administering penicillin (penicillin or benzylpenicillin) in adults with a history of clinical penicillin hypersensitivity
Candida albicans (Monilia) (Dermatophytin-O)	Screen for the detection of nonresponsiveness to antigens in immunocompromised individuals
Cellulose (oxidized regenerated) (Surgicel®)	Temporary packing for the control of capillary, venous, or small arterial hemorrhage
Chondroitin sulfate - sodium hyaluronate (Viscoat®)	Surgical aid in anterior segment procedures, protects corneal endothelium and coats intraocular lens thus protecting it
Corticotropin (Acthar®; H.P. Acthar® Gel)	Diagnostic aid in adrenocortical insufficiency; repository dosage form is used for acute exacerbations of multiple sclerosis or severe muscle weakness in myasthenia gravis; cosyntropin is preferred
Cosyntropin (Cortrosyn® Injection)	Diagnostic test to differentiate primary adrenal from secondary (pituitary) adrenocortical insufficiency
Cyclopentolate (AK-Pentolate®; Cyclogyl®; I-Pentolate®)	Diagnostic procedures requiring mydriasis and cycloplegia
Cyclopentolate and phenylephrine (Cyclomydril® Ophthalmic)	Induce mydriasis greater than that produced with cyclopentolate alone
Dapiprazole (Rêv-Eyes™)	Reverse dilation due to drugs (adrenergic or parasympathomimetic) after eye exams
Dimercaprol (BAL in Oil®)	Antidote to gold, arsenic (except arsine), and mercury poisoning (except nonalkyl mercury); adjunct to edetate calcium disodium in lead poisoning; possibly effective for antimony, bismuth, chromium, copper, nickel, tungsten, or zinc
Dinoprost (Prostin F$_2$ Alpha®)	Abort 2nd trimester pregnancy
Fluorescein sodium (AK-Fluor® Injection; Fluorescite® Injection; Fluorets® Ophthalmic Strips; Fluor-I-Strip®; Fluor-I-Strip-AT®; Fluress® Ophthalmic Solution; Ful-Glo® Ophthalmic Strips)	Demonstrates defects of corneal epithelium; diagnostic aid in ophthalmic angiography
Gelatin, absorbable (Gelfilm® Ophthalmic; Gelfoam® Topical)	Adjunct to provide hemostasis in surgery; used in open prostatic surgery
Histoplasmin (Histolyn-CYL® Injection)	Diagnose histoplasmosis; assess cell-mediated immunity
Hydroxyamphetamine and tropicamide (Paremyd® Ophthalmic)	Diagnostic mydriasis with cycloplegia
Hydroxypropyl methylcellulose (Gonak™; Goniosol®)	Ophthalmic surgical aid in cataract extraction and intraocular implantation; gonioscopic examination
Indocyanine green (Cardio-Green®)	Determine hepatic function, cardiac output, and liver blood flow and for ophthalmic angiography
Methacholine (Provocholine®)	Diagnosis of bronchial airway hyperactivity
Methylene blue (Urolene Blue®)	Antidote for cyanide poisoning and drug-induced methemoglobinemia, indicator dye, chronic urolithiasis. **Unlabeled use:** Has been used topically (0.1% solutions) in conjunction with polychromatic light to photoinactivate viruses such as herpes simplex; has been used alone or in combination with vitamin C for the management of chronic urolithiasis.
Microfibrillar collagen hemostat (Avitene®; Helistat®; Hemotene®)	Adjunct to hemostasis when control of bleeding by ligature is ineffective or impractical
Mumps skin test antigen	Assess the status of cell-mediated immunity
Proparacaine (AK-Taine®; Alcaine®; I-Paracaine®; Ophthetic®)	Anesthesia for tonometry, gonioscopy; suture removal from cornea; removal of corneal foreign body; cataract extraction, glaucoma surgery; short operative procedure involving the cornea and conjunctiva
Proparacaine and fluorescein (Fluoracaine® Ophthalmic)	Anesthesia for tonometry, gonioscopy; suture removal from cornea; removal of corneal foreign body; cataract extraction, glaucoma surgery
Protirelin (Relefact® TRH Injection; Thypinone® Injection)	Adjunct in the diagnostic assessment of thyroid function, and an adjunct to other diagnostic procedures in assessment of patients with pituitary or hypothalamic dysfunction; causes release of prolactin from the pituitary and is used to detect defective control of prolactin secretion
Secretin (Secretin Ferring Powder)	Diagnose Zollinger-Ellison syndrome, chronic pancreatic dysfunction, and some hepatobiliary diseases such as obstructive jaundice resulting from cancer or stones in the biliary tract

DIAGNOSTICS AND SURGICAL AIDS *(Continued)*

Agent	Use
Sermorelin acetate (Geref® Injection; Geref® Diagnostic)	Geref® Diagnostic: For the evaluation of short children whose height is at least 2 standard deviations below the mean height for their chronological age and sex, presenting with low basal serum levels of IGF-1 and IGF-1-BP3. A single intravenous injection of sermorelin is indicated for evaluating the ability of the somatotroph of the pituitary gland to secrete growth hormone (GH). A normal plasma GH response demonstrates that the somatotroph is intact. Geref® injection: Treatment of idiopathic growth hormone deficiency
Sincalide (Kinevac®)	Postevacuation cholecystography; gallbladder bile sampling; stimulate pancreatic secretion for analysis
Skin test antigens, multiple (Multitest CMI®)	Detection of nonresponsiveness to antigens by means of delayed hypersensitivity skin testing
Sodium hyaluronate (AMO Vitrax®; Amvisc®; Amvisc® Plus; Healon®; Healon® GV)	Surgical aid in cataract extraction, intraocular implantation, corneal transplant, glaucoma filtration, and retinal attachment surgery
Succinylcholine (Anectine® Chloride Injection; Anectine® Flo-Pack®; Quelicin® Injection)	Produces skeletal muscle relaxation in procedures of short duration such as endotracheal intubation or endoscopic exams
Thrombin, topical (Thrombinar®; Thrombogen®; Thrombostat®)	Hemostasis whenever minor bleeding from capillaries and small venules is accessible
Thyrotropin Alpha (Thyrogen®)	As an adjunctive diagnostic tool for serum thyroglobulin (Tg) testing with or without radioiodine imaging in the follow-up of patients with well-differentiated thyroid cancer
Trichophyton skin test (Dermatophytin® Injection)	Assess cell-mediated immunity
Tropicamide (Mydriacyl®; Opticyl®; Tropicacyl®)	Short-acting mydriatic used in diagnostic procedures, as well as preoperatively and postoperatively; treatment of some cases of acute ititis, iridocyclitis, and keratitis

HERBAL AND NUTRITIONAL PRODUCTS

TOP HERBAL PRODUCTS

This section contains general information on commonly encountered herbal or nutritional products. A more complete listing of products follows.

Alpha-Lipoic Acid

Synonyms: Alpha-Lipoate; Lipoic Acid; Thioctic acid
Use: Treatment of glaucoma and neuropathies
Mechanism of Action/Effect: Sulfur-containing cofactor normally synthesized in humans; potent antioxidant
Warnings: Use with caution in individuals who may be predisposed to hypoglycemia (including individuals receiving antidiabetic agents).
Drug Interactions: Oral hypoglycemics or insulin
Adverse Reactions: Rash
Dosing: Oral: 20-600 mg/day (common dose: 25-50 mg twice daily)

Androstenedione

Use: Increase strength and muscle mass
Mechanism of Action/Effect: Weak androgenic steroid hormone believed to facilitate faster recovery from exercise and to promote muscle development in response to training
Contraindication: Hypertension
Warnings: Use with caution in individuals with CHF, prostate conditions, and hormone-sensitive tumors. The FDA requires specific labeling on this supplement, noting that these supplements "contain steroid hormones that may cause breast enlargement, testicular shrinkage, and infertility in males, and increased facial and body hair, voice deepening and clitoral enlargement in females."
Drug Interactions: Estrogens and androgenic drugs
Dosing: Oral: 50-100 mg/day (usually about 1 hour before exercising)

Arginine

Synonyms: L-Arginine
Use: Treatment of high cholesterol, poor circulation, inflammatory bowel disease, immunity enhancement, male infertility; promotes lean body mass, surgery and wound healing, sexual vitality and enhancement
Mechanism of Action/Effect: Precursor to nitric oxide; plays a key role in the urea cycle, which is the biochemical pathway that metabolized protein and other nitrogen-containing compounds
Warnings: Use caution in individuals with herpes simplex; may stimulate growth of virus.
Drug Interactions: Nitroglycerin and sildenafil
Dosing: Oral: 3-6 g/day

Bifidobacterium bifidum / Lactobacillus acidophilus

Use:
> *B. bifidum:* Treatment of Crohn's disease, diarrhea, ulcerative colitis; maintenance of anaerobic microflora in the colon
> *L. acidophilus:* Treatment of constipation, infant diarrhea, lactose intolerance; recolonization of the GI tract with beneficial bacteria during and after antibiotic use

Mechanism of Action/Effect: Natural components of colonic flora, used to facilitate recolonization with benign symbiotic organisms; promote vitamin K synthesis and absorption
Drug Interactions: Antibiotics eliminate *B. bifidum* and *L. acidophilus*
Adverse Reactions: No known toxicity or serious side effect
Dosing: Oral: 5-10 billion colony forming units (CFU) per day (dairy free); refrigerate to maintain optimum potency

Bilberry

Synonym: *Vaccinium myrtillus*
Use: Treatment of ophthalmologic disorders (eg, macular degeneration, diabetic retinopathy, cataracts) and vascular disorders (eg, varicose veins, phlebitis)
Mechanism of Action/Effect: Reportedly inhibits a variety of inflammatory mediators, including histamine, proteases, leukotrienes, and prostaglandins; may decrease capillary permeability and inhibit platelet aggregation
Contraindication: Active bleeding (eg, peptic ulcer, intracranial bleeding)
Warnings: Use with caution in individuals with a history of bleeding, hemostatic disorders, or drug-related hemostatic problems. Use with caution in individuals taking

HERBAL AND NUTRITIONAL PRODUCTS *(Continued)*

anticoagulants (eg, warfarin, aspirin, aspirin-containing products, NSAIDs) or anti-platelet agents (eg, ticlopidine, clopidogrel, dipyridamole). Discontinue use prior to dental or surgical procedures (generally at least 14 days before).

Drug Interactions: Oral hypoglycemics, anticoagulants, NSAIDs, aspirin, or insulin (effects may be altered)

Dosing: Oral: 80 mg 2-3 times/day

Black Cohosh

Synonym: *Cimicifuga racemosa*

Use: Treatment of vasomotor symptoms of menopause, premenstrual syndrome (PMS), mild depression, arthritis

Mechanism of Action/Effect: Contains multiple phytoestrogens and salicylic acid (small amounts)

Contraindications: Pregnancy (may stimulate uterine contractions) and lactation; history of estrogen-dependent tumors or endometrial cancer

Warnings: Use with caution in individuals allergic to salicylates (unknown whether the amount of salicylic acid is likely to affect platelet aggregation or have other effects associated with salicylates); those receiving hormone replacement therapy, taking oral contraceptives, or with a history of thromboembolic disease or stroke

Drug Interactions: Oral contraceptives, hormonal replacement therapy

Adverse Reactions: High doses: Nausea, vomiting, headache, hypotension

Dosing: Oral: 20-40 mg twice daily

Chamomile

Synonyms: *Matricaria chamomilla*; *Matricaria recutita*

Use: Topical anti-inflammatory with hypnotic properties; treatment of hemorrhoids, irritable bowel, eczema, mastitis and leg ulcers; cigarette tobacco flavoring

Mechanism of Action/Effect: Antispasmodic; anti-inflammatory; antiulcer; antibacterial and sedative effects also documented

Contraindications: Hypersensitivity to *Asteraceae/Compositae* family or ragweed pollens

Warnings: Use with caution in asthmatics; cross sensitivity may occur in individuals allergic to ragweed pollens, asters, or chrysanthemums.

Drug Interactions: May increase effect of coumarin-type anticoagulants at high doses; may potentiate sedatives (benzodiazepines, barbiturates)

Adverse Reactions: Contact dermatitis, emesis (from dried flowering heads), anaphylaxis, hypersensitivity reactions (especially in atopic individuals)

Dosing:

Tea: ±150 mL H_2O poured over heaping tablespoon (±3 g) of chamomile, covered and steeped 5-10 minutes; tea is used 3-4 times/day for GI upset

Liquid extract: 1-4 mL 3 times/day

Pregnancy Implications: Excessive use should be avoided due to potential teratogenicity.

Chasteberry

Synonyms: Chastetree; *Vitex agnus-castus*

Use: Treatment of acne vulgaris, corpus luteum insufficiency, hyperprolactinemia, insufficient lactation, menopause, menstrual disorders (eg, amenorrhea, endometriosis, premenstrual syndrome)

Mechanism of Action/Effect: Noted to possess significant effect on pituitary function; demonstrated to have progesterone-like effects (may stimulate luteinizing hormone [LH] and inhibit follicle-stimulating hormone [FSH]

Contraindications: Pregnancy and lactation (based on case reports of uterine stimulation and emmenagogue effects)

Warnings: Use with caution in individuals receiving hormonal therapy.

Drug Interactions: Hormonal replacement therapy, oral contraceptives, dopamine antagonists (eg, metoclopramide and antipsychotics)

Dosing: Oral: 400 mg/day in the morning (preferably on an empty stomach)

Chondroitin Sulfate

Use: Treatment of osteoarthritis

Mechanism of Action/Effect: Reported to act synergistically with glucosamine to support the maintenance of strong, healthy cartilage and maintain joint function; inhibits synovial enzymes (elastase, hyaluronidase) which may contribute to cartilage destruction and loss of joint function (studies inconclusive)

Adverse Reactions: No known toxicity or serious side effects.

Dosing: Oral: 300-1500 mg/day

Chromium

Use: Improves glycemic control; increases lean body mass; reduces obesity; improves lipid profile by decreasing total cholesterol and triglycerides, increasing HDL (dosages in excess of >300 mg/day reported to benefit breast cancer, diabetes, and cardiovascular diseases)

Mechanism of Action/Effect: Chromium picolinate is the only active form of chromium. It appears that chromium, in its trivalent form, increases insulin sensitivity and improves glucose transport into cells. The mechanism by which this happens could include one or more of the following: Increase the number of insulin receptors, enhance insulin binding to target tissues, promote activation of insulin-receptor tyrosine dinase activity, enhance beta-cell sensitivity in the pancreas.

Drug Interactions: Any medications that may also affect blood sugars (eg, beta-blockers, thiazides, oral hypoglycemics, and insulin); discuss chromium use prior to initiating

Adverse Reactions: Nausea, loose stools, flatulence, changes in appetite; isolated reports of anemia, cognitive impairment, renal failure

Dosing: 50-600 mcg/day

Coenzyme Q_{10}

Synonym: Ubiquinone

Use: Treatment of angina, chronic fatigue syndrome, CHF, hypertension, muscular dystrophy, obesity, Parkinson's disease, periodontal disease

Mechanism of Action/Effect: Functions as a lipid-soluble antioxidant, providing protection against free radical damage; involved in ATP generation, the primary source of energy in human physiology

Drug Interactions: Drugs which can cause depletion of CoQ_{10}: Hydralazine, thiazide diuretics, HMG-CoA reductase inhibitors, sulfonylureas, beta-blockers, tricyclic antidepressants, chlorpromazine, clonidine, methyldopa, diazoxide, biguanides, haloperidol; CoQ_{10} may decrease response to warfarin

Contraindications: Doxorubicin

Warnings: Controlled trials have not demonstrated benefit in heart failure.

Dosing: Oral: 30-200 mg/day

Cranberry

Synonym: *Vaccinium macrocarpon*

Use: Prevention of nephrolithiasis, prevention and treatment of urinary tract infection

Mechanism of Action/Effect: Although early research indicated that cranberry worked through urinary acidification, current research indicates that a cranberry-derived glycoprotein inhibits *E. coli* adherence to the epithelial cells of the urinary tract.

Dosing: Oral: 300-400 mg twice daily or 8-16 oz/day of 100% cranberry juice

Dehydroepiandosterone

Synonym: DHEA

Use: Treatment of depression, diabetes, fatigue, aging, lupus

Mechanism of Action/Effect: Precursor for the synthesis of over 50 hormones (including estrogen and testosterone); secreted by the adrenal glands, DHEA has been shown to stimulate production of insulin growth factor-1 (IGF-1) and change the response to insulin, decreasing the insulin requirement in individuals with diabetes. Supplementation may also increase circulating testosterone levels.

Contraindications: History of prostate or breast cancer

Warnings: Use with caution in individuals with hepatic dysfunction, diabetes, or those predisposed to hypoglycemia. Blood glucose should be closely monitored in diabetics and the dosage of antidiabetic agents should be closely monitored among health care providers.

Drug Interactions: May interact with androgens, estrogens, corticosteroids, insulin, oral hypoglycemic agents

Adverse Reactions: No known toxicity or serious side effects; long-term human studies have not been conducted

Dosing: Oral: 5-50 mg/day; 100 mg/day has been used in elderly individuals

Dong Quai

Synonyms: *Angelica sinensis*; Chinese angelica

Use: Treatment of anemia, hypertension, menopause, dysmenorrhea, PMS, amenorrhea; improves energy (particularly in females)

Mechanism of Action/Effect: Reported to cause vasodilation and may have hematopoietic properties; rich in phytoestrogens which may demonstrate similar pharmacological effects, but are less potent than pure estrogenic compounds

Contraindications: Active bleeding (eg, peptic ulcer, intracranial bleeding); may alter hemostasis, based on potential interference with platelet aggregation (observed with related species)

Warnings: Use with caution in individuals at risk of hypotension and those who would tolerate hypotension poorly (eg, cerebrovascular or cardiovascular disease); individuals taking antihypertensive medications, hormone replacement therapy, oral contraceptives, or with a history of estrogen-dependent tumors, endometrial cancer, thromboembolic disease, or stroke; individuals with a history of bleeding,

HERBAL AND NUTRITIONAL PRODUCTS *(Continued)*

hemostatic disorders, or drug-related hemostatic problems; those taking anticoagulants (may potentiate effects of warfarin) or antiplatelet agents (eg, ticlopidine, clopidogrel, dipyridamole); and in pregnant and lactating women. May cause photosensitization; avoid prolonged exposure to sunlight or other sources of ultraviolet radiation (ie, tanning booths). Discontinue use prior to dental or surgical procedures (generally at least 14 days before).

Drug Interactions: Antihypertensives, anticoagulants, antiplatelet drugs, hormonal replacement therapy, oral contraceptives, photosensitizing medications

Dosing: Oral: 200 mg twice daily

Echinacea

Synonyms: American Coneflower; Black Susans; Comb Flower; *Echinacea angustifolia*; Indian Head; Purple Coneflower; Scury Root; Snakeroot

Use: Treatment of cold and flu, upper respiratory tract infections, urinary tract infections

Mechanism of Action/Effect: Has antihyaluronidase and anti-inflammatory activity; caffeic acid glycosides and isolutylamides associated with the plant can cause immune stimulation (leukocyte phagocytosis and T-cell activation)

Contraindications: Allergy to sunflowers, daisies, ragweed; autoimmune diseases (eg, collagen vascular disease [lupus, RA], HIV/AIDS), multiple sclerosis, tuberculosis, pregnancy; per Commission E: Parenteral administration is contraindicated, but oral use is not contraindicated during pregnancy

Warnings: May alter immunosuppression; long-term use may cause immunosuppression. Persons allergic to sunflowers may display cross-allergy potential. Use as a preventative treatment should be discouraged.

Drug Interactions: May alter response to immunosuppressive therapy

Adverse Reactions: Tingling sensation of tongue, allergic reactions (rare); may become immunosuppressive with continuous use over 6-8 weeks
Per Commission E: None known for oral and external use

Dosing: Continuous use should not exceed 8 weeks
Capsule: 500 mg 3 times/day on day 1, then 250 mg 4 times/day, standardized to contain 4% echinacosides *(E. angustifolia)* or 4% sesquiterpene esters *(E. purpurea)* per dose
Plant juice: Freshly expressed *(E. purpurea)*: 60 drops 3 times/day with food for 1 day, then 40 drops 3 times/day with food for up to 10 days, standardized to contain not less than 2.4% soluble beta-1,2 D-5 fructofuranosides per dose
Topical: Apply to affected area as needed

Evening Primrose

Synonyms: Evening Primrose Oil; *Oenothera biennis*

Use: Treatment of diabetic neuropathy, endometriosis, hyperglycemia, irritable bowel syndrome, multiple sclerosis, omega-6-fatty acid supplementation, PMS, menopause, rheumatoid arthritis

Mechanism of Action/Effect: Contains high amounts of gamma-linolenic acid, or GLA, an essential omega-6 fatty acid which reportedly reduces generation of arachidonic acid metabolites in short-term use, improving symptoms of various inflammatory and immune conditions; reported to stimulate hormone synthesis

Contraindications: Seizure disorders (may lower seizure threshold, based on animal studies), schizophrenia, active bleeding (may inhibit platelet aggregation), individuals receiving anticonvulsant or antipsychotic medications

Warnings: Use with caution in individuals with a history of bleeding, hemostatic disorders, or drug-related hemostatic problems; individuals taking anticoagulants (eg, warfarin, aspirin, aspirin-containing products, NSAIDs) or antiplatelet agents (eg, ticlopidine, clopidogrel, dipyridamole). Discontinue use prior to dental or surgical procedures (generally at least 14 days before).

Drug Interactions: Anticonvulsants (seizure threshold decreased), anticoagulants, antiplatelet agents

Dosing: Oral: 500 mg to 8 g/day

Feverfew

Synonyms: Altamisa; Bachelor's Buttons; Featherfew; Featherfoil; Nosebleed; *Tanacetum parthenium*; Wild Quinine

Use: Prophylaxis and treatment of migraine headaches; treatment of menstrual complaints and fever

Mechanism of Action/Effect: Active ingredient is parthenolide (~0.2% concentration), which is a serotonin antagonist; also, the plant may be an inhibitor of prostaglandin synthesis and platelet aggregation; may have spasmolytic activity

Contraindications: Pregnancy and lactation; children <2 years of age; allergies to feverfew and other members of Asteraceae, daisy, ragweed, chamomile

Warning: Use with caution in patients taking medications with serotonergic properties.

Drug Interactions: Anticoagulants (eg, aspirin, aspirin-containing products, NSAIDs)

Adverse Reactions: Mouth ulcerations, contact dermatitis, abdominal pain, nausea, vomiting, loss of taste; postfeverfew syndrome on discontinuation (nervousness, insomnia, still joints, headache)

Dosing: 125 mg 1-2 times/day

Garlic

Synonyms: *Allium savitum*; Comphor of the Poor; Nectar of the Gods; Poor Mans Treacle; Rustic Treacle; Stinking Rose

Use: Treatment of hypertension; lowers LDL cholesterol and triglycerides and raises HDL cholesterol; may lower blood glucose and decrease thrombosis; potential anti-inflammatory and antitumor effects

Mechanism of Action/Effect: Allinin garlic is converted to allicin (after the bulb is ground), which is odoriferous and may have some antioxidant activity; ajoene (a byproduct of allicin) has potent platelet inhibition effects; garlic can also decrease LDL cholesterol levels and increase fibrinolytic activity. The LDL benefit of garlic is modest.

Contraindication: Pregnancy

Warnings: Onset of cholesterol-lowering and hypotensive effects may require months. Use with caution in patients receiving treatment for hyperglycemia or hypertension.

Drug Interactions: Iodine uptake may be reduced with garlic ingestion; can exacerbate bleeding in patients taking aspirin or anticoagulant agents; may increase the risk of hypoglycemia; may increase response to antihypertensives

Adverse Reactions: Skin blistering, eczema, systemic contact dermatitis, immunologic contact urticaria, GI upset and changes in intestinal flora (rare) per Commission E, lacrimation, asthma (upon inhalation of garlic dust), allergic reactions (rare), change in odor of skin and breath (per Commission E)

Half-Life Elimination: N-acetyl-S-allyl-L-cysteine: 6 hours

Excretion: Pulmonary and renal

Dosing: Adults: 4-12 mg allicin/day

> Average daily dose for cardiovascular benefit: 0.25-1 g/kg or 1-4 cloves daily in an 80 kg individual in divided doses

> Toxic dose: >5 cloves or >25 mL of extract can cause GI symptoms

Additional Information: 1% as active as penicillin as an antibiotic; number one over-the-counter medication in Germany; enteric-coated products may demonstrate best results.

Ginger

Synonym: *Zingiber officinale*

Pregnancy Risk Factor: Per Commission E, not to be used for morning sickness during pregnancy (some contradictory recommendations exist); high doses may be abortifacient

Use: Antiemetic; digestive aid; treatment of nausea and motion sickness, headaches, colds and flu, osteoarthritis; flavoring agent in beverages and mouthwashes

Mechanism of Action/Effect: Unknown; appears to decrease prostaglandin synthesismay increase GI motility; may have cardiotonic activity and inhibit platelet aggregation (very high doses)

Contraindication: Gallstones (per Commission E)

Warnings: Use with caution in diabetics, patients on cardiac glycosides, and those receiving anticoagulants.

Drug Interactions: May alter response to cardiotonic, hypoglycemic, anticoagulant, and antiplatelet agents

Dosing:

> Prevention of motion sickness or digestive aid: 1-4 g/day (250 mg of ginger root powder 3-4 times/day)

> Per Commission E: 2-4 g/day or equivalent preparations

HERBAL AND NUTRITIONAL PRODUCTS *(Continued)*

Ginkgo Biloba

Synonyms: Kew Tree; Maidenhair Tree

Use: Treatment of tinnitus, visual disorders, traumatic brain injury, vertigo of vascular origin

Europe: Treatment of intermittent claudication, arterial insufficiency, and cerebral vascular disease (dementia)

Per Commission E: Demential syndromes including memory deficits, etc (tinnitus, headache); depressive emotional conditions, primary degenerative dementia, vascular dementia, or both

Mechanism of Action/Effect: Dilates blood vessels and inhibits platelet aggregation; leaf extract contain terpenoids and flavonoids which can allegedly inactivate oxygen-free radicals causing vasodilatation and antagonize effects of platelet activating factor (PAF); fruit pulp contains ginkolic acids which are allergens (seeds are not sensitizing)

Contraindications: Pregnancy, clotting disorders, hypersensitivity to ginkgo biloba preparations (per Commission E)

Warnings: Use with caution following recent surgery or trauma. Effects may require 1-2 months. Controlled studies have not demonstrated consistent efficacy in dementia.

Drug Interactions: Due to effects on PAF, use with caution in patients receiving anticoagulants or platelet inhibitors.

Adverse Reactions: Palpitations, bilateral subdural hematomas, dizziness, seizures (in children), restlessness, urticaria, cheilitis, nausea, diarrhea, vomiting, stomatitis, proctitis, stomach or intestinal upsets, hyphema

Rare (per Commission E): Headache, allergic skin reactions, stomach or GI upset

Onset of Effect: 1 hour

Peak Absorption: 2-3 hours

Duration of Action: 7 hours

Bioavailability: 70% to 100%

Half-life: Ginkgolide A: 4 hours; ginkgolide B: 10.6 hours; bilobalide: 3.2 hours

Dosing: ~40 mg 3 times/day with meals; 60-80 mg twice daily to 3 times/day (depending on indication); maximum dose: 360 mg/day

Cerebral ischemia: 120 mg/day in 2-3 divided doses (24% flavonoid-glycoside extract, 6% terpene glycosides); beneficial effects for cerebral ischemia in the elderly occur after 1 month of use

Ginseng, Panax

Synonyms: Asian Ginseng; *Panax ginseng*

Use: Adrenal tonic; immunosupportive; enhances physical/mental performance and energy levels; adjunct support for chemotherapy/radiation

Mechanism of Action/Effect: Ginsenosides are believed to act via hormone receptors in the hypothalamus, pituitary glands, and other tissues. Ginsenosides stimulate secretion of adrenocorticotropic hormone (ACTH), leading to production of increased release of adrenal hormones, including cortisol. Specific triterpenoid saponins (diols) are claimed to be mediate improvements in endurance and learning. These compounds are also believed to contribute to sedative and antihypertensive properties. A second group (triols) reportedly increase blood pressure and function as central nervous system stimulants. *Panax ginseng* is reported to have immunostimulating effects. *Panax ginseng* has been claimed to facilitate adaptation to stress caused by chemotherapy and radiation.

Contraindications: Renal failure, acute infection, active bleeding (may alter hemostasis), pregnancy and lactation

Adverse Reactions: Mastalgia, vaginal breakthrough bleeding **Note:** Prolonged use or high dosages may cause Ginseng Abuse Syndrome (diarrhea, hypertension, nervousness, dermatologic eruptions, insomnia) and/or palpitations and tachycardia in sensitive individuals

Warnings: Use with caution in individuals with hyper- or hypotension; those with a history of bleeding, hemostatic disorders, or drug-related hemostatic problems; those receiving MAO inhibitors or stimulants (eg, decongestants, caffeine). Discontinue use prior to dental or surgical procedures (generally at least 14 days before).

Drug Interactions: Antihypertensives, MAO inhibitors, central nervous stimulants (caffeine), sympathomimetics, and hormonal therapies; anticoagulant medications, including warfarin, aspirin, aspirin-containing products, NSAIDs, or antiplatelet agents (eg, ticlopidine, clopidogrel, dipyridamole).

Dosing: Oral: 100-600 mg/day in divided doses

Ginseng, Siberian

Synonyms: *Eleutherococcus senticosus*; Siberian Ginseng

Use: Believed to facilitate adaptation to stress and to act as an immune stimulant.; reported to enhance athletic performance and physical endurance, increase mental alertness and amount of quality work performed, and decrease sick days

Contraindication: Active bleeding; hemostasis may be affected

Warnings: Use with caution in individuals with hypertension or those receiving antihypertensive medications (may potentiate effects); individuals at risk of hypotension, elderly , or those who would not tolerate transient hyper- or hypotensive episodes (ie, cerebrovascular or cardiovascular disease); diabetics; those with a history of bleeding, hemostatic disorders, or drug-related hemostatic problems. Discontinue use prior to dental or surgical procedures (generally at least 14 days before). Extensive or prolonged use may heighten estrogenic activity (based on pharmacological activity).

Drug Interactions: Barbiturates, antihypertensives, insulin, oral hypoglycemics, digoxin, stimulants (including OTC); anticoagulants (eg, warfarin, aspirin, aspirin-containing products, NSAIDs) or antiplatelet agents (eg, ticlopidine, clopidogrel, dipyridamole)

Dosing: Oral: 100-200 mg twice daily

Glucosamine

Use: Treatment of osteoarthritis, rheumatoid arthritis, tendonitis, gout, bursitis

Mechanism of Action/Effect: An amino sugar, which is a key component in the synthesis of proteoglycans, a group of proteins found in cartilage which are negatively charged, and attract water so they can produce synovial fluid in the joints; the theory is that supplying the body with these precursors will replenish important synovial fluid, and lead to production of new cartilage. Glucosamine also appears to inhibit cartilage-destroying enzymes (eg, collagenase and phospholipase A2), thus stopping the degenerative processes of osteoarthritis. A third mechanism may be glucosamine's ability to prevent production of damaging superoxide radicals, which may lead to cartilage destruction.

Adverse Reactions: Flatulence, nausea

Warnings: Use caution in patients with diabetes; may cause insulin resistance

Drug Interactions: May increase effect of oral anticoagulants and alter response to insulin or oral hypoglycemics

Dosing: 500 mg 3-4 times/day (sulfate form)

Golden Seal

Synonyms: Eye Balm; Eye Root; *Hydrastis canadensis*; Indian Eye; Jaundice Root; Orange Root; Turmeric Root; Yellow Indian Paint; Yellow Root

Use: Treatment of hemorrhoids, postpartum hemorrhage, mucosal inflammation/gastritis (efficacy not established in clinical studies); produces GI and peripheral vascular activity; used in sterile eyewashes; used as a mouthwash and laxative

Mechanism of Action/Effect: Contains the alkaloids hydrastine (4%) and berberine (6%), which at higher doses can cause vasoconstriction, hypertension, and mucosal irritation. Berberine can produce hypotension.

Contraindications: Pregnancy and lactation

Warnings: Should not be used in patients with hypertension, glaucoma, diabetes, history of stroke, seizures, or heart disease.

Drug Interaction: May interfere with vitamin B absorption

Adverse Reactions: High doses: Stimulation/agitation, nausea, vomiting, diarrhea, mouth and throat irritation, extremity numbness, respiratory failure

Dosing:
Root: 0.5-1 g 3 times/day
Solid form: Usual dose: 5-10 grains

Green Tea

Synonym: *Camellia sinensis*

Use: Platelet-aggregation inhibitor; antioxidant with anticarcinogenic activity; supportive in cancer prevention and cardiovascular disease; may lower cholesterol

Mechanism of Action/Effect: Reportedly has antioxidant properties and protects against oxidative damage to cells and tissues. Demonstrated to increase HDL cholesterol, decrease LDL cholesterol, and decrease triglycerides. Green tea has also been reported to block the peroxidation of LDL, inhibit formation of thromboxane formation, and block platelet aggregation. Human studies have noted a correlation between consumption of green tea and improvement in prognosis in some forms of breast cancer.

Contraindications: Active bleeding (eg, peptic ulcer, intracerebral bleeding)

Warnings: Nondecaffeinated products should be used with caution in individuals with peptic ulcer disease or cardiovascular disease. Use with caution in individuals with a history of bleeding, hemostatic disorders, or drug-related hemostatic problems; those receiving anticoagulants (reported to antagonize the effects of warfarin) or antiplatelet agents (eg, ticlopidine, clopidogrel, dipyridamole). Discontinue use prior to dental or surgical procedures (generally at least 14 days before). Use with caution when taking other stimulants (caffeine, decongestants), unless a caffeine-free product is used. **Note:** Addition of milk to tea may significantly lower the antioxidant potential of this agent.

Drug Interactions: Anticoagulants (eg, warfarin, aspirin, aspirin-containing products, NSAIDs), antiplatelet agents (eg, ticlopidine, clopidogrel, dipyridamole), stimulants (including OTC decongestants)

HERBAL AND NUTRITIONAL PRODUCTS *(Continued)*

Adverse Reactions: If product is not decaffeinated, caffeine may cause gastric irritation, decreased appetite, insomnia, tachycardia, palpitations, and nervousness in sensitive individuals.
Dosing: Oral: 250-500 mg/day

Hawthorn

Synonyms: *Crataegus laevigata; Crataegus monogyna; Crataegus oxyacantha; Crataegus pinnatifida*; English Hawthorn; Haw; Maybush; Whitehorn
Use: Sedative; treatment of cardiovascular abnormalities (eg, arrhythmia, angina), increased cardiac output, increased contractility of heart muscle
Mechanism of Action/Effect: Contains flavonoids, catechin, and epicatechin which may be cardioprotective and have vasodilatory properties; shown to dilate coronary vessels
Contraindications: Pregnancy and lactation
Drug Interactions: Antihypertensives (effect enhanced), ACE inhibitors, digoxin; effects with Viagra® are unknown
Adverse Reactions: Hypotension, bradycardia, hypertension, depression, fatigue, rash, nausea
Dosing: Daily dose of total flavonoids: 10 mg
Per Commission E: 160-900 mg native water-ethanol extract (ethanol 45% v/v or methanol 70% v/v, drug-extract ratio: 4-7:1, with defined flavonoid or procyanidin content), corresponding to 30-168.7 mg procyanidins, calculated as epicatechin, or 3.5-19.8 mg flavonoids, calculated as hyperoside in accordance with DAB 10 (German pharmacopoeia #10) in 2 or 3 individual doses; duration of administration: 6 weeks minimum

Horse Chestnut

Synonym: *Aesculus hippocastanum*
Use: Treatment of varicose veins, hemorrhoids, other venous insufficiencies, deep venous thrombosis, lower extremity edema
Mechanism of Action/Effect: Reportedly functions as an anti-inflammatory, which may be related to quercetin's reported ability to inhibit cyclo-oxygenase and lipoxygenase, the enzymes which form inflammatory prostaglandins and leukotrienes; quercetin is also an inhibitor of phosphodiesterase, which has been correlated to cardiotonic, hypotensive, spasmolytic, antiplatelet, and sedative actions; inhibits platelet aggregation and supports collagen structures
Contraindications: Active bleeding (eg, peptic ulcer, intracranial bleeding)
Warnings: Use with caution in individuals with hepatic or renal impairment, a history of bleeding, hemostatic disorders, or drug-related hemostatic problems. Discontinue use prior to dental or surgical procedures (generally at least 14 days before).
Drug Interactions: Anticoagulants (eg, warfarin, aspirin, aspirin-containing products, NSAIDs) and antiplatelet agents (eg, ticlopidine, clopidogrel, dipyridamole)
Adverse Reaction: GI upset
Dosing:
Oral: 300 mg 1-2 times/day, standardized to 50 mg escin per dose
Topical: Apply 2% escin gel 1-2 times/day to affected area

Kava

Synonyms: Awa; Kew; *Piper methysticum*; Tonga; Kava kava
Use: Treatment of anxiety, stress, and restlessness (per Commission E); sleep inducement
Mechanism of Action/Effect: Contains alpha-pyrones in root extracts; may possess central dopaminergic antagonistic properties
Contraindications: Per Commission E: Pregnancy, endogenous depression
Warnings: Extended continuous intake can cause a temporary yellow discoloration of skin, hair, and nails. In this case, further application must be discontinued. In rare cases, allergic skin reactions occur. Also, accommodative disturbances (eg, enlargement of the pupils and disturbances of the oculomotor equilibrium) have been described.
Drug Interactions: Coma can occur from concomitant administration of alprazolam; may potentiate alcohol or CNS depressants, barbiturates, psychopharmacological agents
Adverse Reactions: Euphoria, depression, somnolence, skin discoloration (prolonged use), muscle weakness, eye disturbances, hepatotoxicity
Dosing: Per Commission E: Do not use for >3 months without medical advice. Herb and preparations equivalent to 60-120 mg kavalactones

Melaleuca Oil

Use: Dermal agent for burns; marketed as fungicidal, bactericidal
Mechanism of Action/Effect: Consists of plant terpenes, pinenes, and cineole, derived from the *Melaleuca alternifolia* tree, the colorless or pale yellow oil can cause CNS depression; may be bacteriostatic

Adverse Reactions: Allergic reactions or dermatitis (rare)
Dosing: Topical: Minimal toxic dose: Infant: <10 mL

Melatonin

Use: Treatment of sleep disorders (eg, jet lag, insomnia, neurologic problems, shift work), aging, cancer, immune system support
Mechanism of Action/Effect: Hormone responsible for regulating the body's circadian rhythm and sleep patterns; release is prompted by darkness and inhibited by light. Secretion appears to peak during childhood, and declines gradually through adolescence and adulthood. Melatonin receptors have been found in blood cells, the brain, gut, and ovaries; may also have a role in regulating cardiovascular and reproductive function through its antioxidant properties.
Contraindications: Immune disorders; pregnancy and lactation
Warnings: Avoid prolonged use. Persistent sleep difficulties may be a sign of medical illness.
Drug Interactions: Medications commonly used as sedatives or hypnotics, or those that induce sedation, drowsiness (eg, benzodiazepines, narcotics); CNS depressants (prescription, supplements such as 5-HTP); other herbs known to cause sedation include kava, valerian
Adverse Reactions: Reduced alertness, headache, irritability, increased fatigue, drowsiness, sedation
Dosing: Sleep disturbances: 0.3-5 mg/day

Red Yeast Rice

Synonym: *Monascus purpureus*
Use: Hypercholesterolemic agent; may lower triglycerides and LDL cholesterol and raise HDL cholesterol
Mechanism of Action/Effect: Eight compounds with HMG-CoA reductase inhibitory activity have been identified, including lovastatin and its active hydroxy acid metabolite.
Contraindications: Pregnancy, or if trying to become pregnant, and lactation (based on pharmacological activity); known hypersensitivity to rice or yeast; children and adults <20 years of age; hepatic disease, history of liver disease, or those who may be at risk of liver disease; serious infection, recent major surgery, other serious disease, or organ transplant individuals; any individual who consumes more than 1-2 alcohol-containing drinks per day
Warnings: Use with caution in individuals currently receiving other cholesterol-lowering medications. HMG-CoA reductase inhibitors have been associated with rare (less than 1% to 2% incidence) but serious adverse effects, including hepatic and skeletal muscle disorders (myopathy, rhabdomyolysis). The risk of these disorders may be increased by concomitant therapy with specific medications. Discontinue use at the first sign of hepatic dysfunction.
Drug Interactions: HMG-CoA reductase inhibitors, other cholesterol-lowering agents, anticoagulants, gemfibrozil, erythromycin, itraconazole, ketoconazole, cyclosporine, niacin, clofibrate, fenofibrate
Adverse Reaction: GI upset
Dosing: Oral: 1200 mg twice daily

SAMe

Synonym: S-Adenosylmethionine
Use: Treatment of depression
Mechanism of Action/Effect: Not defined; functions as a cofactor in many synthetic pathways
Contraindication: Active bleeding (eg, peptic ulcer, intracranial bleeding)
Warnings: Use caution when combining with other antidepressants, tryptophan, or 5-HTP. SAMe is not effective in the treatment of depressive symptoms associated with bipolar disorder.
Drug Interactions: May potentiate activity and/or toxicities of MAO inhibitors, tricyclic antidepressants, or SSRIs; may potentiate the antidepressant effects of 5-HTP, tryptophan, and St John's wort
Adverse Reactions: Dry mouth, nausea, restlessness
Dosing: Oral: 400-1600 mg/day

Sassafras Oil

Synonym: *Sassafras albidum*
Use: Mild counterirritant on the skin (ie, lice or insect bites)
Mechanism of Action/Effect: Contains safrole (up to 80%) which inhibits liver microsomal enzymes; its metabolite may cause hepatic tumors
Adverse Reactions: Primarily related to sassafras oil and safrole: Tachycardia, flushing, hypotension, sinus tachycardia, anxiety, hallucinations, vertigo, aphasia, contact dermatitis, vomiting, fatty changes of liver, hepatic necrosis, mydriasis, diaphoresis; little documentation of adverse effects due to ingestion of herbal tea
Absorption: Orally
Metabolism: Hepatic

HERBAL AND NUTRITIONAL PRODUCTS *(Continued)*

Excretion: Renal primarily
Warnings: Considered unsafe by the FDA; should not be ingested (banned in food by FDA since 1960)
Dosing: Tea can contain as much as 200 mg (3 mg/kg) of safrole.
Toxic: 0.66 mg/kg (based on rodent studies); Lethal: ~5 mL

Saw Palmetto

Synonyms: Palmetto Scrub; *Sabal serrulata; Sabasilis serrulatae; Serenoa repens*
Use: Treatment of benign prostatic hyperplasia
Mechanism of Action/Effect: Liposterolic extract of the berries may inhibit the enzymes 5α-reductase, along with cyclo-oxygenase and 5-lipoxygenase, thus exhibiting antiandrogen and anti-inflammatory effects; does not reduce prostatic enlargement but may help increase urinary flow (not FDA approved)
Contraindications: Pregnancy and lactation
Adverse Reactions: Headache, gynecomastia, stomach problems (rare, per Commission E)
Absorption: Oral: Low
Dosing: Adults: Dried fruit: 0.5-1 g 3 times/day

Schisandra

Synonym: *Schizandra chinensis*
Use: Promoted as an adaptogen/health tonic; hepatic protection and detoxification; increased endurance, stamina, and work performance
Mechanism of Action/Effect: Stimulates hepatic glycogen synthesis, protein synthesis, and increases microsomal enzyme activity; functions as an antioxidant
Contraindication: Pregnancy (based on uterine stimulation in animal studies)
Drug Interactions: Cytochrome P450 enzyme induction may alter the metabolism of many drugs (calcium channel blockers noted to be decreased)
Dosing: Oral: 100 mg twice daily

Soy Isoflavones

Synonym: Isoflavones
Use: Treatment of decreased bone loss, hypercholesterolemia, menopausal symptoms
Mechanism of Action/Effect: Contains plant-derived estrogenic compounds, however, the estrogenic potency has been estimated to be only 1/1000 to 1/100,000 that of estradiol; reported to inhibit bone reabsorption in postmenopausal women and lower serum lipids, including LDL cholesterol and triglycerides, along with increases in HDL cholesterol
Contraindication: History of estrogenic tumors (endometrial or breast cancer)
Warnings: May alter response to hormonal therapy; use with caution in individuals with history of thromboembolism or stroke
Drug Interactions: Weak estrogenic effect; may interact with estrogen-containing medications (close monitoring is recommended)
Dosing: Oral: 500-1000 mg/day soy extract

St John's Wort

Synonyms: Amber Touch-and-Feel; Goatweed; *Hypercium perforatum*; Klamath Weed; Rosin Rose
Use: Treatment of mild-moderate depression, stress, anxiety, insomnia, vitiligo (topical); popular drug for AIDS patients due to possible antiretroviral activity; topically for wound healing
Per Commission E: Psychovegetative disorders, depressive moods, anxiety and/ or nervous unrest; oily preparations for dyspeptic complaints; oily preparations externally for treatment of post-therapy of acute and contused injuries, myalgia, first degree burns
Mechanism of Action/Effect: Active ingredients are xanthones, flavonoids (hypericin) which can act as monoamine oxidase inhibitors, although *in vitro* activity is minimal; majority of activity appears to be related to GABA modulation; may be related to dopamine, serotonin, norepinephrine modulation also
Contraindications: Endogenous depression, pregnancy, children <2 years of age; concurrent use of indinavir or therapeutic immunosuppressants (cyclosporine)
Warnings: May be photosensitizing; use caution with tyramine-containing foods; appears to induce hepatic cytochrome P450 3A3/4 enzymes, potentially reducing effect of many medications.
Drug Interactions: Avoid amphetamines or other stimulants and concurrent use with SSRI or other antidepressants. Use caution with MAO inhibitors, levodopa, 5-hydroxytryptophan, and drugs metabolized by CYP3A3/4. Treatment failure with HIV medications and immunosuppressants has been associated with use.
Adverse Reactions: Sinus tachycardia, photosensitization (especially in fair-skinned person, per Commission E), stomach pains, abdominal pain
Dosing: Based on hypericin extract content: Oral: 300 mg 3 times/day

Valerian

Synonyms: Radix; Red Valerian; *Valeriana edulis; Valeriana wallichi*

Use: Sleep-promoting agent and minor tranquilizer; treatment of anxiety, panic attacks, intestinal cramps, headache

Per Commission E: Restlessness, sleep disorders based on nervous conditions

Mechanism of Action/Effect: May affect neurotransmitter levels (serotonin, GABA, and norepinephrine); also has antispasmodic properties

Drug Interactions: Not synergistic with alcohol; potentiation of other CNS depressants is possible

Adverse Reactions: Cardiac disturbances (unspecified), lightheadedness, restlessness, fatigue, nausea, tremor, blurred vision

Dosing:

Sedative: 1-3 g (1-3 mL of tincture)

Sleep aid: 1-3 mL of tincture at bedtime

Dried root: 0.3-1 g

Vanadium

Use: Treatment of type 1 and type 2 diabetes

Mechanism of Action/Effect: Reported to be a cofactor in nicotinamide adenine dinucleotide phosphate (NADPH) oxidation reactions, lipoprotein lipase activity, amino acid transport, and hematopoiesis; may improve/augment glucose regulation

Warning: Use with caution in diabetics or in those predisposed to hypoglycemia; may alter glucose regulation. Effects of drugs with hypoglycemic activity may be potentiated (including insulin and oral hypoglycemics). Closely monitor blood sugar, dosage of these agents (including insulin) may require adjustment. This should be carefully coordinated among the individual's healthcare providers.

Drug Interactions: Oral hypoglycemics or insulin

Adverse Reactions: No dietary toxicity or serious side effects reported, however industrial exposure has resulted in toxicity.

Dosing: Oral: RDI: 250 mcg 1-3 times/day

HERBAL AND NUTRITIONAL PRODUCTS *(Continued)*

HERBS AND COMMON NATURAL AGENTS

The authors have chosen to include this list of natural products and proposed medical claims. However, due to limited scientific investigation to support these claims, this list is not intended to imply that these claims have been scientifically proven.

Proposed Medicinal Claims

Herb	Medicinal Claim
Agrimony	Digestive disorders
Alfalfa	Source of carotene (vitamin A); contains natural fluoride
Allspice	General health
Aloe	Healing agent
Anise (seed)	Prevent gas
Astragalus	Enhance energy reserves; immune system modulation; adaptogen
Barberry (bark)	Treat halitosis
Bayberry (bark)	Relieve and prevent varicose veins
Bay (leaf)	Relieves cramps
Bee pollen	Renewal of enzymes, hormones, vitamins, amino acids, and others
Bergamot	Calming effect
Bilberry (leaf)	Increases night vision; reduces eye fatigue; antioxidant; circulation
Birch (bark)	Treat urinary problems; used for rheumatism
Blackberry (leaf)	Treat diarrhea
Black cohosh	Relieves menstrual cramps; phytoestrogen
Blueberry (leaf)	Diarrhea
Blue cohosh	Regulate menstrual flow
Blue flag	Treatment of skin diseases and constipation
Boldo (leaf)	Stimulates digestion; treatment of gallstones
Boneset	Treatment of colds and flu
Bromelain	Digestive enzyme
Buchu (leaf)	Diuretic
Buckthorn (bark)	Expels worms; laxative
Burdock (leaf and root)	Treatment of severe skin problems; cases of arthritis
Butternut (bark)	Works well for constipation
Calendula (flower)	Mending and healing of cuts or wounds topically
Capsicum (cayenne)	Normalizes blood pressure; circulation
Caraway (seed)	Aids digestion
Cascara sagrada (bark)	Remedies for chronic constipation
Catnip	Calming effect in children
Celery (leaf and seed)	Blood pressure; diuretic
Centaury	Stimulates the salivary gland
Chamomile (flower)	Excellent for a nervous stomach; relieves cramping associated with the menstrual cycle
Chickweed	Rich in vitamin C and minerals (calcium, magnesium, and potassium); diuretic; thyroid stimulant
Chicory (root)	Effective in disorders of the kidneys, liver, and urinary canal
Cinnamon (bark)	Prevents infection and indigestion; helps break down fats during digestion
Cleavers	Treatment of kidney and bladder disorders; useful in obstructions of the urinary organ
Cloves	General medicinal
Coriander (seed)	Stomach tonic
Cornsilk	Diuretic
Cranberry	Urinary tract health
Cubeb (berry)	Chronic bladder trouble; increases flow of urine
Damiana (leaf)	Sexual impotency
Dandelion (leaf)	Diuretic

Proposed Medicinal Claims *(continued)*

Herb	Medicinal Claim
Dandelion (root)	Detoxify poisons in the liver; beneficial in lowering blood pressure
Dill weed	Digestive health
Dong quai (root)	Female troubles; menopause and PMS symptoms; anemia; blood pressure
Echinacea (root)	Treat strep throat, lymph glands; immune modulating
Eucalyptus (leaf)	Mucolytic
Elder	Antiviral
Elecampane (root)	Cough with mucus
Eyebright	Eyesight
Fennel (seed)	Remedies for gas and acid stomach
Fenugreek (seed)	Allergies, coughs, digestion, emphysema, headaches, migraines, intestinal inflammation, ulcers, lungs, mucous membranes, and sore throat
Feverfew	Migraines; helps reduce inflammation in arthritis joints
Garlic (bulb)	Lowers blood cholesterol; anti-infective
Gentian	Digestive health
Ginger (root)	Antiemetic
Ginkgo biloba	Improves blood circulation to the brain; asthma; vertigo; tinnitus; impotence
Ginseng, Siberian (root)	Resistance against stress; slows the aging process; adaptogen
Goldenseal	Treatment of bladder infections, cankers, mouth sores, mucous membranes, and ulcers
Gota kola	"Memory herb"; nerve tonic; wound healing
Gravelroot (queen of the meadow)	Remedy for stones in the kidney and bladder
Green barley	Antioxidant
Hawthorn	Antioxidant; cardiotonic
Henna	External use only
Hibiscus (flower)	Diuretic
Hops (flower)	Insomnia; used to decrease the desire for alcohol
Horehound	Acute or chronic sore throat and coughs
Horsetail (shavegrass)	Rich in minerals, especially silica; used to develop strong fingernails and hair, good for split ends; diuretic
Ho shou wu	Rejuvenator
Hydrangea (root)	Backaches
Juniper (berry)	Diuretic
Kava (root)	Calm nervousness; anxiety; pain
Kelp	High contents of natural plant iodine, for proper function of the thyroid; high levels of natural calcium, potassium, and magnesium
Lavender (oil)	Wound healing; decrease scarring (topical)
Lecithin	Break up cholesterol; prevent arteriosclerosis
Licorice (root)	Expectorant; used in peptic ulceration; adrenal exhaustion
Malva (flower)	Soothes inflammation in the mouth and throat; helpful for earaches
Marjoram	Beneficial for a sour stomach or loss of appetite
Marshmallow (leaf)	Demulcent
Milk thistle	Liver detoxifier; antioxidant
Motherwort	Nervousness
Mugwort	Used for rheumatism and gout
Mullein (leaf)	High in iron, magnesium, and potassium; sinuses; relieves swollen joints; soothing bronchial tissue
Mustard (seed)	General medicinal
Myrrh (gum)	Removes bad breath; sinus problems
Nettle (leaf)	Remedy for dandruff; antihistaminic qualities
Nettle (root)	Used in benign prostatic hyperplasia (BPH)

HERBAL AND NUTRITIONAL PRODUCTS *(Continued)*

Proposed Medicinal Claims *(continued)*

Herb	Medicinal Claim
Nutmeg	Gas
Oregano (leaf)	Settles the stomach after meals; helps treat colds
Oregon grape (root)	Gallbladder problems
Papaya (leaf)	Digestive stimulant; contains the enzyme papain
Paprika (sweet)	Stimulates the appetite and gastric secretions
Passion (flower)	Mild sedative
Pau d'arco	Protects immune system; antifungal
Peppermint (leaf)	Excellent for headaches; digestive stimulation
Pleurisy (root)	Mucolytic
Poppy seed blue	Excellent in the making of breads and desserts
Prickly ash (bark)	Increases circulation
Psyllium (seed)	Lubricant to the intestinal tract
Red clover	Phytoestrogenic properties
Red raspberry (leaf)	Decreases menstrual bleeding
Rhubarb (root)	Powerful laxative
Rose hips	High content of vitamin C
Saw palmetto (berry)	Used in benign prostatic hyperplasia (BPH)
Scullcap	Nerve sedative
Seawrack (bladderwrack)	Combat obesity; contains iodine
Senna (leaf)	Laxative
Shepherd's purse	Female reproductive health
Sheep sorrel	Diuretic
Slippery elm (bark)	Normalize bowel movement; beneficial for hemorrhoids and constipation
Solomon's seal (root)	Poultice for bruises
Spikenard	Skin ailments such as acne, pimples, blackheads, rashes, and general skin problems
Star anise	Promotes appetite and relieves flatulence
St John's wort	Mild to moderate depression
Summer savory (leaf)	Treats diarrhea, upset stomach, and sore throat
Thyme (leaf)	Ulcers (peptic)
Uva-ursi (leaf)	Diuretic; used in urinary tract health
Valerian (root)	Promotes sleep
Vervain	Remedy for fevers
White oak (bark)	Strong astringent
White willow (bark)	Used for minor aches and pains in the body; aspirin content
Wild alum (root)	Powerful astringent; used as rinse for sores in mouth and bleeding gums
Wild cherry	Cough suppressant
Wild Oregon grape (root)	Chronic skin disease
Wild yam (root)	Used in female reproductive health
Wintergreen (leaf)	Valuable for colic and gas in the bowels
Witch hazel (bark and leaf)	Hemorrhoids
Wormwood	Antiparasitic
Yarrow (root)	Fevers
Yellow dock (root)	Good in all skin problems
Yerba santa	Bronchial congestion
Yohimbe	Natural aphrodisiac
Yucca (root)	Reduces inflammation of the joints

HERB-DRUG INTERACTIONS / CAUTIONS

Herb	Drug Interaction / Caution
Acidophilus/bifidobacterium	Antibiotics (oral)
Activated charcoal	Vitamins or oral medications may be adsorbed.
Alfalfa	Do not use with lupus due to amino acid L-canavanine; causes pancytopenia at high doses; warfarin (alfalfa contains a large amount of vitamin K).
Aloe vera	Caution in pregnancy, may cause uterine contractions; digoxin, diuretics (hypokalemia)
Ashwagandha	May cause sedation and other CNS effects
Asparagus (root)	Causes diuresis
Barberry	Normal metabolism of vitamin B may be altered with high doses.
Birch	If patient is taking a diuretic, instruct them to drink plenty of fluids.
Black cohosh	Estrogen-like component; pregnant and nursing women should probably avoid this herb; also women with estrogen-dependent cancer and women who are taking birth control pills or estrogen supplements after menopause; caution also in people taking sedatives or blood pressure medications
Black haw	Do not give to children <6 years of age (salicin content) with flu or chickenpox due to potential Reye's syndrome; do not take if allergic to aspirin.
Black pepper (*Piper nigrum*)	Antiasthmatic drugs (decreases metabolism)
Black tea	May inhibit body's utilization of thiamine
Blessed thistle	Do not use with gastritis, ulcers, or hyperacidity since herb stimulates gastric juices.
Blood root	Large doses can cause nausea, vomiting, CNS sedation, low BP, shock, coma, and death.
Broom (*Cytisus scoparius*)	MAO inhibitors lead to sudden blood pressure changes.
Bugleweed (*Lycopus virginicus*)	May interfere with nuclear imaging studies of the thyroid gland (thyroid uptake scan)
Cat's claw (*Uncaria tomentosa*)	Avoid in organ transplant patients or patients on ulcer medications, antiplatelet drugs, NSAIDs, anticoagulants, immunosuppressive therapy, intravenous immunoglobulin therapy.
Chaste tree (berry) (*Vitex agnus-castus*)	Interferes with actions of oral contraceptives, HRT, and other endocrine therapies; may interfere with metabolism of dopamine-receptor antagonists
Chicory (*Cichorium intybus*)	Avoid with gallstones due to bile-stimulating properties.
Chlorella (*Chlorella vulgaris*)	Contains significant amounts of vitamin K
Chromium picolinate	Picolinic acid causes notable changes in brain chemicals (serotonin, dopamine, norepinephrine); do not use if patient has behavioral disorders or diabetes.
Cinnabar (root) (*Salviae multorrhizae*)	Warfarin (increases INR)
Deadly nightshade (*Atropa belladonna*)	Contains atropine
Dong quai	Warfarin (increases INR), estrogens, oral contraceptives, photosensitizing drugs, histamine replacement therapy, anticoagulants, antiplatelet drugs, antihypertensives
Echinacea	Caution with other immunosuppressive therapies; stimulates TNF and interferons
Ephedra	Avoid with blood pressure medications, antidepressants, and MAOIs.
Evening primrose (oil)	May lower seizure threshold; do not combine with anticonvulsants or phenothiazines
Fennel	Do not use in women who have had breast cancer or who have been told not to take birth control pills.

HERBAL AND NUTRITIONAL PRODUCTS (Continued)

Herb	Drug Interaction / Caution
Fenugreek	Practice moderation in patients on diabetes drugs, MAO inhibitors, cardiovascular agents, hormonal medicines, or warfarin due to the many components of fenugreek.
Feverfew	Antiplatelets, anticoagulants, NSAIDs
Forskolin, coleonol	Lowers blood pressure (vasodilator); is a bronchodilator and increases the contractility of the heart; inhibits platelet aggregation; increases gastric acid secretion
Foxglove	Digitalis-containing herb
Garlic	Blood sugar-lowering medications, warfarin, and aspirin at medicinal doses of garlic
Ginger	May inhibit platelet aggregation by inhibiting thromboxane synthetase at large doses; *in vitro* and animal studies indicate that ginger may interfere with diabetics; has anticoagulant effect, so avoid in medicinal amounts in patients on warfarin or heart medicines
Ginkgo biloba	Warfarin (ginkgo decreases blood clotting rate); NSAIDs, MAO inhibitors
Ginseng	Blood sugar-lowering medications (additive effects) and other stimulants
Ginseng (American, Korean)	Furosemide (decreases efficacy)
Ginseng (Siberian)	Digoxin (increases digoxin level)
Glucomannan	Patients with diabetes (herb delays absorption of glucose from intestines, decreasing mean fasting sugar levels)
Goldenrod	Diuretics (additive properties)
Gymnema	Blood sugar-lowering medications (additive effects)
Hawthorn	Digoxin or other heart medications (herb dilates coronary vessels and other blood vessels, also inotropic)
Hibiscus	Chloroquine (reduced effectiveness of chloroquine)
Hops	Alcohol or sedative (additive effects); patients with depression (accentuate symptoms) Patients with estrogen-dependent breast cancer should not take hops (contains estrogen-like chemicals).
Horehound	May cause arrhythmias at high doses
Horseradish	In medicinal amounts with thyroid medications
Kava	CNS depressants (additive effects, eg, alcohol, barbiturates, etc); benzodiazepines
Kelp	Thyroid medications (additive effects or opposite effects by negative feedback); kelp contains a high amount of sodium
Labrador tea	Plant has narcotic properties, possible additive effects with other CNS depressants.
Lemon balm	Do not use with Graves disease since it inhibits certain thyroid hormones.
Licorice	Acts as a corticosteroid at high doses (about 1.5 lbs candy in 9 days) which can lead to hypertension, edema, hypernatremia, and hypokalemia (pseudoaldosteronism. Do not use in patients with hypertension; glaucoma; diabetes; kidney or liver disease; or those on hormonal therapy. It may interact with digitalis (due to hypokalemia).
Lobelia	Contains lobeline which has nicotinic activity; may mask withdrawal symptoms from nicotine. It can act as a polarizing neuromuscular blocker.
Lovage	Is a diuretic
Ma huang	MAO inhibitors, digoxin, beta-blockers, methyldopa, caffeine, theophylline, decongestants (increases toxicity)
Marshmallow	May delay absorption of other drugs taken at the same time; may interfere with treatments of lowering blood sugar

Herb	Drug Interaction / Caution
Meadowsweet	Contains salicylates
Melatonin	Acts as contraceptive at high doses; antidepressants (decreases efficacy)
Mistletoe	May interfere with medications for blood pressure, depression, and heart disease
L-phenylalanine	MAO inhibitors
Pleurisy (root)	Digoxin (plant contains cardiac glycosides); also contains estrogen-like compounds; may alter amine concentrations in the brain and interact with antidepressants
Prickly ash (Northern)	Contains coumarin-like compounds
Prickly ash (Southern)	Contains neuromuscular blockers
Psyllium	Digoxin (decreases absorption)
Quassia	High doses may complicate heart or blood-thinning treatments (quassia may be inotropic).
Red clover	May have estrogen-like actions; avoid when taking birth control pills, HRT, people with heart disease or at risk for blood clots, patients who suffer from estrogen-dependent cancer; do not take with warfarin
Red pepper	May increase liver metabolism of other medications and may interfere with high blood pressure medications or MAO inhibitors
Rhubarb (Chinese)	Do not use with digoxin (enhanced effects).
St John's wort	Indinavir, cyclosporine, SSRIs or any antidepressants, tetracycline (increases sun sensitivity); digoxin (decreases digoxin concentration); may also interact with diltiazem, nicardipine, verapamil, etoposide, paclitaxel, vinblastine, vincristine, glucocorticoids, cyclosporine, dextromethorphan, ephedrine, lithium, meperidine, pseudoephedrine, selegiline, yohimbine, ACE inhibitors (serotonin syndrome, hypertension, possible exacerbation of allergic reaction)
Saw palmetto	Acts an antiandrogen; do not take with prostate medicines or HRT.
Squill	Digoxin, quinidine, calcium, laxatives, saluretics, prednisone (long-term); patients with potassium deficiency
Tonka bean	Contains coumarin, interacts with warfarin
Vervain	Avoid large amounts of herb with blood pressure medications or HRT
Wild Oregon grape	High doses may alter metabolism of vitamin B.
Wild yam	May interfere with hormone precursors
Wintergreen	Warfarin, increased bleeding
Sweet woodruff	Contains coumarin
Yarrow	Interferes with anticoagulants and blood pressure medications
Yohimbe	Do not consume tyramine-rich foods. Do not take with nasal decongestants, PPA-containing diet aids, antidepressants, or mood-altering drugs.

HERBAL AND NUTRITIONAL PRODUCTS *(Continued)*

Herbs Contraindicated During Lactation
According to German Commission E

Aloe
  (*Aloe vera*)

Basil
  (*Ocimum basillicum*)

Buckthorn (bark and berry)
  (*Rhamnus frangula,*
  R. cathartica)

Cascara sagrada
  (*Rhamnus purshiana*)

Coltsfoot (leaf)
  (*Tussilago farfara*)

Combination of senna, peppermint
  oil, and caraway oil

Kava (root)
  (*Piper methysticum*)

Petasite (root)
  (*Petasites* spp)

Indian snakeroot
  (*Rauwolfia serpentina*)

Rhubarb (root)
  (*Rheum palmatum*)

Senna
  (*Cassia senna*)

Herbs Contraindicated During Pregnancy
According to German Commission E

Aloe
  (*Aloe vera*)

Autumn crocus
  (*Colchicum autumnale*)

Black cohosh (root)
  (*Cimicifuga racemosa*)

Buckthorn (bark and berry)
  (*Rhamnus frangula,*
  R. cathartica)

Cascara sagrada (bark)
  (*Rhamnus purshiana*)

Chaste tree (fruit)
  (*Vitex agnus-castus*)

Cinchona (bark)
  (*Cinchona* spp)

Cinnamon (bark)
  (*Cinnamomum zeylanicum*)

Coltsfoot (leaf)
  (*Tussliago farfara*)

Echinacea purpurea
  (*Echinacea purpurea*)

Fennel (oil)
  (*Foeniculum vulgare*)

Combination of licorice,
  peppermint, and chamomile

Combination of licorice, primrose,
  marshmallow, and anise

Combination of senna, peppermint
  oil, and caraway oil

Ginger (root)[1]
  (*Zingiber officinale*)

Indian snakeroot
  (*Rauwolfia serpentina*)

Juniper (berry)
  (*Juniperus comunis*)

Kava (root)
  (*Piper methysticum*)

Licorice (root)
  (*Glycyrrhiza glabra*)

Marsh tea
  (*Ledum palustre*)

Mayapple (root)
  (*Podophyllum peltatum*)

Petasite (root)
  (*Petasites* spp)

Rhubarb (root)
  (*Rheum palmatum*)

Sage (leaf)
  (*Salvia officinalis*)

Senna
  (*Cassia senna*)

[1]A subsequent review of the clinical literature could find no basis for the contraindication of ginger, a common spice, during pregnancy (Fulder and Tenne, 1996).

IMMUNIZATION RECOMMENDATIONS

Standards for Pediatric Immunization Practices

Standard 1.	Immunization services are readily available.
Standard 2.	There are no barriers or unnecessary prerequisites to the receipt of vaccines.
Standard 3.	Immunization services are available free or for a minimal fee.
Standard 4.	Providers utilize all clinical encounters to screen and, when indicated, immunize children.
Standard 5.	Providers educate parents and guardians about immunizations in general terms.
Standard 6.	Providers question parents or guardians about contraindications and, before immunizing a child, inform them in specific terms about the risks and benefits of the immunizations their child is to receive.
Standard 7.	Providers follow only true contraindications.
Standard 8.	Providers administer simultaneously all vaccine doses for which a child is eligible at the time of each visit.
Standard 9.	Providers use accurate and complete recording procedures.
Standard 10.	Providers co-schedule immunization appointments in conjunction with appointments for other child health services.
Standard 11.	Providers report adverse events following immunization promptly, accurately, and completely.
Standard 12.	Providers operate a tracking system.
Standard 13.	Providers adhere to appropriate procedures for vaccine management.
Standard 14.	Providers conduct semiannual audits to assess immunization coverage levels and to review immunization records in the patient populations they serve.
Standard 15.	Providers maintain up-to-date, easily retrievable medical protocols at all locations where vaccines are administered.
Standard 16.	Providers operate with patient-oriented and community-based approaches.
Standard 17.	Vaccines are administered by properly trained individuals.
Standard 18.	Providers receive ongoing education and training on current immunization recommendations.

Recommended by the National Vaccine Advisory Committee, April 1992.
Approved by the United States Public Health Service, May 1992.
Endorsed by the American Academy of Pediatrics, May 1992.

The Standards represent the consensus of the National Vaccine Advisory Committee (NVAC) and of a broad group of medical and public health experts about what constitutes the most desirable immunization practices. It is recognized by the NVAC that not all of the current immunization practices of public and private providers are in compliance with the Standards. Nevertheless, the Standards are expected to be useful as a means of helping providers to identify needed changes, to obtain resources if necessary, and to actually implement the desirable immunization practices in the future.

IMMUNIZATION RECOMMENDATIONS *(Continued)*

Recommended Childhood and Adolescent Immunization Schedule
United States, 2005

Vaccine ▼ / Age ►	Birth	1 mo	2 mo	4 mo	6 mo	12 mo	15 mo	18 mo	24 mo	4-6 y	11-12 y	13-18 y
Hepatitis B[1]	HepB #1	only if mother HBsAg(-)	HepB #2		HepB #3						HepB series	
Diphtheria, tetanus, pertussis[2]			DTaP	DTaP	DTaP		DTaP			DTaP	Td	Td
Haemophilus influenzae type b[3]			Hib	Hib	Hib	Hib						
Inactivated poliovirus			IPV	IPV		IPV				IPV		
Measles, mumps, rubella[4]						MMR #1				MMR #2	MMR #2	MMR #2
Varicella[5]						Varicella				Varicella		
Pneumococcal[6]			PCV	PCV	PCV	PCV			PCV	PPV		
Influenza[7]					Influenza (yearly)					Influenza (yearly)		
Vaccines below this line are for selected populations												
Hepatitis A[8]										Hepatitis A series		

☐ Range of recommended ages ■ Preadolescent assessment ☐ Catch-up immunization

This schedule indicates the recommended ages for routine administration of currently licensed childhood vaccines, as of December 1, 2004, for children through age 18 years. Any dose not given at the recommended age should be given at any subsequent visit when indicated and feasible. ☐ Indicates age groups that warrant special effort to administer those vaccines not given previously. Additional vaccines may be licensed and recommended during the year. Licensed combination vaccines may be used whenever any components of the combination are indicated and the vaccine's other components are not contraindicated. Providers should consult the manufacturers' package inserts for detailed recommendations. Clinically significant adverse events that follow immunization should be reported to the Vaccine Adverse Event Reporting System (VAERS). Guidance about how to obtain and complete a VAERS form can be found on the Internet: http://www.vaers.org or by calling 800-822-7967.

[1] **Hepatitis B (HepB) vaccine.** All infants should receive the first dose of hepatitis B vaccine soon after birth and before hospital discharge; the first dose may also be given by age 2 months if the infant's mother is HBsAg-negative. Only monovalent HepB can be used for the birth dose. Monovalent or combination vaccine containing HepB may be used to complete the series. Four doses of vaccine may be administered when a birth dose is given. The second dose should be given at least 4 weeks after the first dose, except for combination vaccines, which cannot be administered before age 6 weeks. The third dose should be given at least 16 weeks after the first dose and at least 8 weeks after the second dose. The last dose in the vaccination series (third or fourth dose) should not be administered before age 24 weeks.

Infants born to HBsAg-positive mothers should receive HepB vaccine and 0.5 mL hepatitis B immune globulin (HBIG) within 12 hours of birth at separate sites. The second dose is recommended at age 1-2 months. The last dose in the vaccination series should not be administered before age 24 weeks. These infants should be tested for HBsAg and anti-HBs at 9-15 months of age.

Infants born to mothers whose HBsAg status is unknown should receive the first dose of the HepB vaccine series within 12 hours of birth. Maternal blood should be drawn as soon as possible to determine the mother's HBsAg status; if the HBsAg test is positive, the infant should receive HBIG as soon as possible (no later than age 1 week). The second dose is recommended at age 1-2 months. The last dose in the vaccination series should not be administered before age 24 weeks.

[2] **Diphtheria, tetanus toxoids, and acellular pertussis (DTaP) vaccine.** The fourth dose of DTaP may be administered as early as age 12 months, provided that 6 months have elapsed since the third dose and the child is unlikely to return at age 15-18 months. The final dose in the series should be given at age ≥4 years. **Tetanus and diphtheria toxoids (Td)** is recommended at age 11-12 years if at least 5 years have elapsed since the last dose of tetanus and diphtheria toxoid-containing vaccine. Subsequent routine Td boosters are recommended every 10 years.

[3] **Haemophilus influenzae type b (Hib) conjugate vaccine.** Three Hib conjugate vaccines are licensed for infant use. If PRP-OMP (PedvaxHIB® or ComVax® [Merck]) is administered at ages 2 and 4 months, a dose at age 6 months is not required. DTaP/Hib combination products should not be used for primary immunization in infants at ages 2, 4, or 6 months, but can be used as boosters following any Hib vaccine. The final dose in the series should be given at age ≥12 months.

[4] **Measles, mumps, and rubella vaccine (MMR).** The second dose of MMR is recommended routinely at age 4-6 years but may be administered during any visit, provided at least 4 weeks have elapsed since the first dose and both doses are administered beginning at or after age 12 months. Those who have not previously received the second dose should complete the schedule by the visit at age 11-12-years.

[5] **Varicella vaccine** is recommended at any visit at or after age 12 months for susceptible children (ie, those who lack a reliable history of chickenpox). Susceptible persons age ≥13 years should receive 2 doses, given at least 4 weeks apart.

[6] **Pneumococcal vaccine.** The heptavalent **pneumococcal conjugate vaccine (PCV)** is recommended for all children age 2-23 months. It is also recommended for certain children age 24-59 months. The final dose in the series should be given at age ≥12 months. **Pneumococcal polysaccharide vaccine (PPV)** is recommended in addition to PCV for certain high-risk groups. See *MMWR*, 2000, 49(RR-9):1-35.

[7] **Influenza vaccine** is recommended annually for children age ≥6 months with certain risk factors (including but not limited to asthma, cardiac disease, sickle cell disease, HIV, and diabetes), healthcare workers, and other persons (including household members) in close contact with persons in groups at high risk (see *MMWR*, 2004, 53(RR-6):1-40), and can be administered to all others wishing to obtain immunity. In addition, healthy children age 6-23 months and close contacts of healthy children age 0-23 months are recommended to receive influenza vaccine, because children in this age group are at substantially increased risk for influenza-related hospitalizations. For healthy persons age 5-49 years, the intranasally administered live, attenuated influenza vaccine (LAIV) is an acceptable alternative to the intramuscular trivalent inactivated influenza vacine (TIV). See *MMWR*, 2004, 53(RR-6):1-40. Children receiving TIV should be administered a dosage appropriate for their age (0.25 mL if 6-35 months or 0.5 mL if ≥3 years). Children age ≤8 years who are receiving influenza vaccine for the first time should receive two doses (separated by at least 4 weeks for TIV and at least 6 weeks for LAIV).

[8] **Hepatitis A vaccine** is recommended for children and adolescents in selected states and regions, and for certain high-risk groups; consult your local public health authority. Children and adolescents in these states, regions, and high-risk groups who have not been immunized against hepatitis A can begin the hepatitis A vaccination series during any visit. The two doses in the series should be administered at least 6 months apart. See *MMWR*, 1999, 48(RR-12):1-37

Additional information about vaccines, including precautions and contraindications for vaccination and vaccine shortages is available at http://www.cdc.gov/nip or from the National Immunization Information Hotline, 800-232-2522 (English) or 800-232-0233 (Spanish). Approved by the Advisory Committee on Immunization Practices (http://www.cdc.gov/nip/acip), the American Academy of Pediatrics (http://www.aap.org), and the American Academy of Family Physicians (http://www.aafp.org).

Reference:
"Recommended Childhood and Adolescent Immunization Schedule — United States, 2005," *MMWR*, 2005, 53(51 & 52):Q1-3.

CATCH-UP SCHEDULE FOR CHILDREN AND ADOLESCENTS WHO START LATE OR WHO ARE >1 MONTH BEHIND

Tables 1 and 2 give catch-up schedules and minimum intervals between doses for children who have delayed immunizations. There is no need to restart a vaccine series regardless of the time that has elapsed between doses. Use the chart appropriate for the child's age.

Table 1. Catch-up Schedule for Children Age 4 Months - 6 Years

Dose 1 (Minimum Age)	Minimum Interval Between Doses			
	Dose 1 to Dose 2	Dose 2 to Dose 3	Dose 3 to Dose 4	Dose 4 to Dose 5
DTaP (6 wk)	4 wk	4 wk	6 mo	6 mo[1]
IPV (6 wk)	4 wk	4 wk	4 wk[2]	
HepB[3] (birth)	4 wk	8 wk (and 16 wk after 1st dose)		
MMR (12 mo)	4 wk[4]			
VAR (12 mo)				
Hib[5] (6 wk)	**4 wk:** If 1st dose given at age <12 mo **8 wk (as final dose):** If 1st dose given at age 12-14 mo **No further doses needed:** If 1st dose given at age ≥15 mo	**4 wk[6]:** If current age <12 mo **8 wk (as final dose):** If current age ≥12 mo and 2nd dose given at age <15 mo **No further doses needed:** If previous dose given at age ≥15 mo	**8 wk (as final dose):** This dose only necessary for children age 12 mo - 5 y who received 3 doses before age 12 mo	
PCV[7] (6 wk)	**4 wk:** If 1st dose given at age <12 mo and current age <24 mo **8 wk (as final dose):** If 1st dose given at age ≥12 mo or current age 24-59 mo **No further doses needed:** For healthy children if 1st dose given at age ≥24 mo	**4 wk:** If current age <12 mo **8 wk (as final dose):** If current age ≥12 mo **No further doses needed:** For healthy children if previous dose given at age ≥24 mo	**8 wk (as final dose):** This dose only necessary for children 12 mo - 5 y who received 3 doses before age 12 mo	

Table 2. Catch-up Schedule for Children Age 7-18 Years

Minimum Interval Between Doses		
Dose 1 to Dose 2	Dose 2 to Dose 3	Dose 3 to Booster Dose
Td: 4 wk	Td: 6 mo	Td[8]: **6 mo:** If 1st dose given at age <12 mo and current age <11 y **5 y:** If 1st dose given at age ≥12 mo and 3rd dose given at age <7 y and current age ≥11 y **10 y:** If 3rd dose given at age ≥7 y
IPV[9]: 4 wk	IPV[9]: 4 wk	IPV[2,9]
HepB: 4 wk	HepB: 8 wk (and 16 wk after first dose)	
MMR: 4 wk		
VAR[10]: 4 wk		

IMMUNIZATION RECOMMENDATIONS *(Continued)*

Footnotes to Table 1 and Table 2

[1]**Diphtheria and tetanus toxoids and acellular pertussis vaccine (DTaP):** The fifth dose is not necessary if the fourth dose was given after the fourth birthday.

[2]**Inactivated polio vaccine (IPV):** For children who received an all-IPV or all-oral poliovirus (OPV) series, a fourth dose is not necessary if third dose was given at age ≥4 years. If both OPV and IPV were given as part of a series, a total of four doses should be given, regardless of the child's current age.

[3]**Hepatitis B vaccine (HepB):** All children and adolescents who have not been immunized against hepatitis B should begin the hepatitis B vaccination series during any visit. Providers should make special efforts to immunize children who were born in, or whose parents were born in, areas of the world where hepatitis B virus infection is moderately or highly endemic.

[4]**Measles, mumps, and rubella vaccine (MMR):** The second dose of MMR is recommended routinely at age 4-6 years, but may be given earlier if desired.

[5]*Haemophilus influenzae* **type b (Hib) conjugate vaccine:** Vaccine is not generally recommended for children age ≥5 years.

[6]**Hib:** If current age <12 months and the first 2 doses were PRP-OMP (PedvaxHIB® or ComVax® [Merck]), the third (and final) dose should be given at age 12-15 months and at least 8 weeks after the second dose.

[7]**Pneumococcal conjugate vaccine (PCV):** Vaccine is not generally recommended for children age ≥5 years.

[8]**Tetanus and diphtheria toxoids (Td):** For children age 7-10 years, the interval between the third and booster dose is determined by the age when the first dose was given. For adolescents age 11-18 years, the interval is determined by the age when the third dose was given.

[9]**IPV:** Vaccine is not generally recommended for persons age ≥18 years.

[10]**Varicella (VAR):** Give 2-dose series to all susceptible adolescents age ≥13 years.

Reporting Adverse Reactions

Clinically significant adverse events that follow vaccination should be reported to the Vaccine Adverse Event Reporting System (VAERS). Guidance on completing a VAERS form is available at http://www.vaers.org or call 800-822-7967.

Disease Reporting

Suspected cases of vaccine-preventable diseases should be reported to state or local health departments. Additional information about vaccines, including precautions and contraindications for vaccination and vaccine shortages, is available at http://www.cdc.gov/nip or from the National Immunization Information Hotline, 800-232-2522 (English) or 800-232-0233 (Spanish).

Recommended Adult Immunization Schedule, by Vaccine and Age Group
United States, October 2004 - September 2005

Vaccine	Age Group (years)		
	19-49	50-64	≥65
Tetanus, diphtheria (Td)*	1 dose booster every 10 years[1]		
Influenza	1 dose annually[2]		1 dose annually
Pneumococcal (polysaccharide)	1 dose[3,4]		1 dose[3,4]
Hepatitis B*	3 doses (0, 1-2, 4-6 months)[5]		
Hepatitis A*	2 doses (0, 6-12 months)[6]		
Measles, mumps, rubella (MMR)*	1 or 2 doses[7]		
Varicella*	2 doses (0, 4-8 weeks)[8]		
Meningococcal (polysaccharide)	1 dose[9]		

☐ For all persons in this group　　■ For persons lacking documentation of vaccination or evidence of disease　　▨ For persons at risk (ie, with medical/exposure indications)

*Covered by the Vaccine Injury Compensation Program.

Recommended Adult Immunization Schedule, by Vaccine and Medical and Other Indications — United States, October 2004 - September 2005

Vaccine	Indication						
	Pregnancy	Diabetes, heart disease, chronic pulmonary disease, chronic liver disease (including chronic alcoholism)	Congenital immunodeficiency, cochlear implants, leukemia, lymphoma, generalized malignancy, therapy with alkylating agents, antimetabolites, CSF† leaks, radiation, or large amounts of corticosteroids	Renal failure/ end-stage renal disease, recipients of hemodialysis or clotting factor concentrates	Asplenia (including elective splenectomy and terminal complement component deficiencies)	HIV‡ infection	Healthcare workers
Tetanus, diphtheria (Td)*,1							
Influenza[2]		A, B			C		
Pneumococcal (polysaccharide)[3,4]		B	D	D	D, E, F	D, G	
Hepatitis B*,5				H			
Hepatitis A*,6		I					
Measles, mumps, rubella (MMR)*,7						J	
Varicella*,8			K				

☐ For all persons in this group　　■ For persons lacking documentation of vaccination or evidence of disease　　▨ For persons at risk (ie, with medical/exposure indications)　　■ Contraindicated

*Covered by the Vaccine Injury Compensation Program.
†Cerebrospinal fluid.
‡Human immunodeficiency virus.

IMMUNIZATION RECOMMENDATIONS *(Continued)*

Special Notes for Medical and Other Indications

I.   Although chronic liver disease and alcoholism are not indications for influenza vaccination, administer 1 dose annually if the patient is ≤50 years, has other indications for influenza vaccine, or requests vaccination.

II. Asthma is an indication for influenza vaccination but not for pneumococcal vaccination.

III. No data exist specifically on the risk for severe or complicated influenza infections among persons with asplenia. However, influenza is a risk factor for secondary bacterial infections that can cause severe disease among persons with asplenia.

IV. For persons <65 years, revaccinate once after ≥5 years have elapsed since initial vaccination.

V.   Administer meningococcal vaccine and consider *Haemophilus influenzae* type b vaccine.

VI. For persons undergoing elective splenectomy, vaccinate ≥2 weeks before surgery.

VII. Vaccinate as soon after diagnosis as possible.

VIII. For hemodialysis patients, use special formulation of vaccine (40 µg/mL) or two 20 µg/mL doses administered at one body site. Vaccinate early in the course of renal disease. Assess antibody titers to hepatitis B surface antigen (anti-HB) levels annually. Administer additional doses if anti-HB levels decline to <10 mIU/mL.

IX. For all persons with chronic liver disease.

X.   Withhold MMR or other measles-containing vaccines from HIV-infected persons with evidence of severe immunosuppression (see *MMWR*, 1998, 47[RR-8]:21-2 and *MMWR*, 2002, 51[RR-2]:22-4).

XI. Persons with impaired humoral immunity but intact cellular immunity may be vaccinated (see *MMWR*, 1999, 48[RR-6]).

Footnotes to Recommended Adult Immunization Schedule

[1]**Tetanus and diphtheria (Td).** Adults, including pregnant women with uncertain history of a complete primary vaccination series, should receive a primary series of Td. A primary series for adults is 3 doses; administer the first 2 doses at least 4 weeks apart and the 3rd dose 6-12 months after the second. Administer 1 dose if the person received the primary series and if the last vaccination was received ≥10 years previously. Consult recommendations for administering Td as prophylaxis in wound management (see *MMWR*, 1991, 40[RR-10]). The American College of Physicians Task Force on Adult Immunization supports a second option for Td use in adults: a single Td booster at age 50 years for persons who have completed the full pediatric series, including the teenage/young adult booster.

[2]**Influenza vaccination.** The Advisory Committee on Immunization Practices (ACIP) recommends inactivated influenza vaccination for the following priority groups, when vaccine is available. *Medical indications:* Chronic disorders of the cardiovascular or pulmonary systems, including asthma; chronic metabolic diseases, including diabetes mellitus, renal dysfunction, hemoglobinopathies, or immunosuppression (including immunosuppression caused by medications or by human immunodeficiency virus [HIV]); and pregnancy during the influenza season. *Occupational indications:* Healthcare workers and employees of long-term care and assisted living facilities. *Other indications:* Residents of nursing homes and other long-term care facilities; persons likely to transmit influenza to persons at high risk (ie, in-home caregivers to persons with medical indications, household/close contacts and out-of-home caregivers of children 0-23 months, household members and caregivers of elderly persons and adults with high-risk conditions); and anyone who wishes to be vaccinated. For healthy persons 5-49 years without high-risk conditions who are not contacts of severely immunocompromised persons in special care units, either the inactivated vaccine or the intranasally administered influenza vaccine (FluMist®) may be administered (see *MMWR*, 2004, 53[RR-6]). **Note:** Because of the vaccine shortage for the 2004-5 influenza season, CDC has recommended that vaccination be restricted to the following priority groups, which are considered to be of equal importance: all children 6-23 months; adults ≥65 years; persons 2-64 years with underlying chronic medical conditions; all women who will be pregnant during the influenza season; residents of nursing homes and long-term care facilities; children 6 months to 18 years on chronic aspirin therapy; healthcare workers involved in direct patient care; and out-of-home caregivers and household contacts of children <6 months. For the 2004-5 season, intranasally administered, live, attenuated influenza vaccine, if available, should be encouraged for healthy persons who are 5-49 years and are not pregnant, including healthcare workers (except those who care for severely immunocompromised patients in special care units) and persons caring for children <6 months (see *MMWR*, 2004, 53:923-4).

[3]**Pneumococcal polysaccharide vaccination.** *Medical indications:* Chronic disorders of the pulmonary system (excluding asthma); cardiovascular diseases; diabetes mellitus; chronic liver diseases, including liver disease as a result of alcohol abuse (eg, cirrhosis); chronic renal failure or nephrotic syndrome; functional or anatomic asplenia (eg, sickle cell disease or splenectomy); immunosuppressive conditions (eg, congenital immunodeficiency, HIV infection, leukemia, lymphoma, multiple myeloma, Hodgkins disease, generalized malignancy, or organ or bone marrow transplantation); chemotherapy with alkylating agents, antimetabolites, or long-term systemic corticosteroids; or cochlear implants. *Geographic/other indications:* Alaska natives and certain American Indian populations. *Other indications:* Residents of nursing homes and other long-term care facilities (see *MMWR*, 1997, 46[RR-8] and *MMWR*, 2003, 52:739-40).

[4]**Revaccination with pneumococcal polysaccharide vaccine.** One-time revaccination after 5 years for persons with chronic renal failure or nephrotic syndrome; functional or anatomic asplenia (eg, sickle cell disease or splenectomy); immunosuppressive conditions (eg, congenital immunodeficiency, HIV infection, leukemia, lymphoma, multiple myeloma, Hodgkins disease, generalized malignancy, or organ or bone marrow transplantation); or chemotherapy with alkylating agents, antimetabolites, or long-term systemic corticosteroids. For persons ≥65 years, one-time revaccination if they were vaccinated ≥5 years previously and were <65 years at the time of primary vaccination (see *MMWR*, 1997, 46[RR-8]).

[5]**Hepatitis B vaccination.** *Medical indications:* Hemodialysis patients or patients who receive clotting factor concentrates. *Occupational indications:* Healthcare workers and public-safety workers who have exposure to blood in the workplace; and persons in training in schools of medicine, dentistry, nursing, laboratory technology, and other allied health professions. *Behavioral indications:* Injection-drug users; persons with more than one sex partner during the previous 6 months; persons with a recently acquired sexually transmitted disease (STD); all clients in STD clinics; and men who have sex with men. *Other*

indications: Household contacts and sex partners of persons with chronic hepatitis B virus (HBV) infection; clients and staff members of institutions for the developmentally disabled; inmates of correctional facilities; or international travelers who will be in countries with high or intermediate prevalence of chronic HBV infection for >6 months (http://www.cdc.gov/travel/ diseases/hbv.htm) (see *MMWR*, 1991, 40[RR-13]).

[6]**Hepatitis A vaccination.** *Medical indications:* Persons with clotting factor disorders or chronic liver disease. *Behavioral indications:* Men who have sex with men or users of illegal drugs. *Occupational indications:* Persons working with hepatitis A virus (HAV)-infected primates or with HAV in a research laboratory setting. *Other indications:* Persons traveling to or working in countries that have high or intermediate endemicity of hepatitis A. If the combined hepatitis A and hepatitis B vaccine is used, administer 3 doses at 0, 1, and 6 months (http://www.cdc.gov/travel/diseases/hav.htm) (see *MMWR*, 1999, 48[RR-12]).

[7]**Measles, mumps, rubella (MMR) vaccination.** *Measles component:* Adults born before 1957 can be considered immune to measles. Adults born during or after 1957 should receive ≥1 dose of MMR unless they have a medical contraindication, documentation of ≥1 dose, or other acceptable evidence of immunity. A second dose of MMR is recommended for adults who 1) were recently exposed to measles or in an outbreak setting, 2) were previously vaccinated with killed measles vaccine, 3) were vaccinated with an unknown vaccine during 1963-1967, 4) are students in postsecondary educational institutions, 5) work in healthcare facilities, or 6) plan to travel internationally. *Mumps component:* 1 dose of MMR vaccine should be adequate for protection. *Rubella component:* Administer 1 dose of MMR vaccine to women whose rubella vaccination history is unreliable and counsel women to avoid becoming pregnant for 4 weeks after vaccination. For women of childbearing age, regardless of birth year, routinely determine rubella immunity and counsel women regarding congenital rubella syndrome. Do not vaccinate pregnant women or those planning to become pregnant during the next 4 weeks. For women who are pregnant and susceptible, vaccinate as early in the postpartum period as possible (see *MMWR*, 1998, 47[RR-8] and *MMWR*, 2001, 50:1117).

[8]**Varicella vaccination.** Recommended for all persons lacking a reliable clinical history of varicella infection or serologic evidence of varicella zoster virus (VZV) infection who might be at high risk for exposure or transmission. This includes healthcare workers and family contacts of immunocompromised persons; persons who live or work in environments where transmission is likely (eg, teachers of young children, child care employees, and residents and staff members in institutional settings); persons who live or work in environments where VZV transmission can occur (eg, college students, inmates, and staff members of correctional institutions, and military personnel); adolescents 11-18 years and adults living in households with children; women who are not pregnant but who might become pregnant; and international travelers who are not immune to infection. **Note:** Approximately 95% of U.S.-born adults are immune to VZV. Do not vaccinate pregnant women or those planning to become pregnant during the next 4 weeks. For women who are pregnant and susceptible, vaccinate as early in the postpartum period as possible (see *MMWR*, 1999, 48[RR-6]).

[9]**Meningococcal vaccine (quadrivalent polysaccharide for serogroups A, C, Y, and W 135).** *Medical indications:* Adults with terminal complement component deficiencies or those with anatomic or functional asplenia. *Other indications:* Travelers to countries in which meningococcal disease is hyperendemic or epidemic (eg, the "meningitis belt" of sub-Saharan Africa and Mecca, Saudi Arabia). Revaccination after 3-5 years might be indicated for persons at high risk for infection (eg, persons residing in areas where disease is epidemic). Counsel college freshmen, especially those who live in dormitories, regarding meningococcal disease and availability of the vaccine to enable them to make an educated decision about receiving the vaccination (see *MMWR*, 2000, 49[RR-7]). The American Academy of Family Physicians recommends that colleges should take the lead on providing education on meningococcal infection and availability of vaccination and offer it to students who are interested. Physicians need not initiate discussion of meningococcal quadrivalent polysaccharide vaccine as part of routine medical care.

Adapted from "Recommended Adult Immunization Schedule – United States, October 2004-September 2005," *MMWR*, 2004, 53(45)Q1-4.

The Recommended Adult Immunization Schedule has been approved by the Advisory Committee on Immunization Practices (ACIP), the American College of Obstetricians and Gynecologists (ACOG), and the American Academy of Family Physicians (AAFP).

This schedule indicates the recommended age groups for routine administration of currently licensed vaccines for persons ≥19 years of age. Licensed combination vaccines may be used whenever any components of the combination are indicated and when the vaccine's other components are not contraindicated. Providers should consult manufacturers' package inserts for detailed recommendations.

Additional information about the vaccines listed above and contraindications for immunization is available at http://www.cdc.gov/nip or from the National Immunization Hotline, 800-232-2522 (English) or 800-232-0233 (Spanish).

IMMUNIZATION RECOMMENDATIONS *(Continued)*

RECOMMENDATIONS OF THE ADVISORY COMMITTEE ON IMMUNIZATION PRACTICES (ACIP)

Recommended Poliovirus Vaccination Schedules for Children

Vaccine	Child's Age			
	2 mo	4 mo	12-18 mo	4-6 y
Sequential IPV [1]/OPV[1]/ OPV[2]	IPV	IPV	OPV	OPV
OPV[1]	OPV	OPV	OPV[3]	OPV
IPV[2]	IPV	IPV	IPV	OPV

[1]Inactivated poliovirus vaccine.

[2]Live, oral poliovirus vaccine.

[3]For children who receive only OPV, the third dose of OPV may be administered as early as 6 months of age.

Adapted from "Poliomyelitis Prevention in the United States: Introduction of a Sequential Vaccination Schedule of Inactivated Poliovirus Vaccine Followed by Oral Poliovirus Vaccine" *MMWR Recomm Rep*, 1997, 46(RR-3).

Recommendations for Measles Immunization

Category	Recommendations
Unimmunized, no history of measles (12-15 mo)	A 2-dose schedule (with MMR) is recommended. The first dose is recommended at 12-15 mo; the second is recommended at 4-6 y
Children 6-11 mo in epidemic situations	Immunize (with monovalent measles vaccine or, if not available, MMR); reimmunization (with MMR) at 12-15 mo is necessary, and a third dose is indicated at 4-6 y
Children 4-12 y who have received 1 dose of measles vaccine at ≥12 mo	Reimmunize (1 dose)
Students in college and other post-high school institutions who have received 1 dose of measles vaccine at ≥12 mo	Reimmunize (1 dose)
History of vaccination before the first birthday	Consider susceptible and immunize (2 doses)
History of receipt of inactivated measles vaccine or unknown type of vaccine, 1963-1967	Consider susceptible and immunize (2 doses)
Further attenuated or unknown vaccine given with IG	Consider susceptible and immunize (2 doses)
Allergy to eggs	Immunize; no reactions likely
Neomycin allergy, nonanaphylactic	Immunize; no reactions likely
Severe hypersensitivity (anaphylaxis) to neomycin or gelatin	Avoid immunization
Tuberculosis	Immunize; vaccine does not exacerbate infection
Measles exposure	Immunize and/or give IG, depending on circumstances
HIV-infected	Immunize (2 doses) unless severely immunocompromised
Personal or family history of seizures	Immunize; advise parents of slightly increased risk of seizures
Immunoglobulin or blood recipient	Immunize at the appropriate interval

MMR = measles-mumps-rubella vaccine; IG = immune globulin; HIV = human immunodeficiency virus.

Adapted from "Report of the Committee on Infectious Diseases," *2003 Red Book*®, 26th ed.

Immunization in HIV-Infected Persons

Vaccination of immunocompromised patients depends on the characteristics of the vaccine and the patient. Vaccines are typically divided into two broad categories: those which contain live virus/bacteria or those which are derived from a component of the organism (or an inactivated organism). Live virus or live bacterial vaccines have been associated with severe complications in immunocompromised patients, and should generally be avoided [(except in selected circumstances (noted below)]. Inactivated, recombinant, subunit, polysaccharide, and conjugate vaccines and toxoids can be administered to all immunocompromised patients. However, it should be recognized that the response to these vaccines may be suboptimal. If indicated, all inactivated vaccines are recommended in usual doses and according to prescribed schedules. Pneumococcal, meningococcal, and Hib vaccines are recommended only for specific subpopulations, including functional or anatomic asplenia.

Special consideration must be given to immunization with measles and/or varicella vaccines. Persons with HIV are at a higher risk for severe complications from measles infection. In patients without severe immunocompromise, measles vaccination in HIV-infected persons has not been reported to cause severe and/or unusual adverse events. MMR vaccination is recommended for all HIV-infected persons who do not have evidence of severe immunocompromise (defined as a low age-specific total CD4$^+$ T-lymphocyte count or a low CD4$^+$ T-lymphocyte count as a percentage of total lymphocytes).

Varicella and/or herpes zoster infections are also associated with an increased risk of severe complications in children with HIV infection. Asymptomatic or mildly symptomatic HIV-infected children receiving varicella vaccination have demonstrated adequate response to the vaccine without evidence of severe and/or unusual events. However, experience has been limited. Varicella vaccine should be considered for children who are classified as CDC class N1 or A1 with age-specific CD4$^+$ T-lymphocyte percentages ≥25%.

HIV-infected persons who are receiving IVIG may not respond to MMR or varicella vaccines (or an individual component) due to the presence of a passively acquired antibody. Measles vaccine should be considered approximately 2 weeks before the next scheduled dose of IVIG (unless otherwise contraindicated). Unless serologic testing confirms the production of specific antibodies, the vaccination should be repeated at the recommended interval. In patients receiving maintenance IVIG therapy, an additional dose of IVIG should be considered if the exposure to measles occurs ≥3 weeks following a standard dose. Persons with cellular immunodeficiency should not receive varicella vaccine; however, persons with humoral immunodeficiency should be vaccinated (including persons with dysgammaglobulinemia or hypogammaglobulinemia).

Summarized/adapted from Atkinson WL, Pickering LK, Schwartz B, et al, "General Recommendations on Immunization. Recommendations of the Advisory Committee on Immunization Practices (ACIP) and the American Academy of Family Physicians (AAFP)," *MMWR Recomm Rep*, 2002, 51(RR-2):1-35.

IMMUNIZATION RECOMMENDATIONS *(Continued)*

Recommendations for Pneumococcal Conjugate Vaccine Use Among Healthy Children During Moderate and Severe Shortages

Age at First Vaccination (mo)	No Shortage[1]	Moderate Shortage	Severe Shortage
<6	2, 4, 6, and 12-15 months	2, 4, and 6 months (defer fourth dose)	2 doses at 2-month interval in first 6 months of life (defer third and fourth doses)
7-11	2 doses at 2-month interval; 12-15 month dose	2 doses at 2-month interval; 12-15-month dose	2 doses at 2-month interval (defer third dose)
12-23	2 doses at 2-month interval	2 doses at 2-month interval	1 dose (defer second dose)
>24	1 dose should be considered	No vaccination	No vaccination
Reduction in vaccine doses used[2]		21%	46%

[1]The vaccine schedule for no shortage is included as a reference. Providers should not use the no shortage schedule regardless of their vaccine supply until the national shortage is resolved.

[2]Assumes that approximately 85% of vaccine is administered to healthy infants beginning at age <7 months; approximately 5% is administered to high-risk infants beginning at age <7 months; and approximately 10% is administered to healthy children beginning at age 7-24 months. Actual vaccine savings will depend on a provider's vaccine use.

Adapted from the Advisory Committee on Immunization Practices, "Updated Recommendations on Use of Pneumococcal Conjugate Vaccine in a Setting of Vaccine Shortage," *MMWR Morb Mortal Wkly Rep*, 2001, 50(50):1140-2.

Recommended Regimens for Pneumococcal Conjugate Vaccine Among Children With a Late Start or Lapse in Vaccine Administration

Age at Examination (mo)	Previous Pneumococcal Conjugate Vaccination History	Recommended Regimen[1]
2-6	0 doses	3 doses 2 months apart, 4th dose at 12-15 months
	1 dose	2 doses 2 months apart, 4th dose at 12-15 months
	2 doses	1 dose, 4th dose at 12-15 months
7-11	0 doses	2 doses 2 months apart, 3rd dose at 12-15 months
	1 or 2 doses before age 7 months	1 dose at 7-11 months, with another dose at 12-15 months (≥2 months later)
12-23	0 doses	2 doses ≥2 months apart
	1 dose before age 12 months	2 doses ≥2 months apart
	1 dose at ≥12 months	1 dose ≥2 months after the most recent dose
	2 or 3 doses before age 12 months	1 dose ≥2 months after the most recent dose
24-59		
Healthy children[2]	Any incomplete schedule	Consider 1 dose ≥2 months after the most recent dose
High risk[3]	<3 doses	1 dose ≥2 months after the most recent dose and another dose ≥2 months later
	3 doses	1 dose ≥2 months after the most recent dose

[1]For children vaccinated at age <1 year, the minimum interval between doses is 4 weeks. Doses administered at ≥12 months should be at least 8 weeks apart.

[2]Providers should consider 1 dose for healthy children 24-59 months, with priority to children 24-35 months, American Indian/Alaska native and black children, and those who attend group child care centers.

[3]Children with sickle cell disease, asplenia, human immunodeficiency virus infection, chronic illness, cochlear implant, or immunocompromising condition.

Adapted from "CDC. Notice to Readers: Pneumococcal Conjugate Vaccine Shortage Resolved," *MMWR Morb Mortal Wkly Rep*, 2003, 52(19):446-7.

POSTEXPOSURE PROPHYLAXIS FOR HEPATITIS B[1]

Exposure	Hepatitis B Immune Globulin	Hepatitis B Vaccine
Perinatal	0.5 mL I.M. within 12 h of birth	0.5 mL[2] I.M. within 12 h of birth (no later than 7 d), and at 1 and 6 mo[3]; test for HB_sAg and anti-HB_s at 12-15 mo
Sexual	0.06 mL/kg I.M. within 14 d of sexual contact; a second dose should be given if the index patient remains HB_sAg-positive after 3 mo and hepatitis B vaccine was not given initially	1 mL I.M. at 0, 1, and 6 mo for homosexual and bisexual men and regular sexual contacts of persons with acute and chronic hepatitis B
Percutaneous; exposed person unvaccinated		
Source known HB_sAg-positive	0.06 mL/kg I.M. within 24 h	1 mL I.M. within 7 d, and at 1 and 6 mo[4]
Source known, HB_sAg status not known	Test source for HB_sAg; if source is positive, give exposed person 0.06 mL/kg I.M. once within 7 d	1 mL I.M. within 7 d, and at 1 and 6 mo[4]
Source not tested or unknown	Nothing required	1 mL I.M. within 7 d, and at 1 and 6 mo
Percutaneous; exposed person vaccinated		
Source known HB_sAg-positive	Test exposed person for anti-HB_s.[5] If titer is protective, nothing is required; if titer is not protective, give 0.06 mL/kg within 24 h.	Review vaccination status[6]
Source known, HB_sAg status not known	Test source for HB_sAg and exposed person for anti-HB_s. If source is HB_sAg-negative, or if source is HB_sAg-positive but anti-HB_s titer is protective, nothing is required. If source is HB_sAg-positive and anti-HB_s titer is not protective or if exposed person is a known nonresponder, give 0.06 mL/kg I.M. within 24 h. A second dose of hepatitis B immune globulin can be given 1 mo later if a booster dose of hepatitis B vaccine is not given.	Review vaccination status[6]
Source not tested or unknown	Test exposed person for anti-HB_s. If anti-HB_s titer is protective, nothing is required. If anti-HB_s titer is not protective, 0.06 mL/kg may be given along with a booster dose of hepatitis B vaccine.	Review vaccination status[6]

[1]HB_sAg = hepatitis B surface antigen; anti-HB_s = antibody to hepatitis B surface antigen; I.M. = intramuscularly; SRU = standard ratio units.

[2]Each 0.5 mL dose of plasma-derived hepatitis B vaccine contains 10 mcg of HB_sAg; each 0.5 mL dose of recombinant hepatitis B vaccine contains 5 mcg (Merck Sharp & Dohme) or 10 mcg (SmithKline Beecham) of HB_sAg.

[3]If hepatitis B immune globulin and hepatitis B vaccine are given simultaneously, they should be given at separate sites.

[4]If hepatitis B vaccine is not given, a second dose of hepatitis B immune globulin should be given 1 month later.

[5]Anti-HB_s titers <10 SRU by radioimmunoassay or negative by enzyme immunoassay indicate lack of protection. Testing the exposed person for anti-HB_s is not necessary if a protective level of antibody has been shown within the previous 24 months.

[6]If the exposed person has not completed a three-dose series of hepatitis B vaccine, the series should be completed. Test the exposed person for anti-HB_s. If the antibody level is protective, nothing is required. If an adequate antibody response in the past is shown on retesting to have declined to an inadequate level, a booster dose (1 mL) of hepatitis B vaccine should be given. If the exposed person has inadequate antibody or is a known nonresponder to vaccination, a booster dose can be given along with one dose of hepatitis B immune globulin.

IMMUNIZATION RECOMMENDATIONS *(Continued)*

PREVENTION OF HEPATITIS A THROUGH ACTIVE OR PASSIVE IMMUNIZATION: RECOMMENDATIONS OF THE ADVISORY COMMITTEE ON IMMUNIZATION PRACTICES (ACIP)

PROPHYLAXIS AGAINST HEPATITIS A VIRUS INFECTION

Recommended Doses of Immune Globulin (IG) for Hepatitis A Pre-exposure and Postexposure Prophylaxis[1]

Setting	Duration of Coverage	IG Dose[2]
Pre-exposure	Short-term (1-2 months)	0.02 mL/kg
	Long-term (3-5 months)	0.06 mL/kg[3]
Postexposure	—	0.02 mL/kg

[1]Infants and pregnant women should receive a preparation that does not include thimerosal.

[2]IG should be administered by intramuscular injection into either the deltoid or gluteal muscle. For children <24 months of age, IG can be administered in the anterolateral thigh muscle.

[3]Repeat every 5 months if continued exposure to HAV occurs.

Recommended Dosages of Havrix®[1]

Vaccinee's Age (y)	Dose (EL.U.)[2]	Volume (mL)	No. Doses	Schedule (mo)[3]
2-18	720	0.5	2	0, 6-12
>18	1440	1.0	2	0, 6-12

[1]Hepatitis A vaccine, inactivated, SmithKline Beecham Biologicals.

[2]Enzyme-linked immunosorbent assay (ELISA) units.

[3]0 months represents timing of the initial dose; subsequent numbers represent months after the initial dose.

Recommended Dosages of VAQTA®[1]

Vaccinee's Age (y)	Dose (units)	Volume (mL)	No. Doses	Schedule (mo)[2]
2-17	25	0.5	2	0, 6-18
>17	50	1.0	2	0, 6

[1]Hepatitis A vaccine, inactivated, Merck & Company, Inc.

[2]0 months represents timing of the initial dose; subsequent numbers represent months after the initial dose.

Adapted from "Prevention of Hepatitis A Through Active or Passive Immunization: Recommendations of the Advisory Committee on Immunization Practices (ACIP)," *MMWR Recomm Rep*, 1999, 48(RR-12):1-37.

RECOMMENDATIONS FOR TRAVELERS

Recommended Immunizations for Travelers to Developing Countries[1]

Immunizations	Length of Travel		
	Brief, <2 wk	Intermediate, 2 wk - 3 mo	Long-term Residential, >3 mo
Review and complete age-appropriate childhood schedule	+	+	+
• DTaP; poliovirus vaccine, and *H. influenzae* type b vaccine may be given at 4-wk intervals if necessary to complete the recommended schedule before departure			
• Measles: 2 additional doses given if younger than 12 mo of age at first dose			
• Varicella			
• Hepatitis B[2]			
Yellow fever[3]	+	+	+
Hepatitis A[4]	+	+	+
Typhoid fever[4]	±	+	+
Meningococcal disease[5]	±	±	+
Rabies[6]	±	+	+
Japanese encephalitis[3]	±	±	+

[1] + = recommended; ± = consider.
[2] If insufficient time to complete 6-month primary series, accelerated series can be given.
[3] For endemic regions, see *Health Information for International Travel* in *Red Book®*. For high-risk activities in areas experiencing outbreaks, vaccine is recommended even for brief travel.
[4] Indicated for travelers who will consume food and liquids in areas of poor sanitation.
[5] For endemic regions of Africa, during local epidemics, and travel to Saudi Arabia for the Hajj.
[6] Indicated for person with high risk of animal exposure, and for travelers to endemic countries.
Adapted from "Report of the Committee on Infectious Diseases," *2003 Red Book®*, 26th ed, 94.

Recommendations for Pre-exposure Immunoprophylaxis of Hepatitis A Virus Infection for Travelers[1]

Age (y)	Likely Exposure (mo)	Recommended Prophylaxis
<2	<3	IG, 0.02 mL/kg[2]
	3-5	IG, 0.06 mL/kg[2]
	Long-term	IG, 0.06 mL/kg at departure and every 5 mo if exposure to HAV continues[2]
≥2	<3[3]	HAV vaccine[4,5] **or** IG, 0.02 mL/kg[2]
	3-5[3]	HAV vaccine[4,5] **or** IG, 0.06 mL/kg[2]
	Long-term	HAV vaccine[4,5]

[1] IG = immune globulin; HAV = hepatitis A virus.
[2] IG should be administered deep into a large muscle mass. Ordinarily, no more than 5 mL should be administered in one site in an adult or large child; lesser amounts (maximum 3 mL) should be given to small children and infants.
[3] Vaccine is preferable, but IG is an acceptable alternative.
[4] To ensure protection in travelers whose departure is imminent, IG also may be given.
[5] Dose and schedule of hepatitis A vaccine as recommended according to age.
Adapted from "Report of the Committee on Infectious Diseases," *2003 Red Book®*, 26th ed, 312.

IMMUNIZATION RECOMMENDATIONS *(Continued)*

Prevention of Malaria[1]

Drug	Adult Dosage	Pediatric Dosage
Chloroquine-Sensitive Areas[2]		
Chloroquine phosphate[3,4]	500 mg (300 mg base), once/week[5]	5 mg/kg base once/week, up to adult dose of 300 mg base[5]
Chloroquine-Resistant Areas[2]		
Mefloquine[4,6,7]	250 mg once/week[5]	<15 kg: 5 mg/kg[5] 15-19 kg: ¼ tablet[5] 20-30 kg: ½ tablet[5] 31-45 kg: ¾ tablet[5] >45 kg: 1 tablet[5]
or		
Doxycycline[4,8]	100 mg/d[9]	2 mg/kg/d, up to 100 mg/d[9]
or		
Atovaquone/proguanil[4,10]	250 mg/100 mg (1 tablet) daily[11]	11-20 kg: 62.5 mg/25 mg[10,11] 21-30 kg: 125 mg/50 mg[10,11] 31-40 kg: 187.5 mg/75 mg[10,11] >40 kg: 250 mg/100 mg[10,11]
Alternative:		
Primaquine[8,12,13]	30 mg base daily	0.5 mg/kg base daily
Chloroquine phosphate[3]	500 mg (300 mg base), once/week[5]	5 mg/kg base once/week, up to adult dose of 300 mg base[5]
plus		
Proguanil[14]	200 mg once/day	<2 y: 50 mg once/day 2-6 y: 100 mg once/day 7-10 y: 150 mg once/day >10 y: 200 mg once/day

[1]No drug regimen guarantees protection against malaria. If fever develops within a year (particularly within the first 2 months) after travel to malarious areas, travelers should be advised to seek medical attention. Insect repellents, insecticide-impregnated bed nets, and proper clothing are important adjuncts for malaria prophylaxis.

[2]Chloroquine-resistant *P. falciparum* occurs in all malarious areas except Central America west of the Panama Canal Zone, Mexico, Haiti, the Dominican Republic, and most of the Middle East (chloroquine resistance has been reported in Yemen, Oman, Saudi Arabia, and Iran).

[3]In pregnancy, chloroquine prophylaxis has been used extensively and safely.

[4]For prevention of attack after departure from areas where *P. vivax* and *P. ovale* are endemic, which includes almost all areas where malaria is found (except Haiti), some experts prescribe in addition primaquine phosphate 26.3 mg (15 mg base)/day or, for children, 0.3 mg base/kg/day during the last 2 weeks of prophylaxis. Others prefer to avoid the toxicity of primaquine and rely on surveillance to detect cases when they occur; particularly when exposure was limited or doubtful.

[5]Beginning 1-2 weeks before travel and continuing weekly for the duration of stay and for 4 weeks after leaving.

[6]In the U.S., a 250 mg tablet of mefloquine contains 228 mg mefloquine base. Outside the U.S., each 275 mg tablet contains 250 mg base.

[7]The pediatric dosage has not been approved by the FDA, and the drug has not been approved for use during pregnancy. However, it has been reported to be safe for prophylactic use during the second or third trimester of pregnancy and possibly during early pregnancy as well (CDC Health Information for International Travel, 2001-2003, 113; BL Smoak, Writer JV, Keep LW, et al, "The Effects of Inadvertent Exposure of Mefloquine Chemoprophylaxis on Pregnancy Outcomes and Infants of US Army Servicewomen," *J Infect Dis*, 1997, 176(3):831-3). Mefloquine is not recommended for patients with cardiac conduction abnormalities. Patients with a history of seizures or psychiatric disorders should avoid mefloquine (*Medical Letter*, 1990, 32:13). Resistance to mefloquine has been reported in some areas, such as Thailand; in these areas, doxycycline should be used for prophylaxis. In children <8 years of age, proguanil plus sulfisoxazole has been used (KN Suh and JS Keystone, *Infect Dis Clin Pract*, 1996, 5:541).

[8]An approved drug, but considered investigational for this condition by the U.S. Food and Drug Administration.

[9]Beginning 1-2 days before travel and continuing for the duration of stay and for 4 weeks after leaving. Use of tetracyclines is contraindicated in pregnancy and in children <8 years of age. Doxycycline can cause gastrointestinal disturbances, vaginal moniliasis, and photosensitivity reactions.

[10]Atovaquone plus proguanil is available as a fixed-dose combination tablet: adult tablets (250 mg atovaquone/100 mg proguanil, *Malarone*) and pediatric tablets (62.5 mg atovaquone/25 mg proguanil, *Malarone Pediatric*). To enhance absorption, it should be taken within 45 minutes after eating (Looareesuwan S, Chulay JD, Canfield CJ, et al, "Malarone (Atovaquone and Proguanil Hydrochloride): A Review of Its Clinical Development for Treatment of Malaria. Malarone Clinical Trials Study Group," *Am J Trop Med Hyg*, 1999, 60(4):533-41). Although approved for once daily dosing, to decrease nausea and vomiting the dose for treatment is usually divided in two.

[11]Shanks GE et al, *Clin Infect Dis*, 1998, 27:494; Lell B, Luckner D, Ndjave M, et al, "Randomised Placebo-Controlled Study of Atovaquone Plus Proguanil for Malaria Prophylaxis in Children," *Lancet*, 1998, 351(9104):709-13. Beginning 1-2 days before travel and continuing for the duration of stay and for 1 week after leaving. In one study of malaria prophylaxis, atovaquone/proguanil was better tolerated than mefloquine in nonimmune travelers (Overbosch D, Schilthuis H, Bienzle U, et al, "Atovaquone-Proguanil Versus Mefloquine for Malaria Prophylaxis in Nonimmune Travelers: Results From a Randomized, Double-Blind Study," *Clin Infect Dis*, 2001, 33(7):1015-21).

[12]Primaquine phosphate can cause hemolytic anemia, especially in patients whose red cells are deficient in glucose-6-phosphate dehydrogenase. This deficiency is most common in African, Asian, and Mediterranean peoples. Patients should be screened for G6PD deficiency before treatment. Primaquine should not be used during pregnancy.

[13]Several studies have shown that daily primaquine, beginning 1 day before departure and continued until 7 days after leaving the malaria area, provides effective prophylaxis against chloroquine-resistant *P. falciparum* (Baird JK, Lacy MD, Basri H, et al, "Randomized, Parallel Placebo-Controlled Trial of Primaquine for Malaria Prophylaxis in Papua, Indonesia," *Clin Infect Dis*, 2001, 33(12):1990-7). Some studies have shown less efficacy against *P. vivax*. Nausea and abdominal pain can be diminished by taking with food.

[14]Proguanil (Paludrine – Wyeth Ayerst, Canada; AstraZeneca, United Kingdom), which is not available alone in the U.S.A. but is widely available in Canada and Europe, is recommended mainly for use in Africa south of the Sahara. Prophylaxis is recommended during exposure and for 4 weeks afterwards. Proguanil has been used in pregnancy without evidence of toxicity (Phillips-Howard PA and Wood D, "The Safety of Antimalarial Drugs in Pregnancy," *Drug Saf*, 1996, 14(3):131-45).

Adapted from "Report of the Committee on Infectious Diseases," *2003 Red Book®*, 26th ed, 760-1.

ADVERSE EVENTS AND VACCINATION

Reportable Events Following Vaccination[1]

Vaccine / Toxoid		Event	Onset Interval
Tetanus in any combination; DTaP, DTP, DTP-Hib, DT, Td, TT	A.	Anaphylaxis or anaphylactic shock	7 days
	B.	Brachial neuritis	28 days
	C.	Any sequela (including death) of above events	Not applicable
	D.	Events described in manufacturer's package insert as contraindications to additional doses of vaccine	See package insert
Pertussis in any combination; DTaP, DTP, DTP-Hib, P	A.	Anaphylaxis or anaphylactic shock	7 days
	B.	Encephalopathy (or encephalitis)	7 days
	C.	Any sequela (including death) of above events	Not applicable
	D.	Events described in manufacturer's package insert as contraindications to additional doses of vaccine	See package insert
Measles, mumps, and rubella in any combination; MMR, MR, M, R	A.	Anaphylaxis or anaphylactic shock	7 days
	B.	Encephalopathy (or encephalitis)	15 days
	C.	Any sequela (including death) of above events	Not applicable
	D.	Events described in manufacturer's package insert as contraindications to additional doses of vaccine	See package insert
Rubella in any combination; MMR, MR, R	A.	Chronic arthritis	42 days
	B.	Any sequela (including death) of above events	Not applicable
	C.	Events described in manufacturer's package insert as contraindications to additional doses of vaccine	See package insert
Measles in any combination; MMR, MR, M	A.	Thrombocytopenic purpura	7-30 days
	B.	Vaccine-strain measles viral infection in an immunodeficient recipient	6 months
	C.	Any sequela (including death) of above events	Not applicable
	D.	Events described in manufacturer's package insert as contraindications to additional doses of vaccine	See package insert
Inactivated polio (IPV)	A.	Anaphylaxis or anaphylactic shock	7 days
	B.	Any sequela (including death) of above events	Not applicable
	C.	Events described in manufacturer's package insert as contraindications to additional doses of vaccine	See package insert
Hepatitis B	A.	Anaphylaxis or anaphylactic shock	7 days
	B.	Any sequela (including death) of above events	Not applicable
	C.	Events described in manufacturer's package insert as contraindications to additional doses of vaccine	See package insert
Haemophilus influenzae type b (conjugate)	A.	Events described in manufacturer's package insert as contraindications to additional doses of vaccine	See package insert
Varicella	A.	Events described in manufacturer's package insert as contraindications to additional doses of vaccine	See package insert
Rotavirus	A.	Intussusception	30 days
	B.	Any sequela (including death) of above events	Not applicable
	C.	Events described in manufacturer's package insert as contraindications to additional doses of vaccine	See package insert
Pneumococcal conjugate	A.	Events described in manufacturer's package insert as contraindications to additional doses of vaccine	See package insert

[1]Effective date: August 26, 2002.
The Reportable Events Table (RET) reflects what is reportable by law (42 USC 300aa-25) to the Vaccine Adverse Event Reporting System (VAERS), including conditions found in the manufacturer's package insert. In addition, individuals are encouraged to report **any** clinically significant or unexpected events (even if you are not certain the vaccine caused the event) for **any** vaccine, whether or not it is listed on the RET. Manufacturers are also required by regulation (21CFR 600.80) to report to the VAERS program all adverse events made known to them for any vaccine.

Adapted from the website http://www.vaers.org/reportable.htm. For further information, contact VAERS at 1-800-822-7967.

IMMUNIZATIONS[1] (VACCINES[2])

Drug	Use	Stability	Dosage and Administration
Anthrax vaccine (adsorbed)[2,3] BioThrax™	Immunization against *Bacillus anthracis*, recommended for individuals who may come in contact with animal products which come from anthrax endemic areas and may be contaminated with *Bacillus anthracis* spores; postexposure prophylaxis in combination with antibiotics, recommended for high-risk persons such as veterinarians and others handling potentially infected animals; routine immunization for the general population is not recommended. The Department of Defense is implementing an anthrax vaccination program against the biological warfare agent anthrax, which will be administered to all active duty and reserve personnel. **Note:** Safety and efficacy not established for adults >65 years of age.	Store under refrigeration at 2°C to 8°C (36°F to 46°F). Do not freeze. Do not mix with other injections or use the same site. Shake well before use; do not use if discolored or contains particulate matter.	SubQ: Children ≥18 years and Adults: Three injections of 0.5 mL each given 2 weeks apart, followed by three additional injections given at 6-, 12-, and 18 months; booster at 1-year intervals Massage site to disperse the vaccine postinjection. It is not necessary to restart the series if a dose is not given on time; resume as soon as practical.
BCG vaccine[5] TheraCys®; TICE® BCG	Immunization against tuberculosis and immunotherapy for cancer; treatment of bladder cancer; strongly recommended for infants and children with negative tuberculin skin tests who are at high risk of intimate and prolonged exposure to persistently untreated or ineffectively treated patients with infectious pulmonary tuberculosis; cannot be removed from the source of exposure; cannot be placed on long-term preventive therapy; and are continuously exposed with tuberculosis who have bacilli resistant to isoniazid and rifampin; recommended for tuberculin-negative infants and children in groups in which the rate of new infections exceeds 1% per year and for whom the usual surveillance and treatment programs have been attempted but are not operationally feasible	Refrigerate; protect from light. Use TICE® BCG within 2 hours of mixing.	Children >1 month and Adults: **Immunization against tuberculosis** (TICE® BCG): 0.2-0.3 mL percutaneous; initial lesion usually appears after 10-14 days consisting of small red papule at injection site and reaches maximum diameter of 3 mm in 4-6 weeks. Conduct postvaccinal tuberculin test (ie, 5 TU of PPD) in 2-3 months; if test is negative, repeat vaccination. **Immunotherapy for bladder cancer:** *Intravesical treatment:* Instill into bladder for 2 hours *TheraCys®:* One dose instilled into the bladder once weekly for 6 weeks followed by one treatment at 3, 6, 12, 18, and 24 months *TICE® BCG:* One dose instilled into the bladder once weekly for 6 weeks followed by once monthly for 6-12 months (should only be given intravesicularly or percutaneously)
Diphtheria and tetanus toxoid[6]	Active immunity against diphtheria and tetanus when pertussis vaccine is contraindicated; tetanus prophylaxis in wound management	Refrigerate.	I.M.: **Children: 6 weeks to 1 year of age:** DT: Three 0.5 mL doses at least 4 weeks apart; administer a reinforcing dose 6-12 months after third injection. **Children >1-6 years:** DT: Two 0.5 mL doses at least 4 weeks apart; reinforcing dose 6-12 months after second injection **Children 4-6 years:** Booster: DT: 0.5 mL; not necessary if all 4 doses were given after fourth birthday; administer doses at 10-year intervals with adult preparation. **Children ≥7 years and Adults:** Td: 2 primary doses of 0.5 mL each, given at an interval of 4-6 weeks; third (reinforcing) dose of 0.5 mL 6-12 months later; booster every 10 years
Diphtheria, tetanus toxoids, and acellular pertussis vaccine[6] Daptacel™; Infanrix®; Tripedia®	Active immunization of children from 6 weeks of age through seventh birthday for prevention of diphtheria, tetanus, and pertussis	Refrigerate at 2°C to 8°C (35°F to 46°F); do not freeze.	I.M. (anterolateral aspect of thigh or deltoid muscle of upper arm): **Children 6 weeks through 6 years of age** (use same product for all 3 doses): Three doses of 0.5 mL, usually given at 2-, 4-, and 6 months of age; may be repeated every 4-8 weeks; booster: fourth dose given at ~15-20 months of age, but at least 6 months after third dose. Fifth dose given at 5-6 years of age, prior to starting school or kindergarten. (If the fourth dose is given at 4 years of age, the fifth dose may be omitted.) **Children ≥7 years and Adults:** Adult Td preparation is the preferred agent.
Diphtheria, tetanus toxoids, acellular pertussis vaccine and *Haemophilus influenzae* b conjugate vaccine (combined)[2,5] TriHIBit®	Active immunization of children 15-18 months of age for prevention of diphtheria, tetanus, pertussis, and invasive disease caused by *H. influenzae* type b	Should be used within 30 minutes of reconstitution.	I.M.: Children >15 months of age: 0.5 mL TriHIBit® vaccine used to reconstitute ActHIB® (*Haemophilus* b conjugate) vaccine. The combination can be used for the DTaP dose given at 15-18 months when Tripedia® was used for the initial doses and a primary series of HIB vaccine has been given.

Drug	Use	Stability	Dosage and Administration
Diphtheria, tetanus toxoids, acellular pertussis, hepatitis B (recombinant), and poliovirus (inactivated) vaccine[5,6] Pediarix™	Active immunization against diphtheria, tetanus, pertussis, hepatitis B virus (all known subtypes), and poliomyelitis (caused by poliovirus types 1, 2, and 3)	Store under refrigeration of 2°C to 8°C (36°F to 46°F). Do not freeze; discard if frozen. Do not administer additional vaccines or immunoglobulins at the same site, or use the same syringe. Shake well prior to use; do not use unless a homogeneous, turbid, white suspension forms.	I.M. (anterolateral aspects of the thigh or the deltoid muscle of the upper arm): **Immunization:** Vaccination usually begins at 2 months, but may be started as early as 6 weeks of age; 0.5 mL; repeat in 6-8 week intervals (preferably 8-week) for a total of 3 doses. **Children previously vaccinated with one or more components and who are also scheduled to receive all vaccine components** (safety and efficacy not established): *Hepatitis B vaccine:* Infants born of HBsAg-negative mothers who received 1 dose of hepatitis B vaccine at birth may be given Pediarix™. Infants who received 1 or more doses of hepatitis B vaccine (recombinant) may be given Pediarix™ to complete the hepatitis B series. *Diphtheria and tetanus toxoids, and acellular pertussis vaccine (DTaP):* Infants previously vaccinated with 1 or 2 doses of Infanrix® may use Pediarix™ to complete the first 3 doses of the series; use of Pediarix™ to complete DTaP vaccination started with products other than Infanrix® is not recommended. *Inactivated polio vaccine (IPV):* Infants previously vaccinated with 1 or 2 doses of IPV may use Pediarix™ to complete the first 3 doses of the series.
Haemophilus b conjugate vaccine[2,6] ActHIB®; HibTITER®; PedvaxHIB®	Routine immunization of children 2 months to 5 years of age against invasive disease caused by *H. influenzae* ; unimmunized children 5 years of age with a chronic illness known to be associated with increased risk of *Haemophilus influenzae* type b disease, specifically, persons with anatomic or functional asplenia or sickle cell anemia or those who have undergone splenectomy, should receive Hib vaccine. *Haemophilus* b conjugate vaccines are not indicated for prevention of bronchitis or other infections due to *H. influenzae* in adults; adults with specific dysfunction or certain complement deficiencies who are at especially high risk of *H. influenzae* type b infection (HIV-infected adults); patients with Hodgkin's disease (vaccinated at least 2 weeks before the initiation of chemotherapy or 3 months after the end of chemotherapy)	Keep in refrigerator; may be frozen (not diluent) without affecting potency. Reconstituted Hib-Imune® remains stable for only 8 hours, whereas HibVAX® remain stable for 30 days when refrigerated.	**Note:** The same brand drug should be used throughout the vaccination series. If vaccine previously used is unknown, infants (2-6 months of age) should be given a primary series of three doses. Have epinephrine 1:1000 available. I.M. Children: 0.5 mL as a single dose administered according to one of the following "brand-specific" schedules (boosters to be given at least 2 months after previous dose): **HibTITER®:** Age at 1st dose: *2-6 months:* 3 doses, 2 months apart; booster in 15 months *7-11 months:* 2 doses, 2 months apart; booster in 15 months *12-14 months:* 1 dose; booster in 15 months *15-60 months:* 1 dose; no booster **PedvaxHIB®:** Age at 1st dose: *2-6 months:* 2 doses, 2 months apart; booster in 12 months *7-11 months:* 2 doses, 2 months apart; booster in 15 months *12-14 months:* 1 dose; booster in 15 months *15-60 months:* 1 dose; no booster **ProHIBIT®:** Age at 1st dose: 15-60 months: 1 dose; no booster

IMMUNIZATIONS[1] (VACCINES[2]) *(Continued)*

Drug	Use	Stability	Dosage and Administration
Hepatitis A vaccine[2,5,6] Havrix®; VAQTA®; Avaxim®; Avaxim®-Pediatric; Epaxal Berna®	Protection against hepatitis A or for populations at risk: travelers to developing countries, household and sexual contact with persons infected with hepatitis A, child day care employees, patients with chronic liver disease, illicit drug users, male homosexuals, institutional workers (eg, institutions for the mentally and physically handicapped persons, prisons, etc), and healthcare workers who may be exposed to hepatitis A virus (eg, laboratory employees); protection lasts for ~15 years		**Note:** Use caution in patients with serious active infection, cardiovascular disease, or pulmonary disorders; treatment for anaphylactic reactions should be immediately available. **Havrix®:** *Children 2-18 years:* 720 ELISA units (administered as 2 injections of 360 ELISA units [0.5 mL]) 15-30 days prior to travel; booster in 6-12 months *Adults:* 1440 ELISA units (1 mL) 15-30 days prior to travel with a booster 6-12 months following primary immunization **VAQTA®:** *Children 2-17 years:* 25 units (0.5 mL) with 25 units (0.5 mL); booster in 6-18 months *Adults:* 50 units (1 mL) with 50 units (1 mL); booster in 6 months
Hepatitis A (inactivated) and hepatitis B (recombinant) vaccine[2,5,6] Twinrix®	Active immunization against disease caused by hepatitis A virus and hepatitis B virus (all known subtypes) in populations desiring protection against or at high risk of exposure to these viruses: travelers to areas of intermediate/high endemicity for **both** HAV and HBV; those at increased risk of HBV infection due to behavioral or occupational factors: patients with chronic liver disease; laboratory workers who handle live HAV and HBV; healthcare workers, police, and other personnel who render first aid or medical assistance; workers who come in contact with sewage; employees of day care centers and correctional facilities; patients/staff of hemodialysis units; male homosexuals; patients frequently receiving blood products; military personnel; users of injectable illicit drugs; close household contacts of patients with hepatitis A and hepatitis B infection	Store in refrigerator at 2°C to 8°C (36°F to 46°F). Do not freeze (discard if frozen). Do not use the same syringe or site as additional vaccines or immunoglobulins. Shake well prior to use; do not dilute.	I.M. (deltoid muscle): Adults: Three doses (1 mL each) given on a 0-, 1-, and 6-month schedule
Hepatitis B immune globulin BayHepB™; Nabi-HB®	Provide prophylactic passive immunity to hepatitis B infection to those individuals exposed; newborns of mothers known to be hepatitis B surface antigen positive; not indicated for treatment of active hepatitis B infections; ineffective in the treatment of chronic active hepatitis B infection	Refrigerate at 2°C to 8°C (36°F to 46°F); do not freeze.	HBIG may be administered at the same time (but at a different site) or up to 1 month preceding hepatitis B vaccination without impairing the active immune response. I.M. (gluteal or deltoid region): **Newborns:** Hepatitis B: 0.5 mL as soon after birth as possible (within 12 hours); may repeat at 3 months in order for a higher rate of prevention of the carrier state to be achieved. At this time, an active vaccination program with the vaccine may begin. **Adults:** Postexposure prophylaxis: 0.06 mL/kg as soon as possible after exposure (ie, within 24 hours of needlestick, ocular, or mucosal exposure or within 14 days of sexual exposure); usual dose: 3-5 mL; repeat at 28-30 days after exposure

Drug	Use	Stability	Dosage and Administration
Hepatitis B vaccine Engerix-B®= Recombivax HB®	Immunization against infection caused by all known subtypes of hepatitis B virus in individuals considered at high risk of potential exposure to hepatitis B virus or HB,Ag-positive materials. Immunity will last~5-7 years.	Refrigerate at 2°C to 8°C (36°F to 46°F); do not freeze. Shake well prior to withdrawal and use.	It is possible to interchange the vaccines for completion of a series or for booster doses; the antibody produced in response to each type of vaccine is comparable, however, the quantity of vaccine will vary. Administer with caution in patients receiving anticoagulant therapy. SubQ injection may be administered in patients at risk of hemorrhage which may result in an increased incidence of local reactions and a reduced therapeutic effect. Refer to specific product labeling for dosing. **I.M.** (deltoid muscle): Adults: Immunization regimen consists of 3 doses (0, 1, and 6 months); first dose given on the elected date; second dose given 1 month later; third dose given 6 months after the first dose **Recombivax HB®**: *Children 11-15 years* (10 mcg/mL adult formulation): First dose of 1 mL given on the elected date, second dose given 4-6 months later **Engerix-B®**: *Children ≥10 years*: (10 mcg/0.5 mL formulation): High-risk children: 0.5 mL at 0, 1, 2, and 12 months; lower-risk children ages 5-10 who are candidates for an extended administration schedule may receive an alternative regimen of 0.5 mL at 0, 12, and 24 months.; if booster is needed, revaccinate with 0.5 mL *Adolescents 11-19 years* (20 mcg/mL formulation): 1 mL at 0, 1, and 6 months. High-risk adolescents: 1 mL at 0, 1, 2, and 12 months; lower-risk adolescents 11-16 years who are candidates for an extended administration schedule may receive an alternative regimen of 0.5 mL (using the 10 mcg/0.5 mL) formulation at 0, 12, and 24 months; if booster is needed, revaccinate with 20 mcg *Adults ≥ 20 years*: High-risk adults (20 mcg/mL formulation): 1 mL at 0, 1, 2, and 12 months; if booster dose is needed, revaccinate with 1 mL

IMMUNIZATIONS[1] (VACCINES[2]) *(Continued)*

Drug	Use	Stability	Dosage and Administration
Immune globulin (intramuscular) BayGam®	Household and sexual contacts of persons with hepatitis A, measles, varicella, and possibly rubella; travelers to high-risk areas outside tourist routes; staff, attendees, and parents of diapered attendees in daycare center outbreaks. For travelers, IG is not an alternative to careful selection of foods and water; frequent travelers should be tested for hepatitis A antibody; immune hemolytic anemia, and neutropenia (with TTP, I.V. route is usually used).	Refrigerate; do not freeze. Do not mix with other medications.	Skin testing should not be performed as local irritation can occur and be misinterpreted as a positive reaction. Immune globulin can interfere with the antibody response to parenterally administered live virus vaccines. I.M.: **Hepatitis A:** *Pre-exposure prophylaxis upon travel into endemic areas (hepatitis A vaccine preferred):* 0.02 mL/kg for anticipated risk 1-3 months; 0.06 mL/kg for anticipated risk >3 months; repeat approximate dose every 4-6 months if exposure continues. *Postexposure prophylaxis:* 0.02 mL/kg given within 2 weeks of exposure **Measles:** Prophylaxis: 0.25 mL/kg/dose (max: 15 mL) given within 6 days of exposure followed by live attenuated measles vaccine in 3 months or at 15 months of age (whichever is later) **Leukemia, lymphoma, immunodeficiency disorders, generalized malignancy, or those receiving immunosuppressive therapy:** 0.5 mL/kg (max: 15 mL). **Poliomyelitis:** Prophylaxis: 0.3 mL/kg/dose as a single dose **Rubella:** Prophylaxis: 0.55 mL/kg/dose within 72 hours of exposure **Varicella:** Prophylaxis: 0.6-1.2 mL/kg (varicella-zoster immune globulin preferred) within 72 hours of exposure **IgG deficiency:** 1.3 mL/kg, then 0.66 mL/kg in 3-4 weeks **Hepatitis B:** Prophylaxis: 0.06 mL/kg/dose (HBIG preferred)
Influenza virus vaccine FluMist™ Fluvirin® Fluzone®	Provide active immunity to influenza virus strains contained in the vaccine; for high-risk persons including those ≥65 years of age; residents of nursing homes and other chronic-care facilities that house persons of any age with chronic medical conditions; adults and children with chronic disorders of the pulmonary or cardiovascular systems (asthma); adults and children who have required regular medical follow-up or hospitalization during the preceding year because of chronic metabolic diseases (including diabetes mellitus), renal dysfunction, hemoglobinopathies, or immunosuppression (including immunosuppression caused by medications); children and adolescents (6 months to 18 years of age) who are receiving long-term aspirin therapy and therefore, may be at risk for developing Reye's syndrome after influenza; women who will be in the 2nd or 3rd trimester of pregnancy during the influenza season. Otherwise healthy children aged 6-23 months, healthy persons who may transmit influenza to those at risk, and others who are interested in immunization to influenza virus should receive the vaccine as long as supply is available.	Store between 2°C to 8°C (36°F to 46°F). Potency is destroyed by freezing; do not use if product has been frozen. Suspension should be shaken well prior to use; inspect for particulate matter and discoloration prior to administration. **Note:** Previous year vaccines should not be used to prevent present year influenza.	I.M.: (deltoid muscle in adults and older children; anterolateral aspect of the thigh in infants and young children): *Previously unvaccinated children <9 years:* 2 doses given >1 month apart **FluShield®, Fluzone®:** *Children 6-35 months:* 0.25 mL (1 or 2 doses) *Children 3-8 years:* 0.5 mL (1 or 2 doses) *Children ≥9 years and Adults:* 0.5 mL (1 dose) **Fluvirin®:** *Children 4-8 years:* 0.5 mL (1 or 2 doses) *Children ≥9 years and Adults:* 0.5 mL (1 dose)

Drug	Use	Stability	Dosage and Administration
Japanese encephalitis virus vaccine (inactivated) JE-VAX®	Active immunization against Japanese encephalitis for children ≥ 1 year of age and adults who plan to spend 1 month or more in endemic areas in Asia (especially persons traveling during the transmission season or visiting rural area); older adults >55 years of age should be considered for vaccination (due to increased risk of developing symptomatic illness after infection) Those planning travel to or residence in endemic areas should consult the Travel Advisory Service (Central Campus) for specific advice; consider vaccination for shorter trips to epidemic areas or extensive outdoor activities in rural endemic areas. Because of the potential for severe adverse reactions, Japanese encephalitis vaccine is not recommended for **all** persons traveling to or residing in Asia.	Refrigerate at 2°C to 8°C. Do not freeze. Discard 8 hours after reconstitution.	Severe adverse reactions may occur within minutes following vaccination or up to 17 days later; most reactions occur within 10 days (majority within 48 hours). Observe vaccinees for 30 minutes after vaccination; warn them of the possibility of delayed generalized urticaria and to remain where medical care is readily available for 10 days following any dose of the vaccine. U.S. recommended primary immunization schedule: **SubQ:** **Children 1-3 years:** Three 0.5 mL doses given on days 0, 7, and 30 **Children >3 years and Adults:** Three 1 mL doses given on days 0, 7, and 30; give third dose on day 14 when time does not permit waiting **Booster:** After 2 years, or according to current recommendation **Note:** Abbreviated schedules should be used only when necessary due to time constraints. Two doses a week apart produce immunity in about 80% of recipients; the longest regimen yields highest titers after 6 months. Travel should not commence ≤10 days after the last dose of vaccine, to allow adequate antibody formation and recognition of any delayed adverse reaction. Advise concurrent use of other means to reduce the risk of mosquito exposure when possible, including bed nets, insect repellents, protective clothing, avoidance of travel in endemic areas, and avoidance of outdoor activity during twilight and evening periods.
Measles, mumps, and rubella vaccines (combined) M-M-R® II	Prophylaxis for measles, mumps, and rubella	Prior to reconstitution, store the powder at 2°C to 8°C (36°F to 46°F) or colder (freezing does not affect potency). Protect from light. Diluent may be stored with powder or at room temperature.	SubQ (outer aspect of the upper arm): Infants >12 months: Administer 0.5 mL, then repeat at 4-6 years of age. If the second dose was not received, the schedule should be completed by the 11- to 12-year-old visit. If there is risk of exposure to measles, single-antigen measles vaccine should be administered at 6-11 months of age with a second dose (of MMR) at >12 months of age. **Note:** MMR vaccine should not be given within 3 months of immune globulin or whole blood. Have epinephrine available during and after administration. Should not be administered to severely immunocompromised persons with the exception of asymptomatic children with HIV (ACIP and AAP recommendation). Severely immunocompromised patients and symptomatic HIV-infected patients who are exposed to measles should receive immune globulin, regardless of prior vaccination status. Defer immunization during any acute illness. Females should not become pregnant within 3 months of vaccination.
Measles virus vaccine (live) Attenuvax®	Immunization for adults born after 1957 without documentation of live vaccine on or after first birthday, physician-diagnosed measles, or laboratory evidence of immunity should be vaccinated, ideally with two doses of vaccine separated by no less than 1 month; for those previously vaccinated with one dose of measles vaccine, revaccination is recommended for students entering colleges and other institutions of higher education, for healthcare workers at the time of employment, and for international travelers who visit endemic areas.	Refrigerate at 2°C to 8°C. Discard if left at room temperature for over 8 hours. Protect from light.	SubQ (outer aspect of upper arm): Children ≥15 months and Adults: 0.5 mL; no routine booster.

IMMUNIZATIONS[1] (VACCINES[2]) *(Continued)*

Drug	Use	Stability	Dosage and Administration
Meningococcal polysaccharide vaccine (groups A, C, Y, and W-135) Menomune®-A/C/Y/W-135	Immunization of children ≥2 years of age and adults in epidemic or endemic areas as might be determined in a population delineated by neighborhood, school, dormitory, or other reasonable boundary; the prevalent serogroup in such a situation should match a serogroup in the vaccine. Individuals at particular high-risk include persons with terminal component complement deficiencies and those with anatomic or function asplenia. For use with travelers visiting areas of a country that are recognized as having hyperendemic or epidemic meningococcal disease. Vaccinations should be considered for household or institutional contacts of persons with meningococcal disease as an adjunct to appropriate antibiotic chemoprophylaxis as well as medical and laboratory personnel at risk of exposure to meningococcal disease.	Store at 2°C to 8°C (35°F to 46°F).	SubQ: One dose (0.5 mL); individuals who are sensitive to thimerosal should receive single-dose pack (reconstituted with 0.78 mL vial without preservative); the need for booster is unknown; have epinephrine 1:1000 available
Mumps virus vaccine (live/attenuated) Mumpsvax®	Mumps prophylaxis by promoting active immunity. **Note:** Trivalent measles-mumps-rubella (M-M-R®) vaccine is the preferred agent for most children and many adults. Persons born prior to 1957 are generally considered immune and need not be vaccinated.	Refrigerate; protect from light. Discard within 8 hours after reconstitution.	SubQ (outer aspect of upper arm): Children ≥15 months and Adults: 0.5 mL; no booster
Plague vaccine	Vaccinate selected travelers to countries where avoidance of rodents and fleas is impossible; laboratory and field personnel working with *Yersinia pestis* organisms possibly resistant to antimicrobials; those engaged in *Yersinia pestis* aerosol experiments or in field operations in areas with enzootic plague where regular exposure to potentially infected wild rodents, rabbits, or their fleas cannot be prevented; prophylactic antibiotics may be indicated following definite exposure, whether or not the exposed persons have been vaccinated.		I.M.: Three doses: First dose 1 mL, second dose (0.2 mL), 1 month later, third dose (0.2 mL), 5 months after the second dose; booster at 1- to 2-year intervals if exposure continues

Drug	Use	Stability	Dosage and Administration
Pneumococcal conjugate vaccine (7-valent) Prevnar®	Immunization of infants and toddlers against active disease caused by *Streptococcus pneumoniae* due to serotypes included in the vaccine	Store refrigerated at 2°C to 8°C (36°F to 46°F).	Use of the pneumococcal conjugate vaccine does not replace the use of the 23-valent vaccine in children >24 months of age with sickle cell disease, asplenia, HIV infection, chronic illness, or if immunocompromised. I.M. **Infants: 2-6 months:** 0.5 mL at approximately 2 month-interval for 3 consecutive doses, followed by a fourth dose of 0.5 mL at 12-15 months of age. The first dose may be given as young as 2 months of age, but is typically given at 6 weeks of age. In case of a moderate shortage of vaccine, defer the fourth dose until shortage is resolved; in case of a severe shortage of vaccine, defer third and fourth doses until shortage is resolved. **Infants and Children (previously unvaccinated):** *7-11 months:* 0.5 mL for a total of 3 doses; 2 doses at least 4 weeks apart, followed by a third dose after the 1-year birthday, separated from the second dose by at least 2 months *12-23 months:* 0.5 mL for a total of two doses, separated by at least 2 months *24-59 months:* *Healthy Children:* 0.5 mL as a single dose. *Children with sickle cell disease, asplenia, HIV infection, chronic illness, or immunocompromising conditions (not including bone marrow transplants with results pending):* Use PPV23 (pneumococcal polysaccharide vaccine, polyvalent) at 12- and 24-months until studies are complete): 0.5 mL for a total of 2 doses, separated by 2 months **Children (previously vaccinated with a lapse in vaccination administration):** *7-11 months:* Previously received 1 or 2 doses PCV7: 0.5 mL dose at 7-11 months of age, followed by a second dose≥2 months later at 12-15 months of age. *12-23 months:* Previously received 1 dose before 12 months of age: 0.5 mL dose, followed by a second dose ≥2 months later.

IMMUNIZATIONS[1] (VACCINES[2]) *(Continued)*

Drug	Use	Stability	Dosage and Administration
Pneumococcal polysaccharide vaccine (polyvalent) Pneumovax® 23; Pneumo 23™	For children >2 years of age and adults who are at increased risk of pneumococcal disease and its complications because of underlying health conditions; older adults, including those ≥65 years of age	Refrigerate.	SubQ, I.M. (deltoid muscle or lateral midthigh): **Children >2 years and Adults:** 0.5 mL; have epinephrine (1:1000) available. **Revaccination** should be considered if: ≥6 years have elapsed since initial vaccination; for patients who received 14-valent pneumococcal vaccine and are at highest risk (asplenic) for fatal infection; at ≥6 years in patients with nephrotic syndrome, renal failure, or transplant recipients; and 3-5 years in children with nephrotic syndrome, asplenia, or sickle cell disease. Use with caution in individuals who have had episodes of pneumococcal infection within the preceding 3 years; may result in increased reactions to vaccine or cause relapse in patients with stable idiopathic thrombocytopenia purpura. **Previously vaccinated with PCV7 vaccine:** *With sickle cell disease, asplenia, immunocompromised or HIV infection:* 0.5 mL at 2 years of age and 2 months after last dose of PCV7; revaccination with PPV23 should be given 5 years for children >10 years of age and every 3-5 years for children <3 years of age; revaccination should be administered <3 years after the previous PPV23 dose *With chronic illness:* 0.5 mL at 2 years of age and 2 months after last dose of PCV7; revaccination with PPV23 is not recommended *Following bone marrow transplant (use of PCV7 under study):* Administer one dose PPV23 at 12- and 24-months following BMT.
Poliovirus vaccine (inactivated) IPOL®	All children should receive four doses of IPV (at age 2 months, age 4 months, between ages 6-18 months, and between ages 4-6 years). OPV supplies are expected to be very limited in the United States after inventories are depleted. ACIP reaffirms its support for the global eradication initiative and use of OPV as the vaccine of choice to eradicate polio where it is endemic. Oral poliovirus vaccine (OPV), if available, may be used only for the following special circumstances: Mass vaccination campaigns to control outbreaks of paralytic polio; unvaccinated children who will be traveling within 4 weeks to areas where polio is endemic or epidemic; children of parents who do not accept the recommended number of vaccine injections (these children may receive OPV only for the third or fourth dose or both; healthcare providers should administer OPV only after discussing the risk for VAPP with parents or caregivers)		**Infants 6-12 weeks of age:** Oral: 0.5 mL; second dose 6-8 weeks after first dose (commonly at 4 months); third dose 8-12 months after second dose (commonly at 18 months) **Older Children and Adults** (adolescents through 18 years of age): SubQ: Two 0.5 mL doses 4-8 weeks apart and a third dose of 0.5 mL, 6-12 months after second dose. Enhanced-potency inactivated poliovirus vaccine (E-IPV) is preferred for primary vaccination of adults, two doses 4-8 weeks apart, a third dose 6-12 months after the second. For adults with a completed primary series and for whom a booster is indicated, either OPV or E-IPV can be given (E-IPV preferred). If immediate protection is needed, either OPV or E-IPV is recommended. **Booster:** All children who have received primary immunization series, should receive a single follow-up dose and all children who have not completed primary series.
Rabies immune globulin (human) BayRab®; Imogam®	Part of postexposure prophylaxis of persons with rabies exposure who lack a history of pre-exposure or postexposure prophylaxis with rabies vaccine or a recently documented neutralizing antibody response to previous rabies vaccination; it is preferable to give RIG with the first dose of vaccine, but it can be given up to 8 days after vaccination. **Note:** RIG should always be administered in conjunction with rabies vaccine (HDCV) regimen (as soon as possible after the first dose of vaccine, up to 8 days). Persons with an adequate titer and those who have been completely immunized with rabies vaccine should not receive RIG, only booster doses of HDCV.	Refrigerate.	I.M. (gluteal muscle): 20 units/kg in a single dose Infiltrate half of the dose locally around the wound; administer the remainder I.M.

Drug	Use	Stability	Dosage and Administration
Rabies vaccine Imovax® Rabies; RabAvert®	**Pre-exposure immunization:** Vaccinate persons with greater than usual risk due to occupation or avocation including veterinarians, rangers, animal handlers, certain laboratory workers, and persons living in or visiting countries for >1 month where rabies is a constant threat. Complete pre-exposure prophylaxis does not eliminate the need for additional therapy with rabies vaccine after a rabies exposure. **Postexposure prophylaxis:** If a bite from a carrier animal is unprovoked and it is not captured and rabies is present in that species and area, administer rabies immune globulin (RIG) and the vaccine as indicated.	Refrigerate at 2°–8°C (36°–46°F); do not freeze. Protect from light. Use reconstituted vaccine immediately.	I.M. (deltoid muscle, in adults and older children; outer aspect of the thigh for younger children): **Pre-exposure prophylaxis:** 1 mL on days 0, 7, and 21–28; prolonging the interval between doses does not interfere with immunity achieved after concluding dose of the basic series. **Postexposure prophylaxis** (Cleanse wound with soap and water first.): *Persons not previously immunized:* 20 units/kg body weight, half infiltrated at bite site if possible, remainder I.M. and 5 doses of rabies vaccine, 1 mL on days 0, 3, 7, 14, and 28 *Persons who have previously received postexposure prophylaxis, pre-exposure series, or have a documented adequate rabies antibody titer:* 1 mL of either vaccine on days 0 and 3; do not administer RIG *Booster* (for occupational or other continuing risk): 1 mL every 2-5 years (or based on antibody titers)
Rubella virus vaccine (live) Meruvax® II	Selective active immunization against rubella; recommended for persons from 12 months of age to puberty; all adults lacking documentation of live vaccine on or after first birthday, or laboratory evidence of immunity should be vaccinated (particularly women of childbearing age; young adults who work in or congregate in hospitals, colleges, and on military bases; susceptible travelers) **Note:** Trivalent measles-mumps-rubella (M-M-R® II) vaccine is the preferred agent for most children and many adults. Persons born prior to 1957 are generally considered immune and need not be vaccinated.	Refrigerate; store at 2°C to 8°C (36°F to 46°F). Discard reconstituted vaccine after 8 hours. Ship using dry ice. Protect from light.	Children ≥12 months and Adults: SubQ (outer aspect of upper arm): 0.5 mL; avoid injection into blood vessel.
Smallpox vaccine[4] Dryvax®	Active immunization against vaccinia virus, the causative agent of smallpox ACIP recommends vaccination of laboratory workers at risk of exposure from cultures or contaminated animals which may be a source of vaccinia or related Orthopoxviruses capable of causing infections in humans (monkeypox, cowpox, or variola). Revaccination is recommended every 10 years. In October 2002, the FDA approved the licensing of the current stockpile of smallpox vaccine. This approval allows the vaccine to be distributed and administered in the event of a smallpox attack.	Store at 2°C to 8°C (36°F to 46°F). Do not freeze.	Using a bifurcated needle, 1 drop of vaccine is introduced into the superficial layers of the skin using a multiple-puncture technique. The skin over the insertion of the deltoid muscle or the posterior aspect of the arm over the triceps are the preferred sites for vaccination. A single-use bifurcated needle should be dipped carefully into the reconstituted vaccine (following removal of rubber stopper). Visually confirm that the needle picks up a drop of vaccine solution. Deposit the drop of vaccine onto clean, dry skin at the vaccination site. Holding the bifurcated needle perpendicular to the skin, punctures are to be made rapidly into the superficial skin of the vaccination site. The puncture strokes should be vigorous enough to allow a trace of blood to appear after approximately 15-20 seconds. Wipe off any remaining vaccine with dry sterile gauze. To prevent transmission of the virus, cover vaccination site with gauze and cover gauze with a semipermeable barrier or clothing. Good handwashing prevents inadvertent inoculation. Dispose of all materials in a biohazard waste container. All materials must be burned, boiled, or autoclaved. If no evidence of vaccine take is apparent after 7 days, the individual may be vaccinated again.

IMMUNIZATIONS[1] (VACCINES[2]) *(Continued)*

Drug	Use	Stability	Dosage and Administration
Tetanus antitoxin	Tetanus prophylaxis or treatment of active tetanus only when tetanus immune globulin (TIG) is not available; tetanus immune globulin (Hyper-Tet®) is the preferred tetanus immunoglobulin for the treatment of active tetanus. May be given concomitantly with tetanus toxoid adsorbed when immediate treatment is required, but active immunization is desirable.	Refrigerate; do not freeze.	**Note:** I.V. Tetanus antitoxin is not the same as tetanus immune globulin. Sensitivity testing should be conducted in all individuals regardless of clinical history. Have epinephrine 1:1000 available. **Prophylaxis:** I.M., SubQ: Children <30 kg: 1500 units Children and Adults ≥30 kg: 3000–5000 units **Treatment:** Children and Adults: Inject 10,000–40,000 units into wound; administer 40,000–100,000 units
Tetanus immune globulin (human) BayTet™	Passive immunization against tetanus (tetanus immune globulin is preferred over tetanus antitoxin for treatment of active tetanus); part of the management of an unclean wound in a person whose history of previous receipt of tetanus toxoid is unknown or who has received less than three doses of tetanus toxoid; elderly may require TIG more often than younger patients with tetanus infection due to declining antibody titers with age.	Refrigerate at 2°C to 8°C (36°F to 46°F). Never administer tetanus toxoid (Td) and TIG in the same syringe (toxoid will be neutralized).	Toxoid may be given at a separate site. Have epinephrine 1:1000 available. Boosters will be necessary. I.M.: **Prophylaxis:** Children: 4 units/kg (some recommend administering 250 units to small children) Adults: 250 units **Treatment:** Children: 500–3000 units (infiltrate some solution locally around the wound) Adults: 3000–6000 units
Tetanus toxoid (adsorbed)	Selective induction of active immunity against tetanus in selected patients. **Note:** Not equivalent to tetanus toxoid fluid. Tetanus and diphtheria toxoids for adult use (Td) is the preferred immunizing agent for most adults and for children after 7 years of age. Young children should receive trivalent DTwP or DTaP (diphtheria/tetanus/pertussis – whole cell or acellular), as part of their childhood immunization program, unless pertussis is contraindicated, then TD is warranted.	Refrigerate; do not freeze.	Have epinephrine 1:1000 available. Avoid injection into a blood vessel. I.M. (midthigh laterally or deltoid): Adults: 0.5 mL; repeat 0.5 mL at 4–8 weeks after the first dose and at 6–12 months after the second dose; booster every 5–10 years
Tetanus toxoid (fluid)	Detection of delayed hypersensitivity and assessment of cell-mediated immunity; active immunization against tetanus in the rare adult or child who is allergic to the aluminum adjuvant (a product containing adsorbed tetanus toxoid is preferred)	Refrigerate.	Have epinephrine 1:1000 available. Anergy testing: Adults: Intradermal: 0.1 mL (Td, TD, DTaP/DTwP recommended): Three doses of 0.5 mL I.M. or SubQ at 4- to 8-week intervals; give fourth dose 6-12 months after third dose; booster: 0.5 mL I.M., S.C every 10 years
Typhoid vaccine Typhim Vi® Vivotif Berna®	**Parenteral:** Promotes active immunity to typhoid fever for patients intimately exposed to a typhoid carrier or foreign travel to a typhoid fever endemic area. **Oral:** Immunization of children >6 years and adults who expect intimate exposure of or household contact with typhoid fever, travelers to areas of the world with a risk of exposure to typhoid fever, and workers in microbiology laboratories with expected frequent contact with *S. typhi*. **Typhoid vaccine:** Live, attenuated typhoid vaccine should not be administered to immunocompromised persons, including those known to be infected with HIV (parenteral inactivated vaccine is a theoretically safer alternative for this group)	Refrigerate, do not freeze; if mistakenly placed in a freezer, remove as soon as possible and place in refrigerator (potency unaffected). Can be used if exposed to temperature ≤80°F.	I.M. (deltoid muscle): Typhim Vi®: Children ≥2 years and Adults: 0.5 mL (25 mg) injection in given at least 2 weeks prior to expected exposure; reimmunization: 0.5 mL single dose every 2 years is currently recommended for repeated or continued exposure **Oral:** Children ≥6 years and Adults: Swallow 1 capsule whole (do not chew) 1 hour before a meal with cold or lukewarm drink on alternate days (day 1, 3, 5, and 7) for a total of 4 doses; booster every 5 years (full course). **Note:** Not all recipients of typhoid vaccine will be fully protected against typhoid fever. Unless a complete immunization schedule is followed, an optimum immune response may not be achieved.

Drug	Use	Stability	Dosage and Administration
Varicella virus vaccine Varivax®	The American Association of Pediatrics recommends that the chickenpox vaccine should be given to all healthy children between 12 months of age to 18 years. Children 12 months of age to 13 years who have not been immunized or who have not had chickenpox should receive 1 vaccination while children 13-18 years of age require 2 vaccinations 4-8 weeks apart. The vaccine has been added to the childhood immunization schedule for infants 12-28 months of age and children 11-12 years of age who have not been vaccinated previously or who have not had the disease. It is recommended to be given with the measles, mumps, and rubella (MMR) vaccine.	Store powder in freezer at -15°C (5°F); may be stored under refrigeration for up to 72 continuous hours prior to reconstitution. Protect from light. Discard vaccine if not used within 72 hours. Store diluent separately at room temperature or in refrigerator.	SubQ: **Children 12 months to 12 years:** 0.5 mL **Children ≥12 years to Adults:** 2 doses of 0.5 mL separated by 4-8 weeks.
Varicella-zoster immune globulin (human)	Passive immunization of susceptible immunodeficient patients after exposure to varicella. Most effective if begun within 96 hours of exposure. There is no evidence that VZIG modifies established varicella-zoster infections. **Restrict administration to:** Patients with neoplastic disease (leukemia, lymphoma); congenital or acquired immunodeficiency; immunosuppressive therapy with steroids, antimetabolites, or other immunosuppressive treatment regimens; newborns or mothers who had onset of chickenpox within 5 days before delivery or within 48 hours after delivery; premature infant (≥28 weeks gestation) whose mother has no history of chickenpox; premature infants (<28 weeks gestation or ≤1000 g VZIG) regardless of maternal history. **One of the following types of exposure to chickenpox or zoster patients may warrant administration:** Continuous household contact; playmate contact (>1 hour play indoors); hospital contact (in same 2-4 bedroom or adjacent beds in a large ward or prolonged face-to-face contact with an infectious staff member of patient); susceptible to varicella-zoster; age <15 years (administer to immunocompromised adolescents and adults and to other older patients on an individual basis). An acceptable alternative to VZIG prophylaxis is to treat varicella, if it occurs, with high-dose I.V. acyclovir.	Refrigerate at 2°C to 8°C.	I.M. (gluteal muscle or large muscle mass): 125 units/10 kg (22 lb); maximum dose: 625 units (5 vials); minimum dose: 125 units; do not administer fractional doses. High-risk susceptible patients who are exposed again more than 3 weeks after a prior dose of VZIG should receive another full dose; there is no evidence VZIG modifies established varicella-zoster infections.

IMMUNIZATIONS[1] (VACCINES[2]) *(Continued)*

Drug	Use	Stability	Dosage and Administration
Yellow fever vaccine YF-VAX®	Induction of active immunity against yellow fever virus, primarily among persons traveling or living in areas where yellow fever infection exists. (Some countries require a valid international Certification of Vaccination showing receipt of vaccine; if a pregnant woman is to be vaccinated only to satisfy an international requirement, efforts should be made to obtain a waiver letter.) The WHO requires revaccination every 10 years to maintain traveler's vaccination certificate.	Do not use vaccine unless shipping case contains some dry ice on arrival; must be shipped on dry ice. Maintain vaccine at continuous temperature of -30°C to 5°C (-22°F to 41°F). Use within 1 hour of reconstitution.	SubQ: 0.5 mL single dose 10 days to 10 years before travel; booster every 10 years

[1]Contact Poison Control Center.

[2]Federal law requires that date of administration, name of vaccine manufacturer, lot number of vaccine, and administering person's name, title, and address be entered into the patient's permanent medical record.

[3]Not commercially available in the U.S.; presently, all anthrax vaccine lots are owned by the U.S. Department of Defense. The Centers for Disease Control (CDC) does not currently recommend routine vaccination of the general public.

[4]The bulk of current supplies have been designated for use by the U.S. military. Bioterrorism experts have proposed immunization of first responders (including police, fire, and emergency workers), but these plans may not be implemented until additional stocks of vaccine are licensed. Recommendations for use in response to bioterrorism are regularly updated by the CDC, and may be found at www.cdc.gov.

[5]For patients at risk of hemorrhage following intramuscular injection, the ACIP recommends "it should be administered intramuscularly if, in the opinion of the physician familiar with the patients bleeding risk, the vaccine can be administered with reasonable safety by this route. If the patient receives antihemophilia or other similar therapy, intramuscular vaccination can be scheduled shortly after such therapy is administered. A fine needle (23 gauge or smaller) can be used for the vaccination and firm pressure applied to the site (without rubbing) for at least 2 minutes. The patient should be instructed concerning the risk of hematoma from the injection."

[6]All serious adverse reactions must be reported to the U.S. Department of Health and Human Services (DHHS) Vaccine Adverse Event Reporting System (VAERS), 1-800-822-7967.

SELECTED ADVERSE EFFECTS

Adverse drug reactions can range from inconvenient to life-threatening. The type of effects, the severity, and frequency of occurrence is dependent on the medication and dosage of the medication being used, as well as the individual's response to the therapy. Early recognition by healthcare providers or patients of these adverse side effects is a major factor if appropriate intervention is to implemented. The following are definitions of selected adverse effects, and examples of some (by no means all) medications associated with these adverse effects.

Name	Description
Acute tubular necrosis	Acute renal failure characterized by direct toxicity to tubular cells. Cellular debris (casts) are a prominent feature of urinary sediment. Usually requires several days of treatment. **Examples of associated drugs:** Aminoglycosides
Ageusia	Loss of sense of taste. **Examples of associated drugs:** Bleomycin, cisplatin, diltiazem
Akathisia	Evidenced by an uncontrollable constant need for motion, pacing, and squirming or restlessness; usually develops within first 2 months of antipsychotic treatment. **Examples of associated drugs:** Phenergan, haldol
Alopecia	Loss of body hair. **Examples of associated drugs:** Chemotherapeutic agents, beta-blockers
Anemia	A condition in which the number of red blood cells, the amount of hemoglobin, and the volume of packed red blood cells of blood is less than normal; manifested by pallor of the skin and mucus membranes, shortness of breath, palpitation of the heart, soft systolic murmurs, lethargy, fatigability, nosebleeds, bleeding gums, easy bruising, hematuria or blood in stool. **Examples of associated drugs:** Amoxicillin, warfarin
Angioedema	Localized swelling of the subcutaneous tissue of face, hands, feet, and genitalia. **Examples of associated drugs:** ACE inhibitors
Anhidrosis	Deficiency of or absence of sweat; since sweating is necessary for cooling, persons with anhidrosis are at increased risk for hyperthermia
Anorexia	Loss of desire for food. **Examples of associated drugs:** CNS stimulants
Anticholinergic effects	Usually used to describe blockade of muscarinic receptors. Symptoms include blurred vision, mydriasis, increased intraocular pressure, headache, flushing, tachycardia, nervousness, constipation, dizziness, insomnia, mental confusion or excitement, dry mouth, altered taste perception, dysphagia, constipation, palpitations, bradycardia, urinary hesitancy or retention, impotence, decreased sweating, susceptibility to heat prostration, thickening or drying of bronchial secretions. **Examples of associated drugs:** Tricyclic antidepressants, antihistamines
Anticoagulant skin necrosis	Occurs early in therapy (3-5) days with oral anticoagulants (eg, warfarin). A paradoxical effect of oral anticoagulant therapy which involves microembolization and necrosis of skin often localized to the abdomen, breast, buttock, and thigh regions. Genetic deficiency of protein C appears to be a risk factor. **Examples of associated drugs:** Oral anticoagulants (eg, warfarin)
Cushing's syndrome	Usually a response to excess levels of circulating glucocorticoids; resembles Cushing's disease (pituitary tumor); characterized by obesity, hyperglycemia, glycosuria, muscle weakness, menstrual irregularities, fluid and electrolyte disturbances, hirsutism, myopathy, and decreased resistance to infection. **Examples of associated drugs:** Prednisone
Disulfiram reaction	Many drugs will produce a disulfiram-type reaction when the patient ingests alcohol. Symptoms includes nausea and/or vomiting, pounding or throbbing headache, systemic flushing, respiratory difficulties (dyspnea, hyperventilation), sweating, excessive thirst, cardiac disturbances (chest pain, palpitations), vertigo, visual disturbances (blurred or double vision), and CNS disturbances (confusion, convulsions). **Examples of associated drugs:** Metronidazole, cephalosporins with MTT side chains
Drug fever	Persistent fever which may be associated with low-grade allergic reaction to a drug entity. Often develops several days after initial defervescence from antibiotics. Other causes of fever related to drugs may be due to dopamine inhibition (see neuroleptic malignant syndrome). **Examples of associated drugs:** Beta-lactams, macrolides
Dysgeusia	Impairment of or perversion of sense of taste
Dystonia	Develops early in therapy – sometimes within hours of first dose. Typically, appears as severe spasms of the muscles of face, neck, tongue, and back. Oculogyric crisis (upward deviation of the eyes) and opisthotonus (tetanic spasm of back muscles cause trunk to arch forward, with head and lower extremities thrown backward. Acute cramping can cause dislocation of joints and laryngeal dystonia can impair respiration (can be fatal, requires emergency treatment). **Examples of associated drugs:** Haldol, phenothiazines
Eosinophilic pneumonitis	Development of interstitial pneumonitis due to eosinophilic infiltrates. Shortness of breath and inflammation are prominent features. **Examples of associated drugs:** Mesalamine
Erythema multiforme	Cutaneous eruption of macules, papules, and/or subdermal vesicles (multiform appearance), including characteristic "target" or "iris" lesions over the dorsal aspect of the hands and forearms. Self-limiting eruptions are termed "minor", while major eruptions may be referred to as Stevens-Johnson syndrome. **Examples of associated drugs:** Phenytoin, sulfonamides

SELECTED ADVERSE EFFECTS (Continued)

Name	Description
Extrapyramidal movement disorders	Movement disorders associated with antipsychotic effects: Dystonia, pseudoparkinsonism, akathisia, tardive dyskinesia. **Examples of associated drugs:** Metoclopramide, haldol, phenothiazines
Hallucinations	**Examples of associated drugs:** Opiates
Hepatotoxicity	Hepatocellular damage or multilobular hepatic necrosis can result in liver dysfunction manifested as jaundice or hepatitis; yellowing of skin or eyes is usually a later manifestation; anorexia, fatigue or malaise, nausea, darkening in color of urine or light colored stool may occur first. **Examples of associated drugs:** Troglitazone
Interstitial nephritis	Acute renal failure characterized by localized inflammatory/allergic reaction, pronounced eosinophilic collection in interstitial cells of kidney. Eosinophils may appear in urine. Usually develops after several days of therapy. **Examples of associated drugs:** Beta-lactams, NSAIDs
Leukopenia / neutropenia	**Examples of associated drugs:** Beta-lactams, procainamide
Methemoglobinemia	Rare reaction in which the hemoglobin molecule is altered, rendering it unable to effectively carry oxygen after exposure to a chemical initiator. Cyanosis, respiratory distress, lactic acidosis, and shock may progress rapidly after exposure. May occur with any route of administration, including topical. **Examples of associated drugs:** Nitrates, local anesthetics
Myositis / rhabdomyolysis	Inflammation/toxicity to muscle cells characterized by muscle pain/stiffness. Pronounced lysis of muscle cells leads to dramatic increase in serum CPK and possible precipitation of myoglobin in urine. **Examples of associated drugs:** HMG CoA reductase inhibitors (particularly when combined with drugs like erythromycin or cyclosporin)
Neuroleptic malignant syndrome	Rare, but may cause 30% to 50% fatality, response to antipsychotic therapy – usually with high-potency drugs. Manifests as extremely rigid musculoskeletal posturing, extremely high fevers, sweating, dysrhythmias, and acute fluctuations of blood pressure and consciousness, respiratory failure and/or cardiac collapse (requires immediate supportive care and withdrawal of antipsychotic medication). **Examples of associated drugs:** Haldol, phenothiazines
Neuromuscular blockade	Weakness, respiratory failure as neuromuscular transmission may be interrupted. Patients with decreased neuromuscular transmission (ie, myasthenia gravis) are at particular risk. **Examples of associated drugs:** Aminoglycosides, macrolides
Neutropenia	Usually associated with antineoplastic medications. A reduction in circulating neutrophils (white blood cells that are essential in fighting infection) means that both severity and incidence of infections are significantly increased. Usually, benign infections such as candidiasis can become systemically life-threatening. **Examples of associated drugs:** Beta-lactams, procainamide, carbamazepine
Opportunistic infection	Many medications reduce the natural resistance to infection and/or mask the more obvious indications of an infection when persons are receiving antineoplastics, antivirals, antibiotics, and glucocorticoids. Symptoms include sore throat, fever, chills, unhealed sores, purulent vaginal discharge, white plaques in mouth, fatigue, and joint pain. **Examples of associated drugs:** Chemotherapeutic agents, broad-spectrum antibiotics, immunosuppressants
Optic neuritis	Blurred vision, altered color discrimination, and constriction of visual fields. **Examples of associated drugs:** Quinidine, cisplatin
Orthostatic hypotension	Reduced muscle tone in the venous wall which causes blood to pool in lower extremity veins when the person assumes an erect position from lying or sitting; blood return to the heart is decreased because of this pooling, resulting in decreased cardiac output, and abrupt fall in blood pressure. **Examples of associated drugs:** Tricyclic antidepressants, beta-blockers
Paradoxical response	A response to a medication that is opposite of the anticipated response or side effects (eg, a paradoxical response to CNS depressants may be CNS excitation such as hyperactivity, aggression, decreased ability to concentrate, etc). **Examples of associated drugs:** Benzodiazepines, phenobarbital
Photophobia	Blocking muscarinic receptors on the sphincter of the iris decreases ability to adapt to bright light with intolerance for any bright light; both artificial lighting and outside sunlight. **Examples of associated drugs:** Anticholinergics
Photosensitization / phototoxicity	Phototoxic and photoallergic reactions result from a combination of a sensitizing agent and ultraviolet light. The sensitizing agent in phototoxic reactions may be systemically ingested or locally applied. The reaction occurs within hours of exposure. Photoallergy results from chemical change to the structure of a sensitizing agent, and may require several days before symptoms appear. **Examples of associated drugs:** Fluoroquinolones, tetracyclines
Postural hypotension	See orthostatic hypotension.
Pseudoparkinsonism	Blocking of dopamine receptors produces symptoms that resemble Parkinson's disease: Bradycardia, facies, drooling, tremors, rigidity, gait disturbance, and stooped posture (usually develops within first month of therapy). **Examples of associated drugs:** Antipsychotic medications, haldol
Pulmonary fibrosis	Restrictive airway disease due to fibrous changes in the lungs, often manifest only after long-term drug administration. **Examples of associated drugs:** Nitrofurantoin, melphalan, amiodarone

Name	Description
Purple toes syndrome	Peripheral ischemia and cyanosis generally localized to the plantar surfaces and sides of the toes which may occasionally progress to necrosis or gangrene. The effect is believed to be caused by cholesterol microemboli. Effects are noted after weeks to months of therapy. **Examples of associated drugs:** Oral anticoagulants
QTc prolongation	Lengthening of the corrected Q-T interval (on ECG) which may predispose to the development of polymorphic ventricular tachycardia (torsade de pointes). **Examples of associated drugs:** Type Ia and III antiarrhythmics, selected fluoroquinolones, erythromycin, thioridazine, mesoridazine
Seizures (drug -induced)	An infrequent, nonspecific effect of a variety of medications, particularly at high concentrations. Drug-induced seizures may occur due to lowering of seizure threshold, blockade of inhibitory neurotransmitters (GABA) or direct neuroexcitatory effects. **Examples of associated drugs:** Tricyclic antidepressants (lower seizure threshold), high-dose beta-lactam or fluoroquinolone antibiotics (GABA blockade); theophylline or accumulation of normeperidine (neuroexcitation)
Serotonin syndrome	Presence of three or more of the following: Altered mental status (40% – primarily confusion or hypomania), agitation, tremor (50%), shivering, diarrhea, hyperreflexia (pronounced) in lower extremities, myoclonus (50%), ataxia or incoordination, fever (50% incidence; temperature >105°F associated with grave prognosis), diaphoresis. **Examples of associated drugs:** Serotonin reuptake inhibitors, MOMA (ecstasy), clomipramine, combinations of many drugs
Stevens-Johnson syndrome (SJS)	Rare reaction; symptoms include widespread lesions of the skin and mucous membranes, fever, malaise, and toxemia; reducing or discontinuing the sulfonamide at the first sign of skin rash may reduce the incidence of SJS. **Examples of associated drugs:** Associated primarily with sulfonamides and associated compounds such as sulfonylureas, thiazide diuretics, and loop diuretics; anticonvulsants
Stomatitis	**Examples of associated drugs:** Chemotherapeutic agents
Sulfite hypersensitivity	Reactions occur within 2-15 minutes after ingestion or inhalation and include nasal pruritus, rhinorrhea, conjunctivitis, generalized urticaria, dyspnea, wheezing, angioedema, flushing, weakness, and anaphylaxis; patients frequently have underlying allergies or asthmatic disease. **Examples of associated drugs:** Sulfite derivatives are common antioxidant preservatives used in foods and medications. Sulfite derivatives include sodium bisulfite, potassium bisulfite, sodium metabisulfite, sodium sulfites, potassium metabisulfite, and sulfur dioxide. Most common food sources are fresh fruits and vegetables, shellfish, soft drinks, beer, wine, dried foods, and fruit drinks. Sympathomimetic medications are very susceptible to oxidation and frequently contain bisulfites in concentrations of 0.3% to 0.75%.
Tardive dyskinesia	Usually develops with long-term therapy – symptoms may be irreversible. Characterized by wormlike, writhing movements of tongue and facial muscles, lip-smacking, or flicking tongue movements; can progress to involuntary movements of digits or limbs. **Examples of associated drugs:** Haldol, phenothiazines
Tendonitis / Achilles' tendon rupture	Pain associated with tendon area, most commonly in the Achilles' region, which may progress to tendon rupture, particularly if the effect is not recognized and therapy is continued. **Examples of associated drugs:** Fluoroquinolone antibiotics
Teratogenic effects	Neonatal abnormalities (physical and mental) that result from impaired development at some stage in the fetal development; specificity of defects depends on several factors, including the period of fetal development when the medication was used (eg, some drugs are teratogenic during the early period of fetal development, some are teratogenic during later periods of development, and some have negative impact on fetal development during any period of the pregnancy). **Examples of associated drugs:** Phenytoin, metronidazole
Thrombocytopenia	**Examples of associated drugs:** H_2 antagonists, beta-lactams
Tyramine reaction	Specific foods in the presence of MAO inhibitors; see Food/Drug Interactions for a list of tyramine-containing foods which the patient taking MAO inhibitors should be advised to avoid. Normally, dietary tyramine is inactivated by MAO (monamine oxidase) in the intestinal wall and by hepatic MAO. In the presence of MAO inhibitors, dietary tyramine is not inactivated, passes without metabolism into the circulation to promote the release of accumulated norepinephrine stores in the sympathetic nerve terminals, thereby causing massive vasoconstriction and acute stimulation of the heart. Reactions can be severe and usually require emergency treatment. **Examples of associated drugs:** MAO inhibitors
Vestibulotoxicity	Form of ototoxicity which affects vestibular function, as opposed to hearing. Primary symptom is ataxia or difficulty maintaining balance. **Examples of associated drugs:** Aminoglycosides
Virilization	Acne, deepening of voice, increased body and facial hair, baldness, clitoral enlargement, increased libido, menstrual irregularities (hair loss, voice changes, and enlargement of clitoris may be irreversible). **Examples of associated drugs:** Minoxidil, phenytoin
Xerostomia	Dry mouth results from blockade of muscarinic receptors on salivary glands. Decreased salivation and excessively dry mouth are extremely uncomfortable but also interfere with mastication and swallowing, resulting in poor nutrition. **Examples of associated drugs:** Clonidine, anticholinergics

DISCOLORATION OF FECES DUE TO DRUGS

Black
Acetazolamide
Alcohols
Alkalies
Aluminum hydroxide
Aminophylline
Aminosalicylic acid
Amphetamine
Amphotericin
Antacids
Anticoagulants
Aspirin
Betamethasone
Bismuth
Charcoal
Chloramphenicol
Chlorpropamide
Clindamycin
Corticosteroids
Cortisone
Cyclophosphamide
Cytarabine
Digitalis
Ethacrynic acid
Ferrous salts
Floxuridine
Fluorides
Fluorouracil
Halothane
Heparin
Hydralazine
Hydrocortisone
Ibuprofen
Indomethacin
Iodine drugs
Iron salts
Levarterenol
Levodopa
Manganese
Melphalan
Methylprednisolone
Methotrexate

Methylene blue
Oxyphenbutazone
Phenacetin
Phenolphthalein
Phenylbutazone
Phenylephrine
Phosphorous
Potassium salts
Prednisolone
Procarbazine
Pyrvinium
Reserpine
Salicylates
Sulfonamides
Tetracycline
Theophylline
Thiotepa
Triamcinolone
Warfarin

Blue
Chloramphenicol
Methylene blue

Dark Brown
Dexamethasone

Gray
Colchicine

Green
Indomethacin
Iron
Medroxyprogesterone

Greenish Gray
Oral antibiotics
Oxyphenbutazone
Phenylbutazone

Light Brown
Anticoagulants

Orange-Red
Phenazopyridine
Rifampin

Pink
Anticoagulants
Aspirin
Heparin
Oxyphenbutazone
Phenylbutazone
Salicylates

Red
Anticoagulants
Aspirin
Heparin
Oxyphenbutazone
Phenolphthalein
Phenylbutazone
Pyrvinium
Salicylates
Tetracycline syrup

Red-Brown
Oxyphenbutazone
Phenylbutazone
Rifampin

Tarry
Ergot preparations
Ibuprofen
Salicylates
Warfarin

White/Speckling
Aluminum hydroxide
Antibiotics (oral)
Indocyanine green

Yellow
Senna

Yellow-Green
Senna

Adapted from Drugdex® — Drug Consults, Micromedex, Vol 62, Denver, CO: Rocky Mountain Drug Consultation Center, 1998.

DISCOLORATION OF URINE DUE TO DRUGS

Black
Cascara
Co-trimoxazole
Ferrous salts
Iron dextran
Levodopa
Methocarbamol
Methyldopa
Naphthalene
Pamaquine
Phenacetin
Phenols
Quinine
Sulfonamides

Blue
Anthraquinone
DeWitt's pills
Indigo blue
Indigo carmine
Methocarbamol
Methylene blue
Mitoxantrone
Nitrofurans
Resorcinol
Triamterene

Blue-Green
Amitriptyline
Anthraquinone
DeWitt's pills
Doan's® pills
Indigo blue
Indigo carmine
Magnesium salicylate
Methylene blue
Resorcinol

Brown
Anthraquinone dyes
Cascara
Chloroquine
Hydroquinone
Levodopa
Methocarbamol
Methyldopa
Methocarbamol
Metronidazole
Nitrofurans
Nitrofurantoin
Pamaquine
Phenacetin
Phenols
Primaquine
Quinine
Rifabutin
Rifampin
Senna
Sodium diatrizoate
Sulfonamides

Brown-Black
Isosorbide mono- or
dinitrate
Methyldopa
Metronidazole
Nitrates
Nitrofurans
Phenacetin
Povidone iodine
Quinine
Senna

Dark
p-Aminosalicylic acid
Cascara
Levodopa
Metronidazole
Nitrites
Phenacetin
Phenol
Primaquine
Quinine
Resorcinol
Riboflavin
Senna

Green
Amitriptyline
Anthraquinone
DeWitt's pills
Indigo blue
Indigo carmine
Indomethacin
Methocarbamol
Methylene blue
Nitrofurans
Phenols
Propofol
Resorcinol
Suprofen

Green-Yellow
DeWitt's pills
Methylene blue

Milky
Phosphates

Orange
Chlorzoxazone
Dihydroergotamine
mesylate
Heparin sodium
Phenazopyridine
Phenindione
Rifabutin
Rifampin
Sulfasalazine
Warfarin

Orange-Red-Brown
Chlorzoxazone
Doxidan
Phenazopyridine
Rifampin
Warfarin

Orange-Yellow
Fluorescein sodium
Rifampin
Sulfasalazine

Pink
Aminopyrine
Anthraquinone dyes
Aspirin
Cascara
Danthron
Deferoxamine
Methyldopa
Phenazopyridone
Phenolphthalein
Phenothiazines
Phenytoin
Salicylates
Senna

Purple
Phenolphthalein

Red
Anthraquinone
Cascara
Chlorpromazine
Daunorubicin
Deferoxamine
Dihydroergotamine
mesylate
Dimethyl sulfoxide
DMSO
Doxorubicin
Heparin
Ibuprofen
Methyldopa
Oxyphenbutazone
Phenacetin
Phenazopyridine
Phenolphthalein
Phenothiazines
Phensuximide
Phenylbutazone
Phenytoin
Rifampin
Senna

Red-Brown
Cascara
Deferoxamine
Methyldopa
Oxyphenbutazone
Pamaquine
Phenacetin
Phenazopyridine
Phenolphthalein
Phenothiazines
Phenylbutazone
Phenytoin
Quinine
Senna

Red-Purple
Chlorzoxazone
Ibuprofen
Phenacetin
Senna

Rust
Cascara
Chloroquine
Metronidazole
Nitrofurantoin
Pamaquine
Phenacetin
Quinacrine
Riboflavin
Senna
Sulfonamides

Yellow
Nitrofurantoin
Phenacetin
Quinacrine
Riboflavin
Sulfasalazine

DISCOLORATION OF URINE DUE TO DRUGS *(Continued)*

Yellow-Brown
Aminosalicylate acid
Bismuth
Cascara
Chloroquine
DeWitt's pills
Methylene blue
Metronidazole
Nitrofurantoin
Pamaquine
Primaquine
Quinacrine
Senna
Sulfonamides

Yellow-Pink
Cascara
Senna

Adapted from Drugdex® — Drug Consults, Micromedex, Vol 62, Denver, CO: Rocky Mountain Drug Consultation Center, 1998.

FEVER DUE TO DRUGS

Most Common

Atropine	Cephalosporins	Procainamide
Amphotericin B	Interferon	Quinidine
Asparaginase	Methyldopa	Salicylates (high doses)
Barbiturates	Penicillins	Streptomycin
Bleomycin	Phenytoin	Sulfonamides

Less Common

Allopurinol	Hydralazine	Nitrofurantoin
Antihistamines	Hydroxyurea	Pentazocine
Azathioprine	Imipenem	Procarbazine
Carbamazepine	Iodides	Propylthiouracil
Cimetidine	Isoniazid	Rifampin
Cisplatin	Mercaptopurine	Streptokinase
Colistimethate	Metoclopramide	Triamterene
Diazoxide	Nifedipine	Vancomycin
Folic acid	NSAIDs	

References

Cunha BA, "Antibiotic Side Effects," *Med Clin North Am*, 2001, 85(1):149-85.

Mackowiak PA and LeMaistre CF, "Drug Fever: A Critical Appraisal of Conventional Concepts. An Analysis of 51 Episodes in Two Dallas Hospitals and 97 Episodes Reported in the English Literature," *Ann Intern Med*, 1987, 106(5):728-33.

Tabor PA, "Drug-Induced Fever," Table 2, "Drugs Implicated in Causing a Fever," *Drug Intell Clin Pharm*, 1986, 20(6):416.

SEROTONIN SYNDROME

Diagnostic Criteria for Serotonin Syndrome

- Recent addition or dosage increase of any agent increasing serotonin activity or availability (usually within 1 day)
- Absence of abused substances, metabolic infectious etiology, or withdrawal
- No recent addition or dosage increase of a neuroleptic agent prior to onset of signs and symptoms
- Presence of three or more of the following: (% incidence)

Agitation (34%)
Abdominal pain (4%)
Ataxia/incoordination (40%)
Diaphoresis (45%)
Diarrhea (8%)
Hyperpyrexia (45%)
Hypertension/hypotension (35%)
Hyperthermia
Hyperreflexia (52%)
Mental status change – cognitive
    behavioral changes:
    Anxiety (15%)
    Euphoria/hypomania (21%)
    Confusion (51%)
    Agitation (34%)
    Disorientation
    Coma/unresponsiveness (29%)

Muscle rigidity (51%)
Mydriasis
Myoclonus (58%)
Nausea (23%)
Nystagmus (15%)
Restlessness/hyperactivity (48%)
Salivation (2%)
Seizures (12%)
Shivering (26%)
Sinus tachycardia (36%)
Tachypnea (26%)
Tremor (43%)
Unreactive pupils (20%)

Drugs (as Single Causative Agent) Which Can Induce Serotonin Syndrome

Specific serotonin reuptake inhibitors (SSRI)
MDMA (Ecstasy)
Clomipramine

Drug Combinations Which Can Induce Serotonin Syndrome[1]

Alprazolam – Clomipramine
Amphetamines – MAO inhibitors
Amphetamines – SSRIs (Citalopram, Fluoxetine, Fluvoxamine, Paroxetine, Sertraline)
Amphetamines – Tricyclic antidepressants
Amitriptyline – Dihydroergotamine
Amitriptyline – Lithium – Trazodone
Amitriptyline – Sertraline
Anorexiants – MAO inhibitors
Bromocriptine – Levodopa/Carbidopa
Buspirone – Nefazodone
Buspirone – SSRIs (Citalopram, Fluoxetine, Fluvoxamine, Paroxetine, Sertraline)
Buspirone – Trazodone
Buspirone – Tricyclic antidepressants
Carbamazepine – Fluoxetine
Citalopram – Moclobemide
Clomipramine – Alprazolam
Clomipramine – Clorgiline
Clomipramine – Lithium
Clomipramine – MAO inhibitors
Clomipramine – Moclobemide
Clomipramine – S-adenosylmethionine
Clomipramine – Tranylcypromine
Clorgiline – Clomipramine
Dextromethorphan – MAO inhibitors
Dextromethorphan – SSRIs (Citalopram, Fluoxetine, Fluvoxamine, Paroxetine, Sertraline)
Dextropropoxyphene – Phenelzine – Trazodone
Dihydroergotamine – Amitriptyline
Dihydroergotamine – Paroxetine

Dihydroergotamine – SSRIs (Citalopram, Fluoxetine, Fluvoxamine, Paroxetine, Sertraline)
Dihydroergotamine – Tricyclic antidepressants
Fentanyl – SSRIs (Citalopram, Fluoxetine, Fluvoxamine, Paroxetine, Sertraline)
Fluoxetine – Carbamazepine
Fluoxetine – Remoxipride
Fluoxetine – Tryptophan
Levodopa/Carbidopa – Bromocriptine
Linezolid - SSRIs (Citalopram, Fluoxetine, Fluvoxamine, Paroxetine, Sertraline)
Linezolid – Tramadol
Linezolid – Tricyclic antidepressants
Lithium – Amitriptyline – Trazodone
Lithium – Clomipramine
Lithium – SSRIs (Citalopram, Fluoxetine, Fluvoxamine, Paroxetine, Sertraline)
Lithium – Tricyclic antidepressants
Lithium – Venlafaxine
Lysergic acid diethylamide (LSD) – SSRIs (Citalopram, Fluoxetine, Fluvoxamine, Paroxetine, Sertraline)
Metoclopramide – Sertraline
Metoclopramide – Venlafaxine
MAO inhibitors – Amphetamines
MAO inhibitors – Anorexiants
MAO inhibitors – Clomipramine
MAO inhibitors – Dextromethorphan
MAO inhibitors – Meperidine
MAO inhibitors – Nefazodone
MAO inhibitors – Serotonin agonists

MAO inhibitors – S-adenosylmethionine
MAO inhibitors – SSRIs (Citalopram, Fluoxetine, Fluvoxamine, Paroxetine, Sertraline)
MAO inhibitors – St John's Wort
MAO inhibitors – Tramadol
MAO inhibitors – Trazodone
MAO inhibitors – Tricyclic antidepressants
MAO inhibitors – Tryptophan
MAO inhibitors – Venlafaxine
Meperidine – MAO inhibitors
Meperidine – Moclobemide
Meperidine – Nefazodone
Meperidine – SSRIs (Citalopram, Fluoxetine, Fluvoxamine, Paroxetine, Sertraline)
Moclobemide – Citalopram
Moclobemide – Clomipramine
Moclobemide – Meperidine
Moclobemide – Pethidine
Moclobemide – SSRIs (Citalopram, Fluoxetine, Fluvoxamine, Paroxetine, Sertraline)
Moclobemide – Tricyclic antidepressants
Nefazodone – Buspirone
Nefazodone – MAO inhibitors
Nefazodone – Meperidine
Nefazodone – Serotonin agonists
Nefazodone – SSRIs (Citalopram, Fluoxetine, Fluvoxamine, Paroxetine, Sertraline)
Nefazodone – Trazodone
Nefazodone – Tramadol
Nefazodone – Valproic Acid
Nortriptyline – Trazodone
Paroxetine – Dihydroergotamine
Paroxetine – Trazodone
Pethidine – Moclobemide
Phenelzine – Trazodone – Dextropropoxyphene
Remoxipride – Fluoxetine
S-adenosylmethionine – Clomipramine
S-adenosylmethionine – MAO inhibitors
S-adenosylmethionine – SSRIs (Citalopram, Fluoxetine, Fluvoxamine, Paroxetine, Sertraline)
S-adenosylmethionine – Tricyclic antidepressants
Selegiline (high-dose) – SSRIs (Citalopram, Fluoxetine, Fluvoxamine, Paroxetine, Sertraline)
Selegiline (high-dose) – Tricyclic antidepressants
Selegiline (high-dose) – Venlafaxine
Serotonin agonists (Sumatriptan, others) – MAO inhibitors
Serotonin agonists (Sumatriptan, others) – Nefazodone
Serotonin agonists (Sumatriptan, others) – SSRIs (Citalopram, Fluoxetine, Fluvoxamine, Paroxetine, Sertraline)
Serotonin agonists (Sumatriptan, others) – TCAs
Serotonin agonists (Sumatriptan, others) – Tramadol
Sertraline – Amitriptyline
Sibutramine – SSRIs (Citalopram, Fluoxetine, Fluvoxamine, Paroxetine, Sertraline)
SSRIs – Amphetamines
SSRIs – Buspirone

SSRIs – Dextromethorphan
SSRIs – Dihydroergotamine
SSRIs – Fentanyl
SSRIs – Linezolid
SSRIs – Lithium
SSRIs – Lysergic acid diethylamide (LSD)
SSRIs – MAO inhibitors
SSRIs – Meperidine
SSRIs – Moclobemide
SSRIs – Nefazodone
SSRIs – S-adenosylmethionine
SSRIs – Selegiline (high-dose)
SSRIs – Serotonin agonists
SSRIs – Sibutramine
SSRIs – St John's Wort
SSRIs – Tramadol
SSRIs – Trazodone
SSRIs – Tricyclic antidepressants
SSRIs – Tryptophan
St John's Wort – MAO inhibitors
St John's Wort – SSRIs (Citalopram, Fluoxetine, Fluvoxamine, Paroxetine, Sertraline)
St John's Wort – Tricyclic antidepressants
Sympathomimetics – Tricyclic antidepressants
Tramadol – Linezolid
Tramadol – MAO inhibitors
Tramadol – Nefazodone
Tramadol – Serotonin agonists
Tramadol – SSRIs (Citalopram, Fluoxetine, Fluvoxamine, Paroxetine, Sertraline)
Tramadol – TCAs
Tranylcypromine – Clomipramine
Trazodone – Buspirone
Trazodone – Lithium – Amitriptyline
Trazodone – MAO inhibitors
Trazodone – Nefazodone
Trazodone – Nortriptyline
Trazodone – Paroxetine
Trazodone – SSRIs (Citalopram, Fluoxetine, Fluvoxamine, Paroxetine, Sertraline) (theoretical)
Tricyclic antidepressants – Amphetamines
Tricyclic antidepressants – Buspirone
Tricyclic antidepressants – Dihydroergotamine
Tricyclic antidepressants – Linezolid
Tricyclic antidepressants – Lithium
Tricyclic antidepressants – MAO inhibitors
Tricyclic antidepressants – Moclobemide
Tricyclic antidepressants – S-adenosylmethionine
Tricyclic antidepressants – Serotonin agonists
Tricyclic antidepressants – SSRIs (Citalopram, Fluoxetine, Fluvoxamine, Paroxetine, Sertraline)
Tricyclic antidepressants – St John's Wort
Tricyclic antidepressants – Sympathomimetics
Tricyclic antidepressants – Tramadol
Tryptophan – Fluoxetine
Tryptophan – MAO inhibitors
Tryptophan – SSRIs (Citalopram, Fluoxetine, Fluvoxamine, Paroxetine, Sertraline)
Valproic acid – Nefazodone

SEROTONIN SYNDROME *(Continued)*

Venlafaxine – Lithium	Venlafaxine – Selegiline (high-dose)
Venlafaxine – MAO inhibitors	

[1]When administered within 2 weeks of each other.

Guidelines for Treatment of Serotonin Syndrome

Therapy is primarily supportive with intravenous crystalloid solutions utilized for hypotension and cooling blankets for mild hyperthermia. Norepinephrine is the preferred vasopressor. Chlorpromazine (25 mg I.M.) or dantrolene sodium (1 mg/kg I.V. – maximum dose 10 mg/kg) may have a role in controlling fevers, although there is no proven benefit. Benzodiazepines are the first-line treatment in controlling rigors and thus, limiting fever and rhabdomyolysis, while clonazepam may be specifically useful in treating myoclonus. Endotracheal intubation and paralysis may be required to treat refractory muscular contractions. Tachycardia or tremor can be treated with beta-blocking agents; although due to its blockade of 5-HTIA receptors, the syndrome may worsen. Serotonin blockers such as diphenhydramine (50 mg I.M.), cyproheptadine (adults: 4-8 mg every 2-4 hours up to 0.5 mg/kg/day; children: up to 0.25 mg/kg/day), or chlorpromazine (25 mg I.M.) have been used with variable efficacy. Methysergide (2-6 mg/day) and nitroglycerin (I.V. infusion of 2 mg/kg/minute with lorazepam) also has been utilized with variable efficacy in case reports. It appears that cyproheptadine is most consistently beneficial.

Recovery seen within 1 day in 70% of cases; mortality rate is about 11%.

References

Gardner DM and Lynd LD, "Sumatriptan Contraindications and the Serotonin Syndrome," *Ann Pharmacother*, 1998, 32(1):33-8

Gitlin MJ, "Venlafaxine, Monoamine Oxidase Inhibitors, and the Serotonin Syndrome," *J Clin Psychopharmacol*, 1997, 17:66-7.

Heisler MA, Guidery JR, and Arnecke B, "Serotonin Syndrome Induced by Administration of Venlafaxine and Phenelzine," *Ann Pharmacother*, 1996, 30:84.

Hodgman MJ, Martin TG, and Krenzelok EP, "Serotonin Syndrome Due to Venlafaxine and Maintenance Tranylcypromine Therapy," *Hum Exp Toxicol*, 1997, 16:14-7.

John L, Perreault MM, Tao T, et al, "Serotonin Syndrome Associated With Nefazodone and Paroxetine," *Ann Emerg Med*, 1997, 29:287-9.

LoCurto MJ, "The Serotonin Syndrome," *Emerg Clin North Am*, 1997, 15(3):665-75.

Martin TG, "Serotonin Syndrome," *Ann Emerg Med*, 1996, 28:520-6.

Mills K, "Serotonin Toxicity: A Comprehensive Review for Emergency Medicine," *Top Emerg Med*, 1993, 15:54-73.

Mills KC, "Serotonin Syndrome: A Clinical Update," *Crit Care Clin*, 1997, 13(4):763-83.

Nisijima K, Shimizu M, Abe T, et al, "A Case of Serotonin Syndrome Induced by Concomitant Treatment With Low-Dose Trazodone, and Amitriptyline and Lithium," *Int Clin Psychopharmacol*, 1996, 11:289-90.

Sobanski T, Bagli M, Laux G, et al, "Serotonin Syndrome After Lithium Add-On Medication to Paroxetine," *Pharmacopsychiatry*, 1997, 30:106-7.

Sporer, "The Serotonin Syndrome: Implicated Drugs, Pathophysiology and Management," *Drug Safety*, 1995, 13(2):94-104.

Sternbach H, "The Serotonin Syndrome," *Am J Psychiatry*, 1991, 146:705-7.

Van Berkum MM, Thiel J, Leikin JB, et al, "A Fatality Due to Serotonin Syndrome," *Medical Update for Psychiatrists*, 1997, 2:55-7.

APOTHECARY / METRIC EQUIVALENTS

Approximate Liquid Measures
Basic equivalent: 1 fluid ounce = 30 mL

Examples:

1 gallon	3800 mL	1 gallon	128 fluid ounces
1 quart	960 mL	1 quart	32 fluid ounces
1 pint	480 mL	1 pint	16 fluid ounces
8 fluid oz	240 mL	15 minims	1 mL
4 fluid oz	120 mL	10 minims	0.6 mL

Approximate Household Equivalents

1 teaspoonful	5 mL	1 tablespoonful	15 mL

Weights

Basic equivalents:

1 oz	30 g	15 gr	1 g

Examples:

4 oz	120 g	1 gr	60 mg
2 oz	60 g	1/100 gr	600 mcg
10 gr	600 mg	1/150 gr	400 mcg
7½ gr	500 mg	1/200 gr	300 mcg
16 oz	1 lb		

Metric Conversions

Basic equivalents:

1 g	1000 mg	1 mg	1000 mcg

Examples:

5 g	5000 mg	5 mg	5000 mcg
0.5 g	500 mg	0.5 mg	500 mcg
0.05 g	50 mg	0.05 mg	50 mcg

Exact Equivalents

1 g	=	15.43 gr		
1 mL	=	16.23 minims		
1 minim	=	0.06 mL		
1 gr	=	64.8 mg		
1 pint (pt)	=	473.2 mL		
1 oz	=	28.35 g		
1 lb	=	453.6 g		
1 kg	=	2.2 lb		
1 qt	=	946.4 mL		

0.1 mg	=	1/600 gr
0.12 mg	=	1/500 gr
0.15 mg	=	1/400 gr
0.2 mg	=	1/300 gr
0.3 mg	=	1/200 gr
0.4 mg	=	1/150 gr
0.5 mg	=	1/120 gr
0.6 mg	=	1/100 gr
0.8 mg	=	1/80 gr
1 mg	=	1/65 gr

Solids[1]

¼ grain	=	15 mg
½ grain	=	30 mg
1 grain	=	60 mg
1½ grains	=	90 mg
5 grains	=	300 mg
10 grains	=	600 mg

[1]Use exact equivalents for compounding and calculations requiring a high degree of accuracy.

AVERAGE WEIGHTS AND SURFACE AREAS

Average Weight and Surface Area of Preterm Infants, Term Infants, and Children

Age	Average Weight (kg)[1]	Approximate Surface Area (m²)
Weeks Gestation		
26	0.9-1	0.1
30	1.3-1.5	0.12
32	1.6-2	0.15
38	2.9-3	0.2
40 (term infant at birth)	3.1-4	0.25
Months		
3	5	0.29
6	7	0.38
9	8	0.42
Year		
1	10	0.49
2	12	0.55
3	15	0.64
4	17	0.74
5	18	0.76
6	20	0.82
7	23	0.90
8	25	0.95
9	28	1.06
10	33	1.18
11	35	1.23
12	40	1.34
Adults	70	1.73

[1]Weights from age 3 months and older are rounded off to the nearest kilogram.

BODY MASS INDEX (BMI)

$$BMI = \frac{weight\ (kg)}{[height\ (m)]^2}$$

See "Obesity Treatment Guidelines for Adults" in Therapy Recommendations section.

BODY SURFACE AREA OF ADULTS AND CHILDREN

Calculating Body Surface Area in Children

In a child of average size, find weight and corresponding surface area on the boxed scale to the left; or, use the nomogram to the right. Lay a straightedge on the correct height and weight points for the child, then read the intersecting point on the surface area scale.

FOR CHILDREN OF NORMAL HEIGHT AND WEIGHT

NOMOGRAM

BODY SURFACE AREA FORMULA
(Adult and Pediatric)

$$BSA\ (m^2) = \sqrt{\frac{Ht\ (in)\ x\ Wt\ (lb)}{3131}} \quad \text{or, in metric: } BSA\ (m^2) = \sqrt{\frac{Ht\ (cm)\ x\ Wt\ (kg)}{3600}}$$

References

Lam TK and Leung DT, "More on Simplified Calculation of Body Surface Area," *N Engl J Med*, 1988, 318(17):1130 (Letter).

Mosteller RD, "Simplified Calculation of Body Surface Area", *N Engl J Med*, 1987, 317(17):1098 (Letter).

IDEAL BODY WEIGHT CALCULATION

Adults (18 years and older) (IBW is in kg)

IBW (male) = 50 + (2.3 x height in inches over 5 feet)

IBW (female) = 45.5 + (2.3 x height in inches over 5 feet)

Children (IBW is in kg; height is in cm)

    a.   1-18 years

$$IBW = \frac{(height^2\ x\ 1.65)}{1000}$$

    b.   5 feet and taller

       IBW (male) = 39 + (2.27 x height in inches over 5 feet)

       IBW (female) = 42.2 + (2.27 x height in inches over 5 feet)

CREATININE CLEARANCE ESTIMATING METHODS IN PATIENTS WITH STABLE RENAL FUNCTION

These formulas provide an acceptable estimate of the patient's creatinine clearance **except** in the following instances.

- Patient's serum creatinine is changing rapidly (either up or down).
- Patients are markedly emaciated.

In above situations, certain assumptions have to be made.

- In patients with rapidly rising serum creatinines (ie, >0.5-0.7 mg/dL/day), it is best to assume that the patient's creatinine clearance is probably <10 mL/minute.
- In emaciated patients, although their actual creatinine clearance is less than their calculated creatinine clearance (because of decreased creatinine production), it is not possible to easily predict how much less.

Infants

Estimation of creatinine clearance using serum creatinine and body length (to be used when an adequate timed specimen cannot be obtained). **Note:** This formula may not provide an accurate estimation of creatinine clearance for infants younger than 6 months of age and for patients with severe starvation or muscle wasting.

$Cl_{cr} = K \times L/S_{cr}$

where:

Cl_{cr} = creatinine clearance in mL/minute/1.73 m^2

K = constant of proportionality that is age specific

Age	K
Low birth weight ≤1 y	0.33
Full-term ≤1 y	0.45
2-12 y	0.55
13-21 y female	0.55
13-21 y male	0.70

L = length in cm

S_{cr} = serum creatinine concentration in mg/dL

Reference

Schwartz GJ, Brion LP, and Spitzer A, "The Use of Plasma Creatinine Concentration for Estimating Glomerular Filtration Rate in Infants, Children and Adolescents," *Ped Clin N Amer*, 1987, 34:571-90.

Children (1-18 years)

Method 1: (Traub SL and Johnson CE, *Am J Hosp Pharm*, 1980, 37:195-201)

Equation:

$$Cl_{cr} = \frac{0.48 \times (height)}{S_{cr}}$$

where

Cl_{cr} = creatinine clearance in mL/min/1.73 m^2

S_{cr} = serum creatinine in mg/dL

Height = height in cm

<u>Method 2</u>: Nomogram (Traub SL and Johnson CE, *Am J Hosp Pharm*, 1980, 37:195-201)

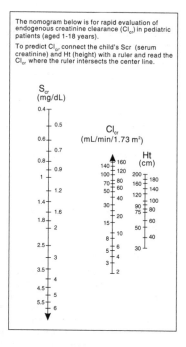

The nomogram below is for rapid evaluation of endogenous creatinine clearance (Cl_{cr}) in pediatric patients (aged 1-18 years).

To predict Cl_{cr}, connect the child's Scr (serum creatinine) and Ht (height) with a ruler and read the Cl_{cr} where the ruler intersects the center line.

Adults (18 years and older)

<u>Method 1</u>: (Cockroft DW and Gault MH, *Nephron*, 1976, 16:31-41)

Estimated creatinine clearance (Cl_{cr}) (mL/min):

$$\text{Male} = \frac{(140 - age) \times BW\ (kg)}{72 \times S_{cr}}$$

$$\text{Female} = male \times 0.85$$

Note: Use of actual body weight (BW) in obese patients (and possibly patients with ascites) may significantly overestimate creatinine clearance. Some clinicians prefer to use an adjusted ideal body weight (IBW) in such cases [eg, IBW + 0.4(ABW-IBW)], especially when calculating dosages for aminoglycoside antibiotics.

<u>Method 2</u>: (Jelliffe RW, *Ann Intern Med*, 1973, 79:604)

Estimated creatinine clearance (Cl_{cr}) (mL/min/1.73 m²):

$$\text{Male} = \frac{98 - 0.8\ (age - 20)}{S_{cr}}$$

$$\text{Female} = male \times 0.90$$

I.V. TO ORAL CONVERSION

1. **Consider drug class and indication. Conversion is acceptable only if the risk and benefit evaluation justifies conversion. Conversion should never be made only because of drug costs. The cost of failed therapy is much higher.**

   Assuming access is available, intravenous dosing rapidly produces effective serum concentrations, suitable when this benefit outweighs the risk of venous irritation/trauma, infection, and cost. Conversion from I.V. to oral is often dependent on the patient's specific clinical situation. As the clinical situation improves, oral administration may be acceptable. In general, changing the route of administration for a drug treating the patient's primary problem is to be approached with more caution than a drug which is a continuation of prior therapy.

2. **Consider pharmaceutical and pharmacokinetic issues.**

   Specifically, adjustments for bioavailability or to standard oral dosing must be made. It should be recognized that standard oral dosing is often a much lower total daily dose as compared to oral dosing (this is particularly true for some antibiotics. In addition, the patient must be able to ingest or receive the drug in the dosage form available. Drugs not available in a liquid dosage form may be difficult to convert.

3. **Consider the patient's ability to absorb drug.**

   The reliability of swallowing or enteral access should be considered. If the patient is receiving medications by an enteral access device such as an enteral feeding tube (eg, PEG, PEJ, or nasogastric), the function of these tubes should be assured. In addition, the functional status of the gastrointestinal tract must be evaluated. Obviously, NPO status normally precludes conversion to oral therapy. However, gastrointestinal motility should be assessed in all patients when a conversion is planned. The presence or suspicion of obstruction, use of multiple promotility agents, or problems with nausea/emesis should be assessed. Agents with complete absorption in ambulatory patients may not be well absorbed in acute illness. For patients receiving continuous enteral feedings, conversion should not be attempted until the patient has demonstrated an ability to tolerate feedings up to their goal rate. In addition, the presence or absence of diarrhea should be assessed as indicators of the patient's potential to absorb medications.

4. **Prospectively identify potential interferences with absorption.**

   Absorption of some medications may be dramatically altered in the presence of enteral feedings or specific electrolytes in the gastrointestinal tract. For example, sucralfate may reduce the absorption of fluoroquinolones to ineffective levels. In this instance, one may consider the replacement with an H_2 antagonist to eliminate potential interferences or selection of comparable nonquinolone antibiotic coverage. Other drug binding agents include bile acid sequestrants and activated charcoal.

5. **Monitoring**

   With any change in the route of administration, consider that a recurrence may require reconsideration of the route.

SPECIFIC MEDICATION GROUPS

Antibiotics

May be readily converted to oral therapy in most situations. Most institutions encourage evaluation of an initial response (3- to 5-day period) prior to oral therapy. In most cases, a lack of clinical improvement over the evaluation period or a recent change in the status should delay prompting to oral therapy.

I.V. Agent	Usual I.V. Dose	Oral Agent (if different)	Common Oral Dose
Ampicillin	1 g q6h	Amoxicillin	500 mg q6h[1]
Ampicillin/ sulbactam	1.5-3 g q6h	Amoxicillin/ clavulanate	500 mg q8h or 875 mg q12h
Azithromycin	500 mg qd		250 mg qd
Cefazolin	1 g q8h	Cephalexin	500 mg q6h
Cefuroxime	750 mg q8h	Cefuroxime axetil	250-500 mg q12h[1,2]
Ciprofloxacin	400-600 mg q12h		500-750 mg q12h
Clindamycin	300-600 mg q8h		300-450 mg orally q6h
Co-trimoxazole	7.5-20 mg/kg		Equivalent # tablets (divide q6h or q12h)
Doxycycline	100 mg q12h		100 mg q12h
Erythromycin	500-1000 mg q6h		500 mg q6h
Fluconazole	100 mg qd		100 mg qd
Gatifloxacin	200-400 mg q24h		200-400 mg q24h
Levofloxacin	500 mg q24h		500 mg q24h
Metronidazole	500 mg q8-12h		500 mg q8h or 250 mg q6h
Ofloxacin	200-400 mg q12h		200-400 mg q12h
Trovafloxacin	100-200 mg qd		100-200 mg qd

[1]Oral dose represents dose reduction.

[2]Poor oral absorption.

Others

- H_2 antagonists – generally converted 1:1 to equivalent dose and scheduled orally.

- Methylprednisolone – may be converted to oral prednisone (each 4 mg methyl-prednisolone = 5 mg prednisone).

- Aminophylline – must be calculated based on infusion rate. However, a simple conversion calculation is possible: Dose in mg/h x 10 = dose of sustained release product to be given every 12 hours (ie, a typical infusion of 30 mg/h = 300 mg of sustained release theophylline q12h or 150 mg q6h of nonsustained release product.

MILLIEQUIVALENT AND MILLIMOLE CALCULATIONS AND CONVERSIONS

DEFINITIONS AND CALCULATIONS

Definitions

mole	=	gram molecular weight of a substance (aka molar weight)
millimole (mM)	=	milligram molecular weight of a substance (a millimole is 1/1000 of a mole)
equivalent weight	=	gram weight of a substance which will combine with or replace 1 gram (1 mole) of hydrogen; an equivalent weight can be determined by dividing the molar weight of a substance by its ionic valence
milliequivalent (mEq)	=	milligram weight of a substance which will combine with or replace 1 milligram (1 millimole) of hydrogen (a milliequivalent is 1/1000 of an equivalent)

Calculations

moles	=	$\dfrac{\text{weight of a substance (grams)}}{\text{molecular weight of that substance (grams)}}$
millimoles	=	$\dfrac{\text{weight of a substance (milligrams)}}{\text{molecular weight of that substance (milligrams)}}$
equivalents	=	moles x valence of ion
milliequivalents	=	millimoles x valence of ion
moles	=	$\dfrac{\text{equivalents}}{\text{valence of ion}}$
millimoles	=	$\dfrac{\text{milliequivalents}}{\text{valence of ion}}$
millimoles	=	moles x 1000
milliequivalents	=	equivalents x 1000

Note: Use of equivalents and milliequivalents is valid only for those substances which have fixed ionic valences (eg, sodium, potassium, calcium, chlorine, magnesium bromine, etc). For substances with variable ionic valences (eg, phosphorous), a reliable equivalent value cannot be determined. In these instances, one should calculate millimoles (which are fixed and reliable) rather than milliequivalents.

MILLIEQUIVALENT CONVERSIONS

To convert mg/100 mL to mEq/L the following formula may be used:

$$\frac{(\text{mg}/100\ \text{mL}) \times 10 \times \text{valence}}{\text{atomic weight}} = \text{mEq/L}$$

To convert mEq/L to mg/100 mL the following formula may be used:

$$\frac{(\text{mEq/L}) \times \text{atomic weight}}{10 \times \text{valence}} = \text{mg/100 mL}$$

To convert mEq/L to volume of percent of a gas the following formula may be used:

$$\frac{(\text{mEq/L}) \times 22.4}{10} = \text{volume percent}$$

Valences and Atomic Weights of Selected Ions

Substance	Electrolyte	Valence	Molecular Wt
Calcium	Ca^{++}	2	40
Chloride	Cl^-	1	35.5
Magnesium	Mg^{++}	2	24
Phosphate	HPO_4^{--} (80%)	1.8	96[1]
pH = 7.4	$H_2PO_4^-$ (20%)	1.8	96[1]
Potassium	K^+	1	39
Sodium	Na^+	1	23
Sulfate	SO_4^{--}	2	96[1]

[1]The molecular weight of phosphorus only is 31, and sulfur only is 32.

Approximate Milliequivalents — Weights of Selected Ions

Salt	mEq/g Salt	mg Salt/mEq
Calcium carbonate [$CaCO_3$]	20	50
Calcium chloride [$CaCl_2 \bullet 2H_2O$]	14	74
Calcium gluceptate [$Ca(C_7H_{13}O_8)_2$]	4	245
Calcium gluconate [$Ca(C_6H_{11}O_7)_2 \bullet H_2O$]	5	224
Calcium lactate [$Ca(C_3H_5O_3)_2 \bullet 5H_2O$]	7	154
Magnesium gluconate [$Mg(C_6H_{11}O_7)_2 \bullet H_2O$]	5	216
Magnesium oxide [MgO]	50	20
Magnesium sulfate [$MgSO_4$]	17	60
Magnesium sulfate [$MgSO_4 \bullet 7H_2O$]	8	123
Potassium acetate [$K(C_2H_3O_2)$]	10	98
Potassium chloride [KCl]	13	75
Potassium citrate [$K_3(C_6H_5O_7) \bullet H_2O$]	9	108
Potassium iodide [KI]	6	166
Sodium acetate [$Na(C_2H_3O_2)$]	12	82
Sodium acetate [$Na(C_2H_3O_2) \bullet 3H_2O$]	7	136
Sodium bicarbonate [$NaHCO_3$]	12	84
Sodium chloride [$NaCl$]	17	58
Sodium citrate [$Na_3(C_6H_5O_7) \bullet 2H_2O$]	10	98
Sodium iodine [NaI]	7	150
Sodium lactate [$Na(C_3H_5O_3)$]	9	112
Zinc sulfate [$ZnSO_4 \bullet 7H_2O$]	7	144

CORRECTED SODIUM

Corrected Na^+ = measured Na^+ + [1.5 x (glucose − 150 divided by 100)]

Note: Do not correct for glucose <150.

WATER DEFICIT

Water deficit = 0.6 x body weight [1 − (140 divided by Na^+)]

Note: Body weight is estimated weight in kg when fully hydrated; **Na^+** is serum or plasma sodium. Use corrected Na^+ if necessary. Consult medical references for recommendations for replacement of deficit.

TOTAL SERUM CALCIUM CORRECTED FOR ALBUMIN LEVEL

[(Normal albumin − patient's albumin) x 0.8] + patient's measured total calcium

MILLIEQUIVALENT AND MILLIMOLE CALCULATIONS AND CONVERSIONS (Continued)

ACID-BASE ASSESSMENT

Henderson-Hasselbalch Equation

$$pH = 6.1 + \log (HCO_3^- / (0.03) (pCO_2))$$

Alveolar Gas Equation

$$PIO_2 = FiO_2 \times (\text{total atmospheric pressure} - \text{vapor pressure of } H_2O \text{ at } 37°C)$$

$$= FiO_2 \times (760 \text{ mm Hg} - 47 \text{ mm Hg})$$

$$PAO_2 = PIO_2 - PACO_2 / R$$

Alveolar/arterial oxygen gradient = $PAO_2 - PaO_2$

Normal ranges:

Children	15-20 mm Hg
Adults	20-25 mm Hg

where:

PIO_2	=	Oxygen partial pressure of inspired gas (mm Hg) (150 mm Hg in room air at sea level)
FiO_2	=	Fractional pressure of oxygen in inspired gas (0.21 in room air)
PAO_2	=	Alveolar oxygen partial pressure
$PACO_2$	=	Alveolar carbon dioxide partial pressure
PaO_2	=	Arterial oxygen partial pressure
R	=	Respiratory exchange quotient (typically 0.8, increases with high carbohydrate diet, decreases with high fat diet)

Acid-Base Disorders

Acute metabolic acidosis:
  $PaCO_2$ expected = 1.5 (HCO_3^-) + 8 ± 2 **or**
  Expected decrease in $PaCO_2$ = 1.3 (1-1.5) x decrease in HCO_3^-

Acute metabolic alkalosis:
  Expected increase in $PaCO_2$ = 0.6 (0.5-1) x increase in HCO_3^-

Acute respiratory acidosis (<6 h duration):
  For every $PaCO_2$ increase of 10 mm Hg, HCO_3 increases by 1 mEq/L

Chronic respiratory acidosis (>6 h duration):
  For every $PaCO_2$ increase of 10 mm Hg, HCO_3 increases by 4 mEq/L

Acute respiratory alkalosis (<6 h duration):
  For every $PaCO_2$ decrease of 10 mm Hg, HCO_3 decreases by 2 mEq/L

Chronic respiratory alkalosis (>6 h duration):
  For every $PaCO_2$ decrease of 10 mm Hg, HCO_3 increases by 5 mEq/L

ACID-BASE EQUATION

H^+ (in mEq/L) = (24 x $PaCO_2$) divided by HCO_3^-

Aa GRADIENT

Aa gradient $[(713)(FiO_2 - (PaCO_2 \text{ divided by } 0.8))] - PaO_2$

Aa gradient	=	alveolar-arterial oxygen gradient
FiO_2	=	inspired oxygen (expressed as a fraction)
$PaCO_2$	=	arterial partial pressure carbon dioxide (mm Hg)
PaO_2	=	arterial partial pressure oxygen (mm Hg)

OSMOLALITY

Definition: The summed concentrations of all osmotically active solute particles.

Predicted serum osmolality =
  2 Na^+ + glucose (mg/dL) / 18 + BUN (mg/dL) / 2.8

The normal range of serum osmolality is 285-295 mOsm/L.

Differential diagnosis of increased serum osmolal gap (>10 mOsm/L)

  Medications and toxins
    Alcohols (ethanol, methanol, isopropanol, glycerol, ethylene glycol)
    Mannitol

Calculated Osm

Osmolal gap = measured Osm – calculated Osm

> 0 to +10: Normal
> >10: Abnormal
> <0: Probable lab or calculation error

For drugs causing increased osmolar gap, see "Toxicology Information" section in this Appendix.

BICARBONATE DEFICIT

HCO_3^- deficit = (0.4 x wt in kg) x (HCO_3^- desired – HCO_3^- measured)

Note: In clinical practice, the calculated quantity may differ markedly from the actual amount of bicarbonate needed or that which may be safely administered.

ANION GAP

Definition: The difference in concentration between unmeasured cation and anion equivalents in serum.

Anion gap = $Na^+ - (Cl^- + HCO_3^-)$
    (The normal anion gap is 10-14 mEq/L)

Differential Diagnosis of Increased Anion Gap Acidosis

Organic anions

> Lactate (sepsis, hypovolemia, seizures, large tumor burden)
> Pyruvate
> Uremia
> Ketoacidosis (β-hydroxybutyrate and acetoacetate)
> Amino acids and their metabolites
> Other organic acids

Inorganic anions

> Hyperphosphatemia
> Sulfates
> Nitrates

Differential Diagnosis of Decreased Anion Gap

Organic cations

> Hypergammaglobulinemia

Inorganic cations

> Hyperkalemia
> Hypercalcemia
> Hypermagnesemia

Medications and toxins

> Lithium

Hypoalbuminemia

RETICULOCYTE INDEX

(% retic divided by 2) x (patient's Hct divided by normal Hct) **or**
(% retic divided by 2) x (patient's Hgb divided by normal Hgb)

Normal index: 1.0
Good marrow response: 2.0-6.0

PEAK AND TROUGH GUIDELINES

Drug	When to Sample	Usual Half-Life	Steady State (Ideal Sampling Time)	Therapeutic Levels*	Potentially Toxic Levels*
Antibiotics					
Gentamicin Tobramycin	30 min after 30 min infusion Trough: <0.5 h before next dose	2 h	15 h	Peak: 4-10 mcg/mL Trough: <2.0 mcg/mL	Peak: >12 mcg/mL Trough: >2 mcg/mL
Amikacin				Peak: 20-35 mcg/mL Trough: <8 mcg/mL	Peak: >35 mcg/mL Trough: >8 mcg/mL
Vancomycin	Peak: 1 h after 1 h infusion Trough: <0.5 h before next dose	6-8 h	24 h	Peak: 30-40 mcg/mL Trough: 5-10 mcg/mL	Peak: >80 mcg/mL Trough: >13 mcg/mL
Anticonvulsants					
Carbamazepine	Trough: Just before next oral dose In combination with other anticonvulsants	15-20 h	7-12 d	4-12 mcg/mL 4-8 mcg/mL	>12 mcg/mL
Ethosuximide	Trough: Just before next oral dose	30-60 h	10-13 d	40-100 mcg/mL	>100 mcg/mL
Phenobarbital	Trough: Just before next dose	40-120 h	20 d	15-40 mcg/mL	>40 mcg/mL
Phenytoin Free phenytoin	Trough: Just before next dose Draw at same time as total level.	Concentration dependent	5-14 d	10-20 mcg/mL 1-2 mcg/mL	>20 mcg/mL
Primidone	Trough: Just before next dose (**Note:** Primidone is metabolized to phenobarb, order levels separately.)	10-12 h	5 d	5-12 mcg/mL	>12 mcg/mL
Valproic acid	Trough: Just before next dose	5-20 h	4 d	50-100 mcg/mL	>150 mcg/mL
Bronchodilators					
Aminophylline (I.V.)	18-24 h after starting or changing a maintenance dose; given as a constant infusion	Nonsmoking adult: 8 h Children and smoking adults: 4 h	2 d	10-20 mcg/mL	>20 mcg/mL
Theophylline (P.O.)	Peak levels: Not recommended Trough level: Just before next dose				
Cardiovascular Agents					
Digoxin	Trough: Just before next dose (levels drawn earlier than 6 h after a dose will be artificially elevated)	36 h	5 d	0.5-2 ng/mL	>2 ng/mL
Lidocaine	Steady-state levels are usually achieved after 6-12 h	1.5 h	5-10 h	1.2-5.0 mcg/mL	>6 mcg/mL

(continued)

Drug	When to Sample	Therapeutic Levels*	Usual Half-Life	Steady State (Ideal Sampling Time)	Potentially Toxic Levels*
Procainamide	Trough: Just before next oral dose I.V.: 6-12 h after infusion started Combined procainamide plus NAPA	4-10 mcg/mL NAPA: 6-10 h 5-30 mcg/mL	Procain: 2.7-5 h >30 (NAPA + procain)	20 h	>10 mcg/mL
Quinidine	Trough: Just before next oral dose	2-5 mcg/mL	6 h	24 h	>10 mcg/mL
Warfarin	Same time of day each draw	See Warfarin monograph.	42 h	5-7 d	See Warfarin monograph.
Other Agents					
Amitriptyline plus nortriptyline	Trough: Just before next dose	120-250 ng/mL		4-80 d	
Cyclosporine		Months post-transplant: Plasma: 50-150 ng/mL Whole blood: 150-450 ng/mL		Variable	
Desipramine		50-300 ng/mL	12-54 h	3-11 d	
Imipramine plus desipramine		150-300 ng/mL	9-24 h	2-5 d	
Lithium		0.6-1.2 mEq/mL (acute)	18-20 h	2-7 d	>3 mEq/mL
Nortriptyline		50-140 ng/mL		4-19 d	

*Due to methodology differences, reference ranges may vary from laboratory to laboratory; check with the laboratory service used for their appropriate levels.

PEDIATRIC DOSAGE ESTIMATIONS

Dosage Estimations Based on Weight:

Augsberger's rule:

$$\frac{(1.5 \times \text{weight in kg} + 10)}{\% \text{ of adult dose}} = \text{child's approximate dose}$$

Clark's rule:

$$\frac{\text{weight (in pounds)}}{150} \times \text{adult dose} = \text{child's approximate dose}$$

Dosage Estimations Based on Age:

Augsberger's rule:

$$\frac{(4 \times \text{age in years} + 20)}{\% \text{ of adult dose}} = \text{child's approximate dose}$$

Bastedo's rule:

$$\frac{\text{age in years} + 3}{30} \times \text{adult dose} = \text{child's approximate dose}$$

Cowling's rule:

$$\frac{\text{age at next birthday (in years)}}{24} \times \text{adult dose} = \text{child's approximate dose}$$

Dilling's rule:

$$\frac{\text{age (in years)}}{20} \times \text{adult dose} = \text{child's approximate dose}$$

Fried's rule for infants (younger than 1 year):

$$\frac{\text{age (in months)}}{150} \times \text{adult dose} = \text{infant's approximate dose}$$

Young's rule:

$$\frac{\text{age (in years)}}{\text{age} + 12} \times \text{adult dose} = \text{child's approximate dose}$$

POUNDS / KILOGRAMS CONVERSION

1 pound = 0.45359 kilograms
1 kilogram = 2.2 pounds

lb	=	kg		lb	=	kg		lb	=	kg
1		0.45		70		31.75		140		63.50
5		2.27		75		34.02		145		65.77
10		4.54		80		36.29		150		68.04
15		6.80		85		38.56		155		70.31
20		9.07		90		40.82		160		72.58
25		11.34		95		43.09		165		74.84
30		13.61		100		45.36		170		77.11
35		15.88		105		47.63		175		79.38
40		18.14		110		49.90		180		81.65
45		20.41		115		52.16		185		83.92
50		22.68		120		54.43		190		86.18
55		24.95		125		56.70		195		88.45
60		27.22		130		58.91		200		90.72
65		29.48		135		61.24				

TEMPERATURE CONVERSION

Celsius to Fahrenheit = ($^\circ$C x 9/5) + 32 = $^\circ$F
Fahrenheit to Celsius = ($^\circ$F − 32) x 5/9 = $^\circ$C

$^\circ$C	=	$^\circ$F		$^\circ$C	=	$^\circ$F		$^\circ$C	=	$^\circ$F
100.0		212.0		39.0		102.2		36.8		98.2
50.0		122.0		38.8		101.8		36.6		97.9
41.0		105.8		38.6		101.5		36.4		97.5
40.8		105.4		38.4		101.1		36.2		97.2
40.6		105.1		38.2		100.8		36.0		96.8
40.4		104.7		38.0		100.4		35.8		96.4
40.2		104.4		37.8		100.1		35.6		96.1
40.0		104.0		37.6		99.7		35.4		95.7
39.8		103.6		37.4		99.3		35.2		95.4
39.6		103.3		37.2		99.0		35.0		95.0
39.4		102.9		37.0		98.6		0		32.0
39.2		102.6								

REFERENCE VALUES FOR ADULTS

Automated Chemistry (CHEMISTRY A)

Test	Values	Remarks
SERUM / PLASMA		
Acetone	Negative	
Albumin	3.2-5 g/dL	
Alcohol, ethyl	Negative	
Aldolase	1.2-7.6 IU/L	
Ammonia	20-70 mcg/dL	Specimen to be placed on ice as soon as collected.
Amylase	30-110 units/L	
Bilirubin, direct	0-0.3 mg/dL	
Bilirubin, total	0.1-1.2 mg/dL	
Calcium	8.6-10.3 mg/dL	
Calcium, ionized	2.24-2.46 mEq/L	
Chloride	95-108 mEq/L	
Cholesterol, total	≤200 mg/dL	Fasted blood required – normal value affected by dietary habits. This reference range is for a general adult population.
HDL cholesterol	40-60 mg/dL	Fasted blood required – normal value affected by dietary habits.
LDL cholesterol	<160 mg/dL	If triglyceride is >400 mg/dL, LDL cannot be calculated accurately (Friedewald equation). Target LDL-C depends on patient's risk factors.
CO_2	23-30 mEq/L	
Creatine kinase (CK) isoenzymes		
CK-BB	0%	
CK-MB (cardiac)	0%-3.9%	
CK-MM (muscle)	96%-100%	
CK-MB levels must be both ≥4% and 10 IU/L to meet diagnostic criteria for CK-MB positive result consistent with myocardial injury.		
Creatine phosphokinase (CPK)	8-150 IU/L	
Creatinine	0.5-1.4 mg/dL	
Ferritin	13-300 ng/mL	
Folate	3.6-20 ng/dL	
GGT (gamma-glutamyltranspeptidase)		
male	11-63 IU/L	
female	8-35 IU/L	
GLDH	To be determined	
Glucose (preprandial)	<115 mg/dL	Goals different for diabetics.
Glucose, fasting	60-110 mg/dL	Goals different for diabetics.
Glucose, nonfasting (2-h postprandial)	<120 mg/dL	Goals different for diabetics.
Hemoglobin A_{1c}	<8	
Hemoglobin, plasma free	<2.5 mg/100 mL	
Hemoglobin, total glycosolated (Hb A_1)	4%-8%	
Iron	65-150 mcg/dL	
Iron binding capacity, total (TIBC)	250-420 mcg/dL	
Lactic acid	0.7-2.1 mEq/L	Specimen to be kept on ice and sent to lab as soon as possible.
Lactate dehydrogenase (LDH)	56-194 IU/L	
Lactate dehydrogenase (LDH) isoenzymes		
LD_1	20%-34%	
LD_2	29%-41%	
LD_3	15%-25%	
LD_4	1%-12%	
LD_5	1%-15%	
Flipped LD_1/LD_2 ratios (>1 may be consistent with myocardial injury) particularly when considered in combination with a recent CK-MB positive result.		
Lipase	23-208 units/L	
Magnesium	1.6-2.5 mg/dL	Increased by slight hemolysis.
Osmolality	289-308 mOsm/kg	
Phosphatase, alkaline		
adults 25-60 y	33-131 IU/L	
adults 61 y or older	51-153 IU/L	
infancy-adolescence	Values range up to 3-5 times higher than adults	

Automated Chemistry (CHEMISTRY A) *(continued)*

Test	Values	Remarks
Phosphate, inorganic	2.8-4.2 mg/dL	
Potassium	3.5-5.2 mEq/L	Increased by slight hemolysis.
Prealbumin	>15 mg/dL	
Protein, total	6.5-7.9 g/dL	
SGOT (AST)	<35 IU/L (20-48)	
SGPT (ALT) (10-35)	<35 IU/L	
Sodium	134-149 mEq/L	
Transferrin	>200 mg/dL	
Triglycerides	45-155 mg/dL	Fasted blood required.
Troponin I	<1.5 ng/mL	
Urea nitrogen (BUN)	7-20 mg/dL	
Uric acid		
male	2-8 mg/dL	
female	2-7.5 mg/dL	

CEREBROSPINAL FLUID

Glucose	50-70 mg/dL	
Protein		
adults and children	15-45 mg/dL	CSF obtained by lumbar puncture.
newborn infants	60-90 mg/dL	

On CSF obtained by cisternal puncture: About 25 mg/dL
On CSF obtained by ventricular puncture: About 10 mg/dL

Note: Bloody specimen gives erroneously high value due to contamination with blood proteins

URINE
(24-hour specimen is required for all these tests unless specified)

Test	Values	Remarks
Amylase	32-641 units/L	The value is in units/L and **not** calculated for total volume.
Amylase, fluid (random samples)		Interpretation of value left for physician, depends on the nature of fluid.
Calcium	Depends upon dietary intake	
Creatine		
male	150 mg/24 h	Higher value on children and during pregnancy.
female	250 mg/24 h	
Creatinine	1000-2000 mg/24 h	
Creatinine clearance (endogenous)		
male	85-125 mL/min	A blood sample must accompany urine specimen.
female	75-115 mL/min	
Glucose	1 g/24 h	
5-hydroxyindoleacetic acid	2-8 mg/24 h	
Iron	0.15 mg/24 h	Acid washed container required.
Magnesium	146-209 mg/24 h	
Osmolality	500-800 mOsm/kg	With normal fluid intake.
Oxalate	10-40 mg/24 h	
Phosphate	400-1300 mg/24 h	
Potassium	25-120 mEq/24 h	Varies with diet; the interpretation of urine electrolytes and osmolality should be left for the physician.
Sodium	40-220 mEq/24 h	
Porphobilinogen, qualitative	Negative	
Porphyrins, qualitative	Negative	
Proteins	0.05-0.1 g/24 h	
Salicylate	Negative	
Urea clearance	60-95 mL/min	A blood sample must accompany specimen.
Urea N	10-40 g/24 h	Dependent on protein intake.
Uric acid	250-750 mg/24 h	Dependent on diet and therapy.
Urobilinogen	0.5-3.5 mg/24 h	For qualitative determination on random urine, send sample to urinalysis section in Hematology Lab.
Xylose absorption test		
children	16%-33% of ingested xylose	

FECES

Fat, 3-day collection	<5 g/d	Value depends on fat intake of 100 g/d for 3 days preceding and during collection.

GASTRIC ACIDITY

Acidity, total, 12 h	10-60 mEq/L	Titrated at pH 7.

REFERENCE VALUES FOR ADULTS *(Continued)*

Blood Gases

	Arterial	Capillary	Venous
pH	7.35-7.45	7.35-7.45	7.32-7.42
pCO_2 (mm Hg)	35-45	35-45	38-52
pO_2 (mm Hg)	70-100	60-80	24-48
HCO_3 (mEq/L)	19-25	19-25	19-25
TCO_2 (mEq/L)	19-29	19-29	23-33
O_2 saturation (%)	90-95	90-95	40-70
Base excess (mEq/L)	-5 to +5	-5 to +5	-5 to +5

HEMATOLOGY

Complete Blood Count

Age	Hgb (g/dL)	Hct (%)	RBC (mill/mm³)	RDW
0-3 d	15.0-20.0	45-61	4.0-5.9	<18
1-2 wk	12.5-18.5	39-57	3.6-5.5	<17
1-6 mo	10.0-13.0	29-42	3.1-4.3	<16.5
7 mo to 2 y	10.5-13.0	33-38	3.7-4.9	<16
2-5 y	11.5-13.0	34-39	3.9-5.0	<15
5-8 y	11.5-14.5	35-42	4.0-4.9	<15
13-18 y	12.0-15.2	36-47	4.5-5.1	<14.5
Adult male	13.5-16.5	41-50	4.5-5.5	<14.5
Adult female	12.0-15.0	36-44	4.0-4.9	<14.5

Age	MCV (fL)	MCH (pg)	MCHC (%)	Plts (x 10³/mm³)
0-3 d	95-115	31-37	29-37	250-450
1-2 wk	86-110	28-36	28-38	250-450
1-6 mo	74-96	25-35	30-36	300-700
7 mo to 2 y	70-84	23-30	31-37	250-600
2-5 y	75-87	24-30	31-37	250-550
5-8 y	77-95	25-33	31-37	250-550
13-18 y	78-96	25-35	31-37	150-450
Adult male	80-100	26-34	31-37	150-450
Adult female	80-100	26-34	31-37	150-450

WBC and Differential

Age	WBC (x 10³/mm³)	Segs	Bands	Lymphs	Monos
0-3 d	9.0-35.0	32-62	10-18	19-29	5-7
1-2 wk	5.0-20.0	14-34	6-14	36-45	6-10
1-6 mo	6.0-17.5	13-33	4-12	41-71	4-7
7 mo to 2 y	6.0-17.0	15-35	5-11	45-76	3-6
2-5 y	5.5-15.5	23-45	5-11	35-65	3-6
5-8 y	5.0-14.5	32-54	5-11	28-48	3-6
13-18 y	4.5-13.0	34-64	5-11	25-45	3-6
Adults	4.5-11.0	35-66	5-11	24-44	3-6

Age	Eosinophils	Basophils	Atypical Lymphs	No. of NRBCs
0-3 d	0-2	0-1	0-8	0-2
1-2 wk	0-2	0-1	0-8	0
1-6 mo	0-3	0-1	0-8	0
7 mo to 2 y	0-3	0-1	0-8	0
2-5 y	0-3	0-1	0-8	0
5-8 y	0-3	0-1	0-8	0
13-18 y	0-3	0-1	0-8	0
Adults	0-3	0-1	0-8	0

Segs = segmented neutrophils.

Bands = band neutrophils.

Lymphs = lymphocytes.

Monos = monocytes.

Erythrocyte Sedimentation Rates and Reticulocyte Counts

Sedimentation rate, Westergren	Children	0-20 mm/hour
	Adult male	0-15 mm/hour
	Adult female	0-20 mm/hour
Sedimentation rate, Wintrobe	Children	0-13 mm/hour
	Adult male	0-10 mm/hour
	Adult female	0-15 mm/hour
Reticulocyte count	Newborns	2%-6%
	1-6 mo	0%-2.8%
	Adults	0.5%-1.5%

REFERENCE VALUES FOR CHILDREN

Chemistry

Albumin	0-1 y	2-4 g/dL
	1 y to adult	3.5-5.5 g/dL
Ammonia	Newborns	90-150 µg/dL
	Children	40-120 µg/dL
	Adults	18-54 µg/dL
Amylase	Newborns	0-60 units/L
	Adults	30-110 units/L
Bilirubin, conjugated, direct	Newborns	<1.5 mg/dL
	1 mo to adult	0-0.5 mg/dL
Bilirubin, total	0-3 d	2-10 mg/dL
	1 mo to adult	0-1.5 mg/dL
Bilirubin, unconjugated, indirect		0.6-10.5 mg/dL
Calcium	Newborns	7-12 mg/dL
	0-2 y	8.8-11.2 mg/dL
	2 y to adult	9-11 mg/dL
Calcium, ionized, whole blood		4.4-5.4 mg/dL
Carbon dioxide, total		23-33 mEq/L
Chloride		95-105 mEq/L
Cholesterol	Newborns	45-170 mg/dL
	0-1 y	65-175 mg/dL
	1-20 y	120-230 mg/dL
Creatinine	0-1 y	≤0.6 mg/dL
	1 y to adult	0.5-1.5 mg/dL
Glucose	Newborns	30-90 mg/dL
	0-2 y	60-105 mg/dL
	Children to adults	70-110 mg/dL
Iron	Newborns	110-270 µg/dL
	Infants	30-70 µg/dL
	Children	55-120 µg/dL
	Adults	70-180 µg/dL
Iron binding	Newborns	59-175 µg/dL
	Infants	100-400 µg/dL
	Adults	250-400 µg/dL
Lactic acid, lactate		2-20 mg/dL
Lead, whole blood		<10 µg/dL
Lipase	Children	20-140 units/L
	Adults	0-190 units/L
Magnesium		1.5-2.5 mEq/L
Osmolality, serum		275-296 mOsm/kg
Osmolality, urine		50-1400 mOsm/kg
Phosphorus	Newborns	4.2-9.0 mg/dL
	6 wk to ≤18 mo	3.8-6.7 mg/dL
	18 mo to 3 y	2.9-5.9 mg/dL
	3-15 y	3.6-5.6 mg/dL
	>15 y	2.5-5.0 mg/dL
Potassium, plasma	Newborns	4.5-7.2 mEq/L
	2 d to 3 mo	4.0-6.2 mEq/L
	3 mo to 1 y	3.7-5.6 mEq/L
	1-16 y	3.5-5.0 mEq/L
Protein, total	0-2 y	4.2-7.4 g/dL
	>2 y	6-8 g/dL
Sodium		136-145 mEq/L
Triglycerides	Infants	0-171 mg/dL
	Children	20-130 mg/dL
	Adults	30-200 mg/dL
Urea nitrogen, blood	0-2 y	4-15 mg/dL
	2 y to adult	5-20 mg/dL
Uric acid	Male	3-7 mg/dL
	Female	2-6 mg/dL

ENZYMES

Alanine aminotransferase (ALT) (SGPT)	0-2 mo	8-78 units/L
	>2 mo	8-36 units/L
Alkaline phosphatase (ALKP)	Newborns	60-130 units/L
	0-16 y	85-400 units/L
	>16 y	30-115 units/L
Aspartate aminotransferase (AST) (SGOT)	Infants	18-74 units/L
	Children	15-46 units/L
	Adults	5-35 units/L
Creatine kinase (CK)	Infants	20-200 units/L
	Children	10-90 units/L
	Adult male	0-206 units/L
	Adult female	0-175 units/L
Lactate dehydrogenase (LDH)	Newborns	290-501 units/L
	1 mo to 2 y	110-144 units/L
	>16 y	60-170 units/L

BLOOD GASES

	Arterial	Capillary	Venous
pH	7.35-7.45	7.35-7.45	7.32-7.42
pCO_2 (mm Hg)	35-45	35-45	38-52
pO_2 (mm Hg)	70-100	60-80	24-48
HCO_3 (mEq/L)	19-25	19-25	19-25
TCO_2 (mEq/L)	19-29	19-29	23-33
O_2 saturation (%)	90-95	90-95	40-70
Base excess (mEq/L)	-5 to +5	-5 to +5	-5 to +5

THYROID FUNCTION TESTS

T_4 (thyroxine)	1-7 d	10.1-20.9 µg/dL
	8-14 d	9.8-16.6 µg/dL
	1 mo to 1 y	5.5-16.0 µg/dL
	>1 y	4-12 µg/dL
FTI	1-3 d	9.3-26.6
	1-4 wks	7.6-20.8
	1-4 mo	7.4-17.9
	4-12 mo	5.1-14.5
	1-6 y	5.7-13.3
	>6 y	4.8-14.0
T_3 by RIA	Newborns	100-470 ng/dL
	1-5 y	100-260 ng/dL
	5-10 y	90-240 ng/dL
	10 y to adult	70-210 ng/dL
T_3 uptake		35%-45%
TSH	Cord	3-22 µU/mL
	1-3 d	<40 µU/mL
	3-7 d	<25 µU/mL
	>7 d	0-10 µU/mL

ANGIOTENSIN AGENTS

ACE Inhibitors: Comparison of Indications and Adult Dosages

Drug	Hypertension	CHF	Renal Dysfunction	Dialyzable	Strengths (mg)
Benazepril (Lotensin®)	10-40 mg/day	Not FDA approved	Cl$_{cr}$ <30 mL/min: 5 mg/day initially Maximum: 40 mg/day	Yes	Tablets 5, 10, 20, 40
Captopril (Capoten®)	25-100 mg/day bid-tid	6.25-100 mg tid Maximum: 450 mg/day	Cl$_{cr}$ 10-50 mL/min: 75% of usual dose Cl$_{cr}$ <10 mL/min: 50% of usual dose	Yes	Tablets 12.5, 25, 50, 100
Enalapril (Vasotec®)	2.5-40 mg/day qd-bid	2.5-20 mg bid Maximum: 20 mg bid	Cl$_{cr}$ 30-80 mL/min: 5 mg/day initially Cl$_{cr}$ <30 mL/min: 2.5 mg/day initially	Yes	Tablets 2.5, 5, 10, 20
Enalaprilat[1]	0.625 mg, 1.25 mg, 2.5 mg q6h Maximum: 5 mg q6h	Not FDA approved	Cl$_{cr}$ <30 mL/min: 0.625 mg q6h	Yes	2.5 mg/2 mL vial
Fosinopril (Monopril®)	10-40 mg/day	10-40 mg/day	No dosage reduction necessary	Not well dialyzed	Tablets 10, 20, 40
Lisinopril (Prinivil®, Zestril®)	10-40 mg/day Maximum: 40 mg/day	5-40 mg/day	Cl$_{cr}$ 10-30 mL/min: 5 mg/day initially Cl$_{cr}$ <10 mL/min: 2.5 mg/day initially	Yes	Tablets 2.5, 5, 10, 20, 30, 40
Moexipril (Univasc®)	7.5-30 mg/day qd-bid Maximum: 30 mg/day	LV dysfunction (post-MI): 7.5-30 mg/day	Cl$_{cr}$ <40 mL/min: 3.75 mg/day initially Maximum: 15 mg/day	Unknown	Tablets 7.5, 15
Perindopril (Aceon®)	4-8 mg/day	4-8 mg/day Maximum: 16 mg/day	Cl$_{cr}$ 30-60 mL/min: 2 mg/day Cl$_{cr}$ 15-29 mL/min: 2 mg qod Cl$_{cr}$ <15 mL/min: 2 mg on dialysis days	Yes	Tablets 2, 4, 8
Quinapril (Accupril®)	10-40 mg/day qd-bid	5-20 mg bid	Cl$_{cr}$ 30-60 mL/min: 5 mg/day initially Cl$_{cr}$ <10-30 mL/min: 2.5 mg/day initially	Not well dialyzed	Tablets 5, 10, 20, 40
Ramipril (Altace®)	2.5-20 mg/day qd-bid	2.5-10 mg/day	Cl$_{cr}$ <40 mL/min: 25% of normal dose	Unknown	Capsules 1.25, 2.5, 5, 10
Trandolapril (Mavik®)	1-4 mg/day Maximum: 8 mg/day qd-bid	LV dysfunction (post-MI): 1-4 mg/day	Cl$_{cr}$ <30 mL/min: 0.5 mg/day initially	No	Tablets 1, 2, 4

Dosage is based on 70 kg adult with normal hepatic and renal function.

[1]Enalaprilat is the only available ACE inhibitor in a parenteral formulation.

Angiotensin II Receptor Blockers: Comparison of Indications and Adult Dosages

Drug	Hypertension	CHF	Renal Dysfunction	Dialyzable	Strengths (mg)
Candesartan (Atacand®)	8-32 mg/day	4-32 mg once daily (not FDA approved)	No dosage adjustment necessary	No	Tablets 4, 8, 16, 32
Eprosartan (Teveten®)	400-800 mg/day qd-bid	Not FDA approved	No dosage adjustment necessary	Unknown	Tablets 400, 600
Irbesartan (Avapro®)	150-300 mg/day	Not FDA approved	No dosage reduction necessary	No	Tablets 75, 150, 300
Losartan (Cozaar®)	25-100 mg qd or bid	Not FDA approved	No dosage adjustment necessary	No	Tablets 25, 50, 100
Olmesartan (Benicar™)	20-40 mg/day	Not FDA approved	No dosage adjustment necessary	Unknown	Tablets 5, 20, 40
Telmisartan (Micardis®)	20-80 mg/day	Not FDA approved	No dosage reduction necessary	No	Tablets 20, 40, 80
Valsartan (Diovan®)	80-320 mg/day	40-160 mg bid	Decrease dose only if Cl_{cr} <10 mL/minute	No	Tablets 40, 80, 160, 320

Dosage is based on 70 kg adult with normal hepatic and renal function.

ANGIOTENSIN AGENTS (Continued)

Comparative Pharmacokinetics of ACE Inhibitors

Drug	Prodrug	Absorption (%)	Serum $t_{1/2}$ (h) Normal Renal Function	Serum Protein Binding (%)	Elimination	Onset of BP Lowering Action (h)	Peak BP Lowering Effects (h)	Duration of BP Lowering Effects (h)
Benazepril	Yes	37		~97	Renal (32%), biliary (~12%)	1	2-4	24
Benazeprilat			10-11 (effective)	~95%				
Captopril	No	60-75 (fasting)	1.9 (elimination)	25-30	Renal	0.25-0.5	1-1.5	~6
Enalapril	Yes	55-75	2	50-60		1	4-6	12-24
Enalaprilat			11 (effective)		Renal (60%-80%), fecal			
Fosinopril		36				1		24
Fosinoprilat			12 (effective)	>99	Renal (~50%), biliary (~50%)			
Moexipril	Yes		1	90	Fecal (53%), renal (8%)		1-2	>24
Moexiprilat			2-10	50				
Perindopril	Yes		1.5-3	60	Renal		3-7	
Perindoprilat			3-10 (effective)	10-20				
Quinapril	Yes	>60	0.8	97	Renal (~60% as metabolite, fecal	1	2-4	24
Quinaprilat			2					
Ramipril	Yes	50-60	1-2	73	Renal (60%), fecal (40%)	1-2	3-6	24
Ramiprilat			13-17 (effective)	56				
Trandolapril	Yes		6	80	Renal (33%), fecal (66%)	1-2	6	≥24
Trandolaprilat			10	65-94				

Comparative Pharmacokinetics of Angiotensin II Receptor Blockers

	Candesartan (Atacand®)	Eprosartan (Teveten®)	Irbesartan (Avapro®)	Losartan (Cozaar®)	Olmesartan (Benicar™)	Telmisartan (Micardis®)	Valsartan (Diovan™)
Prodrug	Yes[1]	No	No	Yes[2]	Yes	No	No
Time to peak	3-4 h	1-2 h	1.5-2	1 h / 3-4 h[2]	1-2 h	0.5-1 h	2-4 h
Bioavailability	15%	13%	60%-80%	33%	26%	42%-58%	25%
Food – area-under-the-curve	No effect	No effect	No effect	9%-10%	No effect	9.6%-20%	9%-40%
Elimination half-life	9 h	5-9 h	11-15 h	1.5-2 h / 6-9 h[2]	13 h	24 h	6 h
Elimination altered in renal dysfunction	Yes[3]	No	No	No	Yes	No	No
Precautions in severe renal dysfunction	Yes	Yes	Yes	Yes	Yes	Yes	Yes
Elimination altered in hepatic dysfunction	No	No	No	Yes	Yes	Yes	Yes
Precautions in hepatic dysfunction	No	Yes	No	No	No	Yes	Yes
Protein binding	>99%	98%	90%	~99%	99%	>99.5%	95%

[1]Candesartan cilexetil: Active metabolite candesartan.

[2]Losartan: Active metabolite E-3174.

[3]Dosage adjustments are not necessary.

ANTIARRHYTHMIC DRUGS

Vaughan Williams Classification of Antiarrhythmic Drugs Based on Cardiac Effects

Class	Drug(s)	Conduction Velocity[1]	Refractory Period	Automaticity
I	Moricizine	↓	↓	↓ (0 on SA node)
Ia	Disopyramide Procainamide Quinidine	↓	↑	↓
Ib	Lidocaine Mexiletine Tocainide	0/↓	↓	↓
Ic	Flecainide Propafenone[2]	↓↓	0	↓
II	Beta-blockers	0	0	↓
III	Amiodarone Bretylium Dofetilide Ibutilide Sotalol[2]	0	↑↑	0
IV	Diltiazem Verapamil[3]	↓	↑	↓

[1]Variables for normal tissue models in ventricular tissue.

[2]Also has type II, beta-blocking action.

[3]Variables for SA and AV nodal tissue only.

Vaughan Williams Classification of Antiarrhythmic Agents and Their Indications / Adverse Effects

Class	Drug(s)	Indication	Route of Administration	Adverse Effects
I	Moricizine	VT	P.O.	Dizziness, nausea, rash, seizures
Ia	Disopyramide	AF, VT	P.O.	Anticholinergic effects, CHF
Ia	Procainamide	AF, VT, WPW	P.O./I.V.	GI, CNS, lupus, fever, hematological, anticholinergic effects
Ia	Quinidine	AF, PSVT, VT, WPW	P.O./I.V.	Hypotension, GI, thrombocytopenia, cinchonism
Ib	Lidocaine	VT, VF, PVC	I.V.	CNS, GI
Ib	Mexiletine	VT	P.O.	GI, CNS
Ib	Tocainide	VT	P.O.	GI, CNS, pulmonary, agranulocytosis
Ic	Flecainide	VT	P.O.	CHF, GI, CNS, blurred vision
Ic	Propafenone	VT	P.O.	GI, blurred vision, dizziness
II	Esmolol	VT, SVT	I.V.	CHF, CNS, lupus-like syndrome, hypotension, bradycardia, bronchospasm
II	Propranolol	SVT, VT, PVC, digoxin toxicity	P.O./I.V.	CHF, bradycardia, hypotension, CNS, fatigue
III	Amiodarone	VT	P.O.	CNS, GI, thyroid, pulmonary fibrosis, liver, corneal deposits
III	Bretylium	VT, VF	I.V.	GI, orthostatic hypotension, CNS
III	Dofetilide	AF	P.O.	Headache, dizziness, VT, torsade de pointes
III	Ibutilide	AF	I.V.	Torsade de pointes, hypotension, branch bundle block, AV block, nausea, headache
III	Sotalol	AF, VT	P.O.	Bradycardia, hypotension, CHF, CNS, fatigue
IV	Diltiazem	AF, PSVT	P.O./I.V.	Hypotension, GI, liver
IV	Verapamil	AF, PSVT	P.O./I.V.	Hypotension, CHF, bradycardia, vertigo, constipation
Miscellaneous	Adenosine	SVT, PSVT	I.V.	Flushing, dizziness, bradycardia, syncope
Miscellaneous	Digoxin	AF, PSVT	P.O./I.V.	GI, CNS, arrhythmias
Miscellaneous	Magnesium	VT, VF	I.V.	Hypotension, CNS, hypothermia, myocardial depression

AF = atrial fibrillation.
PSVT = paroxysmal supraventricular tachycardia.
SVT = supraventricular tachycardia.
VF = ventricular fibrillation.
VT = ventricular tachycardia.
WPW = Wolf-Parkinson-White arrhythmias.

ANTIARRHYTHMIC DRUGS (Continued)

Comparative Pharmacokinetic Properties of Antiarrhythmic Agents

Class	Drug(s)	Bioavailability (%)	Primary Route of Elimination	Volume of Distribution (L/kg)	Protein Binding (%)	Half-Life	Therapeutic Range (mcg/mL)
I	Moricizine	34-38	Hepatic	6-11	92-95	1-6 h	—
Ia	Disopyramide	70-95	Hepatic/Renal	0.8-2	50-80	4-8 h	2-6
	Procainamide	75-95	Hepatic/Renal	1.5-3	10-20	2.5-5 h	4-15
	Quinidine	70-80	Hepatic	2-3.5	80-90	5-9 h	2-6
Ib	Lidocaine	20-40	Hepatic	1-2	65-75	60-180 min	1.5-5
	Mexiletine	80-95	Hepatic	5-12	60-75	6-12 h	0.75-2
	Tocainide	90-95	Hepatic	1.5-3	10-30	12-15 h	4-10
Ic	Flecainide	90-95	Hepatic/Renal	8-10	35-45	12-30 h	0.3-2.5
	Propafenone[1]	11-39	Hepatic	2.5-4	85-95	12-32 h / 2-10 h	—
II	Esmolol			Refer to Beta-Blocker Comparison Chart			
	Propranolol			Refer to Beta-Blocker Comparison Chart			
III	Amiodarone	22-28	Hepatic	70-150	95-97	15-100 d	1-2.5
	Bretylium	15-20	Renal	4-8	Negligible	5-10 h	0.5-2
	Dofetilide	>90%	Renal	3 L/kg	60-70	10 h	—
	Ibutilide	NA	Hepatic	11	40	2-12 h	—
	Sotalol	90-95	Renal	1.6-2.4	Negligible	12-15 h	—
IV	Diltiazem	80-90	Hepatic/Renal	1.7	77-85	4-6 h	0.05-0.2
	Verapamil	20-40	Hepatic	1.5-5	95-99	4-12 h	>50 ng/mL

[1]Top numbers reflect **poor** metabolizers and **bottom** numbers reflect **extensive** metabolizers.

ANTICOAGULANTS, INJECTABLE

Name	Use	Limitation	Dose (SubQ unless otherwise noted)	Average MW (in daltons)
Low Molecular Weight Heparins				
Dalteparin (Fragmin®)	Prophylaxis	Abdominal surgery[1]	2500 units/d	4000-6000
		Abdominal surgery[2]	5000 units/d	
		Hip surgery[1]	5000 units/d postoperatively	
	Treatment	DVT[3]	100 units/kg bid 200 units/kg qd	4000-6000
		Unstable[4] angina Non-Q-wave MI	120 units/kg (max: 10,000 units) q12h for 5-8 d	
Enoxaparin (Lovenox®)	Prophylaxis	Hip or knee replacement	30 mg twice daily[5]	3500-5500
		High-risk hip replacement or abdominal surgery	40 mg once daily	
	Treatment	DVT or PE	1 mg/kg q12h	
		Acute coronary	1 mg/kg q12h	
Tinzaparin (Innohep®)	Treatment	DVT or PE	175 anti-Xa int. units/kg/day	5500-7500
Heparin				
Heparin (Hep-Lock®)	Prophylaxis	Risk of thromboembolic disease	5000 units q8-12h	3000-30,000
	Treatment	Thrombosis or embolization	80 units/kg IVP then 20,000-40,000 units daily as continuous I.V. infusion	
	Treatment[3]	Unstable angina[3]	80 units/kg IVP then 20,000-40,000 units daily as continuous I.V. infusion	
Heparinoid				
Danaparoid (Orgaran® [DSC])	Prophylaxis	Hip replacement	750 units bid	6500
	Treatment[3]		2000 units q12h	
Selective Anti-Xa Inhibitor				
Fondaparinux[6] (Arixtra®)	Prophylaxis	Hip fracture Hip or knee replacement	2.5 mg once daily	1728
Coumarin Derivatives				
Warfarin (Coumadin®)	Prophylaxis	NS	Variable	NS
	Treatment		2-5 mg/d	

NS = not stated.

[1] Patients with low risk of DVT.

[2] Patients with high risk of DVT.

[3] Not FDA approved.

[4] Patients >60 years of age may require a lower dose of heparin.

[5] Patients weighing <100 lb or ≥65 years of age may receive 0.5 mg/kg/dose every 12 hours.

[6] Synthetic pentasaccharide.

ANTICONVULSANTS BY SEIZURE TYPE

Seizure Type	Age	Commonly Used	Alternatives
Primary generalized tonic-clonic	1 mo - 6 y	Carbamazepine, phenytoin, phenobarbital	Valproate
	6-11 y	Carbamazepine	Valproate, phenytoin, phenobarbital, lamotrigine, primidone
Primary generalized tonic-clonic with absence or with myoclonic	1 mo - 18 y	Valproate	Phenytoin, phenobarbital, carbamazepine, primidone
Partial seizures (with or without secondary generalization)	1-12 mo	Phenobarbital	Carbamazepine, phenytoin
	1-6 y	Carbamazepine	Phenytoin, phenobarbital, valproate, lamotrigine, gabapentin, oxcarbazepine (>4 y), primidone
	>6 y	Carbamazepine	Lamotrigine, levetiracetam, oxcarbazepine, phenytoin, phenobarbital, tiagabine, topiramate, valproate, primidone, zonisamide (>16 y)
Absence seizures	<10 y	Ethosuximide, valproate	Clonazepam, acetazolamide, lamotrigine
	>10 y	Valproate	Ethosuximide, acetazolamide, clonazepam
Juvenile myoclonic		Valproate	Phenobarbital, primidone, clonazepam; consider: carbamazepine, phenytoin, acetazolamide
Progressive myoclonic		Valproate	Valproate plus clonazepam, phenobarbital
Lennox-Gastaut and related syndromes		Valproate	lamotrigine, phenobarbital, clonazepam, ethosuximide; consider: steroids, ketogenic diet
Infantile spasms		ACTH, steroids	Valproate; consider: clonazepam, vigabatrin, pyridoxine
Neonatal seizures		Phenobarbital	Phenytoin; consider: clonazepam, primidone, valproate, pyridoxine

ANTIDEPRESSANT AGENTS

Comparison of Usual Dosage, Mechanism of Action, and Adverse Effects

Drug	Initial Dose	Usual Dosage (mg/d)	Dosage Forms	Adverse Effects						Comments
				ACH	Drowsiness	Orthostatic Hypotension	Conduction Abnormalities[1]	GI Distress	Weight Gain	
Tricyclic Antidepressants and Related Compounds[1]										
Amitriptyline	25–75 mg qhs	100-300	T, I	4+	4+	3+	3+	1	4+	Also used in chronic pain, migraine, and as a hypnotic; contraindicated with cisapride
Amoxapine	50 mg bid	100-400	T	2+	2+	2+	2+	0	2+	May cause extrapyramidal symptom (EPS)
Clomipramine[2] (Anafranil®)	25–75 mg qhs	100-250	C	4+	4+	2+	3+	1+	4+	Approved for OCD
Desipramine (Norpramin®)	25–75 mg qhs	100-300	T	1+	2+	2+	2+	0	1+	Blood levels useful for therapeutic monitoring
Doxepin (Sinequan®, Zonalon®)	25–75 mg qhs	100-300	C, L	3+	4+	2+	2+	0	4+	
Imipramine (Tofranil®, Tofranil-PM®)	25–75 mg qhs	100-300	T, C	3+	3+	4+	3+	1+	4+	Blood levels useful for therapeutic monitoring
Maprotiline	25–75 mg qhs	100-225	T	2+	3+	2+	2+	0	2+	
Nortriptyline (Pamelor®)	25–50 mg qhs	50-150	C, L	2+	2+	1+	2+	0	1+	Blood levels useful for therapeutic monitoring
Protriptyline (Vivactil®)	15 mg qAM	15-60	T	2+	1+	2+	3+	1+	1+	
Trimipramine (Surmontil®)	25–75 mg qhs	100-300	C	4+	4+	3+	3+	0	4+	

ANTIDEPRESSANT AGENTS (Continued)

Comparison of Usual Dosage, Mechanism of Action, and Adverse Effects (continued)

Drug	Initial Dose	Usual Dosage (mg/d)	Dosage Forms	Adverse Effects						Comments
				ACH	Drowsiness	Orthostatic Hypotension	Conduction Abnormalities	GI Distress	Weight Gain	
Selective Serotonin Reuptake Inhibitors[3]										
Citalopram (Celexa™)	20 mg qAM	20-60	T	0	0	0	0	3+[4]	1+	
Escitalopram (Lexapro™)	10 mg qAM	10-20	T	0	0	0	0	3+	1+	S-enantiomer of citalopram
Fluoxetine (Prozac®, Prozac Weekly™, Sarafem™)	10-20 mg qAM	20-80	C, L, T	0	0	0	0	3+[4]	1+	CYP2B6 and 2D6 inhibitor
Fluvoxamine[2]	50 mg qhs	100-300	T	0	0	0	0	3+[4]	1+	Contraindicated with pimozide, thioridazine, mesoridazine, CYP1A2, 2B6, 2C19, and 3A4 inhibitors
Paroxetine (Paxil®, Paxil® CR™)	10-20 mg qAM	20-50	T, L	1+	1+	0	0	3+[4]	2+	CYP2B6 and 2D6 inhibitor
Sertraline (Zoloft®)	25-50 mg qAM	50-200	T	0	0	0	0	3+[4]	1+	CYP2B6 and 2C19 inhibitor
Dopamine-Reuptake Blocking Compounds										
Bupropion (Wellbutrin®, Wellbutrin SR®, Wellbutrin XL™, Zyban®)	100 mg bid-tid IR[5] 150 mg qAM-bid SR[6]	300-450[7]	T	0	0	0	1+/0	1+	0	Contraindicated with seizures, bulimia, and anorexia; low incidence of sexual dysfunction IR: A 6-h interval between doses preferred SR: An 8-h interval between doses preferred
Serotonin / Norepinephrine Reuptake Inhibitors[8]										
Duloxetine (Cymbalta®)	40-60 mg qd	40-60	C	1+	1+	0	1+	3+[4]	0	
Venlafaxine (Effexor®, Effexor® XR)	25 mg bid-tid IR 37.5 mg qd XR	75-375	T	1+	1+	0	1+	3+[4]	0	High-dose is useful to treat refractory depression; frequency of hypertension increases with dosage >225 mg/d

Comparison of Usual Dosage, Mechanism of Action, and Adverse Effects (continued)

Drug	Initial Dose	Usual Dosage (mg/d)	Dosage Forms	Adverse Effects						Comments
				ACH	Drowsiness	Orthostatic Hypotension	Conduction Abnormalities	GI Distress	Weight Gain	
5-HT₂ Receptor Antagonist Properties										
Nefazodone	100 mg bid	300–600	T	1+	1+	2+	1+	1+	0	Contraindicated with carbamazepine, pimozide, astemizole, cisapride, and terfenadine; caution with triazolam and alprazolam; low incidence of sexual dysfunction
Trazodone (Desyrel®)	50 mg tid	150–600	T	0	4+	3+	1+	1+	2+	
Noradrenergic Antagonist										
Mirtazapine (Remeron®, Remeron® SolTab®)	15 mg qhs	15–45	T	1+	3+	1+	1+	0	3+	Dose >15 mg/d less sedating, low incidence of sexual dysfunction
Monoamine Oxidase Inhibitors										
Isocarboxazid (Marplan®)	10 mg tid	10–30	T	2+	2+	2+	1+	1+	2+	Diet must be low in tyramine; contraindicated with sympathomimetics and other antidepressants
Phenelzine (Nardil®)	15 mg tid	15–90	T	2+	2+	2+	0	1+	3+	
Tranylcypromine (Parnate®)	10 mg bid	10–60	T	2+	1+	2+	1+	1+	2+	

ACH = anticholinergic effects (dry mouth, blurred vision, urinary retention, constipation); 0 - 4+ = absent or rare - relatively common. T = tablet; L = liquid, I = injectable, C = capsule; IR = immediate release, SR = sustained release.

Important note: A 1-week supply taken all at once in a patient receiving the maximum dose can be fatal.

[1]Not approved by FDA for depression. Approved for OCD.

[2]Flat dose response curve, headache, nausea, and sexual dysfunction are common side effects for SSRIs.

[3]Nausea is usually mild and transient.

[4]IR: 100 mg bid, may be increased to 100 mg tid no sooner than 3 days after beginning therapy.

[5]SR: 150 mg qAM, may be increased to 150 mg bid as early as day 4 of dosing.

[6]To minimize seizure risk, do not exceed IR 150 mg/dose or SR 200 mg/dose.

[7]Do not use with sibutramine; relatively safe in overdose.

ANTIMIGRAINE DRUGS: 5-HT$_1$ RECEPTOR AGONISTS

Pharmacokinetic Differences

Pharmacokinetic Parameter	Almotriptan (Axert™) Oral (6.25 mg)	Eletriptan (Relpax®) Tablets	Frovatriptan (Frova®) Oral	Naratriptan (Amerge®) Oral	Rizatriptan (Maxalt®, Maxalt-MLT®) Tablets	Rizatriptan Disintegrating Tablets	Sumatriptan (Imitrex®) SubQ (6 mg)	Sumatriptan Oral (100 mg)	Sumatriptan Nasal (20 mg)	Zolmitriptan (Zomig®, Zomig-ZMT™) Oral (5 mg)	Zolmitriptan Oral (10 mg)
Onset	<60 min	<2 h	<2 h	30 min	~30 min	~30 min	10 min	30-60 min	<60 min	0.5-1 h	
Duration	Short	Short	Long	Long	Short	Short	Short	Short	Short	Short	
Time to peak serum concentration (h)	1-3	1.5-2	2-4	2-4	1-1.5	1.6-2.5	5-20	1.5-2.5	1	1.5	2-3.5
Average bioavailability (%)	70	50	20-30	70	45	—	97	15	17	40-46	46-49
Volume of distribution (L)	180-200	138	210-280	170	110-140	110-140	170	170	NA	—	402
Half-life (h)	3-4	4	26	6	2-3	2-3	2	2-2.5[1]	2	2.8-3.4	2.5-3.7
Fraction excreted unchanged in urine (%)	40	—	32	50	14	14	22	3	3	8	8

[1]With extended dosing, the half-life extends to 7 hours.

ANTIPSYCHOTIC AGENTS

Antipsychotic Agent	Dosage Forms	I.M./P.O. Potency	Equiv Dosages (approx) (mg)	Usual Adult Daily Maint Dose (mg)	Sedation (Incidence)	Extrapyramidal Side Effects	Anticholinergic Side Effects	Orthostatic Hypotension	Comments
Aripiprazole (Abilify™)	Tab		4	10-30	Low	Very low	Very low	Very low	Low weight gain; activating
Chlorpromazine	Inj, tab	4:1	100	200-1000	High	Moderate	Moderate	Moderate/high	
Clozapine (Clozaril®)	Tab		100	75-900	High	Very low	High	High	~1% incidence of agranulocytosis; weekly-biweekly CBC required; potential for weight gain, lipid abnormalities, and diabetes
Fluphenazine (Prolixin Decanoate®)	Conc, elix, inj, tab	2:1	2	0.5-20	Low	High	Low	Low	
Haloperidol (Haldol®, Haldol® Decanoate)	Conc, inj, tab	2:1	2	0.5-20	Low	High	Low	Low	
Loxapine (Loxitane®, Loxitane® C)	Cap, conc		10	25-250	Moderate	Moderate	Low	Low	
Mesoridazine [DSC]	Inj, liq, tab	3:1	50	30-400	High	Low	High	Moderate	Prolongs QTc; use only in treatment of refractory illness
Molindone (Moban®)	Conc, tab		15	15-225	Low	Moderate	Low	Low	May cause less weight gain
Olanzapine (Zyprexa®, Zyprexa® Zydis®)	Tab		4	5-20	Moderate/high	Low	Moderate	Moderate	Potential for weight gain, lipid abnormalities, diabetes
Perphenazine	Conc, inj, tab		10	16-64	Low	Moderate	Low	Low	
Pimozide (Orap®)	Tab		2	1-20	Moderate	High	Moderate	Low	Contraindicated with CYP3A inhibitors
Quetiapine (Seroquel®)	Tab		125	50-800	Moderate/high	Very low	Moderate	Moderate	Moderate weight gain; potential for lipid abnormalities; diabetes
Risperidone (Risperdal®)	Sol, tab		1	0.5-6	Low/moderate	Low	Very low	Moderate	Low to moderate weight gain; potential for diabetes
Thioridazine	Conc, tab		100	200-800	High	Low	High	Moderate/high	May cause irreversible retinitis pigmentosa at doses >800 mg/d; prolongs QTc; use only in treatment of refractory illness

ANTIPSYCHOTIC AGENTS (Continued)

Antipsychotic Agent	Dosage Forms	I.M./P.O. Potency	Equiv Dosages (approx) (mg)	Usual Adult Daily Maint Dose (mg)	Sedation (Incidence)	Extrapyramidal Side Effects	Anticholinergic Side Effects	Orthostatic Hypotension	Comments
Thiothixene (Navane®)	Cap, conc; powder for inj	4:1	4	5-40	Low	High	Low	Low/moderate	
Trifluoperazine	Inj, tab		5	2-40	Low	High	Low	Low	
Ziprasidone (Geodon®)	Cap, powder for inj	2:1	40	40-160	Low/moderate	Low	Very low	Low/moderate	Low weight gain; contraindicated with QTc-prolonging agents

BENZODIAZEPINES

Agent	Dosage Forms	Relative Potency	Peak Blood Levels (oral) (h)	Protein Binding (%)	Volume of Distribution (L/kg)	Major Active Metabolite	Half-Life (parent) (h)	Half-Life[1] (metabolite) (h)	Usual Initial Dose	Adult Oral Dosage Range
					Anxiolytic					
Alprazolam (Alprazolam Intensol®, Xanax®)	Sol, tab	0.5	1-2	80	0.9-1.2	No	12-15	—	0.25-0.5 tid	0.75-4 mg/d
Chlordiazepoxide (Librium®)	Cap, powder for inj	10	2-4	90-98	0.3	Yes	5-30	24-96	5-25 mg tid-qid	15-100 mg/d
Diazepam (Diastat® Rectal Delivery System, Diazepam Intensol®, Valium®)	Gel, inj, sol, tab	5	0.5-2	98	1.1	Yes	20-80	50-100	2-10 mg bid-qid	4-40 mg/d
Lorazepam (Ativan®, Lorazepam Intensol®)[2]	Inj, sol, tab	1	1-6	88-92	1.3	No	10-20	—	0.5-2 mg tid-qid	2-4 mg/d
Oxazepam (Serax®)	Cap, tab	15-30	2-4	86-99	0.6-2	No	5-20	—	10-30 mg tid-qid	30-120 mg/d
					Sedative / Hypnotic					
Estazolam (ProSom®)	Tab	0.3	2	93	—	No	10-24	—	1 mg qhs	1-2 mg
Flurazepam (Dalmane®)	Cap	5	0.5-2	97	—	Yes	Not significant	40-114	15 mg qhs	15-60 mg
Quazepam (Doral®)	Tab	5	2	95	5	Yes	25-41	28-114	15 mg qhs	7.5-15 mg
Temazepam (Restoril®)	Cap	5	2-3	96	1.4	No	10-40	—	15-30 mg qhs	15-30 mg
Triazolam (Halcion®)	Tab	0.1	1	89-94	0.8-1.3	No	2.3	—	0.125-0.25 qhs	0.125-0.25 mg
					Miscellaneous					
Clonazepam (Klonopin®)	Tab	0.25-0.5	1-2	86	1.8-4	No	18-50 h	—	0.5 mg tid	1.5-20 mg/d
Clorazepate (Tranxene®)	Tab	7.5	1-2	80-95	—	Yes	Not significant	50-100 h	7.5-15 mg bid-qid	15-60 mg
Midazolam	Inj, syr		0.4-0.7[3]	95	0.8-6.6	No	2-5 h	—	NA	

[1]Significant metabolite.

[2]Reliable bioavailability when given I.M.

[3]I.V. only.

NA = not available.

BETA-BLOCKERS

Agent	Adrenergic Receptor Blocking Activity	Lipid Solubility	Protein Bound (%)	Half-Life (h)	Bioavailability (%)	Primary (Secondary) Route of Elimination	Indications	Usual Dosage
Acebutolol (Sectral®)	beta₁	Low	15-25	3-4	40 / 7-fold¹	Hepatic (renal)	Hypertension, arrhythmias	P.O.: 400-1200 mg/d
Atenolol (Tenormin®)	beta₁	Low	<5-10	6-9²	50-60 / 4-fold¹	Renal (hepatic)	Hypertension, angina pectoris, acute MI	P.O.: 50-200 mg/d; I.V.: 5 mg x 2 doses
Betaxolol (Kerlone®)	beta₁	Low	50-55	14-22	84-94	Hepatic (renal)	Hypertension	P.O.: 10-20 mg/d
Bisoprolol (Zebeta®)	beta₁	Low	26-33	9-12	80	Renal (hepatic)	Hypertension, heart failure	P.O.: 2.5-5 mg
Carteolol (Cartrol®)	beta₁, beta₂	Low	20-30	6	80-85	Renal	Hypertension	P.O.: 2.5-10 mg/d
Carvedilol (Coreg®)	beta₁, beta₂, alpha₁	ND	98	7-10	25-35	Bile into feces	Hypertension, heart failure (mild to severe)	P.O.: 6.25 mg twice daily
Esmolol (Brevibloc®)	beta₁	Low	55	0.15	NA / 5-fold¹	Red blood cell	Supraventricular tachycardia, sinus tachycardia	I.V. infusion: 25-300 mcg/kg/min
Labetalol (Normodyne®, Trandate®)	alpha₁, beta₁, beta₂	Moderate	50	5.5-8	18-30 / 10-fold¹	Renal (hepatic)	Hypertension	P.O.: 200-2400 mg/d; I.V.: 20-80 mg at 10-min intervals up to a maximum of 300 mg or continuous infusion of 2 mg/min
Metoprolol (Lopressor®, Toprol-XL®)	beta₁	Moderate	10-12	3-7	50 / 10-fold¹ (Toprol XL®: 77)	Hepatic/renal	Hypertension, angina pectoris, acute MI, heart failure (mild to moderate; XL formulation only)	P.O.: 100-450 mg/d; I.V.: Post-MI 15 mg; Angina: 15 mg then 2-5 mg/hour; Arrhythmias: 0.2 mg/kg
Nadolol (Corgard®)	beta₁, beta₂	Low	25-30	20-24	30 / 5- to 8-fold¹	Renal	Hypertension, angina pectoris	P.O.: 40-320 mg/d
Penbutolol (Levatol®)	beta₁, beta₂	High	80-98	5	≅100	Hepatic (renal)	Hypertension	P.O.: 20-80 mg/d
Pindolol	beta₁, beta₂	Moderate	57	3-4²	90 / 4-fold¹	Hepatic (renal)	Hypertension	P.O.: 20-60 mg/d
Propranolol (Inderal®, various)	beta₁, beta₂	High	90	3-5²	30 / 20-fold¹	Hepatic	Hypertension, angina pectoris, arrhythmias	P.O.: 40-480 mg/d; I.V.: Reflex tachycardia 1-10 mg
Propranolol long-acting (Inderal-LA®)	beta₁, beta₂	High	90	9-18	20- to 30-fold¹	Hepatic	Hypertrophic subaortic stenosis, prophylaxis (post-MI)	P.O.: 180-240 mg/d

Agent	Adrenergic Receptor Blocking Activity	Lipid Solubility	Protein Bound (%)	Half-Life (h)	Bioavail-ability (%)	Primary (Secondary) Route of Elimination	Indications	Usual Dosage
Sotalol (Betapace®, Betapace AF®, Sorine®)	beta$_1$ beta$_2$	Low	0	12	90-100	Renal	Ventricular arrhythmias/ tachyarrhythmias	P.O. 160-320 mg/d
Timolol (Blocadren®)	beta$_1$ beta$_2$	Low to moderate	<10	4	75 7-fold[1]	Hepatic (renal)	Hypertension, prophylaxis (post-MI)	P.O.: 20-60 mg/d P.O.: 20 mg/d

Dosage is based on 70 kg adult with normal hepatic and renal function.

Note: All beta$_1$-selective agents will inhibit beta$_2$ receptors at higher doses.

[1]Interpatient variations in plasma levels.

[2]Half-life increased to 16-27 hours in creatinine clearance of 15-35 mL/minute and >27 hours in creatinine clearance <15 mL/minute.

CALCIUM CHANNEL BLOCKERS

Comparative Pharmacokinetics

Agent	Bioavailability (%)	Protein Binding (%)	Onset (min)	Peak (h)	Half-Life (h)	Volume of Distribution	Route of Metabolism	Route of Excretion
Dihydropyridines								
Amlodipine (Norvasc®)	52-88	97	6 h	6-9	33.8	21 L/kg	Liver, inactive metabolites, not a significant first-pass metabolism/presystemic metabolism	Bile, gut wall
Felodipine (Plendil®)	10-25	>99	3-5 h	2.5-5	10-36	10.3 L/kg	Liver, inactive metabolites, extensive metabolism by several pathways including cytochrome P450, extensive first-pass metabolism/presystemic metabolism	70% urine, 10% feces
Isradipine (DynaCirc®)	15-24	97	120	0.5-2.5	8	2.9 L/kg	Liver, inactive metabolites, extensive first-pass metabolism	90% urine, 10% feces
Nicardipine (Cardene®)	35	>95	20	0.5-2	2-4	ND	Liver, saturable first-pass metabolism	60% urine, 35% feces
Nifedipine (prototype) (Adalat® CC, Procardia®/Procardia XL®)	Immediate/sustained release 45-70/86	92-98	20	Immediate/sustained release 0.5/6	2-5	ND	Liver, inactive metabolites	60%-80% urine, feces, bile
Nimodipine (Nimotop®)	13	>95	ND	≤1	1-2	0.43 L/kg	Liver, inactive metabolites, high first-pass metabolism	Urine
Nisoldipine (Sular®)	4-8	>99	ND	6-12	7-12	4-5 L/kg	Liver, 1 active metabolite (10%), presystemic metabolism	70%-75% kidney, 6%-12% feces
Phenylalkylamines								
Verapamil (prototype) (Calan®)	20-35	83-92	30	1-2.2	3-7	4.5-7 L/kg	Liver	70% urine, 16% feces
Benzothiazepines								
Diltiazem (prototype) (Cardizem®/Cardizem® CD, Dilacor® XR)	40-67	70-80	30-60	Immediate/sustained release 2-3/6-11	Immediate/sustained release 3.5-6/5-7	ND	Liver; drugs which inhibit/induce hepatic microsomal enzymes may alter disposition	Urine
Miscellaneous								
Bepridil	59	>99	60	2-3	24	ND	Liver	70% urine, 22% feces

COMPATIBILITY OF DRUGS

Drug Compatibility Guide

KEY

Y = Compatible
N = Incompatible
Blank = Information about compatibility was not available

	aminophylline	amphotericin B	ampicillin	atropine	calcium gluconate	carbenicillin	cefazolin	cimetidine	clindamycin	diazepam	dopamine	epinephrine	erythromycin	fentanyl	furosemide	gentamicin
aminophylline	■		Y		Y	N	N		N	Y	Y	Y	N	N		
amphotericin B		■	N		N	N		N			N					N
ampicillin	Y	N	■	N	N	Y	Y		N		N		N			N
atropine			N	■				Y		N		N		Y		
calcium gluconate	Y	N	N		■		N		N		Y	N	Y			
carbenicillin	N	N	Y			■	Y	Y		Y	N	N				N
cefazolin	N		Y		N		■	N	Y			N				N
cimetidine		N		Y		Y	N	■	Y			Y	Y		Y	Y
clindamycin	N		N		N	Y		Y	■							Y
diazepam	Y			N			Y			■		N			N	
dopamine	Y	N	N		Y	Y					■					N
epinephrine	N			N	N	N		Y		N		■	N		N	
erythromycin	N		N		Y	N	N	Y				N	■			
fentanyl				Y										■		
furosemide							Y		N		N				■	N
gentamicin		N	N			N	N		Y		Y				N	■
glycopyrrolate				Y							N					
heparin sodium	Y	Y	Y	N	Y			Y	Y	N	Y	Y	N		Y	N
hydrocortisone	Y	Y	N		Y	Y	Y			Y		Y				
hydroxyzine	N			Y						N				Y		
levarterenol	N			N	Y	N	N	Y		N		N			N	
lidocaine	Y	N	Y		Y	Y	N	Y		N	Y	N	Y			
meperidine	N			Y						N		Y		Y		
morphine	N			Y						N				Y		
nitroglycerin	Y									Y				Y		
pentobarbital	Y			N			N	N	N	N			N	N		
potassium chloride	Y	N	Y	Y	Y	Y	Y	Y	Y	Y	N	Y	N	Y		Y
sodium bicarbonate	Y	Y		N	N			Y	N		N	Y				
tetracycline	N	N	N		N	N	N	Y			Y		N		N	
vancomycin	N			Y			Y				Y					
verapamil	Y	N	Y	Y	Y	Y	Y	Y	Y	Y	Y	Y	Y		Y	Y
vitamin B & C complex	N		Y	Y	Y	N	Y	Y	Y	N	Y	Y	N		Y	Y

NOTE: Because the compatibility of two or more drugs in solution depends on several variables such as the solution itself, drug concentration and the method of mixing (bottle, syringe, or Y-site), this table is intended to be used solely as a guide to general drug compatibilities. Before mixing any drugs, the healthcare professional should ascertain if a potential incompatibility exists by referring to an appropriate information source.

COMPATIBILITY OF DRUGS (Continued)

(continued)

KEY Y = Compatible N = Incompatible Blank = Information about compatibility was not available	glycopyrrolate	heparin sodium	hydrocortisone	hydroxyzine	levarterenol	lidocaine	meperidine	morphine	nitroglycerin	pentobarbital	potassium chloride	sodium bicarbonate	tetracycline	vancomycin	verapamil	vitamin B & C complex
aminophylline		Y	Y	N	N	Y	N	N	Y	Y	Y	Y	N	N	Y	N
amphotericin B		Y	Y			N					N	Y	N		N	
ampicillin		Y	N			Y					Y		N		Y	Y
atrophine	Y	N		Y	N		Y	Y		N	Y	N			Y	Y
calcium gluconate		Y	Y		Y	Y					Y	N	N	Y	Y	Y
carbenicillin			Y		N	Y					Y		N		Y	N
cefazolin			Y		N	N				N	Y		N		Y	Y
cimetidine		Y			Y	Y				N	Y		Y	Y	Y	Y
clindamycin		Y	Y							N	Y	Y			Y	Y
diazepam	N	N		N	N	N	N	N		N	N	N			Y	N
dopamine		Y	Y			Y			Y		Y		Y		Y	Y
epinephrine		Y		N	N	Y					N	N			Y	Y
erythromycin		N	Y			Y				N	Y	Y	N	Y	Y	N
fentanyl				Y			Y	Y		N						
furosemide		Y			N				Y		Y		N		Y	Y
gentamicin		N													Y	Y
glycopyrrolate	■		Y			Y	Y	Y		N		N				
heparin sodium		■	N	N	Y	Y	N	N			Y	Y	N	N	Y	Y
hydrocortisone		N	■		Y	Y				N	Y	Y	N	Y	Y	Y
hydroxyzine	Y	N		■			Y	Y	Y	N						N
levarterenol		Y	Y		■					N	Y		Y		Y	Y
lidocaine	Y	Y	Y	Y		■			Y	Y	Y	Y	Y		Y	Y
meperidine	Y	N		Y			■	N		N		N			Y	
morphine	Y	N		Y			N	■		N	Y	N			Y	Y
nitroglycerin						Y			■						Y	
pentobarbital	N		N	N	N	Y	N	N		■		N	N	N	Y	
potassium chloride		Y	Y		Y	Y		Y			■	Y	Y	Y	Y	
sodium bicarbonate	N	Y	Y			Y	N	N		N	Y	■	N	N	Y	N
tetracycline		N	N		Y	Y				N	Y	N	■			Y
vancomycin		N	Y							N	Y	N		■	Y	Y
verapamil		Y	Y	Y	Y	Y	Y	Y	Y	Y	Y			Y	■	Y
vitamin B & C complex		Y	Y	N	Y	Y		Y				N	Y	Y	Y	■

Reprinted from Malseed RT, Goldstein FJ, & Balkon N, *Pharmacology: Drug Therapy and Nursing Management* (4th ed), Philadelphia: JB Lippincott Co (1995). Used with permission.

COMPATIBILITY OF DRUGS IN SYRINGE

Compatibility of Drugs in Syringe

	atropine	butorphanol	chlorpromazine	cimetidine	dimenhydrinate	diphenhydramine	fentanyl	glycopyrrolate	heparin	hydroxyzine	meperidine
atropine	■	Y	Y	Y	M	M	M	Y	M	Y	Y
butorphanol	Y	■	Y	Y	N	Y	Y			Y	M
chlorpromazine	Y	Y	■	N	N	M	M	Y	N	M	M
cimetidine	Y	Y	N	■		Y	Y	Y	Y	Y	Y
dimenhydrinate	M	N	N		■	M	M	N	M	N	M
diphenhydramine	M	Y		Y	M	■		Y		M	M
fentanyl	M	Y	M		M	M	■		M	Y	M
glycopyrrolate	Y		Y	Y	N	Y		■		Y	Y
heparin	M		N		M		M		■		N
hydroxyzine	Y	Y	M	Y	N	M	Y	Y		■	M
meperidine	Y	M	M	Y	M	M	M	Y	N	M	■
metoclopramide	M		M		M	Y	M			M	M
midazolam	Y	Y	Y	Y	N	Y	Y	Y		Y	Y
morphine	M	Y	M	Y	M	M	M	Y	N	Y	N
nalbuphine	Y			Y						Y	
pentazocine	M	Y	M	Y	M	M	M	N	N	Y	M
pentobarbital	M	N	N	N	N	N	N	N		N	N
prochlorperazine	M	Y	Y	Y	N	M	M	Y		M	M
promethazine	M	Y	M	Y	N	M	M	Y	N	M	Y
ranitidine	Y		Y		Y	Y	Y	Y		N	Y
secobarbital				N				N			
thiopental			N		N	N		N			N

KEY
Y = Compatible in a syringe
M = Moderately compatible, inject immediately after combining
N = Incompatible, do not mix in syringe
Blank = Information about compatibility is not currently available

COMPATIBILITY OF DRUGS IN SYRINGE *(Continued)*

(continued)

	metoclopramide	midazolam	morphine	nalbuphine	pentazocine	pentobarbital	prochlorperazine	promethazine	ranitidine	secobarbital	thiopental
atropine	M	Y	M	Y	M	M	M	M	Y		
butorphanol		Y	Y		Y	N	Y	Y			
chlorpromazine	M	Y	M		M	N	Y	M	Y		N
cimetidine		Y	Y	Y	Y	N	Y	Y		N	
dimenhydrinate	M	N	M		M	N	N	N	Y		N
diphenhydramine	Y	Y	M		M	N	M	M	Y		N
fentanyl	M	Y	M		M	N	M	M	Y		
glycopyrrolate		Y	Y		N	N	Y	Y	Y	N	N
heparin	M		N		N			N			
hydroxyzine	M	Y	Y	Y	Y	N	M	M	N		
meperidine	M	Y	M		M	N	M	Y	Y		N
metoclopramide	■	Y	M		M		M	M	Y		
midazolam	Y	■	Y	Y		N	N	Y	N		
morphine	M	Y	■		M	N	M	M	Y		N
nalbuphine		Y		■		N	Y	Y	Y		
pentazocine	M		M		■	N	M	Y	Y		
pentobarbital	N	N	N	N	N	■	N	N			Y
prochlorperazine	M	N	M	Y	M	N	■	M	Y		N
promethazine	M	Y	M	Y	Y	N	M	■	Y		N
ranitidine	Y	N	Y	Y	Y		Y	Y	■		
secobarbital										■	
thiopental			N			Y	N	N			■

Reprinted from Malseed RT, Goldstein FJ, & Balkon N, *Pharmacology: Drug Therapy and Nursing Management* (4th ed), Philadelphia: JB Lippincott Co (1995). Used with permission.

CONTROLLED SUBSTANCES

Drugs (Trade or Other Names)	Medical Uses	Physical Dependence	Psychological Dependence	Tolerance	Duration (h)	Usual Method	Possible Effects	Effects of Overdose	Withdrawal Syndrome
Anabolic Steroids									
Testosterone (cypionate, enanthate) (C-V) (Depo®-Testosterone, Delatestry®)	Hypogonadism	Unknown			14-28 d	Injected	Virilization, acne, testicular atrophy, gynecomastia, aggressive behavior, edema	Unknown	Possible depression
Nandrolone (decanoate, phenpropionate) (C-III) (Nortestosterone, Durabolin, Deca-Durabolin®, Deca)	Anemia, breast cancer				14-21 d				
Oxymetholone (C-III) (Anadrol®-50)	Anemia				24	Oral			
Cannabis									
Marijuana (C-I) (Pot, Acapulco gold, grass, reefer, sinsemilla, Thai sticks)	None	Unknown	Moderate	Yes	2-4	Smoked, oral	Euphoria, relaxed inhibitions, increased appetite, disorientation	Fatigue, paranoia, possible psychosis	Occasional reports of insomnia, hyperactivity, decreased appetite
Tetrahydrocannabinol (C-I, II) (THC, Marinol®)	Antinauseant								
Hashish and hashish oil (C-I) (Hash, hash oil)	None								

CONTROLLED SUBSTANCES (Continued)

Drugs (Trade or Other Names)	Medical Uses	Physical Dependence	Psychological Dependence	Tolerance	Duration (h)	Usual Method	Possible Effects	Effects of Overdose	Withdrawal Syndrome
Depressants									
Chloral hydrate (C-IV) (Noctec, Somnos, Felsules)	Hypnotic	Moderate	Moderate	Yes	5-8	Oral	Slurred speech, disorientation, drunken behavior without odor of alcohol	Shallow respiration, clammy skin, dilated pupils, weak and rapid pulse, coma, possible death	Anxiety, insomnia, tremors, delirium, convulsions, possible death
Barbiturates (C-II, III, IV) (Amytal®, Fiorinal®, Nembutal®, Seconal™, Tuinal®, phenobarbital, pentobarbital)	Anesthetic, anticonvulsant, sedative, hypnotic, veterinary euthanasia agent	High-moderate	High-moderate	Yes	1-16	Oral, injected			
Benzodiazepines (C-IV) (Ativan®, Dalmane®, diazepam, Librium®, Xanax®, Serax®, Valium®, Tranxene® Verstran, Versed®, Halcion®, Paxipam®, Restoril®)	Antianxiety, sedative, anticonvulsant, hypnotic	Low	Low	Yes	4-8	Oral, injected			
Glutethimide (C-II) (Doriden)	Sedative, hypnotic	High	Moderate	Yes	4-8	Oral			
Other depressants (C-I, II, III, IV) (Equanil®, Miltown®, Noludar, Placidyl®, Valmid, methaqualone)	Antianxiety, sedative, hypnotic	Moderate	Moderate	Yes	4-8	Oral			
Hallucinogens									
LSD (C-I) (Acid, microdot)	None	None	Unknown	Yes	8-12	Oral	Illusions and hallucinations, altered perception of time and distance	Longer, more intense "trip" episodes, psychosis, possible death	Unknown
Mescaline and peyote (C-I) (Mescal, buttons, cactus)	None	None	Unknown	Yes	8-12	Oral			
Amphetamine variants (C-I) (2,5-DMA, STP, MDA, MDMA, ecstasy, DOM, DOB)	None	Unknown	Unknown	Yes	Variable	Oral, injected			
Phencyclidine and analogs (C-I, II) (PCE, PCPy, TCP, PCP, hog, loveboat, angel dust)	None	Unknown	High	Yes	Days	Oral, smoked			
Other hallucinogens (C-I) (Bufotenine, ibogaine, DMT, DET, psilocybin, psilocyn)	None	None	Unknown	Possible	Variable	Smoked, oral, injected, sniffed			

Drugs (Trade or Other Names)	Medical Uses	Physical Dependence	Psychological Dependence	Tolerance	Duration (h)	Usual Method	Possible Effects	Effects of Overdose	Withdrawal Syndrome
Narcotics									
Heroin (C-I) (Diacetylmorphine, horse, smack)	None in U.S; analgesic, antitussive	High		Yes	3-6	Injected, sniffed, smoked	Euphoria, drowsiness, respiratory depression, constricted pupils, nausea	Slow and shallow breathing, clammy skin, convulsions, coma, possible death	Watery eyes, runny nose, yawning, lose of appetite, irritability, tremors, panic, cramps, nausea, chills and sweating
Morphine (C-II) (Duramorph®, MS-Contin®, Roxanol™, Oramorph SR™)	Analgesic					Oral, smoked, injected			
Codeine (C-II, III, V) (Tylenol® w/codeine, Empirin® w/codeine, Robitussin® A-C, Fiorinal® w/codeine, APAP w/codeine)	Analgesic, antitussive		Moderate			Oral, injected			
Hydrocodone (C-II, III) (Tussionex®, Vicodin®, Hycodan®, Lorcet®)					3-6	Oral			
Hydromorphone (C-II) (Dilaudid®)					3-6	Oral, injected			
Oxycodone (C-II) (Percodan®, Percocet®, Tylox®, Roxicet®, Roxicodone™)	Analgesic		High		4-5	Oral			
Methadone and LAAM (C-I, II) (Dolophine®, methadone, levo-alpha-acetylmethadol, levomethadyl acetate)	Analgesic, treatment of dependence				12-72	Oral, injected			
Fentanyl and analogs (C-I, II) (Innovar®, Sublimaze®, Alfenta®, Sufenta®, Duragesic®)	Analgesic, adjunct to anesthesia, anesthetic				0.1-72	Injected, transdermal patch			
Other narcotics (C-II, III, IV, V) (Percodan®, Percocet®, Tylox®, opium, Darvon®, Talwin®, buprenorphine, meperidine (pethidine), Demerol®)	Analgesic, antidiarrheal	High-low		Yes	Variable	Oral, injected			

CONTROLLED SUBSTANCES *(Continued)*

Stimulants

Drugs (Trade or Other Names)	Medical Uses	Physical Dependence	Psychological Dependence	Tolerance	Duration (h)	Usual Method	Possible Effects	Effects of Overdose	Withdrawal Syndrome
Cocaine[1] (C-II) (Coke, flake, snow, crack)	Local anesthetic	Possible	High	Yes	1-2	Sniffed, smoked, injected	Increased alertness, excitation, euphoria, increased pulse rate and blood pressure, insomnia, loss of appetite	Agitation, increased body temperature, hallucinations, convulsions, possible death	Apathy, long periods of sleep, irritability, depression, disorientation
Amphetamine/methamphetamine (C-II) (Biphetamine, Desoxyn[2], Dexedrine[2], Obetrol, ice)	Attention deficit disorder, narcolepsy, weight control				2-4	Oral, injected, smoked			
Methylphenidate (C-II) (Ritalin[2])	Attention deficit disorder, narcolepsy					Oral, injected			
Other stimulants (C-I, II, III, IV) (Adipex[2], Didrex[2], Ionamin[2], Melfiat[2], Plegine, Captagon, Sanorex[2], Tenuate[2], Tepanil, Prelu-2[2], Preludin)	Weight control								

[1]Not designated a narcotic under the CSA.

[2]Designated a narcotic under the CSA.

Adapted from U.S. Department of Justice Drug Enforcement Administration, *Drugs of Abuse,* 1996.

CORTICOSTEROIDS

Corticosteroids, Systemic Equivalencies

Glucocorticoid	Pregnancy Category	Approximate Equivalent Dose (mg)	Routes of Administration	Relative Anti-inflammatory Potency	Relative Mineralocorticoid Potency	Protein Binding (%)	Half-life Plasma (min)	Half-life Biologic (h)
Short-Acting								
Cortisone	D	25	P.O., I.M.	0.8	2	90	30	8-12
Hydrocortisone	C	20	I.M., I.V.	1	2	90	80-118	8-12
Intermediate-Acting								
Methylprednisolone[1]	—	4	P.O., I.M., I.V.	5	0	—	78-188	18-36
Prednisolone	B	5	P.O., I.M., I.V., intra-articular, intradermal, soft tissue injection	4	1	90-95	115-212	18-36
Prednisone	B	5	P.O.	4	1	70	60	18-36
Triamcinolone[1]	C	4	P.O., I.M., intra-articular, intrasynovial, soft tissue injection	5	0	—	200+	18-36
Long-Acting								
Betamethasone	C	0.6-0.75	P.O., I.M., intra-articular, intradermal, intrasynovial, soft tissue injection	25	0	64	300+	36-54
Dexamethasone	C	0.75	P.O., I.M., I.V., intra-articular, intradermal, soft tissue injection	25-30	0	—	110-210	36-54
Mineralocorticoids								
Fludrocortisone	C	—	P.O.	10	125	42	210+	18-36

[1]May contain propylene glycol as an excipient in injectable forms.

CORTICOSTEROIDS *(Continued)*

GUIDELINES FOR SELECTION AND USE OF
TOPICAL CORTICOSTEROIDS

The quantity prescribed and the frequency of refills should be monitored to reduce the risk of adrenal suppression. In general, short courses of high-potency agents are preferable to prolonged use of low potency. After control is achieved, control should be maintained with a low potency preparation.

1. Low-to-medium potency agents are usually effective for treating thin, acute, inflammatory skin lesions; whereas, high or super-potent agents are often required for treating chronic, hyperkeratotic, or lichenified lesions.

2. Since the stratum corneum is thin on the face and intertriginous areas, low-potency agents are preferred but a higher potency agent may be used for 2 weeks.

3. Because the palms and soles shave a thick stratum corneum, high or super-potent agents are frequently required.

4. Low potency agents are preferred for infants and the elderly. Infants have a high body surface area to weight ratio; elderly patients have thin, fragile skin.

5. The vehicle in which the topical corticosteroid is formulated influences the absorption and potency of the drug. Ointment bases are preferred for thick, lichenified lesions; they enhance penetration of the drug. Creams are preferred for acute and subacute dermatoses; they may be used on moist skin areas or intertriginous areas. Solutions, gels, and sprays are preferred for the scalp or for areas where a nonoil-based vehicle is needed.

6. In general, super-potent agents should not be used for longer than 3 weeks unless the lesion is limited to a small body area. Medium-to-high potency agents usually cause only rare adverse effects when treatment is limited to 3 months or less, and use on the face and intertriginous areas are avoided. If long-term treatment is needed, intermittent vs continued treatment is recommended.

7. Most preparations are applied once or twice daily. More frequent application may be necessary for the palms or soles because the preparation is easily removed by normal activity and penetration is poor due to a thick stratum corneum. Every-other-day or weekend-only application may be effective for treating some chronic conditions.

Corticosteroids, Topical

	Steroid	Vehicle
Very High Potency		
0.05%	Augmented betamethasone dipropionate	Ointment
0.05%	Clobetasol propionate	Cream, ointment
0.05%	Diflorasone diacetate	Ointment
0.05%	Halobetasol propionate	Cream, ointment
High Potency		
0.1%	Amcinonide	Cream, ointment, lotion
0.05%	Betamethasone dipropionate, augmented	Cream
0.05%	Betamethasone dipropionate	Cream, ointment
0.1%	Betamethasone valerate	Ointment
0.05%	Desoximetasone	Gel
0.25%	Desoximetasone	Cream, ointment
0.05%	Diflorasone diacetate	Cream, ointment
0.05%	Fluocinonide	Cream, ointment, gel
0.1%	Halcinonide	Cream, ointment
0.5%	Triamcinolone acetonide	Cream
Intermediate Potency		
0.05%	Betamethasone dipropionate	Lotion
0.1%	Betamethasone valerate	Cream
0.1%	Clocortolone pivalate	Cream
0.05%	Desoximetasone	Cream
0.025%	Fluocinolone acetonide	Cream, ointment
0.05%	Flurandrenolide	Cream, ointment, lotion, tape
0.005%	Fluticasone propionate	Ointment
0.05%	Fluticasone propionate	Cream
0.1%	Hydrocortisone butyrate[1]	Ointment, solution
0.2%	Hydrocortisone valerate[1]	Cream, ointment
0.1%	Mometasone furoate[1]	Cream, ointment, lotion

Corticosteroids, Topical *(continued)*

	Steroid	Vehicle
0.1%	Prednicarbate	Cream, ointment
0.025%	Triamcinolone acetonide	Cream, ointment, lotion
0.1%	Triamcinolone acetonide	Cream, ointment, lotion
Low Potency		
0.05%	Alclometasone dipropionate[1]	Cream, ointment
0.05%	Desonide	Cream
0.01%	Fluocinolone acetonide	Cream, solution
0.5%	Hydrocortisone[1]	Cream, ointment, lotion
0.5%	Hydrocortisone acetate[1]	Cream, ointment
1%	Hydrocortisone acetate[1]	Cream, ointment
1%	Hydrocortisone	Cream, ointment, lotion, solution
2.5%	Hydrocortisone	Cream, ointment, lotion

[1]Not fluorinated.

INHALANT AGENTS

Medications Commonly Used for Asthma, Bronchospasm, and COPD

Agent	Indications	Onset	Duration	Frequency	Comments
Anticholinergics					
Ipratropium bromide (Atrovent®)	Bronchospasm associated with COPD		6 h	2 puffs qid	Additive bronchodilating effects used with α-, β₂-adrenergic agonists
Bronchodilators					
Albuterol (Proventil®, Proventil® HFA, Ventolin®, Ventolin® HFA)	Prevent exercise-induced bronchospasm; relief and prevention of bronchospasm	5 min	6-8 h	2 puffs q4-6h	
Bitolterol mesylate (Tornalate®)	Prevent and treat bronchial asthma and reversible bronchospasm	5 min	8 h	2 puffs q8h	Contains a high alcohol content that may irritate the airway
Epinephrine (various)	Acute paroxysms of bronchial asthma; treatment of postintubation and infectious croup	1-5 min	Individualize dosing		OTC; shorter-acting and less effective than prescription β-agonists
Formoterol (Foradil® Aerolizer™)	Long-term maintenance of asthma, prevention of bronchospasm in patients ≥5 y; prevention of exercise-induced bronchospasm in patients ≥12 y		12 h	q12h	Not meant to relieve acute asthmatic symptoms
Ipratropium bromide and albuterol sulfate (Combivent®)	Patients with chronic obstructive pulmonary disease (COPD) on a regular aerosol bronchodilator who continue to have evidence of bronchospasm and who require a second bronchodilator			2 puffs qid	Additional doses may be administered; however, total doses should not exceed 12 in 24 hours
Isoetharine HCl (various)	Bronchial asthma and reversible bronchospasm with bronchitis and emphysema	5 min	1-3 h	1-2 puffs q4h	May cause cardiac stimulation
Levalbuterol (Xopenex®)	Bronchospasm in adults and adolescents ≥12 years of age with reversible obstructive airway disease	10-17 min	5-6 h	0.63 mg tid at 6-8 h intervals	
Metaproterenol sulfate (Alupent®)	Bronchial asthma and reversible bronchospasm; acute asthmatic attacks in children ≥6 years of age	5-30 min	4-6 h	2-3 puffs q3-4h (max 12 puffs/d)	Contraindicated in patients with arrhythmias; should not be used with other β-adrenergic aerosol inhalers because of additive effects
Pirbuterol acetate (Maxair™, Maxair™ Autohaler™)	Prevent and reverse bronchospasm with reversible bronchospasm	Within 5 min	4-6 h	2 puffs q4-6h	
Salmeterol (Serevent®, Serevent® Diskus®)	Long-term maintenance treatment of asthma and prevention of bronchospasm in patients >12 years of age	20 min	12 h	Aerosol: 2 puffs q12h Diskus®: 1 inhalation q12h	Not meant to relieve acute asthmatic symptoms
Terbutaline sulfate (various)	Bronchial asthma and reversible bronchospasm with bronchitis or emphysema	5-30 min	6-8 h	2 puffs q4-6h	
Corticosteroids[1]					
Beclomethasone dipropionate (various)	Bronchial asthma		6-8 h	2 puffs q6-8h	Coughing and wheezing are more common
Budesonide (Pulmicort®)	Bronchial asthma		12 h	1-2 puffs q12h	
Dexamethasone Na phosphate (various)	Bronchial asthma		6-8 h	3 puffs q6-8h (max 12 puffs/d)	
Flunisolide (various)	Bronchial asthma		12 h	2 puffs bid (max 4 puffs bid)	

Medications Commonly Used for Asthma, Bronchospasm, and COPD *(continued)*

Agent	Indications	Onset	Duration	Frequency	Comments
Fluticasone (Flonase®, Flovent®)	Maintenance treatment of asthma as prophylactic therapy; also indicated for patients requiring oral corticosteroid therapy for asthma to assist in total discontinuation or reduction of total oral dose; NOT indicated for the relief of acute bronchospasm	—		2-4 puffs qd (44-220 mcg)	May allow weaning from oral steroids in selected patients
Triamcinolone acetonide (Azmacort®)	Bronchial asthma		6-8 h	2 puffs q6-8h (max 16 puffs/d)	Asthma should be reasonably stable before Azmacort® treatment
Miscellaneous					
Cromolyn (Intal®)	Severe bronchial asthma; prevent exercise-induced bronchospasm		6 h	2 puffs qid	Only useful in prophylaxis; has low toxicity and is as effective as theophylline in many patients
Nedocromil sodium (Tilade®)	Mild to moderate bronchial asthma		6 h	2 puffs qid	Must be taken regularly for benefit — even during symptom-free periods

[1]Not indicated for rapid relief of bronchospasm. Dysphonia and oral candidiasis can occur. Long-term use is associated with cataract formation.

INOTROPIC AND VASOCONSTRICTOR COMPARISON

Drug	Hemodynamic Effects			
	CO	TPR	Mean BP	Renal Perfusion
Dobutamine (Dobutrex®)	↑	↓	↑	–
Dopamine (Intropin®)	↑	+/–[1]	–/↑[1]	↑[1]
Epinephrine (Adrenalin®)	↑	↓	↑	↓
Inamrinone (Inocor®)	↑	↓	–	↑
Isoproterenol (Isuprel®)	↑	↓	↓	+/–[2]
Mephentermine (Wyamine®)	↑	–/↑	↑	+/–
Metaraminol (Aramine®)	↓	↑	↑	↓
Methoxamine	–/↓	↑	↑	↓
Milrinone (Primacor®)	↑	↓	–	↑
Norepinephrine (Levophed®)	–/↓	↑	↑	↓
Phenylephrine (Neo-Synephrine®)	↓	↑	↑	↓

↑ = increase.

↓ = decrease.

– = no change.

[1] = dose dependent.

[2]In patients with cardiogenic or septic shock, renal perfusion commonly increases, however, in the normal patient, renal perfusion may be reduced with isoproterenol.

LAXATIVES, CLASSIFICATION AND PROPERTIES

Laxative	Onset of Action	Site of Action	Mechanism of Action
Saline			
Magnesium citrate Magnesium hydroxide (Phillips'® Milk of Magnesia)	30 min to 3 h	Small and large intestine	Attract/retain water in intestinal lumen increasing intraluminal pressure; cholecystokinin release
Sodium phosphate/ biphosphate enema (Fleet® Enema)	2-15 min	Colon	
Irritant / Stimulant			
Cascara Casanthranol Senna (Senokot®)	6-10 h	Colon	Direct action on intestinal mucosa; stimulate myenteric plexus; alter water and electrolyte secretion
Bisacodyl (Dulcolax®) tablets, suppositories	15 min to 1 h	Colon	
Castor oil	2-6 h	Small intestine	
Cascara aromatic fluid extract	6-10 h	Colon	
Bulk-Producing			
Methylcellulose (Citrucel®) Psyllium (Metamucil®) Malt soup extract [DSC]	12-24 h (up to 72 h)	Small and large intestine	Holds water in stool; mechanical distention; malt soup extract reduces fecal pH
Lubricant			
Mineral oil	6-8 h	Colon	Lubricates intestine; retards colonic absorption of fecal water; softens stool
Surfactants / Stool Softener			
Docusate sodium (Colace®) Docusate calcium (Surfak®) Docusate potassium	24-72 h	Small and large intestine	Detergent activity; facilitates admixture of fat and water to soften stool
Miscellaneous and Combination Laxatives			
Glycerin suppository	15-30 min	Colon	Local irritation; hyperosmotic action
Lactulose	24-48 h	Colon	Delivers osmotically active molecules to colon
Docusate/senna (Peri-Colace®)	8-12 h	Small and large intestine	Senna – mild irritant; docusate – stool softener
Polyethylene glycol-electrolyte solution (GoLYTELY®)	30-60 min	Small and large intestine	Nonabsorbable solution which acts as an osmotic agent
Sorbitol 70%	24-48 h	Colon	Delivers osmotically active molecules to colon

LIPID-LOWERING AGENTS

Effects on Lipoproteins

Drug	Total Cholesterol (%)	LDLC (%)	HDLC (%)	TG (%)
Bile-acid resins	↓20-25	↓20-35	→	↑5-20
Fibric acid derivatives	↓10	↓10 (↑)	↑10-25	↓40-55
HMG-CoA RI (statins)	↓15-35	↓20-40	↑2-15	↓7-25
Nicotinic acid	↓25	↓20	↑20	↓40
Probucol	↓10-15	↓<10	↓30	→
Ezetimibe	↓12-13	↓16-18	↑1-4	↓5-6

Lipid-Lowering Agents

Drug	Dose/Day	Effect on LDL (%)	Effect on HDL (%)	Effect on TG (%)
HMG-CoA Reductase Inhibitors				
Atorvastatin	10 mg	-39	+6	-13
	20 mg	-43	+5	-20
	40 mg	-50	+5	-32
	80 mg	-60	+5	-37
Fluvastatin	20 mg	-22	+2	-5
	40 mg	-25	+3	-12
	80 mg	-36	+4	-12
Lovastatin	20 mg	-27	+7	-8
	40 mg	-32	+5	-2
	80 mg	-42	+8	-13
Pravastatin	10 mg	-22	+5	-3
	20 mg	-32	+3	-15
	40 mg	-34	+6	-10
Rosuvastatin	10 mg	-52	+14	-10
	20 mg	-55	+8	-23
	40 mg	-63	+10	-28
Simvastatin	5 mg	-26	+7	-12
	10 mg	-30	+5	-17
	20 mg	-38	+10	-15
	40 mg	-41	+8	-24
	80 mg	-47		
Bile Acid Sequestrants				
Cholestyramine	4-24 g	-15 to -30	+3 to +5	+0 to +20
Colestipol	7-30 g	-15 to -30	+3 to +5	+0 to +20
Colesevelam	6 tablets	-10	+10 to +25	+0 to +10
Fibric Acid Derivative				
Clofibrate	500 mg 4 times	-10	+10 to +25	-40 to -55
Fenofibrate	67-200 mg	-20 to -25	+1 to -34	-30 to -50
Gemfibrozil	600 mg twice daily	-5 to -10[1]	+10 to +20	-40 to -60
Niacin	1.5-6 g	-21 to -27	+10 to +35	-10 to -50
2-Azetidinone				
Ezetimibe	10 mg	-16 to -18	+1 to +4	-5 to -6

[1]May increase LDL in some patients.

Recommended Liver Function Monitoring for HMG-CoA Reductase Inhibitors

Agent	Initial and After Elevation in Dose	6 Weeks[1]	12 Weeks[1]	Periodically
Atorvastatin (Lipitor®)	x		x	x
Fluvastatin (Lescol®)	x		x	x
Lovastatin (Mevacor®)	x	x	x	x
Pravastatin (Pravachol®)	x			x
Simvastatin (Zocor®)	x			x

[1]After initiation of therapy or any elevation in dose.

NARCOTIC / OPIOID ANALGESIC COMPARISON

Dose Equivalents for Opioid Analgesics in Opioid-Naive Adults ≥50 kg[1]

Drug	Approximate Equianalgesic Dose		Usual Starting Dose for Moderate to Severe Pain	
	Oral	Parenteral	Oral	Parenteral
Opioid Agonist				
Morphine[2]	30 mg q3-4h (repeat around-the-clock dosing) 60 mg q3-4h (single dose or intermittent dosing)	10 mg q3-4h	30 mg q3-4h	10 mg q3-4h
Codeine[3]	130 mg q3-4h	75 mg q3-4h	60 mg q3-4h	60 mg q2h (I.M./SubQ)
Hydromorphone[2] (Dilaudid®)	7.5 mg q3-4h	1.5 mg q3-4h	6 mg q3-4h	1.5 mg q3-4h
Levorphanol (Levo-Dromoran®)	4 mg q6-8h	2 mg q6-8h	4 mg q6-8h	2 mg q6-8h (SubQ)
Meperidine[4] (Demerol®; Meperitab®)	300 mg q2-3h	100 mg q3h	NR	100 mg q3h
Methadone (Dolophine®, others)	20 mg q6-8h	10 mg q6-8h	20 mg q6-8h	10 mg q6-8h
Oxymorphone[2] (Numorphan®)	NA	1 mg q3-4h	NA	1 mg q3-4h
Combination Opioid / NSAID Preparations[5]				
Hydrocodone (in Lorcet®, Lortab®, Vicodin®, others)	30 mg q3-4h	NA	10 mg q3-4h	NA
Oxycodone (Roxicodone®, also in Percocet®, Percodan®, Tylox®, others)	30 mg q3-4h	NA	10 mg q3-4h	NA
Opioid Agonist-Antagonist and Partial Agonist				
Buprenorphine (Buprenex®)	NA	0.3-0.4 mg q6-8h	NA	0.4 q6-8h
Butorphanol (Stadol®)	NA	2 mg q3-4h	NA	2 mg q3-4h
Nalbuphine (Nubain®)	NA	10 mg q3-4h	NA	10 mg q3-4h
Pentazocine (Talwin®, others)	150 mg q3-4h	60 mg q3-4h	50 mg q4-6h	NR

Note: Tables vary in the suggested doses that are equianalgesic to morphine. Clinical response is the criterion that must be applied for each patient; titration to clinical response is necessary. Because there is not complete cross tolerance among these drugs, it is usually necessary to use a lower than equianalgesic dose when changing drugs and to retitrate to response.

Caution: Recommended doses do not apply to patients with renal or hepatic insufficiency or other conditions affecting drug metabolism and kinetics.

[1]**Caution:** Recommended doses do not apply for adult patients with body weight <50 kg. For recommended starting doses for adults <50 kg body weight, see following table.

[2]**Caution:** For morphine, hydromorphone, and oxymorphone, rectal administration is an alternate route for patients unable to take oral medications. Equianalgesic doses may differ from oral and parenteral doses because of pharmacokinetic differences. **Note:** A short-acting opioid should normally be used for initial therapy of moderate to severe pain.

[3]**Caution:** Doses >1.5 mg/kg not recommended. 60 mg oral codeine = 650 mg aspirin or acetaminophen.

[4]For short-term treatment of acute pain only.

[5]**Caution:** Doses of aspirin and acetaminophen in combination opioid/NSAID preparations must also be adjusted to the patient's body weight.

NA = not available; NR = not recommended.

NARCOTIC / OPIOID ANALGESIC COMPARISON *(Continued)*

Dose Equivalents for Opioid Analgesics in Opioid-Naive Adults <50 kg[1]

Drug	Approximate Equianalgesic Dose		Usual Starting Dose for Moderate to Severe Pain	
	Oral	Parenteral	Oral	Parenteral
Opioid Agonist				
Morphine[2]	30 mg q3-4h (repeat around-the-clock dosing) 60 mg q3-4h (single dose or intermittent dosing)	10 mg q3-4h	0.3 mg/kg q3-4h	0.1 mg/kg q3-4h
Codeine[3]	130 mg q3-4h	75 mg q3-4h	1 mg/kg q3-4h[5]	NR
Hydromorphone[2] (Dilaudid®)	7.5 mg q3-4h	1.5 mg q3-4h	0.06 mg/kg q3-4h	0.015 mg/kg q3-4h
Levorphanol (Levo-Dromoran®)	4 mg q6-8h	2 mg q6-8h	0.04 mg/kg q6-8h	0.02 mg/kg q6-8h
Meperidine[4] (Demerol®; Meperitab®)	300 mg q2-3h	100 mg q3h	NR	0.75 mg/kg q2-3h
Methadone (Dolophine®, others)	20 mg q6-8h	10 mg q6-8h	0.2 mg/kg q6-8h	0.1 mg/kg q6-8h
Oxymorphone[2] (Numorphan®)	NA	1 mg q3-4h	NR	NR
Combination Opioid / NSAID Preparations[5]				
Hydrocodone (in Lorcet®, Lortab®, Vicodin®, others)	30 mg q3-4h	NA	0.2 mg/kg q3-4h[5]	NA
Oxycodone (Roxicodone®, also in Percocet®, Percodan®, Tylox®, others)	30 mg q3-4h	NA	0.2 mg/kg q3-4h[5]	NA
Opioid Agonist-Antagonist and Partial Agonist				
Buprenorphine (Buprenex®)	NA	0.3-0.4 mg q6-8h	NA	0.4 q6-8h
Butorphanol (Stadol®)	NA	2 mg q3-4h	NA	2 mg q3-4h
Nalbuphine (Nubain®)	NA	10 mg q3-4h	NA	10 mg q3-4h
Pentazocine (Talwin®, others)	150 mg q3-4h	60 mg q3-4h	50 mg q4-6h	NR

Note: Tables vary in the suggested doses that are equianalgesic to morphine. Clinical response is the criterion that must be applied for each patient; titration to clinical response is necessary. Because there is not complete cross tolerance among these drugs, it is usually necessary to use a lower than equianalgesic dose when changing drugs and to retitrate to response.

Caution: Recommended doses do not apply to patients with renal or hepatic insufficiency or other conditions affecting drug metabolism and kinetics.

[1]**Caution:** Doses listed for patients with body weight <50 kg cannot be used as initial starting doses in babies younger than 6 months of age.

[2]**Caution:** For morphine, hydromorphone, and oxymorphone, rectal administration is an alternate route for patients unable to take oral medications. Equianalgesic doses may differ from oral and parenteral doses because of pharmacokinetic differences. **Note:** A short-acting opioid should normally be used for initial therapy of moderate to severe pain.

[3]**Caution:** Doses >1.5 mg/kg not recommended. 60 mg oral codeine = 650 mg aspirin or acetaminophen.

[4]For short-term treatment of acute pain only.

[5]**Caution:** Doses of aspirin and acetaminophen in combination opioid/NSAID preparations must also be adjusted to the patient's body weight.

NA = not available; NR = not recommended.

Comparative Pharmacokinetics

Drug	Onset (min)	Peak (h)	Duration (h)	Half-Life (h)	Average Dosing Interval (h)	Equianalgesic Doses[1] (mg) I.M.	Equianalgesic Doses[1] (mg) Oral
Alfentanil	Immediate	ND	ND	1-2	—	ND	NA
Buprenorphine	15	1	4-8	2-3	—	0.4	—
Butorphanol	I.M.: 30-60; I.V.: 4-5	0.5-1	3-5	2.5-3.5	(3-6)	2	—
Codeine	P.O.: 30-60; I.M.: 10-30	0.5-1	4-6	3-4	(3-6)	120	200
Fentanyl	I.M.: 7-15; I.V.: Immediate	ND	1-2	1.5-6	(0.5-2)	0.1	NA
Hydrocodone	ND	ND	4-8	3.3-4.4	(4-8)	ND	ND
Hydromorphone	P.O.: 15-30	0.5-1	4-6	2-4	(3-6)	1.5	7.5
Levorphanol	P.O.: 10-60	0.5-1	4-8	12-16	(6-24)	2 (A) 1 (C)	4 (A) 1 (C)
Meperidine	P.O./I.M./SubQ: 10-15; I.V.: ≤5	0.5-1	2-4	3-4	(2-4)	75	300
Methadone	P.O.: 30-60; I.V.: 10-20	0.5-1	4-6 (acute); >8 (chronic)	15-30	(6-12)	10 (A) 2-4 (C)	20 (A) 2-4 (C)
Morphine	P.O.: 15-60; I.V.: ≤5	P.O./I.M./SubQ: 0.5-1; I.V.: 0.3	3-6	2-4	(3-6)	10	60[2] (A) 30 (C)
Nalbuphine	I.M.: 30; I.V.: 1-3	1	3-6	5	—	10	—
Oxycodone	P.O.: 10-15	0.5-1	4-6	3-4	(3-6)	NA	20
Oxymorphone	5-15	0.5-1	3-6		(3-6)	1	10[3]
Pentazocine	15-20	0.25-1	3-4	2-3	(3-6)		
Propoxyphene	P.O.: 30-60	2-2.5	4-6	3.5-15	(4-8)	ND	130[4]-200[5]
Remifentanil	1-3	<0.3	0.1-0.2	0.15-0.3	—	ND	ND
Sufentanil	ND	ND	ND	2.5-3	—	0.02	NA

ND = no data available. NA = not applicable. (A) = acute, (C) = chronic.

[1] Based on acute, short-term use. Chronic administration may alter pharmacokinetics and decrease the oral parenteral dose ratio. The morphine oral-parenteral ratio decreases to ~1.5-2.5:1 upon chronic dosing.

[2] Extensive survey data suggest that the relative potency of I.M.:P.O. morphine of 1:6 changes to 1:2-3 with chronic dosing.

[3] Rectal

[4] HCl salt

[5] Napsylate salt

Adapted from Principles of Analgesic Use in the Treatment of Acute Pain and Cancer Pain, 4th ed, Glenview, IL: The American Pain Society, 1999.

NARCOTIC / OPIOID ANALGESIC COMPARISON (Continued)

Comparative Pharmacology

Drug	Analgesic	Antitussive	Constipation	Respiratory Depression	Sedation	Emesis
Phenanthrenes						
Codeine	+	+++	+	+	+	+
Hydrocodone	+	+++		+		
Hydromorphone	++	+++	+	++	+	+
Levorphanol	++	++	++	++	++	+
Morphine	++	+++	++	++	++	++
Oxycodone	++	+++	++	++	++	++
Oxymorphone	++	+	++	+++		+++
Phenylpiperidines						
Alfentanil	++					
Fentanyl	++			+	+	+
Meperidine	++	+	+	++		
Remifentanil	++			++	+++	++
Sufentanil	+++					
Diphenylheptanes						
Methadone	++	++	++	++	+	+
Propoxyphene	+			+	+	+
Agonist / Antagonist						
Buprenorphine	++	N/A	+++	+++	++	++
Butorphanol	++	N/A	+++	+++	++	+
Dezocine	++		+	++	+	++
Nalbuphine	++	N/A	+++	+++	++	++
Pentazocine	++	N/A	+	++	++ or stimulation	++

NONSALICYLATE / NONSTEROIDAL ANTI-INFLAMMATORY AGENTS

Name	Plasma Half-Life (h)	Time to Peak (h)[1]	Usual Duration (h)	Maximum Recommended Daily Dose (mg)	Considerations
Celecoxib (Celebrex®)	11	2-3	12	400	Selective COX-2 inhibitor
Choline magnesium salicylate (Trilisate®, Tricosal®)	2-30	2	8-24	4500	Nonacetylated salicylates: limited antiplatelet effects
Diclofenac potassium immediate release (Cataflam®)	1-2	1	8	200	Less GI distress, less CNS depression
Diclofenac sodium delayed release (Voltaren®)	1-2	2-3	8-12	200	Less GI distress, less CNS depression
Diflunisal (Dolobid®)	8-12	2-3	8-12	1500	
Etodolac (Lodine®)	7	1-2	6-8	1200	Less GI distress
Fenoprofen (Nalfon®)	2-3	1-2	4-6	3200	Increased nephrotoxicity, increased antiplatelet activity
Flurbiprofen (Ansaid®)	3-6	1.5-2	6-12	300	Increased GI distress
Ibuprofen (Motrin®, Advil®)	2	1-2	4-6	3200	Less GI distress, moderately increased nephrotoxicity
Indomethacin (Indocin®)	4.5	3-4	4-6	200	Increased nephrotoxicity, GI distress, and CNS depression
Indomethacin SR, (Indocin® SR)	4.5-6	2-4	6-12	150	
Ketoprofen (Orudis®, Oruvail®)	1-4	0.5-2	4-6	300	
Ketorolac (Toradol®)	5-6	1	6-8	P.O.: 40[2] I.M.: 120	Increased nephrotoxicity and GI distress
Meclofenamate (Meclomen®)	2-3	0.5-1.5	2-4	400	Less hepatic injury, increased GI distress
Mefenamic acid (Ponstel®)	3.5	2-4	2-6	1000	
Meloxicam (Mobic®)	15-20	5-10	>24	15	
Nabumetone (Relafen®)	24	3-6	>24	2000	Less GI distress
Naproxen (Naprosyn®)	9-20	1-2	2-7	1500	Less GI distress
Naproxen sodium (Anaprox®)	12-13	1-2	8-12	1375	
Oxaprozin (Daypro™)	42-50	3-5	>24	1800	Less GI distress
Piroxicam (Feldene®)	30-86	P.O.: 3-5	24	40	Less hepatic injury
Salsalate (Disalcid®)	7-8	2	8-24	3 g	Nonacetylated salicylates: limited antiplatelet effects
Sulindac (Clinoril®)	7 (16)[3]	2-4	12	400	
Tolmetin (Tolectin®)	5	0.5-1	6-8	2000	
Valdecoxib (Bextra®)	8-11	2.25-3	12-24	40	Selective COX-2 inhibitor

Dosage is based on a 70 kg adult with normal hepatic and renal function.

[1] Food decreases the rate of absorption and may delay the time to peak levels.

[2] 150 mg on the first day.

[3] Half-life of active sulfide metabolite.

CYTOCHROME P450 ENZYMES: SUBSTRATES, INHIBITORS, AND INDUCERS

INTRODUCTION

Most drugs are eliminated from the body, at least in part, by being chemically altered to less lipid-soluble products (ie, metabolized), and thus are more likely to be excreted via the kidneys or the bile. Phase I metabolism includes drug hydrolysis, oxidation, and reduction, and results in drugs that are more polar in their chemical structure, while Phase II metabolism involves the attachment of an additional molecule onto the drug (or partially metabolized drug) in order to create an inactive and/or more water soluble compound. Phase II processes include (primarily) glucuronidation, sulfation, glutathione conjugation, acetylation, and methylation.

Virtually any of the Phase I and II enzymes can be inhibited by some xenobiotic or drug. Some of the Phase I and II enzymes can be induced. Inhibition of the activity of metabolic enzymes will result in increased concentrations of the substrate (drug), whereas induction of the activity of metabolic enzymes will result in decreased concentrations of the substrate. For example, the well-documented enzyme-inducing effects of phenobarbital may include a combination of Phase I and II enzymes. Phase II glucuronidation may be increased via induced UDP-glucuronosyltransferase (UGT) activity, whereas Phase I oxidation may be increased via induced cytochrome P450 (CYP) activity. However, for most drugs, the primary route of metabolism (and the primary focus of drug-drug interaction) is Phase I oxidation, and specifically, metabolism.

CYP enzymes may be responsible for the metabolism (at least partial metabolism) of approximately 75% of all drugs, with the CYP3A subfamily responsible for nearly half of this activity. Found throughout plant, animal, and bacterial species, CYP enzymes represent a superfamily of xenobiotic metabolizing proteins. There have been several hundred CYP enzymes identified in nature, each of which has been assigned to a family (1, 2, 3, etc), subfamily (A, B, C, etc), and given a specific enzyme number (1, 2, 3, etc) according to the similarity in amino acid sequence that it shares with other enzymes. Of these many enzymes, only a few are found in humans, and even fewer appear to be involved in the metabolism of xenobiotics (eg, drugs). The key human enzyme subfamilies include CYP1A, CYP2A, CYP2B, CYP2C, CYP2D, CYP2E, and CYP3A.

CYP enzymes are found in the endoplasmic reticulum of cells in a variety of human tissues (eg, skin, kidneys, brain, lungs), but their predominant sites of concentration and activity are the liver and intestine. Though the abundance of CYP enzymes throughout the body is relatively equally distributed among the various subfamilies, the relative contribution to drug metabolism is (in decreasing order of magnitude) CYP3A4 (nearly 50%), CYP2D6 (nearly 25%), CYP2C8/9 (nearly 15%), then CYP1A2, CYP2C19, CYP2A6, and CYP2E1. Owing to their potential for numerous drug-drug interactions, those drugs that are identified in preclinical studies as substrates of CYP3A enzymes are often given a lower priority for continued research and development in favor of drugs that appear to be less affected by (or less likely to affect) this enzyme subfamily.

Each enzyme subfamily possesses unique selectivity toward potential substrates. For example, CYP1A2 preferentially binds medium-sized, planar, lipophilic molecules, while CYP2D6 preferentially binds molecules that possess a basic nitrogen atom. Some CYP subfamilies exhibit polymorphism (ie, multiple allelic variants that manifest differing catalytic properties). The best described polymorphisms involve CYP2C9, CYP2C19, and CYP2D6. Individuals possessing "wild type" gene alleles exhibit normal functioning CYP capacity. Others, however, possess allelic variants that leave the person with a subnormal level of catalytic activity (so called "poor metabolizers"). Poor metabolizers would be more likely to experience toxicity from drugs metabolized by the affected enzymes (or less effects if the enzyme is responsible for converting a prodrug to it's active form as in the case of codeine). The percentage of people classified as poor metabolizers varies by enzyme and population group. As an example, approximately 7% of Caucasians and only about 1% of Orientals appear to be CYP2D6 poor metabolizers.

CYP enzymes can be both inhibited and induced by other drugs, leading to increased or decreased serum concentrations (along with the associated effects), respectively. Induction occurs when a drug causes an increase in the amount of smooth endoplasmic reticulum, secondary to increasing the amount of the affected CYP enzymes in the tissues. This "revving up" of the CYP enzyme system may take several days to reach peak activity, and likewise, may take several days, even months, to return to normal following discontinuation of the inducing agent.

CYP inhibition occurs via several potential mechanisms. Most commonly, a CYP inhibitor competitively (and reversibly) binds to the active site on the enzyme, thus preventing the substrate from binding to the same site, and preventing the substrate from being metabolized. The affinity of an inhibitor for an enzyme may be expressed by an inhibition constant (Ki) or IC50 (defined as the concentration of the inhibitor required to cause 50% inhibition under a given set of conditions). In addition to reversible competition for an enzyme site, drugs may inhibit enzyme activity by binding to sites on the enzyme other than that to which the substrate would bind, and thereby cause a change in the functionality or physical structure of the enzyme. A drug may also bind to the enzyme in an irreversible (ie, "suicide") fashion. In such a case, it is not the concentration of drug at the enzyme site that is important (constantly binding and releasing), but the number of molecules available for binding (once bound, always bound).

Although an inhibitor or inducer may be known to affect a variety of CYP subfamilies, it may only inhibit one or two in a clinically important fashion. Likewise, although a substrate is known to be at least partially metabolized by a variety of CYP enzymes, only one or two enzymes may contribute significantly enough to its overall metabolism to warrant concern when used with potential inducers or inhibitors. Therefore, when attempting to predict the level of risk of using two drugs that may affect each other via altered CYP function, it is important to identify the relative effectiveness of the inhibiting/inducing drug on the CYP subfamilies that significantly contribute to the metabolism of the substrate. The contribution of a specific CYP pathway to substrate metabolism should be considered not only in light of other known CYP pathways, but also other nonoxidative pathways for substrate metabolism (eg, glucuronidation) and transporter proteins (eg, P-glycoprotein) that may affect the presentation of a substrate to a metabolic pathway.

HOW TO USE THE TABLES

The following CYP SUBSTRATES, INHIBITORS, and INDUCERS tables provide a clinically relevant perspective on drugs that are affected by, or affect, cytochrome P450 (CYP) enzymes. Not all human, drug-metabolizing CYP enzymes are specifically (or separately) included in the tables. Some enzymes have been excluded because they do not appear to significantly contribute to the metabolism of marketed drugs (eg, CYP2C18). Others have been combined in recognition of the difficulty in distinguishing their metabolic activity one from another, or the clinical practicality of doing so (eg, CYP2C8/9, CYP3A4). In the case of CYP3A4, the industry routinely uses this single enzyme designation to represent all enzymes in the CYP3A subfamily. CYP3A7 is present in fetal livers. It is effectively absent from adult livers. CYP3A4 (adult) and CYP3A7 (fetal) appear to share similar properties in their respective hosts. The impact of CYP3A7 in fetal and neonatal drug interactions has not been investigated.

The **CYP Substrates table** contains a list of drugs reported to be metabolized, at least in part, by one or more CYP enzymes. An enzyme that appears to play a clinically significant (major) role in a drug's metabolism is indicated by "●", and an enzyme whose role appears to be clinically insignificant (minor) is indicated by "○". A clinically significant designation is the result of a two-phase review. The first phase considered the contribution of each CYP enzyme to the overall metabolism of the drug. The enzyme pathway was considered potentially clinically relevant if it was responsible for at least 30% of the metabolism of the drug. If so, the drug was subjected to a second phase. The second phase considered the clinical relevance of a substrate's concentration being increased twofold, or decreased by one-half (such as might be observed if combined with an effective CYP inhibitor or inducer, respectively). If either of these changes was considered to present a clinically significant concern, the CYP pathway for the drug was designated "major." If neither change would appear to present a clinically significant concern, or if the CYP enzyme was responsible for a smaller portion of the overall metabolism (ie, <30%), the pathway was designated "minor."

The **CYP Inhibitors table** contains a list of drugs that are reported to inhibit one or more CYP enzymes. Enzymes that are strongly inhibited by a drug are indicated by "●". Enzymes that are moderately inhibited are indicated by "◐". Enzymes that are weakly inhibited are indicated by "○". The designations are the result of a review of published clinical reports, available Ki data, and assessments published by other experts in the field. As it pertains to Ki values set in a ratio with achievable serum drug concentrations ([I]) under normal dosing conditions, the following parameters were employed: [I]/Ki ≥1 = strong; [I]/Ki 0.1-1 = moderate; [I]/Ki <0.1 = weak.

The **CYP Inducers table** contains a list of drugs that are reported to induce one or more CYP enzymes. Enzymes that appear to be effectively induced by a drug are indicated by "●", and enzymes that do not appear to be effectively induced are indicated by "○". The designations are the result of a review of published clinical reports and assessments published by experts in the field.

In general, clinically significant interactions are more likely to occur between substrates and either inhibitors or inducers of the same enzyme(s), all of which have been indicated by "●". However, these assessments possess a degree of subjectivity, at times based on limited indications regarding the significance of CYP effects of particular agents. An attempt has been made to balance a conservative, clinically-sensitive presentation of the data with a desire to avoid the numbing effect of a "beware of everything" approach. Even so, other potential interactions (ie, those involving enzymes indicated by "○") may warrant consideration in some cases. It is important to note that information related to CYP metabolism of drugs is expanding at a rapid pace, and thus, the contents of this table should only be considered to represent a "snapshot" of the information available at the time of publication.

CYTOCHROME P450 ENZYMES: SUBSTRATES, INHIBITORS, AND INDUCERS (Continued)

Selected Readings

Bjornsson TD, Callaghan JT, Einolf HJ, et al, "The Conduct of in vitro and in vivo Drug-Drug Interaction Studies: A PhRMA Perspective," J Clin Pharmacol, 2003, 43(5):443-69.

Drug-Drug Interactions, Rodrigues AD, ed, New York, NY: Marcel Dekker, Inc, 2002.

Levy RH, Thummel KE, Trager WF, et al, eds, Metabolic Drug Interactions, Philadelphia, PA: Lippincott Williams & Wilkins, 2000.

Michalets EL, "Update: Clinically Significant Cytochrome P-450 Drug Interactions," Pharmacotherapy, 1998, 18(1):84-112.

Thummel KE and Wilkinson GR, "In vitro and in vivo Drug Interactions Involving Human CYP3A," Annu Rev Pharmacol Toxicol, 1998, 38:389-430.

Zhang Y and Benet LZ, "The Gut as a Barrier to Drug Absorption: Combined Role of Cytochrome P450 3A and P-Glycoprotein," Clin Pharmacokinet, 2001, 40(3):159-68.

Selected Websites

http://www.gentest.com
http://www.imm.ki.se/CYPalleles
http://medicine.iupui.edu/flockhart
http://www.mhc.com/Cytochromes

CYP Substrates

● = major substrate
○ = minor substrate

Drug	1A2	2A6	2B6	2C8/9	2C19	2D6	2E1	3A4
Acetaminophen	○	○		○		○	○	○
Albendazole	○							●
Albuterol								●
Alfentanil								●
Almotriptan						○		○
Alosetron	●			○				○
Alprazolam								●
Aminophylline	●						○	○
Amiodarone	○			●	○	○		●
Amitriptyline	○		○	○	○	●		○
Amlodipine								●
Amoxapine						●		
Amphetamine						○		
Amprenavir				○				●
Aprepitant	○				○			●
Argatroban								○
Aripiprazole						●		●
Aspirin				○				
Atazanavir								●
Atomoxetine					○	●		
Atorvastatin								●
Azelastine	○				○	○	○	○
Azithromycin								○
Benzphetamine			○					●
Benztropine						○		
Betaxolol	●					●		
Bexarotene								○
Bezafibrate								○
Bisoprolol						○		●
Bortezomib	○			○	○	●	○	●
Bosentan				●				●
Brinzolamide								○
Bromazepam								●
Bromocriptine								●
Budesonide								●
Bupivacaine	○					○	○	○
Buprenorphine								●
BuPROPion	○	○	●	○		○	○	○
BusPIRone						○		●
Busulfan								●
Caffeine	●			○		○	○	○
Candesartan				○				
Capsaicin							○	
Captopril						●		
Carbamazepine				○				●
Carisoprodol					●			
Carteolol						○		
Carvedilol	○			●		●	○	○

CYP Substrates *(continued)*

Drug	1A2	2A6	2B6	2C8/9	2C19	2D6	2E1	3A4
Celecoxib				○				○
Cerivastatin								●
Cetirizine								○
Cevimeline						○		○
Chlordiazepoxide								●
Chloroquine						●		●
Chlorpheniramine						○		●
ChlorproMAZINE	○					●		○
ChlorproPAMIDE					○			
Chlorzoxazone	○	○				○	●	○
Cilostazol	○				○	○		●
Cinacalcet	○					○		○
Cisapride	○	○	○	○	○			●
Citalopram						●	○	●
Clarithromycin								●
Clobazam						●		●
Clofibrate								○
ClomiPRAMINE	●					●	●	○
Clonazepam								●
Clopidogrel	○							○
Clorazepate								●
Clozapine	●	○		○		○	○	○
Cocaine								●
Codeine[1]						●		○
Colchicine								●
Cyclobenzaprine	●					○		○
Cyclophosphamide[2]		○	●	○	○			●
CycloSPORINE								●
Dacarbazine	●						●	
Dantrolene								●
Dapsone				○	○		○	●
Delavirdine						○		●
Desipramine	○					●		
Desogestrel					●			
Dexamethasone								○
Dexmedetomidine		●						
Dextroamphetamine						●		
Dextromethorphan		○		○	○	●	○	○
Diazepam	○		○	○	●			●
Diclofenac	○		○	○	○	○		○
Digitoxin								●
Digoxin								○
Dihydrocodeine[1]						●		
Dihydroergotamine								●
Diltiazem				○		○		●
Dirithromycin								○
Disopyramide								●
Disulfiram	○	○	○			○	○	○
Docetaxel								●
Dofetilide								○
Dolasetron				○				○
Domperidone								○
Donepezil						○		○
Dorzolamide				○				○
Doxepin	●					●		●
DOXOrubicin						●		●
Doxycycline								●
Drospirenone								○
Duloxetine	●					●		●
Dutasteride								○
Efavirenz			●					●
Eletriptan								●
Enalapril								●
Enflurane							●	
Eplerenone								●
Ergoloid mesylates								●
Ergonovine								●
Ergotamine								●
Erythromycin				○				●

CYTOCHROME P450 ENZYMES: SUBSTRATES, INHIBITORS, AND INDUCERS (Continued)

CYP Substrates (continued)

Drug	1A2	2A6	2B6	2C8/9	2C19	2D6	2E1	3A4
Escitalopram					●			●
Esomeprazole					●			○
Estazolam								○
Estradiol	●	○	○	○	○	○	○	●
Estrogens, conjugated A/synthetic	●	○	○	○	○	○	○	●
Estrogens, conjugated equine	●	○	○	○	○	○	○	●
Estrogens, conjugated esterified	●		○	○			○	●
Estrone	●		○	○			○	●
Estropipate	●		○	○			○	●
Ethinyl estradiol				○				●
Ethosuximide								●
Etonogestrel								○
Etoposide	○						○	●
Exemestane								●
Felbamate							○	●
Felodipine								●
Fenofibrate								○
Fentanyl								●
Fexofenadine								○
Finasteride								○
Flecainide	○					●		
Fluoxetine	○		●	○	○	●	○	○
Fluphenazine						●		
Flurazepam								●
Flurbiprofen				○				
Flutamide	●							●
Fluticasone								●
Fluvastatin				○		○		○
Fluvoxamine	●					●		
Formoterol		○		○	○			
Fosamprenavir (as amprenavir)				○				●
Fosphenytoin (as phenytoin)				●	●			○
Frovatriptan	○							
Fulvestrant								○
Galantamine						○		○
Gefitinib								●
Gemfibrozil								○
Glimepiride				●				
GlipiZIDE				●				
Granisetron								○
Guanabenz	●							
Halazepam								○
Halofantrine				○		○		●
Haloperidol	○					●		●
Halothane		○	○	○		○	●	○
Hydrocodone[1]						●		
Hydrocortisone								○
Ibuprofen				○	○			
Ifosfamide[3]		○	○	○	○			●
Imatinib	○			○	○	○		●
Imipramine	○		○		●	●		○
Imiquimod	○							○
Indinavir						○		●
Indomethacin				○	○			
Irbesartan				○				
Irinotecan			●					●
Isoflurane							●	
Isoniazid							●	
Isosorbide								●
Isosorbide dinitrate								●
Isosorbide mononitrate								●
Isradipine								●
Itraconazole								●

CYP Substrates *(continued)*

Drug	1A2	2A6	2B6	2C8/9	2C19	2D6	2E1	3A4
Ivermectin								○
Ketamine			●	●				●
Ketoconazole								●
Labetalol						●		
Lansoprazole				○	●			●
Letrozole		○						●
Levobupivacaine	○							○
Levonorgestrel								●
Lidocaine	○	○	○	○		●		●
Lomustine						●		
Lopinavir								○
Loratadine						○		○
Losartan				●				●
Lovastatin								●
Maprotiline						●		
MedroxyPROGESTERone								●
Mefenamic acid				○				
Mefloquine								●
Meloxicam				○				○
Mephenytoin			○	●	●			
Mephobarbital			○	○	●			
Mestranol[4]				●				●
Methadone				○	○	○		●
Methamphetamine						●		
Methoxsalen		○						
Methsuximide					●			
Methylergonovine								●
Methylphenidate						●		
MethylPREDNISolone								○
Metoclopramide	○					○		
Metoprolol					○	●		
Mexiletine	●					●		
Miconazole								●
Midazolam			○					●
Mifepristone								○
Miglustat								●
Mirtazapine	●			○		●		●
Moclobemide					●	●		
Modafinil								●
Mometasone furoate								○
Montelukast				●				●
Moricizine								●
Morphine sulfate						○		
Naproxen	○			○				
Nateglinide				●				●
Nefazodone						●		●
Nelfinavir				○	●	○		●
Nevirapine			○			○		●
NiCARdipine	○			○		○	○	●
Nicotine	○	○	○	○	○	○	○	○
NIFEdipine						○		●
Nilutamide					●			
Nimodipine								●
Nisoldipine								●
Nitrendipine								●
Norelgestromin								○
Norethindrone								●
Norgestrel								●
Nortriptyline	○				○	●		○
Olanzapine	○					○		
Omeprazole		○		○	●	○		○
Ondansetron	○			○		○	○	●
Orphenadrine	○		○			○		○
Oxybutynin								○
Oxycodone[1]						●		
Paclitaxel				●				●
Palonosetron	○					○		○
Pantoprazole					●			○
Paroxetine						●		

CYTOCHROME P450 ENZYMES: SUBSTRATES, INHIBITORS, AND INDUCERS *(Continued)*

CYP Substrates *(continued)*

Drug	1A2	2A6	2B6	2C8/9	2C19	2D6	2E1	3A4
Pentamidine					●			
Pergolide								●
Perphenazine	○			○	○	●		○
Phencyclidine								●
Phenobarbital				○	●		○	
Phenytoin				●	●			○
Pimecrolimus								○
Pimozide	●							●
Pindolol						●		
Pioglitazone				●				●
Pipecuronium				○				
Pipotiazine						●		●
Piroxicam				○				
Pravastatin								○
Prazepam								○
PrednisoLONE								○
PredniSONE								○
Primaquine								●
Procainamide						●		
Progesterone	○	○		○	●	○		●
Proguanil	○				○			○
Promethazine			●			●		
Propafenone	○					●		○
Propofol	○	○	●	●	○	○	○	○
Propranolol	●				○	●		○
Protriptyline						●		
Quazepam								○
Quetiapine						○		●
Quinidine					○		○	●
Quinine	○				○			○
Rabeprazole					●			●
Ranitidine	○				○	○		
Repaglinide				●				●
Rifabutin	●							●
Rifampin		●		●				●
Riluzole	●							
Risperidone						●		○
Ritonavir	○		○			○		●
Rofecoxib				○				
Ropinirole	●							○
Ropivacaine	○		○			○		○
Rosiglitazone				●				
Rosuvastatin				○				○
Saquinavir						○		●
Selegiline	○	○	●	●		○		○
Sertraline				○	○	●		○
Sevoflurane		○	○				●	○
Sibutramine								●
Sildenafil				○				●
Simvastatin								●
Sirolimus								●
Spiramycin								●
Sufentanil								●
SulfaDIAZINE				●			○	○
Sulfamethoxazole				●				○
Sulfinpyrazone				●				○
SulfiSOXAZOLE				●				
Suprofen				○				
Tacrine	●							
Tacrolimus								●
Tamoxifen		○	○	●		●	○	●
Tamsulosin						●		●
Telithromycin	○							●
Temazepam			○	○	○			○
Teniposide								●
Terbinafine	○			○	○			○

CYP Substrates *(continued)*

Drug	1A2	2A6	2B6	2C8/9	2C19	2D6	2E1	3A4
Testosterone			○	○	○			○
Tetracycline								●
Theophylline	●			○		○	●	●
Thiabendazole	○							
Thioridazine					○	●		
Thiothixene	●							
Tiagabine								●
Ticlopidine								●
Timolol						●		
Tinidazole								○
Tiotropium						○		○
TOLBUTamide				●	○			
Tolcapone		○						○
Tolterodine				○	○	●		●
Toremifene	○							●
Torsemide				●				
Tramadol[1]						●		○
Trazodone						○		●
Tretinoin		○	○	○				
Triazolam								●
Trifluoperazine	●							
Trimethadione				○	○		●	○
Trimethoprim				●				●
Trimipramine					●	●		●
Troleandomycin								●
Valdecoxib				○				○
Valproic acid		○	○	○	○		○	
Vardenafil								●
Venlafaxine				○	○	●		○
Verapamil	○			○	○		○	●
VinBLAStine						○		●
VinCRIStine								●
Vinorelbine						○		●
Voriconazole				●	●			○
Warfarin	○			●	○			○
Yohimbine						○		
Zafirlukast				●				
Zaleplon								○
Zidovudine		○		○	○			○
Zileuton	○			○				○
Ziprasidone	○							○
Zolmitriptan	○							
Zolpidem	○			○	○	○		●
Zonisamide						○		●
Zopiclone				●				●
Zuclopenthixol						●		

[1]This opioid analgesic is bioactivated *in vivo* via CYP2D6. Inhibiting this enzyme would decrease the effects of the analgesic. The active metabolite might also affect, or be affected by, CYP enzymes.

[2]Cyclophosphamide is bioactivated *in vivo* to acrolein via CYP2B6 and 3A4. Inhibiting these enzymes would decrease the effects of cyclophosphamide.

[3]Ifosfamide is bioactivated *in vivo* to acrolein via CYP3A4. Inhibiting this enzyme would decrease the effects of ifosfamide.

[4]Mestranol is bioactivated *in vivo* to ethinyl estradiol via CYP2C8/9. See Ethinyl Estradiol for additional CYP information.

CYTOCHROME P450 ENZYMES: SUBSTRATES, INHIBITORS, AND INDUCERS (Continued)

CYP Inhibitors

● = strong inhibitor
◐ = moderate inhibitor
○ = weak inhibitor

Drug	1A2	2A6	2B6	2C8/9	2C19	2D6	2E1	3A4
Acebutolol						○		
Acetaminophen								○
AcetaZOLAMIDE								○
Albendazole	○							
Alosetron	○						○	
Amiodarone	●	◐	○	◐	○	◐		◐
Amitriptyline	○			○	○	○	○	
Amlodipine	◐	○	○	○				○
Amphetamine						○		
Amprenavir					○			●
Anastrozole	○			○				○
Aprepitant				○	○			◐
Atazanavir	○			○				●
Atorvastatin								○
Azelastine			○	○	○	○		○
Azithromycin								○
Bepridil						○		
Betamethasone								○
Betaxolol						○		
Biperiden						○		
Bortezomib	○			○	◐	○		○
Bromazepam							○	
Bromocriptine	○							○
Buprenorphine	○	○				○	○	
BuPROPion						○		
Caffeine	●							◐
Candesartan				○				
Celecoxib						○		
Cerivastatin								○
Chloramphenicol				○				○
Chloroquine						◐		
Chlorpheniramine						○		
ChlorproMAZINE						●	○	
Chlorzoxazone							○	○
Cholecalciferol				○	○	○		
Cimetidine	◐			○	◐	◐	○	◐
Cinacalcet						○		
Ciprofloxacin	●							○
Cisapride						○		○
Citalopram	○		○		○	○		
Clarithromycin	○							●
Clemastine						○		○
Clofazimine								○
Clofibrate		○						
ClomiPRAMINE						◐		
Clopidogrel				○				
Clotrimazole	○	○	○	○	○	○	○	◐
Clozapine	○			○	○	◐	○	○
Cocaine						●		○
Codeine						○		
Cyclophosphamide								○
CycloSPORINE				○				◐
Danazol								○
Delavirdine	○			●	●	●		●
Desipramine		◐	◐			◐	○	◐
Dexmedetomidine	○			○		●		○
Dextromethorphan						○		
Diazepam					○			○

CYP Inhibitors *(continued)*

Drug	1A2	2A6	2B6	2C8/9	2C19	2D6	2E1	3A4
Diclofenac	◐			○			○	●
Dihydroergotamine								○
Diltiazem				○		○		◐
Dimethyl sulfoxide				○	○			
DiphenhydrAMINE						◐		
Disulfiram	○	○	○	○		○	●	○
Docetaxel								○
Dolasetron						○		
DOXOrubicin			◐			○		○
Doxycycline								◐
Drospirenone	○			○	○			○
Duloxetine						◐		
Econazole							○	
Efavirenz				○	○			○
Enoxacin	●							●
Entacapone	○	○		○	○	○	○	○
Eprosartan				○				
Ergotamine								○
Erythromycin	○							◐
Escitalopram						○		
Estradiol	○							
Estrogens, conjugated A/synthetic	○							
Estrogens, conjugated equine	○							
Ethinyl estradiol	○		○		○			○
Ethotoin					○			
Etoposide				○				○
Felbamate					○			
Felodipine				○		○		○
Fenofibrate		○		○	○			
Fentanyl								○
Fexofenadine						○		
Flecainide						○		
Fluconazole	○			●	●			◐
Fluoxetine	◐		○	○	◐	●		○
Fluphenazine	○			○		○	○	
Flurazepam							○	
Flurbiprofen				●				
Flutamide	○							
Fluvastatin	○			◐		○		○
Fluvoxamine	●		○	○	●	○		○
Fosamprenavir (as amprenavir)					○			●
Gefitinib					○	○		
Gemfibrozil	◐			●	●			
Glyburide								○
Grapefruit juice								◐
Halofantrine						○		
Haloperidol						◐		◐
HydrALAZINE								○
HydrOXYzine						○		
Ibuprofen				●				
Ifosfamide								○
Imatinib				○		○		●
Imipramine	○				○	◐	○	
Indinavir				○	○	○		●
Indomethacin				●	○			
Interferon alfa-2a	○							
Interferon alfa-2b	○							
Interferon gamma-1b	○						○	
Irbesartan				◐		○		○
Isoflurane			○					
Isoniazid	○	◐		◐	●	◐	◐	●
Isradipine								○
Itraconazole								●

CYTOCHROME P450 ENZYMES: SUBSTRATES, INHIBITORS, AND INDUCERS (Continued)

CYP Inhibitors (continued)

Drug	1A2	2A6	2B6	2C8/9	2C19	2D6	2E1	3A4
Ketoconazole	●	◑	○	●	◑	◑		●
Ketoprofen				○				
Labetalol						○		
Lansoprazole				○	◑	○		○
Leflunomide				○				
Letrozole		●			○			
Lidocaine	●					◑		◑
Lomefloxacin	○							
Lomustine						○		○
Loratadine					◑	○		
Losartan	○			◑				○
Lovastatin				○		○		○
Mefenamic acid				●				
Mefloquine						○		○
Meloxicam				○				
Mephobarbital					○			
Mestranol	○		○		○			○
Methadone						◑		○
Methimazole	○	○	○	○	○	◑	○	○
Methotrimeprazine						○		
Methoxsalen	●	●		○	○	○		○
Methsuximide					○			
Methylphenidate						○		
MethylPREDNISolone								○
Metoclopramide						○		
Metoprolol						○		
Metronidazole					○			◑
Metyrapone		○						
Mexiletine	●							
Miconazole	◑	●	○	●	●	●	◑	●
Midazolam				○				○
Mifepristone						○		○
Mirtazapine	○							○
Mitoxantrone								○
Moclobemide	○				○	○		
Modafinil	○	○		○	●		○	○
Montelukast				○				
Nalidixic acid	○							
Nateglinide				○				
Nefazodone	○		○			○		●
Nelfinavir	○		○	○	○	○		●
Nevirapine	○					○		○
NiCARdipine				●	◑	◑		●
Nicotine		○					○	
NIFEdipine	◑			○		○		○
Nilutamide					○			
Nisoldipine	○							○
Nitrendipine								○
Nizatidine								○
Norfloxacin	●							◑
Nortriptyline						○	○	
Ofloxacin	●							
Olanzapine	○			○	○	○		○
Omeprazole	○			◑	●	○		○
Ondansetron	○			○		○		
Orphenadrine	○	○	○	○	○	○	○	○
Oxcarbazepine					○			
Oxprenolol						○		
Oxybutynin						○		○
Pantoprazole				◑				
Paroxetine	○		◑	○	○	●		○
Peginterferon alfa-2a	○							

CYP Inhibitors *(continued)*

Drug	1A2	2A6	2B6	2C8/9	2C19	2D6	2E1	3A4
Peginterferon alfa-2b	○							
Pentamidine				○	○	○		○
Pentoxifylline	○							
Pergolide						●		○
Perphenazine	○					○		
Phencyclidine								○
Pilocarpine		○					○	○
Pimozide					○	○	○	○
Pindolol						○		
Pioglitazone				●	○	◐		
Piroxicam				●				
Pravastatin				○		○		○
Praziquantel						○		
PrednisoLONE								○
Primaquine	●					○		○
Probenecid					○			
Progesterone				○	○			○
Promethazine						○		
Propafenone	○			○		○		
Propofol	◐			○	◐	○	○	●
Propoxyphene				○		○		○
Propranolol	○					○		
Pyrimethamine				◐		◐		
Quinidine				○		●		●
Quinine				◐		●		○
Quinupristin								○
Rabeprazole					◐	○		○
Ranitidine	○					○		
Risperidone						○		○
Ritonavir				○	○	●	○	●
Rofecoxib	○							
Ropinirole	○					●		
Rosiglitazone				◐	○	○		
Saquinavir				○	○	○		◐
Selegiline	○	○		○	○	○	○	○
Sertraline	○		◐	○	◐	◐		◐
Sildenafil	○			○	○	○	○	○
Simvastatin				○		○		
Sirolimus								○
Sulconazole	○	○		○	○	○	○	○
SulfaDIAZINE				●				
Sulfamethoxazole				◐				
Sulfinpyrazone				◐				
SulfiSOXAZOLE				●				
Tacrine	○							
Tacrolimus								○
Tamoxifen			○	○				○
Telithromycin						○		●
Telmisartan					○			
Teniposide				○				○
Tenofovir	○							
Terbinafine						●		
Testosterone								○
Tetracycline								◐
Theophylline	○							
Thiabendazole	●							
Thioridazine	○			○		◐	○	
Thiotepa			○					
Thiothixene						○		
Ticlopidine	○			○	●	◐	○	○
Timolol						○		
Tioconazole	○	○		○	○	○	○	
Tocainide	○							
TOLBUTamide				●				
Tolcapone				○				

CYTOCHROME P450 ENZYMES: SUBSTRATES, INHIBITORS, AND INDUCERS *(Continued)*

CYP Inhibitors *(continued)*

Drug	1A2	2A6	2B6	2C8/9	2C19	2D6	2E1	3A4
Topiramate					○			
Torsemide					○			
Tranylcypromine	◐	●		○	◐	◐	○	○
Trazodone						◐		○
Tretinoin				○				
Triazolam				○				
Trimethoprim				◐				
Tripelennamine						◐		
Triprolidine						○		
Troleandomycin								◐
Valdecoxib				○	○			
Valproic acid				○	○	○		○
Valsartan				○				
Venlafaxine			○			○		○
Verapamil	○			○		○		◐
VinBLAStine						○		○
VinCRIStine								○
Vinorelbine						○		○
Voriconazole				○	○			◐
Warfarin				◐	○			
Yohimbine						○		
Zafirlukast	○			◐	○	○		○
Zileuton	○							
Ziprasidone						○		○

CYP Inducers

● = effectively induced
○ = not effectively induced

Drug	1A2	2A6	2B6	2C8/9	2C19	2D6	2E1	3A4
Aminoglutethimide	●				●			●
Amobarbital			●					
Aprepitant				○				○
Bexarotene								○
Bosentan				○				○
Calcitriol								○
Carbamazepine	●		●	●	●			●
Clofibrate			○				○	○
Colchicine				○			○	○
Cyclophosphamide			○	○				
Dexamethasone		○	○	○				○
Dicloxacillin								○
Efavirenz (in liver only)			○					○
Estradiol								○
Estrogens, conjugated A/synthetic								○
Estrogens, conjugated equine								○
Exemestane								○
Felbamate								○
Fosphenytoin (as phenytoin)			●	●	●			●
Griseofulvin	○			○				○
Hydrocortisone								○
Ifosfamide				○				
Insulin preparations	○							
Isoniazid (after D/C)							○	
Lansoprazole	○							
MedroxyPROGESTERone								○
Mephobarbital		○						
Metyrapone								○
Modafinil	○		○					○
Moricizine	○							○
Nafcillin								●
Nevirapine			●					●
Norethindrone					○			
Omeprazole	○							
Oxcarbazepine								●
Paclitaxel								○
Pantoprazole	○							○
Pentobarbital		●						●
Phenobarbital	●	●	●	●				●
Phenytoin			●	●	●			●
Pioglitazone								○
PredniSONE					○			○
Primaquine	○							
Primidone[1]	●		●	●				●
Rifabutin								●
Rifampin	●	●	●	●	●			●
Rifapentine				●				●
Ritonavir (long-term)	○			○				○
Rofecoxib								○
Secobarbital		●		●				
Sulfinpyrazone								○
Terbinafine								○
Topiramate								○
Tretinoin							○	
Troglitazone								○
Valproic acid		○						

[1]Primidone is partially metabolized to phenobarbital. See Phenobarbital for additional CYP information.

TYRAMINE CONTENT OF FOODS

Food	Allowed	Minimize Intake	Not Allowed
Beverages	Milk, decaffeinated coffee, tea, soda	Chocolate beverage, caffeine-containing drinks, clear spirits	Acidophilus milk; alcoholic, nonalcoholic, or reduced-alcohol beer, ale, wine, or malted beverages
Breads/cereals	All except those containing cheese	None	Cheese bread and crackers
Dairy products	Cottage cheese, farmers or pot cheese, cream cheese, ricotta cheese, all milk, eggs, ice cream, pudding (except chocolate)	Yogurt (limit to 4 oz per day)	All other cheeses (aged cheese, American, Camembert, cheddar, Gouda, gruyere, mozzarella, parmesan, provolone, romano, Roquefort, stilton)
Meat, fish, and poultry	All fresh or frozen	Aged meats, hot dogs, canned fish and meat	Chicken and beef liver, dried and pickled fish, summer or dry sausage, pepperoni, dried meats, meat extracts, bologna, liverwurst
Starches — potatoes/rice	All	None	Soybean (including paste)
Vegetables	All fresh, frozen, canned, or dried vegetable juices except those not allowed	Chili peppers, Chinese pea pods	Fava beans, sauerkraut, pickles, olives, Italian broad beans
Fruit	Fresh, frozen, or canned fruits and fruit juices	Avocado, banana, raspberries, figs	Banana peel extract
Soups	All soups not listed to limit or avoid	Commercially canned soups	Soups which contain broad beans, fava beans, cheese, beer, wine, any made with flavor cubes or meat extract, miso soup
Fats	All except fermented	Sour cream	Packaged gravy
Sweets	Sugar, hard candy, honey, molasses, syrups	Chocolate candies	None
Desserts	Cakes, cookies, gelatin, pastries, sherbets, sorbets	Chocolate desserts	Cheese-filled desserts
Miscellaneous	Salt, nuts, spices, herbs, flavorings, Worcestershire sauce	Soy sauce, peanuts	Brewer's yeast, yeast concentrates, all aged and fermented products, monosodium glutamate, vitamins with Brewer's yeast

MATERNAL / FETAL MEDICATIONS

Adapted from Briggs GG, "Medication Use During the Perinatal Period,"
J Am Pharm Assoc, 1998, 38:717-27.

Antibiotics in Pregnancy

Antibiotic	Comments
Antibiotics to Be Avoided	
Aminoglycosides (prolonged use)	Eighth cranial nerve damage (hearing loss, vestibulotoxicity)
Erythromycin estolate	Hepatotoxic in mother
Fluoroquinolones	Potentially mutagenic, cartilage damage, arthropathy, and teratogenicity
Ribavirin	Possibly fetotoxic
Tetracyclines	Staining of deciduous teeth (4th month through term)
Antibiotics Which Are Generally Regarded as Safe	
Aminoglycosides (limited use)	
Cephalosporins	
Clindamycin	
Erythromycin	
Penicillins	

Treatment and Prevention of Infection

Prophylaxis	
Preterm premature rupture of membranes	Ampicillin, amoxicillin, cefazolin, amoxicillin/clavulanate, ampicillin/sulbactam, erythromycin
Prevention of bacterial endocarditis	Ampicillin 2 g and gentamicin 1.5 mg/kg (max 120 mg) within 30 minutes of delivery, followed by 1 g ampicillin (I.V.) or amoxicillin (oral) 6 hours later
Cesarean section	Cefazolin (I.V. or uterine irrigation) or clindamycin/gentamicin
Treatment	
Bacterial vaginosis	Clindamycin (oral or gel) in first trimester (gel has been associated with higher rate of preterm deliveries) Metronidazole (oral) for 7 days or gel for 5 days (after first trimester)
Chorioamnionitis	Ampicillin plus gentamicin (clindamycin, erythromycin, or vancomycin if PCN allergic)
Genital herpes	First episode: Oral acyclovir Near term treatment may reduce Cesarian sections I.V. therapy for disseminated infection
Group B streptococci	Penicillin G 5 million units once, then 2.5 million units q4h Ampicillin 2 g once, then 1 g q4h Clindamycin or erythromycin if PCN allergic
HIV*	*Note: Always consult HIV guidelines (www.hivatis.org) Zidovudine (limits maternal-fetal transmission) Oral dosing during pregnancy/I.V. prior to delivery Other antiretroviral agents – effects unknown Lamivudine during labor used in combination with zidovudine in women who have not received prior antiretroviral therapy
Postpartum endometritis	Ampicillin (vancomycin if PCN allergic) plus clindamycin (or metronidazole) plus gentamicin until afebrile
Pyelonephritis	Ampicillin-gentamicin Cefazolin Co-trimoxazole
Urinary tract infection	Amoxicillin/ampicillin (resistance has increased) Co-trimoxazole Nitrofurantoin Cephalexin
Vaginal candidiasis	Buconizole for 7 days Clotrimazole for 7 days Miconazole for 7 days Terconazole for 7 days

MATERNAL / FETAL MEDICATIONS *(Continued)*

Preterm Labor: Tocolytic Agents

Drug Class	Route	Fetal / Neonatal Toxicities	Maternal Toxicities
Beta-adrenergic agonists			
Ritodrine, terbutaline	Oral, I.V., SubQ	Fetal tachycardia, intraventricular septal hypertrophy, neonatal hyperinsulinemia/ hypoglycemia	Pulmonary, edema, myocardial infarction, hypokalemia, hypotension, hyperglycemia, tachycardia
Magnesium	I.V.	Neurologic depression in newborn (loss of reflexes, hypotonia, respiratory depression); fetal hypocalcemia and hypercalcuria; abnormal fetal bone mineralization and enamel hypoplasia	Hypotension, respiratory depression, ileus/ constipation, hypocalcemia, pulmonary edema, hypotension, headache/dizziness
NSAIDs			
Indomethacin	Oral, P.R.	Ductus arteriosis: premature closure, ricuspid regurgitation, primary pulmonary hypertension of the newborn, PDA; intraventricular hemorrhage, necrotizing enterocolitis, renal failure	GI bleeding, oligohydramnios, pulmonary edema, acute renal failure
Calcium channel blockers			
Nifedipine	Oral	Hypoxia secondary to maternal hypotension	Hypotension, flushing, tachycardia, headache
Nitrates			
Nitroglycerin	I.V./ S.L.	Hypoxia secondary to maternal hypotension	Hypotension, headache, dizziness

Pregnancy-Induced Hypertension[1]

Drug Class	Maternal / Fetal Effects
Antihypertensives Contraindicated in PIH	
Diuretics	Reduction of maternal plasma volume exacerbates disease; use in chronic hypertension acceptable (if no superimposed pregnancy-induced hypertension)
ACE-inhibitors	Teratogenic in second and third trimester; fetal/newborn anuria and hypotension, fetal oligohydramnios; neonatal death (congenital abnormalities of skull and renal failure)
Hypertension Treatment[2]	
Central-acting	
Methyldopa	Relatively safe in second/third trimester
Beta-blockers	
Acebutolol, atenolol, metoprolol, pindolol, propranolol	Increased risk of IUGR
Alpha-/beta-blockers	
Labetolol	See beta-blockers
Vasodilators	
Hydralazine	
Nitrates	
Nitroglycerin	Relatively safe in second/third trimester
Calcium channel blockers	
Nifedipine	

[1]Includes management of pre-eclampsia/eclampsia and HELLP syndrome.
Note: Prevention may include low-dose aspirin (81 mg/day) or calcium supplementation (2 g/day).

[2]All agents must be carefully titrated to avoid fetal hypoxia.

Other Maternal-Fetal Drug Therapy

Drug	Dose / Route
Fetal Lung Maturation	
Betamethasone	Two 12 mg doses I.M. at 24-hour intervals
Dexamethasone	Four 6 mg doses I.M. at 12-hour intervals
Doses repeated weekly up to 34 weeks gestation	
Cervical Ripening	
Oxytocin	I.V. dosing – often ineffective
Hygroscopic cervical dilators	
Dinoprostone (prostaglandin E2)	Gel (0.5 mg) or vaginal insert (10 mg, releasing 0.3 mg/h)
Misoprostol (prostaglandin E1)	Oral tablets inserted intravaginally 25 mcg q3-6h for up to 24 hours. **Note:** Manufacturer issued warning in 2000 emphasizing the risk of this unlabeled use.
Analgesia During Labor	
Meperidine	25-50 mg I.V. q1-2h or 50-100 mg I.M. q2-4h
Fentanyl	50-100 mcg q1h
Butorphanol	No advantage over other agents
Nalbuphine	
Tramadol	
Postpartum Hemorrhage	
Oxytocin	I.V. (usually), I.M., or intramyometrially (I.M.M.)
Methylergonovine	I.M. or intramyometrially (I.M.M.); contraindicated in hypertension
Carboprost (PG F2 alpha)	Pyrexia is common; contraindicated in cardiac, pulmonary, renal, or hepatic disease.
Misoprostil	Rectal administration has been investigated.

MATERNAL / FETAL TOXICOLOGY

Drugs and Chemicals Proven to Be Teratogenic in Humans

Drug / Chemical	Fetal Adverse Effects	Relative Risk for Teratogenicity	Clinical Intervention
Alcohol	**Fetal alcohol syndrome:** Mental retardation, microcephaly, poor coordination, hypotonia, hyperactivity, short upturned nose, micrognathia or retrognathia (infancy) or prognathia (adolescence), short palpebral fissures, hypoplastic philtrum, thinned upper lips, microphthalmia, antenatal/postnatal growth retardation, occasional pathologies of eyes, mouth, heart, kidneys, gonads, skin, muscle, and skeleton	In alcoholic women consuming >2 g/kg/d ethanol over first trimester: 2- to 3-fold higher risk for congenital malformations (about 10%)	To calculate accurate dose of alcohol: **Prospective:** To discontinue exposure; if woman is alcoholic, refer to addiction center **During pregnancy:** To alleviate fears in mild or occasional drinkers who may terminate pregnancy based on unrealistic perception of risk, level 2 ultrasound to rule out visible malformation
Alkylating agents (busulfan, chlorambucil, cyclophosphamide, mechlorethamine)	Growth retardation, cleft palate, microphthalmia hypoplastic ovaries, cloudy corneas, agenesis of kidney, malformations of digits, cardiac defects, multiple other anomalies	Based on case reports, between 10% and 50% of cases were malformed for different drugs. It is possible that adverse outcome was over-represented.	Level 2 ultrasound to rule out visible malformations. Supplement folic acid to women receiving antifolates (eg, methotrexate).
Antimetabolite agents (aminopterin azauridine, cytarabine, 5-FU, 6-MP, methotrexate)	Hydrocephalus, meningoencephalocele, anencephaly, malformed skull, cerebral hypoplasia, growth retardation, eye and ear malformations, malformed nose and cleft palate, malformed extremities and fingers **Aminopterin syndrome:** Cranial dysostosis, hydrocephalus, hypertelorism, anomalies of external ear, micrognathia, posterior cleft palate	Based on case reports 7%-75% of cases were malformed. It is possible that adverse outcome was over-represented.	Level 2 ultrasound to rule out visible malformations.
Carbamazepine	Increased risk for neural tube defects (NTDs)	NTDs estimated at 1% with carbamazepine	Periconceptional folate; maternal and/ or amniotic α-fetoprotein; ultrasound to rule out NTD.
Carbon monoxide	Cerebral atrophy, mental retardation, microcephaly, convulsions, spastic disorders, intrauterine or postnatal death	Based on case reports, when mother is severely poisoned, high risk for neurological sequelae; no increased risk in mild accidental exposures	Measure maternal carboxyhemoglobin levels. Treat with 100% oxygen for 5 hours after maternal carboxyhemoglobin returns to normal because fetal equilibration takes longer. If hyperbaric chamber available, should be used, as elimination half-life of CO is more rapid. Fetal monitoring by an obstetrician; sonographic follow-up.
Lead	Lower scores in developmental tests	Higher risk when maternal lead is >10 µg/dL	**Maternal lead levels >10 µg/dL:** Investigate for possible source of contamination. **Levels >25 µg/dL:** Consider chelation

Drugs and Chemicals Proven to Be Teratogenic in Humans
(continued)

Drug / Chemical	Fetal Adverse Effects	Relative Risk for Teratogenicity	Clinical Intervention
Lithium carbonate	Possibly higher risk for Ebstein's anomaly; no detectable higher risk for other malformations		Women who need lithium should continue therapy, with sonographic follow-up. Patients may need higher doses because of increased clearance rate.
Methyl mercury, mercuric sulfide	Microcephaly, eye malformations, cerebral palsy, mental retardation, malocclusion of teeth	Women of affected babies consumed 9-27 ppm mercury; greater risk when ingested at 6-8 gestational months. Relative risk was not elucidated, but 13/220 babies born in Minamata, Japan, at time of contamination had severe disease.	Good correlation between mercury concentrations in maternal hair follicles and neurological outcome of the fetus. Hair mercury content >50 ppm was used successfully as a cut point for termination. In acute poisoning, the fetus is 4-10 times more sensitive than the adult to methylmercury toxicity.
PCBs	**Stillbirth** **Signs at birth:** White eye discharge, 30% (32/108); teeth present, 8.7% (11/127); irritated/swollen gums, 11% (11/99); hyperpigmentation ("cola" staining), 42.5% (54/127); deformed/small nails, 24.6% (30/122); acne, 12.8% (16/125) **Subsequent history:** Bronchitis or pneumonia, 27.2% (30/124); chipped or broken teeth, 35.5% (38/107); hair loss, 12.2% (14/115); acne scars, 9.6% (11/115); generalized itching, 27.8% (32/1150) **Developmental:** Do not meet milestones; lower scores than unexposed controls; evidence of CNS damage	4%-20% (6/159-8/39)	These figures, which are from cases poisoned by high consumption of PCB-contaminated rice oil, cannot be extrapolated to cases in which maternal poisoning has not been verified. Women working near PCBs (eg, hydroelectric facilities) should use effective protection.
Penicillamine	Skin hyperelastosis	Few case reports; risk unknown	
Phenytoin	**Fetal hydantoin syndrome:** Low nasal bridge, inner epicanthal folds, ptosis, strabismus, hypertelorism, low set or abnormal ears, wide mouth, large fontanels, anomalies and hypoplasia of distal phalanges and nails, skeletal abnormalities, microcephaly and mental retardation, growth deficiency, neuroblastoma, cardiac defects, cleft palate/lip	5%-10% of typical syndrome; about 30% of partial picture. Relative risk of 7 for offspring IQ ≤84.	Neurologist should consider changing to other medications. Keep phenytoin concentrations at lower effective levels. Level 2 ultrasound to rule out visible malformations, vitamin K to neonate. Epilepsy itself increases teratogenic risk.
Systemic retinoids (isotretinoin, etretinate)	Spontaneous abortions; deformities of cranium, ears, face, heart, limbs, liver; hydrocephalus, microcephalus, heart defects. Cognitive defects even without dysmorphology	For isotretinoin: 38% risk. 80% of malformation are CNS.	Treated women should have an effective method of contraception. Pregnancy termination. If diagnosed too late, sonographic follow-up to rule out confirmed malformations.

MATERNAL / FETAL TOXICOLOGY *(Continued)*

Drugs and Chemicals Proven to Be Teratogenic in Humans
(continued)

Drug / Chemical	Fetal Adverse Effects	Relative Risk for Teratogenicity	Clinical Intervention
Tetracycline	Yellow, gray-brown, or brown staining of deciduous teeth, destruction of enamel	From 4 months of gestation and on, occurs in 50% of fetuses exposed to tetracycline; 12.5% to oxytetracycline	If exposure before 14-16 weeks of gestation, no known risk
Thalidomide	Limb phocomelia, amelia, hypoplasia, congenital heart defects, renal malformations, cryptorchidism, abducens paralysis, deafness, microtia, anotia	About 20% risk when exposure to drug occurs in days 34-50 of gestation.	Thalidomide is an effective drug for some forms of leprosy. Treated women should have an effective mode of contraception.
Trimethadione	**Fetal trimethadione syndrome:** Intrauterine growth retardation, cardiac anomalies, microcephaly, cleft palate and lip, abnormal ears, dysmorphic face, mental retardation, tracheoesophageal fistula, postnatal death	Based on case reports: 83% risk; 32% infantile or neonatal death	No need for this antiepileptic to date
Valproic acid	Lumbosacral spina bifida with meningomyelocele; CNS defects, microcephaly, cardiac defects	1.2% risk of neural tube defects	Level 2 ultrasound and maternal α-fetoproteins or amniocentesis to rule out neural tube defects. Epilepsy itself increases teratogenic risk.
Warfarin	**Fetal warfarin syndrome:** Nasal hypoplasia, chondrodysplasia punctata, branchydactyly, skull defects, abnormal ears, malformed eyes, CNS malformations, microcephaly, hydrocephalus, skeletal deformities, mental retardation, optic atrophy, spasticity, Dandy Walker malformations	16% of exposed fetuses have malformation; another 3% hemorrhages; 8% stillbirths	**Prospective:** Switch to heparin for the first trimester. Deliver by a cesarean section. Women should be followed up in a high-risk perinatal unit.

Reprinted with permission from "Drugs and Chemicals Proven to Be Teratogenic in Humans," *Maternal-Fetal Toxicology: A Clinician's Guide*, 2nd ed, Koren G, ed, New York, NY: Marcel Dekker, Inc, 1994, 37-43.

ANTIDEPRESSANT MEDICATION GUIDELINES

The under-diagnosis and under-treatment of depression in nursing homes has been documented in a *Journal of the American Medical Association* paper entitled, "Depression and Mortality in the Nursing Home" [*JAMA*, February 27, 1991, 265(8)]. The Centers for Medicare and Medicaid Services (CMS), formerly known as the Health Care Financing Administration (HCFA), continues to support the accurate identification and treatment of depression in nursing homes.

The surveyor should not urge a facility to use behavioral monitoring charts (documenting quantitatively [eg, number of episodes] and objectively [eg, withdrawn behavior such as, staying in their room, refusal to speak, etc]) when antidepressant drugs are used in nursing homes. Such charts are promoted in the interpretative guidelines for antipsychotic and benzodiazepine and other anxiolytic/sedative drugs, but **not** for antidepressant drugs. These charts may be helpful for monitoring the effects of antidepressant drugs in nursing homes, but they may place additional paperwork burden on the facility, and thus act as a deterrent to the appropriate diagnosis and treatment of this condition.

The following is a list of commonly used antidepressant drugs:

Generic Name	Brand Name
Amitriptyline[1]	Elavil®
Amoxapine	Asendin®
Bupropion	Wellbutrin®
Citalopram[1]	Celexa®
Clomipramine[1]	Anafranil®
Desipramine	Norpramin®
Doxepin[1]	Sinequan®
Fluoxetine	Prozac®
Fluvoxamine	Luvox®
Imipramine[1]	Tofranil®
Maprotiline	Ludiomil®
Mirtazapine	Remeron®
Nefazodone	Serzone®
Nortriptyline	Aventyl®, Pamelor®
Paroxetine	Paxil®
Phenelzine[1]	Nardil®
Protriptyline	Vivactil®
Sertraline	Zoloft®
Tranylcypromine[1]	Parnate®
Trazodone	Desyrel®
Trimipramine[1]	Surmontil®
Venlafaxine	Effexor®

[1]These are not necessarily drugs of choice for depression in the elderly. They are listed here only in the event of their potential use.

ANTIPSYCHOTIC MEDICATION GUIDELINES

Appropriate indications for use of antipsychotic medications are outlined in the Health Care Finance Administration's Omnibus Reconciliation Act (OBRA) of 1987. These regulations require that antipsychotics be used to treat specific conditions (listed below) and not solely for behavior control.

Approved indications include:

- acute psychotic episode
- atypical psychosis
- brief reactive psychosis
- delusional disorder
- Huntington's disease
- psychotic mood disorder (including manic depression and depression with psychotic features)
- schizo-affective disorder
- schizophrenia
- schizophrenic form disorder
- Tourette's disease
- short-term (7 days) for hiccups, nausea, vomiting, or pruritus
- organic mental syndrome with psychotic or agitated features:

    - behaviors are quantitatively and objectively documented
    - behaviors must be **persistent**
    - behaviors are not caused by preventable reasons
    - patient presents a danger to self or others
    - continuous crying or screaming if this impairs functional status
    - psychotic symptoms (hallucinations, paranoia, delusions) which cause resident distress or impaired functional capacity

"Clinically contraindicated" means that a resident with a "specific condition" who has had a history of recurrence of psychotic symptoms (eg, delusions, hallucinations) which have been stabilized with a maintenance dose of an antipsychotic drug without incurring significant side effects (eg, tardive dyskinesia) **should not receive gradual dose reductions**. In residents with organic mental syndromes (eg, dementia, delirium), "clinically contraindicated" means that a gradual dose reduction has been attempted **twice** in 1 year and that attempt resulted in the return of symptoms for which the drug was prescribed to a degree that a cessation in the gradual dose reduction, or a return to previous dose levels was necessary.

If the medication is being used outside the guidelines, the physician must provide justification why the continued use of the drug and the dose of the drug is clinically appropriate.

Antipsychotics should not be used if one or more of the following is/are the **only** indication:

- wandering
- poor self care
- restlessness
- impaired memory
- anxiety
- depression (without psychotic features)
- insomnia
- unsociability
- indifference to surroundings
- fidgeting
- nervousness
- uncooperativeness
- agitated behaviors which do **not** represent danger to the resident or others

Selection of an antipsychotic agent should be based on the side effect profile since all antipsychotic agents are equally effective at equivalent doses. Coadministration of two or more antipsychotics does not have any pharmacological basis or clinical advantage and increases the potential for side effects. See Antipsychotic Agents table in Comparison Charts.

DOSING GUIDELINES

1. Daily dosages should be equal to or less than those listed below, unless documentation exists to support the need for higher doses to maintain or improve functional status.

Generic	Brand	Daily Dose for Patients With Organic Mental Syndrome
Chlorpromazine	Thorazine®	75 mg
Clozapine	Clozaril®	50 mg
Fluphenazine	Prolixin®	4 mg
Haloperidol	Haldol®	4 mg
Loxapine	Loxitane®	10 mg
Mesoridazine	Serentil®	25 mg
Molindone	Moban®	10 mg
Olanzapine	Zyprexa®	5 mg
Perphenazine	Trilafon®	8 mg
Pimozide	Orap™	4 mg
Prochlorperazine	Compazine®	10 mg
Quetiapine	Seroquel®	100 mg
Risperidone	Risperdal®	2 mg
Thioridazine	Mellaril®	75 mg
Thiothixene	Navane®	7 mg
Trifluoperazine	Stelazine® [DSC]	8 mg

2. The dose of prochlorperazine may be exceeded for short-term (up to 7 days) for treatment of nausea and vomiting. Residents with nausea and vomiting secondary to cancer or cancer chemotherapy can also be treated with higher doses for longer periods of time.

3. The residents must receive adequate monitoring for significant side effects such as tardive dyskinesia, postural hypotension, cognitive-behavioral impairment, akathisia, and parkinsonism.

4. Gradual dosage reductions are to be attempted twice in 1 year if prescribed for OMS. If symptoms for which the drug has been prescribed return and both reduction attempts have proven unsuccessful, the physician may indicate further reductions are clinically contraindicated.

5. "Clinically contraindicated" means that a resident **need not undergo** a "gradual dose reduction" or "behavioral interventions" if:

   - The resident has a "specific condition" and has a history of recurrence of psychotic symptoms (eg, delusions, hallucinations), which have been stabilized with a maintenance dose of an antipsychotic drug without incurring significant side effects.

   - The resident has organic mental syndrome (now called "delirium, dementia, and amnestic and other cognitive disorders" by DSM IV) and has had a gradual dose reduction attempted **twice** in 1 year and that attempt resulted in the return of symptoms for which the drug was prescribed to a degree that a cessation in the gradual dose reduction, or a return to previous dose reduction was necessary.

   - The resident's physician provides a justification why the continued use of the drug and the dose of the drug is clinically appropriate. This justification should include: a) a diagnosis, but not simply a diagnostic label or code, but the description of symptoms, b) a discussion of the differential psychiatric and medical diagnosis (eg, why the resident's behavioral symptom is thought to be a result of a dementia with associated psychosis and/or agitated behaviors, and not the result of an unrecognized painful medical condition or a psychosocial or environmental stressor), c) a description of the justification for the choice of a particular treatment, or treatments, and d) a discussion of why the present dose is necessary to manage the symptoms of the resident. This information need not necessarily be in the physician's progress notes, but must be a part of the resident's clinical record.

ANTIPSYCHOTIC MEDICATION GUIDELINES *(Continued)*

Examples of evidence that would support a justification of why a drug is being used outside these guidelines but in the best interests of the resident may include, but are not limited to the following.

- A physician's note indicating for example, that the dosage, duration, indication, and monitoring are clinically appropriate, **and the reasons why they are clinically appropriate**; this note should demonstrate that the physician has carefully considered the risk/benefit to the resident in using drugs outside the guidelines.

- A medical or psychiatric consultation or evaluation (eg, Geriatric Depression Scale) that confirms the physician's judgment that use of a drug outside the guidelines is in the best interest of the resident.

- Physician, nursing, or other health professional documentation indicating that the resident is being monitored for adverse consequences or complications of the drug therapy.

- Documentation confirming that previous attempts at dosage reduction have been unsuccessful.

- Documentation (including MDS documentation) showing resident's subjective or objective improvement, or maintenance of function while taking the medication.

- Documentation showing that a resident's decline or deterioration is evaluated by the interdisciplinary team to determine whether a particular drug, or a particular dose, or duration of therapy, may be the cause.

- Documentation showing why the resident's age, weight, or other factors would require a unique drug dose or drug duration, indication, or monitoring.

- Other evidence you may deem appropriate.

ANXIOLYTIC / HYPNOTIC USE IN LONG-TERM CARE FACILITIES

One of the regulations regarding medication use in long-term care facilities concerns "unnecessary drugs." The regulation states, "Each resident's drug regimen must be free from unnecessary drugs." The Health Care Financing Administration (HCFA), now known as Centers for Medicaid and Medicare Services (CMS), issued the final interpretive guidelines on this regulation (*State Operations Manual: Provider Certification, Transmittal 232,* Washington, DC: HCFA, Department of Health and Human Services, September 1989). The following is a summary of these guidelines as they pertain to anxiolytic/hypnotic agents.

A. **Long-Acting Benzodiazepines**

Long-acting benzodiazepine drugs should not be used in residents unless an attempt with a shorter-acting drug has failed. If they are used, the doses must be no higher than the listed dose, unless higher doses are necessary for maintenance or improvement in the resident's functional status. Daily use should be less than 4 continuous months unless an attempt at a gradual dose reduction is unsuccessful. Residents on diazepam for seizure disorders or for the treatment of tardive dyskinesia are exempt from this restriction. Residents on clonazepam for bipolar disorder, tardive dyskinesia, nocturnal myoclonus, or seizure disorder are also exempt. Residents on long-acting benzodiazepines should have a gradual dose reduction at least twice within 1 year before it can be concluded that the gradual dose reduction is "clinically contraindicated."

Generic	Brand	Maximum Daily Geriatric Dose (mg)
Chlordiazepoxide	Librium®	20
Clonazepam	Klonopin™	1.5
Clorazepate	Tranxene®	15
Diazepam	Valium®	5
Flurazepam	Dalmane®	15
Halazepam	Paxipam®	40
Quazepam	Doral®	7.5

B. **Benzodiazepine or Other Anxiolytic / Sedative Drugs**

Anxiolytic/sedative drugs should be used for purposes other than sleep induction only when other possible causes of the resident's distress have been ruled out and the use results in maintenance or improvement in the resident's functional status. Daily use should not exceed 4 continuous months unless an attempt at gradual dose reduction has failed. Anxiolytics should only be used for generalized anxiety disorder, dementia with agitated states that either endangers the resident or others, or is a source of distress or dysfunction; panic disorder or symptomatic anxiety associated with other psychiatric disorders. The dose should not exceed those listed below unless a higher dose is needed as evidenced by the resident's response. Gradual dosage reductions should be attempted at least twice within 1 year before it can be concluded that a gradual dose reduction is "clinically contraindicated."

ANXIOLYTIC / HYPNOTIC USE IN LONG-TERM CARE FACILITIES *(Continued)*

Short-Acting Benzodiazepines

Generic	Brand	Maximum Daily Geriatric Dose (mg)
Alprazolam	Xanax®	0.75
Estazolam[1]	ProSom®	0.5
Lorazepam	Ativan®	2
Oxazepam	Serax®	30

[1]Primarily used as a hypnotic agent.

Other Anxiolytic and Sedative Drugs

Generic	Brand	Maximum Daily Geriatric Dose (mg)
Chloral hydrate	Noctec®, etc	750
Diphenhydramine	Benadryl®	50
Hydroxyzine	Atarax®, Vistaril®	50

Note: Chloral hydrate, diphenhydramine, and hydroxyzine are not necessarily drugs of choice for treatment of anxiety disorders. CMS lists them only in the event of their possible use.

C. **Drugs Used for Sleep Induction**

Drugs for sleep induction should only be used when all possible reasons for insomnia have been ruled out (ie, pain, noise, caffeine). The use of the drug must result in the maintenance or improvement of the resident's functional status. Daily use of a hypnotic should not exceed 10 consecutive days unless an attempt at a gradual dose reduction is unsuccessful. The dose should not exceed those listed below unless a higher dose has been deemed necessary. Gradual dose reductions should be attempted at least three times within 6 months before it can be concluded that a gradual dose reduction is "clinically contraindicated."

Hypnotic Drugs

Generic	Brand	Daily Geriatric Dose (mg)
Alprazolam[1]	Xanax®	0.25
Chloral hydrate	Noctec®	500
Diphenhydramine	Benadryl®	25
Estazolam	ProSom®	0.5
Hydroxyzine	Atarax®, Vistaril®	50
Lorazepam[1]	Ativan®	1
Oxazepam[1]	Serax®	15
Temazepam	Restoril®	7.5
Triazolam	Halcion®	0.125
Zaleplon	Sonata®	5
Zolpidem	Ambien®	5

[1]Not officially indicated as a hypnotic agent.

Note: Chloral hydrate, diphenhydramine, and hydroxyzine are not necessarily drugs of choice for sleep disorders. CMS lists them only in the event of their possible use.

FEDERAL OBRA REGULATIONS RECOMMENDED MAXIMUM DOSES (Continued)

Anxiolytics[1]

Drug	Brand Name	Usual Daily Dose for Age ≥65	Usual Daily Dose for Age ≤65
Alprazolam	Xanax®	2 mg	4 mg
Chlordiazepoxide	Librium®	40 mg	100 mg
Clorazepate	Tranxene®	30 mg	60 mg
Diazepam	Valium®	20 mg	60 mg
Halazepam	Paxipam®	80 mg	160 mg
Lorazepam	Ativan®	3 mg	6 mg
Meprobamate	Miltown®	600 mg	1600 mg
Oxazepam	Serax®	60 mg	90 mg

[1]**Note:** CMS-OBRA (formerly HCFA-OBRA) guidelines strongly urge clinicians not to use barbiturates, glutethimide, and ethchlorvynol due to their side effects, pharmacokinetics, and addiction potential in the elderly. Also, CMS (formerly HCFA) discourages use of long-acting benzodiazepines in the elderly.

Hypnotics[1]
(Should not be used for more than 10 continuous days)

Drug	Brand Name	Usual Max Single Dose for Age ≥65	Usual Max Single Dose
Alprazolam	Xanax®	0.25 mg	1.5 mg
Amobarbital	Amytal®	105 mg	300 mg
Butabarbital	Butisol®	100 mg	200 mg
Chloral hydrate	Noctec®	750 mg	1500 mg
Chloral hydrate	Various	500 mg	1000 mg
Diphenhydramine	Benadryl®	25 mg	50 mg
Ethchlorvynol	Placidyl®	500 mg	1000 mg
Flurazepam	Dalmane®	15 mg	30 mg
Glutethimide	Doriden®	500 mg	1000 mg
Halazepam	Paxipam®	20 mg	40 mg
Hydroxyzine	Atarax®	50 mg	100 mg
Lorazepam	Ativan®	1 mg	2 mg
Oxazepam	Serax®	15 mg	30 mg
Pentobarbital	Nembutal®	100 mg	200 mg
Secobarbital	Seconal®	100 mg	200 mg
Temazepam	Restoril®	15 mg	30 mg
Triazolam	Halcion®	0.125 mg	0.5 mg

[1]**Note:** CMS-OBRA (formerly known as HCFA-OBRA) guidelines strongly urge clinicians not to use barbiturates, glutethimide, and ethchlorvynol due to their side effects, pharmacokinetics, and addiction potential in the elderly. Also, CMS (formerly known as HCFA) discourages use of long-acting benzodiazepines in the elderly and also discourages the use of diphenhydramine and hydroxyzine.

D. **Miscellaneous Hypnotic / Sedative / Anxiolytic Drugs**

The initiation of the following medications should not occur in any dose in any resident. Residents currently using these drugs or residents admitted to the facility while using these drugs should receive gradual dose reductions. Newly admitted residents should have a period of adjustment before attempting reduction. Dose reductions should be attempted at least twice within 1 year before it can be concluded that it is "clinically contraindicated."

Examples of Barbiturates

Generic	Brand
Amobarbital	Amytal®
Amobarbital/secobarbital	Tuinal®
Butabarbital	Butisol Sodium®
Combinations	Fiorinal®, etc
Pentobarbital	Nembutal®
Secobarbital	Seconal®

Miscellaneous Hypnotic / Sedative / Anxiolytic Agents

Generic	Brand
Ethchlorvynol	Placidyl®
Glutethimide	Doriden®
Meprobamate	Equanil®, Miltown®
Methyprylon	Noludar®

CMS[1] GUIDELINES FOR UNNECESSARY DRUGS IN LONG-TERM CARE FACILITIES

Procedures: Section 483.25(1)(1)

Omnibus Budget Reconciliation Act of 1987. PL100-203, December 22, 1987.

Consider drug therapy "unnecessary" only after determining that the facility's use of the drug is:

- in excessive dose (including duplicate drug therapy)
- for excessive duration
- without adequate monitoring
- without adequate indications of use
- in the presence of adverse consequences which indicate the dose should be reduced or discontinued, or
- any combination of the reasons above

Allow the facility the opportunity to provide a rationale for the use of drugs prescribed outside the preceding guidelines. The facility may not justify the use of a drug prescribed outside the proceeding guidelines solely on the basis of "the doctor ordered it." This justification would render the regulation meaningless. The rationale must be based on sound risk-benefit analysis of the resident's symptoms and potential adverse effects of the drug. Examples of evidence that would support a justification of why a drug is being used outside these guidelines but in the best interests of the resident may include, but are not limited to:

- a physician's note indicating for example, that the dosage, duration, indication, and monitoring, are clinically appropriate, **and the reasons why they are clinically appropriate**; this note should demonstrate that the physician has carefully considered the risk/benefit to the resident in using drugs outside the guidelines
- a medical or psychiatric consultation or evaluation (eg, geriatric depression scale) that confirms the physician's judgment that use of a drug outside the guidelines is in the best interest of the resident
- physician, nursing, or other health professional documentation indicating that the resident is being monitored for adverse consequences or complications of the drug therapy
- documentation confirming that previous attempts at dosage reduction have been unsuccessful
- documentation (including MDS documentation) showing resident's subjective or objective improvement, or maintenance of function while taking the medication
- documentation showing that a resident's decline or deterioration is evaluated by the interdisciplinary team to determine whether a particular drug, or a particular dose, or duration of therapy, may be the cause
- documentation showing why the resident's age, weight, or other factors would require a unique drug dose or drug duration, indication, monitoring, and
- other evidence the survey team may deem appropriate

If the survey team determines that there is a deficiency in the use of antipsychotics, cite the facility under either the "unnecessary drug" regulation or the "antipsychotic drug" regulation, but not both.

Note: The unnecessary drug criterion of "adequate indications for use" does not simply mean that the **physician's order** must include a reason for using the drug (although such order-writing is encouraged). It means that the **resident** lacks a valid clinical reason for use of the drug, as evidenced by the survey team's evaluation of some, but not necessarily all, of the following:

- observation, assessment, and interview of the resident
- plan of care
- progress notes/reports of significant change
- laboratory reports
- professional consults
- drug orders

[1]The Health Care Financing Administration (HCFA) has been renamed **Centers for Medicare and Medicaid Services (CMS).**

FEDERAL OBRA REGULATION RECOMMENDED MAXIMUM DOS

Antidepressants

Drug	Brand Name	Usual Max Daily Dose for Age ≥65	Usual D
Amitriptyline	Elavil®	150 mg	300
Amoxapine	Asendin®	200 mg	400
Desipramine	Norpramin®	150 mg	300 r
Doxepin	Adapin®, Sinequan®	150 mg	300 m
Imipramine	Tofranil®	150 mg	300 m
Maprotiline	Ludiomil®	150 mg	300 m
Nortriptyline	Aventyl®, Pamelor®	75 mg	150 mg
Protriptyline	Vivactil®	30 mg	60 mg
Trazodone	Desyrel®	300 mg	600 mg
Trimipramine	Surmontil®	150 mg	300 mg

Antipsychotics

Drug	Brand Name	Usual Max Daily Dose for Age ≥65	Usual Max Daily Dose	Daily Oral Dose for Residents With Organic Mental Syndromes
Chlorpromazine	Thorazine®	800 mg	1600 mg	75 mg
Chlorprothixene	Taractan®	800 mg	1600 mg	75 mg
Clozapine	Clozaril®	25 mg	450 mg	50 mg
Fluphenazine	Prolixin®	20 mg	40 mg	4 mg
Haloperidol	Haldol®	50 mg	100 mg	4 mg
Loxapine	Loxitane®	125 mg	250 mg	10 mg
Mesoridazine	Serentil®	250 mg	500 mg	25 mg
Molindone	Moban®	112 mg	225 mg	10 mg
Perphenazine	Trilafon®	32 mg	64 mg	8 mg
Promazine	Sparine®	50 mg	500 mg	150 mg
Risperidone	Risperdal®	1 mg	16 mg	2 mg
Thioridazine	Mellaril®	400 mg	800 mg	75 mg
Thiothixene	Navane®	30 mg	60 mg	7 mg
Trifluoperazine	Stelazine®	40 mg	80 mg	8 mg
Trifluopromazine	Vesprin®	100 mg	20 mg	–
Quetiapine	Seroquel®		800 mg	200 mg

OVERDOSE AND TOXICOLOGY

GENERAL STABILIZATION OF THE PATIENT

The recommended treatment plan for the poisoned patient is not unlike general treatment plans taught in advanced cardiac life support (ACLS) or advanced trauma life support (ATLS) courses. In this manner, the initial approach to the poisoned patient should be essentially similar in every case, irrespective of the toxin ingested, just as the initial approach to the trauma patient is the same, irrespective of the mechanism of injury. This approach, which can be termed as routine poison management, essentially includes the following aspects.

- Stabilization: ABCs (airway, breathing, circulation; administration of glucose, thiamine, oxygen, and naloxone)

- History, physical examination leading toward the identification of class of toxin (toxidrome recognition)

- Prevention of absorption (decontamination)

- Specific antidote, if available

- Removal of absorbed toxin (enhancing excretion)

- Support and monitoring for adverse effects

Drug	Effect	Comment
25-50 g **dextrose** ($D_{50}W$) intravenously to reverse the effects of drug-induced hypoglycemia (adult); 1 mL/kg $D_{50}W$ diluted 1:1 (child)	This can be especially effective in patients with limited glycogen stores (ie, neonates and patients with cirrhosis)	Extravasation into the extremity of this hyperosmolar solution can cause Volkmann's contractures
50-100 mg intravenous **thiamine**	Prevent Wernicke's encephalopathy	A water-soluble vitamin with low toxicity; rare anaphylactoid reactions have been reported
Initial dosage of **naloxone** should be 2 mg in adult patients preferably by the intravenous route, although intramuscular, subcutaneous, intralingual, and endotracheal routes may also be utilized. Pediatric dose is 0.1 mg/kg from birth until 5 years of age.	Specific opioid antagonist without any agent properties	It should be noted that some semisynthetic opiates (such as meperidine or propoxyphene) may require higher initial doses for reversal, so that a total dose of 6-10 mg is not unusual for the adults. If the patient responds to a bolus dose and then relapses to a lethargic or comatose state, a naloxone drip can be considered. This can be accomplished by administering two-thirds of the bolus dose that revives the patient per hour or injecting 4 mg naloxone in 1 L crystalloid solution and administering at a rate of 100 mL/hour 0.4 mg/hour)
Oxygen, utilized in 100% concentration	Useful for carbon monoxide, hydrogen, sulfide, and asphyxiants	While oxygen is antidotal for carbon monoxide intoxication, the only relative toxic contraindication is in paraquat intoxication (in that it can promote pulmonary fibrosis)
Flumazenil	Benzodiazepine antagonist	Not routinely recommended due to increased risk of seizures

OVERDOSE AND TOXICOLOGY *(Continued)*

LABORATORY EVALUATION OF OVERDOSE

Unknown ingestion: Electrolytes, anion gap, serum osmolality, arterial blood gases, serum drug concentration

Known ingestion: Labs tailored to agent

ANION GAP

Definition: The difference in concentration between unmeasured cation and anion equivalents in serum

Anion gap = $Na^+ - Cl^- + HCO_3^-$
        (The normal anion gap is 10-14 mEq/L)

DIFFERENTIAL DIAGNOSIS

Increased Anion Gap Acidosis

Organic anions:
    Lactate (sepsis, hypovolemia, seizures, large tumor burden)
    Pyruvate
    Uremia
    Ketoacidosis (β-hydroxybutyrate and acetoacetate)
    Amino acids and their metabolites
    Other organic acids

Inorganic anions:
    Hyperphosphatemia
    Sulfates
    Nitrates

Decreased Anion Gap

Organic cations:
    Hypergammaglobulinemia

Inorganic cations:
    Hyperkalemia
    Hypercalcemia
    Hypermagnesemia

Medications and toxins:
    Lithium

Hypoalbuminemia

TOXINS AFFECTING THE ANION GAP

Drugs Causing Increased Anion Gap (>12 mEq/L)

Nonacidotic
    Carbenicillin   Sodium salts

Metabolic Acidosis

Acetaminophen	Fluoroacetate
(ingestion >75-100 g)	Formaldehyde
Acetazolamide	Fructose (I.V.)
Amiloride	Glycol ethers
Ascorbic acid	Hydrogen sulfide
Benzalkonium chloride	Ibuprofen (ingestion >300 mg/kg)
Benzyl alcohol	Inorganic acid
Beta-adrenergic drugs	Iodine
Bialaphos	Iron
2-Butanone	Isoniazid
Carbon monoxide	Ketamine
Centrimonium bromide	Ketoprofen
Chloramphenicol	Metaldehyde
Colchicine	Metformin
Cyanide	Methanol
Dapsone	Methenamine mandelate
Dimethyl sulfate	Monochloracetic acid
Dinitrophenol	Nalidixic acid
Endosulfan	Naproxen
Epinephrine (I.V. overdose)	Niacin
Ethanol	Papaverine
Ethylene dibromide	Pennyroyal oil
Ethylene glycol	Pentachlorophenol
Fenoprofen	Phenelzine

Phenformin (off the market)
Phenol
Phenylbutazone
Phosphoric acid
Potassium chloroplatinite
Propylene glycol
Salicylates
Sorbitol (I.V.)
Strychnine

Surfactant herbicide
Tetracycline (outdated)
Theophylline
Tienilic acid
Toluene
Tranylcypromine
Vacor
Verapamil

Drugs Causing Decreased Anion Gap (<6 mEq/L)

Acidosis

Ammonium chloride
Bromide
Iodide

Lithium
Polymyxin B
Tromethamine

OSMOLALITY

Definition: The summed concentrations of all osmotically active solute particles

Predicted serum osmolality =

2 Na^+ + glucose (mg/dL) / 18 + BUN (mg/dL) / 2.8

The normal range of serum osmolality is 285-295 mOsm/L.

Differential diagnosis of increased serum osmolal gap (>10 mOsm/L)

Medications and toxins
Alcohols (ethanol, methanol, isopropanol, glycerol, ethylene glycol)
Mannitol

Calculated Osm

Osmolal gap = measured Osm – calculated Osm

0 to +10: Normal
>10: Abnormal
<0: Probable lab or calculation error

Drugs Causing Increased Osmolar Gap
(by freezing-point depression, gap is >10 mOsm)

Ethanol[1]
Ethylene glycol[1]
Glycerol
Hypermagnesemia (>9.5 mEq/L)
Isopropanol[1] (acetone)
Iodine (questionable)

Mannitol
Methanol[1]
Propylene glycol
Severe alcoholic ketoacidosis or
    lactic acidosis
Sorbitol[1]

[1]Toxins increasing both anion and osmolar gap.

Toxins Associated With Oxygen Saturation Gap
(>5% difference between measured and calculated value)

Carbon monoxide
Cyanide (questionable)

Hydrogen sulfide (possible)
Methemoglobin

OVERDOSE AND TOXICOLOGY *(Continued)*

Toxins Eliminated by Multiple Dosing of Activated Charcoal

Acetaminophen	Meprobamate
Amitriptyline	Methotrexate
Atrazine (?)	Methyprylon
Baclofen (?)	Nadolol
Bupropion (?)	Nortriptyline
Carbamazepine	Phencyclidine (?)
Chlordecone	Phenobarbital
Cyclosporine	Phenylbutazone
Dapsone	Phenytoin (?)
Dextropropoxyphene	Piroxicam
Diazepam (desmethyldiazepam)	Propoxyphene
Digitoxin	Propranolol (?)
Digoxin (with renal impairment)	Salicylates (?)
Disopyramide	Theophylline
Glutethimide	Valproic acid
Maprotiline	Vancomycin (?)

The following agents have been studied and have not been demonstrated to result in enhanced elimination:

Amiodarone	Imipramine
Chlorpropamide	Tobramycin

Toxins Eliminated by Forced Saline Diuresis

Barium	Isoniazid (?)
Bromides	Meprobamate
Chromium	Methyl iodide
Cimetidine (?)	Mushrooms (Group I)
Cis-platinum	Nickel
Cyclophosphamide	Potassium chloroplatinite
Hydrazine	Thallium
Iodide	Valproic acid (?)
Iodine	

Toxins Eliminated by Alkaline Diuresis

2,4-D-chlorophenoxyacetic acid	Orellanine (?)
Barbital (serum levels >10 mg/dL)	Phenobarbital
Chlorpropamide	Primidone
Fluoride	Quinolones antibiotic
Iopanoic Acid (?)	Salicylates
Isoniazid (?)	Sulfisoxazole
Mephobarbital	Uranium
Methotrexate	
2-Methyl-4-chlorophenoxyacetic acid (MCPA)	

A urine flow of 3-5 mL/kg/hour should be achieved with a combination of isotonic fluids or diuretics. Alkalinization can be achieved by administration of 44-88 mEq of sodium bicarbonate per liter to titrate a urine pH of 7.5; 20-40 mEq/L of potassium chloride may also be required (potassium should not be administered in patients with renal insufficiency). It should be noted that the efficacy of forced diuresis has only been studied for salicylates and phenobarbital. Although several drugs can exhibit enhanced elimination through an acidic urine (tranylcypromine, quinine, chlorpheniramine, fenfluramine, strychnine, cathinone or khat, amphetamines, phencyclidine, nicotine, bismuth, diethylcarbamazine citrate, ephedrine, flecainide, local anesthetics), the practice of acidifying the urine should be discouraged in that it can produce metabolic acidosis and promote renal failure in the presence of rhabdomyolysis.

D. **Miscellaneous Hypnotic / Sedative / Anxiolytic Drugs**

The initiation of the following medications should not occur in any dose in any resident. Residents currently using these drugs or residents admitted to the facility while using these drugs should receive gradual dose reductions. Newly admitted residents should have a period of adjustment before attempting reduction. Dose reductions should be attempted at least twice within 1 year before it can be concluded that it is "clinically contraindicated."

Examples of Barbiturates

Generic	Brand
Amobarbital	Amytal®
Amobarbital/secobarbital	Tuinal®
Butabarbital	Butisol Sodium®
Combinations	Fiorinal®, etc
Pentobarbital	Nembutal®
Secobarbital	Seconal®

Miscellaneous Hypnotic / Sedative / Anxiolytic Agents

Generic	Brand
Ethchlorvynol	Placidyl®
Glutethimide	Doriden®
Meprobamate	Equanil®, Miltown®
Methyprylon	Noludar®

CMS[1] GUIDELINES FOR UNNECESSARY DRUGS IN LONG-TERM CARE FACILITIES

Procedures: Section 483.25(1)(1)

Omnibus Budget Reconciliation Act of 1987. PL100-203, December 22, 1987.

Consider drug therapy "unnecessary" only after determining that the facility's use of the drug is:

- in excessive dose (including duplicate drug therapy)
- for excessive duration
- without adequate monitoring
- without adequate indications of use
- in the presence of adverse consequences which indicate the dose should be reduced or discontinued, or
- any combination of the reasons above

Allow the facility the opportunity to provide a rationale for the use of drugs prescribed outside the preceding guidelines. The facility may not justify the use of a drug prescribed outside the proceeding guidelines solely on the basis of "the doctor ordered it." This justification would render the regulation meaningless. The rationale must be based on sound risk-benefit analysis of the resident's symptoms and potential adverse effects of the drug. Examples of evidence that would support a justification of why a drug is being used outside these guidelines but in the best interests of the resident may include, but are not limited to:

- a physician's note indicating for example, that the dosage, duration, indication, and monitoring are clinically appropriate, **and the reasons why they are clinically appropriate**; this note should demonstrate that the physician has carefully considered the risk/benefit to the resident in using drugs outside the guidelines

- a medical or psychiatric consultation or evaluation (eg, geriatric depression scale) that confirms the physician's judgment that use of a drug outside the guidelines is in the best interest of the resident

- physician, nursing, or other health professional documentation indicating that the resident is being monitored for adverse consequences or complications of the drug therapy

- documentation confirming that previous attempts at dosage reduction have been unsuccessful

- documentation (including MDS documentation) showing resident's subjective or objective improvement, or maintenance of function while taking the medication

- documentation showing that a resident's decline or deterioration is evaluated by the interdisciplinary team to determine whether a particular drug, or a particular dose, or duration of therapy, may be the cause

- documentation showing why the resident's age, weight, or other factors would require a unique drug dose or drug duration, indication, monitoring, and

- other evidence the survey team may deem appropriate

If the survey team determines that there is a deficiency in the use of antipsychotics, cite the facility under either the "unnecessary drug" regulation or the "antipsychotic drug" regulation, but not both.

Note: The unnecessary drug criterion of "adequate indications for use" does not simply mean that the **physician's order** must include a reason for using the drug (although such order-writing is encouraged). It means that the **resident** lacks a valid clinical reason for use of the drug, as evidenced by the survey team's evaluation of some, but not necessarily all, of the following:

- observation, assessment, and interview of the resident
- plan of care
- progress notes/reports of significant change
- laboratory reports
- professional consults
- drug orders

[1]The Health Care Financing Administration (HCFA) has been renamed **Centers for Medicare and Medicaid Services (CMS)**.

FEDERAL OBRA REGULATIONS RECOMMENDED MAXIMUM DOSES

Antidepressants

Drug	Brand Name	Usual Max Daily Dose for Age ≥65	Usual Max Daily Dose
Amitriptyline	Elavil®	150 mg	300 mg
Amoxapine	Asendin®	200 mg	400 mg
Desipramine	Norpramin®	150 mg	300 mg
Doxepin	Adapin®, Sinequan®	150 mg	300 mg
Imipramine	Tofranil®	150 mg	300 mg
Maprotiline	Ludiomil®	150 mg	300 mg
Nortriptyline	Aventyl®, Pamelor®	75 mg	150 mg
Protriptyline	Vivactil®	30 mg	60 mg
Trazodone	Desyrel®	300 mg	600 mg
Trimipramine	Surmontil®	150 mg	300 mg

Antipsychotics

Drug	Brand Name	Usual Max Daily Dose for Age ≥65	Usual Max Daily Dose	Daily Oral Dose for Residents With Organic Mental Syndromes
Chlorpromazine	Thorazine®	800 mg	1600 mg	75 mg
Chlorprothixene	Taractan®	800 mg	1600 mg	75 mg
Clozapine	Clozaril®	25 mg	450 mg	50 mg
Fluphenazine	Prolixin®	20 mg	40 mg	4 mg
Haloperidol	Haldol®	50 mg	100 mg	4 mg
Loxapine	Loxitane®	125 mg	250 mg	10 mg
Mesoridazine	Serentil®	250 mg	500 mg	25 mg
Molindone	Moban®	112 mg	225 mg	10 mg
Perphenazine	Trilafon®	32 mg	64 mg	8 mg
Promazine	Sparine®	50 mg	500 mg	150 mg
Risperidone	Risperdal®	1 mg	16 mg	2 mg
Thioridazine	Mellaril®	400 mg	800 mg	75 mg
Thiothixene	Navane®	30 mg	60 mg	7 mg
Trifluoperazine	Stelazine®	40 mg	80 mg	8 mg
Trifluopromazine	Vesprin®	100 mg	20 mg	–
Quetiapine	Seroquel®		800 mg	200 mg

FEDERAL OBRA REGULATIONS RECOMMENDED MAXIMUM DOSES *(Continued)*

Anxiolytics[1]

Drug	Brand Name	Usual Daily Dose for Age ≥65	Usual Daily Dose for Age ≤65
Alprazolam	Xanax®	2 mg	4 mg
Chlordiazepoxide	Librium®	40 mg	100 mg
Clorazepate	Tranxene®	30 mg	60 mg
Diazepam	Valium®	20 mg	60 mg
Halazepam	Paxipam®	80 mg	160 mg
Lorazepam	Ativan®	3 mg	6 mg
Meprobamate	Miltown®	600 mg	1600 mg
Oxazepam	Serax®	60 mg	90 mg

[1]**Note:** CMS-OBRA (formerly HCFA-OBRA) guidelines strongly urge clinicians not to use barbiturates, glutethimide, and ethchlorvynol due to their side effects, pharmacokinetics, and addiction potential in the elderly. Also, CMS (formerly HCFA) discourages use of long-acting benzodiazepines in the elderly.

Hypnotics[1]
(Should not be used for more than 10 continuous days)

Drug	Brand Name	Usual Max Single Dose for Age ≥65	Usual Max Single Dose
Alprazolam	Xanax®	0.25 mg	1.5 mg
Amobarbital	Amytal®	105 mg	300 mg
Butabarbital	Butisol®	100 mg	200 mg
Chloral hydrate	Noctec®	750 mg	1500 mg
Chloral hydrate	Various	500 mg	1000 mg
Diphenhydramine	Benadryl®	25 mg	50 mg
Ethchlorvynol	Placidyl®	500 mg	1000 mg
Flurazepam	Dalmane®	15 mg	30 mg
Glutethimide	Doriden®	500 mg	1000 mg
Halazepam	Paxipam®	20 mg	40 mg
Hydroxyzine	Atarax®	50 mg	100 mg
Lorazepam	Ativan®	1 mg	2 mg
Oxazepam	Serax®	15 mg	30 mg
Pentobarbital	Nembutal®	100 mg	200 mg
Secobarbital	Seconal®	100 mg	200 mg
Temazepam	Restoril®	15 mg	30 mg
Triazolam	Halcion®	0.125 mg	0.5 mg

[1]**Note:** CMS-OBRA (formerly known as HCFA-OBRA) guidelines strongly urge clinicians not to use barbiturates, glutethimide, and ethchlorvynol due to their side effects, pharmacokinetics, and addiction potential in the elderly. Also, CMS (formerly known as HCFA) discourages use of long-acting benzodiazepines in the elderly and also discourages the use of diphenhydramine and hydroxyzine.

Drugs and Toxins Removed by Hemoperfusion (Charcoal)

Amanita phalloides (?)

Atenolol (?)

Bromisoval

Bromoethylbutyramide

Caffeine

Carbamazepine

Carbon tetrachloride (?)

Carbromal

Chloral hydrate (trichloroethanol)

Chloramphenicol

Chlorfenvinfos (?)

Chlorpropamide

Clonidine

Colchicine (?)

Creosote (?)

Dapsone

Demeton-S-methyl sulfoxide

Diltiazem (?)

Dimethoate

Disopyramide

Ethylene oxide

Glutethimide

Levothyroxine (?)

Lindane

Liotrix

Meprobamate

Methaqualone

Methotrexate

Methsuximide

Methyprylon (?)

Metoprolol (?)

Nadolol (?)

Orellanine (?)

Oxalic acid (?)

Paraquat

Parathion (?)

Pentamidine

Phenelzine (?)

Phenobarbital

Phenol

Phenytoin

Podophyllin (?)

Procainamide (?)

Quinidine (?)

Rifabutin (?)

Sotalol (?)

Thallium

Thyroglobulin/thyroid hormone

Theophylline

Valproic acid

Verapamil (?)

Continuous arteriovenous hemofiltration has been used to treat lithium, paraquat, N-acetyl-procainamide, and vancomycin ingestions with varying results. It is capable of filtering molecules with a molecular weight up to 50,000 but some substances such as thallium and formaldehyde cannot be removed by this method despite their low molecular weight.

Exchange transfusion is a useful modality to enhance drug elimination in neonatal or infant drug toxicity. Usually double or triple volume exchanges are performed. It has been utilized to treat barbiturate, acetaminophen, iron, caffeine, methyl salicylate, propafenone, ganciclovir, sodium nitrite, lead, phenazopyridine hydrochloride, pine oil, theophylline overdose, and nitrate exposure in pediatric patients. Exchange transfusions (500-2000 mL) volume replacement have also been used to treat adults with 80-150 g ingestions of parathion.

OVERDOSE AND TOXICOLOGY *(Continued)*

TREATMENTS[1]

Drug or Drug Class	Signs / Symptoms	Treatment / Comments
Acetaminophen	Nausea, vomiting, diaphoresis, delirium, fever, coma, vascular collapse, hepatic necrosis, transient azotemia, renal tubular necrosis	Assess severity of ingestion; adult doses ≥140 mg/kg are thought to be toxic. Obtain serum concentration ≥4 hours postingestion and use acetaminophen nomogram to evaluate need for acetylcysteine. Gastric decontamination within 2-4 hours after ingestion. May administer activated charcoal for one dose; this may decrease absorption of acetylcysteine if given within 1 hour of acetylcysteine. For unknown ingested quantities and for significant ingestion, give acetylcysteine orally (diluted 1:4 with juice or carbonated beverage); initial: 140 mg/kg then give 70 mg/kg every 4 hours for 17 doses. I.V. protocols are used in some institutions.
Alpha-adrenergic blocking agents	Hypotension, drowsiness	Give activated charcoal, additional treatment if symptomatic; use I.V. fluids, dopamine, or norepinephrine to treat hypotension. Epinephrine may worsen hypotension due to beta effects.
Aminoglycosides	Ototoxicity, nephrotoxicity, neuromuscular toxicity	Hemodialysis or peritoneal dialysis may be useful in patients with decreased renal function; calcium may reverse the neuromuscular toxicity.
Anticholinergics, antihistamines	Coma, hallucinations, delirium, tachycardia, dry skin, urinary retention, dilated pupils	For life-threatening arrhythmias or seizures. Adults: 2 mg/dose physostigmine, may repeat 1-2 mg in 20 minutes and give 1-4 mg slow I.V. over 5-10 minutes if signs and symptoms recur (relatively contraindicated if QRS >0.1 msec).
Barbiturates	Respiratory depression, circulatory collapse, bradycardia, hypotension, hypothermia, slurred speech, confusion, coma	Repeated oral doses of activated charcoal given every 3-6 hours will increase clearance. Adults: 30-60 g. Assure GI motility, adequate hydration, and renal function. Urinary alkalinization with I.V. sodium bicarbonate will increase renal elimination of longer-acting barbiturates (eg, phenobarbital). Charcoal hemoperfusion may be required in severe overdose.

TREATMENTS[1] *(continued)*

Drug or Drug Class	Signs / Symptoms	Treatment / Comments
Benzodiazepines	Respiratory depression, apnea (after rapid I.V.), hypoactive reflexes, hypotension, slurred speech, unsteady gait, coma	Dialysis is of limited value; support blood pressure and respiration until symptoms subside. Flumazenil: Initial dose: 0.2 mg given I.V. over 30 seconds. If further response is desired after 30 seconds, give 0.3 mg over another 30 seconds. Further doses of 0.5 mg can be given over 30 seconds at 1-minute intervals up to a total of 3 mg. Continuous infusions may be used in rare instances since duration of benzodiazepines is longer than flumazenil.
Beta-adrenergic blockers	Hypotension, bronchospasm, bradycardia, hypoglycemia, seizures	Activated charcoal; treat symptomatically; glucagon, atropine, isoproterenol, dobutamine, or cardiac pacing may be needed to treat bradycardia, conduction defects, or hypotension.
Carbamazepine	Dizziness, drowsiness, ataxia, involuntary movements, opisthotonos, seizures, nausea, vomiting, agitation, nystagmus, coma, urinary retention, respiratory depression, tachycardia, arrhythmias	Use supportive therapy, general poisoning management as needed. Use repeated oral doses of activated charcoal given every 3-6 hours to decrease serum concentrations. Charcoal hemoperfusion may be needed. Treat hypotension with I.V. fluids, dopamine, or norepinephrine. Monitor EKG. Diazepam may control convulsions but may exacerbate respiratory depression.
Cardiac glycosides	Hyperkalemia may develop rapidly and result in life-threatening cardiac arrhythmias, progressive bradyarrhythmias, second or third degree heart block unresponsive to atropine, ventricular fibrillation, asystole	Obtain serum drug level, induce emesis, or perform gastric lavage. Give activated charcoal to reduce further absorption. Atropine may reverse heart block. Digoxin immune Fab (digoxin-specific antibody fragments) is used in serious cases. Each 40 mg of digoxin immune Fab binds with 0.6 mg of digoxin.
Cholinergic	Nausea, vomiting, diarrhea, miosis, CNS depression, excessive salivation, excessive sweating, muscle weakness	Suction oral secretions, decontaminate skin, atropinize patient. Atropine dose must be individualized. Adults: Initial atropine dose: 1 mg; titrate dose upward. Pralidoxime (2-PAM) may need to be added for moderate to severe intoxications.
Cyanide	Myocardial depression, lactic acidosis, hypotension, respiratory depression, shock, and cyanosis despite high oxygen saturation	Cyanide antidote kit: 1) Inhale vapor from 0.3 mL amyl nitrate ampul until I.V. sodium nitrite available; 2) sodium nitrite 300 mg I.V. then 3) sodium thiosulfate 12.5 g I.V. over 10 minutes
Heparin	Severe hemorrhage	1 mg of protamine sulfate will neutralize approximately 90 units of heparin sodium (bovine) or 115 units of heparin sodium (porcine) or 100 units of heparin calcium (porcine).

OVERDOSE AND TOXICOLOGY *(Continued)*

TREATMENTS[1] *(continued)*

Drug or Drug Class	Signs / Symptoms	Treatment / Comments
Hydantoin derivatives	Nausea, vomiting, nystagmus, slurred speech, ataxia, coma	Gastric lavage or emesis; repeated oral doses of activated charcoal may increase clearance of phenytoin. Use 0.5-1 g/kg (30-60 g/dose) activated charcoal every 3-6 hours until nontoxic serum concentration is obtained. Assure adequate GI motility, supportive therapy.
Iron	Lethargy, nausea, vomiting, green or tarry stools, hypotension, weak rapid pulse, metabolic acidosis, shock, coma, hepatic necrosis, renal failure, local GI erosions	If immediately after ingestion and not already vomiting, give ipecac or lavage with saline solution. Give deferoxamine mesylate I.V. at 15 mg/kg/hour in cases of severe poisoning (serum iron >350 µg/mL) until the urine color is normal, the patient is asymptomatic, or a maximum daily dose of 8 g is reached. Urine output should be maintained >2 mL/kg/hour to avoid hypovolemic shock.
Isoniazid	Nausea, vomiting, blurred vision, CNS depression, intractable seizures, coma, metabolic acidosis	Control seizures with diazepam. Give pyridoxine I.V. equal dose to the suspected overdose of isoniazid or up to 5 g empirically. Give activated charcoal.
Nonsteroidal anti-inflammatory drugs	Dizziness, abdominal pain, sweating, apnea, nystagmus, cyanosis, hypotension, coma, seizures (rarely)	Induce emesis. Give activated charcoal via NG tube. Fluid therapy is commonly effective in managing the hypotension that may occur following an acute NSAIDs overdose, except when this is due to an acute blood loss. Seizures tend to be very short-lived and often do not require drug treatment, although, recurrent seizures should be treated with I.V. diazepam. Since many of the NSAIDs undergo enterohepatic cycling, multiple doses of charcoal may be needed to reduce the potential for delayed toxicities. Provide symptomatic and supportive care.
Opioids and morphine analogs	Respiratory depression, miosis, hypothermia, bradycardia, circulatory collapse, pulmonary edema, apnea	Establish airway and adequate ventilation. Give naloxone 0.4 mg and titrate to a maximum of 10 mg. Additional doses may be needed every 20-60 minutes. May need to institute continuous infusion, as duration of action of opiates can be longer than duration of action of naloxone.
Organophosphates (insecticides, pyridostigmine, neostigmine)	Bronchospasm, diarrhea, diaphoresis, ventricular dysrhythmia, fasiculations, flacid paralysis, lethargy, coma	Atropine 2-5 mg every 15 minutes until symptoms abate (0.05 mg/kg children). If severe, may add pralidoxime 1-2 g over 15-30 minutes (20-50 mg/kg children); may repeat every 8-12 hours or continuous infusion 0.5 g/hour (10-20 mg/kg/hour children).

TREATMENTS[1] *(continued)*

Drug or Drug Class	Signs / Symptoms	Treatment / Comments
Phenothiazines	Deep, unarousable sleep, anticholinergic symptoms, extrapyramidal signs, diaphoresis, rigidity, tachycardia, cardiac dysrhythmias, hypotension	Activated charcoal; do **not** dialyze. Use I.V. benztropine mesylate 1-2 mg/dose slowly over 3-6 minutes for extrapyramidal signs. Use I.V. fluids and norepinephrine to treat hypotension. Avoid epinephrine which may cause hypotension due to phenothiazine-induced alpha-adrenergic blockade and unopposed epinephrine B_2 action. Use benzodiazepines for seizure management and to decrease rigidity.
Salicylates	Nausea, vomiting, respiratory alkalosis, hyperthermia, dehydration, hyperapnea, tinnitus, headache, dizziness, metabolic acidosis, coma, hypoglycemia, seizures	Induce emesis or gastric lavage immediately. Give several doses of activated charcoal, rehydrate, and use sodium bicarbonate to correct metabolic acidosis and enhance renal elimination by alkalinizing the urine. Control hyperthermia by cooling blankets or sponge baths. Correct coagulopathy with vitamin K I.V. and platelet transfusions as necessary. Hypoglycemia may be treated with I.V. dextrose. Seizures should be treated with I.V. benzodiazepines (diazepam 5-10 mg I.V.). Give supplemental potassium after renal function has been determined to be adequate. Monitor electrolytes; obtain stat serum salicylate level and follow.
Tricyclic antidepressants	Agitation, confusion, hallucinations, urinary retention, hypothermia, hypotension, tachycardia, arrhythmias, seizures	Give activated charcoal ± lavage. Use sodium bicarbonate for QRS >0.1 msec; alkalinization by hyperventilation has been used in patients on mechanical ventilation; I.V. fluids and norepinephrine may be used for hypotension; benzodiazepines may be used for seizure management.
Warfarin	Internal or external hemorrhage, hematuria	For moderate overdoses, give oral, SubQ, or I.D., or slow I.V. (I.V. associated with anaphylactoid reactions) phytonadione; usual dose: 2.5-10 mg, adjust per prothrombin time. For severe hemorrhage, give fresh frozen plasma or whole blood. See Warfarin monograph.
Xanthine derivatives	Vomiting, abdominal pain, bloody diarrhea, tachycardia, extrasystoles, tachypnea, tonic/clonic seizures	Give activated charcoal orally. Repeated oral doses of activated charcoal increase clearance. Use 0.5-1 g/kg (30-60 g/dose) of activated charcoal every 1-4 hours (depending on the severity of ingestion) until nontoxic serum concentrations are obtained. Assure adequate GI motility, supportive therapy. Charcoal hemoperfusion or hemodialysis can also be effective in decreasing serum concentrations and should be used if the serum concentration approaches 90-100 mcg/mL in acute overdoses.

[1]Consult more specific toxicology references (eg, Leikin JB and Paloucek FP, *Poisoning & Toxicology Handbook*, Hudson, OH: Lexi-Comp Inc, 1998, and Poisondex®) for further information.

ANTICOAGULANT THERAPY GUIDELINES

ATRIAL FIBRILLATION (AF)

The goal of anticoagulation in patients with AF is to prevent stroke and thromboembolic events and to promote thrombus dissolution, if present, prior to elective cardioversion. Anticoagulation in patients with atrial fibrillation is required prior to cardioversion, if the patient has been in AF for more than 48 hours, or if a thrombus is observed by echocardiography. Patients with a longer or unknown duration of AF may undergo transesophageal echocardiography (TEE) to aid in the assessment for anticoagulation therapy. Anticoagulation therapy is maintained for 3-4 weeks prior to cardioversion and continued for 4 weeks after successful cardioversion. It is important that anticoagulation be maintained after cardioversion because even though the atrium is electrically in sinus rhythm, the mechanical force is diminished and the likelihood of clotting is still high. Obviously, if there are other indications for anticoagulation, it should be continued. In the absence of contraindications, daily aspirin should be started after warfarin therapy is completed.

The need for chronic antithrombotic therapy in AF depends on patient risk factors: If the patient has had a previous transient ischemic attack, stroke, systemic embolus; or has hypertension (treated or untreated), poor ventricular function, rheumatic mitral valve disease, or a prosthetic heart valve. Patients with diabetes, coronary artery disease, or thyrotoxicosis are at a high risk for stroke. The risk of stroke in AF is approximately 6 times that of patients without AF and increases with age (>60 years). These risk factors should be considered when deciding on the intensity of oral anticoagulation or when prescribing chronic antithrombotic therapy (see table). Patients with chronic or paroxysmal AF should be on chronic antithrombotic therapy. Warfarin (INR 2.0-3.0) and aspirin (325 mg/day) are considered first-line therapies for the prophylaxis of thromboembolic events in AF.

Recommendations for Atrial Fibrillation

Risk Factors[1]	Age	Recommended Therapy
None	<65 y	Aspirin
	65-75 y	Aspirin or warfarin
≥1	<65 to 75 y	Warfarin
None or ≥1	>75 y	

[1]Risk factors: Prior TIA or stroke, systemic embolus, hypertension (treated or untreated), poor left ventricular function, rheumatic mitral valve disease, or prosthetic heart valve.

HEPARIN THERAPY

Heparin therapy may be initially started to anticoagulate patients with AF. Therapy may be switched to warfarin therapy on the first day if a therapeutic aPTT can be achieved. The aPTT should be evaluated at baseline and every 6 hours following the start of heparin therapy or if dosage adjustments are made. The optimal dose of heparin is achieved when aPTT is maintained between 1.5-2.5 times the patient's baseline aPPT. Please refer to Heparin *on page 739* for dosing information.

WARFARIN THERAPY

The target INR range for warfarin therapy in AF is 2.0-3.0. Patients with mechanical heart valves may require a higher range (see below). In general, patients should not receive loading doses of warfarin (ie, 10 mg/day for 3 days, then 5 mg/day), as the steady-state INR is not achieved more quickly. The intensity of anticoagulation therapy should be monitored closely until the patient has reached a stable PT/INR. Once the patient is stabilized on a fixed dose of warfarin, the PT/INR can be monitored on a monthly basis if the patient demonstrates a stable PT/INR on chronic therapy. If dosage adjustments are made, PT/INR should be evaluated in approximately 2 weeks. Supratherapeutic INR values are managed based on the presence and severity of bleeding (see following table). Patients on warfarin should be warned to seek medical evaluation if they develop a very severe headache, abdominal pain, unusual bleeding, backache, or if they experience significant trauma, particularly head injuries. Please refer to Warfarin *on page 1573* for complete drug information.

Initiation of Oral Anticoagulation Therapy With Warfarin

The dosing of warfarin must be individualized according to the patient's response to the drug as indicated by the PT/INR. Use of a large loading dose may increase the incidence of hemorrhagic and other complications, does not offer more rapid protection against thrombus formation, and is not recommended. Low initiation doses (eg, 2-5 mg/day) are recommended for elderly and/or debilitated patients and those with potential for increased responsiveness to warfarin.

Step 1: Obtain baseline PT/INR.

Begin therapy with warfarin with a dose of 2-5 mg/day with dosage adjustment based on the results of PT/INR determinations. **Note:** Consider using lower dosages (<5 mg) for geriatric or malnourished patients, those with hepatic impairment, or when high risk of bleeding.

For patients on heparin: Since the anticoagulant effect of warfarin is delayed, heparin is preferred initially for rapid anticoagulation. Conversion to warfarin may begin concomitantly with heparin therapy or may be delayed 3-6 days. When warfarin has produced the desired therapeutic range, INR, or prothrombin time, heparin may be discontinued.

Step 2: Check PT/ INR daily.

Day that the PT/INR is stabilized in the therapeutic range: Adjust warfarin dose based on the results of PT/ INR determinations.

Patients stabilized in the therapeutic range: Intervals between subsequent PT/INR determinations should be based upon the physician's judgment of the patient's reliability and response to warfarin in order to maintain the individual within the therapeutic range. Acceptable intervals for PT/INR determinations are normally within the range of 1-4 weeks after a stable dosage has been determined. Most patients are satisfactorily maintained on warfarin at a dose of 2-10 mg/day.

Monitoring – The International Normalized Ratio (INR)

Because PT results are very dependent on the thromboplastin reagent used, a system of standardizing the prothrombin time in oral anticoagulant therapy was introduced by the World Health Organization (WHO) in 1983. It is based upon determination of an INR, which is equivalent to the PT ratio one would obtain if a sensitive reference thromboplastin were used for the PT.

- Thromboplastin sensitivity is determined by the manufacturer and is expressed as an International Sensitivity Index (ISI).

- The INR can be calculated as **INR = (observed PT ratio)^{ISI}.**

- The calculation of the INR from the PT ratio is usually performed by the laboratory.

Reminder:

- Be aware of potential drug interactions and other factors that may affect INR (refer to prescribing information for warfarin).

- Patient/staff education about warfarin is an important part of therapy. Effective therapeutic levels with minimal complications are in part dependent upon cooperative and well-instructed patients who communicate effectively with their physician. Various warfarin patient educational guides are available to health professionals on request.

ANTICOAGULANT THERAPY GUIDELINES *(Continued)*

Management of Supratherapeutic INR

INR	Patient Situation	Action
>3 and ≤5	No bleeding or need for rapid reversal (ie, no need for surgery)	Omit next few warfarin doses and/or restart at lower dose when INR approaches desired range. If only minimally above range, then no dosage reduction may be required.
>5 and <9.0	No bleeding or need for rapid reversal	Omit next 1-2 doses, monitor INR more frequently, and restart at lower dose when INR approaches target range **or** omit dose and give 1-2.5 mg vitamin K orally (use this if patient has risk factors for bleeding).
	No bleeding but reversal needed for surgery or dental extraction within 24 hours	Give vitamin K 2-4 mg orally (expected reversal within 24 hours); give additional 1-2 mg if INR remains high at 24 hours.
>9.0 and <20.0	No bleeding	Stop warfarin, give vitamin K 3-5 mg orally; follow INR closely; repeat vitamin K if needed. Reassess need and dose of warfarin when INR approaches desirable range.
Rapid reversal required (ie, INR >20)	Serious bleeding or major warfarin overdose	Stop warfarin, give vitamin K 10 mg by slow I.V. infusion. May repeat vitamin K every 12 hours and give fresh plasma transfusion or prothrombin complex concentrate as needed. When appropriate, heparin can be given until the patient becomes responsive to warfarin.

WARFARIN INTERACTIONS

Numerous factors, alone or in combination, including travel, changes in diet, environment, physical state, and medication may influence response of the patient to anticoagulants. It is generally good practice to monitor the patient's response with additional PT/INR determinations in the period immediately after discharge from the hospital, and whenever other medications are initiated, discontinued, or taken irregularly. The following factors are listed for reference; however, other factors may also affect the anticoagulant response.

Intensity of warfarin anticoagulation is affected by foods high in vitamin K, alcohol, diseases such as congestive heart failure, and by concomitant drug therapy. Drugs that inhibit or induce P450 2C9 isoenzyme will have the greatest effect on INR (see following table). It is important to note that just as the therapeutic effect of warfarin requires several days to become apparent, treatment with vitamin K may also inhibit the effects of warfarin for several days. Foods high in vitamin K decrease PT/INR and include green leafy vegetables (eg, kale, broccoli, spinach, parsley, collard greens). Acute alcohol consumption can increase PT/INR while chronic ingestion can decrease PT/INR. Drug interactions with warfarin may occur by several mechanisms, including impairment of absorption, induction or inhibition of metabolism, competition for protein-binding sites, and platelet inhibition. Drugs that inhibit or induce P450 2C9 (responsible for metabolism of S-warfarin) may have the greatest effect on INR. Select and important drug-drug interactions are depicted in the following table.

Selected Warfarin Drug Interactions

Drug	Effect on P450	Isoenzyme		
		1A2	2C9	3A4
Amiodarone	Inhibits		X	X
Carbamazepine	Induces			
Ciprofloxacin	Inhibits	X		
Cimetidine				
Dicloxacillin	Induces			
Erythromycin		X		X
Fluconazole	Inhibits		X	
Metronidazole				
Nafcillin	Induces			
Omeprazole	Inhibits			X
Phenobarbital		X	X	
Phenytoin	Induces			
Rifampin				
SSRI				
TMP/SMX (Bactrim®)	Inhibits		X	
Zileuton		X		
Zafirlukast			X	

PROSTHETIC HEART VALVES

Patients with mechanical prosthetic valves require life-long anticoagulation therapy. The optimal intensity of anticoagulation is not established. The risk of thromboembolism is greater in valve patients who have atrial fibrillation (AF); have an enlarged left atrium (>5.5 cm); have a history of systemic embolism, left ventricular systolic dysfunction, coronary artery disease, left atrial thrombus; have ball valve; or have more than one mechanical valve. The risk for thromboembolism is also higher for mechanical valves in the mitral position compared to aortic. These factors should be weighed in each patient before deciding the desired level of anticoagulation to prevent thromboembolism and to avoid bleeding complications. Ranges for anticoagulation intensity in patients with prosthetic valves are described in the following table.

Prosthetic Valves

Valve Location	Type	Recommended INR / Therapy
Mechanical	Mitral – bileaflet or tilting disk	2.5-3.5 or 2.0-3.0 plus aspirin (80-100 mg/day)
	Mitral – cage disk or ball	2.5-3.5 plus aspirin (80-100 mg/day)
	Aortic – bileaflet (eg, St Jude, CarboMedics)	2.0-3.0 if normal left ventricular function, left atrial size, and sinus rhythm 2.5-3.5 or 2.0-3.0 plus aspirin (80-100 mg/day) if AF and high-risk patients
	Mitral or aortic valve and history of systemic embolism despite adequate warfarin therapy	2.5-3.5 plus aspirin (80-100 mg/day)
Bioprosthetic	Mitral or aortic	2.0-3.0 for 3 months after insertion **or** indefinitely if patient has AF; left atrial thrombus or permanent pacemaker, duration uncertain; prior systemic embolism, duration of therapy should be increased to 3-12 months; chronic low-dose aspirin therapy (≤160 mg/day) after warfarin therapy

As a general rule, concomitant warfarin and aspirin therapy should be avoided, except in special situations. For patients with mechanical prosthetic valves who suffer a systemic thromboembolism despite adequate anticoagulation therapy, low-dose aspirin should be added and the INR should be maintained between 2.5 and 3.5. The combination of warfarin and low-dose aspirin in all mechanical valve patients is uncertain; patients at the highest risk for thromboembolism should be considered. For patients who cannot tolerate aspirin, dipyridamole 150 mg/day may be combined with warfarin therapy.

REFERENCES

Guidelines
Proceedings of the American College of Chest Physicians – 6th Consensus Conference on Antithrombotic Therapy, *Chest*, 2001, 119(1 Suppl):1S-370S.

Drug Therapy
Crowther MA, Ginsberg JB, Kearon C, et al, "A Randomized Trial Comparing 5 mg and 10 mg Warfarin Loading Doses," *Arch Intern Med*, 1999, 159:46-8.

ANTIEMETICS FOR CHEMOTHERAPY-INDUCED NAUSEA AND VOMITING

GENERAL PRINCIPLES FOR MANAGING NAUSEA AND VOMITING

1. Prophylaxis is **much** better than treatment of actual vomiting. For agents with a moderate-to-high (30% to 100%) incidence of nausea, patients should be pretreated with an antiemetic. Depending on the antiemetic agent(s) and route(s) of administration, pretreatment may range from 1 hour to 5 minutes prior to administration of the antineoplastic agent(s).

2. Doses and intervals of the antiemetic regimen need to be individualized for each patient. "PRN" regimens should **not** be used. A fixed schedule of drug administration is preferable.

3. If a patient has had no nausea for 24 hours while on their scheduled antiemetic regimen, it is usually possible to switch to a "PRN" regimen. The patient should be advised to resume the fixed schedule at the **first** sign of recurrent nausea, and continue it until they have had at least 24 hours without nausea.

4. Titrate antiemetic dose to patient tolerance.

5. In most cases, combination regimens are required for optimum control of nausea. Do not be afraid to use two or more agents, from different pharmacologic categories, to achieve optimal results.

6. To the extent possible, avoid duplication of agents from the same pharmacologic category.

7. Anticipatory nausea and vomiting can often be minimized if the patient receives effective prophylaxis against nausea from the first cycle of therapy.

8. If anticipatory nausea does develop, an anxiolytic agent is usually the drug of choice.

9. "If it's not broken - **don't** fix it!" Regardless of your own preferences, if the patient's current antiemetic regimen is working, don't change it.

10. For moderately emetogenic regimens, a steroid and dopamine blocker (eg, metoclopramide, prochlorperazine, thiethylperazine) may be the most cost-effective regimen.

11. For highly emetogenic regimens, a steroid and serotonin receptor blocker (eg, dolasetron, granisetron, ondansetron) combination is the preferred regimen.

12. A dopamine blocker (eg, metoclopramide, prochlorperazine, thiethylperazine) is a good first alternative if the serotonin blocker fails.

13. Although most nausea or vomiting develops within the first 24 hours after treatment, delayed reactions (1-7 days after chemotherapy) are not uncommon.

14. Other antiemetics (eg, cannabinoids, antihistamines, or anticholinergics) have limited use as initial therapy. They are best used in combination with more effective agents (steroids, dopamine, or serotonin blockers); or, as second- or third-line therapy.

15. Serotonin blockers are most effective in scheduled prophylactic regimens; rather than in "PRN" regimens to chase existing vomiting.

16. The serotonin blockers appear to have a "ceiling" dose, above which there is little or no added antiemetic effect.

Time Course of Nausea and Vomiting

Drug	Onset (h)	Duration (h)
Azacitidine	1-3	3-4
Carboplatin	2-6	1-48
Carmustine	2-6	4-6
Cisplatin	1-4	12-96
Cyclophosphamide	6-8	8-24
Cytarabine	1-3	3-8
Dacarbazine	1-2	2-4
Dactinomycin	2-5	4-24
Daunorubicin	1-3	4-24
Doxorubicin	1-3	4-24
Ifosfamide	2-3	12-72
Lomustine	2-6	4-6
Mechlorethamine	1-3	2-8
Mitomycin	1-2	48-72
Plicamycin	4-6	4-24
Procarbazine	24-27	Variable
Streptozocin	1-3	1-12

Emetogenic Potential of Single Chemotherapeutic Agents

Very High (>90%)

Cisplatin
Cytarabine (>2 g)
Dacarbazine
Didemnin-B
JM-216
Mechlorethamine
Melphalan (I.V.)
Streptozocin

High (60% to 90%)

Aldesleukin
Amifostine
Carmustine
Cyclophosphamide (>1 g)
Cytarabine (<2 g)
Dactinomycin
Elsamitrucin
Estramustine
Etoposide
Hydroxyurea
Idarubicin
Irinotecan
Lomustine
Mitotane
Mitomycin
Mitoxantrone
Semustine
Toremifene
Tretinoin

Moderate (30% to 60%)

Altretamine
Amonafide
Amsacrine
Asparaginase
Azacytidine
Carboplatin
Cladribine
Cyclophosphamide (<1 g)
Daunorubicin
Dexrazocane
Diazequone
Docetaxel
Doxorubicin
Epirubicin
Ifosfamide
Interferons
Interleukin-6
Mitoguazone
PALA
Pegaspergase
Pentostatin
Plicamycin
Procarbazine
Teniposide
Tomudex
Topotecan
Trimetrexate
Vinblastine
Vinorelbine

Low (10% to 30%)

Floxuridine
Fluorouracil
Flutamide
Gemcitabine
Levamisole
Melphalan (oral)
Methotrexate (high dose)
Steroids
Suramin
Tamoxifen
Thioguanine
Vindesine

Very Low (<10%)

Androgens
Aminoglutethimide
Anastrozole
Bicalutamide
Bleomycin
Busulfan
Chlorambucil
Estrogens
Fludarabine
Goserelin
Homoharringtonine
Leucovorin
Leuprolide
Megestrol
Mercaptopurine
Mesna
Methotrexate (low dose)
Paclitaxel
Thiotepa
Vincristine

ANTIEMETICS FOR CHEMOTHERAPY-INDUCED NAUSEA AND VOMITING *(Continued)*

Drugs With a High Incidence but Low Severity of Nausea / Vomiting

Amonafide	Hydroxyurea
Carboplatin	Interferons
Cyclophosphamide (<1 g)	Mitoguazone
Dexrazoxane	Mitoxantrone
Docetaxel	Tretinoin
Gemcitabine	Vinblastine

Drugs With a Low Incidence but High Severity of Nausea / Vomiting

Lomustine	Semustine
Methotrexate (high dose)	

Potency of Antiemetic Drugs

Potency	Type of Antiemetic Drug
Active against highly emetogenic chemotherapy	Serotonin antagonist Substituted benzamide (high dose)
Active against mildly or moderately emetogenic chemotherapy	Butyrophenone Cannabinoid Corticosteroid Phenothiazine
Minimally active	Anticholinergic agent Antihistamine Benzodiazepine

REPRESENTATIVE ANTIEMETIC REGIMENS

Highly Emetogenic Chemotherapy

Dexamethasone 10-20 mg P.O. or I.V. + a serotonin antagonist daily 15-30 minutes before treatment on each day of chemotherapy

Recommended serotonin antagonist regimens:
Dolasetron 100 mg P.O. once daily
Granisetron 2 mg P.O. once daily
Granisetron 1 mg P.O. every 12 hours
Granisetron 10 mcg/kg I.V. once daily
Granisetron 1 mg I.V. once daily
Ondansetron 0.45 mg/kg I.V. once daily
Ondansetron 24-32 mg I.V. once daily
Ondansetron 0.15 mg/kg I.V. every 8 hours
Ondansetron 8-10 mg I.V. every 8 hours

For continuous infusion therapy, carboplatin, and high-dose (>1 g/m²) cyclophosphamide regimens, the following regimen may be preferred:

Dexamethasone 10 mg P.O. or I.V. + a serotonin antagonist every 12 hours

Recommended serotonin antagonist regimens:
Granisetron 1 mg P.O.
Granisetron 10 mcg/kg I.V.
Ondansetron 10-16 mg I.V.
Ondansetron 16-24 mg P.O.

Moderately Emetogenic Chemotherapy

Dexamethasone 10 mg P.O. or I.V. + a serotonin antagonist daily 15-30 minutes before treatment on each day of chemotherapy

Recommended serotonin antagonist regimens:
Granisetron 1 mg P.O. once daily
Ondansetron 16 mg P.O. once daily
Ondansetron 8-10 mg I.V. once daily

For continuous infusion therapy, the following regimen may be preferred:

Dexamethasone 4 mg P.O. or I.V. + ondansetron 8 mg P.O. or I.V. every 12 hours on each day of chemotherapy

Mildly emetogenic chemotherapy (all agents are given 15-30 minutes before treatment, and may be repeated every 4-6 hours if necessary. With the exceptions of dexamethasone (given over 5-15 minutes) and droperidol (given by I.V. push), intravenous doses should be given over 30 minutes.):

> Dexamethasone 4 mg P.O./I.V./I.M.
> Droperidol 1.25-5 mg I.M./I.V. push
> Haloperidol 2 mg P.O./I.V./I.M.
> Metoclopramide 30 mg P.O./I.V./I.M.
> Prochlorperazine 10-20 mg P.O./I.V./I.M.
> Thiethylperazine 10-20 mg P.O./I.V./I.M.

Delayed Nausea and Vomiting

Dexamethasone + a dopamine or serotonin antagonist. Therapy should start within 12-24 hours of administration of the emetogenic chemotherapy.

> Recommended regimens:
> Dexamethasone
> 8 mg P.O. every 12 hours for 2 days, then 4 mg P.O. every 12 hours for 2 days **or**
> 20 mg P.O. 1 hour before chemotherapy; 10 mg P.O. 12 hours after chemotherapy, then 8 mg P.O. every 12 hours for 4 doses, then 4 mg P.O. every 12 hours for 4 doses

> Recommended dopamine/serotonin antagonist regimens:
> Droperidol 1.25-2.5 mg I.V./I.M. every 4 hours for 4 days
> Metoclopramide 0.5 mg/kg P.O. every 6 hours for 4 days
> Ondansetron 8 mg P.O. every 8 hours for 4 days
> Prochlorperazine 10 mg P.O. every 6 hours for 4 days
> Prochlorperazine 15 mg (sustained release) P.O. 1 hour before chemotherapy, then every 12 hours for 5 doses
> Thiethylperazine 10 mg P.O. every 6 hours for 4 days

Recommended Doses of Serotonin (5HT$_3$) Antiemetics Prophylaxis of Acute Highly Emetogenic Chemotherapy-Induced Nausea / Vomiting

ASCO	ASHP	NCCN	MASCC
Dolasetron			
100 mg P.O.	100-200 mg P.O.	100 mg P.O.	100-200 mg P.O.
1.8 mg/kg[1] I.V.	1.8 mg/kg[1] I.V.	1.8 mg/kg[1] I.V.	1.8 mg/kg I.V.
Granisetron			
2 mg P.O.	2 mg P.O.	2 mg P.O.[2]	2 mg P.O.
10 mcg/kg[3] I.V	10 mcg/kg I.V.	10 mcg/kg[4] I.V.	10 mcg/kg I.V.
Ondansetron			
12-24 mg P.O.	24 mg P.O.	8 mg P.O. bid	12-16 mg P.O.
8 mg I.V.[5]	8 mg I.V.	8 mg I.V.[6]	8 mg I.V.

[1]Or 100 mg
[2]Or 100 mg
[3]Or 1 mg
[4]Maximum: 1 mg
[5]Or 0.15 mg/kg
[6]Maximum: 32 mg/24 hours

ANTIMICROBIAL DRUGS OF CHOICE

Empirical treatment of some common infecting organisms is listed below. These recommendations are based on results of susceptibility studies, clinical trials, and the opinions of *Medical Letter* consultants. The site and severity of the infection, pharmacokinetic characteristics of antibiotics, local resistance patterns, potential drug interactions, and specific patient factors should be taken into account in choosing an appropriate regimen.

Infecting Organism	Drug of First Choice	Alternative Drugs
GRAM-POSITIVE COCCI		
Enterococcus[1]		
endocarditis or other severe infection	Penicillin G or ampicillin + gentamicin or streptomycin[2]	Vancomycin + gentamicin or streptomycin[2]; linezolid; daptomycin[3]; quinupristin/dalfopristin[4]
uncomplicated urinary tract infection	Ampicillin or amoxicillin	Nitrofurantoin; a fluoroquinolone[5]; fosfomycin
Staphylococcus aureus or *epidermidis*		
methicillin-susceptible	A penicillinase-resistant penicillin[6]	A cephalosporin[7,8]; vancomycin; imipenem or meropenem; clindamycin; linezolid; daptomycin[3]; a fluoroquinolone[5]
methicillin-resistant[9]	Vancomycin ± gentamicin ± rifampin	Linezolid; daptomycin[3]; a fluoroquinolone[5]; quinupristin/dalfopristin; a tetracycline[10]; trimethoprim-sulfamethoxazole
Streptococcus pyogenes (group A[11]) and groups C and G	Penicillin G or V[12]	Clindamycin; erythromycin; a cephalosporin[7,8]; vancomycin; clarithromycin[13]; azithromycin; linezolid; daptomycin[3]
Streptococcus, group B	Penicillin G or ampicillin	A cephalosporin[7,8]; vancomycin; daptomycin[3]; erythromycin
Streptococcus, viridans group[1]	Penicillin G ± gentamicin	A cephalosporin[7,8]; vancomycin
Streptococcus bovis	Penicillin G	A cephalosporin[7,8]; vancomycin
Streptococcus, anaerobic or *Peptostreptococcus*	Penicillin G	Clindamycin; a cephalosporin[7,8]; vancomycin
Streptococcus pneumoniae[14] (pneumococcus)		
penicillin-susceptible (MIC <0.1 mcg/mL)	Penicillin G or V[12]; amoxicillin	A cephalosporin[7,8]; erythromycin; azithromycin; clarithromycin[13]; levofloxacin, gatifloxacin or moxifloxacin[16]; meropenem; imipenem or ertapenem; trimethoprim-sulfamethoxazole; clindamycin; a tetracycline[10]; vancomycin
penicillin-intermediate resistance (MIC 0.1-≤2 mcg/mL)	Penicillin G I.V. (12 million units/day for adults); ceftriaxone or cefotaxime	Levofloxacin, gatifloxacin or moxifloxacin[16]; vancomycin; clindamycin
penicillin-high level resistance (MIC >2 mcg/mL)	**Meningitis:** Vancomycin ± rifampin + ceftriaxone or cefotaxime	
	Other Infections: Vancomycin + ceftriaxone or cefotaxime; levofloxacin, gatifloxacin, or moxifloxacin[16]	Linezolid; quinupristin/dalfopristin
GRAM-NEGATIVE COCCI		
Moraxella (Branhamella) catarrhalis	Cefuroxime[7]; a fluoroquinolone[5]	Trimethoprim-sulfamethoxazole; amoxicillin/clavulanate; erythromycin; clarithromycin[13]; azithromycin; a tetracycline[10]; cefotaxime[7]; ceftizoxime[7]; ceftriaxone[7]; cefpodoxime[7]
Neisseria gonorrhoeae (gonococcus)[17]	Ceftriaxone[7]; ciprofloxacin, gatifloxacin, or ofloxacin[15,16]	Cefotaxime[7]; penicillin G

Infecting Organism	Drug of First Choice	Alternative Drugs
Neisseria meningitidis[18] (meningococcus)	Penicillin G	Cefotaxime[7]; ceftizoxime[7]; ceftriaxone[7]; chloramphenicol[19]; a sulfonamide[20]; a fluoroquinolone[5]
GRAM-POSITIVE BACILLI		
*Bacillus anthracis[21] (anthrax)	Ciprofloxacin[16]; a tetracycline[10]	Penicillin G, amoxicillin; erythromycin; imipenem; clindamycin; levofloxacin[16]
Bacillus cereus, subtilis	Vancomycin	Imipenem or meropenem; clindamycin
Clostridium perfringens[22]	Penicillin G; clindamycin	Metronidazole; imipenem, meropenem, or ertapenem; chloramphenicol[19]
Clostridium tetani[23]	Metronidazole	Penicillin G; a tetracycline[10]
Clostridium difficile[24]	Metronidazole (oral)	Vancomycin (oral)
Corynebacterium diphtheriae[25]	Erythromycin	Penicillin G
Corynebacterium, JK group	Vancomycin	Penicillin G + gentamicin; erythromycin
*Erysipelothrix rhusiopathiae	Penicillin G	Erythromycin, a cephalosporin[7,8]; a fluoroquinolone[5]
Listeria monocytogenes	Ampicillin ± gentamicin	Trimethoprim-sulfamethoxazole
ENTERIC GRAM-NEGATIVE BACILLI		
*Campylobacter fetus	A third-generation cephalosporin[8]; gentamicin	Ampicillin; imipenem or meropenem
*Campylobacter jejuni	Erythromycin or azithromycin	A fluoroquinolone[5]; a tetracycline[10]; gentamicin
*Citrobacter freundii	Imipenem or meropenem[26]	A fluoroquinolone[5];ertapenem; amikacin; a tetracycline[10]; trimethoprim-sulfamethoxazole; cefotaxime[7,26]; ceftizoxime[7,26]; ceftriaxone[7,26]; cefepime[7,26] or ceftazidime[7,26]
*Enterobacter	Imipenem or meropenem[26]; cefepime[7,26]	Gentamicin, tobramycin or amikacin; trimethoprim-sulfamethoxazole; ciprofloxacin[16]; ticarcillin/clavulanate[27] or piperacillin/sulbactam[27]; aztreonam[26]; cefotaxime, ceftizoxime, ceftriaxone, or ceftazidime[7,26]
*Escherichia coli[28]	Cefotaxime, ceftriaxone, cefepime, or ceftazidime[7,26]	Ampicillin ± gentamicin, tobramycin or amikacin; gentamicin, tobramycin, or amikacin; amoxicillin/clavulanate[26]; ticarcillin/clavulanate[27]; piperacillin/tazobactam[27]; ampicillin/sulbactam[26]; trimethoprim-sulfamethoxazole; imipenem, meropenem, or ertapenem[26]; aztreonam[26]; a fluoroquinolone[5]; another cephalosporin[7,8]
*Klebsiella pneumoniae[28]	Cefotaxime, ceftriaxone, cefepime, or ceftazidime[7,26]	Imipenem, meropenem, or ertapenem[26]; gentamicin, tobramycin or amikacin; amoxicillin/clavulanate[26]; ticarcillin/clavulanate[27]; piperacillin/tazobactam[27]; ampicillin/sulbactam[26]; trimethoprim-sulfamethoxazole; aztreonam[26]; a fluoroquinolone[5]; another cephalosporin[7,8]
*Proteus mirabilis[28]	Ampicillin[29]	A cephalosporin[7,8,26]; ticarcillin/clavulanate or piperacillin/tazobactam[27]; gentamicin, tobramycin, or amikacin; trimethoprim-sulfamethoxazole; imipenem, meropenem, or ertapenem[26]; aztreonam[26]; a fluoroquinolone[5]; chloramphenicol[19]
*Proteus, indole-positive (including Providencia rettgeri, Morganella morganii, and Proteus vulgaris)	Cefotaxime, ceftriaxone, cefepime, or ceftazidime[7,26]	Imipenem, meropenem, or ertapenem[28]; gentamicin, tobramycin, or amikacin; amoxicillin/clavulanate[26]; ticarcillin/clavulanate[27]; piperacillin/tazobactam[27]; ampicillin/sulbactam[26]; aztreonam[26]; trimethoprim-sulfamethoxazole; a fluoroquinolone[5]

ANTIMICROBIAL DRUGS OF CHOICE (Continued)

Infecting Organism	Drug of First Choice	Alternative Drugs
*Providencia stuartii	Cefotaxime, ceftriaxone, cefepime, or ceftazidime[7,26]	Imipenem, meropenem, or ertapenem[26]; ticarcillin/clavulanate[27]; piperacillin/tazobactam[27]; gentamicin, tobramycin, or amikacin; aztreonam[26]; trimethoprim-sulfamethoxazole; a fluoroquinolone[5]
*Salmonella typhi (typhoid fever)[30]	A fluoroquinolone[5] or ceftriaxone[7]	Chloramphenicol[19]; trimethoprim-sulfamethoxazole; ampicillin; amoxicillin; azithromycin[31]
*Other Salmonella[32]	Cefotaxime[7] or ceftriaxone[7] or a fluoroquinolone[5]	Ampicillin or amoxicillin; trimethoprim-sulfamethoxazole; chloramphenicol[19]
*Serratia	Imipenem or meropenem[26]	Gentamicin or amikacin; cefotaxime, ceftizoxime, ceftriaxone, cefepime, or ceftazidime[7,26]; aztreonam[26]; trimethoprim-sulfamethoxazole; a fluoroquinolone[5]
*Shigella	A fluoroquinolone[5]	Azithromycin; trimethoprim-sulfamethoxazole; ampicillin; ceftriaxone[7]
*Yersinia enterocolitica	Trimethoprim-sulfamethoxazole	A fluoroquinolone[5]; gentamicin, tobramycin, or amikacin; cefotaxime[7]

OTHER GRAM-NEGATIVE BACILLI

Infecting Organism	Drug of First Choice	Alternative Drugs
*Acinetobacter	Imipenem or meropenem[26]	An aminoglycoside; ciprofloxacin[16]; trimethoprim-sulfamethoxazole; ticarcillin/clavulanate,[27] or piperacillin/tazobactam[27]; ceftazidime[26]; minocycline[10]; doxycycline[10]; sulbactam[33]; polymyxin
*Aeromonas	Trimethoprim-sulfamethoxazole	Gentamicin or tobramycin; imipenem; a fluoroquinolone[5]
*Bacteroides	Metronidazole	Clindamycin; imipenem, meropenem or ertapenem; amoxicillin/clavulanate; ticarcillin/clavulanate; piperacillin/tazobactam or ampicillin/sulbactam; cefoxitin[7]; chloramphenicol[19]
Bartonella henselae or quintana (bacillary angiomatosis, trench fever))	Erythromycin	Azithromycin; doxycycline[10]
Bartonella henselae[34] (cat scratch bacillus)	Azithromycin	Erythromycin; ciprofloxacin[16]; trimethoprim-sulfamethoxazole; gentamicin; rifampin
Bordetella pertussis (whooping cough)	Erythromycin; clarithromycin[13]	Azithromycin; trimethoprim-sulfamethoxazole
*Brucella	A tetracycline[10] + rifampin	A tetracycline[10] + streptomycin or gentamicin; chloramphenicol[19] ± streptomycin; trimethoprim-sulfamethoxazole ± gentamicin; ciprofloxacin[16] + rifampin
*Burkholderia cepacia	Trimethoprim-sulfamethoxazole	Ceftazidime[7]; chloramphenicol[19]; imipenem
Burkholderia (Pseudomonas) mallei (glanders)	Streptomycin + a tetracycline[10]	Streptomycin + chloramphenicol[19]; imipenem
*Burkholderia (Pseudomonas) pseudomallei (melioidosis)	Imipenem; ceftazidime[7]	Meropenem; chloramphenicol[19] + doxycycline[10] + trimethoprim-sulfamethoxazole; amoxicillin/clavulanate
Calymmatobacterium granulomatis (granuloma inguinale)	Trimethoprim-sulfamethoxazole	Doxycycline[10] or ciprofloxacin[16] ± gentamicin
Capnocytophaga canimorsus[35]	Penicillin G	Cefotaxime, ceftizoxime, or ceftriaxone[7]; imipenem or meropenem; vancomycin; a fluoroquinolone[5]; clindamycin
*Eikenella corrodens	Ampicillin	Erythromycin; azithromycin; clarithromycin[13]; a tetracycline[10]; amoxicillin/clavulanate; ampicillin/sulbactam; ceftriaxone[7]

Infecting Organism	Drug of First Choice	Alternative Drugs
*Francisella tularensis (tularemia)	Gentamicin or streptomycin either + a tetracycline[10]	Chloramphenicol[19]; ciprofloxacin[16]
*Fusobacterium	Penicillin G; metronidazole	Clindamycin; cefoxitin[7]; chloramphenicol[19]
Gardnerella vaginalis (bacterial vaginosis)	Oral metronidazole[37]	Topical clindamycin or metronidazole; oral clindamycin
*Haemophilus ducreyi (chancroid)	Azithromycin or ceftriaxone	Ciprofloxacin[16] or erythromycin
*Haemophilus influenzae		
meningitis, epiglottitis, arthritis, and other serious infections	Cefotaxime or ceftriaxone[7]	Cefuroxime[7] (not for meningitis); chloramphenicol[19]; meropenem
upper respiratory infections and bronchitis	Trimethoprim-sulfamethoxazole	Cefuroxime[7]; amoxicillin/clavulanate; cefuroxime axetil[7]; cefpodoxime[7]; cefaclor[7]; cefotaxime[7]; ceftizoxime[7]; ceftriaxone[7]; cefixime[7]; a tetracycline[10]; clarithromycin[13]; azithromycin; a fluoroquinolone[5]; ampicillin or amoxicillin
*Helicobacter pylori[38]	Proton pump inhibitor[39] + clarithromycin[13] + either amoxicillin or metronidazole	Bismuth subsalicylate + metronidazole + tetracycline HCl[10] + either a proton pump inhibitor[39] or H$_2$-blocker[39]
Legionella species	Azithromycin or a fluoroquinolone[5] ± rifampin	Doxycycline[10] ± rifampin; trimethoprim-sulfamethoxazole; erythromycin
Leptotrichia buccalis	Penicillin G	A tetracycline[10]; clindamycin; erythromycin
Pasteurella multocida	Penicillin G	A tetracycline[10]; a second- or third-generation cephalosporin[7,8]; amoxicillin/clavulanate; ampicillin/sulbactam
*Pseudomonas aeruginosa		
urinary tract infection	Ciprofloxacin[16]	Levofloxacin[16]; ticarcillin/clavulanate or piperacillin/tazobactam; ceftazidime[7]; cefepime[7]; imipenem or meropenem; aztreonam; tobramycin; gentamicin or amikacin
other infections	Piperacillin/tazobactam or ticarcillin/clavulanate **each** + tobramycin, gentamicin, or amikacin[40]	Ceftazidime,[7] ciprofloxacin[16]; imipenem or meropenem, aztreonam, cefepime[7] **each** + tobramycin, gentamicin, or amikacin
Spirillum minus (rat bite fever)	Penicillin G	A tetracycline[10]; streptomycin
*Stenotrophomonas maltophilia	Trimethoprim-sulfamethoxazole	Minocycline[10]; a fluoroquinolone[5]
Streptobacillus moniliformis (rat bite fever, Haverhill fever)	Penicillin G	A tetracycline[10]; streptomycin
Vibrio cholerae (cholera)[41]	A tetracycline[10]	A fluoroquinolone[5]; trimethoprim-sulfamethoxazole
Vibrio vulnificus	A tetracycline[10]	Cefotaxime[7]; ciprofloxacin[13]
Yersinia pestis (plague)	Streptomycin ± a tetracycline[10]	Chloramphenicol[19]; gentamicin; trimethoprim-sulfamethoxazole; ciprofloxacin[13]
ACID-FAST BACILLI		
*Mycobacterium tuberculosis	Isoniazid + rifampin + pyrazinamide ± ethambutol or streptomycin[19]	A fluoroquinolone[5]; cycloserine[19]; capreomycin[19] or kanamycin[19] or amikacin[19]; ethionamide[19]; para-aminosalicylic acid[19]
*Mycobacterium kansasii	Isoniazid + rifampin ± ethambutol or streptomycin[19]	Clarithromycin[13] or azithromycin; ethionamide[19]; cycloserine[19]
*Mycobacterium avium complex		
treatment	Clarithromycin[13] or azithromycin + ethambutol ± rifabutin	Ciprofloxacin[16]; amikacin[19]
prophylaxis	Clarithromycin[13] or azithromycin ± rifabutin	

ANTIMICROBIAL DRUGS OF CHOICE *(Continued)*

Infecting Organism	Drug of First Choice	Alternative Drugs
Mycobacterium fortuitum/ chelonae complex	Amikacin + clarithromycin[13]	Cefoxitin[7]; rifampin; a sulfonamide; doxycycline[10]; ethambutol; linezolid
Mycobacterium marinum (balnei)[42]	Minocycline[10]	Trimethoprim-sulfamethoxazole; rifampin; clarithromycin[13]; doxycycline[10]
Mycobacterium leprae (leprosy)	Dapsone + rifampin ± clofazimine	Minocycline[10]; ofloxacin[16]; clarithromycin[13]
ACTINOMYCETES		
Actinomyces israelii (actinomycosis)	Penicillin G	A tetracycline[10]; erythromycin; clindamycin
Nocardia	Trimethoprim-sulfamethoxazole	Sulfisoxazole; amikacin[19]; a tetracycline[10]; ceftriaxone; imipenem or meropenem; cycloserine[19]; linezolid
Rhodococcus equi	Vancomycin ± a fluoroquinolone,[5] rifampin, imipenem, or meropenem; amikacin	Erythromycin
Tropheryma whippelii (Whipple's disease)	Trimethoprim-sulfamethoxazole	Penicillin G; a tetracycline[10]; ceftriaxone
CHLAMYDIAE		
Chlamydia trachomatis		
trachoma	Azithromycin	A tetracycline[10] (topical plus oral); a sulfonamide (topical plus oral)
inclusion conjunctivitis	Erythromycin (oral or I.V.)	A sulfonamide
pneumonia	Erythromycin	A sulfonamide
urethritis, cervicitis	Azithromycin or doxycycline[10]	Erythromycin; ofloxacin[16]; amoxicillin
lymphogranuloma venereum	A tetracycline[10]	Erythromycin
Chlamydophilia (formerly Chlamydia) pneumoniae (TWAR strain)	Erythromycin; a tetracycline[10]; clarithromycin[13] or azithromycin	A fluoroquinolone[5]
Chlamydophilia (formerly Chlamydia) psittaci (psittacosis, ornithosis)	A tetracycline[10]	Chloramphenicol[19]
EHRLICHIA		
Anaplasma phagocytophilum (formerly *Ehrlichia phagocytophila*)	Doxycycline[10]	Rifampin
Ehrlichia chaffeensis	Doxycycline[10]	Chloramphenicol[19]
Ehrlichia ewingii	Doxycycline[10]	
MYCOPLASMA		
Mycoplasma pneumoniae	Erythromycin; a tetracycline[10]; clarithromycin[13] or azithromycin	A fluoroquinolone[5]
Ureaplasma urealyticum	Azithromycin	Erythromycin; a tetracycline[10]; clarithromycin[13]; ofloxacin[16]
RICKETTSIOSES		
Coxiella burnetii (Q fever)	Doxycycline[10]	Chloramphenicol[19]; a fluoroquinolone[5]
Orientia tsutsugamushi (scrub typhus)	Doxycycline[10]	Chloramphenicol[19]; a fluoroquinolone[5]
Rickettsia prowazekii (epidemic typhus – louse-borne)	Doxycycline[10]	Chloramphenicol[19]; a fluoroquinolone[5]
Rickettsia rickettsii Rocky Mountain spotted fever)	Doxycycline[10]	Chloramphenicol[19]; a fluoroquinolone[5]
Rickettsia typhi (endemic typhus – murine)	Doxycycline[10]	Chloramphenicol[19]; a fluoroquinolone[5]
SPIROCHETES		
Borrelia burgdorferi (Lyme disease)[43]	Doxycycline[10]; amoxicillin; cefuroxime axetil[7]	Ceftriaxone[7]; cefotaxime[7]; penicillin G; azithromycin; clarithromycin[13]
Borrelia recurrentis (relapsing fever)	A tetracycline[10]	Penicillin G; erythromycin
Leptospira	Penicillin G	A tetracycline[10]; ceftriaxone[7,44]

Infecting Organism	Drug of First Choice	Alternative Drugs
Treponema pallidum (syphilis)	Penicillin G[12]	A tetracycline[10]; ceftriaxone[7]
Treponema pertenue (yaws)	Penicillin G	A tetracycline[10]

*Resistance may be a problem; susceptibility tests should be used to guide therapy.

[1]Disk sensitivity testing may not provide adequate information; beta-lactamase assays, "E" tests, and dilution tests for susceptibility should be used in serious infections.

[2]Aminoglycoside resistance is increasingly common among enterococci; treatment options include ampicillin 2 g I.V. every 4 hours, continuous infusion of ampicillin, a combination of ampicillin plus a fluoroquinolone, or a combination of ampicillin, imipenem, and vancomycin.

[3]Daptomycin should not be used to treat pneumonia.

[4]Quinupristin/dalfopristin is not active against *Enterococcus faecalis*.

[5]Among the fluoroquinolones, levofloxacin, gatifloxacin, and moxifloxacin have excellent *in vitro* activity against *S. pneumoniae*, including penicillin- and cephalosporin-resistant strains. Levofloxacin, gatifloxacin, and moxifloxacin also have good activity against many strains of *S. aureus*, but resistance has become frequent among methicillin-resistant strains. Ciprofloxacin has the greatest activity against *Pseudomonas aeruginosa*. For urinary tract infections, norfloxacin, lomefloxacin, or enoxacin can be used. For tuberculosis, levofloxacin, ofloxacin, ciprofloxacin, gatifloxacin, or moxifloxacin could be used. Ciprofloxacin, ofloxacin, levofloxacin, moxifloxacin, and gatifloxacin are available for intravenous use. None of these agents are recommended for pregnant women. Ciprofloxacin has FDA approval for use in children.

[6]For oral use against staphylococci, cloxacillin or dicloxacillin is preferred; for severe infections, a parenteral formulation of nafcillin or oxacillin should be used. Ampicillin, amoxicillin, carbenicillin, ticarcillin, and piperacillin are not effective against penicillinase-producing staphylococci. The combinations of clavulanate with amoxicillin or ticarcillin, sulbactam with ampicillin, and tazobactam with piperacillin may be active against these organisms.

[7]Cephalosporins have been used as alternatives to penicillins in patients allergic to penicillins, but such patients may also have allergic reactions to cephalosporins.

[8]For parenteral treatment of staphylococcal or nonenterococcal streptococcal infections, a first-generation cephalosporin such as cefazolin can be used. For oral therapy, cephalexin or cephradine can be used. The second-generation cephalosporins cefamandole, cefprozil, cefuroxime, cefotetan, cefoxitin, and loracarbef are more active than the first-generation drugs against gram-negative bacteria. Cefuroxime is active against ampicillin-resistant strains of *H. influenzae*. Cefoxitin and cefotetan are the most active of the cephalosporins against *B. fragilis*, but cefotetan has been associated with prothrombin deficiency. The third-generation cephalosporins cefotaxime, cefoperazone, ceftizoxime, ceftriaxone, and ceftazidime, and the fourth-generation cefepime have greater activity than the second-generation drugs against enteric gram-negative bacilli. Ceftazidime has poor activity against many gram-positive cocci and anaerobes, and ceftizoxime has poor activity against penicillin-resistant *S. pneumoniae*. Cefepime has *in vitro* activity against gram-positive cocci similar to cefotaxime and ceftriaxone and somewhat greater activity against enteric gram-negative bacilli. The activity of cefepime against *Pseudomonas aeruginosa* is similar to that of ceftazidime. Cefixime, cefpodoxime, cefdinir, ceftibuten, and cefditoren are oral cephalosporins with more activity than second-generation cephalosporins against facultative gram-negative bacilli; they have no useful activity against anaerobes or *P. aeruginosa*, and cefixime and ceftibuten have no useful activity against staphylococci. With the exception of cefoperazone (which, like cefamandole, can cause bleeding), ceftazidime and cefepime, the activity of all currently available cephalosporins against *P. aeruginosa* is poor or inconsistent.

[9]Many strains of coagulase-positive and coagulase-negative staphylococci are resistant to penicillinase-resistant penicillins; these strains are also resistant to cephalosporins, imipenem, and meropenem, and are often resistant to fluoroquinolones, trimethoprim-sulfamethoxazole, and clindamycin. Community-acquired MRSA often is susceptible to clindamycin and trimethoprim-sulfamethoxazole.

[10]Tetracyclines are generally not recommended for pregnant women or children younger than 8 years of age.

[11]For serious soft-tissue infection due to group A streptococci, clindamycin may be more effective than penicillin. Group A streptococci may, however, be resistant to clindamycin; therefore, some *Medical Letter* consultants suggest using both clindamycin and penicillin, with or without I.V. immune globulin, to treat serious soft-tissue infections. Surgical debridement is usually needed for necrotizing soft tissue infections due to group A streptococci. Group A streptococci may also be resistant to erythromycin, azithromycin, and clarithromycin.

[12]Penicillin V (or amoxicillin) is preferred for oral treatment of infections caused by nonpenicillinase-producing streptococci, is first choice. For initial therapy of severe infections, penicillin G, administered parenterally, is first choice. For somewhat longer action in less severe infections due to group A streptococci, pneumococci or *Treponema pallidum*, procaine penicillin G, an intramuscular formulation, can be given once or twice daily, but is seldom used now. Benzathine penicillin G, a slowly absorbed preparation, is usually given in a single monthly injection for prophylaxis of rheumatic fever, once for treatment of group A streptococcal pharyngitis and once or more for treatment of syphilis.

[13]Not recommended for use in pregnancy.

[14]Some strains of *S. pneumoniae* are resistant to erythromycin, clindamycin, trimethoprim-sulfamethoxazole, clarithromycin, azithromycin, and chloramphenicol, and resistance to the newer fluoroquinolones is rare but increasing (Davidson R, Cavalcanti R, Brunton JL, et al, "Resistance to Levofloxacin and Failure of Treatment of Pneumococcal Pneumonia," *N Engl J Med*, 2002, 346(10):747-50). Nearly all strains tested so far are susceptible to linezolid and quinupristin/dalfopristin *in vitro*.

[15]Fluoroquinolone-resistant strains of gonococcus are increasingly common (*MMWR, Morb Mortal Wkly Rep*, 2002, 51:1041; Fenton KA, Ison C, Johnson AP, et al, "Ciprofloxacin Resistance in *Neisseria gonorrhoeae* in England and Wales in 2002," *Lancet*, 2003, 361(9372):1867-9.

[16]Usually not recommended for use in children or pregnant women.

[17]Patients with gonorrhea should be treated presumptively for coinfection with *C. trachomatis* with azithromycin or doxycycline.

[18]Rare strains of *N. meningitidis* are resistant or relatively resistant to penicillin. A fluoroquinolone or rifampin is recommended for prophylaxis after close contact with infected patients.

[19]Because of the possibility of serious adverse effects, this drug should be used only for severe infections when less hazardous drugs are ineffective.

[20]Sulfonamide-resistant strains are frequent in the U.S.A; sulfonamides should be used only when susceptibility is established by susceptibility tests.

[21]For postexposure prophylaxis, ciprofloxacin for 4 weeks if given with vaccination, and 60 days if not given with vaccination, might prevent disease; if the strain is susceptible, doxycycline is an alternative

ANTIMICROBIAL DRUGS OF CHOICE *(Continued)*

(Bartlett JG, Inglesby TV Jr, and Borio L, "Management of Anthrax," *Clin Infect Dis*, 2002, 35(7):851-8; *Medical Letter*, 2001, 43:87.

[22]Debridement is primary. Large doses of penicillin G are required. Hyperbaric oxygen therapy may be a useful adjunct to surgical debridement in management of the spreading, necrotizing type of infection.

[23]For prophylaxis, a tetanus toxoid booster and, for some patients, tetanus immune globulin (human) are required.

[24]In order to decrease the emergence of vancomycin-resistant enterococci in hospitals and to reduce costs, most clinicians now recommend use of metronidazole first in treatment of patients with *C. difficile* colitis, with oral vancomycin used only for seriously ill patients or those who do not respond to metronidazole.

[25]Antitoxin is primary; antimicrobials are used only to halt further toxin production and to prevent the carrier state.

[26]In severely ill patients, most *Medical Letter* consultants would add gentamicin, tobramycin, or amikacin.

[27]In severely ill patients, most *Medical Letter* consultants would add gentamicin, tobramycin, or amikacin (but see footnote 40).

[28]For an acute, uncomplicated urinary tract infection, before the infecting organism is known, the drug of first choice is trimethoprim-sulfamethoxazole.

[29]Large doses (6 g or more daily) are usually necessary for systemic infections. In severely ill patients, some *Medical Letter* consultants would add gentamicin, tobramycin, or amikacin.

[30]A fluoroquinolone or amoxicillin is the drug of choice for *S. typhi* carriers (Parry CM, Hien TT, Dougan G, "Typhoid Fever," *N Engl J Med*, 2002, 347(22):1770-82).

[31]Frenck RW Jr, Nakhla I, Sultan Y, et al, "Azithromycin Versus Ceftriaxone for the Treatment of Uncomplicated Typhoid Fever in Children," *Clin Infect Dis*, 2000, 31(5):1134-8.

[32]Most cases of *Salmonella* gastroenteritis subside spontaneously without antimicrobial therapy. Immunosuppressed patients, young children, and the elderly may benefit the most from antibacterials.

[33]Sulbactam may be useful to treat multidrug resistant *Acinetobacter*. It is only available in combination with ampicillin as Unasyn®. *Medical Letter* consultants recommend 3 g I.V. every 4 hours (Urban C, Segal-Maurer S, and Rahal JJ, "Considerations in Control and Treatment of Nosocomial Infections Due to Multidrug-Resistant *Acinetobacter baumannii*," *Clin Infect Dis*, 2003, 36(10):1268-74; Levin AS, Levy CE, Manrique AE, et al, "Severe Nosocomial Infections With Imipenem-Resistant *Acinetobacter baumannii* Treated With Ampicillin/Sulbactam," *Int J Antimicrob Agents*, 2003, 21(1):58-62.

[34]Role of antibiotics is not clear (Conrad DA, "Treatment of Cat-Scratch Disease," *Curr Opin Pediatr*, 2001, 13(1):56-9).

[35]Pers C, Gahrm-Hansen B, Frederiksen W, et al, "*Capnocytophaga canimorsus* Septicemia in Denmark, 1982-1995: Review of 39 Cases," *Clin Infect Dis*, 1996, 23(1):71-5.

[36]For postexposure prophylaxis, doxycycline, or ciprofloxacin begun during the incubation period and continued for 14 days might prevent disease (*Medical Letter*, 2001, 43:87).

[37]Metronidazole is effective for bacterial vaginosis even though it is not usually active *in vitro* against *Gardnerella*.

[38]Eradication of *H. pylori* with various antibacterial combinations, given concurrently with a proton pump inhibitor or H₂-blocker, has led to rapid healing of active peptic ulcers and low recurrence rates (Mégraud F and Marshall BJ, "How to Treat *Helicobacter pylori*. First-line, Second-line, and Future Therapies," *Gastroenterol Clin North Am*, 2000, 29(4):759-73; *Treatment Guidelines*, 2004, 2:9.).

[39]Proton pump inhibitors available in the U.S.A. are omeprazole (Prilosec®, and others) lansoprazole (Prevacid®), pantoprazole (Protonix®), esomeprazole (Nexium®), and rabeprazole (Aciphex®). Available H₂-blockers include cimetidine (Tagamet®, and others), famotidine (Pepcid®, and others), nizatidine (Axid®, and others), and ranitidine (Zantac®, and others).

[40]Neither gentamicin, tobramycin, netilmicin, or amikacin should be mixed in the same bottle with carbenicillin, ticarcillin, mezlocillin, or piperacillin for intravenous administration. When used in high doses or in patients with renal impairment, these penicillins may inactivate the aminoglycosides.

[41]Antibiotic therapy is an adjunct to and not a substitute for prompt fluid and electrolyte replacement.

[42]Most infections are self-limited without drug treatment.

[43]For treatment of erythema migrans, uncomplicated facial nerve palsy, mild cardiac disease, and arthritis, oral therapy is satisfactory; for other neurologic or more serious cardiac disease, parenteral therapy with ceftriaxone, cefotaxime, or penicillin G is recommended. For recurrent arthritis after an oral regimen, another course of oral therapy or a parenteral drug may be given (Wormser GP, Nadelman RB, Dattwyler RJ, et al, "Practice Guidelines for the Treatment of Lyme Disease. The Infectious Diseases Society of America," *Clin Infect Dis*, 2000, 31(Suppl 1):1-14).

[44]Vinetz JM, "A Mountain Out of a Molehill: Do We Treat Acute Leptospirosis, and if so, With What?" *Clin Infect Dis*, 2003, 36(12):1514-5; Panaphot T et al, *Clin Infect Dis*, 2003, 36:1507.

Adapted with permission from "Choice of Antibacterial Drugs," *Treatment Guidelines*, 2004, 2(19):18-23.

ASTHMA

Adapted from National Asthma Education and Prevention Program (NAEPP) Expert Panel Report, "Guidelines for the Diagnosis and Management of Asthma – Update on Selected Topics 2002," NIH Publication No. 02-5075 (www.nhlbi.nih.gov/guidelines/asthma/asthgdln.htm)

MANAGEMENT OF ASTHMA IN ADULTS AND CHILDREN >5 YEARS OF AGE

Goals of Asthma Treatment

- Minimal or no chronic symptoms day or night
- Minimal or no exacerbations
- No limitations on activities; no school/work missed
- Minimal use of inhaled short-acting beta$_2$-agonist (<1 time/day, <1 canister/month)
- Minimal or no adverse effects from medications
- Children >5 years of age and adults only: PEF >80% of personal best

All Patients

- Short-acting bronchodilator: **Inhaled beta$_2$-agonists** as needed for symptoms.
- Intensity of treatment will depend on severity of exacerbation; see "Management of Asthma Exacerbations".
- Use of short-acting inhaled beta$_2$-agonists on a daily basis, or increasing use, indicates the need to initiate or titrate long-term control therapy.

Education

- Teach self-management.
- Teach about controlling environmental factors (avoidance of allergens or other factors that contribute to asthma severity).
- Review administration technique and compliance with patient.
- May use a written action plan to help educate.

Stepwise Approach for Managing Asthma in Adults and Children >5 Years of Age: Treatment[1]

Symptoms[2]	Lung Function[3]	Long-Term Control (Daily Medications)
STEP 4: Severe Persistent		
Day: Continual Night: Frequent	PEF/FEV$_1$ ≤60% PEF variability >30%	• **Preferred treatment:** – **High dose inhaled corticosteroid** AND – **Long-acting inhaled beta$_2$-agonist** AND, if needed – Long-term oral corticosteroid (2 mg/kg/day, generally do not exceed 60 mg/day). (Make repeated attempts to reduce systemic corticosteroids and maintain control with high-dose inhaled corticosteroids.)
STEP 3: Moderate Persistent		
Day: Every day Night: >1 night/week	PEF/FEV$_1$ >60% - <80% PEF variability >30%	• **Preferred treatment:** – **Low-medium dose inhaled corticosteroid** AND – **Long-acting inhaled beta$_2$-agonist** • Alternatives: – Increase inhaled corticosteroids within medium-dose range OR – Low-medium dose inhaled corticosteroids and either leukotriene receptor antagonist or theophylline
		If needed (especially with recurring severe exacerbations): • **Preferred treatment:** – Increase inhaled corticosteroids within medium-dose range, and add long-acting inhaled beta$_2$-agonist • Alternatives: – Increase inhaled corticosteroids in medium-dose range, and add either leukotriene receptor antagonist or theophylline

ASTHMA *(Continued)*

Stepwise Approach for Managing Asthma in Adults and Children >5 Years of Age: Treatment[1]

Symptoms[2]	Lung Function[3]	Long-Term Control (Daily Medications)
STEP 2: Mild Persistent		
Day: >2 days/week but <1 time/day Night: >2 nights/month	PEF/FEV$_1$ ≥80% PEF variability 20%-30%	• **Preferred treatment:** – **Low-dose inhaled corticosteroid** • Alternatives: Cromolyn, leukotriene receptor antagonist, nedocromil, or sustained release theophylline (serum concentration 5-15 mcg/mL)
STEP 1: Mild Intermittent		
Day: ≤2 days/week Night: ≤2 nights/month	PEF/FEV$_1$ ≥80% PEF variability <20%	No daily medication needed. A course of systemic corticosteroids is recommended for severe exacerbations.

[1]Classify severity. The presence of one of the features of severity is sufficient to place a patient in that category. An individual should be assigned to the most severe grade in which any feature occurs. The characteristics noted are general and may overlap because asthma is highly variable. Furthermore, an individual's classification may change over time.

[2]Patients at any level of severity can have mild, moderate, or severe exacerbations. Some patients with intermittent asthma experience severe and life-threatening exacerbations separated by long periods of normal lung function and no symptoms.

[3]PEF is % of personal best and FEV$_1$ is % predicted.

↓ **Step down**
Review treatment every 1-6 months; a gradual stepwise reduction in treatment may be possible.

↑**Step up**
If control is not maintained, consider step up. First, review patient medication technique, adherence, and environmental control.

Notes:

- **The stepwise approach presents general guidelines to assist clinical decision making; it is not intended to be a specific prescription. Asthma is highly variable; clinicians should tailor specific medication plans to the needs and circumstances of individual patients.**

- Gain control as quickly as possible; then decrease treatment to the least medication necessary to maintain control.

- A rescue course of systemic corticosteroids may be needed at any time and at any step.

- Some patients with intermittent asthma experience severe and life-threatening exacerbations separated by long periods of normal lung function and no symptoms. This may be especially common with exacerbations provoked by respiratory infections. A short course of systemic corticosteroids is recommended.

- At each step, patients should control their environment to avoid or control factors that make their asthma worse.

- Antibiotics are not recommended for treatment of acute asthma exacerbations except where there is evidence or suspicion of bacterial infection.

- Consultation with an asthma specialist is recommended for moderate or severe persistent asthma.

- Peak flow monitoring for patients with moderate-severe asthma should be considered.

MANAGEMENT OF ASTHMA IN INFANTS AND YOUNG CHILDREN

All Patients

- Bronchodilator as needed for symptoms ≤2 times/week. Intensity of treatment will depend upon severity of exacerbation (see "Management of Asthma Exacerbations"). Either:
  - Preferred treatment: Inhaled short-acting beta$_2$-agonist by nebulizer or face mask and spacer/holding chamber
    or
  - Alternative treatment: Oral beta$_2$-agonist
- With viral respiratory infection:
  - Bronchodilator q4-6h up to 24 hours (longer with physician consult) but, in general, repeat no more than once every 6 weeks.
  - Consider systemic corticosteroid if current exacerbation is severe or patient has history of severe exacerbations.
- Use of short-acting inhaled beta$_2$-agonist on a daily basis, or increasing use, indicates the need to initiate or titrate long-term control therapy.

Education

- Teach self-management or caregiver management.
- Teach about controlling environmental factors.
- Review administration technique and compliance with patient.
- May use a written action plan to help educate.

Stepwise Approach for Managing Infants and Young Children (≤5 Years of Age) With Acute or Chronic Asthma[1]

Symptoms[2]	Long-Term Control (Daily Medications)
STEP 4: Severe Persistent	
Day: Continual Night: Frequent	• **Preferred treatment:** – **High dose inhaled corticosteroid** **AND** – **Long-acting inhaled beta$_2$-agonist** AND, if needed – Long-term oral corticosteroids (2 mg/kg/day, generally do not exceed 60 mg/day). (Make repeated attempts to reduce systemic corticosteroids and maintain control with high-dose inhaled corticosteroids.)
STEP 3: Moderate Persistent	
Day: Every day Night: >1 night/week	• **Preferred treatment:** – **Low-dose inhaled corticosteroid** **AND** **Long-acting inhaled beta$_2$-agonist** **OR** **Medium-dose inhaled corticosteroid** • Alternatives: – Low-dose inhaled corticosteroid and either leukotriene receptor antagonist or theophylline
	If needed (especially with recurring severe exacerbations): • **Preferred treatment:** – **Medium-dose inhaled corticosteroid and long-acting inhaled beta$_2$-agonist** • Alternatives: – Medium-dose inhaled corticosteroid and either leukotriene receptor antagonist or theophylline
STEP 2: Mild Persistent	
Day: >2 days/week but <1 time/day Night: >2 nights/month	• **Preferred treatment:** – **Low-dose inhaled corticosteroid (with nebulizer or MDI with holding chamber with or without face mask or DPI)** • Alternatives: Cromolyn (nebulizer is preferred or MDI with holding chamber) **OR** Leukotriene receptor antagonist
STEP 1: Mild Intermittent	
Day: ≤2 days/week Night: ≤2 nights/month	No daily medication needed

[1]Classify severity. The presence of one of the features of severity is sufficient to place a patient in that category. An individual should be assigned to the most severe grade in which any feature occurs. The characteristics noted in this figure are general and may overlap because asthma is highly variable. Furthermore, an individual's classification may change over time.

[2]Patients at any level of severity can have mild, moderate, or severe exacerbations. Some patients with intermittent asthma experience severe and life-threatening exacerbations separated by long periods of normal lung function and no symptoms.

↓ Step Down
Review treatment every 1-6 month; a gradual stepwise reduction in treatment may be possible.

↑ Step Up
If control is not achieved, consider step up. But first: review patient medication technique, adherence, and environmental control (avoidance of allergens or other precipitant factors)

ASTHMA *(Continued)*

Notes:

- **The stepwise approach presents guidelines to assist clinical decision making. Asthma is highly variable; clinicians should tailor specific medication plans to the needs and circumstances of individual patients.**

- Gain control as quickly as possible; then decrease treatment to the least medication necessary to maintain control.

- A rescue course of systemic corticosteroid may be needed at any time and step.

- In general, use of a short-acting beta$_2$-agonist on a daily basis indicates the need for additional long-term control therapy.

- There are very few studies on asthma therapy for infants.

- Studies comparing medications in children <5 years of age are not available.

- Consultation with an asthma specialist is recommended for moderate or severe persistent asthma. Consider consultation for patient with mild persistent asthma.

- Initiation of long-term control therapy should be considered in infants and young children who have had >3 episodes of wheezing in the past year that lasted >1 day and affected sleep and who have risk factors for asthma.

- Inhaled corticosteroids improve health outcomes for children with mild-moderate persistent asthma. Monitor growth of children taking corticosteroids by any route. If growth appears slowed, weigh the benefits against the risks.

- Antibiotics are not recommended for treatment of acute asthma exacerbations except where there is evidence or suspicion of bacterial infection.

Management of Asthma Exacerbations: Home Treatment[1]

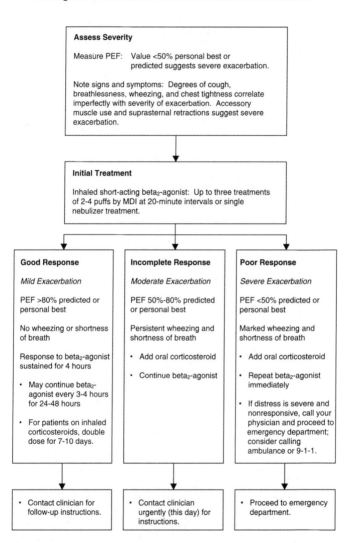

Assess Severity

Measure PEF: Value <50% personal best or
predicted suggests severe exacerbation.

Note signs and symptoms: Degrees of cough,
breathlessness, wheezing, and chest tightness correlate
imperfectly with severity of exacerbation. Accessory
muscle use and suprasternal retractions suggest severe
exacerbation.

Initial Treatment

Inhaled short-acting beta$_2$-agonist: Up to three treatments
of 2-4 puffs by MDI at 20-minute intervals or single
nebulizer treatment.

Good Response

Mild Exacerbation

PEF >80% predicted or
personal best

No wheezing or shortness
of breath

Response to beta$_2$-agonist
sustained for 4 hours

- May continue beta$_2$-
  agonist every 3-4 hours
  for 24-48 hours

- For patients on inhaled
  corticosteroids, double
  dose for 7-10 days.

Incomplete Response

Moderate Exacerbation

PEF 50%-80% predicted
or personal best

Persistent wheezing and
shortness of breath

- Add oral corticosteroid

- Continue beta$_2$-agonist

Poor Response

Severe Exacerbation

PEF <50% predicted or
personal best

Marked wheezing and
shortness of breath

- Add oral corticosteroid

- Repeat beta$_2$-agonist
  immediately

- If distress is severe and
  nonresponsive, call your
  physician and proceed to
  emergency department;
  consider calling
  ambulance or 9-1-1.

- Contact clinician for
  follow-up instructions.

- Contact clinician
  urgently (this day) for
  instructions.

- Proceed to emergency
  department.

[1]Patients at high risk of asthma-related death should receive immediate clinical attention after
initial treatment. Additional therapy may be required.

ASTHMA *(Continued)*

Management of Asthma Exacerbations: Emergency Department and Hospital-Based Care

Initial Assessment
History, physical examination (auscultation, use of accessory muscles, heart rate, respiratory rate), PEF or FEV$_1$, oxygen saturation, and other tests as indicated

FEV$_1$ or PEF >50%
- Inhaled beta$_2$-agonist by metered-dose inhaler or nebulizer, up to three doses in first hour
- Oxygen to achieve O$_2$ saturation ≥90%
- Oral systemic corticosteroids if no immediate response or if patient recently took oral systemic corticosteroid

FEV$_1$ or PEF <50%
(Severe Exacerbation)
- Inhaled high-dose beta$_2$-agonist and anticholinergic by nebulization every 20 minutes or continuously for 1 hour
- Oxygen to achieve O$_2$ saturation ≥90%
- Oral systemic corticosteroid

Impending or Actual Respiratory Arrest
- Intubation and mechanical ventilation with 100% O$_2$
- Nebulized beta$_2$-agonist and anticholinergic
- Intravenous corticosteroid

Repeat Assessment
Symptoms, physical examination, PEF, O$_2$ saturation, other tests as needed

Admit to Hospital Intensive Care
(see box)

Moderate Exacerbation
FEV$_1$ or PEF 50%-80% predicted/personal best
Physical exam: moderate symptoms
- Inhaled short-acting beta$_2$-agonist every 60 minutes
- Systemic corticosteroid or increased dose of inhaled corticosteroid
- Continue treatment 1-3 hours, provided there is improvement

Severe Exacerbation
FEV$_1$ or PEF <50% predicted/personal best
Physical exam: severe symptoms at rest, accessory muscle use, chest retraction
History: high-risk patient
No improvement after initial treatment
- Inhaled short-acting beta$_2$-agonist, hourly or continuous + inhaled anticholinergic
- Oxygen
- Systemic corticosteroid

Good Response
- FEV$_1$ or PEF ≥70%
- Response sustained 60 minutes after last treatment
- No distress
- Physical exam: normal

Incomplete Response
FEV$_1$ or PEF ≥50% but <70%
Mild-to-moderate symptoms

Poor Response
FEV$_1$ or PEF <50%
PCO$_2$ ≥42 mm Hg
Physical exam: symptoms severe, drowsiness, confusion

Individualized decision re: hospitalization (see text)

Discharge Home
- Continue treatment with inhaled beta$_2$-agonist
- Continue course of oral systemic corticosteroid
- Patient education
  - Review medicine use
  - Review/initiate action plan
  - Recommend close medical follow-up

Admit to Hospital Ward
- Inhaled beta$_2$-agonist + inhaled anticholinergic
- Systemic (oral or intravenous) corticosteroid
- Oxygen
- Monitor FEV$_1$ or PEF, O$_2$ saturation, pulse

Admit to Hospital Intensive Care
- Inhaled beta$_2$-agonist hourly or continuously + inhaled anticholinergic
- Intravenous corticosteroid
- Oxygen
- Possible intubation and mechanical ventilation

Improve

Discharge Home
- Continue treatment with inhaled beta$_2$-agonist
- Continue course of oral systemic corticosteroid
- Patient education
  - Review medicine use
  - Review/initiate action plan
  - Recommend close medical follow-up

ESTIMATED COMPARATIVE DAILY DOSAGES FOR INHALED CORTICOSTEROIDS

Adults

Drug	Low Dose	Medium Dose	High Dose
Beclomethasone dipropionate	168-504 mcg	504-840 mcg	>840 mcg
42 mcg/puff	4-12 puffs	12-20 puffs	>20 puffs
84 mcg/puff	2-6 puffs	6-10 puffs	>10 puffs
Beclomethasone dipropionate HFA	80-240 mcg	240-640 mcg	>640 mcg
40 mcg/puff	2-6 puffs	6-16 puffs	>16 puffs
80 mcg/puff	1-3 puffs	3-8 puffs	>8 puffs
Budesonide Turbuhaler	200-600 mcg	600-1200 mcg	>1200 mcg
200 mcg/inhalation	1-3 inhalations	3-6 inhalations	>6 inhalations
Flunisolide	500-1000 mcg	1000-2000 mcg	>2000 mcg
250 mcg/puff	2-4 puffs	4-8 puffs	>8 puffs
Fluticasone	88-264 mcg	264-660 mcg	>660 mcg
MDI: 44, 110, 220 mcg/puff			
DPI: 50, 100, 250 mcg/dose			
Triamcinolone acetonide	400-1000 mcg	1000-2000 mcg	>2000 mcg
100 mcg/puff	4-10 puffs	10-20 puffs	>20 puffs

Children

Drug	Low Dose	Medium Dose	High Dose
Beclomethasone dipropionate	84-336 mcg	336-672 mcg	>672 mcg
42 mcg/puff	2-8 puffs	8-16 puffs	>16 puffs
84 mcg/puff	1-4 puffs	4-8 puffs	>8 puffs
Beclomethasone dipropionate HFA	80-160 mcg	160-320 mcg	>320 mcg
40 mcg/puff	2-4 puffs	4-8 puffs	>8 puffs
80 mcg/puff	1-2 puffs	2-4 puffs	>4 puffs
Budesonide Turbuhaler	200-400 mcg	400-800 mcg	>800 mcg
200 mcg/inhalation	1-2 inhalations	2-4 inhalations	>4 inhalations
Inhalation suspension for nebulization	0.5 mg	1 mg	2 mg
Flunisolide	500-750 mcg	1000-1250 mcg	>1250 mcg
250 mcg/puff	2-3 puffs	4-5 puffs	>5 puffs
Fluticasone	88-176 mcg	176-440 mcg	>440 mcg
MDI: 44, 110, 220 mcg/puff			
DPI: 50, 100, 250 mcg/dose			
Triamcinolone acetonide	400-800 mcg	800-1200 mcg	>1200 mcg
100 mcg/puff	4-8 puffs	8-12 puffs	>12 puffs

Notes:

- **The most important determinant of appropriate dosing is the clinician's judgment of the patient's response to therapy.** The clinician must monitor the patient's response on several clinical parameters and adjust the dose accordingly. The stepwise approach to therapy emphasizes that once control of asthma is achieved, the dose of mediation should be carefully titrated to the minimum dose required to maintain control, thus reducing the potential for adverse effect.
- The reference point for the range in the dosages for children is data on the safety on inhaled corticosteroids in children, which, in general, suggest that the dose ranges are equivalent to beclomethasone dipropionate 200-400 mcg/day (low dose), 400-800 mcg/day (medium dose), and >800 mcg/day (high dose).
- Some dosages may be outside package labeling.
- Metered-dose inhaler (MDI) dosages are expressed as the actuator dose (the amount of drug leaving the actuator and delivered to the patient), which is the labeling required in the United States. This is different from the dosage expressed as the valve dose (the amount of drug leaving the valve, all of which is not available to the patient), which is used in many European countries and in some of the scientific literature. Dry powder inhaler (DPI) doses (eg, Turbuhaler) are expressed as the amount of drug in the inhaler following activation.

ASTHMA *(Continued)*

ESTIMATED CLINICAL COMPARABILITY OF DOSES FOR INHALED CORTICOSTEROIDS

Data from *in vitro* and in clinical trials suggest that the different inhaled corticosteroid preparations are not equivalent on a per puff or microgram basis. However, it is not entirely clear what implications these differences have for dosing recommendations in clinical practice because there are few data directly comparing the preparations. Relative dosing for clinical comparability is affected by differences in topical potency, clinical effects at different doses, delivery device, and bioavailability. The Expert Panel developed recommended dose ranges for different preparations based on available data and the following assumptions and cautions about estimating relative doses needed to achieve comparable clinical effect.

Relative Topical Potency Using Human Skin Blanching

- The standard test for determining relative topical anti-inflammatory potency is the topical vasoconstriction (MacKenzie skin blanching) test.

- The MacKenzie topical skin blanching test correlates with binding affinities and binding half-lives for human lung corticosteroid receptors (see following table) (Dahlberg, et al, 1984; Hogger and Rohdewald 1994).

- The relationship between relative topical anti-inflammatory effect and clinical comparability in asthma management is not certain. However, recent clinical trials suggest that different *in vitro* measures of anti-inflammatory effect correlate with clinical efficacy (Barnes and Pedersen 1993; Johnson 1996; Kamada, et al, 1996; Ebden, et al, 1986; Leblanc, et al, 1994; Gustaffson, et al, 1993; Lundback, et al, 1993; Barnes, et al, 1993; Fabbri, et al, 1993; Langdon and Capsey, 1994; Ayres, et al, 1995; Rafferty, et al, 1985; Bjorkander, et al, 1982, Stiksa, et al, 1982; Willey, et al, 1982.)

Medication	Topical Potency (Skin Blanching)[1]	Corticosteroid Receptor Binding Half-Life	Receptor Binding Affinity
Beclomethasone dipropionate (BDP)	600	7.5 hours	13.5
Budesonide (BUD)	980	5.1 hours	9.4
Flunisolide (FLU)	330	3.5 hours	1.8
Fluticasone propionate (FP)	1200	10.5 hours	18.0
Triamcinolone acetonide (TAA)	330	3.9 hours	3.6

[1]Numbers are assigned in reference to dexamethasone, which has a value of "1" in the MacKenzie test.

Relative Doses to Achieve Similar Clinical Effects

- Clinical effects are evaluated by a number of outcome parameters (eg, changes in spirometry, peak flow rates, symptom scores, quick-relief beta$_2$-agonist use, frequency of exacerbations, airway responsiveness).
- The daily dose and duration of treatment may affect these outcome parameters differently (eg, symptoms and peak flow may improve at lower doses and over a shorter treatment time than bronchial reactivity) (van Essen-Zandvliet, et al, 1992; Haahtela, et al, 1991).
- Delivery systems influence comparability. For example, the delivery device for budesonide (Turbuhaler) delivers approximately twice the amount of drug to the airway as the MDI, thus enhancing the clinical effect (Thorsson, et al, 1994; Agertoft and Pedersen, 1993).
- Individual patients may respond differently to different preparations, as noted by clinical experience.
- Clinical trials comparing effects in reducing symptoms and improving peak expiratory flow demonstrate:
  - BDP and BUD achieved comparable effects at similar microgram doses by MDI (Bjorkander, et al, 1982; Ebden, et al, 1986; Rafferty, et al, 1985).
  - BDP achieved effects similar to twice the dose of TAA on a microgram basis.

Reference

National Asthma Education and Prevention Program (NAEPP), Clinical Practice Guidelines, Expert Panel Report 2, "Guidelines for the Diagnosis and Management of Asthma," NIH Publication No. 97-4051, July 1997.

COMMUNITY-ACQUIRED PNEUMONIA IN ADULTS

The initial site of treatment should be based on a 3-step process:

1. assessment of pre-existing conditions that compromise safety of home care
2. calculation of the pneumonia PORT (Pneumonia Outcome Research Team) Severity Index with recommendation for home care for risk classes I, II, and III, and
3. clinical judgment

Algorithm

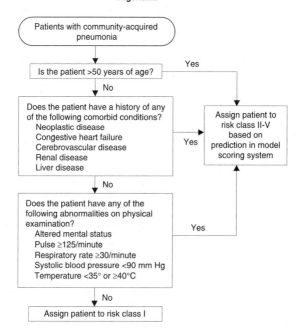

Stratification of Risk Score

Risk	Risk Class	Based on
	I	Algorithm
Low	II	≤70 total points
	III	71-90 total points
Moderate	IV	91-130 total points
High	V	>130 total points

COMMUNITY-ACQUIRED PNEUMONIA IN ADULTS *(Continued)*

Risk-Class Mortality Rates for Patients With Pneumonia

Risk Class	No. of Points	Validation Cohort		Recommended Site of Care
		No. of Patients	Mortality (%)	
I	No predictors	3034	0.1	Outpatient
II	≤70	5778	0.6	Outpatient
III	71-90	6790	2.8	Outpatient or brief inpatient
IV	91-130	13,104	8.2	Inpatient
V	>130	9333	29.2	Inpatient

Epidemiological Conditions Related to Specific Pathogens in Patients With Selected Community-Acquired Pneumonia

Condition	Commonly Encountered Pathogens
Alcoholism	*Streptococcus pneumoniae*, anaerobes
COPD and/or smoker	*S. pneumoniae, Haemophilus influenzae, Moraxella catarrhalis, Legionella* species
Nursing home residency	*S. pneumoniae*, gram-negative bacilli, *H. influenzae, Staphylococcus aureus*, anaerobes, *Chlamydia pneumoniae*
Poor dental hygiene	Anaerobes
Epidemic Legionnaires' disease	*Legionella* species
Exposure to bats or soil enriched with bird droppings	*Histoplasma capsulatum*
Exposure to birds	*Chlamydia psittaci*
Exposure to rabbits	*Francisella tularensis*
HIV infection (early stage)	*S. pneumoniae, H. influenzae, Mycobacterium tuberculosis*
HIV infection (late stage)	Above plus *P. carinii, Cryptococcus, Histoplasma* species
Travel to southwestern United States	*Coccidioides* species
Exposure to farm animals or parturient cats	*Coxiella burnetii* (Q fever)
Influenza active in community	Influenza, *S. pneumoniae, S. aureus, Streptococcus pyogenes, H. influenzae*
Suspected large-volume aspiration	Anaerobes (chemical pneumonitis, obstruction)
Structural disease of the lung (bronchiectasis, cystic fibrosis, etc)	*Pseudomonas aeruginosa, Burkholderia (Pseudomonas) cepacia, S. aureus*
Injection drug use	*S. aureus*, anaerobes, *M. tuberculosis, S. pneumoniae*
Airway obstruction	Anaerobes, *S. pneumoniae, H. influenzae, S. aureus*

COPD = chronic obstructive pulmonary disease.

APPENDIX / TREATMENT / PROPHYLAXIS GUIDELINES

Scoring System: Assignment to Risk Classes II-V

Patient Characteristic	Points Assigned[1]
Demographic factors	
Age	
Male	No. of years
Female	No. of years -10
Nursing home resident	+10
Comorbid illnesses	
Neoplastic disease[2]	+30
Liver disease[3]	+20
Congestive heart failure[4]	+10
Cerebrovascular disease[5]	+10
Renal disease[6]	+10
Physical examination findings	
Altered mental status[7]	+20
Respiratory rate >30 breaths/minute	+20
Systolic blood pressure <90 mm Hg	+20
Temperature <35°C or >40°C	+15
Pulse >125 beats/minute	+10
Laboratory or radiographic findings	
Arterial pH <7.35	+30
BUN >30 mg/dL	+20
Sodium <130 mEq/L	+20
Glucose >250 mg/dL	+10
Hematocrit <30%	+10
pO$_2$ <60 mm Hg[8]	+10
Pleural effusion	+10

[1]A total point score for a given patient is obtained by adding the patient's age in years (age -10, for females) and the points for each applicable patient characteristic.
[2]Any cancer, except basal or squamous cell cancer of the skin, that was active at the time of presentation or diagnosed within 1 year of presentation.
[3]A clinical or histologic diagnosis of cirrhosis or other form of chronic liver disease such as chronic active hepatitis.
[4]Systolic or diastolic ventricular dysfunction documented by history and physical examination, as well as chest radiography, echocardiography, Muga scanning, or left ventriculography.
[5]A clinical diagnosis of stroke, transient ischemic attack, or stroke documented by MRI or computed axial tomography.
[6]A history of chronic renal disease or abnormal blood urea nitrogen (BUN) and creatinine values documented in the medical record.
[7]Disorientation (to person, place, or time; not known to be chronic), stupor, or coma.
[8]In the Pneumonia Patient Outcome Research Team cohort study, an oxygen saturation value <90% on pulse oximetry or intubation before admission was also considered abnormal.

COMMUNITY-ACQUIRED PNEUMONIA IN ADULTS *(Continued)*

Table 1. Initial Empiric Therapy for Suspected Bacterial Community-Acquired Pneumonia (CAP) in Immunocompetent Adults

Patient Variable	Preferred Treatment Options
Outpatient	
Previously healthy	
No recent antibiotic therapy	A macrolide[1] or doxycycline
Recent antibiotic therapy[2]	A respiratory fluoroquinolone[3] alone, an advanced macrolide[4] plus high-dose amoxicillin,[5] or an advanced macrolide plus high-dose amoxicillin-clavulanate[6]
Comorbidities (COPD, diabetes, renal or congestive heart failure, or malignancy)	
No recent antibiotic therapy	An advanced macrolide[4] or a respiratory fluoroquinolone
Recent antibiotic therapy	A respiratory fluoroquinolone[3] alone or an advanced macrolide plus a β-lactam[7]
Suspected aspiration with infection	Amoxicillin-clavulanate or clindamycin
Influenza with bacterial superinfection	A β-lactam[7] or a respiratory fluoroquinolone
Inpatient	
Medical ward	
No recent antibiotic therapy	A respiratory fluoroquinolone alone or an advanced macrolide plus a β-lactam[8]
Recent antibiotic therapy	An advanced macrolide plus a β-lactam or a respiratory fluoroquinolone alone (regimen selected will depend on nature of recent antibiotic therapy)
ICU	
Pseudomonas infection is not an issue	A β-lactam[8] plus either an advanced macrolide or a respiratory fluoroquinolone
Pseudomonas infection is not an issue but patient has a β-lactam allergy	A respiratory fluoroquinolone, with or without clindamycin
Pseudomonas infection is an issue[9]	Either (1) an antipseudomonal agent[10] plus ciprofloxacin, or (2) an antipseudomonal agent plus an aminoglycoside[11] plus a respiratory fluoroquinolone or a macrolide
Pseudomonas infection is an issue but the patient has a β-lactam allergy	Either (1) aztreonam plus levofloxacin,[12] or (2) aztreonam plus moxifloxacin or gatifloxacin, with or without an aminoglycoside
Nursing home	
Receiving treatment in nursing home	A respiratory fluoroquinolone alone or amoxicillin-clavulanate plus an advanced macrolide
Hospitalized	Same as for medical ward and ICU

COPD = chronic obstructive pulmonary disease; ICU = intensive care unit.

[1] Erythromycin, azithromycin, or clarithromycin.

[2] That is, the patient was given a course of antibiotic(s) for treatment of any infection within the past 3 months, excluding the current episode of infection. Such treatment is a risk factor for drug-resistant *Streptococcus pneumoniae* and possibly for infection with gram-negative bacilli. Depending on the class of antibiotics recently given, one or other of the suggested options may be selected. Recent use of a fluoroquinolone should dictate selection of a nonfluoroquinolone regimen, and vice versa.

[3] Moxifloxacin, gatifloxacin, levofloxacin, or gemifloxacin (oral gemifloxacin only, which was approved by the U.S. Food and Drug Administration on April 4, 2003 and which is the only fluoroquinolone approved for multidrug-resistant *S. pneumoniae*; not yet marketed).

[4] Azithromycin or clarithromycin.

[5] Dosage, 1 g P.O. 3 times/day.

[6] Dosage, 2 g P.O. twice daily.

[7] High-dose amoxicillin, high-dose amoxicillin-clavulanate, cefpodoxime, cefprozil, or cefuroxime.

[8] Cefotaxime, ceftriaxone, ampicillin-sulbactam, or ertapenem; ertapenem was recently approved for such use (in once-daily parenteral treatment), but there is little experience thus far.

[9] The antipseudomonal agents chosen reflect this concern. Risk factors for *Pseudomonas* infection include severe structural lung disease (eg, bronchiectasis), and recent antibiotic therapy or stay in hospital (especially in the ICU). For patients with CAP in the ICU, coverage for *S. pneumoniae* and *Legionella* species must always be assured. Piperacillin-tazobactam, imipenem, meropenem, and cefepime are excellent β-lactams and are adequate for most *S. pneumoniae* and *Haemophilus influenzae* infections. They may be preferred when there is concern for relatively unusual CAP pathogens, such as *Pseudomonas aeruginosa*, *Klebsiella* species, and other gram-negative bacteria.

[10] Piperacillin, piperacillin-tazobactam, imipenem, meropenem, or cefepime.

[11] Data suggest that elderly patients receiving aminoglycosides have worse outcomes.

[12] Dosage for hospitalized patients, 750 mg daily.

Table 2. Empiric Antibacterial Selection for Community-Acquired Pneumonia (CAP): Advantages and Disadvantages

Patient Group, Drug(s)	Advantages	Disadvantages
Outpatients		
Macrolides (azithromycin, clarithromycin, and erythromycin)	Active against most common pathogen, including atypical agents.	Macrolide resistance is reported for 20% to 30% of *Streptococcus pneumoniae*, and *in vitro* resistance has emerged during therapy.
	S. pneumoniae resistance *in vitro* may be deceptive, because the M phenotype may not be clinically relevant, and alveolar lining fluid or intracellular levels may be more important than serum levels used to determine *in vitro* activity.	Breakthrough pneumococcal bacteria with macrolide-resistant strains appear to be more common than with β-lactams or fluoroquinolones.
	Clinical trial data have shown consistently good results, including activity against strains resistant *in vitro*.	Erythromycin is poorly tolerated and is less effective against *Haemophilus influenzae*.
	Azithromycin and clarithromycin have the advantage of once-daily therapy and are well tolerated.	
Amoxicillin	Amoxicillin is the preferred drug for oral treatment of susceptible strains of *S. pneumoniae*.	Lacks activity against atypical agents and β-lactamase producing bacteria.
	Active against 90% to 95% of *S. pneumoniae* strains when used at a dosage of 3-4 g/day.	High dosages (3-4 g/day) required to achieve activity against >90% of *S. pneumoniae*
	Standard in many European CAP guidelines for empiric treatment of outpatients, as well as CDC guidelines.	The number of recent publications documenting efficacy is modest.
Amoxicillin-clavulanate	Compared with amoxicillin, spectrum *in vitro* includes β-lactamase producing bacteria, such as most *H. influenzae*, methicillin-susceptible *Staphylococcus aureus*, and anaerobes.	Lacks activity against atypical agents.
	Clinical trials reported to document efficacy.	More expensive and more gastrointestinal intolerance, compared with amoxicillin.
	Standard in many European CAP guidelines for empiric treatment of outpatients, as well as CDC guidelines.	The number of recent publications documenting efficacy is relatively modest.
Oral cephalosporins (cefpodoxime, cefprozil and cefuroxime axetil)	Active against 75% to 85% of *S. pneumoniae* and virtually all *H. influenzae*	All cephalosporins (and all β-lactams) are inactive against atypical agents.
	Clinical trial data support efficacy in outpatients with CAP.	Amoxicillin is more predictably active against *S. pneumoniae* (cefprozil and cefpodoxime are more active than cefuroxime).
Doxycycline	Active against 90% to 95% of strains of *S. pneumoniae*; also active against *H. influenzae*, atypical agents, and category A bacterial agents of bioterrorism.	Very limited recent published clinical data on CAP, and few clinicians use it.
	At least 1 recent report showing good outcomes in hospitalized patients with CAP.	
	Generally well tolerated and inexpensive.	

COMMUNITY-ACQUIRED PNEUMONIA IN ADULTS *(Continued)*

Table 2. Empiric Antibacterial Selection for Community-Acquired Pneumonia (CAP): Advantages and Disadvantages *(continued)*

Patient Group, Drug(s)	Advantages	Disadvantages
Fluoroquinolones (gatifloxacin, levofloxacin, moxifloxacin, and gemifloxacin)	Active against >98% of *S. pneumoniae* strains in United States, including penicillin-resistant strains.	Concern for abuse with risk of increasing resistance by *S. pneumoniae*; this includes clinical failures attributed to emergence of resistance during therapy and selection of resistant strains such as 23F that may be prevalent in selected areas and are usually resistant to macrolides and β-lactams as well.
	Substantial comparative clinical trial data to confirm equivalence or superiority to alternative commonly used regimens, and a meta-analysis of trials showed significantly better outcomes than for β-lactams or macrolides.	Expensive compared with some alternatives, such as doxycycline or erythromycin.
	Active against *H. influenzae*, atypical agents, methicillin-susceptible *S. aureus*, and category A bacterial agents of bioterrorism.	
	Regimens have advantage of once-daily administration and are well tolerated.	
Clindamycin	Active against 90% of *S. pneumoniae*.	Not active against *H. influenzae* or atypical agents.
	Good *in vitro* activity and established efficacy in anaerobic bacterial infections and favored for toxic shock associated with pneumonia due to group A streptococci.	Limited published data on use for CAP.
		High rates of diarrhea and *Clostridium difficile* associated colitis.
Macrolide plus amoxicillin-clavulanate	Macrolide adds activity against atypical agents to spectrum of amoxicillin-clavulanate (described above).	Limited published data for outpatients.
		Requires high dosages of amoxicillin-clavulanate (4 g/day).
		High rates of gastrointestinal intolerance anticipated.
		Unlikely to be effective against fluoroquinolone-resistant strains of *S. pneumoniae*.
		Escalating rates of resistance to both macrolides and penicillin by *S. pneumoniae*.
Hospitalized Patients		
Fluoroquinolones (gatifloxacin, levofloxacin, moxifloxacin, and gemifloxacin)	Broad spectrum of activity against likely agents of CAP (summarized above).	Concern for increasing resistance, as summarized above.
	Extensive published data, including retrospective analysis of hospitalized Medicare patients, showing significantly lower mortality than for macrolides alone or cephalosporins alone.	Clinical failures attributed to resistant strains reported.
	Efficacy in serious infections, including bacteremic pneumococcal pneumonia, established.	

Table 2. Empiric Antibacterial Selection for Community-Acquired Pneumonia (CAP): Advantages and Disadvantages *(continued)*

Patient Group, Drug(s)	Advantages	Disadvantages
	Available in oral and parenteral formulations (except for gemifloxacin, for which only oral formulations are available), facilitating intravenous-to-oral switch.	
Macrolides (azithromycin and erythromycin)	*In vitro* spectrum summarized above.	Retrospective analysis of 14,000 hospitalized Medicare recipients for 1998-1999 shows mortality rate for macrolide alone was significantly greater than that for cephalosporin plus a macrolide or a fluoroquinolone alone.
	Extensive clinical trial data and clinical experience to document efficacy for CAP.	Increasing *in vitro* resistance by *S. pneumoniae*, as summarized above.
	Azithromycin is included as an appropriate choice in many current CAP guidelines, including the guidelines of the American Thoracic Society.	Breakthrough bacteremia due to resistant strains of *S. pneumoniae* is unusual but appears to be more common with macrolides than with other agents.
Cephalosporins (ceftriaxone and cefotaxime)	Considered the parenteral drugs of choice (as well as penicillin G) for CAP caused by susceptible strains of *S. pneumoniae*.	Not active against atypical agents or category A agents of bioterrorism.
	Active *in vitro* against 90% to 95% of *S. pneumoniae*; also active against *H. influenzae* and methicillin-susceptible *S. aureus*.	Retrospective analysis of 14,000 Medicare patients showed higher mortality for cephalosporins alone than for cephalosporins plus macrolides or fluoroquinolones alone.
	Extensive clinical trial experience to document efficacy.	Increasing resistance by *S. pneumoniae*.
Fluoroquinolone plus cephalosporin	May increase antimicrobial activity against *S. pneumoniae*.	No documented benefit, compared with fluoroquinolone alone.
Macrolide plus cephalosporin	Cephalosporin provides better *in vitro* activity against *S. pneumoniae*, and macrolide adds activity against atypical agents.	Data suggesting that the macrolide-cephalosporin combination is superior to monotherapy in pneumococcal bacteremia are uncontrolled and inconsistent (P. Houck, personal communication).
	Retrospective analyses show reduced mortality for this combination, compared with single-agent therapy, in patients with pneumococcal bacteremia and for empiric treatment of pneumonia.	
Penicillin G	Preferred agent (along with ceftriaxone, cefotaxime, and amoxicillin) for proven penicillin-susceptible strains of *S. pneumoniae*.	Limited spectrum of activity against common pulmonary pathogens other than *S. pneumoniae*.
	Published experience to document clinical efficacy is extensive.	

New Agents

Patient Group, Drug(s)	Advantages	Disadvantages
Telithromycin	Active *in vitro* against most *S. pneumoniae*, including macrolide-resistant strains; also active against *H. influenzae* and atypical agents.	Available only in oral formulation.
	Favorable pharmacokinetics.	Clinical trial data are considered preliminary.

COMMUNITY-ACQUIRED PNEUMONIA IN ADULTS *(Continued)*

Table 2. Empiric Antibacterial Selection for Community-Acquired Pneumonia (CAP): Advantages and Disadvantages *(continued)*

Patient Group, Drug(s)	Advantages	Disadvantages
	Clinical trials in CAP show equivalence to high-dose amoxicillin, macrolides, and trovafloxacin, including CAP caused by β-lactam resistant strains of *S. pneumoniae*.	
Gemifloxacin	Most active of the "respiratory fluoroquinolone" against *S. pneumoniae in vitro*.	High rate of rash, especially in women aged <40 years and with use for >10 days.
	Clinical trial data for CAP show good results.	Available only in oral formulation.
Ertapenem	Clinical efficacy for empiric treatment of CAP comparable to ceftriaxone.	Parenteral formulation only.
	Once-daily parenteral dosing.	Inactive against atypical agents and less active than imipenem against *Pseudomonas aeruginosa*.
	In vitro activity against *S. pneumoniae* is similar to ceftriaxone and cefotaxime.	
Linezolid	Active *in vitro* against most gram-positive bacteria, including multidrug resistant *S. pneumoniae* and *S. aureus*.	Lacks established activity against atypical agents.
	Efficacy comparable to ceftriaxone for treatment of pneumococcal pneumonia.	Alternative antimicrobials have more established role in CAP.
	Oral and parenteral formulations.	Concern about abuse, expense, drug-drug interaction, and toxicity.

Note: Durations of therapy are as follows: *S. pneumoniae*, until afebrile for 72 hours; *M. pneumoniae*, duration of therapy for newer agents is not well established; *C. pneumoniae*, numerous clinical trials indicate good clinical response with 7-14 days of treatment; *Legionella*, 10-21 days; pathogens that potentially cause pulmonary necrosis (*S. aureus*, *P. aeruginosa*, *Klebsiella* species, or anaerobes), ≥2 weeks. CDC, Centers for Disease Control and Prevention.

ANTIMICROBIAL TREATMENT

Pathogen-Specific Therapy

S. pneumoniae: Susceptibility of *S. pneumoniae* isolates to cefotaxime and ceftriaxone in nonmeningeal infections should be defined as an MIC of ≤1 mcg/mL, intermediate should be defined as an MIC of 2 mcg/mL, and resistant should be defined as an MIC of ≥4 mcg/mL. Cefotaxime or ceftriaxone are the preferred parenteral agents for treatment of pneumococcal pneumonia without meningitis for strains with reduced susceptibility to penicillin but with MICs of cefotaxime or ceftriaxone of <2 mcg/mL. Amoxicillin is the preferred antibiotic for oral treatment of pneumococcal pneumonia involving susceptible strains.

Initial empiric therapy prior to availability of culture data for a patient ill enough to require admission to a hospital ward can be with a β-lactam plus macrolide combination or a respiratory fluoroquinolone alone. If sufficiently ill to need ICU management and if *Pseudomonas* infection is not a concern, a combination of a β-lactam plus either a macrolide or a respiratory fluoroquinolone should be used. Once culture data are available and it is known that the patient has pneumococcal pneumonia with bacteremia without evidence to support infection with a copathogen, treatment will depend upon *in vitro* susceptibility results. If the isolate is penicillin susceptible, a β-lactam (penicillin G or amoxicillin) alone may be used. If the isolate is penicillin resistant, cefotaxime, ceftriaxone, or a respiratory fluoroquinolone or other agent indicated by *in vitro* testing may be used.

Legionella: Treatment for legionnaires' disease is appropriate when there is epidemiologic evidence of this disease, despite negative diagnostic test results. The preferred treatment for legionnaires' disease for hospitalized patients is azithromycin or a fluoroquinolone (moxifloxacin, gatifloxacin, and levofloxacin; gemifloxacin is only available as an oral formulation). For patients who do not require hospitalization, acceptable antibiotics include erythromycin, doxycycline, azithromycin, clarithromycin, or a fluoroquinolone. Treatment should be initiated as rapidly as is feasible.

Influenza: Early treatment (within 48 hours after onset of symptoms) is effective in the treatment of influenza A using amantadine, rimantadine, oseltamivir, or zanamivir and is effective in the treatment influenza B using oseltamivir and zanamivir. Use of these drugs is not recommended for uncomplicated influenza with a duration of symptoms of >48 hours, but these drugs may be used to reduce viral shedding in hospitalized patients or for influenza pneumonia.

Herpes viruses: Pneumonia caused by varicella zoster virus or herpes simplex virus should be treated with parenteral acyclovir.

Other viruses: There is no antiviral agent with established efficacy for the treatment of adults with pulmonary infections involving parainfluenza virus, respiratory syncytial virus, adenovirus, metapneumovirus, the SARS agent, or Hantavirus.

Empiric Therapy

See Table 1 and Table 2.

Empiric treatment of suspected bacterial superinfection of influenza should provide activity against *S. pneumoniae, Staphylococcus aureus*, and *Haemophilus influenzae* with antibiotics such as amoxicillin-clavulanate, cefpodoxime, cefprozil, cefuroxime, or a respiratory fluoroquinolone.

Fluoroquinolones (gatifloxacin, gemifloxacin, levofloxacin, and moxifloxacin) are recommended for initial empiric therapy of selected outpatients with CAP. Other options (macrolides and doxycycline) are generally preferred for uncomplicated infections in outpatients. Fluoroquinolones (gatifloxacin, gemifloxacin, levofloxacin, and moxifloxacin) may be used as monotherapy for patients with CAP who are admitted to a hospital ward. With the exception of gemifloxacin (no intravenous formulation), they may be used as part of a combination for patients with CAP admitted to an ICU.

A macrolide is recommended as monotherapy for selected outpatients, such as those who were previously well and not recently treated with antibiotics. A macrolide plus a β-lactam is recommended for initial empiric treatment of outpatients in whom resistance is an issue and for hospitalized patients.

Telithromycin may have a role as an alternative to macrolides for treatment of patients with CAP.

COMMUNITY-ACQUIRED PNEUMONIA IN ADULTS *(Continued)*

Special Populations and Circumstances

SARS: Health care workers must be vigilant in recognizing SARS because of important epidemiologic implications, which include the potential for rapid spread to close contacts, including health care workers and household contacts. The major therapeutic intervention is supportive care. Preventive efforts include proper precautions in patients with suspected or established SARS. These include standard precautions (hand hygiene), contact precautions (use of gowns, goggles, and gloves), and airborne precautions (use of negative-pressure rooms and fit-tested N95 respirators).

Elderly patients: Antimicrobial selection for elderly patients with CAP is the same as for all adults with CAP.

Bioterrorism: Physicians should know the clues to bioterrorism and the appropriate mechanisms to alert public health officials in cases of suspected bioterrorism. Recommended diagnostic tests and management guidelines are those of the Johns Hopkins Center for Biodefense Strategies and of the CDC, as modified for the specific outbreak.

References

Bartlett JG, Breiman RF, Mandell LA, et al, "Community-Acquired Pneumonia in Adults: Guidelines for Management. The Infectious Diseases Society of America," *Clin Infect Dis*, 1998, 26(4):811-38.

Mandell LA, Bartlett JG, Dowell SF, et al, "Update of Practice Guidelines for the Management of Community-Acquired Pneumonia in Immunocompetent Adults," *Clin Infect Dis*, 2003, 37(11):1405-33.

DEPRESSION

Criteria for Major Depressive Episode

A. Five (or more) of the following symptoms have been present during the same 2-week period and represent a change from previous functioning; at least one of the symptoms is either (1) depressed mood or (2) loss of interest or pleasure.

1. Depressed mood most of the day, nearly every day

2. Marked diminished interest or pleasure in all, or almost all, activities

3. Significant weight loss (not dieting) or weight gain, or decrease or increase in appetite nearly every day

4. Insomnia or hypersomnia nearly every day

5. Psychomotor agitation or retardation nearly every day

6. Fatigue or loss of energy nearly every day

7. Feelings of worthlessness or excessive or inappropriate guilt (may be delusional) nearly every day

8. Diminished ability to think or concentrate, or indecisiveness

9. Recurrent thoughts of death, recurrent suicidal ideation without a specific plan, or a suicide attempt or a specific suicide plan

B. The symptoms cause clinically significant distress or impairment in social, occupational or other important areas of functioning.

C. The symptoms are not due to the direct physiologic effects of a substance or a general medical condition (eg, hypothyroidism).

Medications That May Precipitate Depression

Anticancer agents	Vinblastine, vincristine, interferon, procarbazine, asparaginase, tamoxifen, cyproterone
Anti-inflammatory & analgesic agents	Indomethacin, pentazocine, phenacetin, phenylbutazone
Antimicrobial agents	Cycloserine, ethambutol, sulfonamides, select gram-negative antibiotics
Cardiovascular/ antihypertensive agents	Clonidine, digitalis, diuretics, guanethidine, hydralazine, indapamide, methyldopa, prazosin, procainamide, propranolol, reserpine
CNS agents	Alcohol, amantadine, amphetamine & derivatives, barbiturates, benzodiazepines, chloral hydrate, carbamazepine, cocaine, haloperidol, L-dopa, phenothiazines, succinimide derivatives
Hormonal agents	ACTH, corticosteroids, estrogen, melatonin, oral contraceptives, progesterone
Miscellaneous	Cimetidine, disulfiram, organic pesticides, physostigmine

Medical Disorders & Psychiatric Disorders Associated With Depression

Endocrine diseases	Acromegaly, Addison's disease, Cushing's disease, diabetes mellitus, hyperparathyroidism, hypoparathyroidism, hyperthyroidism, hypothyroidism, insulinoma, pheochromocytoma, pituitary dysfunction
Deficiency states	Pernicious anemia, severe anemia, Wernicke's encephalopathy
Infections	Encephalitis, fungal infections, meningitis, neurosyphilis, influenza, mononucleosis, tuberculosis, AIDS
Collagen disorders	Rheumatoid arthritis
Systemic lupus erythematosus	
Metabolic disorders	Electrolyte imbalance, hypokalemia, hyponatremia, hepatic encephalopathy, Pick's disease, uremia, Wilson's disease
Cardiovascular disease	Cerebral arteriosclerosis, chronic bronchitis, congestive heart failure, emphysema, myocardial infarction, paroxysmal dysrhythmia, pneumonia
Neurologic disorders	Alzheimer's disease, amyotrophic lateral sclerosis, brain tumors, chronic pain syndrome, Creutzfeldt-Jakob disease, Huntington's disease, multiple sclerosis, myasthenia gravis, Parkinson's disease, poststroke, trauma (postconcussion)
Malignant disease	Breast, gastrointestinal, lung, pancreas, prostate
Psychiatric disorders	Alcoholism, anxiety disorders, eating disorders, schizophrenia

DEPRESSION (Continued)

Somatic Treatments of Depression in the Patient With Medical Illness

Condition	First Choice	Second-Line Options	Alternatives
Thyroid			
Hypothyroid	Thyroid (T)	T_4 or T_3 + antidepressant (SSRIs , TCAs, new generation agents)	ECT, other antidepressants psychostimulants
Hyperthyroid	Antidepressant and antihyperthyroid medications	Select a different group of antidepressants	
Diabetes mellitus	SSRIs, other new generation antidepressants	TCAs (second amine or low-dose tertiary amine) MAOIs	ECT, buspirone, psychostimulants, thyroid supplements, mood stabilizers
Cardiovascular disorders	SSRIs, bupropion	ECT, psychostimulants B-blockers, buspirone	ECT, TCAs, MAOIs, mood stabilizers
Renal disease	Fluoxetine, sertraline	TCAs, other new generation antidepressants, psychostimulants	ECT, anticonvulsants, lithium (if dialysis or CLOSELY monitored)
Hepatic disease (reduced dose ALL)	Sertraline	Other new generation antidepressants, TCAs-secondary amines	TCAs-tertiary amines
HIV	Bupropion, SSRIs, psychostimulants	TCAs	ECT
Transplant	**Closely monitor.** See cardiovascular, renal, liver, pulmonary, new antidepressant agents, TCAs-secondary amines		
Neurologic	Newer generation antidepressants, TCAs-secondary amines	Selegiline, anticonvulsants	Bromocriptine
Malignancy	Newer generation antidepressants, TCAs-secondary amines psychostimulants	TCAs-tertiary amines of pain MAOIs	ECT
Respiratory	Activating antidepressants, buspirone		More sedating antidepressants, ECT
Gastrointestinal	TCAs-secondary amines, new generation antidepressants	TCAs-tertiary amines	ECT

DIABETES MELLITUS MANAGEMENT

OVERVIEW

Diabetes represents a significant health care problem in the United States and world-wide. Of the nearly 16 million Americans with diabetes, the majority (90% to 95%) have type 2 diabetes. Of this number, roughly one-third are undiagnosed. The incidence of type 2 diabetes is increasing around the world. There is strong evidence to support an interaction between a genetic predisposition and behavioral or environmental factors, such as obesity and physical inactivity, in the development of this disease. In individuals at high risk of developing type 2 diabetes, it has been shown that the development of diabetes may be prevented by changes in lifestyle (*N Engl J Med*, 2001, 344:1343-50).

Within the United States, type 1 diabetes is estimated to affect 500,000 to 1 million people, and therefore represents the minority of individuals with diabetes. In addition to type 1 and type 2 diabetes, approximately 2% to 5% of pregnancies are complicated by the development of gestational diabetes, which usually remits following delivery. This occurs in women with no previous history of type 1 or type 2 diabetes. However, women who have had gestational diabetes are at an increased risk for later development of type 2 diabetes. In addition to the causes noted above, diabetes may result from genetic syndromes, surgery (pancreatectomy), chemicals and/or drugs, recurrent pancreatitis, malnutrition, and viral infections.

COMPLICATIONS OF DIABETES

Complications due to diabetes comprise the seventh leading cause of death in the United States. The greatest number of these deaths are related to cardiovascular complications (myocardial infarction, CHF, and stroke), which have been estimated to result in more than 77,000 deaths annually.

In addition to cardiovascular effects, diabetes is the leading cause of new blindness in people 20-74 years of age, and diabetic nephropathy is the most common cause of end-stage renal disease. Mild to severe forms of diabetic neuropathy are common. Neuropathy and circulatory insufficiency combine to make diabetes the most frequent cause of nontraumatic lower-limb amputations. The rate of impotence in diabetic males over 50 years of age has been estimated to be as high as 50% to 60%. Control of hyperglycemia may significantly decrease the rate at which diabetic complications develop, and provides compelling justification for early diagnosis and management of this disorder.

DIAGNOSIS

Diabetes

Diagnosis of diabetes is made by any of the three criteria described below. In the absence of unequivocal hyperglycemia with acute metabolic decompensation, these criteria should be confirmed by repeat testing on a different day. The third method, (OGGT), is not recommended for routine clinical use.

1. Symptoms of diabetes (polydipsia, polyuria, unexplained weight loss) plus casual plasma glucose concentration ≥200 mg/dL (11.1 mmol/L)
   Note: Casual plasma glucose is defined as any time of day without regard to time of last meal.

OR

2. Fasting plasma glucose (no caloric intake for at least 8 hours) ≥126 mg/dL (7 mmol/L)

OR

3. A 2-hour plasma glucose ≥200 mg/dL (11.1 mmol/L) during an oral glucose tolerance test (OGTT)

Intermediate Disorders of Glucose Homeostasis

Impaired fasting glucose:

- FPG ≥110 mg/dL (6.1 mmol/L) and <126 mg/dL (7 mmol/L)

- A 2-hour plasma glucose ≥140 mg/dL (7.8 mmol/L) and <200 mg/dL (11.1 mmol/L)

DIABETES MELLITUS MANAGEMENT *(Continued)*

Gestational Diabetes Mellitus (GDM)

Low risk: Routine screening is not recommended; must fulfill **all** criteria:

- <25 years of age
- normal body weight
- no family history of diabetes (ie, first-degree relatives)
- no history of abnormal glucose metabolism
- no history of poor obstetric outcome
- not a member of an ethnic/racial group with a high prevalence of diabetes (Hispanic, Native American, Asian, African, Pacific Islander)

Average risk: Testing at 24-28 weeks gestation is recommended (oral glucose tolerance test – OGTT).

High risk: Initial screening (OGTT) as soon as feasible; repeat at 24-28 weeks gestation.

- marked obesity
- personal history of GDM
- glycosuria
- strong family history

GOALS

The goals of diabetes treatment include normalization of hyperglycemia, avoidance of hypoglycemia, and slowing the development of diabetic complications. The following table lists guidelines for the evaluation of glucose control and parameters for addressing hyperglycemia.

	Normal	Goal	Action Suggested
Plasma (mg/dL)			
Average preprandial glucose	<110	90-130	<90 or >150
Average bedtime glucose	<120	110-150	<110 or >180
Whole Blood (mg/dL)			
Average preprandial glucose	<100	80-120	<80 or >140
Average bedtime glucose	<110	100-140	<100 or >160
Hb A$_{1c}$ (%)	<6	<7	>8

Consult website (http://diabetes.org) for frequently updated guidelines.

MANAGEMENT

Current American Diabetes Association (ADA) recommendations emphasize a multidisciplinary approach to the management of diabetes, with an emphasis on the participation of the patient and/or caregivers in the monitoring and management of the disease. Consultation with a diabetes educator and dietitian may help to prepare the patient to manage his/her disease and adjust to the necessary changes in diet and lifestyle. Patients must be educated about disease monitoring procedures, including blood glucose self-monitoring equipment and tests. Patients should be encouraged to wear or carry appropriate identification to inform health care providers of the disease in the event of an emergency. Foot care and other issues related to possible complications should be addressed. It is extremely important to educate patients concerning the recognition and management of hypoglycemic symptoms. The management of diabetes is constantly adapting to new information, techniques, and technologies. For the most current information on diabetes diagnosis and management, visit the ADA website at http://diabetes.org.

Pharmacological Algorithm for Treatment of Type 2 Diabetes
(Patients inadequately controlled with diet and exercise)

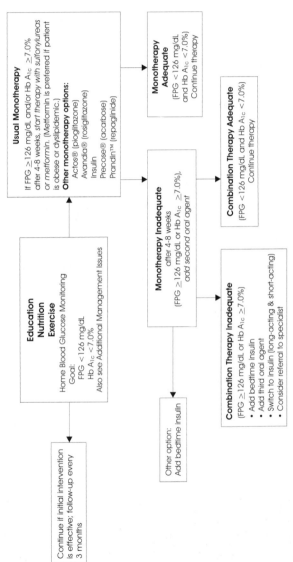

Education
Nutrition
Exercise
Home Blood Glucose Monitoring
Goal:
 FPG <126 mg/dL
 Hb A$_{1c}$ <7.0%
Also see Additional Management Issues

Continue if initial intervention is effective; follow-up every 3 months

Usual Monotherapy
If FPG ≥126 mg/dL and/or Hb A$_{1c}$ ≥7.0% after 4-8 weeks, *start therapy with sulfonylureas or metformin.* (Metformin is preferred if patient is obese or dyslipidemic.)
Other monotherapy options:
 Actos® (pioglitazone)
 Avandia® (rosiglitazone)
 Insulin
 Precose® (acarbose)
 Prandin™ (repaglinide)

Monotherapy Adequate
(FPG <126 mg/dL and Hb A$_{1c}$ <7.0%)
Continue therapy

Monotherapy Inadequate
after 4-8 weeks
(FPG ≥126 mg/dL or Hb A$_{1c}$ ≥7.0%),
add second oral agent

Other option:
Add bedtime insulin

Combination Therapy Adequate
(FPG <126 mg/dL and Hb A$_{1c}$ <7.0%)
Continue therapy

Combination Therapy Inadequate
(FPG ≥126 mg/dL or Hb A$_{1c}$ ≥7.0%)
• Add bedtime insulin
• Add third oral agent
• Switch to insulin (long-acting & short-acting)
• Consider referral to specialist

Modified from DeFronzo RA, "Pharmacological Treatment for Type 2 Diabetes Mellitus," *Ann Intern Med,* 1999, 131:281-303.

DIABETES MELLITUS MANAGEMENT *(Continued)*

Additional Management Issues

Recommendations by the ADA include glycemic control as well as the following:

1. Use an ACEI or ARB in diabetics with micro- or macroalbuminuria to slow the progression of nephropathy, unless contraindicated.

2. Consider statin use in all diabetics, irrespective of lipoprotein levels.

3. Immunize against pneumococcal disease and influenza.

4. Daily ASA use 75-162 mg daily in all diabetics ≥21 years of age, unless contraindicated.

DRUG TREATMENT

Insulin

Insulin therapy is required in type 1 diabetes, and may be necessary in some individuals with type 2 diabetes. Product selection and combination is designed to limit fluctuations in blood glucose values. There is solid scientific documentation of the benefit of tight glucose control, either by insulin pump or multiple daily injections (4-6 times daily). However, the benefits must be balanced against the risk of hypoglycemia, the patient's ability to adhere to the regimen, and other issues regarding the complexity of management. In addition to the educational issues outlined above, patients should be instructed in administration techniques, timing of administration, and sick-day management.

Types of Insulin	Onset (h)	Peak (h)	Duration (h)
Lispro (Humalog®)	0.25	0.5-1.5	6-8
Insulin aspart injection (NovoLog®)	0.25	1-3	3-5
Insulin, regular (Novolin® R)	0.5-1	2-3	8-12
Isophane insulin suspension (NPH) (Novolin® N)	1-1.5	4-12	24
Insulin zinc suspension (Lente®)	1-2.5	8-12	18-24
Isophane insulin suspension and regular insulin injection (Novolin® 70/30)	0.5	2-12	24
Extended insulin zinc suspension (Ultralente®)	4-8	16-18	>36
Insulin glargine (Lantus®)	–	–	24

Oral Agents

A large number of drugs for oral administration have become available for diabetic management. Oral hypoglycemic agents include sulfonylureas, meglitanides, alpha-glucosidase inhibitors, biguanides, and thiazolidinediones (TZDs). The drug classes vary in terms of their magnitude of effect on glycemic control, mechanism of action, and adverse effect profiles. In many cases, the adverse effect profile may influence the selection of a particular drug. The risk of hypoglycemia is higher for drugs which prompt insulin secretion (particularly sulfonylureas or insulin secretagogues). Drug selection is based on patient-specific factors and anticipated tolerance of adverse effects. Contraindications and adverse effect profiles may be compared in the following table.

Contraindications to Therapy and Potential Adverse Effects of Oral Antidiabetic Agents

	Sulfonylureas/ Meglitinide	Metformin (Glucophage®)	Acarbose (Precose®)/ Miglitol (Glyset®)	Pioglitazone (Actos®)/ Rosiglitazone (Avandia®)
Contraindications				
Insulin dependency	A	A	A¹	
Pregnancy/lactation	A	A	A	
Hypersensitivity to the agent	A	A	A	A
Hepatic impairment	R	A	R	A
Renal impairment	R	A	R	
Congestive heart failure		A		R
Chronic lung disease		A		
Peripheral vascular disease		A		
Steroid-induced diabetes	R	R		
Inflammatory bowel disease		A	A	
Major recurrent illness	R	A		
Surgery	R	A		
Alcoholism	R	A		A
Adverse Effects				
Hypoglycemia	Yes	No	No	No
Body weight gain	Yes	No	No	Yes
Hypersensitivity	Yes	No	No	No
Drug interactions	Yes	No	No	Yes/No
Lactic acidosis	No	Yes	No	No
Gastrointestinal disturbances	No	Yes	No	No

¹Can be used in conjunction with insulin. A = absolute; R = relative.

At least two drugs have been withdrawn from the U.S. market due to toxicities. Phenformin was removed many years ago after a number of cases of fatal lactic acidosis were reported. Metformin (a drug similar to phenformin) carries some risk of this reaction, but it is tremendously lower than the risk associated with phenformin. Troglitazone, a prototype thiazolidinedione, was associated with hepatic failure and several deaths, and it was withdrawn shortly after introduction. Currently, marketed drugs from this class appear to have a lower risk of these reactions.

Combination therapy may be necessary to achieve glycemic goals. The risk of additive or additional adverse effects must be balanced with the desire to achieve goals of glycemic control as well as normalization of other metabolic parameters. In particular, weight gain and lipid disturbances may complicate drug treatment.

Effect on Glycemic Control of Oral Hypoglycemic Agents as Monotherapy

Agent	Fasting Blood Glucose (mg/dL)	Postprandial Blood Glucose (mg/dL)	Hb A₁c (%)
Acarbose (Precose®) 25-100 mg 3 times/day	-25	-49	-0.44 to -0.74
Glimepiride (Amaryl®) 1-8 mg/day	-60	NA	-1.5 to 2
Glyburide (Diaβeta®/ Micronase®) 1.25-20 mg/day			
Glyburide (Glynase® PresTab®) 0.75-12 mg/day			
Metformin (Glucophage®) Up to 2500 mg/day	-52	NA	-1.4
Miglitol (Glyset®) 25-50 mg 3 times/day	NA	-35 to -60	-0.3 to -0.82
Nateglinide (Starlix®) 60-120 mg 3 times/day	-54	NA	-0.3 to -0.5
Pioglitazone (Actos®) 15-45 mg/day	-56	NA	-0.3 to 0.9
Repaglinide (Prandin®) 0.25-4 mg 3 times/day	-39.8	-54	-0.6 to -1.9
Rosiglitazone (Avandia®) 4-8 mg/day	-67	NA	-0.3 to 0.7

DIABETES MELLITUS MANAGEMENT *(Continued)*

Class	Key Adverse Effects
Alpha-Glucosidase Inhibitors	GI distress, bloating, flatulence
Acarbose (Precose™)	
Miglitol (Glyset™)	
Biguanide	GI distress (common), lactic acidosis (rare)
Metformin (Glucophage®, Glucophage® XR, Riomet™)	
Secretagogues	Hypoglycemia
Repaglinide (Prandin®)	
Nateglinide (Starlix®)	
Sulfonylureas	Hypoglycemia, allergic reactions, resistance, weight gain
Glimepiride (Amaryl®)	
Glyburide (Diaβeta®, Micronase®, Glynase™ PresTab™)	
Glipizide (Glucotrol®, Glucotrol® XL)	
Older Agents	SIADH (with chlorpropamide)
Acetohexamide	
Chlorpropamide (Diabinese®)	
Tolazamide (Tolinase®)	
Thiazolidinediones	Hepatic dysfunction, hepatic failure, weight gain, edema, CHF, lipid changes
Rosiglitazone (Avandia®)	
Pioglitazone (Actos®)	

2005 ADA Summary of Recommendations for Adults With Diabetes

Glycemic control

A_{1c}	<7%[1]
Preprandial capillary plasma glucose	90-130 mg/dL
Peak postprandial capillary plasma glucose[2]	<180 mg/dL

Blood pressure <130/80 mm Hg

Lipids[3]

LDL	<100 mg/dL
Triglycerides	<150 mg/dL
HDL[4]	>40 mg/dL

Key concepts in setting glycemic goals:

- A_{1c} is the primary target for glycemic control.

- Goals should be individualized.

- Certain populations (children, pregnant women, and elderly) require special considerations.

- Less intensive glycemic goals may be indicated in patients with severe or frequent hypoglycemia.

- More stringent glycemic goals (ie, a normal A_{1c}, <6%) may further reduce complications at the cost of increased risk of hypoglycemia (particularly in those with type 1 diabetes).

- Postprandial glucose may be targeted if A_{1c} goals are not met despite reaching preprandial glucose goals.

Footnotes

[1]Referenced to a nondiabetic range of 4% to 6% using a DCCT-based assay.

[2]Postprandial glucose measurements should be made 1-2 hours after the beginning of the meal, generally peak levels in patients with diabetes.

[3]Current NCEP/ATP III guidelines suggest that in patients with triglycerides ≥200 mg/dL, the "non-HDL cholesterol" (total cholesterol minus HDL) be used. The goal is ≤130 mg/dL.

[4]For women, it has been suggested that the HDL goal be increased by 10 mg/dL.

Comparative Lipid Effects

Parameter	Pioglitazone (Actos®)	Rosiglitazone (Avandia®)
LDL	No significant change	↑ up to 12.1%
HDL	↑ up to 13%	↑ up to 18.5%
Total cholesterol	No significant change	↑
Total cholesterol/HDL ratio	–	–
LDL/HDL ratio	–	No change
Triglycerides	↓ up to 28%	Variable effects

Comparative Pharmacokinetics

Drug	Duration of Action (h)	Daily Dose and Frequency (mg)	Metabolism
First Generation Sulfonylurea Agents			
Acetohexamide	12-24	250-1500 bid	Hepatic (60%) with active metabolite
Chlorpropamide (Diabinese®)	24-72	100-500 qd	Renal excretion (30%) and hepatic metabolism with active metabolites
Tolazamide (Tolinase®)	10-24	100-1000 qd or bid	Hepatic with active metabolites
Tolbutamide	6-24	500-3000 qd-tid	Hepatic
Second Generation Sulfonylurea Agents			
Glimepiride (Amaryl®)	24	1-4 mg qd	Hepatic
Glipizide (Glucotrol®)	12-24	2.5-40 mg qd or bid	Hepatic
Glipizide GITS	24	5-10 qd	Hepatic
Glyburide (DiaBeta®, Glynase®, Micronase®)	16-24	1.25-20 qd or bid	Hepatic with active metabolites
Biguanide			
Metformin (Glucophage®)	12-24	1000-2550 mg/day bid or tid	None; excreted unchanged in urine
Alpha-Glucosidase Inhibitors			
Acarbose (Precose®)	8-12	150-300 mg/day tid	GI tract
Miglitol (Glyset®)	8	50 mg 3 times/day	Renal excretion
Meglitinides			
Nateglinide (Starlix®)	<4	120 mg 3 times/day before meals	Hepatic with active metabolites
Repaglinide (Prandin®)	<4 (single dose)	0.4-4 mg administered with meals 2, 3, or 4 times/day	Hepatic to inactive metabolites

DIABETES MELLITUS MANAGEMENT *(Continued)*

Comparative Thiazolidinedione Pharmacokinetics

Parameter	Pioglitazone (Actos®)	Rosiglitazone (Avandia®)
Absorption	Food slightly delays but does not alter the extent of absorption	Absolute bioavailability is 99% Food ↓ C_{max} and delays T_{max}, but not change in AUC
C_{max}	156-342 ng/mL	–
T_{max}	2 hours	1 hour
Distribution	0.63 ± 0.41 L/kg	17.6 L
Plasma protein binding	>99% to serum albumin	99.8% to serum albumin
Metabolism	Extensive liver metabolism by hydroxylation and oxidation. Some metabolites are pharmacologically active. CYP2C8 and CYP3A4 metabolism	Extensive metabolism via N-demethylation and hydroxylation with no unchanged drug excreted in the urine CYP2C8 and some CYP2C9 metabolism
Excretion	Urine (15% to 30%) and bile	Urine (64%) and feces (23%)
Half-life	3-6 hours (pioglitazone) 16-24 hours (pioglitazone and metabolites)	3.15-3.59 hours
Effect of hemodialysis	Not removed	Not removed

Approved Indications for Thiazolidinedione Derivatives

Indication	Pioglitazone (Actos®)	Rosiglitazone (Avandia®)
Monotherapy	x	x
Combination Therapy – Dual Therapy		
Combination with sulfonylureas	x	x
Combination therapy with Glucophage® (metformin)	x	x
Combination therapy with insulin	x	x
Combination Therapy – Triple Therapy		
Combination therapy with sulfonylureas and Glucophage® (metformin)	–	–

References

American Diabetes Association, "Clinical Practice Recommendations 2005," *Diabetes Care*, 2005, 28(Suppl 1):S1-79.

Colhoun HM, Betteridge DJ, Durrington PN, et al, "Primary Prevention of Cardiovascular Disease With Atorvastatin in Type 2 Diabetes in the Collaborative Atorvastatin Diabetes Study (CARDS): Multicentre Randomised Placebo-Controlled Trial," *Lancet*, 2004, 364(9435):685-96.

Heart Protection Study Collaborative Group, "MRC/BHF Heart Protection Study of Cholesterol Lowering With Simvastatin in 20,536 High-Risk Individuals: A Randomised Placebo-Controlled Trial," *Lancet*, 2002, 360(9326):7-22.

The Diabetes Control and Complications Trial Research Group, "The Effect of Intensive Treatment of Diabetes on the Development and Progression of Long-Term Complications in Insulin-dependent Diabetes Mellitus," *N Engl J Med*, 1993, 329(14):977-86.

The Expert Committee on the Diagnosis and Classification of Diabetes Mellitus, "Report of the Expert Committee on the Diagnosis and Classification of Diabetes Mellitus," *Diabetes Care*, 2002, 25 (Suppl 1).

Tuomilehto J, Lindstrom J, Eriksson JG, et al, "Prevention of Type 2 Diabetes Mellitus by Changes in Lifestyle Among Subjects With Impaired Glucose Tolerance," *N Engl J Med*, 2001, 344(18):1343-50.

UK Prospective Diabetes Study Group, " Intensive Blood Glucose Control With Sulphonylureas or Insulin Compared With Conventional Treatment and Risk of Complications in Patients With Type 2 Diabetes (UKPDS 33)," *Lancet*, 1998, 352(9131):837-53.

GLAUCOMA DRUG THERAPY

Ophthalmic Agent (Brand)	Reduces Aqueous Humor Production	Increases Aqueous Humor Outflow[1]	Average Duration of Action	Strengths Available
Cholinesterase Inhibitors[1]				
Echothiophate (Phospholine Iodide®)	No data	Significant	2 wk	0.03% to 0.25%
Physostigmine	No data	Significant	24 h	0.25%
Direct-Acting Cholinergic Miotics				
Carbachol	Some activity	Significant	8 h	0.75% to 3%
Pilocarpine (various)	Some activity	Significant	5 h	0.5%, 1%, 2%, 3%, 4%
Sympathomimetics				
Apraclonidine (Iopidine®)	Moderate	Moderate	4 h	0.5%, 1%
Brimonidine (Alphagan® P)	Moderate	Moderate	12 h	0.2%
Dipivefrin (Propine®)	Some activity	Moderate	12 h	0.1%
Epinephrine	Some activity	Moderate	18 h	0.25% to 2%
Beta-Blockers				
Betaxolol (Betoptic® S)	Significant	Some activity	12 h	0.5%
Carteolol	Yes	No	12 h	1%
Levobetaxolol [DSC]	Significant	No data	12 h	0.5%
Levobunolol (Betagan®)	Significant	Some activity	18 h	0.5%
Metipranolol (OptiPranolol®)	Significant	Some activity	18 h	0.3%
Timolol (Betimol®, Timoptic®)	Significant	Some activity	18 h	0.25%, 0.5%
Carbonic Anhydrase Inhibitors				
Acetazolamide (Diamox®)	Significant	No data	10 h	250 mg tab; 500 mg cap
Brinzolamide (Azopt®)	Yes	No data	8 h	1%
Dorzolamide (Trusopt®)	Yes	No	8 h	2%
Methazolamide	Significant	No data	14 h	50 mg
Prostaglandin Agonists				
Bimatoprost (Lumigan®)		Yes	≥24 h	0.03%
Latanoprost (Xalatan®)		Yes	≥24 h	0.005%
Travoprost (Travatan®)		Yes	20 h	0.004%
Unoprostone [DSC]		Yes	12 h	0.15%

[1]All miotic drugs significantly affect accommodation.

HEART FAILURE

This chapter outlines a general approach to treatment of chronic systolic heart failure and highlights various aspects of drug therapy in this population. Patient assessment, management, and select drug therapies for heart failure are listed (see following table), followed by general considerations for each class of drugs. Detailed consensus recommendations for the management of chronic heart failure are published (http://www.acc.org/clinical/guidelines/failure/hf_index.htm and *J Heart Lung Transplant*, 2002, 21(2):189-203).

Drug Therapy for Systolic Heart Failure

Drug Therapy[1]	Role	Benefit	Comment
Routine Use			
ACEI	Standard therapy for patients with asymptomatic and symptomatic heart failure (NYHA class I-IV)	Improves morbidity and mortality	• Achieve target or maximum tolerated dose • Optimize diuretic therapy, if needed, prior to initiating ACEI therapy • Ramipril may improve cardiovascular morbidity and mortality in high-risk patients without heart failure
Beta-blockers	Standard therapy for patients with **stable** NYHA class II-III heart failure	Improves morbidity and mortality	• Beneficial effects specific to individual agents • Need close patient contact / follow-up
Diuretics	Standard therapy for the treatment of symptoms of heart failure	Improves symptoms; spironolactone improves mortality in severe (NYHA class IV) heart failure	• Achieve and maintain euvolemia • Combine with standard therapy • Consider spironolactone in severe heart failure
Digoxin	Patients with symptoms despite optimal standard therapy	Improves symptoms and frequency of hospitalizations for heart failure	• No beneficial impact on mortality • No therapeutic range for efficacy (toxicity >2 ng/mL) • Potential for drug interactions
Selected Patients			
Aldosterone antagonist	Recent or current symptoms at rest despite digoxin, diuretics, ACEI and (usually) a beta-blocker	May reduce morbidity and mortality	• Initiate only in patients with S_{cr} <2.5 mg/dL and serum potassium <5.0 mmol/L
Angiotensin-II receptor blockers	Patients intolerant to ACEI	Very limited data showing similar improvements in morbidity and mortality compared to ACEI	• Mechanistically similar to ACEI • Should not be considered equivalent or superior to ACEI
Beta-type natriuretic peptide	Patients with acutely decompensated NYHA Class IV	Short-term symptomatic improvement	Hemodynamic effects/ symptomatic improvement not sustained
Hydralazine/ISDN	Patients intolerant to ACEI	Improves mortality	• Requires frequent daily dosing • No outcome data for combined therapy with standard therapy
Treprostinil	Patients with NYHA Class II-IV pulmonary artery hypertension	Decreases exercise-associated symptoms	Dosage must be carefully and individually titrated

[1]See following information and also individual monographs.

DRUG THERAPY

Angiotensin-Converting Enzyme Inhibitors (ACEIs)

ACEIs improve morbidity and mortality and are "standard therapy" for the treatment of systolic heart failure. All patients with symptomatic or asymptomatic systolic heart failure (NYHA class I-IV) should be on ACEI therapy unless contraindicated. Therapy should be initiated and titrated to the established target dose (see the following table) or to the maximum tolerated dose. Therapy should be continued long-term unless the patient cannot tolerate or develops a contraindication.

Contraindications for therapy include hypotension (systolic pressure <90 mm Hg; diastolic pressure <60 mm Hg), shock, angioedema, anuric renal failure, pregnancy, significant hyperkalemia, and bilateral renal artery stenosis. Patients on diuretic therapy or those with asymptomatic low blood pressure should be monitored more closely for signs of symptomatic hypotension with initiation of ACEI therapy. ACEIs should not be used to treat hemodynamically unstable heart failure. See specific ACEI monographs for drug and dosing information.

Dosing of ACEIs in Heart Failure[1]

ACEI	Initial Dose	Maximum Dose
Captopril	6.25-12.5 mg tid	50 mg tid
Enalapril	2.5 mg bid	10-20 mg bid
Fosinopril	5-10 mg daily	40 mg daily
Lisinopril	2.5-5 mg daily	20-40 mg daily
Quinapril	10 mg bid	40 mg bid
Ramipril	1.25-2.5 mg bid	10 mg daily
Trandolapril	1 mg daily	4 mg daily

[1]Doses are based on clinical trials and national guidelines.

Beta-Blockers

Carvedilol, sustained release metoprolol (CR/XL), and bisoprolol have demonstrated in clinical trials to decrease morbidity and mortality in patients with mild to moderate heart failure (NYHA class II-III) when combined with standard therapy (target doses of ACEI, diuretics, ± digoxin). Other beta-blockers (eg, bucindolol and celiprolol) have no benefit or may tend to increase mortality. Only carvedilol is FDA approved for the treatment of heart failure. (See individual drug monographs for carvedilol, metoprolol, and bisoprolol.)

All patients on standard therapy with **stable** NYHA class II-III systolic heart failure should be on beta-blocker therapy. Beta-blocker therapy may be considered for patients on standard therapy with mild systolic heart failure (NYHA class I). Patients with sympathetic nervous system activation (eg, heart rate >85 beats/minute) may derive greatest benefit. Beta-blocker therapy is not recommended for patients with unstable heart failure and in those who cannot tolerate therapy or where therapy is contraindicated.

Contraindications to beta blockade include bradycardia, 2nd or 3rd degree AV block, hypotension (systolic pressure <90 mm Hg/diastolic pressure <60 mm Hg), decompensated heart failure, and noncompliance. Special consideration should be given in evaluating the risk versus benefit for beta blockade in patients with coexisting conditions, including poorly controlled diabetes, severe COPD, and severe reactive airway disease. These patients should be followed more frequently if beta-blocker therapy is prescribed.

In general, beta-blocker therapy should be initiated at a low dose and titrated slowly, no faster than doubling the dose at weekly intervals to tolerated or target doses (see following table). Therapy should be initiated and titrated by practitioners or clinics with experience and capabilities for close patient contact and follow-up.

During the initiation and titration of beta-blocker therapy it is imperative that patients be frequently monitored for signs of worsening heart failure. Significant weight gain, increasing shortness of breath, edema, paroxysmal nocturnal dyspnea, and dyspnea on exertion may necessitate slowing or decreasing the dose of beta-blocker with dose adjustment of ACEI and diuretic therapies. Patients should be well educated on the potential signs of worsening heart failure, importance of diet and drug compliance, and the need to notify the practitioner or clinic immediately if symptoms of worsening heart failure occur.

HEAD FAILURE *(Continued)*

Initial and Target Doses for Beta-Blocker Therapy in Heart Failure[1]

Beta-Blocker	Starting Dose	Target Dose	Comment
Bisoprolol	1.25 mg/day	10 mg/day	• β_1-selective: possible benefit in patients with reactive airway disease • Inconvenient dosage forms for initial dose titration
Carvedilol	3.125 mg twice daily	25-50 mg twice daily	• FDA approved for heart failure • Nonselective beta-blocker/ α_1-blocker • Possible greater reduction in blood pressure (α-blocking effects) • Convenient dosages
Metoprolol XL/CR	12.5-25 mg/day	200 mg/day	• Compelling data for mortality benefit • β_1-selective: possible benefit in patients with reactive airway disease • Inconvenient dosage forms for initial dose titration • Less potential to decrease blood pressure (no α-blocking properties)

[1]Doses are those used in clinical trials.

Digoxin

Digoxin improves symptoms of heart failure and decreases hospitalizations for heart failure, but does not improve mortality. Digoxin should be used in patients who have symptoms despite optimal standard therapy (ACEIs, diuretics, beta-blockers). There is no compelling evidence for a target therapeutic serum level for digoxin in the treatment of heart failure.

Digoxin should be avoided in patients with sinus and AV block. Caution should be used with digoxin in patients with potential drug interactions, unstable renal function, hypokalemia, and hypomagnesemia.

Diuretics

Therapy should be initiated immediately in patients with heart failure who have signs of volume overload. Patients with mild volume overload can be managed adequately on thiazide diuretics. Patients with more severe volume overload, particularly patients with a creatinine clearance <30 mL/minute, should be started on a loop diuretic. Diuretic therapy should eliminate symptoms of heart failure (eg, edema) and may be monitored and dosed by changes in body weight. Resistance to therapy, as is seen in severe heart failure, may necessitate intravenous diuretic therapy or the use of more than one diuretic. See monographs for individual diuretics.

Diuretic Therapy for Heart Failure

Diuretic	Initial Dose (mg)	Target Dose (mg)	Recommended Maximal Dose (mg)	Comment
Thiazide Diuretics				
Chlorthalidone Hydrochlorothiazide	25 qd	As needed	50 qd	• Postural hypotension, hypokalemia, hyperglycemia, hyperuricemia, rash; rare severe reaction includes pancreatitis, bone marrow suppression, and anaphylaxis
Loop Diuretics				
Bumetanide	0.5-1 qd-bid	As needed	10 qd	• Same as thiazide diuretics
Furosemide	10-40 qd-bid		240 bid	
Torsemide	10-20 mg qd-bid		200 mg qd	
Thiazide-Related Diuretic				
Metolazone	2.5[1]	As needed	10 qd	• Same as thiazide diuretics
Potassium-Sparing Diuretics				
Amiloride	5 qd	As needed	40 qd	• Hyperkalemia (especially if administered with ACEI), rash
Triamterene	50 qd		100 bid	
Aldosterone Antagonist				
Spironolactone	25 qd	As needed	50 qd	• Hyperkalemia (especially if administered with ACEI), gynecomastia • Decreases mortality in severe heart failure (initiate only in patients with S_{cr} <2.5 mg/dL and serum potassium <5.0 mmol/L)

[1]Given as a single test dose initially.

Adapted from U.S. Department of Health & Human Services, the Agency for Healthcare Policy and Research (ACHPR) Publication No. 94-0613, June, 1994.

HEART FAILURE (Continued)

Hydralazine / Isosorbide Dinitrate (ISDN)

The combination of hydralazine (initial dose 10 mg qid up to 75 mg qid) and isosorbide dinitrate (initial dose 5 mg tid up to 40 mg tid) has been shown to improve mortality in patients with heart failure not on ACEI therapy. ACEI therapy is superior compared to hydralazine/ISDN in improving mortality.

The combination of hydralazine/ISDN may be considered in patients intolerant to ACEI therapy. The combination is sometimes added to standard therapy if symptoms or fatigue persist. However, there is little data to suggest that the addition of hydralazine/ISDN to standard therapy further improves morbidity and mortality.

The chronic use of other direct vasodilators may increase morbidity and mortality in this population.

Angiotensin II Receptor Blockers (ARBs)

The renin-angiotensin-aldosterone system plays a key role in the progression of heart failure. For this reason, the role of ARBs in this patient population is being extensively evaluated. Mechanistically, angiotensin II is also produced through non-ACE systems and heart failure patients have "escape" of angiotensin II levels with chronic ACEI therapy. For these reasons, ARB therapy may confer a positive impact on morbidity and mortality by directly blocking the detrimental affects of angiotensin II. It is not established if ARB therapy provides similar mortality benefits as ACEIs or if there is an added benefit in combining an ABR to standard (ACEI) therapy.

In the Evaluation of Losartan in the Elderly (ELITE) trial, losartan and captopril therapy produced similar effects on renal function (primary study endpoint). The risk for cardiovascular events (secondary study endpoint) were significantly decreased in those treated with losartan. A follow-up study (ELITE-II) showed similar cardiovascular events and no differences in hospitalization rates between patients randomized to captopril or losartan. In another ARB trial (RESOLVD), candesartan and enalapril therapy alone and the combination of these two agents were evaluated. The findings of this trial showed no difference in clinical effects overall and a trend for improved left ventricular structure with ARB and ACEI combination therapy. The addition of ARBs to ACEI therapy (as well as other heart failure treatment) did not result in a decrease in mortality, although hospitalization was significantly reduced (ValHeFT) and the combined endpoint of mortality and morbidity was reduced. In a subgroup analysis, patients taking both an ACEI and a beta-blocker at baseline had a higher mortality after valsartan was added. Ongoing studies will give more data on the potential role of ARBs in the treatment of heart failure.

Current recommendations for ARB therapy is in those heart failure patients who are intolerant of ACEI therapy (see drug monographs).

Aldosterone Antagonists

In the RALES study, a large, long-term trial (*N Engl J Med*, 1999, 341:709-17), low-dose spironolactone, when added to prior ACEI therapy in patients with recent or current Class IV symptoms, resulted in a reduced risk of hospitalization and death. Patients who were also receiving digitalis and beta-blockers appeared to demonstrate the most marked effect. Therapy should only be initiated in patients with a serum potassium <5.0 mmol/L and a serum creatinine <2.5 mg/dL. Close monitoring of serum potassium is required.

Eplerenone was recently studied in patients with left ventricular dysfunction after a myocardial infarction. Patients were randomly assigned to eplerenone (25 mg daily initially; goal: 50 mg daily) or placebo in addition to standard treatment (ACEI or ARB, beta-blocker, diuretic, aspirin, statin). Patients were excluded if their creatinine was >2.5 mg/dL, they had a high-normal serum potassium, or they were maintained on a potassium-sparing diuretic. The primary endpoints were death, hospitalization for heart failure, ischemic event (myocardial infarction or stroke), or ventricular arrhythmia. Mean follow-up was 16 months. There were significantly fewer deaths in the eplerenone group. Additional research may help determine its place in therapy.

B-Type Natriuretic Peptide

Infusions of nesiritide have been shown to result in improvement of symptoms in acutely decompensated patients with CHF. Careful monitoring and titration is required and duration of the symptomatic response following infusion has been limited, in most cases, to a few days.

Resources

<u>Guidelines</u>

Hung SA, Baker DW, Chin MH, et al, "ACC/AHA Guidelines for the Evaluation and Management of Chronic Heart Failure in the Adult: A Report of the American College of Cardiology/American Heart Association Task Force on Practice Guidelines (Committee to Revise the 1995 Guidelines for the Evaluation and Management of Heart Failure)," *J Heart Lung Transplant,* 2002, 21(2):189-203. American College of Cardiology Web site available at http://www.acc.org/clinical/guidelines/failure/hf_index.htm.

PHARMACOLOGICAL MANAGEMENT OF PATIENTS WITH HEART FAILURE

HEART FAILURE TREATMENT ALGORITHM

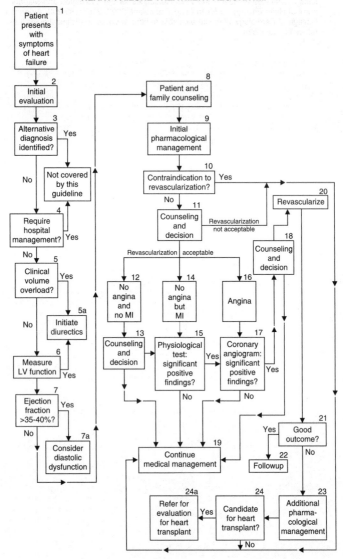

HELICOBACTER PYLORI TREATMENT

Multiple Drug Regimens for the Treatment of *H. pylori* Infection

Drug	Dosages	Duration of Therapy
H₂-receptor antagonist[1]	Any one given at appropriate dose	4 weeks
plus		
Bismuth subsalicylate	525 mg 4 times/day	2 weeks
plus		
Metronidazole	250 mg 4 times/day	2 weeks
plus		
Tetracycline	500 mg 4 times/day	2 weeks
Proton pump inhibitor[1]	Esomeprazole 40 mg once daily	10 days
plus		
Clarithromycin	500 mg twice daily	10 days
plus		
Amoxicillin	1000 mg twice daily	10 days
Proton pump inhibitor[1]	Lansoprazole 30 mg twice daily or Omeprazole 20 mg twice daily	10-14 days
plus		
Clarithromycin	500 mg twice daily	10-14 days
plus		
Amoxicillin	1000 mg twice daily	10-14 days
Proton pump inhibitor[1]	Rabeprazole 20 mg twice daily	7 days
plus		
Clarithromycin	500 mg twice daily	7 days
plus		
Amoxicillin	1000 mg twice daily	7 days
Proton pump inhibitor	Lansoprazole 30 mg twice daily or Omeprazole 20 mg twice daily	2 weeks
plus		
Clarithromycin	500 mg twice daily	2 weeks
plus		
Metronidazole	500 mg twice daily	2 weeks
Proton pump inhibitor	Lansoprazole 30 mg once daily or Omeprazole 20 mg once daily	2 weeks
plus		
Bismuth	525 mg 4 times/day	2 weeks
plus		
Metronidazole	500 mg 3 times/day	2 weeks
plus		
Tetracycline	500 mg 4 times/day	2 weeks

[1]FDA-approved regimen.

Modified from Howden CS and Hunt RH, "Guidelines for the Management of *Helicobacter pylori* Infection," *AJG*, 1998, 93:2336.

HYPERLIPIDEMIA MANAGEMENT

MORTALITY

There is a strong link between serum cholesterol and cardiovascular mortality. This association becomes stronger in patients with established coronary artery disease. Lipid-lowering trials show that reductions in LDL cholesterol are followed by reductions in mortality. In general, each 1% fall in LDL cholesterol confers a 2% reduction in cardiovascular events. The aim of therapy for hyperlipidemia is to decrease cardiovascular morbidity and mortality by lowering cholesterol to a target level using safe and cost-effective treatment modalities. The target LDL cholesterol is determined by the number of patient risk factors (see the following Risk Factors and Goal LDL Cholesterol tables). The goal is achieved through diet, lifestyle modification, and drug therapy. The basis for these recommendations is provided by longitudinal interventional studies, demonstrating that lipid-lowering in patients with prior cardiovascular events (secondary prevention) and in patients with hyperlipidemia but no prior cardiac event (primary prevention) lowers the occurrence of future cardiovascular events, including stroke.

Major Risk Factors That Modify LDL Goals

	Male ≥45 years
	Female ≥55 years
Positive risk factors	Family history of premature coronary heart disease, defined as CHD in male first-degree relative <55 years; CHD in female first-degree relative <65 years
	Cigarette smoking
	Hypertension (blood pressure ≥140/90 mm Hg) or taking antihypertensive medication
	Low HDL (<40 mg/dL [1.03 mmol/L])
Negative risk factors	High HDL (≥60 mg/dL [1.6 mmol/L])[1]

[1]If HDL is ≥60 mg/dL, may subtract one positive risk factor.

Adult Treatment Panel (ATP) III LDL-C Goals and Cutpoints for Therapeutic Lifestyle Changes (TLC) and Drug Therapy in Different Risk Categories

Risk Category	LDL-C Goal	Initiate TLC	Consider Drug Therapy[1]
High risk: CHD[2] or CHD risk equivalents[3] (10-year risk >20%)	<100 mg/dL (optional goal: <70 mg/dL)[4]	≥100 mg/dL[5]	≥100 mg/dL[6] (<100 mg/dL: Consider drug options)[1]
Moderately high risk: 2+ risk factors[7] (10-year risk 10% to 20%)[8]	<130 mg/dL[9]	≥130 mg/dL[5]	≥130 mg/dL (100-120 mg/dL: Consider drug options)[10]
Moderate risk: 2+ risk factors[7] (10-year risk <10%)[8]	<130 mg/dL	≥130 mg/dL	≥160 mg/dL
Lower risk: 0-1 risk factor[11]	<160 mg/dL	≥160 mg/dL	≥190 mg/dL (160-189 mg/dL: LDL-lowering drug optional)

[1]When LDL-lowering drug therapy is employed, it is advised that intensity of therapy be sufficient to achieve at least a 30% to 40% reduction in LDL-C levels.

[2]CHD includes history of myocardial infarction, unstable angina, stable angina, coronary artery procedures (angioplasty or bypass surgery), or evidence of clinically significant myocardial ischemia.

[3]CHD risk equivalents include clinical manifestations of noncoronary forms of atherosclerotic disease (peripheral arterial disease, abdominal aortic aneurysm, and carotid artery disease [transient ischemic attacks or stroke of carotid origin or >50% obstruction of a carotid artery]), diabetes, and 2+ risk factors with 10-year risk for hard CHD >20%.

[4]Very high risk favors the optional LDL-C goal of <70 mg/dL, and in patients with high triglycerides, non-HDL-C <100 mg/dL.

[5]Any person at high risk or moderately high risk who has lifestyle-related risk factors (eg, obesity, physical inactivity, elevated triglyceride, low HDL-C, or metabolic syndrome) is a candidate for therapeutic lifestyle changes to modify these risk factors regardless of LDL-C level.

[6]If baseline LDL-C is <100 mg/dL, institution of an LDL-lowering drug is a therapeutic option on the basis of available clinical trial results. If a high-risk person has high triglycerides or low HDL-C, combining a fibrate or nicotinic acid with an LDL-lowering drug can be considered.

[7]Risk factors include cigarette smoking, hypertension (BP ≥140/90 mm Hg or on antihypertensive medication), low HDL cholesterol (<40 mg/dL), family history of premature CHD (CHD in male first-degree relative <55 years of age; CHD in female first-degree relative <65 years of age), and age (men ≥45 years; women ≥55 years).

[8]Electronic 10-year risk calculators are available at www.nhlbi.nih.gov/guidelines/cholesterol.

[9]Optional LDL-C goal <100 mg/dL.

[10]For moderately high-risk persons, when LDL-C level is 100-129 mg/dL, at baseline or on lifestyle therapy, initiation of an LDL-lowering drug to achieve an LDL-C level <100 mg/dL is a therapeutic option on the basis of available clinical trial results.

[11]Almost all people with zero or 1 risk factor have a 10-year risk <10%, and 10-year risk assessment in people with zero or 1 risk factor thus not necessary.

Any person with elevated LDL cholesterol or other form of hyperlipidemia should undergo evaluation to rule out secondary dyslipidemia. Causes of secondary dyslipidemia include diabetes, hypothyroidism, obstructive liver disease, chronic renal failure, and drugs that increase LDL and decrease HDL (progestins, anabolic steroids, corticosteroids).

Elevated Serum Triglyceride Levels

Elevated serum triglyceride levels may be an independent risk factor for coronary heart disease. Factors that contribute to hypertriglyceridemia include obesity, inactivity, cigarette smoking, excess alcohol intake, high carbohydrate diets (>60% of energy intake), type 2 diabetes, chronic renal failure, nephrotic syndrome, certain medications (corticosteroids, estrogens, retinoids, higher doses of beta-blockers), and genetic disorders. Non-HDL cholesterol (total cholesterol minus HDL cholesterol) is a secondary focus for clinicians treating patients with high serum triglyceride levels (≥200 mg/dL). The goal for non-HDL cholesterol in patients with high serum triglyceride levels can be set 30 mg/dL higher than usual LDL cholesterol goals. Patients with serum triglyceride levels <200 mg/dL should aim for the target LDL cholesterol goal.

ATP classification of serum triglyceride levels:

- – Normal triglycerides: <150 mg/dL
- – Borderline-high: 150-199 mg/dL
- – High: 200-499 mg/dL
- – Very high: ≥500 mg/dL

NONDRUG THERAPY

Dietary therapy and lifestyle modifications should be individualized for each patient. A total lifestyle change is recommended for all patients. Dietary and lifestyle modifications should be tried for 3 months, if deemed appropriate. Nondrug and drug therapy should be initiated simultaneously in patients with highly elevated cholesterol (see LDL Cholesterol Goals and Cutpoints for Therapeutic Lifestyle Changes and Drug Therapy in Different Risk Categories table). Increasing physical activity and smoking cessation will aid in the treatment of hyperlipidemia and improve cardiovascular health.

Note: Refer to the National Cholesterol Education Program reference for details concerning the calculation of 10-year risk of CHD using Framingham risk scoring. Risk assessment tool is available on-line at http://hin.nhlbi.nih.gov/atpiii/calculator.asp?usertype=prof, last accessed March 14, 2002.

Total Lifestyle Change (TLC) Diet

	Recommended Intake
Total fat	25%-35% of total calories
Saturated fat[1]	<7% of total calories
Polyunsaturated fat	≤10% of total calories
Monounsaturated fat	≤20% of total calories
Carbohydrates[2]	50%-60% of total calories
Fiber	20-30 g/day
Protein	~15% of total calories
Cholesterol	<200 mg/day
Total calories[3]	Balance energy intake and expenditure to maintain desirable body weight/prevent weight gain

[1] *Trans* fatty acids (partially hydrogenated oils) intake should be kept low. These are found in potato chips, other snack foods, margarines and shortenings, and fast-foods.

[2] Complex carbohydrates including grains (especially whole grains, fruits, and vegetables).

[3] Daily energy expenditure should include at least moderate physical activity.

DRUG THERAPY

Drug therapy should be selected based on the patient's lipid profile, concomitant disease states, and the cost of therapy. The following table lists specific advantages and disadvantages for various classes of lipid-lowering medications. The expected reduction in lipids with therapy is listed in the Lipid-Lowering Agents table. Refer to individual drug monographs for detailed information.

HYPERLIPIDEMIA MANAGEMENT *(Continued)*

Advantages and Disadvantages of Specific Lipid-Lowering Therapies

	Advantages	Disadvantages
Bile acid sequestrants	Good choice for ↑ LDL, especially when combined with a statin (↓ LDL ≤50%); low potential for systemic side effects; good choice for younger patients	May increase triglycerides; higher incidence of adverse effects; moderately expensive; drug interactions; inconvenient dosing
Niacin	Good choice for almost any lipid abnormality; inexpensive; greatest increase in HDL	High incidence of adverse effects; may adversely affect NIDDM and gout; sustained release niacin may decrease the incidence of flushing and circumvent the need for multiple daily dosing; sustained release niacin may not increase HDL cholesterol or decrease triglycerides as well as immediate release niacin
HMG-CoA reductase inhibitors	Produces greatest ↓ in LDL; generally well-tolerated; convenient once-daily dosing; proven decrease in mortality	Expensive
Gemfibrozil	Good choice in patients with ↑ triglycerides where niacin is contraindicated or not well-tolerated; gemfibrozil is well tolerated	Variable effects on LDL
Ezetimibe	Additional cholesterol-lowering effects when combined with HMG-CoA reductase inhibitors	Effects similar to bile acid sequestrants

Lipid-Lowering Agents

Drug	Dose/Day	Effect on LDL (%)	Effect on HDL (%)	Effect on TG (%)
HMG-CoA Reductase Inhibitors				
Atorvastatin	10 mg	-39	+6	-13
	20 mg	-43	+5	-20
	40 mg	-50	+5	-32
	80 mg	-60	+5	-37
Fluvastatin	20 mg	-22	+2	-5
	40 mg	-25	+3	-12
	80 mg	-36	+4	-12
Lovastatin	20 mg	-27	+7	-8
	40 mg	-32	+5	-2
	80 mg	-42	+8	-13
Pravastatin	10 mg	-22	+5	-3
	20 mg	-32	+3	-15
	40 mg	-34	+6	-10
Rosuvastatin	10 mg	-52	+14	-10
	20 mg	-55	+8	-23
	40 mg	-63	+10	-28
Simvastatin	5 mg	-26	+7	-12
	10 mg	-30	+5	-17
	20 mg	-38	+10	-15
	40 mg	-41	+8	-24
	80 mg	-47		
Bile Acid Sequestrants				
Cholestyramine	4-24 g	-15 to -30	+3 to +5	+0 to +20
Colestipol	7-30 g	-15 to -30	+3 to +5	+0 to +20
Colesevelam	6 tablets	-10	+10 to +25	+0 to +10
Fibric Acid Derivative				
Clofibrate	500 mg 4 times	-10	+10 to +25	-40 to -55
Fenofibrate	67-200 mg	-20 to -25	+1 to -34	-30 to -50
Gemfibrozil	600 mg twice daily	-5 to -10[1]	+10 to +20	-40 to -60
Niacin	1.5-6 g	-21 to -27	+10 to +35	-10 to -50
2-Azetidinone				
Ezetimibe	10 mg	-16 to -18	+1 to +4	-5 to -6

[1]May increase LDL in some patients.

Recommended Liver Function Monitoring for HMG-CoA Reductase Inhibitors

Agent	Initial and After Elevation in Dose	6 Weeks[1]	12 Weeks[1]	Periodically
Atorvastatin (Lipitor®)	x		x	x
Fluvastatin (Lescol®)	x		x	x
Lovastatin (Mevacor®)	x	x	x	x
Pravastatin (Pravachol®)	x			x
Simvastatin (Zocor®)	x			x

[1] After initiation of therapy or any elevation in dose.

DRUG SELECTION

Lipid Profile	Monotherapy	Combination Therapies
Increased LDL with normal HDL and triglycerides (TG)	Resin Niacin[1] Statin	Resin plus niacin[1] or statin Statin plus niacin[1,2]
Increased LDL and increased TG (200-499 mg/dL)[2]	Intensify LDL-lowering therapy	Statin plus niacin[1,3] Statin plus fibrate[3]
Increased LDL and increased TG (≥500 mg/dL)[2]	Consider combination therapy (niacin,[1] fibrates, statin)	
Increased TG	Niacin[1] Fibrates	Niacin[1] plus fibrates
Increased LDL and low HDL	Niacin[1] Statin	Statin plus niacin[1,2]

[1] Avoid in diabetics.

[2] Emphasize weight reduction and increased physical activity.

[3] Risk of myopathy with combination.

Resins = bile acid sequestrants; statins = HMG-CoA reductase inhibitors; fibrates = fibric acid derivatives (eg, gemfibrozil, fenofibrate).

COMBINATION DRUG THERAPY

If after at least 6 weeks of therapy at the maximum recommended or tolerated dose, the patient's LDL cholesterol is not at target, consider optimizing nondrug measures, prescribing a higher dose of current lipid-lowering drug, or adding another lipid-lowering medication to the current therapy. Successful drug combinations include statin and niacin, statin and bile acid sequestrant, or niacin and bile acid sequestrant. At maximum recommended doses, LDL cholesterol may be decreased by 50% to 60% with combination therapy. This is the same reduction achieved by atorvastatin 40 mg twice daily. If a bile acid sequestrant is used with other lipid-lowering agents, space doses 1 hour before or 4 hours after the bile acid sequestrant administration. Statins combined with either fenofibrate, clofibrate, gemfibrozil, or niacin increase the risk of rhabdomyolysis. In this situation, patient education (muscle pain/weakness) and careful follow-up are warranted.

Progression of Drug Therapy in Primary Prevention

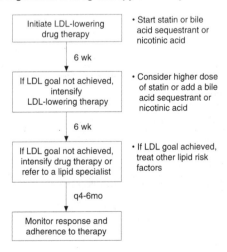

1839

HYPERLIPIDEMIA MANAGEMENT *(Continued)*

References

Guidelines

Gavin JR, Alberti KGMM, Davidson MB, et al, for the Members of the Expert Committee on the Diagnosis and Classification of Diabetes Mellitus, "American Diabetes Association: Clinical Practice Recommendations," *Diabetes Care*, 1999, 22(Suppl 1):S1-S114.

National Cholesterol Education Program, "Third Report of the Expert Panel on Detection, Evaluation, and Treatment of High Blood Cholesterol in Adults (Adult Treatment Panel III)," *JAMA*, 2001, 285:2486-97.

Grundy SM, Cleeman JI, Merz CN, et al, "Implications of Recent Clinical Trials for the National Cholesterol Education Program Adult Treatment Panel III Guidelines," *JACC*, 2004, 44(3):729.

Others

Berthold HK, Sudhop T, and von Bergmann K, "Effect of a Garlic Oil Preparation on Serum Lipoproteins and Cholesterol Metabolism: A Randomized Controlled Trial," *JAMA*, 1998, 279:1900-2.

Bertolini S, Bon GB, Campbell LM, et al, "Efficacy and Safety of Atorvastatin Compared to Pravastatin in Patients With Hypercholesterolemia," *Atherosclerosis*, 1997, 130:191-7.

Blankenhorn DH, Nessim SA, Johnson RL, et al, "Beneficial Effects of Combined Colestipol-Niacin Therapy on Coronary Atherosclerosis and Venous Bypass Grafts," *JAMA*, 1987, 257:3233-40.

Brown G, Albers JJ, Fisher LD, et al, "Regression of Coronary Artery Disease as a Result of Intensive Lipid-Lowering Therapy in Men With High Levels of Apolipoprotein B," *N Engl J Med*, 1990, 323:1289-98.

Capuzzi DM, Guyton JR, Morgan JM, et al, "Efficacy and Safety of an Extended-Release Niacin (Niaspan®): A Long-Term Study," *Am J Cardiol*, 1998, 82:74U-81U.

Coronary Drug Project Research Program, "Clofibrate and Niacin in Coronary Heart Disease," *JAMA*, 1975, 231:360-81.

Dart A, Jerums G, Nicholson G, et al, "A Multicenter, Double-Blind, One-Year Study Comparing Safety and Efficacy of Atorvastatin Versus Simvastatin in Patients With Hypercholesterolemia," *Am J Cardiol*, 1997, 80:39-44.

Davidson MH, Dillon MA, Gordon B, et al, "Colesevelam Hydrochloride (Cholestagel): A New Potent Bile Acid Sequestrant Associated With a Low Incidence of Gastrointestinal Side Effects," *Arch Intern Med*, 1999, 159(16):1893-900.

Davidson M, McKenney J, Stein E, et al, "Comparison of One-Year Efficacy and Safety of Atorvastatin Versus Lovastatin in Primary Hypercholesterolemia," *Am J Cardiol*, 1997, 79:1475-81.

Frick MH, Heinonen OP, Huttunen JK, et al, "Helsinki Heart Study: Primary-Prevention Trial With Gemfibrozil in Middle-Aged Men With Dyslipidemia," *N Engl J Med*, 1987, 317:1237-45.

Garber AM, Browner WS, and Hulley SB, "Clinical Guideline, Part 2: Cholesterol Screening in Asymptomatic Adults, Revisited," *Ann Intern Med*, 1995, 124:518-31.

Johannesson M, Jonsson B, Kjekshus J, et al, "Cost-Effectiveness of Simvastatin Treatment to Lower Cholesterol Levels in Patients With Coronary Heart Disease. Scandinavian Simvastatin Survival Study Group," *N Engl J Med*, 1997, 336:332-6.

Jones P, Kafonek S, Laurora I, et al, "Comparative Dose Efficacy Study of Atorvastatin Versus Simvastatin, Pravastatin, Lovastatin, and Fluvastatin in Patients With Hypercholesterolemia," *Am J Cardiol*, 1998, 81:582-7.

Kasiske BL, Ma JZ, Kalil RS, et al, "Effects of Antihypertensive Therapy on Serum Lipids," *Ann Intern Med*, 1995, 133-41.

Lipid Research Clinics Program, "The Lipid Research Clinics Coronary Primary Prevention Trial Results: I. Reduction in Incidence of Coronary Heart Disease," *JAMA*, 1984, 251:351-64.

Mauro VF and Tuckerman CE, "Ezetimibe for Management of Hypercholesterolemia," *Ann Pharmacother*, 2003, 37(6):839-48.

Multiple Risk Factor Intervention Trial Research Group, "Multiple Risk Factor Intervention Trial: Risk Factor Changes and Mortality Results," *JAMA*, 1982, 248:1465-77.

Pitt B, Waters D, Brown WV, et al, "Aggressive Lipid-Lowering Therapy Compared With Angioplasty in Stable Coronary Artery Disease. Atorvastatin Versus Revascularization Treatment Investigators," *N Engl J Med*, 1999, 341(2):70-6.

Ross SD, Allen IE, Connelly JE, et al, "Clinical Outcomes in Statin Treatment Trials: A Meta-Analysis," *Arch Intern Med*, 1999, 159:1793-802.

Sacks FM, Pfeffer MA, Moye LA, et al, "The Effect of Pravastatin on Coronary Events After Myocardial Infarction in Patients With Average Cholesterol Levels," *N Engl J Med*, 1996, 335:1001-9.

Scandinavian Simvastatin Survival Study, "Randomized Trial of Cholesterol Lowering in 4444 Patients With Coronary Heart Disease: The Scandinavian Simvastatin Survival Study (4S)," *Lancet*, 1994, 344:1383-9.

Schrott HG, Bittner V, Vittinghoff E, et al, "Adherence to National Cholesterol Education Program Treatment Goals in Postmenopausal Women With Heart Disease. The Heart and Estrogen/Progestin Replacement Study (HERS)," *JAMA*, 1997, 277:1281-6.

Shepherd J, Cobbe SM, Ford I, et al, "Prevention of Coronary Heart Disease With Pravastatin in Men With Hypercholesterolemia, The West of Scotland Coronary Prevention Study Group," *N Engl J Med*, 1995, 333:1301-7.

Stein EA, Davidson MH, Dobs AS, et al, "Efficacy and Safety of Simvastatin 80 mg/day in Hypercholesterolemic Patients. The Expanded Dose Simvastatin U.S. Study Group," *Am J Cardiol*, 1998, 82:311-6.

HYPERTENSION

The optimal blood pressure for adults is <120/80 mm Hg. Consistent systolic pressure ≥140 mm Hg or a diastolic pressure ≥90 mm Hg, in the absence of a secondary cause, defines hypertension. Hypertension affects approximately 25% (50 million people) in the United States. Of those patients on antihypertensive medication, only one in three have their blood pressure controlled (<140/90 mm Hg).

Controlling systolic hypertension has been much more difficult than controlling diastolic hypertension. Educating patients in lifestyle management, cardiovascular risk reduction, and drug therapy aids in improving the morbidity and mortality of patients with hypertension.

The Seventh Report of the Joint National Committee (JNC VII) is an excellent reference and guide for the treatment of hypertension (Chobanian AV, Bakris GL, Black HR, et al, "The Seventh Report of the Joint National Committee on Prevention, Detection, Evaluation, and Treatment of High Blood Pressure: The JNC 7 Report," *Jama*, 2003, 289(19):2560-71. For adults, hypertension is classified in stages (see following table).

Adult Classification of Blood Pressure

Category	Systolic (mm Hg)		Diastolic (mm Hg)
Normal	<120	and	<80
Prehypertension	120-139	or	80-89
Hypertension			
Stage 1	140-159	or	90-99
Stage 2	≥160	or	≥100

Adapted from Chobanian AV, Bakris GL, Black HR, et al, "The Seventh Report of the Joint National Committee on Prevention, Detection, Evaluation, and Treatment of High Blood Pressure: The JNC 7 Report," *Jama*, 2003, 289(19):2560-71.

Normal Blood Pressure in Children

Age (y)	Girls' SBP / DBP (mm Hg)		Boys' SBP / DBP (mm Hg)	
	50th Percentile for Height	75th Percentile for Height	50th Percentile for Height	75th Percentile for Height
1	104/58	105/59	102/57	104/58
6	111/73	112/73	114/74	115/75
12	123/80	124/81	123/81	125/82
17	129/84	130/85	136/87	138/88

SBP = systolic blood pressure.

DBP = diastolic blood pressure.

Adapted from the report by the NHBPEP Working Group on Hypertension Control in Children and Adolescents, *Pediatrics*, 1996, 98(4 Pt 1):649-58.

PATIENT ASSESSMENT

- **Cardiovascular Risk Factors:** Hypertension, cigarette smoking, obesity (BMI ≥30), inactive lifestyle, dyslipidemia, diabetes mellitus, microalbuminuria or estimated GFR <60 mL/minute, age (>55 years for men, >65 years for women), family history of premature cardiovascular disease (men <55 years or women >65 years).

  Components of metabolic syndrome include hypertension, obesity, dyslipidemia, diabetes mellitus.

- Identify causes of high BP.

- Assess target-organ damage and CVD.

Target-Organ Disease

Organ System	Manifestation
Cardiac	Clinical, ECG, or radiologic evidence of coronary artery disease; prior MI, angina, post-CABG; left ventricular hypertrophy (LVH); left ventricular dysfunction or cardiac failure, prior coronary revascularization
Cerebrovascular	Transient ischemic attack or stroke
Peripheral vascular	Absence of pulses in extremities (except dorsalis pedis), claudication, aneurysm, peripheral arterial disease
Renal	Serum creatinine ≥130 μmol/L (1.5 mg/dL); proteinuria (≥1+); microalbuminuria, chronic kidney disease
Eye	Hemorrhages or exudates, with or without papilledema; retinopathy

Adapted from Chobanian AV, Bakris GL, Black HR, et al, "The Seventh Report of the Joint National Committee on Prevention, Detection, Evaluation, and Treatment of High Blood Pressure: The JNC 7 Report," *Jama*, 2003, 289(19):2560-71.

HYPERTENSION *(Continued)*

BLOOD PRESSURE MEASUREMENT

At an office visit, patients should be seated quietly for ≥5 minutes in a chair with feet on the floor and arm supported at heart level. At least two measurements should be made. Patients should be given their results and their goal BP.

Ambulatory BP monitoring is useful in evaluating "white coat hypertension" (no end-organ damage), drug resistance, hypotensive symptoms, episodic hypertension, and autonomic dysfunction. Ambulatory BP monitoring correlates better with end-organ damage than office measurements.

Having patients monitor their own BP helps to improve compliance and provides information on response to therapeutic interventions.

Based on these initial assessments, treatment strategies for patients with hypertension are stratified based on their blood pressure and comorbidities (compelling indications).

Management of Blood Pressure

BP Classification	Management: Based upon highest BP category		
	Lifestyle Modification	Initial Therapy Without Compelling Indication	Initial Therapy With Compelling Indication[1]
Normal	Encourage	None	None
Prehypertensive	Yes	None	Treat patients with chronic kidney disease or diabetes to BP goal of <130/80 mm Hg
Hypertension Stage 1	Yes	Thiazide-type diuretic for most; consider ACEI, ARB, β-blocker, CCB, or combination	Drugs for the compelling indications; other antihypertensives as needed
Hypertension Stage 2	Yes	Two drug combos (typically a thiazide-type diuretic and ACEI or ARB or β-blocker or CCB). Use combo cautiously in patients at risk for orthostasis.	Drugs for the compelling indications; other antihypertensives as needed

[1]Compelling Indication: Conditions for which specific classes of antihypertensive drugs have proven beneficial.

Adapted from Chobanian AV, Bakris GL, Black HR, et al, "The Seventh Report of the Joint National Committee on Prevention, Detection, Evaluation, and Treatment of High Blood Pressure: The JNC 7 Report," *Jama*, 2003, 289(19):2560-71.

ACHIEVING BLOOD PRESSURE CONTROL

Treatment of hypertension should be individualized. Lower blood pressure (goal <130/80 mm Hg) should be achieved in patients with diabetes or chronic renal disease. The following Hypertension Treatment Algorithm may be used to select specific antihypertensives based on compelling indications.

Special consideration for starting combination therapy should be made in each patient.

Starting drug therapy at a low dose and titrating upward if blood pressure is not controlled is recommended.

Most patients with hypertension will require two or more drugs to achieve their BP goals.

Adding a second drug from a different class will help when a single drug at reasonable doses has failed to achieve the goal.

If the untreated BP is >20/10 mm Hg away from the goal, consider initiating therapy with two drugs. Use caution in those at risk for orthostasis (eg, diabetics, geriatrics, and those with autonomic dysfunction).

Low-dose aspirin therapy should be considered when BP is controlled; use in uncontrolled hypertension can increase the risk of hemorrhagic stroke.

Lifestyle modification and risk reduction should always be reviewed and reinforced.

MONITORING THERAPY

Generally, monthly follow-up is recommended until BP control is reached.

More frequent monitoring is required for those patients with Stage 2 hypertension or those with complications.

Serum potassium and serum creatinine should be monitored at least twice yearly.

When BP is at goal and stable, follow-up can be maintained every 3-6 months. Treat other cardiovascular risk factors if present.

Hypertension Treatment Algorithm

Begin or continue lifestyle modifications

↓

Not at goal blood pressure (<140/90 mm Hg or <130/80 mm Hg for patients with diabetes or chronic renal disease)

↓

Initial Drug Choice

Hypertension

Stage I
Thiazide-type diuretic for most.
Consider ACEI, ARB, β-blocker,
CCB, or combo.

Stage 2
Two-drug combo for most
(typically thiazide-type diuretic +
ACEI or ARB or β-blocker or CCB)

Compelling Indications

Chronic kidney disease
- ACEI
- ARB

Diabetes mellitus
- ACEI
- ARB
- β-blocker
- CCB
- Diuretic

Heart failure
- ACEI
- Aldosterone blocker
- ARB
- β-blocker
- Diuretic

High coronary risk
- ACEI
- β-blocker
- CCB
- Diuretic

Myocardial infarction
- ACEI
- Aldosterone blocker
- β-blocker

Recurrent stroke prevention
- ACEI
- Diuretic

↓

Not at goal blood pressure

↓   ↓

Optimize dosages or add additional
drugs until goal BP achieved.

Consider consultation with
hypertension specialist.

HYPERTENSION *(Continued)*

Additional Considerations for Specific Therapies

Indication	Drug Therapy
Atrial tachyarrhythmias	β-blocker, CCB (non-DHP)
Chronic kidney disease	
Cl_{cr} <60 mL/min or albuminuria	ACEI or ARB
Cl_{cr} <30 mL/min	Increase loop diuretic
Diabetes	Thiazide diuretic, β-blocker, ACEI, ARB, CCB
Nephropathy	ACEI, ARB
Essential tremor	β-blocker (noncardioselective)
Heart failure	
Ventricular dysfunction (asymptomatic)	ACEI, β-blocker
Ventricular dysfunction (symptomatic)	ACEI, β-blocker, ARB, aldosterone blocker, loop diuretic
Hypertensive women who are pregnant	Methyldopa, β-blocker, vasodilator
Ischemic heart disease	
Angina	β-blocker, CCB (long-acting)
Acute coronary syndromes	β-blocker, ACEI
Migraine	β-blocker (noncardioselective), CCB (long-acting, non-DHP)
Osteoporosis	Thiazide diuretic
Perioperative hypertension	β-blocker
Prostatism (BPH)	Alpha-adrenergic blocking agent
Raynaud syndrome	CCB
Thyrotoxicosis	β-blocker

Note: ACEI = angiotensin-converting enzyme inhibitor; ARB = angiotensin receptor blocker; CCB = calcium channel blocker; DHP = dihydropyridine.

May Have Unfavorable Effects on Comorbid Conditions

Condition	Drug Therapy to Avoid
Angioedema	ACEI
Bronchospastic disease	β-blocker
Gout	Thiazide diuretic
Heart block (second or third degree)	β-blocker, CCB (non-DHP)
Hyponatremia	Thiazide diuretic
Potassium >5 mEq/L before treatment	Potassium sparing diuretic, aldosterone antagonist
Pregnancy or those likely to become pregnant	ACEI, ARB

Note: ACEI = angiotensin-converting enzyme inhibitor; ARB = angiotensin receptor blocker; CCB = calcium channel blocker; DHP = dihydropyridine.

HYPERTENSIVE EMERGENCIES AND URGENCIES

General Treatment Principles in the Treatment of Hypertensive Emergencies

Principle	Considerations
Admit the patient to the hospital, preferably in the ICU. Monitor vital signs appropriately.	Establish I.V. access and place patient on a cardiac monitor. Place a femoral intra-arterial line and pulmonary arterial catheter, if indicated, to assess cardiopulmonary function and intravascular volume status.
Perform rapid but thorough history and physical examination.	Determine cause of, or precipitating factors to, hypertensive crisis if possible (remember to obtain a medication history including Rx, OTC, and illicit drugs). Obtain details regarding any prior history of hypertension (severity, duration, treatment), as well as other coexisting illnesses. Assess the extent of hypertensive end organ damage. Determine if a hypertensive urgency or emergency exists.
Determine goal blood pressure based on premorbid level, duration, severity and rapidity of increase of blood pressure, concomitant medical conditions, race, and age.	Acute decreases in blood pressure to normal or subnormal levels during the initial treatment period may reduce perfusion to the brain, heart, and kidneys, and must be avoided except in specific instances (ie, dissecting aortic aneurysm). Gradually establish a normal (or reasonable) blood pressure over the next 1-2 weeks.
Select an appropriate antihypertensive regimen depending on the individual patient and clinical setting.	Initiate a controlled decrease in blood pressure. Avoid concomitant administration of multiple agents that may cause precipitous falls in blood pressure. Select the agent with the best hemodynamic profile based on the primary treatment goal. Avoid diuretics and sodium restriction during the initial treatment period unless there is a clear clinical indication (ie, CHF, pulmonary edema). Avoid sedating antihypertensives in patients with hypertensive encephalopathy, CVA, or other CNS disorders in whom mental status must be monitored. Use caution with direct vasodilating agents that induce reflex tachycardia or increase cardiac output in patients with coronary heart disease, history of angina or myocardial infarction, or dissecting aortic aneurysm. Preferably choose an agent that does not adversely affect glomerular filtration rate or renal blood flow and also agents that have favorable effects on cerebral blood flow and its autoregulation, especially for patients with hypertensive encephalopathy or CVAs. Select the most efficacious agent with the fewest adverse effects based on the underlying cause of the hypertensive crisis and other individual patient factors.
Initiate a chronic antihypertensive regimen after the patient's blood pressure is stabilized	Begin oral antihypertensive therapy once goal blood pressure is achieved before gradually tapering parenteral medications. Select the best oral regimen based on cost, ease of administration, adverse effect profile, and concomitant medical conditions.

HYPERTENSION (Continued)

Oral Agents Used in the Treatment of Hypertensive Urgencies

Drug	Dose	Onset	Cautions
Captopril[1]	P.O.: 25 mg, repeat as required	15-30 min	Hypotension, renal failure in bilateral renal artery stenosis
Clonidine	P.O.: 0.1-0.2 mg, repeated every hour as needed to a total dose of 0.6 mg	30-60 min	Hypotension, drowsiness, dry mouth
Labetalol	P.O.: 200-400 mg, repeat every 2-3 h	30 min to 2 h	Bronchoconstriction, heart block, orthostatic hypotension

[1]There is no clearly defined clinical advantage in the use of sublingual over oral routes of administration with these agents.

Recommendations for the Use of Intravenous Antihypertensive Drugs in Selected Hypertensive Emergencies

Condition	Agent(s) of Choice	Agent(s) to Avoid or Use With Caution	General Treatment Principles
Hypertensive encephalopathy	Nitroprusside, labetalol, diazoxide	Methyldopa, reserpine	Avoid drugs with CNS-sedating effects.
Acute intracranial or subarachnoid hemorrhage	Nicardipine,[1] nitroprusside	β-blocker	Careful titration with a short-acting agent.
Cerebral infarction	Nicardipine,[1] nitroprusside, labetalol	β-blocker, minoxidil, diazoxide	Careful titration with a short-acting agent. Avoid agents that may decrease cerebral blood flow.
Head trauma	Esmolol, labetalol	Methyldopa, reserpine, nitroprusside, nitroglycerin, hydralazine	Avoid drugs with CNS-sedating effects, or those that may increase intracranial pressure.
Acute myocardial infarction, myocardial ischemia	Nitroglycerin, nicardipine[1] (calcium channel blocker), labetalol	Hydralazine, diazoxide, minoxidil	Avoid drugs which cause reflex tachycardia and increased myocardial oxygen consumption.
Acute pulmonary edema	Nitroprusside, nitroglycerin, loop diuretics	β-blocker (labetalol), minoxidil, methyldopa	Avoid drugs which may cause sodium and water retention and edema exacerbation.
Renal dysfunction	Hydralazine, calcium channel blocker	Nitroprusside, ACE inhibitors, β-blocker (labetalol)	Avoid drugs with increased toxicity in renal failure and those that may cause decreased renal blood flow.
Eclampsia	Hydralazine, labetalol, nitroprusside[2]	Diuretics, diazoxide (diazoxide may cause cessation of labor)	Avoid drugs that may cause adverse fetal effects, compromise placental circulation, or decrease cardiac output.
Pheochromo-cytoma	Phentolamine, nitroprusside, β-blocker (eg, esmolol) only after alpha blockade (phentolamine)	β-blocker in the absence of alpha blockade, methyldopa, minoxidil	Use drugs of proven efficacy and specificity. Unopposed beta blockade may exacerbate hypertension.
Dissecting aortic aneurysm	Nitroprusside and beta blockade	Hydralazine, diazoxide, minoxidil	Avoid drugs which may increase cardiac output.
Postoperative hypertension	Nitroprusside, nicardipine,[1] labetalol		Avoid drugs which may exacerbate postoperative ileus.

[1]The use of nicardipine in these situations is by the recommendation of the author based on a review of the literature.

[2]Reserve nitroprusside for eclamptic patients with life-threatening hypertension unresponsive to other agents due to the potential risk to the fetus (cyanide and thiocyanate metabolites may cross the placenta).

Selected Intravenous Agents for Hypertensive Emergencies

Drug	Dose[1]	Onset of Action	Duration of Action	Adverse Effects[2]	Special Indications
Vasodilators					
Sodium nitroprusside	0.25-10 mcg/kg/min as I.V. infusion[3] (max: 10 min only)	Immediate	1-2 min	Nausea, vomiting, muscle twitching, sweating, thiocyanate and cyanide intoxication	Most hypertensive emergencies; caution with high intracranial pressure or azotemia
Nicardipine hydrochloride	5-15 mg/h I.V.	5-10 min	1-4 h	Tachycardia, headache, flushing, local phlebitis	Most hypertensive emergencies except acute heart failure; caution with coronary ischemia
Fenoldopam mesylate	0.1-0.3 mcg/kg/min as I.V. infusion	<5 min	30 min	Tachycardia, headache, nausea, flushing	Most hypertensive emergencies; caution with glaucoma
Nitroglycerin	5-100 mcg/min as I.V. infusion[3]	2-5 min	3-5 min	Headache, vomiting, methemoglobinemia, tolerance with prolonged use	Coronary ischemia
Enalaprilat	1.25-5 mg every 6 hours I.V.	15-30 min	6 h	Precipitous fall in pressure in high-renin states; response variable	Acute left ventricular failure; avoid in acute myocardial infarction
Hydralazine hydrochloride	10-20 mg I.V. 10-50 mg I.M.	10-20 min 20-30 min	3-8 h	Tachycardia, flushing, headache, vomiting, aggravation of angina	Eclampsia
Diazoxide	50-100 mg I.V. bolus repeated, or 15-30 mg/min infusion	2-4 min	6-12 h	Nausea, flushing, tachycardia, chest pain	Now obsolete; when no intensive monitoring available
Adrenergic Inhibitors					
Labetalol hydrochloride	20-80 mg I.V. bolus every 10 min; 0.5-2 mg/min as I.V. infusion	5-10 min	3-6 h	Vomiting, scalp tingling, burning in throat, dizziness, nausea, heart block, orthostatic hypotension	Most hypertensive emergencies except acute heart failure
Esmolol hydrochloride	250-500 mcg/kg/min for 1 min, then 50-100 mcg/kg/min for 4 min; may repeat	1-2 min	10-20 min	Hypotension, nausea	Aortic dissection, perioperative
Phentolamine	5-15 mg I.V.	1-2 min	3-10 min	Tachycardia, flushing, headache	Catecholamine excess

[1]These doses may vary from those in the *Physicians' Desk Reference* (51st edition).

[2]Hypotension may occur with all agents.

[3]Require special delivery system.

HYPERTENSION *(Continued)*

References

Guidelines

1999 World Health Organization-International Society of Hypertension Guidelines for the Management of Hypertension. Guidelines Subcommittee, *J Hypertens*, 1999, 17:151-83.

Chobanian AV, Bakris GL, Black HR, et al, "The Seventh Report of the Joint National Committee on Prevention, Detection, Evaluation, and Treatment of High Blood Pressure: The JNC 7 Report," *Jama*, 2003, 289(19):2560-71.

National High Blood Pressure Education Program Working Group on Hypertension Control in Children and Adolescents. Update on the 1987 Task Force Report on High Blood Pressure in Children and Adolescents: A Working Group Report From the National High Blood Pressure Education Program, *Pediatrics*, 1996, 98(4 Pt 1):649-58.

National High Blood Pressure Education Program Working Group. 1995 Update of the Working Group Reports on Chronic Renal Failure and Renovascular Hypertension, *Arch Intern Med*, 1996, 156:1938-47.

"The Sixth Report of the National Committee on Detection, Evaluation, and Treatment of High Blood Pressure (JNC-VI)," *Arch Intern Med*, 1997, 157:2413-46.

Others

Appel LJ, Moore TJ, Obarzanek E, et al, "A Clinical Trial of the Effect of Dietary Patterns on Blood Pressure. The DASH Collaborative Research Group," *N Engl J Med*, 1997, 336:1117-24.

Epstein M and Bakris G, "Newer Approaches to Antihypertensive Therapy: Use of Fixed-Dose Combination Therapy," *Arch Intern Med*, 1996, 156:1969-78.

Estacio RO and Schrier RW, "Antihypertensive Therapy in Type II Diabetes: Implications of the Appropriate Blood Pressure Control in Diabetes (ABCD) Trial," *Am J Cardiol*, 1998, 82:9R-14R.

Flack JM, Neaton J, Grimm RJ, et al, "Blood Pressure and Mortality Among Men With Prior Myocardial Infarction. The Multiple Risk Factor Intervention Trial Research Group," *Circulation*, 1995, 92:2437-45.

Frishman WH, Bryzinski BS, Coulson LR, et al, "A Multifactorial Trial Design to Assess Combination Therapy in Hypertension: Treatment With Bisoprolol and Hydrochlorothiazide," *Arch Intern Med*, 1994, 154:1461-8.

Furberg CD, Psaty BM, and Meyer JV, "Nifedipine: Dose-Related Increase in Mortality in Patients With Coronary Heart Disease," *Circulation*, 1995, 92:1326-31.

Glynn RJ, Brock DB, Harris T, et al, "Use of Antihypertensive Drugs and Trends in Blood Pressure in the Elderly," *Arch Intern Med*, 1995, 155:1855-60.

Gradman AH, Cutler NR, Davis PJ, et al, "Combined Enalapril and Felodipine Extended Release (ER) for Systemic Hypertension. The Enalapril-Felodipine ER Factorial Study Group," *Am J Cardiol*, 1997, 79:431-5.

Grim RH Jr, Flack JM, Grandits GA, et al, "Long-Term Effects on Plasma Lipids of Diet and Drugs to Treat Hypertension. The Treatment of Mild Hypertension Study (TOMHS) Research Group," *JAMA*, 1996, 275:1549-56.

Grim RH Jr, Grandits GA, Cutler JA, et al, "Relationships of Quality-of-Life Measures to Long-Term Lifestyle and Drug Treatment in the Treatment of Mild Hypertension Study. The TOMHS Research Group," *Arch Intern Med*, 1997, 157:638-48.

Grossman E, Messerli FH, Grodzicki T, et al, "Should a Moratorium Be Placed on Sublingual Nifedipine Capsules Given for Hypertensive Emergencies and Pseudoemergencies?" *JAMA*, 1996, 276:1328-31.

Hansson L, Zanchetti A, Carruthers SG, et al, "Effects of Intensive Blood Pressure Lowering and Low-Dose Aspirin in Patients With Hypertension: Principal Results of the Hypertension Optimal Treatment (HOT) Randomized Trial. HOT Study Group," *Lancet*, 1998, 351:1755-62.

Kaplan NM and Gifford RW Jr, "Choice of Initial Therapy for Hypertension," *JAMA*, 1996, 275:1577-80.

Kasiske BL, Ma JZ, Kalil RSN, et al, "Effects of Antihypertensive Therapy in Serum Lipids," *Ann Intern Med*, 1995, 122:133-41.

Kostis JB, Davis BR, Cutler J, et al, "Prevention of Heart Failure by Antihypertensive Drug Treatment in Older Persons With Isolated Systolic Hypertension. SHEP Cooperative Research Group," *JAMA*, 1997, 278:212-6.

Lazarus JM, Bourgoignie JJ, Buckalew VM, et al, "Achievement and Safety of a Low Blood Pressure Goal in Chronic Renal Disease: The Modification of Diet in Renal Disease Study Group," *Hypertension*, 1997, 29:641-50.

Lindheimer MD, "Hypertension in Pregnancy," *Hypertension*, 1993, 22:127-37.

Materson BJ, Reda DJ, Cushman WC, et al, "Single-Drug Therapy for Hypertension in Men: A Comparison of Six Antihypertensive Agents With Placebo. The Department of Veterans Affairs Cooperative Study Group on Antihypertensive Agents," *N Engl J Med*, 1993, 328:914-21.

Miller NH, Hill M, Kottke T, et al, "The Multi-Level Compliance Challenge: Recommendations for a Call to Action; A Statement for Healthcare Professionals," *Circulation*, 1997, 95:1085-90.

Neaton JD and Wentworth D, "Serum Cholesterol, Blood Pressure, Cigarette Smoking, and Death From Coronary Heart Disease: Overall Findings and Differences by Age for 316,099 White Men. The Multiple Risk Factor Intervention Trial Research Group," *Arch Intern Med*, 1992, 152:56-64.

Neaton JD, Grim RH, Prineas RJ, et al, "Treatment of Mild Hypertension Study (TOHMS). Final Results," *JAMA*, 1993, 270:721-31.

Oparil S, Levine JH, Zuschke CA, et al, "Effects of Candesartan Cilexetil in Patients With Severe Systemic Hypertension," *Am J Cardiol*, 1999, 84:289-93.

Perloff D, Grim C, Flack J, et al, "Human Blood Pressure Determination by Sphygmomanometry," *Circulation*, 1993, 88:2460-7.

Perry HM Jr, Bingham S, Horney A, et al, "Antihypertensive Efficacy of Treatment Regimens Used in Veterans Administration Hypertension Clinics. Department of Veterans Affairs Cooperative Study Group on Antihypertensive Agents," *Hypertension*, 1998, 31:771-9.

Preston RA, Materson BJ, Reda DJ, et al, "Age-Race Subgroup Compared With Renin Profile as Predictors of Blood Pressure Response to Antihypertensive Therapy," *JAMA*, 1998, 280:1168-72.

Psaty BM, Smith NL, Siscovick DS, et al, "Health Outcomes Associated With Antihypertensive Therapies Used as First-Line Agents. A Systemic Review and Meta-analysis," *JAMA*, 1997, 277:739-45.

Radevski IV, Valtchanova SP, Candy GP, et al, "Comparison of Acebutolol With and Without Hydrochlorothiazide Versus Carvedilol With and Without Hydrochlorothiazide in Black Patients With Mild to Moderate Systemic Hypertension," *Am J Cardiol*, 1999, 84(1):70-5.

Setaro JF and Black HR, "Refractory Hypertension," *N Engl J Med*, 1992, 327:543-7.

SHEP Cooperative Research Group, "Prevention of Stroke by Antihypertensive Drug Treatment in Older Persons With Isolated Systolic Hypertension: Final Results of the Systolic Hypertension in the Elderly Program (SHEP)," *JAMA*, 1991, 265:3255-64.

Sibai BM, "Treatment of Hypertension in Pregnant Women," *N Engl J Med*, 1996, 335:257-65.

Sowers JR, "Comorbidity of Hypertension and Diabetes: The Fosinopril Versus Amlodipine Cardiovascular Events Trial," *Am J Cardiol*, 1998, 82:15R-19R.

Sternberg H, Rosenthal T, Shamiss A, et al, "Altered Circadian Rhythm of Blood Pressure in Shift Workers," *J Hum Hypertens*, 1995, 9:349-53.

"The Hypertension Prevention Trial: Three-Year Effects of Dietary Changes on Blood Pressure. Hypertension Prevention Trial Research Group," *Arch Intern Med*, 1990, 150:153-62.

Trials of Hypertension Prevention Collaborative Research Group, "Effects of Weight Loss and Sodium Reduction Intervention on Blood Pressure and Hypertension Incidence in Overweight People With High-Normal Blood Pressure: The Trials of Hypertension Prevention, Phase II," *Arch Intern Med*, 1997, 157:657-67.

Tuomilehto J, Rastenyte D, Birkenhager WH, et al, "Effects of Calcium Channel Blockade in Older Patients With Diabetes and Systolic Hypertension," *N Engl J Med*, 1999, 340:677-84.

Veelken R and Schmieder RE, "Overview of Alpha-1 Adrenoceptor Antagonism and Recent Advances in Hypertensive Therapy," *Am J Hypertens*, 1996, 9:139S-49S.

White WB, Black HR, Weber MA, et al, "Comparison of Effects of Controlled Onset Extended Release Verapamil at Bedtime and Nifedipine Gastrointestinal Therapeutic System on Arising on Early Morning Blood Pressure, Heart Rate, and the Heart Rate-Blood Pressure Product," *Am J Cardiol*, 1998, 81:424-31.

OBESITY TREATMENT GUIDELINES FOR ADULTS

SUMMARY OF CLINICAL PRACTICE GUIDELINES

National Heart, Lung, and Blood Institute

Note: Weight loss treatment for children and adolescents is not covered by these guidelines.

ASSESSMENT

Assessment of weight involves evaluating body mass index, waist circumference, and the patient's risk factors.

A. Body Mass Index (BMI)

    1. BMI should be calculated for all adults (see table). Those with normal BMI should be reassessed in 2 years. A very muscular person may have a high BMI without the additional health risks.

    2. Overweight is defined as a BMI of 25-29.9 kg/m^2.

    3. Obesity is defined as a BMI of ≥30 kg/m^2.

B. Abdominal Fat

    1. Excess abdominal fat, not proportional to total body fat, is an independent predictor for risk and morbidity.

    2. Waist circumference for men >40 inches or women >35 inches is an increased risk for those with a BMI of 25-34.9.

C. Risk Factors

    1. Coronary heart disease or other atherosclerotic diseases, type 2 diabetes, and sleep apnea are factors associated with a very high risk of developing disease complications and mortality.

    2. Other obesity-associated diseases: Gynecological abnormalities, osteoarthritis, gallstones, stress incontinence.

    3. Cardiovascular risk factors: Cigarette smoking, hypertension, high-risk LDL-cholesterol, low HDL-cholesterol, impaired fasting glucose, family history of premature CHD.

    4. Other risk factors: Physical inactivity, high serum triglycerides.

    Weight loss is recommended for those who are obese and for those who are classified as overweight or have a high waist circumference and two or more risk factors.

Body Mass Index (BMI), kg/m^2
Height (feet, inches)

Weight (lb)	5'0"	5'3"	5'6"	5'9"	6'0"	6'3"
140	27	25	23	21	19	18
150	29	27	24	22	20	19
160	31	28	26	24	22	20
170	33	30	28	25	23	21
180	35	32	29	27	25	23
190	37	34	31	28	26	24
200	39	36	32	30	27	25
210	41	37	34	31	29	26
220	43	39	36	33	30	28
230	45	41	37	34	31	29
240	47	43	39	36	33	30
250	49	44	40	37	34	31

Note: For BMI calculations see "Body Mass Index" in Abbreviations and Measurements section.

TREATMENT

Patients who are overweight or obese, but are not candidates for weight loss or do not wish to lose weight, should be counseled to avoid further weight gain.

- A. Goals of Treatment
    1. Prevent further weight gain.
    2. Reduce body weight. The initial goal is to reduce body weight by 10% from baseline over the suggested time period of 6 months.
    3. Maintain a lower body weight, long term.
- B. Nonpharmacologic treatment should include:
    1. An individually-planned diet which includes a decrease in fat as well as total calories.
    2. An increase in physical activity. Physical activity should be gradually increased to a goal of 30 minutes per day of moderate-intensity activity.
    3. Behavior therapy, which should include tools to help overcome individual barriers to weight loss.

        Nonpharmacologic treatment should be tried for 6 months before starting physician-prescribed drug therapy.
- C. Drug Therapy

    In select patients with BMI ≥30, or BMI ≥27 with 2 or more risk factors, who did not lose weight or maintain weight loss, drug therapy can be started along with dietary therapy and physical activity.
- D. Surgery

    Patients with severe clinical obesity, BMI ≥40 or BMI ≥35 with coexisting conditions, can be considered for weight loss surgery when other methods have failed. Lifelong surveillance after surgery is necessary.

Medications for the Treatment of Obesity

Generic (Trade) Name	Therapeutic Category / Mechanism of Action	Usual Adult Dosage
Orlistat (Xenical®)	Lipase inhibitor; a reversible inhibitor of gastric and pancreatic lipases thus inhibiting absorption of dietary fats by 30% (at doses of 120 mg 3 times/day)	120 mg 3 times/day with each main meal containing fat (during or up to 1 hour after the meal); omit dose if meal is occasionally missed or contains no fat.
Amphetamine	The amphetamines are noncatecholamine sympathomimetic amines with CNS stimulant activity. The anorexigenic effect is probably secondary to the CNS-stimulating effect; the site of action is probably the hypothalamic feeding center.	Long-acting capsule: 10 or 15 mg/day, up to 30 mg/day; Immediate release tablets: 5-30 mg/day in divided doses
Benzphetamine (Didrex®)	Anorexiant; noncatechol sympathomimetic amines with pharmacologic actions similar to ephedrine; anorexigenic effect is probably secondary to the CNS-stimulating effect; the site of action is probably the hypothalamic feeding center	25-50 mg 2-3 times/day, preferably twice daily (midmorning and midafternoon); maximum dose: 50 mg 3 times/day
Diethylpropion (Tenuate®; Tenuate® Dospan®)	Anorexiant; pharmacological and chemical properties similar to those of amphetamines. The mechanism of action of diethylpropion in reducing appetite appears to be secondary to CNS effects, specifically stimulation of the hypothalamus to release catecholamines into the central nervous system; anorexiant effects are mediated via norepinephrine and dopamine metabolism. An increase in physical activity and metabolic effects (inhibition of lipogenesis and enhancement of lipolysis) may also contribute to weight loss.	Tablet: 25 mg 3 times/day before meals or food
Tablet, controlled release: 75 mg at midmorning
Methamphetamine (Desoxyn®)	A sympathomimetic amine related to ephedrine and amphetamine with CNS stimulant activity	5 mg, 30 minutes before each meal; long-acting formulation: 10-15 mg in morning; treatment duration should not exceed a few weeks

OBESITY TREATMENT GUIDELINES FOR ADULTS *(Continued)*

Medications for the Treatment of Obesity *(continued)*

Generic (Trade) Name	Therapeutic Category / Mechanism of Action	Usual Adult Dosage
Phentermine (Adipex-P®, Ionamin®)	Anorexiant; structurally similar to dextroamphetamine and is comparable to dextroamphetamine as an appetite suppressant, but is generally associated with a lower incidence and severity of CNS side effects. Stimulates the hypothalamus to result in decreased appetite; anorexiant effects are most likely mediated via norepinephrine and dopamine metabolism. However, other CNS effects or metabolic effects may be involved.	8 mg 3 times/day 30 minutes before meals or food or 15-37.5 mg/day before breakfast or 10-14 hours before retiring
Sibutramine (Meridia®)	Anorexiant; blocks the neuronal uptake of norepinephrine and, to a lesser extent, serotonin and dopamine	Initial: 10 mg once daily; after 4 weeks may titrate up to 15 mg once daily as needed and tolerated

OSTEOPOROSIS MANAGEMENT

PREVALENCE

Osteoporosis effects 25 million Americans of whom 80% are women. 27% of American women >80 years of age have osteopenia and 70% of American women >80 years of age have osteoporosis.

CONSEQUENCES

1.3 million bone fractures annually (low impact/nontraumatic) and pain, pulmonary insufficiency, decreased quality of life, and economic costs; >300,000 hip fractures per year with a 20% mortality rate and >700,000 vertebral fractures in women.

RISK FACTORS

- Advanced age
- Anorexia/hypogonadism, cancer, chronic renal disease, Cushing's disease, hyper-parathyroidism, hyperprolactinemia, hyperthyroidism (current condition, history of, or use of excessive thyroid supplements), hypogonadism
- Caucasian or Asian race
- Early menopause
- Excessive alcohol intake
- Excessive exercise
- Family history
- Female gender
- History of low calcium intake
- Oophorectomy without hormone replacement
- Sedentary lifestyle
- Smoking
- Use of aluminum-containing antacids (excessive), anticonvulsants, ethanol, heparin or glucocorticoids (large doses or prolonged use), methotrexate or cyclo-sporine

DIAGNOSIS / MONITORING

- DXA bone density scan
- Osteomark™ urine assay*
- History of fracture (low impact or nontraumatic)
- Compressed vertebrae
- Decreased height
- Hump-back appearance
- Excluded secondary causes

*Osteomark™ urine assay measures bone breakdown fragments and may help assess therapy response earlier than DXA bone scan but diagnostic value is uncertain as Osteomark™ does not reveal extent of bone loss. Bone markers may be tested to evaluate effectiveness of antiresorptive urine therapy.

PREVENTION

1. Adequate intake of dietary calcium (eg, dairy products)

2. Increased intake of vitamin D (eg, fortified dairy products, cod, fatty fish)

3. Weight-bearing exercise (eg, walking), as tolerated

4. Calcium supplement: 1000-1500 mg **elemental** calcium daily (divided in 500 mg increments); see table located at the end of this section. Do not administer orally with bran, foods high in oxalates, or whole grain cereals. Calcium carbonate is given with food to enhance bioavailability. Chewable and liquid products are available.

    Adults ≥51 years: Supplement 1200 mg **elemental** calcium.

    Women >65 years on estrogen replacement therapy: Supplement 1000 mg **elemental** calcium.

    Women >65 years not receiving estrogens and men >55 years: Supplement 1500 mg **elemental** calcium.

    - Contraindications: Hypercalcemia, renal calculi, ventricular fibrillation
    - Side effects: Constipation, anorexia; to minimize constipation, add fiber supplement to diet and start with 500 mg/day for several months, then increase to 500 mg twice daily taken at different times than the fiber supplement
    - Drug interactions: May potentiate digoxin toxicity, antagonize effects of calcium channel blockers (eg, verapamil), decrease potassium-binding ability of polystyrene sulfonate, and decrease absorption of tetracycline, atenolol, iron, quinolone antibiotics, alendronate, sodium fluoride, and zinc; high doses of calcium with thiazide diuretics may result in milk-alkali syndrome and hypercalcemia

OSTEOPOROSIS MANAGEMENT *(Continued)*

5. Bisphosphonates: Alendronate 5 mg/day or 35 mg/week, and risidronate 5 mg/day or 35 mg/week are approved for the prevention of osteoporosis in postmenopausal women. Risidronate 5 mg/day is also approved for the prevention of glucocorticoid-induced osteoporosis. Patients must be capable of following specific instructions related to drug administration (see Treatment for administration, side effects, and precautions).

6. Selective estrogen receptor modulators: SERMs are nonsteroidal modulators of estrogen-receptor mediated reactions. The key difference between these agents and estrogen replacement therapies is the potential to exert tissue-specific effects. Due to their chemical differences, these agents retain some of estrogen's beneficial effects on bone metabolism and lipid levels, but differ in their actions on breast and endometrial tissues, potentially limiting adverse effects related to nonspecific hormone stimulation. Among the SERMs, tamoxifen retains stimulatory effects in endometrial tissue, while raloxifene does not stimulate endometrial or breast tissue, limiting the potential for endometrial or breast cancer related to this agent. Raloxifene is the only SERM which has been approved by the FDA for osteoporosis prevention.

    Note: The effects on bone observed with SERMs appear to be less than that observed with estrogen replacement. In one study, the effect of raloxifene on hip bone mineral density was approximately half of that observed with conjugated estrogens. Raloxifene decreases total high-density lipoprotein cholesterol or triglyceride levels. Raloxifene has been shown to reduce the risk of breast cancer, not increase the risk of endometrial cancer, but increase the risk of DVT compared to placebo in postmenopausal women. Finally, SERMs do not block the vasomotor effects observed with menopause, which may limit compliance with therapy.

    Raloxifene: 60 mg/day; may be taken any time of the day without regard to meals but should be stopped 72 hours prior to or during prolonged immobilization due to risk of thromboembolic events (similar to reported risk of HRT) .

    - Contraindications: Active thromboembolic disorder, prolonged immobilization (eg, postoperative recovery, prolonged bedrest)

    - Side effects: Hot flashes (vasomotor symptoms), increased risk of thromboembolism (DVT, PE) and superficial thrombophlebitis, flu-like symptoms (resolve with use), GI upset, vaginitis, UTI

    - Drug interactions: Ampicillin and cholestyramine decrease raloxifene absorption. Avoid ethanol.

7. Estrogens should not be considered first agents for preventing osteoporosis due to increased risk of breast cancer, heart disease, stroke, and deep-vein thrombosis (DVT) found in the Women's Health Initiative study. Estradiol, as well as various combination therapies, including ethinyl estradiol with norethindrone (femhrt®) and ethinyl with norgestimate (Ortho-Prefest®), have been approved for the prevention of osteoporosis.

8. Estrogen: 0.625 mg/day conjugated estrogen **or** its equivalent; initiate therapy slowly and monitor blood pressure in long-term use. In women with an intact uterus, administer with medroxyprogesterone acetate (MPA) 2.5-5 mg/day **or** another oral progesterone; unopposed estrogen can cause endometrial cancer.

    Note: Continuous therapy is preferred; especially useful if bone density is <80% of average and patient has symptoms of estrogen deficiency. Substantial evidence suggests that estrogen therapy increases bone mineralization; bone density increases over 1-2 years, then reaches a plateau. Therapy should be initiated after careful evaluation of risk:benefit ratio. Pretreatment mammogram and gynecological exam are advised along with routine breast exam due to possible increased risk of breast cancer with long-term use.

    - Contraindications: Breast or estrogen-dependent cancer, undiagnosed abnormal genital bleeding, active thrombophlebitis, history of thromboembolism during previous estrogen therapy

      Note: It is important that patients on long-term estrogens avoid cigarette use. Conjugated estrogens (alone or in combination with a progestin) should not be used to prevent coronary heart disease. The HERS trial found that women with coronary disease derived no cardiovascular protection compared to those treated with placebo. In the Women's Health Initiative trial, a conjugated estrogen/progestin combination did not offer protection against heart disease. No cardiovascular benefits were seen, in fact, **more coronary heart disease was observed** in the treatment group.

    - Side effects (more common/severe in women without estrogen for many years): Vaginal spotting/bleeding, nausea, vomiting, breast tenderness/enlargement, amenorrheic (with extended use), hypertension (less severe with lower doses), thromboembolic events (particularly in women who smoke). **Note:** If MPA is also used, it can increase vaginal bleeding, increase weight, edema, and mood changes.

    - Drug interactions: May enhance the effects of hydrocortisone and prednisone; monitor for need to decrease corticosteroid dose. Anticoagulants: Increase potential for thromboembolic events with anticoagulants. CYP3A4 enzyme inducers (eg, carbamazepine, phenobarbital, rifampin) may decrease estrogen plasma concentrations; inhibitors (eg, clarithromycin, erythromycin, itraconazole, ketoconazole, ritonavir) may increase estrogen plasma concentrations. Avoid ethanol, grapefruit juice, St John's wort, black cohosh, dong quai, red clover, saw palmetto, and ginseng.

9. Vitamin D: 400-800 units/day (often satisfied by 1-2 multivitamins or fortified milk) in addition to calcium or a combined calcium and vitamin D supplement, **and/or** >15 minutes direct sunlight/day. Avoid doses ≥1000 int. units/day due to potential toxicity. Symptoms of deficiency include bone and tooth disorders, rickets, and osteomalacia.

    Note: Some older adults, especially those with significant renal or liver disease cannot metabolize (activate) vitamin D and require calcitriol or dosage adjustment per serum calcium level, the active form of vitamin D. Check 1,25 OH vitamin D level to confirm need for calcitriol. If required, administer 0.25 mcg calcitriol orally twice daily.

    *   Contraindications: Hypercalcemia (weakness, headache, drowsiness, nausea, diarrhea), hypercalciuria, renal stones

    *   Side effects: Hypercalcemia (uncommon); monitor 24-hour urine and serum calcium if using >1000 units/day. Overdose symptoms include excessive thirst, dehydration, anorexia, nausea, vomiting, headache, constipation, weakness, weight loss, hypercalcemia, kidney stones, arterial calcium deposits

    *   Drug interactions: Drugs which can cause depletion of vitamin D include cholestyramine, anticonvulsants, corticosteroids, isoniazid, rifampin, H_2-receptor antagonists, and mineral oil. Vitamin A antagonizes some of the activity of vitamin D.

TREATMENT

1. Calcium, vitamin D, exercise, and estrogen: See table.

2. Bisphosphonates: Administer ≥30 minutes before first food or drink (except water) with 6-8 ounces tap water (**not** mineral water) and remain upright (or raise head of bed to at least a 30° angle) to avoid ulcerative esophagitis.

    Note: Bisphosphonates may be useful even when the patient has severe osteoporosis (ie, ≥2.5 standard deviations below average young adult bone density, T-score, or history of low impact or nontraumatic fracture). Increasing bone density of hip and spine has been observed for at least 3 years (ie, no plateau as seen with estrogen). Therapy with calcium and vitamin D is advised (must be given at a different time of day than alendronate):

    Contraindications: Hypocalcemia (must be corrected prior to therapy), abnormalities of the esophagus which delay emptying (ie, stricture, achalasia), inability to stand or sit upright for at least 30 minutes

    *   Alendronate (Fosamax®): Not recommended if Cl_{cr} <35 mL/minute.

        Osteoporosis: **Males/postmenopausal females:** Treatment: 10 mg once daily **or** 70 mg once weekly.

        Glucocorticoid-induced Osteoporosis: Treatment: 5 mg once daily; 10 mg once daily for postmenopausal women not receiving estrogen

        Side effects: Hypocalcemia, hypophosphatemia, GI disturbances, musculoskeletal pain

        Drug interactions: Increased GI effects with >10 mg alendronate and aspirin-containing products; wait at least 30 minutes after taking alendronate before taking any oral medications. Ranitidine can double the bioavailability of alendronate.

    *   Etidronate is not FDA-approved for postmenopausal osteoporosis and can decrease the quality of bone formation; **use alendronate**.

    *   Risedronate (Actonel®): Not recommended if Cl_{cr} <30 mL/minute.

        Osteoporosis: **Postmenopausal females:** 5 mg once daily **or** 35 mg once weekly

        Glucocorticoid-induced Osteoporosis: 5 mg once daily

        Side effects: Flu-like symptoms

        Drug interactions: Administer antacids and calcium supplements at a different time of the day so as not to interfere with absorption of risedronate. Avoid ethanol.

3. Calcitonin is indicated for the treatment of osteoporosis and may also be used as adjunctive therapy for hypercalcemia. Adequate dietary or supplemental calcium and vitamin D is essential. I.M. route is preferred if volume exceeds 2 mL. Administration in the evening may minimize flushing, nausea, and vomiting.

    Hypercalcemia: Initial: 4 units/kg every 12 hours I.M., SubQ; may increase up to 8 units/kg every 12 hours (maximum every 6 hours)

OSTEOPOROSIS MANAGEMENT *(Continued)*

Osteoporosis: **Postmenopausal females:** 100 units/day I.M., SubQ **or** 200 units/day (1 spray) intranasal; 1 spray (200 units) into 1 nostril daily (alternate right and left nostril daily); 5 days on and 2 days off is also effective but alternate day administration is not effective. If used only for pain, can decrease dose once pain is controlled.

- Contraindications: Hypersensitivity to salmon protein or gelatin diluent

- Side effects: Nasal dryness/irritation (periodically inspect), flushing, nausea, vomiting; SubQ 100 units/day: Many side effects including nausea, flushing, anorexia, and the discomfort/inconvenience of injection

4. Raloxifene: Refer to raloxifene information under "Prevention" (above).

5. Teriparatide is indicated for the treatment of osteoporosis in postmenopausal women at high risk of fracture as well as the treatment of primary or hypogonadal osteoporosis in men at high risk of fracture.

- Dose: SubQ: 20 mcg once daily. **Note:** Initial administration should occur under circumstances in which the patient may sit or lie down, in the event of orthostasis.

- Contraindications: Should not be used in patients with a history of skeletal metastases, hyperparathyroidism, or pre-existing hypercalcemia. Metabolic bone disease other than osteoporosis should be excluded prior to initiating therapy.

- Warnings: Should be used with caution in patients with active or recent urolithiasis or in patients at risk of orthostasis patients as well as patients who may not tolerate transient hypotension. Due to concerns for a possible association between long term, high-dose use and osteosarcoma, teriparatide is not recommended for use longer than 2 years, and should be avoided in patients with an increased risk of osteosarcoma.

- Side effects: Transient hypercalcemia may be noted between 4 and 6 hours after a dose. Arthralgia, asthenia, and leg cramps may occur. May be associated with central nervous system effects such as dizziness, depression or vertigo. In addition, teriparatide use has been associated with gastrointestinal effects (nausea, dyspepsia) and rash.

6. Fall prevention: Minimize psychoactive and cardiovascular drugs, monitor BP for orthostasis, administer diuretics early in the day, and check environment for safety hazards.

Calcium Type	Elemental Calcium	Equivalent Elemental Calcium	Brand
Acetate	25%	667 mg = 169 mg	Phos-Lo® gelcaps and tablets
Carbonate	40%	364 mg = 145.6 mg	Florical® capsules and tablets
		400 mg = 160 mg	Mylanta® Children's chewable tablets
		420 mg = 168 mg	Chewable tablets: Alcalak, Amitone®, Titralac™
		500 mg = 200 mg	Chewable tablets: Cal-Gest, Chooz®, Tums®
		650 mg = 260 mg	Cal-Mint chewable tablets
		750 mg = 300 mg	Chewable tablets: Titralac™ Extra Strength, Tums® E-X, Tums® Extra Strength Sugar Free, Tums® Smooth Dissolve
		850 mg = 340 mg	Alka-Mints® chewable tablets
		1000 mg = 400 mg	Tums® Ultra chewable tablets
		1250 mg = 500 mg	Calci-Mix® capsules
			Chewable tablets: Calci-Chew®, Os-Cal® 500, Oysco 500, Oyst-Cal 500
		1250 mg/5 mL = 500 mg	Generic oral solution
		1500 mg = 600 mg	Chewable tablets: Calcarb 600, Caltrate® 600, Nephro-Calci®
Citrate	21%	950 mg = 200 mg	Citracal®
		2376 mg = 500 mg	Citracal® Liquitab effervescent tablets
Glubionate	6.5%	1.8 g = 115 g/5 mL	Various OTC and generic brands available
Gluconate	9%	500 mg = 45 mg	
Lactate	13%	325 mg = 42.25 mg	
Phosphate tribasic	39%	1565.2 mg = 600 mg	Posture®

References

Ashworth L, "Focus on Alendronate. A Nonhormonal Option for the Treatment of Osteoporosis in Postmenopausal Women," *Formulary*, 1996, 31:23-30.

Barrett-Connor E, Grady D, Sashegyi A, et al, "Raloxifene and Cardiovascular Events in Osteoporotic Postmenopausal Women: Four-Year Results From the MORE (Multiple Outcomes of Raloxifene Evaluation) Randomized Trial," *JAMA*, 2002, 287(7):847-57.

Grady D, Ettinger B, Moscarelli E, et al, "Safety and Adverse Effects Associated With Raloxifene: Multiple Outcomes of Raloxifene Evaluation," *Obstet Gynecol*, 2004, 104(4):837-44.

Hully S, Grady D, Bush T, et al, "Randomized Trial of Estrogen Plus Progestin for Secondary Prevention of Coronary Heart Disease in Postmenopausal Women. Heart and Estrogen/Progestin Replacement Study (HERS) Research Group," *JAMA*, 1998, 280(7):605-13.

Johnson SR, "Should Older Women Use Estrogen Replacement," *J Am Geriatr Soc*, 1996, 44:89-90.

Liberman UA, Weiss SR, and Brool J, "Effect of Oral Alendronate on Bone-Mineral Density and the Incidence of Fracture in Postmenopausal Osteoporosis," *N Engl J Med*, 1995, 333:1437-43.

"New Drugs for Osteoporosis," *Med Lett Drugs Ther*, 1996, 38:1-3.

NIH Concensus Development Panel on Optimal Calcium Intake, *JAMA*, 1994, 272:1942-8.

PCA Osteoporosis Prevention and Treatment Video-Teleconference (March 1, April 2 and 3, 1996).

"Writing Group for the Women's Health Initiative Investigators. Risks and Benefits of Estrogen Plus Progestin in Healthy Postmenopausal Women: Principle Results From the Women's Health Initiative Randomized Controlled Trial," *JAMA*, 2002, 288:321-33.

Multiple outcomes of raloxifene trial.

PHARMACOTHERAPY OF URINARY INCONTINENCE

Incontinence Type	Drug Class	Drug Therapy	Adverse Effects and Precautions	Comments
Urge incontinence	Anticholinergic agents	Oxybutynin (2.5-5 mg 2-4 times/day or extended release 5-20 mg once daily), propantheline (7.5-30 mg at least 3 times/day), dicyclomine (10-20 mg twice daily), tolterodine (1-2 mg twice daily; extended release capsule: 2-4 mg once daily)	Dry mouth, visual disturbances, constipation, dry skin, confusion	Anticholinergics are the first-line drug therapy (oxybutynin or tolterodine is preferred). Propantheline and dicyclomine are not considered drugs of choice in older adults.
	Tricyclic antidepressants (TCAs)	Imipramine, desipramine, nortriptyline (25-100 mg/ day)	Anticholinergic effects (as above), orthostatic hypotension, and cardiac dysrhythmia	TCAs are generally reserved for patients with an additional indication (eg, depression, neuralgia) at an initial dose of 10-25 mg 1-3 times/day.
Stress incontinence	Alpha-adrenergic agonists	Pseudoephedrine (15-60 mg 3 times/day)	Anxiety, insomnia, agitation, respiratory difficulty, sweating, cardiac dysrhythmia, hypertension, tremor; should not be used in obstructive syndromes and/or hypertension	Pseudoephedrine is the first-line drug therapy for women with no contraindication (notably hypertension).
Stress or combined urge/stress incontinence	Estrogen replacement agents	Conjugated estrogens (0.3-0.625 mg/day orally or 1 g vaginal cream at bedtime)	Should not be used if suspected or confirmed breast or endometrial cancer, active or past thromboembolism with past oral contraceptive, estrogen, or pregnancy; headache, spotting, edema, breast tenderness, possible depression	Estrogen (oral or vaginal) is an adjunctive therapy for postmenopausal women, as it augments alpha-agonists (eg, pseudoephedrine).
			Give progesterone with estrogen if uterus is present; pretreatment/periodic mammogram, gynecologic, breast exam advised	Progestin (eg, medroxyprogesterone 2.5-10 mg/day) continuously or intermittently; combined oral or vaginal estrogen and PPA in postmenopausal women, if single drug is inadequate; imipramine is an alternative therapy when first-line therapy is inadequate.
	imipramine (10-25 mg 3 times/day)		May worsen cardiac conduction abnormalities, postural hypotension, anticholinergic effects	
Overflow	Alpha-adrenergic antagonists	Terazosin (1 mg at bedtime with first dose in supine position and increase by 1 mg every 4 days to maximum 10 mg/day)	Postural hypotension, dizziness, vertigo, heart palpitations, edema, headache, anticholinergic effects	Possible benefit in men with obstructive symptoms of benign prostatic hyperplasia; monitor postural vital signs with first dose/each dose increase; may worsen female stress incontinence
		Doxazosin (1 mg at bedtime with first dose in supine position and increase by 1 mg every 7-14 days to maximum 8 mg/day)	Same as terazosin (may be smaller incidence of hypotension)	Same as terazosin

Adapted from "Urinary Incontinence," *Clinical Practice Guideline*, 1996, American Medical Directors Association, reprinted with permission. For more information call 1-800-876-2632.

PROPHYLAXIS FOR EXPOSURE TO COMMUNICABLE DISEASES

Disease	Exposure	Prophylaxis / Management
Anthrax	Postexposure inhalational	Doxycycline and ciprofloxacin; 60-day (oral and intravenous) regimens have been recommended.
Invasive *Haemophilus influenzae* disease	Close contact with an infected child for more than 4 hours	Give rifampin 20 mg/kg orally once daily for 4 days (600 mg maximum daily dose) to entire family with at least one household contact <48 months old. Contraindication: Pregnant contacts.
Hepatitis A	Direct contact with an infected child, or sharing of food or utensils	Give 0.02 mL/kg immune globulin (IG) within 7 days of exposure.
Hepatitis B	Needlestick (used needle); mucous membrane exposure with blood or body fluid; direct inoculation of blood or body fluid into open cut, lesion, or laceration	**Known source and employee status unknown: Test patient for HB$_s$Ag and employee for anti-HB$_s$.** If patient is HB$_s$Ag negative and the patient does not have non-A, non-B hepatitis, do nothing. If patient is HB$_s$Ag negative and has non-A, non-B hepatitis, **offer** ISG (optional). If patient is HB$_s$Ag positive, give HBIG and hepatitis B vaccine within 48 hours of exposure. Employee antibody status may not be available for up to a week, so the above should be given as soon as patient's antigen status is known. Occasionally, the patient's antigen status will be unavailable for more than 24 hours. In these cases, HBIG should be given if the patient is high risk (ie, Asian immigrants, institutionalized patients, homosexuals, intravenous drug abusers, hemodialysis patients, patients with a history of hepatitis). If the employee is anti-HB$_s$ negative, give the second and third doses of hepatitis B vaccine. **Known source and employee documented anti-HB$_s$ positive:** If source has non-A, non-B hepatitis, offer ISG (optional). If employee is believed to be anti-HB$_s$ positive due to vaccination, has received 3 doses of vaccine, and has not had an anti-HB$_s$ test done, draw serum for anti-HB$_s$.
Measles	15 minutes or more in the same room with a child with measles from 2 days before the onset of symptoms to 4 days after the appearance of the rash	Children who have not been vaccinated and have not had natural infection should be isolated from the 7th through the 18th day after exposure and/or for 4 days after the rash appears. Those who have not been vaccinated should be vaccinated within 72 hours of exposure if no contraindication exists, or receive immune globulin (IG) 0.25 mL/kg I.M. for immunocompetent individuals and 0.5 mL/kg (maximum: 15 mL) for immunosuppressed individuals. Children who are younger than 15 months of age should be revaccinated at 15 months of age but at least 3 months after receipt of vaccine or IG. Older individuals who have received IG should be vaccinated 3 months later.
Meningococcal disease	Household contact or direct contact with secretions	Household, day care center, and nursery school children should receive rifampin prophylaxis for 2 days. Dosages are given every 12 hours for a total of 4 doses. Dosage is 10 mg/kg/dose for children ages 1 month to 12 years (maximum: 600 mg/dose), 5 mg/kg/dose for infants <1 month of age, and 600 mg/dose for adults. Alternatively, ciprofloxacin 750 mg as a single dose may be used. Contraindication: Pregnant contacts. **Because prophylaxis is not always effective, exposed children should be monitored for symptoms.** **Employee exposure: Anyone who develops a febrile illness should receive prompt medical evaluation. If indicated, antimicrobial therapy should be administered.**

PROPHYLAXIS FOR EXPOSURE TO COMMUNICABLE DISEASES (Continued)

Disease	Exposure	Prophylaxis / Management
Pertussis	Housed in the same room with an infected child or spent 15 minutes in the playroom with the infected child	**Prophylaxis:** Contacts <7 years old who have had at least 4 doses of pertussis vaccine should receive a booster dose of DTP, unless a dose has been given within the past 3 years, and should receive erythromycin 40-50 mg/kg/day orally for 14 days. Contacts <7 years old who are not immunized or who have received less than 4 doses of DTP should have DTP immunization initiated or continued according to the recommended schedule. Children who have received their third dose 6 months or more before exposure should be given their fourth dose at this time. Erythromycin should also be given for 14 days. Contacts ≥7 years of age and above should receive prophylactic erythromycin (maximum: 1 g/day) for 10-14 days. All exposed patients should be watched closely for respiratory symptoms for 14 days after exposure has stopped because immunity conferred by the vaccine is not absolute and the efficacy of erythromycin in prophylaxis has not been established.
Tuberculosis	Housed in the same room with a child with contagious tuberculosis (tuberculosis is contagious if the child has a cough plus AFB seen on smear plus cavitation on CXR)	Place PPD immediately and 10 weeks after exposure. Start on INH. Consult Infectious Diseases if seroconversion occurs.
Varicella-zoster	1 hour or more in the same room with a contagious child from 24 hours before vesicles appear to when all vesicles are crusted, which is usually 5-7 days after vesicles appear. In household exposure, communicability is 48 hours before vesicles appear.	**Immunocompetent** children who have not been vaccinated or had natural infection, should have titers drawn only if they will still be hospitalized for more than 10 days after exposure. If titers are negative, they should be isolated from 10 to 21 days after exposure and/or until all lesions are crusted and dry. If VZIG was given the child should be isolated from 10 to 28 days after exposure. **Immunocompromised** children who have not been vaccinated or had natural infection should first have titers drawn, and then receive VZIG (varicella-zoster immune globulin) **1 vial/10 kg I.M.** up to a maximum of 5 vials as soon as possible but at most 96 hours after exposure. Fractional doses are not recommended. If titers are positive, nothing further need be done. If titers are negative, the child should be isolated from 10 to 28 days after exposure and should be monitored very carefully for the appearance of vesicles so that treatment can be initiated. VZIG is available from the Blood Bank.

TREATMENT OF SEXUALLY TRANSMITTED INFECTIONS

Type or Stage	Drugs of Choice / Dosage	Alternatives
CHLAMYDIAL INFECTION AND RELATED CLINICAL SYNDROMES[1]		
Urethritis, cervicitis, conjunctivitis, or proctitis (except lymphogranuloma venereum)		
	Azithromycin 1 g oral once **or** Doxycycline[2,3] 100 mg oral bid x 7 d	Ofloxacin[3] 300 mg oral bid x 7 d **or** Levofloxacin[3] 500 mg oral once/d x 7 d **or** Erythromycin[4] 500 mg oral qid x 7 d
Infection in pregnancy		
	Azithromycin 1 g oral once **or** Amoxicillin 500 mg oral tid x 7 d	Erythromycin[4] 500 mg oral qid x 7 d
Neonatal ophthalmia or pneumonia		
	Azithromycin 20 mg/kg oral once daily x 3 d	Erythromycin 12.5 mg/kg oral qid x 14 d[5]
Lymphogranuloma venereum		
	Doxycycline[2,3] 100 mg oral bid x 21 d	Erythromycin[4] 500 mg oral qid x 21 d
EPIDIDYMITIS		
	Ofloxacin 300 mg bid x 10 d **or** Levofloxacin 500 mg oral once daily x 10 d	Ceftriaxone 250 mg I.M. once **followed by** doxycycline[2] 100 mg oral bid x 10 d
GONORRHEA[6]		
Disseminated gonococcal infection		
	Ceftriaxone 1 g I.M. or I.V. q24h	Cefotaxime 1 g I.V. q8h **or** Ceftizoxime 1 g I.V. q8h **or** **For persons allergic to β-lactam drugs:** Ciprofloxacin 400 mg I.V. q12h **or** Levofloxacin 250 mg I.V. once daily **or** Ofloxacin 400 mg I.V. q12h **or** Spectinomycin 2 g I.M. q12h
		All regimens should be continued for 24-48 hours after improvement begins, at which time therapy may be switched to one of the following regimens to complete a full week of antimicrobial therapy:
		Cefixime 400 mg oral bid **or** Ciprofloxacin 500 mg oral bid **or** Levofloxacin 500 mg oral once daily **or** Ofloxacin 400 mg oral bid
Gonococcal meningitis and endocarditis		
	Ceftriaxone 1-2 g I.V. q12h	
Urethral, cervical, rectal, or pharyngeal		
	Cefixime 400 mg oral once **or** Ceftriaxone 125 mg I.M. once	Cefpodoxime 400 mg oral once **or** Ciprofloxacin[3,7] 500 mg oral once **or** Ofloxacin[3,7] 400 mg oral once **or** Levofloxacin[3,7] 250 mg oral once **or** Spectinomycin 2 g I.M. once[8]
PELVIC INFLAMMATORY DISEASE		
– parenteral	Cefotetan 2 g I.V. q12h **or** cefoxitin 2 g I.V. q6h **plus** doxycycline[3] 100 mg oral or I.V. q12h, until improved **followed by** doxycycline[3] 100 mg oral bid to complete 14 d[10] **or** Clindamycin 900 mg I.V. q8h **plus** gentamicin 2 mg/kg I.V. once, then 1.5 mg/kg I.V. q8h,[11] until improved **followed by** doxycycline[3] 100 mg oral bid to complete 14 d[10]	Ofloxacin[3] 400 mg I.V. q12h **or** levofloxacin[3] 500 mg I.V. once daily **plus** metronidazole 500 mg I.V. q8h[9] **or** Ampicillin/sulbactam 3 g I.V. q6h **plus** doxycycline[3] 100 mg oral or I.V. q12h **All continued until improved, then followed by** doxycycline[3] 100 mg oral bid to complete 14 d[10]

TREATMENT OF SEXUALLY TRANSMITTED INFECTIONS
(Continued)

Type or Stage	Drugs of Choice / Dosage	Alternatives
– oral	Ofloxacin[3] 400 mg bid x 14 d **or** Levofloxacin[3] 500 mg once daily x 14 d ± metronidazole[9] 500 mg bid x 14 d **or** Ceftriaxone 250 mg I.M. once **followed by** doxycycline[3,12] 100 mg bid x 14 d	Cefoxitin 2 g once **plus** probenecid 1 g oral once **followed by** doxycycline[3,12] 100 mg bid x 14 d
TRICHOMONIASIS	Metronidazole 2 g oral once **or** Tinidazole 2 g oral once	Metronidazole 375 or 500 mg oral bid x 7 d
BACTERIAL VAGINOSIS	Metronidazole 500 mg oral bid x 7 d **or** Metronidazole gel 0.75%[14] 5 g intravaginally once or twice daily x 5 d **or** Clindamycin 2% cream[14] 5 g intravaginally qhs x 3-7 d	Metronidazole 2 g oral once[13] or Flagyl ER® 750 mg once daily x 7 d **or** Clindamycin 300 mg oral bid x 7 d **or** Clindamycin ovules[14] 100 mg intravaginally once daily x 3 d
VULVOVAGINAL CANDIDIASIS	Intravaginal butoconazole, clotrimazole, miconazole, terconazole, or tioconazole[15] **or** Fluconazole 150 mg oral once	Nystatin 100,000 unit vaginal tablet once daily x 14 d
SYPHILIS		
Early (primary, secondary, or latent <1 y)	Penicillin G benzathine 2.4 million units I.M. once[16]	Doxycycline[3] 100 mg oral bid x 14 d
Late (>1 year's duration, cardiovascular, gumma, late-latent)	Penicillin G benzathine 2.4 million units I.M. weekly x 3 wk	Doxycycline[3] 100 mg oral bid x 4 wk
Neurosyphilis[17]	Penicillin G 3-4 million units I.V. q4h or 24 million units continuous I.V. infusion x 10-14 d	Penicillin G procaine 2.4 million units I.M. daily **plus** probenecid 500 mg qid oral, both x 10-14 d **or** Ceftriaxone 2 g I.V. once daily x 10-14 d
Congenital	Penicillin G 50,000 units/kg I.V. q8-12h for 10-14 d **or** Penicillin G procaine 50,000 units/kg I.M. daily for 10-14 d	
CHANCROID[18]	Azithromycin 1 g oral once **or** Ceftriaxone 250 mg I.M. once	Ciprofloxacin[3] 500 mg oral bid x 3 d **or** Erythromycin[4] 500 mg oral qid x 7 d
GENITAL WARTS[19]	Trichloroacetic or bichloroacetic acid, or podophyllin[3] or liquid nitrogen 1-2 times/ wk until resolved **or** Imiquimod 5% 3 times/wk x 16 wk **or** Podofilox 0.5% bid x 3 d, 4 days rest, then repeated up to 4 times	Surgical removal **or** Laser surgery **or** Intralesional interferon
GENITAL HERPES		
First episode	Acyclovir 400 mg oral tid x 7-10 d **or** Famciclovir 250 mg oral tid x 7-10 d **or** Valacyclovir 1 g oral bid x 7-10 d	Acyclovir 200 mg oral 5 times/d x 7-10 d
Severe (hospitalized patients)	Acyclovir 5-10 mg/kg I.V. q8h x 5-7 d	
Suppression of recurrences[20]	Acyclovir 400 mg oral bid **or** Famciclovir 250 mg oral bid **or** Valacyclovir 500 mg - 1 g once daily[21]	Acyclovir 200 mg oral, 2-5 times/d
Episodic treatment of recurrences[22]	Acyclovir 800 mg oral tid x 2 d or 400 mg oral tid x 3-5 d[23] **or** Famciclovir 125 mg oral bid x 3-5 d[23] **or** Valacyclovir 500 mg oral bid x 3 d	

Type or Stage	Drugs of Choice / Dosage	Alternatives
GRANULOMA INGUINALE		
	TMP-SMZ 1 double-strength tablet oral bid for a minimum of 3 wk **or** Doxycycline 100 oral bid for a minimum of 3 wk	Ciprofloxacin 750 mg oral bid for a minimum of 3 wk **or** Erythromycin base 500 mg oral qid for a minimum of 3 wk **or** Azithromycin 1 g oral once per week for a minimum of 3 weeks

[1]Related clinical syndromes include nonchlamydial nongonococcal urethritis and cervicitis.

[2]Or oral tetracycline 500 mg qid.

[3]Not recommended in pregnancy.

[4]Erythromycin ethylsuccinate 800 mg may be substituted for erythromycin base 500 mg; erythromycin estolate is contraindicated in pregnancy.

[5]Pyloric stenosis has been associated with use of erythromycin in newborns.

[6]All patients should also receive a course of treatment effective for *Chlamydia.*

[7]Fluoroquinolones should not be used to treat gonorrhea acquired in Asia, Hawaii, Israel, or other areas where fluoroquinolone-resistant strains of *N. gonorrhoeae* are common.

[8]Recommended only for use during pregnancy in patients allergic to β-lactams. Not effective for pharyngeal infection.

[9]Some clinicians believe the addition of metronidazole is not required.

[10]Or clindamycin 450 mg oral qid to complete 14 days.

[11]A single daily dose of 3 mg/kg is likely to be effective, but has not been studied in pelvic inflammatory disease.

[12]Some experts would add metronidazole 500 mg bid.

[13]Higher relapse rate with single dose, but useful for patients who may not comply with multiple-dose therapy.

[14]In pregnancy, topical preparations have not been effective in preventing premature delivery; oral metronidazole has been used in some studies.

[15]For preparations and dosage of topical products, see *Med Lett Drugs Ther*, 1994, 36:81; single-dose therapy is not recommended.

[16]Some experts recommend a repeat dose after 7 days, especially in patients with HIV infection or pregnant women.

[17]Patients allergic to penicillin should be desensitized and treated with penicillin.

[18]All regimens, especially single-dose ceftriaxone, are less effective in HIV-infected patients.

[19]Recommendations for external genital warts. Liquid nitrogen can also be used for vaginal, urethral, and oral warts. Podofilox or imiquimod can be used for urethral meatus warts. Trichloroacetic or bichloroacetic acid can be used for anal warts.

[20]Some experts recommend discontinue preventive treatment for 1-2 months once a year to reassess the frequency of recurrence.

[21]Use 500 mg once daily in patients with <10 recurrences per year and 500 mg bid or 1 g daily in patients with <10 recurrences per year.

[22]Antiviral therapy is variably effective for episodic treatment of recurrences; only effective if started early.

[23]No published data are available to support 3 days' use.

Adapted from "Sexually Transmitted Diseases Treatment Guidelines 2002," *MMWR Morb Mortal Wkly Rep*, 2002, 51(RR-6).

Adapted from "Drugs for Sexually Transmitted Infections," *Treatment Guidelines From The Medical Letter®*, 2004, 2(26):70-2.

TUBERCULOSIS

Tuberculin Skin Test Recommendations[1]

Children for whom immediate skin testing is indicated:

- Contacts of persons with confirmed or suspected infectious tuberculosis (contact investigation); this includes children identified as contacts of family members or associates in jail or prison in the last 5 years

- Children with radiographic or clinical findings suggesting tuberculosis

- Children immigrating from endemic countries (eg, Asia, Middle East, Africa, Latin America)

- Children with travel histories to endemic countries and/or significant contact with indigenous persons from such countries

Children who should be tested annually for tuberculosis[2]:

- Children infected with HIV or living in household with HIV-infected persons

- Incarcerated adolescents

Children who should be tested every 2-3 years[2]:

- Children exposed to the following individuals: HIV-infected, homeless, residents of nursing homes, institutionalized adolescents or adults, users of illicit drugs, incarcerated adolescents or adults, and migrant farm workers. Foster children with exposure to adults in the preceding high-risk groups are included.

Children who should be considered for tuberculin skin testing at ages 4-6 and 11-16 years:

- Children whose parents immigrated (with unknown tuberculin skin test status) from regions of the world with high prevalence of tuberculosis; continued potential exposure by travel to the endemic areas and/or household contact with persons from the endemic areas (with unknown tuberculin skin test status) should be an indication for repeat tuberculin skin testing

- Children without specific risk factors who reside in high-prevalence areas; in general, a high-risk neighborhood or community does not mean an entire city is at high risk; rates in any area of the city may vary by neighborhood, or even from block to block; physicians should be aware of these patterns in determining the likelihood of exposure; public health officials or local tuberculosis experts should help clinicians identify areas that have appreciable tuberculosis rates

Children at increased risk of progression of infection to disease: Those with other medical risk factors, including diabetes mellitus, chronic renal failure, malnutrition, and congenital or acquired immunodeficiencies deserve special consideration. Without recent exposure, these persons are not at increased risk of acquiring tuberculosis infection. Underlying immune deficiencies associated with these conditions theoretically would enhance the possibility for progression to severe disease. Initial histories of potential exposure to tuberculosis should be included on all of these patients. If these histories or local epidemiologic factors suggest a possibility of exposure, immediate and periodic tuberculin skin testing should be considered. An initial Mantoux tuberculin skin test should be performed before initiation of immunosuppressive therapy in any child with an underlying condition that necessitates immunosuppressive therapy.

---

[1]BCG immunization is not a contraindication to tuberculin skin testing.

[2]Initial tuberculin skin testing is at the time of diagnosis or circumstance, beginning as early as at age 3 months.

Adapted from "Report of the Committee on Infectious Diseases," *2003 Red Book*®, 26th ed, 646.

Table 1. Tuberculosis Prophylaxis
Infection Without Disease (Positive Tuberculin Test)[1]

Specific Circumstances/ Organism	Comments	Regimen
Regardless of age (see INH Preventive Therapy)	Rx indicated	INH (5 mg/kg/d, maximum: 300 mg/d for adults, 10 mg/kg/d not to exceed 300 mg/d for children). Results with 6 months of treatment are nearly as effective as 12 months (65% vs 75% reduction in disease). *Am Thoracic Society* (6 months), *Am Acad Pediatrics*, 1991 (9 months). If CXR is abnormal, treat for 12 months. In HIV-positive patient, treatment for a minimum of 12 months, some suggest longer. Monitor transaminases monthly (*MMWR Morb Mortal Wkly Rep* 1989, 38:247).
Age <35 y	Rx indicated	Reanalysis of earlier studies favors INH prophylaxis for 6 months (if INH-related hepatitis case fatality rate is <1% and TB case fatality is ≥6.7%, which appears to be the case, monitor transaminases monthly (*Arch Int Med*, 1990, 150:2517).
INH-resistant organisms likely	Rx indicated	Data on efficacy of alternative regimens is currently lacking. Regimens include ETB + RIF daily for 6 months. PZA + RIF daily for 2 months, then INH + RIF daily until sensitivities from index case (if available) known, then if INH-CR, discontinue INH and continue RIF for 9 months, otherwise INH + RIF for 9 months (this latter is *Am Acad Pediatrics*, 1991 recommendation).
INH + RIF resistant organisms likely	Rx indicated	Efficacy of alternative regimens is unknown; PZA (25-30 mg/kg/d P.O.) + ETB (15-25 mg/kg/d P.O.) (at 25 mg/kg ETB, monitoring for retrobulbar neuritis required), for 6 months unless HIV-positive, then 12 months; PZA + ciprofloxacin (750 mg P.O. bid) or ofloxacin (400 mg P.O. bid) x 6-12 months (*MMWR Morb Mortal Wkly Rep*, 1992, 41(RR11):68).

INH = isoniazid; RIF = rifampin; KM = kanamycin; ETB = ethambutol
SM = streptomycin; CXR = chest x-ray; Rx = treatment
See also guidelines for interpreting PPD in "Skin Testing for Delayed Hypersensitivity."
[1]Tuberculin test (TBnT). The standard is the Mantoux test, 5 TU PPD in 0.1 mL diluent stabilized with Tween 80. Read at 48-72 hours measuring maximum diameter of induration. A reaction ≥5 mm is defined as positive in the following: positive HIV or risk factors, recent close case contacts, CXR consistent with healed TBc. ≥10 mm is positive in foreign-born in countries of high prevalence, injection drug users, low income populations, nursing home residents, patients with medical conditions which increase risk (see above, preventive treatment). ≥15 mm is positive in all others (*Am Rev Resp Dis*, 1990, 142:725). Two-stage TBnT: Use in individuals to be tested regularly (ie, healthcare workers). TBn reactivity may decrease over time but be boosted by skin testing. If unrecognized, individual may be incorrectly diagnosed as recent converter. If first TBnT is reactive but <10 mm, repeat 5 TU in 1 week, if then ≥10 mm = positive, not recent conversion (*Am Rev Resp Dis*, 1979, 119:587).

TUBERCULOSIS *(Continued)*

Changes From Prior Recommendations on Tuberculin Testing and Treatment of Latent Tuberculosis Infection (LTBI)

Tuberculin Testing

- Emphasis on targeted tuberculin testing among persons at high risk for recent LTBI or with clinical conditions that increase the risk for tuberculosis (TB), regardless of age; testing is discouraged among persons at lower risk

- For patients with organ transplants and other immunosuppressed patients (eg, persons receiving the equivalent of ≥15 mg/day prednisone for 1 month or more), 5 mm of induration rather than 10 mm of induration rather than 10 mm of induration as a cut-off level for tuberculin positivity

- A tuberculin skin test conversion is defined as in increase of ≥10 mm of induration within a 2-year period, regardless of age

Treatment of Latent Tuberculosis Infection

- For human immunodeficiency virus (HIV)-negative persons, isoniazid given for 9 months is preferred over 6-month regimens

- For HIV-positive persons and those with fibrotic lesions on chest x-ray consistent with previous TB, isoniazid should be given for 9 months instead of 12 months

- For HIV-negative and HIV-positive persons, rifampin and pyrazinamide should be given for 2 months

- For HIV-negative and HIV-positive persons, rifampin should be given for 4 months

Clinical and Laboratory Monitoring

- Routine baseline and follow-up laboratory monitoring can be eliminated in most persons with LTBI, except for those with HIV infection, pregnant women (or those in the immediate postpartum period), and persons with chronic liver disease or those who use alcohol regularly

- Emphasis on clinical monitoring for signs and symptoms of possible adverse effects, with prompt evaluation and changes in treatment, as indicated

Adapted from *MMWR*, 2000, 49(RR-6).

Table 2. Recommended Treatment Regimens for Drug-Susceptible Tuberculosis in Infants, Children, and Adolescents

Infection or Disease Category	Regimen	Remarks
Latent tuberculosis infection (positive tuberculin skin test, no disease):		
• Isoniazid-susceptible	9 months of isoniazid once a day	If daily therapy is not possible, directly observed therapy twice a week may be used for 9 months.
• Isoniazid-resistant	6 months of rifampin once a day	
• Isoniazid-rifampin-resistant[1]	Consult a tuberculosis specialist	
Pulmonary and extrapulmonary (except meningitis)	2 months of isoniazid, rifampin, and pyrazinamide daily, followed by 4 months of isoniazid and rifampin[2]	If possible drug resistance is a concern, another drug (ethambutol or aminoglycoside) is added to the initial 3-drug therapy until drug susceptibilities are determined. Directly observed therapy is highly desirable.
		If hilar adenopathy only, a 6-month course of isoniazid and rifampin is sufficient.
		Drugs can be given 2 or 3 times/week under directly observed therapy in the initial phase if nonadherence is likely.
Meningitis	2 months of isoniazid, rifampin, pyrazinamide, and aminoglycoside or ethionamide, once a day, followed by 7-10 months of isoniazid and rifampin once a day or twice a week (9-12 months total)	A fourth drug, usually an aminoglycoside, is given with initial therapy until drug susceptibility is known.
		For patients who may have acquired tuberculosis in geographic areas where resistance to streptomycin is common, capreomycin, kanamycin, or amikacin may be used instead of streptomycin.

[1]Duration of therapy is longer for human immunodeficiency virus (HIV)-infected people, and additional drugs may be indicated.

[2]Medications should be administered daily for the first 2 weeks to 2 months of treatment and then can be administered 2-3 times/week by directly observed therapy.

Adapted from "Report of the Committee on Infectious Diseases," *2003 Red Book*®, 26th ed, 649.

TUBERCULOSIS *(Continued)*

Table 3. Recommended Drug Regimens for Treatment of Latent Tuberculosis Infection in Children

Drug	Interval and Duration	Comments
Isoniazid	Daily for 9 mo Twice weekly for 9 mo	This includes treatment for any child <5 years old who is exposed to household members or other close contacts who are potentially infectious even if skin test is negative
Rifampin	Daily for 4-9 mo	No controlled trials; only to be used in INH intolerant or resistant
Rifampin-pyrazinamide	Daily for 3 mo	No controlled trials; only to be used in INH intolerant or resistant

Modified from *MMWR*, 2000, 14(RR-6).

Table 4. Recommended Drug Regimens for Treatment of Latent Tuberculosis Infection in Adults

Drug	Interval and Duration	Comments	Rating[1] (Evidence)[2] HIV⁻	Rating[1] (Evidence)[2] HIV⁺
Isoniazid	Daily for 9 months[3,4]	In HIV-infected patients, isoniazid may be administered concurrently with nucleoside reverse transcriptase inhibitors (NRTIs), protease inhibitors, or non-nucleoside reverse transcriptase inhibitors (NNRTIs)	A (II)	A (II)
	Twice weekly for 9 months[3,4]	Directly observed therapy (DOT) must be used with twice-weekly dosing	B (II)	B (II)
Isoniazid	Daily for 6 months[4]	Not indicated for HIV-infected persons, those with fibrotic lesions on chest radiographs, or children	B (I)	C (I)
	Twice weekly for 6 months[4]	DOT must be used with twice-weekly dosing	B (II)	C (I)
Rifampin	Daily for 4 months	For persons who cannot tolerate pyrazinamide	B (II)	B (III)
		For persons who are contacts of patients with isoniazid-resistant, rifampin-susceptible TB who cannot tolerate pyrazinamide		
Rifampin plus pyrazinamide	Daily for 2 months	May also be offered to persons who are contacts of pyrazinamide patients with isoniazid-resistant, rifampin-susceptible TB	B (II)	A (I)
		In HIV-infected patients, protease inhibitors or NNRTIs should generally not be administered concurrently with rifampin. Rifabutin can be used as an alternative for patients treated with indinavir, nelfinavir, amprenavir, ritonavir, or efavirenz, and possibly with nevirapine or soft-gel saquinavir[5]		
	Twice weekly for 2-3 months	DOT must be used with twice-weekly dosing	C (II)	C (I)

[1]Strength of recommendation: A = preferred; B = acceptable alternative; C = offer when A and B cannot be given.

[2]Quality of evidence: I = randomized clinical trial data; II = data from clinical trials that are not randomized or were conducted in other populations; III = expert opinion.

[3]Recommended regimen for children <18 years of age.

[4]Recommended regimens for pregnant women. Some experts would use rifampin and pyrazinamide for 2 months as an alternative regimen in HIV-infected pregnant women, although pyrazinamide should be avoided during the first trimester.

[5]Rifabutin should not be used with hard-gel saquinavir or delavirdine. When used with other protease inhibitors or NNRTIs, dose adjustment of rifabutin may be required.

Adapted from *MMWR Recomm Rep*, 2000, 49(RR6).

Table 5. TB Drugs in Special Situations

Drug	Pregnancy[1]	CNS TB Disease	Renal Insufficiency
Isoniazid	Safe	Good penetration	Normal clearance
Rifampin	Safe	Fair penetration Penetrates inflamed meninges (10% to 20%)	Normal clearance
Pyrazinamide	Avoid	Good penetration	Clearance reduced Decrease dose or prolong interval
Ethambutol	Safe	Penetrates inflamed meninges only (4% to 64%)	Clearance reduced Decrease dose or prolong interval
Streptomycin	Avoid	Penetrates inflamed meninges only	Clearance reduced Decrease dose or prolong interval
Capreomycin	Avoid	Penetrates inflamed meninges only	Clearance reduced Decrease dose or prolong interval
Kanamycin	Avoid	Penetrates inflamed meninges only	Clearance reduced Decrease dose or prolong interval
Ethionamide	Do not use	Good penetration	Normal clearance
Para-amino-salicylic acid	Safe	Penetrates inflamed meninges only (10% to 50%)	Incomplete data on clearance
Cycloserine	Avoid	Good penetration	Clearance reduced Decrease dose or prolong interval
Ciprofloxacin	Do not use	Fair penetration (5% to 10%) Penetrates inflamed meninges (50% to 90%)	Clearance reduced Decrease dose or prolong interval
Ofloxacin	Do not use	Fair penetration (5% to 10%) Penetrates inflamed meninges (50% to 90%)	Clearance reduced Decrease dose or prolong interval
Amikacin	Avoid	Penetrates inflamed meninges only	Clearance reduced Decrease dose or prolong interval
Clofazimine	Avoid	Penetration unknown	Clearance probably normal

[1]Safe = the drug has not been demonstrated to have teratogenic effects.

Avoid = data on the drug's safety are limited, or the drug is associated with mild malformations (as in the aminoglycosides).

Do not use = studies show an association between the drug and premature labor, congenital malformations, or teratogenicity.

TUBERCULOSIS *(Continued)*

Table 6. Recommendations for Coadministering Different Antiretroviral Drugs With the Antimycobacterial Drugs Rifabutin and Rifampin

Antiretroviral	Use in Combination with Rifabutin	Use in Combination with Rifampin	Comments
Saquinavir[1]			
Hard-gel capsules (HGC)	Possibly[2], if antiretroviral regimen also includes ritonavir	Possibly, if antiretroviral regimen also includes ritonavir	Coadministration of saquinavir SGC with usual-dose rifabutin (300 mg/day or 2-3 times/week) is a possibility. However, the pharmacokinetic data and clinical experience for this combination are limited.
Soft-gel capsules (SGC)	Probably[3]	Possibly, if antiretroviral regimen also includes ritonavir	The combination of saquinavir SGC or saquinavir HGC and ritonavir, coadministered with 1) usual-dose rifampin (600 mg/day or 2-3 times/week), or 2) reduced-dose rifabutin (150 mg 2-3 times/week) is a possibility. However, the pharmacokinetic data and clinical experience for these combinations are limited. Coadministration of saquinavir or saquinavir SGC with rifampin is not recommended because rifampin markedly decreases concentrations of saquinavir.
Ritonavir	Probably	Probably	If the combination of ritonavir and rifabutin is used, then a substantially reduced-dose rifabutin regimen (150 mg 2-3 times/week) is recommended. Coadministration of ritonavir with usual-dose rifampin (600 mg/day or 2-3 times/week) is a possibility, though pharmacokinetic data and clinical experience are limited.
Indinavir	Yes	No	There is limited, but favorable, clinical experience with coadministration of indinavir[4] with a reduced daily dose of rifabutin (150 mg) or with the usual dose of rifabutin (300 mg 2-3 times/week). Coadministration of indinavir with rifampin is not recommended because rifampin markedly decreases concentrations of indinavir.
Nelfinavir	Yes	No	There is limited, but favorable, clinical experience with coadministration of nelfinavir[5] with a reduced daily dose of rifabutin (150 mg) or with the usual dose of rifabutin (300 mg 2-3 times/week). Coadministration of nelfinavir with rifampin is not recommended because rifampin markedly decreases concentrations of nelfinavir.
Amprenavir	Yes	No	Coadministration of amprenavir with a reduced daily dose of rifabutin (150 mg) or with the usual dose of rifabutin (300 mg 2-3 times/week) is a possibility, but there is no published clinical experience. Coadministration of amprenavir with rifampin is not recommended because rifampin markedly decreases concentrations of amprenavir.

Table 6. Recommendations for Coadministering Different Antiretroviral Drugs With the Antimycobacterial Drugs Rifabutin and Rifampin *(continued)*

Antiretroviral	Use in Combination with Rifabutin	Use in Combination with Rifampin	Comments
Nevirapine	Yes	Possibly	Coadministration of nevirapine with usual-dose rifabutin (300 mg/day or 2-3 times/week) is a possibility based on pharmacokinetic study data. However, there is no published clinical experience for this combination. Data are insufficient to assess whether dose adjustments are necessary when rifampin is coadministered with nevirapine. Therefore, rifampin and nevirapine should be used only in combination if clearly indicated and with careful monitoring.
Delavirdine	No	No	Contraindicated because of the marked decrease in concentrations of delavirdine when administered with either rifabutin or rifampin.
Efavirenz	Probably	Probably	Coadministration of efavirenz with increased-dose rifabutin (450 mg/day or 600 mg/day, or 600 mg 2-3 times/week) is a possibility, though there is no published clinical experience. Coadministration of efavirenz[6] with usual-dose rifampin (600 mg/day or 2-3 times/week) is a possibility, though there is no published clinical experience.

[1]Usual recommended doses are 400 mg twice daily for each of these protease inhibitors and 400 mg of ritonavir.

[2]Despite limited data and clinical experience, the use of this combination is potentially successful.

[3]Based on available data and clinical experience, the successful use of this combination is likely.

[4] Usual recommended dose is 800 mg every 8 hours; some experts recommend increasing the indinavir dose to 1000 mg every 8 hours if indinavir is used in combination with rifabutin.

[5]Usual recommended dose is 750 mg 3 times/day or 1250 mg twice daily; some experts recommend increasing the nelfinavir dose to 1000 mg if the 3-times/day dosing is used and nelfinavir is used in combination with rifabutin.

[6]Usual recommended dose is 600 mg/day; some experts recommend increasing the efavirenz dose to 800 mg/day if efavirenz is used in combination with rifampin.

Updated March 2000 from www.aidsinfo.nih.gov -"Updated Guidelines for the Use of Rifabutin or Rifampin for the Treatment and Prevention of Tuberculosis Among HIV-Infected Patients Taking Protease Inhibitors or Non-nucleoside Reverse Transcriptase Inhibitors," *MMWR,* March 10, 2000, 49(09):185-9.

TUBERCULOSIS *(Continued)*

Table 7. Criteria for Tuberculin Positivity, by Risk Group

Reaction ≥5 mm of Induration	Reaction ≥10 mm of Induration	Reaction ≥15 mm of Induration
HIV-positive persons	Recent immigrants (ie, within the last 5 years) from high prevalence countries	Persons with no risk factors for TB
Recent contacts of tuberculosis (TB) case patients	Injection drug users	
Fibrotic changes on chest radiograph consistent with prior TB	Residents and employees[1] of the following high risk congregate settings: prisons and jails, nursing homes and other long-term facilities for the elderly, hospitals and other healthcare facilities, residential facilities for patients with AIDS, and homeless shelters	
Patients with organ transplant and other immunosuppressed patients (receiving the equivalent of ≥15 mg/day of prednisone for 1 month)[2]	Mycobacteriology laboratory personnel	
	Persons with the following clinical conditions that place them at high risk: silicosis, diabetes mellitus, chronic renal failure, some hematologic disorders (eg, leukemias and lymphomas), other specific malignancies (eg, carcinoma of the head or neck and lung), weight loss of ≥10% of ideal body weight, gastrectomy, and jejunoileal bypass	
	Children <4 years of age or infants, children, and adolescents exposed to adults at high-risk	

[1]For persons who are otherwise at low risk and are tested at the start of employment, a reaction of ≥15 mm induration is considered positive.

[2]Risk of TB in patients treated with corticosteroids increases with higher dose and longer duration.

Modified from *MMWR Morb Mortal Wkly Rep*, 2000, 49(RR-6).

Table 8. Recommendations, Rankings, and Performance Indicators for Treatment of Patients With Tuberculosis (TB)

Recommendation	Ranking[1] (Evidence)[2]	Performance Indicator
Obtain bacteriologic confirmation and susceptibility testing for patients with TB or suspected of having TB	A (II)	90% of adults with or suspected of having TB have 3 cultures for mycobacteria obtained before initiation of antituberculosis therapy (50% of children 0-12 y)
Place persons with suspected or confirmed smear-positive pulmonary or laryngeal TB in respiratory isolation until noninfectious	A (II)	90% of persons with sputum smear-positive TB remain in respiratory isolation until smear converts to negative
Begin treatment of patients with confirmed or suspected TB disease with one of the following drug combinations, depending on local resistance patterns: INH + RIF + PZA **or** INH + RIF + PZA + EMB **or** INH + RIF + PZA + SM	A (III)	90% of all patients with TB are started on INH + RIF + PZA + EMB or SM in geographic areas where >4% of TB isolates are resistant to INH
Report each case of TB promptly to the local public health department	A (III)	100% of persons with active TB are reported to the local public health department within 1 week of diagnosis
Perform HIV testing for all patients with TB	A (III)	80% of all patients with TB have HIV status determined within 2 months of a diagnosis of TB
Treat patients with TB caused by a susceptible organism for 6 months, using an ATS/CDC-approved regimen	A (I)	90% of all patients with TB complete 6 months of therapy with 12 months of beginning treatment
Re-evaluate patients with TB who are smear positive at 3 months for possible nonadherence or infection with drug-resistant bacilli	A (III)	90% of all patients with TB who are smear positive at 3 months have sputum culture/susceptibility testing performed within 1 month of the 3-month visit
Add ≥2 new antituberculosis agents when TB treatment failure is suspected	A (II)	100% of patients with TB with suspected treatment failure are prescribed ≥2 new antituberculosis agents
Perform tuberculin skin testing on all patients with a history of ≥1 of the following: HIV infection, I.V. drug use, homelessness, incarceration, or contact with a person with pulmonary TB	A (II)	80% of persons in the indicated population groups receive tuberculin skin test and return for reading
Administer treatment for latent TB infection to all persons with latent TB infection, unless it can be documented that they received such treatment previously	A (I)	75% of patients with positive tuberculin skin tests who are candidates for treatment for latent TB infection complete a course of therapy within 12 months of initiation

Note: ATS/CDC = American Thoracic Society and Centers for Disease Control and Prevention; EMB = ethambutol; INH = isoniazid; PZA = pyrazinamide; RIF = rifampin; SM = streptomycin.

[1]Strength of recommendation: A = preferred; B = acceptable alternative; C = offer when A and B cannot be given.

[2]Quality of evidence: I = randomized clinical trial data; II = data from clinical trials that are not randomized or were conducted in other populations; III = expert opinion.

Adapted from the Infectious Diseases Society of America, *Clinical Infectious Diseases,* 2000, 31:633-9.

TUBERCULOSIS (Continued)

Table 9. Drug Regimens for Culture-Positive Pulmonary Tuberculosis Caused by Drug-Susceptible Organisms

Initial Phase			Continuation Phase			Range of Total Doses (minimal duration)	Rating[1] (Evidence)[2]	
Regimen	Drugs	Interval and Doses[3] (minimal duration)	Regimen	Drugs	Interval and Doses[3,4] (minimal duration)		HIV-	HIV+
1	INH RIF PZA EMB	Seven days per week for 56 doses (8 wk) or 5 d/wk for 40 doses (8 wk)[5]	1a	INH/RIF	Seven days per week for 126 doses (18 wk) or 5 d/wk for 90 doses (18 wk)[5]	182-130 (26 wk)	A (I)	A (II)
			1b	INH/RIF	Twice weekly for 36 doses (18 wk)	92-76 (26 wk)	A (I)	A (II)[6]
			1c[7]	INH/RPT	Once weekly for 18 doses (18 wk)	74-58 (26 wk)	B (I)	E (I)
2	INH RIF PZA EMB	Seven days per week for 14 doses (2 wk), then twice weekly for 12 doses (6 wk) or 5 d/wk for 10 doses (2 wk)[5], then twice weekly for 12 doses (6 wk)	2a	INH/RIF	Twice weekly for 36 doses (18 wk)	62-58 (26 wk)	A (II)	B (II)[6]
			2b[7]	INH/RPT	Once weekly for 18 doses (18 wk)	44-40 (26 wk)	B (I)	E (I)
3	INH RIF PZA EMB	Three times weekly for 24 doses (8 wk)	3a	INH/RIF	Three times weekly for 54 doses (18 wk)	78 (26 wk)	B (I)	B (II)
4	INH RIF EMB	Seven days per week for 56 doses (8 wk) or 5 d/wk for 40 doses (8 wk)[5]	4a	INH/RIF	Seven days per week for 217 doses (31 wk) or 5 d/wk for 155 doses (31 wk)[5]	273-195 (39 wk)	C (I)	C (II)
			4b	INH/RIF	Twice weekly for 62 doses (31 wk)	118-102 (39 wk)	C (I)	C (II)

Definition of abbreviations: EMB = ethambutol; INH = isoniazid; PZA = pyrazinamide; RIF = rifampin; RPT = rifapentine.

[1] Definitions of evidence ratings: A = preferred; B = acceptable alternative; C = offer when A and B cannot be given; E = should never be given.

[2] Definitions of evidence ratings: I = randomized clinical trial; II = data from clinical trials that were not randomized or were conducted in other populations; III = expert opinion.

[3] When directly observed therapy (DOT) is used, drugs may be given 5 days/week and the necessary number of doses adjusted accordingly. Although there are no studies that compare five with seven daily doses, extensive experience indicates this would be an effective practice.

[4] Patients with cavitation on initial chest radiograph and positive cultures at completion of 2 months of therapy should receive a 7-month (31-week; either 217 doses daily] or 62 doses [twice weekly]) continuation phase.

[5] Five-day/week administration is always given by DOT. Rating for 5 day/week regimens is AIII.

[6] Not recommended for HIV-infected patients with CD4+ cell counts <100 cells/μL.

[7] Options 1c and 2b should be used only in HIV-negative patients who have negative sputum smears at the time of completion of 2 months of therapy and who do not have cavitation on initial chest radiograph. For patients started on this regimen and found to have a positive culture from the 2-month specimen, treatment should be extended an extra 3 months.

Adapted from MMWR, 2003, 52(RR11).

Table 10. Doses[1] of Antituberculosis Drugs for Adults and Children

Drug	Preparation	Adults / Children	Doses Daily	Doses 1x	Doses 2x	Doses 3x
			FIRST-LINE DRUGS			
Isoniazid	Tablets (50 mg, 100 mg, 300 mg); elixir (50 mg/5 mL); aqueous solution (100 mg/mL) for I.V. or I.M injection	Adults (max.)	5 mg/kg (300 mg)	15 mg/kg (900 mg)	15 mg/kg (900 mg)	15 mg/kg (900 mg)
		Children (max.)	10-15 mg/kg (300 mg)	—	20-30 mg/kg (900 mg)	—
Rifampin	Capsule (150 mg, 300 mg) powder may be suspended for oral administration; aqueous solution for I.V. injection	Adults[3] (max.)	10 mg/kg (600 mg)	—	10 mg/kg (600 mg)	10 mg/kg (600 mg)
		Children (max.)	10-20 mg/kg (600 mg)	—	10-20 mg/kg (600 mg)	—
Rifabutin	Capsule (150 mg)	Adults[3] (max.)	5 mg/kg (300 mg)	—	5 mg/kg (300 mg)	5 mg/kg (300 mg)
		Children	Appropriate dosing for children is unknown			
Rifapentine	Tablet (150 mg, film coated)	Adults	—	10 mg/kg (continuation phase) (600 mg)	—	—
		Children	The drug is not approved for use in children			
Pyrazinamide	Tablet (500 mg, scored)	Adults	See table 11	—	See table 11	See table 11
		Children (max.)	15-30 mg/kg (2 g)	—	50 mg/kg (2 g)	—
Ethambutol	Tablet (100 mg 400 mg)	Adults	See table 12	—	See table 12	See table 12
		Children[4] (max.)	15-20 mg/kg daily (1 g)	—	50 mg/kg (2.5 g)	—
			SECOND-LINE DRUGS			
Cycloserine	Capsule (250 mg)	Adults (max.)	10-15 mg/kg/d (1 g in two doses), usually 500-750 mg/d in two doses[5]	There are no data to support intermittent administration		
		Children (max.)	10-15 mg/kg/d (1 g/d)			—

TUBERCULOSIS *(Continued)*

Table 10. Doses[1] of Antituberculosis Drugs for Adults and Children *(continued)*

Drug	Preparation	Adults / Children	Daily	Doses 1x	Doses 2x	Doses 3x
Ethionamide	Tablet (250 mg)	Adults[6] (max.)	15-20 mg/kg/d (1 g/d), usually, 500-750 mg/d in a single daily dose or two divided doses[6]	There are no data to support intermittent administration		
		Children (max.)	15-20 mg/kg/d (1 g/d)	There are no data to support intermittent administration		
Streptomycin	Aqueous solution (1 g vials) for I.M. or I.V. administration	Adults (max.)		See footnote 7		
		Children (max.)	20-40 mg/kg/d (1 g)	–	20 mg/kg	–
Amikacin/ Kanamycin	Aqueous solution (500 mg and 1 g vials) for I.V. or I.M. administration	Adults (max.)		See footnote 7		
		Children (max.)	15-30 mg/kg/d (1 g) I.V. or I.M. as a single daily dose	–	15-30 mg/kg	–
Capreomycin	Aqueous solution (1 g vials) for I.M. or I.V. administration	Adults (max.)		See footnote 7		
		Children (max.)	15-30 mg/kg/d (1 g) as a single daily dose	–	15-30 mg/kg	–
p-Aminosalicylic acid (PAS)	Granules (4 g packets) can be mixed with food; tablets (500 mg) are still available in some countries, but not in the United States; a solution for I.V. administration is available in Europe	Adults	8-12 g/d in 2 or 3 doses	There are no data to support intermittent administration		
		Children	200-300 mg/kg/d in 2-4 divided doses (10 g)	There are no data to support intermittent administration		
Levofloxacin	Tablets (250 mg, 500 mg, 750 mg); aqueous solution (500 mg vials) for I.V. injection	Adults	500-1000 mg daily	There are no data to support intermittent administration		
		Children		See footnote 8		
Moxifloxacin	Tablets (400 mg); aqueous solution (400 mg/250 mL) for I.V. injection	Adults	400 mg daily	There are no data to support intermittent administration		
		Children		See footnote 9		

Table 10. Doses[1] of Antituberculosis Drugs for Adults and Children *(continued)*

Drug	Preparation	Adults / Children	Daily	Doses		
				1x	2x	3x
Gatifloxacin	Tablets (400 mg); aqueous solution (200 mg/20 mL; 400 mg/ 40 mL) for I.V. injection	Adults	400 mg daily	There are no data to support intermittent administration		
		Children		See footnote 10		

[1]Dose per weight is based on ideal body weight. Children weighing >40 kg should be dosed as adults.

[2]For purposes of this document adult dosing begins at age 15 years.

[3]Dose may need to be adjusted when there is concomitant use of protease inhibitors or non-nucleoside reverse transcriptase inhibitors.

[4]The drug can likely be used safely in older children but should be used with caution in children less than 5 years of age, in whom visual acuity cannot be monitored. In younger children EMB at the dose of 15 mg/kg per day can be used if there is suspected or proven resistance to INH or RIF.

[5]It should be noted that, although this is the dose recommended generally, most clinicians with experience using cycloserine indicate that it is unusual for patients to be able to tolerate this amount. Serum concentration measurements are often useful in determining the optimal dose for a given patient.

[6]The single daily dose can be given at bedtime or with the main meal.

[7]Dose: 15 mg/kg per day (1 g), and 10 mg/kg in persons more than 59 years of age (750 mg). Usual dose: 750-1000 mg administered intramuscularly or intravenously, given as a single dose 5-7 days/week and reduced to two or three times per week after the first 2-4 months or after culture conversion, depending on the efficacy of the other drugs in the regimen.

[8]The long-term (more than several weeks) use of levofloxacin in children and adolescents has not been approved because of concerns about effects on bone and cartilage growth. However, most experts agree that the drug should be considered for children with tuberculosis caused by organisms resistant to both INH and RIF. The optimal dose is not known.

[9]The long-term (more than several weeks) use of moxifloxacin in children and adolescents has not been approved because of concerns about effects on bone and cartilage growth. The optimal dose is not known.

[10]The long-term (more than several weeks) use of gatifloxacin in children and adolescents has not been approved because of concerns about effects on bone and cartilage growth. The optimal dose is not known.

TUBERCULOSIS *(Continued)*

Table 11. Suggested Pyrazinamide Doses, Using Whole Tablets, for Adults Weighing 40-90 kg

	Weight (kg)[1]		
	40-55	**56-75**	**76-90**
Daily, mg (mg/kg)	1000 (18.2-25)	1500 (20-26.8)	2000[2] (22.2-26.3)
Thrice weekly, mg (mg/kg)	1500 (27.3-37.5)	2500 (33.3-44.6)	3000[2] (33.3-39.5)
Twice weekly, mg (mg/kg)	2000 (36.4-50)	3000 (40-53.6)	4000[2] (44.4-52.6)

[1]Based on estimated lean body weight
[2]Maximum dose regardless of weight.

Table 12. Suggested Ethambutol Doses, Using Whole Tablets, for Adults Weighing 40-90 kg

	Weight (kg)[1]		
	40-55	**56-75**	**76-90**
Daily, mg (mg/kg)	800 (14.5-20)	1200 (16-21.4)	1600[2] (17.8-21.1)
Thrice weekly, mg (mg/kg)	1200 (21.8-30)	2000 (26.7-35.7)	2400[2] (26.7-31.6)
Twice weekly, mg (mg/kg)	2000 (36.4-50)	2800 (37.3-50)	4000[2] (44.4-52.6)

[1]Based on estimated lean body weight
[2]Maximum dose regardless of weight.

NOTES

NOTES

NOTES

NOTES

NOTES

NOTES

NOTES

Products offered by LEXI-COMP

CLINICIAN'S GUIDE TO LABORATORY MEDICINE
—A Practical Approach by Samir P. Desai, MD and Sana Isa-Pratt, MD

When faced with the patient presenting with abnormal laboratory tests, the clinician can now turn to the Clinician's Guide to Laboratory Medicine: A Practical Approach. This source is unique in its ability to lead the clinician from laboratory test abnormality to clinical diagnosis. Written for the busy clinician, this concise handbook will provide rapid answers to the questions that busy clinicians face in the care of their patients. No longer does the clinician have to struggle in an effort to find this information - it's all here.
Included is a **FREE** copy of Clinician's Guide to Laboratory Medicine - Pocket. Great to carry in your pocket! Perfect for use "in the trenches."

CLINICIAN'S GUIDE TO INTERNAL MEDICINE—A Practical
Approach by Samir P. Desai, MD

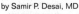

Provides quick access to essential information covering diagnosis, treatment, and management of commonly encountered patient problems in Internal Medicine. Contains up-to-date, clinically-relevant information in an easy-to-read format and is easily accessible. Contains practical approaches that are not readily available in standard textbooks. Contains algorithms to help you establish the diagnosis and select the appropriate therapy. There are numerous tables and boxes that summarize diagnostic and therapeutic strategies. It is an ideal reference for use at the point-of-care. This is a reference companion that will provide you with the tools necessary to tackle even the most challenging problems in Internal Medicine.

CLINICIAN'S GUIDE TO DIAGNOSIS—A Practical Approach
by Samir P. Desai, MD

Symptoms are what prompt patients to seek medical care. In the evaluation of a patient's symptom, it is not unusual for healthcare professionals to ask "What do I do next?" This is precisely the question for which the Clinician's Guide to Diagnosis: A Practical Approach provides the answer. It will lead you from symptom to diagnosis through a series of steps designed to mimic the logical thought processes of seasoned clinicians. For the young clinician, this is an ideal book to help bridge the gap between the classroom and actual patient care. For the experienced clinician, this concise handbook offers rapid answers to the questions that are commonly encountered on a day-to-day basis. Let this guide become your companion, providing you with the tools necessary to tackle even the most challenging symptoms.

Products offered by LEXI-COMP

ORAL SOFT TISSUE DISEASES

by J. Robert Newland, DDS, MS; Timothy F. Meiller, DDS, PhD; Richard L. Wynn, BSPharm, PhD; and Harold L.Crossley, DDS, PhD

Designed for all dental professionals, a pictorial reference to assist in the diagnosis and management of oral soft tissue diseases (over 160 photos). Easy-to-use, sections include: Diagnosis process: obtaining a history, examining the patient, establishing a differential diagnosis, selecting appropriate diagnostic tests, interpreting the results, etc.; white lesions; red lesions; blistering-sloughing lesions; ulcerated lesions; pigmented lesions; papillary lesions; soft tissue swelling (each lesion is illustrated with a color representative photograph); specific medications to treat oral soft tissue diseases; sample prescriptions; and special topics.

ORAL HARD TISSUE DISEASES

by J. Robert Newland, DDS, MS

A reference manual for radiographic diagnosis, visually-cued with over 130 high quality radiographs is designed to require little more than visual recognition to make an accurate diagnosis. Each lesion is illustrated by one or more photographs depicting the typical radiographic features and common variations. There are 12 chapters tabbed for easy access: 1) Periapical Radiolucent Lesions; 2) Pericoronal Radiolucent Lesions; 3) Inter-Radicular Radiolucent Lesions; 4) Periodontal Radiolucent Lesions; 5) Radiolucent Lesions Not Associated With Teeth; 6) Radiolucent Lesions With Irregular Margins; 7) Periapical Radiopaque Lesions; 8) Periocoronal Radiopaque Lesions; 9) Inter-Radicular Radiopaque Lesions; 10) Radiopaque Lesions Not Associated With Teeth; 11) Radiopaque Lesions With Irregular Margins; 12) Selected Readings / Alphabetical Index

DENTAL OFFICE MEDICAL EMERGENCIES

by Timothy F. Meiller, DDS, PhD; Richard L. Wynn, BSPharm, PhD; Ann Marie McMullin, MD; Cynthia Biron, RDH, EMT, MA; and Harold L. Crossley, DDS, PhD

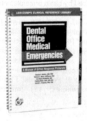

Designed specifically for general dentists during times of emergency. A tabbed paging system allows for quick access to specific crisis events. Created with urgency in mind, it is spiral bound and drilled with a hole for hanging purposes. Contains the following: Basic Action Plan for Stabilization; Allergic / Drug Reactions; Loss of Consciousness / Respiratory Distress / Chest Pain; Altered Sensation / Changes in Affect; Management of Acute Bleeding; Office Preparedness / Procedures and Protocols; Automated External Defibrillator (AED); Oxygen Delivery

Patient Education for Dentistry
(Flip Charts)

A PATIENT GUIDE TO ROOT CANAL THERAPY
Contributor Thom C. Dumsha, M.S., D.D.S., M.Sc.

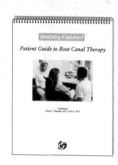

- An ideal tool used to educate and explain to your patients about root canals

- 8 1/2" x 11" colorful tabbed flip chart explaining each of the steps involved in a root canal

- Actual clinical photographs, radiographs, and diagrams

PATIENT GUIDE TO DENTAL IMPLANTS
Contributor Marvin L. Baer, D.D.S., M.Sc.

- An ideal tool used to educate and explain to your patients about dental implants

- 8 1/2" x 11" colorful tabbed flip chart explaining each of the steps involved in:

  1.) Single tooth restoration
  2.) Replacement of several teeth
  3.) Implants supported overdenture (4 implants/2 implants)
  4.) Screw-retained denture

Patient Education for Psychiatry
(Flip Charts)

A PATIENT GUIDE TO MENTAL HEALTH ISSUES

- ▶ Alzheimer's Disease
- ▶ Anxiety (GAD)
- ▶ Bipolar Disorder (BD)
- ▶ Depression
- ▶ Insomnia
- ▶ Obsessive-Compulsive Disorder (OCD)
- ▶ Panic Attacks (PD)
- ▶ Schizophrenia